EMERGENCY MEDICINE

EMERGENCY MEDICINE

Editor

James G. Adams, MD
Professor and Chair
Department of Emergency Medicine
Northwestern University Feinberg School of Medicine
Northwestern Memorial Hospital
Chicago, Illinois

Associate Editors

Erik D. Barton, MD, MS, MBA
Associate Professor of Surgery
Chief, Division of Emergency Medicine
University of Utah School of Medicine
Salt Lake City, Utah

Jamie Collings, MD
Assistant Professor
Residency Director
Department of Emergency Medicine
Northwestern University Feinberg School of Medicine
Northwestern Memorial Hospital
Chicago, Illinois

Peter M. C. DeBlieux, MD
Professor of Clinical Medicine
Director of Resident and Faculty Development
Section of Emergency Medicine
Louisiana State University Health Sciences Center School of Medicine
New Orleans, Louisiana

Michael A. Gisondi, MD
Assistant Professor
Associate Residency Director
Department of Emergency Medicine
Northwestern University Feinberg School of Medicine
Northwestern Memorial Hospital
Chicago, Illinois

Eric S. Nadel, MD
Assistant Professor of Medicine
Harvard Medical School
Residency Director
Harvard Affiliated Emergency Medicine Residency
Brigham and Women's Hospital
Massachusetts General Hospital
Boston, Massachusetts

SAUNDERS
ELSEVIER

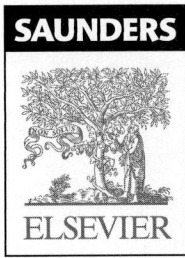

SAUNDERS
ELSEVIER

1600 John F. Kennedy Blvd.
Ste 1800
Philadelphia, PA 19103-2899

EMERGENCY MEDICINE ISBN: 978-1-4160-2872-7

Notice

Knowledge and best practice in this field are constantly changing. As new research and experience broaden our knowledge, changes in practice, treatment, and drug therapy may become necessary or appropriate. Readers are advised to check the most current information provided (i) on procedures featured or (ii) by the manufacturer of each product to be administered, to verify the recommended dose or formula, the method and duration of administration, and contraindications. It is the responsibility of the practitioner, relying on his or her experience and knowledge of the patient, to make diagnoses, to determine dosages and the best treatment for each individual patient, and to take all appropriate safety precautions. To the fullest extent of the law, neither the Publisher nor the Editors assume any liability for any injury and/or damage to persons or property arising out of or related to any use of the material contained in this book.

The Publisher

Library of Congress Cataloging-in-Publication Data
Adams, James, 1962 May 8-
Emergency medicine / James G. Adams ; with contributions by Erik D. Barton . . . [et al.].
– 1st ed.
p. ; cm.
Includes bibliographical references and index.
ISBN 978-1-4160-2872-7
1. Emergency medicine. I. Title.
[DNLM: 1. Emergencies. 2. Emergency Medicine—methods. WB 105 A214e 2008]
RC86.7.A285 2008
616.02'5–dc22 2007026212

Publishing Director: Judith Fletcher
Developmental Editor: Joanie Milnes
Publishing Services Manager: Frank Polizzano
Project Manager: Michael H. Goldberg
Design Direction: Steven Stave

Printed in Canada

Last digit is the print number: 9 8 7 6 5 4 3 2 1

To my immediate and extended family, for their love, support, patience, and encouragement. To my friends, mentors, and colleagues, from whom I continue to learn so much. To the faculty and residents, whose great talent and dedication invigorate me. To the authors and editors of this text, in recognition of their knowledge, skill, wisdom, and generosity.
JGA

To my family, friends, and faculty, who better understand the virtues of patience and without whose support I could never achieve anything great! I am very blessed to be surrounded by such amazing souls. Thanks for being part of this success!
EDB

To my parents, Jan and Wayne Davis and Jimmie Collings, for their enduring love and support in everything I do; and to my amazing husband, Mark Kling, and my precious son Keaton for surviving the process of creating this book and showing me what is really important in life. You make every day worth it!
JC

To my wife, Karen, and children, Joshua and Zachary, whose patience, faith, and love keep me whole. To our patients at Charity Hospital in New Orleans, the LSU Emergency Medicine residents, and our hard working EM faculty, particularly Keith VanMeter, M.D. To Ellen Slaven, M.D., for her educational insights.
PMCD

This is for Derek: I am blessed by your love, support, guidance, and patience each and every day. To my parents, Andrew and Linda, thank you for giving me every opportunity in life and more love than any boy could ask for. Mom, you made me a better doctor. To Toni, Linda, and Ronger, thank you for always believing in us, caring for us, and supporting our dreams. To Mary Catherine Barron, thank you for making me a writer. To Marion Ficke, thank you for helping me to succeed. Family, friends, mentors, and patients: you are with me always.
MAG

To the HAEMR residents and dedicated faculty who keep me motivated and humble as we perpetuate the cycle of teaching and learning. To my colleagues who have shared their experience and wisdom to expand the foundation of our field with this text. To my family and friends who have supported me along the way. To my mother, Harriet, who was always proud and would continue to be so. To Robert and Carole Nadel, and Margie and Bert Paley, for their love and support. To my wife, Marianne, and our children, Josh, Emily, and Henry, for their love, patience, and laughter.
ESN

Contributors

Fredrick M. Abrahamian, DO
Associate Professor of Medicine, David Geffen School of Medicine at UCLA, Los Angeles; Director of Education, Department of Emergency Medicine, Olive View–UCLA Medical Center, Sylmar, California

Mohammed A. Abu Aish, MBBCh, FRCPC
Clinical Fellow, Department of Pediatrics, Faculty of Medicine, University of British Columbia, and Division of Pediatric Emergency Medicine, British Columbia Children's Hospital, Vancouver, British Columbia, Canada

Bruce D. Adams, MD
Clinical Professor of Emergency Medicine, Medical College of Georgia, Augusta, Georgia; Chief, Department of Clinical Investigation, and Faculty Physician, Department of Emergency Medicine, William Beaumont Army Medical Center, El Paso, Texas

James G. Adams, MD
Professor and Chair, Department of Emergency Medicine, Northwestern University Feinberg School of Medicine and Northwestern Memorial Hospital, Chicago, Illinois

Nima Afshar, MD
Clinical Instructor, Department of Medicine, University of California, San Francisco, School of Medicine; Attending Physician, Department of Emergency Medicine, San Francisco General Hospital; Attending Physician, Department of Medicine, San Francisco Veterans Affairs Medical Center, San Francisco, California

Steven E. Aks, DO
Associate Professor of Emergency Medicine, Rush Medical College; Director, Toxikon Consortium, Division of Toxicology, Department of Emergency Medicine, John H. Stroger, Jr., Hospital of Cook County, Chicago, Illinois

Amer Aldeen, MD
Clinical Instructor, Northwestern University Feinberg School of Medicine; Attending Physician, Department of Emergency Medicine, Northwestern Memorial Hospital, Chicago, Illinois

Kostas Alibertis, BA, CCEMT-P
Lead Instructor, Life Support Learning Center, University of Virginia Health System, Charlottesville; Chief, Western Albemarle Rescue Squad, Crozet, Virginia; National Faculty, American Heart Association, Dallas, Texas

Todd L. Allen, MD
Assistant Professor, Division of Emergency Medicine, Department of Surgery, University of Utah School of Medicine; Assistant Program Director, University of Utah Affliated Emergency Medicine Residency, Intermountain Medical Center, Salt Lake City, Utah

Paul J. Allegretti, DO
Associate Professor and Emergency Medicine Residency Program Director, Midwestern University Chicago College of Osteopathic Medicine; Attending Physician, Emergency Medicine, Provident Hospital of Cook County, Chicago, Illinois

Jennifer Anders, MD
Assistant Professor of Pediatrics, Johns Hopkins University School of Medicine; Attending Physician, Pediatric Emergency Medicine, Johns Hopkins Children's Center, Baltimore, Maryland

Phillip Andrus, MD
Assistant Professor, Mount Sinai School of Medicine; Attending Physician, Mount Sinai Hospital, New York, New York

Nicholas Armellino, DO
Attending Physician, Department of Emergency Medicine, Maine Medical Center, Portland, Maine

Chandra D. Aubin, MD, RDMS
Assistant Professor and Assistant Director, Emergency Medicine Residency, Division of Emergency Medicine, Washington University School of Medicine, St. Louis, Missouri

Jennifer Avegno, MD, MA
Clinical Instructor, Department of Emergency Medicine, Louisiana State University Health Sciences Center, New Orleans, Louisiana

John Bailitz, MD
Assistant Professor of Emergency Medicine, Rush Medical College; Assistant Program Director, John H. Stroger, Jr., Hospital of Cook County, Chicago, Illinois

Patricia Baines, MD
Assistant Professor, Emory University School of Medicine; Assistant Medical Director and Director of Patient Ambulatory Care Express (PACE), Grady Health System, Atlanta, Georgia

Aaron E. Bair, MD, MSc
Associate Professor, University of California, Davis, School of Medicine, Sacramento, California

Katherine Bakes, MD
Assistant Professor of Surgery, University of Colorado School of Medicine; Director of Pediatric Emergency Medicine, Denver Health Medical Center, Denver, Colorado

Emily Baran, MD, RDMS
Assistant Professor, Department of Emergency Medicine, Northwestern University Feinberg School of Medicine; Assistant Residency Director, Department of Emergency Medicine, Northwestern Memorial Hospital, Chicago, Illinois

William G. Barsan, MD
Professor and Chair, Department of Emergency Medicine, University of Michigan Medical School, Ann Arbor, Michigan

Craig G. Bates, MD, MS
Clinical Assistant Professor of Emergency Medicine, Case Western Reserve University School of Medicine; Attending Physician, Department of Emergency Medicine, MetroHealth Medical Center, Cleveland, Ohio

Jamil Bayram, MD, MPH
Assistant Professor of Emergency Medicine, Rush Medical College; Director, International Emergency Medicine Fellowship, and Attending Physician, Department of Emergency Medicine, Rush University Medical Center, Chicago, Illinois

Tomer Begaz, MD
Assistant Professor, Medical College of Wisconsin; Faculty Physician, Froedtert Memorial Lutheran Hospital, Milwaukee, Wisconsin

Kip Benko, MD, MS
Clinical Assistant Professor of Emergency Medicine, University of Pittsburgh School of Medicine; Faculty, Presbyterian University Hospital, Pittsburgh, Pennsylvania

Kriti Bhatia, MD
Instructor in Medicine, Harvard Medical School; Attending Physician, Department of Emergency Medicine, Brigham and Women's Hospital, Boston, Massachusetts

Paul D. Biddinger, MD
Assistant Professor of Surgery, Harvard Medical School; Assistant Professor of Public Health Practice, Harvard School of Public Health; Director of Operations and Director of Prehospital Care and Disaster Medicine, Department of Emergency Medicine, Massachusetts General Hospital, Boston, Massachusetts

Andra L. Blomkalns, MD
Associate Professor and Vice Chairman of Education, University of Cincinnati College of Medicine, Cincinnati, Ohio

John M. Boe, MD, MS
Assistant Clinical Professor of Emergency Medicine, Indiana University School of Medicine; Attending Physician, Wishard Memorial Hospital, Indianapolis, Indiana

J. Stephen Bohan, MD, MS
Assistant Professor, Harvard Medical School; Executive Vice Chair, Emergency Medicine, Brigham and Women's Hospital, Boston, Massachusetts

Keith Boniface, MD
Associate Residency Director and Director of Emergency Ultrasound, Department of Emergency Medicine, George Washington University Medical Center, Washington, DC

Laura J. Bontempo, MD
Assistant Professor of Emergency Medicine, Yale University School of Medicine; Emergency Medicine Residency Program Director, Yale–New Haven Hospital, New Haven, Connecticut

Ashley Booth, MD
Assistant Professor and Associate Residency Director, Department of Emergency Medicine, University of Florida College of Medicine Jacksonville, Jacksonville, Florida

Keith Borg, MD, PhD
Assistant Professor and Research Director, Division of Emergency Medicine, Medical University of South Carolina, Charleston, South Carolina

Philip Bossart, MD
Professor, Division of Emergency Medicine, University of Utah School of Medicine, Salt Lake City, Utah

Mark E. Bracken, MD
Assistant Professor, Boston University School of Medicine; Attending Physician, Department of Emergency Medicine, Boston Medical Center, Boston, Massachusetts

William J. Brady, MD
Professor of Emergency Medicine and Internal Medicine, University of Virginia School of Medicine; Operational Medical Director, Charlottesville-Albemarle Rescue Squad, Charlottesville, Virginia

Jeremy Branzetti, MD
Department of Emergency Medicine, Northwestern University Feinberg School of Medicine and Northwestern Memorial Hospital, Chicago, Illinois

Gail Braunholtz, MD
Staff Physician, Rose Medical Center, Denver, Colorado

David F. M. Brown, MD
Assistant Professor, Harvard Medical School; Vice Chair, Department of Emergency Medicine, Massachusetts General Hospital, Boston, Massachusetts

Sean M. Bryant, MD
Assistant Professor, Department of Emergency Medicine, Rush Medical College and John H. Stroger, Jr., Cook County Hospital; Associate Medical Director, Illinois Poison Center, Chicago, Illinois

John H. Burton, MD
Residency Program Director, Department of Emergency Medicine, Albany Medical Center, Albany, New York

Daniel Cabrera, MD
Department of Emergency Medicine, Mayo Clinic College of Medicine, Rochester, Minnesota

Rhonda S. Cadena, MS, MD
University of Cincinnati Emergency Medicine Residency Training Program, University of Cincinnati College of Medicine, Cincinnati, Ohio

Robert Cannon, DO
Clinical Instructor, University of Pittsburgh School of Medicine, and Division of Toxicology, Department of Emergency Medicine, University of Pittsburgh Medical Center–Presbyterian, Pittsburgh, Pennsylvania

David A. Caro, MD
Assistant Professor and Residency Director, Department of Emergency Medicine, University of Florida College of Medicine Jacksonville, Jacksonville, Florida

Christopher R. Carpenter, MD, MSc
Assistant Professor, Division of Emergency Medicine, Washington University School of Medicine; Attending Physician, Barnes-Jewish Hospital, St. Louis, Missouri

Wallace A. Carter, MD
Associate Professor of Emergency Medicine in Medicine, Weill Cornell Medical College of Cornell University; Associate Professor of Clinical Medicine, Columbia University College of Physicians and Surgeons; Program Director, Emergency Medicine Residency, New York–Presbyterian Hospital, New York, New York

Michael Catenacci, MD
Assistant Professor and Assistant Residency Program Director, Department of Emergency Medicine, University of Alabama at Birmingham School of Medicine; Medical Director, Department of Critical Care Transport, UAB Hospital, Birmingham, Alabama

Gar Ming Chan, MD
Assistant Clinical Professor of Emergency Medicine, New York University School of Medicine, New York; Attending Physician, North Shore University Hospital, Manhasset, New York

Andrew K. Chang, MD, MS
Associate Professor, Albert Einstein College of Medicine of Yeshiva University; Attending Physician, Montefiore Medical Center, Bronx, New York

Douglas M. Char, MD, MA
Associate Professor of Emergency Medicine, Washington University School of Medicine; Attending Physician, Barnes-Jewish Hospital and St. Louis Children's Hospital, St. Louis, Missouri

Yi-Mei Chng, MD, MPH
Attending Physician, Kaiser Permanente Santa Clara Medical Center, Santa Clara, California

Richard F. Clark, MD
Professor of Medicine, University of California, San Diego, School of Medicine; Director, Division of Medical Toxicology, UCSD Medical Center; Medical Director, San Diego Division, California Poison Control System, San Diego, California

Kathleen J. Clem, MD
Associate Professor and Chair, Department of Emergency Medicine, Loma Linda University School of Medicine, Loma Linda, California

James E. Colletti, MD
Associate Residency Director, Department of Emergency Medicine, Mayo Clinic College of Medicine, Rochester, Minnesota

Jamie Collings, MD
Assistant Professor and Residency Director, Department of Emergency Medicine, Northwestern University Feinberg School of Medicine and Northwestern Memorial Hospital, Chicago, Illinois

Christopher B. Colwell, MD
Associate Professor, Division of Emergency Medicine, Department of Surgery, University of Colorado Health Sciences Center; Associate Director, Department of Emergency Medicine, Denver Health Medical Center, Denver, Colorado

Jeremy L. Cooke, MD
Assistant Professor, Department of Emergency Medicine, University of California, Davis, School of Medicine, Sacramento, California

Troy P. Coon, MD
Chief of Medical Education, Eisenhower Army Medical Center, Fort Gordon, Georgia

Francis L. Counselman., MD
Chairman and Program Director, Department of Emergency Medicine, Eastern Virginia Medical School, Norfolk, Virginia

D. Mark Courtney, MD
Assistant Professor, Department of Emergency Medicine, Northwestern University Feinberg School of Medicine; Director of Research, Department of Emergency Medicine, Northwestern Memorial Hospital, Chicago, Illinois

Robert Cowan, MD
Attending Physician, Emergency Medicine, Virtua Memorial Hospital, Mount Holly, New Jersey

Chad S. Crystal, MD
Assistant Professor, Clinical Educator Track, Department of Emergency Medicine, Texas A&M University System Health Science Center, College Station, Texas; Attending Physician, Legacy Good Samaritan Hospital, Portland, Oregon

Kirk L. Cumpston, DO
Assistant Professor of Emergency Medicine, Virginia Commonwealth University School of Medicine; Medical Director, Virginia Poison Center, Richmond, Virginia

Rita K. Cydulka, MD, MS
Associate Professor and Vice Chair, Department of Emergency Medicine, Case Western Reserve University School of Medicine; Attending Physician, Department of Emergency Medicine, MetroHealth Medical Center, Cleveland, Ohio

Lynda Daniel-Underwood, MD, MS
Assistant Professor of Emergency Medicine and Assistant Dean for Clinical Site Recruitment, Loma Linda University School of Medicine, Loma Linda, California

Daniel Davis, MD
Associate Professor of Emergency Medicine, University of California, San Diego, School of Medicine, San Diego, California

Jonathan E. Davis, MD
Assistant Professor, Georgetown University School of Medicine; Associate Program Director, Department of Emergency Medicine, Georgetown University Hospital and Washington Hospital Center, Washington, DC

Wyatt W. Decker, MD
Associate Professor of Emergency Medicine and Chair, Department of Emergency Medicine, Mayo Clinic College of Medicine, Rochester, Minnesota

Jorge del Castillo, MD, MBA
Associate Professor of Emergency Medicine, Northwestern University Feinberg School of Medicine, Chicago; Associate Head, Division of Emergency Medicine, Evanston Northwestern Healthcare, Evanston, Illinois

Tara D. Director, MD
Attending Physician, Department of Emergency Medicine, St. Vincent's Catholic Medical Center, New York, New York

Gail D'Onofrio, MD, MS
Professor and Section Chief, Section of Emergency Medicine, Department of Surgery, Yale University School of Medicine, and Adult Emergency Department, Yale–New Haven Hospital, New Haven, Connecticut

Gerard S. Doyle, MD, MPH
Assistant Professor (Clinical Health Sciences), Section of Emergency Medicine, University of Wisconsin School of Medicine and Public Health, Madison, Wisconsin

Jeffrey Druck, MD
Assistant Professor, Assistant Head, Education, and Associate Program Director, Denver Health Residency in Emergency Medicine, Division of Emergency Medicine, Department of Surgery, University of Colorado School of Medicine and University of Colorado Hospital, Aurora, Colorado

Mary Ann Edens, MD
Assistant Professor, Emory University School of Medicine; Director of Emergency Ultrasound, Grady Hospital and Emory Crawford Long Hospital, Atlanta, Georgia

Jonathan A. Edlow, MD
Associate Professor of Medicine, Harvard Medical School; Vice Chairman, Department of Emergency Medicine, Beth Israel Deaconess Medical Center, Boston, Massachusetts

Timothy B. Erickson, MD
Director, Clinical Toxicology, and Assistant Head, Department of Emergency Medicine, University of Illinois at Chicago College of Medicine, Chicago, Illinois

Ugo A. Ezenkwele, MD, MPH
Assistant Professor of Emergency Medicine, New York University School of Medicine; Attending Physician, New York University Medical Center/Bellevue Hospital Center, New York, New York

Jeffrey D. Ferguson, MD, NREMT-P
Assistant Professor of Emergency Medicine, The Brody School of Medicine at East Carolina University; Attending Physician, Pitt County Memorial Hospital, Greenville, North Carolina

Jessica A. Fulton, DO
Assistant Professor of Emergency Medicine, New York University School of Medicine and Bellevue Hospital Center; Consultant, New York City Poison Control Center, New York, New York

Fiona E. Gallahue, MD
Assistant Professor of Emergency Medicine, Weill Medical College of Cornell University, New York; Associate Residency Director, New York Methodist Hospital, Brooklyn, New York

Cynthia Galvan, MD
Department of Emergency Medicine, Northwestern University Feinberg School of Medicine and Northwestern Memorial Hospital, Chicago, Illinois

Manish Garg, MD
Assistant Professor of Emergency Medicine, Temple University School of Medicine; Assistant Residency Program Director, Department of Emergency Medicine, Temple University Hospital, Philadelphia, Pennsylvania

Gus M. Garmel, MD
Clinical Associate Professor, Division of Emergency Medicine, Department of Surgery, Stanford University School of Medicine, Stanford; Co-Program Director, Stanford-Kaiser Emergency Medicine Residency, and Senior Emergency Medicine Physician, The Permanente Medical Group, Kaiser Permanente Medical Center, Santa Clara, California

Chris Ghaemmaghami, MD
Associate Professor of Emergency Medicine and Internal Medicine, University of Virginia Health System, Charlottesville, Virginia

Michael A. Gibbs, MD
Associate Professor, University of Vermont College of Medicine, Burlington, Vermont; Chief of Emergency Services, Maine Medical Center, Portland, Maine

Gregory H. Gilbert, MD
Assistant Clinical Professor, Clerkship Director, and Principles of Medicine Associate Director, Stanford University School of Medicine, Stanford; Attending Physician and Life Flight Medical Director, Stanford University Hospital, Palo Alto, California

Michael A. Gisondi, MD
Assistant Professor and Associate Residency Director, Department of Emergency Medicine, Northwestern University Feinberg School of Medicine and Northwestern Memorial Hospital, Chicago, Illinois

Andy Godwin, MD
Associate Chair, Academic Affairs, Assistant Dean, Simulation Education, and Associate Professor, Department of Emergency Medicine, University of Florida College of Medicine Jacksonville, Jacksonville, Florida

Joshua N. Goldstein, MD, PhD
Instructor in Surgery, Harvard Medical School; Attending Physician, Department of Emergency Medicine, Massachusetts General Hospital, Boston, Massachusetts

Deepi G. Goyal, MD
Associate Program Director, Mayo Emergency Medicine Residency, Mayo School of Graduate Medical Education; Consultant, Department of Emergency Medicine, Mayo Clinic, Rochester, Minnesota

Matthew N. Graber, MD, PhD
Assistant Professor, Department of Emergency Medicine, Emory University School of Medicine; Attending Physician, Department of Emergency Medicine, Grady Memorial Hospital, Atlanta, Georgia

Jill A. Grant, MD, MS
Adjunct Assistant Professor of Military/Emergency Medicine, Uniformed Services University of the Health Sciences F. Edward Hébert School of Medicine, Bethesda, Maryland; Faculty Emergency Physician, Brooke Army Medical Center, Fort Sam Houston, Texas

David D. Gummin, MD
Medical Director, Wisconsin Poison Center, Children's Hospital of Wisconsin, Milwaukee, Wisconsin

David Hackstadt, MD
Clinical Professor, Division of Emergency Medicine, University of South Florida College of Medicine, Tampa, Florida

Azita G. Hamedani, MD, MPH
Associate Professor, University of Wisconsin School of Medicine and Public Health; Director of Quality, Section of Emergency Medicine, University of Wisconsin Hospital and Clinics, Madison, Wisconsin

Benjamin P. Harrison, MD
Assistant Professor, University of Washington School of Medicine, Seattle; Program Director, Madigan–University of Washington Emergency Medicine Residency, Madigan Army Medical Center, Tacoma, Washington

Stephen C. Hartsell, MD
Professor (Clinical) of Surgery and Director, Emergency Medicine Residency Program, Division of Emergency Medicine, Department of Surgery, University of Utah School of Medicine, Salt Lake City, Utah

E. Parker Hays, Jr., MD
Associate Professor of Emergency Medicine, University of North Carolina School of Medicine, Chapel Hill; Residency Director, Carolinas Medical Center, Charlotte, North Carolina

Alan C. Heffner, MD
Clinical Assistant Professor, University of North Carolina School of Medicine, Chapel Hill; Attending Physician, Departments of Emergency Medicine and Internal Medicine, Carolinas Medical Center, Charlotte, North Carolina

Diane B. Heller, MD, JD
Attending Physician, Morristown Memorial Hospital, Morristown, New Jersey

Robin R. Hemphill, MD, MPH
Associate Professor, Department of Emergency Medicine, Vanderbilt University School of Medicine and Vanderbilt Medical Center; Associate Director, Health Care Solutions Group, Nashville, Tennessee

Gregory L. Henry, MD
Clinical Professor, Department of Emergency Medicine, University of Michigan Medical School; CEO, Medical Practice Risk Assessment, Ann Arbor, Michigan; President, Savannah Assurance Limited, Bridgetown, Barbados

H. Gene Hern, MD, MS
Assistant Clinical Professor of Medicine, University of California, San Francisco, School of Medicine, San Francisco; Residency Director, Department of Emergency Medicine, Highland Hospital, Alameda County Medical Center, Oakland, California

Sheryl L. Heron, MD, MPH
Associate Professor, Associate Residency Director, and Assistant Dean of Medical Education and Student Affairs, Emory University School of Medicine, Atlanta, Georgia

Erik P. Hess, MD
Clinical Research Fellow, Department of Epidemiology and Community Medicine, University of Ottawa Faculty of Medicine, Ottawa, Ontario, Canada

Cherri D. Hobgood, MD
Associate Professor of Emergency Medicine, University of North Carolina School of Medicine, Chapel Hill, North Carolina

Russ Horowitz, MD
Instructor, Northwestern University Feinberg School of Medicine; Attending Physician, Emergency Department, Children's Memorial Hospital, Chicago, Illinois

David S. Howes, MD
Professor of Medicine and Pediatrics, University of Chicago Pritzker School of Medicine; Residency Program Director, Section of Emergency Medicine, and Senior Attending Physician, Sections of Emergency Medicine and Pediatric Emergency Medicine, University of Chicago Medical Center, Chicago, Illinois

J. Steven Huff, MD
Associate Professor of Emergency Medicine and Neurology, University of Virginia Health System, Charlottesville, Virginia

Amy Jo Irvin, MD
Attending Physician, Emergency Medicine, Plaza Medical Center, Fort Worth, Texas

Eric Isaacs, MD
Clinical Professor of Medicine, University of California, San Francisco, School of Medicine; Director of Quality Improvement, Department of Emergency Services, San Francisco General Hospital, San Francisco, California

Jennifer L. Isenhour, MD
Adjunct Assistant Professor, Department of Emergency Medicine, University of North Carolina School of Medicine, Chapel Hill; Associate Residency Director, Department of Emergency Medicine, Carolinas Medical Center, Charlotte, North Carolina

Andy Jagoda, MD
Professor, Vice Chair, and Medical Director, Department of Emergency Medicine, Mount Sinai School of Medicine and Mount Sinai Hospital, New York, New York

Edward C. Jauch, MD, MS
Assistant Professor, Department of Emergency Medicine, University of Cincinnati College of Medicine; Attending Physician, University Hospital, Cincinnati, Ohio

Christopher G. Jenson, MD
Attending Physician, Lawrence Memorial Hospital, Lawrence, Kansas

Scott Jolley, MD
Assistant Professor, Division of Emergency Medicine, Department of Surgery, University of Utah School of Medicine; Attending Physician, Intermountain Medical Center, Salt Lake City, Utah

Kerin A. Jones, MD, MS
Assistant Professor, Wayne State University School of Medicine; Associate Residency Directory, Detroit Receiving Hospital, Detroit, Michigan

Randall S. Jotte, MD
Associate Professor, Division of Emergency Medicine, Washington University School of Medicine; Attending Physician, Barnes-Jewish Hospital, St. Louis, Missouri

Karen Jubanyik, MD
Assistant Professor, Section of Emergency Medicine, Department of Surgery, Yale University School of Medicine; Attending Physician, Adult Emergency Department, Yale–New Haven Hospital, New Haven, Connecticut

Christopher S. Kang, MD
Clinical Assistant Professor, University of Washington School of Medicine, Seattle; Research Coordinator and Attending Physician, Department of Emergency Medicine, Madigan Army Medical Center, Tacoma, Washington

Tara Khan, DO
Assistant Staff Attending Physician and Health Services Research Fellow, New York Methodist Hospital, Brooklyn, New York

Tae Eung Kim, MD
Assistant Professor, Department of Emergency Medicine, Loma Linda University School of Medicine; Attending Physician, Loma Linda University Medical Center, Loma Linda, California

Matthew Kippenhan, MD
Assistant Professor, Department of Emergency Medicine, Northwestern University Feinberg School of Medicine; Attending Physician, Northwestern Memorial Hospital, Chicago, Illinois

Niranjan Kissoon, MD, FRCPC
Associate Head and Professor, Department of Pediatrics, University of British Columbia Faculty of Medicine; Senior Medical Director, Acute and Critical Care Programs, BC Children's Hospital, Vancouver, British Columbia, Canada

Frederick Korley, MD
Assistant Professor, Department of Emergency Medicine, Johns Hopkins University School of Medicine and Johns Hopkins Hospital, Baltimore, Maryland

Joshua M. Kosowsky, MD
Assistant Professor, Harvard Medical School; Clinical Director, Department of Emergency Medicine, Brigham and Women's Hospital, Boston, Massachusetts

Ted Koutouzis, MD
Clinical Instructor, Department of Emergency Medicine, Northwestern University Feinberg School of Medicine and Northwestern Memorial Hospital, Chicago, Illinois

Rick G. Kulkarni, MD
Assistant Professor of Surgery, Section of Emergency Medicine, Department of Surgery, Yale University School of Medicine; Medical Director, Adult Emergency Department, Yale–New Haven Hospital, New Haven, Connecticut

Thomas Kunisaki, MD
Associate Professor, Department of Emergency Medicine, University of Florida College of Medicine Jacksonville; Medical Director, Florida Poison Information Center, Jacksonville, Florida

Erin M. Lareau, MD
Instructor, Department of Emergency Medicine, Northwestern University Feinberg School of Medicine, Chicago, Illinois

Erik G. Laurin, MD
Associate Professor, University of California, Davis, School of Medicine, Sacramento, California

Matthew P. Lazio, MD
Department of Emergency Medicine, Northwestern University Feinberg School of Medicine and Northwestern Memorial Hospital, Chicago, Illinois

Eric L. Legome, MD
Assistant Professor of Emergency Medicine, New York University School of Medicine; Director, Emergency Medicine Residency, New York University/Bellevue Hospital Center, New York, New York

Jill F. Lehrman, MD, MPH
Assistant Professor, Department of Emergency Medicine, Northwestern University Feinberg School of Medicine, Chicago, Illinois

Jay Lemery, MD
Assistant Professor, Weill Cornell Medical College of Cornell University; Attending Physician, New York–Presbyterian Hospital, New York, New York

Gretchen S. Lent, MD
Associate Professor, Albert Einstein College of Medicine of Yeshiva University, Bronx, New York; Attending Physician, Torrance Memorial Medical Center, Torrance, California

Matthew R. Levine, MD
Assistant Professor, Department of Emergency Medicine, Northwestern University Feinberg School of Medicine, Chicago, Illinois

Marc Levsky, MD
Attending Physician, Department of Emergency Medicine, Carl R. Darnall Army Medical Center, Fort Hood, Texas

Erica L. Liebelt, MD
Associate Professor of Pediatrics, University of Alabama School of Medicine; Director, Medical Toxicology Services, UAB Hospital and Children's Hospital, Birmingham, Alabama

Jason E. Liebzeit, MD
Assistant Professor of Emergency Medicine, Emory University School of Medicine, Emory Healthcare, and Grady Memorial Hospital, Atlanta, Georgia

Ingrid T. Lim, MD
Attending Physician, Kaiser Permanente San Francisco Medical Center, San Francisco, California

Michelle Lin, MD
Assistant Clinical Professor, Department of Emergency Medicine, University of California, San Francisco, School of Medicine; Associate Program Director, UC San Francisco–San Francisco General Hospital Emergency Medicine Residency, San Francisco General Hospital, San Francisco, California

M. Scott Linscott, MD
Professor of Surgery (Clinical), Division of Emergency Medicine, University of Utah School of Medicine, Salt Lake City, Utah

Heather Long, MD
Assistant Professor, Department of Emergency Medicine, New York University School of Medicine, New York; Fellowship Director, Medical Toxicology, North Shore University Hospital, Manhasset, New York

Troy E. Madsen, MD
Instructor, Division of Emergency Medicine, Department of Surgery, University of Utah School of Medicine and University of Utah Medical Center, Salt Lake City, Utah

Swaminatha V. Mahadevan, MD
Assistant Professor of Surgery, Division of Emergency Medicine, Department of Surgery, Stanford University School of Medicine, Stanford; Associate Chief and Medical Director, Division of Emergency Medicine, Department of Surgery, Stanford University Medical Center, Palo Alto, California

Mamta Malik, MD, MPH
Clinical Instructor, Department of Emergency Medicine, Rush Medical College; Associate Director, International Emergency Medicine Fellowship, and Attending Physician, Department of Emergency Medicine, Rush University Medical Center, Chicago, Illinois

Gerald Maloney, DO
Senior Instructor, Department of Emergency Medicine, Case Western Reserve University School of Medicine; Attending Physician and Staff Toxicologist, Department of Emergency Medicine, MetroHealth Medical Center, Cleveland, Ohio

Rita A. Manfredi, MD
Assistant Clinical Professor of Emergency Medicine, George Washington University School of Medicine, Washington, DC

David E. Manthey, MD
Associate Professor and Director of Undergraduate Medical Education, Wake Forest University School of Medicine, Winston-Salem, North Carolina

Keith A. Marill, MD
Assistant Professor, Harvard Medical School; Attending Physician, Emergency Department, Massachusetts General Hospital, Boston, Massachusetts

Robin A. C. Marshall, MD
Core Faculty, Emergency Medicine Residency, Naval Medical Center Portsmouth, Portsmouth, Virginia

Jorge Martinez, MD, JD
Professor of Clinical Medicine and Residency Program Director, Department of Internal Medicine, and Program Director, Combined LSU Emergency Medicine/Internal Medicine Residency Program, Section of Emergency Medicine, Louisiana State University Health Sciences Center School of Medicine, New Orleans, Louisiana

Joseph P. Martinez, MD
Assistant Dean of Student Affairs and Assistant Professor of Emergency Medicine, University of Maryland School of Medicine, Baltimore, Maryland

Amal Mattu, MD
Associate Professor of Emergency Medicine and Residency Director, Emergency Medicine, University of Maryland School of Medicine, Baltimore, Maryland

Jennifer E. McCain, MD
Assistant Professor of Pediatrics, University of Alabama School of Medicine, Birmingham, Alabama

Maureen McCollough, MD
Associate Professor of Clinical Emergency Medicine and Pediatrics, University of Southern California Keck School of Medicine; Medical Director, Adult and Pediatric Emergency Medicine Departments, Los Angeles County University of Southern California Medical Center, Los Angeles, California

Christy McCowan, MD, MPH
Assistant Professor, Division of Emergency Medicine, Department of Surgery, University of Utah School of Medicine; Associate Medical Director, Emergency Department, and Medical Director, University Health Care Transfer Center, University Health Care, Salt Lake City, Utah

Mark S. McIntosh, MD, MPH
Assistant Professor, Department of Emergency Medicine, University of Florida Health Science Center, Jacksonville, Florida

Catherine McLaren Oliver, MD
Assistant Clinical Professor of Surgery, University of Hawaii John A. Burns School of Medicine; Director of Emergency Ultrasound, Queen's Medical Center, Honolulu, Hawaii

Ron Medzon, MD
Assistant Professor, Boston University School of Medicine; Attending Physician, Department of Emergency Medicine, Boston Medical Center, Boston, Massachusetts

Carl R. Menckhoff, MD
Associate Professor, Department of Emergency Medicine, Medical College of Georgia, Augusta, Georgia

Nathan W. Mick, MD
Assistant Professor, Division of Emergency Medicine, University of Vermont College of Medicine, Burlington, Vermont; Director, Pediatric Emergency Medicine, Maine Medical Center, Portland, Maine

Michael A. Miller, MD
Associate Professor, Department of Military and Emergency Medicine, Uniformed Services University of the Health Sciences F. Edward Hébert School of Medicine, Bethesda, Maryland; Assistant Chief and Medical Toxicologist, Department of Emergency Medicine, Tripler Army Medical Center, Honolulu, Hawaii

Lisa D. Mills, MD
Associate Professor of Emergency Medicine, Louisiana State University Health Sciences Center School of Medicine, New Orleans, Louisiana

Trevor J. Mills, MD, MPH
Chief of Emergency Medicine, Veterans Affairs Northern California Health Care System, Sacramento, California

Raveendra S. Morchi, MD
Assistant Professor and Director of Simulation, Division of Emergency Medicine, Department of Surgery, University of Colorado Health Sciences Center School of Medicine, Denver, Colorado

Thomas Morrissey, MD, PhD
Assistant Professor, Clerkship Director, and Assistant Residency Director, Department of Emergency Medicine, University of Florida College of Medicine Jacksonville, Jacksonville, Florida

Elizabeth Mort, MD, MPH
Vice President, Quality and Safety, Massachusetts General Physicians Organization, and Associate Chief Medical Officer, Massachusetts General Hospital, Boston, Massachusetts

Robert L. Muelleman, MD
Professor and Chairman, Department of Emergency Medicine, University of Nebraska School of Medicine, Omaha, Nebraska

Antonio E. Muñiz, MD
Associate Professor of Emergency Medicine and Pediatrics, University of Texas Health Science Center at Houston; Medical Director, Pediatric Emergency Department, Children's Memorial Hermann Hospital, Houston, Texas

Heather Murphy-Lavoie, MD
Clinical Assistant Professor, Section of Emergency and Hyperbaric Medicine, Department of Medicine, Louisiana State University School of Medicine, New Orleans, Louisiana

Mark B. Mycyk, MD
Assistant Professor, Department of Emergency Medicine, Northwestern University Feinberg School of Medicine; Attending Physician, Northwestern Memorial Hospital and John H. Stroger, Jr., Hospital of Cook County, Chicago, Illinois

Brian K. Nelson, MD
Professor and Residency Program Director, Department of Emergency Medicine, Texas Tech University Health Sciences Center School of Medicine and Thomason Hospital, El Paso, Texas

Lewis S. Nelson, MD
Associate Professor of Emergency Medicine and Director, Fellowship in Medical Toxicology, New York University School of Medicine; Attending Physician, New York University Hospital, New York, New York

Chris Newton, MD
Assistant Program Director, University of Michigan/St. Joseph Mercy Emergency Medicine Residency Program, Ann Arbor, Michigan

Bret Nicks, MD
Associate Professor, Department of Emergency Medicine, Wake Forest University School of Medicine; Assistant Medical Director, Adult Emergency Department, Wake Forest University Baptist Medical Center, Winston-Salem, North Carolina

Robert L. Norris, MD
Associate Professor of Surgery and Emergency Medicine, Stanford University School of Medicine; Chief of Emergency Medicine, Stanford Hospital and Clinics, Stanford, California

Kelly P. O'Keefe, MD
Associate Professor, Division of Emergency Medicine, University of South Florida College of Medicine; Program Director, University of South Florida Emergency Medicine Residency, Tampa General Hospital, Tampa, Florida

Yasuharu Okuda, MD
Assistant Professor, Associate Residency Director, and Director of Simulation Education, Department of Emergency Medicine, Mount Sinai School of Medicine and Mount Sinai Hospital, New York, New York

Michael I. Omori, MD
Assistant Professor, University of South Florida College of Medicine; Attending Physician, Adult Emergency Care Center, Tampa General Hospital, Tampa, Florida

Leigh A. Patterson, MD
Assistant Professor and Residency Director, Department of Emergency Medicine, East Carolina University Brody School of Medicine; Attending Physician, Pitt County Memorial Hospital, Greenville, North Carolina

Richard Paula, MD
Assistant Professor, University of South Florida College of Medicine; Director of Research, Emergency Medicine, Tampa General Hospital, Tampa, Florida

Joseph F. Peabody, MD
Clinical Instructor, Section of Emergency Medicine, Department of Medicine, University of Chicago Pritzker School of Medicine, Chicago; Attending Physician, Department of Emergency Medicine, Lutheran General Hospital, Park Ridge, Illinois

David A. Peak, MD
Instructor, Harvard Medical School; Assistant Residency Director, Harvard-Affiliated Emergency Medicine Residency, and Attending Physician, Massachusetts General Hospital, Boston, Massachusetts

John Nelson Perret, MD
Clinical Assistant Professor, Department of Medicine, Louisiana State University Health Sciences Center School of Medicine, New Orleans; Didactic Curriculum Co-coordinator, Emergency Medicine Residency Program, LSU/Earl K. Long Medical Center, Baton Rouge, Louisiana

Andrew D. Perron, MD
Associate Professor of Emergency Medicine, University of Vermont College of Medicine, Burlington, Vermont; Residency Program Director, Maine Medical Center, Portland, Maine

Robert F. Poirier, MD
Assistant Professor, Division of Emergency Medicine, Washington University School of Medicine; Attending Physician, Department of Emergency Medicine, Barnes-Jewish Hospital, St. Louis, Missouri

Beatrice D. Probst, MD
Associate Clinical Professor of Medicine and Surgery, Loyola University Chicago Stritch School of Medicine; Assistant Director, Emergency Department, Foster G. McGaw Hospital, Maywood, Illinois

Susan B. Promes, MD
Professor of Clinical Medicine and Residency Program Director, Division of Emergency Medicine, University of California, San Francisco, School of Medicine, San Francisco, California

Ryan Pursley, MD
Attending Physician, Department of Emergency Medicine, Sacred Heart Medical Center, Spokane, Washington

Tammie E. Quest, MD
Associate Professor, Department of Emergency Medicine, Emory University School of Medicine, Atlanta, Georgia

James Quinn, MD, MS
Associate Professor of Surgery and Emergency Medicine, Stanford University School of Medicine, Stanford, California

Claudia Ranniger, MD, PhD
Assistant Professor, Director, Medical Simulation Program, and Co-Director, Advanced Life Support Training Programs, Department of Emergency Medicine, George Washington University School of Medicine, Washington, DC

Niels K. Rathlev, MD
Associate Professor, Boston University School of Medicine; Executive Vice Chair, Department of Emergency Medicine, Boston Medical Center, Boston, Massachusetts

Rachel Reisner, MD
Attending Physician, Northwest Community Hospital, Arlington Heights, Illinois

James W. Rhee, MD
Assistant Professor of Medicine and Pediatrics, University of Chicago Pritzker School of Medicine; Attending Physician, Sections of Emergency Medicine and Pediatric Emergency Medicine, and Director of Medical Toxicology, University of Chicago Medical Center, Chicago, Illinois

James V. Ritchie, MD
Captain, Medical Corps, United States Navy; Assistant Professor of Military and Emergency Medicine, Uniformed Services University of the Health Sciences F. Edward Hébert School of Medicine, Bethesda, Maryland; Residency Director, Emergency Medicine, Naval Medical Center Portsmouth, Portsmouth, Virginia

Colleen Roche, MD
Assistant Professor and Associate Residency Director, Department of Emergency Medicine, George Washington University Medical Center, Washington, DC

Matthew T. Robinson, MD
Assistant Professor Clinical Emergency Medicine, University of Missouri School of Medicine; Attending Physician, University Hospital, Columbia, Missouri

Tara Roeder, MD
Attending Physician, Columbus Regional Hospital, Columbus, Indiana

Robert L. Rogers, MD
Assistant Professor of Emergency Medicine and Medicine and Director of Undergraduate Medical Education, University of Maryland School of Medicine, Baltimore, Maryland

Carlo L. Rosen, MD
Assistant Professor, Harvard Medical School; Program Director, Beth Israel Deaconess Medical Center Harvard-Affiliated Emergency Medicine Residency, Beth Israel Deaconess Medical Center, Boston, Massachusetts

Christopher Ross, MD
Assistant Professor, Department of Emergency Medicine, Rush Medical College; Assistant Program Director, Department of Emergency Medicine, John H. Stroger, Jr., Cook County Hospital, Chicago, Illinois

Todd C. Rothenhaus, MD
Department of Emergency Medicine, Tufts University School of Medicine; Chief Medical Information Officer, Caritas Christi Healthcare System, Boston, Massachusetts

Scott E. Rudkin, MD, MBA
Assistant Dean, Continuing Medical Education, and Associate Clinical Professor of Emergency Medicine, University of California, Irvine, School of Medicine, Irvine; Vice Chair, Assistant Program Director, and Director of Medical Informatics, University of California, Irvine, Medical Center, Orange, California

Anne-Michelle Ruha, MD
Assistant Professor, Department of Emergency Medicine, University of Arizona College of Medicine, Tucson; Director, Medical Toxicology Fellowship, Banner Good Samaritan Medical Center, Phoenix, Arizona

Michael S. Runyon, MD
Instructor of Emergency Medicine, University of North Carolina School of Medicine, Chapel Hill; Director of Medical Student Education, Department of Emergency Medicine, Carolinas Medical Center, Charlotte, North Carolina

Annie T. Sadosty, MD
Program Director, Mayo Emergency Medicine Residency, Mayo School of Graduate Medical Education; Consultant, Department of Emergency Medicine, Mayo Clinic, Rochester, Minnesota

David Salzman, MD
Department of Emergency Medicine, Northwestern University Feinberg School of Medicine and Northwestern Memorial Hospital, Chicago, Illinois

Tracy G. Sanson, MD
Assistant Professor and Education Director, Division of Emergency Medicine, University of South Florida College of Medicine; Attending Physician, Tampa General Hospital, Tampa, Florida

Sally A. Santen, MD
Assistant Professor, Office of Teaching and Learning, Department of Emergency Medicine, Vanderbilt University School of Medicine, Nashville, Tennessee

Osman R. Sayan, MD
Assistant Clinical Professor of Medicine, Columbia University College of Physicians and Surgeons; Assistant Residency Director, Emergency Medicine, New York–Presbyterian Hospital/Columbia University Medical Center, New York, New York

Michael J. Schmidt, MD
Assistant Professor, Department of Emergency Medicine, Northwestern University Feinberg School of Medicine; Attending Physician, Department of Emergency Medicine, Northwestern Memorial Hospital, Chicago, Illinois

Kathleen Schrank, MD
Professor of Medicine and Chief, Division of Emergency Medicine, University of Miami Miller School of Medicine; Emergency Medicine Core Faculty, Jackson Memorial Hospital; EMS Medical Director, City of Miami Fire Rescue, Miami, Florida

Theresa Schwab, MD
Attending Physician, Department of Emergency Medicine, Advocate Christ Medical Center, Oak Lawn, Illinois

Wesley H. Self, MD
Department of Emergency Medicine, Northwestern University Feinberg School of Medicine and Northwestern Memorial Hospital, Chicago, Illinois

Clare Sercombe, MD
Attending Physician, Emergency Department, North Memorial Medical Center, Robbinsdale, Minnesota

Rawle A. Seupaul, MD
Assistant Professor of Clinical Emergency Medicine, Indiana University School of Medicine, Indianapolis, Indiana

Ghazala Q. Sharieff, MD
Medical Director, Emergency Care Center, Rady Children's Hospital, San Diego, California

Rahul Sharma, MD, MBA
Instructor, Division of Emergency Medicine, Weill Cornell Medical College of Cornell University; Attending Physician and Co-coordinator, Medical Student Subinternship in Emergency Medicine, New York–Presbyterian Hospital/Weill Cornell Medical Center, New York, New York

Philip Shayne, MD
Associate Professor and Residency Program Director, Emory University School of Medicine, Atlanta, Georgia

Sanjay Shetty, MD
Affiliate Assistant Professor, University of South Florida College of Medicine; Staff Physician, Tampa General Hospital, Tampa, Florida

Robert J. Sigillito, MD
Assistant Professor of Clinical Medicine, Section of Emergency Medicine, Louisiana State University Health Sciences Center School of Medicine, New Orleans, Louisiana

Sandy Sineff, MD
Assistant Professor, Department of Emergency Medicine, Washington University School of Medicine, St. Louis, Missouri

Amandeep Singh, MD
Assistant Clinical Professor of Medicine, Division of Emergency Medicine, Department of Medicine, University of California, San Francisco, School of Medicine, San Francisco; Attending Physician, Department of Emergency Medicine, Highland General Hospital, Alameda County Medical Center, Oakland, California

Ellen M. Slaven, MD
Clinical Assistant Professor of Medicine, Section of Emergency Medicine, Louisiana State University School of Medicine, New Orleans, Louisiana

Mitchell C. Sokolosky, MD
Associate Professor of Emergency Medicine and Director, Emergency Medicine Residency Program, Wake Forest University School of Medicine, Winston-Salem, North Carolina

John C. Southall, MD
Associate Professor, University of Vermont College of Medicine, Burlington, Vermont; Chief, Department of Emergency Medicine, Mercy Hospital, Portland, Maine

Jeremy D. Sperling, MD
Assistant Professor of Medicine, Weill Cornell Medical College; Assistant Director, Emergency Medicine Residency Program, New York–Presbyterian Hospital, New York, New York

Sarah A. Stahmer, MD
Associate Professor, Department of Surgery, Duke University Medical School; Residency Program Director, Division of Emergency Medicine, Duke University Medical Center, Durham, North Carolina

Robert L. Stephen, MD
Assistant Professor, Division of Emergency Medicine, Department of Surgery, University of Utah School of Medicine, Salt Lake City, Utah

Brian A. Stettler, MD
Assistant Professor and Residency Director, Department of Emergency Medicine, University of Cincinnati College of Medicine; Attending Physician, University Hospital, Cincinnati, Ohio

Matthew Strehlow, MD
Clinical Instructor, Stanford University School of Medicine; Director, Clinical Decision Area, and Associate Medicine Director, Division of Emergency Medicine, Stanford University Medical Center, Stanford, California

Jared N. Strote, MD, MS
Assistant Professor, University of Washington School of Medicine; Attending Physician, University of Washington Medical Center, Seattle, Washington

Mark Su, MD
SUNY-Downstate Medical Center, Brooklyn; Director, Fellowship in Medical Toxicology, North Shore University Hospital, Manhasset, New York

D. Matthew Sullivan, MD
Adjunct Assistant Professor, Department of Emergency Medicine, University of North Carolina School of Medicine, Chapel Hill; Director of Finance, Productivity, and Efficiency, and Associate Director of Operations, Department of Emergency Medicine, Carolinas Medical Center, Charlotte, North Carolina

Jeffrey A. Tabas, MD
Associate Professor, University of California, San Francisco, School of Medicine; Attending Physician, Emergency Department, San Francisco General Hospital, San Francisco, California

James K. Takayesu, MD, MSc
Instructor in Surgery, Harvard Medical School; Associate Residency Director, Brigham and Women's Hospital/Massachusetts General Hospital Harvard-Affiliated Emergency Medicine Residency, and Faculty, Emergency Services, Massachusetts General Hospital, Boston, Massachusetts

Asim F. Tarabar, MD, MS
Assistant Professor, Section of Emergency Medicine, Department of Surgery, Yale University School of Medicine; Attending Physician, Adult Emergency Department, Yale–New Haven Hospital, New Haven, Connecticut

Kristine Thompson, MD
Assistant Professor, Mayo College of Medicine, Rochester, Minnesota; Attending Physician, Department of Emergency Medicine, Mayo Clinic, Jacksonville, Florida

Trevonne M. Thompson, MD
Assistant Professor of Medicine and Pediatrics, University of Chicago Pritzker School of Medicine; Attending Physician, Sections of Emergency Medicine and Pediatric Emergency Medicine, and Associate Director of Medical Toxicology, University of Chicago Medical Center, Chicago, Illinois

Tri Chau Tong, MD
Assistant Clinical Professor, Department of Emergency Medicine, University of California, San Diego, School of Medicine and University of California, San Diego, Medical Center, San Diego; Assistant Medical Director, South Coast Medical Center, Laguna Beach, California

David A. Townes, MD, MPH, DTM&H
Associate Professor, Division of Emergency Medicine, and Associate Residency Program Director, University of Washington–Madigan Army Medical Center Residency Program in Emergency Medicine, University of Washington School of Medicine; Attending Physician, Emergency Department, University of Washington Medical Center, Seattle, Washington

T. Paul Tran, MD
Associate Professor of Emergency Medicine, University of Nebraska School of Medicine, Omaha, Nebraska

Victor Tuckler, MD
Director of Toxicology, Department of Medicine, Director, Toxicology Fellowship, and Clinical Instructor, Section of Emergency Medicine, Louisiana State University Health Sciences Center School of Medicine, New Orleans, Louisiana

Jacob W. Ufberg, MD
Associate Professor of Emergency Medicine and Director, Emergency Medicine Residency Program, Temple University School of Medicine; Attending Physician, Temple University Hospital, Philadelphia, Pennsylvania

David Ulick, MD
Attending Physician, Department of Emergency Medicine, Cedars-Sinai Medical Center, Los Angeles, California

Andrew S. Ulrich, MD
Clinical Instructor, Department of Emergency Medicine, Boston University School of Medicine; Residency Director, Emergency Department, Boston Medical Center, Boston, Massachusetts

Guido F. Valdés, MD
Commander, United States Navy Medical Corps; Staff Physician, Emergency Medicine Department, Naval Medical Center, Portsmouth, Virginia

Jon D. Van Roo, MD
Department of Emergency Medicine, Northwestern University Feinberg School of Medicine and Northwestern Memorial Hospital, Chicago, Illinois

Jaime Vasquez, MD
Department of Emergency Medicine, Boston University Medical Center, Boston, Massachusetts

Rais Vohra, MD
Assistant Professor of Emergency Medicine, David Geffen School of Medicine at UCLA, Los Angeles, and Olive View–UCLA Medical Center, Sylmar, California

Michael C. Wadman, MD
Associate Professor and Program Director, Department of Emergency Medicine, University of Nebraska College of Medicine, Omaha, Nebraska

Ernest E. Wang, MD
Assistant Professor, Department of Emergency Medicine, Northwestern University Feinberg School of Medicine, Chicago; Attending Physician, Division of Emergency Medicine, Evanston Hospital, Evanston, Illinois

N. Ewen Wang, MD
Assistant Professor of Pediatrics and Surgery, Stanford University School of Medicine, Stanford; Associate Director, Pediatric Emergency Medicine, Division of Emergency Medicine, Department of Surgery, Stanford University Hospital, Palo Alto, California

Edward John Ward, MD, MPH
Assistant Professor, Rush Medical College and Rush University Medical Center, Chicago, Illinois

Danielle Ware-McGee, MD
Instructor, Department of Emergency Medicine, Northwestern University Feinberg School of Medicine and Northwestern Memorial Hospital, Chicago, Illinois

Beranton Whisenant, MD
Assistant Professor and Director of Research, Department of Emergency Medicine, University of Florida College of Medicine Jacksonville, Jacksonville, Florida

Kurt Whitaker, MD
Instructor of Emergency Medicine, University of Utah School of Medicine, Salt Lake City; Director of Quality Improvement, Department of Emergency Medicine, Intermountain Medical Center, Murray, Utah

Michael E. Winters, MD
Assistant Professor of Emergency Medicine and Medicine, Departments of Emergency Medicine and Medicine, University of Maryland School of Medicine, Baltimore, Maryland

Stephen J. Wolf, MD
Assistant Professor of Surgery, University of Colorado at Denver Health Sciences Center; Director, Residency in Emergency Medicine, Denver Health Medical Center, Denver, Colorado

Richard E. Wolfe, MD
Associate Professor of Medicine, Harvard Medical School; Chief of Emergency Medicine, Beth Israel Deaconess Medical Center, Boston, Massachusetts

Christine Yang-Kauh, MD
Clinical Instructor of Emergency Medicine in Medicine, Weill Medical College of Cornell University, New York; Attending Physician and Assistant Residency Director, Emergency Medicine, New York Methodist Hospital, Brooklyn, New York

Steven M. Zahn, MD
Department of Emergency Medicine, Northwestern University Feinberg School of Medicine and Northwestern Memorial Hospital, Chicago, Illinois

David K. Zich, MD
Assistant Professor of Medicine, Departments of Emergency Medicine and General Internal Medicine, Northwestern University Feinberg School of Medicine and Northwestern Memorial Hospital, Chicago, Illinois

Amy Zosel, MD
Attending Physician, Division of Emergency Medicine, University of Colorado Hospital; Fellow, Rocky Mountain Poison and Drug Center, Denver, Colorado

David N. Zull, MD
Associate Professor, Department of Emergency Medicine, Northwestern University Feinberg School of Medicine; Co-Director, Observation Unit, Department of Emergency Medicine, Northwestern Memorial Hospital, Chicago, Illinois

Preface

It is with gratitude to the talented, energetic teachers of emergency medicine, past and present, that we have created this text. Inspired by their lessons, methods, and insights, we have attempted, within this new textbook, to offer the reader core information for the practice of emergency medicine and communicate this information in a relevant, useful, and interesting way. Great teachers don't just have extensive knowledge. They also have enthusiasm, creativity, and passion. Further, they have the ability to motivate learners, to reinforce their understanding of lessons, to enhance their retention of information, and to ena-ble them to transfer the knowledge to their own practice.

It is these ideal characteristics that we had in mind when we embarked on this text. Admittedly, a textbook cannot really emulate a teacher, but at least we could be inspired by the values. This text uses an abundance of pedagogical tools and devices to maximize the usefulness to the learner. It emphasizes clarity, impact, and ease of use. This book is not just a collection of information. We have attempted to physically instill the spirit and lessons of our great teachers into this work.

Great teachers understand the adult learner. Adult learners—our residents and ourselves—demand engagement, relevancy, and a goal orientation. The best teachers help the learner focus, remember, and apply. Clinical teachers find themselves reaching for a piece of paper to draw an algorithm, create a list, or help a learner construct a table. They engage the learner in lively interaction with guidance through memory aids or compact bites of information that will assist learners to recall and apply the information.

Based on these principles, this text provides no excessive recitation of information in extended prose passages. The chapters are discrete units, broken down into focused passages by subheadings. Information is explained with energy, at a depth sufficient for insight and understanding. This text is intended to be visual. An abundance of figures, tables, algorithms, and photos help emphasize the important messages. The many algorithms force the reader to actively engage the information, consider each decision point, and work through the clinical reasoning.

The chapter topics are not merely academic but are highly relevant to clinical practice for both the expert and the learner. For example, instructions for ultrasound technique are provided in short, focused chapters that are placed alongside related clinical chapters. Other clinical chapters properly include relevant CT findings, for example, but there is also a separate chapter on how to read a head CT. Learners at every level of experience will find information presented in a compelling, approachable way. We hope readers find the text is easy to use, sufficiently detailed, and above all, practical.

This work also attempts to highlight what is new and advanced. Our practice is varied, so the topics across chapters are wide-ranging, covering everything from resuscitation to conversion disorders; from airway management to addiction. Many topics are familiar as core emergency medicine, such as stroke, trauma, and heart failure. Even these core topics are sure to include the latest recommendations and are framed around the best available evidence-based practices. Importantly, new topics are offered such as emergent complications of fertility treatment and management of emergencies in patients who have had bariatric surgery, to name just two examples. Each future edition will attempt to cover the novel emergencies that inevitably result from advancing medical practices and new patterns of disease. "New" information will ultimately become familiar and then be merged as the next generation of emergency situations arise and are highlighted in subsequent editions.

Fortunately, we were able to draw on the abundant talent in the specialty of emergency medicine to create this new work. We sought authors who possessed both content expertise and teaching excellence. They know what the readers want and what the learners need. The authors, collectively, are shining examples of the remarkable teachers in our field. We express deep gratitude and admiration for all who contributed. They understood the novel aims of this text and produced exciting chapters. We have benefited enormously by reading their chapters. It was a joy being their students.

We hope this text will be used by residents to learn and will be accessed by experienced clinicians to recall key information or gain new knowledge. We hope that master teachers will find the work useful for their seminars. The chapters can be efficiently read, perhaps preparing residents to engage in interactive sessions. The work is detailed enough to contain the critical information that must be known by practitioners in the field. All users will hopefully benefit from the authors' creative and expert presentations.

Although a text cannot easily do what great teachers do, such as increase motivation, ensure reinforcement of key messages, test retention, and facilitate transference to clinical practice, we hope that this book will be a useful support for these goals. This work is presented in honor of both the teachers who can accomplish these aims, and the learners who, through their own perseverance and subsequent expertise, will so ably serve their patients.

The Editors wish to acknowledge the following individuals for their assistance, support, and guidance:

Ellen Slaven, M.D., for her educational insights;

Jamie Vasquez, M.D., for editorial assistance;

The faculty and residents at Northwestern University, the Harvard-Affiliated Emergency Medicine residency, LSUHSC New Orleans and University "Charity" Hospital, and the University of Utah;

The staff at Elsevier, including Judy Fletcher, Todd Hummel, Joanie Milnes, and Michael Goldberg, for shepherding this work from concept to physical reality;

Romeo Ines, whose advice, support, and critical analysis were invaluable;

The chapter authors, whose talent, knowledge, and teaching excellence ensured great contributions, as well as Tiffany Osborn, M.D., and Trevor Mills, M.D., whose scholarly contributions and expertise improved this text;

Ron Walls, John Marx, Bob Hockberger, and Michelle Biros for being superb role models, great academic leaders, and exceptional editors.

James G. Adams
Erik D. Barton
Jamie Collings
Peter M. C. DeBlieux
Michael A. Gisondi
Eric S. Nadel

Contents

SECTION I

Resuscitation Skills and Techniques

Chapter **1**

Basic Airway Management

David A. Caro

KEY POINTS

The establishment of a patent airway is the cornerstone of successfully resuscitating and it is a defining proficiency of emergency medicine.

Airway management is a series of clinical decisions based on the patient's ability to oxygenate, ventilate, and protect the airway, as well as the clinician's estimate of the patient's anticipated clinical course.

The failure to evaluate and anticipate airway difficulty is one of the major causes of intubation failure.

A patient who cannot be intubated or oxygenated with a ventilation device requires an immediate surgical intervention.

Emergency airway management is a critical emergency medicine skill. The goal of an emergency intubation is safe, successful intubation of the trachea with an endotracheal tube that allows oxygenation and ventilation while protecting the airway from aspiration. The establishment of a patent airway is the cornerstone of successful resuscitation and a defining proficiency of emergency medicine.

Emergency intubation must occur rapidly, safely, and successfully. The patient has not been preevaluated, may not have been fasted, may have anatomic obstacles that are not readily apparent, and may have unstable hemodynamic parameters. To be successful, the intubator must take these hurdles into account.

The key to emergency intubation is the presence of an arsenal of techniques, tools, and algorithms that the intubator is familiar with and can immediately employ to successfully obtain an airway in the heat of a patient decompensation. Familiarity with the following principles can help ensure safe intubation in the vast majority of patients encountered in clinical practice.

Rapid-sequence intubation (RSI) is the technique of combining sedation and paralysis to create optimal intubating conditions during emergency intubation. RSI has become the standard in emergency airway management, with intubation success rates higher than 99%.[1-6] The emergency airway operator (1) should fully understand the risks and benefits of this technique, (2) should be able to utilize it successfully when indicated, and (3) should know when to deviate from the standard algorithm. RSI is discussed in detail later in this chapter.

Airway Assessment

The first priority in resuscitation is airway analysis and security. The first overriding question for the EP in the resuscitation is, "Do I need to intubate this

The author would like to thank Dr. Ron Walls, Professor, Harvard Medical School, and Chair, Department of Emergency Medicine, Brigham and Women's Hospital, Boston, Massachusetts, for his contributions to this chapter.

patient?" Walls[7,8] describes the following specific indications for intubating a patient:

- Failure to oxygenate or ventilate
- Failure to protect the airway
- Anticipated course that will require intubation

Once one of these indications is identified, the patient requires intubation.[9,10]

The patient's oxygenation status usually can be determined by pulse oximetry. The oximeter reads infrared absorption of hemoglobin, which changes with hemoglobin's oxidation or reduction.[11] Falsely elevated pulse oximetry readings occur with carbon monoxide poisoning.[12-16] Falsely depressed pulse oximetry readings occur with peripheral vasoconstriction, other dyshemoglobinemias, excessive ambient fluorescent lighting, and excessive motion, among other causes.[11,17-22] Concern about misreading should first encourage an alternative site for the probe; and then, if there is still no correction, arterial blood gas analysis. *Oxygenation failure* is defined as the inability to maintain the oxygen saturation greater than 90%.

The patient's ventilatory status usually is measured by clinical features. The patient's respiratory rate is the first sign to be evaluated. Ventilatory problems should be considered for a rate less than 10 breaths/min or more than 20 breaths/min. Next, the depth of and difficulty with breathing should be assessed. Abnormal breathing patterns (e.g., Kussmaul's respirations) are harbingers of impending ventilatory failure and various pathophysiologic states. Use of accessory muscles, the inability to speak in complete sentences, or the presence of abnormal airway sounds should also raise concern. Stridor, an inspiratory, high-pitched sound, signals upper airway obstruction. Wheezing is associated with lower airway constriction from bronchospasm. Finally, the patient's mental status serves to help in the assessment of ventilation. As the carbon dioxide tension increases in the blood, the patient experiences a "CO_2 narcosis" and becomes increasingly drowsy.[7,31-34] It is important for the EP to remember that the decision to intubate is a clinical one. Arterial blood gas analysis is a helpful adjunct, but *a patient whose mental status is waning because of ventilatory insufficiency is in emergency ventilatory failure* and should be intubated immediately to facilitate ventilation.

Airway protection is a complex reflex that involves powerful sensory and motor pathways designed to maintain airway patency at all costs. Stimulation of the pharynx, hypopharynx, and tongue base results in gagging, protective coughing, and voluntary attempts to remove the stimulant if the patient is able to move. *Acute obtundation, however, diminishes a patient's ability to sense irritant stimuli and therefore spontaneously protect the airway.*[10,35,36] This fact is the impetus behind the use of a Glasgow Coma Scale score less than or equal to 8 as a cue to intubate patients with trauma.[35] Such a score indicates that the patient is at risk to aspirate gastric contents or blood, which is associated with a rise in mortality.[37-40]

Traditionally, the gag reflex has been used to determine whether a patient's airway reflexes are intact. Stimulation of a gag in the obtunded or trauma patient, however, may result in unwanted reactions, such as bucking, gagging, coughing, and actual vomiting; additionally, up to 37% of healthy volunteers in several studies did not demonstrate a gag reflex, calling into question the use of this sign to assess the patient's ability to protect the airway.[35,36,41,42] A less invasive approach is to observe for the occurrence of spontaneous swallowing. A patient who swallows spontaneously while recumbent has sensory and motor paths capable of protecting the airway.[43-45] Conversely, *the patient who is not spontaneously swallowing has impairment in the ability to protect the airway.*

Finally, *the patient's anticipated course* serves as an intubation criterion if loss of airway patency or protection is predicted within the near future. For example, a significant thermal or chemical burn of the airway can subsequently cause significant airway edema that eventually will make intubation difficult; early intubation in such cases may protect the airway. Similarly, an asthmatic patient who is beginning to tire despite maximal therapy is frequently intubated before ventilatory failure is complete.

Emergency Airway Algorithms

A specific framework is required to effectively address resuscitation in the acute setting. The Difficult Airway Course: Emergency, a national continuing medical education training course developed by the Airway Management Education Center (AMEC), has treatment algorithms that allow for a standardized approach to these stressful situations, which in turn helps to prevent errors and improve patient safety (Fig. 1-1).

Resuscitation protocols universally include a primary survey designed to identify immediate life threats that would preclude further history or physical examination. The first of these priorities is the airway assessment. As already discussed, the overriding question the EP asks is, "Do I need to intubate this patient?" If the answer is "Yes," a further series of questions and actions must be addressed, as follows.

■ "DOES THIS PATIENT HAVE A 'CRASH' AIRWAY?"

A "crash" airway is one in which the patient is dead (or nearly so). If the answer is "Yes!" the EP should proceed immediately to intubation without delay for administration of sedatives or paralytic agents (Fig. 1-2).

If the patient does not have a crash airway, medications should be used to facilitate intubation. Neuromuscular blockers are one of the classes of medications to consider. With this in mind, the EP considers the next question.

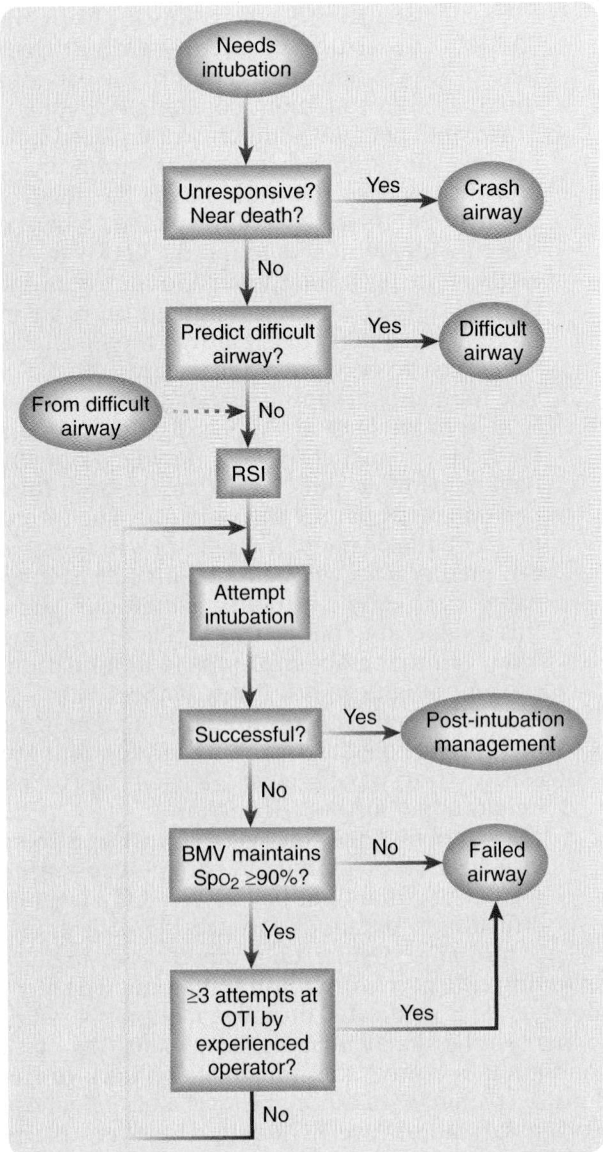
Needs intubation
Unresponsive? Near death?
Yes
Crash airway
No
Predict difficult airway?
Yes
Difficult airway
From difficult airway
No
RSI
Attempt intubation
Successful?
Yes
Post-intubation management
No
BMV maintains Spo2 ≥90%?
No
Failed airway
Yes
≥3 attempts at OTI by experienced operator?
Yes
No

FIGURE 1-1 Main emergency airway management algorithm. BMV, bag-mask ventilation; OTI, orotracheal intubation; RSI, rapid-sequence intubation; SpO_2, pulse oximetry. (Adapted from Walls RM: The emergency airway algorithms. In Walls RM, Luten RC, Murphy MF, Schneider RE [eds]: Manual of Emergency Airway Management, 2nd ed. Philadelphia, Lippincott-Williams & Wilkins, 2004. Copyright 2004: The Airway Course and Lippincott Williams & Wilkins.)

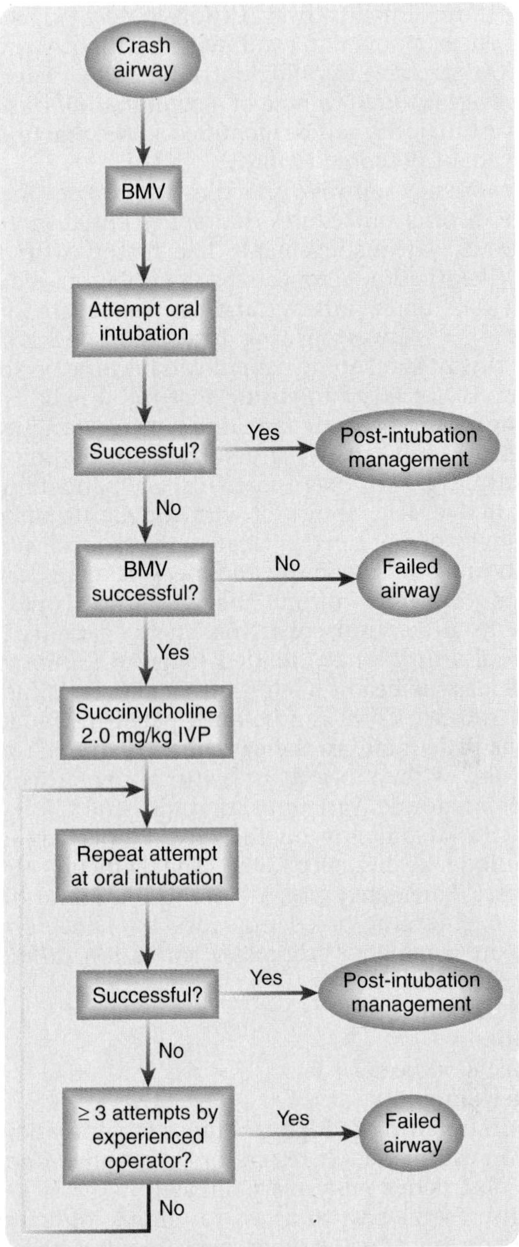
Crash airway
BMV
Attempt oral intubation
Successful?
Yes
Post-intubation management
No
BMV successful?
No
Failed airway
Yes
Succinylcholine 2.0 mg/kg IVP
Repeat attempt at oral intubation
Successful?
Yes
Post-intubation management
No
≥ 3 attempts by experienced operator?
Yes
Failed airway
No

FIGURE 1-2 Crash airway algorithm. BMV, bag-mask ventilation; IVP, intravenous "push." (Adapted from Walls RM: The emergency airway algorithms. In Walls RM Luten RC, Murphy MF, Schneider RE [eds]: Manual of Emergency Airway Management, 2nd ed. Philadelphia, Lippincott-Williams & Wilkins, 2004. Copyright 2004: The Airway Course and Lippincott-Williams & Wilkins.)

■ "IS THIS A DIFFICULT AIRWAY?"

The failure to evaluate and anticipate airway difficulty is one of the major causes of intubation failure.[46,47] The use of paralytic agents in emergency intubation requires "difficult airway" assessment and preparation for an alternative airway in the event that a patient cannot be intubated by standard means. A difficult airway may preclude the use of paralytic agents altogether until the EP can ensure glottic visualization, usually with procedural sedation and topical anesthesia. The approach to the difficult airway is discussed in greater detail in Chapter 2.

Unfortunately, there is no universal definition of a "difficult airway." In some patients, the EP receives an immediate impression that the airway will be difficult. EPs tend to be correct when their initial reaction is that an airway will be difficult.[10,47] The converse is not true. Some otherwise normal-appearing patients have subtle anatomic differences that may make their intubation difficult and are not immediately recognizable by an EP who is not specifically evaluating for difficulty.

Fortunately, a number of studies have demonstrated various clinical cues that can be used to predict the difficult airway. Unfortunately, no clinical sign, either alone or in combination with other signs, is 100% sensitive in ruling out a difficult airway.[1,46-59] However, through the use of a combination of signs, the vast majority can be identified so the practitioner is aware of potential hazards.

Emergency airway difficulty can arise in the three distinct procedures that are essential in emergency airway management. The first is with bag-mask ventilation. Proper mask ventilation requires both an open airway and an adequate mask seal.[10,46,48,50] Airway opening depends on positioning. The airway in a supine patient can become occluded if care is not taken to ensure that the tongue is not falling against the hypopharynx. Large tongues or excessive soft tissue structures surrounding the airway (e.g., in obese patients or patients with obstructive sleep apnea, or with tongue hematomas or angioedema) might create airway obstruction. Positioning of the head and neck is necessary to create the most direct line of airway opening. Patients in cervical collars or elderly patients with cervical arthritis have limited range of motion that precludes the head-tilt, chin-lift maneuver. Difficulty with the mask seal can be anticipated in the edentulous patient and in the patient with an open nasal fracture, with a beard, or with retrognathism or other anatomic variations that do not allow the mask to sit properly on the face. Proper bag-mask technique is discussed later. The Difficult Airway Course: Emergency has developed a useful mnemonic checklist, based on work by Langeron, to evaluate a patient's bag-mask ventilation difficulty; it is **MOANS**[10,48,50]:

- **M**ask seal
- **O**besity
- **A**ge (>50 years)
- **N**eck mobility
- **S**tiff (referring to high resistance to ventilation, as in asthma, adult respiratory syndrome, chronic obstructive pulmonary disease)

The second area to assess for airway difficulty is laryngoscopy. Oral laryngoscopy requires that the mouth be opened and that the various axes the laryngoscope has to navigate be aligned as much as possible. Anatomic obstacles can make laryngoscopy difficult. Large incisors, retrognathism, temporomandibular joint inflammation, tongue swelling, and obesity can all impair oral access with the laryngoscope. The addition of cervical immobility, whether due to cervical arthritis (as with ankylosing spondylitis), fracture, or the possibility of a fracture with placement of a cervical collar, impedes the EP's ability to align the head and neck optimally for intubation.

Laryngoscopy difficulty can generally be assessed by using the mnemonic **LEMON**, which was developed for The Difficult Airway Course: Emergency and validated in a subsequent study in the United Kingdom[46,53-59]:

1. **L**ook to see whether there is any obvious anatomy distortion
2. **E**valuate the airway geometry quickly using the "3-3-2" rule. Three of the patient's fingers, placed side-by-side, should fit into the patient's mouth. If they can, mouth opening is adequate. Three of the patient's fingers, again placed side-by-side, should fit between the mentum (chin) and the angle of the neck (i.e., at the level of the hyoid). Finally, two of the patient's fingers, placed side-by-side, should fit between the angle of the neck and the superior notch on the thyroid cartilage. If these rough measures are in place, the geometry of the airway should enable the larynx to be viewed adequately.[10,48,53-55,59]
3. The **M**allampati score is assessed if the patient is able to perform it. Mallampati described a method to predict ease of laryngoscopy by having patients put themselves in a sniffing position and opening their mouths. The extent to which the posterior pharyngeal wall is visible can predict who will be more difficult to intubate.[10,53-55,59] Some patients' conditions allow this evaluation, but a true Mallampati score often cannot be obtained (due to obtundation, concern about cervical injury, and so on).
4. Are there signs of **o**bstruction? Drooling or inability to tolerate secretions, stridor, and the classic "hot potato voice" are all signs that herald upper airway obstruction.
5. **N**eck mobility plays a key role in the ease of visualization of a larynx. A patient whose neck cannot or should not be moved adds a layer of difficulty to obtaining laryngeal visualization.

The third area of emergency airway assessment is reviewing critical cricothyrotomy anatomy. The technique of RSI is predicated on the practitioner's ability to manage the airway if laryngoscopy fails. Bag-mask ventilation is always the immediate fallback procedure in a patient who cannot be intubated and whose oxygen saturation level is falling. However, in the failed airway scenario (see later discussion), a patient who cannot be intubated or oxygenated with a ventilation device requires an immediate surgical intervention. In the majority of cases, there is not time to consult a surgeon for this management.[2,5,61,62] It is the responsibility of the practitioner using RSI to be familiar with and to be able to use surgical airway techniques and provide a definitive airway in this uncommon but highly stressful scenario.

The discussion of how to perform a cricothyrotomy is left to Chapter 2. However, the EP must recognize the signs of potential difficulty with cricothyrotomy and, potentially, with immediate paralysis of the patient. The mnemonic **SHORT**, developed by Sakles for The Difficult Airway Course: Emergency, allows the EP to readily recall the following factors that may affect cricothyrotomy[10]:

- Prior neck **s**urgery
- Expanding neck **h**ematomas
- **O**besity
- Prior **r**adiation
- **T**umors and abscesses that might distort anatomy

Critical Airway Anatomy

A rational approach to airway analysis and management requires a review of pertinent airway anatomy. First, the EP should examine the patient for facial distortion and the position in which the airway is held. The face is the immediately obvious structure the EP encounters. Specific structures to observe are the nose and nostrils, the lips, and the teeth. Obvious nasal deformities might hinder efforts at mask ventilation. Large nasal turbinates may not allow nasal airway adjuncts to pass. Swollen lips might tip the practitioner to the possibility of angioedema or an allergic reaction. Dentures might help during mask ventilation but may hinder laryngoscopy attempts. Drooling or inability to tolerate secretions may be apparent and is an ominous sign suggesting significant supraglottic irritation or obstruction. The EP should ask the patient to open the mouth or, in an obtunded patient, should carefully perform a jaw-thrust and mouth-opening maneuver to determine how far the mouth can open. Palpation of facial structures involves determining nasal, maxillary, and mandibular stability. Mobility of any of these facial structures may pose a difficulty to managing the airway. Maxillary instability, in particular, should alert the EP to be cautious with any nasal intubation, whether with nasal trumpet, nasogastric tube, or blind nasotracheal intubation, because intracranial misplacement of nasal trumpets and nasotracheal tubes has been reported.[63-67] To avoid having fingers bitten by the patient when assessing maxillary instability, the EP should warn the patient of the maxillary manipulation; if a combative patient requires this examination, an oral airway or bite block can be positioned in the mouth to assure clinician safety.

Next the EP should view the tongue, comparing its size in relation to the oropharynx and evaluating the tongue for lacerations, swelling, foreign bodies, and signs of inflammation. The hard and soft palate, as well as the tonsils, should be similarly evaluated. Enlarged, scarred tonsils should raise the possibility of enlarged palatine tonsils, which might impair ventilation attempts.[68] Inflamed, erythematous tonsils or an inflamed, swollen soft palate alerts the EP to significant upper airway soft-tissue infectious disorders and potential obstruction.

The junction of the oropharynx and nasopharynx marks the superior boundary of the hypopharynx. This is the level at which most airway structures become hidden. The base of the tongue dips into the hypopharynx and ends at the valleculae—small wells formed by the tongue base and the takeoff of the epiglottis. The epiglottis attaches to the anterior airway and enlarges superiorly to create an airway shield for swallowing. It is immediately superior to the glottic opening, the target of laryngoscopy.

The larynx is a cartilaginous structure that houses the vocal cord apparatus. It is shield-shaped, with a distinctive V notch at its anterior-superior border. Posteriorly, the laryngeal cartilage angles sharply cranial then dips caudad, so it is not as tall as the anterior aspect in the midline. The vocal cords originate from the anterior aspect of the laryngeal cartilage and insert posteriorly into the arytenoid cartilages, which are small, pointed, and mobile. The arytenoids sit on the superior surface of the posterior laryngeal cartilage. The larynx encircles the glottis, the opening between the vocal cords. Mucous membrane lines the opening to the glottis, the posterior aspect of the anterior laryngeal cartilage, the entire posterior laryngeal cartilage, and the arytenoids. A set of false cords are created by folds of mucosa overlying the actual vocal cords.

The cricoid ring and the trachea are cartilaginous structures attached to the laryngeal cartilage that create the passageway into the lower respiratory tree. The cricoid cartilage attaches to the laryngeal cartilage via the cricothyroid membrane. This relationship is critical for the EP to keep in mind, because surgical airway control requires the proper identification of this landmark. Also, the cricoid ring is the only completely solid ring that surrounds the airway, which can be used as another landmark and tool in airway management. In young children, the cricoid ring is the narrowest portion of the airway, and the cricothyroid membrane is too small to access. As the patient ages, the glottis becomes the tightest structure.

The trachea leads to the mainstem bronchi. The right mainstem bronchus is oriented with a less acute angle in relation to the axis of the trachea than the left mainstem. It is relatively easy to intubate the right mainstem bronchus, which would hinder bilateral lung insufflation. The bronchi then subdivide into the bronchial tree, ultimately ending in microscopic alveoli.

Pertinent Airway-Related Physiology

Oxygenation is a complex process that begins with the inspiration of ambient air (typically made up of a mixture of gases, 21% of which is oxygen). The inspired breath mixes with tracheal and bronchial air, subsequently diffusing into the lower airways and ultimately into the alveoli. At the alveolus, oxygen must diffuse across the alveolar membrane and into the blood stream. The dissolved oxygen must then bind reduced hemoglobin to be transported to the body's tissues.

The volume of air that is inspired during breathing is the *tidal volume*. The volume of air inspired during the deepest breath a patient can take is the *vital capacity*. The difference between the vital capacity and tidal volume is the *functional residual capacity*, or the reserve left in the lung at typical end-expiration.

The alveolar membrane normally allows rapid and efficient diffusion of oxygen across it. Blood hemoglobin binds oxygen and transports it throughout the body. Hemoglobin-oxygen binding is not linear.

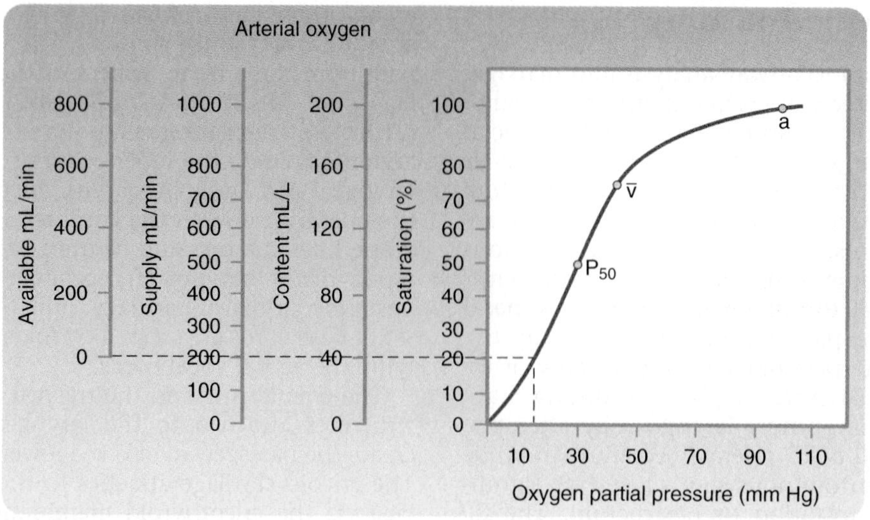

Arterial oxygen
Available mL/min
800
600
400
200
0
Supply mL/min
1000
800
700
600
500
400
300
200
100
0
Content mL/L
200
160
120
80
40
0
Saturation (%)
100
80
70
60
50
40
30
20
10
0
a
v̄
P50
10 30 50 70 90 110
Oxygen partial pressure (mm Hg)

FIGURE 1-3 Oxygen-hemoglobin dissociation curve. Four different ordinates are shown as a function of oxygen partial pressure (the *abscissa*). In order from right to left, they are saturation (%); O_2 content (mL of O_2/0.1 L of blood); O_2 supply to peripheral tissues (mL/min); and O_2 available to peripheral tissues (mL/min), which is calculated as O_2 supply minus the approximately 200 mL/min that cannot be extracted below a partial pressure of 20 mm Hg. Three points are shown on the curve: *a,* normal arterial pressure; $\bar{v}$, normal mixed venous pressure; and P_{50}, the partial pressure (27 mm Hg) at which hemoglobin is 50% saturated. (From: Miller RD [ed]: Miller's Anesthesia, 6th ed. Philadelphia, Churchill Livingstone, 2005.)

Hemoglobin tends to bind oxygen well until the partial pressure of oxygen reaches 60 mm Hg and then rapidly dissociates from the oxygen to allow it to diffuse into the blood and surrounding tissue. An oxygen partial pressure of 60 mm Hg correlates to an oxygen saturation level of 90%. This is an important correlation that should be kept in mind throughout resuscitation. Figure 1-3 shows the relationship between oxygen partial pressure and hemoglobin saturation.

Ventilation refers to the exchange of gas in the lungs. Ventilation is necessary to clear carbon dioxide (CO_2) from the alveoli, creating a carbon dioxide gradient between the alveoli and the blood. CO_2 diffuses rapidly across the alveolar membrane, such that alveolar CO_2 tension approximates capillary and venous CO_2 tension. As long as adequate ventilation occurs, this gradient allows efficient removal of CO_2 from the body.

The inability to expire effectively (e.g., during an exacerbation of asthma or chronic obstructive pulmonary disease) impairs ventilation. Global ventilation failure typically results in climbing CO_2 tension within the blood, resulting in acidosis and cerebral dysfunction. CO_2 is usually in equilibrium with bicarbonate in the serum. A rising CO_2 level shifts this balance to cause a "respiratory" acidosis.

Local or regionalized impairment in ventilation can also occur. Ventilation-perfusion ($\dot{V}/\dot{Q}$) mismatching occurs when an area of the lung is ventilated but not perfused, such as with a pulmonary embolus or during certain shock states. The air in the alveoli cannot draw CO_2 from the blood in this setting. Shunting occurs when blood perfuses alveoli that are not ventilated, emptying CO_2-rich blood into the left heart.

Oxygenation Techniques

A patient breathing room air is receiving 21% oxygen. Patients with a higher oxygen demand should receive supplemental oxygen to raise the fractional percentage of exygen (FiO_2) they receive. The standard nasal cannula can comfortably deliver up to 6 L of oxygen per minute. A nasal cannula set at 2 L/min delivers approximately 23% FiO_2; at 4 L/min, 25% FiO_2; and at 6 L, approximately 27% FiO_2. A Venturi mask can deliver up to 40% FiO_2. A nonrebreather mask with an oxygen reservoir can deliver 15 L/min and will provide an FiO_2 of 65% to 70%. (Of note, the term "100% nonrebreather mask" is a misnomer; the delivery system that the nonrebreather is equipped with cannot provide 100% FiO_2.) Other inert gases (helium, in particular) can be mixed with oxygen and used to replace nitrogen, improving laminar flow and, potentially, better oxygenation for patients with large airway masses or severe bronchoconstriction.[69] Patients who require intubation should be preoxygenated with a nonrebreather mask for as long as possible. The goal of this step is to wash as much nitrogen out of the lung as possible and to replace it with oxygen.[10,70,71] When the patient is paralyzed during RSI, this reservoir will allow for the continued delivery of oxygen at the alveoli for some time, thereby enabling the patient to maintain oxygen saturation while apneic. Preoxygenation for 5 minutes or more allows for this reservoir to develop. Alternatively, if no such time is available, the patient can be asked to take eight vital capacity breaths through the nonrebreather to build as great a reservoir as possible.[10,70,72,73] Not surprisingly, critically ill patients have decreased oxygen reserve and tolerate apnea less well than relatively healthy subjects.[10,70,71,74]

A bag-mask device can also be used to passively oxygenate patients, provided that it has a one-way inhalation port and a true nonrebreather port. A proper seal is essential.[75] Patients with the ability to inspire can draw air through the mask as the EP maintains a tight seal around the nose and mouth. The EP can thereby avoid "assisting" ventilation by this method, decreasing the risk of aspiration. This apparatus offering a tight seal can reach FiO_2 levels higher than 90%.

Positive pressure will, at times, be required to oxygenate a patient before intubation. Continuous positive airway pressure (CPAP) or bilevel positive airway pressure (BiPAP) can provide a constant level of positive-pressure support or two levels of pressure support, respectively, through a tightly fitted mask that fits over the nose or the mouth and nose.[69,76] The positive pressure is used to "stent" the alveoli and small airways to help ventilation in patients experiencing severe dyspnea due to a number of disorders. These modalities are used in an effort to temporize disorders that rapidly "turn around" if concomitant pharmacologic therapy can be effectively applied.

Finally, active bag ventilation and oxygenation may need to be given in patients who are experiencing acute oxygenation failure. Most adult bag-mask devices have reservoirs larger than 1 L and can deliver high-flow oxygen if a good mask seal is maintained.[71,74,77-79] Active bag-mask ventilation and oxygenation are reserved for those whose oxygen saturation is below 90%. Any positive-pressure ventilation not only ventilates the lungs but also insufflates the stomach. Knowledge of this fact is critical to the performance of RSI. A paralyzed patient is at risk for aspiration due to relaxed esophageal sphincter tone, especially if the stomach is distended with air.[37]

■ TECHNIQUE OF BAG-MASK VENTILATION

Bag-mask ventilation is a critical skill that all airway managers must master before learning to perform RSI. Mask ventilation is the airway management modality of choice for any patient who cannot maintain adequate oxygenation with a nonrebreather mask or begins to become desaturated ($FiO_2 < 90\%$) while apneic during an RSI attempt.[10,70,71] It is the fallback method of choice; if it fails, the airway manager is forced to follow the failed airway algorithm. Proper bag-mask technique can provide indefinite oxygenation for patients who can be ventilated with this technique. A brief review is essential.

The bag-mask device comes in neonatal, pediatric, and adult sizes. The mask is made of clear plastic to allow visualization of the mouth and nose during active ventilation. It is usually formed to fit the nose and mouth. The mask has an air-filled balloon attached to the surface that contacts the face, allowing the practitioner to create an airtight seal when the mask is applied correctly. The mask size differs with the size of the device. The mask attaches either to a 90-degree, clear plastic adapter, which then attaches to the bag device; or it can attach directly to the bag device. The bag itself is usually made of rubber or plastic, is compressible, and attaches to an oxygen source. The bag size differs with the size of the device as well. A neonatal bag typically has a 250-mL reservoir; a pediatric bag a 500-mL reservoir; and an adult bag a 1000- to 1500-mL reservoir.

Other devices may be attached to the bag-mask device. One of the most important devices to check for is the presence of a pressure-relief (or "popoff") valve. This valve is attached to the bag adapter to allow air to release from the circuit if the pressure inside the bag-mask reaches or exceeds a certain level.[10,71] It can be set to "pop off" or can be stopped from doing so; different valves are constructed differently, so the EP should consult the manual that comes with the device to ensure understanding of this airway tool before using it.

Another component of the bag that is not readily apparent is the presence of a one-way exhalation valve and port that allow exhaled air to escape, ensuring that none returns into the bag reservoir. These valves also ensure one-way flow of oxygen into the mask and patient. Not all bags are constructed with this type of valve, which becomes important when the bag-mask device is used as a passive oxygenation device. Without this valve, a patient breathing spontaneously with the mask applied to the face will receive very low concentrations of oxygen.[10] Patients receiving supplemental oxygen through a mask with a one-way valve and expiration port can receive above 90% FiO_2 when breathing spontaneously through a properly applied mask.

The application of the bag and mask requires *proper patient positioning* and *correct application of a mask seal.* Ideally, for mask ventilation, the patient should be supine with the head and neck in the "sniffing" position.[10,71] The head is extended at C1 to C2, and the neck is flexed at the cervicothoracic junction. This position allows the airway axes to align as close together as possible. An alternative position is to keep the patient's head neutral but apply a jaw-thrust maneuver to pull the base of the tongue away from the hypopharynx and create a passageway for air to enter. Ventilation adjuncts may have to be used when creating the best position to ventilate. Nasal airways (or nasal "trumpets") can be used in the responsive patient to ensure an adequate opening through which oxygenation and ventilation occur; oral airways can be used in the unresponsive patient to accomplish the same task. It is important to realize that an oral airway should *not* be used in an awake patient because it could stimulate a gag reflex.

A proper mask seal is obtained by first approximating the mask to the patient's face. It is correctly sized if it covers the nose and mouth and the mask balloon can rest on the patient's mentum.[10,71] The mask is then apposed to the facial skin to create a good air seal. A lone operator needs to use a single hand to apply the mask-seal technique; if a second operator is present, the primary operator can concentrate on

Table 1-1 SEDATIVE AGENTS FOR INTUBATION

Agent	Recommended Dose	Time to Onset (sec)	Duration of Action (min)	Relevant Side Effects
Midazolam (benzodiazepine)	0.1-0.3 mg/kg intravenously (IV)	30-60	15-30	Hypotension
Thiopental (barbiturate)	1-6 mg/kg IV	<30	5-10	Hypotension Bronchospasm
Etomidate	0.3 mg/kg IV	15-45	3-12	Myoclonus
Ketamine	1.5 mg/kg IV	45-60	10-20	Laryngospasm Elevated intracranial pressure Sympathomimetic response
Propofol	1.5-3 mg/kg IV	15-45	5-10	Hypotension

a two-handed mask seal application. The single-hand mask seal method is inferior to the double-handed method in generating tidal volume and peak pressure.[10,71,77] The airway manager applies both hands to the mask to appose it to the patient's face. The traditional method of grasping the mask is with the hands in the shape of a C for the left hand and a reverse C for the right hand.[71] The index fingers meet at the part of the mask overlying the mentum, and the thumbs meet at the part of the mask overlying the nose. The long, ring, and small fingers of both hands are then used to raise the mandible to the mask to create a seal.

An alternative method that is not as demanding on the lumbrical muscles of the hands is to apply the mask as previously described, and then apply the thenar eminences of the hand along the nasal part of the mask and place the thumbs parallel to each other, so that they surround the connector and extend onto the part of the mask that covers the mouth. All other fingers are then used to hook the mandible and bring it up to the mask. Moving the thumbs and thenar eminences can allow for any compensation needed to maintain an adequate mask seal.[10]

It is imperative that no seal leak occurs during mask ventilation. A mask seal leak creates a distinctive sound that all practitioners should train themselves to listen for. An inadequate seal mandates a review of technique and equipment. If the mask balloon is popped, another mask must be obtained. Inadequate hand strength or muscle tiring due to prolonged mask seal maintenance may require a personnel switch.

Physiologic Responses to Laryngoscopy and Pharyngeal Stimulation

Physical stimulation of the pharynx causes a physiologic set of responses. Adult patients respond with sympathetic stimulation, resulting in reflex tachycardia and increases in blood pressure and intracranial pressure, among other responses.[10,71] This response is termed the *reflex sympathetic response to laryngoscopy.* Pediatric patients tend to respond with parasympathetic stimulation and can display significant bradycardia in response to pharyngeal manipulation.[10]

Medications, Pharmacology, and Physiologic Responses to Medication Classes

Ideal RSI technique depends on the use of the combination of sedation and paralysis to render a patient optimally relaxed for the procedure. Once the patient has been determined to be "safe" for RSI (i.e., does *not* have a crash airway or a difficult airway), the medications should be chosen.

Multiple sedatives are available for use in RSI. The use of a sedative humanely allows for amnesia and sedation, potentially improving laryngoscopy and intubation.[80] The choice of sedative agent for a given clinical scenario differs according to the pathophysiologic parameters that the EP observes or anticipates to occur during the RSI attempt. Hemodynamic instability, elevated intracranial pressure, and bronchospasm are the most common complicating factors the EP must consider during preparation for sedation. Table 1-1 contains a list of sedative agents used in RSI and their side effect profiles.

Commonly used sedatives in current emergency practice are midazolam (Versed) and etomidate (Amidate). Midazolam doses recommended in the anesthesia literature are 0.1 to 0.3 mg/kg intravenously (IV).[10,71,81] The danger of using midazolam in these doses is the hypotension they generate, especially in critically ill patients. Most practitioners intentionally underdose midazolam in the setting of RSI for this specific reason.[81] Etomidate is given at 0.3 mg/kg IV and does not cause the hypotension seen with midazolam.[82,83] Etomidate does cause a reversible cortisol suppression, however, so is no longer used as a drip for long-term sedation. The effect on cortisol after a single dose has been demonstrated to resolve spontaneously and not have a poor effect on patient outcome.[84]

The paralytic agents commonly used for RSI are depolarizing agents (succinylcholine) and nondepolarizing agents (pancuronium, vecuronium, and

Table 1-2 NONDEPOLARIZING AGENTS FOR INTUBATION

Agent	Recommended Dose	Time to Onset (sec)	Duration of Action (min)	Relevant Side Effects
Rocuronium	1 mg/kg intravenously (IV)	45-60	30-60	—
Norcuronium	0.1 mg/kg IV	90-120	60-75	—
Pancuronium	0.1 mg/kg IV	100-150	120-150	Tachycardia Histamine release

From Walls RM, Luten RC, Murphy MF, Schneider RE (eds): Manual of Emergency Airway Management, 2nd ed. Philadelphia, Lippincott Williams & Wilkins, 2004.

BOX 1-1

Succinylcholine

Dosage

1.5 mg/kg IV (range 1-3 mg/kg)

Mechanism of Action

Depolarizing neuromuscular blockade; succinylcholine binds to acetylcholine receptors, stimulating a continual depolarization and resulting in paralysis

Side Effects

- Hyperkalemia (sometimes fatal in patients with preexisting hyperkalemia)
- Fasciculations
- Increased intraocular pressure
- Increased intragastric pressure
- Bradycardia in children
- Malignant hyperthermia
- Masseter spasm in children (requires nondepolarizing agent—rocuronium, vecuronium, norcuronium—to overcome)

rocuronium). Succinylcholine has been studied extensively and is the classic agent used for RSI. It has a short onset time (approximately 45 seconds), a short duration of action (approximately 5 to 10 minutes), and a wide dosing margin (typical dose for is RSI 1.5 mg/kg, but doses up to 6 mg/kg do not change its pharmacokinetics[71]). Succinylcholine also has some significant side effects, including occasionally significant hyperkalemia, fasciculations, and malignant hyperthermia. Any airway manager who plans to use succinylcholine should be well versed in its mechanism of action as well as its potentially significant and life-threatening side effects (Box 1-1).[85]

Rocuronium has come into favor as a nondepolarizing agent that can provide succinylcholine-like intubating conditions in 45 to 60 seconds provided that the correct dose (1.0 to 1.2 mg/kg IV) is used.[85-89] The benefits of using a nondepolarizing agent include the absence of fasciculations and hyperkalemia. The duration of action of the nondepolarizing agents is much longer than that of succinylcholine, however, rocuronium being the shortest-acting at 45 to 60 minutes.[10,71] See Table 1-2 for a list of commonly used nondepolarizing paralytic agents and their side effect profiles.

Intubation

The process of intubation involves proper patient positioning, EP positioning, tool assembly, and the technique of laryngoscopy. The standard, oral intubation occurs with the patient lying flat and supine, while the positioning of the patient's head is addressed.[71] In the patient with an immobile cervical spine, whether due to trauma, arthritis, or other causes, the head and neck should not be manipulated, and the head should be maintained in a neutral position with in-line stabilization by a person designated for this task.[10,71] If mobility is not an issue, the age of the patient and size of the occiput determine the need for elevation of the patient's shoulders or head. Infants have a relatively large occiput compared with their bodies and therefore will passively flex the head forward when lying flat.[10] This makes a more acute angle that the laryngoscopist has to navigate. The airway axes better align if the infant's shoulders are elevated. The adult's head is relatively smaller and tends to extend at the cervicothoracic junction instead of flexing. This extension counterintuitively moves the laryngeal and pharyngeal axes into alignment that is less parallel; it can be overcome by placing a roll under the adult's head.[10] A key anatomic relationship to keep in mind is that the head is ideally aligned when an imaginary line drawn between the tragus of the ear and the anterior axillary line is parallel to the floor.[10]

Standard orotracheal intubation occurs with the practitioner at the head of the bed looking down at the patient's face from above the head. The EP gently grasps the laryngoscope with the fingertips of the left hand. The laryngoscope's blade should be extended and locked into position. Using the right hand, the EP opens the mouth, with either a scissoring technique with the thumb and index finger or by grasping the mentum and moving it caudally to expose the mouth. The blade of the laryngoscope is then gently inserted into the right side of the mouth and advanced into the pharynx.

The blades most commonly used in emergency intubation are the curved MacIntosh blade and the straight Miller blade. Traditional intubation with the MacIntosh blade begins with the insertion of the blade at the right corner of the mouth. The blade is advanced under direct visualization, is swept to the midline, and concomitantly sweeps the tongue to the patient's left. The tip of the blade is directed into the vallecula, and then the laryngoscope is *pushed* up as a unit. The epiglottis is lifted up because of its connection to the hyoepiglottic ligament, which attaches to the posterior surface of the mucosa behind the hyoid and the base of the epiglottis. Epiglottic lifting exposes the vocal cords and glottis.

Traditional intubation with the Miller blade similarly occurs with insertion of the blade in the right side of the mouth. The blade is brought to the midline by the time it reaches the epiglottis, again under direct visualization. Tongue control is a major issue, with the blade pushing the tongue to the left. The laryngoscope is then *pushed* upward to physically lift the epiglottis and expose the vocal cords.

An alternative method of oral laryngoscopy with the Miller blade is described in the National Emergency Airway Course.[10] The Miller blade is inserted into the right side of the mouth as usual. Instead of beginning the visualization attempt immediately upon insertion, the EP gently inserts the blade blindly as far as it can advance. It is usually possible to insert the blade to the hub of the handle in this manner. At this point, the laryngoscopy actually begins. The EP can look down the blade to see what is exposed, which should be the esophagus. The blade is then gently withdrawn under constant visualization, until either the glottis or epiglottis falls into view. Much less muscular strength is required by this method, and the operator gains the benefit of always starting distal to the glottis and knowing where the airway should lie in relation to the blade tip. The risk—blunt trauma to the arytenoids or vocal cords—is the reason for the emphasis on gentle insertion of the blade. It is important in this or any other laryngoscopic technique that any movement to lift the epiglottis or push up the tongue is the result of *pushing* the handle parallel to its axis towards the ceiling, and not pulling the handle to use the teeth as a fulcrum.

Finally, nasotracheal intubation is another primary option for intubation, although its use is decreasing in favor of directly visualized oral intubation. Nasotracheal intubation requires a spontaneously breathing patient because the patient's breath sounds guide the intubator as to where to place the tube. The practitioner stands on the side of the patient that allows use of the practitioner's dominant hand. Either a standard endotracheal (ET) tube or a directional-tipped ET tube can be prepared for the intubation. The nares should be anesthetized (with benzocaine or tetracaine sprays) and vasoconstricted before the attempt. Pharyngeal anesthesia should also be attempted. The ET tube is introduced into a nostril and directed posteriorly, the curve of the tube being allowed to pass anatomically with the curve of the posterior nasopharynx. Once the tube has navigated the nasopharynx, the operator begins listening through the ET tube for breath sounds. As the glottis is blindly approached, the patient's breath sounds become louder. Once the maximal breath sounds are achieved, the operator attempts to time glottic intubation with a deep inspiration on the part of the patient. Typically, the patient experiences at least some coughing and gagging when the ET tube is passed in this manner.

Putting It Together: Rapid-Sequence Intubation

Rapid-sequence intubation is the technique of combining sedation and paralysis to create the optimal intubating conditions during emergency intubation.[2,6,10,80] The operator must assume that (1) the patient's stomach is full (i.e., the patient has not been fasted), (2) the patient's hemodynamics are potentially unstable, and (3) the patient's condition is critical. The choice of techniques, medications, and instruments is based on a number of these factors.

Walls[10] describes seven checklist points that have been identified to help EPs prepare for emergency intubation with RSI (Box 1-2). Also known as "the 7 Ps," this or a similar checklist can be employed during each intubation that airway managers participate in. The EP should regard this tool as a patient safety device and error minimization instrument. As with any high-stakes activity, the use of memory aids and algorithms can reduce the cognitive load associated with decision-making and allow the practitioner to focus on the specific task at hand.[90]

■ STEP 1: PREPARATION

The first step in the RSI sequence, adequate preparation for the procedure, occurs before the patient enters the ED. A fundamental safety principle is to have all relevant airway equipment in a centralized place that is easily identified and rapidly accessed. The process of creating an "airway cart," if not already stationed in the department, is a good exercise in identifying and centralizing equipment that will prepare the team for intubations. It is also important to train personnel who assist intubations on what is expected of them during RSI. Everyone must be working from the same protocol to minimize the potential for teamwork errors. Preparation begins well before the patient requiring an intubation arrives in the ED.

BOX 1-2

Rapid Sequence Intubation—the "7 Ps"

Preparation
Preoxygenation
Pretreatment
Paralysis with sedation
Protection of airway (Sellick maneuver)
Pass the tube (and confirm)
Postintubation management

Immediate preparation is necessary when the intubation situation arises. Equipment must be assembled, roles assigned to team members, and medications brought out and arranged. It is at this point that the essential equipment must be brought out and checked to ensure proper functioning, and backup equipment prepared. A typical intubation requires, at a minimum, the following equipment:

- Nonrebreather mask attached to high-flow oxygen
- Bag-mask device attached to high-flow oxygen
- Oral and nasal airways ready for use
- Laryngoscope with backup blades identified and accessible
- Proper-sized ET tube with stylet, along with a tube one size smaller
- 10-mL syringe for the endotracheal cuff
- Functioning suction canister with a rigid suction tip (such as a Yankauer)
- Alternative intubating devices (e.g., a gum elastic bougie, a laryngeal mask airway, or a tracheal lightwand)
- Surgical airway equipment

■ STEP 2: PREOXYGENATION

The airway manager should preoxygenate the patient at the same time as the immediate preparation is occurring, even if the current oxygen saturation level is 100%. The goal is to create an oxygen reservoir in the lungs that allows the maximum amount of apneic time while the patient is paralyzed.[10,70] A nonrebreather mask is placed on the patient's face in an effort to reach this goal. If the patient's oxygen saturation level remains less than 90% with the nonrebreather mask, oxygenation should be assisted by bag-mask ventilation. A patient whose oxygen saturation remains below 90% with bag-mask ventilation at this point has a failed airway, which requires an even more rapid approach than usual (see Chapter 2).

■ STEP 3: PRETREATMENT

The third step is pretreatment with medications that have the potential to aid physiologic responses to intubation (Table 1-3). Laryngoscopy invokes physiologic responses that could be detrimental to the critically ill patient. The medications most commonly employed are lidocaine, atropine, fentanyl, and smaller doses of a paralytic (also known as a *defasciculating* doses) given before the true intubating dose.

The typical laryngoscopy in an adult results in sympathetic stimulation, which could be detrimental in certain cases. The pathophysiology in patients with elevated intracranial pressure, aortic dissection, hypertensive emergencies, or acute myocardial infarction would be exacerbated by an increase in sympathetic stimulation.[10,71] Lidocaine, opioids such as fentanyl, atropine, and defasciculating agents all have theoretical benefit in certain medical conditions, and there is a body of literature that indirectly supports their use in critical airway management. Laryngoscopy or succinylcholine dosage in pediatric patients can result in parasympathetic stimulation and resultant bradycardia, leading some experts to call for a pretreatment dose of atropine prior to all intubation attempts in children.[10,71,91]

■ STEP 4: PARALYSIS WITH SEDATION

A combination of sedative and paralytic drugs is administered to improve laryngoscopy and facilitate intubation (see previous discussion). The drugs are "pushed" in tandem, in contrast to the common anesthesia technique of a slow induction to the point of blunted airway reflexes. RSI and the situations that require it mandate medications that give consistent conditions within 45 to 60 seconds.

■ STEP 5: PROTECTION

The airway must be protected with cricoid ring pressure (Sellick maneuver) during the process of paralysis, intubation, and confirmation of endotracheal placement. The cricoid ring is compressed with an assistant's index finger and thumb, in an attempt to compress the underlying esophagus and prevent passive regurgitation of stomach contents into the trachea.[92-94] The amount of force recommended is equivalent to the amount required to create discomfort when one presses with the same fingers on the bridge of one's nose.[10,71]

Table 1-3 PRETREATMENT DRUGS FOR INTUBATION

Agent	Recommended Dose	Proposed Action(s)
Lidocaine	1.5 mg/kg intravenously (IV)	Blunts bronchospasm Blunts reflex response to laryngoscopy
Opioid (fentanyl)	1.5 μg/kg IV	Blunts reflex response to laryngoscopy
Atropine	0.01 mg/kg IV	To avoid bradycardia in children receiving succinylcholine
Depolarizing agent (rocuronium, vecuronium, pancuronium)	One tenth the dose of the nondepolarizing agent	To attempt to prevent fasciculations

■ STEP 6: PASSAGE OF THE TUBE

Laryngoscopy is performed approximately 1 minute after the paralytic agent has been pushed. The ET tube is placed under direct vision through the cords and into the trachea. In an adult male, the tube is typically placed orally to a depth of 24 cm, and in an adult female, typically to 21 cm. A general rule of thumb is that the ET tube should be inserted to at distance that is 3 times the tube size.[10,71] Placement of the ET tube is considered complete once objective verification of placement has occurred, typically by end-tidal CO_2 detection.[95,96]

■ STEP 7: POSTINTUBATION MANAGEMENT

Proper ventilation and medication management are critical once the tube is in place and secured. Please refer to Chapter 3 for a detailed discussion of ventilator management principles.

Summary

Emergency airway management is a combination of techniques and strategies designed to ensure intubation success in critically ill patients. The approach to an airway emergency is necessarily different from the one taken for an elective or urgent case. The airway manager must have a solid foundation in bag-mask technique, which RSI will be the first rescue device. Airway assessment is a critical skill mandating a methodical approach to ensure that the difficult airway is recognized and appropriately planned for. The use of RSI has revolutionized emergency intubation, requiring employment of a set of strategies to deal with routine intubation and intubation of the difficult airway. The management of difficult airways is discussed in the Chapter 2.

REFERENCES

1. Altman KW, Waltonen JD, Kern RC: Urgent surgical airway intervention: A 3 year county hospital experience. Laryngoscope 2005;115:2101-2104.
2. Sagarin MJ, Barton ED, Chng YM, Walls RM: Airway management by US and Canadian emergency medicine residents: A multicenter analysis of more than 6,000 endotracheal intubation attempts. Ann Emerg Med 2005;46: 328-336.
3. Wong E, Fong YT: Trauma airway experience by emergency physicians. Eur J Emerg Med 2003;10:209-212.
4. Butler JM, Clancy M, Robinson N, Driscoll P: An observational survey of emergency department rapid sequence intubation. Emerg Med J 2001;18:343-348.
5. Tayal VS, Riggs RW, Marx JA, et al: Rapid-sequence intubation at an emergency medicine residency: Success rate and adverse events during a two-year period. Acad Emerg Med 1999;6:31-37.
6. Sagarin MJ, Chiang V, Sakles JC, et al: Rapid sequence intubation for pediatric emergency airway management. Pediatr Emerg Care 2002;18:417-423.
7. Walls RM: Airway management. Emerg Med Clin North Am 1993;11:53-60.
8. Walls RM, Luten RC, Murphy MF, Schneider RE (eds): Manual of Emergency Airway Management, 2nd ed. Philadelphia, Lippincott-Williams & Wilkins, 2004.
9. Rabinstein AA, Wijdicks EF: Warning signs of imminent respiratory failure in neurological patients. Semin Neurol 2003;23:97-104.
10. Rodricks MB, Deutschman CS: Emergent airway management: Indications and methods in the face of confounding conditions. Crit Care Clin 2000;16:389-409.
11. Hanning CD, Alexander-Williams JM: Pulse oximetry: A practical review. Brit Med J 1995;311:367-370.
12. Bozeman WP: Pulse oximetry gap in carbon monoxide poisoning. Ann Emerg Med 1998;31:656.
13. Bozeman WP, Hampson NB: Pulse oximetry in CO poisoning: Additional data. Chest 2000;117:295-296.
14. Bozeman WP, Myers RA, Barish RA: Confirmation of the pulse oximetry gap in carbon monoxide poisoning. Ann Emerg Med 1997;30:608-611.
15. Buckley RG, Aks SE, Eshom JL, et al: The pulse oximetry gap in carbon monoxide intoxication. Ann Emerg Med 1994;24:252-255.
16. Wright RO: Pulse oximetry gap in carbon monoxide poisoning. Ann Emerg Med 1998;31:525-526.
17. Hanning CD: Pulse oximeters and poor perfusion. Anaesth Intensive Care 1989;17:238.
18. Hanning CD, Langton JA: Pulse oximeters and poor perfusion. Anaesthesia 1991;46:887.
19. Langton JA, Hanning CD: Effect of motion artefact on pulse oximeters: Evaluation of four instruments and finger probes. Br J Anaesth 1990;65:564-570.
20. Langton JA, Lassey D, Hanning CD: Comparison of four pulse oximeters: Effects of venous occlusion and cold-induced peripheral vasoconstriction. Br J Anaesth 1990;65: 245-247.
21. Wilkins CJ, Moores M, Hanning CD: Comparison of pulse oximeters: Effects of vasoconstriction and venous engorgement. Br J Anaesth 1989;62:439-444.
22. Seidler D, Hirschl MM, Roeggla G: Limitations of pulse oximetry. Lancet 1993;341:1600-1601.
23. Branson RD, Mannheimer PD: Forehead oximetry in critically ill patients: The case for a new monitoring site. Respir Care Clin North Am 2004;10:359-367, vi-vii.
24. Cheng EY, Hopwood MB, Kay J: Forehead pulse oximetry compared with finger pulse oximetry and arterial blood gas measurement. J Clin Monit 1988;4:223-226.
25. Clayton DG, Webb RK, Ralston AC, et al: Pulse oximeter probes: A comparison between finger, nose, ear and forehead probes under conditions of poor perfusion. Anaesthesia 1991;46:260-265.
26. Jorgensen JS, Schmid ER, Konig V, et al: Limitations of forehead pulse oximetry. J Clin Monit 1995;11:253-256.
27. MacLeod DB, Cortinez LI, Keifer JC, et al: The desaturation response time of finger pulse oximeters during mild hypothermia. Anaesthesia 2005;60:65-71.
28. Mannheimer PD, Bebout DE: The OxiMax System: Nellcor's new platform for pulse oximetry. Minerva Anestesiol 2002;68:236-239.
29. Nuhr M, Hoerauf K, Joldzo A, et al: Forehead SpO2 monitoring compared to finger SpO2 recording in emergency transport. Anaesthesia 2004;59:390-393.
30. Sugino S, Kanaya N, Mizuuchi M, et al: Forehead is as sensitive as finger pulse oximetry during general anesthesia. Can J Anaesth 2004;51:432-436.
31. Caroll GC, Rothenberg DM: Carbon dioxide narcosis: Pathological or "pathillogical"? Chest 1992;102:986-988.
32. Forslid A, Ingvar M, Rosen I, Ingvar DH: Carbon dioxide narcosis: Influence of short-term high concentration carbon dioxide inhalation on EEG and cortical evoked responses in the rat. Acta Physiol Scand 1986;127: 281-287.
33. Fothergill DM, Hedges D, Morrison JB: Effects of CO2 and N2 partial pressures on cognitive and psychomotor performance. Undersea Biomed Res 1991;18:1-19.
34. Fowler B, Ackles KN, Porlier G: Effects of inert gas narcosis on behavior—a critical review. Undersea Biomed Res 1985;12:369-402.
35. Mackway-Jones K, Moulton C: Towards evidence based emergency medicine: Best BETs from the Manchester Royal

Infirmary. Gag reflex and intubation. J Accid Emerg Med 1999;16:444-445.
36. Moulton C, Pennycook AG: Relation between Glasgow coma score and cough reflex. Lancet 1994;343: 1261-1262.
37. Li J, Murphy-Lavoie H, Bugas C, et al: Complications of emergency intubation with and without paralysis. Am J Emerg Med 1999;17:141-143.
38. Davis DP, Stern J, Sise MJ, Hoyt DB: A follow-up analysis of factors associated with head-injury mortality after paramedic rapid sequence intubation. J Trauma 2005;59: 486-490.
39. Kozlow JH, Berenholtz SM, Garrett E, et al: Epidemiology and impact of aspiration pneumonia in patients undergoing surgery in Maryland, 1999-2000. Crit Care Med 2003;31:1930-1937.
40. Liebler JM, Benner K, Putnam T, Vollmer WM: Respiratory complications in critically ill medical patients with acute upper gastrointestinal bleeding. Crit Care Med 1991;19: 1152-1157.
41. Leder SB: Gag reflex and dysphagia. Head Neck 1996;18:138-141.
42. Davies AE, Kidd D, Stone SP, MacMahon J: Pharyngeal sensation and gag reflex in healthy subjects. Lancet 1995;345:487-488.
43. Pavlin EG, Holle RH, Schoene RB: Recovery of airway protection compared with ventilation in humans after paralysis with curare. Anesthesiology 1989;70:381-385.
44. Page M, Jeffery HE: Airway protection in sleeping infants in response to pharyngeal fluid stimulation in the supine position. Pediatr Res 1998;44:691-698.
45. Nishino T: Physiological and pathophysiological implications of upper airway reflexes in humans. Jpn J Physiol 2000;50:3-14.
46. Murphy M, Hung O, Launcelott G, et al: Predicting the difficult laryngoscopic intubation: Are we on the right track? Can J Anaesth 2005;52:231-235.
47. Walls RM: Management of the difficult airway in the trauma patient. Emerg Med Clin North Am 1998;16:45-61.
48. Yildiz TS, Solak M, Toker K: The incidence and risk factors of difficult mask ventilation. J Anesth 2005;19:7-11.
49. Levitan RM, Everett WW, Ochroch EA: Limitations of difficult airway prediction in patients intubated in the emergency department. Ann Emerg Med 2004;44:307-313.
50. Langeron O, Masso E, Huraux C, et al: Prediction of difficult mask ventilation. Anesthesiology 2000;92:1229-1236.
51. Gupta S, Pareek S, Dulara SC: Comparison of two methods for predicting difficult intubation in obstetric patients. Middle East J Anesthesiol 2003;17:275-285.
52. Egan TD, Wong KC: Predicting difficult laryngoscopy for tracheal intubation: An approach to airway assessment. Ma Zui Xue Za Zhi 1993;31:165-178.
53. Krobbuaban B, Diregpoke S, Kumkeaw S, Tanomsat M: The predictive value of the height ratio and thyromental distance: Four predictive tests for difficult laryngoscopy. Anesth Analg 2005;101:1542-1545.
54. Merah NA, Wong DT, Ffoulkes-Crabbe DJ, et al: Modified Mallampati test, thyromental distance and inter-incisor gap are the best predictors of difficult laryngoscopy in West Africans. Can J Anaesth 2005;52:291-296.
55. Merah NA, Foulkes-Crabbe DJ, Kushimo OT, Ajayi PA: Prediction of difficult laryngoscopy in a population of Nigerian obstetric patients. West Afr J Med 2004;23:38-41.
56. Juvin P, Lavaut E, Dupont H, et al: Difficult tracheal intubation is more common in obese than in lean patients. Anesth Analg 2003;97:595-600, table of contents.
57. Iohom G, Ronayne M, Cunningham AJ: Prediction of difficult tracheal intubation. Eur J Anaesthesiol 2003;20: 31-36.
58. Karkouti K, Rose DK, Wigglesworth D, Cohen MM: Predicting difficult intubation: A multivariable analysis. Can J Anaesth 2000;47:730-739.
59. Reed MJ, Dunn MJ, McKeown DW: Can an airway assessment score predict difficulty at intubation in the emergency department? Emerg Med J 2005;22:99-102.
60. Reed MJ, Rennie LM, Dunn MJ, et al: Is the "LEMON" method an easily applied emergency airway assessment tool? Eur J Emerg Med 2004;11:154-157.
61. Bair AE, Filbin MR, Kulkarni RG, Walls RM: The failed intubation attempt in the emergency department: Analysis of prevalence, rescue techniques, and personnel. J Emerg Med 2002;23:131-140.
62. Walls RM, Pollack CV Jr: Successful cricothyrotomy after thrombolytic therapy for acute myocardial infarction: A report of two cases. Ann Emerg Med 2000;35:188-191.
63. Arslantas A, Durmaz R, Cosan E, Tel E: Inadvertent insertion of a nasogastric tube in a patient with head trauma. Childs Nerv Syst 2001;17:112-114.
64. Marlow TJ, Goltra DD Jr, Schabel SI: Intracranial placement of a nasotracheal tube after facial fracture: A rare complication. J Emerg Med 1997;15:187-191.
65. Moustoukas N, Litwin MS: Intracranial placement of nasogastric tube: An unusual complication. South Med J 1983;76:816-817.
66. Martin JE, Mehta R, Aarabi B, et al: Intracranial insertion of a nasopharyngeal airway in a patient with craniofacial trauma. Mil Med 2004;169:496-497.
67. Schade K, Borzotta A, Michaels A: Intracranial malposition of nasopharyngeal airway. J Trauma 2000;49:967-968.
68. Fishbaugh DF, Wilson S, Preisch JW, Weaver JM 2nd: Relationship of tonsil size on an airway blockage maneuver in children during sedation. Pediatr Dent 1997;19:277-281.
69. Hess D, Chatmongkolchart S: Techniques to avoid intubation: Noninvasive positive pressure ventilation and heliox therapy. Int Anesthesiol Clin 2000;38:161-187.
70. Benumof JL, Dagg R, Benumof R: Critical hemoglobin desaturation will occur before return to an unparalyzed state following 1 mg/kg intravenous succinylcholine. Anesthesiology 1997;87:979-982.
71. Miller RD: Miller's Anesthesia, 6th ed. Philadelphia, Churchill Livingstone, 2005.
72. Rapaport S, Joannes-Boyau O, Bazin R, Janvier G: [Comparison of eight deep breaths and tidal volume breathing preoxygenation techniques in morbid obese patients]. Ann Fr Anesth Reanim 2004;23:1155-1159.
73. Chiron B, Laffon M, Ferrandiere M, et al: Standard preoxygenation technique versus two rapid techniques in pregnant patients. Int J Obstet Anesth 2004;13:11-14.
74. Mort TC: Preoxygenation in critically ill patients requiring emergency tracheal intubation. Crit Care Med 2005;33: 2672-2675.
75. McGowan P, Skinner A: Preoxygenation—the importance of a good face mask seal. Br J Anaesth 1995;75:777-778.
76. Hore CT: Non-invasive positive pressure ventilation in patients with acute respiratory failure. Emerg Med (Fremantle) 2002;14:281-295.
77. Davidovic L, LaCovey D, Pitetti RD: Comparison of 1- versus 2-person bag-valve-mask techniques for manikin ventilation of infants and children. Ann Emerg Med 2005;46:37-42.
78. Dorges V, Ocker H, Hagelberg S, et al: Optimisation of tidal volumes given with self-inflatable bags without additional oxygen. Resuscitation 2000;43:195-199.
79. Dorges V, Ocker H, Hagelberg S, et al: Smaller tidal volumes with room-air are not sufficient to ensure adequate oxygenation during bag-valve-mask ventilation. Resuscitation 2000;44:37-41.
80. Sivilotti ML, Filbin MR, Murray HE, et al: Does the sedative agent facilitate emergency rapid sequence intubation? Acad Emerg Med 2003;10:612-620.
81. Sagarin MJ, Barton ED, Sakles JC, et al: Underdosing of midazolam in emergency endotracheal intubation. Acad Emerg Med 2003;10:329-338.
82. Oglesby AJ: Should etomidate be the induction agent of choice for rapid sequence intubation in the emergency department? Emerg Med J 2004;21:655-659.
83. Fuchs-Buder T, Sparr HJ, Ziegenfuss T: Thiopental or etomidate for rapid sequence induction with rocuronium. Br J Anaesth 1998;80:504-506.

84. Schenarts CL, Burton JH, Riker RR: Adrenocortical dysfunction following etomidate induction in emergency department patients. Acad Emerg Med 2001;8:1-7.
85. Sparr HJ: Choice of the muscle relaxant for rapid-sequence induction. Eur J Anaesthesiol Suppl 2001;23:71-76.
86. Perry J, Lee J, Wells G: Rocuronium versus succinylcholine for rapid sequence induction intubation. Cochrane Database Syst Rev 2003(1):CD002788.
87. Cheng CA, Aun CS, Gin T: Comparison of rocuronium and suxamethonium for rapid tracheal intubation in children. Paediatr Anaesth 2002;12:140-145.
88. Laurin EG, Sakles JC, Panacek EA, et al: A comparison of succinylcholine and rocuronium for rapid-sequence intubation of emergency department patients. Acad Emerg Med 2000;7:1362-1369.
89. Andrews JI, Kumar N, van den Brom RH, et al: A large simple randomized trial of rocuronium versus succinylcholine in rapid-sequence induction of anaesthesia along with propofol. Acta Anaesthesiol Scand 1999;43:4-8.
90. Agro F, Hung OR, Cataldo R, et al: Lightwand intubation using the Trachlight: A brief review of current knowledge. Can J Anaesth 2001;48:592-599.
91. Turgeon AF, Nicole PC, Trepanier CA, et al: Cricoid pressure does not increase the rate of failed intubation by direct laryngoscopy in adults. Anesthesiology 2005;102: 315-319.
92. Kalinowski CP, Kirsch JR: Strategies for prophylaxis and treatment for aspiration. Best Pract Res Clin Anaesthesiol 2004;18:719-737.
93. Landsman I: Cricoid pressure: Indications and complications. Paediatr Anaesth 2004;14:43-47.
94. Bair AE, Smith D, Lichty L: Intubation confirmation techniques associated with unrecognized non-tracheal intubations by pre-hospital providers. J Emerg Med 2005;28: 403-407.
95. Vukmir RB, Heller MB, Stein KL: Confirmation of endotracheal tube placement: A miniaturized infrared qualitative CO2 detector. Ann Emerg Med 1991;20:726-729.
96. Levitan RM: Patient safety in emergency airway management and rapid sequence intubation: metaphorical lessons from skydiving. Ann Emerg Med 2003;42:81-87.

Chapter 2

Advanced Airway Management

Aaron E. Bair and Erik G. Laurin

KEY POINTS

Advanced airway management is predicated on selecting the right technical approach for a given patient.

Anticipated difficult airway management often relies on a sedated (or "awake") technique.

An organized approach (and backup plan) is essential for success with the unanticipated difficult airway.

Scope

The *cognitive* skills to determine when a patient requires airway support are as important as the *manual* skills to accomplish the task. Currently, rapid-sequence intubation (RSI) is the most frequently used and most successful means of intubating the trachea in emergency medical practice.[1-4] It is clear that combining the use of a paralytic agent with a sedative agent has resulted in more successful laryngoscopy and fewer intubation failures ("failed" airways).[5,6] Complacency can be lethal, however. Every attempt at intubation may be difficult. Therefore, a prepared and practiced backup or contingency plan is vital. The discussion of the various techniques and adjuncts in this chapter reflects their application within an overall strategy.

There are cases in which the use of paralytics (i.e., RSI) is inappropriate owing to (1) a relatively high likelihood of intubation failure with subsequent worsening of the clinical condition by the intubation attempts and (2) the likelihood of failed ventilation. Accordingly, it is important to distinguish the patient who is likely to be difficult to intubate, ventilate, and rescue (often "rescue" means performing a cricothyrotomy). These concepts are emphasized by the mnemonics LEMON, MOANS, and SHORT,[7] which are discussed in Chapter 1. What follows here is an overview of a strategic approach to advanced emergency airway management.

■ PREVALENCE OF DIFFICULT AIRWAYS

The *difficult airway* (case in which intubation is difficult to achieve) in the ED is far less studied, but likely far more common, than in the more controlled environment of the operating suite. Severity of illness and lack of patient preparation make encountering both anticipated and unanticipated difficulty of intubation more likely, with some estimates of incidence as high as 20%.[8] Fortunately, however, intubation failure in the ED is much lower, approximating 1%.[3,9,10] Prevalence of airways requiring rescue from previous failed attempts in the ED is difficult to determine. What is apparent is that rescue devices are not routinely employed although they are commonly available.[11,12]

■ ANTICIPATED DIFFICULTY OF INTUBATION

Multiple predictors related to airway anatomy have been studied in the anesthesia literature, and none has been shown to be useful when used alone for predicting intubation difficulty.[13-18] However, some evidence supports the use of a limited set of assessments in patients undergoing airway management in the ED. The LEMON mnemonic has been proposed for this purpose (Box 2-1; also see Chapter 1).[7,19] If difficulty is predictable and the patient is not a suitable candidate for RSI, the optimal approach depends on prior training of the intubator and availability of advanced airway tools.

■ UNANTICIPATED DIFFICULTY OF INTUBATION

Every patient, in any environment, has the potential for being unexpectedly difficult to intubate. Encountering blood, emesis, mass, an anatomical variant, or evolving traumatic injury can result in a challenging intubation. In this chapter we attempt to organize and briefly define some of the many rescue techniques that might be employed in emergency practice.

BOX 2-1

The LEMON Mnemonic for Possible Difficult Intubation

*L*ook to see if there is obvious abnormality
*E*valuate the 3-3-2 rule
*M*allampati assessment
*O*bstruction of upper airway
*N*eck immobility

The Anticipated Difficult Airway

Only a small fraction of ED patients requiring intubation are actually deemed poor candidates for RSI, even though many patients are expected to be "difficult" to intubate. No discrete threshold has ever been determined at which an RSI is deemed to be "safe" or contraindicated. This situation is due, in part, to the lack of sensitivity of the various tools for predicting difficult airways. Importantly, many ED patients are in extremis and unable to cooperate with a pre-procedural examination.[20] Much of what is discussed in the current literature is based on the anesthesia experience, which generally reflects the "elective" intubation of cooperative patients. Nevertheless, it is often useful to perform a pre-procedural assessment if allowed by time constraints and patient condition. Some evaluation is necessary to enable an accurate estimate of the potential of encountering a difficult airway.

The algorithm presented in Figure 2-1 represents a clinical approach to the difficult airway.[7] The appli-

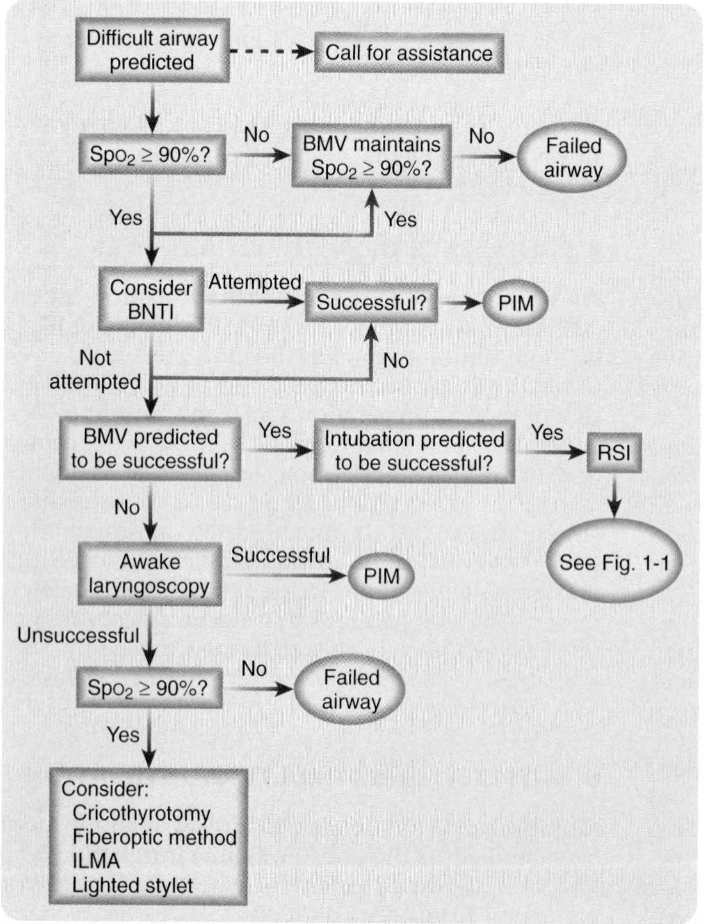
Difficult airway predicted
Call for assistance
$Spo_2 \geq 90\%$?
No
BMV maintains $Spo_2 \geq 90\%$?
No
Failed airway
Yes
Yes
Consider BNTI
Attempted
Successful?
PIM
Not attempted
No
BMV predicted to be successful?
Yes
Intubation predicted to be successful?
Yes
RSI
See Fig. 1-1
No
Awake laryngoscopy
Successful
PIM
Unsuccessful
$Spo_2 \geq 90\%$?
No
Failed airway
Yes
Consider:
Cricothyrotomy
Fiberoptic method
ILMA
Lighted stylet

FIGURE 2-1 Algorithm for managing the difficult airway. BMV, bag-mask ventilation; PIM, post-intubation management; Spo_2, oxygen saturation as measured by pulse oximeter. (Adapted from Walls RM, Luten RC, Murphy MF, Schneider RE [eds]: Manual of Emergency Airway Management, 2nd ed. Philadelphia, Lippincott Williams & Wilkins, 2004.)

cation of such an approach is predicated on the answers to the following key questions:

1. Is there enough time to plan a methodical approach?
2. Despite the identified presence of difficult airway predictors, can RSI be safely employed?
3. Is oxygenation adequate?

Understanding these issues in the context of a given clinical scenario helps in the decision-making process regarding alternative approaches.

■ RAPID-SEQUENCE INTUBATION FOR THE DIFFICULT AIRWAY

RSI is preferred for the vast majority of intubations performed in the ED. It is important to realize that EP familiarity is likely the major determinant in the section of devices and techniques beyond the use of RSI. For this reason, it is prudent for the EP to focus on techniques that are likely to remain familiar through frequent use. The use of optimized and augmented laryngoscopy merits discussion because these concepts are simply extensions of "routine" RSI.

■ OPTIMIZED LARYNGOSCOPY

Routine direct laryngoscopy relies on manipulation of the soft tissues of the hypopharynx and the base of the tongue into the relatively fixed proportions of the mandible. The goal of such manipulation is to allow a direct line of sight to the larynx and vocal cords. This process can be difficult, however, given certain unalterable variables of patient anatomy. The process of optimizing the view is probably the simplest and often least appreciated of the skills of the expert airway manager. The features of optimization are as follows:

Head and neck positioning: In the absence of cervical spine immobilization, active range of neck flexion/extension can often provide markedly better visualization.[21]

External laryngeal manipulation: This is distinct from the familiar cricoid pressure concept (e.g., Sellick's maneuver) but is related to BURP (backward, upward, rightward pressure). The process of laryngeal manipulation is active. It requires that the intubator actively move the larynx to maximize visualization of laryngeal structures. Generally, once the view is optimized, an assistant is needed to maintain the preferred positioning.[22-24]

Facility with various blade types: Laryngoscope blade types come in various sizes and shapes and so have various advantages and disadvantages. In general, two formats are employed with regularity, curved (e.g., MacIntosh) and straight (e.g., Miller). The curved blades are often best for sweeping the tongue laterally. Some patients may be difficult to intubate owing to an elongated or deep epiglottis. In such a patient, a straight blade is probably useful. Although most practitioners have a preferred blade, it is important to maintain facility with both general blade types because they often have offsetting advantages. Additionally, a multitude of variably profiled laryngoscopes with adjunctive prisms and mirrors are available; these are not frequently used in emergency practice, however.

■ AUGMENTED LARYNGOSCOPY

The concept of *augmented laryngoscopy* refers to the use of an assistive device to either extend the view of the intubator (e.g., fiberoptic stylet) or to assist in tube placement through use of a narrow-diameter introducer. Such introducers have been used for decades and come in various formats (e.g., Eschmann, Frova). The leading tip of such introducers is angled anteriorly to provide tactile feedback about the location of the introducer. These devices can be valuable when visualization is limited.

■ ALTERNATIVE TECHNIQUES FOR THE ANTICIPATED DIFFICULT AIRWAY

■ Fiberoptic Devices

As a class, directable and flexible scopes have been available for decades. They have recently been made more portable by replacement of the heavy light source with a battery pack attached to the handle. These devices are consequently more convenient in the harried ED. The majority of the products currently on the market consist of a directable cable mechanism associated with a light source and fiberoptic bundle. Notable issues are (1) the glass fibers that constitute the optics are breakable and (2) small amounts of debris can greatly diminish the viewing quality. Historically, fiberoptic devices were considered too expensive or impractical, but in the future they will likely be increasingly available. To date there is relatively little research on the use of these devices in emergency medicine.[2,25-27] A 1999 survey of emergency medicine training programs in the United States suggested that the majority maintain this type of equipment,[11] but clinical expertise is variable.

■ *Flexible, Directable Fiberoptic Scopes*

Flexible, directable fiberoptic models are portable, with variable diameters and lengths. This equipment varies according to its intended purpose. The nasopharyngoscope is approximately 35 cm in length, in contrast to the bronchoscope, which measures 60 cm.

The goal of the use of such a scope is to directly visualize the glottis via the nares or mouth. Once the cords are visualized, the tip of the fiberoptic scope is advanced into the airway to the level of the carina. The preloaded endotracheal tube (ETT) is then advanced off the scope and into the airway. The efficacy of this technique in awake patients requires

BOX 2-2

Patient Preparation

1. If *nasal* approach is used, adequate topical anesthetic and vasoconstriction can be achieved with various agents through the use of an atomizer.
2. If *oral* approach is used, various spray anesthetic agents can be used in addition to nebulized agents (e.g., lidocaine). Additionally, gargled lidocaine (4%) can be effective, patient cooperation permitting.
3. Antisialogogue (e.g., glycopyrrolate) can be useful to allow better tissue absorption of topical anesthetic agents. This drying agent, however, takes at least 20 minutes to achieve efficacy.
4. Sedation should be used as necessary to achieve reasonable anxiolysis in order to improve patient cooperation.
5. Preoxygenation, as always, is fundamental to procedural sedation and airway management.

adequate preparation of both the patient and the equipment (Box 2-2).

Although a complete tutorial in the technical details of employing flexible fiberoptics is beyond the scope of this chapter, there are a few technique "pearls" worth highlighting (see Tips and Tricks box).

Flexible, Nondirectable Fiberoptic Scopes

Flexible, nondirectable fiberoptic scopes have been designed to be used from within the lumen of the ETT. Like directable scopes, they have disadvantages related to obscuration of view with debris. Additionally, any attempt to direct such a scope relies on manipulation of the associated ETT with visual feedback through either an eyepiece or video monitor. Despite these shortcomings, these devices are attractive because they are generally regarded as more durable than directable scopes, and they are less expensive. An example of this type of device is the TrachView Intubating Videoscope (Parker Medical, Englewood, CO).

Semirigid Fiberoptic Scopes

The semirigid fiberoptic scopes is, conceptually, a semimalleable stylet with internal fiberoptic bundles.[32] These scopes are similar to nondirectable fiberoptic scopes with respect to their image quality and durability. An example of a type of device is the Shikani Optical Stylet (Clarus Medical, LLC, Minneapolis, MN).

Tips and Tricks

TECHNIQUE FOR FLEXIBLE FIBEROPTIC INTUBATION

- Recognize that the procedure will take at least 15 to 20 minutes to accomplish. If the patient cannot tolerate such a wait, use of this technique may be misguided.
- Keep the scope in the anatomic midline at all times during the procedure. Allowing it to stray laterally will often result in poor visualization and inability to pass the cords.
- Keep the slack out of the fiber bundle. If such slack is present, rotation of the body of the scope will not translate into rotation of the tip.
- The use of the working channel in most scopes is essentially worthless for suction.
- If the tube is resistant to passage off the scope and into the airway, the tip is probably caught at the level of the arytenoids. Rotation of the *entire* tube-scope apparatus 45 to 90 degrees will probably overcome the obstruction.
- Further considerations:

Nasal approach: This route may be better tolerated by the patient and will not subject the equipment to breakage by a patient bite. However, the nose is prone to bleeding with passage of the tube. Adequate vasoconstriction is key. Partially intubating the chosen naris with the endotracheal tube can often simplify the procedure by avoiding the obscuring materials in the nasopharynx. Be aware, however, that placing the tube tip too deep makes subsequent scope manipulation very difficult owing to the acute angle required for the scope tip to reach the glottis. Optimally, the tip of the endotracheal tube should be placed at the level of the uvula.

Oral approach: Bite blocks are necessary if there is any possibility that the patient will bite the equipment. Additionally, the EP can use the fiberoptic technique in conjunction with a second provider using a laryngoscope to manipulate the soft tissues of the oropharynx.

Adjunct use: The use of flexible fiberoptic instruments through a laryngeal mask airway or similar device has been well described.[28-31]

Rigid Fiberoptic Scopes

Rigid fiberoptic scopes consist of an imaging bundle enclosed within a rigid L- or J-shaped assembly. This shape is designed for placement into the hypopharynx with subsequent indirect visualization of the glottis. One of the chief advantages of these devices is that limited head, neck, and jaw mobility are less of a concern because of the ability of the user to "look around the corner" of the hypopharynx. Examples in this class are the Bullard Laryngoscope (Circon Corporation, Stanford, CT),[33-35] WuScope Tubular Fiberoptic Laryngoscope (Achi Corporation, San Jose,

Tips and Tricks

USING A GLIDESCOPE VIDEO LARYNGOSCOPE*

- The GlideScope handle stays in midline, requiring no tongue sweep.
- Unlike with the more common laryngoscope, the handle of the GlideScope is *not* used to lift.
- To accommodate the approach to the glottis, the styletted endotracheal tube needs an acute angle (approximately 90 degrees).
- To accommodate advancement of the tube off the stylet, it may help to partially withdraw the stylet during tube advancement. Generally, this last step requires coordination with an assistant.

*Verathon, Inc., Bothell, WA.

CA),[36-39] and Upsherscope (Metropolitan Medical, Inc.).[40,41] These scopes are relatively expensive, however, and their availability in the ED has been limited.[11]

Video Laryngoscopy

Video laryngoscopes utilize either a micro-video camera or more traditional fiberoptic bundles encased in a rather familiar-appearing laryngoscope handle design. The placement of the camera is meant to provide a wide-angle view of the glottis and is somewhat more protected from the various debris issues often encountered with the optics-in-the-tube format. The GlideScope Video Laryngoscope (Verathon, Inc., Bothell, WA) is an example of the micro-video camera design. This device is relatively new with limited ED experience reported. The literature that exists suggests that it can be used with very little motion to the cervical spine and that glottic visualization is generally excellent.[42-45] However, actual intubation may be more of a challenge because it requires an extreme "hockey-stick" angulation of the styletted ETT to reach the glottis. Currently, laryngoscope sizes available correspond roughly to MacIntosh No. 4 and No. 2 (see Tips and Tricks: GlideScope box).

"Awake" Techniques

In the context of the difficult airway, the role of an "awake" technique may be (1) to determine the status of airway landmarks (with consideration of RSI if the landmarks are recognizable) or (2) to perform the intubation in a patient who can maintain spontaneous respirations. Either may be accomplished with direct laryngoscopy. A confirmatory look may also be made with a flexible fiberoptic scope.

The term "awake" is a misnomer. It is important to realize that the better descriptor of this concept would be "sedated." In a patient who is currently maintaining some airway tone and respiratory drive, this approach may be indicated when difficult intubation and ventilation are *both* anticipated.

This approach may be somewhat time-consuming because adequate sedation and topical anesthesia of the airway are required (Box 2-3). However, the advantage is that the patient is able to breathe on his or her own during the attempts to definitively control the airway. It is important to understand the underlying pathologic process with respect to its dynamic impact on the airway. A quick look to determine the risks for RSI may be misleading if rapid swelling from burns or angioedema are evolving during the process. The EP should keep this in mind, because an initial look may be reassuring with subsequent attempts being profoundly disappointing.

BOX 2-3

Patient Sedation and Topical Anesthesia: A Recipe

Nasal (Anesthesia and Vasoconstriction)

Needed *only* if nasal route is anticipated:

Oxymetazoline (0.05%)/lidocaine (1%) 1:1 in mucosal atomizer; 10 mL total.

Use preservative-free (cardiac) lidocaine to avoid rare allergic reaction to preservative.

Provides effective anesthesia and vasoconstriction.

Time: 2-3 minutes.

Oral

Lidocaine (4%) 30 mL gargle and spit.

Time: 1-2 minutes.

Glottis

Lidocaine (1%-4%, preservative-free) 10 mL in nebulizer.

Time: 10 minutes.

Sedation

The goal is only light sedation. Deep procedural sedation defeats the purpose, as airway obstruction, given the clinical situation, is likely to be disastrous.

The Unanticipated Difficult Airway

The concept of an "unanticipated difficult airway" generally presupposes that an attempt at intubation has already been made. As such, it is often a situation that requires a change in strategy. Although failed intubation attempts are uncommon, they do occur, and a rational backup or rescue plan must be in place. Ultimately, the choice of rescue devices is limited by simple availability or by the EP's experience with their use. Here we highlight the various classes of devices that appear promising for use in emergency practice.

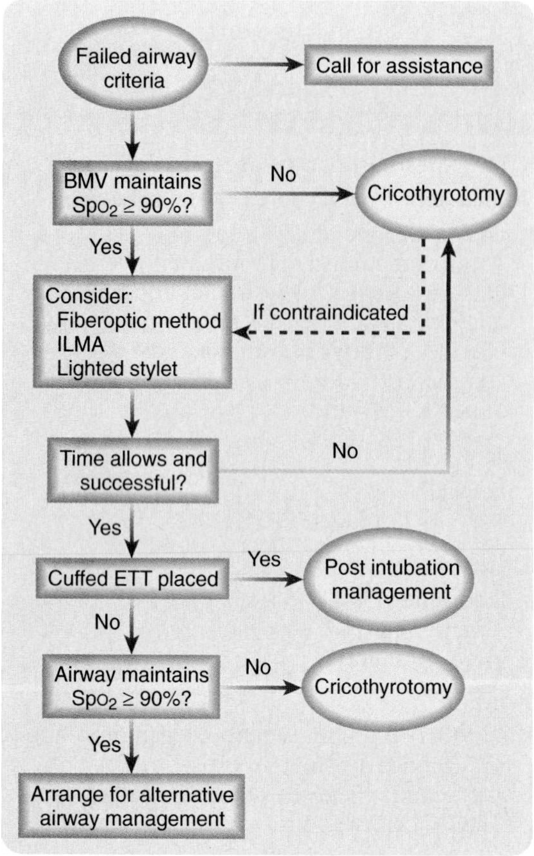
Failed airway criteria
Call for assistance
BMV maintains Spo2 ≥ 90%?
No
Cricothyrotomy
Yes
Consider: Fiberoptic method ILMA Lighted stylet
If contraindicated
Time allows and successful?
No
Yes
Cuffed ETT placed
Yes
Post intubation management
No
Airway maintains Spo2 ≥ 90%?
No
Cricothyrotomy
Yes
Arrange for alternative airway management

FIGURE 2-2 Algorithm for managing failed intubation (the failed airway). Spo_2, oxygen saturation as measured by pulse oximeter. (Adapted from Walls RM, Luten RC, Murphy MF, Schneider RE [eds]: Manual of Emergency Airway Management, 2nd ed. Philadelphia, Lippincott Williams & Wilkins, 2004.)

The difficult airway and failed airway are related but distinct concepts. The difficult airway becomes a failed airway after three unsuccessful attempts at intubation by a skilled operator. From this point, subsequent maneuvers are in large part directed by operator familiarity and skill. However, the key branch point in the decision-making process depends on the adequacy of ventilation. The "Can't intubate, CAN ventilate" scenario is managed differently from the "Can't intubate, can't ventilate" scenario. The following discussions approach each of these scenarios within the concept of the algorithm for managing the failed airway shown in Figure 2-2.

■ "CAN'T INTUBATE, CAN VENTILATE" SCENARIO

Successful ventilation is defined as the ability to maintain oxygen saturations above 90% with bag-mask ventilation. In this situation, the provider has some time to direct further efforts at intubation and take advantage of any opportunity for success as identified on previous attempts. A directed response might include optimizing or augmenting a previous RSI failure with maneuvers previously discussed. Additionally, it may include the use of alternative intubation devices.

■ The Laryngeal Mask Airway

The laryngeal mask airway (LMA) currently has several format variations, one of which is the intubating LMA (ILMA; e.g., Fastrach [LMA Inc., San Diego, CA]) shown in Figure 2-3. This device has been shown to provide adequate ventilation and a good opportunity for success with blind intubation through the LMA.[46-53] Placement of the ILMA is nearly identical to that for a standard LMA, with one notable difference: The metal handle of the ILMA allows easier manipulation of the device and does not require the operator to place fingers inside the patient's mouth to guide placement. Once the ILMA is placed in the hypopharynx and the cuff is inflated, bag ventilations can begin. If ventilations are adequate (which is the case in the majority of patients and implies good ILMA positioning), the proprietary nonkinking ETT can be advanced through the lumen of the ILMA. In reports of its use during surgical anesthesia, such intubation has a high rate of success. The ILMA cuff is then deflated, and the ILMA is removed over the ETT, leaving the ETT in place as a definitive airway. The success rate in ED patients in whom prior intubation attempts have failed, and who often have full stomachs, is so far unpublished and unknown.

■ Tracheal Introducer

The tracheal introducer has been in use since the 1940s. Several products are currently available commercially. The Eschmann tracheal tube introducer has also been known as the "gum elastic bougie." This term, incidentally, is a misnomer, because the introducer is not a bougie (e.g., dilator), nor is it made of gum. Instead, it is a woven Dacron rod 30 cm long that has been coated with resin for durability and added stiffness. Newer products have also arrived on the market (e.g., Frova [Cook Medical, Bloomington, IN]). These introducers are used in conjunction with direct laryngoscopy, especially when the vocal cords cannot be visualized. Their design helps access an extremely anterior trachea and confirm proper placement. One of the design features is an angulated tip, which allows for directable manipulation and tactile feedback: The tip "clicks" as it bumps along the anterior tracheal rings; the absence of clicks suggests esophageal placement. Additionally, if the introducer is in the airway, a "hard stop" is felt as the introducer passes from the trachea into a small-diameter airway. In contrast, if the introducer is mistakenly placed in the esophagus, the operator will be able to advance the introducer without a firm end point, as the introducer enters the stomach.[54-58] Once tracheal placement is confirmed, a standard ETT is advanced over the introducer and into the trachea.

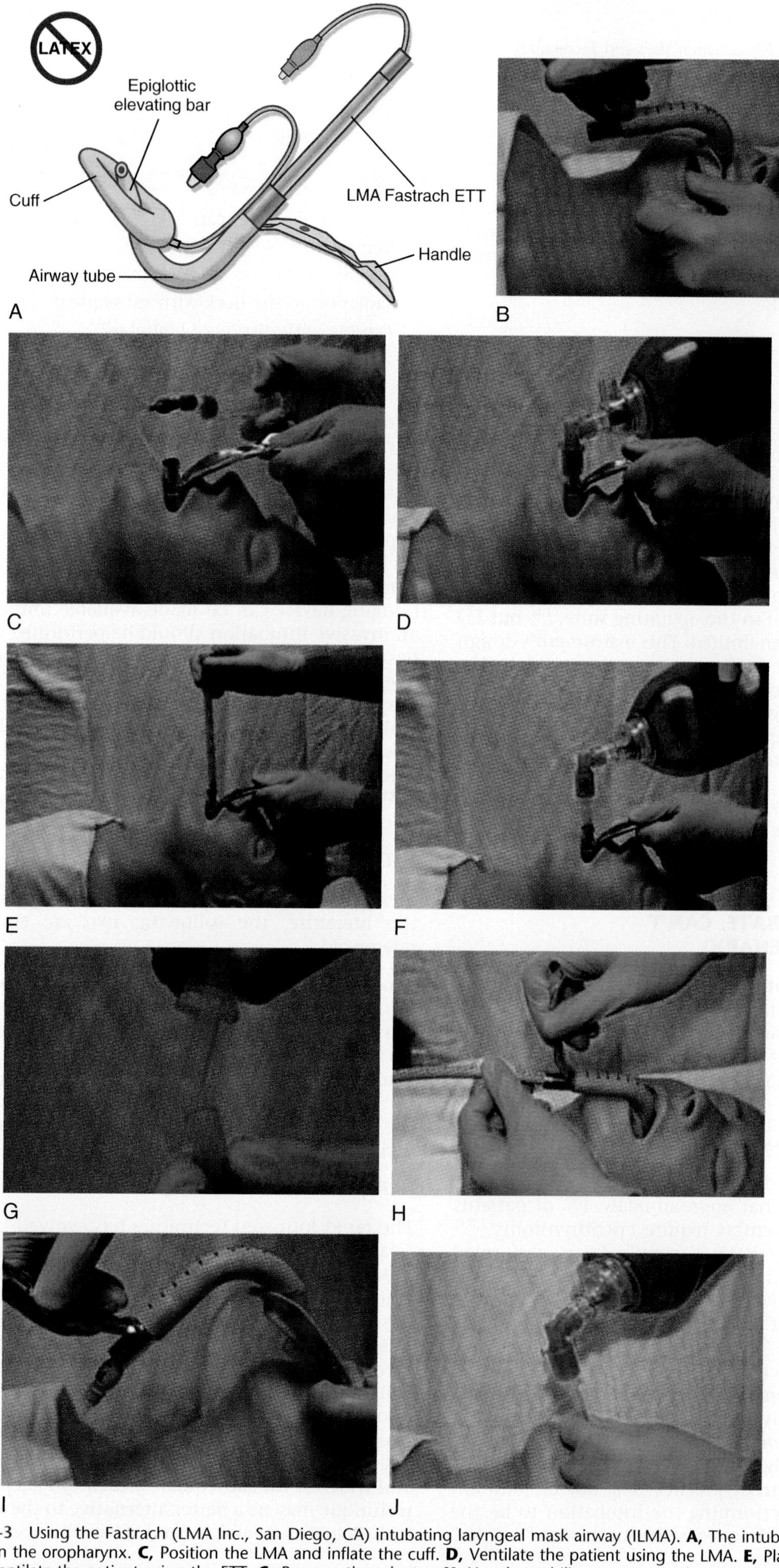
LATEX
Epiglottic elevating bar
Cuff
Airway tube
LMA Fastrach ETT
Handle
A
B
C
D
E
F
G
H
I
J

FIGURE 2-3 Using the Fastrach (LMA Inc., San Diego, CA) intubating laryngeal mask airway (ILMA). **A,** The intubating LMA. **B,** Place the LMA in the oropharynx. **C,** Position the LMA and inflate the cuff. **D,** Ventilate the patient using the LMA. **E,** Place the ETT into the LMA. **F,** Ventilate the patient using the ETT. **G,** Remove the adaptor. **H,** Use the stabilizer to remove the LMA. **I,** Allow the balloon to pass through the lumen of the LMA. **J,** Confirm tube placement, and ventilate the patient.

Blind Nasotracheal Intubation

The overall success rate of blind nasotracheal intubation (BNTI) is lower than that of RSI.[59,60] Additionally, BNTI can be complicated by nasal hemorrhage and induction of vomiting (with the associated risk of aspiration). However, this technique is often an expedient option in patients who still have fairly vigorous spontaneous respirations. See Chapter 1 for further discussion of BNTI.

Light Wand

One of the most successful light wands (lighted stylets), according to the anesthesia literature, is the Trachlight lighted stylet (Laerdal Medical AS). Lightwand intubation does not rely on visualization of any internal structure. Instead, it relies on a transmitted glow of light through the soft tissues of the neck. The skill required for its application relies largely on recognizing midline (i.e., tracheal) placement versus lateral soft tissue placement. The Trachlight has been shown to be useful in the operating suite,[61-65] but ED experience has been limited. This instrument's design and the necessity for a pronounced L curve in the stylet and ETT make it very forgiving of difficult anatomy that might otherwise inhibit direct laryngoscopy. It is important to note that proper tube placement and preparation of the device do take a few minutes. To make it more useful as a rescue device, and more amenable to quick-grab deployment, it should be prepared and stored in a ready-to-use condition.

"CAN'T INTUBATE, CAN'T VENTILATE" SCENARIO

The "Can't intubate, can't ventilate" scenario is a dire circumstance. In this situation, the vast majority of patients require an invasive intubation, unless the expeditious use of a bridging device can convert the situation to "Can't intubate, CAN ventilate."

Invasive Intubation

Studies performed since the common acceptance of ED RSI show that approximately 1% of patients at large trauma centers require cricothyrotomy.[1,3,10] These procedures have generally been performed with an open surgical technique. However, newer developments have provided a percutaneous option. The advantage of this latter option may lie in the familiarity of use, because it relies on the routinely used Seldinger technique.

There are several key considerations with respect to cricothyrotomy. First, one must recognize that providers are often hesitant to perform what may be perceived as a highly problematic and complicated procedure. In current practice it is not uncommon for the person performing the intubation to be the same one who needs to recognize intubation "failure." Additionally, it is this same provider who will need to change course and provide an invasive airway. In this circumstance, overcoming cognitive inertia can be difficult and may contribute to a disastrous delay. Many practitioners say that the most difficult portion of performing a cricothyrotomy is simply making the decision to do so. Such a decision is mandated in a "can't intubate, can't ventilate" scenario. Unless a bridging device can be made available immediately, an invasive intubation should be performed without hesitation. The presence of certain features may influence the actual approach chosen. The EP should keep in mind that certain clinical circumstance may make an invasive airway particularly challenging. The SHORT mnemonic has been proposed for use when one is considering an invasive airway (Box 2-4). Several technical variants of cricothyrotomy are in common use, as discussed here.

> **BOX 2-4**
>
> **Mnemonic for Predicting a Difficult Cricothyrotomy**
>
> *S*urgery (i.e., neck scar)
> *H*ematoma
> *O*besity
> *R*adiation to the neck with subsequent scar
> *T*rauma with disrupted landmarks

Open Surgical Technique

Among the open surgical techniques described in the literature, the following two are commonly referenced:

"Standard" Technique.[66,67] The "standard" technique of open surgical intubation generally involves positioning of the surgeon over the right shoulder of the patient. The incision is midline and vertical, with placement of a tracheal hook into the thyroid cartilage. Cephalad traction is applied, and an incision of the cricothyroid membrane is created. Dilation of the incision is followed by intubation (Fig. 2-4).

Rapid Four-Step Technique[68-72]

The rapid four-step technique has evolved from the "standard" technique for sake of expediency. The procedure is initiated from the head of the gurney, where the intubating operator is most likely to be positioned (Fig. 2-5). If the pertinent anatomy is clearly palpable (step 1), the skin and cricothyroid membrane are incised simultaneously with a No. 20 scalpel in a horizontal orientation (step 2). A blunt hook is then applied along the caudal side of the scalpel; the hook is used to apply traction to the cricoid ring (step 3). Thus, the incision is stabilized and widened for subsequent intubation (step 4). This technique may be a better alternative to the standard technique for several reasons. First, the operator per-

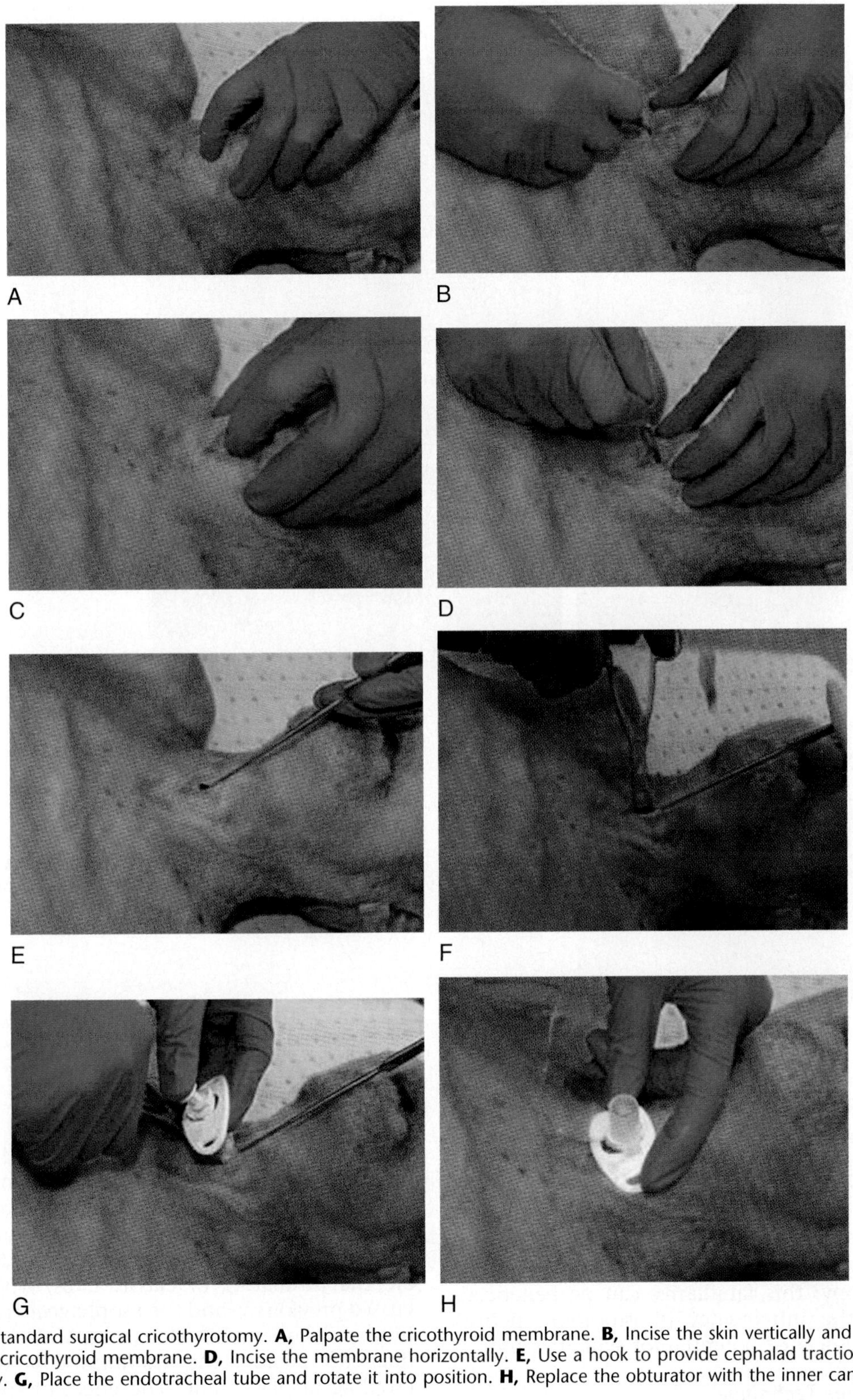
A
B
C
D
E
F
G
H

FIGURE 2-4 Standard surgical cricothyrotomy. **A,** Palpate the cricothyroid membrane. **B,** Incise the skin vertically and in the midline. **C,** Identify the cricothyroid membrane. **D,** Incise the membrane horizontally. **E,** Use a hook to provide cephalad traction. **F,** Dilate the stoma vertically. **G,** Place the endotracheal tube and rotate it into position. **H,** Replace the obturator with the inner cannula.

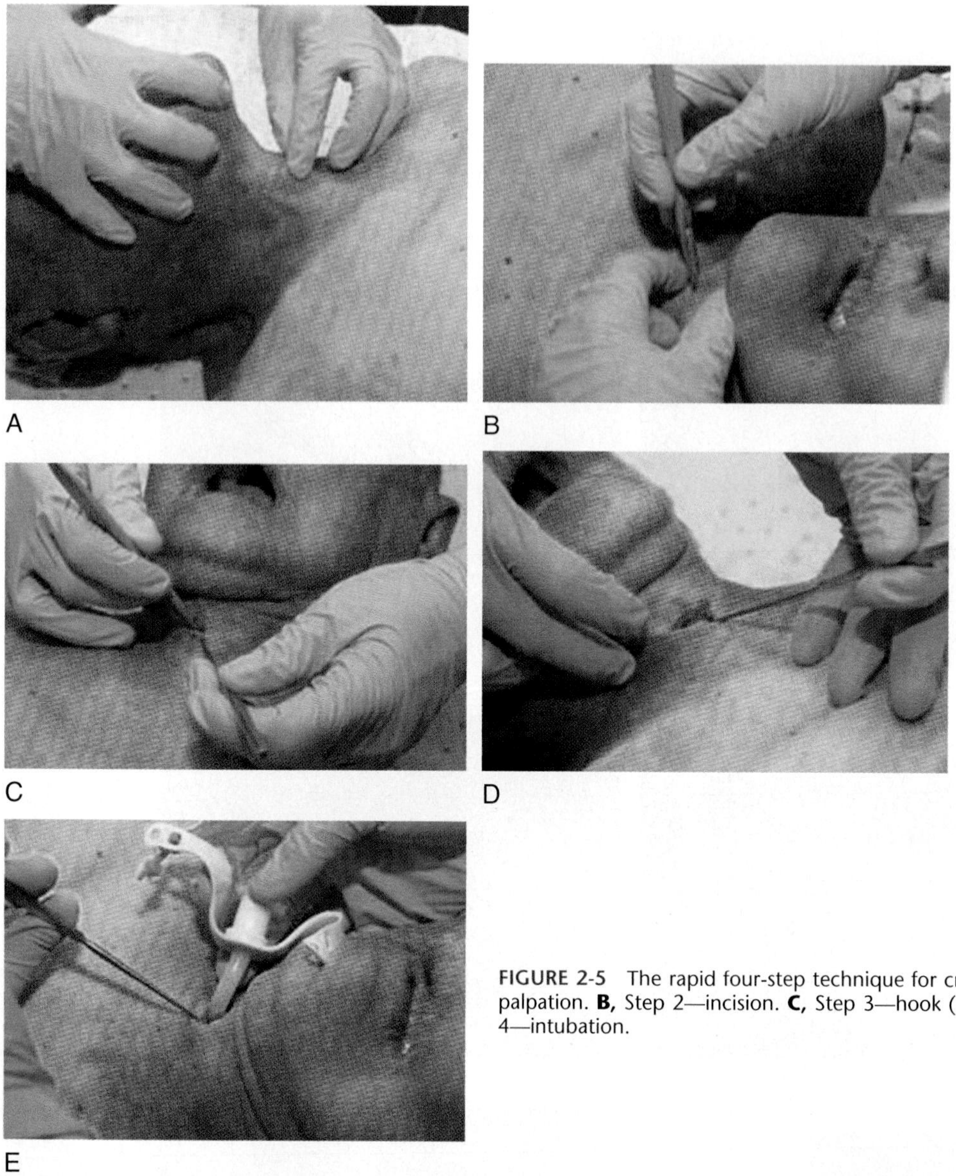
A
B
C
D
E

FIGURE 2-5 The rapid four-step technique for cricothyrotomy. **A,** Step 1—palpation. **B,** Step 2—incision. **C,** Step 3—hook (placement and pull). **D,** Step 4—intubation.

forms the procedure from the head of the bed or gurney instead of having to step around to the side. Second, the traction applied to the cricoid ring obliterates the pretracheal potential space, which may be inadvertently intubated during the standard technique. Third, the operator's hand positioning, when applying cricoid traction, is somewhat similar to that of laryngoscopy; this familiarity can be beneficial, considering the infrequency of procedure performance and associated potential for skill atrophy.

Percutaneous Technique

In contrast to the "open" techniques just described, the percutaneous technique of intubation relies on a wire-through-needle (e.g., Seldinger) method for accessing the airway.[73,74] Technologic advances have resulted in the production of *cuffed* ETTs that can be placed within the airway by using a dilator over a wire (Fig. 2-6).

Bridging Devices

Bridging devices can be rapidly employed to augment ventilation. Generally, they are placed in a supraglottic position. Most of these products do not provide a route for intubation, except for the intubating LMA. Examples of commercially available bridging devices are the intubating or classic LMA, which was discussed previously, and the Esophageal Tracheal Combitube (Tyco-Kendall, Mansfield, MA). A dual-lumen, dual-cuff airway, the Combitube is designed for esophageal placement. The effect of the dual cuffs above and below the glottis is to isolate the laryngeal inlet and allow for directed ventilation. The insertion of the Combitube is meant to be a blind technique. However, a laryngoscope is commonly used to assist in placement. Placement is relatively easy, and ventilation is generally effective.[75-78] Complications related to esophageal injury and mucosal ischemia by the Combitube have been reported.[79]

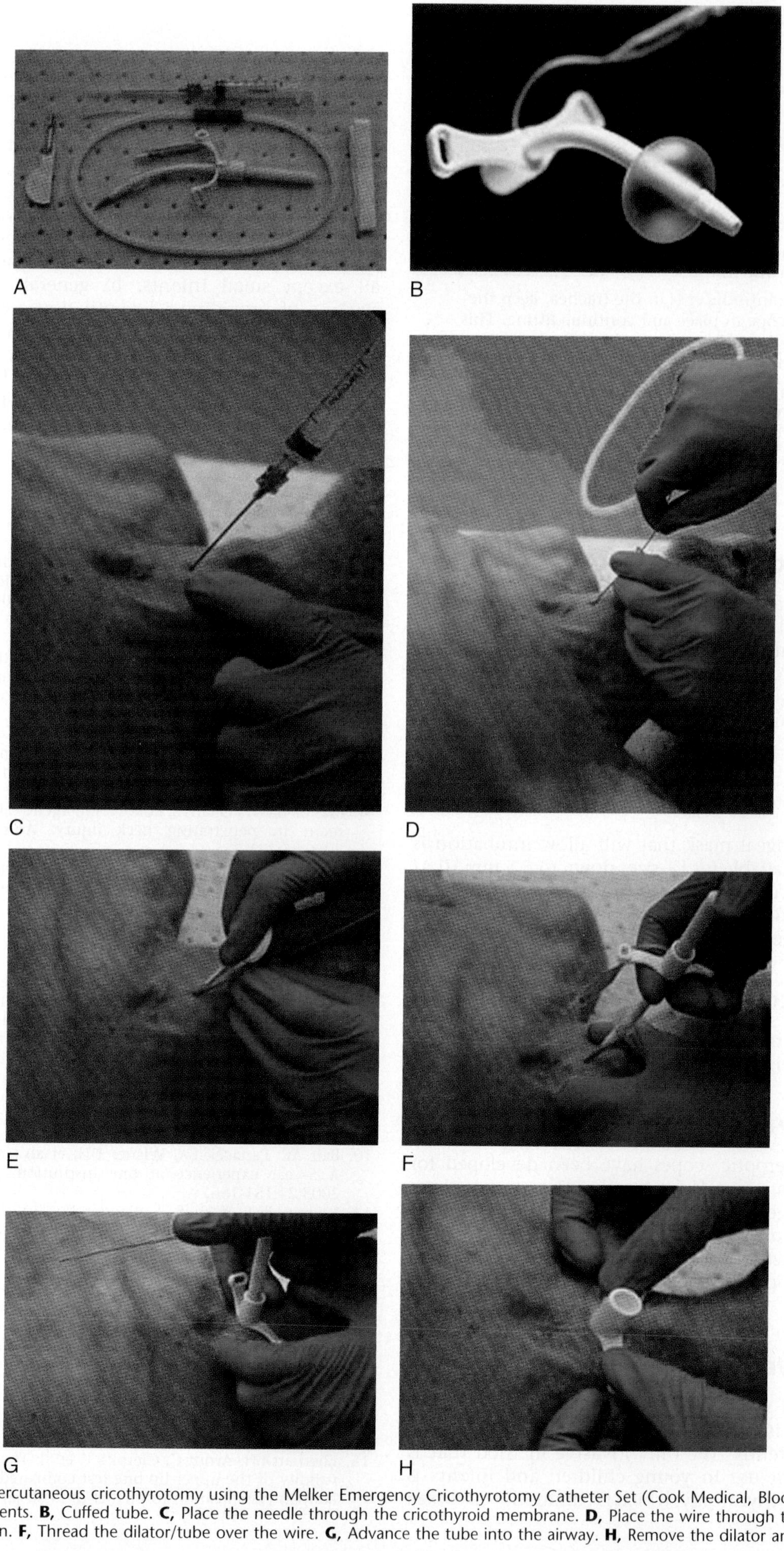

FIGURE 2-6 Percutaneous cricothyrotomy using the Melker Emergency Cricothyrotomy Catheter Set (Cook Medical, Bloomington, IN). **A,** Kit contents. **B,** Cuffed tube. **C,** Place the needle through the cricothyroid membrane. **D,** Place the wire through the needle. **E,** Incise the skin. **F,** Thread the dilator/tube over the wire. **G,** Advance the tube into the airway. **H,** Remove the dilator and wire.

Tips and Tricks

FOR SUCCESS WITH A TRACHEAL INTRODUCER

- Ideally, use a tracheal introducer when the patient's vocal cords are too anterior to be visualized well with direct laryngoscopy.
- Have a helper ready to assist in advancing the tube over the introducer.
- Once the introducer is in the trachea, keep the laryngoscope in place and continue lifting. This will straighten the path for the endotracheal tube to slide over the introducer into the trachea.
- If resistance is met at the level of the glottis, use gentle pressure and rotate the tube 45 to 90 degrees to enable to pass the obstruction.

Pediatric Considerations

Most of the adjunct devices discussed in this chapter have limited or no application in young children. It is likely that some of them may be used in older children and teens as size allows, but very little research has been performed in this area. We offer a brief summary of products that have some applicability in infants and children.

■ CLASSIC LARYNGEAL MASK AIRWAY

A new laryngeal mask that will allow intubation is currently available for ET sizes down to 5.5 mm (ILA/AIR-Q, Mercury Medical, Clearwater, FL). The classic (nonintubating) LMA is available in all sizes appropriate for teens to neonates.

■ GLIDESCOPE FOR CHILDREN

There is currently a small GildeScope available for children weighing in the 2 kg range.

■ FIBEROPTIC SCOPES

Flexible fiberoptic scopes have been developed for very small airways. However, the diameters of these scopes are generally too small to allow easy passage of the ETT off the scope into the airway. This "railroading" method in thinner scopes is more likely to kink the scope, risks breaking the scope, and is prone to failure.

■ INVASIVE CONSIDERATIONS

In children younger than 10 years, an open cricothyrotomy is contraindicated because of airway size issues. Currently, the only invasive method that is available for use in young children and infants is needle cricothyrotomy, which is commonly discussed in the context of jet insufflation. Such high-pressure oxygen has been shown to provide adequate short-term oxygenation with less successful ventilation. The technique does nothing to protect the airway because a cuffed tube is not present in the airway. Various adapted combinations have been described to allow the use of the ventilation bag (with adaptor) and the cricothyrotomy needle. The pressure generated with such a bag is generally inadequate for all except small infants. In general, commercial systems of providing jet ventilation are more reliable. In any case, barotrauma is often a concern. Likewise, egress of the needle from its original placement owing to the high pressure can be an issue. In such a case, manual stabilization of the catheter assembly is prudent until a definitive airway can be established.

REFERENCES

1. Sagarin MJ, Barton ED, Chng YM, Walls RM: National Emergency Airway Registry Investigators: Airway management by US and Canadian emergency medicine residents: A multicenter analysis of more than 6,000 endotracheal intubation attempts. Ann Emerg Med 2005;46:328-336.
2. Bair AE, Filbin MR, Kulkarni RG, Walls RM: The failed intubation attempt in the emergency department: Analysis of prevalence, rescue techniques, and personnel. J Emerg Med 2002;23:131-140.
3. Sakles JC, Laurin EG, Rantapaa AA, Panacek EA: Airway management in the emergency department: A one-year study of 610 tracheal intubations. Ann Emerg Med 1998;31:325-332.
4. Mandavia DP, Qualls S, Rokos I: Emergency airway management in penetrating neck injury. Ann Emerg Med 2000;35:221-225.
5. Li J, Murphy-Lavoie H, Bugas C, et al: Complications of emergency intubation with and without paralysis. Am J Emerg Med 1999;17:141-143.
6. Sivilotti ML, Filbin MR, Murray HE, et al: Does the sedative agent facilitate emergency rapid sequence intubation? Acad Emerg Med 2003;10:612-620.
7. Walls RM, Luten RC, Murphy MF, Schneider RE (eds): Manual of Emergency Airway Management, 2nd ed. Philadelphia, Lippincott Williams & Wilkins, 2004.
8. Orebaugh SL: Difficult airway management in the emergency department. J Emerg Med 2002;22:31-48.
9. Tayal VS, Riggs RW, Marx JA, et al: Rapid-sequence intubation at an emergency medicine residency: Success rate and adverse events during a two-year period. Acad Emerg Med 1999;6:31-37.
10. Bair AE, Panacek EA, Wisner DH, et al: Cricothyrotomy: A 5-year experience at one institution. J Emerg Med 2003;24:151-156.
11. Levitan RM, Kush S, Hollander JE: Devices for difficult airway management in academic emergency departments: Results of a national survey. Ann Emerg Med 1999;33:694-698.
12. Walsh K, Cummins F: Difficult airway equipment in departments of emergency medicine in Ireland: Results of a national survey. Eur J Anaesthesiol 2004;21:128-131.
13. Mallampati SR: Clinical sign to predict difficult tracheal intubation (hypothesis). Can Anaesth Soc J 1983;30:316-317.
14. Mallampati SR, Gatt SP, Gugino LD, et al: A clinical sign to predict difficult tracheal intubation: A prospective study. Can Anaesth Soc J 1985;32:429-434.
15. Eberhart LH, Arndt C, Cierpka T, et al: The reliability and validity of the upper lip bite test compared with the Mallampati classification to predict difficult laryngoscopy: An

external prospective evaluation. Anesth Analg 2005;101: 284-289.
16. Samsoon GL, Young JR: Difficult tracheal intubation: A retrospective study. Anaesthesia 1987;42:487-490.
17. Tse JC, Rimm EB, Hussain A: Predicting difficult endotracheal intubation in surgical patients scheduled for general anesthesia: A prospective blind study. Anesth Analg 1995;81:254-258.
18. Levitan RM, Ochroch EA, Kush S, et al: Assessment of airway visualization: Validation of the percentage of glottic opening (POGO) scale. Acad Emerg Med 1998;5:919-923.
19. Reed MJ, Dunn MJ, McKeown DW: Can an airway assessment score predict difficulty at intubation in the emergency department? Emerg Med J 2005;22:99-102.
20. Levitan RM, Everett WW, Ochroch EA: Limitations of difficult airway prediction in patients intubated in the emergency department. Ann Emerg Med 2004;44:307-313.
21. Levitan RM, Mechem CC, Ochroch EA, et al: Head-elevated laryngoscopy position: Improving laryngeal exposure during laryngoscopy by increasing head elevation. Ann Emerg Med 2003;41:322-330.
22. Benumof JL, Cooper SD: Quantitative improvement in laryngoscopic view by optimal external laryngeal manipulation. J Clin Anesth 1996;8:136-140.
23. Ho AM, Chung DC: Use of external laryngeal manipulation to facilitate laryngoscopy. Ann Emerg Med 2003;41(4):587; author reply 587-588.
24. Knopp RK: External laryngeal manipulation: A simple intervention for difficult intubations. Ann Emerg Med 2002;40:38-40.
25. Mlinek EJ Jr, Clinton JE, Plummer D, Ruiz E: Fiberoptic intubation in the emergency department. Ann Emerg Med 1990;19:359-362.
26. Delaney KA, Hessler R: Emergency flexible fiberoptic nasotracheal intubation: A report of 60 cases. Ann Emerg Med 1988;17:919-926.
27. Schafermeyer RW: Fiberoptic laryngoscopy in the emergency department. Am J Emerg Med 1984;2:160-163.
28. Birmingham B, Mentzer SJ, Body SC: Laryngeal mask airway for therapeutic fiberoptic bronchoscopic procedures. J Cardiothorac Vasc Anesth 1996;10:519-520.
29. Benumof JL: A new technique of fiberoptic intubation through a standard LMA. Anesthesiology 2001;95:1541.
30. Ianchulev SA: Through-the-LMA fiberoptic intubation of the trachea in a patient with an unexpected difficult airway. Anesth Analg 2005;101:1882-1883.
31. Johr M, Berger TM: Fiberoptic intubation through the laryngeal mask airway (LMA) as a standardized procedure. Paediatr Anaesth 2004;14:614.
32. Liem EB, Bjoraker DG, Gravenstein D: New options for airway management: Intubating fibreoptic stylets. Br J Anaesth 2003;91:408-418.
33. Cohn AI, Hart RT, McGraw SR, Blass NH: The Bullard laryngoscope for emergency airway management in a morbidly obese parturient. Anesth Analg 1995;81:872-873.
34. Wackett A, Anderson K, Thode H: Bullard laryngoscopy by naive operators in the cervical spine immobilized patient. J Emerg Med 2005;29:253-257.
35. Watts AD, Gelb AW, Bach DB, Pelz DM: Comparison of the Bullard and Macintosh laryngoscopes for endotracheal intubation of patients with a potential cervical spine injury. Anesthesiology 1997;87:1335-1342.
36. Smith CE, Sidhu TS, Lever J, Pinchak AB: The complexity of tracheal intubation using rigid fiberoptic laryngoscopy (WuScope). Anesth Analg 1999;89:236-239.
37. Smith CE, Pinchak AB, Sidhu TS, et al: Evaluation of tracheal intubation difficulty in patients with cervical spine immobilization: Fiberoptic (WuScope) versus conventional laryngoscopy. Anesthesiology 1999;91:1253-1259.
38. Wu TL, Chou HC: A new laryngoscope: The combination intubating device. Anesthesiology 1994;81:1085-1087.
39. Wu TL, Chou HC: WuScope versus conventional laryngoscope in cervical spine immobilization. Anesthesiology 2000;93:588-589.
40. Pearce AC, Shaw S, Macklin S: Evaluation of the Upsherscope: A new rigid fibrescope. Anaesthesia 1996;51: 561-564.
41. Fridrich P, Frass M, Krenn CG, et al: The UpsherScope in routine and difficult airway management: A randomized, controlled clinical trial. Anesth Analg 1997;85:1377-1381.
42. Cooper RM, Pacey JA, Bishop MJ, McCluskey SA: Early clinical experience with a new videolaryngoscope (GlideScope) in 728 patients. Can J Anaesth 2005;52:191-198.
43. Agro F, Barzoi G, Montecchia F: Tracheal intubation using a Macintosh laryngoscope or a GlideScope in 15 patients with cervical spine immobilization. Br J Anaesth 2003; 90:705-706.
44. Turkstra TP, et al: Cervical spine motion: A fluoroscopic comparison during intubation with lighted stylet, GlideScope, and Macintosh laryngoscope. Anesth Analg 2005; 101(3):910-915; table of contents.
45. Sun DA, Warriner CB, Parsons DG, et al: The GlideScope Video Laryngoscope: Randomized clinical trial in 200 patients. Br J Anaesth 2005;94:381-384.
46. Levitan RM, Ochroch EA, Stuart S, Hollander JE: Use of the intubating laryngeal mask airway by medical and nonmedical personnel. Am J Emerg Med 2000;18:12-16.
47. Pollack CV Jr: The laryngeal mask airway: A comprehensive review for the Emergency physician. J Emerg Med 2001;20:53-66.
48. Foley LJ, Ochroch EA: Bridges to establish an emergency airway and alternate intubating techniques. Crit Care Clin 2000;16:429-444; vi.
49. Parmet JL, Colonna-Romano P, Horrow JC, et al: The laryngeal mask airway reliably provides rescue ventilation in cases of unanticipated difficult tracheal intubation along with difficult mask ventilation. Anesth Analg 1998;87:661-665.
50. Stanwood PL: The laryngeal mask airway and the emergency airway. AANA J 1997;65:364-370.
51. Young B: The intubating laryngeal-mask airway may be an ideal device for airway control in the rural trauma patient. Am J Emerg Med 2003;21:80-85.
52. Ferson DZ, Rosenblatt WH, Johansen MJ, et al: Use of the intubating LMA-Fastrach in 254 patients with difficult-to-manage airways. Anesthesiology 2001;95:1175-1181.
53. Wakeling HG, Bagwell A: The intubating laryngeal mask (ILMA) in an emergency failed intubation. Anaesthesia 1999;54:305-306.
54. Bair AE, Laurin EG, Schmitt BJ: An assessment of a tracheal tube introducer as an endotracheal tube placement confirmation device. Am J Emerg Med 2005;23:754-758.
55. Carley S, Jackson R: Towards evidence based emergency medicine: Best BETs from the Manchester Royal Infirmary. Gum elastic bougies in difficult intubation. Emerg Med J 2001;18:376-377.
56. Combes X, Dumerat M, Dhonneur G: Emergency gum elastic bougie-assisted tracheal intubation in four patients with upper airway distortion. Can J Anaesth 2004;51: 1022-1024.
57. Phelan MP: Use of the endotracheal bougie introducer for difficult intubations. Am J Emerg Med 2004;22:479-482.
58. Morton T, Brady S, Clancy M: Difficult airway equipment in English emergency departments. Anaesthesia 2000;55:485-488.
59. van Elstraete AC, Mamie JC, Mehdaoui H: Nasotracheal intubation in patients with immobilized cervical spine: A comparison of tracheal tube cuff inflation and fiberoptic bronchoscopy. Anesth Analg 1998;87:400-402.
60. van Elstraete AC, Pennant JH, Gajraj NM, Victory RA: Tracheal tube cuff inflation as an aid to blind nasotracheal intubation. Br J Anaesth 1993;70:691-693.
61. Hung O, Pytka S, Morris I, et al: Lightwand intubation. II: Clinical trial of a new lightwand for tracheal intubation in patients with difficult airways. Can J Anaesth 1995;42:826-830.
62. Hung OR, Stewart RD: Lightwand intubation. I: A new lightwand device. Can J Anaesth 1995;42:820-825.

63. Agro F, Hung OR, Cataldo R, et al: Lightwand intubation using the Trachlight: A brief review of current knowledge. Can J Anaesth 2001;48:592-599.
64. Hirabayashi Y, Hiruta M, Kawakami T, et al: Effects of lightwand (Trachlight) compared with direct laryngoscopy on circulatory responses to tracheal intubation. Br J Anaesth 1998;81:253-255.
65. Croinin DF, Coleman MM: The Trachlight compared to laryngeal mask airway assisted intubation. Anaesthesia 2002;57:715-716; author reply 716.
66. Mace S, Hedges J: Cricothyrotomy and translaryngeal jet insufflation. In Roberts JR, Hedges JR (eds): Clinical Procedures in Emergency Medicine, 4th ed. Philadelphia, Saunders, 2004.
67. Walls RM: Cricothyroidotomy. Emerg Med Clin North Am 1988;6:725-736.
68. Brofeldt BT, et al: Evaluation of the rapid four-step cricothyrotomy technique: An interim report. Air Med J 1998;17:127-130.
69. Brofeldt B, Panacek EA, Richards JR: An easy cricothyrotomy approach: The rapid four-step technique. Acad Emerg Med 1996;3:1060-1063.
70. Holmes JF, Panacek EA, Sakles JC, Brofeldt BT: Comparison of 2 cricothyrotomy techniques: Standard method versus rapid 4-step technique. Ann Emerg Med 1998;32:442-446.
71. Bair AE, Laurin EG, Karchin A, et al: Cricoid ring integrity: Implications for cricothyrotomy. Ann Emerg Med 2003; 41:331-337.
72. Davis DP, Bramwell KJ, Vilke GM, et al: Cricothyrotomy technique: Standard versus the rapid four-step technique. J Emerg Med 1999;17:17-21.
73. Chan TC, Vilke GM, Bramwell KJ, et al: Comparison of wire-guided cricothyrotomy versus standard surgical cricothyrotomy technique. J Emerg Med 1999;17:957-962.
74. Eisenburger P, Laczika K, List M, et al: Comparison of conventional surgical versus Seldinger technique emergency cricothyrotomy performed by inexperienced clinicians. Anesthesiology 2000;92:687-690.
75. Davis D, Valentine C, Ochs M, et al: The Combitube as a salvage airway device for paramedic rapid sequence intubation. Ann Emerg Med 2003;42:697-704.
76. Rabitsch W, Schellongowski P, Staudinger T, et al: Comparison of a conventional tracheal airway with the Combitube in an urban emergency medical services system run by physicians. Resuscitation 2003;57:27-32.
77. Agro F, Frass M, Benumof JL, Krafft P: Current status of the Combitube: A review of the literature. J Clin Anesth 2002;14:307-314.
78. Blostein PA, Koestner AJ, Hoak S: Failed rapid sequence intubation in trauma patients: Esophageal tracheal Combitube is a useful adjunct. J Trauma 1998;44:534-537.
79. Vezina D, Lessard MR, Bussières J, et al: Complications associated with the use of the Esophageal-Tracheal Combitube. Can J Anaesth 1998;45:76-80.

Chapter 3

Mechanical Ventilation

Robert J. Sigillito

KEY POINTS

Noninvasive ventilation (NIV) reduces the need for endotracheal intubation.

Rapid titration and adjustment of the noninvasive ventilator to reduce the work of breathing is essential to success of NIV.

Monitoring airway pressures and employment of a low tidal volume strategy minimize the risk of ventilator-induced lung injury.

Appropriate selection of ventilator mode, tidal volume, PEEP, Fio_2, and inspiratory flow rate is essential to minimize work of breathing and enhance correction of hypoxemia.

Correction of hypoxemia is critical; correction of hypercarbia is not.

Scope

Patients with severe respiratory complaints account for about 12% of ED visits.[1] Between 1992 and 1999, ED visits for asthma rose 26%, for pneumonia 12%, and for chest pain 50%.[2] 26% of asthmatic patients who required intubation reported to the ED as their primary source of health care.[3] A thorough knowledge of noninvasive and invasive mechanical ventilation, lung protective ventilation strategies, and methods to enhance patient-ventilator synchrony is essential to the practice of emergency medicine.

Techniques and Methods of Mechanical Ventilation

Mechanical ventilation support may be provided using a noninvasive or invasive approach. Furthermore, each technique may be applied using a variety of ventilator modes. The key differences in ventilatory support are determined by the trigger, the limit, and the cycle. The trigger is the event that starts inspiration: either patient initiated respiratory effort or machine initiated positive pressure. The limit refers to the airflow parameter that is regulated during inspiration: either airflow rate or airway pressure. The cycle terminates inspiration: either a set volume is delivered (volume cycled ventilation), a pressure is delivered for a set period of time (pressure cycled ventilation), or the patient ceases inspiratory effort (pressure support ventilation).

■ MODES OF INVASIVE MECHANICAL VENTILATION

■ Control Mode

Control mode ventilation (CMV) is used almost exclusively in anesthesia, but knowledge of this mode's limitations aids in the comprehension of other modes' features (Fig. 3-1). In control mode, all breaths are triggered, limited, and cycled by the ventilator. The physician selects a tidal volume (Vt), respiratory rate (RR), inspiratory flow rate (IFR),

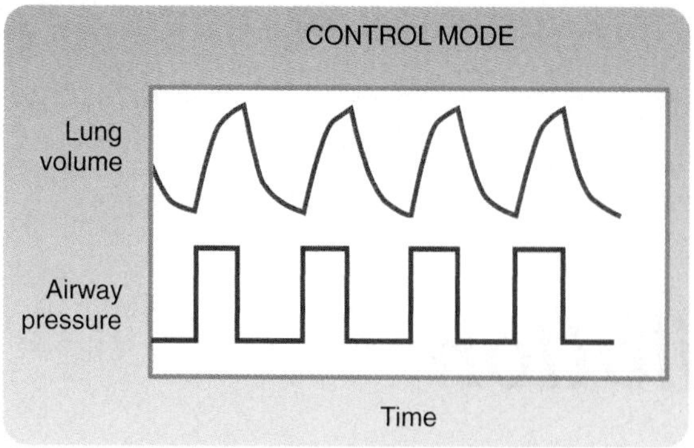
CONTROL MODE
Lung
volume
Airway
pressure
Time

FIGURE 3-1 Control mode. Tidal, respiratory rate, inspiratory flow rate, FiO_2, and PEEP are controlled. There is no synchronization with patient's respiratory effort.

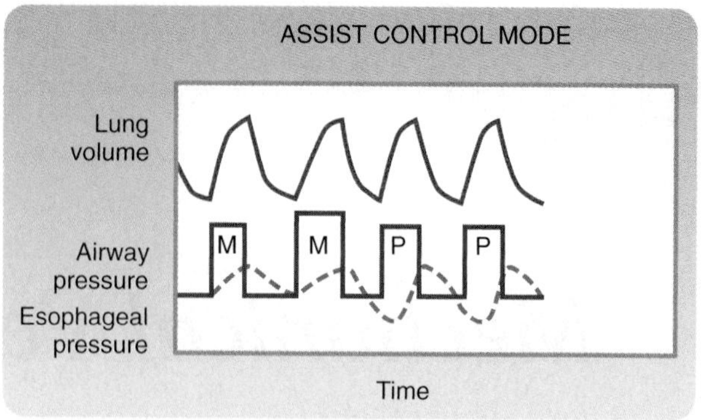
ASSIST CONTROL MODE
Lung
volume
Airway
pressure
Esophageal
pressure
M
M
P
P
Time

FIGURE 3-2 Assist control mode (volume-cycled ventilation). The tidal volume is controlled. A minimum mandatory respiratory rate is set, and synchronized with patient effort. If the patient breathes at a rate higher than the set rate, all breaths are assisted. *Dashed line* represents esophageal/intrathoracic pressure dynamics. The first two breaths represent machine-initiated (M) breaths; the second two breaths represent patient-initiated (P) breaths.

fraction of inspired oxygen (FiO_2), and positive end expiratory pressure (PEEP). The machine then delivers positive pressure, applying as much pressure as is required to deliver the set Vt (the cycle) at the set IFR (the limit). The patient is not able to initiate or terminate a breath. If inspiratory effort were initiated before the machine was triggered to deliver a breath, then regardless of the patient's inspiratory effort, airflow would not occur. Imagine sucking on an empty bottle, and the concept is clearly evident. Furthermore, if exhalation were incomplete, yet the time for the machine to deliver a breath occurred, then the ventilator would provide as much pressure as necessary to cause inhalation. Imagine forcibly exhaling, or coughing, when the ventilator triggers to deliver a breath. This lack of synchrony would cause distress and risk structural lung or airway injury. For these reasons, CMV is never used except in apneic, paralyzed, anesthetized patients.

Assist Control Mode

Assist control (AC) mode usually provides the greatest level of ventilatory assistance (Fig. 3-2). The physician sets Vt, RR, IFR, FiO_2, and PEEP. In contrast to all other modes, *the trigger that initiates inspiration can be either an elapsed time interval (determined by the set RR), or the patient's spontaneous inspiratory effort.* When either occurs, the machine delivers the set Vt. The machine follows a time algorithm that synchronizes the machine with patient-initiated breaths. If the patient is breathing at or above the set RR, then all breaths are patient initiated. If the patient breathes below the set RR, then machine-initiated breaths are interspersed among the patient's breaths. The work of breathing (WOB) is primarily the effort that the patient exerts to cause the airway pressure to drop to the threshold that triggers the ventilator. (Manipulating the ventilator sensitivity sets this threshold.) Further WOB may be performed to a variable degree during inspiration, depending upon how much the respiratory muscles are activated. WOB on the AC mode may be extreme in two situations: when the Vt drawn by the patient is greater than the set Vt,

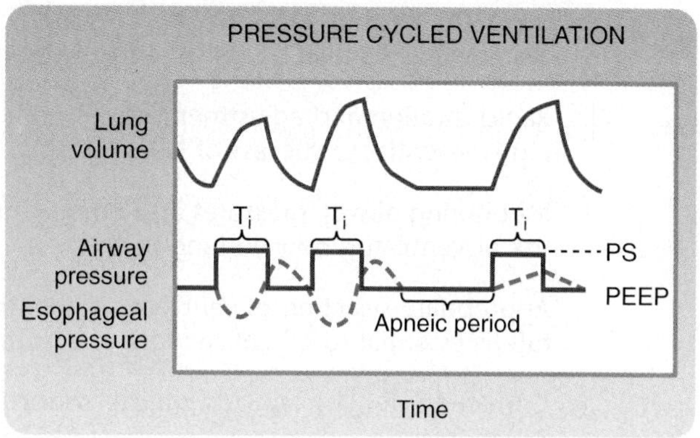
PRESSURE CYCLED VENTILATION
Lung
volume
Airway
pressure
Esophageal
pressure
Ti
Ti
Ti
PS
PEEP
Apneic period
Time

FIGURE 3-3 Assist control mode (pressure-cycled ventilation). Inspiratory pressure support (PS) and inspiratory time (Ti) are controlled. Tidal volume may vary from breath to breath. Minimum mandatory respiratory rate is set and synchronizes with patient effort. *Dashed line* represents esophageal/intrathoracic pressure dynamics. The first two breaths represent patient-initiated breaths; the third breath is a machine-initiated (mandatory) breath. PEEP, positive end expiratory pressure.

and when the patient inspires at a rate that exceeds the set IFR (refer to the section on Enhancing Ventilator Synchrony).

In the majority of situations, AC is used as described earlier, termed volume cycled ventilation (VCV). As an alternative, some ventilators allow pressure cycled ventilation (PCV, not to be confused this with pressure support ventilation, described later) (Fig. 3-3). Instead of IFR, the limit during PCV is a set airway pressure. Instead of Vt, the cycle during PCV is a set inspiratory time (Ti). [On some ventilator models, RR and inspiratory to expiratory (I : E) ratio are set; Ti is then calculated from those settings. On other models, Ti is available as a setting.] Since Vt is not set, the delivered Vt varies slightly from breath to breath, depending on lung compliance, airway resistance, and patient effort. PCV may offer a slight advantage over VCV in clinical scenarios that require control of the I : E ratio; however, a body of literature

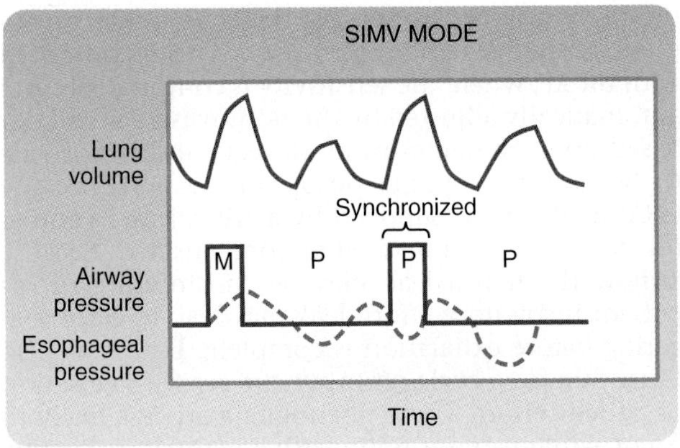
SIMV MODE
Lung volume
Synchronized
Airway pressure
Esophageal pressure
M
P
P
P
Time

FIGURE 3-4 Synchronized intermittent mandatory ventilation (SIMV). Tidal volume is controlled only during machine-assisted breaths. Tidal volume may vary during nonassisted (patient-initiated) breaths. Minimum mandatory respiratory rate is set. If the patient breathes more slowly than the set rate, the machine synchronizes with patient effort (third breath). If the patient breathes faster than the set rate, breaths in excess of the set rate are not assisted (second and fourth breaths). M, mandatory breath; P, patient-initiated breath. *Dashed line* represents esophageal/intrathoracic pressure dynamics.

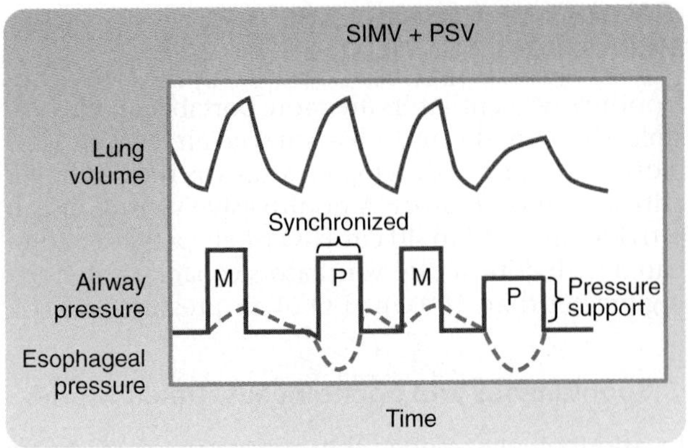
SIMV + PSV
Lung volume
Synchronized
Airway pressure
Esophageal pressure
M
P
M
P
Pressure support
Time

FIGURE 3-5 Synchronized intermittent mandatory ventilation (SIMV) with pressure support (PSV). Tidal volume is controlled during machine-initiated (M) breaths (first and third breaths) and synchronized patient-initiated (P) breaths (second breath). Pressure support is provided whenever the patient initiates a breath over the set rate (fourth breath). Tidal volume may vary during pressure-supported breaths. *Dashed line* represents esophageal/intrathoracic pressure dynamics.

investigating this concept does not exist. Historically PCV was commonly used in neonates and infants, although modern ventilators that precisely measure small Vt are currently more favored. PCV may be the only mode available on some portable and transport ventilators.

■ Synchronized Intermittent Mandatory Ventilation and Pressure Support

Synchronized intermittent mandatory ventilation (SIMV) is probably the most commonly misunderstood mode of mechanical ventilation (Fig. 3-4). The physician sets Vt, RR, IFR, FiO_2, and PEEP, as in AC. In contrast to AC mode, the trigger that initiates inspiration depends upon the patient's RR relative to the set RR. *When the patient breathes at or below the set RR, the trigger can be either elapsed time or the patient's respiratory effort.* In this case, the WOB is equivalent to AC. However, *when the patient breathes above the set RR, the ventilator does not trigger to assist the spontaneous breaths in excess of the set RR.* In fact, the work associated with those breaths may be quite high, because the patient must generate enough negative force to pull air through the ventilator and to overcome the resistance to airflow due to the ventilator circuit tubing and the endotracheal tube. This is in addition to the WOB required due to the underlying disease process.

This limitation of SIMV can be diminished by the addition of pressure support ventilation (PSV) (Fig. 3-5). PSV is inspiratory positive pressure applied during patient initiated breaths that exceed the set RR. The patient initiates and terminates inspiration, thereby determining Vt. Once the patient triggers pressure support, it is maintained until the machine detects cessation of patient effort, indicated by a fall in inspiratory airflow. Vt, IFR, and Ti are not controlled, but are determined by patient effort. The WOB performed during PSV involves triggering the ventilator to deliver the pressure *and maintaining inspiratory effort throughout inhalation.* Contrast this with machine assisted ventilation in AC or SIMV, where WOB involves triggering the ventilator, with lung inflation continuing regardless of whether or not the patient maintains inspiratory effort. WOB during PSV also depends on the set level of pressure support. Insufficient pressure support is associated with a high WOB, leading to a small Vt and a high RR. Adequate pressure support reduces WOB and improves Vt and RR. In our experience, RR seems to be the best index of the adequacy of the level of pressure support. It should be adjusted to maintain an acceptable RR less than 30, but preferably less than 24.

■ Continuous Positive Airway Pressure

Continuous positive airway pressure (CPAP) alone is not a true form of assisted mechanical ventilation, because inspiration is not assisted by increasing airway pressure. Pressure greater than ambient atmospheric pressure is supplied, but is held constant throughout the respiratory cycle. During inhalation, the gradient between the airway and intrathoracic pressure is higher than it would be if breathing ambient air. Conversely, the gradient is lower during exhalation. As a result, inhalation requires slightly less effort than normal breathing, and the airways are held open during exhalation allowing better expiratory airflow. As in SIMV, PSV may be added to CPAP. CPAP with PSV is a form of assisted ventilation, because inspiratory pressure is augmented. As discussed earlier, the patient initiates and terminates each breath, therefore WOB is performed as the patient initiates each breath and maintains inspiratory effort throughout inhalation.

■ MODES OF NONINVASIVE MECHANICAL VENTILATION

Noninvasive ventilators are more portable, made possible through the use of a smaller air compressor/blower but cannot develop pressures as high as larger critical care ventilators. A noninvasive ventilator can provide up to 20 to 40 cm H_2O of air pressure, compared with critical care ventilators capable of delivering greater than 100 cm H_2O of air pressure.

■ Spontaneous and Spontaneous/Timed Modes

In spontaneous mode, the airway pressure cycles between an inspiratory positive airway pressure (IPAP) and expiratory positive airway pressure (EPAP). This is commonly referred to as biphasic (or bilevel, not to be confused with bilevel invasive mode, not discussed here) positive airway pressure (BiPAP), but other proprietary names refer to the same mode. The trigger to switch from EPAP to IPAP is patient inspiratory effort. A variety of ventilator models employ one or several of the following to indicate patient effort: a drop in airway pressure, measured inspired volume (usually 5 to 6 mL), or increases in airflow rate. The limit during inspiration is the set level of IPAP. The inspiratory phase cycles off when the machine senses cessation of patient effort, indicated by decrease in inspiratory flow below a set threshold (typically 60% of the peak inspiratory flow rate), or a maximum inspiratory time is reached (usually 3 seconds). The latter is a safety mechanism to prevent lung hyperinflation from ventilator "runaway," but was not available on early generations of noninvasive ventilators. Vt may vary from breath to breath, dependent primarily on the magnitude and duration of patient effort, but also upon lung compliance. WOB is predominantly related to initiating and maintaining airflow throughout the inspiratory phase. Additional WOB may occur if the patient actively contracts the expiratory muscles.

Spontaneous mode is dependent upon patient effort to trigger inhalation. A patient breathing at a slow, inadequate rate will develop respiratory acidosis. To prevent this adverse consequence, spontaneous/timed (ST) mode allows the machine to trigger by either patient effort or after an elapsed time interval calculated from a set minimum RR. If the patient does not initiate inspiration during the set interval, IPAP is triggered. For machine-initiated breaths, the machine cycles back to EPAP based upon a set inspiratory time. For patient-initiated breaths, the ventilator cycles as it would in spontaneous mode.

Pragmatically, (noninvasive) BiPAP and (invasive) CPAP with PSV are similar, with a few noteworthy differences. First, the trigger for CPAP with PSV is a drop in airway pressure sensed by the ventilator. Some ventilators monitor the airflow in the inspiratory and expiratory limbs of the ventilator circuit, and will trigger if the airflow in the inspiratory limb is greater than the airflow in the expiratory limb. The sensitivity of the trigger is adjustable on a conventional ventilator, by setting the magnitude of the pressure change required to trigger. This is contrasted with BiPAP, where the sensitivity is continuously and automatically adjusted by the noninvasive ventilator based upon the amount of air leak, and is not able to be adjusted by the physician. Second, because CPAP with PSV is supplied by a critical care ventilator, leaks are not tolerated or compensated. Because airflow through a leak may be "misinterpreted" as patient inspiratory effort, leak may lead to early triggering before exhalation is complete. Leak may also cause failure to cycle off in synchrony with cessation of patient effort. These phenomena are less likely to occur while using a noninvasive ventilator. Finally, the nomenclature used for the airway pressure is different. The pressure during the expiratory phase is termed CPAP or PEEP, analogous to EPAP of BiPAP. The pressure during the inspiratory phase is termed CPAP with PSV, analogous to IPAP of spontaneous mode. The distinction is that in CPAP with PSV, the numerical value for pressure support is the equivalent of the difference between IPAP and EPAP.

Selection of a Ventilation Technique and Ventilator Mode

The etiology of respiratory failure is the best predictor of whether a patient will respond to noninvasive technique. The literature supports its application in select patient groups with chronic obstructive pulmonary disease (COPD), asthma, congestive heart failure (CHF), pneumonia, trauma, cancer, neuromuscular disease, and in pediatrics.

Initiation of Noninvasive Ventilation

There are 4 basic steps in the process of initiating a trial of noninvasive ventilatory support. First, the patient must be willing to accept face mask ventilation. Since the patient should remain awake and cooperative during ventilation, the process should be explained before the mask is applied. Initially, provide a FIO_2 of 100%, with 3 to 5 cm H_2O of CPAP. Acceptance may improve if the patient holds the mask against his or her face. The mask is secured with straps once the patient demonstrates acceptance.

Next, after explaining that the pressure will change, switch to BiPAP with 3 to 5 cm H_2O EPAP and 8 to 10 cm H_2O IPAP. Titrate IPAP in 2 to 3 cm H_2O increments until exhaled tidal volume (measured by the ventilator) is in the range of 6 to 10 mL/kg ideal body weight. Further adjustment of IPAP should be directed toward obtaining an RR less than 30.

EPAP is then adjusted to the lowest level that allows synchrony between the patient and ventilator. Understanding this process requires a review of the components of WOB related to triggering the ventilator. The patient activates the inspiratory muscles to decrease the intrathoracic pressure. As the intrathoracic pressure falls below airway pressure, the transpulmonary pressure becomes positive, airflow begins, and the ventilator triggers. In a normal patient, the inspiratory muscle force required to lower the intrathoracic pressure to a level that triggers the ventilator is not great. However, in a patient with high intrinsic positive end expiratory pressure ($PEEP_i$, also known as auto-PEEP), intrathoracic pressure is high at end exhalation. The inspiratory muscle force required to lower the intrathoracic pressure below airway pressure is significantly greater. Thus, the WOB that is performed to trigger the ventilator is proportional to the amount of PEEPi that is present.

While delivering NPPV, it is impossible to measure PEEPi without invasive means. Instead, to detect PEEPi, signs of difficulty triggering the ventilator or signs of expiratory airflow obstruction should be sought. On physical examination, recruitment of the accessory muscles of inspiration suggests that PEEPi is a problem. A useful technique is palpation of the sternocleidomastoid muscle while simultaneously watching the ventilator flow graphs, or listening for the ventilator to trigger. When the muscle is felt to contract before the ventilator triggers, PEEPi may be the culprit. Observation of active abdominal muscle recruitment during exhalation indicates airflow obstruction that is a cause of elevated PEEPi. When elevated PEEPi is suspected, EPAP (or PEEP/CPAP) should be increased in increments of 2 to 3 cm H_2O until the problem is controlled. The maximum safe level of EPAP (or CPAP) that should be employed during NPPV has not been determined in an evidenced-based manner. Typical initial settings range from 0 to 5 cm H_2O; maximum settings described in methods sections of various trials range from 12.5 to 15 cm H_2O. It is prudent to measure the heart rate, blood pressure, and pulse oximetry after each increment in EPAP/CPAP, since high levels may compromise cardiac output. As EPAP is increased, corresponding increasing increments in IPAP are required to maintain adequate tidal volume.

Finally, FiO_2 is adjusted to maintain adequate O_2 saturation. In many clinical situations, continuous pulse oximetry alone is adequate for this purpose. Arterial blood gas determinations are not routinely required, but may be helpful in select patients to assess improvement in respiratory acidosis.

Monitoring Dynamic Pressures during Invasive Ventilation

Mechanical ventilation can cause damage to the lungs on a macroscopic and microscopic level. The direct cause of lung injury is believed to be a combination of overdistention of the alveoli and repetitive alveolar opening/closing with shear of the alveolar wall. The concept of ventilator-induced lung injury (VILI) has evolved to encompass all forms of injury at the organ and alveolar level, including pneumothorax, pneumomediastinum, bronchial rupture, diffuse alveolar damage, and acute respiratory distress syndrome (ARDS). Pressure is measured at the ventilator end of the circuit (the proximal airway) and the measurement used as an index of the pressures within the lung.

■ PEAK INSPIRATORY AIRWAY PRESSURE

The peak inspiratory airway pressure (P_{peak}) is the highest pressure that is generated during inflation of the lung. Since pressure decreases incrementally along the path at each point of resistance, the pressure delivered at the alveolar level may be significantly less than the measured P_{peak}, particularly when there is high resistance to airflow. Therefore, P_{peak} is not an ideal surrogate measurement for alveolar pressure.

■ PLATEAU PRESSURE

Plateau pressure (P_{plat}) is the end inspiratory airway pressure, measured just after airflow has ceased. Because this is a static measurement (there is no airflow), resistance of the circuit and airways do not play a role. Therefore, P_{plat} is a logical surrogate measurement for alveolar pressure. The primary limitation is that compliance is not equal in all regions of the lung. The degree of alveolar distention in healthy regions of the lung may be significantly greater than in heavily diseased lung regions, at the same P_{plat}. P_{plat} in a healthy adult with normal lung compliance undergoing mechanical ventilation is low, usually in the range of 5 to 15 cm H_2O. Patients with alveolar disease (pneumonia, cardiogenic pulmonary edema, acute lung injury [ALI], and ARDS) have poor lung compliance, therefore P_{plat} is typically much higher. Measures to maintain P_{plat} below 30 cm H_2O, the currently recommended limit, are discussed later.

■ INTRINSIC POSITIVE END EXPIRATORY PRESSURE

Positive end expiratory pressure (PEEP) indicates that the measured airway pressure at the end of exhalation is above ambient air pressure. When PEEP is set by the clinician and applied by the ventilator, it is termed extrinsic PEEP ($PEEP_e$). In contrast, $PEEP_i$ arises when exhalation is incomplete, either due to intrathoracic airway obstruction, early airway closure during exhalation, or inadequate exhalation time. The common end point is trapping of air in the lung at the end of exhalation, ultimately leading to increased intrathoracic pressure. $PEEP_i$ can cause problems by several mechanisms. First, because exhalation is incomplete, air is progressively trapped in the lungs leading to early airway closure and dynamic hyperinflation with associated risk of VILI. Second, $PEEP_i$ leads to difficulty triggering the ventilator and increased WOB, discussed previously. Third, $PEEP_i$

can cause patient ventilator dysynchrony if the patient continues active contraction of the respiratory muscles at end exhalation, as the ventilator triggers. Lung inflation may begin while the patient is attempting to complete exhalation. Finally, increased intrathoracic pressure can impede venous return to the heart, leading to hemodynamic instability. Simultaneously, impaired venous return may compromise pulmonary blood flow, increase physiologic dead space, and lead to worsening hypercapnea. Control of $PEEP_i$ is discussed later.

Lung-Protective Ventilator Strategies

Causes of difficulty with mechanical ventilation fall into four general categories:

- high airway pressure during lung inflation
- high $PEEP_I$ due to obstructive airways disease
- patient/ventilator dysynchrony
- equipment failure

CONTROLLING AIRWAY PRESSURE

ARDS, ALI, and Pulmonary Edema

Elevated plateau pressures are encountered in patients with poor lung compliance due to parenchymal lung disease (e.g., pulmonary edema, either cardiogenic or noncardiogenic) or obstructive airways disease with air trapping. The goal is to support the respiratory system while avoiding iatrogenic injury.

Initial studies compared conventional ventilation strategy (Vt 10-15 mL/kg ideal body weight [IBW], with a goal of obtaining normal Pao_2 and $Paco_2$) with a lung protective ventilation strategy (Vt 6 to 8 mL/kg IBW with correction of hypoxia, but allowing hypercapnea in favor of avoiding high airway pressures). The results were conflicting.[4-8] The most recently and largest reported trial, the ARDS Network Trial,[9] prospectively compared a conventional strategy (12 mL/kg Vt and a P_{plat} limit of 50 cm H_2O) with a protective strategy (6 mL/kg Vt and P_{plat} limit of 30 cm H_2O). After enrollment of 861 patients with ARDS and an interim analysis, the trial was stopped early due to a 22% reduction in mortality, 20% fewer days requiring mechanical ventilation, and fewer organ system failures in the group receiving the low Vt strategy.

Mechanical ventilation strategy in patients with other disease processes has not been as extensively studied. The extrapolation of these findings to patients with CHF, ALI, pneumonia, pulmonary fibrosis, lung cancer, and other lung pathology is not based on experimental evidence.

In summary, based on the available literature, employ a lung protective strategy using low Vt, limiting P_{plat} to 30 cm H_2O, and permissive hypercapnea in a patient with ARDS or pulmonary edema, in order to avoid iatrogenic lung injury.

Obstructive Airways Disease

Obstructive airways disease (OAD) exacerbation requiring mechanical ventilation is often associated with air trapping and dynamic hyperinflation of the lungs. High P_{peak} arises as a result of inspiratory airflow limitation, a phenomenon more common in the support of patients with severe asthma than those with COPD. High P_{plat} arises as a result of lung overdistention and consequent diminished compliance. Those patients with both high P_{peak} and P_{plat} comprise a group of high-risk patients with both obstruction and overdistention at high risk for complications including pneumothorax, tension pneumothorax, pneumomediastinum, dysrhythmias, and hemodynamic collapse. There have been no prospective trials comparing ventilation strategies in such patients. It is common practice to employ a strategy of permissive hypercapnea/controlled hypoventilation to eliminate $PEEP_I$ and avoid high P_{plat}. This strategy employs use of a low Vt, low RR, and high IFR to shorten inspiratory time and prolong expiratory time. Although this strategy often leads to hypercapnea, it is considered safer to allow the patient to develop a respiratory acidosis than to ventilate at excessive airway pressures. A lower limit of acceptable pH has not been established, but general recommendations have been to allow pH as low as 7.0 to 7.2. Controlled hypoventilation is required more often in the management of status asthmaticus than in COPD. Evidence in support of controlled hypoventilation comes from retrospective studies. In a report of 26 patients requiring 34 episodes of mechanical ventilation for status asthmaticus, a strategy using an initial RR of 6 to 10 cycles/min, Vt of 8 to 12 mL/kg, and Fio_2 adjusted to obtain normal Pao_2, P_{peak} was maintained below 50 cm H_2O by subsequent reduction of Vt and decreasing IFR. All patients required sedation, and 9 required pharmacologic paralysis to control respiratory rate. All patients survived. Complications included transient hypotension (57%), pneumonia (27%), supraventricular tachycardia (15%), and pneumomediastinum or subcutaneous emphysema (11%).[10] This report led to widespread acceptance of the concept of permissive hypercapnea and controlled hypoventilation in the management of acute asthma exacerbation.[11] Subsequent reports suggest that P_{peak} and P_{plat} are not adequate indicators of pulmonary hyperinflation,[12] and recommend that expiratory volumes be measured in these patients.[13] This latter technique has not gained widespread acceptance.

In sharp contrast, a retrospective study described a series of 18 asthmatic patients ventilated using a conventional approach with rapid correction of Pao_2 and $PaCo_2$ regardless of the airway pressures required. That study demonstrated no mortality attributable to mechanical ventilation. Complications included transient hypotension (35%) and pneumomediastinum/subcutaneous emphysema (5%).

These complication rates are comparable to those reported with use of controlled hypercapnea

■ CONTROLLING INTRINSIC PEEP

Maneuvers directed at elimination of $PEEP_I$ have in common the effect of decreasing inspiratory time, therefore providing more expiratory time. Decreasing RR, Vt and increasing IFR effectively accomplish this goal. Often, this cannot be achieved without sedation, sometimes requiring the addition of pharmacologic paralysis.

■ ENHANCING PATIENT VENTILATOR SYNCHRONY

Some of the commonly under-recognized problems that arise in the support of the critically ill patient fall into the category of patient/ventilator dysynchrony. These situations can markedly increase the WOB, leading to increased CO_2 and lactic acid production, with both respiratory and metabolic acidosis.

■ Difficulty Triggering the Ventilator

In order to trigger a ventilator, a patient must cause either a drop in pressure or increase in airflow at the proximal airway, depending upon the type of ventilator in use. The magnitude of change required to trigger the ventilator is adjusted by setting the sensitivity, usually in the range of –1 to –2 cm H_2O below the level of $PEEP_E$. Difficulty in triggering the ventilator is often difficult to detect. When it becomes obvious by physical examination that the patient is using the accessory muscles of respiration to trigger the ventilator, the problem may be severe. The condition can be detected earlier by inspecting the pressure-volume time curve on the ventilator display, if available. A large negative deflection at the beginning of inhalation suggests that the ventilator sensitivity needs to be increased.

More commonly, high $PEEP_i$ is the cause. The patient must first lower the intrathoracic pressure enough to overcome $PEEP_i$ before the airway pressure can drop to the threshold sensitivity. The solution to this problem is to raise $PEEP_e$ to a level $^1/_2$ to $^3/_4$ of $PEEP_i$, allowing the patient to perform less work to trigger inhalation. This process mandates frequent reassessment of $PEEP_I$ and manipulation of the ventilator during this dynamic period.

■ Autocycling

Autocycling refers to a phenomenon when the ventilator set in AC mode begins to rapidly trigger without the patient initiating respiration. The cause is usually small vacillations in airway pressure that the ventilator "interprets" as patient efforts. Tremors, shivering, voluntary motion, convulsions, and crying all are examples of potential causes. Autocycling should prompt immediate disconnection from the ventilator circuit and ventilation by bag-valve device until the problem is resolved.

■ Rapid Breathing

When attempting to ventilate a patient with OAD, the goal is to eliminate $PEEP_i$. Permissive hypercapnea is best achieved at low respiratory rates, but at the same time hypercapnea leads to increased respiratory drive. This can be typically quelled using a combination of sedation with benzodiazepines and analgesia using opiates. Neuromuscular blockade should be considered a last resort undertaken only after careful consideration of the risk of prolonged paralysis and potential development of neuropathy in critical illness.

■ Overbreathing the Ventilator

Patients who are receiving low Vt ventilation for ARDS or for OAD develop hypercapnea and increased respiratory drive. Overbreathing the ventilator refers to the patient's effort to draw a higher Vt than is set. This can be detected by observing the exhaled Vt, or by finding a negative deflection at the end of inhalation on the pressure-volume time plot. As with controlling rapid breathing, the solution is sedation and analgesia.

■ Straining over the Ventilator

Straining over the ventilator indicates that the patient is attempting to inhale at a flow rate in excess of the set IFR. When it is obvious by examination that the patient is actively inhaling, the problem may be severe. On the pressure-volume time plot, the rise in pressure during inhalation will be concave, rather that convex. Potential solutions are to raise the IFR, to switch modes to pressure support ventilation, or to use sedation and analgesia.

■ Coughing

Coughing is a common problem, arising from increased secretions, airway foreign body (endotracheal tube [ETT]), or the underlying pulmonary disease process. Coughing can lead to autocycling, poor patient comfort, ET tube dislodgment, and rarely airway injury. Placement of the ET tube above the carina should be confirmed. Suctioning and provision of warmed, humidified air is often helpful. If these simple measures fail to provide relief, then aerosolized lidocaine or suppression with opiates may increase patient comfort.

■ EQUIPMENT FAILURE

Whenever a patient decompensates while receiving mechanical ventilation, consideration should be given to equipment failure as the cause. Interruption of oxygen supply, accidentally rotated knobs, disconnected ventilator circuitry, and obstructed tubes are all potential culprits. Immediate action should include disconnection from the ventilator and bag ventilation with 100% O_2. The mnemonic made popular by the American Heart Association Pediatric Advanced Life Support Course is useful to recall the causes of unexpected decompensation: DOPE (*D*islodgment of the ETT, *O*bstruction of the tube, *P*neumothorax, and *E*quipment failure). Confirmation of ETT placement, suctioning via endotracheal catheter, auscultation, chest radiography, and equipment troubleshooting are necessary actions.

REFERENCES

1. McCaig LF, Ly N: National hospital ambulatory medical care survey: 2000 emergency department summary. Adv Data April 22, 2002.
2. Trends in hospital emergency department utilization: United States 1992-99. Vital and Health Statistics 2001 Nov (150) Revised.
3. Moore BB, Wagner R, Weiss KB. A community based study of near-fatal asthma. Ann Allergy Asthma Immunol 2001; 86(2):190-195.
4. Bower RG, Shanholtz CB, Fessler HE, et al: Prospective, randomized, controlled clinical trial comparing traditional versus reduced tidal volume ventilation in acute respiratory distress syndrome patients. Crit Care Med 1999; 27:1492-1498.
5. Stewart TE, Meade MO, Cook DJ, et al: Evaluation of a ventilation strategy to prevent barotrauma in patients at high risk for acute respiratory distress syndrome. N Engl J Med 1998;338:355-361.
6. Brochard L, Roudot-Thoraval F, Roupie E, et al: Tidal volume reduction for prevention of ventilator-induced lung injury in acute respiratory distress syndrome. Am J Respir Crit Care Med 1998;158:1831-1838.
7. Amato MBP, Barbas CSV, Medeiros DM, et al: Effect of a protective ventilation strategy on mortality in the acute respiratory distress syndrome. N Engl J Med 1998;338: 347-354.
8. Amato MBP, Barbas CSV, Medeiros DM, et al: Beneficial effects of the "open lung approach" with low distending pressures in acute respiratory distress syndrome. Am J Respir Crit Care Med 1995;152:1835-1846.
9. The Acute Respiratory Distress Syndrome Network Authors: Ventilation with lower tidal volumes as compared with traditional tidal volumes for acute lung injury and the acute respiratory distress syndrome. N Engl J Med 2000;342:1301-1308.
10. Darioli R, Perre C: Mechanical controlled hypoventilation in status asthmaticus. Am Rev Respir Dis 1984;129: 385-387.
11. Slutsky AS: Mechanical ventilation. American College of Physicians' Consensus Conference. Chest 1993;104: 1833-1859.
12. Williams TJ, Tuxen DV, Scheinkestel CD, et al: Risk factors for morbidity in mechanically ventilated patients with acute severe asthma. Am Rev Respir Dis 1992;146: 607-615.
13. Tuxen DV, Williams TJ, Scheinkestel CD, et al: Use of a measurement of pulmonary hyperinflation to control the level of mechanical ventilation in patients with acute severe asthma. Am Rev Respir Dis 1992;146;1136-1142.

Chapter **4**

Circulatory Assessment and Support

Michael E. Winters

KEY POINTS

Circulatory dysfunction can occur at three levels—the central circulation, the peripheral circulation, and the microcirculation—sometimes with subtle clinical findings.

The initial history and physical examination should focus on detecting signs of hypoperfusion.

Circulatory support is aimed at restoring adequate oxygen delivery.

Endpoints of circulatory resuscitation include clinical signs, mean arterial blood pressure, serum lactate level, central venous pressure, and central venous oxygenation.

Scope

The circulatory system is a complex vascular network that stretches more than 60,000 miles and circulates an average of 8000 liters of blood each day. When circulatory dysfunction occurs, oxygen delivery is impaired. Impaired oxygen delivery leads to progressive cellular dysfunction, which, if not identified and treated, results in organ failure and patient death. In addition to a focused history and physical examination, the EP utilizes a number of invasive and noninvasive modalities to assess and support the circulatory system that are discussed in this chapter.

■ PATHOPHYSIOLOGY

Normal organ function depends on adequate perfusion and oxygen delivery. Although calculation of oxygen delivery requires a complex formula, it is primarily determined by arterial oxygen content and cardiac output. Cardiac output is governed by heart rate, contractility, and loading conditions, whereas arterial oxygen content is a function of the hemoglobin concentration and arterial oxygen saturation. Any process that adversely affects cardiac output and/or arterial oxygen saturation can decrease oxygen delivery and result in circulatory dysfunction.

Abnormalities in heart rate and rhythm alter cardiac output and impair oxygen delivery. Depending on the clinical situation, bradyarrhythmias can cause decreased perfusion and are the result of structural cardiac abnormalities, medication effects, hypoxia, or other metabolic stimuli. Similarly, tachyarrhythmias can decrease ventricular filling and lead to poor cardiac output. Tachyarrhythmias may be due to underlying cardiac disease, medications, or environmental stimuli.

Alterations in ventricular loading can negatively affect cardiac output. Most important is a decrease in intravascular volume. In the normal heart, intravascular volume (preload) is the principal force that governs the strength of ventricular contraction.[1] Intravascular volume depletion can result from loss of plasma, water, or red blood cells. Similarly, marked increases in arteriolar tone (afterload) can impede cardiac output, as in the case of severe hypertension.

In addition to abnormalities affecting cardiac output, circulatory dysfunction can occur with alterations in regional or microcirculatory blood flow. Disorders that affect the arteriolar tone between organs, such as sepsis, result in maldistribution of blood flow and the mismatching of oxygen delivery with oxygen demand. Capillary obstruction, or endothelial impairment, interrupts intraorgan oxygen delivery, potentially resulting in organ failure.

Finally, any process that qualitatively or quantitatively affects hemoglobin or arterial oxygen saturation also impairs oxygen delivery, resulting in circulatory dysfunction.

Anatomy

Figure 4-1 illustrates the anatomy of the circulatory system.

Presenting Signs and Symptoms

Circulatory insufficiency can manifest as a myriad of clinical presentations. Signs and symptoms primarily reflect organ dysfunction secondary to hypoperfu-

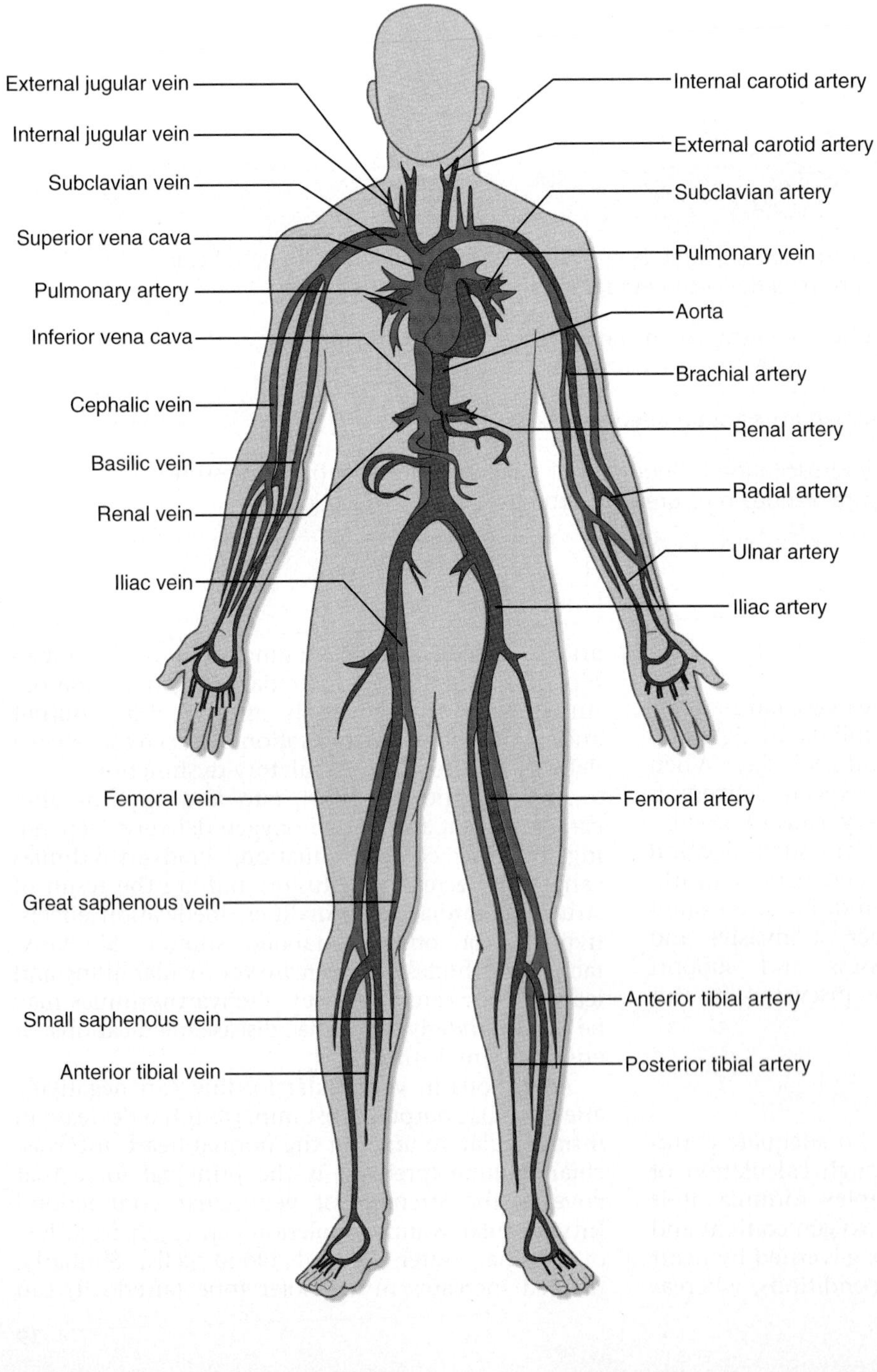
External jugular vein
Internal jugular vein
Subclavian vein
Superior vena cava
Pulmonary artery
Inferior vena cava
Cephalic vein
Basilic vein
Renal vein
Iliac vein
Femoral vein
Great saphenous vein
Small saphenous vein
Anterior tibial vein
Internal carotid artery
External carotid artery
Subclavian artery
Pulmonary vein
Aorta
Brachial artery
Renal artery
Radial artery
Ulnar artery
Iliac artery
Femoral artery
Anterior tibial artery
Posterior tibial artery

FIGURE 4-1 Anatomy of the circulatory system.

sion and decreased oxygen delivery. Classic signs of circulatory dysfunction are reduced blood pressure, abnormal heart rate, tachypnea, hypoxia, mottled extremities, and decreased urine output. The most dramatic classic clinical presentation is the patient in cardiac arrest with complete circulatory failure. Unfortunately, many ED patients with circulatory dysfunction present with vague, nonspecific symptoms. Common *nonspecific* symptoms of circulatory insufficiency are fatigue, malaise, weakness, lightheadedness, dizziness, altered mental status, diaphoresis, dyspnea, and syncope. Circulatory dysfunction should be considered in every patient presenting with vague, undifferentiated symptoms.

Initial Circulatory Assessment

An initial circulatory assessment must be performed on every ED patient within the first several minutes of presentation. This assessment consists of a review of triage vital signs, a focused history, and a physical examination. Emergency ultrasonography should be incorporated into the initial assessment for any patient presenting with profound circulatory dysfunction. The goal of the initial circulatory assessment is to detect signs of organ hypoperfusion and identify any immediate life-threatening circulatory disorders. Life-threatening disorders that require rapid diagnosis and treatment include pulmonary embolism, acute myocardial infarction, cardiac tamponade, tension pneumothorax, aortic dissection, and ruptured abdominal aortic aneurysm.

■ VITAL SIGNS

For nearly all ED patients, circulatory assessment begins with the noninvasive measurement of vital signs. Although blood pressure and heart rate are central to the initial assessment, it is important to also note the respiratory rate and oxygen saturation. Any abnormality in respiratory rate or oxygen saturation may affect arterial oxygen saturation and thus may result in impaired oxygen delivery. Noninvasive vital sign measurements correlate poorly with organ perfusion in critically ill patients but serve as an important component of the initial ED assessment of the circulatory system.[2]

■ Blood Pressure

Blood pressure, the "driving force" for organ perfusion, is determined by cardiac output and arterial tone.[1] It is important to understand that no value for blood pressure is considered normal for every patient. Normal blood pressure values do not always indicate sufficient oxygen delivery. Blood pressure values should be interpreted in the context of the patient's clinical presentation and medical history as well as the treatment received.

Blood pressure is one of the most common measurements in all of clinical medicine, yet it is often incorrectly measured.[3] In the ED, blood pressure is initially obtained in triage with the use of automated blood pressure devices. Automated devices utilize the oscillometric method of blood pressure determination. It is important to note that these devices can be adversely affected by ambient noise and cuff position. In addition, automated devices typically overestimate the true arterial blood pressure in low-flow states. These limitations, combined with the triage environment, often result in inaccurate measurements of blood pressure. Triage blood pressure values have been shown to be an unreliable indicator of true blood pressure. The blood pressure measurement should be repeated at the bedside in any patient demonstrating evidence of circulatory insufficiency.

The auscultatory method has long been considered the gold standard for noninvasive blood pressure measurements. It determines systolic and diastolic pressures on the basis of the detection of Korotkoff sounds. The ideal location is the upper arm; the procedure is as follows:

1. Remove all clothing from the arm and place the blood pressure cuff so that the middle of the cuff is approximately at the level of the right atrium. The lower edge of the cuff should be 2 to 3 centimeters above the antecubital fossa to allow easy palpation and auscultation of the brachial artery.
2. Locate the radial artery. Inflate the blood pressure cuff to approximately 30 mm Hg above the point at which the radial arterial pulse disappears.
3. Place the bell of the stethoscope over the brachial artery, and deflate the cuff at a rate of 2 to 3 mm Hg per second. The appearance of faint, repetitive sounds for at least two consecutive beats is phase I of the Korotkoff sounds. Phase I is the systolic blood pressure. The point at which all sounds disappear is phase V, the diastolic blood pressure.

Always measure bilateral blood pressures during the initial circulatory examination. A difference of greater than 10 mm Hg is significant and may indicate an aortic emergency. Unfortunately, up to 20% of individuals have significant blood pressure differences between their arms.[4] Nevertheless, an aortic emergency must be ruled out in any patient with evidence of circulatory insufficiency and blood pressure discrepancies. Although considered the gold standard, the auscultatory method has several pitfalls. Box 4-1 lists errors commonly made during measurement of blood pressure via the auscultatory method.

■ Heart Rate

Heart rate is an integral component of cardiac output. Circulatory function can be impaired by any tachycardia or bradycardia. As with blood pressure, triage measurements of heart rate can be inaccurate and unreliable. Therefore, the heart rate measurement

BOX 4-1

Pitfalls in Blood Pressure Measurement

Failure to Use Appropriately Sized Blood Pressure Cuff

Falsely elevated blood pressure if cuff too small.

Bladder should be at least 80% the length and 40% the width of the upper arm.

Use thigh cuff if necessary.

Failure to Recognize the Auscultatory Gap

Seen in elderly hypertensive patients with wide pulse pressure.

Results in overestimation of diastolic pressure.

Auscultation should be continued until the cuff is fully deflated.

Hypotensive States

Auscultatory method overestimates blood pressure in low-flow states.

Do not use auscultatory method to monitor unstable patients.

should be repeated in every patient upon initial examination. In addition to the rate, any irregularities in rhythm should be noted. Depending on the etiology, arrhythmias can severely compromise circulatory function and organ perfusion. Studies now indicate that heart rate variability may constitute an early indication of potential circulatory dysfunction.[5] At present, methods to determine heart rate variability remain investigational and require additional research before clinical application.

■ Orthostatic Blood Pressure

Intravascular volume depletion can impair oxygen delivery by decreasing venous return and cardiac output. Symptoms of volume depletion are attributable to reduced cerebral blood flow and include weakness, lightheadedness, unsteadiness, impaired cognition, tremulousness, and syncope. Orthostatic blood pressure measurements can occasionally aid the EP in detecting otherwise unsuspected intravascular volume depletion. Most important, orthostatic blood pressure measurements must be integrated with specific clinical findings. They are not routinely performed because they have significant limitations.

An orthostatic blood pressure response is defined as a reduction in systolic blood pressure of at least 20 mm Hg or in diastolic blood pressure of at least 10 mm Hg within 3 minutes of standing in the patient with symptoms of volume depletion.[6] Obtain orthostatic blood pressure measurements with the patient in the supine and standing positions. For patients who are unable to stand or markedly unsteady, a sitting position may be used. Wait at least 2 minutes before performing a standing blood pressure measurement, because nearly all patients have a brief orthostatic response immediately upon standing. Always measure heart rate with orthostatic blood pressures. In normal patients, heart rate increases anywhere from 5 to 12 beats/min. Increases in heart rate greater than 20 beats/min are abnormal and indicate significant volume depletion.

There are several limitations to orthostatic blood pressure measurements. Numerous conditions in addition to volume depletion impair the postural hemodynamic response and result in orthostatic hypotension. Most notable are the effects of aging and medications. Up to 30% of elderly patients demonstrate an orthostatic response in the absence of volume depletion.[7] In addition, many elderly patients take medications that alter the postural response to changes in position. Classes of medications that can cause orthostatic hypotension are antiadrenergics, antidepressants, antihypertensives, neuroleptics, anticholinergics, and antiparkinsonian drugs. Also, any disorder that causes primary or secondary autonomic dysfunction can lead to orthostatic hypotension.

■ Pulse Pressure

There is increasing evidence that abnormal pulse pressure—the difference between systolic and diastolic blood pressures—is an independent risk factor for cardiovascular morbidity and mortality. To date, studies have primarily examined outpatients with established hypertension. Nevertheless, it is important to determine pulse pressure in the initial circulatory assessment of the ED patient. Often, acute disorders that alter circulatory function manifest as abnormalities in pulse pressure. A narrow pulse pressure indicates reduced stroke volume and thus cardiac output. Life-threatening conditions that result in a narrow pulse pressure include tension pneumothorax, cardiac tamponade, pulmonary embolism, acute myocardial infarction causing cardiogenic shock, and severe volume depletion. A widened pulse pressure results from any process that lowers systemic vascular resistance. Diseases that can manifest as widened pulse pressure include sepsis, anaphylaxis, adrenal insufficiency, and neurogenic shock.

■ HISTORY

A focused history is an essential component of the initial circulatory assessment. Key elements are the history of present illness, past medical history, medications, family history, and social history. With respect to the history of present illness, determine the onset and duration of symptoms, the context in which symptoms developed, any associated symptoms, and any aggravating or alleviating factors. Important associated symptoms include chest pain, dyspnea, palpitations, syncope, and altered mental status. Review the past medical history with attention to any disorder that may impair cardiac output or arterial oxygen content.

Medications can result in a wide array of circulatory abnormalities, through either direct effects or side effects. Two important classes of medications are antiarrhythmic agents and antihypertensive agents. It is crucial to note whether the patient is taking a beta-blocker or calcium channel blocker, either of which can alter the compensatory response to circulatory insufficiency. Always interpret vital signs in the context of the medical history and medication regimen.

Additional key components of the history are the family and social histories. Directly question the patient about a family history of sudden death, premature coronary artery disease, venous thromboembolism, and connective tissue disorders such as Marfan's syndrome. Similarly, question patients about the use of illicit substances known to have circulatory effects, namely cocaine.

■ PHYSICAL EXAMINATION

Physical examination of the circulatory system begins with the general appearance. Observe patient positioning, mental status, skin color, and respiratory pattern. Suspect circulatory abnormalities in any patient who is restless, diaphoretic, delirious, pale, mottled, or tachypneic. In addition, note any distinct clinical features that imply the presence of an underlying condition. Table 4-1 lists the characteristic features of several disorders that can affect the circulatory system.

Examine the head and neck for abnormalities that may suggest circulatory disease. Facial edema denotes impaired venous return and can be due to conditions such as superior vena cava thrombosis and constrictive pericarditis. Examination of the jugular venous pulse provides important information about central venous pressure and the dynamics of the right side of the heart.[8] Place the patient in a 45-degree recumbent position and shine a light tangentially across the neck. The right side is preferred because of its anatomic alignment with the superior vena cava and right atrium. Beginning at the sternal notch, measure the height (in centimeters) of pulsations in the internal jugular vein. Pulsations more than 4 centimeters above the sternal notch are abnormal and are a sign of elevated central venous pressure.[8] Figure 4-2 illustrates jugular venous distention in a young woman with a pericardial effusion.

The cardiopulmonary examination is a quintessential component of circulatory assessment. Begin

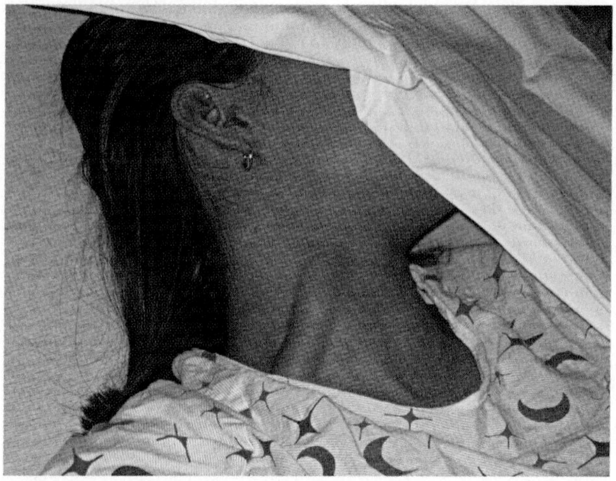

FIGURE 4-2 An example of jugular venous distention in a young woman with a pericardial effusion.

Table 4-1 CHARACTERISTIC APPEARANCE OF CONDITIONS THAT AFFECT THE CIRCULATORY SYSTEM

Condition	Clinical Appearance	Potential Circulatory Implications
Marfan's syndrome	Arachnodactyly Arm span greater than height Longer pubis-to-foot length than pubis-to-head length	Aortic dissection
Osteogenesis imperfecta	Blue sclera	Aortic dissection Aortic aneurysm Aortic valve insufficiency Mitral valve prolapse
Hyperthyroidism	Exophthalmos	Congestive heart failure
Hypothyroidism	Expressionless face Periorbital edema Loss of the lateral third of the eyebrows Dry, sparse hair	Congestive heart failure Pericardial effusion
Hemochromatosis	Bronze pigmentation of skin Loss of axillary and pubic hair	Cardiomyopathy
Turner's syndrome	Short stature Webbed neck "Shield" chest Medial deviation of the extended forearm	Aortic coarctation
Aortic insufficiency	Bobbing of the head with each heartbeat Systolic flushing of the nail beds	—

by observing the rate, depth, and effort of respirations. Tachypnea, accompanied by shallow respirations or accessory muscle use, indicates impending respiratory failure. Auscultate the lungs for asymmetrical breath sounds, rhonchi, rales, and wheezing. Recall that virtually any pulmonary process can adversely affect arterial oxygen content and impair oxygen delivery. Auscultate the heart over the right and left upper sternal edges, the lower left sternal edge, and the cardiac apex. Determine the rate and listen for rhythm irregularities, intensity of heart sounds, murmurs, gallop rhythms, and pericardial rubs. Although difficult in the environment of the ED, attempt to determine whether cardiac murmurs are systolic or diastolic, which may provide valuable information in the patient with acute cardiopulmonary dysfunction. Gallop rhythms are low-frequency sounds so are heard best with the bell of the stethoscope.

Examination of the extremities must be performed in the initial circulatory assessment. Note the color and temperature. Signs of poor perfusion include cold, pale, clammy, mottled skin associated with a delayed capillary refill. Normal capillary refill time is less than 2 seconds. Inspect for symmetrical, or asymmetrical, edema and clubbing of the fingers and toes. Finally, palpate the carotid, radial, femoral, dorsalis pedis, and posterior tibial pulses for rate, amplitude, and regularity.

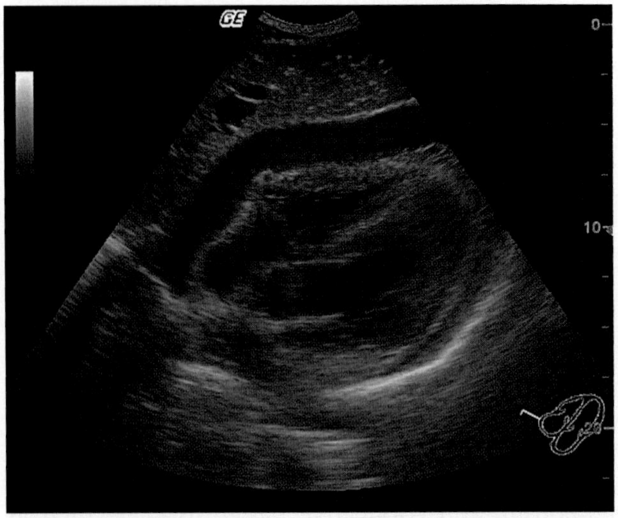

FIGURE 4-3 With bedside ultrasonography, the EP can reliably detect an abdominal aortic aneurysm, hemoperitoneum, or, as shown, pericardial effusion.

■ EMERGENCY ULTRASONOGRAPHY

Ultrasonography has rapidly become an integral component of the ED evaluation and treatment of the circulatory system. With bedside ultrasonography, the EP can reliably detect an abdominal aortic aneurysm, hemoperitoneum, pericardial effusion (Fig. 4-3), or electromechanical dissociation and can approximate central venous pressure.[9,10] In addition, ultrasonography is invaluable in guiding emergency procedures such as intravenous access, pericardiocentesis, and transvenous cardiac pacing.[11] Although assessment of left ventricular ejection is currently outside the scope of emergency ultrasonography, there is now evidence that with additional training, EPs can accurately perform this assessment. Use ultrasonography during the initial assessment of any patient presenting with signs and symptoms of circulatory collapse. Figure 4-4 illustrates proper ultrasonography probe positioning for the subxiphoid, long-axis, and short-axis views in emergency cardiac ultrasonography.

Procedures

Procedures pertinent to circulatory assessment and support center on vascular access and invasive circulatory monitoring. Rapid attainment of intravenous access is required in any patient exhibiting signs and symptoms of hypoperfusion. Invasive circulatory monitoring is used to ensure adequate tissue perfusion and oxygen delivery. Invasive monitoring is indicated in patients who continue to exhibit signs of hypoperfusion despite initial resuscitative measures. Common invasive modalities are arterial blood pressure monitoring, central venous pressure monitoring, and pulmonary artery catheterization. A number of new monitoring modalities have now been developed to further evaluate the adequacy of circulation. New modalities include the esophageal Doppler ultrasound analysis, pulse contour analysis, thoracic bioimpedance, near-infrared retinal spectroscopy, transcutaneous tissue oxygen monitors, central venous oxygen saturation monitoring, and sublingual capnometry.

■ INTRAVENOUS ACCESS

Intravenous access must be established in any patient with signs or symptoms of hypoperfusion. It can be obtained with peripheral or central venous catheters. Despite the physician's desire to perform central venous catheterization during the initial resuscitation, peripheral venous cannulation is preferred. The reader should recall Poiseuille's law: The rate at which intravenous fluids can be infused depends on the radius and length of the catheter. Greater volume can be infused over a shorter time via short peripheral catheters than with a central venous line. Peripheral catheters should be 18 gauge or larger. The external jugular veins and the veins of the antecubital fossa provide rapid and safe access for peripheral venous cannulation.

Central venous catheterization has become a common bedside procedure in emergency medicine. In the United States, more than 5 million central venous catheters are placed each year. Table 4-2 and Boxes 4-2 and 4-3 list indications, contraindications, complications, and tips for central venous access. Figure 4-5 illustrates proper ultrasonography probe

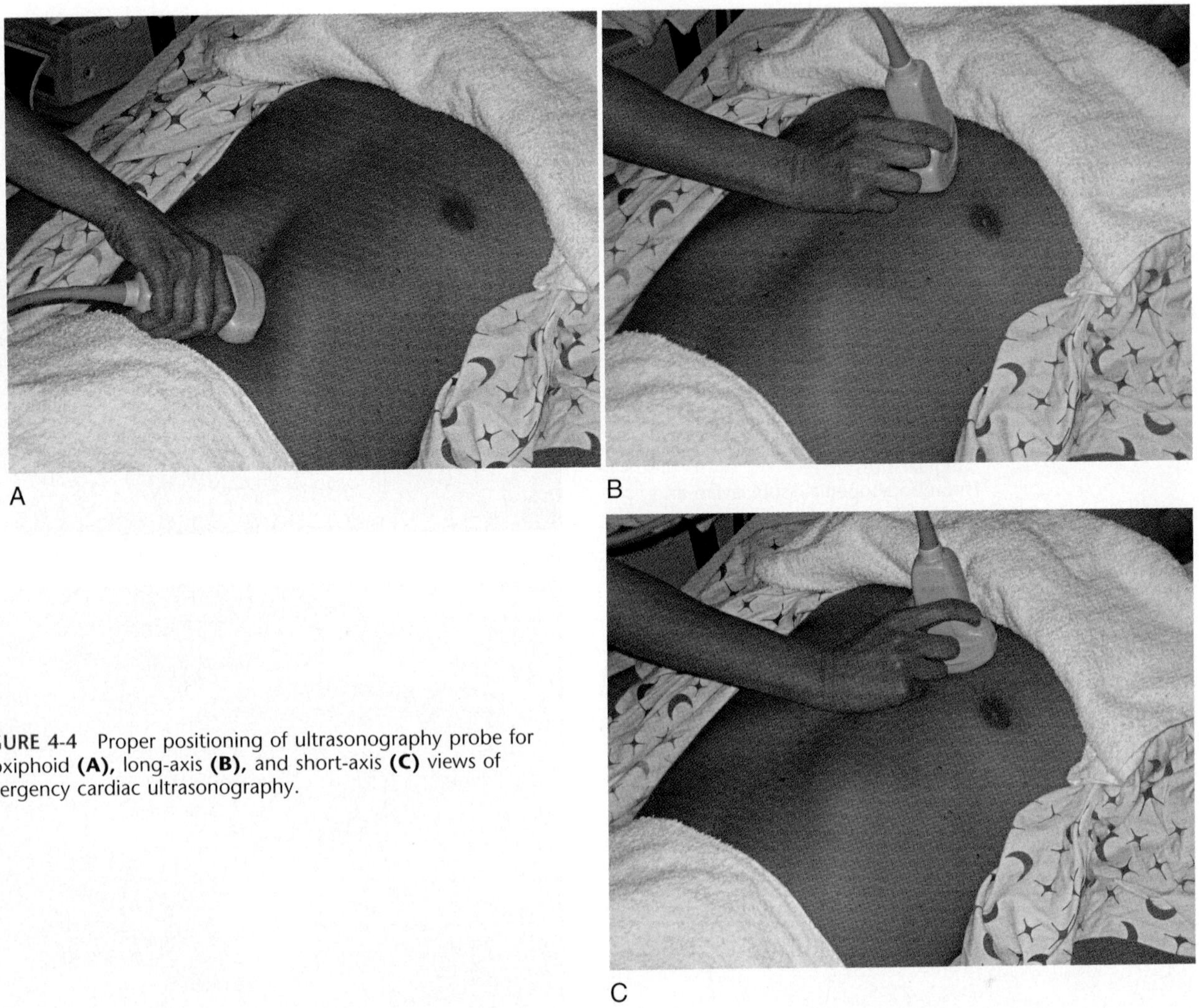
A
B
C

FIGURE 4-4 Proper positioning of ultrasonography probe for subxiphoid **(A)**, long-axis **(B)**, and short-axis **(C)** views of emergency cardiac ultrasonography.

BOX 4-2

Complications of Central Venous Catheterization

Mechanical—5% to 19%:

- Arterial puncture
- Arteriovenous fistula
- Pseudoaneurysm
- Atrial arrhythmias
- Ventricular arrhythmias
- Hematoma
- Catheter malposition
- Pneumothorax (subclavian, internal jugular)
- Embolism (air, thrombus, guidewire)
- Cardiac perforation producing tamponade
- Bladder aspiration (femoral)

Infection—5% to 26%:

- Cutaneous infection
- Catheter-related blood stream infection

Thrombosis—2% to 26%

BOX 4-3

Tips for Decreasing Rate of Complications in Central Venous Catheterization

Use maximal sterile barrier precautions—cap, mask, gown, gloves, and sterile drapes.

Use chlorhexidine-based solutions if available.

Do not allow inexperienced operators (<50 catheterizations) more than three attempts.

Whenever possible, place a *subclavian* central venous catheter—associated with lowest rate of mechanical, infectious, and thrombotic complications.

Use ultrasonographic guidance routinely for internal jugular venous catheterizations.

Do not use topical antibiotic ointments; their use has not been shown to decrease the risk of catheter-related infections.

Table 4-2 INDICATIONS FOR AND CONTRAINDICATIONS TO CENTRAL LINE PLACEMENT

Indications	Failed peripheral venous access Cardiopulmonary arrest Central venous pressure monitoring Transvenous pacemaker insertion Emergency hemodialysis Administration of medications known to irritate peripheral veins
Contraindications	
Absolute	None
Relative	Cutaneous infection at the site of puncture Existing venous thrombosis Existing arteriovenous fistula Coagulopathy—subclavian and internal jugular sites Thrombocytopenia—subclavian and internal jugular sites

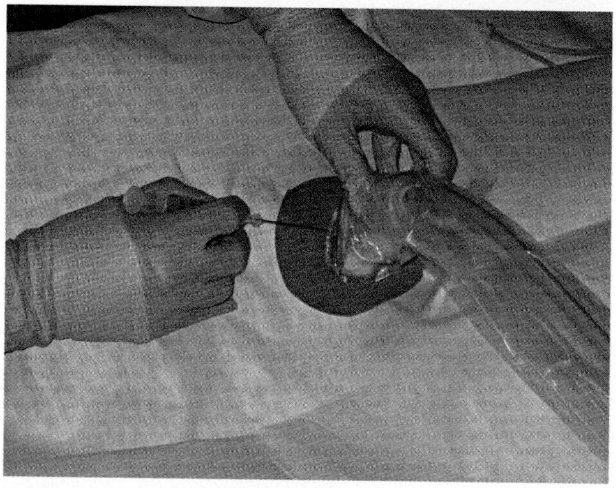

FIGURE 4-5 Proper positioning of ultrasonography probe for internal jugular vein catheterization.

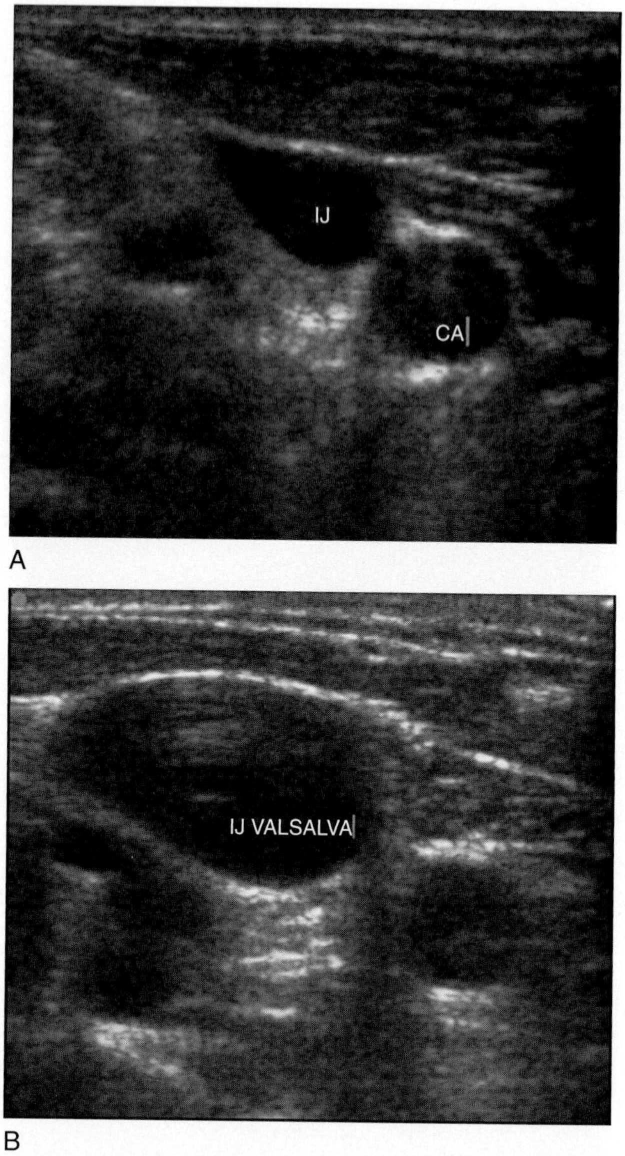
IJ
CA
A
IJ VALSALVA
B

FIGURE 4-6 Ultrasonographic appearance of the internal jugular vein (IJ) at baseline (**A**) and when the patient performs a Valsalva maneuver (**B**). CA, carotid artery.

positioning for use with internal jugular venous catheterization. Figure 4-6 shows the ultrasonographic appearance of the internal jugular vein at baseline; note the engorgement of the vein with the Valsalva maneuver (see Fig. 4-6B).

■ ARTERIAL BLOOD PRESSURE MONITORING

Invasive arterial blood pressure monitoring is required for patients with persistent circulatory dysfunction despite initial resuscitative measures. Primary indications for arterial line placement consist of continuous blood pressure monitoring and the need for frequent blood sampling. Although an arterial line can be placed into any artery, traditional sites are the radial and femoral arteries. Advantages to the radial arterial line include its peripheral position, easy compressibility in the event of unsuccessful cannulation, and the additional blood supply to the hand provided by the ulnar artery. Unfortunately, the radial pulse may not be palpated in markedly hypotensive patients.

Box 4-4 lists available sites and complications of arterial blood pressure monitoring. Figure 4-7 illustrates the proper patient positioning for radial artery cannulation.

■ CENTRAL VENOUS PRESSURE MONITORING

Central venous pressure (CVP) is the intravascular pressure in the central vena cava system, near the junction of the right atrium. Clinically, CVP is used as a marker of volume status and cardiac preload. Normal values for CVP range from 8 to 12 mm Hg. CVP can be estimated by examination of the internal jugular vein or measured invasively with a central venous catheter. Bedside determinations of CVP, however, have been shown to be inaccurate and

BOX 4-4

Sites of, Complications of, and Tips for Arterial Cannulation

Sites of Insertion

Radial artery (most common and preferred)
Femoral artery
Brachial artery
Axillary artery
Ulnar artery
Dorsalis pedis artery

Complications

Thrombosis with arterial occlusion
Hematoma
Infection (catheter-related blood stream infections)
Heparin-induced thrombocytopenia
Anemia (frequent blood sampling)

Tips

Avoid cannulation of the brachial artery, complications of which can be severe:

- Forearm ischemia
- Compartment syndrome
- Median nerve damage

Femoral arterial line has lower rate of catheter malfunction and greater longevity but higher risk of infection.

Wear sterile gown, gloves, and mask, and place a drape.

Give lidocaine without epinephrine for local anesthesia.

Flush line frequently to maintain patency and prevent thrombosis.

unreliable.[12] Direct measurements, through a subclavian or internal jugular vein catheter, provide more reliable results. CVP measurements can be obtained via a femoral central venous catheter; however, values typically differ by 0.5 to 3 mm Hg from those obtained from the superior vena cava.

Several potential pitfalls of the interpretation of CVP limit its overall clinical utility. CVP is affected by venous compliance, arrhythmias, tricuspid valve disease, and any process that alters intrathoracic pressure, such as mechanical ventilation. In addition, CVP depends on the reference point selected for measurement. As a result, normal, or elevated, CVP cannot be taken to indicate adequate circulatory volume and cardiac preload. For the EP, the clinical utility of CVP monitoring lies in the patient with low values. The patient with low CVP readings who is given a fluid challenge and shows an increase in CVP of at least 2 mm Hg has intravascular volume depletion. Such a patient requires additional fluid administration to optimize preload and cardiac output.

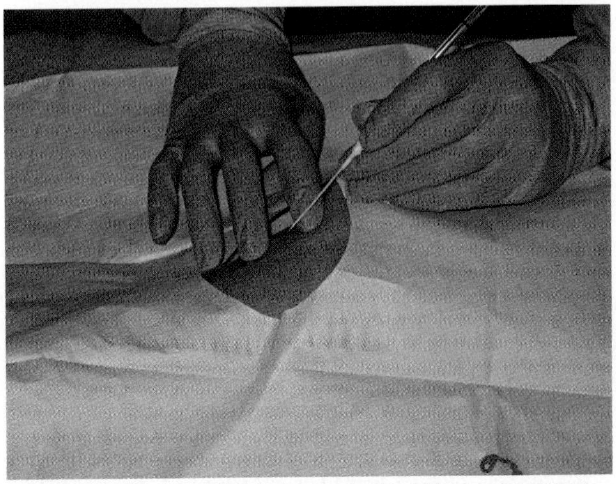

FIGURE 4-7 Proper patient positioning for radial artery cannulation.

■ PULMONARY ARTERY CATHETERIZATION

First described by Swan and colleagues in the early 1970s, pulmonary artery catheterization is considered the gold standard for circulatory monitoring in the critically ill. Circulatory measurements obtained with the pulmonary artery catheter include cardiac output, right ventricular ejection fraction, mixed venous oxygen saturation, and intrapulmonary vascular pressures. From these measurements, oxygen delivery, oxygen consumption, systemic vascular resistance, and left ventricular stroke index can be calculated. With the ability to directly measure oxygen delivery, it would seem that the pulmonary artery catheter would be an invaluable tool for circulatory monitoring in the ED. Unfortunately, the use of the pulmonary artery catheter in such a setting remains controversial. At present, use of the pulmonary artery catheter has not been shown to improve patient morbidity or mortality.[13] In fact, there are studies showing that the use of a pulmonary artery catheter may be detrimental. Complications of insertion of a pulmonary artery catheter include pneumothorax, ventricular arrhythmias, ventricular perforation, and pulmonary artery rupture. Until further evidence is published, a pulmonary artery catheter should not be used in the ED for assessment and support of the circulatory system.

■ ADDITIONAL CIRCULATORY MONITORING MODALITIES

Additional circulatory monitoring modalities are based on the detection of global, or tissue, markers of hypoperfusion. Current ED methods to detect global hypoperfusion include central venous oxygen saturation and serum lactate values. Under normal circumstances, cells extract approximately 25% to 30% of oxygen from the circulation. Blood returning to the central circulation, therefore, has an oxygen saturation ranging from 70% to 75%. When the circulation fails to deliver adequate oxygen, cellular oxygen extraction is increased. This increase is reflected as a decrease in mixed venous oxygen saturation, measured via pulmonary artery catheter. Mixed venous oxygen saturation values less than 70% are associated with decreased perfusion and oxidative impairment of some vascular bed. Central venous oxygen saturation, measured intermittently or continuously via central venous catheter, has been shown to be a reliable surrogate for mixed venous oxygen saturation. Central venous oxygen saturation, as a global marker of hypoperfusion, was used in a landmark study that demonstrated significant improvement in mortality among ED patients with sepsis in whom that marker was used.[14] It is important to recognize that central venous oxygen saturation values should be obtained from either a subclavian or internal jugular central venous catheter.

Serum lactate values are also used as a global marker of hypoperfusion. With persistently impaired oxygen delivery, cells convert to anaerobic metabolism, resulting in the accumulation of lactic acid. A lactate level higher than 2 mmol/liter is considered an indicator of inadequate oxygenation. Despite numerous etiologies for abnormal lactate levels, the clinician should always regard impaired tissue perfusion as the primary cause in the ED patient. Finally, it is the trend in lactate values that is most useful. Serial lactate levels that are increasing portend a worse prognosis and indicate persistent circulatory dysfunction.

Tissue-specific monitors of hypoperfusion include gastric tonometry, sublingual capnometry, near-infrared spectroscopy, and tissue oxygen tension. These circulatory monitoring modalities detect hypoperfusion and impaired oxygen delivery of specific vascular beds. Although promising, these modalities are not currently utilized in the daily practice of emergency medicine and require further prospective investigation. Available noninvasive methods to measure cardiac output include the esophageal Doppler ultrasonography, impedance plethysmography, and pulse-contour analysis. As with tissue-specific monitors of hypoperfusion, noninvasive methods to measure cardiac output require further prospective analysis before their widespread clinical application.

Treatment

Treatment goals for circulatory support are based on restoring adequate oxygen delivery. Methods of restoration consist of improving arterial oxygen content, cardiac output, and peripheral perfusion pressure. General ED therapies are supplemental oxygen, intubation, intravenous fluids, vasopressor medications, inotropic agents, and mechanical support devices such as cardiac pacemakers. Regardless of the therapy chosen, it is important to recognize established endpoints of circulatory resuscitation. First and foremost, patients should exhibit clinical signs of improvement. Examples are improving mental status, increasing urine output, and normalization of vital signs. Additional endpoints of resuscitation are mean arterial blood pressure, serum lactate level, central venous pressure, and central venous oxygen saturation. Mean arterial pressure should be at least 65 mm Hg. Mean arterial pressure, which represents the true perfusion pressure, is superior to systolic blood pressure monitoring. There is no survival benefit to raising mean arterial pressures beyond 65 mm Hg. As discussed, serum lactate values should show a decreasing trend over serial measurements if there is an appropriate response to resuscitation. Persistently elevated lactate values indicate inadequate and incomplete circulatory resuscitation. For patients with a central venous catheter, CVP and central venous oxygen saturation can be followed. CVP should range from 8 to 12 mm Hg, whereas central venous oxygen saturation values should exceed 70%. Box 4-5 summarizes the goals of resuscitation.

■ GENERAL PRINCIPLES

Patients with circulatory dysfunction require rapid assessment that is performed simultaneously with treatment, as follows:

1. Immediately begin cardiac monitoring to determine the patient's heart rate and rhythm regularity.
2. Provide supplemental oxygen to improve arterial oxygen saturation.
3. Maintain a low threshold for intubation. The respiratory muscles are avid consumers of oxygen, thereby limiting oxygen delivery to other vital organs. Early intubation and paralysis of respiratory muscles may be

BOX 4-5

Goals of Resuscitation

Clinical Signs

Improved mental status
Improved capillary refill/skin perfusion

Vital Signs

Urine output 0.5-1.0 mL/kg/hr
Mean arterial pressure > 65 mm Hg
Heart rate < 100 beats/min
Respiratory rate < 20 breaths/min
Oxygen saturation > 95%
Central venous pressure 8-12 mm Hg
(12-15 mm Hg if patient is mechanically ventilated)

Serum Markers of Hypoperfusion

Normalization of serum lactate value
Central venous oxygen saturation > 70%

required in patients with ongoing circulatory compromise.
4. Rapidly establish peripheral intravenous access.
5. Perform an electrocardiogram and obtain a portable chest radiograph within the first several minutes to evaluate for acute myocardial infarction and pneumothorax.
6. Use ultrasonography early to look for myocardial dysfunction, pericardial effusion, hemoperitoneum, and abdominal aortic aneurysm in the patient with persistent hypotension.

■ INTRAVENOUS FLUIDS

Initially acute circulatory failure should be treated with intravenous fluids. In the absence of left ventricular failure, rapid fluid therapy is provided to improve preload and augment cardiac output. For patients without preexisting cardiopulmonary disease, a liter of fluid is infused over 10 minutes. Smaller volumes of fluid are used in patients with existing cardiac disease. Rates of fluid administration in patients with cardiac disease range from 250 to 500 milliliters over 15 minutes. Regardless of the volume chosen, patients are reassessed after every fluid bolus to determine whether additional treatment is needed. Recent studies have shown that there is no mortality benefit to the use of colloid fluids during the initial circulatory resuscitation.[15] Thus, an isotonic crystalloid solution is the first-line intravenous fluid. Fluid therapy is continued until the endpoints of resuscitation are achieved or the patient demonstrates pulmonary edema or evidence of right heart dysfunction. Depending on the etiology of circulatory dysfunction, patients may require several liters of intravenous fluid.

■ TRENDELENBURG POSITIONING

Hypotensive patients are often placed in the Trendelenburg position while resuscitative efforts, such as intravenous access and fluid administration, are initiated. The Trendelenburg position is traditionally thought to increase venous return, thereby augmenting cardiac output. Owing to the capacitance of the venous circulation, however, this assumption is incorrect. The Trendelenburg position does not promote venous return nor increase cardiac output. Hypotensive patients should *not* be put in the Trendelenburg position, which serves to only raise the risk of aspiration in patients with altered mental status.

■ VASOACTIVE THERAPY

Vasopressor agents are indicated when the mean arterial pressure remains below 65 mm Hg despite a fluid challenge of 20 to 40 mL/kg. Vasopressor agents help restore perfusion pressure and maintain cardiac output. These agents exert their effects through stimulation of alpha- and beta-adrenergic receptors. The degree to which these receptors are stimulated depends on the agent. Common vasopressor agents used in emergency medicine are norepinephrine, dopamine, and vasopressin. Less commonly used agents are phenylephrine, epinephrine, and milrinone. The hemodynamic responses to and dosage ranges of these agents are listed in Table 4-3. An important concept to understand is that a rise in blood pressure may not correlate with clinical improvement. Additional markers of hypoperfusion, such as serum lactate level and central venous oxygen saturation, must be considered in the overall circulatory assessment. To date, no available studies clearly support the superiority of one vasopressor agent. The choice of vasopressor agents depends on the acute disease process and underlying comorbidities.

Patients with poor cardiac contractility may require inotropic support. Inotropic agents increase cardiac contractility through stimulation of β_1 receptors, ultimately resulting in rises in intracellular calcium concentration. Although dobutamine is the prototypical inotropic agent, any vasopressor that stimulates β_1

Table 4-3 VASOPRESSOR AGENTS

Agent	Receptor Activation	Circulatory Effects	Dosage Range
Norepinephrine	α_1 (primary) β_1 (secondary)	Vasoconstriction ↑ Heart rate (HR) and contractility (small)	1-30 μg/kg/min
Dopamine	DA_1 β_1 (primary) α_1	Vasodilation ↑ HR and contractility Vasoconstriction	<5 μg/kg/min 5-10 μg/ kg/min 10-20 μg/kg/min
Vasopressin	V_1 (vascular) V_2 (renal) V_3 (pituitary)	Vasoconstriction Antidiuretic effects Adrenocorticotrophic hormone (ACTH) secretion	0.01-0.04 U/min
Epinephrine	α_1/α_2 β_1	Vasoconstriction ↑ HR and contractility	1-10 μg/min
Phenylephrine	α	Vasoconstriction	40-180 μg/kg/min
Dobutamine	β_1 β^2	↑ HR and contractility Vasodilation	2-20 μg/kg/min

Adapted from Holmes CL, Walley KR: The evaluation and management of shock. Clin Chest Med 2003;24:775-789.

receptors increases cardiac contractility. Dopamine, milrinone, and epinephrine are potent inotropic medications. It is important to recognize that dobutamine can also cause peripheral vasodilation in hypovolemic patients. An additional vasopressor medication, such as norepinephrine, should be used in hypotensive patients requiring dobutamine for inotropic support.

■ MECHANICAL CIRCULATORY SUPPORT

Support of the circulatory system may require cardiac pacing. Box 4-6 lists indications for temporary cardiac pacing. Cardiac pacing can be performed by either transcutaneous or transvenous routes. Transcutaneous pacing is noninvasive and the more common method of pacing used in the ED. Proper placement of pacer pads is crucial in this modality. The anterior pacer pad is placed close to the heart, typically the location of the V3 lead on an electrocardiogram; the posterior pad is placed between the spine and the inferior border of the left or right scapula. Once the pads are properly placed, the steps listed in Box 4-7 for initiation of transcutaneous pacing should be followed.

Transvenous pacers are placed through a central venous catheter. The right internal jugular vein and the left subclavian vein are the preferred sites of cannulation. Obtaining proper positioning in the right ventricle can be difficult. Ultrasonography should be used to guide placement of a transvenous pacer. If ultrasonography is not available, the V1 lead of an electrocardiograph machine should be attached to the cathode. Contact with the right ventricle is characterized by prominent ST segment elevation. The ventricular rate is set the same as for transcutaneous pacing. Note that when pacer output is adjusted, the pacing threshold for transvenous pacing is much less than that required for transcutaneous pacing, typically ranging between 1 and 2 mA. When the right ventricle is paced, the surface ECG should demonstrate a pacer spike followed by a QRS complex displaying a left bundle branch block pattern. Box 4-8 lists the complications of emergency transvenous pacing.

BOX 4-6

Indications for Temporary Cardiac Pacing

- Witnessed asystole
- Hemodynamically significant bradycardia
- Symptomatic second- or third-degree atrioventricular block
- Complete atrioventricular dissociation with a ventricular rate < 50 beats/min
- Termination of supraventricular or ventricular tachyarrhythmias

BOX 4-7

Steps and Tips for Transcutaneous Pacing

Step 1—Set the Rate

For bradyarrhythmias, set the rate between 60 and 75 beats/min.

For overdrive pacing, set the rate to exceed the rate of the tachyarrhythmia.

Step 2—Adjust the Output

Pacing threshold for transcutaneous pacing typically ranges from 20 to 140 mA.

Increase the output (mA) until 100% of beats are captured.

Capture is indicated by a spike on the electrocardiogram followed by a wide QRS complex.

Set the output 5 to 10 mA above the threshold value.

Step 3—Provide Analgesia

Tip

Patients with emphysema or pericardial effusion or who are mechanically ventilated require higher pacing threshold values.

BOX 4-8

Complications of Transvenous Pacing

- Arterial puncture
- Hematoma
- Pneumothorax
- Atrial and ventricular arrhythmias
- Myocardial perforation
- Diaphragmatic stimulation

Summary

Assessment of the circulatory system is central to the initial evaluation of every ED patient. Assessment begins with a focused history, physical examination, and noninvasive measurements of blood pressure and heart rate. For many ED patients, additional circulatory assessment and monitoring are not needed. However, patients with evidence of circulatory dysfunction require rapid evaluation and support as follows: Obtain peripheral venous access and administer isotonic crystalloid fluid boluses followed by frequent reassessment. Use ultrasonography early in the evaluation of patients with severe circulatory compromise to exclude pericardial effusion, hemoperitoneum, and abdominal aortic aneurysm. Insert an arterial line for continuous blood pressure monitoring in patients who remain hypotensive despite

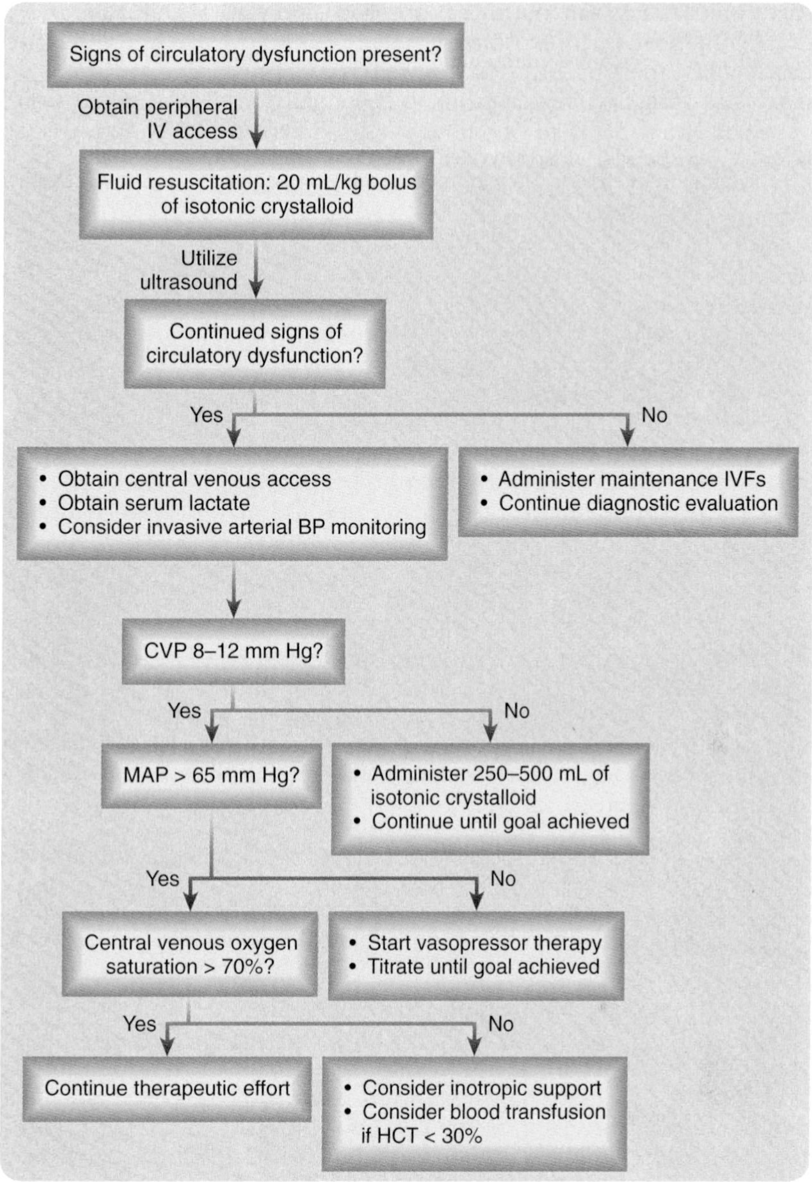
Signs of circulatory dysfunction present?
Obtain peripheral IV access
Fluid resuscitation: 20 mL/kg bolus of isotonic crystalloid
Utilize ultrasound
Continued signs of circulatory dysfunction?
Yes
No
• Obtain central venous access
• Obtain serum lactate
• Consider invasive arterial BP monitoring
• Administer maintenance IVFs
• Continue diagnostic evaluation
CVP 8–12 mm Hg?
Yes
No
MAP > 65 mm Hg?
• Administer 250–500 mL of isotonic crystalloid
• Continue until goal achieved
Yes
No
Central venous oxygen saturation > 70%?
• Start vasopressor therapy
• Titrate until goal achieved
Yes
No
Continue therapeutic effort
• Consider inotropic support
• Consider blood transfusion if HCT < 30%

FIGURE 4-8 A general algorithm for circulatory support. BP, blood pressure; CVP, central venous pressure; HCT, hematocrit; IV, intravenous; IVFs, intravenous fluids; MAP, mean arterial pressure.

initial intravenous fluids. Use global markers of hypoperfusion, such as serum lactate level and central venous oxygen saturation, to detect persistently impaired oxygen delivery. Begin a vasopressor agent for any patient with a mean arterial pressure less than 65 mm Hg despite an adequate fluid challenge. Figure 4-8 illustrates a general algorithm for circulatory support.

REFERENCES

1. Marino PL: The ICU Book, 2nd ed. Baltimore, Williams & Wilkins, 1998.
2. Rady MY, Rivers EP, Nowak RM: Resuscitation of the critically ill in the ED: Responses of blood pressure, heart rate, shock index, central venous oxygen saturation, and lactate. Am J Emerg Med 1996;14:218-225.
3. Pickering TG, Hall JE, Appel LJ, et al: Recommendations for blood pressure measurement in humans and experimental animals. Part 1: Blood pressure measurement in humans: A statement for professionals from the Subcommittee of Professional and Public Education of the American Heart Association Council on High Blood Pressure Research. Circulation 2005;111:697-716.
4. Rogers RL, McCormack R: Aortic disasters. Emerg Med Clin North Am 2004;22:887-908.
5. Barnaby D, Ferrick K, Kaplan DT, et al: Heart rate variability in emergency department patients with sepsis. Acad Emerg Med 2002;9:661-670.
6. Consensus statement on the definition of orthostatic hypotension, pure autonomic failure, and multiple system atrophy. The Consensus Committee of the American Autonomic Society and the American Academy of Neurology. Neurology 1996;46:1470.
7. Carlson JE: Assessment of orthostatic blood pressure: Measurement technique and clinical applications. South Med J 1999;92:167-173.
8. Zipes DP, Braunwald E: Braunwald's Heart Disease: A Textbook of Cardiovascular Medicine, 7th ed. Philadelphia, WB Saunders, 2005.
9. Tang A, Euerle B: Emergency department ultrasound and echocardiography. Emerg Med Clin North Am 2005;23:1179-1194.

10. Ciccone TJ, Grossman SA: Cardiac ultrasound. Emerg Med Clin North Am 2004;22:621-640.
11. Tibbles CD, Porcaro W: Procedural applications of ultrasound. Emerg Med Clin North Am 2004;22:797-815.
12. McGee SR: Physical examination of venous pressure: A critical review. Am Heart J 1998;136:10-18.
13. Shah MR, Hasselblad V, Stevenson LW, et al: Impact of the pulmonary artery catheter in critically ill patients: Meta-analysis of randomized clinical trials. JAMA 2005;294:1664-1670.
14. Rivers E, Nguyen B, Havstad S, et al: Early goal-directed therapy in the treatment of severe sepsis and septic shock. N Engl J Med 2001;345:1368-1377.
15. Roberts I, Alderson P, Bunn F, et al: Colloids versus crystalloids for fluid resuscitation in critically ill patients. Cochrane Database Syst Rev 2004(4):CD000567.

Chapter **5**

Ultrasound-Guided Vascular Access

Emily Baran

KEY POINTS

The static technique uses ultrasound imaging to localize the anatomy prior to and separate from the procedure.

The dynamic technique uses ultrasound for real-time assessment simultaneous with the procedure.

The transverse approach images vessels in their short axis, which is helpful for medial-to-lateral localization.

The longitudinal approach images vessels in their long axis, which is helpful for assessing slope and depth.

A 5- to 10-MHz or higher frequency linear vascular probe is used for this procedure.

The basic procedural steps include: (1) prepare equipment and position the patient, (2) identify and confirm the vein, and (3) cannulate the vein under ultrasound guidance.

Background

Emergency ultrasound is used to facilitate multiple procedures in the ED, such as pericardiocentesis, thoracentesis, arthrocentesis, abscess incision and drainage, lumbar puncture, and foreign body localization. One of the most important uses for procedural ultrasound is in facilitating vascular access for both central and peripheral veins. Ultrasound-guided vascular access has been shown to improve patient safety by reducing the number of attempts, the time to cannulation, and the number of complications.[1-5] In 2001, the Agency for Healthcare Research and Quality listed ultrasound-guided establishment of central venous lines as one of the top practices that should be implemented to improve patient care.[6]

Ultrasound for central venous access is most useful for internal jugular and femoral vein cannulation but can also be used for the subclavian/axillary vein. Ultrasound for peripheral venous access primarily targets the basilic, brachial, and cephalic veins in the arm or the external jugular vein in the neck. Additionally, ultrasound can help guide arterial puncture and insertion of arterial lines.

Technique

Ultrasound-guided procedures can be performed with either static or dynamic techniques. The static technique involves positioning the patient for the procedure, using ultrasound to confirm and localize

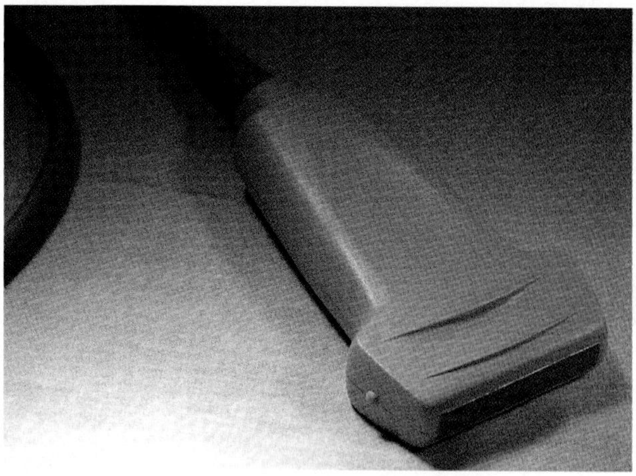

FIGURE 5-1 A 5- to 10-MHz linear vascular probe should be used.

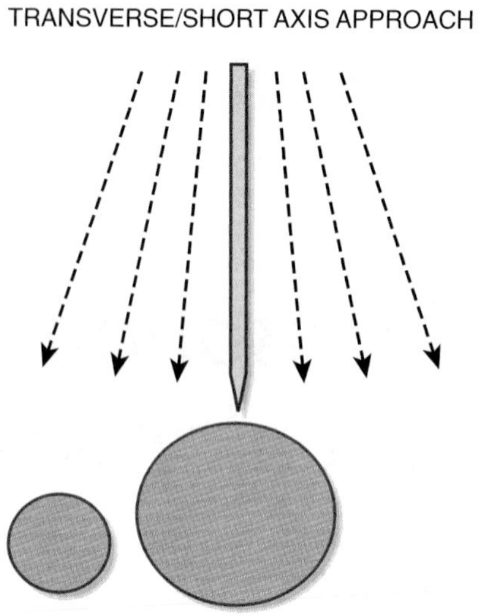
TRANSVERSE/SHORT AXIS APPROACH

FIGURE 5-2 Diagram of the transverse approach.

anatomy, and then proceeding with the procedure as one would without further imaging. The dynamic or real-time approach involves performing ultrasound simultaneously with the procedure and visualizing anatomy on the ultrasound screen during the key parts of the process (e.g., needle entering vessel). Whenever possible, the dynamic approach is preferred for venous access. With the dynamic approach, the operator's nondominant hand is used to scan while the dominant hand performs the procedure. Alternatively, an assistant can scan or hold the probe in position during the procedure.

All ultrasound-guided procedures, including vascular access, should follow standard sterile techniques. A 5- to 10-MHz or higher-frequency linear vascular probe should be used (Fig. 5-1). A sterile ultrasound probe cover should be used for central venous access.

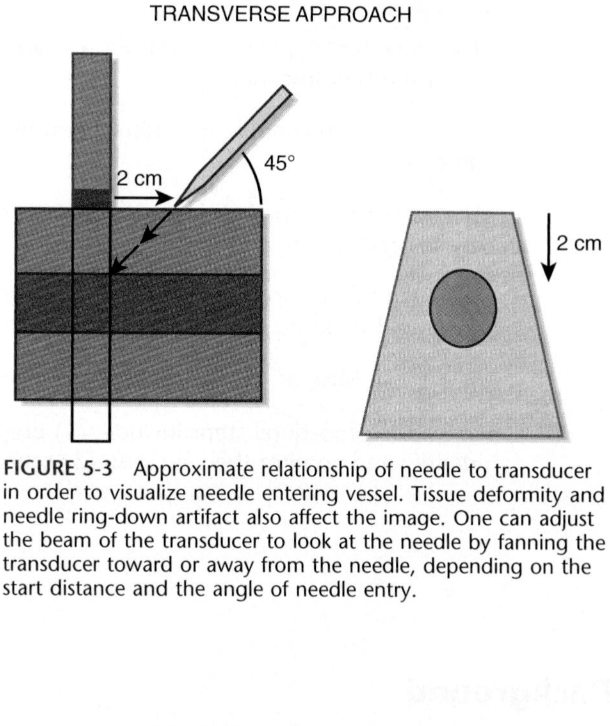
TRANSVERSE APPROACH
45°
2 cm
2 cm

FIGURE 5-3 Approximate relationship of needle to transducer in order to visualize needle entering vessel. Tissue deformity and needle ring-down artifact also affect the image. One can adjust the beam of the transducer to look at the needle by fanning the transducer toward or away from the needle, depending on the start distance and the angle of needle entry.

Approach

Ultrasound-guided venous access can be performed with a transverse or longitudinal approach. In the transverse approach, vessels appear circular, and medial-to-lateral localization is easier (Fig. 5-2). With this approach, the vessel target is placed in the center of the screen. The depth of the vessel should be noted on the screen, and the needle should be placed approximately this distance away from the middle of the transducer. Doing so allows visualization of the needle as it enters the vessel at a 45-degree angle (Fig. 5-3). Fanning the probe towards or away from the needle may be needed to alter the trajectory of the ultrasound beam if a different angle or start distance is used. In the transverse approach, it is important for the operator to keep the probe marker turned to his or her left so that the left side of the screen (screen indicator) is also the operator's left, in case any needle adjustments are needed.

In the longitudinal approach, the vessels appear tubular. The slope and depth of the needle are better appreciated in a longitudinal approach (Fig. 5-4).

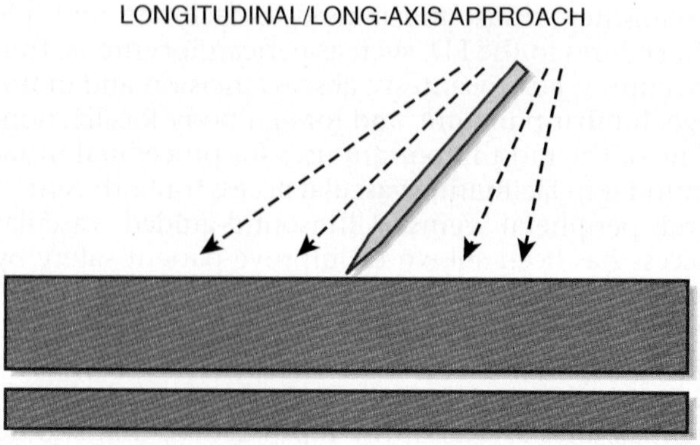
LONGITUDINAL/LONG-AXIS APPROACH

FIGURE 5-4 Diagram of the longitudinal approach.

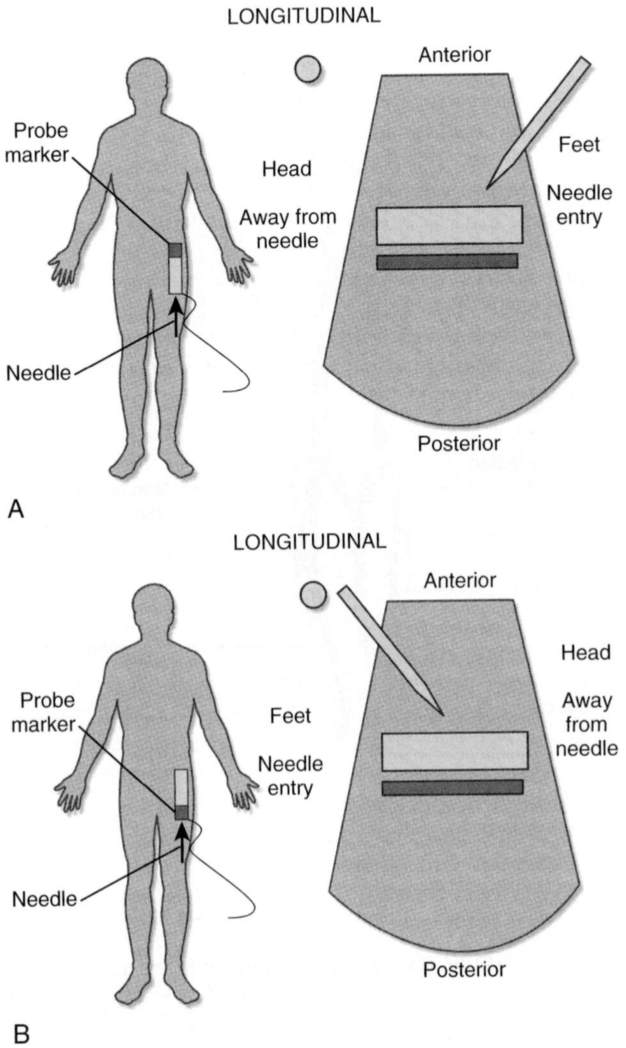
LONGITUDINAL
Anterior
Probe marker
Head
Away from needle
Feet
Needle entry
Needle
Posterior
A
LONGITUDINAL
Anterior
Head
Away from needle
Probe marker
Feet
Needle entry
Needle
Posterior
B

FIGURE 5-5 **A** and **B**, Diagrams demonstrating the orientation of the needle on the screen based on the direction of the probe indicator during the procedure.

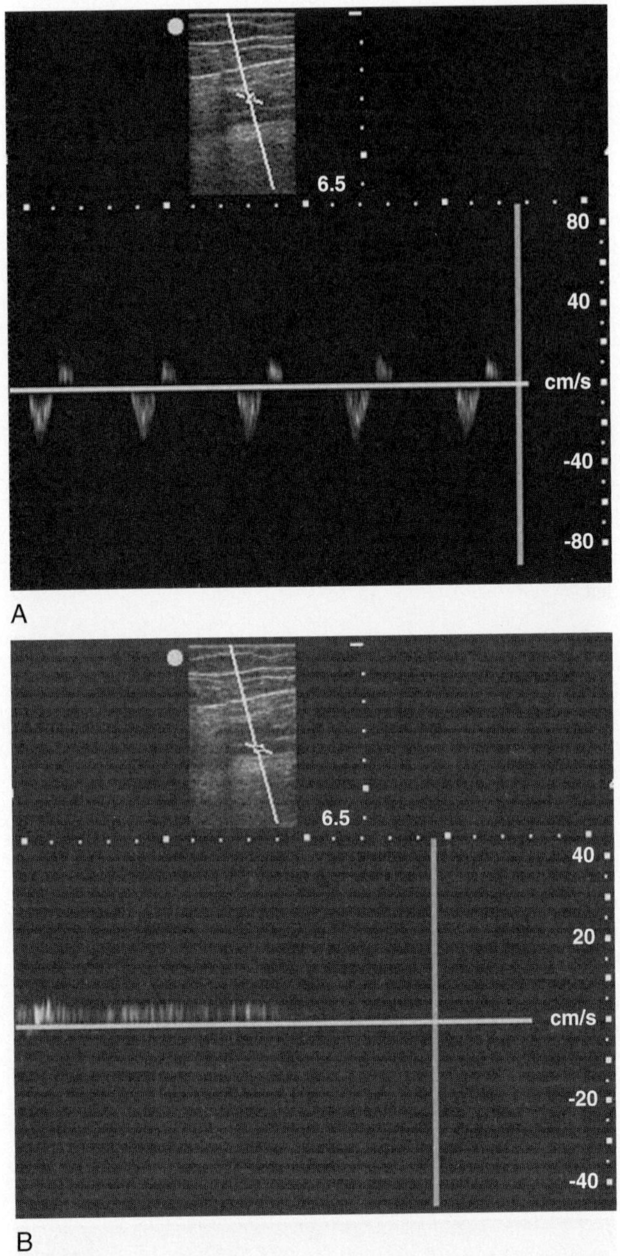
6.5
80
40
cm/s
-40
-80
A
6.5
40
20
cm/s
-20
-40
B

FIGURE 5-6 **A,** Doppler image of a femoral artery. **B,** Doppler image of a femoral vein.

With this approach, the needle can be placed just under the probe and so is better visualized at all depths. The direction of the probe indicator determines which side of the screen the needle will enter from (Fig. 5-5).

Central Venous Access

Patient positioning and anatomy are similar to positioning of the patient for achieving venous access with traditional anatomical approaches. After patient positioning and sterile preparation, the vein should be identified and confirmed. Veins have thin walls, are compressible, and should undulate rather than pulsate. Arteries are more thick-walled, should not compress, and should pulsate. Doppler ultrasound can be used to help differentiate between vein and artery if there is any question (Fig. 5-6). Figure 5-7 demonstrates approximate probe position for the transverse approach of the internal jugular vein. Figure 5-8 shows images of the internal jugular vein in transverse and longitudinal views.

Peripheral Venous Access

For ultrasound-guided peripheral venous access, the patient's arm should be extended and externally rotated to access the medial surface. A tourniquet is helpful to prevent collapse of the vein during cannulation. The basilic vein runs medial to, and the cephalic vein runs lateral to, the brachial vessels (Fig. 5-9). Figure 5-10A and B demonstrate approximate probe position and image at the level of mid-humerus for venous access in the upper extremity. Figure 5-10C shows the longitudinal view of a basilic vein

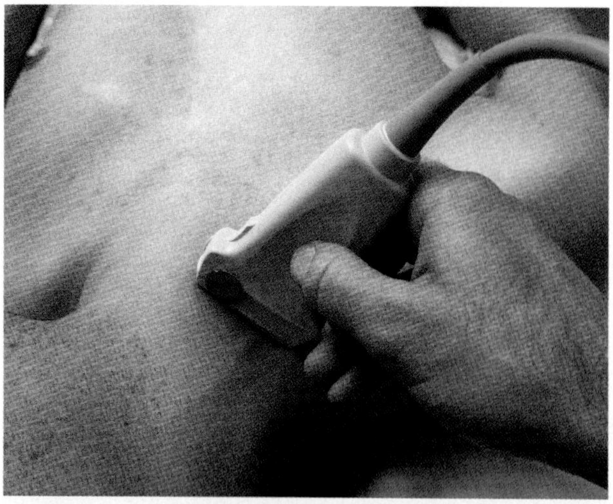

FIGURE 5-7 Approximate probe position for ultrasound imaging of the internal jugular vein. Note: The round sticker indicates that the probe marker is turned to the sonographer's left.

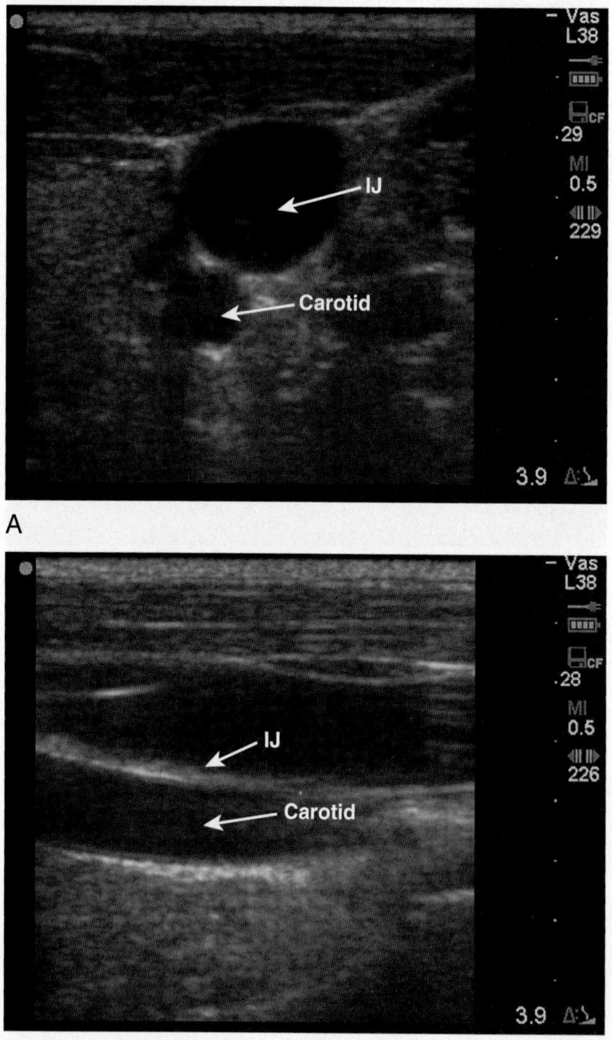

A
IJ
Carotid
Vas
L38
.29
MI
0.5
229
3.9
B
IJ
Carotid
Vas
L38
.28
MI
0.5
226
3.9

FIGURE 5-8 **A,** Transverse view of the internal jugular vein (IJ). Note the depth markers at the right of the screen. **B,** Internal jugular vein, longitudinal view.

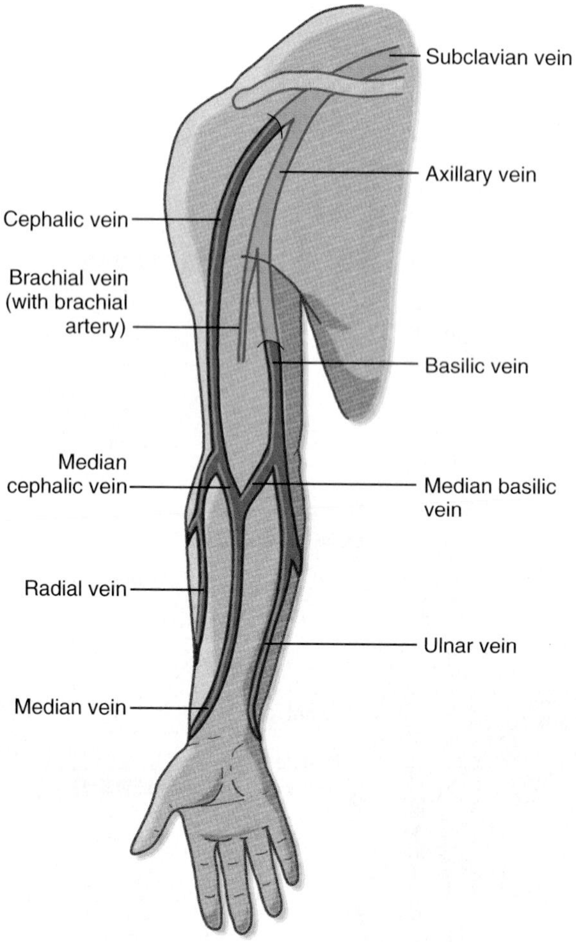

Subclavian vein
Axillary vein
Cephalic vein
Brachial vein (with brachial artery)
Basilic vein
Median cephalic vein
Median basilic vein
Radial vein
Ulnar vein
Median vein

FIGURE 5-9 Venous anatomy of the arm.

with the needle tip entering the vessel. A longer peripheral catheter is needed for these veins, usually 1.88 inches or longer.

Limitations

Ultrasound imaging for venous access can be technically limited by patient obesity or the presence of subcutaneous air. Ultrasound guidance makes venous access easier, but no technique is perfect. Complications seen with the ultrasound-guided approach are similar to those with other approaches to cannulation, including arterial puncture, hematoma, and pneumothorax. The deeper peripheral venous lines have a significant rate of infiltration and should be aspirated or flushed to confirm position before each administration of medication or any contrast agents.

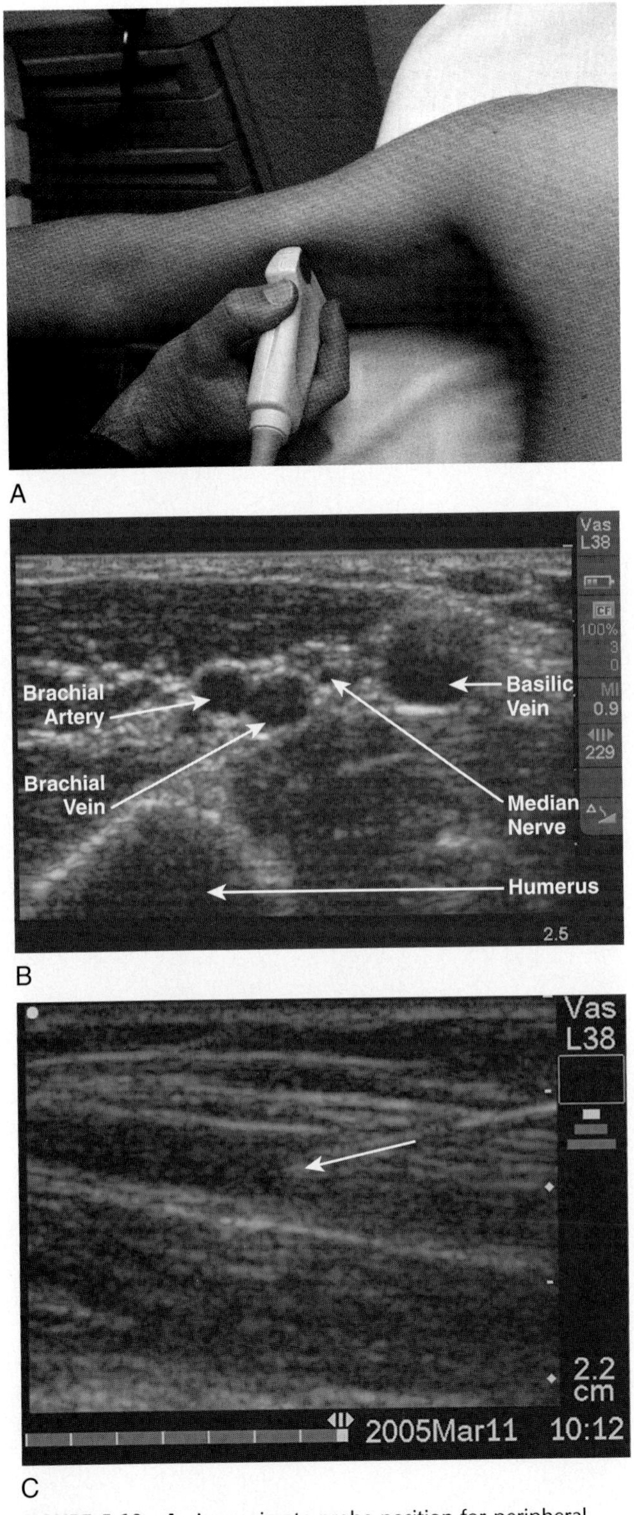
A
Vas
L38
Brachial
Artery
Brachial
Vein
Basilic
Vein
Median
Nerve
Humerus
2.5
B
Vas
L38
2.2
cm
2005Mar11
10:12
C

FIGURE 5-10 **A,** Approximate probe position for peripheral venous access. **B,** Representative transverse image. **C,** Longitudinal view of basilic vein. Note the needle tip in the vessel (*arrow*).

Tips and Tricks

PEARLS AND PITFALLS FOR ULTRASOUND-GUIDED VASCULAR ACCESS

- Make sure to anchor your hand on the patient's body to keep the probe from sliding during the procedure.
- Remember that the probe marker corresponds with the indicator on the monitor screen. For procedures, it is helpful to keep the probe marker turned to your left during the transverse approach, so that the left side of the screen (indicator on monitor) corresponds to your left.
- Always check the depth marker on the screen, and watch the depth of the needle throughout the procedure.
- Fanning or rocking the transducer beam can help accurately identify the needle's location.
- If using a static approach, make sure patient is positioned before scanning and marking the site. Changes in position after ultrasound imaging can cause anatomic relationships to change.
- Make sure to confirm identification of a vein with compression or Doppler imaging to avoid arterial puncture.
- The transverse approach is often easier with smaller vessels and for novice operators.

REFERENCES

1. Leung J, Duffy M, Finckh A: Real-time ultrasonographically-guided internal jugular vein catheterization in the emergency department increases success rates and reduces complications: A randomized, prospective study. Ann Emerg Med 2006;48:540-547.
2. Milling TJ Jr, Rose J, Briggs WM, et al: Randomized, controlled clinical trial of point-of-care limited ultrasonography assistance of central venous cannulation: The Third Sonography Outcomes Assessment Program (SOAP-3) Trial. Crit Care Med 2005;33:1764-1769.
3. Hind D, Calvert N, McWilliams R, et al: Ultrasonic locating devices for central venous cannulation: Meta-analysis. BMJ 2003;327:361.
4. Keyes LE, Frazee BW, Snoey ER, et al: Ultrasound-guided brachial and basilic vein cannulation in emergency department patients with difficult intravenous access. Ann Emerg Med 1999;34:711-714.
5. Costantino TG, Parikh AK, Satz WA, Fojtik JP: Ultrasonography-guided peripheral intravenous access versus traditional approaches in patients with difficult intravenous access. Ann Emerg Med 2005;46:456-461.
6. Shojania KG, Duncan BW, McDonald KM, et al: Making health care safer: A critical analysis of patient safety practices. Evid Rep Technol Assess (Summ) 2001;43:i-x, 1-668.

Chapter 6

Dysrhythmias in Cardiorespiratory Arrest

Jeffrey D. Ferguson, Kostas Alibertis, and William J. Brady

KEY POINTS

- Do not interrupt chest compressions when performing cardiopulmonary resuscitation (CPR).
- Rapid defibrillation can be lifesaving. Patients who have been in cardiac arrest for longer than 3-5 minutes may benefit from CPR prior to defibrillation.
- Amiodarone, epinephrine, and vasopressin can improve the likelihood of return of cardiac activity but might not increase the rate of neurologically-intact survival.
- Resuscitation algorithms are beneficial but key alterations may be needed based on the cause and circumstance of the cardiorespiratory arrest.

Primary cardiac events account for 75% of the episodes of sudden death (Fig. 6-1). Acute dysrhythmia may be the primary event (e.g., sudden ventricular fibrillation) or a secondary process (e.g., acute pulmonary edema with progressive hypoxemia and resultant bradycardia) (Box 6-1). In patients with sudden death from dysrhythmia, the most appropriate term is *sudden cardiac death.* Alternatively, the term *cardiac arrest* can be applied to any cause, including traumatic injury, metabolic disorder, or massive toxic ingestion.

Ventricular fibrillation (VF) and pulseless ventricular tachycardia (VT) result in death unless aggressively and rapidly treated. *Asystole,* the effective absence of cardiac electrical activity, is the true cardiac arrhythmia (i.e., the "absence" of any rhythm). *Pulseless electrical activity* (PEA) applies to a diverse range of rhythms and related clinical scenarios; it is defined as an electrical rhythm (i.e., the cardiac rhythm) with absence of discernible mechanical contraction of the heart and, therefore, no detectable perfusion. A somewhat "dated" term, *electromechanical dissociation,* provides another descriptor for this malignant cardiac presentation—the complete dissociation of electrical and mechanical activity of the cardiovascular system. The cardiac rhythm itself in the PEA state essentially includes any dysrhythmia seen in clinical medicine (with the notable exceptions of VF and pulseless VT), including bradycardic and tachycardic dysrhythmias.

Interestingly, the frequencies of the dysrhythmias differ according to clinical setting (Fig. 6-2). The prehospital population tends to demonstrate a higher rate of VT and VF, yet asystole remains the most common dysrhythmia. In this "less chronically ill" population, PEA is the least common dysrhythmia seen initially in sudden cardiac death. In the hospitalized patient population, asystole remains the most common initial dysrhythmia managed in the patients with cardiopulmonary arrest; PEA is next most often seen, whereas VT and VF are much less common. The more frequent appearance of PEA in the hospitalized

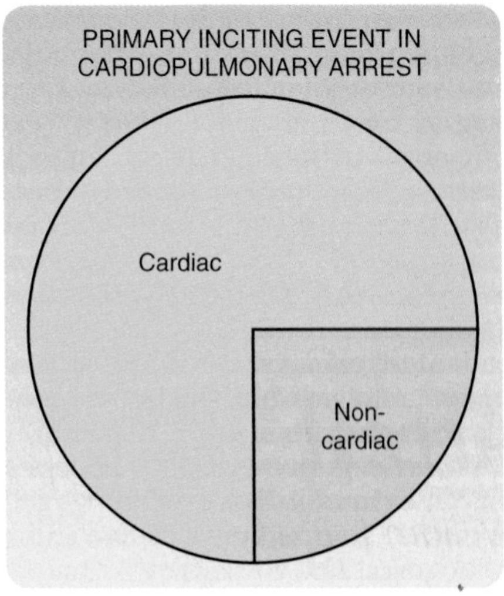
PRIMARY INCITING EVENT IN CARDIOPULMONARY ARREST
Cardiac
Non-cardiac

FIGURE 6-1 Primary inciting event in cardiopulmonary arrest. Sudden death may occur for a range of reasons, including medical and traumatic. Of the medical events, cardiac causes are most common; in fact, 75% of sudden death events are related to cardiac causes. In this setting, acute dysrhythmias are common, whether they represent the primary event (e.g., sudden ventricular fibrillation) or a secondary process related to the primary event (e.g., acute pulmonary edema with progressive hypoxemia and resultant bradycardia).

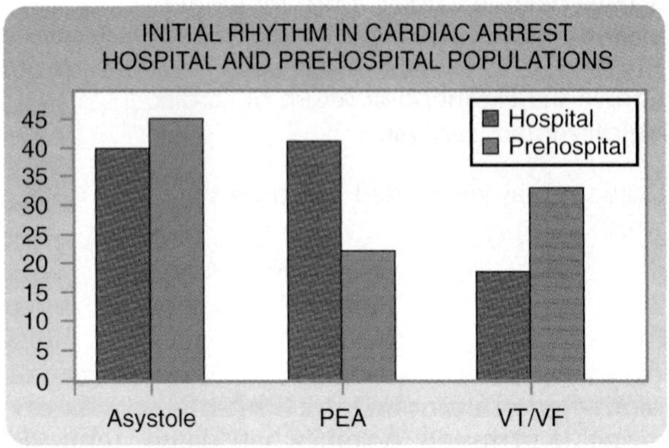
INITIAL RHYTHM IN CARDIAC ARREST
HOSPITAL AND PREHOSPITAL POPULATIONS
Hospital
Prehospital
45
40
35
30
25
20
15
10
5
0
Asystole
PEA
VT/VF

FIGURE 6-2 The cardiac arrhythmias encountered in cardiac arrest in hospitalized and prehospital patient groups. Note the preponderance of asystole in both groups as well as the higher rates of pulseless electrical activity (PEA) in the hospitalized patients and of ventricular fibrillation and ventricular tachycardia (VT/VF) in the prehospital patients.

BOX 6-1

Dysrhythmias Encountered in Sudden Cardiac Death

- Ventricular fibrillation
- Pulseless ventricular tachycardia
- Pulseless electrical activity (electromechanical dissociation)
- Asystole

population is understandable in that inpatients tend to have more comorbidities and active, acute illness than the prehospital group.

General Management

The core concepts of management of cardiorespiratory arrest are reversing any immediately treatable cause, such as a dysrhythmia, and ensuring the basics of airway, breathing, and circulatory support. Advanced life support protocols and guidelines are important but are simply guides to management. In no way is the clinician required to mindlessly follow these various algorithms in sequential order. Individual patient scenarios, clinical features, local medical resources, setting, and expertise are all factors that ultimately form the resuscitation strategy.

Adequate oxygenation and ventilation are paramount and can be performed in many situations with appropriate bag-mask ventilation. Chest compressions in cardiopulmonary resuscitation (CPR) are vital, and adequate perfusion can be produced with proper CPR technique. Not only the success of the resuscitation effort itself but also the effectiveness of the various interventions depends on appropriate circulation and tissue perfusion. Interruptions in chest compressions must be minimized; it has been demonstrated that noncompression periods, even seconds of interruption, are universally followed by segments of minimal to no perfusion of the brain and other vital organs despite subsequent correct CPR performance. Rhythm analysis, pulse determinations, and other periods of no chest compression must be minimized so that perfusion can be sustained.

Each of the management priorities—airway, breathing, and circulation—must be addressed either in sequential fashion (limited personnel available) or simultaneously (multiple personnel available). Certainly, achieving an adequate airway with appropriate oxygenation and ventilation are early, key interventions. Basic airway support with proper bag-mask ventilation is favorable in the early stages of resuscitation.

The "C" in the ABC pneumonic, circulation, is at least as complex as the airway and respiration management. Cardiac rhythm, myocardial contractility, vascular tone, and volume status, among many other considerations, must be addressed.

Electrical Therapy

Electrical therapy—defibrillation and transcutaneous cardiac pacing—can be remarkably successful. Early defibrillation improves survival rates, but only if accomplished within minutes. This therapy is appropriate only for VF and pulseless VT; it is never indicated for asystole or PEA rhythms. Because early defibrillation is important, it precedes airway management. Patients in cardiac arrest and VT or VF should undergo immediate defibrillation by the first person on the scene. Automatic external defibrillators (AEDs) should be available, perhaps even in hospitals. It is reasonable for hospital personnel to know how to use them.

Defibrillators exist in two basic styles, monophasic and biphasic. Most commercially available defibrillators (automatic and manual) are biphasic, although many monophasic models remain in use today. Thus far, neither defibrillator style is associated with higher rates of successful resuscitation or survival to hospital discharge. The biphasic defibrillator has achieved a higher rate of termination of VF and pulseless VT, yet this early benefit has not translated into survival to hospital discharge with a meaningful quality of life. With a monophasic defibrillator, a 360-joule (J) shock should be applied; with a biphasic unit, the equivalent, device-specific maximal emergency should be applied. Devices are engineered to prevent confusion. In either device, a single shock is delivered initially and in subsequent defibrillations. The multiple, "stacked" defibrillatory shocks of the recent past are no longer believed to be beneficial for a number of reasons, including prolonged noncompression time and the poor record of dysrhythmia termination in subsequent shocks with a stacked approach. The goals are to limit the amount of no perfusion when CPR is not in progress and to give the patient a single shock of maximal energy.

The AED is a lifesaving intervention when applied appropriately from both a systems and an individual use perspective. The use of the AED by trained lay rescuers (the Public Access Defibrillation [PAD] program) has demonstrated a markedly shorter time to defibrillation and an improved rate of resuscitation. AED use by nontrained rescuers in a PAD application has anecdotally demonstrated positive outcome, but its use by untrained personnel requires additional investigation at this point. The Targeted First Responder (TFR) application has also demonstrated significant success. The first responder is often a law enforcement officer, a firefighter, or a basic life support emergency medical technician (EMT). Regardless of the trained first responder job classification, the TFR program demonstrated remarkably shorter times to defibrillation with correspondingly higher rates of resuscitation. Relative to traditional advanced list support care

The correct incorporation of CPR and electrical defibrillation into treatment of patients with cardiac arrest is significant. In the recent past, it was believed that the most rapid application of electrical defibrillation was appropriate, providing the VF and pulseless VT patient with the best opportunity of successful resuscitation. Multiple different reviews noted a rather high incidence of post-countershock asystole in patients, particularly those with prolonged cardiac arrest prior to defibrillation. It is now believed that in patients in whom cardiac arrest has lasted more than 3 to 5 minutes (either witnessed or unwitnessed event), five cycles (2 minutes) of CPR should be performed prior to defibrillation. This approach is believed to optimize the chances for successful defibrillation, reduce the likelihood of post-countershock asystole, and increase the rate of a return to a perfusing, stable rhythm.[1,2] If the arrest is witnessed and a device is immediately available, a defibrillatory shock should be delivered as soon as possible.

Transcutaneous pacing is a rapid, minimally invasive means of treating asystole and PEA bradyarrhythmias. Transcutaneous pacing electrodes are applied to the skin of the anterior and posterior chest walls, and pacing is initiated with a portable pulse generator. In an emergency situation, such a pacing technique is more easily and rapidly accomplished than other methods of cardiac pacing. Recommended indications for transcutaneous pacemaker use in cardiac arrest are limited; they are asystole and bradycardic PEA rhythms. The very early use of transcutaneous ventricular pacing is encouraged, although evidence of its benefit is lacking. Transcutaneous pacing is much less effective after the loss of spontaneous circulation or prolonged cardiac arrest.[3,4]

Pharmacologic Therapy

Although numerous medications may be employed in a resuscitation event, the agents of chief importance are epinephrine, vasopressin, atropine, amiodarone, lidocaine, magnesium, calcium, and sodium bicarbonate. The two primary vasopressor agents used in resuscitation are epinephrine and vasopressin.

Epinephrine and vasopressin have been demonstrated to improve rates of return of spontaneous circulation, but not to cause meaningful increases in rates of survival to hospital discharge with intact neurologic status. Epinephrine is a potent adrenergic agonist with both alpha and beta effects. The alpha effects are believed to be responsible for the beneficial impact of this drug—essentially, vasoconstriction that promotes higher perfusion pressures of the coronary and cerebral vascular beds during CPR. The beta effects, largely negative in this setting, increase myocardial work and may also impair subendocardial perfusion. Vasopressin is a nonadrenergic vasopressor with pronounced peripheral vasoconstriction. Coronary and renal vasoconstriction is also encountered with its use, but vasopressin has no direct effect on cardiac contractility. Both vasopressors are indicated in all three cardiac arrest treatment scenarios—VF and pulseless VT, PEA, and asystole. These medications can be used interchangeably in the cardiac arrest scenario; that is, the use of one vasopressor does not preclude future use of the other agent in the same resuscitation.

Atropine is a parasympatholytic drug that enhances both sinoatrial node automaticity and atrioventricular conduction via direct vagolytic action. Atropine exerts a direct influence on the function of the atrioventricular junctional tissue and subjunctional components of the cardiac conduction system. The response to atropine depends on the varying sensitivities of different levels of the conduction system to autonomic stimuli and on other extrinsic factors, such as the degree of systemic perfusion and medication-related issues. In cardiac arrest, atropine should be given to patients with both asystole and PEA, particularly those patients with bradydysrhythmic electrical activity presentations.

Amiodarone and lidocaine are the primary antidysrhythmic agents used in cardiac arrest resuscitation scenarios. Amiodarone has a very broad range of mechanisms, including sodium and calcium blockade, potassium efflux antagonism, and adrenergic blocking effects. In cardiac arrest, its use is indicated for VF and pulseless VT unresponsive to CPR, defibrillation, and initial vasopression. Although amiodarone has demonstrated impressive results in terms of the return of spontaneous perfusion in cardiac arrest, it has not altered the ultimate outcome—meaningful survival to hospital discharge. Lidocaine is a well-known and widely used antidysrhythmic agent of limited efficacy in cardiac arrest. In the Vaughn-Williams classification scheme, lidocaine is a type I agent. Unfortunately, lidocaine has effected no alteration in outcome for patients with out-of-hospital cardiac arrest due to VF and pulseless VT. Furthermore, in comparisons with amiodarone, lidocaine has demonstrated a less favorable rate of respiration of spontaneous circulation with a higher rate of asystole in general and after defibrillation. Like amiodarone, it should be used in patients with VF and pulseless VT that is unresponsive to initial therapies. Lidocaine is best considered an alternative to amiodarone for refractory VF and pulseless VT.

The electrolytes magnesium and calcium play a limited role in resuscitation. Magnesium should be used in patients with polymorphic VT that is believed to be torsades de pointes. Possible secondary indications for magnesium are PEA cardiac arrest potentially resulting from hyperkalemia and cardiorespiratory arrest related to toxemia. Calcium use should be limited to cardiac arrests involving excessive parenteral administration of magnesium, hyperkalemia, and ingestion of cardiotoxic substances.

Sodium bicarbonate is a potent buffer, and there is no evidence supporting its widespread use in cardiac arrest. Sodium bicarbonate can adversely affect perfusion in certain vascular beds, unfavorably alter acid-base status at the tissue and cellular levels, and promote hyperosmolarity and hypernatremia. Like magnesium and calcium, sodium bicarbonate is potentially indicated in several specific clinical scenarios—tricyclic antidepressant overdose, severe metabolic acidosis, hyperkalemia, and prolonged cardiac arrest.

Ventricular Fibrillation and Pulseless Ventricular Tachycardia

Ventricular fibrillation and pulseless ventricular tachycardia are discussed together because they occur in the same clinical settings with similar mechanisms, etiologies, and modes of therapy. The only clinically significant classification system of VF concerns the amplitude of the chaotic waveform deflections, dividing them into coarse (large-amplitude) and fine (small-amplitude) varieties. Regardless of morphology, VF invariably results in death unless prompt therapy is given (Table 6-1).

Ventricular fibrillation is divided into two clinical types. It is considered "primary" in the absence of acute left ventricular dysfunction and cardiogenic shock; this type is noted in approximately 5% of cases of acute myocardial infarction (AMI). The majority of primary VF episodes occur within the first 4 hours of AMI, and 80% are seen within the first 12 hours. VF may represent abrupt reperfusion, but recurrent or ongoing ischemia is more likely. Although there is a brief period of increased inpatient mortality for patients with primary VF, their overall prognosis does not differ from that of patients with AMI without VF. Secondary VF, which occurs at any time in the course of AMI that is complicated by acute heart failure and/or cardiogenic shock, is seen in up to 7% of patients with AMI. Unlike in primary VF, the prognosis for patients with secondary VF is dismal; the in-hospital mortality approaches 60%, and long-term mortality (beyond 5 years) remains poor.

In contrast to VF, VT usually originates from a specific focus in the ventricular myocardium or in the infranodal conduction pathway. *Ventricular tachycardia* is defined as a tachycardia with rapid, wide QRS complexes originating from the infranodal cardiac tissues. VT can be classified from several different perspectives, including the overall clinical presentation (stable vs. unstable), the hemodynamic state (the presence or absence of a pulse), the temporal course (sustained vs. nonsustained), and the morphology (monomorphic vs. polymorphic). In sudden cardiac death, it is most appropriate to consider ventricular tachycardia from the overall clinical presentation, with stress on temporal and hemodynamic factors as well—in this instance, VT is considered pulseless and sustained, and thus unstable. Pulseless VT accounts for a minority of rhythms seen in cardiac arrest and has the most favorable prognosis. This relatively infrequent occurrence in the cardiac arrest scenario results from an early appearance with rapid degeneration into more malignant rhythms, such as VF and asystole.

▪ PATHOPHYSIOLOGY

These two malignant dysrhythmias most often arise from direct myocardial damage (i.e., acute myocardial infarction, myocarditis, cardiomyopathy), medication toxicity, or electrolyte abnormality. The pathophysiology usually involves either a reentry phenomenon or triggered automaticity. A reentry circuit within the ventricular myocardium is the most common source. The properties of a reentry circuit involve two pathways of conduction with differing electrical characteristics. The reentry circuits

Table 6-1 SUGGESTED RESUSCITATIVE APPROACH TO THE PATIENT WITH VENTRICULAR FIBRILLATION OR PULSELESS VENTRICULAR TACHYCARDIA

Time	Treatment Priority	Comments
Minute 0	CPR	Compressions should be done at a rate of 100/min and a ratio of 30 compressions to every 2 breaths. Initial compressions may improve defibrillation efficacy by increasing the amplitude of the VF. Pulse checks and rhythm analysis should be performed no more often than every 2 min. If arrest is witnessed and defibrillator is available, patient should be defibrillated immediately; if arrest is unwitnessed and/or cardiac arrest time is more than 4-5 min, a period of CPR is recommended prior to defibrillation.
Minute 0-2	Defibrillation at 360 J (or biphasic equivalent, 1 shock at highest energy) If no change in ECG, CPR IV access	Because of the increased first shock conversion with biphasic energy and the importance of continuous CPR, 1 high-energy shock is recommended. Medication administration via ET tube, although acceptable, is no longer considered equivalent to IV administration.
Minute 3	Defibrillation at 360 J (or biphasic equivalent, 1 shock at highest energy) Vasopressin 40 IU ET tube placement	Initially, vasopressin or epinephrine may be given interchangeably. ET tube placement is not a priority unless bag-mask ventilation is inadequate. Assessment for correct ET tube placement should include a secondary confirmation device.
Minute 5	Defibrillation at 360 J (or biphasic equivalent, 1 shock at highest energy) Amiodarone 300 mg	CPR should occur over 2-min periods with intervening defibrillation attempts.
Minute 6	Epinephrine 1 mg	Medication dosing frequency in cardiac arrest remains every 3-5 min, with the recognition that peak central levels may vary according to physiologic differences in patients.
Minute 7	Defibrillation at 360 J (or biphasic equivalent, 1 shock at highest energy)	CPR should not be interrupted for periods longer than 15 seconds at a time.
Minute 9	Defibrillation at 360 J (or biphasic equivalent, 1 shock at highest energy) Epinephrine 1 mg	Other medications should be considered in presence of an identified underlying cause for cardiac arrest.
Minute 10	Amiodarone 150 mg	Amiodarone can be repeated in 5 minutes at half the first dose

CPR, cardiopulmonary resuscitation; ECG, electrocardiogram; ET, endotracheal; IV, intravenous; VF, ventricular fibrillation.

that provide the substrate for VT and VF usually occur in a zone of acute ischemia or chronic scar. This dysrhythmia is usually initiated by an ectopic beat, although any of a number of other factors can be the primary initiating event, including acute coronary ischemia, electrolyte disorders, and dysautonomia. Conversely, triggered automaticity of a group of cells can result from various cardiac anomalies, including congenital heart disease, acquired heart ailments, electrolyte disorders, and medication toxicity.

One electrophysiologic model describes these ventricular dysrhythmias with respect to morphology and suggests that the three entities—VF, polymorphic VT (PVT), and monomorphic VT (MVT)—manifest across an electrophysiologic spectrum. This model notes that PVT differs from VF and MVT in frequency, amplitude, and variability, suggesting that MVT, PVT, and VF are states of electrical activity occurring across a spectrum of ventricular dysrhythmia. In this model, MVT is the most highly organized rhythm, and VF the least, and PVT intermediate between the two ends of the spectrum.

■ CLINICAL PRESENTATION

■ Ventricular Fibrillation

Ventricular fibrillation results in a lack of spontaneous perfusion except in the rare case of witnessed, recent onset in which the patient is able to cough, enabling perfusion to continue for a short period. VF is diagnosed electrocardiographically in the pulseless and apneic patient from the lower amplitude and chaotic activity (Fig. 6-3). The "rate" of the deflections is usually between 200 and 500 depolarizations per minute. Morphologically, VF is divided into coarse (see Fig. 6-3A) and fine (see Fig. 6-3B and C). Coarse VF tends to occur early after cardiac arrest and is characterized by high-amplitude, or coarse, wave-

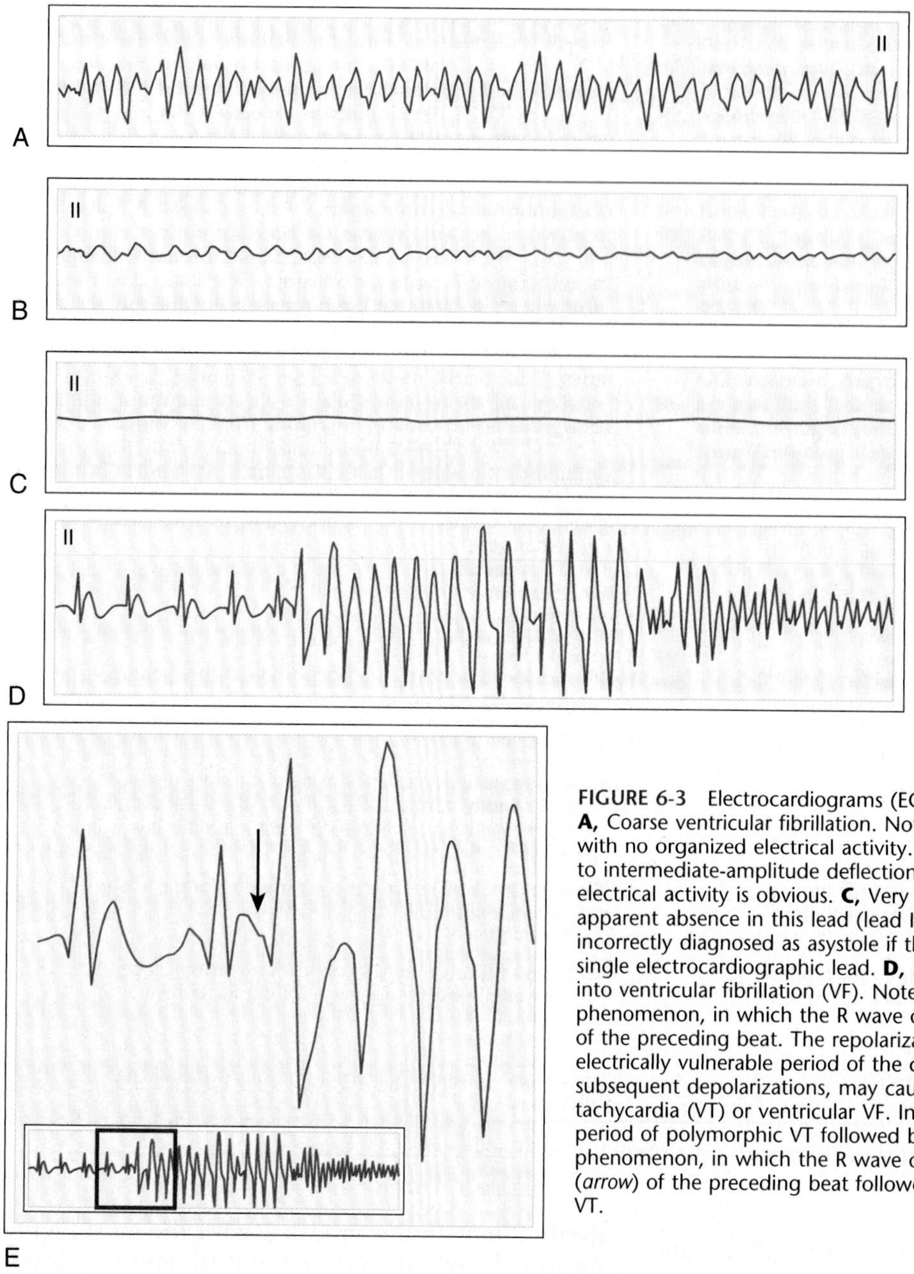

II
A
II
B
II
C
II
D
E

FIGURE 6-3 Electrocardiograms (ECGs) of ventricular fibrillation. **A,** Coarse ventricular fibrillation. Note the large-amplitude deflections with no organized electrical activity. **B,** Ventricular fibrillation with low- to intermediate-amplitude deflections; also, the absence of organized electrical activity is obvious. **C,** Very fine ventricular fibrillation. Note the apparent absence in this lead (lead II) of deflection. This rhythm may be incorrectly diagnosed as asystole if the patient is monitored solely in a single electrocardiographic lead. **D,** Sinus tachycardia with degeneration into ventricular fibrillation (VF). Note the appearance of the R-on-T phenomenon, in which the R wave of an early beats falls on the T wave of the preceding beat. The repolarization period of the ECG cycle is an electrically vulnerable period of the cardiac phase—insults, such as subsequent depolarizations, may cause the development of ventricular tachycardia (VT) or ventricular VF. In this case, the patient has a short period of polymorphic VT followed by coarse VF. **E,** The R-on-T phenomenon, in which the R wave of an early beat falls on the T wave (*arrow*) of the preceding beat followed by a short period of polymorphic VT.

forms with a "better" prognosis relative to fine VF. With continued cardiac arrest, the amplitude dampens, with less dramatic appearance of the dysrhythmia, ultimately producing fine VF (see Fig. 6-3B and C).

Fine VF may be confused with asystole. If the sensing electrode is oriented perpendicular to the primary depolarization vector, the amplitude of the deflections is minimal, mimicking asystole. The mimicking can negatively affect the patient's care if electrical defibrillation is not considered. This potential pitfall is easily avoided if the dysrhythmia is viewed with at least two or three simultaneous or consecutive electrocardiographic leads. In fine VF there is a significantly greater incidence of post-countershock asystole than in coarse VF. In fine VF, a period of CPR prior to defibrillation can reduce the incidence of post-countershock asystole.

■ Ventricular Tachycardia

As previously mentioned, *ventricular tachycardia* is defined as three or more ventricular beats in succession with a QRS complex duration of more than 0.12 sec and a ventricular rate greater than 100 or 120 beats/min (Fig. 6-4). Most instances of VT are characterized by very rapid rates, although patients may present with "slower" versions of VT, particularly if they are using amiodarone.

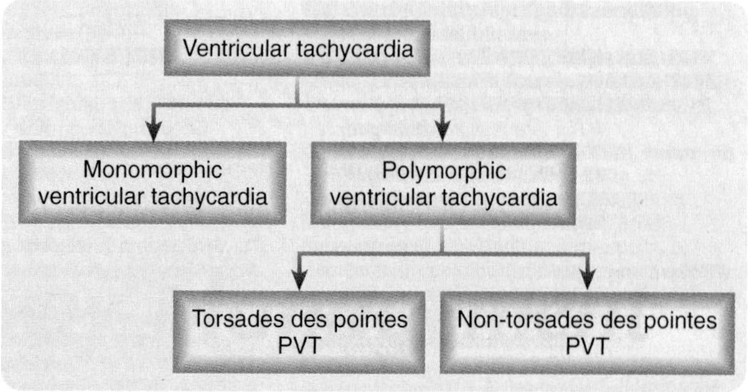
Ventricular tachycardia
Monomorphic ventricular tachycardia
Polymorphic ventricular tachycardia
Torsades des pointes PVT
Non-torsades des pointes PVT

FIGURE 6-4 Morphologic description of ventricular tachycardia (VT). Morphologically, VT can be divided into monomorphic and polymorphic on the basis of the nature of the QRS complex. Polymorphic VT (PVT) can be further subdivided into torsades de pointes (TdP) PVT and non-torsades de pointes PVT; this distinction is made through consideration of not only the morphology of the QRS complex but also other electrophysiologic issues (the repolarization state as manifested by the QT interval). With TdP PVT, QT interval prolongation is noted; this determination obviously can be made only when the patient's electrocardiogram shows a supraventricular rhythm.

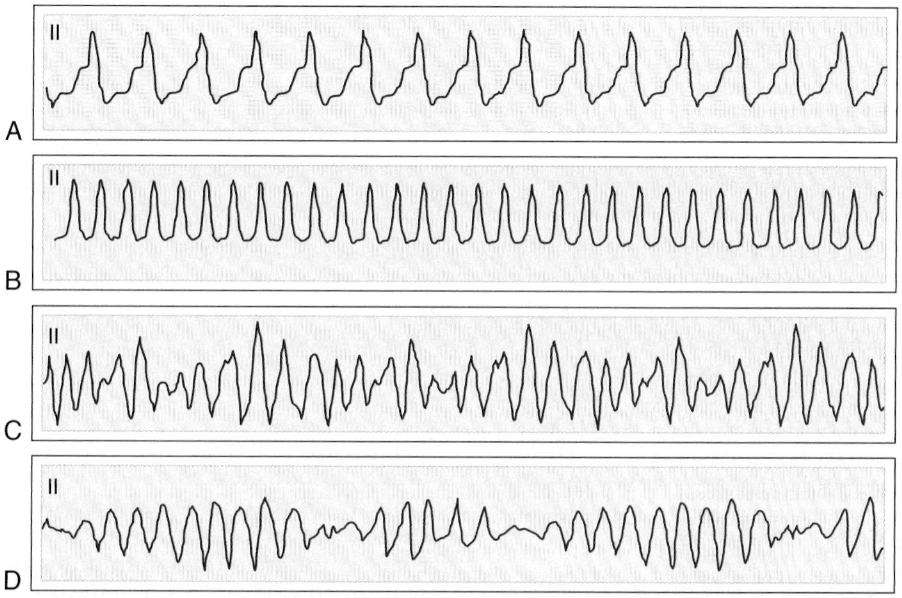
II
A
II
B
II
C
II
D

FIGURE 6-5 Electrocardiograms (ECGs) of ventricular tachycardia. **A,** Monomorphic ventricular tachycardia. Note the very wide QRS complex and rate of approximately 150 beats/min. **B,** Monomorphic ventricular tachycardia. Note the very rapid rate of approximately 240 beats/min. **C,** Polymorphic ventricular tachycardia. The QRS complex is continually changing (potentially in both amplitude and morphology) in any single lead. The QRS complex also tends to be greater than 0.12 seconds, with beat-to-beat variations in the morphology and width; significant variability in the R-R interval and QRS complex axis is noted as well. **D,** Polymorphic ventricular tachycardia, torsades de pointes type (TdP PVT). Note the marked beat-to-beat variation in QRS complex morphology occurring in a gradual pattern. The QRS complex ranges from small to large with an undulating pattern as if it is "twisting about a point"—the torsades de pointes version of polymorphic ventricular tachycardia. TdP PVT has a characteristic appearance—the QRS complex varies in amplitude, appearing to rotate about the isoelectric baseline in a semisinusoidal fashion. Also required for the ECG (and clinical) diagnosis(es) of TdP is the demonstration of abnormal repolarization manifested by QT interval prolongation on the ECG when the patient is in a supraventricular rhythm.

From an electrocardiographic perspective, the morphology of the VT is of importance (Figs. 6-4 and 6-5). Monomorphic VT is identified when each consecutive waveform is of a single morphology—that is, when the beat-to-beat variation in QRS complex morphology is negligible (Fig. 6-5A and B). The rate is usually between 140 and 180 beats/min and very regular. MVT is the most common form of VT, seen in 65% to 75% of patients with VT in the nonhospital setting (Fig. 6-6).[5,6] In patients with MVT, the cause of the dysrhythmia is usually secondary to myocardial scarring from a prior infarct.

Polymorphic VT is characterized by a frequently changing QRS complex (Fig. 6-5C and D). The QRS complex tends to be longer than 0.12 seconds with beat-to-beat variations in the morphology and width. There is significant variability in the R-R interval and QRS complex axis. The rate is usually more rapid than in MVT, ranging from 150 to 300 beats/min, and PVT accounts for 25% to 30% of VT in out-of-hospital cardiac arrests (see Fig. 6-6).[5,6]

The PVT subtype torsades de pointes (TdP) demonstrates polymorphous QRS complexes that vary from beat to beat (Figs. 6-5D and 6-7). The variation is often quite pronounced and easily observed. TdP also has a highly characteristic electrocardiographic pattern; the literal translation of the French term *torsades de pointes*—"twisting of the points"—elegantly describes the appearance of the QRS complex as it varies in amplitude, appearing to rotate

Table 6-2 ETIOLOGIES, PATHOPHYSIOLOGIC EVENT, AND SPECIFIC THERAPIES FOR PULSELESS ELECTRICAL ACTIVITY CARDIAC ARREST

Etiology	Pathophysiologic Event	Potentially Reversible?	Specific Therapy
Profound hypovolemia	Dehydration, hemorrhage	Yes	Volume resuscitation (crystalloid and colloid)
Cardiac tamponade	Obstruction to flow	Yes	Pericardiocentesis
Large acute myocardial infarction	Myocardial dysfunction	No	Volume resuscitation, inotropic and vasopressor support
Tension pneumothorax	Obstruction to flow	Yes	Chest decompression
Massive pulmonary embolism	Obstruction to flow	Yes	Fibrinolysis and embolectomy
Severe sepsis	Poor vascular tone, reduced contractility, increased capillary permeability	No	Volume resuscitation, inotropic and vasopressor support
Anaphylactic shock	Poor vascular tone, reduced contractility, increased capillary permeability	Yes	Volume resuscitation, inotropic and vasopressor support—in particular, early administration of epinephrine
Significant electrolyte abnormality	Myocardial dysfunction	No	Target therapy
Pronounced metabolic acidosis	Myocardial dysfunction	No	Sodium bicarbonate, ventilation
Cardiotoxic ingestion	Myocardial dysfunction	No	Antidote
Hypothermia	Myocardial dysfunction	Yes	Rewarming therapy
Prolonged cardiac arrest	Myocardial malfunction	No	None

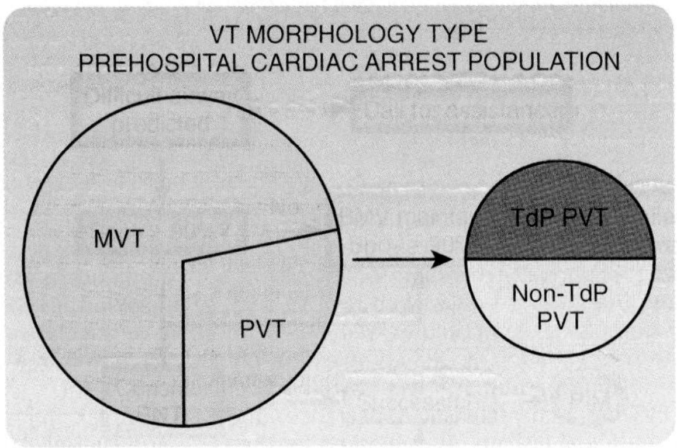
VT MORPHOLOGY TYPE
PREHOSPITAL CARDIAC ARREST POPULATION
MVT
PVT
TdP PVT
Non-TdP
PVT

FIGURE 6-6 The morphologic subtypes of ventricular tachycardia (VT) in prehospital patients with cardiac arrest. Among patients with polymorphic VT (PVT), both non–torsades de pointes PVT and torsades de pointes PVT (TdP PVT) are seen in approximate equal frequency. MVT, monomorphic VT.

about the isoelectric baseline in a semisinusoidal fashion. Also required for the electrocardiographic (and clinical) diagnosis of TdP is the demonstration of abnormal repolarization, manifested as QT interval prolongation on the electrocardiogram (ECG) (Fig. 6-7B.)

■ MANAGEMENT

The resuscitative management of VT is similar to that of VF (Table 6-2). Figure 6-8 presents one acceptable algorithm for the management of VF and pulseless VT. The basic approach includes CPR and electrical defibrillation. If the event is witnessed and the cardiac arrest period is less than 4 to 5 minutes, then immediate defibrillation should occur. If the period of cardiac arrest is unknown or is known to be longer than 5 minutes, then 2 minutes of CPR should be performed prior to defibrillation.

Once defibrillation has occurred, CPR resumes for an additional 2 minutes. If the dysrhythmia persists at electrocardiographic analysis, a vasopressor is administered, either vasopressin or epinephrine. Epinephrine should be used in 1-mg doses, preferably administered via an intravenous (IV) or intraosseous (IO) line. If it is given via an endotracheal tube, a larger dose, 2 to 2.5 mg, should be used. Epinephrine should be readministered every 3 to 5 minutes during the resuscitation. Comparisons of standard-dose, escalating-dose, and high-dose epinephrine strategies have not demonstrated a benefit for any strategy in terms of survival to hospital discharge or intact neurologic recovery. In fact, an analysis of eight trials involving more than 9000 patients showed no epinephrine regimen to be better than another.[7] In certain situations, such as cardiotoxic drug ingestion, higher doses of epinephrine may be required, although this issue is unexplored. Vasopressin is administered via the IV or IO route at a dose of 40 international units (IU). In multiple studies of vasopressin alone or vasopressin versus epinephrine in prehospital and hospital-based populations, no significant difference has been found in restoration of spontaneous circulation, survival to ED admission, or survival to hospital discharge.[8-10] A single dose of vasopressin may be used at either the first or second

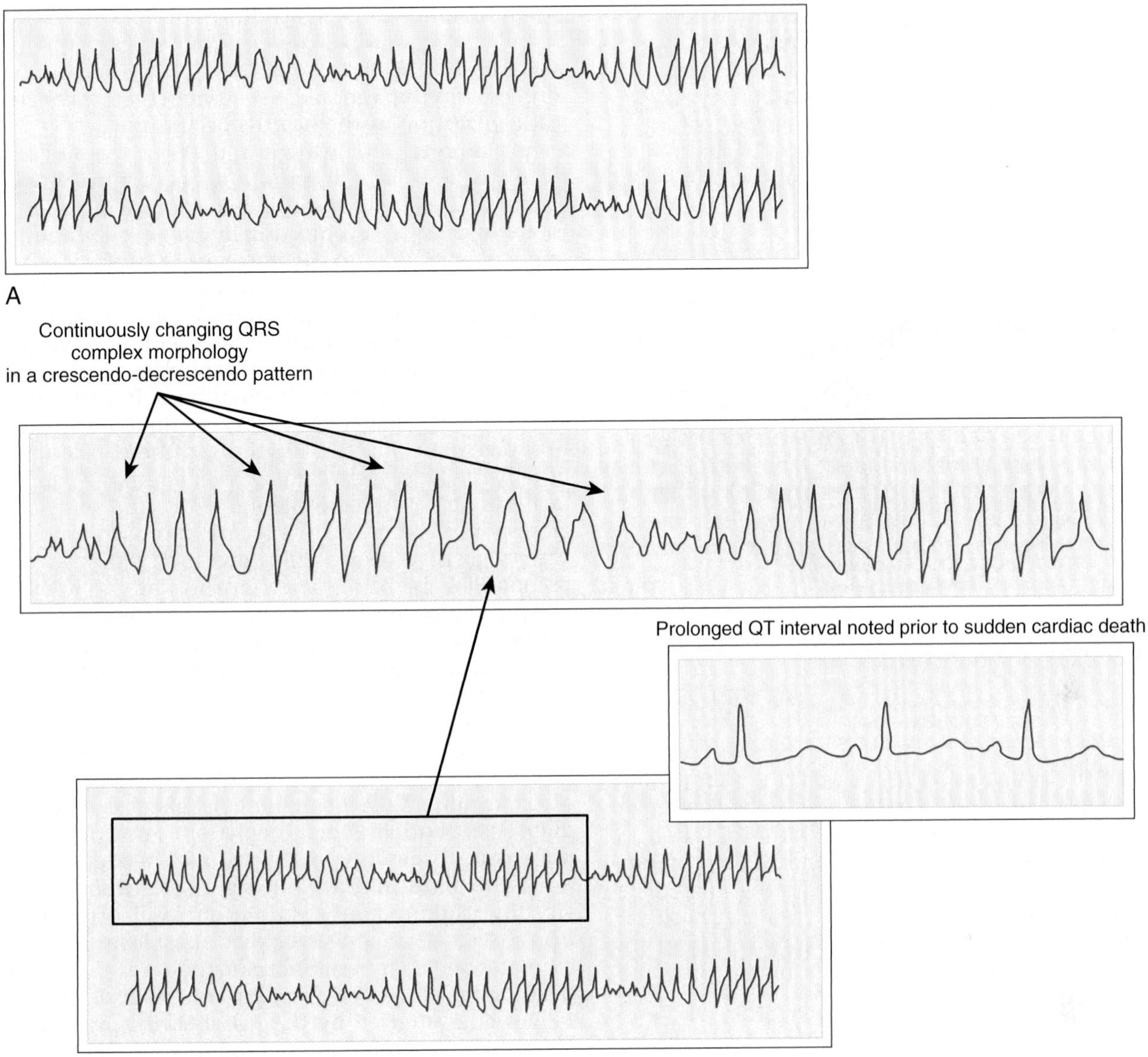
A
Continuously changing QRS complex morphology in a crescendo-decrescendo pattern
Prolonged QT interval noted prior to sudden cardiac death
B

FIGURE 6-7 Torsades de pointes polymorphic ventricular tachycardia (TdP PVT). **A,** The appearance of the QRS complex is characteristic of this subtype of PVT—in any single electrocardiographic lead, it varies in both morphology and amplitude, appearing to rotate about the isoelectric baseline in a semisinusoidal fashion. **B,** Note the polymorphous QRS complexes that vary from beat to beat. The variation is often quite pronounced, with marked variation easily observed in any single lead from one beat to the subsequent beat. TdP also demonstrates a highly characteristic electrocardiographic pattern; the literal translation of the French term *torsades de pointes*—"twisting of the points"—elegantly describes the appearance of the QRS complex as it varies in amplitude, appearing to rotate about the isoelectric baseline in a semisinusoidal fashion. Also required for the diagnosis is the demonstration of abnormal repolarization, manifested as QT interval prolongation on the ECG when the patient is in a supraventricular rhythm (i.e., prior to arrest or after successful resuscitation and return of spontaneous circulation).

vasopressor administration; epinephrine is then used at other times.

After the vasopressor administration, CPR should be continued for 2 minutes, followed by a second defibrillation. If VT and VF persist, amiodarone or lidocaine should be administered. Amiodarone is the preferred agent and should be considered for patients with VF and pulseless VT that are unresponsive to CPR, a vasopressor, and defibrillation. It is administered to the pulseless patient as a bolus dose of 300 mg IV, and can be given in a second dose of 150 mg IV. Amiodarone has demonstrated a benefit over both placebo and lidocaine in this patient group. Although the rates of restoration of spontaneous circulation and survival to hospital admission were greater in the amiodarone-treated patients, the rates of ultimate survival to hospital discharge were no different in the two groups.[11-13]

Polymorphic VT should be managed similarly to pulseless monomorphic VT or VF. CPR, defibrillation, vasopressor, and antidysrhythmic agents are appropriate therapeutic interventions. In two comparisons of MVT with PVT in prehospital patients with cardiorespiratory arrest, MVT occurred (60%) more often

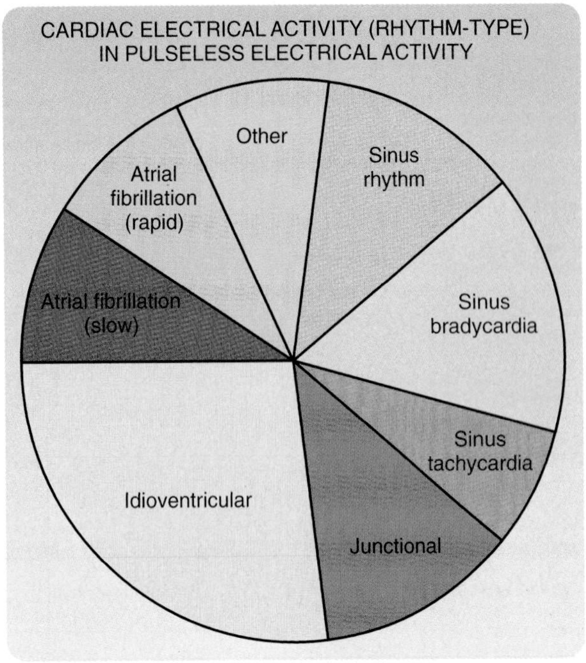
CARDIAC ELECTRICAL ACTIVITY (RHYTHM-TYPE)
IN PULSELESS ELECTRICAL ACTIVITY
Other
Sinus
rhythm
Atrial
fibrillation
(rapid)
Atrial fibrillation
(slow)
Sinus
bradycardia
Sinus
tachycardia
Idioventricular
Junctional

FIGURE 6-8 Distribution of electrical rhythm diagnoses in patients presented with pulseless electrical activity (PEA).

than PVT (15%) and TdP (15%).[5,6] Clinical outcomes were similar in both rhythm groups with similar therapies; the subset of patients with TdP fared as well as the patients with PVT and MVT.[5,6] If sustained, PVT is always unstable, requiring immediate attention. Initial therapy is unsynchronized electrical cardioversion. Antiarrhythmic therapy is warranted, including the use of intravenous magnesium and amiodarone. The patient should be closely observed because the rhythm frequently recurs.

Pulseless Electrical Activity

Pulseless electrical activity (PEA) is a malignant dysrhythmia indicating a very serious underlying medical event, such as profound hypovolemia, massive myocardial infarction, large pulmonary embolism, significant electrolyte disorder, or cardiotoxic overdose. PEA features the unique combination of no discernible cardiac mechanical activity (e.g., a "pulseless" state) with persistent cardiac electrical activity (e.g., the cardiac rhythm). Essentially, any dysrhythmia other than VT or VF may be seen.

■ PATHOPHYSIOLOGY

PEA must be separated into "pseudo" and "true" types. Pseudo-PEA occurs when cardiac electrical activity (i.e., a cardiac rhythm) is demonstrated while a palpable pulse is absent and is diagnosed when myocardial contractions are noted via echocardiography or some other imaging modality. In this presentation, a pronounced decrease in the cardiovascular system's ability to generate "forward flow" is found despite the continued presence of myocardial contractions. In true PEA, cardiac electrical activity in the form of a rhythm is noted, yet absolutely no mechanical contraction of the heart is occurring.

It is important to distinguish the two types of PEA. With pseudo-PEA, a significant pathophysiologic event has impaired the cardiovascular system's ability to perfuse. Such events usually involve profound hypovolemia due to hemorrhage, obstruction to forward flow resulting from massive pulmonary embolism, tension pneumothorax, or cardiac tamponade, and hypocontractile states with poor vascular tone, such as advanced anaphylactic or septic shock or very rapid tachydysrhythmias. In these situations, myocardial contractions continue but perfusion pressure is limited. Rhythms in these situations usually include tachycardias, predominantly sinus tachycardia, or atrial fibrillation with rapid ventricular response. A directed therapeutic approach coupled with aggressive resuscitation gives the patient with pseudo-PEA the best chance for survival.

True PEA occurs with a primary electromechanical uncoupling of the myocytes. From the cardiac electrical perspective, this uncoupling event is usually characterized by abnormal automaticity and disrupted cardiac conduction that results in the continued presence of a cardiac rhythm, albeit a bradydysrhythmia with a slow and/or widened QRS complex. Mechanically, this uncoupling is likely caused by global myocardial energy depletion. Local myocardial tissue issues (hypoxia, acidosis, hyperkalemia, and ischemia) also contribute to this electromechanical dissociation. True electromechanical disassociation is seen in prolonged cardiac arrest states as well as metabolic, hypothermic, and poisoning sudden death scenarios. Another important subtype of true PEA is characterized by the patient with prolonged VF in whom defibrillation produces an electromechanical dissociation state with a broad QRS complex, bradycardic rhythm. In this instance, near-complete exhaustion of energy substrate associated with profound hypoxia and acidosis accounts for this dismal scenario.

The clinical progression of the PEA event usually starts with an altered perfusion that progresses to pseudo-PEA with continued cardiac contractions. The absence of discernible pulse followed by the loss of cardiac mechanical activity yields the development of true PEA.

■ CLINICAL PRESENTATION

Etiologies of PEA are numerous and span all of acute care medicine, including profound hypovolemia, cardiac tamponade, large anterior wall myocardial infarction, tension pneumothorax, massive pulmonary embolism, severe sepsis, anaphylactic reaction with shock, significant electrolyte abnormality (e.g., disorders of potassium), pronounced metabolic acidosis, substantial cardiotoxic ingestion, and hypothermia (see Table 6-2). These presentations

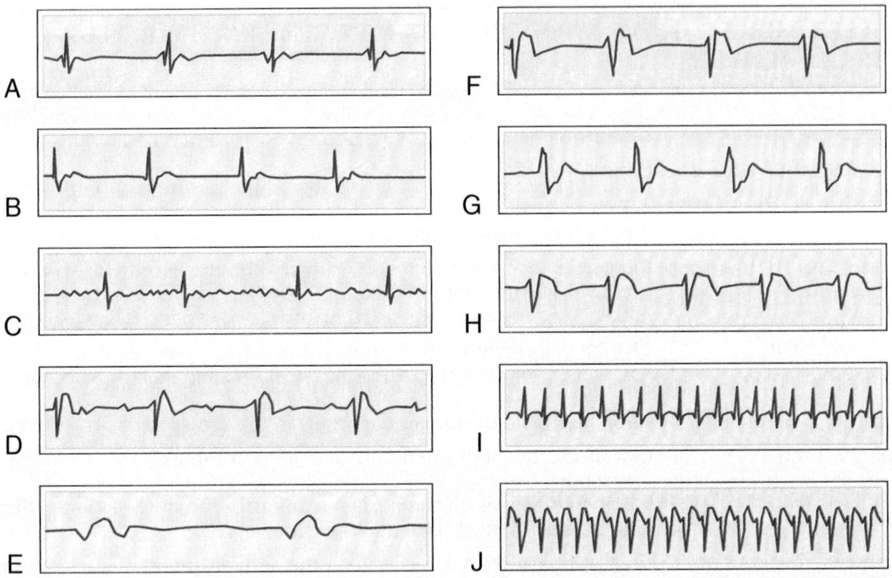
A
B
C
D
E
F
G
H
I
J

FIGURE 6-9 Pulseless electrical activity (PEA). This dysrhythmia requires the absence of detectable mechanical activity of the heart (i.e., the absence of a pulse) with some form of organized electrical activity of the heart (i.e., a rhythm). Any dysrhythmia (other than ventricular fibrillation, ventricular tachycardia, or asystole) can be encountered in this cardiac arrest scenario. The most typical dysrhythmias seen in the PEA presentation are bradycardias with both narrow and wide–QRS complexes. **A,** Sinus bradycardia; **B,** junctional bradycardia; **C,** atrial fibrillation with slow ventricular response; **D,** third-degree atrioventricular block; **E,** idioventricular bradycardia; **F,** idioventricular bradycardia; **G,** idioventricular rhythm; **H,** idioventricular rhythm; **I,** sinus tachycardia; **J,** sinus tachycardia with bundle branch block morphology.

have a final common pathophysiologic denominator of severe hypovolemia (absolute or relative), marked obstruction to flow, and/or profound hypocontractility.

As with the clinical events causing the PEA event, the rhythm presentations are numerous. The dysrhythmias most commonly seen in PEA are idioventricular, junctional, and sinus bradycardias (Figs. 6-8 and 6-9).

Some causes of PEA are reversible if they are recognized early and correctly treated in the initial phases of resuscitation. For instance, a recent history of melena suggests gastrointestinal hemorrhage with profound hypovolemia; recent surgery and dyspnea preceding cardiac arrest suggest pulmonary embolism. A patient with chronic obstructive pulmonary disease or asthma may have a tension pneumothorax, and in a patient with cardiac instrumentation, a pericardial hemorrhagic effusion with tamponade may explain the PEA arrest. Each of these scenarios may represent treatable (and potentially) reversible PEA events.

The electrocardiographic rhythm may be a useful guide to etiology and a key to successful resuscitation. Presentations of tachycardia with rapid, narrow QRS complexes are associated with a better, though still bleak, opportunity for survival. Profound hypovolemia of various causes is the most frequently encountered event in the patient with PEA. In an attempt to maintain cardiac output, the heart increases its rate as its ability to maintain an adequate output declines. This rate increase usually occurs in the form of sinus tachycardia. In patients with atrial fibrillation, a rapid ventricular response is present, creating a presentation that is likely a pseudo-PEA cardiac arrest. Conversely, a slow, wide QRS complex rhythm is a predictor of very poor outcome in the patient with PEA. Prolonged cardiac arrest, profound metabolic disarray, severe overdose, hypothermia, end-stage sepsis, and large anterior wall MI are typical clinical PEA scenarios. In these instances, a true PEA scenario is evolving. Only 2% to 3% of patients with PEA as the initial and/or primary dysrhythmia in cardiac arrest survive to hospital discharge and have a meaningful quality of life.

Electrocardiographic variables may be predictive of successful resuscitation.[14] Rapid rhythm rates are much more frequently associated with a return of spontaneous circulation; for instance, a sinus mechanism with rapid rate (i.e., sinus tachycardia) is seen more often than sinus bradycardia in resuscitated patients. The width of the QRS complex is also potentially predictive of resuscitative outcome. Progressively wider QRS complexes are found in patients with lower likelihood of a restoration of spontaneous perfusion. In this risk prognostication application, an idioventricular rhythm is associated with a lower chance of resuscitation than sinus bradycardia with a normal QRS complex duration. Other electrocardiographic findings encountered in patients with PEA who were successfully resuscitated were the development of P waves and shortened QT intervals.

■ MANAGEMENT

The management of the patient in PEA arrest should focus on both standard resuscitation treatments and

Table 6-3 SUGGESTED RESUSCITATIVE APPROACH TO THE PATIENT WITH PULSELESS ELECTRICAL ACTIVITY

Time	Treatment Priority	Comments
Minute 0	CPR	Compressions should be done at a rate of 100/min and a ratio of 30 compressions to every 2 breaths. Pulse checks and rhythm analysis should be performed no more often than every 2 min. If patient has narrow complex rhythm, assess for occult blood flow (pseudo-PEA).
Minute 1	IV access Vasopressin 40 IU	Medication administration via ET tube, although acceptable, is no longer considered equivalent to IV administration. Initially, vasopressin or epinephrine may be given interchangeably.
Minute 2	ET tube placement Atropine 1 mg	ET tube placement is not a priority unless bag-mask ventilation is inadequate. Assessment for correct ET tube placement should include a secondary confirmation device. Atropine should be administered only in the presence of bradycardic electrical activity.
Minute	Epinephrine 1 mg	CPR should be interrupted only to change compresssions (no longer than 15 seconds). If epinephrine was given initially, vasopressin can now be given; then epinephrine is administered in all subsequent doses.
Minute 5	Supplemental medications	Underlying causes may necessitate the administration of adjunctive medications (see Table 6-2).
Minute 7	Epinephrine 1 mg Atropine 1 mg	Medication dosing frequency in cardiac arrest remains every 3-5 min, with the recognition that peak central levels may vary according to physiologic differences in patients. Atropine should be administered only in the presence of bradycardic electrical activity.
Minute 10	Epinephrine 1 mg Atropine 1 mg	At 10 min, the outcome-related implications should be weighed, because likelihood of patient survival to discharge decreases after this point without restoration of spontaneous circulation.

CPR, cardiopulmonary resuscitation; ET, endotracheal; IV, intravenous; PEA, pulseless electrical activity.

the identification and correction of reversible causes but otherwise is similar to that for patients with VF and pulseless VT (Table 6-3).

Atropine is recommended for bradycardia, given in 1-mg doses every 3 to 5 minutes for a total of 3 mg. The use of atropine is this setting has demonstrated mixed results, with two small series yielding an improved rate of survival to hospital admission with its use[15,16] but a third investigation noting no difference in survival rates.[17]

Asystole

Asystole is the absence of any and all cardiac electrical activity and usually results from a failure of impulse formation in the primary (sinoatrial node) and default pacemaker (atrioventricular node and ventricular myocardium) sites. Asystole can also result from a failure of impulse propagation to the ventricular myocardium from atrial tissues. Ventricular standstill—the absence of ventricular depolarizations with continued atrial electrical activity—is encountered, but most often, atrial and ventricular asystole are present simultaneously, producing the ominous electrocardiographic "flat line."

■ PATHOPHYSIOLOGY

Patients with asystole usually have experienced prolonged cardiac arrest, likely initially manifested as either VT/VF or PEA and ultimately degenerating to a complete cessation of cardiac electrical activity. Asystole can be structurally mediated because of a large myocardial infarction, neurally mediated as seen in aortic stenosis, or functionally mediated as a result of cardiotoxic ingestions or metabolic poisoning. Regardless of the clinical event or responsible mechanism, patients with asystole demonstrate a complete exhaustion of myocardial energy stores. Other characteristics common in asystole are issues similar to those in PEA, such as myocardial hypoxia, acidosis, hyperkalemia, and ischemia.

■ CLINICAL PRESENTATION

The American Heart Association, in its Advanced Cardiac Life Support (ACLS) teaching, describes refractory asystole as "the transition from life to death." Affected patients have likely been in full cardiorespiratory arrest for prolonged periods. Patients presenting with asystole as the initial and/or primary dysrhythmia most often do not survive. At best, 1% to 2% of patients with presumed asystole as the initial and/or primary dysrhythmia in cardiac arrest survive to hospital discharge and have a meaningful quality of life.

In asystole, the ECG demonstrates a flat near-flat or line (Fig. 6-10). Minimal undulations of the electrocardiographic waveform can be seen resulting from electrocardiographic baseline drift. Several pitfalls must be avoided in the apparent asystole presentation, including monitor malfunction, electro-

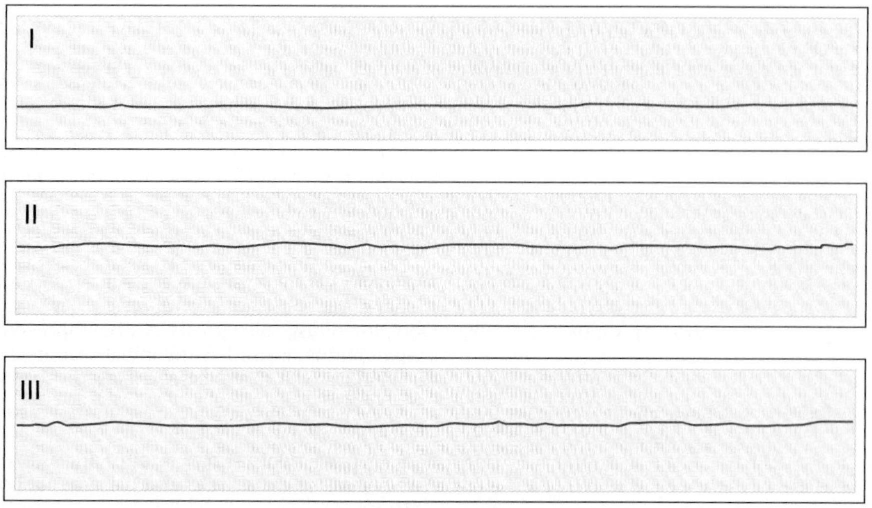
I
II
III

FIGURE 6-10 Asystole. Note the proper determination of asystole in three simultaneous electrocardiographic leads. It is important to view any rhythm with at least two different electrocardiographic leads.

cardiographic lead disconnect, and fine VF with minimal amplitude in the imaging lead. The last potential error can be detected by confirming asystole with at least two leads oriented in perpendicular fashion.

MANAGEMENT

Resuscitation of the patient with asystole should resemble that described in the algorithm for PEA, with the notable exception of the consideration of cardiac pacing (Table 6-4). Although several trials have not demonstrated a benefit of transcutaneous pacing in patients with asystolic arrest,[3,4] it is not unreasonable to consider a short course of cardiac pacing if it is performed very early in the resuscitation. A comment should be made with respect to vasopressor choice: One large study demonstrated a short-term survival benefit of vasopressin over epinephrine in patients with asystole, and this benefit remained apparent at hospital discharge.[10]

Special Arrest Populations and Scenarios

The following situations present unique challenges in resuscitation of the patient in cardiac arrest. Although attention to an acceptable airway, adequate oxygenation and ventilation, and sufficient circulation represent standard priorities in a resuscitation, certain patient characteristics or event scenarios can alter the typical treatment approach. For instance, significant trauma, hypothermic body temperature, and cardiotoxic overdose represent resuscitation scenarios that mandate alterations in the "standard" advanced life support management plans.

TRAUMATIC INJURY

Multiple traumatic causes can lead to cardiac arrest in the setting of trauma. The following pathophysiologic issues can occur individually or in combination and thus lead to cardiorespiratory arrest: (1) severe head injury, (2) profound hypoxia (due to airway obstruction or disruption, pulmonary injury, hemothorax and/or pneumothorax), and (3) diminished cardiac output (exsanguination, tension pneumothorax, pericardial tamponade, and/or myocardial contusion). Prognosis of out-of-hospital cardiac arrest due to trauma is poor, particularly in the setting of blunt injury.[18]

In cases of traumatic arrest for which a clear etiology is not readily apparent, aggressive resuscitation is indicated even though the prognosis is bleak. General trauma management should be performed while specific therapy is aimed at the medical portion of the cardiorespiratory arrest. "Standard" advanced life support interventions aimed at dysrhythmia management should be pursued with the realization that the likelihood of successful resuscitation is minimal. Pulseless VT and VF should be treated with defibrillation immediately upon their recognition. In most traumatic situations, the underlying etiology must be corrected in order for return of circulation to occur.[7] Medical therapies are unlikely to correct the issue and restore spontaneous circulation.

If definitive surgical intervention is available, resuscitative thoracotomy may be a reasonable intervention for a subset of patients. This subset includes any patient with traumatic arrest and any of the following features[7]:

- Witnessed arrest in the ED
- Arrest time less than 5 minutes and penetrating cardiac injury
- Arrest time less than 15 minutes and penetrating thoracic injury
- Any exsanguinating abdominal vascular injury and the presence of secondary signs of life (e.g., pupillary reflexes, spontaneous movement, organized ECG activity)

Thoracotomy allows for internal cardiac massage and defibrillation, relief of pericardial tamponade, direct control of cardiac or thoracic hemorrhage, and cross-clamping of the aorta. Many of these interven-

Table 6-4 SUGGESTED RESUSCITATIVE APPROACH TO THE PATIENT WITH ASYSTOLE

Time	Treatment Priority	Comments
Minute 0	CPR	Compressions should be done at a rate of 100/min and a ratio of 30 compressions to every 2 breaths. Pulse checks and ECG analysis should be performed no more often than every 2 min. ECG findings should be confirmed with use of multiple leads.
Minute 1	TCP IV access Vasopressin 40 IU Atropine 1 mg	Although its use is anecdotal and not recommended by the AHA 2005 guidelines, TCP can be considered early, particularly in a sudden witnessed asystolic event (e.g., Stokes-Adams attack). Medication administration via ET tube, although acceptable, is no longer considered equivalent to IV administration. Outcome of asystolic arrests can be improved when vasopressin, rather than epinephrine, is used as the initial vasopressor. Atropine is given to mediate increased vagal tone.
Minute 2	Assessment for cause ET tube placement	An underlying cause should be considered early in the treatment course so that therapy can be optimized. ET tube placement is not a priority unless bag-mask ventilation is inadequate. Assessment for correct ET tube placement should include a secondary confirmation device.
Minute 4	Epinephrine 1 mg Atropine 1 mg	Although these two vasopressor agents are interchangeable, outcome has been shown to be better when epinephrine is used as the second agent.
Minute 7	Epinephrine 1 mg Atropine 1 mg	Medication dosing frequency in cardiac arrest remains every 3-5 min, with the recognition that peak central levels may vary according to physiologic differences in patients.
Minute 10	Epinephrine 1 mg Atropine 1 mg	At 10 min, the outcome-related implications should be weighed, because likelihood of patient survival to discharge decreases after this point without restoration of spontaneous circulation.

AHA, American Heart Association; CPR, cardiopulmonary resuscitation; ECG, electrocardiogram; ET, endotracheal; TCP, transcutaneous pacing.

tions require a high degree of technical skill and should be attempted only by experienced providers. Nevertheless, the outcome for these patients remains poor.

■ STATUS ASTHMATICUS

More than 4000 deaths occur annually because of asthma. Two general scenarios in the decompensated asthma patient most often account for the cardiac arrest. The first is the sudden onset of a severe exacerbation that rapidly worsens and progresses to full cardiorespiratory arrest. The second involves the patient with progressive bronchospasm that is unresponsive to maximal therapy. Progressive hypoxia and hypercarbia with metabolic and respiratory acidosis account for the ultimate decline. At times in this setting, complications of therapy such as barotrauma cause the hemodynamic decline.

The mainstay of therapy in asthma-induced arrest is overcoming hypoxia and bronchoconstriction. To that end, endotracheal intubation should be rapidly performed, yet barotrauma (primarily pneumothorax) must be avoided.

Decreasing tidal volumes to 4 to 5 mL/kg and reducing the ventilatory rate can avoid excessive increases in lung volumes caused by breath stacking with prolonged inspiratory and expiratory phases. This technique is an extension of controlled hypoventilation, or permissive hypercapnia. If resuscitation is successful with the return of spontaneous perfusion, intravenous administration of sodium bicarbonate is used to maintain a serum pH above 7.20.

External compression of the thorax during the expiratory phase to maximize exhalation has been proposed,[19] yet its use remains controversial and will likely be difficult to coordinate during compressions. Needle or tube thoracostomy decompression should be performed if pneumothorax is detected or suspected. Bilateral decompression for refractory cases is warranted, given the potential for masking of lateralizing signs of pneumothorax.

Standard advanced life support strategies also apply to dysrhythmias. Epinephrine is likely to be the most useful of the standard drug therapies. Correction of acidosis may be necessary to achieve response to sympathomimetic agents via the empirical use of sodium bicarbonate. Addition of isoproterenol, aminophylline, terbutaline, and magnesium may be considered for improved bronchodilation, but their benefit in asthma-induced cardiac arrest has not been reported and is unlikely to achieve success.

■ PREGNANCY

Causes of cardiac arrest specific to the pregnant patient are maternal hemorrhage, toxemia, HELLP (hemolysis, elevated liver enzymes, low platelet count) syndrome, amniotic fluid embolus, and adverse effects of maternal care, including tocolytic and anesthetic therapies. Pregnancy also increases the likelihood of certain nonobstetric causes, including pulmonary embolus, septic shock, cardiovascular diseases such as cardiomyopathy and myocardial infarction, endocrine disorders, and collagen vascular disease. Because of documented increased rates of abuse and homicide among pregnant women, traumatic causes of arrest should also be considered.

Cesarean delivery should be accomplished as soon as cardiac arrest in a pregnant patient is identified. The highest survival rates for infants of more than 24 to 25 weeks' gestational age occur in deliveries performed within 5 minutes of the mother's cardiac arrest. This intervention is most appropriately performed by a multidisciplinary team skilled in emergency obstetrical surgery.[20] Early delivery also may be necessary for the successful resuscitation of the mother. Removal of the fetus allows for decompression of the inferior vena cava and abdominal aorta, thereby improving venous return and cardiac output.

The pregnant patient should be placed in the left lateral decubitus position. Displacement of the gravid uterus should be achieved by elevation of the right hip and lumbar region 15 to 30 degrees from supine. This maneuver is best accomplished with blanket rolls or a commercially available wedge. Manual displacement of the uterus using two hands to lift the uterus and direct it toward the patient's left upper abdomen can be used before the blanket rolls are placed and afterwards to optimize venous return.[20]

No modification of routine advanced life support algorithms is required for the care of the pregnant patient. Owing to increased volumes of distribution, higher doses of medications should be considered if no response is seen to initial dosing, although this recommendation is based solely on anecdote and theory. Venous access and subsequent medication administration should be performed at sites above the diaphragm when possible to avoid failure of the medication to reach central circulation because of decreased venous return. If cardiac arrest occurs in the setting of treatment of eclampsia or premature labor that involves the administration of magnesium, it should be discontinued, and calcium, in the form of 1 g of calcium gluconate, should be administered intravenously.

■ POISONING

Toxidromes—useful means of toxin class identification in the patient with perfusion—may be masked in the setting of cardiac arrest due to prolonged hypoxia and hypoperfusion. Such a confounding factor further complicates the selection of specific antidotes or therapies. Once poisoning is suspected, consultation with a medical toxicologist or poison control center should be sought if feasible.

In the setting of an unknown toxin or mixed ingestion, standard advanced life support algorithms are unlikely to be harmful and probably represent the most appropriate course of action. However, special circumstances apply. For example, a patient with a tricyclic antidepressant overdose might have apparent ventricular tachycardia, but bicarbonate is the treatment of choice. When specific antidotes are required, ACLS is insufficient. If a specific toxin is suspected on the basis of history or clinical signs, the clinician should consider adding targeted therapies. When poisoning is suspected, prolonged resuscitation attempts might be warranted.

■ ELECTRICAL INJURY

The heart, as an electrically driven organ, is particularly sensitive to electrical injury. Alternating current is likely to produce VT through a mechanism similar to the R-on-T phenomenon, and a lightning strike can produce asystole or VT through depolarization of the myocardium by a direct-current shock. In the case of the latter, a patient's spontaneous cardiac activity may return, only to suffer a secondary hypoxic arrest owing to disruption of respiratory drive or thoracic muscle paralysis.

Advanced life support algorithms do not require modification for electrically induced cardiac arrest. The potential for successful resuscitation is higher than for other causes of cardiac arrest, given that patients with electrical injury are typically younger and lack coexisting cardiopulmonary disease. Such patients also often require treatment for trauma and burns, which are common sequelae of electric shock and lightning injury.

■ HYPOTHERMIA

Severe hypothermia causes a marked functional depression of all critical organ systems. This dysfunction can lead to cardiovascular collapse yet may also have a protective effect, allowing for successful resuscitation after prolonged arrest times. Many providers believe that a patient with hypothermia cannot be pronounced dead until rewarming has occurred and resuscitative efforts remain futile. Clinical judgment, however, should still prevail in the decision to attempt resuscitation. In fact, the often quoted maxim "One is not dead until he/she is warm and dead" applies only in select situations and is not a blanket statement for all patients in cardiopulmonary arrest. The two basic types of patient who may actually benefit from rewarming therapy while in cardiorespiratory arrest are the patient in full arrest who has experienced a precipitous decline in body temperature (e.g., fall into a frigid lake in a very cold climate) and the profoundly hypothermic individual with signs of life in whom cardiorespiratory arrest has developed in the ED. In other instances, resuscitation is futile and is therefore not recommended. Furthermore, efforts should be withheld in the presence of obvious lethal injuries, dependent lividity, or obstruction of airways with ice or if chest compressions are impossible owing to advanced freezing. In the patient who has drowned prior to hypothermia, chances of resuscitation are markedly reduced. If resuscitation is pursued in this hypothermic setting, other causes of injury and illness often accompany the hypothermia (e.g., overdose, hypoglycemia, trauma) and should be considered and treated appropriately.

If the decision is made to attempt resuscitation in the patient with complete cardiopulmonary arrest and no signs of life, orotracheal intubation and cardiopulmonary resuscitation with chest compressions should be performed. Further efforts are then guided by core temperature, which should be measured as soon as possible. Needle-type electrodes, if available, are preferred for cardiac monitoring. For severe hypothermia—core temperature lower than 30° C—aggressive active internal rewarming should be undertaken. Measures include warmed, humidified oxygen and intravenous fluids, pleural or peritoneal lavage, and partial or complete cardiopulmonary bypass. A single attempt at defibrillation should be made for VF and pulseless VT. All advanced life support medications should be withheld. The reasons for both of these modifications are that the hypothermic heart will probably remain unresponsive to subsequent shocks and that medications are likely to accumulate to toxic levels in the periphery owing to low-perfusion states, only to "become active" once perfusion has been restored.

For moderate hypothermia—core temperature 30° to 34° C—or once rewarming has raised the core temperature to 30° C, defibrillation should resume according to advanced life support guidelines. Medications may be administered at standard doses, but the interval of administration should be increased. Active internal rewarming should be undertaken or continued. If hypothermia is mild—core temperature higher than 34° C—or when rewarming has raised core temperature to 34°C, standard advanced life support guidelines may be applied. These include decisions regarding termination of resuscitation efforts. If rewarming efforts occur for longer than 45 minutes, volume expansion will likely be necessary owing to vasodilation.

■ SUBMERSION INJURY/NEAR-DROWNING

Cardiac arrest from submersion is usually due to hypoxia, from suffocation, but may also be secondary to head or spinal cord injury. For this reason, early intubation is suggested if feasible and should be performed with manual stabilization of the cervical spine. Aspiration of large volumes of fluid with submersion is rare, but because of pulmonary edema, higher inspiratory and positive end-expiratory pressures may be required to achieve adequate ventilation and oxygenation.

Routine advanced life support algorithms should be used for cardiac arrhythmias without modification. Electrolyte and acid-base disturbances are unlikely causes of cardiac arrest in early presentation of submersion injury and do not warrant empirical therapy. Correction of acidosis should be considered in the patient whose condition deteriorates later, during observation. Prognosis depends on duration of submersion and the severity and duration of hypoxia. Submersion or resuscitative efforts longer than 25 minutes and pulseless arrest on arrival at the ED have been reportedly associated with universal mortality in one pediatric study.[21] A second study correlated the severity of respiratory involvement with mortality, citing 93% mortality for patients presented in arrest.[22] Hypothermia and trauma are common confounders of submersion injury, and appropriate therapy should be applied simultaneously for these conditions if suspected.

REFERENCES

1. Wik L, Hansen TB, Fylling F, et al: Delaying defibrillation to give basic cardiopulmonary resuscitation to patients with out-of-hospital ventricular fibrillation: A randomized trial. JAMA 2003;289:1389-1395.
2. Cobb LA, Fahrenbruch CE, Walsh TR, et al: Influence of cardiopulmonary resuscitation prior to defibrillation in patients with out-of-hospital ventricular fibrillation. JAMA 1999;281:1182-1188.
3. Hedges JR, Syverud SA, Dalsey WC, et al: Prehospital trial of emergency transcutaneous cardiac pacing. Circulation 1987;76:1337-1343.
4. Cummins RO, Graves JR, Larsen MP, et al: Out-of-hospital transcutaneous pacing by emergency medical technicians in patients with asystolic cardiac arrest. N Engl J Med 1993;328:1377-1382.
5. Brady W, Meldon S, DeBehnke D: Comparison of prehospital monomorphic and polymorphic ventricular tachycardia: Prevalence, response to therapy, and outcome. Ann Emerg Med 1995;25:64-70.
6. Brady WJ, DeBehnke DJ, Laundrie D: Prevalence, therapeutic response, and outcome of ventricular tachycardia in the out-of-hospital setting: A comparison of monomorphic ventricular tachycardia, polymorphic ventricular tachycardia, and torsades de pointes. Acad Emerg Med 1999;6: 609-617.
7. ECC Committee, Subcommittees and Task Forces of the American Heart Association: 2005 American Heart Association Guidelines for Cardiopulmonary Resuscitation and Emergency Cardiovascular Care. Circulation 2005; 112(Suppl):IV1-IV203.
8. Stiell IG, Herbert PC, Wells GA, et al: Vasopressin versus epinephrine for inhospital cardiac arrest: A randomized controlled trial. Lancet 2001;358:105-109.
9. Wenzel V, Krismer AC, Arntz HR, et al: A comparison of vasopressin and epinephrine for out-of-hospital cardiopulmonary resuscitation. N Engl J Med 2004;350: 105-113.
10. Guyette FX, Guimond GE, Hostler D, Callaway CW: Vasopressin administration with epinephrine is associated with a return of a pulse in out-of-hospital cardiac arrest. Resuscitation 2004;63:277-282.
11. Kudenchuk PJ, Cobb LA, Copass MK, et al: Amiodarone for resuscitation after out-of-hospital due to ventricular fibrillation. N Engl J Med 1999;346:871-878.
12. Dorian P, Cass D, Schwartz B, et al: Amiodarone as compared with lidocaine for shock-resistant ventricular fibrillation. N Engl J Med 2002;346:884-890.
13. Somberg JC, Biailin SJ, Haffajee CI, et al: Intravenous lidocaine versus intravenous amiodarone for incessant ventricular tachycardia. Am J Cardiol 2002;90:853-859.
14. Aufderheide TP, Thakur RK, Steuven HA, et al: Electrocardiographic characteristics in EMD. Resuscitation 1989; 17:183-193.
15. Steuven HA, Tonsfeldt DJ, Thompson BM, et al: Atropine in asystole: Human studies. Ann Emerg Med 1984;13: 815-817.
16. Brown DC, Lewis AJ, Criley JM: Asystole and its treatment: The possible role of parasympathetic nervous system in cardiac arrest. J Am Coll Emerg Phys 1979;8:448-452.

17. Coon GA, Clinton JE, Ruiz E: Use of atropine for brady-asystolic prehospital cardiac arrest. Ann Emerg Med 1981;10:462-467.
18. Rosemugy AS, Norris PA, Olson SM, et al: Prehospital traumatic cardiac arrest: The cost of futility. J Trauma 1993;35: 468-743.
19. Van der Touw T, Mudiliar Y, Nayyar V: Cardiorespiratory effects of manually compressing the rib cage during tidal expiration in mechanically ventilated patients recovering from acute severe asthma. Crit Care Med 1998;26: 1361-1367.
20. Whitty JE: Maternal cardiac arrest in pregnancy. Obstet Gynecol 2002;45:377-392.
21. Quan L, Kinder D: Pediatric submersions: Prehospital predictors of outcome. Pediatrics 1992;90:909-913.
22. Spilman D: Near-drowning and drowning classification: a proposal to stratify mortality based on the analysis of 1,831 cases. Chest 1997;112:660-665.

Chapter 7

Trauma Resuscitation

Trevor J. Mills

KEY POINTS

Early, systematic evaluation and treatment of patients with trauma can save lives and minimize injury.

Initial trauma resuscitation (the primary survey) concentrates on immediate recognition and treatment of life-threatening injuries.

Subsequent trauma resuscitation (the secondary survey) identifies each injury in a comprehensive fashion.

Perspective

Injury is a leading cause of death and disability worldwide. In the United States, traumatic death is especially significant in young people; in people between 1 and 44 years old, unintentional injury is the primary cause of death.[1] Approximately half of the deaths due to trauma occur on the scene, or before the patients reach the hospital. Another 30% of deaths can occur in the first few hours after the event.

Trauma resuscitation is based on the assumption that all severely injured patients can be initially evaluated and treated by the same set of guidelines. Regardless of specific injury, these guidelines focus on the broader concept of sustaining life by maximizing oxygenation, ventilation, and perfusion—the ABCs of trauma resuscitation.

Pathophysiology

The primary survey prioritizes rapid evaluation of the airway and the respiratory and circulatory systems.

In the traumatized patient, the loss of an airway and/or respiratory failure may be due to direct injury to the head, face, oropharynx, neck, trachea, bronchi, chest, or lungs. Alternatively, airway and respiratory compromise may be caused by an indirect injury that results in loss of muscle control or respiratory drive, aspiration of blood, tissue, teeth, or gastric contents, or air or fat emboli.

Likewise, there are several causes of traumatic shock. This condition is most frequently due to direct hemorrhagic blood loss but may have other indirect etiologies. Shock in the patient with trauma could be due to damage to the heart or great vessels, compression of the heart, or tension pneumothorax. Alternative causes of traumatic shock include transection of the spinal cord, leading to spinal (neurogenic) shock. Traumatic injuries may lead to hypoxia or adrenergic surge, either of which results in acute coronary ischemia, arrhythmias, or cardiogenic shock (Box 7-1).

Clinical Presentation

What appears to be an insignificant injury can sometimes be fatal. Therefore, specific clinical presentations that have a high risk of representing fatal problems have been identified. The American College of Surgeons and many emergency medical services (EMS) systems have adopted criteria for transport of patients to a trauma center.[2] These trauma center

BOX 7-1

Causes of Respiratory Compromise and Shock in Trauma

Causes of Traumatic Airway/Respiratory Compromise

- Direct trauma to the face, oropharynx, neck, trachea, or pulmonary system resulting in airway obstruction or respiratory compromise
- Indirect injury due to brain or spine injury (loss of drive), fat or air pulmonary emboli, or aspiration of blood or gastric contents

Causes of Shock in the Traumatized Patient

- Hemorrhagic shock
- Injury to the heart (cardiac contusion, valve rupture, penetrating trauma)
- Compression of the heart due to tamponade or tension pneumothorax
- Cardiogenic shock (ischemia, arrhythmias)
- Neurogenic or spinal shock

criteria attempt to identify the traumatized patient who has early physiologic changes, readily apparent serious injury (anatomic criteria), or a mechanism with a high likelihood of significant injury (Box 7-2).

Criteria for expedited trauma center evaluation include alteration in mental status, hemodynamic instability or respiratory compromise, evident serious anatomic injuries such as thoracic trauma, multiple long-bone fractures, amputations, paralysis, burns, and pelvic fractures (see Red Flags box). Injury mechanisms with a high likelihood of morbidity require presumptive trauma center evaluation. Examples are penetrating trauma to the head, neck, chest, abdomen, and proximal extremities as well as significant motor vehicle collisions.

■ ALTERNATIVE PRESENTATIONS

Some types of patients have serious injuries but few obvious signs. They include the elderly, the very young, patients with known coagulopathies, and those with reduced physiologic reserve due to chronic disease or acute intoxication. All of these types of patients are at high risk of serious injury with even minor mechanisms. Furthermore, the serious injury may not be readily apparent. The trauma center criteria are an attempt to maximize sensitivity for serious injury but are not perfect. In the decision to route patients to a trauma center, EMS medical control should take age and underlying physiology into consideration.

BOX 7-2

Criteria for Identification of Traumatized Patients with a High Probability of Injury that Requires Transport to a Trauma Center

Physiologic Criteria

- Glasgow Coma Scale score <14
- Respiratory rate <10 or >29 breaths/min
- Systolic blood pressure <90 mm Hg or the pediatric equivalent

Anatomic Criteria (Injuries Need Only Be Suspected)

- Flail chest
- Two or more long-bone fractures
- Amputations proximal to wrist or ankle
- Penetrating trauma to head, neck, chest, or abdomen or to extremity proximal to elbow or knee
- Limb paralysis
- Pelvic fractures
- Combination of significant trauma with burns

Mechanism of Injury

- Ejection from auto
- Death of other person in the same vehicle
- Pedestrian hit by vehicle
- High-speed motor vehicle collision
- Falls of more than 20 ft
- Rollover motor vehicle collision
- Duration of extrication of patient from entrapment longer than 20 min
- Motorcycle crash at speed higher than 20 mph or with separation of patient from motorcycle

RED FLAGS

Early alterations in vital signs
Altered mental status
Patient at either extreme of age
Extrication of patient from entrapment long
Transport time to trauma center long
Weakness or paralysis

Differential Diagnosis

■ TRAUMATIC RESUSCITATION

The differential diagnosis for the patient who requires traumatic resuscitation is extensive, and often involves injuries to one or more anatomic areas.

Head injuries may involve a decreased level of consciousness leading to loss of airway protection or respiratory drive. Head injuries can also result in hemorrhagic shock because both the scalp and face have abundant vascular supply. Because of their proportionally larger heads, children may lose a significant amount of blood into closed intracranial hemorrhages. Scalp injury can cause both adults and children to become hemodynamically unstable from blood loss, so early or immediate closure of wounds is prudent. For further specific evaluation and treatment of head injuries, see Chapter 68.

Injury to the face, including the unstable midface, or trauma to the oropharynx may cause direct airway compromise. Facial injuries can also lead to aspiration of blood, tissue, teeth, and bone. Like head injuries, facial injuries can result in significant hemorrhage because the face has a large vascular supply. Early or prophylactic intubation should be considered if hemorrhage is present.

High spinal injuries may lead to loss of airway control, loss of respiratory drive, or hemodynamic instability due to spinal shock. Paralysis may also make the evaluation of other injuries extremely difficult. Thoracic injuries can result in direct tracheal, pulmonary, or cardiac damage, leading to significant intrathoracic hemorrhage or direct respiratory compromise.

Because the abdominal cavity can hold a large amount of blood, solid organ or vascular injury in the abdomen can easily result in hemodynamic collapse. Pelvic fractures are also a potential site of significant blood loss due to uncontrolled venous bleeding. Finally, even isolated extremity injuries can result in arterial hemorrhage or considerable blood loss in the form of fracture-related hematomas. Fractures may also cause delayed respiratory distress because of fat emboli.

■ MOST THREATENING INJURIES

In each of the major anatomic areas, there are subtle but important clues to potentially life- and limb-threatening injures (Table 7-1).

Diagnostic Testing

■ PRIMARY SURVEY

During the primary survey, diagnosis and treatment rely on the physical examination. Although the execution of the survey should be fluid and may involve multiple individuals performing multiple actions simultaneously, the components of the primary survey can be broken down into six sequential steps: airway, breathing, circulation, disability, exposure, and fingers/Foley (ABCDEF; Fig. 7-1 and Priority Actions box).

The initial evaluation of the airway (A) starts with a question to the patient to evaluate for response (airway patency) and then direct visualization of the facial structures and oropharynx.

Breathing or ventilatory status can then be evaluated through visual examination of the trachea and

Table 7-1 SIGNS OF SIGNIFICANT INJURIES IN THE PATIENT WITH TRAUMA

Anatomic Area	Most Threatening Signs
Head	Cerebrospinal fluid leak Raccoon eyes Battle's sign Hemotympanum Anisocoria
Neck	Expanding hematoma Thrill or murmur Subcutaneous air Trachea deviated from midline Pulsatile hemorrhage
Spine	Paralysis Paresthesias Decreased rectal tone
Chest	Subcutaneous air Multiple rib fractures Sucking chest wound Asymmetrical chest rise
Abdomen	Abdominal wall bruising Distended abdomen
Pelvis	Unstable pelvis Large expanding hematoma Blood at the urethral meatus Scrotal hematoma Bone fragments in vaginal vault or rectum High-riding prostate
Extremities	Pallor Decrease in or absence of pulses Weakness or paralysis

PRIORITY ACTIONS

Primary Survey

A = Airway control

B = Breathing: Maximize ventilation

C = Circulation: Stabilize hemodynamic status

D = Disabilty: Evaluate mental status and perform neurologic examination

E = Exposure: Completely undress and examine patient

F = Fingers and Foley: Perform orogastric, bladder catheter, vaginal, and rectal examinations

Secondary Survey

Head-to-toe physical examination

AMPLIFIED (allergies, medications, past medical history, last meal, immediate events, friends/family report of the event, immunizations, emergency medical technician–obtained history, drugs [current medications]) history

Laboratory tests and radiographs

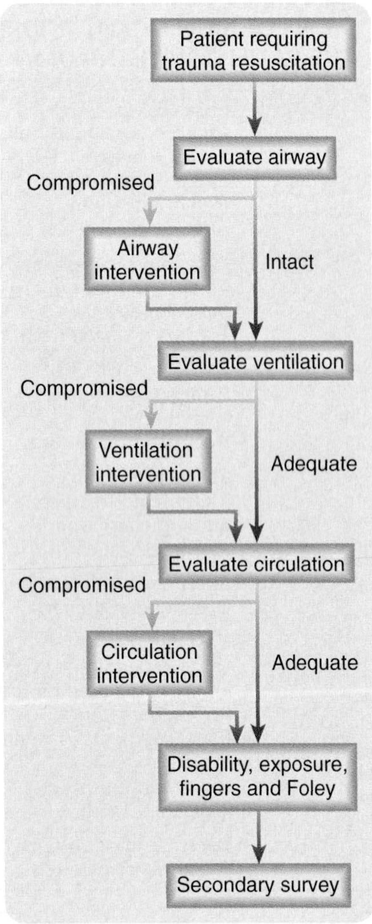
Patient requiring trauma resuscitation
Evaluate airway
Compromised
Airway intervention
Intact
Evaluate ventilation
Compromised
Ventilation intervention
Adequate
Evaluate circulation
Compromised
Circulation intervention
Adequate
Disability, exposure, fingers and Foley
Secondary survey

FIGURE 7-1 Approach to traumatic resuscitation.

thorax, auscultation of all lung fields, and palpation of the chest. Palpation can provide clues to rib injury, open or sucking chest wounds, and subcutaneous air in the neck and chest. Respiratory rate, patient report of chest pain or shortness of breath, and pulse oximetry also contribute to the B phase of the resuscitation.

Evaluation of the circulatory status (C) involves judgment of general appearance, heart rate and blood pressure, extremity pulses, and nail bed capillary refill. If the patient has not been connected on a continuous heart rate and blood pressure monitor, this step can be taken now. It is important to remember that any abnormality found in this initial phase of the resuscitation usually mandates immediate intervention and then reevaluation.

The next step is a brief neurologic examination (for disability; D). At this point, disability assessment does not include a detailed neurologic examination, but instead looks for gross motor movement of all extremities and level of alertness. The most common tool for evaluating global neurologic function is the Glasgow Coma Scale (GCS) (Table 7-2).[3] Three systems are evaluated (eye opening, verbal response, and motor response). The closer each function is to baseline, the higher the score for each system. A GCS score of 13 or higher correlates with a mild brain injury, 9 to 12 with a moderate injury, and 8 or less with a severe brain injury. A GCS score lower than 8 is an indication for immediate secure airway control. Thus the GCS can help with evaluation for the need of intubation as well as provide a marker for serial neurologic examinations and clear communication with consultants regarding patient status.

Table 7-2 GLASGOW COMA SCALE (GCS) SCORING*

Response	Score
Eye opening:	
No eye opening	1
Eye opening to pain	2
Eye opening to verbal command	3
Eyes open spontaneously	4
Verbal:	
No verbal response	1
Incomprehensible sounds	2
Inappropriate words	3
Patient confused	4
Patient oriented	5
Motor:	
No motor response	1
Extension to pain	2
Flexion to pain	3
Withdrawal from pain	4
Patient localizes pain	5
Patient obeys commands	6

*The best of each response is used for the individual score; scores are added for total GCS score.

Completion of the primary survey involves exposure of the entire patient (E) in a way that prevents hypothermia; coordinated in-line cervical spine immobilization should be maintained during this procedure. The F (fingers and Foley) step of the primary survey involves placement of a Foley bladder catheter and orogastric tube, a rectal examination, and a bimanual vaginal examination.

■ SECONDARY SURVEY

The secondary survey comprises a brief, expanded history, a head-to-toe examination, and initiation of the standard trauma radiographic procedures and laboratory tests. If possible, the history should be taken from the patient or the prehospital personnel (e.g., emergency medical technicians [EMTs]) who delivered the patient to the hospital. The key points of the history can be remembered with use of the mnemonic AMPLIFIED, which stands for allergies, medications, past medical history, last meal, immediate events, friends/family report of the event, immunizations, EMT-obtained history, and drugs (current medications).

The head-to-toe examination involves a second review of the airway and pulmonary examination as well as an expanded physical examination to identify further injury.

The advantage of the standard "trauma series" radiographs (cervical spine radiograph, chest radio-

Table 7-3 TRAUMA SERIES RADIOGRAPHS

Structure and View(s)	Advantages	Disadvantages
Cervical spine (anteroposterior [AP], lateral, odontoid)	Inexpensive Good initial screening tool for significant fractures	Not 100% sensitive for fracture detection May miss ligamentous injuries Does not evaluate spinal cord injury
AP chest	Inexpensive Good initial screening tool for significant thoracic and pulmonary injuries	Will miss small pneumothorax May falsely show a widened mediastinum Low sensitivity for cardiac injuries
AP pelvis	Inexpensive Good initial screening tool for major pelvis fractures	Not 100% sensitive for fracture detection

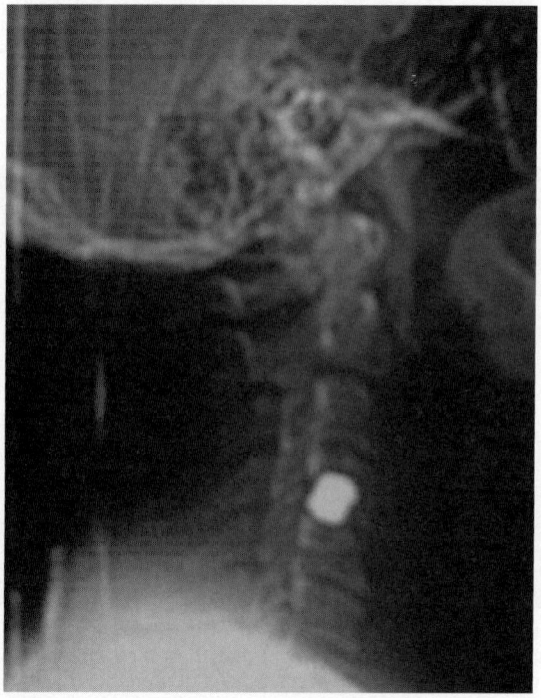

FIGURE 7-2 This case demonstrates the need for the "trauma series" radiographs even in patients with penetrating trauma. Radiograph shows that this patient sustained a gunshot wound to the shoulder, without obvious injury to the neck.

graph, and pelvic radiograph) is to identify life-threatening injuries that may necessitate immediate attention (Table 7-3; Fig. 7-2). Significant cervical spine fractures may lead to airway compromise, loss of ventilatory drive, or spinal shock. The chest radiograph may identify a treatable condition, such as a large pneumothorax, hemothorax, or pulmonary contusion. A pelvic radiograph should identify the open-book pelvis fracture that may lead to hemorrhagic shock. Although each of the three radiographs is important, none of them is comprehensive or the most sensitive imaging modality available. After the secondary survey is complete and the screening films are evaluated, more sensitive and specific imaging modalities should be ordered.

The abdominal cavity can "hide" enough blood to warrant immediate evaluation for intra-abdominal hemorrhage (Table 7-4). The advent of the focused abdominal sonography examination for trauma (FAST) provides the answer to this question. The FAST can be done in the resuscitation area. Because it is faster and less invasive to obtain, the FAST has for the most part replaced diagnostic peritoneal lavage (DPL).[4,5] Likewise, the more sensitive computed tomography (CT) of the abdomen should be reserved for patients with a sufficiently stable hemodynamic status, because CT scanning may be time-consuming and takes the patient out of the resuscitation area.[6]

Blood specimens for laboratory studies may be drawn during the initiation of intravenous (IV) access during the primary survey or can be obtained during the secondary survey. Laboratory tests should include complete blood count, serum chemical analysis, coagulation studies (prothrombin time, partial thromboplastin time), and urinalysis. Two immediately available studies are the urine pregnancy test and finger-stick serum glucose measurement, results of either of which can significantly change the course of the resuscitation. In the setting of altered mental status, a blood alcohol measurement and toxicology screen may also be useful. The serum lactate level can be monitored as a marker of tissue perfusion.[7,8]

After the primary and secondary surveys are completed and the patient is sufficiently resuscitated, the evaluation and treatment plan takes on a much more individualized course.[9]

Special Circumstances

Depending on the specific patient's presentation,[10] injuries, underlying diseases, and age, each injury may necessitate further study (Table 7-5), observation, or surgical intervention.

Treatment (Intervention and Procedures)

The key to maximizing the success of trauma resuscitation is the early diagnosis and treatment of injury. The extent of damage from many significant injuries can be reduced with early intervention, includ-

Table 7-4 DIAGNOSTIC MODALITIES USED IN ABDOMINAL TRAUMA

Modality	Advantages	Disadvantages
Radiographs	Inexpensive Easy to obtain and read Good for identification of foreign objects and projectiles May be useful as screening for free air prior to DPL	Very low sensitivity and specificity for injury in the patient with blunt abdominal trauma
Computed tomography (CT)	High sensitivity High specificity	Patient has to leave resuscitation area
Ultrasonography (US)	Easy and quick	Operator-dependent Variable sensitivity and specificity for organ injury
Diagnostic peritoneal lavage (DPL)	High sensitivity High specificity	Operator-dependent Time-consuming More invasive than CT or US Significant complications (perforated bowel, bleeding, infection)

Tips and Tricks

Intubation

- Prepare equipment.
- Preoxygenate the patient with 100% O_2.
- Evaluate oropharynx.
- Use end-tidal CO_2 detector.
- Have alternative method available.

Chest Tube Placement

- Extend arm on side of chest tube above head.
- Use local anesthesia.
- Have cell saver in pleural evacuation unit (Pleurovac) prior to patient arrival.

IV Access

- Place access site away from injury(ies).
- Consider external jugular vein approach.
- Consider femoral central venous access.

Focused Abdominal Sonography for Trauma (FAST)

- Clamp Foley catheter.
- Perform serial examinations if vital signs change.

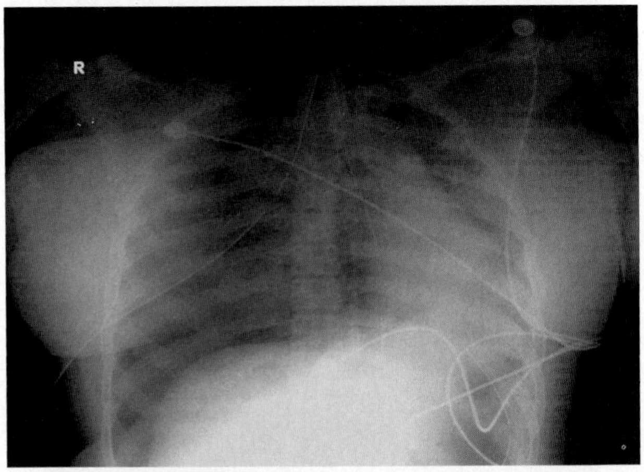
R

FIGURE 7-3 The patient whose radiograph is shown here initially improved with placement of a chest tube, but later had decompensation. This case represents a good reason for the need to restart the ABCs of trauma resuscitation after any change in patient condition or after any intervention.

ing cervical spine immobilization throughout the resuscitation.

During the primary survey, if an indication for intervention is discovered, treatment should be initiated and the primary survey restarted from the beginning (Fig. 7-3). For the severely injured patient, the primary airway intervention is orotracheal intubation using rapid sequence induction (RSI). Indications for airway intervention include airway protection, expected clinical course, and the need for assisted ventilation or airway protection (Box 7-3).

Alternative methods to orotracheal intubation include nasotracheal intubation, cricothyrotomy, laryngeal mask airway, retrograde intubation, and transtracheal jet insufflation. At minimum, 100% oxygen should be administered via a nonrebreather mask to maximize tissue oxygenation.

After the airway is controlled, respiratory status is evaluated. Several alterations in ventilation mandate immediate intervention (Table 7-6).

After airway and breathing are evaluated and stabilized, hemodynamic status should be evaluated. During trauma resuscitation, it is imperative to immediately establish IV access, which can facilitate rapid transfusion and/or administration of blood products (18-gauge IV or larger). Ideal guidelines recommend a minimum of two working IV sites. Alternatives to large-bore peripheral IV access are intraosseous lines,

Table 7-5 ADDITIONAL STUDIES IN TRAUMA PATIENTS DICTATED BY SPECIAL CIRCUMSTANCES

Trauma Presentation	Additional Studies
Altered mental status, head trauma	Head computed tomography (CT) Brain magnetic resonance imaging (MRI) CT angiogram of cerebral vascular system See also Chapter 68 for detailed evaluation of head trauma.
Chest wall trauma	Repeat chest radiography Full upright posteroanterior and lateral chest radiographs CT of the chest Angiogram MRI of the chest See also Chapter 73 for detailed evaluation of chest/thoracic trauma.
Abdominal trauma	CT of the abdomen Focused abdominal sonographic examination for trauma (FAST) Diagnostic peritoneal lavage See also Chapters 74 and 75 for detailed evaluation of abdominal trauma.
Pelvis	Retrograde urethrogram Cystogram CT of abdomen and pelvis
Extremity	Angiography
Neck/back/spine	CT or MRI of the cervical, thoracic, or lumbar spine
Obstetric	Ultrasonography Fetal heart monitoring

Table 7-6 INDICATIONS FOR RESPIRATORY INTERVENTION IN PATIENTS WITH TRAUMA

Indication	Intervention
Tension pneumothorax	Needle decompression
Pneumothorax/hemothorax	Tube thoracostomy
Sucking chest wound	Tube thoracostomy, petroleum jelly (Vaseline) compression dressing
Pulmonary contusion with hypoxia	Intubation

BOX 7-3

Indications for Airway Intervention

- Decreased level of consciousness (Glasgow Coma Scale score <8)
- Extreme agitation
- Presence of or impending airway obstruction
- Presence of or impending compromise of ventilation
- Need for immediate surgical intervention
- Hemodynamic instability

central lines, and venous cutdown lines. In the hypotensive adult patient with trauma, an initial bolus of two liters of warm normal saline or lactated Ringer's is a reasonable starting point. In children, a 20 mL/kg bolus should be used. If the traumatized patient remains hypotensive after the initial bolus, then transfusion of type 0-negative or type-specific blood should be considered. A caveat to this statement is in the patient who has sustained penetrating trauma to the chest or abdomen, in whom a short period of permissive hypotension (on the way to the operating room) may improve survivability by not disrupting an internal tamponade.[5] When possible, manual pressure or military tourniquets should be used in conjunction with fluid or blood resuscitation to temporize hemorrhage.

Once the primary survey is completed and the patient is stabilized, the secondary survey is used to unveil the remaining injuries. Patients may then require specific care of individual injuries or specialty consult as needed.

Disposition

All patients requiring trauma evaluation and treatment because of anatomic or physiologic trauma center criteria (see Box 7-2) must be admitted to the hospital. Patients who meet mechanism criteria only and in whom thorough evaluation identifies no injuries may be candidates for discharge with careful warnings and solid discharge planning.

Documentation

The following categories of information should appear in the documentation for every patient with trauma.

History

- Prehospital history
- Detailed mechanism (speed of vehicle, height of fall, etc.)
- Circumstances (damage to vehicle, type of weapon, etc.)
- Timing of event
- Time to ED
- Concurrent medications
- Drug or alcohol use
- Past medical history
- Last meal
- Immunizations
- Prior operations

Physical Examination

- Primary survey and interventions
- Head-to-toe examination

Studies

- ED interpretation of radiographs
- Results of focused abdominal sonography examination for trauma (FAST) or diagnostic peritoneal lavage (DPL)

Medical Decision-Making

- Reasons to pursue or not pursue work-up of each injury
- Consultation of surgical or other subspecialists

Procedures

- Each procedure (document in full)

Patient Instructions

- Discussion of injuries and potential outcomes with patient and/or patient's family

PATIENT TEACHING TIPS

- Recovery from injuries takes time and often extensive rehabilitation.
- Recidivism for certain injuries is high; consider referrals to specific programs according to circumstances.
- Prevention of further injury, wound care, cast care, etc.
- Warning signs for which patient should seek immediate care.

REFERENCES

1. WISQARS Leading Causes of Death Reports, 1999-2003. Available at http://webapp.cdc.gov/sasweb/ncipc/leadcaus10.html/
2. American College of Surgeons: Advanced Trauma Life Support Program for Doctors, 7th ed. Chicago, American College of Surgeons, 2007.
3. Teasdale G, Jennett B: Assessment of coma and impaired consciousness: A practical scale. Lancet 1974;2(7872): 81-94.
4. Blaivas M, Lyon M, Brannam L, et al: Bedside emergency ultrasonographic diagnosis of diaphragmatic rupture in blunt abdominal trauma. Am J Emerg Med 2004; 22:601-604.
5. Branney S, Moore EE, Cantrill SV, et al: Ultrasound based key clinical pathway reduces the use of hospital resources for the evaluation of blunt abdominal trauma. J Trauma 1997;42:1086-1090.
6. Grieshop N, Jacobson LE, Gomez GA, et al: Selective use of computed tomography and diagnostic peritoneal lavage in blunt abdominal trauma. J Trauma 1995;38:727-731.
7. Asimos AW, Gibbs MA, Marx JA, et al: Value of point of care blood testing in emergent trauma management. J Trauma 2000;24:1101-1108.
8. Lavery RF, Livingston DH, et al: The utility of venous lactate to triage injured patients in the trauma center. J Am Coll Surg 2000;190:656-664.
9. Giannoudis PV: Surgical priorities in damage control in polytrauma. J Bone Joint Surg Br 2003;85:478-483.
10. Shah AJ, Kilcline BA: Trauma in pregnancy. Emerg Med Clin North Am 2003;21:615-629.

Chapter **8**

The Focused Assessment with Sonography for Trauma

Emily Baran

KEY POINTS

- The indication for the focused assessment with sonography for trauma (FAST) is the rapid evaluation of blunt or penetrating trauma to the torso in which there is clinical suspicion for intraperitoneal hemorrhage, pericardial tamponade, and/or hemothorax.
- Standard views used in the FAST are right upper quadrant/hepatorenal (Morrison's pouch), left upper quadrant/splenorenal, pelvic/suprapubic, and subxyphoid cardiac.
- Additional views can include the paracolic gutters and the apical or parasternal cardiac windows.
- The patient is imaged in the supine or in the Trendelenburg position.
- A 2- to 5-MHz curvilinear probe, or a probe with similar frequency and a smaller footprint, should be used.
- The question that a FAST tries to answer is "Does this trauma patient have blood in the peritoneum, pleural spaces, or pericardium?" The results may be positive, negative, or equivocal/inadequate.

Background

The physical examination is surprisingly inaccurate in the setting of abdominal trauma, and indeterminate physical findings are common because of intubation, altered mental status, or neurologic or distracting injuries. Diagnostic peritoneal lavage (DPL) and computed tomography (CT) were the primary methods used to evaluate patients with abdominal trauma until ultrasound imaging began being used, in Japan and Europe in the 1970s and in the United States in the early 1990s. CT provides the best information about site and extent of organ injury and remains the examination of choice in stable patients.

Ultrasound imaging, however, has clear advantages over both CT and DPL because it can be performed at the bedside rapidly, noninvasively, and without radiation exposure. Ultrasound imaging is also easily repeatable. In the setting of trauma, a standard approach has been developed, the focused assessment with sonography for trauma (FAST). This examination has become the standard of care in the evaluation of trauma patients and has been incorporated into the American College of Surgeons' Advanced Trauma Life Support (ATLS) curriculum. The FAST is probably the most universally accepted and studied application of emergency ultrasound. It has proven utility in identifying patients with blunt abdominal trauma who must undergo exploratory laparotomy and decreases the time to surgical intervention.[1-2]

Indication

The indication for performing a FAST is rapid evaluation of blunt or penetrating trauma to the torso in which there is clinical suspicion of intraperitoneal hemorrhage, pericardial tamponade, and/or hemothorax. The clinical question that a FAST tries to answer is "Does this trauma patient have blood in the peritoneum, pleural spaces, or pericardium?"

A simplified algorithm for evaluation of a patient with the FAST is shown in Figure 8-1. The most important pathway is highlighted in red. The FAST's primary purpose should be to rapidly identify free fluid in the hemodynamically unstable trauma patient and, in the setting of intraperitoneal hemorrhage, determine that the patient must be transferred immediately to the operating room for lifesaving intervention. The FAST is an important adjunct to the emergency care of the trauma patient and should complement, not interfere with, basic airway-breathing-circulation evaluation and resuscitation.

Anatomy and Approach

The trauma patient is usually imaged in the supine position. Trendelenburg positioning can be used to improve the sensitivity of the examination. A 2- to 5-MHz abdominal curvilinear probe or similar-frequency probe with a smaller footprint can be used.

In the patient with trauma, free fluid collects in predictable peritoneal recesses. These recesses are examined, in addition to the pericardial space and pleural spaces, during the FAST. The four standard views are right upper quadrant, left upper quadrant, pelvic, and subxiphoid cardiac. Approximate transducer position for each of the views with representative images are demonstrated in Figures 8-2 to 8-7. The depth and gain settings on the machine may have to be adjusted for each of the four views; specifically, more depth is often needed for the subxiphoid cardiac view, and less far-field gain is often used for better pelvic images (see Fig. 8-7).

Clinical studies suggest that the right upper quadrant view is the most sensitive single view for hemoperitoneum, because blood from a pelvic or left upper quadrant source overflows to the perihepatic region (Fig. 8-8). In each standard area, it is important to scan or fan through the entire space to look for free fluid. In the upper quadrant views, it is also important to look above the diaphragm for hemothorax.

Additional ultrasound views for trauma are imaging inferior to the hepatorenal and splenorenal regions

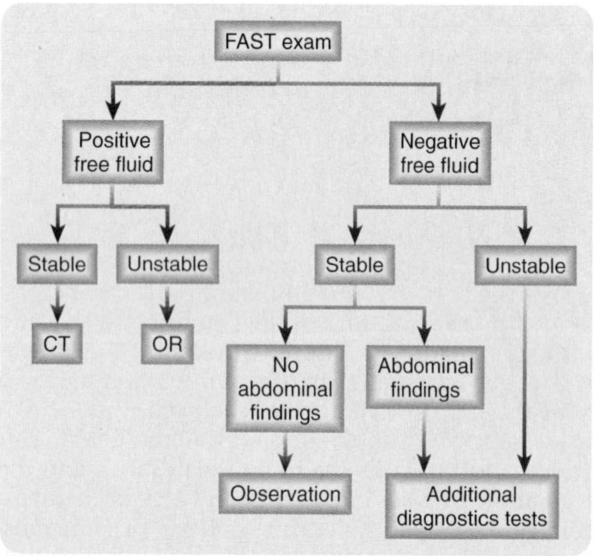
FAST exam
Positive free fluid
Negative free fluid
Stable
Unstable
Stable
Unstable
CT
OR
No abdominal findings
Abdominal findings
Observation
Additional diagnostics tests

FIGURE 8-1 Simplified algorithm for medical decision-making using the focused assessment with sonography for trauma (FAST). The primary purpose of the FAST is to rapidly identify life-threatening injuries and direct appropriate intervention. CT, computed tomography; OR, operating room.

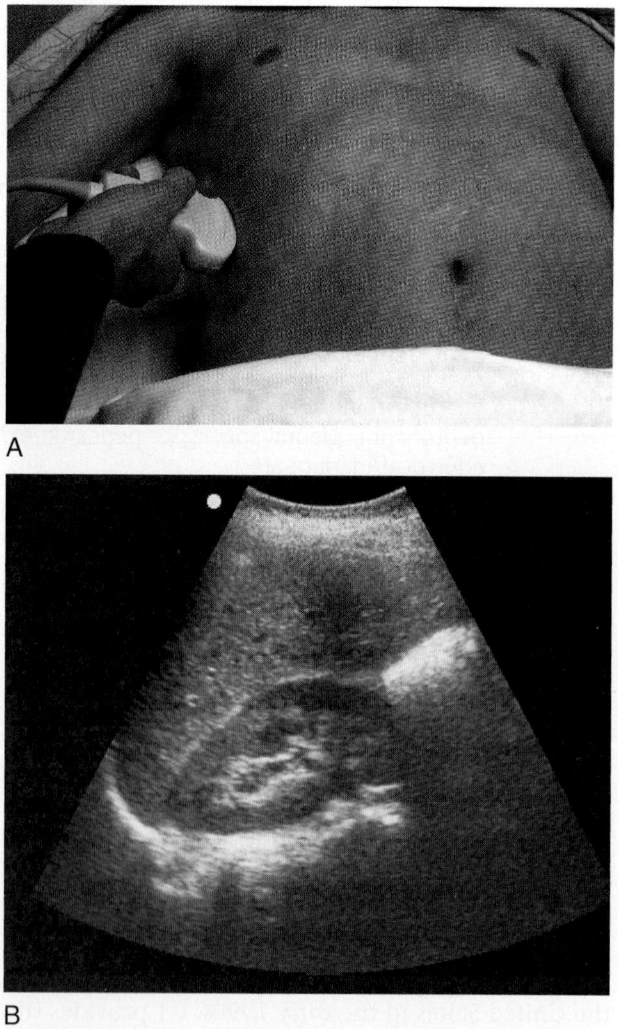
A
B

FIGURE 8-2 **A,** Right upper quadrant view demonstrating approximate probe position (*red sticker* represents probe indicator). **B,** Normal image.

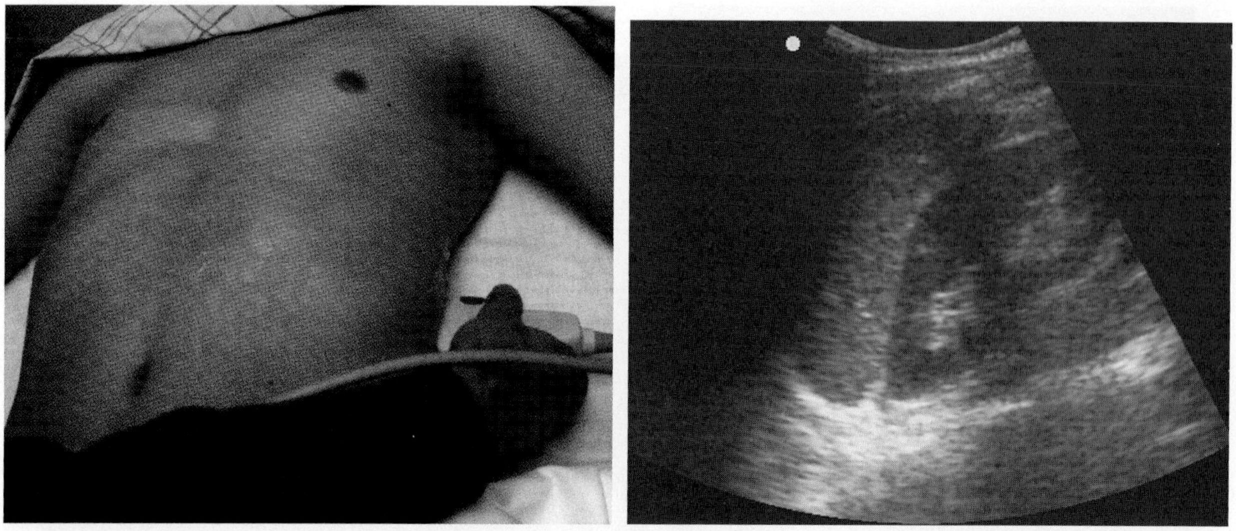

A B

FIGURE 8-3 **A,** Left upper quadrant view demonstrating approximate probe position (*red sticker* represents probe indicator). **B,** Normal image.

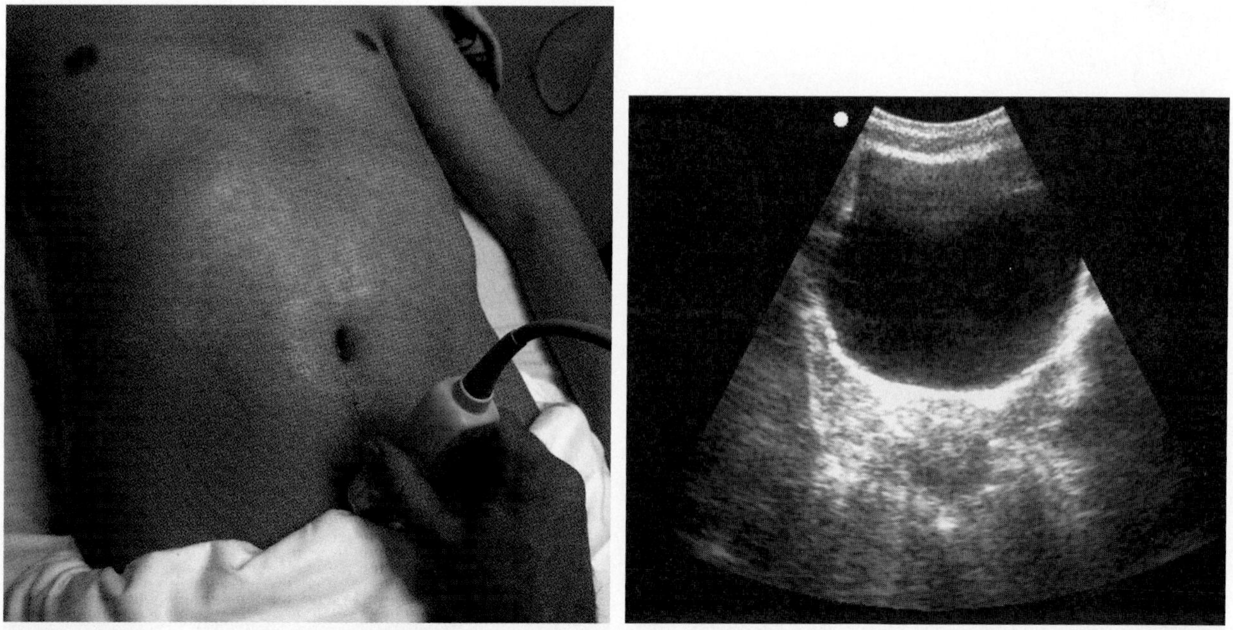

A B

FIGURE 8-4 **A,** Pelvic transverse view demonstrating approximate probe position (*red sticker* represents probe indicator). **B,** Normal image.

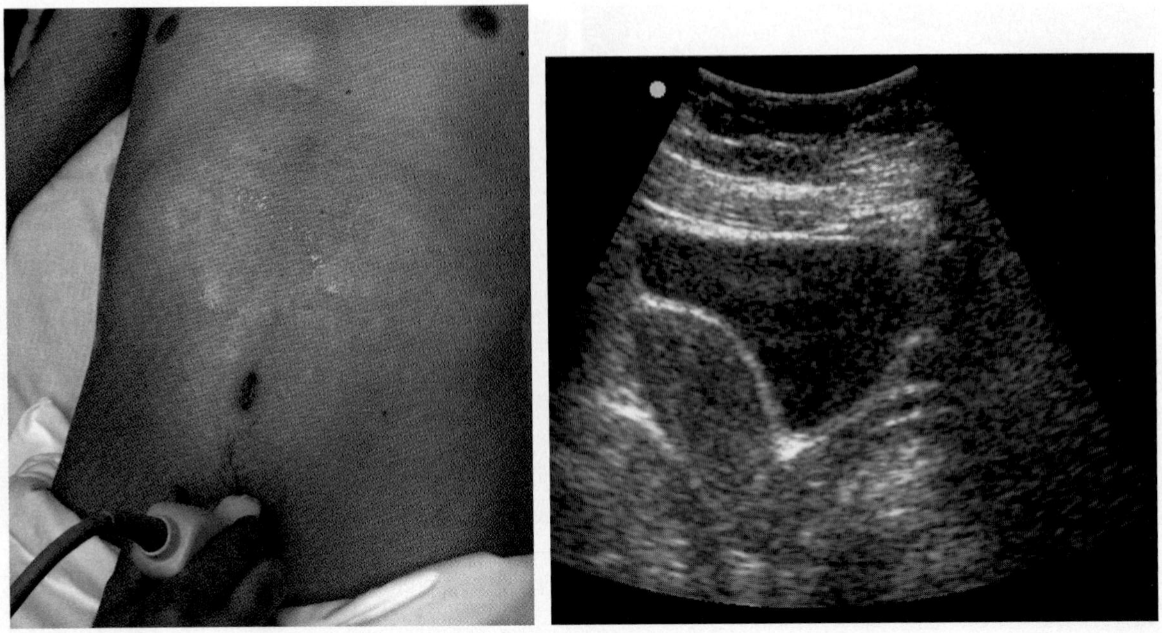

A B

FIGURE 8-5 **A,** Pelvic longitudinal view demonstrating approximate probe position (*red sticker* represents probe indicator). **B,** Normal image.

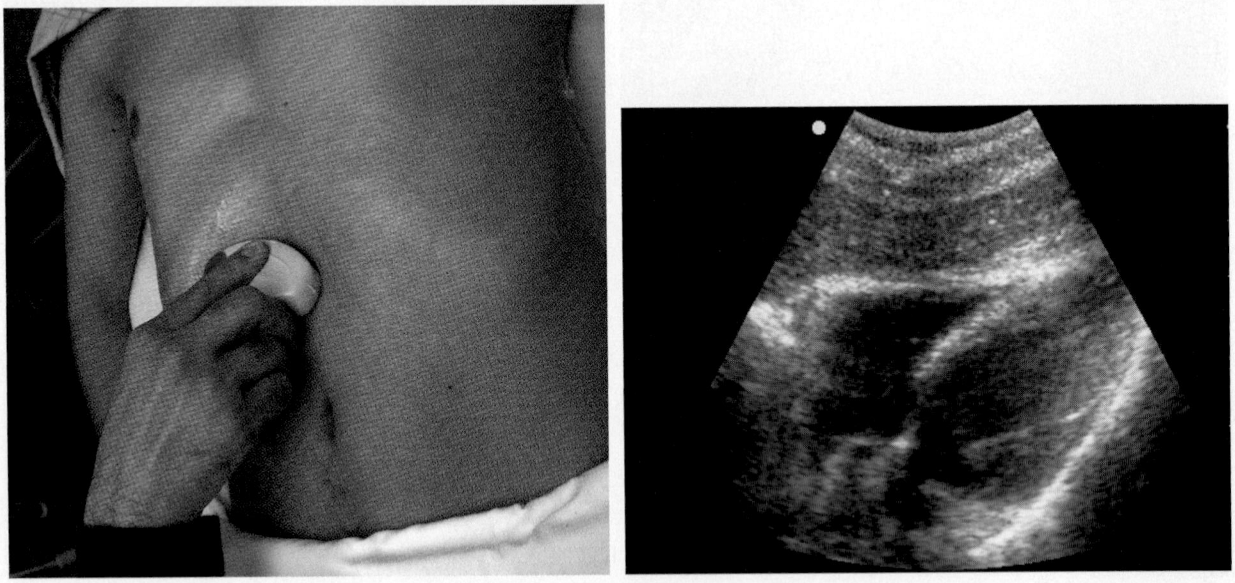

A B

FIGURE 8-6 **A,** Subxiphoid cardiac view demonstrating approximate probe position (*red sticker* represents probe indicator). **B,** Normal image. Note the hand positioning on top of the probe to allow fanning up into chest, bringing the probe handle flat against abdominal wall.

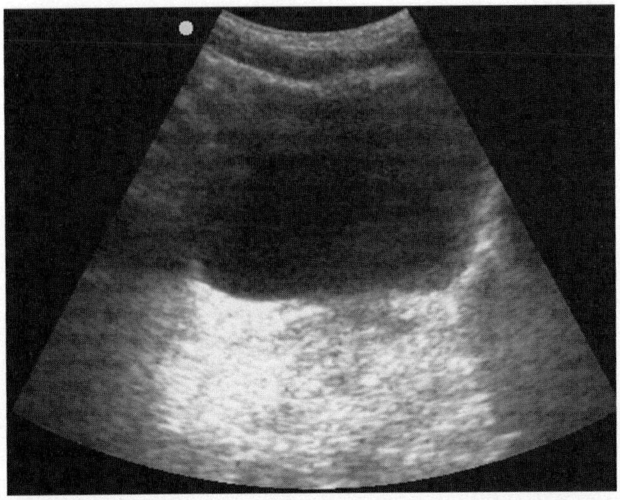

FIGURE 8-7 Pelvic view demonstrating bright acoustic enhancement posterior to bladder. To help visualize free fluid in pelvic view, the far-field gain should be turned down to minimize this artifact.

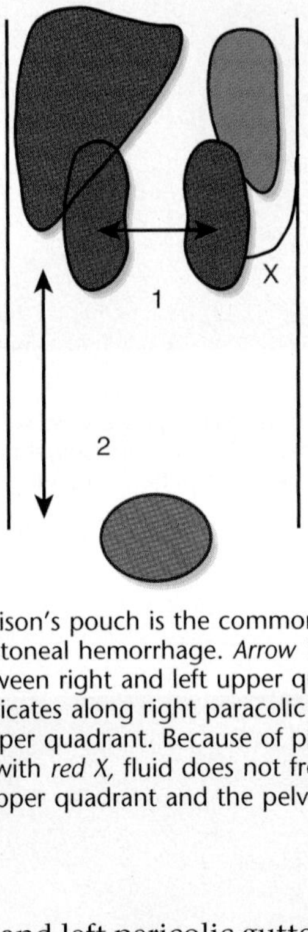
1
X
2

FIGURE 8-8 Morrison's pouch is the common destination for all sources of intraperitoneal hemorrhage. *Arrow 1,* Fluid can spread across midline between right and left upper quadrants. *Arrow 2,* Fluid also communicates along right paracolic gutter between pelvis and right upper quadrant. Because of phrenocolic ligament, marked with *red X,* fluid does not freely communicate between the left upper quadrant and the pelvis.

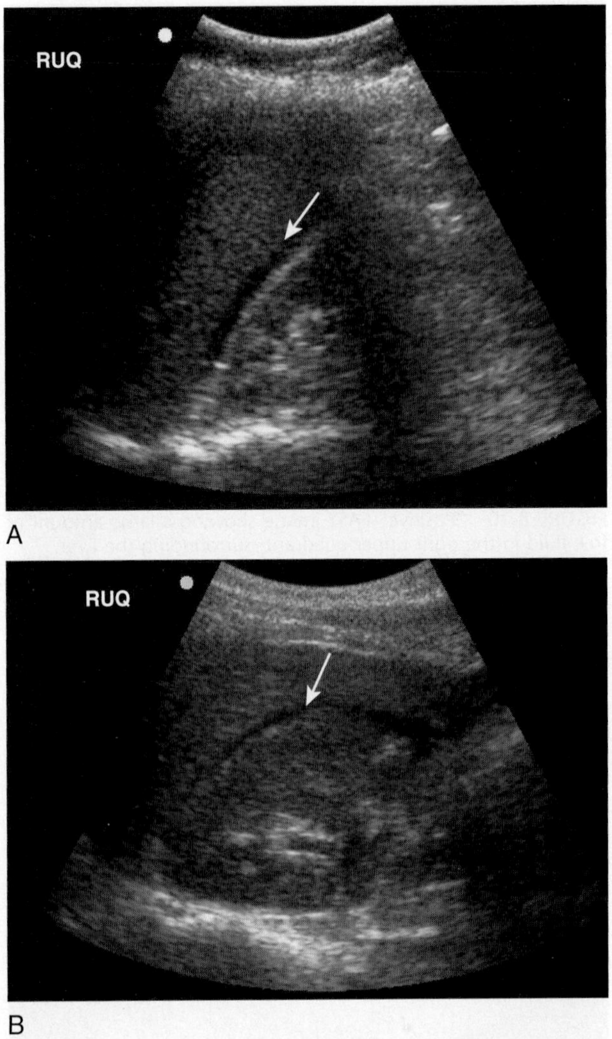
RUQ
A
RUQ
B

FIGURE 8-9 **A** and **B,** "Positive" FAST images demonstrating right upper quadrant view with small anechoic stripe (*arrow*) between the liver and kidney, in Morrison's pouch.

along the right and left pericolic gutters, respectively. Another cardiac view, such as parasternal long axis or apical, can be helpful if the subxiphoid view is technically difficult (owing to body habitus, subcutaneous air, epigastric penetrating wound, or abdominal pain).

Interpretation and Limitations of the FAST

In general, free fluid should appear anechoic or black on ultrasound imaging. Blood gains echoes as it clots, becoming more like surrounding tissue and making identification more difficult. A positive FAST finding is the presence of any free fluid or anechoic area in a place it does not belong. Positive results are demonstrated in Figures 8-9 to 8-13. A negative result consists of no free fluid in all four standard views with technically adequate images. Ultrasound images can be technically difficult to obtain in obese patients and in the setting of subcutaneous air or significant bowel gas. Assessments without adequate views of all four areas should be considered equivocal or inadequate.

An important limitation of the FAST is the presumption that free fluid is blood in the setting of trauma, which can lead to false-positive results, primarily in the setting of preexisting ascites. The other major limitations for trauma ultrasound are that it is insensitive for specific organ injury and is not accurate for determining retroperitoneal hemorrhage, bowel injury, or active bleeding (Box 8-1).

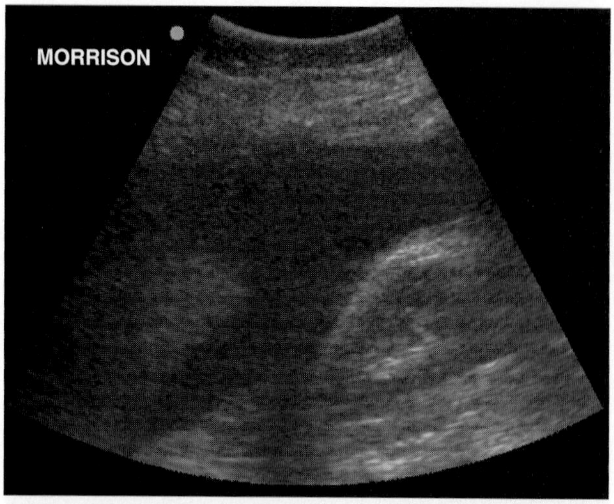
MORRISON

FIGURE 8-10 "Positive" FAST image showing a large amount of free fluid in the right upper quadrant, surrounding the liver.

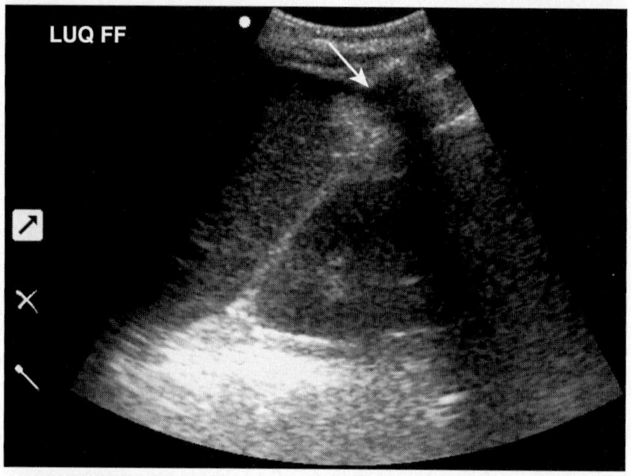
LUQ FF

FIGURE 8-11 Left upper quadrant shows anechoic fluid collection (*arrow*) in subdiaphragmatic space. Note that the splenorenal space is normal.

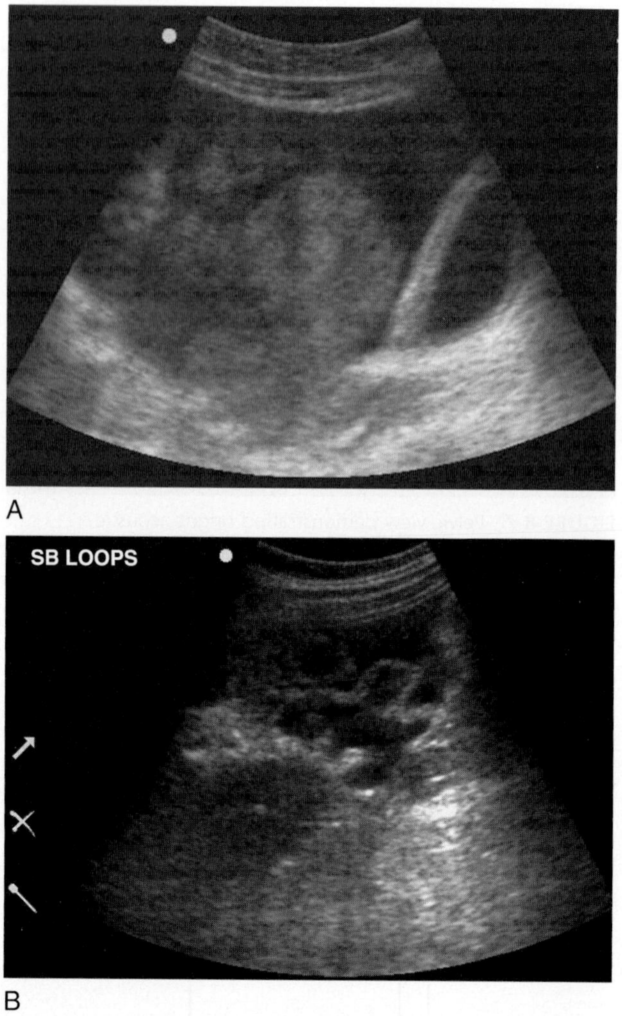
A
SB LOOPS
B

FIGURE 8-12 **A,** Longitudinal pelvic view with large amount of free fluid surrounding the uterus and bowel in the pelvis. **B,** Another pelvic view in same patient, showing small bowel loops floating in free fluid.

BOX 8-1

Limitations of the Focused Assessment with Sonography for Trauma (FAST)

- The diagnosis of free fluid as blood is based on the clinical setting of trauma.
- Subcutaneous air, bowel gas, and obesity can technically limit image acquisition.
- Two hundred to 600 mL of blood is needed for the identification of free fluid, so injuries with small amounts of bleeding can be missed.
- In patients with prior adhesions, blood may not accumulate in areas assessed with standard views.
- FAST is insensitive for specific organ injury.
- FAST does not identify retroperitoneal hemorrhage.

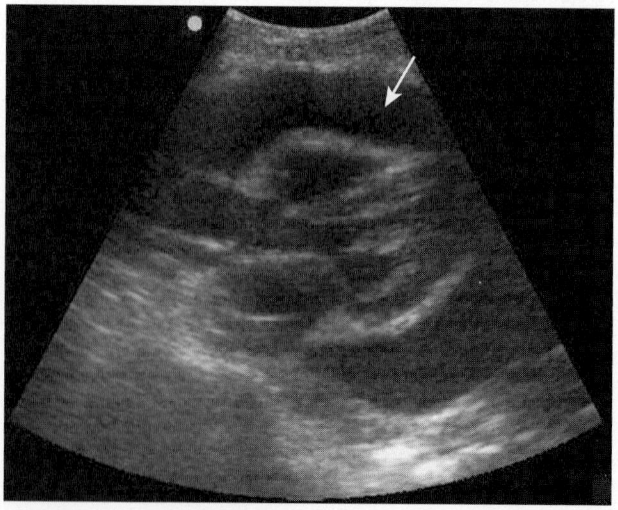

FIGURE 8-13 Subxiphoid cardiac view showing circumferential pericardial effusion (*arrow*).

Tips and Tricks

PEARLS AND PITFALLS OF THE FOCUSED ASSESSMENT WITH SONOGRAPHY FOR TRAUMA (FAST)

- Vary the probe placement to obtain the best window.
- Rotate slightly between ribs to get a clearer image.
- Start more posterior in the left upper quadrant to avoid gas in the splenic flexure.
- Make sure to scan through the entire spleen, especially anteriorly, to look for blood between the spleen and the diaphragm.
- Perinephric fat should be symmetrical; compare with the other side if unclear.
- Obtain pelvic views before insertion of Foley catheter to ensure a full bladder for pelvic windows.
- Decrease the far-field gain in pelvic views to limit "bright" enhancement artifact posterior to the bladder (see Fig. 8-7).
- Readjust depth for the subxyphoid cardiac view; the heart is farther away than it appears.
- Repeat the examination if the clinical situation changes.

REFERENCES

1. Lee BC, Ormsby EL, McGahan JP, et al: The utility of sonography for the triage of blunt abdominal trauma patients to exploratory laparotomy. AJR Am J Roentgenol 2007; 18:415-421.
2. Melniker LA, Leibner E, McKenney MG, et al: Randomized controlled clinical trial of point-of-care, limited ultrasonography for trauma in the emergency department: The first sonography outcomes assessment program trial. Ann Emerg Med 2006;48:227-235.

Chapter 9

Ethics of Resuscitation

Tammie E. Quest

KEY POINTS

- Resuscitation comprises a spectrum of care that includes intravenous fluids, oxygen, antibiotics as well as cardiopulmonary resuscitation in the event of cardiac arrest.
- The ethical principles of autonomy, beneficence, nonmaleficence, and justice must be considered.
- EPs should be prepared to guide patients and families regarding usual outcomes of cardiac arrest in terms of survival and disability.
- When counseling regarding prognosis in patients with underlying chronic progressive medical illness, it may be helpful to say that the best that can be hoped for is that the patient return to the "baseline status" (i.e., his or her condition before admission).
- EPs should be able to recognize and treat the syndrome of imminent death with measures other than cardiopulmonary resuscitation.

Scope

In the United States, patients consent to cardiopulmonary resuscitation (CPR) by default unless they have previously expressed a desire to be treated otherwise. Once a patient is in the hospital setting, the ethical choice to initiate CPR or other life-prolonging or life-sustaining measures after cardiac arrest should be based on the EP's best predictions of the expected medical outcomes and should be measured against the goals and outcomes of the patient and his or her decision-maker(s).

Structure and Function

Cardiopulmonary resuscitation interventions hold a unique position in medicine and society. These are the only procedures that the patient must take steps to refuse in advance, because consent is presumed, even if in the clinician's professional opinion, the intervention is likely not warranted. Ethical dilemmas in regard to this fact are common.

Patient autonomy, nonmaleficence (doing no harm), beneficence (doing good), and justice (being fair) are the guiding principles of medical ethics. In order for a patient to make autonomous decisions about resuscitation, the patient (or decision makers) should be given the best information available to weigh his or her medical care options. The Jonsen model[1] for ethical decision-making suggests that the following four "ethical quadrants" be weighed: medical indications, quality of life, patient preferences, and contextual features.

Medical futility has been defined as having a less than 1% chance of success. The goal of CPR is return of spontaneous circulation (ROSC) after cardiac arrest. In few patients is the likely outcome of ROSC less than 1%; the question is what will the patient be left with after the ROSC. Also, what are the patient's preferences?

On the road to possible death, patients may have a constellation of physical, psychological, and emotional symptoms that may be treated. The majority of patients who are critically ill do not present in active cardiac arrest but are at high risk for it. EPs most often care for patients at "high risk" for cardiac arrest and may find themselves ethically driven to discuss with patients, families, or surrogates the appropriateness of an attempt to reverse death in the event of a cardiopulmonary arrest.

Pathophysiology

Sixty to 70% of cardiac arrests occur outside the hospital.[2] Long-term survival rates for out-of-hospital cardiac arrests vary from 0% to 20%, depending on the cause and length of the resuscitation as well as the patient's pre-arrest health.[3] For patients who have an in-hospital cardiac arrest, survival rates of initial resuscitation can be higher, with a survival-to-discharge rate for all patients of 1 in 8.[4] Survival rates can be much lower for individual patients. The EP should be cognizant that a large number of patients who survive may experience significant additional morbidity as a result of resuscitation, such as anoxic brain injury (Table 9-1). U.S. television programs suggest that the survival of in-hospital cardiac arrest may approach 80%. In reality, the survival rate of in-hospital cardiac arrest varies highly with the patient's underlying medical condition. Discharge survival rates and function in patients with chronic, progressive terminal illness such as end-stage cancer, heart failure, and pulmonary and neurologic diseases, however, tend to be extremely poor. It is an indisputable fact that all people will die physiologically with cardiac arrest. In adults, chest compressions and artificial ventilation are attempts to reverse death (loss of pulse/respirations). In the emergency setting, all patients consent to undergo an attempt at reversal of death called CPR, unless legally contraindicated in writing or in some cases verbally by a decisional patient. Increasingly, the language of "allow natural death" suggests that no attempt be made to restart the heart or support ventilation in the event of physiologic death but that many other measures may be initiated to support comfort (oxygen, fluids, nutrition, pain control).

Presenting Signs and Symptoms

The classic scenario is that patients present to the ED in a terminal cardiac rhythm with little or no chance of survival according to the algorithms for advanced cardiac life support published by American Heart Association guidelines. Choices must be made regarding termination of efforts on the basis of medical futility and/or patient choice, when known by way of legal documents or discussions with family.

■ VARIATIONS

Many more patients present to the ED critically ill with possible impending cardiac arrest or with the signs of active dying (Table 9-2). Decisions must be made quickly regarding which life-extending versus comfort measures will be employed. If a patient is likely to rapidly deteriorate or shows signs of imminent death, a discussion regarding resuscitation should be initiated with the patient or the appropriate surrogate. Table 9-2 lists the signs of active dying

Tips and Tricks

PROGNOSTICATION

The safest prognostication the EP can make about a patient's outcome is: The best we can expect is that the patient returns to his/her baseline, or how he/she was right before this episode.

For example: If the patient has end-stage dementia at baseline and is unable to care for himself, the best outcome of cardiac arrest would be survival to return to the baseline end-staged dementia, and he would still need the same assistance.

Table 9-1 SURVIVAL AFTER IN-HOSPITAL CARDIOPULMONARY RESUSCITATION*

Immediate survival (%)	40.7-43.1
Survival to discharge (%)	13.4-14.6
Predictors of failure to survive to discharge	Sepsis Cancer/metastatic cancer Dementia Coronary artery disease African-American race Serum creatinine level >1.5 mg/dL
Summary recommendations	The authors state, "When talking with patients, physicians can describe the overall likelihood of surviving discharge as 1 in 8 for patients undergoing cardiopulmonary resuscitation and 1 in 3 for patients who survive cardiopulmonary resuscitation."

*51 studies involving 12,000 patients.

Data from Ebell MH, Becker LA, Barry HC, Hagen M: Survival after in-hospital cardiopulmonary resuscitation: A meta-analysis. J Gen Intern Med 1998;13:805-816.

Table 9-2 SIGNS OF ACTIVE DYING IN PATIENTS WITH CHRONIC ILLNESS

	Early	Mid	Late
Recognition	Confinement to bed Loss of both interest in and ability to consume food and drink Cognitive changes: either hypoactive or hyperactive, with delirium or increasing sleepiness	Further decline in mental status—obtunded "Death rattle"—from pooled oral secretions that are not cleared owing to loss of swallowing reflex Fever is common	Coma Cool extremities Altered respiratory pattern—either fast or slow Fever is common Death
Time course	The time to traverse the three stages can be less than 24 hours or up to 10 to 14 days. Once a patient enters the process, it is difficult to accurately predict the time course, which may cause considerable family distress if the dying patient seems to "linger."		

in the setting of chronic progressive incurable illness such as late-stage cancer, dementia, or failure to thrive.

Diagnostic Testing

Prior to the discussion with family and patient about critical illness, the EP can institute several easy interventions that can provide much information for the patient and family. Bedside glucose testing and pulse oxygen saturation measurements may be sought. Arterial blood gas testing with rapid measurement of serum electrolytes (potassium in particular) may yield a quick view of the patient's level of cardiovascular compromise and might help initiate sooner a discussion with the patient or family regarding the possibility of cardiac arrest. Bedside ultrasonography is a minimally invasive way to diagnose potential end-of-life catastrophes such as pericardial tamponade and rupture of a viscus/structure (e.g., abdominal aortic aneurysm). Bedside electrocardiogram (ECG) may detect myocardial infarction. Good clinical information can help guide decision-making.

Interventions and Procedures

Temporizing measures that might "buy time" for discussing the medical and ethical grounds for resuscitation should be considered on a case-by-case basis. They include minimally to noninvasive ventilation techniques, such as biphasic positive airway pressure and oral airway, as well as intravenous fluids, intravenous glucose, and cardioactive medications.

RED FLAGS

EPs should be careful that they are considering the medical facts when advising patients and/or families about resuscitation, and should carefully examine their own biases and prejudices. Depending on the age and previous health or other socioeconomic feature of the patient, a provider may either hold out false hope or may be overly pessimistic.

Treatment and Disposition

Patients who themselves or for whom their decision-makers choose to forgo measures of CPR may chose a comfort approach. The EP should be able to provide comfort measures and support a comfort approach (Table 9-3). Such patients may still need intensive hospital care. In some cases, placement of a patient from the ED to a hospice may be possible. More

Table 9-3 SUPPORT OF A COMFORT APPROACH

Clearly define treatment goals	Once imminent death is recognized, discuss with family and confirm treatment goals. When assuming a comfort approach, make a supportive statement, such as "You are doing the right thing." Discuss with family stopping interventions that do not contribute to comfort.
Provide good palliative care	Use antimuscarinic blockers such as glycopyrrolate, 0.2 mg IV (onset 1 min), atropine, 0.1 mg IV (onset 1 min), atropine eyedrop 1%, sublingual 2 drops (onset 30 min), or hycoscyamine hydrobromide 1.5 mg transdermal (onset 12 hr). Use morphine to control dyspnea or tachypnea. It is very disturbing for the families to see their loved one in a coma breathing at 40 breaths/min; the goal should be to keep the respiratory rate in range of 10-15 breaths/min. Provide excellent mouth and skin care.
Determine disposition	According to symptom burden, patients may require assignment to the intensive care unit to ensure that treatment goals remain on target and medical aspects of palliative care are met (pain/dyspnea control) despite "Allow natural death" or "Do not resuscitate" status.

often, patients are admitted to the hospital and may need intensive care to support their comfort. For the patient who is undergoing advanced life support measures, such as invasive ventilation and cardioactive drugs, a time-limited trial may help the patient and his or her family to feel more comfortable about making decisions regarding goals of care.

REFERENCES

1. Jonsen AR, Siegler M, Winslade WJ: Clinical Ethics: A Practical Approach to Ethical Decisions in Clinical Medicine, 6th ed. New York, McGraw-Hill Medical, 2006.
2. Gillum RF: Sudden coronary death in the United States: 1980-1985. Circulation 1989;79:456-465.
3. Engdahl J, Holmberg M, Karlson BW, et al: The epidemiology of out-of-hospital "sudden" cardiac arrest. Resuscitation 2002;52:235-245.
4. Ebell MH, Becker LA, Barry HC, Hagen M: Survival after in-hospital cardiopulmonary resuscitation: A meta-analysis. J Gen Intern Med 1998;13:805-816.

Chapter 10

Emergency Medical Services and Disaster Medicine

Jennifer Avegno

KEY POINTS

Emergency medical services (EMS) are a heterogeneous group of entities that vary according to urbanization, training procedures, and skill levels of practioners, resources, and scope.

Although EMS research is rapidly developing, controversy exists over the role of EMS interventions and protocols in commonly encountered conditions such as trauma and cardiovascular emergencies.

Disaster medicine encompasses planning, resource allocation, and health care response to any event—natural or human-caused—that overwhelms the resources of a particular locality.

Weapons of mass destruction have the potential to cause severe physical damage and health concerns that require specific, targeted planning and coordination for emergency care personnel.

An emergency medical services (EMS) system can be defined as "a coordinated arrangement of resources (including personnel, equipment, and facilities) organized to respond to medical emergencies, regardless of the cause."[1] The development of modern EMS in the United States has its origins largely in a long tradition of battlefield medicine.[2-6] Although the great London fire of 1666 put in motion events that ultimately led to the establishment of a nascent fire department,[2] it was a surgeon in the Napoleonic military campaign who pioneered the concept of rapid response to injuries on the battlefield.[3] Baron Larrey, the "father of modern prehospital care," developed a systematic approach to combat trauma in which ambulances transported wounded soldiers from the battlefield to medical stations, including field hospitals. In the American Civil War, ambulances were put under organized medical direction. Successive advances in technology and EMS organization in later wars resulted in significantly lower mortality rates for battle combatants who were transported to field hospitals.[5]

Although civilian "rescue societies" and ambulance services existed from the mid-1800s, the most significant nonmilitary advancement of EMS occurred in the 1950s with the establishment of life support training programs through the Chicago Fire Department. From this effort, the basis for the now widely accepted emergency medical technician (EMT) and paramedic training programs was formed.[2] By the 1960s, there were two limited EMS models: ambulance systems with paramedics trained in advanced life support (ALS) techniques, and a separate system of "heartmobiles" with physicians on board to provide care only for cardiac emergencies.[7]

The need for sophisticated, coordinated EMS systems was brought to the national spotlight in 1966 with the publication of the National Academy of Sciences paper titled "Accidental Death and Disability: The Neglected Disease of Modern Society." This paper noted that (1) few people were trained in advanced resuscitation, (2) there were no widely accepted standards for ambulance personnel training, and (3) communication systems and supplies were lacking. These findings spurred a national, organized effort to increase the awareness of traumatic disease and the need for EMS system development.[5] Congress responded with the National Highway Safety Act of 1966 and the EMS Systems Act of 1973, which authorized federal grants to state, local, and regional governments for the development of EMS systems within a specified "systems approach" framework.[8] By 1981, however, guaranteed federal funding for EMS was replaced with state block grants and greater financial insecurity.[4] Currently, nearly 1 million people are certified in some form as emergency response personnel and nearly 20 million patients are treated in the EMS system annually, but heterogeneity in system design, scope, and certification requirements persists.[9]

System Design

EMS systems are, arguably, some of the most complex organizational entities in modern society (Box 10-1). They involve representatives from municipalities of every size, law enforcement, fire and safety, health care, transportation services, and community groups. Federal governing bodies define necessary components of EMS systems but do not directly oversee organization or management. Coordination between agencies is necessary but often difficult to achieve.[1] Ideally, the design of an EMS system is centered on the particular needs of the community it serves, with one standard characteristic: emergency medical personnel act as on-scene "physician surrogates" to provide appropriate life support techniques.[7] Common models categorize different systems in terms of public or private agency control, rural or urban communities, and single-tiered or multitiered systems.

BOX 10-1

Components of EMS Systems

- Manpower
- Training
- Communications
- Transportation
- Emergency facilities
- Critical care units
- Public safety agencies
- Consumer participation
- Access to care
- Patient transfer
- Standardized record-keeping
- Public information and education
- System review and evaluation
- Disaster planning
- Mutual aid

From Archibald S: EMS systems. In EMS Medical Director Curriculum. Available at http://kbems.ky.gov/NR/rdonlyres/C6B3B209-E1DD-4AF5-8AF6-99D4DC1DC9E6/0/EMSCurriculum.pdf/

■ PUBLIC AND PRIVATE AGENCIES

Public EMS systems are usually based in the local fire department organization and are more common in large urban counties or cities. This structure developed in the early days of EMS systems out of logistical concerns: Fire stations were located at tactical points throughout communities and had experience in emergency response. Firefighters could be trained in basic life support (BLS) techniques and thus could function as both fire/safety and emergency medical personnel. Municipal third-service systems are public EMS systems that are not part of a fire or police organization but instead are supported by local government and often are interconnected with fire and police as part of a larger public safety agency. Municipal systems are generally funded through a combination of local taxes, user fees, and patient insurance.

Private EMS systems may be hospital-based, locally owned, or subsidiaries of large national corporations. Depending on the community, these organizations often provide interfacility transfers as well as respond to local 911 calls. In some areas, private firms constitute the designated first or second responders for all calls and also provide routine transports of nonemergency patients (e.g., scheduled patient trips to dialysis or rehabilitation facilities). Financing generally depends on individual patient insurance and user fees, with occasional government subsidies. Hospital-based systems are least common and may be located in one hospital or a larger hospital organization. If they are under the control of a state or county-run hospital, they may operate under public authority in concert with other safety agencies.

Public-private hybrids are quite common. A local government may contract with one or both types of EMS systems for fulfillment of specified emergency medical services in a particular region. For example, fire department personnel may be the designated first responders for all 911 calls, but a private ambulance company may transport all patients from the scene to the hospital. Financing may involve direct patient billing, reimbursement from local government, or a designated fee for services.

■ RURAL AND URBAN SYSTEMS

The design of and challenges faced by EMS systems in rural and urban areas are often significantly different. In general, rural systems developed later than urban systems and are more likely to be staffed with unpaid volunteers. These volunteer-based organizations may be public or private and are usually nonprofit entities. Volunteers are customarily citizens with outside employment who offer their services on an unpaid basis for emergency response, training, and community education. Such systems are funded largely through taxes and municipal support. Volunteer EMS systems face many challenges that are representative of rural systems as a whole; namely, (1) high costs to cover large geographic areas with few citizens, (2) long response times, (3) lower levels of training, and (4) relatively low patient volumes. Urban EMS systems have their own distinct set of difficulties, the principal issues being high patient volumes, traffic congestion, and limited resources.

Evidence suggests that patient morbidity and mortality rates in rural emergency systems are significantly greater than in comparable urban systems. Reasons for this difference include longer response time and on-scene time (period from arrival of responders on the scene to transport of patient away from it), lower patient volumes, and less overall training for first responders.[10-12] Technological advances, such as E911 (enhanced 911; see later), show some promise in significantly reducing emergency responders' transport time to the scene.[13] Adapting specific on-scene protocols and increasing access to highly trained paramedics have also been suggested as possible ways to close the gap between rural and urban adverse outcome rates.[14]

■ SINGLE-TIERED AND MULTITIERED SYSTEMS

EMS systems are further divided by hierarchical types. In single-tiered systems, all dispatched calls are serviced by a single level of first responder and vehicle. Single-tiered models are most commonly seen in urban areas. In contrast, multitiered systems have variable types and levels of personnel, equipment, and vehicles available for response. A typical multitiered model includes both "first responders"—police and fire department personnel at geographically strategic locations throughout the area—and a second response tier consisting of more skilled paramedics and EMS personnel. First responders generally have limited training in basic life support techniques such as lifesaving airway maneuvers, hemorrhage control efforts, and cardiopulmonary resuscitation (CPR). The second response tier usually can perform advanced emergency techniques and provides transport to the hospital.

Other multitiered EMS designs may also be used. Examples are police/fire first response with private ambulance transport; ground first response with air transport; basic life support transport with advanced life support intercept vehicle as needed, and separate advanced life support response and transport vehicles. All systems are designed, in theory, to minimize EMS response, on-scene, and transport times while providing the highest possible quality of patient care. Each agency participating in patient care or transport is responsible for adding documentation to the patient record.

System Organization, Training, and Transport Types

■ DISPATCH AND MEDICAL CONTROL

In the United States, 99% of the population has access to 911 for emergency calls.[7] Most dispatch centers utilize E911, a system whereby the caller's location is shown on the dispatch operator's screen. Although there is formal training for 911 dispatch personnel, no national or regional standards have been developed. Generally, in small communities one operator both answers calls and relays information to EMS units, whereas in larger areas there are often two separate dispatchers for these duties. In comparison, the British emergency dispatch system relies heavily on computer protocols for both triage and information relay to emergency units.[15] A controlled trial of British nonurgent emergency calls found that when a computerized decision tool plus either nurse or paramedic input was used, more than half of callers were identified by triage as not needing an emergency ambulance. However, only 20% of these callers chose to cancel the ambulance, and hospital admission rates for this group were similar to those of callers identified by triage as needing an emergency transport.[16]

Medical direction refers to both on-line (direct) and off-line (indirect) medical control. Physician involvement in EMS medical control developed as physicians spent less time directly in the field and paramedics improved their training and ability to act as physician surrogates. Every EMS system is headed by a medical director, a physician with or without specialty training who has direct authority over system operation, emergency personnel performance, and patient care. Standardized guidelines and requirements for EMS medical direction have been published by the American College of Emergency Physicians (ACEP).[17,18]

On-line medical direction involves direct communication about patient care between on-scene emergency responders and the EMS medical director or a designated representative. Depending on the region, on-line medical control may be provided by a single centralized facility (base station), so that all calls requiring medical control—regardless of their destination—are handled by one institution. In other areas, each receiving hospital may have its own medical control that may handle calls specifically directed toward that facility. Personnel responsible for direct medical control must be knowledgeable about specific protocols or regional system requirements in order to provide accurate information about patient care in the field and as well as appropriate transports.

The evidence basis for improved patient outcomes in on-line medical control is mixed. It has been shown to significantly lengthen on-scene time, and orders given via medical direction rarely deviate from existing protocols.[19-21] The greatest benefits of on-line direction may be in resolving difficult ethical or medicolegal situations on the scene and in notifying receiving hospitals of incoming critical patients so that resources are assembled and ready prior to patient arrival.

Off-line medical direction refers to written protocols that guide common patient interactions as well as continuing education and quality assurance initiatives. EMS systems have specific protocols for commonly encountered situations that, ideally, should improve patient outcomes and reduce on-scene time. Protocols should be developed on the basis of patient history, mechanism of injury, physiologic characteristics, local hospital capability, and transport times.[22] Medical directors should be active in developing and implementing protocols as well as in training responders in the application and quality evaluation of patient records. Research indicates that use of well-developed standing protocols significantly reduces on-scene time and decreases inappropriate treatment in the field.[23] Furthermore, rates of accuracy of responder diagnoses and of agreement between responder and physician assessments of patients are generally high.[24]

Development of protocols for specific patient populations—for example, children, pregnant women, and patients with trauma or cardiovascular problems—is essential for consistent response and delivery of care. Protocols should be continually evaluated and refined on the basis of the experience of the individual EMS system. Deviation from protocols should be reviewed for deficiencies in EMS personnel training or activity, medical direction, or design of the protocol itself.[14] Thus, quality assurance and continuing medical education and training of all those involved in EMS delivery—medical director, dispatch, and responders—are key.

■ RESPONDER PERSONNEL

Prior to the National Academy of Sciences paper on trauma in the 1960s, there were few standardized training programs for EMS personnel. The creation of the U.S. Department of Transportation in 1966 resulted in a formalized, 70-hour curriculum for basic Emergency Medical Technician (EMT) certification. Passage of the EMS act of 1973 provided millions of dollars for EMS training, equipment, and research, and identified the 15 basic elements of all EMS systems (see Box 10-1).[25] However, until recently, heterogeneity of regional systems persisted; a 1996 survey identified more than 40 different types of EMS personnel certification across the country.[26]

In general, EMS personnel are categorized into the following four skill levels:

- First responders
- EMT-Basic (EMT-B)
- EMT-Intermediate (EMT-I)
- EMT-Paramedic (EMT-P)

First responders undergo roughly 50 hours of training in basic first aid, CPR, uncomplicated obstetric deliveries, simple wound and fracture care, and automated external defibrillators (AEDs). EMT-B personnel receive first responder training plus 50 to 60 hours of education in triage, extrication, transfer, oxygen and self-medication assistance, and, possibly, advanced airway techniques. Most American ambulances are staffed with at least one EMT-B. EMT-I requirements often vary by state but generally include IV access and monitoring, and, possibly, advanced airway and life support measures. EMT-Ps undergo EMT-B training plus at least 250 to 500 hours of education, including in-hospital experience; they are skilled in advanced airway and life support techniques, vascular access, monitoring, and medication administration.

Recognition of the wide regional variation in training standards and skill levels led to the development of the National Highway Traffic Safety Administration (NHTSA) National EMS Scope of Practice Model in 2005. This consensus document promotes national standardization in training and education in order to improve consistency within and between agencies, increase public understanding of EMS roles, and move toward a coordinated, national EMS system.[9] The model advocates four separate and sequential levels of certification—emergency medical responder (EMR), EMT, advanced EMT (AEMT), and paramedic—and clearly defines minimum educational levels and skill sets for each.

There is some evidence basis for the current multilevel EMS personnel system. Early EMS research found significantly lower mortality rates for patients with cardiac arrest treated by paramedic responder crews than for those treated by EMT-Bs.[27,28] Outcomes in trauma have also been shown to be significantly higher when ambulance crews with advanced life support are on scene than when BLS personnel are.[29,30] However, an evaluation of British ambulance calls with paramedic and nonparamedic crews found mixed results. There was no significant difference in the type or severity of patient encounters between the two groups, but the on-scene time was significantly longer for crews with a paramedic. Although paramedics had higher skill levels and provided more on-scene interventions, the evaluation's authors suggest that the presence of paramedics on every ambulance may not be warranted.[31]

Vehicles, Equipment, and Types of Transport

Equipment available on emergency transport vehicles varies by both type of vehicle and the skill level of responder personnel on board. Joint guidelines developed by the ACEP and the American College of Surgeons (ACS) detail the minimum necessary supplies for appropriate patient care.[32] Items needed for basic level interventions are ventilation and airway equipment, monitors and defibrillators, immobilization devices, bandages, mobile communication devices, obstetric and pediatric specialty equipment, and infection control and injury prevention measures. Ambulances with advanced life support capability (EMT-I or P) should contain all of the preceding basic equipment plus vascular access materials, advanced airway and ventilation tools, Advanced Cardiac Life Support (ACLS) and other protocol-driven medications, more sophisticated monitoring, and advanced diagnostic equipment (blood glucose meters, pulse oximetry, etc.). In addition, all vehicles should have some measure of extrication equipment for use in patient rescue.

■ AIR MEDICINE TRANSPORTS

Although a full description of air ambulance systems is beyond the scope of this chapter, the method plays a crucial role in the transport and transfer of critically ill patients. Ground emergency transport remains the mainstay of prehospital transports and transfers; however, air medical services can have a significant effect on patient care in selected conditions.[33,34] The benefits of air ambulance transport are largely attributed to increased speeds and higher crew skill levels; however, safety, costs, and limited evidence to support improved outcomes are major concerns.

Review of the literature on selected patient air transports presents mixed evidence for its use. One multiyear retrospective study of blunt trauma showed a significant decrease in mortality for patients transported by helicopter,[35] and other work found a small but significant benefit for trauma patients transported by air.[36] However, several studies have found no difference in patient outcomes for both trauma and non-trauma patient groups[37-39] and that air transport is overused and costly.[36,38,40] The National Association of EMS Physicians has published guidelines about the use of various methods of air transport as well as which patients are most likely to benefit from its use. In general, helicopters are best used for shorter distance (less than 100 miles) transports but are subject to weather concerns. Fixed-wing air craft, which are preferable for distances greater than 100 miles, are less dependent on inclement weather but must land at airports (thereby prolonging transport time). Severely injured trauma patients at some distance from a regional trauma center are most likely to benefit from air transport or transfer; patients who are critically ill as well as those with non-trauma, cardiac, pediatric, and, possibly, obstetric problems may also have better outcomes with air transport in selected situations.[41] In general, use of this resource should be guided by the needs of the particular regional EMS system.

Current Controversies

Research into the influence of EMS systems on patient outcome is a nascent but growing field. Ideally, well-designed studies should investigate the effects of EMS system design, training, personnel, and operation on community needs and patient outcomes. Most studies to date have focused on several broad topics: cardiovascular emergencies, trauma, and response times.

■ CARDIOVASCULAR EMERGENCIES

Some of the earliest organized EMS research focused on cardiac arrest and early CPR and defibrillation. A 20-year review of EMS systems in 29 cities published in 1990 found that systems with a single emergency responder had lower rates of survival in patients with cardiac arrest than two-responder (EMT and paramedic) systems, largely because of the availability of early CPR in the latter.[42] Time to defibrillation has consistently been found to improve outcomes for patients with cardiac arrest,[43,44] although the evidence for prehospital ACLS drug administration is less convincing. Interestingly, a 25-year retrospective review of cardiac arrest with EMS intervention published in 2003 found that survival rates remained stagnant; the authors of the review suggest, however, that improvements in EMS delivery, such as dispatcher-assisted bystander CPR and early defibrillation, balanced adverse temporal trends that otherwise would have increased mortality rates.[45] The development of AEDs has increased the bystander role in the care of patients in cardiac arrest, which is now regarded as an important adjunct to trained EMS response.[46]

■ TRAUMA

Much research on EMS response to trauma focuses on response times and the perceived benefit of "regionalization" of trauma care—that is, linking prehospital systems with participating hospitals, public health agencies, and other care providers within a certain region to achieve optimum system efficiency and outcomes.[47] Regional systems generally have specific protocols governing EMS responder actions and transport to specialized trauma centers when appropriate. A multiyear comparison of a Canadian province before and after regionalization showed significant decreases in mortality, prehospital transport, and time to hospital admission with a regional trauma system. Furthermore, despite more critical injuries in patients transported to designated trauma centers, mortality remained low, largely owing to direct transport from the scene to these facilities.[48]

Despite the advantages of regionalization, the effect of EMS transport to a trauma center may not always be significant. In a small study of patients with critical trauma, those transported to a trauma center by EMS arrived at hospital significantly faster than patients in private vehicles, but demonstrated no significant improvement in mortality rate, complication rates, or length of stay.[49] Prehospital interventions in severely injured patients are also of questionable advantage. No significant benefit has been shown from on-scene ACLS medications and interventions for patients with traumatic cardiac arrest; furthermore, in one retrospective study, strict adherence to ACLS guidelines would have resulted in prehospital termination of efforts in the majority of patients who ultimately survived to hospital discharge.[50] In addition, prehospital intubation has not been shown to improve survival in severe traumatic head injury.[51] Many researchers thus recommend the "scoop and run" approach to traumatized patients rather than delaying transport for possibly unhelpful interventions.[47,49]

■ RESPONSE TIME

EMS response time is often used as a benchmark of overall system performance, with accepted standards of 4 minutes for BLS personnel arrival and 8 minutes for ALS personnel arrival.[52] However, studies of these criteria have shown mixed results. Retrospective and post hoc analyses of urban EMS transports show a possible survival benefit for patients transported to hospitals in 4 minutes or less, although the advantage was nonsignificant for those not in cardiac arrest.[52,53] In patients with trauma, prehospital transport times have been shown to be approximately twice those in urban areas, and there is some suggestion that this delay—particularly if time to hospital exceeds 30 minutes—contributes to significantly higher mortality rates.[10,12] Although the ideal response time for non–cardiac arrest ambulance calls is unknown, limited research suggests ways to better quantify and improve upon service in general. In the United Kingdom, response times are nearly equal in urban and rural areas because of better community saturation with solo responders and a trend toward increasing in-field critical interventions by highly trained paramedics or MDs.[15] Enhanced 911 systems—in which caller location is available instantly—can reduce response times they help plan more direct routes to the scene and decrease the likelihood that ambulance crews will become lost.[13] Furthermore, response times may be maximized in all areas by a strong community-wide first responder presence, strategic ambulance placement based on historical call data, mobile mapping systems or global positioning systems, and adequate fleet maintenance.[5]

From their earliest beginnings as purely military organizations to the complex heterogenous models in place today, emergency medical services have evolved into critical providers of health care. To meet the challenges of the next century, research suggests that they must continue to be adaptive and responsive to patient and community needs.

Disaster Medicine

A *disaster* can be defined as "sudden and extraordinary misfortune that overwhelms the immediate ability to manage or compensate."[2] Growing attention has been focused on this nascent medical specialty with such high-profile disasters as the September 11, 2001, terrorist attacks as well as severe natural disasters, such as hurricanes, earthquakes, and tsunamis. With each successive disaster and its medical and public health response, more is learned and planning can be refined for the next event.

Although the existence of apathy about disaster planning (and resource allocation to this end) is well known, major and minor disasters occur with regular and increasing frequency. In the past 100 years, millions of lives have been lost worldwide from natural disasters. Hurricane-induced flooding in Galveston, Texas, caused more than 6000 deaths in 1900 and Hurricane Katrina–related flooding was responsible for more than 1500 fatalities along the U.S. Gulf Coast in 2005. Flooding of the Yangtze River in China caused 3 million casualties in 1931, and deaths from the Indian Ocean tsunami of 2004 approached 300,000. Over the years, earthquakes, landslides, volcano eruptions, and massive fires have resulted in staggering economic losses, population displacement, disease, and death. Research suggests that losses from natural disasters are likely only to rise in the coming years. The reasons are growing population density, particularly in high-risk areas, and greater hazards due to rapidly expanding technology (i.e., transportation of more dangerous materials, fire threats in high-rise buildings, vulnerable financial and economic infrastructures).

Despite the clear threats from natural disasters, much of the focus of disaster medicine in recent years has been on intentional, human-caused events—namely, terrorism and mass casualty incidents. Even before the devastating terrorist attacks on New York City and Washington, DC, in 2001, researchers predicted that the probability of exactly such an event was extremely high.[54] Even though a mass casualty drill was performed in New York City just 3 days prior to the September 11 attack on the World Trade Center, none of the existing protocols or triage systems proved adequate for the actual event.[55] The subsequent creation of the U.S. Department of Homeland Security (DHS) has provided federal agency support for and focus on expanded research and development into all aspects of disaster planning for human-caused incidents.

■ DEFINITIONS AND CLASSIFICATIONS

In general, disasters are classified according to their relation to hospital setting, inciting event (natural or human-caused), and the anticipated necessary response. Internal events occur solely within a particular hospital or medical center (for example, a power outage or building collapse), whereas external events involve some part of the larger community. This system is most useful in preparing the facility to either receive patients from outside or deal with internal problems; however, many disasters have both internal and external effects, and such a narrow classification scheme is not easily applicable to a

Table 10-1 TERMINOLOGY FOR POTENTIAL INJURY-CREATING EVENT (PICE) MODEL

Potential for Additional Casualties	Degree to which Facility Can Respond with Routinely Available Resources	Geographic Event	PICE Stage
Static	Controlled	Local	0
Dynamic	Disruptive Paralytic	Regional National International	I II III

From Koenig KL, Dinerman N, Kuehl AE: Disaster nomenclature—a functional impact approach: The PICE system. Acad Emerg Med 1996;3:723-727.

variety of situations. In terms of anticipated response, most disasters are classified into one of three categories. Level I disasters are those in which local emergency response teams and organizations are adequate to manage the event alone. Level II incidents require a regional approach and mutual aid from surrounding areas. Level III events overwhelm local and regional efforts and require state or federal support.

Attempts to standardize disaster nomenclature led to creation of the Potential Injury-Causing Event (PICE) model (Table 10-1).[56] This model is based on the assumption that in order to be useful and applicable, any naming system should focus on the disaster's effect on the health care system. Disaster events are categorized by their potential for additional casualties, the ability of the health care system to respond with readily available resources, and the geographic extent of the incident. This nomenclature obviates the need to define internal versus external or natural versus human-caused disasters and instead focuses on defining the event according to response needs, resource capabilities, and rapid reassessments of the situation. A PICE stage 0 classification assumes that no outside aid will be required. Stage I estimates that limited amounts of aid may be needed and puts outside relief agencies on alert. Stage II disasters should be expected to need moderate assistance, and external organizations are put on standby. Stage III requires a large amount of aid and immediate dispatch of outside resources and personnel. For example, the flooding and destruction caused by Hurricane Katrina in 2005 would be classified as dynamic, paralytic, and regional, or PICE stage III, whereas a multivehicle collision in a rural area may be described as static, disruptive, and local, or PICE stage I.

■ DISASTER PLANNING

Although the Joint Commission on Accredited Healthcare Organizations (JCAHO) requires all health care facilities to conduct two disaster drills per year, disaster planning is rarely emphasized or sufficient. Many factors contribute to the inadequacy of most hospital or regional disaster plans, namely, the unexpected and sudden nature of most events (making prospective evaluation impossible), poor record-keeping, faulty assumptions upon which significant parts of the plan are based, and failures of communication and command structures.[57] In order for disaster plans to be effective, they must be based on valid assumptions of what may occur in a variety of event settings. Furthermore, the planning process must involve all systems and organizations that will be affected by the disaster and have a role in its aftermath, and all parties must have a working knowledge of the plan, the chain of command, and their role in it.[58] Critical to the development of an appropriate plan is a hazards analysis of particular events to which a hospital or region is most susceptible. With this approach, organizations can effectively plan for the types of disasters they are most likely to experience.

A good disaster plan should cover both internal agency and external community needs and should focus on all phases of the inciting event: prodrome/mitigation, impact, rescue, and recovery.[2,59] Interhospital plans should involve all departments responsible for patient care and infrastructure and should detail clear policies relating to chain of command and physical control centers, communication and public relations, record-keeping, personnel needs, and equipment and resource supply. External planning should involve all local agencies responsible for citizen protection and care. The Incident Command Structure (ICS) model provides a means to delineate a clear chain of command and management structure during critical events. Developed after a series of devastating California wildfires in the 1970s, this model provides for an overall Incident Commander of any disaster event who oversees predesignated public relations, logistics, finance, supply, and organizational section chiefs. Each section has a variety of personnel with specific duties and areas of focus who report to the chiefs at regular intervals. The ICS is frequently revised and is designed to be flexible, predictable, and accountable, with improved documentation, common language, and cost efficiency.[60]

Frequent rehearsals of disaster plans are of utmost importance. A written plan is useless unless it is thoroughly understood and practiced by all parties involved. Rehearsals should be varied and should include single-agency drills, tabletop exercises with participating community organizations, functional experiences with state and local emergency operations centers, and a full-scale interagency real-time drill. The last should be as realistic as possible, with mock patients, evolving scenarios, and full community-wide participation. Equally important to any disaster plan is the "after-action"—discussion of the drill or real-life event with focus on identification and rectification of problems and appropriate refinement of the plan.

■ DISASTER RESPONSE

Response to a catastrophic event requires rapid mobilization and efficient use of available resources. There should be clear and defined roles for prehospital providers, health care facilities, and all levels of governmental agencies involved in public safety and welfare.

■ Prehospital Disaster Response and Triage

Although fully capable of responding to individual emergency calls, most local EMS systems are often not able to respond adequately to a widespread or overwhelming event.[61] The concept of prehospital triage, used routinely in EMS, is of utmost importance in managing disasters. Unlike routine triage—in which the aim is to identify those few critically ill patients who require immediate, aggressive resource utilization—disaster triage attempts to "do the most good for the most people" and often requires that seriously injured victims receive little to no immediate care. Disaster triage models attempt to rapidly identify the individuals who will benefit most from immediate stabilization with the fewest available resources. Although no civilian triage system has been prospectively validated with outcome data, several well-used models exist.

The simplest method of triage assigns each patient a color-coded tag with opportunities for frequent reassessment (Fig. 10-1). Green tags are given to patients who require minor, nonimmediate medical interventions. Yellow tags indicate potentially serious injuries that are relatively stable and can wait a short time for treatment. Red tags designate life-threatening, but potentially treatable injuries that require immediate medical care. Black tags signify dead or critically ill patients who will not survive without significant use of resources and time unavailable under disaster conditions. For example, victims of a large-scale blast injury with significant head and abdominal injuries who might survive with aggressive neurosurgical intervention and laparotomy in hospital may be tagged "black," because their immediate resuscitative and stabilization needs would require an inordinate use of personnel and equipment, given the number of victims and likelihood of meaningful outcome.

Tag systems are combined with triage models in order to provide specific algorithms for patient classification. Widely used in the United Start, the Simple

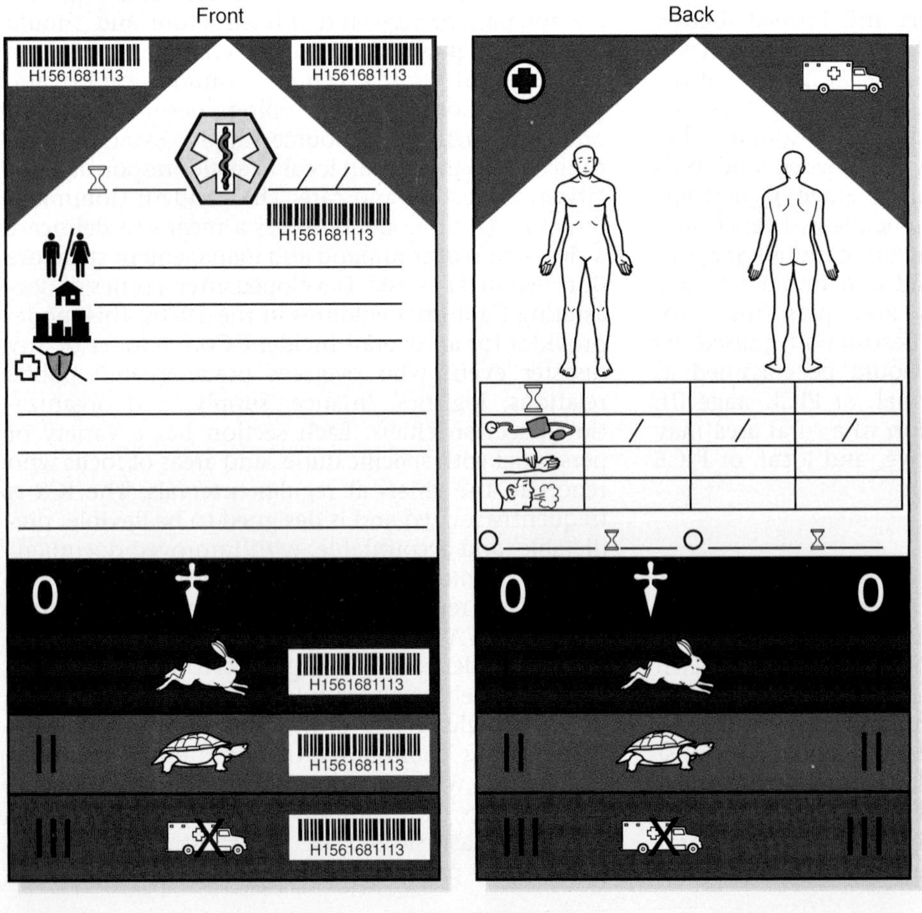
Front
Back
H1561681113
H1561681113
H1561681113
0
0
0
H1561681113
II
H1561681113
II
II
III
H1561681113
III
III

FIGURE 10-1 Example of a simple disaster triage tag.

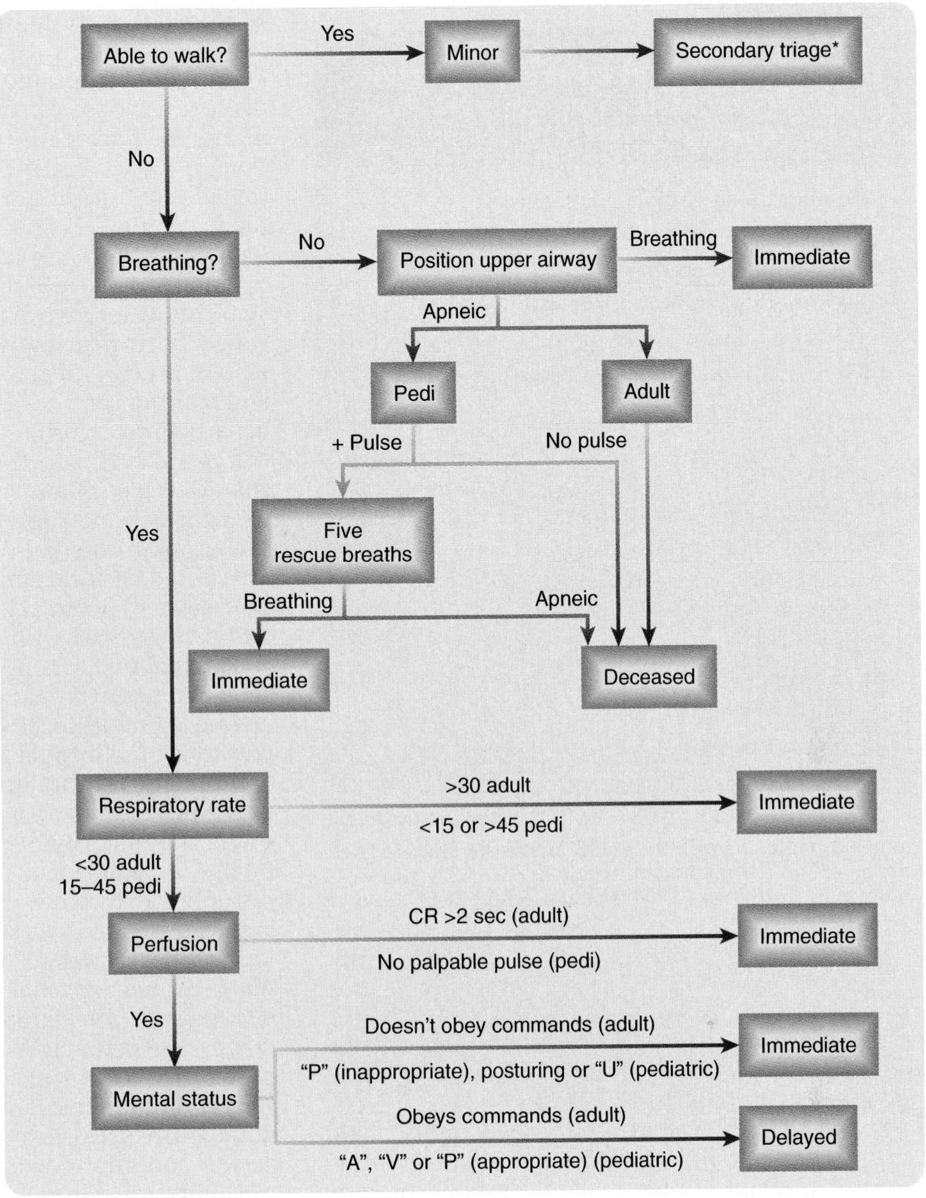
Able to walk?
Yes
Minor
Secondary triage*
No
Breathing?
No
Position upper airway
Breathing
Immediate
Apneic
Pedi
Adult
+ Pulse
No pulse
Yes
Five rescue breaths
Breathing
Apneic
Immediate
Deceased
Respiratory rate
>30 adult
<15 or >45 pedi
Immediate
<30 adult
15–45 pedi
Perfusion
CR >2 sec (adult)
No palpable pulse (pedi)
Immediate
Yes
Mental status
Doesn't obey commands (adult)
"P" (inappropriate), posturing or "U" (pediatric)
Immediate
Obeys commands (adult)
"A", "V" or "P" (appropriate) (pediatric)
Delayed

FIGURE 10-2 Combined START (Simple Triage and Rapid Treatment)/JumpSTART triage algorithm. *Using the JumpStart algorithm, evaluate first all children who did not walk under their own power. A, alert; CR, capillary refill time (seconds); Delayed, treatment may be delayed for hours to days; Immediate, requires immediate life-saving treatment; JS, JumpSTART; P, pain; Pedi, pediatric (patient); U, unresponsive; V, voice.

Triage and Rapid Treatment (START) system triages mass casualty patients according to several simple variables: breathing, ambulation, radial pulse, and ability to follow commands (Fig. 10-2). Patients are categorized as "green" if they are initially ambulatory with minor injuries. "Yellow" victims are those who may be unable to walk but are breathing with respiratory rates less than 30 breaths/min, are well perfused (capillary refill time less than 2 seconds), and can follow simple commands. Patients with respiratory rates higher than 30 breaths/min (with or without airway positioning), delayed capillary refill, and/or inability to follow simple commands are tagged as "red," and their need for immediate lifesaving attention is assessed. Apneic patients are tagged as "black," and no further interventions are performed for them. Refinement of this model has led to specific, but still simple, modifications for pediatric patients.[62]

The Secondary Assessment of Victim Endpoint (SAVE) model was developed as an adjunct to the START system. After primary assessment with START, secondary triage is performed with the use of SAVE in order to assess the following: prognosis if only minimal treatment is performed, and prognosis using only available resources on site or at the disaster medical aid center. Patients are sent to a treatment area only if treatment will reduce morbidity or mortality within the delayed time to definitive care without consuming a disproportionate amount of resources.[63] The SAVE protocol provides specific guidelines based on age, injury location (head, extremity, spine, chest, and abdomen) and type

BOX 10-2

SAVE (Secondary Assessment of Victim Endpoint) Protocol Treatment Priorities (in Descending Order)

- Temporary airway management
- Pressure dressings to bleeding
- Simple pneumothorax
- Treatment of shock after bleeding control
- Advanced airway techniques
- Limb manipulation for vascular supply
- Burns—25% mortality
- Chest trauma
- Spinal injury
- Fasciotomies/amputations
- Open wound care/closure
- Head injury—Glasgow Coma Scale (GCS) score ≥8
- Abdominal trauma
- Head injury—GCS score <8
- Burns—50% mortality
- Burns—75% mortality
- Head injury—GCS score = 3

From Benson M, Koenig KL, Schultz CH: Disaster triage: START, then SAVE—a new method of dynamic triage for victims of a catastrophic earthquake. Prehospital Disaster Med 1996;11: 117-124.

(burns, crush injuries, blunt or penetrating trauma) and suggests treatment priorities in order of likelihood of success (Box 10-2).

The START system has been shown to be taught easily to first responders, with appropriate retention of basic principles after a simple 2-hour training class.[64] However, real-time use of the START system during the terrorist attack in New York City in 2001 proved ineffective. Because of the dynamic nature of the event, the loss of communications, and the fact that rescue personnel were in personal danger, the START system was abandoned.[57] A new refinement of triage methods—the RPM (Respiratory–Pulse–Motor) score—was developed to address some of the imprecision and limitations of the START model. A model was developed through the use of blunt trauma victims that organizes patients into 12 priority categories determined by the sum of coded scores for respiratory rate, pulse, and best motor response. In simulation scenarios, this method improved survival chances in certain types of disasters and locations, but a prospective validation in real time has yet to be performed.[65] International triage systems (Careflight, Triage Save and Sort) are comparable to START in prediction of critical injury, but rigorous studies are needed before any single triage model is deemed superior.[66]

Hospital and Agency Disaster Response

With proper triage and communications, prehospital disaster response can successfully reduce the burden of any mass incident on receiving health care facilities.[59,67] JCAHO requirements mandate that hospitals prepare for both internal and external events; these plans should be easily integrated in the event of a combined internal and external disaster. Internal and external events may involve different roles for ED staff. In an internal disaster, the ED's main focus is generally to treat individuals within the institution who may be injured, leaving the actual management and control of the situation to other in-hospital departments according to the institution's incident command protocol. The possibility of ED evacuation should be part of any hospital plan; it should be well thought out and rehearsed for maximum speed and safety. In an internal disaster, resources and outside aid should be sufficient for patient care and evacuation such that critically ill patients can be treated and/or evacuated with highest priority.[14]

External disasters usually result in the presence of sudden and often overwhelming volumes of patients at one or more local health care facilities. Ideally, controlled prehospital triage should lead to even and appropriate distribution of patients to local hospitals; however, research on a variety of disasters shows that often, the majority of patients do not arrive at hospitals via ambulance. This fact can cause significant disruption of carefully planned dispersion of resources and lead to rapid saturation of closest or most familiar facilities as well as difficulties with patient tracking and timely hospital notification. Hospitals should be prepared for significant communication breakdowns, restricted access, limited outside help, mass influx of victims with a variety of injuries, and personnel limitations. For example, hospitals in the flood zone of Hurricane Katrina suffered prolonged austere conditions owing to protracted physical inaccessibility, primitive communications, and lack of timely outside aid. Although no plan can prepare for every eventuality, flexibility and awareness of available resources are key to success in a significant disaster.

When local and regional resources are overwhelmed in a disaster, national governmental and private agencies may be needed for assistance. The largest and most important source of aid comes from the federal government through the DHS. This department, established after the 2001 terrorist attacks, combined many different government agencies that were responsible in some way for public health or safety. The Emergency Preparedness and Response subdirectorate of DHS combined the Federal Emergency Management Agency (FEMA), the National Disaster Medical Service (NDMS), the FBI, and Energy and Justice Department agencies in order to oversee federal disaster response and training. FEMA has several thousand full-time and reserve employees who are responsible for planning and coordinating a federal response to disaster as well as on-scene deployment of resources. NDMS provides medical assistance to disaster areas in the form of volunteer health care personnel, resources, and infrastructure for care delivery, veterinary and mortuary teams, and pre-event training of first responders. Nongovernmental organizations such as the Red Cross (and internationally, the United Nations) often partner with federal agencies to coordinate response and allocation of resources after catastrophes.

Although FEMA search-and-rescue teams are ideally deployed within 6 hours after disaster declaration and can provide basic scene and patient stabilization, federal resources are often delayed for several days. Evidence suggests that local response to disasters has the most lifesaving potential, because outside aid generally arrives too late for meaningful immediate medical care.[68] New models of disaster response, such as the Medical Disaster Response Project, address this gap by training providers for catastrophic events in which hospitals are severely affected and significant outside aid does not arrive for several days.

■ WEAPONS OF MASS DESTRUCTION AND HAZARDOUS MATERIALS

Traditional disaster medicine developed mainly in response to natural events such as floods, earthquakes, and tornadoes. However, growing sophistication and spread of human-caused events in recent years have brought human-caused catastrophic incidents to the forefront of focus and research. Potential agents available to terrorists include chemical, biologic, nuclear, radiologic, and explosive devices (generally referred to as "weapons of mass destruction" [WMDs]); although the overall likelihood of an attack is low, the consequences may be cataclysmic. For example, 1 gram of botulin toxin has the potential to kill a million people, and effects of nuclear and radioactive agents can reach across continents.[69] The response to WMD events may differ significantly from that to traditional disaster models described previously, with shifting priority on decontamination, agent-specific triage, and special resources and personnel.

Preparing for biologic and chemical attacks is difficult and must be adaptive. Disease surveillance programs that link a community are essential to detection and prompt response, because biologic agents may not be detected for days to weeks.[70] Predisaster emphasis should be put on hazard analysis as well as on training of personnel and stockpiling of antidotes for the agents most likely to be used. In both biologic and chemical attacks, early evacuation and containment of the "hot zone" (the area of maximum contamination) are critical to mitigation of injuries and spread. The hot zone should have clear and strict entry and exit, separate "clean" and "dirty" areas, and continuous monitoring. Primary emphasis should be given to decontamination and safety of first responder personnel, not only to ensure strong medical response but also to limit unintentional dissemination of the contaminant. Accurate risk assessments should be communicated to the public and should be frequently updated.

Traditionally, preparation for WMDs has used the more common hazardous materials exposure (HAZMAT) training methods. These models may not, however, be appropriate.[71] HAZMAT events assume an exposure away from health care facilities, where response teams with maximum personal protection and extensive decontamination equipment work to rescue and decontaminate small numbers of victims. Large-scale exposures to WMDs may encompass public areas and health care facilities, compromising response efforts and calling into question traditional decontamination methods.[72] For example, in the 1995 Japan subway nerve gas attacks, several thousand people were potentially exposed yet fewer than 100 were killed or seriously injured. Nevertheless, thousands of victims arrived at hospitals by private vehicle without having undergone on-scene decontamination, quickly overwhelming the health care facilities and potentially exposing scores of essential medical personnel.[73]

■ THE ROLE OF EMERGENCY PHYSICIANS IN DISASTER MEDICINE

Published ACEP policy advocates a leadership role for emergency physicians (EPs) in all aspects of disaster research, planning, and implementation.[74] The traditional focus of disaster medicine—to do the most good for the greatest number of people—may seem to be at odds with traditional emergency medicine principles—aggressive resource utilization for selected critically ill patients. However, the EP is generally the best-trained individual to coordinate medical control, supervise triage, connect with other municipal and public health agencies, and oversee direct patient care during a catastrophic event. There are several formal disaster medicine fellowships for EM physicians, and disaster training is included in the EM residency curriculum. Advances in research and greater global attention on natural and human-caused disasters create exciting potential for EPs to lead the development of disaster medicine as a discipline.

REFERENCES

1. Narad RA: Coordination of the EMS system: An organizational theory approach. Prehosp Emerg Care 1998;2: 145-152.
2. Dara SI, Ashton RW, Farmer JC, Carlton PK Jr: Worldwide disaster medical response: An historical perspective. Crit Care Med 2005;33(Suppl):S2-S6.
3. McSwain NE Jr: Prehospital care from Napoleon to Mars: The surgeon's role. J Am Coll Surg 2005;200:487-504.
4. Mullins RJ: A historical perspective of trauma system development in the United States. J Trauma 1999;47(Suppl): S8-S14.
5. Boyd DR: The conceptual development of EMS systems in the United States, part I. Emerg Med Serv 1982;11:19-23.
6. Hoff WS, Schwab CW: Trauma system development in North America. Clin Orthop Relat Res 2004;422:17-22.
7. Pozner CN, Zane R, Nelson SJ, Levine M: International EMS systems: The United States: past, present, and future. Resuscitation 2004;60:239-244.

8. Boyd DR: The conceptual development of EMS systems in the Unites States, part II. Emerg Med Serv 1982;11:26-33.
9. National Highway Traffic Safety Administration: The National EMS Scope of Practice Model. (DOT HS 809 898.) Washington, DC: U.S. Department of Transportation/ National Highway Traffic Safety Administration, 2005.
10. Grossman DC, Kim A, Macdonald SC, et al: Urban-rural differences in prehospital care of major trauma. J Trauma 1997;42:723-729.
11. Nathens AB, Brunet FP, Maier RV: Development of trauma systems and effect on outcomes after injury. Lancet 2004;363:1794-1801.
12. Esposito TJ, Maier RV, Rivara FP, et al: The impact of variation in trauma care times: Urban versus rural. Prehospital Disaster Med 1995;10:161-166.
13. Careless J: The importance of rural E9-1-1. Emerg Med Serv 2005;34:56.
14. Marx JA: Rosen's Emergency Medicine: Concepts and Clinical Practice, 5th ed. St. Louis, Mosby, 2002.
15. Black JJ, Davies GD: International EMS systems: United Kingdom. Resuscitation 2005;64:21-29.
16. Dale J, Higgins J, Williams S, et al: Computer assisted assessment and advice for "non-serious" 999 ambulance service callers: The potential impact on ambulance dispatch. Emerg Med J 2003;20:178-183.
17. American College of Emergency Physicians; National Association of EMS Physicians; National Association of State EMS Directors: Position statement: Role of the State EMS Medical Director. Prehosp Emerg Care 2005;9:338.
18. American College of Emergency Physicians: Policy statement: Medical Direction of EMS. Available at http://www.acep.org/webportal/PracticeResources/PolicyStatements/ems/emsmeddir.htm/
19. Erder MH, Davidson SJ, Cheney RA: On-line medical command in theory and practice. Ann Emerg Med 1989;18:261-268.
20. Wuerz RC, Swope GE, Holliman CJ, et al: On-line medical direction: A prospective study. Prehospital Disaster Med 1995;10:174-177.
21. Holliman CH, Wuerz RC, Vazques-de Miguel G, et al: Comparison of interventions of prehospital care by standing orders versus interventions ordered by direct (on-line) medical command. Prehospital Disaster Med 1994;9: 202-209.
22. Blackwell TH: Prehospital care. Emerg Med Clin North Am 1993;11:1-14.
23. Rottman SJ, Schriger DL, Charlop G, et al: On-line medical control versus protocol-based prehospital care. Ann Emerg Med 1997;30:62-68.
24. Wuerz RC, Meador SA: Evaluation of a prehospital chest pain protocol. Ann Emerg Med 1995;26:595-597.
25. Archibald S: EMS systems. In EMS Medical Director Curriculum. Available at http://kbems.ky.gov/NR/rdonlyres/C6B3B209-E1DD-4AF5-8AF6-99D4DC1DC9E6/0/EMSCurriculum.pdf/
26. United States Department of Transportation, National Highway Traffic Safety Administration: EMS Education Agenda for the Future: A systems approach. Prehosp Emerg Care 2000;4:365-366.
27. Eisenberg M, Bergner L, Hallstrom A: Paramedic programs and out-of-hospital cardiac arrest. I: Factors associated with successful resuscitation. Am J Public Health 1979;69: 30-38.
28. Eisenberg M, Bergner L, Hallstrom A: Paramedic programs and out-of-hospital cardiac arrest. II: Impact on community mortality. Am J Public Health 1979;69:39-42.
29. Messick WJ, Rutledge R, Meyer AA: The association of advanced life support training and decreased per capita trauma death rates: An analysis of 12,417 trauma deaths. J Trauma 1992;33:850-855.
30. Jacobs LM, Sinclair A, Beiser A, D'Agostino RB: Prehospital advanced life support: Benefits in trauma. J Trauma 1984;24:8-13.
31. Weston CF, McCabe MJ: Audit of an emergency ambulance service: Impact of a paramedic system. J R Coll Physicians Lond 1992;26:86-89.
32. American College of Emergency Physicians and American College of Surgeons: Equipment for Ambulances. Available at http://www.acep.org/NR/rdonlyres/AE62E47D-4700-4AD8-8A7B-3D168BDFFF29/0/ambulance_equip.pdf/
33. Moylan JA: Impact of helicopters on trauma care and clinical results. Ann Surg 1988;208:673-678.
34. Schneider C, Gomez M, Lee R: Evaluation of ground ambulance, rotor-wing, and fixed-wing aircraft services. Crit Care Clin 1992;8:533-564.
35. Thomas SH, Harrison TH, Buras WR, et al: Helicopter transport and blunt trauma mortality: A multicenter trial. J Trauma 2002;52:13-45.
36. Wills VL, Eno L, Walker C, Gani JS: Use of an ambulance-based helicopter retrieval service. Aust N Z J Surg 2000; 70:506-510.
37. Skogvoll E, Bjelland E, Thorarinson B: Helicopter emergency medical service in out-of-hospital cardiac arrest—a 10-year population-based study. Acta Anaesthesiol Scand 2000;44:972-979.
38. DeWing MD, Curry T, Stephenson E, et al: Cost-effective use of helicopters for the transportation of patients with burn injuries. J Burn Care Rehab 2000;21:535-540.
39. Di Bartolomeo S, Sanson G, Nardi G, et al: Effects of 2 patterns of prehospital care on the outcome of patients with severe head injury. Arch Surg 2001;136:1293-1300.
40. Slater H, O'Mara MS, Goldfarb IW: Helicopter transportation of burn patients. Burns 2002;28:70-72.
41. Thomson DP, Thomas SH; 2002-2003 Air Medical Services Committee of the National Association of EMS Physicians: Guidelines for air medical dispatch. Prehosp Emerg Care 2003;7:265-271.
42. Eisenberg MS, Horwood BT, Cummins RO, et al: Cardiac arrest and resuscitation: A tale of 29 cities. Ann Emerg Med 1990;19:179-186.
43. Bunch TJ, Hammill SC, White RD: Outcomes after ventricular fibrillation out-of-hospital cardiac arrest: Expanding the chain of survival. Mayo Clin Proc 2005;80: 774-782.
44. White RD, Bunch TJ, Hankins DG: Evolution of a community-wide early defibrillation programme experience over 13 years using police/fire personnel and paramedics as responders. Resuscitation 2005;65:279-283.
45. Rea TD, Eisenberg MS, Becker LJ, et al: Temporal trends in sudden cardiac arrest: A 25-year emergency medical services perspective. Circulation 2003;107:2780-2785.
46. Hazinski MF, Idris AH, Kerber RE, et al: Lay rescuer automated external defibrillator ("public access defibrillation") programs: Lessons learned from an international multicenter trial: Advisory statement from the American Heart Association Emergency Cardiovascular Committee; the Council on Cardiopulmonary, Perioperative, and Critical Care; and the Council on Clinical Cardiology. Circulation 2005;111:3336-3340.
47. Liberman M, Mulder DS, Jurkovich GJ, Sampalis JS: The association between trauma system and trauma center components and outcome in a mature regionalized trauma system. Surgery 2005;137:647-658.
48. Sampalis JS, Denis R, Lavoie A, et al: Trauma care regionalization: A process-outcome evaluation. J Trauma 1999; 46:565-579.
49. Cornwell EE 3rd, Belzberg H, Hennigan K, et al: Emergency medical services (EMS) vs non-EMS transport of critically injured patients: A prospective evaluation. Arch Surg 2000;135:315-319.
50. Pickens JJ, Copass MK, Bulger EM: Trauma patients receiving CPR: Predictors of survival. J Trauma 2005;58: 951-958.
51. Davis DP, Peay J, Sise MJ, et al: The impact of prehospital endotracheal intubation on outcome in moderate to severe traumatic brain injury. J Trauma 2005;58:933-939.
52. Pons PT, Haukoos JS, Bludworth W, et al: Paramedic response time: Does it affect patient survival? Acad Emerg Med 2005;12:594-600.
53. Blackwell TH, Kaufman JS: Response time effectiveness: Comparison of response time and survival in an urban

emergency medical services system. Acad Emerg Med 2002;9:288-295.
54. Waeckerle JF: Domestic preparedness for events involving weapons of mass destruction. JAMA 2000;283:252-254.
55. Asaeda G: The day that the START triage system came to a STOP: Observations from the World Trade Center disaster. Acad Emerg Med 2002;9:255-256.
56. Koenig KL, Dinerman N, Kuehl AE: Disaster nomenclature—a functional impact approach: The PICE system. Acad Emerg Med 1996;3:723-727.
57. Auf der Heide E: The importance of evidence-based disaster planning. Ann Emerg Med 2006;47:34-49.
58. Auf der Heide E: Disaster Response: Principles of Preparation and Coordination. St. Louis, Mosby, 1989.
59. Mothershead JL: Disaster planning (updated 1/19/05). Available at www.emedicine.com/
60. Hospital Emergency Incident Command System, 3rd ed, 1998. Available at http://www.heics.com/HEICS98a.pdf/
61. Branas CC, Sing RF, Perron AD: A case series analysis of mass casualty incidents. Prehosp Emerg Care 2000; 4:299-304.
62. Romig L: The JumpSTART Algorithm. Available at http://www.jumpstarttriage.com/TheJumpSTARTAlgorithm.html/
63. Benson M, Koenig KL, Schultz CH: Disaster triage: START, then SAVE—a new method of dynamic triage for victims of a catastrophic earthquake. Prehospital Disaster Med 1996;11:117-124.
64. Risavi BL, Salen PN, Heller MB, Arcona S: A two-hour intervention using START improves prehospital triage of mass casualty incidents. Prehosp Emerg Care 2001;5: 197-199.
65. Sacco WJ, Navin DM, Fiedler KE, et al: Precise formulation and evidence-based application of resource-contained triage. Acad Emerg Med 2005;12:759-770.
66. Garner A, Lee A, Harrison K, Schultz CH: Comparative analysis of multiple-casualty incident triage algorithms. Ann Emerg Med 2001;38:541-548.
67. McDonald CC, Koenigsberg MD, Ward S: Medical control of mass gatherings: Can paramedics perform without physicians on-site? Prehospital Disaster Med 1993;8:327-331.
68. Schultz CH, Koenig KL, Noji EK: A medical disaster response to reduce immediate mortality after an earthquake. N Engl
69. Arnon SS, Schechter R, Inglesby TV, et al: Botulinum toxin as a biological weapon: Medical and public health management. JAMA 2001;285:1059-1070.
70. Flowers LK, Mothershead JL, Blackwell TH: Bioterrorism preparedness. II: The community and emergency medical services systems. Emerg Med Clin North Am 2002;20: 457-476.
71. Macintyre AG, Christopher GW, Eitzen E Jr, et al: Weapons of mass destruction events with contaminated casualties: Effective planning for health care facilities. JAMA 2000;283:242-249.
72. Okumura T, Takasu N, Ishimatsu S, et al: Report on 640 victims of the Tokyo subway sarin attack. Ann Emerg Med 1996;28:129-135.
73. World Health Organization: Public Health Response to Biological and Chemical Weapons: WHO guidance, 2nd ed. Geneva, WHO, 2004.
74. American College of Emergency Physicians: Disaster medical services policy statement. Available at http://www.acep.org/webportal/PracticeResources/PolicyStatements/ems/dismedsvc.htm/

Chapter 11

Procedural Sedation

Andy Godwin and Beranton Whisenant

KEY POINTS

Procedural sedation refers to the technique of administering sedatives or dissociative agents with (procedural sedation and analgesia [PSA]) or without analgesics to induce a state that allows the patient to tolerate unpleasant procedures while maintaining cardiorespiratory function.[1,2]

Procedural sedation and analgesia in the ED is generally intended to create a depressed level of consciousness that allows the patient to maintain airway control and oxygenation without continuous assistance.

Patients must be assessed before sedation to proactively identify potential difficulties associated with disease states and airway maintenance.

When drugs are used in combination, their effects are more than additive, and this effect can be beneficial or can potentiate respiratory depression and cardiovascular instability.

In the presence of liver disease, the metabolism of drugs is altered in many ways and it is difficult to predict effects.

In patients with recent history of opiate and benzodiazepine overuse, propofol may offer advantages over the other agents.

Definitions

Procedural sedation, not including dissociative agents, represents a continuum of sedation ranging across defined levels of consciousness. These varying degrees of awareness have been termed *minimal sedation* (anxiolysis), *moderate sedation, deep sedation,* and *general anesthesia*. See Table 11-1 for the general definitions as defined by the Joint Commission on Accreditation of Healthcare Organizations (JCAHO). Because patients can move from one state or level of awareness to another without warning, serial assessments and close hemodynamic monitoring are advised.

Indications for Procedural Sedation and Analgesia in the ED

Patients often present to the ED with acute injuries or disorders that require timely intervention to reduce both the physical and psychological effects of pain, anxiety, disability, and life-threatening complications. Common indications that may require procedural sedation are listed in Box 11-1.

Patient Monitoring

Individual patient responses to sedatives and analgesics often vary; therefore, constant monitoring is

Table 11-1 GENERAL DEFINITIONS RELATED TO ANESTHESIA*

Parameter	Minimal Sedation	Moderate Sedation	Deep Sedation	General Anesthesia
Responsiveness	Normal responsive to verbal stimulation	Purposeful response to verbal or tactile sedation	Purposeful response after repeated or painful stimulation	Unarousable even with painful stimulation
Airway	Unaffected	No intervention required	Intervention may be required	Intervention often required
Spontaneous ventilation	Unaffected	Adequate	May be inadequate	Frequently inadequate
Cardiovascular function	Unaffected	Usually maintained	Usually maintained	May be impaired
Modified Ramsay sedation scale score	1	2-4	5-7	8

*As defined by the Joint Commission on Accreditation of Healthcare Organizations.

BOX 11-1

Indications for Procedural Sedation and Analgesia in the ED

- Fracture reduction and orthopedic procedures
- Burn and wound débridement
- Laceration repair, especially in pediatrics
- Foreign body removal
- Elective and nonelective cardioversion
- Thoracostomy tube insertion
- Endoscopy
- Awake intubation and mechanical ventilation
- Radiologic studies in the agitated or uncooperative patient

important to identify subtle changes in respiratory effort and hemodynamics. American College of Emergency Physician (ACEP) guidelines recommend that patients selected for PSA undergo continuous cardiac monitoring, continuous pulse oximetry, and documented blood pressure checks every 5 minutes during the procedure and postprocedural period.[2] Box 11-2 provides a list of objective physiologic parameters recommended for safe bedside monitoring. In addition, see Table 11-2 for the 8-point Ramsay sedation scale that was initially validated in intensive care units for the assessment of sedation depth and later modified to correlate with JCAHO sedation definitions.

■ CAPNOMETRY (END-TIDAL CARBON DIOXIDE MONITORING)

Many agents decrease the tidal volume and respiratory rate creating a potential for hypoventilation and apnea. In the majority of patients, pulse oximetry readings correlate well with arterial O_2 saturation values. Unfortunately, oximetry is ineffective in the early detection of hyperventilation hypercarbia, particularly if patients are receiving supplemental

Table 11-2 RAMSAY SEDATION SCALE

Clinical Score	Level of Sedation Achieved
1	Patient agitated, anxious
2	Patient cooperative, oriented, and tranquil
3	Patient responds to commands only
4	Brief response to light glabellar stimuli or loud auditory stimuli
5	Sluggish response to light glabellar tap or loud auditory stimuli
6	No response to a light glabellar tap or loud auditory stimuli

BOX 11-2

Objective Physiologic Parameters for Patient Monitoring

- Vital signs: blood pressure, respiratory rate
- Cardiac rhythm: cardiac monitor
- Oxygenation: pulse oximetry
- Clinical assessment of depth of sedation: modified Ramsay scale
- Ventilatory effort: clinical examination and end-tidal CO_2 monitoring with continuous capnometry

oxygen. Therefore, in patients whose ventilatory status can not be visualized (e.g., covered with a sterile sheet), continuous capnometry should be considered for rapid identification of hypoventilation and apnea.

■ PULSE OXIMETRY

Pulse oximetry may be misleading for a variety of reasons. The EP must be aware of the pitfalls of this modality in order to correctly address changes in oxygenation (Table 11-3).[3,4]

Table 11-3 PITFALLS IN PULSE OXIMETRY

Low-perfusion states	Low cardiac output, vasoconstriction, or hypothermia
Motion artifact	The most common source of error
Nail polish	Black, green, and blue nail polish colors have the same light absorbencies (660 and 940 nm)
Type of probe and location	Ear probes have rapid response time Accuracy of reading depends on the patient's perfusion state and heart rate
Ambient light	Falsely low O_2 saturation values with fluorescent and xenon surgical lamps
Dyshemoglobinemias (carboxyhemoglobin; methemoglobin)	Overestimation of true O_2 saturation
Transient hypoxia consistent with patient's normal sleep patterns	Inherent disadvantage of oximetry with insignificant hypoxic episodes

Data from references 3 and 4.

■ DEPTH OF SEDATION MONITORING

■ Bispectral Index Monitoring

Electroencephalographic (EEG) bispectral index monitoring has been studied for use in the ED as a means to avoid hypercarbia and hypoxic events, and to objectively determine the depth of sedation during PSA. The bispectral index is a statistical numerical value based on the bispectral processing of the last 15 to 30 seconds of the harmonic and phase relation of the frontal lobe EEG data (Fig. 11-1). A score of 90 to 100 represents an awake state; 70 to 80, a moderate sedation state; 60 to 70, a deep sedation state; 40, general anesthesia; and 0, consistent with brain death. These scores can vary with the PSA used and in individual patients.[5] The use of combination PSA agents makes titrating to a predefined bispectral index value difficult owing to the synergistic effect of the agents.[6,7] There is insufficient evidence to recommend routine use of this monitoring in the ED.[2]

Preprocedural Considerations and Risk Assessment

The clinician must obtain and document a complete history and physical examination for a patient administering sedative medications. This step is critical in determining whether the patient is an appropriate candidate for PSA.

The goal of PSA is to effectively alleviate the patient's anxiety, pain, and discomfort to the degree that best facilitates the safe performance of both painful and nonpainful procedures. PSA represents a dynamic continuum, with patients moving from one level of consciousness to the next without any clear

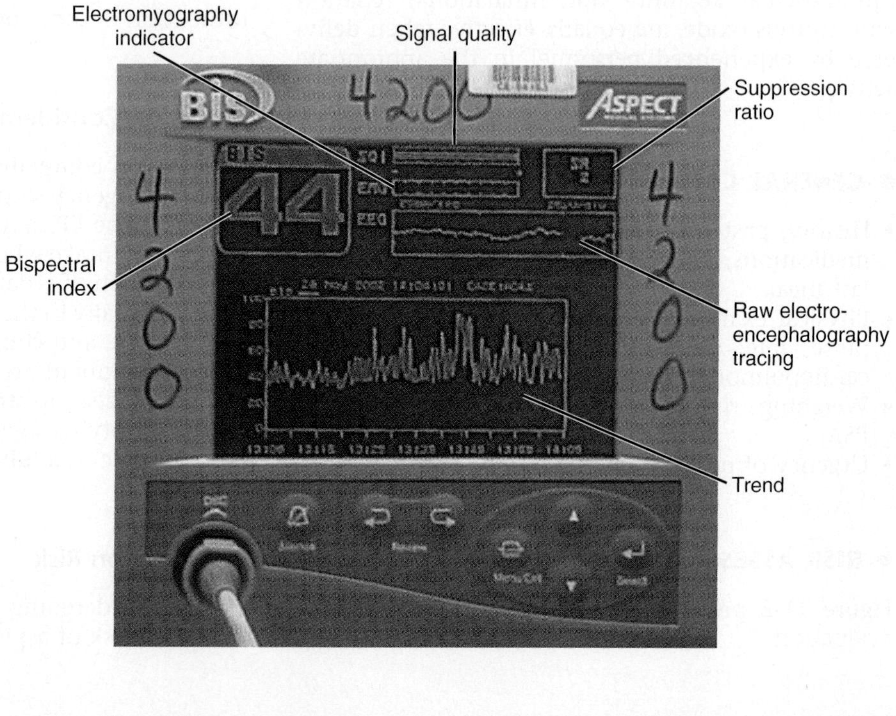
Electromyography indicator
Signal quality
Suppression ratio
Bispectral index
Raw electro-encephalography tracing
Trend
BIS
ASPECT
4200
44

FIGURE 11-1 Screen of a (bispectral electroencephalographic index (BIS) monitor.

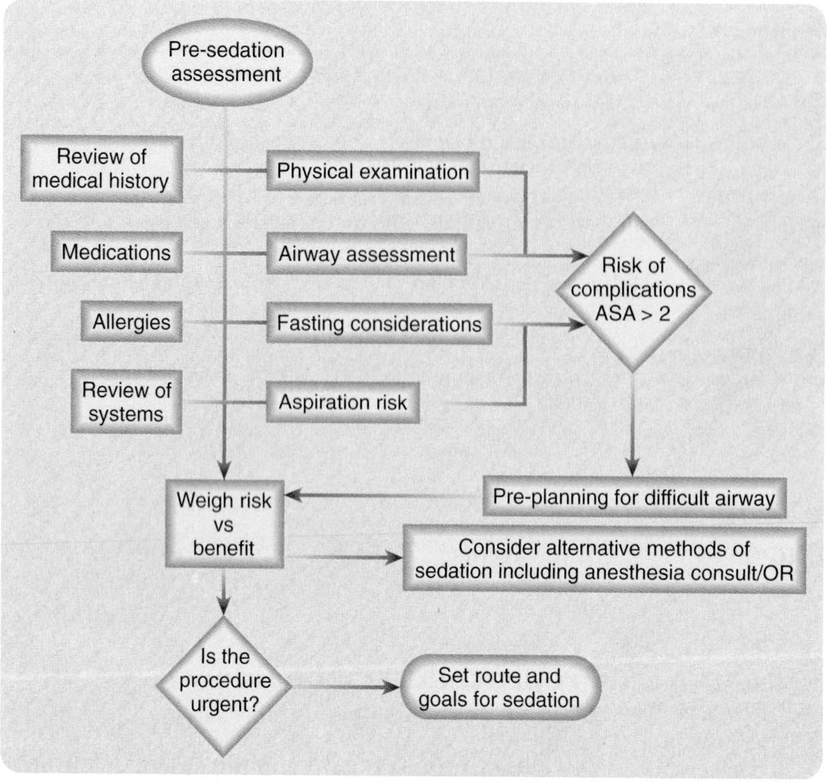
Pre-sedation assessment
Review of medical history
Physical examination
Medications
Airway assessment
Allergies
Fasting considerations
Review of systems
Aspiration risk
Risk of complications ASA > 2
Weigh risk vs benefit
Pre-planning for difficult airway
Consider alternative methods of sedation including anesthesia consult/OR
Is the procedure urgent?
Set route and goals for sedation

FIGURE 11-2 Algorithm for presedation evaluation. ASA, American Society of Anesthesiologists [score]; OR, operating room.

point of transition. The predefined level of sedation should be determined on the basis of the patient's acute disease state, the nature and duration of the therapeutic intervention being planned, and sedation/analgesia goals such as pain control, anxiolysis, and amnesia. In the ED the preferred method of administration for most PSA agents is often intravenous (IV). However selected agents, including intramuscular ketamine and inhalational sedation with nitrous oxide, are equally effective when delivered by experienced personnel in the appropriate setting.

■ GENERAL CONSIDERATIONS

- History: past medical history, anesthesia history, medications, allergies, review of systems, time of last meal.
- Physical examination: vital signs (blood pressure, pulse rate, respiratory rate), pulse oximetry, cardiopulmonary and neurologic examinations.
- Weighing risks against benefits of performing PSA.
- Urgency of performing PSA.

■ RISK ASSESSMENT

Figure 11-2 presents an algorithm for presedation evaluation.

■ Airway Evaluation

An assessment of the patient for potential difficult bag-mask ventilation due to facial, oral, or neck anomalies is important before PSA administration. Use of the mnemonic MOANS and LEMONS has been described as an aid in identifying anatomic and clinical features that may pose potential difficulties in airway management should bag-mask ventilation or intubation become necessary (Box 11-3).[8]

■ Fasting Considerations

There is no compelling evidence to support fasting in the emergency setting for either children or adults. However, the EP may consider a patient's history of recent oral intake when determining the appropriateness of depth of sedation and complexity of a procedure, especially in the patient at higher risk for airway compromise and complications. Prudence and good clinical judgment are paramount.[2]

There is also no strong evidence to support use of gastric emptying agents prior to sedation in either the pediatric or adult population.

■ Aspiration Risk

Patients undergoing procedural sedation are at no increased risk of aspiration because of:

BOX 11-3

Use of the Mnemonics MOANS and LEMON for Preprocedural Airway Assessment for Difficult Airway

MOANS: Difficult Bag-Mask Ventilation

M: Mask seal: bushy beards, distorted lower facial contour

O: Obesity/obstruction: morbidly obese patients (due to increase in upper airway redundant tissue) and patients with disorders that obstruct the upper airway

A: Age greater than 55, resulting in decreased muscular tone of upper airway

N: No teeth, creating difficulty with achieving an adequate mask-seal

S: Stiff: Patients with stiff noncompliant lungs, such as with COPD, asthma, CHF, and pulmonary fibrosis

LEMON: Difficult Intubations

L: Look externally for physical features that may make intubation difficult: small mandible, large teeth, large tongue, short neck

E: Evaluate 3-3-2 rule:

- For mouth opening, 5 cm or at least 3 (patient's) fingerbreadths
- Thyromental distance of 5 cm or 3 fingerbreadths
- 2 fingerbreadths from the hyoid to the thyroid cartilage for evaluation of the position of the larynx in relation to tongue base

M: Mallampati score: the ability to visualize the posterior oropharynx with opening of the mouth

O: Obstruction: upper airway obstruction, stridor, odynophagia, and dysphagia.

N: Neck mobility: immobilization due to cervical trauma, arthropathies

- Maintenance of protective reflexes during PSA
- Brevity of the procedure
- Lack of manipulation of the airway
- Depth of sedation[2]

Neither gastric emptying with pharmacologic agents nor antacid use has been shown to be beneficial.

Pharmacodynamics and Pharmacokinetics of Common Agents

In view of the array of procedures requiring PSA in the ED and the varied underlying clinical disorders, an understanding of the pharmacology of individual agents is important. This knowledge allows the provider to tailor sedation and analgesia to meet individual patients' needs. A number of agents are well suited to the ED environment because of their rapid onset of action, brief recovery period, and minimal untoward effects. It is difficult for a single agent to meet all of the sedative and analgesic goals of an individual patient; therefore a combination of drugs is sometimes used. Table 11-4 details the pharmacology of individual PSA agents,[9-15] and Table 11-5 details the drug effects of commonly used combination regimens.[16-17] A list of reversal agents for PSA can be found in Box 11-4.

BOX 11-4

Reversal Agents for PSA

Naloxone (Narcan)

Opioid antagonist that is used for oversedation and respiratory depression with opioids:

- For partial reversal of oversedation of a PSA opioid agent, a dose of 0.1 to 0.4 mg can be used.
- For complete reversal of sedation 2 mg should be given IV.
- Following reversal with naloxone the patient should be observed for 90 minutes due to risk of re-sedation.

Flumazenil

A reversal agent for benzodiazepine-induced oversedation and hypoventilation.

- Use 1 mg for the reversal of midazolam PSA.
- Onset of action of 1 to 2 minutes with duration of 45 minutes.
- Caution should be used in patients who are long-term users of benzodiazepine, owing to the risk of acute withdrawal.

Table 11-4 PHARMACODYNAMICS AND PHARMACOKINETICS OF COMMON SEDATION AGENTS

Drugs Short-Acting PSA Agents	Summary	Pharmacodynamic and Pharmacokinetics	Recommended Sedative Dose and Clinical Indications	Onset of Action	Recovery Period Duration
Fentanyl	Synthetic opioid 100 times more potent than morphine Analgesic agent Minimal sedative effect Used in combination with anxiolytic agent	Lipid soluble Metabolized by liver to inactive metabolite Side effects: hypotension, hypoxemia, apnea, vomiting, and rare episodes of chest wall rigidity reported when given over less than 2 min	0.5 to 1 μg/kg every 1-2 min and titrate to the desired level of sedation in combination with a sedative	Within 1 min	30-60 min after a single dose of 100 μg
Midazolam	Potent anxiolytic, sedative, and amnesic properties Useful for brief, painless ED procedures Frequently use with an opioid for analgesic effect	Binds to GABA receptors in CNS to exert anxiolysis Drug effect is terminated by redistribution and hepatic metabolism to an active metabolite Active metabolite can accumulate and prolong sedation in patients who are elderly, have renal failure, and/or are taking protease inhibitors Causes respiratory depression and hypotension; should be used with caution in patients with COPD, cardiomyopathy, or hypovolemia	Adult: common dose regimen is 0.05-0.2 mg/kg IV Decrease dose by 30%-50% when combined with an opioid	30 sec-1 min Duration of action 20-40 min	20-40 min
Etomidate	Frequently used to facilitate performance of both painful and nonpainful procedures Has sedative and hypnotic effects Has minimal effect on cardiac and respiratory function	Exerts its sedative and hypnotic effects at the GABA receptors by increasing the number and enhancing the functioning of these receptors Is metabolized by the liver to an nonactive metabolite, but hepatic dysfunction does not affect the rapid recovery period Side effects: myoclonus the most unique side effect; also nausea, vomiting, hiccups, superficial thrombophlebitis, and/or apnea Can cause hypoventilation and apnea when combined with an opioid or other anxiolytic agent Mild (clinically insignificant) adrenocortical suppression after a single IV bolus	Adult: 0.2 mg/kg over 1 min	<1 min	5 min

Methohexital	An effective ultra-short-acting, rapid-recovery PSA agent of the barbiturate class Most frequently use in the ED for short painful procedures such as orthopedic reduction	Rapidly produces a state of unconsciousness, profound amnesia and has no analgesic properties Is frequently combined with opioid for painful procedures Side effects: most common, respiratory depression and apnea Also has a direct myocardial depressant effect and should not be used in hemodynamically unstable patients	Adult: 0.75-1 mg/kg bolus IV administration and can be titrated at 0.5 mg/kg at 3- to 5-min intervals to desired level of sedation	<1 min	5-7 min
Propofol	Ideal for procedures requiring brief periods of sedation Rapid onset of action and rapid recovery makes it an ideal PSA agent for use in the ED A preferred sedative for patients with brain injury	Produces its sedative-hypnotic effects by binding to and mediating upregulation of GABA receptors Metabolized by extensive tissue redistribution and hepatic and extrahepatic metabolism Coadministration with opioid slows metabolic clearance and prolongs the recovery time Side effects: respiratory depression, apnea and hypotension; also, pain at the injection site, hyperlipidemia, and pancreatitis	Adult: A loading dose of 1 mg/kg over 1-2 min followed by a continuous infusion at 1.5-4.5 mg/kg/min or 20-mg aliquots to titrate to the desired effect Elderly patients: continuous infusion of 25 μg/kg/min is preferred without bolus injection to limit respiratory depression/hypotension	<1 min	10 min
Dexmedetomidine	Highly selective α_2-adrenergic agonist with sedative, anxiolytic, and analgesic properties Induces natural sleep to exert its sedative-anxiolytic effects Can be used to sedate patients who are insensitive to the usual doses of benzodiazepines Also used as an effective PSA agent for nonpainful procedures	Acts on α_2-adrenergic receptor in the brain to regulate sleep and respiratory pattern	Adults: loading dose of 0.3-1 μg/kg/min over 5-10 min followed by infusion at 0.5-1.0 μg/kg/hr	Rapid	Short
Remifentanil	Provides excellent sedative and analgesia for brief ED procedures	An ester derivative of fentanyl with ultra-short-acting sedative and analgesic properties Metabolized by esterases present in interstitial tissues and RBCs Metabolism is independent of hepatic or renal dysfunction Side effect: respiratory depression that is responsive to verbal commands	Adult: Infusion at 0.5 μg/kg over 90 min with continuous dosing of 0.25 μg/kg as needed	<1 min	Rapid (3-15 min)

Table 11-4 PHARMACODYNAMICS AND PHARMACOKINETICS OF COMMON SEDATION AGENTS—cont'd

Drugs Short-Acting PSA Agents	Summary	Pharmacodynamic and Pharmacokinetics	Recommended Sedative Dose and Clinical Indications	Onset of Action	Recovery Period Duration
Pentobarbital	Used in the ED for painless diagnostic procedures	A short-acting barbiturate agent with sedative and anticonvulsive properties Exerts its sedative-hypnotic effects at the GABA receptors site and is terminated by hepatic metabolism to an inactive metabolite that is renally excreted Side effects: hypotension, respiratory depression, and bronchospasm; use is contraindicated in intermittent porphyria COPD	Adults: A loading dose of 100-mg slow bolus that may be repeated every 1-3 min; max 200-500 mg Pediatric dose: 2-5 mg/kg; max 100 mg	3-5 min	15-45 min when given IV; 1-2 hr when given IM
Ketamine	Phencyclidine derivation with amnesic, sedative, analgesic properties Agent of choice for pediatric patients	Dissociative effect due to binding to NMDA receptors of the CNS Has bronchodilatory effect on bronchial smooth muscles and is useful in patients with bronchoconstriction Side effects: most common adverse effect is emesis, which can be decreased with the addition of midazolam Emergence phenomena with vivid dreams, hallucinations, and recovery agitation	Adults: 1 mg/kg bolus injection followed by 0.25-0.5 mg/kg every 5-10 min as needed Children: same dose as adults IM dose: 3-4 mg/kg Give glycopyrrolate 0.2 mg concomitantly for hypersalivation	IV: <1 min IM: 5 min	15-20 min
Nitrous oxide	Excellent agent for quick ED procedures	Blended solely with oxygen and has a linear dose-response pattern Advantage: does not requires vascular access Side effects: emesis, dizziness, and headaches Do not use in patients with bowel obstruction, pneumothorax	Gas mixture 50:50 nitrogen and oxygen	3-5 min	3-5 min after cessation of gas

CNS; central nervous system; COPD, chronic obstructive pulmonary disease; GABA, gamma-aminobutyric acid; IM, intramuscular(ly); IV, intravenous(ly); NMDA, *N*-methyl-D-aspartate; PSA, procedural sedation and analgesia; RBCs, red blood cells.

Table 11-5 PEDIATRIC CONSIDERATIONS FOR PROCEDURAL SEDATION AND ANALGESIA (PSA)

Combined PSA Regimens	General Comments	Onset and Duration of Action	Side Effect(s)
Propofol/fentanyl	This combination has a rapid onset of action and rapid recovery period in comparison with other combinations Significant clinical experience lacking in comparison with midazolam/fentanyl	Rapid onset <1 min Rapid recovery (15 min)	Deep sedation with respiratory depression
Etomidate/fentanyl	Frequently used in painful procedures that require brief sedation	Short onset and duration of action	Hypoxic and respiratory depression frequent but short-lived
Midazolam/fentanyl	Has an excellent safety profile when titrated to effect Most commonly used PSA combination in the ED	Short onset of action and a relative prolonged recovery time in comparison with other combination regimens	Hypoxic and respiratory depression Prolonged recovery period with hangover effect lasting up to several hours due to active metabolite
Ketamine/midazolam	Very effective in producing excellent analgesia and sedation for more painful and anxiety-producing therapeutic procedures Can be given as oral midazolam and IM ketamine, so IV access not necessary Has an excellent safety profile	Provides 15-20 min of dissociative sedation	More hypoventilation and hypoxia than with ketamine alone

REFERENCES

1. American College of Emergency Physicians: Clinical policy for procedural sedation and analgesia in the emergency department. Ann Emerg Med 1998;31:663-677.
2. American College of Emergency Physicians: Clinical policy for procedural sedation and analgesia in the emergency department. Ann Emerg 2005;45:177-196.
3. Cote CJ, Goldstein EA, Fuchsman WH, Hoaglin DC: The effect of nail polish on pulse oximetry. Anesth Analg 1989;67:683-686.
4. Tobin MJ: Respiratory monitoring. JAMA 1990;264: 244-251.
5. Miner J, Biros M, Seigel T, Ross K: The utility of the bispectral index in procedural sedation with propofol in the emergency department. Acad Emerg Med 2005;12: 190-196.
6. Barr G, Anderson RE, Samuelsson S, et al: Fentanyl and midazolam anesthesia for coronary bypass surgery: A clinical study of bispectral electroencephalogram analysis, drug concentrations and recall. Br J Anaesth 2000;84: 749-752.
7. Kissin I: Depth of anesthesia and bispectral index monitoring. Anesth Analg 2000;90:1114-1117.
8. Murphy MF, Walls RM: Identification of the difficult and failed airway. In Walls RM, Murphy MF (eds): Manual of Emergency Airway Management, 2nd ed. Philadelphia, Lippincott Williams and Wilkins, 2004.
9. Kennedy RM, Luhmann JD, Luhmann SJ: Emergency department management of pain and anxiety in orthopedic fracture care. Pediatr Drugs 2004;6:11-31.
10. Bahn E, Holt K: Procedural sedation and analgesia: A review and new concepts. Emerg Med Clin North Am 23;2005: 503-517.
11. Beers R, Camponesi E: Remifentanil update: Clinical science and utility. CNS Drugs 2004;18:1085-1104.
12. Buttershill AJ, Keating GM: Remifentanil: A review of its analgesic and sedative use in the intensive care unit. Drugs 2006;66:365-385.
13. Schenart CL: Adrenocortical dysfunction following etomidate induction in emergency department patients. Acad Emerg Med 2001;8:1-7.
14. Green SM, Krauss B: Clinical practice guideline for emergency department ketamine dissociative sedation in children. Ann Emerg Med 2004;44:460-471.
15. Minor JR, Burton JH: Clinical practice advisory: Emergency department procedural with propofol. Ann Emerg Med 2007;50:182–187.
16. Godambe SA, Elliot V, Matheny D, Pershad J: Comparison of propofol/fentanyl vs ketamine/midazolam for brief orthopedic procedural sedation in pediatric emergency department. Pediatr 2003;112:116-123.
17. Muellejans B, Matthey T, Scholpp J, Schill M: Sedation in the intensive care unit with remifentanil/propofol versus midazolam/fentanyl: A randomized, open-label, pharmacoeconomic trial. Crit Care 2006;10:R91.

Chapter 12

Local and Regional Anesthesia

Heather Murphy-Lavoie

KEY POINTS

- Alternatives to local infiltration for anesthesia include topical anesthesia and regional nerve blocks.
- Comfortable wound repair requires adequate anesthesia.
- Local infiltration may be inadequate or suboptimal in certain situations.
- For the safety and efficacy of regional anesthesia, the EP must have a detailed understanding of the local anatomy.

Scope

Adequate anesthesia is essential for many situations in the ED, such as acute wound repair, foreign body removal, abscess drainage, ingrown toenail treatment, and fracture management. In order to achieve anesthesia safely and accurately, the EP must have a thorough understanding of the various agents that can be used, the methods of administration, and the techniques for achieving regional anesthesia.

Selection of Anesthetic Agents

■ MECHANISM OF ACTION

Local anesthetics usually have an aromatic ring structure connected to a tertiary amine by either an ester or an amide link. This link determines which class an agent is in, ester or amide. Local anesthetics work by reversibly binding to and blocking sodium channels on the nerve cells, thereby blocking conduction of the nerve impulse. Their potency, onset, and duration of action are determined by their ability to access these sodium channels and stay bound to them. The higher the lipid solubility of the agent is, the higher the potency. The higher the level of protein binding is, the longer the duration of action. The onset of action is determined by the pKa—the pH at which the agent exists in equal amounts of its ionized and un-ionized forms. The closer the pKa is to physiologic pH, the faster the onset of action.[1] Most local anesthetic agents, when administered, are associated with a burning sensation that lasts several seconds before the onset of anesthesia. Patients should be warned of this feature prior to application (Table 12-1).

■ TOXICITY

Local anesthetic agents have toxic effects primarily on the cardiovascular system and central nervous system (CNS). The severity of toxicity is directly related to the lipid solubility and, therefore, the potency of an agent; thus, bupivacaine is much more likely to cause toxicity than lidocaine. The likelihood of toxicity also rises with increased vascularity and systemic absorption. The absorption rates by anatomic location, from highest to lowest, are as follows:

Intercostal > Intratracheal > Epidural > Brachial plexus > Mucosal > Distal peripheral nerve > Subcutaneous

Table 12-1 TABLE OF AGENTS

Agent	Potency*	Cost per 10 mL†	pKa‡	Onset	Duration (hours)	Maximum Dose (mg/kg)
Lidocaine	2	$0.23	7.8	Fast	2-3	4.5 (7 when given with epinephrine)
Mepivicaine	2	$4.16	7.6	Fast	2-4	4.5 (7 when given with epinephrine)
Tetracaine	4	$18.86	8.2	Moderate	3	3
Ropivacaine	4	$14.91	8.1	Moderate	3-8	3
Bupivacaine	5	$8.18	8.1	Moderate	4-10	2 (3 when given with epinephrine)

*This table assumes requal concentrations of agents conpared (e.g., 1%).
†Internet search (September 2007) includes walgreens.com, vaxserve.com, and San Francisco General Hospital price list.
‡pKa=the pH at which the agent exists in equal amounts of its ionized and un-ionized forms.
Data from references 1 and 2.

The intercostal block has the highest potential for toxicity; therefore, the maximum amount of anesthetic agent recommended for this location is only one tenth of the maximum for peripheral nerve blocks.[1] All sites are associated with a certain degree of risk, especially when accidental intravascular injection is likely.

The signs of CNS toxicity with local anesthetics are shown in Box 12-1.

If exposure is not halted, toxicity can progress to seizures, coma, respiratory depression, and cardiorespiratory arrest. Higher doses have cardiovascular toxicity, leading to tachycardias, sinus arrest, atrioventricular dissociation, hypotension, and full arrest. Premedication with benzodiazepines may blunt the CNS toxicity, so the first sign of toxicity to develop may be cardiovascular collapse.[2,3] Amides are metabolized by the liver; therefore, patients with hepatic dysfunction may be predisposed to systemic toxicity. Esters are metabolized by plasma pseudocholinesterase; therefore patients with pseudocholinesterase deficiency, such as those with myasthenia gravis, are at higher risk for systemic toxicity. In addition, metabolites of prilocaine (a component of EMLA cream) and benzocaine have been associated with methemoglobinemia.

BOX 12-1

Signs of Central Nervous System Toxicity

- Tingling
- Numbness
- Dysarthria
- Lightheadedness
- Vertigo
- Tinnitus
- Metallic taste in mouth
- Difficulty focusing
- Agitation
- Apprehension
- Twitching in face/extremities
- Seizures
- Mental status change/coma

SYSTEMIC AGENTS

Lidocaine

Lidocaine is the most commonly used local anesthetic agent. Its low cost, rapid onset, duration, and toxicity profile make it ideal for most routine applications. The maximum dose of lidocaine is 4 to 4.5 mg/kg (e.g., a 70-kg patient should receive no more than 300 mg, or 30 mL of a 1% solution). The maximum dose can be increased to 7 mg/kg when lidocaine is given with epinephrine, but the increase will also cause an increase in the sympathomimetic side effects (tachycardia and hypertension) and a theoretically higher risk of infection due to diminished blood supply to the affected area. Pain of injection can be reduced either by warming lidocaine to body temperature in a fluid warmer before administration[4] or buffering it with sodium bicarbonate (1 mL sodium bicarbonate to 9 mL of 1% lidocaine).[2,5]

Mepivacaine

Mepivacaine is structurally similar to lidocaine, with a similar onset of action and a slightly longer duration. As with bupivacaine, this longer duration of action is associated with a slightly higher risk of toxicity. The toxicity of mepivacaine is between that of lidocaine and bupivacaine, corresponding to its intermediate duration of action.

Tetracaine

Tetracaine is an ester agent. It is most commonly used in the ED for corneal anesthesia and as a component of LET (lidocaine 4%, epinephrine 0.1%, tetracaine 0.5%, see later).

Ropivacaine

Ropivacaine is a relatively new amide local anesthetic approved by the U.S. Food and Drug Administration

(FDA) in 1996. Being the s-isomer of bupivacaine, ropivacaine is very similar in terms of onset of action, slightly less potent, and slightly shorter duration of action; however, it is associated with a 70% lower likelihood of cardiac toxicity. It also costs almost twice as much as bupivacaine.

■ Bupivacaine

Bupivacaine is slightly more potent than lidocaine and lasts longer, but its onset of action is later. The maximum dose of bupivacaine is 2.5 mg/kg (e.g., a 70-kg patient should receive no more than 175 mg, or 35 mL of a 0.5% solution), which can be increased to 3 mg/kg if this agent is given with epinephrine. Owing to bupivacaine's high potency and protein binding, the risk of systemic toxicity with its use is much greater than with use of lidocaine.

■ ALLERGIC REACTIONS

True allergic reactions to local anesthetics are relatively rare. They are usually secondary to the preservative rather than to the agent itself. Therefore, if an allergy is reported but not verified, the EP should consider using a preservative-free agent, such as cardiac lidocaine from the "code" cart. Other options are switching classes (allergy to esters is more common than to amides, and cross-reactivity is common within the class) and using benzyl alcohol,[6] diphenhydramine,[7] ice, or a normal saline injection. An easy way to determine the class of an agent is to remember that all amides have two *i*'s in their names and the esters only have one. If a patient is truly allergic to lidocaine for instance, none of the anesthetic agents with two *i*'s should be used (diphenhydramine is an exception to this rule of thumb, as it is not classically considered an anesthetic agent).

■ TOPICAL AGENTS

■ LET

LET (lidocaine 4%, epinephrine 0.1%, tetracaine 0.5%) is an excellent and safe topical anesthetic agent. It can be premixed by the hospital pharmacy and stored in the refrigerator for use in the ED. One applies it to wounds by soaking a cotton ball in LET and then securing the cotton ball to the wound for 15 to 30 minutes. Blanching of the skin around the wound indicates that the wound is anesthetized. Additional injected anesthetic may be required, but its application should be much more comfortable for the patient after LET pretreatment. LET should not be used on the ear, nose, penis, or digits because it contains a vasoconstrictor.[8,9]

■ EMLA

EMLA (eutectic mixture of local anesthetics: 2.5% lidocaine and 2.5% prilocaine) is approved by the FDA only for use on intact skin, although its successful use in open wounds has been reported in the medical literature. Approximately 1 hour of topical application of EMLA is needed to achieve local anesthesia, a characteristic that limits its usefulness in emergency cases. Infants younger than 3 months are at a theoretically higher risk for development of methemoglobinemia from EMLA owing to inadequate levels of methemoglobin reductase.[1,8,9]

■ Liposomal Lidocaine

ELA-Max is a relatively new proprietary mixture of 4% liposomal lidocaine approved by the FDA for the temporary relief of pain from minor cuts and abrasions. Its onset of action is much shorter than that of EMLA (only 30 minutes) and it carries no theoretical risk of methemoglobinemia because it does not contain prilocaine. This formulation may replace EMLA for most topical indications.[8,9]

Regional Nerve Blocks

■ INDICATIONS

Regional nerve blocks are used for areas that are not amenable to local infiltration, such as the palms, the soles, and the fat pads of fingers and toes. Other advantages are avoidance of local tissue distortion and the ability to anesthetize large areas with fewer injections and less anesthetic agent, thereby reducing both the likelihood of toxicity and overall discomfort to the patient. Specific examples of indications for regional nerve blocks are for paronychia or felon drainage; treatment of hand, foot, ear, and digit lacerations; débridement of road rash; treatment of nail-bed injuries and ingrown toenails; and dental extraction.

■ GENERAL TECHNIQUE

The EP should explain the procedure to the patient and obtain consent (after carefully documenting any known allergies). The procedure is as follows:

1. Prepare the skin with povidone-iodine or other antiseptic skin solution.
2. Identify the area's landmarks.
3. Induce a superficial skin wheal at the injection site to reduce the discomfort of further manipulation.
4. Advance the needle to the target area while asking the patient to report any paresthesias.
5. If the patient does report paresthesias, indicating that the needle is within the nerve sheath, (a) withdraw the needle 1 to 2 mm, (b) draw back on the syringe, (c) aspirate to ensure that the needle is not in a vessel, and (d) inject the agent slowly.

The agent of choice is usually lidocaine. Bupivacaine may be preferable when longer duration of action is desired.

UPPER EXTREMITY BLOCKS

Median Nerve

The median nerve provides sensation to the palmar surface of the radial half of the hand and the first through fourth fingers (Fig. 12-1). The median nerve is accessed between the palmaris longus tendon and the flexor carpi radialis tendon at the proximal wrist crease (Fig. 12-2). The patient should be instructed to oppose the thumb and fifth digit with the wrist flexed to allow visualization of these landmarks. The needle is inserted perpendicularly between the palmaris longus and the flexor carpi radialis tendon and is then advanced until a "pop" is felt as the flexor retinaculum is penetrated. The needle is then advanced 0.5 cm past the retinaculum, aspiration is performed to verify that the needle is not in a vessel, and 5 mL of anesthetic agent is injected slowly as the needle is withdrawn.

Ulnar Nerve

The ulnar nerve provides sensation to the palmar surface of the ulnar half of the hand and the fourth and fifth fingers (see Fig. 12-1). The ulnar nerve travels very closely to the ulnar artery deep to the flexor carpi ulnaris, so extra care must be taken to avoid intra-arterial injection. The landmarks for this

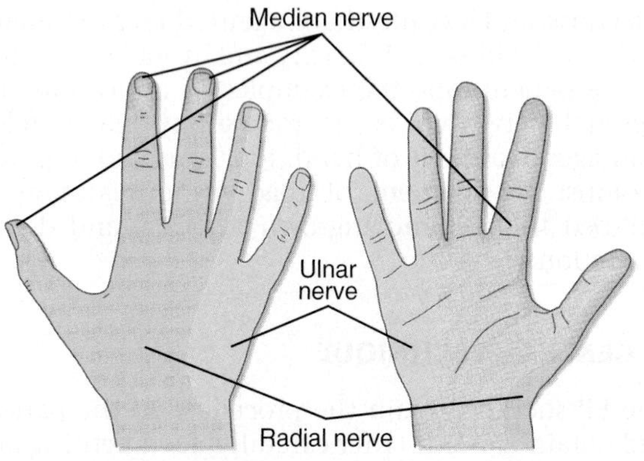
Median nerve
Ulnar nerve
Radial nerve
FIGURE 12-1 Sensory nerve distribution of the hand.

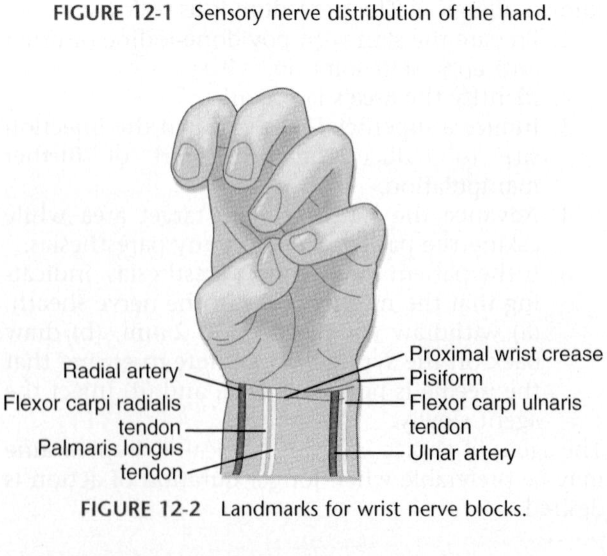
Radial artery
Flexor carpi radialis tendon
Palmaris longus tendon
Proximal wrist crease
Pisiform
Flexor carpi ulnaris tendon
Ulnar artery
FIGURE 12-2 Landmarks for wrist nerve blocks.

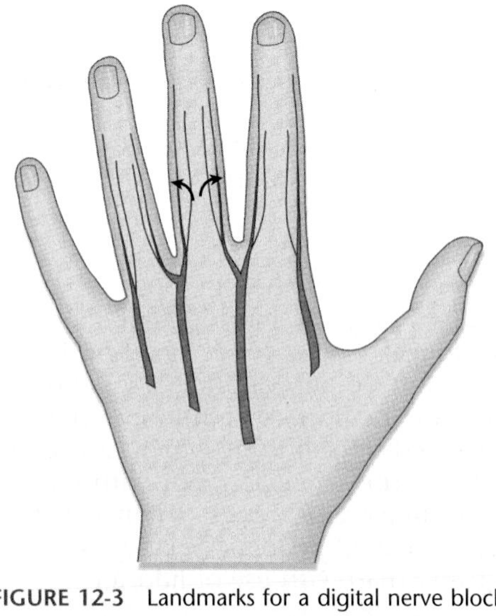
FIGURE 12-3 Landmarks for a digital nerve block.

block are the flexor carpi ulnaris and the proximal wrist crease (see Fig. 12-2). The patient should be instructed to flex the wrist, and the operator should palpate the tendon proximal to the pisiform. With the lateral approach, the needle is advanced 1 to 1.5 cm horizontally under the flexor carpi ulnaris tendon, aspiration is performed to ensure that the needle is not located intra-arterially, and 5 mL of anesthetic agent is slowly injected while the needle is withdrawn.

The ulnar nerve also gives off several subcutaneous branches, which travel from the lateral border of the flexor carpi ulnaris to the dorsal midline. These are blocked with subcutaneous injection of an additional 5 to 10 mL in a superficial ringlike wheal from the lateral aspect of the proximal wrist crease to the dorsal midline (see Fig. 12-2).

Radial Nerve

The radial nerve provides sensation to the dorsal radial aspect of the hand and the first through third fingers (see Fig. 12-1). The radial nerve travels lateral to the radial artery at the wrist and gives off superficial cutaneous branches that travel laterally to the dorsal midline. The landmarks for this block are the proximal wrist crease and the radial pulse (see Fig. 12-2). The needle is inserted perpendicularly just lateral to the radial pulse and 1 to 2 mm below the depth of the artery. Aspiration is performed, and 3 to 5 mL of anesthetic agent is injected as the needle is slowly withdrawn. The subcutaneous branches are blocked with a superficial ring-like wheal starting at the initial injection site and tracking to the dorsal midline (see Fig. 12-2).

Digital Nerves

Each finger has two sets of nerves, called the dorsal and palmar digital nerves, which travel in the 2, 4, 8, and 10 o'clock positions around the digit (Fig. 12-3). These four branch from two root nerves at the metacarpal-metatarsal heads. The most common approach for the digital nerve block is the proximal-most aspect of the finger or toe, where the nerves travel in the most consistent path. A skin wheal is formed on the dorsal surface of the finger or toe. Then the needle is directed to the 2, 4, 8, and 10 o'clock positions, respectively. After aspiration is performed, 0.5 to 1 mL of agent is injected at each site. Epinephrine and other vasoconstricting agents should not be used in this location because of the risk of critical ischemia associated with their use.

Bier Block

A Bier block involves the intravenous injection of regional anesthesia in a tourniqueted extremity. Its use is relatively uncommon in the ED, but its advantage is the concomitant creation of a bloodless field. Peripheral intravenous access should be established in the target extremity at least 10 cm distal to the tourniquet. In addition, access should be established in a back-up extremity in case resuscitation access is needed. Owing to its safely profile, 0.5% lidocaine without epinephrine is the agent of choice. This can be mixed by dilution of 1% lidocaine with equal parts of normal saline. The usual dose is 1.5 to 3 mg/kg.

A pneumatic tourniquet is applied over cotton padding proximal to the problem in the arm. The arm is elevated for at least 3 minutes to exsanguinate it prior to inflation of the tourniquet. With the arm elevated, the cuff is inflated to 250 mm Hg (or, in a child, to 50 mm Hg greater than the systolic pressure). The extremity is then lowered, and the agent is slowly injected. Onset of action is 3 to 5 minutes. Tourniquet time should be carefully monitored and should not exceed 1 hour. If the procedure is brief, the tourniquet should be left in place for at least 30 minutes after the injection of anesthetic to avoid a systemic bolus and a higher risk of toxicity.

At the completion of the procedure and waiting period, the tourniquet should be deflated for 5 seconds and re-inflated for 1 to 2 minutes; this cycle should be repeated three or four times to ensure slow release of the anesthetic into the systemic circulation. The patient should then be monitored for at least 20 minutes for any signs of toxicity.[1]

LOWER EXTREMITY BLOCKS

Femoral Nerve and 3-in-1 Block

The femoral nerve block and the 3-in-1 block (femoral, obturator, and lateral femoral cutaneous nerves) are useful for patients with femur or hip fractures. In view of the proximity of the femoral artery and vein to the target nerve, careful palpation of the pulse and aspiration are crucial to the safety of this procedure. The landmarks for this procedure are the inguinal ligament and the femoral artery (Fig. 12-4). The femoral artery is palpated 1 to 2 cm distal to the inguinal ligament. The operator's nondominant hand is kept on the femoral pulse throughout the procedure to reduce the likelihood of intra-arterial injection. With a perpendicular and slightly cephalad approach, the needle is inserted 0.5 to 1 cm lateral to the pulse until paresthesias are elicited, the patella moves involuntarily, or the needle begins to pulsate laterally. To anesthetize only the femoral nerve, about 10 to 20 mL of agent should be injected. To anesthetize all three nerves, approximately 30 mL of agent should be injected in a cephalad direction into the femoral sheath while distal pressure is maintained to ensure the proximal tracking of the anesthetic agent.[1,3,10]

Sural Nerve

The sural nerve supplies sensation to the heel and lateral foot (Fig. 12-5). The landmarks for this block are the lateral malleolus and the Achilles tendon (Fig. 12-6). The needle is inserted just lateral to the Achilles tendon, 1 cm above the lateral malleolus, and is directed toward the fibula. When contact with the fibula is made, the needle is withdrawn 1 mm, aspiration is performed, and 5 mL of agent is injected as the needle is withdrawn slowly.

Peroneal Nerves (Superficial and Deep)

The superficial peroneal nerve supplies sensation to the dorsum of the foot and toes, whereas the deep peroneal nerve supplies the first webspace (see Fig. 12-5). The landmarks for these blocks are the extensor hallucis longus tendon, the anterior tibialis tendon, and the anterior lip of the tibia (see Fig. 12-6). The superficial peroneal nerve travels anteriorly between the extensor hallucis longus tendon and the lateral malleolus. The deep peroneal nerve travels under the extensor hallucis longus tendon. For superficial peroneal nerve block, the needle is inserted just lateral to the hallucis longus tendon and is directed toward the lateral malleolus. The agent is injected in a ring-like fashion from the extensor hallucis longus to the lateral malleolus. For deep peroneal nerve block, the needle is inserted between the anterior tibialis tendon and the extensor hallucis longus tendon 1 cm above the base of the medial malleolus and is directed 30 degrees laterally under the tendon. Then the needle is advanced until it touches the tibia (less than 1 cm) and withdrawn 1 mm, and then 5 mL of agent is injected while the needle is slowly withdrawn.

Saphenous Nerve

The saphenous nerve provides sensation to the medial aspect of the foot and the arch (see Fig. 12-5). The landmarks for this block are the medial malleolus and the anterior tibialis tendon (see Fig. 12-6). The patient is instructed to dorsiflex the foot to enable the anterior tibialis tendon to be located at the anterior lip of the tibia. The saphenous nerve travels superficially between the anterior tibialis tendon and

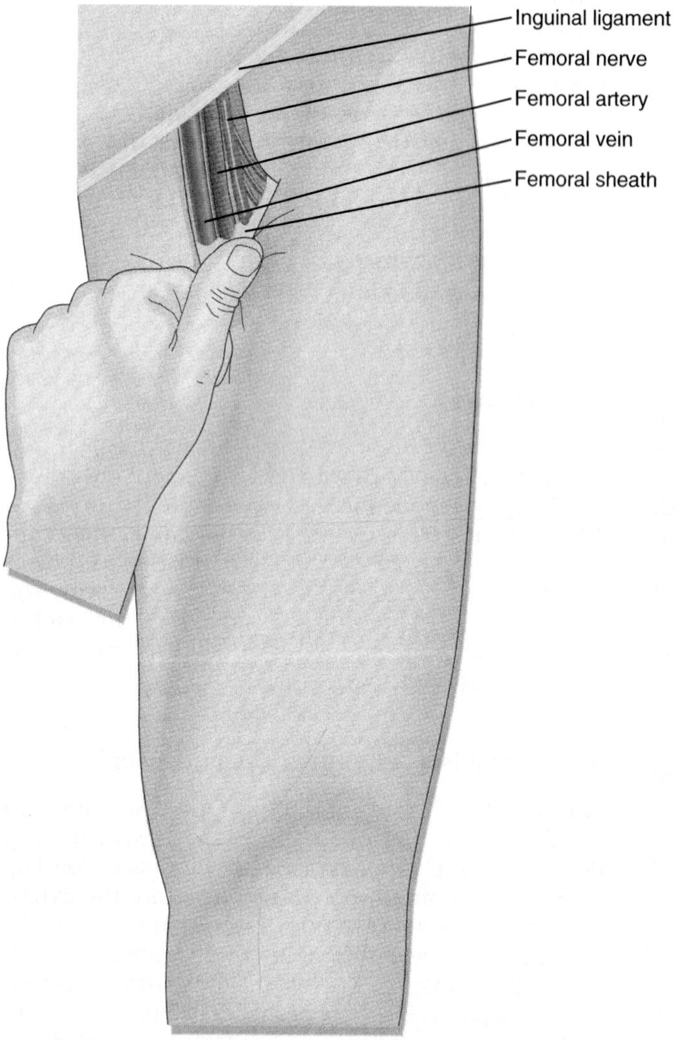
Inguinal ligament
Femoral nerve
Femoral artery
Femoral vein
Femoral sheath

FIGURE 12-4 Landmarks for a femoral nerve or 3-in-1 nerve block.

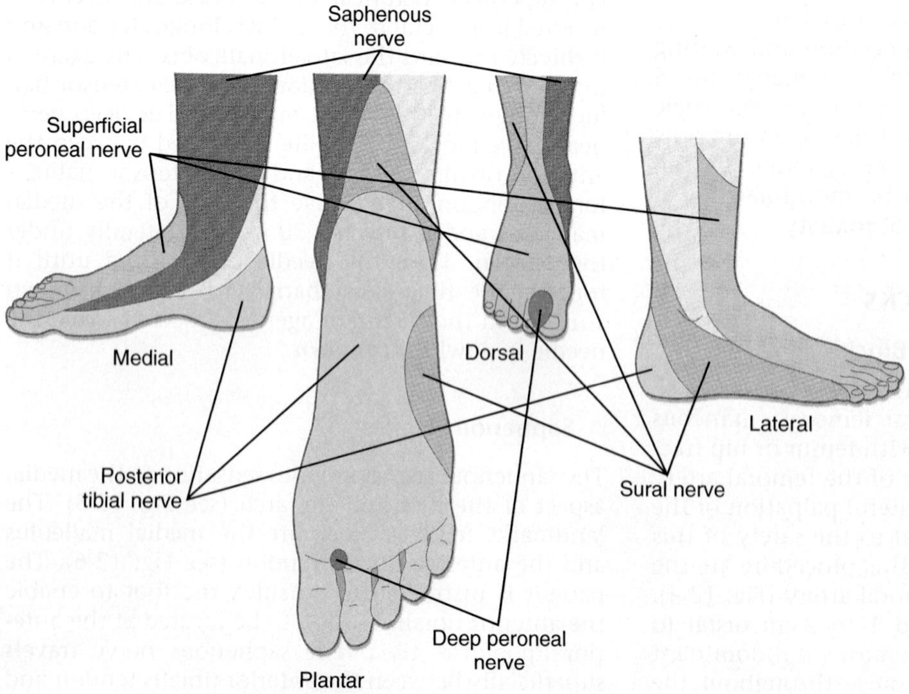
Saphenous nerve
Superficial peroneal nerve
Medial
Dorsal
Lateral
Posterior tibial nerve
Sural nerve
Deep peroneal nerve
Plantar

FIGURE 12-5 Sensory nerve distribution of the ankle.

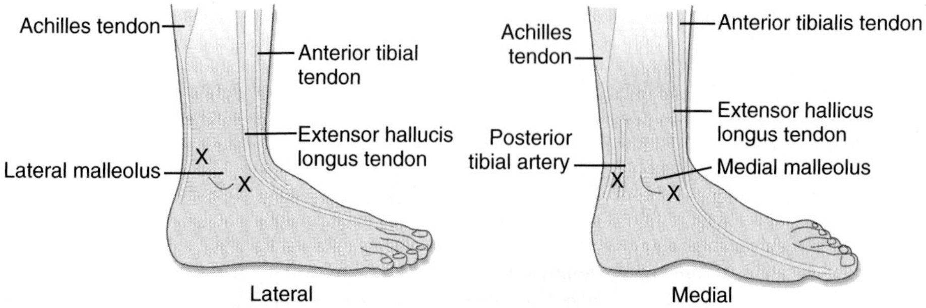
Achilles tendon
Anterior tibial tendon
Extensor hallucis longus tendon
Lateral malleolus
X
X
Lateral
Achilles tendon
Anterior tibialis tendon
Extensor hallicus longus tendon
Posterior tibial artery
Medial malleolus
X
X
Medial

FIGURE 12-6 Landmarks for ankle nerve blocks.

the medial malleolus. The needle is inserted at the anterior lip of the distal tibia, just lateral to the tibialis tendon, and is directed toward the medial malleolus. 5 mL of the agent is injected subcutaneously in a ring-like fashion from the anterior tibialis tendon to the medial malleolus.

■ Posterior Tibial Nerve

The posterior tibial nerve supplies sensation to the distal two thirds of the plantar surface of the foot (see Fig. 12-5). The landmarks for this block are the medial malleolus, the posterior tibial artery, and the Achilles tendon (see Fig. 12-6). The needle is inserted just lateral to the Achilles tendon at a level 1 cm above the medial malleolus. The needle is directed just posterior to the posterior tibial artery toward the posterior aspect of the tibia. It is advanced until it hits the tibia, and then is withdrawn 1 mm. Then 5 mL of agent is injected while the needle is slowly withdrawn.

■ FACIAL/ORAL BLOCKS

■ Supraorbital Nerve

The supraorbital nerve exits the supraorbital notch along the supraorbital rim and supplies sensation to the forehead along with the supratrochlear and infratrochlear nerves (Figs. 12-7 and 12-8). For a nerve block, the supraorbital notch is palpated, and 1 to 3 mL of agent is injected at this location. If inadequate anesthesia is obtained, a subcutaneous wheal is made down the supraorbital rim with 5 mL

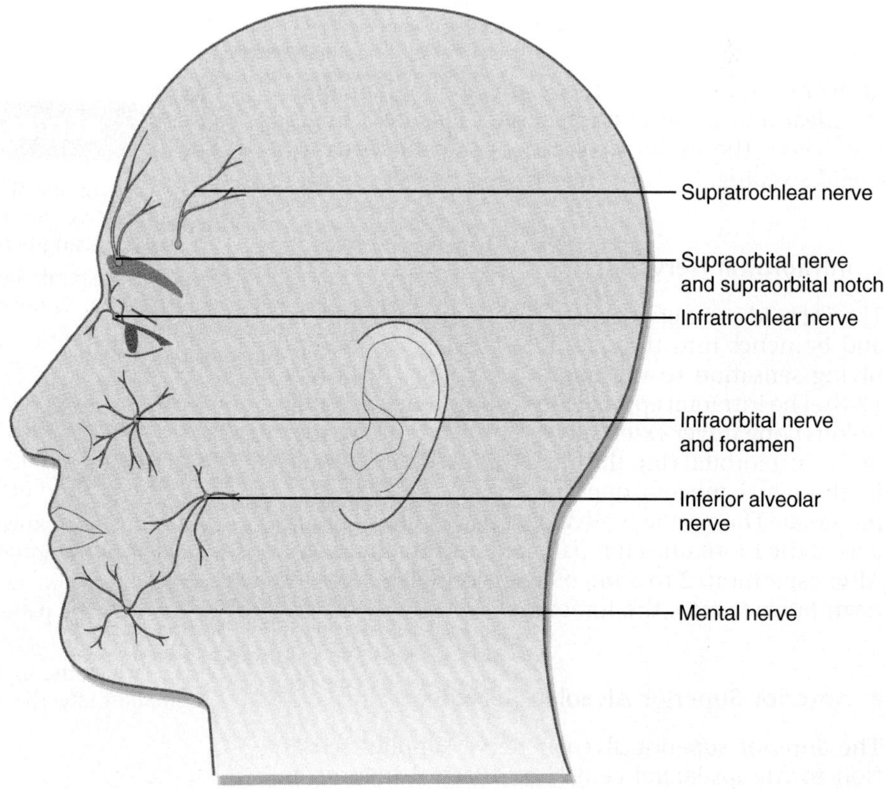
Supratrochlear nerve
Supraorbital nerve and supraorbital notch
Infratrochlear nerve
Infraorbital nerve and foramen
Inferior alveolar nerve
Mental nerve

FIGURE 12-7 Distribution of the facial nerves.

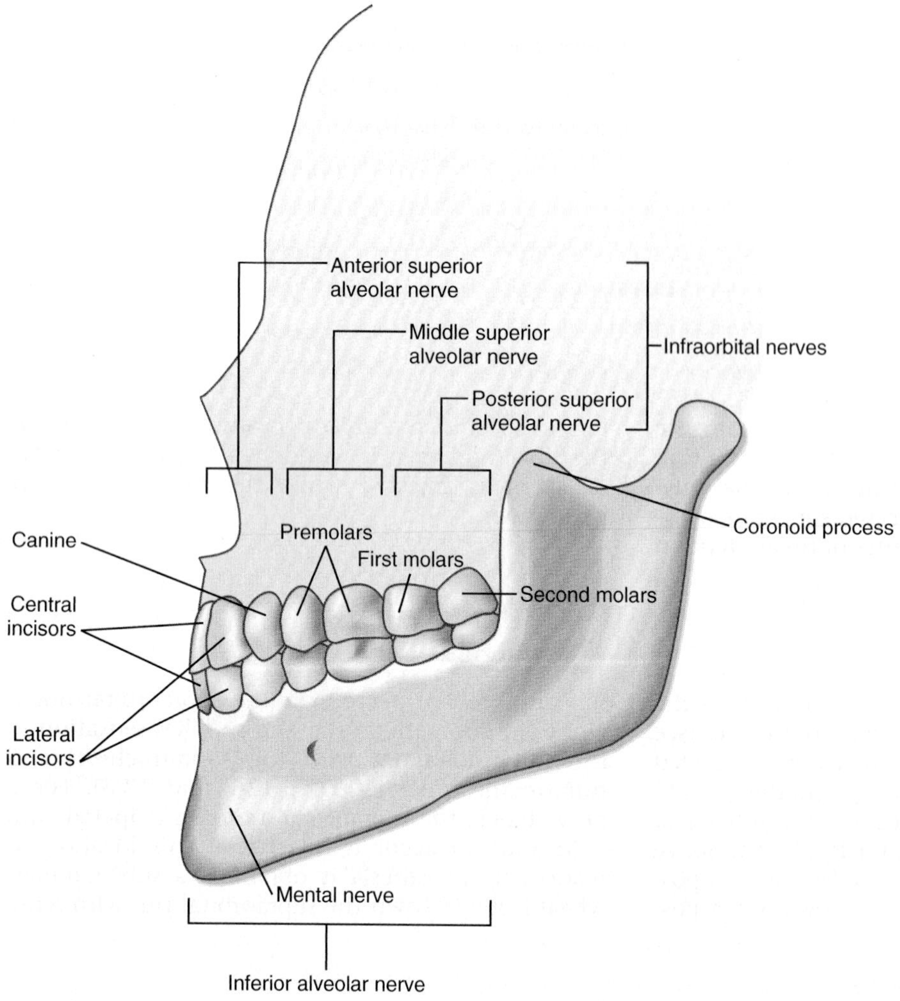
Anterior superior alveolar nerve
Middle superior alveolar nerve
Infraorbital nerves
Posterior superior alveolar nerve
Coronoid process
Canine
Premolars
First molars
Second molars
Central incisors
Lateral incisors
Mental nerve
Inferior alveolar nerve

FIGURE 12-8 Landmarks for facial nerve blocks.

of agent to anesthetize the branches of the supratrochlear and infratrochlear nerves. Placing a finger just below the eyebrow decreases the incidence of eyelid swelling.[2]

■ Infraorbital Nerve

The infraorbital nerve exits the infraorbital foramen and branches into the superior alveolar nerves supplying sensation to the midface (see Figs. 12-7 and 12-8). The intraoral approach is recommended. While holding one finger externally over the inferior border of the infraorbital rim, the operator inserts the needle in the labial mucosa opposite the apex of the first premolar. The needle is advanced parallel to the long axis of the tooth until it is palpated near the foramen. After aspiration, 2 to 3 mL of agent is injected slowly near, but not into, the foramen.

■ Anterior Superior Alveolar Nerve

The anterior superior alveolar nerve supplies sensation to the ipsilateral central and lateral incisors as

RED FLAGS

- Be wary of anesthetic allergy; consider preservative-free agent, crossing an anesthetic class, or using benzoyl alcohol.
- Always aspirate before injecting to avoid accidental intravascular injection.
- Perform a thorough neurologic evaluation prior to initiating local anesthesia.
- Ask the patient to tell you whether paresthesias develop.
- If paresthesias develop, withdraw the needle 1 to 2 mm prior to making the injection.
- Do not use epinephrine or other vasoconstrictive agents for anesthesia of the digits, ear, nose, or penis.
- Monitor the patient closely for any signs of toxicity.
- To reduce the incidence of toxicity, use the smallest effective dose of an anesthetic agent.

Tips and Tricks

- Inject anesthetic agents slowly in increments of no more than 3 mL, and aspirate before injecting.
- Maintain verbal contact with the patient to help screen for dysarthria and mental status changes.
- Use a small needle (27- to 30-gauge for local infiltration, 25- or 27-gauge for nerve blocks).
- Use warmed or buffered lidocaine.
- Use a small-caliber syringe to reduce the pressure and pain of injection.
- Use 1 to 2 mL of anesthetic for digital blocks, 5 mL for most other blocks.

well as the canine tooth and half the upper lip (see Fig. 12-8). For block of this nerve, the needle is inserted with the bevel facing bone superior to the apex of the canine and is directed to the canine fossa. After aspiration, 2 mL of agent is injected (see Fig. 12-8).

■ Posterior Superior Alveolar Nerve

The posterior superior alveolar nerve provides sensation to the ipsilateral maxillary molars (see Fig. 12-8). After the cheek is retracted laterally, the needle is inserted into the mucosal reflection just distal to the distal buccal root of the upper second molar. The needle is advanced along the curvature of the maxillary tuberosity 2 to 2.5 cm, where 2 to 3 mL of agent is injected to effect a nerve block. The operator should beware of the pterygoid plexus and must be sure to perform aspiration, as always, before making an injection.

■ Middle Superior Alveolar Nerve

The middle superior alveolar nerve provides sensation to the ipsilateral premolars and sometimes the first maxillary molars (see Fig. 12-8). For block of this nerve, the needle is inserted with bevel facing bone superior to the apex of the upper, second premolar tooth, and 2 mL of agent is injected.

■ Inferior Alveolar Nerve

The inferior alveolar nerve supplies sensation to the ipsilateral mandibular teeth, lower lip, and chin (see Figs. 12-7 and 12-8). The coronoid process of the mandible is palpated, and the cheek is retracted laterally. A triangle is visualized in the mucosa posterior to the molars. The needle is inserted into this triangle 1 cm above the occlusal surface of the molars. It is advanced until it contacts the mandible. The needle is retracted slightly, aspiration is performed, and 2 mL of agent is slowly injected. If the needle does not contact the mandible and is directed posteriorly toward the parotid gland, a temporary Bell's palsy may be elicited as the facial nerve is unintentionally anesthetized. Injection of more agent while the needle is withdrawn will anesthetize the lingual nerve as well.

FACTS AND FORMULAS

- Names of all amide anesthetic agents contain two *i*'s.
- The maximum dose of lidocaine is 4.5 mg/kg without epinephrine and 7 mg/kg with epinephrine.
- 1 mL of a 1% solution of lidocaine contains 10 mg of lidocaine.

■ Mental Nerve

The mental nerve branches off the inferior alveolar nerve to supply sensation to the ipsilateral chin (see Figs. 12-7 and 12-8). This nerve emerges from the mental foramen inferior to the second premolar (see Fig. 12-8). For mental nerve block, the foramen is palpated. Then, through an intraoral approach, the needle is inserted in the mucobuccal fold and advanced until it can be palpated over the foramen. After aspiration is performed, 1 to 3 mL of agent is slowly injected.

■ Nerve Block of an Individual Tooth (Supraperiosteal Block)

The operator can block the nerve of a single tooth by having the needle enter the mucobuccal fold with the bevel facing the bone and injecting 1 to 2 mL of agent at the apex of the tooth, close to the periosteum. It may take longer than most blocks to achieve complete anesthesia because the agent has to penetrate the cortex of the bone to reach the nerve root (5 to 10 minutes).

■ Ear Block

Several different nerves supply sensation to the ear; therefore, a block requires a superficial skin wheal all around the anterior and posterior auricular face and scalp (see Fig. 12-8).

■ MISCELLANEOUS NERVE BLOCKS

■ Intercostal Nerve Block

The intercostal nerve block is perhaps one of the most dangerous nerve blocks because of both the greater systemic absorption of agent injected in this area and a 1.4% incidence of pneumothorax[11]; however, significant pain relief from rib fractures can be obtained with this method. In most cases opiate

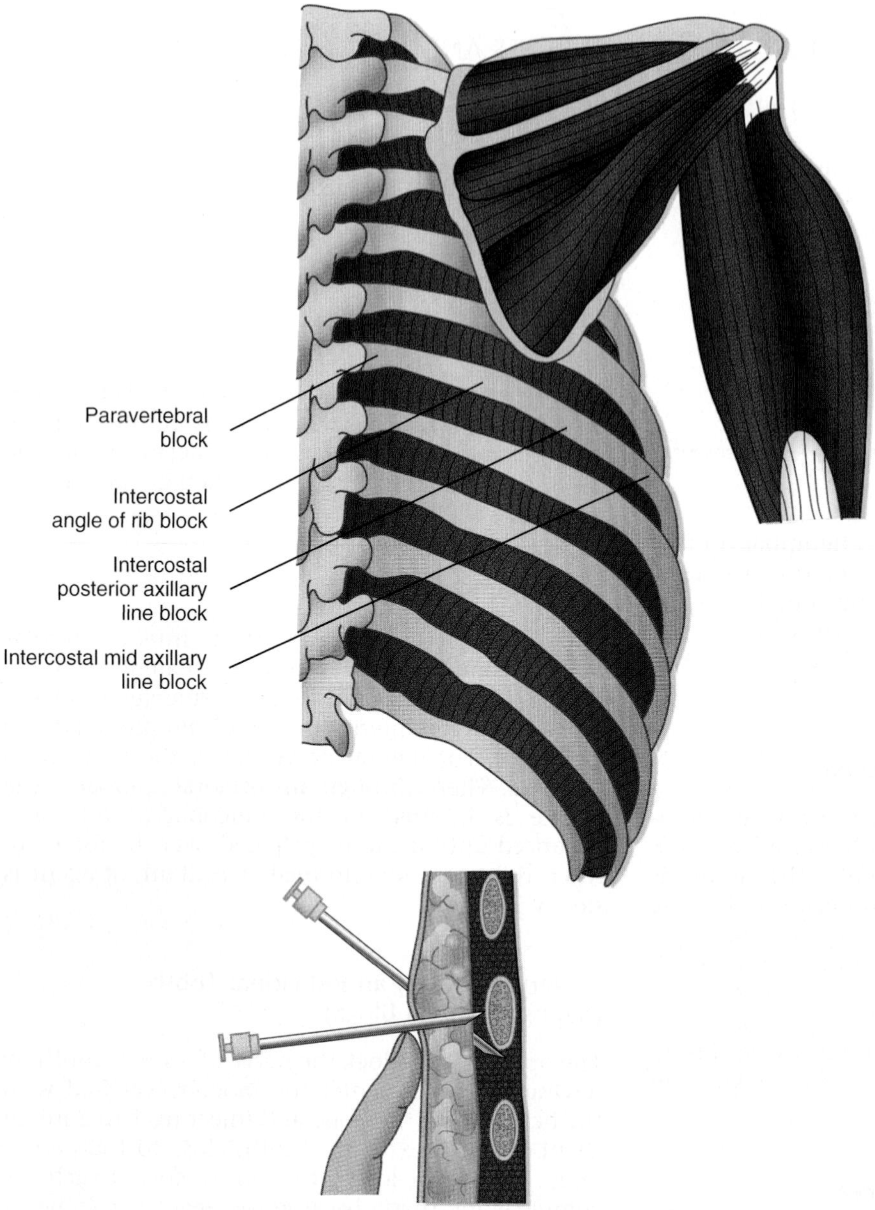
Paravertebral block
Intercostal angle of rib block
Intercostal posterior axillary line block
Intercostal mid axillary line block

FIGURE 12-9 Landmarks for intercostal nerve block.

analgesia is probably a safer method of pain control. The injured rib is palpated posterior to the posterior axillary line, and the skin is retracted superiorly over the rib. The needle is inserted over the rib 5 mm, the retracted skin is released, and the needle is walked gently down the inferior edge of the rib. The needle is then advanced 2 to 3 mm, aspiration is performed, and 2 to 5 mL of agent is injected. If the pain control is inadequate, this procedure can be repeated for two ribs above and two below the injured area (Fig. 12-9).

Hematoma Block

The hematoma of a fracture can be locally anesthetized to relieve the pain associated with relocation of a displaced fracture. This block is most commonly used for metacarpal fractures, for which 2 mL of agent is usually sufficient. In this case, if aspiration of blood confirms placement of the needle within the hematoma, care should be taken to avoid anatomic locations of known vessels (Fig. 12-10).[3]

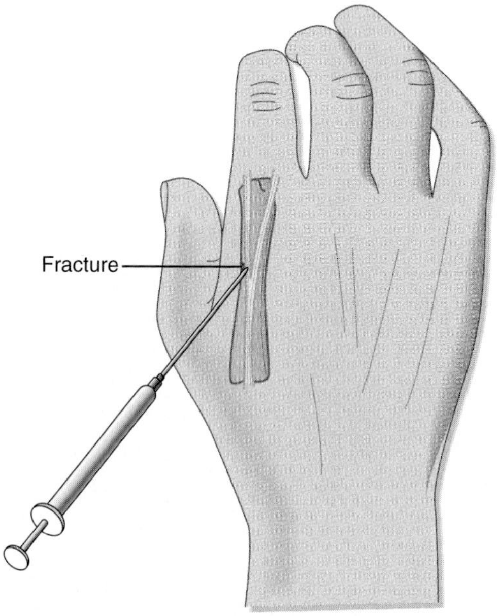
Fracture

FIGURE 12-10 Landmarks for hematoma block.

REFERENCES

1. Crystal C, Blankenship R: Local anesthetics and peripheral nerve blocks in the emergency department. Emerg Med Clin North Am 2005;23:477-502.
2. Salam G: Regional anesthesia for office procedures. Part 1: Head and neck surgeries. Am Fam Physician 2004; 69:585-590.
3. Wedmore I, Johnson T, Czarnik J, et al: Pain management in the wilderness and operational setting. Emerg Med Clin North Am 2005;23:585-601.
4. Waldbillig D, Quinn J, Steill I, et al: Randomized double-blind controlled trial comparing room-temperature and heated lidocaine for digital nerve block. Ann Emerg Med 1995;26:677-681.
5. Brogan G, Giarrusso E, Hollander J, et al: Comparison of plain, warmed and buffered lidocaine for anesthesia of traumatic wounds. Ann Emerg Med 1995;26:121-125.
6. Bartfield J, Jandreau S, Raccio-Robak N: Randomized trial of diphenhydramine versus benzoyl alcohol with epinephrine as an alternative to lidocaine local anesthesia. Ann Emerg Med 1998;32:650-654.
7. Pollack C, Swindle G: Use of diphenhydramine for local anesthesia in "caine"-sensitive patients. J Emerg Med 1989;7:611-614.
8. Zempsky W, Cravero JP: American Academy of Pediatrics Committee on Pediatric Emergency Medicine and Section on Anesthesiology and Pain Medicine: Relief of pain and anxiety in pediatric patients in emergency medical systems. Pediatrics 2004;114:1348-1356.
9. Eidelman A, Weiss J, Lau J, et al: Topical anesthetics for dermal instrumentation: A systematic review of randomized, controlled trials. Ann Emerg Med 2005;46:343-351.
10. Fletcher A, Rigby A, Heyes F: Three–in-one femoral nerve block as analgesia for fractured neck of femur in the emergency department: A randomized controlled trial. Ann Emerg Med 2003;41:227-233.
11. Shanti C, Carlin A, Tyburski G: Incidence of pneumothorax from intercostal nerve block for analgesia in rib fractures. J Trauma 2001;51:536-539.

Chapter 13

Resuscitation in Pregnancy

Susan B. Promes

KEY POINTS

Roll the pregnant patient onto her left side to displace the gravid uterus off the great vessels.

When the uterus is palpable above the umbilicus and the mother is in cardiac arrest, perform an immediate cesarean section.

For an Rh-negative woman who has vaginal bleeding after trauma, administer Rh immunoglobulin (RhoGAM): a 50-µg dose in the first trimester, and a 300-µg dose in the second or third trimester.

Any pregnant woman at more than 24 weeks' gestation who has trauma to the abdomen should undergo fetal monitoring for 4 to 6 hours.

In a pregnant woman, hands for cardiopulmonary resuscitation, chest tubes, and defibrillator paddles should be placed higher on the chest wall. Cardioversion and defibrillation will not harm the fetus.

Scope

Resuscitating a pregnant woman is, thankfully, an infrequent event. Cardiac arrest statistics are hard to quantify, but cardiac arrests reportedly occur in roughly 1 in 30,000 near-term pregnancies.[1] Two lives are on the line. Quick, decisive management is paramount for the livelihood of the mother and her unborn child. Knowing exactly what to do and acting quickly ensures the best possible outcome for the mother and her unborn child.

Anatomy and Physiology

What are generally considered abnormal vital signs in nonpregnant people may actually be within normal range for a pregnant woman. In gravid females, the heart rate and respiratory rate are increased. In the second trimester, blood pressure is decreased by 5 to 15 mm Hg, but it returns to normal near term. Hypoxemia occurs earlier in pregnant patients because of a diminished reserve and buffering capacity. Pregnant patients have a slight respiratory alkalosis that must be taken into account when interpreting arterial blood gas values: P_{CO_2} 30 mm Hg and pH 7.43. Central venous pressure decreases in pregnancy to a third-trimester value of 4 mm Hg.[2]

A pregnant woman has less respiratory reserve and greater oxygen requirements. The gravid uterus pushes up on the diaphragm, resulting in reduced functional residual capacity. Minute ventilation and tidal volume rise, as does maternal oxygen consumption. The basal metabolic rate increases during pregnancy. Greater oxygen demands of the unborn child significantly alter the mother's respiratory physiology, and the mother hyperventilates to meet the demands of the fetus. The pregnant patient at baseline is in a state of compensatory respiratory alkalosis owing to excessive secretion of bicarbonate. A pregnant woman's ability to compensate for acidosis is impaired. Other physiologic changes that may affect resuscitation are airway edema and friability, reduced chest compliance, and higher risk of regurgitation and aspiration.

As the uterus grows, it moves from the pelvis into the abdominal cavity, pushing the contents of the abdominal cavity up toward the chest. In late pregnancy, the gravid uterus compresses the aorta and inferior vena cava and limits the venous return to the heart. Stroke volume is decreased when a near-term pregnant woman is lying on her back and increased when the uterus is moved away from the great vessels. Hence, the woman in the second or third trimester of pregnancy should be placed in the left lateral tilt position or the uterus should be manually displaced to the left to optimize cardiac output. Also during late pregnancy, cardiac output is increased. Pulmonary capillary wedge pressures remain unchanged, as does ejection fraction.

Electrocardiography (ECG) changes are also present during pregnancy. They include left axis deviation, secondary to the diaphragm's moving cephalad and changing the position of the heart. Q waves are present in leads III and aVF, and flattened or inverted T waves are seen in lead III.

During pregnancy blood volume increases, causing a dilution anemia. The average hematocrit value is 32% to 34%. White blood cell counts are higher than normal and platelet counts are lower in pregnancy. Blood urea nitrogen (BUN) and serum creatinine values are lower than normal, as are cortisol values. Erythrocyte sedimentation rates are increased. Albumin and total protein levels are decreased. Fibrinogen levels double in pregnancy, so a patient with disseminated intravascular coagulation (DIC) could have a normal fibrinogen level.

Pregnancy-related changes can be seen on radiographic studies. A chest radiograph of a pregnant woman, for example, shows an increased anteroposterior (AP) diameter, mild cephalization of the pulmonary vasculature, cardiomegaly, and a slightly widened mediastinum. Widening of the sacroiliac joints and pubic symphysis are apparent on imaging of the pelvis. Radiography should not be avoided in a pregnant woman because of concerns about radiation exposure for the fetus, which can simply be shielded. Ultrasonography can be used at the bedside to identify fluid in the abdomen, pelvis, and pericardium and to evaluate fetal activity and heart rate. Fetal well-being is closely linked to the well-being of the mother, so all studies indicated to diagnose and treat the mother should be performed.

Differential Diagnosis

Pregnant women are generally young and healthy. The rare cardiac arrest in a gravid female may be due to venous thromboembolism, severe pregnancy-induced hypertension, amniotic fluid embolism, or hemorrhage. In addition to such pregnancy-related problems, pregnant women are not exempt from common conditions that affect the general population. Trauma and sepsis may lead to cardiopulmonary failure and the need for maternal resuscitation. Box 13-1 lists key etiologic factors leading to cardiac arrest in the pregnant patient.[3]

BOX 13-1

Major Causes of Cardiac Arrest during Pregnancy*

- Venous thromboembolism
- Pregnancy-induced hypertension
- Sepsis
- Amniotic fluid embolism
- Hemorrhage:
  - Placental abruption
  - Placenta previa
  - Uterine atony
  - Disseminated intravascular coagulation
- Trauma
- Iatrogenic:
  - Medication errors
  - Allergic reactions to medications
  - Anesthetic complications
  - Oxytocin administration
  - Hypermagnesemia
- Preexisting heart disease:
  - Congenital
  - Acquired—cardiomyopathy of pregnancy

*Listed in order of decreasing frequency.
From Mallampalli A, Powner DJ, Gardner MO: Cardiopulmonary resuscitation and somatic support of the pregnant patient. Crit Care Clin 2004;20:748.

■ HEMORRHAGE

During routine vaginal delivery, the average blood loss is 500 mL. Excessive blood loss or postpartum hemorrhage complicates 4% of vaginal deliveries.[4] Common causes of hemorrhage around the time of delivery are uterine atony (excessive bleeding with a large relaxed uterus after delivery), vaginal or cervical tears, retained fragments of placenta, placenta previa, placenta accreta, and uterine rupture. Hereditary abnormalities in blood clotting may cause hemorrhage as well, so inquiries about excess bleeding, known disorders, and family history are relevant in a patient with excessive bleeding.

■ Nonhemorrhagic Shock

The causes of nonhemorrhagic obstetrical shock—pulmonary embolism, amniotic fluid embolism, acute uterine inversion, and sepsis—are uncommon, but are responsible for the majority of maternal deaths in the developed world.[5] These conditions must be diagnosed and treated expeditiously. Patients in whom pulmonary embolism is suspected should be started on heparin and then should undergo diagnostic imaging. Treatment of amniotic fluid embolism is supportive, the goals being to maintain maternal oxygenation and support blood pressure. Some case reports describe success with use of cardiopulmonary bypass to treat women suffering from amniotic fluid embolism.

Acute uterine inversion can also cause shock. Cardiovascular collapse complicates approximately half the cases of acute uterine inversion. Classically, the extent of the shock is out of proportion to the blood loss noted. One theory to explain this observation is a parasympathetic reflex causing neurogenic shock from stretching of the broad ligament and/or compression of the ovaries as they are drawn together. Uterine replacement combined with vigorous fluid resuscitation, including blood transfusion as required, should reverse the hypotension.[6]

■ TRAUMA

Traumatic injuries occur commonly in pregnancy and are the leading cause of maternal death, accounting for more than 46% of cases. Motor vehicle crashes, assaults, and falls are the most common causes of injuries. Pregnant women are at increased risk for domestic violence; the police should be notified when warranted.

Fetal outcome is affected when the mother becomes hypotensive or acidotic owing to major injury. However, maternal vital signs and physical symptoms do not predict fetal distress in women with minor trauma. Only cardiotocographic monitoring for a minimum of 4 to 6 hours is useful to predict fetal outcome. Women with even apparently minor falls should undergo fetal monitoring.

In pregnant women suffering blunt trauma, most fetal deaths occur from placental abruption. Classic symptoms are abdominal cramps, vaginal bleeding, uterine tenderness, and hypovolemia (several liters of blood can accumulate in the uterus). None of these findings is sensitive, however, and cannot be relied on, so monitoring is required.

Diagnostic Testing

■ INTERVENTIONS AND PROCEDURES

A fundamental principle in treating pregnant women is that fetal well-being depends on maternal well-being. As with all ED patients, resuscitation starts with the ABCs (airway, breathing, and circulation). Hypoxia should be treated aggressively in this patient population, because when the mother is hypoxic, oxygen is shunted away from the fetus. Aggressive volume resuscitation, administration of vasopressors if needed, and close attention to the patient's body position are all very important in the treatment of hypotension in the pregnant patient. Fetal heart monitoring and, ideally, cardiotocographic monitoring should be initiated as soon as possible for the patient in the second or third trimester of pregnancy.[7]

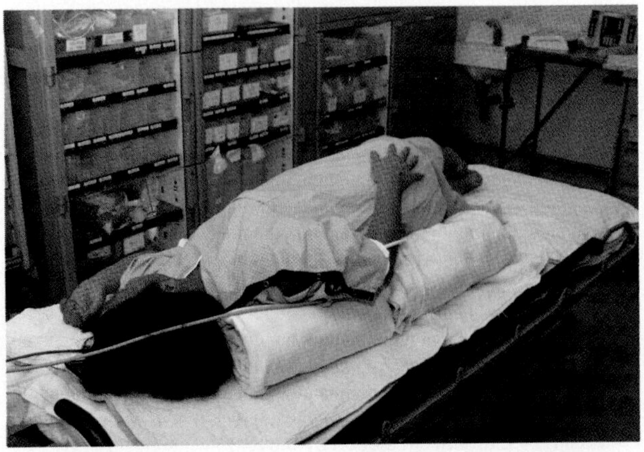

FIGURE 13-1 Blanket roll technique to tilt the patient.

A commercially produced wedge called a Cardiff wedge is available for purchase to aid in the resuscitation of pregnant women. It can be placed under the women's right side to support her back while she lies in the preferred left lateral tilt position. In the absence of a wedge, a "human wedge" can be used; the patient is tilted on the bent knees of a kneeling rescuer. Pillows, towel roll, and blanket roll are readily available in EDs and accomplish the same purpose—angling the woman's back 30 to 45 degrees from the floor (Fig. 13-1). If for some reason the patient must lie on her back, which is not recommended for reasons previously discussed, a member of the health care team should manually displace the uterus to the left so it does not rest on the great vessels.

American Heart Association Basic Life Support (AHA BLS) guidelines should be followed with two modifications:

- Move the uterus off the great vessels.
- Adjust the hand position for CPR superiorly to account for displacement of the thoracic contents superiorly by the gravid uterus.

American Heart Association Advanced Cardiac Life Support (ACLS) guidelines for medications, intubation, and defibrillation for patients in cardiac arrest should be followed in the gravid female with one simple exception—a change in placement of the defibrillation paddles/pads:

- Place one paddle below the right clavicle in the midclavicular line.
- Position the second paddle outside the normal cardiac apex, avoiding the breast tissue.[7]

Defibrillation energy requirements remain the same (Fig. 13-2).[8] Defibrillation will not harm the fetus. ACLS medications should be used as needed. Box 13-2 lists the U.S. Food and Drug Administration (FDA) categories for the various ACLS drug options for pregnancy.

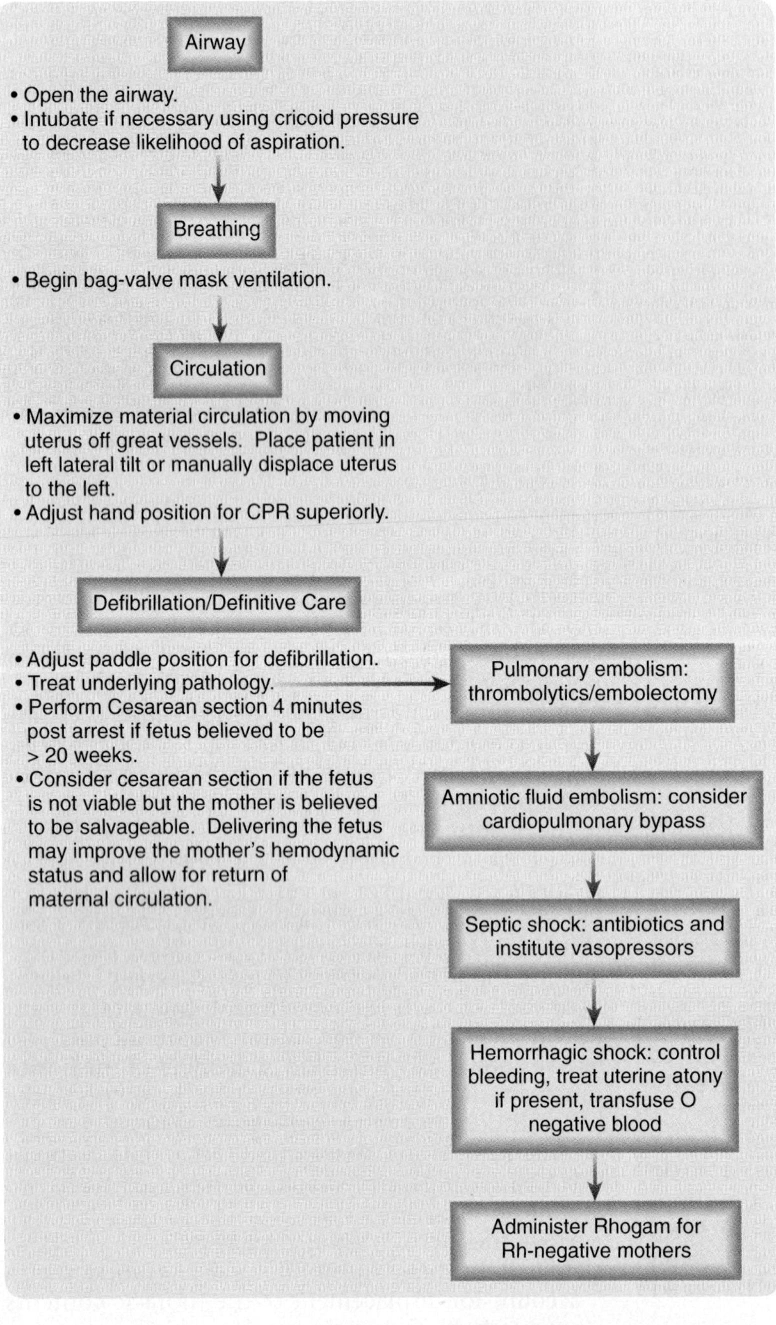
Airway
• Open the airway.
• Intubate if necessary using cricoid pressure to decrease likelihood of aspiration.
Breathing
• Begin bag-valve mask ventilation.
Circulation
• Maximize material circulation by moving uterus off great vessels. Place patient in left lateral tilt or manually displace uterus to the left.
• Adjust hand position for CPR superiorly.
Defibrillation/Definitive Care
• Adjust paddle position for defibrillation.
• Treat underlying pathology.
• Perform Cesarean section 4 minutes post arrest if fetus believed to be > 20 weeks.
• Consider cesarean section if the fetus is not viable but the mother is believed to be salvageable. Delivering the fetus may improve the mother's hemodynamic status and allow for return of maternal circulation.
Pulmonary embolism: thrombolytics/embolectomy
Amniotic fluid embolism: consider cardiopulmonary bypass
Septic shock: antibiotics and institute vasopressors
Hemorrhagic shock: control bleeding, treat uterine atony if present, transfuse O negative blood
Administer Rhogam for Rh-negative mothers

FIGURE 13-2 Algorithm for resuscitation of the pregnant patient. CPR, cardiopulmonary resuscitation.

In pregnant patients with trauma who are in need of a thoracostomy, the chest tube must be placed one or two intercostal spaces higher than normal to avoid diaphragmatic injury. The open supraumbilical approach should be used for diagnostic peritoneal lavage in a pregnant patient, with the gravid uterus palpable on abdominal examination.

■ RADIOGRAPHY

Ultrasonography is an important method for assessment of both mother and the fetus. However, radiographic studies are often required. Shielding can ensure that exposure even with maternal head and chest computed tomography (CT) can be kept below the 1-rad (1000-millirad) limit. Intrauterine exposure to 10 rads (10,000 millirads) produces a small increase in childhood cancers; exposure of 15 rads creates the risk of mental retardation, childhood cancer, and small head. A head or chest radiograph delivers less than 1 millirad to the shielded gravid uterus. A lumbar spine, hip, or kidneys-ureters-bladder radiograph delivers more than 200 millirads. A CT scan of the head delivers less than 50 millirads to the shielded uterus, and a chest CT scan provides an exposure of less than a 1000 millirads. In sum, important radio-

BOX 13-2

Classification of Drugs Used in Pregnancy

The U.S. Food and Drug Administration (FDA) categories for the various Advanced Cardiac Life Support (ACLS) drug options for pregnancy are as follows:

Category B

Definition

Animal studies have revealed no evidence of harm to the fetus, although there are no adequate and well-controlled studies in pregnant women.

OR

Animal studies have shown an adverse effect, but adequate and well-controlled studies in pregnant women have failed to demonstrate a risk to the fetus in any trimester.

Agents

Atropine
Magnesium

Category C

Definition

Animal studies have shown an adverse effect, and there are no adequate and well-controlled studies in pregnant women.

OR

No animal studies have been conducted, and there are no adequate and well-controlled studies in pregnant women.

Agents

Epinephrine
Lidocaine
Bretylium
Bicarbonate
Dopamine
Dobutamine
Adenosine

Category D

Definition

Adequate well-controlled or observational studies in pregnant women have demonstrated a risk to the fetus. However, the benefits of therapy may outweigh the potential risk. For example, the drug may be acceptable if needed in a life-threatening situation or serious disease for which safer drugs cannot be used or are ineffective.

Agent

Amiodarone

graphic studies of the head, neck, and chest can safely proceed if the uterus is shielded.

Fetomaternal Transfusion

After the 12th week of pregnancy, when the uterus rises above the pelvic rim and becomes susceptible to trauma, fetal blood can theoretically cross into the maternal circulation after significant trauma. A 50-μg dose of Rh immunoglobulin (RhoGAM) is used when the mother is Rh-negative. During the second and third trimesters, a 300-μg dose is used, which protects against 30 mL of fetomaternal hemorrhage. The 16-week fetus has about a 30-mL volume of blood, so the entire blood volume is covered by the 300-μg dose.

Pregnant patients in the second or third trimester who suffer major traumatic injury could theoretically have fetomaternal transfusion that exceeds the coverage provided by the 300-μg dose. This situation is rare, occurring in less than 1% of pregnant patients with trauma. In patients with major trauma and advanced pregnancy, the Kleihauer-Betke test should be considered, especially when significant vaginal bleeding is present. The Rh immunoglobulin is effective when administered within 72 hours, so the test does not have to be performed in the ED.

Perimortem Cesarean Section

The likelihood that a perimortem cesarean section will result in a living and neurologically normal infant is related to the interval between onset of maternal cardiac arrest and delivery of the infant.[9,10] The gestational age of the neonate is also critical. If an ED cesarean section is performed, it should be done rapidly. Time is of the essence. Fetal viability outside the uterus is believed to occur at approximately 24 weeks' gestation. In the ED it is not always possible to know the exact gestational age. On the basis of case reports, it is recommended that an ED cesarean section be performed if the gestational age is believed to be more than 20 weeks. At this stage of pregnancy, the fundus is palpable at or above the level of the umbilicus.

The child should be delivered within 5 minutes of maternal cardiac arrest, so the procedure should be initiated within 4 minutes of failed cardiopulmonary resuscitation of the mother. The procedure is summarized in Box 13-3. Maternal cardiopulmonary resuscitation should be maintained throughout the procedure in order to optimize blood flow to the uterus and the mother. Then, once delivery is accomplished, ED personnel should be prepared to resuscitate the neonate. It is important to note that published and anecdotal reports describe return of maternal blood pressure and maternal survival after perimortem cesarean section.[11] Successful resuscitation of a pregnant woman and her unborn child requires a coordinated team approach.

BOX 13-3

Technique of Perimortem Cesarean Section

NOTE: Have suction available for this procedure because bleeding can be excessive.

1. Ideally, while the EP is preparing for the procedure, a catheter is placed in the bladder and the abdominal wall prepared with povidone-iodine. However, *do not* delay the procedure for these activities.
2. Using a No. 10 scalpel, make a midline vertical incision from umbilicus to the publis along the linea nigra.
3. Once the peritoneal cavity is open, use bladder retractors and Richardson retractors to improve access to the uterus.
4. Make a short vertical incision in the lower uterine segment just cephalad to the bladder.
5. Extend the uterine incision cephalad with blunt scissors. Place a hand in the uterus to keep the baby from being cut.
6. Deliver the baby.
7. Suction the mouth and nose, cut and clamp the umbilical cord, and resuscitate the baby.
8. Document Apgar scores at 1, 5, and 10 minutes.
9. If the mother regains vital signs, remove the placenta and repair the uterus and abdominal wall.
10. Consider intramuscular injection of oxytocin into the bleeding uterus.

Conclusion

In the setting of a resuscitation, a pregnant woman poses challenges, given the physiologic and anatomic changes associated with the pregnancy. Remembering these normal adjustments that occur in gravid women is critical. Aortocaval compression must be avoided during resuscitation of the pregnant woman. Appropriately diagnosing the etiology of the patient's medical problem while being mindful of the ABCs of resuscitation is a must. Thankfully, cardiac arrest is an uncommon event in pregnant women. When it occurs later in pregnancy, perimortem cesarean section may improve the outcome of the infant and the mother if performed in a timely manner. As with all resuscitations, a team effort is mandatory, but possibly even more so in this setting because the EP is caring for two patients whose lives are very tenuous and time is of the essence.

REFERENCES

1. Peters CW, Layon AJ, Edwards RK: Cardiac arrest during pregnancy. J Clin Anesth 2005;17:229-234.
2. Shah AJ, Kilcline BA: Trauma in pregnancy. Emerg Med Clin North Am 2003;21:615-629.
3. Mallampalli A, Powner DJ, Gardner MO: Cardiopulmonary resuscitation and somatic support of the pregnant patient. Crit Care Clin 2004;20:748.
4. Miller DA: Obstetric hemorrhage. OBFocus High Risk Pregnancy. Available at http://www.obfocus.com/high-risk/bleeding/hemorrhagepa.htm.
5. Thomas AJ, Greer IA: Non-hemorrhagic obstetric shock. Best Pract Res Clin Obstet Gynaecol 2000;14:19-41.
6. O'Grady JP, Pope CS: Malposition of the uterus. eMedicine [serial online] June 5, 2006: Available at http://www.emedicine.com/med/topic3473.htm/
7. Luppo CJ: Cardiopulmonary resuscitation: Pregnant women are different. AACN Clin Issues 1997;8:574-585.
8. Nanson J, Elcock D, Williams M, Deakin CD: Do physiologic changes in pregnancy change defibrillation energy requirements? Br J Anaesth 2001;87:237-239.
9. Weber CE: Postmortem cesarean section: Review of the literature and case reports. Am J Obstet Gynecol 1971;110:158-165.
10. Oates S, Williams GL, Rees GAD: Cardiopulmonary resuscitation in late pregnancy. BMJ 1988;297:404-405.
11. Katz V, Balderston K, DeFreest M: Perimortem cesarean delivery: Were our assumptions correct? Am J Obstet Gynecol 2005;192:1916-1920.

Chapter **14**

Newborn Resuscitation

Katherine Bakes and Kurt Whitaker

PEDIATRIC CARDIOPULMONARY RESUSCITATION

KEY POINTS

Survival of cardiac arrest is significantly lower in children than in adults.
Sudden infant death syndrome is the most common identifiable cause of pediatric cardiac arrest. The majority of cases occur in children younger than 1 year.
For children aged 1 to 10 years, the following formula can be used to estimate ideal body weight: Weight (kg) = (age [in years] × 2) + 8.
Securing the pediatric airway is the most important and potentially life-saving maneuver of resuscitation.
The latest pediatric advanced life support (PALS) guidelines instituted by the American Heart Association (AHA)[1] emphasize the importance of effective chest compressions, which are defined as follows: (1) adequate rate (100 per minute), (2) adequate depth ($\frac{1}{2}$ to $\frac{1}{3}$ the anteroposterior diameter of the chest), (3) full recoil of the chest, and (4) minimal interruptions.

Perspective

In the pediatric population, primary respiratory arrest is the most commonly trigger for emergency medical life support. Primary pediatric respiratory arrest without cardiac arrest portends a potentially good outcome. This chapter focuses not on this subset of patients but on the pediatric patient presenting without a pulse and in full cardiac arrest.

Although a less common event than in adults, pediatric cardiac arrest represents a more terminal event, with rates of survival to hospital admission, survival to hospital discharge, and good neurologic outcome of survivors being significantly lower in children.

In all pediatric cardiopulmonary arrests in out-of-hospital and in-hospital settings combined, Young and Seidel[2] reported a 13% survival to hospital discharge. However, rates of in-hospital and out-of-hospital survival to discharge are, separately, 24% and 8.4%, respectively, with good neurologic outcome also being worse in victims of out-of-hospital arrest.

In a later study, Donoghue and colleagues[3] performed a review of more than 5000 patients with out-of-hospital pediatric cardiac arrest. In this analysis, 6.7% of patients survived to hospital discharge, 2.2% of whom had "intact" neurologic survival.[3]

Pathophysiology

■ EPIDEMIOLOGY

Seventy-five percent of out-of-hospital pediatric arrests occur at home. Studies have consistently shown that over half of all pediatric cardiac arrests occur in the under one year of age population.

Approximately 30% of out-of-hospital pediatric arrests are witnessed and over half occur in males.

■ CAUSES

Sudden infant death syndrome (SIDS) is the most common identifiable cause of pediatric cardiac arrest, with the majority of cases occurring in the children younger than 1 year. SIDS has decreased since the public health Back to Sleep campaign encouraged parents to place infants on their backs instead of their stomachs. Trauma, sepsis, cardiac etiologies, and near-drowning or submersion injuries are additional causes of cardiac arrest in infants and children.

■ PRESENTING RHYTHMS

Only 8% to 10% of pediatric patients with cardiac arrest present in ventricular fibrillation (VF) or pulseless ventricular tachycardia (VT), compared with up to 80% of adult arrest patients. More than three fourths of pediatric patients present in asystole and another 10% to 15% present with pulseless electrical activity (PEA).

■ PREDICTORS OF OUTCOME

Cardiopulmonary resuscitation performed by a person on the scene (bystander CPR) is an independent predictor of survival of pediatric cardiac arrest. Although reports vary on the percentage of pediatric patients receiving bystander CPR, the benefit of CPR remains clear.

An initial heart rhythm of VF/VT is a positive predictor of outcome, with a reported survival of 30% for patients presenting with such a rhythm, compared with 5% survival for victims presenting in asystole. Infants have a higher rate of presenting in asystole and, thus, a lower survival rate. Near-drowning victims have a greater chance of presenting in VF/VT (20%) and have a higher survival rate (23% survival to discharge, and 6% with good neurologic outcome).

Highlighting the dismal overall prognosis of the patient with pediatric arrest, analysis of seven studies showed that the need for epinephrine was a negative predictor of survival, with no patient surviving after receiving more than two doses of epinephrine.

Anatomy

■ WEIGHT

For weight estimates in children of various ages, the length-based Broeselow-Luten tape can be used. Alternatively, for children 1 to 10 years old, the following formula (age × 2) + 8 kg can be used to estimate ideal body weight:

$$\text{Body weight (kg)} = (\text{age [in years]} \times 2) + 8$$

■ GENERAL CONSIDERATIONS IN THE SETTING OF AN ARREST

Relative to adults, children have a greater ratio of surface area to body volume. Secondary to this feature, hypovolemic shock is often a cause of or contributing factor to an arrest. The pediatric heart compensates via increasing chronotropy, as opposed to increasing inotropy as in adults. This difference in physiology results in a precipitous drop in blood pressure after the pediatric patient in critical condition has reached maximum chronotropic capacity.

■ AIRWAY

The pediatric airway (up to approximately 8 years of age) has anatomically distinct features that make the approach to intubation different relative to intubation in adults; they are as follows:

- The airway is more anterior and superior.
- The airway is more funnel-shaped, with the cricoid ring representing the narrowest portion.
- The epiglottis is relatively larger and more floppy.
- The airway is less rigid and, thus, more prone to obstruction from improper positioning.
- The tongue and adenoid tissue are larger relative to the airway, making visualization of the vocal cords challenging.
- The head is relatively larger, making alignment of the pharyngeal, laryngeal, and tracheal airway axes contingent on head and body positioning (e.g., a roll should be placed under the shoulders of an infant because of the prominent occiput.)

Details are discussed in Chapter 15.

Presenting Signs and Symptoms

Hypotension is a *systolic* blood pressure less than the fifth percentile of normal for age, as follows:

- <60 mm Hg: term neonates (0 to 28 days)
- <70 mm Hg: infants (1 month to 12 months)
- <70 mm Hg + (2 × age in years): children 1 to 10 years
- <90 mm Hg: children ≥10 years of age

Interventions and Procedures

■ AIRWAY

Securing the pediatric airway is the most important and potentially life-saving maneuver in the resuscitation of the arrest victim. Expertise in bag-mask ventilation (BMV) is the most critical airway technique to master because it can provide adequate airway and breathing maintenance while a more definitive airway is prepared. There is evidence to suggest that BMV is superior to endotracheal intubation by first responders in the out-of-hospital setting.[4] As in adults, adjuncts such as oropharyngeal and nasopharyngeal airways should be utilized if BMV is not demonstrating efficacy, although the EP must keep in mind that the nasopharyngeal airway of the small infant can easily become obstructed by secretions. Cricoid pressure should always be applied, with care taken not to mechanically obstruct the malleable pediatric upper airway, and suction devices of various sizes should be readily available.

The latest Pediatric Advanced Life Support (PALS) guidelines state that there is insufficient evidence for the use of laryngeal mask airways. There is mounting evidence, however, that in the hands of experienced users, these devices are effective in multiple settings (i.e., operating room and out-of-hospital airway control).[1]

Although an in-depth discussion of the pediatric airway and pediatric endotracheal intubation is covered elsewhere in this text, the following basic reminders are reiterated here:

Because the smallest portion of the pediatric airway is at the level of the cricoid ring, an uncuffed or deflated cuffed endotracheal tube (ETT) is used in patients younger than 8 years.

- When a cuffed ETT is used, cuff pressures should be kept less than 20 cm H_2O.
- The correct uncuffed ETT size can be estimated using the formula 4+(age in years/4); estimate for cuffed ETT size uses the formula 3+(age in years/4.)
- The depth of the ETT should be roughly three times that of the ETT size at the level of the gum.
- Owing to the large floppy pediatric epiglottis, a straight laryngoscope blade is often used to lift the epiglottis up to facilitate a view of the vocal cords.

■ BREATHING

To avoid gastric insufflation while performing BVM ventilation, the EP should apply cricoid pressure prior to ETT placement, and a nasogastric or orogastric tube should be used after intubation is completed. Furthermore, caution must be taken to insufflate the lungs with enough pressure only to provide adequate chest rise and fall.

In the patient undergoing BMV, the guidelines for ratio of breaths to compressions are as follows:

One rescuer: 2 breaths for every 30 compressions

Two rescuers: 2 breaths per 15 compressions

In both circumstances, each breath should be administered over one second.

In the pulseless victim, after placement of an advanced airway, 8 to 10 breaths/minute should be administered without pauses for compressions. In the intubated patient with a pulse, 12 to 20 breaths/minute should be given. Using the cue "squeeze-release-release" can help the provider pace ventilations to provide adequate breathing support without causing barotrauma.

■ CIRCULATION

The latest PALS guidelines[1] emphasize the importance of effective chest compressions, which would consist of adequate rate (100 per minute), adequate depth (½ to ⅓ the anteroposterior diameter of the chest, full recoil of the chest, and minimal interruptions.

Chest compressions should be instituted in situations of pulseless arrest and in patients with a heart rate less than 60 beats/min with evidence of poor end-organ perfusion.

The patient's rhythm should be checked every 2 minutes, simultaneously with the rotation of providers administering chest compressions.

One should refer to the PALS algorithms as a guide for level of defibrillator charge (J/kg) in the setting of specific rhythm abnormalities in patients with a pulse. Providers should defibrillate the pulseless pediatric patient in VF/VT with 2 J/kg and should follow with uninterrupted CPR for 5 cycles or 2 minutes prior to checking the rhythm. The logic behind not checking the rhythm immediately after defibrillation is that the 90% of patients who show response to this intervention do so after the first shock. Furthermore, there is often latency between achieving a normal rhythm and recovery of pulses, indicating an ongoing need for chest compressions during this adjustment period. If after this period the patient is still in pulseless VF/VT, subsequent doses should be administered at 4 J/kg.

If intravenous access (IV) is not secured at the time of patient arrival at the ED, an intraosseous (IO) line should be placed immediately (Fig. 14-1). This line can be used to administer fluids, blood products, and medications. The EP must remember that an intra-

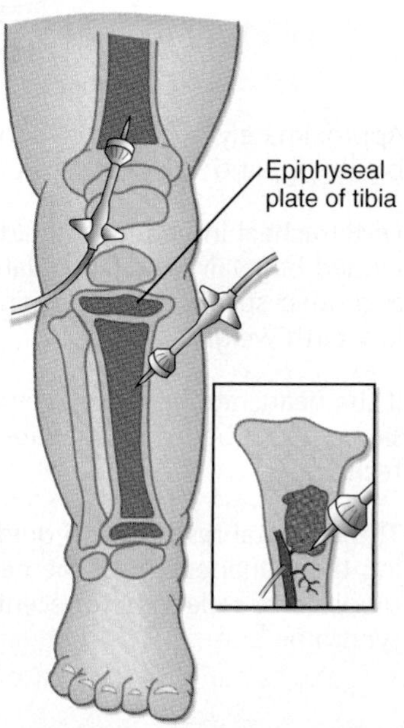
Epiphyseal
plate of tibia

FIGURE 14-1 Placement of an intraosseous line for infusion into the tibia or femur. The upper part of the tibia is the preferred site. For the tibia, the needle is directed toward the foot to avoid the growth plate at the knee.

osseous line is a high-pressure system that requires a pressurized pump or administration by manual syringe.

Resuscitation Medications and Arrest Algorithms

Figures 14-2, 14-3, and 14-4 offer algorithms for resuscitation of children in pulseless arrest, bradycardia, and tachycardia, respectively. Table 14-1 lists medications for resuscitation, and Table 14-2 lists medications for stabilization of the resuscitated patient.

■ EPINEPHRINE

Standard-dose epinephrine for pediatric cardiac arrest is 0.01 mg/kg of the 1:10,000 solution administered IV or IO. Alternatively, a higher dose of epinephrine, at 0.1 mg/kg of a 1:1000 solution, can be administered down the ETT, followed by a saline flush. However, there is mounting evidence that the 1:1000 dose is not helpful and is even potentially harmful if given IV or IO. A prospective randomized trial found that high-dose epinephrine resulted in a statistically significant lower survival outcome than standard-dose epinephrine in in-patient cardiac arrests.[5]

■ VASOPRESSIN

Studies on the use of vasopressin in humans have been mixed. In a piglet model, the combination of epinephrine and vasopressin conferred a better rate of return of spontaneous circulation than either drug given alone.[6] The latest PALS recommendations hold that there is insufficient evidence to recommend the use of vasopressin in pediatric cardiac arrest.

■ AMIODARONE

In the adult population, amiodarone has proved superior to lidocaine in achieving return of spontaneous circulation and survival to hospital admission.[7] Unfortunately, neither drug has demonstrated improvement in survival to hospital discharge. On the basis of the adult literature, however, amiodarone is currently preferred over lidocaine for the treatment of pulseless VT/VF in a child that is refractory to defibrillation and epinephrine.

NEONATAL CARDIOPULMONARY RESUSCITATION

KEY POINTS

Approximately 10% of newborns require assistance after birth to achieve spontaneous breathing, and 1% need even more support.

Endotracheal intubation should be considered for tracheal suctioning for meconium, prolonged bag-valve-mask ventilation or chest compressions, administration of medications, and other special considerations, such as congenital diaphragmatic hernia and extremely low birth weight.

If the heart rate remains below 60 beats/min despite respiratory support, chest compressions should be given at a rate of 100 per minute using the two-finger or chest encircling technique.

The neonatal resuscitation guidelines from the American Heart Association (AHA) regarding the management of the newborn with potential meconium aspiration have been modified to reflect more recent evidence related to outcomes of meconium aspiration syndrome.[8]

Text continued on p. 147.

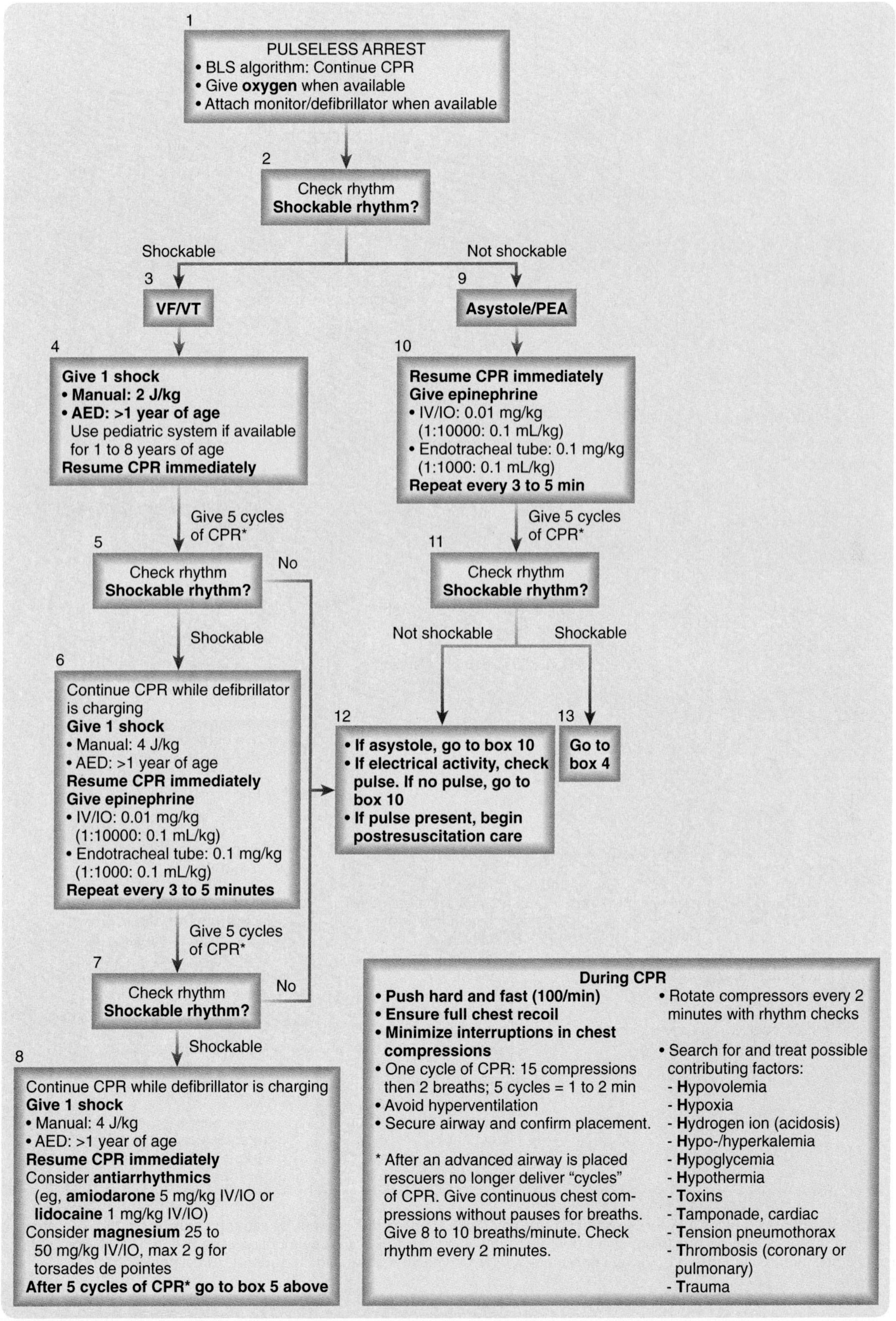
1
PULSELESS ARREST
• BLS algorithm: Continue CPR
• Give **oxygen** when available
• Attach monitor/defibrillator when available
2
Check rhythm
Shockable rhythm?
Shockable
Not shockable
3
VF/VT
4
Give 1 shock
• Manual: 2 J/kg
• AED: >1 year of age
Use pediatric system if available for 1 to 8 years of age
Resume CPR immediately
Give 5 cycles of CPR*
5
Check rhythm
Shockable rhythm?
No
Shockable
6
Continue CPR while defibrillator is charging
Give 1 shock
• Manual: 4 J/kg
• AED: >1 year of age
Resume CPR immediately
Give epinephrine
• IV/IO: 0.01 mg/kg (1:10000: 0.1 mL/kg)
• Endotracheal tube: 0.1 mg/kg (1:1000: 0.1 mL/kg)
Repeat every 3 to 5 minutes
Give 5 cycles of CPR*
7
Check rhythm
Shockable rhythm?
No
Shockable
8
Continue CPR while defibrillator is charging
Give 1 shock
• Manual: 4 J/kg
• AED: >1 year of age
Resume CPR immediately
Consider **antiarrhythmics** (eg, **amiodarone** 5 mg/kg IV/IO or **lidocaine** 1 mg/kg IV/IO)
Consider **magnesium** 25 to 50 mg/kg IV/IO, max 2 g for torsades de pointes
After 5 cycles of CPR* go to box 5 above
9
Asystole/PEA
10
Resume CPR immediately
Give epinephrine
• IV/IO: 0.01 mg/kg (1:10000: 0.1 mL/kg)
• Endotracheal tube: 0.1 mg/kg (1:1000: 0.1 mL/kg)
Repeat every 3 to 5 min
Give 5 cycles of CPR*
11
Check rhythm
Shockable rhythm?
Not shockable
Shockable
12
• If asystole, go to box 10
• If electrical activity, check pulse. If no pulse, go to box 10
• If pulse present, begin postresuscitation care
13
Go to box 4
During CPR
• Push hard and fast (100/min)
• Ensure full chest recoil
• Minimize interruptions in chest compressions
• One cycle of CPR: 15 compressions then 2 breaths; 5 cycles = 1 to 2 min
• Avoid hyperventilation
• Secure airway and confirm placement.
* After an advanced airway is placed rescuers no longer deliver "cycles" of CPR. Give continuous chest compressions without pauses for breaths. Give 8 to 10 breaths/minute. Check rhythm every 2 minutes.
• Rotate compressors every 2 minutes with rhythm checks
• Search for and treat possible contributing factors:
- **H**ypovolemia
- **H**ypoxia
- **H**ydrogen ion (acidosis)
- **H**ypo-/hyperkalemia
- **H**ypoglycemia
- **H**ypothermia
- **T**oxins
- **T**amponade, cardiac
- **T**ension pneumothorax
- **T**hrombosis (coronary or pulmonary)
- **T**rauma

FIGURE 14-2 2005 AHA guidelines for resuscitation of a child with pulseless arrest. AED, automatic external defibrilator; BLS, basic life support; CPR, cardiopulmonary resuscitation; IO, intraosseous(ly); IV, intravenous(ly); PEA, pulseless electrical activity; VF, ventricular fibrillation; VT, ventricular tachycardia. (From Pediatric advanced life support. Circulation 2005;112:IV-167-IV-187.)

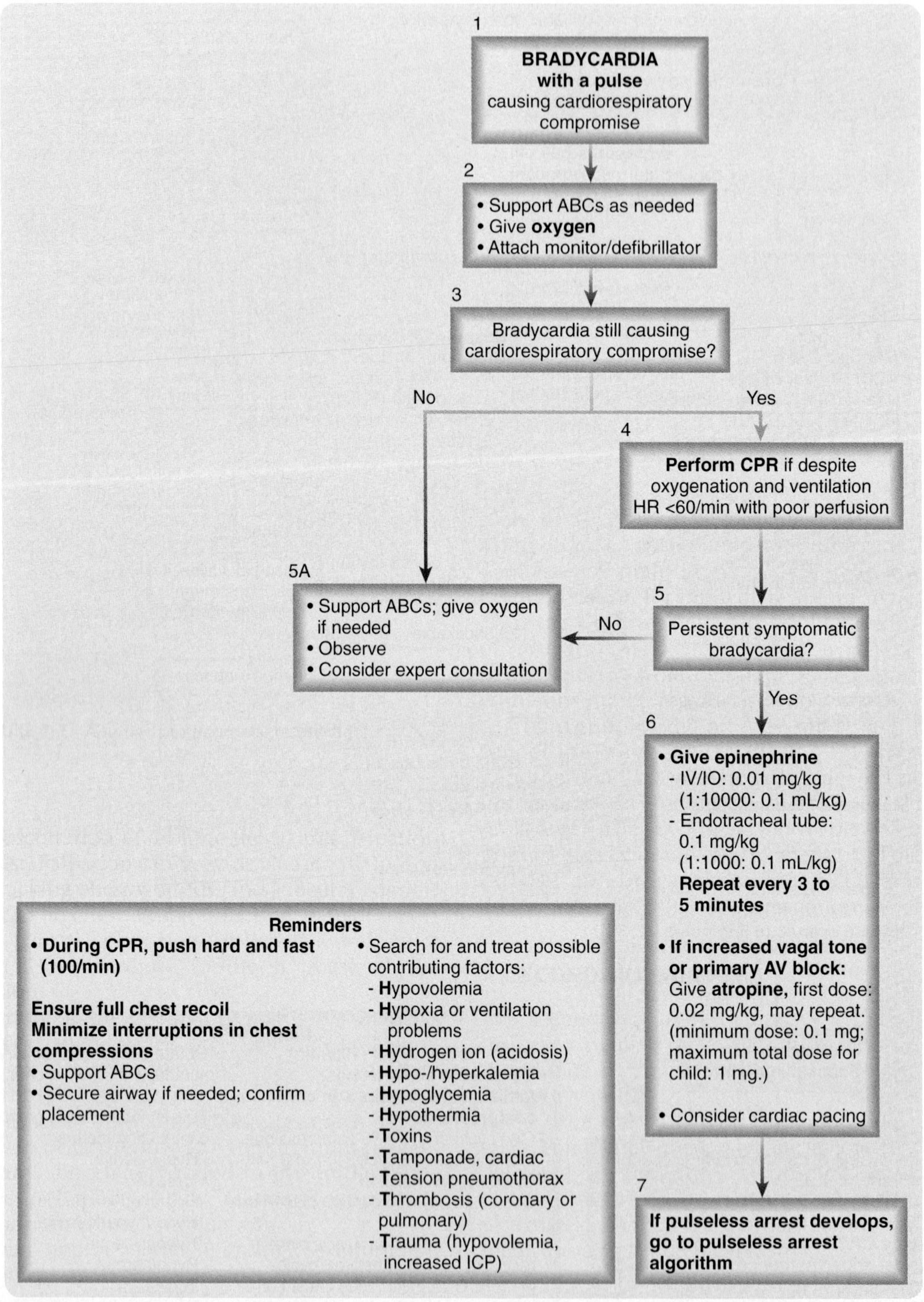
1
BRADYCARDIA with a pulse causing cardiorespiratory compromise
2
• Support ABCs as needed
• Give oxygen
• Attach monitor/defibrillator
3
Bradycardia still causing cardiorespiratory compromise?
No
Yes
4
Perform CPR if despite oxygenation and ventilation HR <60/min with poor perfusion
5A
• Support ABCs; give oxygen if needed
• Observe
• Consider expert consultation
No
5
Persistent symptomatic bradycardia?
Yes
6
• Give epinephrine
- IV/IO: 0.01 mg/kg (1:10000: 0.1 mL/kg)
- Endotracheal tube: 0.1 mg/kg (1:1000: 0.1 mL/kg)
Repeat every 3 to 5 minutes
• If increased vagal tone or primary AV block: Give atropine, first dose: 0.02 mg/kg, may repeat. (minimum dose: 0.1 mg; maximum total dose for child: 1 mg.)
• Consider cardiac pacing
7
If pulseless arrest develops, go to pulseless arrest algorithm
Reminders
• During CPR, push hard and fast (100/min)
Ensure full chest recoil
Minimize interruptions in chest compressions
• Support ABCs
• Secure airway if needed; confirm placement
• Search for and treat possible contributing factors:
- Hypovolemia
- Hypoxia or ventilation problems
- Hydrogen ion (acidosis)
- Hypo-/hyperkalemia
- Hypoglycemia
- Hypothermia
- Toxins
- Tamponade, cardiac
- Tension pneumothorax
- Thrombosis (coronary or pulmonary)
- Trauma (hypovolemia, increased ICP)

FIGURE 14-3 2005 AHA guidelines for resuscitation of a child with bradycardia and a pulse causing cardiorespiratory compromise. ABCs [of resuscitation], airway, breathing, circulation; AV, atrioventricular; CPR, cardiopulmonary resuscitation; HR, heart rate; ICP, intracranial pressure; IO, intraosseous(ly); IV, intravenous(ly). (From Pediatric advanced life support. Circulation 2005;112: IV-167-IV-187.)

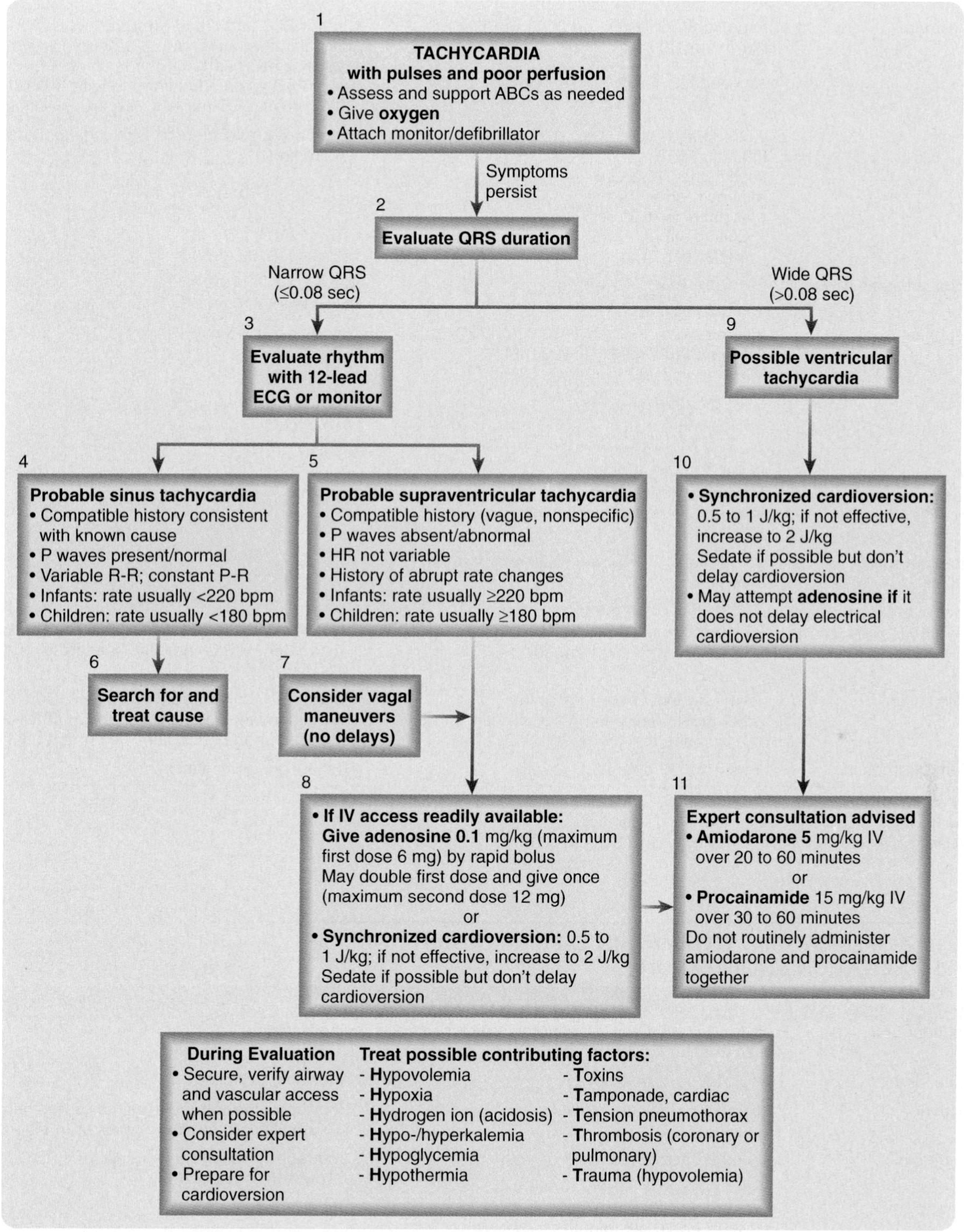
1
TACHYCARDIA
with pulses and poor perfusion
• Assess and support ABCs as needed
• Give oxygen
• Attach monitor/defibrillator
Symptoms persist
2
Evaluate QRS duration
Narrow QRS (≤0.08 sec)
Wide QRS (>0.08 sec)
3
Evaluate rhythm with 12-lead ECG or monitor
9
Possible ventricular tachycardia
4
Probable sinus tachycardia
• Compatible history consistent with known cause
• P waves present/normal
• Variable R-R; constant P-R
• Infants: rate usually <220 bpm
• Children: rate usually <180 bpm
5
Probable supraventricular tachycardia
• Compatible history (vague, nonspecific)
• P waves absent/abnormal
• HR not variable
• History of abrupt rate changes
• Infants: rate usually ≥220 bpm
• Children: rate usually ≥180 bpm
10
• Synchronized cardioversion: 0.5 to 1 J/kg; if not effective, increase to 2 J/kg
Sedate if possible but don't delay cardioversion
• May attempt adenosine if it does not delay electrical cardioversion
6
Search for and treat cause
7
Consider vagal maneuvers (no delays)
8
• If IV access readily available: Give adenosine 0.1 mg/kg (maximum first dose 6 mg) by rapid bolus
May double first dose and give once (maximum second dose 12 mg)
or
• Synchronized cardioversion: 0.5 to 1 J/kg; if not effective, increase to 2 J/kg
Sedate if possible but don't delay cardioversion
11
Expert consultation advised
• Amiodarone 5 mg/kg IV over 20 to 60 minutes
or
• Procainamide 15 mg/kg IV over 30 to 60 minutes
Do not routinely administer amiodarone and procainamide together
During Evaluation
• Secure, verify airway and vascular access when possible
• Consider expert consultation
• Prepare for cardioversion
Treat possible contributing factors:
- Hypovolemia
- Hypoxia
- Hydrogen ion (acidosis)
- Hypo-/hyperkalemia
- Hypoglycemia
- Hypothermia
- Toxins
- Tamponade, cardiac
- Tension pneumothorax
- Thrombosis (coronary or pulmonary)
- Trauma (hypovolemia)

FIGURE 14-4 2005 AHA guidelines for resuscitation of a child with tachycardia, who has pulses and poor perfusion. ABCs [of resuscitation], airway, breathing, circulation; bpm, beats per minute; ECG, electrocardiogram; HR, heart rate; IV, intravenousl(ly). (From Pediatric advanced life support. Circulation 2005;112:IV-167-IV-187.)

Table 14-1 MEDICATIONS FOR PEDIATRIC RESUSCITATION AND ARRHYTHMIAS

Medication	Dose	Remarks
Adenosine	0.1 mg/kg (maximum 6 mg) Repeat: 0.2 mg/kg (maximum 12 mg)	Monitor ECG Rapid IV/IO bolus
Amiodarone	5 mg/kg IV/IO; repeat up to 15 mg/kg Maximum: 300 mg	Monitor ECG and blood pressure Adjust administration rate to urgency (give more slowly when perfusing rhythm present) Use caution when administering with other drugs that prolong QT (consider expert consultation)
Atropine	0.02 mg/kg IV/IO 0.03 mg/kg ET* Repeat once if needed Minimum dose: 0.1 mg Maximum single dose: Child 0.5 mg Adolescent 1 mg	Higher doses may be used with organophosphate poisoning
Calcium chloride (10%)	20 mg/kg IV/IO (0.2 mL/kg)	Slowly Adult dose: 5-10 mL
Epinephrine	0.01 mg/kg (0.1 mL/kg 1 : 10,000) IV/IO 0.1 mg/kg (0.1 mL/kg 1 : 1000) ET* Maximum dose: 1 mg IV/IO; 10 mg ET	May repeat q 3-5 min
Glucose	0.5-1 g/kg IV/IO	$D_{10}W$: 5-10 mL/kg $D_{25}W$: 2-4 mL/kg $D_{50}W$: 1-2 mL/kg
Lidocaine	Bolus: 1 mg/kg IV/IO Maximum dose: 100 mg Infusion: 20-50 µg/kg per minute ET*: 2-3 mg	
Magnesium sulfate	25-50 mg/kg IV/IO over 10-20 min; faster in torsades Maximum dose: 2 g	
Naloxone	<5 y or ≤20 kg: 0.1 mg/kg IV/IO/ET* ≥5 y or >20 kg: 2 mg IV/IO/ET*	Use lower doses to reverse respiratory depression associated with therapeutic opioid use (1-15 µg/kg)
Procainamide	15 mg/kg IV/IO over 30-60 min Adult dose: 20 mg/min IV infusion up to total maximum dose 17 mg/kg	Monitor ECG and blood pressure Use caution when administering with other drugs that prolong QT (consider expert consultation)
Sodium bicarbonate	1 mEq/kg per dose IV/IO slowly	After adequate ventilation

IV, intravenous; IO, intraosseous; ET, via endotracheal tube.
*Flush with 5 mL of normal saline and follow with 5 ventilations.
From Pediatric advanced life support. Circulation 2005;112:IV-167-IV-187.

Table 14-2 MEDICATIONS TO MAINTAIN CARDIAC OUTPUT AND FOR POSTRESUSCITATION STABILIZATION

Medication	Dose Range*	Comment
Inamrinone	0.75-1 mg/kg IV/IO over 5 minutes; may repeat ×2; then 2-20 µg/kg per minute	Inodilator
Dobutamine	2-20 µg/kg per minute IV/IO	Inotrope; vasodilator
Dopamine	2-20 µg/kg per minute IV/IO	Inotrope; chronotrope; renal and splanchnic vasodilator in low doses; pressor in high doses
Epinephrine	0.1-1 µg/kg per minute IV/IO	Inotrope; chronotrope; vasodilator in low doses; pressor in higher doses
Milrinone	50-75 µg/kg IV/IO over 10-60 min then 0.5-0.75 µg/kg per minute	Inodilator
Norepinephrine	0.1-2 µg/kg per minute	Inotrope; vasopressor
Sodium nitroprusside	1-8 µg/kg per minute	Vasodilator; prepare only in D_5W

IV, intravenous; IO, intraosseous.
*Alternative formula for calculating an infusion: Infusion rate (mL/h) = [weight (kg) × dose (mg/kg/min) × 60 (min/h)]/concentration mg/mL.
From Pediatric advanced life support. Circulation 2005;112:IV-167-IV-187.

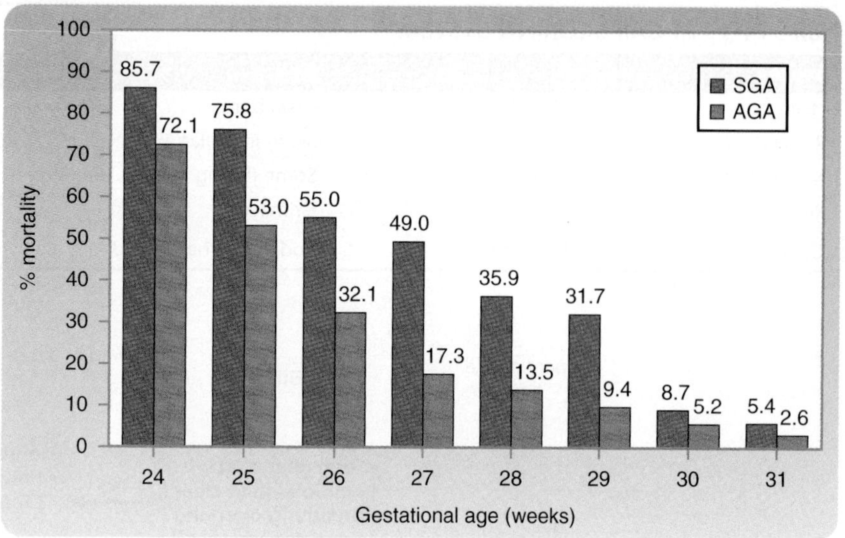

100
90
80
70
60
50
40
30
20
10
0
% mortality
85.7
72.1
75.8
53.0
55.0
32.1
49.0
17.3
35.9
13.5
31.7
9.4
8.7
5.2
5.4
2.6
SGA
AGA
24
25
26
27
28
29
30
31
Gestational age (weeks)

FIGURE 14-5 Percentage mortality for infants who are small for gestational age (SGA) compared with that for infants who are appropriate for gestational age (AGA), shown according to gestational age at birth. Mortality rate of SGA infants was significantly higher than that of AGA infants in the 25th gestational week ($P=.015$) and from 26 to 29 weeks of gestation ($P<.01$). (From Regev RH, Lusky A, Dolfin T, et al: Excess mortality and morbidity among small-for-gestational-age premature infants: A population-based study. J Pediatr 2003;143:186-191.)

Perspective

Approximately 10% of newborns require assistance after birth to achieve spontaneous breathing, and 1% need even more support. The likelihood of survival can be estimated from the gestational age and birth weight (Fig. 14-5).[9]

Survival with Comorbidities

In one study looking at more than 700 neonatal intensive care unit admissions involving infants born at or before 25 weeks of gestation found that among survivors (63%), there was a high incidence of chronic lung disease (51%), high-grade retinopathy of prematurity (32%), intraventricular hemorrhage (44%), nosocomial infection (38%), and necrotizing enterocolitis (11%).[10]

In this same study, only 23% of survivors had no major morbidity, which was defined as chronic lung disease, necrotizing enterocolitis, at least grade 3 intraventricular hemorrhage, or at least grade 3 retinopathy of prematurity.

Anatomy

Anatomic considerations for the neonatal airway are similar to those already discussed for the pediatric patient, with the exception that the structures are even smaller and more anterior and superior, making visualization of the vocal cords an even greater challenge.

The neonatal chest wall is very flexible and can be notably distorted if vigorous inspiratory efforts are made, resulting in inadequate lung expansion and the potential need for positive-pressure ventilatory support.

Presenting Signs and Symptoms

Positive answers to the following four questions identify the baby who does not require post-birth support but can be dried, covered, and kept with the mother if desired[8]:

- Was the baby born after a full-term gestation?
- Is the amniotic fluid clear of meconium and evidence of infection?
- Is the baby breathing or crying?
- Does the baby have good muscle tone?

Apgar scores are measured at 1 minute and 5 minutes after delivery. These scores are used to (1) predict which infants will require resuscitation and (2) identify infants who are at higher risk of neonatal mortality. A score of 7 or higher is reassuring (Table 14-3).

Interventions and Procedures: Resuscitation Steps

Figure 14-6 lists the steps of neonatal resuscitation.

■ AIRWAY

Meconium-stained amniotic fluid occurs in up to 20% of deliveries, and up to 9% of infants with meconium-stained amniotic fluid experience meconium aspiration syndrome (MAS), which carries a modern-day mortality rate of approximately 5%.

MAS occurs when the fetus aspirated meconium before or during birth, leading to obstruction of the airways, atelectasis, severe hypoxia, inflammation, acidosis, and infection.[11] The American Academy of Pediatrics Neonatal Resuscitation Program (NRP)

Table 14-3 APGAR SCORING SYSTEM

Score	0	1	2
Heart rate	Absent	<100 bpm	>100 bpm
Respiration	Absent	Slow, irregular; weak cry	Good; strong cry
Muscle tone	Limp	Some flexing or arms and legs	Active motion
Reflex	Absent	Grimace	Grimace and cough or sneeze
Color	Blue or pale	Body pink; hands and feet blue	Completely pink

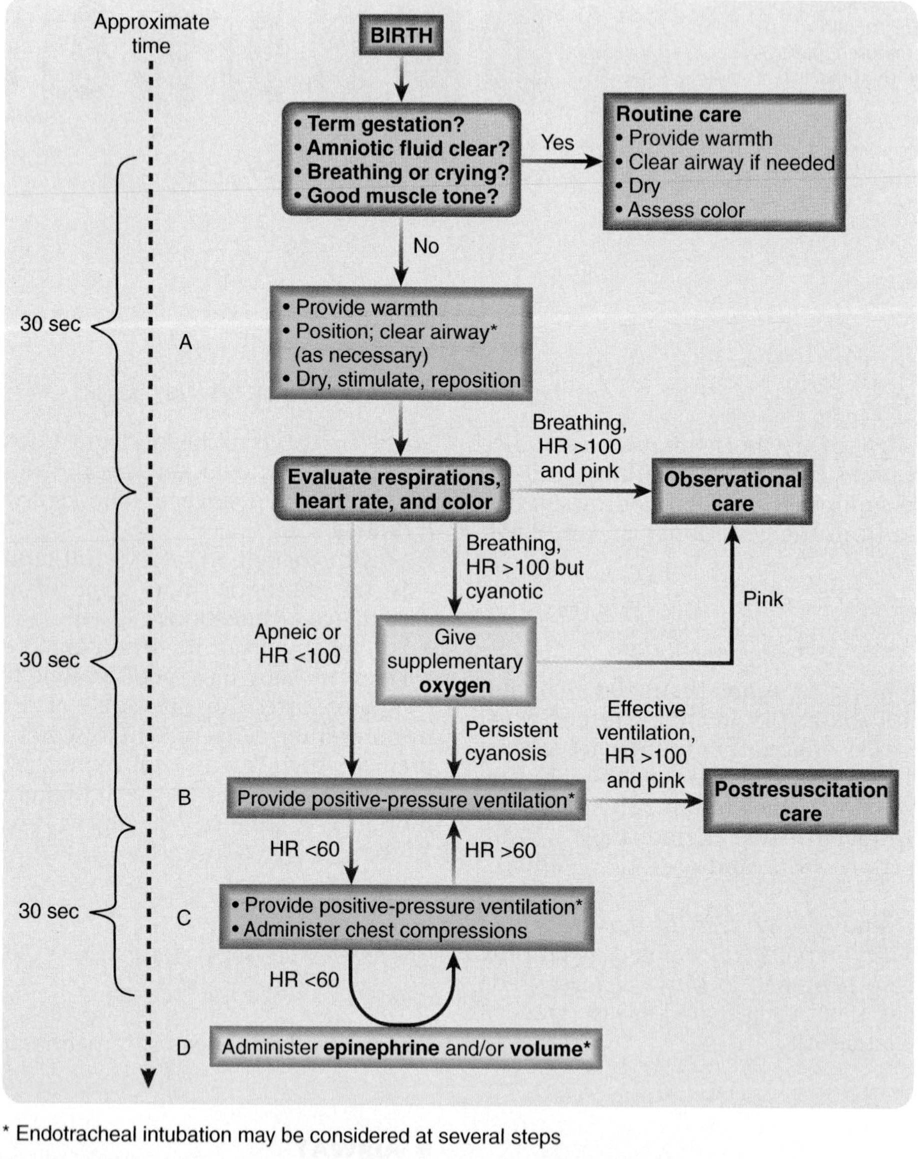
Approximate time
BIRTH
• Term gestation?
• Amniotic fluid clear?
• Breathing or crying?
• Good muscle tone?
Yes
Routine care
• Provide warmth
• Clear airway if needed
• Dry
• Assess color
No
30 sec
A
• Provide warmth
• Position; clear airway* (as necessary)
• Dry, stimulate, reposition
Breathing, HR >100 and pink
Evaluate respirations, heart rate, and color
Observational care
Breathing, HR >100 but cyanotic
Pink
Apneic or HR <100
Give supplementary oxygen
30 sec
Persistent cyanosis
Effective ventilation, HR >100 and pink
B
Provide positive-pressure ventilation*
Postresuscitation care
HR <60
HR >60
30 sec
C
• Provide positive-pressure ventilation*
• Administer chest compressions
HR <60
D
Administer epinephrine and/or volume*
* Endotracheal intubation may be considered at several steps

FIGURE 14-6 2005 AHA guidelines for resuscitation of a neonate. HR, heart rate (beats/min). *Endotracheal intubation may be considered at these steps. (From Neonatal resuscitation guidelines. Circulation 2005;112:IV-188-IV-195.)

guidelines[9] regarding the management of the newborn with potential meconium aspiration have been modified to reflect more recent evidence related to outcomes of meconium aspiration syndrome. There is no distinction between thin and thick meconium, as both have shown to lead to meconium aspiration syndrome.

The nonvigorous newborn with meconium-stained amniotic fluid should no longer be suctioned on the mother's perineum. Avoiding such suctioning prevents undue stimulation, which would lead to breathing and aspiration of meconium prior to endotracheal suctioning.[1] Such a newborn should undergo endotracheal intubation and suctioning of meconium. A

10 F to 14 F suction catheter and meconium aspirator attached to an ETT should be utilized to suction meconium from the airways.

The vigorous newborn of a birth with meconium-stained amniotic fluid should not undergo endotracheal suctioning for any level of meconium staining. Endotracheal suctioning has shown no benefit in this setting, as the meconium has already caused irreversible damage to the lower airways. *Vigorous* is defined as having strong respiratory efforts, good muscle tone, and a heart rate higher than 100 beats/min.[8]

■ BREATHING

Methods to stimulate breathing in neonatal resuscitation are as follows:

- Rubbing the back/spine
- Flicking the soles of the feet
- Vigorously drying the skin

If these measures are not stimulating an adequate change in heart rate, color, or activity, blow-by oxygen (blowing or wafting oxygen) should be administered.

Positive-pressure ventilation via bag-valve-mask at a rate of 40 to 60 breaths/min is indicated for the following situations:

- The infant is apneic after warming, stimulation, and administration of blow-by oxygen.
- The heart rate remains less than 100 beats/min after the preceding methods have been applied.
- The infant has persistent central cyanosis.[9]

As recommended by the AHA, inflation pressures of 30 to 40 cm H_2O should be used in the term infant, and 20 to 25 cm H_2O in the preterm infant.

In the absence of meconium-stained amniotic fluid, laryngeal mask airways may be utilized in the term or near-term infant requiring assisted ventilation, but not chest compressions.

Continuous positive airway pressure (CPAP) delivered via face mask immediately after delivery may be utilized in the neonate with respiratory effort but significant distress. Devices that provide some level of CPAP include standard self-inflating bags, flow-inflating bags, and predetermined CPAP devices such as the Neopuff Infant Resuscitator (Fisher and Paykel, Auckland, NZ). Benefits of CPAP include diminished work of breathing, reduced incidence of apnea, reduced inspiratory resistance, and improved oxygenation. Drawbacks relate to the risk of overdistention, which can result in reduced pulmonary perfusion, diminished cardiac output, and, ultimately, ventilation-perfusion mismatch.

There are no randomized controlled trials comparing the use of CPAP and standard bag-valve-mask devices in the setting of neonatal resuscitation, so there is no formal recommendation for the use of one modality over the other.[13]

Guidelines for endotracheal intubation in neonatal resuscitation are as follows[8]:

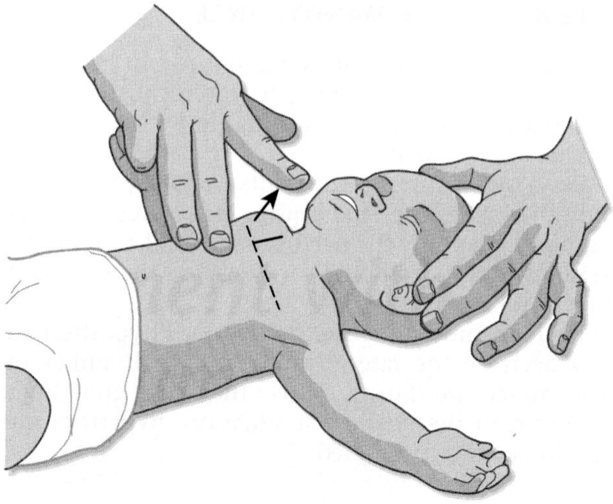
A

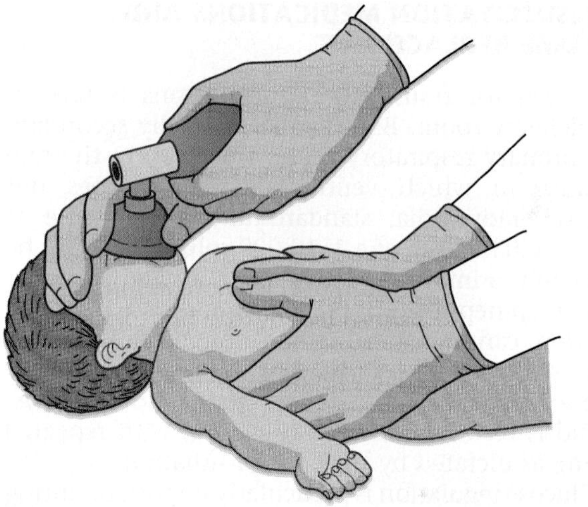
B

FIGURE 14-7 The two-finger **(A)** and chest encircling **(B)** techniques. A 3 : 1 ratio of compressions to ventilations should be used, resulting in approximately 90 compressions and 30 ventilations per minute of cardiopulmonary resuscitation performed.

- Tracheal suctioning is needed for meconium-stained amniotic
- Bag-valve-mask ventilation is prolonged or ineffective.
- Chest compressions are prolonged.
- ETT administration of medications is desired.
- Special considerations, such as congenital diaphragmatic hernia or extremely low birth weight.

■ CIRCULATION

If the heart rate remains below 60 beats/min despite respiratory support, chest compressions should be given at a rate of 100 per minute using the two-finger or chest encircling technique (Fig. 14-7).

■ TEMPERATURE MAINTENANCE

For the term well infant, temperature can be maintained with standard drying followed by swaddling and placement under warming lights or on the mother's warm skin.

Very-low-birthweight infants (<1500 g) require additional warming techniques. AHA guidelines recommend wrapping the newborn in "food-grade heat-resistant plastic wrapping" and placing the newborn under radiant heat.

There is some evidence that induced hypothermia may decrease the rate of death and/or disability in asphyxiated newborns. Thus, the AHA guidelines state that in the post-arrest situation, hyperthermia should be strictly avoided.[8]

■ RESUSCITATION MEDICATIONS AND VOLUME REPLACEMENT

The need for resuscitation medications is rare in the delivery room. Bradycardia is usually secondary to a primary respiratory cause. However, in the rare instance in which ventilatory support does not reverse bradycardia, standard-dose epinephrine at 0.01 to 0.03 mg/kg of a 1:10,000 solution should be preferably administered IV. Alternatively, a higher dose of epinephrine, at 0.1 mg/kg also of a 1: 10,000 solution, can be administered through the ETT until IV access has been established.

If volume replacement is necessary, isotonic crystalloid is recommended at 10 mL/kg, with repeated dosing as dictated by the clinical situation.

Glucose regulation is particularly important during the post-stabilization period in the asphyxiated newborn, whose glycogen stores can be rapidly depleted. A serum glucose level greater than 40 mg/dL should be maintained with the administration of 10% dextrose in water ($D_{10}W$).

Naloxone administration should generally be avoided in the resuscitation of the newborn at the time of delivery, concentrating treatment instead on the support of breathing and circulation. Administration of naloxone to mothers with known opioid addiction can have adverse outcomes and also is not recommended by the AHA.

Bicarbonate is not recommended in the acute resuscitation of the newborn, because of studies showing deleterious effects, including depression of myocardial function, intracellular acidosis, reductions in cerebral blood flow, and risk of intracranial hemorrhage.[14]

■ UMBILICAL VEIN CATHETER PLACEMENT

Immediately after delivery, an umbilical vein catheter may be placed to administer medications and volume resuscitation. The catheter should be placed with sterile technique and by a trained provider (Fig. 14-8). Umbilical vein catheterization can reasonably be attempted up to 1 week after delivery, although the likelihood of cord patency diminishes with time.

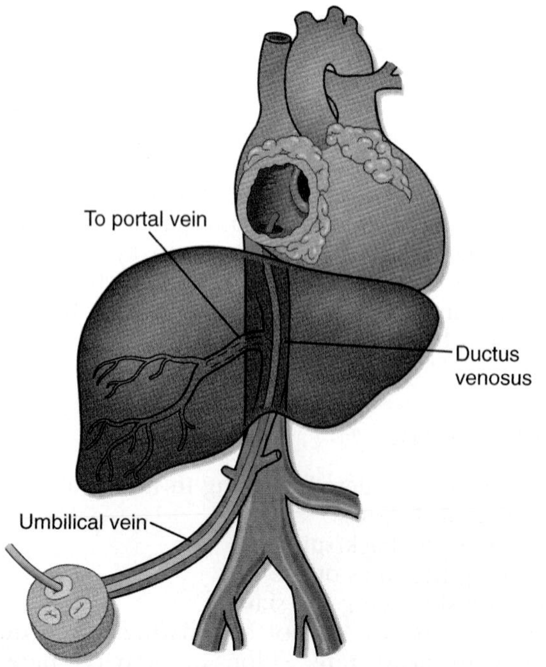

To portal vein
Ductus venosus
Umbilical vein

FIGURE 14-8 Umbilical vein catheterization. The drawing illustrates passage of the catheter from the umbilical vein into the portal vein in the liver and then through the inferior vena cava to the right atrium. The tip of the catheter should be in the inferior vena cava, just at the entrance to the right atrium.

REFERENCES

1. Pediatric advanced life support. Circulation 2005;112: IV-167-IV-187.
2. Young KD, Seidel JS: Pediatric cardiopulmonary resuscitation: A collective review. Ann Emerg Med 1999;33: 195-205.
3. Donoghue AJ, Nadkarni V, Berg RA, et al: CanAm Pediatric Cardiac Arrest Investigators: Out-of-hospital cardiac arrest: An epidemiologic review and assessment of current knowledge. Ann Emerg Med 2005;46:512-522.
4. Gausche M, Lewis RJ, Stratton SJ, et al: Effect of out-of-hospital pediatric endotracheal intubation on survival and neurological outcome: A controlled clinical trial. JAMA 2000;283:783-790.
5. Perondi M, Reis A, Paiva FF, et al: A comparison of high-dose and standard-dose epinephrine in children with cardiac arrest. N Engl J Med 2004;350:1722-1730.
6. Voelckel WG, Lurie KG, McKnite S, et al: Effects of epinephrine and vasopressin in a piglet model of prolonged ventricular fibrillation and cardiopulmonary resuscitation. Crit Care Med 2002;30:957-962.
7. Dorian P, Cass K, Schwartz B, et al: Amiodarone as compared with lidocaine for shock-resistant ventricular fibrillation. N Engl J Med 2002;346:884-890.
8. Neonatal resuscitation guidelines. Circulation 2005; 112IV:188-IV-195.
9. Regev RH, Lusky A, Dolfin T, et al: Excess mortality and morbidity among small-for-gestational-age premature infants: A population-based study. J Pediatr 2003; 143:186-191.
10. Chan K, Ohisson A, Synnes A, et al: Survival, morbidity, and resource use of infants of 25 weeks' gestational age or less. Am J Obstet Gynecol 2001;185:220-226.
11. Velaphi S, Vidyasagar D: Intrapartum and postdelivery management of infants born to mothers with meconium-

stained amniotic fluid: Evidence-based recommendations. Clin Perinatol 2006;33:29-42.
12. Vain NR, Szyld EG, Prudent LM, et al: Oropharyngeal and nasopharyngeal suctioning of meconium-staining neonates before delivery of their shoulders: Multicentre, randomized controlled trial. Lancet 2004;364:597-602.
13. Halamek L, Morley C: Continuous positive airway pressure during neonatal resuscitation. Clin Perinatol 2006;33: 83-98.
14. Wyckoff M, Perlman MB: Use of high-dose epinephrine and sodium bicarbonate during neonatal resuscitation: Is there proven benefit? Clin Perinatol 2006;33:141-151.

Chapter **15**

Pediatric Resuscitation

Ghazala Q. Sharieff and Maureen McCollough

KEY POINTS

Correct positioning is imperative for successful airway management in the child, whose airway is quite anterior.

The use of a cuffed endotracheal tube is acceptable in any child older than a newborn.

Patients in full cardiorespiratory arrest should not receive more than 8-10 breaths per minute during resuscitation.

"Push hard, push fast" is the new recommendation for cardiopulmonary resuscitation. Minimal interruptions between compressions should be the goal of resuscitation.

"Stacked shocks" are no longer recommended for treatment of ventricular fibrillation or pulseless ventricular tachycardia.

Airway Management

■ ANATOMY

The pediatric airway differs from the adult airway in many significant ways (Box 15-1). Therefore, some special techniques are helpful in attempts to intubate a child. Because the occiput is large in a young child, a towel roll should be placed beneath the patient's shoulders and not behind the head as in adults. The shoulder roll helps place the child in a more neutral position. A child's airway is very anterior, and it is imperative that the person performing the intubation is looking up at the airway; if necessary, the operator should squat to make this view possible. Another tip is to raise the bed so that the operator can look up at the airway. A straight blade is recommended in infants, because it helps lift the floppy epiglottis out of the way. An additional tip in infants who have very small mouths is to have an assistant pull the baby's cheek to the side, to allow passage of the laryngoscope and endotracheal tube.[1,2]

■ PHARMACOLOGIC AGENTS FOR RAPID-SEQUENCE INTUBATION IN CHILDREN

Potential combinations of agents that might be used for rapid-sequence intubation are listed in Table 15-1.

■ BAG-VALVE-MASK VENTILATION

Correct mask sizing is vital to proper bag-valve-mask ventilation. The mask should snugly fit from the bridge of the nose to the cleft of chin. A mask that is too large can place pressure on the eyes and cause vagal bradycardia. A mask that is too small will not allow adequate oxygenation and ventilation. The mask should be held using a "CE" grip—the holder's thumb and index grip the mask and the third, fourth, and fifth fingers are placed on the angle of jaw. It is important to avoid pushing on the soft tissue below the mandible, which might cause airway obstruction.

BOX 15-1

Ways in Which the Child's Airway Differs Anatomically from the Adult's Airway

- Prominent occiput can cause airway obstruction; a 1-inch towel roll should be placed below the shoulders
- Dependence on nasopharynx patency; nasal airways should be avoided in children younger than 1 year owing to their larger adenoidal tissue, which can bleed
- Lots of secretions
- Loose primary teeth
- Relatively larger tongues, which can obstruct the airway; an oral or nasal airway may be needed instead
- Epiglottis is U-shaped and floppy; a straight laryngoscope blade should be used to lift the epiglottis directly
- Larynx is more anterior and cephalad
- Cricoid is the smallest area of the airway
- Small tracheal diameter and distance between rings, which make tracheostomy or cricothyrotomy more difficult; the American Heart Association recommends needle cricothyrotomy for difficult airways (see text discussion of this modality)
- Much shorter tracheal length (in newborn, 4-5 cm; in 18-month-old child, 7-8 cm)
- Endotracheal tube may be easily dislodged; position of tube should be reassessed frequently
- Large airways are more narrow, leading to greater resistance
- Ribs more horizontal in very young child, who depends on diaphragm for movement
- Increased risk of gastric dependence*

*Decompress stomach with nasogastric tube to ventilate easier; rough guide to size is 2 × endotracheal tube size.

The rate of bagged breaths per minute is best controlled by having the operator say "squeeze-release-release" as he or she is ventilating the patient. This practice helps decrease the rapid rate of ventilation and resultant adverse effects that often occur in resuscitative events. Patients in full arrest should not receive more than 8 to 10 breaths/min via either bag-valve-mask or endotracheal tube. Complications of bag-valve-mask ventilation include gastric distention, pneumothorax, vomiting, aspiration, and hypoxia.

Appropriate bag size can be chosen as follows:

- For an infant or child up to 5 years: 450-mL bag
- For an older child: 750-mL or adult bag

Table 15-1 CLINICAL SCENARIOS FOR INTUBATION AND RECOMMENDED INDUCTION AGENTS

Clinical Scenario	Induction Agents
Isolated head injury	Propofol Thiopental Etomidate DO NOT USE ketamine!
Status epilepticus	Thiopental Propofol Etomidate Midazolam
Asthma	Ketamine Etomidate DO NOT USE thiopental!
Respiratory failure	Ketamine Etomidate Propofol

Adapted from presentation by Sacchetti A, American College of Emergency Physicians Scientific Assembly, Boston, 2003.

The ED should NOT be stocked with neonatal 250-mL bags, which are inadequate for any child older than a newborn and can cause confusion in resuscitation situations.

Rapid-Sequence Intubation in Children

Intubating timeline and drugs of choice are listed in Tables 15-2 and 15-3. Post-intubation assessment includes confirmation that the endotracheal tube is in correct position. The EP should listen first over the stomach and then over the axillae for breath sounds. A confirmation device, such as an end-tidal carbon dioxide monitor, a carbon dioxide chart (e.g., Pedi-Cap, which should change from purple to yellow with proper tube placement), or an esophageal detector, should be used.[3,4] A nasogastric or orogastric tube should also be placed as soon as possible. Any amount of gastric distention can make it difficult to ventilate and oxygenate a child. A rough rule of thumb for nasogastric and orogastric tube size is 2 times the endotracheal tube size.

■ Principles of Endotracheal Intubation

Recommended endotracheal tube sizes are listed in Box 15-2. With the advent of high-volume, low-pressure endotracheal tubes with cuffs, the dictum of using only uncuffed endotracheal tubes in children younger than 8 years is changing. Therefore, it is possible to use a cuffed endotracheal tube in a child. An uncuffed endotracheal tube smaller than that calculated is typically recommended. Handy formulas for choosing tube size are 4 + (age/4) for uncuffed tube and 3+(age/4) for a cuffed tube. Cuff inflation pressure should be kept less than 20 cm H_2O. Cuffed endotracheal tubes are not recommended for use in newborns.[5,6]

Table 15-2 PARALYTIC AGENTS COMMONLY USED FOR INTUBATION IN CHILDREN*

Agent	Dose (mg/kg)	Onset of Action	Duration of Action (minutes)	Comments
Succinylcholine	1-2	<1 min	<10	Can cause bradycardia Children younger than 10 years should be pretreated with atropine DO NOT USE in children with chronic muscular disorders
Rocuronium	1.0	<1 min	40-60	Causes no change in potassium Does not cause malignant hyperthermia
Vecuronium	0.1 *or* 0.3	2-3 min *or* 60-90 sec	30-40 *or* Up to 100	Priming dose of 0.01 mg/kg may be given intravenously, followed 2-3 min later by the induction agent and a second vecuronium dose at 0.15 mg/kg

*Timed Intubation: When using nondepolarizing agents, it is not necessary to induce the patient immediately. This permits a timed intubation in which the non-depolarizing agent is administered first and begins subclinical muscle relaxation. Approximately 15 seconds later the induction agent is administered. Both agents then therapeutically overlap at about 30-45 seconds after beginning procedure resulting in good intubating conditions.

Table 15-3 INDUCTION AGENTS FOR INTUBATION IN CHILDREN

Drug	Dose (mg/kg)	Onset of Action (seconds)	Duration (minutes)	Blood Pressure Response	Intracranial Pressure Response	Side Effects
Propofol	1-2	10-20	3-14	Decreases	Decreases	Antiepileptic effects DO NOT USE in patients with soy or egg allergies
Etomidate	0.3	20-30	7-14	None	May decrease	Adrenal suppression, myoclonic jerks
Ketamine	Intravenous: 1-2 Intramuscular: 4	15-60	Intravenous: 10-15 Intramuscular: 20-30	Increases	Increases	Bronchial relaxation, myocardial depression
Thiopental	3.0-5.0	20-30	3-5	Decreases	Decreases	Antiepileptic effects Can cause bronchospasm
Midazolam	0.1-0.3	30-60	Intravenous: 30	Decreases	May decrease	Antiepileptic effects

BOX 15-2

Ways of Choosing Endotracheal Tube Size

1. Estimate size according to patient's age:
   - Newborns 3.0 mm or, in large newborn, 3.5 mm
   - Up to 6 months, 3.5-4.0 mm
   - 1 year, 4.0-4.5 mm
   - Older than 1 year:

   Uncuffed tube: 4 + (age/4)
   Cuffed tube: 3 + (age/3)
2. Use a length-based resuscitation tape, such as the Broselow-Luten.
3. Estimate according to patient's finger:
   - Width of child's little finger *nail* is equal to the *internal diameter* of endotracheal tube
   - Width of child's little *finger* is equal to *width of whole* endotracheal tube

Nasotracheal intubations are more complicated in children, for several reasons. The small size of the nares makes passage of the tube difficult, and large adenoids can be lacerated, resulting in profuse bleeding. Additionally, if the child has significant facial fractures or a basilar skull fracture, there is a potential risk of inserting the tube into the cranium.

Incorrect endotracheal tube size can lead to the inability to ventilate if the tube is too small or airway trauma (such as subglottic edema) if the tube is too large. Easy formulas for estimating the depth of endotracheal tube placement are as follows:

3 × tube size; for example, a 4.0-mm tube placed with 12-cm mark at the lips

10 + age in years = number of centimeters of tube to the lips

For premature infants, the following estimations of tube depth based on body weight are helpful:

1 kg: 7 cm
2 kg: 8 cm
3 kg: 9 cm
4 kg: 10 cm

Table 15-4 CHOOSING LARYNGOSCOPE SIZE AND TYPE FOR A CHILD

Age or Weight	Laryngoscope Size	Laryngoscope Type
2.5 kg	0	Straight
0-3 mo	1.0	Straight
3 mo-3 yr	1.5-2.0 *or* 1.5	Straight or curved Wisconsin
3-12 yr	2.0-4.0	Straight or curved

Approximate laryngoscope sizes are listed in Table 15-4. The Broselow-Luten resuscitation tape can also be used to choose size. However, it is important to remember that the actual blade size needed is determined by the individual patient's weight, body habitus, and anatomic variability. It is important to have laryngoscopes available that are one size smaller and one size larger than anticipated.

Once endotracheal tube placement is confirmed, the tube should be secured. It is helpful to place a cervical collar, even in the nontrauma setting, to minimize tube motion. The endotracheal tube can very easily be dislodged, particularly in young infants whose tracheal width is quite small.

Complications of endotracheal tube placement are esophageal intubation, right mainstem intubation, dislodgment, obstruction, barotrauma, trauma to airway, and subglottic stenosis.

Although drug delivery via an endotracheal tube is unpredictable, this approach may be used for patients in whom intravenous access has not been established. The endotracheal tube can be used for administration of the following drugs (which can be remembered with the mnemonic LEAN):

Lidocaine
Epinephrine
Atropine
Naloxone

The endotracheal tube dosage of epinephrine is 10 times the intravenous or intraosseous dosage (0.1 mg/kg [0.1 mL/kg] of a 1:1000 concentration). Lidocaine, atropine, and naloxone are typically administered at 2 to 3 times the intravenous or intraosseous dosage.

Procedure for Rapid-Sequence Intubation

Table 15-5 summarizes the procedure.

Initial Ventilator Settings. Initial ventilator settings are typically chosen through assessment of the height and weight of the patient and the underlying cause of respiratory distress. The following recommendations are for initial ventilatory management. Adjustments should be made according to blood gas measurements, end-tidal CO_2 and pulse oximetry monitors, and patient status.

For children weighing less than 10 kg, a pressure-limited system should be used. The infant should be given sufficient oxygen to relieve cyanosis and maintain normal oxygen saturation (92% to 96%) and/or normal PO_2 (60-90 mm Hg). The following settings should be used:

Rate: 20-60 breaths/min (or the rate that produces a normal $PaCO_2$ value [35-45 mm Hg])
Fraction of inspired oxygen (FIO_2): 100%
Positive end-expiratory pressure (PEEP) value: 3-5 cm H_2O
Peak inspiratory pressure (PIP): 15-35 cm H_2O (or sufficient to produce discernible chest wall movement)
Inspiratory time to expiratory time (I:E) ratio: 1:2 (inspiratory time 0.4-0.7 seconds)

For children weighing greater than 10 kg, a volume-limited system should be used. The initial volume, 10-15 mL/kg, changes to a smaller volume, such as 6-8 mL/kg, particularly in an asthmatic patient. The following settings should be used:

Rate: for infant, 20-30 breaths/min; for a child, 15-20 breaths/min

Table 15-5 PROCEDURE FOR RAPID-SEQUENCE INTUBATION

Time to intubation 5 minutes	Start preoxygenation
Time to intubation 3 minutes	Give any premedication (atropine, lidocaine)
Intubation time	Push induction and paralytic agents
After patient is relaxed	Intubate: Apply cricoid pressure Use BURP (backward, upward, and rightward pressure) technique*
Immediately after intubation	Release cricoid pressure Secure endotracheal tube Place a nasogastric tube

*Too much pressure can occlude the airway!

FiO_2: 100%
PEEP: 3-5 cm H_2O
I:E ratio: 1:2

■ THE DIFFICULT PEDIATRIC AIRWAY

■ Failed Intubation

In the event that endotracheal intubation is unsuccessful, there are several options for airway rescue. The laryngeal mask airway (LMA) has the advantages of being easily placed without the need for laryngoscopy and also has little cardiac effect during the insertion process. Disadvantages include the lack of airway protection from vomiting or aspiration of gastric contents, the requirement that the patient be unconscious or sedated for its placement, and the fact that LMA is not a definitive airway.

Approximate LMA sizes are listed in Table 15-6.

Complications of LMA placement are coughing/bronchospasm, aspiration/regurgitation, airway trauma, lingual nerve palsy, vocal cord paralysis, hypoglossal nerve paralysis, hoarseness, stridor, and pharyngeal or mouth ulcers.

Table 15-6 RECOMMENDED LARYNGEAL MASK AIRWAY (LMA) SIZES

Patient Age and Weight	LMA Size
Neonates to 5 kg	1
Infants/children:	
5-10 kg	1½
10-20 kg	2
20-30 kg	2½
30-50 kg	3
Adults:	
50-70 kg	4
70-100 kg	5
>100 kg	6

■ Needle Cricothyrotomy (Jet Ventilation)

Needle cricothyrotomy should be used when endotracheal intubation is not successful. It is most often indicated in children younger than 10 to 12 years, in whom a surgical airway is technically difficult to perform. Most procedure texts discuss the use of a jet ventilator to ventilate through a needle cricothyrotomy; unfortunately, most EDs do not have access to a jet ventilator. This chapter describes various oxygen setups that can be used in any ED to ventilate with a needle cricothyrotomy without a jet ventilator attachment. The procedure for placing the needle is quite simple, as follows:

1. Identify the cricothyroid membrane; prepare with povidone-iodine solution if possible.
2. Use a 12- to 14-gauge angiocatheter attached to a syringe to puncture the cricothyroid membrane.
3. Direct the catheter at a 45-degree angle caudally (toward the patient's feet). Placement of normal saline in the syringe helps to demonstrate when air is aspirated.
4. Remove the needle from the angiocatheter.

Some experts advocate inserting another 14-gauge angiocatheter into the cricothyroid membrane to allow exhalation; one must make sure to occlude this second angiocatheter while squeezing the bag-mask-valve bag and then free the angiocatheter to allow exhalation.

With these methods, the child can be oxygenated, but ventilation (CO_2 exhalation) is limited.

■ *Methods for Ventilation*

Once the angiocatheter is placed, one of the following methods may be chosen for ventilation:

- Attach the following items to the angiocatheter as follows: a 3-mL syringe barrel, a 7.0 F endotracheal tube adapter, and a bag-valve-mask bag. Turn the wall oxygen (O_2) up to 15 L, and attempt to administer ventilation with the bag and through the angiocatheter.
- Attach a 3.0 F endotracheal tube adapter directly to the angiocatheter and then a bag-valve-mask bag; turn the wall O_2 up to 15 L, and attempt to administer ventilation with the bag and through the angiocatheter.
- Attach one prong of a nasal cannula to the angiocatheter, and use the other prong for oxygen flow (1 second on, 4 seconds off).
- Use an Enk Oxygen Flow Modulator kit (Cook Medical).
- The QuickTrach kit (Rusch, Inc.) can also be used for cricothyrotomy.

■ *Complications*

Complication rates for needle cricothyrotomy range from 10% to 40%. Complications are exsanguinating hematoma, perforation of the esophagus, posterior wall of the trachea, or thyroid, infection, inadequate oxygenation (inadequate ventilation with a rise in CO_2 is inevitable; the goal is good oxygenation), and subcutaneous or mediastinal emphysema.

Vascular Access

■ INTRAVASCULAR ACCESS

Establishment of intravascular access can also be anxiety provoking in children. If the patient is stable, there may be more time for attempts at peripheral access; the unstable patient, however, requires immediate access, which is most commonly obtained via an intraosseous line. With the neonate, there is the unique option of umbilical venous cannulation.

Initial volume resuscitation is with 20 mL/kg of normal saline or lactated Ringer's injection. In newborns, 10 mL/kg is a good starting point. Repeat boluses may be given. However, in cases of hemorrhagic shock, if the blood pressure is not improved after two or three boluses, packed red blood cells should be given, in a dose of 10 mL/kg. The Pediatric

Advanced Life Support (PALS) formula for a blood pressure goal in children notes that the fifth percentile is 70 + (2 × age in years). Because this is only the fifth percentile, the preferred formula is 90 + (2 × age in years).

Vascular access sites are discussed in the following sections.

Peripheral Intravenous Lines

The large peripheral veins, including the antecubital and saphenous, are good options in patients of all ages. A small, 20- to 24-gauge catheter may be necessary. Scalp veins and the external jugular veins are also excellent options if intravenous access placement in the extremities is difficult.

Intraosseous Access

An intraosseous line should be considered when emergency access is necessary and peripheral vascular access is not obtainable. The preferred site for placement of an intraosseous line is the anteromedial surface of the proximal tibia 1 cm inferior to and 1 cm medial to the tibial tubercle. Alternative sites are the distal femur, medial malleolus, distal humerus, and anterior-superior iliac crest. In older children and adults, attempts at intraosseous access may be made in the distal tibia and the distal radius and ulna. In addition to commercially available intraosseous infusion needles, Jamshidi-type bone marrow aspiration needles are often used. Contraindications to placement of an intraosseous vascular line are a current attempt in the same area, cellulitis, fracture in the same bone, and osteogenesis imperfecta (relative contraindication).

The procedure of establishing intraosseous access in the anterior tibia is as follows:

1. The skin over the anterior tibia is sterilized.
2. Starting 1 to 3 cm below the tibial tuberosity (to avoid damaging the growth plate), the needle is directed at a 90-degree angle to the medial surface of the tibia.
3. Once the cortex is passed, the operator must stop pushing, so as to avoid forcing the needle through the other side of the bone.

The following signs help confirm that the needle is in the marrow cavity:

- A sudden decrease in resistance as the needle passes through the cortex.
- The needle stands upright without support.
- When a syringe is attached to the needle, bone marrow may be aspirated. If this is not possible, an infusion flush should be used, because it is common to be unable to aspirate marrow.
- Fluid infuses freely without signs of subcutaneous infiltration.

Any drug or fluid that can be administered intravenously can be rapidly infused through the intraosseous line. The aspirate can be sent for all laboratory studies except complete blood count. Complications of intraosseous infusions, which are rare, include osteomyelitis, compartment syndrome, tibial fracture, and skin necrosis.

Central Venous Access

Indications for central venous access in emergency situations are inability to establish peripheral venous or intraosseous access and for monitoring in the hemodynamically unstable patient.

A 3 or 4 F percutaneous central venous catheter should be used in infants younger than 1 year, and a 4 F to 5.5 F catheter in children 1 year to 12 years. The subclavian, internal jugular, or femoral vein may be accessed with the percutaneous central venous catheter. However, the femoral vein is the easiest and safest central vein to cannulate in emergencies owing to its large diameter and ability to be cannulated while cardiopulmonary resuscitation is in progress. The procedure is as follows:

1. The leg is slightly externally rotated, and the area prepared and draped in sterile fashion.
2. The femoral vein is located medial to the femoral artery. If time permits, the area below the inguinal ligament, medial to the femoral artery, should be infiltrated with 1% lidocaine.
3. In children, the introducer needle is directed at a 30- to 40-degree angle to the skin, starting about 1 cm below the inguinal ligament and aiming toward the contralateral shoulder or umbilicus.
4. Once a flash of blood is obtained, the guidewire is threaded through the introducer.
5. The Seldinger technique is then followed to complete line placement.

Complications of central line placement are bleeding, thrombosis, arterial puncture, pneumothorax, and hemothorax (for subclavian or internal jugular attempts). The use of ultrasonography to improve central venous access has become more popular, including its use in children.

Vascular Cutdown

Surgical venous cutdown may be used when attempts at peripheral, intraosseous, and central venous access fail. The saphenous vein, which courses anterior to the medial malleolus at the ankle, is the preferred site.

1. The lower extremity is immobilized with the foot turned laterally to reveal the saphenous vein.
2. After the area is prepared in a sterile fashion, 1% lidocaine may be injected subcutaneously over the vein, and a tourniquet should be placed proximal to this site.
3. An incision perpendicular to the vein is made, and the vein is isolated by blunt dissection with a curved hemostat.

4. Two silk sutures are looped around the vein; the distal one may be used to ligate the vein.
5. While tension is applied to the proximal suture loop, a venotomy with a No. 11 blade is made by puncturing the lateral wall of the vessel and drawing the scalpel gently upwards. This maneuver avoids complete transection of the vessel.
6. The cannula is then inserted into the vein and secured by tying of the proximal suture loop.
7. It may be necessary to remove the tourniquet while the catheter is being advanced.

Umbilical Vascular Access

In neonates, the umbilical vessels may be directly accessed during the first several days of life. The umbilical vein may be used for blood sampling, fluid or drug infusion, and monitoring of blood pressure and central venous pressure. Anatomically, there are typically two umbilical arteries and one umbilical vein. The vein is usually in the 12 o'clock position and has a thinner wall and wider lumen than the artery. The umbilical vein is often described as resembling a "smiley face."

In emergency situations, the umbilical vein is the preferred vessel to access because the umbilical arteries are often tortuous and difficult to cannulate. The procedure is as follows:

1. The umbilicus is prepared with a bactericidal solution and draped, and a silk suture is placed around the base of the umbilicus stump.
2. The distal end of the stump is cut off, and the stump and vessels are occluded with the silk suture to prevent blood loss.
3. A 3.5 to 5.0 F catheter is flushed with saline and inserted into the lumen of the desired vessel.
4. An umbilical vein catheter should be advanced just to the point where good blood return is obtained.
5. Plain radiographs should be taken to confirm placement.

Complications of umbilical catheters are hemorrhage, infection, air embolism, and perforation of a blood vessel.

Basic Principles of Cardiopulmonary Resuscitation

Single-rescuer cardiopulmonary resuscitation (CPR) providers should activate EMS after 1 minute of rescue breathing and compressions if the patient is younger than 8 years (as the underlying cause is more likely to be respiratory than cardiac). The American Heart Association now recommends "push hard and push fast" with compressions. Infants and children should have a compression rate of at least 100 per minute. In lone-rescuer CPR, the compression-to-ventilation ratio is 30:2. For health care providers or responders trained in CPR, the ratio is 15:2. According to the new PALS guidelines, an adequate compression depth is approximately one third to one half the anterior-posterior diameter of the patient's chest. In infants, the two-thumb method is preferred over the finger method for compressions, and the compression to ventilation ratio is 3:1. There should be full recoil of the chest after each compression.

The effectiveness of CPR is best judged clinically from the presence of a pulse in the femoral area corresponding to chest compressions. Interruptions in compressions should be limited to less than 10 seconds for interventions such as placement of an advanced airway or defibrillation. Interruptions in compressions have shown to decrease the rate of return to spontaneous circulation. Rhythm checks should be performed every 2 minutes or every five cycles of CPR. Once an advanced airway is in place, compressions and breaths should be performed continuously without interruption.

Foreign-body removal maneuvers consist of a sequence of five back blows and five chest thrusts for infants and the Heimlich maneuver for children.

RESUSCITATIVE DRUGS

Epinephrine

The initial intravenous/intraosseous dose of epinephrine for patients in pulseless arrest who are older than neonates is 0.01 mg/kg (0.1 mL/kg) of the 1:10,000 solution. All endotracheal doses are 0.1 mg (0.1 mL/kg) of the 1:1000 solution for pulseless arrest. Note that intravenous epinephrine and endotracheal epinephrine doses have the same number of milliliters; only the concentration of the drug changes. These doses may be administered every 3 to 5 minutes during arrest. There is no evidence-based literature to support the use of high-dose epinephrine. High-dose epinephrine may increase the chances of return of spontaneous circulation (ROSC); however, it does not improve survival to hospital discharge. Therefore, PALS guidelines no longer recommend high-dose epinephrine, except for special circumstances such as beta-blocker overdose.[7] For bradycardia, epinephrine may be given intravenously or intraosseously at 0.01 mg/kg (0.1 mL/kg) of the 1:10,000 solution, or 0.1 mg/kg (0.1 mL/kg) of the 1:1000 solution per endotracheal tube.

Atropine

Atropine increases heart rate and may help improve cardiac output. Atropine is indicated for symptomatic bradycardia that is associated with increased vagal tone or primary atrioventricular block, after oxygenation-ventilation and epinephrine have been given. It is also helpful in decreasing the vagolytic effects of airway manipulation on infants and children during intubation.

The recommended dose of atropine is 0.02 mg/kg, with a minimum dose of 0.1 mg and a maximum single dose of 0.5 mg children and 1.0 mg for adolescents. The initial dose may be repeated once. The total of the two doses should not exceed 1.0 mg for children or 2.0 mg for adolescents. Use of less than 0.1 mg may result in paradoxical bradycardia. The most efficacious dose of endotracheal atropine is unknown, but the current recommended dose is 0.03 mg/kg.

Electrolytes

In infants and small children, the small reserve of endogenous glucose in the form of hepatic glycogen is readily exhausted during stress. Rapid bedside glucose testing, with easily usable equipment that provides accurate results, is mandatory in any location in which resuscitation of a child may occur. Levels of serum glucose and its anaerobic end product, lactate, can be monitored during the resuscitation process. If needed, glucose can be given intravenously or intraosseously in a dose of 2 to 4 mL/kg of 25% dextrose in water ($D_{25}W$). Peripheral vein sclerosis can occur in neonates if high glucose concentrations are used; therefore, the 10% dextrose solution ($D_{10}W$) should be used in neonates. (Range in 2-10 mL.)

Recommended indications for calcium are calcium channel blocker toxicity, hypocalcemia, hyperkalemia, and hypermagnesemia. Calcium chloride in a dose of 20 mg/kg (0.2 mL/kg) is the calcium solution of choice. Magnesium in a dose of 25 to 50 mg/kg (maximum 2 g) may be used for hypomagnesemia or torsades de pointes.

Sodium bicarbonate may be indicated for acidemia after a prolonged arrest when adequate ventilation-oxygen and cardiac compressions are being performed. During CPR, sodium bicarbonate should be given intravenously or intraosseously. The dose of sodium bicarbonate is 1 mEq/kg.

Lidocaine

Lidocaine may be used in ventricular tachycardia (VT) and ventricular fibrillation (VF) or symptomatic ventricular arrhythmias. The initial dosage is a 1-mg/kg bolus (maximum dose 100 mg), followed by a drip at 20 to 50 μg/kg/min. Endotracheal tube dosage is 2 to 3 mg/kg.

Amiodarone

Amiodarone is now recommended for VT without a pulse and for VF. It should be administered as a 5-mg/kg bolus. The dose may be repeated up to a maximum of 15 mg/kg. This agent can also be used for VT with a pulse and for supraventricular tachycardia (SVT), in which case it is administered as 5 mg/kg over 20 to 60 minutes.

Procainamide

Procainamide may also be used for VT with a pulse and for SVT. The dose is 15 mg/kg given over 30 to 60 minutes. Amiodarone and procainamide should not be routinely administered together because hypotension and prolongation of the QT interval may occur.

INTERVENTIONS

Defibrillation is the immediate treatment for witnessed pulseless VT or VF. However, if the time of the arrest in unknown, CPR should be initiated for 2 minutes (5 cycles) prior to defibrillation attempts. "Stacked shocks" are no longer recommended. Instead, each shock should be followed by 2 minutes of CPR.

Synchronized cardioversion energy levels for SVT and unstable tachyarrhythmias are 0.25 to 1.0 J/kg, whereas the unsynchronized cardioversion (defibrillation) for VF or pulseless VT starts at 2 J/kg. Figure 15-1 illustrates an algorithm for potentially lethal arrhythmias.

The management of pulseless electrical activity in children is similar to that in adults. The airway should be controlled, IV access obtained, and CPR initiated. Specific, treatable causes of pulseless electrical activity should be sought; they include hypovolemia, hypoxemia, acidosis, hypothermia, hyperkalemia, tension pneumothorax, cardiac tamponade, toxic ingestions, pulmonary embolus, and myocardial infarction.

Bradycardia in children should initially focus on airway management, because bradycardia is often caused by respiratory disease. Epinephrine is the initial drug of choice. Unlike in adults, atropine is not typically the first-line agent for bradycardia in children. It may be used in bradycardia due to increased vagal tone, cholinergic drug toxicity, or atrioventricular block; in these situations, atropine may be used before epinephrine. However, if there is no response, epinephrine should be given. Pacer placement may be warranted if pharmacologic agents are not successful.

The Broselow-Luten resuscitation tape relates the patient's length to his or her weight and, therefore, to the appropriate drug dosages and equipment sizes. Only a single measurement with the tape offers immediate access to this information.

When cardioversion is being used to convert an unstable rhythm, appropriately sized paddles must be placed in the correct position. The recommended paddle diameter for small children (less than 10 kg) is 4.5 cm; paddles up to 8 cm in diameter are used in larger children and adolescents. If only large paddles are available, they should be placed in the anteroposterior position. Regardless of position, a proper conducting medium must be used, with full paddle contact on the chest wall.

Automatic external defibrillators are being used more commonly and may be effective in children as young as 1 year. Their use is not recommended in infants, however, because of the potential for myocardial damage.

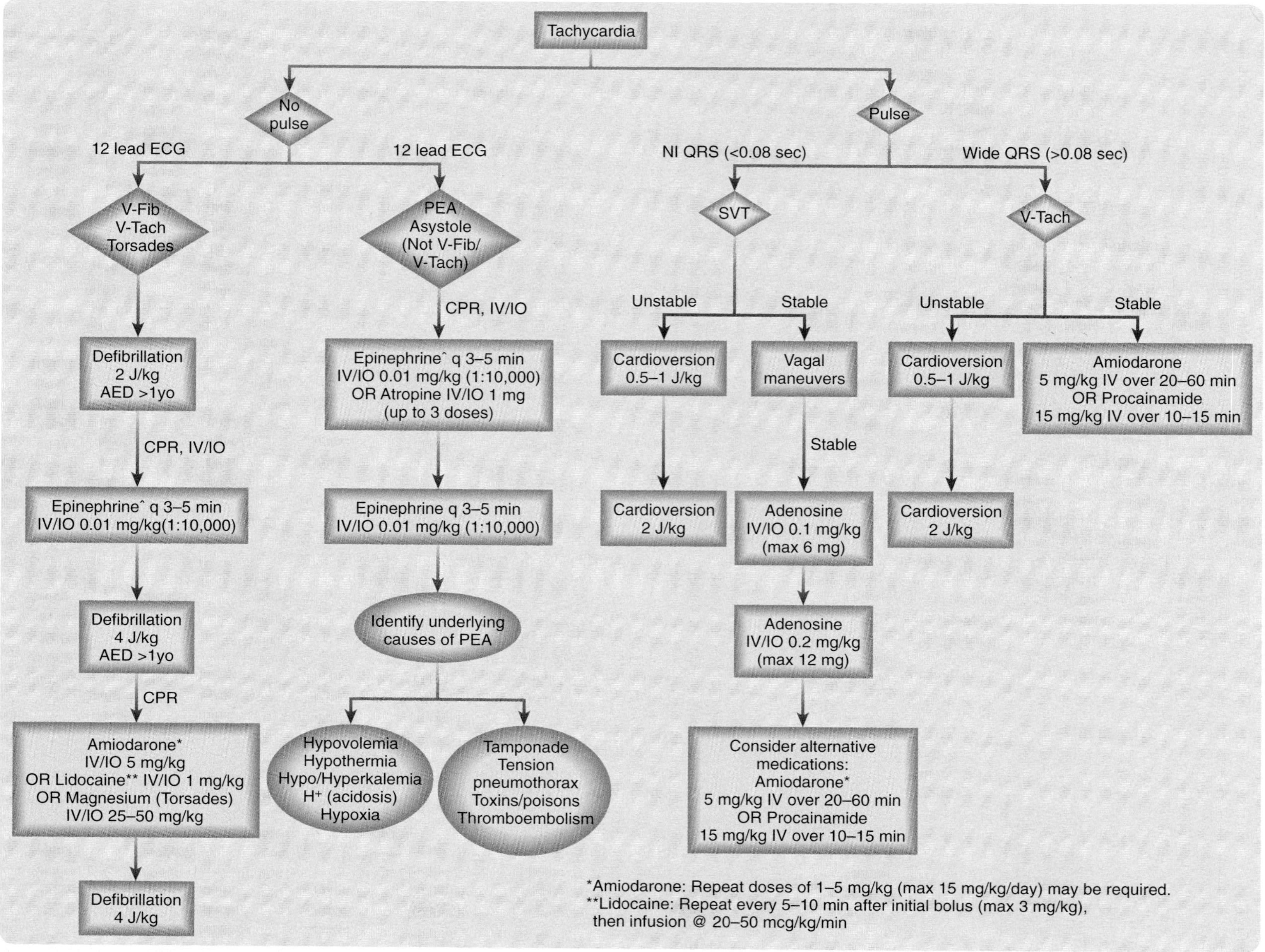
Tachycardia
No pulse
Pulse
12 lead ECG
12 lead ECG
NI QRS (<0.08 sec)
Wide QRS (>0.08 sec)
V-Fib V-Tach Torsades
PEA Asystole (Not V-Fib/ V-Tach)
SVT
V-Tach
CPR, IV/IO
Unstable
Stable
Unstable
Stable
Defibrillation 2 J/kg AED >1yo
Epinephrine^ q 3–5 min IV/IO 0.01 mg/kg (1:10,000) OR Atropine IV/IO 1 mg (up to 3 doses)
Cardioversion 0.5–1 J/kg
Vagal maneuvers
Cardioversion 0.5–1 J/kg
Amiodarone 5 mg/kg IV over 20–60 min OR Procainamide 15 mg/kg IV over 10–15 min
CPR, IV/IO
Stable
Epinephrine^ q 3–5 min IV/IO 0.01 mg/kg(1:10,000)
Epinephrine q 3–5 min IV/IO 0.01 mg/kg (1:10,000)
Cardioversion 2 J/kg
Adenosine IV/IO 0.1 mg/kg (max 6 mg)
Cardioversion 2 J/kg
Defibrillation 4 J/kg AED >1yo
Identify underlying causes of PEA
Adenosine IV/IO 0.2 mg/kg (max 12 mg)
CPR
Amiodarone* IV/IO 5 mg/kg OR Lidocaine** IV/IO 1 mg/kg OR Magnesium (Torsades) IV/IO 25–50 mg/kg
Hypovolemia Hypothermia Hypo/Hyperkalemia H+ (acidosis) Hypoxia
Tamponade Tension pneumothorax Toxins/poisons Thromboembolism
Consider alternative medications: Amiodarone* 5 mg/kg IV over 20–60 min OR Procainamide 15 mg/kg IV over 10–15 min
Defibrillation 4 J/kg
*Amiodarone: Repeat doses of 1–5 mg/kg (max 15 mg/kg/day) may be required.
**Lidocaine: Repeat every 5–10 min after initial bolus (max 3 mg/kg), then infusion @ 20–50 mcg/kg/min

FIGURE 15-1 Tachycardia algorithm. AED, automatic external defibrillator; CPR, cardiopulmonary resuscitation; ECG, electrocardiogram; IO, intraosseously; IV, intravenously; PEA, pulseless electrical activity; SVT, supraventricular tachycardia; V-Fib, ventricular fibrillation; V-Tach, ventricular tachycardia. (Adapted from American Heart Association: PALS Provider Manual. Dallas, American Heart Association, 2005. Courtesy of Stephanie Doniger, MD, Children's Hospital and Health Center/University of California, San Diego.)

REFERENCES

1. Luten R: The pediatric patient. In Walls R, Luten R, Murphy M, et al (eds): Manual of Airway Management. Philadelphia, Lippincott Williams & Wilkins, 2000, pp 143-152.
2. Luten R: The difficult airway in pediatrics. In Walls R, Luten R, Murphy M, et al (eds): Manual of Airway Management. Philadelphia, Lippincott Williams & Wilkins, 2000, pp 112-118.
3. Sharieff GQ, Rodarte A, Wilton N, et al: The self-inflating bulb as an esophageal detector device in children weighing more than twenty kilograms: A comparison of two techniques. Ann Emerg Med 2003;41:623-629.
4. Sharieff GQ, Rodarte A, Wilton N, et al: The self-inflating bulb as an airway adjunct: Is it reliable in children weighing less than 20 kilograms? Acad Emerg Med 2003;10:303-308.
5. Newth CJ, Rachman B, Patel N, Hammer J: The use of cuffed versus uncuffed endotracheal tubes in pediatric intensive care. J Pediatr 2004;144:333-337.
6. Ralston M, Hazinski M, Zaritsky A, et al: Pediatric assessment. In Pediatric Advanced Life Support, Provider Manual. Dallas, American Heart Association, 2006, pp 1-32.
7. American Heart Association: Currents in Emergency Cardiovascular Care 2005-2006;16:1-27.

Chapter 16

Pediatric Trauma

Kurt Whitaker and Katherine Bakes

KEY POINTS

Trauma is the leading cause of death in children.
Pediatric trauma victims have worse outcomes than adult victims.
Head trauma is the leading cause of death and disability, followed by thoracic and abdominal trauma.
Children with life-threatening injuries may have little or no external evidence of trauma.
Pediatric resuscitation equipment should be stored in an easily accessed, clearly labeled area in the ED.
Pediatric medication dosing and treatment algorithms should be posted in the ED, and Broselow-Luten resuscitation tapes should be available.

Scope and Outline

The report of the Institute of Medicine's Committee on Future of Emergency Care, released in June 2006, identified a lack of pediatric emergency services as a significant problem facing the health care system in the United States.[1] Trauma is the leading cause of death and disability in children and young adults.[2]

Pathophysiology

Anatomic characteristics of children predispose them to more significant injuries than adults would experience from similar trauma. The severity of pediatric head injury is at least partially related both to the thin skull and to the larger head-to-body ratio in children. The bones and connective tissues of children are more pliable than those of adults, possibly leading to severe internal injuries with minimal external evidence of significant chest and abdominal trauma. Children have a greater ratio of surface area to volume, resulting in an easier transfer of forces to internal organs. Multiple trauma is common in children because of the smaller distances between vital structures. The sympathetic tone of a child is better than that of an adult, so a child's blood pressure may be maintained despite large volume loss.

Approach and Management

The ABCs of resuscitation (airway, breathing, circulation) should be used to identify the loss of an airway and/or respiratory failure first. Injuries to the airway itself—the oropharynx, trachea, or bronchi—are not the only cause of airway failure. An expanding neck hematoma or aspirated foreign body can have similar effects.

Breathing difficulties in children may be the sequelae of insults to the chest wall, lungs, heart, great vessels, or abdomen as well as neurologic or muscular injuries. They may also result from the loss of ventilatory musculature, as in a cervical spine

Table 16-1 THE AVPU SCALE

Category	Appropriate Response	Inappropriate
Alert	Normal interaction for age	Lethargic, irritable
Verbal	Responds to name	Confused, unresponsive
Painful	Withdraws from pain	Nonpurposeful movement or sound without localization of pain
Unresponsive	No response to verbal or painful stimuli	

injury or respiratory muscle fatigue. Young children may have disordered ventilation secondary to gastric distention because considerable air is gulped into the stomach during crying.

Circulation can be assessed in children through an evaluation of mental status, skin color and temperature, heart sounds, pulses, and capillary refill. Shock should be identified and treated immediately. Children differ from adults in several critical ways. The leading cause of cardiac arrest in children is hypoxemia. Also, normal blood pressure may be maintained in trauma despite severe injury and massive blood loss. Traumatic shock should be presumed to be secondary to blood loss and should be treated with volume restoration. Two intravenous (or intraosseous) lines of the largest bore possible should be established immediately. Two boluses of crystalloid solution, 20 mL/kg each, should be administered. If shock persists, packed red blood cell transfusion should be administered, starting with 10 mL/kg and proceeding as necessary. Other causes of shock—such as tension pneumothorax, pericardial tamponade, neurogenic shock, hypoxemia, metabolic derangements, and toxidromes—should be sought and treated concomitantly with the administration of fluids to restore volume.

Disability must be assessed thoroughly. Mental status is evaluated with the Glasgow Coma Scale (GCS) or an AVPU scale (Table 16-1). Use an age-appropriate examination to evaluate for neurologic deficits.

Exposure of the body immediately after the ABCs have been dealt with is imperative in all pediatric trauma patients. Emergency personnel should briefly expose and roll (with precautions) the patient to assess for initially unapparent injuries, such as the puncture wound to the posterior chest in a victim of assault. Because of the increased ratio of surface area to volume in children, it is important to use blankets and warmed intravenous fluids to maintain normothermia. The family should be present in the room to comfort the child. The EP should communicate with the child while examining him or her.

After exposure, the secondary survey should be performed. An AMPLE (allergies, medications, past medical history, last meal, and events leading up to the patient's arrival in the ED) history should be obtained, and a complete head-to-toe examination performed. Particular attention should be paid to the eyes, ears, mouth, axillae, hands, and genitalia, and a rectal examination should be done. A nasogastric tube and Foley catheter should be placed. As part of the secondary survey, initial radiographs and laboratory studies should be ordered to further investigate any history and physical findings.

PRIORITY ACTIONS

- A=Airway control: bag-valve-mask, endotracheal intubation
- B=Breathing: maximize ventilation
- C=Circulation: stabilize hemodynamic status
- D=Disability: evaluate mental status and perform neurologic examination
- E=Exposure: completely undress and examine patient
- F="Fingers and Foleys": orogastric tube, bladder catheter, vaginal and rectal examinations
- Secondary survey: head-to-toe physical examination and AMPLE (allergies, medications, past medical history, last meal, and events leading up to the patient's arrival in the ED) history
- Laboratory studies and radiographs

Younger children, particularly infants, have little reserve. Time is of the essence in restoring oxygenation, ventilation, and circulation. The ABCs of resuscitation should be repeated if there is any change in the patient's status.

The most common life- and limb-threatening injuries in children, as in adults, are those to the head, chest, and abdomen. In each of these areas, there are subtle but important clues to such injures (Box 16-1).

Diagnostic Testing

■ PRIMARY AND SECONDARY SURVEYS

Primary and secondary surveys should be performed in children as in adults. Particular modalities of testing are discussed in depth in later sections on specific systems and injuries. In the child with multiple trauma or severe injury, basic tests must be ordered as part of the primary and secondary surveys. Cardiac and oxygen saturation monitoring should be instituted. Plain radiographs of the cervical spine, chest, and pelvis should be performed and reviewed immediately at the bedside. A bedside focused abdominal sonography in trauma (FAST) examina-

BOX 16-1

Overview of Pediatric Trauma Management

1. Attend to the ABCs of resuscitation (airway, breathing, circulation) first.
2. Obtain intravenous access, administer oxygen or secure the airway, and connect the patient to a cardiac and oxygen saturation monitor.
3. If the patient is hypotensive or tachycardic, administer normal saline in a 20-mL/kg bolus.
4. Roll the patient, perform a secondary survey, and recheck vital signs.
5. If shock persists, additional intravenous access should be obtained, and a second 20-mL/kg bolus of normal saline should be administered.
6. Abdominal ultrasonography, radiography, and laboratory studies should be performed as indicated.
7. If shock persists, transfuse packed red blood cells at 10 mL/kg, and continue evaluation for and treatment of life-threatening injuries.

Documentation

The following information should be documented:

History

- Prehospital history
- Detailed mechanism of injury (speed of vehicle, height of fall, etc.)
- Circumstances of injury (damage to vehicle, type of weapon, etc.)
- Timing of event
- Time to ED
- Concurrent medications
- Patient's access to medications or exposures to drugs or toxins
- Past medical history
- Last meal
- Immunizations
- Prior surgeries
- Inconsistencies in history between witnesses, particularly when child abuse is suspected

Physical Examination

- Primary survey and interventions
- Head-to-toe physical examination

Laboratory Studies

- ED interpretation of radiographs
- Laboratory studies ordered and their results
- Results of focused abdominal sonography in trauma (FAST) examination or diagnostic peritoneal lavage

Medical Decision-Making

- Reasons to pursue or not pursue work-up of each injury
- Timing of consultation of surgical or other subspecialists

Procedures

Each procedure in full

Patient Instructions

Discussion of injuries and potential outcomes with patient and/or patient's family

tion should be performed to evaluate for free fluid in the abdomen or pericardium. A finger-stick glucose measurement should be performed. Laboratory studies should include a complete blood count (CBC), serum chemistry analysis, coagulation studies, urinalysis, blood type and crossmatch, blood gas measurements, and pregnancy test. Further radiologic testing (e.g., computed tomography [CT], angiography, and magnetic resonance imaging [MRI]) as well as more in-depth laboratory testing (e.g., panel of hepatic function tests, screening for toxins or drugs, pancreatic enzyme measurements) may be ordered as indicated.

There are some pediatric-specific issues in the management of trauma. With younger patients, small tubes should be used for laboratory testing. The clinician should be aware that the hematocrit does not drop immediately in a child, even in the setting of large volume loss. For minimally injured patients, such as those with isolated extremity fractures or low-risk head or abdominal trauma, no laboratory studies are needed, although a hematocrit and urinalysis can be ordered. Toxidromes must be considered, especially in a patient with altered mental status, when the circumstances of the event are suspicious, or when the patient is a teenager.

The ALARA (as low as reasonably achievable) principle should be applied to minimize radiation; for example, the clinician should limit the number of CT scans performed and should make size-based adjustments to the radiation exposure scanning parameters.[3] Some investigators have questioned the need for portable radiographs of the cervical spine, chest, and pelvis to screen for injury in all trauma patients. As with trauma triage, it is advisable to err on the side of caution: These studies should be performed in all seriously injured patients or if there is any uncertainty about the status of the spine, chest, or pelvis. A more focal radiologic screening examination, as indicated by history and physical findings, may be considered in stable patients with normal mental status. The clinician should have a low threshold for performing abdominal CT. Children younger than 2 years old in whom there is suspicion of child abuse must undergo a skeletal radiographic survey.

PEDIATRIC HEAD TRAUMA

KEY POINTS

Head trauma is responsible for 80% of pediatric trauma deaths.

Cervical immobilization is required if head injury is suspected.

The AVPU scale can be used in children as an alternative to the Glasgow Coma Scale score.

Significant alterations in a child's mental status should prompt early airway management and immediate CT of the brain.

Declining mental status with suspected intracranial injury requires immediate neurosurgical evaluation or transfer of the patient to a facility with neurosurgical capabilities.

Scope and Outline

Head injury is the leading cause of death, responsible for 80% of pediatric trauma deaths. Annually in the United States, there are 500,000 ED visits and almost 100,000 hospital admissions due to pediatric head trauma.[4-6] Rates of death from traumatic brain injury are equal in boys and girls until the age 5 years, after which the incidence is higher in males.[6] For the survivors of head trauma, there is high morbidity. Costs of caring for children who are victims of head trauma exceed $1 billion per year. The leading causes of head trauma are falls, motor vehicle collisions, bicycle accidents, auto-pedestrian accidents, diving injuries, sporting accidents, and child abuse.

Pathophysiology

Children have relatively larger heads than adults. The intracranial volume of a 2-year old is approximately 75% that of an adult. The child's skull is thinner and less rigid than the adult's skull, and infants and younger children have open or soft sutures that act as joints. As a result, parenchymal injury may occur in the absence of skull fracture. The supporting musculature of the neck is not well developed in children, resulting in higher-impact speeds from deceleration mechanisms.

Clinical Presentation

Major intracranial injuries may be immediately apparent from the patient's depressed level of consciousness or confusion, or from abnormal neurologic findings. Significant injuries may be present, however, in the patient with completely normal neurologic findings. Loss of consciousness is a poor predictor of intracranial injury.

Early recognition and treatment of mild or moderate severity head injury in a child is as important as, or even more important than, recognition and treatment of serious injuries (see Red Flags: Warning Signs box). Sadly, the EP has little ability to affect the outcome of a child who suffers a gunshot wound to the head and arrives at the ED with bradycardia and a GCS score of 3. However, an epidural hematoma in a mildly confused victim of a car accident will certainly have dire consequences. It is important to screen for other system injuries and to aggressively resuscitate a child with a head injury. Concomitant tracheal injury in a child who fell from a tree and now has a GCS of 6 will lead to hypoxemia and hemodynamic compromise. Such a development will certainly worsen the patient's chances for neurologically intact survival. Strict attention should be paid

RED FLAGS

Warning Signs of Intracranial Injury in Children with Head Trauma

- Prolonged loss of consciousness
- Multiple seizures
- Persistent vomiting
- Amnesia
- Lethargy
- Irritability
- Large cephalohematoma or clinical skull fracture
- Abnormal neurologic findings

to maintaining oxygenation and cerebral perfusion in the head-injured child to avoid secondary injury.

Approach and Management

Physical examination should be performed with attention to neurologic findings. Obvious external head and neck trauma may be an indicator of serious injury, although severe internal injury often exists with minimal—such as a small cephalohematoma—or no external signs. The GCS or AVPU Scale may be used to assess mental status. An age-appropriate neurologic examination may reveal deficits requiring further testing and treatment. The clinician should have a low threshold for managing the airway of a pediatric trauma patient who has altered mentation.

Diagnostic Testing

The goal of diagnostic testing in children in whom intracranial injury is suspected is to identify the patients with injuries that will require intervention before his or her condition worsens. A secondary goal is to avoid unnecessary testing and admission, both to prevent overutilization of resources and avoid unnecessary exposure to radiation. The most commonly used and most widely available options for the evaluation of children with head injuries are plain radiography of the skull, computed tomography of the head, and observation with serial examinations.

■ SKULL RADIOGRAPHS

Historically, plain radiography of the skull was the test of choice. With the wider availability of CT, plain film radiography has a more limited role. Skull films are indicated for suspected child abuse, for suspicion of a foreign body in a scalp wound, and to image a ventriculoperitoneal shunt. Screening skull films may be appropriate in asymptomatic, low-risk infants who would otherwise need sedation for a CT scan.

■ COMPUTED TOMOGRAPHY

Noncontrast CT of the head is the best initial means of screening for intracranial injury in the majority of patients (Boxes 16-2 and 16-3). The clinician should perform emergency CT of the head in all children whose mental status altered from baseline or who have neurologic deficits, after the cervical spine has been immobilized and immediate threats to life have been managed. CT of the head is also required in patients with obvious skull fracture, whether open or closed, or multisystem trauma.

A great deal of controversy exists regarding which patients not fitting into any of these categories should undergo CT of the head. Studies have shown varying results for the predictive value of positive findings of head CT in a child with a history of loss of consciousness, seizures, vomiting, and headache. For simplicity, such well-appearing children should be divided into two categories. Children younger than 2 years are at increased risk of intracranial injury, and the clinician should have a low threshold for ordering CT scans. Children older than 2 years are at somewhat lower risk. However, CT scanning does have its drawbacks: It is expensive and time-consuming, requires transport out of the patient of the direct care area, and may require sedation. Therefore a selective approach to ordering CT is recommended. Although there is a small risk of delayed bleeding after head CT with normal findings in the acute setting, convincing data also indicate that that normal CT findings in the patient being treated in the ED effectively rule out intracranial injury requiring intervention.[7]

BOX 16-2

Indications for Computed Tomography of the Head in Children Older than 2 Years

- Glasgow Coma Scale score less than 15
- Focal neurologic deficits in the setting of trauma
- Clinical signs of skull fracture
- Seizures
- Headache
- History of vomiting

BOX 16-3

Indications for Computed Tomography of the Head in Children Younger than 2 Years

- All of the indications from Box 16-2
- Any loss of consciousness
- Protracted vomiting
- Bulging fontanelle
- Seizure
- Irritability
- Poor feeding
- Suspected abuse
- Scalp hematoma

Specific Injuries

■ INTRACRANIAL INJURIES

All of the intracranial injuries discussed in this section require emergency neurosurgical consultation.

Epidural Hematoma

In children, arterial or venous bleeding can cause epidural hematoma, but the primary source is the middle meningeal artery. There are overlying skull fractures in most patients. The clinician should suspect epidural hematoma in the classic presentation consisting of loss of consciousness, confusion directly after impact followed by a period of lucidity, and then rapid deterioration. Unfortunately, many patients with epidural hematoma have a much more subtle presentation and may have a more slowly developing hematoma.

Subdural Hematoma

The clinician should suspect subdural hematoma in infants and toddlers particularly. Skull fractures are less common in this entity than in epidural hematoma. Bleeding arises from bridging veins. Subdural hematoma may manifest acutely after head trauma or may be found in children presenting with vomiting, poor feeding, seizures, lethargy, and other injuries. Child abuse should be suspected if there is no history of trauma or if the history of trauma is not consistent with the injury. The physician should perform a funduscopic examination to search for retinal hemorrhages in any child younger than 2 years with subdural hematoma.

Subarachnoid Hemorrhage

Subarachnoid hemorrhage may occur in isolation or with other intracranial injuries. Large subarachnoid hemorrhage often results in significant morbidity and mortality. If the hemorrhage is small and isolated, it is usually self-limited and associated with a good outcome.

Parenchymal Contusion, Hemorrhage, or Edema

The child with contusion, hemorrhage, or edema with the parenchyma may have symptoms such as confusion, vomiting, headache, seizures, and focal neurologic deficits. The typical mechanism is a coup/contrecoup.

Diffuse Axonal Injury

Diffuse axonal injury results from major mechanisms of injury. The clinician should suspect this entity in children with profound alterations in mental status or neurologic function in whom CT of the brain does not yield significant findings.

SKULL FRACTURES

The incidence of skull fracture is inversely proportional to age, with the majority occurring in children 2 years and younger.[8] The parietal bone is the most commonly fractured bone in the skull. Skull fracture is a significant risk factor for intracranial injury. Any fracture should be consistent with the story given by the parents, and any suspicious skull fractures, such as those that are bilateral or multiple or that pass through sutures, should prompt a thorough evaluation for child abuse.

Linear fractures occur most commonly. Such fractures are usually associated with hematoma. Neurosurgery consultation should be obtained for linear skull fractures if they are widely diastatic or if concomitant intracranial injury exists.

The patient with a *basilar skull fracture* may (but may not) have Battle's sign, raccoon eyes, hemotympanum, blood in external auditory canal, cerebrospinal fluid rhinorrhea, or abnormal cranial nerve findings. Neurosurgery consultation is required.

Depressed skull fractures may be associated with crepitus or deformity. They can be associated with hematomas as well. The likelihood of intracranial injury rises with the depth of intrusion of the fracture. Neurosurgery consultation is required for a depressed skull fracture.

CONCUSSION

Concussion exists when there is brain insult with transient alteration in mental status. Head CT findings are negative for intracranial injury, although microscopic injury may be present, leaving the brain at risk for second impact syndromes. Concussion may be associated with subtle neuropsychiatric sequelae that can last for extended periods. Table 16-2 summarizes the recommendations for a child's or adolescent's return to sports activity after a concussion.

Disposition

Children with even minor intracranial injury, such as parenchymal contusion, require neurosurgical consultation and admission to the hospital or ED observation unit. Significant intracranial injury, such as major subdural or epidural hemorrhage, must be transferred to a pediatric level I trauma center. Suspected child abuse requires admission of the child to the hospital, notification of the appropriate authorities, and a skeletal survey and formal funduscopic examination. Children with nondisplaced, simple linear skull fractures without intracranial injury may be managed with close monitoring at home and arrangements for 24-hour follow-up with either the primary care provider or in the ED. Those with depressed or basilar skull fractures require neurosurgical consultation and admission. Children with minor head trauma and/or their dependable care-

Table 16-2 RECOMMENDATIONS FOR RETURN TO SPORTS ACTIVITY AFTER CONCUSSION

Grade of Concussion	Definition	Management
1	Transient confusion, no loss of consciousness (LOC), and duration of mental status abnormalities <15 minutes	Return to sports activity same day only if all symptoms resolve within 15 minutes If a second grade 1 concussion occurs, no sports activity until asymptomatic for 1 week
2	Transient confusion, no LOC, and duration of mental status abnormalities ≥15 minutes	No sports activity until asymptomatic for 1 full week If a grade 2 concussion occurs on the same day as a grade 1 concussion, no sports activity until asymptomatic for 2 weeks
3	Concussion involving LOC	
First concussion		No sports activity until asymptomatic for 1 week if LOC is brief (seconds) No sports activity until asymptomatic for 2 weeks if LOC is prolonged (minutes or longer).
Second concussion		No sports activity until asymptomatic for 1 month If an intracranial problem is detected by computed tomography or magnetic resonance imaging, no sports activity for remainder of season, and the athlete should be discouraged from future return to contact sports

Modified from Centers for Disease Control and Prevention: Sports-related recurrent brain injuries—United States. MMWR Morb Mortal Wkly Rep 1997;46:224-227.

RED FLAGS

Pitfalls and Pearls in the Work-up of Head Trauma in Children

- Forces involved in the traumatic event may not be accurately reported.
- Many patients with significant intracranial injury are awake and alert on arrival at the ED.
- History and physical findings are often unreliable in infants and small children.
- Behavior should be recorded as consistent or not with age and with baseline according to parents.
- Loss of consciousness is a poor predictor of intracranial injury in neurologically intact patients.
- Vomiting is an unclear prognosticator of intracranial injury.
- Seizures:
  - Impact seizure is not necessarily associated with intracranial injury.
  - Seizures occurring more than 20 minutes after insult are more worrisome.
- Any neurologic deficit or persistent alteration in appropriate mental status for age mandates immediate computed tomography of the head and a neurosurgical consultation.

givers should receive detailed aftercare precautions and instructions. They should follow up with their primary care provider in 1 to 2 weeks and should be referred at that time for neuropsychiatric testing for any persistent symptoms.

CERVICAL SPINE INJURY

Scope and Outline

Spinal cord injuries are uncommon in children, accounting for less than 2% of injuries found in pediatric trauma patients. Motor vehicle collisions represent the most common mechanism for this injury, and death is usually secondary to brain injury.

Pathophysiology and Anatomy

Mechanisms of fractures of the cervical spine in children are similar to those in adults, although there is a higher risk of ligamentous injuries in children (Box 16-14; Fig. 16-1). Because the pediatric cervical spine is hypermobile, a traumatic injury can cause transient severe ligamentous disruption, leading to brief sensory or motor deficits or electric shocks with rapidly clearing weakness. The initial rapid clearance of symptoms represents the realignment of structures with the counterforce of the injury, drawing the cord back into anatomical position. Unfortunately, this phase can be followed by delayed neurologic deficits precipitated by cord edema after this stretch injury. The delay can be quite significant, with deficits appearing up to 4 days after the inciting event.

Fortunately, documented cases of this type of injury, known as spinal cord injury without radiographic abnormality (SCIWORA), tend not to be subtle in the pre-verbal child, resulting from impressive multiple-trauma mechanisms such as falls from

BOX 16-4

Unique Characteristics of the Pediatric Cervical Spine

- Incomplete ossification of posterior elements
- Physiologic C1-C2 widening
- Absence of lordosis
- Pseudosubluxation at C2-C3 and C3-C4 (see Figure 16-1)
- Hypermobility or ligamentous laxity of the intervertebral ligaments
- Horizontal orientation of the facet joints, allowing increased mobility, which leads to:
  - Loss of normal lordosis
  - Pseudosubluxation of C2 on C3
  - Spinal cord injury without radiographic abnormalities (SCIWORA)
- Accentuated prevertebral soft tissue spaces, which should not exceed two thirds of the C2 body
- Portions of the vertebra are radiolucent or wedge-shaped up to 8 years, leading to widened disk spaces and anterior wedging
- Anatomic fulcrum in children younger than 8 years is between C1 and C3:
  - Most injuries occur in the upper cervical spine
  - After age 8, anatomic fulcrum is between C5 and C6
  - Makes SCIWORA possible

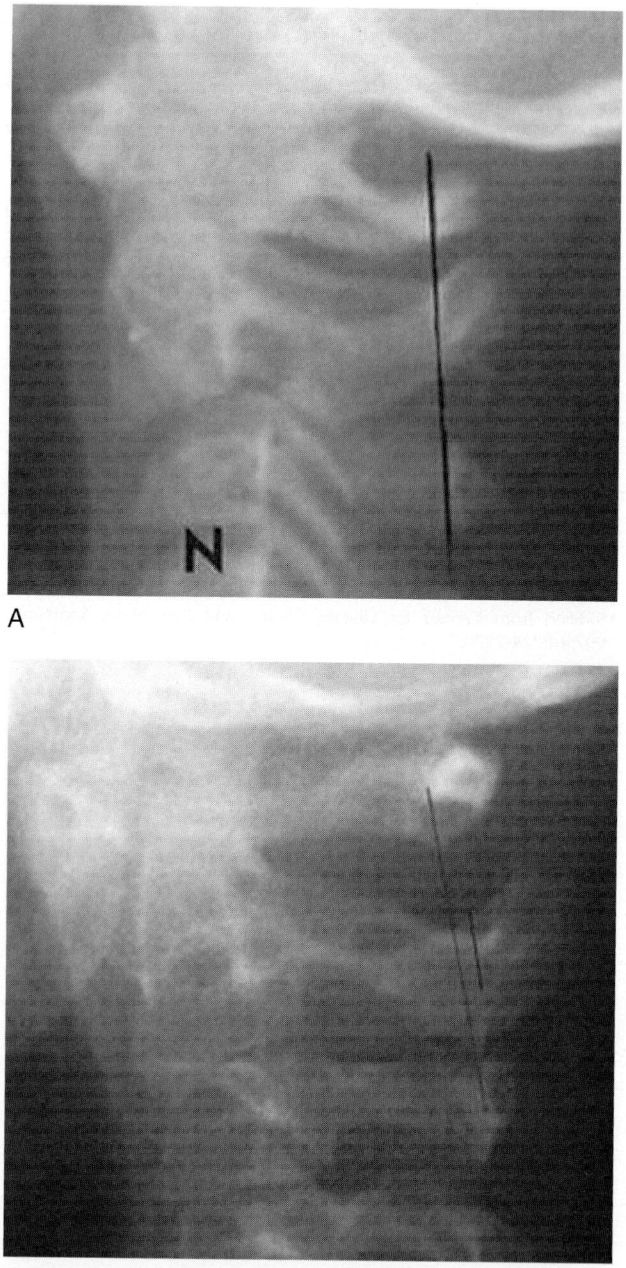
N

A

B

FIGURE 16-1 Radiographs showing psuedosubluxation of the cervical spine. The clinician should draw a line through the corticies of the spinous processes of C1 and C3. If the cortex of the spinous process of C2 is more than 1.5 mm off of this line (called the line of Swischuk), suspect a fracture or ligamentous injury. A, A normal cervical spine with psuedosubluxation. Note that the line of Swischuk is straight, but the anterior and posterior spinal lines have step-offs. B, The cortex of the spinal process of C2 is less than 1.5 mm off of the line of Swischuk.

extreme heights and high-risk mechanism motor vehicle accidents. In the verbal older child, SCIWORA can initially manifest as mild transient neurologic complaints; thus, a heightened awareness of this phenomenon is needed, so that the treating physician takes the necessary steps for diagnosis and treatment.

Diagnostic Testing

■ PLAIN RADIOGRAPHS

More than 3000 children were studied as part of the National Emergency X-Radiography Utilization Study group (NEXUS) multicenter effort.[9] On the basis of these data, the same criteria used to identify spine injuries in the adult have been recommended for the verbal child. Thus, the patient can undergo clinical "clearance" of the cervical spine without radiographs if he or she is awake and has no midline tenderness, focal neurologic deficit, intoxication, or painful/distracting injuries such as fractures, burns, or crush injuries (Boxes 16-5 and 16-6). In the nonverbal child, a more conservative approach is recommended.

Flexion and extension radiographs of the cervical spine are not used in the acute management phase of children in the ED.

BOX 16-5

Indications for Cervical Spine Radiography in Children

- High-risk mechanism: high-speed motor vehicle collision, fall greater than 8 feet, spearing or loading injuries
- History of neurologic abnormality around time of injury
- Distracting injury
- Cervical spine pain
- Cervical spine tenderness
- Abnormal neurologic findings
- Decreased level of consciousness
- Patient unable to communicate reliably (no good data on this population, so most clinicians take more conservative approach)

■ COMPUTED TOMOGRAPHY

There is mounting evidence that the patient with a high mechanism injury, such as a fall from height or a high-speed motor vehicle collision, should undergo CT evaluation of the cervical spine.

■ MAGNETIC RESONANCE IMAGING

Any history of transient neurologic dysfunction requires extended observation or MRI if plain radiographic findings are abnormal secondary to SCIWORA.

BOX 16-6

Tips for Reading Cervical Spine Radiographs in Children

- Look for compression or widening of the intervertebral spaces.
- Prevertebral soft tissue space widening should not be greater than one third to one half the width of the adjacent vertebral body.
- Radiographs may be repeated with adequate inspiratory breath and neck positioning (not in flexion).

Treatment and Disposition

Immobilization with a cervical collar is required for any child with a cervical injury. When such an injury is diagnosed, emergency consultation of a pediatric spine surgeon and admission of the patient to the hospital are mandatory. Blunt spinal cord lesions with neurologic deficits in children are currently treated as those in adults, with the high-dose methylprednisolone protocol within 8 hours after injury, although this practice is controversial.

PEDIATRIC THORACIC TRAUMA

KEY POINTS

Respiratory distress or hypoxemia should prompt a thorough radiographic evaluation.

Gastric decompression should be performed early in any child with respiratory distress or hypoxemia.

Perspective

Trauma to the chest is the second leading cause of death from trauma in children. The majority of cases are the result of blunt mechanisms. Associated injury is the most important mortality factor. The death rate from isolated chest trauma in children is 5%, whereas that from abdominal and chest trauma is 20%, and that from trauma to the head, chest, and abdomen is 39%.[10,11]

Anatomy and Pathophysiology

The thorax of the child is smaller and more compliant than that of an adult. Bones are less dense and less rigid, so that less force is required for intrathoracic injury. Associated abdominal, pelvic, and head injuries are relatively common, and the clinician should suspect concomitant abdominal injuries in victims of chest trauma until proven otherwise. Infants and toddlers depend on diaphragmatic breathing, leading to respiratory depression if mobility of the diaphragm is impaired. In children, the ratio of oxygen consumption to mass is high and functional residual capacity is lower, putting them at risk for sudden respiratory failure with little to no warning.

Clinical Presentation

Patients with major thoracic injuries frequently have significant chest pain, respiratory distress, disordered chest and abdominal movement, hypoxemia, or hemodynamic compromise. They may also have chest deformity, flail chest, crepitus, decreased breath sounds, or sucking chest wounds.

Thoracic injuries account for 5% to 12% of admissions to pediatric trauma centers,[12] but many children evaluated for chest trauma in the ED have much more subtle findings (Box 16-7). Children presenting with chest pain, dyspnea, altered mental status, tachypnea, retractions, hypoxemia, shock, multiple-system trauma, or concern because of a high mechanism should be evaluated for thoracic trauma. Injuries may occur in isolation or in combination with other thoracic or extrathoracic problems. Significant injuries may be present with little or no external evidence.

BOX 16-7

Most Common and Most Lethal Injuries to the Chest in Children

Most Common

Pulmonary contusion
Rib fractures
Pneumothorax
Hemothorax
Cardiac injury
Great vessel injury
Diaphragmatic injury

Most Lethal

Great vessel injury
Cardiac injury
Hemothorax
Rib fracture

Data from Holmes JF, Sokolove PE, Brant WE, Kuppermann N: A clinical decision rule for identifying children with thoracic injuries after blunt torso trauma. Ann Emerg Med 2000; 39:492-499.

Diagnostic Testing

■ CHEST RADIOGRAPH

A chest radiograph is the most useful test in the evaluation of suspected chest trauma, although it is not as sensitive as CT scanning for many diagnoses, such as rib fracture, sternal fracture, pneumothorax, hemothorax, pulmonary contusion, and great vessel injury. However, many rib fractures and pneumothoraces not evident on plain films of the chest do not require any specific intervention.

■ COMPUTED TOMOGRAPHY OF THE CHEST

The best test for defining the extent of intrathoracic injuries is CT. Also, in the case of evaluation of great vessel injury, CT angiography has largely replaced angiography (Box 16-8).

Specific Injuries

■ RIB FRACTURES

Rib fractures are less common in children than in adults. The compliance of the child's rib cage allows transfer of strong forces to internal organs before fracture. Half of significant intrathoracic injuries in children occur without rib fracture. Mortality rises with the number of fractures. Flail rib segments—three or more ribs broken in a segmental fashion—can lead to serious respiratory compromise. The clinician should manage pain aggressively, and early intubation should be considered in a child with flail chest or multiple rib fractures. Otherwise, treatment is supportive. In addition to parenteral pain medication, intercostal nerve block and epidural anesthesia can be effective.

BOX 16-8

Indications for Computed Tomography of Chest in Pediatric Trauma

- Wide mediastinum on chest radiograph
- Thoracic spine fracture
- Superior rib fracture
- Abnormal lung fields
- Unexplained hypotension or hypoxemia
- New cardiac murmur or carotid bruit
- Asymmetric pulses or blood pressures

■ PULMONARY CONTUSION

Pulmonary contusion appears in up to 71% of children with thoracic injuries.[13] Owing to the increased compliance of the rib cage in children, forces are transferred directly to lung parenchyma. Parenchymal hemorrhage and edema lead to alveolar collapse and disorders of gas exchange. Contusions large enough to impair respiratory function may occur without any external signs of trauma. Contusions may be immediately visible on chest radiographs or have a delayed appearance. The radiographic appearance of a pulmonary contusion ranges from minimal hazy opacity to diffuse, dense infiltrate. The sensitivity of chest radiography for pulmonary contusion was 67% in one study, which used CT of the chest as the "gold standard"; however, contusions not visible on chest radiographs were not clinically significant and did not require a change in management.[14] Treatment of pulmonary contusion consists of pain control, pulmonary toilet, and mechanical ventilation when appropriate.

■ PNEUMOTHORAX

Pneumothorax occurs primarily as a result of trauma in children; spontaneous pneumothorax is uncommon but does occur. Signs and symptoms are pain, dyspnea, hemoptysis, tachypnea, retractions, hypoxemia, decreased breath sounds, and tympany. The clinician should also consider pneumothorax in the setting of chest wall abrasion, contusion, laceration, wound, or deformity. Auscultatory lung examination is unreliable, because the small chest cavity in children transmits breath sounds easily even in the presence of pneumothorax.

The primary screening examination is a chest radiograph, performed with the patient supine if the cervical spine has not been evaluated as uninjured. It is an insensitive test for pneumothorax, however, with some estimates of sensitivity as low as 20% to 60%.[15] An upright chest radiograph should be performed if possible. CT scan of the chest is extremely sensitive for detection of pneumothoraces, even very small ones that may need no intervention. Abdominal CT may demonstrate pneumothoraces, but patients with pneumothorax uncommonly need tube thoracostomy (Table 16-3).[13] In adults, ultrasonography at the bedside by EPs and trauma surgeons is comparable is specificity to chest radiography but is more sensitive than chest radiography for the detection of pneumothoraces after trauma.[16]

Table 16-3 TREATMENT OF PNEUMOTHORAX

Size	Treatment
More than 20% of pleural space	Tube thoracostomy
Less than 20% of pleural space	High-flow oxygen Observation Second chest radiography in 3-6 hr Tube thoracostomy if mechanical ventilation or air transport is required

Data from Weissberg D, Refaely Y: Pneumothorax: Experience with 1,199 patients. Chest 2000;117:1279-1285.

■ DIAPHRAGMATIC INJURY

Injury of the diaphragm may result from either penetrating trauma or, more commonly, a major mechanism blunt injury to the abdomen such as a fall from height, a crush injuiy, of a high-speed motor vehicle collision. It is uncommon in children, occurring in about 3% of victims of blunt abdominal trauma. Patients may be asymptomatic, may have chest or abdominal pain, or may present with respiratory failure and shock.

The diagnosis of diaphragmatic injury is difficult. If significant abdominal contents have herniated into the thorax, the diaphragmatic injury may be diagnosed on screening chest radiography. Overall, the sensitivity rates for both chest radiography and chest CT are not good. Sensitivity rates for CT of the chest detecting blunt diaphragmatic rupture have been reported at 42% to 90%.[17-19] One study found that only 50% of patients admitted to a level I trauma center with diaphragmatic injury were correctly diagnosed on admission.[20] Diagnostic peritoneal lavage (DPL) may have some utility in detecting diaphragmatic injury, although it is performed less frequently today than previously. Its sensitivity has been reported at 80% in a select population, although it is not specific.[21] Because of the pressure differential between the abdomen and thorax, any missed defect in the diaphragm will continue to enlarge until it is repaired surgically.

■ CARDIAC CONTUSION

The patient with a cardiac contusion may complain of chest pain or palpitations. External findings are sternal fracture, rib fracture, chest contusion, and, sometimes, no signs of trauma. The most common dysrhythmia is sinus tachycardia. The patient is unlikely to have complications if findings on electrocardiogram (ECG) are normal and troponin is normal over 6 to 12 hours of observation. In one study of pediatric blunt cardiac injury, no hemodynamically stable patient who presented with a normal sinus rhythm subsequently demonstrated a cardiac arrhythmia or cardiac failure.[22] Using any ECG changes, including sinus tachycardia, bradycardia, conduction delays, and atrial or ventricular dysrhythmias, can provide a sensitivity of 100%, a specificity of 47%, and a negative predictive value of 90% in the detection of complications related to blunt cardiac injury that require treatment.[23] Several prospective series have demonstrated that if the admission ECG displays normal sinus rhythm, the risk for development of cardiac complications related to blunt cardiac injury is extremely small.[24,25]

■ COMMOTIO CORDIS

Commotio cordis resulting from blunt chest trauma that caused cardiac arrest has been reported to occur in children. The clinician should apply the normal Pediatric Advanced Life Support (PALS) algorithm for treatment. Commotio cordis may or may not respond to treatment.

■ TRAUMATIC ASPHYXIA

Traumatic asphyxia is unique to children. Findings include cervical and facial petechiae or cyanosis with vascular engorgement and subconjunctival hemorrhage. The syndrome is secondary to blunt, compressing thoracic trauma with airway obstruction and retrograde high pressure in the superior vena cava. Central nervous system injuries, pulmonary contusions, and intra-abdominal injuries are commonly associated with thoracic injuries. Despite the dramatic presentation of traumatic asphyxia, overall prognosis is good for patients who arrive with vital signs.

Disposition

Children with significant thoracic trauma are admitted to the hospital after the trauma surgery team has been consulted. In centers where pediatric trauma care is unavailable, transfer to a pediatric trauma center is recommended. A child with an isolated rib fracture, with a small pneumothorax that is stable on chest radiography after 4 to 6 hours of observation, or in whom a suspected myocardial contusion has been ruled out may be discharged. Any child in whom there is suspicion for child abuse should receive thorough evaluation and should be admitted to the hospital. Police and child protective services should be contacted to investigate, and hospital social workers should be involved.

PEDIATRIC ABDOMINAL TRAUMA

KEY POINTS

- Abdominal trauma is the third leading cause of traumatic death in children.
- Most intra-abdominal injuries are the result of blunt trauma.
- Missed intra-abdominal injuries are a leading cause of preventable death.
- Children in whom intra-abdominal injury is suspected are admitted to a pediatric trauma center.
- Most solid organ injuries are managed nonoperatively.

Perspective

Motor vehicle accidents are the leading cause of abdominal trauma, although falls, sports accidents, and child abuse account for a significant number of injuries. Children struck by motor vehicles—or who as motor vehicle passengers are not properly restrained or are ejected—are at increased risk. Blunt trauma accounts for 90% of all pediatric injuries.[26] Missed intra-abdominal injury in the setting of blunt abdominal trauma is a leading cause of preventable mortality and morbidity in children.

Anatomy and Pathophysiology

The abdomen of a child is smaller than that of an adult, so forces are distributed over a smaller area. Children have less adipose tissue than adults, and the muscular layers of the child's abdomen are thinner and weaker. External forces are efficiently transmitted to abdominal organs. Not surprisingly, in children found to have intra-abdominal injury, multiple-organ injury is common. Injuries to the solid organs, such as the liver, spleen, pancreas, and kidneys, may result in significant hemorrhage.

Hollow viscus injuries rarely result in hemodynamic compromise and are more challenging to diagnose in the ED. Bony injury to the inferior ribs, lumbar spine, or pelvis should raise the suspicion for intra-abdominal injury.

Clinical Presentation

Children with abdominal injuries may present with abdominal pain, vomiting, distention, or abdominal tenderness. They may, however, have none of these findings. Children with altered mental status, hemodynamic instability, respiratory distress, or multiple-system injuries should be presumed to have intra-abdominal injury until proven otherwise. Head injuries, fractures, and even significant soft tissue injuries should be considered distracting injuries in children; thorough abdominal evaluation should be performed for suspicion of abdominal trauma. It is important to remember that significant intra-abdominal injury can occur in children without any external evidence of trauma. An example is the child who receives a handlebar injury to the abdomen at normal bicycling speed. Such a child may have a completely transected pancreas and torn duodenum and yet have no external signs of trauma.

Abdominal trauma in children is a challenge to evaluate and manage, even in the setting of hard evidence of intra-abdominal injury (such as positive FAST examination findings). Most children with blunt trauma do not have intra-abdominal injury, and most patients with solid organ injury do not require surgery. Serious injuries commonly occur in the setting of high mechanism forces, but they also occur in what may be initially reported as minor trauma. The identification of injuries in preverbal children or those who do not have normal mental status is difficult. A high index of suspicion is required, even in the stable patient. The clinician should pay particular attention to injuries from an automobile lap belt or bicycle handlebar.

In a patient with free fluid in the abdomen, the physician should start with a bolus of crystalloid solution. If the patient is stabilized and there are no other threats to life or limb, CT of the abdomen and pelvis should be performed immediately to identify and grade the injury.

Diagnostic Testing

■ LABORATORY VALUES

Routine ordering of a full "trauma panel" of laboratory tests is not recommended for a child with abdominal trauma. In the hypotensive patient, blood typing and crossmatching is the most important laboratory test to order early. In patients with low risk of intra-abdominal injury, the urinalysis may be the only test with relatively high diagnostic yield. Few consistent data are available to support a recommendation for which laboratory tests to order to screen children with low- to moderate-risk trauma for the presence of intra-abdominal injury. White blood cell count and serum alanine and aspartate aminotransferase determinations have been suggested to be useful[27] as have hematocrit and measurements of serum amylase and lipase.

■ THE FAST EXAMINATION

The sensitivity of the FAST examination in pediatric trauma is 55% to 82%.[28-31] Its utility is higher in unstable patients. Finding free fluid on FAST examination in stable pediatric patients rarely leads to operative management; the vast majority of patients with such findings are observed and discharged with some restrictions of activities and good precautions. For this reason, the argument can be made that abdominal ultrasonography is less useful in pediatric trauma. However, one study found that using ultrasonography as a triage tool can reduce the cost of pediatric abdominal evaluation.[32] Furthermore, using this modality allows the clinician to quickly identify significant intraperitoneal fluid, which would require further evaluation and possible laparotomy. In this study, children with a positive ultrasonography who showed response to initial fluid resuscitation underwent abdominal CT; unstable patients underwent laparotomy. This approach allowed for a major reduction in the number of CT scans performed. It has also been suggested—but not proven—that the FAST examination, aside from being a screening tool, is sufficient for the evaluation of the majority of the children sustaining blunt abdominal trauma.[33]

■ COMPUTED TOMOGRAPHY

An abdominal CT should be ordered in any stable patient in whom intra-abdominal injury is suspected or to type and grade the injury in the patient with a positive FAST finding. Intravenous administration of contrast agent is sufficient; oral administration is not necessary (Box 16-9).[34] CT findings also allow the

BOX 16-9

Indications for Computed Tomography of the Abdomen in Pediatric Trauma

- Abdominal pain
- Distracting injury accompanied by the suspicion of abdominal trauma
- Altered mental status
- Hemodynamic instability without identifiable source
- Abdominal tenderness
- Seat belt sign
- Inferior rib fractures
- Thoracolumbar spine fractures
- Pelvic fractures
- Gross hematuria

inpatient trauma service to select the appropriate level of inpatient care and monitoring for the patient.[35] Although CT is excellent for evaluating solid organ injury, it is less sensitive for mesenteric, intestinal, and diaphragmatic injuries. If these latter injuries are suspected, further evaluation—such as admission, serial abdominal examinations, and laboratory tests—are indicated.[36] There are drawbacks, however, to the routine performance of CT in any child in whom intra-abdominal injury is suspected after trauma. CT is expensive, requires transport away from the direct care-giving environment, and may necessitate sedation of the child. In addition, computed risk estimates now suggest that pediatric CT may impose a higher lifetime risk of radiation-induced cancer in children than in adults.[37]

■ DIAGNOSTIC PERITONEAL LAVAGE

Although it has fallen out of favor with the increasing availability of CT and ultrasonography, DPL still plays a role in the management of abdominal trauma. This procedure has excellent sensitivity for intra-abdominal injury and may be of value in unstable pediatric trauma patients with suspected intra-abdominal injury. DPL is also useful in the evaluation of children with penetrating injury to the abdomen, particularly in the stable patient in whom there is a question of a bowel injury, which would not be well evaluated with either the FAST examination or CT of the abdomen.[38]

Specific Injuries

Penetrating injuries to the abdomen must be evaluated by a surgeon. If the wound is suspected of violating the abdominal fascia, surgical exploration is the standard of care.

Blunt injuries to the abdomen may cause a variety of internal damages, and a high index of suspicion is required in their evaluation.

Seat belt sign (SBS) refers to ecchymoses, abrasions, or erythema caused by the restraint of the seat belt across the abdomen during a motor vehicle accident.[39] Its presence carries an increased risk of intra-abdominal injuries, particularly to the intestines and pancreas. Proper, age-appropriate restraint of a child in an automobile is extremely important. Proper seat belt use does not increase the risk of injury, but use of just the lap belt does change the spectrum of injury.[40] Other injuries associated with the use of lap belts are facial fractures and lumbar spine fractures termed Chance fractures.

Solid organ injuries include injuries to the liver, spleen, kidneys, and pancreas. FAST examination findings may or may not be positive in the presence of a solid organ injury. Those that are the result of blunt trauma are increasingly being managed nonoperatively in stable patients. In unstable patients, resuscitation with crystalloid solution followed by administration of blood is attempted. If the patient's condition stabilizes, nonoperative management may still be appropriate, as determined by the pediatric trauma surgeon who has seen and evaluated the patient. Unstable patients in whom FAST examination demonstrates free fluid in the abdomen go directly to surgery. Even if nonoperative management is the plan, admission to a pediatric trauma center, usually to an intensive care unit for at least the first 24 hours, is required.

Hollow viscus injury may occur in penetrating or blunt trauma. In penetrating trauma, enterotomies may occur when a missile or sharp object passes directly through the intestine. In blunt trauma, a portion of viscus—such as the sigmoid or the duodenum—may be crushed against the retroperitoneum and may rupture. Alternatively, a portion of viscus may rupture from sudden increases in intra-abdominal pressure or may be torn by being swung forcefully on the mesentery with a sudden deceleration.

Mesenteric injuries may also occur with similar mechanisms. FAST examination findings are frequently normal in the setting of hollow viscus or mesenteric injury. CT has better sensitivity but still may miss significant hollow viscus injuries because free fluid in the abdomen or air in the peritoneum may not be visualized immediately. Even with a high index of suspicion and admission of the patient for serial examinations and observations, these injuries will sometimes be missed. Patients with hollow viscus injuries are treated in the operating room, as are unstable patients with mesenteric injuries. A stable patient with a mesenteric injury may be admitted to the hospital and observed rather than undergo exploratory laparotomy.

Injuries to the bladder and urethra are uncommon in children. A child with gross hematuria and no CT evidence of kidney injuries should undergo retrograde urethrography to evaluate for rupture of the bladder or a torn urethra. Injuries to the urinary collecting system require emergency evaluation by a pediatric urologist.

Disposition

Children who have abdominal trauma and suspicion for intra-abdominal injury and in whom results of ED evaluations are otherwise negative for injury are generally admitted to the hospital for observation. The child who has no other indication for admission and in whom abdominal CT findings are normal may be considered for discharge from the ED if he or she is free of pain, tolerates a regular diet, and has a responsible adult parent or guardian who can monitor the child's status and return him or her immediately to the ED if it changes.

REFERENCES

1. Institute of Medicine, Committee on the Future of Emergency Care in the U.S. Health System: Hospital-Based

Emergency Care: At the Breaking Point. Washington, DC: National Academies Press, 2006.
2. National Center for Injury Prevention and Control: WISQARS Leading Causes of Death Reports, 1999-2004. Available at http://webappa.cdc.gov/sasweb/ncipc/leadcaus10.html/
3. Frush DP, Donnelly LF, Rosen NS: Computed tomography and radiation risks: What pediatric health care providers should know. Pediatrics 2003;112:951-957.
4. Kraus JF, Rock A, Hemyari P: Brain injuries among infants, children, adolescents, and young adults. Am J Dis Child 1990;144:684-691.
5. Rivara FP: Childhood injuries. III: Epidemiology of non-motor vehicle head trauma. Dev Med Child Neurol 1984;26:81-87.
6. Childhood injuries in the United States. Division of Injury Control. Center for Environmental Health and Injury Control, Centers for Disease Control. Am J Dis Child 1990;144:627-646.
7. Schutzman SA, Greenes DS: Pediatric minor head trauma. Ann Emerg Med 2001;37:65-74.
8. Muhonen MG, Piper JG, Menezes AH: Pathogenesis and treatment of growing skull fractures. Surg Neurol 1995;43:367-373.
9. Hoffman JR, Mower WR, Wolfson AB, et al: Validity of a set of clinical criteria to rule at injury to the cervical spine in patients with blunt trauma. National Emergency X-Radiography Utilization Study Group. N Engl J Med 2000;343: 94-99.
10. Balci EA, Kazez A, Eren S, et al: Blunt thoracic trauma in children: Review of 137 cases. Eur J Cardiothorac Surg 2004;26:387-392.
11. Peclet MH, Newman KD, Eichelberger MR, et al: Thoracic trauma in children: An indicator of increased mortality. J Pediatr Surg 1990;25:961-965.
12. Bliss D, Silen M: Pediatric thoracic trauma. Crit Care Med 2002;30:S409-S415.
13. Holmes JF, Brant WE, Bogren HG, et al: Prevalence and importance of pneumothoraces visualized on abdominal computed tomographic scan in children with blunt trauma. J Trauma 2001;50:516-520.
14. Kwon A, Sorrells DL Jr, Kurkchubasche AG, et al: Isolated computed tomography diagnosis of pulmonary contusion does not correlate with increased morbidity. J Pediatr Surg 2006;41:78-82.
15. Bridges KG, Welch G, Silver M, et al: CT detection of occult pneumothorax in multiple trauma patients. J Emerg Med 1993;11:179-186.
16. Kirkpatrick AW, Sirois M, Laupland KB, et al: Hand-held thoracic sonography for detecting post-traumatic pneumothoraces: The Extended Focused Assessment with Sonography for Trauma (EFAST). J Trauma. 2004;57: 288-295.
17. Murray JG, Caoili E, Gruden JF, et al: Acute rupture of the diaphragm due to blunt trauma: Diagnostic sensitivity and specificity of CT. AJR 1996;166:1035-1039.
18. Shapiro MJ, Heiberg E, Durham RM, et al: The unreliability of CT scans and initial chest radiographs in evaluating blunt trauma induced diaphragmatic rupture. Clin Radiol 1996;51:27-30.
19. Killeen KL, Mirvis SE, Shanmuganathan K: Helical CT of diaphragmatic rupture caused by blunt trauma. AJR 1999;173:1611-1616.
20. Nchimi A, Szapiro D, Ghaye B, et al: Helical CT of blunt diaphragmatic rupture. AJR 2005;184:24-30.
21. Voeller GR, Reisser JR, Fabian TC, et al: Blunt diaphragm injuries: A five-year experience. Am Surg 1990;56:28-31.
22. Dowd MD, Krug S: Pediatric blunt cardiac injury: Epidemiology, clinical features, and diagnosis. Pediatric Emergency Medicine Collaborative Research Committee: Working Group on Blunt Cardiac Injury. J Trauma 1996;40:61-67.
23. Healey MA, Brown R, Fleiszer D: Blunt cardiac injury: Is this diagnosis necessary? J Trauma Inj Infect Crit Care 1990;30:137-146.
24. Foil MB, Mackersie RC, Furst SR, et al: The asymptomatic patient with suspected myocardial contusion. Am J Surg 1990;160:638-643.
25. Illig KA, Swierzewski MJ, Feliciano DV, Morton JH: A rational screening and treatment strategy based on the electrocardiogram alone for suspected cardiac contusion. Am J Surg 1991;162:537-543.
26. Potoka DA, Saladino RA: Blunt abdominal trauma in the pediatric patient. Clin Pediatr Emerg Med 2005;6:23-31.
27. Isaacman DJ, Scarfone RJ, Kost SI, et al: Utility of routine laboratory testing for detecting intra-abdominal injury in the pediatric trauma patient. Pediatrics 1993;92: 691-695.
28. Coley BD, Mutabagani KH, Martin LC: Focused abdominal sonography for trauma (FAST) in children with blunt abdominal trauma. J Trauma 2000;48:902-906.
29. Soundappan SV, Holland AJ, Cass DT, Lam A: Diagnostic accuracy of surgeon-performed focused abdominal sonography (FAST) in blunt paediatric trauma. Injury 2005;36: 970-975.
30. Suthers SE, Albrecht R, Foley D: Surgeon-directed ultrasound for trauma is a predictor of intra-abdominal injury in children. Am Surg 2004;70:164-167.
31. Tas F, Ceran C, Atalar MH, et al: The efficacy of ultrasonography in hemodynamically stable children with blunt abdominal trauma: A prospective comparison with computed tomography. Eur J Radiol 2004;51:91-96.
32. Partrick DA, Bensard DD, Moore EE: Ultrasound is an effective triage tool to evaluate blunt abdominal trauma in the pediatric population. J Trauma 1998;45:57-63.
33. Akgur FM, Aktug T, Olguner M, et al: Prospective study investigating routine usage of ultrasonography as the initial diagnostic modality for the evaluation of children sustaining blunt abdominal trauma. J Trauma 1997;42: 626-628.
34. Shankar KR, Lloyd DA, Kitteringham L, Carty HM: Oral contrast with computed tomography in the evaluation of blunt abdominal trauma in children. Br J Surg 1999;86:1073-1077.
35. Neish AS, Taylor GA, Lund DP, Atkinson CC: Effect of CT information on the diagnosis and management of acute abdominal injury in children. Radiology 1998;206: 327-331.
36. Graham JS, Wong AL: A review of computed tomography in the diagnosis of intestinal and mesenteric injury in pediatric blunt abdominal trauma. J Pediatr Surg 1996;31:754-756.
37. Brenner DJ, Elliston, CD Hall EJ, Berdon W: Estimated risk of radiation-induced fatal cancer from pediatric CT. AJR 2001;176:297-301.
38. Meyer DM, Thal ER, Coln D, Weigelt JA: Computed tomography in the evaluation of children with blunt abdominal trauma. Ann Surg 1993;217:272-276.
39. Campbell DJ, Sprouse LR 2nd, Smith LA, et al: Injuries in pediatric patients with seatbelt contusions. Am Surg 2003;69:1095-1099.
40. Sokolove PE, Kuppermann N, Holmes JF: Association between the "seat belt sign" and intra-abdominal injury in children with blunt torso trauma. Acad Emerg Med 2005;12:808-813.

SECTION II

Special Considerations in the Pediatric Patient

Chapter 17

General Approach to the Pediatric Patient

Antonio E. Muñiz

KEY POINTS

Each stage of childhood development brings about unique changes in anatomic, physiologic, and developmental features that affect assessment and management.

Although growth and development occur simultaneously, they are discrete and separate processes. *Growth* refers to an increase in the number of cells and results in an increase in physical size. *Development* is the gradual and successive increase in abilities or skills that is predominantly age-specific and reflects neurologic, emotional, and social maturation.

Parents or caregivers must be considered during every interaction with a child, especially if the child is seriously injured or ill. A child's anxiety and fear often reflect what he or she feels or sees in the parent(s)/caregiver(s).

Family presence during invasive procedures and resuscitation can be a positive experience for some parents/caregivers, especially those of children with chronic illnesses.

General Approach

Children account for about 30% of all ED visits; of these, 80% are initially evaluated in a general rather than a pediatric ED.[1,2] The environment should be child friendly and child safe.

The following suggestions constitute a general approach to a child in the ED:

- Allow the parent or caregiver to stay with the child whenever possible.
- Ask what name to use for the child, and then address the child by name.
- Talk with the family using nonmedical terminology, especially when discussing planned interventions, findings, and treatments. Use language that children will comprehend.
- Always provide privacy no matter how young the child.
- Observe the patient's level of consciousness, activity level, interaction with the environment and caregiver, position of comfort, skin color, respiratory rates and efforts, and level of discomfort before touching him or her. Compare assessment findings with the parents' or caregivers' description of the child's normal behaviors, such as eating and sleeping habits, activity level, and level of consciousness.
- Be honest with the child and parent or caregiver. Parents or caregivers require reassurance about and explanations of the situation and the anticipated plan of treatment.
- Acknowledge and compliment good behavior, and encourage and praise the child. Provide rewards such as stickers or books.
- Allow the child to make simple age-appropriate choices and to participate in the treatment plan. For example, ask the child which arm to use for measuring blood pressure.
- Encourage play during the examination and any procedures. Use diversion and distraction techniques: Encourage the child to blow bubbles and blow the hurt away. Ask the child to sing a

favorite song, and sing along or have the parents or caregivers do so. Have the child picture a favorite place and describe it in detail with all five senses.

Give the child permission to voice his or her feelings. Tell the child it is okay to cry. Sympathy is essential.

- Assess for pain using age-appropriate assessment tools. Elicit from the parents or caregivers the child's typical response to pain.
- Be cautious about what you say in the presence of an apparently unconscious child.

The Family

The parents and other significant caregivers play a fundamental role in the child's health care experience.[3] The child is not the only person who needs attention. Communicating effectively with the parents or caregivers is critical to obtain an accurate history and consent for treatment.[3] When the child suffers from pain because of illness or injury, the parents or caregivers experience almost equal anxiety and emotional stress. The parent's or caregiver's reaction to the child's condition will directly affect how the child behaves.

Innate parental or caregiver instincts may evoke powerful emotional reactions. Such reactions are affected by guilt, fear, anxiety, disbelief, shock, anger, and loss of control.[3] Abandoning a child to a stranger's care, not understanding what will occur next, and worrying about a child's condition leave parents or caregivers feeling defenseless. The fear of the unknown, fear of separation, fear of the possibility of significant morbidity or death, and fear of a strange environment may add stress to the parents' or caregivers' attitudes about the illness or injury of the child. A parent's or caregiver's own anxiety and response to the event may negatively influence his or her ability to console the child, to understand information communicated by the healthcare providers, to participate in decision-making for the child's care, and to recall information given at discharge.[3]

Parents or caregivers in emotional shock from a child's acute illness or injury react differently. They may be very quiet, uncommunicative, and withdrawn, and may be unaware of the presence of others. They may appear to ignore and may not answer questions. Alternatively, some parents or caregivers become very demanding, offensive, or rude. Such people, like parents or caregivers who react in other ways, need confident, competent care providers who are able to enlist them in the medical process.

■ FAMILY PRESENCE

Evidence now suggests that presence of the child's family during invasive procedures and resuscitation can be positive, especially in children with chronic illnesses.[4] Although many family members and health care providers support the concept of family presence, parents or caregivers frequently are not given the option to remain with the child during invasive procedures.[5] Many providers are concerned that family presence will impede caring for the child, that it will be distracting to the members of the team providing care, and that it will increase stress among the team.[5,6] Contrary to this belief, studies show that family members do not interfere with health care providers and that the family benefits in a variety of ways from the experience.[7-10] There is also evidence that children feel less stress when parents or caregivers are allowed to remain during procedures.[11] In addition, when institutions have incorporated family presence into their practice, staff members have remained supportive.[12] Family members who were present for procedures reported that they would do so again and that their grieving behavior was positively affected by the experience.[4]

Before a family member is offered the choice to be present during an invasive procedure, a health care provider must assess whether the family can cope with what they will experience during the events. A family member who appears out of control or too emotional may be distracting and disruptive to the health care providers during the procedure. In this case, it may not be advisable to offer the opportunity for family presence. A designated member of the staff who functions to support the family and serve as a patient and caregiver advocate should stay with the family whether or not they decide or are allowed to be present with the child.

The choice to remain present during invasive or resuscitation procedures must be made by the parent or caregiver.[13,14] If the parent or caregiver prefers not to stay with the child, ED personnel must respect that decision and continue to provide appropriate support and explanations.[14] If the parent or caregiver chooses to stay with the child, the health care team must ensure that the he or she is given a clear explanation of the procedure and expected responses.

Before escorting family members into the room of a child who is undergoing a procedure or resuscitation, the health care provider supporting them must prepare them for what they will see. The family should be instructed about where they should stand while in the room, and if possible, they should have the opportunity to touch the child. The health care provider supporting the family should offer an ongoing account of activities in a gentle, calm, and directive voice. Should the resuscitation efforts or procedure not result in positive changes in the child's condition, the health care provider supporting the family must remember that his or her role is to support family presence and to avoid any derogatory comments.

Growth and Development

Although growth and development occur simultaneously, they are discrete and separate processes. *Growth*

Table 17-1 DEVELOPMENTAL MILESTONES

Age	Milestones
Newborn	Prone: Lies in flexed attitude, turns head from side to side, head lags on ventral suspension. Supine: Generally lies flexed with mildly increased muscle tone. Visual: Fixates to bright lights and close objects in the line of vision, "doll's-eye" movement of eyes on turning of the body. Reflexes: Moro, stepping and placing, grasping, rooting, startle, and Babinski. Social: Visual preference for human faces.
1 month	Prone: Legs are more extended; child holds chin up, turns head, head is lifted momentarily to plane of body on ventral suspension. Supine: Tonic neck posture predominates; is supple and relaxed, head lags on lifting to sitting position, has tight grasp. Visual: Follows a moving object or person, watches a person. Social: Body movements in cadence with voice, smiles responsively, becomes alert in response to voice.
4 months	Prone: Lifts head and chest in vertical axis with legs extended, rolls front to back. Supine: Symmetrical posture predominates, hands in midline, reaches and grasps objects and brings them to mouth. Sitting: No head lag on pull to sitting position, head steady, enjoys sitting with full truncal support, tracks objects through a 180-degree horizontal arc. Standing: When held erect, pushes with feet. Adaptive: When held erect, pushes with feet. Reflexes: Lacks Moro reflex. Language: Coos, says "aah." Social: Laughs out loud, may show displeasure if social contact is broken, is excited at sight of food, waves at toys.
6 months	Prone: Rolls over, may pivot. Supine: Lifts head, rolls over, makes squirming motions. Sitting: Sits unsupported but falls on hands, and back is rounded. Standing: May support most of weight, bounces actively. Adaptive: Resists the pull of a toy, reaches out for and grabs large objects, transfers object from hand to hand, grasps using radial palm, rakes at a pellet. Motor: Helps hold the bottle during feeding. Language: Babbles, giggles, or laughs when tickled. Social: Responds more to emotions, enjoys looking at a mirror, responds to changes in emotional content, turns to a voice, clicks tongue to gain notice.
9 months	Sitting: Sits up alone with no support. Standing: Pulls to standing position. Adaptive: Grasps objects with thumb and forefinger, pokes at things with forefinger, picks up a pellet with assisted pincer movement, uncovers a hidden toy, attempts to retrieve a dropped object, release object by other person. Motor: Crawls or creeps, walks holding onto furniture. Language: Makes repetitive sounds, such as "mama" and "dada"; imitates speech. Social: Plays pat-a-cake or peek-a-boo, waves bye-bye, tries to find hidden objects, responds to name, begins to respond to "no" and to one-step commands.
1 year	Motor: Walks with one hand held, walks holding onto furniture, takes several steps. Adaptive: Picks up a pellet with unassisted pincer movement of forefinger and thumb, releases a held object to other person on request or gesture, points to a desired objects, tries to build a tower of 2 cubes. Motor: Drinks from a cup with help. Language: Has 3 simple words, understands approximately 10 words. Social: Plays simple games, makes postural adjustment to dressing, follows simple commands.
2 years	Motor: Walks up and down stairs with one hand held, jumps and runs well, stands on either foot alone for 1 second, climbs on furniture, kicks and throws a ball. Adaptive: Handles spoon well, is able to turn a doorknob, makes circular scribbling, imitates a horizontal stroke, folds paper once imitatively, can build a tower of 6 to 7 cubes, points to named objects or pictures. Language: Puts 3 words together, uses pronouns. Social: Listens to stories with pictures, turns pages of book, observes pictures, helps to undress self, often tells immediate experiences, verbalizes toilet needs.
3 years	Motor: Goes up stairs alternating feet, rides a tricycle, stands momentarily on one foot. Adaptive: Can construct a block tower of more than 9 cubes, makes vertical and horizontal strokes on a paper but does not join them to make a cross, copies a circle, holds crayon with fingers. Language: Composes sentences of 3 to 4 words, has a vocabulary of 900 words. Social: Knows own age and sex, counts 3 objects, knows first and last names, plays simple games, helps in dressing self, washes hands.
4 years	Motor: Hops on one foot, throws ball overhead, uses scissors to cut out pictures, climbs well, runs and turns without losing balance, stands on one leg for at least 10 seconds, catches ball bounced to him/her. Adaptive: Copies cross and square, draws people with 2 to 4 parts besides the head, knows the days of the week. Language: Counts 4 pennies, tells a story, learns and sings simple songs, has a vocabulary of more than 1500 words, easily composes sentences of 4 to 5 words, can use the past tense, knows the days of the week, can ask up to 500 questions a day. Social: Plays with several children with beginning of social interaction and role-playing, goes to toilet alone.
5 years	Motor: Skips smoothly, can catch a ball. Adaptive: Draws a triangle from copy, names heavier of 2 weights, knows right and left hand, draws person with at least 8 details. Language: Names 4 colors, repeats sentences of 10 syllables, has vocabulary of more 2100 words, counts 10 pennies, prints first name, tells age. Social: Dresses and undresses, asks questions about meanings of words, engages in domestic role-playing.

refers to an increase in the number of cells and leads to an increase in physical size. *Development* is the gradual and successive increase in abilities or skills performance along a predetermined path, often referred to as developmental milestones or tasks (Table 17-1). Development is predominantly age specific and reflects neurologic, emotional, and social maturation. Although there is cross-cultural similarity in the sequence and timing of developmental milestones, cultures exert an all-pervasive influence on developing children.

REFERENCES

1. American College of Emergency Physicians Policy Statement: The role of the emergency physician in the care of children. Ann Emerg Med 1990;19:435-436.
2. Nelson DS, Walsh K, Fleisher GR: Spectrum and frequency of pediatric illness presenting to a general community hospital emergency department. Pediatrics 1992;90:5-10.
3. Horowitz L, Kassam-Adams N, Bregstein J: Mental health aspects of emergency medical services for children: Summary of a consensus conference. Acad Emerg Med 2001;8:1187-1196.
4. Henderson DP, Knapp J: Report of the National Consensus Conference on Family Presence during Pediatric Cardiopulmonary Resuscitation and Procedures. Pediatr Emerg Med 2005;21:789-791.
5. MacLean SL, Guzzetta CE, White C, et al: Family presence during cardiopulmonary resuscitation and invasive procedures: Practice of critical care and emergency nurses. J Emerg Nursing 2003;29:208-221.
6. Williams JM: Family presence during resuscitation: To see or not to see? Nursing Clin North Am 2002;37:211-220.
7. Hanson C, Strawser D: Family presence during cardiopulmonary resuscitation: Foote Hospital emergency department's nine-year perspective. J Emerg Nurs 1992;18:104-106.
8. Sacchetti A, Carraccio C, Leva E, et al: Acceptance of family member presence during pediatric resuscitations in the emergency department: Effects of personal experience. Pediatr Emerg Care 2000;16:85-87.
9. Bauchner H, Waring C, Vinci R: Parental presence during procedures in an emergency room: Results from 50 observations. Pediatrics 1991;87:544-548.
10. Boie ET, Moore GP, Brummett C, Nelson DR: Do parents want to be present during invasive procedures performed on their children in the emergency department? A survey of 400 parents. Ann Emerg Med 1999;34:70-74.
11. Wolfram RW, Turner ED, Philput C: Effects of parental presence during young children's venipunctures. Pediatr Emerg Care 1997;13:325-328.
12. Doyle CJ, Post H, Burney RE, et al: Family participation during resuscitation: An option. Ann Emerg Med 1987;16:673-675.
13. Boudreaux ED, Francis JL, Layacano T: Family presence during invasive procedures and resuscitations in the emergency department: A critical review and suggestions for future research. Ann Emerg Med 2002;40:193-205.
14. Eichhorn DJ, Meyers TA, Guzzetta CE, et al: During invasive procedures and resuscitation: Hearing the voice of the patient. Am J Nursing 2001;101:48-55.

Chapter 18

The First Weeks of Life

John Nelson Perret

KEY POINTS

Congenital heart and gastrointestinal anomalies commonly manifest during the first month of life.

A complete set of vital signs, including weight (undressed), are required for the proper evaluation of the neonatal patient.

The majority of neonates who have experienced an apparent life-threatening event (ALTE) have a normal appearance at the time of presentation to the ED.

An echocardiogram is the most definitive test that can be performed in the ED to distinguish between pulmonary and cardiac causes of cyanosis. If an echocardiogram is unavailable, a hyperoxia-hyperventilation test or "100% oxygen challenge test" should be conducted.

Administration of intravenous prostaglandin E_1 is frequently associated with apnea, fever, and, occasionally, shock; the EP should be prepared to intubate if such complications arise.

Two thirds of the deaths that occur in the first year of life do so in the first month.[1] The leading causes of neonatal death are preterm birth, low birth weight, birth defects, maternal pregnancy complications, respiratory distress syndrome, and placenta or cord complications.[2]

Figure 18-1 summarizes the initial evaluation and management of the seriously ill infant in the ED.

Newborns are presented to the ED with a multitude of issues, ranging from life-threatening conditions to benign findings. An understanding of age-appropriate norms helps the EP identify infants with significant illness.

The Normal Neonate

■ WEIGHT

A normal neonate may lose up to 10% of birth weight during the first week of life. By the end of the second week, the infant should have returned to birth weight, often a little above it. The weight gain from this point through the first month should be about 30 grams (1 ounce) per day. It is essential that an accurate weight (undressed) of any neonate is measured in the ED.

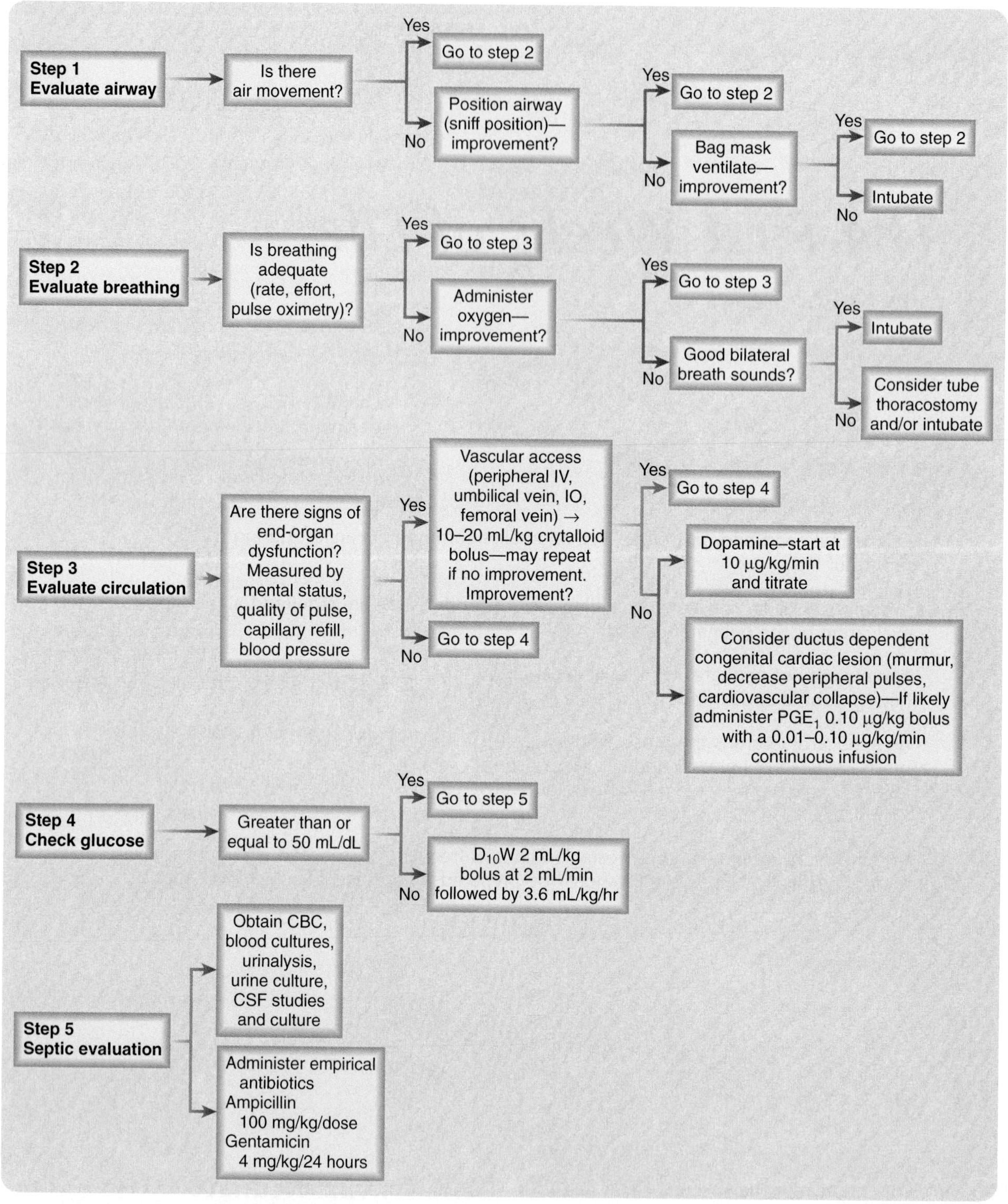
Step 1
Evaluate airway
Is there air movement?
Yes
Go to step 2
No
Position airway (sniff position)—improvement?
Yes
Go to step 2
No
Bag mask ventilate—improvement?
Yes
Go to step 2
No
Intubate
Step 2
Evaluate breathing
Is breathing adequate (rate, effort, pulse oximetry)?
Yes
Go to step 3
No
Administer oxygen—improvement?
Yes
Go to step 3
No
Good bilateral breath sounds?
Yes
Intubate
No
Consider tube thoracostomy and/or intubate
Step 3
Evaluate circulation
Are there signs of end-organ dysfunction? Measured by mental status, quality of pulse, capillary refill, blood pressure
Yes
Vascular access (peripheral IV, umbilical vein, IO, femoral vein) → 10–20 mL/kg crytalloid bolus—may repeat if no improvement. Improvement?
Yes
Go to step 4
No
Dopamine–start at 10 μg/kg/min and titrate
Consider ductus dependent congenital cardiac lesion (murmur, decrease peripheral pulses, cardiovascular collapse)—If likely administer PGE1 0.10 μg/kg bolus with a 0.01–0.10 μg/kg/min continuous infusion
No
Go to step 4
Step 4
Check glucose
Greater than or equal to 50 mL/dL
Yes
Go to step 5
No
D10W 2 mL/kg bolus at 2 mL/min followed by 3.6 mL/kg/hr
Step 5
Septic evaluation
Obtain CBC, blood cultures, urinalysis, urine culture, CSF studies and culture
Administer empirical antibiotics
Ampicillin
100 mg/kg/dose
Gentamicin
4 mg/kg/24 hours

FIGURE 18-1 The initial evaluation and management of the seriously ill neonate. CBC, complete blood count; CSF, cerebrospinal fluid; $D_{10}W$, 10% dextrose in water; IV, intravenous; IO, intraosseous.

FEEDING

There is much variability among neonates regarding feeding schedules. The same child can show significant variability within a 24-hour period. The average neonate eats between 6 and 9 times a day. Feeding intervals may range between 2 and 4 hours. Breastfed infants tend to eat more often than formula-fed infants.

SLEEPING

Newborns sleep 16 to 18 hours per day with almost equal amounts of day and night sleep. Awake periods are generally about 1 to 2 hours in duration.

CRYING

Crying peaks at about 6 weeks of age, with an average of 3 hours per day. This behavior tends to "cluster," occurring mostly in the late afternoon and early evening. By 3 months of age the average crying time per day drops to 1 hour.

VITAL SIGNS

A normal neonatal pulse is in the range of 120 to 160 beats/min but certainly rises if the child is stimulated. The heart rate slows during sleep.

The normal respiratory rate is between 40 and 60 breaths/min. Some irregularity and pauses of less than 20 seconds are normal in the neonatal period. Respiratory pauses should not be associated with any color change or hypotonia, however. Because of this irregularity in respiratory rate, accurate measurements can be obtained only if breaths are counted for at least 30 seconds.

Obtaining a blood pressure in the newborn can be frustrating and time-consuming. Oscillometric devices, such as the Dinamap, facilitate the procedure but lack some accuracy. The pressure can be measured on the calf as well as the arm. The size of the cuff is very important: The bladder of the cuff should cover two thirds of the length and three quarters of the circumference of the extremity. It is easier to use a Doppler probe when using a sphygmomanometer. A systolic blood pressure less than 60 mm Hg is abnormal in a neonate.

TEMPERATURE

The core temperature for an infant is the same as the adult. Fever is generally recognized as a temperature greater than 38°C or 100.4°F. Any temperature less than 36.1°C or 97°F should raise concern for hypothermia. Owing to a limited thermoregulatory ability, the neonate should be examined and treated in a warm ambient environment. This should be done in a radiant warmer if the neonate is to be undressed for a prolonged period. See Table 18-1 for normal neonatal vital signs.

Table 18-1 NORMAL VITAL SIGNS IN THE NEONATE

Heart rate	120-160 beats/min
Respiratory rate	40-60 breaths/min
Blood pressure	Systolic pressure >60 mm Hg
Temperature	36.1-38°C or 97-100.4°F

Apnea and Apparent Life-Threatening Event

The 1986 National Institutes of Health Consensus Development Conference on Infantile Apnea and Home Monitoring defined *apparent life-threatening event* (ALTE) as "an episode that is frightening to the observer and is characterized by some combination of apnea (central or occasionally obstructive), color change (usually cyanotic or pallid but occasionally erythematous or plethoric), marked change in muscle tone (usually marked limpness), choking, or gagging."[3]

The conventional definition of *apnea* is absence of breathing for 20 seconds or for a shorter period if associated with clinical signs such as cyanosis, hypotonia, and bradycardia. Because periods of apnea up to 30 seconds have been observed in normal healthy asymptomatic term and preterm infants, duration of apnea does not seem as clinically important as apnea associated with signs and symptoms.[4] Apnea should be distinguished from the normal periodic breathing of the newborn, which is characterized by irregular breathing and episodes of pauses. This latter pattern is more commonly seen in premature infants during sleep.

The majority of neonates who have had an ALTE have a normal appearance at the time of presentation to the ED. The EP should not be complacent because of this normal appearance. A comprehensive history and a thorough physical examination should be performed. One study showed that history and physical examination were helpful in diagnosing the etiology of ALTE in 70% of cases.[5] The history should comprise a detailed description of the event, a prenatal and perinatal history, a review of systems, and a family history (especially child deaths, neurologic diseases, cardiac diseases, and congenital problems). Box 18-1 lists essential questions for the caregivers of such an infant. A detailed physical examination, with particular attention paid to the neurologic, respiratory, cardiac, and developmental components, is essential. Evidence of child abuse should be sought, including a funduscopic examination for retinal hemorrhage.

ALTEs and apnea are clinical presentations that have many causes, as summarized in Table 18-2. The most common organ systems involved (in order of decreasing frequency) are gastrointestinal, neurologic, respiratory, cardiac, metabolic, and endocrine.

BOX 18-1

Historical Questions to Ask the Caregiver of the Infant Who Has Had an Apparent Life-Threatening Event (ALTE) or Apnea

1. What was the appearance of the infant when found?
2. Were any interventions (cardiopulmonary resuscitation) necessary?
3. How long did the event last?*
4. Was the infant awake or asleep when the event occurred?
5. What was the infant's body position?
6. Was the infant alone in the bed?
7. When was the last time the infant ate?
8. Has the infant been sick or well in the time before the event?
9. Is there any history of trauma?
10. Is there a family history of sudden infant death syndrome or ALTE?
11. What are the prenatal history and perinatal history?

*A trick the EP can use to help the caregiver answer this question is as follows: (1) the EP asks the caregiver to look at him or her; (2) the EP says "Go"; and (3) the caregiver says "Stop" when he/she thinks the time that has passed matches the time at which the event ended.

There is no published standard for diagnostic testing in the ED evaluation of apnea or ALTE. Diagnostic testing is best guided by the history and physical examination. Laboratory tests have been shown to be contributory to the diagnosis only 3.3% of the time if results of the history and physical examination were noncontributory.[5] A study of patients with ALTE demonstrated a correlation between anemia and ALTE, especially recurrent ALTE.[6] All infants who had a severe episode of apnea or a significant ALTE should be admitted for monitoring and further diagnostic evaluation.

Excessive Crying and Irritability

Crying peaks in infancy at 6 weeks of age with an average crying time of 3 hours per day. More of the crying time is clustered in the late afternoon and evening. The average crying time for infants less than 3 months of age is 1.6 hours per day, divided over an average of five episodes.[7] Forty percent of the infants cry for 30 minutes or more, 75% of these having the longest crying spells between 6 and 12 PM.[7] Box 18-2 lists important questions to ask the caregiver of the afebrile infant with excessive crying. Table 18-3 lists possible physical findings in these infants.

The first differentiation the clinician must make is whether the crying is an acute single episode or has been an ongoing problem for some time. The latter describes colic, which affects a large subgroup of

Table 18-2 ETIOLOGIES OF APPARENT LIFE-THREATENING EVENT (ALTE)

Gastrointestinal	Gastroesophageal reflux Aspiration, choking, swallowing abnormalities Volvulus Intussusception Infection
Neurologic	Seizure disorder Infection Congenital malformations of the brain (e.g., type II Chiari malformation) Intraventricular hemorrhage Neuromuscular disorders Apnea of prematurity Central hypoventilation syndrome (Ondine's curse) Brain tumors Vasovagal reflex Brainstem infarction Drugs
Respiratory	Infection (respiratory syncytial virus, mycoplasma, pertussis, croup) Congenital airway abnormalities (Pierre Robin syndrome, laryngotracheomalacia) Vocal cord abnormalities Obstructive sleep apnea
Cardiovascular	Arrhythmias (long QT syndrome, Wolff-Parkinson-White syndrome) Congenital heart disease Myocarditis
Metabolic or endocrine	Inborn errors of metabolism Glucose and electrolyte disorders
Other	Sepsis Medication or drug toxicity Child abuse Munchausen by proxy syndrome

BOX 18-2

Historical Questions to Ask the Caregiver of an Afebrile Infant with Acute and Excessive Crying

1. Was the crying gradual or sudden in onset?
2. Is this the first episode?
3. How long has the child been crying?
4. Can the child be consoled?
5. Were there any potential inciting events (trauma, immunizations)?
6. Has the child been sick or had a fever?
7. Has here been any change in feeding pattern or stooling?
8. Did the infant have any significant birth or perinatal problems?

excessively crying infants. Historically, colic has been described by the rule of threes—crying for 3 hours a day, for at least 3 days a week, for 3 weeks. There have been scores of theories as to the etiology of colic, ranging from physiologic disturbances (cow's milk allergies, gastrointestinal reflux, hypocontractile gallbladder, and other gastrointestinal disturbances) to infant temperament and maternal response, to deficiencies in parenting practices.[8] No single cause has been found.

No pharmacologic agent has been identified as both safe and efficacious for the treatment of colic. Simethicone is safe, but studies have shown it to be no better than placebo.[9] Anticholinergic agents have been found to be more effective than placebo[10] but are associated with apnea and should not be used in infants younger than 6 months. Many other interventions have been proposed for colic, such as having the infant in a car, specific ways to hold the infant, use of white noise, crib vibrators, and herbal teas. None has been shown to be particularly beneficial. The EP should reassure parents that there is no ideal treatment for colic, that their child is normal, that the infant will outgrow the colic, and that colic has no long-term sequelae.

Diagnostic testing guided by history and physical findings make the diagnosis in 20% of crying infants.[11] Up to 39% of the final diagnoses in afebrile infants with acute prolonged crying are made on follow-up.[11] A suggested approach to the ED evaluation of the excessively crying child is shown in Figure 18-2.

Table 18-3 POTENTIAL PHYSICAL EXAMINATION ABNORMALITIES IN THE CRYING INFANT

	Finding(s) and Possible Diagnoses
Inspection	
General	Ill appearance: Sepsis, meningitis, other infectious process Dehydration Congenital heart disease (cardiogenic shock), supraventricular tachycardia Volvulus, bowel perforation, incarcerated hernia, intussusception, appendicitis Intracranial hemorrhage (traumatic/nontraumatic) Hypoglycemia, inborn error of metabolism
Skin	Trauma, abscess, cellulitis
Eyes, ears, nose, throat	Corneal abrasion, foreign body, teething
Abdomen, genitourinary structures	Hernia, hair tourniquet on penis, paraphimosis
Extremities/clavicles	Fracture deformity (accidental/nonaccidental), digit hair tourniquet
Palpation	
Head	Trauma, fontanelle (dehydration, increased intracranial pressure)
Chest	Clavicular fracture
Abdomen	Tenderness/peritoneal signs: Volvulus, bowel perforation, appendicitis, intussusception, incarcerated hernia
Genitourinary structures	Testicular torsion
Extremities/clavicles	Trauma, fracture, soft tissue infection
Auscultation	
Heart	Decreased pulses (congenital heart disease, septic shock)
Lungs	Murmur: Congenital heart disease Tachycardia: Supraventricular tachycardia, congestive heart failure Stridor: Upper airway obstruction Wheezing: Airway foreign body, bronchiolitis Rales: Pneumonia, congestive heart failure
Abdomen	Hypoactive/hyperactive or absence of bowel sounds: Volvulus, intussusception, appendicitis, incarcerated hernia

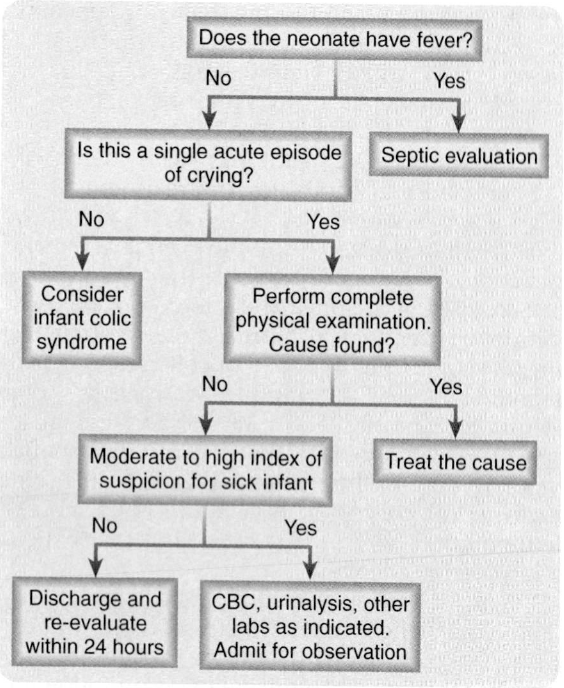
Does the neonate have fever?
No
Yes
Is this a single acute episode of crying?
Septic evaluation
No
Yes
Consider infant colic syndrome
Perform complete physical examination. Cause found?
No
Yes
Moderate to high index of suspicion for sick infant
Treat the cause
No
Yes
Discharge and re-evaluate within 24 hours
CBC, urinalysis, other labs as indicated. Admit for observation

FIGURE 18-2 Evaluation of the crying neonate. CBC, complete blood count.

Cyanosis

Cyanosis in the neonate may be persistent or transient, central or peripheral (acrocyanosis), an emergency or nonemergency. An infant with cyanosis or a history of cyanosis should undergo a rapid evaluation and initiation of treatment for correctable causes.

Cyanosis is the result of either deoxygenated hemoglobin or abnormal hemoglobin (methemoglobin). Cyanosis occurs with the presence of 4 to 5 grams of deoxygenated (unsaturated or reduced) hemoglobin per 100 mL of blood. This is an absolute quantity and not a percentage of unsaturated hemoglobin—therefore, a cyanotic, polycythemic infant with a hemoglobin value of 18 g/100 mL might have no tissue hypoxia if the total amount of unsaturated hemoglobin is only 5 g/100 mL, because the oxygen content of the blood would still be adequate. Conversely, an anemic infant with a hemoglobin value of 7 g/100 mL would have severe tissue hypoxia because at least 4 to 5 g/100 mL of the total is deoxygenated hemoglobin.

The EP can best evaluate cyanosis clinically by looking at the tongue and mucous membranes. Duskiness or blueness in these areas defines central cyanosis, a pathologic condition. In peripheral or acrocyanosis, the extremities are blue but the oral mucosa and tongue remain pink; this pattern is frequently a normal finding in the neonate but can be associated with pathologic oxygenation.

An easy method of classifying cyanosis is by causative organ system (Table 18-4). The cardiac and respiratory systems are responsible for the large majority of cases of neonatal cyanosis. Distinguishing between the two categories of causes can be difficult but is absolutely necessary for optimal management of the patient.

An echocardiogram is the most definitive test that can be performed in the ED to distinguish between pulmonary and cardiac causes of cyanosis. If unavailable, the next best test would be the hyperoxia-hyperventilation test (also called the "100% oxygen challenge test"), which is performed as follows:

1. A blood gas measurement is performed with the infant on room air.
2. The patient is administered 100% oxygen, and the blood gases are measured again.

If the hypoxia is secondary to pulmonary disease, the Pa_{O_2} value usually rises to more than 150 mm Hg with 100% oxygen. If the hypoxia is secondary to right-to-left cardiac shunting from congenital heart disease, the Pa_{O_2} value does not significantly rise when the infant is receiving 100% oxygen. Occasionally, enough intrapulmonary right-to-left shunting occurs in lung disease to prevent the rise in Pa_{O_2} with simple administration of 100% oxygen. In these cases, the infant can be manually ventilated with 100% oxygen, and the Pa_{O_2} rises if the source of cyanosis is in the lungs. In many instances, these results are clinically obtained by the infant's response to oxygen during the initial resuscitation.

The initial treatment of any neonate with cyanosis includes adequate supplemental oxygenation, ventilation, and intravascular volume challenge with 10 to 20 mL/kg of normal saline. If there is no response to volume resuscitation, vasopressor support with dopamine, 5 to 20 μg/kg/min, should be administered.

If the cyanotic neonate continues to show signs of inadequate tissue oxygenation after the initial resuscitation, then prostaglandin E_1 (alprostadil) should be given intravenously starting at 0.1 μg/kg/min. Administration of prostaglandin is frequently associated with apnea, fever, and occasionally shock; the EP should be prepared to intubate the infant if such complications arise. One study has shown that aminophylline, 6 mg/kg bolus prior to administration of prostaglandin E_1, followed by 2 mg/kg intravenously every 8 hours for 72 hours, significantly reduces apnea.[12]

Although rare, methemoglobinemia is still a possibility in the cyanotic neonate. This syndrome may be inherited or acquired. The acquired form is secondary to drugs and toxins such as nitrites, anesthetics, and aniline dyes as well as to diarrhea and acidosis.

Difficulty Breathing

Respiratory distress involves a spectrum of clinical findings from apnea, dyspnea, tachypnea, stridor, nasal flaring, grunting, chest retractions, wheezing, and rales to simple nasal congestion and periodic breathing.

Table 18-4 CAUSES OF NEONATAL CYANOSIS

Respiratory	
Upper airway	Choanal atresia Macroglossia Glossoptosis (secondary to micrognathia) Laryngomalacia Laryngeal web or cyst Vascular anomalies (e.g., cystic hygromas, rings) Subglottic stenosis (commonly secondary to intubation) Foreign body
Lower airway	Pneumonia Bronchiolitis Pulmonary edema Atelectasis Bronchopulmonary dysplasia
Systemic	Sepsis Trauma Poisons
Cardiac	Cyanotic congenital heart diseases Transposition of the great vessels (most common neonatal) Tetralogy of Fallot Truncus arteriosus Tricuspid atresia Total anomalous pulmonary venous return Ebstein's anomaly
Gastrointestinal	Gastroesophageal reflux
Neurologic	Seizures Central hypoventilation syndrome (Ondine's curse) Spinal muscular atrophy type I (Werdnig-Hoffmann) Botulism Congenital myopathies
Hematologic	Methemoglobinemia

The differential diagnosis of pulmonary causes of respiratory distress in the neonate can be divided into those syndromes that manifest in the first hours of life and those that can manifest anytime during the first 28 days. The former group includes transient tachypnea of the newborn (TTN), respiratory distress syndrome (RDS), persistent pulmonary hypertension of the newborn (PPHN), and meconium aspiration syndrome (MAS). These are not discussed further because they are almost certainly diagnosed and treated in the nursery, not the ED.

A list of potential causes of respiratory distress that can occur anytime during the first 28 days is given in Box 18-3. The majority of causes are pulmonary, cardiac, or infectious. Diagnostic testing includes a complete blood count, serum glucose measurement, metabolic profile, blood cultures, arterial blood gas measurements, urinalysis, urine culture, chest radiography, and electrocardiogram (ECG).

■ PNEUMONIA

Pneumonia is the most common and most serious infectious cause of respiratory distress in the first 28 days of life. It occurs in up to 10% of preterm neonates and is associated with significant morbidity and mortality.

Neonatal pneumonia is transmitted in one of three ways—transplacental, during birth (perinatal), or postnatal (hospital-acquired or community-acquired infection). From a clinical perspective, neonatal pneumonia can be divided into early-onset and late-onset types (Table 18-5).

Early-onset pneumonia usually manifests within 3 days of birth and is caused by organisms transferred from the mother to the infant via the placenta or from organisms aspirated from the amniotic fluid before or during birth. The organisms most commonly associated with early-onset pneumonia are group B streptococci, *Escherichia coli,* other Enterobacteriaceae, and herpes simplex virus.

Late-onset pneumonia may occur during the nursery stay or after hospitalization. It can be caused by organisms that colonized the neonate in the birthing process or by organisms from infected persons or contaminated equipment. Common bacterial etiologic agents in late-onset pneumonia are *Staphylococcus aureus, Streptococcus pyogenes,* and *Streptococcus pneumoniae. E. coli* and other gram-negative organisms are still significant in the differential diagnosis. *Chlamydia trachomatis* and *Ureaplasma urealyticum* are associated with "afebrile pneumonia of infancy." Respiratory syncytial virus is a common viral cause of pneumonia in neonates.

The clinical presentation of pneumonia in the neonate can be atypical. The signs of respiratory distress are generally present but may be absent. Gastrointestinal symptoms, such as vomiting, abdominal

BOX 18-3

Etiologic Considerations in the Infant with Difficulty in Breathing

Respiratory system
- Infectious
  - Pneumonia
  - Bronchiolitis
  - Laryngotracheitis
  - Viral upper respiratory tract infection
- Congenital structural
  - Choanal atresia
  - Laryngotracheomalacia
  - Laryngeal webs
  - Laryngeal cysts
  - Laryngocoeles
  - Hemangiomas
  - Foreign body
- Acquired structural
  - Pneumothorax
  - Chest wall injury/rib injury

Cardiovascular
- Congenital heart disease
  - Cyanotic
  - Non-cyanotic
- Hypovolemia
- Anemia

Metabolic
- Hypoglycemia
- Acidosis

Neurologic
- Central nervous system hemorrhage
- Muscle disease

Drugs

Sepsis

distention, and poor feeding, may predominate. General systemic signs such as lethargy, ill appearance, poor feeding, and jaundice may be the initial complaints. The classic radiographic appearance is that of bilateral alveolar densities with air bronchograms.[13] However, the chest radiograph may be normal in up to 15% of cases.[14]

Empirical antibiotic coverage consists of intravenous ampicillin 100 mg/kg per dose every 12 hours. Intravenous gentamicin is given according to gestational age. For infants born after 35 weeks of gestation, the dose is 4 mg/kg every 24 hours; for those born between 30 and 35 weeks of gestation, the dose is 3.5 mg/kg every 24 hours.[15] In cases of late onset neonatal pneumonia, some authorities would recommend using intravenous vancomycin 15 mg/kg every 12 hours instead of ampicillin until culture results are available.[16] If herpes simplex virus pneumonia is suspected, intravenous acyclovir 20 mg/kg every 8 hours (in infants with normal renal function) should be started.[17] All neonates with pneumonia should be admitted to the hospital.

STRIDOR

Stridor is a symptom of upper airway obstruction. It is caused by anatomic narrowing of the airway from either intrinsic or extrinsic causes. It may be a fixed narrowing that is not worsening and therefore not dangerous, or it may be a progressive narrowing that requires immediate airway control.

The phase of respiration in which the stridor occurs helps localize the site of the lesion. Inspiratory stridor points to a lesion above the glottis, such as laryngomalacia. Biphasic stridor occurs from lesions at the level of the glottis or the subglottic area; the most common lesions in this area are vocal cord paralysis and subglottic stenosis. Expiratory stridor localizes the lesion to the area below the thoracic inlet. Tracheomalacia is a lesion that causes expiratory stridor.

Table 18-5 CAUSES OF NEONATAL PNEUMONIA

Onset of Pneumonia	Bacterial Causes	Viral Causes
Early	Group B streptococci (most common) *Escherichia coli* *Klebsiella* *Staphylococcus aureus* *Streptococcus pneumoniae* *Listeria monocytogenes* *Mycobacterium tuberculosis* *Ureaplasma urealyticum*	Herpes simplex virus (most common) Adenovirus Enteroviruses Cytomegalovirus Rubella
Late	*S. aureus* *Streptococcus pyogenes* *S. pneumoniae* *E. coli* *Klebsiella* *Chlamydia trachomatis*	Respiratory syncytial virus (most common) Rhinovirus Adenovirus Enterovirus Influenza Parainfluenza

Table 18-6 DIFFERENTIAL DIAGNOSIS FOR STRIDOR IN THE NEONATE

Intrinsic lesions	Larynx: Laryngomalacia Infection (laryngitis) Vocal cord paralysis Laryngeal web Laryngocele or laryngeal cyst Laryngotracheal esophageal cleft Foreign body Trachea: Tracheomalacia Tracheal stenosis Tracheoesophageal fistula Subglottic hemangioma Tracheal web
Extrinsic compression	Vascular ring Anomalous innominate artery Mediastinal mass Esophageal foreign body
Other	Macroglossia Gastroesophageal reflux

The initial goal of the physical examination is an assessment of the level of respiratory distress. Vital signs, pulse oximetry readings, work of breathing, skin color, and activity of the child should be observed. If respiratory distress is present, it is best not to manipulate the child too much unless emergency airway interventions are necessary. Otherwise, the EP should perform the physical examination in conjunction with an otorhinolaryngologist or pediatric surgeon, who can obtain a surgical airway immediately in a controlled setting (operating suite).

The stridorous infant without severe distress should be examined by the EP. Radiographs of the chest and soft tissues of the neck are indicated. The definitive diagnostic test is direct laryngoscopy by a pediatric otorhinolaryngologist. Table 18-6 lists the differential diagnosis for neonatal stridor.

Laryngomalacia is the most common cause of stridor in infants. Stridor due to laryngomalacia starts soon after birth and is exacerbated by crying, agitation, and a supine position. This disorder is generally benign and self-limiting. The stridor worsens with upper respiratory tract infections, occasionally necessitating hospital admission for supportive care. Less than 10% of patients with laryngomalacia have significant respiratory or feeding problems that mandate epiglottoplasty or tracheotomy.

Vocal cord paralysis is the next most common cause of neonatal stridor.[18] It can be unilateral or bilateral. Unilateral cord paralysis usually requires conservative treatment, such as monitoring oxygen saturation and observing for aspiration secondary to an incompetent glottis. Half of infants with bilateral vocal cord paralysis need tracheotomy. The majority of vocal cord paralysis cases are idiopathic. A central nervous system cause should be sought in bilateral vocal cord paralysis.

The neonate with stridor should be admitted to the hospital unless the EP is certain that the child is stable and the cause of the stridor is not progressing.

■ ACYANOTIC CARDIAC CONDITIONS

Acyanotic cardiac conditions can manifest as tachypnea in the first month of life. They include three ductus-dependent obstructive left-sided heart lesions (coarctation of the aorta, critical aortic stenosis, and hypoplastic left ventricle), tachycardias, and neonatal myocarditis. The respiratory distress in cardiac conditions frequently manifests as tachypnea without labored breathing and associated with diaphoresis when feeding.

Coarctation of the aorta, critical aortic stenosis, and hypoplastic left ventricle cause tachypnea by increasing pulmonary blood flow secondary to left-to-right shunting. Diagnosis is made from the following findings: decrease to absence of peripheral pulses, wet lungs, evidence of systemic hypoperfusion, and, occasionally, a heart murmur. The only nonoperative way to maintain adequate systemic circulation is to keep the ductus arteriosus patent by administration of a continuous infusion of prostaglandin E_1 (alprostadil). The initial dose is 0.1 μg/kg/min IV with a maintenance dose titrated to the lowest dose effective in maintaining patency.[19] The EP should be ready to treat the side effects—apnea, hypotension, fever, and seizure—but should not allow appearance of the side effects to influence discontinuation of this lifesaving treatment.[20]

Fever

Fever is defined as a rectal temperature equal to or higher than 38°C or 100.4°F. The majority of febrile illnesses in infants are self-limiting viral infections. However 10% to 20% of febrile infants younger than 3 months have a *serious bacterial infection,* defined as bacterial meningitis, bacteremia, urinary tract infection, pneumonia, skin or soft tissue infection, bacterial enteritis, septic arthritis, or osteomyelitis. Bacteremia is twice as likely to occur in the first month of life as in the second month.[21]

The neonate's immature immune system lacks the ability to localize and contain infection. The immature neurologic system does not allow the newborn to show specific signs of serious underlying disease. The birth process exposes the infant to an array of bacterial and viral pathogens. The most common bacterial pathogens in the first 28 days of life are group B streptococci and *E. coli.* Other bacteria may be gram-negative organisms (e.g., *Klebsiella, Enterobacter, Salmonella*) or gram-positive (*S. aureus, Enterococcus,* other streptococcal species, and *Listeria monocytogenes*). Herpes simplex virus and the enteroviruses can also cause febrile illness in the neonate.

Authorities agree that all febrile children younger than 28 days should undergo a septic evaluation

BOX 18-4

Septic Work-up for Febrile Infant Less than 28 Days Old

1. Complete blood count with differential
2. Blood culture
3. Urinalysis—catheter or suprapubic
4. Urine culture
5. Lumbar puncture—cell count, glucose, protein, Gram stain
6. Cerebrospinal fluid culture
7. Chest radiograph (if symptoms of respiratory infection)
8. Stool for white blood cell count and culture and sensitivity (if diarrhea present)

BOX 18-6

Empirical Antibiotic Therapy for Term Neonates 8 to 28 Days Old with Fever

Ampicillin
200 mg/kg/day divided q6h (50 mg/kg/dose)
and
Gentamicin 4 mg/kg/day once-daily dosing
OR
Ampicillin
200 mg/kg/day divided q6h (50 mg/kg/dose)
and
Cefotaxime
150 mg/kg/day divided q8h (50 mg/kg/dose)

Box 18-4 and should be admitted to the hospital for parenteral antibiotics. Outpatient protocols with and without antibiotics have been published for infants older than 1 month.

Empirical antibiotic treatment for neonatal sepsis consists of either ampicillin and gentamicin or ampicillin and cefotaxime (Boxes 18-5 and 18-6). If neonatal meningitis is suspected, ampicillin and cefotaxime are preferred. Some authorities would add gentamicin as a third antibiotic in suspected meningitis when no organisms are seen on Gram stain of the cerebrospinal fluid.[22]

Does the neonate with fever but an identifiable viral source of infection (e.g., respiratory syncytial virus) need a septic evaluation and empirical antibiotic therapy? Several studies have shown that the risk for serious bacterial infection is less in infants in whom a viral infection can be identified than in infants in whom such identification is not possible, yet the risk remains as high as 7% in certain groups who are "viral positive."[23-26] Therefore, a septic evaluation should be performed in any child 1 to 28 days old with fever despite an identifiable viral infection. Empirical antibiotics should be given to this group until culture results are available.

Herpes simplex virus infection should be strongly considered in febrile infants with seizures and abnormal cerebrospinal fluid results. Skin lesions and abnormal liver function values should further increase suspicion for this disorder. An infant with suspected herpes simplex virus infection should receive acyclovir 60 mg/kg/day in 3 divided doses (20 mg/kg/dose).

BOX 18-5

Empirical Antibiotic Therapy for Term Neonates Younger Than 7 Days with Fever

Ampicillin
200 mg/kg/day divided q12h (100 mg/kg/dose)
and
Gentamicin 4 mg/kg/day once-daily dosing
OR
Ampicillin
200 mg/kg/day divided q12h (100 mg/kg/dose)
and
Cefotaxime
100 mg/kg/day divided q12h (50 mg/kg/dose)

Gastrointestinal Complaints

■ VOMITING

Vomiting is defined as *forceful* diaphragmatic and abdominal wall contraction with simultaneous relaxation of the stomach, gastroesophageal sphincter, and esophagus, and closure of the gastric pylorus. *Regurgitation,* or "spitting up," is a *nonforceful reflux* of milk or gastric contents into the mouth. Regurgitation is generally a benign disorder but occasionally can be associated with gastroesophageal reflux disease (GERD), which can have serious consequences such as apnea. The causes of vomiting can be divided into anatomic and nonanatomic categories (Table 18-7).

The appearance of the vomitus is important. Bilious vomit suggests obstruction below the ampulla of Vater. Undigested milk may simply be regurgitation but could be caused by gastrointestinal obstruction above the ampulla of Vater. Bloody vomitus requires a search for upper gastrointestinal bleeding.

A healthy-appearing infant with appropriate weight gain and normal vital signs who is vomiting requires no diagnostic testing. Abdominal radiographs should be performed if there is a concern

Table 18-7 CAUSES OF NEONATAL VOMITING

Anatomic causes	Esophagus, trachea, great vessels: Stricture Web Tracheoesophageal fistula Laryngeal cleft Double aortic arch Stomach and duodenum: Pyloric stenosis Duodenal atresia (usually noted on first day of life) Small and large intestine: Volvulus secondary to malrotation Incarcerated hernia Hirschsprung's disease (secondary to obstipation) Necrotizing enterocolitis Genitourinary: Testicular torsion
Nonanatomic causes	Infection: Septicemia Meningitis Urinary tract infection Gastroenteritis Otitis media? Increased intracranial pressure: Cerebral edema Subdural hematoma Hydrocephalus Brain tumor Congenital adrenal hyperplasia (salt-losing variety) Inborn errors of metabolism Renal disease

about obstruction. In dehydrated and toxic infants, complete blood count, serum glucose and electrolyte measurements, and a septic evaluation should be performed.

If the infant is moderately or severely dehydrated, intravenous 0.9% sodium chloride should be given in a 20 mL/kg bolus. Oral rehydration may be tried in a mildly dehydrated infant. Nasogastric decompression is required for intestinal obstruction. Empirical therapy with ampicillin and gentamicin or ampicillin and cefotaxime should be administered for suspected sepsis.

Infants with regurgitation may be managed as outpatients. Children younger than 28 days with true vomiting should be admitted to the hospital for further evaluation and treatment

■ DIARRHEA

Diarrhea is defined as an increase in both the number and the looseness or wateriness of stools. Even in the neonatal period, diarrhea tends to be self-limited and without significant morbidity. Viral infections are common, with rotavirus being the most frequent cause. Other viral causes of diarrhea are enterovirus, enteric adenovirus, and coronavirus. Bacterial diarrhea that occurs in neonates is caused by the same organisms as in other age groups. They include *Salmonella, Shigella, Campylobacter, E. coli, Vibrio, Yersinia,* and *Clostridium difficile.*

Salmonella gastroenteritis is potentially dangerous in the neonate because of its association with systemic sepsis. Bacteremia may occur in 30% to 50% of neonates infected with this organism. Diarrhea from *Salmonella* is usually watery with mucus and may appear bloody. This organism is an enteroinvasive bacteria (i.e., it invades the intestinal mucosa), so a methylene blue smear of a stool specimen will reveal white blood cells. Neonates with *Salmonella* gastroenteritis should be treated with cefotaxime 50 mg/kg per dose.

Necrotizing enterocolitis is one of the more dangerous causes of neonatal diarrhea. It is classically seen in the premature infant but can occur in the term neonate. Incidence is also higher in infants with congenital heart disease.[27] The diarrhea is typically bloody and is associated with other symptoms, such as decreased feeding, vomiting, ileus, and abdominal distention. If not treated, symptoms progress to bradycardia, hypothermia, apnea, hypotension, and death. The diagnostic radiographic findings are pneumatosis intestinalis (air in the bowel wall) and air in the portal vein. Intestinal perforation leads to pneumoperitoneum. Treatment involves cessation of oral feedings, nasogastric decompression, intravenous fluids, and antibiotics (ampicillin, cefotaxime, clindamycin).

Neonatal Jaundice

Jaundice is the yellow color that results from the accumulation of bilirubin, a breakdown product of the hemoglobin molecule. It is most noticeable in the sclera and skin and can generally be detected when

BOX 18-7

Criteria for Physiologic Jaundice

- Jaundice occurs after the 24 hours of life.
- Serum bilirubin level rises no faster than 0.5 mg/dL/hr or 5 mg/dL/day.
- Total bilirubin value does not exceed 15 mg/dL in a term neonate or 10 mg/dL in a preterm neonate.
- There is no evidence of acute hemolysis.
- Jaundice does not persist longer than 10 days in a term neonate or 21 days in a preterm neonate.*

*Breastfed infants may remain jaundiced up to 2 weeks longer.

the serum bilirubin level reaches about 5 mg/dL. In almost all newborns, the bilirubin level is 2 to 3 mg/dL in the first few days of life. Around 60% of full-term infants and 80% of premature infants have clinical jaundice. Jaundice can be normal (physiologic) or abnormal (nonphysiologic). Box 18-7 lists the criteria for physiologic jaundice.

Hemoglobin degrades to form unconjugated bilirubin. This unconjugated (indirect bilirubin) is lipid soluble and binds to albumin. The bilirubin that is not bound to albumin can cross the blood-brain barrier and injure the brain (kernicterus). Albumin-bound unconjugated bilirubin is transported to the liver and converted to water-soluble conjugated bilirubin (direct bilirubin). Conjugated bilirubin is excreted into the bile and then into the gut. Most bilirubin is eliminated from the gut in the stool.

Physiologic jaundice usually becomes visible on the second or third day of life. It is thought to be secondary to the higher breakdown of red blood cells in neonates and a transient slowing of conjugation processes in the liver. It peaks at levels between 5 and 12 mg/dL on the third or fourth day of life and then starts to decline. Risk factors for higher levels of physiologic hyperbilirubinemia include family history of neonatal jaundice, breastfeeding, bruising and cephalohematoma, maternal age greater than 25 years, Asian ethnicity, prematurity, weight loss, and delayed bowel movement. *Jaundice in the first 24 hours of life is always abnormal.*

Breast milk jaundice develops after the seventh day of life and peaks during the second or third week. It is postulated that a glucuronidase in the breast milk causes increased enterohepatic absorption of the unconjugated bilirubin. Because of its late onset, breast milk jaundice is almost never a neurologic threat.

Laboratory tests are indicated in a jaundiced infant unless the EP is absolutely sure that the jaundice is physiologic. A total serum bilirubin measurement (of both direct and indirect components) and a complete blood count are required. A Coombs test for autoimmune hemolysis is indicated if the maternal blood type is Rh negative and the infant blood type is Rh positive, or if the maternal blood type is O and the fetal blood type is A, B, or AB. A reticulocyte count is useful for evaluating hemolytic anemia. Because jaundice can be the initial manifestation of hypothyroidism, measurements of serum thyroid-stimulating hormone and thyroxine may be helpful. If the neonate appears ill—has lethargy, decreased feeding, temperature instability, difficulty breathing—a septic evaluation is indicated. Measurement of glucose-6-phosphate dehydrogenase (G6PD), hemoglobin electrophoresis, and tests for pyruvate kinase deficiencies and galactosemia should be reserved for the pediatrician.

The early treatment of hyperbilirubinemia ensures adequate hydration and feeding. The breastfed infant should be fed more often, to promote stooling and excretion of bilirubin. Further management of hyperbilirubinemia may involve phototherapy or exchange transfusion. Initiation of these therapies depends on several factors, including the total serum bilirubin level and the infant's birth weight and age. Some preterm infants are at higher risk for neurologic sequelae and mandate a lower threshold for initiation of phototherapy. This complicated group of higher-risk infants includes those with perinatal asphyxia, acidosis, hypoxia, hypothermia, hypoalbuminemia, meningitis, intraventricular hemorrhage, hemolysis, hypoglycemia, and signs of kernicterus.

The American Academy of Pediatrics has practice guidelines for the treatment of neonatal jaundice.[28] Only well-appearing neonates with clearly physiologic or breast milk jaundice and a serum bilirubin level below the guideline limits for phototherapy should be discharged. Close follow-up and monitoring should be arranged for such infants at the time of discharge. All other infants should be admitted for further testing.

REFERENCES

1. Stoll BJ, Kliegman RM: The newborn infant. In Behrman RE, Kliegman RM, Jenson HB (eds): Nelson Textbook of Pediatrics, 17th ed. Philadelphia, WB Saunders, 2004, p 523.
2. National Center for Health Statistics: 1999 period linked birth/infant death data. Prepared by March of Dimes Perinatal Data Center, 2002. http://www.cdc.gov/nchs/data/nvsr52/nvsr52_03.pdf.
3. National Institutes of Health: National Institutes of Health Consensus Development Conference on Infantile Apnea and Home Monitoring Consensus Statement. Pediatrics 1987;79:292-299.
4. Baird T: Clinical correlates, natural history and outcome of neonatal apnoea. Semin Neonatol 2004;9:205-211.
5. Brand DA, Altman RL, Purtill K, Edwards KS: Yield of diagnostic testing in infants who have had an apparent life-threatening event. Pediatrics 2005;115:885-893.
6. Pitetti RD, Lovallo A, Hickey R: Prevalence of anemia in children presenting with apparent life-threatening events. Acad Emerg Med 2005;12:926-931.
7. Michelsson K, Rinne A, Paajanen S: Crying, feeding and sleeping patterns in 1 to 12-month-old infants. Child Care Health Dev 1990;16:99-111.

8. Long T: Excessive infantile crying: A review of the literature. J Child Health Care 2001;5:111-116.
9. Metcalf TJ, Irons TG, Sher LD, Young PC: Simethicone in the treatment of infant colic: A randomized, placebo-controlled, multicenter trial. Pediatrics 1994;94:29-34.
10. Lucassen PL, Assendelft WJ, Gubbels JW, et al: Effectiveness of treatments for infantile colic: Systematic review [published erratum appears in BMJ 1998;317:171]. BMJ 1998; 316:1563-1569.
11. Poole S: The infant with acute, unexplained, excessive crying. Pediatrics 1991;88:450-455.
12. Lim DS, Kulik TJ, Kim DW: Aminophylline for the prevention of apnea during prostaglandin E_1 infusion. Pediatrics 2003;112:e27-e29.
13. Haney PJ, Bohlman M, Sun CC: Radiographic findings in neonatal pneumonia. AJR Am J Roentgenol 1984; 143:23-26.
14. Mathur NV, Garg K, Kumar S: Respiratory distress in neonates with special reference to pneumonia. Indian Pediatr 2002;39:529-537.
15. Hansen A, Forbes P, Arnold A, O'Rourke E: Once-daily gentamicin dosing for the preterm and term newborn: Proposal for a simple regimen that achieves target levels. J Perinatol 2003;23:635-639.
16. Speer ME: Neonatal pneumonia. UpToDate 2005.
17. American Academy of Pediatrics: Herpes simplex. In Pickering LK (ed): Red Book: 2003 Report of the Committee on Infectious Disease, 26th ed. Elk Grove Village, IL, American Academy of Pediatrics, 2003, p 344.
18. Mancuso RF: Stridor in neonates. Pediatr Clin North Am 1996;43:1339-1356.
19. Schamberger MS: Cardiac emergencies in children. Pediatr Ann 1996;25:339-344.
20. Brierley J: Congenital cardiac emergencies. Hosp Med 2005;66:46-50.
21. Berman S: Acute fever in infants younger than three months. In Pediatric Decision Making, 4th ed. Philadelphia, Mosby, 2003.
22. Byington CL, Rittichier KK, Bassett KE, et al: Serious bacterial infections in febrile infants younger than 90 days of age: The importance of ampicillin-resistant pathogens. Pediatrics 2003;111:964-968.
23. Byington CL, Enriquez FR, Hoff C, et al: Serious bacterial infections in febrile infants 1 to 90 days old with and without viral infections. Pediatrics 2004;113:1662-1666.
24. Melendez E, Harper MB: Utility of sepsis evaluation in infants 90 days of age or younger with fever and clinical bronchiolitis. Pediatr Infect Dis J 2003;22:1053-1056.
25. Antonow JA, Hansen K, McKinstry CA, et al: Sepsis evaluations in hospitalized infants with bronchiolitis. Pediatr Infect Dis J 1998;17:231-236.
26. Levine DA, Platt SL, Dayan PS, et al: Risk of serious bacterial infection in young febrile infants with respiratory syncytial virus infections. Pediatrics 2004;113:1728-1734.
27. McElhinney DB, Hedrick HL, Bush DM: Necrotizing enterocolitis in neonates with congenital heart disease: Risk factors and outcomes. Pediatrics 2000;106:1080-1087.
28. American Academy of Pediatrics, Provisional Committee for Quality Improvement and Subcommittee on Hyperbilirubinemia: Practice parameter: Management of hyperbilirubinemia in the healthy term newborn. [erratum in Pediatrics 1995;95(3):458-61]. Pediatrics 1994;94:558-565.

Chapter **19**

Infants and Toddlers

Mark McIntosh

KEY POINTS

Intussusception, trauma, and ingestion should be considered when the etiology of persistent vomiting is unclear. Vomiting does not always imply infectious gastroenteritis.

Bilious emesis or peritonitis in small children requires emergency surgical consultation.

Oral rehydration therapy is indicated for mild to moderate dehydration due to gastroenteritis.

Young children have less respiratory reserve and progress to respiratory distress and failure more rapidly than older children or adults.

Hypoxemia and hypoventilation may result in cardiopulmonary arrest in infants and toddlers.

The cough reflex can be induced by stimulation of pulmonary or extrapulmonary chemical receptors.

Physical abuse is the leading cause of serious head injury in young children.

When the cause of altered mental status is not obvious, the EP should maintain a high level of suspicion for abuse, accidental toxin ingestion or exposure, intussusception, infection, and nonconvulsive seizure activity.

Vomiting

■ SCOPE

Vomiting in children is usually caused by a self-limiting condition but may be the result of a severe, life-threatening illness. A systematic approach based on age-specific considerations is critical to the appropriate diagnosis and treatment of infants and toddlers who are presented with vomiting. The EP should consider an expanded differential diagnosis in a child who comes to the ED with vomiting but no diarrheal illness.

■ EPIDEMIOLOGY

Episodes of acute gastroenteritis in children younger than 5 years lead to 2 to 3 million physician visits annually.[1] The majority of these children have uneventful clinical courses.

■ PATHOPHYSIOLOGY

Vomiting, the forceful expulsion of gastric contents through the mouth, is coordinated by the vomiting center in the reticular formation of the medulla. This

Documentation

INFANT OR TODDLER IN THE ED

Document consideration of life-threatening diagnoses.

Create a word picture of the child: minor or serious illness; for example:

"Child is playful, interactive, and taking bottle or fluids well."

"Well-hydrated, non-toxic, and no evidence of trauma, sepsis, meningitis, or distress."

"Alert, good tone, moving all extremities."

"Appropriately cries but can be consoled by caregivers."

vomiting center integrates and responds to afferent pathways from higher cortical centers in the brain and visceral afferents from receptors in the gastrointestinal tract and other organs. Specifically, the chemoreceptor trigger zone in the floor of the fourth ventricle monitors chemical abnormalities in the blood and cerebrospinal fluid. Drugs such as chemotherapeutic agents and metabolic aberrations (e.g., uremia, diabetic ketoacidosis) act at the level of the chemoreceptor trigger zone. A basic understanding of these major pathways is essential for developing diagnostic and treatment strategies for infants and toddlers with vomiting.

■ CLINICAL PRESENTATION

A review of the expansive list of potential causes of vomiting emphasizes the importance of developing an organized approach to achieve an accurate diagnosis. The EP should first elicit an AMPLIFIEDD history (Box 19-1) and perform a thorough "head-to-toe" physical examination focusing on the age of the infant or toddler. Associated evidence of bowel obstruction or peritonitis and signs or symptoms suggestive of extraintestinal disease should be sought. Hydration status (Box 19-2) should be assessed, and a risk of future dehydration established through quantification of the frequency and amount of vomitus and diarrhea, if present. At the onset of the clinical encounter, the EP should clarify whether child has had bilious or nonbilious vomiting. Bilious emesis in infants should be attributed to intestinal obstruction unless proven otherwise and requires immediate surgical consultation.[2] Bilious vomiting due to malrotation with volvulus, leading to bowel ischemia, is associated with high rates of morbidity and mortality.

The child should be assessed for abnormal behavior and appearance, such as a decrease in activity or level of consciousness, which might indicate more serious illness. Vital signs should be reviewed for clues of systemic disease. A bulging fontanel suggests increased intracranial pressure due to meningitis, trauma, or intracranial mass or bleeding. Retinal hemorrhages or scleral icterus, suggestive of non-accidental trauma or hepatobiliary disease, respectively, should be sought. An unusual odor may be the first clue of an inborn error of metabolism. Marked abdominal distention, peristaltic waves, increased bowel sounds, palpable masses, bloody stools, and guarding all point to an intra-abdominal disorder. The child should be undressed and examined to exclude torsion of the testis and the ambiguous genitalia associated with congenital adrenal hyperplasia. The skin should be examined for rashes that raise suspicion for an infectious etiology or even sepsis. The child should be evaluated for unusual contusions or musculoskeletal injury that may evidence trauma.

■ DIFFERENTIAL DIAGNOSIS

The list of potential causes of vomiting in infants is extensive but can be conveniently organized according to age-related categories (Table 19-1). Young infants, from birth to the first few months of life, commonly experience reflux exacerbated by overfeeding. However, many other serious medical conditions may initially manifest as vomiting, including infectious causes such as sepsis, meningitis, urinary tract infections, and hepatitis. These conditions must be differentiated from urgent and emergency surgical conditions such as pyloric stenosis, incarcerated hernia, intussusception, and malrotation with volvulus. Older infants and children experience some of the same diseases, although intussusception is the most common cause of intestinal obstruction among those 3 months to 5 years old, whereas appendicitis is the most common condition requiring surgical intervention.[3,4]

■ DIAGNOSTIC TESTING

The large numbers of potential causes of vomiting make routine laboratory and radiographic evaluation impractical. History and physical finding should direct the choice of testing for each patient. For most common conditions causing vomiting, laboratory testing is not indicated. A bedside finger-stick (or heel-stick) glucose measurement should be performed in any child with an alteration in mental status. Serum electrolytes should be measured in children with dehydration requiring intravenous rehydration. A serum bicarbonate level lower than 17 mEq/L appears to be the most useful laboratory value for predicting the likelihood of 5% dehydration.[5,6] Electrolyte abnormalities are associated with pyloric stenosis as well as metabolic and renal diseases. An elevated white blood cell count is associated with bacterial infections and sepsis but lacks sensitivity and specificity. Cerebrospinal fluid analysis should be performed if there is suspicion of meningitis or encephalitis. Drug screening may be necessary to

BOX 19-1

The "AMPLIFIEDD" History for an Infant or Toddler with Vomiting

Allergies: to medications or foods (protein intolerance to cow milk, soy, gluten)

Medications: prescription, over-the-counter, or "natural remedies"

Past medical history:

- Chronic or previous illness: metabolic or endocrinopathy, recent unresolved illness
- Prior surgery, suggesting abdominal adhesions, shunt infection, or obstruction
- Newborn screen: identify abnormalities
- Appropriate developmental milestones?

Last "feed, pee, poop, sleep":

- Feed: diet, amount, and frequency; correct formula preparation; recent changes; types of solids
- Pee and poop: urine output and characterization of stooling pattern (diarrhea, blood, mucus)
- Sleep pattern: waking with intermittent episodes of pain (intussusception)

Immediate events (history of the present illness and review of systems)—OLD CAARS:

- *O*nset of vomiting
- *L*ocation of pain (e.g., abdomen or head)
- *D*uration and frequency of vomiting: estimate ongoing volume loss by quantifying number and quantity of vomiting or diarrheal episodes
- *C*haracterize the emesis:
  - Contents: undigested gastric contents (reflux), bilious (postampullary obstruction), feculent (colonic obstruction), blood or "coffee ground" (gastritis, ulcer, Mallory Weiss tear)
  - Force of vomiting: Projectile (pyloric stenosis), non-projectile (reflux, postfeed regurgitation)
- *A*ggravating factors: What factors exacerbate the vomiting (early morning: central nervous system mass; feeding: food allergen, after ingestion of toxin)?
- *A*lleviating factors: What factors relieve the vomiting (keeping child in upright position: reflux)?
- *R*ecurrent: similar episodes suggestive of recurring disorders (pyloric stenosis, cyclical vomiting, inborn error of metabolism, malrotation with intermittent volvulus)
- *S*ystem review: inquire about fever, trauma, neurologic symptoms (headache, vertigo, visual symptoms), diarrhea (infectious gastroenteritis), ingestion of toxins

Family/social history:

- Infectious contacts, travel
- Characterize caretaker-infant interactions: identify risk for child abuse

Immunizations: up to date?

EMT history: elicit history from emergency medical personnel for potential trauma, ingestion, abuse, or toxin exposure

Doctor: name of primary care physician or specialist to contact for additional information and help

Documents: obtain prior medical records

BOX 19-2

Key Objective Physical Findings for Assessing Dehydration

Presence of two findings indicates >5% dehydration; presence of three or more findings indicates >10% dehydration:

- Capillary refill time >2 seconds
- Dry mucous membranes
- Absence of tears
- Abnormally lethargic or listless appearance

Adapted from Gorelick M, Shaw K, Murphy K: Validity and reliability of clinical signs in the diagnosis of dehydration in children. Pediatrics 1997;99:e6.

confirm an ingestion. Urinalysis, liver function test, and serum lipase and ammonia measurements should be considered when the differential diagnosis is broadened.

Diagnostic imaging is also dictated by clinical findings. Computed tomography (CT) of the head should be performed to evaluate for closed-head injury, intracranial tumor, or hydrocephalus. Plain radiographs may be used to assess for bowel obstruction. An upper gastrointestinal (GI) series is the preferred radiographic modality for diagnosing malrotation with volvulus.[7] Diagnostic ultrasonography is the modality of choice for diagnosing pyloric stenosis and intussusception.[8] Ultrasonography and abdominal CT are used to investigate potential appendicitis when the diagnosis is in question. In children with equivocal findings for appendicitis,

Table 19-1 DIFFERENTIAL DIAGNOSIS OF CAUSES OF VOMITING IN INFANTS AND CHILDREN USING THE "HEAD-TO-TOE" MEMORY TOOL

	Infants	Toddlers
Head	Meningitis/encephalitis Central nervous system (CNS) mass Head injury Hydrocephalus (i.e., shunt malfunction) Otitis media Oral ingestion (overdose) "Spitting up"	Meningitis/encephalitis CNS mass Head injury Hydrocephalus Otitis media Oral ingestion (overdose) Cyclic vomiting Psychogenic
Chest	Post-tussive emesis due to reactive airways Respiratory infection (pneumonia)	Posttussive emesis due to reactive airways Respiratory infection (pneumonia)
Abdomen Gastrointestinal tract	Gastroesophageal reflux disease Gastroenteritis Nutrient intolerance Rumination Obstruction: Pyloric stenosis Intussusception Malrotation Incarcerated hernia Hirschsprung's disease Peritonitis	Peptic ulcer disease Gastroenteritis Obstruction: Intussusception Malrotation Incarcerated hernia Hirschsprung's disease Appendicitis Meckel's diverticulum Peritonitis
Adrenal glands	Congenital adrenal hyperplasia	Adrenal Insufficiency
Renal system	Uremia Obstruction Urinary tract infection or pyelonephritis Renal insufficiency	Uremia Obstruction Urinary tract infection or pyelonephritis Renal insufficiency
Liver	Hepatitis Inborn errors of metabolism	Hepatitis Inborn errors of metabolism
Pancreas	Diabetic ketoacidosis Pancreatitis	Diabetic ketoacidosis Pancreatitis
Other	Sepsis	Sepsis

ultrasonography using the graded-compression technique should be performed, followed by focused abdominal CT if ultrasonographic findings are normal.[9] Similarly, implement protocols for appropriate use of ultrasonography and CT for evaluation of intra-abdominal pathology such as trauma, intra-abdominal mass, or nephrolithiasis.

■ TREATMENT

Initial management of the vomiting infant or toddler should focus on stabilization if signs and symptoms are consistent with shock. Persistent vomiting, severe dehydration, and electrolyte abnormalities necessitate treatment in parallel with other diagnostic testing. Rehydration is accomplished with intravenous 20-mL/kg boluses of isotonic saline that are repeated as indicated. Treatment should be directed toward the underlying cause.

A surgeon should be consulted immediately for infants presenting with bilious vomiting. Malrotation with volvulus is a surgical emergency requiring rapid response to prevent infarction of the bowel. Timely surgical consultation is also the standard of care for other conditions, such as peritonitis, incarcerated hernia, and pyloric stenosis. In selected cases the radiologist may be able to successfully reduce the intussuscepted bowel with an air or contrast enema, although surgical "backup" is required in case such treatment fails or complications occur. Children with ileus or bowel obstruction should undergo decompression with nasogastric suctioning.

Most infants and children with vomiting do well with oral rehydration alone. Administration of an antiemetic may serve as a successful adjunct to suppress vomiting and allow for oral rehydration. Intravenous and oral ondansetron (a selective [5-HT_3] receptor antagonist) have been successfully used in the ED in infants and children with gastroenteritis.[10,11]

Oral rehydration therapy (ORT) should be administered in children with mild to moderate dehydration due to gastroenteritis (Box 19-3).[12] A meta-analysis of randomized control trials involving 1545 children younger than 15 in 11 countries compared ORT with intravenous hydration. This study concluded that enteral rehydration by the oral or nasogastric route is as effective as if not better than intravenous rehydration.[13]

BOX 19-3

Oral Rehydration Therapy

Rehydration Phase

1. Replace fluid deficit over 4 hours using rehydrating solution (Rehydralyte, Pedialyte).
2. Administer oral rehydration solution (ORS) in frequent, small amounts: no more than 5 mL every 1 to 2 minutes using syringe, spoon, cup, or nasogastric tube. Goal: 50 mL/kg in mild dehydration, 100 mL/kg in moderate dehydration.
3. Replace ongoing losses from diarrhea (10 mL/kg/watery stool) and vomiting (2 mL/kg/episode of emesis) with ORS.
4. Avoid giving nonphysiologic foods like sports drinks, juices, tea, and colas during this phase.

Maintenance Phase

Begin realimentation with goal to return to unrestricted age-appropriate diet.

Data from Practice parameter: The management of acute gastroenteritis in young children. American Academy of Pediatrics, Provisional Committee on Quality Improvement, Subcommittee on Acute Gastroenteritis. Pediatrics 1996;97:428-429.

■ DISPOSITION

The infant or toddler with a self-limiting condition and no evidence of systemic illness or dehydration can be discharged. The parents or caregiver should be given clear plans for follow-up and instructions for outpatient oral rehydration as indicated. The EP should confirm that the caretaker understands that he or she should return the child to the ED if there is any progression of illness.

Infants or children with persistent vomiting, abnormal electrolyte values, or a more complex diagnosis requiring further medical or surgical management should be admitted. The EP should communicate a concise summary of diagnostic and therapeutic interventions and any ongoing concerns to consultants prior to transferring the patient to their care.

PARENT TEACHING TIPS

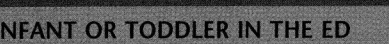

INFANT OR TODDLER IN THE ED

- Confirm that parents understand diagnosis, treatment, follow-up plans, and any symptoms that warrant immediate return to the ED.
- Reinforce that parents are always welcome to return to the ED with any concern.

Cough

■ SCOPE

Cough is usually a symptom of minor respiratory infection in infants and toddlers, although it may also appear in more serious illnesses, which must be recognized early and appropriately treated. Respiratory difficulties in this age group can rapidly progress to respiratory failure, the most common cause of cardiopulmonary arrest in children. Young children have higher metabolic demands and less respiratory reserve than older children or adults and so progress to distress and even failure more rapidly when hypoxia or hypoventilation occurs.

■ EPIDEMIOLOGY

Young children with respiratory symptoms are commonly presented to the ED. Respiratory infections encompass a wide variety of conditions that lack definitive end-point criteria by which to facilitate disease surveillance. A syndromic surveillance study of 39 EDs in New York City showed that, of all children presenting for evaluation and treatment, 5.8% were diagnosed with viral "colds," 13.3% with other respiratory illnesses, and 4.9% with asthma.[14]

Aspiration can also induce cough, leading to respiratory compromise. Foreign body obstruction after aspiration or ingestion with external compression of the upper airway can be immediately life-threatening. The most common products aspirated by young children are food products such as peanuts, nuts, candy, and hot dogs.[15]

■ PATHOPHYSIOLOGY

A cough is produced by a complex reflex arc that facilitates the clearance of secretions and inhaled particles that are irritating to the respiratory tract. The cough reflex may also be initiated by a variety of extrapulmonary disorders through stimulation of receptors in the esophagus, stomach, diaphragm, pericardium, or external ear. Therefore, the causes of cough encompass a broad differential diagnosis consisting of respiratory and nonrespiratory problems.

The upper airways of young children are narrow and more susceptible than the adult's to obstruction from excessive secretions, localized edema, foreign bodies, external compression, or mechanical constriction. The chest wall is more compliant in the young child than in older children or adults, making the diaphragm less effective (a reason for paradoxic breathing or "see-saw respirations").

■ CLINICAL PRESENTATION

Cough can be classified as either an acute or chronic symptom. The most common and most life-threatening coughs manifest an acute onset.

An AMPLIFIEDD history should be obtained to gather the essential data for reaching an accurate

BOX 19-4

The AMPLIFIEDD History for an Infant or Toddler with Cough

Allergies to medications, food, or environmental allergens

Medications: prescription, over-the-counter, or "natural remedies"

Past medical history:

- Birth history suggestive of prematurity
- Eczema
- Asthma, previous pulmonary infections
- Congenital heart disease

L—Relation of cough to "last" feed or associated with any feed

Immediate events (history of present illness and review of systems)—OLD CAARS:

- *O*nset: rapid or gradual? Age and conditions at onset of cough (e.g., present since birth)? Nocturnal cough or cough resolves at night
- *L*ocation: seems to originate from lower vs. upper airway?
- *D*uration: How long has the cough been present?
- *C*haracter: paroxysmal (pertussis), barking (croup), staccato (chlamydial pneumonia), loud-honking (psychogenic), brassy (tracheitis)
- *A*lleviating factors: What mitigates the cough (bronchodilators, antihistamines)?
- *A*ggravating factors: What aggravates the cough (triggers: allergens, smoke, cold, exercise)?
- *R*ecurrent: episodes of wheezing?
- *S*ystem review: Is cough associated with upper respiratory symptoms, fever, choking episode, chest pain, weight loss?

Family/social history:

- History of asthma, allergic or atopic disease, cystic fibrosis, immune deficiency
- Travel
- Smokers in home
- Exposure to pets

Immunizations up to date?

EMT history: elicit history from emergency medical personnel for potential trauma, ingestion, abuse, or toxin exposure

Doctor: name of primary care physician or specialist to contact for additional information and help

Documents: obtain prior medical records

diagnosis (Box 19-4). The timing and progression of symptoms should be established. Acute-onset coughing associated with a choking episode suggests foreign body aspiration. Rapid onset of cough may also be associated with anaphylaxis or trauma involving the airway, whereas a more gradual onset of cough with fever is more consistent with respiratory infection. Mild symptoms followed by rapid decompensation can occur with tracheitis or epiglottitis. Children with psychogenic cough often have a loud, honking type of cough that is absent during sleep. A primarily nocturnal cough may reflect reactive airway disease or sinusitis.

The caretaker should be asked to characterize the quality of the cough. A "barking" or "seal-like" cough reflects croup, whereas a paroxysmal cough followed by an inspiratory "whoop" is heard with pertussis. Triggers associated with the cough can give key diagnostic clues. Cough due to asthma is often triggered by exercise, cold exposure, allergens, or smoke. Children who have gastroesophageal reflux or the less common condition tracheoesophageal fistula cough during or after feeding.

The EP should focus on key elements of the past medical, family, and social histories. Premature infants with neonatal respiratory distress syndrome are at risk for bronchopulmonary dysplasia and chronic lung disease. Infants or toddlers with cough since birth may have a congenital anomaly causing an anatomic obstruction, such as a vascular ring or airway stenosis. A child with a family history of asthma or atopy has a higher risk for chronic cough due to reactive airway disease. A family history of cystic fibrosis can raise suspicion for this inherited, autosomal recessive disorder. Systemic factors associated with cough, such as headache and fever suggesting sinusitis or cough with weight loss suggestive of tuberculosis, should be reviewed. Cough with nasal congestion is often associated with a viral upper respiratory infection, but a protracted cough in a child with more systemic signs of illness may indicate a bacterial infection.

The infant or toddler with a cough should be assessed immediately for signs of respiratory compromise or failure. The general appearance and behavior of the child provide a rapid assessment of the work of breathing and the potential for respiratory failure. Evaluation for signs of distress is accomplished through inspection for tachypnea, nasal flaring, use of accessory muscles, or paradoxic ("see-saw") breathing.

The EP should characterize the sounds of the respiratory cycle. Prolongation of the inspiratory component of the respiratory cycle associated with stridor reflects extrathoracic obstruction. Prolongation of the expiratory cycle reflects intrathoracic obstruction and produces wheezing.

In children with respiratory distress, treatment should be initiated in parallel with a "head-to-toe" physical examination. The EP should evaluate for nasal congestion, rhinorrhea, or foreign body and listen for subtle inspiratory stridor or wheezing. Auscultation should be performed for rales, which can be associated with pneumonia, pulmonary edema, or chronic lung diseases such as bronchopulmonary dysplasia. Murmurs or extra heart sounds suggest cardiac disease. The abdominal examination may

Table 19-2 DIFFERENTIAL DIAGNOSIS OF COUGH IN INFANTS AND TODDLERS

	Acute Cough	Chronic Cough
Upper airway	Nasal congestion/postnasal drip Nasal foreign body Allergic rhinitis Acute viral upper respiratory infection (e.g., croup) Sinusitis/tonsillitis Epiglottitis Tracheitis Foreign body (aspiration, esophageal) Allergy/anaphylaxis Trauma Chemical irritation (e.g., smoke, fumes)	Laryngotracheomalacia Airway malformation (e.g., stenosis, webs) Tracheoesophageal fistula Cystic mass Tumors (e.g., polyp, hemangioma) Vascular compression (e.g., sling, rings)
Lower airway	Asthma/reactive airways (cough variant) Pneumonia (viral, bacterial, atypical—e.g., *Chlamydia,* tuberculosis) Pertussis Viral (e.g., bronchiolitis) Passive smoking Pulmonary edema (e.g., cardiogenic)	Chronic lung disease: Cystic fibrosis Bronchopulmonary dysplasia Pulmonary sequestration Bronchiectasis Tumors (mediastinal) Chronic infection (tuberculosis, fungal, parasitic) Interstitial lung disease
Other (cardiac, gastrointestinal)	Pulmonary edema Pulmonary emboli	Recurrent aspiration (gastroesophageal reflux) Psychogenic Granulomatous disease Medications (e.g., angiotensin-converting enzyme inhibitors) Foreign body in otic canal

show a liver edge consistent with hyperinflatio n or hepatomegaly seen in congestive heart failure. Skin findings consistent with eczema should raise the suspicion of asthma.

■ DIFFERENTIAL DIAGNOSIS

It is helpful to classify the causes of cough as acute or chronic, with emphasis on anatomic location, either along the pulmonary tree and/or with extrapulmonary involvement (Table 19-2).

Cough with stridor usually reflects some form of upper airway obstruction. Associated fever suggests an infectious process, whereas the acute onset of stridor in an otherwise healthy child should prompt concern for foreign body aspiration or inhalation of a chemical or environmental irritant. In infants and toddlers with chronic stridorous cough and no clearly associated infection, congenital airway malformations and vascular compression, including such anomalies as laryngomalacia, tracheal stenosis, and vascular rings or slings, should be considered.

■ INTERVENTIONS AND PROCEDURES

The child's anxiety should be alleviated and empirical therapy (such as the administration of supplemental oxygen and bronchodilators) should be initiated. In the case of acute respiratory decompensation, the airway should be secured to achieve adequate ventilation and oxygenation.

For complete airway obstruction in infants younger than 1 year, back blows and chest thrust are recommended; the Heimlich maneuver is reserved for older children.[16] Immediate laryngoscopy may enable the EP to directly visualize and remove an obstructing foreign body.[17] Children who have partial airway obstruction and adequate oxygenation and ventilation should be prepared for intraoperative bronchoscopic removal of a foreign body with general anesthesia.

■ DIAGNOSTIC TESTING

Thorough history and physical examination are generally adequate to make a diagnosis in most clinical situations of infants or toddlers presenting with cough. Pulse oximetry should be used to evaluate for hypoxemia. A screening chest radiograph should be ordered in children with focal auscultatory findings or if the diagnosis is uncertain.

When a nonradiopaque foreign body aspiration is suspected, right and left lateral decubitus radiographs may show air trapping. If no air trapping is noted and clinical findings are suggestive of aspiration, fluoroscopy or bronchoscopy should be performed.

Few laboratory tests are useful in the initial evaluation of the young child with a cough. Selective testing is dictated by history and physical examination in the pursuit of a specific diagnosis. A complete blood count with differential analysis may suggest diagnosis on occasion; findings of the differential

Documentation

INFANT OR TODDLER WITH A COUGH

Record consideration of foreign body aspiration as appropriate.

At time of discharge, document a repeat pulmonary examination that includes no evidence of respiratory distress, a respiratory rate within a normal range for age, and adequate oxygen saturation.

PARENT TEACHING TIPS

INFANT OR TODDLER WITH A COUGH

- Bringing the child back for any evidence of shortness of breath or distress
- Reinforcement of the importance of close follow-up
- Children with persistent cough will need further urgent evaluations

analysis could include a marked lymphocytosis with pertussis, eosinophilia in an allergic processes or parasitic disease, or neutrophilia in bacterial infection. Rapid assays are available to test nasopharyngeal aspirates or swab specimens for respiratory syncytial virus (RSV), influenza, and pertussis. The EP should arrange for sweat testing (pilocarpine iontophoresis method) in patients with history, signs, or symptoms suggestive of cystic fibrosis. The results of the tuberculin skin test may support the diagnosis of tuberculosis.

Other radiographic studies that may prove useful in selected children with cough are barium swallow (for tracheoesophageal fistula) and CT of the sinuses (sinusitis), neck (trauma), or chest (mediastinal mass, bronchiectasis, pulmonary sequestration). Many institutions are using magnetic resonance imaging (MRI) to evaluate for congenital vascular anomalies. In addition to cases of airway foreign body, bronchoscopy may be indicated for the evaluation of airway masses, atypical pneumonias, and airway anomalies. Specialists should be consulted early so they can help guide the diagnostic approach.

TREATMENT AND DISPOSITION

The underlying cause of the cough should be treated if known. Early in the ED visit, the child should receive oxygen, the complicated or failed airway should be secured, and pharmacotherapeutic measures, such as bronchodilators, steroids, anticholinergics, and antibiotics (if appropriate), should be instituted.

Proper disposition requires the consideration of multiple factors. For discharge to home, young children must demonstrate adequate oral intake, tolerance of secretions, oxygenation, and ventilation without evidence of an excess work of breathing. Admission or transfer to a pediatric specialty center is dictated by severity of illness and institutional resources. All transfers should be performed by personnel skilled in pediatric airway management.

Altered Level of Consciousness

SCOPE

The infant or toddler with an altered level of consciousness or self-awareness may have a life-threatening illness that requires immediate recognition and treatment to prevent permanent central nervous system (CNS) dysfunction.

EPIDEMIOLOGY

An altered level of consciousness in this pediatric age group is caused by nonstructural etiologies (e.g., infection, metabolic abnormalities, or toxin ingestions) or primary structural disease of the CNS (e.g., hemorrhage or tumors). Physical abuse is the leading cause of serious head injury in young children. Shaken baby syndrome most often involves children younger than 2 years and can be easily misdiagnosed.[18]

PATHOPHYSIOLOGY

A normal level of consciousness requires proper function and communication of the cerebral cortex and the reticular activating system. Normal neuronal activity involves a multifaceted balance of water, electrolytes, metabolic substrates, and neurotransmitter concentrations within a tightly controlled environment of temperature, pH, and osmolality. Any alteration of this environment resulting from insufficient blood flow, electrolyte imbalance, lack of substrate, presence of toxins, abnormal concentration of metabolic waste products, or loss of temperature results in the final common pathway of CNS dysfunction and an altered level of consciousness.

CLINICAL PRESENTATION

The history and physical examination should be directed toward potential life-threatening conditions that require immediate intervention to prevent progression of disease and long-term sequelae. Emergency conditions such as hypoxia, hypotension, extremes of temperature, hypoglycemia, seizure activity, and increased intracranial pressure should be diagnosed and treated. Once these issues have been excluded, the EP should perform an AMPLIFIEDD history (Box 19-5). Also, all available caretak-

BOX 19-5

The AMPLIFIEDD History for an Infant or Toddler with Altered Level of Consciousness

Allergies: to medications, environmental allergens

Medications: prescription, over-the-counter, "natural remedies"

Past medical history:
- Birth history
- Congenital anomaly
- Chronic disease (e.g., inborn error of metabolism, endocrinopathy)
- Infections
- Seizures

Last "feed, pee, poop": feeding, stool, and urine pattern; use of formula (dilution?)

Immediate events (history of present illness and review of systems): OLD CAARS
- *O*nset: rapid or gradual
- *L*ocation: evidence for localized pain?
- *D*uration and progression of symptoms
- *C*haracterize change in level of consciousness: lethargy, irritable, excessive crying
- *A*lleviating factors: Can child be consoled?
- *A*ggravating factors: Does movement of child cause apparent discomfort (e.g., meningitis, peritonitis, injury)?
- *R*ecurrence of symptoms: ever had similar presentation?
- *S*ystem review: trauma, seizure activity, fever, vomiting, diarrhea, recent infection, shortness of breath, change in behavior (e.g., colicky pain, paroxysmal crying), rash, irritability

Family/social history:
- Inherited disorders
- Day care: Who cares for child?

Immunizations up to date?

EMT history: elicit history for potential trauma, ingestion, abuse, or toxin exposure

Doctor: name of primary care physician or specialist to contact for additional information and help

Documents: obtain prior medical records

ers and EMS personnel should be interviewed. The EP should ask questions about the risk for accidental or nonaccidental trauma, infection, ingestion, or toxin exposure while identifying signs or symptoms suggestive of systemic disease.

Once the primary survey has been completed and emergency interventions have been performed, a "head-to-toe evaluation" should be performed with the infant or toddler completely undressed. Alterations in level of consciousness can be subtle or profound. The EP should:

- Pay close attention to pupillary responses, which generally remain intact with metabolic insults but may be absent with structural lesions, toxin exposures, or severe asphyxia.
- Note the eye position (e.g., deviation of conjugate gaze away from brainstem lesions and toward cerebral lesions).
- Identify abnormalities in the respiratory pattern that may reflect CNS insults or metabolic conditions such as metabolic acidosis.
- Evaluate motor strength, tone, and reflexes and characterize activity that may be consistent with seizures, cerebrate or decerebrate posturing.
- Look for signs of trauma, such as scalp contusions and lacerations, hemotympanum, postauricular or periorbital hematomas, retinal hemorrhages, cerebrospinal fluid otorrhea, and a bulging anterior fontanel suggestive of increased intracranial pressure.
- Note odors, which may give clues to inborn errors of metabolism or other metabolic disorders (e.g., the smell of acetone in the child with diabetic ketoacidosis).
- Identify physical findings that may signify systemic CNS illness, such as infection (e.g., vesicular or purpuric rashes), intussusception (e.g., abdominal mass or blood in stool), liver (e.g., jaundice, icterus), or cardiopulmonary disease (e.g., hypoxia, rales, or hepatomegaly).

■ DIFFERENTIAL DIAGNOSIS

A comprehensive differential diagnosis for alterations in consciousness in infants and toddlers can be generated with the "head-to-toe" memory tool (Fig. 19-1; Table 19-3). Possible causes involve essentially every organ system. When the underlying cause of altered mental status is not obvious, a high level of suspicion should be maintained for abuse, accidental toxin ingestion or exposure, intussusception, infection, or nonconvulsive seizure activity.

■ INTERVENTIONS AND PROCEDURES

The ABCs of resuscitation—airway, breathing, and circulation—should be assessed rapidly, and any interventions necessary to promote ventilation, volume resuscitation, and termination of seizure activity should be instituted immediately. If indicated, broad-spectrum antibiotics should be administered early. The child should be connected to a cardiorespiratory monitor, pulse oximetry started, rapid bedside glucose testing performed, and antidotes for toxin exposure or poisonings (e.g., naloxone for opioid ingestion) considered.

Table 19-3 DIFFERENTIAL DIAGNOSIS OF ALTERED LEVEL OF CONSCIOUSNESS IN INFANTS AND TODDLERS USING THE "HEAD-TO-TOE" MEMORY TOOL

Head		Seizure (postictal state) Infection: Meningitis Encephalitis Abscess Ventriculoperitoneal shunt malfunction or infection Closed-head injury: Epidural, subdural, or intraparenchymal hematoma Concussion Cerebral edema Vascular: Ischemic or hemorrhagic infarction Subarachnoid hemorrhage Venous thrombosis Central nervous system tumor
Mouth		Toxin ingestion or exposure Sedatives Anticholinergics Tricyclic antidepressants Salicylates Alcohols Precipitant of methemoglobinemia Carbon monoxide Heavy metals
Neck		Hypothyroidism Hyperthyroidism Parathyroidism (hypercalcemia, hypocalcemia)
Chest	Pulmonary	Respiratory failure Asphyxia Hypoxia secondary to pulmonary disease
	Cardiac	Hypotension (congenital heart disease, dysrhythmias, congestive heart failure) Anemia
Abdomen	Gastrointestinal tract	Intussusception Dehydration secondary to vomiting or diarrhea
	Liver	Inborn errors of metabolism Reye's syndrome Hepatic encephalopathy
	Pancreas	Hypoglycemia Diabetic ketoacidosis
	Kidney/urinary tract	Electrolyte disorders: Hyponatremia Hypernatremia Hypermagnesemia Hypomagnesemia Uremia Metabolic acidosis or alkalosis Infection: pyelonephritis with urosepsis
	Adrenal glands	Cortisol deficiency
Other		Sepsis Hypothermia Hyperthermia

Table 19-4 LABORATORY AND RADIOGRAPHIC TESTING IN INFANTS AND TODDLERS WITH ALTERED LEVEL OF CONSCIOUSNESS

	Laboratory Testing	Radiographic Testing
Routine	Rapid bedside glucose measurement Bedside urine dipstick test Complete blood count Electrolyte measurements Blood urea nitrogen and serum creatinine measurements Urinalysis	Chest radiograph
Selective	Arterial blood gas measurements (ventilation/oxygenation) Toxicology screening Liver function testing Serum ammonia and lactate measurements (inborn errors of metabolism) Collect samples for acylcarnitine profile, quantitative plasma amino acid, qualitative urine organic acids (inborn errors of metabolism) Serum osmolality (measured and calculated) Blood and urine cultures Cerebrospinal fluid analysis and culture Ethanol level Lead level Serum cortisol measurement Thyroid profile	Cranial computed tomography (CT) Abdominal ultrasonography Abdominal CT Skeletal survey Magnetic resonance imaging of head Barium or air contrast enema Shunt series

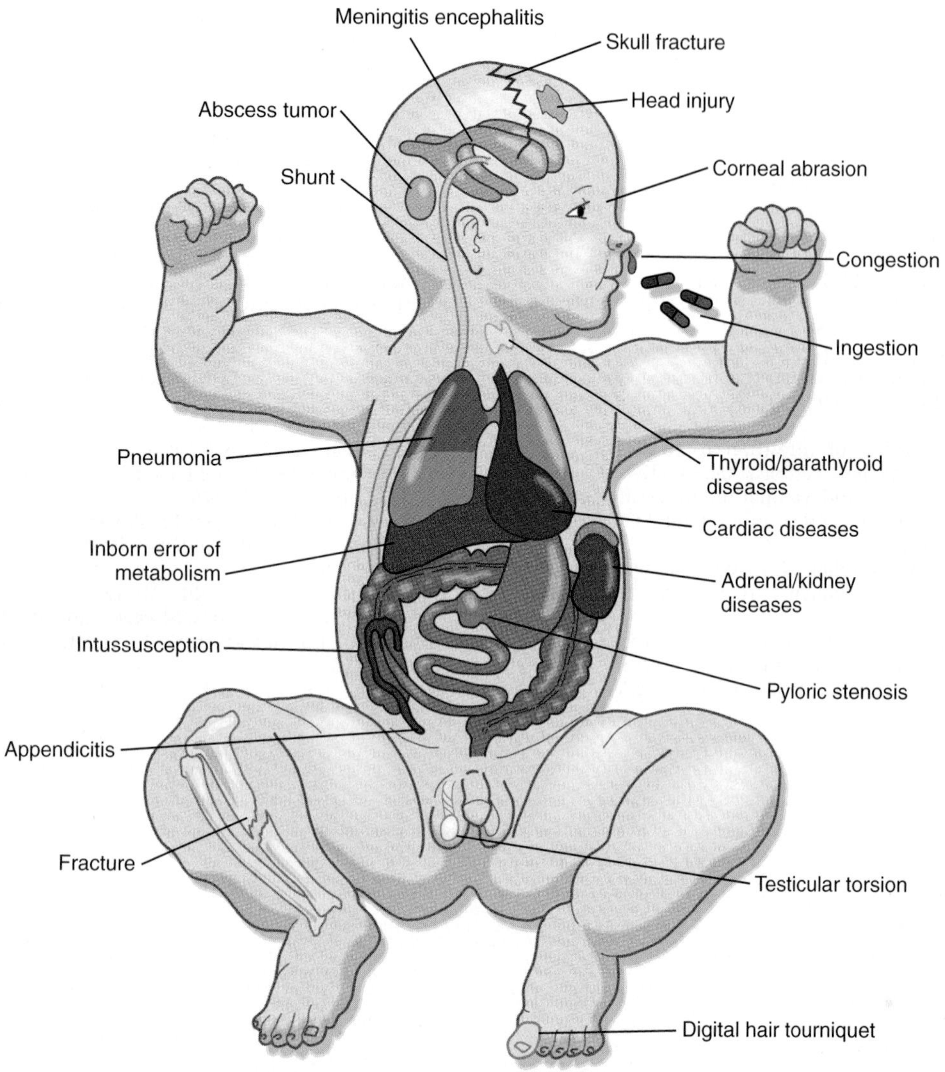
Meningitis encephalitis
Skull fracture
Head injury
Abscess tumor
Shunt
Corneal abrasion
Congestion
Ingestion
Pneumonia
Thyroid/parathyroid diseases
Cardiac diseases
Inborn error of metabolism
Adrenal/kidney diseases
Intussusception
Pyloric stenosis
Appendicitis
Fracture
Testicular torsion
Digital hair tourniquet

FIGURE 19-1 Head-to-toe differential diagnosis.

■ DIAGNOSTIC TESTING

Perform laboratory and radiographic testing using a systematic, comprehensive approach (Table 19-4). In the critically ill infant or toddler without a definitive diagnosis, routine testing for sepsis, trauma, and metabolic derangements should be supplemented with selective tests as dictated by the progression of the clinical course, by the response to initial interventions, and by history and physical findings.

> *Tips and Tricks*
>
> **INFANT OR TODDLER WITH ALTERED LEVEL OF CONSCIOUSNESS**
>
> Perform rapid bedside glucose testing on arrival.
>
> If underlying etiology is not clear, consider following diagnoses: intussusception, accidental ingestion, environmental exposures, nonaccidental trauma.

■ TREATMENT AND DISPOSITION

When a definitive diagnosis is not established in a child with altered level of consciousness upon arrival at the ED, supportive care should be instituted to assist ventilation, adequate circulation maintained, and potentially life-threatening conditions, such as sepsis or electrolyte abnormalities, treated. When an etiology is diagnosed, appropriate treatment should be given. Unless an easily recognizable and reversible cause is found, all children with altered level of consciousness should be admitted to a pediatric intensive care unit.

REFERENCES

1. Glass R, Lew J, Gangarosa R, et al: Estimates of morbidity and mortality rates for diarrheal diseases in American children. J Pediatr 1991;118:S27-S33.
2. Godbole P, Stringer M: Bilious vomiting in the newborn: How often is it pathologic? J Pediatr Surg 2002;37:909-911.
3. Parashar U, Holman R, Cummings K: Trends in intussusception-associated hospitalizations and deaths among US infants. Pediatrics 2000;106:1413-1421.
4. Bundy D, Byerley J, Liles E, et al: Does this child have appendicitis? JAMA 2007;298:438-451.
5. Steiner M, Dewalt D, Byerley J: Is this child dehydrated? JAMA 2004;291:2746-2754.
6. Vega R, Avner J: A prospective study of the usefulness of clinical and laboratory parameters for predicting percentage of dehydration in children. Pediatr Emerg Care 1997;13:179-182.
7. Strouse P: Disorders of intestinal rotation and fixation ("malrotation"). Pediatr Radiol 2004;34:837-851.
8. Vasavada P: Ultrasound evaluation of acute abdominal emergencies in infants and children. Radiol Clin North Am 2004;42:445-456.
9. Kwok M, Kim M, Gorelick M: Evidence-based approach to the diagnosis of appendicitis in children. Pediatr Emerg Care 2004;20:690-698.
10. Reeves J, Shannon M, Fleisher G: Ondansetron decreases vomiting associated with acute gastroenteritis: A randomized, controlled trial. Pediatrics 2002;109:e62.
11. Ramsook C, Sahagun-Carreon I, Kozinetz C, et al: A randomized clinical trial comparing oral ondansetron with placebo in children with vomiting from acute gastroenteritis. Ann Emerg Med 2002;39:397-403.
12. Practice parameter: The management of acute gastroenteritis in young children. American Academy of Pediatrics, Provisional Committee on Quality Improvement, Subcommittee on Acute Gastroenteritis. Pediatrics 1996;97:424-435.
13. Fonseca B, Hodgate A, Craig J: Enteral vs. intravenous rehydration therapy for children with gastroenteritis: A meta-analysis of randomized controlled trials. Arch Pediatr Adolesc Med 2004;158:483-490.
14. Heffernan R, Mostashari F, Das D, et al: Syndromic surveillance in public health practice, New York City. Emerg Infect Dis 2004;10:858-864.
15. Black R, Johnson D, Matlack M: Bronchoscopic removal of aspirated foreign bodies in children. J Pediatr Surg 1994;29:682-684.
16. American Academy of Pediatrics Committee on Pediatric Emergency Medicine: First aid for the choking child. Pediatrics 1993;92:477-479.
17. Rubio Q, Munoz Saez M, Povatos Serran E, et al: Magill forceps: A vital forceps. Pediatr Emerg Care 1995;11:302-303.
18. Committee on Child Abuse and Neglect. American Academy of Pediatrics: Shaken Baby Syndrome: rotational cranial injuries—technical report. Pediatrics 2001;108:206-210.

SECTION III

Head and Neck Injuries

Chapter 20

Eye Emergencies

Kriti Bhatia and Rahul Sharma

KEY POINTS

Eye emergencies can be classified into three major types: the red eye, the painful eye, and visual loss.
Nausea and vomiting can be the only symptoms of acute angle-closure glaucoma, especially in elderly patients.
Topical anesthetics should not be prescribed for a painful eye disorder because their use may lead to corneal ulcers.
Close follow-up with an ophthalmologist is essential for most eye emergencies.

Approximately 2% of ED visits involve complaints associated with the eye or vision.[1] Eye emergencies can be categorized as the red eye, the painful eye, or visual loss. This chapter discusses the various disorders that fall into each category. Table 20-1 summarizes the differential diagnosis and priority actions to be taken for any patient presenting to the ED with an eye complaint.

Anatomy

Light passes through the cornea and then through an opening in the iris called the pupil. The iris is responsible for controlling the amount of light that enters the eye by dilating and constricting the pupil. This light then reaches the lens, which refracts the light rays onto the retina. The anterior chamber is located between the lens and the cornea and contains aqueous humor that is produced by the ciliary body. This fluid maintains pressure and provides nutrients to the lens and cornea. This fluid is reabsorbed from the anterior chamber into the venous system through the canal of Schlemm. The vitreous chamber, located between the retina and the lens, contains a gelatinous fluid called vitreous humor. Light rays pass through the vitreous humor before reaching the retina. The retina lines the back of the eye and contains photoreceptor cells called rods and cones. Rods help vision in dim light, and cones help vision in color. The cones are located in the center of the retina in an area called the macula. The fovea is a small depression in the center of the macula that contains the highest concentration of cones. The optic nerve is located behind the retina; it is responsible for transmitting the signals from the photoreceptor cells to the brain (Fig. 20-1).

The extraocular muscles (Fig. 20-2) help in the stabilization of the eye. Six extraocular muscles assist in horizontal, vertical, and rotational movements. These muscles are controlled by impulses from cranial nerves III, IV, and VI, which tell the muscles to relax or contract.

Glaucoma

■ SCOPE

More than 3 million Americans suffer from glaucoma, the leading cause of preventable blindness in the United States.[2] The term *glaucoma* refers to a

Table 20-1 DIFFERENTIAL DIAGNOSIS AND PRIORITY ACTIONS FOR EYE COMPLAINTS IN THE ED

Eye pain?	
Does the patient have any visual changes, history of trauma, or associated neurologic complaints?	Separate the etiologies into traumatic and atraumatic. Perform a complete eye examination, including visual acuity assessment, slit-lamp examination, and measurement of intraocular pressure (IOP).
Decreased visual acuity?	
Does the patient have any risk factors for central retinal vessel occlusion or glaucoma? Is there any history of recent infection or trauma? Does the patient also have a headache or any associated neurologic complaints?	Perform a complete eye examination, including visual acuity assessment, slit-lamp examination, and measurement of IOP, and a neurologic examination.
Eye trauma?	
Does the patient have any evidence of increased IOP or decreased visual acuity?	Consider computed tomography (CT) of the orbits with possible emergency lateral canthotomy and immediate ophthalmologic consultation.
Red eye?	
Is there any evidence of infection, trauma, foreign body, or systemic illness?	Perform complete eye examination, including visual acuity assessment and IOP measurement, and treat with appropriate medications (see Table 20-2).

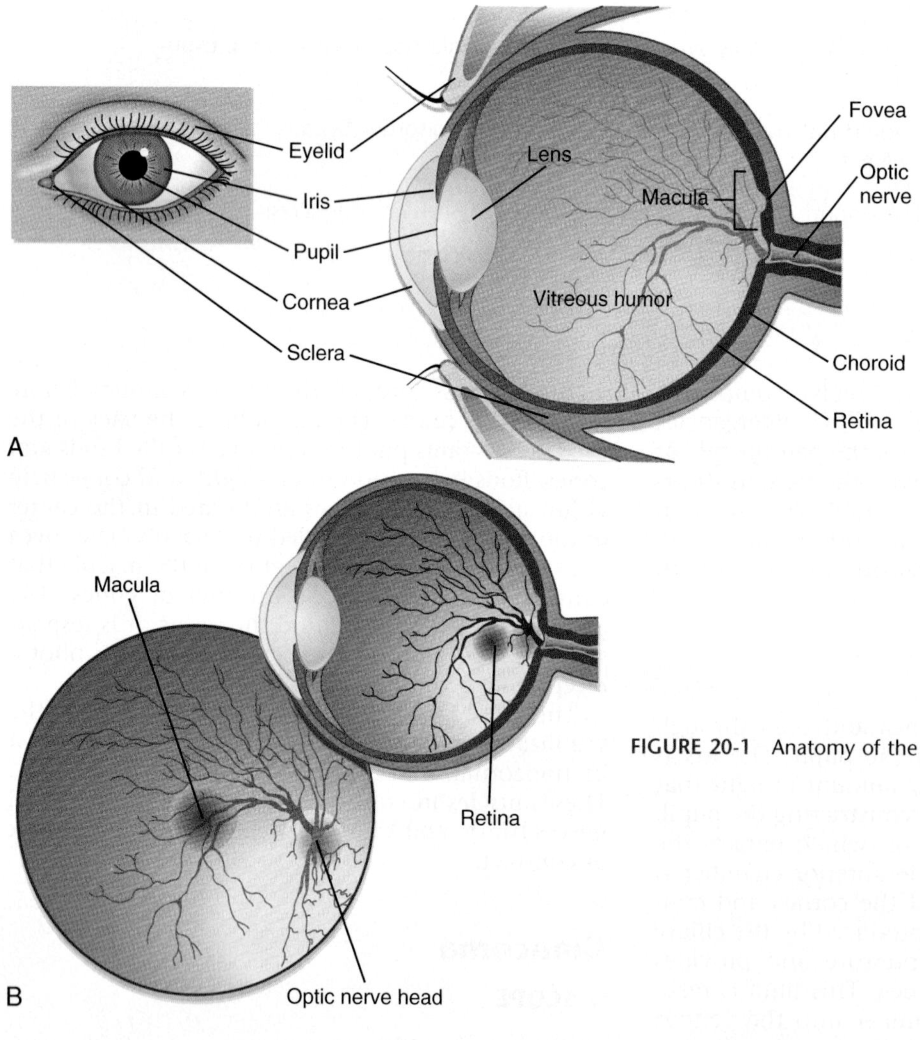
Eyelid
Iris
Pupil
Cornea
Sclera
Lens
Macula
Vitreous humor
Fovea
Optic
nerve
Choroid
Retina
A
Macula
Retina
Optic nerve head
B

FIGURE 20-1 Anatomy of the eye (**A**) and retina (**B**).

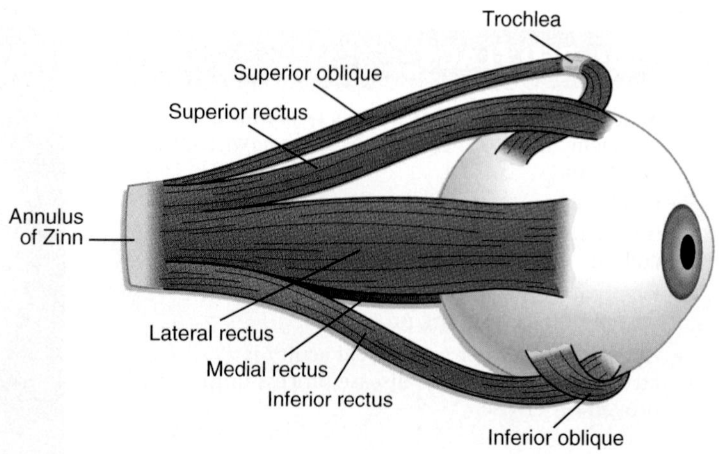
Trochlea
Superior oblique
Superior rectus
Annulus of Zinn
Lateral rectus
Medial rectus
Inferior rectus
Inferior oblique

FIGURE 20-2 Extraocular muscles. (Courtesy of Ted Montgomery, OD, www.tedmontgomery.com/the_eye/)

group of disorders that damage the optic nerve, leading to loss of vision. There are two main classifications of glaucoma, open-angle and angle-closure. Acute angle-closure glaucoma is more common in white persons and women. African Americans, patients older than 65 years, and people with diabetes and ocular trauma are at increased risk for open-angle glaucoma. The differentiation between the two types of glaucoma lies in the mechanism of obstruction of the outflow (see later). This discussion focuses mainly on acute angle-closure glaucoma.

When the angle of the anterior chamber is reduced, outflow of aqueous humor is blocked, resulting in elevated intraocular pressure (IOP) with ultimate visual compromise. Patients with a shallow anterior chamber, hyperopic (farsighted) eyes, and eyes with lens abnormalities such as cataracts are more prone to acute angle-closure glaucoma. Pupillary dilation, caused by events such as presence in a dark room, is the most significant event that can cause an acute attack of glaucoma, because the flaccid iris can be pushed against the trabecular meshwork, causing obstruction.

■ PRESENTING SIGNS AND SYMPTOMS

Patients with acute angle-closure glaucoma may present with sudden onset of headache or eye pain. Occasionally, nausea and vomiting from vagal stimulation can be the dominant symptoms. Shortly after the onset of pain, blurry vision or halos in the visual field may occur.

The classic physical findings are unilateral eye injection, especially at the limbus, a nonreactive, midsize pupil; shallow anterior chamber; corneal edema or haziness; and high IOP (usually 60 to 90 mm Hg). If the attack has been prolonged, ischemia of the ciliary body reduces aqueous humor production with a resultant decrease in IOP. This process is especially important because the ultimate damage depends on the duration of the attack rather than the severity of pressure elevation.

With open-angle glaucoma, disease progression is usually insidious, bilateral, slowly progressive, and painless.

■ DIAGNOSTIC TESTING

Physical examination holds the key to the diagnosis of glaucoma. The EP should suspect disease in the appropriate setting. Visual acuity should be recorded in both eyes. Examination of the eye should include a search for the classic signs of glaucoma already described, including a mid-dilated pupil in the affected eye and corneal haziness. The slit-lamp should be used to estimate the depth of the anterior chamber. If this depth is less than one fourth of the corneal thickness, the anterior chamber angle is very narrow. It is important to measure anterior chamber depth in both eyes; a shallow angle in only one eye argues against acute angle-closure glaucoma. IOP is usually measured with a tonometer: The cornea is flattened, and pressure is determined through measurement of the force needed to flatten it and of the area flattened.

■ TREATMENT

Acute angle-closure glaucoma is an ophthalmologic emergency. Because outcome is contingent on the duration of IOP elevation, treatment should be started immediately. Therapy is geared toward decreasing aqueous production, increasing aqueous outflow, and reducing vitreous volume to lower the IOP. Topical beta-blockers such as the nonselective agent timolol decrease aqueous production. Because these topical agents are systemically absorbed, potential systemic contraindications should be considered before they are administered. Pilocarpine is a direct-acting parasympathomimetic miotic agent that mechanically promotes aqueous outflow. Systemic therapy with acetazolamide, a carbonic anhydrase inhibitor that limits aqueous humor formation, and

RED FLAGS

- Acute angle-closure glaucoma may manifest as headache alone or headache as the overwhelming symptom.
- Unless a search for central retinal artery occlusion is undertaken, the patient may have further embolic events before the diagnosis is apparent.
- Even painless eye conditions can result from serious and devastating processes.
- Always assume that poor visual acuity is attributable to a serious disease process until proven otherwise.

mannitol, which creates an osmotic gradient between the vitreous and the blood to cause vitreous volume reduction, are additional components of therapy. Surgical therapy is definitive.

■ DISPOSITION

Disposition of the patient is made in conjunction with the consulting ophthalmologist. Indications for admission include intractable nausea and vomiting and need for careful monitoring to administer systemic agents.

Central Retinal Artery Occlusion

■ SCOPE

Retinal artery occlusion affects less than 1 person per 100,000 annually.[3,4] It is most commonly caused by an embolus from the carotid artery that lodges in a distal branch of the ophthalmic artery. Central retinal artery occlusion most commonly affects elderly patients and men. Although most emboli are formed from cholesterol, they may also be calcific, fat, or bacterial from cardiac valve vegetations.

■ PATHOPHYSIOLOGY

The visual complaints and deficits resulting from retinal artery disease are caused by ischemia. In addition to the embolic causes already described, low-flow states and vasospasm may have the same visual consequences.

■ PRESENTING SIGNS AND SYMPTOMS

Sudden, painless visual loss is the classic presentation in central retinal artery occlusion. Sometimes patients report transient visual loss prior to complete compromise. Visual loss is usually profound. Examination can often elicit an afferent pupillary defect (when light is shined into the abnormal eye, the pupil of the affected eye paradoxically dilates instead of constricting). Funduscopic examination typically demonstrates a pale retina with a cherry-red spot at the fovea (Fig. 20-3). Complete evaluation involves auscultation of the carotid arteries for bruits, palpation of the temporal artery for tenderness, and cardiac auscultation and pulse palpation to detect atrial fibrillation.

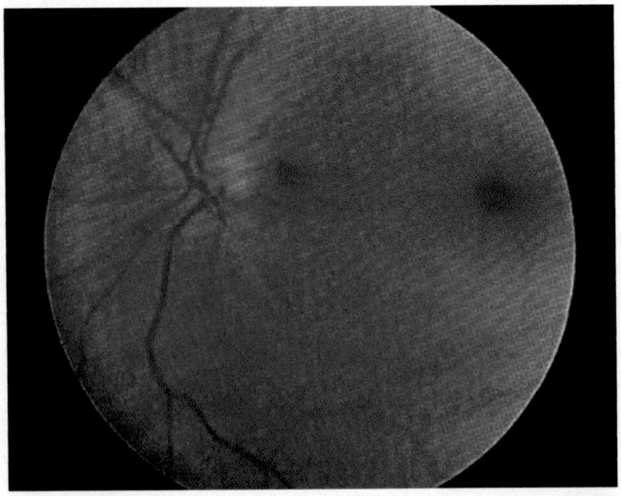

FIGURE 20-3 Central retinal artery occlusion. (Courtesy of Ted Montgomery, OD, www.tedmontgomery.com/the_eye/)

■ DIFFERENTIAL DIAGNOSIS

Sudden, painless visual loss can also result from central retinal vein occlusion, temporal arteritis, ischemic optic neuropathy, amaurosis fugax, retinal detachment, or vitreous hemorrhage. If there is associated pain, arterial dissection should be part of the differential diagnosis. The presence of a headache, temporal artery tenderness, and elevated erythrocyte sedimentation rate (ESR) suggests temporal arteritis. Amaurosis fugax, a unilateral transient obstruction of a retinal artery, does not cause visual loss lasting more than 15 minutes. Ischemic optic neuropathy causes optic disc pallor and elevation. Retinal detachment and vitreous hemorrhage cause visual disturbances such as floaters in addition to visual loss—the occurrence of which is variable with a detached retina. Vitreous hemorrhage causes absence of the normal red reflex of the fundus. A neurologic cause such as cerebral infarct must also be considered.

■ TREATMENT

Treatment must be initiated immediately because visual loss is generally irreversible after 2 hours of ischemia. Regardless, the outcome is generally poor. Several approaches may be used. Intermittent globe massage can be performed in an effort to dislodge the clot and propel it distally: Moderate pressure is applied for 5 second and then released for 5 seconds, and the cycle is repeated. The use of anterior chamber paracentesis for visual loss is based on the principle

Documentation

- Visual acuity should be documented for every eye complaint, no matter how minor.
- Both eyes should be examined and compared even if the complaint is monocular.
- The eye examination should be thorough, including eversion of both eyelids and inspection for foreign bodies.

that decreased IOP allows for better perfusion of the retinal artery and may propel the clot distally. Intravenous acetazolamide can be administered for the same purpose. Inhaled carbogen (mixture of 95% oxygen, 5% carbon dioxide) can be used to dilate the vasculature, thereby increasing retinal Po_2.

Other treatment options are intra-arterial thrombolysis and hyperbaric oxygen; studies have showed limited improvement in visual outcome with early administration of both of these treatment modalities, however.[5-8] One retrospective study reported found that even with thrombolysis, vision did not improve to better than 20/300 in the affected eye.[5] Another study investigated the outcomes of 32 patients with central retinal artery occlusion, 17 of whom received fibrinolysis.[4] This study found that all but 6 of the treated patients reported improvement in their visual compromise, and only 5 of the untreated patients had any improvement. In this study, patients with up to 24 hours of symptoms were treated.

Patients with sudden visual loss are admitted to the hospital so the underlying cause can be sought.

Central Retinal Vein Occlusion

■ Scope

Patients older than 50 years who have cardiovascular disease, hypertension, glaucoma, venous stasis, hypercoagulable conditions, collagen vascular diseases, or diabetes are at risk for central retinal vein occlusion.[1]

■ PATHOPHYSIOLOGY

There are two types of retinal vein occlusion, ischemic and nonischemic. The ischemic type is also known as hemorrhagic retinopathy, and the nonischemic type is also called venous stasis retinopathy. The presentation and physical findings differ according to the type of occlusion involved.

■ PRESENTATION

Typically, patients with ischemic retinal vein occlusion report acute and relatively profound decrease in visual acuity. Those with the nonischemic type present with progressively blurry vision that is worse in the mornings. An afferent pupil defect is found in the ischemic type. Funduscopic examination shows an edematous optic disc and macular, dilated retinal veins, retinal hemorrhage, and cotton-wool spots. Sometimes, these findings are called the "blood and thunder" appearance of the fundus (Fig. 20-4).

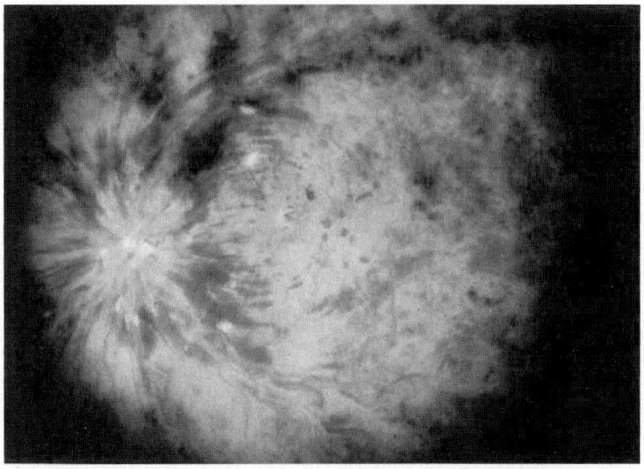

FIGURE 20-4 Central retinal vein occlusion. (From Noble J: Textbook of Primary Care Medicine, 3rd ed. St. Louis, Mosby, 2001.)

■ DIFFERENTIAL DIAGNOSIS

The processes that must be considered in the assessment of a patient with possible central retinal vein occlusion are the same as those for central retinal artery occlusion. Branch retinal vein occlusion may also occur distal to an arteriovenous crossing, with hemorrhages developing distal to the occlusion site.

■ DIAGNOSTIC TESTING

No specific diagnostic test can identify central retinal vein occlusion. Diagnosis is based on careful clinical history and physical examination, which exclude other processes that also cause painless visual loss.

■ TREATMENT

No effective therapeutic regimen exists for central retinal vein occlusion. The EP should arrange for immediately ophthalmologic consultation. A search for a cause should be performed in order to protect the contralateral eye from the same problem. Prognosis largely depends on the type of retinal venous occlusion—nonischemic vein occlusion, unless there is extensive macular involvement, offers a better outcome than the ischemic type. Spontaneous resolution may occur in some cases.

Although no specific treatment exists, a number of interventions have been proposed and practiced. However, these have not been based on evidence of efficacy. Laser photocoagulation, for example, cauterizes leaking vessels with the aim of halting further visual loss.[9] This procedure can be especially helpful

PRIORITY ACTIONS

1. Determine whether the patient's complaint is monocular or binocular.
2. Determine whether the complaint is trauma-related.
3. Always ask whether the patient wears contact lenses or glasses.
4. Always check visual acuity.
5. Determine whether physical findings are monocular or binocular.
6. Involve an ophthalmologist in treatment of a patient with an eye complaint as soon as possible if there is reasonable suspicion of a vision-compromising process, such as acute angle-closure glaucoma or central retinal artery occlusion.

in branch retinal vein occlusions. With nonischemic vein occlusion, attempts to reduce macular edema can be helpful. The reduction is accomplished with administration of topical corticosteroids. Studies have been conducted to determine the benefit of steroids in both forms of retinal vein occlusion. Jonas and colleagues[10] conducted a prospective, comparative, nonrandomized clinical interventional study evaluating the visual outcomes in 32 patients with central retinal vein occlusion after intravitreal administration of triamcinolone acetate. The study included patients with both ischemic and nonischemic forms of retinal vein occlusion. These researchers found that the medication resulted in temporary (up to 3 months) improvement in visual outcome but also raised IOPs. Anticoagulants are not recommended because they may propagate hemorrhaging.

Optic Neuritis

■ SCOPE

Optic neuritis is inflammation of the optic nerve. Visual loss occurs because of focal demyelination of the optic nerve. Most affected patients are between 15 and 40 years old. This disorder can be associated with numerous diseases, including sarcoidosis, systemic lupus erythematosus, measles, leukemia, syphilis, and alcoholism; however, it is most commonly associated with multiple sclerosis. In fact, up to a third of patients with optic neuritis are eventually diagnosed with multiple sclerosis, and approximately two thirds of patients with multiple sclerosis have optic neuritis. Optic neuritis can also be idiopathic.

■ PATHOPHYSIOLOGY

Optic neuritis results from an autoimmune reaction, ultimately causing demyelinating inflammation. In idiopathic and multiple sclerosis–related optic neuritis, lesions are characterized by areas of loss of myelin sheath with preservation of axons. In acute disease, remyelination may occur. In chronic disease, owing to accumulation of scar tissue, the process is irreversible. Lesions in multiple sclerosis–associated optic neuritis are pathologically the same as those in the brain.

■ PRESENTING SIGNS AND SYMPTOMS

Symptoms of optic neuritis are usually unilateral. Patients complain of pain, especially with eye movement. Visual loss, which can range from minimal loss to complete loss of light perception, usually occurs over a number of hours or days. Patients may also experience dulling of color vision, worse vision after exertion or exposure to steam, brief light flashes, and central scotoma. Afferent pupillary defect is always present. Funduscopic examination may show disc pallor, swelling, or elevation. However, because up to two thirds of cases are retrobulbar, the fundus can appear normal.

■ DIFFERENTIAL DIAGNOSIS

Any condition that causes visual disturbance along with eye pain must be considered in the differential diagnosis of optic neuritis. Orbital cellulitis can cause this clinical picture but does not include an afferent pupillary defect; furthermore, inspection alone should allow for differentiation between the two diseases. Glaucoma can also cause the combination of ocular pain and visual impairment. Physical examination, including assessment of pupil size and reactivity as well as corneal inspection, allows for distinction between glaucoma and optic neuritis.

■ DIAGNOSIS

Unilateral, ocular pain with visual compromise should always raise clinical suspicion for optic neuritis. If no afferent pupillary defect in found on physical examination, another diagnosis is almost assured. Although imaging is usually not indicated, magnetic resonance imaging (MRI) provides adequate visualization of the optic nerve.

■ TREATMENT AND DISPOSITION

Ophthalmologic and neurologic consultations should be obtained if optic neuritis is suspected. The goals of treatment are to restore visual acuity and to prevent propagation of the underlying disease process. The Optic Neuritis Treatment Trial was a randomized, 15-center clinical trial involving 457 patients performed to evaluate both the benefit of corticosteroid treatment of optic neuritis and the relationship of this entity with multiple sclerosis. Use of intravenous steroids in conjunction with oral steroids reduced the short-term risk of development of multiple sclerosis as determined by MRI evaluation. There was no reported long-term immunity from or benefit for multiple sclerosis, however. The study concluded that although intravenous steroids have only minimal, if any, effect on the patient's ultimate visual acuity, they do expedite recovery from optic neuritis. Use of oral steroids alone is associated with higher recurrence of optic neuritis. The dosage regimen recommended on the basis of study results was methylprednisolone 250 mg every 6 hours for 3 days followed by oral prednisone 1 mg/kg/day for 11 days.[11]

Retinal Detachment

Retinal detachment is a true ophthalmologic emergency. Unfortunately, it is also relatively common, affecting 1 in 300 people. Before the introduction of and improvement in a number of treatment modalities, this entity was uniformly blinding. Early diagnosis and treatment are imperative for preservation of vision. Retinal detachment may be associated with vascular disorders, congenital malformations, metabolic disarray, trauma, shrinking of the vitreous, myopia, and degeneration, and, less commonly, with diabetic retinopathy and uveitis. It is generally more common in older patients. There are three different types of retinal detachment, each associated with different conditions.

■ PATHOPHYSIOLOGY AND ANATOMY

The retina has two layers, the inner neuronal layer and the outer pigment epithelial layer (the choroid). *Retinal detachment* refers to separation of the two layers. *Rhegmatogenous* retinal detachment, the most common of the three types, is caused by a tear or hole in the neuronal layer that leads to extrusion of fluid from the vitreous cavity into the potential space between the two retinal layers. This is the most common type of detachment, being more common in patients older than 45 years and in patients with severe myopia. When caused by trauma, this type of detachment can affect any age group. *Exudative* retinal detachment is caused by leakage of fluid or blood from within the retina itself. Predisposing factors for this type include hypertension, vasculitis, and central retinal venous occlusion. *Traction* retinal detachment results from formation and subsequent contraction of fibrous bands in the vitreous.

■ PRESENTING SIGNS AND SYMPTOMS

Retinal detachment can occasionally be asymptomatic. More commonly, patients complain of flashes of light, floaters, or fine dots or cobwebs in their visual fields. Visual acuity correlates with extent of macular involvement. Vision loss is generally sudden in onset and starts peripherally, with propagation to the central visual field. Retinal detachment is painless. A large detachment may cause an afferent pupillary defect. On examination, the detached retina may appear gray or translucent or may seem out of focus (Fig. 20-5). Retinal folds may be seen. Visual field defects are variable, depending on the involvement of the retina and macula. Left untreated, all cases of retinal detachment progress to involve the macula, resulting in complete loss of vision in the affected eye.

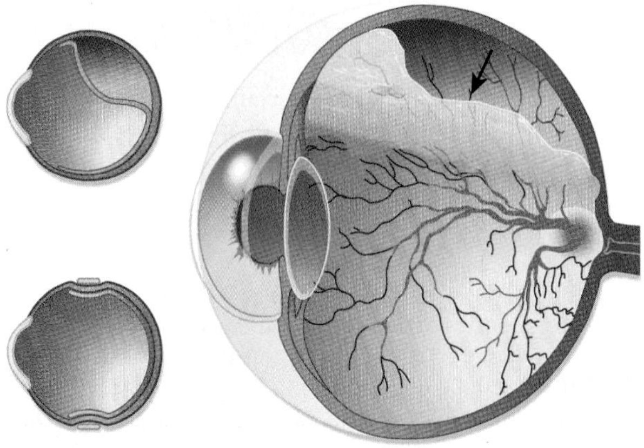

FIGURE 20-5 Retinal detachment. (Courtesy of Ted Montgomery, OD, www.tedmontgomery.com/the_eye)

■ DIFFERENTIAL DIAGNOSIS

Vitreous hemorrhage, which results from bleeding into either the preretinal space or the vitreous cavity itself, can be difficult to distinguish from retinal detachment. Complaints with this disorder range from floaters or cobwebs in the visual field to severe, painless loss of vision. Vitreous hemorrhage without concomitant retinal detachment should not, however, cause an afferent pupillary defect. Ophthalmoscopy usually demonstrates discoloration (ranging from reddish to black) with fundal structural details difficult to discern. Therapy for vitreous hemorrhage consists of bedrest with head elevation followed by possible interventional procedures such as laser photocoagulation and cryotherapy.

All macular disorders can cause painless vision loss. They manifest as loss of central vision with peripheral vision preservation as well as findings of retinal abnormalities. A careful history and physical examination can exclude macular degeneration as a cause of central visual loss. Funduscopic examination in age-related macular degeneration shows the presence of drusen—small, yellow masses scattered on the retina. A gray-green subretinal neovascular membrane may also be seen. Inflammatory processes involving the retina often cause inflammatory proteins to fill the vitreous, making it appear cloudy.

■ TREATMENT

The sooner treatment is initiated for retinal detachment, the greater the chance of visual preservation

Tips and Tricks

- Perform slit-lamp examination prior to fluorescein examination, to prevent false-positive results of assessment for corneal abrasions.
- Apply local anesthetic (e.g., tetracaine) to facilitate a slit-lamp examination.
- A cotton-tipped applicator can be used to evert the upper eyelid.
- Never send a patient home with topical anesthetic eyedrops, which can raise the risk for further injury.

and recovery. After detachment, retinal ischemia ensues because of loss of the choroidal blood supply. Patients with suspected or confirmed retinal breaks or detachments require emergency ophthalmologic consultation. Laser photocoagulation or cryotherapy is often used to create small burns around the area of detachment to prevent further leakage of fluid between the retinal layers. Intraocular gas is sometimes used to tamponade the tear. These procedures are approximately 95% effective in halting the disease process.[12] Surgical repair may be necessary to repair the tear and simultaneously remove the traction forces at work on the retina.

Temporal Arteritis

Temporal arteritis, an inflammatory condition that occurs from a generalized vasculitis of medium and large arteries, typically affects patients older than 50 years. This condition is also called *giant cell arteritis*. There is a female preponderance. Temporal arteritis occurs in as many as 1 of every 2000 people. Although mortality is not affected by the condition, it can cause blindness. Up to 75% of patients with visual compromise due to temporal arteritis would eventually have contralateral visual impairment if not treated. Temporal arteritis is commonly, though not uniformly, associated with polymyalgia rheumatica.

■ PATHOPHYSIOLOGY

Vessels affected by giant cell arteritis are infiltrated with lymphocytes, plasma cells, and multinucleated giant cells in patches or segmental patterns. A cell-mediated immune response is thought to account for the vascular changes seen with this disorder. Inflammation of the branches of the ophthalmic artery, especially the posterior ciliary artery, leads to ischemic optic neuritis, compromising vision. The central retinal artery is also often affected. Inflammation of the temporal artery causes the classic headache associated with this diagnosis.

■ PRESENTING SIGNS AND SYMPTOMS

Unilateral headache, jaw or tongue claudication, constitutional symptoms including anorexia and malaise, and visual impairment are common presenting symptoms of temporal arteritis. Occasionally, visual loss is preceded by amaurosis fugax. Patients with polymyalgia rheumatica may also complain of pain and stiffness in the shoulders or hips.

Examination may demonstrate tenderness and decreased pulsations over the involved temporal artery. Funduscopic findings may be normal or may consist of optic disc edema or pallor, scattered cotton-wool spots, flame-shaped retinal hemorrhages, and distended retinal veins. An afferent pupillary defect may be present. Evaluation of vision often detects horizontal field defects and involvement of the extraocular muscles.

■ DIFFERENTIAL DIAGNOSIS

For patients who do not have visual complaints, a differential diagnosis for headache must be investigated. Migraines, tension headaches, and subarachnoid hemorrhage may mimic temporal arteritis. Palpation of the temporal artery along with a careful history, including questions about jaw symptoms, may allow for the distinction. Because temporal arteritis is a medical emergency associated with high morbidity if not recognized and treated promptly, it must be definitively excluded on the basis of history and physical or laboratory findings before the patient's symptoms are attributed to another entity. Acute angle-closure glaucoma is also high on the differential diagnosis list, whether or not visual symptoms are present. Occasionally, headache can be the dominant symptom of glaucoma. In glaucoma, however, physical examination should find a mid-dilated, nonreactive pupil with corneal haziness and a shallow anterior chamber.

■ DIAGNOSIS

Although temporal arteritis can rarely be accompanied by a normal ESR, this parameter is almost always elevated. The upper limit of normal ESR increases with age. A rough approximation of the upper limit of normal for men is age in years divided by 2. For women it is age in years plus 10, with the sum divided by 2, or half the age in years plus 5. Elderly patients with new-onset headaches, visual loss, and elevated ESR should always be treated for temporal arteritis. Generally, the ESR is higher than 80 mm/hr in the presence of temporal arteritis. Temporal biopsy confirms presence of the disease. Early on, however, biopsy findings may be normal.

■ TREATMENT

Treatment of temporal arteritis should never be delayed to await biopsy because outcome is contingent upon early medical treatment. Initial treatment should be given with prednisone 60 to 80 mg or high-dose intravenous methylprednisolone. The exact duration and regimen of steroid therapy are determined on a case-by-case basis. Generally, treatment is continued until symptoms improve and ESR begins to normalize. It has also been suggested that methotrexate, infliximab, and aspirin may also halt progression of visual symptoms, but further studies are necessary to establish practice patterns.[13]

Orbital Cellulitis and Periorbital Cellulitis

Without proper treatment, orbital cellulitis causes blindness and death in approximately 20% of patients. Because the venous drainage of the orbital regions occurs through communicating vessels into the brain via the cavernous sinus, infection can progress rapidly with devastating consequences. Differentiating orbital from periorbital (preseptal) cellulitis can be difficult but is important because the outcomes of the two entities, and therefore their treatments, are different.

■ ANATOMY AND PATHOPHYSIOLOGY

Orbital cellulitis is inflammation of any of the tissues within the orbit posterior to the orbital septum, whereas *preorbital cellulitis* is confined to the tissues anterior to the septum. Making this distinction is extremely important for management. Owing to the gravity of the potential consequences of orbital cellulitis and the fact that most cases of orbital cellulitis have a concomitant periorbital component, the EP evaluating an infected, erythematous orbit should always assume that the patient has orbital cellulitis until it can be definitively excluded.

Approximately 75% of orbital and periorbital cellulitides have identifiable antecedent causes. Sinusitis is the most common predisposing condition. Because the inferior, medial, and superior walls of the orbit lie adjacent to the sinuses, it is easy to understand how extension of infection may occur. The ethmoid sinus most commonly involved. Infection from trauma or surgery with direct inoculation and hematogenous spread from other sources of bacteremia are other methods of acquiring the infection. The pathogen involved is contingent upon the mode of infection. Aerobic, non–spore-forming organisms are most frequently the culprits. Anaerobic organisms tend to be causative when infection results from chronic sinusitis.

■ PRESENTING SIGNS AND SYMPTOMS

Patients with infection limited to the periorbital tissues typically present with erythema, edema, and warmth of the external eye tissues. Although usually unilateral, infection can be bilateral. There may be constitutional symptoms, including fever and malaise. The presence of ocular pain, ophthalmoplegia, and pain with extraocular movement suggests orbital involvement. Patients with orbital infection may also have decreased visual acuity and pupillary paralysis. They may have elevated IOPs, preseptal (periorbital) cellulitis, conjunctival injection, and proptosis (Fig. 20-6).

■ DIFFERENTIAL DIAGNOSIS

Signs of periorbital infection can be similar to those of allergic periorbital swelling, especially when there is bilateral involvement. With allergy, there may be cobblestoning on the interior aspect of the upper lid, and the condition should improve with administration of diphenhydramine or another antihistamine. It can be difficult to distinguish orbital cellulitis from subperiosteal and orbital abscesses and even from cavernous sinus thrombosis, which carries a dismal prognosis. With subperiosteal abscesses, the globe is often displaced by the abscess; the displacement should be obvious on inspection. Orbital abscesses are located in the postseptal tissues. They may cause obvious pus, significant ophthalmoplegia, and exophthalmos as well as globe displacement. Cavernous sinus thrombosis typically starts unilaterally and progresses to contralateral involvement. Examination should detect dilation of the episcleral vessels and venous engorgement of the fundus; the pupil may be fixed and dilated. Depending on the time course, orbital neoplasm with associated inflammation may cause similar symptoms.

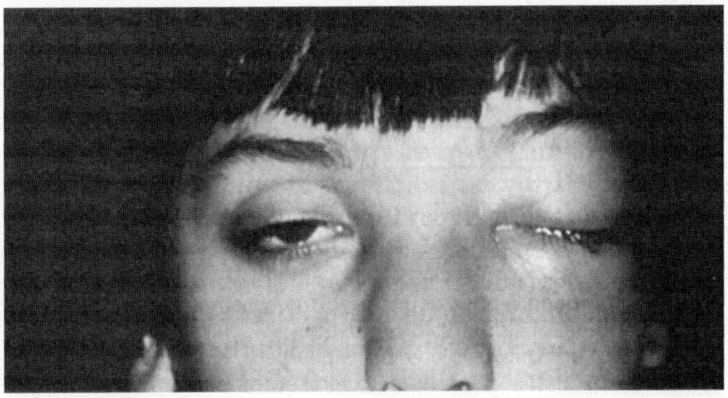

FIGURE 20-6 Orbital cellulitis. (From Long SS, Pickering LK, Prober CG [eds]: Principles and Practice of Pediatric Infectious Diseases, 2nd ed. Philadelphia, Churchill Livingstone, 2003.)

■ DIAGNOSTIC PROCEDURES

In many cases, it may be possible to exclude orbital involvement on the basis of the history and physical examination alone. If there is any doubt or the suspicion of another entity or complication such as abscess is present, computed tomography (CT) is the diagnostic modality of choice. It is not necessary to use intravenous contrast. MRI is another acceptable mode of diagnosis.

■ TREATMENT AND DISPOSITION

In adults, preorbital infection should be treated with oral antibiotics and close outpatient follow-up should be arranged. An antibiotic that provides coverage for staphylococci, streptococci, and Enterobacteriaceae is appropriate. Orbital cellulitis should be treated with broad-spectrum intravenous antibiotics; the patient should be admitted to the hospital; and consideration should be given to incision and drainage if imaging reveals a collection. For periorbital infection in children, there should be a lower threshold for admission. Patients with mild periorbital cellulitis can be discharged with arrangements for extremely close outpatient follow-up. For patients with more involved cases, including any underlying comorbidities, admission for observation should be seriously considered.

The Red Eye

An injected, red eye signals an inflammatory reaction. Fortunately, most inflammation is self-limited and can be treated on an outpatient basis. The specific cause, treatment, course, and prognosis, as well as the impact on vision, depend on the underlying cause (Table 20-2).

This discussion focuses on conjunctivitis, the diagnosis for 30% of patients presenting to the ED with ocular complaints. When there is corneal involvement as well, the process is called *keratoconjunctivitis*.

■ PATHOPHYSIOLOGY AND ANATOMY

An eye appears red because of dilation of blood vessels. Ciliary injection, caused by dilation of branches of the anterior ciliary arteries, indicates corneal, iris, or ciliary body inflammation. Conjunctival injection results from the more posterior, superficial conjunctival vessels. Because of the conjunctiva's more superficial location, vascular dilation causes more dramatic injection there than in the ciliary body.

Conjunctivitis refers to inflammation of the mucous membrane that lines the anterior sclera and inner eyelids. The conjunctiva is a key player in maintaining lubrication of the eye. Infection can result in scarring and abnormal tear formation in the affected eye.

Conjunctivitis can have a viral, bacterial, fungal, toxic, chemical, or allergic cause. The presentation and treatment differ with the underlying etiology. Sometimes it may be difficult to determine the underlying cause.

■ SIGNS AND SYMPTOMS

Generally, bilateral conjunctivitis signifies an infectious or allergic cause. However, this is not always the case. Viral infection is the most common cause of conjunctivitis. Adenovirus infection, which is highly contagious, is extremely common. Patients have significant injection, itching, irritation, and watery discharge. They may have accompanying preauricular adenopathy. Patients often have associated mild systemic symptoms because the conjunctivitis occurs in concert with a viral syndrome. Epidemic keratoconjunctivitis, which may cause pseudomembranes, is caused by adenovirus types 8 and 19; this is the classic pink eye. Patients are contagious for up to 2 weeks.

Herpes simplex conjunctivitis manifests as unilateral conjunctival injection with clear discharge. Patients complain of foreign body sensation and photophobia. With gross inspection alone, it may be impossible to distinguish herpes simplex from other viral causes. Patients may have facial or lid vesicles. This infection can spread rapidly, causing corneal damage, which manifests as a dendritic pattern on fluorescein examination. Depending on the location, size, and depth of corneal involvement, patients may have decreased visual acuity.

Herpes zoster ophthalmicus is caused by activation of the virus along the ophthalmic branch of the trigeminal nerve. The vesicular rash is present along the involved dermatome, resulting in forehead and upper eyelid lesions. Lesions on the tip of the nose, called Hutchinson's sign, signify involvement of the nasociliary branch of the fifth nerve. The presence of Hutchinson's sign indicates a much higher likelihood of ocular involvement (76% risk compared with 34% risk in the absence of such lesions). Fluorescein examination may show punctate, ulcerated, or dendritic corneal lesions (Fig. 20-7).

Patients with bacterial conjunctivitis present with conjunctival erythema, foreign body sensation, purulent drainage, and morning crusting of the eye. They usually do not have photophobia or loss of visual acuity. The most common causative organisms are *Staphylococcus, Streptococcus,* and *Haemophilus* (although with immunization, this last pathogen is decreasingly seen).

Gonococcal infection usually results in unilateral conjunctival injection, copious purulent discharge, and edema and erythema of the lids. The patient populations usually affected are infants, health care workers, and sexually active young adults. The amount of discharge helps distinguish gonococcal infection from other bacterial pathogens. Patients may have associated urethral discharge or arthritis.

Table 20-2 TREATMENT OF EYE INFLAMMATION (RED EYE) ACCORDING TO CAUSE

Feature	Conjunctivitis	Scleritis	Acute Angle-Closure Glaucoma	Acute Anterior Uveitis	Superficial Keratitis	Traumatic Iritis	Foreign Body
Ocular pain	Mild	Moderate to severe	Moderate to severe	Moderate	Moderate to severe	Moderate to severe	Moderate to severe
Visual acuity	Usually normal	May be reduced	Severely reduced	Mildly reduced	Moderately to severely reduced	Mildly reduced	May be reduced
Cornea	Clear	Clear	Hazy	Can be hazy	Hazy	Can be hazy	Clear or abrasion
Pupil	Normal	Normal Constricted if uveitis present	Dilated unreactive to light	Constricted with poor response to light	Normal Constricted if uveitis present	Constricted, weakly dilating	Normal if no globe penetration
Discharge	Yes	No	No	Minimal	Not usual, except with infectious cause	No	Not usual unless superinfection present
Hyperemia	Diffuse	Focal or diffuse	Diffuse	Diffuse	Diffuse	Perilimbal	Focal or diffuse
Intraocular pressure (IOP)	Normal	Normal	Increased	Usually normal but can increase if not treated	Normal	Can be increased	Normal
Treatment	Pain medications Antibiotics if bacterial, antiviral if herpes, ocular decongestants if allergic Supportive care with artificial tears if viral	Pain medications; steroid therapy in consultation with ophthalmologist Eye shield to protect the eye	Decrease in IOP, pain medications	Pain medications, steroid therapy in consultation with ophthalmologist, cycloplegics	Antibiotics if superinfection present, pain medications	Cycloplegics and steroids in consultation with ophthalmologist	Pain medications, removal of foreign body, tetanus status check/update, antibiotics if corneal abrasion present

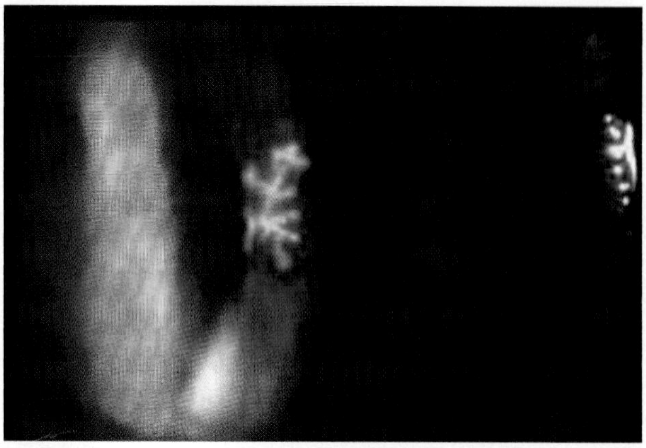

FIGURE 20-7 Herpes zoster ophthalmicus. (From www.emedicine.com.)

Pseudomonas aeruginosa infection should be suspected in patients who are immunosuppressed or wear contact lenses. Usually, a sticky, mucopurulent, yellow-green discharge is present. The cornea should be carefully inspected for ulceration because corneal perforation with progression of the infection is a major concern with this organism.

Fungal pathogens that cause conjunctivitis include *Actinomyces, Aspergillus, Candida, Coccidioides,* and *Mucor* (in diabetic patients). These should be considered in any immunosuppressed patient as well as any patient who has sustained eye trauma with vegetable matter. Examination may show a corneal infiltrate with underlying endothelial plaque and hypopyon, which is the presence of pus cells in the anterior chamber.

Chlamydial conjunctivitis is fairly common, especially in sexually active young adults. It is also a common cause of neonatal conjunctivitis. Patients may have associated gonococcal disease and thus should be asked about urethral discharge and arthritis. Patients with chlamydial conjunctivitis present with scant seropurulent eye discharge and fair to moderate conjunctival injection. Preauricular adenopathy is occasionally associated with this disorder.

Allergic conjunctivitis gives rise to significant pruritus and chemosis. Generally there is an associated clear discharge, in varying amounts. Cobblestoning may be seen on the inner eyelids.

■ DIAGNOSIS

Diagnosis of conjunctivitis is based on history, physical examination, and appropriate exclusion of other causes of red eye. It is important, in the correct setting, to perform a thorough examination to rule out both other causes of red eye and potential complications of conjunctivitis such as corneal ulceration. When there is concern for particularly virulent pathogens, Gram stain and cultures may be necessary.

■ TREATMENT AND DISPOSITION

Some basic tenets should be followed in the treatment of conjunctivitis, with separate consideration for the specific cause as detailed later.

Often, treatment is supportive. Cold compresses help with swelling and lid discomfort. Broad-spectrum antibiotic drops are used for bacterial conjunctivitis and often to prevent superinfection with other organisms. Erythromycin is appropriate for uncomplicated cases. A fluoroquinolone that provides coverage against *Pseudomonas* should be given to contact lens wearers. Topical corticosteroids should be prescribed only after consultation with an ophthalmologist and should never be used in a patient with suspected or confirmed herpes infection. Artificial tears alleviate keratitis and photophobia.

■ Adenovirus

Adenovirus infection requires supportive care, with cool compresses, decongestants, and lubricants, as well as topical antibiotics to prevent superinfection. Owing to the high transmissibility of adenovirus, care should be taken to prevent contamination of the other eye and of others. Cases of adenovirus conjunctivitis can be managed on an outpatient basis.

■ Herpes Simplex Conjunctivitis

Ophthalmologic consultation is indicated immediately for patients with herpes simplex conjunctivitis. The ophthalmologist may consider mechanical débridement. Topical antivirals such as vidarabine 3% and trifluridine 1% are prescribed in consultation with an ophthalmologist.

■ Herpes Zoster Ophthalmicus

The EP should consult an ophthalmologist about a patient with herpes zoster ophthalmicus. Systemic antiviral agents are indicated early in the disorder. Corticosteroid therapy may be considered in consultation with the ophthalmologist.

■ Uncomplicated Bacterial Conjunctivitis

Supportive care with warm compresses and lubricants should be given as needed for bacterial conjunctivitis. Topical antibiotics should be prescribed. The multiple choices include erythromycin, sulfacetamide 10%, gentamicin 0.3%, polymyxin B–neomycin–bacitracin (Neosporin), and ciprofloxacin. Use of neomycin solutions is associated with a relatively high incidence of hypersensitivity. Coverage against *Pseudomonas* should be included for contact lens wearers.

■ Gonococcal Conjunctivitis

Gonococcal conjunctivitis should be considered a systemic condition. Affected patients require emergency ophthalmologic consultation, and hospital admission is usually indicated. Treatment involves topical and parenteral antibiotic therapy and frequent eye irrigation to prevent corneal perforation. In some situations, patients are given one dose of intramuscular ceftriaxone and are then discharged after receiving topical antibiotics, instructions for eye rinsing, and arrangements for close follow-up.

■ Chlamydial Conjunctivitis

Like gonococcal infection, chlamydial conjunctivitis requires systemic therapy. Treatment involves oral and topical antibiotics. In neonates, systemic therapy is effective for concomitant pneumonitis.

■ Fungal Conjunctivitis

For a patient with fungal conjunctivitis, the EP should consult with an ophthalmologist about prescribing an appropriate topical agent, such as natamycin 5% suspension. Patients with this eye disorder require close follow-up.

■ Allergic Conjunctivitis

Patients with allergic conjunctivitis need supportive care with compresses and ocular decongestants. Diphenhydramine therapy can also be effective.

Corneal Abrasions

Corneal abrasions are one of the most common ocular injuries, accounting for 10% of ED visits related to ocular complaints. They result from scraping away of the corneal epithelium through contact with a foreign body or application of a moving force, such as rubbing over a closed lid. Most corneal abrasions heal spontaneously without long-term sequelae; on occasion, scarring, however, and permanent epithelial damage, ensue. Corneal abrasions are more common in contact lens wearers.

■ PATHOPHYSIOLOGY

Abrasions are defects in the corneal surface that are typically limited to the epithelial layer. Sometimes, the bulbar conjunctiva is also affected. Severe injuries can involve the deeper, thicker stromal layer of the cornea.

■ PRESENTING SIGNS AND SYMPTOMS

Common complaints of patients with corneal abrasions include photophobia, foreign body sensation, pain, and tearing. Conjunctival injection and blepharospasm may or may not be seen. Depending on the location and size of the abrasion, patients may also complain of decreased visual acuity. Fluorescein examination demonstrates the abrasion as a staining

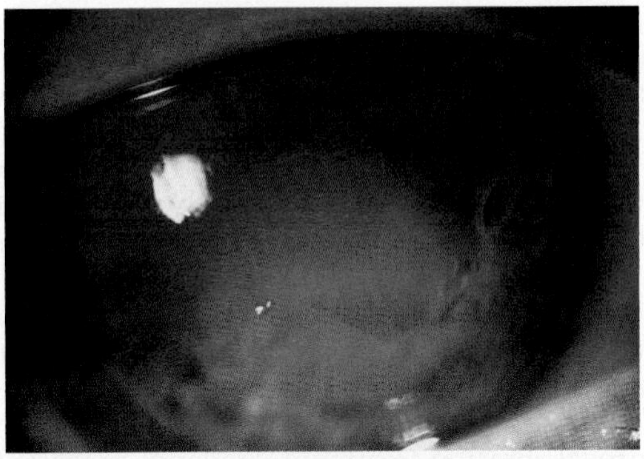

FIGURE 20-8 Corneal abrasions. (From Goldman L, Ausiello D [eds]: Cecil Medicine, 23rd ed. Philadelphia, Saunders, 2007.)

defect (Fig. 20-8). If a linear abrasion is noted, the EP should carefully search for a retained foreign body on the inner side of upper eyelid. Corneal ulceration should be excluded with a slit-lamp examination, especially in contact lens wearers. A topical anesthetic should be administered to facilitate the examination.

■ DIFFERENTIAL DIAGNOSIS

All entities that cause eye pain should be included in the differential diagnosis for corneal abrasion. Because erythema and changes in visual acuity may or may not be present, the differential diagnosis has to be tailored to the individual case. Examination and measurement of IOPs should eliminate glaucoma as a cause of the symptoms. Slit-lamp examination demonstrates cells and flare in the anterior chamber in a patient with iritis. Lack of infiltrate and ulcer morphology excludes corneal ulcer. The EP should carefully look for a foreign body in order to eliminate it as a cause of the complaints.

■ TREATMENT

Providing comfort for the patient is the goal of treatment for corneal abrasion. Although topical antibiotics may be administered to facilitate evaluation, patients should never be discharged with such medications. Continued use of topical ocular anesthetics may cause injury through loss of protective reflexes and drying of the eye. Systemic analgesia should be prescribed as needed. Studies have suggested that topical nonsteroidal anti-inflammatory drugs (NSAIDs) also provide relief and may reduce the need for oral narcotic agents. A cycloplegic agent such as homatropine provides relief from photophobia and blepharospasm.

The practice of routinely prescribing topical antibiotics for corneal abrasions to prevent corneal ulceration is not clearly evidence-based, although some studies have suggested that it is beneficial. For example, a prospective study investigating the incidence of corneal ulceration in close to 35,000 patients diagnosed with corneal abrasions demonstrated that none of the patients who received antibiotics had ulceration. Contact lens wearers should be treated with agents that provide coverage against *Pseudomonas*. Eye patching should be avoided, especially in contact lens wearers and patients whose abrasions were cause by organic material, because it may encourage infection. Evidence suggests that patching may be harmful, but current data are not available. Patients with abrasions should discontinue contact lens wear during the healing period.

Tetanus prophylaxis is a long-standing component of corneal abrasion treatment. Evidence suggests that this practice is not routinely indicated. In the absence of infection, corneal perforation, or devitalized tissue, there is no benefit to routine administration of a tetanus booster. However, current Centers for Disease Control and Prevention (CDC) guidelines recommend a tetanus booster within 5 years if the event causing the corneal abrasion involved a dirty instrument such as vegetable matter and within 10 years if the corneal injury was caused by a clean, uncontaminated vector.[14,15] Patients with corneal abrasions can be discharged with arrangements for close outpatient follow-up.

Corneal Ulcers

Generally, corneal ulcers are infectious in etiology. A corneal ulcer is an ophthalmologic emergency because the diagnosis carries the risk of permanent visual impairment and eye perforation. Risk factors for corneal ulcer include eye trauma, known infection, contact lens wear, and immunosuppression.

■ PATHOPHYSIOLOGY

Even seemingly minor trauma to the cornea can create a break, which serves as a port of entry for bacteria. Conditions such as lack of lubrication and malnutrition make the cornea more susceptible to injury.

■ PRESENTING SIGNS AND SYMPTOMS

Corneal ulcers cause significant eye pain, ciliary injection, tearing, foreign body sensation, blurry vision, and photophobia. Eyelid swelling and purulent drainage may be present. Depending on the location and extent of the lesion, visual acuity may be decreased. Inspection may show eyelid swelling and erythema. Large ulcers can be seen as round or oval white spots on the cornea with the naked eye. Fluorescein and slit-lamp examinations demonstrate a corneal defect, usually with sharply demarcated borders and a gray appearance to the infiltrated ulcer base. On anterior chamber examination, hypopyon or flare consistent with iritis is often seen. With the exception of the classic dendritic lesions seen with herpes simplex virus infection, there are no pathognomonic signs or symptoms to diagnose the etiology of the ulcer seen on examination (Fig. 20-9).

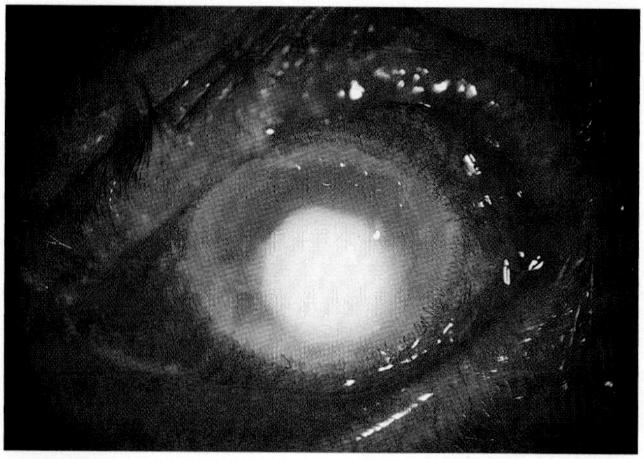

FIGURE 20-9 Corneal ulcers. (From Auerbach PS [ed]: Wilderness Medicine, 5th ed. Philadelphia, Mosby, 2007.)

■ DIFFERENTIAL DIAGNOSIS

The same conditions that must be considered in the differential diagnosis for patients with corneal abrasions must be considered for those with corneal ulcers.

■ TREATMENT AND DISPOSITION

Immediate ophthalmologic consultation should be obtained for a patient with corneal ulcer. Some ophthalmologists advocate discharge with follow-up the next day. A cycloplegic agent such as homatropine is given for comfort. Frequent topical antibiotic therapy should be prescribed. The typical regimen involves administration of the drop every 1 to 2 hours until the follow-up appointment the next day.

Ocular Foreign Bodies

Corneal foreign bodies are generally superficial and they do not cause long-term morbidity. However, if they are allowed to remain in place for a long enough time, infection, tissue necrosis, and scarring may occur.

■ PATHOPHYSIOLOGY

Objects, especially those projected with considerable force, may become embedded in the corneal epithelium or deeper into the stroma. The irritation triggers a cascade of events including vascular dilation, which manifests as conjunctival injection and lid edema.

■ PRESENTING SIGNS AND SYMPTOMS

Typical symptoms of ocular foreign body include pain, photophobia, tearing, conjunctival injection, and foreign body sensation. Examination may show conjunctival injection, a visible foreign body, corneal epithelial defect, and corneal edema. White blood cell mobilization may occur and can be detected as

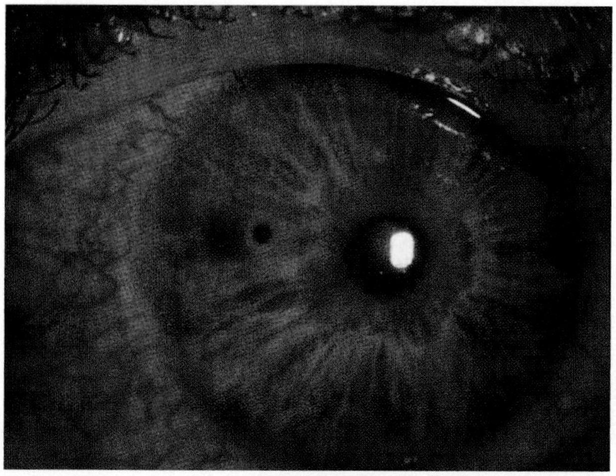

FIGURE 20-10 Rust ring seen after removal of metallic foreign body. (Courtesy of Ted Montgomery, OD, www.tedmontgomery.com/the_eye/)

anterior chamber flare and presence of cells. Visual acuity can be decreased. Metallic foreign bodies can cause visible rust rings (Fig. 20-10).

■ DIFFERENTIAL DIAGNOSIS

The conditions that may mimic corneal abrasion and corneal ulceration must also be considered in the patient with ocular foreign body. Application of topical anesthesia blunts or obliterates the pain and photophobia associated with superficial corneal processes. This response can be helpful in distinguishing among various eye disorders.

■ DIAGNOSIS

Diagnosis of ocular foreign body is based on history and physical findings. If there is concern about a foreign body that is not visible, especially an intraocular foreign body, CT should be obtained. MRI is contraindicated if it is possible that the foreign body is metallic. Ultrasonography can be used to visualize a superficial foreign body, but this modality is limited by type of particle as well as possible obscuration of findings by processes such as subconjunctival hemorrhage. A Seidel test should be performed to look for corneal rupture if deep projection is suspected. The lids should be everted and a possible lodged foreign body sought.

■ TREATMENT AND DISPOSITION

Treatment consists first of removal of the foreign body. Topical anesthesia should be used, and a cycloplegic agent considered. Superficial foreign bodies are removed with a spud or needle. A cotton-tipped applicator should be used with great caution because it may propagate abrasion owing to its large surface area. The foreign body should be removed under magnification with the slit-lamp. The EP should approach the foreign body with the removal device held parallel to the surface of the eye to avoid inadvertent perforation. Retained rust rings after removal of a metallic foreign body must be removed with a rust ring drill; an ophthalmologist should be consulted for this maneuver.

After foreign body removal, the patient should be given topical antibiotics. Patching of the eye for comfort is not necessary and is strictly contraindicated in the presence of severe corneal injury because it may foster infection. Pain control should be adequate, and arrangements should be made for prompt follow-up.

Intraocular Foreign Body

More than three fourths of intraocular foreign bodies enter the eye through the cornea. Suspicion of such a foreign body is based on patient complaints as well as history. Injuries associated with mechanical grinding, drilling, and hammering should raise the possibility of intraocular foreign body. Intraorbital and intracranial injury should always be considered in the patient with intraocular injury.

The extent and process of eye damage depend on the object involved and the area penetrated. Because of gravity, the inferior aspect of the eye is more commonly injured. The composition of the object involved affects local tissue reaction. Inert substances such as glass cause less reaction than organic materials. Metallic and magnetic substances are most common.

Patient presentations also vary according to the factors just described. Patients often complain of discomfort or pain deep within the eye. Presence of obvious abnormalities on inspection, such as conjunctival injection, is variable. Visual acuity is also contingent upon the area involved. Careful slit-lamp and funduscopic examinations should be performed to search for the object. An abnormally shaped pupil is suspicious for globe rupture.

CT is the imaging modality of choice if it is necessary to search for the injury or to more closely ascertain its specifics. Ultrasonography can be helpful with relatively superficial objects. Plain radiographs cannot distinguish between intraocular and extraocular positions of a foreign body. MRI cannot be used if there is any suspicion the foreign body may be metallic.

■ DIFFERENTIAL DIAGNOSIS

If the eye with the foreign body appears externally normal, inspection alone excludes several painful eye disorders, such as iritis. Application of topical anesthetics should not affect the pain caused by intraocular foreign body—in contrast to the pain of a corneal foreign body or abrasion. A careful examination can exclude glaucoma as the cause of the patient's symptoms.

■ TREATMENT

An ophthalmologist consultation should be sought immediately. The patient should not eat or drink, and antibiotics and pain medications should be administered. Tetanus status should be updated as necessary. Generally, intraocular foreign bodies are surgically removed. The technique and approach are chosen by the ophthalmologist. The patient with an intraocular foreign body should be admitted to the hospital.

Ocular Burns

Ocular burns, which include burns to the sclera, conjunctiva, cornea, and lids, can be damaging to visual integrity as well as cosmesis. Burns may be chemical, thermal, or from radiation exposure. The method and extent of damage vary with the cause.

■ PATHOPHYSIOLOGY

Burns cause tissue damage by denaturing and coagulating cellular proteins and through vascular ischemia. Thermal burns usually cause superficial epithelial destruction, but deep penetration can occur. Radiation injury causes punctuate keratitis, which is extremely painful. Patients with radiation ocular burns report exposure to sun lamps, tanning booths, high altitudes, or welder's arcs. Acidic burns cause coagulation necrosis, which serves as a barrier, limiting the extent of penetration. Alkaline chemicals can cause devastating injury. Such a chemical causes liquefaction necrosis that continually penetrates and dissolves tissue until the chemical is removed. At pH values greater than 11.5, damage is generally irreversible.

■ PRESENTING SIGNS AND SYMPTOMS

Patients usually complain of eye pain and limited visual acuity. Examination in the acute phase often shows corneal cloudiness and scleral whitening. The eye may be erythematous or whitened. There may be findings consistent with anterior chamber reaction, chemosis, and vascular engorgement. Radiation burn or ultraviolet keratitis causes intense pain, tearing, photophobia, blepharospasm, and foreign body sensation. Physical findings include punctate lesions on the corneal epithelium, conjunctival injection, and decreased visual acuity. Thermal burns are almost always limited to the corneal epithelium.

■ DIFFERENTIAL DIAGNOSIS

The history of exposure usually leads to a clear diagnosis. Radiation burns are not always so clear-cut because symptoms develop 6 to 10 hours after exposure to the light source. Other conditions to consider are iritis, glaucoma, corneal ulcer, corneal abrasion, and retained foreign body. Slit-lamp and fluorescein examinations allow for differentiation among the various entities.

■ DIAGNOSIS

Type of chemical burn can be diagnosed with determination of pH of the affected eye. Findings depend on concentration of the chemical and duration of exposure to it. Most burns can be diagnosed from history alone. Radiation burns can be a bit more challenging to diagnose owing to extreme patient discomfort. Providing adequate topical analgesic should enable examination.

■ TREATMENT AND DISPOSITION

The most important component of treatment for chemical burns is copious irrigation. Eye irrigation should be started immediately—with no waiting even for measurement of visual acuity. After irrigation for 30 minutes, the pH should be checked. The EP should not withhold irrigation or delay initiation even if the patient underwent prehospital irrigation. Irrigation should continue until a normal pH is recorded. Once a normal pH is obtained, the measurement should be repeated 10 to 15 minutes later to confirm neutrality. Topical anesthetics and manual lid retraction may be necessary for proper irrigation.

After adequate irrigation, a complete examination of the eye, including slit-lamp examination and determination of visual acuity, should be performed. Patients with minor burns can be discharged home with topical antibiotics, oral analgesics, and cycloplegics as necessary with arrangements for follow-up in 24 hours. An ophthalmologist should be consulted for all but the most minor ocular burns. Severe burns may cause secondary glaucoma, which is treated in consultation with the ophthalmologist. Patients with severe burns require admission for monitoring, including IOP measurements, and adequate analgesia.

Most thermal burns, which are relatively minor and restricted to the lid and corneal epithelium, can be treated the same as corneal abrasions. Initial irrigation may provide relief. Topical antibiotics, oral pain medications, and cold compresses should be provided. Patients can be discharged with outpatient follow-up. An ophthalmologist should be consulted for more severe burns.

Radiation burns are treated with cycloplegic agents and topical antibiotics. Eye patching can be considered for comfort. Oral pain medications should be prescribed. *Topical anesthetics delay healing and can lead to corneal ulcer formation.* Follow-up in 24 hours should be arranged.

Retrobulbar Hematoma

Retrobulbar hematoma is bleeding in the potential space surrounding the globe. It results from blunt trauma as well as from retrobulbar injection and operative intervention. This entity can compromise vision, so immediate recognition and intervention are warranted. Bleeding typically results from injury to the infraorbital artery or one of its branches. Accumulation of blood results in an increase in pressure, ultimately compressing blood vessels and other structures. The compression leads to optic nerve and central retinal artery ischemia. With trauma, concomitant orbital wall fractures serve to decompress the hemorrhage, thereby sparing vision.

■ PRESENTING SIGNS AND SYMPTOMS

Severe eye pain, nausea, vomiting, diplopia, and decreases in both visual acuity and eye movement are common complaints at presentation in a patient with retrobulbar hematoma. Physical findings include proptosis, decreased ocular motility, visual loss, elevated IOP, and hemorrhagic chemosis. An afferent pupillary defect is common (Fig. 20-11).

■ DIAGNOSIS

Clinical examination suggests the diagnosis. If there is doubt about the diagnosis, CT can be performed to demonstrate the hematoma.

■ TREATMENT

The rate of development of retrobulbar hematoma dictates the treatment. If the condition develops over minutes, the eye must be decompressed immediately via lateral canthotomy (Fig. 20-12). If the process is slower and develops over hours, conservative management can be effective. This consists of head elevation, ice packs to reduce swelling, intravenous acetazolamide and mannitol, and topical beta-blockers. Progress is monitored through serial measurements of IOPs and pupillary reactivity. An ophthalmologist should be notified for consultation as soon as the diagnosis is suspected. Patients with

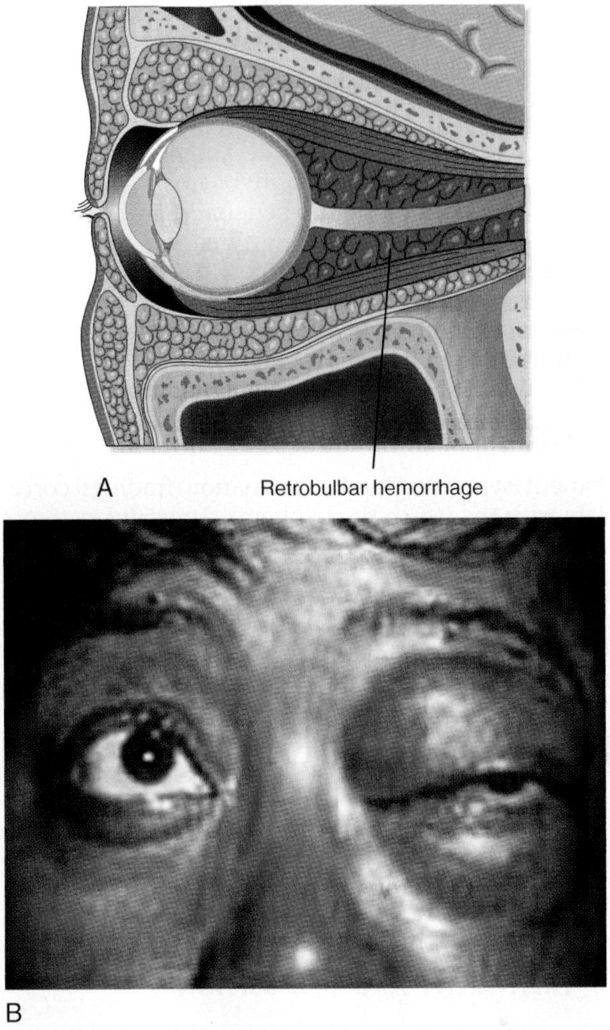
A
Retrobulbar hemorrhage
B

FIGURE 20-11 **A** and **B,** Retrobulbar hematoma. (**B** from Pacific University: Online Optometry Education. Available at http://www.opt.pacificu.edu/ce/catalog/10310-SD/Trauma%20Pictures/Retrobulbar%20Heme.jpg.)

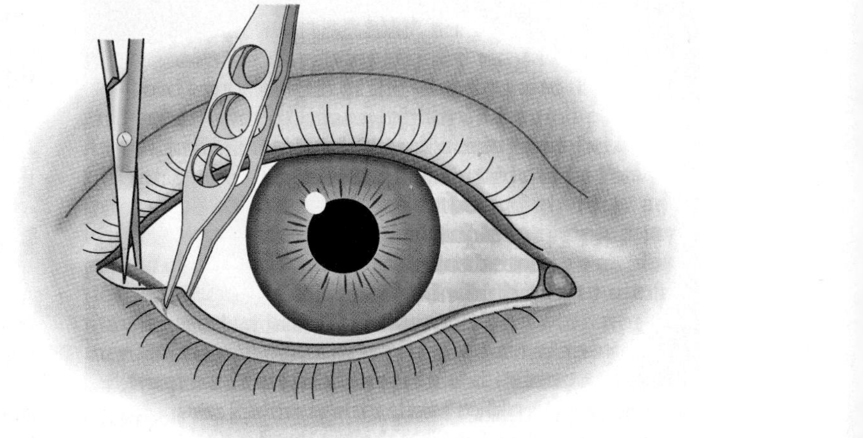

FIGURE 20-12 Lateral canthotomy.

retrobulbar hematoma are admitted to the hospital to monitor progress.

Hyphema

Accumulation of blood in the anterior chamber is called *hyphema.* Traumatic hyphemas, which can occur from both blunt and penetrating mechanisms, are generally caused by a ruptured iris root vessel. Spontaneous hyphemas are most commonly associated with sickle cell disease and neovascularization of diabetes. Even small hyphemas can signal significant injury.

■ PRESENTING SIGNS AND SYMPTOMS

Patient symptoms and examination findings correlate with the size of the hyphema. Typically, patients complain of eye pain, decreased visual acuity, and photophobia. If the patient is upright, the hyphema usually layers out in the inferior portion of the anterior chamber. Depending on the size of the hyphema, it can be seen with either the naked eye or a slit-lamp examination. If the hyphema is large, IOP can be elevated. Generally, there is no afferent pupillary defect (Fig. 20-13).

■ DIAGNOSIS

Diagnosis is made by visualization of blood in the anterior chamber.

■ TREATMENT AND DISPOSITION

All patients with hyphemas should be seen by an ophthalmologist. The goal is to stop damage to the visual process by preventing or curbing elevations of IOP. The patient's head should be elevated to allow inferior settling of the red blood cells. This settling will prevent trabecular meshwork clogging. The pupil should be dilated to avoid "pupillary play"—movements of the iris to accommodate changing light conditions; this step should be taken with consultation from the ophthalmologist. Dilation does not block drainage of aqueous humor in normal eyes. Topical beta-blockers should be used to lower IOP. Topical alpha-agonists, topical carbonic anhydrase inhibitors, and systemic acetazolamide or mannitol may also be considered. Adequate should be given analgesia, with care taken to avoid aspirin and other antiplatelet agents.

Surgery may be necessary if IOP elevation is refractory to medical therapy or to remove a large clot. Almost all patients with hyphema are admitted to the hospital for bedrest and observation. Consultation with an ophthalmologist may determine that a patient with an extremely small hyphema can receive outpatient management. The major complication of hyphema is rebleeding after 2 to 5 days, when the initial clot loosens, resulting in potentially severe elevations in IOP. This is the rationale behind hospital admission.

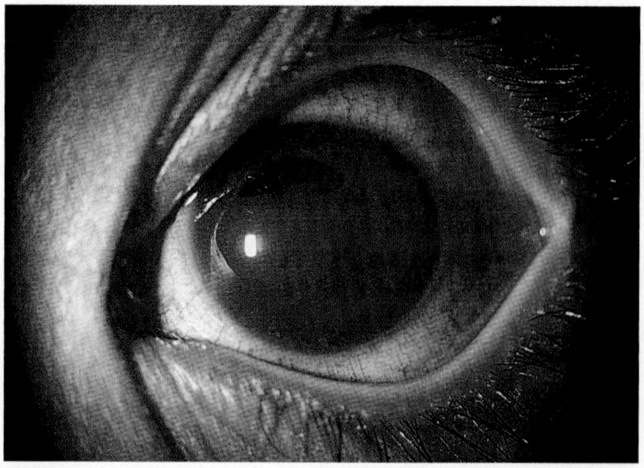

FIGURE 20-13 Hyphema. (From Auerbach PS [ed]: Wilderness Medicine, 5th ed. Philadelphia, Mosby, 2007.)

Orbital Wall or Blow-out Fractures

Blunt force to the orbital region can raise intraorbital pressure, relief of which is accomplished by fracture of the orbital walls. The inferior and medial walls are most frequently involved. Orbital contents slip into the corresponding sinus, the maxillary sinus for inferior wall fractures and the ethmoid sinus for medial wall fractures. Concomitant facial injuries should be sought in a patient with an orbital wall or blow-out fracture (Fig. 20-14).

■ PRESENTING SIGNS AND SYMPTOMS

Presentation in orbital wall or blow-out fracture can be highly variable, ranging from mild swelling and ecchymosis to impairment of vision. Patients may have tenderness with palpation of the orbit. Subcutaneous orbital emphysema can often be found by examination. Inferior wall fractures can cause entrapment of the inferior rectus and inferior oblique muscles and orbital fat. Patients may have restricted upward gaze and diplopia, anesthesia of the ipsilateral cheek and upper lip, and ptosis. Epistaxis and diplopia can be seen with medial wall fractures. On rare occasion, orbital emphysema can have a mass effect, compressing the optic nerve and causing blindness.

■ DIAGNOSIS

A Waters view radiograph can show indirect signs of fracture: cloudy sinus, a bulge extending from the orbit into the maxillary sinus (the teardrop sign), or an air-fluid level in the maxillary sinus. CT is the diagnostic study of choice because it demonstrates the fracture as well as the other injuries.

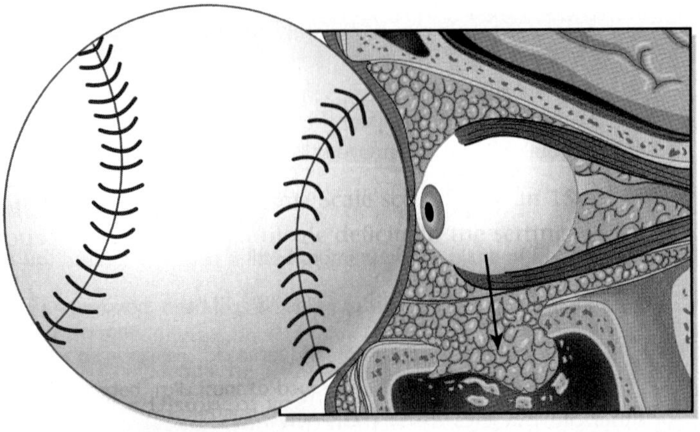

FIGURE 20-14 Orbital wall/blow-out fracture.

■ TREATMENT AND DISPOSITION

Immediate surgery is not necessary. Indications for surgical repair include muscle entrapment and cosmetic deformity with significant enophthalmos. Surgery is delayed to allow for abatement of swelling and a better examination. The preferred time frame for operative repair is 10 to 14 days, which optimizes the balance of reduced swelling with the absence of scar tissue formation. Administration of prophylactic antibiotics for an orbital wall or blow-out fracture without evidence of sinus infection is controversial. Data are inadequate for a definitive recommendation, as review of 214 studies to examine this very question found.[16,17]

Ruptured Globe

Globe rupture involves a full-thickness defect in the cornea and/or sclera. Penetrating mechanisms are almost always involved. Rarely, enough force is generated by a blunt injury that transmission of the force results in eventual rupture. This entity is a true ophthalmologic emergency and always requires surgical intervention.

Sharp objects and objects traveling at considerable velocity have the potential to perforate the globe directly. Any projective injury can cause globe rupture. Significant blunt force can result in globe compression with resultant IOP increases sizeable enough to tear the sclera. Such injuries typically occur where the sclera is the thinnest, such as at muscle insertion sites or sites of previous surgery.

■ PRESENTING SIGNS AND SYMPTOMS

Patients with globe rupture complain of eye pain and decreased visual acuity. Because this entity is associated with a high rate of concomitant orbital floor fractures, patients may report diplopia. Rupture may not be easily apparent on examination. Finding of a shallow anterior chamber on slit-lamp examination, hyphema, and an irregular (teardrop) pupil are possible findings. A Seidel test can identify wound leaks from the anterior chamber.

■ DIAGNOSIS

Diagnosis is not always easy. History and the physical findings described lead to the diagnosis. Although not always indicated, CT can detect occult tears as well as retained foreign bodies. Plain radiographs may show foreign bodies.

■ TREATMENT AND DISPOSITION

Direct pressure should never be applied to a globe that is suspected or confirmed to be ruptured, because of the risk of extrusion of intraocular contents. A protective eye shield should be placed, and an ophthalmologist should be contacted immediately. The patient's tetanus status should be checked and updated if necessary, and a dose of prophylactic antibiotics should be given to prevent endophthalmitis. Because skin flora is typically involved in infections of a rupture globe, cefazolin or ciprofloxacin plus clindamycin are good choices. Adequate antiemetics should be given to prevent Valsalva maneuvers. Surgery is performed expeditiously, and all patients with globe rupture are admitted to the hospital.

Traumatic Iritis

Blunt ocular trauma can contuse and irritate the iris, with resultant ciliary spasm. Symptoms usually start 1 to 4 days after the injury.

■ PRESENTING SIGNS AND SYMPTOMS/DIAGNOSIS

Eye pain and photophobia are the most common patient complaints in traumatic iritis. Patients report impaired vision. Evaluation shows perilimbal conjunctival injection, cells and flare in the anterior chamber, and a constricted, weakly dilating pupil.

■ TREATMENT AND DISPOSITION

Treatment involves administration of a long-acting cycloplegic agent such as homatropine 5%, a topical

PATIENT TEACHING TIPS

- The patient with a red eye should seek evaluation by the primary care physician because this disorder has several benign and serious causes.
- If the pain worsens, visual acuity decreases, a discharge appears, or a fever occurs, the patient should immediately return to the ED for reevaluation.
- Patients at high risk for eye problems (e.g., those with diabetes) should be encouraged to obtain yearly eye examinations. More information for patients with diabetes is available from the American Diabetes Association (www.diabetes.org).

steroid chosen in consultation with an ophthalmologist, and oral analgesics. Patients can be discharged with arrangements for ophthalmologic follow-up.

REFERENCES

1. Bruncette DD: Ophthalmology. In Marx JA, Hockberger RS, Walls RM (eds): Rosen's Emergency Medicine, vol II, 5th ed. St. Louis, CV Mosby, 2002, p 908.
2. Tham CC, Lai JS, Leung DY, et al: Acute angle-closure glaucoma. Ophthalmology 2005;112:1479-1480.
3. Rumelt S, Brown GC: Update on treatment of retinal arterial occlusions. Curr Opin Ophthalmol 2003;14:139-141.
4. Atebara NH, Brown GC, Cater J: Efficacy of anterior chamber paracentesis and carbogen in treating acute nonarteritic central retinal artery occlusion. Ophthalmology 1995; 102:2029-2035.
5. Pettersen JA, Hill MD, Demchuk AM, et al: Intra-arterial thrombolysis for retinal artery occlusion: the Calgary experience. Can J Neurol Sci 2005;32:507-511.
6. Weber J, Remonda L, Mattle HP, et al: Selective intra-arterial fibrinolysis of acute central retinal artery occlusion. 1998;29:2076-2079.
7. Beiran I, Goldenberg I, Adir Y, et al: Early hyperbaric oxygen therapy for retinal artery occlusion. Eur J Ophthalmol 2002;11:345-350.
8. Rumelt S, Dorenboim Y, Rehany U: Aggressive systematic treatment for central retinal artery occlusion. Am J Ophthalmol 1999;128:733-738.
9. Jonas JB, Akkoyun I, Kamppeter B, et al: Branch retinal vein occlusion treated by intravitreal triamcinolone acetonide. Eye 2005;19:65-71.
10. Horio N, Horiguchi M: Retinal blood flow and macular edema after radial optic neurotomy for central retinal vein occlusion. Am J Ophthalmol 2006;141:145-146.
11. Chan CK, Lam DS: Optic neuritis treatment trial: 10 year follow-up results. Am J Ophthalmol 2004;138:695.
12. Quintyn JC, Benouaich X, Pagot-Mathis V, Mathis A: Retinal detachment, a condition little known to patients. Retina 2006;26:1077-1078.
13. Brown SM, Raflo GT, Harper DK, et al: Temporal arteritis management. Am J Ophthalmol 2006;113:1059-1060.
14. Mukherjee P, Sivakumar A: Tetanus prophylaxis in superficial corneal abrasions. Emerg Med J 2003;20:62-64.
15. Benson WH, Snyder IS, Granus V, et al: Tetanus prophylaxis following ocular injuries. J Emerg Med 1993; 11:677-683.
16. Martin B, Ghosh A, Mackway-Jones K: Antibiotics in orbital floor fractures. Emerg Med J 2003;20:66.
17. Westfall CT, Shore JW: Isolated fractures of the orbital floor: Risk of infection and the role of antibiotic prophylaxis. Ophthalmic Surg 1991;22:409-411.

Chapter 21

Ear Emergencies

Thomas Morrissey

KEY POINTS

- Ears are exquisitely sensitive organs. Treating pain is important in care and will facilitate the examination.
- Simple otitis externa can be treated with topical medications and débridement.
- Many cases of uncomplicated otitis media resolve spontaneously. Use of a "rescue" antibiotic prescription has been shown to decrease unnecessary antibiotic use and improve patient/parent satisfaction.
- Subtle malalignments or malformations in repair of ear trauma can have profound cosmetic consequences.
- Pain from teeth, pharynx, the temporomandibular joint, or cranial/cervical neuropathies can be referred to the ear.
- Hearing loss must be categorized as conductive or sensorineural. Conductive lesions can often be diagnosed clinically. Sensorineural hearing loss requires urgent referral to an otolaryngologist to improve the chances of recovery of hearing.

Anatomically, the ear is divided into three areas. The *external ear* extends outward from the tympanic membrane and comprises the external auditory canal and the external structures. Its primary function is to guide sound waves into the "business end" of the ear. The external location places it at high risk for traumatic injuries, environmental exposure, obstruction, and infection.

The *middle ear* extends inward from the tympanic membrane to the oval and round windows. The main function of the middle ear is to transfer mechanical energy from the outside world, through the ossicles in the middle ear, to the organ of Corti in the inner ear. Here, the energy is translated into signals that the brain interprets as sound. The enclosed nature of the middle ear predisposes it to fluid accumulation, infection, and barotrauma.

The *inner ear* is composed of the cochlea, the vestibule (saccule and utricle), and semicircular canals, the structures responsible for sound transduction and balance. Although dysfunction of this portion of the ear accounts for some visits to the ED, significant treatment of this area is rarely given by EPs. Recognition of injury to this area allows the EP to educate patients about processes and prognosis and to implement precautions that may limit further damage until referral to an otolaryngologist can be made.

The ear is surrounded by the middle cranial fossa superiorly, the mastoid air cells posteriorly, cranial vault medially, and the temporomandibular joint and parotid glands anteriorly. Evaluation of these structures is a necessary part of the ear exam.

Ear Pain

Ear pain may be referred or may occur from infections, trauma, or foreign body affecting the ear.

INFECTIONS

Ear pain is commonly rooted in infection. Any portion of the ear can become infected. The disease state is categorized by the portion of the ear that is primarily affected.

Otitis Externa

Infections of the outer ear canal (external otitis, otitis externa) most often begin when breakdown of the natural barriers allow infectious organisms to gain a foothold. This commonly occurs in the summer months, when warm weather and frequent water sports lead to excessive ear moisture, which washes out cerumen and alkalinizes the normally acidic environment—hence the term "swimmer's ear." Cotton-swab trauma can be the inciting event, especially in diabetic patients.

The most common pathogens are *Pseudomonas aeruginosa* (frequently found in pools) and *Staphylococcus aureus*. Less common causes include chemical or contact dermatitis and fungal infections. The spectrum of disease ranges from mild (with minimal pain and canal inflammation) to severe (complete canal occlusion and exquisite pain). Further extension results in an invasive or systemic disease state called *necrotizing external otitis* (formerly "malignant otitis externa" [MOE]; see later).

Diagnosis of external otitis is made from the history and physical examination. Complaints of pain or pruritus and findings of canal irritation and edema clinch the diagnosis. Thick greenish discharge suggests *Pseudomonas* as the offending organism, whereas golden crusting implicates *S. aureus*. Other colored or black discharge may indicate fungal infections. Small abscesses can form in the external ear canal and cause obstruction, leading to otitis externa. These often require incision and drainage as well as standard treatment for otitis externa.

Treatment

Treatment consists of débridement/aural toilet and antibiotics. Despite a relative lack of controlled studies, the American Academy of Otolaryngology–Head and Neck Surgery Foundation (AAO-HNSF) has released clinical practice guidelines based on evidence available as of 2005 (Fig. 21-1; see also Patient Teaching Tips box).[1] They are summarized here:

1. Clinicians should distinguish acute external otitis (AEO) from other causes of otalgia, otorrhea, and inflammation of the external ear canal. Diagnostic criteria include rapid onset (2-3 days) and duration of less than 3 weeks. Symptoms of ear canal inflammation include otalgia, itching or fullness, and signs of inflammation, which include tenderness of the pinna or tragus, or visual evidence of canal erythema, edema, or otorrhea.
2. Patients should be assessed for factors that may complicate the disease or treatment. Examples are tympanic membrane perforation, presence of tympanostomy tubes, immunocompromising states such as diabetes mellitus and human immunodeficiency virus, and prior radiotherapy. These factors are important because they raise the level of needed treatment and heighten suspicion for more invasive disease states, such as necrotizing otitis externa (see later). All of these guidelines pertain to patients older than 2 years with normal states of health.
3. Attention should be paid to assessment and treatment of pain. Mild to moderate pain usually responds to acetaminophen or a nonsteroidal anti-inflammatory drug (NSAID) alone or in combination with an opioid.
4. Topical preparations should be used as first-line agents in the treatment of acute uncomplicated otitis externa. Systemic antimicrobial therapy should not be used unless there is extension outside the ear canal or the presence of specific host factors that would indicate the need for systemic therapy. Topical therapy produces drug concentrations 100 to 1000 times that available with systemic administration, which overwhelms resistance mechanisms. No clear evidence points to the superiority of one particular treatment. Antiseptic and acidifying agents (such as aluminum acetate and boric acid) appear to work as well as antibiotic-containing solutions (such as solutions that contain cortisone and neosporin or a fluoroquinolone). The presence of corticosteroids in the drops decreases the duration of pain by about 1 day.[2]
5. Make sure the patient is able to instill the drops into the ear canal correctly. Canal edema or detritus may prevent the drops from entering the canal. Debris can be removed by aural toilet or irrigation. The placement of a compressed cellulose or ribbon gauze wick into the canal will enable drops to penetrate into the canal. Wick placement can often be very difficult due to pain and limited patient cooperation. The inner two thirds of the external auditory canal consists of epithelium directly over periosteum and is extremely sensitive to pain. The added inflammation exacerbates the pain. Within 1 to 2 days the canal edema should subside, and the wick falls out or can be removed.
6. Pain and swelling often limit visualization of the tympanic membrane. If the EP cannot be sure the membrane is intact, a non-ototoxic, pH-balanced preparation should be prescribed. Antibiotics that get into the middle ear space can be absorbed through the round or oval window into the inner ear space. As of December 2005, the only topical preparations approved by the U.S. Food and Drug Administration (FDA) for middle ear exposure were ofloxacin and ciprofloxacin/dexamethasone.
7. If the symptoms have not improved in 48 to 72 hours, the patient should be reassessed to confirm the diagnosis and exclude other causes.

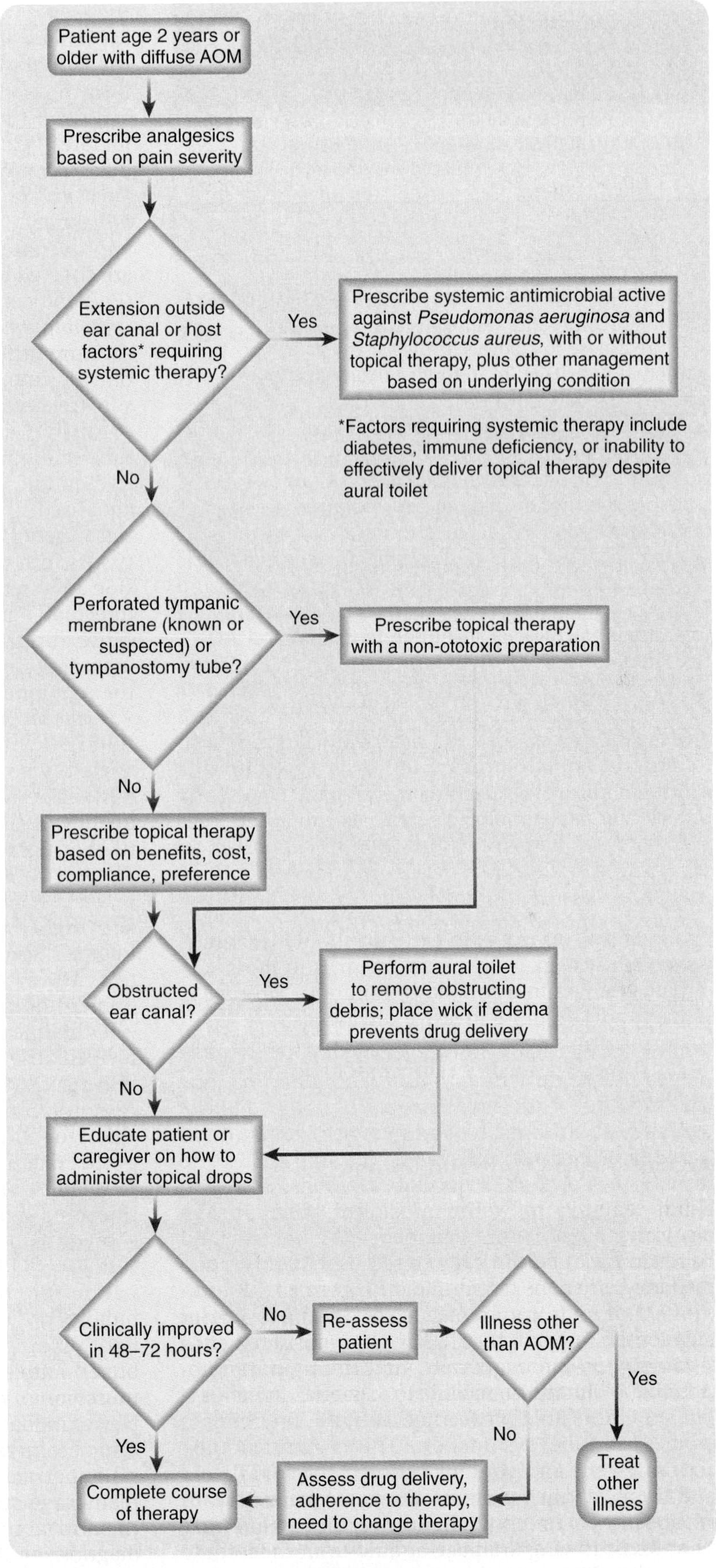
Patient age 2 years or older with diffuse AOM
Prescribe analgesics based on pain severity
Extension outside ear canal or host factors* requiring systemic therapy?
Yes
Prescribe systemic antimicrobial active against *Pseudomonas aeruginosa* and *Staphylococcus aureus*, with or without topical therapy, plus other management based on underlying condition
*Factors requiring systemic therapy include diabetes, immune deficiency, or inability to effectively deliver topical therapy despite aural toilet
No
Perforated tympanic membrane (known or suspected) or tympanostomy tube?
Yes
Prescribe topical therapy with a non-ototoxic preparation
No
Prescribe topical therapy based on benefits, cost, compliance, preference
Obstructed ear canal?
Yes
Perform aural toilet to remove obstructing debris; place wick if edema prevents drug delivery
No
Educate patient or caregiver on how to administer topical drops
Clinically improved in 48–72 hours?
No
Re-assess patient
Illness other than AOM?
Yes
Treat other illness
No
Yes
Complete course of therapy
Assess drug delivery, adherence to therapy, need to change therapy

FIGURE 21-1 Algorithm of treatment for diffuse acute otitis media (AOM). (From Rosenfeld RM, Brown L, Cannon CR, et al: Clinical practice guideline: Acute otitis externa. Otolaryngol Head Neck Surg 2006;134;S4-S23.)

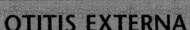

PATIENT TEACHING TIPS

OTITIS EXTERNA

- Most patients with otitis externa can be managed as outpatients. Follow-up in 1 to 2 days is indicated if a wick is placed for treatment, if the patient is started on oral antibiotic therapy, or if the pain does not begin to resolve in 24 to 36 hours.
- Patients should discontinue the use of the drops after full resolution of their symptoms. Continued use of antibiotics (especially neomycin) can predispose to changes in the ear canal environment and can foster fungal infections or sensitivity reactions.
- Patients must avoid getting water in the ear during the healing process. Cotton balls soaked in petroleum jelly work well as earplugs. Any water that gets into the ear can be removed by gentle blow-drying.
- Patients with evidence of significant immunocompromise or failure to improve in 1 to 2 days should be considered for admission to the hospital to be evaluated for more extensive disease.
- Drying the ear after swimming or showering helps prevent otitis externa. Placing drops of acetic acid (vinegar) and rubbing alcohol in the ear two or three times a week during periods of heavy water exposure (summer vacation) helps dry the ear and restore the acidic environment that protects against otitis externa.

Significant decreases in ear pain should usually be seen within 1 day of treatment, and most pain resolves in 4 to 7 days. Failure to improve may indicate more invasive disease (e.g., necrotizing otitis), inability of drops to reach the canal (wick needed), or noncompliance with therapy.

Otitis Media (Acute and Chronic)

Fluid accumulation in the middle ear (medial to the tympanic membrane) is termed *otitis media.* Fluid collections can be clinically sterile, as in barotrauma-mediated effusions or chronic otitis media with effusion (OME), or can result from infectious causes (acute otitis media [AOM]). Infection-mediated effusions may be serous (usually viral in origin) or suppurative (primary or secondary bacterial infection). The common link between all of these processes is eustachian tube dysfunction. The eustachian tube acts as a vent and conduit between the middle ear and the posterior pharynx, allowing equalization of air pressures between the middle ear and ambient air as well as allowing drainage of fluid from the middle ear cavity. After infections (primarily upper respiratory infections [URIs]), edema can cause blockage of the tube. Air is easily absorbed through the middle ear tissues, leading to a relative negative pressure in the middle ear. This negative pressure draws fluid into the enclosed cavity. Native or invasive bacteria can work their way into this enclosed area and proliferate.[3,4] Common bacterial pathogens are the same bugs commonly found in sinus infections, including *Streptococcus pneumoniae,* nontypable *Haemophilus influenzae,* and *Moraxella catarrhalis.* Currently, approximately 60% to 70% of *S. pneumoniae* species are covered by the polyvalent pneumococcal vaccine (Pneumovax).[5,6]

Barotrauma refers to rapid development of relative pressure differences between the middle ear and the outside environment. Rapid rises in middle ear pressure (relative to outside, such as in ascent while flying or diving) usually forces air out of the eustachian tube and equalizes pressure. A relative drop in relative middle ear pressure (during descent) that is not equalized (by collapsed or obstructed eustachian tubes) generates a vacuum force that draws fluid from tissues into the middle ear space. The resultant effusion may remain sterile or may become secondarily infected. Very rapid changes in pressure can even cause direct trauma to the tympanic membrane, including rupture or hemorrhage within the layers of the membrane itself.

Acute otitis media is primarily a disease of children. In early childhood the eustachian tubes are not angled downward and do not drain well spontaneously. The relatively small tube size and higher frequency of URIs in children 6 to 24 months old lead to the highest incidence of OM in this age group. There is another increase in incidence of OM at 5 to 6 years, which coincides with entrance into school and higher frequency of URIs. Craniofacial abnormalities seen with some developmental disorders (e.g., Down syndrome) also predispose to the development of middle ear effusions.

Otitis media is one of the most common reasons for pediatric physician visits, with estimates that $5 billion are spent as direct or indirect costs annually. A significant proportion of cases are probably misdiagnosed, and guidelines have been issued to ensure proper diagnosis and thus curb wasting of resources.[7] "Visualization of the tympanic membrane with identification of a middle ear effusion and inflammatory changes is necessary to establish the diagnosis with certainty."[7] Effusions are signified on physical examination by bulging of the tympanic membrane, bubbles or fluid levels behind the membrane, loss of light reflex (opacification or cloudiness of the membrane), and (most definitively) loss of tympanic membrane mobility on pneumatic insufflation. Newer modalities, such as acoustic reflectometry and tympanometry, also demonstrate middle ear effusions but are not available in many EDs. Tympanic membrane injection (common in crying children) or the presence of fluid alone is not enough to make the diagnosis of AOM. Accompanying fever, pain, purulent drainage, or other systemic signs point to acute infection.

Chronic otitis media is defined as (1) the chronic presence of middle ear effusion in the absence of acute signs of infection or (2) chronic complications from otitis media, including persistent perforation of the tympanic membrane.

The role of infectious organisms in chronic otitis media is unclear. It was originally thought to be a noninfectious entity, but studies have shown the presence of bacteria (and bacterial DNA, mRNA, and bacterial proteins) in a biofilm model of chronic otitis media.[8] Current guidelines offer the option of a trial of antibiotics (typically amoxicillin) or watchful waiting as treatment.[7]

Treatment

American physicians have historically treated otitis media with antibiotics, whereas European physicians are typically less likely to do so. A 2005 study compared immediate antibiotic treatment with "watchful waiting" in *nonsevere* otitis media.[9] In the "watchful waiting" group, 66% of children had complete resolution of symptoms with no antibiotic treatment, no adverse outcomes, cost savings, and similar patient satisfaction.

Several treatment options have been issued or recommendations made by the American Academy of Pediatrics for acute otitis media as follows:[7]

1. Pain management must be addressed in patients with AOM. Particular attention should be paid to pain management in the first 24 hours of any treatment regimen.
2. Observation without the use of antibacterial agents is an option for the first 2 to 3 days in selected children. In children younger than 6 months, antibiotic treatment is recommended if the disease is suspected (even if diagnosis is uncertain). Children between 6 months and 2 years can be treated without antibiotics if the diagnosis is uncertain and the child is not febrile or in severe pain. A child older than 2 years can be treated without antibiotics even if the diagnosis is certain, provided that the patient is not febrile or in severe pain. The child must be otherwise healthy and in a sound social environment with an adult capable of watching the child closely and returning to the physician if the condition deteriorates.
3. If antimicrobial treatment is chosen, the first-line agent should be amoxicillin 80 to 90 mg/kg/day. In treatment failures, or cases in which broader beta-lactamase coverage is desired, amoxicillin 90 mg/kg with clavulanate 6.4 mg/kg in two divided doses can be used. Penicillin-allergic patients (non–type 1) can be treated with a third-generation cephalosporin (cefdinir, cefpodoxime, cefuroxime, or ceftriaxone). For patients with severe type 1 penicillin allergy, alternative treatments include azithromycin, clarithromycin, erythromycin-sulfisoxazole, and sulfamethoxazole-trimethoprim. Treatment is aimed at common pathogens, including *S. pneumoniae,* nontypable *H. influenzae,* and *M. catarrhalis. Mycoplasma* species may also cause otitis media, often causing blister formation on the tympanic membrane (bullous myringitis). Multiple virus species can cause otitis media and are obviously unaffected by antibiotics.
4. Failure of response in 2 to 3 days should prompt initiation of or change in antibiotic treatment. If amoxicillin fails, alternatives include amoxicillin-clavulanate, cephalosporin (ceftriaxone), macrolides, and sulfa preparations.

Some authorities have suggested a compromise between meeting patient expectations and decreasing the inappropriate overuse of antibiotics.[10,11] Patients can be given a "rescue prescription," which they should have filled only if no improvement occurs in 2 to 3 days.

In the face of clear clinical improvement, continued presence of a middle ear effusion should not be mistaken as an indicator for continued antibiotic therapy. Nearly 50% of patients retain an effusion 1 month after clinical resolution, and up to 25% still have an effusion at 3 months. The current guidelines suggest that children who are not otherwise at risk for speech, language, or learning problems can be managed with watchful waiting for 3 months without deleterious sequelae.[12] Children at higher risk for learning disorders (including those with previous hearing loss, speech or language disorders, autism, developmental delay, or visual impairment) require early referral for evaluation and treatment of chronic ear complications.

Chronic otitis media is typically not an emergency. The American Academies of Family Physicians, Pediatrics and Otolaryngology–Head and Neck Surgeons has recently issued guidelines to direct the diagnosis and treatment of otitis media with effusion; they are summarized as follows:[12]

1. Pneumatic otoscopy should be used to identify the presence of effusion.
2. History and physical examination, searching for acute signs and symptoms of inflammation/infection, should be used to distinguish this disorder from AOM.
3. OME should be managed with watchful waiting for 3 months in children who are not at risk for speech, language, or other learning disabilities.
4. Hearing tests (referral to an otolaryngologist) should be performed if the disease lasts longer than 3 months, or earlier if any language, learning, or hearing problems are suspected.
5. Antihistamines and decongestants are ineffective and should not be used as treatment; antimicrobial agents and steroids do not have long-term efficacy and should not be used for routine management.

Middle ear effusions in adults should be able to be explained clinically (e.g., post-URI) and should resolve within a few weeks. Any other circumstances require otolaryngologic referral to evaluate for other nasopharyngeal disease, such as an obstructing tumor.

PATIENT TEACHING TIPS

OTITIS MEDIA

- Most patients with otitis media can be treated as outpatients.
- If antibiotic therapy is chosen, patients should be counseled to take the entire course of antibiotic therapy.
- Patients should follow up with their primary physicians or return to the ED if no improvement occurs in 1 to 3 days.
- Patients should be warned of the signs and symptoms of intratemporal and intracranial complications (headache, neck stiffness, vomiting, altered mental status).
- Patients should also be apprised of the risks of risks of otitis media with effusion and must be sure to follow up with their primary physicians to alleviate the risk of hearing deficits.

Necrotizing (Malignant) Otitis Externa

Necrotizing otitis externa (formerly known as malignant otitis externa) is aggressive extension of infection from the auditory canal to the skull base and other nearby bony structures. This complication occurs nearly exclusively in immunocompromised hosts, with elderly diabetic patients accounting for most of the affected population. This disease can be the presenting complaint in undiagnosed diabetic patients, and all patients with the appearance of a progressive ear infection need prompt evaluation for diabetes. The emergence of widespread human immunodeficiency virus infection now puts children at risk for a condition that was once almost exclusively an adult disease.[13]

Necrotizing otitis externa may be difficult to distinguish from simple otitis externa at early stages, but exquisite otalgia and otorrhea unresponsive to topical measures point to the former diagnosis. The pain often extends to the temporomandibular joint and gets worse with chewing. Granulation tissue is often seen at the inferior portion of the canal, where the cartilage and bone meet, at the site of the fissures of Santorini. Inflammation of bony structures from the osteomyelitis can cause nerve palsies (facial nerve most frequently involved). Progression of the infection inward can lead to catastrophic complications such as brain or epidural abscess, sinus thrombophlebitis, and meningitis. Evaluation with computed tomography (CT) or magnetic resonance imaging (MRI) can show the extent of the invasive process and can be helpful in evaluation for intracranial complications, but arranging for such an evaluation should not delay initiation of treatment.

More than 95% of cases of necrotizing otitis externa are caused by *P. aeruginosa,* and antibiotic therapy should be aimed at this organism. Since the introduction of semisynthetic penicillins, antipseudomonal cephalosporins, and antipseudomonal fluoroquinolones, mortality from this disorder has decreased from 50% to 10%. Empirical treatment with ciprofloxacin 400 mg intravenously (IV) every 8 hours is reasonable. Alternative treatments are an antipseudomonal penicillin (e.g., ticarcillin/clavulanate [Timentin] 3.1 g IV every 6 hours) and cephalosporins (e.g., ceftazidime 1 to 2 g every 8 hours).

Ramsay-Hunt Syndrome

The combination of ear pain, ipsilateral facial paralysis, and vesicular lesions indicate Ramsay-Hunt syndrome, also known as herpes zoster oticus. This reactivation of latent varicella-zoster infection in the geniculate ganglion and spread to the eighth cranial nerve (and frequently cranial nerves V, IX, and X) results in both auditory and vestibular dysfunction.[14]

Physical examination usually demonstrates vesicular lesions in the ear canal, but the variable course and innervation of the nervous structures may lead to involvement of the anterior tongue, soft palate, pinna, and face. Owing to the proximity of the ear to the eye, evaluation for ocular involvement is necessary. The disease tends to be self-limiting and mortality is extremely rare, but deficits in nerve function and facial paralysis are common, and patients with such paralysis are much less likely to recover than those with Bell's palsy.

Treatment is aimed at shortening the duration of the outbreak and controlling symptoms. Acyclovir and steroids are often used. No clear prospective studies have been undertaken. In light of the known safety and effectiveness of anti–varicella zoster or anti–herpes simplex drugs, acyclovir (800 mg five times a day) or famciclovir (500 mg three times a day) should be strongly considered, along with added prednisone.[15] Aggressive analgesia is often needed for pain control. Vestibular symptoms can be treated with meclizine or diphenhydramine. Cranial nerve VII palsies can occur, leading to inability to close eye, and can cause drying and abrasions. Use of a moisturizer/lubricant opthalmic ointment (Lacri-Lube) or other measures to moisten and protect the eye are often needed.

Mastoiditis

All cases of otitis media are accompanied by some subclinical fluid collection in the mastoid air cells, often seen on CT scan. Further blockage of the communicating spaces by mucosal edema and inflammation generates pus under pressure in the mastoid air spaces and results in what we know as clinically significant mastoiditis. Left untreated, the chronic inflammation results in abscess formation and resorption of trabecular bone.

This process can further extend outward or inward. Outward extension leads to subperiosteal abscess formation. This development is associated with the classic findings for mastoiditis (tenderness and erythema over the mastoid process, outward bulging of the pinna, loss of the postauricular crease, and fluctuance behind the ear). Inward extension leads to potentially catastrophic complications such as erosion into the cranial vault, meningitis, and brain abscess formation.

Mastoiditis is a clinical diagnosis, and physical findings should prompt CT evaluation to delineate the extent of the process. Treatment consists of supportive care and resuscitation, administration of antibiotics and otolaryngology/ENT consultation for surgical drainage. Antibiotic coverage should initially be broad spectrum, including coverage against common otitis media pathogens, anaerobes, and pseudomonas and bacteroides species.

Trauma

External ear trauma can be classified into contusions/ecchymosis, seromas/hematomas, and lacerations/tears/avulsions. Fluid collections and anatomic disruptions require directed attention because of the propensity for necrosis or disfigurement if managed inappropriately.

Blunt trauma can cause blood to collect in the fascial plane between the cartilage and the perichondrium. The cartilage is an avascular structure that derives its nutritional support from the blood supply of the perichondrium, and the separation of the two starves the cartilage. Furthermore, neocartilage formation in the fluid collection space leads to scarring and deformation ("cauliflower ear"). Fluid collections can be drained by either needle aspiration or open evacuation. For cosmetic purposes, collections that form lateral (external) to the cartilage layer can be drained through a medial approach. A drainage incision can be made through the medial skin and then through the cartilage, allowing the blood to be expressed. This avoids an incision in the external auricle.

An important therapeutic treatment is a compression dressing to hold the potential spaces closed and prevent further fluid buildup. Gentle compression can be achieved by packing the ear canal with dry cotton and packing the rest of the auricle with a conforming material (gauze or foam). Several layers of gauze should be cut to shape and placed between the posterior auricle and the skull. Gauze roll can then be wrapped around the head to compress the entire bandage into place. Elastic bandage should be used as a compression material only with caution, because overly tight compression can lead to ear necrosis. Follow-up within 24 hours is needed to check for reaccumulation of fluid, which would need to be redrained.

Lacerations and avulsions need special repair techniques because of the cosmetic importance of ears. As with all facial wound repairs, minimal débridement (minimizing tissue loss) and alignment of visually eye-catching lines (pinna edge, vermilion border, nares rim) are key to aesthetic repair. Complex disruptions with significant tissue loss can be managed conservatively with referral for plastic or reconstructive repair at a later date.

Through-and-through lacerations of the pinna necessitate alignment and repair of underlying cartilage. Use of deep sutures should be minimized (one or two usually suffice). Closure of the overlying skin can then be used to realign the pinna rim first, followed by closure of the remainder of the defect. Compression packing should be used to prevent reaccumulation of fluid.

Earlobe clefts are common. Most often, abrupt traction to earrings causes either a partial or complete tear of the earlobe. Wound repair should align the anatomical shape, with minimal débridement. Referral for outpatient plastic surgery may be indicated, even for primary repair, because of difficulties in fostering a good cosmetic outcome following healing.

Foreign Body

Direct visualization of the foreign body in an ear is critical to identification of the object and aids in the choice of removal method. A small amount of lidocaine or mineral oil instilled into the ear anesthetizes or immobilizes most insects in the ear canal within about a minute.

Methods of foreign body removal are as follows:

- *Irrigation:* An IV catheter without needle (18- to 20-gauge) can be used with a 10- to 20-mL syringe. Irrigating the superior portion of the canal seems to provide the best results. The force generated is well below that needed to perforate a normal tympanic membrane. Materials that swell when wet (vegetables, cellulose, wood) should not be removed by this method because of the risk of further swelling.
- *Forceps:* Small forceps (alligator forceps) can be used to grasp irregularly shaped or malleable objects. They work extremely well for insect removal.
- *Cyanoacrylate:* A small amount of cyanoacrylate (e.g., Super Glue) can be applied to the blunt end of a cotton-tipped applicator and held against the impacted object for about 60 seconds, thus gluing the foreign body to the applicator and allowing its gentle removal. This method should not be attempted in the moving, uncooperative patient, in whom the foreign body could be glued into the ear canal.
- *Right-angle probe:* A small probe can sometimes be worked behind the object and used to pull it forward. This works best for loose or pliable objects.
- *Suction:* A flanged end of thin plastic tubing (or a premade suction device) can sometimes grasp smooth, regularly shaped objects (beads) or pieces of insects for removal.

If removal of a foreign body from the ear canal is difficult or impossible, the patient in most cases can be treated with pain/anxiety medications and followed up in an otolaryngologic clinic in 12 to 24 hours. Exceptions to this statement are lodged button batteries (risk of caustic damage from leakage) and signs of advanced infection (redness, fever, uncontrollable pain); these cases require an otolaryngologic consultation in the ED.

Sudden Hearing Loss

Anatomically and physiologically, there are two parts to the "hearing" process. *Conduction* refers to the mechanical transmission of sound waves from the external environment through the outer and middle ear to the round window. The *sensorineural component* refers to the transduction of sound waves to electrical (neural) impulses and the delivery of these impulses to the brain, where they can be interpreted as sound. Hearing can be impaired by dysfunction in either or both of these pathways. The first step in evaluating hearing complaints (and the primary guide to treatment) is to ascertain the location and extent of the hearing loss. History and physical examination provide nearly all the information needed to guide ED treatment of hearing loss. History must include details about the timing of hearing loss, laterality, previous episodes, associated symptoms (tinnitus, vertigo, or pain), preceding events (diving, plane rides, trauma), potential placement of a foreign body, environmental noise exposures, and potential ototoxic drugs.

Tuning fork tests provide the best clues to distinguish between conductive and sensorineural hearing loss. They key component of the test is to compare how well the ear hears conduction through bone compared with conduction through air. A 512-Hz fork should be used, because lower-frequency tuning forks can often be "felt" through the air, thus confounding interpretation of results.

The *Weber test* compares the two ears to each other (Fig. 21-2). A vibrating fork is placed midline on the top of the head or between the front top teeth (some patients find this intolerable). The patient is asked which ear hears the vibrations better. The EP should remember that outside sounds (from air conduction) suppress perception of vibratory conduction, so an ear that is hearing outside sounds normally dampens the sensation of the bone conduction vibrations from the fork. Thus, an ear with a conductive hearing defect will "hear" the fork vibrating through bone "louder" than the other ear. So if the fork is heard louder in one ear, either that ear has a conductive deficit or the other ear has a neural deficit.

The *Rinne test* evaluates each ear independently (Fig. 21-3). Normally, air conduction is more sensitive than bone conduction, and one should be able to hear a vibrating fork longer through the air than through bone. The handle of a vibrating fork is placed on the mastoid process of the side being evaluated. Then the vibrating end is held near the ear canal. Normally functioning ears hear the air conduction louder and longer than the bone conduction. A simple technique is to hold the base of the fork against the mastoid process as the sound dissipates. When the patient indicates when he or she can no longer hear the vibrations, the vibrating tip is quickly moved near the ear canal. If the patient can still hear the vibrations through the air, the result is considered normal. Perception of sound better through bone conduction indicates a conductive deficit. Lack of hearing either bone or air conduction points to sensorineural hearing loss.

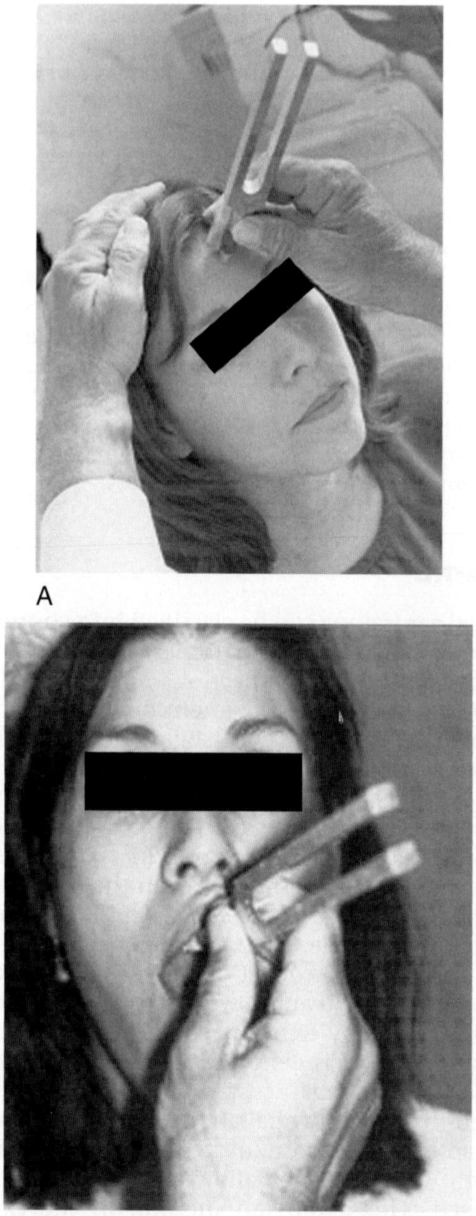

A

B

FIGURE 21-2 The Weber test compares hearing in the two ears to each other. A vibrating tuning fork is held midline against the patient's forehead (**A**) or teeth/gums (**B**). The patient is asked if one ear hears the fork more loudly. Unequal sound perception indicates a conductive deficit in the loud ear or a neural deficit in the quiet ear.

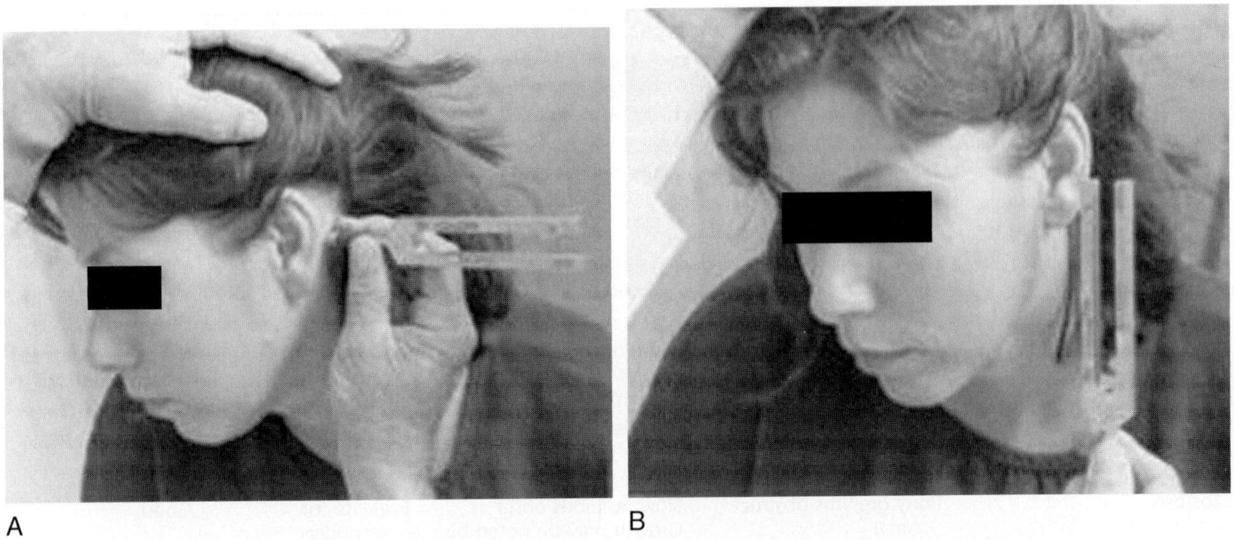
A
B

FIGURE 21-3 The Rinne test compares air and bone conduction in each ear independently. A vibrating tuning fork is held against the mastoid process (bone conduction; **A**) until the vibrations can no longer be heard. The still vibrating tip is then moved near the canal opening to see if the patient can still hear the vibration through air conduction (**B**). Longer or louder hearing through air conduction is normal. Longer or louder hearing through bone conduction indicates a conductive hearing deficit.

■ TREATMENT

Treatment options for hearing loss are limited in the ED environment, and are governed by physical findings (Table 21-1).

Tympanic membrane perforations cause conductive hearing deficits, with losses being greater in the low-frequency range. Traumatic perforations usually occur in the pars flaccida (the portion inferior to the malleolar fold). Perforations usually heal spontaneously but require urgent referral to an otolaryngologist for follow-up. Larger perforations are more likely to require such specialist interventions as patching. All patients with perforations need clear counseling about the importance of keeping the affected ear clean and dry.

Fluid collections in the middle ear dampen the vibrations of the ossicles and decrease sound wave transmission, resulting in a relative conductive hearing deficit. Acute middle ear fluid collections may respond to decongestants alone. If there is evidence of infection (otitis media), antibiotics may be added to the treatment regimen. Solid masses may be seen behind the tympanic membrane but are not usually treatable in the ED. All patients with chronic fluid collections and masses require referral to an otolaryngologist because studies have indicated a connection between increased duration of middle ear disease and extent of sensorineural hearing loss.[16,17]

Sensorineural hearing loss may stem from several causes but there are few emergency treatment options. The patient can be counseled about the variable recovery rate, and some prognosis may be given on the basis of the suspected cause of the lesion. Viral causes and inflammatory or autoimmune causes may respond to steroid treatment started in the first few days. Steroids have been regarded as standard therapy for sensorineural hearing loss suspected to be of viral etiology, although no controlled trials have shown significant benefit.[18,19] Steroids should be prescribed with caution, and care must be taken to rule out infections, which may worsen with steroid treatment. Steroids should be given only if prompt follow-up is ensured. Antiviral agents (acyclovir, famciclovir, valacyclovir) are also commonly prescribed because of the possible role of herpes simplex virus type 1 as an etiologic agent in sensorineural hearing loss. There has been no clear evidence, however, to show a better outcome with steroids plus antiviral agents than with steroids alone.[20-22]

Patients with suspected perilymph fistulas need absolute bed rest with head elevation to avoid raising intracranial pressure (and increasing cerebrospinal fluid flow through the fistula). Some patients may require admission and sedation for this goal to be achieved.

Other causes of sensorineural hearing loss are not likely to be identified in the ED. These cases need expedited follow-up with an otolaryngologist for MRI and audiometry. Many patients receive relief from the reassurance that their hearing loss is not a life-threatening event, but the EP should be cautious not to give an overly optimistic picture, because hearing often does not return after this type of hearing loss.

Table 21-1 LESIONS THAT CAUSE HEARING LOSS

	Description of Pathology	Onset/Course	Actions/ Treatment	Prognosis
Conductive Lesions				
Foreign body	Mass in external canal blocks sound conduction	Acute onset ± associated with pain, drainage, or odor	Removal (in ED if possible) Evaluate for secondary infection Evaluate for TM perforation	Excellent
Otitis externa	Edema and detritus obstruct external canal	Rapid onset Associated with pain, edema, swelling Drainage and odor often present	Aural toilet to remove debris Topical (± oral) antibiotics Evaluate for necrotizing otitis	Excellent if treated appropriately
Exostosis	Bony growths obstruct canal Often seen with prolonged exposure to cold water (divers)	Slow insidious onset Growth may be noted by others No pain or drainage unless causes complete obstruction	Evaluate for secondary infection Reassurance ENT referral	Good
Tympanosclerosis	Frequent TM perforations or infections lead to scarring of TM; decreased mobility impairs sound conduction	Slow onset after perforations, trauma, or infections	ENT referral Reassurance	Variable
Perforated TM	Disruption of TM integrity results in impaired sound transmission to ossicles	Acute onset May follow direct trauma or sudden barotrauma May have sudden relief from pain if due to otitis media	Treat eliciting cause if possible (e.g., acute otitis media) Counsel on importance of keeping water out of ear canal Use of pH-balanced otic suspensions if needed for concomitant infection ENT referral	Good
Sterile effusion (barotrauma)	Fluid in middle ear dampens conduction through ossicles	Often coincident with flying or diving, or after URI May be intermittent as bubbles in effusion equalize	Decongestants Evaluate for infectious etiology Follow-up	Excellent
Acute otitis media	Pus (or fluid) in middle ear dampens conduction through ossicles	Acute to subacute onset, often after URI Often associated with pain ± fever	Antibiotics (viral origin unless strongly suspected) Decongestants Pain control	Excellent if treated appropriately
Cholesteatoma	Trapped stratified squamous epithelium grows to produce mass in middle ear that interferes with ossicle conduction May destroy ossicles or erode into surrounding structures	Slow onset Often history of prior perforations or chronic infections May be associated with focal neurologic symptoms	ENT referral	Variable
Glomus tumor	Vascular tumor occupies middle ear space Interferes with ossicle conduction	Slow onset May be associated with rushing pulsatile sensation	ENT referral	Variable

Table 21-1 LESIONS THAT CAUSE HEARING LOSS—cont'd

	Description of Pathology	Onset/Course	Actions/ Treatment	Prognosis
Cancer	Squamous cell most common Obstructs external canal	Slow onset Often noticed first by others Painless unless causes complete canal occlusion and otitis externa	ENT referral Evaluate for secondary infection	Variable
Sensorineural Lesions				
Perilymph fistula (inner ear barotrauma)	Disruption of round or oval window allows leak of perilymph into middle ear	Sudden onset of hearing loss often with tinnitus and vertigo Often follows straining or abrupt pressure change	Turning in the direction of fistula exacerbates symptoms Complete bed rest with elevation of head of bed to avoid increases in cerebrospinal fluid pressure (may require hospitalization of very symptomatic or non-compliant patients) May require tympanostomy and patch of oval or round window	Variable
Viral cochleitis	Cochlear inflammation	Rapid onset Often follows URI	Steroids often used, though no good data to support better outcome If hearing loss does not resolve, may be helped by hearing aid or cochlear implant	Variable
Presbycusis	Natural hearing loss associated with aging May be related to previous occupational or recreational noise exposures	Slow onset Usually symmetrical and involves high frequencies Often associated with tinnitus	Hearing aid may help with both hearing loss and tinnitus	Variable
Acoustic neuroma	Benign schwannoma of eighth cranial nerve	Slow onset Usually unilateral May be associated with tinnitus and vertigo May be associated with facial hyperesthesias or facial muscle twitching	May require surgical excision if symptoms debilitating	Variable
Ototoxic agents*	Direct toxicity to inner ear structures	Variable onset Loss usually begins in high-frequency range Often history of exposure to ototoxic drugs May be associated with tinnitus	Stop offending agent Thought not to be a problem with ear drops because inflammation in middle ear prevents passage through round or oval windows	Variable; extent of hearing loss at the time offending agent is stopped is usually permanent (except ASA, chloroquine, quinine)
Multiple sclerosis	Multiple demyelinating lesions interfere with nerve conduction	May be associated with other neurologic findings May wax and wane	Standard treatment for multiple sclerosis (steroids, cytotoxic agents)	Variable

Table 21-1 LESIONS THAT CAUSE HEARING LOSS—cont'd

	Description of Pathology	Onset/Course	Actions/ Treatment	Prognosis
Stroke/cerebrovascular accident	Focal ischemic lesion to auditory nerve or auditory cortex May be microcirculatory deficiency from diabetes mellitus or hypertension	Sudden onset Often associated with other neurologic deficits	Treat risk factors for cerebrovascular accident (ASA, anticoagulants, glycemic control, blood pressure control)	Variable
Meningitis	Infection gains access to inner ear through central nervous system–perilymph connection Inflammation damages organ of Corti	Follows clinical picture of meningitis	Treat infection Steroids may limit inflammation and damage Hearing aid or cochlear implant may be needed	Variable
Ménière's disease	Endolymphatic hydrops Abnormal homeostasis of inner ear fluids (presumed clinical diagnosis because definitive diagnosis only made histologically)	Episodic spells of vertigo often lasting hours Associated with sensation of aural fullness, tinnitus and SNHL, or auditory distortion Usually most prominent at low-frequency ranges	Reduce salt, caffeine, nicotine (vasoconstrictors) intake Diuretics and beta-histidines (histamine H_1 agonists) May be helped with hearing aids Patients with debilitating disease may be candidates for cochlear destruction or other surgical therapies	Variable
Chronic noise exposure	Direct mechanical damage to cochlear structures/hair cells	Slow onset Usually most profound at high frequency	Prevention measures (ear plugs) Stop exposure	Usually permanent
Skull trauma	Interruption of eighth cranial nerve, often from temporal bone fractures or gunshot wound Ossicle disruption Concussive forces transmitted to inner ear fluids cause shearing effects on organ of Corti	Sudden onset after trauma	Possible surgical repair If some retained hearing, lesion is likely to be ossicle disruption If "dead ear," likely due to nerve disruption	Variable with ossicle disruption Poor with damage to nerve or organ of Corti
Autoimmune causes	Vascular or neuronal inflammatory changes	Bilateral asymmetrical SNHL May be fluctuating or progressive May be associated with other systemic autoimmune findings	Outpatient autoimmune evaluation (antinuclear antibodies, erythrocyte sedimentation, rheumatoid factor, and especially cochlear autoantibodies) Steroids and cytotoxic agents may slow progression	Variable

ASA, acetylsalicylic acid (aspirin); ENT, ear-nose-throat specialist (i.e., otolaryngologist); SNHL, sensorineural hearing loss; TM, tympanic membrane; URI, upper respiratory infection.

*Ototoxic drugs: aminoglycosides (listed in order of most to least ototoxic: gentamycin, tobramycin, amikacin, neomycin), erythromycin, vancomycin, tetracycline, chemotherapeutic agents (5-fluorouracil, bleomycin, nitrogen mustard), ASA, chloroquine, and quinine.

REFERENCES

1. Rosenfeld RM, Brown L, Cannon CR, et al: Clinical practice guideline: Acute otitis externa. Otolaryngol Head Neck Surg 2006;134;S4-S23.
2. Van Balen FA, Smith WM, Zuithoff NP, Verhuij TJ: Clinical efficacy of three common treatments in acute otitis externa in primary care: Randomized controlled trial. BMJ 2003;327:1201-1205.
3. Rovers MM, Schilder AG, Zielhuis GA, Rosenfeld RM: Otitis media. Lancet. 2004;363:465-473.
4. Daly KA, Giebink GS: Clinical epidemiology of otitis media. Pediatr Infect Dis J 2000;19:S31-S36.
5. Klein JO: Microbiology. In Bluestone CD, Klein JO (eds): Otitis Media in Infants and Children, 3rd ed. Philadelphia, WB Saunders, 2001.
6. Hausdorff WP, Yothers G, Dagan R, et al: Multinational study of pneumococcal serotypes causing acute otitis media in children. Pediatr Infect Dis J 2002;21:1008-1016.
7. American Academy of Pediatrics Subcommittee on Management of Acute Otitis Media: Diagnosis and management of acute otitis media. Pediatrics 2004;113:1451-1465.
8. Ehrlich GD, Veeh R, Wang X, et al: Mucosal biofilm formation on middle-ear mucosa in the chinchilla model of otitis media. JAMA 2002;287:1710-1715.
9. McCormick DP, Chonmaitree T, Pittman C, et al: Nonsevere acute otitis media: A clinical trial comparing outcomes of watchful waiting versus immediate antibiotic treatment. Pediatrics 2005;115:1455-1465.
10. Cates C: An evidence based approach to reducing antibiotic use in children with acute otitis media: Controlled before and after study. BMJ 1999;318:715-716.
11. Siegel RM, Kiely M, Bien JP, et al: Treatment of otitis media with observation and a safety-net antibiotic prescription Pediatrics 2003;112:527-531.
12. American Academy of Family Physicians, American Academy of Otolaryngology–Head and Neck Surgery and American Academy of Pediatrics Subcommittee on Otitis Media with Effusion. Otitis media with effusion. Pediatrics 2004;113:1412-1429.
13. Rubin Grandis J, Branstetter BF 4th, Yu VL: The changing face of malignant (necrotizing) external otitis: Clinical, radiological and anatomic correlations. Lancet Infectious Diseases 2004;4:34-39.
14. Sweeney CJ, Gilden DH: Ramsay Hunt syndrome. J Neurol Neurosurg Psychiatry 2001;71:149-154.
15. Murakami S, Hato N, Horiuchi J, et al: Treatment of Ramsay Hunt syndrome with acyclovir-prednisone: Significance of early diagnosis and treatment. Ann Neurol 1997; 41:353-357.
16. Mehta RP, Rosowski JJ, Voss SE, et al: Determinants of hearing loss in perforations of the tympanic membrane. Otol Neurotol 2006;27:136-143.
17. Radaelli de Zinis LO, Campovecchi C, Parrinello G, Antonelli AR: Predisposing factors for inner ear hearing loss associated with chronic otitis media. Int J Audiol 2005;44(:593-598.
18. Wei BP, Mubiru S, O'Leary S: Steroids for idiopathic sudden sensorineural hearing loss. Cochrane Database Syst Rev 2006;(1):CD003998.
19. Slattery WH, Fisher LM, Iqbal Z, Liu N: Oral steroid regimens for idiopathic sudden sensorineural hearing loss. Otolaryngol Head Neck Surg 2005;132:5-10.
20. Stokroos RJ, Albers FW, Tenvergert EM: Antiviral treatment of idiopathic sudden sensorineural hearing loss: A prospective randomized double-blind clinical trial. Acta Otolaryngol 1998;118:488-495.
21. Uri N, Doweck I, Cohen-Kerem R, Greenberg E: Acyclovir in the treatment of idiopathic sudden sensorineural hearing loss. Otolaryngol Head Neck Surg 2003;128:544-549.
22. Tucci DL, Farmer JC Jr, Kitch RD, Witsell DL: Treatment of sudden sensorineural hearing loss with systemic steroids and valacyclovir. Otol Neurotol 2002;23:301-308.

Chapter 22

Dental Emergencies

Kip Benko

KEY POINTS

Adults have 32 permanent teeth. Children have 20 primary teeth.

A tooth consists of (1) the enamel, which is the outermost, hard protective layer, (2) the underlying porous dentin, which cushions the tooth during mastication and carries nutrients from the pulp to the enamel, (3) the pulp, which contains the neurovascular supply of the tooth, and (4) the cementum and the periodontal ligament, which anchor the tooth into the alveolar bone.

The use of bupivacaine in the form of a dental nerve block is an effective means of obtaining relief from severe odontalgia. A dental block should also be performed before manipulation of any significantly traumatized tooth.

Radiographs are usually not necessary for most dental complaints, but they can be useful when one must search for a tooth fragment, an avulsed or intruded tooth, or a mandible fracture.

Any exposed dentin or pulp of an acutely fractured tooth should be covered. The covering aids in pain control and may prevent the need for a root canal.

Subluxated or luxated teeth should be splinted if they are significantly loosened in order to prevent aspiration and maximize potential viability.

Avulsed teeth should be placed in a storage medium immediately by emergency medical services or ED personnel so as to maximize potential viability.

Scope and Outline

■ PERSPECTIVE

Patients generally understand that definitive care of a dental emergency must be provided by a dentist or oral surgeon, but a lack of financial resources, inability to contact a dentist, severe pain, or acute trauma leads patients to the ED first. Treating dental emergencies in the ED can be difficult and challenging but can also be immensely satisfying when the EP has a general understanding of dental anatomy and understands some simple techniques required to relieve pain and preserve teeth. EPs are called upon to treat dental problems, and it is essential to have a diagnostic and treatment plan to facilitate patient care.

■ EPIDEMIOLOGY AND ETIOLOGY

The incidence of dental complaints presenting to EDs appears to be rising, which may reflect the increasing use of EDs as primary care facilities.[1] Injuries involving the younger population are most often secondary to falls or accidents, whereas those in older age groups are most often secondary to motor vehicle accidents, falls, or assaults.[2] Traumatic dental injuries usually involve the permanent anterior dentition, but adult dentoalveolar injuries are often associated with fractures of the mandible and face. Patients who have both mandibular condyle and body fractures are more likely to have related tooth injury than patients with either isolated body fractures or condyle fractures.[2]

Structure and Function

■ THE STOMATOGNATHIC SYSTEM

The muscles of mastication are responsible for opening and closing the mouth and are those most frequently associated with temporomandibular disorders (TMDs). The clinician should be knowledgeable about the position of the muscles in order to perform an examination properly and to recognize the origin of certain painful conditions. The muscles that close the mouth are those most often associated with TMDs; they are the masseter, the temporalis, and the medial pterygoid muscles (Fig. 22-1).[3] The contraction of this group of muscles bilaterally serves to move the condyle superiorly and posteriorly, causing the mouth to close. The opening muscles are the anterior digastric, posterior digastric, mylohyoid, geniohyoid, and infrahyoid muscles (Fig. 22-2). The lateral pterygoid muscles are responsible for anterior translation and lateral movement of the mandible (Fig. 22-3). Unilateral contraction causes lateral movement away from the side of the muscle contraction, whereas bilateral contraction causes protrusion of the mandible.

Each side of the mandible consists of the horizontal body and the ascending ramus, which are connected by the angle. The bodies of the mandible are connected by the symphysis in the midline. The ascending ramus gives rise superiorly to two processes, the condylar process and the coronoid process (Fig. 22-4). The mandibular condyle, along with the mandibular fossa and the articular eminence of the temporal bone, make up the temporomandibular joint (TMJ). The TMJ provides for both hinge and gliding actions. Between the mandibular condyle and the articular eminence lies the meniscus, a fibrous collagen disk. A ligamentous joint capsule surrounds the TMJ and serves to limit condylar movement. TMJ pain may be caused by a number of conditions, both traumatic and nontraumatic.

■ TEETH

■ Names

The adult dentition normally consists of 32 teeth, of which 8 are incisors, 4 are canines, 8 are premolars, and 12 are molars. From the midline to the back of

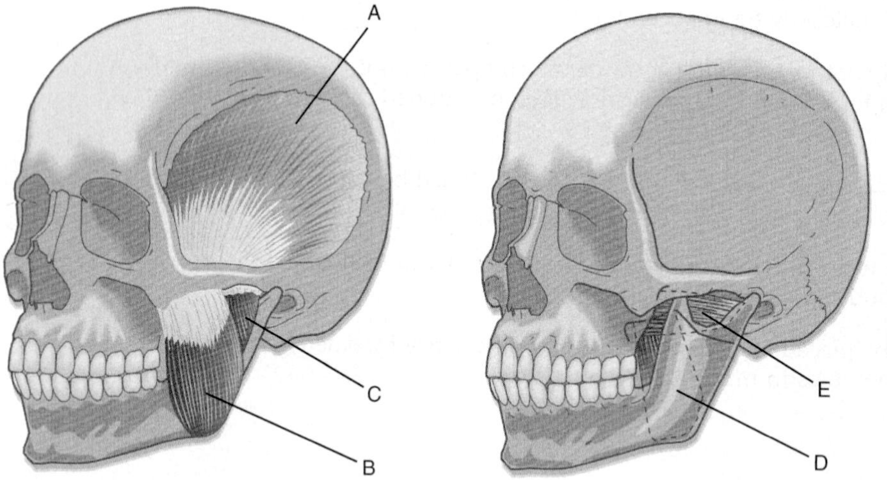
A
C
B
E
D

FIGURE 22-1 Muscles responsible for closing and excursive mandibular movements. Sagittal skull views illustrating the anatomic positions of the following muscles: *A,* Temporalis; *B,* superfici masseter; *C,* deep masseter; *D,* medial pterygoid; *E,* lateral pterygoid. (From King R, Montgomeny M, Redding S [eds]: Oral-Facial Emergencies—Diagnosis and Management. Portland, OR, JBK Publishing, 1994.)

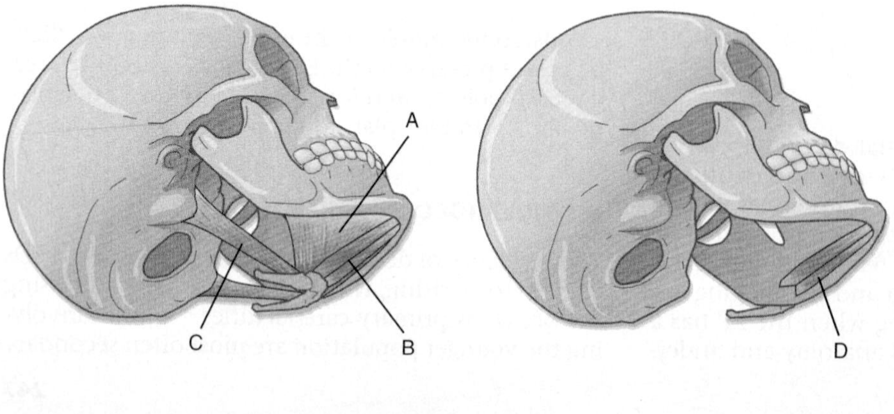
A
C
B
D

FIGURE 22-2 Muscles responsible for mandibular opening. Oblique skull views illustrating the anatomic positions of the following muscles: *A,* Mylohyoid; *B,* anterior belly of the digastric; *C,* posterior belly of the digastric. *D,* geniohyoid. (From King R, Montgomeny M, Redding S [eds]: Oral-Facial Emergencies—Diagnosis and Management. Portland, OR, JBK Publishing, 1994.)

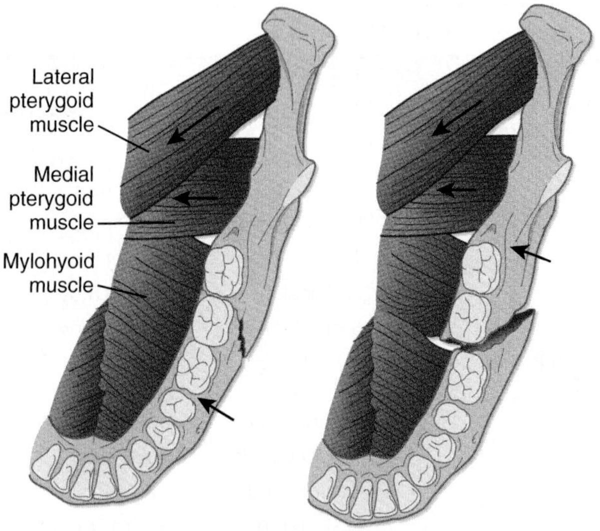
Lateral
pterygoid
muscle
Medial
pterygoid
muscle
Mylohyoid
muscle

FIGURE 22-3 Axial view of the floor of the mandible. *Arrows* indicate the direction of pull of the lateral pterygoid, medial pterygoid, and mylohyoid muscles. View 2 shows how contraction of the pterygoids displaces a fracture. (From Eisele D, McQuone S [eds]: Emergencies of the Head and Neck. St. Louis, Mosby, 2000.)

the mouth on each side there is a central incisor, a lateral incisor, a canine (eye tooth), two premolars, and three molars, the last of which is the troublesome wisdom tooth (Fig. 22-5).

■ Numbers

The adult teeth are numbered from 1 to 32, with the No. 1 tooth being the right upper wisdom tooth and the No. 16 tooth being the left upper wisdom tooth. The left lower wisdom tooth is No. 17, and the right lower wisdom tooth No. 32.

■ Identification of Teeth

There are numerous classification and numbering systems of the teeth; however, it is probably best for EPs to simply describe the location and type of tooth in question, for example, "the upper (or maxillary) right second premolar" or "the left lower (or mandibular) canine." This approach removes any question when the EP is discussing a case with a consultant.

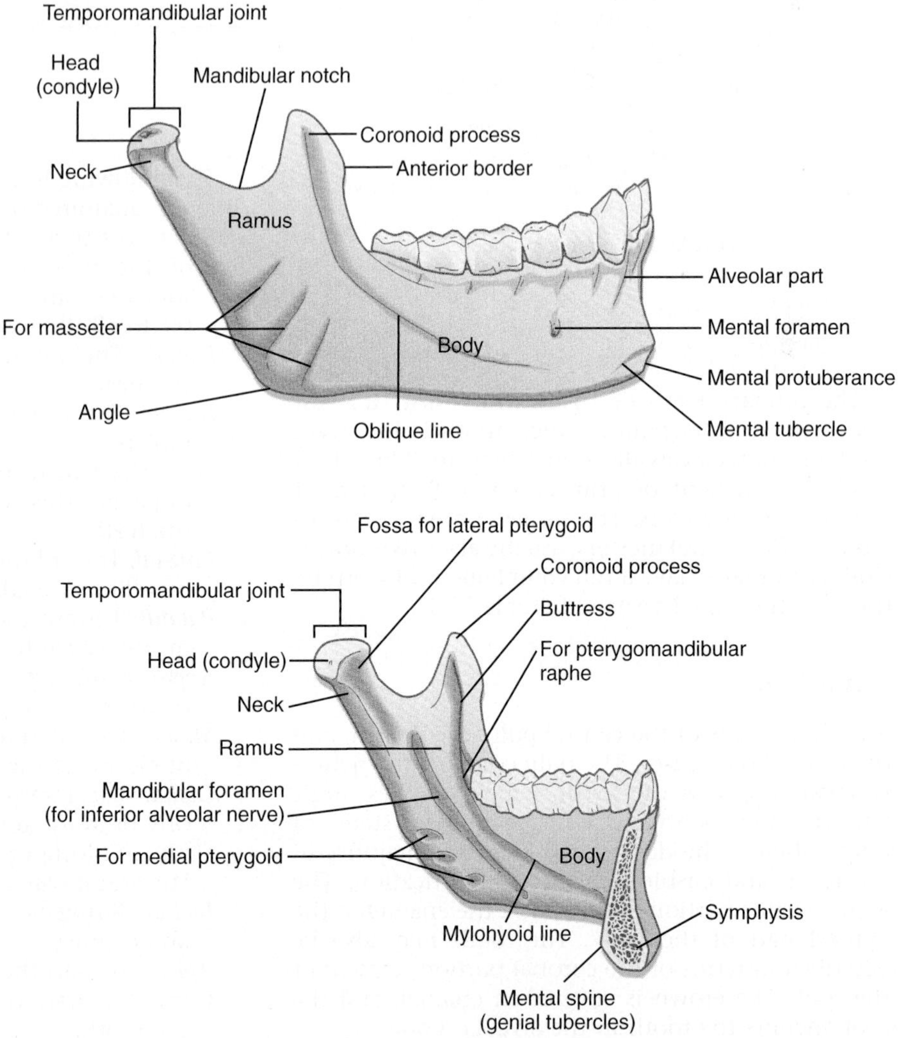
Temporomandibular joint
Head
(condyle)
Mandibular notch
Coronoid process
Neck
Anterior border
Ramus
Alveolar part
For masseter
Mental foramen
Body
Mental protuberance
Angle
Oblique line
Mental tubercle
Fossa for lateral pterygoid
Coronoid process
Temporomandibular joint
Buttress
For pterygomandibular
raphe
Head (condyle)
Neck
Ramus
Mandibular foramen
(for inferior alveolar nerve)
For medial pterygoid
Body
Symphysis
Mylohyoid line
Mental spine
(genial tubercles)

FIGURE 22-4 Anatomy of the mandible. *Top,* View from lateral (buccal) perspective. Bottom, View from medial (lingual) perspective. (Redrawn from Grant JC: Grant's Atlas of Anatomy, 5th ed. Baltimore, Williams & Wilkins, 1962.)

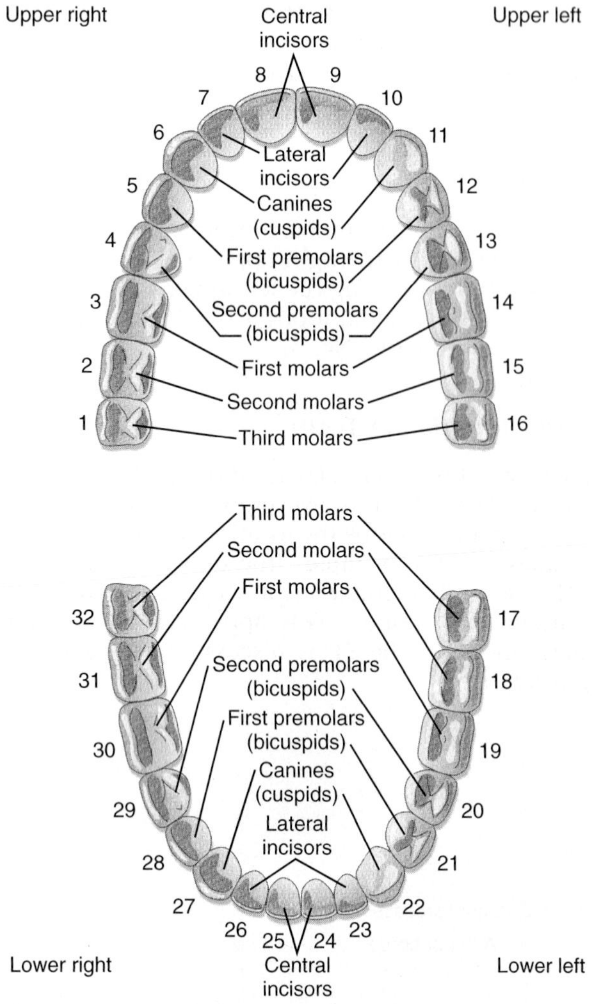
Upper right
Central incisors
Upper left
8
9
7
10
6
11
Lateral incisors
5
12
Canines (cuspids)
4
13
First premolars (bicuspids)
3
14
Second premolars (bicuspids)
2
15
First molars
Second molars
1
16
Third molars
Third molars
Second molars
First molars
32
17
31
Second premolars (bicuspids)
18
First premolars (bicuspids)
30
19
Canines (cuspids)
29
20
Lateral incisors
28
21
27
22
26
25
24
23
Lower right
Central incisors
Lower left

FIGURE 22-5 Adult dentition.

Table 22-1 TOOTH NAMES

Tooth Designation	Name of Tooth	Appearance in the Mouth
Baby (Primary) Teeth		
A	Central incisor	4-14 mos
B	Lateral incisor	8-18 mos
C	Canine tooth	14-24 mos
D	First molar	10-20 mos
E	Second molar	20-36 mos
Adult (Permanent) Teeth		
1	Central incisor	5-9 yrs
2	Lateral incisor	6-10 yrs
3	Canine tooth	8½-14 yrs
4	First premolar (bicuspid)	9-14 yrs
5	Second premolar (bicuspid)	10-15 yrs
6	First molar (6-year molar)	5-9 yrs
7	Second molar (12-year molar)	10-15 yrs
8	Third molar (wisdom tooth)	17-25 yrs

The primary teeth or "baby teeth" also are best described by determining which tooth is involved, not by its official classification. There are 20 teeth in a full complement of primary teeth, 8 incisors, 4 canines, and 8 molars. The earliest primary teeth to erupt are the central incisors, usually at 4 to 8 months. Children usually have a full complement of teeth by the time they are 3 years old (Table 22-1).

■ Anatomy

A tooth consists of the central pulp, the dentin, and the enamel (Fig. 22-6). The pulp contains the neurovascular supply of the tooth, which supplies nutrients to the dentin, a microporous system of microtubules. The dentin makes up the majority of the tooth and cushions it during mastication. The white, visible portion of the tooth, the enamel, is the hardest part of the body. The tooth may also be described in terms of the coronal portion (crown) or the root. The crown is covered in enamel, and the root anchors the tooth in the alveolar bone.

The following terminology is used to describe the different anatomic surfaces of the tooth:

Facial: The part of the tooth that faces the opening of the mouth. This surface is visible when someone smiles. This is a general term applicable to all the teeth.

Labial: The facial surface of the incisors and canines.

Buccal: The facial surface of the premolars and molars.

Oral: The part of the tooth that faces the tongue or palate. This is a general term applicable to all the teeth.

Lingual: Toward the tongue; the oral surface of the mandibular teeth.

Palatal: Toward the palate; the oral surface of the maxillary teeth.

Approximal/interproximal: The contacting surfaces between two adjacent teeth.

Mesial: The interproximal surface facing anteriorly or closest to the midline.

Distal: The interproximal surface facing posteriorly or away from the midline.

Occlusal: Biting or chewing surface of the premolars and molars.

Incisal: Biting or chewing surface of the incisors and canines.

Apical: Toward the tip of the root of the tooth.

Coronal: Toward the crown or the biting surface of the tooth.

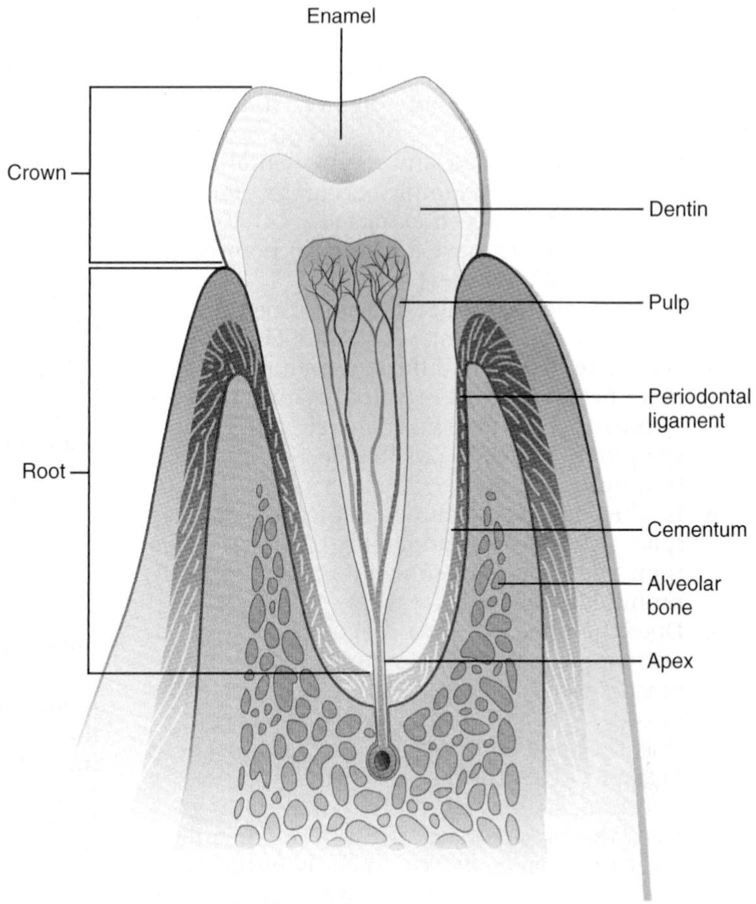
Enamel
Crown
Dentin
Pulp
Periodontal ligament
Root
Cementum
Alveolar bone
Apex

FIGURE 22-6 Dental anatomy.

■ THE PERIODONTIUM

The periodontium is the attachment apparatus. It consists of the gingival and periodontal subunits. These subunits maintain the integrity of the entire dentoalveolar unit. The gingival subunit consists of the gingival tissue and the junctional epithelium. The periodontal subunit consists of the periodontal ligament, the alveolar bone, and the cementum of the root of the tooth (see Fig. 22-6). The gingival sulcus is that space between the attached gingiva and the tooth. The mucobuccal fold is that area of mucosa where the attached gingiva gives rise to the looser buccal mucosa. The mucobuccal fold is the area penetrated when most dental nerve blocks are performed.

Presenting Signs and Symptoms

The patient's signs and symptoms can be elicited by means of a thorough history. If the patient has sustained trauma, it is important to ascertain the following information:

1. When did the incident occur? This is important in the evaluation of avulsed permanent teeth, because the decision to reimplant a tooth is based largely on the duration of the avulsion.
2. Were any teeth found at the scene?
3. Did the patient have any symptoms suggestive of tooth aspiration, such as coughing or choking at the scene?
4. Has the patient been using alcohol or any other sedatives or recreational drugs that may have made aspiration more likely?
5. Does the patient have amnesia, which may suggest a loss of consciousness?
6. Does the patient complain of pain? Do the teeth feel as if they are touching normally? Is the pain associated with occlusion? Mandibular fractures typically worsen with jaw movement, and patients complain that their bite is off. Pain from TMJ injuries is often referred to the ear. Fractured teeth often hurt more with inspiration of air or contact with cold substances. Luxated or subluxated teeth hurt during mastication or chewing.
7. Did the patient take any over-the-counter analgesics or apply any substances to decrease the pain? Over-the-counter topical anesthetics can cause sterile abscesses when applied directly to the pulp.[3]
8. Is the tooth a permanent or a primary tooth? Avulsed primary teeth are managed differently from permanent teeth.

9. Does the patient have a history of bleeding disorders or allergies?

Additional historical information must be obtained if the complaint does not involve trauma, as follows:

1. Has the patient had any recent dental work? Dry sockets, for example, occur several days after a tooth has been extracted.
2. Does the patient have a history of poor dentition or multiple caries?
3. Is the patient having difficulty opening the mouth, which suggests a TMJ problem?
4. Has there been any difficulty swallowing? Has there been a change in voice or any shortness of breath? Has there been any swelling? These symptoms suggest a possible deep space infection or hematoma.
5. Is the patient immunocompromised? Deep space infections spread rapidly to the mediastinum and cavernous sinus in an immunocompromised patient.
6. Does the patient have a coagulopathy secondary to aspirin, warfarin, or other anticoagulants, or symptoms or history suggestive of a bleeding disorder?
7. Was the time course of the problem insidious or rapid? Has the patient had symptoms of infection, such as fever, chills, or vomiting?
8. Does the patient have a history of rheumatic fever or valvular disease, such as mitral valve prolapse[4]? Does the patient have artificial joints, valves, or shunts? These may predispose to endocarditis or infection of the implant/shunt if dental infection is present.

Differential Diagnosis

The differential diagnosis is fairly straightforward when one is dealing with dental complaints. Trauma to the teeth usually consists of fracture, subluxation (loose but nondisplaced tooth), luxation (loose displaced tooth), intrusion, or complete avulsion. Lacerations to the oral soft tissues can be challenging to find, and good lighting is essential. Trauma to the surrounding maxillofacial structures and mandible must also be considered. The final diagnosis is determined primarily by a meticulous physical examination, with radiography sometimes serving a confirmatory role.

Nontraumatic dental emergencies usually result from poor oral hygiene, recent dental instrumentation, or infection. Uncomplicated tooth pain (odontalgia) is often pulpitis, and further diagnostic testing is not necessary in the ED. The other consideration is periodontal or pulpal infection or abscess. Nonodontogenic sources may cause referred pain to the dentition. Referred pain from the sinuses or the TMJ also must be considered, especially for nonlocalizable pain (Table 22-2). A patient who has undergone recent dental instrumentation or extraction may present to the ED with dry socket, hematoma, or hemorrhage.

Interventions and Procedures

■ PHYSICAL EXAMINATION

The physical examination of the oral cavity must be meticulous. Injuries to the dentition are easily missed because of more impressive traumatic findings or by a casual examination. Likewise, the nooks and crannies of the mouth can hide fairly large abscesses, injuries, or foreign bodies.

Simple observation and discussion with the patient can often provide clues to the diagnosis. The EP should pay attention to voice change, muffling, drooling, and other signs of airway involvement. External inspection may disclose injuries such as mandibular dislocations and fractures that often result in asymmetry, swelling, or deformity of the face. Abscesses or deep space infections will cause swelling over the involved space, although such swellings can be subtle; therefore, the face should be viewed from multiple angles. The opening of the mouth should be smooth and complete, with no limitations or hesitations. Erythema, warmth, or drainage is indicative of possible abscess, cellulitis, or hematoma formation. The face should be palpated for fractures, tenderness, and crepitus. The entire mandible and midface should be palpated, with particular attention to the maxilla, zygomas, mandibular condyles, and coronoid processes. The TMJ should be palpated throughout the range of motion. There should be no clicks, pops, or pain as the joint moves.

Palpation of the neck should pay particular attention to the area along and beneath the length of the mandibular body. The oral cavity should be examined for any bleeding, swelling, tenderness, fractures, abrasions, or lacerations, and each tooth should be percussed and accounted for. A tongue blade should be used to assess the entire mucobuccal fold region. The EP should palpate the cheek and the floor of the mouth with the thumb of a gloved hand inside the patient's oral cavity. Each tooth should be percussed with a tongue blade for sensitivity and palpated with gloved fingers for mobility. Blood in the gingival crevice (the area where the gingiva meets the enamel) suggests a traumatized tooth or a fractured jaw. The teeth should meet symmetrically and evenly during biting, and the patient should be able to exert firm pressure on a tongue blade when biting with the molars. The inability to crack a tongue blade bilaterally when it is twisted between the molars (the tongue blade test) suggests a mandibular fracture (Fig. 22-7).

■ AIRWAY MANAGEMENT

Any patient presenting with maxillofacial trauma or infection is at risk for airway compromise. Airway assessment should always precede evaluation of the surrounding structures. If definitive airway management is required, the integrity of the surrounding

Table 22-2 DIFFERENTIAL DIAGNOSIS OF OROFACIAL PAIN

Odontogenic Pain	Dental Caries
	Reversible pulpitis Irreversible pulpitis Pulpal necrosis and abscess Tooth eruption Pericoronitis Postrestorative pain Postextraction discomfort Postextraction alveolar osteitis Bruxism Cervical erosion Deep space odontogenic infection Deep space hematoma Alveolar osteitis Periapical abscess Dentoalveolar abscess Oral hemorrhage
Periodontal pathology	Gingivitis Periodontal disease Periodontal abscess Acute necrotizing gingivostomatitis
Orofacial trauma	Dental fractures: subtle enamel cracks, Ellis fractures Dental subluxation, luxation, intrusion, and avulsion Facial fractures Alveolar ridge fractures Soft tissue lacerations Traumatic ulcers Mandible/maxilla fracture Mucosa/tongue lacerations
Infection	Oral candidiasis Herpes simplex, types 1 and 2 Varicella-zoster, primary and secondary Herpangina Hand, foot, and mouth disease Sexually transmitted diseases Mycobacterial infections Mumps
Malignancies	Squamous cell carcinoma Kaposi's sarcoma Lymphoma Leukemia Graft-versus-host disease Melanoma
Other etiologies	Cranial neuralgia Stomatitis and mucositis: uremia, vitamin deficiency, other Erythema migrans Pyogenic granuloma Ulcerative disease: lichen planus, cicatricial pemphigoid, pemphigus vulgaris, erythema multiforme Crohn's disease Behçet's syndrome

Adapted from Tintinalli JE, Kelen GD, Stapczynski JE (eds): Emergency Medicine: A Comprehensive Study Guide, 5th ed. New York, McGraw-Hill, 2000.

maxillofacial structures may be compromised. Bag-mask ventilation may be very difficult to perform in a patient who has sustained severe midface and mandibular trauma because of the loss of normal bony support. Mandibular fractures can result in the loss of tongue support, which can result in airway obstruction. Bleeding tongue and oral mucosa lacerations can likewise cause airway obstruction and make intubation difficult. Rapid-sequence intubation can be performed in most patients with maxillofacial trauma; however, if any of the preceding conditions are encountered, consideration must be given to an alternative airway.

■ HEMORRHAGE CONTROL

Bleeding from the oral cavity is common and is often associated with dental procedures. The EP is often the first one to see the problem when it occurs in a delayed manner. First, the EP should ascertain whether the bleeding is from recent dental instrumentation or was spontaneous. Spontaneous bleeding from the oral cavity that is not secondary to recent instrumentation suggests advanced periodontal disease or a systemic process.

Bleeding from the gingiva after scaling or other routine dental procedures is usually controllable with

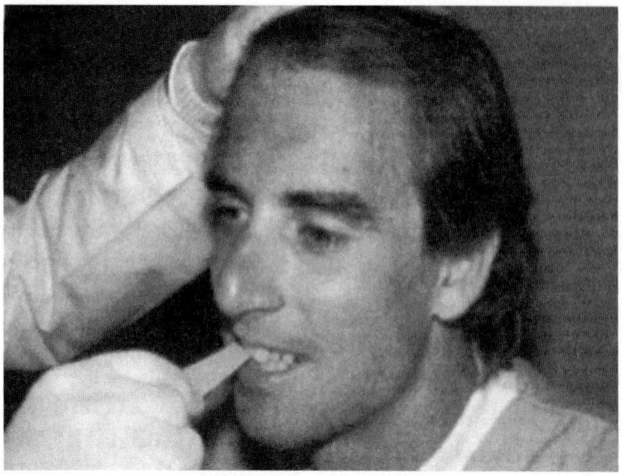

FIGURE 22-7 Tongue blade test.

direct pressure. Gingival bleeding that persists suggests a coagulopathy, alcoholism, medications, and so on. Much more common than gingival bleeding is postextraction bleeding, usually from the molars. Patients with such problems usually present after normal office hours and after they have failed to stop the bleeding at home. The EP has a number of options to stop the bleeding. A systematic approach should be taken, as follows:

1. Apply direct pressure. Any excessive clot should be removed and the area should be anesthetized with local infiltration of lidocaine or bupivacaine with epinephrine. The epinephrine provides vasoconstriction and the anesthetic enables the patient to bite harder. Next, insert a dental roll gauze or dental tampon into the space that was left by the extracted tooth. Dental roll gauze fits nicely into the extraction space and thus helps increase direct pressure. Use a folded-up 2-inch×2-inch gauze pad if dental rolls are unavailable. Cover the dental roll gauze with 2-inch×2-inch gauze pads and have the patient bite hard on it for 10 to 15 minutes. It also helps to soak the dental rolls in epinephrine or phenylephrine.
2. If bleeding persists, insert a coagulating agent (Gelfoam, Surgicel, HemCon) into the socket and then, if possible, loosely close the gingiva surrounding the socket with fast-absorbing suture. Instruct the patient to bite down on gauze placed over the sutures. If there is not enough gingival tissue to close, simply place the coagulating agent into the socket and have the patient bite down into gauze placed over the bleeding socket.
3. Topical thrombin, which can usually be obtained from the operating room, is also very effective in stopping oozing blood, but it is very expensive. Simply spraying the topical thrombin onto the site and then having the patient bite into gauze usually works well.
4. Low-temperature cautery is also very effective, although it can be destructive to tissue if not used carefully. Battery-operated thermal cautery units, which are often used for nail trephination, are available in many EDs. Anesthetize the gingiva prior to using the cautery.
5. If the preceding measures are not effective in controlling bleeding, call a specialist. It is also reasonable to consider the use of fresh frozen plasma or platelets if a coagulopathy is determined to be present.

If bleeding can be controlled, the patient may be discharged. He or she should be instructed not to eat or drink anything for several hours and then to have only cold liquids and soft foods.

■ PAIN MANAGEMENT

Severe tooth pain (odontalgia), as anyone who has had it knows, can be debilitating. Often the quickest relief is found in the ED. The ability to perform dental nerve blocks is invaluable and rewarding.

The use of bupivacaine in dental block anesthesia affords the patient the luxury of 8 to 12 hours of relative comfort until he or she can follow up with a dentist. Likewise, the use of narcotics is minimized because the patient's pain has been relieved. The use of topical anesthesia, in the form of 20% benzocaine or 5% lidocaine, is also a valuable aid, as both agents decrease the pain of intraoral injection. It behooves the EP to be able to use them properly.[5]

■ DIAGNOSTIC TESTING

The routine evaluation and treatment of most patients with dental emergencies presenting to the ED can be performed without radiographic studies or laboratory evaluation. Unlike the definitive treatment in the dentist's or oral surgeon's office, the ED treatment of tooth fractures or alveolar ridge fractures is usually not changed by information gained from radiographs. Radiographs can be helpful, however, if a tooth fragment is missing and thought to be aspirated or embedded in the lip or oral mucosa somewhere. Intruded teeth are also not always apparent, and radiographs can help distinguish between an intruded tooth and an avulsed tooth.

A panoramic facial radiograph (Panorex) view and a Towne's view are probably the most useful and cost-effective radiographs for evaluating mandibular trauma in the ED.[6] The panoramic radiograph of the mandible shows the mandible in its entirety and demonstrates fractures in all regions, including the symphysis.[6] Occasionally, however, a such a radiograph can miss overriding anterior fractures; if such fractures are likely, computed tomography (CT) scan is indicated. The Towne's view allows better visualization of the condyles than the panoramic radiograph. A coronal CT scan is more definitive and is often used in preoperative evaluation, but is seldom necessary for the diagnosis of isolated mandibular trauma. CT should be obtained if multiple facial fractures are suspected or if the initial radiographic findings for the mandible are equivocal and the clinical suspicion is high.[6,7] If the patient is immobilized, mandibular films or CT scanning may be obtained. Mandibular films may miss the symphysis, and if the clinician is concerned about a symphysis fracture, either occlusal films or a CT scan should be obtained.

Dental abscesses or infections are best treated by antibiotics, incision and drainage, or both. Although panoramic radiographic views can visualize sizable periapical abscesses, their routine use in the ED is not warranted because their results would not change the treatment and disposition of the patient.[3] Bite-wing radiographs, obtained in the dentist office, are the standard for diagnosing small periapical abscesses and caries. Deep space infections of the head and neck are often difficult to localize by physical examination, and CT scanning has become the modality of choice to delineate collections of abscess or cellulitis of the face and neck.[8]

Routine blood tests, such as cell counts and serum chemistry analysis, are not useful for the majority of patients with dental emergencies and should be considered on an individual basis. Bleeding times and coagulation profiles are unnecessary in routine cases of postextraction or traumatic intraoral bleeding, but they should be considered if the patient is undergoing anticoagulation therapy or the history is compatible with a bleeding disorder.

Treatment and Disposition

■ TRAUMA

■ Fractured Teeth

Injury to the maxillary central incisors accounts for between 70% and 80% of all tooth fractures. The morbidity associated with dental fractures can be significant and includes failure to erupt, abscess, loss of space in the dental arch, color change of the tooth, ankylosis, and root resorption. The following principles apply to the ED evaluation and management of dental trauma:

1. Identify all fracture fragments and mobile teeth, and note whether a mandible fracture is open or closed. Radiographs should be taken if there is intrusion of fragments into the mucosa of the alveolar bone. Obtain chest radiography if there is any concern about aspiration of a tooth or tooth fragment.
2. The dentition is much more easily manipulated if the patient is not in significant discomfort. Tooth infiltration and dental block anesthesia should be part of the EP's armamentarium. Narcotic and nonnarcotic alternatives, although helpful after treatment is completed, do not usually offer the patient enough comfort to allow performance of most dental manipulations.
3. Administer tetanus booster if indicated.

ED management of fractured teeth depends on the extent of fracture with regard to the pulp, the extent of development of the apex of the tooth, and the age of the patient.[9] There are many classification systems for describing injured dentition, such as the Ellis system; however, most dentists and maxillofacial surgeons do not use this nomenclature. The most easily understood method of classification is based on description of the injury.[10]

■ *Crown Fractures*

Crown fractures may be divided into complicated and uncomplicated categories. Uncomplicated crown fractures involve the enamel alone or the enamel and dentin in combination.

Uncomplicated crown fractures through the enamel only are usually not sensitive to forced air, temperature, or percussion and usually pose no real threat to the dental pulp. ED treatment is not necessary but may consist of smoothing the sharp edges off with an emery board if they are significantly bothersome to the patient. The patient should be reassured that the dentist can restore the tooth with bonding composites and resins. Follow-up is important because pulp necrosis and color change can occur, although rarely (0 to 3% of cases) (Figs. 22-8 and 22-9).[11]

Uncomplicated fractures that extend through the enamel and dentin are at higher risk of pulp necrosis and need more aggressive treatment (Fig. 22-10; see Fig. 22-8). The risk of pulp necrosis in these patients is 1% to 7% but increases as time until treatment extends beyond 24 hours.[12] Affected patients usually have sensitivity to forced air, percussion, and extremes of temperature. Physical findings are notable for the yellowish tint of the dentin in contrast to the white hue of the enamel. Fractures that are close to the pulp reveal a slight pink coloration. The dentin is porous and allows the oral flora to pass into the pulp chamber, possibly allowing inflammation and infection. This process occurs predominantly after 24 hours but may do so earlier if the fracture is closer to the pulp. Patients younger than 12 years have a higher pulp-to-dentin ratio than adults and therefore are at higher risk for pulp contamination. Dentin fracture in a younger patient should be treated more aggressively, and the patient should be seen by a dentist within 24 hours.[12]

The two primary reasons to treat dental fractures in the ED are (1) to cover the exposed dentin and prevent inflammation and infection and (2) to provide pain relief. If a tooth is properly covered in the ED, a dentist can later rebuild it using modern composites. A tooth nerve block should be performed prior to covering the tooth. Dressings that may be considered for covering tooth fractures include calcium hydroxide paste, zinc oxide paste, glass ionomer composites, and cyanoacrylates.[13-15] Some emergency medicine texts support the use of glass ionomer cements in the ED; however, this issue is controversial in the dental community. The ease of use, affordability, and inherent properties of calcium hydroxide paste make it an attractive option in the ED. It is watertight, dries on contact with saliva, is

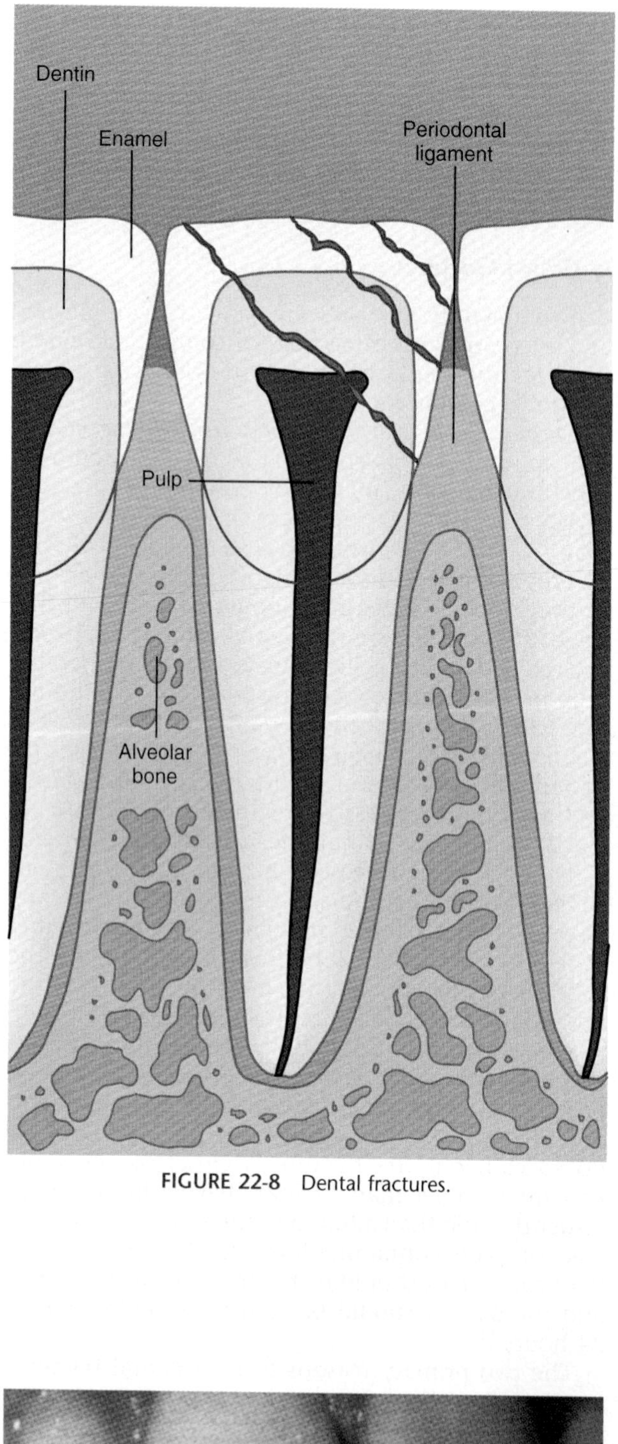
Dentin
Enamel
Periodontal ligament
Pulp
Alveolar bone

FIGURE 22-8 Dental fractures.

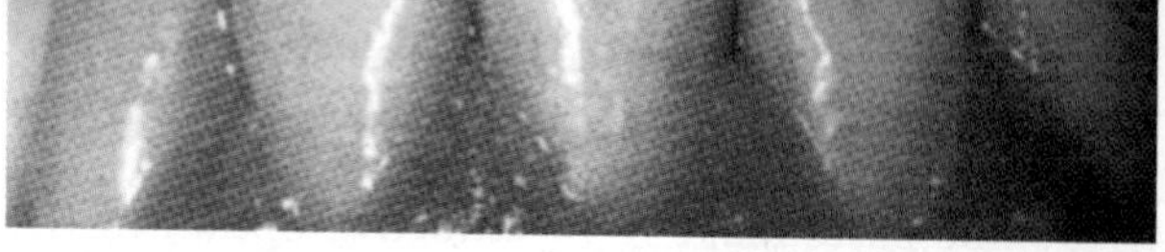

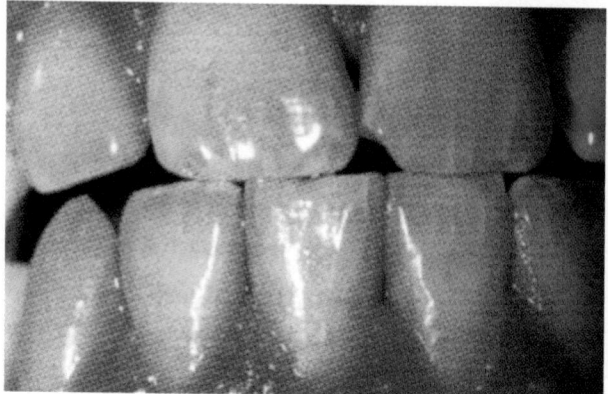

FIGURE 22-9 Enamel fractures.

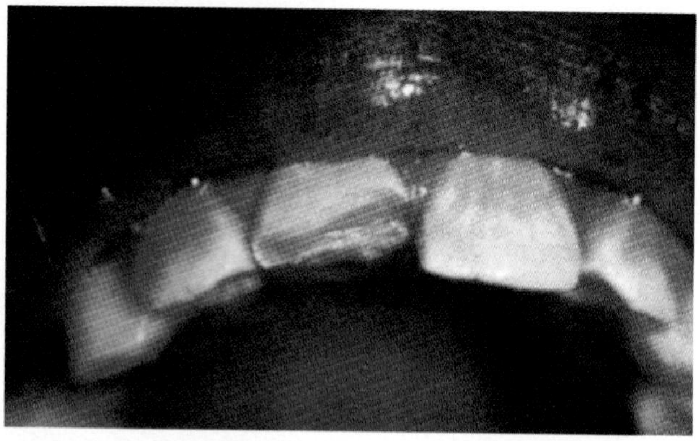

FIGURE 22-10 Dentin fracture.

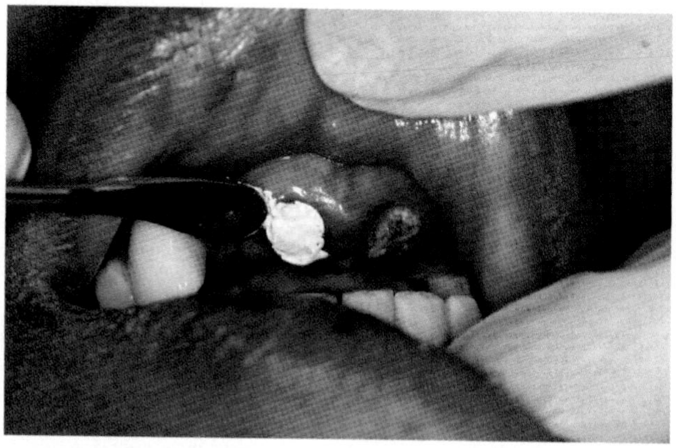

FIGURE 22-11 Calcium hydroxide paste.

durable, and is pH neutral (Fig. 22-11). Composites that are applied with a bonding light are beyond the scope of most emergency medicine practice. Bone wax is sometimes used but is not recommended because it is slightly porous and cannot be used as a base in rebuilding the tooth. Skin adhesives have been used in fracture repair, but they last only a short time inside the mouth and cannot be used as a base in tooth restorations. Their use will probably become more commonplace if clinical studies corroborate their usefulness.

Many patients sustaining dentin fractures eventually require a root canal or other definitive endodontic therapy; however, the timely application of an appropriate dressing in the ED can prevent contamination of the pulp and might prevent the need for a root canal. Even if it does not save the pulp, such a dressing will eliminate the majority of the pain because the dentin is no longer exposed to the air. The EP should make sure to remind the patient that anterior tooth trauma may disrupt the neurovascular supply, possibly resulting in pulp necrosis, color change, or root resorption.

Complicated fractures of the crown involving the pulp are true dental emergencies (Fig. 22-12; see Fig. 22-8). They lead to pulp necrosis at least 10% to 30% of the time, even with rapid, appropriate dental treatment.[11] Such fractures are distinguished by the pink-red tinge of the pulp. They are usually severely

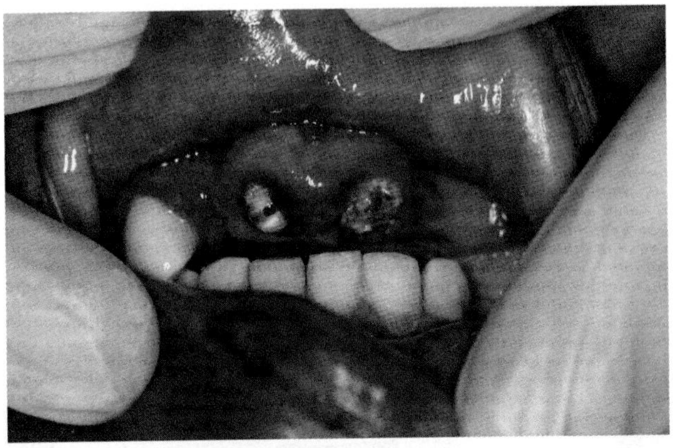

FIGURE 22-12 Pulp fracture.

painful, but occasionally there is a lack of sensitivity secondary to a disruption of the neurovascular supply of the tooth. Immediate management involves referral to a dentist, endodontist, or oral surgeon. These fractures usually require pulpectomy (complete pulpal removal) or, in the case of primary teeth, pulpotomy (partial pulp removal) as definitive treatment.[12] The longer the pulp is exposed, the greater the chance of abscess development. If a dentist cannot see the patient immediately, the EP should relieve the pain with a supraperiosteal infiltration and cover the pulp with one of the dressings previously described. If bleeding is brisk, it can usually be controlled by having the patient bite into a gauze pad soaked with epinephrine or phenylephrine. Alternatively, injecting a small amount of lidocaine with epinephrine into the pulp will stop bleeding and poses no threat to the tooth because the pulp needs to be removed anyway.

If the exposure was prolonged, some authorities would advocate antibiotic prophylaxis with penicillin or clindamycin, although the effectiveness of the approach has never been proven.[16] With regard to antibiotic prophylaxis in dental fractures, it is important to remember the following assumptions: It is uncertain when many patients will be able to secure follow-up. Delayed fracture care and poor gingival health raise the risk of pulp necrosis and, potentially, the development of abscess. Therefore, although it is not customary or standard to prescribe antibiotics in patients with dentin or pulp fractures, it should be considered if the patient has the preceding two risk factors.

■ Luxation and Subluxation

In *subluxation,* a tooth is mobile but not displaced, whereas a luxated tooth has been removed, either completely or partially, from its socket. Luxation injuries are further divided as follows:

Extrusive luxation: The tooth is displaced in a direction toward the crown (Fig. 22-13).

Intrusive luxation: The tooth is forced apically toward the root of the tooth; it may be associ-

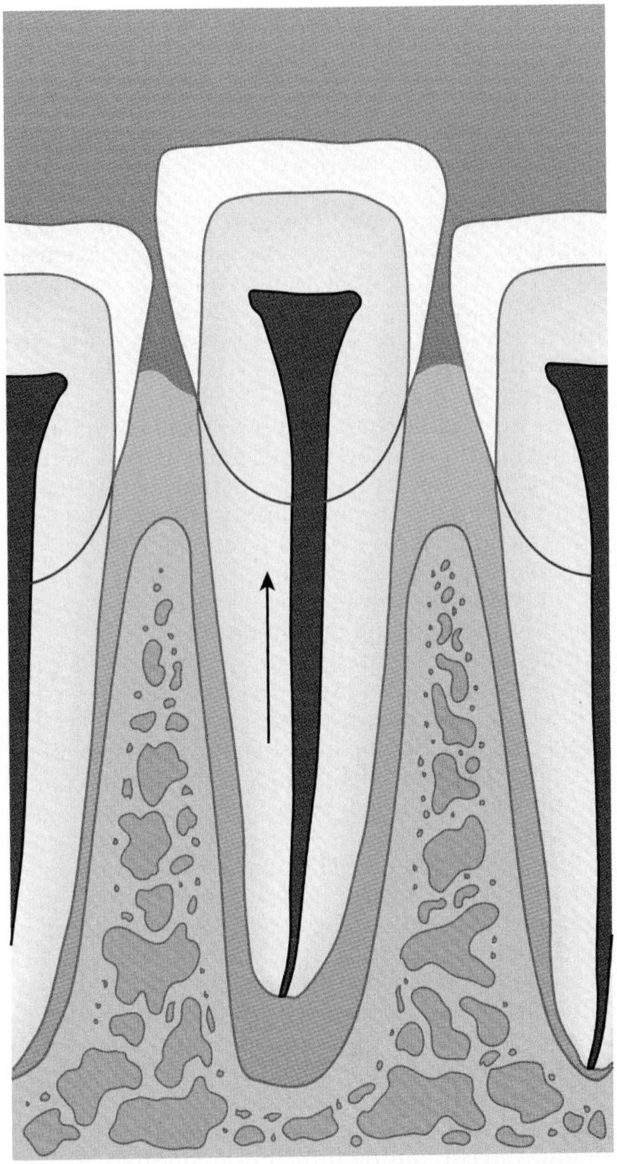

A

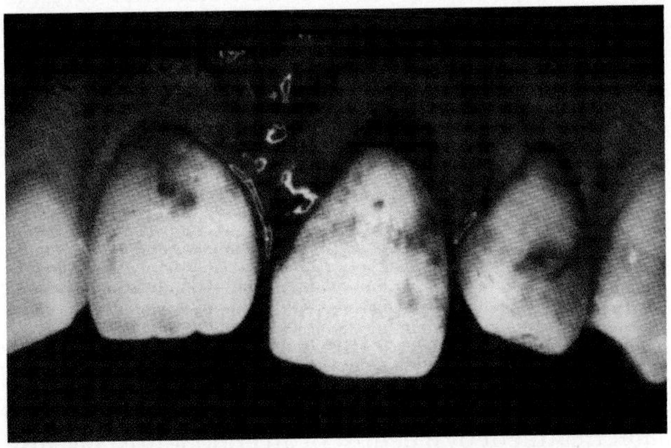

B

FIGURE 22-13 **A** and **B**, Extrusive luxation.

ated with a crushing or fracture of the apex of the tooth (Fig. 22-14).

Lateral luxation: The tooth is displaced facially, mesially, lingually, or distally (Fig. 22-15).

Complete luxation: A complete avulsion; the tooth that is completely out of the socket (Fig. 22-16).

Teeth that are minimally mobile and minimally displaced do well with conservative management alone. The traumatized tooth will firm up as the alveolar ligament binds to the alveolar bone. The patient should be instructed to eat only a soft diet for 1 to 2 weeks and to follow up with his or her dentist as soon as possible.

Grossly mobile teeth, however, require some form of stabilization in the ED. Fixation is best accomplished by the dental professional with enamel bonding materials or wire splinting, which are usually not practical in the ED. Many different techniques are available to the EP, although one must be aware of the concern for aspiration of teeth, or even the splint, if the splinting technique fails.

Temporizing splinting techniques available for use by EPs include periodontal paste and self-cure composites. At this time, the tissue glues do not have the properties required to firmly splint teeth, although this situation may change and tissue glue in combination with splinting wire may eventually be a good option.

Coe-Pak, a commercially available form of periodontal paste, is a very sticky dressing that becomes firm after application (Fig. 22-17). Self-cure composite is another reasonable splinting option in the ED. Self-cure composite does not require etching acids or bonding lights and is easy to use (Fig. 22-18). The disadvantage of self-cure composite is that it is rigid and inflexible and tends to pop off with slight trauma to the teeth before the patient sees a dentist. Both splinting techniques are easily removed by the dentist or oral surgeon during formal restoration.

Teeth that are luxated in the horizontal or axial planes or teeth that are slightly extruded can also can be splinted with the preceding techniques. Teeth do not need to be in perfect alignment before the patient is discharged from the ED.

■ Intrusion and Avulsion

Intruded teeth have been forced into the alveolar bone and often cause disruption of the attachment apparatus or fracture of the supporting alveolar bone. Such teeth are often immobile and, therefore, do not require immobilization in the ED, but often do need later treatment by a dentist or an endodontist because of pulp necrosis. Radiographs should be obtained in the ED if there is uncertainty about whether a tooth is fractured, avulsed, or intruded. The dentist should manage intruded teeth within 24 hours if possible, because intruded adult teeth are often associated with alveolar bone fractures. Permanent teeth usually need to be repositioned by the dentist, whereas

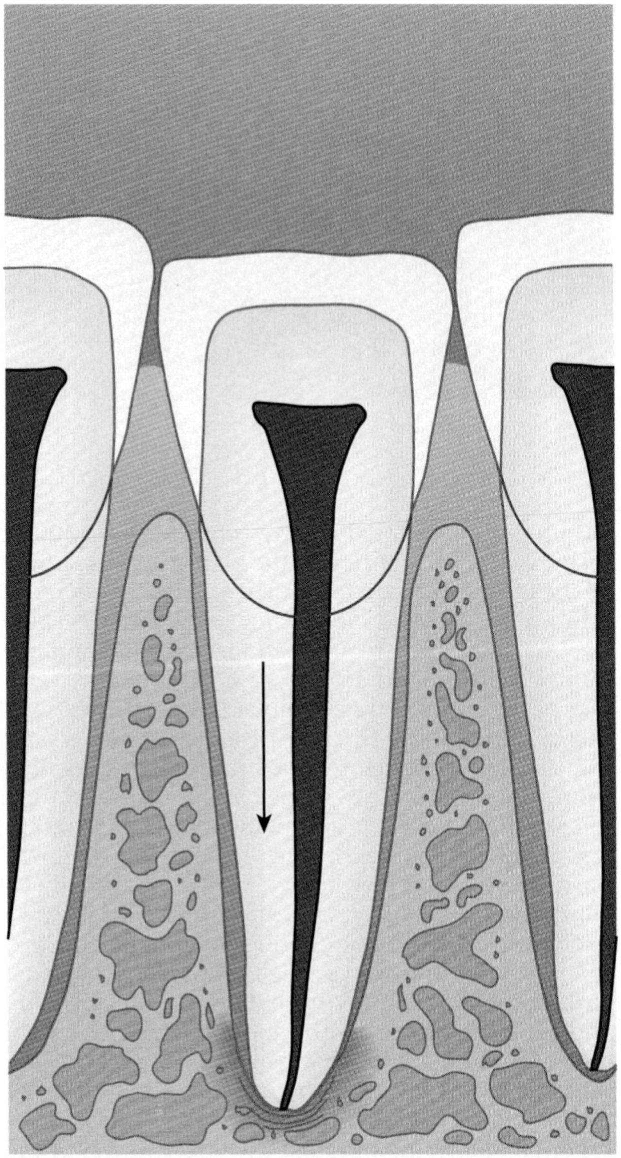

A

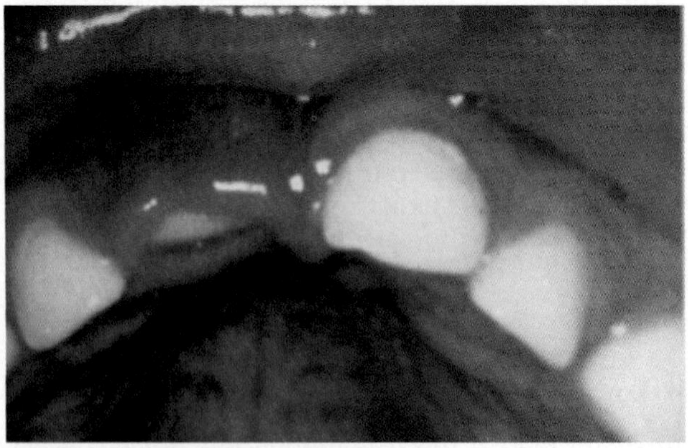

B

FIGURE 22-14 A and **B**, Intrusive luxation.

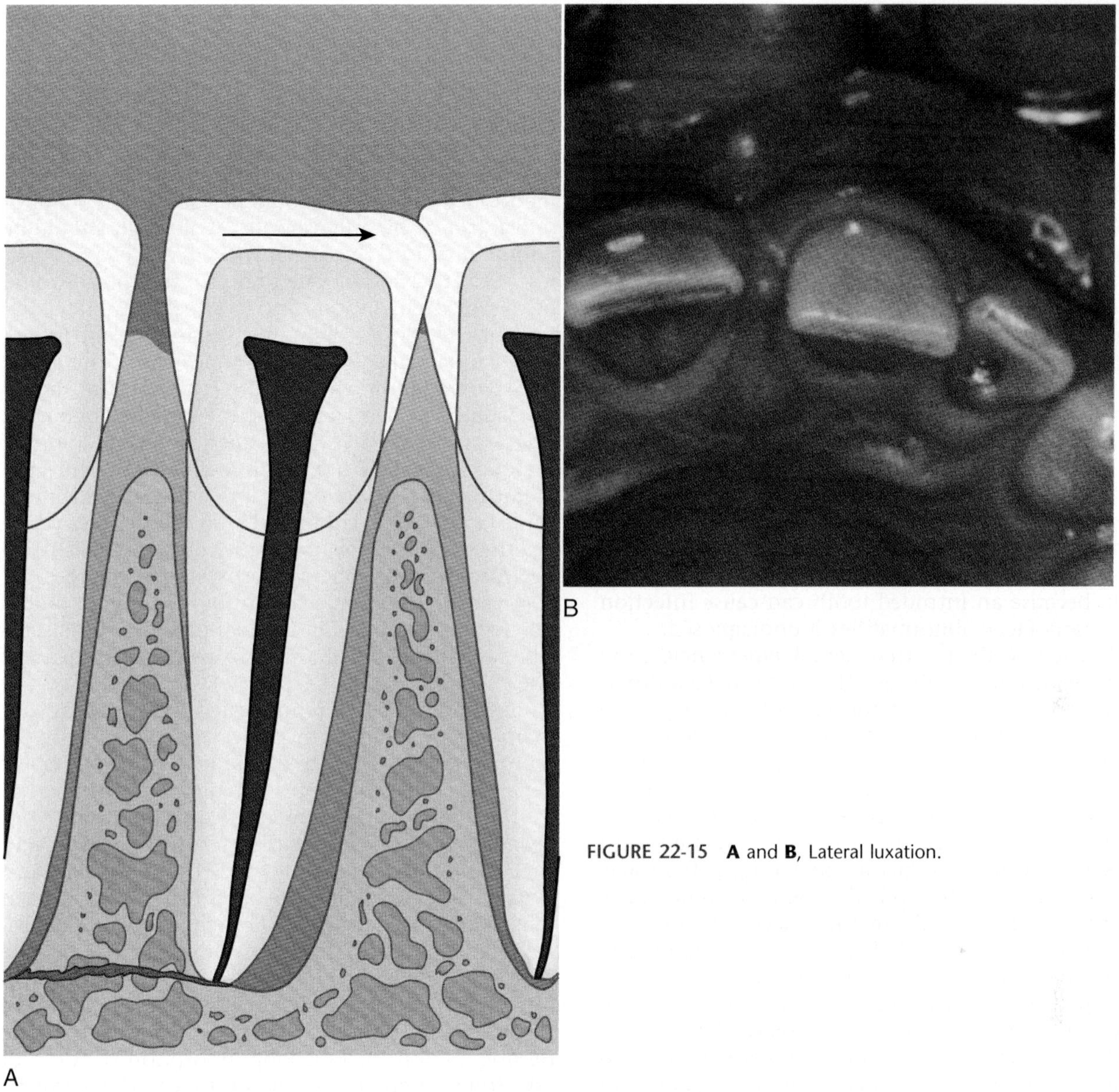
A
B

FIGURE 22-15 **A** and **B**, Lateral luxation.

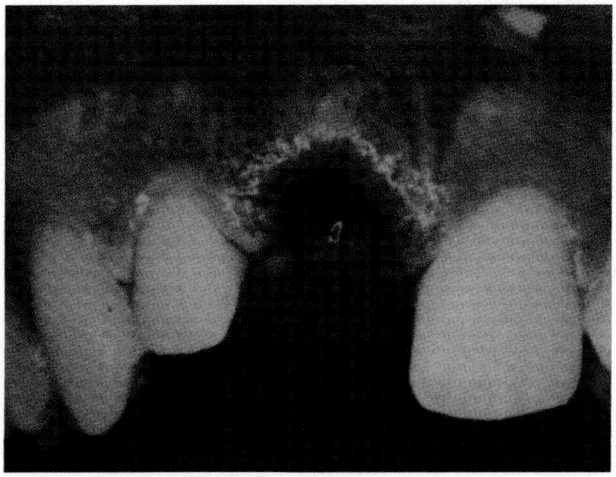

FIGURE 22-16 Avulsion.

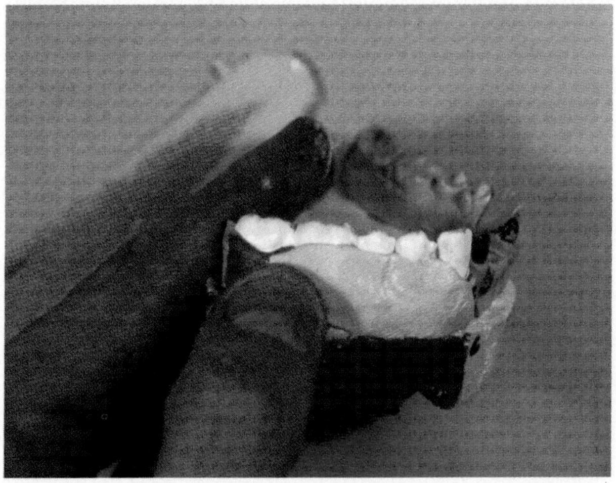

FIGURE 22-17 Periodontal paste.

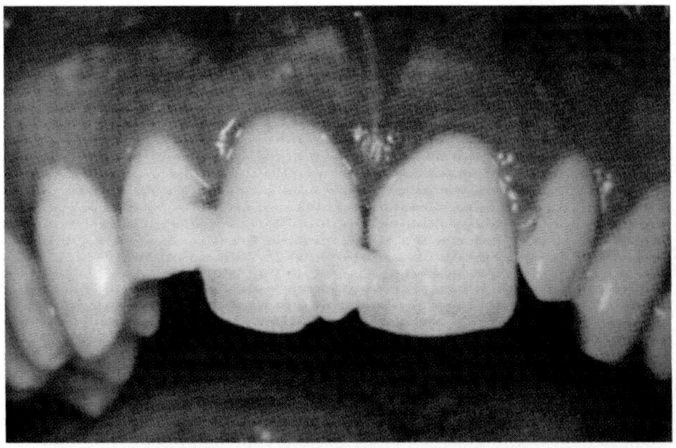

FIGURE 22-18 Self-cure composite.

primary teeth are usually given a trial period to erupt on their own before interventions are taken. The EP should always consider the possibility of an intruded tooth if there is a new abnormal space in the dentition, because an intruded tooth can cause infection and craniofacial abnormalities if undiagnosed.

Avulsed teeth are true dental emergencies and provide an opportunity for the EP to make a difference in the outcome of the patient. Missing teeth may be intruded, aspirated, fractured, swallowed, or embedded in the oral mucosa. A panoramic radiograph, facial films, or a chest radiograph should be considered to look for fragments of fractured teeth or an avulsed tooth. The management of avulsed teeth depends on multiple factors, including patient age, periodontal health, and duration of time since avulsion. Primary teeth are not replaced because they can fuse to the underlying alveolar bone and cause craniofacial abnormalities or infection and also may interfere with normal eruption of the permanent teeth. Parents should be reassured that prosthetic teeth can be worn until the permanent teeth erupt, if desired, although this is usually not necessary.

Time since avulsion is the most important determinant in the decision whether to reimplant an avulsed tooth. Generally, the longer the tooth is out of the socket, the higher the incidence of periodontal ligament necrosis and subsequent reimplantation failure.[16] Periodontal ligament cells generally die within 1 hour if not placed in an appropriate transport medium.[17] Many studies have been conducted on the various transport media used to keep the cells of the periodontal ligament viable. Milk, Hank's balanced salt solution, EMT Toothsaver (commercial formulation of Hank's solution), saliva, water, and Gatorade have all been studied. Cell culture formulations have been developed that cause periodontal ligament cells to not only remain viable, but also to proliferate; however, they are not practical for ED use. To date, milk and Hank's solution (generic or commercial formulation) are best for prehospital as well as ED use. They each preserve the periodontal ligament for at least 8 hours, although reimplantation should take place as rapidly as is reasonably possible.

The tooth should be placed in some sort of transport medium immediately after avulsion if possible, as even 5 to 10 minutes of exposure to the air will begin to cause desiccation and death of periodontal ligament cells. Saline is less optimal than the media mentioned earlier but should be used before water or saliva, if it is the only option.[18] The tooth should be reimplanted into the socket at the scene by paramedics, but if they are unable to do so, the tooth should be reimplanted as soon as possible in the ED. Preparation of the socket, including suctioning and irrigation, can take place while the tooth is soaking in the transport medium. The patient's tetanus status should be updated as necessary, and the patient discharged home on a soft diet. The American Association of Endodontists does not recommend the routine use of antibiotics for fractures or avulsions, although some writers recommend antibiotics effective against mouth flora (penicillin or clindamycin) to decrease the inflammatory resorption of the root.[12,14] If possible, treatment with antibiotics should probably be tailored to the individual patient after discussion with the consultant who will see the patient later.

The prognosis of a reimplanted tooth depends on many factors, the most critical being the time to reimplantation. The age of the patient, the stage of development of the root (younger is better), and the overall health of the gingiva are also important. It is always better to keep a native tooth if possible, and that should be the goal of the EP presented with an avulsed or fractured tooth. A tooth that has been reimplanted usually loses the majority of its neurovascular supply and undergoes pulp necrosis, but the periodontal ligament attaches, and the tooth will remain a functional unit, obviating an implant or a prosthesis. Complications that can be expected after reimplantation include some resorption of the root and some discoloration of the tooth. These can be managed by the follow-up dentist.

■ Alveolar Bone Fractures

Trauma to the anterior teeth may result in fractures of the alveolar ridge, which is the tooth-bearing portion of the mandible or maxilla. Alveolar ridge fractures often occur in multi-tooth segments and vary in the number of teeth involved, the amount of mobility present, and the amount of displacement of the affected segment. Dental bite-wing radiographs obtained in the dental office confirm the diagnosis, and facial films or a panoramic radiograph may show a fracture line apical to the roots of the involved teeth.

Treatment consists of rigid splinting of the affected segment, which should be performed urgently by an oral surgeon or a dentist. It ideally should be done within 24 hours, but the urgency depends on the extent, the mobility, and the displacement of the affected segment. The role of the EP is to diagnose the injury, identify any avulsed or fractured teeth, and preserve as much of the alveolar bone and surrounding mucosa as possible. Alveolar bone that is lost, débrided, or missing is difficult for the specialist to repair properly.[14]

Alveolar Osteitis (Dry Socket)

Dry socket pain is severe and often requires intervention other than pain medication. Alveolar osteitis is a localized osteomyelitis that occurs when exposed alveolar bone becomes inflamed. This typically occurs when a clot that is present after a tooth extraction becomes dislodged or dissolves, most commonly 3 to 4 days after a tooth extraction. The examination is unremarkable with the exception of the missing clot, which is not always obvious to the untrained eye. Smoking, drinking from a straw, periodontal disease, and hormone replacement therapy are all risk factors predisposing a patient to dry socket. This complication occurs after 2% to 5% of all extractions, although the rate increases if the extraction was especially traumatic or involves an impacted third molar.[3,11]

Patients presenting with dry socket usually have no response to nonsteroidal anti-inflammatory drugs or narcotics but experience immediate relief from a dental nerve block. After a dental block, the socket can be irrigated, suctioned, and packed appropriately. The socket may be packed with gauze that is impregnated with eugenol or a local anesthetic. Gauze tends to dry out and loosen, so it usually needs to be replaced in 24 to 36 hours. The socket also may be packed with a slurry of hemostatic gauze and eugenol (or lidocaine). The hemostatic gauze acts as a matrix to hold the anesthetic in place. A commercial paste for dry sockets (Dry Socket Paste) also can be applied to the socket; it has the advantages of staying in place longer than gauze and not drying out.

Antibiotics can be given in alveolar osteitis, but this is not a common practice, and dry socket heals completely once the socket has been covered. Such agents should be prescribed only after consultation with the patient's dentist or oral surgeon.[11]

DENTAL INFECTIONS

Dental infections run the gamut from minor, easily managed infections to abscesses to severe, life-threatening deep space infections that require airway management and operative intervention. Dental infections seen in the ED most commonly are secondary to pulp infection or inflammation or to periodontal disease. Disease of the periodontium usually is a chronic condition, but over time, abscesses develop and require emergency treatment.

Diseases of the pulp can be secondary to trauma or operations, but clearly the most common cause is bacterial invasion after the carious destruction of the enamel. As enamel is destroyed, caries development progresses rapidly through the dentin and into the pulp chamber, causing an inflammatory reaction known as pulpitis. If the erosion caused by the bacteria is large enough to drain the developing inflammation, the patient may remain asymptomatic for a long time. When the drainage becomes blocked, the process progresses to the pulp and periapical space, causing exquisite tenderness. Periapical abscesses follow the path of least resistance, which may be through the alveolar bone and gingiva and into the mouth or into the deep structures of the neck (Fig. 22-19). If the infection has progressed apically through the alveolar bone and there is localized swelling and tenderness at the base of the tooth, incision and drainage in the ED are indicated. Antibiotics effective against oral flora should be prescribed.

In the ED, the differentiation between periapical abscesses and pulpitis is very difficult, and dental bite-wing radiographs are seldom available. Therefore, some physicians begin antibiotics in the patient who has not undergone recent dental instrumentation but complains of tooth pain and has percussion tenderness. Routine antibiotics for tooth pain that is caused by pulpitis, instrumentation, or localized abscess are not recommended by the dental societies, and a recent study in the emergency medicine literature suggests that the use of antibiotics for undifferentiated dental pain is not necessary.[19,20] Antibiotics have been recommended for odontogenic infections that have spread outside the immediate periapical area or have associated systemic signs, such as fever, swelling, and trismus. A supraperiosteal infiltration (tooth nerve block) should be performed in most cases, not only to provide immediate and long-acting relief but also because it reduces the need for narcotic analgesics even after the anesthetic has worn off.

Periodontal disease, unlike pulpal disease, is usually asymptomatic unless accompanied by abscess or ulcerations. *Periodontal disease* is infection of the gingiva, periodontal ligament, or the alveolar bone, which essentially make up the attachment apparatus of the tooth. *Gingivitis* is an inflammation of the gingiva caused by bacteria; in advanced cases, the

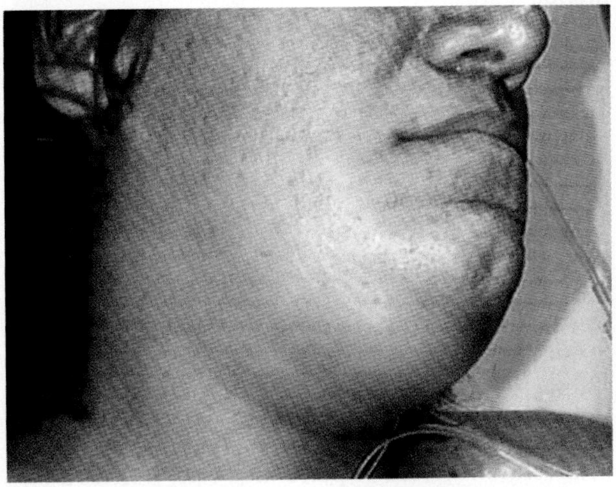

FIGURE 22-19 Ludwig's angina.

gingiva may be reddened, painful, and inflamed. In chronic disease, abscess formation occurs as organisms become trapped in the periodontal pocket. The purulent collection usually drains through the gingival sulcus. However, it can become invasive and involve the supporting tissues, the alveolar bone, and the periodontal ligament (periodontitis). Periodontal abscesses that are not draining adequately through the gingival sulcus should be drained in the ED. Antibiotics should be prescribed, and saline rinses are encouraged to promote drainage, but chlorhexidine rinses can be substituted for saline in more severe disease.

Pericoronitis usually occurs when the wisdom teeth erupt and the gingiva overlying the erupting teeth becomes traumatized and inflamed. The gingiva overlying the crown may entrap bacteria and occasionally become infected, but usually the patient presents with pain from inflamed gingival tissue. Rarely, however, the localized infection can spread to deeper tissues, such as the pterygomandibular or submasseteric space. Clinically, patients with spread of the periocoronal infection present with trismus secondary to irritation of the masseter and pterygoid muscles. If pericoronal infection is localized, saline rinses and oral antibiotics are prescribed with dental follow-up in 24 to 48 hours.

■ Deep Space Infections of the Head and Neck

It is not unusual for odontogenic infections to spread to the various potential spaces of the head and neck. Presenting signs and symptoms are varied but usually consist of pain, swelling, difficulty with swallowing or speech, trismus, fever, and chills.

Certain teeth allow infectious spread to particular deep spaces of the head and neck, but rapid spread of these infections can make localizing the exact space difficult. Maxillary extension, likewise, is possible and can spread to several different spaces and potentially to the cavernous sinus. Cavernous sinus involvement is usually associated with periorbital cellulitis as well as meningeal signs or a change in mental status.

Deep space infections can rapidly become severe and life-threatening. The submandibular space connects to the sublingual space, and bilateral involvement of the sublingual spaces can result in a condition known as Ludwig's angina, an airway-compromising deep space infection that may require airway intervention.

The management of complicated odontogenic head and neck infections focuses primarily on airway management, surgical drainage, and antibiotics. CT scanning has become the imaging modality of choice for deep space infections of the head and neck and should be utilized to localize and delineate collections of abscess or cellulitis that cannot be precisely determined from physical examination.[8] Airway intervention should be performed early if there is any question of compromise. The EP should administer intravenous antibiotics and obtain surgical consultation early in the evaluation and treatment of the patient.

The bacteria usually isolated from deep space infections of the head and neck typically consist of mixed *Staphylococcus/Streptococcus* or mixed aerobic/anaerobic flora. Almost half the isolates from odontogenic infections are resistant to beta-lactam antibiotics.[21] Drugs of choice include penicillin G plus metronidazole or extended-spectrum penicillins such as ampicillin-sulbactam, ticarcillin-clavulanate, and piperacillin-tazobactam. These combination antibiotics are effective against beta-lactamase–producing bacteria as well as common oral anaerobes such as *Bacteroides fragilis.* Clindamycin is an effective choice for penicillin allergic patients but it should be combined with a cephalosporin such as cefotetan or cefoxitin for resistant organisms. It is prudent to remember that antibiotics are adjunctive therapy only and are not a substitute for surgical therapy.

REFERENCES

1. Waldrop R, Ho B, Reed S: Increasing frequency of dental patients in the urban ED. Am J Emerg Med 2000; 18:687-689.
2. Bringhurst C, Herr RD, Aldous JA: Oral trauma in the emergency department. Am J Emerg Med 1993;11: 486-490.
3. King R, Montgomery M, Redding S (eds): Oral-Facial Emergencies—Diagnosis and Management. Portland, OR, JBK Publishing, 1994.
4. Dajani AS, Taubert KA, Wilson W, et al: Prevention of bacterial endocarditis: Recommendations by the American Heart Association. JAMA 1997;277:1794-1801.
5. Jastak T, Yagiela J, Donaldson D (eds): Local Anesthesia of the Oral Cavity. Philadelphia, WB Saunders, 1995.
6. Druelinger L, Guenther M, Marchand EG: Radiographic evaluation of the facial complex. Emerg Med Clin North Am 2000;18:393-410.
7. Markowitz BL, Sinow JD, Kawamoto HK Jr, et al: Prospective comparison of axial computed tomography and standard and panoramic radiographs in the diagnosis of mandibular fractures. Ann Plast Surg 1999;42:163-169.
8. Lazor JB, Cunningham MJ, Eavey RD, et al: Comparison of computed tomography and surgical findings in deep neck infections. Otolaryngol Head Neck Surg 1994;111: 746-750.
9. Rauschenberger CR, Hovland EJ: Clinical management of crown fractures. Dent Clin North Am 1995;39:25-51.
10. Ellis SG: Incomplete tooth fracture: Proposal for a new definition. Br Dent J 2001;190:424-428.
11. Dale RA: Dentoalveolar trauma. Emerg Med Clin North Am 2000;18:521-538.
12. McTigue D: Diagnosis and management of dental injuries in children. Pediatr Clin North Am 2000;47:1067-1084.
13. Rauschenberger CR, Hovland EJ: Clinical management of crown fractures. Dent Clin North Am 1995;39:25-51.
14. Blatz M: Comprehensive treatment of traumatic fracture and luxation injuries in anterior permanent dentition. Pract Proced Aesthet Dent 2001;13:273-279.
15. Bakland LK, Milledge T, Nation W: Treatment of crown fractures. J Calif Dent Assoc 1996;24:45-50.
16. Barrett EJ, Kenny DJ: Avulsed permanent teeth: A review of the literature and treatment guidelines. Endod Dent Traumatol 1997;13:6153-6318.
17. Marino TG, West LA, Liewehr F, et al: Determination of periodontal ligament cell viability in long shelf-life milk. J Endod 2000;26;699-702.

18. Olson BD, Mailhot JM, Anderson RW, et al: Comparison of various transport media on human periodontal ligament cell viability. J Endod 1997;23:676-679.
19. Ashman S: Oral cavity and dental emergencies. In Eisele D, McQuone D (eds): Emergencies of the Head and Neck. St. Louis, Mosby, 2000.
20. Runyon MS, Brennan MT, Batts JJ, et al: Efficacy of penicillin for dental pain without overt infection. Acad Emerg Med 2004;11:1268-1271.
21. Gilbert DN, Moellering RC, Elipoulos GM, et al: Sanford Guide to Antimicrobial Therapy. Sperryville, VA, Antimicrobial Therapy, 2005.

Chapter **23**

Pharynx and Throat Emergencies

H. Gene Hern

KEY POINTS

- Viruses cause most cases of pharyngitis but the modified Centor criteria is a scoring system that can improve the detection of group A beta-hemolytic *Streptococcus* pharyngitis.
- Consider corticosteroids in patients with pharyngitis for symptomatic relief of tonsillar hypertrophy.
- Unilateral pain and swelling may indicate peritonsillar abscess (consider ultrasonography).
- Consider epiglottitis in circumstances when the physical findings do not match the patient's pain and other symptoms. Visualize the epiglottitis to rule out the disease.
- Ludwig's angina manifests as bilateral submandibular swelling, fever, and an elevated or protruding tongue.
- A suppurative thrombophlebitis, Lemierre's syndrome, located within the internal jugular vein, is a complication of nearby infections in the pharynx or mastoid space.
- Retropharyngeal abscesses occur in children younger than 6 years secondary to infected lymph nodes and in adults from local or hematogenous spread. Such abscesses require imaging to make the diagnosis, because physical findings are notoriously unreliable in this disease.

Pharynx Emergencies

The oropharynx plays a vital role in the health of every patient. It is not only the entry point for food and nutrition. Oxygen and carbon dioxide must also move through the oropharynx every minute to maintain metabolic homeostasis. Any disease process that interferes with the function of the oropharynx has the potential to cause significant morbidity and perhaps death of the patient.

The most obvious potential complication is airway compromise. Restrictive spaces such as the hypopharynx and larynx (with the narrow vocal cords and superior epiglottis) provide ample opportunity for even mild inflammation or edema to significantly alter the normal airflow through this region. In addition the proximate location of the great vessels of the carotid artery and internal jugular veins provides fertile ground for infections or complications from airway procedures such as peritonsillar abscess drainage. The fascial planes in the oropharynx reach toward vital structures, infection of which may have disastrous results. Deep fascial planes track posteriorly toward the vertebral column, inferiorly into the mediastinum, and superiorly near the cavernous sinus, providing opportunities for cervical vertebral osteomyelitis, mediastinitis, and cranial nerve problems.

Anatomy

The pharynx anatomy resembles an inverted cone with the narrowest part where it attaches to the esophagus at the level of the cricoid cartilage and the widest part attaching to the base of the skull. The pharynx has abundant immunologic tissue to help fight infection—the palatine tonsils, adenoids, and lingual tonsils—which may predispose the host to dangerous circumstances (e.g., airway compromise) if the inflammatory response is too dramatic.

Acute Pharyngitis and Tonsillitis

Inflammation of the oropharynx, pharyngitis, is a predominantly infectious disease. Pharyngeal pain and dysphagia are the more common complaints in outpatient clinics and EDs alike. Although pharyngitis is usually a benign disease, the immunologic response to the infection occasionally causes severe complications both in immediate proximity to the tissues of the airway and also systemically. The local inflammation may cause straightforward complications like otitis media but may also produce more dramatic complications, such as dehydration, tissue edema, and airway compromise.

Pharyngeal irritation and inflammation produce throat pain that is worsened by swallowing. Occasionally, this pain may radiate to the ears or feel "pressure-like," because the eustachian tubes may also be blocked or swollen. The tonsils and pharynx may be erythematous with or without tonsillar enlargement, exudates, petechiae, or lymphadenopathy.

■ ETIOLOGY

Viruses cause most cases of pharyngitis. Even the most common cause of bacterial pharyngitis in children, group A beta-hemolytic *Streptococcus* (GABHS), is responsible for only 30% of cases. Among adults, *Streptococcus* species account for only 23% of cases, *Mycoplasma* (9%) and *Chlamydia* (8%) species also being significant.[1]

■ PRESENTING SIGNS AND SYMPTOMS

■ Viral Pharyngitis

In addition to the characteristic pharyngeal pain and dysphagia, pharyngitis with a viral cause may also produce low-grade fevers, cough, rhinorrhea, myalgias, or headaches. Viral pharyngitis may cause exudates as well, although cervical adenopathy is less common. Common viral causes are rhinoviruses, adenoviruses, Epstein-Barr virus (EBV), herpes simplex virus (HSV), influenza virus, and parainfluenza virus. Less common viruses that may cause pharyngitis are respiratory syncytial virus, cytomegalovirus, and primary human immunodeficiency virus (HIV) infection.

Documentation

CONSIDERATIONS

- Visualization of airway, including in patients with suspected epiglottitis or supraglottitis
- Work of breathing and use of accessory muscles.
- Patient ability to take fluids by mouth
- Discussion with patient and family, with confirmation of their understanding, of the need for close observation and what symptoms to return for
- Arranged follow-up

Pharyngitis in young adults may be due to infectious mononucleosis, an infection caused by EBV. Infectious mononucleosis often causes thick tonsillar exudates or membranes and manifests other systemic symptoms and signs. Splenomegaly (50%) is often present, and generalized lymphadenopathy is usually present. Palatal petechiae and periorbital edema also may be seen.

Also a disease of young adults, herpes simplex virus (HSV) infection may produce a painful and characteristic pharyngitis. HSV pharyngitis characteristically produces painful vesicles on erythematous bases. These vesicles occur in the pharynx, lips, gums, or buccal mucosa. Fever, lymphadenopathy, and tonsillar exudates may also be present and may last for 1 to 2 weeks. HSV pharyngitis may be either a primary infection or a reactivation of prior infection. In addition, bacterial superinfection of affected tissues may occur.

■ Bacterial Pharyngitis

The most common cause of bacterial pharyngitis among children is GABHS. It is less commonly implicated in patients older than 15 years. During epidemics, the incidence may double. Characteristic symptoms include tonsillar exudates, high fevers (more than 38.3° C), tender cervical adenopathy, and pharyngeal erythema. Headache, nausea, and abdominal pain may also be found. GABHS pharyngitis usually lacks the traditional symptoms of viral infections (cough, rhinorrhea, myalgias). This infection occasionally produces a fine sandpaper-like rash that is termed *scarlet fever*.

Mycoplasma pneumoniae pharyngitis occurs in crowded conditions, may be associated with epidemics, and typically produces a mild pharyngitis. Symptoms include exudates and a hoarse voice; there may also be lower respiratory symptoms such as cough and occasional dyspnea.

Chlamydia pneumoniae pharyngitis resembles *M. pneumoniae* pharyngitis in its occurrence in epidemic and crowded conditions. The pharyngitis is classically described as severe and persistent with tenderness in the deep cervical lymph nodes and occasional associated sinusitis.

Gonococcal and *Chlamydia trachomatis* pharyngitis have varying presentations from exudative to nonexudative, from mildly symptomatic to severely symptomatic, and from transient to persistent. These infections result from orogenital sexual transmission, and asymptomatic carriers may unknowingly spread the disease.

DIAGNOSTIC TESTING

Viral Pharyngitis

Diagnostic testing for viral pharyngitis is limited to only a few different specific causes. EBV may be diagnosed with a few different tests. Peripheral blood smears of up to 75% of patients with EBV demonstrate atypical mononuclear cells. An EBV mononucleosis spot test may have positive results in up to 95% of adults and 90% of children, but the result may not be positive for the first test during the first few days of illness. EBV immunoglobulin (Ig) M antibodies develop in 100% of cases but tests for them also may be initially negative.

Herpes pharyngitis is diagnosed with serologic tests, herpes culture, or cytopathologic tests of lesion scrapings. Primary HIV pharyngitis may be diagnosed with serologic testing using Western blot analysis and the enzyme-linked immunosorbent assay (ELISA). New rapid HIV tests using buccal swabs have also been shown to be effective in an ED setting.

Bacterial

Diagnostic testing for GABHS is a subject of some controversy. Although the diagnosis of GABHS is important in preventing many serious complications of streptococcal pharyngitis, including rheumatic fever, accurately diagnosing GABHS pharyngitis is notoriously difficult. The only valid method of diagnosing acute GABHS infection is with antistreptolysin O titers collected during acute disease and upon recovery. However, this method is far from practical in the ED setting. Throat cultures have a sensitivity of near 90% for detecting *Streptococcus pyogenes* in the pharynx, but the accuracy may vary with recent antibiotic use as well as culture and collection techniques.

Rapid diagnostic testing for GABHS detects antigens using varying techniques, including latex agglutination, enzyme-linked or optical immunoassay, and DNA luminescent probes. Specificities are reported to be higher than 90% and sensitivities to range from 60% to 95%.[2] A positive result appears to reliably indicate the presence of GABHS in the pharynx, but a number of factors must be considered. Some patients with a positive result may be asymptomatic carriers, and results of rapid tests may be negative in patients with low bacterial counts.

In addition to cultures and rapid streptococcal tests, clinical criteria have been proposed to aid in the diagnosis of GABHS pharyngitis. The best known are the Centor criteria and the McIsaac modifications to those criteria. As shown in Box 23-1, the modified Centor criteria give 1 point each to temperature higher than 38° C, swollen tender anterior cervical nodes, tonsillar swelling or exudates, absence of symptoms of upper respiratory infection (cough, coryza, etc.), and patient age between 3 and 15 years. If the patient is older than 45 years, 1 point is deducted from the total score. If the score is 1 point or zero, no further testing or treatment is warranted. For scores of 2 to 3 points, further testing may be indicated, such as culture or a rapid streptococcal test. For scores of 4 or more, no further testing is required, and the patient may be started on antibiotics for GABHS pharyngitis.[3,4]

Two recent guidelines—Infectious Disease Society of America (IDSA) and American Society of Internal Medicine (ASIM)—have proposed slightly different approaches to patients with pharyngitis. In children, the guidelines are similar in proposing the following approach: (1) use a rapid test on all children, (2) treat those who have positive results, (3) perform a throat culture on those with negative rapid test results, and (4) treat those with positive culture results. The guidelines have suggested different approaches to adults with pharyngitis, however. The IDSA guidelines are similar to the pediatric recommendations for all adults.[5] The ASIM, however allows two additional approaches for adults, including performing a rapid test on all adults with a Centor score of 2 or 3 and treating those with a positive rapid test result as well as treating empirically all patients with a score

BOX 23-1

Clinical Diagnosis of "Strep" Pharyngitis

The modified Centor criteria are a scoring system that can increase the detection of group A beta-hemolytic *Streptococus* (GABHS) pharyngitis.

1 point each is assigned to the following features:

- Temperature >38° C
- Swollen tender anterior cervical nodes
- Tonsillar swelling or exudates
- Absence of symptoms of an upper respiratory infection (cough, coryza, etc.)
- Age between 3 and 15 years; if the patient is older than 45 years, a point is deducted from the total score

If the score is 1 or zero, no treatment is needed.

For a score of 2 or 3, further testing may be indicated, such as cultures and rapid streptococcal tests.

For a score of 4 or more, no further testing is required, and the patient may be given antibiotics for GABHS pharyngitis.

of 4 or more. The final approach endorsed by the ASIM suggests testing no adult but treating all adults with a Centor score of 3 or 4 empirically.[6] A recent analysis comparing the different recommendations found that an approach using throat cultures had a sensitivity of 100%; an approach using rapid streptococcal tests or clinical criteria alone had sensitivities of around 75%. Furthermore, the specificity of clinical criteria alone was less than 50%, suggesting that many adults were given antibiotics for pharyngitis unnecessarily.[7]

Diagnostic testing for other causes of bacterial pharyngitis requires either culture on special media (Thayer-Martin agar for gonococcal infection) or specialized antigen or serologic testing. *Mycoplasma* infection may be detected with culture, serologic testing, or rapid antigen testing. Antigen detection as well as culture or serologic testing may also be used for chlamydial infection.

■ DIFFERENTIAL DIAGNOSIS

In addition to the infectious causes of pharyngitis mentioned in this chapter, a number of other infectious and noninfectious causes must be considered in the differential diagnosis of patients with pharyngitis. Among dangerous infections, deep space infections such as retropharyngeal abscesses, peritonsillar abscesses, and epiglottitis must be considered. Noninfectious but potentially serious diseases in the differential diagnosis include drug or allergic reactions, foreign body or caustic ingestion, angioedema, and chemical or thermal burns.

■ TREATMENT

Luckily, most cases of pharyngitis are acute and self-limiting. Supportive care with analgesics and antipyretics and, perhaps, topical anesthetics (lozenges or sprays) help with symptoms. Even most infectious causes of pharyngitis rarely cause serious complication.

Among viral causes of pharyngitis, few allow for specific treatment. HSV infection may be treated with acyclovir, famciclovir, or valacyclovir, all of which produce similar earlier resolution of symptoms without eradicating the etiologic agent. Infectious mononucleosis has no effective antiviral agent, although some important aspects of disposition of patients with this disease remain important. Patients with suspected infectious mononucleosis should be advised against contact sports for 6 to 8 weeks out of concern for potential serious splenic injury. Patients with infectious mononucleosis for whom tonsillar edema and hypertrophy severely limit adequate oral hydration secondary to dysphagia may receive corticosteroids (dexamethasone 6 to 10° mg intramuscularly) to aid in symptomatic relief.

Of all bacterial causes of pharyngitis, GABHS is the most common and the most often studied. Regardless of the diagnostic strategy employed, antimicrobial therapy directed at streptococcal species will likely be very effective. There are two main reasons to treat GABHS pharyngitis—the improvement of symptoms and the decrease in rate of complications. Patients who receive antibiotics in the first 2 to 3 days of symptoms are likely to improve 1 to 2 days faster with antibiotics than without. In terms of complications, the most feared complication of GABHS is acute rheumatic fever. Treating with antibiotics within the first 9 days of infection decreases the rate of rheumatic fever after GABHS infection. However, the incidence of acute rheumatic fever has fallen drastically in the last few decades so that the number of patients one would need to treat (NNT) to prevent one case of rheumatic fever has risen from 63 to now more than 4000. This change is due to the amount of antibiotics prescribed for GABHS over the years, the presence of less virulent strains of bacteria, and improved living conditions. Antibiotic use also limits transmission to others. Antibiotic therapy also limits the rate of suppurative complications of GABHS pharyngitis, including peritonsillar abscesses, retropharyngeal and other deep space infections, otitis, and mastoiditis but has no effect on the incidence of post-streptococcal glomerulonephritis.

Penicillin remains an effective choice for GABHS pharyngitis; 1.2 million units of benzathine penicillin or a 10-day course of 500 mg penicillin VK orally twice a day both effectively treat pharyngitis and reduce symptoms. The intramuscular route may be more effective in treating streptococcal pharyngitis because of compliance issues but is associated with more severe allergic reactions. Alternative regimens include macrolide antibiotics (such as erythromycin and azithromycin) and clindamycin. Oral cephalosporins have been shown to have slightly better cure rates than penicillins and may be used for a shorter time (5 days).

Mycoplasmal pharyngitis may be treated with a course of macrolide antibiotics, tetracycline, or doxycycline. *C. pneumoniae* pharyngitis is treated for 10 days with doxycycline, trimethoprim-sulfamethoxazole, or a macrolide. *C. trachomatis* pharyngitis may require repeated courses or prolonged use of antibiotics.

Corticosteroids given in conjunction with antibiotics decrease the duration of symptoms in patients

PATIENT TEACHING TIPS

- When to take antibiotics
- When to take pain medicine
- To return to the ED for the following problems:
  - Increased difficulty breathing
  - Increased difficulty swallowing
  - Worsening pain
  - Confusion or changes in thinking
  - Worsening fever

with pharyngitis without increasing complication rates. Steroids are particularly useful in patients with profound tonsillar hypertrophy and edema or with severe dysphagia and mild dehydration. By reducing the inflammatory response and significantly reducing pain, steroids allow patients to swallow with comfort sooner.

Peritonsillar Abscess and Cellulitis

■ BACKGROUND

Peritonsillar cellulitis and peritonsillar abscess exemplify the continuum of peritonsillar infections best characterized as peritonsillitis. Peritonsillar infections represent the most common deep infection of the head and neck region. These infections occur more commonly in teenagers and young adults, but they can manifest at any age. The infection begins most commonly when tonsillitis spreads beyond the boundary of tonsillar capsule and invades the potential space between the lateral aspect of the tonsillar capsule and the superior constrictor muscle of the pharynx. The local spread of infection begins as a cellulitis but progresses to abscess formation if left untreated. Predisposing factors include chronic tonsillitis, dental infections, smoking, and infectious mononucleosis. Peritonsillitis can occur in patients who have previously undergone a complete tonsillectomy.

■ PRESENTING SIGNS AND SYMPTOMS

Symptoms of peritonsillitis begin with the symptoms of tonsillitis and progress over a few days into increasing pain and unilateral symptoms. Patients with peritonsillitis often complain of dysphagia, odynophagia-related drooling, trismus, and referred otalgia on the affected side. In addition patients describe voice changes (hoarseness or a "hot potato" voice) from decreased movement of the palate. They may also describe recurrent bouts of pharyngitis or trials of antibiotics without resolution of symptoms.

■ Signs

On physical examination, the patient may have trismus, which may prevent clear visualization of the pharynx but may respond to benzodiazepines. Erythematous mucosa as well as purulent exudates may be present. The distinguishing features of a peritonsillar abscess include predominant unilateral swelling. Classically, displacement of the infected tonsil and often of the soft palate toward the midline occurs, resulting in the deviation of the uvula to the contralateral side.

■ DIAGNOSTIC TESTING

Although it is often difficult to distinguish peritonsillar cellulitis from peritonsillar abscess,[8] a number of modalities exist to aid the diagnosis. For patients who cannot lie down or who are unable to cooperate with needle aspiration, intraoral ultrasonography is a useful test.[9] Computed tomography (CT) is helpful in delineating the extent and scope of the abscess but it may be difficult for the patient to lie supine during the study.

When an acute infectious cause is not evident, CT or ultrasonography should be used to evaluate for other causes of tonsillar and peritonsillar disease, such as lymphoma, other neoplasms, and internal carotid artery aneurysm.

■ TREATMENT AND DISPOSITION

Pending airway obstruction requires emergency aspiration of a peritonsillar abscess. For less urgent conditions, the classic recommendation was incision and drainage. Needle aspiration, with or without ultrasonographic guidance, provides a diagnosis, induces less pain, and is easier to perform than traditional incision and drainage. Approximately 10% of needle-aspirated abscesses require a second aspiration.[8]

Patients should also receive antibiotics (penicillin or clindamycin) and steroids for relief of the pain and swelling.

■ Disposition

Most cases of peritonsillitis can be safely treated and discharged home with antibiotics and steroids and close follow-up in 24 to 48 hours. For patients with severe dehydration or severe trismus requiring intravenous hydration, a brief inpatient stay may be required. Any patient with tissue edema and potential airway compromise must be admitted for observation and potential aggressive airway management.

Epiglottitis and Supraglottitis

■ BACKGROUND

Inflammation and edema of the epiglottis may result in rapid and life-threatening airway obstruction if not identified and treated effectively. In addition, the tissues immediately adjacent to the epiglottis (arytenoids, false vocal cords, and pharyngeal wall) may also become edematous, resulting in a similar infection known as supraglottitis. The presentations of the two diseases may be remarkably similar although their populations may be somewhat different. Until the introduction of the *Haemophilus influenzae* type B (Hib) vaccine in the mid 1980s, epiglottitis was a disease of children. The annual incidence decreased dramatically to a very low 0.3 to 0.6 per 100,000 children.[10] Adult epiglottitis appears to be on the rise. One study showed a 31% rise in the incidence of adult epiglottitis over an 18-year period.[11] Incidence rates for adults cluster near 3 per 100,000 with a case fatality-rate reported as high as 7%. Lower overall

Table 23-1 PRESENTING SYMPTOMS OF EPIGLOTTITIS OR SUPRAGLOTTITIS IN CHILDREN

	FREQUENCY (%)	
Sign or Symptom	**Age <2 years**	**Age >2 years to <18 years**
Fever	100	99
Difficulty breathing	97	94
Irritability	89	94
Change in voice or cry	82	96
Stridor	92	88
Retractions	88	78

Table 23-2 PRESENTING SIGNS AND SYMPTOMS OF EPIGLOTTITIS OR SUPRAGLOTTITIS IN ADULTS

Sign or Symptom	Frequency (%)
Muffled voice	54-79
Pharyngitis	57-73
Fever	54-70
Tenderness of anterior neck	79
Dyspnea	29-37
Drooling	22-39
Stridor	12-27

bacteremia rates in adults than in children with epiglottitis suggest that adults may have more viral etiologies as well as other, noninfectious, causes. The noninfectious causes include trauma, caustic ingestion, and thermal injuries from illicit drug inhalation. Of organisms recovered in blood cultures, Hib still predominates but *Streptococcus* and *Staphylococcus* species may be isolated as well.

■ PRESENTING SIGNS AND SYMPTOMS

■ Children

Epiglottitis in children produces a dramatic progression from a relatively well child to a toxic-appearing one; 85% of patients are sick for less than 24 hours. The child appears anxious, may be sitting forward in a tripod position, and may have difficult with secretions (Table 23-1).

■ Adults

The mean presenting age of adults with epiglottitis is between 42 and 50 years. Unlike children, adults present after 2 to 3 days of symptoms. They complain of odynophagia and throat pain rather than the drooling and stridor seen in pediatric patients. This difference is thought to be due to the larger and more rigid trachea and lack of generous lymph tissue in adults. The pharyngeal pain may be disproportionate to the clinical findings seen. Fever is frequently absent in adults until the later stages. Additionally, the epiglottitis or supraglottitis in an adult is frequently misdiagnosed as "strep" pharyngitis, with the true diagnosis made later (Table 23-2).

■ DIFFERENTIAL DIAGNOSIS

The differential diagnosis for epiglottitis includes pharyngitis, peritonsillar abscess, and even life-threatening causes (retropharyngeal abscess, Ludwig's angina). If the symptoms are consistent with the visible physical findings, the diagnosis of pharyngitis or peritonsillar abscess may be appropriate. However, if the symptoms are out of proportion to the physical findings, the more dangerous diseases must be excluded. Other life-threatening diseases are angioedema, foreign body aspiration, laryngospasm, and caustic ingestion. One rare disease that is occasionally confused with epiglottitis is adult botulism. The blockade of cholinergic nerve transmissions characteristically produces an inflamed and painful pharynx, and the muscular paralysis may produce a muffled voice, leading to a confusion of this problem with epiglottitis.

■ DIAGNOSTIC TESTING

Patients with any sign of respiratory distress (drooling, aphonia, or stridor) should be moved to a critical care room and plans should be made for obtaining a surgical airway if needed. Any attempt at direct laryngoscopy to visualize the epiglottis should be made only if the personnel and equipment are available to secure a surgical airway, cricothyrotomy, or tracheostomy.

A lateral radiograph of patients with suspected epiglottitis have a sensitivity approaching 90% compared with direct laryngoscopy. Findings on a lateral radiograph may include an edematous and thickened epiglottis (thumb shaped, or thumb sign) (Fig. 23-1), a disappearance of the vallecula, swelling of the epiglottic folds or arytenoids, and edema of the retropharyngeal spaces. Adults with normal radiographic findings and suspected epiglottitis must undergo laryngoscopy, either direct or indirect. No attempt should be made to visualize the epiglottis in pediatric patients in the ED. Children should be taken to the operating room for direct laryngoscopy, with surgical staff present to obtain a surgical airway, if needed.

■ TREATMENT

All patients with suspected epiglottitis should be treated with extreme caution because their disease may suddenly progress to complete airway obstruction without warning. Endotracheal intubation must be performed under direct visualization either with a laryngoscope or with a fiberoptic bronchoscope or laryngoscope. At all times, equipment and

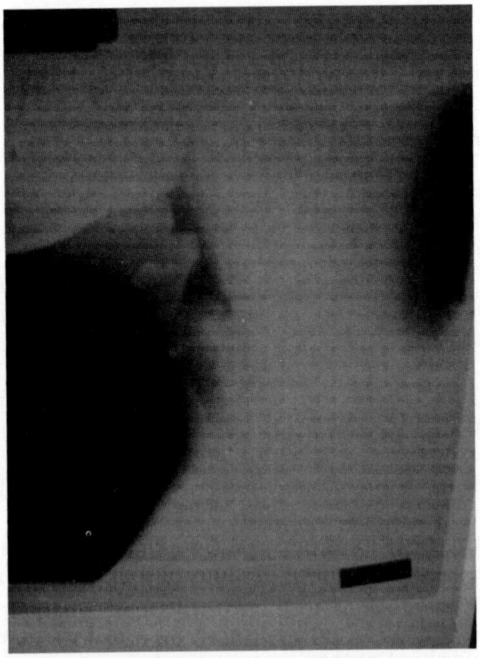

FIGURE 23-1 Classic radiograph of epiglottitis with thumb sign indicating a swollen epiglottis.

personnel for an emergency cricothyrotomy must be available.

Patients should receive broad-spectrum antibiotic treatment including effectiveness against *H. influenzae* as well as other common bacterial pathogens. Ampicillin-sulbactam and ceftriaxone are both acceptable first-line agents. Corticosteroids and racemic epinephrine have not been conclusively proven to be of benefit in these patients.

■ DISPOSITION

All patients in whom epiglottitis or supraglottitis is suspected should be admitted. Adults without respiratory distress (drooling, stridor, or dyspnea) may be admitted without intubation and observed, but in a carefully monitored setting. The vast majority of children with suspected epiglottitis should be intubated in the operating room and then admitted to the intensive care unit (ICU) for intravenous antibiotics. Rarely, a child with epiglottis may not require intubation. However, the decision not to intubate such a child is made only in consultation with the pediatric anesthesiologist and intensivist after they have evaluated the patient. Children with epiglottis who are not intubated should always be admitted to an ICU setting because they have a very high potential to deteriorate rapidly.

Ludwig's Angina

■ BACKGROUND

First described in 1836, *Ludwig's angina* is a fast-spreading, potentially lethal infection of the submandibular, sublingual, and submental spaces. These spaces effectively function as one unit because infection can spread easily between them. True Ludwig's angina involves all of the submandibular spaces, although serious and life-threatening infections can occur with infection of only some of the spaces. Mortality of this disease approached 50% before the advent of antibiotics and surgical decompression but is now commonly reported less than 10%.[12]

■ ETIOLOGY

Approximately 80% of cases involve patients with odontogenic disease. Patients with infection or recent extraction of the second or third molars are particularly at risk because the roots of these teeth extend below the mylohyoid ridge. Abscesses located here can easily perforate the lingual plate of the mandible, allowing for direct spread of the infection to the submandibular spaces. Other predisposing conditions are deep lacerations or trauma to the floor of the mouth, mandibular fractures, and salivary calculi.

■ PRESENTING SIGNS AND SYMPTOMS

On presentation, patients with Ludwig's angina appear ill and anxious. Males predominate slightly over females by a ratio of 3:2. The classic symptoms are tooth pain (79%), swelling of the neck and/or chin (71%), dysphagia (52%), neck pain (33%), respiratory symptoms (dyspnea, tachypnea, stridor) (27%), and dysarthria (18%).

Physical findings in almost all patients comprise bilateral submandibular swelling, fever, and an elevated or protruding tongue (Figs. 23-2 to 23-4). Trismus is found in approximately half of all patients. Complications of Ludwig's angina can be disastrous, with infection spreading to the mediastinum, pericardium, or pleural cavity as well as the lungs and great vessels.

PRIORITY ACTIONS

- Move patients with potential airway compromise to critical care rooms.
- Prepare for emergency airway procedure.
- In pediatric patients with possible epiglottitis, laryngoscopy should not be attempted until personnel skilled in emergency airway techniques are present.
- Initiate antibiotic therapy early in patients with serious infections.
- Appropriate imaging should be performed for patients with serious infections such as retropharyngeal abscess or supraglottitis when their pain is out of proportion to physical findings.

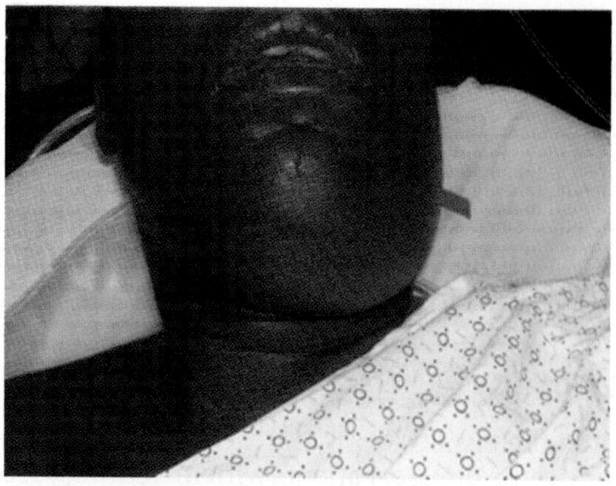

FIGURE 23-2 Submandibular swelling in Ludwig's angina.

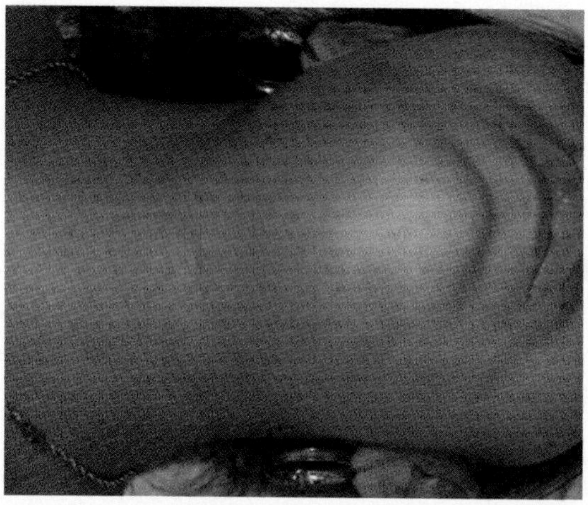

FIGURE 23-3 Submandibular redness and swelling in Ludwig's angina.

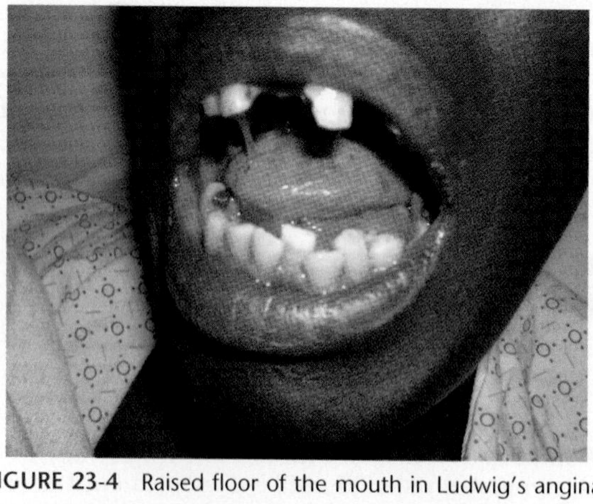

FIGURE 23-4 Raised floor of the mouth in Ludwig's angina.

■ DIFFERENTIAL DIAGNOSIS

The differential diagnosis in a patient with suspected Ludwig's angina should also include Lemierre's syndrome (a septic thrombophlebitis of the internal jugular vein). It is distinguished from Ludwig's angina by its unilateral nature. Tumors of the floor of the mouth can be distinguished from Ludwig's angina because of their tendency to be much slower-growing. Mandibular abscesses are usually unilateral and produce less swelling of the floor of the mouth.

■ DIAGNOSTIC TESTING

Because Ludwig's angina is predominantly a clinical diagnosis, diagnostic testing commonly delineates the extent of infection, not whether it is present. Soft tissue lateral neck radiographs may be helpful in showing edema of the soft tissues and air in soft tissue spaces. If the patient is able to lay supine for a short while, a helical CT scan (Fig. 23-5) may be helpful in delineating the progression of the abscess and allow more accurate surgical débridement. If there is any question about the safety of having the patient lie supine, the airway must be secured first. At all times, the utmost caution is required in these patients, and securing the airway will likely involve the capabilities of an anesthesiologist, otorhinolaryngologist, or general surgeon. No airway maneuvers may be attempted until the equipment and personnel capable of obtaining a surgical airway are present at the bedside.

■ TREATMENT AND DISPOSITION

The treatment of patients with Ludwig's angina predominantly involves airway protection through nasal (fiberoptic), oropharyngeal, or surgical techniques, antibiotic therapy, and surgical débridement. The antibiotic chosen should have broad-spectrum coverage because up to 50% of cases have polymicrobial involvement. Although streptococci, staphylococci, and *Bacteroides* are the commonly cultured organisms, other species identified are *Klebsiella, H. influenzae, Proteus,* and *Pseudomonas* species. Once the airway is protected, 50% of cases of Ludwig's angina resolve with only antibiotics. All patients with this disorder should be admitted to an ICU for further monitoring as well as for fluid resuscitation in case the clinical picture deteriorates into one of bacteremia and sepsis. ICU observation is required for patients with milder cases who are not immediately intubated because the progression to airway compromise and obstruction may be rapid.

Lemierre's Syndrome

■ BACKGROUND

A particularly dangerous and intractable complication of nearby infections, Lemierre's syndrome is a suppurative thrombophlebitis located within the internal jugular vein. This dangerous but fortunately rare complication of nearby infections in the pharynx or mastoid may produce septic emboli.

■ ETIOLOGY

Lemierre's syndrome is often caused by *Fusobacterium necrophorum,* a gram-negative anaerobe that produces

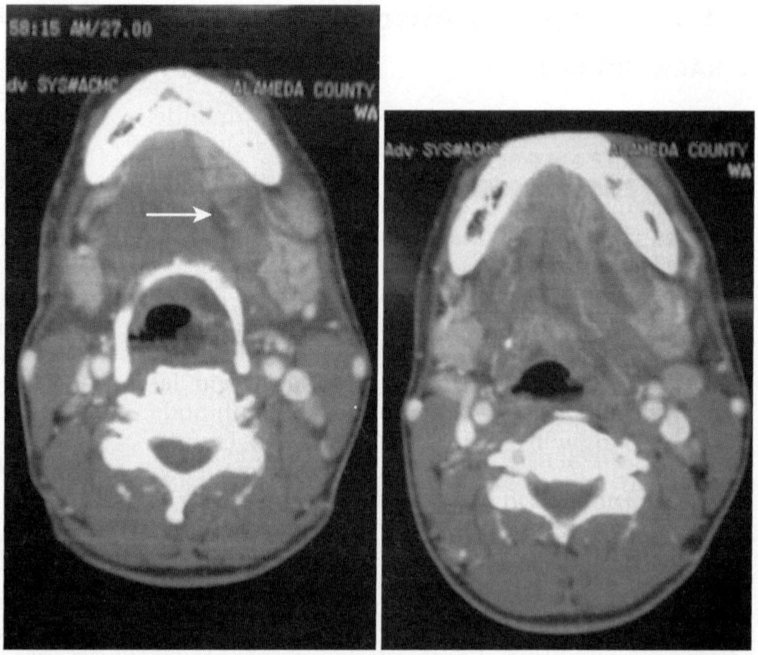
A
B

FIGURE 23-5 **A,** Computed tomography (CT) scan of Ludwig's angina showing infection in the submandibular spaces (*arrow*). **B,** CT scan of Ludwig's angina showing infection in the submandibular spaces.

endotoxin. *F. necrophorum* can colonize the upper respiratory, gastrointestinal, and genitourinary tracts. Other organisms may also cause this particular variant of septic thrombophlebitis, including *Bacteroides melaninogenicus, Eikenella corrodens,* and non–group A streptococci.

■ PRESENTING SIGNS AND SYMPTOMS

Signs and symptoms of Lemierre's syndrome may resemble those of other localized infections, including fever, swelling, tenderness, and pain with range of motion of the neck. This disorder, however, also causes obstruction of normal blood flow in the affected internal jugular vein. Unilateral swelling, edema, and induration in the tissues occur on the affected side, regardless whether they are actually infected.

■ DIFFERENTIAL DIAGNOSIS

When considering the diagnosis of Lemierre's syndrome, one must also consider Ludwig's angina and other deep space infections in the neck and parapharyngeal tissues. Whether from odontogenic, lymphatic, or other sources, deep space infections in the neck and pharynx must be taken very seriously.

■ DIAGNOSTIC TESTING

Lemierre's syndrome is a diagnosis that, when suspected requires confirmatory testing to document the involvement of the internal jugular vein. Soft tissue lateral neck radiographs may be helpful in showing edema of the soft tissues and air in soft tissue spaces but lack the specific information about vein involvement needed to make the diagnosis of Lemierre's syndrome. The diagnosis is made most commonly via a contrast-enhanced CT scan of the neck. In addition, magnetic resonance imaging may also delineate the extent of involvement of the jugular vein. Both modalities also provide information about the surrounding anatomy, including distortion of nearby tissues and localized pockets of infection that must be drained. Other tests that may aid in the diagnosis of Lemierre's syndrome are duplex ultrasonography, retrograde venography, and gallium scanning. If there is any question about the safety of having the patient lie supine, the airway must be secured first.

■ TREATMENT AND DISPOSITION

Treatment of Lemierre's syndrome must include both heparin and antibiotics. The thrombus provides a nidus of ongoing infection and, subsequently, septic emboli. Anticoagulation effectively limits the progression of thrombus and, in turn, limits the creation of further septic emboli. Broad-coverage antibiotics should be administered. Prolonged high-dose broad-spectrum antimicrobial therapy is recommended because of the high risk of septic emboli and endocarditis. Close consultation with an infectious disease specialist would be helpful in such cases. Patients with Lemierre's syndrome clearly must be admitted, and consultation with a vascular surgeon may be helpful if a thrombectomy is considered.

Retropharyngeal Abscess

■ BACKGROUND

Although retropharyngeal abscesses predominantly occur in children, adults may also be affected. Pediatric patients possess prominent lymph nodes in the retropharyngeal area. These nodes predispose children to abscesses in the retropharyngeal spaces because the nodes can become infected and progress to cellulitis and abscess formation. These nodes atrophy by age 6, and the incidence of retropharyngeal abscesses drops precipitously.

The etiology of cases in the nonpediatric population differs greatly from that of the local lymph node infections in children younger than 6 years. The etiology of adult retropharyngeal abscesses ranges from the extension of other pharyngeal infections (such as parotitis, peritonsillar abscess, tonsillitis, Ludwig's angina, and dental infections) to recent dental instrumentation and other trauma (fish bones or dental instruments), to hematologic spread of systemic infections.[13]

■ MICROBIOLOGY

The microbiology of retropharyngeal abscesses reveals a diverse array of causative bacteria. Although the preponderance of abscess are polymicrobial (up to 86%), some species predominate. The majority of aerobic pathogens are *Streptococcus* and *Staphylococcus* species, and *Bacteroides fusiformis* and *Peptostreptococcus* species dominate the anaerobic isolates. Tuberculous and fungal etiologies must also be considered.

■ PRESENTING SIGNS AND SYMPTOMS

The patient with a retropharyngeal abscess has a sore throat as well as any number of other symptoms, including dysphagia, drooling, odynophagia, neck pain, and a muffled voice. Dysphonia commonly sounds like a duck "quack" (cri du canard). Patients may complain of a feeling of a lump in the throat and may prefer to lie supine or with the neck extended to keep the swelling in the posterior pharynx from compressing their upper airway. In the pediatric population, many case series have described the mean presenting age as 3 years old. It is uncommon for children in this age group to describe these symptoms, and the more common presenting complaints are related to feeding, fever, and stridor.[14]

On physical examination, only a minority of adult patients (37%) have visible swelling of the posterior pharynx.[15] Other physical findings are cervical lymphadenopathy, torticollis, and trismus. Palpating the neck or moving the larynx and tracheal side to side (tracheal "rock" sign) may induce pain. Pain and other symptoms out of proportion to the physical findings require further diagnostic testing and evaluation.

■ DIFFERENTIAL DIAGNOSIS

Other possible diagnoses to consider in patients in whom retropharyngeal abscess is being considered are other pharyngeal infections, including pharyngitis, peritonsillar abscess, and infectious mononucleosis. Abrasions or caustic burns to the posterior pharynx might produce similar symptoms of dysphagia and odynophagia. Other causes of retropharyngeal swelling and pain are cervical fractures, hematomas, and other causes of tissue edema, such as tendinitis. Finally, the distinction between a true abscess and cellulitis may be difficult and is sometimes accomplished only through imaging.

■ DIAGNOSTIC TESTING

Imaging of retropharyngeal abscesses involves two main types of radiologic tests, plain lateral neck radiographs and CT scans. Early studies of normal lateral radiographs suggest that the upper limit of normal for retropharyngeal spaces is 7 mm at C2 and 22 mm at C6. Anything beyond 7 mm is considered pathologic for both children and adults. In addition, retropharyngeal abscesses displace the larynx and esophagus anteriorly. If there is still a question about the extent of involvement or the distinction between cellulitis and abscess, a CT scan of the neck (Fig. 23-6) or magnetic resonance imaging (Fig. 23-7) will easily elucidate the exact anatomic extension of the abscess. Of course, patients must be stable enough to lie flat for the time it takes to complete the study. Intraoral ultrasonography is another modality with great potential for distinguishing between abscess and cellulitis of the pharynx.[16]

■ TREATMENT AND DISPOSITION

Retropharyngeal infections require broad-spectrum intravenous antibiotics. The antibiotics must be effective against anaerobes as well as gram-positive and gram-negative species. Although most retropharyngeal abscesses require surgical drainage, selected cases

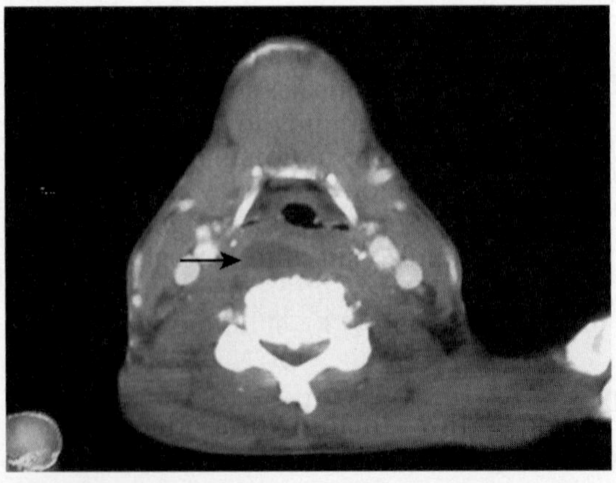

FIGURE 23-6 Computed tomography scan of a retropharyngeal abscess (*arrow*).

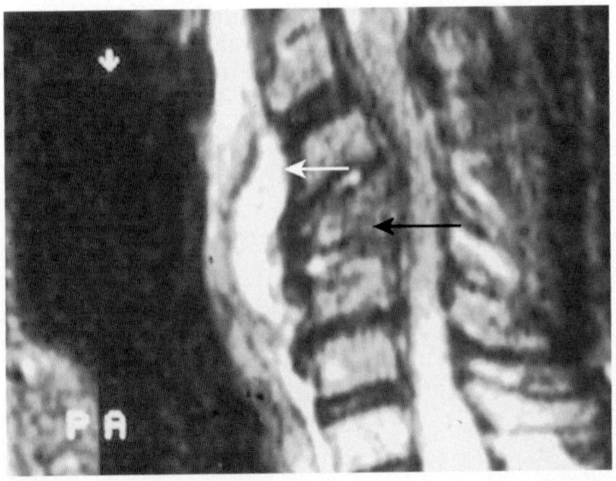

FIGURE 23-7 Magnetic resonance imaging of retropharyngeal abscess (*white arrow*). Note extension into vertebral bodies (osteomyelitis) (*black arrow*).

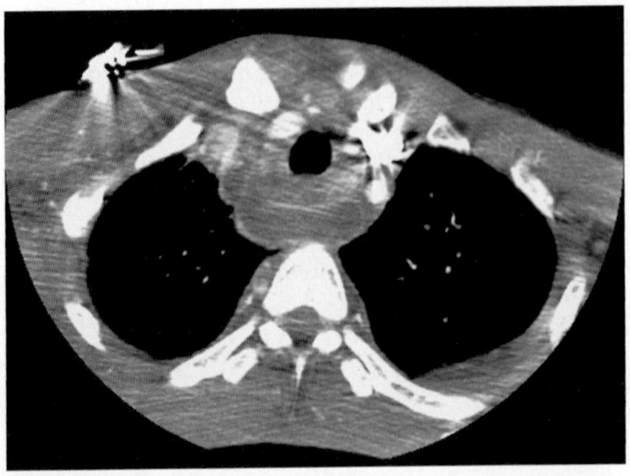

FIGURE 23-9 Computed tomography scan showing inferior extension of a retropharyngeal abscess into the mediastinum.

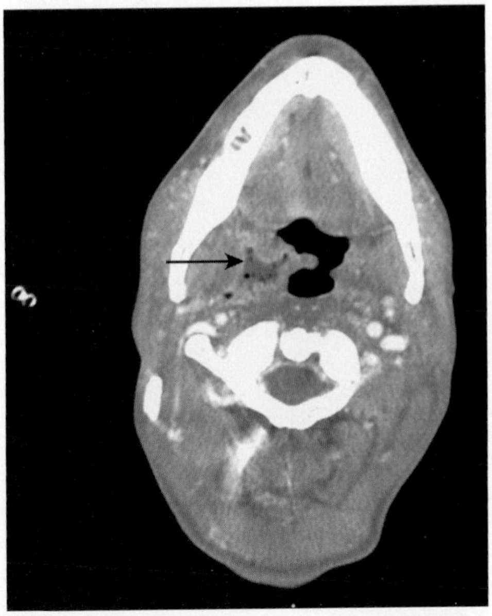

FIGURE 23-8 Computed tomography scan of extension of a retropharyngeal abscess (*arrow*) extending laterally and inferiorly.

RED FLAGS

- Do not miss the diagnosis of acute epiglottitis or supraglottitis. In children this disease occurs more quickly than in adults.
- Do not give ampicillin to patients with suspected infectious mononucleosis, because it may cause an uncomfortable rash.
- Do not miss abscesses. Deep space neck infections and abscesses are difficult to diagnose unless considered and imaged.
- When the pharyngeal pain is out of proportion to the physical findings, exclude more serious causes, such as epiglottitis and deep space infections.

may occasionally be managed with intravenous antibiotics alone.[17] Even if surgical drainage is deferred, admission of the patient to a monitored bed after thorough airway evaluation is required.

Complications from retropharyngeal abscesses include spread of infection inferiorly or laterally (Fig. 23-8) into the mediastinum (Fig. 23-9), pericardium, and nearby vascular structures. Osteomyelitis (see Fig. 23-7), transverse myelitis, and epidural abscesses have also been reported.

REFERENCES

1. Bisno AL: Acute pharyngitis. N Engl J Med 2001;344: 205-211.
2. Bisno AL, Gerber MA, Gwaltney JM Jr, et al: Diagnosis and management of group A streptococcal pharyngitis: A practice guideline. Infectious Diseases Society of America. Clin Infect Dis 1997;25:574-583.
3. Centor RM, Witherspoon JM, Dalton HP, et al: The diagnosis of strep throat in adults in the emergency room. Medical Decision Making 1981;1:239-246.
4. McIsaac WJ, White D, Tannenbaum D, Low DE: A clinical score to reduce unnecessary antibiotic use in patients with sore throat. CMAJ 1998;158:75-83.
5. Bisno AL, Gerber MA, Gwaltney JM, et al: Practice guidelines for the diagnosis and management of group A streptococcal pharyngitis. Clin Infect Dis 2002;35: 113-125.
6. Cooper RJ, Hoffman JR, Bartlett, JG, et al: Principles of appropriate antibiotic use for acute pharyngitis in adults: Background. Ann Intern Med 2001;134:509-517.
7. McIsaac WJ, Kellner JD, Aufricht P, et al: Empirical validation of guidelines for the management of pharyngitis in children and adults. JAMA 2004;291:1587-1595.
8. Spires JR, Owens JJ, Woodson GE, Miller RH: Treatment of peritonsillar abscess: A prospective study of aspiration vs incision and drainage. Arch Otolaryngol Head Neck Surg 1987;113:984-986.
9. Lyon M, Blaivas M: Intraoral ultrasound in the diagnosis and treatment of suspected peritonsillar abscess in the emergency department. Acad Emerg Med 2005;12:85-88.
10. Frantz TD, Rasgon BM: Acute epiglottitis: Changing epidemiologic patterns. Otolaryngol Head Neck Surg 1993;109: 457-460.
11. Mayo-Smith MF, Spinale JW, Donskey CJ, et al: Acute epiglottitis: An 18-year experience in Rhode Island. Chest 1995;108:1640-1647.

13. Bansal A, Miskoff J, Lis RJ: Otolaryngologic critical care. Crit Care Clin 2003;19:55-72.
13. Goldenberg D, Golz A, Joachims HZ: Retropharyngeal abscess: A clinical review. J Laryngol Otol 1997;111: 546-550.
14. Thompson JW, Cohen SR, Reddix P: Retropharyngeal abscess in children: A retrospective and historical analysis. Laryngoscope 1988;98:589-592.
15. Tannebaum RD: Adult retropharyngeal abscess: A case report and review of the literature. J Emerg Med 1996;14: 147-158.
16. Ben-Ami T, Yousefzadeh DK, Aramburo MJ: Pre-suppurative phase of retropharyngeal infection: Contribution of ultrasonography in the diagnosis and treatment. Pediatr Radiol 1990;21:23-26.
17. Craig FW, Schunk JE: Retropharyngeal abscess in children: Clinical presentation, utility of imaging, and current management. Pediatrics. 2003;111:1394-1398.

Chapter 24

Maxillofacial Disorders

Laura J. Bontempo

KEY POINTS

- Temporomandibular joint dislocation is usually readily reduced in the ED after the patient has been pretreated with analgesic and antispasmodic agents.
- Epistaxis may be the presenting complaint of a patient with a more serious systemic illness, such as a clotting disorder.
- When visible blood loss from the nasopharynx has been stopped, the clinician should examine the oropharynx for ongoing occult blood loss.
- Posterior epistaxis accounts for about 10% of nasal hemorrhages and can result in large volumes of blood loss.
- Any abnormal neurologic or ocular physical findings in a patient with sinusitis mandate further investigation to assess for central nervous system extension of the disease.

Temporomandibular Joint Disease

■ SCOPE

The temporomandibular articulations are unique within the body in that there are bilateral joints which are nearly continuously in use. As such, the temporomandibular joint (TMJ) is subject to both pain (TMJ syndrome) and dislocation. It is roughly estimated that more than 10 million people in the United States alone have symptomatic TMJ disorders.[1]

■ PATHOPHYSIOLOGY

TMJ syndrome pain is likely due to excessive strain on the muscles of mastication with resultant strain on the capsular ligaments of the TMJ.[2] The result is that the mandibular condyle does not articulate properly in its joint. The patient feels pain and senses an occlusal disturbance.

When in normal position, with the mandible open, the condyle moves anteriorly and inferiorly. When the mandible closes, the condyle moves posteriorly and superiorly, returning to its original location (Fig. 24-1).

Patients with TMJ dislocation present with an inability to close the mouth. TMJ dislocation results when the mandibular condyle moves anterior to the temporal eminence. The temporal eminence is the anterior portion of the mandibular fossa (see Fig. 24-1). Once the dislocation occurs, the muscles of mastication spasm, resulting in trismus and inability of the patient to return the mandibular condyle to its anatomic position. The dislocation usually results from excessive opening of the mouth, such as occurs with yawning or laughing. TMJ dislocation can also be the result of trauma or dystonic drug reactions.

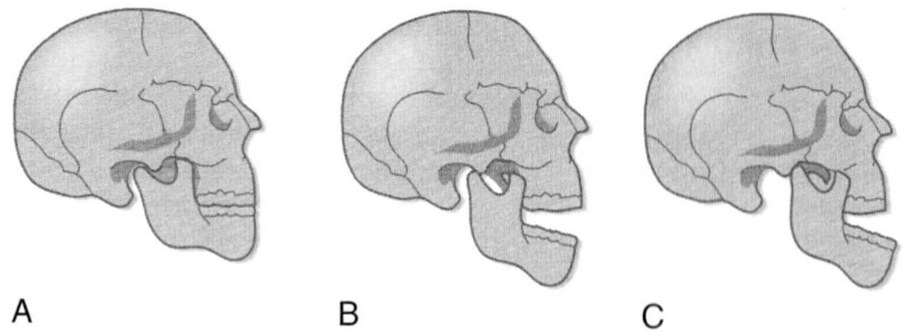

FIGURE 24-1 Anatomic drawing of the mandible in open, (**A**), closed, (**B**), and dislocated (**C**), positions.

BOX 24-1

Pain Presentation of TMJ Syndrome

Dull or throbbing in character
Unilateral more common than bilateral
Preauricular location
Worsens during the day
Exacerbated by chewing

PRESENTING SIGNS AND SYMPTOMS

Unilateral pain in the region of the TMJ and clicking or crepitance that is exacerbated by chewing are the classic presenting complaints of a patient with TMJ syndrome (Box 24-1). The dull or throbbing pain is localized to the preauricular region and typically worsens during the day. If a click is present, the patient hears it when jaw opening is initiated. The pain may also radiate to the neck or temporal region.

Physical examination should include evaluation of the muscles of mastication through intraoral and external palpation. Palpation finds muscular spasm and tenderness. Palpation of the TMJ or muscles of mastication may reproduce the patient's symptoms and trigger significant pain. The patient may have great pain with any attempts at jaw range of motion. Physical findings are also notable for reduced jaw opening and possible lateral deviation of the jaw. If the TMJ dislocation is unilateral, the mandible deviates away from the affected side.

DIFFERENTIAL DIAGNOSIS

When considering the diagnosis of TMJ syndrome, the EP must rule out odontogenic causes. If the possibility of an intraoral etiology remains after carefully performed history and physical examination, the patient should be referred to a dentist for a full dental evaluation. This evaluation can be done concurrently with the start of TMJ treatment.

Central nervous system (CNS) disorders must also be ruled out in the evaluation of a patient with symptoms suggestive of TMJ syndrome. The clinician must be especially careful to address this possibility when the presenting complaints include CNS-related symptoms, such as headache and vertigo. A detailed neurologic examination must be performed. Except for possible hyperesthesias immediately around the TMJ, there should be no abnormalities in the neurologic findings for patient with TMJ syndrome.

DIAGNOSTIC TESTING

An atraumatic TMJ dislocation does not require imaging unless attempts at reduction are unsuccessful. However, in the case of trauma, a panoramic radiographic evaluation of the mandible or a TMJ radiograph series should be performed to assess for a fracture.

TREATMENT AND DISPOSITION

Temporomandibular Dislocation

TMJ reduction is performed in the ED and is usually readily accomplished. Controlling the patient's pain and masseter spasm facilitates the procedure. Intravenous analgesics (e.g., morphine 5 mg as needed) and antispasmodics (e.g., diazepam 5 to 10 mg titrated to patient response) should be given before reduction is attempted.

Once the patient is comfortable, the clinician faces the patient and grasps the mandible inferiorly with the fingers of both hands. The clinician's thumbs should be heavily wrapped in gauze for protection, and then placed on the occlusive surfaces of the mandibular molars. Downward pressure is applied to move the mandibular condyle inferior to the temporal eminence. The mandible is then pushed posteriorly (Fig. 24-2). Once the condyle is posterior to the temporal eminence and pressure is released, the condyle returns to its anatomic position in the mandibular fossa. At the time of reduction, the masseter muscles may contract forcefully, causing the patient to inadvertently clench the jaw. The clinician must be aware of this possibility, ensuring that his or her thumbs are guarded during the procedure and removing the thumbs from the occlusive surface of the molars as quickly as possible.

When reduction of the TMJ has been accomplished, the patient needs to avoid excessive mouth opening to prevent a recurrent dislocation, and may be discharged home. Post-reduction pain can be treated with analgesics and antispasmodics. Advising a soft diet for 2 weeks will also minimize the patient's discomfort. The patient should follow up with an oromaxillofacial surgeon within 2 weeks.

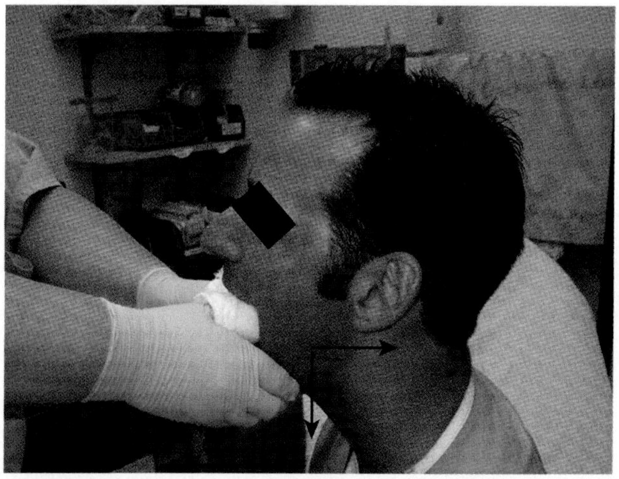

FIGURE 24-2 Proper technique for reduction of a dislocated temporomandibular joint.

PATIENT TEACHING TIPS

TEMPOROMANDIBULAR JOINT DISLOCATION

- Avoid excessive mouth opening to prevent a recurrence of the dislocation; this includes laughing and yawning.
- Take pain medications and muscle relaxants as prescribed. These drugs may cause sedation.
- Eat a soft diet for 2 weeks.
- Follow up with an oromaxillofacial surgeon within 2 weeks.
- Return to the emergency department if your pain is not controlled or if you are unable to fully close your mouth, which may indicate a recurrent dislocation.

PATIENT TEACHING TIPS

TEMPOROMANDIBULAR JOINT SYNDROME

- Take anti-inflammatory and pain medications as prescribed.
- Apply warm compresses to the region in front of your ear for 15 minutes 3 times per day.
- Benzodiazepines may have been prescribed to control muscle spasm. These drugs may cause sedation.
- Eat only soft foods until symptoms resolve.
- Avoid chewing gum.
- See your dentist for follow-up to evaluate whether bruxism is the cause of your condition.
- See your doctor or return to the emergency department if your pain is not controlled or if you are unable to fully open or close your mouth, which may indicate a dislocation of your jaw.

■ Temporomandibular Joint Syndrome

The management of TMJ syndrome is primarily directed at improving the patient's comfort. This is accomplished through analgesia, muscle relaxation, and behavioral modifications.

Pain should be addressed with anti-inflammatory agents (e.g., ibuprofen 600 mg by mouth every 6 hours or naproxen 500 mg by mouth every 12 hours) and narcotic pain medications (e.g., oxycodone 5 to 10 mg by mouth every 6 hours). Warm compresses should also be applied to the TMJ region for 15 minutes three times per day. Benzodiazepines are used to relieve masseter muscle spasm (e.g., diazepam 5 mg by mouth every 8 hours). Behavioral modifications include minimizing masseter muscle use through a soft diet and cessation of gum chewing.

If bruxism is suspected, dental follow-up should be arranged, and a bite appliance can be considered. To date, experimentation with the use of botulinum toxin to reduce masseter muscle contractility and strength has yielded mixed results.[3,4]

The patient with TMJ syndrome can be discharged home with instruction to follow up with the primary care physician and dentist.

Epistaxis

■ SCOPE

The true incidence of epistaxis is unknown because many patients do not seek medical attention. However, from 1992 to 2001, epistaxis accounted for 4,503,000 ED visits, or 0.46% of all visits during that 10-year period. Epistaxis affects both adults and children, with higher incidences in children and elderly patients. Specifically, there is a bimodal peak in ED visits for epistaxis. The first peak occurs in patients younger than 10 years, and the second peak occurs in patients 70 to 79 years old.[5]

The majority of patients presenting to the ED with epistaxis can be managed by the EP and discharged home; only 6% of patients require admission.[5]

■ PATHOPHYSIOLOGY

The nasal mucosa is a vascularly rich area supplied by three arteries. Any disruption of this mucosa can result in bleeding. Although epistaxis can be caused by trauma, this is not the most common cause. Bleeding more commonly results from upper respiratory infections, a dry environment, nasal foreign bodies, allergic rhinitis, or nasal mucormycosis (Box 24-2). Additionally, epistaxis may be the presenting symptom of a systemic bleeding disorder.

BOX 24-2

Risk Factors for Epistaxis

Alcoholism
Allergic rhinitis
Anticoagulant use
Barotrauma
Blood dyscrasia
Diabetes mellitus
Endometriosis
Intranasal drug use
Intranasal neoplasm
Low-humidity environment
Nasal foreign body
Nasal polyps
Platelet inhibitor use
Pregnancy
Recent otorhinoloaryngologic surgery
Septal deviation
Sinusitis
Trauma, including nose picking
Upper respiratory infection

ANATOMY

The nasal mucosa is a vascularly rich area whose blood supply coming from branches of both the internal and external carotid arteries. The anterior and posterior ethmoidal arteries, which are branches of the internal carotid artery, supply blood to the septum and the superior lateral region of the nose. The sphenopalatine artery, another branch of the internal carotid artery, supplies the inferoposterior portion of the septum as well as the turbinates and meati. The superior labial artery, from the external carotid artery, and the greater palantine artery, a branch of the internal carotid artery, supply the anterior septum and floor of the nasal cavity.

Kiesselbach's plexus is an anatomic region of vessels on the anterior portion of the nasal septum. Its blood supply is from the sphenopalatine artery, the anterior and posterior ethmoidal arteries, and the greater palatine artery. Another name for Kiesselbach's plexus is Little's area.

Epistaxis can be divided into two general categories, anterior nasal bleeds and posterior nasal bleeds. Anterior nasal bleeds most commonly arise from Kiesselbach's plexus. Functionally, epistaxis is considered anterior when the site of bleeding can be visualized in the anterior portion of the nasopharynx. Posterior nasal hemorrhage cannot be directly visualized and occurs in the posterior or superior parts of the nose.

PRESENTING SIGNS AND SYMPTOMS

Epistaxis may manifest as a minor bleed with small quantities of blood dripping from the nares, or a major bleed with the patient vomiting blood. Approximately 90% of epistaxis is anterior, and the bleeding source is unilateral. Many patients, however, present with blood from both nares because blood from the unilateral bleeding source travels around the septum and exits on the other side.

Patients with both anterior and posterior bleeds may arrive at the ED with various home treatments in progress. All foreign bodies (cotton, tissues, tampons) should be removed from the nose after the patient's arrival to better assess the location and quantity of bleeding. If the patient has to wait before being seen, he or she can apply direct pressure to the area by squeezing the soft tissue portion of the nose with the fingers. The nares are successfully compressed when a change in the patient's voice is heard.

Obtaining a detailed history is often the key to figuring out the cause of the patient's epistaxis. Hypertension, although not a risk factor for epistaxis itself, is a risk factor for larger quantities of blood loss once epistaxis has begun.[6,7] The patient's antihypertensive agent (i.e., beta-blocker) can mask the early stages of shock by limiting the tachycardia a patient can mount. Most importantly, the possibility of a blood dyscrasia must be addressed. The clinician must know whether the patient has recurrent epistaxis, easy bruising, or other sources of bleeding (such as when shaving or brushing the teeth) or is taking a platelet inhibitor or anticoagulant medication. Past medical history is important in the patient who has hepatic disease, atherosclerosis, Rendu-Osler-Weber disease (hemorrhagic telangiectasias), diabetes mellitus, or cancer with ongoing chemotherapy treatment; each of these conditions is a risk factor for epistaxis.[8,9] Women are more prone to epistaxis during pregnancy.

Trauma, nose picking, recent otorhinolaryngologic surgery, nasal foreign body, an upper respiratory infection, nasal polyps, and exposure to a low humidity environment all predispose to epistaxis. Each of these entities must be addressed in the patient's history. Family medical history may demonstrate recurrent epistaxis among multiple family members. In the absence of a hereditary bleeding disorder, this history suggests familial idiopathic epistaxis. A social history must also be obtained to identify alcoholism, intranasal drug use, or domestic violence.

The physical examination of patient with epistaxis must focus on the nasopharynx and oropharynx; however, a complete examination is helpful. A skin examination may reveal ecchymosis or petechiae (suggestive of a systemic bleeding disorder), spider angiomas or caput medusa (suggestive of hepatic disease), or signs of trauma. Cardiac examination may demonstrate an irregular heartbeat, prompting the clinician to inquire further about anticoagulant medications.

Concurrent with examining the nasal mucosa, the posterior oropharynx must also be examined. The patient may have occluded the nares with a nasal packing or by compression, but may continue to have significant blood loss into the oropharynx. The patient swallows this blood, and without careful examination, the ongoing loss may not be evident until hematemesis or hemodynamic instability develops.

Alternatively, a patient may present with the chief complaint of hemoptysis. If a patient has a low-volume nasal bleed with blood flowing posteriorly into the oropharynx, coughing of gross blood may be the presenting sign of epistaxis.

DIFFERENTIAL DIAGNOSIS

Mechanical causes of epistaxis, such as trauma, nose picking, nasal foreign bodies and nasogastric or nasotracheal intubation, directly disrupt the nasal mucosa. Blood dyscrasias, hepatic disease, platelet inhibitors, and anticoagulant medications result in decreased blood clotting and predispose the host to bleeding. Infectious causes include sinusitis, rhinitis, mucormycosis, and upper respiratory infections that result in nasal congestion and vasodilation.[9] In women, both endometriosis and pregnancy must be considered as causes. Environmental factors also play a role in the incidence of epistaxis. Presentations to the ED for the treatment of epistaxis are more common in winter months.[5] This fact is proposed to be due to lower ambient humidity and subsequent drying of the nasal membranes during this season. Barotrauma can also incite epistaxis.

In patients presenting with larger-volume hemorrhage, hematemesis may be the presenting complaint. Once the emesis has been controlled, examination of the oropharynx shows blood entering superiorly from the nasal cavity. The clinician can then work to localize the source of bleeding in the nose without being misled into investigating a gastrointestinal source.

DIAGNOSTIC TESTING

Laboratory tests have a limited role in the patient with epistaxis. Patients who present with a low- or moderate-volume anterior bleed, who have no known blood dyscrasia, and who are not taking anticoagulant medications do not require any laboratory studies.[10]

If, however, the patient's history or physical examination raises concern about a systemic cause of the epistaxis, studies should be ordered as appropriate for the clinician's specific suspicions. These studies may include prothrombin time, activated partial thromboplastin time, coagulation factor levels, bleeding time, vitamin K level, and liver function tests.[9] In patients exhibiting signs of shock, the hematocrit should be checked to obtain a starting value with which to compare serial measurements.

BOX 24-3

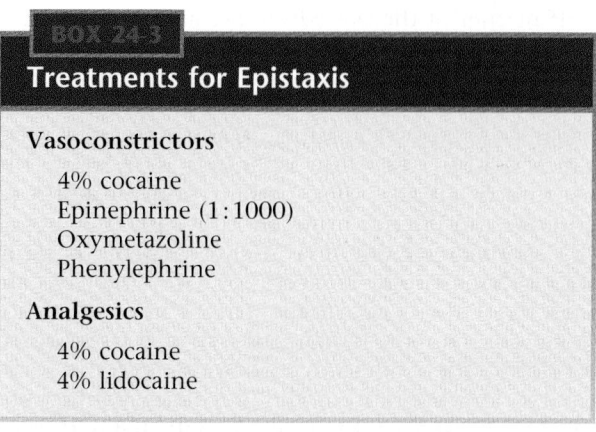

Treatments for Epistaxis

Vasoconstrictors

- 4% cocaine
- Epinephrine (1:1000)
- Oxymetazoline
- Phenylephrine

Analgesics

- 4% cocaine
- 4% lidocaine

INTERVENTIONS AND TREATMENT

Standard supplies for treatment of epistaxis include suction with a Frazier tip, nasal speculum, bayonet forceps, cotton-tipped applicators, silver nitrate cautery sticks, packing material, nasal tampons, gelatin foam (Gelfoam) or oxidized cellulose (Surgicel), a posterior nasal balloon with syringe, and a good light source. Universal precautions should be followed at all times. The clinician must also wear eye protection owing to the risk of ocular exposure during management of the epistaxis.

In the absence of massive epistaxis, the initial step is to evacuate intranasal clots and apply a topical vasoconstrictor and analgesic to the mucosa (Box 24-3). This can be achieved by soaking cotton pledgets in a combined vasoconstrictor and topical analgesic solution. If cotton is not available, rolled 2-inch ×2-inch gauze can be used. The analgesic is added to improve patient comfort during any necessary interventions once vasoconstriction has occurred. These medications are left in contact with the mucosa for 5 to 10 minutes, and then can be removed.

After removal of the pledgets, the nasal cavity and oropharynx are inspected. If the source of bleeding is identified in the nose and the oropharynx is dry, anterior epistaxis has been confirmed. For anterior epistaxis in which vasoconstriction has mostly controlled the bleeding, chemical cautery with silver nitrate is an excellent first choice. The silver nitrate cautery stick is applied directly to the area of bleeding from peripheral to central and from superior to inferior. This method minimizes the quantity of blood that comes between the cautery stick and the nasal mucosa. Nitric acid is formed, which coagulates the contacted tissue. Septal damage from silver nitrate can occur. For this reason, the cautery stick should not be in contact with the nasal mucosa for more than 15 seconds, and bilateral septal coagulation should be avoided. Bilateral coagulation can lead to septal ischemia, necrosis, and perforation.

Another approach to anterior epistaxis is to apply a topical hemostatic packing agent, such as gelatin foam or oxidized cellulose, directly to the bleeding area.

If neither of the preceding measures is successful, direct compression of the mucosa through packing of the anterior nasal cavity is necessary. This can be accomplished with a nonadherent ribbon gauze packing or a nasal tampon. If nonadherent ribbon gauze is to be used, the technique is to insert the packing in an accordion pattern from posterior to anterior and inferior to superior. If septal bowing to the contralateral side is seen after packing, packing the other naris may be necessary. *Nasal tampons* are preformed nasal packs that expand when exposed to fluid. The tampon is lubricated with a water-based lubricant, then directed posteriorly into the nasal cavity. The tampon should be placed gently but firmly and quickly into the nasal cavity. If it is inserted too slowly, the first part may expand from contact with blood before insertion is complete; this makes further insertion more difficult for both the patient and clinician. If, after insertion, the tampon is not fully expanded, saline or a vasoconstrictive agent (see Box 24-1) can be dripped into the nasal cavity until expansion is achieved. Pain medication may be necessary owing to the discomfort from the nasal pack.

Bleeding from posterior epistaxis is more challenging to control. By definition, the bleeding site is not readily visualized, making compression and treatment more difficult. The most rapid method for controlling posterior epistaxis is the insertion of a posterior balloon device. Typically this device has a double-balloon design, one balloon to tamponade the posterior nasal cavity and the other for the anterior nasal cavity. After the device is lubricated, it is inserted into the nasal cavity to its hub. The posterior balloon is inflated, and the hub is then drawn out away from the nose until resistance is met. The resistance indicates that the posterior balloon has set in the posterior nasal cavity and is not in the pharynx. Next, the anterior balloon is inflated. The quantity of saline required to fill each balloon varies by device but typically it is 7 to 10 mL for the posterior balloon and 15 to 30 mL for the anterior balloon.[9]

If a posterior balloon device is not available, a Foley catheter can be used in its place. For an average-sized adult, a 12F to 14F catheter with a 30-mL balloon is used. The catheter is inserted through the nose until the noninflated balloon can be seen in the posterior oropharynx. The balloon is then inflated with 10 mL of saline, and the catheter is slowly withdrawn from the nose until resistance is met. While traction is maintained, the anterior nasal cavity is packed with ribbon gauze. The catheter is secured by placement of a padded umbilical clamp or other equivalent device around the catheter where it exits the nostril. Securing the catheter properly is extremely important. If the catheter is allowed to migrate posteriorly, the inflated balloon descends into the oropharynx and possibly the trachea, resulting in airway obstruction. Using a Foley catheter for control of posterior epistaxis is only a temporary technique, and the catheter should be exchanged for a safer double-balloon device as soon as possible.

PATIENT TEACHING TIPS

EPISTAXIS

- Avoid nose blowing, bending over, and straining.
- Be sure to open your mouth when you sneeze.
- Avoid any activity that puts you at risk for nasal injury.
- If you live or work in a dry environment, use humidifiers and saline nasal spray to help keep the interior of your nose moist.
- Take pain medications as needed.
- Do not take aspirin or aspirin products.
- Follow up with an otorhinolaryngologist in 48 to 72 hours.
- Take your antibiotics as prescribed. It is important that you continue to take antibiotics as long as your nasal packing or balloon is in place.
- Do not put anything into your nose.
- If bleeding recurs, compress your nose by squeezing the bottom half of it with your thumb and index finger. Hold this compression for 10 minutes. If bleeding continues beyond this time, see your doctor or return to the emergency department.
- See your doctor or return to the emergency department if you develop a fever or rash.

For the patient who presents with massive epistaxis, use of nasal tampons and balloons is the fastest way to minimize or stop the bleeding. Bilateral anterior tampons are placed, and then the oropharynx examined. If active bleeding continues into the oropharynx, one tampon is removed and replaced with a posterior balloon device. If significant bleeding continues, the second tampon is removed and a second posterior balloon is inserted. Immediate otorhinolaryngology consultation is then necessary. Bilateral posterior balloons should be in place for the minimal amount of time possible. Intravenous access should be obtained and fluid resuscitation begun for any patient with significant blood loss or vital signs indicative of shock.

Epistaxis that persists despite the preceding interventions requires otorhinolaryngologic consultation. Additional management options include arterial ligation or embolization and endoscopy for direct visualization and cauterization.[11]

■ DISPOSITION

The hemodynamically stable patients with anterior epistaxis, in whom hemostasis has been achieved and maintained, should be discharged home. The patient is instructed to avoid nose blowing, bending over, straining, closed-mouth sneezing, and any activity that raises the risk for nasal trauma. In dry environments, humidifiers and saline nasal spray are recommended to help keep the nasal mucosa moist. Pain medications are prescribed as needed for patient comfort; however, aspirin products are avoided. Any patient with anterior packing or recurrent epistaxis must follow up with an otorhinolaryngologist in 48 to 72 hours.

Patients with nasal packing or balloons should be treated with anti-staphylococcal antibiotics to minimize the risk of sinusitis and toxic shock syndrome.[12] Drug choices include amoxicillin-clavulanate potassium 875 mg two times per day and cephalexin 500 mg four times per day. Packings should be left in place for 3 to 5 days, and antibiotics continued until the packing is removed. Nasal packings containing antibiotics are also available; these products have been shown to inhibit the growth of nasal flora and may supplant the need for additional systemic antibiotics.

Patients with posterior epistaxis require admission. If a posterior balloon were to become dislodged and migrate posteriorly, airway compromise could occur. Additionally, such a patient may have a drop in PaO_2 and a rise in their $PaCO_2$ after placement of posterior packing. Bradycardia and other cardiac dysrhythmias have also been reported. The mechanism of these events is unclear.

Sinusitis

■ SCOPE

Sinusitis is an inflammatory disease of the paranasal sinuses. Each year approximately 37 million Americans seek medical treatment for sinusitis. It is a complication of upper respiratory infections (URIs) in 5% to 10% of cases in children and 0.5% to 2% of cases in adults. The actual number of people affected by sinusitis may be significantly higher than reported owing to the multitude of over-the-counter sinus medications available. It is estimated that 16% of the adult U.S. population is affected annually.[13]

In 1996, the Task Force on Rhinosinusitis proposed that the term *sinusitis* be replaced by the term *rhinosinusitis* because rhinitis (inflammation of the lining of the nose) almost always accompanies sinusitis.[14] Rhinosinusitis most commonly occurs as a complication of a URI. For this text, the term *sinusitis* will be used, acknowledging that although rhinosinusitis is a more accurate description of the pathophysiology involved, this term is not yet in widespread use.

Sinusitis, as defined by the Task Force on Rhinosinusitis, can be divided into five subcategories (Table 24-1). *Acute* sinusitis has symptoms of 4 weeks' or less duration. In *subacute* sinusitis, symptoms are present for more than 4 weeks but less than 12 weeks. *Chronic* sinusitis involves symptoms for 12 weeks or longer. *Recurrent acute* sinusitis is defined as more than four episodes of acute sinusitis within 1 year. An *acute exacerbation* of chronic sinusitis is an acute infection superimposed on chronic sinusitis.

■ ANATOMY

There are four pairs of paranasal sinuses: the frontal, maxillary, sphenoid, and ethmoid. The sinuses' names indicate the facial bones in which they are located. The maxillary and ethmoid sinuses are present in humans at the time of birth. The frontal sinuses develop around age 7 years, and the sphenoid sinuses around age 10 years. Maxillary sinusitis is most common followed by ethmoid, frontal, then sphenoid sinusitis.

Each sinus drains through an ostium, which communicates with the nose. The sphenoid sinuses drain into the nose above the superior turbinate. The posterior ethmoid sinuses empty into superior meatus in the nose. The frontal, maxillary, and anterior ethmoid sinuses empty into the medial meatus, between the middle and inferior turbinates. This region is termed the ostiomeatal complex. Obstruction of this complex is a critical step in the development of sinusitis.

The anatomy of the ethmoid sinus deserves special mention. This sinus is divided into anterior and posterior portions, each composed of multiple air cells. The blood supply to these air cells connects with the ophthalmic blood vessels as well as the cavernous sinus. Ethmoid sinusitis, therefore, poses a risk of extension of infection into the orbit and central nervous system. The optic nerve, cavernous sinus, and carotid artery are also adjacent to the sphenoid sinus. Infection in the sphenoid sinus may spread to involve these structures.

Each sinus is lined with ciliated epithelium and mucous goblet cells. Healthy sinuses have relatively

Table 24-1 TASK FORCE ON RHINOSINUSITIS CLINICAL FORMS OF SINUSITIS

Type	Definition
Acute	Symptoms present ≤4 weeks
Subacute	Symptoms >4 weeks but <12 weeks
Chronic	Symptoms ≥12 weeks
Recurrent acute	>4 acute episodes within 1 year
Acute exacerbation of chronic	Acute infection superimposed on chronic disease

From Report of the Rhinosinusitis Task Force Committee Meeting. Alexandria, Virginia, August 17, 1996. Otolaryngol Head Neck Surg 1997;117:S1-S68.

few mucus-producing goblet cells, and the cilia beat the mucous produced by the goblet cells toward the ostium of the sinus. The patent ostium allows for the free flow of mucus and air from the sinus. When an ostium is occluded, these normal processes are interrupted, and new mucus-producing cells develop.

PATHOPHYSIOLOGY

The paranasal sinuses are air-filled pockets of bone within the skull that are lined with ciliated epithelium and mucous goblet cells. Each sinus drains through a sinus ostium, which exits into the nose. When this ostium becomes blocked, air and mucus no longer flow freely from the sinus. Therefore, any process that obstructs the ostia and/or causes ciliary dysfunction results in mucostasis.[15]

When the sinus epithelium becomes damaged, as can occur from a viral URI, ciliary dysfunction and inflammation result. When sinus drainage is obstructed, air resorption within the sinus creates a lower PaO_2, and continued metabolism lowers the pH. This hypoxic, hypercarbic, acidic environment aids bacterial growth.[16] Once bacterial infection occurs, mucous viscosity increases, further inhibiting sinus drainage. Bacteria can be introduced into the affected sinus through nose blowing, coughing, or, in the case of maxillary sinusitis, dental infection.

There are many causes of ostial obstruction and ciliary dysfunction. A viral URI with rhinitis is the most common infectious cause. Fungal rhinitis may also cause mucosal edema and inflammation, resulting in ostial obstruction. This is more common in immunocompromised hosts. Allergic rhinitis, another common cause of obstruction, leads to sinusitis. The sinusitis results from ostial obstruction and the subsequent cascade of events described previously. The allergen itself does not cause sinus inflammation.

Noninfectious causes include congenital diseases that inhibit ciliary function, such as cystic fibrosis and Kartagener's syndrome; autoimmune diseases, such as Wegener's granulomatosis and sarcoidosis; anatomic obstruction, such as nasal polyps or nasal tumors; and facial trauma, which directly disrupts sinus drainage.[16] Nasal foreign bodies, including nasogastric and nasotracheal tubes, may cause direct ostial obstruction. Up to 95% of patients with nasal intubation experience sinusitis.

The infectious organisms causing sinusitis can be viral, bacterial, or fungal. Viral causes are the most common, and multiple viruses are known to cause sinusitis; the most common types are rhinovirus, parainfluenza, and influenza.[17] The most common bacterial pathogens of acute sinusitis, recurrent acute sinusitis, and acute exacerbations of chronic sinusitis in an immunocompetent host are *Streptococcus pneumoniae, Haemophilus influenzae,* and *Moraxella catarrhalis*. Sinusitis pathogens more commonly found in immunocompromised hosts are *Pseudomonas aeruginosa, Rhizopus, Aspergillus, Candida, Histoplasma, Blastomyces, Coccidioides,* and *Cryptococcus*. *P. aeruginosa* is also a common pathogen in patients with cystic fibrosis.[16]

The pathogens of chronic sinusitis include those of acute bacterial sinusitis plus group A streptococci, *Staphylococcus aureus, P. aeruginosa,* and fungi.

BOX 24-4

Task Force on Rhinosinusitis Diagnostic Criteria for Acute Sinusitis

Major Criteria

- Facial pain or pressure
- Fever
- Hyposmia or anosmia
- Nasal congestion
- Nasal obstruction
- Purulent nasal discharge

Minor Criteria

- Cough
- Dental pain
- Ear pain or pressure
- Fatigue
- Halitosis
- Headache

From Report of the Rhinosinusitis Task Force Committee Meeting. Alexandria, Virginia, August 17, 1996. Otolaryngol Head Neck Surg 1997;117:S1-S68.

PRESENTING SIGNS AND SYMPTOMS

In order to standardize the diagnosis of acute sinusitis, the Task Force on Rhinosinusitis set forth the major and minor clinical criteria for the diagnosis (Box 24-4).[18] The diagnosis of acute sinusitis can be made when a patient has two major or one major and two minor criteria for longer than 7 days but less than 4 weeks.

It is very difficult to differentiate early sinusitis from a URI, and since viral URIs are the most common event precipitating sinusitis, the two may be present concurrently. For this reason, the Task Force on Rhinosinusitis recommends considering the diagnosis of acute bacterial sinusitis if symptoms worsen after 7 days or persist beyond 10 days.

The signs and symptoms of chronic sinusitis include those of acute sinusitis but are often more vague and less severe. Nasal obstruction, nasal discharge, and a chronic cough are prominent features. By definition, these symptoms must be present for more than 12 weeks.

Physical examination of the nose shows mucosal erythema and edema. Purulent nasal secretions may also be seen. Purulent secretions have the highest positive predictive value for sinusitis of any physical finding.[19] The nasal cavities must also be thoroughly inspected for foreign bodies, especially in children.

Sinus tenderness to percussion may be present on examination, although this finding is neither sensitive nor specific. Additionally, assessing percussion tenderness is possible only for the maxillary and frontal sinuses because of their anatomic location. Transillumination of the frontal and maxillary sinuses is likely not helpful in the ED. This technique is neither sensitive nor specific, and it is not possible to differentiate a fluid-filled sinus from a congenitally small sinus after a single evaluation. The clinician must examine the oral cavity for signs of posterior pharyngeal mucopurulent secretions and for evidence of a dental infection, which can be the source of maxillary sinusitis. Periorbital edema may also be found.

Acute or chronic frontal sinusitis can lead to erosion through the frontal bone and a resultant subperiosteal abscess known as Pott's puffy tumor. In addition to signs and symptoms of sinusitis, patients with this disorder present with a severe localized headache, swelling of the forehead, fever, and, possibly, orbital abnormalities. These infections are most commonly polymicrobial. Frontal sinusitis can also lead to osteomyelitis through direct spread or through thrombophlebitis of the diploic veins. Complications of frontal sinusitis are most common during the second and third decades of life.[20]

Pansinusitis leads to orbital complications in 60% to 80% of patients. Preseptal cellulitis is the most common complication. Clinical findings suggestive of preseptal cellulitis are periorbital edema without an associated vision change or limitation of ocular mobility. Orbital cellulitis, orbital subperiosteal abscesses, and orbital abscesses are other complications of pansinusitis; they manifest as periorbital edema, proptosis, orbital pain, and limitations of ocular mobility, as found by examination of extraocular muscle functions.

Intracranial complications of sinusitis, such as an intracranial abscess, meningitis, epidural abscess, subdural empyema, and cavernous sinus thrombosis, are serious complications of the disease. As of 2002, 18% of brain abscesses were a complication of sinus disease.[21] Disease can progress intracranially through direct extension or via thrombophlebitis of the diploic veins. Any focal neurologic deficits found on examination must raise concern for intracranial extension of sinusitis. Patients with subdural empyema present with system toxicity, nuchal rigidity, and photophobia as well as cranial nerve deficits. The EP must maintain a high index of suspicion. A prior review of patients found that headache and fever without other neurologic abnormalities were the most common presentations of early intracranial complications of sinusitis.

■ DIAGNOSTIC TESTING

The diagnosis of uncomplicated acute sinusitis does not require any diagnostic testing. Plain films of the sinuses should not be obtained. Interpretation of plain sinus film findings is controversial, and it is unclear whether such findings correlate with clinical disease.[16]

Computed tomography (CT) of the sinuses is useful when initial medical treatments for sinusitis have been unsuccessful and the diagnosis of chronic sinusitis is considered. The CT scan shows the extent of sinus disease, the extent of ostiomeatal complex obstruction, and any underlying anatomic abnormalities not found on physical examination. When a CT of the sinuses is obtained to evaluate for chronic sinusitis, coronal views with bone windows should be ordered. No contrast agent is needed.

For any patient in whom intracranial or extracranial complications of sinusitis are suspected, CT or magnetic resonance imaging (MRI) should be obtained. The study should image the brain, orbits, and/or sinus, depending on the clinical suspicion.

Routine laboratory tests are not useful in the management of sinusitis. Nasal cytology and nasal-sinus biopsies may be performed by otorhinolaryngologists. Evaluation for systemic disorders predisposing to sinusitis, such as cystic fibrosis, immunodeficiency, and, possibly gastroesophageal reflux disease, can be made on a nonemergency basis.

■ TREATMENT

Acute sinusitis of less than 7 days' duration is much more likely to be due to a viral rather than bacterial pathogen. For this reason, antibiotic treatment should be initiated only for a patient who meets criteria for the diagnosis of acute sinusitis and in whom symptoms persist beyond 7 days.

First-line antibiotic therapy is amoxicillin. If there is a high incidence of beta-lactamase–positive *H. influenzae* or *M. catarrhalis* in the area of patient care, adults should be treated with amoxicillin–potassium clavulanate. Alternative first-line agents are certain second- and third-generation cephalosporins. Azithromycin or clarithromycin are also first-line treatment choices. Third or fourth generation quinolone antibiotics are also appropriate agents for acute bacterial sinusitis therapy, although they cannot be used in children. The clinician should tailor the antibiotic choice to the specific resistance patterns of his or her practice environment. See Box 24-5 for doses and duration of treatment.

Previously, sulfamethoxazole-trimethoprim was a popular antimicrobial agent for the treatment of sinusitis. However, as increasing resistance to this combination has emerged in the pathogens *S. pneumoniae, H. influenzae,* and *M. catarrhalis,* its clinical utility has become limited.

Acute bacterial sinusitis should be treated with antibiotics for 10 to 14 days (except azithromycin, as noted previously). The patient should be reassessed 3 to 5 days after antibiotic treatment has begun. If there is no improvement, the concern for resistant organisms is raised, and the antibiotic choice should be changed. Chronic sinusitis is treated with a 21-day

BOX 24-5

Antibiotic Choices for Acute and Chronic Sinusitis

Amoxicillin 45 mg/kg per dose PO every 12 hr; maximum dose: 1000 mg every 12 hr
Amoxicillin–potassium clavulanate 875 mg PO twice daily
Cefuroxime 500 mg PO twice daily
Cefpodoxime 400 mg PO twice daily
Azithromycin 250 mg daily for 5 days
Clarithromycin 500 mg PO twice daily
Levofloxacin 500 mg PO daily
Gatifloxacin 400 mg PO daily

Treat acute sinusitis for 10 days, unless otherwise noted. Treat chronic sinusitis for a minimum of 21 days.

course of antibiotics, although data supporting the optimum duration of treatment are minimal.[22,23]

Topical and oral alpha-adrenergic decongestants are often prescribed for patients with sinusitis to induce vasoconstriction and reduce nasal mucosal swelling, thereby improving ostial patency and sinus drainage. There are, however, no controlled clinical trials examining the efficacy of these agents.[16] Topic sprays, such as oxymetazoline hydrochloride 2 sprays in each nostril every 12 hours, or oral decongestants, such as pseudoephedrine hydrochloride 60 mg every 6 hours, should be considered on the basis of the risk-to-benefit profile of the individual patient. Decongestant nasal sprays should not be used for longer than 5 days owing to the risk of rebound nasal congestion (rhinitis medicamentosa).

Other adjunctive therapies for the treatment of sinusitis have been proposed. Unfortunately, there are few controlled trials to determine which of these therapies is effective.[16] Intranasal corticosteroids are known to reduce nasal congestion and therefore may improve ostial patency; these agents have very few identified side effects, so their benefits likely outweigh their risks. Fluticasone and mometasone, used as two 50-μg sprays in each nostril daily, are available topical steroids. H_1 antihistamines have not been proven to offer any benefit in the treatment of sinusitis. Guaifenesin is an expectorant that decreases sputum viscosity. It has been shown to improve the ease of sputum expectoration in respiratory infections but has not been shown to aid in the management of sinusitis. Saline nose drops prevent crusting of nasal secretions and facilitate the elimination of nasal secretions. Use of hypertonic saline may additionally reduce mucosal edema. Several studies have shown better symptomatic outcome in patients who used hypertonic saline nose drops than in those using normal saline nose drops. Saline nose drops, normal or hypertonic, may be a useful adjunct to aid in the symptoms of sinusitis.

Any patient with evidence of ocular or intracranial extension of sinus disease requires immediate otorhinolaryngologic, ophthalmologic, and/or neurosurgical consultation. Broad-spectrum intravenous antibiotic therapy, such as with a third-generation cephalosporin and vancomycin, must be started.[21] However, because many of these complications require surgical intervention, the antibiotic choice should be made in conjunction with the surgical service. The patient with this complication must be admitted to the hospital.

REFERENCES

1. Annino DJ Jr, Goguen LA: Pain from the oral cavity. Otolaryngol Clin North Am 2003;36:1127-1135, vi-vii.
2. Molina OF, dos Santos J Jr, Nelson SJ, Nowlin T: Profile of TMD and bruxer compared to TMD and nonbruxer patients regarding chief complaint, previous consultations, modes of therapy, and chronicity. Cranio 2000;18:205-219.
3. Schwartz M, Freund B: Treatment of temporomandibular disorders with botulinum toxin. Clin J Pain 2002;18(Suppl):S198-S203.
4. Qerama E: A double-blind, controlled study of botulinum toxin A in chronic myofascial pain. Neurology 2006;67:241-245.
5. Pallin DJ, Chng YM, McKay MP, et al: Epidemiology of epistaxis in US emergency departments, 1992 to 2001. Ann Emerg Med 2005;46:77-81.
6. Tan LK, Calhoun KH: Epistaxis. Med Clin North Am 1999;83:43-56.
7. Lubianca-Neto JF, Bredemeier M, Carvalhal EF, et al: A study of the association between epistaxis and the severity of hypertension. Am J Rhinol 1998;12:269-272.
8. Jackson KR, Jackson RT: Factors associated with active, refractory epistaxis. Arch Otolaryngol Head Neck Surg 1988;114:862-865.
9. Kucik CJ, Clenney T: Management of epistaxis. Am Fam Physician 2005;71:305-311.
10. Thaha MA, Nilssen ELK, Holland S, et al: Routine coagulation screening in the management of emergency admission for epistaxis: Is it necessary? J Laryngol Otol 2000;114:38-40.
11. Moreau S, De Rugy MG, Babin E, et al: Supraselective embolization in intractable epistaxis: Review of 45 cases. Laryngoscope 1998;108:887-888.
12. Frazee TA, Hauser MS: Nonsurgical management of epistaxis. J Oral Maxillofac Surg 2000;58:419-424.
13. Anand VK: Epidemiology and economic impact of rhinosinusitis. Ann Otol Rhinol Laryngol 2004;193:S3-S5.
14. Lanza DC, Kennedy DW: Adult rhinosinusitis defined. Otolaryngol Head Neck Surg 1997;117:S1-S7.
15. Dykewicz MS: Rhinitis and sinusitis. J Allergy Clin Immunol 2003;111(Suppl):S520-S529.
16. Slavin RG, Spector SL, Bernstein IL: The diagnosis and management of sinusitis: A practice parameter update. J Allergy Clin Immunol 2005;116(Suppl):S13-S47.
17. Evans KL: Recognition and management of sinusitis. Drugs 1998;56:59-71.
18. Report of the Rhinosinusitis Task Force Committee Meeting. Alexandria, Virginia, August 17, 1996. Otolaryngol Head Neck Surg 1997;117(3 Pt 2):S1-S68.
19. Lacroix JS, Ricchetti A, Lew D, et al: Symptoms and clinical and radiological signs predicting the presence of pathogenic bacteria in acute rhinosinusitis. Acta Otolaryngol 2002;122:192-196.
20. Goldberg AN: Complications of frontal sinusitis and their management. Otolaryngol Clin North Am 2001;34:211-225.

21. Jones NS, Walker JL, Bassi S, et al: The intracranial complications of rhinosinusitis: Can they be prevented? Laryngoscope 2002;112:59-63.
22. Snow V, Mottur-Pilson C, Hickner JM; American Academy of Family Physicians; American College of Physicians–American Society of Internal Medicine; Centers for Disease Control; Infectious Diseases Society of America: Principles of appropriate antibiotic use for acute sinusitis in adults. Ann Intern Med 2001;134:495-497.
23. Williams JW Jr, Aguilar C, Cornell J, et al: Antibiotics for acute maxillary sinusitis. Cochrane Database Syst Rev 2003;(2): CD000243.

SECTION **IV**

Gastrointestinal Diseases

Chapter 25

Approach to the Patient with Abdominal Pain

Jared N. Strote and David A. Townes

KEY POINTS

- Approximately 20% of patients evaluated for abdominal pain in the ED require hospital admission for intervention or observation.
- Up to 25% of such patients are discharged from the ED without identification of a clear cause of their abdominal pain.
- Most stable patients with undifferentiated abdominal pain should be reexamined within 24 hours of discharge.
- Abdominal pain may be the presenting symptom of pathologic processes outside the abdomen, including diseases of the thorax, pelvis, and head.

Scope

This chapter reviews a diagnostic approach to acute, nontraumatic abdominal pain in adult ED patients. Presentations of abdominal pain associated with trauma, with pregnancy, and in children are discussed elsewhere. This chapter focuses on a general approach to diagnosis of the infectious, inflammatory, vascular, and mechanical causes of abdominal pain. Many organs and systems in the abdomen can cause pain; the symptoms are often similar, and the distinguishing features subtle (Tables 25-1 and 25-2).[1,2] Recognizing these sometimes subtle features that distinguish surgical emergencies, life-threatening crises, and urgent, treatable disorders is an essential role of the EP.

Anatomy

The abdomen is bordered superiorly by the diaphragm and inferiorly by the brim of the pelvis. Dividing the abdomen based on the location of pain and tenderness can aid in the development of a differential diagnosis (Fig. 25-1). Clinical symptoms present in one of four quadrants (right upper, right lower, left upper, left lower), or in epigastric, periumbilical, or suprapubic regions.

Pathophysiology of Abdominal Pain

Abdominal pain may be categorized by innervation pattern as visceral, parietal (somatic), or referred pain (Table 25-3).

Visceral pain is caused by stimulation of autonomic nerves in the visceral peritoneum that surrounds abdominal organs; such stimulation results from distention, inflammation, or ischemia of the organ wall or capsule. Patients may have difficulty describing visceral pain, which can be dull, intermittent, vague,

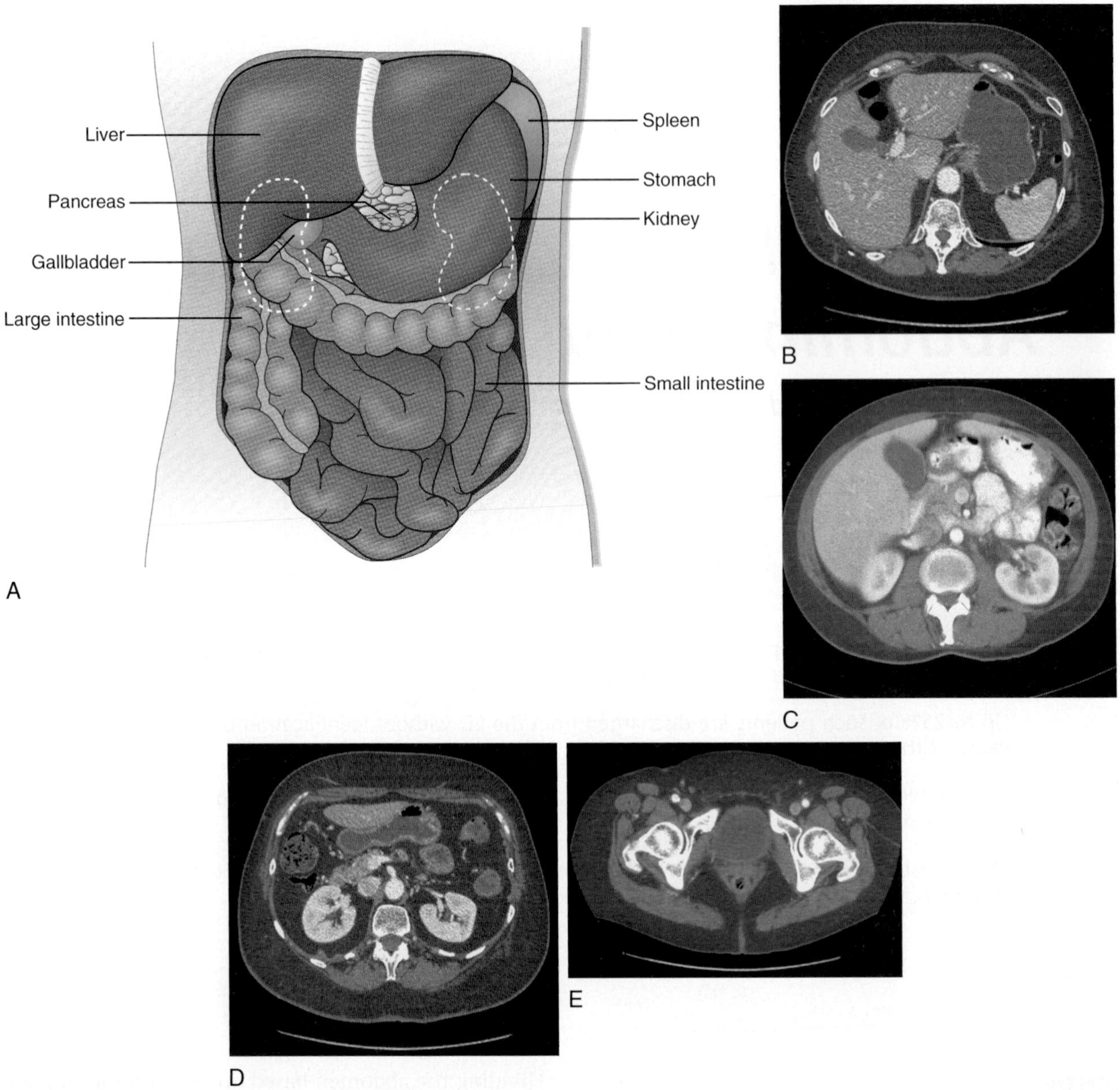
Liver
Pancreas
Gallbladder
Large intestine
Spleen
Stomach
Kidney
Small intestine
A
B
C
D
E

FIGURE 25-1 **A,** Anatomy of the abdomen. **B,** Computed tomography (CT) of the liver and spleen. **C,** CT of the gallbladder and kidneys. **D,** CT of the kidneys. **E,** CT of the bladder and rectum.

Table 25-1 ABDOMINAL PAIN IN THE ED*

Frequency of abdominal pain as ED chief complaint (annual)	6.7%[1]
Patients requiring admission	18.3%[2]
Patients requiring surgery	9.3%[2]

*Superscript numbers indicate chapter references.

Table 25-2 CAUSES FOR ED EVALUATION OF ABDOMINAL PAIN, BY SYSTEM

Cause	Frequency (%)
Undifferentiated (no conclusive diagnosis)	24.9
Gastrointestinal (nonsurgical)	18.4
Gynecologic	11.7
Urinary	11.5
Gastrointestinal (surgical)	7.6
Other	6.4
Unspecified	8.9

Data from Powers RD, Guertler AT: Abdominal pain in the ED: Stability and change over 20 years. Am J Emerg Med 1995;12:301-303.

Table 25-3 CATEGORIES OF ABDOMINAL PAIN

Type	Location	Inciting Stimulus
Visceral	Poorly localized Often midline	Distention Inflammation Ischemia
Parietal	Well-localized Focal	Chemical or infectious irritants
Referred	Remote from cause	Inflammation Trauma Ischemia

or colicky. Visceral irritation is often poorly localized to the midline. Examples of conditions that manifest as visceral pain are bowel ischemia and early appendicitis.

Parietal or somatic pain results from stimulation of peripheral nerves in the parietal peritoneum, generally caused by chemical or infectious irritation. In contrast to visceral pain, parietal pain tends to be sharp, constant, and better localized to the area of the underlying problem. Parietal pain may be present with such diseases as pancreatitis, cholecystitis, and late appendicitis.

Referred pain describes any pain that is perceived in an area remote from the site of the inciting pathologic process. One common example of referred pain is shoulder discomfort caused by diaphragmatic irritation by peritoneal blood or lower lobe pneumonia. Abdominal discomfort may therefore be a symptom of disease localized outside the abdomen, most commonly arising from the thorax, pelvis, retroperitoneum, or head.

Abdominal pain may also be a symptom of systemic disease rather than the result of nerve irritation, as in the cases of *Streptococcus* pharyngitis or hyperglycemia.

History

Box 25-1 lists the key historical questions to ask a patient with abdominal pain.

Physical Examination

▪ VITAL SIGNS

Vital signs provide an objective assessment of hemodynamic stability. Significant vital sign abnormalities may not occur until late in a disease process.

An elevation in temperature is neither sensitive nor specific for most intra-abdominal disease. Fever should raise suspicion of infectious or surgical processes, however, even in the absence of leukocytosis or focal tenderness; such conditions must be convincingly excluded through appropriate testing. Elderly or immunocompromised patients may present

Documentation

History
- Onset, quality, intensity, location, radiation
- Migration
- Modifiers
- Prior episodes

Review of Systems
- Genitourinary
- Gynecologic
- Gastrointestinal
- Cardiovascular
- Pulmonary

Physical Examination
- Vital signs, general appearance
- Cardiac, pulmonary, genitourinary, back, skin, and vascular examinations
- Abdominal examination: visual inspection, auscultation, percussion, palpation, masses, guarding, signs of peritonitis

Clinical Course
- Key studies
- Treatment and response
- Repeat abdominal examinations
- Repeat vital signs
- Toleration of oral hydration challenge

Decision-Making
- Broad differential diagnosis considered
- Likely diagnoses suspected
- Life-threatening diagnoses considered

Discharge Instructions (for Patients Discharged Home)
- Strict return precautions
- Close follow-up for repeat examinations

BOX 25-1

Key Historical Questions for the Patient with Abdominal Pain

Onset, Location, Radiation, Progression, Quality, and Intensity of the Pain

- When did the pain begin?
- Was the onset of the pain sudden or gradual?
- Where did the pain begin? Has it moved or migrated?
- Does the pain radiate? Has the pattern of radiation changed?
- Has the pain been constant or intermittent?
- What type of pain is it? How would you describe the pain?
- How intense or severe is the pain (use a pain scale of 1 to 10)?
- Has the pain become worse, become better, or remained the same?

Alleviating and Aggravating Factors

- What makes the pain better or worse?
- Does eating or drinking affect the pain?
- Is there a position that is most comfortable?
- Is it difficult to find a comfortable position?
- Does urinating, defecating, or vomiting affect the pain?
- Have you taken any medication since the pain began?

Associated Symptoms

Has the pain been associated with any of the following symptoms? If so, when did these symptoms first occur?

- Fever
- Diarrhea
- Constipation
- Nausea
- Vomiting
- Dysuria
- Urinary frequency, urgency
- Vaginal bleeding, discharge
- Shortness of breath
- Chest pain
- Change in appetite, weight loss
- Syncope
- Hematemesis
- Melena
- Hematochezia

Additional Questions

- Have you ever had this pain before? If so, when? What tests did you have? Was a cause ever identified?
- What brought you to the ED this time?
- What do you think might be causing the pain?
- Have you had other abdominal problems or surgery in the past?

with hypothermia rather than hyperthermia. A rectal temperature should be obtained in any nonneutropenic patient who cannot reliably use an oral thermometer.

▪ GENERAL APPEARANCE

Behavioral responses to pain differ widely among patients. General appearance is not helpful in identifying severity of pain, acuity, or risk. Only a sufficient history and physical examination performed by an experienced clinician ensures proper risk stratification.

▪ ABDOMINAL EXAMINATION

The priority goals of the patient examination are to (1) rapidly assess hemodynamic stability, and (2) continuously collect information necessary to refine the differential diagnosis. Assessment of patient history, vital signs, and abdominal assessment is the prudent order, which avoids delayed recognition of catastrophic diagnoses.

Early, adequate analgesia improves the ability to obtain an optimal examination. Parenteral narcotics do not mask signs of the acute surgical abdomen; analgesia should not be withheld.

A proper examination always begins with complete exposure of the abdomen of a supine patient. Scars from operations or injuries provide additional information about prior procedures. Skin findings may demonstrate recent trauma or indicate a dermatologic cause for the pain.

The abdomen should be auscultated for the presence of borborygmi. Auscultation may reveal hyperactive sounds in cases of bowel obstruction or hypoactive sounds in patients with peritonitis. Bowel sounds should not be recorded as "absent" unless no borborygmi are heard for 2 minutes. There is no clinical significance in differentiating hypoactivity from absence of bowel sounds in a potentially unstable surgical patient; the EP should not take the time necessary to make the distinction of "absent" sounds. Many practitioners use auscultation as a preliminary means to palpate the abdomen, by applying varying pressures with the stethoscope while observing patient responses. Rebound tenderness is a nonspecific peritoneal sign, which causes significant distress in patients with true peritonitis; it should be avoided if peritonitis is obvious on percussion or minimal palpation.[3,4]

Palpation is best performed in a patient comfortably lying supine with the knees bent. It is useful to ask the patient to point to the area causing discomfort. The examiner's hand should be placed softly on the patient's mid-abdomen, without pressing initially, to establish trust and prepare the patient for any differences in skin temperature. Palpation should be slow and deep, starting away from the area identified as the most painful. Traditionally, tenderness is described as localized to one of four quadrants. Although this description is broadly useful to communicate with other physicians, more specific localization often improves the predictive value of the examination (e.g., right pelvic vs. McBurney's point tenderness within the right lower quadrant).

Tips and Tricks

- Perform serial abdominal examinations, and document the patient's course and symptom progression. Abdominal disease evolves.
- Obtain a pregnancy test early for a female; even in reliable populations, "unlikely" pregnancies occur.
- Maintain a high index of suspicion for serious disease in elderly or immunocompromised patients. Presentations in these populations are often "atypical."
- Always consider cardiac causes for pain in the elderly.
- Use the patient's symptoms as a discharge diagnosis when a specific disease entity cannot be reliably identified (e.g., "vomiting" rather than "gastroenteritis").

▪ RECTAL AND GENITAL EXAMINATIONS

The digital rectal examination has low sensitivity and specificity for most intra-abdominal disorders. Limited indications for the use of this examination in the evaluation of abdominal pain are summarized in Box 25-2.

A genital examination should be performed in all patients with abdominal pain or tenderness below the umbilicus as well as in all patients with a genitourinary complaint. Although genital examination has been classically recommended for all patients presenting with abdominal pain, this procedure may be selectively deferred, on the basis of physician judgment, in patients with isolated upper quadrant symptoms and a dependable history that does not suggest a genitourinary process. The experienced cli-

BOX 25-2
Indications for Digital Rectal Examination

A digital rectal examination should be performed to evaluate for:

- Prostatic tenderness in a male with urinary tract symptoms
- Rectal disease in a patient with rectal pain or bleeding
- Occult gastrointestinal bleeding
- Fecal impaction or foreign body in a patient with constipation

nician recognizes that patients with ovarian torsion, testicular torsion, and genitourinary infections, for example, sometimes present primarily with abdominal pain (Box 25-3). Prudence, thoroughness, and clinical judgment guide the scope of the examination.

Differential Diagnosis

Owing to the wide range of medical and surgical causes of abdominal pain, no one diagnostic algorithm can be universally applied. Detailed historical information, repeated physical examinations, and appropriate study results should be used to narrow the differential diagnosis and exclude life-threatening processes. Particular care should be taken with pediatric, elderly (Table 25-4), and immunocompromised patients. Risks in these populations are twofold: (1) there is a greater likelihood of significant occult disease and (2) atypical presentations of common and uncommon diseases may occur.

Up to one quarter of patients with abdominal pain are discharged from the ED without a definitive diagnosis. While immediate life-threatening conditions can be excluded with proper evaluation and observation in the ED, some potentially disastrous conditions may be slow to develop. Repeated examinations in the outpatient setting are often needed (Box 25-4).

Clinical Presentation

Boxes 25-4 through 25-6 and Tables 25-5 through 25-8 describe the clinical findings for abdominal pain due to different disorders.[5]

BOX 25-3

Symptoms and Signs of Peritoneal Pain

Pain with movement
Hypoactive bowel sounds
Percussion tenderness
Localized tenderness
Involuntary guarding
Rigidity
Hemodynamic instability (late finding)

Table 25-4 CAUSES OF ABDOMINAL PAIN IN PATIENTS OLDER THAN 70 YEARS

Cause	Frequency (%)
Cholecystitis	26.0
Malignancy	13.2
Bowel obstruction	10.7
Undifferentiated	9.6
Gastroduodenal ulcer	8.4
Diverticular disease	7.0
Incarcerated hernia	4.8
Pancreatitis	4.1
Appendicitis	3.5
Other	12.7

Adapted from Fenyo G: Acute abdominal disease in the elderly: Experience from two series in Stockholm. Am J Surg 1982;143:751-754.

BOX 25-4

Undifferentiated Abdominal Pain

- A large percentage of patients with abdominal pain who present to the ED are discharged without a specific diagnosis.
- Serious medical (and sometimes surgical) causes of abdominal pain cannot be completely excluded in one visit.
- Patients who are discharged with abdominal pain of uncertain cause should be reevaluated by a physician or should return to the ED within 24 hours for reexamination.
- Patients should return immediately for persistent vomiting, fever, or worsening pain.

BOX 25-5

Masses Commonly Palpated on Abdominal Examination

Abdominal wall hematoma
Aorta (pulsatile)
Bladder distention
Hernia
Liver
Spleen
Stool impaction
Tumor
Uterus (gravid, fibroids)

BOX 25-6

Common Causes of Diffuse Peritonitis

Perforation of air-filled structure (appendix, ulcer, gallbladder)
Gangrene from strangulated/ischemic bowel
Spread from genitourinary sources
Rupture of abscess (hepatic, splenic, appendiceal, diverticular, tubo-ovarian)
End-stage liver disease (spontaneous bacterial peritonitis)

Table 25-5 EXTRA-ABDOMINAL SIGNS SUGGESTIVE OF INTRA-ABDOMINAL PROCESSES

Finding	Consideration
Asymmetrical lower extremity pulses	Aortic aneurysm or dissection
Heme-positive stool	Gastrointestinal bleeding
Nonreproducible shoulder pain	Diaphragmatic irritation
Bowel sounds on chest auscultation	Hiatal/diaphragmatic hernia
Flank ecchymosis	Hemorrhagic pancreatitis

Table 25-6 TYPICAL PROGRESSION OF PAIN: EXAMPLES

Maximal intensity at onset	Aortic dissection or rupture Other arterial dissection or rupture Renal colic
Rapid onset	Acute myocardial infarction Bowel perforation Intra-abdominal bleeding Mesenteric infarction Pulmonary embolus Ovarian torsion Ruptured aorta Ruptured ectopic pregnancy Ruptured spleen Testicular torsion Other ruptures, perforations, and mechanical causes
Gradual onset	Appendicitis Bowel obstruction Colitis Constipation Cystitis, pyelonephritis Diverticulitis Gastroesophageal reflux disease Hernia Mesenteric ischemia Pancreatitis Salpingitis Other inflammatory disorders Other intra-abdominal infections Other mechanical causes
Intermittent	Biliary colic Disorders that cause intermittent smooth muscle spasm Intussusception Ovarian or testicular torsion

Table 25-7 COMMON MODIFIERS OF ABDOMINAL PAIN

Modifier	Differential Diagnosis
Worse with eating	Biliary disease Gastric ulcer Ischemic bowel Pancreatitis Small bowel obstruction
Worse with movement	Peritonitis
Worse with breathing	Hugh-Fitz-Curtis syndrome Liver abscess Pulmonary embolus Splenic enlargement
Improved with eating	Duodenal ulcer
No position of comfort	Nephrolithiasis Pancreatitis

Diagnostic Testing

A urine pregnancy test should be ordered for any woman of childbearing age who presents with abdominal pain. This inexpensive, rapid, point-of-care test is more reliable than the combination of history and physical examination to confirm an undiagnosed pregnancy.[6]

Readily available abdominal/pelvic computed tomography (CT) has revolutionized the approach to abdominal pain. Patients are no longer commonly admitted for routine observation. Elderly patients, patients with coexisting illness, and patients whose findings signal a risk for intra-abdominal disease typically undergo CT. The decision to order CT is based on results of the history and physical examination, not laboratory findings.

The financial cost and radiation exposure involved with CT lead many authorities to argue that the modality is overused, yet the drive for diagnostic accuracy ensures its continued common use. Still, CT does not replace patient evaluation. In fact, key actions must be triggered by initial evaluations, such as notification of the surgical service when a patient has a potential surgical catastrophe, such as mesenteric ischemia, aortic dissection, or rupturing aneurysm. Further, CT does not have perfect sensitivity. Serious disease can be present even with apparently negative CT results. Although this modality remains an essential diagnostic tool, its findings must be properly integrated with clinical decision-making and cannot replace it.

CT also can cause complications. Anaphylactoid reactions to contrast material should be treated as allergic reactions. Renal insufficiency can be minimized by patient hydration. Metformin should be withheld for 96 hours for patients taking this medication.

Treatment

Intravenous access must be established to allow collection of blood specimens, provision of analgesia,

Table 25-8 **DIFFERENTIAL DIAGNOSIS BASED ON COMMON LOCATION OF PAIN**

Location of Pain	Differential Diagnosis
Right upper quadrant	Biliary tract disease (cholelithiasis, cholecystitis, cholangitis) Liver disease (hepatitis, hepatomegaly, hepatic abscess) Right lower lobe pneumonia
Left upper quadrant	Abdominal aortic aneurysm Angina/myocardial infarction Gastritis, peptic ulcer disease Left lower lobe pneumonia Pancreatitis Splenic enlargement, rupture, infarction, aneurysm
Right lower quadrant	Appendicitis Ectopic pregnancy Endometriosis Hernia Nephrolithiasis Ovarian cyst, torsion Pelvic inflammatory disease Psoas abscess Regional enteritis
Left lower quadrant	Abdominal aortic aneurysm Diverticulitis Ectopic pregnancy Endometriosis Hernia Nephrolithiasis Ovarian cyst, torsion Pelvic inflammatory disease Psoas abscess Regional enteritis
Generalized	Abdominal aortic aneurysm Black widow spider bite Diabetic ketoacidosis Early appendicitis Gastroenteritis Intestinal obstruction Mesenteric ischemia Sickle cell crisis *Streptococcus* pharyngitis

and administration of fluids and other medications. Large-bore catheters are required for intravenous contrast studies and for rapid resuscitation with crystalloid or blood products. Patients with potential surgical disease should not be given anything by mouth.

Early and adequate pain control is required. Narcotic analgesics are most commonly used and have no significant effect on physical examination accuracy or patient outcome.[7,8] Intravenous ketorolac is specific for prostaglandin-mediated pain, such as smooth muscle spasm in ureteral, biliary, or pelvic disease. Ketorolac has antipyretic properties, is nonsedating, and does not cause addiction. It should *not* be used, however, in patients with renal insufficiency, bleeding, or nonsteroidal medication allergy, or those in whom there is a likelihood of urgent surgery or other invasive procedures. Oral ibuprofen may be as beneficial for outpatient treatment, although patients with kidney stones may require narcotic supplementation for breakthrough pain.

Dehydration is common in patients presenting with abdominal pain, from both decreased intake and losses due to vomiting and diarrhea. Intravenous hydration often results in dramatic symptomatic improvement in patients with benign causes of abdominal pain. Additional fluid administration is required for patients who have fever or are awaiting an intravenous contrast study or surgery.

Disposition

Figure 25-2 summarizes the disposition of patients presenting to the ED with abdominal pain.

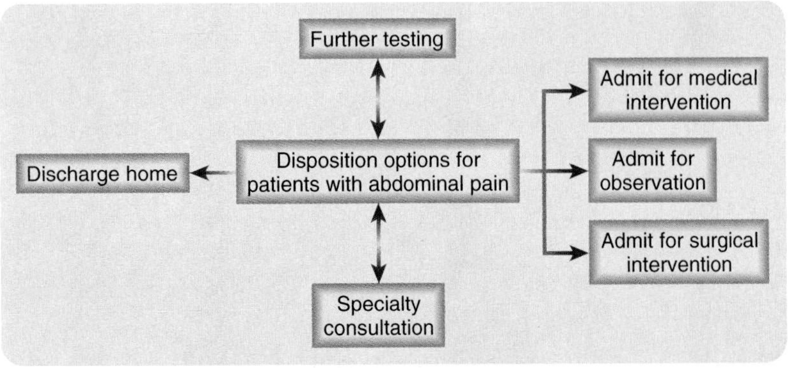
Further testing
Admit for medical intervention
Discharge home
Disposition options for patients with abdominal pain
Admit for observation
Admit for surgical intervention
Specialty consultation

FIGURE 25-2 Diagram of disposition options for patients with abdominal pain.

REFERENCES

1. McCaig LF, Burt CW: National Hospital Ambulatory Medical Care Survey: 2003 Emergency Department Summary. Advance Data from Vital and Health Statistics, no 358. Hyattsville, MD, National Center for Health Statistics, 2005, p 18.
2. Powers RD, Guertler AT: Abdominal pain in the ED: Stability and change over 20 years. Am J Emerg Med 1995;12:301-303.
3. Silen W: Cope's Early Diagnosis of the Acute Abdomen, 21st ed. New York, Oxford University Press, 2005, pp 33-34.
4. Liddington M, Thomson W: Rebound tenderness test. Brit J Surg 1991;78:795-796.
5. Fenyo G: Acute abdominal disease in the elderly: Experience from two series in Stockholm. Am J Surg 1982;143:751-754.
6. Strote J, Chen G: Patient self assessment of pregnancy status in the emergency department. Emerg Med J 2006;23:554-557.
7. Thomas S, Silen W, Cheema F, et al: Effects of morphine analgesia on diagnostic accuracy in emergency department patients with abdominal pain: A prospective, randomized trial. J Am Coll Surg 2003;196:18-31.
8. Neighbor ML, Baird CH, Kohn MA: Changing opioid use for right lower quadrant abdominal pain in the emergency department. Acad Emerg Med 2005;12:1216-1220.

Chapter 26

Esophageal Disorders

Chad S. Crystal and Marc Levsky

KEY POINTS

Esophagitis refers to inflammation or infection of the esophageal mucosa that may lead to malignancy, hemorrhage, or perforation.

Esophagitis may be caused by the reflux of gastric contents, infectious organisms, corrosive agents, irradiation, or direct contact with swallowed pills.

Candida species, cytomegalovirus, and herpes simplex virus are the organisms that frequently infect the esophagus of an immunosuppressed patient.

The most dangerous esophageal foreign body is the disk (button) battery, which can cause a chemically induced perforation in as little as 4 hours.

Esophageal perforation leads to rapidly progressive mediastinitis, overwhelming sepsis, and death.

Perforation initially manifests as mild, nonspecific symptoms that lead to misdiagnosis in over 50% of cases.

Emergency primary closure of spontaneous esophageal perforation (Boerhaave's syndrome) reduces mortality from 90% to 30%.

Anatomy

The esophagus is a muscular tube approximately 25 cm long that extends from the pharynx to the stomach. Two sphincters keep the esophagus closed between swallows, the upper esophageal sphincter (cricopharyngeus muscle) and the lower esophageal sphincter. The lower sphincter functions with a resting pressure of 25 mm Hg. The entire esophageal lumen is lined with stratified squamous epithelium. The esophagus is prone to perforation because it lacks the thick serosal covering found elsewhere in the gastrointestinal tract.

Reflux Esophagitis

■ SCOPE

Gastroesophageal reflux disease (GERD) describes a constellation of symptoms or complications that result from the reflux of gastric contents into the esophagus. Approximately 40% of adults in the United States suffer from symptoms of GERD at least once per month.[1] Complications of GERD include esophageal strictures, Barrett's esophagus, and esophageal adenocarcinoma. The incidence of esophageal adenocarcinoma in the United States is increasing 4% to 10% per year.[2]

Reflux esophagitis is a disease in which patients with symptoms of GERD also have endoscopic evidence of esophageal inflammation. A number of conditions and lifestyle choices increase the risk of reflux esophagitis: pregnancy, obesity, scleroderma, spinal cord injury, cigarette smoking, and the use of coffee, alcohol, and certain medications (beta-blockers, calcium channel blockers, nitrates, nonsteroidal anti-inflammatory drugs).

■ PATHOPHYSIOLOGY

Several factors promote the development of reflux esophagitis: an incompetent lower esophageal sphincter, increased sensitivity of the esophageal mucosa to digestive acids, impaired clearing of esophageal contents, and delayed gastric emptying. Any gastric acid, bile, or pepsin passively regurgitated into the esophagus irritates the mucosa and may cause erosions and ulcerations. In cases of persistent reflux, a columnar lining may replace the normal squamous epithelium; this premalignant condition is called *Barrett's esophagus*. Studies have demonstrated a clear relationship between Barrett's esophagus and the development of esophageal adenocarcinoma.

■ CLINICAL PRESENTATION

The most common complaint of patients with GERD is "heartburn," a painful burning sensation located in the mid-chest that may radiate to the back, neck, or arms. This typically retrosternal pain is often indistinguishable from that of cardiac ischemia. Diaphoresis and dyspnea may be noted as well.

Heartburn is more severe when patients are supine, bend forward, wear tight clothing, or consume large meals. The pain may last from minutes to hours and may resolve spontaneously or with antacids. Patients often complain of the bitter, metallic taste of regurgitated gastric contents. Additional common symptoms are upper abdominal discomfort, nausea, bloating, and satiety.

Complaints of dysphagia should prompt endoscopic evaluation for underlying strictures or adenocarcinoma. Other less common symptoms of GERD are odynophagia, cough, hoarseness, wheezing, and hematemesis. Chest pain from associated esophageal spasm may be relieved with nitrates, further confounding diagnostic accuracy.

■ DIAGNOSTIC TESTING

GERD should be diagnosed only after other, life-threatening causes of chest pain have been convincingly excluded (Box 26-1). A thorough history should be obtained in concert with immediate electrocardiography. Physical examination, laboratory testing, and radiographic imaging aid only in the exclusion of alternate diagnoses. Cardiac stress testing may be required in certain patient populations. Emergency upper endoscopy is indicated only if rare, life-threatening complications are suspected.[3]

A reported clinical response to proton pump inhibitors (PPIs) or histamine H_2 receptor antagonists is often used to make the presumptive diagnosis of GERD, but there is no evidence to support this practice.[4,5]

BOX 26-1

Differential Diagnosis for Reflux Esophagitis

- Acute coronary syndrome
- Pulmonary embolism
- Pneumothorax
- Pneumomediastinum
- Peptic ulcer disease
- Pill esophagitis
- Infectious esophagitis
- Aortic dissection
- Pericarditis
- Pneumonia
- Pancreatitis
- Biliary tract disease
- Esophageal perforation
- Dyspepsia

■ TREATMENT

Lifestyle modifications may reduce symptoms by decreasing the frequency and amount of gastric reflux. Examples of low-cost, low-risk recommendations are summarized in the Patient Teaching Tips box for this section of the chapter.

Acid-suppressive medications do not prevent reflux; they improve GERD symptoms by raising the pH of

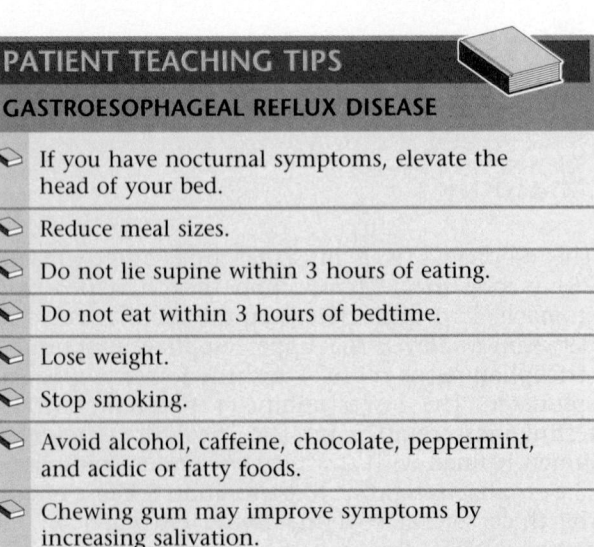

PATIENT TEACHING TIPS

GASTROESOPHAGEAL REFLUX DISEASE

- If you have nocturnal symptoms, elevate the head of your bed.
- Reduce meal sizes.
- Do not lie supine within 3 hours of eating.
- Do not eat within 3 hours of bedtime.
- Lose weight.
- Stop smoking.
- Avoid alcohol, caffeine, chocolate, peppermint, and acidic or fatty foods.
- Chewing gum may improve symptoms by increasing salivation.

Table 26-1 EQUIVALENT DOSAGES FOR HISTAMINE H_2 RECEPTOR ANTAGONISTS

Drug	Recommended Dose
Cimetidine	400 mg twice daily *OR* 800 mg at bedtime
Ranitidine	150 mg twice daily *OR* 300 mg at bedtime
Famotidine	20 mg twice daily *OR* 40 mg at bedtime
Nizatidine	150 mg twice daily *OR* 300 mg at bedtime

the refluxed material. These medications should be used for 2 to 4 weeks before any reassessment of symptoms. Recurrence is a common problem in patients with reflux, and many require long-term maintenance therapy.

H_2 receptor antagonists have similar efficacy with equivalent dosing schedules (Table 26-1).[6] These agents have been previously recommended as first-line therapy; however, cost-effectiveness analyses suggest that PPIs are superior to ranitidine, cimetidine, and placebo.

PPIs provide rapid symptom relief in patients with severe reflux esophagitis refractory to H_2 receptor antagonists.[7] Success rates for PPIs approach 90%, and all agents have equal efficacy at appropriate doses (Table 26-2). Once-daily dosing before breakfast is sufficient for the control of mild to moderate GERD; twice-daily dosing should be considered for those with severe or refractory symptoms.

Gastroprokinetic agents (cisapride) and *coating agents* (sucralfate) are less effective than PPIs but may be useful in selected patients as second-line agents.

Table 26-2 EQUIVALENT DOSAGES FOR PROTON PUMP INHIBITORS

Drug	Recommended Dose
Omeprazole	20 mg before breakfast *OR* 20 mg twice daily*
Lansoprazole	30 mg before breakfast *OR* 30 mg twice daily*
Rabeprazole	20 mg before breakfast *OR* 20 mg twice daily*
Pantoprazole	40 mg before breakfast *OR* 40 mg twice daily*
Esomeprazole	20 mg or 40 mg before breakfast

*Second doses should be taken before dinner.

BOX 26-2

Most Threatening and Most Common Features of Reflux Esophagitis

Most Threatening

Progressive dysphagia

Gastrointestinal bleeding

Unexplained weight loss

Most Common

Heartburn

Regurgitation

Postprandial pain

■ DISPOSITION

Admission to an inpatient or observation unit is indicated when life-threatening causes of the patient's presenting complaints cannot be excluded in the ED (Box 26-2).

Patients with known reflux esophagitis should be admitted for suspected esophageal perforation, significant bleeding, obstruction, volume depletion, or intractable pain. Discharged patients should be referred to their primary care physicians or gastroenterologists for follow-up care.

Infectious Esophagitis

■ SCOPE

Infection of the esophageal mucosa, known as *infectious esophagitis,* may result from a variety of conditions that compromise host immunity. Esophageal infections generally occur either in the settings of acquired immune deficiency syndrome (AIDS), cancer, neutropenia, and diabetes mellitus or as an adverse outcome of chronic immunosuppressive medications (especially corticosteroids) or broad-spectrum antibiotics.

Candida species, cytomegalovirus (CMV), and herpes simplex virus (HSV) are the organisms that most commonly infect the esophagus.[8]

■ CLINICAL PRESENTATION

Candidal esophagitis may manifest as retrosternal pain, dysphagia, and odynophagia. *Candida* is the etiology of odynophagia in up to 50% of immunosuppressed patients.[9] Other symptoms of esophageal candidiasis are nausea, vomiting, fever, abdominal pain, and anorexia. Oral candidiasis (thrush) is not consistently present in patients with endoscopically confirmed candidal esophagitis. Systemic candidal infections may be seen in cases of significant immunosuppression.

HSV esophagitis manifests as odynophagia, dysphagia, nausea, and vomiting. Oropharyngeal ulcerations

BOX 26-3

Differential Diagnosis for Infectious Esophagitis

Acute coronary syndrome
Pulmonary embolism
Pneumothorax
Pneumomediastinum
Peptic ulcer disease
Aortic dissection
Pericarditis
Pneumonia
Pancreatitis
Biliary tract diseas e
Esophageal perforation
Systemic infection

PRIORITY ACTIONS

Esophagitis

For patients with chest pain or other symptoms of cardiopulmonary disease:

1. Check electrocardiogram upon arrival.
2. Establish intravenous access.
3. Provide supplemental oxygen.
4. Apply telemetry monitor.
5. Obtain chest radiograph.
6. Administer analgesics.

and white exudates may indicate HSV infection, although oral lesions are neither sensitive nor specific enough to enable a definitive diagnosis to be made.

CMV esophagitis may cause weight loss, fever, and other constitutional symptoms.

Box 26-3 lists the differential diagnosis for infectious esophagitis.

■ DIAGNOSTIC TESTING

Patients in whom infectious esophagitis is suspected need to be admitted to facilitate diagnosis by upper endoscopy. Biopsies, cultures, and other related testing may be deferred to the inpatient setting. Identification of the causative organism is not a goal of care in the ED.

■ TREATMENT

Esophageal candidiasis requires systemic therapy; topical agents are ineffective. Treatment should begin with oral fluconazole, 100 mg to 200 mg daily for 2 to 3 weeks; this regimen is efficacious in 80% to 90% of cases.

Patients in whom infectious esophagitis is suspected should receive empirical treatment for *Candida.* Endoscopy may be reserved for those whose symptoms do not improve within 3 to 4 days. Treatment failures will likely be the result of either primary infection or coinfection with an unrelated organism.

Esophagitis due to HSV or CMV requires systemic antiviral therapy.

Tips and Tricks

THE "GI COCKTAIL" FOR ESOPHAGITIS

- Coating agents are often used to lessen the pain of GERD or esophagitis. The "GI cocktail" is a coating agent commonly used in the ED. The cocktail generally consists of a preparation of aluminum and magnesium hydroxide (e.g., Maalox or Mylanta), viscous lidocaine, and belladonna phenobarbital (Donnatal).
- Belladonna phenobarbital acts primarily as an antispasmodic and often causes nausea and vomiting. Its use should be reserved only for patients experiencing abdominal cramping.
- Doses for each component of "the GI cocktail" should be explicitly ordered: for example, Maalox 45 mL by mouth (PO), viscous lidocaine 20 mL PO, and belladonna phenobarbital 10 mL PO.
- Some studies suggest that "the GI cocktail" is no better than monotherapy with a liquid antacid alone.

■ DISPOSITION

All cases of infectious esophagitis require EP consultation with infectious disease and gastroenterology specialist to arrange for expedited testing. The need for confirmatory studies or the suspicion of systemic infection mandates hospital admission. Outpatient management should be reserved for the stable patient for whom urgent follow-up has been scheduled with a primary care or subspecialty physician.

Pill Esophagitis

■ SCOPE

Pill esophagitis refers to damage of the esophageal mucosa by prolonged direct contact with a caustic medication. The majority of cases involve potassium chloride, quinidine, emepronium bromide (Cetiprin), alendronate sodium (Fosamax), nonsteroidal anti-inflammatory drugs, vitamin supplements, or antibiotics.

Documentation

ESOPHAGITIS

Documentation should reflect a thorough search for potential complications of esophagitis as well as a consideration of alternate causes of the presenting symptoms. The most critical medicolegal issue to document is the rationale for excluding cardiac ischemia.

■ CLINICAL PRESENTATION

Symptoms begin shortly after the patient takes the medication and commonly involve nausea, vomiting, severe retrosternal pain, odynophagia, and difficulty handling secretions. Patients are more likely to experience pill esophagitis if they take their medications with minimal fluids, while recumbent, or immediately before bedtime.

■ DIAGNOSTIC TESTING

A presumptive diagnosis of pill esophagitis can be made when the history and patient presentation are classic. No further diagnostic evaluation is needed. If other esophageal disease is suspected (e.g., strictures, perforation), additional testing is indicated. Upper endoscopy is the most sensitive method of detecting pill-induced mucosal injury.

■ TREATMENT

Analgesics and coating agents may provide temporary symptomatic relief. Conversion of the offending medication to a liquid preparation often prevents recurrence. Another preventive measure is drinking water prior to and with medication, preferably in a fully upright position. Frequent use of sucralfate may promote healing of the injured mucosa.

Acid-suppressive medication has not been shown to decrease symptoms or repair injured mucosa in cases of pill esophagitis. PPIs may be useful for patients who suffer from coexistent GERD.

■ DISPOSITION

Most patients with pill esophagitis may be discharged with adequate pain management and follow-up. Patients who are unable to swallow owing to severe odynophagia or suspected stricture must be admitted for intravenous hydration, pain control, and gastroenterology consultation.

Esophageal Foreign Bodies

■ SCOPE

Foreign bodies are uncommon, but potentially life-threatening causes of esophageal erosion, perforation, and infection. The most dangerous esophageal foreign body is the disk (button) battery, which can cause a chemically induced perforation in as little as 4 to 6 hours (Box 26-4). Patients with esophageal foreign bodies are most commonly children (80%) between 1 and 4 years of age.[10] A significant proportion of adults with esophageal foreign bodies suffer from psychiatric illness.

BOX 26-4

Most Threatening and Most Common Features of Esophageal Foreign Bodies

Most Threatening

In Children

Disk batteries

Sharp objects

In Adults

Disk batteries

Sharp objects (psychiatric patients)

Packets of narcotics

Toothpicks

Most Common

In Children

Coins (coronal lie)

Marbles

Buttons

Toys

In Adults

Food boluses

Bones

Dentures

■ PATHOPHYSIOLOGY

Foreign objects tend to lodge in one of four areas of anatomic narrowing in the esophagus: the upper esophageal sphincter, the aortic crossover, the left mainstem bronchus crossover, and the lower esophageal sphincter. The upper sphincter is the most common site for impaction in children (75%), and the lower sphincter is the most common location in adults (70%).[11]

Upper esophageal sphincter foreign bodies may compress the airway and cause respiratory distress. Erosions from a foreign body occasionally involve the adjacent aorta, leading to rapid and fatal hemorrhage.

Abnormal areas of esophageal narrowing that predispose individuals to foreign body impaction include strictures, malignancies, dysmotility disorders (achalasia), and scleroderma. Such abnormal narrowings are often the cause of food impaction in adults.

BOX 26-5

Differential Diagnosis for Esophageal Foreign Bodies

In Children

Perforation
Abrasion or laceration
Airway foreign body
Esophagitis
Epiglottitis
Globus hystericus
Reactive airway disease

In Adults

Perforation
Abrasion or laceration
Spasm
Esophagitis
Diverticulum
Malignancy
Myocardial infarction
Globus hystericus

RED FLAGS

Esophageal Foreign Bodies

Drooling
Stridor
Wheezing
Access to a dangerous object
Psychiatric illness

■ CLINICAL PRESENTATION

Adults with esophageal impaction generally present after a known and intentional ingestion with symptoms of dysphagia, foreign body sensation, chest pain, and vomiting. Impaction commonly involves a large, poorly chewed food bolus.

Children with esophageal foreign bodies may present with an acute onset of drooling or respiratory distress of unknown etiology. Other common symptoms associated with esophageal foreign bodies in children are retrosternal pain, dysphagia, coughing, gagging, wheezing, anorexia, and a refusal to drink fluids. Unwitnessed ingestions account for approximately 40% of esophageal foreign bodies in children.[12] Parental suspicion of an ingested object may prompt an ED evaluation, even in the asymptomatic child. Box 26-5 lists the differential diagnosis for esophageal foreign bodies.

PRIORITY ACTIONS

Esophageal Foreign Bodies

1. Address airway compromise.
2. Check electrocardiogram upon arrival.
3. Establish intravenous access.
4. Provide supplemental oxygen.
5. Apply telemetry monitor.
6. Determine potential objects involved.
7. Obtain chest radiograph for a high-risk object.
8. Obtain computed tomography if plain radiograph findings are negative.
9. Gastroenterology consultation for dangerous foreign bodies.

■ DIAGNOSTIC TESTING

A diagnostic algorithm for the evaluation of a suspected esophageal foreign body is presented in Figure 26-1. Dangerous esophageal foreign bodies should undergo emergency removal by upper endoscopy. Foreign bodies found to be in the stomach will likely pass through the remainder of the gastrointestinal tract without intervention. Oral fluid challenges should be attempted when a foreign body is not identified on plain radiographs; inability to tolerate fluids should prompt further evaluation using computed tomography or endoscopy.

■ TREATMENT

Endoscopy is the preferred method for definitively removing or advancing an esophageal foreign body, especially when the presence or nature of the foreign body is uncertain. Endoscopy allows for direct visualization of sharp or otherwise dangerous foreign objects that pose a significant risk of perforation. Although endoscopy is costly and requires the availability of a specialty consultant, this technique can be performed in the ED and may prevent hospital admission at some centers. Upper endoscopy is relatively contraindicated in cases of narcotic "body packing," because unintentional rupture of a packet can cause swift hemodynamic instability and potential death.

Strategies for advancing an esophageal foreign body into the stomach may be less difficult, less invasive, and less costly than endoscopic removal.

Two medications may be used to relax the lower esophageal sphincter and promote advancement of the foreign body: intravenous glucagon 1 to 2 mg in adults, 0.02 to 0.03 mg/kg in children (not to exceed 0.5 mg); and sublingual nitroglycerin 0.4 mg in adults. Both of these regimens can be complicated by significant hypotension or vomiting. The addition of a gas-forming agent or oral meat tenderizer is con-

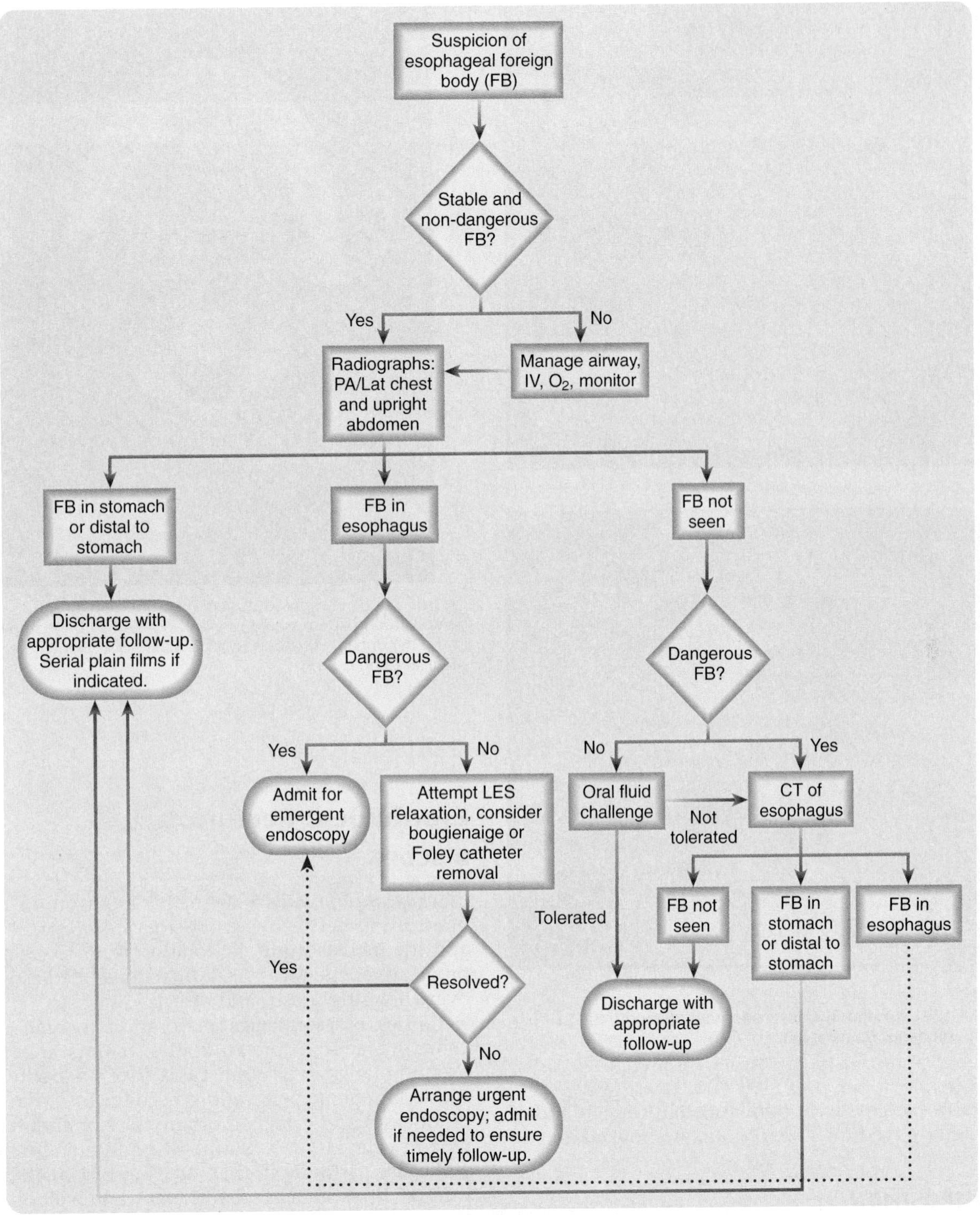

Suspicion of esophageal foreign body (FB)
Stable and non-dangerous FB?
Yes
No
Manage airway, IV, O_2, monitor
Radiographs: PA/Lat chest and upright abdomen
FB in stomach or distal to stomach
FB in esophagus
FB not seen
Discharge with appropriate follow-up. Serial plain films if indicated.
Dangerous FB?
Yes
No
Admit for emergent endoscopy
Attempt LES relaxation, consider bougienaige or Foley catheter removal
Resolved?
Yes
No
Arrange urgent endoscopy; admit if needed to ensure timely follow-up.
Dangerous FB?
No
Yes
Oral fluid challenge
Not tolerated
CT of esophagus
Tolerated
FB not seen
FB in stomach or distal to stomach
FB in esophagus
Discharge with appropriate follow-up

FIGURE 26-1 Diagnostic algorithm for the evaluation of a suspected esophageal foreign body. CT, computed tomography; IV, intravenous; LAT, lateral; LES, lower esophageal sphincter; PA, posterior.

traindicated because of an increased risk of perforation.

Foreign bodies may also be guided into the stomach by *bougienage,* the advancement of a rubber dilator from the oropharynx into the esophagus. Removal of the foreign body may be attempted by similarly passing a urinary catheter distal to the object with use of fluoroscopic guidance, inflating the balloon, and using the inflated distal catheter to withdraw the object. Foreign body advancement via bougienage and removal using a urinary catheter should be attempted only by skilled operators; complications include airway compromise and esophageal perforation. When reserved for relatively low-risk foreign bodies, these techniques have success rates of 84% to 98%.

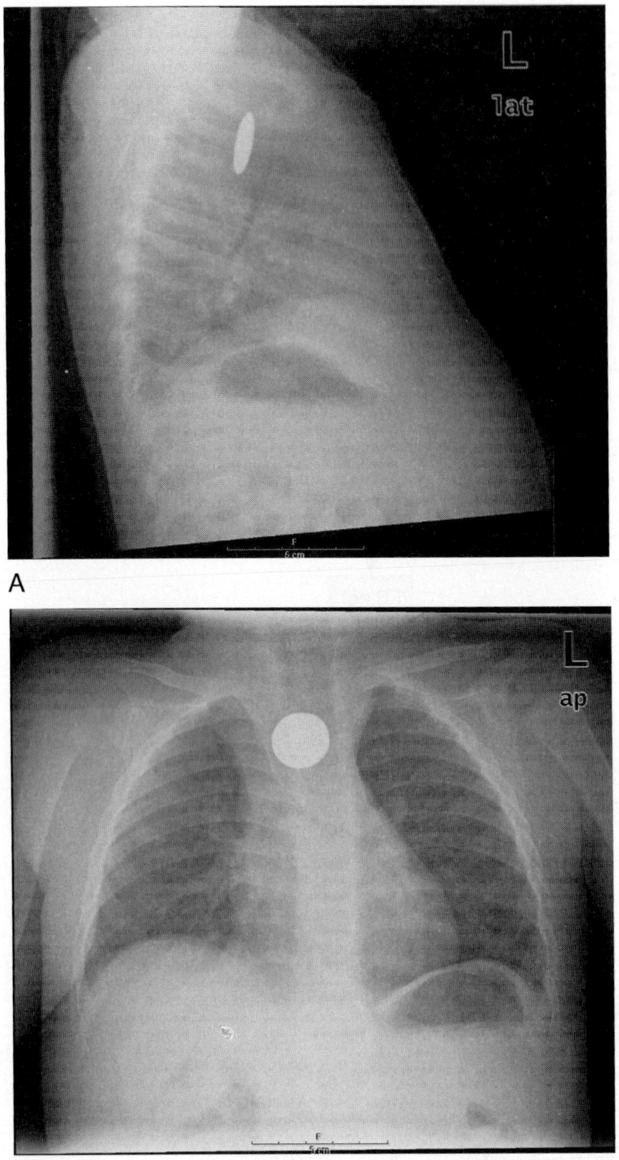
L
lat
A
L
ap
B

FIGURE 26-2 **A** and **B,** Chest radiograph demonstrating a coin in the esophagus (coronal lie).

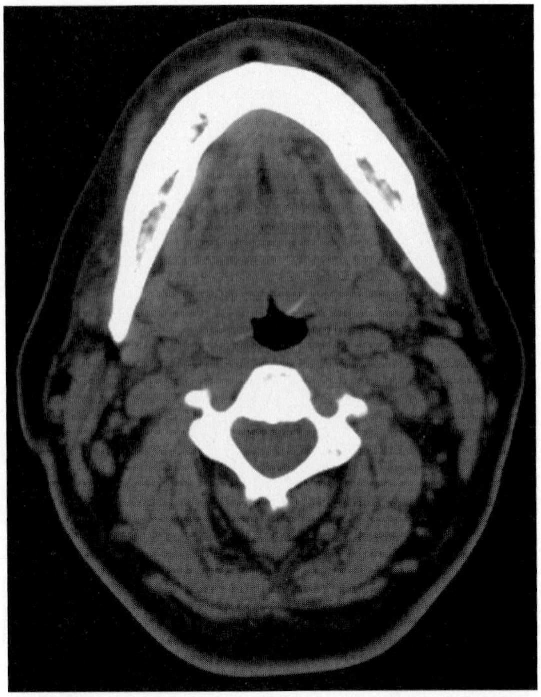

FIGURE 26-3 Computed tomography of esophagus demonstrating an impacted foreign body: A fish bone impacted in the hypopharynx. (Courtesy of E. Wolf, MD, Montefiore Medical Center, Bronx, NY.)

Stable patients with nondangerous foreign bodies can be observed for several hours without harm.

■ DISPOSITION

Patients with dangerous foreign bodies such as disk batteries and sharp objects should undergo emergency endoscopy. Patients with unresolved but low-risk foreign bodies should be referred for endoscopy within 24 hours if they are able to tolerate oral liquids.

Adults with foreign bodies that resolve under observation should be referred for outpatient evaluation of potential structural or neuromuscular diseases of the esophagus. Children with resolved foreign bodies may be discharged for follow-up by a primary care provider. Serial radiographs may be needed to document passage of the foreign object (Figs. 26-2 and 26-3).

Esophageal Perforation

■ SCOPE

Esophageal perforation is defined as a transmural communication between the upper gastrointestinal tract and the mediastinum. Perforation leads to a rapidly progressive chemical and infectious mediastinitis, overwhelming sepsis, and death.

Causes of esophageal perforation include iatrogenic procedures, foreign bodies, trauma, esophagitis, and malignancy. Some cases have no identifiable cause. Iatrogenic perforations account for up to 85% of all cases and carry a mortality rate of about 15%. One in every 10,000 routine diagnostic endoscopies will cause perforation; that rate rises to 1 in 10 when interventions such as sclerotherapy and balloon dilation are performed. Iatrogenic perforations may occur at any anatomic location.

Boerhaave's syndrome, or "spontaneous" esophageal perforation, is most commonly the result of forceful retching or vomiting. Other conditions associated with this syndrome are childbirth, coughing, seizures, asthma exacerbations, and the Valsalva maneuver. Even with treatment, this entity has a mortality rate greater than 30%. Most cases of Boerhaave's syndrome occur in the left posterolateral portion of the esophagus because of the relatively thin muscularis layer and lack of external structural support in that area.[13]

■ CLINICAL PRESENTATION

Esophageal perforation classically manifests as mild, nonspecific symptoms that lead to an initial misdiagnosis in more than half of patients. Pain is the presenting symptom in 70% to 90% of cases, although variability in location makes this feature difficult to interpret. Pain may be felt in the chest, neck, abdomen, or upper back and may be increased with deep breathing or swallowing. Other common symptoms are dyspnea, odynophagia, vomiting, and hematemesis.

Physical examination may reveal subcutaneous emphysema of the neck or upper chest in approximately 60% of patients. Hamman's crunch is a classic but uncommon auscultatory finding attributed to mediastinal emphysema.

Late presentations of esophageal perforation will be complicated by findings of septic shock: fever, tachypnea, tachycardia, and hypotension.

RED FLAGS

Esophageal Perforation
History of instrumentation
History of forceful vomiting
Progressive chest pain
Dyspnea
Sepsis
Hematemesis

■ DIAGNOSTIC TESTING

A diagnostic algorithm for the evaluation of suspected esophageal perforation is presented in Figure 26-4. Chest radiographs often demonstrate nonspecific findings. Contrast-enhanced fluoroscopic swallow studies should be performed in patients who can sit erect and tolerate liquids. Computed tomography of the esophagus is an alternative method of confirming the presence, but not the location, of a suspected perforation. Laboratory studies are of little diagnostic value, because their results are often initially normal and later demonstrate only nonspecific leukocytosis and acidosis.

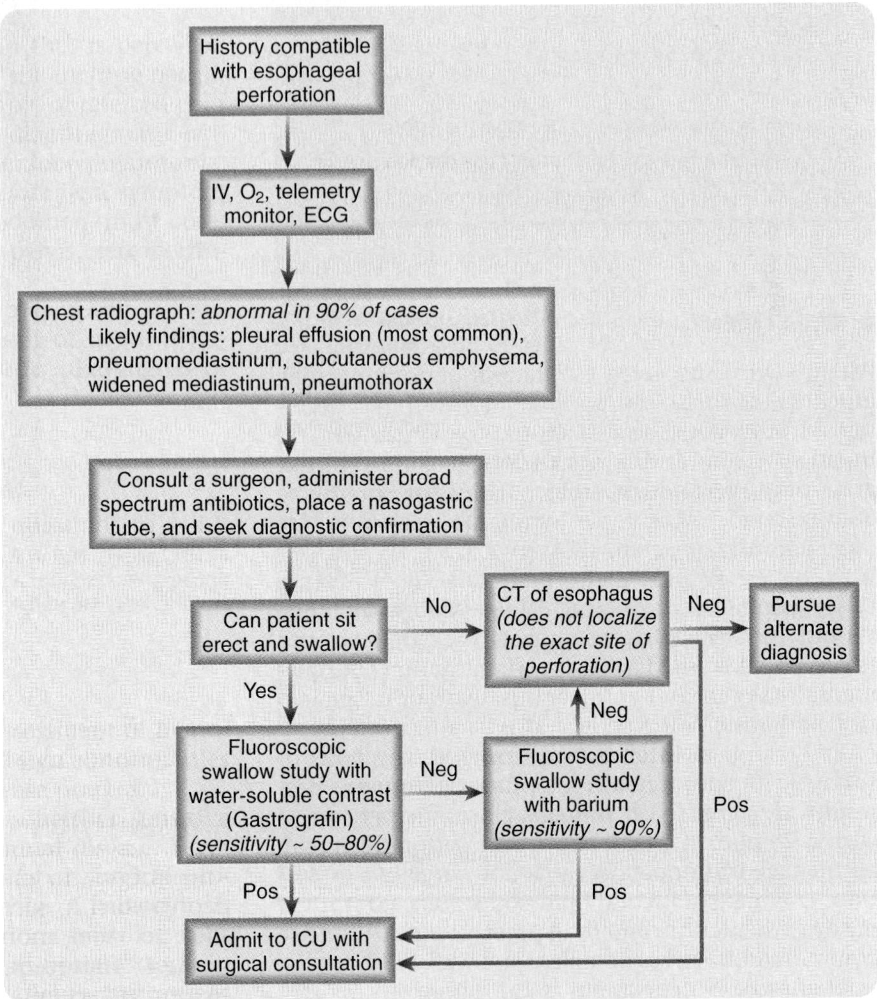
History compatible with esophageal perforation
IV, O2, telemetry monitor, ECG
Chest radiograph: abnormal in 90% of cases
Likely findings: pleural effusion (most common), pneumomediastinum, subcutaneous emphysema, widened mediastinum, pneumothorax
Consult a surgeon, administer broad spectrum antibiotics, place a nasogastric tube, and seek diagnostic confirmation
Can patient sit erect and swallow?
No
CT of esophagus (does not localize the exact site of perforation)
Neg
Pursue alternate diagnosis
Yes
Neg
Fluoroscopic swallow study with water-soluble contrast (Gastrografin) (sensitivity ~ 50–80%)
Neg
Fluoroscopic swallow study with barium (sensitivity ~ 90%)
Pos
Pos
Pos
Admit to ICU with surgical consultation

FIGURE 26-4 A diagnostic algorithm for the evaluation of suspected esophageal perforation. CT, computed tomography; ECG, electrocardiogram; ICU, intensive care unit; IV, intravenous.

Documentation

ESOPHAGEAL PERFORATION

Esophageal perforation is a potentially lethal condition that is frequently misdiagnosed on initial presentation.

Document the presence or absence of risk factors for esophageal perforation in all patients with chest pain, most notably any recent instrumentation or vomiting.

Record the time of surgical consultation, ordering and interpretation of radiographic studies, and the initiation of antibiotic therapy.

PRIORITY ACTIONS

Esophageal Perforation

1. Address airway compromise.
2. Check electrocardiogram upon arrival.
3. Establish intravenous access.
4. Provide supplemental oxygen.
5. Apply telemetry monitor.
6. Obtain chest radiograph.
7. Consult thoracic surgeon.
8. Administer antibiotics.
9. Gastric decompression (nasogastric tube).
10. Confirmation by fluoroscopy or computed tomography.

■ TREATMENT

Patients with suspected esophageal perforation may quickly deteriorate. Appropriate monitoring is necessary. Intravenous access should be obtained and broad-spectrum antibiotics that treat gram-positive, gram-negative and anaerobic organisms should be administered. Acceptable empirical regimens are piperacillin/tazobactam (Zosyn) 3.375 g IV and ceftriaxone 2 g IV plus metronidazole (Flagyl) 500 mg IV or clindamycin 900 mg IV. A nasogastric tube should be placed to decompress the stomach and reduce further mediastinal contamination. Supplemental oxygen and intravenous hydration, analgesics, and antiemetics should also be administered.

Early surgical intervention improves the odds of survival in spontaneous esophageal rupture. Best results are achieved if primary closure is performed within 24 hours.[14] Small, iatrogenic perforations may be managed nonoperatively at the surgeon's discretion. Drainage of pleural fluid collections, continued nasogastric suction, and total parenteral nutrition are common adjunctive therapies. The use of PPIs is postulated to be beneficial but is still unproven.

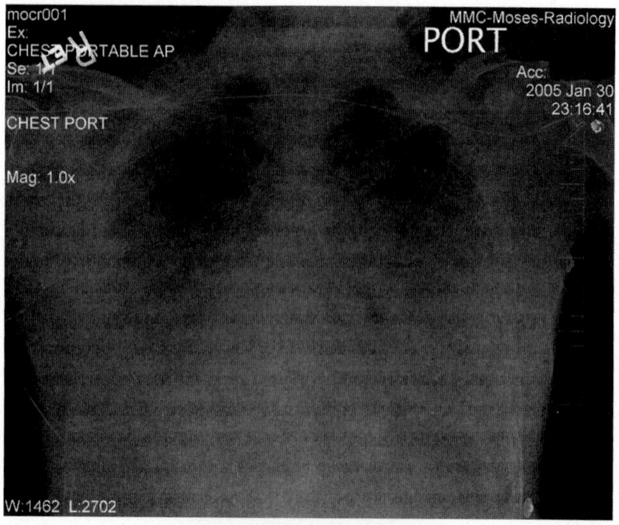
mocr001
Ex:
CHEST PORTABLE AP
Im: 1/1
CHEST PORT
Mag: 1.0x
MMC-Moses-Radiology
PORT
Acc:
2005 Jan 30
23:16:41
W:1462 L:2702

A

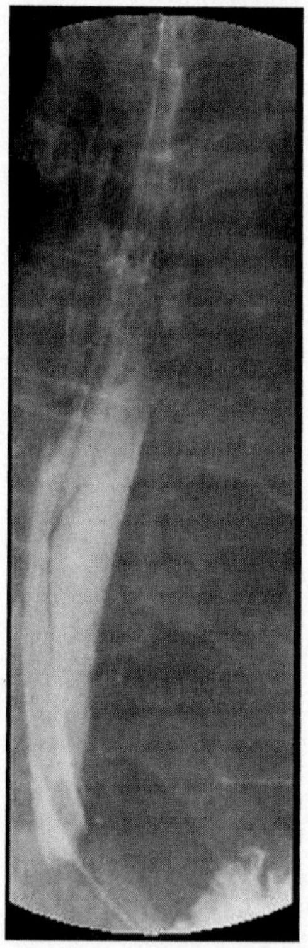

B

FIGURE 26-5 **A** and **B,** Chest radiographs demonstrating pneumomediastinum and bilateral pleural effusions. (Courtesy of E. Wolf, MD, Montefiore Medical Center, Bronx, NY.)

■ DISPOSITION

All patients in whom the diagnosis of esophageal perforation is suspected or confirmed should be admitted to a monitored unit under the care of a thoracic surgeon or a general surgeon experienced in esophageal repair (Figs. 26-5 through 26-7).

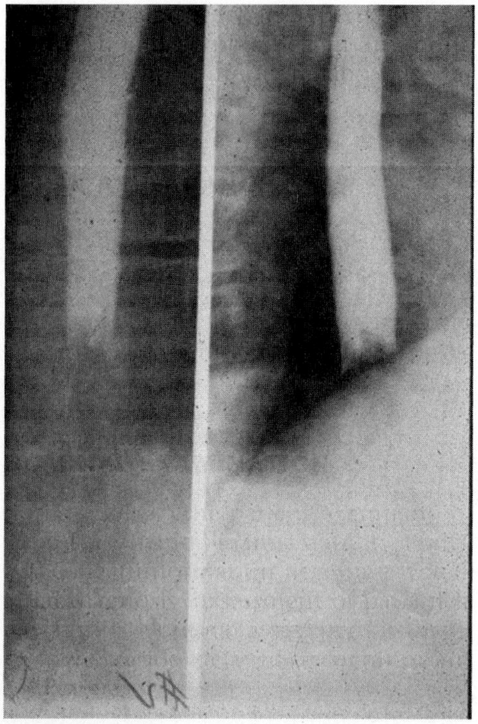

FIGURE 26-6 Fluoroscopic swallow study showing extravasation of contrast agent (as seen from left side of the film). (Courtesy of E. Wolf, MD, Montefiore Medical Center, Bronx, NY.)

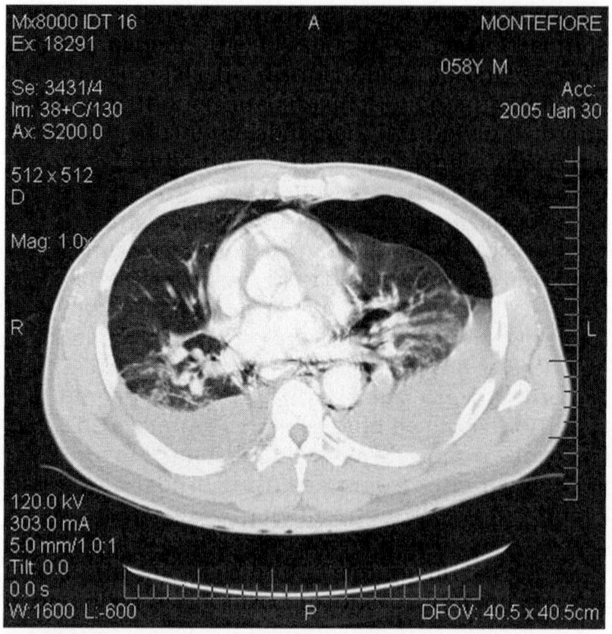
Mx8000 IDT 16
Ex: 18291
A
MONTEFIORE
058Y M
Se: 3431/4
Im: 38+C/130
Ax: S200.0
Acc:
2005 Jan 30
512 x 512
D
Mag: 1.0x
R
L
120.0 kV
303.0 mA
5.0 mm/1.0:1
Tilt: 0.0
0.0 s
W:1600 L:-600
P
DFOV: 40.5 x 40.5cm

FIGURE 26-7 Esophageal computed tomography scan demonstrating typical fluid collections in the setting of perforation.

BOX 26-6

Differential Diagnosis for Esophageal Perforation

Myocardial infarction
Pulmonary embolism
Pneumothorax
Pneumomediastinum
Peptic ulcer disease
Aortic dissection
Pericarditis
Pneumonia
Pancreatitis
Mallory-Weiss tear

REFERENCES

1. Camilleri M, Dubois D, Coulie B, et al: Prevalence and socioeconomic impact of upper gastrointestinal disorders in the United States: Results of the US upper gastrointestinal study. Clin Gastroenterol Hepatol 2005;3:543-552.
2. Ofman J: Decision making in gastroesophageal reflux disease: What are the critical issues? Gastroenterol Clin North Am 2002;31:S67-S76.
3. DeVault KR, Castell DO; American College of Gastroenterology: Updated guidelines for the diagnosis and treatment of gastroesophageal reflux disease. Am J Gastroenterol 2005;100:190-200.
4. Fass R, Ofman JJ, Gralnek IM, et al: Clinical and economic assessment of the omeprazole test in patients with symptoms suggestive of gastroesophageal reflux disease. Arch Intern Med 1999;159:2161-2168.
5. Juul-Hansen P, Rydning A, Jacobsen CD, Hansen T: High-dose proton-pump inhibitors as a diagnostic test of gastro-oesophageal reflux disease in endoscopic-negative patients. Scand J Gastroenterol 2001;36:806-810.
6. Sontag SJ: The medical management of reflux esophagitis: Role of antacids and acid inhibition. Gastroenterol Clin North Am 1990;19:683-712.
7. Chiba N, De Gara CJ, Wilkinson JM, et al: Speed of healing and symptom relief in grade II to IV gastroesophageal reflux disease: A meta-analysis. Gastroenterology 1997; 112:1798-1810.
8. Baden LR, Maguire JH: Gastrointestinal infections in the immunocompromised host. Infect Dis Clin North Am 2001;15:639-670.
9. Wheeler RR, Peacock JE Jr, Cruz JM, Richter JE: Esophagitis in the immunocompromised host: Role of esophagoscopy in diagnosis. Rev Infect Dis 1987;9:88-96.
10. Chen MK, Beierle EA: Gastrointestinal foreign bodies. Pediatr Ann 2001;30:736-742.
11. Stack LB, Munter DW: Foreign bodies in the gastrointestinal tract. Emerg Med Clin North Am 1996;14:493-521.
12. Uyemura MC: Foreign body ingestion in children. Am Fam Physician 2005;72:287-291.
13. Vial CM, Whyte RI: Boorhaave's syndrome: Diagnosis and treatment. Surg Clin North Am 2005;85:515-524.
14. Zwischenberger JB, Savage C, Bidani A: Surgical aspects of esophageal disease. Am J Respir Crit Care Med 2001; 164:1037-1040.

Chapter **27**

Diseases of the Stomach

Danielle Ware-McGee

KEY POINTS

Dyspepsia, gastritis, peptic ulcer disease, and gastric carcinoma represent a progressive spectrum of illness.

Helicobacter pylori is the causative agent of 90% of duodenal ulcers and 60% of gastric ulcers; it is a precursor to gastric carcinoma and is the only bacterium listed as a class I carcinogen.

In the absence of *H. pylori,* use of nonsteroidal anti-inflammatory drugs (NSAIDs) is the cause of peptic ulcer disease in up to 60% of patients.

The ED presentations of acute dyspepsia and acute coronary syndrome are often indistinguishable. The primary diagnostic goal of the EP is to exclude acute coronary syndrome through risk stratification and appropriate testing.

For the hemodynamically stable patient with peptic ulcer disease without perforation, first-line treatment should consist of a 6-week trial of a proton pump inhibitor with or without antibiotic therapy for *H. pylori.*

Serologic testing for *H. pylori* is more cost-effective than empirical treatment without testing.

All ED patients with dyspepsia require referral for outpatient endoscopy to exclude malignant disease.

Scope

Dyspepsia refers to chronic or recurrent pain of gastroduodenal origin centered in the upper abdomen. Dyspepsia affects 25% to 40% of people in industrialized nations, who regularly experience pain accompanied by any or all of the following associated symptoms: bloating, fullness, early satiety, nausea, anorexia, heartburn, regurgitation, and belching.[1] Patients who experience dyspepsia and have endoscopic evidence of gastric mucosal inflammation are said to have *gastritis;* those with ulcerations of the stomach or duodenal lining have *peptic ulcer disease* (PUD). Dyspepsia, gastritis, peptic ulcer disease, and the long-term complication *gastric carcinoma* represent a progressive spectrum of illness.

Dyspepsia accounts for 2% to 5% of annual visits to primary care physicians in the United States, and more than 1 billion healthcare dollars are spent on prescription medications for this disorder each year.[1] PUD chronically affects large portions of the U.S. population and leads to impressive health expenditures, because many affected patients drop out of the work force. More than 7000 American deaths are attributed to PUD each year.

In up to 60% of patients diagnosed with dyspepsia, results of endoscopic evaluation are nondiagnostic.[1] The remaining 40% generally have one of three causative diagnoses: PUD, gastroesophageal reflux disease (GERD), or gastric cancer.[2] The broad differential diagnosis of recognized causes of PUD is summarized in Table 27-1.

Table 27-1 DIFFERENTIAL DIAGNOSIS OF PEPTIC ULCER DISEASE

Cardiovascular	Acute myocardial infarction Dissecting aneurysm Angina pectoris Pericarditis Ischemic bowel disease
Gastrointestinal	
Esophageal	Gastroesophageal reflux disease Erosive esophagitis Esophageal spasm esophageal stricture Schatzki's ring Esophageal cancer
Stomach	Gastritis Gastroparesis Gastric lymphoma/carcinoma
Other	Biliary tract disease Cholelithiasis Pancreatitis Pancreatic carcinoma Infiltrative disorders—sarcoidosis and Crohn's disease High small bowel obstruction Subphrenic abscess Early appendicitis Hypercalcemia Hyperkalemia

From Ferri FF: Ferri's Clinical Advisor 2007: Instant Diagnosis and Treatment. St. Louis, Mosby, 2006.

Duodenal ulcers occur three to four times more frequently than gastric ulcers worldwide, men being affected more commonly than women for both ulcer types. The male-to-female ratio for duodenal ulcer (4:1) is higher than that for gastric ulcer (2:1). Such distributions are mainly observed in the developing countries of Africa and Asia. In westernized societies, there has been a more equal distribution of both ulcer types between the sexes over the past few decades, although the mechanisms underlying these epidemiologic changes are unknown.[3]

Pathophysiology

The stomach is anatomically subdivided into three parts: the fundus, the corpus (body), and the antrum (Fig. 27-1).[4] This subdivision reflects differences in function. The fundus serves as a reservoir for ingested meals, the body as the initial location of peristalsis, and the antrum as the site of food agitation with gastric secretions.[5] Endocrine functions arise from the antrum, while exocrine functions occur at the fundus and body.[5]

The mucosal cells of the fundus and corpus contain simple columnar cells that secrete a protective alkaline mucus, which lines the gastric lumen (Fig. 27-2). More than half of the gastric lumen contains gastric pits that further subdivide into gastric glands. The necks and bases of these glands contain parietal and histamine-producing cells.[5] G cells in the gastric antrum release the hormone gastrin, which stimulates enterochromaffin-like cells in the gastric corpus to release histamine, the agent that causes parietal cells to secrete acid. Gastrin also directly stimulates parietal cells and promotes the growth of

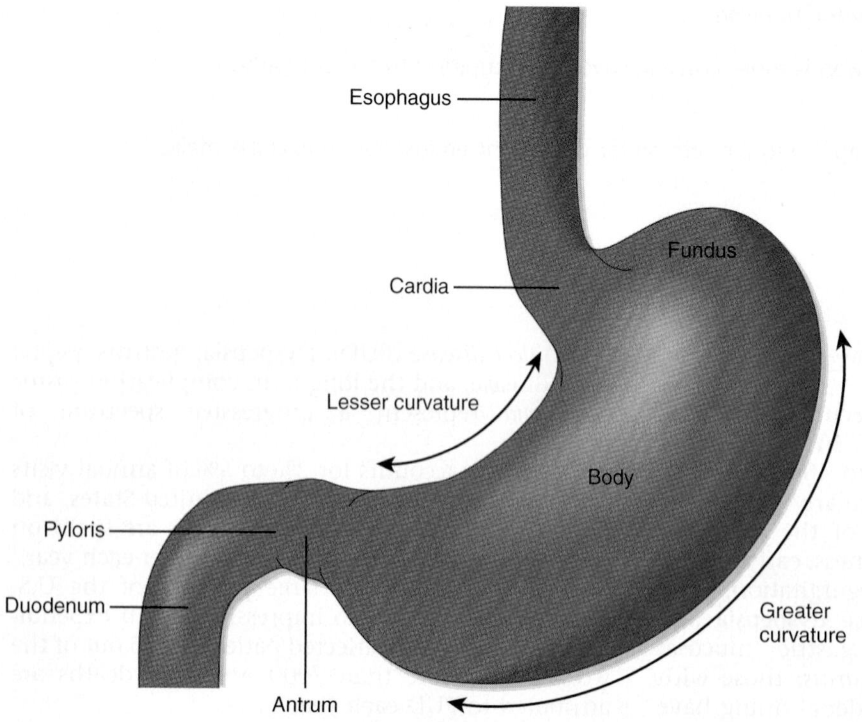
Esophagus
Fundus
Cardia
Lesser curvature
Body
Pyloris
Duodenum
Greater
curvature
Antrum

FIGURE 27-1 Divisions of the stomach. (From Zuidema G: Shackelford's Surgery of the Alimentary Tract, 4th ed. Philadelphia, Saunders, 1995.)

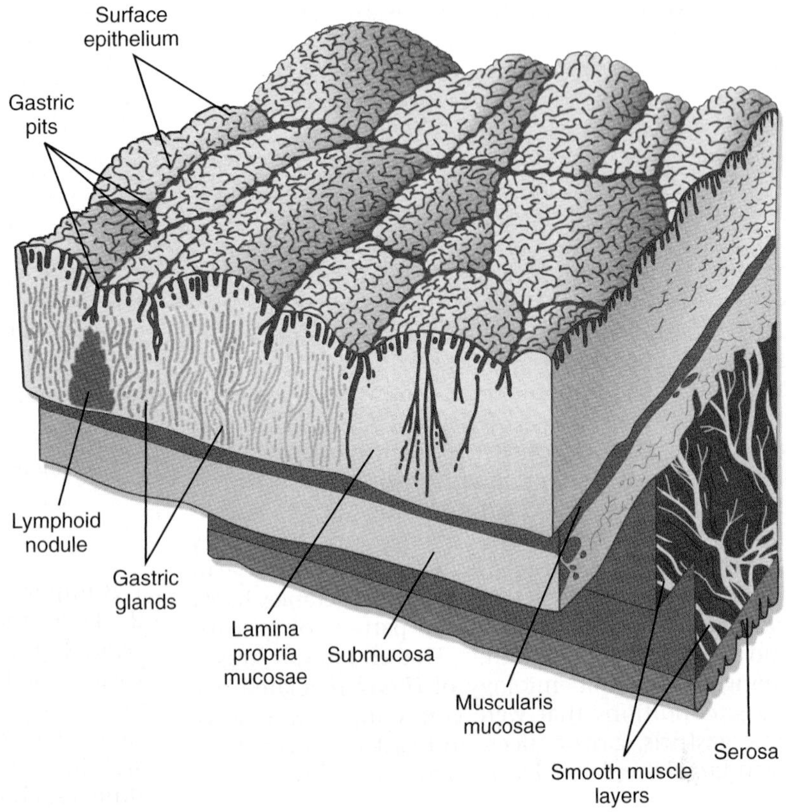
Surface
epithelium
Gastric
pits
Lymphoid
nodule
Gastric
glands
Lamina
propria
mucosae
Submucosa
Muscularis
mucosae
Smooth muscle
layers
Serosa

FIGURE 27-2 Surface of the gastric mucosa. (From Zuidema G: Shackelford's Surgery of the Alimentary Tract, 4th ed. Philadelphia, Saunders, 1995.)

enterochromaffin-like and parietal cells.[6] G cells, enterochromaffin-like cells, and parietal cells are all regulated by release of the inhibitory peptide somatostatin.[6]

PUD is not simply a result of hyperactive parietal and mast cells—instead, it results from a complex interplay of factors that disrupt the delicate balance between the production of protective barrier agents, such as bicarbonate-rich mucus, and the hypersecretion of these acid-producing cells. Endoscopic evaluation is essential for an accurate diagnosis. Small ulcers and erosions can be difficult to differentiate, but any mucosal defect at least 3 mm in diameter with any depth is defined as a chronic ulcer.[7]

The recognition of *Helicobacter pylori* (*H. pylori*) as the causative agent of 90% of duodenal ulcers and 60% of gastric ulcers has led to a paradigm shift in the understanding and management of PUD.[8]

■ *Helicobacter pylori* INFECTION

H. pylori infects at least 50% of the population worldwide and is recognized as an important risk factor for the development of gastric adenocarcinoma and lymphoma. Infection is likely acquired in childhood and, in the absence of antimicrobial therapy, persists for the lifetime of the individual.[9] Risk factors for the acquisition of *H. pylori* include sharing of a bed in childhood, a large number of siblings, lower socioeconomic status, and the lack of a fixed hot water supply.[10] Although it is still unclear whether transmission occurs person to person, three different mechanisms for such transmission have been postulated: fecal-oral, through saliva, and by vomitus.[10]

Case variations of gastritis represent different stages of *H. pylori* infection that may ultimately lead to ulcer disease.[3] In the United States, *H. pylori* infection has a prevalence of up to 1% per year, with an age-related prevalence higher in patients who do not have ulcer disease.[2] In individuals with *H. pylori* infection, the estimated lifetime risk for PUD is approximately 15%.[11]

H. pylori causes acute dyspepsia characterized by epigastric pain, nausea, vomiting, and halitosis. This initial phase of illness is associated with achlorhydria—a relative lack of hydrochloric acid in digestive juices—which can continue for several months. Symptoms usually last only several weeks and then disappear, although the organism loiters within the stomach. Gastritis persists throughout life in various locations, shifting from an antrum-predominant pattern to a corpus-predominant pattern or a pangastritis.[10] The chronic phase of the disease is usually benign, but in susceptible individuals, complications such as gastric or duodenal ulcer may arise.

If sufficiently virulent, *H. pylori* gastritis leads to a destruction of the gastric mucosa, prompting the development of intestinal metaplasia. The rate of gastric acid secretion declines, fostering conditions beneficial to the colonization of the gastric lumen by fecal organisms. *H. pylori* eventually disappears, because the organism is ill-equipped to compete with a growing number of other organisms and is unable to thrive on metaplastic cells in the absence of hyperacidic conditions.[10] Despite its eventual demise, the initial invasion of the stomach lumen by *H. pylori* incites conditions that favor the evolution of noncardia gastric cancer.[10]

Although *H. pylori* induces an acute inflammatory gastritis, this host immunologic response is generally not sufficient to clear infection. In addition, infection with one strain of *H. pylori* does not protect against subsequent co-infection with a different strain. Infection with multiple strains is quite common and occurs more frequently in developing countries. Polyclonal infection allows DNA to be exchanged between different strains, which could promote the spread of genes encoding important virulence factors or resistance to antibiotics.[12] In the last century, Western populations with *H. pylori* infection experienced a reduction in the rate of corpus gastritis that led to a change in frequency of the different *H. pylori*–related diseases. The year-round availability of fresh fruits and vegetables likely prompted these changes in the pattern of gastritis and gastric acid secretion.[13] The end result was a change in the epidemiology of *H. pylori*–related diseases; conditions that were common, such as atrophic gastritis, gastric ulcer, and gastric cancer, have been largely replaced by duodenal ulcer.[13]

■ OTHER INFECTIOUS CAUSES

Although most common, *H. pylori* is not the sole infectious cause of PUD. *Helicobacter heilmannii*, another spiral nonspirochetal bacteria, has been associated with *H. pylori*–negative duodenal ulcers. It is much rarer than *H. pylori*, is less pathogenic, and can be easily differentiated by routine histology.[7] Domestic animals such as dogs, cats, pigs, and monkeys are thought to transmit *H. heilmannii* to human gastric mucosa.[7] Treatment strategies similar to those for *H. pylori* are successful in eradicating this organism.[7]

Additional infectious agents are cytomegalovirus (CMV), herpes simplex virus type 1 (HSV-1), tuberculosis, and syphilis. CMV was first associated with peptic ulcers in renal transplant recipients and is the only organism to be significantly associated with peptic ulceration in persons positive for human immunodeficiency virus (HIV).[7] The ulcers in these patients are usually gastric and numerous. The diagnosis is confirmed by the finding of intranuclear inclusion bodies and/or cytomegalovirus DNA in the gastric mucosa on biopsy specimens taken from the base of the ulcer.[7] HSV-1–induced viruses are usually located in the antrum and often occur in immunocompetent individuals.[7]

■ DRUG-RELATED CAUSES

In the absence of *H. pylori*, use of nonsteroidal anti-inflammatory drugs (NSAIDs) is the cause of PUD in up to 60% of patients.[7] Because gastroduodenal damage does not occur in all patients taking NSAIDs, it is important to identify those at increased risk (Box 27-1). Factors associated with higher rates of NSAID-related gastrointestinal complications are a prior history of PUD or hemorrhage, age more than 65 years, prolonged use of high-dose NSAIDs, use of more than one NSAID, concomitant use of corticosteroids or anticoagulants, and serious comorbid illness such as cardiovascular disease, renal or hepatic impairment, diabetes, or hypertension.[14]

Other drugs have been found to cause PUD, including potassium chloride, nitrogen-containing bisphosphonates, and immunosuppressive medications such as mycophenolate and floxuridine.[7] Additionally, there have been reports of an association of duodenal ulcer and perforation with the use of crack cocaine and/or methamphetamine.[7] Focal tissue ischemia induced by mucosal vasoconstriction may explain the perforation of ulcers in these cases.[7]

BOX 27-1

Drugs Associated with Peptic Ulcer Disease (PUD)

The following agents are associated with PUD; those marked with an asterisk (*) are associated with a higher rate of perforation.

Nonsteroidal anti-inflammatory drugs
Potassium chloride
Bisphosphonates
Mycophenolate
Floxuridine
Crack cocaine*
Amphetamines*

■ ZOLLINGER-ELLISON SYNDROME

Zollinger-Ellison syndrome (ZES) is caused by gastrin-secreting tumors called *gastrinomas*. More 90% of patients with gastrinomas eventually have peptic ulceration.[7] Less than half of patients with PUD due to ZES have *H. pylori*—the absence of *H. pylori* infection and NSAID use should heighten suspicion for ZES.[7]

Approximately 0.1 to 3 persons per million experience gastrinomas each year. The incidence in the United States ranges from 0.1% to 1% of patients who present with PUD.[15] The most common functional pancreatic tumor in patients with multiple endocrine neoplasia type I (MEN-I) is gastrinoma, and approximately 20% of patients with ZES also have MEN-I.[15] The mean age at presentation is 50 years, but patients with ZES range in age from 7 to 90 years.[15] Patients with both MEN-I and ZES become symptomatic at an earlier age and usually present with PUD in the third decade of life.[7,15] The male-to-female ratio of patients with ZES ranges from 2:1 to 3:2.[15]

Patients with ZES commonly present with symptoms of PUD, such as epigastric pain, nausea, and vomiting. Alternatively, severe diarrhea may be the only presenting symptom.[15] The cause of the diarrhea consists of direct injury to the small intestinal mucosa, inactivation of pancreatic lipase, and precipitation of bile acids and gastric acid hypersecretion.[15] Several factors that should raise the suspicion for ZES are recurrent, multiple, and atypically located ulcers (e.g., in the jejunum or distal to the duodenal bulb), refractory or complicated ulcers, and hypercalcemia.[7,15] Recurrent ulcers occur frequently after gastric surgery for PUD, such as antrectomy and vagotomy. Perforated ulcer remains a common complication, with 7% of patients with ZES presenting with perforation of the jejunum.[15]

Patients with ZES have elevated fasting serum gastrin concentrations (>100 pg/mL) and basal gastric acid hypersecretion (>15 mEq/hr). The secretin stimulation test is the best method to distinguish ZES from other conditions causing elevations of serum gastrin.[15] Despite the fact that 50% of gastrinomas are not evident on imaging studies, computed tomography (CT), magnetic resonance imaging (MRI), radionuclide octreotide scanning, endoscopic ultrasonography, and the selective arterial secretin injection test are the recommended imaging studies for localization of this disorder.[15]

All patients with sporadic gastrinoma who have resectable metastatic disease should undergo exploratory laparotomy for potential curative resection. Surgery may be the most effective treatment for metastatic gastrinoma if the tumor can be completely excised.[15] Gastric acid hypersecretion can be controlled in virtually all patients with the use of histamine H_2 receptor antagonists or omeprazole, thereby rendering total gastrectomy unnecessary in patients showing response to these agents.[15]

IDIOPATHIC ULCERS

Once all known etiologic factors are excluded, there remains a group of peptic ulcers that are idiopathic. The etiology of idiopathic PUD is poorly understood but thought to include a genetic predisposition, altered acid secretion, rapid gastric emptying, defective mucosal defense mechanisms, psychological stress, and smoking.[7] Blood group O and nonsecretor status are genetic traits associated with duodenal ulcer disease, and the presence of both factors raises the risk of the disease by 150%.[7] The management of idiopathic peptic ulcers is challenging; these ulcers are more resistant to standard therapy and are associated with more frequent complications. Those that relapse may require long-term maintenance therapy.[7]

Treatment

MEDICAL TREATMENT

Regardless of the cause of dyspepsia, the ED presentation of acute gastroduodenal illness is quite recognizable. Dyspepsia or PUD should be suspected in patients complaining of midepigastric pain, nausea, vomiting, early satiety, substernal chest burning, and a bitter, foul taste in the mouth. Similar symptoms may indicate acute coronary syndrome, however, so the primary goal of ED management is the exclusion of life-threatening cardiac disease through appropriate risk stratification and testing. For patients in whom acute coronary syndrome can be excluded in favor of a diagnosis of dyspepsia, empirical treatment strategies and referral for diagnostic testing are appropriate.

In a hemodynamically stable patient whose symptoms are not severe enough to warrant admission, three options are available for management of dyspepsia not due to NSAIDs. The first option is a single, short-term trial of empirical antiulcer therapy (with a proton pump inhibitor [PPI]) in a setting in which follow-up is ensured.[16] Regardless of response, all such trials should be stopped after about 6 weeks, and an evaluation performed if symptoms recur; further investigation is warranted earlier if symptoms do not respond in 2 weeks.[16] The second option is a definitive endoscopic evaluation, especially in patients older than 50 years with new onset of dyspepsia, anemia, gastrointestinal bleeding, anorexia, early satiety, or weight loss.[16] The urgency for definitive diagnosis stems from a risk that gastric ulcers harbor malignancy in this population.[16] The third option is noninvasive testing for *H. pylori,* followed by the outpatient prescription of antibiotics in *H. pylori*–positive subjects.

Same-day serologic testing for *H. pylori* may not be available in many EDs. The cost-effectiveness of empirical antibiotic therapy against *H. pylori* is unproven, however; *H. pylori*–positive patients with true PUD are likely to show a favorable response, but dyspeptic patients without ulcer have a variable response to antibiotics compared with placebo.[16] Serologic testing for *H. pylori* prior to antibiotic

PRIORITY ACTIONS

- Keep the differential diagnosis of dyspepsia broad. Investigate other potential causes of symptoms, especially atypical acute coronary syndrome.
- Hemodynamically unstable patients mandate prompt resuscitation, intensive care unit monitoring, and gastroenterology consultation.
- All patients with severe pain should have an upright chest radiograph to exclude free air secondary to perforation.
- All patients with dyspepsia should have a digital rectal examination to assess for occult or fresh blood in the stool.
- Perform serial examinations of patients with dyspepsia to exclude the possibility of perforation and to assess the benefit of therapeutic interventions.

administration is warranted and may be best reserved for patients for whom definitive aftercare with a primary provider has been arranged.

Patients with known *H. pylori* disease who are either treatment naïve or were inadequately treated should start a regimen of either bismuth-metronidazole-tetracycline combination plus PPI or PPI plus clarithromycin and either metronidazole or amoxicillin.[16] When *H. pylori* is a consideration, endoscopy should be delayed for 4 to 8 weeks after discontinuation of antibiotics, PPI, and bismuth, so that infection status can be more reliably assessed at biopsy.[16]

The EP should communicate with the patient's primary provider if serologic testing was performed or empirical therapy for *H. pylori* was started, so that the outpatient provider can arrange further diagnostic evaluations. Additionally, the EP should confirm with the patient that he or she understands the treatment plan, the seriousness of the diagnosis, and which lifestyle modifications would aid in healing. Specifically, patients should be educated about the negative effects of smoking, excessive alcohol use, failure to follow up, and medication noncompliance. Lastly, patients should decrease or avoid the use of NSAIDs.[16] If NSAID therapy must continue, the addition of a PPI will allow most duodenal and gastric ulcers to heal in a timely fashion.[7,16] Patients with healed NSAID-induced ulcers are among those at highest risk of further gastroduodenal injury, leading to serious complications such as perforation and bleeding.[14]

Symptomatic management may include the short-term use of aluminum and/or magnesium hydroxide (e.g., Maalox or Mylanta) 30 to 45 mL orally at the time of ED presentation, before meals, and before bedtime. The addition of 10 to 20 mL of oral viscous lidocaine may reduce symptoms while the patient is in the ED. There is no role for anticholinergic agents as part of the "GI cocktail" used for the ED treatment of dyspepsia. Narcotic medications and/or histamine H_2 receptor antagonists can provide additional relief in the outpatient setting.

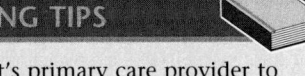

PATIENT TEACHING TIPS

- Involve the patient's primary care provider to ensure follow-up and to tailor a cohesive treatment plan to fit the individual patient.
- Educate patients about the dangers of smoking, excessive use of alcohol and caffeine, and medication noncompliance.
- Provide information about various smoking cessation aids, such as nicotine supplements and bupropion.
- Stress the importance of abstaining from use of nonsteroidal anti-inflammatory drugs.
- Provide well-written, clear, concise anticipatory discharge instructions. Every patient should leave the ED with an understanding of the dangers of worsening pain, hematemesis, melena, or hematochezia.
- Follow-up with both an internist and a gastroenterologist should be arranged for ill patients.

■ SURGICAL TREATMENT

Surgery is rarely necessary, given that medical therapies for PUD are so effective. Indications for elective surgical treatment of PUD are (1) protracted and failed medical therapy, and (2) suspicion of malignancy.[17] For the rare nonhealing benign ulcer in the stomach, resection is indicated for management of symptoms and prevention of malignancy.[17]

Profuse bleeding was a prior indication for surgery, but endoscopic therapy (whether by electrocautery, heater probe, or injection sclerotherapy) controls bleeding in the majority of cases (Fig. 27-3).[17] Surgery is indicated for those cases in which bleeding is not controlled with endoscopy or is recurrent. A further discussion of gastrointestinal bleeding is found in Chapter 28.

When surgery is being considered, some well-established risk factors increase the likelihood of a fatal outcome. They are the presence of severe comorbidity, perforation of more than 24 hours in duration, and the presence of hypotension on presentation.[17] Conservative management with nasogastric suction, circulatory support, and antibiotics should be employed in elderly patients with these risk factors.[17]

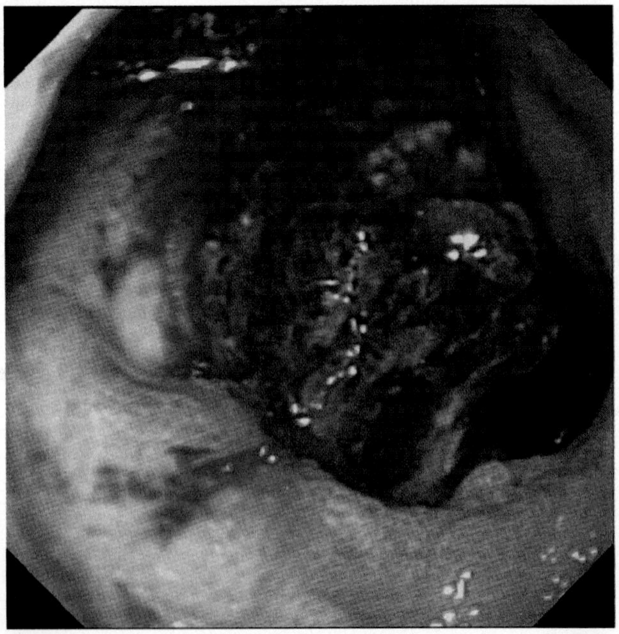

FIGURE 27-3 Endoscopic appearance of a duodenal bulb ulcer with a fresh adherent clot. (From Feldman M, Friedman LS, Brandt LJ [eds]: Sleisenger & Fordtran's Gastrointestinal and Liver Disease: Pathophysiology/Diagnosis/Management, 8th ed. Philadelphia, Saunders, 2006.)

Sequelae of Peptic Ulcer Disease

■ GASTRIC CANCER

Gastric cancer is the second most common cause of cancer-related death worldwide. It is the third most common cancer in southeastern Europe and South America, and globally, it is the fourth most common form of cancer.[18] In comparison with the rest of the world, western Europe and the United States have a relatively low incidence of gastric cancer, the highest incidences being reported in Japan, China, and South America.[18] Gastric cancer rates remain quite high among some subgroups of African Americans, Hispanics, and Native Americans. In the United States, the mean age at diagnosis is 48 years, and the male-to-female ratio is 1 : 1.[18]

Although there are well-established genetic factors that predispose one to gastric cancer, such as blood type A, the main causative agents are environmental.[19] *H. pylori* infection promotes apoptosis in infected cells, starting a metaplastic path of destruction. Inhibition of E-cadherin protein synthesis by *H. pylori* is also associated with development of gastric cancer.[19] The International Agency for Research on Cancer has classified *H. pylori* as a class I carcinogen, the only bacterial agent with this distinction.[18]

Diets high in salt and *N*-nitrosamines and low in the antioxidants typically found in fresh fruits and vegetables have been strongly associated with a higher prevalence of gastric cancer. The prognosis of gastric cancer is poor, with 5-year survival rates less than 25%.[18] Improved survival seen in Japanese populations has been attributed to aggressive screening programs that have led to identification of earlier-stage lesions. Such screening programs are less common in the United States.

ED patients with suspected dyspepsia must have urgent outpatient follow-up for endoscopic screening for gastric malignancy (Fig. 27-4).

■ GASTRIC OUTLET OBSTRUCTION

Chronic peptic ulcers in either the stomach or duodenum may cause scarring and may impair gastric emptying, a condition known as *gastric outlet obstruction* (Fig. 27-5). In adults, PUD is the major cause of benign gastric outlet obstruction—more than 95% of cases are associated with duodenal or pyloric channel ulceration.[20] The resolution of gastric outlet obstruction after the eradication of *H. pylori* has been demonstrated in several studies. Symptomatic improvement can be seen a few weeks after the start of antimicrobial therapy for *H. pylori,* and the benefits seem to persist on long-term follow-up.[20]

Treatment of gastric outlet obstruction should start with the pharmacologic eradication of *H. pylori,* even when stenosis is considered to be fibrotic or when there is some gastric stasis. If this noninvasive treatment is unsuccessful, NSAID use may be the underlying cause.[20] Dilation or surgery should be reserved for patients who show no response to medical therapy.

ED patients with signs or symptoms of gastric outlet obstruction should be admitted for gastroenterology consultation and further management.

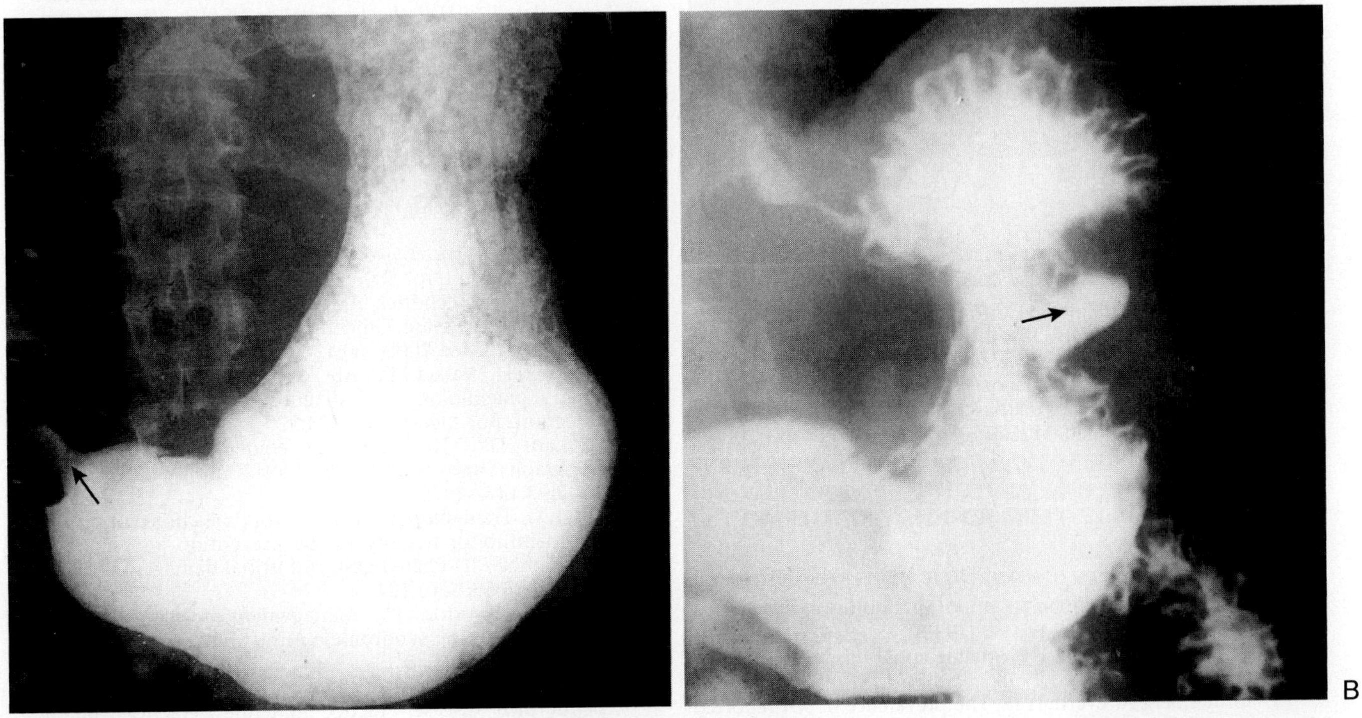

A B

FIGURE 27-4 Radiologic and endoscopic examples of gastric cancer. **A,** Pyloric (gastric outlet) obstruction (*arrow*). **B,** Large greater curve ulcer within a mass (*arrow*).

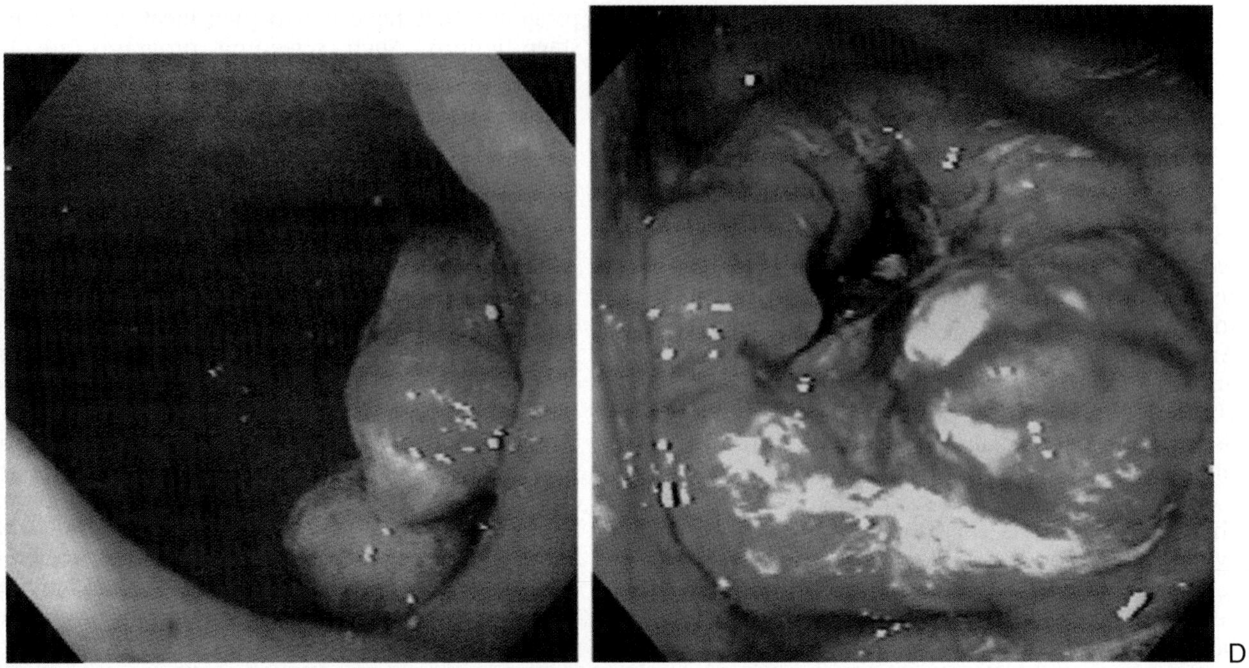

C D

FIGURE 27-4, cont'd **C,** Polypoid gastric cancer. Trilobed polyp at the angularis. **D,** Exophytic gastric cancer. Circumferential masslike lesion involving the gastric body and collapsing the antrum. (From Feldman M, Friedman LS, Brandt LJ [eds]: Sleisenger & Fordtran's Gastrointestinal and Liver Disease: Pathophysiology/Diagnosis/Management, 8th ed. Philadelphia, Saunders, 2006.)

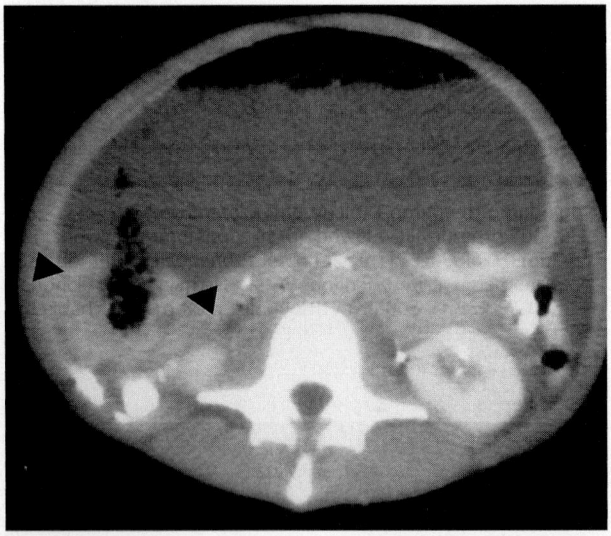

FIGURE 27-5 Gastric outlet obstruction—cancer of the antrum. Markedly distended stomach with air-fluid level on computed tomography. In this case, a mass in the distal antrum can be seen (*arrowheads*). (From Grainger RG, Allison DJ, Dixon AK [eds]: Grainger & Allison's Diagnostic Radiology: A Textbook of Medical Imaging, 4th ed. St. Louis, Churchill Livingstone, 2001.)

REFERENCES

1. Friedman LS: *Helicobacter pylori* and nonulcer dyspepsia. N Engl J Med 1998;339:1928-1930.
2. Fisher RS, Parkman HP: Management of nonulcer dyspepsia. N Engl J Med 1998;339:1376-1381.
3. Sonnenberg A, Everhart JE: The prevalence of self-reported peptic ulcer in the United States. Am J Public Health 1996;86:200-205.
4. Modlin IM, Moss SF, Kidd M, et al: Gastroesophageal reflux disease: Then and now. J Clin Gastroenterol 2004;38: 390-402.
5. Chang EB, Sitrin MD, Black DD: Gastric physiology. In Gastrointestinal, Hepatobiliary, and Nutritional Physiology. Philadelphia, Lippincott-Raven, 1996, pp 53-73.
6. Calam J, Baron JH, ABC of the upper gastrointestinal tract: Pathophysiology of duodenal and gastric ulcer and gastric cancer. Brit Med J 2001;323:980-982.
7. Quan CS, Talley NJ: Management of peptic ulcer disease not related to *Helicobacter pylori* or NSAIDs. Am J Gastroenterol 2002;97:2950-2961.
8. Ford AC, Delaney BC, Forman D, et al: Eradication therapy in *Helicobacter pylori* positive peptic ulcer disease: Systematic review and economic analysis. Am J Gastroenterol 2004;99:1833-1855.
9. Pinto-Santini D, Salama NR: The biology of *Helicobacter pylori* infection, a major risk factor for gastric adenocarcinoma. Cancer Epidemiol Biomarkers Prev 2005;14: 1853-1858.
10. Axon A: *Helicobacter pylori*: What do we still need to know? J Clin Gastroenterol 2006;40:15-19.
11. Peterson WL, Fendrick AM, Cave DR, et al: *Helicobacter pylori*–related disease: Guidelines for testing and treatment. Arch Intern Med 2000;160:1285-1291.
12. Logan RPH, Walker MM: ABC of the upper gastrointestinal tract: Epidemiology and diagnosis of *Helicobacter pylori* infection. Brit Med J 2001;323:920-922.
13. Graham DY: The changing epidemiology of GERD: Geography and *Helicobacter pylori*. Am J Gastroenterol 2003;98:1462-1470.
14. Singh G, Triadafilopoulos G: Appropriate choice of proton pump inhibitor therapy in the prevention and management of NSAID-related gastrointestinal damage. Int J Clin Pract 2005;59:1210-1217.
15. Meko JB, Norton JA: Management of patients with Zollinger-Ellison syndrome. Annu Rev Med 1995:46: 395-411.
16. Soll AH: Consensus conference: Medical treatment of peptic ulcer disease. Practice guidelines. Practice Parameters Committee of the American College of Gastroenterology. JAMA 1996;275:622-629.

17. Jamieson GG: Current status of indications for surgery in peptic ulcer disease. World J Surgery 2000;24:256-258.
18. Zivny J, Wang TC, Yantiss RK, et al: Role of therapy or monitoring in preventing progression to gastric cancer. J Clinical Gastroenterology 2003:36(5):S50-S60; discussion S61-S62.
19. Chan AO, Luk JM, Hui WM, et al: Molecular biology of gastric carcinoma: From laboratory to bedside. J Gastroenterol Hepatol 1999;14:1150-1160.
20. Gisbert JP, Pajares JM: *Helicobacter pylori* infection and gastric outlet obstruction—prevalence of the infection and role of antimicrobial treatment. Aliment Pharmacol Therapeut 2002;16:1203-1208.

Chapter **28**

Gastrointestinal Bleeding

Sheryl L. Heron and Patricia Baines

KEY POINTS

Morbidity and mortality from gastrointestinal (GI) bleeding increases significantly if aggressive resuscitation is not initiated immediately in the ED.

Assessment and management of GI bleeding are predicated on the site of the hemorrhage—that is, whether the bleeding is from an upper or lower GI tract source.

A gastroenterology consultation should be obtained immediately to arrange for diagnostic/therapeutic endoscopy or colonoscopy for cases of active bleeding.

Causes of GI bleeding in children vary considerably with age; most cases are benign and self-limiting, although Meckel's diverticulum, midgut volvulus, and intussusception can result in massive rectal bleeding.

Scope

Demographic risk factors for patients with gastrointestinal bleeding (GI) include older age, male gender, and the use of alcohol, tobacco, aspirin or nonsteroidal anti-inflammatory drugs (NSAIDs).[1] The risk of bleeding is significantly higher in elderly patients who have recently started a regimen of NSAIDs or regular-dose aspirin than in long-term users of these agents. Additional independent risk factors are unmarried status, cardiovascular disease, difficulty with activities of daily living, use of multiple medications, and use of oral anticoagulants.[2]

Intensive resuscitation in the ED significantly decreases mortality in patients who present with *hematemesis* (vomiting blood), *hematochezia* (red bloody stools), or *melena* (black tarry stools).[3] The predictive pneumonic BLEED (ongoing *b*leeding, *l*ow systolic blood pressure, *e*levated prothrombin time, *e*rratic mental status, unstable comorbid *d*isease) applied at the initial ED evaluation can predict hospital outcomes for patients with acute upper or lower GI hemorrhage.[4]

Lower GI bleeding afflicts 20 to 27 of every 100,000 persons annually in the United States.[5] The rate of lower GI bleeding increases more than 200-fold from the third to the ninth decade of life, with 25% to 35% of all cases occurring in elderly patients.[6]

Pediatric GI bleeding is fairly common worldwide, however the incidence of severe GI bleeding in U.S. children is rare.[7] Lower GI bleeding is a more common complaint in the practice of general pediatrics, accounting for 10% to 15% of referrals to a pediatric gastroenterologist.[8,9] In most children, bleeding is not life-threatening and ceases spontaneously, requiring only supportive care.[8] The age of the child guides the clinician toward specific diagnoses.

Pathophysiology

■ UPPER GASTROINTESTINAL BLEEDING

Upper GI bleeding is defined as bleeding from a source proximal to the ligament of Treitz, which is located at the junction of the duodenum and jejunum. Upper GI bleeding accounts for three quarters of GI tract

Tips and Tricks

Patients who present with upper gastrointestinal bleeding should be instructed to avoid nonsteroidal anti-inflammatory drugs (NSAIDs).[32,33] Studies have shown that the risk of recurrent bleeding is significantly higher in long-term users of NSAIDs or regular-dose aspirin, especially if patients are elderly. For short-term users of NSAIDs or aspirin, cotreatment with proton pump inhibitors (but *not* with histamine H_2 blockers) may reduce the risk of bleeding to less than the risk of non-users.[16]

RED FLAGS

- Use of nonsteroidal anti-inflammatory drugs
- Coagulopathies
- Long-term alcohol use
- Neoplasms
- Prior aortic surgery
- Recent nosebleeds

Data from Swaim M, Wilson J: GI emergencies: Rapid therapeutic responses for older patients. Geriatrics 1999;54:20.

hemorrhage, with duodenal and gastric ulcers as the specific sources in more than half of patients with an upper tract cause.

Hematochezia is generally a symptom of lower GI bleeding but may be associated with brisk upper tract hemorrhage. Upper GI bleeding sources are identified in 11% of patients in whom lower GI bleeding was initially suspected.[1] Melena most commonly results from bleeding proximal to the jejunum and should be considered a marker of upper GI bleeding.

Variceal hemorrhage is the most serious complication of portal hypertension and occurs in one third of patients with esophageal varices.[10] The extent of severe bleeding depends on portal pressure, variceal size, and variceal wall thickness.[11] Esophageal varices should be suspected in any alcoholic with unexplained anemia or obvious GI bleeding.

One study has noted a decline in the frequency of peptic ulcer disease in patients with upper GI bleeding and reported that the proportion of bleeding ulcers with a nonvisible vessel is now 20%, which is less than previously reported.[12] Such decline may be related to improved treatment of *Helicobacter pylori* infection.

In children, the pathophysiology of bleeding is determined by the specific causes of hemorrhage for each age group.[13]

LOWER GASTROINTESTINAL BLEEDING

Lower GI bleeding refers to bleeding that originates from an intestinal source distal to the ligament of Treitz. The majority of patients with hematochezia bleed from a colonic source. Diverticular disease, angiodysplasia, and neoplasm are the leading causes of lower GI bleeding in adults. Anal fissure and hemorrhoids are the most benign causes of lower GI bleeding.

Comorbid illnesses and decreased physiologic reserve make elderly patients more vulnerable to adverse consequences of acute blood loss and prolonged hospitalization.[14] Specifically, hematochezia is more commonly associated with syncope, dyspnea, altered mental status, stroke, falls, fatigue, and acute anemia in older patients. Poor prognostic indicators also include continued bright red rectal bleeding, excessive transfusions, orthostasis, shock, and altered mental status on admission.[6]

Ulcerative colitis accounts for the majority of cases of massive lower GI bleeding in young adults in the second or third decade of life. Diverticulosis and arteriovenous malformation are found in older adults.[9]

The independent risk factors listed earlier are useful prognostic indicators, yielding poorer outcomes for patients with either upper or lower tract bleeding.[2] Specifically, use of over-the-counter NSAIDs may represent an important cause of peptic ulcer disease and ulcer-related hemorrhage in those with upper GI bleeding.[15,16]

Although most causes of lower GI bleeding in children are self-limiting and benign, it is imperative to consider Meckel's diverticulum, midgut volvulus, and intussusception in appropriate age groups.[9]

Clinical Presentation

Patients with GI bleeding can be rapidly assessed by their reported volume of blood loss and initial hemodynamic status. Massive hemorrhage is associated with signs or symptoms of hemodynamic instability, including tachycardia (heart rate greater than 100 to 120 beats/min), systolic blood pressure less than 90 to 100 mm Hg, symptomatic orthostasis, syncope, ongoing bright red or maroon hematemesis, transfusion requirements in the first 24 hours, and inability to stabilize the patient.[17]

Vital signs and postural changes should be assessed. An increase of 20 beats/min or more in pulse or a decrease of 20 mm Hg in systolic blood pressure between supine and upright positions indicates loss of more than 20% of blood volume in normal adult patients.[6] Tachycardia, low blood pressure, reduced urine output, and conjunctival pallor in patients presenting with GI bleeding are signs that mandate immediate volume replacement. Hypovolemic shock implies at least a 40% loss of blood volume. Note that vital sign abnormalities are unreliable in pediatric and elderly patients.

History should focus on quantity, frequency, and duration of bleeding (differentiating between melena and hematochezia) to characterize the nature of the GI bleeding as well as an assessment of comorbid status, including other GI disorders, anticoagulant use, syncope, weight loss, alcohol intake, and cardiovascular disease.

In addition to continuous monitoring of vital signs, physical examination should include assessments of mental status, skin (for jaundice or pallor), and pulmonary and cardiovascular compromise (especially in the elderly due to ischemia from blood loss) as well as a thorough abdominal examination for distention, tenderness, or masses. Digital rectal examination and stool testing for gross or occult blood should be performed in every patient with GI bleeding.

Complaints associated with lower GI bleeding include hematochezia or melena, although patients may have additional findings, such as anemia, lightheadedness, hypovolemia, weakness, malaise, chest pain, and dyspnea. It is important to note that patients with lower GI bleeding may be asymptomatic and may present with complaints seemingly unrelated to intestinal bleeding (e.g., fatigue, weight loss); dramatic presentations consisting of massive rectal bleeding in acutely ill and unstable patients are less common.[18]

Delayed black tarry stools may occur from a source of bleeding in the small bowel or ascending colon and may not be noted by the patient until several days after bleeding has stopped.[19]

A thorough history and complete physical examination are important for the evaluation of a child with GI bleeding. Bright red blood that coats but is not mixed with stool suggests an anorectal source. Hematochezia indicates bleeding from the distal small bowel or proximal colon. Bloody diarrhea usually suggests colonic bleeding. Currant-jelly stools indicate the vascular congestion and hyperemia seen with intussusception.

Food allergy may lead to GI bleeding from food-induced colitis and may result in dehydration in infants younger than 3 months.[8] Anal fissures are common in infants and produce red streaks or spots of blood in the diaper.[9] Other causes of dark stool are iron, charcoal, flavored gelatin, red fruits, bismuth, and food dyes. Maternal blood swallowed by neonates during delivery may be diagnosed with the Apt test.[8]

Differential Diagnosis

The most common causes of upper GI bleeding in adults are listed in Table 28-1, and causes of lower GI bleeding in adolescents and adults are listed in Table 28-2.

The exact cause of GI bleeding is less important to the EP than the differentiation between upper and lower tract sources. It is of note, however, that a patient with massive lower GI bleeding and recent surgery should be considered to have an aortoenteric fistula until proven otherwise.[6]

Table 28-1 CAUSES OF UPPER GASTROINTESTINAL BLEEDING

More common	Peptic ulcer disease Gastritis Esophagitis Varices Mallory-Weiss tears
Less common	Gastric cancer Dieulafoy's lesion Portal gastropathy Gastric antral vascular atresia

From Maltz C: Acute gastrointestinal bleeding. Best Practice of Medicine 2003:1-23. http://merck.microdex.com/index.asp?page=bpm_brief &article_id=BPM01GA08.

Table 28-2 CAUSES OF LOWER GASTROINTESTINAL (GI) BLEEDING

Adolescents	Upper GI bleed Inflammatory bowel disease Polyps Meckel's diverticulum Infectious diarrhea Anal fissures Hemorrhoids
Adults	Upper GI bleed Diverticulosis Angiodysplasia Cancer Ischemic bowel disease Polyps Inflammatory bowel disease Infectious diarrhea Foreign body

From Akhtar AJ: Lower gastrointestinal bleeding in elderly patients. J Am Med Dir Assoc 2003;4:320-322.

■ DIFFERENTIAL DIAGNOSIS FOR PEDIATRIC GI BLEEDING

Table 28-3 lists the differential diagnosis for upper GI bleeding and lower GI bleeding according to patient age. Maternal blood ingestion is the most common cause of suspected GI bleeding in neonates; blood is swallowed during either delivery or breastfeeding (from a fissure in the mother's breast). Other causes of GI bleeding in neonates are bacterial enteritis, milk protein allergies, intussusception, anal fissures, lymphonodular hyperplasia, and erosions of the esophageal, gastric, and duodenal mucosa.

Mucosal injuries presumably result from a dramatic rise in gastric acid secretion and laxity of gastric sphincters in infants. Maternal stress in the third trimester has also been proposed to increase maternal gastrin secretion and enhance infantile peptic ulcer formation.

Some drugs are implicated in neonatal GI bleeding, including NSAIDs, heparin, and tolazoline, which are used for persistent fetal circulation. Indomethacin, administered to maintain a patent ductus arteriosus in neonates, may cause GI bleeding through intestinal vasoconstriction and platelet dysfunction.

Table 28-3 CAUSES OF GASTROINTESTINAL (GI) BLEEDING IN CHILDREN, BY AGE

Age Group	Causes of Upper GI Bleeding	Causes of Lower GI Bleeding
Neonates	Hemorrhagic disease of the newborn Swallowed maternal blood Stress gastritis Coagulopathy	Anal fissure Necrotizing enterocolitis Malrotation with volvulus
Infants (1 mo-1 yr)	Esophagitis Gastritis	Anal fissure Intussusception Gangrenous bowel Milk protein allergy
Infants (1-2 yrs)	Peptic ulcer disease Gastritis	Polyps Meckel's diverticulum
Children (2-12 yrs)	Esophageal varices Gastric varices	Polyps Inflammatory bowel disease Infectious diarrhea Vascular lesions

From Arensman R, Abramson L: Gastrointestinal bleeding: Surgical perspective. Emedicine. www.emedicine.com/ped/topic3027.htm.

Maternal medications can also cross the placenta and incite gastrointestinal problems in the developing fetus and neonate on delivery. Aspirin, cephalothin, and phenobarbital are well-known causes of coagulation abnormalities in neonates. Stress ulcers in newborns are associated with dexamethasone, which is used for fetal lung maturation.

Rarer causes of GI bleeding in a neonate are volvulus, coagulopathies, arteriovenous malformations, necrotizing enterocolitis (especially in preterm infants), Hirschsprung's enterocolitis, and Meckel's diverticulitis.[7]

In infants, GI mucosal lesions and irritations are the most common causes of bleeding. They include esophagitis, gastritis, duodenitis, ulcers, colonic polyps, and anorectal disorders. Intussusception is a common and important cause of GI bleeding in this age group. The incidence of intussusception is greatest in infants aged 3 months to 1 year, but it can occur in children up to 5 years. About 80% of all cases of intussusception occur in infants younger than 2 years.

Other causes of infantile GI bleeding are infectious diarrhea, midgut volvulus, Meckel's diverticulum, arteriovenous malformation, and GI duplication. Rare causes include foreign body ingestions, variceal disease, irritable bowel disease, and acquired thrombocytopenia.

Older children may present with any of the preceding conditions, but duodenal ulcer, Mallory-Weiss tear, and nasopharyngeal bleeding are important causes of bleeding in this age group. Less common causes are gastritis or ulcers induced by salicylates or NSAIDs, Henoch-Schönlein purpura, caustic ingestions, hemolytic-uremic syndrome, inflammatory bowel disease, and vasculitis. In adolescents older than 12 years, the most common causes of upper GI bleeding are duodenal ulcers, esophagitis, gastritis, and Mallory-Weiss tears.[7]

Diagnostic Testing

■ NASOGASTRIC ASPIRATION

Historically, nasogastric aspiration has been used to determine whether bleeding originated from the upper GI tract in patients with melena—a bloody aspirate confirmed an upper tract source, whereas an aspirate testing negative for blood represented either resolved bleeding or a more distal site of hemorrhage. In some studies, however, nasogastric aspiration was noted to be insensitive for detection of upper GI bleeding in patients *without* active hematemesis, and a negative result provided little information about the etiology of bleeding.[20,21] Aspirates testing positive for blood confirmed only that the bleeding was proximal to the pylorus, requiring patients to undergo endoscopy for further differentiation.

A nasogastric aspirate of more than 1 liter of fresh blood, or an inability to obtain a clear aspirate through lavage with more than 1500 mL of saline, should alert the physician to massive upper GI bleeding that requires immediate gastroenterologic or surgical intervention.

■ UPPER ENDOSCOPY

Esophagogastroduodenoscopy (upper endoscopy) is now the diagnostic choice for establishing the source of upper GI bleeding. The overwhelming majority of existing data suggest that early endoscopy is a safe and effective procedure in all risk groups.[10,22] Patients without active hematemesis may benefit from immediate upper endoscopy by a gastroenterologist to confirm the site of bleeding, rather than undergoing the potential additional discomfort and morbidity associated with nasogastric tube placement. Endoscopy is both diagnostic and therapeutic in many cases.

■ TAGGED RED BLOOD CELL STUDIES

An advanced modality for the detection of the source of GI bleeding is radionuclide imaging, such as radioisotopic imaging with technetium Tc99m sulfur colloid– or technetium pertechnetate–labeled red cells. Technetium Tc99m red blood cell imaging is a useful test in the management of acute GI bleeding, particularly if bleeding has been occurring for more than 3 hours and other modalities have failed to identify a source. Limitations of this test are poor detection of bleeding in the foregut, with the highest sensitivities noted for bleeding in the colon.[23] A technetium Tc99m sulfur colloid–labeled red blood cell study requires active bleeding at a rate of more than 0.1 mL/min for visualization. Radionuclide imaging has not been widely tested in the ED setting and is still reserved for inpatient use at most institutions.

■ ARTERIOGRAPHY

Angiography is appropriate for initial testing in patients with massive bleeding.[24] When bleeding cannot be identified and controlled by endoscopy, intraoperative enteroscopy or arteriography may help localize the bleeding source, facilitating segmental resection of the bowel.[25] Mesenteric angiography can detect bleeding at a rate of 0.5 mL/min or greater.[26] Either angiography or angiographic computed tomography may be used to identify aortoenteric fistula.

Intra-arterial injection with vasopressin or other vasoconstrictors at the site of bleeding can control hemorrhage; embolization is an option when intra-arterial injection is unsuccessful.[27,28]

■ DISTAL COLONIC IMAGING

Colonoscopy has a high diagnostic yield and low rate of perforation in patients with lower GI bleeding. Colonoscopy is best performed after colonic cleansing and in patients with slow bleeds. Proctosigmoidoscopy is used in patients with mild rectal bleeding to determine whether stool above the rectum contains blood. Barium enema is not useful in the acute setting but can be ordered after an acute bleed has resolved.[29]

■ LABORATORY TESTING

Initial laboratory studies that should be ordered include a complete blood cell count, coagulation studies, and blood type and crossmatch for patients with active bleeding or unstable vital signs. Serial hematocrit measurements are more useful than one isolated test, although marked changes in hematocrit typically lag behind actual blood loss. A blood chemistry panel, liver profile, and lipase measurement should be performed. Stool evaluation for leukocytes, bacteria, ova, parasites, and *Clostridium difficile* should be considered in patients with bloody diarrhea.[8] Electrocardiograms and cardiac enzymes are necessary for patients at risk of early coronary artery disease or those older than 50 years to screen for ischemia secondary to blood loss.

Procedures

The proper technique for the safe placement and use of nasogastric tubes and gastroesophageal balloon tamponade tubes (e.g., Blakemore-Sengstaken tube) is discussed in Chapter 42.

Treatment

Figure 28-1 presents an algorithm for treatment of gastrointestinal bleeding. Insert two 18-gauge or larger intravenous lines and administer 0.9% normal saline or lactated Ringer's injection upon the patient's arrival.[26] Quickly evaluate hemodynamic status and determine the extent of blood on fluid resuscitation necessary. Standard resuscitative measures for the management of shock should precede or occur in parallel with definitive diagnostic testing. Management should otherwise be directed toward the underlying source of bleeding. One should note that in 80% of cases, lower GI bleeding stops spontaneously.[14]

If the patient is hemorrhaging, the EP should consult a gastroenterologist and surgeon. Upper endoscopy is the diagnostic and therapeutic procedure of choice for acute upper GI bleeding. Surgery is indicated for patients with active bleeding when medical therapy proves ineffective and continued hemorrhage requires more than 5 units of blood within the first 4 to 6 hours.[18,19,26,30] Bowel resection may be required for pronounced lower GI bleeding.

In the absence of consultants, massive esophageal hemorrhage due to variceal bleeding may be temporarily treated with the placement of a gastroesophageal balloon tamponade device (Blakemore-Sengstaken tube). Although this is an uncommon procedure, EPs in remote practice locations should be familiar with the indications and proper use of such potentially life-saving devices.

Octreotide acetate is a synthetic analogue of somatostatin that should be administered intravenously for all patients with suspected upper GI bleeding from esophageal varices, to cause splanchnic vasoconstriction and reduction in portal hypertension. The loading dose is 25 to 50 μg intravenously, followed by 25 to 50 μg/hr intravenous infusion.

Comorbidities, such as coagulopathies, hyperkalemia, and cardiac ischemia, should be identified and treated. The EP should consider the administration of fresh frozen plasma, platelets, recombinant factor VIIa (NovoSeven), or desmopressin (DDAVP) as appropriate.

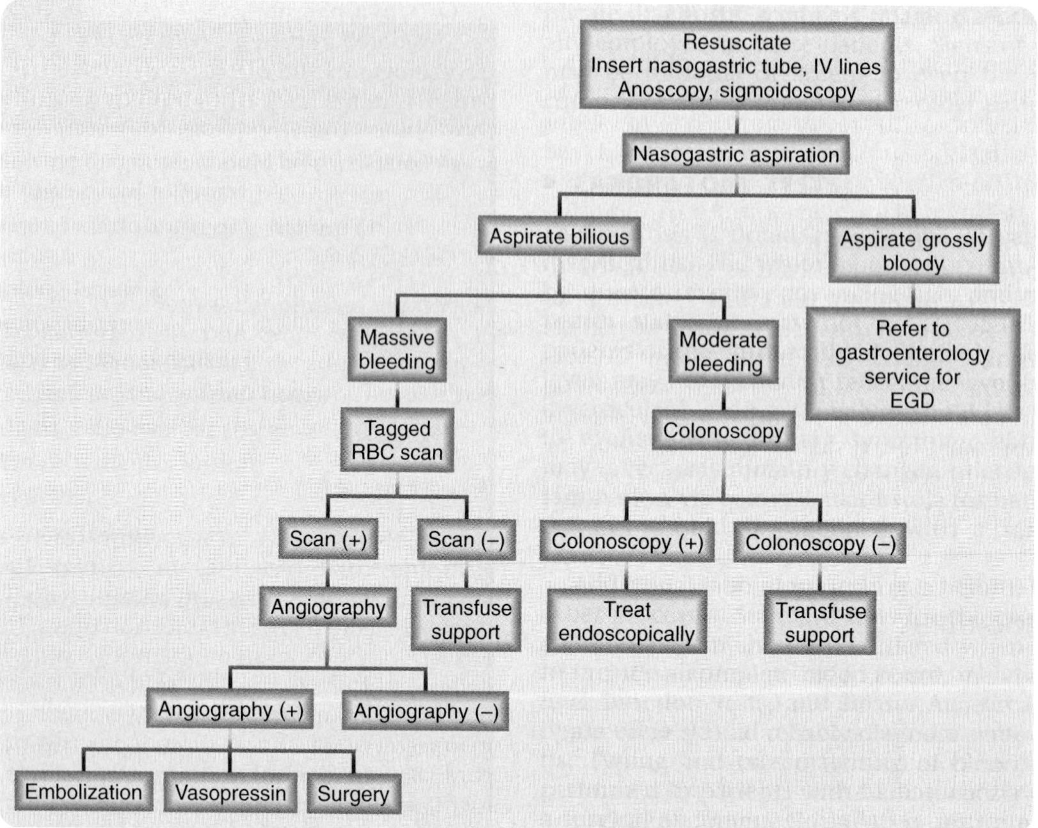
Resuscitate
Insert nasogastric tube, IV lines
Anoscopy, sigmoidoscopy
Nasogastric aspiration
Aspirate bilious
Aspirate grossly bloody
Massive bleeding
Moderate bleeding
Refer to gastroenterology service for EGD
Tagged RBC scan
Colonoscopy
Scan (+)
Scan (–)
Colonoscopy (+)
Colonoscopy (–)
Angiography
Transfuse support
Treat endoscopically
Transfuse support
Angiography (+)
Angiography (–)
Embolization
Vasopressin
Surgery

FIGURE 28-1 Management of lower gastrointestinal hemorrhage. EGD, esophagogastroduodenoscopy; IV intravenous; RBC, red blood cell; (+), positive test results; (–), negative test results. (Adapted from Hoedema RE, Luchtefeld MA: The management of lower gastrointestinal hemorrhage. Dis Colon Rectum Nov 2005;48:2010-2024.)

PATIENT TEACHING TIPS

- Patients should stop drinking alcohol and seek an alcohol cessation program immediately if needed.
- Patients who use nonsteroidal anti-inflammatory agents should receive concomitant therapy with a proton pump inhibitor.
- Patients with gastric ulcers should be re-examined 6 to 8 weeks after the initial bleeding episode.
- Patients should maintain daily intake of synthetic bulk-forming agents.
- Surveillance colonoscopy should be performed every 3 years in patients with colon polyps and adenomatous changes, or every 5 years in those with hyperplastic polyps.

Data from Swaim M, Wilson J: GI emergencies: Rapid therapeutic responses for older patients. Geriatrics 1999;54:20.

Disposition

Most patients who present to the ED with GI bleeding should be admitted for further evaluation and treatment. Patients who require transfusions, have severe anemia or continued bleeding, or are unstable should be admitted to the intensive care unit. Admission to a hospital ward is reserved for stable patients with melena or a history of resolved bleeding with normal physical findings and no significant comorbidity. Stable patients with melena and symptoms of suspected or known cardiac disease must be admitted to a telemetry unit.

Patients with normal physical findings, trace heme-positive stool, and stable vital signs may be sent home with close follow-up. Patients with reported hematochezia but normal-appearing stool and no evidence of hemodynamic compromise may be managed as outpatients with arrangements for urgent colonoscopy and primary care referral.[26]

Patients who have anal fissures, hemorrhoids, or other rectal causes of bleeding can be discharged with conservative therapy and reassurance. A detailed discussion of the management of anorectal disorders can be found in Chapter 36.

Instruct patients to return to the ED if they experience signs and symptoms of recurrent bleeding, fatigue, chest discomfort, dyspnea, or near-syncope.[31]

REFERENCES

1. Peura DA, Lanza FL, Gostout CJ, Foutch PG: The American College of Gastroenterology Bleeding Registry: Preliminary findings. Am J Gastroenterol 1997;92:924-928.

2. Kaplan RC, Heckbert SR, Koepsell TD, et al: Risk factors for hospitalized gastrointestinal bleeding among older persons. J Am Geriatr Soc 2001;49:126-133.
3. Baradarian R, Ramdhaney S, Chapalamadugu R, et al: Early intensive resuscitation of patients with upper gastrointestinal bleeding decreases mortality. The Am J Gastroenterol 2004;99:619-622.
4. Kollef MH, O'Brien JD, Zuckerman GR, Shannon W: BLEED: A classification tool to predict outcomes in patients with acute upper and lower gastrointestinal hemorrhage. Crit Care Med 1997;25:1125-1132.
5. Brackman MR, Gushchin VV, Smith L, et al: Acute lower gastroenteric bleeding retrospective analysis (the ALGEBRA study): An analysis of the triage, management and outcomes of patients with acute lower gastrointestinal bleeding. Am Surg 2003;69:145-149.
6. Akhtar AJ: Lower gastrointestinal bleeding in elderly patients. J Am Med Dir Assoc 2003;4:320-322.
7. Hsai R, Wang N, Halpern J, Loret de Mola O: Pediatrics, gastrointestinal bleeding. Emedicine. www.emedicine.com/emerg/topic381.htm.
8. Leung AK, Wong AL: Lower gastrointestinal bleeding in children. Pediatr Emerg Care 2002;18:319-323.
9. Arensman R, Abramson L: Gastrointestinal bleeding: Surgical perspective. Emedicine. www.emedicine.com/ped/topic3027.htm.
10. Dam JV, Brugge WR: Endoscopy of the upper gastrointestinal tract. N Engl J Med 1999;341:1738-1748.
11. Roberts L, Kamath P: Pathophysiology of variceal bleeding. Gastrointest Endosc Clin North Am 1999;2:167-174.
12. Boonpongmanee S, Fleischer DE, Pezzullo JC, et al: The frequency of peptic ulcer as a cause of upper-GI bleeding is exaggerated. Gastrointest Endosc 2004;59: 788-794.
13. Lazzaroni M, Petrillo M, Tornaghi R, et al: Upper GI bleeding in healthy full-term infants: A case-control study. The Am J Gastroenterology. 2002;97(1):89-94.
14. Swaim M, Wilson J: GI emergencies: Rapid therapeutic responses for older patients. Geriatrics. 1999;54:20-22; 25-26; 29-30.
15. Wilcox CM, Shalek KA, Cotsonis G: Striking prevalence of over-the-counter nonsteroidal anti-inflammatory drug use in patients with upper gastrointestinal hemorrhage. Arch Intern Med 1994;154:42-46.
16. Pilotto A, Franceschi M, Leandro G, et al: The risk of upper gastrointestinal bleeding in elderly users of aspirin and other non-steroidal anti-inflammatory drugs: The role of gastroprotective drugs. Aging Clin Exp Res 2003;15: 494-499.
17. Peter D, Dougherty J: Evaluation of the patient with gastrointestinal bleeding: An evidence based approach. Emerg Med Clin North Am 1999;17:239-261.
18. Hoedema RE, Luchtefeld MA: The management of lower gastrointestinal hemorrhage. Dis Colon Rectum 2005;48: 2010-2024.
19. Vernava AM 3rd, Moore BA, Longo WE, Johnson FE: Lower gastrointestinal bleeding. Dis Colon Rectum 1997;40: 846-858.
20. Cuellar RE, Gavaler JS, Alexander JA, et al: Gastrointestinal tract hemorrhage: The value of a nasogastric aspirate. Arch Intern Med 1990;150:1381-1384.
21. Witting MD, Magder L, Heins AE, et al: Usefulness and validity of diagnostic nasogastric aspiration in patients without hematemesis. Ann Emerg Med 2004;43:525-532.
22. Spiegel BM, Vakil NB, Ofman JJ: Endoscopy for acute nonvariceal upper gastrointestinal tract hemorrhage: Is sooner better? A systematic review. Arch Intern Med 2001;161: 1393-1404.
23. Howarth DM, Tang K, Lees W: The clinical utility of nuclear medicine imaging for the detection of occult gastrointestinal haemorrhage. Nucl Med Commun 2002;23:591-594.
24. Suzman MS, Talmor M, Jennis R, et al: Accurate localization and surgical management of active lower gastrointestinal hemorrhage with technetium-labeled erythrocyte scintigraphy. Ann Surg 1996;224:29-36.
25. Manning-Dimmitt LL, Dimmitt SG, Wilson GR: Diagnosis of gastrointestinal bleeding in adults. Am Fam Physician 2005;71:1339-1346.
26. Cagir B: Lower gastrointestinal bleeding: Surgical perspective. Emedicine. www.emedicine.com/med/topic2818.htm.
27. Gady JS, Reynolds H, Blum A: Selective arterial embolization for control of lower gastrointestinal bleeding: Recommendations for a clinical management pathway. Curr Surg 2003;60:344-347.
28. Khanna A, Ognibene SJ, Koniaris LG: Embolization as first-line therapy for diverticulosis-related massive lower gastrointestinal bleeding: Evidence from a meta-analysis. J Gastrointest Surg 2005;9:343-352.
29. Zuckerman GR, Prakash C: Acute lower intestinal bleeding. Part II: Etiology, therapy, and outcomes. Gastrointest Endosc 1999;49:228-238.
30. Messmann H: Lower gastrointestinal bleeding—the role of endoscopy. Dig Dis 2003;21:19-24.
31. Zuccaro G Jr: Management of the adult patient with acute lower gastrointestinal bleeding. Am College of Gastroenterology Practice Parameters Committee. Am J Gastroenterol 1998;93:1202-1208.
32. Thomas J, Straus WL, Bloom BS: Over-the-counter nonsteroidal anti-inflammatory drugs and risk of gastrointestinal symptoms. Am J Gastroenterol 2002;97:2215-2219.
33. Blot WJ, McLaughlin JK: Over the counter non-steroidal anti-inflammatory drugs and risk of gastrointestinal bleeding. J Epidemiol Biostat 2000;5:137-142.

Chapter 29

Mesenteric Ischemia

Kelly P. O'Keefe and Tracy G. Sanson

KEY POINTS

Severe abdominal pain out of proportion to physical findings should always raise the suspicion of mesenteric ischemia, especially in elderly patients.

The presence of atrial fibrillation, cardiovascular disease, or recent myocardial infarction increases the likelihood of mesenteric ischemia.

No serum marker is sensitive or specific enough to establish or exclude bowel ischemia.

Bloody diarrhea is a late finding that indicates mucosal sloughing—do not wait for the appearance of melena to make the diagnosis of mesenteric ischemia.

Patient survival improves with early mesenteric angiography and/or surgical intervention.

Scope

Mesenteric ischemia is a lack of adequate blood flow and oxygenation to the mesentery and intestines. Mesenteric ischemia is difficult to diagnose early, yet is deadly when advanced. The clinical course consists of bowel ischemia, infarction, sepsis, and death. Mesenteric ischemia accounts for 0.1% of all hospital admissions. Cases of mesenteric vein thrombosis are more difficult to estimate accurately but have been reported at 2 per 100,000 admissions over 20 years at one center. The incidence of acute ischemia is probably increasing because of our aging population and the prolonged survivability of patients with severe cardiovascular disease. In one study, mesenteric ischemia accounted for 1% of ED visits for abdominal pain in geriatric patients.[1-3]

The overall mortality of mesenteric ischemia is between 60% and 93%, rising once bowel wall infarction has occurred. Patients with an early presentation of nonobstructive mesenteric ischemia have mortality rates of 50% to 55%, whereas patients with mesenteric vein thrombosis have a 15% mortality at 30 days.[1-3]

Patients with advanced age, atherosclerosis, thromboembolic disease, atrial fibrillation, and processes leading to chronic low-flow states are at risk for the development of acute mesenteric ischemia (Tables 29-1 and 29-2).[1]

Acute mesenteric ischemia refers to the precipitous onset of hypoperfusion caused by occlusive or nonocclusive obstruction to either arterial or venous blood flow. Acute hypoperfusion occurs in 65% of cases and carries a mortality rate exceeding 60%. *Occlusive arterial obstruction* is most commonly caused by embolic or thrombotic obstruction of the superior mesenteric artery (SMA). *Occlusive venous obstruction* occurs with thrombosis or segmental strangulation—mesenteric venous thrombosis is the main cause of mesenteric ischemia in younger patients without cardiovascular disease. Nonocclusive arterial obstruction, or *nonocclusive mesenteric ischemia,* is often due to vasoconstriction of the splanchnic system.

Chronic mesenteric ischemia, or "intestinal angina," refers to a pattern of pain typically brought on after eating, which is usually episodic and recurrent, is sometimes constant, and lasts for up to 3 hours at a time. Mesenteric arterial atherosclerotic disease is

Table 29-1 RISK FACTORS FOR ISCHEMIC BOWEL DISEASES*

Risk Factor	Arterial Thrombosis	Embolus	Mesenteric Vein Thrombosis	Nonobstructive Mesenteric Ischemia
Advanced age	+	+	+	+
Atherosclerosis	+			
Aortic dissection	+			
Aortic aneurysm	+	+		
Low cardiac output	+	+		+
Congestive heart failure				+
Shock				+
Severe dehydration	+		+	
Cardiac arrhythmias, especially atrial fibrillation		+		+
Severe cardiac valvular disease		+		
Recent myocardial infarction	+			+
Intra-abdominal malignancy			+	
Abdominal trauma			+	
Intra-abdominal infection			+	
Intra-abdominal inflammatory conditions			+	
Parasitic infection (ascariasis)			+	
Hypercoagulable states (venous thrombosis)			+	
Sickle cell anemia			+	
Recent cardiac surgery	+	+		+
Recent abdominal surgery			+	
Vascular aortic prosthetic grafts proximal to the superior mesenteric artery		+		
Hemodialysis				+
Vasculitis	+		+	
Drugs that cause vasoconstriction:				
Digitalis				+
Cocaine				+
Amphetamines				+
Pseudoephedrine				+
Vasopressin			+†	+
Estrogen therapy			+	
Pregnancy			+	
Decompression sickness			+	
Blast lung due to systemic air embolism		+		

*A plus sign (+) indicates that the factor is a risk for the disease subtype.
†Especially after sclerotherapy.
Data from references 1, 2, 4, 7.

generally the cause of chronic mesenteric ischemia, with a process similar to that of coronary artery disease and resultant angina pectoris.

Colonic ischemia occurs much less frequently than small bowel ischemia. Colonic ischemia often resolves spontaneously and without sequelae, but can lead to significant morbidity and, in some cases, death.

Pathophysiology

Acute arterial embolism causes a dramatic cessation of blood flow, with rapid progression from ischemia to infarction. As the bowel wall necroses, release of intraluminal bacteria leads to peritonitis, sepsis, and toxin-mediated hypotension.

Thrombotic arterial ischemia occurs late in the course of severe mesenteric atherosclerotic disease to the three major sources of intestinal blood supply: the celiac artery, the SMA, and the inferior mesenteric artery (IMA). Symptoms typically manifest when two of the three vessels are significantly stenosed or completely obstructed.

Nonocclusive infarction, which represents 25% of all cases of acute ischemia, is most often caused by

Table 29-2 INCIDENCE OF ISCHEMIC BOWEL DISEASES

Disease	Incidence (%)*
Superior mesenteric artery (SMA) embolism: The SMA is susceptible to embolism due to large vessel caliber and narrow angle of departure from the aorta. The proximal SMA is most commonly obstructed within 6-8 cm of the aorta.	50
Nonocclusive ischemia	25
SMA thrombosis	20
Mesenteric venous thrombosis	5

*Percentage of all cases of acute mesenteric ischemia.

splanchnic hypoperfusion and vasoconstriction. Risk factors for nonocclusive disease include advanced age, acute myocardial infarction, acute cardiac decompensation, and heart failure. Diuretics contribute to a decrease in splanchnic perfusion in patients with profound heart disease, whereas medications such as digoxin and alpha-blockers cause regional vasoconstriction and may add to a low-flow state. Cocaine can cause splanchnic vasoconstriction and should be suspected as a cause of mesenteric ischemia in younger patients.

Bowel perfusion is generally preserved during periods of hypotension; therefore nonobstructive mesenteric ischemia represents a failure of normal autoregulatory systems.[2,5,6] Patients with chronic renal failure may have bowel ischemia after hemodialysis, likely from hypoperfusion that promotes a preferential shunting of blood from the splanchnic circulation to preserve flow to the cardiac and cerebrovascular systems.

Although acute mesenteric vein thrombosis accounts for a small portion of ischemic bowel disease cases (5%-10%), the ease of diagnosis with computed tomography (CT) has allowed for identification of a greater number of patients with vein thrombosis. Symptoms are even less specific than those of arterial obstruction and manifest over a longer time before bowel infarction. Thrombus due to hypercoagulable states develops first in the smaller vessels, later progressing into the larger veins; clots caused by cirrhosis, neoplasm, or local injury (operative, trauma) start at the site of obstruction and evolve peripherally.[4]

Anatomy

The celiac artery arises anteriorly from the abdominal aorta at the level of the 12th thoracic vertebra. The celiac artery branches into the common hepatic, splenic, and left gastric arteries. These vessels supply their corresponding organs with significant redundancies, so ischemia to these areas is rare.

The SMA comes off the aorta 1 cm below the celiac artery and terminates as the ileocolic artery. This latter vessel supplies the majority of the blood delivered to the small intestine as well as some flow to the pancreas, right colon, and transverse colon.

The IMA originates from the aorta 7 cm distal to the SMA. It provides blood to the distal transverse colon, descending colon, and rectum.

There is a significant array of collateral blood vessels and flow patterns. The small intestine is especially vulnerable to ischemia, however, because the terminal arterioles enter the intestinal wall without collateral pathways.[4] Splanchnic blood flow requirements vary continuously but can account for up to 35% of cardiac output.

Venous drainage of the system occurs via the superior mesenteric vein (SMV), which empties into the portal vein.

Clinical Presentation

■ CLASSIC PRESENTATION

Soon after ischemia begins, patients present with severe abdominal pain that is clearly out of proportion to the physical findings, which consist of a soft abdomen that is not tender to palpation. The description and location of pain vary over time. As the disease progresses, infarction develops and symptoms may temporarily remit. Over the next several hours, bowel necrosis leads to signs of peritonitis: The abdomen becomes rigid, distended, and very painful, with decreased bowel sounds. The intestinal mucosa begins to slough, and rectal bleeding occurs. The stool contains occult blood in 60% of patients. The bowel may perforate, as signaled by findings of hypotension and sepsis.

Clues to the diagnosis of various ischemic bowel diseases are as follows:

- Acute abdominal pain followed by a rapid and forceful evacuation of the bowels (vomiting or diarrhea) strongly suggests an embolic phenomenon in the SMA.
- Long-standing abdominal pain (weeks to months), which is then followed by acute worsening, suggests intestinal angina and SMA thrombosis.
- Patients with risk factors for nonobstructive mesenteric ischemia may present with unexplained

Documentation

- Onset, severity, and duration of symptoms
- Presence of melena or hematochezia
- Risk factors
- Vital signs
- Findings of cardiac, full abdominal, genitourinary, and rectal examinations
- ED course: times of discussions with consultants, discussions with family, availability of testing, treatments, delays

RED FLAGS

- Pain out of proportion to physical findings
- Pain not responsive to narcotics
- Rectal bleeding (late finding)

abdominal distention or gastrointestinal bleeding; pain is totally absent in up to 25% of these patients, and unexplained distention may herald infarction.

- A patient with a history of deep venous thrombosis is at risk for SMV thrombosis, which tends to develop less acutely than other causes of ischemia, with a presentation over several days.[4]
- Bowel ischemia promotes acidosis, lethargy, and confusion in the elderly; altered mental status complicates up to 30% of cases.

■ VARIATIONS IN PRESENTATION

In patients with nonobstructive mesenteric ischemia, there are variations in the severity and location of pain, which complicate early diagnosis. A heightened level of suspicion is necessary for patients with significant risk factors.

Mesenteric vein thrombosis may be totally asymptomatic and may be diagnosed as an incidental finding in patients undergoing CT of the abdomen for reasons other than abdominal pain. Blockage of the inferior mesenteric arteries may be silent owing to adequate collateral circulation.

Patients with mesenteric atherosclerosis may present with symptoms of abdominal angina, classically manifested as postprandial pain. As a result, the patient develops fear of eating, early satiety, weight loss, and altered bowel habits. This syndrome occurs in up to 50% of patients who eventually have thrombotic mesenteric ischemia.[2]

Differential Diagnosis

Few diagnoses portend a more serious course and risk of mortality than mesenteric ischemia. Patients at risk for ischemia are generally also at risk for aortic disease. Other items in the differential diagnosis are listed in Box 29-1.

BOX 29-1

Differential Diagnosis for Ischemic Bowel Disease, Listed in Order of Urgency

Abdominal aortic aneurysm: rupture or expansion
Perforated ulcer or viscus
Ruptured ectopic pregnancy (woman of childbearing age)
Incarcerated or strangulated hernia
Septic shock
Intussusception
Volvulus
Salpingitis or tubo-ovarian abscess
Torsion of ovary or testicle
Appendicitis
Pelvic mass or torsion
Pancreatitis
Diverticulitis
Ruptured ovarian cyst
Renal colic
Biliary colic
Also consider atypical presentations for:
- Inferior wall myocardial infarction
- Pulmonary embolism
- Pneumonia
- Diabetic ketoacidosis
- Acute glaucoma

Diagnostic Testing

■ ANGIOGRAPHY

Mesenteric angiography provides direct visualization of the vasculature and is the preferred method of evaluation for the patient with suspected bowel ischemia (Table 29-3).[4] Angiography is both sensitive (74%-100%) and specific (100%); the test also differentiates between occlusive and nonocclusive disease. Patients who undergo angiography in a timely fashion have better survival; mortality rates of 70% to 90% are observed when bowel infarction has occurred.[4]

Angiography allows for administration of thrombolytic or vasodilatory therapy concomitant with the diagnostic procedure, thereby improving mortality. The diagnostic and therapeutic advantages of angiography should be weighed against concerns for dye administration in patients susceptible to renal insufficiency, availability of an interventional radiologist, stability of the patient, and delays in surgical intervention (Fig. 29-1).

Tips and Tricks

- Suspect the disease, especially in the elderly.
- Do not delay obtaining imaging or consultations by waiting for laboratory test results.
- Rectal findings are often normal.
- Elevated serum amylase value may suggest bowel infarction, *not* pancreatitis.

Table 29-3 ANGIOGRAPHY FINDINGS IN ISCHEMIC BOWEL DISEASE

Disease	Findings
Superior mesenteric artery (SMA) embolus	Filling defect(s) with obstruction of distal flow Secondary vasoconstriction
Nonobstructive mesenteric ischemia	Narrowing of the origins of the SMA branches Irregularities in SMA branches Spasm of the mesenteric arcades Impaired filling of the intramural vessels
SMA thrombus	Occlusion of the proximal SMA Secondary distal vasoconstriction Absence of collateral flow
Superior mesenteric vein (SMV) thrombus	Thrombus, with partial or complete occlusion Failure to visualize the SMV or portal vein Slowness or absence of filling of the mesenteric veins Failure of the arterial arcades to empty Prolonged blush in the involved segment

Data from Burns BJ, Brandt LJ: Intestinal ischemia. Gastroenterol Clin North Am 2003;32:1127-1143.

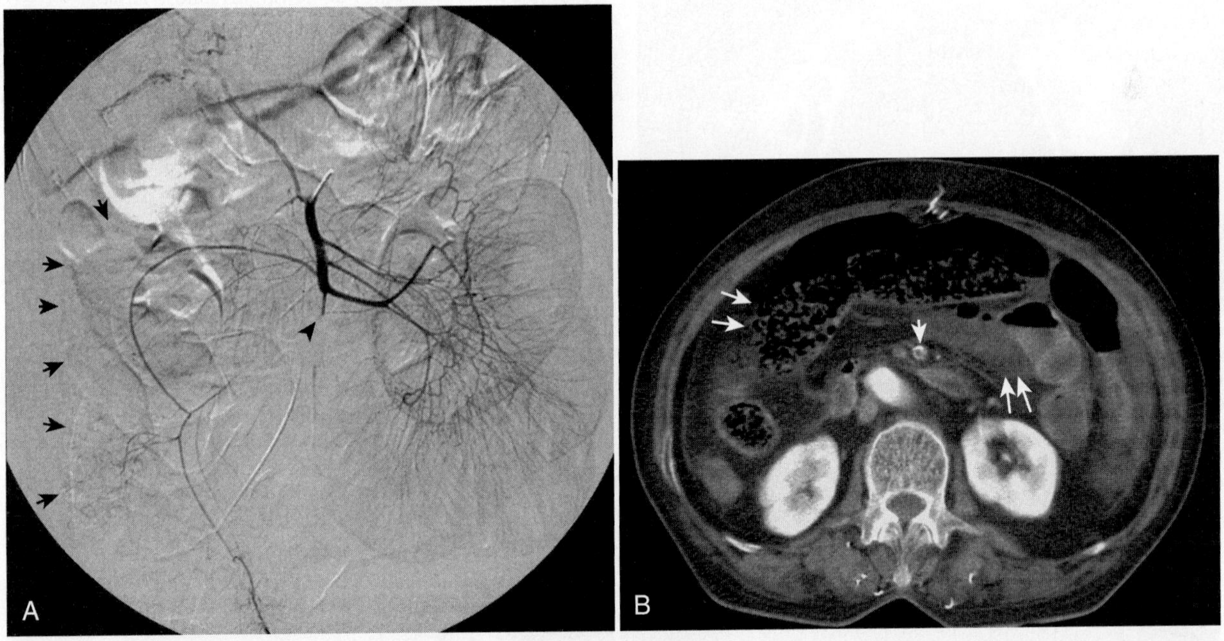
A
B

FIGURE 29-1 Acute intestinal infarction in a patient with a history of atrial fibrillation. **A,** Selective superior mesenteric artery (SMA) angiogram demonstrates abrupt cutoff of the vessel (*arrowhead*), indicating occlusion of the vessel by an embolus, and poor perfusion of the affected small bowel loop (*arrows*). **B,** Small embolus in the SMA (*thick arrow*) is easily detected on the arterial phase of contrast-enhanced computed tomography. Note poor perfusion of affected bowel wall (*thin arrows*), suggesting bowel necrosis. (From Kim AY, Ha HK: Evaluation of suspected mesenteric ischemia: Efficacy of radiologic studies. Radiol Clin North Am 2003;41:327-342.)

With the exception of CT scans for suspected mesenteric vein thrombosis, all other imaging tests are fraught with error and diagnostic delays. CT should not be considered an alternative to angiography for the definitive diagnosis of mesenteric ischemia. It is reasonable to obtain a CT scan while awaiting the arrival of a surgeon and interventional radiologist, but such testing and consultation should be arranged in parallel rather than after CT.

■ COMPUTED TOMOGRAPHY

Early CT findings of acute arterial ischemia are poorly sensitive and nonspecific; late findings identify disease in cases of prolonged ischemia and likely necrosis (Table 29-4; Figs. 29-2 through 29-6). CT is the imaging test of choice only for mesenteric vein thrombosis, for which it has a diagnostic accuracy of 90%.[4] Angiography may be avoided when the diag-

Table 29-4 COMPUTED TOMOGRAPHY FINDINGS IN ISCHEMIC BOWEL DISEASE

Disease	Findings
Arterial ischemia:	
Early	Bowel wall thickening Luminal dilation Pneumatosis
Late	Mesenteric and portal venous gas
Mesenteric vein thrombosis	Lack of opacification of the mesenteric veins after intravenous administration of contrast agent Central lucency in superior mesenteric vein lumen Congestion of collateral veins Thickened mesentery Bowel wall thickening

Data from Burns BJ, Brandt LJ: Intestinal ischemia. Gastroenterol Clin North Am 2003;32:1127-1143.

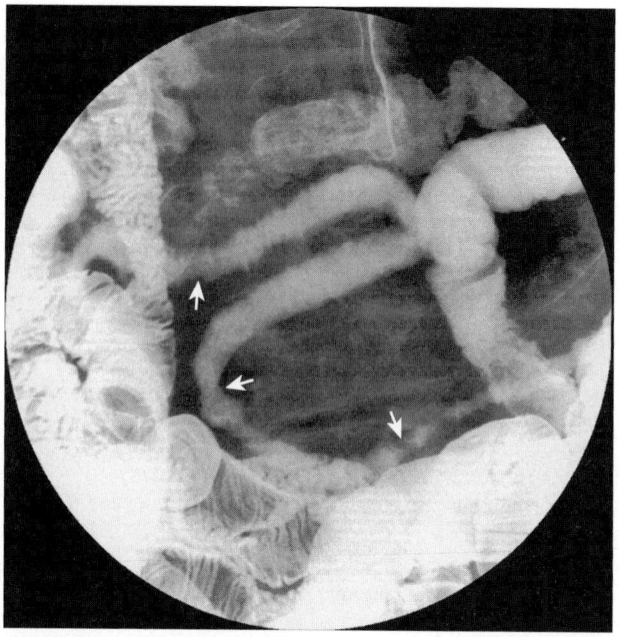

FIGURE 29-3 Barium study of intestinal ischemia. Spot film from a small bowel series demonstrates diffuse luminal narrowing of distal small intestine with prominent thickening of the valvulae conniventes and shallow thumbprinting (*arrows*) in a patient with superior mesenteric vein thrombosis. These findings disappeared after conservative treatment. (From Kim AY, Ha HK: Evaluation of suspected mesenteric ischemia: Efficacy of radiologic studies. Radiol Clin North Am 2003;41:327-342.)

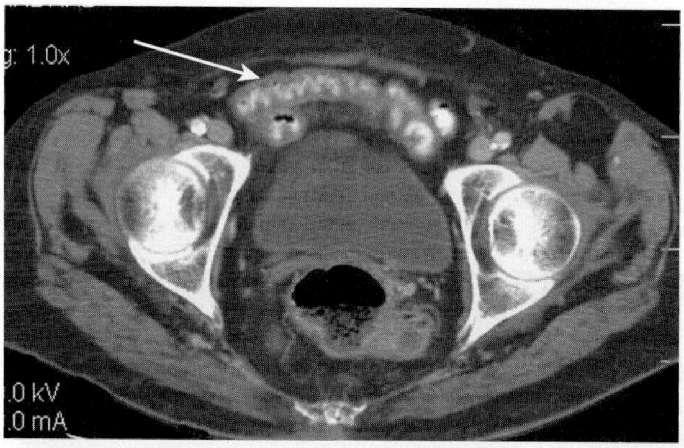

FIGURE 29-2 Pneumatosis intestinalis. Computed tomography scan shows intramural gas in the bowel wall caused by bowel infarction from a superior mesenteric artery embolus. (From Hendrickson M, Narpast TR: Abdominal surgical emergencies in the elderly. Emerg Med Clin North Am 2003;21:937-969.)

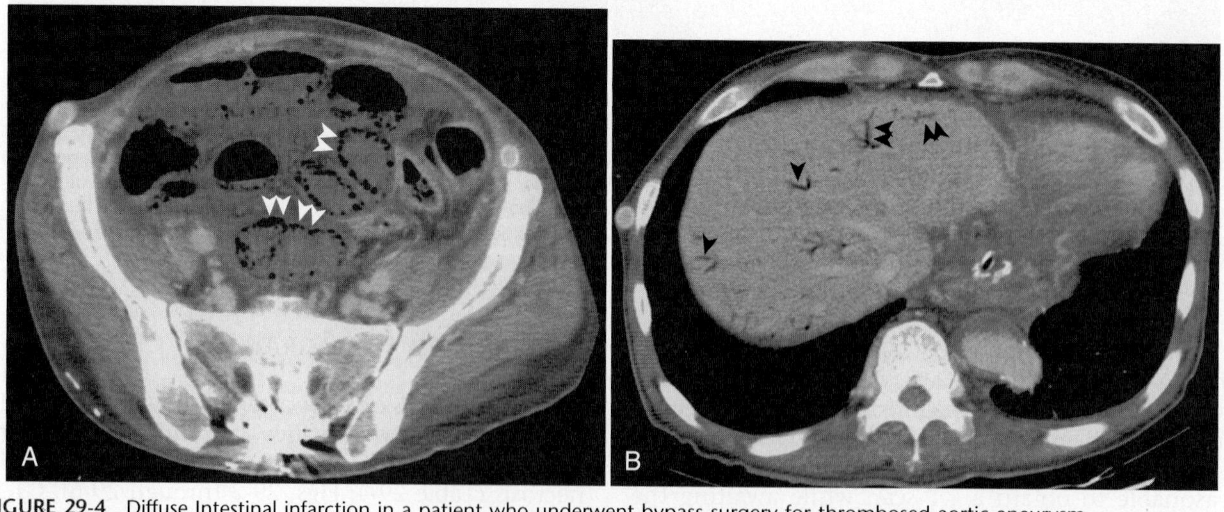
A
B

FIGURE 29-4 Diffuse Intestinal infarction in a patient who underwent bypass surgery for thrombosed aortic aneurysm. **A,** Extensive pneumatosis (*arrowheads*) of the small bowel, both linear and cystic in appearance, is well visualized on computed tomography scan. **B,** Branching pattern of gas in the periphery of the liver is demonstrated in intrahepatic portal veins. (From Kim AY, Ha HK: Evaluation of suspected mesenteric ischemia: Efficacy of radiologic studies. Radiol Clin North Am 2003;41:327-342.)

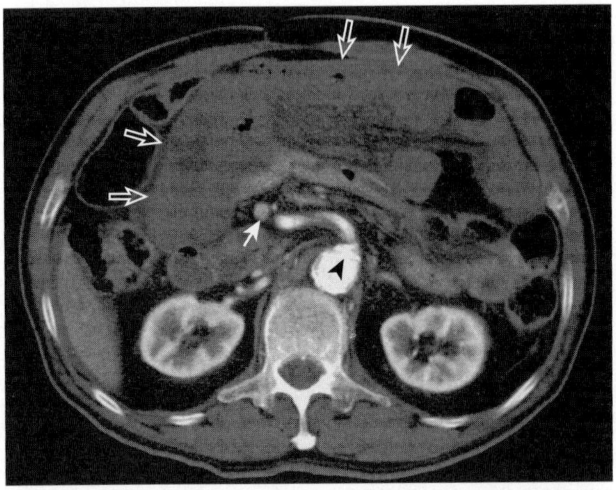

FIGURE 29-5 Diffuse intestinal infarction in an 80-year-old man with sudden onset of abdominal pain. Contrast-enhanced computed tomography scan shows diffuse bowel wall thickening of the small intestine with obvious lack of enhancement (*open arrows*). Completely occluded proximal superior mesenteric artery (*solid white arrow*) and calcified vascular plaques near its origin site (*black arrowhead*) are also seen. (From Kim AY, Ha HK: Evaluation of suspected mesenteric ischemia: Efficacy of radiologic studies. Radiol Clin North Am 2003;41:327-342.)

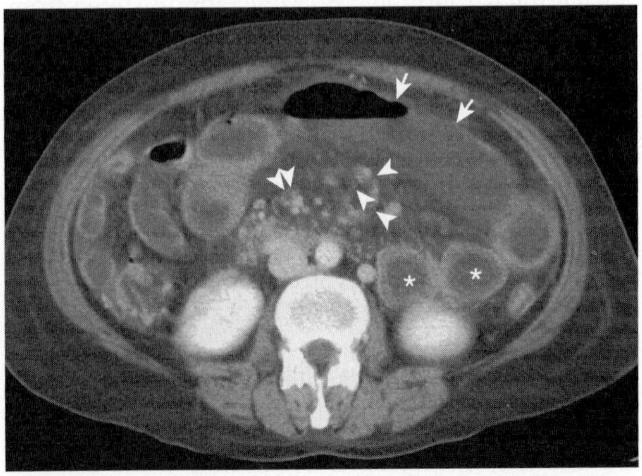

FIGURE 29-6 Intestinal infarction resulting from superior mesenteric vein (SMV) thrombosis. Contrast-enhanced computed tomography scan shows multiple thrombi in tributaries of the SMV (*black arrowheads*) and prominent engorgement of mesenteric vessels. Distended small bowel loops present mural stratification (target sign, indicated by *asterisks* [*]) with poor enhancement of affected bowel (*white arrows*), which were surgically confirmed to be transmural hemorrhagic infarction. (From Kim AY, Ha HK: Evaluation of suspected mesenteric ischemia: Efficacy of radiologic studies. Radiol Clin North Am 2003;41:327-342.)

nosis of SMV thrombosis is confirmed by CT, although catheter placement may be required for purposes of papaverine infusion.

■ OTHER IMAGING MODALITIES

Magnetic resonance angiography (MRA) with gadolinium enhancement is useful for the evaluation of the

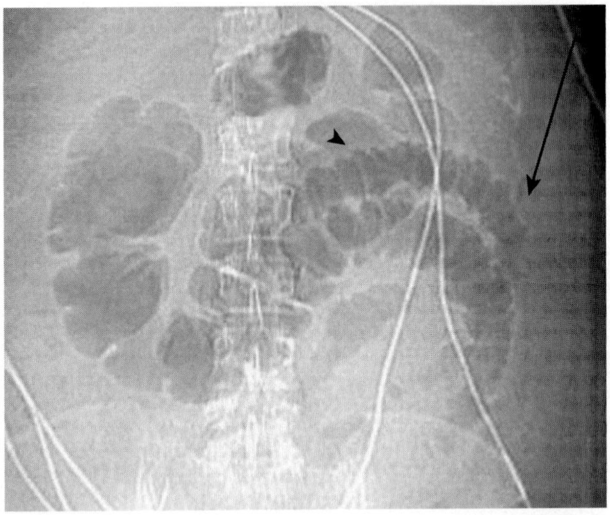

FIGURE 29-7 Thumbprinting in patient who had superior mesenteric vein thrombosis and bowel ischemia (*arrowhead*). Normal concave pattern of the small bowel; convex thumbprinting with wall thickening (*long arrow*). (From Hendrickson M, Narpast TR: Abdominal surgical emergencies in the elderly. Emerg Med Clin North Am 2003; 21: 937-969.)

proximal celiac trunk and SMA. MRA less accurately identifies disease of the IMA, peripheral vessel disease, and nonobstructive mesenteric ischemia. Findings are similar to those of CT. In the future, rapid MRA may replace angiography for the diagnosis of ischemic bowel disease.

Duplex ultrasonography can assess flow in the SMA and detect thrombosis there or in the portal vein. Ultrasonography is frequently limited by the patient's symptoms, condition, and abdominal distention. It is accurate only for the evaluation of proximal vessel disease; false-negative results are common in cases of nonobstructive mesenteric ischemia or distal disease.[4]

Plain radiographs have no role in the evaluation of acute ischemic disease. Plain film findings are usually normal early in the course of illness. Late findings suggest mucosal edema and hemorrhage, including bowel wall thickening, ileus, and thumbprinting (Fig. 29-7). Thumbprinting describes the appearance of the bowel wall, from edema, as if a thumb had been pressed into it, causing an indentation. Pneumatosis intestinalis, the presence of gas in the bowel wall, may also be seen. Late findings are associated with a poor prognosis.

Laboratory Studies

No laboratory studies are confirmatory for mesenteric ischemia. Delaying diagnostic imaging by waiting for laboratory results decreases survival.

Laboratory abnormalities are nonspecific and occur late in disease (Box 29-2); their absence in no way rules out acute ischemia.[4,7,9]

A serum amylase elevation is commonly noted with bowel infarction, sometimes leading to an incorrect diagnosis of pancreatitis. The EP should beware

BOX 29-2

Laboratory Abnormalities of Late-Stage Mesenteric Ischemia

Leukocytosis (white blood cell count >15,000 cells/mm^3)
Metabolic acidemia
Elevated serum lactate
Elevated D-dimer
Elevated serum and peritoneal amylase (with normal lipase)
Bacteremia

Data from references 4, 6, 9.

of the presence of an amylase elevation when the serum lipase value is normal.

Treatment

Early surgical and interventional radiology consultation is a high priority in the patient with suspected mesenteric ischemia. Initial ED management should include volume resuscitation, treatment of contributing cardiac abnormalities (dysrhythmias, heart failure, hypotension), and administration of broad-spectrum antibiotics. Antibiotic administration decreases the infectious complications of bowel infarction when given early in suspected ischemia.[4]

Blood tests, radiographs, and CT may be ordered to exclude other etiologies during the wait for surgical consultation and angiography. Placement of a nasogastric tube reduces abdominal distention and may improve symptoms; nothing should be given by mouth. Placement of a Foley catheter allows monitoring of urinary output. Blood typing and cross-matching should be performed, with the expectation that the patient will undergo surgery. Central venous pressure monitoring may be useful to ensure adequate volume resuscitation in the critically ill patient.

Surgical exploration is mandatory when peritonitis is present, to remove necrotic bowel and restore blood flow via arterial bypass or embolectomy. A "second-look" procedure is generally performed 12 to 24 hours after the first operation to evaluate for additional bowel loss.

PRIORITY ACTIONS

- Administer intravenous hydration, oxygen, and antibiotics.
- Apply telemetry monitoring and obtain electrocardiogram.
- Consider early angiography and surgical consultation.

PATIENT TEACHING TIPS

- The EP should have an early discussion with the patient and family regarding severity of illness, need for aggressive approach to diagnosis and treatment
- Determine the patient's and the family's desive for full resuscitation efforts given the mortality rate

When peritonitis is not present, thrombolytic agents and administration of vasodilators (papaverine) are useful measures that may avoid surgery. Thrombolytics given within 12 hours of the onset of symptoms may completely resolve a partially obstructing or distal thrombus.

Vasospasm may become irreversible if not addressed early, leading to bowel necrosis even after surgical embolectomy or thrombolysis. Papaverine is infused for vasodilation via the angiography catheter at 30 to 60 mg/hr, for all causes of ischemic bowel disease. Papaverine is routinely and safely administered from the preoperative period to several days after surgery. Vasodilation may be used as monotherapy in patients with minor emboli or those who have major emboli but for whom surgery poses a high risk. Reperfusion of vascular structures distal to the obstruction must be demonstrated by angiography.

The placement of intravascular stents has demonstrated some success in selected cases of SMA thrombosis. Mesenteric vein thrombectomy is similarly useful in certain cases of mesenteric vein thrombosis.

Anticoagulation is routinely administered postoperatively to patients with mesenteric vein thrombosis. Immediate heparinization after surgery decreases the chance of thrombus recurrence from 25% to 13%, prevents disease progression, and reduces mortality from 50% to 13%.[8]

In patients with mesenteric vein thrombosis and no signs of peritonitis, anticoagulation may be attempted in lieu of surgery. If deemed successful after close observation, anticoagulation therapy is generally continued for 3 to 6 months.

Disposition

Critical care admission is required for all patients with ischemic bowel disease, regardless of whether they are to receive surgical or medical management.

REFERENCES

1. Boley SJ, Brandt LJ, Sammartano RJ: History of mesenteric ischemia: The evolution of a diagnosis and management. Surg Clin North Am 1997;77:275-288.

2. Klempnauer J, Grothues E, Bektas H, et al: Long term results after surgery for acute mesenteric ischemia. Surgery 1997;121:239-243.
3. Bugliosi TF, Meloy TD, Vukov LF: Acute abdominal pain in the elderly. Ann Emerg Med 1990;19:1383-1386.
4. Burns BJ, Brandt LJ: Intestinal ischemia. Gastroenterol Clin North Am 2003;32:1127-1143.
5. Sudhakar CB, Al-Hakeem M, McArthur JD, et al: Mesenteric ischemia secondary to cocaine abuse: Case reports and literature review. Am J Gastroenterol 1997;92:1053-1054.
6. Diamond S, Emmett M, Henrich WL: Bowel infarction as a cause of death in dialysis patients. JAMA 1986;256: 2545-2547.
7. Sanson TG, O'Keefe KP: Evaluation of abdominal pain in the elderly. Emerg Med Clin North Am 1996;14:615-627.
8. Grieshop RJ, Dalsing MC, Cikrit DF, et al: Acute mesenteric vein thrombosis: Revisited in a time of diagnostic clarity. Am Surg 1992;57:573.
9. Martinez JP, Hogan GJ: Mesenteric ischemia. Emerg Med Clin North Am 2004;22:909-928.
10. Hendrickson M, Narpast TR: Abdominal surgical emergencies in the elderly. Emerg Med Clin North Am 2003;21: 937-969.
11. Kim AY, Ha HK: Evaluation of suspected mesenteric ischemia: Efficacy of radiologic studies. Radiol Clin North Am 2003;41:327-342.

Chapter **30**

Diverticulitis

Kelly P. O'Keefe and Tracy G. Sanson

KEY POINTS

- Diverticulitis is an acute inflammatory process due to injury and bacterial proliferation in an existing diverticulum.
- Patients with diverticular disease may present to the ED with inflammation manifested as abdominal pain or, less commonly, with hematochezia.
- Diverticulitis without evidence of peritonitis may be treated outside the hospital.
- Perforation of a diverticulum or abscess formation must always be considered in patients who exhibit peritoneal findings on examination.
- Surgical consultation is required in cases of peritonitis or significant hematochezia.

Definitions

A *diverticulum* is a saclike protrusion from the wall of the intestines that commonly occurs in the large bowel; *diverticula* is the plural form. *Diverticulosis* connotes the presence of diverticula. *Diverticulitis* refers to a symptomatic inflammatory process involving these structures, which may be characterized as simple (uncomplicated) or complicated. Diverticular hemorrhage is a complication that usually occurs without evidence of inflammatory changes and represents the most common cause of massive lower gastrointestinal bleeding.

Scope

The prevalence of diverticulosis is related to age, ranging from 5% at 40 years to 65% by 85 years. Approximately 70% of patients with diverticula are asymptomatic, while the remainder of patients experience at least one major complication. Twenty percent have diverticulitis and 10% have episodes of bleeding from their diverticula.[1] Diverticulitis accounts for 6% of ED visits for acute abdominal pain in the elderly, occurring more frequently than appendicitis in this age group.[2]

FACTS AND FORMULAS

65% of patients age 85 or older have diverticular disease

Pathophysiology

▪ DIVERTICULOSIS

Diverticula are thought to arise from defects in the muscularis layer of the intestines (Fig. 30-1). Abnormalities in muscle tone and in response to intestinal stimulation result in shortening of the bowel, increased intraluminal pressures, and the eventual development of saclike protrusions at points of weak-

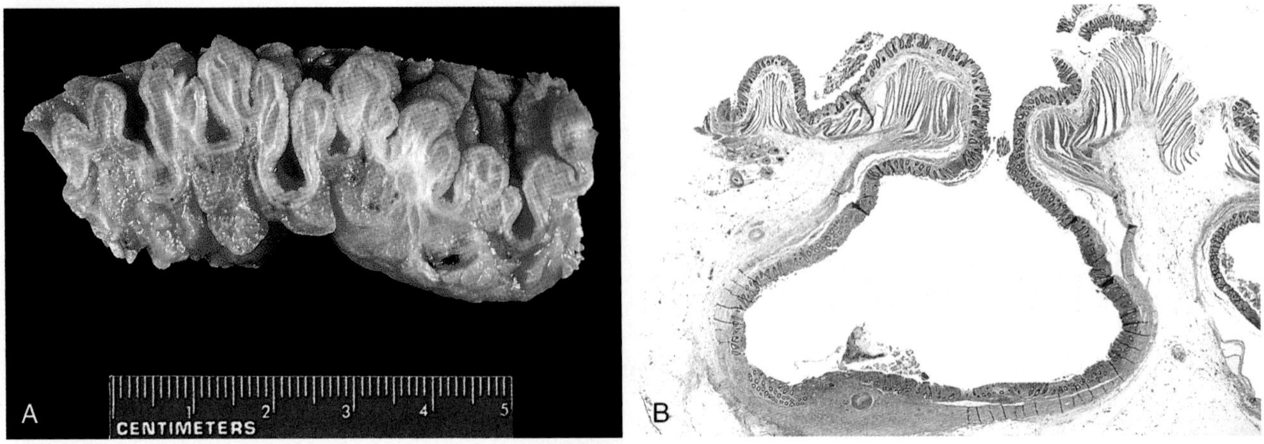
A
CENTIMETERS
1
2
3
4
5
B

FIGURE 30-1 Diverticulosis. **A,** Section through the sigmoid colon, showing multiple saclike diverticula protruding through the muscle wall into the mesentery. The muscularis propria in between the diverticular protrusions is markedly thickened. **B,** Low-power photomicrograph of diverticulum of the colon, showing protrusion of mucosa and submucosa through the muscle wall. A dilated blood vessel at the base of the diverticulum was a source of bleeding; some blood clot is present within the diverticular lumen. (From Kumar V, Fausto N, Abbas A: Robbins & Cotran Pathologic Basis of Disease, 7th ed. Philadelphia, Saunders, 2005.)

ness. If stool is caught in these sacs, it becomes inspissated and hardened, causing abrasions of the mucosa that lead to inflammation. The same process can occur from pressure differentials alone, without the presence of trapped fecal material.

Diverticula generally form at a site of focal weakness in the wall of the bowel, such as the location of blood vessel penetration (vasa recta). Mucosal and submucosal layers herniate through the muscular layer of the intestine, leaving only a covering of serosa. This leads to an inherent weakness in the diverticular sac relative to the normal bowel.[3] Blood vessels that are subject to stretching and thinning of their media become protected only by thinned layers of mucosa, predisposing to weakness and rupture of the vascular tissue.[1]

The left side of the colon is the most common site for diverticulosis in patients with westernized diets and lifestyle. Right-sided diverticula occur more frequently in certain Asian populations. Right-sided diverticula have a higher rate of hemorrhage due to anatomic differences in their development.[4] Small bowel diverticula occur most commonly in the duodenum, where they are predominately asymptomatic. About 20% of small bowel diverticula occur in the jejunum or ileum; these develop complications at rates three times those of duodenal diverticula.[5]

A low-fiber diet and constipation may contribute to the development of diverticular disease. High-fiber diets that prevent constipation clearly lead to fewer relapses of diverticulitis and less frequent complications. A lack of physical activity and advanced age are both believed to increase the incidence of the disease. Men and women are affected equally.[3]

▪ DIVERTICULITIS

Diverticulitis arises from the perforation of a diverticulum (Table 30-1).[6] Damage is initiated by the blockage of the colonic opening of the diverticulum or by direct contact with food and fecal particles lodged in the affected portion of the bowel. Increased intraluminal or direct local pressure causes erosion of the diverticular wall. This leads to inflammatory changes, focal necrosis, and eventual perforation. The process is generally mild and limited by local pericolic fat and mesentery. Virtually all cases of diverticulitis involve a perforation of the intestines, with the course of the resultant illness determined by the extent of this perforation. *Complicated diverticulitis* refers to regional spread of the inflammatory process by the formation of larger abscesses, fistula with adjacent organs, or peritonitis (Fig. 30-2).[1,6,7] Patients with purulent peritonitis have a mortality rate of 6%, which rises to 35% when fecal soilage of the peritoneal cavity occurs.[7] Patients with diverticular disease occasionally have segmental colitis of the sigmoid colon, likely from fecal stasis or localized ischemia. The effects can be mild or may resemble those of inflammatory bowel disease.[1]

Table 30-1 CLASSIFICATION OF SEVERITY OF COLONIC DIVERTICULITIS

Stage	Definition
1	Small, confined pericolic abscesses
2	Larger purulent collections
3	Generalized suppurative peritonitis
4	Fecal peritonitis

Adapted from Hinchey EG, Schaal PGH, Richards GK: Treatment of perforated diverticular disease of the colon. Adv Surg 1978;85-109.

Presenting Signs and Symptoms

The classic presentation of diverticulitis involves several days of worsening left lower quadrant abdominal pain. Low-grade fever commonly develops but is not uniformly present. The patient typically reports

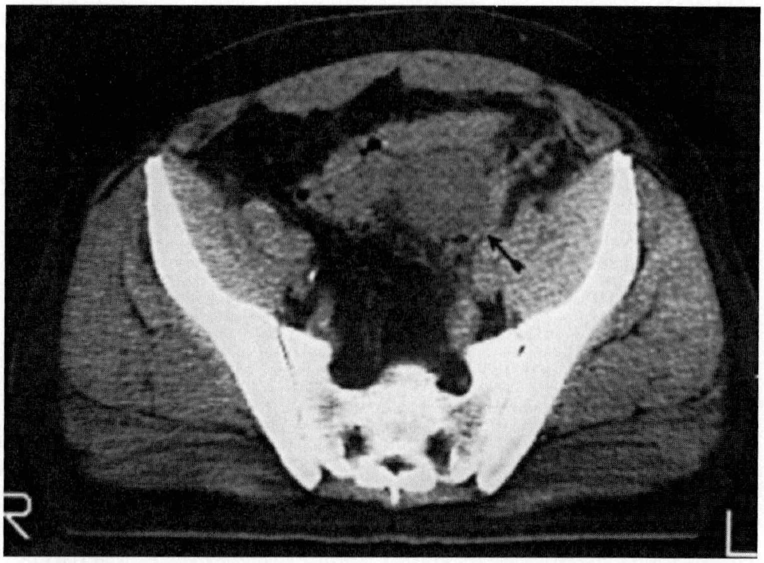
R
L

FIGURE 30-2 A computed tomography scan showing air-filled diverticula in a contracted segment of sigmoid colon lying just anterior to a paracolic abscess, indicated by a circumscribed area of uniform low density (*arrow*). (From Feldman M, Friedman LS, Sleisinger MH, Scharschmidt BF [eds]: Sleisenger & Fordtran's Gastrointestinal and Liver Disease: Pathophysiology/Diagnosis/Management, 7th ed. Philadelphia, Saunders, 2002.)

similar past episodes of pain and fever. Other common symptoms are nausea, vomiting, constipation (50%), and diarrhea (40%). Urinary symptoms (dysuria, urgency, frequency) caused by local inflammation of the bladder occur in only 10% of patients.

Ninety percent of all diverticular fistulas arise from the sigmoid portion of the colon. Classically involved organs are the bladder, vagina, skin, and noncontiguous bowel. Colovesicular fistulas occur more commonly in men than women owing to the interposition of the uterus between the colon and bladder; fistulas involving the ureter or fallopian tubes are unusual.

Intestinal obstruction is a rare complication of diverticular disease and generally arises from the small bowel rather than the large bowel. Obstructions result from chronically diseased bowel and adhesion formation. Recurrent attacks of acute disease can cause strictures and narrowing of the lumen of the colon as well, but subsequent complete obstruction of the large bowel is unusual.

Diverticular bleeding manifests as painless hematochezia that is generally self-limited. The onset can be voluminous, with the blood being maroon or bright red. Bleeding commonly occurs without other signs of inflammation, and therefore, the abdominal findings may be unremarkable. Only 5% of patients with diverticular bleeding present with massive, hemodynamically significant gastrointestinal hemorrhage. These patients are typically older than 60 years and have comorbid conditions.

Complications from diverticulosis of the small bowel are unusual compared with those from disease of the colon. Rarely reported problems include massive gastrointestinal hemorrhage from an arteriovenous malformation located in the submucosa of a jejunal diverticulum, a diverticulum-induced ileoabdominal fistula, and cases of small bowel obstruction and volvulus.[5,8-10]

Duodenal diverticula have been associated with a higher rate of common bile duct stones identified on endoscopic retrograde cholangiopancreatography.[11] This finding may be due to higher rates of bacterial contamination in the biliary system in patients with small bowel diverticula.[12] Rarely, congenital intraluminal diverticula may lead to recurrent abdominal pain and obstructive symptoms.

Jejuno-ileal diverticula occur in 1% of the population and may cause malabsorption from chronic bacterial overgrowth. Other symptoms are early satiety, bloating, and chronic upper abdominal discomfort.[5,13]

RED FLAGS

- Hospitalize patients with signs and symptoms of systemic illness, even without clear peritonitis.
- Consider risk factors for abdominal aortic aneurysm and mesenteric ischemia.
- Rectal findings can be negative or normal in a patient with episodic diverticular bleeding.

Differential Diagnosis

Box 30-1 presents the differential diagnosis for suspicion of diverticulitis.

Diagnostic Testing

■ HISTORY AND PHYSICAL EXAMINATION

A focused history and physical examination are important to making the diagnosis of diverticular disease. Essential historical elements are bowel habits, diet, elucidation of classic symptoms, and prior occurrence. Physical examination should assess for

BOX 30-1

Differential Diagnosis for Suspicion of Diverticulitis

The following diagnoses should be considered in order of urgency, as follows:

- Abdominal aortic aneurysm: rupture or expansion
- Mesenteric ischemia
- Perforated ulcer
- Ruptured ectopic pregnancy
- Incarcerated or strangulated hernia
- Salpingitis, tubo-ovarian abscess
- Ovarian or testicular torsion
- Appendicitis
- Pelvic mass torsion
- Ischemic colitis
- Inflammatory bowel disease
- Pancreatitis
- Ruptured ovarian cyst
- Renal colic
- Biliary colic
- Also, atypical presentations for inferior wall myocardial infarction, pulmonary embolism, pneumonia, diabetic ketoacidosis, and acute glaucoma

hemodynamic stability, the presence of peritonitis, and occult hemorrhage. Complete abdominal, genitourinary, and rectal examinations must be documented.

Fever is often absent in elderly patients, and a rectal temperature may be required for the detection of fever in this population. Dementia, polypharmacy, and other causes of altered mental status may complicate diagnostic accuracy; imaging should be liberally employed in these patients. Signs of peritonitis may be minimal or absent in even the most fully competent and communicative older patient.

Documentation

- Length of symptoms, onset, severity
- Prior occurrence, history of diverticulosis
- Melena or hematochezia
- Risk factors, bowel habits
- Vital signs
- Findings of cardiac, abdominal, genitourinary, rectal, and vascular examinations
- Document multiple repeat examinations
- ED course: times of consultations, discussions with family and consultants, availability of testing, delays
- Document and address other potentially lethal diagnoses (abdominal aortic aneurysm, mesenteric ischemia)

▪ LABORATORY TESTS

Leukocytosis is noted in only half of patients with diverticulitis. The white blood cell count is affected by disease severity, advancing age, and underlying health status; it may not be elevated in elderly patients or the chronically ill. Similarly, hemoglobin levels may not accurately reflect the severity of recent diverticular bleeding. Urinalysis should be performed to evaluate any urinary symptoms; abnormalities may reflect inflammatory changes, infection, or contamination via colovesicular fistula formation. Blood cultures should be obtained with a suspicion of sepsis.

Additional laboratory testing is helpful to exclude other processes. Standard tests for the evaluation of abdominal pain should be ordered when indicated, to include a complete blood count, metabolic panel, liver function tests, and lipase. An elevated serum lipase value should reliably diagnose acute pancreatitis. Typing and crossmatching of blood should be performed in patients with hematochezia or signs of a surgical abdomen. Coagulation tests are also indicated for bleeding patients, for those taking anticoagulant medications, and for critically ill patients at risk for disseminated intravascular coagulopathy. A pregnancy test is required in any woman of childbearing age who complains of abdominal pain.

▪ IMAGING

Plain radiographs of the chest and abdomen are useful to evaluate for the presence of other processes but do not assist in the diagnosis of diverticular disease. Free air is occasionally present in the patient with a perforated diverticulum. Evidence of an ileus or obstruction may be seen in complicated disease.

Computed tomography (CT) of the abdomen and pelvis is the test of choice for confirming the diagnosis of diverticulitis, assessing severity and complications, and directing intervention. CT findings for and complications in diverticular disease are listed in Box 30-2.

Contrast enema studies are less expensive than CT and are better able to evaluate the lumen of the colon. They are generally performed with water-soluble agents rather than barium, given the high likelihood of perforation in diverticulitis. Contrast enema studies provide little information, however, about complications of diverticular disease.

Compression ultrasonography is a relatively new diagnostic procedure for diverticular disease. Ultrasonography may be used to serially assess fluid collections or to assist in the transrectal or transvaginal drainage of abscesses.

BOX 30-2

Computed Tomography (CT) in Diverticulitis

CT Features of Acute Diverticulitis*

Increased soft tissue density with pericolic fat changes (98%)
Colonic diverticula (84%)
Bowel wall thickening (70%)
Soft tissue fluid collections/abscess (35%)

Complications of Diverticulitis Found on CT

Peritonitis (diffuse inflammatory changes, scattered loculated fluid collections)
Fistula formation
Bowel obstruction

Diverticular disease is indistinguishable from carcinoma of the colon in up to 10% of patients.

*Data from Young-Fadok T, Pemberton JH: Clinical manifestations and diagnosis of colonic diverticular disease. UpToDate March 2005. Available at www.uptodate.com/

PRIORITY ACTIONS

- Establish IV access for the management of diverticulitis.
- Obtain pertinent history and examination, including rectal and genitourinary.
- Consider life-threatening conditions in the differential diagnosis.
- Obtain surgical consultation if there is evidence of peritonitis.
- Arrange for radiographic and laboratory analysis.

Colonoscopy and flexible sigmoidoscopy have limited roles in the evaluation of diverticulitis in the acute setting. All patients with diverticulitis should be referred for outpatient colonoscopy when their acute illness has subsided. These modalities allow for direct visualization of the colonic lumen and biopsy of any lesions. Colonoscopy remains an important initial diagnostic procedure for patients with acute diverticular bleeding.

Surgical Consultation

Surgical consultation should be obtained immediately for patients with peritonitis or a vascular catastrophe. Consultants should be notified early in the evaluation of elderly or immunocompromised patients as well as of patients with indications of complicated disease. Twenty-five percent of patients with a new diagnosis of diverticulitis present with complicated disease and require surgical intervention.

BOX 30-3

Antibiotics for Diverticulitis

Antibiotic therapy should be directed against the usual colonic flora, particularly gram-negative rods and anaerobes (particularly *Escherichia coli* and *Bacteroides fragilis*). Suitable regimens are as follows:

Piperacillin-tazobactam
Ticarcillin-clavulanate
Ampicillin, gentamycin, and metronidazole
Imipenem-cilastin
Ampicillin-sulbactam (outpatient)
Quinolone and metronidazole (outpatient)
Sulfamethoxazole-trimethoprim and metronidazole (outpatient)
Cefazolin and metronidazole (outpatient)*

*Clindamycin is an acceptable alternative to metronidazole for the coverage of anaerobes.
Data from Bugliosi TF, Meloy TD, Vukov LF: Acute abdominal pain in the elderly. Ann Emerg Med 1990;19:1383-1386.

Patients with uncomplicated disease may require only follow-up with a surgeon on an outpatient basis. One third of these patients eventually require surgery.[7]

Treatment and Disposition

The majority of patients presenting with acute, uncomplicated diverticulitis show response to bowel rest and antibiotics (Box 30-3).[7] The remaining patients require various levels of intervention, ranging from percutaneous drainage of abscesses to laparoscopic or other surgical procedures. The surgical mortality rate ranges from 1% to 5%, depending on comorbidities and severity of disease.

Fluid resuscitation is needed in patients with dehydration, peritonitis, complicated disease, and significant bleeding. Patients with evidence of peritonitis or other disease complications require surgical consultation and admission.

Patients with uncomplicated diverticulitis can be considered for discharge on the basis of hydration status, ability to tolerate oral fluids, pain level, comorbidities, immune function, home support, age, reliability of follow-up, and ability to obtain antibiotics

Tips and Tricks

- Signs of serious disease/peritonitis may be masked in elderly patients
- Right-sided diverticulitis is often confused with appendicitis
- Patients with signs of localized peritonitis require admission

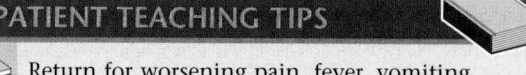

PATIENT TEACHING TIPS

- Return for worsening pain, fever, vomiting, bloody stool
- Treatment of constipation: avoid frequent narcotic use
- Complications of disease: abscess, perforation, fistula, bleeding
- Need for antibiotic treatment
- Complications of pain medications (constipation)
- Dietary considerations: high-fiber diet shown to decrease complications of diverticular disease

and take them as required. Those with high fevers and significant leukocytosis should be admitted because of suspicion of bacteremia or undetected complications. Patients with complex underlying medical diseases should undergo a period of inpatient observation if there is any concern that the disease may progress to perforation or sepsis.

▪ ANALGESIA

Pain medication is necessary in most patients with acute diverticulitis. Narcotic analgesics may slow recovery because they promote constipation; patients should be warned to limit the use of these medicines or use adjunctive bulk laxatives. Patients with significant pain should be admitted. Titration of pain medication should begin in the ED as indicated by the patient's reported pain scale, not based on the timing of examination by the consultant surgeon. Fentanyl is easily titrated in parenteral doses of 25 to 50 μg, is short-acting, and causes minimal histamine release or hemodynamic instability.

▪ OTHER TREATMENT

Bowel rest is a mainstay of treatment for diverticulitis. Patients with complicated disease should take nothing by mouth. Nasogastric decompression should be used in patients with symptomatic ileus. Candidates for outpatient treatment should be restricted to consumption of clear liquids for several days; the diet should be cautiously advanced as tolerated.

REFERENCES

1. Young-Fadok T, Pemberton JH: Clinical manifestations and diagnosis of colonic diverticular disease. UpToDate March 2005. Available at www.uptodate.com/
2. Bugliosi TF, Meloy TD, Vukov LF: Acute abdominal pain in the elderly. Ann Emerg Med 1990;19:1383-1386.
3. Young-Fadok T, Pemberton JH: Epidemiology and pathophysiology of colonic diverticular disease. UpToDate March 2005. Available at www.uptodate.com/
4. Meyers MA, Alonso DR, Gray GF, et al: Pathogenesis of bleeding colonic diverticulosis. Gastroenterology 1976;71: 577-583.
5. Milovic V, Caspary WF, Stein J: Small bowel diverticula. UpToDate Nov 2004. Available at www.uptodate.com/
6. Hinchey EJ, Schaal PGH, Richards GK: Treatment of perforated diverticular disease of the colon. Adv Surg 1978;12:85-109.
7. Young-Fadok T, Pemberton JH: Treatment of acute diverticulitis—1. UpToDate Dec 2004. Available at www.uptodate.com/
8. Chin NW, Lai CLD, Harisiadis SA, et al: Congenital arteriovenous malformation rupturing into a true jejunal diverticulum. Am J Gastroenterol 1989;84:972-974.
9. Eriguchi N, Aoyagi S, Nakayama T, et al: Ileo-abdominal wall fistula caused by a diverticulum of the ileum. J Gastroenterol 1998;33:272-275.
10. Chiu KW, Changchien CS, Chush SIC: Small bowel diverticulum: Is it a risk for small bowel volvulus? J Clin Gastroenterol 1994;19:176-177.
11. Leivonen MK, Halttunen JA, Kivilaakso EO: Duodenal diverticula at endoscopic retrograde cholangiopancreatography: Analysis of 123 patients. Hepatogastroenterology 1996;43:961-966.
12. Miyazawa Y, Okinaga K, Nishida K, et al: Recurrent common bile duct stones associated with periampullary duodenal diverticula and calcium bilirubinate stones. Int Surg 1995;80:120-124.
13. Palder SB, Frey CB: Jejunal diverticulosis. Arch Surg 1988;123:889-894.

Chapter **31**

Inflammatory Bowel Disease

Michael I. Omori and Michael A. Gisondi

KEY POINTS

Acute exacerbations of inflammatory bowel disease are characterized by abdominal pain, nausea, vomiting, diarrhea, and gastrointestinal bleeding.

Life-threatening complications include bowel obstruction, hemorrhagic shock, toxic megacolon, malabsorption, abscess formation, and sepsis.

Treatment with analgesics, intravenous hydration, electrolyte replacement, and antibiotics should occur in parallel with appropriate diagnostic imaging and specialty consultation.

Hypersensitivity reactions can result from long-term immunomodulator and anti-inflammatory therapies.

Scope

Approximately 1 million people in the United States suffer from inflammatory bowel disease (IBD). The two major forms of IBD are Crohn's disease and ulcerative colitis. The incidence of ulcerative colitis remains greater than that of Crohn's disease, though this demographic difference has been lessening in recent decades. Each disease may relapse and remit many times throughout life, inciting exacerbations that often require emergency care and hospitalization.

IBD has a familial predilection, with an absolute risk of 7% among first-degree relatives.[1,2] Up to a fifth of patients with IBD have an affected first-degree family member, whereas spouses of IBD patients rarely have the disease. Ashkenazi Jewish populations continue to have the highest documented incidences per capita of any group in the world.

The age of onset for IBD is bimodal. The greatest numbers of new cases are diagnosed in patients 15 to 35 years of age; classically, a second peak is observed during the sixth decade of life.[3] Advances in diagnostic testing have likely contributed to an overall rise in the number of new cases of IBD as well as to the identification of the disease in younger patients.

Pathophysiology

■ CROHN'S DISEASE

■ Pathology

Crohn's disease is characterized by segmental, transmural, granulomatous inflammatory changes that can occur anywhere along the gastrointestinal tract. Though disease of the terminal ileum is present in the majority of cases, approximately 20% of patients demonstrate only colonic involvement. The finding of "skip lesions" between areas of normal bowel is classic for Crohn's disease, as is "cobblestoning" of the intestinal mucosa. Chronic inflammation commonly leads to bowel stenosis.

■ Epidemiology

The yearly incidence of Crohn's disease is between 1 and 7 cases per 100,000 people in the United States, and between 10 and 100 new cases per 100,000 people worldwide. Women have a 20% to 30% higher incidence than men. Crohn's disease is more common among white and Latino people in the United States than in African Americans, Native Americans, and Asian Americans.

Genetic mutations and chromosomal variants have been linked to the development of Crohn's disease. Specific alterations in the NOD-2 gene are associated with a 20-fold increase in likelihood of Crohn's with ileal predilection.[4-7] Patients with Crohn's disease may be HLA-B27–positive.

The *cold chain hypothesis* suggests that the rise in incidence of Crohn's disease over the last century has been associated with the development of home refrigeration techniques. Bacteria that thrive in refrigerated foods, such as *Yersinia* and *Listeria,* are thought to play a role in the stimulation of immune and inflammatory responses that ultimately lead to Crohn's disease.[8] Exacerbations of Crohn's disease may be worsened during periods of higher physiologic or mental stress.[9]

■ Clinical Presentation

Patients with Crohn's disease typically present with abdominal pain, fever, diarrhea, and weight loss. Perianal abscesses and fistulae are common. Complications include bowel obstruction, fissures, gastrointestinal bleeding, malignancy, malabsorption, malnutrition, and hypocalcemia.

Crohn's disease is associated with an increased risk of demyelinating diseases as well as with higher incidences of inflammatory processes such as asthma, arthritis, bronchitis, psoriasis, and pericarditis.[10,11] Approximately 20% of patients with Crohn's disease experience one or more of the following conditions during their lifetimes: ankylosing spondylitis, uveitis, episcleritis, hepatitis, cholelithiasis, pancreatitis, primary sclerosing cholangitis, cholangiocarcinoma, nephrolithiasis, and erythema nodosum (Fig. 31-1; Box 31-1).

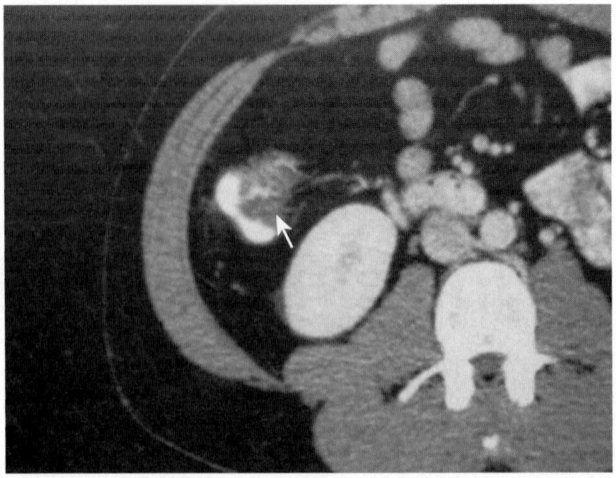

FIGURE 31-1 Computed tomography scan showing terminal ileitis in Crohn's disease.

BOX 31-1

Differential Diagnosis: Colitis

Inflammatory bowel disease:
- Crohn's disease
- Ulcerative colitis
- Indeterminate colitis

Infectious colitis:
- *Shigella*
- *Amoeba*
- *Giardia*
- *Escherichia coli* O157:H7
- *Yersinia*
- *Campylobacter*
- *Entamoeba histolytica*
- Viral infections
- Mycotic infections

Pseudomembranous colitis (*Clostridium difficile*)
- Diverticulitis
- Sarcoidosis
- Tuberculosis

Proctitis (including sexually transmitted etiologies)
- Collagenous colitis
- Food intolerance

■ ULCERATIVE COLITIS

■ Pathology

Ulcerative colitis is an inflammatory disease confined to the mucosal layer of the colon and rectum only. Areas of inflammation are continuous, not segmental; patients commonly experience ascending disease throughout the colon. Isolated rectal involvement is present in a minority of patients.

■ Epidemiology

The yearly incidence of ulcerative colitis in the United States is 8 per 100,000 people, with a disease prevalence of 246 cases per 100,000 people.[12,13] Ulcerative colitis is most commonly found in North American and northern European white populations. The etiology of this disease is unknown.

■ Clinical Presentation

Ulcerative colitis causes bloody, purulent, mucoid diarrhea. Findings of fever, weight loss, dehydration, anemia, and hypoalbuminemia are common. Patients may be categorized as having mild disease (60%), moderate disease (25%), or severe disease (15%). Severe disease is defined as six or more bowel movements per day.

Significant lower gastrointestinal bleeding is the most common complication. Patients may also have

Table 31-1 FEATURES OF CROHN'S DISEASE AND ULCERATIVE COLITIS

Finding	Crohn's Disease	Ulcerative Colitis
Location		
Colonic	Common	Common
Rectal	Common	Common
Extracolonic	Common	Never
Ileal	Common	Never
Presentation		
Fever	Common	Common
Diarrhea	Common	Common
Vomiting	Variable	Occasional
Abdominal pain	Common	Variable
Hematochezia	Variable	Common
Weight loss	Common	Common
Perianal disease	Common	Never
Pathologic Findings		
Continuity	Discontinuous	Continuous
Inflammation	Transmural	Mucosal
Oral ulcers	Variable	Never
Fissures	Common	Never
Fistulas	Variable	Rare
Cobblestoning	Common	Never
Strictures	Common	Rare
Laboratory Findings		
Perinuclease-staining antineutrophil cytoplasmic antibody (p-ANCA) positivity	Uncommon	Common
Anti-*Saccharomyces cerevisiae* antibody (ASCA) positivity	Common	Uncommon

toxic megacolon, a loss of colonic muscular tone that can result in luminal diameters greater than 6 cm.

Patients with ulcerative colitis may also have concurrent arthritis, uveitis, erythema nodosum, pyoderma gangrenosum, and progressive liver disease (Fig. 31-2; Table 31-1).

Diagnostic Testing

■ IMAGING MODALITIES

Most cases of IBD diagnosed in the ED are found through computed tomography (CT) of the abdomen in patients with severe, unexplained abdominal pain. A presumptive diagnosis of IBD can be based on typical CT findings coupled with the appropriate clinical presentation. CT enterography has been shown to have 100% sensitivity and 95% specificity for small bowel lesions associated with Crohn's disease.[14] CT enterography is superior to standard CT of the abdomen and pelvis in patients with a high

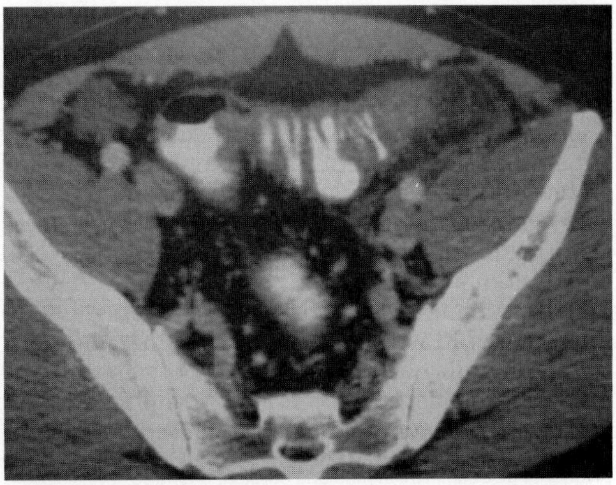

FIGURE 31-2 Computed tomography scan showing colonic wall thickening in ulcerative colitis.

pretest probability of Crohn's disease (i.e., first-degree family members of IBD patients). Confirmation of the diagnosis is made by histologic examination of tissue biopsy specimens obtained through inpatient endoscopy or surgery.

Patients who present to the ED with an exacerbation of known IBD do not always require CT. Plain films are generally sufficient to exclude complications such as bowel obstruction and rare perforations. CT may be used to identify abscesses or other intra-abdominal disease in patients with peritoneal findings or sepsis.

Other imaging modalities are best employed outside the ED. Barium and air-contrast radiographic studies frequently demonstrate classic radiographic evidence of IBD; they are useful tests for obese patients who exceed the weight limit of standard CT scanners. Upper and lower endoscopy allows for direct visualization and biopsy of suspected lesions. Technology that enables patients to swallow tiny endoscopy cameras in capsules (e.g., PillCam) represents a promising, minimally invasive method to visualize bowel mucosa.

■ LABORATORY TESTS

Laboratory studies have limited value in the ED evaluation of IBD. Most tests serve to exclude complications or alternative diagnoses. The complete blood count can provide a baseline hemoglobin level. Leukocytosis is a nonspecific finding in chronic IBD; marked elevations in the white blood cell count may correlate with new abscess formation or sepsis. A serum chemistry panel is needed to exclude hypokalemia and hypocalcemia in patients with severe diarrhea. Liver function tests may be indicated in patients with suspected hepatobiliary processes. Hypoalbuminemia is often present.

Serologic markers may be used to differentiate Crohn's disease from ulcerative colitis. The presence of p-ANCAs (perinuclease-staining antineutrophil cytoplasmic antibodies) is sensitive and predictive for ulcerative colitis, whereas the detection of ASCA (anti-*Saccharomyces cerevisiae* antibodies) markers likely predicts Crohn's disease. These serologic tests are not indicated for use in the ED, but their results may be reported in the medical record as part of a previous outpatient evaluation.

Treatment

■ GENERAL MANAGEMENT

Symptomatic management should occur in parallel with diagnostic testing. Exacerbations of IBD are often marked by significant pain, fever, diarrhea, anorexia and dehydration; symptom severity is pronounced in the patient with chronic disease who presents to the ED. Analgesics, antiemetics, and intravenous hydration should be administered upon the patient's arrival. Nasogastric tube decompression may provide substantial relief. Identification and treatment of electrolyte imbalances, concurrent infections, and blood loss should precede hospital admission.

Immunomodulator, anti-inflammatory, and antibiotic agents should be given in consultation with the patient's gastroenterologist. These medications often require long-term administration and dose adjustments that create complex drug regimens. Treatment algorithms for Crohn's disease and ulcerative colitis are summarized in Figures 31-3 and 31-4.

■ COMMON MEDICATIONS

Sulfasalazine is a first-line oral agent used in the treatment of mild to moderate IBD. Colonic bacteria cleave the drug into 5-aminosalicylic acid (5-ASA) and sulfapyridine. 5-ASA acts directly on intralumi-

Condition	Treatment
Colitis or ileocolitis	Oral 5-ASA drug or metronidazole and/or ciprofloxacin —*Continued activity*→ Prednisone —*Continued activity or steroid dependence*→ Immunomodulator —*Continued activity*→ Surgery or infliximab
Ileitis	Prednisone —*Continued activity*→ Immunomodulator —*Continued activity*→ Surgery or infliximab
Fistula	TPN or immunomodulator or infliximab —*Failure to close*→ Surgery
Abscess	Antibiotics, drainage, and resection
Obstruction due to inflammation	IV fluids, nasogastric suction, parenteral steroids —*Failure to respond*→ Surgery
Obstruction due to scarring	IV fluids, nasogastric suction —*Failure to respond*→ Surgery
Perianal disease	Antibiotics and surgical drainage
Disease in remission	Maintenance with oral 5-ASA drugs or immunomodulators

FIGURE 31-3 Treatment algorithm for Crohn's disease. 5-ASA, 5-aminosalicylic acid; IV, intravenous; TPN, total parenteral nutrition. (From Goldman L, Ausiello D [eds]: Cecil's Textbook of Medicine, 22nd ed. Philadelphia, Saunders, 2003.)

Condition	Treatment
Proctitis	5-ASA enemas or 5-ASA suppositories or oral 5-ASA drugs or corticosteroid enemas —*Continued activity*→ Prednisone or immunomodulators —*Continued activity*→ Colectomy
Mild to moderate pancolitis	Oral 5-ASA drugs —*Continued activity*→ Prednisone —*Continued activity or steroid dependence*→ Immunomodulators or colectomy
Severe or fulminant pancolitis	Parenteral steroids —*Continued activity*→ Cyclosporine or colectomy
Disease in remission	Maintenance with oral 5-ASA drugs

FIGURE 31-4 Treatment algorithm for ulcerative colitis. 5-ASA, 5-aminosalicylic acid. (From Goldman L, Ausiello D [eds]: Cecil's Textbook of Medicine, 22nd ed. Philadelphia, Saunders, 2003.)

nal lesions without systemic absorption. Although the mechanism of action is still unclear, 5-ASA likely inhibits leukocyte chemotaxis as well as prostaglandin and leukotriene production. Sulfapyridine is a toxic byproduct responsible for a variety of dose-related adverse effects (nausea, vomiting, diarrhea, headache, abdominal pain, arthralgias) and hypersensitivity reactions (rash, bone marrow suppression, fever, pancreatitis, liver disease, nephrotoxicity). Sulfasalazine at doses of 4 g or more per day should produce a clinical response within 2 to 4 weeks. Oral, enema, and suppository preparations are available.

Oral steroids improve mild to moderate IBD symptoms within days to weeks. Prednisone 40 mg/day is an acceptable starting dose; equivalent parenteral administration should be reserved for severe disease or for patients who cannot tolerate oral medications. Long-term corticosteroid therapy at a low maintenance dose is often required. Patients with small bowel obstruction due to terminal ileitis may have a response to early treatment with steroids, reducing the need for surgical intervention (Fig. 31-5).

Patients with Crohn's disease can benefit from maintenance therapy with azathioprine or its active metabolite, 6-mercaptopurine (6-MP). These immunomodulator drugs inhibit lymphocytic proliferation and the subsequent activation of inflammatory cascades. Onset of action is 3 to 5 months in most cases. Adverse effects include pancreatitis, leukopenia, hepatitis, and lymphoma.

Infliximab (Remicade) is an inhibitor of tumor necrosis factor that is administered intravenously for the control of severe, refractory Crohn's disease. Complications of infliximab therapy are sepsis, hepatotoxicity, pneumonia, lupus-like syndrome, hypersensitivity reactions, lymphoma, leukopenia, and demyelinating disease. Infliximab, as well as cyclosporine, may be beneficial in the treatment of patients awaiting surgical intervention.

Antibiotics are sometimes needed to treat infectious perianal disease in patients with Crohn's disease. The utility of these agents in ulcerative colitis is unproven. Metronidazole and ciprofloxacin are most commonly used.

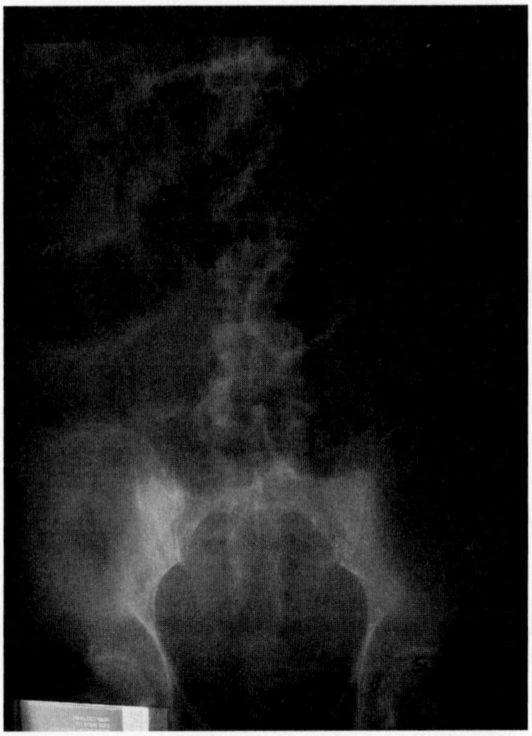

FIGURE 31-5 Plain radiograph showing small bowel obstruction due to terminal ileitis.

■ SURGERY

Seventy-five percent of patients with Crohn's disease require surgery within the first 20 years of initial diagnosis. Urgent surgical consultation is indicated for patients presenting to the ED with severe exacerbations of IBD. Emergency consultation should be obtained for patients with suspected life-threatening complications, including abscess formation, obstruction, and perforation. Intravenous hydration, nasogastric decompression, and broad-spectrum antibiotic therapy should be given in preparation for surgery.

Disposition

Hospital admission is required for moderate to severe exacerbations of IBD. Patients with systemic infection or potentially life-threatening complications must be managed as inpatients. Discharge should be reserved for patients with mild disease in whom oral hydration and pain control are easily attained. Medication changes and disposition should be decided in consultation with a gastroenterologist.

REFERENCES

1. Tysk C, Lindberg E, Jarnerot G, Floderus-Myrhed B: Ulcerative colitis and Crohn's disease in an unselected population of monozygotic and dizygotic twins: A study of heritability and the influence of smoking. Gut 1988,29: 990-996.
2. Orholm M, Munkholm P, Langhoz E, et al: Familial occurrence of inflammatory bowel disease. N Engl J Med 1991;324:84-88.
3. Ekbom A, Helmick C, Zack M, Adami HO: The epidemiology of inflammatory bowel disease: A large, population-based study in Sweden. Gastroenterology 1991;100: 350-358.
4. Satsangi J, Welsh KI, Bunce M, et al: Contribution of genes of the major histocompatibility complex to susceptibility and disease phenotype in inflammatory bowel disease. Lancet 1996;347:1212-1217.
5. Satsangi J, Parkes M, Louis E, et al: A genome-wide search identifies potential new susceptibility loci for Crohn's disease. Inflam Bowel Dis 199;5:271-278.
6. Hugo JP, Laurent-Pig P, Gower-Rousseau C, et al: Mapping of a susceptibility locus for Crohn's disease. Inflam Bowel Dis 1999;5:271-278.
7. Hugot JP, Chamaillard M, Zomali H, et al: Association of NOD 2 leucine-rich repeat variants with susceptibility to Crohn's disease. Nature 2001;411:599-603.
8. Hugot JP, Alberti C, Berrebi D, et al: Crohn's disease: The cold chain hypothesis.
9. Vidal A, Gómez-Gil E, Sans M, et al: Life events and inflammatory bowel disease relapse: A prospective study of patients enrolled in remission. Am J Gastroenterol 2006;101:1-7.
10. Gupta G, Gelfand JM, Lewis JD: Increased risk for demyelinating diseases in patients with inflammatory bowel disease. Gastroenterology 2005;129:819-826.
11. Bernstein CN, Wajda A, Blanchard JF: The clustering of other chronic inflammatory diseases in inflammatory bowel disease: A population-based study. Gastroenterology 2005;129:827-836.
12. Loftus EV, Silverstein MD, Sandborn WJ, et al: Ulcerative colitis in Olmsted County, Minnesota, 1940-1993: Incidence, prevalence, and survival. Gut 2000;46:336-343.
13. Loftus EV: Clinical epidemiology of inflammatory bowel disease: Incidence, prevalence, and environmental influences. Gastroenterology 2004;126:1504-1517.
14. Boudiaf M, Jaff A, Soyer P, et al: Small-bowel diseases: Prospective evaluation of multi-detector row helical ct enteroclysis in 107 consecutive patients: CT enteroclysis is a fast, well-tolerated, and reliable imaging modality for the depiction of small-bowel diseases. Radiology 2004;233: 338-344.

Chapter 32

Constipation

Kathleen Schrank

KEY POINTS

In most patients, constipation has an idiopathic, nonemergent cause that is treatable and is often related to lifestyle habits such as dietary fiber intake, fluid intake, and toileting.

The treatment goal consists of initial cleansing, a maintenance plan, and preventive lifestyle changes.

A wide range of dangerous conditions can mimic constipation, such as bowel obstruction.

A wide range of underlying conditions, such as malignancy, can cause constipation, so primary care follow-up is needed.

An osmotic agent is a proper first-line treatment choice, followed by stimulant use if needed.

Although there is an age-related increase in incidence, constipation is common at all ages, with a reported prevalence ranging from 2% to 27%,[1] depending on the definition used. Of greatest concern to the EP is the patient with *acute onset of symptoms, severe pain, vomiting, fever, gastrointestinal bleeding, significant weight loss, or other atypical symptoms that may indicate serious underlying disease.*

Typical Patient Settings of Constipation and Underlying Causes

Neonates: For constipation in neonates, the EP should consider serious underlying illness, such as Hirschsprung's disease, intestinal pseudo-obstruction, or hypothyroidism.

Children: Constipation is more common in boys and often occurs at the time of toilet training or initial school entrance, when children withhold defecation for psychosocial reasons. The child gets into a vicious circle of difficult passage of hard stool leading to withholding defecation, leading to worsened stool hardening and more painful defecation. Fecal soiling (encopresis) is a common result and frequent presenting symptom.

Adolescents: Constipation is more common in girls, with the predominant symptom of straining to stool. Typically this is a functional problem arising from learned behavior and suppression of urge to defecate, primarily for social reasons. An underlying eating disorder or surreptitious opiate use should be considered.[2]

Adults: Typically, constipation in an adult has a functional cause, including irritable bowel syndrome. Extreme functional constipation (<2 stools per month) is almost exclusively seen in women. Young women with chronic constipation have a higher incidence of unnecessary abdominal surgery (appendectomy, ovarian cystectomy, hysterectomy) for reasons that are unclear but likely related to pain. For acute constipation, obstruction, new medications, and (less likely) sudden lifestyle changes should be considered.

Elderly institutionalized patients: Mental confusion, immobility, poor oral intake, limited toileting opportunities, and medications all contribute to a high prevalence of chronic constipation and high risk for fecal impaction in this population. Impaction is the most common cause of fecal incontinence and may also lead to stercorous ulceration or perforation.

Structure and Function

▪ DEFINITIONS

To the physician, *constipation* usually means a reduced frequency of bowel movements (less than three per week in western society) and/or difficult passage of hard stool. Clinically, a large amount of feces can be felt on digital rectal examination, seen on plain radiographs, or both. To the patient, "constipation" may mean reduced frequency or amount of stool, passage of hard stool, difficulty passing even soft stool, straining, a feeling of incomplete evacuation, or any combination thereof. An individual's perception of what is normal is also highly variable and often deeply ingrained, with many people believing inappropriately that less than one stool per day is a serious problem, although in fact it is medically quite normal.

▪ CATEGORIZATION OF CHRONIC FUNCTIONAL CONSTIPATION BY BOWEL TRANSIT TIME OR PROBLEM

Normal transit time: The majority of constipated patients seen by general clinicians (and about 30% of refractory cases referred to specialists) actually have normal transit times.[1] Their constipation is often perceptual and tends to respond to high-fiber diets and general measures.

Slow transit time (colonic inertia): Slow transit time may be due to overall slowing (pancolonic inertia) or to sigmoid spasm (paradoxic hypermotility of left colon with excessive and uncoordinated segmental contractions, resulting in poor distal propulsion); both may be aggravated by diet. Most patients with severe and chronic constipation requiring specialty referrals have slow transit times. The typical patient reports passage of hard and infrequent stools. There may be a primary dysfunction of the colonic smooth muscle or its innervation, or hormonal imbalance. Colonic manometry findings are abnormal, and often the gastrocolic reflex is markedly diminished.

Dyssynergic or obstructive defecation: Disordered defecatory function, with difficulty expelling stool from the rectum, is also often multifactorial and usually an acquired dysfunction. The patient reports straining even with soft stool. This problem contributes to about 25% of constipation cases in adults (often combined with slow transit time) and is also common in children.

The last category (also called anismus, outlet obstruction, or pelvic floor dyssynergy) is underrecognized—an important fact because this disorder often fails to respond to fiber or laxatives but may respond to retraining and biofeedback. Chronically ignoring the urge to defecate produces rectal distention and eventual muscular incoordination. The pelvic floor musculature may contract poorly or dyssynergistically, the internal sphincter may not relax upon rectal distention, the external sphincter may have markedly increased tone with inability to relax voluntarily, and continued rectal distention may result in habituation and diminished rectal sensitivity. In acute presentations of this condition, painful rectal conditions such as thrombosed hemorrhoids or anal fissures may also produce rectal dysfunction and therefore constipation.

▪ CATEGORIZATION BY CAUSE

Box 32-1 and Tables 32-1 to 32-3 list the various causes of constipation—gastrointestinal (GI) and systemic disorders, medications, and underlying causes in children.

▪ Anatomic and Structural Disorders

The patient should be examined for abdominal or rectal masses (neoplasm, fecaloma, abscess, hernias, closed/trapped loop of bowel, rectocele) that may cause blockage. Anatomic and muscular anomalies,

BOX 32-1

Gastrointestinal Causes of Constipation

- Anal fissure
- Anal stenosis
- Anorectal dyssynergy
- Chronic poor toileting habits
- Diverticular disease
- Functional constipation
- Hemorrhoids
- Hernias (incarcerated)
- Inflammatory bowel disease
- Intussusception
- Irritable bowel syndrome
- Obstructing lesion
- Perirectal/perianal abscess
- Rectal pain from any cause
- Rectocele
- Strictures/adhesions
- Tumors/neoplasms
- Volvulus

Table 32-1 SYSTEMIC CAUSES OF CONSTIPATION

Central nervous system/ neurogenic disorders	Amyotrophic lateral sclerosis Autonomic neuropathies Cerebral palsy Chagas' disease Cerebrovascular accident Delirium Dementia Hirschsprung's disease Intestinal pseudo-obstruction Multiple sclerosis Myotonic dystrophy Neurofibromatosis Parkinson's disease Shy-Drager syndrome Spinal cord lesions: Cauda equina syndrome Meningomyelocele Spinal cord injury Trauma to nervi erigentes
Endocrine/metabolic disorders	Adrenal insufficiency Amyloidosis Celiac disease Cushing's syndrome Cystic fibrosis Diabetes Glucagonoma Hypercalcemia Hyperparathyroidism Hypokalemia Hypomagnesemia Hypophosphatemia Hypothyroidism Multiple endocrine neoplasia type IIB Panhypopituitarism Pheochromocytoma Porphyria Pregnancy Uremia
Psychiatric disorders	Anorexia/bulimia Chronic psychoses Defecation avoidance Depression
Lifestyle/nutritional problems	Dehydration from any cause Immobility Inadequate dietary fiber intake Inadequate toileting opportunities
Collagen vascular disorders	Dermatomyositis Systemic lupus erythematosus Systemic sclerosis
Other	Intra-abdominal abscess Pelvic mass

Table 32-2 MEDICATIONS THAT CAUSE CONSTIPATION

Analgesics	Narcotics Nonsteroidal anti-inflammatory drugs
Anticholinergics	Antidepressants Antihistamines Antiparkinsonian agents Antipsychotics Antispasmodics
Cation-containing agents	Aluminum (antacids, sucralfate) Barium sulfate Calcium (antacids, supplements) Iron
Other	Anticonvulsants Antihypertensives (diuretics, clonidine) Calcium channel blockers Ganglionic blockers Nicotine Opiates Vinca alkaloids Serotonin type 3 receptor antagonists

Table 32-3 ADDITIONAL CAUSES OF CONSTIPATION IN INFANTS AND CHILDREN

Anorectal disorders	Abscess Anal fissure/pain Anal stenosis Anteriorly displaced anus Imperforate anus Intussusception at anal canal Rectocele Skin tags
Neuromuscular disorders	Cerebral palsy Down syndrome Gastroschisis Ganglioneuromatosis Hirschsprung's disease Hypoganglionosis Intestinal neuronal dysplasia Intestinal pseudo-obstruction Meningomyelocele Myotonic dystrophy Neurofibromatosis Prune belly syndrome Spina bifida
Gastrointestinal disorders	Cow's milk protein intolerance Intussusception Obstruction (any cause) Strictures Volvulus
Metabolic/endocrine disorders	Celiac disease Cystic fibrosis Diabetes Electrolyte disorders Hypothyroidism
Other	Behavioral/defecation withholding Drugs/medications Inadequate dietary intake Maternal drugs Sexual abuse history

especially in infants (e.g., Hirschsprung's disease, imperforate anus, prune belly syndrome), should be sought. Other structural causes are acquired strictures from enterocolitis or inflammatory bowel disease, intussusception, volvulus, adhesions, and acute painful rectal disease. Lower spinal cord injury (cauda equina, lumbosacral spine) may produce constipation and/or incontinence; high spinal cord injuries usually leave colonic reflexes intact, although digital rectal stimulation is often needed to initiate defecation.

■ Medications

The medications (prescription, nonprescription, and alternative) that the patient is taking should be established, because so many cause or exacerbate constipation. Classic scenarios include elderly patients taking multiple prescription drugs, recreational users of opiates, and patients with acute painful injuries who were prescribed opiates without stool softeners.

■ Systemic Illnesses

A long list of metabolic, endocrine, and neurogenic disorders may secondarily produce constipation. These conditions are usually obvious from the history, physical examination, and basic laboratory studies, so extensive diagnostic searches are rarely needed in the ED setting. Diabetes (long-standing with autonomic dysfunction), hypothyroidism, hypokalemia, and hypercalcemia (the most common metabolic causes) should be considered. Scleroderma and dermatomyositis commonly cause constipation. Central or peripheral nervous system diseases readily lead to constipation, because colorectal motor functions are coordinated by both enteric nerves and extrinsic innervation from parasympathetic and sympathetic systems. The prevalence of constipation in multiple sclerosis is high, being exacerbated by immobility, medications, and poor intake.

■ Functional Disorders

In the vast majority of patients, constipation has an idiopathic functional cause, often related to lifestyle habits such as dietary fiber intake, fluid intake, and toileting. Contributing factors include psychosocial stressors and unintentionally learned rectal dysfunction. Hormonal contributions are unclear, but constipation is common in pregnancy,[3] and many women report experiencing constipation prior to menstruation. Chronic laxative abuse is generally thought to cause chronic functional constipation, but evidence is lacking. *Irritable bowel syndrome* is a common functional dysmotility disorder characterized by abdominal pain, bloating, and variable diarrhea or constipation, with no structural lesions found; concomitant rectal dyssynergy is common.[4,5]

Presenting Signs and Symptoms

There should be no "red flags" in uncomplicated functional constipation.

Treatment and Disposition

■ ED MANAGEMENT CONSIDERATIONS

Suspected *obstruction* or *perforation* warrants immediate surgical consultation and admission. Patients with small bowel obstruction or ileus with vomiting usually need nasogastric suctioning (with addition of an intravenous [IV] histamine H_2 blocker to prevent metabolic alkalosis). Large bowel obstruction may benefit from colonoscopy with decompression. Laxative agents are contraindicated.

Patients with *pseudo-obstruction* usually need inpatient care unless they are known to have chronic intermittent pseudo-obstruction and this bout is mild. Note that neostigmine is a prokinetic agent effective in acute megacolon from pseudo-obstruction. It is a cholinesterase inhibitor and therefore should not be used if the patient has bradycardia, hypotension, active bronchospasm, or a serum creatinine value more than 3 mg/dL. There is little evidence for the use of other prokinetics in acute pseudo-obstruction, and none should be tried if there is any suspicion of obstruction, perforation, or peritonitis.

For patients with *uncomplicated constipation,* the starting point in the ED focuses on volume repletion and electrolyte correction as needed, followed by a bowel regimen appropriate for the level of fecal loading, plus any treatment specific to contributing causes. The EP should also consider whether the constipation appears to be due to pelvic floor dyssynergia rather than the more usual functional causes. The clinician should keep in mind what problem bothers the patient the most (infrequency, straining, or hard stool) and that the patient's expectations often include prescription "cures" and an unrealistic assumption of rapidly becoming "normal." Patient education is vital.

■ MANAGEMENT FOR PATIENTS WITH UNCOMPLICATED CONSTIPATION

- Initial cleansing (usually laxatives, both oral and rectal)
- Maintenance plan (increase fluid and fiber intake, consider laxatives or softeners)
- Behavioral modification (diet, toilet habits, exercise)
- Other interventions tailored to the underlying cause

Most patients are sent home with a management plan and education, but initial cleansing in the ED with serial reexaminations should be considered if suspicion remains about serious underlying cause or if there is a question whether the patient may be able to perform the initial steps. A myriad of products are available for constipation (Table 32-4). They should be chosen on the basis of their safety and cost as well as patient preference. The patient should start with osmotic laxatives such as polyethylene glycol (PEG) (or just bulk agents if the constipation is mild), but recommendations for a stimulant laxative (e.g., glycerin suppository) should be added if the simpler treatment fails. Review of the literature shows that good evidence supports the use of polyethylene glycol, moderate evidence supports lactulose and

Table 32-4 **THERAPEUTIC AGENTS FOR CONSTIPATION**

Medication	Type	Adult Dose (Oral Unless Noted)	Side Effects	Cost, Type, Pregnancy Category*	Comments
Polyethylene glycol (PEG)	Osmotic laxative	Maintenance: PEG solution without electrolytes 17 g in 8 oz fluid per day Initial cleansing: PEG-electrolyte solution 500 mL bid for 1-2 days	Minimal bloating Diarrhea, volume loss	$$$ OTC Preg C	May reduce effect or absorption of some oral drugs
Lactulose	Osmotic laxative	Maintenance: 15-30 mL 1-2 times/day Initial cleansing: 20-30 g q2h to effect	Flatulence, cramps, nausea, bloating	$$ Rx Preg B	Colonic fermentation to short-chain fatty acids Use with caution in diabetes (check serum glucose) Contains galactose and fructose
Sorbitol 70%	Osmotic laxative	Maintenance: 15-30 mL/day Initial cleansing: 30-150 mL Enema: 120 mL of 25%-30% solution	Flatulence, bloating	$$ Rx Preg C	Reduces effectiveness of other drugs Use with caution in severe CHF or renal failure
Anthraquinones	Stimulant laxatives		Nausea, cramps, melanosis coli	$ OTC Preg B	Avoid in CHF Reduces effectiveness of warfarin
Senna		1-2 tablets/day at bedtime			
Cascara		5 mL or two 150-mg tablets daily			
Bisacodyl	Stimulant laxative	2-3 5-mg tablets/day Suppository 10 mg daily	Cramps, nausea, urolithiasis	$ OTC Preg C	Reduces effect of warfarin, antacids
Castor oil	Stimulant laxative	15-30 mL once	Cramps, severe diarrhea	$ OTC Preg X	May precipitate premature labor Avoid in CHF
Magnesium citrate	Saline laxative	Maintenance: 15-45 mL/day Initial cleansing: 150-300 mL once	Hypermagnesemia in renal failure	$ OTC Preg B	Avoid in renal failure, ostomy ↓ effects of digoxin, tetracyclines, indomethacin
Magnesium hydroxide	Saline laxative	15-30 mL once-twice per day	Hypermagnesemia in renal failure	$ OTC Preg B	Avoid in renal failure, ostomy
Sodium phosphate	Saline laxative	Oral: 10-25 mL in 12 oz fluid Enema: One bottle	Hypermagnesemia in renal failure	$ OTC Preg B	Avoid in renal failure, ostomies
Mineral oil	Lubricant laxative	15-45 mL every night	Impairs absorption of fat-soluble vitamins Lipoid pneumonia Nausea	$ OTC Preg C	Avoid in impaired swallowing or GERD
Fiber:	Bulk agent	Take with liberal fluids Can divide doses	Bloating, flatulence	$ OTC	Titrate dosage upward gradually Impairs absorption of some medications if taken within 30-60 minutes
Psyllium		15-60 g/day		Preg B	
Methylcellulose		15-60 g/day			
Polycarbophil		5-20 g/day		Preg A	

Table 32-4 **THERAPEUTIC AGENTS FOR CONSTIPATION—cont'd**

Medication	Type	Adult Dose (Oral Unless Noted)	Side Effects	Cost, Type, Pregnancy Category*	Comments
Docusates	Stool softener		Possible hepatotoxicity	$$ OTC Preg C	Poor efficacy for long-term use
Docusate sodium		50-200 mg/day			
Docusate calcium		240 mg/day			
Lubiprostone	Activates chloride channels	24 μg twice daily taken with food	Nausea Headache	$$$ Rx Preg C	Avoid if history of bowel obstruction Avoid in children, renal failure, or hepatic failure
Glycerine suppository	Osmotic	3 g	Rectal irritation	$ OTC	
Enemas:				$	
Phosphate		120 mL	May affect serum phosphate and calcium	OTC	Avoid in renal failure
Tap water		100-200 mL	Absorbed if retained		
Saline		100-200 mL	Fluid overload		Avoid in CHF

*Relative cost indicated by number of $ ($ to $$$).
CHF, congestive heart failure; OTC, over-the-counter agent; Preg, pregnancy category (as determined by U.S. Food and Drug Administration); Rx, prescription drug.

psyllium, and little evidence exists for or against other agents.[6] General measures (education, increased fluid intake, exercise, and a dedicated time set aside for bowel movements) are often useful, but there is little evidence available to evaluate this approach.

■ GENERAL CATEGORIES OF THERAPEUTIC AGENTS

■ Bulk Agents

Bulk agents are first-line maintenance treatment for functional constipation with normal or slow transit time. Bulk agents act to increase fecal water content and stool volume, reduce transit time, and improve stool consistency. Bran fiber in foods and psyllium are natural products, whereas synthetics include methylcellulose and polycarbophil. Increased fluid intake must accompany use of the fiber. Fiber may cause increased gas (bloating, flatulence), but this effect is less likely if intake is gradually increased. Switching to a different bulk agent may resolve gas complaints.

■ Stool Softeners

Sodium or calcium docusate decreases surface tension and allows stool to mix with fluids but does not induce defecation. These agents are not suitable for long-term use owing to tachyphylaxis but are very useful in the short term while a patient is taking constipating medications (e.g., opiates) or for the patient who should avoid straining during defecation.

■ Emollient Laxatives

Lubricant agents such as mineral oil penetrate and soften stool. Mineral oil can be given orally or by enema. It may be aspirated and will cause lipoid pneumonia, however, so should not be used in patients with esophageal dysmotility, dysphagia, or gastroesophageal reflux disease.

■ Osmotic Laxatives

Osmotic laxatives, which are hyperosmotic agents, generally provide excellent relief of constipation and may be used in small doses for the long term if needed. Large volumes of PEG are used for procedural preparation or initial cleansing of large fecal loads, but most cases of constipation respond to one packet (17 g) daily, which may be continued as a maintenance dosage; PEG without electrolytes is more palatable. Lactulose and sorbitol are nonabsorbable sugars degraded by colonic bacteria to acids that increase stool acidity and osmolarity, leading to fluid accumulation in the colon to speed defecation. They may be given orally or as enemas. Lactulose is excellent for long-term use in small doses but should be used with caution in diabetic patients and avoided altogether in patients consuming galactose-free diets. Karo syrup is used in infants as an osmotic laxative.

■ Stimulant Laxatives

The most rapidly acting agents, the stimulant laxatives, are given either orally or per rectum. They are likely to cause some cramping. Saline cathartics exert osmotic effects to increase intraluminal water content.

Although relatively nonabsorbable, magnesium preparations should be avoided in patients with renal failure because they may cause hypermagnesemia or sodium and water retention. Castor oil is hydrolyzed to ricinoleic acid, which stimulates intestinal secretion and motility. Bisacodyl also causes fluid accumulation and increased motor activity. The anthraquinones (cascara, senna, aloe) are converted to active states by intestinal microorganisms and increase fluid and electrolyte accumulation in the distal bowel. This group of agents may decrease the effectiveness of other drugs, such as warfarin.

Melanosis coli results from the long-term use of stimulant laxatives but is benign and reversible. There is actually little evidence that long-term use of these agents results in severe chronic constipation,[7] which has been a long-standing belief, but they are nevertheless not recommended for frequent long-term use.

■ OTHER GENERAL MEASURES

Although little study of the efficacy of the general measures described here has been performed, the following recommendations are not harmful and often help:

- Higher intake of fluids (1.5 liters daily) and fiber
- Avoidance of caffeine
- Greater physical mobility and exercise (brisk daily walk)

Dietary fiber sources are primarily bran and grains, but dried fruits, fiber-rich citrus juices, many vegetables, and even popcorn also contribute fiber. Retraining bowel habits may also help; patients must allow an unhurried time (20 minutes or so) to visit the toilet, especially after a meal (breakfast is ideal), to take advantage of the gastrocolic reflex, and they should respond to the urge to defecate.

■ OTHER POSSIBILITIES

Concomitant treatment of underlying causes of constipation is essential. Treatment of anal fissures, hemorrhoids, or painful rectal problems improves overall bowel function. Although they are generally not prescribed from an ED setting, the EP must be aware of other potential treatments.[8] Lubiprostone is a recently approved option for treatment of chronic idiopathic constipation in adults. It activates GI chloride channels to increase intestinal fluid secretion. This softens the stool, reduces colonic transit time, and promotes spontaneous bowel movements, usually within 24 hours after the first dose.[9] Prokinetic, prosecretory agents such as misoprostol and colchicines have had some success in severe chronic constipation. Other prokinetic agents, such as neurotrophin 4, are in clinical trials. Alvimopan is a peripherally-acting mu-opiod receptor antagonist currently in clinical trials; it does not inhibit the analgesic effect of opiods and is effective in the treatment of delayed colonic transit caused by necessary opiod therapy. Cholinergic agents such as bethanechol have met with little success and may have side effects.

Patients with *pelvic floor dyssynergia* often do not have a good response to bulk agents or other laxatives but may improve significantly with behavioral modification and biofeedback training[10]; botulinum toxin injections into the puborectalis muscle may help, but controlled trials have not yet been done. In the past, surgical interventions for rectal dysfunction have had limited success and are rarely done now, although surgery may relieve specific defects, such as rectoceles, and is the mainstay for treatment of Hirschsprung's disease.

Constipation due to a medication requires careful review of the necessity for the offending drug, planned duration of use, and alternatives. For drugs that must be continued, increased fiber and addition of stool softeners may suffice, along with daily PEG or lactulose if needed. Bulk agents may affect the bioavailability of some medications, mainly if the two classes are taken within 30 to 60 minutes of each other. The EP must communicate clearly to the patient that the constipation is a side effect from medication, which needs to be discussed with the primary care physician to ensure improvement or a change of medication.

■ FOLLOW-UP CARE

Follow-up primary care visits are adequate discharge planning for most patients. Outpatient studies of colorectal structure (e.g., colonoscopy) are appropriate for those older than 50 years as cancer screening and are similarly appropriate for patients of any age with alarming signs or symptoms (acute and unexplained onset, weight loss, bleeding, iron deficiency anemia). However, structural studies do not provide assessment of functional constipation. Clinical response to treatment is better judged with ongoing care, and few patients need actual functional studies. The EP rarely will order them, but functional studies for refractory cases include marker studies (patient ingests radiopaque markers, and plain radiographs are obtained to assess their expulsion in 5 days), colonic manometry, anorectal manometry, defecography, and balloon expulsion testing.[11]

■ PATIENT EDUCATION

Patients are often frightened and disturbed by symptoms that the physician may take lightly. Reassurance about and discussion of constipation are invaluable. As appropriate, the EP should explain that cancer or other serious disease is highly unlikely but that compliance with the plan of care is essential. The patient should be taught about "normal" bowel function and general measures to improve it, and should set reasonable goals. The EP must also ensure that patients know how to use recommended items, especially suppositories or enema.[12]

PATIENT TEACHING TIPS

FUNCTIONAL CONSTIPATION

General Concepts

- Bowel goals: bowel movements 3 or more times per week, pain free, with minimal straining.
- Daily bowel movements are *not* needed.
- There is a wide variation in "normal" and healthy bowel habits.
- Long-term prognosis is excellent.
- Serious underlying diseases such as cancer are *not* likely.
- If your constipation is long-standing, a return to "normal" bowel habits may take several weeks.
- Regular exercise (walking) may help stimulate defecation.
- Follow-up with a primary care physician is crucial to see how you are doing and to see if other tests may be needed.
- Keep a "bowel diary" (brief description of diet, fluid intake, bowel movements, problems) for 1 to 2 weeks to review with your primary care doctor.

Laxatives and Enemas

- Short-term use of strong laxatives for the next few days is OK as initial cleansing.
- Small daily doses of osmotic laxatives like lactulose may be needed for a few weeks, along with bowel retraining.
- Avoid long-term use of strong laxatives unless your primary care doctor advises them.

Bowel Retraining

- Visit the toilet every day after the meal of your choice (breakfast is best), and sit for 15-20 minutes.
- Relax, do not hurry, and do not strain.
- Try for about the same time every day.
- Do respond to the urge to defecate.

Dietary Habits

- Drink fluids (water and juice, not caffeine or alcohol) liberally to stay well hydrated.
- Gradually increase your fiber intake (bran, high-fiber cereals, fruits, vegetables, or fiber products).
- Note whether milk or milk products aggravate your symptoms.

REFERENCES

1. Lembo A, Camilleri M: Chronic constipation. N Engl J Med 2003;349:1360-1368.
2. Youssef N, Sanders L, Di Lorenzo C: Adolescent constipation: Evaluation and management. Adolesc Med Clin 2004;15:37-52.
3. Wald A: Constipation, diarrhea, and symptomatic hemorrhoids during pregnancy. Gastroenterol Clin North Am 2003;32:309-322, vii.
4. Laine C, Goldmann D, Wilson J: In the clinic: Irritable bowel syndrome. Ann Internal Med 2007;147: ITC7-1-ITC7-16.
5. Schoenfeld P: Efficacy of current drug therapies in irritable bowel syndrome: What works and does not work. Gastroenterol Clin North Am 2005;34:319-335, viii.
6. Ramkumar D, Rao S: Efficacy and safety of traditional medical therapies for chronic constipation: Systematic review. Am J Gastroenterol 2005;100:936-971.
7. Wald A: Is chronic use of stimulant laxatives harmful to the colon? J Clin Gastroenterol 2003;36:386-389.
8. American College of Gastroenterology Constipation Task Force: An evidence-based approach to the management of. Am J Gastroenterol 2005;100:S1-S4.
9. Johansen J, Ueno R: Lubiprostone, a locally acting chloride channel activator, in adult patients with chronic constipation. Aliment Pharmacol Ther 2007;25:1351-1361.
10. Locke G 3rd, Pemberton J, Phillips S: AGA technical review on constipation. American Gastroenterology Association. Gastroenterology 2000;119:1766-1778.
11. Rao S: Constipation: Evaluation and treatment. Gastroenterol Clin North Am 2003;32:659-683.
12. Wald A: Patient information: Constipation. UpToDate 2007:15.3. Available at www.utdol.com/ and www.patients.uptodate.com

Chapter **33**

Hernias

Chandra D. Aubin

KEY POINTS

Smaller defects in the abdominal wall are more likely to manifest as incarceration or strangulation.

Reduction of a hernia should not be attempted if there is suspicion of strangulation.

Hernias with signs or symptoms suggestive of bowel obstruction or ischemia are true surgical emergencies and require immediate surgical consultation for operative repair.

Manual reduction can be aided by placement of the patient in a supine or Trendelenburg position, application of ice to the hernia site prior to reduction, and administration of analgesics and/or anxiolytics.

Postoperative complications of herniorrhaphy include wound infection, seroma, hematoma, ileus, small bowel obstruction, recurrence of hernia, erosion of preperitoneal mesh into intra-abdominal organs, fistula formation, genitourinary trauma, and chronic pain secondary to nerve injury.

Definitions

Hernias are congenital or acquired defects in the abdominal wall that allow protrusion of intra-abdominal contents through the pathologic opening. The characteristic presentation consists of pain and swelling at the hernia site. Intra-abdominal hernias, which can occur spontaneously or after surgery or trauma, are caused by defects in the diaphragm, mesentery, or ligamentous structures.

Incarcerated hernias are those in which abdominal contents have become trapped in the opening (non-reducible). Bowel incarceration can manifest as pain, vomiting, or frank obstruction.

Strangulated hernias involve a compromise of the blood supply to the hernia contents. Strangulation can manifest as fever, ischemia, or necrosis of the hernia contents and, occasionally, erythema or necrosis of the skin overlying the hernia. Smaller defects in the abdominal wall are more likely to manifest as incarceration or strangulation.

Reduction—replacement of hernia contents back into the abdominal cavity—is the immediate treatment for a hernia. Reduction of a hernia is accomplished by gentle pressure over the area of herniation. Reduction is assisted by supine or Trendelenburg position, analgesia, and procedural sedation to relax the musculature of the abdominal wall. Reduction should not be attempted if there is suspicion of necrosis of the hernia contents. Definitive hernia treatment is surgical repair.

Scope

Herniorrhaphy (also known as hernioplasty, the surgical repair of a hernia) is a very common procedure in the United States. Approximately 800,000 inguinal hernia repairs were performed in the United States in 2003; mesh was used in 90% of the cases.[1]

Of groin hernias, inguinal hernias (96%) are much more common than femoral hernias (4%). The male-to-female ratio for inguinal hernias is 9:1, and that for femoral hernias is 1:4. In elderly women, femoral hernias are as common as inguinal hernias. The incidence of strangulation increases with advancing age.

Operative mortality for a strangulated hernia is 5% to 10% in patients older than 80 years, compared with 3% for elective repair. Mortality increases to 19% when there is bowel necrosis.

The incidence of postoperative intra-abdominal hernias is increasing due to the higher number of Roux-en-Y gastric bypass procedures performed each year; postoperative hernias are observed in 2.5% to 4.5% of patients undergoing bariatric surgery.

Incisional hernias of the abdominal wall occur in up to 11% of all other postoperative patients and in up to 23% of patients with postoperative wound infections. Trocar site hernias after laparoscopic surgery are reported in up to 6% of patients. Parastomal hernia formation occurs in 28% of ileostomies and 48% of colostomies. Morbidity depends on the location and contents of the hernias as well as the development of incarceration or strangulation.

Nomenclature

Table 33-1 and Box 33-1 summarize the nomenclature of hernias, and Figures 33-1 through 33-8 illustrate some of the types.

BOX 33-1

Eponyms Associated with Hernia

Richter's hernia (partial enterocele): Herniation of only the anterior surface of the intestinal wall through the hernia defect; accounts for 10% of strangulated hernias.

Amyand's hernia: Acute appendicitis in the sac of an inguinal hernia.

Garengeot's hernia: Acute appendicitis in the sac of a femoral hernia.

Littre's hernia: Strangulated Meckel's diverticulum in a hernia sac.

Maydl's hernia: Internal hernia with double-loop strangulation.

Chilaiditi's syndrome: Symptomatic interposition of intra-abdominal contents between the liver and the diaphragm; can become incarcerated.

Canal of Nuck: The portion of the processus vaginalis that accompanies the round ligament through the inguinal canal in women; may contain hernia contents or, rarely, hydrocele in women.

Romberg-Howship sign: Lancinating pain along the inner side of the thigh to the knee, or down the leg to the foot, caused by compression of the obturator nerve in cases of incarcerated obturator hernia.

Pathophysiology

In comparison with controls, patients in whom incisional or recurrent hernias develop may exhibit abnormal synthesis of type I and type III collagen.[2] A higher incidence of incisional hernia formation is seen with wound infection, with obesity, and in patients with multiple comorbid conditions. The use of synthetic mesh and "tension-free" repair techniques have reduced rates of hernia recurrence.

Clinical Presentation

The classic presentation of an abdominal wall hernia is pain and swelling at the hernia site. Symptoms are more pronounced with increased intra-abdominal pressure, such as occurs with standing, coughing, and straining. Occasionally, patients note the acute onset of symptoms after heavy lifting or during sports. Many patients observe that the swelling ("lump" or "knot") resolves when they are supine or with pressure over the area.

Inguinal hernias can manifest as scrotal pain, groin mass, or swelling. Incarcerated hernias typically feature a painful lump or knot on the abdominal wall or in the scrotum. The hernia is very tender to palpation and is not reduced by gentle pressure.

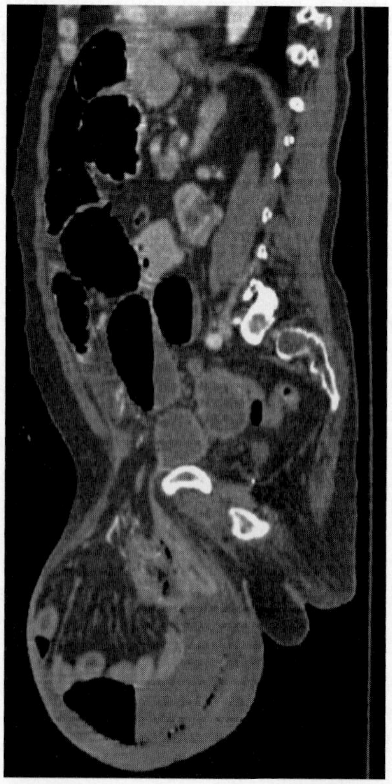

FIGURE 33-1 Infarcted inguinal hernia.

Table 33-1 NOMENCLATURE OF HERNIAS

Groin hernias	
Inguinal hernia (Fig. 33-1)	Physical examination cannot accurately distinguish between indirect and direct inguinal hernias
Indirect	Occurs through the inguinal canal Inguinal canal contents include ilioinguinal nerve, genital branch of genitofemoral nerve, spermatic cord in men (vas deferens, testicular artery, and vein) and round ligament in women 65% of inguinal hernias are indirect
Direct	Weakness of aponeurosis of transversus abdominis and transversalis fascia in Hesselbach's triangle (medial border of which is the lateral aspect of the rectus abdominis, superior border is the epigastric artery, inferior border is the inguinal ligament)
Femoral hernia	Occurs through femoral canal, inferior to the inguinal ligament, medial to the femoral vein More common in elderly, parous women
Sportsman's hernia	Syndrome of persistent groin pain in athletes; likely due to recurrent or persistent groin strain, osteitis pubis, or a nonpalpable hernia More common in kicking sports
Abdominal wall hernias	
Anterior (Fig. 33-2)	
Epigastric hernia	Occurs through the linea alba, the midline between xiphoid line and umbilicus
Umbilical hernia	Caused by an abnormally large or weak umbilical ring Umbilical hernia usually closes spontaneously in infancy but does not heal in adulthood Rarely incarcerates in children Worsened by pregnancy, obesity, or cirrhosis with ascites
Spigelian hernia (Fig. 33-3)	A lateral ventral hernia through the Spigelian zone: transversalis fascia between the lateral margin of rectus abdominis muscle, medial margins of external and internal obliques, and the transversus abdominis muscles Accounts for 1%-2% of all hernias
Ventral or incisional hernia (Fig. 33-4)	Trocar sites: Difficult to recognize on physical examination Dangerous cause of early postoperative small bowel obstruction Can be Richter type (incarceration of one intestinal wall) Iliac crest bone graft sites Parastomal hernias
Traumatic	Due to blunt or penetrating trauma "Handlebar" hernia: Can occur in any location on the abdominal wall, from a fall on a bicycle handlebar, with tear of abdominal wall muscles Has also been reported in the thorax from a tear of intercostal muscles (similar hernias have been reported from severe coughing)
Congenital abdominal wall defects	Surgical emergencies in the neonate: Immediate management: Cover abdominal contents with warm moist saline gauze, insert nasogastric tube, administer intravenous fluids and antibiotics, obtain surgical consultation Types: Gastroschisis: intact umbilical cord, evisceration of bowel through a defect usually to the right of the cord; no membrane covering Omphalocele: herniation of the bowel, liver, and other organs into the intact umbilical cord; membrane present unless ruptured
Posterior (lumbar) hernias (Fig. 33-5)	Bounded superiorly by the 12th rib, inferiorly by the iliac crest, posteriorly by the erector spinae muscles, and anteriorly by the posterior border of the external oblique muscle Types: Inferior or petit: just superior to iliac crest (point up) Superior or Grynfeltt: just below the 12th rib, inverted triangle (point down)
Diaphragmatic hernias	
Congenital hernia (Fig. 33-6)	Eventration: thin diaphragm with normal but widely spaced muscle fibers Posterolateral: through the foramen of Bochdalek Anterior, retrosternal, or parasternal: through the foramen of Morgagni Peritoneopericardial
Acquired hernia	Hiatal: sliding or fixed Paraesophageal Acquired eventration: due to phrenic nerve injury and paralysis Traumatic

Table 33-1 NOMENCLATURE OF HERNIAS—cont'd

Pelvic wall and floor hernias	
Sciatic hernia (Fig. 33-7)	Protrusion of peritoneal sac and contents through greater or lesser sciatic foramen
Obturator hernia (Fig. 33-8)	Protrusion of pre-peritoneal fat or intestine through obturator foramen
Perineal hernia	Protrusion of viscous through pelvic floor (rare)
Prolapse	Weakness of pelvic floor muscles can cause cystocele, rectocele, and uterine or rectal prolapse
Intra-abdominal hernias	
Spontaneous	
Transmesenteric hernia	Through sigmoid mesocolon, broad ligament, or falciform ligament
Transomental hernia	Hernia beneath a mesenteric or peritoneal fold (no disruption of peritoneum) Locations: Epiploic foramen of Winslow Paraduodenal Superior ileocecal fossa Internal supravesicular
Postoperative	Transmesenteric and transomental hernias are most common, especially after Roux-en-Y procedures May occur through falciform ligament from trocar puncture during laparoscopic cholecystectomy Retroanastomotic—may occur behind the anastomosis

RED FLAGS

Symptoms that suggest hernia complications (obstruction, incarceration, or strangulation) are:

- Diffuse rather than localized pain and tenderness with guarding or rebound
- Nausea or vomiting
- Markedly tender, nonreducible hernia
- Fever
- Erythema or necrosis of the skin overlying the hernia

If small bowel is incarcerated in the hernia sac, the patient may present with nausea and vomiting. Incarcerated omentum or preperitoneal fat may give rise to only a localized painful mass.

Over time, as the incarceration persists, swelling of the hernia contents eventually compromises blood supply, and strangulation ensues. The presentation varies with the contents of the hernia. Patients with incarcerated intestine leading to intestinal ischemia or necrosis may present with fever and peritonitis. Prolonged incarceration with necrosis of hernia contents may cause erythema or necrosis of the skin overlying the hernia.

Long-standing hernias may feature very large defects in the abdominal wall. In general, larger defects are less likely to manifest as strangulation. A large hernia may be chronically incarcerated or nonreducible. With time, fibrous adhesions develop that prevent spontaneous reduction when the patient is supine.

Less typical presentations include ill-defined abdominal pain, nausea, and vomiting but without an obvious mass on the abdominal wall. This presentation is more likely to occur with intra-abdominal hernias, in obese patients, or in patients who are unable to give an adequate history.

The incidence of postoperative internal hernias is rising because of the increase in bariatric operations in the United States, particularly with Roux-en-Y gastric bypass.[3] Postoperative complications of hernia repair include wound infection, seroma or hematoma, ileus or small bowel obstruction, recurrence of hernia, and, in rare cases, erosion of preperitoneal mesh into intra-abdominal organs with associated fistula formation.[4] Complications of inguinal hernia repair are chronic pain due to nerve disruption or entrapment and, rarely, testicular ischemia.

Traumatic diaphragmatic disruption from penetrating trauma should be suspected when the trajectory of the gunshot wound or location of the stab wound potentially crosses the diaphragm. Although rare, diaphragmatic disruption can occur after significant blunt trauma and is more common on the left side. Traumatic diaphragmatic disruption is difficult to diagnose in the acute stage because of nonspecific signs, but it should be suspected when there is proximate injury and pain out of proportion to physical findings. Standard imaging techniques, including chest and abdominal computed tomography (CT), may miss small diaphragmatic injuries, and laparoscopy, thoracoscopy, or surgical exploration may be required.

Diaphragmatic disruption has also been described after forceful coughing or vomiting. Delayed presentations of diaphragmatic hernias consist of complaints of chest pain, dyspnea, or abnormal chest radiographs or CT scans (with or without abdominal symptoms). The use of multidetector CT scanning

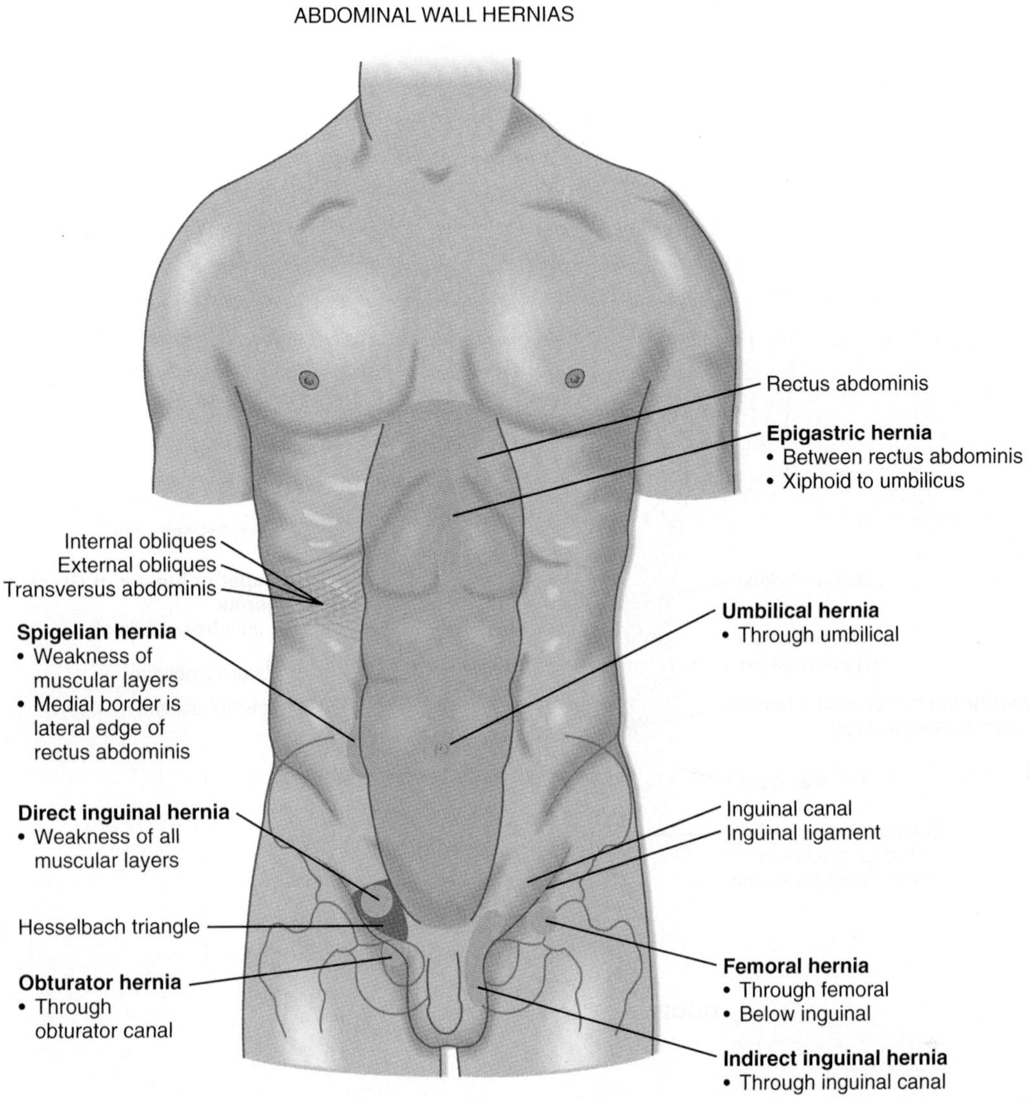
ABDOMINAL WALL HERNIAS
Rectus abdominis
Epigastric hernia
• Between rectus abdominis
• Xiphoid to umbilicus
Internal obliques
External obliques
Transversus abdominis
Spigelian hernia
• Weakness of muscular layers
• Medial border is lateral edge of rectus abdominis
Umbilical hernia
• Through umbilical
Direct inguinal hernia
• Weakness of all muscular layers
Inguinal canal
Inguinal ligament
Hesselbach triangle
Obturator hernia
• Through obturator canal
Femoral hernia
• Through femoral
• Below inguinal
Indirect inguinal hernia
• Through inguinal canal

FIGURE 33-2 Anterior abdominal wall hernias.

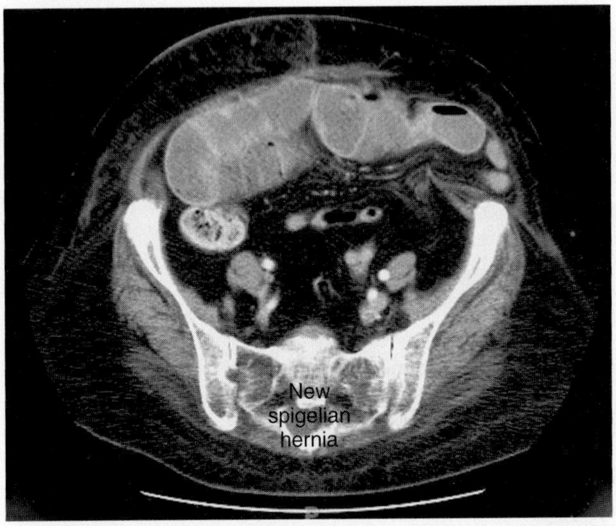
New spigelian hernia

FIGURE 33-3 Spigelian hernia.

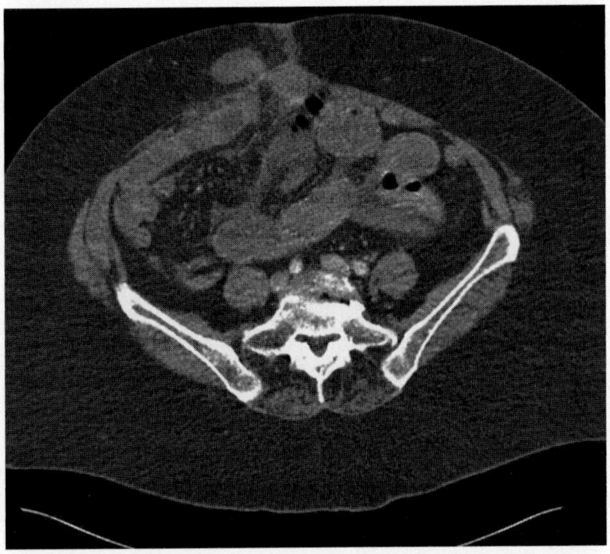

FIGURE 33-4 Ventral hernia with small bowel obstruction.

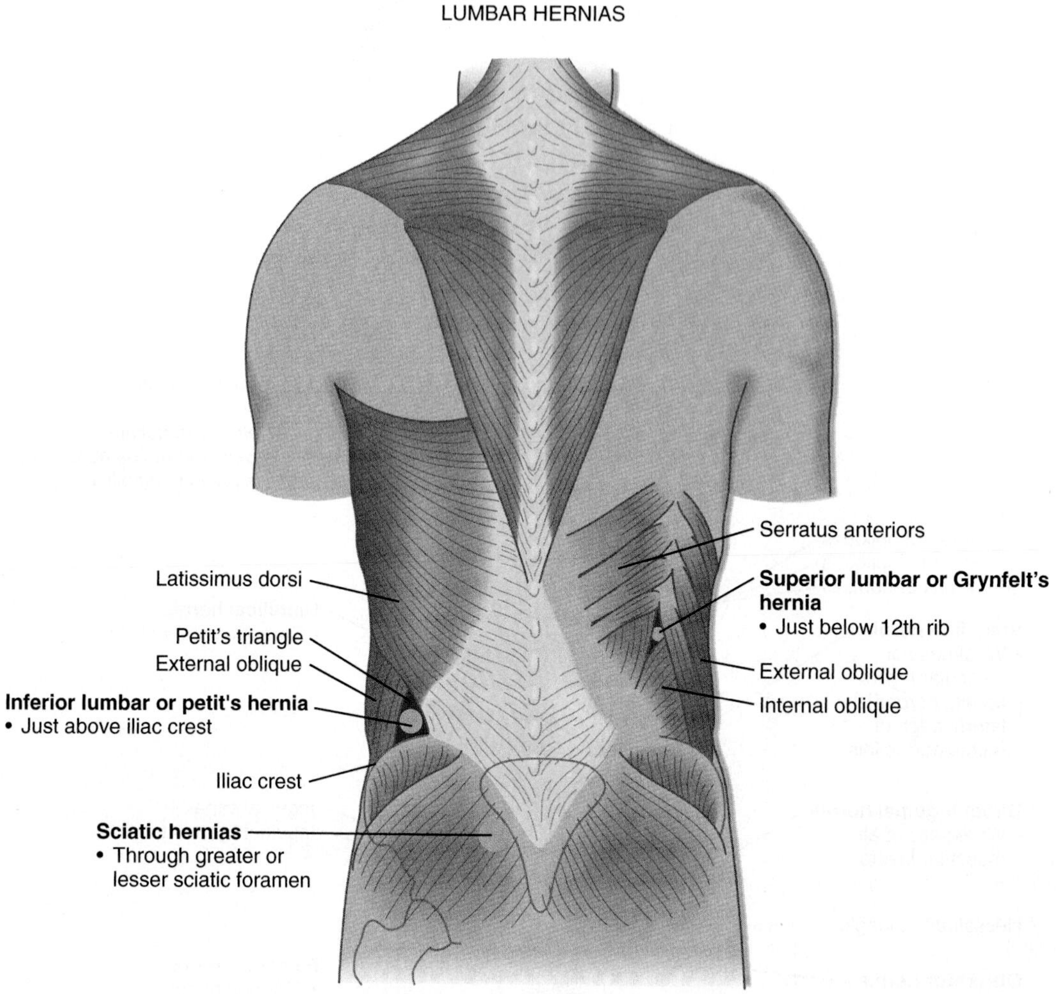
LUMBAR HERNIAS
Serratus anteriors
Latissimus dorsi
Superior lumbar or Grynfelt's hernia
• Just below 12th rib
Petit's triangle
External oblique
External oblique
Internal oblique
Inferior lumbar or petit's hernia
• Just above iliac crest
Iliac crest
Sciatic hernias
• Through greater or lesser sciatic foramen

FIGURE 33-5 Locations of lumbar hernias.

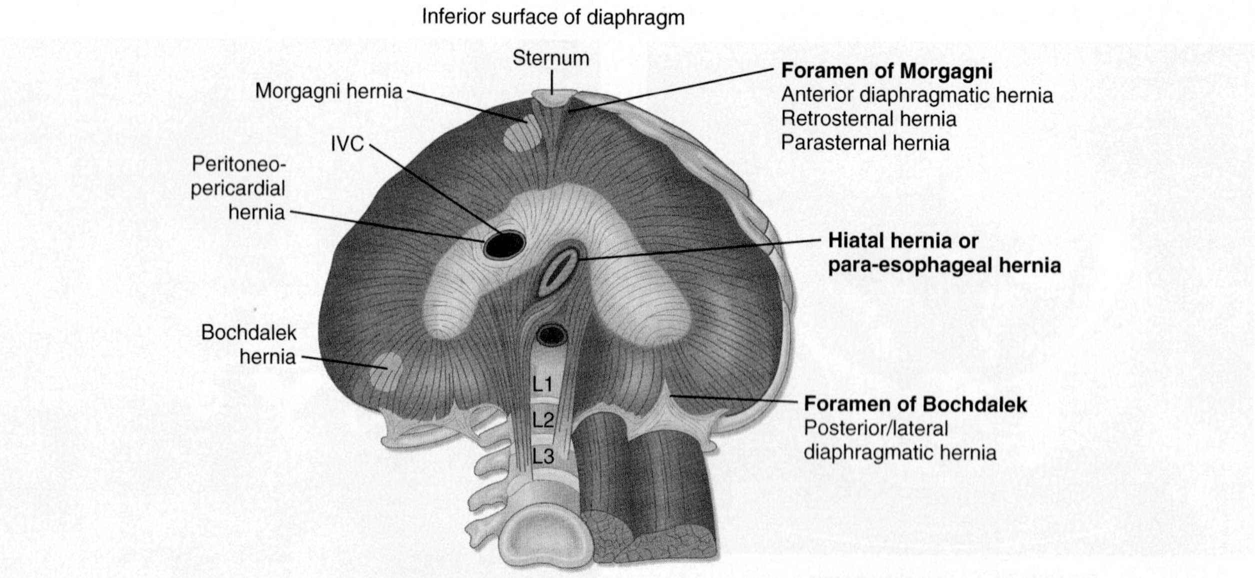
Inferior surface of diaphragm
Sternum
Morgagni hernia
Foramen of Morgagni
Anterior diaphragmatic hernia
Retrosternal hernia
Parasternal hernia
IVC
Peritoneo-pericardial hernia
Hiatal hernia or para-esophageal hernia
Bochdalek hernia
L1
L2
L3
Foramen of Bochdalek
Posterior/lateral diaphragmatic hernia

FIGURE 33-6 Locations of diaphragmatic hernias.

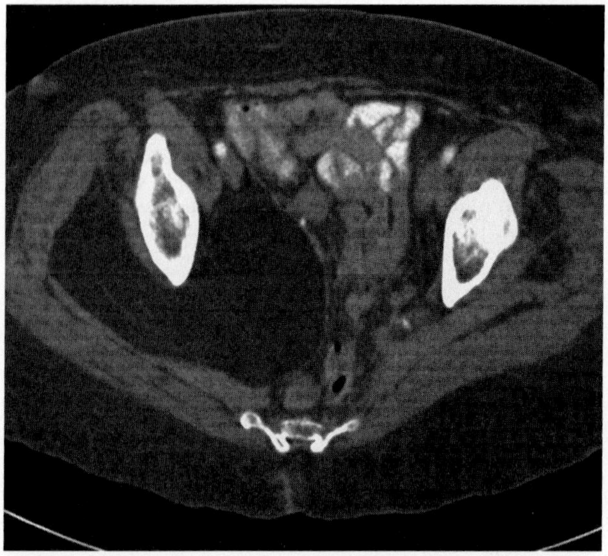

FIGURE 33-7 Sciatic lipoma.

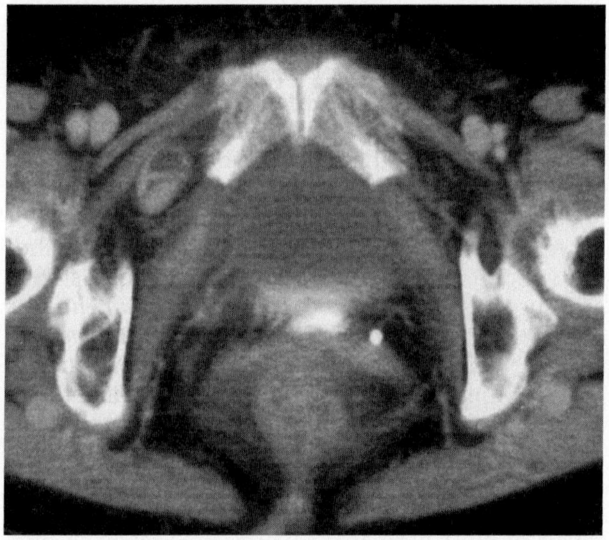

FIGURE 33-8 Obturator hernia with bowel obstruction.

has improved the detection of diaphragmatic hernias.

Differential Diagnosis

The differential diagnosis of abdominal wall hernias includes other masses of the abdominal wall, such as lipomas and rectus sheath hematomas. Abdominal wall or intra-abdominal hernias should be considered a potential cause in patients presenting with signs and symptoms of small bowel obstruction. In patients with prior abdominal surgery, either open or laparoscopic, careful examination of the incisions,[5] trocar sites,[6] and parastomal areas[7] should be performed to detect masses or abdominal wall defects. To facilitate detection of the hernia, the examiner should hold his or her fingertips over the incision while the patient coughs or strains.[8]

Inguinal hernias should be considered in the evaluation of the patient presenting with scrotal pain or swelling. Detection of inguinal hernias is improved by examination of the patient in a standing position and by insertion of the examiner's finger into the inguinal canal through the use of the loose skin of the scrotum. This technique allows direct palpation of the inguinal ring. Having the patient cough or strain allows the examiner to palpate the hernia bulging against the examining finger. Other causes of scrotal pain, masses, or swelling are testicular torsion, tumor, orchitis, epididymitis, lipoma, hydrocele, and varicocele.[9]

Congenital anatomic fistulas of the urachus or omphalomesenteric duct can manifest in children or adults as umbilical pain, swelling, mass, erythema, or discharge and can be confused with an umbilical hernia.

Obturator or other rare pelvic floor hernias should be considered in the differential diagnosis of patients with chronic atypical pelvic pain; CT should be obtained.

Diagnostic Testing

In the majority of cases, physical examination alone enables the identification of abdominal wall or inguinal hernias. When physical examination is not sufficient, ultrasonography, CT, and, occasionally, magnetic resonance imaging (MRI) can assist in the identification of hernias and serve to further delineate their contents.

Ultrasonography is the imaging modality of choice in the evaluation of scrotal swelling or masses, because it allows differentiation of the testicles, spermatic cord, hydrocele, or varicocele separately from the hernia contents. This modality can assist in the diagnosis of abdominal wall hernias through the identification of bowel loops within the hernia sac. Color flow Doppler imaging can detect the presence or absence of blood flow in some cases, aiding in the diagnosis of strangulation.[10]

CT can identify intra-abdominal and abdominal wall hernias as well as delineate the contents of the hernia sac and signs of ischemia, perforation, or abscess formation. Plain abdominal films have limited utility in the diagnosis and evaluation of hernias. Laparoscopy may be necessary to assist in the diagnosis of difficult cases when findings of other modalities are unrevealing.

Pediatric Considerations

Omphalocele occurs in 2 to 3 per 10,000 births. Historically, gastroschisis occurred less frequently than omphalocele, but recent trends show an increase in the incidence of gastroschisis worldwide (and in the United States). *Gastroschisis* occurs more commonly with younger maternal age and is associated with fewer congenital anomalies than omphalocele. Ultrasonography has led to more frequent prenatal diagnosis, but cesarean delivery has not been shown to improve outcomes over vaginal delivery in infants with abdominal wall defects.

Congenital diaphragmatic hernias occur in 1 in 2500 births. The mortality rate is high owing to pulmonary hypoplasia and the development of pulmonary hypertension. Ultrasonography allows prenatal diagnosis and identification of infants with a potential for poor prognosis. Prognosis worsens when the liver is located intrathoracically and the total lung volume is less than the total head volume. In utero repair of diaphragmatic hernias has been performed, although better outcomes than those with conventional treatment have not been observed.[11]

Percutaneous placement of a fetal endoluminal tracheal occlusion balloon may improve survival by preventing egress of pulmonary fluid needed to stimulate lung growth.[12] This treatment is still controversial because of a higher incidence of preterm labor. Stabilization of the infant with congenital diaphragmatic hernia consists of intravenous fluid resuscitation, nasogastric tube insertion, intubation with gentle ventilation/permissive hypercapnia (to avoid barotraumas), and surgical consultation. The use of nitric oxide and surfactant has not been demonstrated to improve outcomes in infants with congenital diaphragmatic hernias.

Late presentations of congenital diaphragmatic hernias have been described in children and adults. Cases typically involve respiratory difficulty; tension gastrothorax has been reported. Unrecognized diaphragmatic hernias can be exacerbated by pregnancy, presenting with incarceration and bowel obstruction in addition to respiratory distress.

Indirect inguinal and umbilical hernias are extremely common in children—parents may bring an infant or child to the ED when the lump or bulge is first noted. Incarceration or strangulation is uncommon but can occur. The clinical presentation in children is similar to that in adults. Physical examination of the scrotum and groin is mandatory in the evaluation of the crying or vomiting infant. Ultrasonography is used more often than CT for the evaluation of hernias in children.

Treatment

Reduction of the hernia is attempted through application of slow gentle pressure over the hernia contents, directing the contents towards the defect in the abdominal wall. Reduction can be facilitated by placing the patient in supine or Trendelenburg position and administering analgesia, which may decrease intra-abdominal pressure and relax abdominal musculature. Some authorities advocate placing a cool pack of ice over the area to decrease swelling and provide slow continuous pressure. Procedural sedation should be used when the patient has significant tenderness and anxiety.

To reduce a hernia through a small defect, it may be wise to pull on the hernia instead of pushing. Imagine a balloon trying to pass through a small hole—direct pressure on the balloon flattens the mass rather than pushing it through the hole. Instead, applied pressure at the defect in the abdominal wall (the base of the hernia) with accompanying traction on the herniated contents can narrow the sac and facilitate passage. The EP should apply a horizontal pressure with the tips of the fingers to narrow the base of the herniated contents while gently pulling the herniated mass. Pulling on the hernia from the base may be more successful than pushing.

Reduction should not be attempted when the patient has signs of peritoneal irritation, fever, or erythema or necrosis of the skin overlying the hernia. These signs signal the possibility of necrotic bowel, reduction of which could lead to diffuse peritonitis and abscess formation. When there is suspicion of bowel ischemia or necrosis, antibiotics that cover intra-abdominal pathogens should be administered, and surgical consultation obtained.

Patients with signs of volume depletion or sepsis should receive fluid resuscitation with normal saline. Urine output should be monitored via catheter placement to help to guide fluid replacement. A nasogastric tube should be placed in patients with signs of bowel obstruction.

The current surgical trend is toward laparoscopic repair of most hernias.[13] Laparoscopic repair of incisional hernias tends to decrease perioperative pain and recovery time, and complication and recurrence rates are similar to those with open repair.[14] Laparoscopic inguinal hernia repair has a slightly higher incidence of bladder and vascular injuries than open repair.[15]

Postoperative complications of hernia repair include bowel injury, hemorrhage, wound infection, and recurrence. The use of prosthetic mesh has decreased hernia recurrence, although mesh is problematic when wound infection occurs. Late complications of the use of prosthetic mesh in hernia repair consist of fibrosis and erosion into adjacent structures, including bowel and bladder, and, occasionally, fistula formation.[16]

Other complications of inguinal hernia repair are entrapment of the genitofemoral or ilioinguinal nerves, persistent pain syndromes, and, in male patients, injuries to the vas deferens and testicles with resultant alterations in fertility.[17] Repair of abdominal wall hernias can injure cutaneous nerves

PRIORITY ACTIONS

- Analgesia, fluid resuscitation, attempts at manual reduction of the hernia, procedural sedation as necessary
- Surgical consultation for incarceration, signs of small bowel obstruction, bowel ischemia, or necrosis

and give rise to persistent abdominal wall pain syndromes.[18]

Disposition

Hernias with signs or symptoms suggestive of *bowel obstruction or ischemia* are *true surgical emergencies* that require immediate surgical attention.

Emergency repair of *incarcerated or strangulated hernias* is associated with higher morbidity and mortality than elective repair, especially in elderly patients or patients with multiple medical comorbidities.[19] Complications include higher incidence of bowel ischemia and necrosis, wound infection and dehiscence, intra-abdominal compartment syndrome, sepsis and respiratory compromise, and higher incidence of hernia recurrence.[20]

Patients with *easily reducible hernias* may be discharged for surgical follow-up and elective hernia repair. Repair is generally recommended for symptomatic hernias in otherwise healthy patients. Patients who have multiple medical problems and for whom surgery poses a high risk may not be suitable candidates for elective hernia repair, especially when the fascial defect is large and less likely to become incarcerated. The decision about timing of hernia repair should be made by the patient in conjunction with the primary care physician and the surgeon. Elective repair of symptomatic hernias in elderly patients should be considered.

Unrepaired hernias may gradually enlarge over time, and some become incarcerated. Patients with *incarcerated hernias* that cannot be reduced should be admitted for urgent surgical reduction and repair, because some hernias progress to ischemia of the hernia contents.

PATIENT TEACHING TIPS

- A *hernia* is a defect in the abdominal wall that allows the intestines or abdominal fat to bulge through the opening. Hernias do not typically heal spontaneously and may enlarge over time. They may be repaired by surgery.
- Sometimes the contents of the hernia may become trapped or incarcerated. This development is potentially dangerous, because the blood supply to the contents of the hernia may be cut off. You should return to the Emergency Department if your hernia suddenly becomes larger or more painful, or if you develop fever, nausea, vomiting, or redness over your hernia; if any of those things happen, your hernia would need to be treated right away.

REFERENCES

1. Carbajo MA, Martin del Olmo JC, Blanco JI, et al: Laparoscopic treatment versus open surgery in the solution of major incisional and abdominal wall hernias with mesh. Surg Endosc 1999;13:250-252.
2. Si Z, Bhardwaj R, Rosch R, et al: Impaired balance of type I and type III procollagen mRNA in cultured fibroblasts of patients with incisional hernia. Surgery 2002;131:324-331.
3. Garza E Jr, Kuhn J, Arnold D, et al: Internal hernias after laparoscopic Roux-en-Y bypass. American J Surg 2004; 188:796-800.
4. Eckhauser A, Torquati A, Youssef Y, et al: Internal hernia: Postoperative complication of Roux-en-Y gastric bypass surgery. Am Surg 2006;72:581-584;discussion 584-585.
5. Cassar K, Munro A: Surgical treatment of incisional hernia. Brit J Surg 2002;89:534-545.
6. Tonouchi H, Ohmori Y, Kobayashi M, Kusunoki M: Trocar site hernia. Arch Surg 2004;139:1248-1256.
7. Carne PW, Robertson GM, Frizelle FA: Parastomal hernia. Brit J Surg 2003;90:784-793.
8. Yahchouchy-Chouillard E, Aura T, Picone O, et al: Incisional hernias. I: Related risk factors. Dig Surg 2003; 20:3-9.
9. Rubenstein RA, Dogra VS, Seftel AD, Resnick MI: Benign intrascrotal lesions. J Urol 2004;171:1765-1772.
10. Toms AP, Dixon AK, Murphy JMP, Jamieson NV: Illustrated review of new imaging techniques in the diagnosis of abdominal wall hernias. Brit J Surg 1999;86:1243-1249.
11. Moyer V, Moya F, Tibboel R, et al: Late versus early surgical correction for congenital diaphragmatic hernia in newborn infants. Cochrane Database Syst Rev 2002;(3):CD001695.
12. Harrison MR, Keller RL, Hawgood SB, et al: A randomized trial of fetal endoscopic tracheal occlusion for severe fetal congenital diaphragmatic hernia. N Engl J Med 2003;13:1916-1924.
13. Bax T, Sheppard BC, Crass RA: Surgical options in the management of groin hernias. Am Fam Physician 1999;59: 893-906.
14. Zanghi A, Di Vita M, Lomenzo E, et al: Laparoscopic repair versus open surgery for incisional hernias: A comparison study. Ann Ital Chir 2000;71:663-667.
15. McCormack K, Scott NW, Go PM, et al: EU Trialists Collaboration: Laparoscopic techniques versus open techniques for inguinal hernia repair. Cochrane Database Syst Rev 2003;(1):CD001785.
16. Scott NW, McCormack K, Graham P, et al: Open mesh versus non-mesh repair of femoral and inguinal hernia. Cochrane Database Syst Rev 2002;(4):CD002197.
17. Ridgeway PR, Shah J, Darzi AW: Male genital tract injuries after contemporary inguinal hernia repair. Brit J Urol 2002;90:272-276.
18. Poobalan AS, Bruce JM, Smith WC, et al: A review of chronic pain after inguinal herniorrhaphy. Clin J Pain 2003;19:48-54.
19. Kulah B, Duzgan AP, Moran M, et al: Emergency hernia repairs in elderly patients. Am J Surg 2001;182:455-459.
20. Alvarez Perez JA, Baldonedo RF, Bear IG, et al: Emergency hernia repairs in elderly patients. Int Surg 2003;88: 231-237.

Chapter **34**

Appendicitis

Rita A. Manfredi and Claudia Ranniger

KEY POINTS

- Appendicitis is the most common abdominal surgical emergency in the United States.
- Physical signs and symptoms vary with the location of the appendix.
- Children, pregnant women, and elderly patients may exhibit subtle clinical findings.
- No single diagnostic test can reliably confirm or exclude appendicitis.
- Early surgical consultation should not be delayed for diagnostic testing.
- Narcotic analgesia does not interfere with diagnostic accuracy.
- Prophylactic antibiotic therapy, properly timed, decreases postoperative infection rates.

Scope

Appendicitis is the most common cause of acute abdominal pain that requires surgical intervention. Although only 1% of patients presenting to the ED with abdominal pain have appendicitis, disturbing rates of missed diagnosis and subsequent morbidity continue to occur. Appendicitis should be included in the differential diagnosis for any patient presenting to the ED with abdominal pain.

The lifetime risk of appendicitis is approximately 9% in men and 7% in women.[1] A "classic" presentation of appendicitis is the exception rather than the norm. Symptoms are frequently atypical, and subtle presentations are common.

Anatomy

The appendix is a tubular structure that arises from the cecum and consists primarily of smooth muscle and an abundance of lymphoid tissue. The average adult appendix can reach a length of 10 cm and a luminal width of 6 to 7 mm. Innervation from sympathetic and vagus nerves accounts for referred pain to the umbilicus when inflammatory changes are present. The location of the appendix (retrocecal, 65%; pelvic, 31%; subcecal, 2%) determines the clinical presentation and the risk for development of perforated appendicitis.[2]

Pathophysiology

Acute appendicitis develops from luminal obstruction, which promotes bacterial overgrowth and distention. Obstruction of the appendiceal lumen is commonly caused by fecal stasis and fecaliths; other obstructive masses are lymphoid hyperplasia, vegetable matter, fruit seeds, intestinal worms, inspissated radiographic barium, and tumors (e.g., carcinoid). Luminal obstruction creates a closed space in which bacterial overgrowth leads to fluid and gas accumulation. Organisms are typically polymicrobial, with a predominance of anaerobic and gram-negative species.[2]

As the appendix distends, normal circulatory supply is impaired and inflammatory changes worsen. Ischemia, infarct, and perforation can ensue. Progression of an inflamed appendix from gangrene to perforation is variable, with a mean duration of abdominal symptoms between 2 days (gangrene) and 3 days (perforation).

Clinical Presentations

CLASSIC

The pain of acute appendicitis starts as diffuse, poorly localized, periumbilical discomfort (*visceral pain*) that localizes to McBurney's point in the right lower quadrant over 12 to 24 hours (*peritoneal pain*). McBurney's point is located one third of the distance from the right anterior superior iliac crest to the umbilicus. The appendix is located within 5 cm of McBurney's point in only 50% of patients.

Once the pain is perceived in the right lower quadrant, sudden movements cause severe discomfort consistent with localized peritonitis. Associated symptoms often include anorexia, nausea, and vomiting. Diarrhea is uncommon, although patients may report an increasing urge to defecate (the "downward urge"). Bowel movements or the passage of flatus do not relieve the pain, however.

Up to 50% of patients have a normal body temperature on initial presentation to the ED.[3] Patients with significant inflammation prefer to remain still in an effort to minimize peritoneal irritation. The right leg may be flexed at the hip to further decrease peritoneal stretch (Table 34-1). Palpation of the abdomen generally reveals localized right lower quadrant tenderness. Rebound tenderness, voluntary and involuntary guarding, and rigidity may be observed, depending on the extent of appendiceal inflammation.

Physical signs and symptoms vary with the location of the appendix. If the appendix is *retrocecal,* pain and tenderness may localize to the flank and not to the right lower quadrant. A *retroileal* appendix in men or boys may irritate the ureter, with resulting radiation of pain to the testicle. The gravid uterus of a pregnant patient may displace the appendix superiorly, causing right upper quadrant or flank pain. A *pelvic* appendix may irritate the bladder or rectum, inciting dysuria, suprapubic pain, or a more pronounced urge to defecate. If the appendix is low-lying, isolated rectal tenderness may be the only sign.[2]

Table 34-1 SPECIAL MANEUVERS THAT SUGGEST APPENDICITIS

Rovsing's sign	With the patient in the supine position, palpation of the left lower quadrant causes pain in the right lower quadrant
Psoas sign	With the patient in the left lateral decubitus position, extension of the right hip increases pain in the right lower quadrant (when an inflamed appendix is overlying the right psoas muscle)
Obturator sign	With the patient in the supine position, internal rotation of a passively flexed right hip and knee increases right lower quadrant pain

VARIATIONS

Children

Appendicitis is the most common condition requiring emergency abdominal surgery in children. Up to 8% of children who present to the ED with abdominal pain have appendicitis. The incidence of appendicitis rises with age, but the likelihood of perforation is highest in infants. Appendicitis most frequently presents in patients between 10 and 20 years old.

In the vast majority of children, the diagnosis of appendicitis is made only after perforation occurs. This fact may be due to a child's inability to describe the pain and/or the physician's misattribution of symptoms to other childhood diseases or gastroenteritis. As a result of perforation, worsening peritonitis in children might manifest as lethargy, inactivity, and hypothermia.[4]

Elderly

Elderly patients often present late in the course of the disease and are three times more likely than the general population to have perforated appendicitis. The elderly have a higher incidence of early perforation because of anatomic changes that occur with age in the appendix, such as thinner mucosal lining, decreased lymphoid tissue, a narrowed appendiceal lumen, and atherosclerosis.[5] The majority of older patients with acute appendicitis are afebrile and do not have leukocytosis. When clinical presentation, laboratory findings, and imaging results are equivocal, a low threshold for surgical consultation and inpatient observation must be considered for elderly patients with abdominal pain.

Pregnant Women

Appendicitis is the most common extrauterine surgical emergency during pregnancy. The diagnosis of appendicitis in pregnancy is difficult because the appendix migrates upward as the uterus enlarges, so the location of pain or tenderness is variable. Early symptoms of appendicitis, particularly nausea and vomiting, are common in pregnancy. Leukocytosis is also a normal finding in pregnancy and does not aid in the differentiation of appendicitis.

There appears to be a protective effect of pregnancy on the development of appendicitis, especially in the third trimester.[2] Maternal death from appendicitis is extremely rare; however, perforation and subsequent peritonitis cause fetal mortality to rise to 30% and maternal mortality to 2%. The use of ultrasonography may differentiate obstetric causes of abdominal pain from appendicitis without the need for imaging studies that employ radiation. Once the diagnosis of appendicitis has been made in a pregnant patient, urgent surgical exploration should be performed.[6]

■ Nonpregnant Women

Gynecologic causes of lower abdominal pain often mimic appendicitis.[7] Up to 45% of women who appear to have appendicitis on clinical examination are found to have a normal appendix at surgery. The highest percentage of misdiagnosis occurs in women of childbearing age.

Differential Diagnosis

The differential diagnosis for acute appendicitis is extensive and includes all causes of an acute abdomen (Table 34-2). Given that atypical presentations in children, pregnant women, and the elderly are not uncommon, a high index of suspicion and early surgical consultation are critical.[8]

Diagnostic Testing

No single diagnostic test can reliably confirm or exclude the diagnosis of appendicitis. Diagnostic testing should not delay surgical consultation for patients with worrisome findings on examination. Even though the use of CT scanning is now the norm, it remains proper to engage the surgeon immediately for a patient with an acute abdomen and also when appendicitis is the most likely clinical diagnosis (Box 34-1).

BOX 34-1

Diagnostic Considerations

Laboratory Testing

- Exclude pregnancy in women of childbearing age.
- The combination of white blood cell count >10,000 cells/mm^3 and C-reactive protein value >10 mg/L has higher positive predictive value.
- Urinalysis results may be abnormal in up to 50% of patients with appendicitis.

Imaging Studies

Computed Tomography (CT)

- Abdominal-pelvic and focused appendiceal study protocols are available.
- Use oral/rectal/intravenous administration of contrast agents as needed; discuss with radiologist.

Ultrasonography

- Preferred modality for children, pregnant women, and nonpregnant women in whom there is high concern for pelvic disease.

Plain Radiographs

- Not indicated for evaluation of appendicitis.
- Useful to exclude pneumoperitoneum, bowel obstruction, and foreign body.

Magnetic Resonance Imaging

- Consider for patients in whom CT is contraindicated and other studies are nondiagnostic.

Table 34-2 DIFFERENTIAL DIAGNOSIS FOR ACUTE APPENDICITIS

Women	Pelvic inflammatory disease/salpingitis Ruptured ovarian cyst Ovarian/adnexal torsion Endometriosis Ectopic pregnancy Tuboovarian abscess
Men	Testicular torsion Epididymitis/orchitis
Men and women	Nephrolithiasis Urinary tract infection/pyelonephritis Diverticulitis Inflammatory bowel disease (terminal ileitis in Crohn's disease) Infectious enteritis/colitis Incarcerated hernia Mesenteric adenitis
Elderly patients	Diverticulitis Mesenteric ischemia Vascular disease

The goals of testing are to improve accuracy and speed of diagnosis, exclude alternative causes of abdominal pain, and reduce the rate of appendectomies performed in patients who are found to have a normal appendix (negative appendectomy rate). Traditionally, a negative appendectomy rate of approximately 15% to 20% is tolerated to minimize the number of patients with missed appendicitis.

■ LABORATORY TESTING

Elevations in the white blood cell (WBC) count, percentage of bands, absolute neutrophil count, and C-reactive protein (CRP) level have each been associated with a greater likelihood of appendicitis. Taken individually, however, these tests have a poor negative predictive value. When they are used in combination, a WBC higher than 10,000 cells/mm^3 and a CRP value exceeding 10 mg/L have been associated with positive likelihood ratios between 8 and 23 for the prediction of appendicitis in adults.[9]

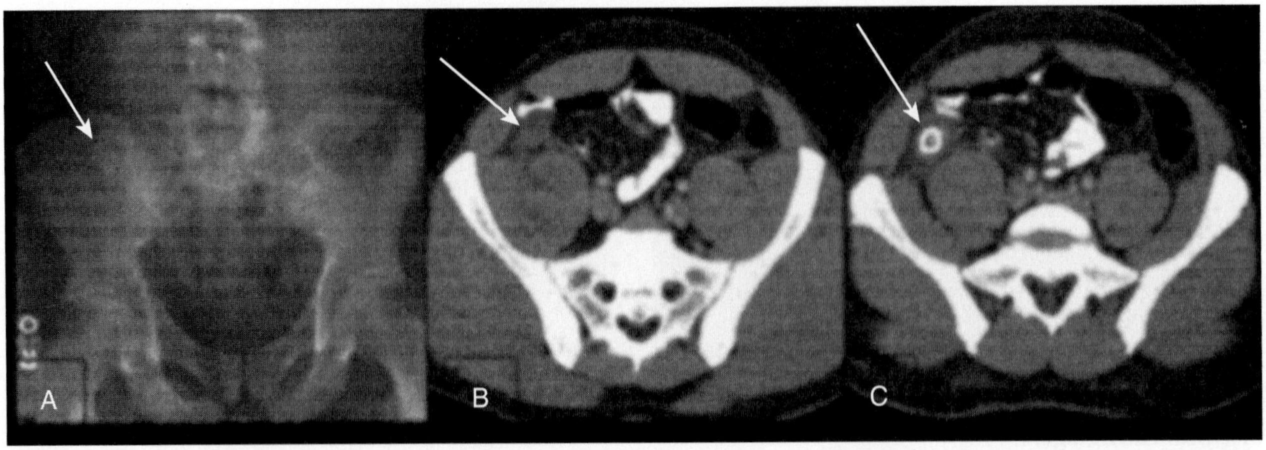
A
B
C

FIGURE 34-1 Plain abdominal radiography and computed tomography demonstrating appendicitis. **A,** The plain film shows an appendiceal fecalith overlying the iliac crest. Computed tomography with oral contrast demonstrates an enlarged, fluid filled appendix (**B**) and a fecalith with periappendiceal inflammation (**C**).

CRP values increase with duration of symptoms. Patients who present early in the disease process may have a normal CRP value.

In children, elevations of WBC count and CRP are poor predictors of disease. An elevated WBC count has a sensitivity of 19% to 60% and a specificity of 53% to 100%; a CRP greater than 10 mg/L has a sensitivity of 48% to 75% and a specificity of 57% to 82%.[4]

It is imperative to exclude pregnancy early in the assessment of a woman of childbearing age by checking a urine or serum quantitative human chorionic gonadotropin (HCG) level.

An abnormal urinalysis result must be interpreted with caution for a patient with suspected appendicitis and a low likelihood of cystitis. Abnormal urinalysis results (including more than 4 red blood cells [RBCs] per high power field [HPF], more than 4 WBCs per HPF, or proteinuria greater than 0.5 g/L) is observed in 36% to 50% of patients with acute appendicitis.[10] These findings are more common in women, in patients with perforated appendicitis, and in patients in whom the appendix is located near the urinary tract. No upper limit of urinary WBC or RBC counts has been defined for appendicitis.

■ IMAGING

■ Plain Radiographs

Plain abdominal radiography is *not* indicated for the evaluation of potential appendicitis. Barium-enhanced imaging (via oral or rectal administration) demonstrates equally poor sensitivity because of the nonfilling of the appendix and therefore has no role in the diagnosis of acute appendicitis. Plain radiographs should be performed only to exclude suspected pneumoperitoneum, bowel obstruction, or foreign body.

■ Helical Computed Tomography

High-resolution helical computed tomography (CT) is the diagnostic test of choice for suspected appendicitis (Fig. 34-1). CT findings in appendicitis include an appendiceal diameter greater than 7 to 10 mm, wall enhancement, wall thickening greater than 3 mm, and periappendiceal fat stranding.[11] The sensitivity and specificity of helical CT for appendicitis are 94% and 95%, respectively.[12]

CT has been shown to reduce the negative appendectomy rate in adults to as low as 2% in some trials. In the elderly, who often present with atypical symptoms, the use of helical CT aids in early diagnosis and has reduced the rate of perforated appendicitis from 72% to 51%.[13]

The intravenous (IV), rectal, and/or oral administration of a contrast agent to enhance CT imaging in patients with suspicion of appendicitis is controversial. Selection of CT technique should be made in consultation with the radiologist who will read the scans, and should be based on patient body habitus and duration of symptoms. Contrast agent administered enterally or IV enhances the appendiceal wall, lumen, and periappendiceal fat, improving visualization of adjacent intraperitoneal organs. An intravenously administered contrast agent can provide valuable information in patients with little visceral fat but may cause allergic reactions or exacerbate renal insufficiency.[14] An enterally administered contrast agent is particularly useful in the identification of perforation, but oral administration of a contrast agent may exacerbate nausea, and 1 to 2 hours are required for the contrast agent to traverse the gut prior to imaging. Recent studies of CT using either limited rectal administration of a contrast agent or no rectal contrast at all for appendicitis indicate similar sensitivity and specificity to those reported by studies using triple-contrast administration protocols; judicious use of these protocols may reduce diagnostic delays and avoid potential contrast agent–related morbidity.[15]

Radiation exposure may be limited to 300 millirads by using a focused appendiceal (right lower quadrant) CT study. Such protocols may be desirable for children and pregnant women, in whom large radiation exposure is a concern, but it may miss other intra-abdominal disease.

In children, the sensitivity of helical CT for appendicitis is 94% to 97% and the specificity is 87% to 99%.[4] A relative paucity of intra-abdominal fat in children decreases the visualization of periappendiceal inflammatory changes. Triple-contrast agent protocols should be used to maximize diagnostic yield.

Ultrasonography

Graded compression ultrasonography is conducted by applying pressure at and around the point of maximal tenderness. Ultrasonographic findings in appendicitis include an enlarged, concentrically layered, and noncompressible appendix more than 6 mm in diameter with periappendiceal fluid, hyperechoic fat, and hypervascularity in advanced cases (Fig. 34-2). Ultrasonography for appendicitis demonstrates a sensitivity of 86% and a specificity of 81% in nongravid adults.[12] Accuracy is reduced by a thick abdominal wall and intestinal tract; consequently, ultrasonography is best used in thin patients and in children. It is the initial imaging test of choice in pregnant women and children, in whom one wishes to avoid radiation exposure. In these populations, higher sensitivities and specificities are attained with ultrasonography than with CT. Ultrasonography is of added benefit when lower abdominal pain may be of pelvic etiology in women of childbearing age.

In children, the sensitivity of ultrasonography for the diagnosis of appendicitis ranges from 71% to 92%. A serial diagnostic approach in which CT is used after nondiagnostic ultrasonography increases the sensitivity and specificity of diagnosis to 94% to 99% and 89% to 94%, respectively.[4]

Magnetic Resonance Imaging

Magnetic resonance imaging (MRI) findings in appendicitis consist of a thickened appendiceal wall, a dilated lumen filled with high-intensity material, and periappendiceal enhancement on T_2-weighted images. The utility of MRI in diagnosis of appendicitis is curtailed by its limited availability, higher cost, and longer image acquisition time. MRI may be appropriate in patients in whom radiation exposure is contraindicated and ultrasonography is nondiagnostic.

Nuclear Medicine

Studies using labeled WBCs, immunoglobulin, and monoclonal antibodies show sensitivities of 89% to 93% and specificities of 87% to 100% for the diagnosis of appendicitis. These nuclear medicine studies are most useful in cases of atypical, subacute, occult disease in which CT is contraindicated and ultrasonography is nondiagnostic.[16]

Treatment

Early surgical consultation should be obtained whenever appendicitis is suspected (Box 34-2). Delays of surgery raise the risk of appendiceal rupture, peritonitis, and sepsis. The EP must maintain high suspicion for appendicitis in children, pregnant women, and elderly patients with abdominal pain, because these populations have atypical presentations and are at higher risk for perforation. *Surgical consultation should not be delayed for testing, and testing should be undertaken only when the clinical diagnosis is in question.*

Intravenous administration of isotonic crystalloid should be initiated as indicated, particularly if pro-

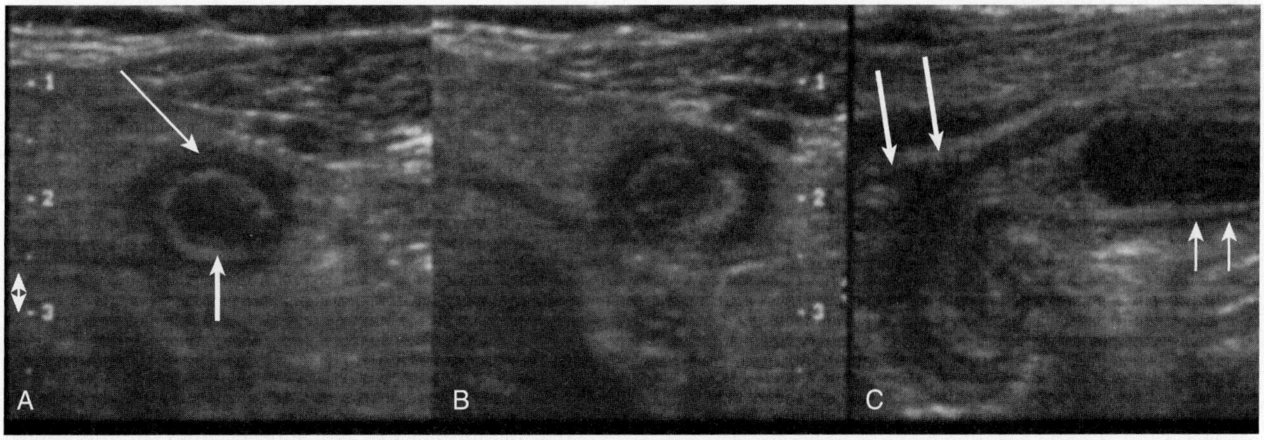
A
B
C

FIGURE 34-2 Transabdominal ultrasonography in a 37-year-old woman with pelvic pain. **A,** A cross-sectional view of the dilated appendix (*large arrow*) with periappendiceal fluid (*small arrow*). **B,** Compression yields minimal change in appendiceal diameter and causes significant pain. **C,** The longitudinal appendix (*small arrows*) and its origin at the cecum (*large arrows*).

Table 34-3 OPTIONS FOR PREOPERATIVE ANTIBIOTICS IN SUSPECTED APPENDICITIS

Adults	
Uncomplicated (nonperforated) appendicitis	Cefoxitin or cefotetan
Perforated or gangrenous appendicitis	A carbapenem Ticarcillin-clavulanate Piperacillin-tazobactam Ampicillin-sulbactam A fluoroquinolone (ciprofloxacin, levofloxacin) + metronidazole
Children	
	Ampicillin + gentamycin + metronidazole Ampicillin + gentamycin + clindamycin A carbapenem Ticarcillin-clavulanate Piperacillin-tazobactam

BOX 34-2

ED Treatment of Patients with Suspected Appendicitis

Immediate resuscitation with isotonic fluids
Advise patient to abstain from oral intake
Early surgical consultation (do not delay for diagnostic testing)
Parenteral antibiotics to reduce the risk of perioperative infections
Pain control with narcotic analgesia
Nausea control with parenteral medications

BOX 34-3

Disposition of Patients with Undifferentiated Abdominal Pain

Admit for observation if:
- There is a high suspicion of appendicitis or other urgent intra-abdominal process despite negative test results.
- Poor follow-up is likely.
- Oral intake is impaired.

Discharge home if:
- Good follow-up can be arranged and there are no impediments to obtaining care.
- The patient is able to tolerate oral fluids

Discharge considerations:
- Instruct the patient to return to the ED for increasing pain, fever, nausea, vomiting, or anorexia.
- Do not prescribe narcotic analgesics.
- Do not prescribe antibiotics.

longed vomiting, anorexia, or fever has been reported. In anticipation of surgery, the patient should be advised not to eat or drink.

Control of pain and nausea is both medically rational and humane. Narcotic administration does not decrease the sensitivity of the physical examination in either adults or children.[17-19] Analgesia with morphine sulfate, hydromorphone, or fentanyl is appropriate. An antiemetic, such as ondansetron, promethazine, prochlorperazine, or metoclopramide, may also be required.

Prophylactic administration of antibiotics has been shown to reduce perioperative infection rates in both simple (nonperforated) and complicated (perforated or gangrenous) appendicitis, with an overall odds ratio of 0.33.[20] Their administration should be timed in consultation with the surgeon so that high antibiotic tissue levels coincide with the surgical procedure. The antibiotics should be effective against both skin flora and common appendiceal pathogens, including *Escherichia coli, Klebsiella, Proteus,* and *Bacteroides* species (Table 34-3).

Disposition

The patients in whom the presentation is a concern despite normal laboratory and imaging results should be admitted for observation and serial abdominal examinations (Box 34-3). Patients with undifferentiated abdominal pain, a low risk of appendicitis, and negative diagnostic evaluation results may be considered for discharge if their clinical symptoms improve and they are able to tolerate oral fluids. Arrangements should be made for close follow-up for such patients, who should be given specific instructions to return to the ED if their symptoms worsen. Antibiotics should not be prescribed for discharged patients with undifferentiated abdominal pain. Narcotic analgesics may mask disease progression and are not recommended.

REFERENCES

1. Addis DG, Shaffer N, Fowler BS, Tauxe RV: The epidemiology of appendicitis and appendectomy in the United States. Am J Epidemiol 1990;132:910-925.
2. Prystowsky J, Pugh C, Nagle A: Appendicitis. Curr Prob Surg 2005;42:694-742.

3. Humes DJ, Simpson J: Acute appendicitis. BMJ 2006;333:530-534.
4. Kwok MY, Kim MK, Gorelick MH: Evidence-based approach to the diagnosis of appendicitis in children. Pediatr Emerg Care 2004;20;10:690-698.
5. Watters JM, Blakslee JM, March RJ, Redmond ML: The influence of age on the severity of peritonitis. Can J Surg 1996;39:142-146.
6. Andersen B, Nielsen TF: Appendicitis in pregnancy: Diagnosis, management and complications. Acta Obstet Gynecol Scand 1999;78:758-762.
7. Paulson EK, Kalady MF, Pappas TN: Clinical practice: Suspected appendicitis. N Engl J Med 2003;348:236-242.
8. Kamin RA, Nowicki RA, Courtney DS, Powers RD: Pearls and pitfalls in the emergency department evaluation of abdominal pain. Emerg Med Clin North Am 2003;21:61-72, vi.
9. Anderson RE: Meta-analysis of the clinical and laboratory diagnosis of appendicitis. Brit J Surg 2004;91:28-37.
10. Puskar D, Bedalov G, Fridrih S, et al: Urinalysis, ultrasound analysis, and renal dynamic scintigraphy in acute appendicitis. Urology 1995;45:108-112.
11. Choi D, Park H, Lee Y, et al: The most useful findings for diagnosing acute appendicitis on contrast-enhanced helical CT. Acta Radiol 2003;44:574-582.
12. Terasawa T, Blackmore C, Bent S, et al: Systematic review: Computed tomography and ultrasonography to detect acute appendicitis in adults and adolescents. Ann Intern Med 2004;141:537-546.
13. Storm-Dickerson T, Horattas M: What have we learned over the past 20 years about appendicitis in the elderly? Am J Surg 2003;185:198-201.
14. Pinto Leite N, Pereira J Cunha R, et al: CT evaluation of appendicitis and its complications: Imaging technique and key diagnostic findings. AJR 2005;185:406-417.
15. Anderson B, Salem L, Flum D: A systematic review of whether oral contrast is necessary for the computed tomography diagnosis of appendicitis in adults. Am J Surg 2005;190:474-478.
16. Annovazzi A, Bagni B, Burroni L, et al: Nuclear medicine imaging of inflammatory/infective disorders of the abdomen. Nucl Med Commun 2005;26:657-664.
17. Wolfe J, Smithline H, Phipen S, et al: Does morphine change the physical examination in patients with acute appendicitis? Am J Emerg Med 2004;22:280-285.
18. Green R, Bulloch B, Kabani A, et al: Early analgesia for children with acute abdominal pain. Pediatrics 2005:116: 978-983.
19. McHale PM, LoVecchio F: Narcotic analgesia in the acute abdomen—a review of prospective trials. Eur J Emerg Med 2001;8:131-136.
20. Andersen BR, Kallehave FL, Andersen HK: Antibiotics versus placebo for prevention of postoperative infection after appendectomy. Cochrane Database System Rev 2005;(3):CD001439.

Chapter 35

Bowel Obstructions

Keith Boniface

KEY POINTS

Partial small bowel obstructions have little risk for strangulation and are generally managed nonoperatively.

Complete small bowel obstructions are at high risk for strangulation and typically require surgical treatment.

Closed-loop bowel obstructions have a higher likelihood of concomitant vascular compromise and strangulation.

Strangulation may lead to bowel wall necrosis, perforation, peritonitis, sepsis, and death. Fever in a patient with bowel obstruction suggests strangulation and perforation.

Plain radiographs should be used initially to evaluate cases of suspected bowel obstruction. Computed tomography may be necessary to confirm the diagnosis when plain radiographic findings are nondiagnostic.

Obstructions that complicate the first 30 days after laparotomy are often managed nonoperatively, whereas obstructions that occur after laparoscopy generally require surgery.

Scope

Bowel obstructions develop from a mechanical blockage to normal intestinal transit. Blockages may result from intraluminal matter (i.e., foreign bodies), intramural wall thickening (tumors, inflammation), or extraluminal compression (hernias, masses, adhesions). Bowel proximal to the obstruction progressively dilates, leading to pain, obstipation (inability to pass flatus), and vomiting. Dehydration and electrolyte abnormalities ensue. As the bowel wall becomes edematous, increasing pressure causes collapse of the capillary bed and resultant tissue ischemia, a condition known as *strangulation.* Strangulation may lead to bowel wall necrosis, perforation, peritonitis, sepsis, and death. In patients with small bowel obstruction, strangulation has an incidence of 5% to 42% and a mortality of 20% to 37%.[1]

Obstruction can be *partial,* allowing some intestinal contents to progress through the area of narrowing, or *complete.* The patient with a complete obstruction has a low likelihood of spontaneous resolution and high likelihood of bowel strangulation, whereas the patient with a partial obstruction can usually be managed nonoperatively because of the lower risk of bowel strangulation. The central dilemma in caring for patients with small bowel obstruction is to identify those at risk of strangulation so as to ensure timely surgical intervention.

Pathophysiology

Bowel obstructions can be divided into *simple* obstructions (bowel occlusion at one location, with intact blood supply) and *closed-loop* obstruction (occluded loop of bowel at two adjacent points, which may or may not involve a vascular pedicle). Closed-loop obstructions are most commonly caused by entrapment of bowel in a hernia (*incarceration*) or, less commonly, by volvulus. Closed-loop bowel obstructions have a higher likelihood of concomitant vascular compromise and strangulation, thus warranting a more aggressive management approach.

Large bowel obstructions are at increased risk of perforation if a closed-loop obstruction is present or if the ileocecal valve is functional (preventing proximal decompression into the small bowel). The most likely sites of perforation are at the cecum (especially if the diameter is larger than 10 cm) or at the site of a primary tumor.

Volvulus, or axial twisting of the bowel, represents a special category of closed-loop obstruction. Volvulus occurs most commonly at either the cecum or the sigmoid colon and much less commonly at the transverse colon, small bowel, or stomach. Sigmoid volvulus, which is responsible for 50% to 75% of all cases of colonic volvulus, is more common in elderly and institutionalized patients. Cecal volvulus is found in younger patients who may have an anatomic predisposition owing to abnormal fixation of the right colon.

Clinical Presentation

Bowel obstructions manifest as colicky abdominal pain that precedes the onset of nausea and vomiting, abdominal distention, constipation, and obstipation. Proximal small bowel obstructions tend to have minimal distention and early intractable vomiting, because the bowel proximal to the obstruction has minimal capacity to distend. Conversely, distal small bowel obstructions manifest as abdominal distention, colicky abdominal pain, and obstipation before the onset of vomiting. Large bowel obstruction may be preceded by changes in stool caliber and progressive abdominal distention when it is caused by a slow-growing tumor or may be sudden in onset in the setting of volvulus.

Physical examination may detect signs of volume depletion, tachycardia, and hypotension. Fever suggests strangulation and perforation. The abdomen is variably distended and tympanitic, depending on the level of obstruction. Scars from prior surgery can provide valuable clues to the etiology of the obstruction. Bowel sounds tend toward high-pitched rushes of "tinkling" borborygmi; a silent abdomen is an ominous sign of perforation and peritonitis. Tenderness may be present, but localized tenderness and peritoneal signs indicate perforation. The examination should include a search for hernias.

Rectal examination should be performed to exclude stool impaction in the elderly. Occult blood may be detected in cases of strangulated obstruction, intussusception, or an obstructing mass. A rectal mass may be identified as the cause of large bowel obstruction.

Differential Diagnosis

The differential diagnosis of suspected bowel obstruction is similar to that of undifferentiated abdominal pain (see Chapter 25). Many abdominal disorders may cause a functional ileus that can be mistaken clinically for bowel obstruction.

Potential causes of mechanical small or large bowel obstruction are summarized in Table 35-1.

Diagnostic Testing

■ LABORATORY TESTING

Laboratory abnormalities are not diagnostic for bowel obstruction but, rather, may indicate complications of obstruction. A complete blood count, for example, may demonstrate leukocytosis with left shift in the patient with strangulation; serum chemistry evaluations may show dehydration, hypokalemia, and acid-base disturbances; the serum lactate concentration can be elevated in the setting of strangulation but its measurement is neither sensitive nor specific.[2]

■ RADIOGRAPHS

Plain supine and upright radiographs of the abdomen are the most commonly ordered initial diagnostic study for bowel obstruction because of the widespread availability and low cost of radiographic evaluation.

Small bowel obstruction appears on radiographs as air-fluid levels and dilated loops of bowel. Air in the distal colon and rectum implies early or partial small bowel obstruction. As obstruction progresses, small bowel dilation and air fluid levels become more prominent, and the distal bowel decompresses and collapses.

Ileus is distinguished from mechanical obstruction by the presence of air-fluid levels at uniform height

Table 35-1 CAUSES OF MECHANICAL BOWEL OBSTRUCTION

Causes of small bowel obstruction	Adhesions Inflammatory bowel disease Neoplasms Hernias Abscess Intussusception Foreign bodies
Causes of large bowel obstruction	Neoplasms Volvulus Diverticulitis Metastatic cancer (extrinsic compression) Stricture Hernia Fecal impaction Adhesions

across an upright image of the abdomen; in obstruction, air-fluid levels are classically at variable heights.

Plain radiography is less useful for closed-loop obstructions, which are detected only from the subtle finding of a paucity of intestinal gas in the region of an often fluid-filled closed loop.

Sigmoid volvulus is characterized by a massively distended loop of large bowel arising out of the pelvis, sometimes described as a "bent inner-tube," with accompanying proximal large bowel dilation. (Large bowel is identified by its widely spaced haustral markings that do not completely traverse the bowel lumen.) A competent ileocecal valve prevents decompression into the small bowel, leading to massive dilation of the large bowel.

Cecal volvulus appears as a coffee bean–shaped loop of bowel projecting from the right lower quadrant into the upper abdomen, often with a collapsed distal large bowel and accompanying small bowel dilation that can be mistaken for a primary small bowel obstruction.

Large bowel obstruction resulting from mechanical causes must be differentiated from pseudo-obstruction, a colonic motility disorder that is treated nonoperatively. Enemas of water-soluble contrast agent (used instead of barium to avoid chemical peritonitis in the setting of perforation) can differentiate obstruction from pseudo-obstruction. A contrast agent enema improves the sensitivity and specificity for mechanical obstruction from 84% and 72% to 96% and 98%, respectively, using a criterion standard of laparotomy findings and clinical follow-up.[3] In addition, a contrast agent enema is helpful in confirming the diagnosis of sigmoid and cecal volvulus, with a tapering "bird's beak" appearance at the end at the column of contrast agent as it reaches the base of the colonic twist.

Studies evaluating the effectiveness of plain radiography for obstruction are limited by their methodology. Researchers have used combinations of discharge diagnosis, surgical reports, enteroclysis, and clinical follow-up as criterion standards. A review of these studies shows that plain radiographs are of limited value because they are diagnostic in only 50% to 60% of cases[4] and have a reported sensitivity of 46% to 76%.[5] A study of plain radiographs interpreted by gastrointestinal radiologists had a sensitivity of 66%; 21% of studies reported as showing normal bowel were actually images of obstructions.[6] Despite limitations related to false-negative interpretations, plain radiography is still recommended as the initial test of choice in the evaluation of possible bowel obstruction, because the classic radiographic findings, when present, are useful for quickly confirming the diagnosis.

Computed tomography (CT) has supplanted the ED use of contrast-enhanced radiography to confirm suspected bowel obstruction when initial plain radiographs are nondiagnostic (typically in cases of low-grade or intermittent obstruction).

■ COMPUTED TOMOGRAPHY

CT of the abdomen is commonly used for the diagnosis of bowel obstruction (1) to confirm a clinically suspected obstruction not identified by plain radiograph, (2) to determine the level, severity, and cause of the obstruction, (3) to characterize a closed-loop obstruction, (4) to demonstrate signs of strangulation,[7] and (5) to identify alternative causes of acute abdominal pain when obstruction is not present.

CT has a sensitivity of 64% to 100% and a specificity of 71% to 100% for the diagnosis of bowel obstruction.[8] Signs of small bowel obstruction on CT consist of small bowel dilation to a caliber of 2.5 cm or more with a distinct transition zone and a collapsed distal bowel lumen. The "small bowel feces sign"—the presence of intraluminal particulate material in dilated small bowel—can be helpful in confirming the diagnosis of small bowel obstruction.[9] CT correctly identifies the cause of obstruction in 73% to 95% of patients.[10]

A completely fluid-filled closed-loop obstruction is more easily diagnosed on CT than on plain radiography. Characteristics of closed-loop obstruction include a C- or U-shaped configuration of the dilated loops, a radial distribution of the dilated loops toward the site of obstruction, radial distribution of dilated loops and engorged mesenteric vessels toward the site of obstruction (the "beak and whirl" sign), and the presence of two collapsed bowel lumens adjacent to the site of obstruction.[1]

For the diagnosis of strangulation, CT has a sensitivity of 68% to 85% and a specificity exceeding 90%.[1,11] Strangulation is suggested by a characteristic configuration of the obstructed loop, bowel wall thickening and enhancement, mesenteric vascular changes, gas in the bowel wall, and presence of ascites. One study found that the presence of two out of four clinical criteria (tachycardia, leukocytosis, fever, and tenderness) increased the specificity of CT criteria.[12]

CT enteroclysis (delivery of contrast agent to the small bowel via a tube so as to bypass the pylorus) combines the anatomic information provided by CT with the intraluminal detail of enteroclysis. Although this technique is more labor-intensive because of the need to intubate the small bowel, it may play a role in the future evaluation of small bowel obstructions.[13] CT enteroclysis is a useful test for confirming the diagnosis of superior mesenteric artery syndrome, a rare cause of proximal small bowel obstruction that occurs after rapid weight loss.

Orally administered water-soluble contrast agent can be helpful in the distinction of a partial small bowel obstruction from a complete obstruction. Meta-analysis has shown that the identification of oral contrast agent in the right colon 4 to 24 hours after administration predicts the success of conservative management with a pooled positive likelihood ratio of 25, and that the absence of contrast agent predicts failure of conservative therapy with a pooled negative likelihood ratio of 0.03.[14]

[illegible]

12. [illegible] et al. [illegible] management of patients with [illegible] small bowel obstruction [illegible]

13. [illegible] laparoscopic small bowel obstruction [illegible] management. Surg Endosc [illegible]

14. Franklin ME Jr, Gonzalez JJ Jr, Miter DB, et al. Laparoscopic diagnosis and treatment of intestinal obstruction. Surg Endosc 2004;18:26–30.

15. [illegible] Kaplan O, et al. [illegible] Dis Colon Rectum [illegible]

[illegible]

8. Lazarus DE, Slywotsky C, Bennett GL, et al. Frequency and relevance of the "small-bowel feces" sign on CT in patients with small-bowel obstruction. AJR 2004;183:1361–1366.

9. Maglinte DDT, Reyes BL, Harmon BH, et al. Reliability and role of plain film radiography and CT in the diagnosis of small bowel obstruction. AJR 1996;167:1451–1455.

10. Frager D, Baer JW, Medwid SW, et al. Detection of intestinal ischemia in patients with acute small-bowel obstruction due to adhesions or hernia [illegible]

■ SURGICAL MANAGEMENT OF SMALL BOWEL OBSTRUCTION

[illegible]

REFERENCES

[illegible]

Chapter **36**

Anorectal Disorders

John M. Boe and Tara Roeder

KEY POINTS

- Structures proximal to the dentate line are insensate, but tissue distal to this boundary can be painful when damaged by trauma, infection, or inflammation.
- An anoscope should be used to directly visualize internal anatomy if abnormalities are suspected.
- Internal hemorrhoids cannot be distinguished from normal rectal tissue by digital rectal examination. Anoscopy is required to visualize suspected internal hemorrhoids.
- Thrombosed external hemorrhoids are treated with elliptical incision rather than linear incision and drainage.
- Fissures that are not properly treated may become chronic and develop the "classic triad" consisting of sentinel pile, deep ulcer, and enlarged anal papillae.
- Pain that subsides between bowel movements is classic for anal fissures.
- Any patient with suspected rectal perforation due to a foreign body (insertion or removal) should undergo proctosigmoidoscopy performed by a gastroenterologist or colorectal surgeon prior to discharge.

Anatomy

The anorectum marks the end of the digestive tract as it transitions from the endodermal tissues of the colon and intestine to the ectodermal tissues of the skin. The rectum is the portion of the digestive tract extending distally from the rectosigmoid junction, at approximately the level of the S3 sacral vertebral body to the dentate line. At the dentate line, the endodermal tissue transitions to ectodermal tissue. The first 1 to 2 cm is considered the anal canal. This tissue, the anoderm, is squamous in origin but contains no hair follicles or sweat glands. At the anal verge, this tissue transforms to more normal external skin marked by hair follicles, apocrine glands, and subcutaneous tissue.

Just proximal to the dentate line, the tissue of the rectum takes on a pleated appearance, forming the rectal ampulla. These pleats create multiple crypts and the anal valves with their insertion at the dentate line. Proximal to the crypts are the columns of Morgagni, where the epithelium of the anoderm transitions to that of the rectum.

Because of the varying embryonic origins of the anorectal region, the vasculature and innervation demonstrate distinct areas of function. The superior, middle, and inferior hemorrhoidal arteries supply blood to the anorectum; they arise, respectively, from the inferior mesenteric, internal iliac, and internal pudendal arteries. Likewise, the venous drainage of the rectum is divided between the superior hemorrhoidal vein (which drains into the portal system) and the inferior hemorrhoidal vein (which drains into the caval system).

Sensory perception of the rectum is supplied by the pudendal nerve, which arises from pelvic branches of the S3 and S4 nerve roots. Structures proximal to the dentate line are insensate, whereas tissue distal to this boundary can be painful when damaged by trauma, infection, or inflammation.

Fecal continence is maintained by motor innervation that arises from the S2 to S4 nerve roots. Defecation is the result of concomitant parasympathetic and sympathetic simulation as well as voluntary contraction of the abdominal muscles.

Examination

To examine the anorectum, the EP puts the patient in the lateral decubitus position (Sims' position) or a knee-to-chest position on the examination table. The anorectal skin, hygiene, and any anatomic abnormalities are inspected. The EP has the patient bear down (Valsalva's maneuver) to accentuate rectal prolapse or prolapse of internal hemorrhoids. The skin of the anorectum is spread to identify fissures that may be hidden in the folds. A 360-degree digital rectal examination is performed, note being made of the prostate in males and the cervix in females. The sample of stool on the withdrawn glove is assessed for gross or occult blood. If abnormalities are suspected, an anoscope is used to directly visualize internal anatomy.

Cryptitis

▪ PATHOPHYSIOLOGY

Anal crypts are small pockets of epithelium located between the anal papillae at the proximal end of the anal canal (the mucocutaneous junction). These crypts have tiny glands that secrete a small drop of mucous as the sphincter muscles contract, easing the passage of stool. Cryptitis occurs when these crypts become inflamed and the mucosal lining of their roofs becomes denuded. Possible causes of cryptitis are as follows:

- Repeated watery stools that can cause trauma or deposits in the crypts
- Direct trauma from large, hard stools
- Inflammation from adjacent structures
- External sources of infection, such as parasites or foreign bodies.

If left untreated, cryptitis can lead to perirectal abscesses, anal fissure, or anal fistula.

▪ PRESENTING SIGNS AND SYMPTOMS

The presenting signs and symptoms of cryptitis are anal pain (rectalgia), which is described as burning or dull in nature and exacerbated with bowel movements, as well as anal spasm, pruritus, and occasional bleeding.

▪ DIFFERENTIAL DIAGNOSIS

The differential diagnosis for cryptitis includes hemorrhoids, anal fissure, anorectal abscess, and proctitis.

▪ DIAGNOSTIC TESTING AND EXAMINATION

- Palpation of hypertrophied (indurated) papillae adjacent to the crypt.
- Classic "pearl of pus" beading from the crypt at the dentate line on anoscopy

▪ TREATMENT

Treatment of cryptitis consists of bulk laxatives to promote well-formed stools and decrease trauma and warm sitz baths. Patients with advanced disease should receive outpatient surgical referral for excision of the gland.

Hemorrhoids

▪ PATHOPHYSIOLOGY

Hemorrhoidal plexuses provide a vascular cushion to the area surrounding the anus. The hemorrhoidal vessels are one of three layers of submucosal tissue that support the anal canal, aiding with continence and defecation. As this tissue deteriorates and weakens, the hemorrhoidal veins may prolapse or may become engorged or thrombosed.

The internal hemorrhoidal veins are located above the dentate line. Their blood supply is from the superior hemorrhoidal plexus, draining into the portal system by way of the superior rectal veins and the inferior mesenteric vein. They also communicate with the external hemorrhoidal veins. Internal hemorrhoids are covered by transitional or columnar epithelium mucosa without pain fibers. They are nearly always in the same positions: left lateral (9 o'clock), right posterolateral (5 o'clock), and right anterolateral (2 o'clock). They are classified into four categories according to severity of presentation (Table 36-1).

The external hemorrhoidal veins are located below the dentate line. Their blood supply is from the in-ferior hemorrhoidal plexus, draining into the iliac and pudendal venous systems. They are covered by anoderm (modified squamous epithelium) with sensory nerve endings that contain pain receptors.

▪ PRESENTING SIGNS AND SYMPTOMS

The most common symptom of hemorrhoids is painless bleeding with defecation (blood on stool or toilet paper). If the hemorrhoid is thrombosed, strangulated, or prolapsed, there is also pain with defecation. The lesion is detected as a curvilinear mass at the anus.

Table 36-1 CLASSIFICATION OF INTERNAL HEMORRHOIDS

Severity of Presentation (Degree)	Presentation
First	No prolapse; painless bleeding
Second	Prolapse with straining, and spontaneous reduction Mild discomfort and bleeding
Third	Prolapse with straining, which requires manual reduction Some throbbing pain, itching, bleeding, and mucous discharge
Fourth	Permanent prolapse that cannot be reduced Pain and bleeding common Potential for thrombosis and strangulation

Prolapsed hemorrhoids also cause mucous discharge and pruritus ani. A thrombosed external hemorrhoid appears as a dark blue, firm, tender mass distal to the anal verge. A prolapsed, strangulated internal hemorrhoid appears as a purplish, tender mass covered by mucosa and emerging from the anal verge. A strangulated internal hemorrhoid is often associated with a thrombosed external hemorrhoid.

▪ DIFFERENTIAL DIAGNOSIS

The differential diagnosis for hemorrhoids consists of anal fissure, rectal prolapse, perianal condyloma, abscess, fistula, rectal varices, tumors, and manifestations of inflammatory bowel disease.

▪ DIAGNOSTIC TESTING AND EXAMINATION

The diagnostic criteria for hemorrhoids are as follows:

- Prolapse of hemorrhoids noted on rectal examination when the patient bears down
- Internal hemorrhoids are not palpable, so anoscopy is required to visualize them

▪ TREATMENTS

As a rule, most hemorrhoids should be treated conservatively, as follows:

- Warm sitz baths for 15 minutes three times a day
- Increase in dietary fiber
- Stool softeners and bulk laxatives (those causing liquid stool, which could lead to cryptitis, should be avoided)
- 0.2% topical nitroglycerin ointment to treat pain by decreasing sphincter spasm
- Topical anesthetics and steroid creams, though controversial, provide anecdotal pain relief
- Judicious use of narcotics (stool softeners should also be used if narcotics are prescribed)

Excision of a nonthrombosed hemorrhoid should never be attempted.

Acutely thrombosed external hemorrhoids can be excised in the ED. Rather than performing a simple incision and drainage, the EP should excise the roof of the thrombosed hemorrhoid as an ellipse. Excision of thrombosed hemorrhoids should never be performed in the ED in children or in adults who are immunocompromised or pregnant, patients receiving anticoagulation therapy, and patients with portal hypertension.

▪ Excision Procedure

Thrombosed external hemorrhoids can be excised as follows:

1. Put the patient in a prone or left lateral decubitus position.
2. Using a 27-gauge needle, infiltrate bupivacaine with epinephrine into the overlying skin and the skin underneath the clot.
3. Make an elliptical incision in the overlying skin (distal to the anal verge).
4. Excise the clot or clots through this opening.
5. To control bleeding, place a small piece of gauze or absorbable gelatin sponge (Gelfoam) into this opening and cover with a pressure dressing.

The patient should remove the dressing in 6 hours, at the time of the first sitz bath.

▪ DISPOSITION

Most patients with hemorrhoids can be discharged home. Immediate surgical consultation should be obtained for patients with strangulated fourth-degree internal hemorrhoids or bleeding hemorrhoids and severe anemia.

Patients with second-degree, third-degree, or nonstrangulated fourth-degree internal hemorrhoids should be referred to an outpatient surgeon for possible sclerotherapy, rubber band ligation, infrared coagulation, or excisional hemorrhoidectomy.

Patients who have undergone ED excision of thrombosed external hemorrhoids should be referred for follow-up with a surgeon.

Anal Fissure

▪ PATHOPHYSIOLOGY

Anal fissure, also called fissure in ano, is a superficial linear tear of the anoderm that begins at or just below the dentate line and extends distally toward the anal verge. Anal fissures are the most common cause of painful rectal bleeding; they are also the most common cause of rectal bleeding in infants.

Ninety-nine percent of fissures in men and 90% of fissures in women are in a posterior midline location. Posterior midline anal fissures are typically caused by passage of a large, hard stool through a tight anus.

The posterior midline is affected most because of weaker skeletal muscle and the acute angle of the rectum on the anus posteriorly.

Anterior midline fissures are most common in postpartum women. Anal fissures in other areas can be caused by receptive anal intercourse or insertion of foreign bodies, or may be manifestations of diseases such as Crohn's disease, cancer, tuberculosis, human immunodeficiency virus (HIV), and syphilis.

Fissures that are not properly treated may become chronic and develop the "classic triad" consisting of sentinel pile, deep ulcer, and enlarged anal papillae. The ulcerating fissure causes edema and irritation of the surrounding tissue. Proximally, the result is hypertrophied papillae. Distally, the result is formation of a *sentinel pile*—fibrotic tissue that may be confused with an external hemorrhoid. The sentinel pile may eventually develop into a skin tag.

▪ PRESENTING SIGNS AND SYMPTOMS

In infants, anal fissures are signified by small amounts of bright red blood on the stool or diaper. Children with anal fissures have painful defecation and "constipation" because of refusal to defecate due to pain.

Adults describe a sharp, cutting, or burning pain with defecation that can persist as a nagging, dull pain for several hours but usually subsides between bowel movements. A small amount of bright red blood may be noted on the stool or toilet paper. Sphincter spasm may also occur, causing further pain.

▪ DIFFERENTIAL DIAGNOSIS

The differential diagnosis of anal fissure includes hemorrhoids, proctitis, cryptitis, perianal abscess, and primary syphilis (chancre).

▪ DIAGNOSTIC TESTING AND EXAMINATION

Diagnosis of anal fissure must be made by physical examination, which should be done very carefully to avoid further spasm and pain. Application of a topical anesthetic such as lidocaine jelly may be necessary to facilitate the examination. Gentle retraction of the buttocks and the perianal skin with the patient bearing down may expose the distal end of the fissure. The sentinel pile may also be visualized in this manner.

Because of the severe pain and spasm, the patient may not be able to tolerate a digital rectal examination. If such an examination is performed, surrounding hypertrophic papillae may be palpated.

If the fissure is not located in the midline, the differential diagnosis, and consequent testing, must be expanded to include more serious diseases such as cancer, HIV, Crohn's disease, sexually transmitted diseases, and tuberculosis.

▪ TREATMENT

Medical treatments that are most common and most effective for anal fissures are as follows:

- Warm sitz baths for 15 minutes, three times a day
- A high-fiber diet
- Topical anesthetics such as lidocaine jelly
- Oral analgesics (narcotics increase constipation and so should be avoided)
- Topical nitroglycerin ointment 0.2%, which may reduce sphincter spasm but is associated with higher recurrence rates
- Topical calcium channel blockers (e.g., nifedipine and diltiazem), which are also associated with higher recurrence rates

Chronic fissures for which medical treatment fails are often successfully repaired through a lateral internal sphincterotomy, which is performed by a surgeon. Patients with non-midline fissures should be referred for further diagnostic testing, including ulcer biopsy and anal cultures.

Anorectal Abscess

▪ PATHOPHYSIOLOGY

Anorectal abscesses are caused primarily by infection of obstructed anal glands, ducts, and crypts. Abscesses are polymicrobial with both anaerobic and aerobic bacteria. Other causes of anorectal abscess are immunosuppression, atypical infection (e.g., tuberculosis, actinomycosis, lymphogranuloma venereum), inflammatory bowel disease (Crohn's disease), trauma (e.g., foreign body), surgery (e.g., anorectal, genitourinary, and gynecologic procedures), malignancy (e.g., rectal carcinoma, leukemia, and lymphoma), radiation, and anal fissures. Anorectal abscesses are classified according to location. The four main types are perianal (most common), ischiorectal, intersphincteric, and supralevator (least common).

▪ PRESENTING SIGNS AND SYMPTOMS

General complaints in patients with anal abscess are pain, swelling, and, occasionally, fever. Signs and symptoms of perianal abscess are a tender, erythematous, fluctuant mass at the anal verge and pain that worsens with sitting or defecating. The patient is usually afebrile.

If large, an ischiorectal abscess may manifest as a lateral perianal swelling. The patient has severe buttock pain but typically there are little to no cutaneous findings. Fever and leukocytosis are also present.

With intersphincteric abscess, there is constant rectal pressure, and the patient has severe rectal pain with sitting or straining. An erythematous, painful rectal mass is present, along with fever and leukocytosis.

Signs and symptoms of supralevator abscess are severe rectal or gluteal pain with no external skin signs, urinary retention, fever, and leukocytosis. A tender mass is detected on rectal or vaginal examination.

▪ DIFFERENTIAL DIAGNOSIS

The differential diagnosis for anal abscess consists of strangulated internal or thrombosed external hemorrhoid, anal fistula, anal fissure, sentinel pile, gonococcal proctitis, and rectal duplication in infants.

▪ DIAGNOSTIC TESTING AND EXAMINATION

- Classic history and physical examination findings
- Abdominal examination to evaluate for intra-abdominal involvement
- Perianal examination to evaluate for perianal abscess and cellulitis
- Rectal examination to evaluate for deeper abscesses
- Vaginal examination to evaluate for deeper abscesses
- Bedside glucose measurement to evaluate for diabetes mellitus
- Abdominal/pelvic computed tomography (CT) or ultrasonography to identify deep abscesses when suspected

▪ TREATMENT

▪ Perianal Abscess

Patients who do not have a complicating disorder (see later) and whose perianal abscesses measure 10 cm or smaller may be treated with incision and drainage in the ED. Elliptical or cruciate incisions are recommended for better drainage, and procedural sedation may be required. Post-incision care consists of sitz baths, stool softeners, and a high-fiber diet.

Abscesses in immunocompromised patients (diabetes, HIV, transplant, chemotherapy) should be treated in the operating room with general anesthesia.

Antibiotics should be prescribed only if there is surrounding cellulitis or the patient is immunocompromised.

▪ Ischiorectal Abscess

Superficial ischiorectal abscesses may be drained in the ED (although there is a high recurrence rate). Deeper abscesses, however, must be drained in the operating room. If there are signs of systemic involvement (fever or leukocytosis), intravenous (IV) antibiotics should be used at the time of drainage, and oral antibiotics should be added to the post-incision care regimen.

▪ Intersphincteric Abscess

The patient with an intersphincteric abscess should undergo urgent drainage in the operating room and should be given IV antibiotics.

▪ Supralevator Abscess

Emergency surgery should be performed in the operating room for any patient with a supralevator (muscle) abscess, and IV antibiotics should be prescribed.

▪ DISPOSITION

The patient with a simple perianal abscess that has been drained in the ED can be discharged. Arrangement should be made for packing changes and/or wound checks in the ED or with the patient's primary care physician in 48 hours. Surgical consultation should be obtained for patients with all other anorectal abscesses.

Anal Fistula

▪ PATHOPHYSIOLOGY

Anal fistula, also called fistula in ano, is considered a chronic variant of a poorly healed anorectal abscess. *Fistulas* are tracts between the anal canal (or rectum) and the skin that are lined with epithelial or granulation tissue. Although anal fistulas typically arise from an anorectal abscess, they can also be associated with inflammatory bowel disease, malignancies, infection (sexually transmitted diseases, actinomycosis, tuberculosis, and diverticulitis), anal fissures, or foreign bodies.

▪ PRESENTING SIGNS AND SYMPTOMS

Presenting signs and symptoms of anal fistula are a bloody-tinged, malodorous discharge and rectal pain that improves with an increased discharge. An abscess may be located at the opening of the fistula. The fistula can be palpated as a cord leading to the sphincter.

▪ DIFFERENTIAL DIAGNOSIS

The differential diagnosis of anal fistula consists of abscess, hemorrhoid, anal fissure, and gonococcal proctitis.

▪ DIAGNOSTIC TESTING AND EXAMINATION

- Anal and rectal examinations with classic findings
- Abdominal/pelvic computed tomography demonstration of a fistula tract
- Transanal ultrasonography (with or without hydrogen peroxide injected into the tract)

BOX 36-1

Causes of Proctitis

- Autoimmune inflammatory bowel disorders
- Crohn's disease
- Ulcerative colitis
- Radiation
- Sexually transmitted disease [STD]–related infections: gonorrhea, chlamydia, syphilis (usually secondary), herpes simplex virus types 1 and 2, lymphogranuloma venereum, amebiasis (oral-anal inoculation)
- Non-STD infections: *Campylobacter, Entamoeba histolytica, Salmonella, Clostridium difficile*
- Trauma
- Idiopathic

- Endoluminal magnetic resonance imaging (MRI) is the most accurate imaging modality

■ TREATMENT

Treatment of anal fistula consists of surgical excision to eliminate the fistula, prevent recurrent disease, and preserve sphincter function. Stable patients may be referred for urgent outpatient consultation.

Proctitis

■ PATHOPHYSIOLOGY

Proctitis is defined as inflammation of the rectal mucosa. It can involve actual loss of mucosal cells as well as damage to the endothelium of the small arterioles supplying the mucosa. The condition may improve spontaneously, depending on the cause, or may progress with resulting tissue ischemia, mucosal friability, bleeding, ulcers, strictures, and fistula formation. The causes of proctitis are listed in Box 36-1.

■ PRESENTING SIGNS AND SYMPTOMS

Signs and symptoms of proctitis are fecal urgency, sensation of rectal fullness, rectalgia, pruritus, rectal bleeding (spotting), and mucoid or purulent rectal discharge. The patient may also describe a change in bowel habits (diarrhea or constipation) and abdominal pain. Ulcers, vesicles or pustules, and strictures may be found on rectal examination.

■ DIFFERENTIAL DIAGNOSIS

The differential diagnosis of proctitis consists of anal fistula, anal fissure, rectal foreign body, diverticulosis, and vulvovaginitis.

■ DIAGNOSTIC TESTING AND EXAMINATION

Anoscopy in a patient with proctitis identifies erythema, friability, bleeding, edema, ulcers, and vesicles; rectosigmoidoscopy demonstrates similar findings. The following laboratory tests should be performed:

- Stool: culture; testing for ova, parasites, fecal leukocytes, and *Clostridium difficile* toxin
- Gonorrhea and chlamydia cultures and Gram stain of anorectal swabs
- Venereal Disease Research Laboratory (VDRL) or rapid plasma reagin test if syphilis is suspected

■ TREATMENT

Most cases of proctitis can be treated medically. The underlying etiology, if known, should also be treated. All forms of the disorder may benefit from the following measures:

- Sitz baths
- Antispasmodic agents
- Low-residue diet
- Stool softeners

Anorectal Foreign Bodies

■ PATHOPHYSIOLOGY

The structure of the rectum and distal colon predisposes a foreign body to migrate cephalad after insertion. A delay in presentation may also allow for the development of edema, further complicating removal of a foreign body. Foreign bodies with smooth contours and a diameter near that of the rectum or colon may become "vacuum locked" in place, with attempts at removal causing collapse of the rectum or colon distal to the object.

■ PRESENTING SIGNS AND SYMPTOMS

Although anorectal foreign bodies are often the subject of humor and medical lore, ED management of an anorectal foreign body is actually quite rare. Because of the social stigmas involved, patients are reluctant to come to the ED and are often not forthcoming about their actual complaint. The patient has frequently attempted to remove the foreign body prior to presentation, causing further damage or complicating the removal.

Although the majority of patients give an accurate history,[1] some present with vague complaints of abdominal pain or an unlikely story about how the object became lodged in the rectum. In the ED, every effort must be made to ascertain the type, shape, number, and composition of a retained foreign body, as well as how long it has been in the anorectum, prior to its removal.

RED FLAGS

Foreign Bodies

- Type: glass, food, metallic, sharp
- Shape
- Number of objects present
- Time of insertion (delays in presentation promote edema)

▪ DIFFERENTIAL DIAGNOSIS

Objects lodged in the anorectum may have been self-inserted, inserted as a result of a sexual assault, iatrogenically inserted (e.g., rectal thermometer), or swallowed.

▪ DIAGNOSTIC TESTING AND EXAMINATION

The shape, composition, surface, contour, and orientation of a foreign body influence the ultimate method of its removal. Most foreign bodies can be classified as low-lying, and therefore palpable in the rectal ampulla, or high-lying foreign bodies—at or proximal to the rectosigmoid junction.[2]

Examination and diagnostic testing should include the following:

- Thorough palpation of the abdomen (identify masses, peritonitis)
- Flat and upright radiographs of the abdomen
- Digital rectal examination (if the object is not sharp)

Anoscopy to visualize the foreign body should be considered.

▪ TREATMENT

Treatment of an anorectal foreign body is based on the results of the abdominal and rectal examinations as well as the plain radiographs (Fig. 36-1). Patients with palpable, low-lying foreign bodies can undergo conscious sedation and local anesthesia for attempted removal in the ED. Patients with high-lying foreign bodies or signs of perforation should be managed operatively.

▪ Foley Catheter Removal of Anorectal Foreign Body

A Foley catheter can be used to break the suction caused by insertion of an object with a diameter similar to that of the colon or rectum; the procedure is as follows:

1. Put the patient in the lithotomy position.
2. Pass one or more Foley catheters beyond the foreign body.
3. Insufflate air to break suction.

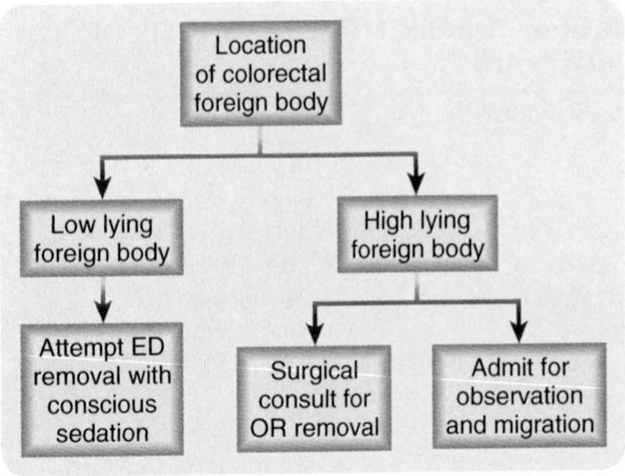
Location
of colorectal
foreign body
Low lying
foreign body
High lying
foreign body
Attempt ED
removal with
conscious
sedation
Surgical
consult for
OR removal
Admit for
observation
and migration

FIGURE 36-1 Treatment algorithm for colorectal foreign body. OR, operating room.

4. Inflate the Foley balloons.
5. While grasping the foreign body with gentle traction using either hands or forceps, slowly remove the catheter(s) with moderate pressure.

▪ DISPOSITION

A patient who underwent successful removal of a low-lying foreign body may be discharged from the ED. For any patient with suspected rectal perforation, proctosigmoidoscopy should be performed by a gastroenterologist or colorectal surgeon prior to disposition.

Pruritus Ani

Pruritus ani is a recurrent and unpleasant itching sensation in the anal canal or perianal, perineal, vulvar, scrotal, or buttocks areas. Approximately 1% to 5% of the population seeks medical attention for this condition during their lifetimes. More men than women experience the disorder, which is more common in the fifth and sixth decades of life.[3] Because of the social stigmas involved, many patients attempt self-treatment prior to presentation. The condition is often poorly understood and improperly treated by health care providers.

▪ PATHOPHYSIOLOGY

In 50% of cases of pruritus ani, the cause is unknown. Potential etiologies (especially malignancy) must be excluded before symptoms can be classified as idiopathic (Table 36-2).

▪ PRESENTING SIGNS AND SYMPTOMS

Patients typically describe an itching sensation that is worse at night and during the summer months. As the patient scratches, the perianal skin is further irritated, and the condition worsens. Physical findings

Table 36-2 DIFFERENTIAL DIAGNOSIS OF PRURITUS ANI

Anorectal disease	Fissures Proctitis Hemorrhoids Abscess Fistula Malignancy
Dermatologic disease	Lichen planus Lichen sclerosis Lichen atrophicus Eczema Psoriasis Seborrhea
Infectious disease	*Candida albicans* dermatophytes *Staphylococcus aureus* *Corynebacterium minutissimum* Group A [beta]-hemolytic streptococci Human papillomavirus Herpes simplex *Enterobius vermicularis* *Sarcoptes scabiei* Pinworms
Medications	Colchicines Quinidine Mineral oil Neomycin
Systemic disease	Diabetes mellitus Renal failure Lymphoma
Foods	Tomatoes Citrus fruits Nuts Chocolate Coffee Tea Cola Beer
Irritants	Fecal contamination Excess moisture Soap Aggressive anal wiping Scented toilet paper

Data from Jones DJ: ABC of colorectal disease: Pruritus ani. BMJ 1992;305:575-577.

vary with the duration of the condition; they include:

- Erythema
- Whitening or cracking of the perianal skin
- Bleeding in severe cases

▪ DIFFERENTIAL DIAGNOSIS

See Table 36-2.[4] Fecal contamination of the perianal skin is the most common cause of pruritus ani.

▪ DIAGNOSTIC TESTING AND EXAMINATION

Evaluation should include a careful history of potential exposures, examination of the perianal skin, digital rectal examination, anoscopy, and directed testing to exclude specific suspected causes.

▪ TREATMENT

Most cases of pruritus can be treated conservatively, with the following measures:

- Gentle cleansing and attention to hygiene of the perianal skin
- Modifications of diet and medications
- Brief courses of topical steroids (long-term steroid therapy should be avoided as it may thin the perianal skin and further exacerbate the condition)
- An oral antipruritic medication, such as hydroxyzine
- Daily application of topical capsaicin cream (0.006%), which has been shown to be effective in reducing or eliminating symptoms[5,6]

The patient should also be referred to his or her primary care physician for evaluation of chronic symptoms, biopsy, and other testing.

Proctalgia Fugax

▪ PATHOPHYSIOLOGY

Proctalgia fugax is a severe, episodic anal pain. The disorder is poorly understood and difficult to treat. The pathophysiology of this condition is unclear, although it is believed to be caused by spasm of either the anal sphincter or the muscles of the pelvic floor.

▪ PRESENTING SIGNS AND SYMPTOMS

Proctalgia fugax is usually characterized by sudden episodes of intense pain around the anal ring that can occur at any time and may last from 20 minutes to several hours. Typically, the pain occurs at night and often wakes the patient. The sensation may be associated with an urge to pass stool or flatus. Some patients may experience only one episode in their lifetime. The lifetime prevalence of this condition is 14%.[7]

▪ DIFFERENTIAL DIAGNOSIS

Other conditions that commonly cause rectal pain should be considered in the differential diagnosis of proctalgia fugax, such as anal fissure, hemorrhoids, perirectal abscess, and proctitis.

▪ TREATMENT AND DISPOSITION

No specific treatment exists for proctalgia fugax. Anecdotal evidence supports the use of benzodiazepines, topical anesthetics,[7] and botulinum toxin.[8] Hot packs or direct anal pressure have also been recommended.[9]

Patients with recurrent disease should be referred to a gastroenterologist.

Hidradenitis Suppurativa

PATHOPHYSIOLOGY

Perianal hidradenitis suppurativa is a disease of the skin and subcutaneous tissues arising from occlusion of the apocrine glands with keratin. It tends to be chronic, recurrent, and primarily localized to areas with the highest density of apocrine sweat glands (groin, axilla, and mammary regions). Sequelae include inflammation, infection, and eventual rupture of the gland with secondary cellulitis of the surrounding tissues. The disease ultimately leads to formation of chronic draining sinuses.[10]

PRESENTING SIGNS AND SYMPTOMS

Patients with the early stages of perianal hidradenitis suppurativa typically present with a painful boil in the perianal region. Classically, the abscess is deep and round without any central necrosis or fluctuance. The patient may describe similar episodes that resolved spontaneously. Later, more chronic stages of the disease may manifest as open draining fistulas and sinuses (Box 36-2).

DIFFERENTIAL DIAGNOSIS

The differential diagnosis of perianal hidradenitis suppurativa consists of carbuncles, lymphadenitis, infected sebaceous cysts, noninflamed cysts, other infectious processes (abscesses, fistulas), and Crohn's disease.

TREATMENT

Medical treatment for perianal hidradenitis suppurativa consists of weight loss, smoking cessation (if applicable), and the use of antibiotics. Clindamycin 300 mg twice daily has been shown to be effective in suppression,[10-12] but the disease often returns when antibiotics are stopped; topical clindamycin cream is similarly effective. Retinoids may also be tried. Acitretin 25 mg twice daily decreases keratin production and has been shown to reduce the number of outbreaks. Hormonal therapy may also be effective; finasteride was shown to induce remission in a small case study.[10]

Surgical drainage provides only short-term relief, because the condition has a 100% recurrence rate.[11,12] Radical excision of the inflamed apocrine tissue carries a recurrence rate of 25%.[12]

BOX 36-2

Characteristics of Hidradenitis Suppurativa

- Age of onset: puberty
- Female-to-male ratio: 3:1
- Associated conditions: acne, comedones, obesity, hirsutism
- Sites affected (in descending order of frequency): axillary, inguinal, perianal and perineal, mammary and inframammary, buttock, pubic region, chest, scalp, retroauricular, eyelid

DISPOSITION

All patients with perianal hidradenitis suppurativa should be referred to a dermatologist for long-term management.

Pilonidal Disease

PATHOPHYSIOLOGY

Pilonidal disease is a common disorder that generally affects young adults—those between the ages of 15 and 24 years—with a 3:1 male predominance. Pilonidal disease often causes a considerable amount of suffering, inconvenience, and time away from work. An estimated 40,000 to 70,000 patients are treated annually, mostly as outpatients.[13] Approximately 50% of patients with this condition present to an EP with an acute pilonidal abscess.[14]

The term *pilonidal* is the combination of the words *pilus* meaning "hair" and *nidus* meaning "nest." The condition is believed to arise from hairs in the natal cleft that, because of their location, grow inward rather than out. The shafts of these hairs penetrate the skin, leading to a condition of chronic inflammation and eventual infection. Chronic infection results in the formation of sinus tracts and recurrent disease.

PRESENTING SIGNS AND SYMPTOMS

The presenting signs and symptoms of pilonidal disease usually are pain and swelling in the sacrococcygeal region with inability to sit on one side of the buttocks, or perhaps inability to tolerate a sitting position at all. Systemic involvement is rare. Physical examination usually demonstrates either a tender fluctuant mass over the coccyx or sacrum or a larger area of inflammation with multiple draining tracts.

DIFFERENTIAL DIAGNOSIS

Other diseases that manifest as infection or fistula must be excluded, such as rectal or perirectal abscess, Crohn's disease, and hidradenitis suppurativa.

DIAGNOSTIC TESTING AND EXAMINATION

The classic clinical presentation of pilonidal disease is sufficient for diagnosis. Imaging is not useful for a typical presentation of this condition.

▪ TREATMENT AND DISPOSITION

Treatment is both medical and surgical. ED treatment generally consists of incision and drainage of the abscess. Simple incision and drainage results in healing in 58% of patients within 10 weeks; of those patients, 40% have no further symptoms, and 20% experience only minor symptoms.[15] Antibiotics should be prescribed to treat any secondary cellulitis. In one study, metronidazole 500 mg orally four times a day for 14 days resulted in more rapid healing than no antibiotics.[15]

Patients with pilonidal disease can be discharged from the ED with arrangements or instructions for follow-up with a surgeon.

REFERENCES

1. Busch BB, Starling JR: Rectal foreign bodies: Case reports and a comprehensive review of the world's literature. Surgery 1986;100:512-519.
2. Eftaiha M, Hambrick E, Abcarian H: Principles of management of colorectal foreign bodies. Arch Surg 1977;112: 691-695.
3. Fry RD: Hemorrhoids, fissures, and pruritus ani. Surg Clin North Am 1994;74:1289-1292.
4. Jones DJ: ABC of colorectal diseases: Pruritus ani. BMJ 1992;305:575-577.
5. Lysy J, Sistiery-Ittah M, Israelit Y, et al: Topical capsaicin—a novel and effective treatment for idiopathic intractable pruritus ani: A randomised, placebo controlled, crossover study. Gut 2003;52:1323-1326.
6. Anand P: Capsaicin and menthol in the treatment of itch and pain: Recently cloned receptors provide the key. Gut 2003;52:1233-1235.
7. Peleg R, Shvartzman P: Low-dose intravenous lidocaine as a treatment for proctalgia fugax. Reg Anesth Pain Med 2002;27:97-99.
8. Katsinelos P, Kalomenopoulou M, Christodoulou K, et al: Treatment of proctalgia fugax with botulinum A toxin. Eur J Gastroenterol Hepatol 2001;13:1371-1373.
9. Vincent C: Anorectal pain and irritation. Prim Care 1999;26:53-66.
10. Slade D, Powell B, Mortimer P: Hidradenitis suppurativa: Pathogenesis and management. Brit J Plast Surg 2003; 56:451-461.
11. Mortimer P, Lunniss P: Hidradenitis suppurativa. J Roy Soc Med 1999;93:420-422.
12. Rubin R, Chinn B: Perianal hidradenitis suppurativa. Surg Clinics North Am 1994;74:1317-1325.
13. Surrell J: Pilonidal disease. Surg Clin North Am 1994; 74:1309-1315.
14. Jones DJ: ABC of colorectal diseases. Pilonidal sinus. BMJ 1992;305:410-412.
15. Allen-Mersh T: Pilonidal sinus: Finding the right track for treatment. Br J Surg 1990;77:123-132.

Chapter 37

Hepatic Disease

Richard Paula

KEY POINTS

Causes of jaundice are best categorized by the fraction of measured bilirubin implicated in disease—unconjugated or conjugated hyperbilirubinemia.
The possibility of cerebral edema should be considered in patients with advanced liver disease who present with nausea, vomiting, and mental status changes.
Because of the uncertain relationship of measured serum ammonia and cerebral ammonia concentration, patients with known or suspected hepatic encephalopathy should be treated for hyperammonemia regardless of the measured level.
The prevalence of spontaneous bacterial peritonitis is high in cirrhotic patients, with rates of 3.5% in those with no symptoms to 30% in patients who present to a hospital for any reason and undergo paracentesis.
Hepatitis B virus immune globulin effectively prevents transmission of hepatitis B virus if administered within 72 hours of exposure; it should be given for any high-risk exposure.
Pyogenic liver abscesses are best treated with a combination of antibiotics and percutaneous drainage. Antibiotics alone are insufficient treatment.

Scope

Chronic liver disease accounts for 70,000 hospitalizations annually in the United States and is one of the top ten leading causes of death. Almost half of the 40,000 deaths per year in the United States are related to alcohol abuse. Although the majority of deaths are due to chronic liver disease and cirrhosis, 2000 deaths per year are associated with fulminant hepatic failure.[1] Many of the patients in these cases die while awaiting liver transplantation. Hepatitis B and hepatitis C infections account for 40% of chronic liver disease, although many of these cases are exacerbated by concomitant alcohol abuse.

Liver disease is debilitating and deadly because the liver is intimately involved in many physiologic functions. The liver (1) synthesizes coagulation factors, cholesterol, bile, and glycogen, (2) conjugates bilirubin, and (3) detoxifies exogenous chemicals such as alcohol as well as endogenous metabolic byproducts such as ammonia. The loss of any of these functions significantly impairs homeostasis.

Common Signs and Symptoms of Liver Disease

■ JAUNDICE

The most common and immediately apparent evidence of liver disease is jaundice, which often manifests without any other symptoms. Jaundice, one of the most recognized human disease states, is documented in pre-biblical writings.

Jaundice begins to appear when the serum bilirubin level reaches 3 mg/dL in white persons, and at higher levels in darker-skinned persons. Jaundice does not require treatment in adults as it does in neonates, but rather, the etiology of the jaundice in adults should be investigated.

Causes of jaundice are often categorized according to the type of bilirubin implicated in disease, unconjugated or conjugated hyperbilirubinemia. In context with associated symptoms, knowledge of the fractionations of bilirubinemia aid in narrowing the differential diagnosis.

Pancreatic and biliary cancers associated with jaundice may manifest as pain.[2] Patients with cirrhosis from chronic hepatitis are likely to describe painless jaundice but also complain of fatigue, pruritus, and constitutional symptoms. Patients who are acutely ill with jaundice, nausea, emesis, and fever should be tested for causes of acute hepatitis; similar presentations without fever occur in toxic ingestions.

■ NAUSEA

Nausea is a common extrahepatic symptom that may complicate hepatitis, toxic liver injury, cholestasis, and many other causes of acute or chronic liver disease. Nausea management is sometimes the sole reason that a patient with acute hepatitis requires hospital admission.

Particular attention should be given to the patient with known liver disease who presents with nausea, emesis, and mental status changes; the EP should consider the possibility of cerebral edema, especially in the patient with advanced liver disease.

■ NEUROPSYCHIATRIC SIGNS AND SYMPTOMS

Mental status changes in the setting of liver disease should be aggressively treated. The degree of encephalopathy is directly correlated to that of liver dysfunction. Patients with a sudden change in mental status and acute hepatic insufficiency usually have an advanced stage of disease that will often progress to acute, fulminant liver failure.

Cerebral edema often occurs in tandem with encephalopathy owing to elevated ammonia levels; immediate treatment with ammonia-clearing agents (e.g., lactulose) is required. Note that lactulose is less effective in treating mental status changes associated with acute liver failure than those associated with chronic disease. Caregivers of patients with chronic hepatic insufficiency often titrate lactulose dosing in accordance with cognitive function.

■ HEPATOMEGALY

In hepatomegaly, the liver becomes significantly enlarged and easily palpable owing to sudden edema from hepatitis or the appearance of fatty infiltrates with alcohol binging. If the enlargement is significant enough to cause portal hypertension, the spleen is often enlarged and palpable as well. As the liver scars and liver cells are replaced by fibrous tissue in cirrhosis, the organ shrinks and eventually becomes small and nodular. The presence or absence of hepatomegaly on examination is an unreliable estimate of liver function and should not be used to exclude a particular diagnosis.[3,4]

■ RASH

Many patients with liver disease complain of skin irritation. Hepatitis has been associated with livedo reticularis, a lacy, erythematous rash caused by capillary spasm. Dermatitis caused by autoimmune hepatitis that promotes jaundice has an intense pruritic component. Patients with liver disease may be unable to control scratching, and infections develop in the self-induced excoriations. Lastly, patients may complain of a "rash" that represents ecchymosis due to coagulopathy; such bruising without reported trauma should raise a concern for advanced liver disease.

Signs and Symptoms of Advanced Liver Disease

■ ENCEPHALOPATHY

Mental status changes may occur with either acute or chronic liver disease. The pathophysiology of hepatic encephalopathy is not completely understood, but it is clear that pronounced encephalopathy is associated with poor outcomes. Although many chemical markers have been implicated as the cause of hepatic encephalopathy, most studies identify two important factors, gamma-aminobutyric acid (GABA) and ammonia.

Serum GABA levels are elevated in cirrhosis. Administration of a GABA receptor antagonist (flumazenil) results in transient but significant improvements in the cirrhotic patient's mental status.

The second and more easily measurable toxicity results from increased ammonia (NH_3) concentration. Serum ammonia concentration rises as liver function declines, with intermittent fluctuations in chronically ill patients. Many factors affect ammonia production, including changes in diet, constipation, hepatorenal syndrome, and gastrointestinal bleeding. Ammonia readily crosses the blood-brain barrier; in patients with hepatic encephalopathy, ammonia causes cerebral toxicity, which promotes mental status decline and eventual coma.[5-7]

Ammonia is clearly toxic, and in animal models, ammonia infusions alone have been directly linked to development of cerebral edema. In the setting of acute liver failure, ammonia levels higher than 200 μg/dL are strongly associated with the development of cerebral edema and herniation.[8-10] In patients with advanced liver disease and cirrhosis, however, mental status may not correlate directly with measured ammonia levels. Ammonia tends to accumulate in the brain, and although blood levels may be normal, the patient may still have enough ammonia in the cerebrospinal fluid to induce encephalopathy.

Owing to the uncertain relationship of measured serum ammonia and cerebral ammonia concentration, patients with known or suspected hepatic encephalopathy should be treated for hyperammonemia regardless of measured serum levels. There is no convincing evidence to suggest that arterial sampling for ammonia measurement is superior to venous measurements.[7]

■ Treatment

The ED management of hepatic encephalopathy consists of appropriate airway control and resuscitation followed by the administration of ammonia-lowering agents. Lactulose (15 to 45 mL once or twice daily) is the most common treatment of choice in the United States, although sodium benzoate has been shown to be equally effective and less expensive.[11] Lactulose is a nonabsorbable disaccharide that decreases intestinal transit time through a direct cathartic effect, thus lowering intestinal bacterial loads. Lactulose also lowers intestinal pH, which favors competitive non–ammonia-producing bacteria. Lactulose may be given orally, by nasogastric tube, or, in severely obtunded patients, as a retention enema.[12]

Neomycin is a poorly absorbed aminoglycoside used as secondary treatment to further reduce intestinal bacterial counts. Even though it is poorly absorbed, neomycin does cause systemic toxicity and should be used only when lactulose is ineffective. Mannitol (0.5 to 1 g/kg) effectively reduces cerebral edema and improves survival in patients with hepatic encephalopathy due to acute liver failure.[8,13]

The following therapies have been shown to be ineffective and should be avoided: hyperventilation,[8,14] corticosteroids,[8,13] and terlipressin.[15]

■ ASCITES

Ascites is the abnormal accumulation of peritoneal fluid, a common feature of advanced liver disease. The exact pathogenesis of ascites has not been found. Multiple theories focus on the interaction of the liver with various other organ systems. The combination of portal hypertension and decreased albumin production contribute significantly to the accumulation of ascitic fluid.

Ascites associated with cirrhosis has a poor prognosis. One episode of ascites has a 3-year mortality rate of 50%, and recurrent ascites has the same 50% mortality at 1 year.[16,17] Comorbid conditions contribute to mortality, including the development of hepatocellular carcinoma, gastrointestinal hemorrhage, coma, and infection.

One important infectious cause of death in patients with ascites is spontaneous bacterial peritonitis (SBP). The prevalence of SBP is high in cirrhotic patients, with rates of 3.5% in asymptomatic patients to 30% in patients who present to a hospital for any reason and undergo paracentesis.[18,19]

Ascites itself may cause morbidity, because paracentesis for the relief of tense ascites has been known to improve cardiac function for 30 years.[20] Reduction of intra-abdominal hypertension and resolution of an effective abdominal compartment syndrome improve venous return to the heart.[21]

Patients who present with symptomatic ascites require paracentesis. Given the high rate of occult SBP in these patients, peritoneal fluid should always be sent for analysis. Previously it was thought that large-volume paracentesis was associated with complications and should be avoided, but this common misperception has been disproved. Large-volume (>5 L) paracentesis is safe and is associated with shorter hospitalization than diuretic therapy in patients with refractory ascites.[22,23]

Complications of paracentesis are rare, even in thrombocytopenic patients. Most complications involve bleeding or persistent leakage from the puncture site and occur within 24 hours. Patients with such complications should be admitted for observation.[24,25]

Controversy exists regarding volume expansion with colloids in conjunction with paracentesis. Studies have not demonstrated any short-term improvements in mortality or morbidity with the use of plasma expanders, although some alterations in renal function, such as elevations in blood urea nitrogen (BUN) and decreased sodium levels (both of which are associated with worse prognosis), have been observed. Albumin is the least expensive, safest, and usually most effective colloid for intravascular volume expansion and should be used for paracentesis volumes of 5 L or larger.[26,27]

Paracentesis is improved when ultrasonography is used to identify ascites and guide the paracentesis. In one study, paracentesis with ultrasonographic guidance was successful in 95% of patients, compared with 65% of procedures without such guidance.[28]

Outpatient treatment for ascites should center on dietary sodium restriction in combination with diuretics. Management by a primary care physician includes frequent checks of potassium and sodium levels, both of which have been implicated in morbidity in these patients. Patients with recurrent ascites should be referred for surgical evaluation for a possible transjugular intrahepatic portosystemic shunt (TIPS) procedure.

■ SPONTANEOUS BACTERIAL PERITONITIS

Symptoms of SBP are often vague. Although abdominal pain and fever are common, both may be absent. Patients may complain only of increased fatigue, myalgias, worsening ascites, or mental status decline.

SBP is thought to be caused by translocation of intestinal flora, although this long-held premise is now under question. Previously, SBP was almost entirely associated with gram-negative bacteria, mostly *Escherichia coli;* a growing number of patients with SBP now present with gram-positive organisms.[29]

Diagnosis is confirmed by culture of peritoneal fluid aspirated on paracentesis. SBP is likely if peritoneal fluid neutrophil counts are greater than 250 cells/μL. Peritoneal fluid lactate levels may be even more accurate.[26,27]

Patients with suspected SPB should have as much fluid drained as possible. Empirical antibiotic treatment should begin as soon as the diagnosis is considered. SBP in cirrhotic patients carries a mortality rate of 20% to 40%, with a 1-year survival rate of only 40%.[26] Treatment should begin with a third-generation cephalosporin, such as ceftriaxone or cefotaxime. Quinolones should not be used, because bacterial resistance to these agents is high and will worsen if the incidence of gram-positive infections continues to rise.

■ CIRRHOSIS

Continued liver injury results in irreparable damage, with permanent loss of liver function and subsequent chronic disease states. Cirrhosis is the common end point of many chronic liver diseases, characterized by the replacement of functioning hepatocytes with physiologically inactive fibrotic tissue. Patients with cirrhosis may present with any number of symptoms or clinical conditions related to end-stage liver disease.

■ PORTAL HYPERTENSION

Portal hypertension occurs when intraportal pressures are elevated 10 mm Hg above normal throughout the portal system. The cause is multifactorial, and the disorder can occur with conditions other than cirrhosis.

Parasite infections are an extremely common cause of reversible portal hypertension in developing countries. Parasites, commonly schistosomiasis, cause chronic inflammatory states in the portal sinusoids, leading to granuloma formation and fibrosis.

Portal hypertension develops in patients with cirrhosis because of increased intrahepatic resistance to greater portal flow. Numerous cellular disorders occur simultaneously in cirrhotic patients with increased portal pressures: Lack of intrahepatic vasodilation is caused by fibrocyte deposition and decreased nitric oxide production within the liver. Increased portal flow results from higher cardiac output and splanchnic flow associated with extrahepatic nitric oxide production. The greater pressure causes deposition of peritoneal fluid and a redirection of blood flow. As these forces coincide, blood is rerouted around the liver to compensate. Collateral flow increases as the portal pressure rises; pressures greater than 12 mm Hg promote the formation of *varices*—chronically dilated veins in the collateral bed that shunt blood flow away from the liver. Varices occur in the following locations

Abdominal wall: Varices of the abdominal wall are called caput Medusa, so named for their serpentine appearance. They arise from dilation of abdominal wall and umbilical veins.

Rectum: Hemorrhoids represent a form of rectal varices. They are often friable and subject to significant bleeding.

Esophagus: Esophageal varices are a common source of gastrointestinal bleeding in patients with portal hypertension. Bleeding may be massive and difficult to control owing to concomitant coagulopathy.

■ HYPONATREMIA

Cirrhotic patients have impaired free water excretion. Low sodium levels, found in a third of all patients with cirrhosis, contribute to ascites, frequent falls, and cognitive decline. Hyponatremia is associated with a decreased response to diuretic therapy and a poor overall prognosis.[30]

■ HEPATORENAL SYNDROME

Hepatorenal syndrome exists as a chronic debilitating state or as rapidly progressive and terminal condition. This syndrome occurs when kidney function declines in the setting of liver failure. All patients with cirrhosis have some degree of renal insufficiency; most continue to decline slowly, whereas others will rapidly progress to renal failure.

Hepatorenal syndrome is diagnosed in a patient with cirrhosis who also has a rise in creatinine levels to more than 1.5 mg/dL in conjunction with a serum sodium level less than 130 mEq/L. SBP, acute alcoholic hepatitis, and hypotension are common precipitants of this syndrome. Although hepatorenal syndrome frequently develops in patients being treated for SBP, there is some evidence that administering albumin as a component of SBP management reduces the likelihood of this development.

Liver transplantation is the only therapy that has been shown to reduce mortality in patients with fulminant hepatorenal syndrome.[31]

Infectious Causes of Liver Disease

■ HEPATITIS A VIRUS

Hepatitis A virus (HAV) is a single-stranded RNA enterovirus in the disease-producing family Picornaviridae, which also includes polio. Also known as "epidemic hepatitis" owing to its ability to spread swiftly and suddenly, HAV occurs in an average 60,000 cases annually worldwide. Transmission is fecal-oral, as in settings such as day care, or through sexual contact. It may also be transmitted by contaminated water or food sources; shellfish is a common vector, although seemingly innocuous food sources, such as imported lettuce, have been implicated in outbreaks as well.[32,33]

Symptoms and Signs

Incubation may be as long as 30 days. Symptoms include anorexia, nausea, emesis, diarrhea, fever, and eventual jaundice.

Diagnostic Testing

Serum IgM titers are diagnostic for HAV injection.

Treatment and Prognosis

Treatment for HAV is supportive. Most infections are subclinical, and full recovery is expected in more than 99.5% of those infected. A vaccine is commercially available for HAV and is recommended for persons traveling to endemic areas. HAV immune globulin may be used up to 2 weeks after exposure; it is generally reserved for high-risk patients, such as those with preexisting infectious hepatitis (other than HAV), elderly patients, and immunocompromised patients.

Disposition

Patients with HAV may need to be admitted to the hospital for parenteral control of vomiting and administration of fluids. Liver function values are often markedly elevated, although this finding is not an indication for admission.

HEPATITIS B VIRUS

Hepatitis B virus (HBV) is a double-stranded DNA virus that has a cross-species reservoir. It infects human, ducks, and squirrels. HBV is transmitted person to person through sexual contact, blood exposure, transfusion, and perinatal vertical transmission. It is highly virulent: Infection may be caused by a small number of virions. HBV is easily passed through contaminated needles, either from needle sharing among drug abusers or through occupational exposure in health care workers.

More than 1 million individuals have chronic HBV in the United States, and approximately 500 million are infected worldwide. From 1990 to 2004, the overall incidence of reported acute HBV infection declined 75% through vaccination efforts, from 8.5 to 2.1 per 100,000 persons.[34-36]

Symptoms and Signs

Acute infection with HBV causes anorexia, nausea, emesis, diarrhea, fever, and eventual jaundice. Levels of serum alanine aminotransferase (ALT) and aspartate aminotransferase (AST) may both rise to more than 10,000 U/L with constitutional symptoms that precede the appearance of jaundice.

Diagnostic Testing

HBV infection can be defined as acute, chronic, or carrier. If the patient has not been immunized against HBV and has not previously shown signs of the disease, the presence of hepatitis B surface antigen (HBsAg) and expected symptoms confirms the diagnosis of acute infection.

Treatment and Prognosis

Prognosis for HBV infection varies widely, although most individuals (90% to 95%) recover completely. Up to 10% of patients enter a chronic infectious state and are at risk for cirrhosis and hepatocellular carcinoma. Approximately 2% die of fulminant hepatic failure.

Multiple drug regimens exist for the treatment of HBV, most notably peginterferon alfa-2b with or without lamivudine. Such regimens have never been shown to be effective in the acute setting, and recommendations are to withhold treatment until evidence of ongoing viral replication is present.

HBV immune globulin (HBV-IG) effectively prevents transmission if given within 72 hours of exposure and should be administered in high-risk exposures. Centers for Disease Control and Prevention (CDC) guidelines recommend administration of HBV-IG and HBV vaccine to unvaccinated health care workers exposed to patients known to have HBV, and HBV-IG for high-risk exposures to persons with unknown HBV status. Nonoccupational post-exposure prophylaxis should follow similar recommendations (e.g., sexual assault or coincident with HIV post-exposure prophylaxis).

Disposition

Patients with HBV infection may require admission for parenteral control of vomiting and administration of fluids. Evidence of possible hepatic failure is reflected in prolongation of the prothrombin time (PT), which should be measured if HBV is suspected. Liver function values are often markedly elevated, but this finding is not an indication for admission.

HEPATITIS C VIRUS

An RNA virus that is extremely complex and diverse, hepatitis C virus (HCV) has at least six distinct genotypes and 50 subtypes. This genetic diversity complicates development of a vaccine against it. HCV infection is the leading cause of liver transplantation; chronic infection commonly causes cirrhosis and hepatocellular carcinoma.[35] Transmission occurs through sexual contact and through sharing needles with infected individuals.

HCV transmission peaked in the United States in the 1980s prior to its discovery, with an estimated 250,000 new cases per year in that decade. Infection rates have dropped to approximately 40,000 annually. Carriers with chronic HCV infection number almost 3 million.[37] The prevalence of HCV among trauma patients is 15% to 20%.[38,39]

Diagnosis

Unlike acute infection with HAV or HBV, acute HCV infection is much more likely to pass without symptoms—up to 80% of infected persons are asymptomatic. HCV can produce a flu-like illness that is easily ignored. It is ultimately diagnosed with anti-HCV antibody screening, which is confirmed by polymerase chain reaction (PCR) for HCV RNA.

Treatment and Prognosis

HCV is much more destructive than either HAV or HBV. Approximately 15% of infected persons fully recover, but 15% have cirrhosis, and 5% eventually have hepatocellular carcinoma. HCV accounts for 50% of cases of cirrhosis diagnosed in the United States.

Treatment with various drug regimens is available, although none is recommended for use in suspected infection in the ED. Viral replication must be verified and serotyped in order to guide treatment. Neither vaccine prophylaxis nor post-exposure prophylaxis is currently available.

Disposition

Patients with HCV may have to be admitted to the hospital for parenteral control of vomiting and administration of fluids. Evidence of possible hepatic failure is reflected in prolongation of the PT, which should be measured if HCV is suspected. Liver function values are often markedly elevated, although this finding is not an indication for admission.

AMEBIASIS

Amebic liver infections are of growing concern in the United States, although the infection is much more prevalent in the developing world. Amebiasis affects 50 million persons worldwide and is estimated to cause 50,000 to 100,000 deaths per year.[40]

Amebiasis frequently manifests as colitis. It is unknown what percentage of cases progress to abscess formation, although approximately a third of patients with abscesses have prodromal nausea, emesis, diarrhea, and bloating.[41,42] Solitary abscess formation is common with amebic abscesses, as opposed to the multiple foci often seen with pyogenic abscesses. Amebic abscesses have a predilection for males, with a 10:1 ratio of infection; such gender bias is not seen with pyogenic abscesses.

Diagnosis

Most patients diagnosed with amebic liver abscesses in the United States are seen in the southwestern states and are males of Mexican origin.[43] Symptoms may mimic those of cholecystitis, with right upper quadrant abdominal pain, fever, chills, and nausea. In one series, 20% of patients with amebiasis presented with isolated pulmonary complaints.[43]

Abscesses are easily seen on ultrasonography. The ultrasonographic appearance in combination with acute symptoms makes the diagnosis in at least two thirds of patients.[42,44,45] Computed tomography (CT) is sensitive as well and should be used when the diagnosis is in question.

E. histolytica–specific antibodies should be ordered if amebic abscess is suspected.

Treatment and Prognosis

Metronidazole remains the first-line treatment (a high-dose schedule consisting of 750 mg three times daily for 10 days provides a 90% cure rate).[46] Aspiration has traditionally been recommended for abscesses larger than 5 cm, although results of studies examining this practice are equivocal.[47,48]

Disposition

Patients with amebic abscesses smaller than 5 cm are at low risk for rupture. If they are able to tolerate oral fluids and medications, such patients should be discharged after being started on high-dose metronidazole therapy with arrangements for appropriate follow-up.

When the diagnosis of amebic abscess cannot be confirmed in the ED by serologic testing, the patient should be admitted in order to exclude a potential pyogenic abscess.

PYOGENIC LIVER ABSCESSES

Liver abscesses in the United States and worldwide are most often due to amebiasis, although pyogenic abscesses represent a more serious condition. Pyogenic abscesses were diagnosed in 3000 patients per year in one European study.[49]

Patients with pyogenic abscesses are more ill, have multiple abscesses, and suffer a worse prognosis than those with amebic abscesses. Unlike those with amebic abscesses, approximately 50% of patients have multiple pyogenic abscesses, either from hematogenous spread (from infections such as diverticulitis) or through direct extension from suppurative cholangitis (now thought to be the most common cause).

Bacterial causes of pyogenic abscess are diverse, including *E. coli, Klebsiella, Staphylococcus aureus,* and various anaerobes.

Patients with pyogenic abscesses are much less likely to have the classic symptoms of liver abscess seen in amebic infections, such as right upper quadrant pain, fever, nausea, and vomiting.

Diagnosis

Because the causes of pyogenic abscesses are so varied, affected patients do not present in a uniform fashion. Right upper quadrant tenderness and hepatomegaly are noted in approximately 50% of cases.[50] Patients commonly show signs of systemic disease, such as fever, malaise, weight loss, and anorexia.

Liver function values may or may not be elevated and should not be used to exclude the diagnosis. Ultrasonography and CT are both excellent imaging modalities, with sensitivities of 85% and 95%, respectively.[50,51]

Treatment and Prognosis

Pyogenic liver abscesses are treated with a combination of antibiotics and drainage. Catheter drainage and needle aspiration are used with similar success rates of 60% to 90%, although these two options have not been compared directly. The largest published trials have demonstrated success rates exceeding 95% with ultrasonography-guided aspiration without catheter placement followed by broad-spectrum intravenous antibiotics (to cover gram-positive, gram-negative, and anaerobic organisms).[52,53] Antibiotic therapy without abscess drainage is generally unsuccessful.

Disposition

Even with appropriate therapy, the mortality rate of pyogenic abscess is 5% to 10%. Any patient with a suspected pyogenic abscess must be admitted to the hospital.

PARASITIC INFECTIONS

The most common parasitic infections of the liver are schistosomiasis (which commonly affects the portal and mesenteric circulation) and clonorchiasis (found in the biliary tree). Both parasites are very common outside the United States—an estimated 1 in 30 persons worldwide are infected with *Schistosoma* and 25% of all Asian immigrants to the United States are infected with *Clonorchis sinensis*. These parasites cause portal hypertension in a large percentage of patients in developing countries and often go undetected for years owing to lack of symptoms.

Diagnosis

Patients with parasitic infections exhibit symptoms based on the number of parasites causing infection. Those with a smaller number of organisms are asymptomatic or may have only malaise and diarrhea. With higher numbers of parasites, more constitutional symptoms are present, such as fever, chills, and weight loss.

ED patients presenting with hepatobiliary symptoms after travel to Asia should be considered at high risk for parasitic infections. Ultrasonography and CT may show indirect signs of infection, such as biliary stones and dilation; these imaging methods are not helpful for identifying the organisms themselves.[54]

Treatment and Prognosis

Praziquantel is effective for both clonorchiasis and schistosomiasis, with effective cure rates of 60% to 95%.[55] Reversal of portal hypertension is observed in 95% of children and 85% of adults with these parasitic diseases.[56]

Disposition

Patients with suspected acute parasitic disease should be admitted to the hospital because of a significant risk of mortality from *Schistosoma japonicum*. Chronic infection may be managed with supportive care and outpatient follow-up.

Noninfectious Liver Disorders

ALCOHOLIC LIVER DISEASE

Alcohol consumption is responsible for half of all chronic liver disease in the United States.[1] Alcohol may poison the liver acutely or may damage hepatocytes through repeated insult, permanently destroying hepatic architecture and eventually causing cirrhosis. Alcohol consumption causes fatty accumulation in the liver that displaces hepatocytes; the accumulation is normally reversible, but if the liver is subject to repeated insult, the fatty accumulation slowly becomes permanent. Chronic fatty liver is subject to inflammatory changes that induce scarring and permanent replacement of functional hepatocytes with lipocytes and fibrous tissue. Smaller numbers of hepatocytes cannot handle the physiologic requirements of the body. This pathologic progression is significantly accelerated by coexisting HCV or HBV infection.[57] Women are much more prone to alcohol-induced hepatic injury.[58]

Acute hepatitis due to alcohol consumption is termed *alcoholic hepatitis* or *alcohol steatohepatitis*. Steatohepatitis, so named from the overwhelming fatty infiltration seen with alcohol metabolism, is associated with impairment of liver function. Acute alcoholic hepatitis is common among heavy, chronic, binge-type alcohol users.

Diagnosis

Patients with alcoholic hepatitis often admit to heavy alcohol use and may appear jaundiced or may complain of dark urine. Constitutional symptoms are common—weakness, nausea, emesis, and malaise.

Patients often display signs of chronic liver insufficiency, including asterixis and spider angiomas.

Treatment and Prognosis

Treatment is mostly supportive, although as with other forms of liver disease, both coagulopathy and mental status changes should be aggressively treated. The mortality rate in hospitalized patients with alcoholic hepatitis is approximately 10%.[59] Higher mortality is observed when patients have concomitant encephalopathy and coagulopathy; immediate liver transplantation may be required for their survival.

Corticosteroid use in hospitalized patients with alcoholic hepatitis is controversial. During the 1980s and early 1990s, a number of studies were published proclaiming significant reductions in mortality with the use of corticosteroids (particularly convincing was one study of the use of prednisolone in 1992).[60] However, a carefully performed meta-analysis published in 1995 that examined 12 controlled trials did not find benefit.[61] The use of corticosteroids should be reserved for the inpatients and should not be initiated in the ED.

Disposition

Admission to the hospital is necessary for patients with acute alcoholic hepatitis owing to high mortality rates and a significant need for transfusion, vasopressors, and aggressive resuscitation.

AUTOIMMUNE LIVER DISORDERS

The two major immunologic causes of liver disease are autoimmune hepatitis and primary biliary sclerosis. Patients with immune-related liver disease are mostly female and show signs of autoimmune disease as well as liver disease. The clinical signs regularly include myalgias, polyarthritis, rash, and findings consistent with other autoimmune disorders, such as Sjögren's syndrome and systemic lupus erythematosus (SLE).

Patients with autoimmune liver disorders have progressive disease and an untreated survival rate of 10% to 50% in 5 years. As the disease advances, the patient exhibits signs of liver insufficiency similar to those in other patients with chronic liver disease.[62,63]

These diseases are difficult to detect and differentiate from other forms of chronic liver disease—such differentiation is not a goal of ED care.

Management of patients with autoimmune liver disorders is complicated by immunosuppressive drugs used in treatment (prednisone and azathioprine are most commonly prescribed). When caring for patients in the ED, the clinician must consider complications of immunosuppressive therapy and must administer stress-dose corticosteroids when required.

Prognosis has improved with liver transplantation, providing a 10-year survival rate of 75%; recurrence is seen in 42% of patients.[64]

Table 37-1 DRUGS THAT CAUSE LIVER DISEASE

Anesthetics	Halothane Enflurane Isoflurane
Antimicrobials	Sulfonamides Dapsone Pyrazinamide Ketoconazole Isoniazid Rifampin
Anticonvulsants	Phenytoin Valproic acid Carbamazepine Felbamate
Analgesics	Acetaminophen Diclofenac Sulindac Etodolac Oxaprozin
Miscellaneous	Nicotinic acid Labetalol Flutamide Disulfiram Propylthiouracil (PTU) Nefazodone

From Lewis J: Drug-induced liver disease. Med Clin North Am 2000;84:1275-1311.

DRUG-INDUCED LIVER DISEASE

Many pharmaceutical and naturally occurring substances can cause catastrophic liver injury (Table 37-1). The presentation of drug-induced liver disease varies from benign jaundice to fulminant hepatic failure. Almost 40% of cases of acute hepatic failure in the United States are caused by drug-induced injury; almost half of these cases are due to acetaminophen alone.[65,66]

PREGNANCY-ASSOCIATED LIVER DISEASE

Approximately 5 out of 1000 pregnancies in the United States are complicated by liver disease. The two main disease states are HELLP syndrome (hemolysis, elevated liver enzymes, and low platelets; seen in 1 to 6 in 1000 pregnancies) and acute fatty liver of pregnancy (AFLP; seen in 1 in 13,000 pregnancies).[67,68]

HELLP Syndrome

HELLP syndrome is a serious condition that affects 20% of pregnant women with preeclampsia. It occurs when oxidative stressors associated with microangiopathic hemolytic anemia lead to multisystem organ dysfunction and hepatic malfunction. As opposed to eclampsia, the HELLP syndrome usually occurs in older multiparous women. Most of the cases are diagnosed in the third trimester but can occur earlier or even after delivery. HELLP can be observed without significant hypertension or proteinuria.[69] The most severe complications of HELLP syndrome are coagulopathy and eventual disseminated intravascular coagulation.

Diagnosis

Women with HELLP syndrome most commonly complain of nausea, vomiting, or right upper quadrant pain. Jaundice is rare but its presence should trigger an evaluation. One classification scheme focuses on the extent of dysfunction as measured by a combination of abnormal laboratory values: serum ALT or AST greater than 150 U/L, platelet count less than 100,000 cells /mm^3, and serum lactate dehydrogenase (LDH) level more than 600 IU/L. Lactate dehydrogenase has become an important prognostic indicator—levels exceeding 1400 IU/L are associated with greater morbidity.[70]

Treatment and Prognosis

The prognosis for women diagnosed with HELLP is very good, but a mortality rate of 1% to 4% is still observed.[61,70] Definitive treatment consists of delivery. Corticosteroids are recommended by the National Institutes of Health (NIH) to encourage fetal lung maturity and allow for earlier delivery. Corticosteroids given to the postpartum mother may shorten time to recovery and decrease hospital stay.[71,72]

Acute Fatty Liver of Pregnancy

Though much more rare than HELLP, AFLP is more devastating. It is common in the third trimester but can also occur earlier or after delivery. The pathophysiology of AFLP is similar to that of HELLP. Liver biopsy differentiates the disease from HELLP by demonstration of fatty infiltration and necrosis not unlike those seen in alcoholic steatohepatitis. AFLP can recur with subsequent pregnancies and is also associated with metabolic disorders in the fetus.[73]

Diagnosis

Emesis, right upper quadrant pain, and jaundice are common complaints with AFLP. Laboratory abnormalities demonstrate some important differences from HELLP syndrome, such as elevated serum bilirubin and normal platelet count. AFLP may also progress to disseminated intravascular coagulation, and thrombocytopenia can occur.

Treatment and Prognosis

Definitive treatment for AFLP is delivery. The prognosis is much worse if the disease is left untreated, with a maternal death approaching 20%. Liver transplantation improves survival rates.

Care of the Patient with Liver Transplantation

More than 36,000 patients living in the United States have undergone liver transplantation.[74] Transplantation patients present to the ED with common complaints, such as fever and abdominal pain, that carry a high morbidity in this population. Almost 70% of liver transplant recipients who present to an ED require hospitalization.[75]

Transplant recipients are immunosuppressed, and any fever must be taken seriously. Serious febrile illnesses associated with liver transplantation are bacteremia and pneumonia; otitis media is common. Immunosuppressive medications also raise the risks for viral and fungal infections.

The most common infection seen in the first few months after transplantation is cytomegalovirus, which manifests as fever, arthralgias, and malaise. Other viral infections, such as herpes simplex virus, varicella-zoster virus, and herpes zoster virus are also common but are not as serious as cytomegalovirus.[74] Infections with fungi such as *Candida* should be suspected.

Serious infections may be present in the absence of fever or leukocytosis. Half of liver transplant recipients with an eventual diagnosis of a serious infection had neither a fever nor an elevated white blood cell count.

Other complications seen in liver transplant recipients are due to vascular or structural problems surrounding and within the transplant. Hepatic artery stenosis and hepatic artery thrombosis are each present in approximately 10% of liver transplant recipients, often because of rejection. Either stenosis or thrombosis of the hepatic artery can manifest as abdominal pain, and both are accurately detected with ultrasonography.[75] The portal system may also be affected; ultrasonography should be used to evaluate the portal system at the time the arterial system is examined, because another 10% of liver transplant recipients have portal vein or hepatic vein thrombosis. Magnetic resonance venography is needed to confirm suspected portal or hepatic vein thrombosis.

Liver Function Tests

Liver function may be indirectly measured through a variety of laboratory tests. Laboratory abnormalities are neither specific nor sensitive and can therefore be misleading; however, certain abnormalities can help guide the astute physician toward further diagnostic testing in search of a specific diagnosis.

ALANINE AMINOTRANSFERASE AND ASPARTATE AMINOTRANSFERASE

Called aminotransferases, both ALT and AST are concentrated intrahepatocyte enzymes (although AST exists in measurable quantities elsewhere in the body as well). Any hepatocyte necrosis elevates these enzymes. The often quoted 2:1 ratio of AST to ALT in alcoholic liver disease is not supported by the literature.[76,77]

Table 37-2 **CAUSES OF HYPERBILIRUBINEMIA**

Type	Cause	Clinical Features and Biochemical Abnormalities
Unconjugated hyperbilirubinemia	Hemolysis	Decreased hemoglobin and haptoglobin levels Increased reticulocyte count
	Gilbert's syndrome	None
	Hematoma reabsorption	Increased creatine kinase and lactic dehydrogenase levels
	Ineffective erythropoiesis	—
Conjugated hyperbilirubinemia	Bile duct obstruction	Preceded by marked increase in aminotransferase levels Presence of suggestive symptoms (right upper quadrant pain, nausea, fever)
	Hepatitis (various causes)	Concomitant moderate to marked increase in aminotransferase levels
	Cirrhosis	Aminotransferase levels may be normal or only slightly increased Presence of other physical and instrumental signs of chronic liver disease
	Autoimmune cholestatic diseases (primary biliary cirrhosis, primary sclerosing cholangitis)	Marked increase in alkaline phosphatase (ALP) levels with normal or mildly increased aminotransferase levels Presence of other autoimmune diseases or associated diseases (e.g., inflammatory bowel disease)
	Total parenteral nutrition	Increased ALP and gamma-glutamyl-transferase levels
	Drug toxins	Concomitant increase in ALP levels
	Vanishing bile duct syndrome	Can be associated with drug reactions or occur with orthotopic liver transplantation

From Giannini E, Testa R, Savarino V: Liver enzyme alteration: A guide for clinicians. CMAJ 2005;172:367-379.

Chronic disease states such as HCV, alcoholic cirrhosis, and autoimmune hepatitis often have persistent elevations in ALT and AST, although normal values should not be used to exclude the possibility of disease. More than 15% of patients with biopsy-proven chronic HCV have aminotransferase elevations.[78]

ALKALINE PHOSPHATASE AND GAMMA-GLUTAMYL TRANSFERASE

Both alkaline phosphatase (AP) and gamma-glutamyl transferase (GGT) are markers of cholestasis. However, AP is present at significant levels in many other organ systems—bone, intestine, and placenta. AP values are elevated in normal pregnancy and with metastatic disease in bone (e.g., prostate cancer). Children also have physiologically normal elevations in AP during growth. GGT is much more highly concentrated in the liver and can be used in conjunction with AP to determine whether an abnormality is intrahepatic or extrahepatic.

PROTHROMBIN TIME

Prothrombin time measures the activity of certain clotting factors from both the intrinsic and extrinsic pathways. The liver is the primary site for manufacture of these clotting factors, and decreases in synthesis by an impaired liver can be inferred from a prolonged PT. Vitamin K is a cofactor in clotting factor synthesis, and medications that block its absorption, such as warfarin, prolong PT values.

BILIRUBIN

Bilirubin exists in two distinct forms, conjugated (direct) and unconjugated (indirect). Bilirubin is a byproduct of hemoglobin metabolism. Unconjugated bilirubin exists in the serum bound to albumin in a water-insoluble state. It is transported to the liver, where it is conjugated with glucuronide, in preparation for excretion into the bile.

Understanding this process of bilirubin metabolism helps focus the differential diagnosis of patients with hyperbilirubinemia and/or jaundice (Tables 37-2 and 37-3). Unconjugated hyperbilirubinemia results from increased production of bilirubin (hemolysis) or from decreased uptake in the liver (as seen in various inherited conditions). Conjugated hyperbilirubinemia results from loss of excretory capacity, which can occur from intrahepatic diseases (such as drug reactions, hepatitis, and cirrhosis) or from biliary obstruction. Obstructive jaundice occurs from a lesion that blocks the excretion of bile through the biliary ducts, either proximally at the hepatic duct or more distal at the common bile duct.[76,79]

Table 37-3 GUIDE TO INTERPRETATION OF HEPATIC FUNCTION PANEL RESULTS

	LIKELY TEST RESULTS							
Suspected Hepatic Disorder	**Total Protein**	**Albumin**	**AST**	**ALT**	**AST:ALT Ratio**	**ALP**	**Total Bilirubin**	**Direct Bilirubin**
Acute hepatitis	↔	↔	↑↑ to ↑↑↑	↑↑ to ↑↑↑	<1	↔ to ↑	↑↑ to ↑↑↑	↑↑ to ↑↑↑
Acute alcoholic hepatitis	↔	↔	↑ to ↑↑	↑	1 to >2	↔ to ↑	↑↑ to ↑↑↑	↑↑ to ↑↑↑
Chronic hepatitis	↑ to ↑↑	↓ to ↓↓	↑ to ↑↑	↑ to ↑↑	<1 to 1	↔ to ↑	↑ to ↑↑	↑ to ↑↑
Chronic alcoholic disease	↑ to ↑↑	↓ to ↓↓	↑ to ↑↑	↑ to ↑↑	>1	↔ to ↑	↑ to ↑↑	↑ to ↑↑
Diffuse intrahepatic cholestasis	↔ to ↑↑	↔ to ↓↓	↑ to ↑↑	↑ to ↑↑	1	↑↑ to ↑↑↑	↑ to ↑↑	↑ to ↑↑
Extrahepatic obstruction	↔ to ↑↑	↔ to ↓↓	↑ to ↑↑	↑ to ↑↑	1	↑↑ to ↑↑↑	↑ to ↑↑	↑ to ↑↑
Focal intrahepatic disease	↔ to ↓↓	↔ to ↓↓	↑ to ↑↑	↑ to ↑↑	1	↑↑ to ↑↑↑	↔	↔ to ↑

ALP, alkaline phosphatase; ALT, alanine aminotransferase; AST, aspartate aminotransferase; ↔, within reference limits; ↑, slightly increased; ↓, slightly decreased; ↑↑, moderately increased; ↓↓, moderately decreased; ↑↑↑, markedly increased; ↓↓↓, markedly decreased.
Modified from Burke M: Liver function: Test selection and interpretation of results. Clin Lab Med 2002;22:377-390.

REFERENCES

1. Centers for Disease Control and Prevention (CDC): Deaths and hospitalizations from chronic liver disease and cirrhosis–United States, 1980-1989. MMWR Morb Mortal Wkly Rep 1993;41:969-973.
2. Modolell I: Vagaries of clinical presentation of pancreatic and biliary tract cancer. Ann Oncol 1999;10(Suppl 4):82-84.
3. Zoli M: Physical examination of the liver: Is it still worth it? Am J Gastroenterol 1995;90:1428-1432.
4. Tucker WN: The scratch test is unreliable for detecting the liver edge. J Clin Gastroenterol 1997;25:410-414.
5. Basile AS, Jones EA: Ammonia and GABA-ergic neurotransmission: Interrelated factors in the pathogenesis of hepatic encephalopathy. Hepatology 1997;25:1303-1305.
6. Lockwood AH, Bolomey L, Napoleon F: Blood-brain barrier to ammonia in humans. J Cereb Blood Flow Metab 1984;4:516-522.
7. Lockwood AH: Blood ammonia levels and hepatic encephalopathy. Metab Brain Dis 2004;19:345-349.
8. Polson J, Lee WM: American Association for the Study of Liver Disease: AASLD position paper: The management of acute liver failure. Hepatology 2005;41:1179-1197.
9. Clemmensen JO, Larsen FS, Knodrup J, et al: Cerebral herniation in patients with acute liver failure is correlated with arterial ammonia concentration. Hepatology 1999;29: 648-653.
10. Blei AT, Olafsson S, Therrien G, et al: Ammonia induced brain edema and intracranial hypertension in tars after portacaval anastomosis. Hepatology 1994;19:1437-1444.
11. Sushma S, Dasarathy S, Tandon RK, et al: Sodium benzoate in the treatment of acute hepatic encephalopathy: A double-blind randomized trial. Hepatology 1992;16: 138-144.
12. Alba L, Hay JE, Angulo P, et al: Lactulose therapy in acute liver failure. J Hepatol 2002;36:33A.
13. Canalese J, Gimson AES, Davis C, et al: Controlled trial of dexamethasone and mannitol for the treatment of fulminant hepatic failure. Gut 1982;23:625-629.
14. Ede RJ, Gimson AE, Bihari D, Williams R: Controlled hyperventilation in the prevention of cerebral edema in fulminant hepatic failure. J Hepatol 1986;2:43-51.
15. Shawcross D: Worsening of cerebral hyperemia by the administration of terlipressin in acute liver failure with severe encephalopathy. Hepatology 2004;39:471-475.
16. Moreau R: Clinical characteristics and outcome of patients with cirrhosis and refractory ascites. Liver Int 2004; 24:457-464.
17. D'Amico G, Morabito A, Pagliaro L, et al: Survival and prognostic indicators in compensated and decompensated cirrhosis. Dig Dis Sci 1986;31:468-475.
18. Jepsen P: Prognosis of patients with liver cirrhosis and spontaneous bacterial peritonitis. Hepatogastroenterology 2003;50:2133-2136.
19. Evans LT: Spontaneous bacterial peritonitis in asymptomatic outpatients with cirrhotic ascites. Hepatology 2003; 37:897-901.
20. Guazzi M: Negative influences of ascites on the cardiac function of cirrhotic patients Am J Med 1975;59:165-170.
21. Malbrain M, Chiumello D, Pelosi P, et al: Incidence and prognosis of intraabdominal hypertension in a mixed population of critically ill patients: A multiple-center epidemiological study. Crit Care Med 2005;33:315-322.
22. Gines P, Arroyo V, Quintero E, et al: Comparison of paracentesis and diuretics in the treatment of cirrhotics with tense ascites: Results of a randomized study. Gastroenterology 1987;93:234-241.
23. Choi CH: Efficacy and safety of large volume paracentesis in cirrhotic patients with spontaneous bacterial peritonitis: A randomized prospective study. Taehan Kan Hakhoe Chi 2002;8:52-60.
24. Peltekian KM: Cardiovascular, renal, and neurohumoral responses to single large-volume paracentesis in patients with cirrhosis and diuretic-resistant ascites. Am J Gastroenterol 1997;92:394-399.
25. Webster ST: Hemorrhagic complications of large volume abdominal paracentesis. Am J Gastroenterol 1996;91: 366-368.
26. Ginès P, Arroyo V, Rodés J: Pathophysiology, complications, and treatment of ascites. Clin Liver Dis 1997;1:129-155.
27. Gines P, Tito L, Arroyo V, et al: Randomized comparative study of therapeutic paracentesis with and without intravenous albumin in cirrhosis. Gastroenterology 1988;94: 1493-1502.
28. Naxeer S, Dewbre H, Miller A: Ultrasound assisted paracentesis performed by emergency physicians vs the traditional technique: A prospective randomized study. Am J Emerg Med 2005;23:363-367.
29. Cholongitas E, Papatheodoridis GV, Lahanas A, et al: Increasing frequency of gram-positive bacteria in spontaneous bacterial peritonitis. Liver Int 2005;25:57-61.
30. Arroyo V: Prognostic value of spontaneous hyponatremia in cirrhosis with ascites. Am J Dig Dis 1976;21:249-256.
31. Cardenas A: Hepatorenal syndrome: A dreaded complication of end-stage liver disease. Am J Gastroenterol 2005;100:460-467.
32. U.S. Food and Drug Administration, Center for Food Safety and Applied Nutrition: Hepatitis A virus. In: Foodborne Pathogenic Microorganisms and Natural Toxins Handbook. Available at http://vm.cfsan.fda.gov/~mow/chap31.html/

33. Kemmer N, Miskovsky E: Hepatitis A. Infect Dis Clin North Am 2000;14:605-615.
34. Lin K, Kerchner J: Hepatitis B. Am Fam Physician 2004;69:75-82.
35. Hayashi P, Bisceglie A: The progression of hepatitis B and C infections to chronic liver disease and hepatocellular carcinoma: Epidemiology and pathogenesis. Med Clin North Am 2005;89:371-389.
36. Diehl A: Alcoholic liver disease. Clin Liver Dis 1998;2: 103-118.
37. Boyer J, Chang E, Collyar D, et al: NIH Consensus Statement: Management of Hepatitis C: 2002. Available at http://consensus.nih.gov/2002/2002HepatitisC2002116html.htm.
38. Brillman JC: Prevalence and risk factors associated with hepatitis C in ED patients Am J Emerg Med 2002;20: 476-480.
39. Caplan E, Preas M, Micheal A, et al: Seroprevalence of human immunodeficiency virus, HBV, HCV, and RPR in a trauma population. J Trauma 1995;39:533-538.
40. World Health Organization: Amoebiasis. Weekly Epidemiological Record 1997;72:97-99.
41. Hai AA: Amoebic liver abscess: Review of 220 cases. Int Surg 1991;76:81-83.
42. Hughes MA, Petri WM Jr: Amebic liver abscesses. Infect Dis Clin North Am 2000;14:565-582.
43. Hoffner R, Kilaghbian T, Esekogwu V, et al: Emergency department presentation of amebic liver abscesses. Acad Emerg Med 1999;6:470-474.
44. Sharma MP: Amoebic liver abscess. Trop Gastroenterol 1993;14:3-9.
45. Ralls PW: Focal inflammatory disease of the liver. Radio Clin North Am 1998:36:377-389.
46. Maltz G: Amebic liver abscesses: A 15 year experience. Am J Gastroenterol 1991;86:704-710.
47. Tandon A: Needle aspiration in large amoebic liver abscess. Trop Gastroenterol 1997;18:19-21.
48. Blessmann J, Binh HD, Hung DM, et al: Treatment of amoebic liver abscess with metronidazole alone or in combination with ultrasound-guided needle aspiration: A comparative prospective and randomized study. Trop Med Int Health 2003;8:1030-1040.
49. Hansen PS, Schonheyder HC: Pyogenic hepatic abscess: A 10-year population-based retrospective study. APMIS 1998;106:396-402.
50. Johannsen E: Pyogenic liver abscesses. Infect Dis Clin North Am 2000;14:547-563.
51. Seeto RK, Rockey DC: Pyogenic liver abscess: Changes in etiology, management, and outcome. Medicine (Baltimore) 1996;75:99-113.
52. Giorgio A, Tarantino L, Mariniello N, et al: Pyogenic liver abscesses: 13 years of experience in percutaneous needle aspiration with US guidance. Radiology 1995;195: 122-124.
53. Ch Yu S, Hg Lo R, Kan PS, Metreweli C: Pyogenic liver abscess: Treatment with needle aspiration. Clin Radiol 1997;52:912-916.
54. Elliott D: Schistosomiasis: Pathophysiology, diagnosis, and treatment. Gastroenterol Clin 1996;25:599-625.
55. Lun ZR: Clonorchiasis: A key foodborne zoonosis in China. Lancet Infect Dis 2005;5:31-41.
56. Homeida MA: Association of the therapeutic activity of praziquantel with the reversal of periportal fibrosis induced by *S. mansonii.* Am J Trop Med Hygiene 1991;45:360-365.
57. Lieber CS: Biochemical factors in alcoholic liver disease. Semin Liver Dis 1993;6:136-147.
58. Saunders JB, Davis M, Williams R: Do women develop alcoholic liver disease more readily than men? Br Med J 1981;282:1140-1143.
59. Fujimoto M, Uemura M, Kojima H: Prognostic factors in severe alcoholic liver injury. Nara Liver Study Group. Alcohol Clin Exp Res 1999;23(Suppl):33S-38S.
60. Ramond MJ, Poynard T, Rueff B, et al: A randomized trial of prednisolone in patients with severe alcoholic hepatitis. N Engl J Med 1992;326:507-512.
61. Christensen E, Gluud C: Glucocorticoids are ineffective in alcoholic hepatitis: A meta-analysis adjusting for confounding variables. Gut 1995;37:113-118.
62. Krawitt EL: Autoimmune hepatitis. N Engl J Med 2006;354: 54-66.
63. Mabee C, Thiele D: Mechanisms of autoimmune liver disease. Clin Liver Dis 2000;4:431-445.
64. Duclos-Vallee JC, Sebagh M, Rifai K, et al: A 10 year follow up study of patients transplanted for autoimmune hepatitis: Histological recurrence precedes clinical and biochemical recurrence. Gut 2003;52:893-897.
65. Lewis J: Drug-induced liver disease. Med Clin North Am 2000;84:1275-1311.
66. Schiodt FV, Atillasoy E, Shakil AO, et al: Etiology and prognosis for 295 patients with acute liver failure. Liver Transpl Surg 1999;5:29-34.
67. Steingrub J: Pregnancy associated severe liver dysfunction. Crit Care Clin 2004;20:763-776.
68. Kaplan M: Acute fatty liver of pregnancy. N Engl J Med 1985;313:367-370.
69. Martin J, Magann F, Blake P: Analysis of 454 pregnancies with severe pre-eclampsia/eclampsia HELLP syndrome using the 3-class system of classification. Am J Obstet Gynecol 1993;68:386-391.
70. Murphy D, Stirrat G: Mortality and morbidity associated with early onset pre-eclampsia. Hypertens Pregnancy 2000;19:221-231.
71. Yalcin O: Effects of post partum corticosteroids in patients with HELLP syndrome. Int J Gynaecol Obstet 1998;61:141-148.
72. Magann E, Perry K, Meydrech E, et al: Postpartum corticosteroids: Accelerated recovery from the syndrome of hemolysis, elevated liver enzymes and low platelets. Am J Obstet Gynecol 1994;171:1154-1158.
73. Knox T, Olans L: Liver disease in pregnancy. N Engl J Med 1996;335:569-576.
74. U.S. Organ Procurement and Transplantation Network (OPTN): Annual Report 2005. Available at www.optn.org/
75. Dodd GD 3rd, Memel DS, Zajko AB, et al: Hepatic artery stenosis and thrombosis in transplant recipients: Doppler diagnosis with resistive index and systolic acceleration time. Radiology 1994;192:657-661.
76. Pinto H, Babtisti A: Nonalcoholic steatohepatitis: Clinicopathological comparison with alcoholic hepatitis in ambulatory and hospitalized patients. Dig Dis Sci 1996;41:172-179.
77. Kew M: Serum aminotransferase concentration as evidence of hepatocellular damage. Lancet 2000;355:591-592.
78. Gholson C, Morgan K: Chronic hepatitis C with normal aminotransferase levels: A clinical histologic study. Am J Gastroenterol 1997;92:1788-1792.
79. Burke M: Liver function: Test selection and interpretation of results. Clin Lab Med 2002;22:377-390.

Chapter 38

Pancreatitis

Mitchell C. Sokolosky

KEY POINTS

Pancreatitis is an inflammatory condition of the pancreas that results from premature activation of pancreatic enzymes.
Elevations in serum pancreatic enzyme values confirm the diagnosis in suspected cases.
Gallstones and alcohol use are the most common causes of acute pancreatitis.
Most patients with acute pancreatitis require hospitalization for supportive care.
The spectrum of illness ranges from mild (edematous) to severe (necrotizing) disease.
Necrotizing pancreatitis requires aggressive management in the intensive care unit and carries significant rates of morbidity and mortality.

Scope

More than 200,000 patients with acute pancreatitis are admitted to U.S. hospitals each year.[1] Eighty percent of these patients suffer from mild disease and demonstrate an overall mortality rate of only 1%. Approximately 20% of patients have severe necrotizing pancreatitis, however, which carries a mortality rate up to 25%.[2,3] The estimated incidence of pancreatitis in the United States is 79.8 per 100,000.[4] Men are affected more commonly than women, and most patients present between 40 and 60 years of age.[5]

Pathophysiology

The pancreas is a retroperitoneal organ with a primary role in digestion, exhibiting both exocrine (i.e., pancreatic enzymes) and endocrine (i.e., insulin and glucagon) functions. *Pancreatitis* is an inflammatory condition of the pancreas that arises from premature activation of pancreatic enzymes. The exact pathogenesis of this disease is unclear. Both acute and chronic forms exist.

Acute pancreatitis is most often caused by gallstones or alcohol use. Other etiologies are hyperlipidemia, hypercalcemia, medications, toxins, trauma, surgery, sphincter of Oddi dysfunction, invasive diagnostic procedures (endoscopic retrograde cholangiopancreatography), and hereditary causes. Approximately 20% of cases are idiopathic, with occult microlithiasis thought to be the underlying cause in half of these.[6] Acute pancreatitis can be classified histologically as edematous or necrotizing, corresponding to clinically mild or severe disease, respectively. Pancreatic necrosis (nonviable tissue) carries significant morbidity and mortality, especially if infection is present.

Chronic pancreatitis is often a progressive disorder with irreversible lesions, such as glandular fibrosis, distortion of the pancreatic duct, and strictures. Long-standing alcohol abuse is the most common cause of chronic pancreatitis.

Standard definitions and terminology for acute pancreatitis (Table 38-1) have been proposed to establish an exact vocabulary across institutions and within the literature.[7]

Table 38-1 DEFINITIONS OF ACUTE PANCREATITIS TERMINOLOGY

Acute pancreatitis	Acute inflammation of the pancreas
Mild acute pancreatitis	Minimal organ dysfunction responsive to fluid administration
Severe acute pancreatitis	One of the following: local complications (pancreatic necrosis, pancreatic pseudocyst, pancreatic abscess), organ failure, ≥3 Ranson criteria, APACHE II score ≥8
Acute fluid collections	Fluid collection in or near the pancreas, without a defined wall, occurring early in course of disease
Acute pseudocyst	Fluid collection containing pancreatic secretions, with a defined wall
Pancreatic necrosis	Nonviable pancreatic tissue diagnosed by contrast enhanced computed tomography scan
Pancreatic abscess	Collection of purulent material in or near the pancreas

APACHE II, Acute Physiology and Chronic Health Evaluation, version 2.

Presenting Signs and Symptoms

■ CLASSIC

Pancreatitis manifests as severe, upper abdominal pain that may radiate to the back. The onset of pain is rapid, typically over an hour or less. The pain is constant and is often worsened by lying flat and partially relieved by sitting up. Fever, nausea, vomiting, and anorexia may be present. Jaundice is rare. Abdominal examination usually demonstrates a soft, tender epigastrium without peritoneal signs. Distention may be present secondary to a concomitant ileus.

■ VARIATIONS

Painless pancreatitis may be encountered in the postoperative period after major surgery or in association with peritoneal dialysis or legionnaires' disease. Although rare, ecchymoses in the flanks (Grey Turner's sign) or in the periumbilical area (Cullen's sign) may be present in patients with hemorrhagic pancreatitis. Diaphragmatic irritation from an inflamed pancreatic tail may produce hiccups and pleural effusions. Patients with necrotizing pancreatitis may present in shock or coma.

BOX 38-1

Nonpancreatic Causes of Serum Amylase Elevation

- Abdominal aortic aneurysm
- Anorexia nervosa, bulimia
- Appendicitis
- Burns
- Cerebral trauma
- Drugs (azathioprine, sulfonamides, tetracycline, furosemide, valproic acid)
- Hepatitis
- Idiopathic hyperamylasemia
- Intestinal obstruction
- Ketoacidosis
- Macroamylasemia
- Mesenteric infarction
- Ovarian cysts
- Perforated bowel
- Peritonitis
- Pneumonia
- Renal failure
- Ruptured ectopic pregnancy
- Salivary diseases
- Salpingitis

Differential Diagnosis

Differential diagnosis for pancreatitis includes peptic ulcer disease with or without perforation, gastritis, biliary colic, acute cholecystitis, aortic dissection, mesenteric ischemia, myocardial infarction, and renal colic.

Diagnostic Testing

■ LABORATORY TESTS

No biochemical marker is considered the "gold standard" for the diagnosis or assessment of severity of acute pancreatitis.[8] Serum amylase and lipase measurements remain important diagnostic assays for acute pancreatitis. Other useful prognostic tests are a complete blood count; measurements of blood urea nitrogen and serum electrolyte, creatinine, glucose, and triglyceride levels; and liver function tests.

The total serum amylase has a reported sensitivity of 83% and specificity of 88% for acute pancreatitis.[9] Nonpancreatic causes of elevated serum amylase levels are listed in Box 38-1. Amylase levels rise within 6 to 12 hours of onset and usually remain elevated for 3 to 5 days. A normal amylase value would generally exclude the diagnosis of acute pancreatitis except in cases involving hyperlipidemia, acute exacerbations of chronic pancreatitis, or markedly delayed

BOX 38-2

Nonpancreatic Causes of Serum Lipase Elevation

Acute cholecystitis
Acute renal failure
Bone fracture
Crush injury
Diabetic ketoacidosis
Extrahepatic biliary obstruction
Fat embolism
Intestinal infarction
Intestinal obstruction
Liver diseases
Mumps
Pancreatic hyperenzymemia
Peptic ulcer disease
Perforated bowel
Postcholecystectomy syndrome
Type I or IV hyperlipoproteinemias

presentations (in which amylase levels may have normalized). Acute pancreatitis should not be excluded on the basis of a normal or mildly elevated amylase value when clinical suspicion of this diagnosis is high. Serum amylase values cannot be used to estimate the severity or determine the etiology of acute pancreatitis.

The serum lipase level is more sensitive (92%) and specific (96%) than total amylase for acute pancreatitis.[9] This measurement has greater sensitivity in acute alcoholic pancreatitis. It is useful in delayed clinical presentations because the serum lipase value stays elevated longer than the serum amylase value. However, serum lipase is not as specific for acute pancreatitis as once thought. The value is elevated in as many disorders as the amylase value (Box 38-2). As with serum amylase values, serum lipase values cannot be used to estimate the severity or determine the etiology of acute pancreatitis.

Controversy exists whether measurements of serum amylase, serum lipase, or both, should be ordered in a patient in whom pancreatitis is suspected. Within 24 hours after onset of symptoms, both enzyme values have high sensitivity and specificity for acute pancreatitis. Simultaneous evaluation of these two serum enzymes has not been shown to increase overall diagnostic accuracy, and the extent of pancreatic enzyme elevation does not correlate with severity of disease. The serum lipase value is thought to have higher diagnostic accuracy because it remains elevated longer than serum amylase. The diagnosis of acute pancreatitis should not rely solely on elevations of serum enzymes above the arbitrary limits of normal laboratory levels, but instead should be made on the basis of the onset of clinical symptoms, because the sensitivities of these enzyme values change with the timing of their measurements.[9]

The *urinary dipstick test* for detecting pancreatic amylase in the urine has demonstrated a sensitivity of 97%. This test for amylase may therefore be a useful point-of-care screening test for acute pancreatitis in the ED.[10]

C-reactive protein (CRP) is currently the best available serum marker to assess the severity of acute pancreatitis.[4] A cutoff level of >150 mg/L is now accepted as a proven predictor of severity. However, CRP levels must be monitored after hospital admission, since it takes 48 to 72 hours for the value to peak, making it less useful in the ED.

Hemoconcentration has been identified as an early marker for pancreatic necrosis. In one study, an admission hematocrit value of 47% or higher and a failure of the value to decrease at 24 hours after admission were associated with the development of pancreatic necrosis.[11]

An increase in *serum alanine aminotransferase (ALT)* level to more than 150 IU/L is suggestive of gallstone pancreatitis.[12] A lower value does not exclude the diagnosis, however.

There is no role for the measurement of isoamylases, immunoreactive trypsinogen, macroamylases, or elastase estimations in the routine management of acute pancreatitis in the ED.[13]

IMAGING

Plain abdominal radiographs are rarely useful except to exclude other causes of abdominal pain such as perforation and obstruction. Positive findings in acute pancreatitis include the presence of a "sentinel loop" (an area of focal ileus) or a "colon cutoff sign" (a paucity of colonic air distal to the splenic flexure, caused by functional spasm of the descending colon due to pancreatic inflammation). Pancreatic calcifications can be seen on radiographs in chronic pancreatitis.

Computed tomography (CT) of the abdomen can aid in the diagnosis of acute pancreatitis and its complications as well as assess the severity of disease. CT of the abdomen enhanced with an intravenously administered contrast agent is considered the gold standard for the noninvasive diagnosis of pancreatic necrosis.[14] Affected portions of the pancreas do not show normal contrast enhancement (Fig. 38-1). CT can diagnose complications such as pseudocysts (Fig. 38-2), phlegmons, and abscesses.

Ultrasonography has a limited role in the diagnosis of pancreatitis. Findings positive for acute pancreatitis include a diffusely enlarged, hypoechoic pancreas. Ultrasonography is very useful for imaging the biliary tract and diagnosing gallstones.

Magnetic resonance imaging (MRI) has been used in the diagnosis and management of acute pancreatitis. This modality is superior to CT in its categorization of fluid collections, necrosis, abscess, hemorrhage, and pseudocysts.[15]

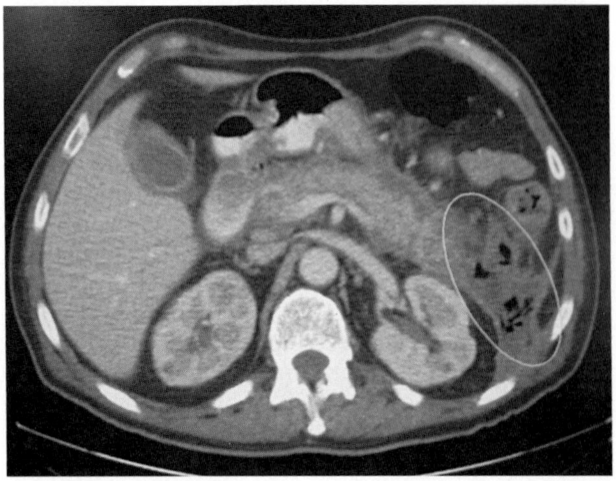

FIGURE 38-1 Necrotic portions of the pancreas (*circled*) with gas suggest infection.

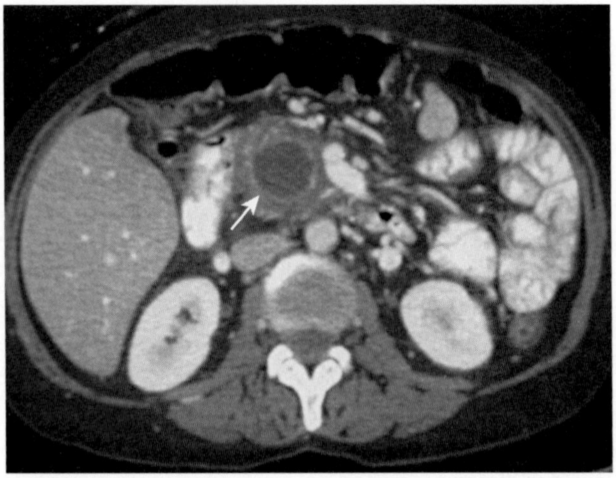

FIGURE 38-2 Computed tomography can diagnose complications such as pseudocysts (*arrow*).

Table 38-2 **COMPUTED TOMOGRAPHY (CT) SEVERITY INDEX SCORE FOR PANCREATITIS***

Grade†	CT Findings	Score
A	Normal pancreas	0
B	Focal or diffuse enlargement of pancreas, contour irregularities, heterogeneous attenuation, no peripancreatic inflammation	1
C	Grade B plus peripancreatic inflammation	2
D	Grade C plus single fluid collection	3
E	Grade C plus multiple fluid collections or gas	4
Percent Necrosis Present on CT		**Score**
0		0
<33%		2
33%-50%		4
>50%		6

*Severity Index Score = Grade Score + Percent Necrosis Score. Maximum score = 10; severe disease = 6 or higher.
†Severity of the acute inflammatory process.

■ Criteria for Determining Severity

CT of the abdomen is also considered the gold standard for determining severity of disease.[18] A CT Severity Index Score can be calculated on the basis of CT findings, with a score of 6 or higher indicating severe disease (Table 38-2).[16]

Although not as accurate as the CT system, scoring systems that use clinical criteria may also estimate severity. The most commonly used clinical scores for determining severity of acute pancreatitis are Ranson's criteria and the second version of the Acute Physiology and Chronic Health Evaluation (APACHE II).

Ranson's score is based on 11 prognostic signs (Box 38-3).[17] Five of the signs are measured on admission, and six are measured 48 hours later. Mortality estimates are based on the number of signs present. Mortality is less than 0.9% when three or fewer signs are present; mortality is 100% when more than six signs are noted.

The APACHE II score is based on 12 physiologic variables, age, and previous health.[18] The APACHE II score is probably the best clinical predictor of severity of acute pancreatitis.[19] A severity score can be assessed on admission and recalculated daily. (A calculator is available at www.sfar.org/scores2/apache22.html.) An APACHE II score higher than 8 indicates severe disease. The disadvantage of the APACHE II score is its complexity. An APACHE III score, developed to improve accuracy, does not appear to be more useful than APACHE II in differentiating mild from severe disease.[20]

Treatment

There is no specific treatment for pancreatitis other than supportive care. Aggressive hydration, pain management, and monitoring are the mainstays of treatment. Nasogastric tubes are not indicated in all patients but may be helpful in those with significant

BOX 38-3

Ranson's Criteria and Score

Criteria

Findings at admission:

- Age >55 yrs
- Serum glucose >200 mg/dL
- Serum lactic dehydrogenase >350 IU/L
- Serum aspartate aminotransferase >250 U/L
- White blood cell count >16,000 cells/mm^2

Findings obtained 48 hours after admission:

- Hematocrit fall >10%
- Blood urea nitrogen rise >5 mg/dL
- Serum calcium <8 mg/dL
- Pa_{O_2} <60 mm Hg
- Base deficit >4 mEq/L
- Estimated fluid sequestration >6 L

Score

Mortality increases with the number of criteria present:

Number of Criteria	*Mortality*
0-2:	1%
3 or 4:	15%
5 or 6:	40%
>7:	100%

vomiting or in whom enteral feeding is indicated. Anticholinergic agents, once given to decrease gastric secretions, are no longer recommended. Endoscopic retrograde cholangiopancreatography is usually indicated within 24 to 48 hours of presentation in patients with severe pancreatitis due to gallstones.

Narcotic analgesia is often needed to control the pain of acute pancreatitis. Controversy exists over which narcotic to use. Morphine has historically been avoided because of the potential to cause sphincter of Oddi spasm and a subsequent worsening of symptoms.[21] Meperidine is often used in place of morphine, but there is no conclusive evidence to support using meperidine rather than other narcotics.[22] In fact, meperidine has several disadvantages, including the potential formation of neurotoxic metabolites, muscle fibrosis if given intramuscularly, and a short duration of action. The administration of adequate doses of narcotic analgesia is probably more important than the particular choice of narcotic used.

Management of necrotizing pancreatitis includes admission to the intensive care unit and prevention of infection with prophylactic antibiotics. Intravenous imipenem-cilastatin (Primaxin I.V.) is considered the antibiotic of choice.[23] Infected necrotizing pancreatitis is considered uniformly fatal without intervention and should be suspected in patients with clinical evidence of sepsis. Urgent surgical consultation should be obtained if infection is suspected, because aggressive surgical debridement (necrosectomy) is the treatment of choice.[8] Drainage options for patients with pancreatic necrosis who will not undergo surgery (poor surgical candidates or patients whose infection is well contained) are expanding and include both percutaneous therapy (interventional radiology) and endoscopic therapy. The treatment of sterile necrosis remains supportive.

Disposition

Most patients with acute pancreatitis require hospital admission. Patients with acute necrotizing pancreatitis must be admitted to the intensive care unit. Mild cases of pancreatitis may be managed on an outpatient basis if the patient's pain is controlled and he or she is tolerating liquids. Patients who are discharged home require proper follow-up and written discharge instructions. Alcoholic patients with pancreatitis are encouraged to stop drinking and seek detoxification treatment.

REFERENCES

1. Russo MW, Wei JT, Thiny MT, et al: Digestive and liver disease statistics. Gastroenterology 2004;126:1448-1453.
2. Uhl W, Warshaw, Imrie C, et al: IAP guidelines for the surgical management of acute pancreatitis. Pancreatology 2002;2:565-573.
3. Dervenis C, Johnson CD, Bassi C, et al: Diagnosis, objective assessment of severity, and management of acute pancreatitis. Int J Pancreatol 1999;25:195-210.
4. Go VLW: Etiology and epidemiology of pancreatitis in the United States. In Bradley EL III (ed): Acute Pancreatitis: Diagnosis and Therapy. New York, Raven Press, 1994, pp 235-239.
5. Lankisch PG, Burchard-Reckert S, Petersen M, et al: Morbidity and mortality in 602 patients with acute pancreatitis seen between the years 1980-94. Z Gastroenterol 1996;34:371-377.
6. Ros E, Navarro S, Bru C, et al: Occult microlithiasis in "idiopathic" acute pancreatitis: Prevention of relapses by cholecystectomy or ursodeoxycholic acid therapy. Gastroenterology 1991;101:1701-1709.
7. Bradley EL III: A clinically based classification system for acute pancreatitis. Summary of the International Symposium on Acute Pancreatitis, 11-13 September 1992, Atlanta, GA. Arch Surg 1993;128:586-590.
8. Baron HB, Morgan DE: Acute necrotizing pancreatitis. N Engl J Med 1999;340:1412-1417.
9. Dominguez-Munoz JE: Diagnosis of acute pancreatitis: Any news or still amylase? In Buchler M, Uhl E, Friess H, Malfertheiner P (eds): Acute Pancreatitis: Novel Concepts in Biology and Therapy. London, Blackwell Science, 1999, pp 171-180.
10. Hedstrom J, Svens E, Kenkimaki P: Evaluation of new urinary amylase test strip in the diagnosis of acute pancreatitis. Scand J Clin Lab Invest 1998;58:611-616.
11. Baillargeon JD, Ramagopal V, Tenner SM, et al: Hemoconcentration as an early risk factor for necrotizing pancreatitis. Am J Gastroenterol 1998:93:2130-2134.
12. Tenner S, Dubner H, Steinberg W: Predicting gallstone pancreatitis with laboratory parameters: A meta-analysis. Am J Gastroenterol 1994;89:1863-1866.
13. Thomson HJ, Obekpa PO, Smith AN, et al: Diagnosis of acute pancreatitis: A proposed sequence of biochemical investigation. Scand J Gastroenterol 1987;22:719-724.
14. Balthazar EJ, Freeny PC, Van Sonnenberg E: Imaging and intervention in acute pancreatitis. Radiology 1994; 193:297-306.

15. Arvanitakis M, Delhaye M, Maertelaere V, et al: Computed tomography and magnetic resonance imaging in the assessment of acute pancreatitis. Gastroenterology 2004;126: 715-723.
16. Balthazar EJ, Robinson DL, Megibow AJ, Ranson JH: Acute pancreatitis: Value of CT in establishing prognosis. Radiology 1990;174:331-336.
17. Ranson JH, Pasternack BS: Statistical methods for quantifying the severity of clinical acute pancreatitis. J Surg Res 1977;22:79-91.
18. Knaus WA, Draper EA, Wagner DP, et al: APACHE II: A severity of disease classification system. Crit Care Med 1985;13:818-829.
19. Larvin M, McMahon MJ: APACHE-II score for assessment and monitoring of acute pancreatitis. Lancet 1989;2: 201-205.
20. Williams M, Simms HH: Prognostic usefulness of scoring systems in critically ill patients with severe acute pancreatitis. Crit Care Med 1999;27:901-907.
21. Isenhour HL, Mueller BA: Selection of narcotic analgesics for pain associated with pancreatitis. Am J Health Syst Pharm 1998;55:480-486.
22. Voorthuizen T, Helmers JH, Tjoeng MM, et al: Meperidine outdated as analgesic in acute pancreatitis. Ned Tijdschr Geneeskd 2000;144:656-658.
23. Pederzoli P, Bassi C, Vesentini S, Campedelli A: A randomized multi-center clinical trial of antibiotic prophylaxis of septic complications in acute necrotizing pancreatitis with imipenem. Surg Gynecol Obstet 1993;176:480-483.

Chapter 39

Biliary Disease

Sanjay Shetty

KEY POINTS

During their reproductive years, women have twice the incidence and prevalence of biliary disease seen in men. After menopause, the incidences of biliary disease in women and men are comparable.

Higher cholesterol content in the bile is associated with a greater risk for gallstone formation. Cholesterol is the primary constituent in up to 80% of all gallstones.

Ultrasonography is the preferred modality for evaluating potential biliary stones, with a sensitivity of 97% and a specificity of 95%.

Acalculous cholecystitis is seen in patients with traumatic injuries, burns, and human immunodeficiency virus as well as in those who are receiving total parenteral nutrition. Rates of perforation, gangrene, and death are higher in acalculous cholecystitis than in acute calculous cholecystitis.

Cholecystoscintigraphy is the most sensitive test for diagnosing acute cholecystitis. Patients with fever or leukocytosis in whom ultrasonographic evidence for cholecystitis is equivocal should be admitted for cholecystoscintigraphy and possible endoscopic retrograde cholangiopancreatography.

Charcot's triad of fever, jaundice, and right upper quadrant pain is seen in less than one third of cases of cholangitis.

Cholelithiasis

■ SCOPE

Approximately 1 million of the 20 million Americans who have cholelithiasis have symptoms of biliary disease each year.[1] In the United States, 500,000 patients undergo cholecystectomy annually for definitive treatment of gallbladder symptoms. Complications of cholelithiasis are acute cholecystitis, ascending cholangitis, acute pancreatitis, and adenocarcinoma of the gallbladder; the combined mortality from these complications is 5000 to 10,000 deaths per year.

During their reproductive years, women have twice the incidence and prevalence of biliary disease seen in men. This difference is likely attributed to estrogen, which stimulates low-density lipoprotein (LDL) receptors and increases the uptake of cholesterol.[2] Higher cholesterol content in the bile is associated with a greater risk for gallstone formation. After menopause, the incidences of biliary disease in women and men are comparable.

The frequency of cholelithiasis varies among different ethnic groups. Some populations of Native Americans have very high incidences of gallbladder disease, but the condition is relatively uncommon in

BOX 39-1

Risk Factors for Gallstone Formation

- Increasing age
- Female gender
- Westernized diet
- Total parenteral nutrition
- Diabetes mellitus
- Hyperlipidemia
- Clofibrate use
- Cystic fibrosis with pancreatic insufficiency
- Ileal resection
- Biliary infection
- Hemolysis
- Cirrhosis

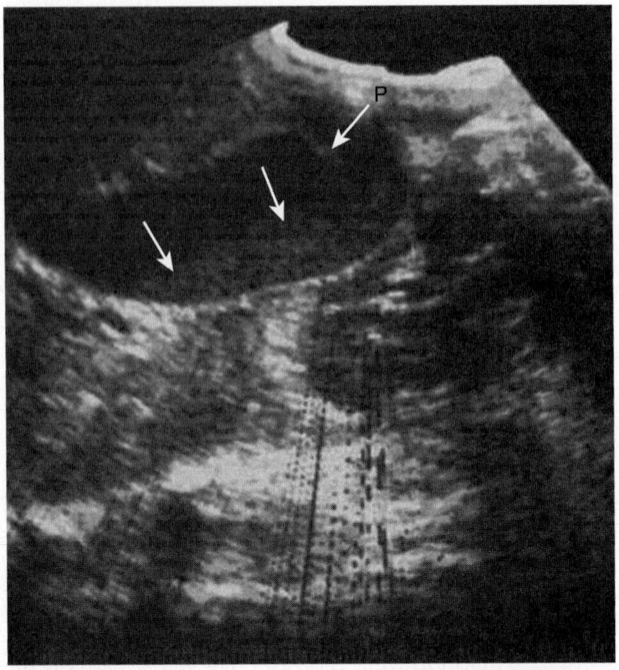
P

FIGURE 39-1 Ultrasonogram demonstrating biliary sludge (*arrows*). P, polyp. (From Berk RN, Ferrucci JT Jr, Leopold GR: Radiology of the Gallbladder and Bile Ducts: Diagnosis and Intervention. Philadelphia, WB Saunders, 1983, p 206.)

Africans. Other classic risk factors are described by the "five Fs": *female, fat, flatulent, forty (years of age),* and *fertile (multiple gestations).* Pediatric and adolescent patients with a history of sickle cell disease or other hemolytic disorders are at high risk for gallbladder disease as well. In patients with multiple risk factors, the probability of gallstone development is 1% to 2% per year (Box 39-1).

■ PATHOPHYSIOLOGY

Bile is primarily composed of cholesterol, lecithin, bile salts, bilirubin, and electrolytes (i.e., calcium, carbonate, and phosphate). Once these solutes exceed their solubility, they form crystals. Crystals trapped in biliary mucus produce sludge and aggregate to form stones. Cholesterol is the primary constituent of 60% to 80% of all gallstones. Calcium bilirubinate salts predominate in another 10% to 20% of stones; cholesterol and calcium bilirubinate are present in relatively equal quantities in the remainder of calculi (Fig. 39-1).

Biliary stasis is thought to play a significant role in stone formation. Both filling and emptying of the gallbladder are impaired in patients with gallstones. Patients in whom stone dissolution has been performed exhibit decreased gallbladder emptying after physiologic stimuli.[3] Factors such as fasting, high progesterone levels (as seen in pregnancy), chronic somatostatin excess, and sympathetic denervation from high spinal cord injury all promote biliary stasis and subsequent gallstone formation.[1]

One of the main complications of gallstones is calculus migration to the common bile duct, termed *choledocholithiasis.* Common duct stones cause a ball-valve action at the lower portion of the duct,[4] leading to biliary stasis and ineffective gallbladder contraction (Fig. 39-2).

■ CLINICAL FINDINGS

Biliary colic refers to the pain caused by dilation of the biliary ducts after gallstone impaction at the cystic duct or ampulla of Vater.[1] Patients with biliary colic classically present with intermittent, right upper quadrant (RUQ) cramping associated with nausea or vomiting. Pain may also be localized to the epigastrium and may radiate to the right scapular tip. Exacerbations usually last from 30 minutes to several hours, with days or months occurring between episodes. Approximately 66% of patients have a recurrent episode of biliary colic within 2 years and about one in six have a complication of gallstone disease.[1]

Laboratory test results in patients with symptomatic cholelithiasis should be normal, except for a mild elevation of serum alkaline phosphatase. Only 20% of gallstones are seen on plain abdominal radiographs.

Ultrasonography is the preferred modality for evaluating potential biliary stones. A meta-analysis of studies demonstrated that this modality has a sensitivity of 97% and specificity of 95% for the diagnosis of cholelithiasis.[5] Common findings on ultrasonography are hyperechoic stones with hypoechoic shadowing, biliary sludge, and stone mobility with changes in patient positioning (Fig. 39-3). Stones within the biliary duct (choledocholithiasis) are more difficult to visualize on ultrasonography, but more than 6 mm of dilation of the common bile duct suggests the presence of a suspected but otherwise unidentified stone.

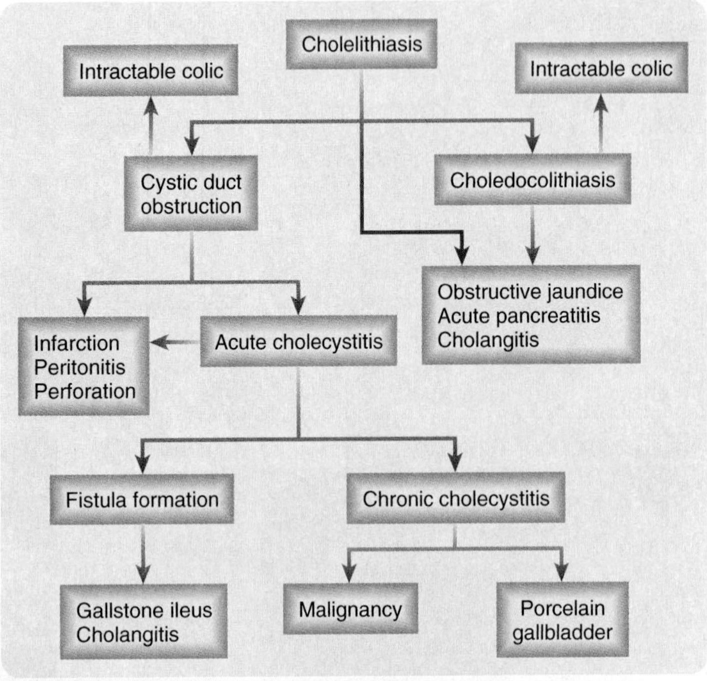
Cholelithiasis
Intractable colic
Intractable colic
Cystic duct obstruction
Choledocolithiasis
Obstructive jaundice
Acute pancreatitis
Cholangitis
Infarction
Peritonitis
Perforation
Acute cholecystitis
Fistula formation
Chronic cholecystitis
Gallstone ileus
Cholangitis
Malignancy
Porcelain gallbladder

FIGURE 39-2 Complications of gallstones.

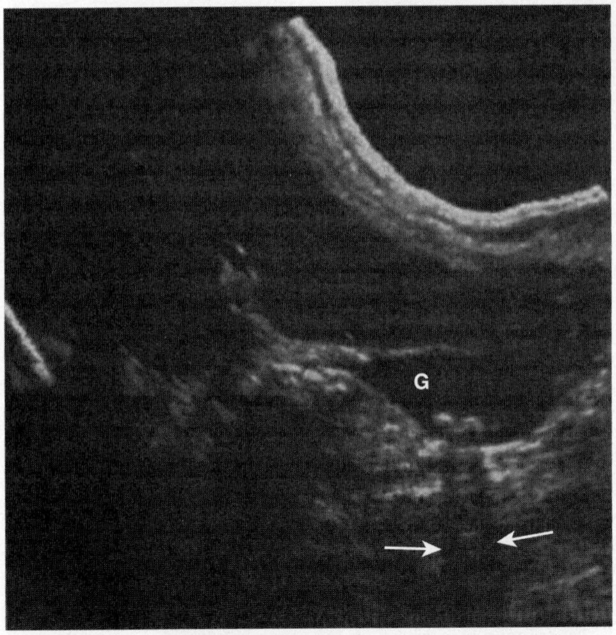
G

FIGURE 39-3 Cholelithiasis shown by ultrasonography. G, gallbladder. (From Berk RN, Ferrucci JT Jr, Leopold GR: Radiology of the Gallbladder and Bile Ducts: Diagnosis and Intervention. Philadelphia, WB Saunders, 1983, p 255.)

Computed tomography (CT) is less sensitive than ultrasonography for the diagnosis of acute biliary disease.[6] CT may offer valuable information about surrounding anatomy if there are confounding clinical signs or symptoms, if ultrasonography does not demonstrate a suspected calculus, or if an alternative diagnosis is as likely as biliary disease (Fig. 39-4).

■ DIFFERENTIAL DIAGNOSIS

The differential diagnosis for cholelithiasis is extensive (see discussion of RUQ pain in Chapter 25). Patients with acute pancreatitis of uncertain etiology should be evaluated for potential choledocholithiasis.

Muscular strain can produce deceptively similar abdominal tenderness but should be diagnosed only after intra-abdominal disease has been sufficiently excluded.

■ MANAGEMENT

Patients presenting to the ED with symptoms suggestive of biliary colic and without prior history of biliary disease should undergo blood tests to exclude alternative diagnoses and complications (complete blood count, comprehensive metabolic profile, measurements of serum amylase and lipase, and urinalysis). A pregnancy test should also be ordered for women of childbearing age. RUQ ultrasonography is the imaging modality of choice; CT is reserved for patients with persistent abdominal pain and negative ultrasonography findings (Fig. 39-5).

For those without contraindications to nonsteroidal anti-inflammatory drugs (NSAIDs), ketorolac (Toradol) is an effective parenteral treatment for biliary colic (60 mg intramuscularly [IM] or 30 mg intravenously [IV]). Opiates can be used for analgesia as well, although morphine may cause constriction of the sphincter of Oddi and could potentially worsen pain from an impacted stone. (This classic teaching about the use of morphine has been questioned in several studies, however.) Nausea and vomiting are treated with metoclopramide (Reglan) 10 mg IV or

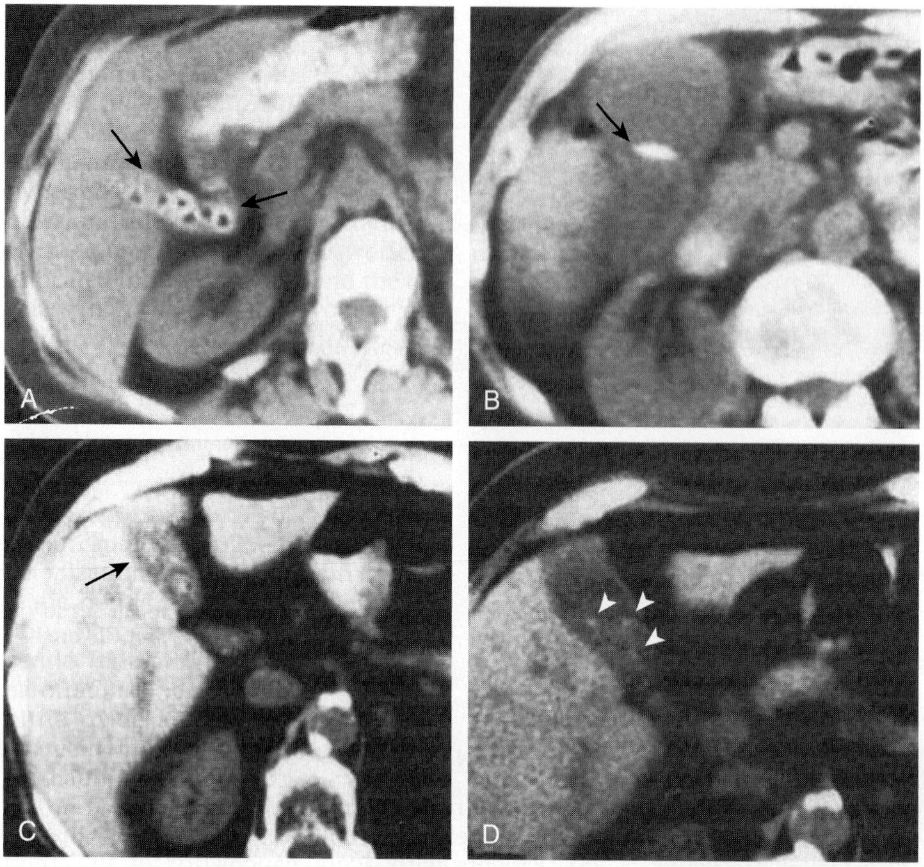

A
B
C
D

FIGURE 39-4 **A** to **D**, Computed tomography scans showing cholelithiasis in four different patients. (From Berk RN, Ferrucci JT Jr, Leopold GR: Radiology of the Gallbladder and Bile Ducts: Diagnosis and Intervention. Philadelphia, WB Saunders, 1983, p 215.)

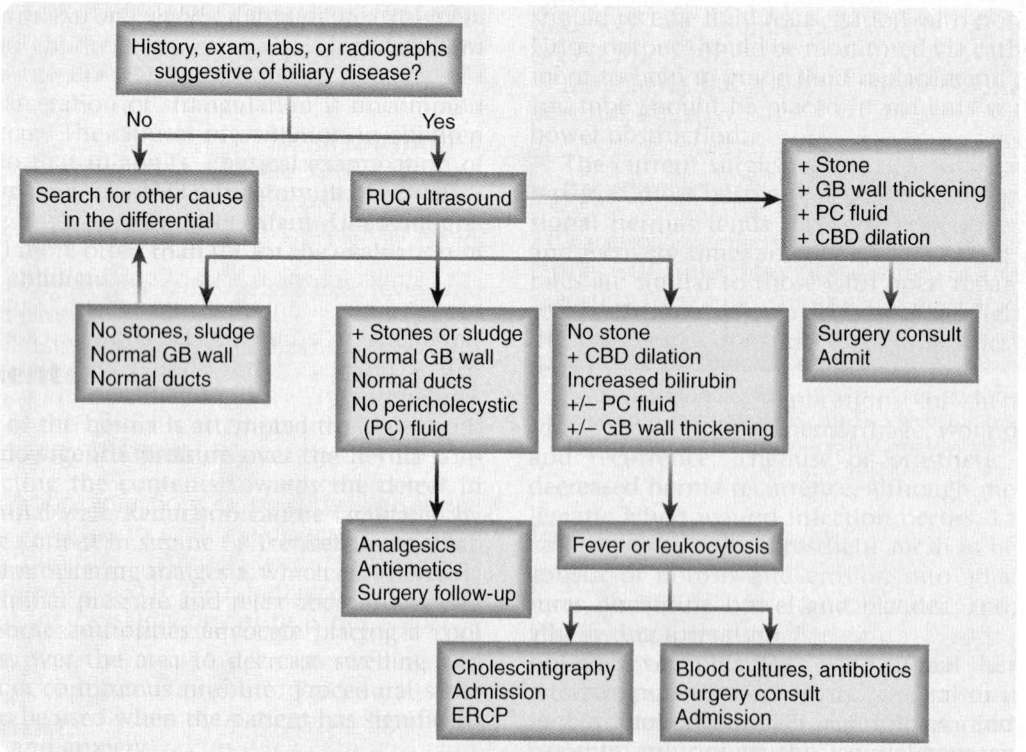

History, exam, labs, or radiographs suggestive of biliary disease?
No
Yes
Search for other cause in the differential
RUQ ultrasound
+ Stone
+ GB wall thickening
+ PC fluid
+ CBD dilation
No stones, sludge
Normal GB wall
Normal ducts
+ Stones or sludge
Normal GB wall
Normal ducts
No pericholecystic (PC) fluid
No stone
+ CBD dilation
Increased bilirubin
+/– PC fluid
+/– GB wall thickening
Surgery consult
Admit
Analgesics
Antiemetics
Surgery follow-up
Fever or leukocytosis
Cholescintigraphy
Admission
ERCP
Blood cultures, antibiotics
Surgery consult
Admission

FIGURE 39-5 Treatment algorithm for right upper quadrant (RUQ) pain. CBD, common bile duct; ERCP, endoscopic retrograde cholangiopancreatography; GB, gallbladder; +, with; –, without; ±, with or without.

PATIENT TEACHING TIPS

BILIARY COLIC

- Avoid greasy, fatty foods.
- Use prescribed analgesics and antiemetics as needed.
- Return to the ED if you have intractable pain, vomiting, fever, or chills.
- Make a follow-up appointment with a surgeon.

ondansetron (Zofran) 4 mg as an orally disintegrating tablet, IM, or IV.

■ DISPOSITION

Patients with uncomplicated biliary colic whose symptoms have improved can be safely discharged with surgical follow-up. Discharge instructions should recommend avoidance of fatty and greasy foods and advise immediate return to the ED for intractable pain or vomiting, fever, or jaundice.

Patients with intractable pain, vomiting, fever, or jaundice should be admitted for further management by a surgeon or gastroenterologist (see Documentation box).

Cholecystitis

■ SCOPE

Acute cholecystitis is inflammation of the gallbladder caused by obstruction of the cystic or common bile duct. Bacterial colonization may accompany this process, but often the bile is sterile.[1]

Persistent inflammation and fibrosis of the gallbladder with poor motor and absorptive function characterizes *chronic cholecystitis*. Patients are usually asymptomatic but may report multiple attacks of colic.

Acalculous cholecystitis is seen in patients with traumatic injuries, burns, and human immunodeficiency virus as well as those who are receiving total parenteral nutrition. Men are more commonly affected. Acalculous cholecystitis accounts for 5% to 10% of cases of acute cholecystitis and is associated with a higher rate of perforation and gangrene than calculous cholecystitis. The mortality for this disorder is twice as high as that for acute calculous cholecystitis.[7]

■ PATHOPHYSIOLOGY

Inflammation of the gallbladder wall causes the clinical findings seen in cholecystitis. Pressure of stones against the wall can cause irritation and ischemia in calculous disease. In patients with acalculous disease, biliary stasis is thought to be the main cause of gallbladder inflammation. Additional factors are poor gallbladder contractility due to systemic illness and lack of cholecystokinin-induced functions caused by decreased oral intake.

■ CLINICAL FINDINGS

The pain of cholecystitis is similar to that of cholelithiasis in location and radiation. Localized pain is caused by peritoneal irritation due to gallbladder inflammation, whereas the visceral pain of cramping and bloating is caused by gallbladder contraction against an impacted cystic duct.

In contrast to the relatively brief episodes of colic associated with cholelithiasis, patients with acute cholecystitis complain of constant pain that lasts 30 to 60 minutes and worsens with movement. Nausea and flatulence are common to both disorders, although persistent common bile duct impaction usually promotes vomiting. Patients appear ill and cannot take deep breaths.

Physical examination demonstrates RUQ tenderness with voluntary guarding and a positive Murphy's sign (arrest of respiration during deep palpation over the gallbladder). The presence of fever suggests bacterial infection, as does a leukocytosis with neutrophilic predominance. Jaundice indicates an obstructed common bile duct.

■ DIFFERENTIAL DIAGNOSIS

The differential diagnosis is essentially the same as that for cholelithiasis. When fever is present, retrocecal appendicitis, perforated peptic ulcer, or intestinal obstruction should be considered. Associated jaundice may suggest ascending cholangitis.

Mirizzi's syndrome is characterized by partial common hepatic duct obstruction from an impacted gallstone in the cystic duct.[8] The pain in Mirizzi's syndrome, which mimics that of acute cholecystitis, occurs when partially obstructed stones erode into the common hepatic duct and create a single cavity.[9]

■ COMPLICATIONS

Emphysematous cholecystitis results from gas-producing bacteria such as *Escherichia coli, Clostridium perfringens,* and anaerobic streptococci. Patients often appear ill, and gas shadows may be seen on plain radiographs. Male diabetics are commonly affected, and treatment consists of broad-spectrum antibiotics and surgical drainage.

Stones may erode through an inflamed and necrotic wall causing *gallbladder perforation.* These stones may travel into the peritoneal cavity or, more commonly, may erode and form adhesions between nearby structures. More than half of patients with gallbladder perforation present with fever and a palpable RUQ mass.[4] Bile peritonitis can develop. Mortality for these patients is 30%.[10] Treatment consists of antibiotics and percutaneous or surgical drainage.

Patients with chronic calculous disease may present with a locally contained abscess or cholecystoenteric fistula. *Porcelain gallbladder* also results from chronic inflammation of the gallbladder and is a risk factor for *carcinoma of the gallbladder.*

■ MANAGEMENT

Patients' oral intake should be restricted (nothing by mouth) in case emergency surgery is necessary. IV fluids should be started, and blood specimens should be collected and sent for complete blood count, basic serum chemistry tests, liver function tests, clotting factor measurement, and blood type and crossmatch.

Specimens for blood culture should be obtained from febrile patients, who should then receive antipyretics. Empirical antibiotics should be given, to cover *E. coli, Klebsiella, Streptococcus faecalis,* and anaerobic organisms. An acceptable combination regimen consists of a third- or fourth-generation cephalosporin (e.g., ceftazidime) with metronidazole.

Abdominal radiographs can be used to exclude intestinal obstruction but are of limited value in acute cholecystitis. RUQ ultrasonography is highly sensitive for diagnosing cholelithiasis but less sensitive for choledocholithiasis. Pericholecystic fluid (Fig. 39-6), gallbladder wall thickening (>3 mm), common bile duct dilation (>6 mm), or dilated intrahepatic and extrahepatic biliary ductal dilation are highly suggestive of acute cholecystitis.

Although not readily available in the ED, cholecystoscintigraphy (Fig. 39-7) is a more sensitive test for diagnosing acute cholecystitis. In a retrospective

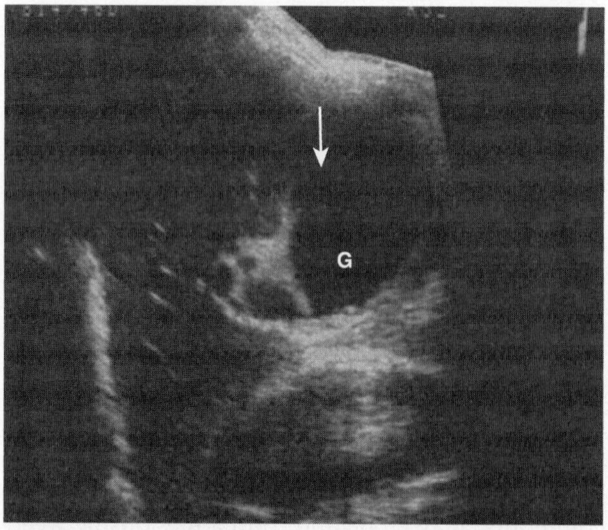
G

FIGURE 39-6 Ultrasonogram demonstrating pericholecystic fluid (*arrow*). G, gallbladder. (From Berk RN, Ferrucci JT Jr, Leopold GR: Radiology of the Gallbladder and Bile Ducts: Diagnosis and Intervention. Philadelphia, WB Saunders, 1983, p 213.)

review of 170 patients who presented to an ED with RUQ pain, cholecystoscintigraphy had a diagnostic sensitivity of 86%, compared with 48% for ultrasonography, in acute cholecystitis.[11] Furthermore, cholecystoscintigraphy results were positive in 87% of patients in whom initial ultrasonographic findings were negative (Fig. 39-8). A previous study reported the sensitivities of cholecystoscintigraphy and ultrasonography for the diagnosis of cholecystitis to be 98% and 67%, respectively.[12]

CT of the abdomen should be reserved for patients in whom a broader differential diagnosis is being considered. A retrospective study of 123 patients who underwent both CT and RUQ ultrasonography demonstrated a sensitivity of only 39% for CT in biliary disease.[6] Ultrasonography had a sensitivity of 83% in that study and suggested the correct diagnosis in 7 of 8 patients who were misdiagnosed from CT findings (Fig. 39-9).

Pain control can be achieved with opiates, and nausea can be treated with metoclopramide 5 or 10 mg IV or ondansetron 4 mg IV. In patients with intractable nausea, vomiting, or pain, an impacted common bile duct stone should be suspected, and the patients should be admitted. EP consultation with surgery and/or gastroenterology specialists will help facilitate their definitive inpatient management via cholecystectomy or endoscopic retrograde cholangiopancreatography (ERCP) for removal.

Cholangitis

■ SCOPE

Cholangitis may be caused by infection (bacterial, viral, tuberculin), autoimmune reaction (graft-versus-host disease after bone marrow transplantation), or idiopathic disease (primary sclerosing cholangitis). Approximately 80% of cases are caused by obstructing gallbladder stones, with a reported mortality of 5%.[13]

Primary sclerosing cholangitis (PSC) is characterized by progressive fibrosis of intrahepatic or extrahepatic biliary ducts (Fig. 39-10). The etiology of this condition is immune-mediated, although it is unclear whether PSC is a primary event or is secondary to an underlying infectious cause. More than 70% of patients with PSC have concomitant irritable bowel disease. Men between the ages of 25 and 60 years are most commonly affected. Ursodeoxycholic acid can slow progression of the disease, and liver transplantation can improve mortality; there is otherwise no effective treatment, and cirrhosis is the ultimate result.

■ PATHOPHYSIOLOGY

E. coli, Klebsiella, Streptococcus, Clostridium, and *Bacteroides* are the common bacterial organisms inciting cholangitis. Infection usually spreads retrograde from the intestines owing to obstruction. Resulting damage

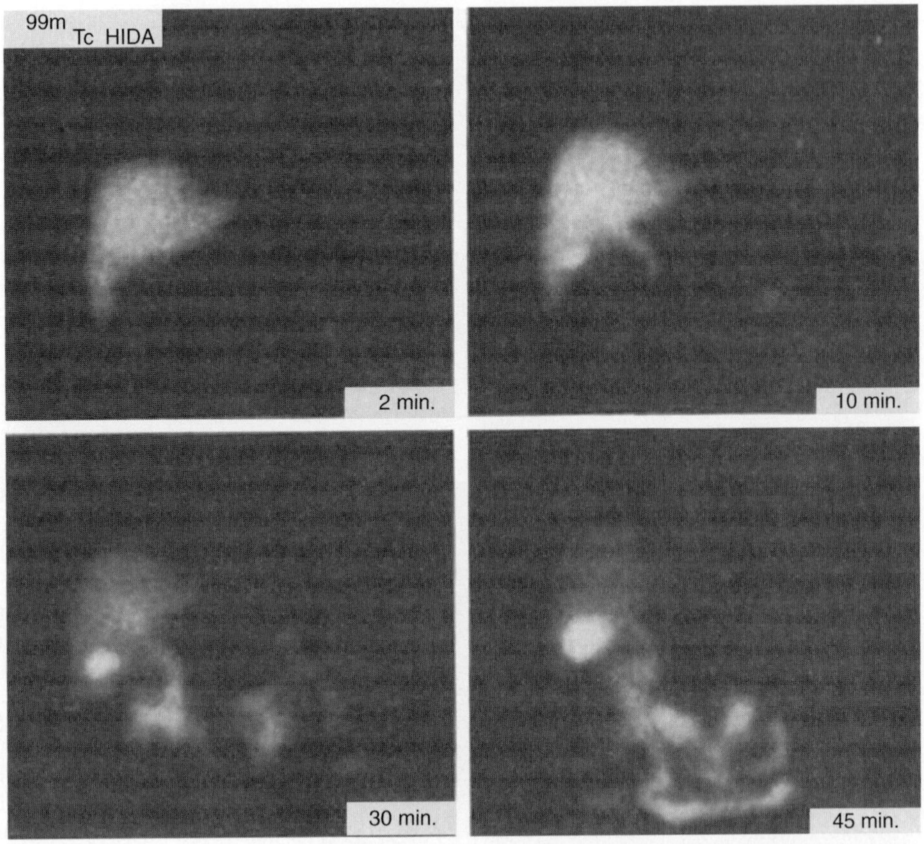
99m Tc HIDA
2 min.
10 min.
30 min.
45 min.

FIGURE 39-7 Normal cholecystoscintigram. (From Berk RN, Ferrucci JT Jr, Leopold GR: Radiology of the Gallbladder and Bile Ducts: Diagnosis and Intervention. Philadelphia, WB Saunders, 1983, p 265.)

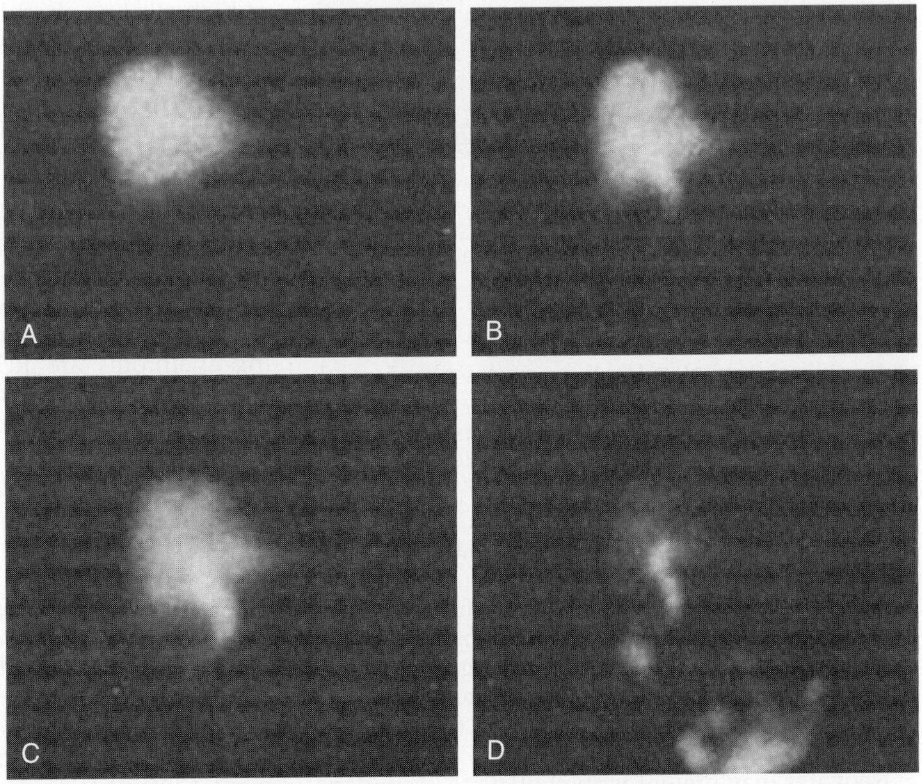
A
B
C
D

FIGURE 39-8 **A** to **D,** Abnormal cholecystoscintigram. (From Berk RN, Ferrucci JT Jr, Leopold GR: Radiology of the Gallbladder and Bile Ducts: Diagnosis and Intervention. Philadelphia, WB Saunders, 1983, p 273.)

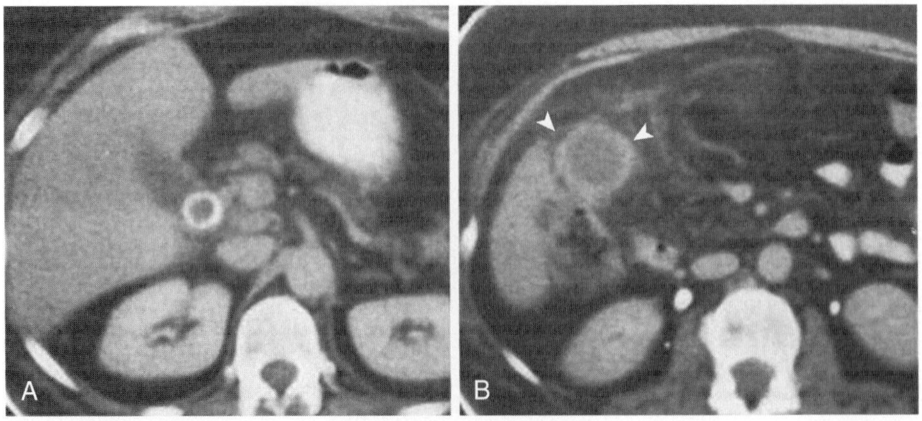
A
B

FIGURE 39-9 **A** and **B,** Cholelithiasis with cholecystitis on computed tomography. (From Berk RN, Ferrucci JT Jr, Leopold GR: Radiology of the Gallbladder and Bile Ducts: Diagnosis and Intervention. Philadelphia, WB Saunders, 1983, p 255.)

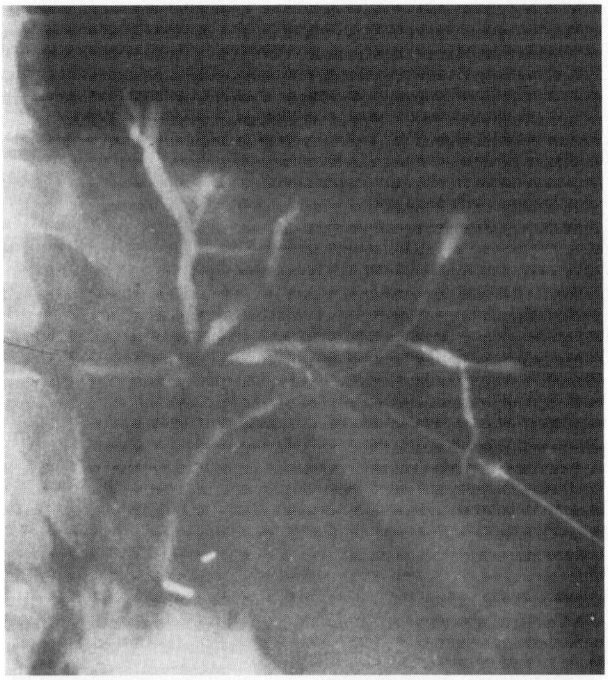

FIGURE 39-10 Primary sclerosing cholangitis demonstrated on endoscopic retrograde cholangiopancreatography. (From Berk RN, Ferrucci JT Jr, Leopold GR: Radiology of the Gallbladder and Bile Ducts: Diagnosis and Intervention. Philadelphia, WB Saunders, 1983, p 320.)

to the biliary ductal epithelium causes fibrosis and ductal loss. This sequence of events may also be seen without biliary obstruction in patients who have undergone sphincteroplasty or a biliary anastomosis to the duodenum (sump syndrome).[4] Cholangitis is associated with infection by the Chinese liver fluke (*Clonorchis sinensis*) and secondary bacterial superinfection.

Patients with acquired immunodeficiency syndrome (AIDS) may present with cholangitis with or without obstruction.[14] The infectious organisms associated with this and other immunodeficiency disorders are cytomegalovirus, cryptosporidia, *Cryptococcus,* and *Candida albicans.*[15]

Neonates may present with cholangitis secondary to cytomegalovirus or reovirus type III.

Cholangitis may also be seen in patients with failing liver transplants from graft incompatibility or hepatic arterial thrombosis.[16] Rejection leading to cholangitis is also seen in patients receiving allogeneic bone marrow transplantation.[17] Progressive biliary ductal necrosis leads to eventual cirrhosis.

■ CLINICAL FINDINGS

Charcot's triad—fever, jaundice, and RUQ pain—is seen in less than one third of cases of cholangitis. The addition of mental obtundation and hypotension to the triad constitutes *Reynold's pentad.*

Patients with infectious cholangitis are usually older, appear ill, and may not complain of RUQ pain. Younger patients with diabetes can also present with nonspecific complaints. In such cases, the finding of high alkaline phosphatase and bilirubin levels on screening comprehensive metabolic panels should heighten suspicion for biliary disease. Both ultrasonography and CT are poorly sensitive for diagnosis of ductal stones and biliary duct dilation, so diagnosis should be made on clinical grounds, and empirical treatment started early.

In contrast, the majority of patients with PSC are asymptomatic until cirrhosis has ensued. Many patients with ulcerative colitis are initially diagnosed after routine screening demonstrates an elevated serum alkaline phosphatase value. Common presenting symptoms are RUQ pain, jaundice, pruritus, weight loss, and fatigue. The serum alkaline phosphatase level is commonly three times above normal.[4] The serum bilirubin value may be normal or elevated.

■ MANAGEMENT

Management of patients with suspected cholangitis is similar to that of patients with cholecystitis. Elevations in white blood cell count, serum bilirubin, and serum alkaline phosphatase in this clinical setting are suggestive of an infectious cholangitis. Elevations of serum amylase and lipase imply pancreatic involvement. Clotting factor levels and blood type and crossmatch should be known before invasive interventions are undertaken. Blood cultures should be performed in febrile patients.

Aggressive fluid resuscitation is warranted for hypotensive patients. Central venous pressure monitoring should be considered for elderly patients during their ED stay.

Early, empirical antibiotic therapy is paramount to initial treatment. Multiple protocols are used in the United States; the EP should tailor antibiotic choices to institutional preferences and local resistance patterns. Combination therapy with an extended-spectrum cephalosporin, metronidazole, and ampicillin, single-agent or combination fluoroquinolones, and ureidopenicillins alone or with metronidazole are accepted regimens.[18] Although fluoroquinolones are thought to have greater biliary penetration, they do not change the mortality of this disease.[19]

Patients with PSC, unless presenting with concomitant signs of infection, do not experience improvement with antibiotics. Also, performing blood cultures to identify an organism and tailor antibiotic therapy does not improve mortality in these patients.

■ DISPOSITION

Patients with infectious cholangitis should be admitted for biliary drainage. ERCP with sphincterotomy is the treatment with the lowest mortality. Percutaneous transhepatic cholangiography (PTC) with drainage is a consideration for patients in whom ERCP fails. Emergency surgery, although not first-line therapy, can be performed via open or laparoscopic approaches. Choledochotomy, decompression, and insertion of a T tube can be performed but are associated with a mortality of 40%. If emergency ERCP or PTC cannot be arranged in the ED, surgical consultation should be obtained. Hypotensive and obtunded patients should be admitted to an intensive care setting.

Tumors of the Biliary Tree and Gallbladder

■ CONSIDERATIONS

Papillomas and adenomas are benign tumors of the gallbladder. Papillomas are small, usually multiple tumors that contain cholesterol esters and are not precancerous lesions. Adenomas, semisolid masses found at the fundus, are normally solitary. Both tumors are asymptomatic and can be distinguished from gallstones ultrasonographically because of their fixed position with movement of the patient.

Carcinoma of the gallbladder is an uncommon malignancy associated with chronic cholecystitis and porcelain gallbladder (Fig. 39-11). It is most commonly an adenocarcinoma that arises in the fundus or neck. Physical examination usually demonstrates an elderly patient with jaundice, RUQ pain, and weight loss. An abdominal mass may be palpable.

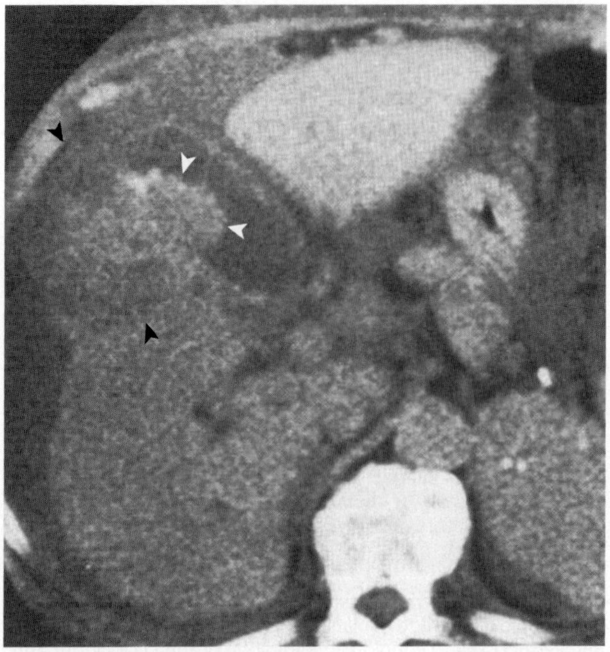

FIGURE 39-11 Computed tomography scan showing gallbladder carcinoma (*arrows*). (From Berk RN, Ferrucci JT Jr, Leopold GR: Radiology of the Gallbladder and Bile Ducts: Diagnosis and Intervention. Philadelphia, WB Saunders, 1983, p 256.)

Both ultrasonography and CT have a sensitivity of 60% to 70% for detecting carcinoma[20]; when results are positive, they usually show a mass in the lumen. Spread via venous and lymphatic systems prevents early detection, and metastasis is present at the time of diagnosis in 50% of cases.[21] One-year survival after diagnosis is observed in just 14% of patients.[22]

Cholangiocarcinoma refers to malignancy anywhere from the intrahepatic ducts to the common bile duct. It is an adenocarcinoma that spreads along and through the duct wall, with extension to lymph nodes, peritoneum, gallbladder, and liver in 50% of patients. Associations with primary biliary cirrhosis, primary sclerosing cholangitis, ulcerative colitis, and *C. sinensis* infestation are documented. One study found that the risk of bile duct carcinoma significantly decreases 10 years after cholecystectomy.[23]

■ CLINICAL FINDINGS

Patients most commonly present to the ED with painless jaundice and pruritus, symptoms that suggest an obstructing mass in the distal biliary tree. Pain is present in only one third of patients and generally is mild.[4] Those with malignancy have associated malaise and weight loss. Hepatomegaly without splenomegaly is often noted. Fever is uncommon, but if it is present, concurrent cholangitis should be considered.

■ MANAGEMENT

A thorough search for the cause of jaundice in an older patient should be initiated on presentation.

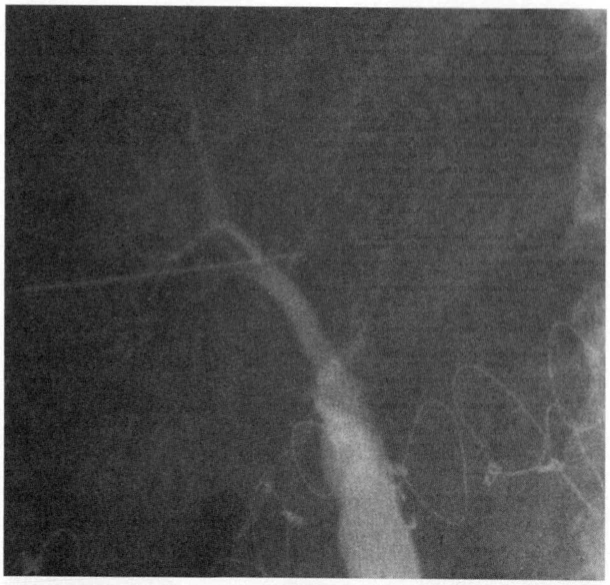

FIGURE 39-12 Primary biliary cirrhosis demonstrated by endoscopic retrograde cholangiopancreatography. (From Berk RN, Ferrucci JT Jr, Leopold GR: Radiology of the Gallbladder and Bile Ducts: Diagnosis and Intervention. Philadelphia, WB Saunders, 1983, p 320.)

Pruritus can be treated with diphenhydramine 25 to 50 mg orally, IM, or IV or hydroxyzine 25 mg orally or IM. A complete blood count will exclude hemolytic anemia as a potential cause. Liver function tests show elevations of serum bilirubin and alkaline phosphatase. Increased International Normalized Ratio (INR) values suggest that a primary liver dysfunction is causing the jaundice.

Ultrasonography and CT demonstrate intrahepatic biliary ductal dilation in jaundiced patients but may not show the actual mass. Depending on the tumor's location along the biliary tree, the common duct may be normal or may be dilated proximal to the mass.

■ DISPOSITION

Patients with jaundice and findings suspicious for a tumor should be admitted to a medical service for ERCP and biopsy.

Primary Biliary Cirrhosis

Intrahepatic bile ducts are progressively destroyed in primary biliary cirrhosis (PBC) (Fig. 39-12). The etiology of this disease is unknown, but the final mechanism involves immune-mediated biliary duct destruction via cytotoxic T cells. Viruses, bacteria, and defective immune regulation have been theorized to incite this cascade.

The disease is found in all races, with a 90% female preponderance. Patients are diagnosed from age 20 to 80 years, although the majority of cases are found in patients 40 to 60 years old. A genetic predisposition is likely, because family members of patients with PBC have a higher prevalence of mitochondrial antibodies associated with the disease. A medical history of an autoimmune disorder such as rheumatoid arthritis, systemic lupus erythematous, or mixed connective tissue disorder has an association with PBC.

Documentation

- Reported changes in stool color, vomiting
- Prior history of gallstones
- Family history of gallstones
- Presence of Murphy's sign on physical examination
- Improvement in pain, tolerance of oral fluids, and patient teaching prior to discharge
- Return precautions, referral to a surgeon

Patients are normally asymptomatic but may present with pruritus or xanthomas. Chronic RUQ pain is an infrequent complaint, and jaundice is not an early feature of this disease. Patients may remain asymptomatic for many years after ductal destruction has begun, but for those with symptoms and jaundice, the average survival time without treatment is 7 years.

The most common laboratory abnormality is an elevation of alkaline phosphatase and gamma glutamyl transpeptidase values. The total serum cholesterol value is usually elevated, and the serum bilirubin value only mildly elevated (usually less than 2 mg/dL).[4] Complications of the disease result from liver cirrhosis (i.e., ascites, bleeding esophageal varices, coagulopathy).

Diagnosis is suggested by antimitochondrial antibodies in the serum and confirmed by liver biopsy. Treatment is initially aimed at controlling itching and steatorrhea. Vitamin D and calcium supplements are necessary because of the bile deficiency.

The only drug shown to improve mortality in patients with PBC is ursodeoxycholic acid.[24] Hepatic transplantation is the best treatment option to extend life, with a 5-year survival of 60% to 70%.[25] Patients with cirrhotic complications should be considered for transplantation. Those who are diagnosed early or who have a serum total bilirubin value of 9 mg/dL or higher should be referred promptly to a transplant center.

REFERENCES

1. Schiff ER, Sorrell MF, Maddey WC (eds): Schiff's Diseases of the Liver, 8th ed, vol 1. Philadelphia, Lippincott-Raven, 1999.
2. Everson GT, McKinley C, Kern F Jr: Mechanisms of gallstone formation in women: Effects of exogenous estrogen (Premarin) and dietary cholesterol on hepatic lipid metabolism. J Clin Invest 1991;87:237-246.
3. Pauletzki J, Althaus R, Holl J, et al: Gallbladder emptying and gallstone formation: A prospective study on gallstone recurrence. Gastroenterology 1996;111:765-771.

4. Sherlock S, Dooley J (eds): Diseases of the Liver and Biliary System, 10th ed. Oxford, UK, Blackwell Science Ltd, 1997, p 612.
5. Shea JA, Berlin JA, Escarce JJ, et al: Revised estimates of diagnostic test sensitivity and specificity in suspected biliary tract disease. Arch Intern Med 1994;154: 2573-2581.
6. Harvey RT, Miller WT Jr: Acute biliary disease: Initial CT and follow-up US versus initial US and follow-up CT. Radiology 1999;13:831-836.
7. Glenn F, Becker CG: Acute calculous cholecystitis. Ann Surg 1982;195:131-136.
8. Mirizzi PL: Sindrome del conducto hepatico. J Int Chir 1948;8:731.
9. Csendes A, Diaz JC, Burdiles P, et al: Mirizzi syndrome and cholecystobiliary fistula: A unifying classification. Br J Surg 1989;76:1139.
10. Roslyn JJ, Thompson JE Jr, Darvin H, DenBesten L: Risk factors for gallbladder perforation. Am J Gastroenterol 1987,82:636-640.
11. Kalimi R, Gecelter GR, Caplin D, et al: Diagnosis of acute cholecystitis: Sensitivity of sonography, cholescintigraphy, and combined sonography-cholescintigraphy. J Am Coll Surg 2001;193:609-613.
12. Zeman RK, Burrell MI, Cahow CE, Caride V: Diagnostic utility of cholescintigraphy and ultrasonography in acute cholecystitis. Am J Surg 1981;141:446-451.
13. What if it's acute cholangitis? Drug Ther Bull 2005; 43:62-64.
14. Cello JP: Acquired immunodeficiency syndrome cholangiopathy: Spectrum of disease. Am J Med 1989;86:539.
15. Cockerill FR 3rd, Hurley DV, Malagelada JR, et al: Polymicrobial cholangitis and Kaposi's sarcoma in blood product transfusion-related acquired immune deficiency syndrome. Am J Med 1986;80;1237-1241.
16. Sebagh M, Farges O, Kalil A, et al: Sclerosing cholangitis following human orthotopic liver transplantation. Am J Surg Pathol 1995;19:81-90.
17. Dilly SA, Sloane JP: An immunohistological study of human hepatic graft-versus-host disease. Clin Exp Immunol 1985; 62:545-553.
18. Yusoff IF, Barkun JS, Barkun AN: Diagnosis and management of cholecystitis and cholangitis. Gastroenterol Clin North Am 2003;32:1145-1168.
19. Hanau LH, Steigbigel NH: Acute (ascending) cholangitis. Infect Dis Clin North Am 2000;14:521-546.
20. Oikarinen H, Paivansalo M, Lahde S, et al: Radiological findings in cases of gallbladder carcinoma. Eur J Radiol 1993;17:179-183.
21. Donohue JH, Nagorney DM, Grant CS, et al: Carcinoma of the gallbladder: Does radical resection improve outcome? Arch Surg 1990;125:237-241.
22. Gainant A, Cucchiaro G: Surgical treatment of 724 carcinomas of the gallbladder: Results of the French Surgical Association Survey. Ann Surg 1994;219:275-280.
23. Ekbom A, Hsieh CC, Yuen J, et al: Risk of extrahepatic bile duct cancer after cholecystectomy. Lancet 1993;342: 1262-1265.
24. Heathcote EJ, Lindon KD, Poupon R, et al: Combined analysis of French, American, and Canadian randomized controlled trials of ursodeoxycholic acid therapy in primary biliary cirrhosis. Gastroenterology 1995;108 (4, Suppl 3): A1082.
25. Tzakis AG, Carcassonne C, Todo S, et al: Liver transplantation for primary biliary cirrhosis. Semin Liver Dis 1989;9: 144-148.

Chapter 40

Emergency Biliary Ultrasonography

Emily Baran

KEY POINTS

The indication for emergency biliary ultrasound is the clinical suspicion of biliary disease in a patient presenting with acute abdominal pain.

The gallbladder should be identified with the main lobar fissure, portal triad, or superior pole of kidney as landmarks.

Both transverse and longitudinal views through the axis of the gallbladder should be obtained.

Imaging of the common bile duct with measurements should be obtained.

The presence or absence of an ultrasonographic Murphy's sign should be documented.

Background

Abdominal pain is a common chief complaint in the emergency department. Evaluation of acute upper or right-sided abdominal pain with emergency ultrasound can help differentiate biliary disease from other potential etiologies. Emergency biliary ultrasound is a limited, focused examination that can be performed rapidly at the bedside. It has been shown to be accurate and is useful for clinical decision-making.[1-4]

Indication

The indication for performing biliary emergency ultrasound is clinical suspicion for biliary disease in a patient presenting with acute abdominal pain.

Probe and Positioning

A 2- to 5-MHz curvilinear abdominal probe should be used. The patient is usually supine. Elevating the head of the bed, asking the patient to take slow deep breaths, and left lateral decubitus positioning can facilitate visualization of the gallbladder.

Anatomy and Approach

The first goal in biliary ultrasound is to correctly identify the gallbladder. This organ is a small cystic structure in the right upper quadrant that can easily be confused with loops of bowel or vascular structures. Anatomically, it lies between the right and left lobes of the liver and anterior to the kidney.

Imaging should begin in the right upper quadrant under the costal margin in the midclavicular line (Fig. 40-1). The probe indicator is pointed toward the patient's head and is rotated between ribs if necessary. Images by convention place the neck of gallbladder on the left of the screen. It is important to keep the inferior margin of the liver as an acoustic window. It may be necessary to move more superior into the rib spaces or more medial or lateral, depending on the individual patient's anatomy. The gallbladder connects to the portal triad by an echogenic

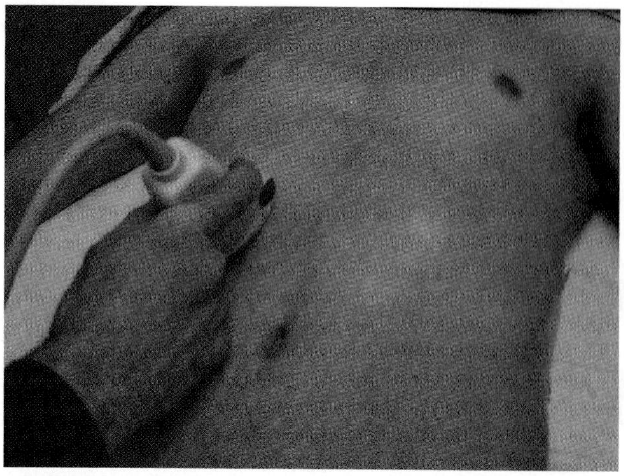

FIGURE 40-1 Initial probe positioning for right upper quadrant imaging (*red sticker* represents probe indicator). The optimal approach varies from patient to patient and may involve variations in both patient positioning—supine, semi-erect, or left lateral decubitus—and in probe positioning—epigastric, subcostal, intercostal, or right flank.

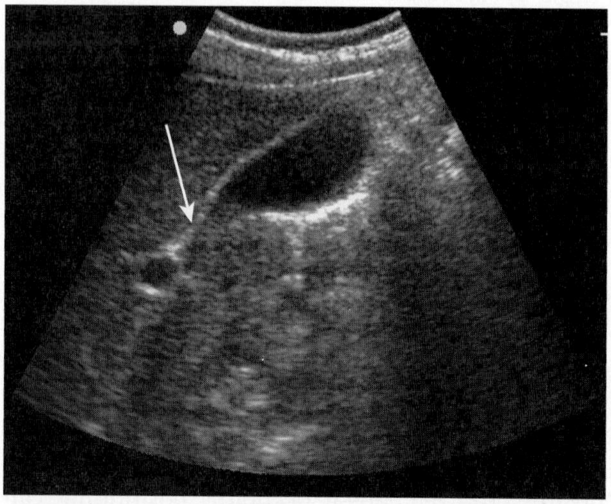

FIGURE 40-2 Main lobar fissure view. Image identifying the pear-shaped cystic structure in liver window as gallbladder using landmark of the main lobar fissure (*arrow*), a bright (echogenic) line connecting to the portal triad.

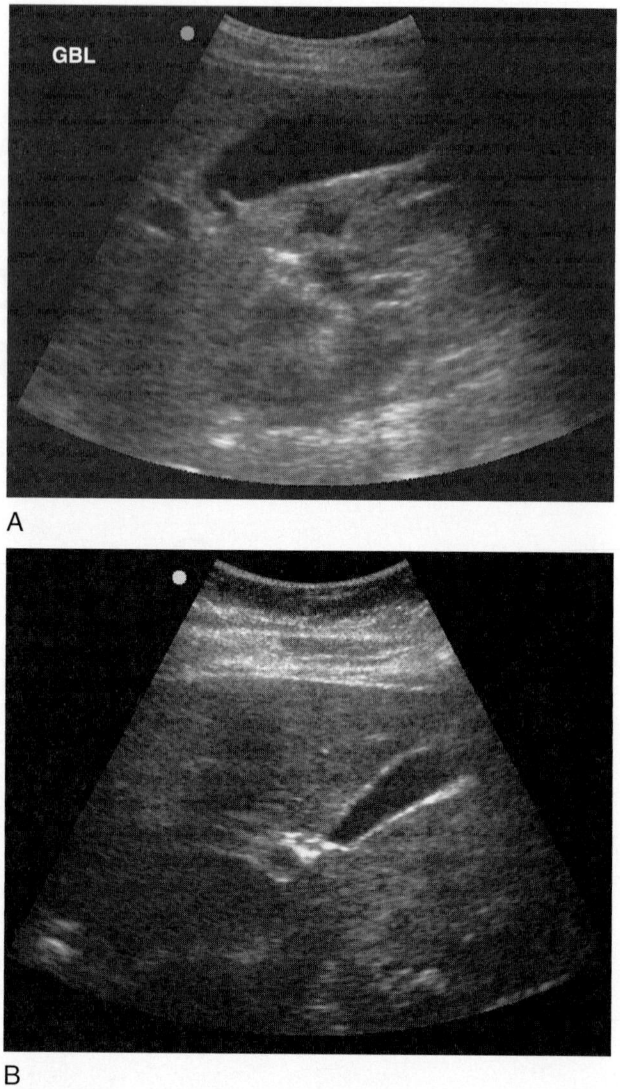
GBL
A
B

FIGURE 40-3 **A and B,** Normal longitudinal views of the gallbladder. Note the S-curved appearance of the neck, which is a normal variation.

(bright) line, the main lobar fissure (Fig. 40-2). Once the gallbladder is correctly identified by anatomic landmarks, it should be scanned from edge to edge in both longitudinal and transverse planes, with special attention paid to the neck and dependent areas. Longitudinal and transverse planes are defined with respect to axis of the structure being imaged, not in relation to true anatomic planes. Figure 40-3 demonstrates normal longitudinal gallbladder views.

Gallstones have a characteristic appearance on ultrasonography. They are hyperechoic (bright-appearing) balls of variable size, shape, and number that create posterior acoustic shadowing (Fig. 40-4). They are usually found in the dependent areas of the gallbladder, frequently collecting at folds or in gallbladder neck (Fig. 40-5). Gallstones are mobile and should move with changes in a patient's position.

The gallbladder is a fluid-filled structure that can create posterior enhancement artifact, which can make the posterior wall difficult to measure accurately. Measurements of the gallbladder wall should be of the anterior wall and should be made in transverse orientation.

The common bile duct (CBD) is identified by location of the portal triad. The larger portal vein is accompanied by the CBD and hepatic artery. In a transverse view, this duct is generally lateral to the hepatic artery. If this view of the portal triad were to be compared with the silhouette of the head of a famous cartoon mouse, the CBD would be the ear on the left of the screen (Fig. 40-6). In longitudinal view, the CBD should appear almost collapsed and running anterior to the portal vein (Fig. 40-7). Measurements of the CBD are taken from inner wall to inner wall and generally should be less than 4 mm, although

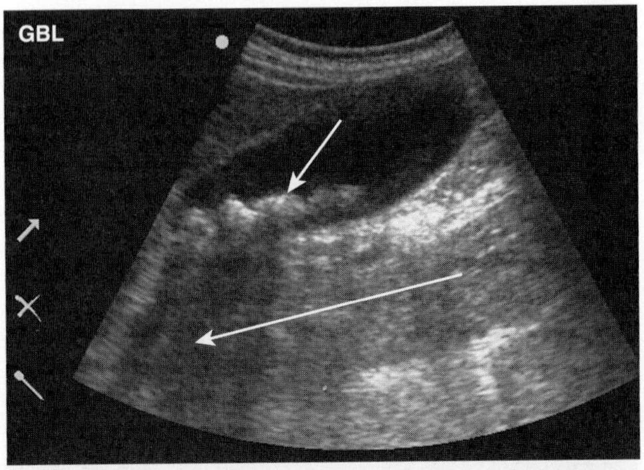
GBL

A

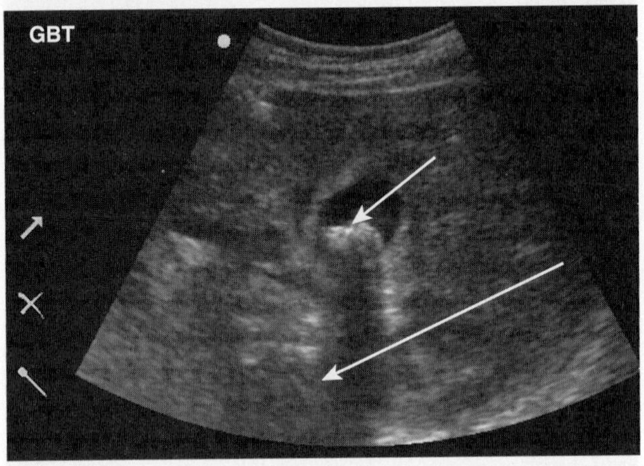
GBT

B

FIGURE 40-4 Multiple echogenic gallstones (*short arrows*) with posterior shadowing (*long arrows*) seen in longitudinal (**A**) and transverse (**B**) views.

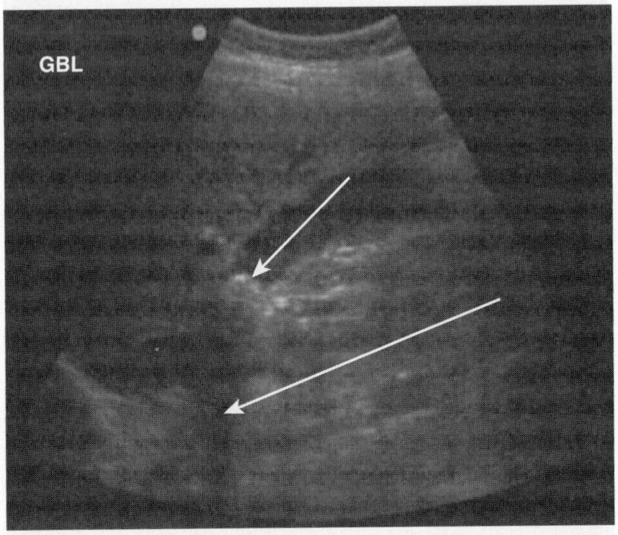
GBL

FIGURE 40-5 A large gallstone (*short arrow*) in the neck of the gallbladder. The *long arrow* shows shadowing.

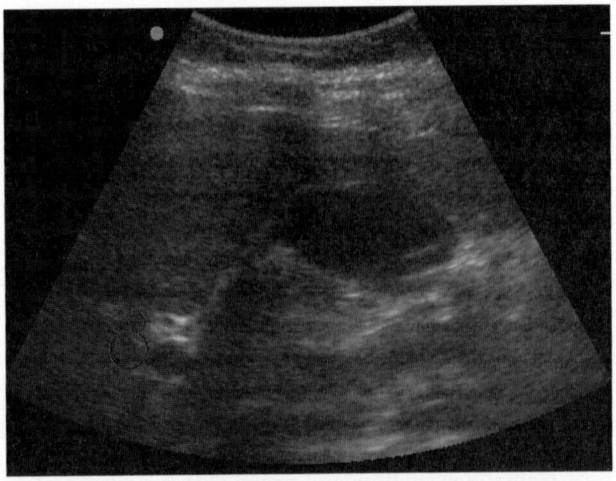

FIGURE 40-6 Transverse (cartoon mouse head) view of the common bile duct (CBD). The duct is the green "ear" on the left of the screen, the red "ear" is the hepatic artery, and the "face" is the portal vein.

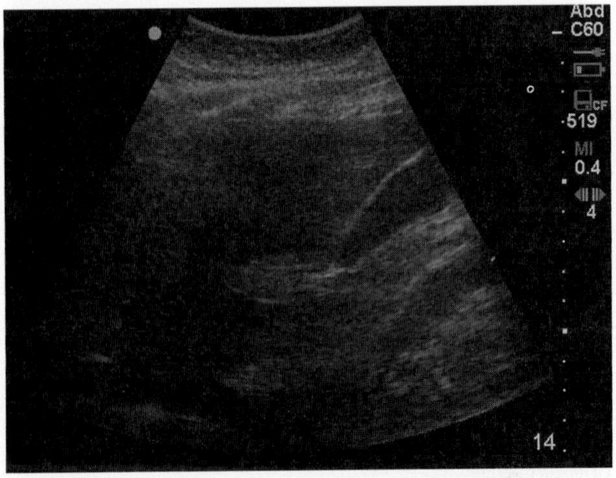
Abd
C60
519
MI
0.4
4
14

FIGURE 40-7 Longitudinal view of the common bile duct running parallel and anterior to the portal vein.

normal CBD diameter may measure as much as 1 mm for every decade of a patient's age.

Pathologic findings in the liver, pancreas, and other right upper quadrant structures are beyond the scope of emergency biliary ultrasound.

Box 40-1 summarizes the pearls and pitfalls for emergency ultrasound for biliary disease.

Interpretation and Limitations

In the presence of gallstones, several ultrasound findings support the diagnosis of cholecystitis. The first and most important is the sonographic Murphy's sign, which is tenderness with direct compression of the gallbladder by the ultrasound probe that reproduces the patient's abdominal pain. The tenderness should be present with the probe pressing over the gallbladder and not in other locations in the abdomen.

BOX 40-1

Pearls and Pitfalls for Emergency Biliary Ultrasound

- Try to keep liver edge as an acoustic window but vary patient position and probe placement to get best view.
- Make sure to correctly identify gallbladder by using anatomic landmarks such as the main lobar fissure and portal triad.
- Gallstones may hide in folds and dependent areas so it is important to fan through the entire gallbladder in two planes (side to side in long-axis and fundus to neck in short-axis).
- Gallstones shadow and move with gravity when the patient changes position. Polyps should not.
- Absence of color-flow Doppler signal can help distinguish common bile duct from hepatic artery.

Additional findings consistent with cholecystitis (Box 40-2) are thickening of the gallbladder wall to more than 3 to 4 mm, increased transverse diameter of the gallbladder to more than 4 to 5 cm, and the presence of pericholecystic fluid (Fig. 40-8). Common bile duct dilation to more than 4 mm in the setting of gallstones suggests choledocholithiasis with obstruction (Fig. 40-9). In the appropriate clinical setting, the presence of gallstones and the sonographic Murphy's sign should prompt a diagnosis of cholecystitis.

Emergency biliary ultrasound may be technically limited by obesity, bowel gas, or significant abdominal tenderness. Failure to identify or adequately image the gallbladder should prompt additional imaging studies. The primary limitation of emergency biliary ultrasound is that it is a focused examination not intended to identify all diseases of the right upper quadrant.

BOX 40-2

The "Magic Number 4" Findings for Ultrasonographic Diagnosis of Cholecystitis

- Anterior gallbladder wall >3-4 mm
- Transverse gallbladder measurement >4-5 cm
- Common bile diameter >4 mm

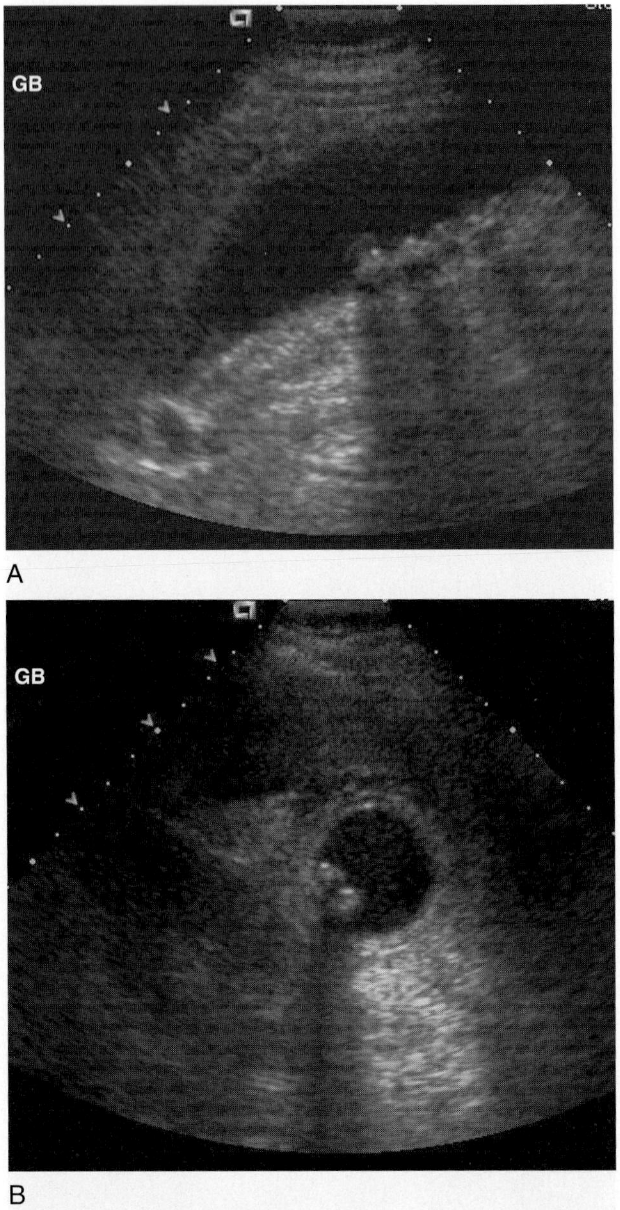
GB
A
GB
B

FIGURE 40-8 Longitudinal (**A**) and transverse (**B**) views of the gallbladder demonstrate multiple stones and a thickened wall with intramural edema. These findings are consistent with the diagnosis of cholecystitis.

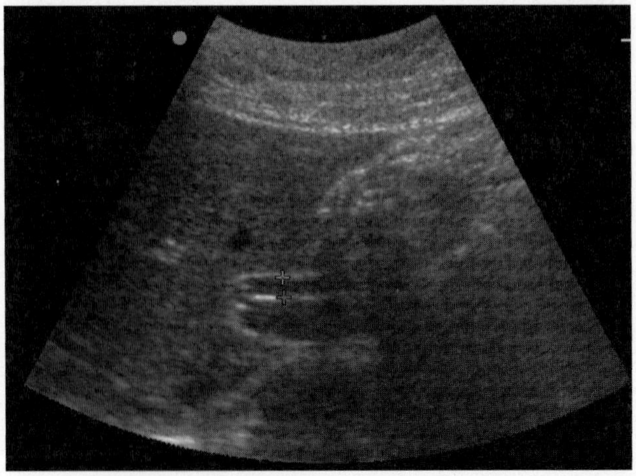

FIGURE 40-9 Dilated common bile duct.

REFERENCES

1. Rosen CL, Brown DF, Chang Y, et al: Ultrasonography by emergency physicians in patients with suspected cholecystitis. Am J Emerg Med 2001;19:32-36.
2. Schlager D, Lazzareschi G, Whitten D, Sanders AB: A prospective study of ultrasonography in the ED by emergency physicians. Am J Emerg Med 1994;12:185-189.
3. Kendall JL, Shimp RJ: Performance and interpretation of focused right upper quadrant ultrasound by emergency physicians. J Emerg Med 2001;21:7-13.
4. Blaivas M, Harwood RA, Lambert MJ: Decreasing length of stay with emergency ultrasound examination of the gallbladder. Acad Emerg Med 1999;6:1020-1023.

Chapter 41

Pediatric Abdominal Disorders

Russ Horowitz

KEY POINTS

The most common presentation in Meckel's diverticulum is painless rectal bleeding.
The most common cause of intestinal obstruction in patients up to the age of 6 years is intussusception, which often causes intermittent bouts of severe pain.
Henoch-Schönlein purpura is a vasculitis that causes abdominal pain, purpura, and arthritis.
Infants with bilious emesis may have malrotation with volvulus, necrotizing enterocolitis, sepsis, or small bowel obstruction.
In up to 90% of children younger than 2 years with appendicitis, the appendix has perforated by the time of diagnosis.

Abdominal Masses

Obstructive uropathy and renal cysts are the most likely causes of abdominal distention in infancy. Abdominal tumors are slow-growing and usually manifest incidentally (e.g., when a parent or physician feels an abdominal mass). The two most common malignancies are Wilms' tumor and neuroblastoma. The majority of affected children are younger than 5 years. Wilms' tumor arises from the renal parenchyma and in most cases is asymptomatic. Neuroblastoma develops from the adrenal gland or along the sympathetic chain, so may manifest as either a midline or flank mass. It is an aggressive malignancy and often has metastasized at diagnosis. Ultrasonography and computed tomography (CT) are useful for investigation of abdominal lesions. A pediatric surgeon and oncologist should be consulted early for management of abdominal tumors.

Gastrointestinal Bleeding

As a general rule, gastrointestinal (GI) bleeding is usually not as severe in children as in adults. In particular, the vast majority of cases of neonatal GI bleeding are benign. The first step in evaluation is to confirm, with a guaiac filter test for occult blood, that the suspicious material found in the stool or diaper is actually blood. Children routinely consume both foods (watermelon) and liquids (antibiotics such as cefdinir, fruit punch and other juices) that turn the stool red and may falsely lead both parents and health care workers to believe that there is GI blood loss. The benign pink or orange urate crystals in the urine of some neonates and young children are sometimes taken for blood when seen in diapers. Urinary tract infections and urethral prolapse may also deposit blood in the diaper that could be confused with GI blood.

Upper GI bleeding produces dark brown, black, or simply heme-positive stool. However, because of fast transit time in neonates, some upper GI bleeding may be bright red. The most common caused is swallowed maternal blood, acquired either during delivery or as a result of breastfeeding from irritated or cracked nipples.

Esophageal varices are rare in children. In contrast to adults, in whom primary hepatic disease is the leading cause, the most likely causes of varices in children are splanchnic and portal vein obstructions. Varices may develop secondary to umbilical vein catheterization, dehydration, sepsis, or omphalitis. Less commonly to blame are hepatic parenchymal conditions such as biliary cirrhosis secondary to biliary atresia, cystic fibrosis, α_1-antitrypsin deficiency, and hepatitis. Early onset of inflammatory bowel disease occurs in the teenage years and is uncommon in younger children.

Perirectal skin breakdown and external rectal fissures both produce blood-streaked stools and are easily identifiable on physical examination. Sitz baths and stool softeners are useful to treat rectal fissures.

ED management of GI bleeding is directed at fluid and blood resuscitation.

Meckel's Diverticulum

Meckel's diverticulum is the most common omphalomesenteric remnant. The most common presentation is painless rectal bleeding, which occurs from ulceration of the diverticulum or neighboring mucosa by the ectopic tissue. The ectopic tissue is gastric in origin in more than 80% of cases but may be pancreatic as well. Symptoms usually occur within the first 2 years of life, and the majority of affected children present by age 20 years (Box 41-1). Meckel's diverticulum can act as a lead point in intussusception. The diagnostic study of choice is a radio-labeled bleeding study called a Meckel's scan. Definitive therapy is surgical excision.

BOX 41-1

Meckel's Diverticulum—the Rule of 2s

- 2% of the population is affected.
- 2% of patients with Meckel's diverticula have a complication.
- 2 inches is the usual length.
- 2 feet from the ileocecal valve is the usual location.
- 2 times as common in males as females.

Intussusception

Intussusception occurs when one loop of intestine invaginates into another. Intussusception of the mesentery can also occur, causing edema and vascular congestion. It is the most common cause of intestinal obstruction in children less than 6 years old. The ileocolic region is most often involved. Intussusception usually manifests in children 6 to 18 months old, with a peak occurrence at 10 to 12 months. The vast majority of cases in children younger than 3 years are idiopathic. One etiologic theory is that inflammation of Peyer's patches within the intestine acts as a lead point for the intussusception. In children older than 5 years, a true lead point is found more than 75% of the time. Lead points include polyps, lymphoma, Meckel's diverticula, surgical adhesions, and mucosal inflammation secondary to vasculitis.

This condition is often preceded by a viral illness, and the patient may have a low-grade fever at the time of evaluation. Presenting symptoms are vomiting and episodic, crampy abdominal pain. Initially children return to baseline status between episodes, but as the condition persists, they may become lethargic. Screaming episodes lasting up to 10 to 15 minutes with hip and knee flexion are routine. The episodes increase in frequency and duration over time, with subsequent shortening of the asymptomatic intervals. The classic triad of symptoms—vomiting, abdominal pain, and "currant jelly stools"—is seen in less than one third of patients. However, more than 75% have two of these findings. Early on, stools test guaiac negative, but with time, they test positive. Frank blood secondary to bowel ischemia mixed with mucus gives the stool a currant jelly appearance. Some children present only with lethargy. The most commonly confused entity is constipation because of the similar pattern of colicky abdominal pain. These two conditions can easily be differentiated with a plain abdominal radiograph.

History is the best guide to the diagnosis of intussusception. On abdominal palpation, there may be an empty right lower quadrant because the cecum has rotated out of its standard position. The actual intussusception may be palpated as a sausage-shaped mass in the right upper quadrant. Normal physical findings should not dissuade the examiner from proceeding with investigation, because most children appear normal between episodes. No laboratory studies support the diagnosis, and guaiac test–positive stool is a late finding. Abdominal radiographic findings are most often normal, but a mass may be seen in the right upper quadrant.

Contrast agent enemas are both diagnostic and therapeutic. Intussusceptions that cannot be reduced via enema must be reduced surgically. Up to 10% of cases recur, most often within 24 hours. After reduction, the child must be admitted to the hospital for a 24-hour observation period.

Children who present with a history and physical findings suspicious for intussusception must be evaluated quickly, because the passage of time increases both the edema and the difficulty of reduction. A pediatric surgeon should be contacted before the child undergoes attempted enema reduction, in case of failure or perforation. Ileoileal intussusceptions may be difficult to visualize and reduce via enema unless there is significant reflux of contrast material. Such intussusceptions are associated with Henoch-Schönlein purpura, in which the vasculitis acts as a lead point.[1]

Henoch-Schönlein Purpura

Henoch-Schönlein purpura is a vasculitis that predominately affects the capillaries and small vessels. It manifests most commonly in school-age children with the classic triad consisting of abdominal pain, purpura, and arthritis. Elevations of immunoglobulin A (IgA) in the blood are found, along with immune complex deposition in the skin and glomeruli. There is no known etiology, but Henoch-Schönlein purpura has often been found to occur after an upper respiratory infection. Recurrences are seen in up to 50% of cases.

Abdominal pain occurs in half of patients and is most often colicky in nature. The EP should strongly consider intussusception in children with guaiac test–positive or frankly bloody stools accompanied by severe pain. The subtype of intussusception associated with Henoch-Schönlein purpura is often ileoileal, which is difficult to visualize and reduce with a contrast enema. CT is the method of choice for identification, and reduction must often be achieved surgically.

The rash is petechial, purpuric, and usually located on the buttocks and lower extremities. It is seen in dependent areas, so the scrotum and hands may also be affected. In younger children, the rash is displayed on the dorsal surfaces of the extremities, trunk, and head. The lesions are palpable, looking and progressing like common bruises.

The arthritis occurs in two thirds of patients and most often involves the large joints of the lower extremities. The knees and ankles may be edematous as well as tender to palpation and with movement. Joint pain may be so severe as to interfere with ambulation. Renal involvement occurs in 25% to 50% of patients and usually manifests as microscopic hematuria and proteinuria.

Diagnosis of Henoch-Schönlein purpura is made from the characteristic rash and accompanying symptoms. Results of complete blood count and clotting studies are normal.

Nonsteroidal anti-inflammatory drugs (NSAIDs) are the traditional therapy for the arthralgias seen in Henoch-Schönlein purpura. Use of corticosteroids for the management of abdominal pain and renal involvement is controversial. Treatment usually is given on an outpatient basis, but substantial discomfort may require inpatient management. Severe abdominal pain, especially in conjunction with guaiac test–positive or grossly bloody stools merits an evaluation for intussusception.[2,3]

Gastroesophageal Reflux

Gastroesophageal reflux (GER) is caused by a loose esophageal sphincter with retrograde passage of food into the esophagus. It usually manifests in the first few weeks after birth as emesis during or soon after cessation of feeding. The emesis may be blood-streaked but should never be bilious. Some children who are eventually diagnosed with GER may have previously been incorrectly labeled as having colic, feeding difficulties, or formula intolerance.

Symptoms of GER range from small "wet burps" to discomfort during feedings with arching of the back. One particularly severe form of reflux is Sandifer's syndrome, in which the child has opisthotonic movements and unusual head and neck positioning. The head movements may be an attempt to reduce pain by elongating the esophagus and protecting the airway from aspiration. Complications of GER include failure to thrive, apnea, laryngospasm, and aspiration pneumonia. Reflux esophagitis may be the culprit in children with guaiac test–positive stools or iron deficiency anemia. In most cases, GER spontaneously resolves by 1 year. Diagnosis is most often made from a careful history. Esophageal pH probe, nuclear milk scan, barium swallow study, and direct feeding under fluoroscopic observation are all diagnostic options.

Nonpharmacologic interventions are often sufficient to relieve the majority of cases of GER. Smaller-volume feedings with breaks for burping are often helpful. Caregivers should be instructed to keep children semi-upright for 30 to 45 minutes after feedings. Thickening of feedings with cereal reduces crying and improves symptoms. Ranitidine, a histamine blocker, reduces gastric acid. Metoclopramide is a stimulator of esophageal and gastric motility. GER that is severe and resistant to medical therapy may require surgical intervention with a Nissen fundoplication. This procedure involves wrapping and surgically fixing a portion of the stomach around the esophagus.

Pyloric Stenosis

Pyloric stenosis, which results from hypertrophy of the antrum of the stomach, has no known cause. The male-to-female ratio is 5:1, and familial incidence is present in up to 50% of patients. Children are usually presented at 2 to 5 weeks of age and rarely after 3 months. They feed normally at first, but vomiting in the midst of or soon after feeds then develops. The emesis begins as mild and small amounts and then progresses to voluminous and projectile. It is never bilious but can be blood-streaked. The patient appears to vomit the entire amount but then ravenously refeeds. After eating, peristaltic waves may be visible across the abdomen. If the condition continues, the child loses weight and becomes dehydrated, with sunken eyes, loose skin, and lethargy. Electrolyte analysis shows a hypochloremic, hypokalemic metabolic alkalosis. As the child continues to vomit, hydrogen and chloride are expelled. The kidneys attempt to maintain normal pH by eliminating potassium and hydrogen ions.

Careful examination, especially in a thin, dehydrated child with prolonged illness, may detect the pylorus, or "olive." Palpation of an "olive" provides definitive diagnosis. In cases in which the pylorus is not palpated, identification is made with either ultrasonography or an upper GI radiographic series. Ultrasonography is the preferred method, because in addition to its high rate of accuracy, it involves no radiation exposure. However, accuracy of ultrasonography is highly operator dependent. Ultrasonographic diagnosis is made by visualization of a thickened pylorus. An upper GI radiographic series will demonstrate a "string sign" as the contrast agent squeezes through a narrowed pylorus.

Surgery is the treatment of choice for pyloric stenosis. However, the diagnosis of this disorder does not represent a surgical emergency. ED management consists of rehydration and electrolyte correction before surgical intervention. Differential diagnosis includes gastroesophageal reflux, overfeeding, and gastritis.

Malrotation with Volvulus

Early in embryonic development, the intestine rotates around the superior mesenteric artery. The duodenum and cecum become widely displaced and fixed into position by peritoneal attachments called Ladd's bands. They are loosely connected by a broad mesentery. In cases of malrotation, the cecum and duodenum do not separate but remain closely aligned. They are only loosely fixed into position, and the mesentery does not fan out. This narrow stretch of mesentery, which contains the superior mesenteric artery, crosses over the duodenum. It can easily twist on itself, causing duodenal obstruction and arterial compression. The result is ischemia with the potential for intestinal necrosis within 1 to 2 hours.

The common presentation is acute onset of abdominal pain with bilious emesis. There may or may not be abdominal distention, depending on the anatomic level of the obstruction. Malrotation must be high on the differential diagnosis list whenever bilious emesis is present. Children are usually presented within the first year of life, with the majority of cases occurring within the first week to month. Older children may have a history of intermittent episodes of vomiting and abdominal pain that suddenly become more severe. Bloody stools should raise the level of concern for bowel ischemia and impending gangrene. Patients are often quite ill and may be in shock at presentation. A loop of small bowel overlying the liver is apparent on plain abdominal radiographs. Distal bowel gas is limited or absent. The "double bubble" sign can be visualized on an upright film; it is produced by a dilated stomach and duodenum. An upper GI radiographic series, the diagnostic study of choice, demonstrates abnormal anatomy with a coiled-spring appearance to the jejunum in the right upper quadrant.

All children with bilious emesis need immediate evaluation by a surgeon. Malrotation with midgut volvulus is a surgical emergency because bowel infarction can occur rapidly.

The differential diagnosis of bilious emesis is short but never benign (Box 41-2). In addition to malrotation, sepsis, small bowel obstruction and necrotizing enterocolitis are included.[4]

BOX 41-2

Differential Diagnosis of Bilious Emesis and the Associated Radiographic Findings

- Small bowel obstruction: air-fluid levels
- Necrotizing enterocolitis: pneumatosis intestinalis
- Malrotation: small bowel overlying liver and absence of distal bowel gas
- Sepsis

Data from Long FR, Kramer SS, Markowitz RI, et al: Radiographic patterns of intestinal malrotation in children. Radiographics 1996;16:547-556.

Necrotizing Enterocolitis

Necrotizing enterocolitis (NEC) is mostly a disease of premature infants and usually occurs in the intensive care unit. However, up to 10% of infants with NEC are born at full term, and presentation in the ED is a possibility. Signs and symptoms range from feeding intolerance and vomiting to pneumatosis intestinalis (air within the intestinal wall), perforation, shock and disseminated intravascular coagulation. Most affected newborns have vomiting, which may or may not be bilious. Clinical presentation may be limited to guaiac test–positive stools and feeding intolerance, but in severe cases, the infants have massively distended, rigid abdomens and are in shock. Gas within the biliary tract is present in 10% to 30% of cases. With improved survival of premature infants, children may be presented with the sequelae of NEC, such as strictures, obstruction, fistulas, and short gut syndrome.

Appendicitis

Appendicitis typically begins with diffuse or periumbilical abdominal pain. Within 8 to 24 hours, vomiting begins, and the pain migrates to the right lower quadrant. Abdominal pain, vomiting, and fever are the classic symptom triad for the disease. Although in adult studies the pain precedes other symptoms, this may not be the case in many children with appendicitis. Up to one third of pediatric cases do not follow this order, and vomiting is often reported as the first sign. Fever is routinely low-grade; a temperature above 39° C reduces the likelihood of appendicitis or suggests perforation.

The position of the appendix dramatically affects the location of the pain and symptoms. A normally placed appendix produces pain at McBurney's point. A low-lying pelvic appendix may irritate the sigmoid colon and mimic enteritis with diarrhea. A retrocecal appendix may produce flank or posterior pain and may be confused with pyelonephritis or septic arthritis of the hip. Movement on the way to the hospital or simply walking increases the discomfort. Patients may walk hunched over, may limp, or may have a shuffling gait. They experience distress when jumping or put weight preferentially on the left leg. Although anorexia is a classic finding, children can be enticed by their favorite foods and may even want to eat. Palpation should be gentle, and the right lower quadrant should be examined last to allow evaluation of nontender regions and gain the patient's confidence. Bowel sounds are usually normal or hypoactive. An external genital examination must be performed to rule out testicular disorders and incarcerated hernias.

Appendicitis is particularly difficult to identify early in the course of illness and in the very young (Box 41-3). Approximately 90% of patients younger than 2 years with appendicitis have perforated appendix at the time of diagnosis. Children have a thinner appendiceal wall and a less well-developed omentum. Therefore, rupture occurs more readily and results in more diffuse bacterial dissemination. Pediatric cases of appendiceal perforation have more severe and diffuse peritonitis than adult cases. Although the mortality from appendicitis has improved dramatically, the rate of perforation has not changed significantly in the past few decades.[5]

BOX 41-3

Special Considerations in Children with Suspected Appendicitis

- Vomiting may be the first sign.
- Children may not experience anorexia and may actually request food.
- Most young children have perforation at the time of diagnosis.
- Children younger than 2 years have generalized symptoms such as irritability and tachypnea.
- Thin appendiceal walls and loose omentum make perforation more likely and serious in children.
- Ultrasonography is useful in evaluation of thin children but is very operator dependent.

Complete blood count showing a leukocytosis and left shift is supportive of the diagnosis, but many children have normal white blood cell (WBC) counts.[6] Most patients with appendicitis have an elevated WBC count in the range of 11,000 to 15,000 cells/mm^3. An appendix in close proximity to the ureter can produce a sterile pyuria and mild hematuria. A positive urine gram stain response and the presence of leukocyte esterase and nitrites can help differentiate a true urinary tract infection from appendicitis-related problems.

In the case of perforation, pain initially resolves but then becomes more generalized with peritoneal symptoms. It may be most severe in both lower quadrants as the pus settles. Young children may simply have nonspecific symptoms, such as fussiness, inconsolable crying, irritability, and grunting respirations. Once perforation occurs, the child may have poor perfusion, tachycardia, high fever (≥39° C), and even septic shock. Bowel sounds are absent; the abdomen is rigid with rebound tenderness and involuntary guarding. The WBC count is dramatically elevated with a significant left shift.

A fecalith is visible on plain abdominal radiographs in 8% to 10% of patients with appendicitis. A number of other findings can be seen on plain films, including a scoliosis concave toward the right side, a sentinel loop overlying the appendix indicating an area of inflammation, air within the appendix, a mass in the right lower quadrant (more often in cases of abscesses), and loss of the psoas shadow on the right.

Ultrasonography is a useful tool for evaluating thin patients. The classic finding known as the "target sign" is a fecalith inside a large, inflamed appendix. In obese children, visualization and diagnosis become more challenging. Sensitivity and specificity of ultrasonography exceed 90%, but diagnosis is very operator-dependent, and ruptured appendices are notoriously difficult to identify. No diagnosis can be made if the appendix is not visualized. Ultrasonography is helpful in differentiating appendicitis from other causes of abdominal pain, such as ovarian cysts, but cannot exclude conditions such as mesenteric adenitis. CT is the modality of choice with sensitivity and specificity of more than 95%, particularly with a triple-contrast method (oral, intravenous, and rectal administration). This technology is helpful at diagnosing inflammatory bowel disease and mesenteric adenitis. Admission for serial abdominal examinations is warranted for a child with a compelling history and physical findings but equivocal laboratory findings.

A surgeon should be involved early in the ED evaluation of a child with suspected appendicitis, because imaging may be avoided in classic presentations. Pain must be addressed, and numerous studies have shown that narcotics do not affect the diagnostic accuracy of the examination. Surgeons may choose to evaluate the patient before analgesia is given, but pain medication should not be withheld indefinitely pending a surgical assessment. Signs of shock should be aggressively addressed, and suspected ruptures should receive broad antibiotic coverage.

Hirschsprung's Disease

Hirschsprung's disease is caused by the absence of ganglion cells in the myenteric plexus of the colon. Without ganglion cells, that segment is under constant contraction. The proximal region dilates to compensate, with resultant constipation. Patients present with complaints of chronic constipation, abdominal distention, and vomiting. Physical examination demonstrates palpable stool in the abdomen with a tight anal sphincter but absence of stool in the rectal vault. There is a 4:1 male preponderance. Eighty percent of affected patients are diagnosed within the first year of life. The most serious complications are toxic megacolon, perforation, and enterocolitis. Dilated colon, fecal impaction, and air-fluid levels are visible on abdominal radiographs. Diagnosis is made from the finding of aganglionosis on biopsy or anal manometry. A barium enema without bowel preparation shows a narrowed colonic segment and a dramatically dilated proximal segment. In uncomplicated cases, outpatient surgical evaluation is indicated. Resection of the aganglionic segment is curative.

The vast majority of cases of constipation are functional and are tied to behavioral and psychological causes. Pathologic causes are rare and, in addition to Hirschsprung's disease, include cystic fibrosis, and hypothyroidism.

Biliary Tract Disease

Gallstones are an unusual condition in healthy children. The most common type, pigment stones, usually develop in children with underlying hemolytic conditions, such as sickle cell disease and hereditary spherocytosis. Cholesterol stones are more prevalent in adolescent girls, obese children, patients with cystic fibrosis, and patients who depend on total parenteral nutrition. Because of the large percentage of pigment stones, up to 50% of cases of cholelithiasis in children are visible on abdominal radiographs, contrasting with 10% to 15% in adults.

Acalculous cholecystitis (gallbladder inflammation in the absence of gallstones) is actually more common in children than cholelithiasis. Causes include Kawasaki's disease, bacterial infections such as typhoid, shigellosis, scarlet fever, and viral infections such as hepatitis.

Acute cholangitis usually manifests in children with a history of biliary surgery, such as for choledochal cysts and biliary atresia. The clinical picture is similar to that in adults, with right upper quadrant pain, fever, and vomiting. Treatment is inpatient admission for therapy with broad-spectrum antibiotics such as ampicillin, gentamicin, and metronidazole.

Milk Protein Allergy

Milk protein allergy manifests as blood-streaked, mucous stools in young infants exposed to cow's milk–based formulas. There may be significant flatus and mild discomfort with feeding. However, most children appear nontoxic and otherwise well. Edema, inflammation, and discrete ulcerations are present in the intestinal mucosa. This condition is best described with consumption of milk protein but may occur with any formula, including soy. The treatment is to change to a formula with a different protein source. Symptoms should resolve within one week of complete withdrawal of the offending agent.[7]

REFERENCES

1. Bajaj L, Roback MG: Postreduction management of intussusception in a children's hospital emergency department. Pediatrics 2003;112:302-307.
2. Ronkainen J, Koskimies O, Ala-Houhala M, et al: Early prednisone therapy in Henoch-Schönlein purpura: A randomized, double-blind, placebo-controlled trial. J Pediatr 2006;149:241-247.
3. Huber AM, King J, McClain P, et al: A randomized, placebo-controlled trial of prednisone in early Henoch Schönlein purpura. BMC Med 2004;2:7.
4. Long FR, Kramer SS, Markowitz RI, et al: Radiographic patterns of intestinal malrotation in children. Radiographics 1996;16:547-556.
5. Nance ML, Adamson WT, Hedrick HL: Appendicitis in the young child: A continuing diagnostic challenge. Pediatr Emerg Care 2000;16:160-162.
6. Wang LT, Prentiss KA, Simon JZ, et al: The use of white blood cell count and left shift in the diagnosis of appendicitis in children. Pediatr Emerg Care 2007;23:69-76.
7. Fiocchi A, Restani P, Bernardini R, et al: A hydrolysed rice-based formula is tolerated by children with cow's milk allergy: A multi-centre study. Clin Exp Allergy 2006;36:311-316.

Chapter **42**

Gastrointestinal Devices and Procedures

Kerin A. Jones

KEY POINTS

Nonfunctional feeding tubes can be safely replaced in the ED with the use of a commercial tube or by making a few simple alterations to a standard Foley catheter to prolong its longevity.

Gastroesophageal balloon tamponade tubes are used only for life-threatening variceal bleeding that is refractory to standard, first-line, endoscopic treatment. There is no absolute contraindication to the use of such tubes as a heroic, life-saving measure.

Scope

EPs should be proficient in nasogastric tube (NGT) placement, the replacement of various types of feeding tubes, gastric lavage, and the use of gastroesophageal balloon tamponade. This chapter reviews the indications, contraindications, and special considerations for each of these important gastrointestinal (GI) procedures.

Nasogastric Tubes

■ LEVIN TUBE

A Levin tube is a single-lumen tube with multiple distal openings for suction, referred to as "eyes." Indications for its use include short-term gastric evacuation or decompression, diagnostic aspiration of gastric contents, and infusion of therapeutic agents. The Levin tube has a relatively large internal diameter, making it ideal for rapid decompression or drug infusion. Levin tubes are not intended for long-term gastric suctioning because they may cause invagination of the stomach wall into the distal eyes, resulting in gastric lining injury or tube obstruction. Levin tubes are not used for gastric lavage. Intermittent suction may be set at a level lower than 40 mm Hg.

■ SALEM SUMP TUBE

The Salem sump is a double-lumen tube with multiple distal suction eyes. The second lumen allows for venting during suction, which prevents invagination and subsequent gastric injury. The Salem sump tube may be used for indications similar to those for the Levin tube as well as for long-term gastric evacuation. Intermittent suction may be at a pressure less than 120 mm Hg.[1]

■ INDICATIONS AND CONTRAINDICATIONS

Box 42-1 lists the indications for and contraindications to the use of NGTs in the ED.

■ INSERTION PROCEDURE

Inserting an NGT may cause the patient to cough, vomit, retch, sneeze, or bleed (epistaxis being most common). The EP should wear protective apparel—

Tips and Tricks

INSERTING A NASOGASTRIC TUBE

- Warming the tube will make it more pliable and easier to advance along the curvature from the nasopharynx into the oropharynx.
- Flexing the patient's neck can help direct the tube from the oropharynx into the esophagus.
- If choking, gagging, or muffling of the voice occurs, withdraw the tube to the oropharynx only. Do not remove the tube completely, or it must be repassed through the nasopharynx into the oropharynx, which is usually the most difficult and painful part of the procedure.
- The tube can coil within the patient's mouth; if problems occur placing or verifying placement of the tube, always check the mouth.
- In an unconscious patient, elevating the jaw will move the trachea anteriorly, a maneuver that can relieve pressure on the esophagus, making it easier to pass the tube.[4]
- A lubricated, soft, nasopharyngeal airway may be inserted nasally if neither naris appears to be amenable to placement of the larger, more rigid NGT. The nasopharyngeal airway may be used to dilate the nasal passage for a few minutes and then removed to allow another attempt at placing the NGT. Alternatively, a smaller NGT may be passed through the nasopharyngeal airway into the esophagus.

BOX 42-1

Indications for and Contraindications to Nasogastric Tubes (NGTs)

Indications

In gastrointestinal bleeding: to monitor blood loss, which may help differentiate upper from lower tract source of the bleed
In intubated patients, to decrease the risk of pulmonary aspiration, treat gastric distention, and deliver medications
Decompression of intestinal obstruction
Treatment of paralytic ileus, intractable vomiting
Treatment of gastric outlet obstruction and distention
In trauma patients, to evaluate for transdiaphragmatic hernia; deviation of NGT may be seen on chest radiograph in patient with aortic dissection

Relative Contraindications

Facial fractures: trauma patients with suspected cribriform plate or midfacial fractures are susceptible to intracranial placement of NGT
Severe coagulopathy
Ingestions likely to cause upper gastrointestinal perforation, such as alkali and highly volatile substances
Esophageal strictures

gloves, gown, and mask—when placing an NGT. The patient should be placed in either an upright or Fowler's position.

1. Estimation of Tube Length

The length of tube to be inserted, to place drainage eyes in the proper location in the stomach (Fig. 42-1), can be estimated by adding the following three measurements together[2]:

a: Measurement from the patient's xiphoid process to the earlobe.
b: Measurement from the earlobe to the tip of the nose.
c: 15 cm

2. Nares Patency Check, Anesthesia, and Vasoconstriction

The EP should check the nares for patency by direct visualization or by having the patient sniff or blow out of each nostril with the other naris occluded. Topical anesthetic spray or ointment should be used to decrease the discomfort and gagging associated with tube placement. The more patent nostril should be anesthetized 5 minutes prior to tube insertion.

Lidocaine (4%) is the most commonly used anesthetic, but many other agents, including tetracaine, butyl aminobenzoate, and benzocaine, are available. Nebulized 4% lidocaine given via bronchodilator has been shown to be more effective than topical lidocaine in reducing the pain associated with NGT insertion[3]; 2.5 mL of 4% lidocaine placed in a nebulizer face mask equals 100 mg lidocaine.

Vasoconstrictors may also be used 3 to 5 minutes prior to the procedure to decrease traumatic bleeding. Phenylephrine (Neo-Synephrine 0.5%) or oxymetazoline (Afrin 0.05%) is typically used. Vasoconstrictors must be used with caution in hypertensive patients.

3. Lubrication of Tube

Once the naris has been treated with an anesthetic and vasoconstrictor, the tube is lubricated with water-soluble lidocaine jelly or viscous lidocaine.

4. Insertion of Tube

The tube is inserted into the naris along the floor of the nose inferior to the lower turbinates. The tube should be inserted at close to a 90-degree angle with the face and directed parallel to the floor of the nose

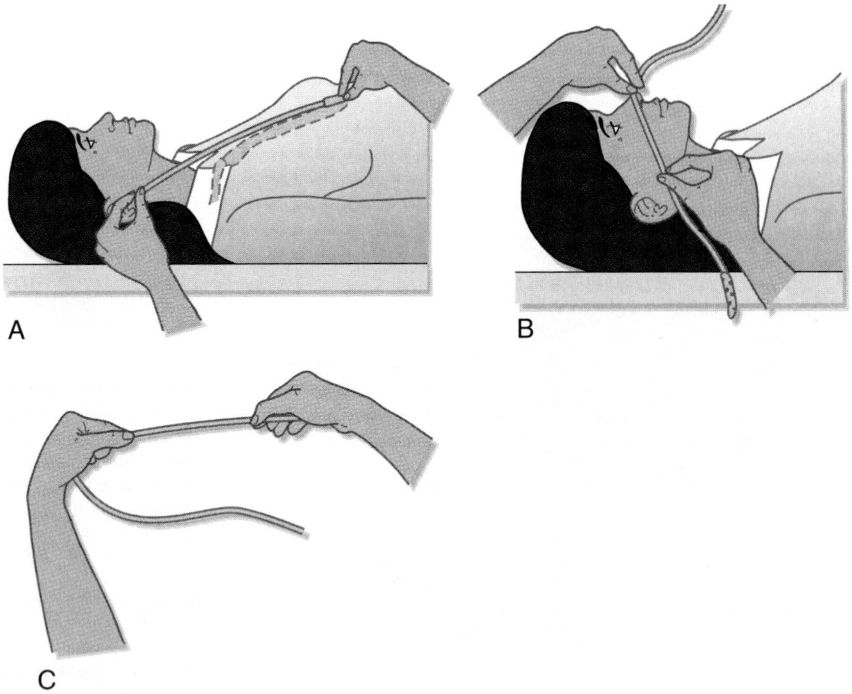
A
B
C

FIGURE 42-1 To estimate the length of nasogastric tube to be inserted, add together the measurement from the patient's xiphoid process to the earlobe (**A**), plus the measurement from the earlobe to the tip of the nose (**B**), plus 15 cm (**C**). (From Samuels LE: Nasogastric and feeding tube placement. In Roberts JR, Hedges JR [eds]: Clinical Procedures in Emergency Medicine, 4th ed. Philadelphia, Saunders, 2004, pp 794-816.)

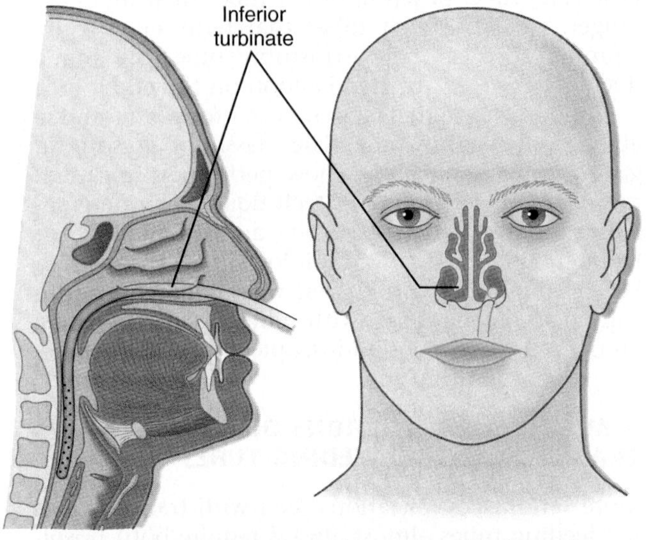
Inferior
turbinate

FIGURE 42-2 The nasogastric tube is passed parallel to the floor of the nose posteriorly and usually passes inferior to the inferior turbinate. The tube should not be directed cephalad. (From Samuels LE: Nasogastric and feeding tube placement. In Roberts JR, Hedges JR [eds]: Clinical Procedures in Emergency Medicine, 4th ed. Philadelphia, Saunders, 2004, pp 794-816.)

(posteriorly), not cephalad (Fig. 42-2). Gentle pressure should be used to advance the tube past the nasopharynx and into the oropharynx. Once the tube is in the posterior pharynx, the patient is asked to swallow or take a sip of water to aid in smooth passage of the tube into the esophagus. Then the tube is quickly advanced to the premeasured length to minimize discomfort. Care should be taken not to use excessive force in placing an NGT so as to avoid mucosal injury.

■ Alternative Approaches with Difficult Tube Insertions

An NGT may be placed by direct visualization using a laryngoscope and McGill forceps. The tube is inserted via the nose into the nasopharynx. The mouth is opened, and a laryngoscope is used to directly visualize the hypopharynx. With Magill forceps, the NGT is grasped and inched into the esophagus under direct visualization.

Alternatively, digital placement of an NGT can be accomplished in a paralyzed, sedated, and intubated patient. The EP places the second and third fingers in the posterior pharynx of the patient and depresses the tongue. He or she then passes the tube through the nose into the posterior pharynx, using the fingers in the pharynx to direct the tube into proper location (Fig. 42-3).[4]

■ Verifying Tube Placement

Radiographic verification is the most sensitive test to detect proper placement, but is not the standard of care. Methods that are normally used to verify tube placement are as follows:

- Insufflation of air causing or resulting in borborygmi (gurgling) sounds heard over the epigastrium verifies that the tube is in the stomach.
- Aspiration of gastric fluid; a pH less than 4 is correlated with a 95% chance that the tip of the tube is in the stomach.
- In a conscious patient, normal clear speech without coughing is suggestive of proper tube placement.[5]

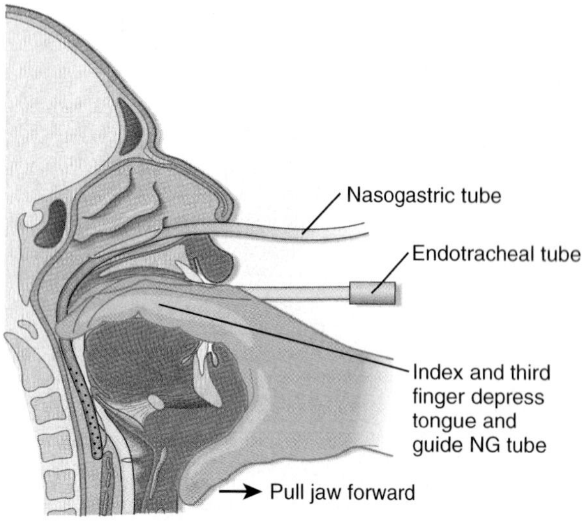
Nasogastric tube
Endotracheal tube
Index and third finger depress tongue and guide NG tube
Pull jaw forward

FIGURE 42-3 Digital placement of a nasogastric tube in a paralyzed, sedated, intubated patient. (From Samuels LE: Nasogastric and feeding tube placement. In Roberts JR, Hedges JR [eds]: Clinical Procedures in Emergency Medicine, 4th ed. Philadelphia, Saunders, 2004, pp 794-816.)

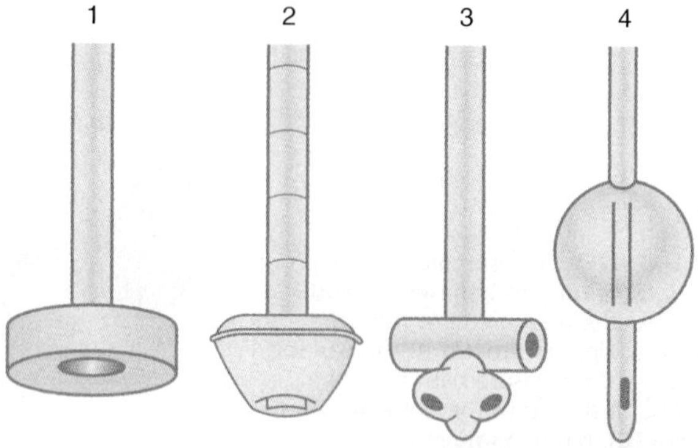
1
2
3
4

FIGURE 42-4 Types of gastrostomy tubes. 1, Polyurethane catheter with collapsible foam flange (CORPAK MedSystems, Wheeling, IL). 2, Silicone catheter (American Endoscopy, Bard Interventional Products, Billerica, MA). 3, Latex catheter with a movable external bolster and an internal mushroom- or de Pezzer–type flange on the end (American Endoscopy). 4, Balloon (Foley) catheter (Wilson-Cooke Co., Winston-Salem, NC). (From Samuels LE: Nasogastric and feeding tube placement. In Roberts JR, Hedges JR [eds]: Clinical Procedures in Emergency Medicine, 4th ed. Philadelphia, Saunders, 2004, pp 794-816.)

■ Securing the Nasogastric Tube

Once the tube is inserted and its location verified, it can be taped into place. Silk tape is usually torn into a butterfly configuration, one end of the tape placed on the nose and the torn ends of the tape wrapped around the tube in opposite directions. Tincture of benzocaine can be used on the skin prior to tape placement to more securely adhere both tube and tape.

■ COMPLICATIONS

Available literature reports a complication rate between 0.5% and 1.5% to placement of NGTs. Common complications are as follows[6]:

- Epistaxis
- Tracheal/bronchial placement
- Pneumothorax
- Intracranial placement
- Esophageal or pharyngeal perforation
- Gastric or duodenal rupture
- Esophageal obstruction or rupture
- Gastrothorax and tension gastrothorax
- Pulmonary aspiration; the NGT may induce a hypersalivation response, a depressed cough reflex, or a mechanical/physiologic impairment of the glottis.[7-9]

Transabdominal Feeding Tubes

Feeding tubes are placed to provide long-term nutritional support for many reasons. They are classified both by the location of their terminal lumen and by the method of placement. Gastrostomy tubes have a terminal lumen located within the stomach and are now typically placed via a percutaneous endoscopic technique; thus they are called PEG (percutaneous, endoscopically placed gastrostomy) tubes (Fig. 42-4). Several manufacturers make various types of PEG tubes. The other most frequently encountered feeding tube is a J-tube, or jejunostomy tube. Such tubes are longer, smaller-caliber tubes that terminate in the jejunum. Unlike the gastrostomy tube, the J-tube does not have an inflated balloon on the end.

Various techniques may be used to place a transabdominal feeding tube. The classic open surgical gastrostomy procedure is now performed less commonly than percutaneous techniques. The percutaneous tubes can be placed by a gastroenterologist through endoscopy or a radiologist via fluoroscopy. Fewer complications are seen with the radiographically placed tubes than with tubes placed either via an open technique or endoscopically (Fig. 42-5).[10,11]

■ MAJOR COMPLICATIONS OF TRANSABDOMINAL FEEDING TUBES

More serious complications seen with transabdominal feeding tubes almost always require both hospitalization and gastroenterology and/or surgery consultation. These include intestinal complications such as obstruction, perforations, GI bleeding, volvulus, and gastric outlet obstruction. Serious infections include bacteremia, pulmonary aspiration, sepsis, peritonitis, advanced local cellulitis, and necrotizing fasciitis.[12-15] Other complications of gastrostomy tubes are prolapse with and without intestinal obstruction, extraluminal position of the tube, and fistula formation.[16] Patients may also demonstrate minor and major electrolyte abnormalities and, rarely, pneumothorax.

■ REPLACING A TUBE

Transabdominal feeding tubes must be replaced (Fig. 42-6) for many reasons, including expulsion, mal-

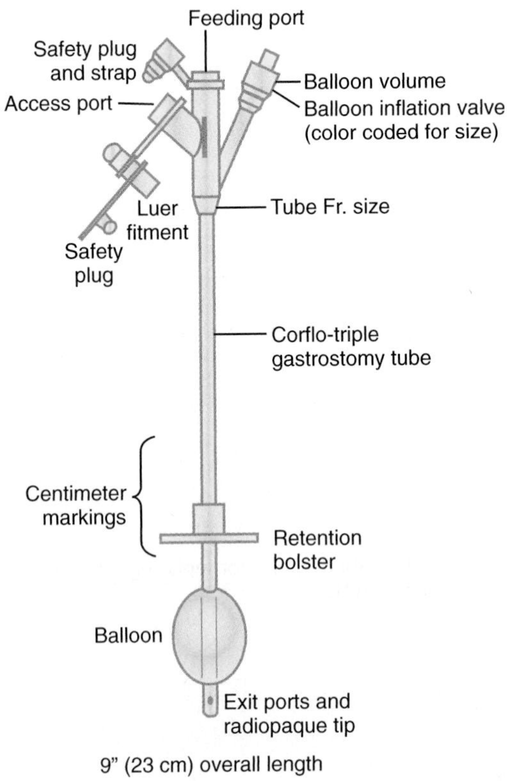
Feeding port
Safety plug and strap
Access port
Balloon volume
Balloon inflation valve (color coded for size)
Luer fitment
Safety plug
Tube Fr. size
Corflo-triple gastrostomy tube
Centimeter markings
Retention bolster
Balloon
Exit ports and radiopaque tip
9" (23 cm) overall length

FIGURE 42-5 A user-friendly gastrostomy tube from CORPAK MedSystems (Wheeling, IL). The tube is packaged with lubricant, a prefilled syringe for inflating the balloon, and an extension set. The color-coded inflation valve indicates tube size (12-24 F). The silicone tube uses a retention balloon and a movable bolster, similar in design to a Foley catheter. Note that the retention bolster is designed to prevent inward migration of the tube and is not to be an anchoring device sutured to the skin. (From Samuels LE: Nasogastric and feeding tube placement. In Roberts JR, Hedges JR [eds]: Clinical Procedures in Emergency Medicine, 4th ed. Philadelphia, Saunders, 2004, pp 794-816.)

function, leakage, tube deterioration resulting in cracks or fissures, and aneurysmal dilations of the tube. It is important that a patient's tube be correctly identified with respect to type, size, and manufacturer prior to an attempt at replacement. A dislodged tube should be replaced as quickly as possible to maintain patency of the feeding tube tract.

■ REMOVING A NONFUNCTIONAL TUBE

If the nonfunctioning tube was placed under fluoroscopic guidance by a radiologist, it can usually be removed by deflation of the balloon and gentle retraction. Some devices have a flange rather than a balloon; these flanges can usually be collapsed with slow, gentle traction. If resistance is met, consultation with gastroenterology, invasive radiology, or surgery specialists is required.

If the tube was placed by a gastroenterologist or a surgeon, it may have been altered at the time of placement with an anchoring device or an internal component that prevents the tube from becoming dislodged from the gastrostomy tract. Such a tube cannot be removed by gentle traction alone; the internal component must be removed endoscopically.

An alternative method is as follows: The tube is lifted off the abdominal wall skin to allow the tube to be cut as close to the skin as possible. The internal component is then pushed into the GI tract so it is free to pass through the intestines to be eliminated rectally. Most internal components pass within 2 weeks. There have been reported cases of intestinal obstruction, perforation, and, rarely, death with this method.[17,18] The internal component is less likely to pass without complications in children than in adults.[19] If this technique is used, reliable patient follow-up is needed to obtain serial abdominal radiographs. Radiographs should be taken within 1 week to monitor the progress of the component through the GI tract. If the internal component has not passed within 1 to 2 weeks, impaction has likely occurred, and endoscopic removal should be considered. Endoscopic removal is also advised in patients with special GI conditions such as intestinal obstruction, pseudo-obstruction, pyloric stenosis, intestinal stricture, history of radiation, and inflammatory bowel disease.[20]

■ FOLEY CATHETERS VERSUS COMMERCIAL FEEDING TUBE PRODUCTS AS REPLACEMENTS

Both commercially available feeding tubes and Foley catheters can be used to replace a dislodged feeding tube. Commercial feeding tubes are more expensive than Foley catheters. Studies have found that when a silicone Foley catheter is used with a retention disk and ring, efficacy and complication rate are similar to those for commercial replacement gastrostomy tubes. The retention disk and ring are used to prevent distal migration of the tube into the GI tract.[21] However, many institutions do not stock silicone Foley catheters.

■ Foley Catheters Used as Replacement Feeding Tubes

A few simple modifications to a standard Foley catheter can maximize its longevity as a feeding tube as well as reduce the chance of complications. An external bolster, or anchor, is used with a Foley catheter to replace a feeding tube, to prevent ingress of the tube into the ostomy and distal migration into the GI tract. An external bolster may be constructed by cutting a 3-cm section from a large rubber catheter. The outer bolster should be secured approximately 1 cm from the skin to prevent moisture trapping and maceration.[22] The construction is as follows:

1. Cut a 3-cm section from the proximal segment of a Foley catheter to be used as a bolster, the end without the balloon. A silicone catheter is preferred to a latex one (Fig. 42-7A).
2. Fold this segment in half and make a diagonal cut on each side of the fold to create a diamond-

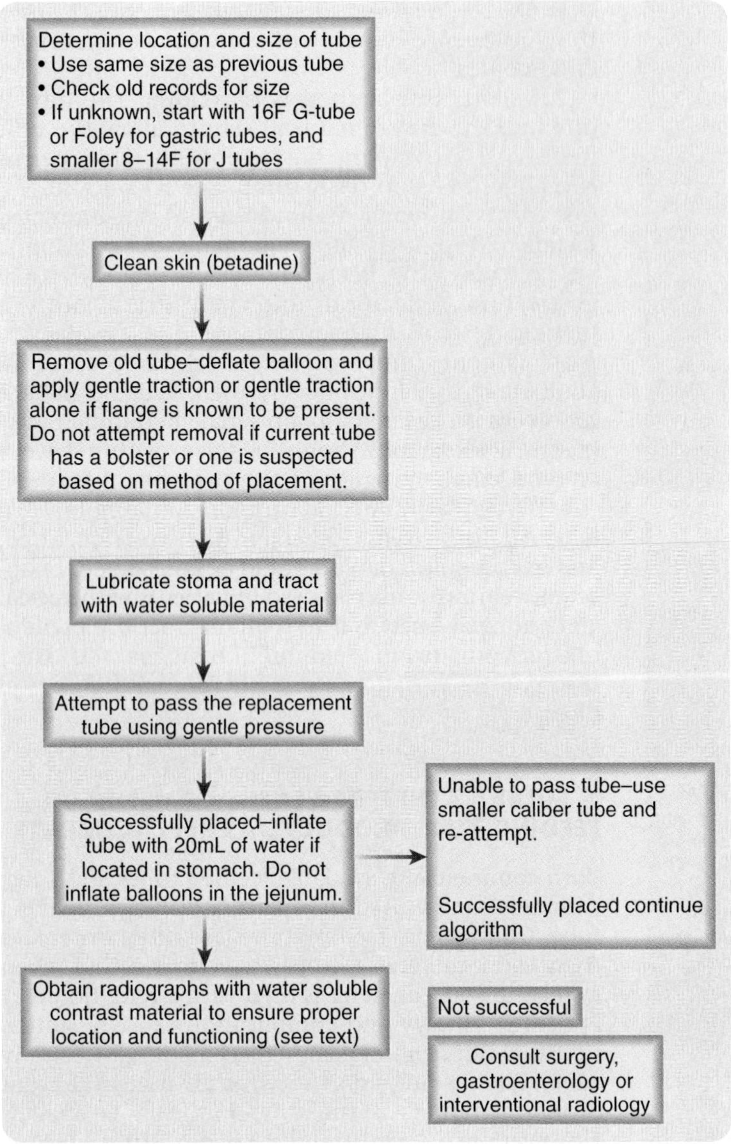

Determine location and size of tube
• Use same size as previous tube
• Check old records for size
• If unknown, start with 16F G-tube or Foley for gastric tubes, and smaller 8–14F for J tubes
Clean skin (betadine)
Remove old tube–deflate balloon and apply gentle traction or gentle traction alone if flange is known to be present. Do not attempt removal if current tube has a bolster or one is suspected based on method of placement.
Lubricate stoma and tract with water soluble material
Attempt to pass the replacement tube using gentle pressure
Successfully placed–inflate tube with 20mL of water if located in stomach. Do not inflate balloons in the jejunum.
Unable to pass tube–use smaller caliber tube and re-attempt.
Successfully placed continue algorithm
Obtain radiographs with water soluble contrast material to ensure proper location and functioning (see text)
Not successful
Consult surgery, gastroenterology or interventional radiology

FIGURE 42-6 Steps for replacing a transabdominal feeding tube.

shaped opening in the middle of each side of the 3-cm segment of tubing. Cut the holes slightly smaller than the tube to be inserted and used as the feeding tube to ensure a snug fit of the bolster on the replacement tube (see Fig. 42-7B and C).

3. Insert a hemostat through the two holes created in the bolster.
4. Grab the proximal end of the replacement tube with the hemostat and pull the tube through the bolster (see Fig. 42-7D).
5. Advance the bolster to its proper location about 1 cm above the skin of the abdomen (see Fig. 42-7E).[21,23]

■ Verifying Tube Location

There is no standard method for verifying tube placement. The safest and most conservative approach is to obtain radiographic confirmation when a feeding tube is replaced. Radiographic confirmation should be obtained in the following circumstances:

- Replacement of a recently placed feeding tube (less than 3 months) because the tract may not be mature.
- When tube replacement was difficult.
- When gastric material cannot be aspirated after placement.
- When the patient is unable to communicate about symptoms such as pain with tube placement and use.

Radiographic confirmation can be accomplished with fluoroscopy or by injection of water-soluble contrast material into the tube followed by plain radiography. Typically 20 to 30 mL of the contrast material is injected into the tube via a catheter-tip syringe. An abdominal film should be obtained within 1 to 2 minutes. Generally a flat-plate abdomi-

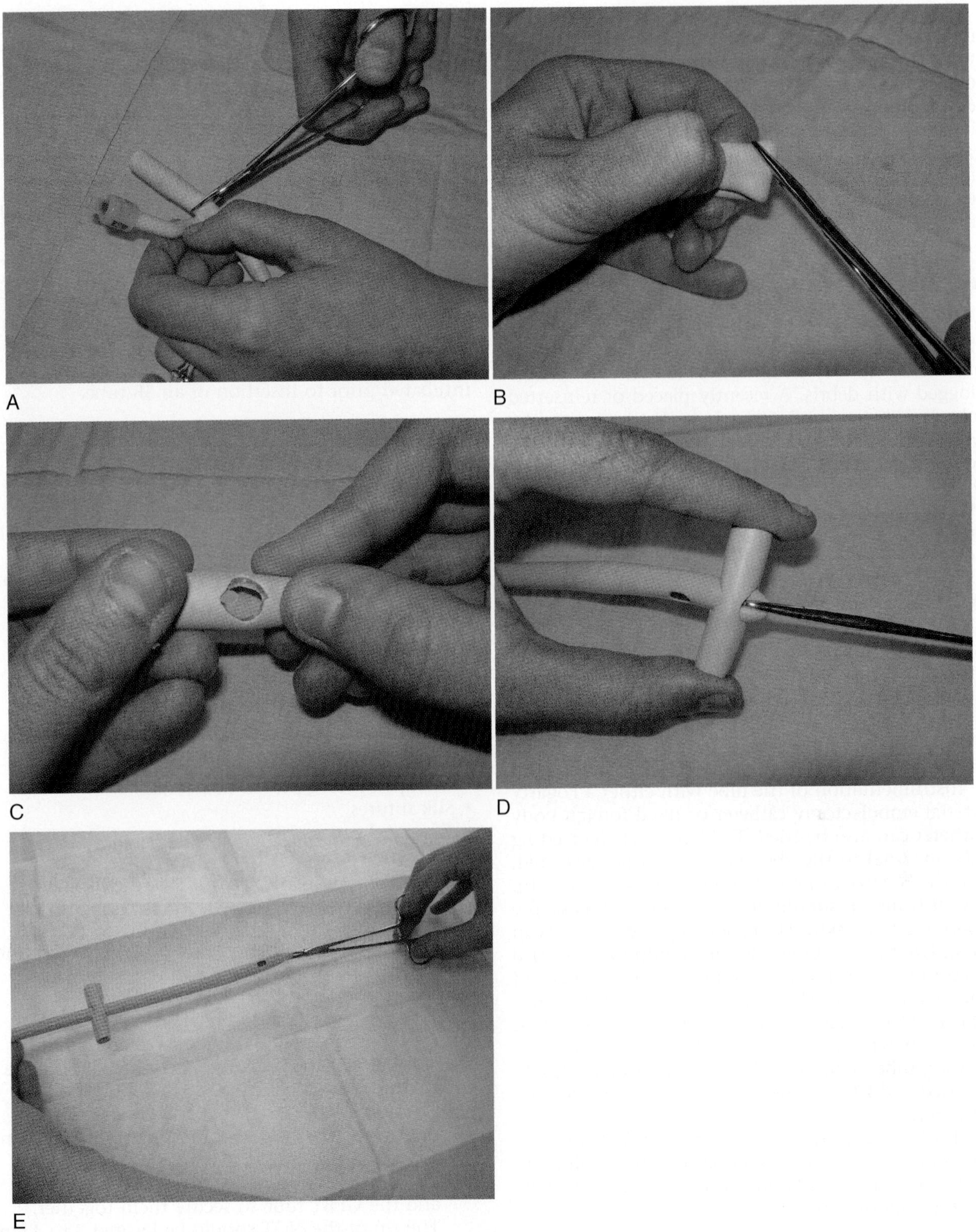
A
B
C
D
E

FIGURE 42-7 Modifying a Foley catheter for use as a replacement feeding tube.

nal view is sufficient to verify tube placement. If the tube insertion was very difficult or malposition is suspected, a two-view abdominal film may be required to ensure proper tube location. Proper location of the replaced tube is indicated by (1) ease of injection of the contrast material and (2) visualization of the gastric and intestinal walls as they are outlined by the contrast material. If extravasation of the dye is seen outside the stomach or intestine, tube malposition is verified.

■ CLOGGED FEEDING TUBES

Larger-diameter feeding tubes are less likely to become clogged than smaller tubes. A tube can become obstructed from kinking, or the lumen can become clogged with debris. A recently placed or reinserted tube is prone to kinking. A kink can be treated by withdrawing the tube a few centimeters and then advancing it again. Contrast-enhanced radiographs should be obtained whenever significant tube manipulation has occurred, to evaluate for patency and proper location. A persistently clogged tube needs to be removed and replaced.

If a feeding tube is clogged by debris, the following approaches can be used to unclog the tube:

- Milk the external part of the tube backwards to attempt to expel the debris.
- Irrigate with small aliquots of carbonated beverages.
- Irrigate with small aliquots of warm water at high pressure; use a small syringe (5-10 mL) with manual injection.

Instrumentation of the tube with either a Fogarty arterial embolectomy catheter or nasal foreign body catheter can also be tried. The length of the feeding tube external to the abdomen should be measured, and the Fogarty catheter inserted only to this length. An instrument should *never* be inserted past the abdominal wall skin. The balloon on the catheter can be inflated in the tube if an obstruction is met, and then further advanced to probe the entire length of the external tube. The catheter should not be withdrawn with the balloon inflated, as this action might cause removal of the feeding tube. In a 10 F or 12 F feeding tube, a No. 4 embolectomy catheter should be used; a 14 F tube requires a No. 5 embolectomy catheter.[24]

If a feeding tube has been unclogged by force or instrumentation, radiographs should be obtained to verify proper tube placement as well as to evaluate for tube perforation.

Gastroesophageal Balloon Tamponade

Variceal bleeding is a leading cause of significant morbidity and mortality in patients with cirrhosis. Sengstaken and Blakemore first described the use of a double-balloon tamponade system to control variceal bleeding in 1950. The Sengstaken-Blakemore (SB) tubes are not advocated as primary or secondary therapy for cirrhotic patients; they are used as rescue therapy for life-threatening variceal bleeding.

Two gastroesophageal balloon tubes are in general use. The SB tubes have three lumens—a gastric balloon, an esophageal balloon, and a gastric aspiration port. The Minnesota tube has a fourth lumen for esophageal aspiration.

The indication for gastroesophageal balloon tamponade is severe, acute, variceal bleeding that is refractory to available first-line therapy, such as sclerotherapy and vasoconstrictor therapy. Relative contraindications are esophageal strictures, recent esophageal surgery, and decreased level of consciousness without airway protection. A patient with a decreased level of consciousness should always be intubated prior to insertion of an SB tube.

■ PROCEDURE

The following equipment is needed:

- Gloves and personal protective equipment
- Gastroesophageal balloon tamponade (GEBT) tube
- NGT if the tamponade tube does not have an esophageal aspiration lumen
- Traction device
- Manometer or sphygmomanometer
- Y-tube connector
- Emesis basin
- Water-soluble lubricant
- Suction device with connectors
- Tubing to connect to suction
- Clamps or nonserrated hemostats
- Silk sutures
- Tape and gauze

The procedure is as follows:

1. If needed, intubate patient prior to placement of the tube.
2. Check balloons for patency and leaks prior to use: Use 100-mL increments of air to inflate the gastric balloon, and check the pressure with a sphygmomanometer after each increment. These pressure measurements should be recorded for each 100-mL air increment and will be used to compare pressure readings once the tube has been inserted (step 12). The pressure in the gastric balloon should not increase more than 15 mm Hg with insufflation of each 100 mL of air.
3. If NGT is to be inserted, tie a suture around it and the GEBT tube to secure them together. The tip of the NGT should be located 3 to 4 cm proximal to the esophageal balloon.
4. Lubricate the tube(s) with a water-soluble lubricant.
5. Position the patient either upright angled at 45 degrees or in left lateral decubitus position.
6. Anesthetize the posterior pharynx or nasopharynx with topical anesthetic spray or nebulized lidocaine (see previous discussion on NGT insertion).

7. Place an NGT and evacuate the stomach prior to placing a GEBT tube, to decrease the chance of emesis and aspiration. Once the gastric contents have been evacuated, remove this NGT.
8. Deflate all balloons and either clamp the ends of the tubes or place plugs in each lumen if provided by the manufacturer.
9. Pass the tube to a minimum level of 50 cm as marked on the tube.
10. Connect suction to the gastric and esophageal lumens to check for contents as well as decrease the likelihood of aspiration.
11. Confirm proper tube placement with radiographs even if gastric contents or blood is evacuated. The tip of the tube/balloon should be located below the diaphragm if properly placed.
12. Remove clamps/plugs, and inflate the gastric balloon slowly with 100-mL increments of air. Check the pressure of the gastric balloon after each injection; with each 100-mL of air insufflated, the pressure should not be more than 15 mm Hg higher than the pressure measurements previously obtained for the same volume of air (step 2). If the pressure rises by more than 15 mm Hg, the balloon may be located in the esophagus and not in the stomach. If this occurs, deflate the balloon and obtain another radiograph to ensure proper tube location prior to resuming air insufflation. Generally, 400 to 500 mL of air must be insufflated to obtain the proper pressure; check the manufacturer's recommendation for the tube being used.
13. Once proper pressure is obtained, clamp/plug the lumens of the gastric balloon and the air inlet.
14. Gently pull back on the GEBT tube until it snugs up against the diaphragm and applies pressure at the gastroesophageal junction.
15. Secure the GEBT tube to the traction device to be used with a small amount of tension applied to the GEBT tube to keep constant pressure on the lower esophageal sphincter. The traction devices may be an orthopedic trapeze apparatus or another device provided by the manufacturer.
16. If the tube was passed nasally, place the sponge rubber cuffs, provided by the manufacturer, into each nostril or pad the nostrils with gauze to prevent pressure ulcers.
17. Once the tube is properly located and secured, lavage the stomach with room-temperature water to assess for active bleeding. Attach the gastric lumen to high-pressure, intermittent suction.
18. If blood continues to be aspirated from the gastric lumen, the esophageal balloon can be inflated to a minimum pressure level to control the bleeding or to a maximum pressure advised by the manufacturer (typically 30-45 mm Hg). Clamp/plug the lumen of the esophageal balloon once a desired pressure level is obtained.
19. Frequent manometer readings of the esophageal balloon should be obtained to decrease the risk of complications.
20. If bleeding continues, the most likely source is gastric; the tension on the gastric balloon may be gradually increased to help control the bleeding.
21. Obtain radiographs any time the position of the tube comes into question.
22. Once the bleeding is controlled, attempts should be made to decrease the pressure in the esophageal balloon by increments of 5 mm Hg every 3 hours until a pressure of 25 mm Hg is reached (or as recommended by the manufacturer). Typically, a pressure of 25 mm Hg can be maintained for 12 to 24 hours if the bleeding is controlled.
23. If the esophageal balloon requires inflation at pressures greater than 30 mm Hg, the balloon should be deflated every 6 hours for 5-minute intervals to prevent complications such as mucosal ischemia and necrosis.
24. To prevent vomiting and aspiration, the esophagus must be aspirated continuously even if the esophageal balloon is not inflated. The gastric balloon will preclude passage of secretions into the stomach. Aspirate with either an esophageal aspiration port in a Minnesota tube, or an NGT with its tip located in the esophagus next to the GEBT tube. The volume of oral and esophageal secretions can total up to 1500 mL/day.

BOX 42-2

Complications of Gastroesophageal Balloon Tamponade

Major Complications

Aspiration pneumonia (most common)
Airway obstruction
Asphyxiation
Esophageal mucosal ischemia and necrosis
Esophageal perforation
Duodenal rupture
Tracheobronchial rupture
Mediastinitis
Migration of balloon, causing one of the preceding complications

Minor Complications

Pressure necrosis of the nose and lips
Gastroesophageal ulceration
Emesis
Epistaxis
Oral and tongue pressure necrosis
Lacerations

25. Once the GEBT tube is properly inserted and bleeding has been controlled, the tube should not be disturbed for 12 to 24 hours.
26. If bleeding cannot be controlled, further therapies are indicated, such as emergency surgery, endoscopic interventions, and angiographic embolization.

■ COMPLICATIONS

Use of GEBT tube is associated with many minor and major complications (Box 42-2). Such tubes should be used only when life-threatening bleeding occurs and other available modalities have failed. Approximately 8% to 16% of patients treated with GEBT tubes have a major complication, with reported mortality rates of 3%.[25-27]

REFERENCES

1. Ikard RW, Federspiel CF: A comparison of Levin and sump nasogastric tubes for postoperative gastrointestinal decompression. Am Surg 1987;53:50-53.
2. Hanson RL: Predictive criteria for length of nasogastric tube insertion for tube feeding. JPEN J Parenter Enteral Nutr 1979;3:160-163.
3. Spektor M, Kaplan J, Kelley J, et al: Nebulized or sprayed lidocaine as anesthesia for nasogastric intubations. Acad Emerg Med 2000;7:406-408.
4. Rosenberg H: The difficult NG intubation: Tips and techniques. Emerg Med 1988;20:95.
5. Metheny N, Reed L, Wiersema L, et al: Effectiveness of pH measurements in predicting feeding tube placement: An update. Nurs Res 1993l;42:324-331.
6. Bankier AA, Wiesmayr MN, Henk C, et al: Radiographic detection of intrabronchial malpositions of nasogastric tubes and subsequent complications in intensive care unit patients. Intensive Care Med 1997;23:406-410.
7. Slater RG: Tension gastrothorax complicating acute traumatic diaphragmatic rupture. J Emerg Med 1992; 10:25-30.
8. Roubenoff R, Ravich WJ: Pneumothorax due to nasogastric feeding tubes: Report of four cases, review of the literature, and recommendations for prevention. Arch Intern Med 1989;149:184-188.
9. Alessi DM, Berci G: Aspiration and nasogastric intubation. Otolaryngol Head Neck Surg 1986;94:486-489.
10. Wollman B, D'Agostino HB, Walus-Wigle JR, et al: Radiologic, endoscopic, and surgical gastrostomy: An institutional evaluation and meta-analysis of the literature. Radiology 1995;197:699-704.
11. Wollman B, D'Agostino HB: Percutaneous radiologic and endoscopic gastrostomy: A 3-year institutional analysis of procedure performance. AJR Am J Roentgenol 1997; 169:1551-1553.
12. Cataldi-Betcher EL, Seltzer MH, Slocum BA, Jones KW: Complications occurring during enteral nutrition support: A prospective study. JPEN J Parenter Enteral Nutr 1983;7:546-552.
13. Rombeau JL, Twomey PL, McLean GK, et al: Experience with a new gastrostomy-jejunal feeding tube. Surgery 1983;93:574-578.
14. Torosian MH, Rombeau JL: Feeding by tube enterostomy. Surg Gynecol Obstet 1980;150:918-927.
15. Ponsky JL, Gauderer MW, Stellato TA, Aszodi A: Percutaneous approaches to enteral alimentation. Am J Surg 1985;149:102-105.
16. Wolf EL, Frager D, Beneventano TC: Radiologic demonstration of important gastrostomy tube complications. Gastrointest Radiol 1986;11:20-26.
17. Korula J, Harma C: A simple and inexpensive method of removal or replacement of gastrostomy tubes. JAMA 1991;265:1426-1428.
18. Coventry BJ, Karatassas A, Gower L, Wilson P: Intestinal passage of the PEG end-piece: Is it safe? J Gastroenterol Hepatol 1994;9:311-313.
19. Yaseen M, Steele MI, Grunow JE: Nonendoscopic removal of percutaneous endoscopic gastrostomy tubes: Morbidity and mortality in children. Gastrointest Endosc 1996; 44:235-238.
20. Tintinalli JE, Kelen GD, Stapczynsky KS; American College of Physicians: Emergency Medicine: A Comprehensive Study Guide, 6th ed. New York, McGraw-Hill, 2004.
21. Kadakia SC, Cassaday M, Shaffer RT: Comparison of Foley catheter as a replacement gastrostomy tube with commercial replacement gastrostomy tube: A prospective randomized trial. Gastrointest Endosc 1994;40:188-193.
22. Strodel WE: Complications of percutaneous gastrostomy. In Ponsky JL (ed): Techniques of Percutaneous Gastrostomy. New York, Igaku-Shoin, 1988.
23. Kadakia SC, Cassaday M, Shaffer MT: Prospective evaluation of Foley catheter as a replacement gastrostomy tube. Am J Gastroenterol. 1992;87(11):1594-1597.
24. Bentz ML, Tollett CA, Dempsey DT: Obstructed feeding jejunostomy tube: A new method of salvage. JPEN J Parenter Enteral Nutr 1988;12:417-418.
25. Hermann RE, Traul D: Experience with the Sengstaken-Blakemore tube for bleeding esophageal varices. Surg Gynecol Obstet 1970;130:879-885.
26. Bauer JJ, Kreel I, Kark AE: The use of the Sengstaken-Blakemore tube for immediate control of bleeding esophageal varices. Ann Surg 1974;179:273-277.
27. Panés J, Terés J, Bosch J, Rodés J: Efficacy of balloon tamponade in treatment of bleeding gastric and esophageal varices. Results in 151 consecutive episodes. Dig Dis Sci 1988;33:454-459.

Chapter **43**

Complications of Bariatric Surgery

Robert F. Poirier

KEY POINTS

- Roux-en-Y gastric bypass is the most commonly performed bariatric procedure in the United States.
- Pulmonary embolism is the most common cause of death after bariatric surgery, although dumping syndrome, wound infections, anastomotic leaks, strictures, and stomal ulcerations are common complications.
- Acute gastric distention is a rare but potentially deadly early postoperative complication that requires decompression.
- A nasogastric tube could perforate the pouch site in patients who have had recent surgery.
- Abdominal pain without vomiting in the early postoperative weeks might represent a small bowel obstruction or internal hernia.

Scope

The prevalence of morbid obesity has risen at least fourfold since 1986.[1] To be considered morbidly obese, one must have either a body mass index (BMI) greater than 40 or a BMI of 35 to 40 with comorbidities.[2] More than 11 million Americans currently have BMI levels that make them eligible for bariatric surgery.[3]

Morbid obesity promotes the development of diabetes mellitus, hypertension, dyslipidemia, and obstructive sleep apnea. Premature death from obesity now rivals the mortality rates associated with smoking, with more than 300,000 deaths attributable to obesity per year.[4]

Bariatric surgery is the most effective treatment for morbid obesity and its associated comorbidities. Five-year mortality is reduced 89% for severely obese patients who undergo weight loss surgery.[5,6] New laparoscopic surgical techniques have contributed to the growing demand for and acceptance of bariatric surgery. Approximately 4925 bariatric procedures were performed in 1990, compared with an estimated 171,200 in 2005.

Women are more likely than men to choose bariatric surgery. It is estimated that men make up 36% of the morbidly obese population in the United States, although they account for fewer than 20% of patients choosing weight loss surgery each year. The typical demographic profile of a bariatric surgery patient is a woman 35 to 49 years of age with private insurance who belongs to a higher socioeconomic class.

Recent trends suggest that higher-risk, older patients are undergoing bariatric procedures with greater frequency; surprisingly, they demonstrate postoperative morbidity and mortality rates similar to those in the general population.[7] Overall, in-hospital mortality rates are between 0.1% and 0.2%, and 30-day mortality rates have been reported between 0.3% and 2%.

Complications of bariatric surgery are common and generally require presentation to an ED. Up to 20% of patients are admitted for a postoperative complication within 1 year of the bariatric procedure; this rate increases to 40% within 3 years. The potential postoperative complications of the various bariatric procedures have predictable timing and clinical presentations.[8]

Types of Bariatric Surgery: Roux-en-Y and Gastric Banding

The two most common types of bariatric surgery in the United States are the Roux-en-Y gastric bypass (80%) and adjustable gastric banding (10%). Adjustable gastric banding has continued to gain popularity since its initial federal approval in 2001.[7]

Caloric restriction and malabsorption are the principal means of weight loss. In the United States, weight loss procedures that combine both restrictive and malabsorptive components are the most popular. Roux-en-Y gastric bypass, biliopancreatic diversion, and duodenal switch are examples of techniques that employ both malabsorption and restriction. In Europe, the preference is for purely restrictive bariatric procedures.

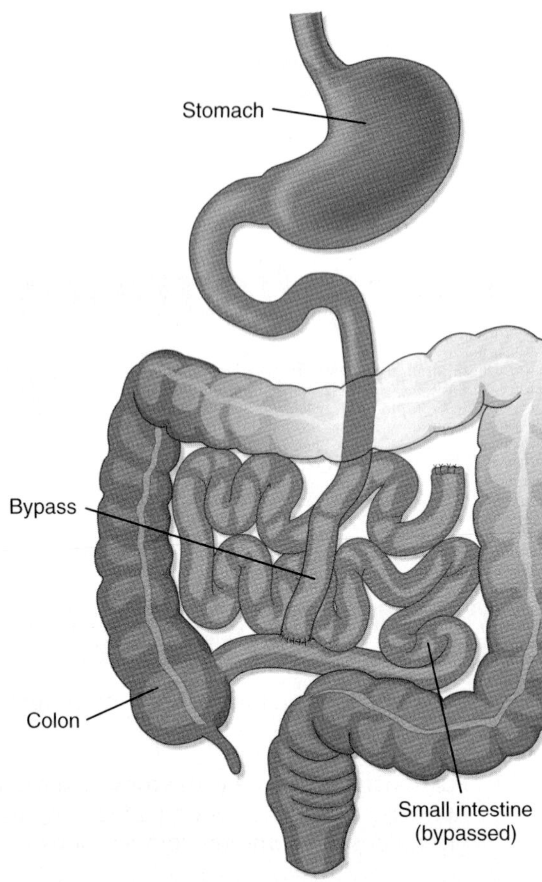
Stomach
Bypass
Colon
Small intestine
(bypassed)

FIGURE 43-1 Jejunoileal bypass.

■ MALABSORPTION

Surgical techniques that induced malabsorption were the first attempted. Malabsorptive techniques were thought to be the most effective method of achieving rapid and sustained weight loss. Surgeons initially connected the proximal jejunum to a distal portion of the ileum or ascending colon in a procedure known as the jejunoileal bypass (Fig. 43-1). This technique resulted in severe diarrhea, dangerous metabolic derangements, arthropathy, renal calculi, gallstones, liver disease, and short bowel syndrome. Gastric bypass has been shown to be a more effective malabsorptive procedure with fewer side effects than jejunoileal bypass. Malabsorptive procedures still in current use include Roux-en-Y gastric bypass, biliopancreatic diversion, duodenal switch, and isolated intestinal bypass.

■ RESTRICTION

Purely restrictive procedures are less effective than malabsorptive techniques.[6] Restrictive surgeries act by reducing oral intake through induction of early satiety. However, some areas of the stomach easily dilate over time, causing gradual increases in perceived hunger and subsequent food intake. Restrictive procedures are more successful when the lesser-curve gastric pouch is 15 mL or less.[4] Restrictive weight loss procedures such as vertical banded gastroplasty and isolated partial gastrectomy (sleeve gastrectomy) have fallen out of favor. Laparoscopic adjustable gastric banding (LAGB) appears to be the most common and most effective restrictive technique currently performed.[9]

■ ROUX-EN-Y GASTRIC BYPASS

The Roux-en-Y gastric bypass creates a gastric pouch from the proximal portion of the lesser curvature of the stomach that can hold about 15 to 30 mL of fluid and food (Fig. 43-2). A portion of the distal small bowel is connected to this pouch to create a concurrent malabsorptive process.

Early postoperative complications of Roux-en-Y include obstruction of the bypassed small bowel segment, obstruction of the Roux limb, anastomotic leak, and intraperitoneal bleeding. Pulmonary embolism remains the most common cause of postoperative death, followed by complications resulting from anastomotic leaks. Other complications are pneumonia, myocardial infarction, renal failure secondary to rhabdomyolysis, and nutritional deficiencies.[10]

Late complications generally involve only nutritional deficiencies. Clinical manifestations include anemia (iron deficiency), osteopenic fractures (calcium deficiency), fatigue and lower extremity edema (protein-calorie malnutrition), chronic pain

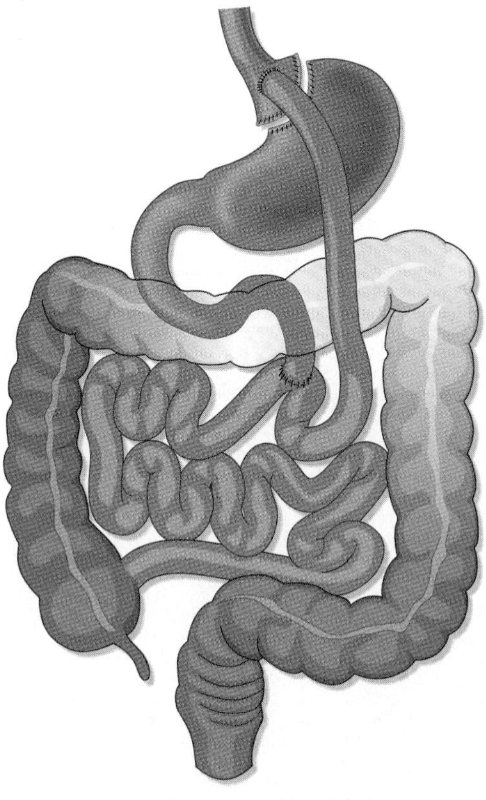

FIGURE 43-2 Roux-en-Y gastric bypass.

and proximal muscle weakness (vitamin D deficiency), visual deficits (vitamin A deficiency), and vague neurologic symptoms (thiamine, folate, and vitamin B_{12} deficiencies).

Complications of Open versus Laparoscopic Procedures

Wound infections and incisional hernias are more common in open bariatric procedures (7% and 9%, respectively) than in laparoscopic procedures (3% and 0.5%, respectively). Patients who have undergone laparoscopic gastric bypass have a slightly higher rate of early small bowel obstruction, anastomotic stenosis, and gastrointestinal hemorrhage. Pulmonary embolism, pneumonia, and anastomotic leaks have similar incidences after both open and laparoscopic procedures.

Specific Clinical Presentations

Persistent, severe vomiting can be caused by anastomotic strictures. Strictures can usually be treated by endoscopic balloon dilation but occasionally require surgical revision. Some nausea and vomiting are common during the immediate postoperative period, but if vomiting persists, an anastomotic stricture may have formed.

Obstruction of the Roux limb requires percutaneous decompression. Patients with such an obstruction present with nausea, vomiting, abdominal pain, and distention. Diagnosis may require computed tomography (CT).

The occurrence of acute fever and tachycardia within weeks of a Roux-en-Y procedure suggests anastomotic leak with or without abscess formation. The abdominal examination of morbidly obese patients is unreliable, and diagnosis is therefore best accomplished through imaging studies. CT of the abdomen and pelvis with oral and intravenous (IV) administration contrast agent is the modality of choice. If the patient is unable to undergo CT because of the weight limitations of the CT table, an upper gastrointestinal radiographic series should be obtained.

Esophageal reflux occurs infrequently after this procedure but may represent damage to the lower esophageal sphincter or impaired gastric emptying secondary to a distal obstruction.

Diarrhea with malodorous flatulence may result from a short Roux limb and usually spontaneously resolves. Persistent diarrhea after weight stabilization, however, should raise suspicion of bacterial overgrowth in the bypassed tract.

Constipation may result from decreased fiber intake.

Cholelithiasis may develop during the period of initial rapid weight loss. Biliary colic and cholecystitis are high on the differential diagnosis list for abdominal pain in patients with ongoing reductions in weight.

Bleeding may occur at any anastomotic site but is most common and dangerous at the gastrojejunostomy area. Upper endoscopy is the most reliable way to confirm blood loss from this site. Bleeding at other anastomotic sites (jejunojejunostomy and transected gastric remnant) is usually self-limited and managed nonoperatively.[10]

LAPAROSCOPIC ADJUSTABLE GASTRIC BANDING

LAP-BAND (INAMED Health, Santa Barbara, CA) is an adjustable device that is laparoscopically secured around the upper portion of the stomach (Fig. 43-3). The band is connected by a tube to a port implanted under the skin. Surgeons may adjust the extent of constriction (restriction) of the LAP-BAND by injecting saline into the subcutaneous port. Increased restriction limits food intake; adjustments can be made in response to adverse symptoms or patient preference, thereby allowing some control over the weight loss process. Operative risks for LAGB are less than those for Roux-en-Y gastric bypass.

Complications

Patients who undergo LAGB are often discharged within 24 hours of surgery. Immediate postoperative vomiting is usually caused by *gastric wall edema* under the band. Inflation of the band during surgery increases the likelihood of gastric wall edema. IV hydration is required until the edema subsides.

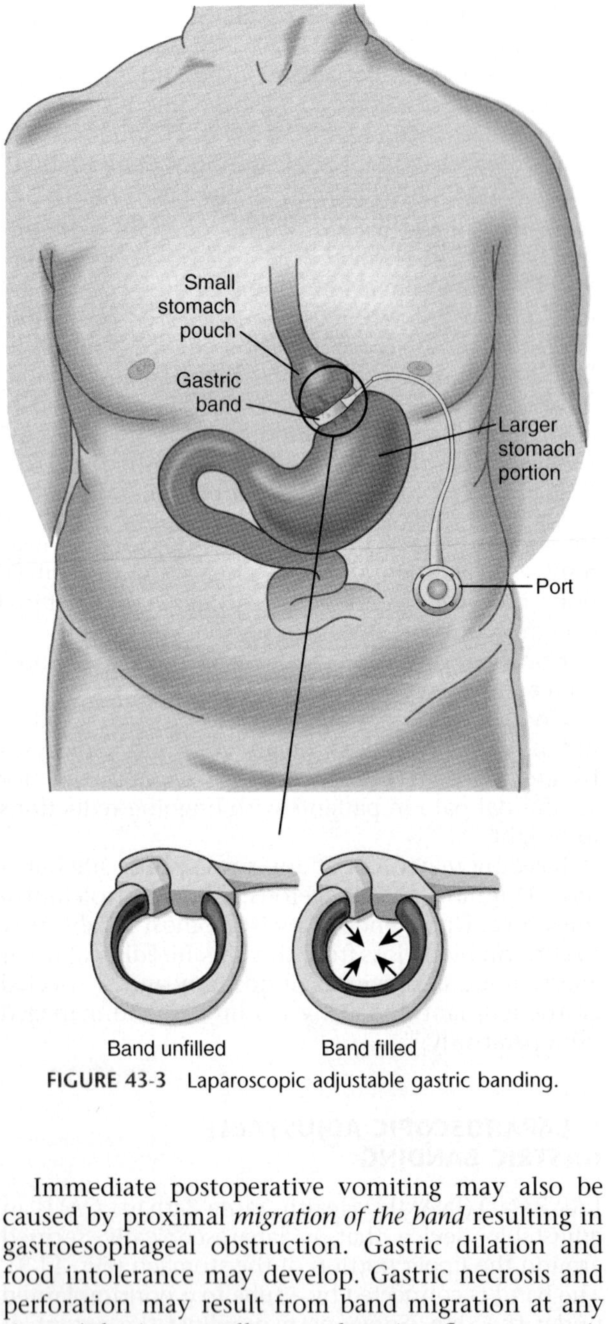
Small
stomach
pouch
Gastric
band
Larger
stomach
portion
Port
Band unfilled
Band filled

FIGURE 43-3 Laparoscopic adjustable gastric banding.

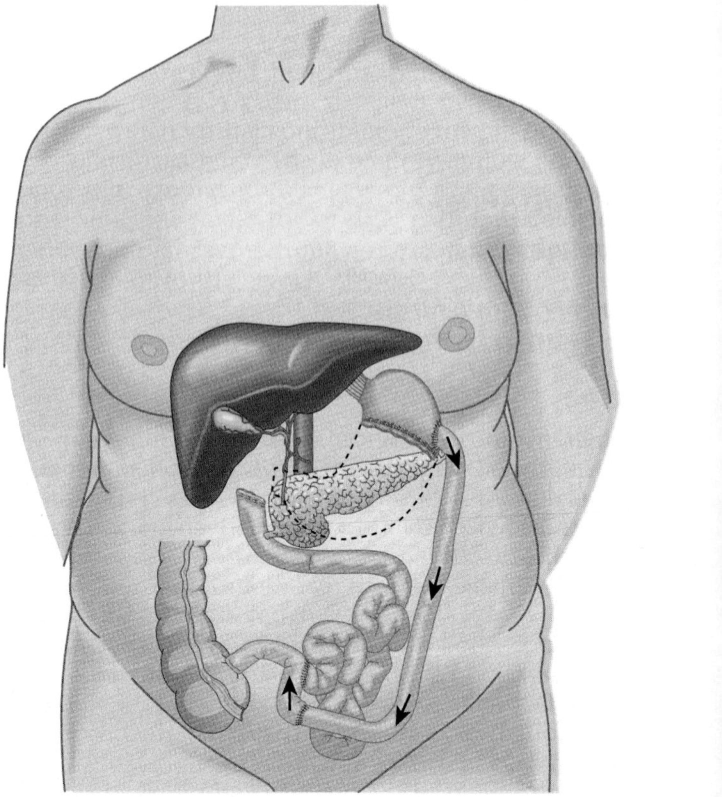

FIGURE 43-4 Biliopancreatic diversion.

Immediate postoperative vomiting may also be caused by proximal *migration of the band* resulting in gastroesophageal obstruction. Gastric dilation and food intolerance may develop. Gastric necrosis and perforation may result from band migration at any time. A barium swallow study using fluoroscopy is the preferred method of diagnosing band migration. An abdominal CT scan may also demonstrate movement of the band.

Any patient with signs of *obstruction* after LABG should have immediate deflation of the band. EPs can easily deflate an adjustable gastric band by accessing the subcutaneous port. A large-bore needle should be used to remove the 5 mL of saline that the reservoir can store. Fluoroscopy may be required if the port cannot be accessed easily at the bedside. A barium swallow study and surgical consultation should be obtained after any band deflation.

Erosion may lead to fistula, abscess, and sepsis. *Device malfunction* can cause port infections, tube leakage, tube disconnection, and skin ulceration. Plain radiographs, abdominal CT scans, and upper endoscopy may all aid in the diagnosis of gastric erosion and device malfunction.

■ BILIOPANCREATIC DIVERSION

Biliopancreatic diversion is popular in Italy (Fig. 43-4). A distal gastrectomy with a long Roux-en-Y limb is generally performed. This procedure is particularly effective for the severely obese patient (BMI>50), causing significant weight loss and morbidity reduction. Less bacterial overgrowth occurs in the bypassed intestine because it is continuously exposed to bile and pancreatic enzymes. Serious complications can result, however, particularly the metabolic abnormalities and nutritional deficiencies seen after malabsorptive procedures. Hepatic dysfunction can occur in 2% of patients undergoing biliopancreatic diversion.

■ DUODENAL SWITCH AND SLEEVE GASTRECTOMY

The duodenal switch procedure is similar to biliopancreatic diversion, but the jejunum is connected to the proximal duodenum rather than the ileum (Fig. 43-5). This operation is also known as the biliopancreatic diversion–duodenal switch (BPD-DS) procedure. It is considered an improvement on the biliopancreatic diversion alone.

A linear (sleeve) gastrectomy is also performed during the duodenal switch, leaving a restrictive

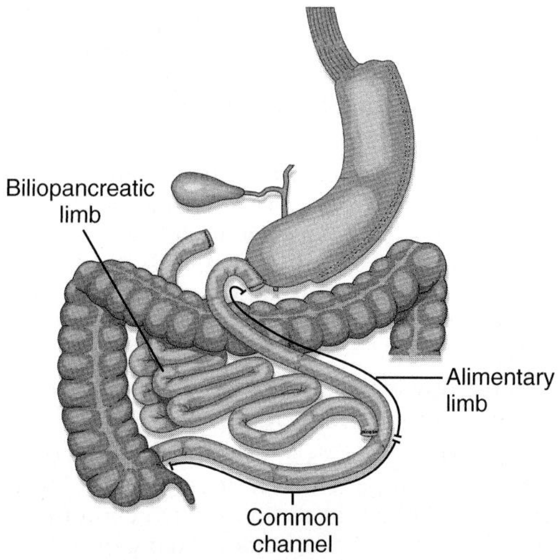
Biliopancreatic limb
Alimentary limb
Common channel
FIGURE 43-5 Duodenal switch.

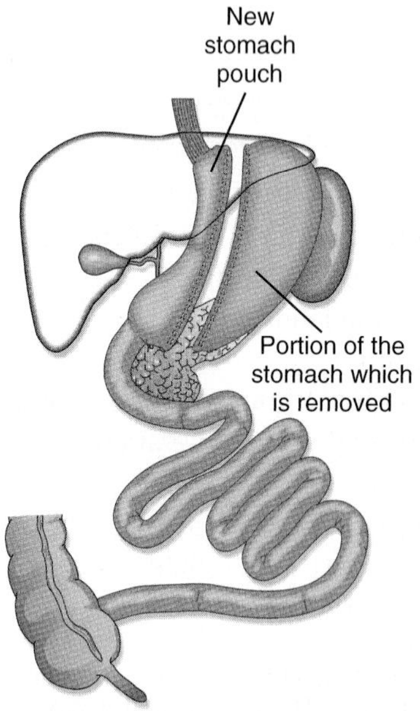
New stomach pouch
Portion of the stomach which is removed
FIGURE 43-6 Sleeve gastrectomy.

pouch of the lesser curvature. The BPD-DS with sleeve gastrectomy allows gastric emptying to be somewhat regulated through the preservation of a functioning pylorus. The risk of dumping syndrome is subsequently reduced.

Some surgeons prefer to perform only a sleeve gastrectomy in high-risk patients (Fig. 43-6). This simple restrictive procedure avoids anastomoses of the gastrointestinal tract. Side effects such as nutritional deficiencies are rare because only mild malabsorption results from sleeve gastrectomy alone.

Complications of Bariatric Surgery

■ GENERAL COMPLICATIONS

■ Pulmonary Embolism

Pulmonary embolism is the leading cause of death after bariatric surgery. Though the postoperative incidence of deep vein thrombosis (DVT) and pulmonary embolism is only 2%, almost one third of affected patients die. The incidence of DVT and pulmonary embolism has not diminished despite the use of pneumatic compression stockings, low-molecular-weight heparin, and various other prophylactic measures. Early postoperative ambulation may be the most important preventive measure in the bariatric population. Lower extremity duplex Doppler ultrasonography for DVT and helical pulmonary CT scanning for pulmonary embolism are the preferred diagnostic studies. If weight limitations prevent a patient from having a CT scan, ventilation-perfusion scintigraphy should be considered.

■ Wound Infections, Seromas, and Dehiscence

Wound infections occur in 10% to 15% of patients undergoing open procedures and in 3% to 4% in those treated by laparoscopic techniques. Seromas commonly occur in up to 40% of patients. Although wound infections may appear superficial, deep extensions may be present in the morbidly obese. Patients with wound infections and fever should undergo contrast-enhanced CT of the abdomen to exclude deep infections.

■ Intraperitoneal Fluid Collections and Peritonitis

Intraperitoneal fluid collections, abscesses, and peritonitis occur in less than 2% of patients undergoing bariatric procedures. Anastomotic leaks are the most common cause of fluid collections in the early postoperative period. Clinical signs are often subtle, and diagnosis cannot be made by physical examination alone. Patients may present with low-grade fevers, tachycardia, and mild tachypnea. An early surgical consultation should be obtained to facilitate the most efficient evaluation and treatment, because life-threatening sepsis may ensue. Poor cardiopulmonary reserve in morbidly obese patients may allow for rapid clinical deterioration. Some institutions advocate CT-guided aspiration during initial imaging.

■ Incisional Hernia

Incisional hernias occur in up to 9% of patients after open Roux-en-Y gastric bypass. Rarely are incisional hernias seen in those who undergo laparoscopic procedures. Physical examination alone confirms the diagnosis.

■ Gallstones

The incidence of cholelithiasis is 1% to 3% after bariatric surgery. Rapid weight loss is known to promote the formation of gallstones. Most surgeons perform a prophylactic cholecystectomy for patients with

BOX 43-1

Top 10 Complications of Bariatric Surgery

1. Dumping syndrome
2. Vitamin and mineral deficiencies
3. Nausea and vomiting
4. Staple line failure
5. Infection
6. Bowel obstruction and anastomotic stenosis
7. Gastric and stomal ulceration
8. Bleeding
9. Iatrogenic splenic injury
10. Perioperative death (pulmonary embolus, sepsis, myocardial infarction)

From Abell TL, Minocha A: Gastrointestinal complications of bariatric surgery: Diagnosis and therapy. Am J Med Sci 2006;331:214-218.

Tips and Tricks

- Consult the surgeon and/or gastroenterologist early for patients with previous bariatric surgery.
- Do not place a nasogastric tube in patients who have undergone gastric bypass without consultation from the surgeon or gastroenterologists. Blind placement of such a tube may result in perforation of the pouch site, particularly in the immediate postoperative period.
- Laparoscopy is often required for definitively diagnosis of internal hernias.
- Small gastric pouches limit the amount of oral contrast agent patients can ingest for a CT scan. They should be told to sip as much contrast agent as they feel comfortable taking over 3 hours before imaging. The scan is then performed, regardless of the amount of contrast ingested.[10]

known cholelithiasis. Distorted anatomy after gastric bypass often precludes successful endoscopic retrograde cholangiopancreatography (ERCP). Symptomatic biliary disease in patients who have undergone Roux-en-Y procedure usually requires surgical intervention or percutaneous drainage.

PROCEDURE-SPECIFIC COMPLICATIONS

Box 43-1 lists the most common gastrointestinal complications of bariatric surgery.[11]

Anastomotic (Staple-Line) Leak

Anastomotic leak most often occurs in the immediate postoperative period, although some leaks are not apparent until weeks after surgery. The incidence is 6% for patients with first procedures, but it rises fivefold to tenfold in patients who undergo revision of the initial procedure. Leaks are difficult to diagnose owing to initially nonspecific signs and symptoms: low-grade fever, abdominal tenderness, tachypnea/respiratory insufficiency, tachycardia, left shoulder pain, and anxiety. An upper gastrointestinal radiographic series or abdominal CT confirms the diagnosis by demonstrating the extravasation of oral contrast agent (Gastrografin). The most common site of the leak is the gastrojejunostomy anastomosis. Interventional or surgical management is required. Early antibiotic therapy is recommended.

Acute Gastric Distention

Acute gastric distention is a rare, potentially deadly, early postoperative complication. Patients may present with pain, nausea, vomiting, abdominal distention, bloating, hiccups, tachycardia, shortness of breath, or referred left shoulder pain. Abdominal plain films or abdominal CT scans usually demonstrate a large air-fluid level in a dilated stomach. Obstruction or edema at the enteroenterostomy site is often the cause of this complication and is best evaluated by CT. Treatment includes percutaneous fine-needle decompression, drainage via gastrectomy tube, or surgery for cases of recurrence or rupture. A nasogastric tube should not be used because of possible perforation.

Stomal Stenosis/Anastomotic Strictures

The incidence of anastomotic strictures occurring at the gastrojejunostomy site varies from 2% to 11%. Patients often present with progressive, postprandial, epigastric pain, and vomiting. Patients are initially unable to tolerate solid foods, with characteristic progression to poor liquid tolerance over time. Plain radiographs and CT of the abdomen are usually unremarkable. Upper endoscopy both diagnoses and treats this condition. Repeated endoscopic balloon dilation of the stricture is often required. Fluoroscopy-guided balloon dilation is an alternative treatment.

Stomal Ulceration

Stomal ulceration causes severe dyspepsia, burning retrosternal pain and vomiting. Abdominal plain films, CT scans, and other upper gastrointestinal radiographic studies are not useful for diagnosis of this complication. Endoscopy is the diagnostic modality of choice. Proton pump inhibitors treat stomal ulceration, and antibiotics are prescribed if the patient is found to have co-infection with *Helicobacter pylori*.

PATIENT TEACHING TIPS

- The American Society for Bariatric Surgery has excellent educational resources at their website, www.asbs.org/
- The patient should return to the hospital if nausea, vomiting, or fast heart rate develops.
- Blood glucose levels can fluctuate widely after weight loss surgery and require close monitoring.
- Patients must adhere to postoperative diet instructions in order to prevent potential complications.

Small Bowel Obstruction and Internal Hernia

Abdominal pain without vomiting in the early postoperative weeks might represent a small bowel obstruction or internal hernia. Small bowel obstructions and internal hernias are difficult to differentiate and have a combined incidence of 5% within the first few postoperative weeks. Small bowel obstructions are more common after open bariatric surgery because of adhesion formation; internal hernias are more common after laparoscopic surgery. The Roux limb or pancreaticobiliary limb may herniate through potential spaces created during surgery. Patients present with nonspecific symptoms, including abdominal cramping, periumbilical pain, and nausea. Vomiting is uncommon because there are only minimal secretions in the small gastric pouch. Abdominal plain films are nondiagnostic, because dilated loops of bowel are not commonly seen. Upper gastrointestinal studies and abdominal CT are often unable to distinguish between obstruction and hernia. Surgeons may perform early laparoscopy to prevent potential bowel strangulation.

Dumping Syndrome

A common complication, dumping syndrome occurs in almost half of patients undergoing gastric bypass. Typical symptoms are bloating, abdominal cramping, nausea, diaphoresis, and lightheadedness; symptoms are more pronounced after the eating of food with high concentrations of refined sugar. Effects are self-limiting and diminish as the patient becomes more selective with the diet.

Disposition

Patients who present to the ED with systemic or gastrointestinal symptoms after bariatric surgery often have a postoperative complication that mandates hospital admission. They generally need CT, upper gastrointestinal radiographic series, and/or endoscopy. Discharge should be considered only for patients who have been evaluated in consultation with a surgeon and/or gastroenterologist, who have stable vital signs and minimal pain, and who can easily tolerate oral fluids.

REFERENCES

1. Sturm R: Increases in clinically severe obesity in the United States, 1986-2000. Arch Intern Med 2003;163:2146-2148.
2. Gastrointestinal surgery for severe obesity: Proceedings of a National Institutes of Health Consensus Development Conference. Am J Clin Nutr 1992;55(Suppl):487S-619S.
3. Trus TL, Pope GD, Finlayson RG: National trends in utilization and outcomes of bariatric surgery. Surg Endosc 2005;19:616-620.
4. Crookes PF: Surgical treatment of morbid obesity. Ann Rev Med 2006;57:243-264.
5. Christou NV, Sampalis JS, Liberman M, et al: Surgery decreases long-term mortality, morbidity, and health care use in morbidly obese patients. Ann Surg 2004;240: 416-423.
6. Buchwald H, Avidor Y, Braunwald E, et al: Bariatric surgery: A systematic review and meta-analysis. JAMA 2004;292: 1724-1737.
7. Santry HP, Gillen DI, Lauderdale DS: Trends in bariatric surgical procedures. JAMA 2005;294:1909-1924.
8. Zingmond DS, McGory ML, Ko CY: Hospitalization before and after gastric bypass surgery. JAMA 2005;294:1918-1924.
9. Kelly J, Tarnoff M, Shikora S, et al: Best practice recommendations for surgical care in weight loss surgery. Obesity Res 2005;13:227-233.
10. Edwards ED, Jacob BP, Gagner M, et al: Presentation and management of common post–weight loss surgery problems in the emergency department. Ann Emerg Med 2006;47:160-166.
11. Abell TL, Minocha A: Gastrointestinal complications of bariatric surgery: Diagnosis and therapy. Am J Med Sci 2006;331:214-218.

SECTION V

Pulmonary Diseases

Chapter **44**

Asthma and Chronic Obstructive Pulmonary Disease

Rita K. Cydulka and Craig G. Bates

ASTHMA

KEY POINTS

Asthma is a chronic inflammatory condition that can be controlled.
Indications of inadequate asthma control include frequent use of short acting β-agonist agents, wheezing, cough, and nighttime symptoms.
ED treatment of asthma exacerbation includes targeted history and physical examination, aerosolized β-agonist agents, and systemic steroids with objective measures of response to therapy. Anticholinergic agents should be added in patients with a severe exacerbation.

Scope

Asthma is a chronic inflammatory disorder characterized by increased responsiveness of the airways to multiple stimuli. Many cells and cellular elements, such as mast cells, eosinophils, T lymphocytes, macrophages, neutrophils, and epithelial cells, play a role in the development of the inflammatory response.[1] The inflammation causes recurrent episodes of wheezing, breathlessness, chest tightness, and coughing, particularly at night or in the early morning. These episodes are associated with airflow obstruction that is reversible either spontaneously or with treatment. Although patients appear clinically to recover completely, evidence suggests that some asthmatic patients have chronic airflow limitation. The recognition that asthma is a chronic inflammatory disorder of the airways has significant implications for the diagnosis, management, and potential prevention of its acute exacerbation.

Asthma affects approximately 4% to 5% of the population in the United States.[2] Although it is the most common chronic disease of childhood, with a prevalence of 5% to 10%, it also affects 7% to 10% of the elderly. Epidemiologic studies suggest that asthma is underdiagnosed and undertreated in all age groups. Part of the problem is that the transient nature of asthma allows many patients to tolerate intermittent respiratory symptoms before seeking medical care. Another important factor resulting in underdiagnosis of asthma is the sometimes nonspecific nature of the symptoms.

About half of cases of asthma develop before age 10 years and another third before age 40 years. The 2:1 male-to-female preponderance of asthma in childhood equalizes by age 30 years.[3] The average asthmatic patient has 15 days of restricted activity each year and spends 5.8 days in bed. Approximately 2 million ED visits, 484,000 hospitalizations, and more than 4000 deaths per year are attributed to asthma. In the United States alone, the estimated direct and indirect cost of asthma in all age groups was 6.2 billion dollars in 1990.[4]

Pathophysiology

All asthmatic patients have hyperresponsive airways that narrow when exposed to various stimuli: allergic, infectious, pharmacologic, environmental, occupational, exercise-related, and emotional.

Allergic asthma occurs when inhaled allergens bind to immunoglobulin (Ig) E molecules bound to mast cells in the lining of the tracheobronchial tree. During the early response, various mediators are released, causing greater vascular permeability, mucosal edema, and contraction of bronchial smooth muscles. A second wave of reaction, the late response, is seen hours to days later; it involves the accumulation of inflammatory cells in the bronchial mucosa, thus perpetuating the reaction. The release of mediators and the regulation of the inflammatory process in asthma are complex, redundant, and self-perpetuating.[5]

Although several theories attempt to explain the pathophysiologic changes that occur in nonallergic asthma, none adequately explains all clinically observed phenomena. Research suggests that even patients without atopy have pathophysiology similar to that in atopic patients.[5] Respiratory infections, particularly viral infections, may precipitate bronchospasm. Viruses cause mucosal inflammation and lower the firing threshold of the subendothelial vagal receptors, resulting in enhanced airway reactivity that may last up to 8 weeks, even in nonasthmatic persons. Pharmacologic agents, such as aspirin and nonsteroidal anti-inflammatory compounds, coloring agents, and beta-blockers, also induce acute asthma. Sulfating agents, which are used widely as food preservatives and antioxidants in pharmaceutical products, also can exacerbate asthma.

A large variety of occupational dusts and fumes may provoke acute airway obstruction. Patients with occupational asthma classically give a cyclic history; they are symptom-free during weekends, vacations, and upon arrival at work. Exercise may also stimulate an asthma attack. Exercise-induced bronchospasm is usually noted within 5 to 20 minutes after the completion of exercise and is related to thermal changes in the respiratory tree. Exercising in a cold, dry environment causes a more marked response than exercising in a warm, humid environment. Finally, endocrine factors, such as variations in progesterone and estradiol levels, also influence asthma exacerbations, probably through modification of vagal efferent activity.

Most patients with asthma seem to display an exaggerated bronchoconstriction response to a variety of exogenous and endogenous stimuli, and inflammation plays a key role. The final common pathway is as follows[1]:

- Airway narrowing
- Bronchial wall edema
- Bronchial smooth muscle contraction
- Mucosal plugging
- Enhanced airway reactivity and airway wall remodeling resulting in increased airway resistance
- Decreased forced expiratory volumes and flow rates
- Lung hyperinflation
- Increased work of breathing
- Ventilation-perfusion mismatch

Presenting Signs and Symptoms

When presenting to the ED, many patients relay the history of asthma, but some do not. Patients presenting with a severe asthma attack may be in obvious respiratory distress, with rapid breathing and loud wheezing, but patients with mild exacerbation may present with cough and end-expiratory wheezing. The classic symptoms of asthma consist of the triad dyspnea, wheezing, and cough, but physical findings during asthma exacerbation can be variable. Early symptoms include a sensation of chest constriction and cough. As the exacerbation progresses, wheezing becomes apparent, expiration becomes prolonged, and use of accessory respiratory muscles may become evident. Patients may sit upright or lean forward to try to decrease the work of breathing. The use of accessory muscles of inspiration indicates diaphragmatic fatigue, whereas the appearance of paradoxical respirations reflects impending ventilatory failure. Alteration in mental status heralds respiratory arrest.

■ VARIATIONS IN PRESENTING SIGNS AND SYMPTOMS

Patients with asthma exacerbation may present simply with cough or a feeling of chest tightness. At the other end of the spectrum are patients with a "silent chest," which reflects very severe airflow obstruction and air movement insufficient to promote a wheeze.

A subset of asthmatic patients experiences the sudden onset of severe symptoms. These individuals tend to respond rapidly to treatment but appear to be at significant risk for a fatal outcome.[6-9]

Differential Diagnosis

Wheezing, coughing, and dyspnea may be present in many common conditions, including pneumonia, bronchitis, croup, bronchiolitis, chronic obstructive pulmonary disease, congestive heart failure, pulmonary embolism, allergic reactions, and upper airway obstruction from edema or a foreign body. Less common conditions with similar presenting symptoms are cystic fibrosis, hypersensitivity pneumonitis, carcinoid syndrome, and exposure to odors, dust, and gas. A careful history and physical examination should help differentiate asthma from these other conditions.

Diagnostic Testing

As for all patients who present to the ED for care, a directed history and physical examination should be performed. Key historical points should be elicited, such as duration and onset of the current attack, identification of precipitating causes, type and amount of medications used before arrival in the ED, response to prior therapy, including current or previous use of corticosteroids, frequency of ED visits and hospitalizations, previous need for intubation or ventilation, history of concurrent medications and allergies, and history of concurrent medical problems. At some point during the patient's ED stay, an effort should be made to evaluate both the severity of the obstruction and the adequacy of ongoing asthma control (Table 44-1).

The physical examination should focus on observing respiratory effort and accessory muscle use and on listening for wheezing or other abnormal breath sounds and prolongation of the expiratory phase. Although wheezing results from the movement of air through narrowed airways, the intensity of the wheeze may not correlate with the severity of airflow obstruction. Tachycardia and tachypnea are usually present in acute asthma, but vital signs normalize very quickly as airflow obstruction is relieved.[10] Therefore, a normal heart rate and respiratory rate are not reliable indicators of the degree or relief from obstruction.

Bedside spirometry provides a rapid, objective assessment of patients and helps both indicate the effectiveness of and guide therapy. Sequential measurements help EPs assess the severity of the problem and determine the response to therapy. Although forced expiratory volume in 1 second (FEV_1) and the peak expiratory flow rate (PEF) measure the extent of large airway obstruction, patient cooperation is essential for these tests to be reliable. When possible, management decisions should be guided by a patient's personal best PEF or FEV_1 value or, if unknown, a percentage of the predicted value in addition to other physiologic and historical factors.[1]

Pulse oximetry is a useful and convenient method for accessing oxygenation and monitoring oxygen saturation during treatment. Analysis of arterial blood gases (ABGs) is not indicated in the majority of patients with mild to moderate asthma exacerbation but is helpful if there is concern for hypoventilation with carbon dioxide retention and respiratory acidosis. Patients with the latter problems almost always have clinical evidence of severe attacks, or spirometry demonstrating a PEF or FEV_1 less than 25% of predicted value.[11,12] Practitioners should be aware that a normal or slightly elevated $Paco_2$ (e.g., 42 mm Hg or higher) indicates extreme airway obstruction and fatigue and may herald the onset of acute ventilatory failure.[11,12]

Routine radiography is unnecessary but is indicated if there is concern for the possibility of pneumothorax, pneumomediastinum, pneumonia, or other medical conditions. In up to a third of asthmatic patients requiring admission, an abnormality is demonstrated on chest radiographs.[13]

A routine complete blood cell count is not indicated and would likely show modest leukocytosis secondary to administration of β_2-agonist therapy or corticosteroid treatment. In patients taking theophylline prior to ED presentation, a serum theophylline level should be determined. Routine electrocardiogram (ECG) is also unnecessary; ECG abnormalities noted include right ventricular strain, abnormal P waves, or nonspecific ST-T wave abnormalities, which resolve with treatment. Older patients, especially those with coexisting heart disease, should have cardiac monitoring during treatment. Asthma severity index scores have failed to predict outcome better than clinical judgment.

Table 44-1 CLASSIFICATION OF ASTHMA SEVERITY: CLINICAL FEATURES BEFORE TREATMENT

	Symptoms	Nighttime Symptoms	Lung Function
Step 4: Severe persistent	Continual symptoms Limited physical activity Frequent exacerbations	Frequent	FEV_1 or PEF<60% of predicted value PEF variability >30%
Step 3: Moderate persistent	Daily symptoms Daily use of inhaled short- acting β_2-agonist Exacerbations affect activity Exacerbations >2 times a week; may last days	>1 time a week	FEV_1 or PEF>60% but <80% of predicted value PEF variability >30%
Step 2: Mild persistent	Symptoms >2 times a week but >1 time a day Exacerbations may affect activity	3-4 times a month	FEV_1 or PEF≥80% of predicted value PEF variability 20%-30%
Step 1: Mild intermittent	Symptoms <2 times a week Asymptomatic and normal PEFR between exacerbations Exacerbations brief (from a few hrs to a few days; intensity may vary)	≤2 times a month	FEV_1 or PEF≥80% of predicted value PEF variability <20%

FEV_1, forced expiratory volume in 1 minute; PEFR, peak expiratory flow rate.
Adapted from National Institutes of Health, National Heart, Lung and Blood Institute, National Asthma Education and Prevention Program: Expert Panel Report 3: Guidelines for the Diagnosis and Management of Asthma. (NIH Publication No. 08-4051) Bethesda, MD, U.S. Department of Health and Human Services, August 2007.

Use of exhaled nitric oxide measurements, and other serum and urine markers, for detection of severity of asthma exacerbation is currently under investigation.[14-17]

Interventions, Procedures, and Treatment

The goal of treatment of acute asthma in the ED is to rapidly reverse airflow obstruction by repetitive or continuous administration of inhaled β_2-agonists, ensure adequate oxygenation, and relieve inflammation. The National Asthma Education and Prevention Program (NAEPP) Expert Panel has developed guidelines for emergency treatment of asthma (Fig. 44-1),[1] as have other organizations around the world. The following types of medications have been shown to be effective for the treatment of acute asthma: β_2 agonists, anticholinergics, and glucocorticoids (Table 44-2).[1] Magnesium should be considered in patients with severe obstruction. Current evidence does not support the use of heliox (helium-oxygen mixture) or ketamine, even when the aforementioned medications fail to relieve bronchospasm. Mast cell–stabilizing agents, methylxanthines, and leukotriene modifiers are currently reserved for maintenance therapy only.

■ PHARMACEUTICALS

■ β_2-Agonist Agents

β_2-agonists are the preferred initial rescue medications for acute bronchospasm. In addition to bronchodilation, these drugs inhibit mediator release and promote mucociliary clearance.[1]

The most common side effect of β_2-agonist drugs is skeletal muscle tremor. Patients may also experience nervousness, anxiety, insomnia, headache, hyperglycemia, palpitations, tachycardia, and hypertension. Despite earlier concerns about the potential cardiotoxicity of these agents, clinical experience has not revealed significant problems. Arrhythmias and evidence of myocardial ischemia are rare, especially in patients without prior history of coronary artery disease.

Aerosol therapy with β_2-agonist drugs produces excellent bronchodilation with minimal systemic absorption and few side effects. Aerosol delivery may be achieved with a metered-dose inhaler (MDI) with a spacing device or a compressor-driven nebulizer.[18] A spacing device attached to the inhaler can improve drug deposition when patient technique is inadequate. Even with optimum technique, however, a maximum of 15% of the drug dose is retained in the lungs, regardless of the aerosol method used. Dry-powder delivery devices and MDIs using hydrofluoroalkane as propellant have replaced chlorinated fluorocarbon (CFC)–driven devices. Aerosol treatments may be administered every 15 to 20 minutes or on a continuous basis.[19] Subcutaneous administration of terbutaline or epinephrine may be used in patients unable to coordinate aerosolized or MDI treatments or to tolerate aerosolized medications.[20]

Intravenous β_2-agonist infusions offer no advantage over aerosolized or MDI-delivered agents and carry potential risk.[21]

Salmeterol xinafoate is indicated only as maintenance therapy, should never be used more frequently than twice per day, and is to be avoided for treatment of acute exacerbations.[1]

■ Corticosteroids

Corticosteroids, which are highly effective drugs in asthma exacerbation, are a cornerstone of treatment.[22] They are thought to produce beneficial effects by restoring β_2-agonist responsiveness and reducing inflammation. The onset of the anti-inflammatory effects of corticosteroids is delayed at least 4 to 8 hours after their intravenous or oral administration.

Data indicate that corticosteroids, administered within 1 hour of a patient's arrival in the ED, reduce the need for hospitalization of a patient with an asthma exacerbation.[22] Although evidence for what constitutes the optimal dose in acute asthma is lacking, experts agree that an initial dose of prednisone 40 to 60 mg, or an intravenous bolus of methylprednisolone 60 to 125 mg IV in patients unable to tolerate oral medications, is usually adequate. No advantage has been demonstrated for higher doses.[23] Additional doses should be given every 4 to 6 hours until significant subjective and objective improvement is achieved. Patients who are being discharged home after ED treatment should be prescribed a 3- to 10-day nontapering "burst" of oral steroids, prednisone 40 to 60 mg per day or its equivalent.

Current recommendations favor maintaining all patients with mild persistent asthma or more severe asthma with inhaled corticosteroids.[1] Therefore, consideration should be given to discharging any patient with mild persistent or more severe asthma with maintenance inhaled corticosteroid therapy in addition to the burst of oral steroids.[24]

■ Anticholinergics

Aerosolized ipratropium bromide, 0.5 mg, should be administered to patients with severe exacerbation of asthma. Ipratropium is a synthetic quaternary derivative that is available as both a nebulized solution and in an MDI (18 mg/puff) and is well tolerated (see Table 44-2). Clinical trials indicate that adding ipratropium to β_2-agonist agents offers mild additional improvement in bronchodilation and significantly decreases the need for hospitalization.[25] Side effects include dry mouth, thirst, and difficulty swallowing. Less commonly, tachycardia, restlessness, irritability, confusion, difficulty in micturition, ileus, blurring of vision, and an increase in intraocular pressure are noted.

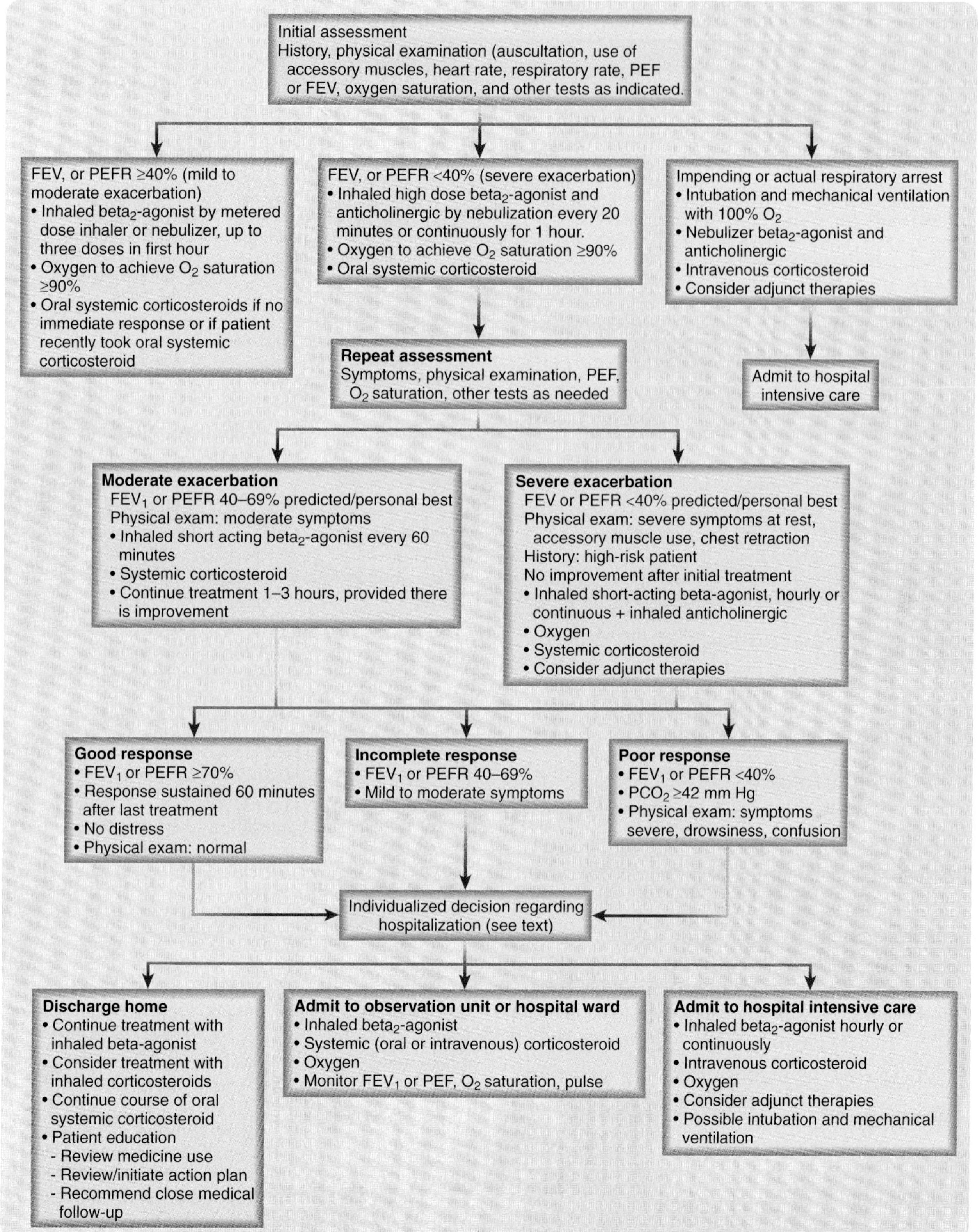
Initial assessment
History, physical examination (auscultation, use of accessory muscles, heart rate, respiratory rate, PEF or FEV, oxygen saturation, and other tests as indicated.
FEV, or PEFR ≥40% (mild to moderate exacerbation)
• Inhaled beta$_2$-agonist by metered dose inhaler or nebulizer, up to three doses in first hour
• Oxygen to achieve O_2 saturation ≥90%
• Oral systemic corticosteroids if no immediate response or if patient recently took oral systemic corticosteroid
FEV, or PEFR <40% (severe exacerbation)
• Inhaled high dose beta$_2$-agonist and anticholinergic by nebulization every 20 minutes or continuously for 1 hour.
• Oxygen to achieve O_2 saturation ≥90%
• Oral systemic corticosteroid
Impending or actual respiratory arrest
• Intubation and mechanical ventilation with 100% O_2
• Nebulizer beta$_2$-agonist and anticholinergic
• Intravenous corticosteroid
• Consider adjunct therapies
Repeat assessment
Symptoms, physical examination, PEF, O_2 saturation, other tests as needed
Admit to hospital intensive care
Moderate exacerbation
FEV_1 or PEFR 40–69% predicted/personal best
Physical exam: moderate symptoms
• Inhaled short acting beta$_2$-agonist every 60 minutes
• Systemic corticosteroid
• Continue treatment 1–3 hours, provided there is improvement
Severe exacerbation
FEV or PEFR <40% predicted/personal best
Physical exam: severe symptoms at rest, accessory muscle use, chest retraction
History: high-risk patient
No improvement after initial treatment
• Inhaled short-acting beta-agonist, hourly or continuous + inhaled anticholinergic
• Oxygen
• Systemic corticosteroid
• Consider adjunct therapies
Good response
• FEV_1 or PEFR ≥70%
• Response sustained 60 minutes after last treatment
• No distress
• Physical exam: normal
Incomplete response
• FEV_1 or PEFR 40–69%
• Mild to moderate symptoms
Poor response
• FEV_1 or PEFR <40%
• PCO_2 ≥42 mm Hg
• Physical exam: symptoms severe, drowsiness, confusion
Individualized decision regarding hospitalization (see text)
Discharge home
• Continue treatment with inhaled beta-agonist
• Consider treatment with inhaled corticosteroids
• Continue course of oral systemic corticosteroid
• Patient education
- Review medicine use
- Review/initiate action plan
- Recommend close medical follow-up
Admit to observation unit or hospital ward
• Inhaled beta$_2$-agonist
• Systemic (oral or intravenous) corticosteroid
• Oxygen
• Monitor FEV_1 or PEF, O_2 saturation, pulse
Admit to hospital intensive care
• Inhaled beta$_2$-agonist hourly or continuously
• Intravenous corticosteroid
• Oxygen
• Consider adjunct therapies
• Possible intubation and mechanical ventilation

FIGURE 44-1 Management of asthma exacerbations: ED and hospital-based care. (Adapted from National Institutes of Health, National Heart, Lung and Blood Institute, National Asthma Education and Prevention Program: Expert Panel Report 3: Guidelines for the Diagnosis and Management of Asthma. [NIH Publication No. 08-4051.] Bethesda, MD, U.S. Department of Health and Human Services, August 2007.)

Table 44-2 MEDICATIONS USED TO TREAT ASTHMA EXACERBATIONS

	DOSAGES		
Medication	**Adult Dose**	**Child Dose***	**Comments**
Short-Acting Inhaled β_2-Agonists			
Albuterol:			
Nebulizer solution (5.0 mg/mL, 2.5 mg/3 mL, 1.25 mg/3 mL, 0.63 mg/3 mL)	2.5-5 mg every 20 min for 3 doses, then 2.5-10 mg every 1-4 hrs as needed, or 10-15 mg/hr continuously	0.15 mg/kg (minimum dose 2.5 mg) every 20 min for 3 doses, then 0.15-0.3 mg/kg up to 10 mg every 1-4 hrs as needed, or 0.5 mg/kg/hr by continuous nebulization	Only selective β_2-agonists are recommended For optimal delivery, dilute aerosols to minimum of 3 mL with gas flow of 6-8 L/min
MDI (90 μg/puff)	4-8 puffs every 20 min up to 4 hrs, then every 1-4 hrs as needed	4-8 puffs every 20 min for 3 doses, then 1-4 hrs inhalation maneuver Use spacer/holding chamber	As effective as nebulized therapy if patient is able to coordinate
Bitolterol:			
Nebulizer solution (2 mg/mL)	See albuterol dose	See albuterol dose Thought to be half as potent as albuterol on a mg basis	Use has not been studied in severe asthma exacerbations Do not mix with other drugs
MDI (370 μg/puff)	See albuterol dose	See albuterol dose	Use has not been studied in severe asthma exacerbation
Levalbuterol (R-albuterol) nebulizer solution (0.63 mg/3 mL, 1.25 mg/3 mL)	1.25-2.5 mg every 20 min for 3 doses, then 1.25-5 mg every 1-4 hrs as needed, or 5-7.5 mg/hr continuously	0.075 mg/kg (minimum dose 1.25 mg) every 20 min for 3 doses, then 0.075-0.15 mg/kg up to 5 mg every 1-4 hrs as needed, or 0.25 mg/kg/hr by continuous nebulization	0.63 mg of levalbuterol is equivalent to 1.25 mg of racemic albuterol for both efficacy and side effects
Pirbuterol MDI (200 μg/puff)	See albuterol dose	See albuterol dose Thought to be half as potent as albuterol on a mg basis	Use has not been studied in severe asthma exacerbations
Systemic (Injected) β_2-Agonists			
Epinephrine 1:1000 (1 mg/mL)	0.3-0.5 mg every 20 min for 3 doses SC	0.01 mg/kg up to 0.3-0.5 mg every 20 min for 3 doses SC	No proven advantage of systemic therapy over aerosol
Terbutaline (1 mg/mL)	0.25 mg every 20 min for 3 doses sq	0.01 mg/kg every 20 min for 3 doses, then every 2-6 hrs as needed SC	No proven advantage of systemic therapy over aerosol
Anticholinergics			
Ipratropium bromide:			
Nebulizer solution (0.25 mg/mL)	0.5 mg every 30 min for 3 doses then every 2-4 hrs as needed	0.25 mg every 20 min for 3 doses, then every 2 to 4 hrs	May mix in same nebulizer with albuterol Should not be used as first-line therapy; should be added to β_2-agonist therapy
MDI (18 μg/puff)	4-8 puffs as needed	4-8 puffs as needed	Dose delivered from MDI is low, and its use has not been studied in asthma exacerbations
Ipratropium with albuterol:			
Nebulizer solution (each 3-mL vial contains 0.5 mg ipratropium bromide and 90 μg of albuterol)	3 mL every 30 min for 3 doses, then every 2-4 hrs as needed	1.5 mL every 20 min for 3 doses, then every 2-4 hrs	Contains EDTA to prevent discoloration This additive does not induce bronchospasm
MDI (each puff contains 18 μg ipratropium bromide and 90 μg of albuterol)	4-8 puffs as needed	4-8 puffs as needed	

Table 44-2 MEDICATIONS USED TO TREAT ASTHMA EXACERBATIONS—cont'd

	DOSAGES		
Medication	**Adult Dose**	**Child Dose***	**Comments**
Short-Acting Inhaled β_2-Agonists			
Systematic Corticosteroids†			
Prednisone, methylprednisolone, prednisolone	40-80 mg/day in 1 or 2 divided doses until PEF reaches 70% of predicted value or patient's personal best	1 mg/kg (maximum=60 mg/day) in 2 divided doses until PEF reaches 70% of predicted value or patient's personal best	For outpatient "burst," use 40-60 mg in single dose or 2 divided doses for adults (children: 1-2 mg/kg/day; maximum 60 mg/day) for 3-10 days

MDI, metered-dose inhaler; SC, subcutaneously.
EDTA, ethylenediaminetetraacetic acid; MDI, metered-dose inhaler; PEF, peak expiratory flow.
*Children ≤12 years old.
†Note: No advantage has been found for higher-dose corticosteroids in severe asthma exacerbations, nor is there any advantage for intravenous administration over oral therapy, provided that gastrointestinal transit time or absorption is not impaired. The usual regimen is to continue the frequent multiple daily doses until the patient achieves a forced expiratory volume (FEV) or PEF of 50% of predicted value or patient's personal best—which usually occurs within 48 hrs—and then to lower the dosage to twice daily. Therapy after a hospitalization or ED visit may last 3 to 10 days. For corticosteroid courses of 1 week or less, there is no need to taper the systemic corticosteroid dose. For slightly longer courses (e.g., up to 10 days), there is probably no need to taper, especially if patients are concurrently taking inhaled corticosteroids. If the follow-up systemic corticosteroid therapy is to be given once daily, one study indicates that it may be more clinically effective to give the dose in the afternoon at 3 PM, with no increase in adrenal suppression.[91]

Magnesium

Intravenous magnesium sulfate is indicated in the management of acute, very severe asthma—that is, in a patient with an FEV_1 less than 25% of predicted, but not in those with mild or moderate asthma exacerbation.[26-28] The dose is 1 to 2 g intravenously over 30 minutes. Later studies indicate that inhaled magnesium may also be a helpful adjunct in the treatment of a severe exacerbation.[29,30] Magnesium is not a substitute for standard therapy regimens.

Heliox, Ketamine, and Halothane

Helium is not indicated for use in mild or moderate asthma exacerbation, although several studies have demonstrated its effectiveness in very severe asthma.[31] Several investigators have reported success with ketamine[32,33] and halothane in cases in which all other treatment modalities have failed. Controlled trials substantiating these claims are lacking.

Mast Cell Modifiers

Neither cromolyn nor nedocromil, both of which modulate mast cell mediator release and eosinophil recruitment, is indicated for treatment of acute bronchospasm.

Leukotriene Modifiers

Leukotriene modifiers improve lung function, diminish symptoms, and diminish the need for short-acting β_2-agonists.[1] They are recommended as alternative to low-dose inhaled corticosteroid therapy in patients with mild persistent asthma and as steroid-sparing agents with inhaled corticosteroids in those with moderate persistent asthma. Several leukotriene modifiers—montelukast, zafirlukast, and zileuton—are currently available as oral tablets for the treatment of asthma. Although intravenous montelukast has been demonstrated to cause rapid bronchodilation when used as adjuvant therapy for acute asthma in a single trial, recommending its use in the treatment of acute bronchospasm in the ED would be premature.[34]

Theophylline

Although theophylline is no longer considered a first-line treatment for acute asthma,[35] some patients who present for treatment may be using it at home. Some data suggest that this agent has an anti-inflammatory mechanism of action. When used in combination with inhaled β_2-agonists, theophylline appears to increase the toxicity, but not the efficacy, of treatment. The most common side effects of theophylline are nervousness, nausea, vomiting, anorexia, and headache. At plasma theophylline levels greater than 30 μg/mL, there is a risk of seizures and cardiac arrhythmias.

MECHANICAL VENTILATION

When it appears that the patient needs more than the aforementioned treatments, noninvasive positive-pressure ventilation (NPPV) may be attempted (see later discussion for COPD). A single study suggested that bilevel positive airway pressure ventilation (BiPAP) may improve lung function and decrease the need for hospitalization.[36] Data showing that BiPAP reduces the need for intubation and mechanical ventilation are lacking.[37,38]

If the patient begins to exhibit signs of acute ventilatory failure with progressive hypercarbia and acidosis or becomes exhausted or confused, intubation and mechanical ventilation are needed to prevent respiratory arrest. Mechanical ventilation can eliminate the work of breathing and enable the patient to rest. It does not relieve the airflow obstruction. Direct, controlled oral intubation by an experienced physician is preferred.

The potential complications of mechanical ventilation in asthmatic patients are numerous: barotrauma, hemodynamic impairment, mucous plugging leading to increased airway resistance, atelectasis, and pulmonary infection. Air trapping and increased residual volume [intrinsic positive end-expiratory pressure (intrinsic PEEP)] may be partially avoided by utilizing controlled mechanical hypoventilation or permissive hypoventilation[37,38]—that is, using low inspiratory volumes and pressures and allowing adequate time for the expiratory phase. One can achieve the goal of ventilatory support—maintenance of adequate arterial oxygen saturation (90% or more)—without concern about "normalizing" the hypercarbic acidosis. All patients requiring mechanical ventilation should be admitted to an intensive care unit.

Disposition

Disposition decisions for patients after treatment for asthma exacerbation are rarely straightforward. A number of subjective and objective factors should be considered, as follows:

- Does the patient feel that the wheezing air exchange has improved?
- Does auscultation confirm improvement or lack thereof?
- Has a significant improvement in FEV_1 or PEF been noted?
- What is the patient's health care history?
- Is the patient usually compliant with care plans and medication regimens?
- Does the patient have access to prompt follow-up?
- Does the patient usually require hospitalization after an exacerbation?

Unfortunately, a formula for successful discharge without risk of early relapse does not yet exist, and up to 25% of patients treated in the ED for asthma return within 3 weeks.[39-42]

Because some degree of residual airflow obstruction, airway lability, and inflammation persists after treatment and discharge from the ED, a postdischarge treatment plan must be formulated.

Addition of a short, nontapering course of oral steroids to the scheduled use of a β_2-agonist bronchodilator reduces relapse rates among discharged patients. Patients with chronic asthma, who are not using controller medications at home, should be prescribed and educated about the daily use of either inhaled corticosteroids or leukotriene modifiers, in addition to their rescue medications.[43] Data indicate that relying on the primary care physician to prescribe these controllers at follow-up is inadequate.[24]

Current guidelines suggest that patients with a *good response* to treatment, as demonstrated by complete resolution of symptoms and a PEF or FEV_1 value greater than 70% of predicted, can be safely discharged home. Patients with a *poor response* to treatment, as defined by persistent symptoms, a PEF or FEV_1 value less than 50% of predicted, and persistent wheezing and dyspnea at rest, should be admitted. Many patients with an *incomplete response* to treatment, as defined by some persistence of symptoms and a PEF or FEV_1 value between 50% and 70% of predicted, may be discharged home safely, provided that they have no risk factors for death from asthma.[1] Patients who do not show adequate improvement over several hours because they are in the late phase of the exacerbation as well as those with significant risk factors for death from asthma should be admitted to either an observation unit or the hospital. Most patients have an incomplete response to treatment and fall into this "gray zone" of disposition decisions.

Studies indicate that the majority of asthmatic patients admitted to an observation unit where strict care protocols are followed can be successfully treated and discharged.[44,45]

Early follow-up care is indicated to monitor disease resolution and to review the long-term medication and care plans for the ongoing management of asthma. High relapse rates, despite the routine use of steroids, strongly suggest the need for follow-up within days of the ED visit. Ideally, education of the patient begins in the ED and a written plan of action that addresses both routine care and care of worsening symptoms is developed either in the ED or at follow-up. ED personnel should provide basic education about asthma and help connect the patient with a primary care provider or asthma specialist while providing discharge instructions. Review of the patient's discharge medication, inhaler technique, and the use of peak flow monitoring are just some of the issues EPs can teach and emphasize.

CHRONIC OBSTRUCTIVE PULMONARY DISEASE

KEY POINTS

Chronic obstructive pulmonary disease (COPD) is a chronic lung disease with significant societal costs; its prevalence is likely underestimated.

Acute exacerbations of COPD are usually triggered by respiratory irritant or infection that initiates an inflammatory cascade.

ED evaluation of potential acute exacerbations must include evaluation for other life-threatening causes of dyspnea such as cardiac ischemia, pneumonia, pulmonary embolism, and congestive heart failure.

ED management of COPD exacerbation includes oxygen, inhaled bronchodilators, antibiotics, corticosteroids, and in serious cases, noninvasive positive pressure ventilation or intubation.

Scope

Chronic obstructive pulmonary disease (COPD) is a heterogeneous disease that encompasses clinical entities such as emphysema and chronic bronchitis.[46] Although a variety of guidelines address the definition and diagnosis of COPD, a major issue is that most guidelines include a combination of clinical terms and anatomic pathology that limits their utility for EPs. The American Thoracic Society defines COPD as a disease state characterized by the presence of airflow obstruction due to chronic bronchitis or emphysema. *Chronic bronchitis* is defined as the presence of chronic productive cough for 3 months in each of 2 successive years in a patient in whom other causes of chronic cough have been excluded. *Emphysema* is defined as abnormal permanent enlargement of the air spaces distal to the terminal bronchioles accompanied by destruction of their walls and without obvious fibrosis.[47] A potentially more useful definition for EPs comes from the Global Initiative for Chronic Obstructive Lung Disease (GOLD), which states that COPD is a disease state characterized by airflow limitation that is not fully reversible.[48] The airflow limitation is usually both progressive and associated with an inflammatory response of the lungs to noxious particles or gases, such as tobacco smoke in particular. This definition encompasses chronic bronchitis, emphysema, bronchiectasis, and, to a lesser extent, asthma and is more flexible in that it acknowledges that most COPD patients have a combination of the different diseases.

Lack of agreement among definitions of COPD, combined with delayed diagnosis in many patients, makes prevalence estimates difficult. For example, although close to 24 million Americans have evidence of impaired lung function, only 14 million people are diagnosed with COPD, indicating that the condition remains underdiagnosed.[49,50]

COPD accounted for 1.5 million ED visits and 726,000 hospitalizations in 2000.[51] Total costs for COPD in the United States were $37.2 billion in 2004.[52] COPD was the fourth leading cause of death in the United States in 2002, with 120,000 victims—more than half of whom were female.[53] Of note, the prevalence of COPD in women has doubled in the past few decades but remained stable in men.[54]

Pathophysiology

■ CHRONICALLY COMPENSATED COPD

In industrialized countries, 80% to 90% of the risk of COPD is from cigarette smoking. Tobacco smoke is the major risk factor for development of COPD, but only 15% of smokers experience COPD. Other factors in COPD development in addition to smoking are occupational dust, chemical exposure, and air pollution.

The lung reacts to irritants like tobacco smoke by increasing the number of macrophages and neutrophils in the airways, lung interstitium, and alveoli. In susceptible individuals, these inflammatory cells release proteases that, if left unchecked, eventually break down lung parenchyma and stimulate mucus secretion. Cells that normally secrete surfactant and protease inhibitors are replaced by mucus-secreting cells. At the alveolar and bronchiolar level, there is a loss of elastic recoil caused by tissue destruction and, also, collapse and narrowing of the smaller airways due to loss of surfactant-producing cells. At the bronchial level, irritants cause pooling of mucus and resultant colonization by bacteria.

■ ACUTE EXACERBATIONS

Acute exacerbations of COPD are usually triggered by an event, such as infection or other respiratory irritant, that starts an inflammatory cascade. In more than 75% of patients with acute exacerbations an infectious agent is found.[55] In addition, it is likely that up to 50% of acute exacerbations are bacterial in nature.[56] Other important triggers for exacerbations are oxidative stress, lower temperatures,[57] and medications. Beta-blockers, sedatives, and narcotics are the medications that most frequently contribute to exacerbations. Regardless of the specific trigger or triggers, inflammatory mediators cause bronchoconstriction and pulmonary vasoconstriction.

Another aspect of the pathophysiology of acute exacerbation is the potential for acute respiratory acidosis. When high levels of inspired oxygen are administered during management of a COPD exacerbation, the vasoconstriction that normally shunts blood away from inadequately ventilated areas is reversed, leading to worsening ventilation-perfusion mismatch and acute rises in the level of arterial CO_2 concentration. Contrary to previous dogma, there is no significant role for the hypoxic drive in this process.

The overall clinical picture during acute exacerbations of COPD is caused by bronchospasm, inflammation, and mucus hypersecretion that results in airway narrowing, worsening ventilation-perfusion mismatch, and hypoxemia. The work of breathing increases during an exacerbation as a result of greater airway resistance and hyperinflation. This increase creates a higher oxygen demand by respiratory muscles, which further contributes to the physiologic stress on the patient.[58] The expiratory airflow limitation is not significantly increased in acute exacerbations, and the majority of the pathophysiologic manifestations are from ventilation-perfusion mismatch.[59]

Presenting Signs and Symptoms

■ CLASSIC

The presentation of the chronically compensated patient depends largely on the stage of the patient's disease. Very early on in the course of the disease, patients often do not carry the diagnosis of COPD and have subtle findings, such as mild exertional dyspnea and a chronic cough that is frequently identified as a "smoker's cough."

Acute exacerbations produce signs and symptoms that represent the impact on multiple body systems. See Table 44-3 for signs and symptoms of both chronically compensated COPD and acute exacerbations of COPD.

■ VARIATIONS

Because COPD represents a wide range of severity of disease, it has a variety of different presentations. The biggest variations are to be found at the extremes of disease.

Table 44-3 SIGNS AND SYMPTOMS OF CHRONIC OBSTRUCTIVE PULMONARY DISEASE (COPD)

Type of COPD	Symptom(s)	Signs
Chronically compensated COPD: Earlier stages of disease (not likely to carry a COPD diagnosis yet) Later stages of disease	Mild to moderate exertional dyspnea Chronic cough, frequently with small-volume hemoptysis Increasing exertional dyspnea	Mild tachypnea Wheezing with forced expiration Prolonged expiratory phase (pursed-lip breathing) Increasing tachypnea End-expiratory wheezing with normal breathing Use of accessory respiratory muscles Weight loss due both to reduced caloric intake and increased caloric demands from work of breathing Plethora from secondary polycythemia Barrel chest (predominantly emphysematous disease) Decreased breath sounds globally (predominantly emphysematous disease) Coarse crackles or rhonchi from increased secretions (predominantly bronchitic disease)
Acute exacerbations	Symptoms Rest dyspnea Exertional dyspnea that inhibits normal activities Increase in coughing frequency and/or change in appearance of sputum Apprehension	Tachypnea at rest Use of accessory respiratory muscles Diffuse expiratory wheezing with normal breathing Tachycardia and hypertension Cyanosis Altered mental status

Early on in the course, patients may simply have a persistent cough without notable dyspnea. It is important to identify such patients and secure follow-up care. Patients may also note a dry cough that is triggered by deep breaths and may or may not be associated with wheezing and dyspnea. This symptom suggests an episode of bronchitis that could be an exacerbation of underlying lung disease in at-risk patients.

Patients in late stages of COPD pose a new set of challenges. Patients with significant airway obstruction may not generate enough air movement to wheeze and have a "silent chest." Such patients need aggressive management to avoid progressive respiratory failure. The patient with a significantly enlarged chest from emphysematous changes may be difficult to auscultate. Finally, patients with severe hypoxemia and/or hypercapnia may present primarily with symptoms of altered mentation.

Differential Diagnosis

The differential diagnosis of acute dyspnea is quite large. Because many of these conditions are life-threatening, it is critical to differentiate between them so appropriate treatment can be initiated.

The EP must resist the temptation to automatically diagnose COPD as the sole cause of dyspnea in a patient with a history of COPD. Patients with COPD frequently have serious comorbidities, which may be unrecognized and which are playing a role in their ED visit. It is also important for the EP to continue to keep an open mind to the possibility of alternative diagnoses at all times during the ED course if the patient is not showing the expected response to standard treatment for COPD.

ASTHMA

Asthma and COPD coexist in some patients, and both diseases involve the presence of airway obstruction, with some key differences. In the ED setting, the key point is that the initial stabilizing actions for severe presentations of either disease do not vary greatly.

CONGESTIVE HEA\RT FAILURE

Congestive heart failure (CHF) can pose a significant diagnostic challenge for EPs because it can manifest similarly to other causes of acute dyspnea and also coexists with other chronic causes of dyspnea, such as COPD. Patients with a history of both conditions who present with acute dyspnea may have exacerbations of one or even both conditions at the same time.

Historical elements are minimally helpful in discriminating among patients. Although studies indicate that the presence of orthopnea (likelihood ratio [LR] 2.0) and dyspnea with exertion (LR 1.3) are more commonly associated with CHF, both symptoms are common in either disease.[60]

Physical examination can be of some assistance in clarifying the differentiation between CHF and COPD. The presence of jugular venous distention is helpful in pointing toward CHF, and evidence has shown that hepatojugular reflux is probably more reliable.[61] To check hepatojugular reflux, the EP puts the head of the bed at 45 degrees and presses on the patient's upper abdomen for 10 seconds. The result is positive if the venous pulsations rise at least 3 cm over baseline. Wheezing can be present in both CHF and COPD and therefore does not have high diagnostic certainty.

The chest radiograph is most useful when there is evidence of significant interstitial edema. The absence of this finding does not rule out CHF, however, because patients with chronic lung disease are less likely to have the classic chest radiographic findings of CHF.[61]

The brain natriuretic peptide (BNP) assay shows great promise in assisting the diagnosis of CHF. In one study it was more accurate than any other single variable (including history, physical examination, chest radiographs, and ECG) in determining whether CHF was present.[62] It is most helpful if the value is very high (>500 pg/mL) or very low (<100 pg/mL).[63,64] A number of disease states other than CHF can cause elevation of the BNP value; in particular, the presence of COPD with associated cor pulmonale elevates the BNP value to a lesser degree than left-sided failure.[65]

PULMONARY EMBOLISM

The diagnosis of pulmonary embolism (PE) must be considered in any dyspneic patient, particularly when risk factors for venous thromboembolism are present. A recent study found that 25% of patients with a severe COPD exacerbation of unknown origin actually had a PE.[66] Key risk factors include older age, recent surgery or trauma, prior venous thromboembolism, hereditary thrombophilia such as factor V Leiden, malignancy, smoking, and use of estrogen-containing hormone replacement therapy. The classic presentation of PE, consisting of pleuritic chest pain, dyspnea, tachycardia, and hypoxia, is not frequently encountered in the ED, but at least one of these elements is almost always present. Some historical clues to possible PE are sudden onset of symptoms and syncope or near syncope in combination with risk factors as listed previously.

The physical examination offers no clues to the diagnosis of PE in 28% to 58% of cases.[67] The diagnosis is based on a combination of the initial clinical impression of a patient's risk level with results of additional testing such as the D-dimer assay or pulmonary imaging. Patients with significant underlying asthma or COPD are frequently not good candidates for ventilation-perfusion scans because of preexisting ventilation and perfusion abnormalities that will reduce the utility of the test by increasing the likelihood of an intermediate-probability result. D-dimer testing may be of some assistance in patients with sufficiently low pretest probability, as determined by various clinical decision rules in the literature. The EP must be aware of the many disease processes that cause false-positive results, which make the utility of the D-dimer questionable in many acutely ill patients. It is of highest utility in a population that is low-risk for PE and has a lower severity of symptoms—which is not likely to include the patient presenting with a COPD exacerbation.

■ ACUTE CORONARY SYNDROMES

Dyspnea can be the main presenting complaint for patients with acute coronary syndromes. Among elderly patients diagnosed with acute coronary syndromes in the Global Registry of Acute Coronary Events (GRACE) registry, dyspnea was the dominant symptom in 49.3%.[68] An ECG should be obtained in essentially all patients who present to an ED with significant dyspnea. Clinical judgment will guide further cardiac evaluation.

■ PNEUMOTHORAX

COPD is a risk factor for spontaneous pneumothorax, and the primary diagnostic tool is the chest radiograph. The EP should also look for clinical clues, such as asymmetrical chest wall excursion and asymmetry in breath sounds or, in more severe cases, tracheal deviation and hemodynamic instability.

■ PNEUMONIA

Pneumonia commonly coexists with a COPD exacerbation. Clues such as the presence of fever and asymmetric rales on chest auscultation are helpful, but the chest radiograph remains the most useful tool for this diagnosis. The EP should be wary of the accuracy of oral temperatures in patients with tachypnea.[69]

Diagnostic Testing

■ HISTORY

The history should focus on determining the severity of disease in order to predict critical outcomes such as the need for admission and mechanical ventilation. Key historical elements include fever, changes in sputum production, hemoptysis, exercise tolerance, orthopnea, current medications, and compliance with these medications. The EP should remember to consider key elements of the differential diagnosis while taking a history and should remain alert for alternative causes of the patient's dyspnea. The presence of symptoms such as chest pain and leg swelling as well as clarification of how acute in onset the symptoms were will help include or exclude other life-threatening diseases. Important historical questions to ask the patient with possible COPD for the purpose of risk stratification are listed in Box 44-1.

BOX 44-1

Important Historical Questions for Risk-Stratification of Patients with Chronic Obstructive Pulmonary Disease

- How many times have you visited the ED in the past year? When was the last time?
- How many times have you been admitted to the hospital in the past year? When was the last time?
- Have you ever been intubated or on bilevel positive airway pressure ventilation (BiPAP)?
- Do you use oxygen at home? If so, how many liters per minute, and how many hours per day?
- Are you taking prednisone on a regular basis?
- Does this feel like your usual COPD exacerbation?
- How bad is this attack?

Physical Examination

Upon entering the room, the EP should observe the patient's overall level of distress and body position. Patients with significantly increased work of breathing or in the tripod position should have immediate and aggressive intervention.

The patient's respiratory rate should then be assessed; very high or very low respiratory rates are ominous. Next, the patient's use of accessory muscles and the proportion of the expiratory phase in breathing should be evaluated. The expiratory phase will lengthen in direct proportion to the degree of airway obstruction. The length of the patient's sentences provides a simple method of determining severity of illness and can be used for more objective reassessments after treatment is initiated.

Assessment of the patient's overall mental status should follow. Before being spoken to, is the patient awake and alert appearing or drowsy? When asked questions, does the patient respond quickly and do the answers make sense? Mental status is an important clue to the level of hypoxia or hypercapnia present.

Next, the EP should observe the chest wall movement. Is it symmetrical? Is there evidence of abdominal breathing or are they retracting? On auscultation, are there wheezes, rales, or rhonchi, and where are they located? The EP should be wary of a "silent chest," which implies poor air movement. Wheezing can occur due to CHF as well, and asymmetrical auscultation findings suggest other diagnoses, such as pneumothorax and pneumonia.

The remainder of the physical examination should focus on findings that suggest alternative diagnoses. The EP should seek signs of CHF, such as gallop rhythms, jugular venous distention, and symmetrical lower extremity edema. Asymmetrical lower extremity edema and calf tenderness would suggest deep venous thrombosis.

Imaging and Laboratory Testing

■ CHEST RADIOGRAPHS

Chest radiographs should be obtained in all patients presenting with anything but a very mild acute exacerbation of COPD. Evidence has shown that clinical criteria are unreliable for accurately predicting which patients need radiography.[70] The chest radiograph provides valuable information about alternative diagnoses, such as pneumonia, CHF, pneumothorax, and aortic dissection.[48]

■ PULSE OXIMETRY

Pulse oximetry provides a simple and noninvasive method of monitoring hypoxemia in COPD exacerbations. Pulse oximeters provide accurate estimates of arterial $Pa{O_2}$ as long as the $Sa{O_2}$ (arterial oxygen percent saturation) is greater than approximately 90%; with an $Sa{O_2}$ value below this level, the hemoglobin-oxygen dissociation curve becomes quite steep and the correlation is far less reliable. Evidence indicates that an $Sa{O_2}$ value of 92% correlates with a $Pa{O_2}$ value greater than 60 mm Hg.[71]

■ ARTERIAL BLOOD GAS ANALYSIS

Arterial blood gas (ABG) measurements are not routinely required in COPD exacerbations, although they can be helpful in patients with altered mental status, severe distress, or acidosis. ABG analysis can be helpful for estimating the severity of exacerbations or predicting the future need for mechanical ventilation or BiPAP.[72] Patients with simultaneous hypoxemia and hypercapnia are at greatest risk for development of respiratory failure. *It is important to remember that the decision to initiate mechanical ventilation should be based on clinical grounds and should not be delayed to obtain ABG results.* ABG values can provide clues to questions about issues such as patient fatigue but can never replace the decision-making ability of an experienced EP.

Venous blood gas (VBG) values may be used to screen for hypercapnia. However, although correlation between arterial and venous pH is good, agreement for $p{CO_2}$ is only fair. Data indicate that venous $p{CO_2}$ is 5.8 mm Hg higher than arterial; however, the confidence interval was wide and the correlation was not consistent.[73] This same study indicated that when a cutoff of 45 mm Hg is used, VBG measurements are 100% sensitive and 57% specific in detecting hypercapnia.[73]

■ SPIROMETRY

Unlike in asthma, acute spirometry is not of significant utility in assessing acute exacerbations of COPD. Spirometry in COPD is most useful in the primary care setting to follow disease progression over time. Its use in diagnosing or assessing acute exacerbation is not recommended by either the American College of Physicians or the American College of Chest Physicians. The FEV_1 value is only weakly correlated with $p{CO_2}$ and pH and has no correlation with arterial $p{O_2}$ in acute exacerbations.[74] Although many ED studies use spirometry to track clinical changes in COPD, it is important to realize that doing so may provide an incomplete picture of patient status.

■ ADDITIONAL LABORATORY TESTING

There are no data to support or refute the use of routine laboratory testing such as complete blood count or serum chemistry panels in COPD exacerbations. The need will be dictated mainly by the potential alternative diagnoses, such as CHF or pneumonia. A serum chemistry panel is helpful if an ABG measurement has been ordered, because the former provides a more reliable bicarbonate measurement for clarifying the acuity of a respiratory acidosis and also assists in diagnosing other acid-base disorders that may be present. A serum chemistry panel should also be ordered in patients complaining of vomiting or weakness and in patients who are taking diuretics or have a history of renal failure. Because of the frequently significant comorbidities present in patients with COPD who are sick enough to require admission, laboratory tests for cardiac markers and brain natriuretic peptide (BNP) are often indicated. Other indications for testing are discussed in the section on differential diagnosis.

Interventions, Procedures, and Treatment

The ED goals for treating acute exacerbations of COPD are as follows:

- Rule out other life-threatening causes of dyspnea
- Ensure adequate oxygenation and ventilation
- Manage reversible airway obstruction
- Treat any infectious component of the exacerbation
- Determine appropriate patient disposition
- Provide a discharge plan of care that will minimize the risk of recurrences

A concise summary of ED management for acute exacerbations of COPD can be found in Table 44-4. The rest of this section supplies additional detail on the different components of management.

Table 44-4 BASIC APPROACH TO ACUTE EXACERBATIONS OF COPD

Intervention	Comments and Cautions
Initiate O_2 to maintain saturation value >92%	Observe closely for CO_2 retention
Initiate continuous cardiac monitoring and pulse oximetry	—
Albuterol 2.5-5 mg via nebulizer	Can give continuously (10-15 mg/hr) or every 20-60 min Alternatively, give 4-10 puffs via MDI with spacer
Ipratropium 0.5 mg via nebulizer	Little data on frequency of administration—typically given once in ED visit Can be mixed with albuterol nebulizer Alternatively give 4-6 puffs via MDI with spacer
Prednisone 60 mg PO or methylprednisolone (Solu-Medrol) 125 mg IV	PO and IV routes likely equivalent in patients who are well enough to tolerate PO
Administer antibiotics	Many options; common choices are macrolides such as azithromycin (add ceftriaxone if patient being admitted) and quinolones such as moxifloxacin Local resistance patterns and patient's prior antibiotic usage are important considerations
Consider NPPV on seriously ill patients who do not yet need intubation	NPPV is most effective at reducing need for intubation if initiated early
Chest radiograph	Seek out alternative diagnoses Perform radiograph as soon as possible in course, because can be done without disrupting lifesaving care
Electrocardiography	Most useful for patients with chest pain, arrhythmias, severe exacerbations Strongly consider for all patients
Directed laboratory testing	Arterial blood gas analysis for severe disease, altered mental status, significant hypoxia, or suspicion of acidosis Theophylline measurement as appropriate Electrolyte measurements for renal failure, vomiting, or weakness Brain natriuretic peptide assay if differential diagnosis unclear D-dimer test as appropriate
Further diagnostic imaging	Chest computed tomography for pulmonary embolism if differential diagnosis in doubt
Disposition determination	If good response to therapy in a mild exacerbation, consider discharge home For patients with moderate exacerbations, consider admission to ED observation unit if available Patients with severe illness and/or multiple significant comorbidities will probably need hospital admission—use likelihood of need for ventilatory support to guide disposition to intensive care unit vs. hospital floor Patients requiring NPPV should be admitted to a closely monitored setting, which in most hospitals means at least a stepdown-care bed

IV, intravenous(ly); MDI, metered-dose inhaler; NPPV, noninvasive positive-pressure ventilation; PO, by mouth.

■ OXYGEN

Appropriate use of supplemental oxygen is a key component of COPD exacerbation management. Oxygen has a number of benefits during exacerbations, including relief of pulmonary vasoconstriction, decrease of right heart workload, and reduction of myocardial ischemia. The effects on the heart allow an increase in oxygen delivery to tissues above and beyond simple rises in the hemoglobin oxygen saturation.

The challenge is to maintain appropriate oxygenation while not provoking acute CO_2 retention. For most patients, targeting an oxygen saturation value of just over 92% (a reasonable surrogate for a pO_2 of 60 mm Hg) provides a good balance between these two issues.[48] Whether this saturation value is maintained with oxygen administered via a nasal cannula or Venturi-type mask is not important, as long as the saturation values are closely monitored to avoid delivering too little or too much oxygen.

■ INHALED MEDICATIONS

After oxygen, inhaled β_2-agonists and anticholinergics are the primary treatment modality in COPD exacerbations, because there is usually a small reversible component of the airflow obstruction.

The prototypical β_2-agonist for COPD is albuterol, delivered either by nebulizer or by MDI with a spacer. Side effects include tremor, palpitations, tachycardia, headache, mild hypokalemia, nausea, and vomiting. Evidence has shown that the two delivery methods are likely comparable but that severely dyspneic patients may tolerate nebulized medications better.[75] Albuterol can be given continuously via nebulizer or given intermittently. The American Thoracic Society guidelines advise that β_2-agonists may be used every 30 to 60 minutes, but more frequent use or continuous administration is well tolerated and may have some benefit. There is, however, little literature on continuous administration of β_2-agonists in COPD treatment. Decreasing the treatment interval from 60 minutes to 20 minutes has not been shown to improve FEV_1; however, patients with a lower starting FEV_1 appear to have more benefit with shorter treatment intervals.[76] It is important to realize the limitations of the FEV_1 value in assessing acute exacerbations; the EP should instead rely on the overall clinical picture to guide treatment. Evidence suggests that 2.5-5 mg per dose is adequate for management of COPD exacerbation.[77]

Ipratropium bromide, a quaternary anticholinergic compound, is delivered either by nebulizer or by MDI with a spacer. Side effects include tremor and dry mouth. Both it and albuterol have comparable clinical effects, and when used together, these two agents improve clinical outcomes and shorten ED lengths of stay.[78]

Long-acting inhaled anticholinergics, such as tiotropium, have no place in the acute management of COPD. They have demonstrated better efficacy, however, than 4 times daily ipratropium in the chronic management of COPD.[79]

■ CORTICOSTEROIDS

The use of corticosteroids in the ED, followed by an outpatient course of treatment, improves oxygenation and airflow, and, most importantly, decreases the rate of treatment failures.[80,81] Current literature, although limited, supports a longer course of treatment than is traditionally done for asthma. A tapering of the dosage over 7 to 14 days most likely sufficiently balances the risks of corticosteroid use with the advantages of decreased treatment failures. There is no evidence that courses of corticosteroids longer than 14 days confer added benefits. Despite common practice, there is no strong clinical evidence that courses less than 14 days require a tapering dose.

Administration of corticosteroids in the ED has not been shown to affect the rate of hospitalization. This finding is probably due to the approximately 6-hour delay before onset of the action of corticosteroids administered in the ED.[82] Nevertheless, it is important to administer these medications in the ED as soon as possible and before transferring the patient to an inpatient unit, because doing so will probably decrease the overall hospital length of stay.

In patients who can tolerate oral intake, there is probably no advantage to intravenous administration of corticosteroids, but data specifically addressing this clinical question are limited.

■ ANTIBIOTICS

The use of antibiotics in acute exacerbations of COPD is recommended in all current guidelines despite some conflicting evidence as to their efficacy. A review of 11 randomized trials showed an overall benefit to antibiotic use, with greater efficacy in more severe exacerbations.[72] Antibiotics shorten the duration of the exacerbation and accelerate recovery of peak expiratory flow rates.

The choice of antibiotic has been studied with particular concern about recent increases in betalactamase-producing strains of bacteria. There is evidence that newer extended-spectrum quinolones achieve better clinical outcomes at lower overall costs than nonquinolone therapy in patients with high risk for treatment failure (severe underlying lung disease, more than 4 exacerbations per year, COPD duration >10 years, elderly, and significant comorbid illnesses).[83] There is also evidence that newer antibiotics, such as azithromycin, ciprofloxacin, and amoxicillin-clavulanate, are associated with lower hospitalization and clinical failure rates while costing less overall than older antibiotics (such as cephalosporins and trimethoprim-sulfamethoxazole).[84] The selection of an antibiotic must take into account factors such as prior antibiotic treatment in the past 3 months, severity of illness, and community resistance patterns.

The ideal duration of antibiotic treatment is not clear. Data suggest that 5 days of antibiotics are likely sufficient,[85] but studies on the optimal duration of treatment with extended-spectrum macrolides and quinolones are lacking.

■ METHYLXANTHINES

Despite a number of guidelines that still recommend their use, methylxanthines such as aminophylline are of no significant benefit to patients with acute exacerbations of COPD and should not be used.[86]

■ NONINVASIVE POSITIVE-PRESSURE VENTILATION

NPPV involves application of positive-pressure ventilation via face mask and has significantly fewer complications than endotracheal intubation and mechanical ventilation. NPPV can be applied in one of two modes, continuous positive airway pressure (CPAP) or BiPAP. Both modes can have oxygen bled into the system.

CPAP delivers a continuous level of positive pressure throughout the respiratory cycle and is analogous to positive end-expiratory pressure (PEEP) in mechanical ventilation. CPAP improves respiratory mechanics by increasing the mean airway pressure, improving functional residual capacity, and opening underventilated and collapsed alveoli. The overall effect is to enhance gas exchange and oxygenation. CPAP is usually initiated at a low level and titrated upwards to a typical maximum of 15 cm H_2O to allow adequate oxygenation with as low an FIO_2 (fraction of inspired oxygen) value as possible.

BiPAP provides different levels of positive pressure for inspiration (IPAP) and expiration (EPAP). This is analogous to pressure support and PEEP in mechanical ventilation. BiPAP provides the same benefits of continuously applied positive pressure as CPAP, but also theoretically reduces the work of breathing by providing a pressure boost for inspiration. BiPAP can be time-triggered to a certain number of breaths per minute or flow-cycled to allow the patient to trigger the device. The IPAP is typically started at around 8 cm H_2O and titrated upwards to a typical maximum of 20 cm H_2O. The EPAP is typically started around 4 cm H_2O and titrated upwards to a typical maximum of 15 H_2O. The settings should be balanced to allow physiologic tidal volumes (5-7 mL/kg) and maximal oxygenation with a minimum FiO_2 while still maintaining patient comfort.

To be successful candidates for NPPV, patients must be alert, breathing spontaneously, and able to cooperate with instructions. This modality can be used with extreme care in patients with mild decreases in level of consciousness.[87] A good rule of thumb is that a patient who cannot constantly keep his or her head up independently will not likely succeed with NPPV. Adequate staffing levels and continuous monitoring of heart rate, pulse oximetry, and intermittent blood pressure measurements must be present to safely and successfully utilize NPPV for a patient. NPPV is most likely to be successful when a partnership exists among the patient, nursing, respiratory therapy, and physician that involves effective communication in all directions before and during initiation of treatment. It is also most likely to be successful if initiated early in the patient's stay in the ED.

As with mechanical ventilation, the EP must be alert for hemodynamic changes and desaturations that may indicate loss of mask seal, intrinsic PEEP (also called auto-PEEP), pneumothorax, and patient intolerance. Gastric distention with resultant restriction of diaphragmatic excursion or vomiting is another potential complication of NPPV.

Contraindications to NPPV are altered mental status, impaired airway-protection mechanisms, apnea, cardiovascular instability, and pneumothorax. In addition, any craniofacial abnormality (prior surgery, trauma, etc.) that impairs the ability to obtain a reliable mask seal would preclude NPPV.

In patients with COPD, NPPV has been shown to significantly decrease both the need for intubation and overall patient mortality and to generate significant improvements in pH, pCO_2, and respiratory rate.[88,89] The delivery method (CPAP vs. BiPAP) has not been shown to make a significant difference in outcomes to date.

NPPV should be considered in patients with the following clinical features as long as the contraindications previously discussed are not present:

- Difficulty maintaining oxygen saturations >90% with a nonrebreather mask
- Moderate to severe dyspnea
- Respiratory rate >25 breaths/min
- Moderate acidosis (pH 7.30-7.35)

ENDOTRACHEAL INTUBATION AND MECHANICAL VENTILATION

The decision to intubate a patient with COPD is largely based on clinical judgment and experience. Some patients obviously need intubation (respiratory arrest, decline with NPPV) but in other patients the need is far less apparent. As mentioned previously, ABG values can assist in the decision to intubate, but the ultimate decision must always be based on an assessment made with the EP standing in front of the patient. *Intubation decisions should not be delayed in critically ill patients to wait for ABG results.* There are general guidelines to assist in this decision-making process, but they are just tools that will not make the final decision, and some of the guidelines are vague; they are listed in Box 44-2.[48]

Once the EP has determined that a patient with COPD requires intubation, there are a few special considerations to think about. In general, the largest size tube that can fit safely between the cords should be used (8-8.5 in men, 7.5-8 in women) to decrease overall airway resistance. The EP must also carefully consider the expected difficulty of intubation before administering paralytic agents. Effective bag-valve-mask ventilation can be difficult in patients with COPD owing to higher airway resistance and lung hyperinflation. Other potential comorbidities such as obesity can also make intubation difficult. Patients with COPD are commonly difficult to preoxygenate adequately, a feature that significantly reduces the time available for direct laryngoscopy. Consider an "awake" look, using a combination of topical anesthesia of the airway and sedation, but not full induction, before employing full rapid-sequence intubation

BOX 44-2

General Criteria for Intubation in Acute Exacerbations of Chronic Obstructive Pulmonary Disease

- Severe dyspnea with use of accessory muscles
- Respiratory rate greater than 35 breaths/min
- Life-threatening hypoxemia ($pO_2 < 40$ mm Hg or $pO_2/FiO_2 < 200$)
- Severe acidosis (pH < 7.25) and hypercapnia ($pCO_2 > 60$ mm Hg)
- Respiratory arrest
- Somnolence or significant impairment of mental status
- Cardiovascular complications (hypotension, shock, heart failure)
- Other complications (metabolic abnormalities, sepsis, pneumonia, pulmonary embolism, barotrauma, massive pleural effusion)
- Failure of noninvasive positive-pressure ventilation

is an alternative. Ketamine in initial doses of 0.5 to 1 mg/kg IV has some properties that make it an attractive option in this situation because it preserves airway protection reflexes and also has bronchodilation properties. Additional doses can be given as necessary.[2] A full discussion of these issues is outside the scope of this chapter.

The management of hypotensive episodes in patients recently intubated for COPD is the same as that for other intubated patients, but some causes are more common in COPD. In particular, the patient with COPD must be evaluated for a pneumothorax versus the auto-PEEP phenomena, as follows: First, remove the ventilator and use manual bag ventilation. Frequently this maneuver rapidly (within 1 minute) resolves auto-PEEP. The EP should look for clues to pneumothorax, such as tracheal deviation, asymmetrical breath sounds, and distended neck veins. Another common cause is dehydration from increased respiratory insensible losses; this condition should respond to bolus administration of fluids. Finally, many patients who are critically ill are driving their bodies with stimulation from the sympathetic nervous system. Inducing anesthesia blunts this stimulation and therefore can result in circulatory instability. The easiest way to manage this issue consists of anticipation and prevention—using smaller doses of medications or selecting medications with minimal hemodynamic effects, such as etomidate. If this problem still occurs, it can be managed with volume resuscitation and, if needed, vasopressors if volume resuscitation alone is not effective.

Disposition and Follow-Up

The decision to admit or discharge the patient with a COPD exacerbation is multifactorial and involves issues that may not be clinical. The response to ED management is the most useful indicator of disposition. EPs must consider whether the patient will be able to receive the maintenance care necessary at home—i.e., outpatient management will almost certainly fail in a patient with an oxygen requirement who was not already receiving oxygen. Clinicians also must estimate the likely clinical course: Is this patient showing a clear trend toward improvement, or is the course in doubt? The availability of rapid and reliable follow-up care can allow safe discharge of potentially sicker patients. Unfortunately, the absence of such care is more frequently encountered in the ED environment; patients whose social issues, such as limited access to care, put them at high risk for a return ED visit should be admitted.

Evidence has shown that the following factors put patients at higher risk for relapse within 2 weeks after an ED visit[90]:

- Number of ED or clinic visits in the past year (≥5 visits)
- Amount of activity limitation prior to arrival
- Initial respiratory rate over 16 breaths/min
- Patients who were taking oral corticosteroids before arriving in the ED

Patients at higher risk for relapse need more careful discharge planning that includes reliable follow-up.

REFERENCES

1. National Institutes of Health, National Heart, Lung and Blood Institute, National Asthma Education and Prevention Program: Expert Panel Report 3: Guidelines for the Diagnosis and Management of Asthma. [NIH Publication NO. 08-4051.] Bethesda, MD, U.S. Department of Health and Human Services, August 2007.
2. National Center for Health Statistics. Health, United States. Hyattsville, Maryland: Public Health Service, 2000.
3. Moorman JE, Rudd RA, Johnson CA, et al: MMWR Surveillance Summaries. National Surveillance for Asthma—United States, 1980-2004. Centers for Disease Control. http://www.cdc.gov/mmwr/preview/mmwrhtml/ss5608.al.htm
4. Weiss KB, Gergen PJ, Hodgson TA: An economic evaluation of asthma in the United States. N Engl J Med 1992; 326:862-866.
5. Bousquet J, Jeffery PK, Busse WW, et al: Asthma: From bronchoconstriction to airways inflammation and remodeling. Am J Respir Crit Care Med 2000;161:1720-1745.
6. Robin ED: Unexpected, unexplained sudden death in young asthmatic subjects. Chest 1989;96:790-793.
7. Wasserfallen JB: Sudden asphyxic asthma: A distinct entity? Am Rev Respir Dis 1990;142:108-111.
8. Brooks SM, Hammad Y, Richards I, et al: The spectrum of irritant-induced asthma: Sudden and not-so-sudden onset and the role of allergy. Chest 1998;113:42-49.
9. Barr RG, Woodruff PG, Clark S, Camargo CA Jr: Sudden-onset asthma exacerbations: Clinical features, response to therapy, and 2-week follow-up. Multicenter Airway Research Collaboration (MARC) investigators. Eur Respir J 2000; 15:266-273.
10. Carden DL, Nowak RM, Sarkar D, Tomlanovich MC: Vital signs including pulsus paradoxus in the assessment of acute bronchial asthma. Ann Emerg Med 1983;12: 80-83.
11. Martin TG, Elenbaas RM, Pingleton SH: Use of peak expiratory flow rates to eliminate unnecessary arterial blood gases in acute asthma. Ann Emerg Med 1982;11:70-73.
12. McFadden ER Jr: Clinical physiologic correlates in asthma. J Allergy Clin Immunol 1986;77:1-5.
13. White CS: Acute asthma: Admission chest radiography in hospitalized adult patients. Chest 1991;100:14-16.
14. Shome GP, Starnes JD, Shearer M, et al: Exhaled nitric oxide in asthma: Variability, relation to asthma severity, and peripheral blood lymphocyte cytokine expression. J Asthma 2006;43:95-99.
15. Redington AE: Modulation of nitric oxide pathways: Therapeutic potential in asthma and chronic obstructive pulmonary disease. Eur J Pharmacol 2006;533:263-276.
16. Taylor DR: Nitric oxide as a clinical guide for asthma management. J Allergy Clin Immunol 2006;117:259-262.
17. Spergel JM, Fogg MI, Bokszczanin-Knosala A: Correlation of exhaled nitric oxide, spirometry and asthma symptoms. J Asthma 2005;42:879-883.
18. Cates CJ, Rowe BH: Holding chambers versus nebulisers for beta-agonist treatment of acute asthma. Cochrane Database Syst Rev 2000;(2):CD000052.
19. Camargo C Jr, Spooner C, Rowe B: Continuous versus intermittent beta-agonists in the treatment of acute asthma. Cochrane Database Syst Rev 2003;4:CD001115.
20. Cydulka R, Davison R, Grammer L, et al: The use of epinephrine in the treatment of older adult asthmatics. Ann Emerg Med 1988;17:322-326.
21. Travers A, Jones AP, Kelly K, et al: Intravenous beta2-agonists for acute asthma in the emergency department. Cochrane Database Syst Rev 2001;(2):CD002988.
22. Rowe BH, Spooner C, Ducharme FM, et al: Early emergency department treatment of acute asthma with systemic corticosteroids. Cochrane Database Syst Rev 2001;(1): CD002178.

23. Emerman CL, Cydulka RK: A randomized comparison of 100-mg vs 500-mg dose of methylprednisolone in the treatment of acute asthma. Chest 1995;107:1559-1563.
24. Cydulka RK, Tamayo-Sarver JH, Wolf C, et al: Inadequate follow-up controller medications among patients with asthma who visit the emergency department. Ann Emerg Med 2005;46:316-322.
25. Rodrigo GJ, Castro-Rodriguez JA: Anticholinergics in the treatment of children and adults with acute asthma: A systematic review with meta-analysis. Thorax 2005; 60:740-746.
26. Rowe BH, Camargo CA Jr: The use of magnesium sulfate in acute asthma: Rapid uptake of evidence in North American emergency departments. J Allergy Clin Immunol 2006;117:53-58.
27. Silverman RA, Osborn H, Runge J, et al: IV magnesium sulfate in the treatment of acute severe asthma: A multicenter randomized controlled trial. Chest 2002; 122:489-497.
28. Cheuk DK, Chau TC, Lee SL: A meta-analysis on intravenous magnesium sulphate for treating acute asthma. Arch Dis Child 2005;90:74-77.
29. Kokturk N, Turktas H, Kara P, et al: A randomized clinical trial of magnesium sulphate as a vehicle for nebulized salbutamol in the treatment of moderate to severe asthma attacks. Pulm Pharmacol Ther 2005;18:416-421.
30. Blitz M, Blitz S, Hughes R, et al: Aerosolized magnesium sulfate for acute asthma: A systematic review. Chest 2005;128:337-344.
31. Rodrigo GJ, Rodrigo C, Pollack CV, Rowe B: Use of helium-oxygen mixtures in the treatment of acute asthma: A systematic review. Chest 2003;123:891-896.
32. Howton JC: Randomized, double-blind, placebo-controlled trial of intravenous ketamine in acute asthma. Ann Emerg Med 1996;27:170-175.
33. Lau TT, Zed PJ: Does ketamine have a role in managing severe exacerbation of asthma in adults? Pharmacotherapy 2001;21:1100-1106.
34. Camargo CA Jr, Smithline HA, Malice MP, et al: A randomized controlled trial of intravenous montelukast in acute asthma. Am J Respir Crit Care Med 2003;167:528-533.
35. Parameswaran K, Belda J, Rowe BH: Addition of intravenous aminophylline to beta2-agonists in adults with acute asthma. Cochrane Database Syst Rev 2000;(4):CD002742.
36. Soroksky A, Stav D, Shpirer I: A pilot prospective, randomized, placebo-controlled trial of bilevel positive airway pressure in acute asthmatic attack. Chest 2003;123: 1018-1025.
37. Oddo M, Feihl F, Schaller MD, Perret C: Management of mechanical ventilation in acute severe asthma: Practical aspects. Intensive Care Med 2006;32:501-510.
38. Austan F, Polise M: Management of respiratory failure with noninvasive positive pressure ventilation and heliox adjunct. Heart Lung 2002;31:214-218.
39. Rowe BH, Spooner CH, Ducharme FM, et al: Corticosteroids for preventing relapse following acute exacerbations of asthma (Cochrane Review). In The Cochrane Library. Oxford, Update Software, 2004.
40. Emerman CL, Cydulka RK, Crain EF, Rowe BH, et al: Prospective multicenter study of relapse after treatment for acute asthma among children presenting to the emergency department. J Pediatr 2001;138:318-324.
41. Emerman CL, Woodruff PG, Cydulka RK, et al: Prospective multicenter study of relapse following treatment for acute asthma among adults presenting to the emergency department. MARC investigators. Multicenter Asthma Research Collaboration [see comments]. Chest 1999;115: 919-927.
42. Cydulka RK, Shah M: Follow-up and prevention of relapse in adults after disposition from the ED. In Brenner BE (ed): Emergency Asthma. New York, Marcel Dekker, 1999, pp 527-532.
43. Frey U: Predicting asthma control and exacerbations: Chronic asthma as a complex dynamic model. Curr Opin Allergy Clin Immunol 2007;7:223-230.
44. Rydman RJ, Roberts RR, Albrecht GL, et al: Patient satisfaction with an emergency department asthma observation unit. Acad Emerg Med 1999;6:178-183.
45. Rydman RJ, Isola ML, Roberts RR, et al: Emergency Department observation unit versus hospital inpatient care for a chronic asthmatic population: A randomized trial of health status outcome and cost. Med Care 1998;36:599-609.
46. Petty TL: COPD in perspective. Chest 2002;121(Suppl 5):116S-120S.
47. Standards for the diagnosis and care of patients with chronic obstructive pulmonary disease. American Thoracic Society. Am J Respir Crit Care Med 1995;152:S77-S121.
48. NHLBI/WHO Workshop Report: Global Initiative for Chronic Obstructive Lung Disease (GOLD): Global Strategy for the Diagnosis, Management and Prevention of Chronic Obstructive Pulmonary Disease. Bethesda, MD, National Institutes of Health, National Heart, Lung, and Blood Institute, April 2001; updated 2005.
49. Mannino DM, Homa DM, Akinbami L, et al: Chronic obstructive pulmonary disease surveillance—United States, 1971-2000. MMWR Surveill Summ 2002;51:1-16.
50. Barnes PJ: Chronic obstructive pulmonary disease. N Engl J Med 2000;343:269-280.
51. National Center for Health Statistics: National Hospital Ambulatory Care Medical Survey. Hyattsville, MD, US Department of Health and Human Services, CDC, NCHS, 2000.
52. National Heart Lung and Blood Institute, Morbidity and Mortality Chartbook, 2004, Bethesda, MD, NIH, 2004.
53. National Center for Health Statistics. Report of Final Mortality Statistics, 2002. Deaths: Final Data for 2002 National Vital Statistics Report Volume 53, no. 2, 2004.
54. National Heart, Lung, and Blood Institute. NHLBI Morbidity and Mortality Chartbook, 2000. Bethesda, MD, NIH, Deaths: Final Data for 2002 National Vital Statistics Report Volume 53, no. 2, 2004.
55. Seth S: Infectious etiology of acute exacerbation of chronic bronchitis. Chest 2000;117(Suppl):380S-385S.
56. Sethi S, Murphy TF: Bacterial infection in chronic obstructive pulmonary disease in 2000: A state-of-the-art review. Clin Microbiol Rev 2001;14:336-363.
57. Donaldson G, Seemungal T, Jeffries D, et al: Effect of temperature on lung function and symptoms in chronic obstructive pulmonary disease. Eur J Respir Dis 1999; 13:844-849.
58. Palm KH, Decker WW: Acute exacerbations of chronic obstructive pulmonary disease. Emerg Med Clin North Am 2003;21:333-352.
59. Barbera JA, Roca J, Ferrer A, et al: Mechanisms of worsening gas exchange during acute exacerbations of chronic obstructive pulmonary disease. Eur Respir J 1997; 10:1285-1291.
60. Badgett RG, Lucey CR, Mulrow CD: Can the clinical examination diagnose left-sided heart failure in adults? JAMA 1997;277:1712-1719.
61. Mulrow CD, Lucey CR, Farnett LE: Discriminating causes of dyspnea through clinical examination. J Gen Intern Med 1993;8:384-392.
62. Dao Q, Krishnaswamy P, Kazanegra R, et al: Utility of B-type natriuretic peptide in the diagnosis of congestive heart failure in an urgent-care setting. J Am Coll Cardiol 2001;37:379-385.
63. Silver MA, Maisel A, Yancy CW, et al: BNP Consensus Panel 2003: A clinical approach for the diagnostic, prognostic, screening, treatment monitoring, and therapeutic roles of natriuretic peptides in cardiovascular diseases. Congest Heart Fail 2004;10(Suppl 3):S1-S30.
64. McCullough PA, Omland T, Maisel AS: B-type natriuretic peptides: A diagnostic breakthrough for clinicians. Rev Cardiovasc Med 2003;4:72-80.
65. Jason P, Keang LT, Hoe LK: B-type natriuretic peptide: Issues for the intensivist and pulmonologist. Crit Care Med 2005;33:2094-2103.
66. Tillie-Leblond I, Marquette CH, Perez T, et al: Pulmonary embolism in patients with unexplained exacerbation of

chronic obstructive pulmonary disease: Prevalence and risk factors. Ann Intern Med 2006;144:390-396.
67. Sadosty AT, Boie ET, Stead LG: Pulmonary embolism. Emerg Med Clin North Am 2003;21:363-384.
68. Brieger D, Eagle K, Goodman S, et al: Acute coronary syndromes without chest pain, an underdiagnosed and undertreated high-risk group: Insights from the Global Registry of Acute Coronary Events. Chest 2004;126:461-469.
69. Tandberg D, Sklar D: Effect of tachypnea on the estimation of body temperature by an oral thermometer. N Engl J Med 1983;308:945-946.
70. Emerman CL, Cydulka RK: Evaluation of high-yield criteria for chest radiography in acute exacerbation of chronic obstructive pulmonary disease. Ann Emerg Med 1993; 22:680-684.
71. Kelly A, McAlpine R, Kyle E: How accurate are pulse oximeters in patients with acute exacerbations of chronic obstructive airways disease? Respir Med 2001;95:336-340.
72. McCrory D, Brown C, Gelfand S, et al: Management of acute exacerbations of COPD: A summary and appraisal of published evidence. Chest 2001;119:1190-1209.
73. Kelly A, McAlpine R: Venous pCO2 can be used to screen for significant hypercarbia in emergency patients with acute respiratory distress. J Emerg Med 2002;22:15-19.
74. Emerman CL, Connors AF, Lukens TW, et al: Relationship between arterial blood gases and spirometry in acute exacerbations of chronic obstructive pulmonary disease. Ann Emerg Med 1989;18:523-527.
75. Turner M, Patel A, Ginsburg S, et al: Bronchodilator delivery in acute airflow obstruction—a meta-analysis. Arch Intern Med 1997;157:1736-1744.
76. Emerman CE, Cydulka RK: Effect of different albuterol dosing regimens in the treatment of acute exacerbation of chronic obstructive pulmonary disease. Ann Emerg Med 1997;29:474-478.
77. Nair S, Thomas E, Pearson SB, et al: A randomized controlled trial to assess the optimal dose and effect of nebulized albuterol in acute exacerbations of COPD. Chest 2005;128:48-54.
78. Shrestha M, O'Brien T, Haddox R, et al: Decreased duration of emergency department treatment of chronic obstructive pulmonary disease exacerbations with the addition of ipratropium bromide to beta-agonist therapy. Ann Emerg Med 1991;120:1206-1209.
79. van Noord JA, Bantje TA, Eland ME, et al: A randomized controlled comparison of tiotropium and ipratropium in the treatment of chronic obstructive pulmonary disease. The Dutch Tiotropium Study Group. Thorax 2000; 55:289-294.
80. Thompson W, Nielson C, Carvalho P, et al: Controlled trial of oral prednisone in outpatients with acute COPD exacerbation. Am J Respir Crit Care Med 1996;154:407-412.
81. Aaron SD, Vandemheen KL, Hebert P, et al: Outpatient oral prednisone after emergency treatment of chronic obstructive pulmonary disease. N Engl J Med 2003;348: 2618-2625.
82. Bullard M, Liaw S, Tsai Y, et al: Early corticosteroid use in acute exacerbation of chronic airflow obstruction. Am J Emerg Med 1996;14:139-143.
83. Balter MS, La Forge J, Low DE, et al; Chronic Bronchitis Working Group; Canadian Thoracic Society; Canadian Infectious Disease Society: Canadian guidelines for the management of acute exacerbations of chronic bronchitis. Can Respir J 2003;10(Suppl B):3B-32B.
84. Destache C, Dewan N, O'Donohue W, et al: Clinical and economic considerations in the treatment of acute exacerbations of chronic bronchitis. J Antimicrob Chemother 1999;43:107-113.
85. McCarty J, Pierce P: Five days of cefprozil versus 10 days of clarithromycin in the treatment of an acute exacerbation of chronic bronchitis. Ann Asthma Immunol 2001; 87:327-334.
86. Barr RG, Rowe BH, Camargo CA: Methylxanthines for exacerbations of chronic obstructive pulmonary disease: Meta-analysis of randomised trials. BMJ 2003;327:643-646.
87. Scala R, Naldi M, Archinucci I, et al: Noninvasive positive pressure ventilation in patients with acute exacerbations of COPD and varying levels of consciousness. Chest 2005;128:1657-1666.
88. Lightowler JV, Wedzicha JA, Elliott MW, et al: Non-invasive positive pressure ventilation to treat respiratory failure resulting from exacerbations of chronic obstructive pulmonary disease: Cochrane systematic review and meta-analysis. BMJ 2003;326:185-187.
89. Keenan SP, Sinuff T, Cook DJ, et al: Which patients with acute exacerbation of chronic obstructive pulmonary disease benefit from noninvasive positive-pressure ventilation? Ann Intern Med 2003;138(11):861-870.
90. Kim S, Emerman CL, Cydulka RK, et al; MARC Investigators: Prospective multicenter study of relapse following emergency department treatment of COPD exacerbation. Chest 2004;125:473-481.
91. Beam WR, Weiner DE, Martin RJ: Timing of prednisone and alterations of airways inflammation in nocturnal asthma. Am Rev Respir Dis 1992;146:1524-1530.

Chapter 45

Lung Infections

David S. Howes and Joseph F. Peabody

KEY POINTS

- A wide variety of infectious agents, including bacteria, viruses, and fungi, cause pneumonia.
- Diagnosis and treatment of pneumonia are determined through assessment of patient risks, other elements of the history, diagnostic studies, and physical examination.
- Chest radiography is an important diagnostic tool and can offer valuable clues to etiology. Other laboratory and sputum studies may also be useful.
- The causative agent is typically not known at presentation, so institution of carefully selected empirical antibiotic therapy is paramount.
- Supplemental oxygen and ventilatory assistance should be provided immediately if the patient has respiratory impairment.
- Age, comorbid diseases, and clinical and laboratory data guide disposition decisions for a patient with pneumonia, such as intensive care unit (ICU) admission.
- The patient who is suspected to be highly infectious or who could be a victim of bioterrorism should be isolated immediately.

Scope

Pneumonia is one of the most common infectious diseases encountered in the ED. When combined with influenza, pneumonia ranks as the sixth leading cause of death in the United States and the most common cause of infection-related mortality.[1-4]

Pneumonia is typically defined as an infection of the lung parenchyma with associated symptoms of cough, fever, and abnormal breath sounds on physical examination. Usually an infiltrate is seen on chest radiographs.

There are many potential pathogens for this disease, and a thorough history and physical examination will be very important to selection of the appropriate empirical antibiotic coverage in the patient with pneumonia.

Structure and Function

The lungs are constantly exposed to potential pathogens by both organisms in inspired air and those living in the oropharynx and upper respiratory tract. Owing to multiple layers of defenses, the lower respiratory tract usually remains sterile. Many protective mechanisms—the cough and gag reflexes, upper airway particle filtration, proper mucociliary clearance, and humoral and cellular immunologic defenses at the alveolar level—play an important role in guarding the lungs against infection.

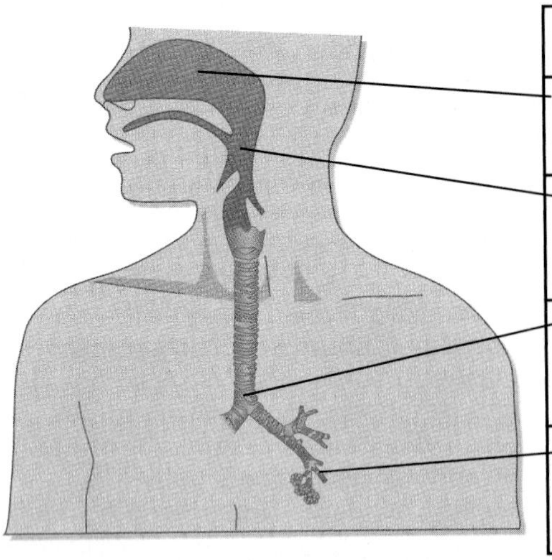

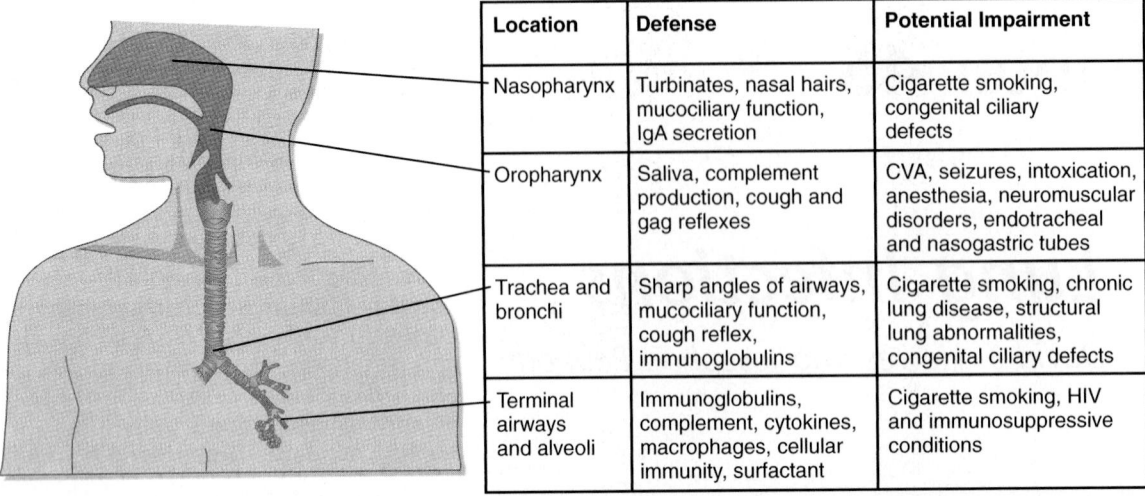

Location	Defense	Potential Impairment
Nasopharynx	Turbinates, nasal hairs, mucociliary function, IgA secretion	Cigarette smoking, congenital ciliary defects
Oropharynx	Saliva, complement production, cough and gag reflexes	CVA, seizures, intoxication, anesthesia, neuromuscular disorders, endotracheal and nasogastric tubes
Trachea and bronchi	Sharp angles of airways, mucociliary function, cough reflex, immunoglobulins	Cigarette smoking, chronic lung disease, structural lung abnormalities, congenital ciliary defects
Terminal airways and alveoli	Immunoglobulins, complement, cytokines, macrophages, cellular immunity, surfactant	Cigarette smoking, HIV and immunosuppressive conditions

FIGURE 45-1 Host defenses against infection. CVA, cerebrovascular accident; HIV, human immunodeficiency virus; IgA, immunoglobulin A. (Redrawn from Donowitz G, Mandell G: Acute pneumonia. In Mandell GL, Bennett JE, Doline R [eds]: Mandell, Douglas, and Bennett's Principles and Practice of Infectious Disease, 6th ed. Philadelphia, Elsevier, 2005, pp 819-841.)

Risks

Pneumonia typically occurs when there is a breach of the protective defenses just described or exposure to a heavy inoculation of organisms or to very virulent organisms. The lung's defenses can be impaired at multiple levels. Aspiration can result when altered levels of consciousness due to neurologic insult or alcohol or drug intoxication impairs the gag reflex. Upper airway defenses are often bypassed by endotracheal tubes or tracheostomy. Smoking and chronic lung disease can impair mucociliary function. Bronchial obstruction due to tumor or lymphadenopathy can lead to obstruction and pneumonia. Immunologic impairment due to human immunodeficiency virus (HIV), chemotherapy, splenectomy, or advanced age also predisposes to pneumonia. The elderly are particularly vulnerable because of impairments at many of these levels and a higher incidence of comorbid conditions[4] (Fig. 45-1).

Presenting Signs and Symptoms

The classic presenting symptoms of pneumonia are fever, cough, purulent sputum, and shortness of breath. Patients may also have several nonrespiratory symptoms such as sweats, chills, confusion, headache, fatigue, nausea, and myalgias. Infants often have decreased intake, lethargy, and, apnea. Patients of advanced age are less likely to present with typical symptoms, often having only weakness or altered mental status.

A goal-directed, reasonably comprehensive history is very important in the evaluation of the patient with pneumonia. Historical clues such as recent hospitalizations, risks for aspiration, recent travel, animal or environmental exposures, recent antibiotic exposure, HIV status or risks, alcoholism, and comorbid illnesses can point toward specific etiologies and guide proper choice of initial empirical therapy (Table 45-1).[5,6]

RED FLAGS

- Look for key clues in the history and physical findings that would suggest a pneumonia caused by an unusual or resistant organism.
- Maintain a high suspicion for aspiration pneumonia in the elderly and in the patient with altered mental status or recent cerebrovascular accident.

Pathogens

Community-acquired pneumonia is often defined as pneumonia in a patient who has not been hospitalized and has not resided in a long-term care facility for more than 14 days before the appearance of symptoms.[2] With the growing prevalence of mixed-organism infections, drug-resistant pathogens, and patients with comorbid illnesses, however, this definition has become somewhat blurred. Guidelines from the American Thoracic Society (ATS), Centers for Disease Control and Prevention (CDC), and Infectious Diseases Society of America (IDSA) now address treatment of patients at increased risk for pseudomonal infection, those with significant comorbidities, and those at risk for infection with drug-resistant *Streptococcus pneumoniae* (DRSP).

The most common etiologic agent causing pneumonia is *S. pneumoniae,* which represents about two thirds of all cases (Table 45-2).[2] Other bacterial pathogens that are often isolated are *Mycoplasma pneu-*

Table 45-1 EPIDEMIOLOGIC CONDITIONS RELATED TO SPECIFIC PATHOGENS WITH SELECTED COMMUNITY-ACQUIRED PNEUMONIA

Condition	Commonly Encountered Pathogens
Alcoholism	*Streptococcus pneumoniae*, oral anaerobes
Chronic obstructive pulmonary disease and/or smoking	*S. pneumoniae, Haemophilus influenzae, Moraxella catarrhalis, Legionella* spp., *Chlamydia pneumoniae*
Poor dental hygiene	Oral anaerobes
Aspiration/lung abscess	Oral anaerobes
Exposure to bats or to soil enriched with bird droppings	*Histoplasma capsulatum*
Exposure to birds	*Chlamydia psittaci*, avian influenza (poultry exposure)
Exposure to rabbits	*Francisella tularensis*
Exposure to farm animals or parturient cats	*Coxiella burnetti* (Q fever)
Human immunodeficiency virus (HIV) infection:	
Early	*S. pneumoniae, H. influenzae, Mycobacterium tuberculosis*
Late	Above plus *Pneumocystis jirovecii* (*carinii*), *Cryptococcus, Histoplasma*
Travel to or residence of southwestern United States	*Coccidioides* spp.
Travel to or residence of Asia	*Burkholderia pseudomallei*, severe acute respiratory syndrome (SARS)
Influenza active in community ("flu season")	Influenza, *S. pneumoniae, S. aureus, H. influenzae*
Structural lung disease (e.g., bronchiectasis)	*Pseudomonas aeruginosa, Burkholderia cepacia, Staphylococcus aureus*
Injection drug use	*S. aureus*, skin anaerobes, *M. tuberculosis, S. pneumoniae*
Endobronchial obstruction	Anaerobes, *S. pneumoniae, H. influenzae, S. aureus*
Recent hospitalization or nursing home residence	Drug-resistant *S. pneumoniae* (DRSP), gram-negative bacilli, *S. aureus*
In context of bioterrorism	*Bacillus anthracis* (anthrax), *Yersinia pestis* (plague), *F. tularensis* (tularemia)

Modified from File T, Niederman M: Antimicrobial therapy of community-acquired pneumonia. Infect Dis Clin North Am 2004;18:993-1016.

Table 45-2 ETIOLOGY OF COMMUNITY-ACQUIRED PNEUMONIA

Pathogen	Prevalance(%)
Streptococcus pneumoniae	20-60
Haemophilus influenzae	3-10
Staphylococcus aureus	3-5
Gram-negative bacilli	3-10
Miscellaneous (includes *Moraxella catarrhalis*, group A streptococci, and *Neisseria meningitidis*, each accounting for 1%-2% of cases)	3-5
Legionella spp.	2-8
Mycoplasma pneumoniae	1-6
Chlamydia pneumoniae	4-6
Viruses	2-15
Aspiration	6-10

From Niederman M: Review of treatment guidelines for community acquired pneumonia. Am J Med 2004;117, 52S (5) is Clin N Am, 18 (2004) p 997(3).

moniae, Chlamydia pneumoniae, Haemophilus influenzae, and *Legionella pneumophila* (often called "the atypical organisms"). Community-acquired pneumonia is also caused by several viruses, including influenza, parainfluenza, and respiratory syncytial virus (RSV). Other pathogens, such as *Pseudomonas aeruginosa*, DRSP, and methicillin-resistant *Staphylococcus aureus* (MRSA) should also be considered in nursing home patients and patients who recently have been hospitalized or have taken broad-spectrum antibiotics. Multiple other organisms may be considered on the basis of history of specific exposures, travel, and lung or immunosuppressive diseases.

Special Populations

■ CHILDREN

Pneumonia and acute bronchiolitis are the most common lower respiratory tract infections in chil-

Table 45-3 TYPICAL PATHOGENS IN PEDIATRIC PNEUMONIA AND RECOMMENDED TREATMENT[8]

Age of Child	Usual Pathogens (in General Order of Predominance)	EMPIRICAL ANTIBIOTIC TREATMENT RECOMMENDED	
		Outpatient	Inpatient
Birth-3 wks	Group B streptococci Gram-negative enteric bacteria Viral causes	Most require inpatient therapy	IV ampicillin and IV gentamicin with or without IV cefotaxime
3 weeks-3 mos	*Chlamydia trachomatis* Viral causes *Streptococcus pneumoniae* *Bordetella pertussis* (rare) *Staphylococcus aureus* (rare)	PO erythromycin or PO azithromycin	(Admit if hypoxia, respiratory distress, or sepsis) IV erythromycin Add IV cefotaxime for signs of sepsis
3 mos-5 yr	Viral causes *S. pneumoniae* *Mycoplasma pneumoniae* (less likely here)	PO amoxicillin	IV ceftriaxone or IV cefotaxime
5-18 yr	Viral causes *M. pneumoniae* *S. pneumoniae*	PO erythromycin, azithromycin, or clarithromycin Consider PO doxycycline if patient >8 yr	IV erythromycin or IV azithromycin Add IV ceftriaxone or IV cefuroxime for sepsis, lobar infiltrate, or effusion

IV, intravenous; PO, oral.
From McIntosh K: Community acquired pneumonia in children. N Engl J Med 2002;346:429-437.

dren. They are caused by a variety of viruses and bacteria, with the prevalence varying by age group[7,8] (Table 45-3). As in adults, *S. pneumoniae* is the predominant organism causing pneumonia except in the newborns, in whom group B streptococci and gram-negative bacilli dominate. *H. influenzae* type b remains an important pneumonia-causing bacterial pathogen in the developing world. It has been nearly eliminated in the United States through immunization practices. Pneumococcal vaccines also appear to be lowering the incidence of invasive pneumococcal disease and pneumonia, but more data are needed.[9] Many viruses, mainly influenza, parainfluenza, and RSV, can also cause pneumonia in children. Most children with pneumonia present with cough, fever, and abnormal lung findings. Signs of tachypnea and increased work of breathing are often present and may be the only signs of disease in infants.[7]

Acute bronchiolitis is typically caused by the RSV or parainfluenza viruses and predominantly affects children younger than 2 years. It can be difficult to distinguish from pneumonia because the clinical features are similar. Bronchiolitis is seasonal, frequently occurring in the winter and early spring months. The affected infant typically has sneezing, rhinorrhea, cough, wheezing, fever, and, possibly, respiratory distress. Chest examination typically demonstrates diffuse fine crackles and expiratory wheezes. Grunting respirations, cyanosis, retractions, and use of accessory muscles are signs of respiratory distress. Antibiotics are not typically indicated in patients with acute bronchiolitis, and treatment is primarily supportive. Bronchodilator therapy with nebulized albuterol or racemic epinephrine may be effective.

Pertussis (whooping cough) is a lower respiratory tract infection worthy of special mention. Caused by the organism *Bordetella pertussis,* it usually affects young children and adolescents. The incidence of the disease has markedly decreased because of immunization. Pertussis manifests in three distinct stages. The first (catarrhal) stage consists of a mild cough, conjunctivitis, and coryza lasting up to 2 weeks. The second stage consists of severe paroxysms of coughing often followed by strong inhalations of air, producing the characteristic "whoop." This stage can last up to 4 weeks. The third (convalescent) stage consists of a chronic cough. The disease is important to identify because multiple complications, such as complete airway obstruction, secondary pneumonia, seizures, and encephalitis, can occur. Treatment is with oral erythromycin or azithromycin. Close contacts of the patient should receive prophylactic antibiotics.[7]

■ THE PATIENT WITH HIV

Pneumonia is one of the most common serious bacterial illnesses affecting patients with HIV. In addition to the common community-acquired pathogens, patients with HIV are more susceptible to opportunistic infections with *Pneumocystis carinii,* pulmonary tuberculosis, and recurrent bacterial pneumonia. Antibiotic chemoprophylaxis, highly active antiretroviral therapy (HAART), and preventive vaccines appear to be significantly improving the incidence and morbidity and mortality of pneumonia in patients with HIV.[10]

■ ASPIRATION PNEUMONIA

Aspiration of oral or gastric contents can occur in the setting of altered mental status or dysfunction of swallowing reflexes due to neurologic impairment such as stroke. Aspiration is typically "silent," and a high index of clinical suspicion is needed for the proper diagnosis to be made. Aspiration can lead to a chemical pneumonitis and a bacterial aspiration pneumonia more than 60% of the time.[4] Abscesses and empyema can occur in more advanced cases. The pathogens involved are typically those found in the oropharynx. Patients who have been recently hospitalized or who reside in nursing homes may be colonized with *S. aureus* or gram-negative bacilli that can cause aspiration pneumonia. Treatment with clindamycin or piperacillin-tazobactam is typically indicated.

■ INFLUENZA

Influenza is one of the most common and most serious viral infections causing pneumonia. Influenza has a seasonal occurrence, typically from December to April. Bacterial superinfections can occur with pneumonia due to influenza, most commonly with *S. pneumoniae* or *S. aureus*. Rapid identification tests are available to assist in diagnosis. Antiviral therapy with amantadine or rimantadine (for influenza A) or oseltamivir (for influenza A and B) may lessen symptoms and quicken recovery if started within 48 hours of illness onset.

Evaluation and Diagnostic Testing

The patient with pneumonia should undergo a complete initial assessment of vital signs, including pulse oximetry and evaluation of respiratory rate.

■ CHEST RADIOGRAPHS

Most authorities agree that chest radiographs (posteroanterior [PA] and lateral, if possible) should be obtained in all patients with suspected pneumonia. The radiographs help confirm the diagnosis of pneumonia and provide possible clues to the causative agent (see Table 45-4). The radiographs will also demonstrate associated conditions, such as lung abscess, bronchial obstruction, and pleural effusion (Figs. 45-2 to 45-4). Computed tomography (CT) may be necessary for further evaluation of complex infiltrates with pleural effusions or suspected masses or abscesses. Although typical radiologic patterns are expected with certain infections (Table 45-4), it is important to remember that multiple factors, such as age, immune status, hydration status, and underlying lung disease, can alter the radiographic appearance of pneumonia.[11]

■ SPUTUM STUDIES

Sputum gram stain and culture should be performed only if a good-quality specimen can be obtained, transported, and processed appropriately. Strong consideration for sputum studies should be made for severe pneumonia and in those patients who are critically ill.[12,13] Sputum cultures should routinely be ordered in cases of suspected hospital-acquired pneumonia, health care–associated pneumonia (HCAP), and ventilator-associated pneumonia (VAP).[14] In the ED setting, sputum studies may be particularly useful in rapid testing for influenza or RSV in peak seasons to help select appropriate antiviral therapy and avoid unnecessary antibiotic use.

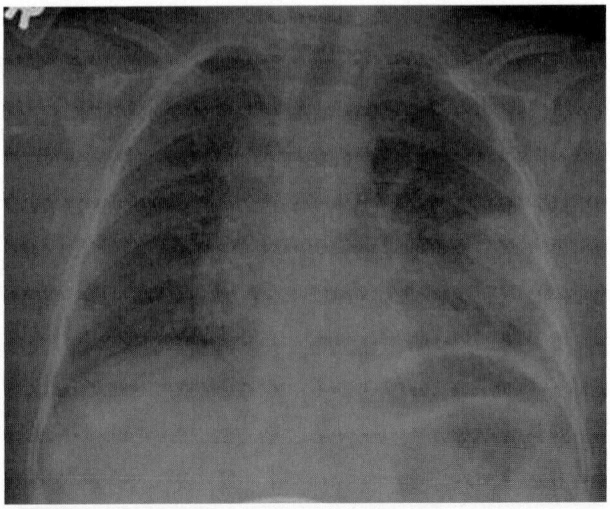

FIGURE 45-2 Chest radiograph of a 33-month-old child showing a left lower lobe infiltrate and a small effusion.

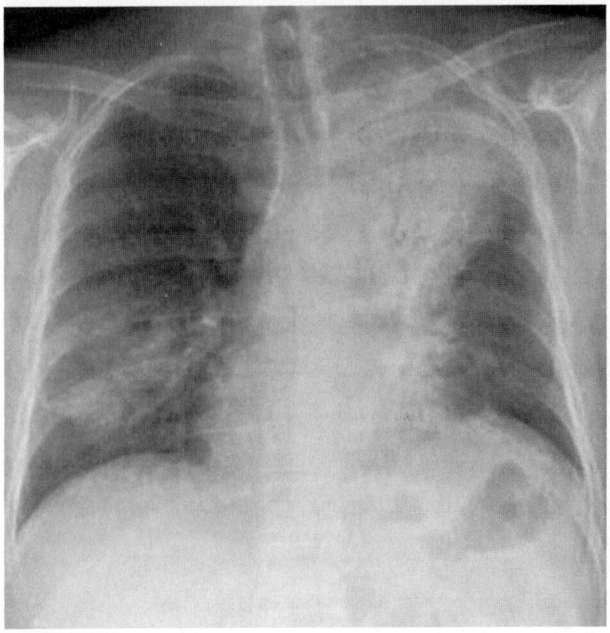

FIGURE 45-3 Chest radiograph of an adult with extensive lobar infiltrate and air bronchograms.

■ BLOOD CULTURES

The IDSA/ATS combined guidelines recommend obtaining two sets of blood cultures in patients admitted with pneumonia prior to the start of antibiotic therapy. However, in a 2005 study of 414 ED patients presenting with pneumonia, Kennedy and colleagues found that blood culture results rarely altered antibiotic therapy decisions. Identification of

Table 45-4 ETIOLOGIC AGENTS OF PNEUMONIA AND COMMON RADIOGRAPHIC PATTERNS

Radiographic Pattern	Pathophysiology	Typical Pathogens
Lobar or multilobar infiltrate with air bronchograms	Edema fluid/inflammatory reaction in the alveoli occurring initially in the periphery of the lung Larger bronchi usually remain patent, causing air bronchograms	Bacterial pneumonias (*Streptococcus pneumoniae, Klebsiella, Legionella*)
Interstitial infiltrates	Edema and inflammatory cellular infiltrate in the interstitial tissue surrounding small airways and vessels	*Mycoplasma pneumoniae, Pneumocystis jirovecii (carinii),* viral pneumonias
Bronchopneumonia	Diffuse patchy infiltrates and peribronchial thickening due to large and intermediate airway involvement	*Staphylococcus aureus,* gram-negative organisms, fungi
Abscesses	Abscess cavity, isolated or within areas of consolidation	*S. aureus, Pseudomonas,* anaerobes
Cavitary masses	Inflammation and necrosis of lung parenchyma	*Mycobacterium tuberculosis, Nocardia, Aspergillus, Actinomyces*

From Tarver R, Teague S, Heitkamp D, et al: Radiology of community acquired pneumonia. Radiol Clin North Am 2005;43:497-512.

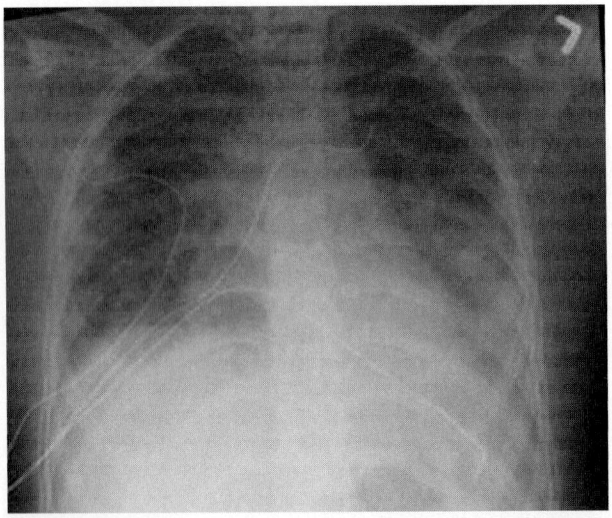

FIGURE 45-4 Chest radiograph of a child showing an interstitial infiltrate.

resistant organisms requiring a broadening of antibiotic therapy was found in only 1% of patients.[15] Obtaining routine blood cultures in patients admitted with pneumonia continues to be recommended.

■ OTHER STUDIES

Complete blood count and basic serum chemistry studies are typically performed in patients with pneumonia who must be admitted to the hospital. The blood count can identify disorders such as lymphopenia (possibly indicating HIV), neutropenia, and anemia, helping to guide appropriate therapy. Electrolyte and glucose abnormalities are often found in patients with pneumonia and testing for them may provide prognostic information. Measurements of blood urea nitrogen and serum creatinine value are important in determining the level of nursing care and appropriate antibiotic dosing for each patient. Urinary studies such as antigen testing for *Legionella* and *S. pneumoniae* may be useful. Bronchoscopy may be considered in patients with HIV, patients who are immunosuppressed, and patients in whom an unusual infection is suspected. Thoracentesis may be necessary if a pleural effusion is present and freely flowing. Ultrasonography may be beneficial in identifying free-flowing effusions and to guide sampling of the fluid for cell count, cultures, pH, and fluid analysis.[13]

Treatment

After decisions about respiratory, hemodynamic, and ventilatory support, the most important decision in treating the patient with pneumonia is the selection of timely and appropriate initial antibiotic therapy. Multiple factors, such as suspected likely infectious causes, severity of illness, recent antibiotic therapy, patient disposition, antibiotic allergies, and comorbid illnesses, all contribute to the selection of the optimum antimicrobial therapy.

As already described, the ATS and IDSA have issued detailed guidelines for the treatment of community-acquired pneumonia. Several studies have demonstrated a lower mortality among hospitalized patients treated within guideline-recommended antimicrobial regimens.[5] In a 2004 study of 420 patients with pneumonia, Mortensen and colleagues[16] found significantly lower 30-day mortality in patients who received antimicrobial therapy in concordance with the ATS or IDSA guidelines.

The recommendations of the guidelines are summarized in Box 45-1. The guidelines group recommendations according to site of therapy (outpatient, inpatient, or ICU), severity of disease, comorbid illnesses, and risks for resistant organisms or *Pseudomonas aeruginosa.*

Ideally, antibiotic therapy should be started in the ED as soon as the diagnosis is made.

BOX 45-1

Recommended Empirical Antibiotics for Community-Acquired Pneumonia

Outpatient Treatment

1. Previously healthy and no use of antimicrobials within the previous 3 months:
   A macrolide (strong recommendation; level I evidence)
   Doxycycline (weak recommendation; level III evidence)
2. Presence of comorbidities such as chronic heart, lung, liver, or renal disease; diabetes mellitus; alcoholism; malignancies; asplenia; immunosuppressing conditions or use of immunosuppressing drugs; or use of antimicrobials within the previous 3 months (in which case an alternative from a different class should be selected):
   A respiratory fluoroquinolone (moxifloxacin, gemifloxacin, or levofloxacin [750 mg]) (strong recommendation; level I evidence)
   A β-lactam **plus** a macrolide (strong recommendation; level I evidence)
3. In regions with a high rate (>25%) of infection with high-level (MIC ≥16 μg/mL) macrolide-resistant *Streptococcus pneumoniae*, consider use of alternative agents listed above in (2) for patients without comorbidities (moderate recommendation; level III evidence)

Inpatients, Non-ICU Treatment

A respiratory fluoroquinolone (strong recommendation; level I evidence)

A β-lactam **plus** a macrolide (strong recommendation; level I evidence)

Inpatients, ICU Treatment

A β-lactam (cefotaxime, ceftriaxone, or ampicillin-sulbactum) **plus** either azithromycin (level II evidence) **or** a respiratory fluoroquinolone (level I evidence) (strong recommendation) (for penicillin-allergic patients, a respiratory fluoroquinolone and aztreonam are recommended)

Special Concerns

If *Pseudomonas* is a consideration:

An antipneumococcal, antipseudomonal β-lactam (piperacillin-tazobactam, cefepime, imipenem, or meropenem) plus either ciprofloxacin or levofloxacin (750 mg)

or

The above β-lactam plus an aminoglycoside and azithromycin

or

The above β-lactam plus an aminoglycoside and an antipneumococcal fluoroquinolone (for penicillin-allergic patients, substitute aztreonam for above β-lactam) (moderate recommendation; level III evidence)

If community-acquired methicillin-resistant *Staphylococcus aureus* is a consideration, add vancomycin or linezolid (moderate recommendation; level III evidence)

ICU, intensive care unit; MIC, minimal inhibitory concentration.
From Mandell LA, Wunderink RG, Anzueto A, et al: Infectious Diseases Society of America/American Thoracic Society consensus guidelines on the management of community-acquired pneumonia in adults. Clin Infect Dis 2007;44:S27–S72.

PRIORITY ACTIONS

- Provide immediate supplemental oxygen and/or ventilatory assistance to the patient with suspected pneumonia as needed.
- A mask should be placed over the face and nose of any patient with suspected pneumonia to prevent spread of disease to other patients waiting for evaluation.
- Antibiotic therapy should be ideally initiated in the ED as soon as the diagnosis is made.

■ HEALTH CARE–ASSOCIATED PNEUMONIA

In the current era of shorter hospital stays and expanded home and long-term care facility treatment, the EP frequently encounters patients at risk for health care–associated pneumonia (HCAP). In 2005, a joint committee of the ATS and IDSA published an additional set of guidelines for the evaluation and treatment of HCAP. They also apply to hospital-acquired pneumonia (HAP) and ventilator-associated pneumonia (VAP). The guidelines emphasize that HCAP can be caused by a wide variety of bacteria, including multidrug-resistant pathogens, gram-negative organisms, and MRSA, and is often polymicrobial. It is recommended that sputum cultures be obtained in all such patients, prior to antibiotic therapy if possible. The recommendations for initial empirical antibiotic therapy are summarized in Table 45-5. The commission also recognized the variability of bacterial pathogens from one institution to another and recommended that local microbiologic data be taken into account in the selection of antibiotic therapy.[18]

Patient Disposition

There are several validated prediction tools to guide admission decisions for patients with pneumonia. These tools all evaluate important patient characteristics, such as age, vital signs, radiographic and laboratory data, and comorbidities, and identify patients at increased risk for 30-day mortality.

In 1997 the Pneumonia Patient Outcomes Research Team (PORT)[17] published a prediction rule to identify patients at low risk for death from pneumonia within 30 days; it is now known as the PORT Criteria or Pneumonia Severity Index. A 2005 comparison of three prediction guidelines by Aujesky and colleagues[18] found the Pneumonia Severity Index to be the most accurate in identifying low-risk and high-risk patients with pneumonia. The system was developed through analysis of data from thousands of patients with community-acquired pneumonia and was validated in more than 50,000 patients. Patients are divided into five classes based on increasing risk of mortality. Class I (mortality 0.1%-0.4%) is assigned on the basis of an age of 50 years or less and key information from the history and physical examination. Other classes are identified with a point system calculated from the presence of historical data and physical and laboratory findings (Box 45-2).[17]

Class I and class II patients are considered at very low risk (30-day mortality <1%) and can likely be treated as outpatients. Many patients in class III (30-day mortality <2.8%) might also be candidates for outpatient treatment. Patients in class IV or class V

PATIENT TEACHING TIPS

- Encourage outpatients to finish their course of antibiotics, even if they start to feel better earlier, because not finishing the full course of medicine could lead to incomplete treatment of the infection and clinical relapse.
- Because most respiratory infections are spread by means of droplets, the patient with pneumonia should be told to wash hands frequently, not share utensils or cups, and cover the mouth when coughing to prevent spread of the infection to close contacts. The patient may wish to wear a mask over the mouth and nose when around others who have chronic lung disease or are immunosuppressed.
- The patient should be encouraged to return to the ED if he or she experiences worsening of symptoms or increasing shortness of breath.

Table 45-5 INITIAL EMPIRICAL ANTIBIOTIC THERAPY RECOMMENDATIONS FOR HEALTH CARE–ASSOCIATED PNEUMONIA

Situation	Potential Pathogens	Recommended Antibiotic
No known risk factors for multidrug-resistant pathogens,* early onset (<5 days hospitalization)	*Streptococcus pneumoniae, Haemophilus influenzae,* methicillin-resistant *Streptococcus aureus* (MRSA), antibiotic-sensitive gram-negative organisms (*Escherichia coli, Klebsiella, Enterobacter, Proteus, Serratia*)	Ceftriaxone *OR* Advanced fluoroquinolone *OR* Ampicillin/sulbactam *OR* Ertapenem
Late-onset disease (≥5 days) or risk factors present for multidrug-resistant pathogens*	As above plus: *Pseudomonas* *Klebsiella* (extended-spectrum beta-lactamase [ESBL]) *Acinetobacter* (ESBL) MRSA *Legionella*	Antipseudomonal cephalosporin (cefepime, ceftazidime) *OR* Antipseudomonal carbipenem (imipenem or meropenem) *OR* Piperacillin/tazobactam *plus* antipseudomonal fluoroquinolone (ciprofloxacin or levofloxacin) *OR* Aminoglycoside (amikacin, gentamicin, tobramycin) *plus* linezolid or vancomycin†

*Risks include antimicrobial therapy in preceding 90 days, current hospitalization of 5 days or more, high frequency of antibiotic resistance in the institution or community, hospitalization for 2 days or more in the preceding 90 days, residence in a nursing home or extended-care facility, home infusion therapy, long-term dialysis within 30 days, home wound care, a family member with multidrug-resistant pathogens, and immunosuppressive diseases/therapy.

†If MRSA is a risk factor or has a high incidence locally.

From American Thoracic Society: Guidelines for the management of adults with hospital-acquired, ventilator-associated, and healthcare-associated pneumonia. Am J Respir Crit Care Med 2005;171;388-416.

BOX 45-2

Summary of Risk Class Assignment for Patients with Pneumonia Based on the Pneumonia Severity Index (PORT Criteria)

Step 1

Does patient have one or more of the following features?

- Age >50 years
- Neoplastic disease
- Congestive heart failure
- Cerebrovascular disease
- Renal disease
- Liver diseases
- Altered mental status
- Pulse ≥125 beats/min
- Respiratory rate ≥30 beats/min
- Systolic blood pressure <90 mm Hg
- Temperature <35° or ≥40° C

No: Assign to risk class I.

Yes: Go to Step 2.

Step 2

Assign points to patient's risk score according to presence of the following characteristics:

Characteristic	**Point(s) Assigned**
Age:	
Men	Age in years (1 point for each year)
Women	Age in years (1 point for each year) –10
Nursing home residency	+10
Coexisting Illnesses	
Neoplastic disease	+30
Liver disease	+20
Congestive heart failure	+10
Cerebrovascular disease	+10
Renal disease	+10
Physical Findings	
Altered mental status	+20
Respiratory rate ≥30 breaths/min	+20
Systolic blood pressure <90 mm Hg	+20
Temperature <35° or ≥40° C	+15
Pulse ≥125 beats/min	+10
Laboratory and Radiographic Findings	
Arterial pH<7.35	+30
Blood urea nitrogen ≥30 mg/dL	+20
Sodium <130 mmol/L	+20
Blood glucose ≥250 mg/dL	+10
Hematocrit <30%	+10
Pao_2 <60 mm Hg or pulse oximetry value <90%	+10
Pleural effusion	+10

Step 3

Use the total points accumulated in Step 2 to assign the patient to the corresponding risk class, as follows:

- ≤70—class II
- 71-90—class III
- 91-130—class IV
- >130—class V

Data from references 17 and 18.

are at much higher risk (30-day mortality 8.5%-31.1%) and should probably be admitted.[18]

It must be emphasized that this prediction rule is only a guideline. Many other factors, such as unique comorbidities, psychosocial factors, ability to take oral medications, and patient and caregiver reliability must also be considered in the decision to admit the patient to the hospital or discharge. Patients demonstrating signs of shock or respiratory distress should be treated in an ICU setting.

REFERENCES

1. Centers for Disease Control and Prevention (CDC): Pneumonia and influenza death rates—United States, 1979-1994. MMWR Morb Mortal Wkly Rep 1995;44:535-537.
2. Bartlett J, Dowell S, Mandell L, et al: Practice guidelines for the management of community acquired pneumonia in adults. Clin Infect Dis 2000;31:347-382.
3. File T, Niederman M: Antimicrobial therapy of community-acquired pneumonia. Infect Dis Clin North Am 2004;18: 993-1016.
4. Donowitz G, Mandell G: Acute pneumonia. In Mandell GL, Bennett JE, Doline R (eds): Mandell, Douglas, and Bennett's Principles and Practice of Infectious Disease, 6th ed. Philadelphia, Elsevier, 2005, pp 819-841.
5. Niederman M: Review of treatment guidelines for community acquired pneumonia. Am J Med 2004;117:51S-57S.
6. Fine M, Smith M, Carson C, et al: Prognosis and outcomes of patients with community acquired pneumonia: A meta-analysis. JAMA 1996;275:134-141.
7. Fleisher FR: Infectious disease emergencies. In Fleisher GR, Ludwig S, Henretig FM, et al (eds): Textbook of Pediatric Emergency Medicine, 5th ed. Philadelphia, Lippincott Williams & Wilkins, 2006, pp 783-851.
8. McIntosh K: Community acquired pneumonia in children. N Engl J Med 2002;346:429-437.
9. Lucero M, Dulalia VE, Parreno RN: Pneumococcal conjugate vaccines for preventing vaccine-type invasive pneumococcal disease and pneumonia with consolidation on x-ray in children under two years of age. Cochrane Database Syst Rev 2004;(1):CD 004977.
10. Feldman C: Pneumonia associated with HIV infection. Curr Opin Infect Dis 2005;18:165-170.
11. Tarver R, Teague S, Heitkamp D, et al: Radiology of community acquired pneumonia. Radiol Clin North Am 2005;43:497-512.
12. Mandell LA, Wunderink PG, Anzueto A, et al: Infectious Diseases Society of America/American Thoracic Society consensus guidelines on the management of community-acquired pneumonia in adults. Clin Infect Dis 2007;44: S27-S72.
13. Mandell L, Bartlett J, Dowell S, et al: Update of practice guidelines for the management of community-acquired pneumonia in immunocompetent adults. Clin Infect Dis 2003;37:1405-1433.
14. American Thoracic Society: Guidelines for the management of adults with hospital-acquired, ventilator-associated, and healthcare-associated pneumonia. Am J Respir Crit Care Med 2005;171:388-416.
15. Kennedy M, Bates D, Wright S, et al: Do emergency department blood cultures change practice in patients with pneumonia? Ann Emerg Med 2005;46:393-400.
16. Mortensen E, Restrepo M, Anzueto A, et al: Effects of guideline-concordant antimicrobial therapy on mortality among patients with community-acquired pneumonia. Am J Med 2004;117:726-731.
17. Fine M, Auble T, Yealy D, et al: A prediction rule to identify low-risk patients with community acquired pneumonia. N Engl J Med 1997;336:243-250.
18. Aujesky D, Auble T, Yealy D, et al: Prospective comparison of three validated prediction rules for prognosis in community-acquired pneumonia. Am J Med 2005;118: 384-392.

Chapter **46**

Pneumothorax

David E. Manthey and Bret Nicks

KEY POINTS

- Primary pneumothoraces occur in patients without clinically apparent lung disease and can be classified as spontaneous or traumatic.
- Chronic obstructive pulmonary disease is the most common cause of secondary pneumothorax.
- The ability of the physical examination to detect a pneumothorax is limited.
- Standard posteroanterior and lateral chest radiographs are the only routine examination needed. Expiratory films add little.
- Treatment of a pneumothorax is based on its cause, size, and stability, the symptomatology of the patient, and the presence or absence of underlying lung disease. It includes observation, catheter aspiration, and tube thoracostomy in the ED.

Scope

Under normal conditions, the parietal and visceral pleura are in close apposition with only a small potential space between them. The presence of free air in the intrapleural space implies a *pneumothorax*. As there are many etiologies for pneumothoraces, the classification categories primary and secondary are commonly used.

Primary pneumothoraces occur in individuals without clinically apparent lung disease. They can occur spontaneously or from penetration of the intrapleural space by trauma. Secondary pneumothoraces occur in patients with underlying lung disease.

Primary spontaneous pneumothorax occurs at a rate of 10 to 18 cases per 100,000 per year in men and 5 cases per 100,000 in women. It has a peak incidence in young adults (20-30 years). Factors associated with primary spontaneous pneumothorax are male gender, cigarette smoking, mitral valve prolapse, Marfan's syndrome, and changes in ambient pressure. Physical exertion does not appear to be a precipitating factor in patients without apparent lung disease. Familial patterns also suggest an inherited association with primary spontaneous pneumothorax.[1] Patients with a spontaneous pneumothorax have a 30% recurrence rate within 2 years after air evacuation only; patients who have experienced two pneumothoraces have about an 80% chance of recurrent pneumothorax.

Traumatic pneumothoraces are subdivided into iatrogenic (due to a medical intervention or procedure) and noniatrogenic (due to direct or indirect trauma unrelated to a medical intervention).

Secondary pneumothoraces make up one third of spontaneous pneumothoraces and occur with underlying pulmonary disease (Box 46-1). Of note, chronic obstructive pulmonary disease (COPD) is the most common cause of secondary spontaneous pneumothorax. Recurrences are common, so recurrence prevention treatment is indicated after the first episode.

BOX 46-1

Etiologies for Secondary Pneumothoraces

- Airway diseases:
  - Chronic obstructive pulmonary disease: most common cause of secondary spontaneous pneumothorax
  - Asthma
  - Cystic fibrosis: 8% to 20% of patients with this disease experience a pneumothorax in their lifetimes
- Infections:
  - Human immunodeficiency virus infection—*Pneumocystis carinii* pneumonia
  - Lung abscess
  - Necrotizing bacterial pneumonia
  - Tuberculosis
- Interstitial lung diseases:
  - Sarcoidosis
  - Pulmonary fibrosis
  - Pneumoconiosis
  - Tuberous sclerosis
- Connective tissue diseases:
  - Rheumatoid arthritis
  - Scleroderma
  - Marfan's syndrome
  - Ehlers-Danlos syndrome
- Cancer
  - Primary (lung)
  - Metastatic
- Catamenial pneumothorax

Pathophysiology

The pleural space lies between the parietal and visceral pleura and is normally negatively pressured at −5 mm Hg with fluctuations of 6 to 8 mm Hg between inspiration and expiration. With the loss of the normal negative pressure, the affected lung collapses. A primary spontaneous pneumothorax occurs when a subpleural bleb, most commonly in the lung apex, ruptures into the pleural space. In secondary spontaneous pneumothorax, rupture of the visceral pleura and alveolar barrier is most commonly due to the underlying pulmonary disease process.

Open chest wounds occur when the diameter of the chest wall defect is greater than two thirds the size of the trachea. At this point, air preferentially enters the pleural cavity during inspiration (negative intrathoracic pressure) via the chest wall defect instead of the trachea. This leaves the lungs without oxygenation or ventilation. A *tension pneumothorax* occurs when a one-way valve develops from the injured lung, by which air enters the pleura during inspiration but cannot escape during expiration. Tension physiology occurs when the increased intrathoracic pressure (>15-20 mm Hg) compresses the great vessels and pericardium and limits the return of venous blood flow from the body and the lungs to the heart, thereby causing hypotension. The increased intrapleural pressure also compresses the contralateral lung, causing hypoxia and asphyxia.

Presenting Signs and Symptoms

■ CLASSIC

Classically, the symptoms of primary spontaneous pneumothorax are sudden onset of ipsilateral, pleuritic chest pain and associated dyspnea. The pain typically begins at rest and is worsened with deep inspiration. It may eventually become a dull persistent ache that does not vary with respiration. Profound dyspnea is rare in the absence of a tension pneumothorax or underlying parenchymal disease. Physical findings correlate with the degree of symptoms. Sinus tachycardia is the most common physical finding, with other classic signs—decreased breath sounds, hyperresonance to percussion, unilateral enlargement of the hemithorax, absence of tactile fremitus, and decreased excursion volumes—occurring less frequently and in larger pneumothoraces. Cough is not a common complaint in pneumothorax.

Symptoms may resolve in 24 hours without resolution of the pneumothorax. Many patients (45%) may delay seeking medical care for 48 hours.

The ability of auscultation to detect hemothorax, pneumothorax, or hemopneumothorax associated with penetrating trauma had a sensitivity of 58%, a specificity of 98%, and a positive predictive value of 98% in one study.[2] Auscultation can miss up to 600 mL of hemothorax, a pneumothorax up to 28%, and a combined hemopneumothorax up to 800 mL and 28%.[2] Physical examination alone is not sensitive enough to exclude the diagnosis of pneumothorax.

Table 46-1 lists the differential diagnosis for pneumothorax.

■ VARIATIONS

■ Tension Pneumothorax

The patient with a tension pneumothorax exhibits extreme dyspnea, hypotension, and cyanosis. Physical findings are hyperresonance, hyperinflation, and absence of breath sounds on the affected side with deviation of the trachea (at the sternal notch) away from the affected side. Tachycardia usually consists of a pulse of 120 to 130 beats/min. Patients with this presentation should undergo immediate tube thoracostomy (or needle thoracostomy if a chest tube is not immediately available) without waiting for a confirmatory radiograph.

Table 46-1 DIFFERENTIAL DIAGNOSIS FOR PNEUMOTHORAX

Pulmonary embolism	Perform a risk stratification based on Wells or Charlotte criteria If result of stratification is not low probability and D-dimer test result is negative, proceed to computed tomography–pulmonary angiogram Chest radiograph may show infarcted lung
Pleurisy	Look for underlying disease process (connective tissue, pneumonia) Pleura-based diseases (pneumonia, tumor, effusion) often have radiographic findings
Pneumonia	Chest radiography will be helpful Clinical examination and history may suggest pneumonia because of cough (uncommon in pneumothorax), upper respiratory symptoms, fever, or immunosuppression
Pericarditis	Look for underlying disease process Check electrocardiogram (ECG) for classic but not common PR segment depression and/or widespread ST elevation Does position affect the pain (less with leaning forward, less with lying back)? Consider ultrasonography to diagnose effusion
Myocardial infarction	Assess for appropriate risk factors Evaluate with ECG and cardiac marker measurements if suspicious ECG findings associated with a pneumothorax include axis deviation, decreased voltage, and T-wave inversion
Aortic dissection	Typically, interscapular back pain with tearing sensation Check chest radiograph for widened mediastinum, apical capping, left-sided pleural effusion, blurring of aortic knob, or displacement of trachea or esophagus to anatomic right Consider checking bilateral arm pressures Look for neurologic deficit or end-organ ischemia
Musculoskeletal pain	Is the pain reproducible with palpation and use of the muscle group? Is there a history consistent with muscle injury? Are the chest radiography and ECG findings normal?
Pneumomediastinum	Subcutaneous emphysema on physical examination? Mediastinal, pericardiac, or prevertebral air on chest radiograph? Typically occurs during a Valsalva maneuver or exertion

■ Secondary Pneumothoraces

Patients with pneumothoraces due to underlying lung disease may experience extreme dyspnea secondary to the deflation of one lung and the limited capacity and function of the remaining lung. Classically, symptoms do not resolve without intervention. Owing to the underlying lung disease (most commonly COPD), lung findings may be abnormal, with hyperinflation and decreased lung sounds.

Diagnostic Testing

■ RADIOGRAPHY

The primary evaluation tool is the standard posteroanterior chest radiograph. The EP should look for loss of lung markings in the periphery as well as a pleural line that runs parallel to the chest wall and does not extend outside the chest cavity (Fig. 46-1). A lateral radiograph contributes to the diagnosis in 14% of cases.[3] There is no evidence that an expiratory radiograph adds any value even in small apical pneumothoraces.[4] The sensitivity for flat anteroposterior chest radiography, compared with computed tomography (CT) as the gold standard, has been found to be 75.5% (95% confidence interval [CI] = 61.7%-86.2%), and the specificity 100% (95% CI = 97.1%-100%).[5]

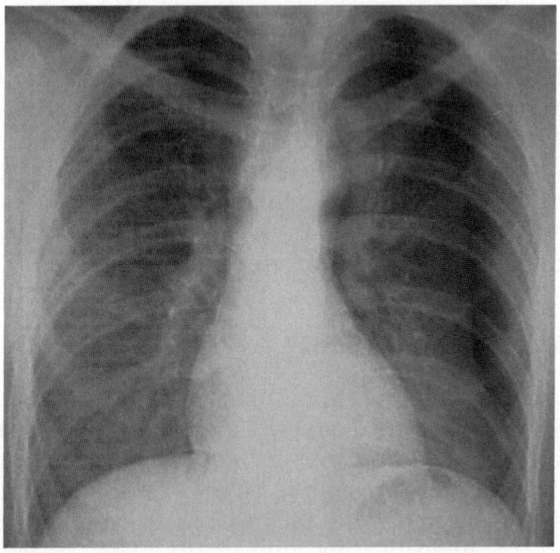

FIGURE 46-1 Radiograph of pneumothorax showing the absence of lung markings in the periphery and the pleural line following the curvature of the chest wall.

The shift of the mediastinum away from a pneumothorax on a chest radiograph can be a normal phenomenon, occurring without tension physiology. In critically ill patients, in whom the radiograph can only be taken in the supine position, the EP should look for the "deep sulcus" sign, a deep lateral costophrenic angle (Fig. 46-2). Diaphragmatic depression

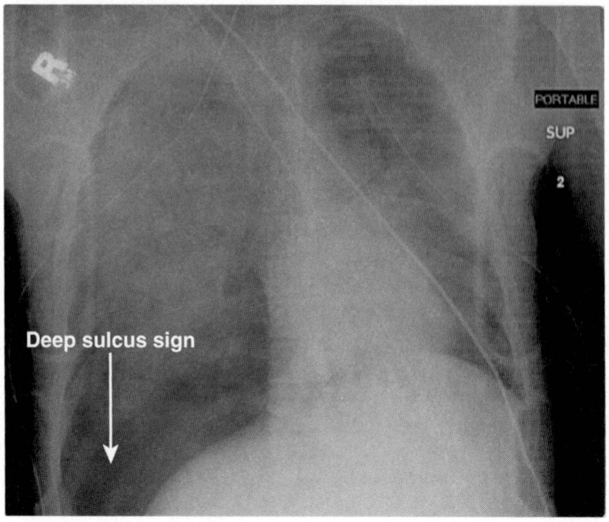
PORTABLE
SUP
Deep sulcus sign

FIGURE 46-2 Deep sulcus sign.

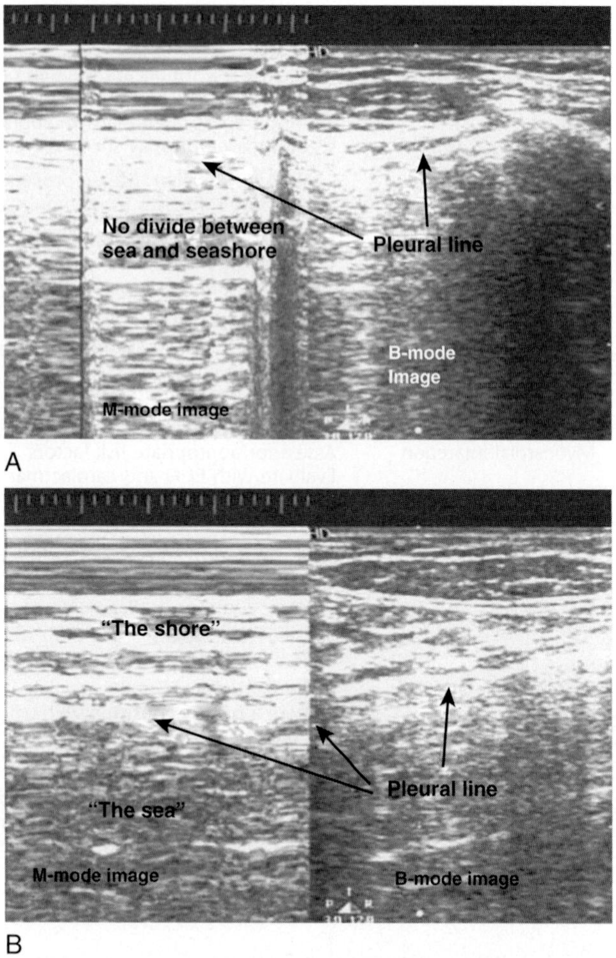
No divide between sea and seashore
Pleural line
B-mode Image
M-mode image
A
"The shore"
Pleural line
"The sea"
M-mode image
B-mode image
B

FIGURE 46-3 Ultrasonograms of abnormal (**A**) and normal (**B**) pleura with M-mode and B-mode imaging. (Courtesy of Christopher L. Moore, MD, Yale University School of Medicine.)

or ipsilateral transradiancy (fewer lung markings, clearer image) may also be seen.[6]

Large bullae can be mistaken for a pneumothorax. In a pneumothorax, the pleural line runs parallel with the chest wall, whereas bullae more commonly have a medially concave appearance and are limited to a single lobe. A chest CT scan helps differentiate these entities.

Pleural adhesions may alter the appearance of the pneumothorax by tethering the lung to the chest wall. Clothing, hair, and skin folds may appear as visceral pleural lines but often continue beyond the chest wall.

In most cases, a radiograph is sufficient to identify a pneumothorax. If it is not, EPs should consider additional modalities if they strongly suspect a pneumothorax, particularly if the patient is unstable, there is underlying lung disease (and thus no reserve if a pneumothorax is missed), or when the patient is undergoing positive pressure ventilation.

ULTRASONOGRAPHY

Normal lung shows a shimmering echogenic stripe of both the parietal and visceral pleura on ultrasonography. A sliding sign at the pleural stripe can be seen with the movement of the visceral pleura in relation to the parietal pleura. Doppler mode can be used to identify this movement. The "seashore analogy" refers to the movement of the lung (ocean) against the stationary chest wall (shore). A comet tail reverberation can be seen distal to the pleura when there is no pneumothorax. The sliding sign of the pleural stripe and the comet tail reverberation are lost with a pneumothorax[7] (Fig. 46-3).

The sensitivity for ultrasonography has been found to be 98.1% (95% CI = 89.9%-99.9%) and the specificity was 99.2% (95% CI = 95.6%-99.9%), making it more sensitive than a flat plate anteroposterior radiograph as would be utilized in a trauma patient.[5] The use of ultrasonography as part of a focused assessment with sonography for trauma (FAST) examination has not been established, but we would advocate for its use in the unstable patient with suspected pneumothorax or in the patient undergoing positive-pressure ventilation. Although an algorithm for determining the size of the pneumothorax has been suggested, it has not been validated.

COMPUTED TOMOGRAPHY

CT is more accurate than radiography in the detection of pneumothoraces, detecting between 25% and 40% of pneumothoraces after lung biopsy that were not visualized on postprocedure chest radiographs.[8] Up to 50% of traumatic pneumothoraces may be occult.[9] CT can detect other problems, such as pulmonary blebs, vascular abnormalities, contusions, infiltrates, and tumors. There is no consensus on when chest CT scan should be used in the evaluation of a primary spontaneous pneumothorax after chest radiography findings are negative. Chest CT is best used in patients with a second pneumothorax to look for underlying lung disease or if there is a persistent

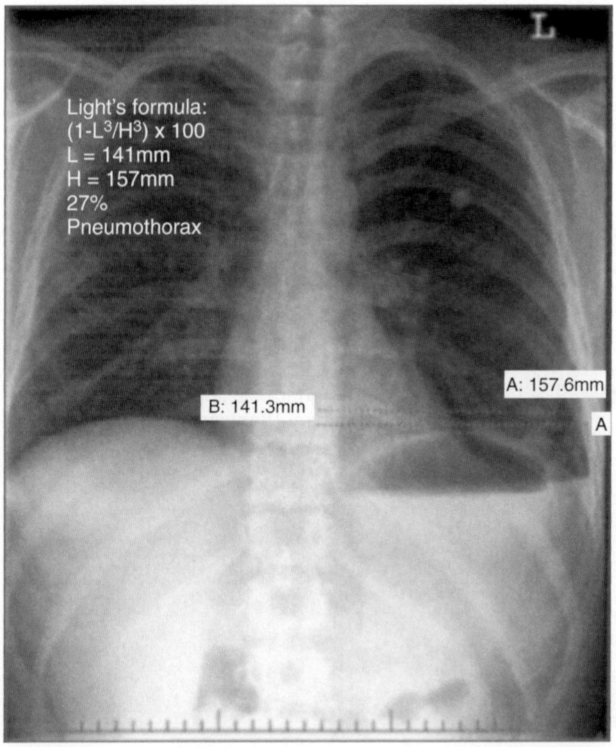
Light's formula:
(1-L³/H³) x 100
L = 141mm
H = 157mm
27%
Pneumothorax
A: 157.6mm
B: 141.3mm
A
L

FIGURE 46-4 Light's formula being applied in a patient with a left-sided pneumothorax.

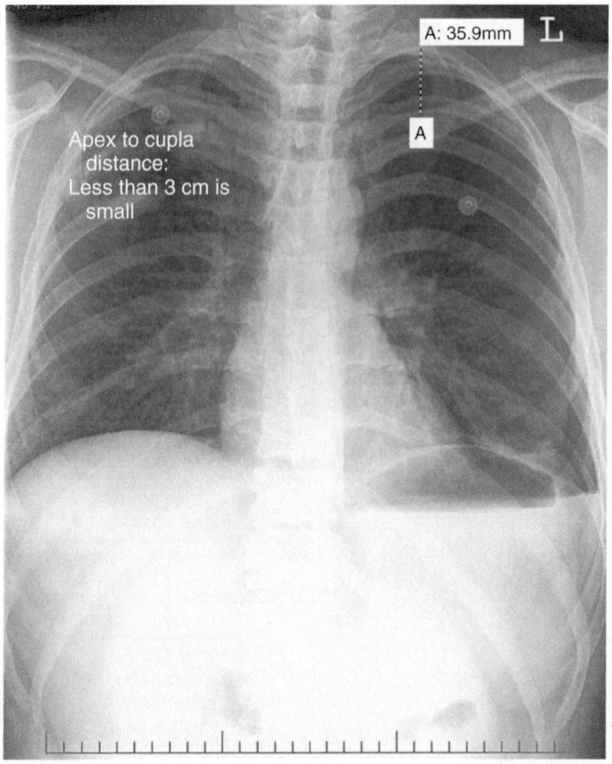
A: 35.9mm
L
A
Apex to cupla
distance:
Less than 3 cm is
small

FIGURE 46-5 Apex-to-cupula measurement performed in a patient with a left-sided pneumothorax.

air leak. We suggest consideration of chest CT in symptomatic high-risk patients with suspected occult pneumothorax, such as those who have underlying lung disease, are undergoing positive-pressure ventilation, or have just undergone lung biopsy.

■ DETERMINING SIZE OF THE PNEUMOTHORAX

Light's formula (Fig. 46-4) is used to estimate the percentage of lung tissue affected by the pneumothorax. The formula is as follows:

$$\text{Percentage pneumothorax} = \frac{1 - L^3}{H^3} \times 100$$

where *H* is the diameter of the hemithorax, and *L* is the diameter of the "collapsed" lung, as measured on a chest radiograph. This diameter is measured at the widest point of the pneumothorax in relation to the lung tissue. Less than 20% is considered a small pneumothorax.

Another method is to measure from the apex of the lung to the cupula of the thoracic cavity on an upright posteroanterior radiograph (Fig. 46-5). Less than 3 cm is considered small. Both of these methods are used to direct treatment.

CT-directed size classification allows grading of occult pneumothoraces. *Minuscule* refers to air collections less than 1 cm thick that appear on fewer than 5 contiguous 10-mm slices. *Anterior* pneumothoraces are air collections more than 1 cm thick that appear on 5 or more contiguous 10-mm slices and do not extend to the midcoronal line (Fig. 46-6). *Anterolateral* pneumothoraces extend to the midcoronal line or beyond.

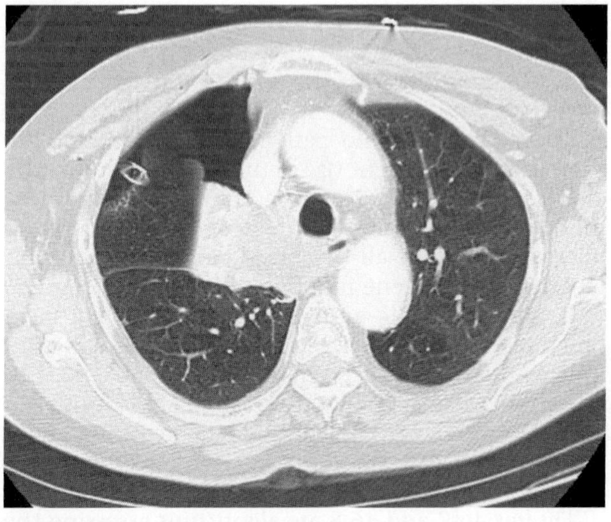

FIGURE 46-6 CT scan of the chest showing anterior pneumothorax and chest tube.

Treatment

Oxygen should be administered to all patients with pneumothorax because it helps in the resorption of the pneumothorax and increases oxygenation of the

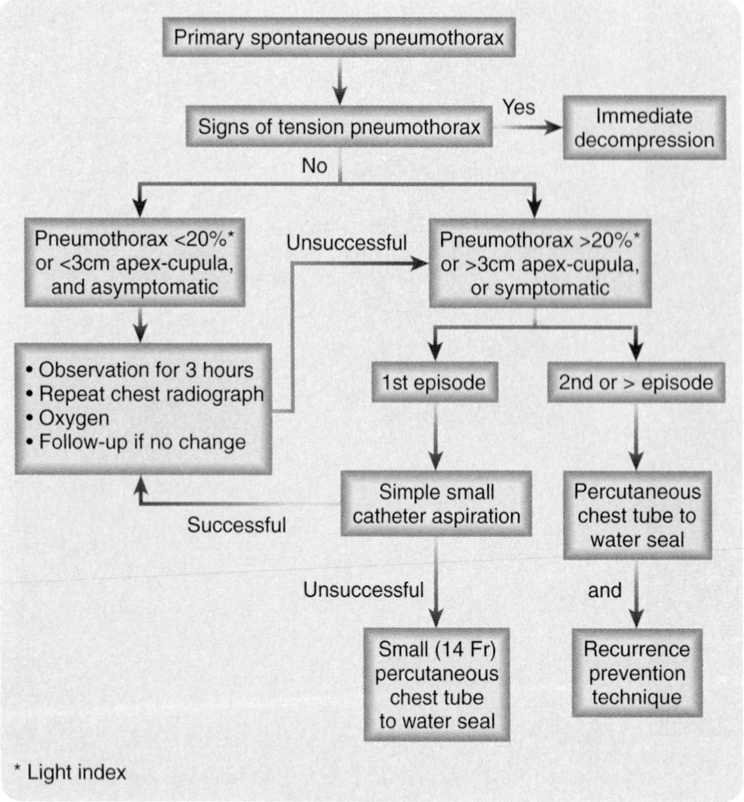

Primary spontaneous pneumothorax
Signs of tension pneumothorax
Yes
Immediate decompression
No
Pneumothorax <20%* or <3cm apex-cupula, and asymptomatic
Unsuccessful
Pneumothorax >20%* or >3cm apex-cupula, or symptomatic
• Observation for 3 hours
• Repeat chest radiograph
• Oxygen
• Follow-up if no change
1st episode
2nd or > episode
Simple small catheter aspiration
Percutaneous chest tube to water seal
Successful
Unsuccessful
and
Small (14 Fr) percutaneous chest tube to water seal
Recurrence prevention technique
* Light index

FIGURE 46-7 Algorithmic approach to the treatment of primary spontaneous pneumothorax.

available alveoli in the noncollapsed lung. The untreated resorption rate is 1% to 2% per day, which increases fourfold with the administration of 100% oxygen.[10]

The stability of the patient, the severity of the symptoms, the current size of the pneumothorax, the change in size over time, the etiology of the pneumothorax (iatrogenic), and the severity of underlying lung disease must all be considered in the decision whether to intervene in a pneumothorax.

A stable patient with pneumothorax has been described as one who has a respiratory rate less than 24 breaths/min, a heart rate between 60 and 120 beats/min, a normal blood pressure, and an oxygen saturation greater than 90% when breathing room air and who can speak in full sentences between breaths.[9]

Figures 46-7 and 46-8 are algorithms assessing the need for intervention in the patient with a primary spontaneous pneumothorax or traumatic pneumothorax, respectively. Patients with bilateral pneumothoraces are treated with aspiration or chest tube placement.

Patients with secondary pneumothoraces should be admitted. Treatment can still be based on clinical stability and size of pneumothorax. The clinically stable patient with a small pneumothorax can be observed or treated with a chest tube. The patient who is not at risk for large air leaks and has a small pneumothorax can be treated with aspiration using a small-bore catheter. The clinically unstable patient or the stable patient with a large pneumothorax should be treated with a chest tube.

Chest tube sizes for patients with spontaneous pneumothoraces are recommended as follows: Catheter (simple) aspiration seems to be as effective as chest tube treatment in the first episode of a primary spontaneous pneumothorax. The clinically stable patient with a large pneumothorax is treated with aspiration using a small-bore catheter (<14F) or with a 16F to 22F chest tube. The clinically unstable patient with a large primary pneumothorax can also be treated with a 16F to 22F chest tube. A larger (24F-28F) chest tube should be used for the patient requiring positive-pressure ventilation, the patient at risk for large pleural air leaks (bronchopleural fistula), and the unstable patient with a secondary spontaneous pneumothorax. In traumatic pneumothoraces, a 28F to 36F chest tube should be used because of the risk for associated hemothorax.

Postprocedure monitoring and radiographs should be performed to assess the success of the intervention and the position of the chest tube (Fig. 46-9).

■ TENSION PNEUMOTHORAX

Emergency needle aspiration is usually performed by emergency medical services personnel when a tension pneumothorax is suspected. In an ED setting, placement of a chest tube more reliably and more definitively addresses the problem in a relatively short time.

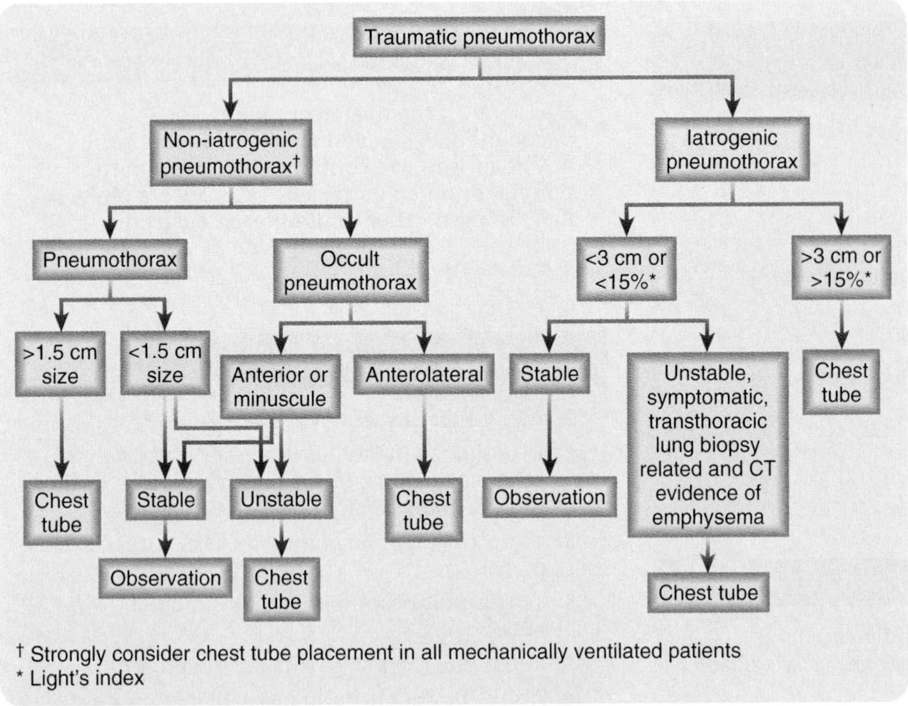
Traumatic pneumothorax
Non-iatrogenic pneumothorax†
Iatrogenic pneumothorax
Pneumothorax
Occult pneumothorax
<3 cm or <15%*
>3 cm or >15%*
>1.5 cm size
<1.5 cm size
Anterior or minuscule
Anterolateral
Stable
Unstable, symptomatic, transthoracic lung biopsy related and CT evidence of emphysema
Chest tube
Chest tube
Stable
Unstable
Chest tube
Observation
Observation
Chest tube
Chest tube
† Strongly consider chest tube placement in all mechanically ventilated patients
* Light's index

FIGURE 46-8 Algorithmic approach to the treatment of traumatic pneumothorax. *According to Light's formula. †Chest tube placement should be strongly considered in all mechanically ventilated patients. (Adapted from Baumann MH: Non-spontaneous pneumothorax. In Light RW, Lee YCG [eds]: Textbook of Pleural Diseases. London, Arnold, 2003, pp 464-474.)

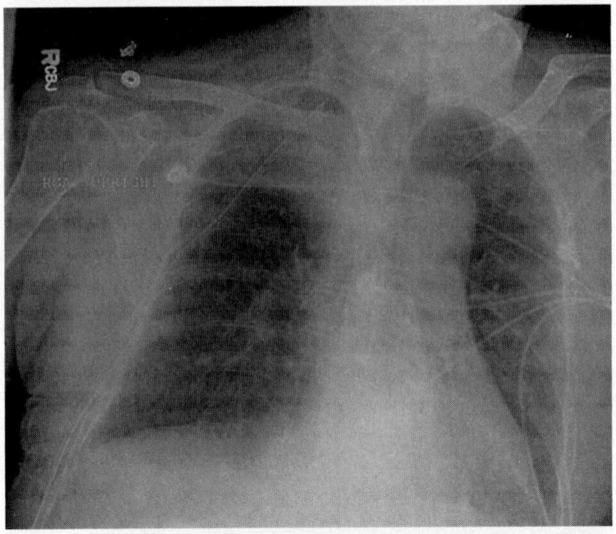

FIGURE 46-9 Properly placed chest tube.

FACTS AND FORMULAS

Light's formula (see Fig. 46-4):

$$\text{Percentage pneumothorax} = \frac{1 - L^3}{H^3} \times 100$$

where H is the diameter of the hemithorax and L is the diameter of the collapsed lung, as measured on a chest radiograph

Apex-to-cupula measurement (see Fig. 46-5): Measure from the apex of the lung to the cupola of the thoracic cavity on an upright posteroanterior radiograph. Less than 3 cm is considered small.

■ OPEN PNEUMOTHORAX

An open pneumothorax should be taped on three sides using a material that will be airtight. An airtight seal can be accomplished with petrolatum (Xeroform) gauze or the aluminum foil in which the gauze is packaged. Securing only three sides prevents the development of a tension pneumothorax by allowing the escape of air from the pleural space via this one-way valve.

■ HEIMLICH VALVE

A Heimlich valve is a one-way valve that can be attached to the end of a chest tube. Because suction has not been proven to aid in the reexpansion or outcome of a pneumothorax, it is not recommended; instead, a water seal or Heimlich valve is used.[11] The Heimlich valve allows the patient to ambulate unrestricted. It should not be used in patients with underlying lung disease or other medical problems that prevent them from tolerating a recurrence of the pneumothorax. Complications of this method include obstruction of the valve with fluid and disconnection.

■ COMPLICATIONS

Complications of the pneumothorax itself include those due to hypoxia, hypercapnia, and hypotension.

Reexpansion lung injury is rare but most commonly occurs after reexpansion of a large pneumothorax. Risk factors appear to include collapse of the lung for longer than 72 hours, a large pneumothorax,

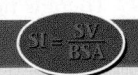

BOX 46-2

Complications

- Intercostal vessel hemorrahge
- Lung parenchymal injury
- Tube malfunction
  Air leak
  Development of tension pneumothorax
- Reinflation pulmonary injury
- Infection of wound site
- Entry into wrong body cavity
- Subcutaneous tube insertion

Documentation

- Document the presence of underlying lung disease to establish the primary versus secondary status of pneumothorax.
- In the case of primary pneumothorax, document whether or not it was traumatic.
- Document estimated size of pneumothorax as well as method of intervention.
- If patient is being discharged, document arrangement for close follow-up within 12 to 48 hours.

rapid reexpansion, and use of negative pleural pressure suction greater than 20 cm H_2O.[14]

Persistent air leaks occur when the volume of air escaping into the pleural space is higher than the volume of air being removed by the drainage device. This complication is more common with a secondary pneumothorax due to underlying lung disease. Most such air leaks resolve spontaneously within a week (75% in primary pneumothorax, 61% in secondary pneumothorax). If an air leak persists beyond 7 days, surgical intervention should be considered.

Complications that can occur during chest tube placement or catheter aspiration include intercostal vessel hemorrhage, lung parenchymal injury, and tube malfunction (Box 46-2).

Prevention of Recurrence

Interventions such as pleurodesis to prevent recurrence of a pneumothorax should be considered in the following situations[13,14]:

- First spontaneous pneumothorax with a persistent air leak
- Second ipsilateral spontaneous pneumothorax
- First contralateral pneumothorax
- Bilateral spontaneous pneumothoraces
- First episode of a secondary pneumothorax

RED FLAGS

Decisions on the treatment options for a pneumothorax should include the input of the physician who will continue care, either in the hospital or on an outpatient basis. Such a physician may be a general or cardiothoracic surgeon.

PRIORITY ACTIONS

1. Administer oxygen.
2. Determine whether tension pneumothorax physiology exists. If it is present, proceed to tube thoracostomy without delay for imaging.
3. Close an open pneumothorax with a three-sided dressing.
4. Obtain posteroanterior and lateral chest radiographs.
5. Determine the size of the pneumothorax.
6. Assess the patient for underlying lung disease, adhesions, etc.

- In patients who will continue activities that put them at risk for complications (diving or flying)

Disposition

The disposition of the patient with pneumothorax is detailed in the algorithms (see Figs. 46-6 and 46-7). The patient with a primary spontaneous pneumothorax who has been treated with observation or with catheter aspiration can be discharged if the pneumothorax does not increase over 3 to 6 hours and the symptoms do not worsen.

PATIENT TEACHING TIPS

- The patient must stop smoking.
- There is no limitation on physical activity.
- The patient with a primary spontaneous pneumothorax has a 30% recurrence rate within 2 years after air evacuation only; the patient who has had two pneumothoraces has an ≈80% chance of recurrence.
- Safety regulations state that a patient cannot fly for 3 weeks after treatment, and diving is also contraindicated.
- Patients sent home after observation should be followed up within 12 to 48 hours to document resolution of the pneumothorax.
- Patients should return to the ED immediately for recurrence of symptoms

In patients with a secondary (associated with underlying lung disease) spontaneous pneumothorax, the treatment algorithm is altered by the underlying lung disease. Clinically stable patients, regardless of the duration of symptoms, should not be monitored in the ED or treated with catheter aspiration and discharged; they should all be admitted for observation, simple aspiration, or tube thoracostomy.[9]

REFERENCES

1. Abolnik IZ: On the inheritance of primary spontaneous pneumothorax. Am J Med Genet 1991;40:155.
2. Chen SC, Markmann JF, Kauder DR, Schwab CW: Hemopneumothorax missed by auscultation in penetrating chest injury. J Trauma 1997;4286-4289.
3. Glazer HS, Anderson DJ, Wilson BS, et al: Pneumothorax: Appearance on lateral chest radiographs. Radiology 1989;173:707-711.
4. Schramel FM, Golding RP, Haakman CD, et al: Expiratory chest radiographs do not improve visibility of small apical pneumothoraces by enhanced contrast. Eur Respir J 1996;9:406-409.
5. Blaivas M, Lyon M, Duggal S: A prospective comparison of supine chest radiography and bedside ultrasound for the diagnosis of traumatic pneumothorax. Acad Emerg Med 2005;12:844-849.
6. Tocino IM, Miller MH, Fairfax WR: Distribution of pneumothorax in the supine and semirecumbent critically ill adult. AJR 1985;144:901-905.
7. Goodman TR, Traill ZC, Phillips AJ, et al: Ultrasound detection of pneumothorax. Clin Radiol 1999;54:736-739.
8. Bungay HK, Berger J, Traill ZC, et al: Pneumothorax post CT-guided lung biopsy: A comparison between detection on chest radiograph and CT. Br J Radiol 1999; 72:1160-1163.
9. Baumann MH, Strange C, Heffner JE, et al: Management of spontaneous pneumothorax: An American College of Chest Physicians Delphi Consensus Statement. Chest 2001;119:590-602.
10. Northfield TC: Oxygen therapy for spontaneous pneumothorax. BMJ 1971;4:86-88.
11. So Sy, Yu Dy: Catheter drainage of spontaneous pneumothorax: Suction or no suction, early or late removal? Thorax 1982;37:46-48.
12. Beng ST, Mahdevan M: An uncommon life-threatening complication after chest tube drainage of pneumothorax in the ED. Am J Emerg Med 2004;22:615-619.
13. Baumann MH: Non-spontaneous pneumothorax. In Light RW, Lee YCG (eds): Textbook of Pleural Diseases. London, Arnold, 2003, pp 464-474.
14. Henry M, Arnold T, Harvey J, et al: BTS guidelines for the management of spontaneous pneumothorax. Thorax 2003;58(Suppl II);ii39-ii52.

Chapter **47**

Pleural Effusion

Bret Nicks and David E. Manthey

KEY POINTS

The most common cause of pleural effusions in developed countries is congestive heart failure.

Pulmonary embolism should be considered in pulmonary effusions of uncertain etiology.

ED therapeutic thoracentesis is indicated for relief of acute respiratory or cardiovascular distress.

Diagnostic thoracentesis should be used in the ED to diagnose immediate life-threatening conditions in toxic-appearing patients.

Scope

Approximately 1 million pleural effusions are diagnosed in the United States each year.[1] The clinical importance of pleural effusions ranges from incidental manifestations of cardiopulmonary diseases to symptomatic infectious or malignant diseases requiring urgent evaluation and treatment. The normal pleural space contains approximately 1 mL of fluid, representing the balance between hydrostatic and oncotic forces in the visceral and parietal pleural vessels and lymphatic drainage. Pleural effusions result from disruption of this balance.

The classic work of Light and colleagues[2] in 1972 demonstrated that 99% of pleural effusions could be classified into two general categories, transudative and exudative (Box 47-1). A basic difference is that transudates, in general, reflect a systemic process, whereas exudates usually signify underlying local pleuropulmonary disease.[2]

Transudative pleural effusions are usually caused by a disorder in the normal hydrostatic and oncotic pressures in the lung. Congestive heart failure is the most common cause of transudative effusion and remains the most common cause of pleural effusions in developed countries. Left ventricular dysfunction causes increased pressure in the pulmonary veins, resulting in a higher capillary hydrostatic pressure in the visceral pleura that drives fluid into the pleural space. When the amount of fluid entering the pleural space overwhelms the ability of the lymphatic system to remove it, a pleural effusion develops.[3] Therefore, any process that decreases left ventricular output (cardiomyopathy, pericardial effusion, myocardial infarction) can cause a pleural effusion. A second mechanism for the formation of transudative effusions is a loss of plasma oncotic pressure due to a decrease in proteins within the vascular system. Cirrhosis leads to hypoalbuminemia, and nephrotic syndrome leads to protein loss, both resulting in diminished capillary oncotic pressures. The loss of oncotic pressure, which keeps fluid in the capillaries and absorbs it from the pleural space, will cause an effusion, or an accumulation of fluid in that space. There is also some evidence that microdefects in the diaphragm may allow fluid to transgress from the abdominal cavity to the pleural cavity when the pressures in the abdominal cavity are increased. This

BOX 47-1

Light Criteria for Classification of Pleural Effusions

In 1972, Light and coworkers[2] developed the currently accepted benchmark in classifying pleural fluid, as follows:

- Pleural fluid protein–to–serum protein ratio >0.5 : 1
- Pleural fluid lactate dehydrogenase (LDH)-to-serum LDH ratio >0.6 : 1
- Pleural fluid LDH greater than two-thirds the upper limit of normal for serum LDH (a cutoff value of 200 IU/L was used previously)

Pleural fluid is classified as an exudate if it meets *any one* of the aforementioned criteria. Conversely, if all three characteristics are absent, the fluid is classified as a transudate. These researchers achieved a diagnostic sensitivity of 99% and specificity of 98% for classification of an exudate.

occurs in disease states associated with ascites or in patients undergoing continuous ambulatory peritoneal dialysis (CAPD).

Exudative effusions form as a result of inflammation of the pleura, which is often caused by lung disease. Transudates can also progress to an exudate over time due to inflammation. Exudative effusions are most commonly associated with infections; however, malignancy and collagen vascular disorders are frequently identified as underlying etiologies. Table 47-1 lists the common causes of pleural effusions. Malignancy-related pleural effusions occur from obstruction of the lymphatic flow out of the lung, and these effusions follow the mechanism for transudates, but they are classified as exudates because of the presence of high levels of lactate dehydrogenase (LDH).

Table 47-1 CAUSES OF PLEURAL EFFUSIONS

Transudates	Atelectasis (early) Congestive heart failure Cirrhosis Glomerulonephritis Hypoalbuminemia Myxedema Nephrotic syndrome Peritoneal dialysis Pulmonary embolism Superior vena cava syndrome
Exudates	
Infectious	Bacterial infection Bronchiectasis Fungal infection Lung abscess Parasitic infection Traumatic hemothorax Tuberculosis Viral illness
Malignancies	Lymphoma Mesothelioma Primary lung cancer Pulmonary metastasis
Connective tissue disease	Rheumatoid arthritis Systemic lupus erythematosus
Abdominal/gastrointestinal disorders	Pancreatitis Subphrenic abscess Esophageal rupture
Other	Atelectasis (chronic) Chylothorax Drug reactions (amiodarone) Postpartum state Pulmonary infarction/embolism Uremia

Pathophysiology

Under normal physiologic conditions, the parietal and visceral pleura are in close apposition with only a small potential space between them. This potential space contains a small amount of pleural fluid (1 mL) to minimize friction from the continuous movement of the appositional lining. The accumulation of pleural fluid can usually be explained by either increased pleural fluid formation or decreased pleural fluid absorption, or perhaps a combination of the two.

Pleural effusions caused by an increase in pleural fluid formation can be further subdivided into elevation of hydrostatic pressure (e.g., congestive heart failure), decreased colloid osmotic pressure (e.g., cirrhosis, nephrotic syndrome), increased capillary permeability (e.g., infection, neoplasm), passage of fluid through openings in diaphragm (e.g., ascites), and reduction of pleural space pressures (e.g., atelectasis). An effusion caused by decreased pleural fluid absorption can be qualified further as either lymphatic obstruction or elevation of systemic venous pressures resulting in impaired lymphatic drainage (e.g., superior vena cava [SVC] syndrome).

The presence of fluid in the normally negative-pressure environment of the pleural space has a number of consequences for respiratory physiology. Pleural effusions produce a restrictive ventilatory defect and also decrease total lung capacity, functional residual capacity, and forced vital capacity. They may cause ventilation-perfusion mismatches and, when large enough, compromise cardiac output.[3]

Presenting Signs and Symptoms

In many cases, pleural effusions are asymptomatic when discovered. Physical findings, which do not usually manifest until an effusion exceeds 300 mL, are usually due to the underlying disease process.

Dyspnea, the most common symptom associated with pleural effusion, is related more to distortion of the diaphragm and chest wall during respiration than to hypoxemia. Less common symptoms of pleural effusions are mild, nonproductive cough and chest pain. Pleuritic chest pain indicates inflammation of the parietal pleura, because the visceral pleura is not innervated. In many patients, drainage of pleural fluid alleviates symptoms despite limited improvement in gas exchange. Findings on lung examination such as decreased breath sounds, dullness to percussion, pleural friction rub, egophony, and reduced tactile fremitus have all been described. However, auscultation can miss up to 600 mL of fluid in the lung.[4]

The EP should assess for clues that point to the cause of the effusion. If a patient complains of fever, weight loss, and progressively worsening cough with associated dyspnea, an oncologic or infectious etiology is likely. Constant chest wall pain may reflect chest wall invasion by bronchogenic carcinoma or malignant mesothelioma. Pleuritic chest pain suggests either pulmonary embolism or an inflammatory pleural process. An effusion can mimic the classic symptoms of acute coronary syndrome, such as chest pain, dyspnea, and shoulder pain.

Diagnostic Testing

■ RADIOGRAPHY

The erect posteroanterior and lateral chest radiographs are still the most important initial tools in the diagnosis of a pleural effusion. On upright and lateral decubitus films, loss of the costophrenic angle is seen. With increasing size of pleural effusion, the hemidiaphragm is obscured (Fig. 47-1), and a mass effect with shift of the mediastinum away from the affected side is seen. If a film is taken with the patient supine, one may see only a nonspecific haze over the affected hemithorax, as the fluid layers posteriorly. To confirm that the fluid is free flowing, lateral decubitus films with the affected side down are often obtained. In very large effusions, the affected side is opacified, and the decubitus film is not helpful. In adults, the minimum amount of fluid required for identification of effusion on an upright film is approximately 400 mL, whereas lateral decubitus films (with the affected side down) may detect as little as 50 mL of fluid accumulation. A lateral decubitus film with the affected side up may facilitate evaluation of the underlying lung for atelectasis, mass, or infiltrates.[5]

Mediastinal shift contralateral to the effusion (observed with effusions >1000 mL) with concomitant displacement of the trachea is an important clue to obstruction of a lobar bronchus by an endobronchial lesion, which can be due to malignancy or, less commonly, obstruction by a foreign body.

Subpulmonic effusions are an uncommon presentation of pleural effusions, seen when fluid accumulates between the lower lung lobe and diaphragm. The fluid collection may mimic an elevated hemidiaphragm in upright imaging (Fig. 47-2). Upwards of 400 mL of fluid can collect in the subpulmonic region before the posterior costophrenic sinus is filled. Evidence of an elevated hemidiaphragm with steep lateral peaks, obscuring of pulmonary vessels below the level of the diaphragm on lateral projection, or a flat appearance of the posterior aspect of the hemidiaphragm on lateral projection is suspicious for a subpulmonic effusion.[6]

■ ULTRASONOGRAPHY

Ultrasonography is effective for visualizing an effusion and determining whether the fluid is free flowing

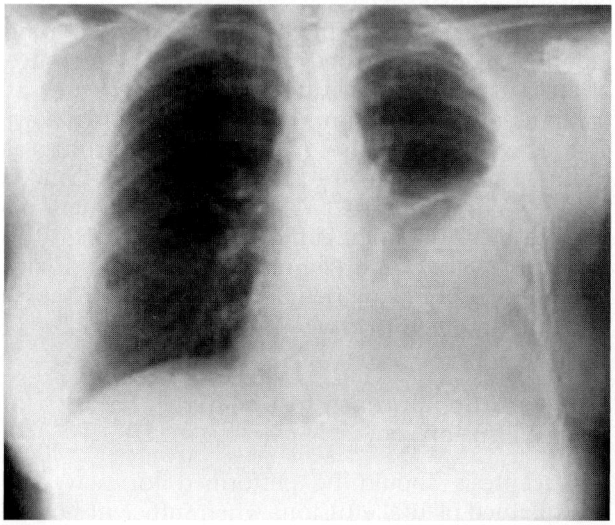

FIGURE 47-1 A large parapneumonic effusion on an upright chest radiograph.

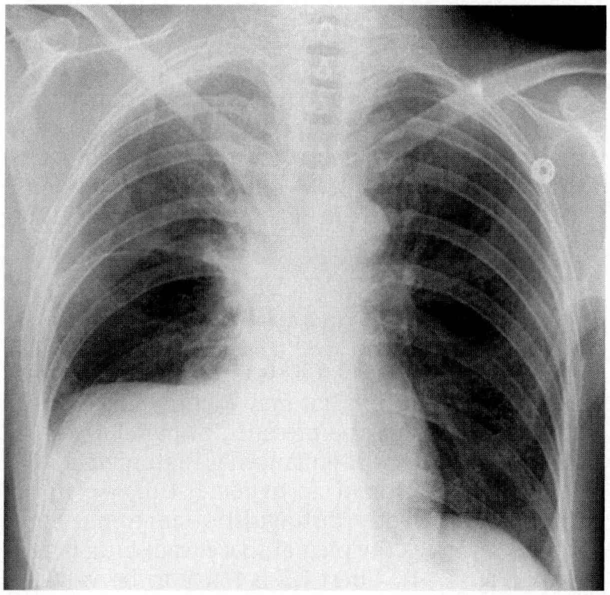

FIGURE 47-2 A subpulmonic effusion may mimic the surface of the diaphragm without blunting the costophrenic angle.

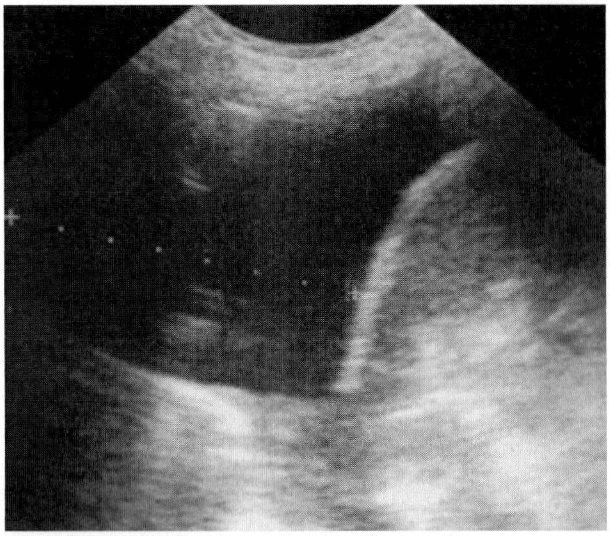

FIGURE 47-3 Upright bedside ultrasonogram of a large pleural effusion.

or loculated (Fig. 47-3).[7] In a prospective study, Piccoli and coworkers[8] compared ultrasonography, physical examination, and radiography in patients with suspected effusions. Agreement of physical examination with radiographic findings was 76%; kappa = 0.52. When compared with the chest ultrasonography, a physical examination showed a sensitivity of 69% and a specificity of 77%. Ultrasonography may help distinguish a large solid chest mass from an effusion and can be used to guide thoracentesis. Ramnath and associates[9] suggested early use of ultrasonography to identify complicated effusions (loculations or organization) because patients whose effusions were treated aggressively with decortication had significantly shorter hospital stays than those whose effusions were treated with tube thoracostomy. The same study showed that in children with effusions but no ultrasonographic evidence of organization, outcomes for those receiving treatment with intravenous antibiotics and drainage were similar to outcomes for those receiving aggressive treatment such as thoracoscopy or decortication. The major advantage of ultrasonography over conventional radiography is its ability to differentiate between solid and liquid components and, thus, to assist in identifying pleural fluid loculations.

■ COMPUTED TOMOGRAPHY

Computed tomography (CT) is rarely needed to diagnose a pleural effusion but may identify an underlying mass. In adults, the presence of parietal pleural thickening on contrast-enhanced CT is a specific, but insensitive indicator of an exudate. Cross-sectional imagery more clearly distinguishes anatomic compartments such as the pleural space from lung parenchyma (Fig. 47-4). Chest CT is likely to be valuable for management decisions in complicated effusions—distinguishing empyema from lung abscess, detecting pleural masses, outlining loculated fluid collections, or identifying additional problems, such as contusions, blebs, and infiltrates.

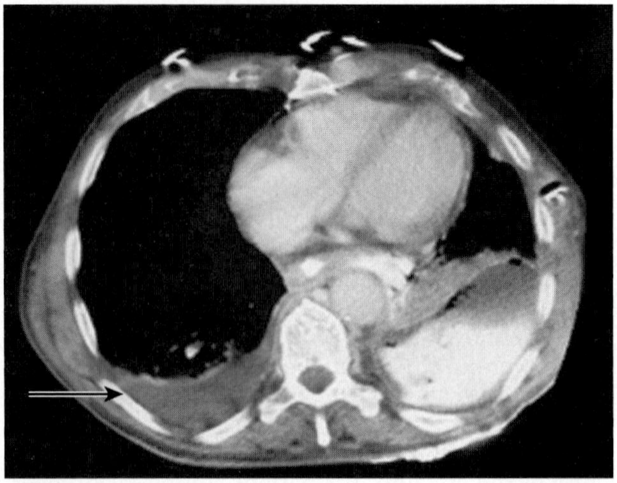

FIGURE 47-4 A pleural effusion seen on chest computed tomography.

■ PLEURAL FLUID ANALYSIS

Ideally, the evaluation of a pleural effusion should begin with a diagnostic thoracentesis and proceed to classification of the pleural fluid as either a transudate or an exudate. The currently accepted benchmark for classifying pleural fluid, developed by Light and coworkers,[2] is shown in Box 47-1. This analysis requires comparison of the pleural fluid and serum protein and LDH levels. Pleural fluid is classified as an exudate if it meets *any one* of the ratio criteria listed. Conversely, if all three criteria are absent, the fluid is classified as a transudate. With these guidelines, the original study by Light and coworkers[2] reported a diagnostic sensitivity of 99% and a specificity of 98% for an exudate. A number of later studies used modifications to the Light criteria, but had poorer diagnostic accuracy.[10]

Normal pleural fluid pH has been estimated to be around 7.64. A pH below 7.30 suggests the presence of an inflammatory or infiltrative process,[11] such as parapneumonic effusion, empyema, malignancy, connective tissue disease, tuberculosis, or esophageal rupture. According to the current American College of Chest Physicians (ACCP) consensus statement on the treatment of parapneumonic effusions, pH is the preferred pleural fluid chemistry test for classifying the category of a parapneumonic effusion for subsequent management (Table 47-2).[12,13]

■ Diagnostic Approach to Unilateral Pleural Effusion

Thoracentesis should be performed for new and unexplained pleural effusions when sufficient fluid is present to allow a safe procedure. Conventional wisdom holds that if a 10-mm layer of fluid is visible

Table 47-2 FLUID ANALYSIS OF PLEURAL EFFUSIONS

Exudates	Protein content >3 g/dL High lactate dehydrogenase (LDH) content Pleural fluid–to–serum LDH ratio >0.6 : 1 Pleural fluid–to–serum protein ratio >0.5 : 1
Differential clues	Gross blood in the pleural fluid suggests tumor, trauma, or infarction. Pleural fluid amylase elevation is associated with pancreatic disease, esophageal rupture, or malignancy. Pleural fluid pH is normally >7.30; pH <7.2 suggests an infectious process, such as empyema. Consider pulmonary emboli as the cause for loculated pleural effusions, particularly if the pleural fluid predominantly contains lymphocytes.

on a radiograph, sufficient fluid is present for thoracentesis to be successful. Treatment of the underlying disorder is generally all that is required for effusions caused by renal, cardiac, or rheumatologic diseases.

■ Diagnostic Approach to Pleural Effusion Associated with Malignancy

Malignancy-induced pleural effusions should undergo therapeutic thoracentesis as needed. If effusions are undiagnosed, cytologic evaluation is required for patients with oncologic risks. Completion of evaluation may require CT assessment and subsequent tissue biopsy.

■ Diagnostic Approach to Parapneumonic Pleural Effusions

Parapneumonic effusion and empyema are treated initially with empirical antibiotics according to the patient's age and the organisms and sensitivities commonly present in the community. Parapneumonic effusion usually progresses through three stages. The *exudative* stage is associated with capillary leak during the first 3 days; the *fibrinopurulent* stage is associated with bacterial invasion of the pleura between 3 and 7 days; and the *organizational* stage is characterized by fibroblast growth, occurring for 2 to 3 weeks if the effusion is not treated properly. Lack of early diagnosis and drainage of empyema, especially in younger children, may worsen the disease course. In a hospitalized patient with complicated parapneumonic effusion, antibiotics are administered intravenously and a thoracostomy tube is left in place until the patient is afebrile and improving clinically. Oral antibiotics are frequently continued for weeks after these procedures.

PRIORITY ACTIONS

- Identify the cause of the pleural effusion.
- Therapeutic thoracentesis is recommended for symptomatic patients.
- Assess respiratory status prior to and after any intervention.
- Inform patients about the complications associated with pleural effusions and thoracentesis.

Interventions and Procedures

Thoracentesis is an elective procedure requiring informed consent. Sterile technique and procedural experience lower the incidence of complications.

Drainage of a pleural effusion is indicated for the following reasons:

- Diagnostic or therapeutic purposes
- Evaluation of complicated parapneumonic effusions or empyema
- Symptomatic relief of dyspnea
- Need for evaluation of underlying lung parenchyma

■ POSITIONING

Ideally for thoracentesis, the patient should sit at the edge of the bed, lean forward slightly, and rest on an adjustable table. If the patient cannot sit up owing to hemodynamic status, mental status, or the presence of tubes and indwelling lines, the thoracentesis can be done with the patient supine. In that case, the patient should turn onto the side with the effusion and move so as to bring his or her back to the edge of the bed.

■ PROCEDURE

A diagnostic thoracentesis is used to determine the etiology of a pleural effusion, whereas a therapeutic thoracentesis is performed to relieve symptoms of

Documentation

- Identify the size and location of the effusion.
- Consider the cause and duration of the effusion.
- Discuss the appropriate intervention and associated risks.
- Assess respiratory function before and after any intervention.
- Ensure appropriate outpatient follow-up or inpatient evaluation.

respiratory insufficiency caused by a large pleural effusion. Therapeutic thoracentesis may be repeated if indicated; however, more definitive therapy such as sclerosis is usually needed to treat recurrent symptomatic pleural effusions. If more than 1 L to 1.5 L of fluid is removed at one time, re-expansion pulmonary edema and post-thoracentesis shock should be considered in the postprocedural period. Supplemental oxygen should be provided, as post-thoracentesis decreases in arterial oxygenation have been reported. The magnitude and duration of this decline roughly correlate with the amount of fluid removed. If removal of a large volume of fluid is anticipated, concurrent fluid resuscitation should be considered to blunt post-thoracentesis shock. Depending on the causative physiologic process, however, reaccumulation of pleural fluid may occur.

With appropriate positioning, the patient is prepared in a standard sterile fashion. The effusion can be identified along the posterior infrascapular line with either clinical examination (auscultation and percussion) or bedside ultrasonography. Ultrasonography is recommended because it identifies not only the level of effusion but also the subdiaphragmatic organs that should be avoided.[7] As the angiocatheter is advanced, the neurovascular bundles located on the inferior aspect of the ribs should be avoided. Aspiration of fluid can continue until enough fluid is obtained for diagnostic purposes or therapeutic relief.

Needle thoracentesis is adequate for both diagnostic and therapeutic evaluation of most parapneumonic pleural effusions. When the effusion has progressed to the fibrinopurulent or organizational stage, needle thoracentesis is often inadequate. Thoracoscopy offers the advantages of visual evaluation of the pleura, direct tissue sampling, and therapeutic intervention such as dissecting loculations and pleurodesis. Medical thoracoscopy and video-assisted thoracoscopic surgery (VATS) is currently indicated for the diagnosis of pleural effusions that remain undiagnosed after less invasive tests.

■ CONTRAINDICATIONS

Procedural contraindications for pleurocentesis or thoracostomy are listed in Table 47-3. Absolute contraindications consist of coagulopathy, known adhesions, and history of pleurodesis. If the patient is symptomatic and coagulopathic, correction of coagulopathy and ultrasonography guidance are recommended to minimize bleeding risks. *Pleurodesis* is introduction of a chemical or medication (talc, tetracycline, or bleomycin sulfate) into the chest cavity. It triggers an inflammatory reaction over the surface of the lung and inside the chest cavity, causing the pleura to adhere to each other and preventing or reducing further accumulation of pleural fluid. Thoracentesis should be avoided in patients who are at increased risk of adverse reactions owing to unstable angina or arrhythmia or known medical noncompliance including lack of established outpatient care. Relative contraindications include mechanical ventilation due to increased risk of lung collapse and difficulty with positioning. In intubated patients, therefore, the use of ultrasonography or CT for thoracentesis or postponing the procedure is recommended if the indication is not urgent. Patients with known bullous lung disease are at increased risk for postprocedural pneumothorax. Placement of the thoracentesis needle through a concurrent chest wall infection should be avoided, as this may seed the pleural space. A postprocedure radiograph should always be obtained to assess for pneumothorax.

Table 47-3 CONTRAINDICATIONS TO THORACENTESIS

Absolute contraindications	Coagulopathy Adhesions/pleurodesis Known medical noncompliance or lach of established outpatient care Dysrhythmia
Relative contraindications	Mechanical ventilation Bullous disease Concurrent chest wall infection

Adverse Outcomes

Adverse outcomes associated with pleural effusions can be characterized as iatrogenic or pathologic. Thoracentesis can predispose patients to pneumothorax, acute reexpansion pulmonary edema (RPE), shock, subsequent fluid reaccumulation, bleeding, infection, and solid organ injury. If untreated, the parapneumonic effusion can progress into a fibrinopurulent empyema, frequently requiring surgical intervention.

If the patient complains of increasing respiratory distress within the first hour after thoracentesis, RPE, or pneumothorax may be occurring, and an emergency chest radiograph should be obtained. RPE is a syndrome associated with hypotension and hypoxemia. It is thought to be a result of combined alveolar-capillary membrane disruption initiated by distention, reperfusion-mediated injury, and increased

PATIENT TEACHING TIPS

- Possible complications of pleural effusions include pneumothorax, respiratory failure caused by massive fluid accumulation, septicemia, bronchopleural fistula, and pleural thickening.
- Follow-up is recommended for all patients undergoing thoracentesis. Some experts recommend serial chest radiographs to ensure clearing. Some perform computed tomography after the plain radiographs show clearing.

Table 47-4 MANAGEMENT OF PATIENTS WITH PARAPNEUMONIC EFFUSIONS

Pleural Anatomy	Pleural Fluid Microbiology	Pleural Fluid Chemical Analysis	Perform Drainage?
Minimal effusion: <10 mm on lateral decubitus radiograph No loculations	Unknown culture and Gram stain results	Unknown pH	No
Small-moderate effusion: >10 mm but $<\frac{1}{2}$ hemithorax on lateral decubitus radiograph No loculations	Negative culture and Gram stain results	pH >7.20	No
Large effusion: $>\frac{1}{2}$ hemithorax *or* associated loculations *or* pleural thickening	Positive culture or Gram stain results	pH <7.20	Yes
Other	Purulent	pH <7.0	Yes

pulmonary flow. Risk factors include previous atelectasis and rapid reexpansion of the lung parenchyma. Typically, the patient with significant RPE becomes symptomatic within 15 minutes to 2 hours of the rapid reexpansion of the lung. Treatment is based on adequate oxygenation and circulation, typically with positive end-expiratory pressure (PEEP). Concern about the potential for RPE after thoracentesis is important, because mortality of patients with this condition is consistently 15% to 20% despite mechanical ventilation.[14,15]

Treatment and Disposition

Not all effusions require immediate drainage. Table 47-4 summarizes findings dictating the appropriateness of intervention. After thoracentesis is performed, stable patients can be discharged after an appropriate observation period, 3 to 6 hours. Patients who have exudative effusions or who require further evaluation or stabilization should be admitted.

Close outpatient follow-up and management are required for all patients evaluated for pleural effusion, whether or not they underwent thoracentesis.

RED FLAGS

- Lack of early diagnosis and drainage of empyema, especially in younger children, which may worsen the disease course
- Failure to recognize pneumothorax after thoracentesis
- Development of constrictive pleural fibrosis in inadequately treated infectious or hemorrhagic effusions

REFERENCES

1. Celli RB: Diseases of the diaphragm, chest wall, pleura and mediastinum. In Cecil RL, Goldman L, Claude Bennett JC (eds): Cecil Textbook of Medicine, 21st ed. Philadelphia, Saunders, 2000.
2. Light RW, MacGregor MI, Luchsinger PC, et al: Pleural effusions: The diagnostic separation of transudates and exudates. Ann Intern Med 1972;77:507-513.
3. Guyton AC: Pulmonary circulation, pulmonary edema, and pleural fluid. In Guyton AC, Hall JE (eds): Textbook of Medical Physiology, 11th ed. Philadelphia, Saunders, 2006.
4. Tu CY, Hsu WH, Hsia TC, et al: Pleural effusions in febrile medical ICU patients: Chest ultrasound study. Chest 2004;126:1274-1280.
5. Blackmore CC, Black WC, Dallas RV, Crow HC: Pleural fluid volume estimation: A chest radiograph prediction rule. Acad Radiol 1996;3:103-109.
6. Desai SR, Wilson AG: Pleura and pleural disorders. In Hansell DM, Armstrong P, Lynch DA, et al (eds): Imaging of Diseases of the Chest, 3rd ed. London, Mosby, 2000.
7. Rosenberg ER: Ultrasound in the assessment of pleural densities. Chest 1983;84:283-285.
8. Piccoli M, Trambaiolo P, Salustri A, et al: Bedside diagnosis and follow-up of patients with pleural effusion by a hand-carried ultrasound device early after cardiac surgery. Chest 2005;128:3413-3420.
9. Ramnath RR, Heller RM, Ben-Ami T, et al: Implications of early sonographic evaluation of parapneumonic effusions in children with pneumonia. Pediatrics 1998;101:68-71.
10. Tarn AC, Lapworth R: Biochemical analysis of pleural fluid: What should we measure? Ann Clin Biochem 2001;38:311-322.
11. Good JT Jr, Taryle DA, Maulitz RM, et al: The diagnostic value of pleural fluid pH. Chest 1980;78:55-59.
12. Colice GL, Curtis A, Deslauriers J, et al: Medical and surgical treatment of parapneumonic effusions: An evidence-based guideline [AACP consensus statement]. Chest 2000; 118:1158-1171.
13. Heffner JE, Brown LK, Barbieri C, DeLeo JM: Pleural fluid chemical analysis in parapneumonic effusions: A meta-analysis. Am J Respir Crit Care Med 1995;151:1700-1708.
14. Ravin CE, Dahmash NS: Re-expansion pulmonary edema. Chest 1980;77:709-710.
15. Mahfood S, Hix WR, Aaron BL, et al: Re-expansion pulmonary edema. Ann Thorac Surg 1997;63:1206-1207.

Chapter **48**

The Lung Transplant Patient in the Emergency Department

Robert L. Rogers

KEY POINTS

All lung transplant recipients with respiratory complaints should be assessed for the possibility of rejection and parenchymal lung infection. In most cases, the assessment requires admission to the hospital.

Pneumonia and lung allograft rejection may be subtle.

Lung rejection is common and can occur anytime after transplantation.

Transplanted lungs are highly susceptible to pneumonia, and cytomegalovirus pneumonia is the most common opportunistic pulmonary infection after lung transplantation.

Rejection and pulmonary infection are frequently indistinguishable, and patients should be admitted to the hospital to address both entities.

Scope

The lung transplant recipient who comes to the ED poses significant challenges because complications of the surgical procedure, infectious complications, mechanical complications, and the threat of lung allograft rejection may be present. In addition, potent immunosuppressive regimens may mask serious or life-threatening infectious diseases in the organ transplant recipient. This chapter provides information to arm the EP with the knowledge necessary to take care of this complex group of patients.

More than a thousand lung transplants are performed yearly in the United States. Survival rates have been rising in recent years because of technological advances in surgical technique and immunobiology. Current survival rates 1 year after transplantation exceed 76%.[1] Multiple conditions lead to the need to perform lung transplantation, including cystic fibrosis, end-stage chronic obstructive lung disease, and interstitial lung disease (Box 48-1).[2]

The number of patients who have undergone solid organ transplantation is growing every year. In 2006 alone, 28,930 organ transplantations were performed in the United States.[2] This figure represents a large number of patients who may sometime present to an ED for medical care. In addition, survival rates are rising. In 1998, the 1-year, 3-year, and 5-year survival rates were 70.7%, 54.8%, and 42.6%, respectively, for lung transplant recipients. Although survival rates for lung transplantation lag behind those for other solid organ transplantations, enhancements in immunotherapy will likely advance the field of lung transplantation even further.[3,4]

BOX 48-1

Reasons for Lung Transplantation

- Emphysema/chronic obstructive pulmonary disease
- Cystic fibrosis
- Idiopathic pulmonary fibrosis
- Primary pulmonary hypertension
- $Alpha_1$ antitrypsin deficiency
- Lung retransplantation (rejection, graft failure)
- Sarcoidosis
- Bronchiectasis
- Pulmonary fibrosis
- Occupational lung disease

From United Network for Organ Sharing, 2007, www.unos.org.

BOX 48-2

Clinical Findings in Acute Lung Allograft Rejection

- Nontoxic-appearing patient
- Leukocytosis
- Dry, nonproductive cough
- Fever
- Shortness of breath
- Hypoxia
- Abnormal chest radiograph
- Abnormal lung physical examination findings

Transplantation—The Procedure

Lung transplantation can be accomplished in various ways. Options for patients undergoing lung transplantation are single lung, double lung, combined heart and lung, and lobar transplantations.[5] The type of transplant depends on the recipient's disease and on the particular transplant center where the procedure is performed. Single lung transplantation requires a lateral thoracotomy incision, whereas double lung transplantation requires a double thoracotomy ("clamshell") incision. In addition, the heart may also be transplanted along with one or both lungs. In some cases, a lobar segment of donor lung may be transplanted. The surgical procedure includes anastomosis of the pulmonary arteries and veins as well as the bronchus.

ED Presentation

Patients who have undergone lung transplantation should be considered high risk when they present to an ED for evaluation. Because many patients live far from the center where their surgery was performed, they are likely to go the nearest ED when problems arise. In a retrospective review of 131 lung and heart/lung transplant patients who visited an ED, the most common presenting complaints were fever (37%), shortness of breath (13%), gastrointestinal symptoms (10%), and chest pain (9%).[6]

ED presentations of lung transplant recipients are commonly related to known complications of the surgical procedure and immunosuppression. It should not be forgotten, however, that disease unrelated to the transplant may also be present.

Differential Diagnosis

Patients who have undergone lung transplantation may present to the ED with a myriad of complaints. Among the most important complications are acute or chronic allograft rejection and infectious complications. In addition, patients in the early postoperative period are at risk for mechanical complications such as bronchial dehiscence.

■ REJECTION

Lung allograft rejection is one of the most feared life-threatening complications of lung transplantation, requiring retransplantation in some cases. The majority of transplant recipients experience at least one episode of rejection after transplantation. Patients who experience repeated episodes of allograft rejection are at increased risk of chronic rejection and bronchiolitis obliterans syndrome.[7-9]

The clinical presentation of lung allograft rejection can be nonspecific (Box 48-2). Patients may report a dry cough, subjective fevers, and varying degrees of shortness of breath. Any or all of these symptoms can occur in combination. Episodes of rejection cannot be distinguished from pulmonary infection on clinical grounds alone.[7] The important point for EPs is that symptoms of allograft dysfunction or rejection may be subtle. In addition, patients may not appear ill or seem to have anything more than a viral upper respiratory tract infection.[10,11]

The chest radiograph in patients with lung rejection may show many different findings. During the first 6 months after transplantation, chest radiographs may show pleural effusions, interstitial edema, or perihilar infiltrates. Episodes of rejection occurring after this time tend not to lead to abnormalities on the chest radiograph. Thus, a normal chest radiograph would not rule out the presence of underlying rejection. In the ED, chest radiographs may help in the evaluation of entities that would require immediate therapy, such as a pneumothorax and large pleural effusion.[10,11]

Diagnosis of lung allograft rejection is usually not accomplished in the ED. Patients are generally admitted for fiberoptic bronchoscopy and biopsy. Treatment of suspected lung transplant rejection begins with clinical suspicion. The patient's pulmonologist and/or lung transplant surgeon should be contacted in all cases of suspected rejection. Treatment of this potentially life-threatening entity should ensue before results of bronchoscopy are available. The biopsy helps determine the degree of tissue rejection and inflammation. The main ED treatment for patients with rejection is high-dose intravenous corticosteroids. Patients are usually given intravenous methylprednisolone in a dose of 0.5 to 1.0 g/day for 3 days, the first dose given in the ED. Resolution of symptoms is usually rapid if rejection is present. The therapy is then switched to oral corticosteroids. It is essential that the ED diagnosis and treatment of these patients occur with input from the patient's transplant physician.[9]

■ INFECTIOUS COMPLICATIONS

Despite advances in immunosuppression, infection is a common complication after any solid organ transplantation, particularly of the lung.[12-14] The most common infection is pneumonia, but any opportunistic infection can occur. Pneumonia is more common because the lung is in close contact with the environment.

Infectious complications after organ transplantation have been extensively studied and are related to multiple factors, the most important being the time since transplantation. Infections in organ recipients can be broken down into three time periods. EPs should consider the time since transplantation when deciding what types of infections may be present.

During the first month after transplantation, nosocomial infections predominate. Wound infections, urinary tract infections, pneumonia, and vascular access infections are common in this period. Infections that usually do *not* occur in the first month after transplantation are most of the opportunistic infections, in particular *Pneumocystis* and *Nocardia* infections.[15]

Infections that occur 1 to 6 months after solid organ transplantation include many of the opportunistic infections, such as *Pneumocystis carinii* and *Listeria monocytogenes*. In addition, immunomodulating viruses (particularly cytomegalovirus [CMV]) become important pathogens. Other immunomodulating viruses are Epstein-Barr virus (EBV), hepatitis B virus (HBV), hepatitis C virus (HCV), and human immunodeficiency virus (HIV).[15]

Infections that occur after the first month of transplantation may be associated with chronic or progressive infection with HBV, HCV, CMV, or EBV. Such infection may be associated with significant injury to the affected transplanted organ. Patients who experience chronic or recurrent bouts of organ rejection are invariably exposed to higher and prolonged periods of immunosuppressive therapy and thus are exposed to more opportunistic pathogens (Fig. 48-1).[15]

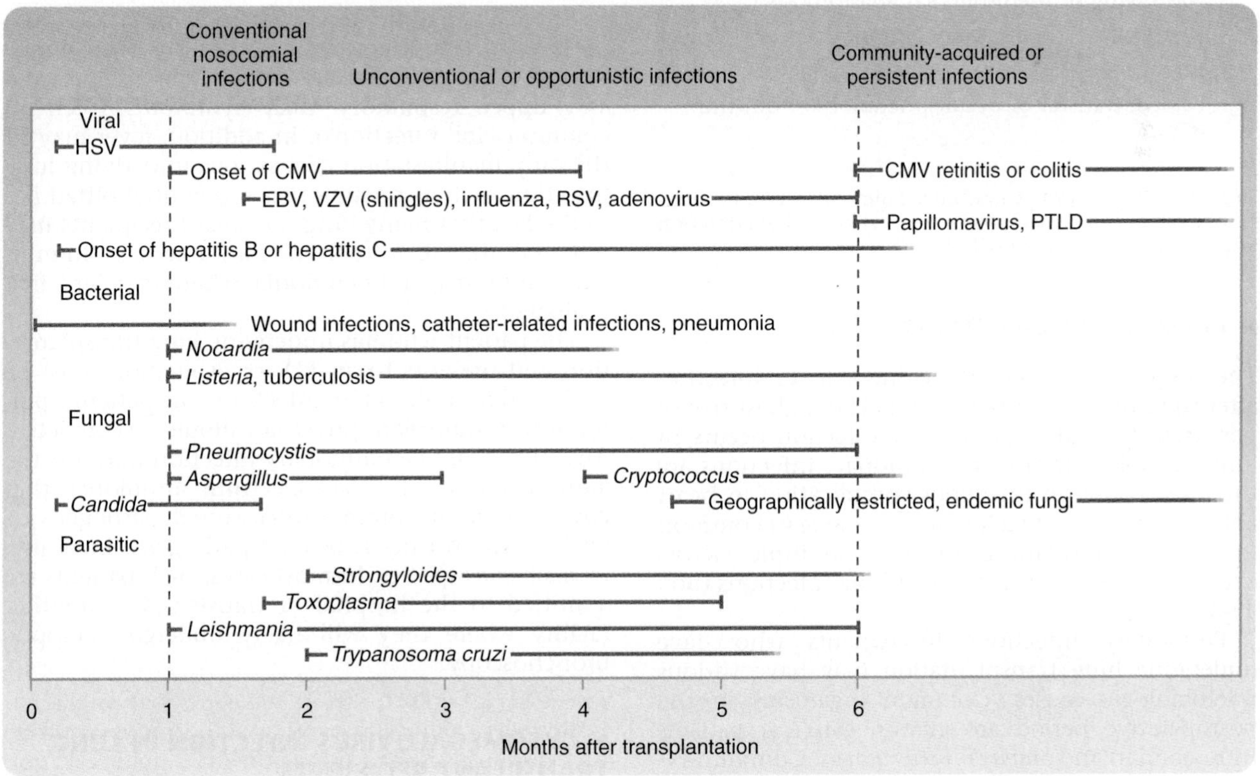

Conventional nosocomial infections
Unconventional or opportunistic infections
Community-acquired or persistent infections
Viral
HSV
Onset of CMV
CMV retinitis or colitis
EBV, VZV (shingles), influenza, RSV, adenovirus
Papillomavirus, PTLD
Onset of hepatitis B or hepatitis C
Bacterial
Wound infections, catheter-related infections, pneumonia
Nocardia
Listeria, tuberculosis
Fungal
Pneumocystis
Aspergillus
Cryptococcus
Candida
Geographically restricted, endemic fungi
Parasitic
Strongyloides
Toxoplasma
Leishmania
Trypanosoma cruzi
0
1
2
3
4
5
6
Months after transplantation

FIGURE 48-1 Time course and likely diseases in patients with lung transplants: Infection, acute rejection, and chronic rejection. CMV, cytomegalovirus; EBV, Epstein-Barr virus; HSV, herpes simplex virus; PTLD, post-transplantation lymphoproliferative disorder; RSV, respiratory syncytial virus; VZV, varicella-zoster virus.

Table 48-1 DIFFERENTIAL DIAGNOSIS OF FEVER AND PULMONARY INFILTRATES IN ORGAN TRANSPLANT RECIPIENTS ACCORDING TO THE ABNORMALITY ON CHEST RADIOGRAPHS AND RATE OF PROGRESSION OF THE ILLNESS

	CAUSE	
Radiographic Abnormality	*Acute Illness**	*Subacute or Chronic Illness**
Consolidation	Bacteria (including *Legionella*) Thromboembolism Hemorrhage Pulmonary edema	Fungi *Nocardia asteroides,* tumor Tuberculosis Viruses, drug reactions, radiation, *Pneumocystis carinii*
Peribronchovascular abnormality	Pulmonary edema Leukoagglutinin reaction Bacteria Viruses (influenza)	Viruses, *P. carinii,* irradiation, drug reactions (occasionally *N. asteroides,* tumor, fungi, tuberculosis)
Nodular infiltrate†	Bacteria (including *Legionella*) Pulmonary edema	Fungi *N. asteroides* Tuberculosis *P. carinii*

**Acute illness* develops and requires medical attention in less than 24 hours. *Subacute* or *chronic illness* develops over a period of several days to a week.
†*Nodular infiltrate* is one or more focal defects more than 1 cm^2 in area on chest radiographs with well-defined borders, surrounded by aerated lung. Multiple tiny nodules are seen in a wide variety of disorders (e.g., cytomegalovirus, varicella-zoster virus infection) and are not included here.
Adapted from Shreeniwas R, Schulman LL, Berkmen YM, et al: Opportunistic bronchopulmonary infections after lung transplantation: Clinical and radiographic findings. Radiology 1996;200:349–356.

BOX 48-3

Factors Contributing to Risk of Pulmonary Infections in Lung Transplant Recipients

- Impairment in cough due to lung denervation
- Narrowing of the bronchial anastomosis
- Disruption of pulmonary lymphatics
- Impairment of the mucociliary "escalator"
- Passive transfer of occult pneumonia from the donor

From Kotloff R, Ahya V, Crawford S. Pulmonary complications of solid organ and hematopoietic stem cell transplantation. Am J Respir Crit Care Med 2004;170:22-48.

■ PULMONARY INFECTIONS

The lungs are particularly vulnerable to infection after solid organ transplantation. The highest risk of post-transplantation pulmonary infection occurs in lung transplant recipients. Pulmonary infections are the most common infectious complication in heart and lung transplant recipients,[12-14] and least common in kidney transplant recipients.[16] Multiple factors explain this higher incidence of lung infections (Box 48-3).

Pulmonary infections in patients who have undergone lung transplantation may have various microbiologic causes. Common organisms in the postoperative period are gram-negative organisms (nosocomial) and *Staphylococcus aureus.* Community-acquired bacterial pneumonia tends to occur later in the post-transplantation period.[16] Organisms included in this category are *Haemophilus influenzae, Streptococcus pneumoniae,* and *Legionella* species. Infections with *Pseudomonas aeruginosa* occur in the majority of cases of lung transplantation–associated bronchiolitis obliterans syndrome. Patients with this syndrome commonly present with recurrent episodes of purulent bronchitis and pneumonia.[14] Other infections to consider are fungal pneumonia and tuberculosis (Table 48-1).

Clinically, pulmonary infections may not cause the typical symptoms seen in healthy outpatients. Symptoms may be subtle and include a dry cough and upper respiratory tract symptoms (seen in common viral infections). In addition, fever may be the only manifestation of a serious underlying lung infection such as pneumonia. A potential pitfall lies in the fact that many lung transplant recipients may not look that ill initially or may not have fulminant symptoms of pneumonia when they are first evaluated.

The patient who has undergone lung transplantation and presents to an ED for evaluation must be evaluated for pulmonary infection. The patient's pulmonary or transplant physician should be contacted. Any suspicion of a pulmonary infection warrants the administration of broad-spectrum antibiotics that cover common community-acquired pathogens as well as health care–associated pathogens, including *Pseudomonas* species. In most cases, such patients are admitted to the hospital or transferred to another facility where they will likely undergo fiberoptic bronchoscopy.

■ CYTOMEGALOVIRUS INFECTION IN LUNG TRANSPLANT RECIPIENTS

Infection with CMV remains one of the most important and lethal of all infections in solid organ recipi-

BOX 48-4

Clinical Findings in Cytomegalovirus Disease

- Fever
- Malaise
- Myalgia
- Cough
- Dyspnea
- Unexplained leukopenia

ents.[16] This virus, which has been referred to as the "troll of transplantation," is the second most common infection in lung transplant recipients, after bacterial pneumonia.[17] The overall likelihood of CMV infection and/or disease in a lung transplant patient is approximately 50% and is related to the CMV status of the donor and recipient.[18]

Cytomegalovirus infection generally manifests in the 1 to 3 months after transplantation. Any episode of acute rejection raises the patient's risk for continued CMV infection secondary to the required, ongoing immunosuppression. The clinical presentation may range from asymptomatic viremia to overwhelming sepsis and multiorgan failure. True clinical disease may manifest as a "mononucleosis-like" syndrome, with fever, malaise, and leukopenia (Box 48-4). There may also be organ-specific involvement in the lungs (pneumonitis), gastrointestinal system (colitis and hepatitis), and central nervous system. Over time, CMV infection leads to a high level of immunosuppression and the subsequent development of chronic allograft dysfunction and loss.[16,19,20]

Pneumonitis is the most common presentation of CMV disease after lung transplantation.[21] Additional features are hepatitis, gastroenteritis, and colitis. Clinically, CMV pneumonitis may look like acute rejection. Patients with either acute lung allograft rejection or CMV pneumonitis may present with low-grade fever, nonproductive cough, and shortness of breath. Further inpatient workup is generally required to distinguish between the two disorders. Diagnosis of CMV pneumonitis is made through serologic testing and results of bronchoscopy and is beyond the scope of this chapter. As many as 10% to 15% of patients with CMV pneumonitis may be initially asymptomatic. In addition, a prodrome consisting of fever, malaise, and myalgias frequently precedes the onset of pneumonitis (cough and dyspnea). Radiographically, the disease may appear as opacities, nodules, or lobar infiltrates on chest radiographs.[22,23]

Treatment of CMV infection may start in the ED. Although diagnoses of CMV infection may not be established on presentation, a presumptive diagnosis is frequently made, and empirical therapy started. Intravenous ganciclovir has been the traditional antiviral treatment of cytomegalovirus infections.[24] Standard treatment of CMV consists of a 2- to 3-week course of this agent. In some cases, ganciclovir is combined with CMV hyperimmune globulin. Much of the time, these therapies are started once the patient has been admitted.[24]

All lung transplant recipients still within the vulnerable period of 1-3 months after surgery should be evaluated carefully for CMV disease in the ED. It should be assumed that any lung transplant recipient who has undergone transplantation less than 3 months previously and who has fever, cough, or other suspicious findings may have active CMV disease. In many cases therapy is started in the ED in consultation with the patient's physician.

Diagnostic Testing

Diagnostic imaging in the ED is usually limited to plain film chest radiography and occasionally computed tomography (CT). EPs should maintain a low threshold for obtaining a CT scan of the chest in lung transplant recipients. CT has been shown far superior to chest radiography in detecting subtle cases of pneumonia in such patients.[25]

Immunosuppressive Therapy and the Lung Transplant Recipient

Transplant recipients undergo long-term immunosuppressive therapy and are prone to multiple drug side effects, drug-drug interactions, and higher risk of opportunistic infections. EPs must use caution when prescribing any new medication to such patients in the ED, because potentially serious drug side effects and drug-drug interactions may result. It is best to discuss any medication issue in a transplant recipient with the patient's physician and/or a pharmacist.

Medications commonly used in the lung transplant patient are calcineurin inhibitors (such as cyclosporine), cell cycle inhibitors, and corticosteroids. Most patients are maintained on a combination of these classes of medications. Table 48-2 lists these medications and their side effects.

Many commonly used medications may interfere with drugs used for long-term immunosuppression. Many medications are known to increase blood levels (and thus lead to toxicity) of certain medications, like cyclosporine (Neoral) and tacrolimus (Prograf). In particular, erythromycin, doxycycline, and azole antifungal agents (ketoconazole, fluconazole, itraconazole) all raise serum concentrations of cyclosporine and tacrolimus. In contrast, other medications, such as isoniazid, rifampin, and rifabutin, lower blood levels of these two immunosuppressants and may put the patient at risk for organ rejection. Medications such as sulfonamides, ganciclovir, and acyclovir may all potentiate the bone marrow

Table 48-2 DRUGS COMMONLY USED IN SOLID ORGAN TRANSPLANT RECIPIENTS

Drug	Mechanism of Action	Adverse Effect(s)
Corticosteroids (prednisone)	Inhibits expression of genes encoding proinflammatory cytokines	Cushingoid, infection, hypertension, edema, osteoporosis, bone necrosis, psychiatric disease
Azathioprine	Inhibitor of purine synthesis	Leukopenia, thrombocytopenia, anemia, hepatotoxicity, increased risk of malignancy
Mycophenolate (Cellcept)	Inhibits purine synthesis	Nausea, vomiting, diarrhea, dyspepsia, leukopenia, anemia
Cyclosporin (Sandimmune, Neoral); causes renal vasoconstriction and ischemia	Calcineurin inhibitor (impairs T-cell function)	Nephrotoxicity (acute or chronic renal failure, renal vasoconstriction), Infections, hypertension, hyperkalemia, increased lipids and glucose, gout, hypomagnesemia, tremor, encephalopathy, thrombotic thrombocytopenic purpura (TTP), hirsutism, gingival hyperplasia, hepatotoxicity
Tacrolimus (FK-506, Prograf)	Calcineurin inhibitor	Same as cyclosporine except much less risk of TTP
Sirolimus	Inhibit cell proliferation (T cells)	Infections, thrombocytopenia, anemia, leukopenia, hyperlipidemia, edema, diarrhea, headaches
Cyclophosphamide	Interferes with B-cell and T-cell proliferation and function	Leukopenia, hemorrhagic cystitis, bladder cancer, syndrome of inappropriate antidiuretic hormone secretion (SIADH)
OKT3-monoclonal (used to treat rejection)	Targets CD3+ T cells and impairs their function Transiently activates T cells	"Cytokine release syndrome" (fever, tachycardia, hypotension), pulmonary edema, aseptic meningitis
ATGAM-polyclonal	Bind to peripheral lymphocytes	Anaphylaxis, serum sickness, fever, rash
Interleukin-2 (IL-2) receptor antibodies (daclizumab, basiliximab)	Bind to IL-2 receptor	Rare hypersensitivity syndrome

toxicity of azathioprine and mycophenolate mofetil.[26-29]

Treatment and Disposition

All patients with suspected lung transplant rejection or infection should be admitted to the hospital for further diagnostic testing and evaluation. The importance of appreciating the subtle nature of these complications cannot be overemphasized. In addition, it is wise to seek consultation with the patient's pulmonary physician or surgeon to discuss all transplant recipients who present to the ED. A safe way to evaluate any lung transplant recipient presenting to the ED for care is to assume that infection and/or rejection is present until proven otherwise (Box 48-5).

Infectious disease complications can best be understood in terms of the time since the lung transplantation was performed. The highest incidence of CMV infection occurs in the first 1 to 3 months. CMV infection has a high morbidity and mortality and must be aggressively treated.

Lastly, lung transplant recipients are maintained on multiple immunosuppressive medications that interfere with many commonly used medications, such as antibiotics, and also have common adverse effects. EPs should never take it upon themselves to add a drug to a transplant recipient's regimen or alter the dose of an immunosuppressant without first consulting with the patient's physicians.

By having an understanding of the subtleties of rejection and pneumonia and of the importance

PRIORITY ACTIONS

- Do not assume that patients with allograft rejection or pneumonia will manifest obvious symptoms.
- Admit patients to the hospital if rejection and/or infection is suspected.
- Discuss every lung transplant recipient who presents to the emergency department with his or her pulmonary physician and/or lung transplant surgeon.
- Institute therapy with broad-spectrum antibiotics if any pulmonary symptoms are present or pneumonia is suspected.
- Treat suspected rejection with high-dose intravenous corticosteroids in conjunction with consultation.

BOX 48-5

Key Pitfalls in Evaluation of the Lung Transplant Recipient

- Relying on a normal chest radiograph to exclude underlying pulmonary infection and/or rejection
- Failure to discuss evaluation and treatment options with the patient's physician
- Failure to appreciate that symptoms of lung allograft rejection may be subtle

of drug side effects and interactions in lung transplant recipients, the EP will be in a better position to take care of this complex group of patients in the ED.

REFERENCES

1. Hertz M, Taylor D, Trulock E: The Registry of the International Society for Heart and Lung Transplantation: Nineteenth Official Report. J Heart Lung Transplant 2002; 21:950-970.
2. United Network of Organ Sharing (UNOS). www.optn.org/latestdata/rptdata.asp.
3. Hosenspud J, Bennett L, Keck B, et al: The Registry of the International Society for Heart and Lung Transplantation: Fifteenth official report—1998. J Heart Lung Transplant 1998;17:656.
4. Lin HM, Kauffman HM, McBride MA, et al: Center-specific graft and patient survival rates: 1997 United Network for Organ Sharing (UNOS) report. JAMA 1998;280: 1153-1160.
5. Boujoukos AJ: Management of Patients with Heart and Lung Transplants, 5th ed. Philadelphia, Elsevier Saunders, 2005.
6. Sternbach G, Varon J, Hunt S: Emergency department presentation and care of heart and heart/lung recipients. Ann Emerg Med 1992;21:1140.
7. De Vito D, Hoffman L, Iacono A: Are symptom reports useful for differentiating between acute rejection and pulmonary infection after lung transplantation? Heart Lung 2004;33:372.
8. Palmer S, Burch L, Davis R: The role of innate immunity in acute allograft rejection after lung transplantation. Am J Respir Crit Care Med 2003;168:628.
9. Chakinala M, Trulock E: Acute allograft rejection after lung transplantation: Diagnosis and therapy. Chest Surg Clin North Am 2003;13:525.
10. Millet B, Higenbottam T, Ferrari L: The radiographic appearances of infection and acute rejection of the lung after heart-lung transplantation. Am Rev Respir Dis 1989; 140:62.
11. Otulana B, Higenbottam T, Scott J: Lung function associated with histologically diagnosed acute lung rejection and pulmonary infection in heart-lung transplant recipients. Am Rev Respir Dis 1990;142:329.
12. Maurer J, Tullis E, Grossman R, et al: Infectious complications following isolated lung transplantation. Chest 1992; 101:1056.
13. Cisneros J, Munoz P, Torre-Cisneros J, et al: Pneumonia after heart transplantation: A multi-institutional study. Clin Infect Dis 1998;27:324.
14. Kramer M, Marshall S, Starnes V, et al: Infectious complications in heart-lung transplantation: Analysis of 200 episodes. Arch Intern Med 1993;153:2010.
15. Fishman J, Rubin R: Infection in organ-transplant recipients. N Engl J Med 1998;338:1741.
16. Kotloff R, Ahya V, Crawford S: Pulmonary complications of solid organ and hematopoietic stem cell transplantation. Am J Respir Crit Care Med 2004;170:22.
17. Zamora M: Cytomegalovirus and lung transplantation. Am J Transplant 2004;4:1219.
18. Zamora M: Controversies in lung transplantation: Management of cytomegalovirus infection. J Heart Lung Transplant 2002;21:841.
19. Duncan S, Paradis I, Yousem S, Similo S: Sequelae of cytomegalovirus pulmonary infections in lung allograft recipients. Am Rev Respir Dis 1992;146:1419.
20. Sia I, Patel R: New strategies for prevention and therapy of cytomegalovirus infection and disease in solid-organ transplant recipients. Clin Microbiol Rev 2000;13:83.
21. Shreeniwas R, Schulman LL, Berkmen YM, et al.: Opportunistic bronchopulmonary infections after lung transplantation: Clinical and radiographic findings. Radiology 1996; 200:349.
22. Collins J, Muller N, Kazerooni E: CT findings of pneumonia after lung transplantation. Am J Roentgenol 2000;175: 811.
23. Franquet T, Lee K, Muller N: Thin-section CT findings in 32 immuno-compromised patients with cytomegalovirus pneumonia who do not have AIDS. Am J Roentgenol 2003;181:1059.
24. Harbison M, De Girolami P, Jenkins R, Hammer S: Ganciclovir therapy of severe cytomegalovirus infections in solid-organ transplant recipients. Transplantation 1988; 46:82.
25. Macori F, Iacari V, Falchetto Osti M, et al: Assessment of complications in patients with lung transplantation with high resolution computed tomography. Radiol Med 1998;96:42.
26. Lake K, Canafax D: Important interactions of drugs with immunosuppressive agents used in transplant recipients. J Antimicrob Chemother 1995;36(Suppl):11.
27. Michalets E: Update: Clinically significant cytochrome P-450 drug interactions. Pharmacotherapy 1998;18:84.
28. Mignat C: Clinically significant drug interactions with new immunosuppressive agents. Drug Safety 1997;16:267.
29. Knoop C, Haverich A, Fischer S: Immunosuppressive therapy after human lung transplantation. Eur Respir J 2004;23:159.

SECTION **VI**

Cardiac Diseases

Chapter 49

Cardiac Imaging and Stress Testing

Andra L. Blomkalns and Rhonda S. Cadena

KEY POINTS

Cardiac imaging and stress testing are key components of any comprehensive patient evaluation for possible acute coronary syndromes or coronary heart disease.
Rest imaging evaluates for ischemia existing at the time of presentation, whereas stress testing evaluates for exercise-induced ischemia.
Rest nuclear imaging can be a useful tool for risk stratification and diagnosis in patients with active or recent chest discomfort.
Exercise and pharmacologic stress testing further stratifies risk and examines for stress-induced ischemia.
Echocardiography can be used to assess global cardiac function and may be performed with the patient at rest or under stress.
Electron beam computed tomography is a new imaging technology that may prove useful in the ED environment.
Several protocols using various combinations of cardiac biomarkers, imaging modalities, stress testing, and time courses of evaluation have proved successful in a variety of ED environments across the country.
Individual institutions and their EDs should develop their own custom protocols to make them most beneficial and feasible in their specific environments.

Background and Scope

Patients with symptoms of chest discomfort or related symptoms present a significant challenge for the EP.[1] Frequently patients have one or two risk factors and some but not all of the "classic" ischemia symptoms, and their electrocardiography (ECG) findings are nondiagnostic. These patients carry up to a 10% chance of significant cardiac disease and need an appropriate risk stratification and diagnostic evaluation. As EPs, our goal is not to diagnose coronary heart disease (CHD) but, rather, to stratify patients' risk and identify those at risk for imminent cardiac ischemia and hence poor outcomes.

EPs use several methods and modalities to evaluate this very heterogenous patient group. Aside from comprehensive history and physical examination, standard adjuncts include ECG, cardiac biomarker measurements, and some sort of cardiac imaging. ECG, although often considered the principal diagnostic tool in cardiac evaluation, indicates only gross electrical derangements caused by dead or dying muscle tissue. Cardiac biomarkers, such as creatine kinase MB fraction (CK-MB) and troponin, indicate more serious myocardial necrosis or cell death. Cardiac imaging can more directly reflect cardiac tissue undergoing ischemia, whether performed with the patient at rest or under stress. Our goal is to familiarize the reader with common cardiac imaging modalities used in the ED for the evaluation of this difficult and high-morbidity population.

In this chapter, we review the most common and established cardiac imaging modalities of echocardiography and myocardial perfusion nuclear imaging. Examples of how these modalities can be incorporated into protocolized patient evaluation are also presented. Lastly, we briefly highlight the new and promising cardiac imaging capabilities of CT and magnetic resonance imaging (MRI).

Echocardiography

■ TWO-DIMENSIONAL ECHOCARDIOGRAM

A two-dimensional (2D) echocardiogram can provide real-time visualization of the anatomy and physiology of the heart to give an abundant amount of diagnostic information in patients presenting to the ED. In patients with chest pain, 2D echocardiogram is a sensitive bedside test that can be an important tool guiding diagnosis, therapeutic interventions, and final disposition of the patient. Among the many causes of chest pain, findings are seen with 2D echocardiography that enable the physician to diagnose cardiac ischemia, acute pulmonary embolism, pericardial effusion, aortic dissection, pericarditis, hypertrophic cardiomyopathy, mitral valve prolapse, and aortic stenosis (Box 49-1).

BOX 49-1

Conditions Detected by Echocardiography

- Cardiac ischemia
- Hypertrophic cardiomyopathy
- Aortic dissection
- Pericarditis
- Mitral valve prolapse
- Aortic stenosis
- Acute pulmonary embolism
- Pericardial effusion

An important tool for 2D echocardiography in the ED includes its role in the diagnosis of myocardial ischemia (Fig. 49-1). In the healthy heart, increases in heart rate and myocardial contractility are seen with cardiac stress. In myocardial ischemia, segmental changes can be seen with 2D echocardiography, including decreased wall thickness during stress, decrease or no change in ejection fraction, and wall motion abnormalities. Regional wall motion abnormalities can be seen in acute myocardial ischemia or infarction with a sensitivity of 90% to 95% with transmural infarcts or 80% to 90% in subendocardial infarcts and a specificity of 80% to 90%.[2] Two-dimensional echocardiography can be performed in patients who have active chest pain or within minutes after its cessation. In patients with active chest pain and no ischemic ECG changes, 2D echocardiography has been shown to be more sensitive (91% vs. 40%) with a higher negative predictive value (NPV) (98% vs. 88%) in predicting myocardial ischemia or need for revascularization than ECG.[3] However, sensitivity of

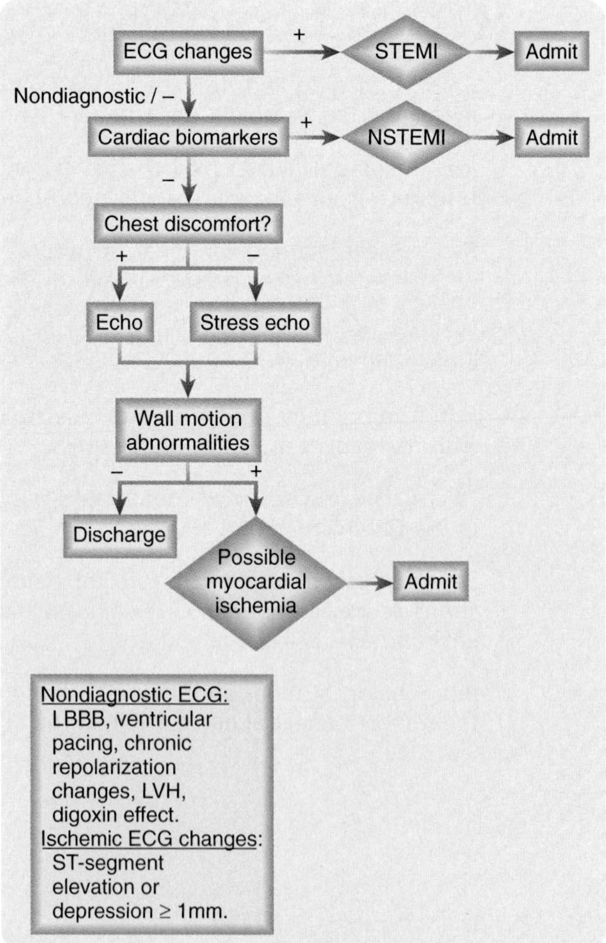
ECG changes
+
STEMI
Admit
Nondiagnostic / –
Cardiac biomarkers
+
NSTEMI
Admit
–
Chest discomfort?
+
–
Echo
Stress echo
Wall motion abnormalities
–
+
Discharge
Possible myocardial ischemia
Admit
Nondiagnostic ECG:
LBBB, ventricular pacing, chronic repolarization changes, LVH, digoxin effect.
Ischemic ECG changes:
ST-segment elevation or depression ≥ 1mm.

FIGURE 49-1 An example of the potential role of echocardiography in the evaluation of patients presenting to the ED with chest pain. ECG, electrocardiography; echo, echocardiography; LBBB, left bundle branch block; LVH, left ventricular hypertrophy; NSTEMI, non-ST-segment elevation myocardial infarction; STEMI, ST-segment elevation myocardial infarction.

2D echocardiography for detecting transient wall motion abnormalities due to acute ischemia diminishes as time between resolution of chest discomfort and acquisition of images increases.[4]

■ STRESS ECHOCARDIOGRAM

In a patient with a history of chest pain and no ischemic ECG changes, a stress echocardiogram is a useful test for risk stratification. In this test, an echocardiogram is performed immediately after the patient undergoes physical stress through the use of a treadmill or bike (upright or supine). If the patient is unable to perform physical stress, pharmacologic stress with the infusion of dobutamine, dipyridamole, or adenosine is used. Dobutamine is an adrenergic-stimulating agent that raises myocardial oxygen demand by increasing contractility, blood pressure, and heart rate. Atropine can be administered in 0.25-mg increments every 3 minutes to a maximum of 2 mg if the study endpoint is not achieved after maximum dobutamine dose.

Rarely, dobutamine can cause distressing symptoms, such as nausea, vomiting, headache, tremor, and anxiety. The vasodilator agents dipyridamole and adenosine cause heterogenous myocardial perfusion, which is sufficient in some patients to cause functional myocardial ischemia. Endpoints for termination of stress include attainment of 85% of age-predicted heart rate, new wall motion abnormalities, ECG changes diagnostic for ischemia, symptoms of severe angina, hemodynamic instability, significant hypertension, ventricular arrhythmia, and significant adverse effects of dobutamine.[5]

The greatest diagnostic benefit of stress echocardiography is in patients with intermediate pretest probability of having coronary artery disease. This includes patients with coronary risk factors (hypertension, smoking history, diabetes) and atypical angina, patients with typical angina, and patients with abnormal baseline ECG findings. Studies have shown that these patients can safely be discharged with outpatient follow-up if results of a stress echocardiogram are negative; this test has NPVs of 98.8% for all cardiac events (hospital admission for angina and revascularization procedure) and 99.6% for hard cardiac events (cardiac death and nonfatal myocardial infarction).[6]

In patients with high pretest probability of having coronary artery disease, stress echocardiography has prognostic benefits, with negative results suggesting decreased mortality and hard cardiac events,[7] but does not lower the post-test probability enough to warrant discharge from the ED. In patients with a low pretest probability, the procedure has a higher false-negative rate and therefore would not be beneficial in determining the immediate disposition of these patients.[1] Patients with no ischemic ECG changes and with negative cardiac biomarker values can be referred for outpatient stress echocardiography.

Myocardial Perfusion Imaging

Myocardial perfusion imaging (MPI) involves the injection of a radioisotope such as thallous chloride Tl 201 (thallium) or technetium Tc 99m sestamibi and imaging of its uptake and diffusion through cardiac tissue. This technique can be used for patients at rest to determine active ischemia or those with stress to determine exercise-induced ischemia.

MPI has gained wide acceptance for the diagnosis of myocardial ischemia in a variety of patient populations traditionally difficult to diagnose, such as women, asymptomatic diabetic patients, patients with existing ECG abnormalities like left bundle branch block (LBBB), and patients with severe renal disease. Gated single photon emission computed tomography (SPECT) and attenuation correction has made MPI even more valuable in the ED setting. Several landmark trials show the high NPV of MPI in the ED evaluation of chest discomfort (Table 49-1).[8-12] Although thallium imaging is older and more established, the diffusion kinetics of sestamibi make it more desirable in the ED setting.

Exercise Testing

Graded exercise testing is a popular method of cardiac stress testing in both inpatient and outpatient settings. Many of the early ED accelerated diagnostic protocols use this test after the initial risk stratification using cardiac biomarkers and ECG. Selection criteria for exercise testing are more restrictive than for other imaging modalities. Patients must be able to walk on a treadmill, and ECG findings should be normal or should show no new changes. Agents such as dobutamine can be used in lieu of exercise, but these have not been studied as extensively in the ED setting. Although exercise testing is being slowly supplanted by studies offering more detailed functional information, it is still a major tool in many centers.

The safety of requiring a potentially unstable patient to exercise was called into question by early critics of treadmill testing. Initial studies responsible for the popular implementation of exercise testing in

Tips and Tricks

- Meet the patient's expectations by explaining the process and time requirements of a comprehensive risk stratification protocol.
- Even after a negative rest protocol result, be sure to emphasize to the patient the need to pursue further stress testing.
- Determine the patient's ability to exercise before sending him/her for an exercise study. Many patients cannot exercise sufficiently for adequate results and ultimately need pharmacologically induced stress to maintain their heart rate in the appropriate range.

Table 49-1 NEGATIVE PREDICTIVE VALUE (NPV) OF REST MYOCARDIAL PERFUSION IMAGING USING TECHNETIUM Tc 99m SESTAMIBI, SINGLE PHOTON EMISSION COMPUTED TOMOGRAPHY (SPECT) IN THE ED*

Study and Year†	Study Population	NPV	Notes
Varetto et al (1993)[8]	64 patients with chest pain thought to be ischemic and nondiagnostic ECG findings	100%	None of the 34 patients with negative scans had adverse events in the 18-month follow-up period; 3 patients had false-positive results.
Hilton et al (1994)[9]	102 patients with "typical angina" and nondiagnostic ECG findings	99%	Of 70 patients with normal scan results, one 70-year-old woman with known CAD had recurrent symptoms; a subsequent catheterization showed advancing multivessel CAD. Predictors of cardiac events included three or more cardiac risk factors (risk ratio 3.3) and abnormal scan results (risk ratio 13.9).
Hilton et al (1996)[10]	150 patients with "typical" chest pain and nondiagnostic ECG findings	100%	None of the 87 patients with negative scans had adverse events in the 90-day follow-up period; one of these 87 patients presented 6 months later with similar symptoms and underwent successful coronary angioplasty.
Kontos et al (1997)[11]	532 low- to moderate-risk patients	99%	Positive scan result was the most important independent predictor of MI or revascularization (odds ratio 14; 95% CI 7.3-25).
Kontos et al (1999)[12]	620 low- to moderate-risk patients	99%	Sensitivity for predicting revascularization or significant coronary disease was higher for perfusion imaging than for serial troponin I measurements.

CAD, coronary artery disease; CI, confidence interval; ECG, electrocardiography; MI, myocardial infarction.
*Sestamibi in all these studies was injected during symptoms of chest pain.
†Superscript numbers indicate chapter references.

Table 49-2 MEDICAL COLLEGE OF VIRGINIA CHEST PAIN CENTER PROTOCOL

Level	Risk for Acute Myocardial Infarction	Risk for Acute Coronary Syndrome	Strategy	Patient Disposition
1	Very high	Very high	Fibrinolysis/percutaneous coronary intervention	Coronary care unit (CCU)
2	High	High	Acetylsalicylic acid, heparin, nitroglycerin, IIb/IIIa	CCU
3	Moderate	Moderate	Cardiac biomarker measurement+nuclear imaging	9-hr observation
4	Low	Moderate or low	Nuclear imaging	Home with outpatient stress test
5	Very low	Very low	As needed	Home

the ED environment have found the method to have an NPV of 98% to 100% and a negligible rate of adverse outcomes.[13] These data support the notion that exercise testing is safe and provides useful risk stratification information for appropriately selected patients.

Classic Examples of Accepted Protocols That Utilize Cardiac Imaging and Echocardiography

Each institution should develop cardiac evaluation protocols on the basis the risk profile of its population and the availability of imaging modalities and in collaboration with emergency medicine, radiology, and cardiology physicians. Specific protocols and imaging modalities vary among locations and institutions. Table 49-2 and Figures 49-2 and 49-3 show some examples of established, accepted, and often duplicated protocols currently in use.[14]

Magnetic Resonance Imaging

Current research continues to explore new and hopefully more effective imaging strategies for the evaluation of patients with chest discomfort in the ED. MRI can determine both myocardial perfusion and regional wall motion abnormalities, including transient stunning after an ischemic event. Several studies have shown its utility in the diagnosis of acute coro-

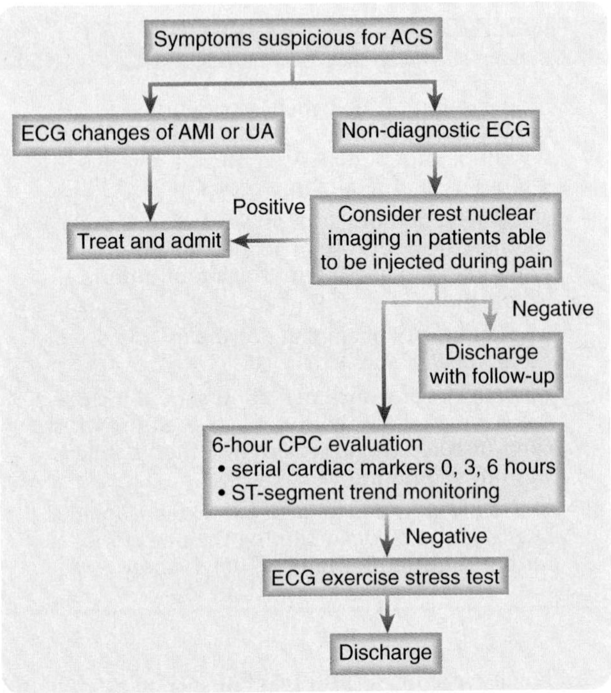
Symptoms suspicious for ACS
ECG changes of AMI or UA
Non-diagnostic ECG
Treat and admit
Positive
Consider rest nuclear imaging in patients able to be injected during pain
Negative
Discharge with follow-up
6-hour CPC evaluation
• serial cardiac markers 0, 3, 6 hours
• ST-segment trend monitoring
Negative
ECG exercise stress test
Discharge

FIGURE 49-2 University of Cincinnati "Heart ER" strategy. ACS, acute coronary syndrome; AMI, acute myocardial infarction; CPC, chest pain center; ECG, electrocardiography; UA, unstable angina. (From Blomkalns AL, Gibler WB: Chest pain unit concept: Rationale and diagnostic strategies. Cardiol Clin 2005;23:411-421.)

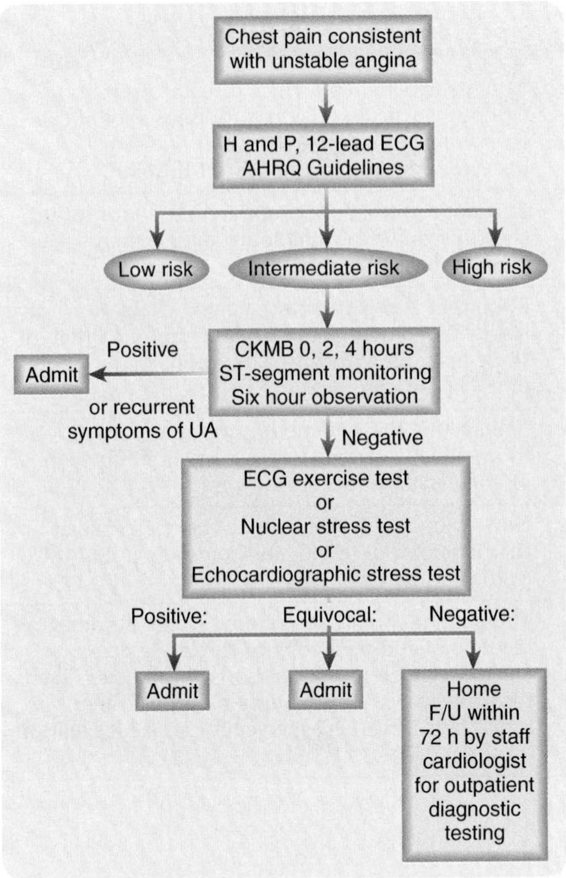
Chest pain consistent with unstable angina
H and P, 12-lead ECG
AHRQ Guidelines
Low risk
Intermediate risk
High risk
CKMB 0, 2, 4 hours
ST-segment monitoring
Six hour observation
Positive
Admit
or recurrent symptoms of UA
Negative
ECG exercise test
or
Nuclear stress test
or
Echocardiographic stress test
Positive:
Equivocal:
Negative:
Admit
Admit
Home F/U within 72 h by staff cardiologist for outpatient diagnostic testing

FIGURE 49-3 Mayo Clinic strategy. AHRQ, Agency for Healthcare Research and Quality; CKMB, creatinine kinase MB fraction; ECG, electrocardiography; F/U, follow-up; H and P, history and physical examination; UA, unstable angina. (From Blomkalns AL, Gibler WB: Chest pain unit concept: Rationale and diagnostic strategies. Cardiol Clin 2005;23:411-421.)

nary syndrome, and recent clinical trials demonstrate its potential value in identifying atherosclerotic lesions and vulnerable plaques.[15,16] We currently believe that limited availability and high cost preclude MRI as a standard, acceptable modality until further studies demonstrate a decisive advantage over nuclear imaging or echocardiography.[17]

Electron Beam Computed Tomography and CT Coronary Angiography

Electron beam computer tomography (EBCT), also known as "ultrafast" CT, has emerged as a highly sensitive means by which to detect calcium in the atherosclerotic lesions of coronary arteries. Secondly, CT coronary angiography using the 64-slice scanners can accurately visualize coronary arteries in a large majority of patients. CT also imparts additive advantage of being able to visualize other potentially significant diagnoses, such as pulmonary embolism and aortic dissection ("triple rule-out"). Although both of these modalities show promise, their utility for the ED risk stratification of patients with possible cardiac ischemia in comparison with traditional stress testing is uncertain. The results from ongoing studies will help determine the optimal role of CT in cardiac evaluation.[18]

FACTS AND FORMULAS

$SI = \frac{SV}{BSA}$

The myocardium takes up technetium-99m sestamibi proportional to blood flow; unlike thallium-201, the sestamibi redistributes minimally after injection. This feature allows for delayed imaging after the initial radioisotope injection.

Contemporary 64-slice computed tomography (CT) scanners generate images with the spatial resolution of 0.4 mm and a temporal resolution of 83 to 165 msec. Although traditional coronary angiography has a spatial resolution of 0.15 mm and a temporal resolution of 0.33 sec, CT angiography can yield sufficient diagnostic data in many patients. In order to facilitate adequate imaging for CT angiography, patients must undergo beta-blocker therapy to achieve a heart rate of approximately 60 beats/min.

PATIENT TEACHING TIPS

- Patients experiencing chest discomfort with or without classic associated symptoms should call their emergency response system (i.e., 911) instead of driving to the nearest hospital.
- In order to provide appropriate risk stratification, chest discomfort evaluation protocols may take several hours to complete.
- Even after a negative rest imaging evaluation result, the patient should follow up for further stress imaging with his or her primary care physician or cardiologist.
- Therapeutic lifestyle modifications and attention to modifiable cardiac risk factors should be part of any evaluation protocol.
- Nuclear imaging does include the use of radiation that is safe, well-tested, and routinely used for cardiac evaluation.
- The patient should keep copies of his/her imaging records, including a copy of the latest electrocardiogram, in a personal health file. These records can be tremendously useful to other physicians if further emergency cardiac evaluation is required.

Documentation

- A description of the patient's presenting symptoms should include onset, duration, severity, location, quality, context, associated symptoms, and modifying factors.
- Documentation of past family history of early coronary heart disease or acute coronary syndromes provides useful risk stratification information.
- A social history of smoking or the use of cocaine should be documented.
- Nuclear imaging documentation should include the last episode of the patient's presenting with chest discomfort, particularly whether the media was injected during pain.
- The clinician needs to justify an extended period of evaluation by documenting the need for further risk stratification and observation.

Pitfalls

- For nuclear imaging, the best results are obtained if the radionuclide is injected while the patient is having symptoms.
- Many protocols for stress testing preclude proximate caffeine ingestion. Make sure to note the patient's prior caffeine intake and to have him/her avoid the inadvertent ingestion of any caffeine-containing product (regular or decaffeinated coffee, tea, soft drinks, and chocolate) during the initial evaluation phase.
- The pharmacy or nuclear medicine department regulates the supply of any nuclear imaging agent. If these agents are unused for a time, they expire and must be discarded. Additional preparation or acquisition of fresh agent may cause delay in the workup of an individual patient.
- Even if the cardiac imaging and evaluation results are negative, alternative diagnoses such as aortic dissection, peptic ulcer disease, and pulmonary embolism should be considered. Patients should leave the ED with some ideas as to what may be causing their symptoms.
- Two nuclear imaging studies, such as a technetium Tc 99m sestamibi scan and a ventilation/perfusion ($\dot{V}/\dot{Q}$) lung scan cannot be performed within the same 24-hour period. If the differential diagnosis includes pulmonary embolism, alternative and complementary imaging modalities may have to be used.
- Exercise and pharmacologic stress studies require that the patient's heart rate rise to appropriate levels. The EP should be cautious about starting beta-blocker therapy in patients who will undergo stress studies in the ED. Although beta blockade is a standard treatment in patients with myocardial ischemia, it can hamper the physician's ability to perform risk stratification for low-risk patients because it causes nondiagnostic stress evaluations.

Summary

Cardiac imaging is an important component in the evaluation of patients presenting to the ED with chest discomfort. The astute clinician should understand the benefits and limitations of each modality and should incorporate appropriate imaging into the framework of the institution, its resources, and its physician collaborators.

REFERENCES

1. Conti A, Sammicheli L, Gallini C, et al: Assessment of patients with low-risk chest pain in the emergency department: Head-to-head comparison of exercise stress echocardiography and exercise myocardial SPECT. Am Heart J 2005;149:894-901.
2. Kabalgoitia M IM: Diagnostic and prognostic use of stress echo in acute coronary syndromes including emergency department imaging. Echocardiography 2000;17:479-493.
3. Kontos MC, Arrowood JA, Paulsen WHJ, et al: Early echocardiography can predict cardiac events in emergency department patients with chest pain. Ann Emerg Med 1998;31:550-557.
4. Sasaki H, Charuzi Y, Beeder C, et al: Utility of echocardiography for the early assessment of patients with nondiagnostic chest pain. Am Heart J 1986;112:494-497.
5. Armstrong WF, Pellikka PA, Ryan T, et al: Stress echocardiography: Recommendations for performance and interpretation of stress echocardiography. J Am Soc Echocardiogr 1998;11:97-104.
6. Bedetti G, Pasanisi EM, Tintori G, et al: Stress echo in chest pain unit: The SPEED trial. Int J Cardiol 2005;102:461-467.

7. Elhendy A, Mahoney DW, Burger KN, et al: Prognostic value of exercise echocardiography in patients with classic angina pectoris. Am J Cardiol 2004;94:559-563.
8. Varetto T, Cantalupi D, Altieri A, et al: Emergency room technetium-99m sestamibi imaging to rule out acute myocardial ischemic events in patients with nondiagnostic electrocardiograms. J Am Coll Cardiol 1993;22:1804-1808.
9. Hilton TC, Thompson RC, Williams HJ, et al: Technetium-99m sestamibi myocardial perfusion imaging in the emergency room evaluation of chest pain. J Am Coll Cardiol 1994;23:1016-1022.
10. Hilton TC, Fulmer H, Abuan T, et al: Ninety-day follow-up of patients in the emergency department with chest pain who undergo initial single-photon emission computed tomographic perfusion scintigraphy with technetium 99m-labeled sestamibi. J Nucl Cardiol 1996;3:308-311.
11. Kontos MC, Jesse RL, Schmidt KL, et al: Value of acute rest sestamibi perfusion imaging for evaluation of patients admitted to the emergency department with chest pain. J Am Coll Cardiol 1997;30:976-982.
12. Kontos MC, Jesse RL, Anderson FP, et al: Comparison of myocardial perfusion imaging and cardiac troponin I in patients admitted to the emergency department with chest pain. Circulation 1999;99:2073-2078.
13. Amsterdam EA, Kirk JD, Diercks DB, et al: Exercise testing in chest pain units: Rationale, implementation, and results. Cardiol Clin 2005;23:503-516.
14. Blomkalns AL, Gibler WB: Chest pain unit concept: Rationale and diagnostic strategies. Cardiol Clin 2005;23:411-421.
15. Fayad ZA: MR imaging for the noninvasive assessment of atherothrombotic plaques. Magn Reson Imaging Clin North Am 2003;11:101-113.
16. Kwong RY, Schussheim AE, Rekhraj S, et al: Detecting acute coronary syndrome in the emergency department with cardiac magnetic resonance imaging. Circulation 2003;107:531-537.
17. Soman P, Bokor D, Lahiri A: Why cardiac magnetic resonance imaging will not make it. J Comput Assist Tomogr 1999;23(Suppl 1):S143-S149.
18. McCord J, Amsterdam EA: Newer imaging methods for triaging patients presenting to the emergency department with chest pain. Cardiol Clin 2005;23:541-548.

Chapter **50**

Congestive Heart Failure

Joshua M. Kosowsky

KEY POINTS

Acute decompensated heart failure (ADHF) often manifests as symptoms of volume overload, acute diastolic dysfunction, and low cardiac output.

Identifying and addressing the precipitants of the decompensation are as important as treating the decompensation itself.

Measurements of B-type natriuretic peptide (BNP) (or NT-proBNP; see later) can assist with the diagnosis, but it is important to understand the limitations of this test.

For patients in respiratory distress, noninvasive support with continuous positive airway pressure (or bilevel positive airway pressure) reduces the need for endotracheal intubation.

Not all patients with ADHF are truly volume overloaded; overaggressive diuresis risks hypotension and worsening renal function.

Nitrates remain the cornerstone of therapy for patients in whom an acute reduction in cardiac preload and afterload is desired.

Inotropic therapy should not be routinely instituted unless the patient is in cardiogenic shock.

Scope and Outline

With the aging of the U.S. population and improved survival after myocardial infarction, the prevalence of heart failure is on the rise.[1] At the same time, advances in medical therapy are allowing patients with heart failure to live longer. There were more than 5 million Americans with heart failure in 2007, and it is estimated that by 2037, that number will top 10 million. Heart failure contributes to nearly 300,000 deaths a year, and costs associated with treatment of heart failure exceed $30 billion annually. Heart failure accounts for more than 1 million inpatient admissions a year and represents the primary reason for hospitalization among the growing elderly population. Approximately 4 of every 5 patients hospitalized for heart failure present initially to the ED.

Evidence-based literature for ED management of heart failure lags behind that of other emergency conditions, such as acute coronary syndrome and stroke. The number of large, randomized, controlled,

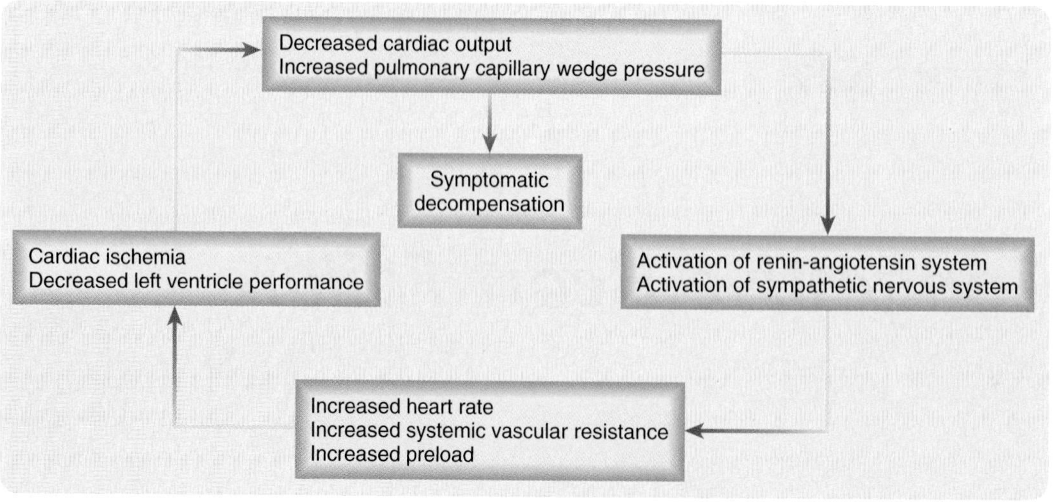
Decreased cardiac output
Increased pulmonary capillary wedge pressure
Symptomatic decompensation
Cardiac ischemia
Decreased left ventricle performance
Activation of renin-angiotensin system
Activation of sympathetic nervous system
Increased heart rate
Increased systemic vascular resistance
Increased preload

FIGURE 50-1 Pathophysiology of heart failure.

clinical trials is small, and most practice guidelines, such as those from the Heart Failure Society of America (HFSA) and the European Society of Cardiology (ESC), rely heavily on consensus statements.[2,3] The America Heart Association and the American Association of Cardiology (ACC/AHA) Guidelines for the Evaluation and Management of Heart Failure have little to say on the subject of ED management.[4] On the other hand, data from the Acute Decompensated Heart Failure National Registry (ADHERE), a large national registry of inpatient admissions, have provided important insights into the clinical characteristics and actual patterns of care of these patients.[5] A clinical policy from the American College of Emergency Physicians on critical issues in the evaluation and management of ED patients with heart failure has recently been published.[6]

In addition to the paucity of controlled clinical trial data, there remains confusion about terminology. *Heart failure* refers to the clinical syndrome that can result from any structural or functional cardiac disorder that impairs the ability of the ventricle to fill with or eject blood. Causes of chronic heart failure are numerous and diverse (Box 50-1), but in the United States, the majority of cases arise as a consequence of coronary artery disease and long-standing hypertension. The term *acute heart failure* is reserved for the presence of acute signs and symptoms of heart failure in an individual without previously known structural or functional cardiac disease. Examples of acute heart failure are massive ST-elevation myocardial infarction, acute papillary muscle rupture, and fulminant myocarditis. Much more commonly, a patient presents to the ED with worsening symptoms of known chronic heart failure, in common parlance a "heart failure exacerbation." The term *acute decompensated heart failure* (ADHF) has been adopted to describe this phenomenon, whereby a patient with an established diagnosis of heart failure experiences increasing signs and symptoms of the disease after a period of relative stability.

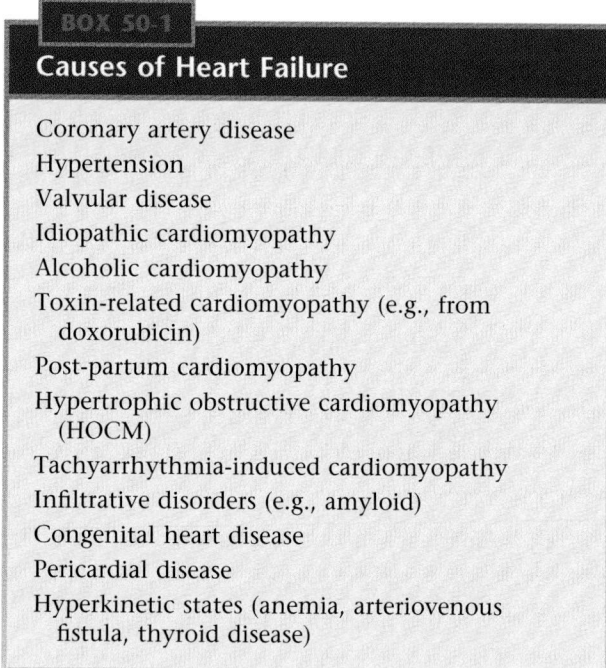

BOX 50-1

Causes of Heart Failure

- Coronary artery disease
- Hypertension
- Valvular disease
- Idiopathic cardiomyopathy
- Alcoholic cardiomyopathy
- Toxin-related cardiomyopathy (e.g., from doxorubicin)
- Post-partum cardiomyopathy
- Hypertrophic obstructive cardiomyopathy (HOCM)
- Tachyarrhythmia-induced cardiomyopathy
- Infiltrative disorders (e.g., amyloid)
- Congenital heart disease
- Pericardial disease
- Hyperkinetic states (anemia, arteriovenous fistula, thyroid disease)

Pathophysiology

In patients with chronic heart failure, inadequacy of cardiac function sets in motion a common set of compensatory mechanisms, based on the Frank-Starling relation and characterized by elevated sympathetic tone, fluid and salt retention, and ventricular remodeling. These adaptations can allow heart failure to remain stable (or "compensated") for a time but also provide the final common pathway for decompensation—a downward spiral that can accelerate in response to a particular precipitant or stress (Fig. 50-1). High circulating levels of aldosterone, vasopressin, epinephrine, and norepinephrine can become maladaptive when tachycardia and vasoconstriction compromise the intrinsic performance of the left

Table 50-1 SYNDROMES OF ACUTE DECOMPENSATED HEART FAILURE

	Systemic Volume Overload	Acute Diastolic Dysfunction	Low-Output Failure
Frequency	High	High	Low
Onset	Gradual	Rapid	Gradual
Characteristics	Congestive	Congestive/ischemic	Poor perfusion
Example	Diuretic noncompliance	Hypertensive crisis	End-stage cardiomyopathy

BOX 50-2

Common Precipitants of Acute Decompensate Heart Failure

Medication non-compliance/dietary indiscretion
Myocardial ischemia/infarction
Cardiac arrhythmia (e.g., atrial fibrillation)
Pulmonary and other infections
Administration of inappropriate medications
Anemia
Alcohol withdrawal
Thyrotoxicosis

ventricle (LV) and worsen myocardial oxygen balance. Deteriorating LV function can result in further neurohormonal activation and self-perpetuation of this adverse cycle. An acute decompensation can develop over a period of minutes, hours, or days and can range in severity from mild symptoms of volume overload or decreased cardiac output to frank pulmonary edema or cardiogenic shock.

■ PRECIPITATING FACTORS

Although ADHF represents a final common pathway, it is generally triggered by one or more specific precipitants (Box 50-2). Noncompliance with medications or dietary restrictions and myocardial ischemia are believed to be the most common causes of clinical cardiac decompensation. Other cardiovascular precipitants are arrhythmia (atrial fibrillation in particular), valvular dysfunction, and hypertensive crisis, but ADHF can also arise as a consequence of noncardiac conditions, such as infections, anemia, alcohol withdrawal, uncontrolled diabetes, and thyroid disease.

The heterogeneity of ADHF presentations reflects, to some extent, the relative contributions of volume overload, acute diastolic dysfunction, and low cardiac output (Table 50-1).[7] Volume overload, which usually occurs in the setting of medication noncompliance and/or dietary indiscretion, is classically associated with gradually worsening congestive symptoms. Acute diastolic dysfunction can occur in the setting of myocardial ischemia, tachyarrhythmia, or uncontrolled hypertension and typically manifests as flash pulmonary edema. Nearly half of all patients admitted to the hospital for ADHF have mild or no impairment of systolic function.[5] Manifestations of low cardiac output (i.e., hypoperfusion) generally do not manifest except in patients with advanced LV dysfunction.

Prehospital Care

Even before patients reach the hospital, ADHF is associated with significant morbidity and mortality, including malignant arrhythmias and prehospital cardiac arrest. With few exceptions, the safety and efficacy of prehospital medications have been poorly studied. Prehospital therapy for decompensated heart failure should be undertaken with particular caution in light of the relatively high number of inaccurate diagnoses made in the field. As many as 50% of patients with assumed heart-associated respiratory distress are diagnosed with a different condition once they arrive in the hospital. Despite these concerns, evidence suggests that prehospital therapy for presumed heart failure can prevent serious complications and improve survival, particularly for critically ill patients.

Nitroglycerin appears to be the safest and most effective of the prehospital medications used for presumed pulmonary edema.[8] The role of other medications for heart failure in the prehospital setting is less clear. Early administration of furosemide appears to have very little benefit and may result in short-term complications. The prehospital use of morphine sulfate for presumed pulmonary edema is associated with a higher rate of endotracheal intubation, particularly among patients who turn out to have been misdiagnosed in the field.

Emergency Department Evaluation

The approach to the patient with ADHF begins with stabilization of respiratory and hemodynamic status and the rapid exclusion or treatment of reversible life-threatening conditions. Clinical evaluation and empirical therapy begin simultaneously, with supplemental oxygen, cardiac monitoring, pulse oximetry, and intravenous access. Patients with clinical signs of exhaustion or cyanosis despite supplemental oxygen require respiratory support with either invasive or noninvasive means. Those with hypotension, obtundation, cool extremities, or other signs of poor perfusion should be presumed to be in or near cardiogenic shock, and managed accordingly. Once the initial

Table 50-2 SENSITIVITY, SPECIFICITY, AND POSITIVE LIKELIHOOD RATIO OF SELECTED CLINICAL FINDINGS FOR ACUTE DECOMPENSATED HEART FAILURE

	Sensitivity (%)	Specificity (%)	Positive Likelihood Ratio (:1)
Past Medical History			
Heart failure	60	90	4.4
Myocardial infarction	40	87	3.1
Coronary artery disease	52	70	1.8
Symptoms			
Paroxysmal nocturnal dyspnea	41	84	2.6
Orthopnea	50	77	2.2
Edema	51	76	2.1
Signs			
Third heart sound	13	99	11
Abdominojugular reflux	24	96	6.4
Jugular venous distention	39	97	5.1
Peripheral edema	50	78	2.3
Rales	60	78	2.8
Wheezing	22	58	0.52
Diagnostic Findings			
Atrial fibrillation	26	93	3.8
Pulmonary venous congestion	54	96	12.0
Cardiomegaly	74	78	3.3

Modifed from Wang CS, FitzGerald JM, Schulzer M, et al: Does this dyspneic patient in the emergency department have congestive heart failure? JAMA 2005;294:1944-1956.

resuscitation is under way, further efforts should be made to establish the diagnosis of ADHF and identify an underlying cause of the acute decompensation.

Most patients with ADHF present with some degree of dyspnea. However, ADHF can closely mimic many other cardiac, respiratory, and systemic diseases. Historical features such as a history of orthopnea, paroxysmal nocturnal dyspnea, and/or peripheral edema make the diagnosis of ADHF more likely. The most valuable single piece of historical information to elicit from patients is a prior history of heart failure, myocardial infarction, or coronary artery disease. For example, patients presenting to the ED with acute dyspnea are approximately six times more likely to have ADHF if they have previously experienced heart failure (Table 50-2).[9]

Older patients often lack typical signs and symptoms of heart failure, which may be obscured by the aging process itself or by the presence of coexisting medical conditions. Nonspecific symptoms, such as weakness, lethargy, fatigue, anorexia, and lightheadedness, may actually be manifestations of decreased cardiac output.

Vital signs provide a sense of the severity of illness and can suggest etiologic factors for decompensation. Hyperthermia or hypothermia may indicate sepsis or thyroid disease. In the absence of rate-controlling pharmacologic agents, tachycardia is nearly universal in decompensated heart failure. Bradycardia should raise concern for high-degree atrioventricular block, hyperkalemia, drug toxicity (digoxin, calcium channel, beta blocker), or severe hypoxia. Hypertension is commonly seen in patients with both systolic and diastolic dysfunction. Hypotension may represent baseline blood pressure (BP) for patients with end-stage cardiomyopathy but otherwise should raise the possibility of cardiogenic or another type of shock.

The diagnostic utility of the physical examination is well-documented for chronic heart failure but less so for ADHF. In ADHF, the physical findings may be misleading owing to the rapidly evolving clinical situation. Generally speaking, jugular venous distention, abdominojugular reflux, pedal edema, and an audible third heart sound are specific but insensitive indicators of heart failure, whereas the presence of pulmonary rales has only moderate specificity for heart failure (see Table 50-2).[9]

Diagnostic Studies

■ LABORATORY TESTS

The majority of patients who present with complaints suggestive of ADHF need laboratory testing. A complete blood count (CBC) is useful for ruling out anemia as an alternative cause for dyspnea or as a precipitant of ADHF. An elevated white blood cell

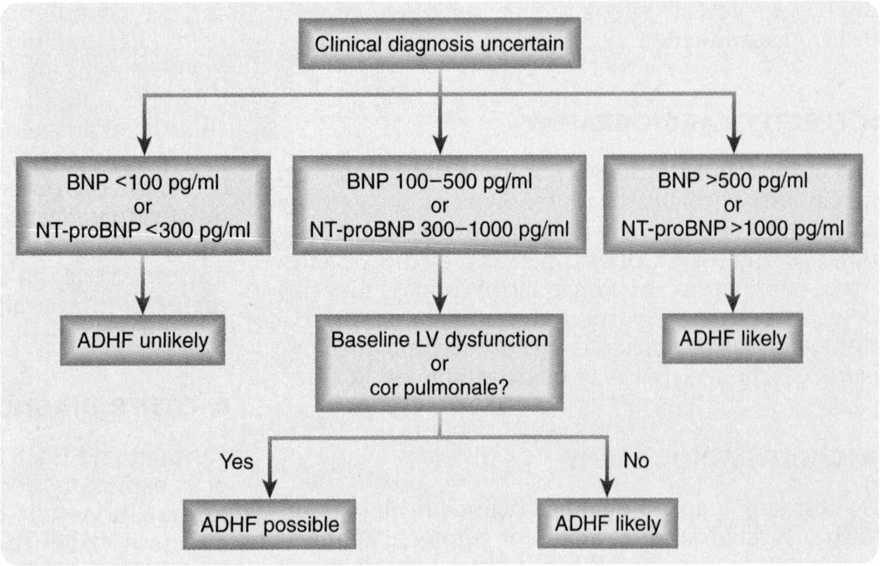
Clinical diagnosis uncertain
BNP <100 pg/ml
or
NT-proBNP <300 pg/ml
BNP 100–500 pg/ml
or
NT-proBNP 300–1000 pg/ml
BNP >500 pg/ml
or
NT-proBNP >1000 pg/ml
ADHF unlikely
Baseline LV dysfunction
or
cor pulmonale?
ADHF likely
Yes
No
ADHF possible
ADHF likely

FIGURE 50-2 Interpretation of natriuretic peptide levels. ADHF, acute decompensated heart failure; BNP, B-type natriuretic peptide; NT-proBNP, inactive *N*-terminal fragment of BNP.

count may suggest the presence of an infectious process, especially if bands are present; however, this finding has not been well studied in the patient with suspected ADHF. Serum chemistry analysis is important for assessing renal function and overall fluid and electrolyte balance in patients who are generally undergoing diuretic therapy already and are likely require additional diuresis.

■ MARKERS OF CARDIAC ISCHEMIA

Elevations of cardiac troponins may be found in up to one third of patients with ADHF and help identify patients with worse short-term prognosis. In any individual case, it remains a clinical determination as to whether biomarker elevations (1) reflect an acute coronary syndrome (i.e., unstable plaque causing ischemia and myocardial cell death and leading to worsening heart failure) or (2) simply reflect the severity of heart failure (i.e., derangements in myocardial oxygen balance leading to "demand ischemia" and myocardial cell death). Information from the history (e.g., onset of symptoms, comparison to prior episodes) may be helpful in this regard.

■ B-NATRIURETIC PEPTIDE AND NT-proBNP

B-type natriuretic peptide (BNP) is a counterregulatory hormone produced by cardiac myocytes in response to increased end-diastolic pressure and volume, as occurs in the setting of heart failure. ProBNP is released into the circulation and cleaved into biologically active BNP and an inactive *N*-terminal fragment, NT-proBNP, which has a half-life three to six times that of BNP. Plasma levels of BNP and NT-proBNP correlate with the degree of LV overload, severity of clinical heart failure, and both short- and long-term cardiovascular mortality.

Plasma levels of BNP and NT-proBNP have been shown to be useful in distinguishing between cardiac and noncardiac causes of dyspnea.[10,11] Acutely dyspneic patients with plasma BNP levels lower than 100 pg/mL or NT-proBNP levels lower than 300 pg/mL are very unlikely to have ADHF (90% to 99% sensitivity), whereas those with BNP levels greater than 500 pg/mL or NT-proBNP levels greater than 1000 pg/mL are very likely to have ADHF (87% to 95% specificity). Intermediate levels must be interpreted in clinical context (Fig. 50-2).

Interpretation of BNP levels must take into account baseline LV dysfunction and other known or suspected conditions associated with left and/or right ventricular pressure overload that may result in BNP elevations. Patients with advanced age or renal insufficiency tend to have higher BNP and NT-proBNP levels, whereas those with high body mass index tend to have lower levels. Although BNP and NT-proBNP measurements retain discriminatory power in these subpopulations, the optimal cutoff points for diagnosing ADHF may vary. The duration of symptoms also plays a role; for example, in the setting of flash pulmonary edema, these substances may not be extremely elevated.

In general, EPs are about 80% accurate in distinguishing between cardiac and noncardiac causes of dyspnea on clinical grounds. Supplementing clinical acumen with routine BNP or NT-proBNP measurement does increase diagnostic accuracy overall, but as demonstrated in the Breathing Not Properly Multinational Study, the improvement is rather marginal.[12] For example, in clear-cut cases, very high or very low values are unlikely to have an effect on diagnosis, but in less clear-cut cases, intermediate results are more likely to do so.

BNP and NT-proBNP levels also carry modest prognostic information.[13] Although admission levels correlate only modestly with short-term outcomes, discharge levels are strong independent predictors of death or readmission.

ELECTROCARDIOGRAPHY

The electrocardiogram (ECG) is likely to be abnormal in patients with heart failure. Signs of pre-existing conditions such as hypertrophy, myocardial infarction, or dilated cardiomyopathy may be present. Atrial fibrillation or other arrhythmias may be detected. A large proportion of heart failure exacerbations are either precipitated or accompanied by cardiac ischemia that may be detectable on ECG.

CHEST RADIOGRAPHY

A chest radiograph should be obtained in all patients with suspected ADHF to assess for pulmonary congestion and to allow for the differential diagnosis of other lung diseases. Findings on chest radiograph in ADHF include cardiomegaly, vascular redistribution (e.g., cephalization, fullness of hilar vessels), interstitial edema, and pulmonary edema. Pleural effusions in heart failure tend to be bilateral or localized to the right side. Although the presence of pulmonary congestion is associated with a very high likelihood of ADHF, it should be noted that as many as 1 in 5 patients with ADHF do not have evidence of congestion on chest radiograph. Among individuals with underlying pulmonary emphysema, congestion may appear atypical or not at all, and patients with long-standing congestive heart failure (CHF) may have scant radiographic evidence of congestion owing to well-developed pulmonary lymphatics. Cardiomegaly may be absent in acute heart failure, particularly in the setting of acute diastolic dysfunction.

CARDIAC ECHOCARDIOGRAPHY

Echocardiography is considered the gold standard for assessing the status of LV function, distinguishing between systolic and diastolic failure and identifying regional wall motion abnormalities. Perhaps more important in the ED setting, echocardiography can assist in diagnosing or excluding potentially reversible causes of acute cardiac decompensation, such as pericardial tamponade, massive pulmonary embolus, ruptured chordae tendineae, and ruptured ventricular septum. As a practical matter, emergency echocardiography is generally not required in most instances of ADHF, particularly if a patient has recently undergone echocardiography and now has a clear precipitant for decompensation.

PULMONARY ARTERY (SWAN-GANZ) CATHETERIZATION

Invasive hemodynamic monitoring is usually unnecessary for the diagnosis and management of ADHF, and its routine use is not recommended. In the absence of pulmonary disease or disproportionate right heart failure, clinical estimation or measurement of right atrial pressure usually correlates with left-sided filling pressures. Compared with standard clinical management, hemodynamically guided therapy is not associated with improvement in short- or long-term outcome. On the other hand, right heart catheterization remains a reasonable option in patients with cardiogenic shock or when there is uncertainty about a patient's hemodynamics after careful clinical evaluation and initial therapy.

OTHER DIAGNOSTIC MODALITIES

Elevated end-tidal CO_2 concentrations and reduced peak expiratory flow rates are more commonly seen exacerbations of chronic obstructive pulmonary disease (COPD) than in ADHF. However, in neither case is there a cutoff value that can be used to accurately distinguish between cardiac and respiratory causes of dyspnea. Another noninvasive means proposed for aiding in the diagnosis of ADHF is impedance cardiography, in which real-time estimates of cardiac output and pulmonary capillary wedge pressure are derived through the use of the principles of thoracic bioimpedance. Although the technology has been available for some time, data as to the overall utility of this diagnostic tool in the ED setting are limited.

Treatment

PRIORITIES OF TREATMENT

As for any ill patient in the ED, the initial focus of attention is on the airway. Although most patients in respiratory distress can be managed with supplemental oxygen and noninvasive ventilatory support (see later), the presence of agonal respirations or profoundly depressed mental status mandates emergency endotracheal intubation. In general, airway management should be accomplished with rapid-sequence intubation (RSI), because prolonged episodes of intubation risk further cardiac decompensation and cardiopulmonary arrest. Most induction agents (thiopental, fentanyl, and midazolam) are associated with a significant risk of hypotension for patients with ADHF, whereas induction with etomidate is generally considered safe. Keeping the patient in an upright position as long as possible before intubation may assist in maximizing preoxygenation.

All patients with ADHF who present in respiratory distress should receive supplemental oxygen and should be positioned upright, if possible, to improve respiratory dynamics and maximize oxygen delivery to vital organs. Practice guidelines recommend early application of monitors, such as pulse oximetry, noninvasive BP, and continuous cardiac monitoring, to provide early warning of further decompensation.

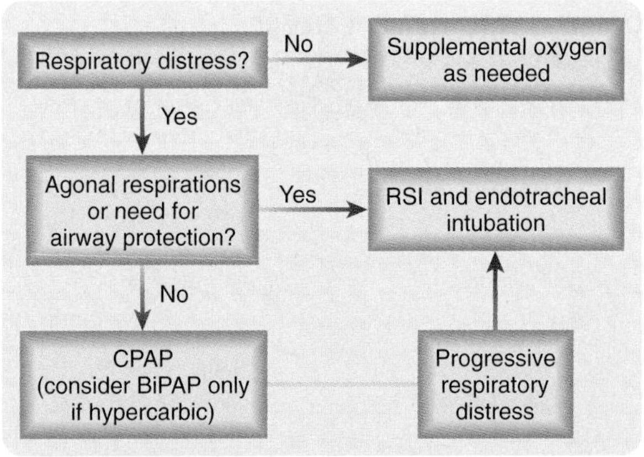
Respiratory distress?
No
Supplemental oxygen as needed
Yes
Agonal respirations or need for airway protection?
Yes
RSI and endotracheal intubation
No
CPAP (consider BiPAP only if hypercarbic)
Progressive respiratory distress

FIGURE 50-3 Algorithm for ventilatory support in acute decompensation heart failure. BiPAP, bilevel positive airway pressure; CPAP, continuous positive airway pressure; RSI, rapid-sequence intubation.

■ NONINVASIVE RESPIRATORY SUPPORT

For patients with ADHF and respiratory distress in whom intubation is not immediately required, noninvasive respiratory support via continuous positive airway pressure (CPAP) or bilevel positive airway pressure (BiPAP) should be employed (Fig. 50-3). Although the decision to initiate noninvasive respiratory support may depend on a variety of factors, the presumption is that the earlier therapy is instituted, the greater the likelihood of averting intubation. Success also depends on appropriate patient selection. Patients with a history of cardiac arrest, unstable cardiac rhythms, or cardiogenic shock are generally believed not to be candidates for a noninvasive approach. Likewise, in the setting of severe myocardial ischemia or infarction, full ventilatory support to decrease the myocardial oxygen demand associated with respiratory effort may be preferable.

CPAP improves lung mechanics by recruiting atelectatic alveoli, improving pulmonary compliance, and reducing the work of breathing. At the same time, particularly for patients with heart failure, CPAP improves hemodynamics by reducing preload and afterload, thereby enhancing LV performance. In patients with ADHF, nasal or face mask–applied CPAP achieves better oxygenation, lower heart rate, and lower BP than supplemental oxygen therapy alone. Pooled data from several randomized, controlled clinical trials suggest that the use of CPAP (at 5-10 mm Hg) for patients with respiratory distress due to ADHF reduces the frequency of endotracheal intubation and may be associated with a lower mortality.[14]

BiPAP combines, which the physiologic advantages of CPAP during expiration with additional ventilatory assistance during inspiration, plays an important role in improving gas exchange for patients with hypercarbia. However, at present, there is little evidence to suggest an advantage of BiPAP over CPAP for patients with ADHF and pure hypoxemic respiratory failure.

If there are signs of progressive respiratory failure in spite of noninvasive support, endotracheal intubation and mechanical ventilation should be instituted.

■ PHARMACOLOGIC THERAPY

The twin objectives of pharmacologic therapy for ADHF are relief of pulmonary congestion and improvement in systemic tissue perfusion. Strategies to achieve these goals involve reducing preload and enhancing LV function while aiming to maintain or even improve myocardial oxygen balance (Table 50-3).

■ Diuretics

Diuretics constitute the mainstay of therapy for patients with volume overload. Although their use is widely recommended as initial therapy for patients with ADHF and generally accepted to be both safe and effective, it should be noted that this practice has not been evaluated in randomized, placebo-controlled trials. It is also important to recognize that not all patients who present with ADHF are, in fact, volume overloaded. For example, patients with acute diastolic dysfunction may benefit more from redistribution of circulating volume (e.g., with a vasodilator) than from diuresis per se. Thus, the indiscriminate use of diuretics carries the risk of over-diuresis, with detrimental effects on systemic perfusion in general and renal function in particular.

Evidence from in vitro and in vivo experiments suggests that direct vascular effects of diuretics may contribute in minor ways to their mechanism of action and that these effects are not necessarily altogether advantageous, in potentially promoting activation of the sympathetic and renin-angiotensin systems. Studies comparing the acute effects of diuretics and nitrates have tended to emphasize the more favorable overall hemodynamic effects of the latter group (see later).

Depending on a patient's clinical condition, state of hydration, and previous use of diuretics, an initial intravenous (IV) dose of furosemide, 20 to 200 mg, is generally administered. For patients undergoing long-term diuretic therapy, a common strategy is to begin with the usual daily dose given as an IV bolus, and to double the dose if there is inadequate diuresis. Although giving repeated IV boluses is common practice, patients with ongoing diuretic requirements may benefit from continuous IV furosemide infusions from the standpoint of both efficacy and safety.[15] In cases of refractory volume overload, substituting a more potent loop diuretic, such as torsemide or bumetanide, or combining furosemide with a thiazide agent, such as metolazone or chlorothiazide, may be effective.

Although not all patients with ADHF require bladder catheterization, monitoring of urinary output

Table 50-3 PHARMACOLOGIC THERAPY FOR ACUTE DECOMPENSATED HEART FAILURE

Therapy	Action(s)	Indications	Cautions or Adverse Effects	Dosing
Oxygen	Improvement in systemic and myocardial oxygen balance	Hypoxia and/or dyspnea	Respiratory depression (chronic obstructive pulmonary disease)	Titrate to pulse oximetry
Morphine	Relief of anxiety	Pulmonary edema	Respiratory depression Hypotension	2- to 4-mg intravenous (IV) boluses
Furosemide	Preload reduction	Volume overload	Hypotension Prerenal azotemia	Start at 20- to 40-mg (or daily oral dose) IV bolus
Nitroglycerin	Preload and afterload reduction Anti-ischemic	Dyspnea Myocardial ischemia	Hypotension Tolerance	Start 10-20 μg/min IV and titrate upward
Nitroprusside	Afterload reduction	Severe hypertension; refractory pulmonary edema	Hypotension Myocardial ischemia Cyanide toxicity	Start at 0.1-0.2 μg/kg/min IV, and titrate upward
Nesiritide	Preload and afterload reduction	Dyspnea	Hypotension ?Impact on renal function Mortality	2-μg/kg bolus, 0.01 μg/kg/hr
Dobutamine	Positive inotropy Afterload reduction	Low-output heart failure Refractory pulmonary edema	Tachycardia Arrhythmia Hypotension Bronchoconstriction	Start at 2.5 μg/kg/min IV, and titrate upward
Milrinone	Positive inotropy Afterload reduction	Low-output heart failure Refractory pulmonary edema	Arrhythmia Hypotension	Give a 50-μg/kg bolus over 10 minutes; then start at 0.375 μg/kg/min IV, and titrate up

should be attempted in any patient for whom diuresis is a chosen as a treatment strategy.

Nitrates

Nitrates are recommended for the treatment of ADHF, whether of ischemic or nonischemic origin. At low doses, nitroglycerin induces venodilation (preload reduction); at high doses, nitroglycerin causes arteriodilation (afterload reduction) as well as dilation of the coronary arteries. Significantly, in patients with severe underlying LV dysfunction, afterload reduction appears to predominate over preload reduction, even at moderate doses of nitroglycerin.

Beyond this theoretically favorable profile, experience has shown that nitrates are both safe and effective for the treatment of ADHF, particularly in the context of acute diastolic dysfunction, as in pulmonary edema.[16] However, few studies have rigorously addressed the role of nitrate therapy in terms actual of clinical outcomes. In the Vasodilation in the Management of Acute Congestive Heart Failure (VMAC) trial, intravenous nitroglycerin resulted in better dyspnea scores among patients with ADHF than placebo during early therapy, but the study was not powered to demonstrate differences in morbidity or mortality.[17]

Single doses of sublingual nitroglycerin (0.4 mg) can be given repeatedly every five to ten minutes provided an adequate BP. In the hospital setting, however, continuous IV administration of nitroglycerin is more convenient and allows for titration (typically starting at 10-20 μg/min and ranging up to 100 μg/min) to specific clinical or hemodynamic endpoints. Alternative formulations for administering nitrates have been described but offer no clear advantages. The hemodynamic effects of transdermal nitroglycerin are comparable to those of IV nitroglycerin but this agent is less amenable to rapid titration and may be less effective in patients with poor skin perfusion.

Hypotension with standard nitrate therapy is generally mild and transient. Severe or persistent hypotension should raise suspicion for hypovolemia, stenotic valvular disease such as aortic stenosis, cardiac tamponade, right ventricular infarction, or recent use of sildenafil (Viagra). If these conditions are known or suspected, nitrates should be avoided or used with extreme caution. Nitrate therapy may not be particularly effective in patients with massive peripheral edema. In such cases, aggressive diuretic therapy is more likely to be of benefit.

Sodium nitroprusside is recommended for patients with marked systemic hypertension, severe mitral or aortic valvular regurgitation, or pulmonary edema not responsive to standard nitrate therapy. Nitroprusside profoundly dilates resistance vessels, rapidly reducing BP and afterload. Typically, nitroprusside is started at a dose of 0.1 to 0.3 μg/kg/min and the dose is increased as needed to improve clinical and hemodynamic status, maintaining a systolic BP above

90 mm Hg or a mean arterial pressure above 65 mm Hg. In patients with renal failure, long-term use of nitroprusside carries the potential for cyanide toxicity as metabolites of the agent accumulate.

Nesiritide

Nesiritide (recombinant BNP) is the only pharmacologic therapy for dyspnea associated with ADHF that has been approved by the U.S. Food and Drug Administration (FDA) in recent years. Like other natriuretic peptides, BNP has intrinsic vasodilatory as well as mild diuretic and natriuretic properties. When administered in supraphysiologic doses as nesiritide (2 μg/kg bolus, followed by continuous infusion at 0.01 μg/kg/hr), favorable hemodynamic, natriuretic, and neurohormonal effects are observed.

Randomized, controlled trials have shown nesiritide to be more effective than placebo in improving hemodynamics in patients with ADHF. In the VMAC trial, pulmonary capillary wedge pressure was lower in patients randomly assigned to treatment with nesiritide than in patients assigned to receive nitroglycerin, although dyspnea scores at 3 and 24 hours were not significantly different between the two groups.[17] Studies have yet to show differences in more durable outcomes, such as of length of hospital stay and hospital costs.

Potential risks associated with nesiritide have come to light. Pooled data from several trials suggest an association between nesiritide and adverse events, specifically worsening renal function and death.[18,19] With data from prospective studies addressing these questions yet to emerge, the routine use of nesiritide for ADHF has fallen off dramatically.

Angiotensin-Converting Enzyme Inhibitors

The beneficial effects of angiotensin-converting enzyme (ACE) inhibitors in chronic heart failure have been appreciated for more than two decades. Although not formally recommended by consensus guidelines for treatment of ADHF, ACE inhibitors do exert potentially hemodynamic and renal effects in the acute setting, and small studies have demonstrated their safety and efficacy as treatment for ADHF.

ACE inhibitors are contraindicated in the context of pregnancy, hyperkalemia, or a history of ACE inhibitor–induced angioedema. For patients with evidence of poor systemic perfusion, an ACE inhibitor should be used cautiously because they may not tolerate vasodilation. Unlike nitrates, ACE inhibitors have a relatively prolonged duration of action, making their dosage less easily titratable.

Inotropic Therapy

Outside the setting of cardiogenic shock (see later), inotropic therapy is not routinely recommended for the treatment of ADHF. Although short-term inotropic therapy may improve hemodynamic performance and acute symptoms, the impact on outcomes is considerably less sanguine. All conventional inotropic agents are associated with undesirable chronotropic effects, arrhythmogenesis, and/or myocardial ischemia. One of the largest randomized placebo-controlled trials ever conducted in patients with ADHF, the Outcomes of a Prospective Trial of Intravenous Milrinone for Exacerbations of Chronic Heart Failure (OPTIME-CHF), showed no difference in mortality or readmission rate for patients receiving inotropic therapy but significantly higher rates of adverse events, particularly sustained hypotension and new atrial arrhythmias.[20]

Nevertheless, for patients who present with severe signs and symptoms of low-output failure, or who show no response to standard therapy, short-term treatment with inotropic agents may still be considered, as long as the EP understands the expected hemodynamic effects of inotropic agents and clear goals for therapy are established.

Digoxin has a very limited role in the ED management of heart failure. The inotropic effects of digoxin are modest and unpredictable, and they are delayed for at least 90 minutes after intravenous loading.

Morphine

Morphine, one of the oldest drugs still in use for the treatment of ADHF, remains an important adjunct for treating the anxiety and discomfort associated with pulmonary edema. The predominant hemodynamic effects of morphine appear to be mediated through the central nervous system. Morphine can be administered safely to most patients at low doses (2 to 4 mg IV); however, because of its sedative properties and potential to depress respirations, caution should be exercised in administering morphine to a patient with chronic pulmonary insufficiency or suspected acidosis. Although some retrospective studies in patients with pulmonary edema have shown an association between administration of morphine and higher rates of endotracheal intubation, it is not clear that the link is causative.

Investigational Drugs

A number of newer drugs for ADHF have been under investigation, focused primarily on treatment of patients with systolic dysfunction; they range from vasopressin antagonists and endothelin antagonists to calcium sensitizers and novel natriuretic peptides. However, none of these agents has been shown in a prospective placebo-controlled, randomized clinical trial to improve outcomes, and no new agents have been approved by the FDA.

Vasopressin antagonists, such as conivaptan and tolvaptan, have shown some promise in promoting diuresis in patients with ADHF, but outcomes data are lacking. The endothelin-1 antagonist tezosentan has been demonstrated to be a potent vasodilator and modulator of the renin-angiotensin-aldosterone system; controlled trials comparing tezosentan with placebo have shown better hemodynamics with the agent but no significant difference in outcomes. Levosimendan is the best studied of the calcium sensitizers, a novel class of inotropic agents that modify the configuration of troponin, enhancing contractility without increasing myocardial oxygen demand. In two randomized controlled studies of patients with severe low-output ADHF, levosimendan was associated with a 6-month mortality benefit compared with dobutamine, but it is not clear how much of this difference was simply due to the adverse affects of conventional inotropic therapy. Finally, novel natriuretic peptides, such as carperitide and ularitide, have been investigated in several small trials, which reported results similar to those seen with nesiritide.

■ Beta-Blockers

Long-term beta-blocker therapy provides an important survival benefit for patients with systolic heart failure. In contrast, administration of beta-blockers to patients with acute systolic dysfunction can cause life-threatening clinical deterioration. Although there has been no study specifically addressing the use of beta-blockers in the setting of ADHF, institution of beta-blocker therapy is generally not recommended in the setting of ADHF, and long-term beta-blocker therapy should either be temporarily discontinued or administered cautiously at a reduced dose in a patient with ADHF. On the other hand, in the context of ongoing ischemia, tachycardia, and severe hypertension, beta-blockers may be considered, particularly in individuals who are known to have relatively preserved systolic function.

■ ULTRAFILTRATION

A novel approach to the problem of volume overload involves ultrafiltration of peripheral blood to remove excess fluid and electrolytes. Although typically reserved for patients with renal failure or cases unresponsive to diuretics, evidence from the Ultrafiltration vs IV Diuretics for Patients Hospitalized for Acute Decompensated CHF (UNLOAD) trial, demonstrated that as an alternative to diuretic therapy, ultrafiltration resulted in greater fluid loss and lower rates of rehospitalization.[21] The major limitation of this approach in the ED is the practicality of instituting therapy in the acute setting.

Special Circumstances

■ CARDIOGENIC SHOCK

Heart failure with cardiogenic shock is most commonly encountered in the setting of acute ST-segment elevation myocardial infarction. Although mortality remains high, referral for emergency cardiac catheterization and revascularization is of proven benefit in this setting. Other potentially reversible causes of cardiogenic shock, such as acute valvular dysfunction, ventricular septal wall rupture, and pericardial tamponade, must be excluded or addressed promptly. Noncardiac causes of shock, such as hypovolemia, sepsis, poisoning, and massive pulmonary embolism, must also be considered.

Aside from addressing reversible causes of shock, the overarching goal in treating patients who present with cardiogenic shock should be to restore and maintain perfusion of vital organs. Patients who present in shock with normal BP or only mild hypotension often have favorable response to dobutamine (starting at 2 to 3 μg/kg/min). Compared with dopamine, dobutamine is associated with a lower incidence of arrhythmias, less peripheral vasoconstriction, and more consistent reduction in LV filling pressure for a comparable rise in cardiac output. Dopamine is required for patients who have severe hypotension (systolic BP $<$ 70 to 80 mm Hg) in the presence of volume overload or after bolus administration of saline. At moderate doses (4 to 5 μg/kg/min), dopamine improves cardiac output without causing excessive systemic vasoconstriction. If the patient can be stabilized with dopamine, dobutamine can then be added and the dose of dopamine lowered, with the goal of reducing myocardial oxygen demand. In extreme cases, norepinephrine can be added to increase systolic pressure to acceptable levels ($\geq$80 mm Hg). However, because of the adverse effects on renal and mesenteric perfusion, the use of high-dose dopamine or norepinephrine should be considered only as a temporizing measure until a definitive therapy can be substituted.

For patients with a potentially reversible condition, referral for intra-aortic balloon counterpulsation (IABC) should be considered as a bridge to definitive management. For example, IABC can be an effective temporizing measure in anticipation of coronary revascularization or cardiac valve repair. Patients least likely to benefit from the IABC are those with multiple previous infarctions, massive irreversible myocardial necrosis, aortic dissection, or advanced stages of cardiogenic shock, and elderly patients with peripheral vascular disease (because of complications from insertion of the device).

It is important for the EP to distinguish acute cardiogenic shock from low-output ADHF, the latter condition tending to manifest more subacutely in patients with preexisting, end-stage, systolic heart failure. Management of these patients can be extremely challenging, and optimal treatment may require the involvement of a heart failure specialist. Attempts to aggressively treat these patients can lead to rapid decompensation. Frequently, the key to management is identifying the cause of decompensation.

■ ATRIAL FIBRILLATION

Atrial fibrillation is seen in approximately one third of patients presenting with ADHF; its coprevalence is due to overlapping preconditions, such as hypertension and coronary artery disease, and to the atrial remodeling that occurs in heart failure. In the context of normal ventricular function, loss of synchronized atrial contractions is of minimal hemodynamic significance. However, in patients who have abnormal systolic or diastolic function, the loss of "atrial kick" can have profound consequences, particularly when atrial fibrillation is accompanied by a rapid ventricular response, thereby reducing filling time and increasing myocardial oxygen demand.

When assessing the patient with rapid atrial fibrillation and ADHF, it is often difficult to attribute cause and effect. New-onset rapid atrial fibrillation may be the precipitant of ADHF, but more commonly, atrial fibrillation is a response to worsening heart failure (e.g., via neurohormonal activation and/or increased atrial stretch). This distinction can often be made only clinically, and in either case, management focuses on the treatment of both conditions.

Management of atrial fibrillation in the context of ADHF should focus on treating the underlying cause of ADHF and controlling the ventricular rate to allow for better ventricular filling and improved myocardial oxygen balance. In general, digoxin, diltiazem, and amiodarone are considered acceptable agents for rate control in patients with LV systolic dysfunction. Caution should be exercised in the use of any beta-blocker or calcium channel blocker for rate control because of the potential that negative inotropic effects will worsen existing systolic dysfunction. Cardioversion, whether electrical or chemical, is a reasonable treatment alternative for truly unstable atrial fibrillation, but maintaining sinus rhythm may not be possible if the underlying heart failure is not addressed.

■ RENAL DYSFUNCTION

In part owing to common preconditions such as diabetes and hypertension, and in part because of the effects of diuretics and low cardiac output on renal function, heart failure and renal insufficiency frequently coexist. Approximately 1 in 5 patients who present with ADHF have creatinine levels greater than 2.0 mg/dL. For patients presenting with ADHF, preexisting renal insufficiency is associated with greater morbidity and mortality, and worsening of renal function over the course of treatment is associated with poorer outcomes.

Among patients undergoing hemodialysis, heart failure is the most common cause of ED visits. In these patients, ADHF is most often due to volume overload between dialysis treatments. Although hemodialysis is the obvious treatment of choice for these patients, it may not always be immediately available, and so ED treatment is directed at stabilizing the patients until hemodialysis can be performed. Because of their direct vascular effects, diuretics may still play a role in managing anuric patients with ADHF, but vasodilator therapy is generally most effective.

Disposition

The vast majority of patients who present to the ED with ADHF are admitted to the hospital.[5] Discharge from the ED without adequate treatment may be associated with recurrent visits and short-term morbidity and mortality. ADHF is often a dynamic entity: One patient may appear dramatically ill at presentation but respond rapidly to treatment, whereas another patient may go on to experience serious complications after a period of apparent stability. For any individual patient, identifying and addressing the precipitant of the decompensation is critical to making the correct disposition.

The Heart Failure Society of America has established criteria for discharge of patients with heart failure (Table 50-4). However, these guidelines have not been prospectively studied. It should be noted that previously published criteria from the U.S.

Table 50-4 HEART FAILURE SOCIETY OF AMERICA RECOMMENDATIONS FOR DISCHARGE OF ED PATIENTS WITH HEART FAILURE

Admission is recommended	Severe acute decompensated heart failure (ADHF): Hypotension Worsening renal function Altered mental status Dyspnea at rest Arrhythmia with hemodynamic compromise, including new-onset atrial fibrillation Acute coronary syndrome
Admission should be considered	Worsening congestion (pulmonary or systemic) Significant electrolyte disturbance Associated comorbidities: Pneumonia Pulmonary embolism Diabetic ketoacidosis Transient ischemic attack/cerebrovascular accident New-onset heart failure

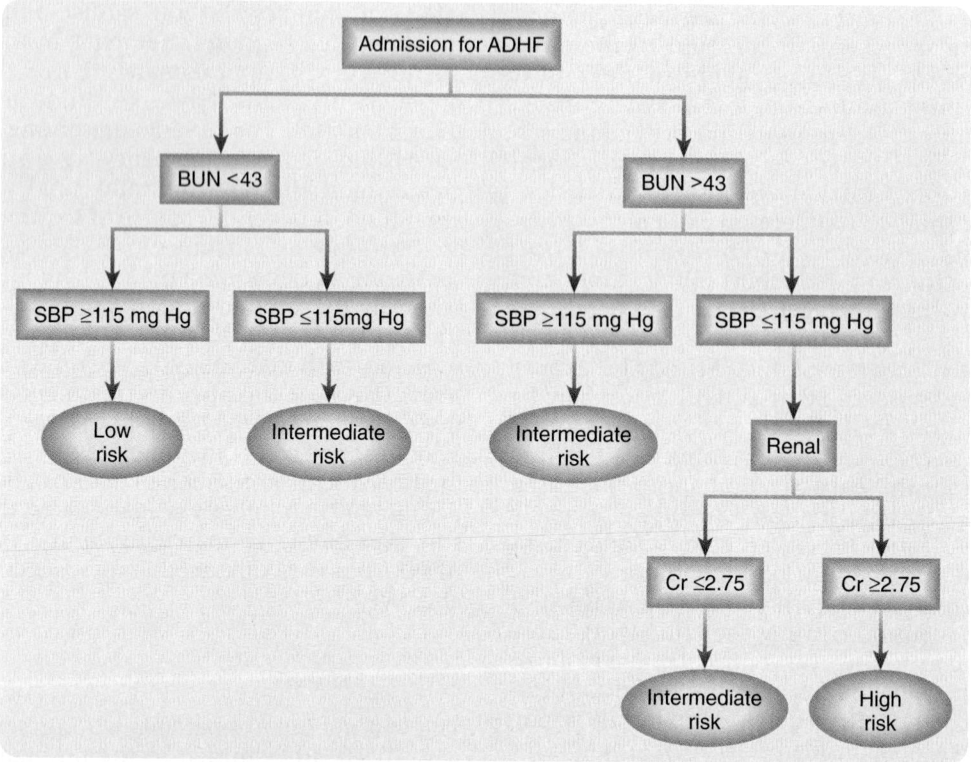
Admission for ADHF
BUN <43
BUN >43
SBP ≥115 mg Hg
SBP ≤115mg Hg
SBP ≥115 mg Hg
SBP ≤115 mg Hg
Low risk
Intermediate risk
Intermediate risk
Renal
Cr ≤2.75
Cr ≥2.75
Intermediate risk
High risk

FIGURE 50-4 Risk stratification among patients hospitalized for acute decompensated heart failure (ADHF). BUN, blood urea nitrogen; Cr, [serum] creatinine; SBP, systolic blood pressure.

Agency for Health Care Policy and Research failed to account for more than 30% of 30-day mortality.[22] Thus, although published criteria and guidelines can help with triage, the significant rate of morbidity, even among seemingly low-risk patients, mandates that clinical judgment be incorporated into the decision-making process.

Although there are no formal guidelines for disposition within the hospital, the majority of patients with ADHF are admitted to telemetry units. On average, in-hospital mortality for patients admitted with ADHF is in the range of 4%, and median length of stay exceeds 4 days.[5] Among patients admitted with more advanced stages of heart failure, inpatient mortality approaches 10%. Clinical correlates of major complications or death during hospitalization include hypotension, tachypnea, ECG abnormalities, hyponatremia, renal insufficiency, elevations in troponin and BNP, and poor initial diuresis. However, even patients without any of these risk factors have measurable rates of inhospital morbidity and mortality. A risk stratification tool derived from the ADHERE registry has been developed to help clinicians determine the mortality risk of patients who present with ADHF (Fig. 50-4).[23]

For the patient who is ultimately discharged home, consultation with the patient's primary care physician or cardiologist is imperative. Depending on what precipitated the patient's decompensation, the outpatient drug regimen may require some adjustment. Intensive outpatient follow-up has been shown to be successful in preventing repeat visits to the ED. Referral to an outpatient heart failure program, where available, can reduce the frequency of ED visits and hospitalizations.

■ OBSERVATION UNITS

Assignment of patients with ADHF to ED observation units has been advanced as a safe and cost-effective means of treating such patients without the need for hospital admissions. Advantages of care in these units over outpatient management include the ability to monitor for response to therapy and for development of any potentially serious adverse events. Small studies have suggested that utilization of ED-based heart failure observation units can result in lower rates of recidivism. Although there is a growing interest in this field, no randomized studies have been performed to date to substantiate their use.

REFERENCES

1. Rosamond W, Flegal K, Friday G, et al: Heart disease and stroke statistics—2007 update: A report from the American Heart Association Statistics Committee and Stroke Statistics Subcommittee. Circulation 2007;115:e119-e121.
2. Heart Failure Society of America: Executive summary: HFSA 2006 Comprehensive Heart Failure Practice Guideline. J Card Fail 2006;12:10-38.
3. Nieminen MS, Bohm M, Cowie MR, et al: Executive summary of the guidelines on the diagnosis and treatment of acute heart failure: The Task Force on Acute Heart Failure of the European Society of Cardiology. Eur Heart J 2005;26:384-416.

4. Hunt SA, Abraham WT, Chin MH, et al: American College of Cardiology; American Heart Association Task Force on Practice Guidelines; American College of Chest Physicians; International Society for Heart and Lung Transplantation; Heart Rhythm Society: ACC/AHA 2005 Guideline Update for the Diagnosis and Management of Chronic Heart Failure in the Adult: A report of the American College of Cardiology/American Heart Association Task Force on Practice Guidelines (Writing Committee to Update the 2001 Guidelines for the Evaluation and Management of Heart Failure): developed in collaboration with the American College of Chest Physicians and the International Society for Heart and Lung Transplantation: endorsed by the Heart Rhythm Society. Circulation 2005;112: e154-e235.
5. Adams KF Jr, Fonarrow GC, Emerman CL, et al: Characteristics and outcomes of patients hospitalized for heart failure in the United States: Rationale, design, and preliminary observations from the first 100,000 cases in the Acute Decompensated Heart Failure National Registry (ADHERE). Am Heart J 2005;149:209-216.
6. American College of Emergency Physicians Clinical Policies Subcommittee (Writing Committee) on Acute Heart Failure Syndromes, Silvers SM, Howell JM, et al: Clinical policy: Critical issues in the evaluation and management of adult patients presenting to the emergency department with acute heart failure syndromes. Ann Emerg Med 2007;49:627–629.
7. Felker GM, Adams KF Jr, Konstam MA, et al: The problem of decompensated heart failure: Nomenclature, classification, and risk stratification. Am Heart J 2003;145:S18-S25.
8. Hoffman JR, Reynolds S: Comparison of nitroglycerin, morphine and furosemide in treatment of presumed prehospital pulmonary edema. Chest 1987;92:586-593.
9. Wang CS, FitzGerald JM, Schulzer M, et al: Does this dyspneic patient in the emergency department have congestive heart failure? JAMA 2005;294:1944-1956.
10. Maisel AS, Krishnaswamy P, Nowak RM, et al: Rapid measurement of B-type natriuretic peptide in the emergency diagnosis of heart failure. N Engl J Med 2002;347: 161-167.
11. Januzzi JL Jr, Camargo CA, Anwaruddin S, et al: The *N*-terminal Pro-BNP Investigation of Dyspnea in the Emergency department (PRIDE) study. Am J Cardiol 2005;95: 948-954.
12. McCullough PA, Nowak RM, McCord J, et al: B-type natriuretic peptide and clinical judgment in emergency diagnosis of heart failure: Analysis from Breathing Not Properly (BNP) Multinational Study. Circulation 2002;106: 416-422.
13. Maisel A, Hollander JE, Guss D, et al: Primary results of the Rapid Emergency Department Heart Failure Outpatient Trial (REDHOT): A multicenter study of B-type natriuretic peptide levels, emergency department decision making, and outcomes in patients presenting with shortness of breath. J Am Coll Cardiol 2004;44:1328-1333.
14. Masip J, Roque M, Sanchez B, et al: Noninvasive ventilation in acute cardiogenic pulmonary edema: Systematic review and meta-analysis. JAMA 2005;294:3124-3230.
15. Salvador DR, Rey NR, Ramos GC, Punzalan FE: Continuous infusion versus bolus injection of loop diuretics in congestive heart failure. Cochrane Database Syst Rev 2005;(3): CD003178.
16. Cotter G, Metzkor E, Kaluski E, et al: Randomised trial of high-dose isosorbide dinitrate plus low-dose furosemide versus high dose furosemide plus low-dose isosorbide dinitrate in severe pulmonary edema. Lancet 1998;351: 389-393.
17. Publication Committee for the VMAC Investigators (Vasodilatation in the Management of Acute CHF): Intravenous nesiritide vs nitroglycerin for treatment of decompensated congestive heart failure: A randomized controlled trial. JAMA 2002;287:1531-1540.
18. Sackner-Bernstein JD, Kowalski M, Fox M, Aaronson K: Short-term risk of death after treatment with nesiritide for decompensated heart failure: A pooled analysis of randomized controlled trials. JAMA 2005;293:1900-1905.
19. Sackner-Bernstein JD, Skopicki HA, Aaronson KD: Risk of worsening renal function with nesiritide in patients with acutely decompensated heart failure. Circulation 2005; 111:1487-1491.
20. Cuffe MS, Califf RM, Adams KF, et al: Short-term intravenous milrinone for acute exacerbation of chronic heart failure: A randomized controlled trial. JAMA 2002;287: 1541-1547.
21. Costanzo MR, Guglin ME, Saltzberg MT, et al: UNLOAD Trial Investigators: Ultrafiltration versus intravenous diuretics for patients hospitalized for acute decompensated heart failure. J Am Coll Cardiol 2007;49:675-683.
22. Graff L, Orledge J, Radford MJ, et al: Correlation of the Agency for Health Care Policy and Research congestive heart failure admission guideline with mortality: Peer review organization voluntary hospital association initiative to decrease events (PROVIDE) for congestive heart failure. Ann Emerg Med 1999;34:429-437.
23. Fonarow GC, Adams KF Jr, Abraham WT, et al: Risk stratification for in-hospital mortality in acutely decompensated heart failure: Classification and regression tree analysis. JAMA 2005;293:572-580.

Chapter **51**

Bradyarrhythmias

Sarah A. Stahmer and Robert Cowan

KEY POINTS

Look at the patient first, then the heart rhythm. A "slow heart rate" is relative to the patient's age, clinical condition, and comorbidities.

Determine whether the cause is extrinsic or intrinsic to the conduction system.

Assess the functionality of the key elements of the conduction system: sinoatrial and atrioventricular nodes and the infranodal conduction system.

Know the vascular supply of the conduction system to determine significance of bradyarrhythmias and conduction blocks in the setting of acute myocardial infarction.

Identify risk of failure of the conduction system and the "backup," for example, a stable escape rhythm, atropine, a pacemaker.

Scope and Outline

Bradycardia, defined as a heart rate of less than 60 beats/min, is of concern only when an underlying pathologic condition exists. *Bradyarrhythmia* (or bradydysrhythmia), a pathologic bradycardia, is signaled by compromised cardiac output or abnormalities of the conduction system (Table 51-1).

In additional to structural and ischemic causes of bradycardia, drugs and medications play important roles. Beta-blockers, calcium channel blockers, and digoxin frequently precipitate bradycardia. Profound bradycardias or atrioventricular (AV) nodal blockade in the setting of therapeutic doses of medications usually indicates underlying nodal disease. Many class I and class III antiarrhythmics predispose patients to sinus node dysfunction and AV conduction block. In addition, antihypertensive medicines that diminish central sympathetic output, such as reserpine and clonidine, can cause bradycardia, as can antidepressants, antipsychotics, and antiseizure medications that depress sinoatrial and/or AV nodal function. Exposures to organophosphates and cholinesterase inhibitors typically manifest as bradyarrhythmia due to excessive cholinergic stimulation.[1-3]

Causes of blocks occurring at the level of the AV node or infranodal conduction tissue are varied and largely reflect the actions of medications, ischemia, or infiltrative diseases of the heart (Table 51-2).

Specific Bradyarrhythmias

■ SINUS BRADYCARDIA

For the diagnosis of sinus bradycardia, the following three electrocardiographic findings must be present (Fig. 51-1):

1. There must be visible P waves at a rate less that 60 beats/min.

Table 51-1 EXTRINSIC CAUSES OF BRADYARRHYTHMIAS

Type	Common	Uncommon
Drugs	α_2 agonists Amiodarone and sotalol Beta-blocking agents Calcium channel blockers Cholinergic agents Class Ia antiarrhythmic agents Class Ic antiarrhythmic agents Class III antiarrhythmic agents Digoxin Opioids Organophosphates Sedatives/hypnotics Tricyclic antidepressants	Amantadine Carbamazepine Chloroquine Cimetidine Clonidine Lithium Phenothiazines Phenytoin Physostigmine Propoxyphene Reserpine Thioridazine
Situational reflex	Cough syncope Maxillofacial reflex Micturition syncope Neurocardiogenic syncope Oculocardiac reflex	Defecation syncope Pain syncope Swallow syncope Vomiting
Metabolic	Hyperkalemia Hypokalemia Hypothyroidism	Hypercalcemia Hypermagnesemia
Ischemia/infarction	Inferior wall ischemia/infarction is associated with bradycardia and/or atrioventricular nodal conduction delays that are due to abnormal sensitivity to parasympathetic stimulation and are responsive to atropine	—
Other	Hypothermia Hypoxia Obstructive sleep apnea	—

Pharmacologic data from Ford M: Clinical Toxicology. Philadelphia, WB Saunders, 2001, pp 23-25.

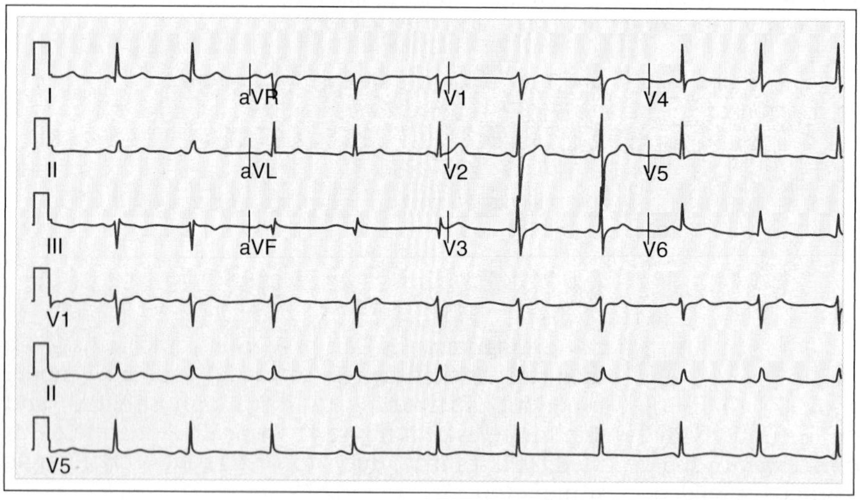
I
aVR
V1
V4
II
aVL
V2
V5
III
aVF
V3
V6
V1
II
V5

FIGURE 51-1 A sinus bradycardia with a ventricular response rate of 59 beats/min. There is a P wave for every QRS complex, with normal PR intervals.

2. The morphology of the P wave must be consistent with a sinus beat (upright in leads I and II).
3. Each P wave must be followed by a QRS complex with a fixed PR interval.

■ Cause

Sinus bradycardia is caused by slowed automaticity of the sinus node. The slowing can be from intrinsic causes, such as fibrosis and ischemia, but more commonly has an extrinsic cause, such as a medication or increased vagal tone. Sinus bradycardia and specifically transient asymptomatic bradycardia are common in the normal healthy population.[4]

■ Clinical Presentation

Most patients who present with sinus bradycardia have no symptoms and the rhythm is incidental. Those who do have symptoms may present with syncope, hypotension, or vague complaints such as weakness and lack of energy. Because so many patients are asymptomatic, it is often difficult to be certain

Table 51-2 INTRINSIC CAUSES OF BRADYARRHYTHMIAS

Ischemia/infarct	Anterior wall myocardial infarction: Type II second-degree heart block Third-degree heart block Inferior wall myocardial infarction: Sinus bradycardia Type I second-degree heart block Third-degree heart block
Infection	Bacterial: Diphtheria Endocarditis Lyme disease Parasitic: Chagas' disease Viral: Hepatitis Mononucleosis Mumps Rubella Varicella
Malignancy	Lymphoma Sarcoma
Rheumatologic	Reiter's syndrome Rheumatoid arthritis Systemic lupus erythematosus Systemic sclerosis
Other	Amyloid Lev's disease (the spread of fibrosis and calcification from the adjacent cardiac skeleton) Lenègre's disease (an idiopathic fibrotic degeneration of the His-Purkinje system) Sarcoid

that the bradycardia is the true cause of the patient's symptoms unless the bradycardia is profound.

Treatment

If the symptoms are mild, the management should focus on reversing the cause, such as withholding the offending medication, treating nausea and/or pain, and monitoring the patient. Atropine (0.5 to 1.0 mg repeated up to 3 mg total dose) is often effective for reflex-induced bradycardias.

SINOATRIAL BLOCK

Recognition

Sinoatrial block is very difficult to differentiate from sinus bradycardia and sick sinus syndrome (SSS). In SA block, the sinus node fires normally but there is a problem with the impulse propagation through the atria. The nature of the block is classified as first, second, or third degree. First-degree SA block represents a delay from the impulse generation to the depolarization of the atria. Because there is no electrocardiographic manifestation of the impulse generation, the delay is imperceptible and is not evident on a 12-lead electrocardiogram (ECG). There are two types of second-degree AV block, both of which can be identified on ECG. With type 1, a gradual lengthening of the delay to atrial depolarization appears as a gradual shortening of the P-P interval until a P-QRS-T complex is dropped. With type 2, the delay to P wave formation is fixed, but occasional impulses do not trigger atrial depolarizations, leading to randomly dropped P-QRS-T complexes. The first P wave after the dropped beat is a multiple of the baseline P-P interval. In third-degree SA block, the sinus node impulses never make it to the atrial tissues, and the ECG shows a junctional escape rhythm without P waves. Third-degree SA block is difficult to distinguish from a sinus pause (Fig. 51-2).[2,5]

PRIORITY ACTIONS

1. Determine whether the patient is hemodynamically compromised by the bradyarrhythmia. If the patient is hypotensive, then determine whether it is due to the absolute heart rate, loss of atrioventricular (AV) synchrony, or associated conditions that will cause a relative bradycardia to be symptomatic, such as dehydration or left ventricular dysfunction.
2. Establish intravenous (IV) access.
3. If the absolute ventricular response rate is determined to be inappropriate for clinical condition, the following interventions may be helpful:
   a. Atropine 1 mg IV up to 3 mg; may be effective for sinus bradycardia, Mobitz type I second-degree AV block (particularly if in the setting of inferior wall myocardial infarction).
   b. Glucagon 1 mg IV; may be effective for beta-blocker and calcium channel blocker toxicity.
   c. Calcium gluconate; may be effective for calcium channel blocker toxicity or hyperkalemia.
4. Indications for temporary transvenous pacemaker placement are as follows. Access should generally be obtained via the right internal jugular in order to reduce the risk of complication and to ensure safe placement and stability.
   a. Symptomatic bradycardia.
   b. Unresponsiveness to pharmacologic therapy.
   c. Alternating bundle branch block.
   d. Bifascicular block with first-degree AV block.
   e. Mobitz type II second-degree AV block.
   f. Third-degree AV block.

Causes

Sinoatrial block is a variant of SSS, and its causes are the same as those of SSS (see later). Rather than being caused by medications, SA block is usually caused by structural defects that result from ischemia, fibrosis, or inflammation.[4]

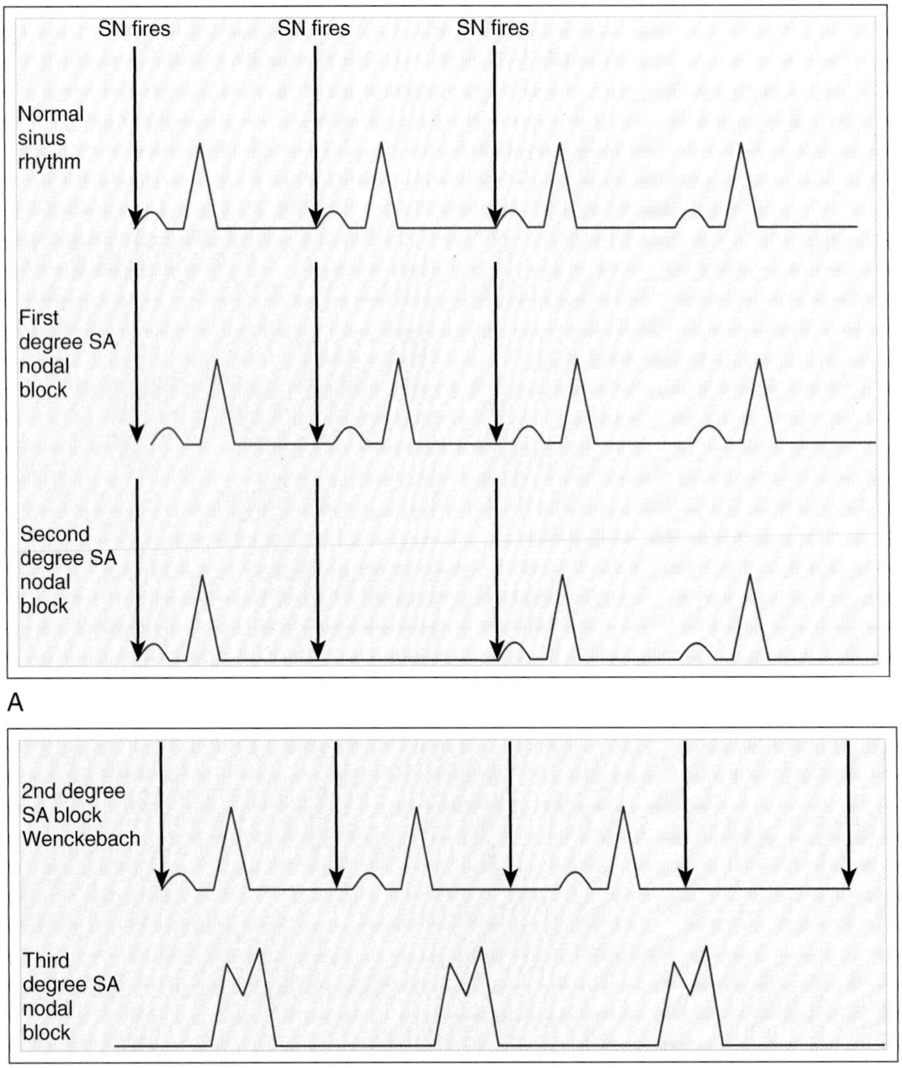
SN fires
SN fires
SN fires
Normal sinus rhythm
First degree SA nodal block
Second degree SA nodal block
A
2nd degree SA block Wenckebach
Third degree SA nodal block
B

FIGURE 51-2 **A** and **B,** Sinoatrial (SA) block. SN, sinus node.

Clinical Presentation

First-degree SA block is clinically silent. Higher degrees of SA block are likely to be symptomatic, depending on the severity of he block and the heart rate.

Treatment

Therapy depends on the severity of symptoms and severity of block. Patients with third-degree SA block are more likely to require intervention because their heart rates are dependent on a junctional escape rhythm. If there is no identifiable and reversible cause of symptomatic SA block in an individual patient, pacemaker therapy may be necessary.

SICK SINUS SYNDROME

Recognition

Sick sinus syndrome is a group of diseases characterized by dysfunction of the sinus node that can have a variety of ECG appearances.[2] The most common ECG appearance is that of severe, inappropriate sinus bradycardia.[4,6] *Sinus arrest* is a prolonged period (>2.5 sec) without any atrial activity. The ECG shows an isoelectric pause without P waves, the duration of which is variable and may be accompanied by either a junctional or ventricular escape beat. Sinus pause can be differentiated from SA exit block, in that the pause in SA exit block is a multiple of prior P-P intervals but sinus pause is not (see Figs. 51-2 and 51-3). The final form of SSS is that of tachycardia-bradycardia syndrome in which there are alternating periods of severe bradycardia interrupted by paroxysms of supraventricular tachycardia, usually atrial fibrillation.

Causes

The causes of SSS are varied. Bradyarrhythmias due to increased vagal tone and effects of medications, such as digoxin and beta-blockers, may have a similar clinical presentation, but they are usually transient

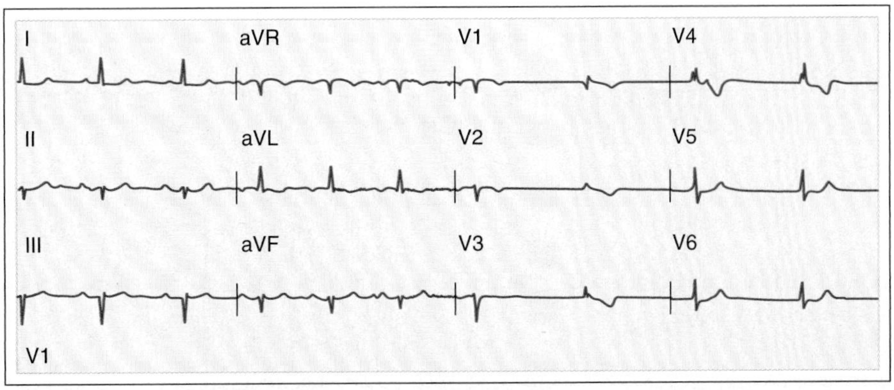
I
aVR
V1
V4
II
aVL
V2
V5
III
aVF
V3
V6
V1

FIGURE 51-3 Sick sinus syndrome. There are many variants to this syndrome, but all have the common feature of abrupt dysfunction of the sinus node. This electrocardiogram (ECG) shows a normal sinus rhythm with abrupt absence of P waves. This rhythm may indicate sinus arrest or third-degree sinus node block, both which are impossible to distinguish on a 12-lead ECG.

and therefore not deemed SSS.[6] The true cause of SSS is an anatomic dysfunction of the SA node and surrounding tissues. Congenital forms of this disease have also been associated with congenital prolonged QT syndrome. Acquired causes include ischemia (inferior wall myocardial infarction [MI]) and idiopathic fibrosis as well as infiltrative and inflammatory processes such as pericarditis, amyloidosis, hemochromatosis, and other rheumatologic diseases.[7]

Clinical Presentation

Manifestations of SSS arise from inadequate cardiac output and may include congestive heart failure or syncope from either profound bradycardia or rapid atrial fibrillation. Other symptoms are often less easily recognized, may be cryptic, and may represent acute or chronic cerebral hypoperfusion. These symptoms include "slight personality changes, fleeting memory losses, nocturnal wakefulness . . . , slurred speech, pareses, errors in judgement, dizziness and syncopal attacks."[6] Because the arrhythmia tends to episodic, its diagnosis is often difficult to make during routine ED observation. Halter monitoring is often invaluable.

Treatment

SSS often responds temporarily to medication with agents such as atropine and isoproterenol, but this is not a practical long-term therapeutic strategy. These agents may be lifesaving in the case of prolonged sinus pauses and should be used in an emergency, but the definitive therapy is a permanent pacemaker. Because there is often associated AV conduction disease, current recommendations are for implantation of ventricular pacing devices rather than isolated atrial pacing.[6]

FIRST-DEGREE ATRIOVENTRICULAR CONDUCTION BLOCK

Recognition

First-degree AV block is defined as a fixed PR interval longer than 200 msec, with each P wave followed by a QRS complex. Because there is no dysfunction in the sinus node and each impulse is conducted to the ventricle, this rhythm often does not cause bradycardia by itself. However, it is often seen in conjunction with other bradycardic rhythms, such as Mobitz type I second-degree AV block (Fig. 51-4).[6]

Cause

First-degree AV block is caused by delayed conduction through the atria to the ventricle. The impulse is generated in the sinus node in a normal manner, but the conduction does not reach the ventricle as quickly, with the delay occurring within the AV node rather than in the atrial tissue. First-degree AV block can be due to prior MI, to medications such as beta-blockers, calcium channel blockers, and digoxin, or to increased vagal tone. It is often seen in the setting of an inferior wall MI, which is discussed later.

Clinical Presentation

Most patients with this isolated AV block have no symptoms, and it is often an incidental finding. However, patients with very prolonged PR intervals and underlying congestive heart failure may have symptoms arising from loss of AV synchrony.[8] The development of first-degree AV block in a patient with systemic disorders that can involve the heart, such as infiltrative processes and infections, may be the first sign of conduction system disease.

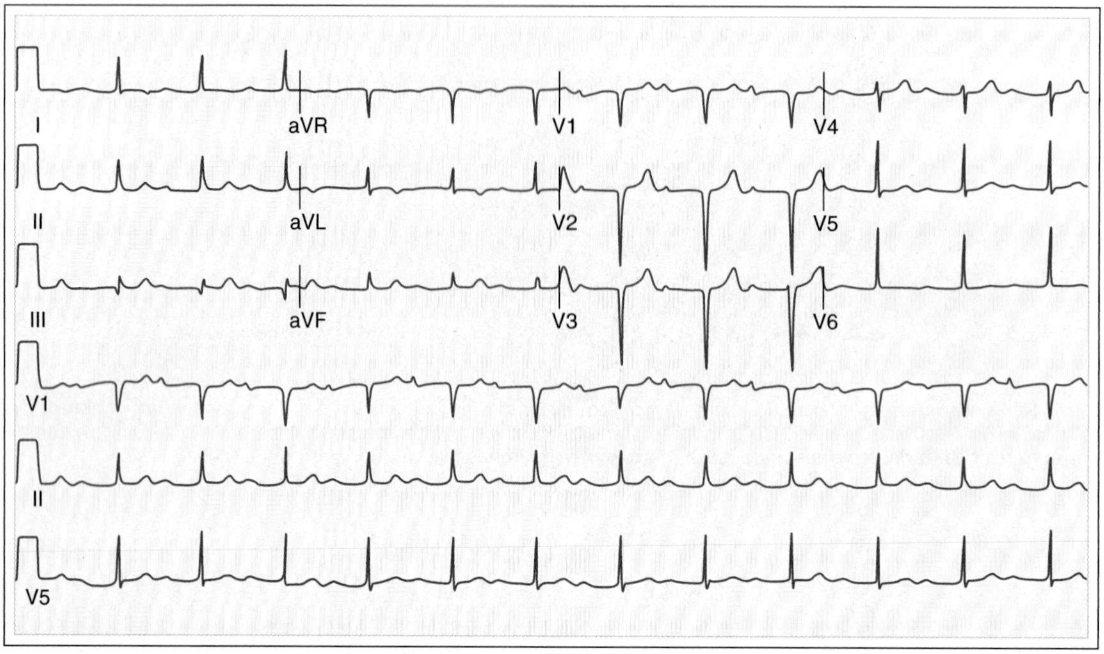
I
aVR
V1
V4
II
aVL
V2
V5
III
aVF
V3
V6
V1
II
V5

FIGURE 51-4 First-degree atrioventricular (AV) block. The rhythm is sinus with a P wave before every QRS complex. The PR interval is prolonged to more than 200 msec, indicating delayed conduction through the AV node.

RED FLAGS

Bradycardia is relative. When the cardiac stroke volume is normal, there can be perfectly adequate perfusion (e.g., blood pressure and cerebral perfusion), even at ventricular response rates in the 30s. When a patient is symptomatic with a bradyarrhythmia, the cause is often multifactorial and attention must be paid to optimizing the stroke volume with fluids, reversing ischemia or adding inotropic agents in addition to increasing the heart rate.

Bradyarrythmias in the hemodynamically compromised patient are rarely overlooked. In the asymptomatic patient, the electrocardiogram (ECG) may provide the only clues to serious life-threatening disease. One example is the "stable" febrile intravenous drug user whose admission ECG shows a type I second-degree heart block—which is the only clue to aortic ring abcess. Another example is the patient with an ST-elevation myocardial infarction that is quickly recognized, but the presence of complete atrioventricular block or significance of a "new" bundle branch block goes unrecognized.

Patients with bradyarrhythmias should be carefully screened for active ischemia of the inferior wall, where the changes can be particularly subtle. Conversely, conduction abnormalities can be easily overlooked in patients with ST segment elevations in the inferior leads.

■ Treatment

For most cases of isolated first-degree AV block, no therapy is required because the patients are asymptomatic. When the block is due to medication overdose, withholding the offending agent may be all that is necessary. Any symptoms associated with first-degree AV block are due to loss of AV synchrony (which is rare), and dual-chamber pacemakers may be indicated.

■ SECOND-DEGREE ATRIOVENTRICULAR CONDUCTION BLOCK

Second-degree AV block is a term encompassing all conduction delays that occur between the atria and the ventricles. Ventricular activation still occurs from above the AV node, but there is some delay in either the AV node or the infranodal conduction pathway. The sinus node is functional, and regular P waves are present. The ventricular response pattern and clinical significance of the block are largely determined by the location. There are two different types, referred to as Mobitz type I and Mobitz type II second-degree heart block. Type I represents a block higher in the AV node, whereas the type II block is lower in the AV node or His bundle.

■ Type I Second-Degree Atrioventricular Block

■ *Recognition*

The key ECG feature of Mobitz type I second-degree AV block, also known as Wenckebach's block, is a

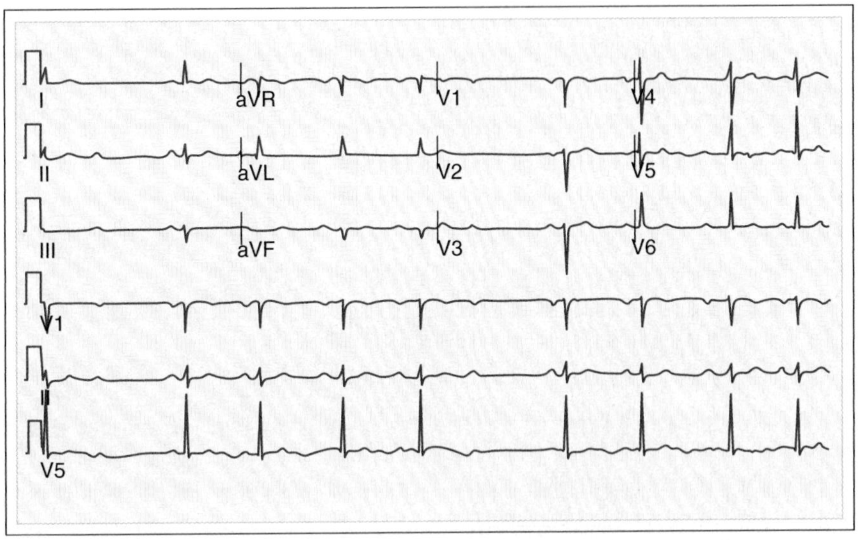
I
aVR
V1
V4
II
aVL
V2
V5
III
aVF
V3
V6
V1
II
V5

FIGURE 51-5 Mobitz type I second-degree heart block. This is sinus rhythm at 70 beats/min with a slower ventricular rate due to progressive delay in atrioventricular (AV) nodal conduction and, finally, a dropped beat. Note that the PR interval after the dropped beat is shorter than the PR interval just before the dropped beat. The hallmark feature of this type of second-degree AV block is the presence of a normal sinus rhythm with progressive delay in AV nodal conduction.

progressive lengthening of the PR interval leading up to a dropped QRS complex. The PR interval of the first-conducted QRS complex after a nonconducted beat has the shortest or a relatively normal PR interval. The P-P interval of this rhythm is stable, meaning that as the PR interval lengthens, the RR interval will actually shorten. One of the most noticeable features of second-degree AV block is that the ECG shows an overall irregular appearance because of the dropped QRS complexes. Classic Wenckebach's block with a steady progression of PR intervals culminating in a dropped beat is present less than 50% of the time.[2,9] The hallmark is that the first PR interval after the dropped beat is the shortest (Fig. 51-5).

Cause

Mobitz type I heart block is caused by a conduction abnormality in the AV node or proximal conduction system. In humans, studies showed that most Wenckebach's blocks arise from blocks above the His bundle.[10,11] For this reason, the QRS complexes are most often narrow.

Clinical Presentation

Whether a patient with this rhythm has symptoms depends on the absolute ventricular response rate and the patient's stroke volume. The rate is usually not slow enough to cause hypotension unless there is a coexisting sinus bradycardia or significantly reduced ejection fraction from active or preexisting cardiac disease.

Treatment

In patients with minimal symptoms or symptoms due to reversible conditions, the best approach is conservative management with observation alone and/or withdrawal of the offending agent when appropriate. As noted earlier, hemodynamic compromise is usually related to a reduced stroke volume and not the absolute heart rate. In patients for whom an increase in rate may be beneficial, atropine may by effective, pacemaker support being reserved for those with refractory symptoms.

Type II Second-Degree Atrioventricular Conduction Block

Recognition

The diagnosis of Mobitz type II heart block is determined by the presence of an intact sinus pacemaker with intermittent failure to conduct to the ventricles. Some P waves are followed by a QRS complex, and some are not. This finding places the rhythm into the category of a second-degree AV block. The next step is to focus on the PR intervals. In contrast to Mobitz type I conduction delays, in which the PR interval invariable, the PR interval in type II block is fixed. It may be normal or prolonged (in the setting of first-degree AV block), but it must be constant from beat to beat—except when there is total failure to conduct (e.g., a P wave and no QRS). The level of the block is infranodal because the disease is in the His-Purkinje fibers, and there is usually a preexisting bundle branch block (BBB) in the conducted beats. It is the failure of the remaining "viable" path to conduct that creates the total AV block for that one beat. The concern with Mobitz II blocks is that this "all-or-none" response in the remaining fascicle is unpredictable. Persistent failure to conduct puts the patient in compete heart block, and the escape rhythms in this case are usually ventricular—slow, wide, and unstable (Fig. 51-6).

Causes

Type II AV block usually indicates significant intrinsic disease of the conduction system, either acute ischemia or progressive degenerative changes. It is rarely

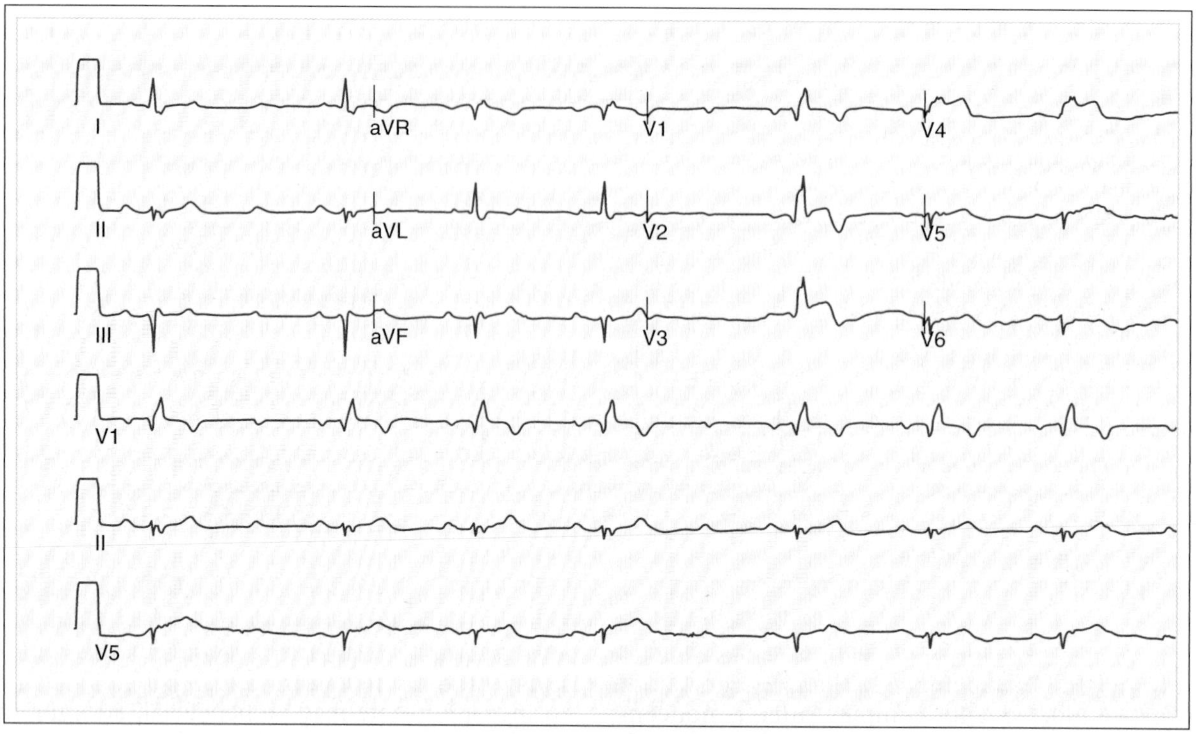
I
aVR
V1
V4
II
aVL
V2
V5
III
aVF
V3
V6
V1
II
V5

FIGURE 51-6 Mobitz type II second-degree atrioventricular block.

caused by medication effects, vagal tone, or hyperresponsiveness.

Treatment

Consideration of the cause as well as the level of AV block is paramount in determining treatment. As opposed to Mobitz I block, type II AV block is likely to be irreversible and to progress to complete heart block. Therefore, early transvenous pacemaker placement is usually required, often with the need for permanent pacing.

2:1 Atrioventricular Block

A variation of second-degree AV block is 2:1 AV block. Initially the ECG shows an overall regular appearance of the QRS complexes because every other QRS complex is blocked. Because of the 2:1 relationship, it is difficult to distinguish between Mobitz I and Mobitz II AV blocks. As noted previously, the distinction is important because the two types are treated differently. As always, if the patient is persistently hypotensive, the distinction is irrelevant because he or she requires a pacemaker; in the stable patient, however, the ECG and the response to simple maneuvers may be helpful in sorting out the differences.

The factors distinguishing between Mobitz type I and II in 2:1 AV block are the QRS morphology and the response to vagal maneuvers. The EP should remember that Mobitz I block is located higher in the conduction system, at the level of the AV node. The infranodal conduction is normal, and the QRS complex should be narrow. Vagal maneuvers may transiently increase the severity of block. Mobitz type II blocks are associated with disease in the His-Purkinje system, and there is often an underlying BBB. These blocks are unaffected by vagal maneuvers. When a BBB is present in the setting of 2:1 AV block, the patient should be assumed to have significant infranodal disease that may progress to complete heart block without warning (Fig. 51-7).

THIRD-DEGREE ATRIOVENTRICULAR BLOCK (COMPLETE HEART BLOCK)

Recognition

Because of its severity, this is the rhythm to consider first when facing a bradyarrhythmia. The ventricular rate is typically very slow, but the actual rate varies according to the inherent rate of the escape rhythm. In this rhythm, there is no connection between the atria and the ventricles, and as such, there is evidence of independent activity. It is important to "march out" the P waves to see whether they are regular, because some are most likely buried within or are part of the QRS complex or T wave. It should be apparent that there is no fixed relationship between the P waves and the QRS complexes. The QRS complexes can be narrow or wide, depending on the location of the escape pacemaker. Junctional escape pacemakers are faster (50 to 60 beats/min), narrow, and relatively stable compared with a ventricular escape rhythm, which is slow (30 to 40 beats/min),

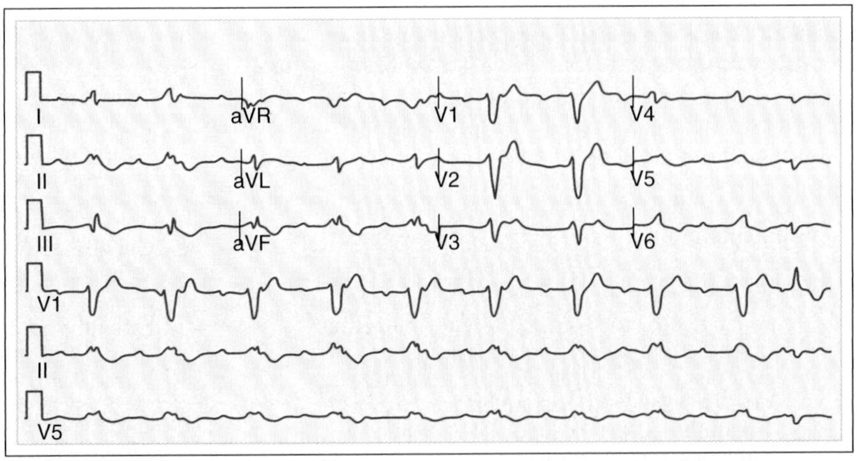
I
aVR
V1
V4
II
aVL
V2
V5
III
aVF
V3
V6
V1
II
V5

FIGURE 51-7 2:1 atrioventricular (AV) block. This electrocardiogram shows an underlying sinus rhythm at 110 beats/min. The ventricular rate is regular and exactly half of the atrial rate. This entity can be distinguished from complete heart block by the fact that each QRS is followed by a P wave with a fixed PR interval. This could represent either Mobitz type I or type II AV block, but the wide QRS suggests disease lower in the conduction system, which therefore should be treated as Mobitz type II block.

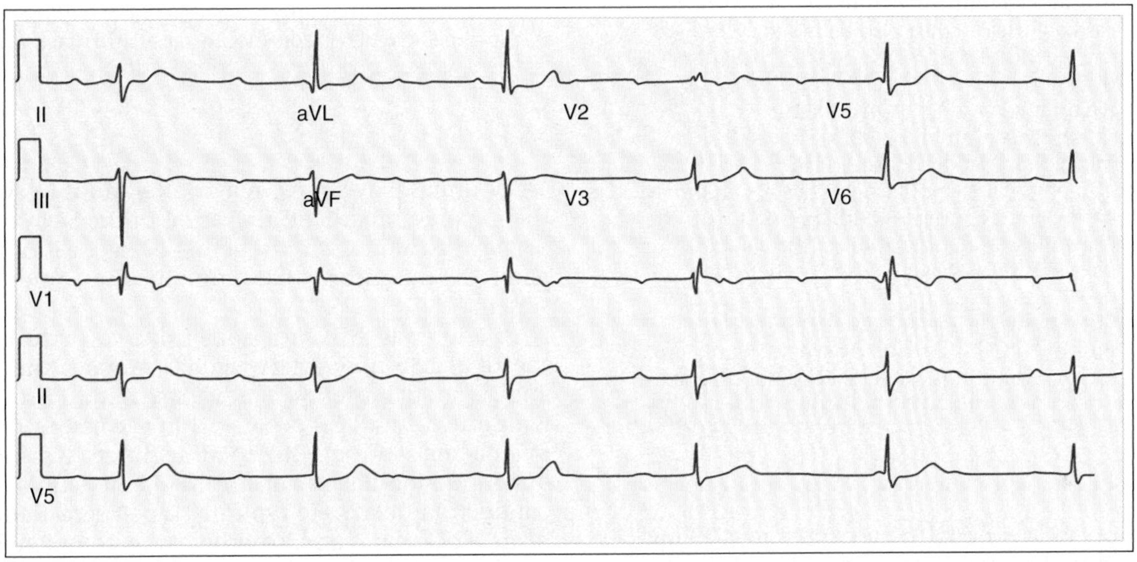
II
aVL
V2
V5
III
aVF
V3
V6
V1
II
V5

FIGURE 51-8 Complete atrioventricular (AV) block. This electrocardiogram (ECG) shows an underlying sinus rhythm that is regular at approximately 80 to 90 beats/min. As with the previous ECG (Fig. 51-7), the ventricular rhythm is slow and regular with no apparent relationship between the P waves and the QRS complexes. The QRS complex is wide and in a left bundle branch pattern, suggesting lack of AV conduction with a ventricular escape rhythm.

wide, and unstable. Often the most helpful feature of the ECG for this rhythm is that the QRS complexes should be absolutely regular. This is a rhythm initiated by a slower pacemaker that has spontaneous automaticity that has "escaped" the influence of the overriding sinus rhythm. Escape rhythms fire automatically at its inherent rate and are regular. Any irregularity in the escape rhythm suggests a high-grade incomplete AV block or an inherently unstable escape rhythm (Fig. 51-8).

■ Cause

Third-degree heart block is caused by a complete interruption of the connection between the atria and ventricles. The level of the block can be at any point within the conduction system. Blocks at the level of the AV node are generally accompanied by escape rhythms that arise from nodal tissues. They are faster, with rates ranging from 40 to 60 bpm, have a narrow QRS complex and tend to be stable. Blocks lower in the conduction system generally occur in patients with serious conduction system disease, such that an acute block at the level of one bundle results in complete heart block because the other bundle is already diseased. The resultant pacemaker tends to be slower with a wide QRS and is less stable.

■ Clinical Presentation

Complete heart block occurs in multiple clinical settings and has variable significance. Nodal block (occurring in the AV node and accompanied by a junctional escape rhythm) occurs in the setting of acute MI, in particular inferior wall MI. Studies have shown that in this setting, there is no significant

Documentation

Bradyarrhythmias are a symptom, not a disease. Often the underlying cause is clearly identified, and documentation is fairly simple—for example, the patient has taken an overdose of his or her blood pressure pill. When the cause is less clear, the documentation must clearly include or exclude those variables that must be considered in the workup and treatment:

- A detailed history of the present illness that helps determine the hemodynamic significance is critical: Did the patient pass out? Is there exertional fatigue or angina? Precipitating factors such as head turning, tight ties, new medications, and poor intake are important clues.
- Risk factors such as cardiac disease will not be overlooked, but the nature and extent of the cardiac disease must also be noted: What is the ejection fraction? Is there any valvular disease or coronary artery disease, and if so, what valve/vessel(s) is involved?
- The history should include a detailed medication list and dosing history.
- The physical examination in the asymptomatic patient rarely provides clinical clues, with the exception of identification of cardiac murmurs or evidence of systemic disease that may involve the heart.
- The electrocardiogram (ECG), and often multiple ECGs, particularly when the patient reports symptoms, often specify the diagnosis.

PATIENT TEACHING TIPS

There are specific conditions that cause bradycardia in which the patient has the ability to exacerbate symptoms and so should be given guidelines to avoid doing so if possible. These generally fall into the category of extrinsic causes of bradycardia:

- Cough, micturition bradycardia/syncope: Patients should be advised to seek treatment to minimize triggers and to have access to support rails. Patients should lie down when lightheaded, and should call 911 for persistent or particularly severe symptoms.
- Patients with carotid sinus hypersensitivity should avoid wearing tight ties and buttoned collars.
- Patients with documented sensitivity to medications that affect the sinus node and/or the atrioventricular node should report this fact when being prescribed any new medications.

infarction of AV nodal tissue and the AV block is often temporary. In contrast, anterior AMI is associated with infranodal block that has a wide QRS complex. In this setting, the block has been shown to be caused by infarction of the conduction system and is irreversible.[10] Complete heart block is also seen in the presence of medication overdose, in particular with a calcium channel blocker, or severe overdose with a beta-blocker.

■ Treatment

Treatment of complete heart block is twofold. The first goal is to ensure hemodynamic stability through use of atropine and/or pacemaker support. Secondary goals are to correct the underlying cause; examples are reperfusion therapies for acute MI and gastric decontamination or antidote therapies for poisonings.

Bradycardia and Acute Myocardial Infarction

Acute MI manifests as significant bradyarrhythmias approximately 25% to 30% of the time.[12,13] These arrhythmias may simply reflect alterations in sympathetic/parasympathetic activation of the SA/AV node or may be the result of ischemia or necrosis of those parts of the heart that contain the conduction system.

Inferior wall MIs are usually due to occlusion of the right coronary artery, which supplies the sinus and AV nodal arteries. Bradyarrhythmias associated with inferior wall MI occur within the first few hours of ischemia and are due to sinus node dysfunction or conduction delays within the AV node. AV nodal conduction delays are typically type I second-degree heart blocks but can also progress to complete heart block. Sinus bradycardia and/or AV nodal blockade have also been attributed to enhanced responsiveness to parasympathetic stimulation seen in association with inferior wall MI. This responsiveness has been attributed to a higher density of cardiac afferent receptors in the inferoposterior portions of the heart. Sinus bradycardia, first-degree AV block, and type I second-degree AV blocks have been observed in up to 40% of patients in the early stages of inferior wall MI. Compete heart block is rarely sudden and usually is the end-stage of a progression of AV nodal conduction delays. The escape rhythm is usually stable, with a narrow QRS complex and rates exceeding 40 beats/min (Fig. 51-9).[12,13]

Bradyarrhythmias in the setting of an inferior wall MI rarely require intervention and, in fact, may be cardioprotective. When a patient with inferior wall MI is hemodynamically unstable, the clinician must first determine whether the heart rate is the primary cause of the hypotension. More often than not, hypotension is due to reduction in stroke volume, particularly in the setting of right ventricular infarct pathophysiology, or a treatment effect from medications that reduce preload, such as nitroglycerin and morphine. Fluids alone usually stabilize the patient's

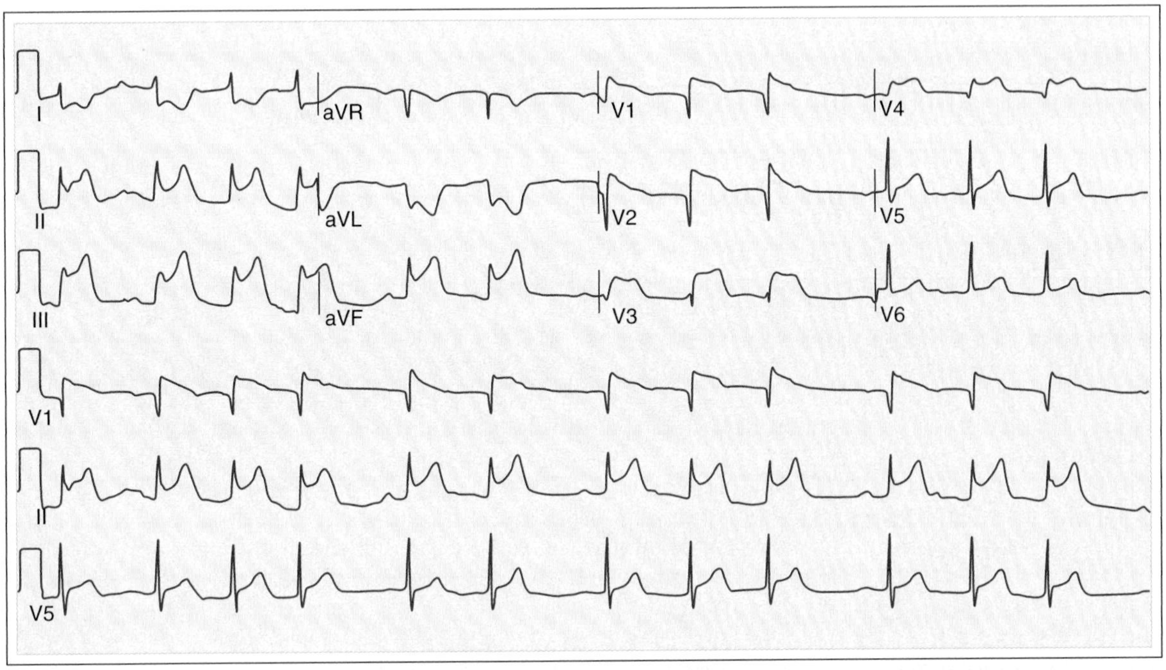
I
aVR
V1
V4
II
aVL
V2
V5
III
aVF
V3
V6
V1
II
V5

A

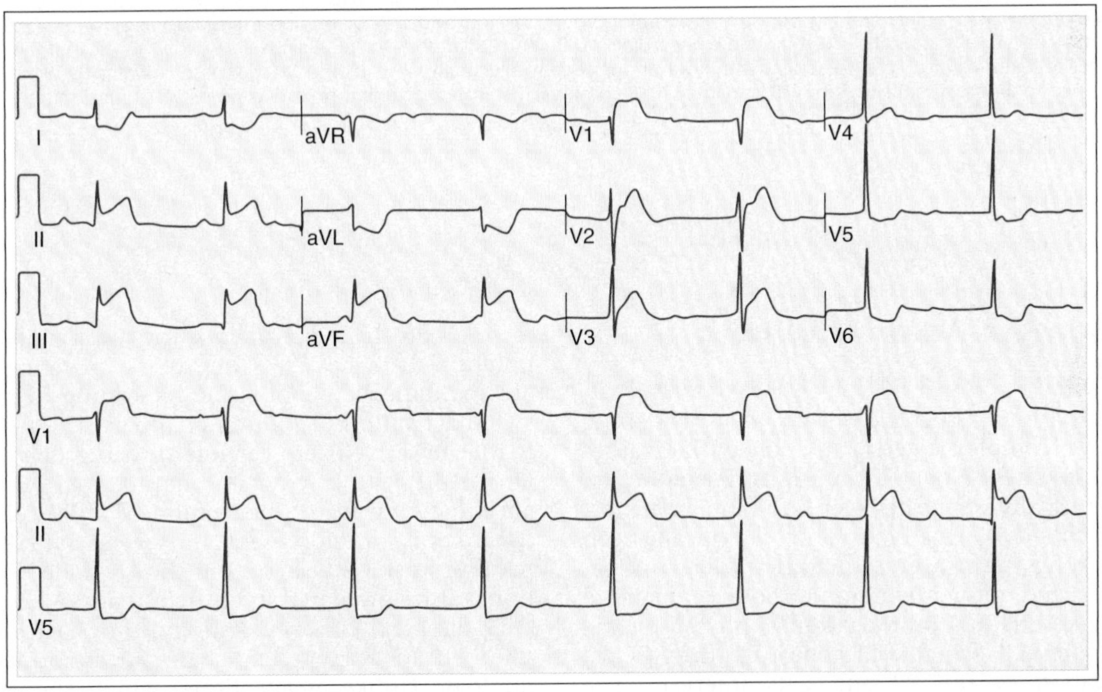
I
aVR
V1
V4
II
aVL
V2
V5
III
aVF
V3
V6
V1
II
V5

B

FIGURE 51-9 **A,** Inferior wall myocardial infarction (MI) and second-degree atrioventricular (AV) block. This electrocardiogram (ECG) shows ST elevations in the inferolateral leads consistent with an inferior/lateral wall MI. The rhythm is a normal sinus rhythm with a Mobitz type I second-degree heart block. There is progressive prolongation of the PR interval, the interval following the blocked beat being shorter than the PR interval immediately preceding the blocked beat. This conduction disturbance may be responsive to atropine. **B,** Inferior wall MI and third-degree AV block. This ECG shows ST elevation in the inferior leads consistent with an inferior wall MI. The rhythm is regular and slow. The lead II rhythm strip shows that there is no fixed relationship between the P waves and the QRS complex. Additionally, it is possible to "march out" the P waves, meaning that this ECG shows complete heart block in the setting of an inferior wall MI.

blood pressure. For hemodynamically compromising bradycardias, atropine is an excellent initial therapy, particularly in the first 6 hours of presentation. Doses should be administered in 0.5-mg increments with a maximal dose of 0.04 mg/kg. Doses less than 0.5 mg should be avoided because of the risk of paradoxical bradycardic response. When atropine is ineffective, transcutaneous or transvenous pacing is indicated. The primary focus in such patients must remain on restoring perfusion to the heart.

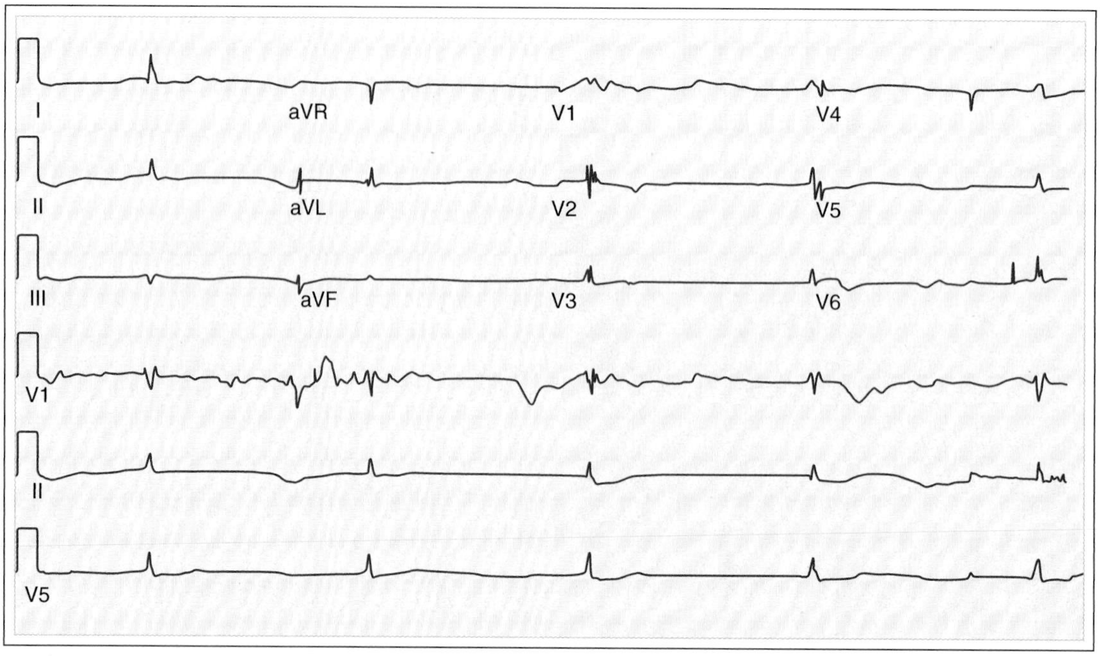
I
aVR
V1
V4
II
aVL
V2
V5
III
aVF
V3
V6
V1
II
V5

FIGURE 51-10 Hyperkalemia. This electrocardiogram (ECG) is from a 52-year-old man who complained of 1 week of generalized weakness. The patient's blood pressure was initially 117 mm Hg systolic/54 mm Hg diastolic, then dropped to 71/37. The ECG shows a very slow rhythm that is regular and has a wide QRS complex. There are no obvious P waves, and the morphology of the QRS complexes is not typical for a right or left bundle branch block. Differential diagnosis includes sinus arrest with an escape rhythm and electrolyte abnormalities. After treatment with intravenous calcium gluconate, insulin, and 5% dextrose in water (D_5W), the heart returned to a normal sinus rhythm with a narrow QRS complex. The patient's serum potassium value was found to be 7.1 mEq/L.

Bradycardia Associated with a Wide QRS Complex

Bradyarrhythmia associated with a "new" widening of the QRS complex suggests an etiology that causes diffuse slowing of depolarization and conduction and that usually implicates agents that block the fast sodium channels. This bradycardia is typically seen in poisonings from agents such as tricyclic antidepressants and diphenhydramine. Sodium channel blockade results in a prolongation of phase 0 of the action potential, which will appear on the ECG as prolongation of the PR and QRS intervals. The right heart and bundle branch are particularly vulnerable to these effects, which manifest as right axis deviation and widened terminal R in lead AVR on the 12-lead ECG. Other causes of diffuse slowing are hyperkalemia, hypothyroidism, and hypothermia.[3]

Hyperkalemia is a common electrolyte disorder seen in the ED. As has been previously discussed, cardiac cells are permeable only to potassium in the resting state. In hyperkalemia, the resting membrane potential becomes "less negative"; therefore, there are spontaneous depolarizations leading to progressive inactivation of sodium channels. The net result is that fewer cells are capable of being depolarized. On the 12-lead ECG, there may be loss of P wave amplitude owing to inactivation of atrial cells. Bradycardia is often present in severe hyperkalemia because of slowed phase 0 in the SA node. Conduction is also slowed in the ventricles, causing a widened QRS complex. One key distinguishing factor is that often the QRS complexes have an abnormal morphology. Unlike escape beats, which should have either a normal morphology (junctional escape) or the morphology of a right or left BBB, hyperkalemic rhythms may have a generally wide QRS termed *nonspecific intraventricular conduction delay*. These QRS complexes may be much wider than 120 msec and have delayed conduction throughout depolarization, which is seen on the ECG as a symmetrically wide QRS complex (Fig. 51-10).

FACTS AND FORMULAS

Sinus bradycardia SB (adults) = 60 beats/min.

Sinoatrial exit block: Pause is due to a nonconducted sinus beat, and pause duration is a multiple of the observed P-P interval.

Sinus pause or arrest: Duration of pause is variable and not a multiple of the P-P interval.

Junctional escape rhythm: Ventricular response rate 40 to 60 beats/min. No P waves. Regular narrow QRS complex (unless there is preexisting bundle branch block [BBB]).

Idioventricular rhythm: Ventricular response rate is 30 to 45 beats/min. No P waves. Regular wide QRS complex (usually does not appear as a typical right or left BBB pattern).

First-degree heart block: Normal sinus rhythm (NSR) with PR interval longer than 200 msec.

Second-degree heart block:

Type I (Wenckebach's block): NSR with progressive P-R prolongation with a nonconducted beat. PR interval of the conducted beat following the blocked beat is the shortest interval of the sequence. QRS complex is usually narrow.

Type II: NSR with fixed PR intervals. Random sinus beats are nonconducted to the ventricle. QRS complex is often wide.

Third-degree heart block: NSR with P waves visible. Ventricular response rate is regular but slower than atrial rate. QRS rate and width dependent on site of escape rhythm. Junctional escape rate is 40 to 60 beats/min, and QRS is narrow. Ventricular escape rhythm is 30 to 45 beats/min, and the QRS is wide.

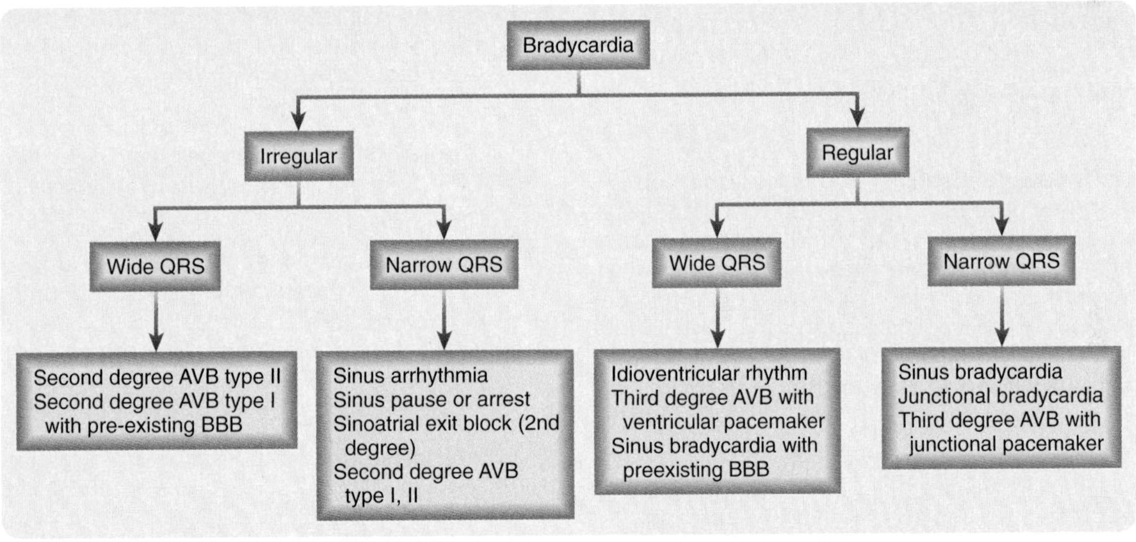
Bradycardia
Irregular
Regular
Wide QRS
Narrow QRS
Wide QRS
Narrow QRS
Second degree AVB type II
Second degree AVB type I with pre-existing BBB
Sinus arrhythmia
Sinus pause or arrest
Sinoatrial exit block (2nd degree)
Second degree AVB type I, II
Idioventricular rhythm
Third degree AVB with ventricular pacemaker
Sinus bradycardia with preexisting BBB
Sinus bradycardia
Junctional bradycardia
Third degree AVB with junctional pacemaker

FIGURE 51-11 Bradycardia flow chart. AV, atrioventricular; BBB, bundle branch block.

REFERENCES

1. Chung EK: Principles of Cardiac Arrhythmias, 3rd ed. Baltimore, Williams & Wilkins, 1983, pp 72-74.
2. Ufberg JW, Clark JS: Bradydysrhythmias and atrioventricular conduction blocks. Emerg Med Clin North Am 2006;24:1-9.
3. Meighem CV, Sabbe M, Knockaert D: The clinical value of the ECG in noncardiac conditions. Chest 2003;125: 1561-1576.
4. Da Costa D, Brady WJ, Edhouse J: ABC of clinical electrocardiography: Bradycardias and atrioventricular conduction block. BMJ 2002;324:535-538.
5. Kaushik V, Leon AR, Forrester JS Jr, Trohman RG: Bradyarrhythmias, temporary and permanent pacing. Crit Care Med 2000;28(Suppl):N121-N128.
6. Ferrer I: Cardiac arrhythmias. Part 3: The sick sinus syndrome. Circulation 1973;47;635-641.
7. Sondheimer HM, Lorts A: Cardiac involvement in inflammatory disease: Systemic lupus erythematosus, rheumatic fever, and Kawasaki disease. Adolesc Med 2001;12: 69-78.
8. Mangrum MJ, Dimarco J: The evaluation and management of bradycardia. N Engl J Med 2000;342:703-709.
9. Denes P, Levy L, Pick A, et al: The incidence of typical and atypical A-V Wenckebach periodicity. Am Heart J 1975; 89:26-31.
10. Rotman M, Wagner GS, Wallace AG: Bradyarrhythmias in acute myocardial infarction. Circulation 1972;45: 703-722.
11. Barold SS, Hayes DL: Second-degree atrioventricular block: A reappraisal [review]. Mayo Clin Proc 2001;76:44-57.
12. Brady WJ, Harrigan RA: Diagnosis and management of bradycardia and atrioventricular block associated with acute coronary ischemia. Emerg Med Clin North Am 2001;19:371-383.
13. Lamas G, Muller JE, Turi ZG, et al: A simplified method to predict occurrence of complete heart block during acute myocardial infarction. Am J Cardiol 1986;57: 1213-1218.

Chapter 52

Tachycardias

Keith A. Marill

KEY POINTS

Tachydysrhythmia may be due to intrinsic cardiologic disease or external stimulation.

Noncardiologic causes, such as hypoxia, inadequate perfusion, metabolic derangements, or toxicity due to medications or other agents, should always be considered.

The higher the tachycardiac heart rate, the greater the likelihood of instability.

Patients with ventricular tachycardia may not necessarily appear unstable.

If there is uncertainty, wide QRS complex tachycardia should be assumed to be ventricular in origin.

The most effective treatment for ventricular tachycardia is electrical cardioversion. However, antidysrhythmic medicines may also be necessary to prevent recurrence.

All ostensibly healthy young patients with syncope should be assessed for valvular disease, left ventricular hypertrophy, Wolff-Parkinson-White syndrome, abnormal QT interval or T wave morphology, and Brugada's syndrome.

Scope

Heart rhythms with rapid rates, or tachydysrhythmias, have a range of causes and associated incidences, morbidities, and mortality. Atrial fibrillation (AF) occurs in up to 5% of people older than 65 years. Conversely, sustained ventricular tachycardia (VT) is rare, accounting for less than 0.1% of ED visits. Morbidity ranges from temporary lightheadedness to syncope and deterioration to ventricular fibrillation (VF), or embolization and subsequent permanent disability due to ischemic stroke. Mortality from atrial tachydysrhythmias is generally low. Mortality from VT is approximately 5%, and that from VF ranges from 80% to more than 90%, depending on the clinical circumstances.[1,2] A particular exception to the low mortality associated with atrial tachydysrhythmias is AF or flutter with rapid ventricular excitation via a bypass tract, such as in Wolff-Parkinson-White (WPW) syndrome.[3]

Mechanisms

Tachycardia is defined as a rhythm with at least three consecutive beats occurring at a rate higher than 100 beats per minute (beats/min). The primary mechanisms for tachycardia are enhanced automaticity, reentry, and triggered beats. Sometimes, a combination of these mechanisms is required for both initiation and maintenance of the tachydysrhythmia.

The normal progression of depolarization in the heart begins with the sinus node, followed by the atria, the atrioventricular (AV) node, the His-Purkinje system, and the ventricles. Sinus and AV nodal tissue depolarization are mediated primarily by calcium channels, and depolarization of the other cardiac tissue is mediated by sodium channels. Repolarization is mediated predominantly by potassium channels.

Automaticity is a characteristic of cardiac tissue wherein the cells depolarize at a periodic rate according to the tissue subtype. Sinus node tissue normally has the fastest intrinsic rate, and thus the sinus node serves as the pacemaker of the heart. Abnormal tachycardia occurs when other foci or circuits supersede the sinus node rate.

Enhanced automaticity occurs when there is an acceleration of the normal periodicity of cells. This may be either a normal physiologic response to increased sympathetic tone or fever or a pathologic response to an overdose of a medicine such as digoxin or theophylline, a stimulant such as an amphetamine or cocaine, or other extrinsic factors. An automatic tachycardia occurs when an ectopic focus of tissue develops a heart rate greater than the sinus rate and paces the heart.

Reentry refers to a microscopic or macroscopic circular pattern of myocardial depolarization. A wave of excitation passes around the circuit, depolarizing the cells until it arrives at the beginning, and the process repeats itself. Reentry can occur if the circuit is sufficiently long or there is a slow-conducting portion that allows enough time for cells to have recovered from their refractory period before the wave of excitation returns (Fig. 52-1). The reentrant rhythm becomes the cardiac pacemaker if it is sufficiently fast to outpace the sinus node.

Tachydysrhythmias can also be initiated or triggered by small depolarizing ion movements that occur during or after normal cellular repolarization. These ion movements are termed *early after-depolarizations* (EADs) and *delayed after-depolarizations* (DADs), respectively. They can trigger a new wave of excitation in the myocardial tissue prior to the normal sequence of depolarization from the sinus node. Unlike early beats due to enhanced automaticity, these beats have a close correlation with the preceding beat and its repolarization phase. Some tachydysrhythmias employ multiple dysrhythmic mechanisms. For example, an EAD may initiate a reentrant tachycardia.

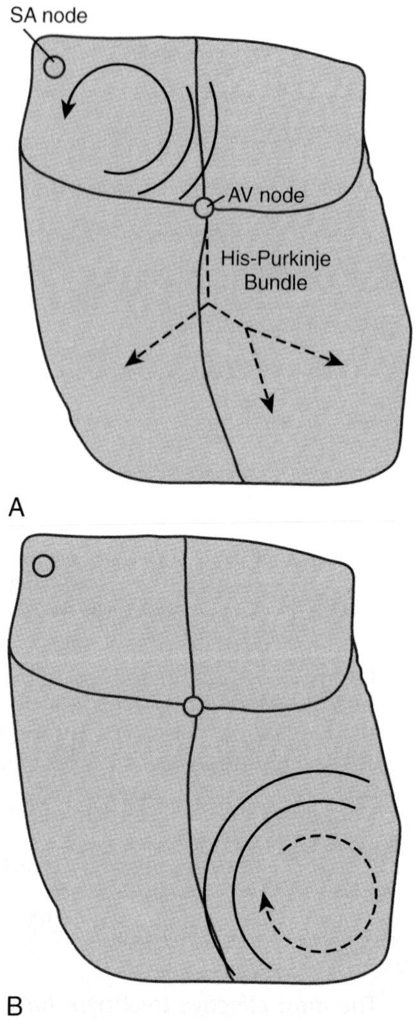
SA node
AV node
His-Purkinje
Bundle
A
B

FIGURE 52-1 Schematic diagrams of cardiac conduction depicting the four heart chambers and the sinoatrial (SA) and atrioventricular (AV) nodes. Normal His-Purkinje conduction is represented by dotted lines with arrows representing conduction through the bundle branches below the AV node. Reentrant waves of cardiac depolarization are represented by semicircular lines with arrows. Conduction through atrial or ventricular myocardial tissue is shown by arcs representing wavelets emanating from the source of excitation. **A,** Typical atrial flutter. **B,** Ventricular tachycardia.

Presenting Signs and Symptoms

Patients with tachydysrhythmias may be entirely asymptomatic or may present with a range of symptoms. They may be lightheaded or may experience palpitations, chest discomfort, shortness of breath, transient syncope, or sudden death.

Signs of tachycardia include a rapid pulse and heart sounds. An irregularly irregular pulse is often detectable with AF, and atrial flutter or atrial tachycardia (AT) with variable AV conduction. VT may be associated with retrograde ventriculoatrial conduction, or there may be AV dissociation. If there is VT with AV dissociation, signs of dissociation may be difficult to discern but can include variable intensity of the first heart sound and/or arterial or jugular venous pulsations. Tachycardia can lead to congestive heart failure (CHF) due to inadequate diastolic filling, myocardial ischemia, or other mechanisms. If CHF occurs, there may be typical signs such as jugular venous distention, rales on pulmonary auscultation, and dependent edema.

The primary findings to assess in the diagnosis of a tachycardiac electrocardiogram (ECG) are as follows:

- The presence, periodicity, and morphology of P waves

- The relationship of the P waves, if any, to the QRS complexes
- The morphology of the QRS complexes and other waves as compared with a prior tracing, if available

The response of the ECG tracing to vagal maneuvers and other therapies such as adenosine may also uncover the underlying rhythm diagnosis.

Differential Diagnosis

A variety of noncardiologic conditions can cause syncope and other symptoms that may suggest a tachydysrhythmia. Inadequate vital organ oxygenation may be due to anemia, hemoglobin malfunction, or respiratory failure. Metabolic derangements include hypoglycemia, hyperthyroidism, dehydration, and fever. A hyperadrenal state due to acute excitement or agitation or, uncommonly, to pheochromocytoma can lead to sinus tachycardia. Neurologic events such as seizure and cerebrovascular accident can cause tachycardia and altered consciousness, which can be confused with a primary tachydysrhythmia. Intoxication with stimulants and anticholinergics can manifest similarly. Overdose with prescription medicines such as antihypertensive agents can cause tachycardia and hypotension.

Primarily nondysrhythmic cardiopulmonary conditions should also be considered in the differential diagnosis. Valvular disease, particularly that involving the aortic site, can lead to tachycardia, chest discomfort, or inadequate cardiac output with subsequent syncope. Hypertrophic obstructive cardiomyopathy can cause inadequate cardiac output if subaortic hypertrophy obstructs cardiac outflow, and pulmonary embolism can lead to pulmonary vasospasm and obstruction to flow. Conditions leading to tamponade, such as pericardial effusion and tension pneumothorax, compromise cardiac output by impairing diastolic filling.

Treatment

The primary emergency therapies for tachydysrhythmias include medicines to slow electrical conduction or to increase the cellular refractory period in the AV node or other groups of cardiac cells (Table 52-1). The goal of therapy is to terminate and suppress the abnormal rhythm or to slow the response in the remainder of the heart. Electrical therapy, including synchronized cardioversion and defibrillation, is used in potentially or frankly unstable patients. Electrical therapy has the advantages of high efficacy and safety, but shocks are painful and do not prevent recurrence of the tachydysrhythmia. Patients with higher heart rates, regardless of the underlying rhythm, have compromised diastolic filling and cardiac output. These patients should be treated more aggressively with early electrical therapy. The EP should understand and use antidysrhythmic medicines but should minimize the use of multiple agents in a single patient. Use of multiple drugs increases the likelihood of drug interactions and compromised cardiac output.

Specific Tachycardias

Primary tachycardiac conditions can be divided most simply into those of supraventricular and ventricular origins (Box 52-1; Fig. 52-2; see also Fig. 52-1). Supraventricular tachycardia (SVT) must involve tissue above the ventricles but may also involve ventricular tissue in a tachycardiac circuit, whereas VT involves only ventricular tissue below the AV node. The remainder of the chapter deals with the diagnosis and treatment of specific tachycardiac conditions.

SUPRAVENTRICULAR TACHYCARDIAS

Irregular Supraventricular Tachycardias

Atrial Fibrillation

The most common cause of an irregularly irregular heart beat, AF is particularly common in the elderly as well as in patients with preexisting cardiopulmonary disease. The mechanism is rapid, quasiperiodic, chaotic reentry within the atria. Consequently, the AV node is bombarded with atrial excitation waves at a high irregular rate. Signal conduction through the AV node is limited by the refractory period of the nodal tissue. The AV node cannot conduct until the cells have recovered from depolarization and are ready to fire again. This determines the rate of the irregular ventricular response to AF.

The clinician can usually diagnose AF at the bedside by feeling the pulse, listening to the heart

BOX 52-1
Major Tachydysrhythmias

Supraventricular Tachycardias
Irregular
- Atrial fibrillation
- Multifocal atrial tachycardia

Regular
- Sinus tachycardia
- Atrial flutter
- Atrial tachycardia
- Atrioventricular (AV) tachycardia
- AV nodal reentrant tachycardia
- Junctional tachycardia

Ventricular Tachycardias
Monomorphic ventricular tachycardia
Polymorphic ventricular tachycardia
- Normal QT interval
- Prolonged QT interval
  - Acquired vs. congenital

Table 52-1 SELECT TACHYDYSRHYTHMIA MEDICATIONS

Class	Primary Mechanism of Action	Medicine	Adult Initial Dosage (IV)	Comments	Adverse Effects
IA	Na and K channel blockade: QRS and QT prolongation	Procainamide	10-15 mg/kg at 20 mg/min	Follow with slow infusion at 1-4 mg/min	Stop if QRS widening >50% or hypotension occurs
IB	Na channel blockade, particularly during ischemia	Lidocaine	1-2 mg/kg at 50 mg/min Load may be repeated to a maximum of 3 mg/kg	Follow with slow infusion at 1-4 mg/min	Confusion, seizures, bradycardia
IC	Na channel blockade	Flecainide	2 mg/kg		Slowing atrial fibrillation/flutter may yield 1:1 AV conduction Heart block, hypotension, ventricular dysrhythmias, CNS confusion
II	Beta-adrenergic receptor blockade	Metoprolol	5 mg every 5 min up to 15 mg		Hypotension, bradycardia, CHF, exacerbation of bronchospasm
		Propranolol	0.25-0.5 mg every 5 min, may increase to 1 mg/kg every 5 min if tolerated, up to 0.20 mg/kg		
		Esmolol	0.5 mg/kg over 1 min followed by 0.05 mg/kg/min for 4 min Second bolus with infusion 0.1 mg/kg/min, if necessary	Short half-life (≈2-9 min)	
III	K channel blockade: QT prolongation	Amiodarone	150 mg over 10 min Bolus may be repeated if necessary	Follow with infusion 1 mg/min for 6 hrs, then 0.5 mg/min	Hypotension, bradycardia Pregnancy class D drug
		Ibutilide	1 mg over 10 min, or 0.01 mg/kg if body weight <60 kg Bolus may be repeated once, if necessary	Pretreatment with magnesium may be helpful to increase efficacy and reduce chance of torsades de pointes	Torsades de pointes (≈2%)
		Sotalol	1-1.5 mg/kg		Hypotension, bradycardia Torsades de pointes rare after IV sotalol bolus (≈0.1%)
IV	Calcium channel blockade	Diltiazem	0.25 mg/kg or 10-20 mg over 2 min Second dose up to 0.35 mg/kg may be given		Hypotension, bradycardia, AV block
		Verapamil	2.5-10 mg over 2 min May be repeated every 15 min up to a total dose of 20 mg		
Other	Adenosine receptor activation: AV and SA nodal block	Adenosine	6-12 mg fast push followed immediately by normal saline flush	Short half-life (≈6-9 sec)	Transient bradycardia, PVCs, flushing, dyspnea, chest pressure
		Magnesium	1-2 g over 5 min or more		Potential CNS or respiratory depression
	Enhanced vagal tone: AV nodal block	Digoxin	0.25-0.5 mg	Slow-onset AV conduction block	Bradycardia with sinus or AV block, ventricular dysrhythmias, nausea and vomiting

AV, atrioventricular; CHF, congestive heart failure; CNS, central nervous system; IV, intravenous; K, potassium; Na, sodium; PVC, premature ventricular contraction; SA, sinoatrial.

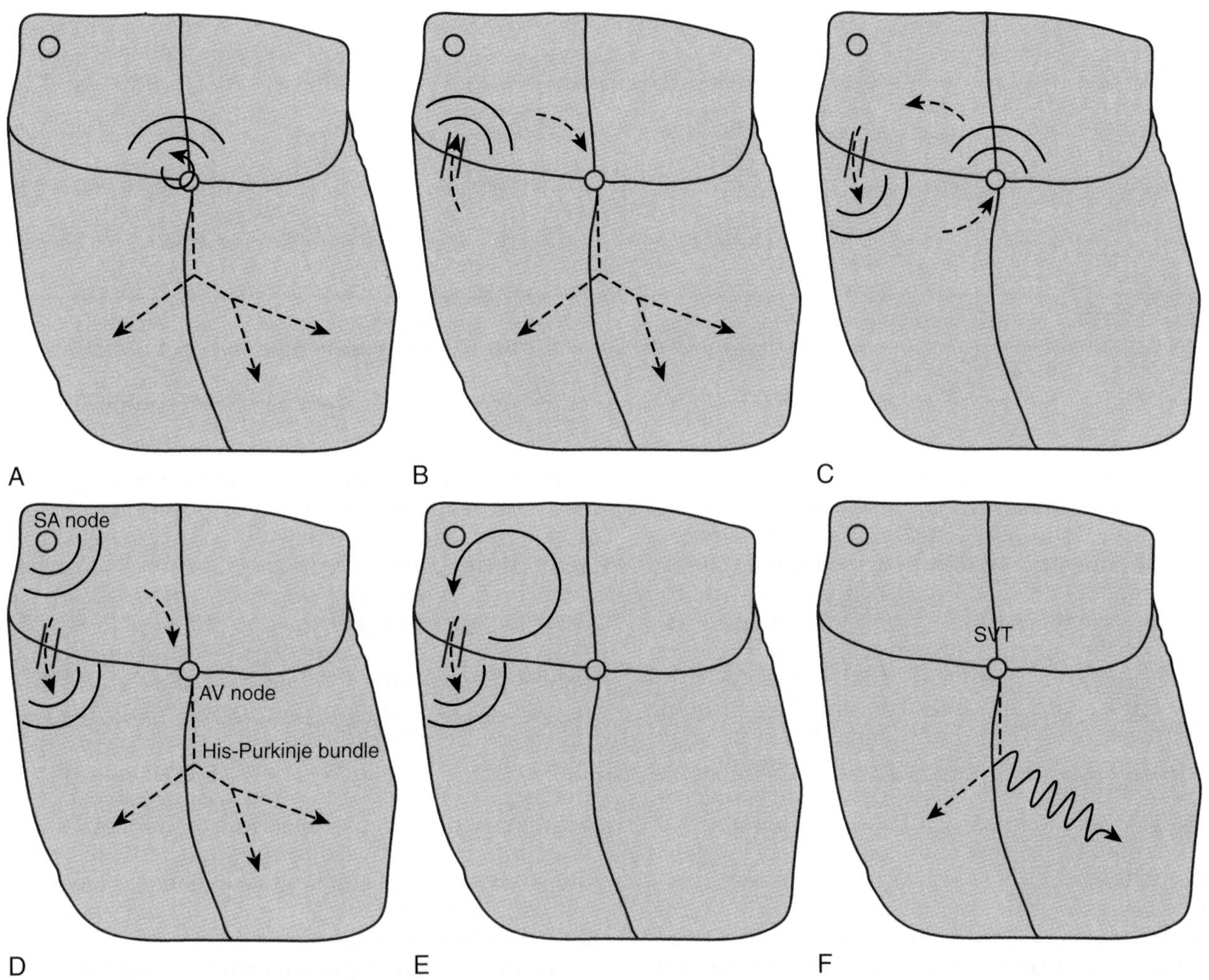
A
B
C
SA node
AV node
His-Purkinje bundle
D
E
SVT
F

FIGURE 52-2 **A,** Atrioventricular (AV) nodal reentrant tachycardia (AVNRT). **B,** Atrioventricular reentrant tachycardia (orthodromic). **C,** Atrioventricular reentrant tachycardia (antidromic). **D,** Normal sinus rhythm and Wolff-Parkinson-White syndrome. SA, sinoatrial. **E,** Atrial fibrillation or flutter with rapid accessory pathway conduction. **F,** Supraventricular tachycardia (SVT) with aberrancy.

sounds, and observing a single-lead cardiac monitor. The ECG may show fine or course, irregular undulations of the baseline and absence of regular P waves. The QRS complex is usually normal; however, if the ventricular response is rapid, the QRS may be transiently widened owing to intermittent aberrant conduction through the His-Purkinje system (Fig. 52-3). This finding, termed Ashman's phenomenon, can occur when areas of the His-Purkinje tissue have a longer refractory period than the AV node. Such bursts of wide QRS complex tachycardia can be confused with nonsustained VT, but on close inspection, the rhythm remains irregularly irregular.

The most common treatment issue for patients with AF in the emergency setting is control of the ventricular rate. Depending on the function of the patient's AV node, the ventricular rate may range up to approximately 150 beats/min in adults. Ventricular rates this fast allow insufficient time for diastolic filling of the heart. The rate can be slowed with a variety of agents that act to lengthen the refractory period of the AV nodal tissue, such as calcium channel blockers,[4] beta-blockers,[5] magnesium,[6] digoxin, and amiodarone. Digoxin is less useful in the emergency setting because it takes a few hours to work, but the other agents must be used carefully because they can decrease blood pressure to varying degrees. The calcium channel blocker diltiazem usually provides excellent rate control with minimal loss of blood pressure. Beta-blockers may cause a greater loss of blood pressure and must be used with caution in patients with CHF or pulmonary disease. There is no indication for the administration of adenosine in patients with AF. The diagnosis should be made on the basis of history, physical and ECG findings, and the response to adenosine, which only transiently blocks AV nodal conduction and has no lasting therapeutic benefit.

If a patient with AF has a rapid ventricular response and associated hypotension, consider emergency cardioversion. It is unusual for AF alone to cause hypotension, so the possibility of other additional causative conditions that can be corrected, such as dehydration, occult hemorrhage, and the metabolic conditions previously mentioned, should also be considered. Nevertheless, cardioversion can be accomplished by

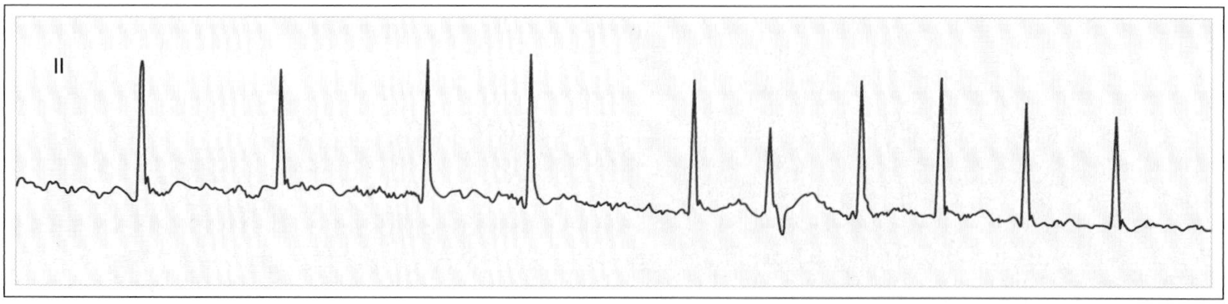
II

FIGURE 52-3 Electrocardiogram showing atrial fibrillation with no clear P waves and irregularly irregular ventricular response. Note that the QRS is widened in a single beat after a relatively short R-R interval. This is Ashman's phenomenon, which occurs because the His-Purkinje system is still partly refractory to excitation.

electrical, chemical, or combined therapies. For the patient with cardiovascular instability, emergency direct current cardioversion (DCCV) is most effective and safe. The patient should be sedated if clinical circumstances allow, and treatment begun with 100 joules (J) of energy with a biphasic or monophasic pulse. A short-acting benzodiazepine such as midazolam is often the first choice for sedation because it is safe and effective, and has amnestic properties as well. The defibrillator should be set to the synchronized mode to synchronize the pulse, if possible, with the QRS deflection, even though the QRS waves occur irregularly. If the initial shock is unsuccessful, the energy of the pulse can be escalated as needed.

Cardioversion can also be accomplished chemically when circumstance allow. Agents that increase the refractory period of the atrial tissue are used to break the reentrant microcircuits within the atria. Vaughn-Williams class III and class I medicines that can accomplish this goal include ibutilide, amiodarone, procainamide, propafenone, and flecainide.[7,8] These agents can terminate AF alone and can increase the likelihood of cardioversion of AF with subsequent DCCV. However, their use entails some risk. There is an approximately 2% to 5% chance of causing torsades de pointes (TdP) after infusion because these agents variably increase the duration of the depolarized phase and the associated QT interval in the ventricles as well as the atria. The newly developed agent vernakalant may be less likely to cause TdP because of its action to block the ultrarapid potassium channels located primarily in the atria. Hypokalemia and hypomagnesemia raise the risk of TdP. Pretreatment with magnesium may be protective, even with normal serum electrolyte levels.[9] Cardioversion is also associated with a risk of embolic stroke.

AF is associated with an unsynchronized, quivering motion of the atrial wall. As a result, there is stasis of blood in the atria and a risk of spontaneous clot formation. AF is an important cause of embolic stroke, with the embolism emanating from the left atrium. Long-term anticoagulation with warfarin has been found to reduce the likelihood of embolic stroke.

In the acute setting, clot may form within 48 hours after the onset of AF. Cardioversion of AF may cause a new clot to embolize into the systemic circulation. If the patient can clearly discern when he or she is in AF, and symptoms have begun within the preceding 1 to 2 days, it may be safe to perform cardioversion without anticoagulation. However, if there is any uncertainty about the time of onset of the tachydysrhythmia or it occurred more than 48 hours ago, the patient should not undergo immediate cardioversion. Instead, the cardiology service should be consulted and a transesophageal echocardiogram should be performed to search for atrial clot formation, or cardioversion should be deferred until the patient is adequately anticoagulated.[10] The only exception would be cardiovascular instability due to AF that requires emergency DCCV.

The disposition of patients with AF depends on a number of factors, including the patient's age, comorbid illnesses and social and outpatient medical support, the adequacy of ventricular rate control, the plans for cardioversion, and the state of anticoagulation. If the patient requires ongoing adjustment of medications to control a rapid ventricular response, attempted cardioversion is planned, or new anticoagulation is initiated, hospitalization should be considered. The EP should make this decision in concert with the patient and the consulting cardiologist.

Multifocal Atrial Tachycardia

Multifocal AT (MFAT) is a relatively uncommon tachydysrhythmia that primarily affects older patients with chronic lung diseases such as chronic obstructive pulmonary disease (COPD), and it appears to be related to methylxanthine administration.[11] The mechanism is uncertain, but MFAT is thought to occur as a result of delayed afterdepolarizations in the atrial tissue triggering ectopic beats. The diagnosis is made on the basis of the following ECG criteria: at least three consecutive P waves with different morphologies, variable PP and PR intervals, and heart rate greater than 100 beats/min. Treatment of MFAT is centered on treating the underlying pulmonary disease and possible hypoxia. Antidysrhythmic agents are poorly effective in slowing the atrial rate or the

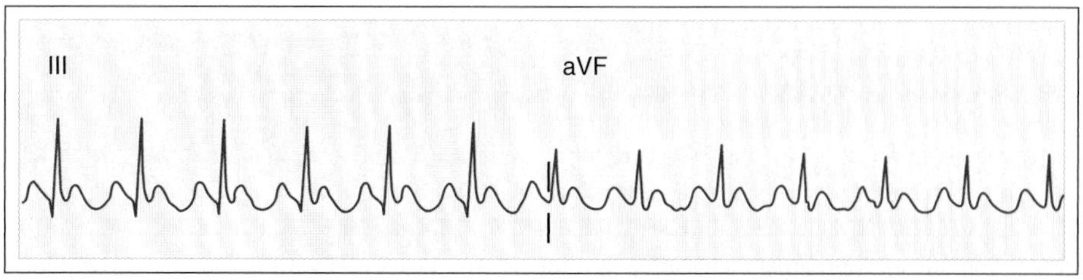
III
aVF

FIGURE 52-4 Electrocardiogram showing atrial flutter with 2:1 conduction and a regular ventricular rate of 150 beats/min.

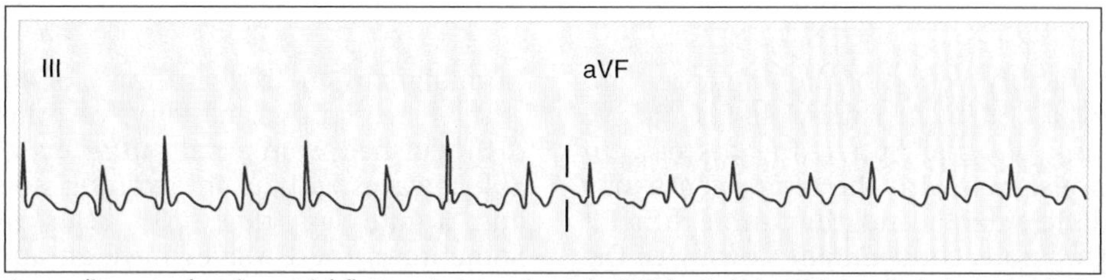
III
aVF

FIGURE 52-5 Electrocardiogram showing atrial flutter at approximately 260 beats/min with regularly irregular 3:2 conduction (3 flutter waves per 2 QRS complexes). Note the variable flutter to QRS conduction interval (Wenckebach pattern) and alternating QRS complex morphology. These findings suggest that the heart rate is on the cusp of the refractory period of both the atrioventricular node and the His-Purkinje system.

ventricular response or in terminating MFAT. Nevertheless, a carefully administered trial of a calcium channel blocker or amiodarone is reasonable. Generally, beta-blockers should be avoided if there is any evidence of bronchospasm. Magnesium therapy, particularly in combination with potassium replacement, may slow the rate or terminate the tachydysrhythmia. Patients usually require admission to treat the pulmonary disease.

Regular Supraventricular Tachycardias

Sinus Tachycardia

Sinus tachycardia may be due to a wide variety of physiologic, pathologic, or pharmacologic causes. If necessary, treatment is usually directed toward the underlying cause. In some settings, such as CHF or acute myocardial infarction (MI), treatment of sinus tachycardia with beta-blockers may improve cardiac hemodynamics and outcome. Sinus tachycardia is often part of the differential diagnosis of other regular tachydysrhythmias. Identifying characteristics of sinus tachycardia are (1) regularly occurring identical P waves with a leftward inferior axis in the frontal plane and (2) gradual onset and offset of the tachycardiac rate.

Atrial Flutter

Atrial flutter can occur as a result of a variety of cardiopulmonary and metabolic derangements, often in association with atrial dilation. Patients with atrial flutter also tend to experience AF, but atrial flutter is less common overall. The mechanism of atrial flutter is a macro-reentrant circuit in the right atrium (see Fig. 52-1A). The most common variant of atrial flutter is termed "typical atrial flutter," which involves a counterclockwise wave of roughly circular excitation when viewed from a position facing the front of the patient. The flutter pathway is constrained in the inferior portion of the circular loop by anatomical structures, and it travels between the tricuspid annulus anteriorly and the inferior vena cava and coronary sinus posteriorly. This segment of the pathway, the isthmus, contains the relatively slower-conducting tissue in the reentrant loop. Atypical atrial flutter most commonly travels over the same pathway, but in the opposite direction.

The rate of atrial flutter waves ranges from 250 to 350 beats/min. The diagnosis is made from the ECG tracing, which demonstrates typical sawtooth-shaped flutter waves at the appropriate rate, generally most prominent in the inferior limb leads (II, III, and aVF) and lead V_1. The flutter waves tend to be identical and to recur regularly, and there is no isoelectric or flat ECG segment between the waves (Figs. 52-4 and 52-5). As in AF, the refractory period of the AV node usually controls the ventricular response to atrial flutter. The most common response is 2:1 AV conduction; however, higher, lower, or variable ratios of conduction are also possible. The ratio of conduction depends on the atrial flutter rate, the health of the AV node, and any modifying physiologic, metabolic, or pharmacologic factors. Because atrial flutter most commonly manifests as flutter waves at 300 beats/min, 2:1 AV conduction, and a ventricular response rate of 150 beats/min, atrial flutter should be the first diagnosis considered in all patients who present with a regular tachycardia at 150 beats/min. It is important to remember, however, that pharmacologic agents can slow the rate of atrial flutter and decrease or increase AV nodal conduction, altering the usual characteristics.

The management of atrial flutter is similar to that of AF but can be a bit more difficult. Agents that

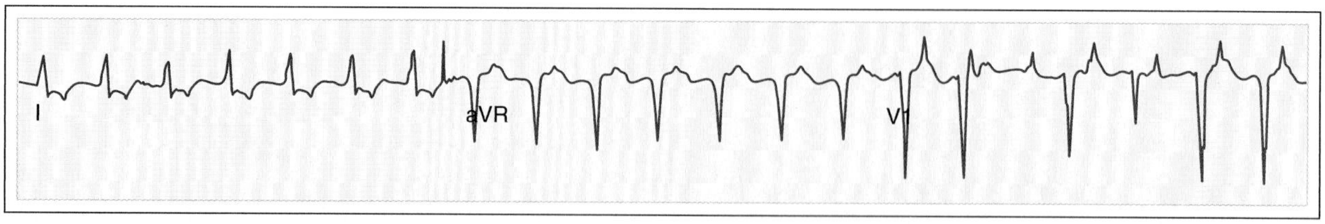
I
aVR
V1

FIGURE 52-6 Electrocardiogram showing atrial tachycardia at a rate of 163 beats/min with first-degree heart block and mostly 1 : 1 atrioventricular (AV) conduction with a single nonconducted beat (see lead V_1). The abnormal rightward P wave axis in lead I is not consistent with sinus rhythm. The rhythm is too slow for atrial flutter, and dropped beats would not be expected with a reentrant rhythm involving the AV node and ventricles.

lengthen the refractory period of the AV node tend to gradually decrease the ventricular response rate to AF. In the setting of atrial flutter, the decrease in ventricular response rate with the same agents may be stepwise and incremental and, thus, more difficult to control. Furthermore, concomitant slowing of the atrial flutter waves may paradoxically allow greater efficiency of AV nodal conduction. For example, slowing flutter from 280 beats/min to 180 beats/min could lead to an augmentation of the ventricular response from 2:1 conduction at 140 beats/min to 1:1 conduction at 180 beats/min.

Ventricular rate control in atrial flutter can usually be achieved with a calcium channel antagonist such as diltiazem, a beta-blocker, or digoxin. Both electrical cardioversion and chemical cardioversion have a high success rate. Synchronized DCCV should start with 50 J and the shock should be repeated with higher energy if the first is ineffective. Chemical cardioversion can be achieved with a variety of agents, including class III antidysrhythmics such as ibutilide and amiodarone, class I agents such as procainamide, and the beta-blocker esmolol. Rate control should generally be achieved prior to attempted chemical cardioversion. These agents can slow the atrial flutter rate with an adverse enhancement of the conduction ratio as previously described or, in the case of procainamide or quinidine, the agent's vagolytic properties may independently enhance AV nodal conduction.

Cardioversion of atrial flutter is associated with thromboembolism, although the association is likely weaker than that with cardioversion of AF.[10] For this reason, cardioversion of atrial flutter should probably not be undertaken in the ED unless the indication is an emergency because of cardiovascular instability, the combined duration of atrial flutter and AF is less than 48 hours, the patient has been adequately anticoagulated prior to presentation, or the patient is newly anticoagulated and there is no evidence of atrial thrombus on transesophageal echocardiography. The decision to hospitalize patients with atrial flutter involves weighing issues similar to those described for AF.

Atrial Tachycardia

Regular AT is a relatively uncommon tachydysrhythmia. It may be due to cardiopulmonary disease with dilated atria and a reentrant mechanism, toxicity from digoxin, methylxanthines, or adrenergic agents with increased automaticity, or other causes. AT is distinguished from atrial flutter by separate identifiable P waves with an intervening isoelectric baseline and a rate less than 200 beats/min (Fig. 52-6). Sometimes, the P waves have an abnormal upward or rightward axis or the onset of tachycardia is abrupt. These characteristics would distinguish the rhythm from sinus tachycardia. Finally, as discussed later, unlike reentrant atrial rhythms that involve the AV node, AT would not be expected to terminate with agents that slow AV nodal conduction. As with atrial flutter, decreasing AV nodal conduction dynamics might slow the ventricular response to the rhythm and facilitate the diagnosis. It would not generally terminate the rhythm because the origin of the tachycardia is contained entirely within the atria.

Treatment of AT begins with an assessment of underlying causes. Digoxin toxicity should be suspected if AT is accompanied by high-grade AV block. Tachycardia in digoxin toxicity results from altered intracellular calcium dynamics and increased excitability, whereas high-grade AV block results from enhanced vagal tone. When there is no evidence of underlying toxicity, ventricular rate control and electrical or chemical cardioversion for AT should be approached as for AF and flutter. If the patient shows evidence of drug toxicity or uncontrolled pulmonary disease or has new tachycardia, admission for further treatment should be considered.

Reentrant Supraventricular Tachycardia

The nomenclature of reentrant supraventricular tachycardias can be confusing. They are often termed "paroxysmal" because of their abrupt onset, or they may be called supraventricular tachycardia. More precisely, they comprise two major subtypes of SVT, atrioventricular reentrant tachycardia (AVRT) and AV nodal reentrant tachycardia (AVNRT). Reentrant SVTs are moderately common in both children and adults, and most commonly are not associated with other cardiopulmonary disease.

Mechanistically, the two major subtypes of reentrant SVT are distinguished by the route of the reentrant pathway. AVRT uses a macroreentrant circuit with atrial and ventricular segments, and connecting segments that comprise the AV node and an accessory conducting tract or, rarely, two accessory conducting tracts (see Fig. 52-2B and C). The AV nodal segment usually serves as the necessary slow-conducting portion of the reentrant circuit.

Many patients have at least two discrete segments that can conduct the input wave of excitability from the right atrium into the AV node. The conducting properties of these inputs may differ, and often there are both a fast-conducting input or pathway and a relatively slow-conducting one. Usually, conduction to the AV node is via the fast pathway. AVNRT uses a small macroreentrant circuit comprising the AV node, right atrial tissue, and connecting fast and slow pathway segments to form a full circle of conduction (see Fig. 52-2A).

Within each subtype of reentrant SVT, the direction of the wave of excitation can vary. In AVRT, the wave of excitation most commonly proceeds down the AV node and normally through the His-Purkinje system, and it returns in a retrograde direction up the accessory tract to the atria to complete the circuit; this is termed *orthodromic conduction* (see Fig. 52-2B). *Antidromic conduction* occurs when the wave of excitation proceeds in the opposite direction, down the accessory pathway, and returns in retrograde fashion up the AV node (see Fig. 52-2C). In this case, conduction down the His-Purkinje system and normal near-simultaneous excitation of the ventricles do not occur. Rather, the ventricles are activated from the terminus of the accessory tract, and the wave of excitation must propagate across the ventricular myocardium similar to excitation from a premature ventricular contraction (PVC). Consequently, it takes longer to excite the entire ventricular muscle mass, and the corresponding QRS wave is widened with antidromic conduction.

Reentrant SVTs are usually easily diagnosed from the ECG. The most common finding is a narrow QRS complex tachycardia at rate of 120 to 250 beats/min. The atria are activated in a retrograde direction from the AV node or an accessory tract. In AVRT, retrograde P waves that are inverted in V_1 and the inferior leads may be observed just after the QRS complex (Fig. 52-7). In AVNRT, retrograde excitation of the atria is often simultaneous with ventricular excitation, and retrograde P waves are not observed because they are hidden or "buried" within the QRS complex (Fig. 52-8). In this case, P waves appear to be absent.

Reentrant SVT may manifest as a wide QRS complex primarily for two reasons. Normal rapid conduction down the His-Purkinje system leads to near-simultaneous excitation and depolarization of the ventricular myocardium and a narrow QRS complex on the ECG. If the left or right bundle of the Purkinje system fails to conduct, the QRS complex is widened and displays bundle branch block (BBB) morphology (see Fig. 52-2F). This can occur because of intrinsic conduction system disease and a chronic BBB, or the failure may be rate-dependent and occur only during tachycardia. The other reason for a widened QRS complex is AVRT with antidromic conduction antegrade down the accessory pathway (see Fig. 52-2C). This path does not utilize the His-Purkinje system, and a widened QRS complex without typical BBB morphology would be expected.

Particularly in children, reentrant supraventricular tachycardias are usually well tolerated. Patients with more rapid heart rates are more prone to cardiovascular instability, including hypotension and presyncope. Patients may also feel palpitations, dyspnea, and chest pain, which can be due to myocardial ischemia.

From an ED perspective, it is usually not important to distinguish AVRT from AVNRT. The acute treatment and prognosis for the two conditions are the same. Vagal maneuvers[12] should be attempted or drugs administered to slow conduction and increase the refractory period through the AV nodal tissue so

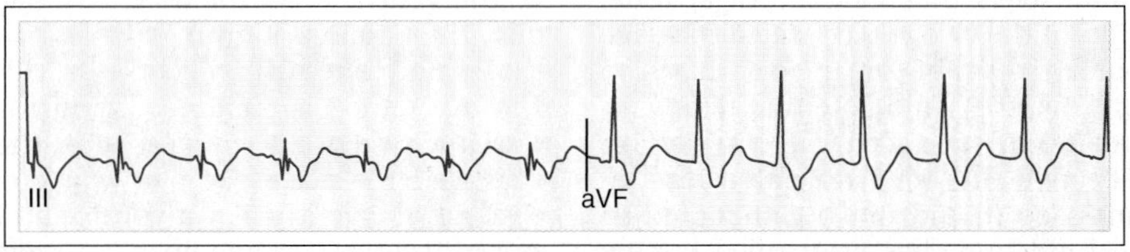
III
aVF

FIGURE 52-7 Electrocardiogram showing atrioventricular reentrant tachycardia (AVRT) with retrograde P waves (inverted in the inferior leads) following the QRS complexes. This strip demonstrates the more common orthodromic conduction variant of AVRT. The ventricles are depolarized normally, and then the signal travels up through the bypass tract to depolarize the atria from bottom to top.

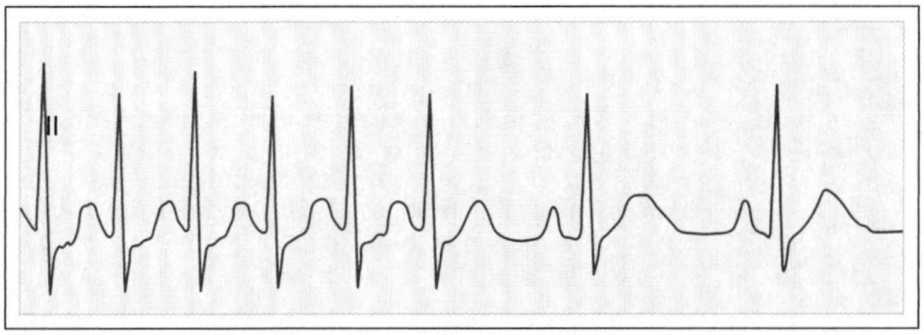
II

FIGURE 52-8 Electrocardiogram showing atrioventricular nodal reentrant tachycardia (AVNRT) at 180 beats/min with spontaneous termination to normal sinus rhythm. During tachycardia, retrograde atrial depolarization occurs simultaneously with ventricular depolarization. Thus, retrograde P waves are buried within the QRS complexes.

BOX 52-2

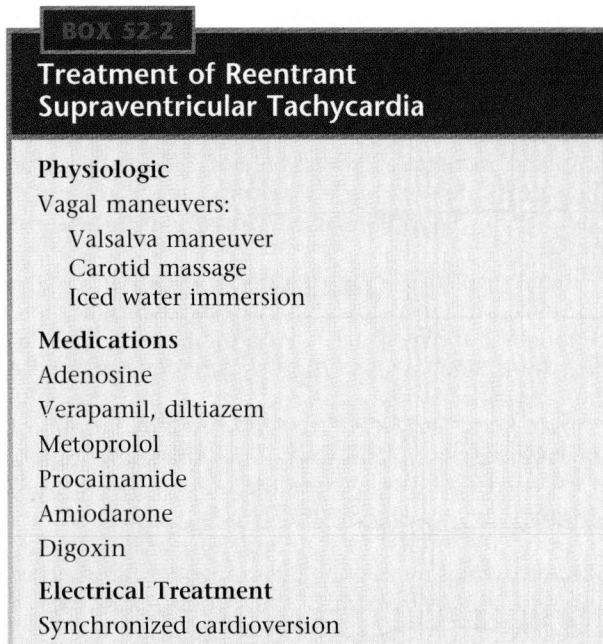

Treatment of Reentrant Supraventricular Tachycardia

Physiologic

Vagal maneuvers:

- Valsalva maneuver
- Carotid massage
- Iced water immersion

Medications

Adenosine

Verapamil, diltiazem

Metoprolol

Procainamide

Amiodarone

Digoxin

Electrical Treatment

Synchronized cardioversion

that the node is refractory to excitation and conduction when the reentrant wave approaches it. Agents such as adenosine and calcium channel blockers act directly on the nodal tissue, whereas other interventions, such as vagal maneuvers, digoxin, and beta-blockers, may alter vagal or adrenergic tone (Box 52-2). Adenosine may be the optimal medicine because it is highly effective and safe, with an ultrashort (9-second) half-life in serum. Rapid clearing, however, can be a disadvantage if the tachydysrhythmia is recurrent. In this case, the calcium channel blocker verapamil may be useful because it is equally effective for termination and may prevent recurrent episodes.[13] Verapamil should not be used in infants, however, because of the risk of cardiovascular collapse.[14]

Physiologic maneuvers that increase vagal tone, such as immersion of the face in iced water, massage of the carotid bulb, and Valsalva maneuver may also be effective, but have the same potential disadvantage of tachycardia recurrence. Iced water immersion may be more effective and better tolerated in children. Carotid massage should not be attempted in adults until a carotid bruit has been ruled out by auscultation. As for other supraventricular tachydysrhythmias, synchronized DCCV should be reserved for patients who demonstrate cardiovascular instability. Most patients can be discharged home after termination of reentrant SVT. Hospitalization should be considered for the patient whose tachydysrhythmia is recurrent or associated with cardiovascular instability.

Preexcitation (Wolff-Parkinson-White) Syndrome

When a patient has an accessory pathway of myocardial fiber connecting the atria and ventricles and there is evidence of antegrade conduction down this pathway, the patient has preexcitation or Wolff-Parkinson-White (WPW) syndrome. The syndrome is uncommon, is usually diagnosed in children or young adults, and is most commonly not associated with other cardiopulmonary disease. Patients may present in normal sinus rhythm or with a variety of supraventricular tachydysrhythmias, including AVRT in 80% of cases, AF in 15% to 30%, and atrial flutter in 5%. Approximately 85% of AVRT episodes have an orthodromic direction of activation, and 15% are antidromic.

The diagnosis can be made while the patient is in normal sinus rhythm if the following ECG characteristics are observed: (1) shortened PR interval (<120 msec), (2) widened QRS complex beyond 120 msec, and (3) atypical initiation of the QRS complex with a "delta wave" morphology (Fig. 52-9). There are often associated ST-T wave abnormalities, with the T wave inverted with respect to the delta wave and QRS complex. These three diagnostic abnormalities are easily understood from an electrophysiologic perspective (see Fig. 52-2D).

In normal sinus rhythm, the wave of excitation can propagate down both the AV node and the accessory pathway. Because the accessory pathway does not contain slow-conducting tissue, the wave traverses the accessory pathway and reaches the ventricular myocardium before traversing the AV node. The shortened PR interval and early delta wave upstroke of the QRS wave are due to "preexcitation" of the ventricle via the accessory pathway. Eventually, the atrial excitation wave also traverses the AV node, and once this occurs, it will move rapidly through the specialized rapid-conducting His-Purkinje system. In the meantime, the wave that has traversed the accessory pathway propagates slowly through the ventricular myocardium because it does not utilize the Purkinje fibers for rapid transmission. Consequently, the QRS deflection arrives early with a delta wave, but the latter portion normalizes owing to the influence of normal AV nodal conduction.

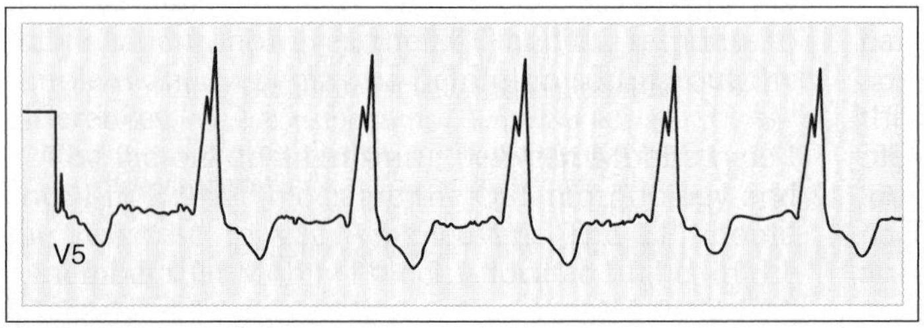
V5

FIGURE 52-9 Electrocardiogram showing Wolff-Parkinson-White (WPW) syndrome with normal sinus rhythm. Note the shortened PR interval, widened QRS wave with slurred upstroke, and abnormal inverted T wave. These findings in lead V_5 are diagnostic of WPW syndrome with an accessory conduction tract, likely in the left lateral position.

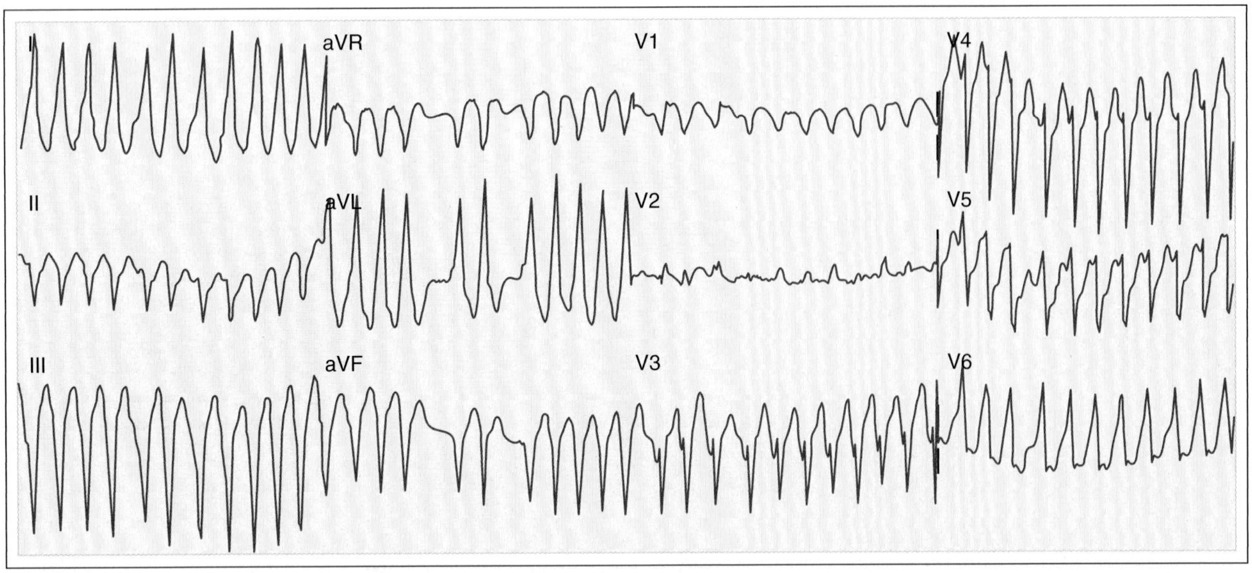
I
aVR
V1
V4
II
aVL
V2
V5
III
aVF
V3
V6

FIGURE 52-10 Electrocardiogram showing atrial fibrillation with wide QRS complexes and a rapid variable ventricular response rate consistent with Wolff-Parkinson-White syndrome. This is a dangerous condition that requires immediate attention and treatment. The risk of conversion to ventricular fibrillation and cardiovascular collapse is inversely associated with the length of the shortest R-R interval.

Because of the atypical pattern of ventricular depolarization, repolarization changes in the form of ST-T abnormalities are expected.

Patients with WPW syndrome are predisposed to AVRT as well as AF and atrial flutter. The pathway of conduction of the AF wavelets from the atria to the ventricles depends on the relative refractory period of the accessory pathway as compared with the AV node. The slow-conducting cells of the AV node have a long refractory period, and the refractory period of the accessory conducting tissue is usually shorter. Consequently, the AV node remains refractory when the accessory pathway tissue is repolarized and ready for conduction. In WPW syndrome, AF usually conducts down the accessory pathway with a rapid ventricular response rate that is determined by the refractory period of the accessory conducting tissue (Fig. 52-10; see Fig. 52-2E). Similar to the situation with normal sinus rhythm, the ventricles are activated from the ectopic accessory pathway terminus, and an irregularly irregular wide QRS complex tachycardia results.

Perhaps the greatest concern regarding patients with WPW syndrome is the higher risk of sudden cardiac death. This risk is inversely associated with the minimum refractory period of the accessory conducting tissue.[3] The mechanism of sudden cardiac death is thought most commonly to be AF with accessory tract conduction and a dangerously high ventricular response rate that causes ischemia and electrical instability, and degenerates to VF.

It is important to remember that, like the AV node and other cardiac tissue, accessory pathways have dynamic electrophysiologic properties that may vary with the hormonal, physiologic, or pharmacologic milieu. However, in this respect, accessory pathway tissue behaves more like myocardium and less like AV nodal tissue, which is highly sensitive to vagal stimulation. Depending on the current milieu, conduction in many patients with WPW syndrome may variably occur primarily down the accessory pathway or the AV node in normal sinus rhythm, and this variation even occasionally occurs in AF (Fig. 52-11).

Treatment of AF in patients with WPW syndrome must be approached differently. The usual treatment of AF is to administer agents that increase the refractory period of the AV node and slow AV nodal conduction. Because conduction is primarily down the accessory pathway in WPW syndrome, treatment must be directed toward lengthening the refractory period of the accessory pathway tissue, not the AV node. Paradoxically, agents that block AV nodal conduction, such as beta-blockers, calcium channel blockers, adenosine, and digoxin, may also cause vasodilation, decrease contractility, or have other effects that reflexively increase adrenergic tone or stimulate and enhance accessory pathway conduction. For this reason, these agents should not be used.

The preferred pharmacologic agents for WPW syndrome with AF and a rapid ventricular response are the class IA antidysrhythmic procainamide[15] and, possibly, class III medicines such as amiodarone and sotalol. These antidysrhythmics are used to decrease the ventricular response rate, and they may also terminate AF. Nevertheless, they have multiple potential dangers and must be used with caution. All of these antidysrhythmic agents can decrease blood pressure. When administered intravenously, amiodarone blocks AV nodal conduction, so the concerns already described with other AV nodal blocking

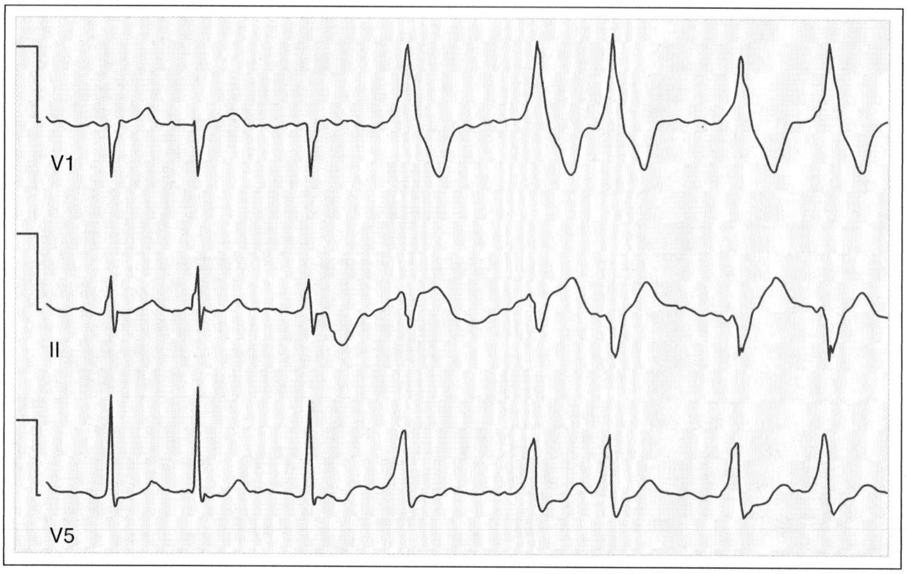
V1
II
V5

FIGURE 52-11 Electrocardiogram showing atrial fibrillation with Wolff-Parkinson-White syndrome and variable conduction down the AV node and His-Purkinje system with a resulting narrow QRS complex as well as down the accessory pathway with a slurred upstroke, wide QRS complex. The slow ventricular response rate suggests that this accessory pathway has a relatively long refractory period and a more benign prognosis.

agents may be applicable.[16] The safest and most effective treatment for patients with WPW syndrome and AF with a rapid ventricular response is synchronized DCCV. The EP should consider using DCCV with prior sedation before administering antidysrhythmics in patients with ventricular response greater than 150 beats/min or borderline low blood pressure.

For patients with WPW syndrome, the principles of treatment for AVRT are similar to those for AF. AV nodal blocking agents should not be used to treat presumed antidromic wide QRS complex AVRT, because the underlying rhythm could be misdiagnosed atrial flutter or tachycardia with accessory pathway conduction. AV nodal blocking agents could be used to treat orthodromic AVRT with a narrow QRS complex, but subsequent AF with rapid accessory pathway conduction remains a potential concern. It may be wiser to use the class IA or class III antidysrhythmics described previously or to proceed directly to DCCV.

Patients with WPW syndrome and rapid antegrade bypass tract conduction are at higher risk of cardiovascular decompensation than other patients with SVT. In particular, patients with recurrent unstable tachycardias should be admitted. Nevertheless, the decision to admit or discharge most patients should be made individually in consultation with the cardiologist.

Junctional Tachycardia

Junctional tachycardia is an uncommon dysrhythmia associated with toxic stimulation of the AV node by digoxin, methylxanthines, or other stimulants, or with cardiac disease such as inferior MI, acute rheumatic fever, or myocarditis. The most common mechanism is enhanced automaticity of the nodal tissue. The heart sounds are usually regular. If there is simultaneous antegrade ventricular and retrograde atrial activation, the right atrium may contract against a closed tricuspid valve, leading to large "cannon" jugular venous waves. The ECG presentation is a narrow complex tachycardia up to a rate of approximately 130 beats/min without synchronous preceding P waves. P waves may be present with evidence of AV dissociation. Alternatively, there may be retrograde nodal to atrial conduction with abnormal P waves with a superior axis occurring after the QRS deflection. P waves may be absent if atrial depolarization occurs simultaneously with the ventricles.

Digoxin toxicity is an important cause of junctional tachycardia. In particular, digoxin toxicity should be suspected when the rapid ventricular response to AF becomes regular during digoxin treatment. Diagnosis and treatment should focus on identifying and addressing the underlying cause, including reversal of toxicity, if any. Digoxin immune Fab fragments (Digibind) may be necessary for cardiovascular instability associated with digoxin toxicity, and DCCV should be avoided if possible. Most patients require admission until the underlying disease or toxicity is resolved.

VENTRICULAR TACHYCARDIAS

Premature Ventricular Contractions and Nonsustained Ventricular Tachycardia

Premature ventricular contractions (PVCs) are common. They can occur chronically with no associated cardiac disease or can develop in association with acute cardiopulmonary or metabolic derangements. Some specific causes are

- Cardiac ischemia, which may be due to local coronary artery disease or systemic hypoxia
- Heart failure with increased myocardial stretching
- Inflamed myocardium
- Electrolyte imbalance
- A vast array of medicines and toxins

There is a spectrum of frequency of ventricular ectopy. PVCs may occur singly in isolation, or there may be a PVC every second or third beat, termed bigeminy or trigeminy, respectively. Three or more ventricular beats in a row at a rate greater than 100 beats/min is defined as VT. If the consecutive ventricular beats spontaneously resolve or terminate within 30 seconds, then the VT is nonsustained (NSVT).

All of the major dysrhythmic mechanisms described, including enhanced automaticity, triggered beats, and reentry, may be involved in the formation of PVCs and NSVT. Irregular cardiac contractions interspersed with a regular rhythm can be heard on cardiac auscultation or felt on examination of the pulse. However, the diagnosis is usually made by examining the ECG tracing. The QRS deflections are wide because the ectopic ventricular beats generally do not utilize the specialized Purkinje conduction system, and the T wave is usually large and inverted with respect to the QRS complex. No premature P wave precedes the ventricular beat, but there may be a visible or hidden inverted retrograde P wave following it. Patients may be asymptomatic, or they may feel palpitations and discomfort from the ectopic beats. If the frequency of ectopic ventricular beats or rate of NSVT is sufficiently high, there may be hemodynamic compromise with hypotension, presyncope, or CHF.

Chronic ventricular ectopy generally does not require emergency treatment, and suppression of chronic ventricular ectopy after MI does not lower the mortality.[17] Patients with chronic PVCs may be at variably higher risk of sudden death, depending on other clinical factors, but even so, it is often unclear whether the increased risk is directly attributable to the ectopy or to underlying cardiac disease. EPs must commonly manage new ventricular ectopy in association with acute MI or other severe systemic disease. The greatest concern is that PVCs may induce sustained VT or VF. Theoretically, this could occur if the ectopic ventricular depolarization occurs during the vulnerable period or upstroke of the T wave of the preceding beat (R on T phenomenon).

The risk of VF and sudden death is elevated during an acute MI, but this risk is not decreased with routine suppressive class I antidysrhythmic therapy.[18] Conversely, beta-blockade with metoprolol may not affect the occurrence of PVCs or NSVT but does lower the rate of VF and death.[19] Suppression of new ventricular ectopy should be considered if the PVCs or tachydysrhythmias are symptomatic, contributing to hemodynamic instability, or the patient has already experienced sustained VT or VF. The first priority is to search for reversible causes of ventricular ectopy, such as hypoxia, potassium, magnesium, or other electrolyte imbalance, or drug toxicity. After reversible causes are addressed, the most commonly used agents include beta-blockers, amiodarone, lidocaine, and procainamide. The class I effect of myocardial sodium channel blockade may be particularly prominent for lidocaine in an ischemic and acidotic local cellular environment. Evidence suggests that amiodarone may be effective when lidocaine fails.[20] The antidysrhythmics should be given as a loading dose followed by a sustained infusion, and the patient monitored closely for adverse effects. The patient should be admitted to a cardiac care unit.

■ Monomorphic Ventricular Tachycardia

VT is considered *sustained* if it is continuous for at least 30 seconds. If the QRS complex has primarily a single morphology, the VT is *monomorphic*, whereas if the QRS complex varies, the VT is *polymorphic*. Monomorphic VT is an uncommon condition underlying the chief complaint in approximately 1 of every 10,000 ED visits. The mechanism in the majority of cases is reentry within the ventricular myocardium, where the slow-conducting segment of the reentrant loop is associated with a scar from a prior MI (see Fig. 52-1B). The scar tissue serves to enable and fix the location of the VT circuit within the myocardium. Other causes of monomorphic VT that are less commonly encountered in the ED are dilated cardiomyopathy, hypertrophic cardiomyopathy, prior surgical repair of congenital heart disease with myocardial scar, arrhythmogenic right ventricular dysplasia, right ventricular outflow tract VT, and fascicular tachycardia.

Patients with VT may present with palpitations, lightheadedness, chest discomfort, dyspnea, or more progressive cardiovascular compromise. The heart sounds and pulse are regular and rapid. Approximately half the patients have separate atrial activity with AV dissociation, evidence of which can occasionally be detected on physical examination as variable intensity of the first heart sound or arterial or jugular venous pulsations. The ECG tracing demonstrates a regular wide QRS complex tachycardia without preceding P waves. Nevertheless, it can be difficult to differentiate VT from SVT with a wide QRS complex due to aberrant or antegrade accessory pathway conduction. The next section addresses this issue specifically. Ultimately, the diagnosis can be most accurately determined when synthesizing combined information from the medical history, physical exam, and ECG.

Treatment of monomorphic VT depends on the patient's cardiovascular status. The patient's condition can be categorized as pulseless, unstable, or stable. Pulseless VT should receive the same treatment as VF: immediate chest compressions and initial shock using unsynchronized 200 J with a biphasic or monophasic waveform as soon as defibrillation is available.

Patients are unstable if they have a pulse but also symptoms of lightheadedness, chest pain, dyspnea, other signs of inadequate vital organ perfusion, or frank hypotension. Patients with unstable VT should undergo cardioversion with synchronized 100 J with a biphasic or monophasic waveform. An awake patient should receive pre-sedation as long as it would not significantly delay DCCV.

Patients with stable VT may initially be treated with medical or electrical therapy. The primary principle of treatment with class I or III antidysrhythmics is to prolong the refractory period of the ventricular myocardium so that the cells remain refractory when the reentrant wave of excitation returns. Amiodarone is recommended by the American Heart Association, and procainamide and sotalol can be used as alternatives when cardiac output seems to be clinically preserved. Lidocaine is no longer recommended for this purpose. Unfortunately, neither amiodarone nor lidocaine immediately increases the refractory period of normal myocardium after intravenous (IV) administration. Both are unlikely to terminate VT within 20 minutes of treatment.[1,21] However, amiodarone may become more effective at both terminating and preventing VT over the ensuing hours after administration.[20] Procainamide and racemic sotalol do prolong the refractory period soon after administered and are more likely to terminate VT. However, procainamide blocks cardiac sodium channels, and the *l* isomer of sotalol is a beta-blocker; thus both agents can cause a decrease in cardiac contractility and subsequent hemodynamic instability. IV sotalol is not currently available in the United States. Other agents that have been used in this situation are pure beta-blockers and magnesium. Neither has been proven to be effective, however, and pure beta-blockers may cause hypotension.

The safest and most effective treatment of stable monomorphic VT remains DCCV. Initial DCCV should be particularly considered in patients with ventricular rates greater than 150 beats/min, who are at higher risk for compromised cardiac output and hemodynamic collapse. Cardioversion with synchronized 100 J with a biphasic or monophasic waveform should be administered after appropriate sedation. If the patient already has an implanted internal cardioverter defibrillator (ICD), overdrive pacing or synchronized cardioversion may be administered by the device automatically, or manually at the bedside by the electrophysiologist. Suppressive treatment with antidysrhythmics should be considered if the VT is recurrent. Over a period of hours, IV amiodarone or procainamide is likely to be the most effective of the agents currently available in the United States. If procainamide is used, it should be loaded slowly over approximately 1 hour, and the patient monitored closely for hypotension. Generally, infusion of multiple antidysrhythmics should be avoided because it might increase the likelihood of adverse effects. Most patients who present with monomorphic VT should be admitted for observation and further treatment.

Wide QRS Complex Tachycardia: Differentiating Supraventricular from Ventricular Tachycardia

Wide QRS complex tachycardia may be due to a SVT with aberrant His-Purkinje conduction or antegrade conduction down an accessory pathway or to VT. Diagnosis of the underlying mechanism is important for a number of reasons. The optimal short- and long-term treatment and prognosis may vary considerably depending on the mechanism involved. History, physical, and ECG findings can be used to make the diagnosis (Box 52-3). In the ED, the pretest probability favors VT by a ratio of 2 : 1 to 3 : 1.

BOX 52-3

Diagnosing Regular Wide QRS Complex Tachycardia: Predictors Suggestive of Ventricular Tachycardia

Past Medical History

Prior ventricular tachycardia

Prior myocardial infarction

Age >35 years

Male sex

Physical Findings

Variable first heart sound or jugular venous pulsation

Electrocardiographic Findings

Frontal axis –90 to –180 degrees

QRS interval >140 msec (right bundle branch block [BBB]) or >160 msec (left BBB), or RS interval >100 msec

Positive or negative concordance across the precordial leads

Wide QRS morphology grossly different from QRS morphology in sinus rhythm

Atrioventricular dissociation (including fusion or capture beats)

Diagnostic Intervention Findings

No response to a 12-mg bolus of adenosine

No single historical factor has been found to be both sensitive and specific for diagnosing VT. Nevertheless, age greater than 35 years and male sex are sensitive for VT, and a prior history of MI or coronary artery bypass graft (CABG), recent angina, or congestive heart failure (CHF) is a specific predictor of VT.[22] The primary underlying theme for all of these predictors is a greater likelihood of coronary artery disease and prior infarction with scar formation. In fact, the strongest single historical predictor of VT is a history of MI, which has a positive likelihood ratio of 13 : 1 to 20 : 1 and a negative likelihood ratio of 0.36.[22,23]

A number of approaches may be used to diagnose wide QRS complex tachycardia from the physical examination. Perhaps the first and most important principle to remember is that apparent hemodynamic stability does not rule out VT. Atrioventricular dissociation is present about half of the time with VT.[24] When it is present, the atria are contracting independently of the ventricles, so the atria may either contract during ventricular diastole and assist cardiac output or contract against closed valves during ventricular systole with a large retrograde venous pulsation. The EP can look for beat-to-beat variation of the first heart sound or the systolic blood pressure, or large "cannon" jugular venous waves. Unfortunately, even under controlled experimental conditions, none of these findings is both sensitive and specific.[25] Under clinical conditions, in which about half of patients have some form of retrograde ventricular-atrial conduction, these tests for physical evidence of AV dissociation can approach a sensitivity for VT of only 50% at best.

Vagal maneuvers, such as carotid sinus massage or Valsalva maneuver, can be performed to increase vagal tone and alter AV nodal conduction. Depending on the type of SVT, vagal maneuvers could terminate a reentrant rhythm involving the AV node, or temporarily decrease the ventricular response to a purely atrial rhythm such as atrial flutter. Termination of wide QRS complex tachycardia with vagal maneuvers would suggest a supraventricular rhythm because most forms of VT are not responsive. Temporary slowing of the ventricular response to an atrial tachydysrhythmia could be diagnostic.

A similar principle of brief increased refractoriness of the AV node underlies the use of adenosine to diagnose and treat wide QRS complex tachycardia. The combined response to a 12-mg bolus of adenosine—either tachycardia termination or transient ventricular slowing—has a sensitivity of 87% and a specificity approaching 100% for an underlying SVT.[26] Considered in a reverse fashion, "nonresponse" to a 12-mg bolus of adenosine would have a positive likelihood ratio of about 8 and a negative likelihood ratio less than 0.1 for VT. This test is useful for diagnosis, but is it safe?

The primary safety concern is the administration of adenosine to patients with atrial flutter and antegrade accessory pathway conduction, with subsequent transient acceleration of this conduction and the ventricular response. This and other destabilizing scenarios have been reported after the administration of adenosine to patients with wide QRS complex tachycardia due to SVT and VT. Adenosine should never be given to patients with a rapid, irregularly irregular wide QRS complex tachycardia, because this presentation may actually be AF with accessory pathway conduction, and acceleration of the ventricular response has been reported in this situation too. Nevertheless, the adverse affects previously described after adenosine administration to patients with regular wide QRS complex tachycardia are rare. Multiple consecutive case series have found no greater rate of adverse effects with adenosine than with other antidysrhythmic medicines.[26,27] Adenosine should be used as a diagnostic and therapeutic agent for regular wide QRS complex tachycardia when the history, physical, and ECG findings suggest a supraventricular origin. The EP should ensure that the adenosine is used properly—given as a 12-mg rapid bolus dose followed immediately by a normal saline bolus flush, with the cardioverter defibrillator immediately available in the event of destabilization.

A number of ECG findings can be used to diagnose wide QRS complex tachycardia. Possible differentiating characteristics include heart rate, frontal axis of the QRS deflection, concordance across the precordial leads, QRS duration, morphology of the QRS complex, AV dissociation, and capture or fusion beats. On average, wide QRS complex tachycardia due to SVT has a faster heart rate than that due to VT.[24] This difference has been slightly augmented in the recent past with the implantation of ICDs. The patient with VT may have already received an ICD, which is preferentially programmed to treat rapid VT, usually greater than 160 to 180 beats/min. It cannot be programmed to treat slower VT because of the risk of inappropriate pacing or shocks of sinus tachycardia. Nevertheless, there is still too much overlap in the heart rate of SVT and VT to use it as a firm differentiating factor. Regardless of the underlying rhythm, higher heart rates are associated with compromised cardiac output due to inadequate diastolic filling and greater electrical instability. Immediate DCCV should be considered for patients with rapid wide QRS tachycardia, regardless of the presumed etiology.

Because of the common ectopic left ventricular origin of the rhythm in VT, there may be abnormal upward and rightward propagation of the excitation wave. In fact, the QRS axis may point in any of the four quadrants in VT, but an upward and rightward QRS axis is highly unusual for SVT. This finding, with a negative QRS deflection in leads I and aVF, is insensitive (24%) but highly specific (100%) for VT (Fig. 52-12).[28] An abnormal QRS vector that points toward

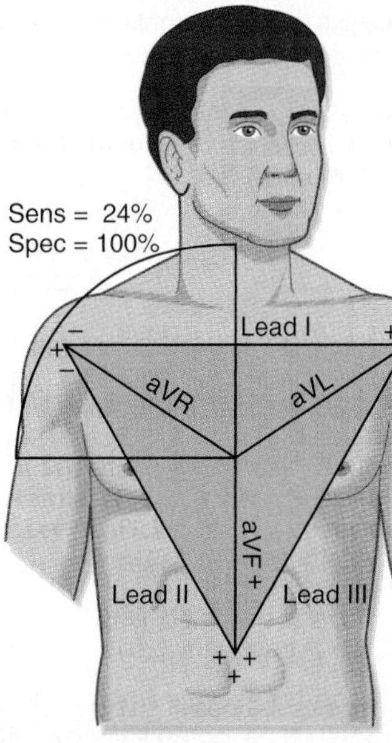
Sens = 24%
Spec = 100%
Lead I
aVR
aVL
aVF
Lead II
Lead III

FIGURE 52-12 Diagram of the chest with the six electrocardiogram limb leads superimposed. The QRS complex depolarization can be viewed as primarily positive in one of four quadrants, and the right upward quadrant is specifically identified in this diagram. Normal QRS depolarization is most commonly in the direction of the left lower quadrant. When the QRS complex points to the right upward quadrant, it is highly abnormal and suggestive of ventricular tachycardia.

or away from all of the precordial leads simultaneously is also indicative of VT. A QRS deflection that is primarily positive in all of the precordial leads is defined as positive concordance. Primarily negative QRS deflections in all precordial leads are defined as negative concordance. Either of these findings is also insensitive (10%) but specific (85%) for VT.[28]

On average, the duration of initial depolarization as recorded by the QRS wave is longer in VT than in wide QRS complex SVT. A QRS duration greater than 140 msec with a right BBB (RBBB) pattern or a QRS duration greater than 160 msec with a left BBB (LBBB) pattern is insensitive but more than 90% specific for VT.[28] Brugada and colleagues[29] modified this concept and found that an RS interval greater than 100 msec in the precordial leads has a sensitivity of 66% and a specificity of 98% for VT (Fig. 52-13). Unfortunately, the high specificity of these findings is not applicable if the patient has received a medicine that widens the QRS, such as a class I antidysrhythmic.

QRS morphology may be helpful, particularly if an old ECG is available. QRS morphology with tachycardia similar to a previous BBB morphology noted in sinus rhythm may suggest, but does not prove, SVT.[30] The distinction of RBBB versus LBBB itself is not helpful, but various morphologic variants within these two categories can at least theoretically be helpful.[23,24,29]

When present, the most definitive evidence of VT is AV dissociation. In SVT an atrial contraction is associated with each ventricular beat. AV dissociation is defined by atrial activity that is separate and independent of ventricular contractions (Fig. 52-14). AV dissociation is present in about half of VT episodes, and it can be seen on the ECG in half of these cases, or about one quarter of all VT episodes. Thus, AV dissociation has a sensitivity of about 25% and specificity approaching 100% for VT. Dissociated P waves should be sought in the V_1 rhythm strip, where they are usually most easily seen. The key is to find two candidate P waves. Then one can look an equal distance on each side of these two for a third deflection. If there are three consecutive deflections that "march out," they are likely P waves; this identification can be confirmed by "marching out" more on the ECG. Fusion beats represent fusion of supraventricular excitation mediated by the His-Purkinje system and local ventricular excitation. Capture beats signify complete ventricular depolarization by a supraventricular signal and usually have a narrow QRS complex. Both of these phenomena also suggest AV dissociation and VT (Figs. 52-15 and 52-16).

Severe hyperkalemia can also cause wide QRS complex tachycardia. Clues to this diagnosis include a history of renal failure or other medical causes of hyperkalemia, and an ECG with very wide and bizarre QRS complexes (Fig. 52-17). Once the condition is diagnosed, it should be confirmed with a serum potassium measurement and treated with IV calcium, insulin, glucose, and bicarbonate. Patients who overdose with cyclic antidepressants or other sodium channel blocking agents may present with a wide

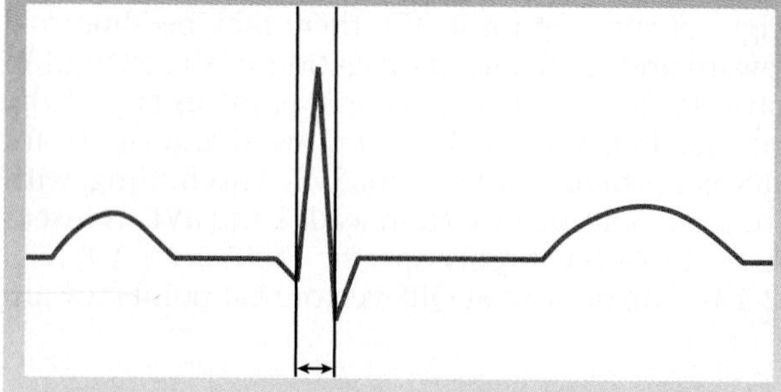

The RS interval begins with the upstroke of the R wave and ends with the nadir of the S wave.

FIGURE 52-13 How to measure the RS interval (*double arrow*). The RS interval begins with the upstroke of the R wave and ends with the nadir of the S wave.

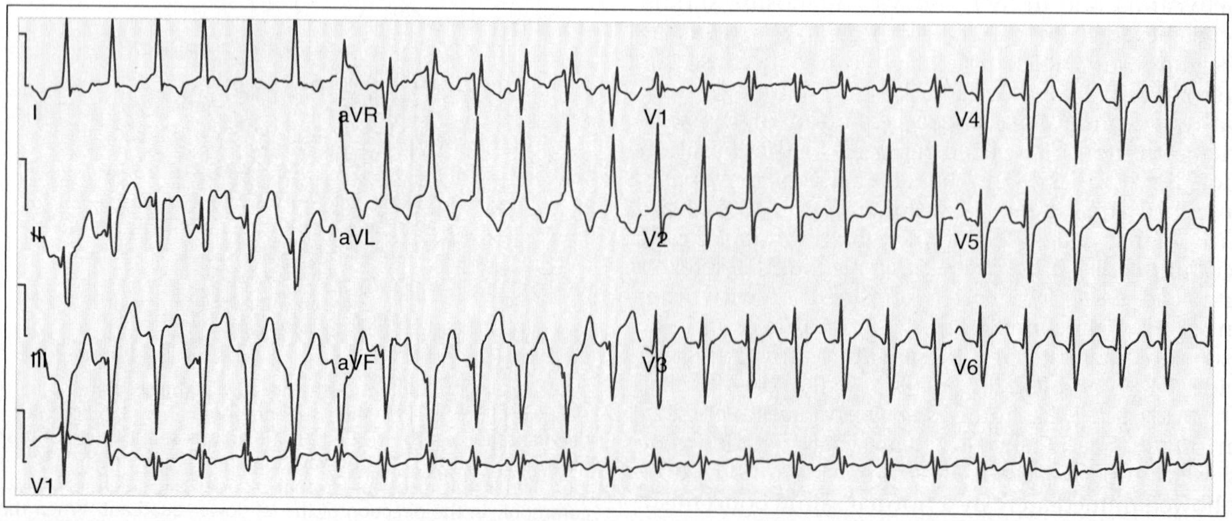
I
aVR
V1
V4
II
aVL
V2
V5
III
aVF
V3
V6
V1

FIGURE 52-14 Electrocardiogram showing ventricular tachycardia with atrioventricular dissociation. Although the QRS complexes are relatively narrow, there is clear evidence of atrioventricular dissociation in the V_1 rhythm strip.

QRS complex tachycardia. An important electrocardiographic clue to this diagnosis is right axis deviation of the terminal 30 msec of the QRS complex. Patients with suspected overdose should be treated with a continuous IV sodium bicarbonate infusion. Patients with acute respiratory distress due to pulmonary disease and with an underlying BBB may appear to have a primary tachydysrhythmic condition. Addressing the airway, with intubation if necessary, may slow the heart rate, expose the P waves, and clarify the rhythm.

Finally, in a significant proportion of cases, it may not be possible to make a definitive ED diagnosis. Some cases of VT may utilize the bundle branches as part of the reentrant limb, mimicking aberrant conduction, and excitation of the ventricles via an accessory pathway may give an ECG appearance of VT. When the diagnosis is in doubt, the safest approach is to sedate the patient, perform cardioversion, and leave the definitive diagnosis for the electrophysiologist.

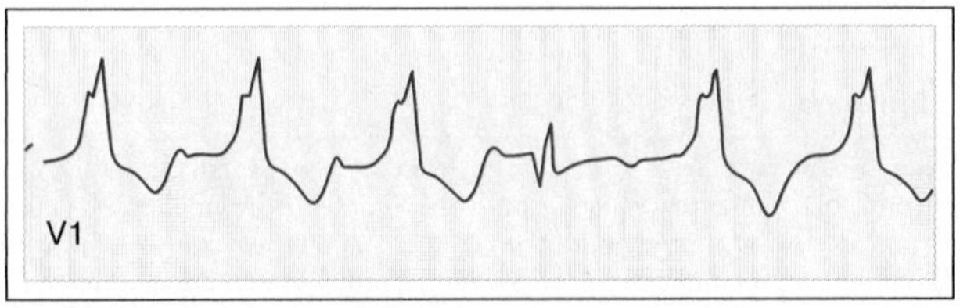
V1

FIGURE 52-15 Electrocardiogram showing ventricular tachycardia with a single capture beat.

■ Polymorphic Ventricular Tachycardia

Polymorphic VT is defined as VT with varying QRS wave morphology (Fig. 52-18). A specific type of polymorphic VT characterized by sinusoidal variation of the QRS deflection occurs when there is a long QT interval during sinus rhythm (Fig. 52-19). This tachydysrhythmia is termed torsades de pointes (TdP), or "twisting of the points" (Fig. 52-20). There are a number of causes of polymorphic VT and TdP, which itself is an important cause of sudden cardiac death. Fortunately, the tachydysrhythmia is rare.

Polymorphic VT in the setting of a normal QT interval is most often associated with acute cardiac ischemia. It is a rare but important indicator of ongoing ischemia. The most important treatment is revascularization therapy. Pending revascularization, suppression of the dysrhythmia can be attempted with lidocaine or amiodarone.

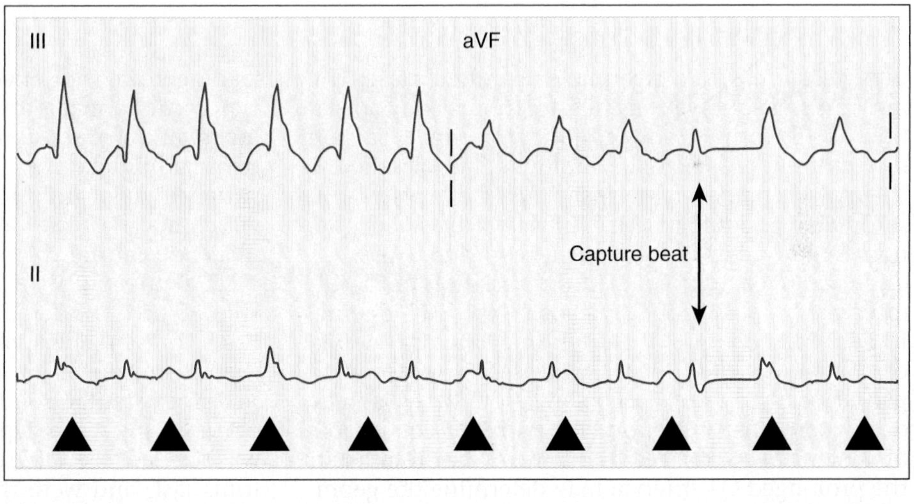
III
aVF
Capture beat
II

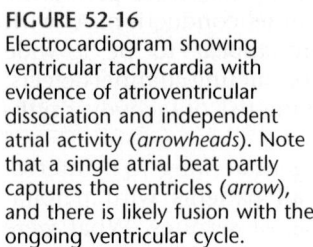

FIGURE 52-16 Electrocardiogram showing ventricular tachycardia with evidence of atrioventricular dissociation and independent atrial activity (*arrowheads*). Note that a single atrial beat partly captures the ventricles (*arrow*), and there is likely fusion with the ongoing ventricular cycle.

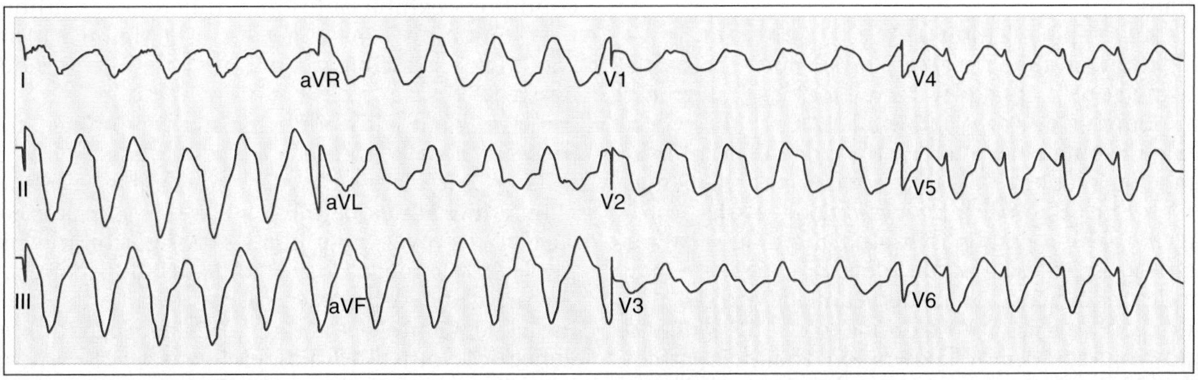
I
aVR
V1
V4
II
aVL
V2
V5
III
aVF
V3
V6

FIGURE 52-17 A 50-year-old man was found lying down, with lethargy and shortness of breath. He was a hemodialysis patient who had missed dialysis for a week. His serum potassium level was 8.4 mEq/L. Note the marked wide and bizarre QRS complexes with right upward frontal plane axis on his electrocardiogram.

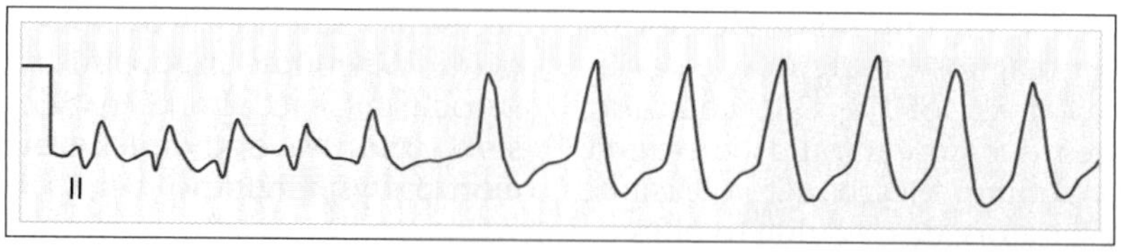
II

FIGURE 52-18 When the electrocardiogram shows polymorphic ventricular tachycardia (VT), the setting and the underlying QT interval should be considered. When this condition occurs in association with a normal QT interval, there is often acute ischemia, and the treatment is focused on the ischemic process. When undulating polymorphic VT occurs in association with a prolonged QT interval in sinus rhythm, the diagnosis is torsades de pointes.

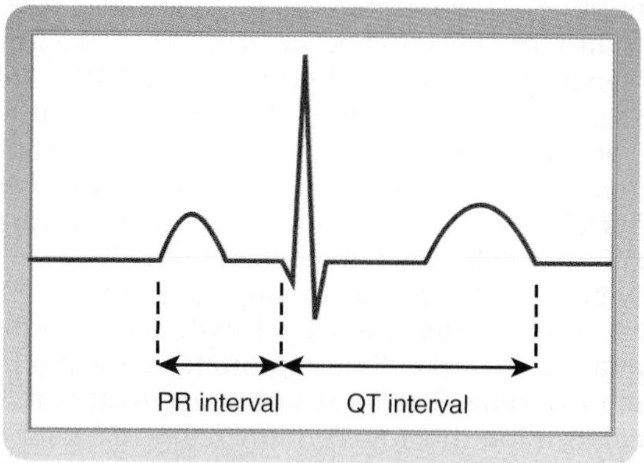
PR interval
QT interval

FIGURE 52-19 Defining the QT interval. The QT interval starts at the beginning of the Q wave, or R wave if no Q wave is present, and ends when the T wave returns to the baseline.

Table 52-2 SUGGESTED QTc VALUES* FOR DIAGNOSING QT PROLONGATION

	QTc Values by Age Group or Gender		
	1-15 Years	**Men**	**Women**
Normal	<0.44	<0.43	<0.45
Borderline	0.44-0.46	0.43-0.45	0.45-0.47
Prolonged (top 1%)	>0.46	>0.45	>0.47

*The QTc values ($sec^{1/2}$) are derived from the measured QT interval in seconds divided by the square root of the RR interval in seconds.

From Moss AJ: Measurement of the QT Interval and the risk associated with QTc interval prolongation: A review. Am J Cardiol 1993;72:23B-25B.

Polymorphic VT in association with a long QT interval can have a congenital or acquired cause. The mechanisms involved in the initiation and propagation of this form of polymorphic VT termed TdP are not entirely understood. Prolongation of the QT interval itself may not cause TdP but may lead to secondary phenomena that initiate TdP. Such phenomena are increased QT dispersion and EADs. *QT dispersion* refers to the maximum variation in the QT interval observed in the 12 leads on the ECG tracing. If the QT interval and corresponding refractory period of the myocardium have increased heterogeneity, partial and abnormal depolarization of cells may occur, particularly after on EAD with subsequent loss of synchrony. Spiral reentrant waves can result, but the prolonged QT interval may determine the geometry and appearance of polymorphic VT as opposed to frank VF.

Cellular repolarization and the QT interval vary as a function of the preceding heart rate. Thus, the measured QT interval is corrected for heart rate, most commonly using Bazett's formula. After puberty, on average, women have a slightly longer QT interval than men (Table 52-2), and a variety of medicines can prolong the QT interval. Patients with a prolonged QT interval are asymptomatic unless TdP or another tachydysrhythmia develops, which may manifest as syncope or sudden cardiac death.

Congenital long QT syndrome with TdP is due to a growing number of known ion channelopathies (Table 52-3). The most common defects are deficient potassium channel conduction and augmentation of sodium channel conduction leading to a prolonged QT interval. Other genetic abnormalities associated with polymorphic VT and sudden cardiac death are rare calcium channel defects, ion channel defects leading to a shortened QT interval, and Brugada's syndrome, which is attributed primarily to premature inactivation of sodium channel conduction. As with hemoglobinopathies, there appear to be a wide variety of myocardial ion-conducting channel defects, which manifest with a varying risk of tachydysrhythmias and mortality.

The possibility of congenital long QT interval should be considered in all patients with palpitations, presyncope, syncope, or seizures. What were the circumstances of the event, and has the patient had prior similar events? Did the onset of symptoms occur during rest, sleep, or activity or after the patient was startled (see Table 52-3)? How long did the symptoms last, and were there any associated symptoms of chest pain or shortness of breath? Many of these conditions exhibit autosomal inheritance, although new mutations are common. The family history should be assessed for recurrent syncope and sudden death.

In a patient with sinus rhythm, the physical findings are usually normal. However, analysis of the ECG QT interval and T wave morphology is critical. Different channelopathies tend to be associated with specific T wave abnormalities. Assess for the morphology of Brugada's syndrome, a RBBB pattern in the precordial chest leads with associated downsloping ST segment elevation (Fig. 52-21). Search for evidence of other cardiologic causes of syncope, including preexcitation and WPW, ventricular hypertrophy, and other tachydysrhythmias or bradydysrhythmias. Serum electrolytes, including potassium,

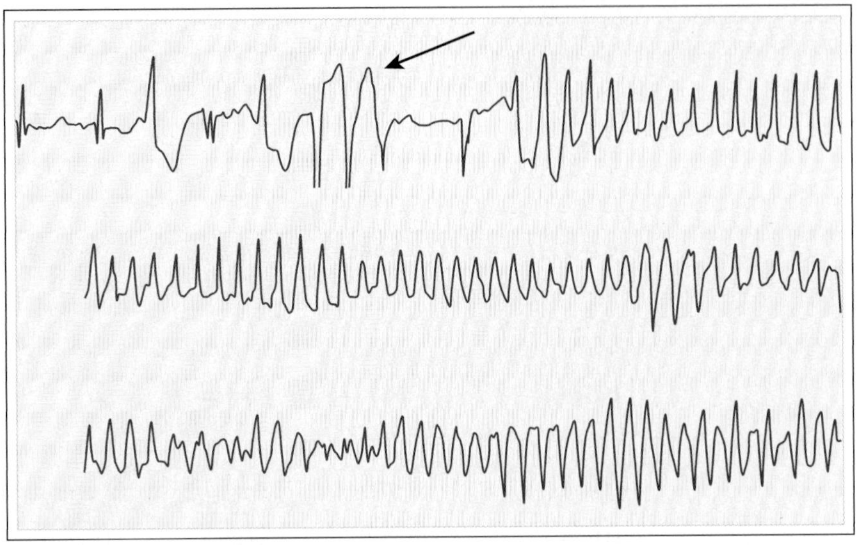

FIGURE 52-20 Electrocardiogram showing torsades de pointes. Note the classic pattern of initiation with a series of early ventricular beats (*arrow*) that fall in the vulnerable period of the prolonged QT interval. (From Stahmer SA, Cowan R: Tachydysrhythmias. Emerg Med Clin North Am 2006;24:11-40, v-vi.)

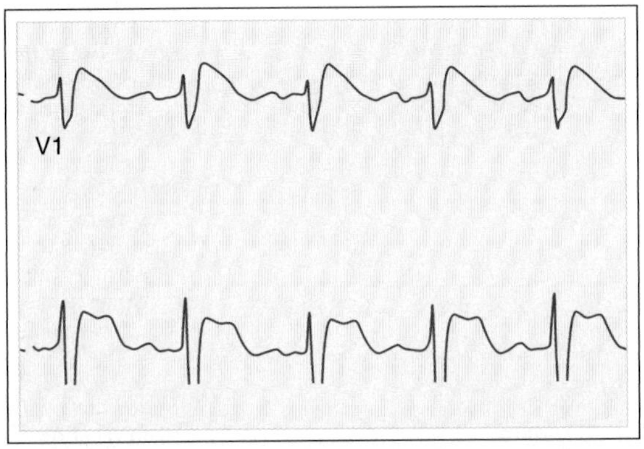
V1

FIGURE 52-21 Electrocardiographic tracings from septal precordial leads with incomplete right bundle branch block and downsloping ST segment elevation consistent with Brugada's syndrome.

calcium, and magnesium, should be measured, and treatment should be given as needed.

Acquired long QT syndrome is due to toxicity from medicines that either prolong the QT interval or block the metabolism of QT-prolonging agents (Table 52-4). Medicines that prolong the QT interval act by altering ion channel flow, such as by disrupting the outward potassium repolarizing current. Women are more prone to acquired long QT syndrome, perhaps in part because of their longer baseline QT interval. Acute symptoms are similar to the congenital form of disease.

The treatment of TdP involves immediate unsynchronized defibrillation if the patient is unstable or pulseless. An initial dose of 200 J should be used for biphasic defibrillation, or 360 J for a monophasic waveform. Synchronized DCCV is not generally recommended because of the variability of the QRS waveform and potential failure to synchronize. Magnesium should be administered to terminate TdP and possibly to prevent recurrences. Increasing the heart rate reduces the QT interval. The heart rate can be increased with external or internal pacing, or with administration of isoproterenol. Class I and III antidysrhythmic agents are generally contraindicated because they may further prolong the QT interval and increase QT dispersion. Removal of the offending agent should be considered for the patient with acquired QT prolongation, although this step is usually not feasible. Patients with polymorphic VT and TdP require admission to a monitored unit for further evaluation and treatment.

Perspective and Summary

ED disposition of the patient with a tachydysrhythmia depends on the diagnosis, if known, symptoms of cardiovascular instability including presyncope, chest pain, or shortness of breath during tachycardia, the patient's underlying cardiovascular health, and his or her social support and medical follow-up. Patients with known recurrent supraventricular tachydysrhythmias that are hemodynamically well tolerated can usually be discharged with close follow-up. Generally, patients with a new-onset, undiagnosed, or ventricular tachydysrhythmia should be admitted.

The long-term and definitive care of patients with dysrhythmias has advanced remarkably. Definitive catheter ablation can be performed on selected patients with AF, atrial flutter, AVT, AVNRT, and VT. ICDs are commonly implanted in patients with ventricular tachydysrhythmias or low ejection fraction after MI. Patients may also require adjunctive oral antidysrhythmic therapy to minimize ICD shocks. The EP should expect to see more patients with intracardiac devices and advanced treatments in the future. Optimal ED care of these patients will require sound understanding of the clinical issues, familiarity with new technologies, and close collaboration with cardiology colleagues.

Table 52-3 KNOWN GENETIC TACHYDYSRHYTHMIAS

Syndrome Type	Name	Abnormal Gene	Abnormal Protein	Functional Alteration	Circumstances Associated with Sudden Cardiac Death	Comments
Long QT syndromes (LQTSs)*						
	LQTS1	*KCNQ1*	Slow K channel	Decreased K flow	Physical (swimming) or emotional stress	43% of LQTS cases
	LQTS2	*KCNH2 (HERG)*	Rapid K channel	Decreased K flow	Arousal (acoustic), sleep, or rest; not exercise	45% of LQTS cases
	LQTS3	*SCN5A*	Na channel	Increased Na flow	Rest or sleep	7% of LQTS cases
	LQTS4	*ANKB*	Ankyrin anchoring protein			Associated with bradycardia, AF, biphasic T waves
	LQTS5	*KCNE1*	Slow K channel	Decreased K flow		
	LQTS6	*KCNE2*	Rapid K channel	Decreased K flow		
	LQT7 (Anderson's syndrome)	*KCNJ2*	K channel	Decreased K flow		Associated with periodic paralysis and skeletal abnormalities
	Timothy's syndrome	*Cav1.2*	L-type Ca channel	Increased Ca flow		Associated with childhood SCD and with central nervous system, structural cardiac, and other abnormalities
Short QT syndromes						
		KCNQ1	Slow K channel	Increased K flow		Associated with familial AF and SCD
		KCNH2	Rapid K channel	Increased K flow		Associated with familial AF and SCD (including infants)
Brugada's syndrome		*SCN5A*†	Na channel	Decreased Na flow	Rest or sleep	SCD more common in males and often manifests in the 3rd or 4th decade of life
Catecholaminergic polymorphic VT						
	Autosomal dominant CPVT	*RyR2*	Cardiac ryanodine receptor	Intracellular Ca movement	Physical or emotional stress	May manifest as bidirectional or polymorphic VT in childhood
	Autosomal recessive CPVT	*CASQ2*	Calsequestrin	Intracellular Ca storage	Physical or emotional stress	May manifest as bidirectional or polymorphic VT in childhood

AF, atrial fibrillation; Ca, calcium; CPVT, catecholaminergic polymorphic VT; K, potassium; Na, sodium; SCD, sudden cardiac death; VT, ventricular tachycardia.

*A single mutation (heterozygous state) in any of the genes responsible for LQTS1 through LQTS7 results in an autosomal dominant form of illness (Romano-Ward syndrome). Two mutations (homozygous state) in LQTS1 or LQTS5 result in a more severe autosomal recessive illness with associated deafness (Jervell and Lange-Nielsen syndrome).

†Defects in SCN5A have been identified in only 20%-30% of cases.

Table 52-4 CAUSES OF ACQUIRED LONG QT SYNDROME

Medications	Antidysrhythmic agents: Class IA: quinidine, procainamide, disopyramide Class III: sotalol, ibutilide, dofetilide, amiodarone Class IV: bepridil (removed from market) Antihistamines: Terfenadine Astemizole (both removed from the market) Antihyperlipidemic agents: Probucol Antimicrobial agents: Antimalarials: halofantrine, chloroquine Macrolides: erythromycin, clarithromycin Ketoconazole Pentamidine Gastrointestinal medications: Cisapride Psychotropic drugs: Cyclic antidepressants Phenothiazines Haloperidol, droperidol Methadone, levomethadyl Risperidone Other medications: Arsenic trioxide (antineoplastic agent) Diuretics (cause of hypokalemia and hypomagnesemia) Organophosphates
Metabolic	Hypokalemia, hypomagnesemia, and hypocalcemia Liquid protein diet Anorexia
Other contributing factors	Female gender Bradycardia, and recent conversion from atrial fibrillation Congestive heart failure Cerebrovascular accident Subclinical ion channel polymorphisms

REFERENCES

1. Marill KA, Greenberg GM, Kay D, et al: Analysis of the treatment of spontaneous sustained stable ventricular tachycardia. Acad Emerg Med 1997;4:1122-1128.
2. Eisenberg MS, Mengert TJ: Cardiac resuscitation. N Engl J Med 2001;344:1304-1313.
3. Klein GJ, Bashore TM, Sellers TD, et al: Ventricular fibrillation in the Wolff-Parkinson-White syndrome. N Engl J Med 1979;301:1080-1085.
4. Schreck DM, Rivera AR, Tricarico VJ: Emergency management of atrial fibrillation and flutter: Intravenous diltiazem versus intravenous digoxin. Ann Emerg Med 1997;29:135-140.
5. Demircan C, Cikriklar HI, Engindeniz Z, et al: Comparison of the effectiveness of intravenous diltiazem and metoprolol in the management of rapid ventricular rate in atrial fibrillation. Emerg Med J 2005;22:411-414.
6. Chiladakis JA, Stathopoulos C, Davlouros P, et al: Intravenous magnesium sulfate versus diltiazem in paroxysmal atrial fibrillation. Int J Cardiol 2001;79:287-291.
7. Volgman AS, Carberry PA, Stambler B, et al: Conversion efficacy and safety of intravenous ibutilide compared with intravenous procainamide in patients with atrial flutter or fibrillation. J Am Coll Cardiol 1998;31:1414-1419.
8. Martinez-Marcos FJ, Garcia-Garmendia JL, Ortega-Carpio A, et al: Comparison of intravenous flecainide, propafenone, and amiodarone for conversion of acute atrial fibrillation to sinus rhythm. Am J Cardiol 2000;86:950-953.
9. Kalus JS, Spencer AP, Tsikouris JP, et al: Impact of prophylactic i.v. magnesium on the efficacy of ibutilide for conversion of atrial fibrillation or flutter. Am J Health Syst Pharm 2003;60:2308-2312.
10. Scholten MF, Thornton AS, Mekel JM, et al: Anticoagulation in atrial fibrillation and flutter. Europace 2005;7:492-499.
11. McCord J, Borzak S: Multifocal atrial tachycardia. Chest 1998;113:203-209.
12. Lim SH, Anantharaman V, Teo WS, et al: Comparison of treatment of supraventricular tachycardia by Valsalva maneuver and carotid sinus massage. Ann Emerg Med 1998;31:30-35.
13. DiMarco JP, Miles W, Akhtar M, et al: Adenosine for paroxysmal supraventricular tachycardia: Dose ranging and comparison with verapamil. Assessment in placebo-controlled, multicenter trials. Ann Intern Med 1990;113:104-110.
14. Kirk CR, Gibbs JL, Thomas R, et al: Cardiovascular collapse after verapamil in supraventricular tachycardia. Arch Dis Child 1987;62:1265-1266.
15. Boahene KA, Klein GJ, Yee R, et al: Termination of acute atrial fibrillation in the Wolff-Parkinson-White syndrome by procainamide and propafenone: Importance of atrial fibrillatory cycle length. J Am Coll Cardiol 1990;16:1408-1414.
16. Boriani G, Biffi M, Frabetti L, et al: Ventricular fibrillation after intravenous amiodarone in Wolff-Parkinson-White syndrome with atrial fibrillation. Am Heart J 1996;131:1214-1216.
17. Echt DS, Liebson PR, Mitchell LB, et al: Mortality and morbidity in patients receiving encainide, flecainide, or placebo. The Cardiac Arrhythmia Suppression Trial. N Engl J Med 1991;324:781-788.
18. Teo KK, Yusuf S, Furberg CD: Effects of prophylactic antiarrhythmic drug therapy in acute myocardial infarction: An overview of results from randomized controlled trials. JAMA 1993;270:1589-1595.
19. Ryden L, Ariniego R, Arnman K, et al: A double-blind trial of metoprolol in acute myocardial infarction: Effects on ventricular tachyarrhythmias. N Engl J Med 1983;308:614-618.
20. Scheinman MM, Levine JH, Cannom DS, et al: Dose-ranging study of intravenous amiodarone in patients with life-threatening ventricular tachyarrhythmias. Circulation 1995;92:3264-3272.
21. Marill KA, deSouza IS, Nishijima DK, et al: Amiodarone is poorly effective for the acute termination of ventricular tachycardia. Ann Emerg Med 2006;47:217-224.
22. Baerman JM, Morady F, DiCario LA, et al: Differentiation of ventricular tachycardia from supraventricular tachycardia with aberration: Value of the clinical history. Ann Emerg Med 1987;16:40-43.
23. Griffith MJ, de Belder MA, Linker NJ, et al: Multivariate analysis to simplify the differential diagnosis of broad complex tachycardia. Br Heart J 1991;66:166-174.
24. Wellens HJ, Bar FW, Lie KI: The value of the electrocardiogram in the differential diagnosis of a tachycardia with a widened QRS complex. Am J Med 1978;64:27-33.
25. Garratt CJ, Griffith MJ, Young G, et al: Value of physical signs in the diagnosis of ventricular tachycardia. Circulation 1994;90:3103-3107.
26. Marill KA, Wolfram S, DeSouza IS, et al: Adenosine for wide-complex tachycardia: Efficacy and safety [abstract]. Acad Emerg Med 2004;11:502.

27. Herbert ME, Votey SR: Adenosine in wide-complex tachycardia. Ann Emerg Med 1997;29:172-174.
28. Akhtar M, Shenasa M, Jazayeri M, et al: Wide QRS complex tachycardia. Ann Intern Med 1988;109:905-912.
29. Brugada P, Brugada J, Mont L, et al: A new approach to the differential diagnosis of a regular tachycardia with a wide QRS complex. Circulation 1991;83:1649-1659.
30. Halperin BD, Kron J, Cutler JE, et al: Misdiagnosing ventricular tachycardia in patients with underlying conduction disease and similar sinus and tachycardia morphologies. West J Med 1990;152:677-682.

Chapter 53

Pericarditis, Pericardial Tamponade, and Myocarditis

Amal Mattu and Joseph P. Martinez

KEY POINTS

- The classic presentation of acute pericarditis is sharp, pleuritic retrosternal chest pain that radiates to one or both trapezius ridges and changes with body position.
- The hallmark electrocardiographic findings of pericarditis include diffuse ST-segment elevation with PR-segment depression in the same leads.
- High-dose aspirin or nonsteroidal anti-inflammatory drugs with the addition of colchicine is effective treatment in most cases of acute pericarditis.
- Steroids should be avoided in the early treatment of first-time pericarditis, as their use may actually increase the chances of recurrence.
- Large pericardial effusions often cause severe tachypnea and dyspnea; however, the oxygen saturation levels are usually normal.
- Jugular venous distention is typical in cases of pericardial tamponade, but it may be absent in the presence of hypovolemia or if tamponade developed rapidly.
- The hallmark echocardiographic finding in patients with pericardial tamponade is the presence of a large effusion with diastolic collapse of the right heart chambers.
- The classic presentation of acute myocarditis includes low-grade fever, tachypnea, and tachycardia out of proportion to the fever.

Scope

Although the greatest concern in patients who present with chest pain is usually the vascular causes of chest pain—acute coronary syndrome, pulmonary embolism, and aortic dissection—other less common, but potentially deadly, illnesses must be considered, including pericarditis, pericardial tamponade, and myocarditis.

Acute pericarditis is often subclinical, so the incidence is uncertain. However, rough estimates range from 2% to 6%,[1] and this disorder may be responsible for as many as 1 of every 1000 hospital admissions.[2] Although acute pericarditis is usually not deadly, it can be painfully disabling if not treated appropriately.

Pericardial tamponade is a potentially deadly result of a pericardial effusion. Such an effusion can develop from pericardial inflammation or cardiac trauma. Unfortunately, the presenting features of tamponade can mimic those of other diseases, leading to initial misdiagnosis.

Acute myocarditis is relatively uncommon, but it is a devastating condition that can occur and progress quickly, with little warning. The initial presentation can vary from mild, viral-type symptoms to fulminant cardiogenic shock.

Pericarditis

■ ANATOMY AND PATHOPHYSIOLOGY

The *pericardium* is the layer of tissue surrounding the heart. It consists of two layers, a serous inner layer (visceral pericardium) and a fibrocollagenous outer layer (parietal pericardium). The pericardium completely encloses the ventricles and the right atrium; a portion of the left atrium remains outside the sac. A thin layer of plasma fluid (usually 15 to 30 mL) separates the visceral and parietal pericardial layers and acts as a lubricant. The main function of the pericardium appears to be to provide ligamentous stability to withstand forces against the heart. It also provides some shielding for the heart. Despite these apparent functions, however, the majority of patients who undergo pericardiectomy do not appear to suffer any decrease in cardiac performance or other ill effects.

Pericarditis refers to inflammation of the layers of the pericardium. There are many possible causes of pericarditis (Box 53-1), but in most cases, the cause is unknown. In the majority of these idiopathic cases, the presumed cause is viral, although most attempts to prove a viral cause have a low yield. The most common viral cause is coxsackievirus B. Other types of infections can also cause acute pericarditis, and the most common cause of pericarditis worldwide is tuberculosis.[3] Other common causes of pericarditis are connective tissue diseases, post–myocardial infarction state, malignancies, irradiation, aortic dissection, certain medications, and cardiac trauma or surgery.

BOX 53-1

Causes of Pericarditis

Viral infections:
- Coxsackievirus B (most common)
- Coxsackievirus A
- Echovirus
- Human immunodeficiency virus
- Influenza virus
- Epstein-Barr virus
- Adenovirus
- Varicella virus

Bacterial infections:
- *Staphylococcus*
- *Pneumococcus*
- *Mycoplasma*
- *Streptococcus*
- *Meningococcus*
- Tuberculosis
- *Salmonella*
- *Haemophilus*
- *Rickettsia*

Parasitic infections:
- Toxoplasmosis
- Amebiasis

Fungal infections:
- *Histoplasma*
- *Aspergillus*
- *Blastomyces*

Connective tissue diseases:
- Systemic lupus erythematosus
- Rheumatoid arthritis
- Sarcoidosis
- Amyloidosis
- Scleroderma

Post–myocardial infarction (MI):
- Early post-MI pericarditis
- Delayed (4-6 weeks) pericarditis (Dressler's syndrome)

Malignancies:
- Primary: mesothelioma, angiosarcoma
- Metastatic (more common): breast, lung, melanoma, lymphoma, leukemia

Radiation therapy

Thoracic aortic dissection

Medications:
- Hydralazine
- Procainamide
- Methyldopa
- Penicillin
- Cromolyn sodium
- Dantrolene
- Methysergide
- Anticoagulants (heparin, warfarin)

Cardiac trauma

Cardiac surgery

■ PRESENTING SIGNS AND SYMPTOMS

■ Classic

Chest pain is the typical presenting complaint of patients with acute pericarditis. Classically, the chest pain is sharp, retrosternal, and pleuritic, and it radiates to one or both trapezius ridges because the phrenic nerve, which traverses the pericardium, innervates these muscles.[4] Typically the pain also changes with body position, improving when the patient sits up and leans forward, and worsening when the patient lies supine.

The physical examination of the patient with acute pericarditis is usually nondiagnostic. Although some researchers report the presence of a friction rub in up to 85% of patients at some point in the course of the disease,[5] the presence of a friction rub at the time of initial presentation is unreliable. When the friction rub is present, it is best heard at the left sternal border at end-expiration with the patient leaning forward. The rub typically is described as consisting of three components that correspond to atrial systole, ventricular systole, and rapid diastolic filling. The friction rub is thought to be caused by rubbing of the inflamed layers of the pericardium against each other.

■ Typical Variations

The typical presentation of acute pericarditis may not always be present. Although chest pain is the most common symptom, patients sometimes present with dyspnea as the primary complaint. When the chest pain is present, it is not always positional or pleuritic, and it may not always radiate to the trapezius ridge. Patients may also complain of cough, upper respiratory symptoms, nausea, or vomiting, which may mislead the physician to an alternative diagnosis. Patients with bacterial infections are likely to present with complaints of fever, and patients with tuberculous pericarditis are likely to report a chronic cough, weight loss, and night sweats.

Although the presence of a triphasic friction rub is classic, it actually occurs in only half of patients with pericarditis.[6] The physical findings may also be notable for hypotension and jugular venous distention in the presence of pericardial tamponade (discussed later).

■ DIFFERENTIAL DIAGNOSIS, DIAGNOSTIC CRITERIA, AND TESTING

A thorough differential diagnosis of a patient presenting with chest pain is described elsewhere in Chapter 57. However, the most important initial consideration should always be the deadly causes of chest pain: pericarditis, acute coronary ischemia/infarction, thoracic aortic dissection, and pulmonary embolus. Table 53-1 lists some historical and physical examination features that are helpful in distinguishing among these diagnoses. The distinction among these causes of chest pain is critical in terms of treatment: Patients with pulmonary embolism or myocardial infarction often require treatment with anticoagulants and thrombolytics, medications that can be deadly in patients with acute pericarditis or aortic dissection.

The diagnosis of acute pericarditis is based primarily on the clinical presentation. In many cases, electrocardiography (ECG) is helpful in confirming the diagnosis. A sound knowledge of the electrocardiographic findings of acute pericarditis is critical as well as some findings that help in diagnosing pericarditis versus myocardial infarction (see Table 53-1). Classically, pericarditis evolves through four electrocardiographic stages (Table 53-2). The first stage of acute pericarditis is characterized by diffuse ST segment elevation, most prominent in the mid- and lateral precordial leads, with PR segment depression or downsloping (Fig. 53-1). The only leads in which these changes should *not* occur are in aVR and V1. PR segment elevation in lead aVR is occasionally taught to be a reliable indication of pericarditis (rather than myocardial infarction). However, this finding is neither sensitive nor specific, and it may actually be seen in some cases of acute myocardial infarction as well (Fig. 53-2). The ST segments should be concave upwards; a convex upward ("tombstone") morphology virtually excludes the diagnosis of pericarditis and rules in acute myocardial infarction. ST segment depression may be present in leads aVR and V1 in a patient with pericarditis but should never be present in any of the other 10 leads. In fact, the presence of ST segment depression in any of the other 10 leads should be considered the "reciprocal" changes of an acute myocardial infarction.

During the second stage of pericarditis, the ST segments and PR segments normalize and the T waves often flatten. During the third stage, the T waves invert. During the fourth and final stage, the ECG findings normalize. These changes generally progress over the course of days to weeks. The ECG changes in the second and third stages usually occur in the same leads in which the initial stage abnormalities occurred.

Although the ECG abnormalities noted are typically described as "classic" for acute pericarditis, physicians should be aware that these findings are typical only for acute *viral* pericarditis. Other forms of pericarditis less commonly caused PR segment depression and occasionally caused less pronounced ST segment elevation. In these cases, the diagnosis must be made based purely on the clinical presentation rather than on ECG findings.

Laboratory studies are rarely helpful in the diagnosis of acute pericarditis. Patients may have an elevated white blood cell count owing to pain and/or infection. Other serum markers of inflammation, including erythrocyte sedimentation rate and C-reactive protein value, are often elevated but such elevations are nonspecific. Cardiac biomarkers may be minimally elevated but should not demonstrate the rise and fall that are typical of myocardial infarction. Chest radiography is also rarely helpful in the diagnosis of acute pericarditis; it is mainly used to evaluate for alternative causes of chest pain (e.g., pneumonia, aortic dissection).

Echocardiography can be useful in distinguishing between acute pericarditis and acute myocardial infarction. Echocardiograms in pericarditis lack the focal wall motion abnormalities that are typical of echocardiograms in myocardial infarction. Echocardiography is also useful to look for evidence of a pericardial effusion, a potential complication of acute pericarditis (see later). If a large pericardial effusion is present, a pericardiocentesis (ultrasonography guided in the stable patient) can be used to obtain fluid for testing for infections and cytology.

Table 53-1 DIFFERENTIAL DIAGNOSIS FOR ACUTE PERICARDITIS

	Acute Pericarditis	Acute Myocardial Ischemia/Infarction	Aortic Dissection	Pulmonary Embolus
Chest pain description	Sharp, pleuritic, positional	Pressure, squeezing, tightness	Sharp, maximal intensity at onset	Sharp, pleuritic, abrupt onset
Chest pain radiation	Trapezius ridge	Usually to left arm, jaw, neck, or shoulder; may also radiate to right side	Straight to midscapular area of back	Not typical
Response to nitroglycerin	Not typical	Improves	Not typical	Not typical
Vital signs	Tachycardia and fever common	Fever not typical; blood pressure and heart rate are variable	Hypertension common	Occasionally low-grade fever, tachycardia and hypoxia common
Other physical examination findings	Friction rub common during course, though less common on initial presentation	Fourth heart sound is "classic" in cases of cardiac ischemia; third heart sound if heart failure present	Occasional pulse deficits	Occasional leg swelling or tenderness if embolus originated in the legs
Electrocardiographic findings	(see Table 53-2) Early: diffuse ST segment elevation and PR segment depression Absence of reciprocal ST segment depression ST-to-T wave amplitude ratio in V6>0.25 Sinus tachycardia common; bradycardia and atrioventricular (AV) blocks uncommon	ST segment elevation or depression typically in anatomic distribution corresponding to involved coronary vessel ST-to-T wave amplitude ratio in V6<0.25 Tachycardia or bradycardia and AV blocks not uncommon	Left ventricular hypertrophy if chronic hypertension present Variable ST segment or T wave changes Sinus tachycardia common	Sinus tachycardia common; bradycardia and AV blocks uncommon Large emboli often associated with T wave inversions, most commonly in right precordial leads and less commonly in inferior leads ST segment elevation possible but uncommon
Chest radiography findings	Usually normal; cardiomegaly if large pericardial effusion present	Cardiomegaly if chronic left ventricular hypertrophy present; evidence of heart failure may be present	Cardiomegaly common if chronic left ventricular hypertrophy present; wide mediastinum common	Usually normal; most common abnormalities are elevated hemidiaphragm, atelectasis, small pleural effusion
Cardiac biomarkers	Levels usually normal; mild elevations not uncommon	Elevations typical in myocardial infarction	Levels normal	Large emboli occasionally associated with mild elevations of troponin or brain natriuretic peptide

■ TREATMENT

Treatment of the patient with acute pericarditis should be targeted at the underlying cause. The majority of patients with viral, rheumatologic, post-traumatic, or idiopathic pericarditis are effectively treated with high-dose aspirin (2 to 4 g daily) or nonsteroidal anti-inflammatory drugs (NSAIDs). Ibuprofen is effective in most cases and has fewer side effects than other NSAIDs; the pain usually improves significantly within days with ibuprofen therapy. If the patient's symptoms persist, an alternative NSAID is indicated. Indomethacin is often used for severe cases because of its stronger anti-inflammatory effect, although it should be avoided in patients with a history of ischemic heart disease because it may decrease coronary blood flow.[4,7] Evidence now suggests that the addition of colchicine (1.0 to 2.0 mg for the first day, then 0.5 to 1.0 mg/day for 3 months) to the standard regimen is effective at hastening resolution of acute symptoms and also preventing recurrence rates, regardless of the cause of pericarditis.[8] Colchicine is also effective in cases of recurrent pericarditis.[9,10] The use of corticosteroids is generally reserved for recurrent cases of pericarditis that are unresponsive to aspirin or NSAIDs plus colchicine.

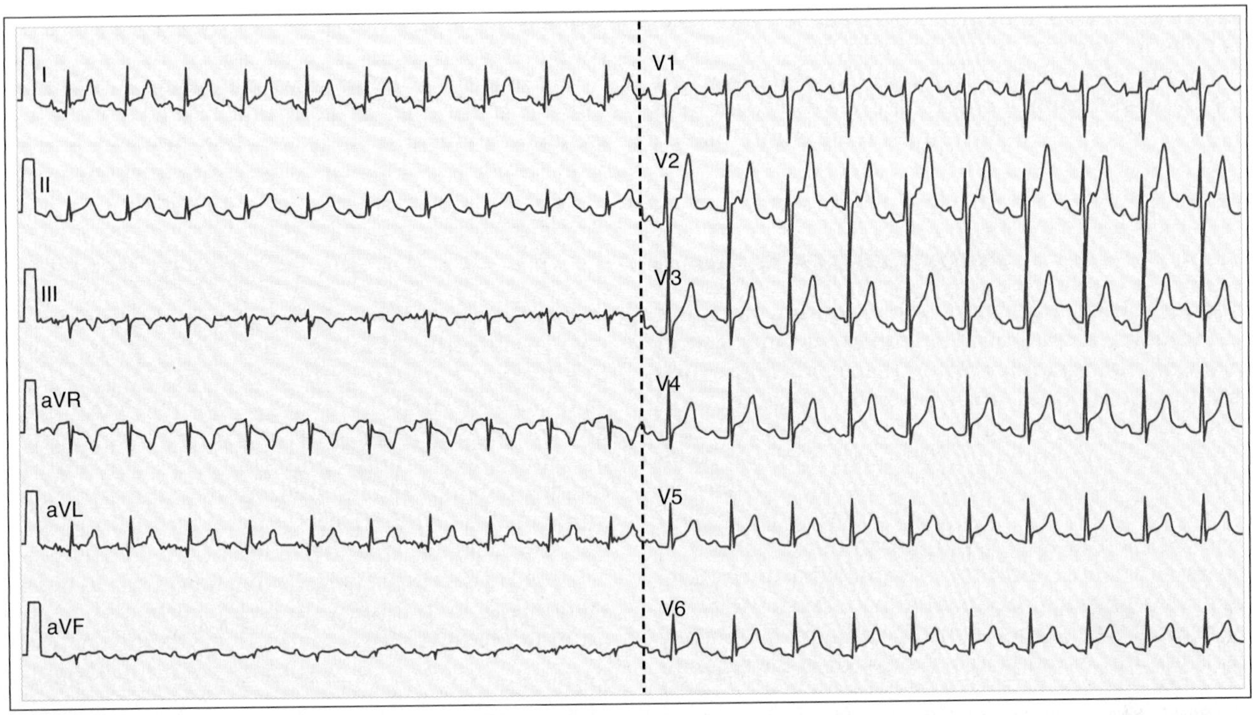
I
II
III
aVR
aVL
aVF
V1
V2
V3
V4
V5
V6

FIGURE 53-1 Acute pericarditis. The electrocardiogram demonstrates diffuse ST segment elevation with PR segment depression in multiple leads.

Table 53-2 ELECTROCARDIOGRAPHIC STAGES OF ACUTE PERICARDITIS

Stage I	Diffuse ST segment elevation and PR segment depression (except in leads V1 and aVR)
Stage II	Resolution of ST segment and PR segment changes T wave flattening in same leads
Stage III	T wave inversions in same leads
Stage IV	Normalization of electrographic abnormalities

Initiation of steroids early in the course of first-time pericarditis may actually be an independent risk factor for recurrence.[8]

Patients with bacterial or other nonviral infectious causes of pericarditis should be treated aggressively with antimicrobial therapy. Large infected pericardial effusions require drainage as well. Treatment for neoplastic causes of pericarditis should be targeted at treating the underlying malignancy. Patients with uremic pericarditis require urgent hemodialysis.

■ DISPOSITION

The majority of patients with acute pericarditis can be treated as outpatients, with symptoms generally resolving within 2 weeks. Outpatient management is suitable for patients with mild symptoms, hemodynamic stability, and ability to tolerate oral medications. Reasonable indications for admission include fever or suspicion of bacterial cause of pericarditis, immunosuppression, pericarditis associated with trauma, presence of moderate-to-large pericardial effusion, and hemodynamic instability. A history of active anticoagulant use is generally considered a poor prognostic factor, warranting admission as well.[4]

Pericardial Tamponade

■ ANATOMY AND PATHOPHYSIOLOGY

Trauma or inflammation of the pericardium can cause the accumulation of fluid within the intrapericardial space. Normally the pericardium is capable of stretching and accommodating two liters of fluid or more when the fluid accumulates very slowly.[11] However, if the fluid accumulates more rapidly than the pericardium's distensibility, especially in the case of trauma, in the presence of a fibrotic pericardium, or if the volume of pericardial fluid is excessive, significant intrapericardial pressure results and can produce pericardial tamponade.

Pericardial tamponade develops when intrapericardial fluid produces sufficient pressure to compress the cardiac chambers. The compression of the chambers impairs ventricular diastolic filling and stroke volume. Initial compensatory mechanisms, especially tachycardia, may temporarily sustain cardiac output. However, as pericardial fluid continues to increase, the compensatory mechanisms begin to fail, resulting in diminished cardiac output, hypotension, and full cardiovascular collapse.

The typical causes of pericardial tamponade include any disorder that causes acute or chronic pericardial inflammation as well as conditions in

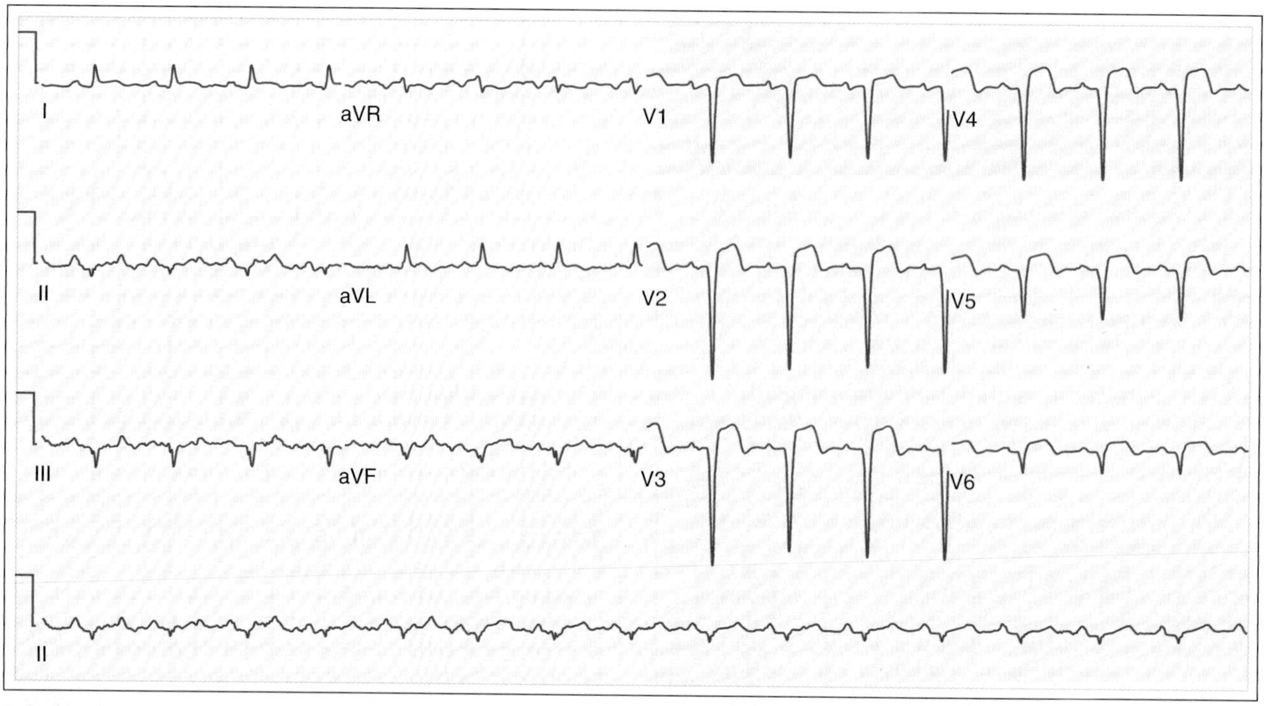
I
aVR
V1
V4
II
aVL
V2
V5
III
aVF
V3
V6
II

FIGURE 53-2 Acute myocardial infarction. The electrocardiogram demonstrates ST segment elevation in multiple leads with concurrent Q waves. PR segment elevation is present in lead aVR, a finding that is often mistakenly taught to be specific for acute pericarditis.

which a patient sustains penetrating trauma to the heart or cardiac surgery. The conditions previously noted as causing pericarditis are common precipitants of pericardial tamponade. The composition of the intrapericardial effusion varies according to the precipitating cause; in bacterial pericarditis, for example, the effusion is often pus, and in cardiac trauma or cardiac surgery, it is often blood and clots. Regardless of the composition of the effusion, the physiology that leads to pericardial tamponade as well as the immediate treatment are similar.

■ PRESENTING SIGNS AND SYMPTOMS

■ Classic

The typical symptoms associated with a large pericardial effusion are nonspecific. Malaise, generalized weakness, ascites, and edema are common in patients with subacute or chronic effusions as a result of poor cardiac function.[12] Many other symptoms are related to compression by the effusion of adjacent mediastinal structures. Dyspnea and cough are common and may be related to displacement or compression of bronchial structures or lung tissue by the effusion. Dyspnea on exertion is common as well, resulting from impairment of venous return and cardiac output. Patients often report a sense of dysphagia, which is due to esophageal compression. Hiccups may occur as a result of esophageal compression and involvement of the phrenic and vagus nerves. Hoarseness may result from compression of the recurrent laryngeal nerve.[12]

Physical findings are also often nonspecific. Tachycardia and tachypnea are common. Despite the presence of tachypnea and dyspnea, however, oxygen saturation levels are usually normal because the effusion itself does not impair alveolar air exchange. Lung sounds are usually normal as well. Finding hypoxia or focal abnormalities on the lung examination should suggest a superimposed pulmonary condition or an alternative diagnosis. Fevers are common if the underlying cause is infectious. Pericardial friction rubs are reportedly common if the underlying cause is inflammatory,[13] although diminished heart sounds are also common because of reduced cardiac function and because the effusion attenuates their transmission.

When a pericardial effusion produces pericardial tamponade, additional findings are notable. Decreased cardiac function produces hypotension and shock. Jugular venous distention is typically present because of impaired venous return. Pulsus paradoxus (drop in systolic blood pressure of more than 10 mm Hg during normal inspiration) is also typical, although its presence has limited specificity for pericardial tamponade. Several other conditions that are associated with hypotension and/or dyspnea can also produce pulsus paradoxus, including massive pulmonary embolism, hemorrhagic shock, and obstructive lung disease.[12] Death is usually preceded by pulseless electrical activity.[14]

■ Typical Variations

Although the symptoms and physical findings already noted are common, certain conditions may produce unexpected findings in the presence of pericardial tamponade. Patients who have severe hypothyroidism or uremia or who take atrioventricular-nodal blocking agents (e.g., calcium channel blockers, beta-blockers, digoxin) may present with a relative bradycardia. Jugular venous distention is typical in pericardial tamponade as well, but it is often absent in patients who are hypovolemic or in whom pericardial tamponade developed very quickly (e.g., after cardiac trauma). Overt hypotension may be absent as well in the patient with a history of severe antecedent hypertension.[12,15]

■ DIFFERENTIAL DIAGNOSIS, DIAGNOSTIC CRITERIA, AND TESTING

A complete differential diagnosis of hypotension and shock is beyond the scope of this chapter. However, the EP should have a sound grasp of the distinguishing features of the conditions that produce the combination of hypotension and jugular venous distension. All of these conditions can be life-threatening unless diagnosis and initiation of treatment are rapid. Table 53-3 summarizes the key distinguishing features among these diagnoses.

The primary means of diagnosing pericardial tamponade is via two-dimensional echocardiography. A pericardial effusion is easily seen in most patients on the subcostal or parasternal views (Fig. 53-3). An echo-free space should be visible throughout the cardiac cycle when the pericardial effusion is at least 25 mL.[3] The presence of a pericardial effusion in combination with hypotension and echocardiographic evidence of early diastolic right ventricular collapse and late diastolic right atrial collapse is diagnostic of pericardial tamponade. In approximately 25% of cases, the left atrium also demonstrates collapse, a very specific sign of tamponade. The left ventricle rarely demonstrates collapse except in specific conditions such as localized postoperative tamponade.[12] Other echocardiographic findings that may be found during pericardial tamponade are a dilated inferior vena cava without inspiratory collapse and beat-to-beat swinging of the heart within the pericardial fluid (when the effusion is large).[3]

Other imaging studies can be helpful in evaluating these patients as well. Computerized tomography (CT) and magnetic resonance imaging (MRI) are very accurate in detecting pericardial effusions as well as diagnosing alternative conditions. However, they should not be used in patients with borderline or overt hemodynamic instability because of the need to remove such patients from the ED for the procedures. Chest radiography is primarily used to evaluate the patient for alternative diagnoses as well, for example, pneumonia or pulmonary edema. In the presence of a large pericardial effusion, cardiomegaly is a nearly universal finding (Fig. 53-4). The chest radiograph is particularly helpful in this setting if prior radiographs are available that demonstrate a normal-sized heart. When comparison with prior radiographs shows massive cardiomegaly to be *new*, this finding is highly suggestive of a large pericardial effusion.

ECG can be helpful in the diagnosis of large pericardial effusions. The most common abnormality is tachycardia, especially in the presence of tamponade. Low voltage is common as well and is caused by attenuation of the electrical impulse as it passes through the effusion before reaching the ECG electrodes. Although low voltage is nonspecific, the presence of *new* low voltage (in comparison with prior

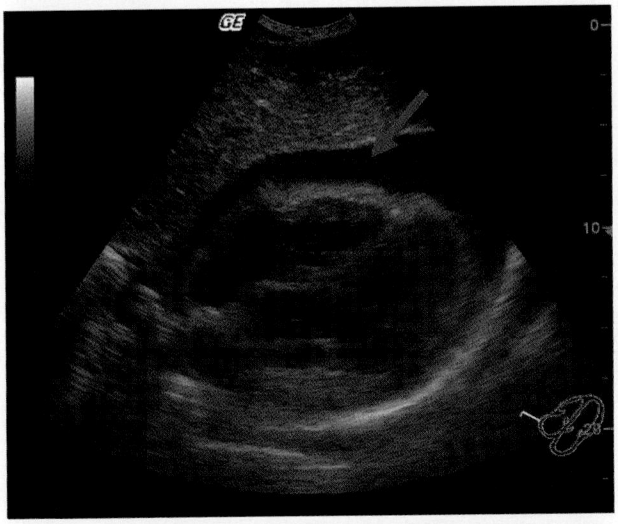

FIGURE 53-3 Large pericardial effusion. The ultrasonogram is a subcostal four-chamber view of the heart demonstrating a large pericardial effusion (*arrow*). The patient also had dynamic changes consistent with pericardial tamponade—right atrial and right ventricular diastolic collapse. (Courtesy Dr. Brian Euerle, Director of Emergency Ultrasound, Emergency Medicine Residency, University of Maryland School of Medicine.)

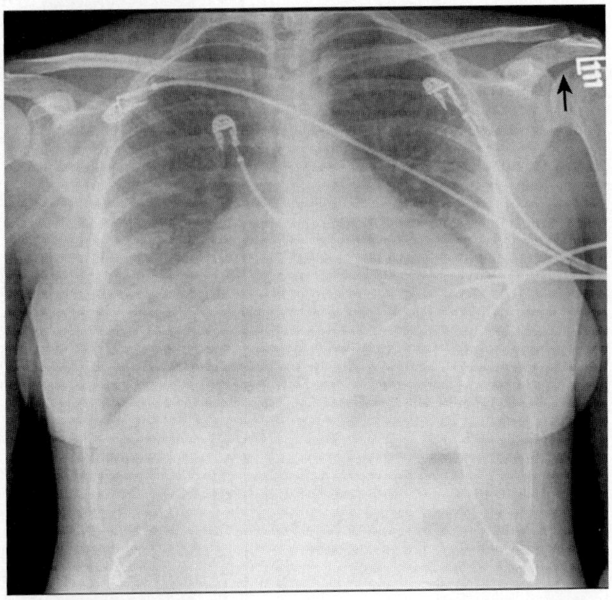

FIGURE 53-4 Large pericardial effusion. The chest radiograph demonstrates massive cardiomegaly, a nearly universal finding in patients with large pericardial effusions.

Table 53-3 DIFFERENTIAL DIAGNOSIS FOR HYPOTENSION WITH JUGULAR VENOUS DISTENTION

	Pericardial Tamponade	Massive Pulmonary Embolism	Large Acute Left Ventricular Myocardial Infarction with Cardiogenic Shock	Acute Right Ventricular Myocardial Infarction	Acute Aortic or Mitral Valve Insufficiency	Superior Vena Cava Syndrome
Key presenting features	Generalized weakness, dyspnea with exertion and at rest, dysphagia	Risk factors for thromboembolic disease, dyspnea	Consistent with acute myocardial infarction	Consistent with acute myocardial infarction	Commonly occurs in patients with risk factors for bacterial endocarditis Acute aortic insufficiency may occur in presence of blunt chest trauma or aortic dissection; acute mitral insufficiency may occur in the first week after myocardial infarction	Facial plethora, distended veins in upper chest and neck, hoarseness not uncommon Historical features consistent with pulmonary malignancy are typical
Onset of symptoms	Usually gradual; primary exception is in the presence of cardiac trauma	Abrupt	Abrupt	Abrupt	Abrupt	Gradual
Heart sounds	Diminished first and second heart sounds; tachycardia, rub may be present	Tachycardia common, otherwise usually normal	Third heart sound (S_3) common; possibly fourth heart sound (S_4)	Usually normal; possibly S_4	S_3 common In acute aortic insufficiency, new diastolic murmur at upper sternal border In acute mitral insufficiency, new systolic murmur from apex to axilla	Usually normal
Lung sounds	Tachypnea; otherwise usually normal	Tachypnea; may have focal wheezes but commonly normal	Tachypnea, rales consistent with pulmonary edema	Tachypnea is variable; otherwise usually normal	Tachypnea, rales consistent with pulmonary edema (generally more prominent with acute mitral insufficiency)	Usually normal, although tachypnea and other findings consistent with underlying lung disease (malignancy, chronic smoking, etc.) are common

Oxygenation	Usually normal	Hypoxia common	Hypoxia common	Usually normal	Hypoxia common	Usually normal, although hypoxia consistent with underlying lung disease (malignancy, chronic smoking, etc.) is common
Echocardiographic findings	Pericardial effusion; right atrial and ventricular diastolic collapse	Right ventricular distention and dysfunction	Regional wall motion hypokinesis	Regional wall motion hypokinesis	Valvular dysfunction and regurgitant blood flow (primarily found when Doppler echocardiography used)	Nonspecific
Chest radiograph findings	Except in the presence of rapidly developing pericardial tamponade (e.g., cardiac trauma), cardiomegaly is nearly universal and is often massive with large effusions	Usually normal; most common abnormalities are elevated hemidiaphragm, atelectasis, small pleural effusion	Pulmonary edema	Usually normal	Pulmonary edema (generally more prominent with acute mitral insufficiency)	Upper lobe malignancy is common
Electrocardiographic findings	Low voltage and tachycardia are typical; electrical alternans is less common	Tachycardia and new T wave inversions are common; less common are rightward axis, tall R wave in V1 ("right heart strain"), $S_1Q_3T_3$ pattern	Changes consistent with acute myocardial infarction: ST segment elevations and/or depressions, new T wave inversions	Changes consistent with acute myocardial infarction usually in inferior leads (less commonly in lateral leads); ST segment elevations noted on right precordial leads (i.e., when a right-sided electrocardiogram is performed)	Nonspecific; in post-infarction mitral insufficiency, Q waves from recent infarction are typically found in the inferior leads	Nonspecific

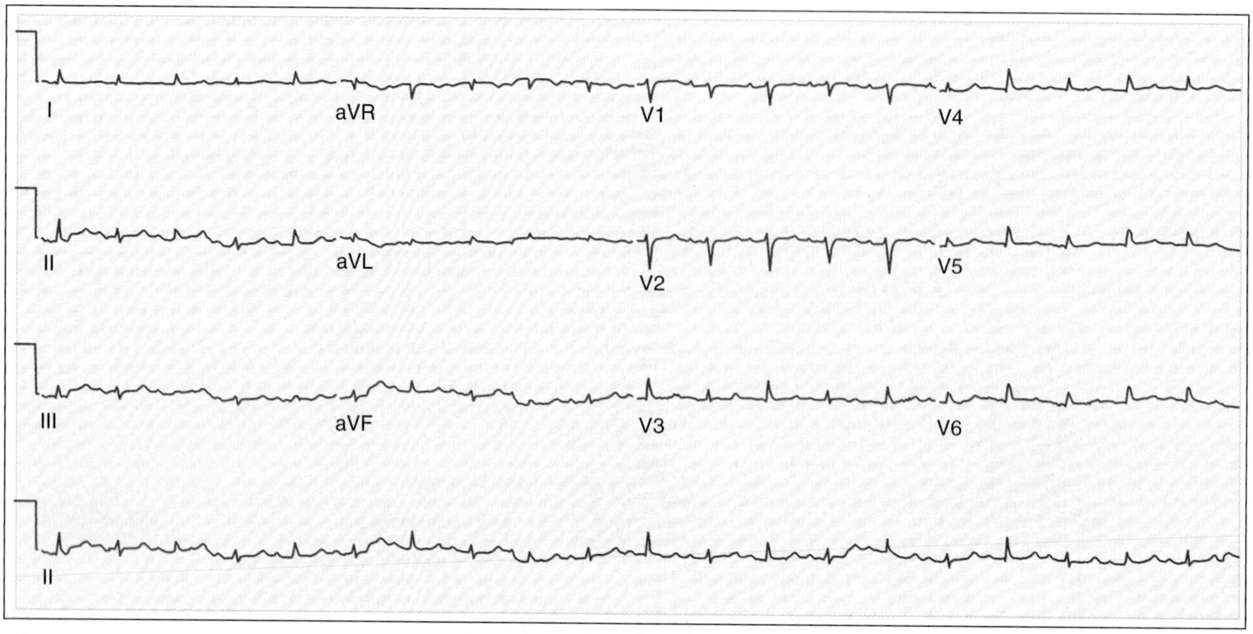
I
aVR
V1
V4
II
aVL
V2
V5
III
aVF
V3
V6
II

FIGURE 53-5 Large pericardial effusion. The electrocardiogram demonstrates the three classic findings in a patient with a large pericardial effusion: sinus tachycardia, low voltage, and electrical alternans.

ECG) is much more specific for large pericardial effusions. The third "classic" ECG abnormality is electrical alternans. *Electrical alternans* refers to beat-to-beat variation in the amplitudes of the ECG complexes (Fig. 53-5) and is attributed to the "swinging" of the heart back and forth within the pericardial fluid. Electrical alternans is present in less than one third of cases of pericardial tamponade. Although none of these three findings individually is completely diagnostic of large pericardial effusions, the combination of all three is very highly specific.

■ TREATMENT

The initial management of the patient with pericardial tamponade should focus on the typical ABCs of resuscitation. Certain caveats should be made, however. Although the primary pathophysiologic abnormality underlying hemodynamic compromise in pericardial tamponade is ventricular filling, the benefit of volume infusion to improve filling is controversial. Animal studies have shown variable results in terms of the hemodynamic benefit of volume infusion,[12,16] which may improve systemic perfusion only in patients with hypovolemia. Strong supporting data in humans are lacking, however. In patients with traumatic pericardial tamponade, large-volume infusions may actually precipitate further deterioration.[17] Strong evidence supporting specific inotropic agents is lacking as well, although theoretically agents that reduce the elevated vascular resistance,[12] such as dobutamine and milrinone, would seem ideal. Mechanical ventilation should generally be avoided as well except in the presence of respiratory failure; the positive airway pressure associated with mechanical ventilation decreases venous return and cardiac output.

The treatment of pericardial tamponade is drainage of the intrapericardial fluid (*pericardiocentesis*). Drainage is best performed via needle aspiration under echocardiographic, CT, or fluoroscopic guidance. For the patients who has rapid cardiac decompensation or is in cardiac arrest, the EP should perform emergency pericardiocentesis without waiting for imaging guidance. The procedure is performed with a 16- or 18-gauge needle, most commonly inserted into the left paraxiphoid area of the chest. The needle is pointed downwards at an approximately 30-degree angle to the chest in order to bypass the left costal margin, aimed toward the left shoulder. The needle should be inserted and advanced slowly until the pericardium is penetrated and fluid is aspirated. The use of a sheathed needle can facilitate the process: Once the pericardium has been penetrated, the core of the needle can be removed with the sheath left in the pericardial space to assist with further fluid removal.[12] Some researchers have advocated attaching ECG leads to the hub of the needle so that when the pericardium is penetrated, an injury pattern (i.e., ST segment elevation) will be noted.[18] However, a recent review recommends against this practice because of likelihood of misleading results.[12]

In the patient with acute cardiac decompensation, aspiration of even 10 to 20 mL of blood should be sufficient to produce some hemodynamic improvement. However, once full cardiac arrest has occurred, pericardiocentesis has a limited success rate. Potential complications of pericardiocentesis include cardiac chamber puncture or laceration, coronary vessel injury, pneumothorax, ventricular dysrhythmias, pneumopericardium, and delayed infection.[19]

BOX 53-2

Causes of Myocarditis

Viral infections (most common):
- Coxsackievirus (most common virus)
- Echovirus
- Human immunodeficiency virus
- Influenza virus
- Parainfluenza virus
- Epstein-Barr virus
- Adenovirus
- Varicella virus
- Cytomegalovirus
- Herpesvirus
- Rabies virus
- Poliovirus
- Hepatitis A, B, C, or D virus
- Rubella virus
- Mumps virus
- Rubeola virus

Bacterial infections:
- *Staphylococcus*
- *Borrelia* (Lyme disease)
- *Legionella*
- *Corynebacterium diphtheriae*
- Tuberculosis
- *Mycoplasma*
- *Streptococcus*
- *Meningococcus*
- *Chlamydia* (*pneumoniae* and *psittaci*)
- *Enterococcus*

Parasitic infections:
- Toxoplasmosis
- Trypanosomiasis
- Trichinosis
- Echinococcosis
- Chagas' disease

Medications/toxins:
- Methyldopa
- Penicillin
- Hydrochlorothiazide
- Sulfamethoxazole
- Lithium
- Doxorubicin
- Cyclophosphamides
- Zidovudine
- Acetaminophen
- Lead
- Arsenic
- Carbon monoxide
- Cocaine
- Ethanol
- Interleukin-2
- Anabolic steroids
- Radiation therapy

Connective tissue diseases:
- Systemic lupus erythematosus
- Rheumatoid arthritis
- Dermatomyositis
- Sarcoidosis

Miscellaneous:
- Giant cell arteritis
- Kawasaki's disease
- Cardiac transplant rejection
- Peripartum state

These complications are more common in the setting of emergency pericardiocentesis, which is performed without imaging guidance.

Pericardiocentesis is less likely to be successful in patients with clotted hemopericardium, who will therefore require surgical drainage. Surgical drainage is also required in patients in whom intrapericardial bleeding is present (e.g., postoperative pericardial tamponade, traumatic pericardial tamponade, pericardial tamponade with aortic dissection). In these patients, pericardiocentesis is temporizing at best; in conjunction with surgical drainage, definitive repair of the bleeding sites is required.

Additional therapy should focus on the underlying cause of pericardial inflammation that led to pericardial tamponade. Patients with uremia should undergo urgent hemodialysis. Patients with underlying infections should receive appropriate supportive and antimicrobial therapy. Patients with malignant pericardial tamponade should receive appropriate antineoplastic therapy once they are hemodynamically stable in order to prevent or minimize recurrences.

■ DISPOSITION

Patients with pericardial tamponade should be admitted to an intensive care setting for definitive therapy and close hemodynamic monitoring. If surgical therapy is indicated, emergency surgical consultation is mandatory. When surgical therapy is not planned, cardiology consultation is most appropriate for the performance of pericardiocentesis under echocardiographic guidance. Nephrology consultation is also appropriate for urgent hemodialysis in patients with uremia.

Myocarditis

■ ANATOMY AND PATHOPHYSIOLOGY

Myocarditis is an inflammatory condition causing myocardial damage, usually due to infectious, immunologic, or toxin-mediated conditions (Box 53-2). Myocarditis can manifest as mild constitutional symptoms, moderate cardiopulmonary symptoms, or fulminant cardiopulmonary decompensation leading

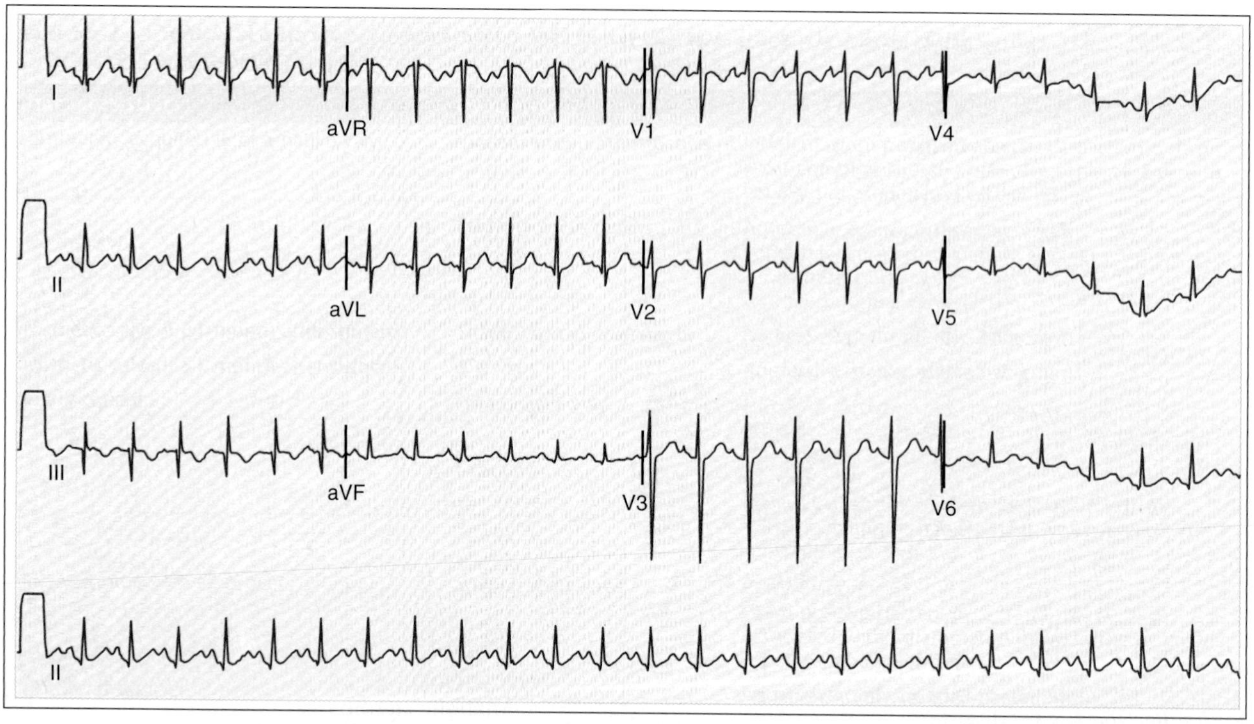
I
aVR
V1
V4
II
aVL
V2
V5
III
aVF
V3
V6
II

FIGURE 53-6 Sinus tachycardia (rate 150 beats/min) in a patient with myocarditis.

to death. In the majority of adult cases, the myocardial damage is believed to be caused by autoimmune processes that are often triggered by viral or other infections,[20] whereas in neonates and infants, injury of the myocytes is believed to occur more often because of direct injury by the pathogen itself.[21]

Approximately 10% of postmortem examinations demonstrate some degree of histologic evidence of myocarditis. However, most of the patients have not been clinically symptomatic prior to death.[22] Conversely, among patients *clinically* diagnosed with myocarditis, only one third have histologic findings consistent with the disease. Even among cases that progress to dilated cardiomyopathy, only 40% of patients have microscopic evidence of myocarditis. Consequently, the actual incidence of myocarditis is unknown.[23]

■ PRESENTING SIGNS AND SYMPTOMS

■ Classic

The clinical manifestations of myocarditis usually begin days to weeks after the acute infection, especially when viruses are implicated as the cause. However, only 50% of patients report a recent upper respiratory or gastrointestinal viral type of infection.[23] Initial symptoms are nonspecific and constitutional in nature: low fevers, fatigue, malaise, myalgias, and arthralgias. These mild symptoms are often the reason for initial misdiagnosis or delays in proper diagnosis of this condition. Cardiopulmonary symptoms, especially mild dyspnea and chest pain, are common as well. The chest pain can be pleuritic, sharp, and positional, much like pericarditis; or substernal and squeezing, much like typical ischemic pain. Patients with congestive heart failure may report more significant dyspnea as well as cough, orthopnea, paroxysmal nocturnal dyspnea, and edema. Less commonly patients may present after a syncopal episode, usually the result of a bradydysrhythmia.

The physical findings are often notable for low-grade fevers, tachypnea, and tachycardia. Classically, the patient presents with a "tachycardia out of proportion to the fever"—extreme tachycardia without obvious hypovolemia or high fever (Fig. 53-6). Patients may also experience bradycardia if a high-grade arterioventricular block develops (Fig. 53-7). Evidence of congestive heart failure is often present as well: jugular venous distention, bibasilar rales on lung examination, a third heart sound (S_3) on cardiac examination, and peripheral edema. Patients with advanced or fulminant myocarditis may present with full cardiogenic shock.

■ Typical Variations

Pediatric patients also tend to present early with nonspecific symptoms, including fevers, viral upper respiratory symptoms, and poor feeding. In more severe cases, the infant or neonate may be presented with severe tachycardia, tachypnea, sweating while feeding, respiratory distress, and cyanosis or other signs of poor perfusion. Tachydysrhythmias and bradydysrhythmias, especially involving high-grade atrioventricular block, are common as well. Severe

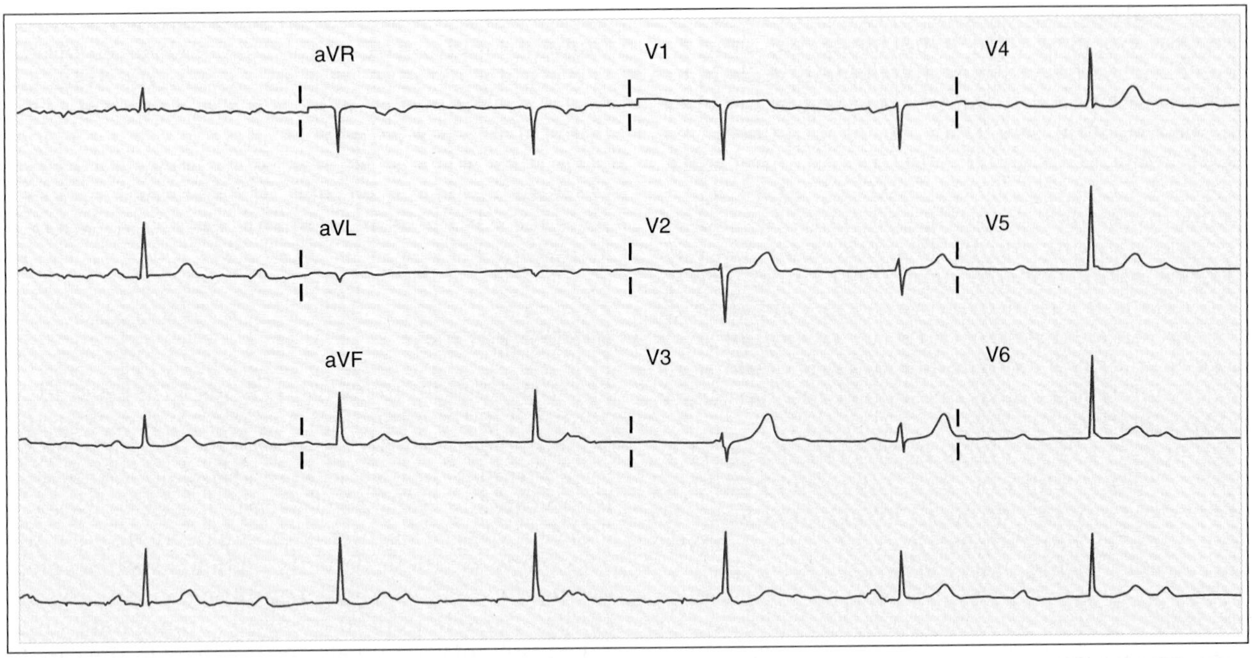
aVR
V1
V4
aVL
V2
V5
aVF
V3
V6

FIGURE 53-7 Sinus rhythm with atrioventricular (AV) dissociation and high-grade AV block in a patient with myocarditis.

myocarditis in the very young often also manifests as pulmonary edema, cardiogenic shock, and multi-organ hypoperfusion.

■ DIFFERENTIAL DIAGNOSIS, DIAGNOSTIC CRITERIA, AND TESTING

The differential diagnosis of myocarditis is extremely broad because of the nonspecific nature of the initial presentation. Patients who initially present with cardiopulmonary symptoms have a slightly more limited differential diagnosis, but initial consideration should as always be focused on the most deadly diseases that produce chest pain and/or dyspnea: acute coronary syndrome, aortic dissection, pulmonary embolism, acute pericarditis/pericardial tamponade, esophageal rupture, cardiogenic pulmonary edema, and pneumonia.

The initial diagnostic evaluation should be prompted by clinical suspicion. The finding of cardiopulmonary complaints, unexplained tachycardia, or evidence of congestive heart failure upon examination in young patients should prompt consideration of myocarditis. ECG and chest radiography are appropriate initial tests in these patients. Although there is no specific or single *diagnostic* ECG abnormality, the majority of patients with myocarditis have at least *some* ECG abnormality. The most common abnormalities are sinus tachycardia (see Fig. 53-6) and nonspecific ST segment/T wave changes. Other abnormalities that may occur in cases of myocarditis are conduction abnormalities (new fascicular blocks, new bundle branch blocks, and atrioventricular blocks), atrial or ventricular tachydysrhythmias and bradydysrhythmias, overt ischemic changes (T wave inversions, ST segment changes), and Q wave formation. The ischemic changes are often indistinguishable from those seen in true cardiac ischemia or myocardial infarction. If the pericardium is also involved, producing myopericarditis, PR segment depression with concurrent ST segment elevation may be found. If a pericardial effusion develops, low voltage may occur. The ECG findings are rarely completely normal.

Plain chest radiograph findings are often normal in mild or early cases of myocarditis. However, most patients with cardiopulmonary complaints manifest some radiographic signs of congestive heart failure: cardiomegaly, pulmonary vascular redistribution, interstitial edema, and frank pulmonary edema. Pleural effusions may be present as well.

Laboratory studies typically ordered in the ED include evaluations of markers of inflammation and cardiac biomarkers. Inflammatory markers, such as white blood cell count, erythrocyte sedimentation rate, and C-reactive protein value, are expected to be elevated but unfortunately, such elevations are nonspecific. Measurements of markers are sometimes used to follow the course of the disease after the diagnosis is made. Cardiac biomarkers, including troponin and creatinine phosphokinase values, are also sometimes elevated. The initial elevations of cardiac biomarkers are often indistinguishable from those expected in acute myocardial infarction. Serial measurements of cardiac biomarkers can be helpful, however, because the levels do not tend to rise and fall as quickly in myocarditis as in myocardial infarction.

Echocardiography may also be helpful in the ED, especially when there is confusion in distinguishing between myocarditis and acute coronary syndrome. Echocardiography in patients with acute coronary syndrome (with active ischemia) usually demonstrates focal wall hypokinesis. Patients with myocarditis can also have focal hypokinesis, but they are more likely to have diffuse hypokinesis and multichamber dilation as well.[23] The echocardiogram can also demonstrate evidence of complications, for example, pericardial effusion or intracardiac thrombus.

Endomyocardial biopsy is generally considered the "gold standard" for the diagnosis of myocarditis. Evidence of microscopic myocardial inflammation with various levels of necrosis is generally used to diagnose and categorize stages of myocarditis.[23,24] However, biopsy is not feasible in the ED. Additionally, recent reports have questioned the sensitivity and specificity of the test.[23,25]

Other tests that can be ordered by the EP are viral cultures, blood cultures, and other immunologic studies. These tests are rarely helpful in the acute setting but they may of use to the inpatient physicians during the hospital course.

■ TREATMENT

Close attention should be paid to the ABCs of resuscitation, because patients with fulminant myocarditis can decompensate rapidly. The mainstay of treatment for myocarditis is primarily supportive, focusing on hemodynamic support and management of complications. Congestive heart failure and hypoxia should be treated as usual, with high-flow oxygen, preload and afterload reduction, and diuretics. The patient's fluid status must also be monitored closely because of the risk of congestive heart failure. Bradydysrhythmias should be managed as usual. Patients with high-degree atrioventricular blocks often require pacemaker placement. Tachydysrhythmias should generally be managed as usual, although preference should be given to titratable medications because drugs with negative inotropic effects can precipitate unpredictable hemodynamic collapse in these patients with myocarditis, whose status is tenuous. Intramural thrombi noted on echocardiography should be treated with anticoagulation. The benefit of prophylactic anticoagulation is uncertain, especially given the risk that these patients have for hemopericardium. Additional myocardial workload reduction can be obtained through fever reduction and correction of anemia.[23]

Patients in shock should be treated aggressively. Adequate perfusion should be obtained in hypotensive patients through the use of vasopressors (e.g., dopamine, norepinephrine) and positive inotropic agents (e.g., dobutamine). Ventricular assist devices, intra-aortic balloon counterpulsation, and cardiopulmonary bypass have been used successfully in some patients during the wait for clinical improvement or cardiac transplantation.[23]

Antiviral therapy may be helpful during the patient's hospital course if a viral cause of myocarditis has been determined. Other therapies should be focused on the determined underlying condition (e.g., Lyme carditis, toxin-induced myocarditis). Immunosuppressive medications have been employed successfully in some patients in the later stages of illness, but this experience appears to be anecdotal only.[26] The use of corticosteroids lacks good evidence of benefit as well. High-dose intravenous gamma globulin has been used successfully in some pediatric patients, with improvement in ventricular function at 1 year.[23]

■ DISPOSITION

Patients in whom myocarditis is suspected should be admitted to the hospital. Cardiac monitoring should be started in order to assess for the development of dysrhythmias, and close hemodynamic monitoring is indicated as well. Critical care, infectious disease, and cardiology consultants should be involved in the care plans for these patients. Patients with severely decompensated cardiac conditions may require cardiac transplantation; therefore, appropriate surgical consultants should also be involved in the care of patients with severe myocarditis.

REFERENCES

1. Mast HL, Haller JO, Schiller MS, et al: Pericardial effusion and its relationship to cardiac disease in children with acquired immunodeficiency syndrome. Pediatr Radiol 1992;22:548.
2. Lorell BH: Pericarditis. In Braunwald E (ed): Heart Disease, 5th ed. Philadelphia, WB Saunders, 1997, p 1478.
3. Aikat S, Ghaffari S: A review of pericardial diseases: Clinical, ECG and hemodynamic features and management. Cleve Clin J Med 2000;67:903.
4. Lange RA, Hillis LD: Acute pericarditis. N Engl J Med 2004;351:2195.
5. Zayas R, Anguita M, Torres F, et al: Incidence of specific etiology and role of methods for specific etiologic diagnosis of primary acute pericarditis. Am J Cardiol 1995;75:378.
6. Spodick DH: Pericardial rub: prospective, multiple observer investigation of pericardial friction in 100 patients. Am J Cardiol 1975;35:357.
7. Schifferdecker B, Spodick DH: Nonsteroidal anti-inflammatory drugs in the treatment of pericarditis. Cardiol Rev 2003;11:211.
8. Imazio M, Bobbio M, Cecchi E, et al: Colchicine in addition to conventional therapy for acute pericarditis. Circulation 2005;112:2012.
9. Adler Y, Finkelstein Y, Guindo J, et al: Colchicine treatment for recurrent pericarditis: A decade of experience. Circulation 1998;97:2183.
10. Millaire A, de Groote P, Decoulx E, et al: Treatment of recurrent pericarditis with colchicine. Eur Heart J 1994;15:120.
11. Reddy PS, Curtiss EI, O'Toole JD, et al: Cardiac tamponade: Hemodynamic observations in man. Circulation 1978;58:265.
12. Spodick DH: Acute cardiac tamponade. N Engl J Med 2003;349:684.
13. Spodick DH: Pericardial rub: Prospective, multiple observer investigation of pericardial friction in 100 patients. Am J Cardiol 1975;35:357.
14. Cooper JP, Oliver RM, Currie P, et al: How do the clinical findings in patients with pericardial effusions influence the success of aspiration? Br Heart J 1995;73:351.
15. Ramsaran EK, Benotti JR, Spodick DH: Exacerbated tamponade: Deterioration of cardiac function by lowering excessive arterial pressure in hypertensive cardiac tamponade. Cardiology 1995;86:77.

16. Cogswell TL, Bernath GA, Keelan MH Jr, et al: The shift in the relationship between intrapericardial fluid pressure and volume induced by acute left ventricular pressure overload during cardiac tamponade. Circulation 1986;74:173.
17. Hashim R, Frankel H, Tandon M, et al: Fluid resuscitation-induced cardiac tamponade. Trauma 2002;53:1183.
18. Harper RJ: Pericardiocentesis. In Roberts JR, Hedges JR (eds): Clinical Procedures in Emergency Medicine, 4th ed. Philadelphia, Saunders, 2004, p 316.
19. Tsang TS, Oh JK, Seward JB: Diagnosis and management of cardiac tamponade in the era of echocardiography. Clin Cardiol 1999;22:446.
20. Klingel K, Hohenadl C, Canu A, et al: Ongoing enterovirus-induced myocarditis is associated with persistent heart muscle infection: Quantitative analysis of virus replication, tissue damage, and inflammation. Proc Natl Acad Sci U S A 1992;89:314.
21. Ledford DK: Immunologic aspects of cardiovascular disease. JAMA 1992;268:2923.
22. See DM, Tilles JG: Viral myocarditis. Rev Infect Dis 1991;13:951.
23. Brady WJ, Ferguson JD, Ullman EA, et al: Myocarditis: Emergency department recognition and management. Emerg Med Clin N Am 2004;22:865.
24. Lieberman EB, Herskowitz A, Rose NR, et al: A clinico-pathologic description of myocarditis. Clin Immunol Immunopathol 1993;68:191.
25. Baughman KL: Diagnosis of myocarditis: Death of Dallas criteria. Circulation 2006;113:593.
26. Mason JW, O'Connell JB, Herskowitz A, et al: A clinical trial of immunosuppressive therapy for myocarditis. N Engl J Med 1995;333:269.

Chapter **54**

Cardiac Valvular Emergencies

Todd C. Rothenhaus

KEY POINTS

Asymptomatic patients with previously undetected heart murmur should be referred for further evaluation.

It is important to consider valvular heart disease in patients presenting with dyspnea, chest pain, syncope, hypotension, shock, or new onset of atrial fibrillation.

Echocardiography is recommended for symptomatic patients with signs of valvular abnormality on examination as well as for asymptomatic patients with diastolic or continuous murmurs.

Absence of a detectable murmur does not rule out significant valvular dysfunction, especially in the patient with shock, decreased cardiac output, or a prosthetic heart valve.

Patients with acquired valvular dysfunction should be given prophylaxis against bacterial endocarditis before undergoing procedures known to potentially result in bacteremia.

Scope

Despite advances in the prevention of rheumatic fever and in our understanding of atherosclerotic heart disease, the advent of diagnostic echocardiography, and more than 40 years of experience with valve replacement surgery, valvular heart disease remains a common problem. The incidence of rheumatic fever in developed countries is declining, but rheumatic heart disease remains the most common cause of valvular heart disease worldwide. As a result, valvular disorders are more common in immigrants than in American-born people. As average life expectancy has risen in the United States, however, calcific degeneration of the cardiac valves has become more prevalent. This inflammatory damage to cardiac valves, although of much later onset than rheumatic heart disease and pathologically similar to atherosclerosis, has become an increasingly common cause of valvular heart disease in developed nations. In the last two decades, the incidence and success of cardiac valve replacement surgery have increased dramatically, making patients with prosthetic valves common in the ED. Valve replacement surgery is relatively safe and effective, but complications from prosthetic valves do occur.

Until recently, little high-quality data existed on the medical management of valvular heart disease. In 1998 the American College of Cardiology and the American Heart Association jointly published comprehensive guidelines for the management of patients with valvular disorders.[1] Despite the publication of these guidelines and significant research on valvular disease and cardiac valve replacement, little literature has been written on the management of the *acute* presentations of valvular disorders.

Patients with acute or severe life-threatening valvular heart disease are nearly always treated surgically. Although the management of the patient with severe valvular heart disease has traditionally been the purview of cardiologists, cardiothoracic surgeons, and anesthesiologists, the care of patients suffering acute valvular disorders almost always begins in the ED, making competent management of acute valvular heart disease an important skill for the EP.

Presenting Signs and Symptoms

The hallmark of most cardiac valvular disorders is a slow progression of disease with symptom-free intervals between initial valve injury (e.g., rheumatic fever, congenital lesion), the onset of detectable murmur, and the ultimate development of symptoms. Although progression of valvular disease occurs slowly, acute decompensation during the asymptomatic phase is difficult to predict and can occur without warning. It is important to consider the development of acute valvular decompensation in patients who have (or have not) been previously diagnosed with valvular heart disease. Likewise, a search for murmurs and other signs of valvular disease should be undertaken in patients who present with signs or symptoms typical of valvular disease, including dyspnea, chest pain, syncope, and hypotension.

Patients with valvular heart disease present to the ED in a number of ways. They may present with completely asymptomatic disease that is noted only on routine cardiac auscultation for an unrelated complaint or with symptoms and signs attributable to a valvular disorder. In the latter case, the EP must try to determine whether valvular heart disease is significant enough to be the cause of symptoms. Valvular heart disease may mimic a number of more common disorders, including myocardial infarction and congestive heart failure. Finally, patients may rarely present in extremis, with severe pump failure and shock. They are among the sickest patients the EP may be called upon to manage. Because proper diagnosis and therapy can be lifesaving for such patients, it is imperative that the EP attempt to delineate the particular valvular disorder before taking specific steps to give hemodynamic support. For example, although afterload reduction may significantly improve cardiac output in patients with regurgitant lesions, vasodilators (or even modest attempts at blood pressure control) in patients with aortic stenosis may lead to hypotension, a reduction in coronary perfusion pressure, and the development of acute ischemia. In the absence of diagnosed valvular abnormality or an equivocal clinical evaluation, emergency echocardiography may be required.

Pathophysiology

There are four principal cardiac valvular disorders: aortic stenosis, aortic regurgitation, mitral stenosis, and mitral regurgitation. Valvular lesions rarely exist in complete isolation. Multiple valves may be diseased, or a single valve may exhibit elements of both stenosis and regurgitation, especially as disease progresses. In most cases, one symptom complex nearly always predominates, and management is usually dictated by the most severe valvular abnormality.[2]

Cardiac murmurs result from (1) increased blood flow across a normal valve, (2) turbulent flow across a narrow or irregular orifice, or (3) regurgitant flow across a diseased valve or other cardiac defect. Murmurs are classically divided into systolic, diastolic, and continuous. Systolic murmurs are further subclassified into holosystolic (pansystolic), midsystolic, early systolic, and late systolic. Diastolic and continuous murmurs are nearly always pathologic and require investigation, even in the absence of symptoms. Although most systolic murmurs merit investigation, especially those associated with symptoms, the majority of systolic murmurs do not signify valvular disease. A summary of the typical findings in the major valvular abnormalities appears in Table 54-1.

Clinical Evaluation and Diagnostic Testing

Evaluation of the patient with potential cardiovascular disease begins with a thorough cardiac examination. Auscultation of the heart, even in a busy ED, is essential in patients with complaint of dyspnea, chest pain, or syncope, even in the absence of abnormal vital signs or hemodynamic instability. In patients with routine chest pain, cardiac examination may indicate potential valvular abnormalities that may guide further testing. For example, routine cardiac stress testing is relatively contraindicated in patients with significant aortic or mitral stenosis because it would raise the risk for acute decompensation, syncope, or even sudden death.

Careful cardiac examination may help diagnose the nature and severity of the murmur, although determination of the magnitude of valvular abnormality with cardiac examination alone is far less reliable than with echocardiography. Clinical evaluation had been determined to accurately diagnose moderate to severe mitral stenosis in more than 90% of patients.[3]

Murmurs other than midsystolic ejection murmurs that are detected in asymptomatic patients require follow-up echocardiography and cardiologic evaluation. In patients who present with cardiopulmonary symptoms, the detection of *any* new murmur warrants further investigation.

Electrocardiography (ECG) is essential in the evaluation of patients with suspected valvular abnormalities. Evidence of left ventricular hypertrophy, atrial abnormalities, conduction disturbance, and arrhythmias suggests potential valvular heart disease. Conversely, completely normal ECG findings reduce the likelihood of significant valvular abnormality.

Chest radiography may be helpful in cases of suspected valve disease and should be performed in patients who present with symptoms suggestive of valvular abnormality, to evaluate cardiac size and contour and to check for the presence of pulmonary congestion. Any evidence of heart failure, cardiomegaly, or calcification of the aorta or cardiac

Table 54-1 CHARACTERISTICS OF MAJOR CARDIAC VALVULAR ABNORMALITIES

Valvular Abnormality	Timing	Loudest	Radiation	First Heart Sound	Second Heart Sound	Associated Findings
Aortic stenosis	Systolic (mid to late)	Upper right sternal border	Carotid arteries	Normal	Single or paradoxically split	Distal pulses delayed and diminished Sustained left ventricular (LV) impulse
Mitral stenosis	Diastolic (rumble)	Apex	Little or none	Loud or normal	Normal	Opening snap
Aortic regurgitation	Diastolic (blowing)	Upper right sternal border	Neck	Soft	Normal	Wide pulse pressure Displaced LV impulse
Mitral regurgitation:						
Acute	Systolic (holosystolic)	Apex with diaphragm of stethoscope	Axilla	Soft or none	Normal or split	Jugular venous distention Apical thrill
Chronic	Systolic (holosystolic)	Base of heart	Neck or head	Soft	Normal or split	
Mitral valve prolapse	Systolic (mid to late)	Apex	None	Normal	Normal	Mid-systolic click

valves on chest radiography merits further investigation.

Two-dimensional echocardiography with color flow Doppler imaging has become the mainstay of investigation of cardiac murmurs. Echocardiography is used to determine the site and severity of valvular abnormalities and to detect secondary lesions or coexisting abnormalities such as thrombus formation and vegetation. Echocardiography is indicated for the evaluation of *asymptomatic* murmurs detected on auscultation, including continuous or diastolic murmurs, holosystolic or late systolic murmurs, grade 3 or higher midsystolic murmurs, and murmurs associated with abnormal findings on physical examination, ECG, or chest radiography. Echocardiography is also recommended for all *symptomatic* patients with possible valvular abnormality as well as for all patients with suspected bacterial endocarditis.[4]

In the patient in whom valvular abnormality is suspected, echocardiography is by far the best diagnostic tool. Limited ED echocardiography performed by the EP is adequate for the detection of the presence or absence of pericardial effusion and semi-qualitative assessment of contractility.[5] However, echocardiography for valvular assessment requires color flow Doppler imaging and particular expertise to determine the extent of stenosis and/or regurgitation and is best performed by an experienced echocardiologist. In the patient in extremis who has no history of valvular disorder or if physical findings are equivocal, bedside echocardiography by the EP should still be considered, especially to rule out other causes of cardiac dysfunction, such as cardiomyopathy (global hypokinesis) and pericardial effusion with tamponade. Bedside echocardiography can also be used to assess right ventricular dysfunction (pulmonary embolism) and hypovolemia (flat inferior vena cava) as well as other causes of shock, including abdominal hemorrhage.[6]

Differential Diagnosis

The differential diagnosis of valvular heart disease is broad and includes a number of other life-threatening disorders, such as acute myocardial infarction, acute decompensated congestive heart failure, and thoracic aortic dissection (Table 54-2). In the presence of recent myocardial infarction, valvular disorders may be mimicked by other structural complications, such as pericardial effusion with tamponade and rupture of the intraventricular septum or free wall. Patients sustaining blunt trauma may rarely present with traumatic aortic injury and, although rare, acute traumatic valvular injury as well. Acute valvular disorder should be considered in all cases of cardiogenic shock.[7]

Specific Valvular Disorders

■ AORTIC STENOSIS

Aortic stenosis most commonly results from progressive, premature calcification of a congenital bicuspid aortic valve, occurring at about the fifth decade of life, or through atherosclerosis of a normal valve, which most commonly occurs much later. Calcific degeneration of the aortic valve results from an inflammatory process similar to coronary artery disease, beginning with intimal injury and progressing through fusion of valve leaflets and stenosis of the aortic valve orifice. When rheumatic heart disease

Table 54-2 DIFFERENTIAL DIAGNOSIS AND PRIORITY ACTIONS

Chest pain	Is there a murmur associated with chest pain? Order ECG and evaluate for acute myocardial infarction resulting in papillary muscle dysfunction or rupture of the cordae tendineae. Obtain chest x-ray and consider thoracic aortic dissection in all patients with chest pain and murmur of aortic regurgitation. If the patient has had recent myocardial infarction, consider emergent echocardiography to rule out rupture of the intraventricular septum or free wall.
Dyspnea	Is there a murmur associated with dyspnea? Consider valvular abnormality in all patients with acute decompensated congestive heart failure (CHF). Consider pericarditis or myocarditis in patients with signs of CHF. Consider pulmonary embolism.
Syncope	Is there a murmur associated with syncope? Order ECG and consider severe aortic stenosis in all patients who present with syncope.
Trauma	Is there a murmur associated with trauma? Consider traumatic aortic injury in all patients who present with a history of trauma and signs or symptoms of aortic insufficiency. Consider traumatic valvular injury in patients with blunt trauma who present with unexplained hypotension or CHF.
Hypotension or shock	Is the patient in shock? Consider acute valvular decompensation in all patients who present with hypotension or cardiogenic shock. Perform bedside echocardiogram to rule out pericardial effusion with tamponade, global hypokinesis, and severe volume depletion. Consider cardiology consultation or emergency echocardiogram in patients with cardiogenic shock if valvular disease is suspected.
Fever	Is there a murmur associated with fever? Consider endocarditis in all patients with fever and either a murmur or a history of intravenous drug abuse.
Abdominal or back pain	Is there a murmur in association with abdominal pain? Consider ultrasonography to evaluate for hypovolemia, abdominal hemorrhage, and ruptured abdominal aortic aneurysm.

is the culprit, the aortic valve commonly exhibits both stenosis and regurgitation and is usually associated with concomitant mitral valve disease.[8]

Progression of aortic stenosis is usually quite slow, with symptoms taking decades to manifest in most cases. Medical management aims at delaying valve replacement until it becomes necessary. Sudden death is rare in patients with aortic stenosis before the development of symptoms. However, progression of stenosis can be unpredictable, and once it becomes significant, acute symptoms can develop quickly and without warning. Once symptoms manifest, valve replacement is necessary. Mean survival with uncorrected aortic stenosis is less than 3 years.

Aortic stenosis causes an increase in the pressure gradient across the aortic valve. Higher ventricular end-systolic pressure leads to increased left atrial pressure, ultimately resulting in symptoms of pulmonary congestion and dyspnea. Ventricular hypertrophy develops, raising myocardial oxygen demand and ultimately resulting in angina from subendocardial ischemia even in the absence of significant coronary artery disease. As the valve orifice size decreases, forward flow diminishes as well. When stenosis is less severe, cardiac output can be maintained. However, progressive stenosis leads to an inability to maintain cardiac output, first with exertion and ultimately at rest. As a result, syncope, especially with exertion, is a common presentation in aortic stenosis.

Aortic stenosis can usually be detected on cardiovascular examination. Auscultation reveals a systolic murmur associated with diminished and delayed carotid pulses (parvus et tardus), a sustained left ventricular impulse on palpation, and diminution or absence of the aortic component of the second heart sound (S_2). Parvus et tardus may not be readily apparent in the elderly owing to decreased compliance of the aging vasculature.

Management of patients with hemodynamically significant aortic stenosis is based on the primary symptom manifested. Patients with dyspnea and evidence of pulmonary vascular congestion should be treated with digoxin and the extremely judicious use of diuretics, because significant reduction in preload can severely worsen cardiac output and result in hypotension. In patients who present with chest pain or suspected ischemia, nitrates may be *carefully* employed, with consideration of how they will affect preload. Beta-blockers, although indicated in cases of suspected ischemia, should be used extremely cautiously in suspected aortic stenosis and should be avoided in patients with evidence of pulmonary congestion. Other drugs that act to depress contractility, such as calcium channel blockers, are not indicated.

As stated earlier, once symptoms develop in aortic stenosis, valve replacement is recommended within 1 month. Admission for all patients with symptomatic aortic stenosis is justified, to monitor for further decompensation and to facilitate further evaluation and management.

■ MITRAL STENOSIS

Mitral stenosis nearly always results from previous rheumatic fever. In fact, a history of rheumatic fever can be elicited in up to 60% of patients who present with mitral stenosis. A period of 20 to 40 years may transpire between the occurrence of rheumatic fever and the onset of symptoms. The ratio of women to men with mitral stenosis is 2:1. Mitral stenosis can also result from severe degenerative calcification, especially in the elderly. Fibrosis, calcification, and fusion of the mitral valve leaflets lead to a progressive rise in left atrial pressure, resulting in pulmonary vascular congestion. Dyspnea is the cardinal symptom of significant mitral stenosis.

In patients with mitral stenosis, cardiac output is significantly reduced by tachycardia, which shortens diastole and reduces the time for left ventricular filing. As a result, symptoms commonly occur at first with exercise, pregnancy, infection, or stress. As mitral stenosis worsens, left atrial pressure continues to rise, leading to atrial dilation and, commonly, atrial fibrillation in up to 40% of patients. When atrial fibrillation occurs with a rapid ventricular response, acute dyspnea and severe sudden pulmonary edema may result. Calcium channel blockers or beta-blockers may be administered to control the ventricular rate. In patients who are unstable, rapid heparinization and electrical cardioversion are indicated. In more stable patients who have had atrial fibrillation for more than 24 to 48 hours before presentation, cardioversion should be preceded by heparinization as well as by transesophageal echocardiography to rule out atrial thrombus before any attempts are made to restore normal sinus rhythm.

Patients who present with symptoms of pulmonary congestion and who are in sinus rhythm or atrial fibrillation with a well-controlled ventricular rate may be treated with preload reduction and diuretics. However, special care should be given to reducing preload gradually so as to not precipitate hypotension. Mitral stenosis is commonly associated with concomitant valvular disorders, most commonly aortic and tricuspid regurgitation. Hence, a careful search for other valvular abnormalities is warranted once mitral stenosis is confirmed. Patients with mild or moderate mitral stenosis may be managed medically for quite some time, until treatment with either balloon valvotomy or valve replacement becomes necessary.[9] Percutaneous valvotomy, although rarely definitive, has become an effective temporizing measure and is frequently employed as a bridge to surgery in critically ill patients or as a substitute for valve replacement in patients who have significant contraindications to surgery or who do not wish to have surgery. In patients who present in extremis, both cardiology and cardiothoracic surgery consultations are recommended.

■ AORTIC REGURGITATION

There are a number of etiologies for aortic regurgitation, including rheumatic heart disease, endocarditis, congenital (bicuspid) aortic valve, calcific degeneration, idiopathic dilation of the aortic root, and Marfan's syndrome. Most importantly, thoracic aortic dissection and traumatic aortic injury may manifest as evidence of acute aortic regurgitation if either involves the aortic valve.

Cardiac examination in patients with aortic regurgitation usually shows a murmur in diastole associated with a widened pulse pressure and displaced left ventricular impulse. Aortic regurgitation leads to an increase in both ventricular volume and afterload. When aortic regurgitation occurs gradually, the myocardium has time to compensate through progressive hypertrophy and dilation. When aortic regurgitation occurs suddenly, however, left ventricular end-diastolic pressure (and hence left atrial pressure) and end-diastolic volume rise abruptly, leading to decreases in stoke volume and cardiac output. Patients with acute aortic regurgitation commonly present in extremis with an unfortunate combination of pulmonary edema and systemic hypotension. To make matters worse, cardiac examination is often unhelpful in cases of acute aortic regurgitation, because pressure equilibrium between the aorta and the left ventricle leads to a short and soft diastolic murmur. Emergency bedside echocardiography with color flow Doppler imaging may be necessary to establish the diagnosis.

The goal of treatment in patients with aortic regurgitation is to minimize regurgitant volume and maximize cardiac output. In patients with aortic regurgitation, the magnitude of regurgitant volume is determined by both the pressure gradient across the diseased valve and the duration of diastole. Reduction of backflow may be significantly decreased by raising the heart rate and thus minimizing time in diastole.[10] In addition, multiple studies have shown that afterload reduction increases cardiac output and systemic oxygen delivery.[11] Hydralazine and sodium nitroprusside, which have both been studied in aortic regurgitation, may be administered to increase cardiac output and decrease regurgitant flow. Preexisting hypotension must be corrected with the administration of fluids and inotropic agents before vasodilator therapy is started. Intra-aortic balloon counterpulsation, which reduces afterload, would at first glance seem to be a good idea. However, it relies on an intact aortic valve during diastole and so is absolutely contraindicated in patients with aortic insufficiency.

■ MITRAL REGURGITATION

Mitral regurgitation occurs most commonly from myxomatous degeneration of the mitral valve apparatus. Degeneration of the mitral valve, which is more common in males and the elderly, is thought to be due to a genetic abnormality that results in a defect in the collagen making up the mitral valve, resulting in stretching of the valve leaflets and chordae tendineae. Mitral regurgitation may also develop acutely, especially in cases of acute myocardial infarction (through papillary muscle dysfunction, rupture of chordae tendineae cordis) or from infective endocarditis. Patients with mitral regurgitation usually exhibit a holosystolic murmur in association with a first heart sound (S_1) that is soft or absent, and, frequently, a normal second heart sound (S_2).

Regurgitation through the mitral valve apparatus leads to an increase in preload and an associated decrease in afterload. The amount of regurgitation, which is determined both by the size of the regurgitant orifice and the pressure gradient across the damaged valve, in turn determines the severity of pulmonary congestion and systemic circulation impairment. Anatomically, the actual size of the mitral valve orifice (in contrast to the aortic valve) is not fixed but in fact can be significantly modulated by changes in both preload and myocardial contractility. Efforts to decrease the actual size of regurgitant orifice include the use of inotropic agents to enhance contractility and of venodilators to reduce preload. Although one might think that reduction of preload could actually worsen regurgitant flow across the diseased mitral valve, studies have shown that the primary effect of preload reduction is a decrease in the size of the ventricle and, hence, of the regurgitant mitral valve orifice.[10]

Afterload reduction also improves forward flow and diminishes regurgitant volume by allowing blood to preferentially enter the systemic circulation during systole. In contrast to patients with aortic regurgitation, patients with mitral regurgitation commonly benefit from intra-aortic balloon counterpulsation. Thus the goal of therapy in mitral regurgitation is to decrease both preload and afterload while enhancing contractility.

BOX 54-1

American Heart Association Guidelines for Antibiotic Prophylaxis for Infective Endocarditis

Endocarditis Prophylaxis Recommended

High-risk category:

- Prosthetic cardiac valve(s)
- Previous bacterial endocarditis
- Complex cyanotic congenital heart disease (e.g., single ventricle states, transposition of the great arteries, tetralogy of Fallot)
- Surgically constructed systemic pulmonary shunts or conduits

Moderate-risk category:

- Most other congenital cardiac malformations
- Acquired valvular dysfunction (e.g., rheumatic heart disease)
- Hypertrophic cardiomyopathy
- Mitral valve prolapse *with* valvular regurgitation

Endocarditis Prophylaxis Not Recommended

Isolated secundum atrial septal defect

Surgical repair of atrial septal defect, ventricular septal defect, or patent ductus arteriosus (without residua beyond 6 months)

Previous coronary artery bypass graft surgery

Mitral valve prolapse *without* valvular regurgitation

Physiologic, functional, or innocent heart murmurs

Previous Kawasaki's disease without valvular dysfunction

Previous rheumatic fever without valvular dysfunction

Cardiac pacemakers or implantable defibrillators

From Dajani AS, Taubert KA, Wilson W, et al: Prevention of bacterial endocarditis: Recommendations by the American Heart Association. Circulation 1997;96:358-366.

■ MITRAL VALVE PROLAPSE

Mitral valve prolapse results when one or both mitral valve leaflets are sufficiently lax to result in abnormal protrusion into the left atrium during systole. Although this abnormality was once thought quite common, estimates of mitral valve prolapse based on newer diagnostic criteria suggest that less than 2.5% of the population is affected. Symptoms include chest pain, palpitations, anxiety, and dyspnea. Physical examination reveals a midsystolic click, frequently in association with a late systolic murmur. Patients with a suspicion of mitral valve prolapse should follow up with a cardiologist or primary care physician and should probably undergo echocardiography. Antibiotic prophylaxis for bacterial endocarditis is not recommended unless a murmur of mitral regurgitation is appreciated (Box 54-1).[12]

■ PROSTHETIC VALVE DISORDERS

Valve replacement surgery is a common procedure that has been significantly refined over the past 40 years. With advances in prosthetic development, surgical technique, and anesthetic management, valve replacement is well tolerated even in quite elderly patients. Prosthetic heart valves are divided into two broad classes, mechanical and biologic.

Mechanical valves have evolved considerably since their introduction in 1965, with the *Starr-Edwards* ball valve. Shortly thereafter, in 1969, disk valves were introduced with the introduction of the *Björk-Shiley* valve. Discontinued in the United States after more than 360,000 implantations, the *Björk-Shiley* valve is still frequently encountered in patients alive today. The traditional, modern mechanical valve remains the bileaflet *St. Jude* valve, which was introduced in 1977 and has that has undergone more than 600,000 implantations.

Biologic valves were developed to obviate the long-term systemic anticoagulation required for mechanical valves. The most common biologic valve in the United States is the porcine heterographic *Carpentier-Edwards* valve, which was introduced in 1977 and has undergone more than 400,000 implantations. In long-term studies, patients undergoing valve replacement with a mechanical valve generally enjoy better long-term survival and a longer period without the need for reoperation. However, complications from long-term anticoagulation do remain, and biologic valves make sense for many patients.

Complications associated with prosthetic valves are generally uncommon but include valvular deterioration, thrombosis, embolism, bleeding complications from anticoagulation, and endocarditis. Malfunction of a prosthetic valve may occur from thrombus or tissue ingrowth. Early complications from valve replacement surgery include mechanical dysfunction, loosening, periprosthetic regurgitation, and perioperative myocardial infarction. Valve complication should be considered in any patient with a prosthetic valve who presents with symptoms of dyspnea, syncope, or angina or with neurologic signs or symptoms. Absence of a murmur does not rule out prosthetic valve dysfunction. Cardiology consultation and admission for further evaluation are warranted.

■ PREGNANCY

Valvular heart disease is an uncommon complication of pregnancy that generally manifests in the first trimester as total blood volume and heart rate increase. Unfortunately, many of the symptoms and signs of valvular heart disease, including dyspnea, fatigue, and palpitations, are common complaints in pregnancy. Furthermore, a systolic flow murmur, often quite loud, is often appreciated in pregnancy. Cardiac echocardiography is often necessary to distinguish valvular heart disease from symptoms and signs of early pregnancy.[13]

Treatment and Disposition

In all patients with valvular heart disease, the goals of the EP are to (1) identify the problem, (2) determine whether valvular abnormality is the cause of the symptoms or presentation, and (3) optimize the hemodynamic status of patients who have suffered acute decompensation.

Asymptomatic patients with previously undetected heart murmur should undergo a thorough cardiopulmonary evaluation, including physical examination, ECG, and chest radiography. If evaluation detects an innocent murmur in an asymptomatic patient, no further evaluation is necessary, and routine follow-up with the patient's primary care physician is appropriate. If evaluation reveals a potentially significant murmur in an otherwise asymptomatic patient, echocardiography and referral to a cardiologist are recommended.

It is critical to consider valvular heart disease as a cause of symptoms in all patients presenting with dyspnea, chest pain, syncope, or other cardiopulmonary symptoms, such as cough, hemoptysis, presyncope, and lightheadedness. Echocardiography is recommended for all symptomatic patients in whom physical examination shows signs of valvular abnormality, as are admission and cardiology consultation.

Valvular abnormality should be considered in all patients presenting in acute heart failure or cardiogenic shock. As stated previously, absence of detectable murmur on physical examination does not rule out significant valvular dysfunction, especially in the patient with shock, decreased cardiac output, or a prosthetic heart valve. Emergency echocardiography should be strongly considered.

Management of patients with an acute valvular decompensation requiring stabilization and hemodynamic support is similar to that of any critically ill patient. First, attention should be paid to control of the airway and adequacy of ventilation. Determination of circulation includes assessment of pulse, blood pressure, and systemic oxygen delivery. Skin color, temperature, capillary refill time, and measurement of arterial base deficit or serum lactate should be assessed. Maneuvers should then be undertaken to improve forward cardiac output to meet systemic oxygen demand.

Optimization of oxygen delivery in cases of acute valvular disorders requires a thorough understanding that maximizing cardiac output and systemic oxygen delivery does not necessarily mean increasing blood pressure. Similarly, patients with pulmonary congestion may not all benefit from significant reduction of circulating volume or preload. In most patients with acute valvular decompensation, there is evidence of pulmonary vascular congestion without hypotension. In general, all patients who are hypotensive should benefit from volume infusion unless they exhibit overt signs or symptoms of pulmonary edema. However, this statement may be less true for patients with mitral regurgitation, in whom greater preload may result in an increase in mitral orifice size and, thus, and in regurgitant volume. Once volume status has been optimized, further therapy is dictated by the type and severity of the valvular lesion. Emergency echocardiography should be strongly considered. In patients in whom an acute coronary syndrome is a possibility, emergency diagnostic cardiac catheterization may be appropriate.

Disposition

There is little rationale for discharging patients from the ED with newly abnormal cardiac examination findings or suspected valvular abnormality who have presented with symptoms ascribable to valvular disease. The timing for definitive management, both surgical and medical, for nearly all valvular disorders begins with the onset of symptoms, and admission of patients for further evaluation is indicated. For selected patients with equivocal cardiac examination findings, cardiology consultation or echocardiography prior to ED discharge may be warranted.

Patients who present with evidence of congestive heart failure or unstable vital signs in the presence of valvular disorder are at high risk for further acute decompensation. Admission of such patients to the intensive care unit for monitoring and further management is recommended.

REFERENCES

1. Bonow RO, Carabello B, de Leon AC Jr, et al: ACC/AHA guidelines for the management of patients with valvular heart disease: A report of the American College of Cardiology/American Heart Association Task Force on Practice Guidelines (Committee on Management of Patients with Valvular Heart Disease). J Am Coll Cardiol 1998;32:1486-588.
2. Boon NA, Bloomfield P: The medical management of valvular heart disease. Heart 2001;87:395-400.
3. Rahimtoola SH, Durairaj A, Mehra A, Nuno I: Current evaluation and management of patients with mitral stenosis. Circulation 2002;106:1183-1188.
4. Cheitlin MD, Alpert JS, Armstrong WF, et al: ACC/AHA Guidelines for the Clinical Application of Echocardiography: A report of the American College of Cardiology/American Heart Association Task Force on Practice Guidelines (Committee on Clinical Application of Echocardiography). Circulation 1997;95:1686-1744.
5. American College of Emergency Physicians: ACEP emergency ultrasound guidelines—2001. Ann Emerg Med 2001;38:470-481.
6. Randazzo MR, Snoey ER, Levitt MA, Binder K: Accuracy of emergency physician assessment of left ventricular ejection fraction and central venous pressure using echocardiography. Acad Emerg Med 2003;10:973-977.
7. Hollenberg SM, Kavinsky CJ, Parrillo JE: Cardiogenic shock. Ann Intern Med 1999;131:47-59.
8. Carabello BA: Evaluation and management of patients with aortic stenosis. Circulation 2002;105:1746-1750.
9. Carabello BA: Modern management of mitral stenosis. Circulation 2005;112:432-437.
10. Judge TP, Kennedy JW, Bennett LJ, et al: Quantitative hemodynamic effects of heart rate in aortic regurgitation. Circulation 1971;44:355-367.
11. Miller RR, Vismara LA, DeMaria AN, et al: Afterload reduction therapy with nitroprusside in severe aortic regurgitation: Improved cardiac performance and reduced regurgitant volume. Am J Cardiol 1976;38:564-567.
12. Dajani AS, Taubert KA, Wilson W, et al: Prevention of bacterial endocarditis: Recommendations by the American Heart Association. Circulation 1997;96:358-366.
13. Elkayam U, Bitar F: Valvular heart disease and pregnancy. Part I: Native valves. J Am Coll Cardiol 2005;46:223-230.

Chapter **55**

Endocarditis

Osman R. Sayan and Wallace A. Carter

KEY POINTS

Endocarditis is an inflammation of the endothelial lining of the heart. It is usually focal and commonly occurs at points of endocardial injury. Heart valves, especially the mitral and aortic valves, are the most common sites of involvement.

Most sites of endocarditis become seeded with bacteria during episodes of transient bacteremia and thus become symptomatic. This is known as infective endocarditis.

The initial symptoms are often vague—low-grade fever, malaise, and weakness.

Presentations can vary from direct structural cardiac injury to conduction system disturbances to embolic phenomena to cardiogenic or septic shock.

Suspicion of infective endocarditis should be raised by the presence of well-known risk factors, such as acquired or congenital valvular or structural heart disease, a prosthetic valve, implanted medical devices, injection drug use, and previous history of endocarditis.

Laboratory testing is often not useful for the EP, but at least three sets of blood cultures performed over time are critical for diagnosis of infective endocarditis as well as for guiding subsequent therapy.

The most useful initial diagnostic test is echocardiography.

In the acutely ill patient, prompt resuscitation, antibiotics, and surgical consultation are imperative.

In the stable patient with subacute disease, the time to antibiotic therapy is less critical, and the performance of serial blood cultures more important.

Nearly all patients with infective endocarditis are admitted to the hospital. Only the most stable patient with no complications in whom the diagnosis of infective endocarditis is being entertained but not confirmed may be discharged with very close follow-up care.

Despite medical advances, the overall mortality for both native valve and prosthetic valve infective endocarditis still ranges from 20% to 25%.[1]

Prevention of the disease is most important. The American Heart Association has issued guidelines for antibiotic prophylaxis in patients at risk for endocarditis.

Scope

Endocarditis is an inflammation of the endothelium, or inner lining, of the heart and/or heart valves. The disrupted endothelium is very susceptible to seeding with infectious agents such as bacteria, viruses, and fungi. This entity is known as *infective endocarditis* (IE). Known to medical science for more than 400 years, IE remains an illness that is difficult to diagnose and treat and that can still have significant morbidity and mortality.

Published reports regarding the overall incidence of IE over the last 30 years have conflictingly cited both a stable incidence and a rising incidence.[1-3] Mortality ranges from 5% to 50% or higher. Why is there such variation in the statistics? Infective endocarditis is a diverse and evolving disease entity—one that is strongly influenced by the characteristics of both the human and microbial populations being studied (Table 55-1).

In the developed world, IE has undergone a remarkable change over the last century. In the developing world, however, it has remained rather unchanged.

Table 55-1 STATISTICS FOR INFECTIVE ENDOCARDITIS (IE) IN THE DEVELOPED WORLD

Median age of IE patients in the pre-antibiotic era	30-40 years of age
Median age of IE patients in the antibiotic era	47-69 years of age
Mean male-to-female ratio	1.7:1
Incidence of community-acquired native-valve IE (Western Europe/USA)	1.7-6.2 cases per 100,000 person-years
Incidence of IE among persons with known mitral valve prolapse	100 cases per 100,000 person-years
Incidence of IE among injection drug users	150-2000 cases per 100,000 person-years
Prosthetic valve IE	7-25% of all cases of IE
Overall mortality for both native and prosthetic valve IE	20-25%
Mortality with viridans group Streptococci and *Streptococcus bovis* IE	4-16%
Mortality with enterococci IE	15-25%
Mortality with Q fever IE	5-37%
Mortality with *Staphylococcus aureus* IE	25-47%
Mortality with *Pseudomonas aeruginosa*, enterobacteriacaea, or fungi IE	more than 50%

Adapted from Mylonakis E, Calderwood SB: Infective endocarditis in adults. N Engl J Med 2001;345:1318-1330.

We are indebted to Dr. Ahmet R. Sayan (Cardiology) for his critical appraisal of this manuscript.

Much of this difference is a result of the influence of advances in health care (e.g., antibiotics, disease prevention, medical devices, the resulting longevity of populations) as well as the complications that arise from these advances (e.g., nosocomial infections and resistant organisms).[4,5]

Unfortunately, the tremendous advances made in health care have not translated into the gains we have seen in other infectious diseases in the last 50 to 80 years. Untreated IE has a mortality of nearly 100%. Treated IE is still associated with a mortality rate of 20-25%.[5] The overall incidence of IE in the developed world has remained unchanged.[1] Why has the advent of antibiotics, advanced critical care and surgical techniques, and medical devices such as prosthetic valves not made a difference in this statistic? There are several reasons.

First, with a low prevalence, no pathognomonic signs or symptoms, and no single diagnostic front-line test, IE remains difficult to diagnose. Therefore, many cases are missed and/or manifest when the disease is advanced. Second, despite the effective control of rheumatic heart disease in the developed world, new risk factors have arisen to fill the void. Degenerative heart disease in the growing elderly population has replaced rheumatic fever as the major cause of valvular disease. The same intravascular medical devices that have improved survival for patients (valvular prosthesis, cardiac pacemakers, long-term indwelling vascular catheters, etc.) predispose them to the development of IE (whether or not they have had IE in the past). Third, other high-risk groups have increased in number—the elderly, patients receiving critical care, and patients with immunocompromise (because of acquired immunodeficiency syndrome [AIDS], diabetes mellitus, end-stage renal disease, chemotherapy, etc.). Risky social behaviors, such as body piercing and injection drug use, are practiced more today than in the early 20th century. Finally, and most concerning of all, a burgeoning antibiotic resistance is making treatment of IE more challenging and sometimes unachievable.[6]

Because prevention and early diagnosis of this disease are the keys to reducing the morbidity and mortality related to IE, EPs must play an important role in this process. We must be vigilant. The subtle symptoms manifesting in a patient with IE risk factors should alert us to include this condition in the differential diagnoses. We must not forget to educate patients at high risk for IE and provide IE prophylaxis to those in whom it is warranted.

Pathophysiology

The term endocarditis literally means inflammation of the inner lining or endothelium of the heart and/or lining of heart valves. Local or systemic stressors, such as trauma, blood-borne contaminants (talc from injection drug use), inflammation, and abnormal blood turbulence, induce injury to the endothelium.

Clinically relevant endocarditis results from the formation of a fibrin and platelet cap on the area of altered surface endothelium. Most commonly, a sterile cap forms at a site of endothelial injury. IE occurs when microbes adhere to these sites of sterile endothelial injury during transient periods of bacteremia, fungemia, or viremia. Colonization occurs, followed by microbial multiplication and growth of each cap into a vegetation (Figs. 55-1 and 55-2). Because of their direct contact with the blood stream, these infections cause a continuous albeit low-level presence of microbes in the blood. The clinical manifestations of endocarditis are quite varied. It is this variation in manifestations that often makes endocarditis difficult to identify. Clinical manifestations can be immunologic, infectious, or embolic.

Microbiology of Infective Endocarditis

Although the microbiology of IE can predict the course of a patient's illness and guide therapy, the actual infecting organism is only rarely known to the EP. The EP needs to know the microbes that cause IE (Box 55-1) and the local resistance patterns so as to make sound choices regarding empirical antibiotic treatment regimens. This section discusses the organisms most commonly associated with IE.[6] Certain patient characteristics and clinical scenarios are associated with certain microorganisms (Table 55-2). These scenarios may guide the EP's empirical antibiotic choice; these regimens are discussed later in this chapter (see Box 55-8).

■ BACTERIA

■ Viridans Group Streptococci

Streptococcus viridans, formerly a species name, is actually a group of gram-positive cocci. This group has been the most common cause of IE, although

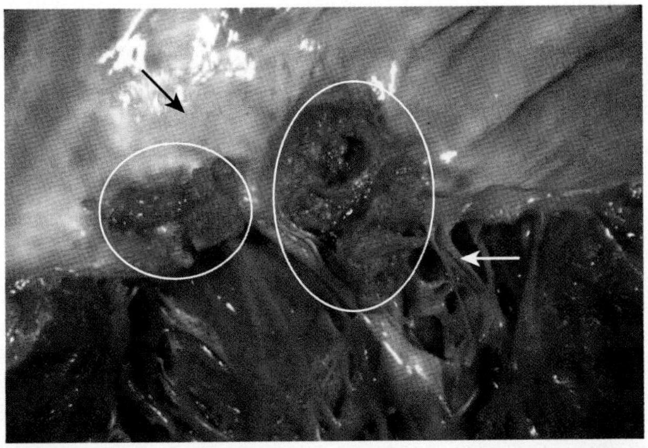

FIGURE 55-1 Large vegetations (*circles*) at edge of this mitral valve (*black arrow*). Chordae tendineae (*white arrow*) connect the mitral valve to papillary muscles in the left ventricle. (Courtesy of Charles C. Marboe, MD.)

BOX 55-1

Microorganisms that Cause Infective Endocarditis

Most Common

Staphylococcus aureus

Viridans group Streptococci

Enterococci

Less Common

Streptococcus bovis

Streptococcus pneumoniae

Staphylococcus epidermidis

Pseudomonas aeruginosa

Culture-negative bacteria:

- *Abiotrophia* spp
- *Bartonella* spp (usually *henselae* or *quintana*)
- *Brucella* spp (usually *melitensis* or *abortus*)
- *Chlamydia* spp (usually *psittaci*)
- *Coxiella burnetii* (Q fever)
- HACEK group of gram-negative bacteria*
- *Legionella* spp
- *Tropheryma whippelii*

Fungi

**Haemophilus* species, *Actinobacillus actinomycetemcomitans, Cardiobacterium hominis, Eikenella corrodens,* and *Kingella kingae.*

Adapted from Baddour LM, Wilson WR, Bayer AS, et al; Committee on Rheumatic Fever, Endocarditis, and Kawasaki Disease; Council on Cardiovascular Disease in the Young; Councils on Clinical Cardiology, Stroke, and Cardiovascular Surgery and Anesthesia; American Heart Association; Infectious Diseases Society of America: Infective endocarditis: Diagnosis, antimicrobial therapy, and management of complications. A statement for healthcare professionals from the Committee on Rheumatic Fever, Endocarditis, and Kawasaki Disease, Council on Cardiovascular Disease in the Young, and the Councils on Clinical Cardiology, Stroke, and Cardiovascular Surgery and Anesthesia, American Heart Association: endorsed by the Infectious Diseases Society of America. Circulation 2005;111: e394-e434.

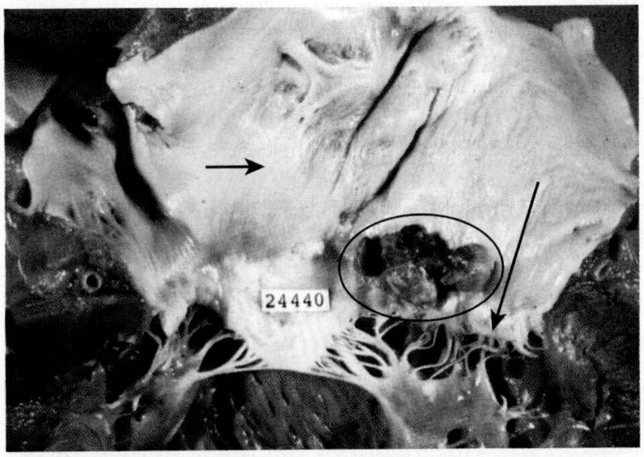
24440

FIGURE 55-2 Large vegetation (*black circle*) in a patient with endocarditis. *Short arrow* indicates the endocardial surface of the dilated left atrium, and *long arrow* indicates the edge of the mitral valve and chordae tendineae. (Courtesy of Charles C. Marboe, MD.)

Table 55-2 CHARACTERISTICS OF PATIENTS WITH INFECTIOUS ENDOCARDITIS (IE) AND THE ASSOCIATED MICROORGANISMS

Characteristic(s)	Organism	Course/Facts*
Community-acquired IE of a native valve	Viridans group Streptococci	Indolent gram-positive bacteria Most common cause(s) of native valve endocarditis Usually seeds damaged cardiac tissue
	Staphylococcus aureus	Aggressive gram-positive bacterium Some new case series identify *S. aureus* as new most common cause of IE Can seed normal valves
Prosthetic valve IE<1 month after surgery	*Staphylococcus epidermidis*	Aggressive gram-positive bacterium
Prosthetic valve IE>1 month after surgery	*S. aureus*	Aggressive gram-positive bacterium
Elderly patient	Enterococci	Usually a subacute presentation Difficult to treat because of intrinsic antibiotic resistance GI flora Typically affects older men after genitourinary manipulation or middle-aged women after obstetric procedures
Elderly patient with GI process	*Streptococcus bovis*	Can be aggressive Gram-positive bacterium Associated with inflammatory bowel disease, colonic polyps, and colon cancer
Injection drug user	*S. aureus*	Aggressive gram-positive bacterium Most common cause of tricuspid valve IE Usually multiple-valve involvement Often oxacillin-resistant
	Viridans group Streptococci	Indolent gram-positive bacteria Usually cause left-sided IE in injection drug users
	Pseudomonas aeruginosa	Aggressive gram-negative bacterium Usually multiple-valve involvement
	Fungi	Patient usually very ill Large vegetations often embolize Surgical intervention commonly needed
Patient is critically ill, is being treated in intensive care unit, or is immunocompromised	Fungi	Patient usually very ill Rare Large vegetations often embolize Surgical intervention commonly needed
	P. aeruginosa	Aggressive gram-negative bacterium Rare Usually multiple-valve involvement

GI, gastrointestinal; IE, infectious endocarditis.

*Data from Baddour LM, Wilson WR, Bayer AS, et al: Committee on Rheumatic Fever, Endocarditis, and Kawasaki Disease; Council on Cardiovascular Disease in the Young; Councils on Clinical Cardiology, Stroke, and Cardiovascular Surgery and Anesthesia; American Heart Association; Infectious Diseases Society of America: Infective endocarditis: Diagnosis, antimicrobial therapy, and management of complications. A statement for healthcare professionals from the Committee on Rheumatic Fever, Endocarditis, and Kawasaki Disease, Council on Cardiovascular Disease in the Young, and the Councils on Clinical Cardiology, Stroke, and Cardiovascular Surgery and Anesthesia, American Heart Association: endorsed by the Infectious Diseases Society of America. Circulation 2005;111: e394-e434.

later case series have shown that *Staphylococcus aureus* may be more common.[6] These streptococci usually seed previously damaged cardiac tissue. The clinical presentation is usually more insidious, with patients experiencing malaise, weakness, and low-grade fever.

■ *Staphylococcus aureus*

Studies have now identified *S. aureus* rather than the viridans group of streptococci as the most common cause of IE.[1] This organism can infect normal valvular endothelium—that is, endothelium without antecedent damage or disease—and usually causes aggressive valve destruction. It is associated with injection drug use as well as with prosthetic valve endocarditis that occurs more than 1 month after surgery. Increasing drug resistance is making *S. aureus* a more formidable organism to treat.

■ *Staphylococcus epidermidis*

Staphylococcus epidermidis is an organism associated with prosthetic valve endocarditis, especially that occurring within 1 month of surgery. The course of IE due to this organism is usually aggressive.

■ *Streptococcus bovis*

Infective endocarditis due to *Streptococcus bovis* occurs more commonly in the elderly and often originates from a gastrointestinal (GI) source. It is commonly associated with GI polyps, inflammatory bowel disease, or GI malignancy.

Streptococcus pneumoniae

Streptococcus pneumoniae is an aggressive organism, often causing an acute, fulminant illness. It can infect normal heart valves, most often the aortic valve, with a high risk for formation of perivalvular abscesses or pericarditis. Pneumococcal endocarditis can occur in association with pneumococcal pneumonia and meningitis in a grouping called *Austrian's triad.*

Enterococci

Enterococci are normal flora of the GI tract and, occasionally, the anterior urethra. IE due to one of these organisms usually runs a subacute course, but cure is often difficult because of the bacteria's intrinsic resistance to antibiotics. There is a high relapse rate after standard therapy. Typically this problem presents in older men after genitourinary manipulation and in middle-aged women after obstetric procedures.

Pseudomonas aeruginosa

A rare cause of IE, *Pseudomonas aeruginosa* is an aggressive gram-negative bacterium. Infective endocarditis due to this organism usually complicates the course of critically ill patients and injection drug users.

Culture-Negative Bacteria

The "culture-negative" bacteria group infrequently causes IE. These bacteria are characterized as "culture-negative" because they are either slow to grow in routine media, require special media to grow, or are not culturable. The clinician must ask that blood cultures be held for prolonged incubation periods (14-21 days), request special culture media on the basis of clinical suspicion, or utilize the serologic and polymerase chain reaction assays available for some of these bacteria. A list of the culture-negative bacteria is provided in Box 55-1.

The HACEK bacteria (*Haemophilus* species, *Actinobacillus actinomycetemcomitans, Cardiobacterium hominis, Eikenella corrodens,* and *Kingella kingae*) are normal bacteria that commonly colonize the human oropharynx. Interestingly, Petti and colleagues[7] have called into question the categorization of HACEK organisms as "culture-negative." These researchers identified all positive blood culture results over a 16-month period at four centers. Of 15,826 positive blood cultures, a HACEK organism was isolated from 16 (0.1%). The mean and median time to detection of HACEK isolates were 3.4 and 3 days, respectively. These findings very closely paralleled 12-year data from Duke University Medical Center as well as later case reports. Petti and colleagues[7] assert that modern culture techniques allow for the identification of all HACEK-positive cultures within the standard incubation period for blood cultures of 5 days and that the cost of tens of thousands of blood cultures held for prolonged incubation periods (14-21 days) is not justified. Fortunately, the decision about blood cultures is made by the inpatient service, not the EP.

FUNGI

Fungi are rarely a cause of endocarditis, but fungal IE has a high mortality. *Candida* species are responsible for most cases of fungal IE. *Aspergillus* species are also seen. Fungal IE tends to occur in patients with cardiac abnormalities, medical devices (prosthetic valves, long-term indwelling vascular catheters), some level of compromised immunity (human immunodeficiency virus, malignancy, organ transplantation), and injection drug users.[8] Fungal IE usually produces large vegetations and is an indication for surgical intervention.

Presenting Signs and Symptoms

Infective endocarditis can vary greatly in the severity of its presentation. Depending on the extent of the injury, location of injury, microorganism involved, and comorbidities in the patient, IE can be an insidious chronic or subacute disease or an aggressive, rapidly debilitating process. EPs are challenged to make the diagnosis when the presentation is subtle—often ascribing symptoms to a more benign diagnosis, such as a nonspecific viral syndrome. EPs are also challenged to make the diagnosis when the presentation is acute and critical—often diagnosing congestive heart failure (CHF), sepsis, heart block, or stroke but failing to identify the underlying cause (endocarditis), which will continue to cause morbidity and possibly mortality if not treated directly.

EPs must rely on maintaining high clinical suspicion in situations associated with IE. Patients at high risk for IE are listed in Box 55-2. In these patients, presentations of sepsis, embolization, or cardiac failure/shock should warrant an evaluation for endocarditis. By understanding the pathophysiology of this disease, the clinician can predict the signs and symptoms that might be seen with IE.

CLASSIC TRIAD

The triad consisting of fever, heart murmur, and anemia has classically been ascribed to the diagnosis of IE. Unfortunately, the sensitivity and specificity of these characteristics for diagnosing endocarditis are poor. The clinician must combine these findings with high-risk patient characteristics (see Box 55-2).

BOX 55-2

Risk Factors for Infective Endocarditis

- Acquired or congenital valvular and structural heart disease, including mitral valve prolapse, rheumatic heart disease, and hypertrophic cardiomyopathy
- Prosthetic valves, including bioprosthetics
- Implantable medical devices (cardiac pacemakers, long-term indwelling vascular catheters, implantable defibrillators)
- Injection drug use
- Poor dental hygiene
- Long-term hemodialysis
- Diabetes mellitus
- Previous history of endocarditis
- Immunocompromised states

Adapted from Mylonakis E, Calderwood SB: Infective endocarditis in adults. N Engl J Med 2001;345:1318-1330.

■ ORGAN-SPECIFIC CLINICAL FINDINGS

Most commonly, patients with IE present with symptoms of malaise and fatigue in the setting of low-grade fever. Most of this probably reflects the immunologic response to constant bacteremia. Patients may complain of generalized weakness with anorexia and weight loss. Without high clinical suspicion, these patients can often be diagnosed with a nonspecific viral syndrome.

■ Vascular Signs and Symptoms

Septic embolization of the vasa vasorum (blood vessels that feed large blood vessels) can lead to the formation of mycotic aneurysms in any of the body's larger arteries. Patients can present with pain, lightheadedness, altered mental status, and even syncope from the vascular insufficiency and/or hemorrhage that may occur at any of the sites of involvement.

Signs and symptoms that may be seen with involvement of specific vascular sites are as follows:

- Central nervous system (CNS) arteries—headache, focal neurologic deficits, confusion
- Sinus of Valsalva—pleuritic chest pain, muffled heart tones
- Hepatic artery—right upper quadrant pain, hematemesis
- Splenic artery—abdominal pain, intra-abdominal hemorrhage
- Renal arteries—flank pain, hematuria
- Intestinal arteries—abdominal pain, intraabdominal hemorrhage, melena, hematochezia.

■ Cardiac Signs and Symptoms

Cardiac symptoms of IE include chest pain, shortness of breath, lightheadedness, and even syncope. These symptoms can come from a variety of heart-specific processes.

Valvular damage can lead to valvular insufficiency (and murmur). This may progress to CHF and even frank cardiogenic shock. This is especially true with left-sided valve involvement. With right-sided valve endocarditis, right heart failure with hepatosplenomegaly and peripheral edema might be evident.

Intracardiac abscess formation causes clinical compromise in a number of ways depending on the cardiac structure involved. Erosion into the conduction system can lead to all manner of heart blocks, including complete heart block. Involvement of the valvular annulus can cause valvular incompetence and heart failure, or may lead to erosion into the pericardial space and cardiac tamponade. Cardiac wall abscess can give rise to septal or free wall rupture or valvular compromise by papillary muscle rupture.

Embolization of endocarditis vegetations to the coronary arteries can cause diffuse myocarditis via diffuse seeding of the myocardium. Myocardial infarction may occur through direct intraluminal embolization and coronary artery occlusion or through embolic seeding of the coronary vasovasorum and the formation of coronary mycotic aneurysms.

■ Pulmonary Signs and Symptoms

Pulmonary complaints need not be present in IE. Common pulmonary symptoms are dyspnea and cough. Pulmonary complaints related to embolization may accompany right-sided IE—tricuspid or pulmonic valve endocarditis. Patients may present with pneumonia due to pulmonary septic emboli. Ventilation-perfusion mismatching may develop from pulmonary embolization. Left-sided endocarditis can lead to pulmonary congestion secondary to cardiac failure and acute pulmonary edema.

■ Neurologic and Psychiatric Signs and Symptoms

Endocarditis can manifest as a myriad of neurologic and psychiatric signs and symptoms. Most of these are the direct result of CNS embolization. Presentations may include headache, complex behavioral changes, confusion, seizure, and stroke. The diagnosis of IE can be hard to make because of the large differential diagnosis list for these symptoms. The pathophysiology is usually the result of embolization of the CNS by septic emboli resulting in microinfarction or macroinfarction, abscess formation, and/or meningitis.

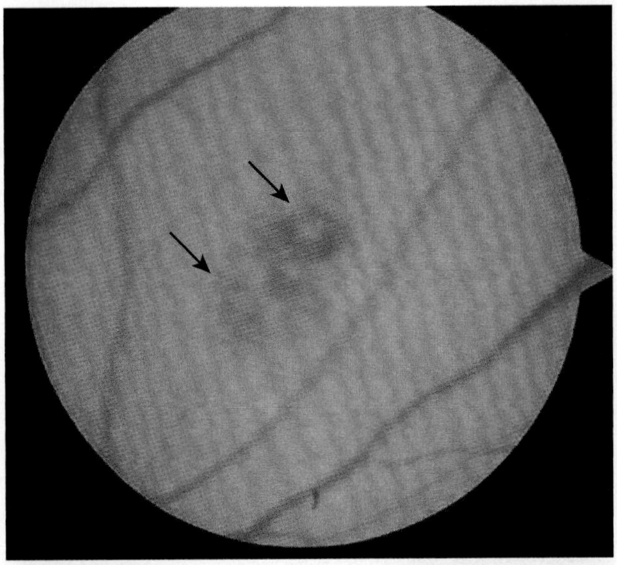

FIGURE 55-3 Roth's spots. Septic microemboli to the retinal arteries result in infarction. Ischemic cotton-wool centers are surrounded by hemorrhagic halos. These spots are *not* pathognomonic for endocarditis. (From Mandell GL, Bennett JE, Dolin R [eds]: Principles and Practice of Infectious Diseases, 6th ed. Philadephia, Churchill Livingstone, 2005).

■ Ophthalmologic Signs and Symptoms

The eye is not immune to possible involvement in endocarditis. Both embolic and immune phenomena can affect the optic nerves, ophthalmic vessels, conjunctivae, and retina. Presenting complaints may include painless conjunctival hemorrhages, visual field cuts, and even frank monocular blindness. Emboli can cause infarction of the ophthalmic or retinal vessels, leading to vision loss. Hemorrhages with pale cotton-wool centers known as Roth's spots can be visualized on the retina of patients with IE (Fig. 55-3). EPs should be aware that these spots are not pathognomonic for IE but rather, if seen, should raise suspicion of this disease. Painless subconjunctival hemorrhages (Fig. 55-4), petechiae involving the conjunctivae, can also be present and are again nonspecific.

■ Hematopoietic Signs and Symptoms

Weakness and fatigue can result from anemia, which can be associated with IE. Usually the anemia is normocytic and mild. IE can also stimulate an immune response marked by leukocytosis and splenomegaly.

■ Gastrointestinal Signs and Symptoms

Nausea and vomiting are very nonspecific symptoms. In the IE patients, these may accompany complications such as myocardial infarction, pulmonary edema, and processes that increase intracranial pressure. Abdominal pain in IE may be a manifestation of a nonspecific ileus, mesenteric ischemia from mesenteric emboli, or mycotic aneurysms of the splanchnic vasculature.

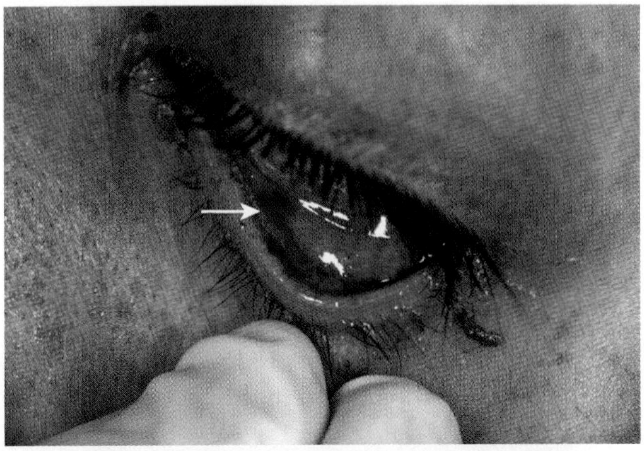

FIGURE 55-4 Subconjunctival hemorrhage (*arrow*) in patient with *Viridans group Streptococci* endocarditis. (Courtesy of Marc E. Grossman, MD, FACP.)

■ Renal Signs and Symptoms

Emboli to the kidneys can result in abscess formation, ischemia, and infarction. The resultant flank pain, pyuria, and/or hematuria may easily be misdiagnosed as renal colic from urolithiasis or pyelonephritis. Hematuria can also be a manifestation of glomerulonephritis from immune complex deposition related to IE.

■ Dermatologic Signs and Symptoms

The skin can give great clues to the presence of IE. Classic findings are Janeway lesions, Osler's nodes, and splinter hemorrhages.

Janeway lesions are small, painless hemorrhages with a macular or slightly nodular character (Fig. 55-5). They are found on the thenar and hypothenar eminences of the palms and soles. The histologic findings are usually consistent with septic microemboli. Bacteria have been cultured from these lesions. Janeway lesions are usually present for days to weeks before healing. They are most often associated with acute IE from *S. aureus*.

Osler's nodes are small, tender, red to purple nodules. They are most often found on the pulp of the distal phalanges of the fingers and toes, the soles, and the thenar and hypothenar eminences of the palms (Fig. 55-6). Preceding the appearance of the nodes, patients often experience neuropathic pain. Although these nodes were initially believed to be purely immunologic in nature, reports have now isolated bacteria from them. It has been postulated that early microembolization with microabscess formation is followed by an immune-mediated hypersensitivity vasculitis. Osler's nodes can appear at any point in the course of IE and can last a few hours to several days. They tend to be associated with subacute IE.

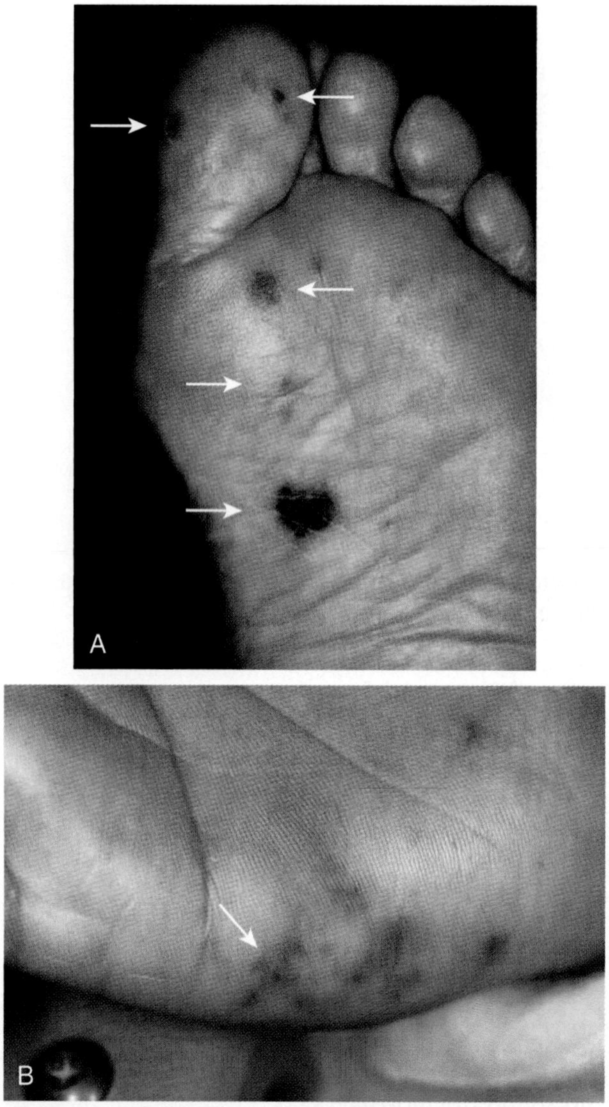
A
B

FIGURE 55-5 Janeway lesions. These nontender, often hemorrhagic, lesions (*arrows*) are most commonly associated with *Staphylococcus aureus* endocarditis. They result from septic microembolization. The lesions are usually macular to slightly nodular and involve the soles (**A**) and the thenar hypothenar eminences of the palms (**B**). (From Mandell GL, Bennett JE, Dolin R [eds]: Principles and Practice of Infectious Diseases, 6th ed. Philadephia, Churchill Livingstone, 2005. **B**, courtesy of Marc E. Grossman, MD, FACP.)

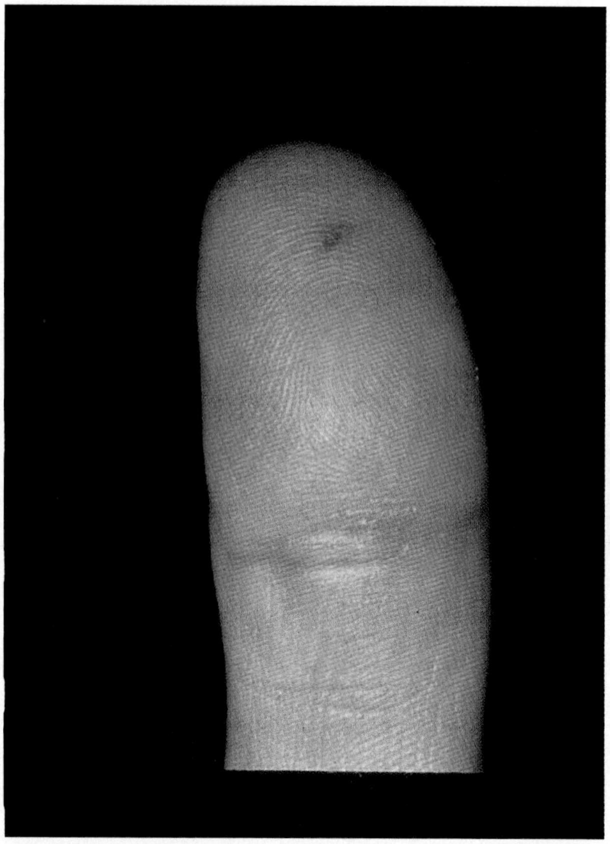

FIGURE 55-6 Osler's nodes. (From Cohen J, Powderly WG [eds]: Infectious Diseases, 2nd ed. Philadephia, Mosby, 2004.)

Splinter hemorrhages are linear petechiae visible on the nail beds of affected patients (Fig. 55-7). They do not blanch when pressure is applied to the nail and are better seen if a bright light is shone directly into the distal tip of the digit.

Differential Diagnosis

Owing to the many clinical manifestations of IE, the differential diagnosis list is overwhelmingly large. Broad areas include infectious/febrile illnesses as well as cardiovascular, neurologic, psychiatric, gastrointestinal, renal, dermatologic, and immunologic disorders (Box 55-3). Most interestingly, the presentations of IE have many causes. The EP can make a diagnosis without the realization that the underlying cause is IE. For example, a cerebrovascular accident or myocardial infarction may be secondary to the embolization or mycotic aneurysms of IE; this fact is important, because the treatment must also focus on treating IE.

The *most common* illness in the differential diagnosis list for IE is febrile illness of any source. Viral syndromes, pneumonia, and urinary infections may cause fever, weakness, behavioral abnormalities, and even hemodynamic instability.

The *most life-threatening* entities are aortic catastrophes, myocardial infarction (with or without acute valve failure), complete heart block, massive pulmonary embolism, cerebrovascular accident, and sepsis.

As mentioned frequently in this chapter, high clinical suspicion guided by knowledge of risk factors (see Box 55-2) is the key to including IE in this long, complex differential diagnosis list.

Diagnosis

Contributing to the complexity of IE is the fact that there is neither a single rapid test to diagnose the disorder nor any routine ancillary test that hints at the diagnosis. Some physical findings might clue the

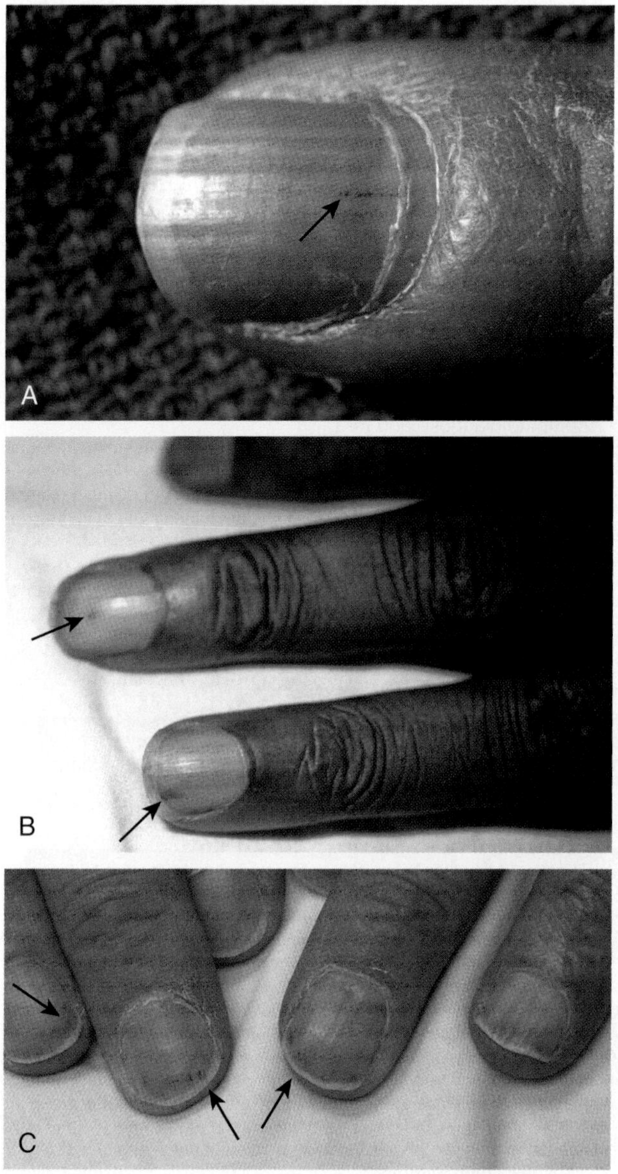
A
B
C

FIGURE 55-7 **A** to **C**, Splinter hemorrhages. These appear as narrow, red to reddish-brown hemorrhages beneath the nails that tend to run in the direction of nail growth. Most commonly caused by trauma, splinter hemorrhages are associated with endocarditis and may represent vessel damage from vasculitis or microemboli. (**A** and **B** courtesy of Marc E. Grossman, MD, FACP; **C** used with permission from Johns Hopkins University and obtained online from www.vasculitis.med.jhu.edu/typesof/polyangiitis.html/)

EP to this diagnosis, but they are nonspecific. For the EP, the most important tool for diagnosing IE is *clinical suspicion.* Elements of history known to identify patients at high risk for endocarditis must trigger this suspicion, which should lead the EP to focus on physical findings typical of endocarditis. With a high suspicion for IE based on history and physical findings, the EP must order serial blood cultures and an echocardiogram to confirm the diagnosis. A diagnostic algorithm is shown in Figure 55-8.

The most accepted diagnostic schema for IE is the *modified Duke criteria* (Box 55-4).[9] Unfortunately for the EP, this approach relies heavily on blood culture and echocardiography, results of which are rarely available to EPs at the outset of care. With recent efforts to bring ultrasonography skills to the ED bedside, echocardiography may become more readily available as an initial evaluation tool, but for now, the procedure requires cardiology consultation and

BOX 55-3

Partial Differential Diagnosis for Infective Endocarditis

Aortic catastrophes
Cardiac tamponade
Cerebrovascular accident
Central nervous system abscess(es)
Complete heart block
Delirium of any cause
Epilepsy
Hematologic disorders (e.g., anemia, platelet disorders)
Infarction:
- Bowel
- Central nervous system
- Intestinal
- Liver
- Myocardial, acute
- Renal
- Spleen

Infection:
- Chronic (e.g., tuberculosis, human immunodeficiency virus)
- Intra-abdominal
- Respiratory (e.g., pneumonia)
- Urinary tract (e.g., pyelonephritis)
- Viral

Intestinal vascular insufficiency
Malignancy
Meningitis
Mental illness (e.g., depression, psychosis)
Pericarditis, acute
Pulmonary edema, acute
Pulmonary embolism
Rheumatic fever, acute
Rheumatologic/immunologic disorders (e.g., vasculitides)
Rupture
- Arterial aneurysm
- Myocardial wall

Septic shock
Toxidromes or medication-related disorders
Urolithiasis
Valvular dysfunction, acute

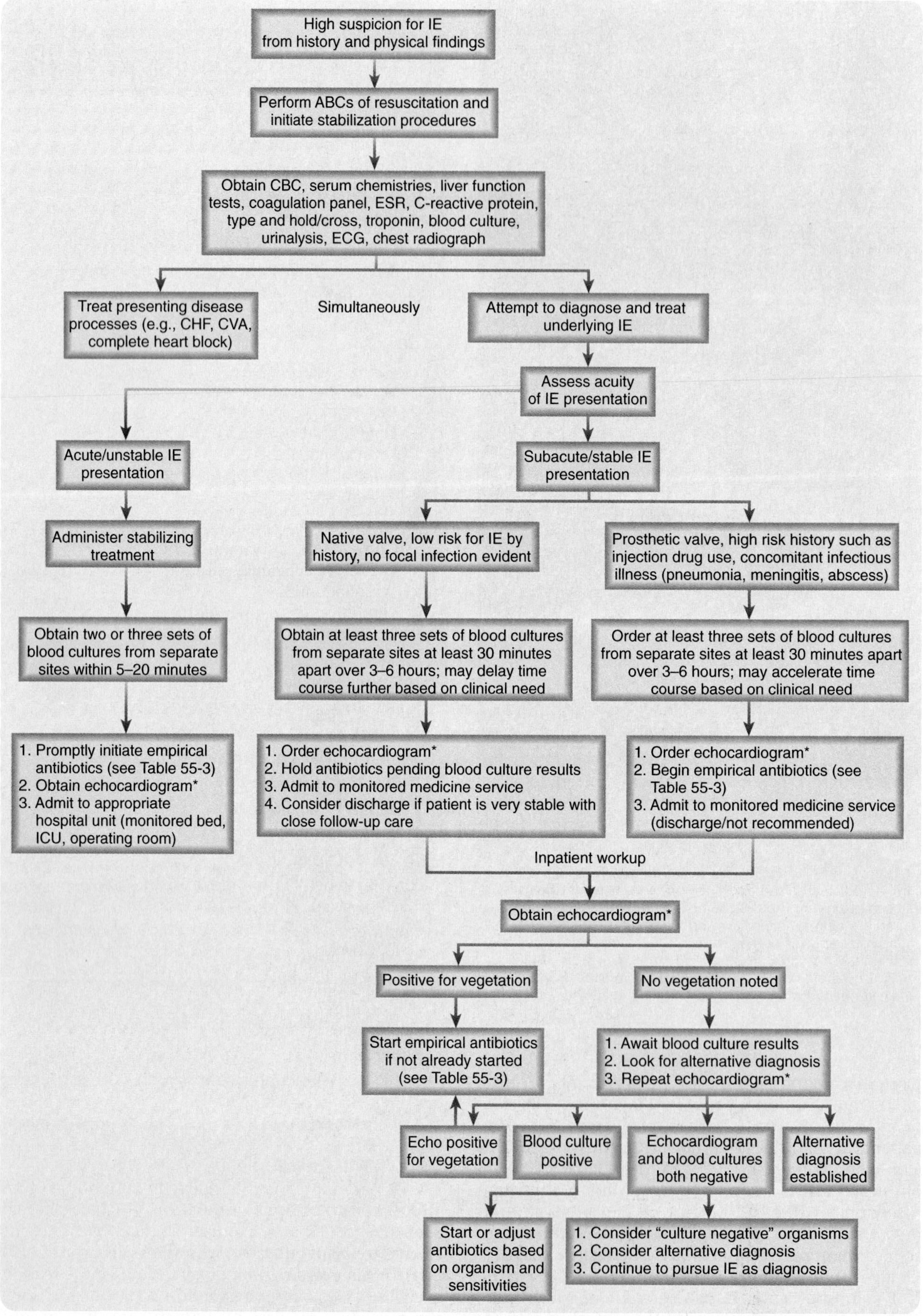
High suspicion for IE from history and physical findings
Perform ABCs of resuscitation and initiate stabilization procedures
Obtain CBC, serum chemistries, liver function tests, coagulation panel, ESR, C-reactive protein, type and hold/cross, troponin, blood culture, urinalysis, ECG, chest radiograph
Treat presenting disease processes (e.g., CHF, CVA, complete heart block)
Simultaneously
Attempt to diagnose and treat underlying IE
Assess acuity of IE presentation
Acute/unstable IE presentation
Subacute/stable IE presentation
Administer stabilizing treatment
Native valve, low risk for IE by history, no focal infection evident
Prosthetic valve, high risk history such as injection drug use, concomitant infectious illness (pneumonia, meningitis, abscess)
Obtain two or three sets of blood cultures from separate sites within 5–20 minutes
Obtain at least three sets of blood cultures from separate sites at least 30 minutes apart over 3–6 hours; may delay time course further based on clinical need
Order at least three sets of blood cultures from separate sites at least 30 minutes apart over 3–6 hours; may accelerate time course based on clinical need
1. Promptly initiate empirical antibiotics (see Table 55-3) 2. Obtain echocardiogram* 3. Admit to appropriate hospital unit (monitored bed, ICU, operating room)
1. Order echocardiogram* 2. Hold antibiotics pending blood culture results 3. Admit to monitored medicine service 4. Consider discharge if patient is very stable with close follow-up care
1. Order echocardiogram* 2. Begin empirical antibiotics (see Table 55-3) 3. Admit to monitored medicine service (discharge/not recommended)
Inpatient workup
Obtain echocardiogram*
Positive for vegetation
No vegetation noted
Start empirical antibiotics if not already started (see Table 55-3)
1. Await blood culture results 2. Look for alternative diagnosis 3. Repeat echocardiogram*
Echo positive for vegetation
Blood culture positive
Echocardiogram and blood cultures both negative
Alternative diagnosis established
Start or adjust antibiotics based on organism and sensitivities
1. Consider "culture negative" organisms 2. Consider alternative diagnosis 3. Continue to pursue IE as diagnosis

is not often available during the first few hours of care.

According to the modified Duke criteria (see Box 55-4), an echocardiogram positive for IE along with presence of three minor criteria would allow the EP to actually make a "definite diagnosis" of IE in the ED. In all other cases, positive echocardiogram results enable the diagnosis to be "possible IE" as the clinician awaits the results of blood cultures or serologic analysis. It must be emphasized that normal echocardiogram findings would not eliminate the diagnosis of IE, especially in the setting of high clinical suspicion (high-risk patient, strongly suggestive presentation). Evaluation should continue until the diagnosis of IE is "rejected" according to the modified Duke criteria. This often means the establishment of an alternative diagnosis or the finding of sterile blood cultures after appropriate incubation procedures (proper media and incubation times) and resolution of illness.

Diagnostic Testing

Many diagnostic tests exist to help the EP evaluate and manage the patient with possible IE. Many of these tests assist in identifying the complications of this disease process.

■ LABORATORY TESTS

Although not diagnostic when performed alone, some laboratory tests can be useful in diagnosing and managing the patient with endocarditis in the ED.

The *complete blood cell count* is less useful than one might think. Leukocytosis is present only in some cases. Normochromic normocytic anemia may be seen.

An elevated *erythrocyte sedimentation rate* or *C-reactive protein value* can be a good although nonspecific clue. Both findings are markers for an ongoing inflammatory process and are nearly always present in patients with IE.

Urinalysis often shows proteinuria and sometimes hematuria. Proteinuria may occur from the immunologic effects of endocarditis. Chronic infection/inflammation leads to formation of immune complexes and their deposition in the glomeruli. Depending on the duration of this illness, the patient may present with glomerulonephritis and renal insufficiency.

Renal function can be affected in IE. A *serum creatinine measurement* is not useful for the diagnosis of IE, but is for its management. Antibiotic dosing and intravenous contrast for computed tomography (CT) are dependent on a patient's renal function.

Less useful for the EP, but part of the modified Duke criteria for IE, are serologic tests. *Rheumatoid factor* may occasionally be found in patients with IE, particularly those with long-standing, indolent cases. *Serologic assays* can detect the presence of bacteria such as *Coxiella, Brucella, Bartonella, Legionella*, and *Chlamydia*. *Polymerase chain reaction (PCR) testing* for specific DNA or RNA from blood, urine, or surgically excised tissue can be used when the potential pathogen is slow growing or cannot be cultured by conventional methods.[10]

■ MICROBIOLOGY

Perhaps the most useful test for the diagnosis and management of IE is *serial blood cultures*. Unfortunately, the results of these are often not available to the EP. At least three sets of blood culture specimens should be collected at intervals of least 30 minutes and over 3 to 6 hours. IE results in a constant, low-grade bacteremia. Therefore, there is no need to obtain blood culture specimens only during temperature spikes. Serial blood culture specimens obtained over hours to days (in the absence of antibiotic therapy) should all yield positive results as long as the proper 10 mL per culture bottle is obtained. In the interest of identifying endocarditis caused by more fastidious organisms, it is recommended that blood cultures be held for 14 to 21 days before being labeled "negative" (see earlier, Culture-Negative Bacteria).

The EP must remember that antecedent antibiotic treatment can also result in negative blood culture results, so the history should include questions about such treatment.[10] In the stable patient with a history of antecedent antibiotic therapy, serial blood culture specimens should be collected over a longer time (even days) before initiation of antibiotic therapy for the IE.

The *caveat* to serial blood culture timing is that withholding antibiotics should be the strategy in the *stable* patient who has no other indications for antibiotics. *In the unstable or acutely ill patient, antibiotics should be given as early as possible.*

FIGURE 55-8 Diagnostic algorithm for the ED management of patient in whom infective endocarditis (IE) is suspected. ABCs of resuscitation, airway, breathing, and circulation; CBC, complete blood count; CHF, congestive heart failure; CVA, cerebrovascular accident; ECG, electrocardiogram; ESR, erythrocyte sedimentation rate; ICU, intensive care unit. *Echocardiography can be performed via either the transthoracic (TTE) or transesophageal (TEE) technique. TEE is more invasive but is more sensitive for detecting vegetations and complications of IE, such as perivalvular abscesses; it is recommended for prosthetic valves; for situations in which optimal visualization by TTE will be difficult, such as emphysema and morbid obesity; for high suspicion of infective endocarditis (IE) but normal TTE findings; and for high suspicion of a complication of IE, such as perivalvular abscess. Normal findings with either technique do not exclude IE if clinical suspicion is high. Echocardiograms can be repeated in an attempt to identify problems such as vegetations and abscesses, which may not be noted initially.

BOX 55-4

Modified Duke Diagnostic Criteria for Infective Endocarditis

Stratification of Patients

The modified Duke diagnostic criteria stratify patients with suspected infective endocarditis (IE) into one of three categories, as follows; the major and minor criteria are listed below.

A **diagnosis of "definite" endocarditis** is made in a patient with *one* of the following:

- Histologic and/or microbiologic evidence of infection at surgery or autopsy
- 2 major criteria
- 1 major criterion and 3 minor criteria
- 5 minor criteria

A **diagnosis of "possible" endocarditis** is made in a patient with *one* of the following:

- 1 major criterion and 1 minor criterion
- 3 minor criteria

A **diagnosis of endocarditis is "rejected"** in a patient with *one* of the following:

- Negative findings at surgery or autopsy in a patient who received antibiotic therapy for ≤4 days
- A firm alternative diagnosis
- Resolution of illness with antibiotic therapy for ≤4 days
- Failure to meet criteria for "possible" endocarditis

Major Criteria

Blood Culture Results Positive for IE

1. Typical microorganisms for infective endocarditis from two separate blood cultures in the absence of a primary focus:
   - Viridans group Streptococci
   - *Streptococcus bovis*
   - HACEK group of bacteria*
   - Community-acquired *Staphylococcus aureus* or *Enterococcus*
2. Persistently positive blood culture results, defined as recovery of a microorganism consistent with infective endocarditis from *one* of the following:
   - Blood culture specimens obtained more than 12 hours apart
   - All of 3 *or* a majority of 4 or more separate blood culture specimens, the first and last of which have been obtained at least 1 hour apart
3. Single positive blood culture result for *Coxiella burnetii* or anti–phase 1 immunoglobulin G antibody titer >1:800.

Evidence of Endocardial Involvement

1. Positive echocardiogram results for infective endocarditis:
   - *Transesophageal echocardiography* recommended in patients who have prosthetic valves, who have been rated as having at least "possible IE" by clinical criteria, or who have complicated IE (paravalvular abscess).
   - *Transthoracic echocardiography* recommended as first test in other patients.

   Definition of positive echocardiogram result is presence of *one* of the following;
   - Oscillating intracardiac mass, on valve or supporting structures, or in the path of regurgitant jets, or on implanted material, in the absence of an alternative anatomical explanation
   - Abscess
   - New partial dehiscence of prosthetic valve
2. New valvular regurgitation. An increase or change in a preexisting murmur is not sufficient evidence.

Minor Criteria

Predisposition: Predisposing heart condition or intravenous drug use

Fever: Body temperature >38.0° C (100.4° F)

Vascular phenomena: Major arterial emboli, septic pulmonary infarcts, mycotic aneurysms, intracranial hemorrhage, conjunctival hemorrhages, Janeway lesion

Immunologic phenomena: Glomerulonephritis, Osler's nodes, Roth's spots, rheumatoid factor

Microbiologic evidence: Positive blood culture result but not meeting major criteria as noted above (excluding single positive culture result for coagulase-negative staphylococci and organisms that do not cause endocarditis) *OR* serologic evidence of active infection with organism consistent with IE.

**Haemophilus* species, *Actinobacillus actinomycetemcomitans, Cardiobacterium hominis, Eikenella corrodens,* and *Kingella kingae.*
Data from Li IS, Sexton DJ, Mick N, et al: Proposed modifications to the Duke criteria for the diagnosis of infective endocarditis. Clin Infect Dis 2000;30:633-638.

■ ELECTROCARDIOGRAPHY

The acquisition of an electrocardiogram (ECG) is often prompted by abnormalities in vital signs, presenting symptoms, or clinical instability. If the EP suspects IE, an ECG must be performed. Abnormalities found on ECG can be caused by endocarditis, but as with other findings for this diagnosis, these abnormalities are nonspecific. The pathologic findings that can be associated with endocarditis are acute myocardial infarction (due to coronary artery involvement), complete heart block, atrioventricular block, and bundle branch blocks. Infarction can occur from direct embolization to the coronary arteries or coronary mycotic aneurysm formation. Conduction abnormalities can result from direct extension of infection into the conduction system. Most commonly, the ECG in a patient with endocarditis is normal or reveals a sinus tachycardia.

■ ECHOCARDIOGRAPHY

Echocardiography, the most important diagnostic tool available to the EP for early identification of endocarditis, should be performed in all cases of suspected IE.[6] This procedure is a major criterion for the modified Duke criteria (see Box 55-4). Any one of the following echocardiogram findings is diagnostic for IE[9]:

- Oscillating intracardiac mass—on a valve or supporting structures, in the path of regurgitant jets, or on implanted material—without an alternative anatomic explanation (Fig. 55-9)
- Annular or intracardiac abscess
- New partial dehiscence of prosthetic valve
- New valvular regurgitation

■ Transthoracic Echocardiography

Easily done at the bedside, transthoracic echocardiography (TTE) should be the initial screening modality. It can identify valvular damage and valvular vegetations as well as assess cardiac function and pulmonary pressures.

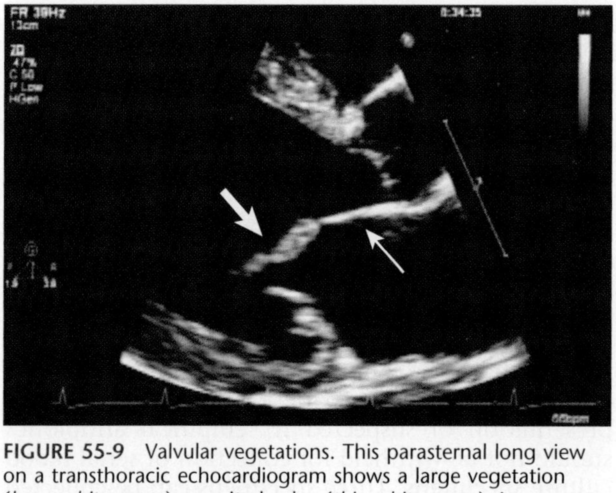

FIGURE 55-9 Valvular vegetations. This parasternal long view on a transthoracic echocardiogram shows a large vegetation (*large white arrow*) on mitral valve (*thin white arrow*). Large arrow is in left ventricle and thin arrow is in left atrium. (Courtesy of Mark Goldberger, MD.)

■ Transesophageal Echocardiography

Although requiring more preparation and being more invasive than TTE, transesophageal echocardiography (TEE) has greater specificity. It can visualize smaller vegetations as well as myocardial involvement such as abscesses and prosthetic valve vegetations. TEE is recommended for patients with the following findings:

- TTE result is negative, but there is high clinical suspicion for IE.
- TTE result is positive, but there is concern for the presence of a high-risk complication of IE, such as large and/or mobile vegetations, significant valvular insufficiency, or suggestion of perivalvular extension.
- TTE result is suboptimal owing, for example, to morbid obesity, mechanical ventilation, emphysema, or chest wall deformity.
- Prosthetic valve(s) are in place.

For patients with high clinical suspicion for IE, a normal echocardiogram result is not enough to stop treatment. TTE or TEE can be used subsequently to assess the response to treatment or the progression of disease.[6]

■ RADIOGRAPHY

Chest radiographs are routinely obtained in most patients presenting with cardiopulmonary symptoms and/or fever. No specific finding on chest radiograph is pathognomonic for IE. Multiple bilateral pulmonary infiltrates might be a clue that septic emboli may be present (Fig. 55-10A).

Computed tomography (CT) is an excellent tool in the evaluation of symptoms that may be associated with IE. The discovery of ischemic or infectious foci or abscesses, especially multiple lesions, should raise the suspicion of a septic focus—such as infective endocarditis. Contrast-enhanced CT is preferred for differentiating mass lesions with necrotic centers from abscesses.

Chest CT may better identify multiple septic emboli, effusions, or pulmonary abscesses (see Fig. 55-10B). Brain CT for the evaluation of the patient with neurologic or neuropsychiatric symptoms may demonstrate ischemic or infectious foci. Contrast-enhanced abdominopelvic CT might identify ischemia or infarction of the intestines, liver, spleen, or kidneys (Fig. 55-11).

For identifying the presence of mycotic aneurysms or peripheral embolization, conventional angiography remains the gold standard, although screening may be undertaken with CT angiography or magnetic resonance angiography.

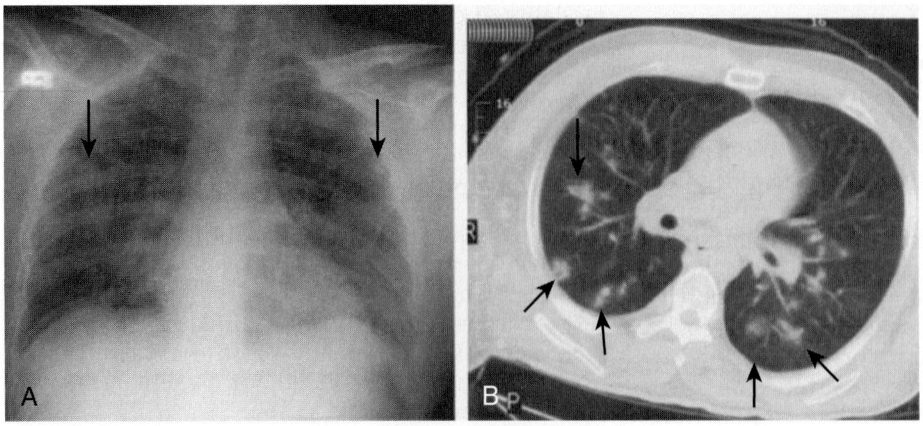
A
B

FIGURE 55-10 Septic emboli. **A,** A chest radiograph shows two nodular densities (*arrows*). In this case, they are foci of infection from embolization of infected vegetations. **B,** This noncontrast CT scan of the chest demonstrates multiple small infiltrates (*arrows*) due to septic embolization.

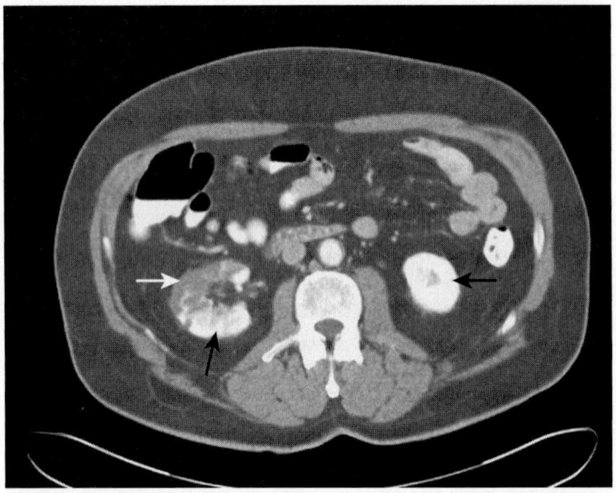

FIGURE 55-11 Renal infarction. Contrast-enhanced abdominopelvic CT scan demonstrates patchy uptake of intravenous contrast agent by the right kidney. Grey areas (*white arrow*) within the anterolateral aspect of the midpole of the right kidney represent infarction caused by septic emboli from infective endocarditis. This contrasts with the rather homogeneously white, well-perfused left kidney and posterior aspect of the right kidney and posterior aspect of the right kidney (*black arrows*). (Courtesy of Jeffrey Newhouse, MD.)

■ LUMBAR PUNCTURE

Lumbar puncture is not helpful in making the diagnosis of IE but is mandatory for diagnosing a potentially serious complication—bacterial meningitis. Meningitis can result from the continuous bacteremia of IE. Lumbar puncture allows the EP to diagnose meningitis and, ultimately, identify the causative organism.

Treatment

■ APPROPRIATE RESUSCITATION

Emergency treatment always begins with the cardinal ABCs of resuscitation—airway, breathing, and circulation. Patients with issues in any of these areas must be stabilized by the usual methods. Supplemental oxygen and/or endotracheal intubation should be used as needed. Circulatory instability due to either cardiogenic or septic shock should be corrected with volume and/or pressor support. Refractory cardiogenic shock may require the use of an intra-aortic balloon counterpulsation device (contraindicated in aortic insufficiency) or emergency heart surgery.

■ EMPIRICAL ANTIBIOTIC THERAPY

Antibiotics are the keystone of IE treatment, and the proper choice of regimen depends on the causative organism. Identification of the specific organism and its resistance pattern allows for a properly tailored antibiotic regimen, which minimizes overuse of extended-spectrum agents. With this in mind, EPs should make every effort to obtain serial blood cultures before starting antibiotic treatment. At least three sets (aerobic and anaerobic) of blood culture specimens should be obtained. The sets should be obtained at least 30 minutes apart and over 3 to 6 hours.

The urgency for empirical antibiotic therapy varies by patient subgroup. In stable patients with subacute presentations and native valves who present with signs and symptoms most consistent with a viral syndrome, antibiotic therapy can be withheld for hours and even days to allow for proper culture results to be obtained. Patients with the same stable, subacute presentation and viral syndrome–type symptoms but with a prosthetic valve or a history of injection drug use should be admitted and should receive appropriate empirical antibiotic therapy after the 3- to 6-hour collection of serial blood culture specimens. In the patient with a concomitant infectious process such as meningitis, pneumonia, or abscess and in whom the diagnosis of IE is being entertained, the serial blood culture specimens should be collected but over the shorter time to allow sooner initiation of appropriate empirical antibiotic therapy to cover both the identified infection and the possible IE. Finally, in the patient with acute, unstable presentation of suspected IE, empirical antibiotics should not be withheld for collection of serial blood culture specimens. Three specimens can be collected over 5 to 20 minutes to allow expeditious antibiotic treatment.

BOX 55-5

Clinical Scenarios to Help Tailor an Empirical Antibiotic Regimen for a Patient with Suspected Infective Endocarditis

Important factors in choosing an antibiotic are as follows:

- Acuity of presentation
- Native valve endocarditis
- Prosthetic valve endocarditis
- Endocarditis in injection drug user
- Recent or current use of antibiotics
- Recent hospitalization
- Antibiotic allergies
- Renal function
- Relapse of previously treated endocarditis
- Regional prevalence of certain organisms and resistance patterns

Unfortunately for the EP, the causative organism is rarely known because culture results are often not available yet. As with many infections, the EP must choose an empirical regimen. So how does the EP choose the empirical regimen? There are a group of organisms known to cause IE (see Box 55-1). Certain of these organisms are more common depending on the clinical scenario (see Table 55-2). Armed with this knowledge, the EP can tailor the empirical antibiotic regimen to the clinical scenario presented. Examples of such scenarios are native valve involvement, prosthetic valve involvement, injection drug use, history of allergy to antibiotics, prolonged hospitalization, ICU admission, and high prevalence of resistant organisms (Box 55-5). All of these factors would influence the antibiotic regimen chosen.

Should the empirical regimen include antibiotics that cover all possible organisms and all resistance patterns? Actually, because most patients with IE have stable, subacute presentations, the EP is not forced to achieve a perfect match of organism and antibiotic. Changes can be made in 2 to 3 days, when the organisms and resistance patterns become known. In contrast, for unstable, acute cases, EPs should maximize coverage to ensure that they account for all possibilities of organism and resistance. Morbidity and mortality could be influenced by failure to properly treat early.

Initial antibiotic therapy should always be parenteral and bactericidal.[1] Owing to growing antibiotic resistance, combination therapy with two or more agents should be used. Recommended empirical antibiotic regimens are listed in Table 55-3.

For complex cases, it is advisable to seek the expertise of an infectious disease specialist. In addition, patients with confirmed IE require prolonged antibiotic administration and will likely be discharged with a long-term central intravenous catheter such as Groshong catheter, or peripherally inserted central catheter (PICC line).

■ CARDIAC PACING

Any hemodynamically unstable patient who presents with complete heart block, irrespective of cause, warrants at least temporary cardiac pacing. In the setting of IE, in which high-degree heart block is unlikely to be a temporary condition, a transvenous pacemaker is preferable to transthoracic pacing.

■ ANTICOAGULATION

Anticoagulation is not a therapeutic regimen for endocarditis. It neither prevents the formation nor the embolization of vegetations. In the setting of native valve IE, anticoagulation should be avoided, as it affords no benefit and might cause harm by converting CNS infarcts from bland to hemorrhagic.

Understanding the risks of anticoagulation in the setting of IE, what does the EP do with patients who would normally require anticoagulation? An excellent example would be the patient with IE and an anticoagulation-requiring prosthetic valve. The recommendation is that anticoagulation should be continued, barring the presence of acute hemorrhages, CNS infarction/hemorrhage, or mycotic aneurysm. Any complaint that may result from these should be fully investigated in order to best inform decisions regarding anticoagulation. We recommend that any patient with possible CNS involvement undergo CT imaging of the brain. Any patient with unexplained abdominal/flank pain should undergo contrast-enhanced abdominal CT imaging to evaluate for the presence of a mycotic aneurysm. Visual complaints warrant a complete funduscopic examination. If contraindications are identified, the temporary discontinuation of anticoagulation is appropriate even with a prosthetic valve.[1,10,11] In these circumstances, close consultation with the appropriate specialty services is recommended.

Patients on warfarin should be switched to intravenous, unfractionated heparin in the event that cardiac surgery is required.

Aspirin has not been shown to prevent embolic events but is likely associated with an increased risk of bleeding. It therefore has no role in early management of patients with infective endocarditis.[12]

■ SURGICAL THERAPY

There are both early and late indications for surgical intervention in the management of IE. Keeping this fact in mind, the EP should obtain early cardiothoracic surgery consultation for any patient with early indications. The only true indication for early, emergency surgical intervention is severe CHF/cardiogenic shock secondary to valvular insufficiency. Intra-aortic balloon counterpulsation devices can be used to tem-

Table 55-3 EMPIRICAL ANTIBIOTIC REGIMEN FOR PRESUMED INFECTIOUS ENDOCARDITIS*†**

Suspected native valve IE with subacute presentation‡	Penicillin G 200–400 units/kg (normal adult dose 12–20 million units/day) IV divided q4h, *or* ampicillin 200 mg/kg/day (normal adult dose 12 g/day) IV divided q4h *plus* Nafcillin or oxacillin 200 mg/kg/day (normal adult dose 12 g/day) IV divided q4h *plus* Gentamicin 1 mg/kg IV or IM q8h (adjust for peak serum concentration of 3-4 μg/mL and trough of <1 μg/mL)§,¶
Suspected native valve IE with the following characteristics: Patient with penicillin allergy *or* Acute presentation *or* History of injection-drug use *or* From region with high incidence of IE due to *Staphylococcus aureus*, especially oxacillin-resistant *S. aureus*	Vancomycin 15 mg/kg IV q12h (adjust for 1 hr peak serum concentration of 30-45 μg/mL and trough of 10-15 μg/mL)¶ *plus* Gentamicin 1 mg/kg IV or IM q8h (adjust for peak serum concentration of 3-4 μg/mL and trough of <1 μg/mL)§,¶
Suspected prosthetic valve IE	Vancomycin 15 mg/kg IV q12h (adjust for 1 hr peak serum concentration of 30-45 μg/mL and trough of 10-15 μg/mL)¶ *plus* Gentamicin 1 mg/kg IV or IM q8h (adjust for peak serum concentration of 3-4 μg/mL and trough of <1 μg/mL)§,¶ *plus* Rifampin 20 mg/kg/day (normal adult dose 900 mg/day) PO divided q8h¶

IE, infectious endocarditis; IM, intramuscular(ly); IV, intravascular(ly); PO, oral(ly).
*Empiric therapy must be designed on the basis of clinical and epidemiologic clues.
†Duration of therapy varies with the microorganism and its drug sensitivities, the presence of prosthetic devices, and the response to therapy.
‡Penicillin G or ampicillin is added to this regimen because nafcillin/oxacillin and gentamicin may not be adequate coverage of enterococci.
§Aminoglycosides such as gentamicin should not be given as single daily doses.
¶Doses of vancomycin and gentamicin should be adjusted for reduced renal function as well as measured serum concentration values.
¶Rifampin increases warfarin requirement for anticoagulation.
**Pediatric dose should not exceed the normal adult dose.
Data from Baddour LM, Wilson WR, Bayer AS, et al; Committee on Rheumatic Fever, Endocarditis, and Kawasaki Disease; Council on Cardiovascular Disease in the Young; Councils on Clinical Cardiology, Stroke, and Cardiovascular Surgery and Anesthesia; American Heart Association; Infectious Diseases Society of America: Infective endocarditis: Diagnosis, antimicrobial therapy, and management of complications. A statement for healthcare professionals from the Committee on Rheumatic Fever, Endocarditis, and Kawasaki Disease, Council on Cardiovascular Disease in the Young, and the Councils on Clinical Cardiology, Stroke, and Cardiovascular Surgery and Anesthesia, American Heart Association: endorsed by the Infectious Diseases Society of America. Circulation 2005;111:e394-e434.

porize all forms of cardiogenic shock except shock due to aortic valve insufficiency. In the case of aortic valve incompetence, valve replacement becomes imperative. The presence of an annular or aortic abscess (with or without a conduction system disturbance), a sinus or aortic true or false aneurysm, or a paravalvular leak of a prosthetic valve warrants surgical intervention, but need not be performed as an emergency procedure if the patient is otherwise stable.

Other potential indications for surgery in the patient with IE are failure of antibiotic therapy, vegetations larger than 10 mm on echocardiography, fungal endocarditis, early prosthetic valve endocarditis (within the first 2 months after surgery), and recurrent embolization despite medical therapy.[11]

■ REMOVAL OF MEDICAL HARDWARE

Blood culture specimens should be obtained via any long-term indwelling intravascular catheters. These devices should then be removed. Decisions to remove prosthetic valves or pacemaker wires are complex and would be made in consultation with cardiology, cardiothoracic surgery, and/or infectious disease specialists.

Disposition

All patients with suspected or confirmed IE should be admitted. The only ED patients with IE who may be discharged home are those with uncomplicated status with low risk for IE (native valves, immunocompetent, no injection drug use, no comorbidities) in whom the diagnosis of IE is not clear, presentation is stable/subacute, and follow-up is very well defined. The patient with a nondiagnostic transthoracic echocardiogram may undergo TEE as an outpatient, and the serial blood culture results can be followed by his or her personal physician.

Otherwise, the disposition of all other patients with potential or confirmed IE is driven by the following factors:

- Need for further evaluation (diagnosis or extent of involvement not certain)
- Severity of illness
- Need for surgical or mechanical support (e.g., mechanical ventilation, intra-aortic balloon counterpulsation device)
- Need for intravenous antibiotic therapy
- Reliability of the patient
- Availability of close follow-up

Immediate operative care should be strongly considered if surgical criteria are met. Patients in critical condition who do not require surgery should be admitted to the intensive care unit. Most other patients with presumed IE can be admitted to a medical service with cardiac monitoring for further evaluation, initiation of intravenous antibiotic therapy, and arrangement for further outpatient care.

Nonbacterial Thrombotic Endocarditis

Endocarditis is not always associated with infection. In association with some disease states, vegetations composed of bland, platelet-fibrin aggregates may adhere to the endocardium. Eventually, fibrosis of these lesions occurs. These vegetations are usually sterile but may become seeded with infectious organisms. Illnesses associated with nonbacterial thrombotic endocarditis (NBTE) include malignancies, severe burns, hypercoagulable states (e.g., antiphospholipid syndrome and disseminated intravascular coagulopathy), uremia, and connective tissue diseases like systemic lupus erythematosus.[13]

It stands to reason that the clinical manifestations of NBTE are related mainly to embolic phenomena and, occasionally, valvular dysfunction. Without infectious vegetations, the generalized immune response and the localized destruction and infectious seeding of other organs do not occur. The indication for surgical intervention most commonly is valvular dysfunction, although patients may undergo surgery to prevent embolic events.

Endocarditis Prophylaxis

For more than 50 years, the American Heart Association (AHA) has set forth recommendations in an effort to prevent IE. Antimicrobial regimens were recommended for planned, potentially contaminated procedures (dental, respiratory, gastrointestinal, and genitourinary) in an effort to prevent IE in at-risk populations. Unfortunately, these guidelines lacked good evidence to support their efficacy and were so complex that their implementation was difficult. In April 2007, the AHA released new guidelines in an effort to address these issues.[14]

Rather than provide prophylaxis to patients at risk for development of IE, the 2007 guidelines have moved to recommend that antimicrobial prophylaxis be administered only to patients at *highest risk for an adverse outcome* from IE (Box 55-6), reducing the group of eligible patients greatly. The procedures for which prophylaxis is recommended are listed in Box 55-7, and the antimicrobial regimens in Table 55-4.

EPs may encounter difficulty managing the expectations of patients who previously were recommended to receive IE prophylaxis but now are not. The rationale for the changes lies in the lack of solid scientific evidence to support the claim that IE prophylaxis is actually effective. It has been shown that the bacteremia resulting from daily activities such as tooth brushing and eating is more likely to result in IE than that associated with dental procedures. Therefore, even if 100% effective, prophylaxis probably prevents only an extremely small number of cases of IE. The cost of prophylaxis is borne financially[15] and through adverse drug reactions. As a result, the AHA is now emphasizing the maintenance of optimal oral health and hygiene as the means to reduce the

BOX 55-6

American Heart Association Recommendations for Prevention of Infective Endocarditis

Cardiac conditions associated with the highest risk of adverse outcome from endocarditis for which antibiotic prophylaxis is recommended are as follows:

- Prosthetic cardiac valves
- Previous infective endocarditis
- Congenital heart disease (CHD)*:
  - Unrepaired cyanotic CHD, including palliative shunts and conduits
  - Completely repaired congenital heart defect with prosthetic material or device, whether placed by surgery or by catheter intervention, during the first 6 months after the procedure†
  - Repaired CHD with residual defects at the site or adjacent to the site of a prosthetic patch or prosthetic device (which inhibits endothelialization)
- Cardiac valvulopathy in a cardiac transplantation recipient

*Except for the conditions listed here, antibiotic prophylaxis is no longer recommended for any other form of CHD.
†Prophylaxis is recommended because endothelialization of prosthetic material occurs within 6 months after the procedure.
Adapted from Wilson W, Taubert KA, Gewitz M, et al: Prevention of infective endocarditis: Guidelines from the American Heart Association. A guideline from the American Heart Association Rheumatic Fever, Endocarditis, and Kawasaki Disease Committee, Council on Cardiovascular Disease in the Young, and the Council on Clinical Cardiology, Council on Cardiovascular Surgery and Anesthesia, and the Quality of Care and Outcomes Research Interdisciplinary Working Group. J Am Dent Assoc 2007;138:739-745, 747-760.

BOX 55-7

ED Procedures Requiring Antimicrobial Prophylaxis against Infective Endocarditis in High-Risk Patients

Patients at high risk of an adverse outcome from infective endocarditis (see Box 55-6) should receive antimicrobial prophylaxis (see Table 55-4) for the following procedures:

Dental Procedures

- *All dental procedures* that involve manipulation of gingival tissue or the periapical region of teeth or perforation of the oral mucosa.

The following procedures and events do not need prophylaxis: routine anesthetic injections through noninfected tissue, taking of dental radiographs, placement of removable prosthodontic or orthodontic appliances, placement of orthodontic brackets, shedding of deciduous teeth, and bleeding from trauma to the lips or oral mucosa.

Otorhinolaryngologic/Respiratory Procedures

- Any surgical procedure that involve incision of respiratory mucosa (e.g., peritonsillar abscess incision and drainage, cricothyroidotomy, tracheotomy, tonsillectomy, and/or adenoidectomy)
- Bronchoscopy with a procedure that involves incision of respiratory mucosa

Minor Surgical Procedures

- Any surgical procedure that involves infected skin, skin structure, or musculoskeletal tissue (e.g., incision and drainage of an abscess)

NOTE: Prophylaxis for gastrointestinal procedures is no longer recommended.

NOTE: Prophylaxis for genitourinary procedures is recommended only if the patient is known to have enterococcal colonization or urinary tract infection at the time of instrumentation.

Modified from Wilson W, Taubert KA, Gewitz M, et al: Prevention of infective endocarditis: Guidelines from the American Heart Association. A guideline from the American Heart Association Rheumatic Fever, Endocarditis, and Kawasaki Disease Committee, Council on Cardiovascular Disease in the Young, and the Council on Clinical Cardiology, Council on Cardiovascular Surgery and Anesthesia, and the Quality of Care and Outcomes Research Interdisciplinary Working Group. J Am Dent Assoc 2007;138:739-745, 747-760.

Table 55-4 ANTIBIOTIC PROPHYLAXIS REGIMENS FOR DENTAL PROCEDURES*†

		Single Dose to Be Administered 30-60 Minutes Prior to Procedure	
Patient	Antibiotic Agent	Adults	Children
Can take oral medications	Amoxicillin	2 g PO	50 mg/kg PO
Cannot take oral medication	Ampicillin *OR* Cefazolin or ceftriaxone	2 g IM or IV 1 g IM or IV	50 mg/kg IM or IV 50 mg/kg IM or IV
Is allergic to penicillins and able to take oral medication	Cephalexin‡§ *OR* Clindamycin *OR* Azithromycin or clarithromycin	2 g PO 600 mg PO 500 mg PO	50 mg/kg PO 20 mg/kg PO 15 mg/kg PO
Is allergic to penicillins and unable to take oral medication	Cefazolin or ceftriaxone§ *OR* Clindamycin	1 g IM or IV 600 mg IM or IV	50 mg/kg IM or IV 20 mg/kg IM or IV

IM, intramuscular(ly); IV, intravenous(ly); PO, oral(ly).

*If a resistant Enterococcus spp or resistant *Staphylococcus aureus* is suspected, consultation with an infectious disease specialist should be considered.

†These regimens may be used for ear/nose/throat, respiratory, and contaminated skin/musculoskeletal procedures as well.

‡Other first- or second-generation oral cephalosporins in appropriate doses can be substituted for cephalexin.

§Cephalosporins should not be used in patients with a history of anaphylaxis, angioedema, or urticaria in association with penicillin or penicillin-related drugs.

Adapted from Wilson W, Taubert KA, Gewitz M, et al: Prevention of infective endocarditis: Guidelines from the American Heart Association. A guideline from the American Heart Association Rheumatic Fever, Endocarditis, and Kawasaki Disease Committee, Council on Cardiovascular Disease in the Young, and the Council on Clinical Cardiology, Council on Cardiovascular Surgery and Anesthesia, and the Quality of Care and Outcomes Research Interdisciplinary Working Group. J Am Dent Assoc 2007;138:739-745, 747-760.

incidence of IE related to daily activities as well as dental procedures.[14]

REFERENCES

1. Mylonakis E, Calderwood SB: Infective endocarditis in adults. N Engl J Med 2001;345:1318-1330.
2. Tleyjeh IM, Steckelberg J, Murad HS, et al: Temporal trends in infective endocarditis: A population-based study in Olmstead County, Minnesota. JAMA 2005;293:3022-3028.
3. Fowler VG Jr, Miro JM, Hoen B, et al: *Staphylococcus aureus* endocarditis: A consequence of medical progress. JAMA 2005;293:3012-3021.
4. Verheul HA, van der Brink RB, van Vreeland T, et al: Effects of change in management of active infective endocarditis on outcome in a 25-year period. Am J Cardiol 1993;72: 682-687.
5. Habib G: Management of infective endocarditis. Heart 2006;92:124-130.
6. Baddour LM, Wilson WR, Bayer AS, et al; Committee on Rheumatic Fever, Endocarditis, and Kawasaki Disease; Council on Cardiovascular Disease in the Young; Councils on Clinical Cardiology, Stroke, and Cardiovascular Surgery and Anesthesia; American Heart Association; Infectious Diseases Society of America: Infective endocarditis: Diagnosis, antimicrobial therapy, and management of complications. A statement for healthcare professionals from the Committee on Rheumatic Fever, Endocarditis, and Kawasaki Disease, Council on Cardiovascular Disease in the Young, and the Councils on Clinical Cardiology, Stroke, and Cardiovascular Surgery and Anesthesia, American Heart Association: endorsed by the Infectious Diseases Society of America. Circulation 2005;111:e394-e434.
7. Petti CA, Bhally HS, Weinstein MP, et al: Utility of extended blood culture incubation for isolation of *Haemophilus, Actinobacillus, Cardiobacterium, Eikenella* and *Kingella* organisms: A retrospective multicenter evaluation. J Clin Microbiol 2006;44:257-259.
8. Pierrotti LC, Baddour LM: Fungal endocarditis, 1995-2000. Chest 2002;122:302-310.
9. Li IS, Sexton DJ, Mick N, et al: Proposed modifications to the Duke criteria for the diagnosis of infective endocarditis. Clin Infect Dis 2000;30:633-638.
10. Bayer AS, Bolger AF, Taubert KA, et al: Diagnosis and management of infective endocarditis and its complications. Circulation 1998;98:2936-2948.
11. Bonow RO, Carabello B, De Leon AC, et al: ACC/AHA Guidelines for the Management of Patients with Valvular Heart Disease: A report of the American College of Cardiology/American Heart Association Task Force on Practice Guidelines (Committee on Management of Patients with Valvular Heart Disease). J Am Coll Cardiol 1998;32: 1486-1588.
12. Chan KL, Dumesnil JG, Cujec B, et al: A randomized trial of aspirin on the risk of embolic events in patients with infective endocarditis. J Am Coll Cardiol 2003;42: 775-780.
13. Eiken PW, Edwards WD, Tazelaar HD, et al: Surgical pathology of nonbacterial thrombotic endocarditis in 30 patients, 1985-2000. Mayo Clin Proc 2001;76:1204-1212.
14. Wilson W, Taubert KA, Gewitz M, et al: Prevention of infective endocarditis: Guidelines from the American Heart Association. A guideline from the American Heart Association Rheumatic Fever, Endocarditis, and Kawasaki Disease Committee, Council on Cardiovascular Disease in the Young, and the Council on Clinical Cardiology, Council on Cardiovascular Surgery and Anesthesia, and the Quality of Care and Outcomes Research Interdisciplinary Working Group. J Am Dent Assoc 2007;138:739-745, 747-760.
15. Agha Z: Is antibiotic prophylaxis for bacterial endocarditis cost-effective? Med Decis Making 2005;25:308-320.

Chapter 56

Pediatric Cardiac Emergencies

Nathan W. Mick

KEY POINTS

Congenital heart disease typically is diagnosed in utero or prior to discharge from the newborn nursery, but delayed presentations occur typically within the first 2 weeks of life when the ductus arteriosus closes.

Congenital heart disease should be considered in a neonate who is in shock or has congestive heart failure or cyanosis.

Subtle signs of cardiac disease in children include sweating, irritability, and poor feeding.

Echocardiography is used for the diagnosis of structural congenital heart disease.

Prostaglandin E_1 can be lifesaving in cases of ductal-dependent congenital heart disease.

Scope

The spectrum of congenital pediatric cardiac disorders includes structural congenital heart disease (CHD) and rhythm disturbances such as supraventricular tachycardia (SVT), the long QTc syndrome, and congenital complete heart block.

Structural CHD occurs in approximately 8 in 1000 live births.[1] Most congenital lesions are diagnosed in utero or in the newborn nursery, but a significant proportion may not manifest until 1 to 2 weeks of life, when the ductus arteriosus closes. In fact, a significant proportion of CHD is diagnosed after hospital discharge. A normal newborn examination does not rule out potentially significant and lethal lesions, and a high index of suspicion is critical to ensure timely diagnosis.[2] Many risk factors for the development of CHD have been identified (Box 56-1); they include a family history of CHD, maternal diabetes (associated with ventricular septal defect [VSD], hypertrophic cardiomyopathy, and transposition of the great arteries), and fetal drug exposure (e.g., Ebstein's anomaly with maternal lithium therapy). Pediatric cardiac disease may be challenging because it may mimic more common illnesses, such as sepsis.

Rhythm disturbances are also important causes of pediatric cardiac disease and can occur in the presence of structural heart disease or in structurally normal hearts. Supraventricular tachycardia is the most common pediatric cardiac arrhythmia and includes atrioventricular nodal reentrant tachycardia, atrioventricular reentrant tachycardia, and preexcitation conditions such as the Wolf-Parkinson-White syndrome. Congenital complete heart block is associated with maternal connective tissue disease and the presence of anti-Ro/SSA and anti-La-SSB antibodies. The long QTc syndrome may be congenital or acquired; the congenital form is estimated to occur in 1 in 7000 to 1 in 10,000 live births.[3] Congenital long QTc syndrome may occur in an autosomal dominant form (Romano-Ward syndrome) or an autosomal recessive form (Jervell and Lange-Nielsen syndrome) associated with sensorineural hearing loss.

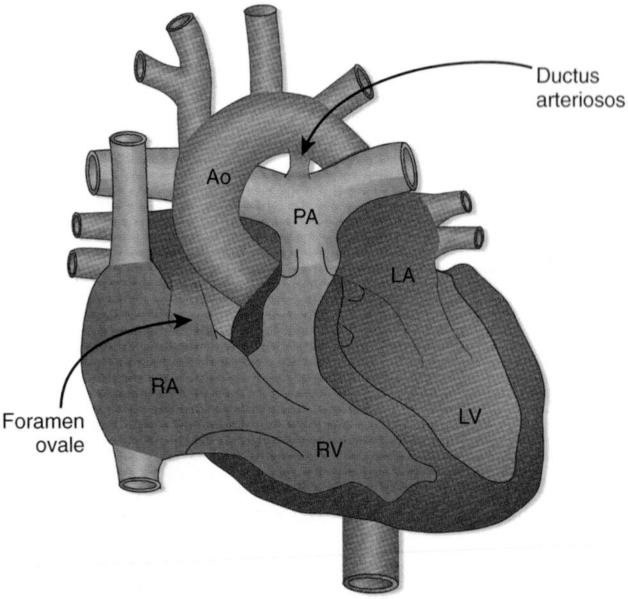
Ductus
arteriosos
Ao
PA
LA
RA
Foramen
ovale
LV
RV

FIGURE 56-1 Normal fetal circulatory anatomy. Ao, aorta; LA, left atrium; LV, left ventricle; PA, pulmonary artery; RA, right atrium; RV, right ventricle.

BOX 56-2

Congenital Heart Lesions that Depend on Patency of the Ductus Arteriosus

Right-to-Left Shunting Critical for Relief of Left-Sided Obstruction

- Hypoplastic left heart syndrome
- Total anomalous pulmonary venous return with obstruction
- Critical coarctation of the aorta
- Interrupted aortic arch
- Congenital aortic stenosis

Left-to-Right Shunting Critical for Relief of Right-Sided Obstruction

- Tetralogy of Fallot with severe right outflow tract obstruction
- Tricuspid atresia
- Pulmonic atresia
- Ebstein's anomaly

BOX 56-1

Risk Factors for the Development of Congenital Heart Disease

- Family history: Risk for CHD is increased with one affected parent or sibling, and is three times greater if two close relatives have CHD.
- Maternal diabetes is associated with hypertrophic cardiomyopathy, ventricular septal defect, transposition of the great arteries.
- Maternal phenytoin use is associated with aortic stenosis and pulmonic stenosis.
- Maternal lithium use is associated with Ebstein's anomaly.
- Fetal alcohol syndrome is associated with atrial septal defect and ventricular septal defect.

Anatomy and Pathophysiology

Fetal circulatory anatomy is designed to transport oxygenated blood from the placenta to the systemic circulation while bypassing the lungs (Fig. 56-1). Fetal oxygenation occurs at the placenta, and the blood is returned to the right atrium after bypassing the liver through the ductus venosus. Most of the oxygen-rich blood is shunted across the foramen ovale into the left atrium and is then delivered to the systemic circulation via the aorta. Some flow travels from the right atrium into the right ventricle and enters the pulmonary arteries. The pulmonary vasculature is constricted, and flow is shunted through the ductus arteriosus, mixing with blood in the aorta to supply the systemic circulation.

Birth results in a complex series of changes resulting from expansion and oxygenation of the lungs. Oxygenation of the lungs leads to a marked decrease in pulmonary vascular resistance and a subsequent increase in pulmonary blood flow. Increasing pulmonary blood flow results in greater blood return to the left atrium, which functionally closes the foramen ovale (the foramen may remain "probe-patent" into adulthood). The decrease in pulmonary vascular resistance is coupled with an increase in systemic vascular resistance, and ductal flow reverses to become left-to-right. The blood traversing the ductus arteriosus is now highly oxygenated, a change that typically stimulates closure by 48 hours of life. In certain cases, the ductus arteriosus does not close until 1 to 2 weeks of life, and so-called ductal-dependent cardiac lesions may manifest at this time (Box 56-2). The increased pressure and volume demands on the left ventricle (LV) stimulate growth of the LV, and the decreased load on the right ventricle (RV) from decreased pulmonary vascular resistance results in a decrease in right ventricular mass.

Clinical Presentation

■ CLASSIC PRESENTATIONS

Infants with previously undiagnosed structural CHD typically are presented to the ED with shock, congestive heart failure, cyanosis, or a combination of these symptoms. Left-sided obstructive lesions such as the hypoplastic left heart syndrome and coarctation of the aorta manifest as shock as the ductus arteriosus closes and the blood supply to the systemic circulation dwindles. Shock can also be the presentation of

Table 56-1 DIFFERENTIAL DIAGNOSIS OF SHOCK IN INFANTS

Type of Shock	Possible Causes
Hypovolemic	Hemorrhage Dehydration
Cardiogenic	Critical coarctation of the aorta Interrupted aortic arch Congenital aortic stenosis Hypoplastic left heart syndrome Arrhythmia Myocarditis Cardiac tamponade Pulmonary embolism Tension pneumothorax
Distributive	Sepsis Spinal cord trauma Anaphylaxis Heavy metal poisoning

total anomalous pulmonary venous return with obstruction. Evidence of poor perfusion, such as lethargy, mottled extremities, tachycardia, and tachypnea, is typically present. Sepsis and other noncardiac conditions (e.g., salt-wasting crisis in congenital adrenal hyperplasia) can cause similar presentations. Shock may also be the presentation of supraventricular tachycardia or complete heart block that has become decompensated (Table 56-1).

Congestive heart failure (CHF) is a common manifestation of both structural heart disease and congenital rhythm disturbances. Although respiratory distress, tachypnea, and rales may be present, subtler signs such as poor feeding and hepatomegaly may be the only manifestations of CHF. Peripheral edema as a manifestation of CHF is rare in infants. Acyanotic heart diseases with large left-to-right shunts, such as congenital aortic stenosis, interrupted aortic arch, and coarctation of the aorta, manifest as CHF as blood preferentially flows into the low-resistance pulmonary bed (Box 56-3). Total anomalous pulmonary venous return and VSD can also manifest as CHF owing to volume overload of the right ventricle.

BOX 56-3

Differential Diagnosis of Congestive Heart Failure in Infants

- Critical coarctation of the aorta
- Interrupted aortic arch
- Congenital aortic stenosis
- Hypoplastic left heart syndrome
- Large ventricular septal defect
- Truncus arteriosus
- Unrecognized supraventricular tachycardia
- Cardiac tamponade
- Myocarditis

Table 56-2 DIFFERENTIAL DIAGNOSIS OF CENTRAL CYANOSIS IN INFANTS

Cardiac Causes	
Right-to-left shunting	Tetralogy of Fallot Tricuspid atresia Pulmonary atresia Transposition of the great arteries with intact ventricular septum Ebstein's anomaly Truncus arteriosus Eisenmenger's syndrome
Pulmonary Causes	
Right-to left-shunting	Persistent pulmonary hypertension of the newborn
Ventilation-perfusion mismatch	Transient tachypnea of the newborn Congenital cystic adenomatoid malformation Pneumonia Congenital diaphragmatic hernia Hyaline membrane disease Pneumothorax Pleural effusion Hemothorax
Hypoventilation	Neonatal asphyxia Intraventricular hemorrhage Seizure Encephalitis Meningitis Sedative agents Botulism Neonatal myasthenia Croup Bronchiolitis Laryngotracheomalacia
Hematologic Causes	
Hemoglobinopathies	Carboxyhemoglobinemia Methemoglobinemia

Rhythm abnormalities such as sustained SVT and congenital complete heart block also can manifest as CHF from poor forward flow.

Cyanosis can be the first manifestation of CHD in infants, and severe lesions are typically diagnosed in utero or in the newborn nursery. Some lesions may escape detection, however, manifesting later in the neonatal period. Central cyanosis affecting the lips, mucous membranes, and trunk represents decreased arterial oxygen saturation and is always pathologic. The differential diagnosis of central cyanosis is presented in Table 56-2. Peripheral cyanosis limited to the extremities or circumoral regions is a normal newborn finding but can also be caused by non-CHD causes such as sepsis, cold exposure, and poor cardiac output.

Rhythm abnormalities such as SVT, long QTc syndrome, hypertrophic cardiomyopathy, and congenital complete heart block may manifest as syncope, especially in older children. Syncope is a common

Table 56-3 DIFFERENTIATING "INNOCENT" MURMURS FROM PATHOLOGIC MURMURS

	Innocent	Pathologic
Grade (out of 6)	1-2	3 or higher
Quality	Soft	Harsh or pansystolic
Second heart sound	Normally split	Single or fixed split
Other heart sounds	No clicks	Click present
Pulse findings	Normal	Decreased femoral pulses
Other abnormal findings	Absent	Present

pediatric presentation and typically has a benign prognosis, although documenting normal electrocardiogram (ECG) findings is important as a screen for more ominous causes of fainting. Although rare, sudden cardiac death as a first manifestation of the long QTc syndrome occurs in 9% of affected children and may be an underappreciated cause of sudden infant death syndrome.[4]

■ TYPICAL VARIATIONS

Although shock, CHF, cyanosis, and syncope are the common presentations of CHD, the signs and symptoms that bring a pediatric patient to the attention of a health care provider may be more protean. CHD, either structural or arrhythmogenic, should be considered in a child presenting with sweating during feeding, failure to thrive, irritability, chest pain (in older children), unexplained hypertension, or a new murmur. Murmurs are common in the pediatric age group, occurring in up to 60% of newborns, the vast majority of whom have structurally normal hearts.[5] Most "innocent" murmurs of infancy and childhood are due to either peripheral pulmonary stenosis (PPS) or Still's murmurs. PPS murmurs are grade 1 to 2 of 6, midsystolic, high-pitched ejection murmurs best heard over the pulmonary area. Still's murmurs are grade 1 to 2 of 6, low-pitched systolic ejection murmurs best heard at the left lower sternal border that vary with heart rate and decrease in intensity with the Valsalva maneuver. Characteristics that differentiate between "innocent" and pathologic murmurs are presented in Table 56-3.

Differential Diagnosis

■ LESION-SPECIFIC PRESENTATIONS

■ Lesions Manifesting as Decreased Pulmonary Blood Flow

■ *Tetralogy of Fallot*

Tetralogy of Fallot, the most common structural CHD occurring outside the neonatal period, consists of the following anatomic abnormalities: a large ventricular septal defect, varying degrees of right ventricular outflow tract obstruction, an overriding aorta and right ventricular hypertrophy. Time of presentation is linked to the severity of right ventricular outflow tract obstruction and, thus, to the amount of pulmonary blood flow, with severe obstruction causing cyanosis in the newborn and earlier age at presentation. Less severe obstruction (a "pink" tet) may delay diagnosis or an infant may be presented to the ED with "tet spells," in which the child becomes episodically more cyanotic, reflecting worsening of the right ventricular outflow tract obstruction and decreased pulmonary blood flow.

Physical findings consist of a right ventricular heave and a single second heart sound (no pulmonic valve component). A harsh systolic ejection murmur, reflecting right ventricular outflow tract obstruction, may be present. The murmur characteristically softens as the severity of obstruction worsens and more blood is shunted across the VSD.

■ *Tricuspid Atresia*

Tricuspid atresia is characterized by complete absence of the tricuspid valve, a hypoplastic right ventricle, and the presence of a VSD. The size of the VSD determines the amount of pulmonary blood flow. Large VSDs may allow relatively normal pulmonary blood flow and delay the presentation. In these cases, because the left ventricle is the only functioning pumping chamber, fluid overload may occur, and affected infants and children may be presented with heart failure and hepatomegaly. Infants with small VSDs are dependent on the ductus arteriosus for pulmonary blood flow and are presented in the neonatal period with cyanosis as the ductus arteriosus closes. Blood returning to the heart enters the right atrium and flows across the foramen ovale (which remains patent) to enter the systemic circulation. A murmur of pulmonic stenosis may be present if the flow across the pulmonary valve is enough to be detected on auscultation.

■ *Pulmonary Atresia*

Pulmonary atresia with intact ventricular septum is associated with a hypoplastic right ventricle and is dependent on an atrial septal defect (ASD) and right-to-left shunting. Pulmonary blood flow depends on the ductus arteriosus, so affected patients are presented in the neonatal period with cyanosis as the ductus arteriosus closes. Physical examination typically demonstrates a single second heart sound (no pulmonic component), and if a murmur is present, it is typical of tricuspid regurgitation.

Lesions Manifesting as Increased Pulmonary Blood Flow

Total Anomalous Pulmonary Venous Return

Total anomalous pulmonary venous return (TAPVR) occurs as a result of the embryologic failure of the pulmonary veins to form a connection to the left atrium. The pulmonary veins can dump into the superior vena cava (supracardiac connection), into the portal vein (infracardiac connection), or into the right atrium via the coronary sinus. Obstruction of any of these anomalous connections leads to pulmonary congestion, respiratory distress, and varying levels of heart failure. Cyanosis may develop because of the decrease in oxygenated blood returning to the heart. Physical findings may indicate heart failure, and TAPVR with obstruction is characterized by a fixed, widely split second heart sound.

Truncus Arteriosus

Truncus arteriosus is defined as the presence of a single trunk arising from the heart that functions as both the aorta and the pulmonary artery. A single semilunar valve is present and overrides a VSD, allowing for complete mixing of systemic blood and pulmonary blood. As pulmonary vascular resistance falls after birth, more and more blood travels into the low-resistance pulmonary circuit, and heart failure develops. Affected infants who were not diagnosed in the newborn nursery typically are presented when heart failure develops. Physical findings include a wide pulse pressure and a systolic ejection murmur representing increased flow across the semilunar valve. A single second heart sound may also be found.

Transposition of the Great Arteries

Transposition of the great arteries (TGA) is a common congenital defect in which the pulmonary and systemic circuits are arranged in parallel rather than in series. TGA may be associated with VSD or ASD, but more commonly, no other defect is present, and mixing of oxygenated and deoxygenated blood occurs only at the ductus arteriosus. Infants with TGA are cyanotic at birth owing to right-to-left shunting, and the cyanosis gets worse as the ductus arteriosus closes. If therapy to keep the ductus arteriosus open (see later) is not instituted promptly, hypoxemia, acidosis, and death quickly ensue. In TGA without associated VSD or ASD, there may be no other telltale signs on physical examination. Children with TGA and an associated VSD or ASD may be presented later in the newborn period with heart failure, and a VSD murmur may be heard.

Hypoplastic Left Heart Syndrome

Hypoplastic left heart syndrome involves a severely hypoplastic left ventricle and small, atretic mitral and aortic valves. The right ventricle is the default pumping chamber to both the lungs and the systemic circulation, and all systemic circulation crosses from the pulmonary artery through the ductus arteriosus to supply the body. Cyanosis from birth is the rule, and typically the lesions are diagnosed in utero or in the nursery. As the ductus arteriosus closes, all blood returning to the heart goes to the lungs, and heart failure develops from volume overload. The pathway to the systemic circulation is also compromised, and shock develops. Physical findings include tricuspid and pulmonic murmurs from increased flow. Hepatomegaly may be apparent as failure develops.

ACYANOTIC STRUCTURAL CONGENITAL HEART DISEASE

Coarctation of the Aorta

Coarctation of the aorta refers to congenital narrowing of the aorta, most commonly at the level of the ductus arteriosus. Infants with coarctation have a normal oxygen saturation value and typically no cyanosis. When the ductus arteriosus is open, blood is able to bypass the obstruction, and few symptoms are present. As the ductus arteriosus closes, the systemic circulation may be compromised by the narrowed aorta. "Critical" coarctation occurs when the narrowing is severe, and these infants are presented when the ductus arteriosus closes with signs of shock. If the narrowing is less severe, children may be presented later in life. Physical findings consistent with coarctation include normal or increased blood pressure in the upper extremities and decreased perfusion to the lower extremities. Four-extremity blood pressures should be measured in any child in whom the diagnosis of coarctation of the aorta is being entertained. Frequently there is a harsh systolic ejection murmur in the left axilla and back.

Congenital Aortic Stenosis

Congenital aortic stenosis typically results when an aortic valve is congenitally bicuspid rather than tricuspid. It is estimated to occur in 1% to 2% of the population. Most infants with aortic stenosis are asymptomatic, and problems do not develop until later in life.[6] Affected children may be diagnosed as part of an evaluation for a heart murmur. If the stenosis is severe, symptoms may develop in infancy. Typically, critical congenital aortic stenosis manifests as the ductus arteriosus closes, the presentation consisting of heart failure due to increased pulmonary blood flow and signs of systemic hypoperfusion. A murmur may not be appreciable because of poor cardiac output. Physical findings include signs of shock with poor peripheral perfusion.

CONGENITAL RHYTHM DISTUBANCES

Supraventricular Tachycardia

Supraventricular tachycardia is characterized by a narrow complex elevated heart rhythm that is regular. Atrioventricular reentrant tachycardia (AVRT), including the Wolff-Parkinson-White syndrome, and atrioventricular nodal reentrant tachycardia (AVNRT) are the two most common forms of SVT in children. AVRT is more common in infants and younger children, with AVNRT rising in frequency after 2 years of age. The majority of children with SVT have structurally normal hearts, although SVT is associated with CHD in about 25% of cases.[7] Infants may be presented with respiratory distress, poor feeding, and irritability, and the rhythm abnormality may not be recognized until heart failure develops. Older children may be presented with syncope, chest pain, palpitations, or lightheadedness. Sudden cardiac death is rare with SVT unless there is underlying structural heart disease. Physical findings include tachycardia, hypotension, and signs of heart failure.

Long QTc Syndrome

Many patients with long QTc syndrome are asymptomatic, although syncope, palpitations, lightheadedness, or cardiac arrest may bring affected children to medical attention. Among those who have symptoms, a significant proportion have exercise-related complaints. The long QTc syndrome may actually cause some cases of sudden infant death syndrome. Family history of sudden cardiac death may be elicited. Autosomal recessive forms of congenital long QTc syndrome are associated with sensorineural hearing loss. Anderson syndrome is a rare autosomal dominant form of long QTc syndrome associated with hypokalemic periodic paralysis, facial dysmorphisms, and cardiac arrhythmias. Torsades de pointes is the classic rhythm abnormality occurring in long QTc syndrome and the baseline electrocardiogram may demonstrate bradycardia or atrioventricular block. The physical examination may demonstrate signs of associated syndromic abnormalities.

Congenital Complete Heart Block

Congenital complete heart block may manifest at any time during childhood, although many cases are diagnosed in utero. The common finding is bradycardia. In infants diagnosed after birth, physical findings include cannon waves in the neck (from atrial contraction against closed tricuspid valves) and signs of poor perfusion. A maternal history of connective tissue disease, particularly systemic lupus erythematosus, is sometimes present. Congenital complete heart block in older patients may manifest as syncope or sudden cardiac death.

Diagnostic Testing

The evaluation of the infant in critical condition with suspected cardiac disease should focus on excluding noncardiac causes of the patient's symptoms while attempting to confirm a cardiac lesion. The distinction between sepsis and decompensated cardiac disease is often difficult, and it is advisable to rule out sepsis in critically ill children and begin treatment with empirically chosen antibiotics. A complete sepsis evaluation consists of a complete blood count, blood culture, urinalysis, urine culture, and cerebrospinal fluid examination for meningitis. In the presence of cardiac disease, polycythemia from chronic hypoxia may be noted. A thorough physical examination is critical to evaluate for sources of possible infection (indicating possible sepsis) or ambiguous genitalia (seen with salt-wasting crisis from congenital adrenal hyperplasia).

ELECTROCARDIOGRAM

A 12-lead electrocardiogram should be performed on every infant and child in whom heart disease is suspected. If structural CHD is part of the differential diagnosis, a 15-lead electrocardiogram (includes leads V_3R, V_4R, and V_7) may give added information. Correct interpretation of pediatric ECG values can be challenging because most normal adult values are abnormal in the newborn period. Normal ECG parameters in children are presented in Table 56-4, whereas Tables 56-5 and 56-6 list ECG findings associated with specific cardiac lesions.[8] SVT typically manifests as a narrow-complex tachycardia with a regular rhythm. Heart rates are generally higher than 220 beats/min, and P waves may be visible. SVT with aberrant conduction (presenting as a wide-complex tachycardia) is rare in the pediatric population, and a wide-complex tachycardia should be considered ventricular in origin until proven otherwise. Long QTc syndrome manifests as a QTc interval that is prolonged (>440 msec). Acquired causes of a prolonged QTc, such as electrolyte abnormality (hypocalcemia, hypokalemia, hypomagnesemia) and drug effect (erythromycin, trimethoprim, etc.), should be ruled out.

CHEST RADIOGRAPH

A chest radiograph is useful in the evaluation of suspected cardiac disease because it allows assessment of heart size, pulmonary vascular markings, and situs of the aortic arch. Heart size can help differentiate between a cardiac lesion and sepsis.[9] An enlarged heart may be seen with left-sided obstructive lesions such as congenital aortic stenosis, interrupted aortic arch, and critical coarctation of the aorta. Certain CHD lesions have specific radiographic findings, such as the egg-on-a-string pattern seen in transposition of the great arteries and the boot-shaped heart in tetralogy of Fallot (Fig. 56-2). Structural CHD can be

Table 56-4 NORMAL PEDIATRIC ELECTROCARDIOGRAPHIC PARAMETERS

			LEAD V1		LEAD V6	
Age	Heart Rate (beats/min)	Normal QRS Axis (mean)	Mean R Wave Amplitude, mm (98th percentile)	Mean S Wave Amplitude, mm (98th percentile)	Mean R Wave Amplitude, mm (98th percentile)	Mean S Wave Amplitude, mm (98th percentile)
0-7 days	95-160	+30 to −180 (+110)	13.3 (25.5)	7.7 (8.8)	4.8 (11.8)	3.2 (9.6)
1-3 wk	105-180	+30 to +180 (+110)	10.6 (20.8)	4.2 (10.8)	7.6 (16.4)	3.4 (9.8)
1-6 mo	110-180	+10 to +125 (+70)	9.7 (19)	5.4 (15)	12.4 (22)	2.8 (8.3)
6-12 mo	110-170	+10 to +125 (+60)	9.4 (20.3)	6.4 (18.1)	12.6 (22.7)	2.1 (7.2)
1-3 yr	90-150	+10 to +125 (+60)	8.5 (18)	9 (21)	14 (23.3)	1.7 (6)
4-5 yr	65-135	0 to +110 (+60)	7.6 (16)	11 (22.5)	15.6 (25)	1.4 (4.7)
6-8 yr	60-130	−15 to +110 (+60)	6 (13)	12 (24.5)	16.3 (26)	1.1 (3.9)
9-11 yr	60-110	−15 to +110 (+60)	5.4 (12.1)	11.9 (25.4)	16.3 (25.4)	1.0 (3.9)
12-16 yr	60-110	−15 to +110 (+60)	4.1 (9.9)	10.8 (21.2)	14.3 (23)	0.8 (3.7)
>16 yr	60-100	−15 to +110 (+60)	3 (9)	10 (20)	10 (20)	0.8 (3.7)

Table 56-5 PHYSICAL, CHEST RADIOGRAPH, AND ELECTROCARDIOGRAM FINDINGS IN CONGENITAL HEART DISEASE

Condition	Physical Findings	Chest Radiograph Findings	Electrocardiogram Findings
Truncus arteriosus	SEM, wide pulse pressure, single S_2	Increased PBF	Biventricular hypertrophy, LAE
Transposition of the great arteries	None	Normal or increased PBF	RVH
Total anomalous pulmonary venous return	Fixed split S_2	Increased PBF, small heart	RVH
Hypoplastic left heart syndrome	TS, PS murmur	Increased PBF	RVH
Tricuspid atresia	±PS murmur	Decreased PBF	LVH, RAE
Pulmonary atresia	±TR murmur, single S_2	Decreased PBF, large heart	LVH
Tetralogy of Fallot	PS murmur, single S_2	Decreased PBF, boot-shaped heart	RVH
Coarctation of the aorta	SEM, pulse differential between upper and lower extremities	Rib notching late	LVH
Aortic stenosis	SEM	Increased PBF	LVH

±, sometimes present, sometimes not; LAE, left atrial enlargement; LVH, left ventricular hypertrophy; PBF, pulmonary blood flow; PS, pulmonic stenosis; RAE, right atrial enlargement; RVH, right ventricular hypertrophy; S_2, second heart sound; SEM, systolic ejection murmur; TR, tricuspid regurgitation; TS, tricuspid stenosis.

broken down into lesions that cause an increase in pulmonary blood flow and lesions with decreased pulmonary blood flow; the presence of increased pulmonary vascular markings on radiograph can aid in diagnosis (Box 56-4). The aorta is normally left-sided, and a right-sided aortic arch can be seen with tetralogy of Fallot, TGA, and truncus arteriosus.

■ HYPEROXIA TEST

Useful in distinguishing cardiac from pulmonary sources of cyanosis, the hyperoxia test hinges on the premise that supplemental oxygen does not increase the PaO_2 value in the presence of an intracardiac shunt to the same degree that it does in isolated

Table 56-6 ELECTROCARDIOGRAM (ECG) FINDINGS IN CONGENITAL RHYTHM DISTURBANCES

Condition	Findings
Supraventricular tachycardia	Regular R-R interval Heart rate >220 beats/min Narrow QRS complex
Long QTc syndrome	QTc interval >440 msec Resting ECG may show bradycardia or atrioventricular (AV) block
Congenital complete heart block	AV dissociation, bradycardia

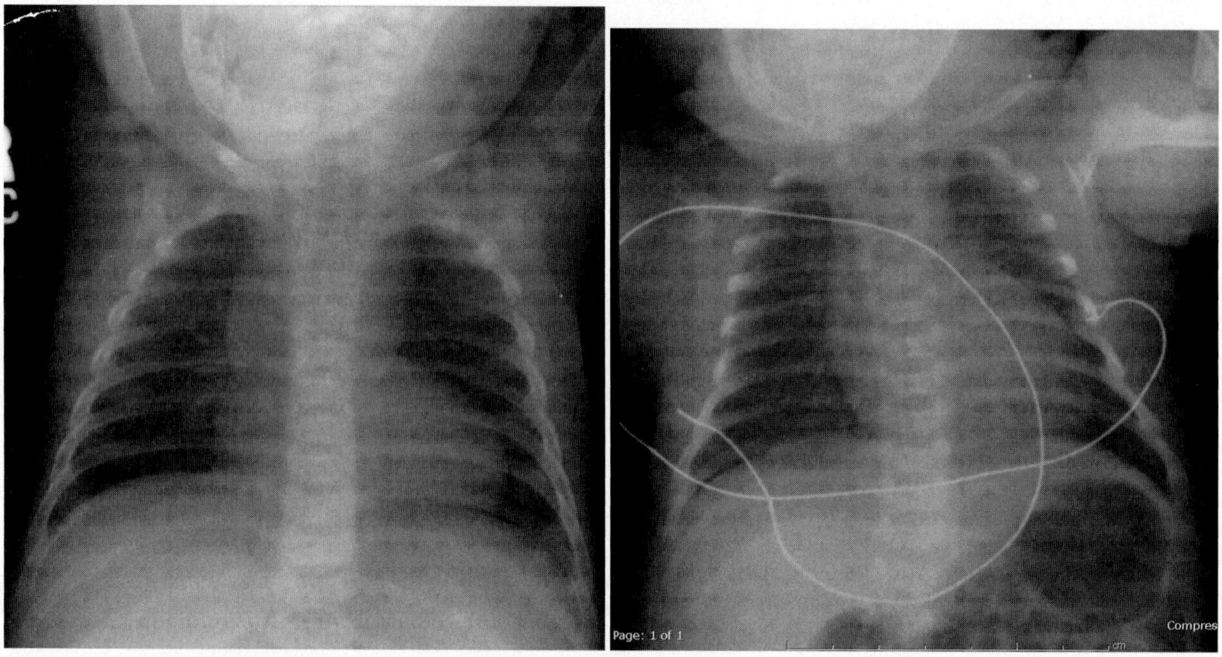
Page: 1 of 1

A B

FIGURE 56-2 Classic chest radiographic findings in congenital heard disease. **A,** Tetralogy of Fallot (boot-shaped heart). **B,** Transposition of the great vessels (egg-on-a-string). (From Multimedia Library, Children's Hospital Boston. **A,** http://www.childrenshospital.org/cfapps/mml/index.cfm?CAT=media&MEDIA_ID=1420; **B,** http://www.childrenshospital.org/cfapps/mml/index.cfm?CAT=media&MEDIA_ID=1355.)

pulmonary disease (see Tips and Tricks box). The child with TGA or severe right ventricular outflow tract obstruction (i.e., tetralogy of Fallot, pulmonary atresia, tricuspid atresia) typically has $Pa{O_2}$ values less than 60 mm Hg during hyperoxia. In lesions such as truncus arteriosus, TAPVR, and hypoplastic left heart syndrome, which involve intracardiac mixing, $Pa{O_2}$ values range between 75 and 150 mm Hg. It is critical to understand that some pulmonary lesions cause right-to-left shunting (persistent pulmonary hypertension of the newborn) or severe ventilation-perfusion mismatch (meconium aspiration syndrome, pneumonia) and the $Pa{O_2}$ value may not rise above 150 mm Hg with hyperoxia.

> *Tips and Tricks*
>
> **THE HYPEROXIA TEST**
>
> Have the patient breathe 100% oxygen for 10 minutes (hyperoxia) and then draw a post-ductal arterial blood gas specimen.
>
> Pulmonary disease is suggested if the $Pa{O_2}$ with 100% oxygen is greater than 150 mm Hg.
>
> If the $Pa{O_2}$ value is below 150 mm Hg during hyperoxia, a cyanotic cardiac lesion should be suspected.

■ ECHOCARDIOGRAPHY

Echocardiography is the definitive test for suspected structural heart disease. Any infant with central cyanosis, cardiac enlargement on chest radiograph, a suspicious murmur, or a pulse differential across the ductus arteriosus or whose $Pa{O_2}$ fails to rise with the hyperoxia test should be evaluated with echocardiography. This modality also allows for evaluation of

BOX 56-4

Lesion-Specific Presentations Based on Pulmonary Blood Flow

Congenital Lesions Causing Increased Pulmonary Blood Flow or Left-to-Right Shunting

- Total anomalous pulmonary venous return
- Tricuspid atresia
- Transposition of the great arteries
- Truncus arteriosus
- Hypoplastic left heart syndrome
- Isolated atrial septal defects
- Isolated ventricular septal defects

Congenital Lesions Causing Decreased Pulmonary Blood Flow or Right-to-Left Shunting

- Tetralogy of Fallot
- Tricuspid atresia
- Pulmonary atresia

heart function and pericardial fluid in acquired conditions such as myocarditis. Echocardiography should also be considered in the evaluation for suspected SVT, because a significant proportion of cases are associated with structural CHD.

Treatment

■ INTERVENTIONS

The initial management of the infant or child with suspected cardiac disease who is presented in extremis should focus on cardiopulmonary support, establishment of intravenous (IV) access, and appropriate monitoring. Intubation may be required, and rapid-sequence intubation should be considered the method of choice for management of the pediatric airway. Because the presentation of decompensated pediatric cardiac disease is similar to that of sepsis, empirical treatment with broad-spectrum antibiotics (ampicillin 100 to 200 mg/kg/day and gentamicin 5 to 6 mg/kg/day; *or* ceftriaxone 100 mg/kg if the child is older than 28 days) should be started after appropriate specimens for blood, urine, and cerebrospinal fluid cultures are obtained. If shock does not respond to fluid resuscitation (normal saline 20 mL/kg IV to a total of 60 mL/kg), inotropes such as dopamine (start 5 μg/kg/min titrated to effect) or dobutamine (0.5 μg/kg/min) may be added.

If a neonate is in shock and does not promptly improve to IV fluid administration, CHD may be present; a neonatologist should be called and prostaglandin E_1 treatment should be considered, even presumptively. Prostaglandin E_1 infusion can be lifesaving in infants with ductal-dependent pulmonary or systemic blood flow. The infusion should be started at 0.1 μg/kg/min and increased or decreased according to clinical response. Side effects include flushing, diarrhea, fever, and apnea. Many such patients require intubation, especially those who are being transferred to another hospital.

BOX 56-5

Management Approach for Congenital Long QTc Syndrome

If first electrocardiogram (ECG) shows QTc >440 msec, a second ECG should be performed. Results of second ECG dictate actions to be taken, as follows:

- Normal QTc: No action needed.
- QTc 440-500 msec: Evaluation (ECG screening of family, genetic testing, Holter monitoring). Also, beta-blocker therapy should be considered.
- QTc >500 msec: Evaluation as above and initiation of beta-blocker therapy.

■ TET SPELLS

Hypercyanotic tet spells should be treated with supplemental oxygen, morphine (0.1 mg/kg), and knee-chest positioning. If these measures fail, and in consultation with a pediatric cardiologist, consideration can be given to phenylephrine infusion (0.1 μ/kg/min titrated to effect) to increase systemic vascular resistance and drive more blood flow across the right ventricular outflow tract obstruction.

■ SUPRAVENTRICULAR TACHYCARDIA

Treatment of SVT depends on the clinical stability of the child. If there are signs of decompensation (hypotension, poor perfusion), immediate synchronized cardioversion with 0.5 to 1 J/kg should be performed. In the more stable child, vagal maneuvers (i.e., application of ice to the face or the Valsalva maneuver) may be attempted. Once IV access is obtained, adenosine (0.1 mg/kg to maximum dose of 6 mg) should be administered via rapid IV bolus if vagal maneuvers fail. If there is no response to the first dose, the second dose should be 0.2 mg/kg to a maximum of 12 mg, given in the same manner.

■ LONG QTc SYNDROME

The mainstay of therapy in patients diagnosed with congenital long QTc syndrome is beta-blocker therapy, which should be given in consultation with a pediatric cardiologist (Box 56-5). Treatment of torsades de pointes associated with long QTc syndrome should consist of cardioversion (0.5-1 J/kg) if the patient is unstable. Magnesium sulfate (25-50 mg/kg IV) is the antiarrhythmic agent of choice for treatment of torsades.

Disposition

Any child presented in extremis with a new diagnosis of CHD should be admitted to an intensive care unit setting in a hospital with pediatric cardiology until stabilized. Children who are less ill may be managed on an appropriately monitored floor. Outpatient management may be appropriate for children in whom structural heart disease is suspected on the basis of a murmur but who have no other symptoms.

Patients with SVT who are asymptomatic, who have no signs of heart failure, and in whom the SVT converted to a normal sinus rhythm in the ED can be considered for outpatient management if appropriate follow-up with a pediatric cardiologist can be arranged. Patients presented with symptomatic long QTc syndrome (resuscitated arrest, torsades de pointes) should be admitted to a monitored bed. Most other cases can be managed with outpatient pediatric cardiology follow-up. The child with congenital complete heart block, when diagnosed, should be admitted to a monitored setting because of the risk of hemodynamic compromise.

REFERENCES

1. Hoffman JI, Christianson R: Congenital heart disease in a cohort of 19,502 births with long-term follow-up. Am J Cardiol 1978;42:641.
2. Keuhl KS, Loffredo CA, Ferencz C: Failure to diagnose congenital heart disease in infancy. Pediatrics 1999;103:743.
3. Schwartz PJ: The long QTc syndrome. Curr Probl Cardiol 1997;22:297.
4. Garson A Jr, Dick M, Fournier A, et al: The long QTc syndrome in children: An international study of 287 patients. Circulation 1993;87:1866.
5. Braudo M, Rowe RD: Auscultation of the heart—early neonatal period. Am J Dis Child 1961;101:575.
6. Roberts WC: The congenitally bicuspid aortic valve: A study of 85 autopsy cases. Am J Cardiol 1970;26:72.
7. Tanel RE, Walsh EP, Triedman JK, et al: Five-year experience with radiofrequency catheter ablation: Implications for management of arrhythmias in pediatric and young adult patients. J Pediatr 1997;131:878.
8. Robertson J, Shilkofski N (eds): The Harriet Lane Handbook: A Manual for Pediatric House Officers, 17th ed. Philadelphia, Mosby, 2005.
9. Pickert CB, Moss MM, Fiser DH: Differentiation of systemic infection and congenital obstructive left heart disease in the very young infant. Pediatr Emerg Care 1998;14:263.

SUGGESTED READINGS

Brickner ME, Hillis LD, Lange RA: Congenital heart disease in adults: First of two parts. N Engl J Med 2000;342:256.

Brickner ME, Hillis LD, Lange RA: Congenital heart disease in adults: Second of two parts. N Engl J Med 2000;342:334.

Burton DA, Cabalka AK: Cardiac evaluation in infants. Pediatr Clin North Am 1994;41:991.

Hoke TR, Donohue PK, Bawa PK, Mitchell RD: Oxygen saturation as a screening test for critical congenital heart disease: A preliminary study. Pediatr Cardiol 2002;23:403.

McNamara DG: Value and limitations of auscultation in the management of congenital heart disease. Pediatr Clin North Am 1990;37:93.

Okelly S, Bove E: Hypoplastic left heart syndrome. Br Med J 1997;314:87.

Schwartz PJ, Priori SG, Dumaine R, et al: A molecular link between the sudden infant death syndrome and the long QTc syndrome. N Engl J Med 2000;343:262.

Schwartz PJ, Stramba-Badiale M, Segantini A, et al: Prolongation of the QTc interval and the sudden infant death syndrome. N Engl J Med 1998;338:1709.

VanRoekens CN, Zuckerberg AL: Emergency management of hypercyanotic crises in tetralogy of Fallot. Ann Emerg Med 1995;25:256.

Chapter 57

Chest Pain

Matthew Strehlow and Jeffrey Tabas

KEY POINTS

Observation and repeated testing are extremely valuable in the patient with chest pain whose diagnosis is unclear.

"Rapid rule-out" of acute myocardial infarction can be performed with serial cardiac marker testing after an appropriate interval from symptom onset (6 hours for creatine kinase–MB fraction or 8 hours for troponin I or T), although shorter intervals may be acceptable if immediate stress testing is performed.

Normal cardiac marker values do not exclude unstable angina.

Consider life-threatening diagnoses other than acute myocardial infarction in the patient with chest pain, including aortic dissection, which is frequently missed and often manifests atypically.

Chest Pain

Every year 5.7 million people present to U.S. EDs complaining of chest pain, which accounts for roughly 5% of ED visits and is the second most common reason for presentation. The differential diagnosis of chest pain ranges from benign causes, such as muscle strain, to the immediately life-threatening, such as acute coronary syndrome, pulmonary embolism, and aortic dissection. Although the focus in patients with chest pain remains appropriately on life-threatening causes, a majority of patients have benign or indeterminate diagnoses after ED evaluation. In one study of ED patients with symptoms consistent with acute cardiac ischemia, only 8% had acute myocardial infarction (AMI) and 9% had unstable angina.[1] Another investigation of patients presenting to the ED with nontraumatic chest pain found that 4% were diagnosed with AMI, 7.5% had unstable angina or stable coronary disease, and less than 1% had pulmonary embolism or aortic dissection.[2] Given the potentially lethal nature of conditions that manifest as chest pain and the lack of sensitivity or specificity, in many instances, of the history and physical examination, the EP must have an organized approach, a complete differential diagnosis, and a thorough understanding of the assessment and management of this common complaint.

■ ANATOMY

In the differential diagnosis of the patient with chest pain, one must consider the five groups of structures in the thorax: cardiac (heart and pericardium), pulmonary (lungs and pleura), gastrointestinal (esophagus and upper abdominal contents), vascular (aorta and great vessels), and musculoskeletal (chest wall). Chest discomfort is experienced through three distinct pathways, as follows:

Visceral pain, from internal structures such as the heart, lungs, esophagus, and aorta, may be difficult for the patient to define or localize. It is experienced as discomfort or a vague sensation, and is often difficult to pinpoint.

Somatic pain, from chest wall structures and the parietal pleura, is often easier to describe and localize. Somatic pain may be sharp or stabbing and exacerbated by movement or position.

Referred pain, from irritation or inflammation of upper abdominal contents, is a form of visceral pain that may be perceived in the chest wall, shoulder or upper back.

A differential diagnosis based on the anatomic structures within the chest is given in Table 57-1.

PRESENTING SIGNS AND SYMPTOMS

Most patients with nontraumatic chest pain warrant high triage priority and an early electrocardiogram (ECG) (recommended within 10 minutes) to evaluate for AMI. Patient stabilization, evaluation of the history, physical examination, and diagnostic and therapeutic interventions proceed simultaneously. As assessment continues, interventions are refined (Box 57-1). Importantly, the history and physical findings alone are inadequate to definitively establish or exclude a diagnosis of cardiac etiology.

The EP should keep the following points and issues in mind during assessment of a patient with chest pain:

- Use the term "discomfort" as opposed to "pain" to facilitate communication.
- Do not ascribe partially reproducible pain to a musculoskeletal cause. Pain arising from inflammation of the pericardium (secondary to AMI or pericarditis) or inflammation of the pleura (pulmonary embolism, pneumonia, or pleurisy) can be partially reproduced by palpation.
- Substantial evidence suggests that responses to treatments such as sublingual nitroglycerin or a "GI cocktail" do not differentiate the etiology of the chest pain.
- Chest pain that is completely pleuritic (present only on inspiration) or completely reproducible significantly decreases suspicion for cardiac etiologies and raises suspicion for pulmonary or musculoskeletal etiologies. Partially pleuritic (worse with inspiration) or partially reproducible chest pain has much less predictive value.
- Do not overestimate the value of low-risk features when high-risk features are present (i.e., pain that is completely pleuritic but radiates to the left arm should still raise concern for possible acute coronary syndrome).
- The history and physical examination of patients with nonspecific chest pain are inadequate to justify discharge without further evaluation.

Table 57-1 DIFFERENTIAL DIAGNOSIS OF CHEST PAIN

Heart	Myocardial infarction Unstable angina Pericarditis Myocarditis Valvular disease (especially aortic stenosis)
Lungs	Pneumonia/other infections Pneumothorax Pulmonary embolus Exacerbation of chronic obstructive pulmonary disease or asthma Tumor
Aorta	Dissection Aneurysm Aortitis
Gastrointestinal	
Esophagus	Esophagitis (e.g., candidal) Gastroesophageal reflux disease (GERD) Spasm (nutcracker esophagus) Foreign body Rupture (Boerhaave's syndrome)
Upper abdomen	Cholecystitis Pancreatitis Duodenal ulcer Hepatic disease Biliary disease Subphrenic abscesses
Chest wall	Costochondritis (Tietze's disease) Contusion Rib fracture Muscle strain or tear Varicella zoster

Acute Coronary Syndrome

Several risk stratification systems have been proposed for acute coronary syndrome. These systems have been shown to help with risk stratification, enabling triage decisions. They have never been shown to

BOX 57-1

Approach to the Patient with Chest Pain

Initial Assessment (<10 minutes)

- ABCs: airway, breathing, and circulation
- Patient appearance
- Vital signs, O_2 saturation
- Electrocardiogram (ECG)
- Directed history and physical examination

If patient appears ill, history raises concerns, vital signs are abnormal, or the ECG shows evidence of ischemia, the following actions should be taken:

- Establishment of intravenous access, O_2 administration, and cardiac monitoring
- Immediate subsequent assessment (as follows)

Subsequent Assessment

- Aspirin 325 mg orally (unless ischemia is excluded or aspirin is contraindicated)
- Complete history and physical examination
- Radiographic, laboratory, and further electrocardiographic evaluation as indicated

improve the ability to formulate discharge decisions in comparison with practitioner judgment. The American College of Cardiology and American Heart Association have published criteria to determine a patient's risk of coronary artery disease (CAD) and adverse outcomes for acute coronary syndrome.[3] These guidelines are cumbersome and more appropriately applied to patients with documented disease than to the undifferentiated ED patient. A simplified approach to stratifying risk is to determine whether the patient has *definite* acute coronary syndrome, *probable* acute coronary syndrome, or *possible* acute coronary syndrome, as follows[4]:

- Patients with *definite* acute coronary syndrome are those with (1) ECG changes diagnostic of ischemia or infarction *or* (2) diagnostic elevation of serum cardiac markers *or* (3) evidence of new heart failure or shock *directly attributable* to an acute ischemic event.
- Patients with *probable* acute coronary syndrome are those in whom there is high suspicion for acute coronary syndrome without definitive criteria. An example is the patient with a classic history for acute coronary syndrome or whose cardiac marker values are slightly elevated but still below the diagnostic cutoff and who does not have clear ECG evidence of ischemia.
- Patients with *possible* acute coronary syndrome constitute the majority of patients with chest pain. They have atypical histories, their ECG findings are normal or unchanged from previous studies, or suspected alternative etiologies triggering their symptoms.

This chapter is focused on patients with *possible* acute coronary syndrome. After chest radiography, a substantial proportion of such patients require further testing and observation, such as serial cardiac biomarker testing or other tests to evaluate for alternate diagnoses.

The challenge for the EP lies in determining when and which patients with *possible* acute coronary syndrome can be safely discharged home. At this time no definitive answer exists. A critical error, however, is failure to identify features that warrant further evaluation. Characteristics such as advanced age, known coronary artery disease, diabetes, pain similar to that of a prior myocardial infarction, worsening of typical angina, pressure-like or squeezing discomfort, and radiation of pain to the neck, left shoulder, or left arm have all been shown to increase the likelihood of AMI.

■ PRESENTING SIGNS AND SYMPTOMS

The classic presentation for AMI is discomfort that feels like an elephant sitting on one's chest, radiates to the left shoulder, arm, or jaw, and is associated with shortness of breath, nausea, or diaphoresis. Patients may describe their discomfort with a clenched fist against their chest, known as Levine's sign. Physical examination demonstrates tachycardia, diaphoresis, and, if the infarction has compromised left ventricular function, findings of acute heart failure, such as hypoxia, tachypnea, elevated jugular venous pulsations, and bilateral rales. The classic presentation for unstable angina is a sense of discomfort or pressure that is similar to that of AMI but transient in nature. Patients experience similar associated symptoms typically brought on by exertion and relieved with rest or nitroglycerin. In practice, these classic presentations are the exception rather than the norm.

Risk factors for coronary artery disease predict a patient's risk for development of ischemic heart disease over many years but are only moderately predictive of acute coronary syndrome in the ED. Most important, it is well established that a lack of cardiac risk factors by itself does not place a patient at low risk for acute cardiac events.

Historical and examination features that raise or lower the likelihood of acute coronary syndrome are described in the Tables 57-2 and 57-3. It is important to remember that the presence of lower-likelihood features does not exclude the diagnosis of acute coronary syndrome. One study of patients with AMI found that 22% had sharp/stabbing pain and 13% partially pleuritic pain.[5]

The physical examination should be thorough, and findings suggestive of an alternative diagnosis

Table 57-2 CLINICAL FEATURES OF PATIENTS WITH CHEST PAIN THAT RAISE THE LIKELIHOOD OF ACUTE MYOCARDIAL INFARCTION

Features with high likelihood ratio (>2.0)	Age >60 years (2.2) Diabetes (2.4) Radiation of pain to either or both arms, shoulder, or jaw (3.0) Findings of congestive heart failure (3.0) Similarity to previous acute myocardial infarction or angina (4.0) Ischemia on electrocardiography (from 5 to 50)
Features with moderate likelihood ratio (1.5 to 2.0)	Smoking history (1.5) Family history of premature cardiac death (1.5) History of myocardial infarction (2.0) Chest pain as the chief complaint (2.0) Nausea or vomiting (2.0) Sweating (2.0) Male gender (1.6)

may be helpful but are often not adequately specific to exclude acute coronary syndrome. For example, in 7% of patients with AMI, the pain is fully reproduced by palpation.[5]

■ DIAGNOSTIC TESTING

Thirty percent to 50% of patients with AMI present with diagnostic ECG findings, 40% to 70% with nonspecific ECG findings, and 1% to 10% with normal ECG findings. Nonspecific or unchanged ECG findings do not affect the likelihood of acute coronary syndrome. Although a normal electrocardiogram does not exclude acute coronary syndrome, it significantly decreases the likelihood. Comparing the electrocardiogram with previous or serial electrocardiograms can improve sensitivity and specificity. A right-sided ECG is recommended in all patients with inferior ST changes, and a posterior lead ECG is recommended if ST depression is present in the septal leads, V_1 through V_3. Electrocardiography helps guide not only diagnosis but also therapy decisions (i.e., the presence of ST segment elevation in AMI is a primary criterion for thrombolytic therapy). As with all tests, it is imperative to interpret ECG findings in context.

An understanding of cardiac biomarkers is pivotal to excluding possible AMI in the ED. Currently, *acute myocardial infarction* is defined as the rise and fall of serum cardiac biomarkers in the presence of at least one of three other findings: ischemic symptoms, a pattern of progressive ischemic changes on an ECG, or coronary artery reperfusion.

Table 57-3 FEATURES OF CHEST PAIN THAT LOWER THE LIKELIHOOD OF ACUTE MYOCARDIAL INFARCTION*

Feature	Frequency in Patients with Acute Ischemia (%)
Pleuritic pain	13
Pain that is reproducible with palpation or movement	7
Sharp, stabbing pain	22
Pain that lasts seconds or is constant for 24 hours or longer[3]	NA

*Likelihood ratio around 0.3.
NA, not available.

Creatine kinase–MB fraction (CK-MB) is an enzyme present at higher percentages in cardiac muscle than in skeletal muscle and is relatively specific for cardiac muscle damage. False-positive results occur in renal failure and with large amounts of skeletal muscle injury, such as that seen in rhabdomyolysis. The CK-MB index improves the specificity of the biomarker by comparing the ratio of CK-MB with total CK. Levels higher than 5% are consistent with AMI, whereas those from 3% to 5% are indeterminate. The presence of CK-MB is detectable in blood 3 to 8 hours after myocardial infarction and returns to normal within 48 to 72 hours (Table 57-4). CK-MB subforms, $CK\text{-}MB_1$ and $CK\text{-}MB_2$, rise earlier than CK-MB and are detectable at 1 to 3 hours after injury, achieving a sensitivity of 92% at 6 hours. Unfortunately, laboratory testing for $CK\text{-}MB_1$ and $CK\text{-}MB_2$ is not widely available.

Cardiac troponins are more sensitive and specific than CK-MB for cardiac muscle damage. Troponins, regulatory proteins found in cardiac muscle, are composed of three subunits: I, T, and C. Cardiac subunits I and T are genetically distinct from skeletal muscle forms, and no cross-reactivity occurs on immunoassays. Within 2 to 8 hours of AMI, troponin levels are abnormal and remain so for 7 to 10 days (see Table 57-3). Detectable troponin at a value below the diagnostic cutoff for AMI still portends a higher risk for adverse outcomes.[6] Nonspecific elevations, especially for troponin T, can occur with renal dysfunction, pulmonary embolism, septic shock, decompensated heart failure, myocardial contusion, pericarditis, and myocarditis.

Myoglobin is a heme protein in skeletal and cardiac muscle that rises rapidly within 2 to 4 hours and returns to normal within 24 to 36 hours. Its utility is limited by inadequate sensitivity and specificity, and its measurement is primarily used in combination with measurements of CK-MB and troponin as a

Table 57-4 CHARACTERISTICS OF CARDIAC MARKER LEVELS AFTER MYOCARDIAL INFARCTION (MI)*

Cardiac Marker	Time of Rise (hours after MI)	Time of Peak (hours after MI)	Time of Return to Baseline (after MI)	Time of Second Measurement (hours after MI)
Myoglobin	<3	4-9	<24 hours	—
Creatine kinase–MB form (CK-MB)	3-8	9-30	1-3 days	6-10
CK-MB subforms	1-3	4-6	18-24 hours	6-10
Troponin T	2-6	10-24	10-15 days	8-12
Troponin I	2-6	10-24	7-10 days	8-12

*The American College of Emergency Physicians (ACEP) recommends an initial cardiac marker measurement and a second measurement at the given intervals for rapid exclusion of MI in low- to moderate-risk patients. It is unclear whether a second measurement is needed if the time between symptom onset and the patient's presentation to the ED exceeds the recommended interval for the second measurement. See Fesmise FM, Decker WW, Diercks DB, et al: Clinical policy: Critical issues in the evaluation and management of adult patients with non-ST-segment elevation acute coronary syndromes. Ann Emerg Med 2006;48:270-301.

point-of-care "triple marker" assay. Studies have demonstrated that specificity can be improved through evaluation of the rate of myoglobin elevation (delta myoglobin) over 1 to 2 hours. It is recommended that delta myoglobin cutoff values of 25% to 40% be used to indicate abnormality. Other cardiac markers are being investigated, and their roles are being determined.

Recommendations, based on the best available evidence and consensus, argue against using a single cardiac marker value within 6 hours of symptom onset to exclude AMI. For patients presenting more than 6 to 8 hours after onset of the most recent episode of pain, a single negative cardiac marker value is often adequate to exclude AMI (but not unstable angina) in patients with possible acute coronary syndrome. A period of observation, which includes repeated ECG and serum cardiac marker testing, can be used to rapidly rule out AMI at 6 hours from symptom onset with CK-MB and 8 hours with troponins (see Table 57-4). There is some evidence that a more accelerated testing approach is appropriate when such testing was followed immediately by stress imaging. In fact, one investigation found it was safe to test patients with chest pain on an exercise treadmill immediately, without obtaining initial cardiac marker values. The patients involved in this study, however, were at extremely low risk, with normal or near-normal ECG findings, no evidence of heart failure, and the ability to exercise, and they were found to have only a 1% rate of AMI.[7]

■ OBSERVATION UNITS AND PROTOCOLS

Increases in resource utilization, costs, and medicolegal concerns associated with patients presenting to the ED with chest pain have led to the advent of rapid assessment protocols (RAPs) and chest pain units. These strategies aim to lower admission rates and cost of care while minimizing the inappropriate discharge of patients with unrecognized acute coronary syndrome. Approaches vary widely in these strategies, and most published methodologies involve immediate stress testing of low- to moderate-risk patients after a period of observation with serial ECGs and cardiac marker testing. Protocol-driven strategies increase the number of patients evaluated, accelerate the rate of evaluation, lower the number of missed events, and may save overall costs.

After a period of observation, repeat cardiac marker testing, and either continuous or intermittent electrocardiographic monitoring, patients in whom ECG findings are unremarkable and cardiac biomarker results are negative undergo stress testing. Guidelines recommend that the stress test be performed within 72 hours of ED discharge; a majority of published reports describe stress testing prior to discharge.[8]

The most common adjunctive test is the continuous-ECG treadmill stress test (TST). Patients with normal TST testing results under these circumstances have been found to have acceptably low rates of missed ischemia and adverse events. Unfortunately, a reasonable percentage of patients are poor candidates for an ECG TST (18% in one study) owing either to an inability to ambulate at a moderate (2.5-mph) pace or to the presence of confounding baseline ECG findings, such as left ventricular hypertrophy, left bundle branch block, ventricular-paced rhythm, or preexcitation syndrome. ECG TST also has a 5% to 25% nondiagnostic rate, depending on the patient population and protocol used. Patients in whom the ECG TST cannot be used must undergo stress imaging studies. Patients with nondiagnostic or abnormal ECG TST results should receive further evaluation, which usually requires admission.

Although the percentage of low risk chest pain patients diagnosed with acute coronary syndrome during their hospital evaluation is low, 0.5% to 5%, the admission rate of patients who have been evaluated in a chest pain unit ranges from 10% to 50%. Patients discharged after a rapid assessment protocol or chest pain unit evaluation should receive outpatient follow-up soon.

■ TREATMENT

Patients with possible acute coronary syndrome should receive aspirin. Patients in whom concern for the syndrome is greater may require nitrates or beta-blockade. Nitrates have never been shown to improve outcomes in acute coronary syndrome, and recently, the response to nitrates has been shown to lack predictive value in the diagnosis of acute coronary syndrome. Their use in these low-likelihood patients should be weighed against the risk of hypotension or even headache. Beta-blockade has been shown to be of benefit in patients with acute coronary syndrome. Therapies such as heparin, clopidogrel, and glycoprotein IIb/IIIa inhibitors have been shown to be of benefit primarily in patients with *definite* acute coronary syndrome and should not be used in this low-likelihood group.[4]

■ DISPOSITION

It is important to acknowledge that the clinician cannot obtain perfect sensitivity in the assessment of patients with any disease. An analysis of multiple studies on acute coronary syndrome found that clinicians missed fewer AMIs when they admitted more patients.[9] Clearly, there is a limit to this strategy, although evidence does suggest that providing resources to increase the number of patients undergoing evaluation may reduce the proportion of acute coronary syndrome that is missed. This appears to be a cost-effective approach but depends on multiple factors that may be outside the clinician's and even the institution's control. Even when clinicians are confident of an alternative diagnosis, subsequent adverse cardiac events may occur, with a 2.8% rate documented in one large study.[10] The acceptable "miss rate" depends on the following factors:

- Risk aversion of the clinician
- Risk aversion of the patient
- Resources available
- Perceived risk of litigation for an adverse outcome even when care is appropriate

Even patients with chest pain who undergo thorough evaluation that yields unremarkable findings experience a low but meaningful rate of adverse events. On the basis of these considerations, clinicians must decide the level of acceptable risk for missed acute coronary syndrome while realizing there is a finite rate of adverse outcomes. It is best for the EP to explain these risks to the patient, clearly document the reasoning, clearly document the patient's understanding, provide appropriate discharge instructions, and document the recommendations for follow-up.

Aortic Dissection

Aortic dissection is a tear of the intimal lining of the aorta. It is a distinct entity from dilated aortic aneurysm, which involves a pathologic dilation of the intima, media, and adventitia, and from traumatic aortic injury. The reported incidence is 2.9 cases per 100,000 patients per year, corresponding to roughly 5000 new adult cases per year in the United States. Missing or incorrectly diagnosing this condition can be fatal, especially if anticoagulation or fibrinolysis is initiated. Risk factors for aortic dissection include hypertension, Marfan's disease, pregnancy, valvular disease, syphilis, and cocaine use.

■ PRESENTING SIGNS AND SYMPTOMS

The classic presentation for aortic dissection is acute (with maximal intensity at onset), severe, tearing chest pain that radiates to the back in patients with a history of hypertension. On exam, patients may exhibit pulse deficits or an aortic insufficiency murmur. Unfortunately, the classic presentation is the exception and the clinical spectrum broad (Table 57-5). Symptoms frequently mimic more common disorders, and the clinician must maintain a high index of suspicion.[11]

No single finding or combination of findings has been determined to be sensitive or specific enough to direct the evaluation for aortic dissection. Given that the diagnosis is frequently missed, the EP should have a low threshold for evaluating the patient for aortic dissection when it is part of the differential diagnosis. Aortic dissection should be considered in a patient with any of the following features:

- Severe chest pain
- Pain that occurs in more than one anatomic distribution (chest and back, chest and abdomen)
- Pain accompanied by a focal neurologic complaint

Table 57-5 FREQUENCY OF SYMPTOMS AND PHYSICAL FINDINGS IN PATIENTS WITH AORTIC DISSECTION

Feature	Frequency (%)
Symptoms	
Pain	95
Abrupt onset	85
Severe or worst ever	90
Tearing or ripping	50
Location in chest	75
Location in chest and back or back alone	50
Syncope	10
Physical Findings	
Hypertension	50
Hypotension	5
AI murmur	30
Pulse deficit (pulse differences in four extremities)	15

■ DIAGNOSTIC TESTING

Chest radiography alone is insufficient to exclude aortic dissection. However, normal chest radiography findings significantly decrease the level of suspicion, if they are truly normal; only 12% of chest radiographs in patients who do have aortic dissection are *retrospectively* considered normal.[11] In 78% of patients with aortic dissection, chest radiography demonstrates either a widened mediastinum or abnormal aortic contour. If possible, the EP should inform the radiologist that aortic dissection is under consideration to direct the examination of the radiograph toward the pertinent abnormalities.

The following features are found on chest radiographs of patients with aortic dissection:

- Wide mediastinum or abnormal aorta (in 78% of cases)
- Normal mediastinum and aorta (12.5%)
- Wide paraspinal shadow
- Pleural effusion
- Tracheal shift
- Calcification displacement
- "Lump" distal to vessels

Electrocardiography is neither sensitive nor specific for the diagnosis. In fact, as many as one in six patients with aortic dissection have evidence of ischemia or AMI on an ECG—presumably resulting from occlusion of the coronary vessels by an intimal flap or thrombosis—and 70% have normal or nonspecific findings.

Helical computed tomography (CT) or echocardiography provides definitive testing for aortic dissection. Either diagnostic test is 95% to 100% sensitive; echocardiography is preferred when the patient is unstable because it can be performed in the critical care setting. Transthoracic echocardiography is extremely sensitive for abnormalities of the aortic

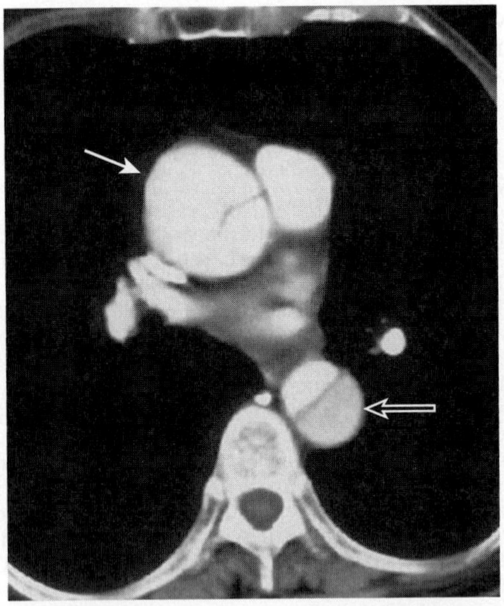

FIGURE 57-1 Computed tomography scan of aortic dissection. *Solid arrow* at ascending aorta and *outline arrow* at descending aorta show large area of false lumen.

root and ascending aorta, whereas the transesophageal approach is required to exclude involvement of the arch or descending aorta (Fig. 57-1).

■ TREATMENT

The goal of initial ED treatment of aortic dissection is to decrease shearing stress on the aorta with negative inotropic and chronotropic agents, such as intravenous beta-blockers or calcium channel blockers. Further blood pressure control can be achieved with intravenous nitroprusside or nitroglycerin. Desired values are a heart rate of 50 to 60 beats/min and a systolic blood pressure of 100 to 110 mm Hg.

■ DISPOSITION

Once aortic dissection is confirmed, ED medical management proceeds in parallel with emergency surgical evaluation, and if surgery is deemed appropriate, arrangements for intervention should not be delayed.

Cocaine-Associated Chest Pain

The U.S. Department of Health and Human Services reported in 2002 that 33 million people 12 years and older (14.4% of the U.S. population) reported using cocaine at least once in their lifetimes. Cocaine abuse is not limited to a specific subset of the population and is frequently seen in ED patients, as demonstrated by an urban ED report that 2% of the institution's patients 60 years and older tested positive for cocaine.[12]

■ PATHOPHYSIOLOGY

Chest pain, the most common complaint of ED patients with cocaine-associated visits, results from myocardial ischemia, trauma, pulmonary damage, and probably nonspecific vasospasm. Cocaine raises the risk of myocardial ischemia through multiple factors including alpha-adrenergic receptor–mediated coronary vasoconstriction, platelet aggregation, direct myocardial toxicity, accelerated atherosclerosis, and increased myocardial oxygen demand. Therefore, acute coronary syndrome may be present in individuals who would otherwise be considered to have a very low risk for the disorder.

■ PRESENTING SIGNS AND SYMPTOMS

Inquiry should be made about recent cocaine use in all patients presenting to the ED with chest pain. Patients who have used cocaine recently often present with chest pain and significant elevations in blood pressure. They may be "jittery" and somnolent at the same time after having binged on "crack." Studies have documented the incidence of AMI in patients with cocaine-associated chest pain to be approximately 6%. One study found that patients presenting with cocaine-associated AMI were young (mean age 38 years), tobacco smokers (91%), and nonwhite (72%), and had used cocaine within the proceeding 24 hours (88%).[13] Nevertheless, a significant proportion of patients with cocaine-associated chest pain are older and their risk of myocardial ischemia, although greatest in the first hours after the drug use, remains elevated for at least 2 weeks after discontinuation of the drug.

■ DIFFERENTIAL DIAGNOSIS

Chest pain or dyspnea associated with cocaine use may stem from a variety of causes. In addition to acute coronary syndrome, aortic dissection has been reported to be associated with cocaine use.[14] Barotrauma after smoking crack cocaine results from deep inhalation followed by Valsalva maneuver or severe cough, leading to pneumothoraces, pneumomediastinum, and pneumopericardium. Pulmonary diseases associated with smoking cocaine include noncardiogenic pulmonary edema, pneumonia, asthma, interstitial lung disease, bronchiolitis obliterans–organized pneumonia (BOOP), parenchymal hemorrhage, and pulmonary vascular disease. Musculoskeletal trauma may also occur.

■ DIAGNOSTIC TESTING

The initial evaluation of a patient with chest pain is the same whether or not cocaine is involved. The EP should obtain laboratory testing of blood, an ECG, and chest radiography for similar indications. ECG findings do not depend on whether the AMI is cocaine related. In both those with and those without cocaine-related AMIs, ECG findings are normal in 1% to 10%, nondiagnostic but abnormal in 30% to 50%, and diagnostic in 50% to 60%. Nonspecific abnormalities and normal variations often found in young persons, such as J point elevation and left ventricular hypertrophy, are common.

Testing for the myocardial markers CK-MB and troponins is the cornerstone of evaluation for AMI in cocaine-associated chest pain. Troponins are the markers of choice because, unlike CK-MB, they are not affected by recent cocaine use. The extent to which skeletal muscle breakdown from cocaine use affects the diagnostic accuracy of CK-MB measurement is not established.

Stress testing in patients with cocaine-associated chest pain after appropriately timed myocardial marker testing to evaluate for AMI is considered safe. The utility of exercise electrocardiography, myocardial perfusion, or stress echocardiography may be limited, however, given the low rate of reversible coronary artery lesions in these patients (2%-14%) and the significant false-positive rate.

■ TREATMENT AND DISPOSITION

Initial therapy (cardiopulmonary monitoring and aspirin) in patients with cocaine-associated chest pain is similar to that for patients with typical chest pain. In addition, the use of short-acting benzodiazepines, for example, lorazepam 1 mg intravenously repeated as necessary, in combination with nitroglycerin is recommended to counteract the sympathomimetic effects of cocaine. Hypertension usually responds to the preceding treatments. Additional blood pressure control is occasionally required because of suspicion of end-organ damage. Beta-adrenergic blockade raises the theoretical concern of worsening hypertension due to vasospasm from unopposed alpha-adrenergic stimulation. In this case, labetalol, which has mild alpha-adrenergic antagonist properties, would be a logical choice. Finally, for patients with evidence of cardiac ischemia or infarction, cardiac catheterization is beneficial and is preferred to thrombolytics, which should be used with caution.

There is some controversy regarding disposition of patients with cocaine-associated chest pain. The EP should maintain a low threshold for evaluation for aortic dissection if symptoms are severe and persist. For patients in whom findings are unremarkable—no ECG evidence of ischemia, no elevation of serial cardiac markers, and symptoms that resolve with treatment during observation—many authorities would argue that discharge is safe. There is preliminary evidence that this population is at low risk for subsequent complications. Until this issue is studied systematically, however, whether patients with cocaine-associated chest pain should be admitted for further evaluation is unclear.

REFERENCES

1. Pope JH, Aufderheide TP, Ruthazer R, et al: Missed diagnoses of acute cardiac ischemia in the emergency department. N Engl J Med 2000;342:1163-1170.
2. Kohn MA, Kwan E, Gupta M, et al: Prevalence of acute myocardial infarction and other serious diagnoses in patients presenting to an urban emergency department with chest pain. J Emerg Med 2005;29:383-390.
3. Braunwald E, Antman EM, Beasley JW, et al: ACC/AHA 2002 guideline update for the management of patients with unstable angina and non-ST-segment elevation myocardial infarction—summary article: a report of the American College of Cardiology/American Heart Association task force on practice guidelines (Committee on the Management of Patients With Unstable Angina). J Am Coll Cardiol 2002;40:1366-1374.
4. Tabas J, McNutt E: Treatment of patients with unstable angina and non-ST elevation myocardial infarction. Emerg Med Clin North Am 2005;23:1027-1042.
5. Lee TH, Cook EF, Weisberg M, et al: Acute chest pain in the emergency room: Identification and examination of low-risk patients. Arch Intern Med 1985;145:65-69.
6. Morrow DA, Cannon CP, Rifai N, et al: Ability of minor elevations of troponins I and T to predict benefit from an early invasive strategy in patients with unstable angina and non-ST elevation myocardial infarction: Results from a randomized trial. JAMA 2001;286:2405-2412.
7. Kirk JD, Turnipseed S, Lewis WR, et al: Evaluation of chest pain in low-risk patients presenting to the emergency department: The role of immediate exercise testing. Ann Emerg Med 1998;32:1-7.
8. Braunwald E, Antman EM, Beasley JW, et al: ACC/AHA guideline update for the management of patients with unstable angina and non-ST-segment elevation myocardial infarction—2002: summary article: a report of the American College of Cardiology/American Heart Association Task Force on Practice Guidelines (Committee on the Management of Patients With Unstable Angina). Circulation 2002;106:1893-1900.
9. Graff LG, Dallara J, Ross MA, et al: Impact on the care of the emergency department chest pain patient from the chest pain evaluation registry (CHEPER) study. Am J Cardiol 1997;80:563-568.
10. Miller CD, Lindsell CJ, Khandelwal S, et al: Is the initial diagnostic impression of "noncardiac chest pain" adequate to exclude cardiac disease? Ann Emerg Med 2004;44:565-74.
11. Hagan PG, Nienaber CA, Isselbacher EM, et al: The International Registry of Acute Aortic Dissection (IRAD): New insights into an old disease. JAMA 2000;283:897-903.
12. Rivers E, Shirazi E, Aurora T, et al: Cocaine use in elder patients presenting to an inner-city emergency department. Acad Emerg Med 2004;11:874-877.
13. Hollander JE, Hoffman RS, Burstein JL, et al: Cocaine-associated myocardial infarction: Mortality and complications. Cocaine-Associated Myocardial Infarction Study Group. Arch Intern Med 1995;155:1081-1086.
14. Hsue PY, Salinas CL, Bolger AF, et al: Acute aortic dissection related to crack cocaine. Circulation 2002;105:1592-1595.

Chapter **58**

Emergencies Associated with Permanently Implanted Cardiac Devices

Daniel Cabrera, Amy Jo Irvin, and Wyatt W. Decker

KEY POINTS

Chest compressions should not be performed in the patient with an implanted left ventricular assist device (LVAD) who is in cardiac arrest, because the device may shear the aorta.

A hand pump should always accompany all patients with an LVAD, and the family should be trained in its use.

A magnet may disable the shocking function of implantable cardioverter-defibrillators (ICDs).

A magnet changes most pacemakers to a continuous, preset rate, usually about 80 beats/min.

When a magnet is moved away from a pacemaker the device returns to the previously programmed, baseline function. ICDs may need to be reprogrammed after exposure to a magnet.

This chapter focuses on the evaluation and management of emergencies related to left ventricular assist devices (LVADs), implantable cardioverter-defibrillators (ICDs), and pacemakers.

Left Ventricular Assist Devices

The LVAD was initially developed more than 20 years ago to "bridge" patients to heart transplantation. It is a battery-operated, mechanical pump that is surgically implanted to help maintain and augment the pumping ability of the heart. Increasing problems with limited organ availability for transplantation and greater numbers of patients with heart failure have expanded the use of these devices. Currently, an estimated 4.7 million Americans have heart failure with an aggregate 5-year survival rate of 50%.[1] The high mortality and poor quality of life for patients with late-stage heart failure has led to further study and proposed uses for the LVAD; the device has now been approved as a therapy for patients with end-stage heart failure who are not candidates for heart transplantation because of age or other medical comorbidities.[2] Currently nearly 700 patients have undergone LVAD implantation as destination therapy for severe heart failure,[3] but an estimated 30,000 to 60,000 patients per year could be eligible for the procedure.[4]

RED FLAGS

In ED Treatment of the Patient with a Left Ventricular Assist Device

- Check for signs of infection in the pocket and the driveline.
- Signs and symptoms of right-sided heart failure can indicate device malfunction.
- Look for evidence of thromboembolic disease.

PRIORITY ACTIONS

In the Patient with a Left Ventricular Assist Device

- Institute continuous cardiac monitoring in all patients.
- Do not start chest compression in the patient with cardiac arrest who has an LVAD.
- Start manual pumping in the patient with hardware failure.

PATIENT TEACHING TIPS

FOR THE PATIENT WITH A LEFT VENTRICULAR ASSIST DEVICE

- The patient must be aware of the type of device implanted and must carry contact information for the implanting surgical team.
- The patient must carry backup batteries and the manual pump for the implanted device.
- The patient should avoid long periods with the device on battery power.

Tips and Tricks

FOR THE ED TREATMENT OF THE PATIENT WITH A LEFT VENTRICULAR ASSIST DEVICE

- Assume that the patient has severe right ventricular failure and no left ventricular reserve.
- Be aware of the type-specific devices common in the local population.
- Stock troubleshooting manuals and batteries in the ED for devices common in the local population.
- Excercise caution with fluid amounts used for volume resuscitation.

FUNCTIONING

An LVAD consists of a stroke-volume generator pump, an outflow tract efferent from the left ventricle, an inflow tract afferent to the ascending aorta, and a battery support system. Currently, three devices are approved by the U.S. Food and Drug Administration (FDA) for destination therapy: the Thoratec LVAD, the HeartMate VE/XVE, and the Novacor LVAS.[5] The pump itself is pneumatically or electronically driven. With internal devices, the pump mechanism is implanted into the upper abdomen and a skin-tunneled driveline connects with the exterior, permitting electrical connections and pneumatic venting. With external apparatuses, the entire hardware, with the exception of the inflow and outflow tracts, is outside the chest cavity. The battery life varies among devices but in general lasts for 4 to 6 hours, and should be accompanied by a backup. Systemic anticoagulation is required with some but not all devices, varying with the material used for the inflow and outflow tracts.

INDICATIONS

Patients awaiting cardiac transplantation and those with New York Heart Association class IV heart failure (and who are ineligible for transplant) are candidates for LVAD implantation. The Randomized Evaluation of Mechanical Assistance for the Treatment of Congestive Heart Failure (REMATCH) trial compared patients with optimal medical management alone and those with medical management and implantation of a HeartMate VE LVAD. The study, conducted over 2 years, showed a relative lower risk of death of 48% during the follow-up period for the LVAD group than in the medical management group.[2] The FDA approved the LVAD device in 2002 as destination therapy for patients with heart failure. Further follow-up has continued to show better survival in the LVAD recipients as well as improved quality of life.[6]

COMPLICATIONS

As growing numbers of patients are undergoing LVAD implantation, it will be important for EPs to understand the major complications of these devices. The problems with LVADs can be divided into broad categories (Box 58-1). Hardware malfunction can occur at a combined rate of about 0.87 events/patient/year.[7] It is paramount for the EP to know that chest compressions should never be used in patients with an LVAD because the trauma from the compressions can shear the outflow tract from the aorta, causing massive hemorrhage. Advanced Cardiac Life Support (ACLS) protocols can otherwise be followed during resuscitation of the patient with an LVAD.

Major Device Failure

A life-threatening emergency, major device failure is caused basically by outflow or inflow disconnections or by pump mechanical failure. Patients present in cardiogenic shock or cardiac arrest.[7] The in extremis nature of such an event requires prompt and aggressive cardiac life support and emergency consultation with the cardiovascular surgical team.

Minor Device Failure

Minor device failure is a broad category related to malfunctions of the external hardware. Commonly the patient presents with a nonfunctioning device secondary to a discharged battery or an external circuitry error.[5] In all such cases, the pumping function of the LVAD must be supported manually until the battery or the control panel can be replaced. Before hospital discharge all patients undergoing LVAD implantation and their family members are taught how to disengage the device and attach a hand pump to continue blood flow through the LVAD. The hand pump should be carried with the patient at all times. Information about how to engage the hand pump system can be found on websites for each of the devices.[3]

Thromboembolic and Bleeding Events

Patients usually require systemic anticoagulation, with an International Normalized Ratio (INR) value of 2.5 to 3.0, and aspirin for anti-inflammatory purposes. Those experiencing thromboembolic complications like cerebrovascular vascular accident and peripheral emboli will benefit from standard treatments. Of note, there is no evidence related to the use of thrombolysis in this population, but the risks appear to outweigh the benefits. In the advent of bleeding, the cardiovascular team in charge of the patient must be contacted prior to anticoagulation reversal. Caution must be taken in the volume resuscitation of such patients, given the tenuous function of the ventricles.

Infections

Infectious complications of the LVAD components are common. Patients with such infections must be admitted to the hospital for intravenous antibiotic therapy. Frequently, débridement and mobilization of the components (e.g., the driveline) must be performed.

BOX 58-1

Categories of Complications of Left Ventricular Assist Devices

- Major device failure (e.g., outflow tract disconnection)
- Minor device failure (e.g., battery dysfunction)
- Thromboembolic events
- Bleeding events
- Infection

Implantable Cardioverter-Defibrillators

The implantable cardioverter-defibrillator (ICD) is the first line of therapy for prevention of sudden cardiac death, which is commonly the result of ventricular fibrillation (VF) or ventricular tachycardia (VT).[8,9] The first internal defibrillator was implanted in 1980 by Mirowski and Mower. Since then, the technology and indications have grown enormously. More than 100,000 devices are implanted in the United States every year.[10] Given this situation, EPs are facing a growing number of patients presenting to EDs with ICD-related complaints.

FUNCTIONING

Current ICDs correspond to third-generation devices, which are small (40 mL) and reliable and contain sophisticated electrophysiologic analysis algorithms. They can store and report a large number of variables, such as electrocardiograms, defibrillation logs, energies, lead impedance, and battery charge.[11] Usually they are implanted in the left infraclavicular area using a transvenous technique, like pacemakers.

The usual ICD unit consists of a case containing the battery, circuitry, and pulse generator, a right ventricular apex lead for sensing and defibrillation, and an atrial lead. Most current devices, for biventricular pacing, can be equipped with a coronary venous lead. The diagnostic and treatment functions are configured during the device placement, with determination of the defibrillatory threshold (DFT)

PRIORITY ACTIONS

In the Patient with an Implantable Cardioverter-Defibrillator

- Patients with ICD-related complaints must have prompt transport by emergency medical services (EMS) to the closest ED.
- Always place the patient with an ICD in a monitored bed.
- In case of a disabled or malfunctioning ICD, the defibrillator patches must been placed in the anteroposterior (AP) position during the monitoring (away from the ICD pocket).
- Gather focused clinical and technical information about the device, and contact the electrophysiologist taking care of the patient.
- Obtain an AP chest radiograph and measurements of cardiac biomarkers and serum electrolytes.
- The patient will most probably need admission to a monitored bed.

RED FLAGS

In the ED Treatment of the Patient with an Implantable Cardioverter-Defibrillator

- Chest pain prior to ICD discharge can be a sign of ischemia leading to ventricular tachycardia/ventricular fibrillation (VT/VF).
- Amiodarone and class 1 antidysrhythmic agents raise the defibrillary threshold, and recent changes in the dose or interactions with other medications can cause ICD defibrillation failure.
- A history of syncope may represent a successfully treated VT/VF.

Tips and Tricks

FOR THE ED TREATMENT OF THE PATIENT WITH AN IMPLANTABLE CARDIOVERTER-DEFIBRILLATOR

- The ICD does not prevent, but only treats ventricular fibrillation/ventricular tachycardia (VT/VF). Always look for reversible causes of VT/VF: ischemia, hypokalemia, hypomagnesemia, proarrhythmic drugs.
- If the ICD does not deactivate when a magnet is placed over it, try to place the magnet in the opposite corner of the ICD or, if the patient is very obese, use two magnets.
- Always assume that the ICD is permanently disabled after being exposed to a magnet.
- The most common cause of death in the patient with an ICD is pulseless electrical activity.
- Always look for mechanical lead complications (fracture or dislodgement) on the chest radiograph, especially after the patient has experienced trauma or been given cardiopulmonary resuscitation.
- Patients receiving multiple shocks may require at least mild sedation (e.g., benzodiazepines).
- ST abnormalities on the electrocardiogram are attributable to ICD shocks only if they occur soon after the shock event.

necessary for the specific patient.[10,11] Typically the ICD is set to deliver energies 5 to 10 J above the DFT. According to these specifications, the battery life of the modern lithium-silver-vanadium device is approximately 8 years but depends largely in the frequency of the shocks delivered.

The ICD detects the atrial and ventricular electrical signals for analysis. If the sensed rhythm fulfills the criteria for VT/VF after the preprogrammed algorithm is completed, the device decides the appropriate tier of treatment, which can be (1) antitachycardia pacing (ATP), generally for monomorphic tachycardias; (2) low-energy defibrillation (±2 J synchronized with the R wave); or (3) high-energy defibrillation, delivering the shocks as a biphasic wave. These energies can be felt by the patient as sensations varying from discomfort to frank pain.[11]

Approximately 50% of the patients experience an ICD discharge in the first 2 years of use. To lower the incidence of ventricular and supraventricular arrhythmias, a considerable portion of these patients receive adjunctive pharmacologic therapy, usually with amiodarone, sotalol, and statins.[12]

The algorithmic criteria for delivering a shock are largely based in the rate, duration, polarity, and waveform of the signal sensed. After the ICD delivers a shock, there are three possible scenarios: successful defibrillation, continuation of the VT/VF, or conversion to another rhythm—usually pulseless electrical activity PEA or asystole. After an efficacious shock, the patient's heart returns to a prior stable rhythm. If the patient continues in VT/VF, the device delivers five more rescue shocks, after which it reanalyzes the waveform.[8,10] In case of post-defibrillation (or primary) bradycardia or asystole, the ICD can display anti-bradycardic features similar to those of a VVI pacemaker.

Up to 25% of the patients can experience an *inappropriate shock,* defined as a shock delivered for a rhythm different from a sustained VT or VF. The most common causes of inappropriate shocks are supraventricular tachycardias (e.g., atrial fibrillation, paroxysmal supraventricular tachycardia [PSVT], or sinus tachycardia) that are read as VT.[8] Another common cause is the misread of T waves as part of the QRS complex, duplicating the sensed rate. Occasionally the leads can suffer mechanical damage, such as insulation defects or lead fracture, causing electronic noise to be mistakenly detected as VT/VF. These problems are partially solved in modern "noncommitted" apparatuses, which can reanalyze the appropriateness of the rhythm after charging but before shocking.

There are several reports of ICD dysfunction related to electromagnetic fields (EMFs). Currently there is no evidence that EMFs from daily life artifacts can interfere significantly with defibrillators. However, it is recommended that patients with ICDs avoid placing their cell phones closer than 15 cm from the device and avoid metal detectors or antitheft devices.[10] Magnetic resonance imaging is contraindicated in patients with ICDs, given the risk of mechanical torque, thermal injury, and deprogramming.

■ INDICATIONS

The major and commonly accepted indications for ICD use are summarized in Box 58-2. In recent years the indications and uses have expanded, outpacing the current published guidelines.[9,13] The early trials showing significant reduction in secondary prevention of sudden cardiac death have been followed by publications with similar results in primary prevention on selected populations with structural heart

BOX 58-2

Commonly Accepted Indications for Placement of an Implantable Cardioverter-Defibrillator

As secondary prevention in patients with structural heart disease and a previous episode of ventricular tachycardia (VT) or fibrillation (VF)

As primary prevention in patients with:

- Ischemic heart disease and decreased ejection fraction
- Congestive heart failure and ejection fraction <35%
- Syncope with structural heart disease, and inducible VT/VF
- Certain cardiac abnormalities: congenital long QT syndrome, Brugada's syndrome, hypertrophic cardiomyopathy, arrhythmogenic right ventricular dysplasia

In patients with congestive heart failure and intraventricular conduction delays who are candidates for cardiac resynchronization

PATIENT TEACHING TIPS

FOR THE PATIENT WITH AN IMPLANTABLE CARDIOVERTER-DEFIBRILLATOR

- The occurrence of more than one shock makes urgent medical attention mandatory; the patient should call 911.
- If the ICD is firing more than once daily, the patient must avoid driving.
- The patient should always carry the identification card for the ICD as well as contact information (emergency phone number) for the treating cardiologist.
- Pain or swelling in the pocket area could be a sign of infection; the patient should seek medical care as soon as possible.

disease and low ejection fraction (EF), and also in other specific cardiac abnormalities.

■ APPROACH TO COMPLICATIONS RELATED TO THE IMPLANTATION PROCEDURE

During the early days of the ICDs, with large abdominal cases and pericardial leads, the morbidity and mortality of the procedure was considerable. With later use of the transvenous technique, the perioperative mortality rate for ICD placement is less than 0.8%.[8] Nevertheless, there may be infectious, lead-related, thromboembolic, and mechanical complications.

The rate of pocket or lead infection has been reported between 2% and 7%.[14] The most common pathogens are cutaneous flora, usually *Staphylococcus aureus* and *S. epidermidis*. During the first year after ICD implantation, infections related to the device are primarily due to the procedure; after that period they are likely due to secondary seed. From the clinical perspective, common infectious signs and symptoms in patients with ICDs are notoriously absent and patients may present with only vague complaints. The diagnosis of a delayed hardware infection requires a high index of suspicion, given the absence of a confirmatory ancillary test. Almost without exception, suspected or proven hardware infections require hospital admission, long-term intravenous antibiotic therapy, and removal of the device.[14]

Modern lead systems are extremely reliable but are still prone to fracture, malposition, dislodgment, and insulation damage. These defects commonly lead to electrical noise that can precipitate inappropriate shocks. In the evaluation of a patient with suspected lead malfunction, a chest radiograph is required for confirmation of proper positioning and integrity of the leads.[8,11,14] Contacting the implanting team for replacement of the lead is the only alternative possible for hardware failure. Problems related to the battery, pulse generator, and circuitry are extraordinarily rare.

Thromboembolic complications can be seen in as many as 30% of patients with ICDs, usually involving the cephalic and subclavian veins and generally not leading to ICD malfunction. An affected patient presents with unilateral arm swelling, pain, discoloration, and paresthesias, requiring radiographic evaluation with ultrasonography, venography, or computed tomography (CT). Standard treatment with heparin and warfarin has a good outcome.[14]

There are many mechanical complications related to placement, which may manifest early or in a delayed fashion. A considerable number of patients experience some degree of tricuspid regurgitation, approximately 10% of which are clinically significant. Also, there is a theoretical risk of fibrosis of the apical lead, which could increase the defibrillatory threshold, making the shocks ineffective. Later presentations with life-threatening mechanical complications, such as cardiac perforation, cardiac tamponade, hemothorax, pneumothorax, and air embolism, are very rare.[14]

■ APPROACH TO PROBLEMS RELATED TO FUNCTION

In a patient with complaints related to the ICD functioning, the EP should consider that the majority of such patients have severe structural heart disease with poor ejection fraction, and many of them are in end-stage congestive heart failure (CHF).[10] They can present with a myriad of symptoms (Box 58-3). The evaluation of a patient with an ICD must start by

BOX 58-3

Clinical Presentation of Patients with Problems Related to Functioning of Implantable Cardioverter-Defibrillators

- Cardiac arrest
- Unstable with ongoing shocks and arrhythmias (electrical storm)
- Stable, complaining about recent isolated or repetitive shocks
- Stable, complaining about other cardiorespiratory symptoms

placing the patient in a monitored setting with external defibrillator capacities.[12,15]

Cardiac Arrest

The causes of death in this population are PEA after VT/VF (29%), defibrillation failure (26%), primary PEA (16%), and refractory VT/VF (13%).[15] When a patient presents with VT/VF cardiac arrest, the most likely scenario is that VT/VF occurred and the ICD correctly sensed and delivered the shocks but failed to achieve defibrillation. It is critical that the EP recognize and treat correctable causes of VT/VF. Common causes are ongoing ischemia, electrolyte disturbances (especially hypokalemia and hypomagnesemia), and the arrhythmic effect of drugs.[8] Many such patients present with non–VT/VF cardiac arrest in the context of end-stage CHF; in these cases, disabling the device could be helpful in the resuscitative efforts. Disabling can be accomplished by placing a magnet over the surface of the case pocket. It is very important to remember that after a magnet is placed over the device, it must be assumed that the device is permanently disabled and reprogramming is needed. Standard ACLS protocols must be followed both for VT/VF and non-VT/VF causes of cardiac, the only difference being that the external defibrillator paddles/patches should not be placed over the ICD case.

Unstable with Ongoing Shocks

The management of an unstable patient must be based on the functioning of the ICD. Patients presenting with sustained VT with pulse, appropriately shocked by the device, represent an in extremis population. The most critical intervention is delivery of higher-energy shocks with an external defibrillator (disabling the ICD or not), and rapid correction of the cause of the VT.[8,10]

Patients also can present with hypotension caused by repetitive inappropriate shocks secondary to supraventricular tachycardias. In that case the treatment must start by decreasing the rate of the tachycardia using usual pharmacologic treatment (e.g., beta-blockers or calcium channel blockers). If this measures fails, the next step is to disable the ICD. A considerable proportion of patients arrive at the ED in unstable bradycardia; in this setting, the VVI function of the device will be helpful; however, prompt recognition of the cause (commonly, end-stage CHF) and standard ACLS treatment are mandatory.

Stable with Recent Shocks

The most common complaint of a patient with an ICD is isolated or repetitive shocks.[12] The most important first step is to determine whether or not the shocks were appropriate.[8] The patient should be placed in a monitored setting where the heart rhythm can be recorded, follow by chest radiograph to evaluate for possible hardware failure (e.g., lead fracture) and basic laboratory tests to look for ischemia or electrolyte disturbances. Any signs or symptoms surrounding the moment of the shock (e.g., chest pain, shortness of breath, or chest trauma) should be noted. It is also important to inquire about new drugs or dose changes (especially for amiodarone). Arrhythmias discovered during the monitoring as well as metabolic causes of VT/VF must be treated in the usual fashion.

Occasionally, patients complain of hearing a beep from the device. Some models can emit a beep in case of battery discharge or other causes of malfunction. Stable patients presenting with repetitive shocks or with disabled devices require electrophysiologic consultation for ICD interrogation, so that the underlying rhythms can be evaluated and the ICD can be reprogrammed.[8] Almost all such patients need admission to a monitored bed and further evaluation for causes of the VT/VF. However, patients who have experienced isolated appropriate shocks but have no change in cardiopulmonary status, no evidence of ischemia, and no electrolyte abnormalities can be discharged from the ED for follow-up with an electrophysiologist.

Stable with Other Cardiorespiratory Symptoms

Patients can present to the ED with cardiorespiratory complains not clearly related to the ICD functioning, such as chest pain, shortness of breath, and dizziness. Evaluation should be performed in order to ensure that the symptoms are not related to device malfunctioning. It appears reasonable to regard a syncopal event as the equivalent of an appropriate shock.

Pacemakers

The pacemaker has two basic units, the pulse-generator (often related to as the pacemaker) and the lead or leads. Pacemaker emergencies can be broadly divided into the following categories: device failure/malfunction, device complication, and acute cardiac emergencies in which the device is functioning as intended.

Device failure/malfunction can be further categorized into the following four key areas[16]:

1. Failure to capture, in which the pulse generator *is* sending an appropriate electrical impulse but it is not resulting in a heart beat
2. Failure to pace in which the device is not generating an electrical impulse
3. Failure to sense, in which the pacemaker is firing inappropriately in spite of a normal cardiac rhythm
4. Pacemaker-induced tachycardua

PRIORITY ACTIONS

In the Patient with a Pacemaker

- Asses the patient with the ABCs of resuscitation (airway, breathing, circulation), and intervene as appropriate.
- Initiate cardiac rhythm monitoring and obtain a 12-lead electrocardiogram.
- Assess patients for the four primary pacemaker malfunctions:

  Failure to capture
  Failure to pace
  Failure to sense
  Pacemaker-induced tachycardia
- Use a magnet to assess for failure to pace.

Documentation

IN THE PATIENT WITH A PACEMAKER

- Document date of insertion, make, and model of the pacemaker (if available; this information is often carried by the patient).
- Document key rhythm strips.
- Document response to any interventions, especially a rhythm strip with a magnet in place.

Device complications can include infections, thromboembolic disease, and migratory fractured leads.

■ PRESENTING SIGNS AND SYMPTOMS

The presentation of pacemaker emergencies varies from asymptomatic (defective on routine electrocardiography [ECG], for example) to full cardiac arrest. Intermediate presentations include palpitations, anxiety, and lightheadedness. Device complications such as infection and thrombosis can manifest the expected features. In the case of infection (fever, chills) soreness over the pulse generator wires may be noted.[17] With thrombosis, neck and arm vein distention, headache, and dyspnea may be prominent features.[18]

■ Differential Diagnosis

Patients with suspected pacemaker malfunction should be connected to a cardiac monitor and should undergo 12-lead ECG. This latter step will be of key importance in assessing the cardiac rhythm and identifying any malfunction.

In failure to capture, pacemaker spikes are present, but no related QRS complex or pulse is found (Fig. 58-1). Potential causes include lead dislodgment or malposition[19] and inflammation at the electrode tip. A chest radiograph can assist in assessing lead placement.

Tips and Tricks

FOR THE ED TREATMENT OF A PATIENT WITH A PACEMAKER

- Understand pacemaker nomenclature (Table 58-1).
- Look for the presence of pacemaker spikes on electrography (ECG); they can be very subtle or, rarely, not visible.
- The presence of a bundle branch block pattern on ECG should alert the clinician to the possibility of a paced rhythm.
- Know how and when to use a magnet.

Table 58-1 NORTH AMERICAN SOCIETY OF PACING AND ELECTROPHYSIOLOGY/BRITISH PACING AND ELECTROPHYSIOLOGY GROUP GENERIC PACEMAKER CODE (NBG CODE)

I: Chamber Paced	II: Chamber Sensed	III: Response to Sensing	IV: Rate Modulation and Programmability	V: Antitachycardia Features
O—None	O—None	O—None	O—None	O—None
A—Atrium	A—Atrium	I—Inhibited	I—Inhibited	P—Antitachycardiac pacing
V—Ventricle	V—Ventricle	T—Triggered	M—Multiple	S—Shock
D—Dual	D—Dual	D—Dual	C—Communicating	D—Dual
			R—Rate modulation	

From Munter DW: Assessment of implanted pacemaker/AICD devices. In Roberts JR, Hedges JR (eds): Clinical Procedures in Emergency Medicine, 4th ed. Philadelphia, Saunders, 2004, p 258.

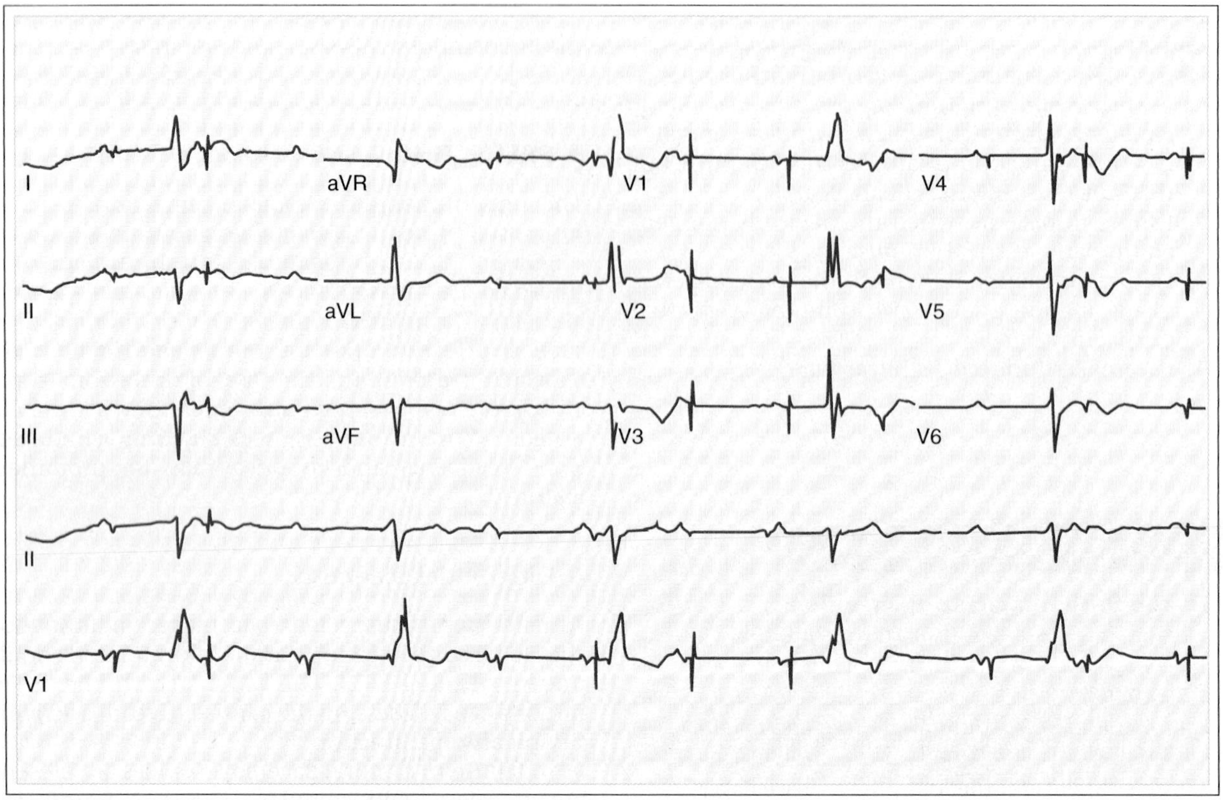
I
aVR
V1
V4
II
aVL
V2
V5
III
aVF
V3
V6
II
V1

FIGURE 58-1 Electrocardiogram depicting failure to sense and failure to capture.

RED FLAGS

- Look for neck and upper extremity venous distention as a sign of superior vena cava syndrome.
- Look for the classic findings of Beck's triad—distended neck veins, muffled heart sounds, and hypotension—in a patient with cardiac tamponade due to a lead perforation of the myocardium.
- Runaway pacemaker syndrome is a rare complication that may respond to placement of a magnet over the pacemaker.
- Using a magnet on an implantable cardioverter-defibrillator, however, may disable the device.

In failure to pace, pacemaker spikes are absent from the ECG, in spite of an abnormal or slow native rhythm (see Fig. 58-1). Causes include lead fracture, battery depletion, failure of the pulse generator, and oversensing. Battery failure is usually a gradual process detected on routine examination. Failure of the pulse generator can result from an internal malfunction, blunt trauma, and a number of iatrogenic causes, including magnetic resonance imaging (MRI), radiation therapy, and electrocautery.[19,20]

Oversensing can occur when a pacemaker interprets non-QRS activity as a QRS complex. Examples of such activities are large P or T waves, shivering of skeletal muscles, vibrations, and some medical procedures, such as lithotripsy and MRI.

Failure to sense occurs when the pacemaker fires regardless of appropriate native cardiac activity. It can be caused by lead dislodgment (most common), lead fracture, development of scar tissue at the site of the lead contact, battery depletion, or an unusually low-amplitude cardiac signal. [21]

Rarely patients present with a pacemaker-induced tachycardia, also known as runaway pacemaker syndrome. This condition is seen most often with older, dual-chamber pacemaker models. The cycle is initiated by an atypical conduction through the heart, such as a retrograde P wave that sets up a reentry circuit, in which the pacemaker fires rapid ventricular beats in response to a perceived atrial beat. As pacemakers have become more sophisticated, this condition has become far less common.

Interventions

The majority of pacemakers are equipped with a magnetic switch that will put the device into synchronized pace mode at a set rate (typically 80 or 100 beats/min). A ring magnet made for this purpose should be held over the pulse generator. Although there are device-specific magnets, any pacemaker

PATIENT TEACHING TIPS

FOR THE PATIENT WITH A PACEMAKER

- Discuss the importance of regularly scheduled checkups for the device as well as the patient.
- Warn of possible interference with device by medical imaging and/or procedures.

magnet will usually suffice.[16] Of note, in patents with ICDs, the shocking function may be disabled by a magnet. The magnet should be placed while the patient is connected to a cardiac rhythm monitor, and once it is placed, ECG should be repeated. In patients with a symptomatic native bradycardia, the placement of a magnet may be lifesaving and should be maintained until the permanent pacemaker is repaired or a temporary transvenous pacemaker has been placed. A magnet is also first-line intervention for pacemaker-associated tachycardia, as it may break the rhythm. Should this approach fail in the unstable patient, external pacing and, ultimately, lead exposure and cutting may be needed.

Patients who have pacemaker failure to sense or failure to capture should be stabilized medically. Then a careful history should be obtained and physical examination, ECG, and chest radiograph should be performed. Such patients will then need evaluation by a cardiologist, often as an inpatient. Likewise, patients in whom there are concerns about infection or thrombosis need further evaluation and cardiology consultation.

REFERENCES

1. 2001 Heart and Stroke Statistical Update. Dallas, American Heart Association, 2000.
2. Rose ER, Gelijns AC, Moskowitz AJ, et al: Long-term use of a left ventricular assist device for end-stage heart failure. N Engl J Med 2001;345:1435-1443.
3. Deng MC, Edwards LB, Hertz MI, et al: Mechanical circulatory support device database of the International Society for Heart and Lung Transplantation: Third Annual Report-2005. J Heart Lung Transplant 2005;24:1182-1187.
4. Copeland JG: Multicenter bridge to transplantation with the HeartMate assist device: Evaluation from another perspective. J Thorac Cardiovasc Surg 2003;125:228-230.
5. Shinn JA: Implantable left ventricular assist devices. J Cardiovasc Nurs 2005;20(Suppl):S22-S30.
6. Park SJ, Tector A, Piccioni W, et al: Left ventricular assist devices as destination therapy: A new look at survival. J Thorac Cardiovasc Surg 2005;129:9-17.
7. Dembitsky WP, Tector AJ, Park S, et al: Left ventricular assist device performance with long-term circulatory support: Lessons from the REMATCH trial. Ann Thorac Surg 2004;78:2123-2130.
8. Stevenson WG, Chaitman BR, Ellenbogen KA, et al; Subcommittee on Electrocardiography and Arrhythmias of the American Heart Association Council on Clinical Cardiology; Heart Rhythm Society: Clinical assessment and management of patients with implanted cardioverter-defibrillators presenting to nonelectrophysiologists. Circulation 2004;110:3866-3869.
9. Gregoratos G, Abrams J, Epstein AE, et al; American College of Cardiology/American Heart Association Task Force on Practice Guidelines American College of Cardiology/American Heart Association/North American Society for Pacing and Electrophysiology Committee: ACC/AHA/NASPE 2002 guideline update for implantation of cardiac pacemakers and antiarrhythmia devices: Summary article. A report of the American College of Cardiology/American Heart Association Task Force on Practice Guidelines (ACC/AHA/NASPE Committee to Update the 1998 Pacemaker Guidelines). J Cardiovasc Electrophysiol 2002;13:1183-1199.
10. Arnsdorf MF, Ganz LI: General principles of the implantable cardioverter-defibrillator. In Rose BD (ed): UpToDate. Waltham, MA, UpToDate, 2006.
11. DiMarco JP: Implantable cardioverter-defibrillators. N Engl J Med 2003;349:1836-1847.
12. Klein RC, Raitt MH, Wilkoff BL, Beckman KJ: Analysis of implantable cardioverter defibrillator therapy in the Antiarrhythmics Versus Implantable Defibrillators (AVID) trial. J Cardiovasc Electrophysiol 2003;14:940-948.
13. Goldberger Z, Lampert R: Implantable cardioverter-defibrillators: Expanding indications and technologies. JAMA 2006;295:809-818.
14. Pavia S, Wilkoff B: The management of surgical complications of pacemaker and implantable cardioverter-defibrillators. Curr Opin Cardiol 2001;16:66-71.
15. Mitchell LB, Pineda EA, Titus JL, et al: Sudden death in patients with implantable cardioverter defibrillators: The importance of post-shock electromechanical dissociation. J Am Coll Cardiol 2002;39:1323-1328.
16. Munter DW: Assessment of implanted pacemaker/AICD devices. In Roberts JR, Hedges J (eds): Clinical Procedures in Emergency Medicine, 4th ed. Philadelphia, Saunders, 2003.
17. Phibbs B, Marriott HJL: Complications of permanent transvenous pacing. N Engl J Med 1985;312:1428-1432.
18. Ferguson R, McCaughan B, May J, et al: Venous occlusion: A rare complication of transvenous cardiac pacing. Aust N Z J Surg 1992;62:977-980.
19. Hayes DL, Vlietstra RE: Pacemaker malfunction. Ann Intern Med 1993;119:828-835.
20. McCann WJ: Pacemaker malfunction associated with blunt trauma. New York State Med J 1978;78:645.
21. Karkal SS, Syverud S: Permanent pacemaker malfunction: A primer for the emergency physician. Emerg Med Rep 1991;12:61-72.

Chapter 59

Acute Coronary Syndrome

David F. M. Brown

KEY POINTS

Acute coronary syndrome occurs as a spectrum of diseases that includes unstable angina pectoris, non–ST-segment elevation myocardial infarction, and ST-segment elevation myocardial infarction.

Acute coronary syndrome classically presents as chest tightness or pressure with associated dyspnea, nausea, and diaphoresis.

Acute coronary syndrome is diagnosed through a careful history and analysis of the 12-lead electrocardiogram.

Treatment for the spectrum of acute coronary syndromes involves oxygen, aspirin, beta-blockers, nitrates, and anticoagulants.

Patients with non–ST-segment elevation myocardial infarction also benefit from clopidogrel and glycoprotein IIb/IIIa receptor inhibitors.

Patients with ST-segment elevation myocardial infarction require early revascularization therapy with either fibrinolysis or primary percutaneous coronary intervention.

Complications of acute coronary syndrome include congestive heart failure/cardiogenic shock (due to infarction or acute valvular incompetence) and rhythm disturbances (ventricular tachycardia, ventricular fibrillation, atrial fibrillation, and atrioventricular nodal block, among others).

Perspective and Epidemiology

Ischemic heart disease occurs as the result of coronary artery disease and does not discriminate on the basis of gender, ethnicity, or race. Ischemic heart disease remains the leading cause of death in the United States, accounting for more than half a million deaths annually—despite the marked advances over the past 5 decades in the prevention as well as the diagnosis and treatment of coronary artery disease. Advances include reduction in smoking rates; improvements in the management of diabetes, hypertension, and hyperlipidemia; utilization of aspirin and other antiplatelet agents as both primary and secondary prevention; and improvements in the acute management of acute coronary syndrome. The last factor has evolved significantly, beginning with the advent of cardiac monitoring and the development of external cardiac defibrillators in the 1950s and progressing to widespread utilization of external cardiac massage and cohorting of patients with acute coronary syndrome within coronary care units in the 1960s. Pharmacologic developments in the management of acute coronary syndrome began with the use of beta-blockers and aspirin and advanced rapidly to include more sophisticated antiplatelet and anticoagulant agents.

The 1980s brought the widespread use of fibrinolytic therapy, ushering in the reperfusion era of therapy for acute coronary syndrome. Also in the 1980s, coronary angiography was first performed in the setting of acute myocardial infarction (MI), demonstrating occlusion of the infarct-related artery and the subsequent development of mechanical interventions to open the artery, beginning with balloon angioplasty and evolving to more sophisticated techniques such as stenting, thrombectomy, and atherectomy. All of these advances have led to a significant decline in the overall age-adjusted mortality of ischemic heart disease, primarily owing to a diminution in both the incidence and case-fatality rate of acute MI.

Nonetheless, the burden of acute coronary syndrome remains significant both from a health care perspective and from an economic perspective. Approximately 1 million acute MIs occur in the United States annually, and 20% of the affected patients die before reaching the hospital, primarily from arrhythmias within first hours of symptoms.[1] Many survivors of acute MI are left with impaired cardiac function, which adversely affects their ability to perform activities of daily living and their quality of life. Approximately 6 million annual ED visits in the United States are made for the evaluation of chest pain, and as many as one in three of the patients are ultimately found to have acute coronary syndrome.[2] The annual cost of providing care for patients with acute coronary syndrome, both immediately and then later for those who survive, is more than $100 billion dollars.[3] Finally, despite advances in diagnostic techniques, 2% to 5% of patients with acute MI are discharged from the ED because their disease is not identified.[4] These "missed MI" patients represent the highest mean payments for emergency medicine–related medical malpractice claims.

Definitions

Angina pectoris or, simply, angina is defined as transient and episodic discomfort in the chest occurring as the result of myocardial ischemia. Chronic stable angina can be reproduced with a specific level of physical or emotional stress and reliably resolves with rest, relief of the stress, or nitroglycerin therapy.

Unstable angina pectoris (UAP) is defined as angina of new onset that occurs at rest or in a crescendo pattern (with longer duration or intensity or with increasingly less exertion). If the angina is occurring at rest, it must be of at least 20 minutes' duration to be characterized as unstable. Pathophysiologically, UAP is characterized by the presence of an unstable coronary atherosclerotic plaque with thrombosis and partial obstruction of the involved coronary artery but without myocardial cell death. In contrast, chronic stable angina is generally related to fixed stable atherosclerotic lesions without rupture or thrombosis. Variant (or Prinzmetal's) angina also occurs at rest but is due to coronary vasospasm rather than an unstable coronary atherosclerotic plaque. It may manifest as ST-segment elevation on an electrocardiogram (ECG), mimicking ST-segment elevation myocardial infarction, but generally responds to nitroglycerin with resolution of acute ECG abnormalities.

Myocardial infarction is defined as myocardial necrosis. Clinical criteria for the presence of an acute, evolving or recent MI, which have been laid out jointly by the American College of Cardiology and the European Society of Cardiology, focus on any evidence of myocardial cell death. The exact definition of an *acute or evolving MI* is as a rise above the upper limit of normal and subsequent fall in levels of cardiac biomarkers specific for myocardial necrosis (troponin or the MB fraction of creatine kinase MB [CK-MB]) with at least one of the following[5]:

- Symptoms consistent with acute coronary syndrome
- Electrocardiographic evidence of myocardial ischemia, specifically ST-segment elevation or depression or T wave inversions
- Development of pathologic Q waves on ECG
- Percutaneous coronary artery intervention

Myocardial infarction is further classified as ST-elevation MI (STEMI) and non–ST-elevation MI (NSTEMI). A STEMI is present when the patient has (1) cardiac biomarkers for necrosis as previously defined and (2) new or presumed new ST-segment elevation in two or more contiguous ECG leads. The cutoff point for ST-segment elevation is 0.1 mV.[6] Contiguous leads are defined in the chest leads as V_1 through V_6, and in the frontal plane as the sequence aVL, I, inverted aVR, II, aVF, and III. Patients who meet the clinical criteria for STEMI and a left bundle branch block (LBBB) not known to be old or who have ECG evidence of an isolated true posterior MI are also considered, for treatment algorithm purposes, to have STEMI. NSTEMI is present when the patient meets the criteria for MI as previously defined but exhibits no evidence of ST segment elevation, new LBBB, or ECG evidence of an isolated posterior wall MI.

Acute coronary syndrome is the clinical manifestation of acute myocardial ischemia resulting from the presence of an unstable coronary plaque. As such, acute coronary syndrome is represented by the full spectrum STEMI, NSTEMI, and UAP, which compose a continuum of similar clinical and pathophysiologic features. STEMI and NSTEMI are differentiated by the findings on 12-lead ECG, whereas UAP is identical to NSTEMI except that the cardiac biomarkers remain normal in the former. Given that a laboratory result is the only distinguishing feature between the patient with UAP and the patient with NSTEMI, the patients are treated identically upon presentation to the initial health care provider.

Pathophysiology

The pathophysiology of acute myocardial ischemia is related to an imbalance between myocardial oxygen supply and demand. Specifically, myocardial ischemia occurs when coronary perfusion is insufficient to meet myocardial oxygen consumption needs. Myocardial oxygen needs depend on heart rate, afterload conditions, and contractility of the myocardium. Insufficient coronary perfusion is generally due to atherosclerosis of the coronary arteries. In patients with chronic stable angina, fixed atherosclerotic lesions partially obstruct flow of blood to the myocardium; when demand for oxygen increases (for example, because of exercise), flow may become insufficient to meet the demand, leading to myocardial ischemia and anginal symptoms.

The pathophysiology of acute coronary syndrome begins when an atherosclerotic plaque within a coronary artery becomes unstable owing to plaque rupture or hemorrhage into the plaque. The atherosclerotic plaque need not be causing critical stenosis prior to becoming unstable. Plaque rupture or hemorrhage exposes the lipid-rich core of the plaque and the basement membrane proteins of the blood vessel wall. As part of the resultant inflammatory cascade, platelets adhere to the core of the ruptured plaque and start to release platelet agonists—adenosine diphosphate, thrombin, and epinephrine. The agonists induce platelet activation, which is characterized by the expression of 50,000 to 80,000 glycoprotein (GP) IIb/IIIa receptors on the surface of each platelet. Fibrinogen, freely circulating in the blood stream, is a bivalent molecule with binding sites on each end that are specific for the GP IIb/IIIa receptor. Fibrinogen thus facilitates platelet aggregation because each strand cross-links two platelets. The resultant platelet-fibrinogen web is further stabilized by thrombin, which is released by activated platelets and by activation of the coagulation cascade. Thrombin cross-links and modifies fibrinogen to the more stable fibrin.

As the platelet-fibrin aggregation grows, it traps red and white blood cells moving through the coronary artery, and a thrombus forms. At the same time, the inflammatory process leads to the release of vasoactive mediators, which may induce vasospasm, further compromising coronary blood flow. If this process leads to complete occlusion of the epicardial coronary artery at the site of plaque rupture, an STEMI will result. If the thrombus is partially obstructing coronary blood flow and generating microemboli to smaller coronary arterioles, which in turn may become obstructed or spasmed, NSTEMI (if there is myocardial cell death as evidence by a rise in cardiac biomarkers) or UAP (if biomarkers remain normal) results.

Much less commonly, acute coronary syndrome occurs because of primary vasospasm rather than primary plaque rupture. Generally the result of sympathetic overstimulation by endogenous epinephrine or serotonin, the vasospasm may lead to platelet activation and thrombus formation in the microenvironment of the coronary vasospasm even in the absence of underlying coronary artery atherosclerosis. Coronary vasospasm is more likely to cause UAP than MI.

Clinical Presentation

■ CLASSIC HISTORICAL FEATURES

Patients with acute coronary syndrome classically present with chest discomfort in the substernal (precordial) area. Classically, this discomfort is described as pain, pressure, or tightness and may begin at rest or during exertion. It may also be located in the left or right anterior chest and may radiate to the shoulder, neck, jaw, arm, or back. Characteristically, the duration of discomfort ranges from several minutes to an hour. It is rare for discomfort related to acute coronary syndrome to last only seconds or to persist continuously for hours. Associated symptoms that may be present are dyspnea, nausea, vomiting, diaphoresis, weakness, dizziness, and fatigue.

■ ATYPICAL PRESENTATIONS

The EP should beware of atypical presentations of acute coronary syndrome, which are common and portend a markedly worse clinical outcome. The quality of the chest discomfort cannot be relied on to exclude acute coronary syndrome. Patients whose discomfort is sharp or stabbing in quality or is pleuritic, palpable, or positional in nature make up a significant minority of patients with acute coronary syndrome. Furthermore, any of the associated symptoms listed previously can manifest either alone or together without chest discomfort and still represent acute coronary syndrome. Presentation in this fashion (without chest discomfort) is referred to as an *anginal equivalent* and requires the same clinical management as cases manifesting more classically. Other atypical presentations include isolated back, neck, jaw, or arm discomfort, epigastric pain or burning, indigestion, isolated dyspnea, and generalized weakness. Elderly patients are particularly likely to have atypical presenting symptoms, in particular weakness and altered mentation. Other populations with acute

RED FLAGS

- Many patients with acute coronary syndrome, particularly the elderly, have atypical presentations.
- Normal electrocardiogram findings do not exclude acute coronary syndrome.
- A single set of "negative" cardiac biomarker values does not exclude acute myocardial infarction.

coronary syndrome who are likely to present atypically are women, non-white patients, and diabetic patients. All of these groups are much more likely to be misdiagnosed initially than the overall population with acute coronary syndrome.

Physical Examination

The physical examination is often unrevealing in patients with acute coronary syndrome, most of the findings being related to complications of acute coronary syndrome. The vital signs should be carefully evaluated and followed for evidence of arrhythmia, respiratory compromise, and cardiogenic shock. Jugular venous distention, rales, and a third heart sound (S_3) are signs of congestive heart failure complicating acute coronary syndrome. When these signs are coupled with altered mental status and hypotension, cardiogenic shock is likely.

Physical findings can also help suggest an alternative diagnosis. For example, fever and signs of consolidation on lung examination are suggestive of pneumonia rather than acute coronary syndrome, whereas unilateral absence of breath sounds suggests pneumothorax as the most likely diagnosis. Although chest wall tenderness is suggestive of a musculoskeletal etiology, acute coronary syndrome should not be excluded as a diagnosis solely on the basis of chest discomfort that is reproducible on palpation.

Differential Diagnosis

The differential diagnosis of acute coronary syndrome includes a host of other diseases that can manifest as chest pain or dyspnea: stable angina, pericarditis, myocarditis, pulmonary embolus (PE), aortic dissection, pneumonia, pleurisy, pneumothorax, Boerhaave's syndrome, esophageal reflux, esophageal spasm, gastritis, biliary colic, pancreatitis, peptic ulcer disease, musculoskeletal pain, and herpes zoster. One of the historical features that tends to favor a diagnosis of acute coronary syndrome is chest pressure or tightness rather than a sharp pain, which is more commonly associated with pericarditis, pleurisy, pneumothorax, PE, and aortic dissection. In addition, the chest discomfort in acute coronary syndrome tends to gradually worsen, unlike the pain of PE or aortic dissection, which is generally worst at the onset and then persistently severe. Pain of a pleuritic nature tends to favor PE, pleurisy, or pneumothorax, whereas pain that is worse on palpation tends to suggest a chest wall musculoskeletal cause. Discomfort that is positional in nature tends to favor pericarditis or gastrointestinal causes rather than acute coronary syndrome. However, it is very important to remember that a significant percentage of patients with acute coronary syndrome have pleuritic, positional, or palpable chest pain and that these historical features cannot be used to exclude the diagnosis.[7]

Although the differential diagnosis of chest discomfort is long and includes entities from several different organ systems, some bear special mention because of the risk they pose to patients. In each patient with chest discomfort, the EP should consider and reasonably exclude aortic dissection, PE, pneumonia, pneumothorax, and Boerhaave's syndrome. This does not mean that these diagnoses must be excluded by definitive diagnostic techniques. They may be reasonably excluded on the basis of the history and physical findings, but this thought process should be documented clearly in the medical record.

Diagnostic Testing

■ ELECTROCARDIOGRAM

The 12-lead ECG remains the most important diagnostic test for patients with suspected acute coronary syndrome. In addition to providing diagnostic information, the ECG can be used to assess the progression of the syndrome and the response to therapeutic interventions. In addition, ECG findings determine treatment pathways and assist with disposition decisions. The ECG in patients with suspected acute coronary syndrome should be carefully and systematically analyzed for evidence of ST-segment elevation, ST-segment depression, T wave inversion, and pathologic Q waves as signs of myocardial ischemia or infarction. In addition, rate, rhythm, and intervals along with QRS morphology should be studied for evidence of complications of acute coronary syndrome. Finally, evidence of noncardiac causes of chest pain should be sought on the ECG, in particular findings suggestive of PE and pericarditis.

It important to remember that many patients with confirmed acute coronary syndrome have normal or nondiagnostic ECG findings. Even in patients with acute MI, the ECG findings can be normal in a small

PRIORITY ACTIONS

1. Immediate 12-lead electrocardiogram for all patients presenting with chest pain or anginal equivalent.
2. Prompt revascularization for patients with ST-segment elevation myocardial infarction ("door-to-needle" time less than 30 minutes or "door-to-balloon" time less than 90 minutes).
3. Administration of aspirin to patients with acute coronary syndrome; the only contraindication to this action is a true aspirin allergy.
4. Early recognition and treatment of electrical and mechanical complications of acute coronary syndrome.
5. Admission to a telemetry unit or coronary care unit for all patients with acute coronary syndrome.

percentage of cases. In addition, the ECG represents only one static point in time, and acute coronary syndrome is a dynamic process. Hence, a single nondiagnostic ECG cannot be relied upon to exclude the diagnosis of acute coronary syndrome, and the history elicited from the patient remains more important than ECG findings, particularly when they are negative or nondiagnostic. Nonetheless, specific ECG findings of myocardial ischemia or infarction are often present and are very helpful in determining treatment and disposition.

Electrocardiographic Findings in ST-Segment Elevation Myocardial Infarction

The initial ECG abnormality that occurs in patients with epicardial coronary artery occlusion is peaked hyperacute T waves in the distribution supplied by the infarct-related artery (IRA). T waves become tall and sharply peaked within minutes of IRA occlusion (Fig. 59-1A). Peaked T waves may also be seen in patients with hyperkalemia, pericarditis, early repolarization, and LBBB. In the next several minutes, ST-segment elevation becomes evident on the ECG (see Fig. 59-1B). Diagnostic ST-segment elevation must be at least 1 mm above the baseline, which generally is considered to be the T-P segment. Most typically, this ST elevation is convex or domed, although less commonly it may be straight or even, rarely, concave. Concave ST-segment elevations are more characteristic of other conditions associated with ST-segment elevation (Box 59-1).

In addition to the clinical situation, a factor distinguishing STEMI from other conditions is the dynamic nature of the ST segment changes with STEMI; serial ECG commonly show waxing and waning ST segment elevation. Hours to days later, the ST segments return toward baseline, the T waves invert, and pathologic Q waves develop in the areas of the ECG that correspond to the IRA. The location of the ST elevations and other findings on the ECG generally correspond to anatomic locations of the myocardium and the associated IRA. Anterior infarctions exhibit ST elevation in leads V_1 through V_4 (Fig. 59-2). Findings in leads V_1 and V_2 indicate involvement of the septum. MIs with these findings are caused by occlusion of the left anterior descending (LAD) coronary artery. When there are additional ST elevations in leads V_5, V_6, I, and aVL, the location of the LAD occlusion is likely proximal to the first diagonal branch, causing an anterolateral infarction (see Fig. 59-1B). Inferior infarctions are characterized by ST elevations in leads II, III, and aVF (Fig. 59-3A) and are due most commonly to right coronary artery (RCA) occlusion. Reciprocal ST depressions may be present in leads I and aVL.

Inferior MIs are may be associated with concomitant right ventricular (RV) infarction, which can be evident on right-sided ECG leads, particularly in RV_4 and RV_5 (see Fig. 59-3B). Inferior MIs are also frequently associated with posterior wall involvement, which is seen on ECG as ST depressions in leads V_1 through V_3 and, on occasion, early R wave progression with tall R waves in leads V_1 through V_3 (Fig. 59-4).

Isolated posterior MIs, the rarest of transmural MIs, are the most easily misdiagnosed, because the 12-lead ECG may show ST depressions in V_1 through V_3 and sometimes V_4 and V_5, often with tall R waves in V_1 through V_3 but without evidence of ST elevations (Fig. 59-5). This situation can be confused with anterior wall ischemia. Electrocardiographic clues to the diagnosis of isolated posterior wall MI include horizontal (rather than sloping) ST depressions with prominent R waves and tall upright T waves in leads V_1 through V_3. Occasionally, isolated posterior wall MIs manifest with a nondiagnostic 12-lead ECG (Fig. 59-6A), with small pathognomonic ST-segment elevations evident only when extended ECG leads are placed inferior to the tip of the left scapula (V_8) and in the left paraspinal line at the same level (V_9) (see Fig. 59-6B). Posterior wall MIs are the result of occlusion of the posterior descending coronary artery or the posterior left ventricular branch, either of which can arise from the RCA (more commonly) or the left circumflex coronary artery.

Lateral wall MIs, characterized by ST-segment elevation in some or all of leads I, aVL, V_5, and V_6, may be associated with anterior MI as previously described or with inferior or posterior MI or may occur in isolation. This is because the lateral wall of the heart is variably supplied with blood by the LAD, the RCA, and the left circumflex artery. Isolated lateral wall MIs are most commonly associated with left circumflex artery occlusion; the ECG may show reciprocal ST depressions in leads II, III, and aVF (Fig. 59-7).

Text continued on p. 655.

BOX 59-1

Differential Diagnosis of ST-Segment Elevation on ECG

- ST-segment elevation myocardial infarction
- Pericarditis
- Benign early repolarization
- Left bundle branch block
- Left ventricular hypertrophy
- Left ventricular aneurysm
- Paced ventricular rhythms
- Prinzmetal's angina
- Hyperkalemia
- Hypothermia with Osborne waves
- Intracranial hemorrhage
- Brugada's syndrome
- Normal variant

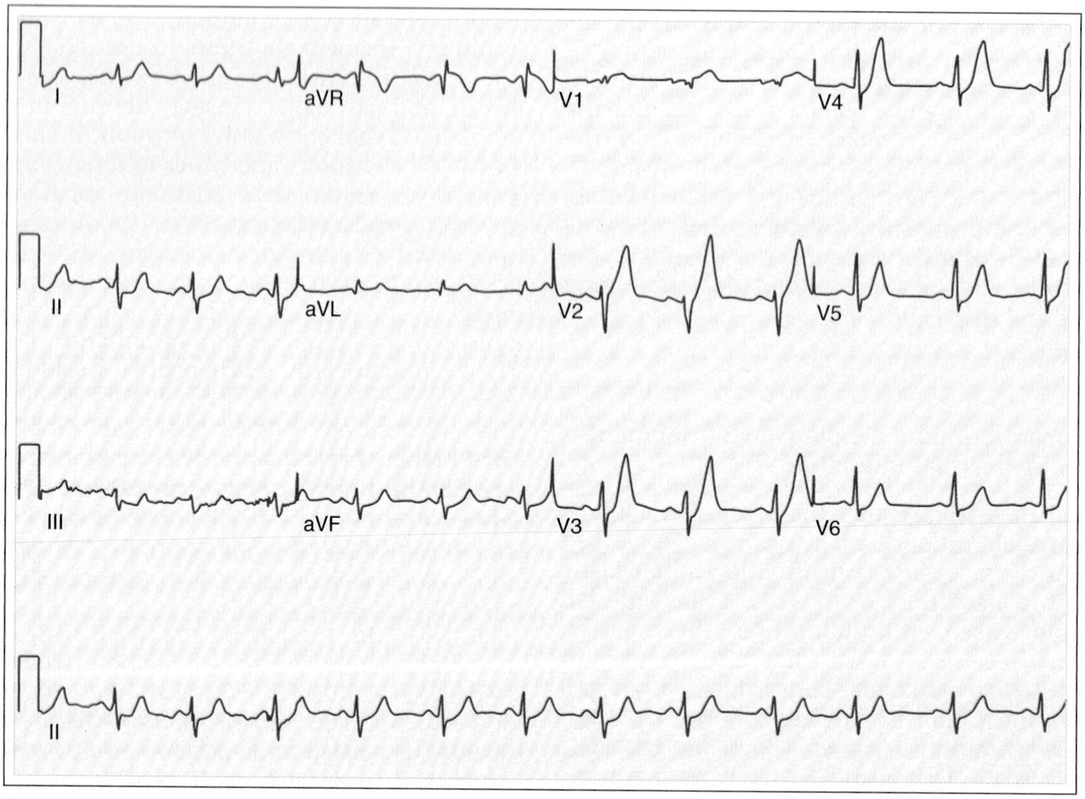
I
aVR
V1
V4
II
aVL
V2
V5
III
aVF
V3
V6
II

A

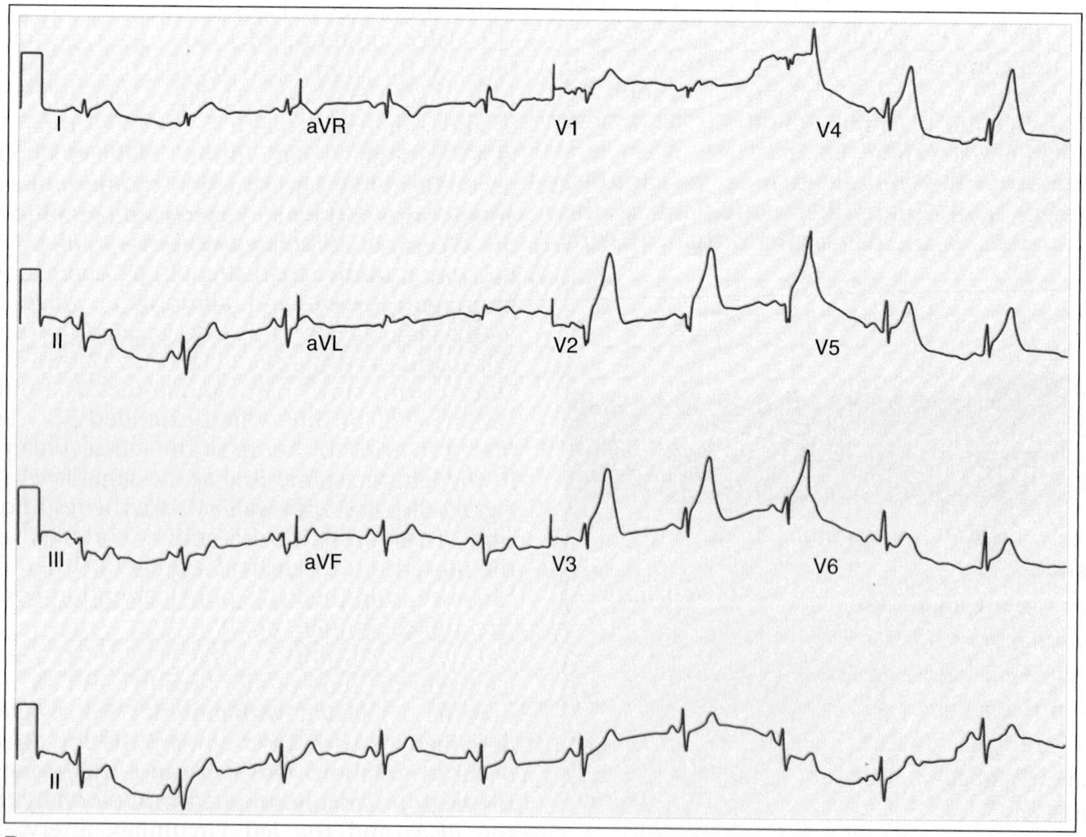
I
aVR
V1
V4
II
aVL
V2
V5
III
aVF
V3
V6
II

B

FIGURE 59-1 **A,** Initial electrocardiogram (ECG) obtained shortly after onset of symptoms shows hyperacute peaked T waves in leads V_2 through V_5, consistent with early transmural injury current. **B,** A second ECG obtained several minutes later shows hyperacute T waves and ST-segment elevation in the precordial leads along with ST-segment elevation in leads 1 and aVL, consistent with acute anterolateral myocardial infarction due to proximal occlusion of the left anterior descending coronary artery.

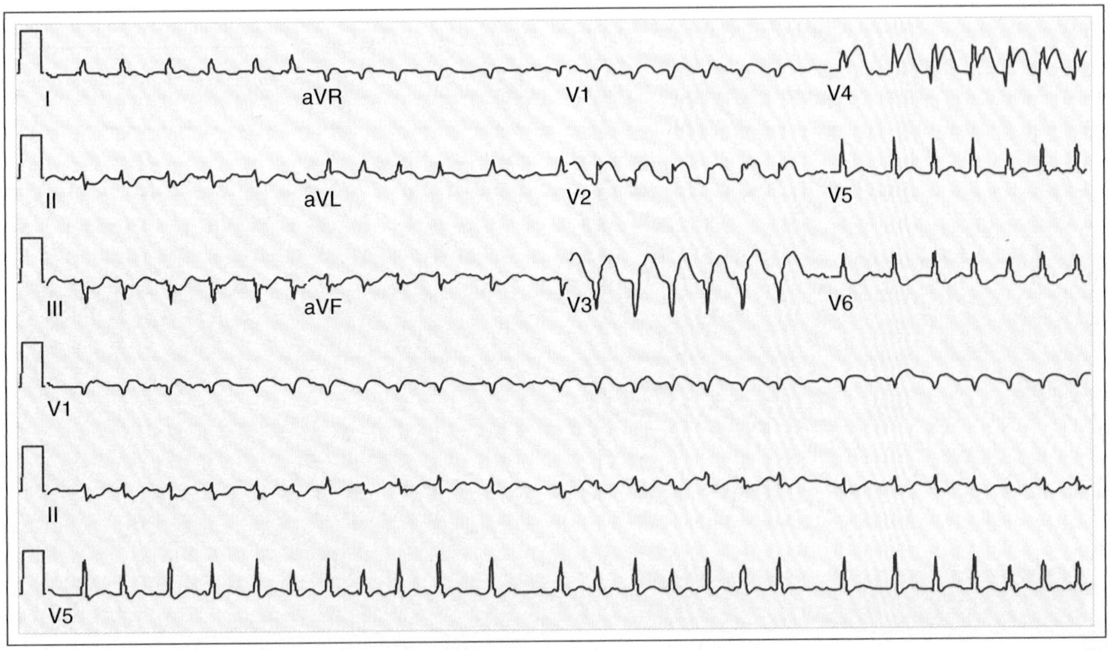
I
aVR
V1
V4
II
aVL
V2
V5
III
aVF
V3
V6
V1
II
V5

FIGURE 59-2 12-lead electrocardiogram shows ST segment elevation in leads V_1 through V_4, consistent with an acute anteroseptal myocardial infarction. Note that there is also rapid atrial fibrillation.

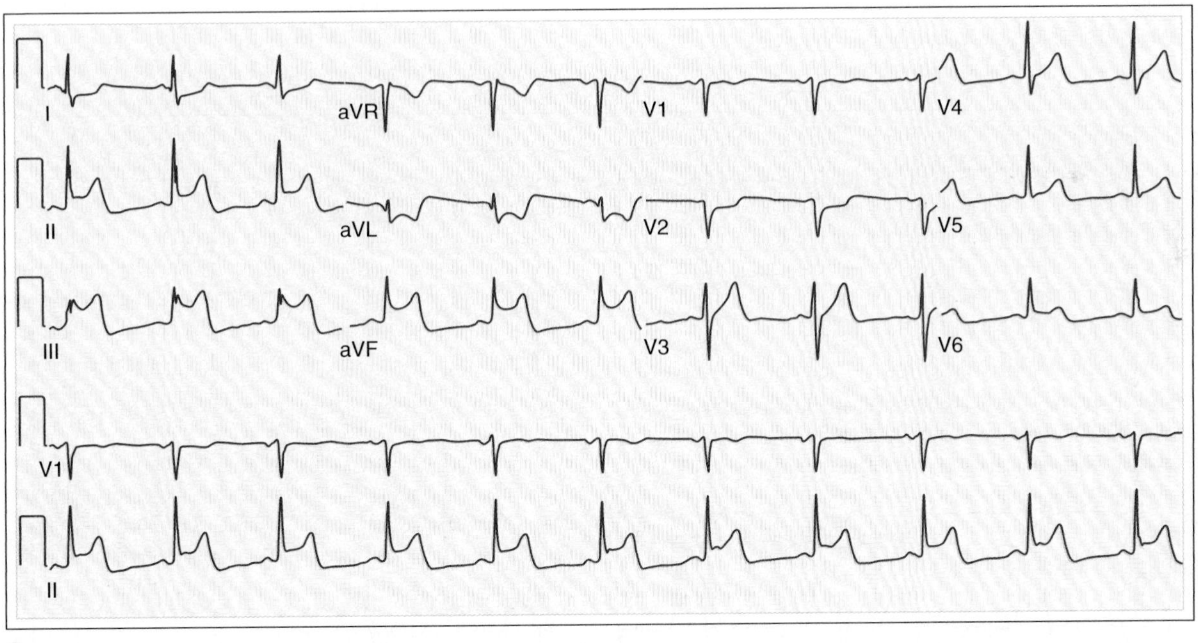
I
aVR
V1
V4
II
aVL
V2
V5
III
aVF
V3
V6
V1
II

A

FIGURE 59-3 **A,** 12-lead electrocardiogram shows ST elevation in leads II, II, and aVF, consistent with acute inferior myocardial infarction (MI). Note the reciprocal ST depressions in leads I and aVL.

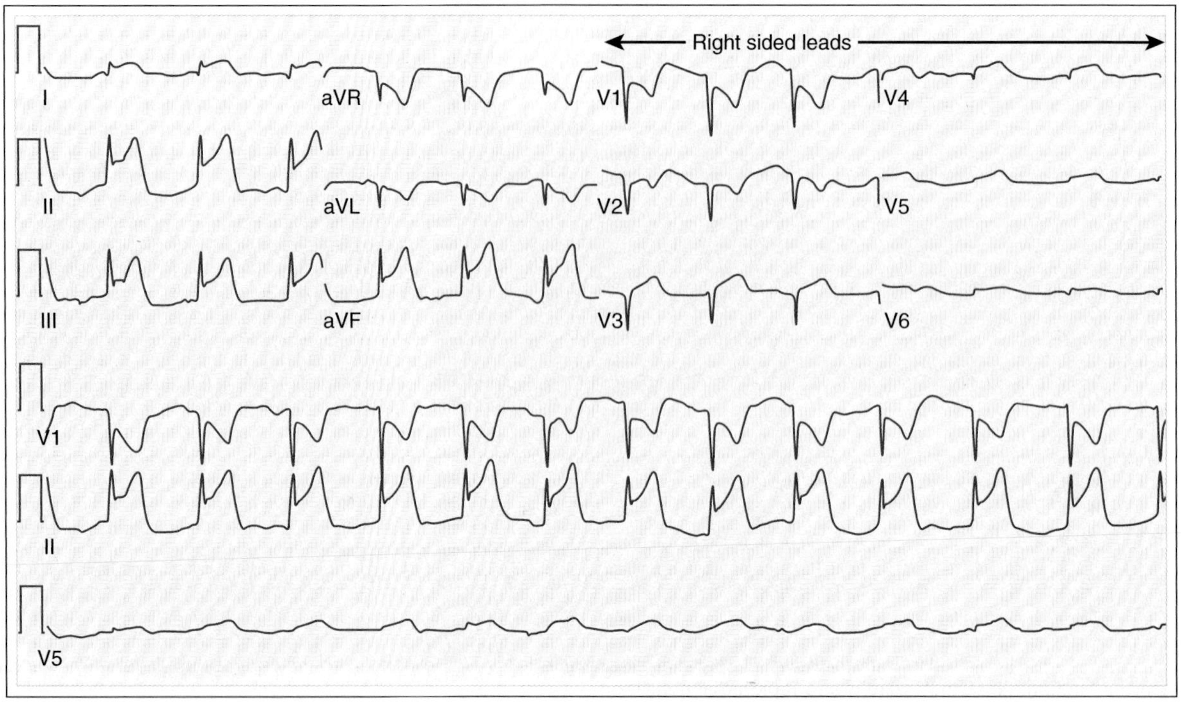
Right sided leads
I
aVR
V1
V4
II
aVL
V2
V5
III
aVF
V3
V6
V1
II
V5

B

FIGURE 59-3, cont'd **B,** Right-sided precordial leads in a patient with an acute inferior ST-segment elevation MI show ST-segment elevation in leads RV_4 and RV_5, consistent with concomitant right ventricular infarction.

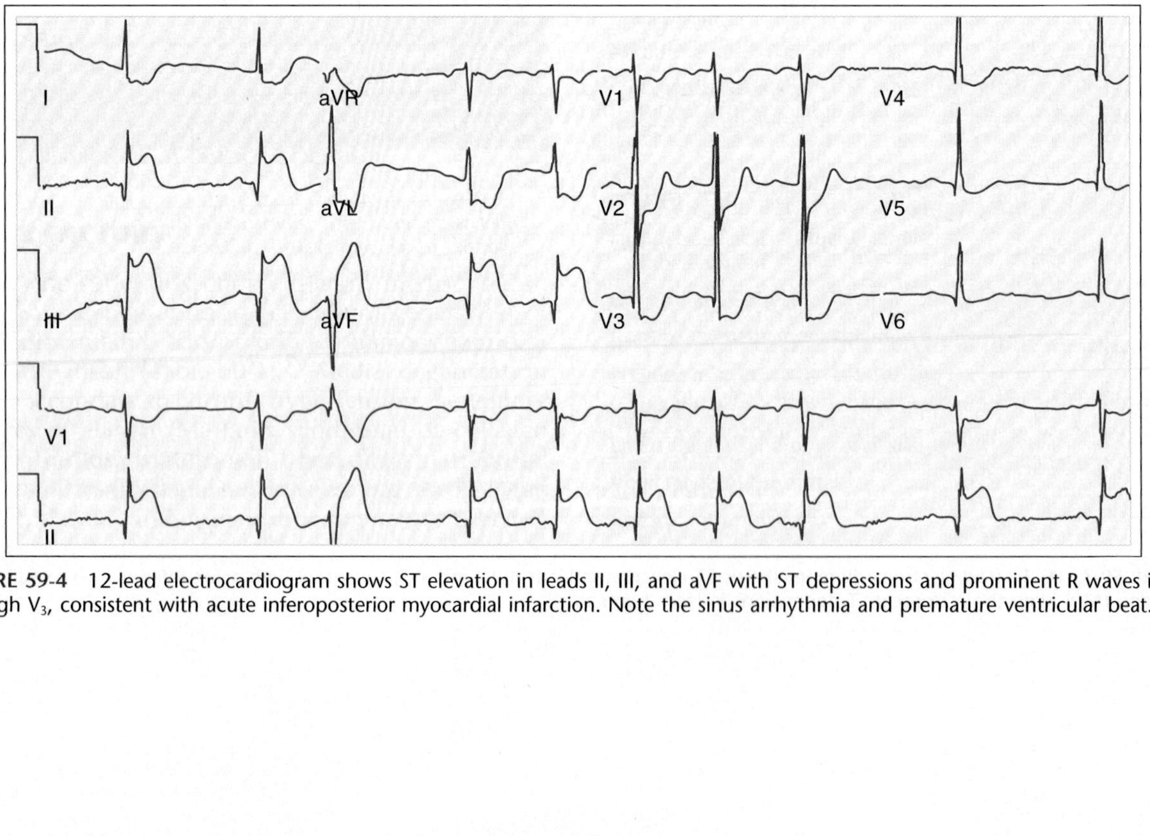
I
aVR
V1
V4
II
aVL
V2
V5
III
aVF
V3
V6
V1
II

FIGURE 59-4 12-lead electrocardiogram shows ST elevation in leads II, III, and aVF with ST depressions and prominent R waves in V_1 through V_3, consistent with acute inferoposterior myocardial infarction. Note the sinus arrhythmia and premature ventricular beat.

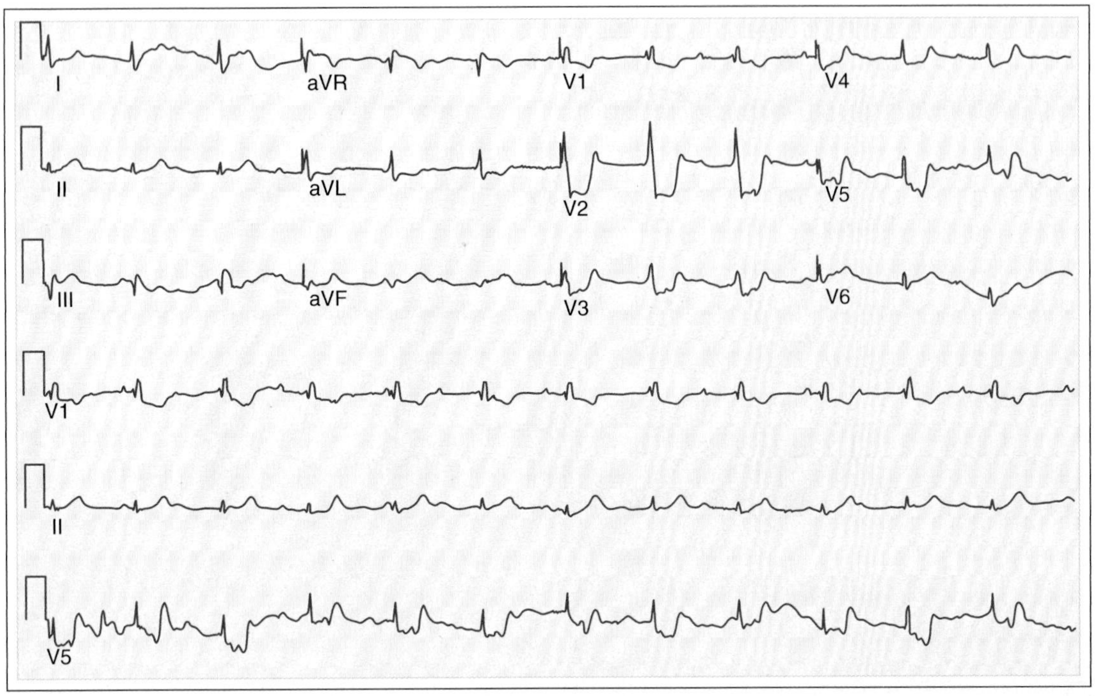
I
aVR
V1
V4
II
aVL
V2
V5
III
aVF
V3
V6
V1
II
V5

FIGURE 59-5 12-lead electrocardiogram shows ST depressions in leads V_1 through V_4 with prominent R waves in V_1 and V_2, consistent with isolated acute posterior myocardial infarction. Note that there is also complete heart block.

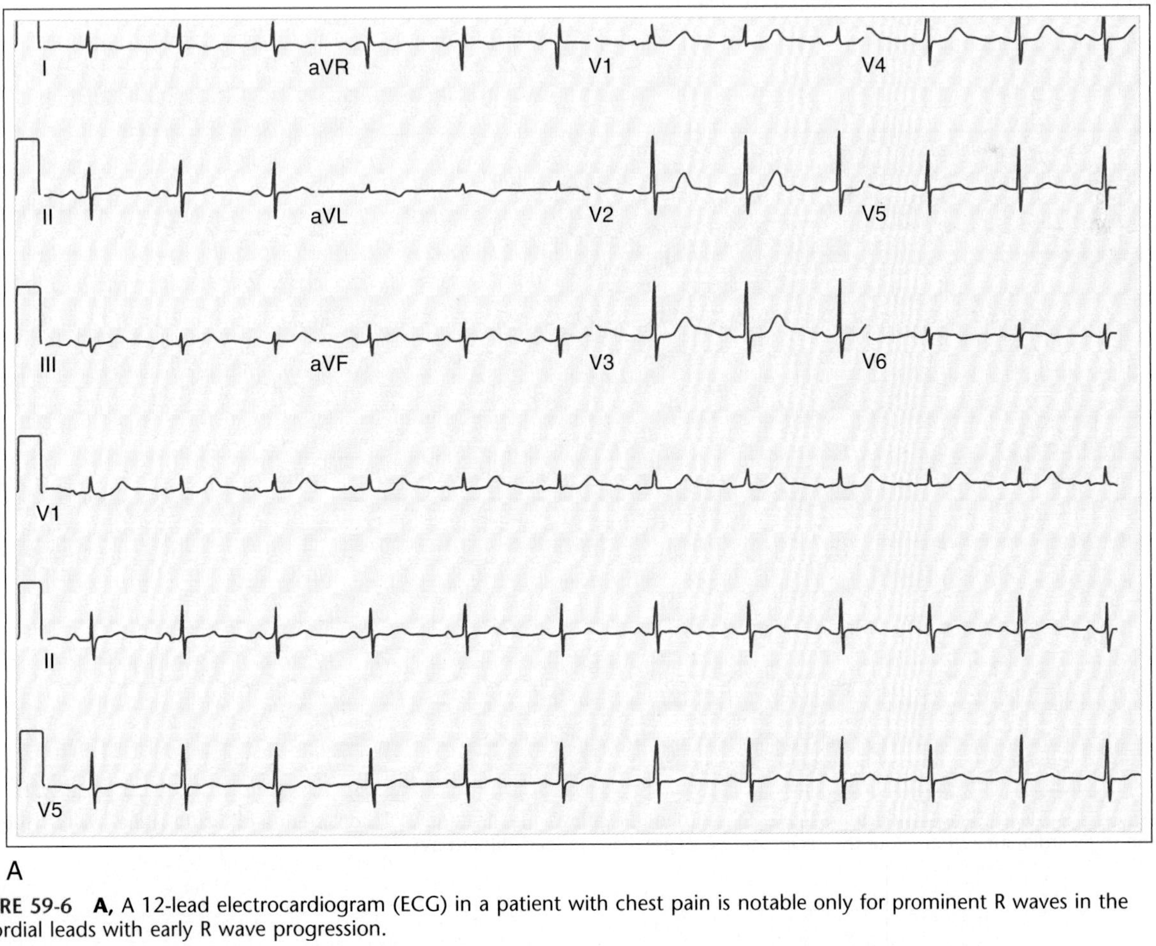
I
aVR
V1
V4
II
aVL
V2
V5
III
aVF
V3
V6
V1
II
V5

A

FIGURE 59-6 **A,** A 12-lead electrocardiogram (ECG) in a patient with chest pain is notable only for prominent R waves in the precordial leads with early R wave progression.

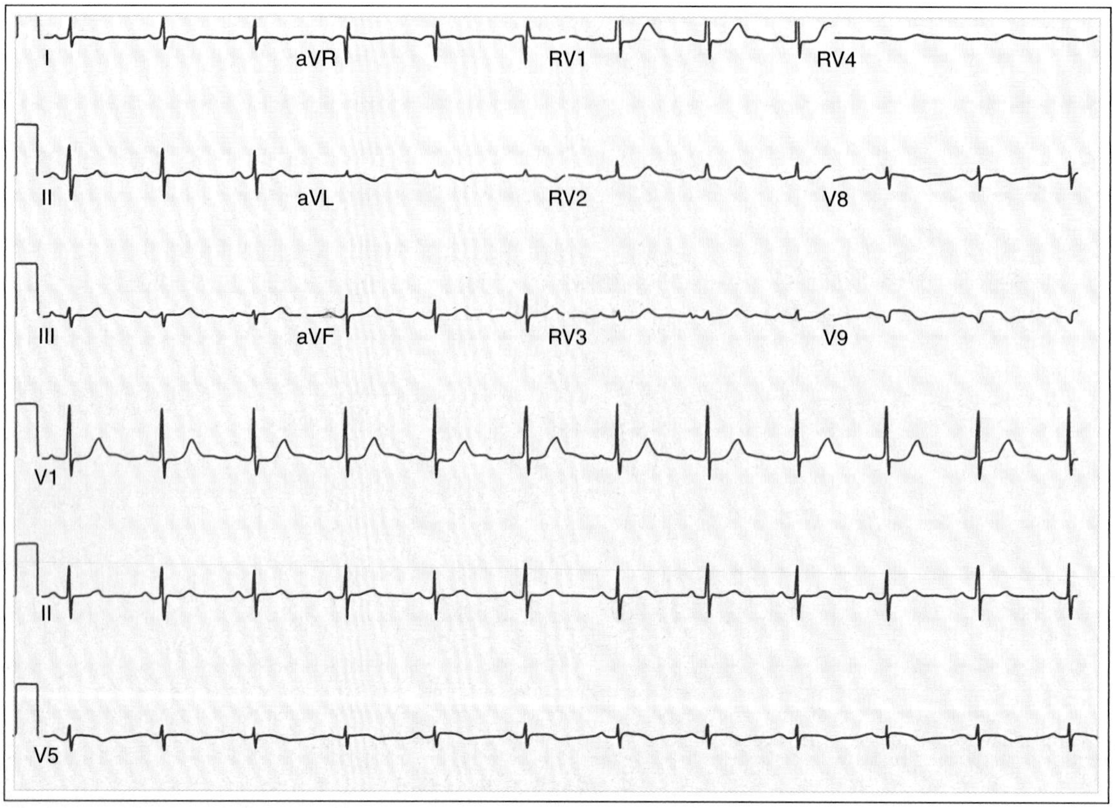
I
aVR
RV1
RV4
II
aVL
RV2
V8
III
aVF
RV3
V9
V1
II
V5

B

FIGURE 59-6, cont'd **B,** Extending the ECG to include right-sided and posterior leads demonstrates ST elevation in leads V_8 and V_9, consistent with isolated acute posterior myocardial infarction.

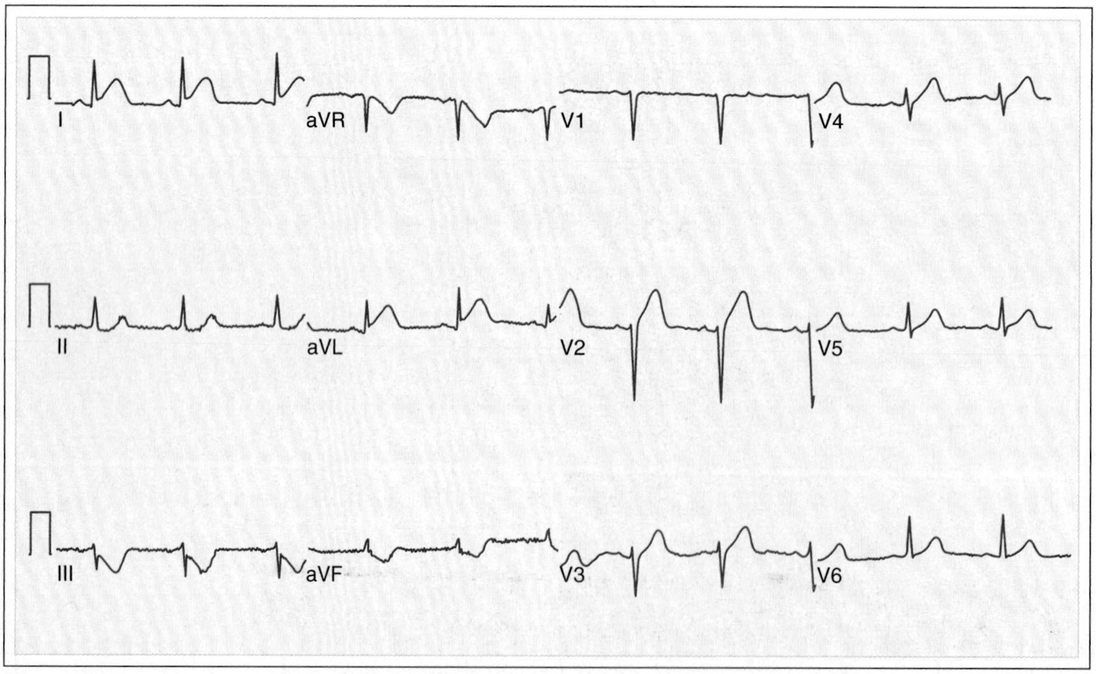
I
aVR
V1
V4
II
aVL
V2
V5
III
aVF
V3
V6

FIGURE 59-7 12-lead electrocardiogram shows ST segment elevation in leads I and aVL, consistent with acute lateral wall ST segment elevation myocardial infarction. Note the reciprocal ST depressions in leads III and aVF.

■ Electrocardiographic Findings in Non–ST-Segment Elevation Acute Coronary Syndrome

In the clinical setting of NSTEMI, the ECG may be normal or unchanged from baseline, though more commonly it will show ST-segment depressions, T-wave abnormalities, or both in the area of the ECG representing the area of ischemia or infarction in the heart (Fig. 59-8). As mentioned, ST-segment depressions in the precordial leads may also represent true posterior wall transmural infarction. In addition, ST depressions may also represent reciprocal changes with STEMI occurring in another location; this is most commonly seen in the lateral leads in the patient with an inferior STEMI or in the inferior leads in the patient with a lateral STEMI (see Fig. 59-7). T wave inversions are nonspecific findings, particularly when seen in isolation (without ST-segment depressions), but do suggest acute coronary syndrome in the right clinical setting, particularly when comparison with prior tracings shows that the findings are new. Note that T waves are normally inverted in leads aVR and V_1 and are variably inverted in leads III, aVF, aVL, and V_2.

One important subgroup of T wave inversions occurs in the precordial leads. The changes may be symmetrical deep T wave inversions (Fig. 59-9A) or more subtle biphasic T wave changes. This pattern, referred to as Wellen's syndrome, represents an unstable lesion in the LAD. Without prompt appropriate treatment, this lesion may lead to an anterior STEMI (see Fig. 59-9B). The differential diagnosis of inverted T waves includes not only acute coronary syndrome but also left ventricular hypertrophy, LBBB, pericarditis, myocarditis, pulmonary embolism, Wolfe-Parkinson-White syndrome, ischemic or hemorrhagic stroke, hypokalemia, and persistent juvenile pattern. These findings may also be normal variants.

Occasionally, patients with chronically inverted T waves present with new upright T waves in the setting of chest pain or anginal equivalent. This finding, referred to as *pseudonormalization* of the T waves, is highly suggestive of acute coronary syndrome.

■ CARDIAC BIOMARKERS

Numerous cardiac biomarkers become elevated in the setting of myocardial cell death and so are indicators of myocardial infarction. The most sensitive and specific of these at present are troponins, which are detectable in the serum 4 to 10 hours after onset of MI. As such, a single "negative" troponin value cannot be used to exclude MI. In addition to troponins, the MB fraction of creatine kinase (CK-MB), and myoglobins, are also useful and widely used. However, none of the cardiac biomarker measurements currently available is an adequate test for unstable angina (without MI). For a complete discussion of cardiac biomarkers, see Chapter 57.

■ OTHER TESTS

Cardiac ultrasonography, nuclear imaging, and stress testing can be very important in confirming the diagnosis of acute coronary syndrome or in suggesting an alternate etiology for the presenting symptoms. Most recently, contrast-enhanced multidetector computed tomography (CT) of the coronary arteries has been suggested to have a role in the evaluation of patients with chest pain. These tests are discussed in detail in Chapter 49.

Chest radiography findings are usual normal or unchanged from baseline in patients with acute coronary syndrome. However, the chest film can be useful to assess for other causes of chest pain, including

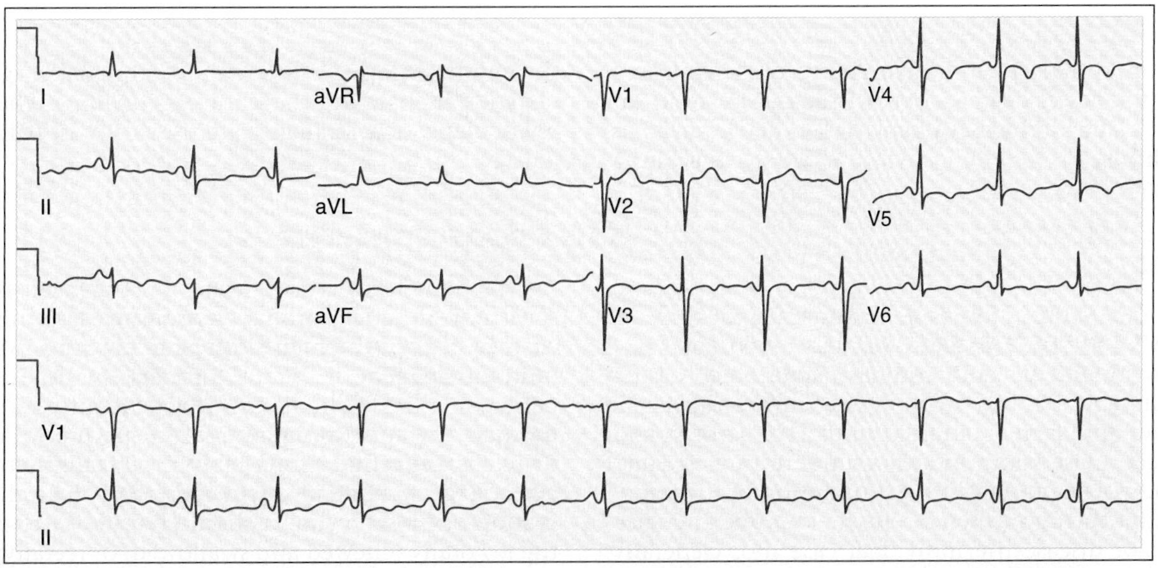
I
aVR
V1
V4
II
aVL
V2
V5
III
aVF
V3
V6
V1
II

FIGURE 59-8 12-lead electrocardiogram shows T wave inversions in leads V_3 through V_6 and ST-segment depression with T wave inversions in leads II, III, and aVF, consistent with non–ST elevation acute coronary syndrome.

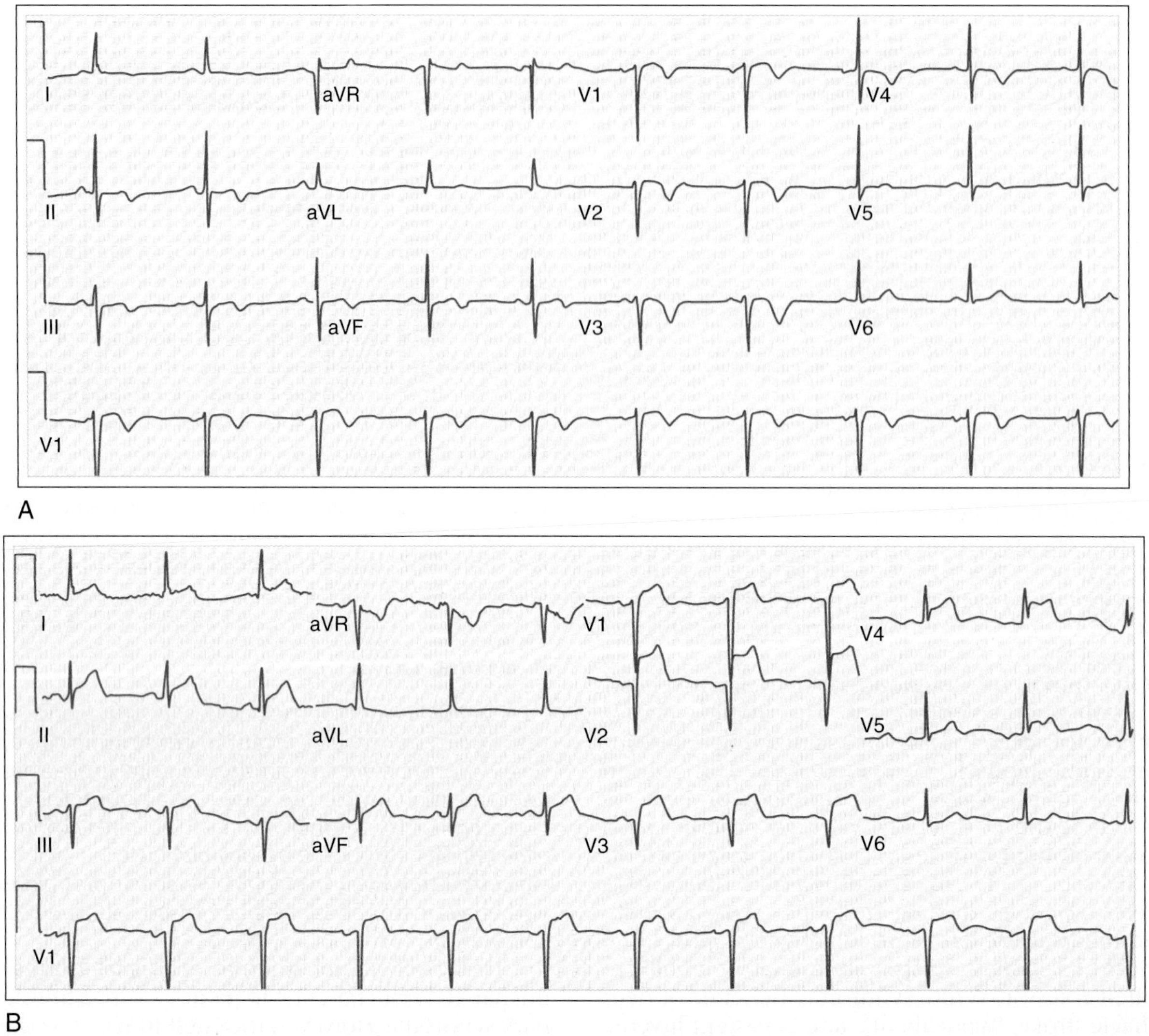
I
aVR
V1
V4
II
aVL
V2
V5
III
aVF
V3
V6
V1
A
I
aVR
V1
V4
II
aVL
V2
V5
III
aVF
V3
V6
V1
B

FIGURE 59-9 **A,** 12-lead electrocardiogram (ECG) in a woman with resolved chest pain. The deep symmetrical-precordial T wave inversions represent Wellen's syndrome. **B,** ECG from the same patient obtained 30 minutes later, now with recurrent chest pain. Note the anterior ST-segment elevation consistent with acute occlusion of the left anterior descending coronary artery.

pneumothorax, pneumonia, Boerhaave's syndrome, and, to a lesser degree, aortic dissection. In addition, chest radiography is valuable when acute coronary syndrome is complicated by congestive heart failure.

Treatment

Figures 59-10 and 59-11 are treatment algorithms for STEMI and non-STE acute coronary symptoms.

Treatment of acute coronary syndrome is time-sensitive and aimed at improving myocardial tissue oxygen supply, reducing myocardial oxygen demand, protecting ischemic myocardium, restoring coronary blood flow, and preventing reocclusion of the artery. Specific therapy depends on where along the spectrum of disease the individual case lies. Generally, unless contraindicated, all patients receive aspirin, oxygen, beta-blocker therapy, nitrates, and antithrombin therapy. Use of other antiplatelet agents depends in part on the clinical situation, whereas revascularization strategies are used only in patients with STEMI.

■ PLATELET INHIBITORS

Aspirin remains the cornerstone of therapy across the spectrum of acute coronary syndrome. It is highly cost-effective and remains one of a few drugs with a mortality benefit in acute coronary syndrome. In patients with STEMI, aspirin independently reduces mortality by approximately 23%.[8] Aspirin is an antiplatelet agent that irreversibly inactivates platelet cyclooxygenase and also reduces endothelial cell formation of prostacyclin. It should be administered in the ED orally (chewed and swallowed) or rectally; the standard dose is 162 to 325 mg. The EP should take care to avoid using enteric-coated preparations in the

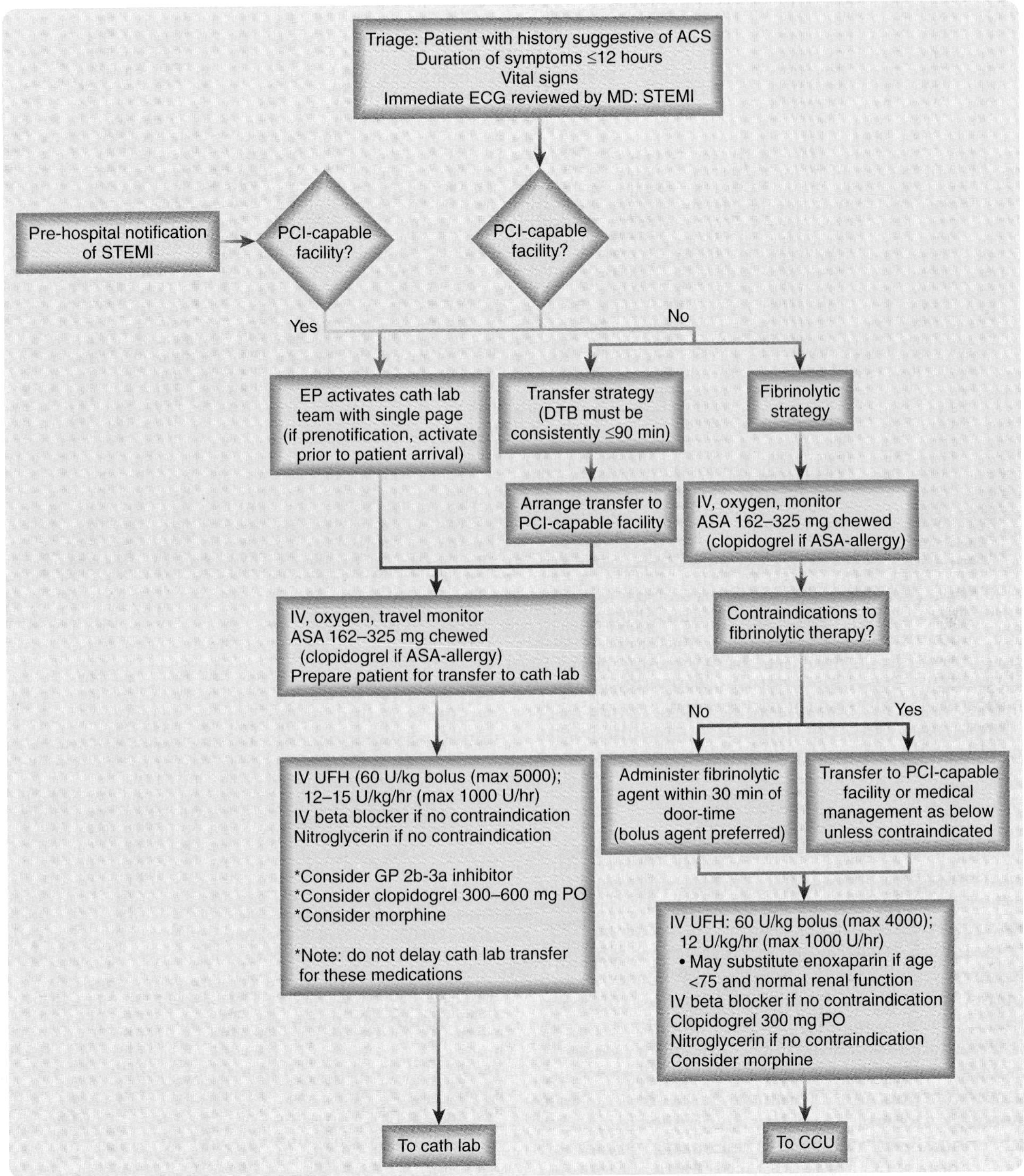
Triage: Patient with history suggestive of ACS
Duration of symptoms ≤12 hours
Vital signs
Immediate ECG reviewed by MD: STEMI
Pre-hospital notification of STEMI
PCI-capable facility?
PCI-capable facility?
Yes
No
EP activates cath lab team with single page (if prenotification, activate prior to patient arrival)
Transfer strategy (DTB must be consistently ≤90 min)
Fibrinolytic strategy
Arrange transfer to PCI-capable facility
IV, oxygen, monitor
ASA 162–325 mg chewed
(clopidogrel if ASA-allergy)
IV, oxygen, travel monitor
ASA 162–325 mg chewed
(clopidogrel if ASA-allergy)
Prepare patient for transfer to cath lab
Contraindications to fibrinolytic therapy?
No
Yes
IV UFH (60 U/kg bolus (max 5000);
12–15 U/kg/hr (max 1000 U/hr)
IV beta blocker if no contraindication
Nitroglycerin if no contraindication
*Consider GP 2b-3a inhibitor
*Consider clopidogrel 300–600 mg PO
*Consider morphine
*Note: do not delay cath lab transfer for these medications
Administer fibrinolytic agent within 30 min of door-time (bolus agent preferred)
Transfer to PCI-capable facility or medical management as below unless contraindicated
IV UFH: 60 U/kg bolus (max 4000);
12 U/kg/hr (max 1000 U/hr)
• May substitute enoxaparin if age <75 and normal renal function
IV beta blocker if no contraindication
Clopidogrel 300 mg PO
Nitroglycerin if no contraindication
Consider morphine
To cath lab
To CCU

FIGURE 59-10 Assessment/treatment algorithm for ST-segment elevation myocardial infarction (STEMI). ACS, acute coronary syndrome; cath lab, catheterization laboratory; CCU, cardiac care unit; DTB, door-to-balloon time; ECG, electrocardiogram; GP, glycoprotein; IV, intravenous; PCI, percutaneous coronary intervention; UFH, unfractionated heparin.

acute treatment of acute coronary syndrome. The only true contraindication for aspirin in ACS is a history of severe allergic reaction.

Clopidogrel is one of two currently available thienopyridines, a class of drugs that inhibits adenosine diphosphate (ADP)–mediated platelet aggregation. These drugs are more potent platelet inhibitors than aspirin. Ticlopidine, the other drug in this class, is generally not used because of its slow onset of action and concerns about its adverse effects, which include neutropenia and, rarely, agranulocytosis. Clopidogrel has been shown to improve clinical outcomes in

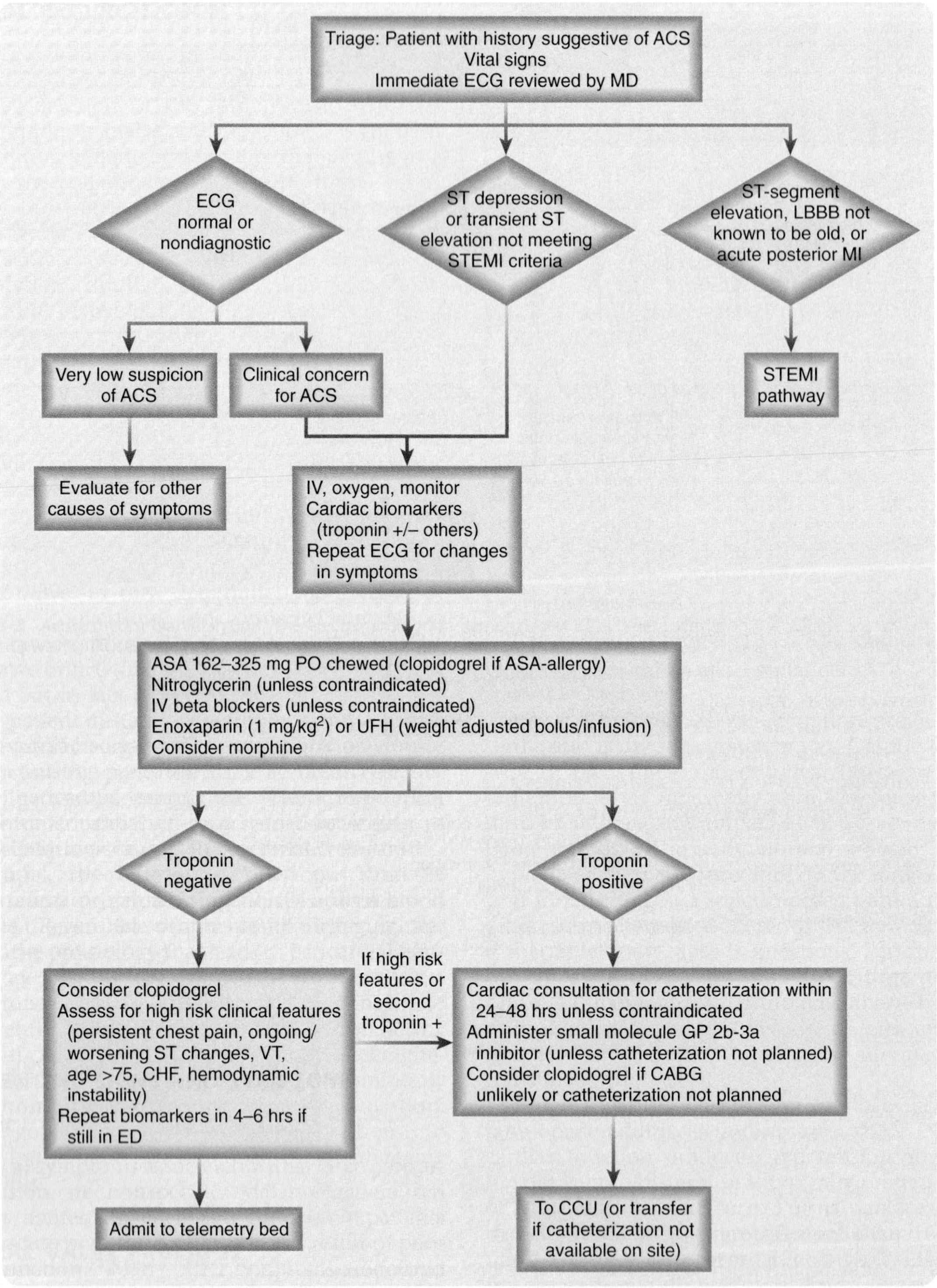
Triage: Patient with history suggestive of ACS
Vital signs
Immediate ECG reviewed by MD
ECG normal or nondiagnostic
ST depression or transient ST elevation not meeting STEMI criteria
ST-segment elevation, LBBB not known to be old, or acute posterior MI
Very low suspicion of ACS
Clinical concern for ACS
STEMI pathway
Evaluate for other causes of symptoms
IV, oxygen, monitor
Cardiac biomarkers (troponin +/– others)
Repeat ECG for changes in symptoms
ASA 162–325 mg PO chewed (clopidogrel if ASA-allergy)
Nitroglycerin (unless contraindicated)
IV beta blockers (unless contraindicated)
Enoxaparin (1 mg/kg2) or UFH (weight adjusted bolus/infusion)
Consider morphine
Troponin negative
Troponin positive
If high risk features or second troponin +
Consider clopidogrel
Assess for high risk clinical features (persistent chest pain, ongoing/ worsening ST changes, VT, age >75, CHF, hemodynamic instability)
Repeat biomarkers in 4–6 hrs if still in ED
Cardiac consultation for catheterization within 24–48 hrs unless contraindicated
Administer small molecule GP 2b-3a inhibitor (unless catheterization not planned)
Consider clopidogrel if CABG unlikely or catheterization not planned
Admit to telemetry bed
To CCU (or transfer if catheterization not available on site)

FIGURE 59-11 Assessment/treatment algorithm for non–ST-segment elevation myocardial infarction. ACS, acute coronary syndrome; CABG, coronary artery bypass grafting; CCU, cardiac care unit; CHF, congestive heart failure; ECG, electrocardiogram; GP, glycoprotein; IV, intravenous; LBBB, left bundle branch block; MI, myocardial infarction; STEMI, ST-segment-elevation myocardial infarction; UFH, unfractionated heparin; VT, ventricular tachycardia.

patients with NSTE acute coronary syndrome, particularly in patients who undergo percutaneous coronary intervention (PCI).[9,10] Clinical benefit is demonstrable within 24 hours of dosing but has been associated with a small increase in bleeding for those who undergo coronary artery bypass grafting (CABG) within 5 days of discontinuation of clopidogrel.[9] The traditional loading dose of clopidogrel has been 300 mg orally, but 600 mg appears to be equally safe and may be more efficacious. Clopidogrel (300 to 600 mg orally) should be administered to all patients with acute coronary syndrome and a documented aspirin allergy as well as to those in whom a noninterventional approach is planned.[11] Clopidogrel should also be administered to patients with NSTE acute coronary syndrome in whom emergency CABG is deemed unlikely[11]; this feature may be best determined in consultation with a cardiologist. For patients with STEMI, clopidogrel 300 mg is indicated as an adjunct to fibrinolytic therapy.[12] In patients with STEMI who will undergo PCI, it is reasonable to administer clopidogrel 300 to 600 mg.

Glycoprotein (GP) IIb/IIIa receptor blockers inhibit the final common pathway of platelet aggregation, namely, the cross-linking of two platelets by one strand of fibrinogen, a bivalent molecule with two binding sites specific for the GP IIb/IIIa receptor. As already mentioned, activated platelets have 50,000 to 80,000 receptors on their cell surfaces, so in the absence of GP IIb/IIIa inhibitors, a complete platelet-fibrinogen web can rapidly develop. With proper dosing, however, platelet inhibition of more than 85% can be attained. As such, GP IIb/IIIa inhibitors are the most potent platelet inhibitors available. Despite this fact, GP IIb/IIIa inhibitors have been shown to provide benefit only in the subgroup of patients with acute coronary syndrome who undergo PCI.

Three GP IIb/IIIa inhibitors are currently available in the United States: abciximab, eptifibatide, and tirofiban. Abciximab, the first agent developed, is a unique chimeric monoclonal antibody to the GP IIb/IIIa receptor. It binds to the receptor by steric hindrance in a noncompetitive fashion and has a long half-life, with antiplatelet effects persisting for 24 hours after discontinuation of infusion. Eptifibatide and tirofiban, referred to as "small molecule GP IIb/IIIa inhibitors," are derived from the poisonous venoms of two different vipers and bind competitively to the receptor. As such, they can both prevent fibrinogen from initially binding to, and also displace bound fibrinogen from, the GP IIb/IIIa receptor. These drugs are renally cleared and have shorter half-lives, with antiplatelet effects persisting for several hours after discontinuation of infusion.

Glycoprotein IIb/IIIa inhibitors have been shown to provide benefit in patients with acute coronary syndrome treated with PCI. There are also data showing benefit in troponin-positive patients who test positive for troponins, but not in patients who test negative or who are managed medically. As such, current recommendations for use of this class of drugs are as follows[11]: GP IIb/IIIa inhibitors should be administered, along with aspirin and a heparin preparation, to patients with acute coronary syndrome in whom PCI is planned. This is true even when clopidogrel is also given. There is no compelling evidence that administration of GP IIb/IIIa inhibitors must occur in the ED, but it is reasonable to administer them to patients with in acute coronary syndrome who test positive for troponins and have no contraindication to cardiac catheterization.

■ BETA-BLOCKING AGENTS

Beta-blockers are an important first-line therapy for patients with acute coronary syndrome. These agents act by reducing the effects of catecholamines on the heart, slowing the heart rate and reducing myocardial contractility, thereby lowering myocardial demand for oxygen. They are also potent antiarrhythmic agents, lessening the likelihood of ventricular and atrial tachyarrhythmias. Beta-blockers have been shown to decrease mortality in patients with acute MI and should be administered intravenously in the ED to all patients without clear contraindications to their use. The goal is to bring the heart rate down to approximately 60 beats/min as tolerated. Several different agents are available, including metoprolol, atenolol, propranolol, and the ultrashort-acting esmolol. Metoprolol is most commonly used; it is administered in 5-mg increments by slow IV "push" up to a total of 15 mg. This can be followed by 25 to 50 mg given orally. Atenolol is longest-acting and so is generally not the best choice for ED use.

Propranolol is not selective for β_1-adrenergic receptor blockade but has been used effectively for many years. It can be administered intravenously in 1-mg increments titrated to the desired effect. Esmolol is ultrashort-acting and must be administered by intravenous bolus followed by continuous infusion. Its ED utility is generally limited to patients in whom there is a strong suspicion that beta-blockers will not be tolerated, such as those with chronic obstructive pulmonary disease or mild to moderate congestive heart failure. Beta-blockers are contraindicated in patients with AV nodal block, bradycardia, hypotension, asthma, and acute severe congestive heart failure.

■ NITRATE PREPARATIONS

Nitrates may be administered in a number of forms to patients with acute coronary syndrome. Most commonly, sublingual nitrate tablets of 0.3 or 0.4 mg are given first, followed by intravenous, oral, or transdermal preparations as tolerated and as needed for ongoing symptoms. It is important to remember that although they do reduce symptoms of chest pain, nitrates have not been shown to reduce mortality. Because they may cause hypotension, which then contraindicates the administration of beta-blockers, it is important to utilize nitrates judiciously in the ED. In addition, nitrates are contraindicated in the setting of acute RV infarction, hypotension, and use of phosphodiesterase inhibitor drug (e.g., sildenafil) within 24 to 48 hours.

■ OXYGEN

Supplemental oxygen should be administered to all patients with acute coronary syndrome, even if the initial oxygen saturation value is normal. This step is particularly important in patients treated with nitrates, which cause pulmonary arterial dilation, thereby impairing the ability of the lung to autoregulate pulmonary blood flow. Treatment with oxygen reduces the areas of the lungs that are poorly oxygenated, giving less opportunity for shunting and resultant hypoxia.

ANTICOAGULANTS

Anticoagulant (or antithrombin) therapy is indicated for patients with acute coronary syndrome who have no contraindications to its use. These agents are particularly useful in patients with recurrent anginal symptoms, "positive" cardiac biomarker values, or ischemic ECG changes. Available agents include unfractionated heparin (UFH), low-molecular-weight heparin (LMWH), fondaparinux, and direct thrombin inhibitors. The heparins (UFH and LMWH) work by activating antithrombin III, which in turn inhibits thrombin and factor Xa. LMWH also can directly inhibit factor Xa. Fondaparinux inhibits factor Xa as its principal mechanism of anticoagulation, and direct thrombin inhibitors, as their name suggests, act directly on thrombin. The net result of therapy with all the drugs in this class is to prevent the conversion of fibrinogen to fibrin, thereby avoiding clot propagation. These drugs are contraindicated in patients with active bleeding. In addition, heparin and LMWH are contraindicated in patients with a known history of heparin-induced thrombocytopenia.

Unfractionated heparin has a synergistic salutary effect on ischemic outcomes when combined with aspirin in patients with acute coronary syndrome, particularly patients with MI. Several LMWH preparations have shown efficacy in patients with acute coronary syndrome, but only enoxaparin has demonstrated an improvement over UFH. Therefore, enoxaparin is the LMWH of choice in the treatment of acute coronary syndrome. Current guidelines recommend the administration of UFH or enoxaparin to patients with acute coronary syndrome in conjunction with antiplatelet therapy.[11] For NSTE acute coronary syndrome, enoxaparin (1 mg/kg given subcutaneously twice daily) is the preferred agent unless urgent CABG is planned.[11] UFH is dosed as an intravenous bolus of 60 U/kg (maximum 4000 U) followed by an infusion of 12 U/kg/hr (maximum 1000 U/hr).[6,11] UFH use must be monitored by serial prothrombin time (PTT) determinations; this monitoring is not necessary in patients treated with enoxaparin. Either drug should be discontinued immediately if there is evidence of bleeding or if thrombocytopenia develops.

Fondaparinux is a relative newcomer to the class of anticoagulant drugs. It is a pentasaccharide molecule that represents the terminal five saccharide moieties of heparin. Principally a factor Xa inhibitor, this agent is administered as a subcutaneous injection, with dose reductions required in patients with renal insufficiency. Fondaparinux already has indications for the treatment of venous thromboembolic disease, and data now suggest that it is similar to enoxaparin in terms of safety and efficacy for the treatment of non-STE acute coronary syndrome.[13] The most recent published guidelines recommend fondaparinux as an acceptable alternative to UFH, or enoxaparin in patients with non-ST-elevation ACS.[11]

Direct thrombin inhibitors (DTIs) offer theoretical advantages over heparins in that they do not work through the intermediary antithrombin III to inhibit thrombin. Nevertheless, there are no convincing data that DTIs provide clinical benefits over UFH or LMWH in ED patients with acute coronary syndrome. At present, ED use of currently available DTIs, argatroban, hirudin, and bivalirudin, should be limited to patients with a history of heparin-induced thrombocytopenia.

MORPHINE

Morphine sulfate is an opioid analgesic agent that has fallen out of favor in the treatment of acute coronary syndrome. There is no compelling evidence in favor of its use, and reports suggest that its sedative effects are associated with an increased risk of respiratory compromise and aspiration. In addition, this agent may cause hypotension through arterial and venous dilation. Morphine has a small role in the management of pain that is refractory to other anti-ischemic therapy and in anxiety reduction for patients in whom anxiety is a prominent feature. It should be delivered intravenously in 3- to 5-mg increments.

ANGIOTENSIN-CONVERTING ENZYME INHIBITORS

Angiotensin-converting enzyme (ACE) inhibitors have a limited role in the treatment of patients with acute coronary syndrome. This class of drugs, which causes afterload reduction, includes captopril, lisinopril, and enalapril. The principal acute adverse effect is hypotension. It is clear that ACE inhibitors are beneficial in the subset of patients with acute or preexisting left ventricular dysfunction. They are also useful as adjunctive therapy for patients with STEMI that is being treated with fibrinolytic therapy. However, no compelling data support the use of ACE inhibitors in the ED, and because there are other agents with stronger indications, specifically beta-blockers, that may also lower the blood pressure, it is reasonable to defer the administration of ACE inhibitors to the inpatient setting. If they are administered, it is preferable to start with a low dose and increase it as tolerated by the blood pressure. Renal function should be monitored during the initial phases of therapy with ACE inhibitors.

REVASCULARIZATION THERAPY

Patients with STEMI who present to the ED within 12 to 24 hours of symptom onset require urgent revascularization therapy. This can be accomplished mechanically with primary PCI or pharmacologically with fibrinolytic therapy. Although fibrinolytic therapy remains the most common strategy worldwide, the utilization of primary PCI for STEMI has been growing rapidly in the United States and has been deemed a preferable approach in terms of safety and efficacy. If a primary PCI strategy is chosen, the IRA must be opened within 90 minutes of patient arrival at the health care system in order to achieve maximal efficacy.[5] This interval includes time spent at the initial hospital if transfer to a PCI-capable facility is necessary. If the "door-to-balloon" target time of 90 minutes cannot be routinely achieved, a fibrinolytic strategy is preferable, particularly for those patients who present early (within 3 hours of symptom onset).[5]

For patients in cardiogenic shock or in those with contraindications to fibrinolytic therapy, primary PCI should be performed as soon as possible. In addition, patients in whom fibrinolytic therapy fails, as evidenced by ongoing anginal symptoms and ongoing ST-segment elevations an hour or more after therapy, should be referred for rescue PCI, which should be performed as soon as possible. Patients with STEMI who are treated with primary PCI should also receive aspirin, clopidogrel, and UFH. It is reasonable to administer a GP IIb/IIIa inhibitor to these patients as well; abciximab is the preferred agent in this setting.

None of these adjunctive therapies, however, should delay the transfer of the patient from the ED to the cardiac catheterization laboratory, which is the first priority. A number of validated strategies should be employed to decrease the "door-to-balloon" time.[14] Those that specifically affect the ED are (1) empowering the EP to activate the entire cardiac catheterization laboratory team with a single phone call, (2) increasing, where possible, the capacity to obtain prehospital ECG tracings in patients with chest pain, with activation of the catheterization laboratory team while the patient is still en route to the hospital, and (3) providing prompt feedback from a multidisciplinary quality improvement team to all clinical providers involved in the care of the patient.[12]

Fibrinolytic therapy remains an important treatment option for patients with STEMI, particularly those who present to community hospitals that do not have PCI capability. Rapid initiation of treatment is the standard of care, with a target goal "door-to-needle" time of less than 30 minutes. Fibrinolytic therapy is indicated for patients who present with symptoms consistent with acute coronary syndrome within 12 hours of symptom onset, meet ECG criteria (Box 59-2), and do not have an absolute contraindication to the therapy (Box 59-3). The presence of relative contraindications (Box 59-4) must be weighed against the risk of treatment delay if primary PCI is not readily available. Advanced age alone is *not* a contraindication, and although elderly patients treated with fibrinolytic therapy do have a higher incidence of hemorrhage, they also have a significantly higher mortality rate, which can be mitigated with therapy.

Several fibrinolytic agents are available. They include streptokinase, which is not fibrin-specific and is administered as an IV infusion of 1.5 million units

BOX 59-2

ECG Criteria for Fibrinolytic Therapy

- ST segment elevation of 0.1 mV or more in two or more contiguous leads
- Left bundle branch block not known to be old
- ST segment depressions and prominent R waves in leads V_1 through V_4

BOX 59-3

Absolute Contraindications to Fibrinolytic Therapy

- Prior history of intracranial hemorrhage
- Known malignant intracranial neoplasm
- Known cerebrovascular lesion (e.g., arteriovenous malformation)
- Suspected aortic dissection
- Active bleeding (excluding menses) or known bleeding diathesis
- Significant closed-head or facial trauma within previous 3 months
- Ischemic stroke within previous 3 months (except if within 3 hours)

BOX 59-4

Relative Contraindications to Fibrinolytic Therapy

- History of chronic, severe, poorly controlled hypertension
- Uncontrolled hypertension on presentation (systolic blood pressure higher than 180 mm Hg or diastolic blood pressure higher than 110 mm Hg)
- Prior ischemic stroke more than 3 months earlier
- Traumatic or prolonged (>10 minutes) cardiopulmonary resuscitation or major surgery within less than 3 weeks
- Recent (within 2 to 4 weeks) internal bleeding
- Noncompressible vascular punctures
- Pregnancy
- Active peptic ulcer
- Current use of anticoagulants

over an hour, and tissue plasminogen activator (tPA), which is fibrin-specific and is delivered as a bolus followed by two separate weight-adjusted infusions. Considerable data suggest that the bolus-administered fibrinolytic agents reteplase ([recombinant plasminogen activator [rPA]) and tenecteplase are safer and easier than the infused fibrinolytic drugs with equivalent clinical efficacy; costs are similar to those of tPA. Both of these newer agents are highly fibrin-specific, and the bolus administration lends itself to prehospital use if that is a consideration. Dosing of rPA is a double bolus of 10 U intravenously at time zero and again at 30 minutes; weight adjusting is not necessary. Tenecteplase is administered in a weight-tiered fashion as a single bolus of 30 to 50 mg based on known or estimated patient weight.

All patients with STEMI treated with fibrinolytic therapy should also receive aspirin, clopidogrel, and intravenous beta-blockers in the absence of contraindications. If a fibrin-specific agent is administered, UFH should be given in a dose of 60 U/kg (maximum of 4000 U) and an infusion of 12 U/kg/hr (maximum 1000 U/hr). Data now suggest that enoxaparin can be safely and effectively substituted for UFH in patients with normal renal function who are younger than 75 years.[15] If streptokinase is administered, either heparin preparation should be withheld.

There is considerable interest in combination pharmacologic therapy for STEMI. The most promising combination has been half-dose fibrinolytic therapy coupled with a GP IIb/IIIa inhibitor, which has been shown to provide better angiographic outcomes in the IRA at 90 minutes. However, large-scale clinical trials have failed to show a mortality benefit of this combination, although they have suggested that it achieves reductions in the risk of recurrent MI and the need for rescue angioplasty.[16] At present, combination therapy, because it is more expensive and cumbersome to administer, should be considered for use only in those facilities whose remote locations make transfer of a patient for rescue PCI very difficult.

Disposition

All patients with acute coronary syndrome should be admitted to a hospital bed equipped with cardiac monitoring. In some institutions, patients with "negative" initial troponin test values and nondiagnostic ECG findings who are deemed to be at low risk for acute coronary syndrome may be admitted to ED-based or cardiology-based chest pain observation units, where the remainder of the diagnostic and therapeutic evaluation may occur. In most hospitals, however, patients with suspected acute coronary syndrome are admitted as inpatients and generally to a cardiac intensive care unit. Cardiac consultation is indicated. Patients with STEMI who are managed with primary PCI go directly from the ED to the cardiac catheterization laboratory and thereafter to a cardiac intensive care unit.

REFERENCES

1. Spertus JA, Radford MJ, Every NR, et al: Challenges and opportunities in quantifying the quality of care for acute myocardial infarction: Summary from the Acute Myocardial Infarction Working Group of the American Heart Association/American College of Cardiology First Scientific Forum on Quality of Care and Outcomes Research in Cardiovascular Disease and Stroke. Circulation 2003;107: 1681-1691.
2. McCaig LF, Nawar EW: National hospital ambulatory medical care survey: 2004 emergency department summary. Adv Data 2006;372:1-29.
3. Weinstein MD, Stason WB: Cost-effectiveness of interventions to prevent or treat coronary heart disease. Annu Rev Public Health 1985;6:41-63.
4. Storrow AB, Gibler WB: Chest pain centers: Diagnosis of acute coronary syndrome. Ann Emerg Med 2000;35: 449-461.
5. Alpert JS, Thygesen K, Antman E, Bassand JP: Myocardial infarction redefined—a consensus document of the joint European Society of Cardiology/American College of Cardiology Committee for the redefinition of myocardial infarction. J Am Coll Cardiol 2000;36: 959-969.
6. Antman EM, Anbe, DT, Armstrong PW, et al: American College of Cardiology; American Heart Association; Canadian Cardiovascular Society: ACC/AHA guidelines for the management of patients with ST-elevation myocardial infarction—executive summary. A report of the American College of Cardiology/American Heart Association Task Force on Practice Guidelines (Writing Committee to revise the 1999 guidelines for the management of patients with acute myocardial infarction). J Am Col Cardiol 2004;44: 671-719.
7. Lee TH, Cook EF, Weisberg M, et al: Acute chest pain in the emergency room: Identification and examination of low-risk patients. Ann Intern Med 1985;145:65-69.
8. Randomised trial of intravenous streptokinase, oral aspirin, both or neither among 17,187 cases of suspected acute myocardial infarction: ISIS-2. ISIS-2 (Second International Study of Infarct Survival) Collaborative Group. Lancet 1988;2(8607):349-360.
9. Yusuf S, Zhao F, Mehta SR, et al: Clopidogrel in Unstable Angina to Prevent Recurrent Events Trial Investigators: Effects of clopidogrel in addition to aspirin in patients with acute coronary syndromes without ST-segment elevation. N Engl J Med 2001;345:494-502.
10. Mehta SR, Yusuf S, Peters RJ, et al: Clopidogrel in Unstable Angina to Prevent Recurrent Events Trial (CURE) Investigators: Effects of pretreatment with clopidogrel and aspirin followed by long-term therapy in patients undergoing percutaneous coronary intervention: The PCI-CURE study. Lancet 2001;358:527-533.
11. Anderson JL, Adams CD, Antman EM, et al: ACC/AHA 2007 guidelines for the management of patients with unstable angină/non ST-elevation myocardial infarction: A report of the American College of Cardiology/American Heart Association Task Force on Practice Guidelines (Writing Committee to Revise the 2002 Guidelines for the Management of Patients With Unstable Angina/Non ST-Elevation Myocardial Infarction). Circulation 2007;116: e148-e304.
12. Sabatine MS, Cannon CP, Gibson CM, et al: Clopidogrel as Adjunctive Reperfusion Therapy (CLARITY)-Thrombolysis in Myocardial Infarction (TIMI) 28 Investigators: Addition of clopidogrel to aspirin and fibrinolytic therapy for myocardial infarction with ST-segment elevation. New Engl J Med 2005;352:1179-1189.
13. Yusuf S, Mehta SR, Chrolavicius S, et al: Fifth Organization to Assess Strategies in Acute Ischemic Syndromes Investigators: Comparison of fondaparinux and enoxaparin in acute coronary syndromes. N Engl J Med 2006;354: 1464-1476.

14. Bradley E, Herrin H, Wang Y,et al: Strategies to reduce the door-to-balloon time in acute myocardial infarction. N Engl J Med 2006;355:2308-2320.
15. Antman EM, Morrow DA, McCabe CH, et al: Enoxaparin versus unfractionated heparin with fibrinolysis for ST-elevation myocardial infarction. N Engl J Med 2006; 354:1477-1488.
16. Topol EJ; GUSTO V Investigators: Reperfusion therapy for acute myocardial infarction with fibrinolytic therapy or combination reduced fibrinolytic therapy and platelet glycoprotein IIb/IIIa inhibition: the GUSTO V randomised trial. Lancet 2001;357:1905-1914.

SECTION VII

Vascular Diseases

Chapter **60**

Aortic Dissection

Nima Afshar and Chris Newton

KEY POINTS

Aortic dissection is deadly and difficult to diagnose. It is suspected less than half the time at initial presentation.

Ninety percent of patients with aortic dissection have sudden, severe, or unrelenting pain in the chest and/or upper back.

When a patient has chest pain with a pulse deficit or any acute neurologic deficit, aortic dissection is the most likely diagnosis.

D-dimer may be a sensitive biomarker for ruling out dissection. CT angiography is the study of choice for making the diagnosis.

The systolic blood pressure in patients with aortic dissection should be maintained at less than 120 mm Hg regardless of the patient's baseline blood pressure, unless symptoms or signs of organ malperfusion occur. Beta-blockers are the first-line antihypertensives.

Scope

A patient in the ED whose proximal aorta has dissected has about a 2% chance of dying every hour during the first 12 hours after presentation and almost a 50% chance of dying within 48 hours without surgical treatment.[1,2] Unfortunately, this disease is often difficult to diagnose. A study of three academic EDs found that the diagnosis was suspected during initial presentation in only 43% of cases.[3]

The incidence is 3 per 100,000 people per year.[4,5] A typical large urban ED sees several cases per year.[3] About 1 in 350 patients presenting to an ED with chest pain has aortic dissection.[4-6]

Aortic dissection is longitudinal cleavage of the aortic wall by blood, creating a false lumen that may propagate. The disease was first described in detail by Morgagni in 1761. In 1955, with the advent of cardiopulmonary bypass, DeBakey successfully repaired a dissected descending aorta, providing the first cure. The proximal aorta was first repaired and medical management was established in the 1960s, setting the stage for the modern approach to this disease.

Pathophysiology

▪ MECHANISM

The aorta dissects by two possible mechanisms (Fig. 60-1). The classic mechanism is an intimal tear, which is usually transverse and extends through the very thin tunica intima into the tunica media. Under pulsatile force, blood enters a layer of the media, dissecting longitudinally and usually in a distal direction. The other major mechanism is rupture of the vasa vasorum, usually of a penetrating branch within the tunica media, with consequent bleeding into the media. Progression then occurs in the same fashion, either with or without secondary tearing through the intima into the aortic lumen. The aorta usually tears

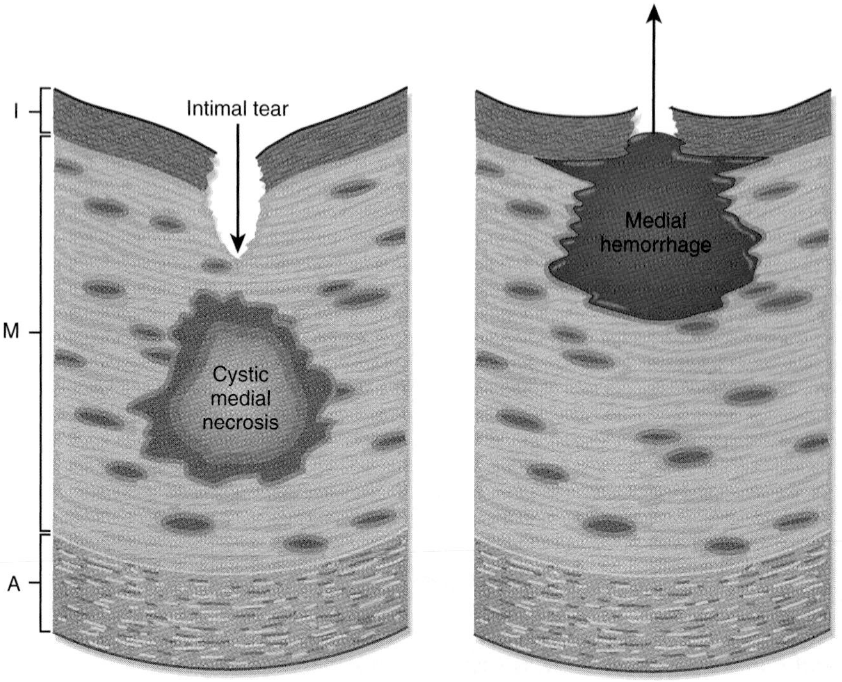
I
M
A
Intimal tear
Cystic medial necrosis
Medial hemorrhage

FIGURE 60-1 Two mechanisms for aortic dissection. A, adventitia; I, intima; M, media. (From Zipes DP, Libby P, Bonow RO, Braunwald E [eds]: Braunwald's Heart Disease: A Textbook of Cardiovascular Medicine, 7th ed. Philadelphia, Elsevier, 2005.)

near tethering points, where the vessel undergoes the greatest flexion stress during cardiac contractions. Thus the most common location of dissection initiation is the first few centimeters of the ascending aorta, the next most common being the origin of the descending aorta just distal to the left subclavian artery.

Major complications of aortic dissection, in order of mortality risk, are (1) rupture through the thin remaining outer wall, (2) proximal propagation, which can cause coronary occlusion, acute aortic regurgitation, or cardiac tamponade, and (3) occlusion or dissection of branch arteries.

■ RISK FACTORS

Those who suffer dissection either are predisposed to it by a weakened aorta, specifically degeneration of the tunica media, and/or suffer a hemodynamic or traumatic insult (Table 60-1).[7-9] Medial degeneration can be secondary to chronic hypertension, hereditary diseases of elastin (Marfan's syndrome) or collagen (Ehlers-Danlos syndrome), hereditary structural abnormalities (bicuspid aortic valve and aortic coarctation), chronic inflammation, and aneurysm of any cause, which increases wall tension according to Laplace's law.

Hemodynamic stress on the aorta is produced by hypertension and shear force (dP/dt)*, or the force of blood ejected from the left ventricle. A hypercontractile, tachycardic heart produces the greatest shear force. These factors may contribute to the initiation of dissection and strongly determine whether or not a dissection propagates. Exacerbations of hypertension, cocaine intoxication, and third-trimester pregnancy are examples of states that can cause hemodynamic stress on the aorta leading to dissection.

Table 60-1 RISK FACTORS FOR AORTIC DISSECTION

Risk Factors	Prevalence (%)
Common Factors	
Hypertension	70
Family history of aortic dissection or aneurysm	10-20
Aortic aneurysm (known)	13
Prior aortic dissection	5
Marfan's syndrome	5 (50% in patients <40 yrs)
Aortic valve disease: atrioventricular replacement, bicuspid aortic valve	9
Iatrogenic: cardiac surgery, cardiac catheterization	4
Uncommon Factors	
Cocaine or methamphetamine use	
Pregnancy	
Weightlifting	
Ehlers-Danlos syndrome—vascular type	
Coarctation of the aorta	
Chronic inflammation: Giant cell (temporal) arteritis; Takayasu's arteritis; Tertiary syphilis	
Trauma	

Data from references 7-9.

$^{*}\ \frac{dP}{dt} = \frac{\text{change in blood pressure}}{\text{change in time}}$

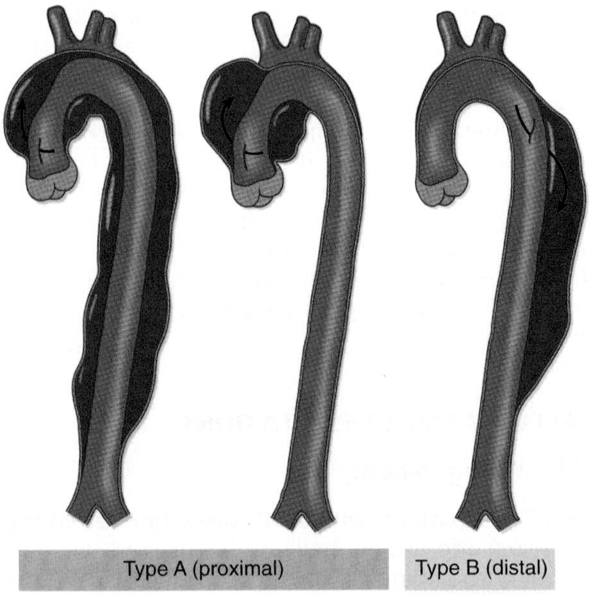
Type A (proximal)
Type B (distal)

FIGURE 60-2 Classification of aortic dissection. Type A and type B represent the two subtypes of dissection under the Stanford classification system. Subtypes of the older DeBakey classification system are types I, II, and III. (From Zipes DP, Libby P, Bonow RO, Braunwald E [eds]: Braunwald's Heart Disease: A Textbook of Cardiovascular Medicine, 7th ed. Philadelphia, Elsevier, 2005.)

Traumatic etiologies include medical procedures, such as aortic catheterization and cardiac surgery, and deceleration events (e.g., falls and motor vehicle collisions), although in blunt trauma, aortic rupture is far more common than dissection.

Classification

Sixty percent of aortic dissections involve the ascending aorta, either alone or with other parts of the aorta; they are type A in the now standard Stanford classification. The 40% that do not involve the ascending aorta are type B (Fig. 60-2). This distinction has important prognostic and therapeutic implications.

Clinical Presentation

■ HISTORY

Dissection of the aorta is usually extremely painful, so acute pain is a chief complaint in nearly 95% of cases (Table 60-2).[7,10-14] Aortic pain is sudden and maximal at onset, with intensity often proportional to the length of dissection. The location of pain is midline and, classically, correlates with the location of dissection: a dissection of the ascending aorta results in chest pain, dissection of the arch results in neck or jaw pain, and a dissection of the descending aorta results in back and sometimes abdominal pain. Thus pain may migrate as the dissection propagates. However, there is considerable variability in presenting symptoms and major overlapping of symptoms in type A and type B dissections.[3,8]

The typical patient is 50 to 70 years old with a history of poorly controlled hypertension. He (2:1 male-to-female ratio) presents with intense chest and/or back pain and is likely to describe it as sharp rather than tearing. The pain does not respond to nitroglycerin. The patient is not dyspneic unless he is suffering one of the cardiac complications of dissection.

Table 60-2 SYMPTOMS, SIGNS, AND FINDINGS IN AORTIC DISSECTION

	Prevalence (%)
History	
Pain:	
Any	94
Sudden	90
Severe	90
Migrating	25
Tearing/ripping	≈35
Chest pain	67
Back pain	50
Abdominal pain	25
Syncope	12
Physical Findings	
High blood pressure	50
Hypotension or shock	15
Diastolic murmur	33
Pulse deficit	30
Focal neurologic deficit	15
Study Results	
Chest radiograph:	
Wide mediastinum	≈60
Abnormal aortic contour	≈60
Normal	15
Electrocardiography:	
Myocardial infarction (ST elevation or new Q waves)	5
Myocardial ischemia (ST depression or T wave inversion)	15

Data from references 7;10-14.

■ PHYSICAL EXAMINATION

The patient appears in obvious pain and often has elevated blood pressure (see Table 60-2). On cardiac examination, the EP may hear a fourth heart sound (S_4), which is due to left ventricular hypertrophy, caused by chronic hypertension. The patient must be examined for two life-threatening complications of type A dissection with retrograde propagation: aortic regurgitation and cardiac tamponade. Aortic regurgitation occurs audibly in a third of cases and manifests as a decrescendo early diastolic murmur, best heard at the left lower sternal border with the patient sitting up, leaning forward, and holding the breath at end-expiration; peripheral pulses can be bounding if the pulse pressure is wide. Cardiac tamponade may manifest as distant heart sounds but more often tachycardia and jugular venous distention occur and are followed by hypotension.

Peripheral pulses should also be examined. If the false lumen is occluding one of the subclavian arteries, there is usually a focal, palpably weak pulse, a finding specific for aortic dissection.[11] Blood pressure should be measured in both arms—a difference of 20 mm Hg or more between extremities should alert the EP to the possibility of subclavian occlusion. It must be remembered, though, that nearly 20% of hypertensive patients have a blood pressure differential of at least 10 mm Hg between extremities.[15] Lower extremity pulses should be evaluated, as frank ischemia of the lower extremities occurs in nearly 10% of cases of aortic dissection.[13]

A thorough neurologic examination should be performed in suspected cases. Fifteen percent of patients with aortic dissection have a focal neurologic deficit, and in the setting of severe acute chest or abdominal pain, this finding is also highly specific for the disease.[11] Potential neurologic deficits in aortic dissection include stroke due to carotid occlusion, spinal cord syndromes due to spinal or intercostal arterial occlusion, and peripheral neuropathy due to neuronal ischemia or compression of a peripheral nerve by the false lumen.

■ ELECTROCARDIOGRAPHY

Electrocardiography (ECG) findings are usually unremarkable even though the patient reports severe pain. To the EP, this situation may seem incongruent. Nonspecific ECG findings in a patient with severe chest pain might alert an astute clinician to consider aortic dissection.

Patients at risk for aortic dissection may have long-term, poorly controlled hypertension. Therefore, ECG might reveal left ventricular hypertrophy with high-amplitude QRS complexes and typical ST-T strain patterns. Low-amplitude QRS complexes or electrical alternans may occur in the presence of cardiac tamponade.

A minority of patients have ischemic ECG changes, which can be due to demand ischemia or partial occlusion of a coronary artery. About 5% of aortic dissections completely occlude a coronary artery, predominantly the right coronary artery. The occlusion usually causes an ST elevation myocardial injury pattern in the inferior leads. With any MI, especially an inferior MI, the EP ideally should assess the mediastinum and aorta on a chest radiograph before anticoagulants are given and especially before thrombolysis is begun. The patient should be asked specifically about pain radiating to the back, which is uncommon in MI.

■ CHEST RADIOGRAPH

The chest radiograph classically shows a wide mediastinum, predominantly on the right in dissection of the ascending aorta and on the left in dissection of the descending aorta (Fig. 60-3). The physician's subjective impression, rather than formal measurements, is the best indicator of whether the mediastinum is wide. A widened mediastinum is not a sensitive indicator of aortic dissection. It probably occurs in about 60% of cases, but some reports note widened mediastinum in less than 20%.[3,10] Other abnormalities of the aorta, such as inward displacement of intimal calcification and a double aortic shadow, may be observed. Pleural effusion may also occur, usually on the left.

■ ALTERNATIVE PRESENTATIONS

■ The Young Patient

About 7% of patients with aortic dissection are young (<40 years) and usually have no history of hypertension or other known medical problems.[7] These patients nearly always have occult structural cardiovascular disease.

The most important structural vascular disease is Marfan's syndrome, which has a prevalence of 1 in 10,000 and occurs in all races. Marfan's syndrome accounts for half of aortic dissections in patients younger than 40 years.[7] It is caused by an autosomal dominant mutation in the gene for a type of fibrillin, a protein that makes up part of the elastic fibers in connective tissue of the aorta, lens, and periosteum. Patients are typically tall with long digits, scoliosis, pectus excavatum, and visual problems due to lens dislocation (Fig. 60-4). Most importantly, however, they invariably develop thoracic aneurysms, usually in the ascending aorta, early in life. If their aneurysms are not repaired, most patients will die from aortic dissection or rupture.

Other young patients without a history of severe hypertension who are nevertheless at risk for dissection are those with bicuspid aortic valves and those experiencing acute insults such as cocaine use and trauma. Family history of aortic aneurysms and dissection, beyond syndromes usually associated with aortic pathology, is a newly recognized risk factor seen in 10% to 20% of patients with dissection.[9]

■ Abdominal Pain

Abdominal pain is one of the complaints in about 25% of patients with aortic dissection and is the primary complaint in 5% of patients[13]; such patients invariably have dissection of the descending aorta. The pain is usually midline but can be referred to the flank, often on the left. The pain is typically out of proportion to physical findings.

■ Painless Dissection

About 6% of patients with aortic dissection do not have pain. Half of these patients have had prior cardiovascular surgery, which potentially disrupts tho-

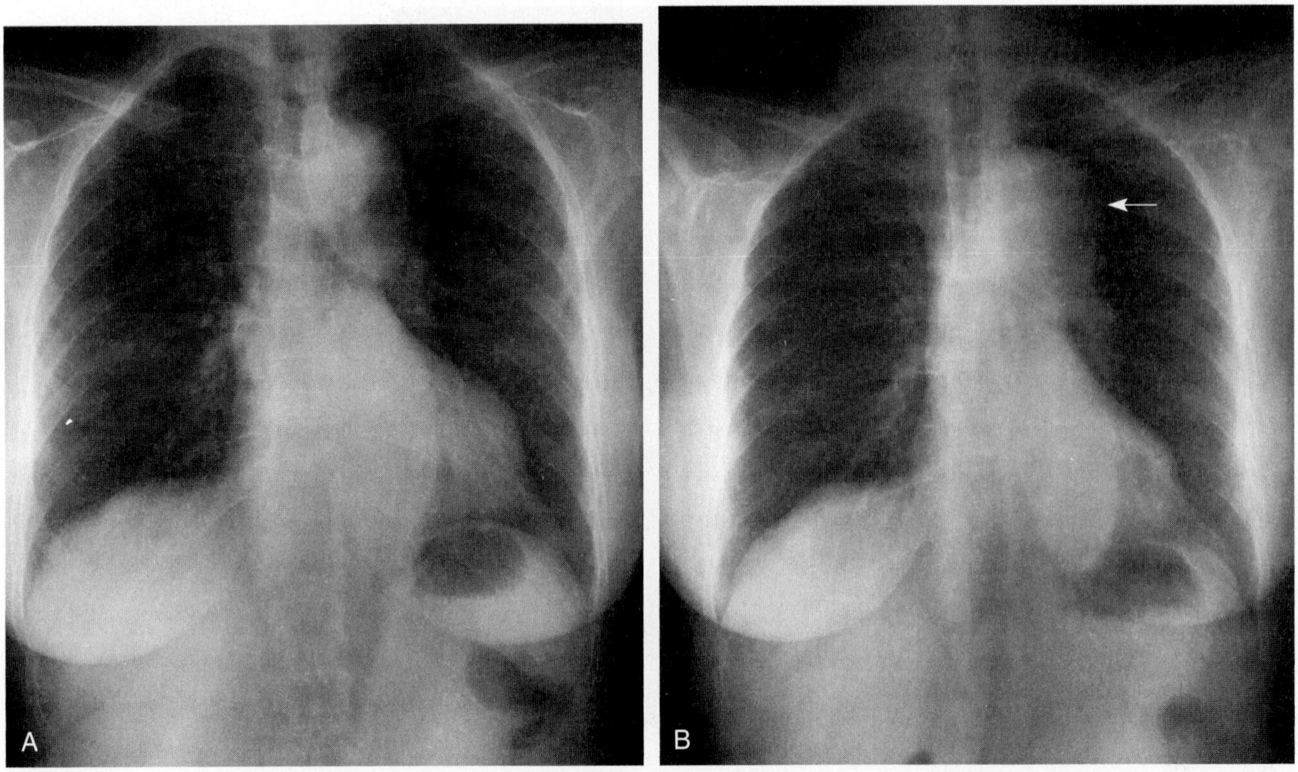
A
B

FIGURE 60-3 Chest radiographs of aortic dissection. **A,** Chest radiograph from 3 years prior, which shows that the patient's cardiac structures are normal. **B,** Current chest radiograph of the same patient showing interval enlargement of the aortic knob (*arrow*). (From Zipes DP, Libby P, Bonow RO, Braunwald E [eds]: Braunwald's Heart Disease: A Textbook of Cardiovascular Medicine, 7th ed. Philadelphia, Elsevier, 2005.)

racic nerves. One third present with syncope, 20% with heart failure, and more than 10% with stroke.[14] There are numerous reports of patients presenting with painless spinal cord syndromes as well.[1] In these difficult cases, picking up clues such as a diastolic murmur, pulse deficit, and an abnormal mediastinum on chest radiograph are critical to making the correct diagnosis.

Differential Diagnosis

■ AORTIC DISSECTION VERSUS ACUTE CORONARY SYNDROME AND PULMONARY EMBOLISM

Aortic dissection often manifests as chest pain (in up to 75% of cases in recent large studies). For any patient with chest pain, the EP must think of three difficult diagnoses that are life-threatening: acute coronary syndrome, pulmonary embolism, and aortic dissection. Acute coronary syndrome often causes a pressure-like pain that is more crescendo than sudden; ECG often shows ischemic changes, and in the absence of complete coronary occlusion, the pain is usually responsive to nitroglycerin. In fact, one distinguishing feature of both pulmonary embolism and aortic dissection is that in the first several hours of either, the pain typically does not resolve. In pulmonary embolism, the pain is usually pleuritic and associated with significant pulmonary symptoms or signs. Other diagnoses to consider are pericarditis/cardiac tamponade, spontaneous pneumothorax, and esophageal rupture.

■ COMBINATION OF FINDINGS

In one prospective study, the absence of aortic pain (sudden and tearing), of a pulse or blood pressure differential, and of mediastinal or aortic widening on chest radiography had a sensitivity of 96% for ruling out the diagnosis of aortic dissection. Conversely, the presence of a pulse deficit or a focal neurologic deficit, with positive likelihood ratios of 47 and 33, respectively, markedly raised the probability of aortic dissection.[11]

Diagnosis

■ GENERAL APPROACH AND D-DIMER

After history, physical examination, ECG, and chest radiography, the clinician must decide whether or not aortic dissection is a reasonable possibility (Fig. 60-5). If so, additional testing is required. The serum biomarker D-dimer may be useful for excluding the diagnosis. A recent meta-analysis found that it was 97% sensitive for aortic dissection; and in a prospective validation substudy of 65 consecutive patients with type A dissection D-dimer—at a cut-off value

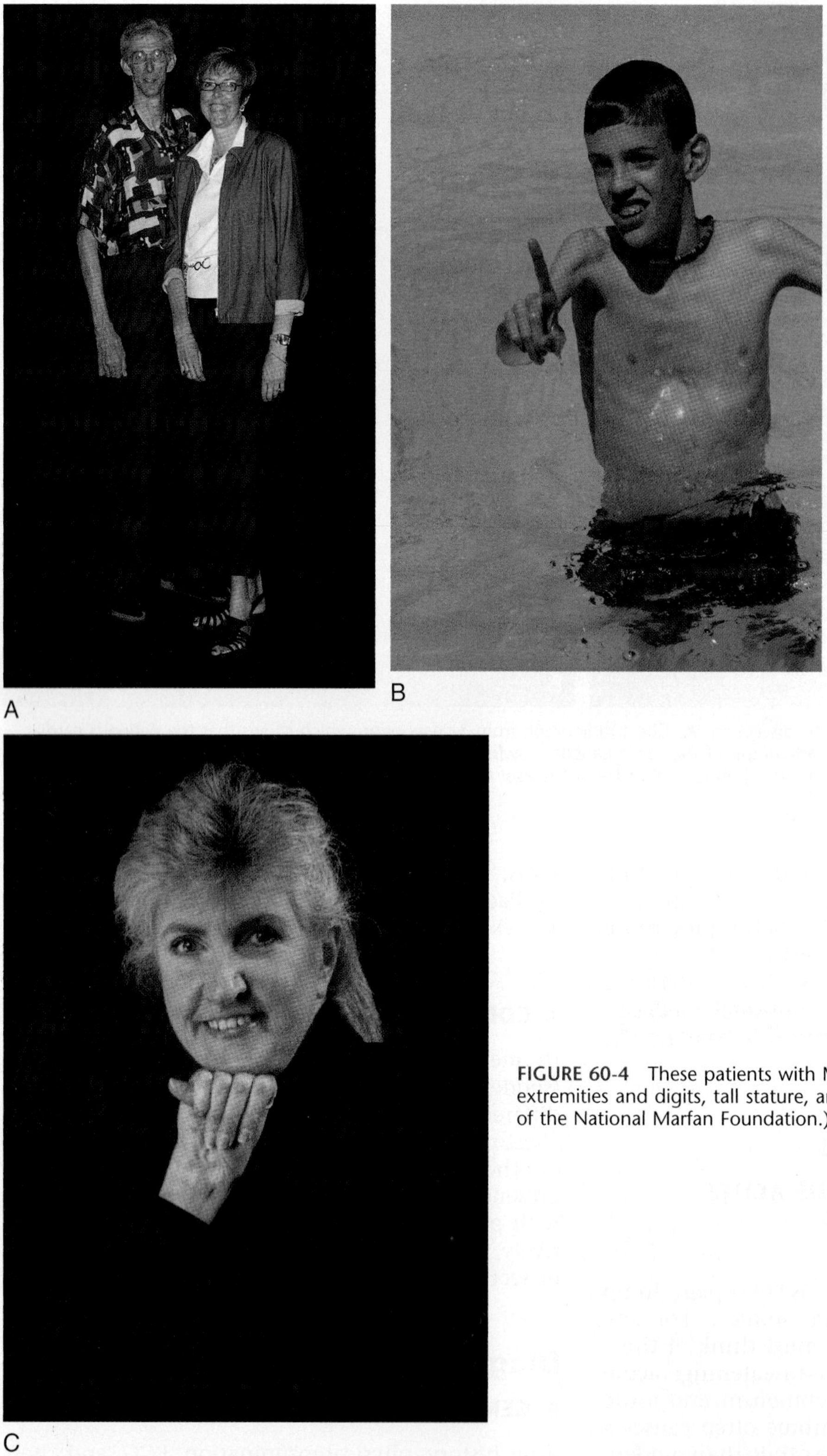

FIGURE 60-4 These patients with Marfan's syndrome have long extremities and digits, tall stature, and pectus carinatum. (Photos courtesy of the National Marfan Foundation.)

commonly used for pulmonary embolism—was false negative in only one case. However, the studies have been small, and as of early 2008 D-dimer has yer to be incorporated as a standard diagnostic tool in this setting. Thus, currently, the next step is advanced imaging of the aorta (Table 60-3).[17-19] Of note, with very strong suspicion for aortic dissection, the clinician should consider contacting a cardiothoracic surgeon while waiting for the imaging study.

■ COMPUTED TOMOGRAPHY

The study of choice is computed tomography (CT) angiography of the aorta (Fig. 60-6). It is immediately

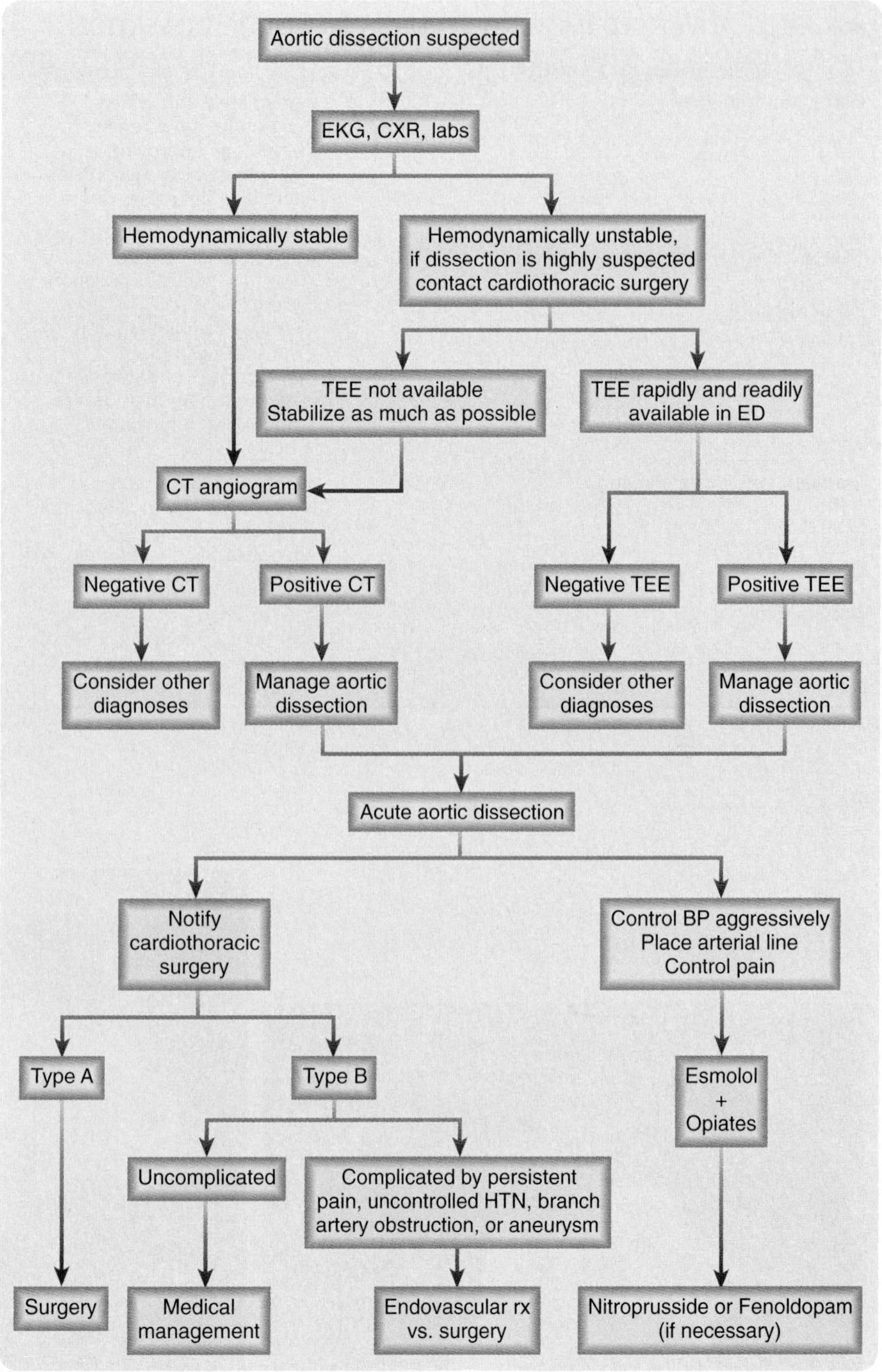
Aortic dissection suspected
EKG, CXR, labs
Hemodynamically stable
Hemodynamically unstable, if dissection is highly suspected contact cardiothoracic surgery
TEE not available Stabilize as much as possible
TEE rapidly and readily available in ED
CT angiogram
Negative CT
Positive CT
Negative TEE
Positive TEE
Consider other diagnoses
Manage aortic dissection
Consider other diagnoses
Manage aortic dissection
Acute aortic dissection
Notify cardiothoracic surgery
Control BP aggressively Place arterial line Control pain
Type A
Type B
Esmolol + Opiates
Uncomplicated
Complicated by persistent pain, uncontrolled HTN, branch artery obstruction, or aneurysm
Surgery
Medical management
Endovascular rx vs. surgery
Nitroprusside or Fenoldopam (if necessary)

FIGURE 60-5 Algorithm for diagnosis and treatment of aortic dissection. CT, computed tomography; CXR, chest radiograph; ECG, electrocardiography; labs, laboratory tests; TEE, transesophageal echocardiography.

available in most EDs and can be interpreted quickly by a radiologist. It is highly sensitive for dissection, especially as CT technology advances—in fact, a 2005 study reported that multidetector CT was 100% accurate in suspected acute aortic disease.[18] Moreover, when its results are negative for dissection, CT frequently shows alternative serious disease to explain the patient's symptoms. With the latest-generation scanners, it may soon be possible to assess in detail the pulmonary arteries, coronary arteries, and aorta with a single study. CT is often more readily available in the ED than is transesophageal echocardiography (TEE), and most patients are able to undergo CT to enable the diagnosis to be made.

■ TRANSESOPHAGEAL ECHOCARDIOGRAPHY

Generally performed by a cardiologist, TEE is an alternative technique in patients with hemodynamic instability or renal failure, both of which are relative contraindications to CT (Fig. 60-7). TEE is as sensitive as CT for type A aortic dissection but may be slightly less sensitive for type B lesions[17]; TEE has the advan-

Table 60-3 ADVANCED IMAGING STUDIES FOR AORTIC DISSECTION

Study	Sensitivity (%)	Advantages	Disadvantages
Computed tomography	93-100	Immediately and widely available; rapid results Technology improving—sensitivity now near 100% Alternative diagnoses often made	Uses large amount of contrast agent Often misses site of intimal tear
Transesophageal echocardiography	88-98	Safe: done at bedside, no contrast agent or radiation exposure Identifies intimal tear: aids surgical planning Can diagnose tamponade, aortic regurgitation, heart failure, and, often, myocardial ischemia	Requires skilled operator—may create delay Blind spots: proximal arch and distal aorta
Magnetic resonance imaging	95-100	Highly accurate No contrast agent or radiation exposure Alternative diagnoses often made	Slow: patient far from ED for prolonged period Expensive, often unavailable
Aortography	87	Able to image/treat coronary arteries, so may be study of choice when patient has ST elevation	Invasive, uses large amount of contrast agent Time-consuming

Data from references 17-19.

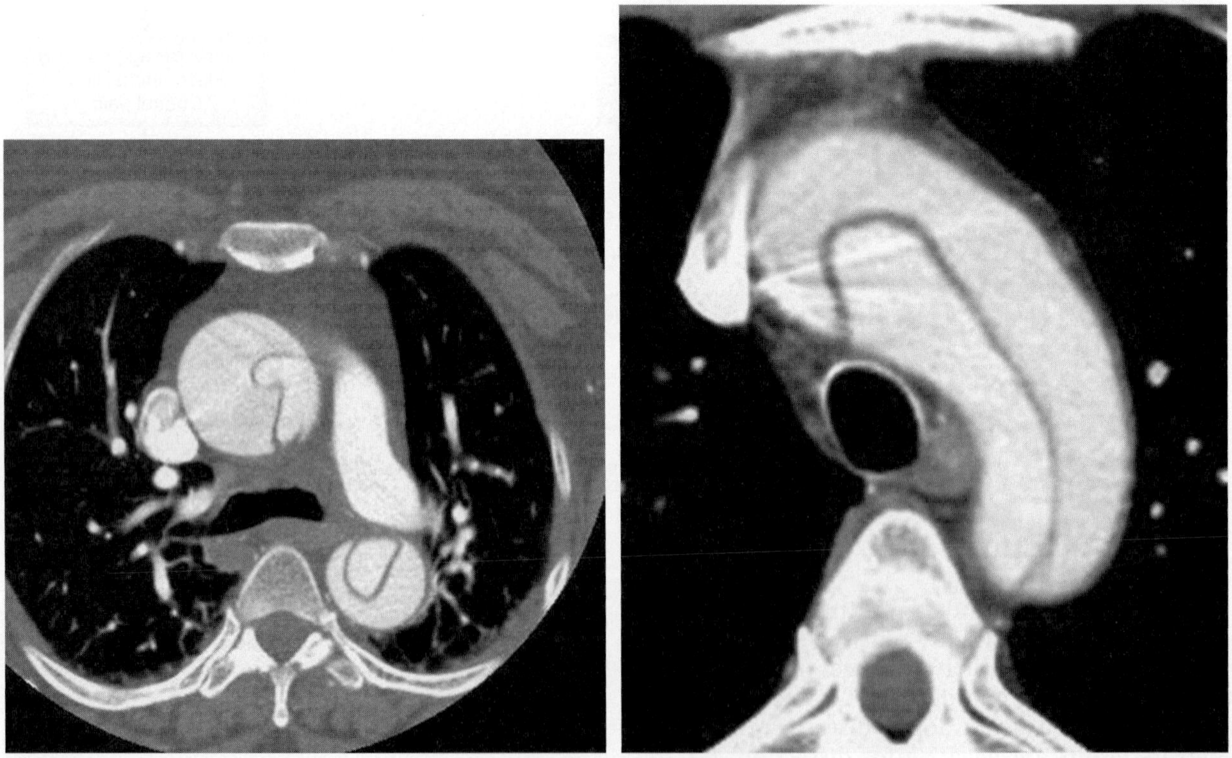

A B

FIGURE 60-6 Computed tomography scans of aortic dissection. The first axial scan (**A**) shows aortic dissection, demonstrated as serpiginous lucencies in the ascending and descending aorta. The second scan (**B**) shows dissection of the aortic arch. (Courtesy Leslie Quint, University of Michigan.)

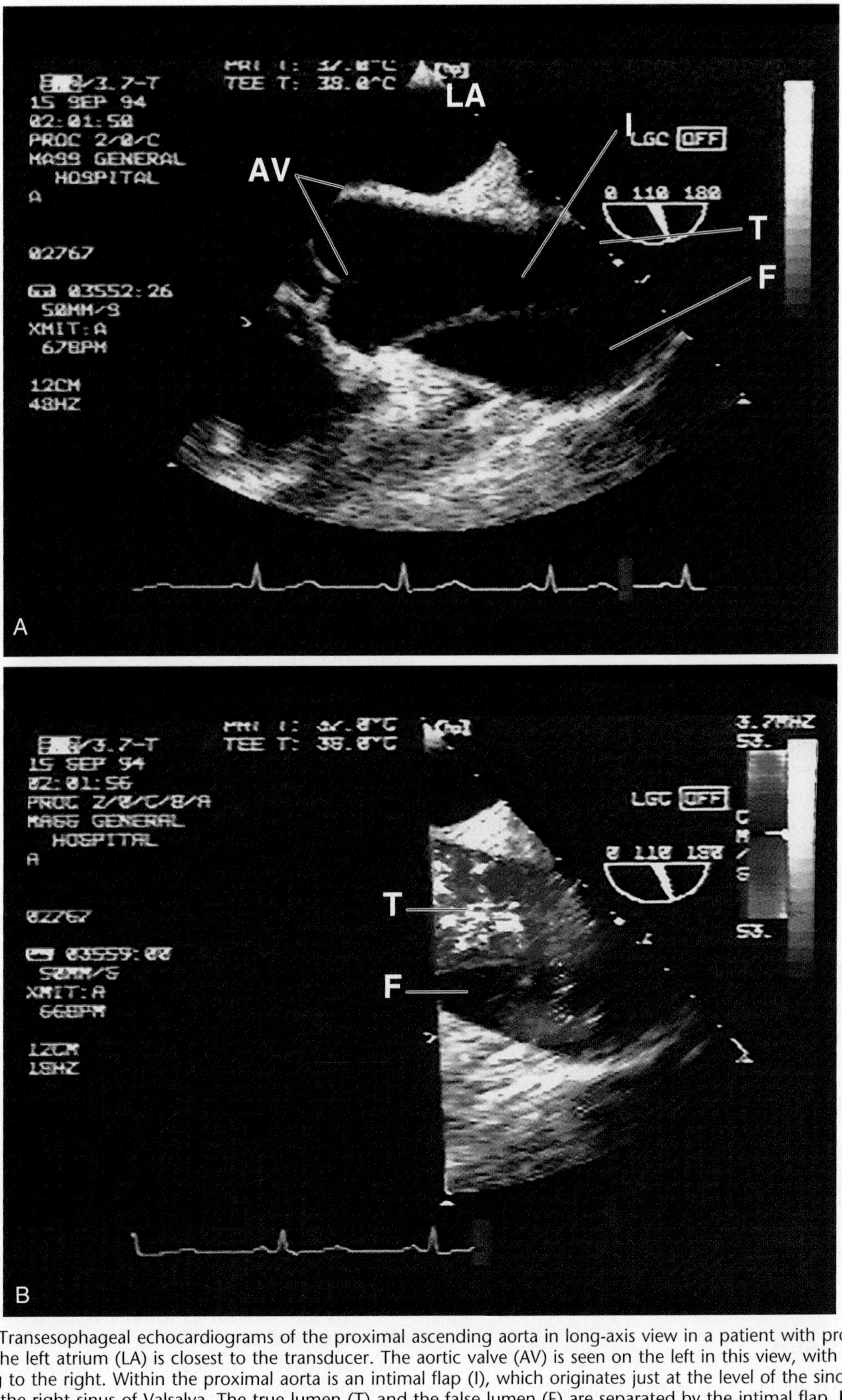
LA
AV
I
T
F
A
T
F
B

FIGURE 60-7 Transesophageal echocardiograms of the proximal ascending aorta in long-axis view in a patient with proximal aortic dissection. **A,** The left atrium (LA) is closest to the transducer. The aortic valve (AV) is seen on the left in this view, with the ascending aorta extending to the right. Within the proximal aorta is an intimal flap (I), which originates just at the level of the sinotubular junction above the right sinus of Valsalva. The true lumen (T) and the false lumen (F) are separated by the intimal flap. **B,** The addition of color flow Doppler imaging in the same view confirms the presence of two distinct lumina. The true lumen (T) fills completely with brisk blood flow (bright blue), while minimal retrograde flow (dark orange) is seen in the false lumen (F). (From Zipes DP, Libby P, Bonow RO, Braunwald E [eds]: Braunwald's Heart Disease: A Textbook of Cardiovascular Medicine, 7th ed. Philadelphia, Elsevier, 2005.)

tage of assessing the aortic valve and pericardial space for complications of type A dissection. It may also detect focal ventricular wall motion abnormalities suggesting myocardial ischemia as the cause of the patient's symptoms. Finally, unlike CT, TEE usually identifies the exact location of the intimal tear and assesses overall cardiac function, which aids operative planning and risk assessment. Thus cardiothoracic surgeons may request the study even when dissection has already been diagnosed.

■ MAGNETIC RESONANCE IMAGING

Magnetic resonance imaging (MRI) is useful in stable patients who have renal failure, especially when a type B dissection is suspected or TEE cannot be performed. However, MRI is slow and the patient must remain in the MRI suite, usually far from the ED, which can be risky in the setting of a potential life-threatening disease.

■ ANGIOGRAPHY

Conventional angiography of the aorta is invasive and is rarely needed for diagnosis of aortic dissection. A possible exception is in those rare patients with ST-elevation myocardial infarction in whom aortic dissection is still a concern. In such a case, the interventional cardiologist may perform an angiogram of the aorta as part of the cardiac catheterization procedure, thereby ruling out dissection without delaying coronary angiography and potential revascularization. However, even in this time-sensitive situation, many cardiologists prefer CT, as cannulating a dissected aorta is not without risk.

Management

Table 60-4 summarizes the intravenous hypertensive agents used in treatment of aortic dissection.[20,21]

■ IMMEDIATE CONSULTATION

For any thoracic aortic dissection, the clinician should consult a cardiothoracic surgeon immediately. A cardiology consultation may be needed as well, either for admission of a patient with type B dissection or for a pre-operative TEE, if needed, in a patient with type A dissection.

■ ED APPROACH

The main goal of ED care is to identify the disease and then manage the patient's blood pressure and heart rate to minimize aortic shear force. The goal for systolic blood pressure is 100 to 120 mm Hg and the goal for the heart rate is 60 to 80 beats/min. Note that the blood pressure goal is independent of the patient's baseline blood pressure, unlike the approach to most hypertensive emergencies. Therefore the clinician must watch for of signs of iatrogenic end-organ malperfusion. Very short-acting antihypertensives should be used, administered as drips to precisely titrate the dose to effect.

A minimum of two peripheral intravenous (IV) lines will be needed, along with an arterial line for continuous blood pressure monitoring. If possible, the arterial line is placed in the right radial artery so it is less likely to be affected by the dissection occluding the upstream artery.

The EP must remember that aortic pain is very severe and so adequate analgesia with intravenous opioids should be provided. This step helps reduce blood pressure.

■ ANTIHYPERTENSIVE THERAPY

Beta-blockers are the first-line antihypertensive agents in patients with aortic dissection because they most effectively reduce both blood pressure and shear force. The ideal beta-blocker is esmolol because of its short half-life and, thereby, its titratability. Blood pressure control with beta-blockers may be limited by bradycardia or a plateau effect; therefore, a second antihypertensive agent is often needed, invariably a vasodilator.

The standard second-line agent is nitroprusside, which is extremely short-acting and universally effective. Fenoldopam, a highly selective dopamine agonist, has become a favored alternative in some centers because, unlike nitroprusside, it maintains or improves renal perfusion, including perfusion during aortic cross-clamping, while lowering peripheral vascular resistance. To avoid dangerous reflex tachycardia, vasodilators should be started only after the heart rate has been controlled pharmacologically.

■ NATURAL HISTORY AND DEFINITIVE MANAGEMENT

Type A aortic dissection requires emergency thoracic surgery, as the mortality rate in patients who do not have surgery increases hourly and is 50% to 80% at 1 month. Typically, the surgeon excises the segment of aorta containing the intimal tear(s) and replaces it with a graft, often leaving some dissected aorta in place. The aortic valve often needs to be replaced as well. With surgery, survival in type A dissection is improved remarkably, to more than 95% at 1 year.[22]

Type B dissection is usually treated medically, with 90% survival at 1 month. Type B dissection that is complicated by persistent pain, uncontrolled hypertension, branch artery obstruction, or aneurysm has traditionally required surgery. However, endovascular stent placement and balloon fenestration have become therapeutic options; malperfusion syndromes can be reversed in the vast majority of cases, and the false lumen can often be obliterated, thus reducing the chances of aneurysm development and progression as well as of other future complications.[23-25]

Table 60-4 INTRAVENOUS ANTIHYPERTENSIVE DRUGS FOR AORTIC DISSECTION

Medication	Mechanism	Pharmacokinetics	Dosing	Notes
Cardiac Inhibitors				
Esmolol	Beta (β_1) blocker	Onset: <1 min Duration: 10-20 min Metabolism: blood	Load 500 μg/kg, then 25-50 μg/kg/min drip; titrate by 25-50 μg/kg/min every 5-10 min Maximum: 200 μg/kg/min	Drug of choice Effective reduction of shear force Highly titratable
Labetalol	Beta (β_1/β_2) and alpha (α_1) blocker (7:1 β:α ratio)	Onset: 2-5 min Peak effect: 5-15 min Duration: 2-4 hours Metabolism: Mostly blood (no dose change in liver/kidney disease)	Bolus 20 mg, then: Give further boluses 40-80 mg q 10 min *or* Start drip at 1-2 mg/min and titrate Maximum total dose: 300 mg	Beta and alpha blockade may obviate a second agent Also has β_2 agonist activity, which limits negative effect of nonspecific beta-adrenergic antagonism on the lungs Not as titratable as esmolol
Diltiazem	Calcium channel blocker Negative chronotropy>>negative inotropy Vasodilation	Onset: 3 min Duration: 1-3 hr Metabolism: Likely in liver (no dose change)	Bolus 20 mg, then 5-15 mg/hr drip Second 25-mg bolus may be given if needed	Use when beta-blockers are contraindicated Blood pressure reduction occurs via vasodilation
Vasodilators				
Nitroprusside	Nitric oxide–mediated vasodilation	Onset: seconds Duration: 2 min Metabolism: Blood (but toxic metabolites excreted by kidney)	Start drip at 0.5 μg/kg/min and titrate Maximum: 3 μg/kg/min—larger doses confer high risk for cyanide toxicity	Extremely potent; highly titratable Vasodilators cause reflex tachycardia: should be started only after cardiac inhibition established When used in chronic kidney disease, there is higher risk of renal failure and cyanide toxicity
Fenoldopam	Dopamine agonist Vasodilation: Renal and peripheral arteries Natriuresis	Onset: 5 min Peak effect: 15 min Duration: 30-60 min Metabolism: Liver (no dose change)	Start drip at 0.1 μg/kg/min; titrate by 0.05-0.1 μg/kg/min every 15 min Maximum: 0.8 μg/kg/min; higher doses associated with adverse effects	Enhances renal perfusion: ideal in acute or chronic renal failure Attenuates renal failure during aortic cross-clamping: preferred by some surgeons Much slower-acting than nitroprusside

Data from references 20 and 21.

■ THE UNDIFFERENTIATED CHEST PAIN PATIENT

In the patient with aortic dissection, aspirin should be avoided because it could cause excessive surgical bleeding and may raise the risk of aortic rupture. Nitroglycerin, in the absence of beta-blockade, should also be avoided as it could cause reflex tachycardia. Because acute corouary disease is far more common than dissection, many patients with undifferentiated chest pain receive aspirin and/or nitroglycerin at the initial encounter from either paramedics or ED care-givers. However, if the patient's presentation strongly suggests aortic dissection, it is prudent to wait until after imaging studies have ruled at the diagnosis before initiating these therapies. Anticoagulation should be avoided if dissection is even being considered.

Disposition

All patients with newly diagnosed aortic dissection should be admitted to the intensive care unit. Patients with type A dissection may go to the operating room first. In the ED, these patients need ICU-level care and should be in a resuscitation bay with a 1:1 nurse-to-patient ratio to ensure adequate monitoring of blood pressure and response to therapy (see "Red Flags" box).

RED FLAGS

- One third of patients with aortic dissection do not have chest pain at presentation.
- Aortic dissection occurs more commonly in winter, even in temperate climates.
- 40% of patients with dissection have a normal mediastinal width on chest radiograph.
- Beware of pseudohypotension, which is a low blood pressure reading due to occlusion of an extremity by a dissected vessel wall.
- An ischemic ECG does not rule out aortic dissection. Always consider dissection in the patient with an inferior ST elevation MI: most ascending aortic dissections involve the right aortic wall and occasionally the right coronary artery will be occluded.

REFERENCES

1. Khan IA, Nair CK: Clinical, diagnostic, and management perspectives of aortic dissection. Chest 2002;122:311-328.
2. Hirst AE Jr, Johns VJ Jr, Kime SW Jr: Dissecting aneurysm of the aorta: A review of 505 cases. Medicine 1958;37:217-279.
3. Sullivan PR, Wolfson AB, Leckey RD, Burke JL: Diagnosis of acute thoracic aortic dissection in the emergency department. Am J Emerg Med 2000;18:46-50.
4. Meszaros I, Morocz J, Szlavi J, et al: Epidemiology and clinicopathology of aortic dissection. Chest 2000;117: 1271-1278.
5. Clouse WD, Hallett JW, Schaff HV, et al: Acute aortic dissection: Population-based incidence compared with degenerative aortic aneurysm rupture. Mayo Clin Proc 2004;79: 176-180.
6. Burt CW: Summary statistics for acute cardiac ischemia and chest pain visits to United States EDs, 1995-1996. Am J Emerg Med 1999;17:552-559.
7. Januzzi JL, Isselbacher EM, Fattori R, et al: Characterizing the young patient with aortic dissection: Results from the International Registry of Acute Aortic Dissection (IRAD). J Am Coll Cardiol 2004;43:665-669.
8. Neinaber CA, Eagle KA: Aortic dissection: New frontiers in diagnosis and management. Part I: From etiology to diagnostic strategies. Circulation 2003;108:628-635.
9. Hasham SN, Lewin MR, Tran VT, et al: Nonsyndromic genetic predisposition to aortic dissection: A newly recognized, diagnosable, and preventable occurrence in families. Ann Emerg Med 2004;43:79-82.
10. Klompas M: Does this patient have an acute thoracic aortic dissection? JAMA 2002;287:2262-2272.
11. Von Kodolitsch Y, Schwartz AG, Nienaber CA: Clinical prediction of acute aortic dissection. Arch Intern Med 2000;160:2977-2982.
12. Hagan PG, Nienaber CA, Isselbacher EM, et al: The International Registry of Acute Aortic Dissection (IRAD): New insights into an old disease. JAMA 2000;283:897-903.
13. Upchurch GR, Nienaber C, Fattori R, et al: Acute aortic dissection presenting with primarily abdominal pain: A rare manifestation of a deadly disease. Ann Vasc Surg 2005;19:367-373.
14. Park SW, Hutchison S, Mehta RH, et al: Association of painless acute aortic dissection with increased mortality. Mayo Clin Proc 2004;79:1252-1257.
15. Pesola GR, Pesola HR, Lin M, et al: The normal difference in bilateral indirect blood pressure recordings in hypertensive individuals. Acad Emerg Med 2002;9:342-345.
16. Sodeck G, Domanovits H, Schillinger M, et al: D-dimer in ruling out acute aortic dissection: A systematic review and prospective cohort study. Eur Heart J 2007;28:3067-3075.
17. Moore AG, Eagle KA, Bruckman D, et al: Choice of computed tomography, transesophageal echocardiography, magnetic resonance imaging, and aortography in acute aortic dissection: International Registry of Acute Aortic Dissection (IRAD). Am J Cardiol 2002;89:1235-1238.
18. Hayter R, Rhea JT, Small A, et al: Suspected aortic dissection and other aortic disorders: Multi-detector row CT in 373 cases in the emergency setting. Radiology 2005;238: 841-852.
19. Shiga T, Wajima Z, Apfel CC, et al: Diagnostic accuracy of transesophageal echocardiography, helical computed tomography, and magnetic resonance imaging for suspected thoracic aortic dissection. Arch Intern Med 2006;166:1350-1356.
20. Veron J, Marik PE: The diagnosis and management of hypertensive crises. Chest 2000;118:214-227.
21. Mosby's Drug Consult 2005: Handheld Software on CD-ROM, 3rd ed. St. Louis, Mosby, 2005.
22. Tsai T, Fattori R, Trimarchi S, et al: International Registry of Acute Aortic Dissection: Long-term survival in patients presenting with type A acute aortic dissection: Insights from the International Registry of Acute Aortic Dissection. Circulation 2006;114:350-356.
23. Nienaber CA, Eagle KA: Aortic dissection: New frontiers in diagnosis and management. Part II: Therapeutic management and follow-up. Circulation 2003;108:772-778.
24. Dialetto G, Covino FE, Scognamiglio G, et al: Treatment of type B aortic dissection: Endoluminal repair or conventional medical therapy? Eur J Cardiothorac Surg 2005;27: 826-830.
25. Moon MC, Pablo Morales J, Greenberg RK: Complicated acute type B dissection and endovascular repair: Indications and pitfall. Perspect Vasc Surg Endovasc Ther 2007;19:146-159.

Chapter **61**

Abdominal Aortic Aneurysm

Danielle Ware-McGee and Jamie Collings

KEY POINTS

Abdominal aortic aneurysms (AAAs) continue to be a significant cause of morbidity and mortality (50% for ruptured AAAs), and the key to mortality reduction is early diagnosis.

The risk of rupture relates linearly to the maximum cross-sectional diameter of the aneurysm.

Elective repair of nonruptured AAAs lowers this mortality significantly and warrants a high level of vigilance by health care providers to diagnose this condition in its potentially curative stages.

Histologically, AAAs develop as a result of a complex interplay of immunologically mediated proteases and antiproteases that cause destruction of elastin and collagen in the arterial wall.

Many risk factors promote the development of AAAs, but the most important are smoking, male gender, and family history.

Classically, patients with impending AAA rupture present with the triad of abdominal pain, pulsatile abdominal mass, and shock.

The two current operative approaches for the repair of AAAs are open surgery and endovascular repair; the better approach for each patient depends on several clinical variables and specific patient characteristics.

Perspective

At present, abdominal aortic aneurysm (AAA) ranks 13th on the list of the leading causes of death in the United States. The word *aneurysm* derives from a Greek word meaning "widening." Sakalihasan and colleagues[1] further define aneurysm as a permanent and irreversible localized dilation of a vessel.[1] AAA continues to be such a difficult diagnosis because vague symptoms that carry large differential diagnoses, such as back or abdominal pain, often herald this diagnosis in its early (virtually asymptomatic) and potentially curative stages. AAA affects approximately 5% of elderly men and is responsible for a significant number of deaths in Western countries.[2]

Epidemiology

Once the AAA ruptures, death is a certainty in more than 65% of cases,[1] with some reports giving mortality rates as high as 90%.[3] Low rates of postmortem examinations and the high likelihood that some of these deaths have been erroneously attributed to a cardiac etiology severely hamper gathering true estimates of mortality related to ruptured AAAs.[2] A ruptured AAA is a life-threatening condition that mandates rapid surgical repair. However, elective repair of an AAA lowers the mortality to less than 5%.[3,4]

Thus, there is an obvious benefit to diagnosing and treating these aneurysms before they rupture. Given that this disease affects 4% to 7% of adults 65 years or older, the onus falls more and more on physicians to accomplish this task as the population ages.[3]

Risk Factors

There is an abundance of research on the identification of risk factors that potentiate the development and growth of AAAs (Box 61-1). Besides male gender, age, and hypertension, every study on the subject of AAAs singles out long-term tobacco smoking as the most important risk factor.[2] The occurrence of AAAs in tobacco smokers is more than four times that in life-long nonsmokers.[1] Lederle and associates[5] compared relative risks for different diseases in long-term cigarette smokers and found that the risk for development of AAAs is five-fold higher than that of cerebrovascular disease and three-fold higher than that of coronary artery disease.[1] Smoking not only raises the risk for development of AAAs but also increases the annual growth rate of existent AAAs, with some studies reporting a rate of 2.83 mm per year in smokers compared with 2.53 mm per year for nonsmokers.[1,6] However, the exact means by which smoking enhances aneurysm formation remain a mystery.

In addition to tobacco smoking, there are other risk factors. Atherosclerosis is so highly associated with AAA development and expansion that the American Heart Association (AHA) guidelines on the treatment of AAAs mandate that blood pressure and fasting serum lipid values be strictly monitored and controlled in patients with AAAs.[7] The AHA further recommends that patients with aneurysms or a family history be offered smoking cessation interventions.[7] Despite the importance of atherosclerosis, additional factors are likely present because not every atherosclerotic patient has an AAA.[1] Many authorities cite a possible causal link between development of AAAs and chronic obstructive pulmonary disease (COPD). Researchers blame tobacco smoking–induced elastin degradation for this proposed association.[7] A review of the literature notes that patients with COPD undergoing long-term treatment with corticosteroids have a much higher AAA expansion rate than COPD patients not taking steroids.[7] Hence, steroid use and coexisting disease are more likely responsible for the high prevalence of AAAs among patients with COPD.[7] Lastly, from a genetic standpoint, several screening studies suggest that male first-degree relatives of people with COPD are most at risk. Female first-degree relatives appear to be at similar risk, but the data are less certain.[7] Familial aneurysms differ from nonfamilial aneurysms mainly in that they may develop at an earlier age.[7] There are likely existing genetic polymorphisms that account for familial clustering of abdominal aortic aneurysms, but this clustering could also result from exposure to common environmental factors, such as tobacco smoke.[1]

BOX 61-1

Risk Factors for Development of Abdominal Aortic Aneurysm

Smoking
Male gender
Age
Family history—especially male first-degree relatives
Hypertension
Dyslipidemia

Principles of Disease

Finding a unifying definition for AAAs that encompasses the various classification schemes surrounding their size, shape, and location is an arduous task. Simplistically, most AAAs occur infrarenally and are defined as aortic diameter greater than 3 cm.[1,2] Most screening studies have defined AAAs on the basis of measurements in the anteroposterior dimension.[7] At baseline, women have slightly smaller normal aortic diameters than men. This fact becomes important only when one is deciding at which size larger aneurysms should be repaired in women and men. However, this difference in normal aortic diameter between the sexes is not substantial enough to warrant changing the size limit of 3 cm that is currently used to characterize a small AAA.[7] Lastly, the dilation must encompass the three layers of the vascular wall; otherwise, the dilation is a *pseudoaneurysm*.[1]

Additionally, most aneurysms are *fusiform*—they are circumferential with respect to artery.[1] *Saccular* aneurysms affect only a part of the circumference.[1] *Inflammatory* aneurysms demonstrate extensive perianeurysmal and retroperitoneal fibrosis as well as dense adhesions to neighboring organs.[1] Furthermore, aneurysms are classified on the basis of their location in reference to the renal arteries. *Juxtarenal* aneurysms arise distal but in very close proximity to the renal arteries.[7] An aneurysm originating from one or both renal arteries is known as a *pararenal* aneurysm.[7] *Suprarenal* aneurysms affect the superior mesenteric and celiac arteries; they become type IV *thoracoabdominal* aneurysms if they extend upward to the crus of the diaphragm.[7]

On a histologic level, elastin and collagen are the main proteins involved in AAA growth and rupture, respectively. Early on in aneurysm formation, elastic fibers are lost, fragmented, and/or attenuated, contributing to the development of the actual wall of the aneurysm.[1,8] However, once the concentration of medial elastin is severely decreased, the collagen-rich adventitial tissue constitutes the artery's last mode of resistance.[1,8] Degradation of this collagen-rich tissue is the eventual cause of rupture.[1,8] Recent research has focused on the role of matrix metalloproteinases (MMPs) in the degradation of elastin and collagen (see later).

The natural history of all arterial aneurysms encompasses gradual and/or sporadic growth in their diameter and the accretion of mural thrombus.[7] These features contribute to rupture, thromboembolic ischemic events, and the compression or erosion of adjacent structures, which are the three most common complications of arterial aneurysms.[7] The risk of AAA rupture relates linearly to the maximum cross-sectional diameter of the aneurysm. Estimates place the risk of rupture at 1% to 3% per year for AAAs measuring up to 5 cm, at 11% per year for 5- to 7-cm aneurysms, and near 20% per year for aneurysms larger than 7 cm.[9]

Clinical Features

Only 50% of patients present with the classic clinical triad of AAA symptoms: abdominal pain, pulsatile abdominal mass, and shock indicating aneurysm rupture.[9] Interestingly enough, younger patients are more apt to be symptomatic at the time of diagnosis. Pain in the hypogastric area or lower back is the most common complaint in patients with symptomatic AAAs. Usually the pain is steady and aggravating in nature, lasts for hours to days, and is unaffected by movement or position.[7] There are some variations on this theme, such as abdominal or flank pain that radiates into the scrotum, groin, buttocks, or legs. Additionally, the extent of shock varies according to the location and size of the rupture and the amount of delay before the patient is examined.[1] The symptoms may masquerade as those of renal colic, diverticulitis, or a gastrointestinal hemorrhage, thereby leading to a fatal misdiagnosis.[7] AAAs that rupture anterolaterally dramatically violate the peritoneal cavity and are most often associated with sudden death. Patients with ruptured AAAs who reach a physician tend to have ruptures of the posterolateral wall in the retroperitoneal space. Some of these patients are fortunate enough that their bodies temporarily tamponade a small tear so they suffer relatively small initial blood loss.[1] A few of these patients with contained ruptures may even present with flank ecchymosis, a physical finding known as Grey Turner's sign.[7] However, AAAs are not contained for long, and even these patients suffer the deleterious effects of a larger rupture if they fail to seek medical attention early or the physician they encounter fails to recognize the signs of impending rupture.[1]

Conversely, nonruptured aneurysms are sometimes found by accident. The astute clinician can often find them on physical examination. Palpation of AAAs is safe and has not been reported to precipitate rupture.[7] Abdominal palpation is moderately sensitive for the detection of AAAs that meet the size criteria necessary for surgical intervention, but even large aneurysms may be difficult to palpate, especially in obese patients. However, in the case of AAAs that are smaller or have already ruptured, physical examination alone is not nearly precise enough.[7] Not infrequently, patients with nonruptured AAAs present only after suffering complications such as various thromboembolic events or after thorough evaluation for chronic vague abdominal and back pain.[7]

Lastly, another clinical triad to be wary of is that found in patients with inflammatory aneurysms. It consists of chronic abdominal pain, weight loss, and elevated erythrocyte sedimentation rate.[7] Patients with inflammatory aneurysms tend to be smokers and most have peripheral vascular disease and coronary artery disease. Compared with patients with noninflammatory atherosclerotic aneurysms, those with inflammatory aneurysms are more likely to be symptomatic at presentation, to have more of a retroperitoneal inflammatory reaction, and to have a higher surgical mortality rate.[7] This propensity for a retroperitoneal inflammatory reaction explains why many patients with this condition present with ureterohydronephrosis.[1]

Table 61-1 lists the differential diagnosis entities for AAA along with priority actions for each.

Diagnostic Strategies

Prior to the 1970s, standard plain radiographs were the only means by which to follow the expansion rate of aneurysms. Plain films are useful for this purpose, however, only when the aneurysm has mural calcification that can be easily seen on radiographs. Additionally, the film may show obscuration of the psoas margin by a soft tissue mass and, possibly, extension of mural calcification into a periaortic soft tissue mass, hinting at a possible ruptured aneurysm.[7] It is not the current standard of care to use plain radiographic studies for follow-up surveillance of AAAs, but quite a few such lesions are initially discovered an incidental findings on plain abdominal films obtained for other purposes.[7]

Before the introduction of B-mode ultrasonography in the 1970s and computed tomography (CT) in the 1980s, plain films and physical examination were the limits of a physician's diagnostic capabilities for discovering or monitoring AAAs.[7] Thus, physicians had a difficult time accurately selecting patients for surgical intervention before their AAAs ruptured.[7] As mentioned earlier, several studies have confirmed the linear association between AAA diameter and annual expansion rate. An observed rate of growth that surpasses these estimates is indicative of a "growth spurt" that may necessitate early elective aneurysm

Table 61-1 DIFFERENTIAL DIAGNOSIS OF ABDOMINAL AORTIC ANEURYSM AND PRIORITY ACTIONS

Alternative Diagnosis	Priority Actions and Comments
Myocardial infarction	Pursue a thorough cardiac work-up, and if the diagnosis is in doubt, be sure to consult both cardiothoracic surgery and cardiology specialists before initiating thrombolytic and/or anticoagulant therapy.
Ischemic bowel	Assuming there are no clinical signs of rupture and the patient is hemodynamically stable, obtain a computed tomography (CT) scan to allow definitive diagnosis.
Acute appendicitis	If patient is hemodynamically stable, obtain both an immediate surgical consultation and a CT scan.
Gastrointestinal bleed	This diagnosis usually is not subtle and is fairly easy to make at the bedside with a rectal examination and/or nasogastric lavage; be wary of aortoenteric fistula.
Pancreatitis	Although a relatively common diagnosis and one that usually requires medical treatment only, pancreatitis is still a life-threatening entity. Be sure to obtain a serum lipase measurement to screen for this diagnosis.
Bowel obstruction	If bowel obstruction is a concern, an acute abdominal radiographic series will aid in its quick diagnosis.
Peptic ulcer disease, perforated ulcer	Upright bedside chest radiography to evaluate for free air should be a routine part of the work-up for AAA to quickly rule out or rule in peptic ulcer disease and perforated ulcer.
Cholelithiasis	On the basis of the patient's clinical symptoms, it may be prudent to order a hepatic function test at presentation.
Diverticulitis	If the abdominal examination raises enough concern for diverticulitis, an immediate surgical consultation is mandatory; if the patient is hemodynamically stable enough for CT, the diagnosis is easily made.
Gastritis	Although part of the differential diagnosis for AAA, gastritis is more of a diagnosis of exclusion, after life-threatening possibilities have been evaluated and/or treated.
Cauda equina, epidural abscess, vertebral osteomyelitis	Consider obtaining erythrocyte sedimentation rate measurement, magnetic resonance imaging, and neurosurgical consultation.
Urinary tract infection (females), pyelonephritis, nephrolithiasis	Urinalysis and CT scan are useful in differentiating these possibilities.
Musculoskeletal pain	Often a diagnosis of exclusion.

Tips and Tricks

- At baseline, women have slightly smaller normal aortic diameters than men (1.9 vs. 2.3 cm); however, this difference in normal aortic diameter between the sexes is not substantial enough to warrant changing the upper limit of 3 cm that is used to characterize a small abdominal aortic aneurysm (AAA).
- Patients who undergo emergency surgery for AAAs and are found to have intact, symptomatic aneurysms still have a mortality of 20% to 25%, compared with 5% for those undergoing elective repair.
- In stable patients with abdominal or back pain in whom AAA is high on the differential diagnosis, the EP should choose the type of CT scan allowing diagnosis of the most likely cause; sometimes rapid abdominal CT without oral contrast is most beneficial.

repair. Katzen and associates[3] define this "growth spurt" as an increase of 1 cm per year. Fortunately, the diagnostic armamentarium of today's physician includes ultrasonography, CT, and magnetic resonance imaging (MRI) or magnetic resonance arteriography (MRA) to aid in estimating aneurysm diameter and/or expansion rate.

Ultrasonography is an excellent choice for diagnosing AAAs, for several reasons (Fig. 61-1A). First, it is an easy, cheap, and accurate diagnostic modality that can evaluate the aorta in the transverse, longitudinal, and anteroposterior dimensions. For these reasons, it is an ideal modality for initial evaluation, surveillance, and population screening with a sensitivity ranging from 92% to 99% and a diagnostic specificity of nearly 100%.[7] Also, ultrasonography provides the EP with a rapid, accurate mode of bedside assessment in the hypotensive patient with suspected AAA who is too unstable to leave the ED for CT or MRI/MRA. However, ultrasonography does have its limitations. Despite its efficacy in ascertaining the size of infrarenal aortic aneurysms, it is an unreliable mode of imaging for pararenal, juxtarenal, and suprarenal aneurysms and for imaging the common and

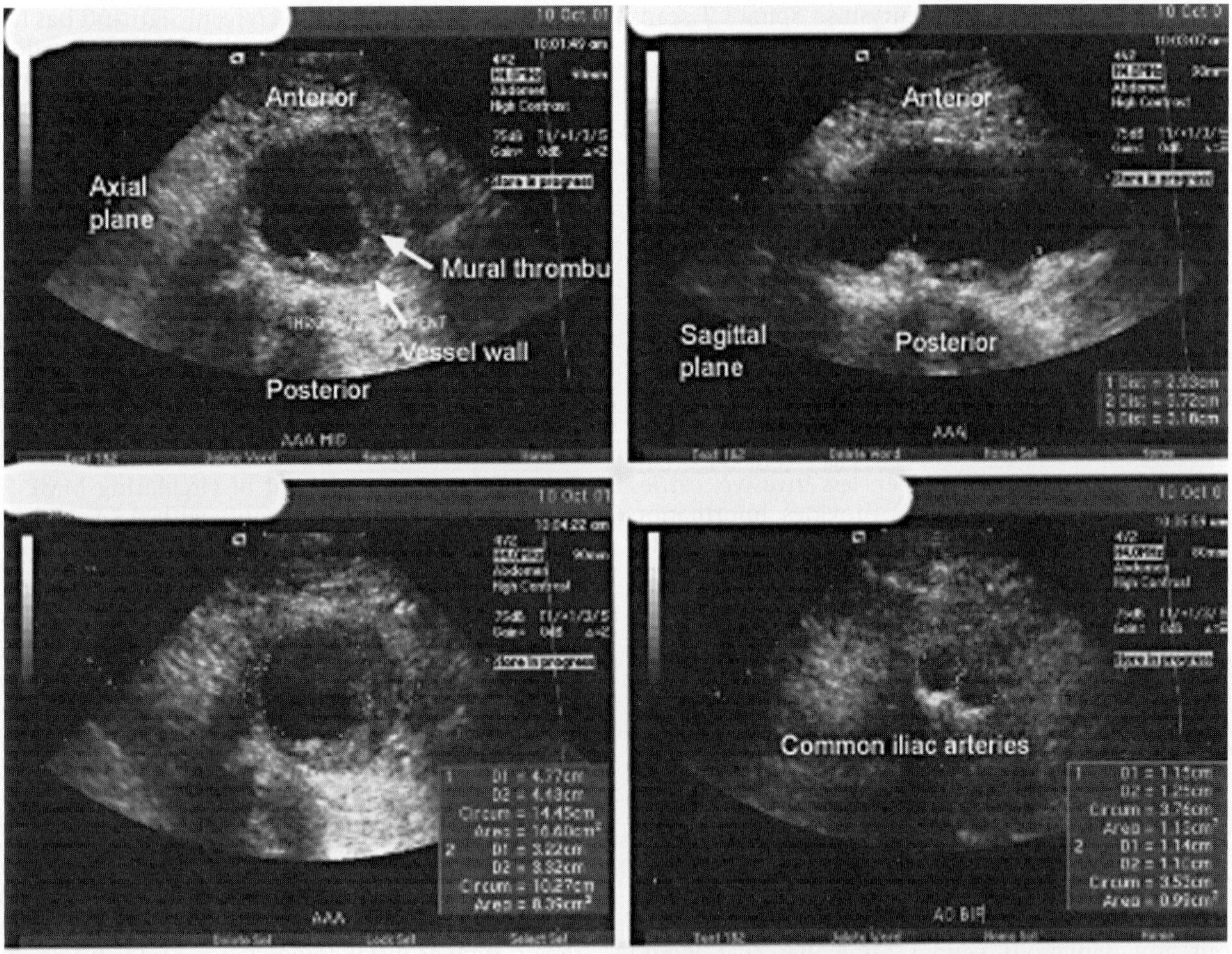
Anterior
Axial plane
Mural thrombu
Vessel wall
Posterior
Anterior
Sagittal plane
Posterior
Common iliac arteries

A

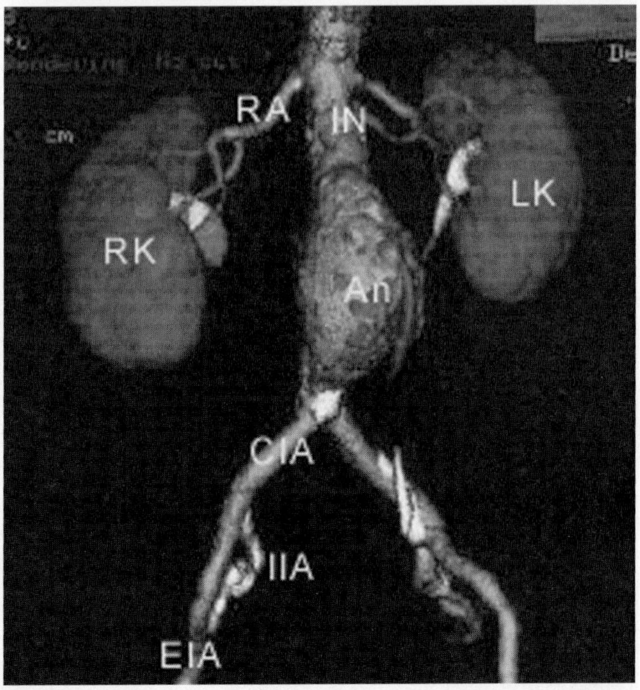
RA
IN
LK
RK
An
CIA
IIA
EIA

B

FIGURE 61-1 **A,** Ultrasonography demonstrates an abdominal aortic aneurysm. Note the posterior mural thrombus within the aneurysm sac. **B,** Three-dimensional computed tomography scan illustrates the presence of an infrarenal abdominal aortic aneurysm (An). CIA, common iliac artery; EIA, external iliac artery; IIA, internal iliac artery; IN, infrarenal neck; LK, left kidney; RA, renal artery; RK, right kidney. (From Townsend CM, Beauchamp RD, Evers BM, Mattox K [eds]: Sabiston Textbook of Surgery: The Biological Basis of Modern Surgical Practice, 17th ed. Philadelphia, Saunders, 2004.)

internal iliac arteries for aneurysms.[7] Spiral CT scans of the abdomen and pelvis with three-dimensional reconstruction are far superior to ultrasonography for this purpose and are most physicians' first choice for diagnostic purposes (see Figure 61-1B).[7] However, MRI and MRA can provide the same information as CT and can do so without the use of nephrotoxic agents. Thus, MRI and MRA are viable, albeit more costly, options for patients with contraindications to iodinated contrast dye who are stable enough to leave the ED for an extended period of time.

Prior to the advent of CT, transcatheter arteriography was the "gold standard" for the preoperative assessment of AAAs despite its inability to determine the exact size of an aneurysm in the presence of a mural thrombus.[7] CT has several advantages over this technique in that it is cheaper, less invasive, carries a lower radiation dose, and provides information about the aorta and surrounding structures simultaneously. Hence, CTA and MRA have become the current gold standard for the preoperative and postoperative evaluation of AAAs.[7] Thus, arteriography is now reserved for resolution of explicit anatomic questions about variant artery anatomy, the arterial supply to a horseshoe kidney, or the severity of occlusive disease.[7]

Serial CT scans can be used preoperatively to give the vascular team charged with repairing the AAA several pieces of important information, especially if endovascular repair is being considered. CT can adequately visualize the proximal neck (the transition between the normal and aneurysmal aorta) and map out any dangerous venous anomalies that would make access difficult.[1] CT can also measure the thickness of a mural thrombus as well as display the presence of blood within a thrombus.[1] Blood within the thrombus is known as the crescent sign and has been highly touted by some as a reliable sign of pending rupture.[1,7,9] Another important marker of aneurysm rupture is extravasation of contrast material. Lastly, CT can demonstrate a contained rupture by showing clear evidence of draping of the posterior aspect of the aorta over the adjacent vertebral body, sometimes concomitant vertebral body erosion may be seen (Fig. 61-2).[9]

Currently, many researchers are actively investigating markers of rupture other than size. Much research revolves around the use of MMPs. These are zinc- and calcium-dependent enzymes that are produced by smooth muscle and inflammatory cells, and several of these proteinases may participate in abdominal aortic aneurysm formation. McMillan and Pearce[10] found the amount of circulating MMP-9 is significantly higher in patients with AAA. Lindholt and associates[11] then noted an impressive association with the size and expansion rate of these aneurysms prompting many to theorize that serum levels of MMP may soon become a standard part of physicians' diagnostic arsenal.[1]

An approach to the diagnosis and management of AAAs is shown in Figure 61-3.

Management

The single most compelling reason to repair AAAs is to prevent fatal rupture. Besides rupture, there are other rare complications that mandate emergency repair, such as distal embolization and fistulous connections between the aorta and adjacent structures.[2,3,7] Once an AAA is identified, the obvious next step is to identify its size via ultrasonography, CT, or

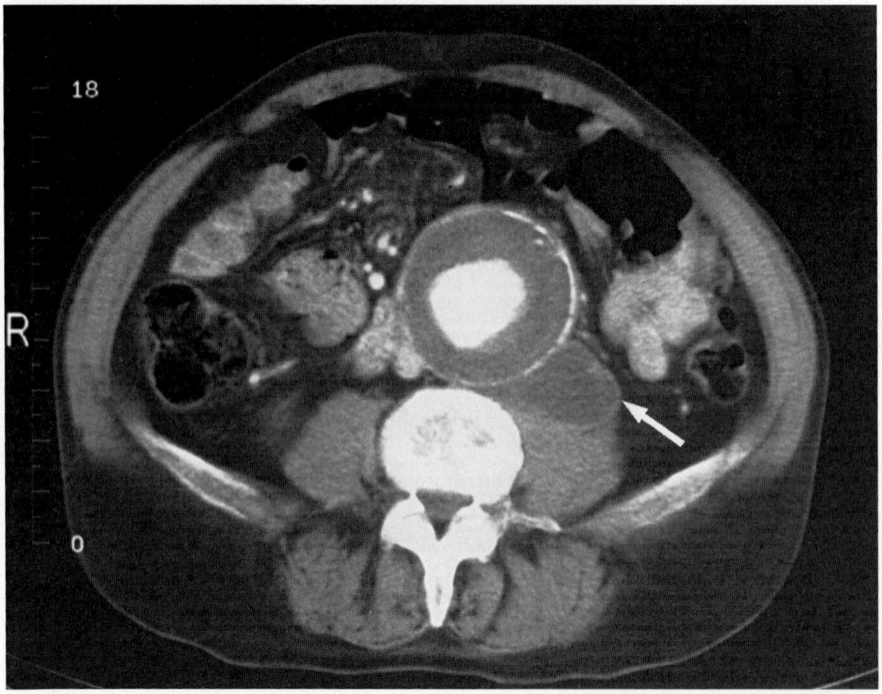
18
R
0

FIGURE 61-2 Computed tomography scan of ruptured abdominal aortic aneurysm, with calcification of the aortic wall and intraluminal thrombus. The patent lumen enhances with the administration of contrast material, but the periaortic hematoma (*arrow*) does not. (Courtesy of Richard Rensio, MD; from Marx JA, Hockberger RS, Walls RM [eds]: Rosen's Emergency Medicine: Concepts and Clinical Practice, 6th ed. Philadelphia, Mosby, 2006.)

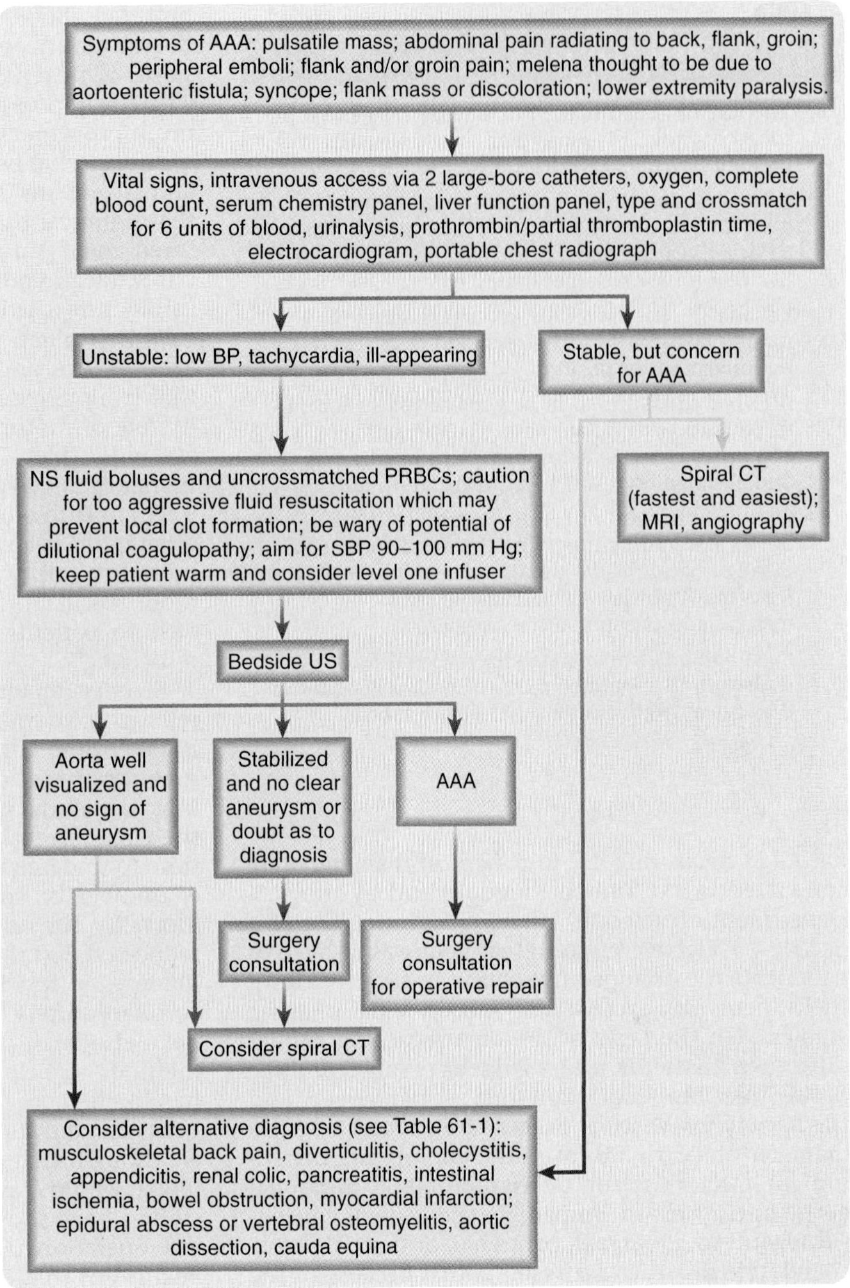
Symptoms of AAA: pulsatile mass; abdominal pain radiating to back, flank, groin; peripheral emboli; flank and/or groin pain; melena thought to be due to aortoenteric fistula; syncope; flank mass or discoloration; lower extremity paralysis.
Vital signs, intravenous access via 2 large-bore catheters, oxygen, complete blood count, serum chemistry panel, liver function panel, type and crossmatch for 6 units of blood, urinalysis, prothrombin/partial thromboplastin time, electrocardiogram, portable chest radiograph
Unstable: low BP, tachycardia, ill-appearing
Stable, but concern for AAA
NS fluid boluses and uncrossmatched PRBCs; caution for too aggressive fluid resuscitation which may prevent local clot formation; be wary of potential of dilutional coagulopathy; aim for SBP 90–100 mm Hg; keep patient warm and consider level one infuser
Spiral CT (fastest and easiest); MRI, angiography
Bedside US
Aorta well visualized and no sign of aneurysm
Stabilized and no clear aneurysm or doubt as to diagnosis
AAA
Surgery consultation
Surgery consultation for operative repair
Consider spiral CT
Consider alternative diagnosis (see Table 61-1): musculoskeletal back pain, diverticulitis, cholecystitis, appendicitis, renal colic, pancreatitis, intestinal ischemia, bowel obstruction, myocardial infarction; epidural abscess or vertebral osteomyelitis, aortic dissection, cauda equina

FIGURE 61-3 Algorithm for diagnosis and treatment of abdominal aortic aneurysm (AAA). BP, blood pressure; CT, computed tomography; MRI, magnetic resonance imaging; PRBCs, packed red blood cells; SBP, systolic blood pressure; US, ultrasonography.

MRI/MRA to discern whether immediate intervention or periodic surveillance is warranted. One prospective but nonrandomized study demonstrated that observation alone is safe until an aneurysm undergoes a growth spurt or attains a threshold diameter of 5.0 cm.[7,12] Aneurysms with a diameter of this size or larger weaken the aortic wall, which is then at higher risk of rupture.[7] In addition, if the patient is a woman with smaller native vessels, one must remember that the relative size representing aneurysmal disease may be less than the conventional range of 5 to 5.5 cm.[7]

However, the caveat in successful watchful waiting is patient cooperation. Valentine and coworkers[13] studied 101 patients with aneurysms less than 5.0 cm in diameter and did not find ruptures among patients who adhered to their follow-up program but did find a 10% rupture rate among patients who complied poorly. If continued surveillance is recommended, measures should be taken to promote lifestyle and dietary modification. Patients who smoke should be strongly encouraged to stop, because tobacco smoke increases the rate of AAA expansion. Such patients should be offered any and all available smoking cessation aids, such as nicotine replacement and bupropion.[7] Additionally, patients undergoing AAA surveillance should have rigorous monitoring and treatment of blood pressure and cholesterol levels, as currently recommended for patients with atherosclerosis.[7]

Prospective randomized trials comparing early intervention with expectant observation for infrare-

RED FLAGS

- The rate of abdominal aortic aneurysms (AAAs) in tobacco smokers is more than four times that in lifelong nonsmokers.
- Estimates place the risk of rupture at 1% to 3% per year for AAAs 4 to 5 cm in diameter, at 6% to 11% per year for those 5 to 7 cm, and nearly 20% per year for those larger than 7 cm.
- Usually the pain is steady and aggravating in nature, lasts for hours to days, and is unaffected by movement or position.
- Another clinical triad to be wary of that is found in patients with inflammatory aneurysms comprises chronic abdominal pain, weight loss, and elevated erythrocyte sedimentation rate.
- One complication of AAA is rupture into the bowel, commonly involving the duodenum, and exsanguination is the usual fatal result, but slow leaks may manifest as melena and may masquerade as peptic ulcer disease.
- Even patients who are stabilized with fluid resuscitation should be monitored closely because they are at high risk for rapid deterioration.

nal AAAs measuring 4.0 to 5.4 cm in diameter were conducted in the United Kingdom and by the U.S. Department of Veterans Affairs (VA) during the past decade.[14,15] Elective surgical treatment was delayed in patients in the nonoperative cohort in each trial until their aneurysms exceeded 5.4 cm on serial imaging studies.[7] On the basis of the data regarding gender differences in the UK trial, a guidelines subcommittee of the American Association for Vascular Surgery and the Society for Vascular Surgery now recommends a diameter of 4.5 to 5.0 cm as the appropriate threshold for elective repair of asymptomatic infrarenal aortic aneurysms in women.[7,16] The general consensus regarding suprarenal, pararenal, or type IV thoracoabdominal aortic aneurysms is that because of the higher risk of surgical complications with these aneurysms, elective intervention should be considered at a slightly larger diameter than with infrarenal aortic aneurysms.[7]

Once an aneurysm has met criteria for repair, the vascular surgeon can choose between open and endovascular repair when determining operative approach. The most important factor determining the utility of either approach is patient selection. Generally, most researchers advocate open surgical repair for younger, low-risk patients, whereas endovascular repair is preferred for older, higher-risk patients.[3] Studies have shown a lower 30-day mortality for endovascular repair (roughly 1.2%) than for open surgery (4.6%).[3] Further study is required to determine whether there is a long-term survival advantage. However, it is quite clear that both approaches decrease the risk of death from AAA rupture.[3] As far as emergency repair for ruptured abdominal aortic aneurysms is concerned, the mortality rate depends on the hemodynamic status of patients at the time of surgery. By contrast with the improvement in mortality for elective repair, no improvement in operative mortality of ruptured aneurysms has been reported during the past decades, and it remains 30% to 70%.[1] The clinical variables that significantly influence the mortality rate for ruptured aneurysm repair include a low initial hematocrit value, hypotension that requires resuscitation, cardiac arrest, a high Acute Physiological and Chronic Health Evaluation (APACHE) score, and advanced age.[7] Prance and coworkers[17] specifically suggested that five preoperative risk factors predict the mortality rate of ruptured abdominal aortic aneurysms: (1) age older than 76 years, (2) serum creatinine value higher than 190 μmol/L, (3) hemoglobin value below 9 g/dL, (4) loss of consciousness, and (5) electrocardiographic evidence of ischemia. In this study, the mortality rate was 100% in patients with three or more risk factors and decreased to 48%, 28%, and 18% in patients with two, one, or no risk factors, respectively.[17]

Elective repair has demonstrated such a drastic reduction in mortality compared with emergency intervention because patients undergoing elective AAA repair are not suffering the catastrophic physiologic demands of sudden, rapid, high-volume loss at the time of repair. Additionally, they have also had time to undergo a thorough preoperative evaluation. A number of studies have demonstrated that the mortality rate for open aortic aneurysm repair can be reduced to less than 2% in a setting in which approximately 5% to 15% of patients undergo preliminary coronary artery intervention.[18] Numerous studies have also been performed to elicit risk stratification methods to help the surgeon identify markers that herald higher morbidity and mortality risks in patients requiring intervention. Many of the researchers thought that patients 60 years or older at time of repair would have higher risks. However, multiple studies have shown that the mortality rate for elective operations is so much lower than for ruptured aneurysms that octogenarians should be offered surgical repair. Generally, AAA repair should be offered regardless of age.[7,19,20] Patient race has also been considered. Study results do not agree, some suggesting race plays no role and others suggesting that the mortality rate for elective AAA repair is higher among African Americans.[7,21,22] Surprisingly, gender has proved to be more influential. According to larger, population-based data sets in various states and countries, the mortality rate for both elective and ruptured aneurysm repair may be as much as 50% higher in women than in men.[7]

Future Therapy

Given the delineation of the role MMPs play in aneurysm development and rupture, a fair amount of research has begun in efforts to find inhibitors of these proteases and the utility of such agents in the treatment of small asymptomatic AAAs. Tetracyclines are potentially effective treatment for this purpose. Protracted administration of doxycycline has been associated with reduced plasma matrix metalloproteinase (MMP-9) levels, but the long-term effects of this medication on rate of aneurysm growth have yet to be determined.[1,7] Interestingly, the hydroxymethyl glutaryl coenzyme A (HMG CoA) reductase inhibitors have been found to decrease the expression of MMP in addition to their effects on cholesterol. Perhaps, in time, statins will prove useful adjuncts to the prevention and or treatment of AAAs.[1,7] Lastly, nonsteroidal anti-inflammatory drugs (NSAIDs) and beta-blockers are being studied as possible medical treatments to prohibit the development of AAAs or inhibit their expansion rate.[1,7]

Complications

As mentioned, AAAs are the 13th cause of death in the United States. Consequently they are also associated with several other complications. First, as many as 13% of patients with aortic aneurysms have multiple aneurysms elsewhere,[7] with some studies finding that more than 20% of patients with thoracic aortic aneurysms have concomitant AAAs.[7] Thus, the patient in whom an aneurysm is discovered at any level should undergo a thorough examination of the entire aorta.[7] Another less common complication is aortocaval fistula. The overall prevalence of aortocaval fistula is 3% to 6% of all ruptured aortic aneurysms.[1] The clinical features of an acute aortocaval fistula usually consist of lower extremity swelling, engorged veins, and high-output cardiac failure.[9] In fact, the development of high-output congestive heart failure and the perception of continuous abdominal noise is pathognomonic of an aortocaval fistula.[1]

There are other even more rare complications of AAA. One is rupture into the bowel usually involving the duodenum.[9] Exsanguination is the common fatal result, but slow leaks may manifest as melena and masquerade as peptic ulcer disease.[9] The incidence of this complication is very low, and it is found less than 0.1% of the time at autopsy. However, aortoduodenal fistula occurs more commonly after previous repair, with an incidence rate of 0.5% to 2.3%.[9] Furthermore, exceptionally large or inflammatory aortic aneurysms occasionally can be associated with early satiety or gastric outlet symptoms because of duodenal compression. Lastly, infectious or "mycotic" aneurysms are worthy of mention. Such an aneurysm may arise by one of two means. It may occur secondary to infection of a preexisting aneurysm[7] or the aortic wall itself may become infected, and an aneurysm, usually saccular in nature, may develop consequently.[7] Primary aortic infections are most commonly caused by *Staphylococcus* and *Salmonella*.[7,23] Tuberculosis has been responsible for infection of aortic pseudoaneurysms.[7]

PATIENT TEACHING TIPS

- Lifestyle modification is essential to the treatment of abdominal aortic aneurysms (AAAs) as well as to the limitation of their progression; patients must be instructed to stop smoking and must be given help to do so.
- Many patients can avoid the complications of AAA rupture by developing long-lasting relationships with a primary care provider and adhering to their prescribed surveillance programs.
- Patients should be educated about the early clinical signs of the rare but deadly complications of aortocaval and aortoenteric fistulas so that they can seek medical attention early if such fistulas develop.
- Diameter is the best predictor for AAA rupture, and follow-up interval depends on size: <3.5 cm, 36 months; 4 cm, 24 months; 4.5 cm, 12 months; 5 cm, 3 months.
- No reduction in mortality occurs if patients with AAAs <5.5 cm undergo surgical repair, even those with low operative risk.
- If discharged after an incidentally found aneurysm, the patient should be cautioned to return if abdominal, back, or flank pain occurs.

Disposition

Any patient diagnosed with a ruptured AAA or a symptomatic intact AAA needs surgical intervention immediately, as previously discussed. Such a patient is treated in the surgical intensive care unit if he or she survives the operative repair. The disposition of patients in whom the diagnosis is made incidentally (asymptomatic) depends on the size of the aneurysm, and such patients should be referred for possible elective repair or screening. The patient with an asymptomatic aneurysm larger than 5.5 cm should be referred to a surgeon immediately and should undergo preoperative testing. The recommended screening intervals for patients with smaller baseline AAA diameters are as follows: less than 3.5 cm, 36 months; 4.0 cm, 24 months; 4.5 cm, 12 months; and 5 cm, 3 months. The risks of rupture for AAAs according to diameter are as follows: less than 4 cm, 0% per year; 4.0 to 5.5 cm, 0.6% to 1% per year; 5.5 to 5.9 cm, 4.4% per year; 6.0 to 6.9 cm, 10.2% per year; and 7 cm or greater, 32.5% per year. In patients with AAA, the aorta is believed to increase 0.5 cm in diameter every year, and these patients will eventually need surgery.

REFERENCES

1. Sakalihasan N, Limet R, Defawe OD: Abdominal aortic aneurysm. Lancet 2005;365:1577-1589.
2. Golledge J, Muller J, Daugherty A, Norman P: Abdominal aortic aneurysm: Pathogenesis and implications for

management. Arterioscler Thromb Vasc Biol 2006;26: 2605-2613.
3. Katzen BT, Dake MD, MacLean AA, Wang DS: Endovascular repair of abdominal and thoracic aortic aneurysms. Circulation 2005;112:1663-1675.
4. Noel AA, Gloviczki P, Cherry KJ Jr, et al: Ruptured abdominal aortic aneurysms: The excessive mortality rate of conventional repair. J Vasc Surg 2001;34:41-46.
5. Lederle FA, Nelson DB, Joseph AM: Smokers' relative risk for aortic aneurysm compared with other smoking-related diseases: A systematic review. J Vasc Surg 2003;38: 329-334.
6. Brady AR, Thompson SG, Fowkes FG, et al: Abdominal aortic aneurysm expansion: Risk factors and time intervals for surveillance. Circulation 2004;110:16-21.
7. Hirsch AT, Haskal ZJ, Hertzer NR, et al: ACC/AHA 2005 practice guidelines for the management of patients with peripheral arterial disease (lower extremity, renal, mesenteric, and abdominal aortic): A collaborative report from the American Association for Vascular Surgery/Society for Vascular Surgery, Society for Cardiovascular Angiography and Interventions, Society for Vascular Medicine and Biology, Society of Interventional Radiology, and the ACC/AHA Task Force on Practice Guidelines (Writing Committee to Develop Guidelines for the Management of Patients With Peripheral Arterial Disease): endorsed by the American Association of Cardiovascular and Pulmonary Rehabilitation; National Heart, Lung, and Blood Institute; Society for Vascular Nursing; TransAtlantic Inter-Society Consensus; and Vascular Disease Foundation. Circulation 2006;113: e463-e654.
8. Dobrin PB, Mrkvicka R: Failure of elastin or collagen as possible critical connective tissue alterations underlying aneurysmal dilatation. Cardiovasc Surg 1994;2:484-488.
9. Schwartz SA, Taljanovic MS, Smyth S, et al: CT findings of rupture, impending rupture, and contained rupture of abdominal aortic aneurysms. Am J Roentgenol 2007;188: W57-W62.
10. McMillan WD, Pearce WH: Increased plasma levels of metalloproteinase-9 are associated with abdominal aortic aneurysms. J Vasc Surg 1999;29:122-127.
11. Lindholt JS, Jørgensen B, Shi GP, Henneberg EW: Relationships between activators and inhibitors of plasminogen, and the progression of small abdominal aortic aneurysms. Eur J Vasc Endovasc Surg 2003;25:546-551.
12. Brown PM, Pattenden R, Gutelius JR: The selective management of small abdominal aortic aneurysms: The Kingston study. J Vasc Surg 1992;15:21-27.
13. Valentine RJ, Decaprio JD, Castillo JM, et al: Watchful waiting in cases of small abdominal aortic aneurysms: Appropriate for all patients? J Vasc Surg 2000;32:441-450.
14. Brown LC, Powell JT: Risk factors for aneurysm rupture in patients kept under ultrasound surveillance. UK Small Aneurysm Trial Participants. Ann Surg 1999;230:289-297.
15. United Kingdom Small Aneurysm Trial Participants: Long-term outcomes of immediate repair compared with surveillance of small abdominal aortic aneurysms. N Engl J Med 2002;346:1445-1452.
16. Brewster DC, Cronenwett JL, Hallett JW Jr, et al: Guidelines for the treatment of abdominal aortic aneurysms: Report of a subcommittee of the Joint Council of the American Association for Vascular Surgery and Society for Vascular Surgery. J Vasc Surg 2003;37:1106-1117.
17. Prance SE, Wilson YG, Cosgrove CM, et al: Abdominal aortic aneurysms: Selecting patients for surgery. Eur J Vasc Endovasc Surg 1999;17:129-132.
18. McFalls EO, Ward HB, Moritz TE, et al: Coronary-artery revascularization before elective major vascular surgery. N Engl J Med 2004;351:2795-804; erratum in: N Engl J Med 2005;95:19.
19. Kazmers A, Perkins AJ, Jacobs LA: Outcomes after abdominal aortic aneurysm repair in those > or =80 years of age: Recent Veterans Affairs experience. Ann Vasc Surg 1998;12:106-112.
20. O'Hara PJ, Hertzer NR, Krajewski LP, et al: Ten-year experience with abdominal aortic aneurysm repair in octogenarians: Early results and late outcome. J Vasc Surg 1995; 21:830-838.
21. Collins TC, Johnson M, Daley J, et al: Preoperative risk factors for 30-day mortality after elective surgery for vascular disease in Department of Veterans Affairs hospitals: Is race important? J Vasc Surg 2001;34:634-640.
22. Heller JA, Weinberg A, Arons R, et al: Two decades of abdominal aortic aneurysm repair: Have we made any progress? J Vasc Surg 2000;32:1091-1100.
23. Fiessinger JN, Paul JF: Inflammatory and infectious aortitis. Rev Prat 2002;52:1094-1099.

Chapter **62**

Aortic Emergency Ultrasound

Emily Baran and Mary Ann Edens

KEY POINTS

Aortic emergency ultrasound is performed for clinical suspicion of abdominal aortic aneurysm.

The aorta should be clearly differentiated from the inferior vena cava by means of anatomical landmarks.

Transverse and longitudinal views should be obtained from epigastrium to bifurcation; measurements should be taken from outside wall to outside wall in the transverse view.

Representative images of the proximal, middle, and distal aorta should be obtained.

A 2- to 5-MHz curvilinear abdominal probe (see Chapter 5) should be used.

The patient should be placed supine.

Aortic emergency ultrasound should answer the following questions: Is the aorta dilated more than 3 cm at any point? and Is there an intimal flap (suggesting aortic dissection) within the lumen of the aorta?

Because most abdominal aortic aneurysms are infrarenal, the aorta must be adequately imaged from diaphragm to bifurcation to rule out aneurysm.

Background

Ruptured abdominal aortic aneurysm (AAA) is a vascular emergency carrying high morbidity and mortality. Emergency ultrasound (EUS) of the aorta has been shown to decrease both time to diagnosis and time to surgery.[1] In addition, ultrasound performed by EPs has been shown to be 100% sensitive for the detection of AAA.[2-4]

Indication

The indication for performing aortic EUS is rapid evaluation of patients with abdominal, flank, or back pain in whom there is a clinical suspicion for AAA. The examination should answer the following questions:

- Is the aorta dilated more than 3 cm at any point?
- Is there an intimal flap within the lumen of the aorta?

Anatomy and Approach

The patient should be in the supine position. A 2- to 5-MHz curvilinear abdominal probe is generally used. Imaging should begin in the epigastric area just below the xiphoid process, and the aorta should be fol-

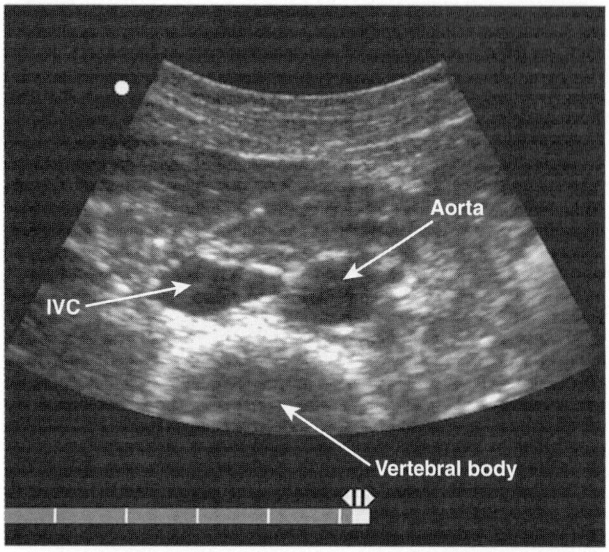
Aorta
IVC
Vertebral body

FIGURE 62-1 Normal transverse view of the aorta. Note the two vascular structures just anterior to the shadowing vertebral body. The thicker-walled aorta lies to the left of midline on the right of the screen and is not compressible; the thin-walled inferior vena cava (IVC) adjacent to it is compressible.

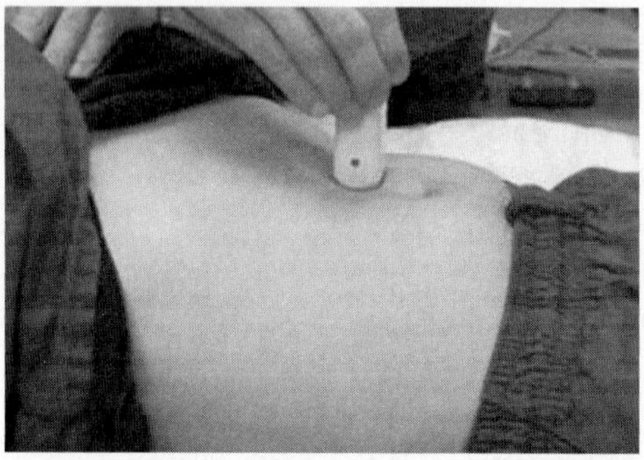

FIGURE 62-2 Transducer placement for the short-axis view of the aorta. Note that the probe indicator is directed to the patient's right.

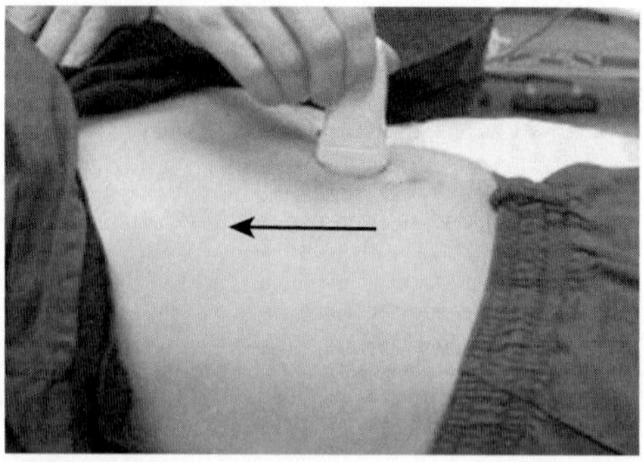

FIGURE 62-3 Transducer placement for the long-axis view of the aorta. *Arrow* shows the direction of the probe indicator.

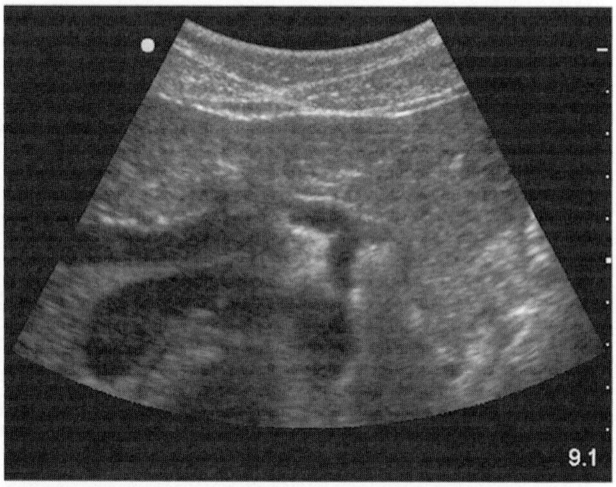
9.1

FIGURE 62-4 Transverse view of the aorta at the subxiphoid area demonstrating the first branch of the abdominal aorta. This image of the celiac axis as it branches into the splenic and common hepatic arteries is often referred to as the "seagull sign."

lowed all the way to its bifurcation at or just below the umbilicus. The aorta is more readily identified in the transverse plane from its relationship with the vertebral body and inferior vena cava (IVC) (Fig. 62-1). The aorta should be to the left (patient's) of midline, should pulsate, and should be noncompressible. The IVC should be to the right (patient's) of midline, may undulate but does not pulsate, and should be easily compressible.

To image the aorta in transverse view, the operator holds the transducer with the probe indicator turned to the patient's right (Fig. 62-2). Once the aorta is located, the transducer is held at right angles to the skin and slowly slid down the abdomen. Steady gentle pressure and a rocking motion can help disperse bowel gas and improve images.

To image the long axis of the aorta, the operator places the curvilinear probe in the midline with the probe indicator toward the patient's head (Fig. 62-3). The transducer is then angled slightly to the left to locate the aorta. As for the transverse view, the transducer should be held at right angles to the skin and slowly slid down the abdomen. Also, anatomic landmarks such as the branches of the celiac or superior mesenteric artery can be used to help identify the aorta (Figs. 62-4 and 62-5).

Interpretation

A normal aorta should be less than 3 cm in diameter. Any dilation to more than 3 cm indicates an aortic aneurysm (Fig. 62-6). This measurement should be made on the short-axis view of the aorta to avoid inaccurate oblique measurements. Measurements should be taken from outside wall to outside wall. Most aneurysms are found infrarenally, but an aneurysm can be located anywhere along the aorta. It is also important to remember that a normal measurement in one portion of the aorta does not rule out an aneurysm in another portion.

An intimal flap within the lumen of the aorta indicates an aortic dissection (Fig. 62-7). The diameter of the aorta may be greater than 3 cm, but it does not have to be for a dissection to be present.

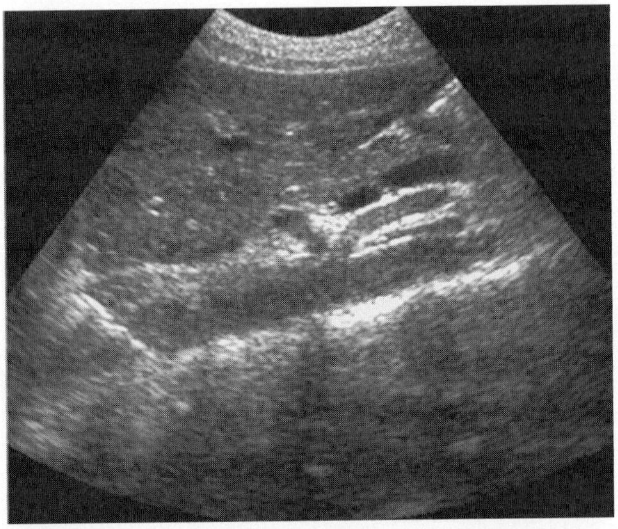

FIGURE 62-5 Longitudinal view of the aorta with superior mesenteric artery coursing parallel and anterior to it.

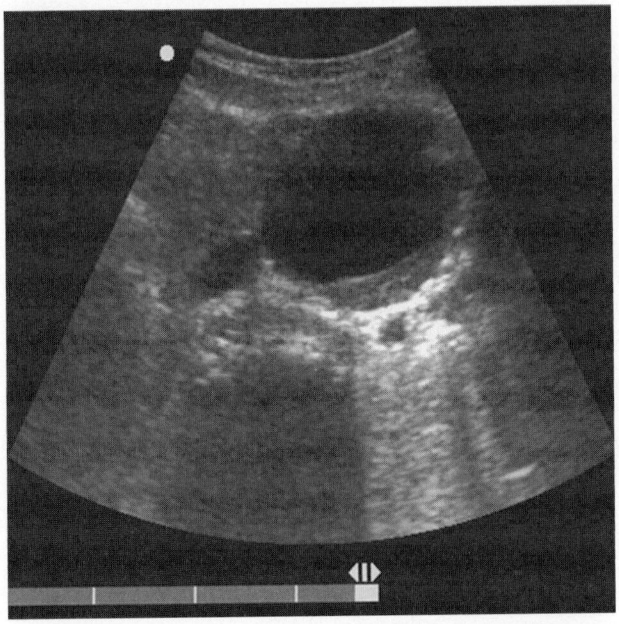

FIGURE 62-6 Transverse view of an abdominal aortic aneurysm. Note the presence of a posterior mural thrombus.

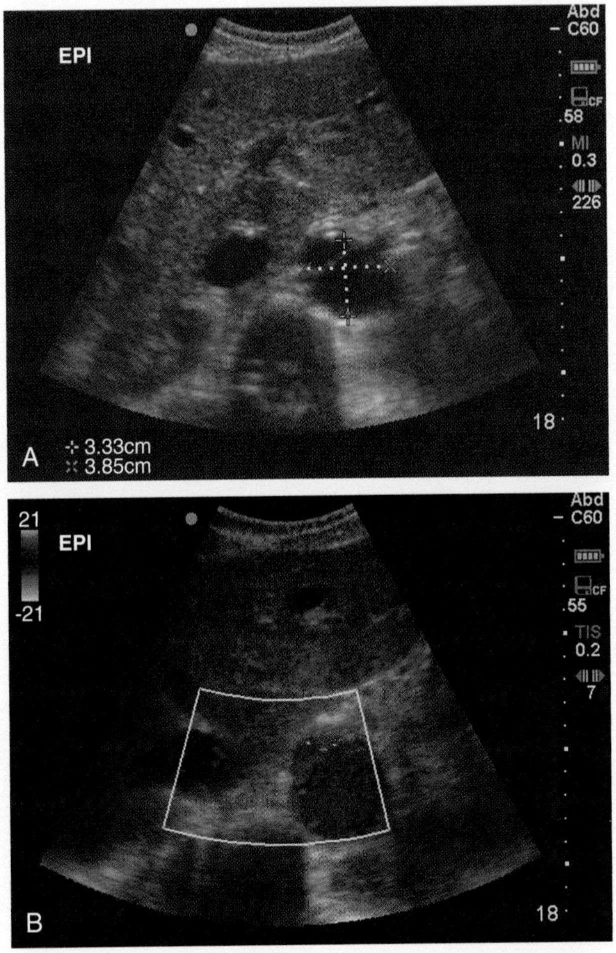
EPI
Abd
- C60
.58
MI
0.3
226
18
A
3.33cm
3.85cm
21
-21
EPI
Abd
- C60
.55
TIS
0.2
7
18
B

FIGURE 62-7 Intimal flap within aorta on two-dimensional (**A**) and color Doppler (**B**) ultrasonography.

Limitations

Aortic EUS may be technically limited by obesity, bowel gas, or significant abdominal tenderness. It is a focused examination that should be performed rapidly at the bedside if there is suspicion for AAA, and results should be interpreted within the clinical context. Inadequate or equivocal findings should prompt additional diagnostic testing.

Tips and Tricks

- Absence of free intraperitoneal fluid does not rule out aortic rupture. Most patients with symptomatic abdominal aortic aneurysms who present to the ED have contained retroperitoneal bleeding that cannot be reliably identified by emergency ultrasound.
- Compression can be used to distinguish the aorta from the inferior vena cava. Although the two structures can look alike, the inferior vena cava collapses with pressure and the aorta does not.
- Measurements are best taken in the transverse or short-axis view. Measuring in the longitudinal view can result in an inaccurate oblique value.
- Gentle anterior-posterior pressure can help imaging by dispersing bowel gas.

REFERENCES

1. Plummer D, Clinton J, Matthew B: Emergency department ultrasound improves time to diagnosis and survival in ruptured AAA [abstract]. Acad Emerg Med 1998;5:147.
2. Tayal VS, Graf CD, Gibbs MA: Prospective study of accuracy and outcome of emergency ultrasound for abdominal aortic aneurysm over two years. Acad Emerg Med 2003; 10:867-871.
3. Kuhn M, Bonnin RL, Davey MJ, et al: Emergency department ultrasound scanning for abdominal aortic aneurysm: Accessible, accurate, and advantageous. Ann Emerg Med 2000;36:219-223.
4. Costantino TG, Bruno EC, Handly N, Dean AJ: Accuracy of emergency medicine ultrasound in the evaluation of abdominal aortic aneurysm. J Emerg Med 2005;29:455-460.

Chapter **63**

Peripheral Arterial Disease

Christopher Ross and Theresa Schwab

KEY POINTS

Findings during the patient review of systems can indicate the presence of peripheral arterial disease.
Intermittent claudication is the earliest clinical manifestation of pathologically significant peripheral arterial disease.
The ankle-brachial index can help confirm a clinical suspicion of occlusive arterial disease.
Ischemic rest pain signals critical, limb-threatening disease.
The classic presentation of acute arterial occlusion in described by the six "Ps": pain, polar (cold) sensation, paresthesia, paralysis, pallor, and pulselessness.
Treatment of nonischemic peripheral arterial disease consists of risk factor modification, exercise programs, and medications aimed at platelet inhibition.
Prompt initiation of therapy is the most important aspect of treatment of acute limb ischemia, and patients should immediately receive a heparin bolus followed by an infusion before diagnostic testing is begun.
Treatment of ischemic peripheral arterial disease depends on whether the extremity is viable, nonviable, or threatened.
Viable: Angiography should be performed to assess disease severity; surgery or intra-arterial thrombolytic therapy can be performed.
Limb-threatening: Immediate surgical intervention is required.
Nonviable: Primary amputation is required.

Scope

In the United States, more than 25 million people suffer with at least one of the clinical manifestations of atherosclerosis. In a significant proportion of patients, the disease is occult but is nevertheless an important indicator of significant cardiovascular events.[1] Systemic atherosclerotic disease with damage to end organs other than the heart continues to be associated with high morbidity and mortality, and surprisingly little research is being done on it.

The most common term used to describe atherosclerotic vascular disease of the lower extremities is *peripheral arterial disease* (PAD). There is a 2% to 3%

BOX 63-1

Risk Factors for Lower Extremity Peripheral Arterial Disease

- Age 70 years and older
- Age 50 to 69 years with history of smoking or diabetes
- Age less than 50 years with diabetes and one other atherosclerotic risk factor (smoking, dyslipidemia, hypertension, or hyperhomocysteinemia)
- Leg symptoms with exertion (suggestive of claudication) or ischemic rest pain
- Abnormal lower extremity pulse findings
- Known atherosclerotic coronary, carotid, or renal artery disease

Data from Hirsch AT, Haskal ZJ, Hertzer NR, et al: American Association for Vascular Surgery/Society for Vascular Surgery; Society for Cardiovascular Angiography and Interventions; Society for Vascular Medicine and Biology; Society of Interventional Radiology; ACC/AHA Task Force on Practice Guidelines: ACC/AHA 2005 guidelines for the Management of Patients with Peripheral Arterial Disease (lower extremity, renal, mesenteric, and abdominal aortic): A collaborative report from the American Associations for Vascular Surgery/Society for Vascular Surgery, Society for Cardiovascular Angiography and Interventions, Society for Vascular Medicine and Biology, Society of Interventional Radiology, and the ACC/AHA Task Force on Practice Guidelines (writing committee to develop guidelines for the management of patients with peripheral arterial disease): Summary of recommendations. J Am Coll Cardiol 2006;47: 1239-1312.

prevalence of PAD by age 50 years, which rises to 20% for those over age 75.[2] Of this patient population, 10% has classic claudication, 50% has atypical leg pain associated with exertion, and the remaining 40% does not have exercise leg pain.[3] Women have a relative risk of 0.7 in comparison with men. African American subjects have the highest relative risk of PAD (2.5), followed by Hispanic subjects (1.5), in comparison with a white population.

Risk Factors

Box 63-1 lists the risk factors for PAD.[4] The risk factor with the highest correlation of PAD is cigarette smoking. Compared with nonsmokers, smokers have a 1.7- to 5.6-fold increase in development and progression of atherosclerosis in the peripheral vasculature.[5] In patients with symptomatic PAD, smoking increases this risk 8 to 10 times.[6] The risk increases in a powerful dose-dependent manner according to the number of cigarettes smoked per day and the number of years of smoking. Diabetes increases the risk of PAD, 3.5 times in men and 8.6 times in women.[7] Diabetic patients are also 7 to 15 times more likely to require amputation. Hypertension is associated with lower extremity PAD, but this association is generally weaker than that with coronary artery disease and cerebrovascular disease. The Framingham Heart Study found that the risk for development of intermittent claudication was 2.5-fold and 4-fold higher in men and women, respectively, who had hypertension, and that this risk was proportional to the severity of the hypertension.[7] Genetic predisposition represents an important risk factor for atherosclerosis, accounting for as much as 50% of the risk in some studies.[8] Patients who have PAD also have a high incidence of coronary heart disease (CHD), and in general, patients have a 2 to 4 times higher incidence of CHD and cerebrovascular disease if PAD is also present.[5]

Progression of Disease

Of patients in whom PAD develops in association with symptoms of intermittent claudication, 5% to 10% will require revascularization in the subsequent 5-year period. Over the same interval, about 5% of patients will have critical leg ischemia, 1% to 4% of whom will need amputation.[9] It should be noted that there is both wide geographic as well as wide ethnic variation in the outcome of PAD. White persons are more likely to receive aortoiliac surgery and less likely to undergo lower extremity amputation than other ethnic groups.[10] This discrepancy cannot be explained by the higher prevalence of risk factors in other ethnic groups.

Mortality

The mortality rate for patients with PAD was around 30% in 1990. This number has dropped significantly with both risk factor modification and medical treatments. Not surprisingly, the primary cause of death in this patient population is cardiac disease.[11]

Pathophysiology

Atherosclerosis was originally thought to be primarily lipoprotein accumulation but is now better understood, fundamentally, as chronic inflammatory disease of the arterial system.[12] It is believed that this inflammation is involved in all stages of atherosclerosis. The inflammatory process leads to plaque disruption and thrombosis, and the plaques that are vulnerable are characterized by a large lipid core, a thin fibrous cap, and inflammatory cells at the thinnest portion of the cap surface (Fig. 63-1).[13] Plaque rupture has been shown to be critical in the development of acute coronary syndromes, but the importance of this event in PAD is not known at this time.

The vascular smooth muscle cell is important in the development of atherosclerosis. Once activated, the cell migrates into the intima and begins to proliferate and secrete matrix proteins and enzymes. This step has been shown to be important in the development of stenosis both in the atherosclerotic

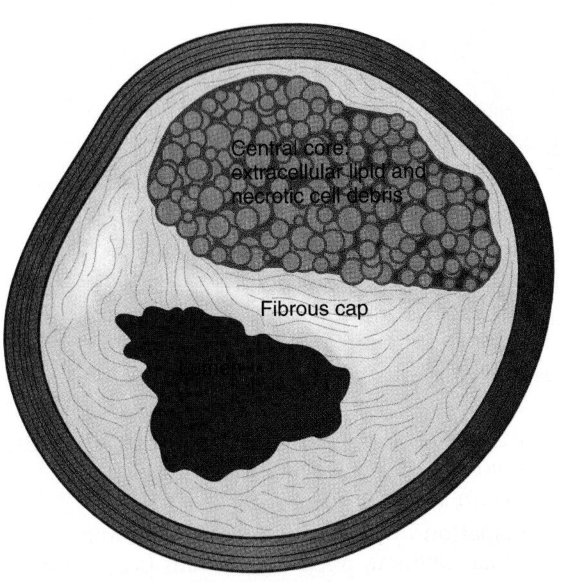
Central core:
extracellular lipid and
necrotic cell debris
Fibrous cap

FIGURE 63-1 Cross-section of a human artery with an advanced atherosclerotic plaque. The fibrous cap is a layer of smooth muscle cells and fibrous tissue that separates the necrotic core of the plaque from the lumen.

vessel and in vessels that have been stented.[14,15] In addition, the vessel often constricts rather than dilates, narrowing the lumen even more.[16]

■ THROMBOEMBOLISM

More than 80% of arterial emboli originate in the heart and travel to the extremities, the lower extremities being much more affected than the upper. Potential sources of emboli from the heart include atrial thrombus from atrial fibrillation and left ventricular thrombus due to hypokinesis after myocardial infarction. The frequencies with which emboli lodge in various areas are as follows[17]:

Femoral arteries: 28%
Arm vessels: 20%
Aortoiliac vessels: 18%
Popliteal arteries: 17%
Visceral vessels: 9%

More than a third of patients with embolic disease present with skin manifestations, which are the most common physical finding.[18]

Because of the size of most emboli, the femoral and popliteal arteries are involved more often than the larger aortic and iliac vessels. Atrial fibrillation can lead to thrombosis of the left atrium and is present in 60% to 75% of cases of embolic events. Valvular heart disease (aortic and mitral) accounts for approximately 5% to 10% of cases of thromboembolic disease. The amount of tissue destruction depends on the size of the vessel, the extent of obstruction, and the amount of collateral circulation that can compensate. Once the embolus has lodged in the vessel wall, further propagation can occur either distally or proximally via thrombosis, which can further exacerbate ischemia.

■ ATHEROEMBOLISM

Debris from atherosclerotic plaques can break off in proximal vessels and give rise to atheroemboli. These emboli can consist of cholesterol, calcium, and infectious and/or platelet aggregates. Atheroemboli are less likely to produce symptoms of acute arterial occlusion. The atheroembolus is usually irregularly shaped and nondistensible, leading to incomplete occlusion. A single atheroembolic event can be thought of as an indicator of potentially more serious subsequent disease that has the potential for extensive tissue loss. If there is simultaneous evidence of both venous and arterial embolism, a patent foramen ovale should be considered.

■ INFLAMMATION

Irradiation, drugs, trauma, or bacterial or fungal invasion can result in an inflammatory arterial injury. Infectious causes lead to direct invasion of the vessel wall and are usually related to intravenous drug abuse, infective endocarditis, or generalized sepsis.

■ TRAUMA

Blunt injury to vessel walls can lead to intimal disruption, which can then cause obstruction and thrombosis. Usually it takes hours to days for complete occlusion to become manifest. Arterial lacerations can be partial or complete, and either type can cause distal ischemia and infarction. Partial arterial lacerations continue to bleed because of the intact portion of the vessel, and this bleeding can result in hematoma formation outside the vessel and thrombosis within the vessel. The hematoma can cause progressive pain, deformity, nerve compression, and subsequent vascular compromise. Complete arterial lacerations actually bleed very little acutely owing to the spasm of the transected ends. Eventually, however, the spasm relaxes, which can lead to delayed bleeding, and the thrombus on the distal side may separate and move distally.

■ VASOSPASM

Abnormal vasomotor responses in distal small arteries can cause ischemic symptoms without tissue loss.

■ ARTERIOVENOUS FISTULAS

Sometimes there may be communication between the arterial and venous systems, which can cause vascular distention, tortuosity, aneurysm formation, and alteration in hemodynamics that are favorable for thrombosis formation. The fistulas result in elevation of the local venous system, which can lead to skin breakdown in the form of dermatitis and ulceration.

Presenting Signs and Symptoms

Key components of the vascular review of symptoms and family history are listed in Box 63-2. Physical findings in peripheral arterial disease are listed in Box 63-3.

■ SPECIFIC CLINICAL FINDINGS

■ Intermittent Claudication

The primary symptom of lower extremity atherosclerotic disease is intermittent claudication. *Claudication* may be defined as fatigue, discomfort, aching, or pain that occurs in specific limb muscle groups during effort owing to exercise-induced ischemia. Intermittent claudication has three major clinical features: it is consistent and reproducible from day to day, symptoms resolve within a couple of minutes after cessation of exercise, and discomfort occurs again at the same distance once the patient resumes the activity.[19] The symptoms usually occur gradually and may be absent or minimal even in a patient with significant disease. The gradual onset of symptoms can often lead the patient to assume that they are the result of aging or arthritis. The pain may also be felt in the thigh, hip, and buttock as the level of the obstruction moves proximally. If many of the vessels are involved, the most distal muscle group is affected first, followed by proximal migration as the patient continues to walk. The pain is primarily unilateral at onset but may be bilateral if an occlusion of the distal aorta occurs. Progressive arterial insufficiency causes development of collateral circulation, which will allow the patient's symptoms not to progress despite worsening of the culprit artery. As described, there is some correlation between where the patient experiences symptoms and the location of the diseased arterial portion, as follows:

Symptoms in the foot: Tibial and peroneal artery
Symptoms in the calf: superficial femoral artery or popliteal artery
Symptoms in the thigh: common femoral artery or aorta and iliac artery

BOX 63-2

Key Findings of the Vascular Review of Systems

- Any exertional limitation of the lower extremity muscles or any history of walking impairment. These limitations may be described as fatigue, aching, numbness, or pain. The primary site(s) of discomfort in the buttock, thigh, calf, or foot should be recorded along with the relation of such discomfort to rest or exertion.
- Any poorly healing of nonhealing wounds of the legs or feet.
- Any pain at rest localized to the lower leg or foot and its association with the upright or recumbent positions.
- Postprandial abdominal pain that reproducibly is provoked by eating and is associated with weight loss.

Data from Hirsch AT, Haskal ZJ, Hertzer NR, et al: American Association for Vascular Surgery/Society for Vascular Surgery; Society for Cardiovascular Angiography and Interventions; Society for Vascular Medicine and Biology; Society of Interventional Radiology; ACC/AHA Task Force on Practice Guidelines: ACC/AHA 2005 guidelines for the Management of Patients with Peripheral Arterial Disease (lower extremity, renal, mesenteric, and abdominal aortic): A collaborative report from the American Associations for Vascular Surgery/Society for Vascular Surgery, Society for Cardiovascular Angiography and Interventions, Society for Vascular Medicine and Biology, Society of Interventional Radiology, and the ACC/AHA Task Force on Practice Guidelines (writing committee to develop guidelines for the management of patients with peripheral arterial disease): Summary of recommendations. J Am Coll Cardiol 2006;47: 1239-1312.

BOX 63-3

Key Components of the Vascular Physical Examination in a Patient with Possible Peripheral Arterial Disease

- Measurement of blood pressure in both arms and notation of any interarm asymmetry.
- Palpation of the carotid pulses and notation of the carotid upstroke and amplitude and presence of bruits.
- Auscultation of the abdomen and flank for bruits.
- Palpation of the abdomen, and notation of the presence of the aortic pulsation and its maximal diameter.
- Palpation of pulses at the brachial, radial, ulnar, femoral, popliteal, dorsalis pedis, and posterior tibial sites.
- Auscultation of both femoral arteries for the presence of bruits.
- Assessment of pulse intensity, which should be recorded numerically as follows: O, absent; 1, diminished; 2, normal; 3, bounding.
- Inspection of the feet, evaluating the color, temperature, and integrity of the skin and intertriginous areas, and recording of the presence of ulceration.
- Documentation of the presence of symmetry, edema, and venous distention of the lower extremities
- Recording of additional findings suggestive of severe peripheral arterial disease, including distal hair loss, trophic skin changes, and hypertrophic nails should be recorded.

Symptoms in buttocks and hips: aorta and iliac artery

Rest Pain

Ischemic rest pain can be a symptom of severe to critical limb ischemia. The pain typically occurs at night when the patient is supine, and the patient may awaken from sleep with pain in the toes or forefoot. The pain is usually worse in a single extremity and is relieved by dependency. The patient may either stand up or hang the legs over the edge of the bed for relief. In this scenario, the physical examination may show marked pallor with elevation of the legs, marked rubor with dependency, and delayed venous filling times. Usually by the time rest pain occurs, there is severe arterial insufficiency in multiple arterial segments. Another condition that commonly manifests as leg pain is peripheral neuropathy.

After rest pain, progression of disease causes necrosis of tissue, generally between two toes. Eventually the ulcers may coalesce or progress to dry gangrene over the tips of the toes or at pressure points. Peripheral gangrene with an arterial cause may be difficult to differentiate from that with a venous cause. A patient with arterial ischemia presents with severe ischemic changes followed by edema because the limb is kept in a dependent position. In venous gangrene, however, the edema occurs first, before the onset of frank ischemic changes.

Clinical signs and symptoms of atheromatous embolization may be nonspecific and manifest in a variable fashion according to the number and size of emboli, site of origin, and end organ affected. The clinical spectrum ranges from a nonspecific systemic illness to a catastrophic event such as an ischemic leg. Skin manifestations are the most common finding in atheromatous embolization, appearing in approximately a third of cases. Livedo reticularis is a red-blue netlike mottling of the skin the represents embolization to the skin. Generally this manifestation is seen on the legs, buttocks, and thighs, and rarely in the arm. "Blue toe syndrome" is a commonly seen condition consisting of a painful, patchy distribution of erythema and cyanosis on the toes. Peripheral pulses are usually palpable in patients with this condition, thus demonstrating the proximal embolization, not a local watershed of ischemia from atherosclerosis. The gastrointestinal tract is an often overlooked area of involvement that has been shown to be involved in about a fifth of presentations. Patients may complain of nausea, vomiting, abdominal pain, melena, or hematochezia. Stools may be heme positive, and intestinal ischemia can progress to infarction in some cases.

Acute Arterial Embolization

The patient with acute arterial embolization commonly complains of a sudden onset of pain and coldness distally, on the side of occlusion (Fig. 63-2). As ischemia progresses, the classic presentation of acute arterial occlusion becomes evident, described by the six "Ps," as follows:

Pain
Polar (cold) sensation
Paresthesia
Paralysis
Pallor
Pulselessness

As peripheral nerves become ischemic, paresthesias, numbness, and then paralysis develop sequentially. Sensory peripheral nerves are affected first, with decreases in proprioception and light touch, and then the larger pain and motor fibers become involved, leading to loss of sensation, weakness, and paralysis. Paralysis is usually a bad prognostic sign for reversibility of the ischemia. The limb may become pale and pulseless as the ischemia continues. The signs of ischemia can be seen distal to the level of arterial occlusion. During the first 8 hours after the ischemic insult, the extremity looks pale owing to the spastic nature of the arterial tree surrounding the region. Twelve to 24 hours after the injury, the extremity may become cyanotic and mottled. As arterial flow ceases, venous drainage also slows or stops, leading to profound stasis, which further aggravates

RED FLAGS

- The risk of peripheral arterial disease increases in a powerful dose-dependent manner with the number of cigarettes smoked per day and the number of years of smoking.
- Ischemic fissures, decubitus ulcers of the ankles and heels, and ischemic ulcers correlate with arterial insufficiency.
- More than a third of patients with embolic disease present with skin manifestations, making them the most common physical finding.
- In contrast to patients with ischemia pain, those with peripheral neuropathy usually have bilateral leg pain that is not relieved by dependency as well as neurologic signs, such as decreased deep tendon reflexes and loss of touch and vibratory sensation.
- Sensory peripheral nerves are affected first, with decreases in proprioception and light touch; then the larger pain and motor fibers become involved, leading to loss of sensation, weakness, and then paralysis.
- Attempt at limb salvage in a patient with hard neurologic findings indicative of prolonged ischemia may endanger the life of the patient because of the severe metabolic changes that occur after revascularization.
- Acute extremity ischemia is associated with high rates of limb loss (30%) as well as of hospital morbidity and mortality (20%).

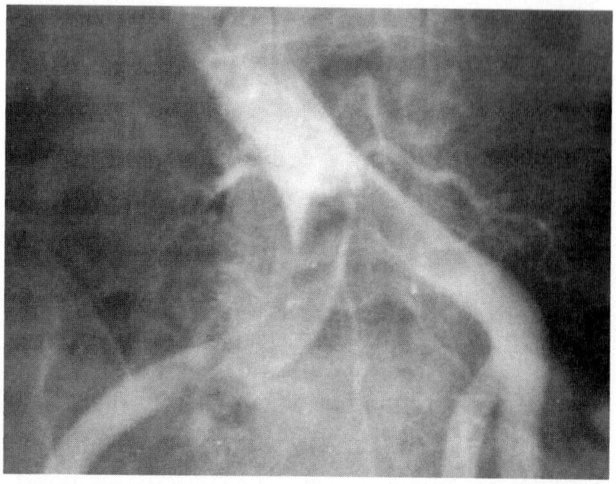

FIGURE 63-2 Large saddle clot at bifurcation of the aorta at the iliac vessels. This clot not only can give symptoms by itself but can embolize more distally.

BOX 63-4

Ankle-Brachial Index (ABI) Measurements

ABI measurements must be obtained properly for accuracy and reliability, in the following sequence:

1. Arm systolic pressure should always be measured with the Doppler flowmeter, because measurement by auscultation can be inaccurate.
2. Pressure must be recorded in both arms and both tibial arteries at the ankle.
3. Systolic pressure is measured at the point at which flow is first detected, not at the point at which it is lost during inflation.
4. Measure the absolute levels of blood pressure and the ankle/brachial index.

the damage. On careful examination, the cold part of the extremity can easily be demarcated from its warmer proximal portion. As mentioned earlier, the ischemia is unlikely to be reversible if the affected limb is paralyzed.

Diagnostic Testing

BLOOD PRESSURE

Because blood flow is diminished, the most common sensor used is the Doppler flowmeter, which has the advantage of being able to measure pressure in any artery in which flow can be detected. Calculating the ankle-brachial index (ABI) is an accurate way to diagnose patients with PAD. An ABI is a simple and relatively inexpensive test to confirm the clinical suspicion of occlusive arterial disease and provides a measure of the severity of peripheral vascular disease.[20] Calculation of the ABI is performed by measuring the systolic blood pressure by Doppler probe in the brachial, posterior tibial, and dorsalis pedis arteries. The highest of the measurements of the ankle and feet is divided by the highest in the upper extremity. The ABI in normal individuals is 1.0 or greater; values higher than 1.3 usually indicate a calcified vessel that is noncompressible. An ABI less than 0.9 has a 95% sensitivity (100% specificity) for PAD (Box 63-4).

IMAGING

Duplex Ultrasonography

The term duplex ultrasonography refers to B-mode real-time imaging and pulsed Doppler analysis of the velocity of flowing blood in arteries and veins. Flowing blood, velocity of sound in tissue, and the difference between frequency of transmitted and reflected sound are all incorporated in the detailed analysis of arterial flow. Arterial duplex ultrasonography provides a "roadmap" of stenosis of the arteries of the lower extremities. The sensitivity and specificity of duplex ultrasonography studies in detecting occlusions and stenoses is 95%, with a specificity of 98%.[21] The utility of obtaining duplex ultrasonography in the ED is limited because most decisions about patient care are based on history and physical findings.

Computed Tomography Angiography

Computed tomography angiography (CTA) is a vascular imaging technique that can assess many vascular diseases rapidly and safely. Multidetector CT scanning can give very-high-quality resolution compared with the single-detector scanners from the not so distant past. CTA has the following advantages over regular angiography: (1) the images can be reconstructed from multiple angles and in multiple planes, (2) the soft tissues and other anatomical structures are better identified, and (3) the technique is less invasive with fewer complications and lower cost.[22] CTA does, however, expose patients to radiation and potentially nephrotoxic dye loads. PAD is commonly multifocal; thus, both arterial inflow and runoff should be imaged in their entirety. Studies have shown 100% concordance of CTA with angiography as well as that CTA better visualizes other portions of distal vessels that are not seen with traditional angiography.[23]

Magnetic Resonance Angiography

Magnetic resonance angiography (MRA) of the peripheral vasculature can be performed quickly and accurately. MRA has two distinct advantages over

CTA: Contrast agents are not nephrotoxic, and images are obtained without exposure to radiation. The quality of MRA is now so good that it has virtually surpassed angiography for evaluating stable patients with PAD to determine what type of intervention is most appropriate.[24] MRA not only can assess vessel occlusion and stenosis but also can evaluate the arterial wall for evidence of atherosclerosis.[25] MRA investigations require prolonged study times and transport from the ED, limiting their usefulness in emergency situations.

Diagnostic Angiography

The past 100 years of performing angiograms has led to advances in the refinement of radiopaque contrast materials, contrast delivery systems (including catheters, guidewires, and injectors), catheterization techniques, and imaging equipment. Catheter-based angiography yields images of the vascular lumen. Any condition that requires luminal evaluation for diagnosis or characterization is best assessed with this technique. Catheter-based angiography is very important in the evaluation of atherosclerotic, thrombotic, and embolic occlusions, because it provides access for some definitive modalities and is indispensable before most percutaneous and surgical procedures related to lower extremity atherosclerotic disease. The contrast materials used today are much safer and more tolerable than previous agents. One adverse effect of contrast administration, renal toxicity, has not been reduced by use of the low-osmolality agents. Contrast agent–induced renal impairment can be reduced by identifying patients at risk for renal impairment, attempting to correct comorbid conditions, limiting the amount of contrast agent given, and ensuring appropriate hydration of the patient.

Digital subtraction angiography (DSA) acquires the image, converts it with an image intensifier, and then transfers it to a monitor, which then saves it in a digital format. DSA is a computer-assisted radiographic technique that subtracts images of bone and soft tissue to permit viewing of the cardiovascular system. Those structures that do not change during injection are canceled out, resulting in the "disappearance" of structures like bone, soft tissues, and air. Improved hardware, software, and speed of the techniques combined with better outcomes from interventions mean DSA is heavily relied on for vascular disease. Need for lower concentrations of iodinated contrast agents or use of non-nephrotoxic agents also make it a more desirable imaging technique than regular angiography.[26] The major attributes of DSA that contribute to its importance are high resolution, ability to selectively evaluate individual vessels, and ability to access direct physiologic information of the tissues. Despite the diagnostic paradigm shift away from angiography, DSA is a cornerstone technology in PAD intervention and will likely remain so for the foreseeable future.[20]

Treatments

The spectrum of PAD ranges from asymptomatic to critical limb ischemia, and CAD and other atherosclerotic vascular disorders may coexist with PAD (Box 63-5). Indications for urgent interventions are (1) incapacitating claudication that interfere with work or lifestyle and (2) limb salvage in persons with limb-threatening ischemia, as manifested by rest pain, nonhealing ulcers, and/or infection or gangrene.

The therapy for PAD may involve medical, percutaneous, and/or surgical approaches, depending on the progression and extent of the disease.

TREATMENT OF ISCHEMIC PERIPHERAL ARTERIAL DISEASE

When arterial blood flow is insufficient to meet the metabolic demands of resting muscle or tissue, limb-threatening ischemia results. This is the most common indication for emergency arterial reperfusion. The affected patient presents with rest pain, ischemic ulcers, gangrene, or a pulseless cold extremity. The selected group of patients requires immediate assessment of their vascular system. Arteriography provides the most useful information in the setting of acute arterial occlusion, because in addition to providing information on anatomy, it can distinguish between embolism and thrombosis. An embolism has a sharp cutoff of contrast agent with a reverse meniscus sign; a thrombosis usually has a more

BOX 63-5

Categories of Acute Limb Ischemia

Viable: *The extremity is not immediately threatened.* The patient does not complain of ischemic rest pain, there is no neurologic deficit, and the skin capillary circulation appears adequate. Physical examination demonstrated pulses with either palpation or Doppler flowmeter.

Threatened viability: Reversible ischemia has occurred, and the extremity is salvageable without major amputation if the arterial obstruction is promptly relieved. The affected patient has ischemic rest pain with mild transient or incomplete neurologic symptoms. The pulses are not detected by Doppler flowmeter.

Major, irreversible ischemic change: Frequently requires major amputation of the affected limb. The affected patient presents with profound sensory loss and muscle paralysis, absence of capillary flow, or evidence of more advanced ischemia (muscle rigor or marbled skin). No pulses can be palpated or detected by Doppler flowmeter.

tapered cutoff. Diffuse atheromatous disease is also usually found around a thrombotic occlusion.

Prompt initiation of therapy is the most important aspect of treatment of acute limb ischemia. Patients should immediately receive a heparin bolus followed by an infusion. This initial therapy prevents clot propagation and inhibits thrombosis distal to the lesion(s), where there is low flow or stasis. Heparin should be administered before diagnostic testing is obtained.[41] Subsequent therapy depends on whether the extremity is viable, threatened, or nonviable.

Patients with Viable Extremities

The patient found to have an ischemic but viable extremity on clinical examination should undergo urgent arteriography. Such a patient may undergo thrombolysis as an alternative to surgical intervention. One study has found limb salvage rates of approximately 70% for both thrombolytic therapy and surgical intervention in this patient population.[42] The important thing for the EP to remember is that thrombolytic therapy is limited by the length of time available to dissolve the thrombus and the severity of the ischemia. Thrombolytics are given at the site of occlusion through the catheter used for the angiogram. This method has been shown to have a better outcome with fewer bleeding complications than intravenous administration. Both urokinase and tissue plasminogen activator have been studied and appear similar on outcome measures. Patients who have ischemic symptoms for less than 14 days and are treated with thrombolytics have better amputation-free survival and shorter hospital stays than the surgical group; patients with ischemic symptoms for longer than 14 days have a better outcome with surgical intervention. Also, in patients who have received thrombolytic therapy and go on to require surgical intervention, the magnitude of the surgical procedure is less than in patients who have not received thrombolytics.

The surgeon and interventional radiologist help decide on the optimal therapy for the patient with limb ischemia and a viable extremity according to (1) the location and length of the lesion, (2) the etiology (embolus vs. thrombus), (3) the duration of symptoms, and (4) the suitability of the patient for surgery. In general, smaller, more distal emboli are best treated with thrombolytics, whereas a large embolus at a more proximal location is best be treated with embolectomy.[43]

Patients with Threatened Extremities

Patients with threatened extremities should undergo immediate surgical revascularization. The vast majority of such patients have an embolic event. Irreversible changes, including necrosis, may occur within 4 to 6 hours of the initial insult, leaving a fairly small therapeutic window. The small amount of time available makes thrombolytic therapy of limited utility.

Surgery usually reveals an embolus that can be removed by embolectomy. After the embolectomy, most surgeons perform an intraoperative arteriogram to assess distal blood flow. If small distal emboli are found after the embolectomy, intraoperative thrombolytic therapy may be considered. If ischemia has been prolonged, a compartment syndrome may result once the blood flow is restored. Therefore, oral anticoagulation should be instituted after the procedure to prevent subsequent embolization.[41]

Patients with Nonviable Extremities

If clinical evaluation of the patient's extremity reveals nonviability, the patient should proceed with prompt amputation. Angiography is not normally required to make this diagnosis, and the clinical findings dictate the level of amputation. In general, surgeons try to preserve as many joints as possible in order to decrease the work of ambulating with a prosthesis. If amputation is not performed in an expedient manner, the patient may have complications, such as sepsis, acute renal failure, rhabdomyolysis, hyperkalemia, and cardiovascular collapse.

TREATMENT OF PERIPHERAL ARTERIAL DISEASE

Nonischemic Peripheral Arterial Disease

Patients who have nonischemic PAD should start exercise programs and risk factor modification along with antiplatelet therapy.[27]

Ischemic Peripheral Arterial Disease

Immediate heparin bolus followed by heparin infusion should be given to a patient with ischemic PAD before arteriography is performed to determine viability of the affected extremity.[28,29]

Patients with Viable Extremities

Urgent arteriography must be performed. Once the anatomy has been defined, vascular surgeons can determine whether surgical or an intra-arterial thrombolytic therapy is needed, depending on the location and length of the lesion, etiology (embolus versus thrombus), duration of symptoms, and suitability of the patient for surgery[29,30] (Figs. 63-3 and 63-4).

Patients with Threatened Extremities

Patients with threatened extremities should receive immediate surgical intervention. Most have an embolic event, and irreversible changes including necrosis may occur within 4 to 6 hours, leaving a small therapeutic window. Small window makes thrombolytic therapy of limited utility[30,31] (Figs. 63-5 and 63-6).

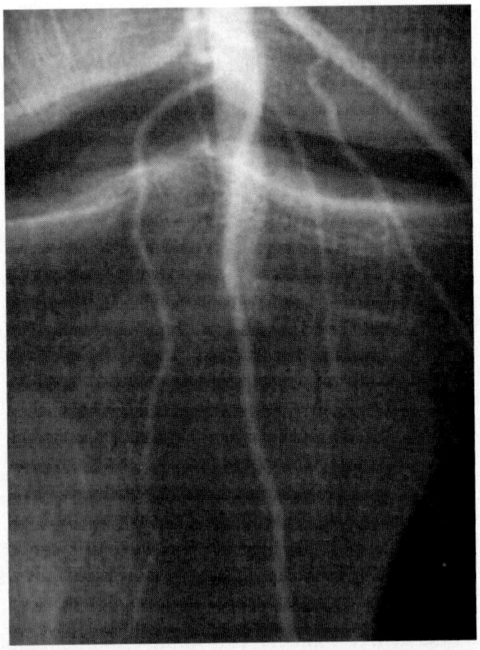

FIGURE 63-3 Popliteal artery reveals a sharp end to contrast material in a patient with a painful, acutely ischemic leg. See Figure 63-4.

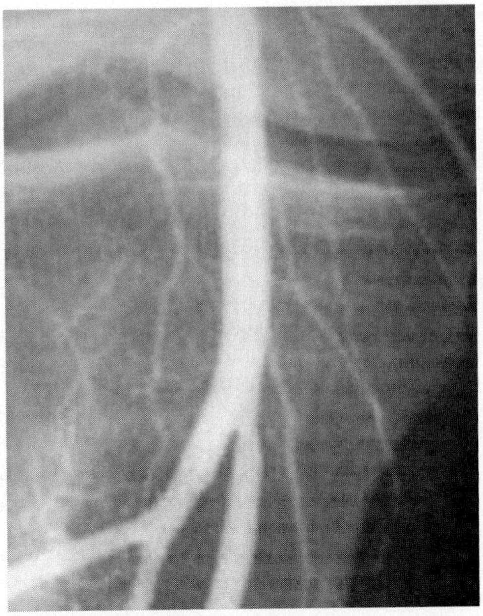

FIGURE 63-4 Leg of the same patient as in Figure 63-3 after administration of a thrombolytic agent. Note the resumption of normal flow distal to the previous obstruction.

Patients with Nonviable Extremities

If clinical evaluation of the patient shows that the extremity is nonviable, the patient should proceed with prompt amputation as discussed previously.[28]

Disposition

Vascular diseases are common, and prompt treatment can diminish disability and death. Preservation of individual health (better functional status and survival) and achievement of public health goals (e.g., diminished rates of amputation and fewer cardiovascular ischemic events and death) can be achieved by the establishment of an accurate vascular diagnostic assessment and treatment plan. Patients with nonischemic PAD can be discharged with instructions for risk factor modification and follow-up with a vascular surgeon. Any patient with signs of ischemic PAD should be admitted as part of evaluation and treatment.

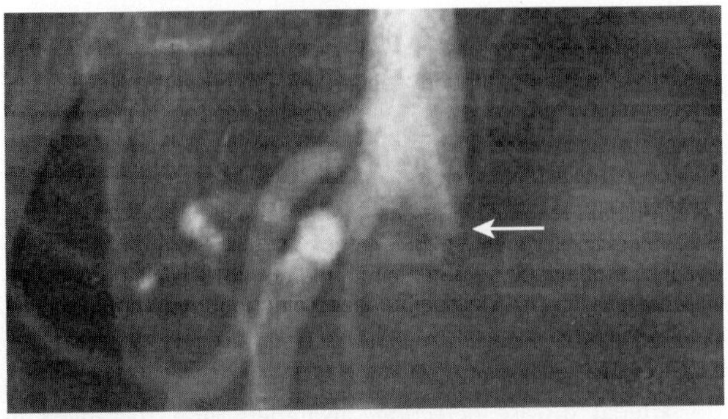

FIGURE 63-5 Angiogram of a patient with embolic disease at the proximal femoral artery as it bifurcates to the deep femoral system. Note the abrupt cutoff of contrast material. See Figure 63-6.

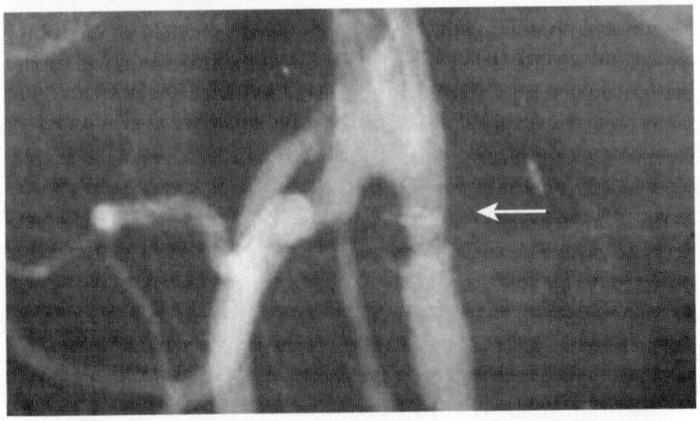

FIGURE 63-6 Angiogram of the same patient as in Figure 63-5 after thrombectomy. Note the resolution of flow and the absence of visible clot.

PATIENT TEACHING TIPS

- Physicians must educate patients on the importance of pain as a symptom of significant arterial disease and the need for immediate evaluation to save a limb.
- Modification of risk factors, especially smoking, can not only arrest the progress the disease but may, in some cases, reverse some of the clinical effects.
- Patients with peripheral arterial disease must also undergo testing for associated coronary artery disease because of the close association of the two disease processes.

REFERENCES

1. Faxon DP, Creager MA, Smith SC Jr, et al: Atherosclerotic Vascular Disease Conference: Executive summary: Atherosclerotic Vascular Disease Conference proceeding for healthcare professionals from a special writing group of the American Heart Association. Circulation 2004;109: 2595-2604.
2. Criqui MH, Fronek A, Klauber MR, et al: The sensitivity, specificity, and predictive value of traditional clinical evaluation of peripheral arterial disease: Results from noninvasive testing in a defined population. Circulation 1985;71: 516-522.
3. Hirsch AT, Criqui MH, Treat-Jacobson D, et al: Peripheral arterial disease detection, awareness, and treatment in primary care. JAMA 2001;286:1317-1324.
4. Hirsch AT, Haskal ZJ, Hertzer NR, et al: American Association for Vascular Surgery/Society for Vascular Surgery; Society for Cardiovascular Angiography and Interventions; Society for Vascular Medicine and Biology; Society of Interventional Radiology; ACC/AHA Task Force on Practice Guidelines. ACC/AHA 2005 guidelines for the Management of Patients with Peripheral Arterial Disease (lower extremity, renal, mesenteric, and abdominal aortic): A collaborative report from the American Associations for Vascular Surgery/Society for Vascular Surgery, Society for Cardiovascular Angiography and Interventions, Society for Vascular Medicine and Biology, Society of Interventional Radiology, and the ACC/AHA Task Force on Practice Guidelines (writing committee to develop guidelines for the management of patients with peripheral arterial disease): Summary of recommendations. J Am Coll Cardiol 2006;47:1239-1312.
5. Criqui MH, Denenberg JO, Langer RD, Fronek A: The epidemiology of peripheral arterial disease: Importance of identifying the population at risk. Vasc Med 1997;2: 221-226.
6. Meijer WT, Hoes AW, Rutgers D, et al: Peripheral arterial disease in the elderly: The Rotterdam Study. Arterioscler Thromb Vasc Biol 1998;18:185-192.
7. Kannel WB, McGee DL: Update on some epidemiologic features of intermittent claudication: The Framingham Study. J Am Geriatr Soc 1985;33:13-18.
8. Rockson SG, Cooke JP: Peripheral arterial insufficiency: Mechanisms, natural history, and therapeutic options. Adv Intern Med 1998;43:253-277.
9. Ouriel K: Peripheral arterial disease. Lancet 2001;358(9289): 1257-1264.
10. Brothers TE, Robison JG, Sutherland SE, Elliott BM: Racial differences in operation for peripheral vascular disease: Results of a population-based study. Cardiovasc Surg 1997;5:26-31.
11. Criqui MH, Langer RD, Fronek A, et al: Mortality over a period of 10 years in patients with peripheral arterial disease. N Engl J Med 1992;326:381-386.
12. Mullenix PS, Andersen CA, Starnes BW: Atherosclerosis as inflammation. Ann Vasc Surg 2005;19:130-138.
13. Davies MJ, Richardson PD, Woolf N, et al: Risk of thrombosis in human atherosclerotic plaques: Role of extracellular lipid, macrophage, and smooth muscle cell content. Br Heart J 1993;69:377-381.
14. Rivard A, Andres V: Vascular smooth muscle cell proliferation in the pathogenesis of atherosclerotic cardiovascular diseases. Histol Histopathol 2000;15:557-571.
15. Morice MC, Serruys PW, Sousa JE, et al: A randomized comparison of a sirolimus-eluting stent with a standard stent for coronary revascularization. N Engl J Med 2002; 346:1773-1780.
16. Lafont A, Topol EJ: Arterial Remodelling: A Critical Factor in Restenosis. Boston, Academic, 1997.
17. Brewster DC, Chin AK, Fogarty TJ: Arterial Thromboembolism, 3rd ed. Philadelphia, WB Saunders, 1989.
18. Falanga V, Fine MJ, Kapoor WN: The cutaneous manifestations of cholesterol crystal embolization. Arch Dermatol 1986;122:1194-1198.
19. Imparato AM, Kim GE, Davidson T, Crowley JG: Intermittent claudication: Its natural course. Surgery 1975;78: 795-799.
20. Olin JW, Kaufman JA, Bluemke DA, et al: Atherosclerotic Vascular Disease Conference: Writing Group IV: Imaging. Circulation 2004;109:2626-2633.
21. Whelan JF, Barry MH, Moir JD: Color flow Doppler ultrasonography: Comparison with peripheral arteriography for the investigation of peripheral vascular disease. J Clin Ultrasound 1992;20:369-374.
22. Bluemke DA, Chambers TP: Spiral CT angiography: An alternative to conventional angiography. Radiology 1995;195:317-319.
23. Rubin GD, Schmidt AJ, Logan LJ, Sofilos MC: Multi-detector row CT angiography of lower extremity arterial inflow and runoff: Initial experience. Radiology 2001;221: 146-158.
24. Grist TM: MRA of the abdominal aorta and lower extremities. J Magn Reson Imaging 2000;11:32-43.
25. Shinnar M, Fallon JT, Wehrli S, et al: The diagnostic accuracy of ex vivo MRI for human atherosclerotic plaque characterization. Arterioscler Thromb Vasc Biol 1999;19: 2756-2761.
26. Oliva VL, Denbow N, Therasse E, et al: Digital subtraction angiography of the abdominal aorta and lower extremities: Carbon dioxide versus iodinated contrast material. J Vasc Interv Radiol 1999;10:723-731.
27. Gardner AW, Poehlman ET: Exercise rehabilitation programs for the treatment of claudication pain: A meta-analysis. JAMA 1995;274:975-980.
28. Yeager RA, Moneta GL, Taylor LM Jr, et al: Surgical management of severe acute lower extremity ischemia. J Vasc Surg 1992;15:385-391; discussion 392-383.
29. Jackson MR, Clagett GP: Antithrombotic therapy in peripheral arterial occlusive disease. Chest 2001;119(Suppl): 283S-299S.
30. Huettl EA, Soulen MC: Thrombolysis of lower extremity embolic occlusions: A study of the results of the STAR Registry. Radiology 1995;197:141-145.
31. Kessel DO, Berridge DC, Robertson I: Infusion techniques for peripheral arterial thrombolysis. Cochrane Database Syst Rev 2004(1):CD000985.

Chapter 64

Hypertensive Crisis

Philip Shayne and Tara D. Director

KEY POINTS

Hypertension is a serious and undertreated medical problem that is common in ED patients.

A severely elevated blood pressure is rarely an emergency, and no level of hypertension in and of itself defines an emergency.

Evaluation of an elevated blood pressure focuses on target organ systems.

Emergencies in hypertension involve evidence of organ damage and require immediate stabilization.

Urgencies in hypertension involve underlying target organ disease in immediately stable patients at higher risk of short-term complications.

Severely elevated blood pressure alone usually does not require aggressive therapy.

Often the most important intervention for patients with elevated blood pressure is to establish good primary care.

Scope

Is severely increased blood pressure an emergency? More than a quarter of all adults in the United States have hypertension.[1] Less than two thirds of U.S. adults with hypertension are aware of their condition, less than half are currently under treatment for it, and only 30% have their blood pressure under control. Elevated blood pressures contribute to morbidity from heart disease, stroke, renal disease, and peripheral vascular diseases, the main causes of death and disability in the developed world.[2] ED patients are at least equally exposed to hypertension, and the uninsured populations who receive a disproportionate amount of their care in the ED have higher prevalence and poorer control of elevated blood pressures. In inner-city public EDs, as many as 20% of the adult census has been found to present with a blood pressure exceeding 140 mm Hg systolic and 90 mm Hg diastolic (140/90).[3-5]

EPs evaluate and treat hypertension in a variety of contexts, ranging from the compliant patient with well-controlled blood pressure to the asymptomatic patient with increased blood pressure to the critically ill patient with increased blood pressure and acute target organ deterioration. Many patients with severely elevated blood pressures have a combination of long-standing, poorly treated hypertension and acute aggravating conditions such as pain, anxiety, and intoxication. Although a major public health risk, an elevated blood pressure is rarely a crisis in the ED. Evidence-based national guidelines exist for the evaluation and treatment of hypertension,[6,7] but there is no good evidence to guide the acute treatment of a patient with severely elevated blood pressure. Instead, the EP relies on an understanding of the disease process, its associated complications, and the health care support available to the patient.

Structure and Function

Hypertension is multifactorial, encompassing genetic and environmental causes. The hallmark of the disease is an elevated peripheral vascular resistance with normal to low cardiac output.[8] The mechanism of the disease probably represents an imbalance in the autoregulation of the renin-angiotensin system. Mechanical stresses on the vascular endothelium resulting from the elevated pressures create an inflammatory process leading to fibrinoid necrosis and scarring of arterioles.

Hypertensive disease manifests in organ systems where arteriole damage leads to ischemic damage or hemorrhage. These *target organs* include the brain, heart, and kidneys (Box 64-1). Persistently elevated blood pressures can trigger or exacerbate crises in these organs. Rapid and progressive target organ damage due to severely elevated blood pressure defines a *hypertensive emergency*.[9,10]

Less commonly, hypertension is the primary crisis. Rising systemic pressures cause an inflammatory endovaculitis; further damage and aggravation from adrenergic stimulation and vasoconstriction accelerate the elevated blood pressure. The multiorgan disease resulting from an overwhelmed autoregulatory function is called *malignant-accelerated hypertension*. Inflammatory changes of the cerebrovasculature produces serious alteration in mental status called *hypertensive encephalopathy*.

The normal autoregulation of the systemic blood pressure complicates the management of severe hypertension. Normotensive individuals are able to maintain steady perfusion of vital organs as their systemic blood pressures vary with normal stresses. As long as the mean arterial pressure (MAP) is maintained within a normal range, perfusion pressures to organs such as the brain remain constant. In chronically hypertensive individuals, the range in which the body is able to maintain normal organ perfusion pressures is increased, and less elastic arterioles are unable to vasodilate or constrict in order to adjust for suddenly normalized blood pressures. Dropping the MAP down to a level considered normal for the nonhypertensive person can make the chronically hypertensive individual relatively hypotensive. This problem prevents such an individual from adequately perfusing vital organs and may even precipitate an ischemic crisis.

BOX 64-1

Hypertensive Emergencies

Primary

- Hypertensive encephalopathy
- Malignant-accelerated hypertension

Secondary

Cerebrovascular Accidents

- Thromboembolic stroke
- Hemorrhagic stroke
- Subarachnoid hemorrhage

Cardiovascular Crises

- Myocardial infarction
- Acute coronary syndromes
- Cardiogenic pulmonary edema
- Aortic dissection
- Uncontrollable arterial bleeding

Renal Crises

- Acute renal failure
- Glomerular nephritis
- Severe hypertension after kidney transplantation

Other Emergencies

- Preeclampsia/eclampsia
- Perioperative hypertension
- Catecholamine excess

Clinical Presentation

The presence or risk of target organ deterioration determines the urgency with which a blood pressure must be treated. As already mentioned, hypertensive emergency is the acute and progressive decompensation or damage of vital organ function caused by an elevated blood pressure. The patient with a hypertensive emergency must be carefully evaluated and monitored, and his or her blood pressure must be controlled. The treatment should be dictated by the clinical situation, not by the severity of blood pressure elevation. No degree of hypertension in and of itself defines an emergency. The absolute level of the patient's blood pressure does not warrant immediate or aggressive treatment; rather, the patient's symptoms determine the intervention (Fig. 64-1).

FACTS AND FORMULAS

Mean arterial blood pressure (MAP) =

$$\frac{\text{systolic pressure} + (2 \times \text{diastolic pressure})}{3}$$

Cerebral perfusion pressure (CPP) = MAP − Intracranial pressure (ICP)

Pulse pressure (dP/dt) = (systolic pressure − diastolic pressure) ÷ heart rate

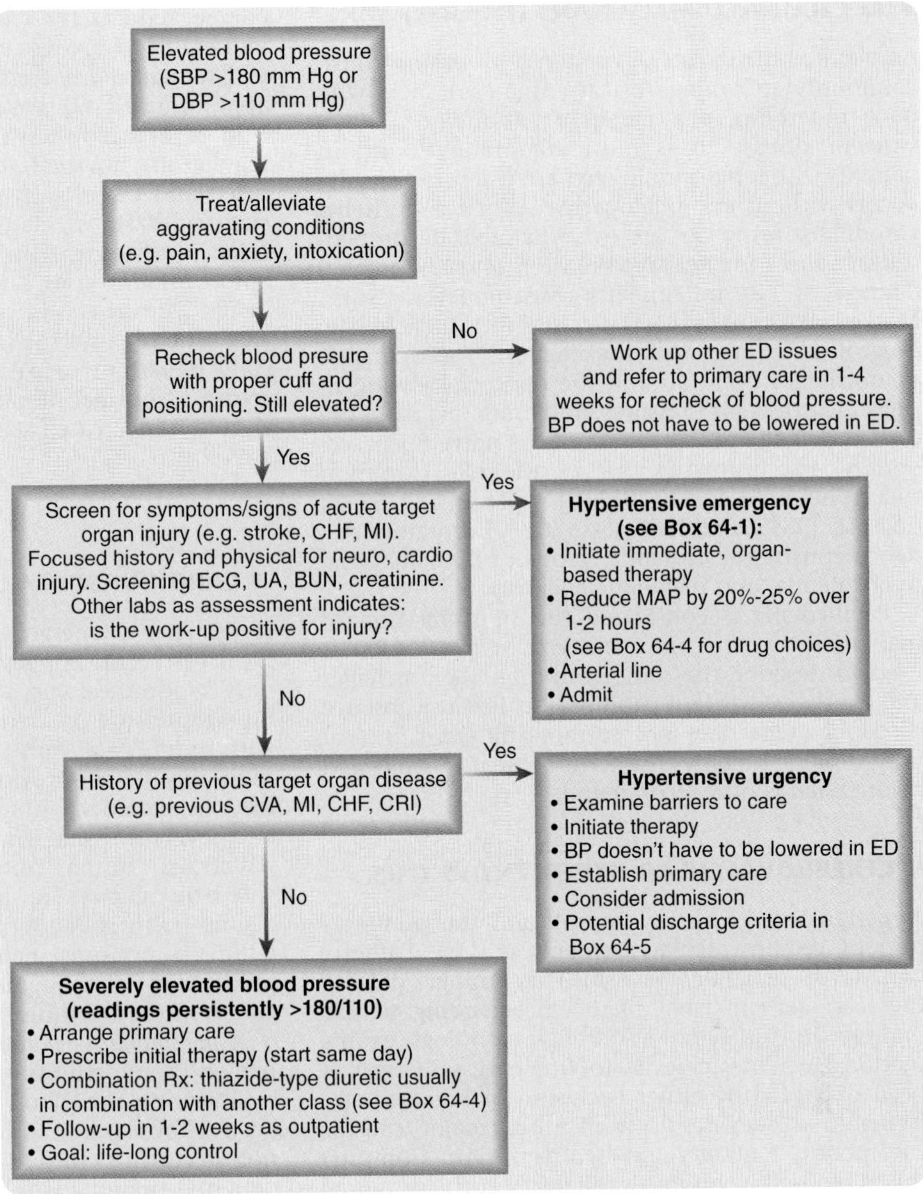
Elevated blood pressure
(SBP >180 mm Hg or
DBP >110 mm Hg)
Treat/alleviate
aggravating conditions
(e.g. pain, anxiety, intoxication)
Recheck blood presure
with proper cuff and
positioning. Still elevated?
No
Work up other ED issues
and refer to primary care in 1-4
weeks for recheck of blood pressure.
BP does not have to be lowered in ED.
Yes
Screen for symptoms/signs of acute target
organ injury (e.g. stroke, CHF, MI).
Focused history and physical for neuro, cardio
injury. Screening ECG, UA, BUN, creatinine.
Other labs as assessment indicates:
is the work-up positive for injury?
Yes
Hypertensive emergency
(see Box 64-1):
• Initiate immediate, organ-
based therapy
• Reduce MAP by 20%-25% over
1-2 hours
(see Box 64-4 for drug choices)
• Arterial line
• Admit
No
History of previous target organ disease
(e.g. previous CVA, MI, CHF, CRI)
Yes
Hypertensive urgency
• Examine barriers to care
• Initiate therapy
• BP doesn't have to be lowered in ED
• Establish primary care
• Consider admission
• Potential discharge criteria in
Box 64-5
No
Severely elevated blood pressure
(readings persistently >180/110)
• Arrange primary care
• Prescribe initial therapy (start same day)
• Combination Rx: thiazide-type diuretic usually
in combination with another class (see Box 64-4)
• Follow-up in 1-2 weeks as outpatient
• Goal: life-long control

FIGURE 64-1 Management of patient with severely elevated blood pressure (BP). BUN, blood urea nitrogen; CHF, congestive heart failure; CVA, cerebrovascular accident; CRI, chronic renal insufficiency; DBP, diastolic BP; ECG, electrocardiogram; MAP, mean arterial pressure; MI, myocardial infarction; Rx, therapy; SBP, systolic BP; UA, urinalysis.

■ HYPERTENSIVE ENCEPHALOPATHY

The triad severe hypertension, altered mental status, and (often) papilledema characterizes *hypertensive encephalopathy,* which may be accompanied by lethargy, confusion, headache, visual disturbances, and seizures. Somnolence, stupor, nausea, or vomiting may also occur. Retinopathy may or may not be present. The diagnosis is confirmed if mentation improves with lowering of the blood pressure. The mechanism is cerebral overperfusion—in effect, the pressure overwhelms the brain's ability to autoregulate cerebral blood flow. Overperfusion results in vasodilation and increased permeability of cerebral blood vessels, which lead in turn to the development of cerebral edema. If not adequately treated, hypertensive encephalopathy can progress to cerebral hemorrhage, coma, and death.

Hypertensive encephalopathy is most likely to occur in previously normotensive individuals who experience a rapid rise in blood pressure, such as children with acute glomerulonephritis and young women with preeclampsia or eclampsia. People with chronic hypertension usually experience a more gradual rise in blood pressure and therefore are less likely to have cerebrovascular decompensation. Hypertensive encephalopathy produces characteristic findings on computed tomography (CT). CT scans show a posterior leukoencephalopathy that predominantly affects the white matter of the parieto-occipital regions bilaterally. CT is useful in excluding other causes of altered mental status, such as intracranial bleeding.

■ ACCELERATED-MALIGNANT HYPERTENSION

Accelerated-malignant hypertension occurs most commonly in young African American men who have underlying renal parenchymal disease or renovascular disease. It is most commonly found in patients with long-standing hypertension and usually occurs without encephalopathy.[8] When endothelial vasodilator responses are overwhelmed, decompensation causes further hypertension and endothelial damage, and an inflammatory vasculopathy results. Marked elevation of blood pressure and characteristic eyeground findings make the diagnosis. Flame-shaped hemorrhages occur around the optic disk owing to high intravascular pressures, and "soft" exudates are caused by ischemic infarction of the nerve fibers secondary to occlusion of supplying arterioles. Common symptoms are headache (85%), visual blurring (55%), nocturia (38%), and weakness (30%). Laboratory evidence consists of azotemia, proteinuria, hematuria, hypokalemia, and metabolic alkalosis.

Papilledema is considered the sine qua non of malignant hypertension; *accelerated hypertension* is used to describe the same condition (hemorrhages and exudates) without papilledema. Because absence of papilledema does not connote different clinical prognosis or therapy, the term *accelerated-malignant hypertension* is now recommended.

■ CEREBROVASCULAR HYPERTENSIVE CRISIS

Hypertension frequently complicates the presentation of cerebrovascular accidents (CVAs). Patients with CVAs generally have focal neurologic deficits that can be somewhat predicted according to the brain territory affected. A thorough neurologic examination elucidates clues as to which vessel flow has been disrupted by either occlusion or hemorrhage. Ischemic strokes result from three major causes: thrombotic, embolic, and hypoperfusion. Compromised blood flow produces cell death at the center of the ischemic region and reversibly damaged neurons in the periphery, also known as the penumbra. The penumbra's viability depends on its perfusion. Hemorrhagic stroke is caused by either intracranial or subarachnoid bleeding. Intracranial pressure rises and cerebral perfusion diminishes at the site of the hematoma. Therefore, maintaining cerebral perfusion is key in both hemorrhagic and occlusive CVAs, and an understanding of cerebrovascular physiology is helpful in determining the best treatment strategy.

Cerebral blood flow (CBF) is a function of the cerebral perfusion pressure (CPP), which is equal to the mean arterial pressure minus the intracranial pressure (ICP): $CPP = MAP - ICP$. Vasoconstriction and vasodilation of the cerebral vasculature maintain a steady CBF. However, cerebral autoregulation fails at approximately 25% above or below the MAP. In addition, changes in ICP or brain injury can result in loss of the brain's ability to autoregulate blood flow. Increased ICP, commonly seen with hemorrhage or edema, reduces the CPP and makes the brain more vulnerable to changes in MAP. In normal individuals, CBF remains fairly constant for an MAP ranging from approximately 60 mm Hg to 150 mm Hg. When the MAP decreases to less than the lower limits of autoregulation, however, the brain becomes hypoperfused and cerebral hypoxia occurs, with symptoms such as dizziness, nausea, and syncope. In chronically hypertensive individuals, the lower limit of autoregulation rises, and autoregulation might fail at MAP values that are well tolerated in nonhypertensive individuals. This situation suggests that chronically hypertensive patients cannot tolerate a rapid return to normal blood pressures and that the MAP should be decreased acutely by no more than 20% to 25%.

■ CARDIOVASCULAR HYPERTENSIVE CRISIS

Hypertensive emergencies involving the heart and great vessels are congestive heart failure, acute coronary syndromes, and aortic aneurysm or dissection. Blood pressure is frequently elevated in patients with *acute pulmonary edema,* particularly when a high-output state is the cause, such as volume overload in patients with renal failure, thyrotoxicosis, and severe anemia. Transient diastolic dysfunction, which may or may not be a direct result of the elevated blood pressure, also causes acute pulmonary edema with hypertension and congestive heart failure. Symptoms include tachypnea, tachycardia, pulmonary rales, jugular venous distention, and a gallop in the third heart sound (S_3).

Acute coronary syndromes are also frequently accompanied by hypertension. Reducing myocardial work by lowering the blood pressure and heart rate has been demonstrated to reduce infarct size in patients not receiving thrombolytic therapy. Classically, patients present with symptoms of chest pain, dyspnea, diaphoresis, nausea, and lightheadedness.

Acute aortic dissection is thought to occur via aortic dilation or high blood pressures superimposed on a structural weakness of the arterial wall, resulting in a tear of the intimal layer. Pulsatile pressure extends the dissection by separating the layers of the arterial wall. Historical series report a mortality of 1% to 2% per hour. The stresses that extend the dissection are thought to be related as much to the aortic pulse wave or pulse pressure (the difference between systolic and diastolic pressures) as it is to MAP. Heart rate, myocardial contractility, and the MAP all contribute to increased pulse pressure. Affected patients include elderly persons with hypertension or atherosclerotic disease and patients with connective tissue disorders. The hallmark symptom is acute, severe retrosternal pain radiating to the back or intrascapular pain. Patients may also have pulse deficits, neurologic symptoms, or ischemic symptoms in involved organs such as the gut, kidney, and heart.

■ RENOVASCULAR HYPERTENSIVE CRISIS

The kidney is unique in being both a target organ and the cause of many hypertensive emergencies. Hypertension causes 30% of cases of end-stage renal disease (ESRD), making it the second most common cause after diabetes. Patients with chronic hypertensive may have nephrosclerosis after 10 to 15 years; it manifests as damage to the medial layer of capillaries, reduced kidney size, and nonnephrotic levels of proteinuria without hematuria. By contrast, malignant hypertension damages the intimal layer of the renal capillary bed and may lead to enlarged kidneys, a cellular urinary sediment, hematuria, and severe proteinuria.

Severe hypertension in a young patient raises the possibility of intrinsic acute renal disease, such as glomerulonephritis. Immunoglobulin A (IgA) nephropathy has surpassed post-streptococcal glomerulonephritis in frequency as a cause of glomerulonephritis in adults, and Henoch-Schönlein purpura is the most likely cause of acute glomerular disease in children.

Renal artery stenosis is present in only 1% of unselected hypertensive patients but in 4% of blacks and 32% of whites who have severe hypertension (diastolic blood pressure >125 mm Hg with retinopathy). It is also more common among patients whose hypertension is rapidly progressive. Occasionally, a rare but devastating acute renal failure may occur, owing to intrarenal vasculitis. This is common in the setting of scleroderma and may be responsive to angiotensin-converting enzyme ACE) inhibitors.

■ CATECHOLAMINE EXCESS

The most familiar drugs causing hypertension in EDs today are sympathomimetic drugs such as phenylephrine, cocaine, and methamphetamine. Tyramine can induce a hypertensive crisis in patients taking a monoamine oxidase inhibitor (MAOI), and hypertension can complicate withdrawal syndromes involving alcohol, benzodiazepines, clonidine, or beta-blockers. Pheochromocytomas can cause intermittent hypertensive crisis and may produce many clinical findings besides hypertension, such as headache, sweating, palpitations, pallor, nausea, and, rarely, seizures. Some patients with pheochromocytomas may have paroxysms of low blood pressure as well.

■ HYPERTENSION IN PREGNANCY

Hypertension in pregnancy is addressed in a separate chapter. Emergencies related to hypertension in pregnancy include eclampsia and preeclampsia. In pregnant women between 20 weeks' gestation and 2 weeks postpartum who have any degree of hypertension (≥140/90 mm Hg) or an increase of more than 30/15 mm Hg above their baseline blood pressures accompanied by peripheral edema and proteinuria have *preeclampsia*. Hypertension is important mainly as a symptom of the underlying disorder rather than a cause. Preeclampsia is important to recognize because it can progress suddenly to *eclampsia,* defined as the occurrence of convulsions in patients with such blood pressure factors. Additional symptoms are headache, visual changes, epigastric pain, oliguria, facial and extremity edema, and the HELLP (hemolysis, elevated liver enzymes, low platelets) syndrome. Eclampsia can rapidly progress to coma or death. Magnesium infusion is more effective than other anticonvulsants in this setting. Definitive treatment consists of delivery of the fetus, so the EP usually collaborates with an obstetrician early in the patient's progress through the ED.

Differential Diagnosis

Patients often present with elevated blood pressure and nonspecific symptoms. The EP must make a prospective decision about the etiology of the symptoms to determine management of blood pressure. If a hypertensive patient's chest pain is possibly anginal, immediate control of blood pressure via parenteral therapy might be necessary. However, if the EP determines that the pain is noncardiovascular, the patient might not need immediate treatment for the blood pressure elevation. The assessment of the patient determines the need to treat.

The concept of the *hypertensive urgency,* in reference to markedly elevated, *asymptomatic* blood pressures requiring rapid intervention, is no longer widely used. In most patients without acute, progressive target organ disease, the severely elevated blood pressure can be managed on an outpatient basis. However, certain patients are at higher risk of near-term complications from their uncontrolled hypertension. This group includes the elderly, the frail, and especially patients with history of previous end-organ disease (e.g., history of stroke, heart failure, renal insufficiency); these patients do require increased vigilance and possible aggressive intervention.

Diagnostic Testing

The clinical evaluation determines the nature, severity, and management of patients in hypertensive crisis. When a patient with markedly elevated blood pressure presents to the ED, accurate measurement of blood pressure is the first step. Blood pressures that are initially elevated in the ED frequently drop spontaneously by the time second readings are obtained.[11,12] Any intervention should be based on the composite of several blood pressure measurements. To obtain an accurate measurement, the clinician should seat the patient with the arm at the level of the heart, cover at least 80% of the arm circumference with the cuff bladder, and evaluate pressures in both arms. Blood pressure measurement with an automated cuff is inaccurate in patients with atrial fibrillation and other heart rhythm irregularities. Appropriate pain

BOX 64-2

Drugs that Elevate Blood Pressure or Interfere with Effectiveness of Antihypertensive Agents

Oral contraceptives
Steroids
Nonsteroidal anti-inflammatory drugs
Nasal decongestants
Cold remedies
Appetite suppressants
Tricyclic antidepressants
Monoamine oxidase inhibitors

management and relief of underlying causes (e.g., hypoxia, bladder distention) may resolve hypertension. Certain medications, over-the-counter preparations, or illicit drugs may transiently exacerbate hypertension (Box 64-2).

If the patient's blood pressure is persistently elevated, the history should be started with an assessment of symptoms that might be consistent with target organ compromise. Details include the duration and severity of preexisting hypertension, success with previous blood pressure regimens, and any history of disease of target organs (cardiovascular, cerebrovascular, renovascular, and great vessels). The physical examination should be aim toward identifying signs of target organ damage. A fundoscopic examination finding of retinal hemorrhage or papilledema sufficiently diagnoses accelerated-malignant hypertension. The cardiovascular examination focuses on identifying signs of heart failure (e.g., increased jugular venous pressure, pulmonary rales, and S_3). The neurologic examination assesses the level of consciousness, the visual fields, and the presence or absence of focal motor and sensory deficits.

The patient's symptoms direct the EP's diagnostic evaluation. For example, dyspnea or signs of heart failure indicate chest radiography, and neurologic findings a CT scan of the head. Box 64-3 summarizes some common symptoms and their associated end organs. Few studies have assessed the prognostic value of laboratory testing in asymptomatic patients with severely elevated blood pressure.[13] However, blood pressures persistently higher than 180/110 in asymptomatic patients warrant a brief assessment of target organ function. Renal failure is clinically silent, so measurement of serum creatinine level and a urinalysis probe for evidence of renal failure or nephritis. Electrocardiography (ECG) is useful in assessing the baseline level of left ventricular hypertrophy, ischemia, or infarction. The finding of left ventricular hypertrophy on ECG carries a poor prognosis and necessitates more vigilant follow-up. When renovascular disease or hypercortisolism is the suspected cause of hypertension, a serum sample should be collected for measurement of plasma renin activity and aldosterone level before medications are administered. A urine screen for cocaine and amphetamines may help confirm extrinsic causes. The value of obtaining a chest radiography or complete blood count in the ED patient who has hypertension without relevant symptoms is likely to be low (see Box 64-3).

BOX 64-3

Common Symptoms of Hypertension

Neurologic
Headache
Visual changes
Altered mental status
Seizures
Nausea

Cardiovascular
Chest pain
Back pain
Dyspnea

Renal
Oliguria
Anuria
Proteinuria

Treatment

■ HYPERTENSIVE EMERGENCY

The goal of therapy in a hypertensive crisis is to reduce the mean MAP by 20% to 25% over 1 to 2 hours. The ideal drug for treating hypertensive emergencies easily controls blood pressure through rapid onset, rapid maximal effect, and rapid offset.[4,14-16] These characteristics are found only in parenteral agents. Table 64-1 summarizes the most commonly used medications and their doses.

Nitroprusside is the classic agent for patients with hypertensive emergencies. It decreases both preload

PRIORITY ACTIONS

For Severely Elevated Blood Pressure

- Recheck blood pressure with correct method in both arms.
- Evaluate and treat aggravating conditions (e.g., pain, anxiety, intoxication).
- Evaluate for evidence of target organ damage.
- Elicit history of target organ disease.
- Therapy based on underlying disease.
- Reevaluate continuously for signs of response to therapy or deterioration.

Table 64-1 PARENTERAL DRUGS FOR TREATMENT OF HYPERTENSIVE EMERGENCIES

Drug	Dose*	Onset of Action	Duration of Action	Adverse Effects[†]	Special Indications
Vasodilators					
Sodium nitroprusside	0.25-10 μg/kg/min as IV infusion[‡] (maximal dose for 10 min only)	Immediate	1-2 min	Nausea, vomiting, muscle twitching, sweating, thiocyanate and cyanide intoxication	Most hypertensive emergencies; should be used with caution in patients with high intracranial pressure or azotemia
Nicardipine hydrochloride	5-15 mg/hr IV	5-10 min	1-4 h	Tachycardia, headache, flushing, local phlebitis	Most hypertensive emergencies except acute heart failure; should be used with caution in patients with coronary ischemia
Fenoldopam mesylate	0.1-0.3 μg/kg per min IV infusion	<5 min	30 min	Tachycardia, headache, nausea, flushing	Most hypertensive emergencies; should be used with caution in patients with glaucoma
Nitroglycerin	5-100 μg/min as IV infusion[‡]	2-5 min	3-5 min	Headache, vomiting, methemoglobinemia; tolerance with prolonged use	Coronary ischemia
Enalaprilat	1.25-5 mg every 6 h IV	15-30 min	6 hr	Precipitous fall in pressure in high-renin states; response variable	Acute left ventricular failure; should be avoided in patients with acute myocardial infarction
Hydralazine hydrochloride	10-20 mg IV 10-50 mg IM	10-20 min 20-30 min	3-8 hr	Tachycardia, flushing, headache, vomiting, aggravation of angina	Eclampsia
Diazoxide	50-100 mg IV bolus repeated, or 15-30 mg/min infusion	2-4 min	6-12 hr	Nausea, flushing, tachycardia, chest pain	Now obsolete; when no intensive monitoring available
Adrenergic Inhibitors					
Labetalol hydrochloride	20-80 mg IV bolus every 10 min 0.5-2.0 mg/min IV infusion	5-10 min	3-6 hr	Vomiting, scalp tingling, burning in throat, dizziness, nausea, heart block, orthostatic hypotension	Used in most hypertensive emergencies except acute heart failure
Esmolol hydrochloride	250-500 μg/kg/min for 1 min, then 50-100 μg/kg/min for 4 min; sequence may be repeated	1-2 min	10-20 min	Hypotension, nausea	Aortic dissection, perioperative
Phentolamine	5-15 mg IV	1-2 min	3-10 min	Tachycardia, flushing, headache	Catecholamine excess

IM, intramuscular; IV, intravenous.
*These doses may vary from those in the Physicians' Desk Reference (51st edition).
[†]Hypotension may occur with all agents.
[§]Require special delivery system.
From The sixth report of the Joint National Committee on prevention, detection, evaluation, and treatment of high blood pressure. Arch Intern Med 1997;157:2413–2446.

and afterload without causing significant reflex tachycardia through arteriovenous vasodilation. Nitroprusside has a quick onset of action, and its effect lasts for only 2 to 5 minutes after it is discontinued. Hemodynamics should be closely monitored with its use to prevent inadvertent hypotension. Thiocyanate toxicity may occur if the drug is used over a period of days, particularly in patients with renal failure. It is contraindicated in pregnancy. Because there is no oral form, the patient must be switched to a different antihypertensive agent once control is achieved. Despite the many benefits of nitroprusside, other agents are often better suited for individual hypertensive crises.

Nicardipine is a rapid-acting parenteral calcium channel blocker. It has a predictable and smooth onset of action but is relatively long-acting. Esmolol is a beta-blocking agent that is both rapid in onset and of short duration, making it easy to titrate. Labetalol, an easily titratable medication, combines alpha- and beta-blockade, making it more potent than esmolol and therefore better able to maintain a consistent cerebral perfusion pressure. Additionally, labetalol has a longer half-life, enabling administration of miniboluses instead of a constant infusion but making it more difficult to titrate down.

Care should be taken with use of beta-blockers in patients with asthma, chronic obstructive pulmonary disease (COPD), acute congestive heart failure, cocaine abuse, or other contraindications to beta-blockade. Fenoldopam is a parenteral dopaminergic receptor blocking agent with an excellent efficacy and safety profile. This agent holds some promise as being equivalent to nitroprusside in efficacy without the rare side effects associated with nitroprusside's cyanide moiety and perhaps with less overshoot hypotension, but it is costly. Other options are enalaprilat, a parenteral ACE inhibitor, and phentolamine, a pure alpha-blocking agent.

■ CEREBROVASCULAR CRISIS

Blood pressure control in *cerebrovascular hypertensive emergencies* should be undertaken with caution.[17] Parenteral drugs that have a short half-life, are easily titrated, and have minimal effect on cerebral vasculature are ideal. Because labetalol does not dilate cerebral capacitance vessels, it is theoretically attractive for use in intracerebral disorders. Caution should be used with direct vasodilators, such as nitroprusside, in the setting of focal brain injury, because they can extend an area of ischemia. Although nicardipine is safe and widely used, some calcium-channel blockers have been linked to a rise in the intracrebral pressure and therefore are not favored for use in patients with brain injury.

The treatment of elevated blood pressure in the setting of *ischemic cerebrovascular accidents* is controversial. When systemic blood pressure is reduced, cerebral autoregulation may fail, extending the ischemic penumbra surrounding the infarct and leading to extension of stroke. Alternatively, infarction may lead to edema, elevated ICP, and further reduction of CBF. The current American Stroke Association guidelines recommend lowering the blood pressure in patients with stroke only when the MAP is higher than 130 mm Hg or the systolic blood pressure is higher than 220 mm Hg.[17]

Theoretically, treatment for elevated blood pressure in patients with *hemorrhagic cerebrovascular accidents* and *subarachnoid hemorrhage* should be more aggressive than for patients with ischemic strokes. The rationale is to decrease the risk of ongoing bleeding from ruptured small arteries and arterioles; however, the relationship between rebleeding and systemic blood pressure is unproven.[18] As with ischemic CVAs, overly aggressive treatment of hypertension may worsen brain injury by decreasing CPP when the ICP is raised. The American Stroke Association guidelines for blood pressure control in patients with hemorrhagic stroke are similar to those for patients with ischemic stroke: The blood pressure should be lowered only when the MAP is higher than 130 mm Hg or the systolic blood pressure higher than 220 mm Hg. Nimodipine, an oral calcium channel blocker, may be given to reduce the incidence of vasospasm and rebleeding after *subarachnoid hemorrhages,* but the agent is not recommended for blood pressure control.

■ CARDIOVASCULAR CRISIS

Nitroglycerin is favored for the treatment of severe hypertension complicating *cardiac ischemia*. A direct vasodilator, nitroglycerin affects the venous vasculature more than the arterial. The agent dilates the coronary arteries and, in contrast to nitroprusside, promotes a favorable redistribution of blood flow to ischemic areas. Beta-blockers are also effective and recommended therapy for acute coronary syndromes. The goal of treatment for patients with *acute coronary syndromes* is reduction of blood pressure to normal if evidence of ischemia persists.[19] However, careful blood pressure reduction requires intensive patient monitoring; overly vigorous blood pressure lowering may worsen ischemia because coronary perfusion depends on diastolic blood pressure.

Most critical cases of *congestive heart failure* are treated with a combination of nitroglycerin, furosemide, and an ACE inhibitor. For patients with pulmonary edema and hypertension, sublingual nitroglycerin should be initiated while intravenous nitroglycerin is being prepared. Captopril should be given orally or sublingually, or enalaprilat intravenously. If systemic fluid overload is present, intravenous furosemide should administered. However, up to 25% of patients with heart failure and severely elevated blood pressure may have "dry failure," in which a pressure natriuresis makes them fluid depleted. Further diuresis may exacerbate the process and continue to stimulate the renin-angiotensin axis. The decision to use furosemide should be based on a clinical judgment of whole-body fluid status. Although beta-blockers have been found to improve survival in patients with chronic congestive heart failure, the use of these agents in patients with acute pulmonary edema may precipitate immediate worsening via negative inotropic effects and bradycardia. Intravenous nesiritide improves hemodynamic function and symptoms in decompensated heart failure and has a modest antihypertensive effect,[20] but this agent is not well studied in the setting of hypertensive crisis.

In *aortic dissection,* beta-blockers should be initiated before nitroprusside to avoid the latter agent's potential adverse effect, reflex tachycardia.[21] Alternatively, labetalol is a unique parenteral agent that achieves its maximal effect within minutes and then remains effective for several hours. This feature allows titration with small boluses, thus avoiding the constant monitoring and high cost required with use of nitroprusside.

■ RENOVASCULAR CRISIS

Fenoldopam may achieve better outcome than nitroprusside in patients with hypertension and *acute renal failure.* Although malignant hypertension may precipitate acute renal failure by injuring the kidney's microvasculature, this causal chain is often reversed in chronic renal failure when long-term renal damage manifests as severe hypertension. Because this distinction cannot be made in the ED, all patients with such findings should undergo blood pressure lowering. Both nitroprusside and labetalol are excellent choices in this setting. ACE inhibitors definitely improve prognosis of patients with chronic hypertension and mild proteinuria, but these agents should be used cautiously in hyperkalemic patients with acute uremia. Nitroprusside may cause thiocyanate poisoning when used over several days in patients with renal failure, so it should be given briefly or to patients who will undergo dialysis soon.

Treatment with an ACE inhibitors may reverse high blood pressure dramatically in patients with unilateral stenosis, but it may provoke acute renal failure and severe hyperkalemia in patients with bilateral stenosis, particularly if they are taking supplemental potassium or a potassium-sparing diuretic. This complication can be completely reversed by discontinuation of the ACE inhibitor.

■ CATECHOLAMINE EXCESS

Patients with severe hypertension due to *pheochromocytoma* are commonly treated with the pure alpha-blocker phentolamine, given intravenously. It may be accompanied by a beta-blocker if needed for tachycardia. Administration of beta-blockers alone in the presence of any sympathomimetic agent (e.g., cocaine) may leave the alpha receptors "open," with subsequent worsening of hypertension.[22] Thus, an attractive alternative to beta-blockers is labetalol, a beta-blocker with some alpha-antagonist properties. However, the alpha- and beta-blockade with labetalol may not be equally effective.[23] Additionally, benzodiazepines are useful adjuncts in cocaine-induced catecholamine excess. They decrease both central and peripheral sympathomimetic outflow stimulated by the cocaine, thereby lowering heart rate, psychomotor hyperactivity, and blood pressure.

■ HYPERTENSION IN PREGNANCY

The mainstay of antihypertensive treatment for hypertensive crisis in pregnancy in many institutions is hydralazine, administered intravenously in boluses of 10 to 20 mg every 10 to 20 minutes, in addition to magnesium therapy for seizure control. If the hypertension is refractory to hydralazine, second-line agents are diazoxide and beta-blockers. Calcium channel blockers have been studied for treatment of

RED FLAGS

Diagnosing a hypertensive emergency when one does not exist: Patients with hypertensive emergencies have evidence of acute end-organ dysfunction.

Reducing the blood pressure too quickly or to too low a level: In patients with chronic hypertension whose autoregulation curve has been reset, this can lead to cerebral or cardiac ischemia.

Lowering a patient's blood pressure acutely without an urgent indication.

Failing to diagnose hypertension or preeclampsia in pregnant patients with blood pressures exceeding 140/90 mm Hg or with an increase in blood pressure of more than 30/15 mm Hg.

Neglecting to match the antihypertensive agent with the clinical scenario.

Tips and Tricks

- Elevated triage blood pressures often spontaneously improve without treatment. Recheck abnormal readings.
- An initially elevated blood pressure might resolve with proper cuff size or treatment of pain, urinary retention, or hypoxia.
- If no emergency is anticipated and immediate parenteral therapy is not required, give the patient a dose of the medications he/she was supposed to have taken.
- Become comfortable with a small number of parenteral agents; in most instances, any one will work.
- Be sure to question patient about use of cocaine or other sympathomimetic drugs.

chronic hypertension in pregnant patients, but they may not be effective with proteinuric hypertension.

Disposition

All patients with hypertensive emergencies require admission to a monitored setting. Such patients generally require emergency involvement of an appropriate specialist for management of a neurologic, cardiovascular, or renovascular crisis. Close blood pressure monitoring, preferably with an arterial line, is indicated. Patients with preeclampsia/eclampsia require emergency obstetric consultation.

Most patients presenting with elevated blood pressures are not in crisis. Very few asymptomatic patients with markedly increased blood pressure are likely to experience a near-term adverse event. Very high blood pressures might be seen in patients with chronic hypertension as a consequence of discontinuing prior therapy or as a result of other easily reversible causes, such as anxiety, pain, drug use, and dietary change.[24,25] There is no evidence that the absolute level of a patient's blood pressure warrants immediate or aggressive treatment. Rather, in the patient with asymptomatic, elevated blood pressure but no evidence of target organ disease, the most important intervention is to ensure proper follow-up. The goal should be lifelong control of the blood pressure.

When the elevated blood pressure may be the artifact of a systemic process such as pain or infection, the best strategy is to refer the patient for reevaluation of blood pressure once the primary problem has resolved. If the patient has discontinued his or her blood pressure medications, the EP should restart the regimen, evaluate the barriers to compliance, and contact a primary care physician to ensure reevaluation in a week. The hypertension guidelines recommend a thiazide-type diuretic as an initial agent, usually in combination with a drug from another class.[6,26] The second agent may be from a number of categories and is best chosen in relation to any compelling indications in the patient's history (Box 64-4).

In principle, in the patient who has never had a blood pressure elevation before, the blood pressure should be rechecked on another visit before the diagnosis of hypertension can be made. However, the latest national guidelines recommend that patients with readings persistently higher than 180/110 in the ED be immediately (same day) started on combination therapy.[6] In the best scenario, the EP also contacts a primary physician and provides follow-up within about a week.

There is an intermediate group of patients who have severely elevated blood pressure and known target organ disease but without active decompensation. An example is a severely hypertensive patient with a previous history of myocardial infarction or stroke. The patient with known target organ disease may be considered at higher risk for a hypertension-related adverse event in the short term. However, there is no good evidence base for the best management of these patients. A treatment strategy should be initiated from the ED, although the blood pressure does not necessarily need to be lowered during the visit. Such patients do require a higher level of vigilance. It may be reasonable to treat them as outpatients, although some may need to be held for short-term observation if their medication compliance or blood pressure monitoring is uncertain; the decision depends on a clinical judgment (Box 64-5).

In practical terms, hypertensive emergencies require immediate (within 1 to 2 hours) decrease in

BOX 64-4

Initial Drug Choices for Hypertension

Use unless contraindicated; start with a low dose of a long-acting once-daily drug and titrate the dose; low-dose combinations might be appropriate.

Uncomplicated Hypertension
Diuretics
Beta-blockers

Diabetes Mellitus (Type 1) with Proteinuria
Angiotensin-converting enzyme (ACE) inhibitors

Heart Failure
ACE inhibitors
Diuretics

Isolated Systolic Hypertension (Older Person)
Diuretics preferred
Long-acting dihydropyridine calcium antagonist

Myocardial Infarction
Beta-blockers (without intrinsic sympathomimetic activity)
ACE inhibitors (with systolic dysfunction)

BOX 64-5

Discharge Criteria for "Hypertensive Urgency"

1. Likely to be compliant with established primary care
2. Known to have hypertension
3. Has a reversible precipitating cause (e.g., medication noncompliance or adverse drug effect)
4. Able to resume a previously effective medication regimen
5. Can be seen for follow-up within 7 days

PATIENT TEACHING TIPS

- Uncontrolled hypertension causes profound and irreversible internal injuries over the long term, many of which are asymptomatic.
- Transient blood pressure elevation is rarely dangerous, and management decisions must be based on evidence of extended hypertension.
- Many medications with different convenience and side-effect profiles are available from which the primary care provider can find a good choice for the individual patient.
- Adherence to a medication regimen is essential for healthy living.
- Chest pains, difficulty in breathing, severe and new headaches, and focal numbness or weakness are possible signs of heart or brain injury and should be evaluated by a doctor immediately.

Documentation

- Ensure that any elevated blood pressure is noted and addressed.
- Make sure to document any change in blood pressure with treatment.
- Document possible etiology of elevated blood pressure.
- List past medical history of target organ disease.
- List current antihypertensive agents and any recent changes in medications or noncompliance with therapy.
- Explain how the elevated blood pressure was assessed.
- Document patient counseling for medications, reasons to return to the ED, and primary care follow-up.

blood pressure, hypertensive urgency requires initiation of a strategy to decrease and monitor blood pressure over 24 to 48 hours, and uncontrolled severe hypertension requires therapy to decrease blood pressure within 1 week. Stratification of individual cases within these categories involves careful clinical evaluation and understanding of target organ disease and treatment strategies.

REFERENCES

1. Wang TJ, Vasan RS: Epidemiology of uncontrolled hypertension in the United States. Circulation 2005;112:1651-1662.
2. Prospective Studies Collaboration: Age-specific relevance of usual blood pressure to vascular mortality: A meta-analysis of individual data for one million adults in 61 prospective studies. Lancet 2002;360:1903-1913.
3. Karras DJ, Ufberg JW, Heilpern KL, et al: Elevated blood pressure in urban emergency department patients. Acad Emerg Med 2005;12:835-843.
4. Zampaglione B, Pascale C, Marchisio M, Cavallo-Perin P: Hypertensive urgencies and emergencies: Prevalence and clinical presentation. Hypertension 1996;27:144-147.
5. Chiang WK, Jamshahi B: Asymptomatic hypertension in the ED. Am J Emerg Med 1998;16:701-7-4.
6. Chobanian AV, Bakris GL, Black HR, et al; Joint National Committee on Prevention, Detection, Evaluation, and Treatment of High Blood Pressure, National Heart, Lung, and Blood Institute, National High Blood Pressure Education Program Coordinating Committee: The Seventh Report of the Joint National Committee on Prevention, Detection, Evaluation, and Treatment of High Blood Pressure: The JNC 7 report. JAMA 2003;289:2560-2572.
7. Decker WW, Godwin SA, Hess EP, et al; American College of Emergency Physicians Clinical Policies Subcommittee (Writing Committee) on Asymptomatic Hypertension in the ED: Clinical policy: Critical issues in the evaluation and management of adult patients with asymptomatic hypertension in the emergency department. Ann Emerg Med 2006;47:237-249.
8. Kaplan NM, Norman M, Lieberman E: Clinical Hypertension, 9th ed. Philadelphia, Lippincott Williams & Wilkins, 2005.
9. Shayne PH, Pitts SR: Severely increased blood pressure in the emergency department [see comment]. Ann Emerg Med 2003;41:513-529.
10. Gilmore RM, Miller SJ, Stead LG: Severe hypertension in the emergency department patient. Emerge Med Clin North Am 2005;23:1141-1158.
11. Pitts SR, Adams RP: Emergency department hypertension and regression to the mean. Ann Emerg Med 1998;31:214-218.
12. Dieterle T, Schuurmans MM, Strobel W, et al: Moderate-to-severe blood pressure elevation at ED entry: Hypertension or normotension? Am J Emerg Med 2005;23:474-479.
13. Karras DJ, Kruus LK, Cienki JJ, et al: Evaluation and treatment of patients with severely elevated blood pressure in academic emergency departments: A multicenter study. Ann Emerg Med 2006;47:230-236.
14. Varon J, Marik PE: The diagnosis and management of hypertensive crises. Chest 2000;118:214-227.
15. Kaplan NM: Management of hypertensive emergencies. Lancet 1994;344:1335-1338.
16. Grossman E, Ironi AN, Messerli FH: Comparative tolerability profile of hypertensive crisis treatments. Drug Saf 1998;19:99-122.
17. Adams HP Jr, Adams RJ, Brott T, et al; Stroke Council of the American Stroke Association: Guidelines for the early management of patients with ischemic stroke: A scientific statement from the Stroke Council of the American Stroke Association. Stroke 2003;34:1056-1083.
18. Broderick JP, Adams HP Jr, Barsan W, et al: Guidelines for the management of spontaneous intracerebral hemorrhage: A statement for healthcare professionals from a special writing group of the Stroke Council, American Heart Association. Stroke 1999;30:905-915.
19. First International Study of Infarct Survival (ISIS-1) Collaborative Group: Randomized trial of intravenous atenolol among 16,027 cases of suspected acute myocardial infarction. ISIS-1. Lancet 1986;2:57-66.
20. Publication Committee for the VMAC Investigators: Intravenous nesiritide vs nitrogylcerin for treatment of decompensated heart failure. Activation of the neurohumoral axis. JAMA 2002;287:1531-1540.
21. Pretre R, Von Segesser LK: Aortic dissection. Lancet 1997;349:1461-1464.
22. Ramoska E, Sacchetti AD: Propranolol-induced hypertension in treatment of cocaine intoxication. Ann Emerg Med 1985;14:1112-1113.
23. Boehrer JD, Moliterno DJ, Willard JE, et al: Influence of labetalol on cocaine-induced coronary vasoconstriction in humans. Am J Med 1993;94:608-610.

24. Viskin S, Berger M, Ish-Shalom M, et al: Intravenous chlorpromazine for the emergency treatment of uncontrolled symptomatic hypertension in the pre-hospital setting: Data from 500 consecutive cases. Isr Med Assoc J 2005;7:812-815.
25. Grossman E, Nadler M, Sharabi Y, et al: Antianxiety treatment in patients with excessive hypertension. Am J Hypertens 2005;18:1174-1177.
26. Psaty BM, Smith NL, Siscovick DS, et al: Health outcomes associated with antihypertensive therapies used as first-line agents: A systematic review and meta-analysis. JAMA 1997;277:739-745.

Chapter **65**

Pulmonary Embolism

D. Mark Courtney

KEY POINTS

Appropriate testing for pulmonary embolism (PE) requires both (1) understanding of pretest probability for each patient and (2) knowledge of diagnostic test characteristics used at the EP's specific institution.

Pretest probability less than 10% along with a negative result of a D-dimer test result that has a sensitivity of at least 95% is sufficient to rule out PE in most settings.

The finding of right heart strain on echocardiography or electrocardiography, decreased oxygenation saturation, and elevated brain natriuretic peptide and troponin values may predict worse short-term and long-term outcomes in patients with diagnosed PE.

Treatment for PE consists of heparin with initiation of warfarin therapy.

Treatment of shock associated with PE comprises intravenous fluid therapy, vasopressor administration, respiratory support, and thrombolytic therapy.

PE represents a spectrum of severity determined by size of clot and baseline cardiopulmonary disease.

The probability of mortality increases steeply once right ventricular dysfunction and hypotension occur.

Diagnosis of PE as a cause of shock requires thinking of PE as a potential cause and a stepwise approach to simultaneous testing and resuscitation.

Scope and Outline

The annual incidence of diagnosed pulmonary embolism (PE) is approximately 1.5 new cases per 1000 persons and is relatively similar among western populations.[1] Dyspnea and chest discomfort are the most typical symptoms of PE, and these chief complaints are responsible for more than 10 million annual patient visits to U.S. EDs.[2] Physicians evaluate large numbers of patients for PE, because symptoms can be vague and severity may range from asymptomatic to shock and subsequent cardiac arrest.[3]

Proliferation of testing strategies for PE and medical-legal concerns related to missing the diagnosis has lead to a dramatic increase in rate of testing. Physicians have become aware that patients previously not thought to have "classic" risk factors may still have PE. To deal with these challenges, the practicing EP must aim to:

- Recognize the potential for PE to exist in the appropriate settings.
- Perform the optimal test on the basis of pretest probability and specific test characteristics.
- Be capable of estimating prognosis for each patient after the diagnosis is made, and institute appropriate therapy.

Structure and Function

PE is part of the continuum of venous thromboembolic disease that most often starts with deep venous thrombosis (DVT) in the leg. Patients with DVT often are found to have concurrent PE when evaluated with imaging tests, and many patients with PE have concurrent DVT. The treatment is similar for both. Risk factors for venous thromboembolic disease include the triad described by Virchow: hypercoagulability, venous stasis, and injury. These factors are most commonly thought of as occurring at the level of the veins, but it is helpful to also think of them as occurring at the level of the patient. For instance, injury to the vein *or* the patient and stasis of flow in the vein *or* of the patient may elevate the risk. Table 65-1 lists several risk factors for venous thromboembolic disease. Understanding risk factors is critical to recognizing the potential for PE.

Embolism to the pulmonary vasculature may result in large bilateral central clots with severe obstruction of flow (so-called saddle embolism), medium clot in lobar or segmental branches, or small clot in the peripheral vasculature. Clot in the pulmonary vasculature activates local inflammation, leading to vasoconstriction and some pulmonary hypertension with the resultant symptoms dyspnea and, possibly, chest pain.

Clinical Presentation

Dyspnea and chest pain form the most common presentations of PE. Chest pain in the absence of *any* shortness of breath or *any* respiratory signs or symptoms is not a typical presentation. Other symptoms can be associated with PE, including syncope, cough, flank pain, abdominal pain, and even fever (Box 65-1). The severity of symptoms in a given patient is a function of (1) the baseline cardiopulmonary status of the patient and (2) the size of the clot.[4] This is why occasionally, large clots are tolerated fairly well in young patients with no cardiopulmonary disease, whereas much smaller clot may result in hypotension, hypoxemia, and deterioration in patients with preexisting cardiopulmonary disease. Older patients with PE often have a worse clinical presentation and

Table 65-1 RISK FACTORS FOR PULMONARY EMBOLISM

Risk Factors	Specific Note(s)
Previous history of pulmonary embolism (PE) or deep venous thrombosis	Inquire about the setting and circumstance of prior venous thromboembolism (VTE)
Recent trauma or surgery	In general, trauma requiring admission, or surgery requiring general anesthesia within the previous month
Cancer	In general, patients with currently treated cancer or palliative care
Age	Risk rises significantly after age 50-60 years
Oral contraceptives	Especially third-generation formulations
Hormone replacement therapy	
Pregnancy	Risk rises along with duration of pregnancy to peak at term, then decreases over 4-6 weeks post partum
Immobility	Includes casts/splints as well as permanent limb or generalized body immobility
Factor V Leiden mutation	Heterozygous carrier state exists in 3%-7% Homozygous mutation is less common and confers 3 times greater risk of VTE relative to normal genotype
Antiphospholipid antibody syndrome	Very potent risk factor Associated with large and recurrent PE May be associated with anticardiolipin antibodies, cerebrovascular accident, myocardial infarction, and first-trimester miscarriage
Prothrombin mutation	
Hyperhomocysteinemia	Can occur from inadequate folate and B vitamin intake as well as genetic mutation in methyltetrahydrofolate reductase
Deficient levels of clotting factors	Protein C, protein S, antithrombin III
Congestive heart failure	
Chronic obstructive pulmonary disease	
Air travel	Primary risk with travel > 5000 km and concurrent other risk factors
Obesity	Risk elevated at body mass index (BMI) > 25 and even higher if BMI > 29

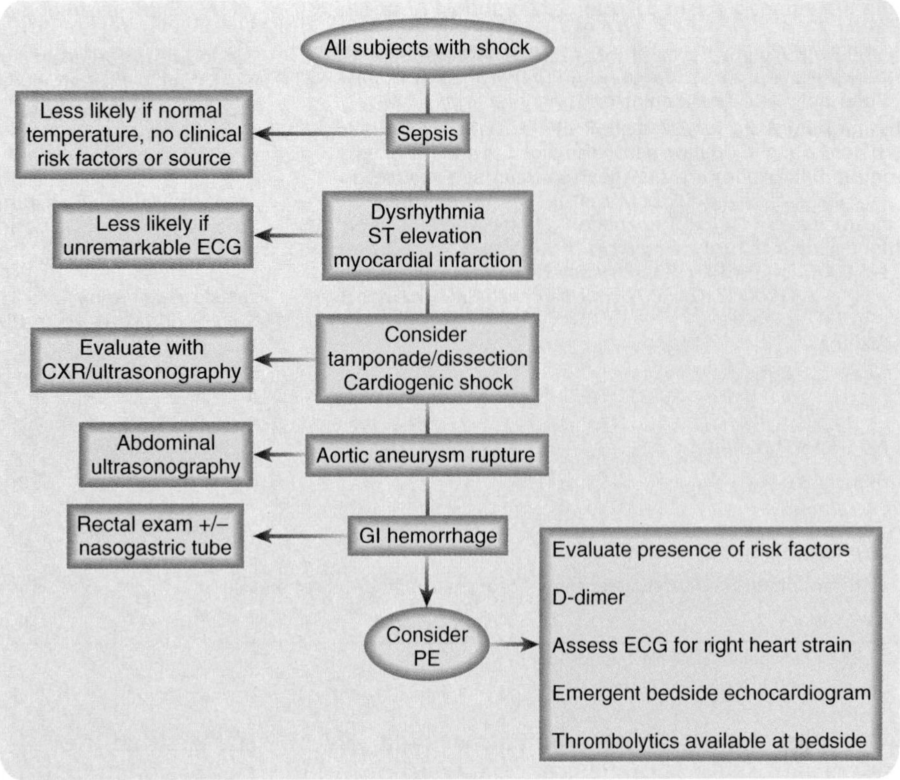
All subjects with shock
Sepsis
Less likely if normal temperature, no clinical risk factors or source
Dysrhythmia ST elevation myocardial infarction
Less likely if unremarkable ECG
Consider tamponade/dissection Cardiogenic shock
Evaluate with CXR/ultrasonography
Aortic aneurysm rupture
Abdominal ultrasonography
GI hemorrhage
Rectal exam +/– nasogastric tube
Consider PE
Evaluate presence of risk factors
D-dimer
Assess ECG for right heart strain
Emergent bedside echocardiogram
Thrombolytics available at bedside

FIGURE 65-1 Stepwise approach to shock with consideration of pulmonary embolism (PE) as possible cause. CXR, chest radiograph; ECG, electrocardiography; GI, gastrointestinal.

BOX 65-1

Signs and Symptoms in Patients with Diagnosed Pulmonary Embolism

- Dyspnea
- Pleuritic chest pain
- Substernal chest pain
- Syncope
- Cough
- Anxiety
- Hemoptysis
- Dizziness/lightheadedness

outcome, largely as a result of having worse cardiopulmonary status at baseline rather than simply being elderly.

Shock may be a primary presentation of PE. Patients may not be able to provide a history of PE symptoms or risk factors and may not be sufficiently stable to leave the ED for imaging, yet consideration of PE with empiric treatment may be warranted. A rapid bedside evaluation to search for clues of non-PE diagnoses can be done promptly and is described in Figure 65-1. A common mistake is to attribute shock to a primary cardiac cause even though electrocardiography (ECG) shows no significant ischemic changes and no significant dysrhythmia, and the chest radiograph shows no evidence of pulmonary vascular congestion or cardiomegaly. If patients can be stabilized with intravenous fluids and possibly vasopressors, computed tomography (CT) should be done. If not, emergency bedside echocardiography to look for signs of massive PE should be performed as an alternative way of confirming the diagnosis of PE.

The other end of the spectrum is the diagnosis in patients with relatively mild symptoms. Despite the fact that patients may have PE with normal oxygen saturation, no known risk factors, and no pulmonary symptoms, this combination is very uncommon. Strict attention to details such as oxygen saturation after walking, physician-obtained respiratory rate, examination of the legs, and serial assessments help to either reassure physicians that the patient has such a low probability of PE that testing is unwarranted or provide evidence to justify an evaluation for PE.

Differential Diagnosis

Because of the vague yet common nature of dyspnea and chest pain, the differential diagnosis for patients with these symptoms is broad. Nevertheless, a targeted diagnostic approach should be used rather than a "chest pain work-up" that attempts to test for every diagnosis possible without regard to pretest probability or negative consequences of "overtesting." This issue is particularly important in PE, because the tests are not 100% sensitive or specific and the consequences of a false-positive diagnosis may involve 6 months of oral anticoagulation with high direct and indirect costs to the patient and society. The consequences are especially important for young patients

Table 65-2 DIAGNOSES THAT SHOULD BE CONSIDERED ALONG WITH PULMONARY EMBOLISM

Diagnoses	Means of Rapidly Obtaining Clues
Potentially Life-Threatening	
Myocardial ischemia/cardiogenic shock/dysrhythmia/congestive heart failure	ECG/CXR
Pneumothorax	CXR
Cardiac tamponade	Bedside cardiac ultrasonography
Pneumonia	CXR
Esophageal rupture	CXR
Pulmonary malignancy (metastatic or primary)	CXR, history
Asthma	Physical examination, history
Aortic dissection	History
Pericarditis	ECG
Non–Life-Threatening	
Bronchitis	History
Chest wall pain	History
Pleuritis/pleurisy	History
Gastroesophageal reflux disease, esophageal spasm, peptic ulcer disease	History
Panic attack	History

CXR, chest radiograph; ECG, electrocardiography.

who must follow activity limitations and older patients at risk for falls, medication interaction, and bleeding.

Table 65-2 lists potential alternative diagnoses in patients evaluated in the ED for PE and clues to assist rapid decision-making. It is not surprising that many of these alternatives are common entities, such as pneumonia, bronchitis, asthma, musculoskeletal pain, gastroesophageal reflux or spasm, and anxiety/panic attack. Many of the potentially life-threatening alternative diagnoses can be evaluated with a chest radiograph, ECG, bedside cardiac ultrasonography, and cardiac enzyme testing in the patient's first hour in the ED.

It is most helpful to think of PE as a continuum of cardiopulmonary stress. Even in normotensive patients, in-hospital or 30-day mortality rates for diagnosed PE are approximately 8% to 13%.[5-9] This mortality in patients with PE but without shock is higher than that for patients with acute myocardial infarction.[10] When early signs of right heart dysfunction occur, the mortality rate begins to take a steep curve upward. These signs are followed by compensated shock, which may initially respond to intravenous fluid. Later, as left-sided filling is decreased owing to septal shift into the left ventricle as well as decreased filling of the left atrium, overt shock is present, and mortality exceeds 30%. If untreated, cardiac arrest occurs, with pulseless electrical activity as the most likely first rhythm.

Diagnostic Testing

Pretest probability is the level of likelihood of a particular diagnosis prior to performance of any tests. It is typically calculated either with a scoring system or by the physician's own "gestalt" estimation. Despite the fact that there is debate over the relative accuracies of gestalt and structured means of pretest probability assessment, the American College of Emergency Physicians (ACEP) practice guideline of 2003 recommended pretest probability assessment for patients being evaluated for PE.[11]

Two structured systems based on derivation in North American populations have been published (Fig. 65-2). The most common is the Canadian score derived by Wells and colleagues,[12] which produces a score for an individual patient that can be used to estimate ranges of pretest probability. Another is the Charlotte criteria, which are composed of objective criteria to identify high-risk patients in whom PE should not be ruled out on the basis of a D-dimer test result alone.[13] Widespread use of these scoring systems has been limited by difficulty in physician recall as well as the fact that they provide ranges of probability rather than an exact estimate. An alternative to these structured pretest probability systems is unstructured or implicit estimation systems, in which physicians arrive at their own pretest probability on the basis of their own experience and the overall integration of clinical information for a particular patient. This approach is commonplace but imprecise and subject to variability.

The most typical means of evaluating for PE (Fig. 65-3) is to determine whether the pretest probability is sufficiently low (Charlotte criteria "safe," Wells score ≤4, or unstructured estimate "low risk") and then to use a sensitive D-dimer blood test that detects the presence of fibrin breakdown products. If the D-dimer test result is negative in such a low-risk patient, the post-test probability of PE is below a sufficient test threshold (<1% to 2%) and PE can be safely excluded from the differential diagnosis for the patient.[14,15]

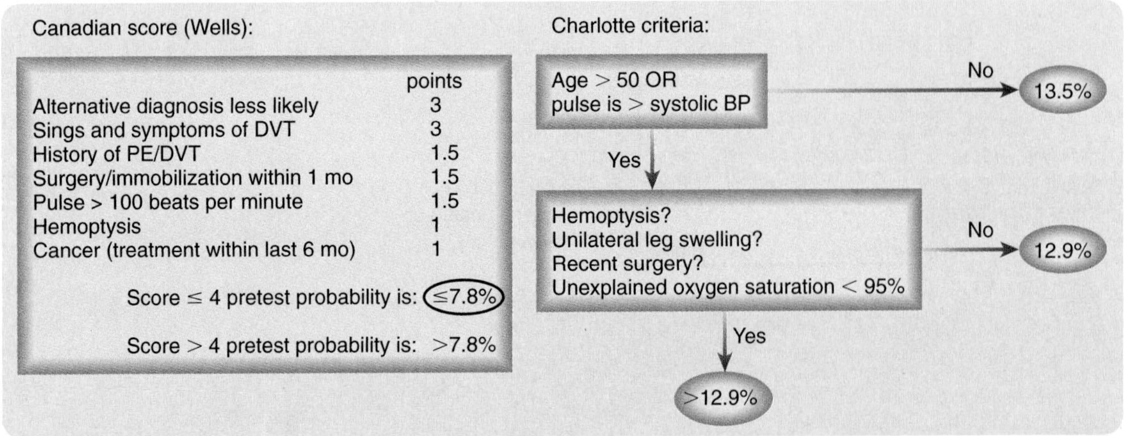
Canadian score (Wells):
points
Alternative diagnosis less likely 3
Sings and symptoms of DVT 3
History of PE/DVT 1.5
Surgery/immobilization within 1 mo 1.5
Pulse > 100 beats per minute 1.5
Hemoptysis 1
Cancer (treatment within last 6 mo) 1
Score ≤ 4 pretest probability is: ≤7.8%
Score > 4 pretest probability is: >7.8%
Charlotte criteria:
Age > 50 OR
pulse is > systolic BP
No
13.5%
Yes
Hemoptysis?
Unilateral leg swelling?
Recent surgery?
Unexplained oxygen saturation < 95%
No
12.9%
Yes
>12.9%

FIGURE 65-2 Structured pretest probability methods (resultant pretest probability in *circles*). BP, blood pressure; DVT, deep venous thrombosis; PE, pulmonary embolism.

Table 65-3 OVERVIEW OF DIAGNOSTIC PERFORMANCE OF D-DIMER TESTS

Pretest Probability	Type Of D-Dimer Test	Approximate Sensitivity	Approximate Specificity	Likelihood Ratio for Negative Result	Probability of Pulmonary Embolism After a Negative Result (Post-Test Probability)
≤10%	Quantitative: enzyme-linked immunoassay or turbidimetric tests	94%	55%	0.1	≤1.2%
≤5%	Qualitative: whole blood agglutination or immunofiltration tests	85%	60%	0.25	≤1.3%

Typically, two types of D-dimer tests are available for ED testing: (1) quantitative (enzyme-linked immunosorbent assay [ELISA] or immunoturbidimetric test, results of which are typically considered positive at levels >500 ng/mL) and (2) qualitative (whole blood agglutination or immunofiltration tests that return a binary result of positive or negative). Benefits of the quantitative tests include higher sensitivity. Benefits of the qualitative tests include rapid results because they may be performed at the bedside. Table 65-3 describes how the two different types of D-dimer tests may be used to rule out PE. The values given in the table are estimates of diagnostic test performance; actual sensitivity/specificity and likelihood ratio values will vary with the individual tests, thus emphasizing the importance of the clinician's familiarity with the specific test at his or her institution. Latex agglutination tests for PE have fallen out of favor owing to low sensitivity, and their use should be discouraged.

Unfortunately, 30% to 60% of patients without PE have false-positive results on D-dimer testing because of the low specificity of these blood tests. Confirmation of the presence or absence of PE must be confirmed with an imaging test, usually a CT scan of the pulmonary arteries or a ventilation-perfusion ($\dot{V}/\dot{Q}$) scan. If the imaging findings are negative in these low-risk patients, PE can be considered sufficiently excluded (see Table 65-3).

The decision to test for PE should always assume that if screening tests such as the D-dimer blood test have positive results, more definitive tests will be undertaken. It is critical to explain this assumption to patients so that they are not surprised and displeased when a false-positive D-dimer result requires them to stay in the ED for imaging (which occurs in nearly half of patients). It is also important for the EP initiating further tests for PE to consider the possible consequences of contrast agent reaction, volume overload from osmotic effects of contrast agent, concerns about testing in pregnant patients, and the overall safety of leaving the ED for the tests.

For these reasons as well as the significant negative effect that false-positive diagnosis may have for the patient—months of anticoagulation—attempts to reduce testing in very-low-risk patients have been proposed. One such method is the PE rule-out criteria (PERC). It was derived in a multicenter U.S. sample and provides simple, easy-to-apply, clinical criteria that, when satisfied, indicate that the baseline probability of PE is below a test threshold (<1.8%) and testing in this setting has the potential to cause more

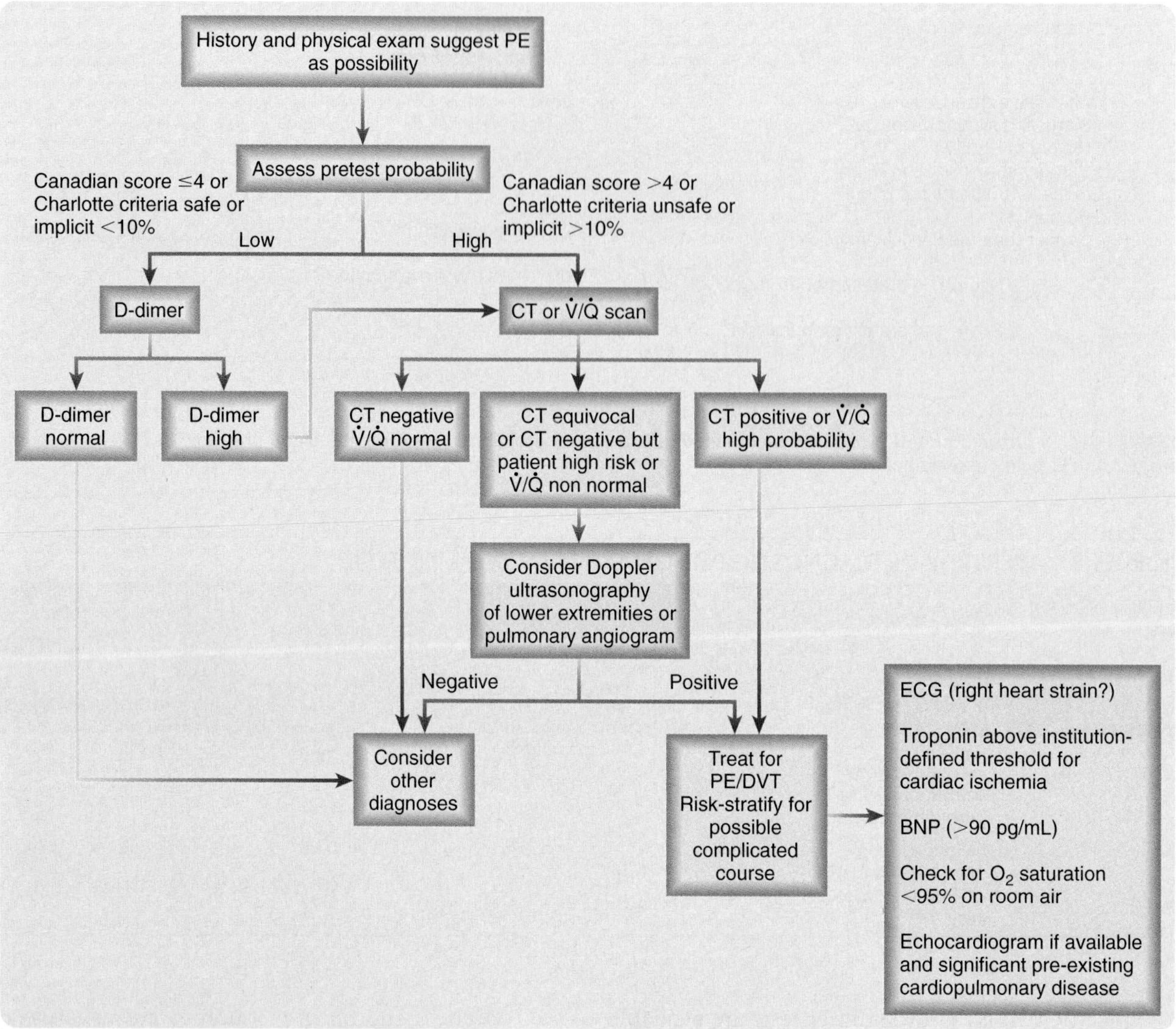
History and physical exam suggest PE as possibility
Assess pretest probability
Canadian score ≤4 or Charlotte criteria safe or implicit <10%
Low
High
Canadian score >4 or Charlotte criteria unsafe or implicit >10%
D-dimer
CT or V̇/Q̇ scan
D-dimer normal
D-dimer high
CT negative V̇/Q̇ normal
CT equivocal or CT negative but patient high risk or V̇/Q̇ non normal
CT positive or V̇/Q̇ high probability
Consider Doppler ultrasonography of lower extremities or pulmonary angiogram
Negative
Positive
Consider other diagnoses
Treat for PE/DVT Risk-stratify for possible complicated course
ECG (right heart strain?)
Troponin above institution-defined threshold for cardiac ischemia
BNP (>90 pg/mL)
Check for O2 saturation <95% on room air
Echocardiogram if available and significant pre-existing cardiopulmonary disease

FIGURE 65-3 Typical algorithmic approach to ruling out pulmonary embolism (PE). CT, computed tomography; DVT, deep venous thrombosis.

harm than benefit. These criteria are only an attempt to support clinician judgment when probability of PE is already very low, and are not intended to replace or dictate individual patient-based decision-making. Patients who meet the PERC but for other reasons are thought to need testing for PE should undergo evaluation (Fig. 65-3; Box 65-2).

CT has largely supplanted the use of ventilation-perfusion scans because of the usual positive/negative result scans produce as well as the fact that other chest diseases may be seen with CT. Sensitivity and specificity of chest CT angiography has improved with the advent of the multidetector CT scanner with higher spatial resolution and lower image acquisition time. Overall, well-accepted sensitivity and specificity data are lacking owing to differences in equipment used, image acquisition technique, and image interpretation, but spiral CT is generally accepted to have a sensitivity of more than 90% and a specificity of more than 90%. One systematic review based on

BOX 65-2

Pulmonary Embolism Rule-out Criteria

- Age < 50 years
- Pulse < 100 beats/min
- Oxygen saturation > 94%
- No hemoptysis
- No clinical evidence of deep venous thrombosis (DVT)
- No hormone use
- No recent surgery or trauma
- No history of pulmonary embolism or DVT

3500 patients and 15 studies reported a pooled negative predictive value of 99.1% and a likelihood ratio for a negative result of 0.07.[16] Newer CT machines with 16- and 64-detector systems and sophisticated post-image processing will become more commonplace and will improve upon the diagnostic accuracy of current imaging. Even with these newer machines, however, pretest probability assessment and D-dimer testing will be important to avoid unnecessary radiation exposure in a large number of patients with a very low likelihood of PE.

Ventilation-perfusion scanning is an alternative to CT for patients who have contrast agent allergy or renal insufficiency. It is important to remember that in patients who are high risk according to pretest probability assessment and who have low or indeterminate ventilation-perfusion scan results, PE cannot be assumed to have been ruled out. These patients need anticoagulation and further testing, most typically duplex Doppler ultrasonography of the lower extremities.

Controversy exists regarding the optimal approach in pregnant patients. The radiation dose estimated from CT of the chest is low (250 mrad) and with shielding of the abdomen and pelvis, only a small fraction of it would be expected to reach the fetus; this fraction is probably significantly lower than the threshold of teratogenicity, which is estimated at 5 rad. However, no longitudinal data exist to determine clearly what the optimal strategy should be. Ventilation-perfusion scans have been used over a long period in pregnant patients and are thought to pose almost no risk to the fetus. However, as ventilation-perfusion scans are done less and less, the availability of technicians and experienced nuclear medicine physicians may decline and limit the availability of ventilation-perfusion scans in the future.

Regardless of the imaging method available or chosen, it should be emphasized that both CT and ventilation-perfusion scanning involve very low rates of radiation to the fetus. The EP must discuss the issue with the patient, obstetrician, radiologist, and family before any tests are ordered, noting the pretest probability of disease, the extremely low probability of radiation-associated negative effects, and the significant morbidity of undiagnosed PE. Tests should be performed if there is appropriate concern for PE. The use of D-dimer testing is problematic in pregnant patients, in whom the likelihood of a false-positive result increases with progression of the pregnancy. It has been advocated that an elevated cutoff point for a quantitative D-dimer test in a low-risk patient may be adequate to rule out PE. No prospective management trials have been conducted, however, to clarify a potential role of the D-dimer test in pregnancy. If it is used in early pregnancy, when the likelihood of a false-positive result is lowest, a normal value in a low-risk scenario may be sufficient to rule out PE. Patients who are otherwise at low risk for PE should not be automatically assumed to have high pretest probability just because they are pregnant.

Treatment of Pulmonary Embolism without Shock

The defining characteristic of the EP role is to perform simultaneous treatment and evaluation. Oxygen should be given to patients with suspicion for PE. Correction of local hypoxemia assists in decreasing reflexive vasoconstriction in the pulmonary vasculature. Patients who are considered to be at high risk for PE with high pretest probability should be treated empirically with anticoagulation while awaiting test results, provided that they have no contraindications to such therapy. Low-molecular-weight heparin (LMWH) has become standard therapy and, despite being more costly than unfractionated heparin, has benefit in achieving appropriate anticoagulation rapidly without the need to monitor coagulation values and is also associated with a lower likelihood of heparin-induced thrombocytopenia with thrombosis. Some studies have suggested that LMWH may have somewhat higher efficacy in terms of time to thrombus resolution and recurrence in DVT patients.[17] Unfractionated heparin is still a safe and effective treatment and may be especially useful if a shorter period of anticoagulation is desired with the ability to cease therapy rapidly. Unfractionated heparin and LMWH do not act to breakdown existing thrombus but, rather, to reduce thrombus propagation and extension. Endogenous mechanisms of antithrombin and plasmin activation are responsible for gradually effecting thrombus breakdown. The dose of enoxaparin, the most commonly used LMWH, is 1 mg/kg given subcutaneously every 12 hours. The dose of unfractionated heparin is 80 U/kg given as a bolus intravenously and then 18 U/kg/hr as an intravenous (IV) infusion, titrated to achieve a prethrombin time between 71 and 90 (2.3 to 3 times normal).

Risk Stratification

It is critical to assess likelihood for further deterioration. It is possible to gather data in the ED to estimate a patient's likelihood of right heart strain and early shock. ECG is the starting point, in which careful attention to the presence of T wave inversion in leads V_1 through V_4, incomplete or complete right bundle branch block, an S wave in lead I, a Q wave in lead III, and inverted T wave in III may all be evidence of right heart strain. The pulse oximetry value, when less than 95%, is an important predictor of 30-day mortality in normotensive patients with PE presenting to the ED.[7] Other means of risk stratification are measurements of blood levels of brain natriuretic peptide (BNP) and troponin. Although these measurements are not specific for PE and not helpful in the diagnosis, emerging studies show that when troponin and BNP are normal in PE patients, the probability of a complicated course is reduced. The most accepted means of risk stratification is echocardiography. This modality is not often available as an emergency procedure in many EDs, but it

BOX 65-3

Echocardiographic Signs of Severe Pulmonary Embolism

- Right heart dysfunction
- Hypokinesis
- Dilation
- Tricuspid regurgitation
- Elevated pulmonary artery pressure
- Impediments to left ventricular (LV) output
- Septal shift
- Decreased LV filling

is a rapid means of identifying right heart strain (Box 65-3).

Treatment of Patients with Confirmed Pulmonary Embolism and Shock

The American College of Emergency Physicians, in a 2003 practice guideline statement, recommended considering fibrinolytic therapy for hemodynamically unstable patients with confirmed PE as a class B recommendation (moderate level of certainty).[11] It has not been shown to provide mortality benefit, but in selected samples of subjects with PE and shock, fibrinolytic therapy has been associated with better perfusion and improved right heart function. Alternatives to pharmacologic fibrinolysis are catheter-based techniques of thrombus fragmentation and surgical embolectomy. These methods are unlikely to be available outside of dedicated interventional radiology and cardiovascular surgery centers and are highly operator-dependent. There is no conclusive evidence that they are superior to pharmacologic approaches.

When fibrinolytic agents have been studied in patients without overt shock but with right ventricular dysfunction, these drugs have been associated with decreased need to escalate therapy with vasopressors as well as with lower rates of intubation and need for additional thrombolytic treatment.[18] The on-label use of fibrinolytic therapy for PE approved by the U.S. Food and Drug Administration (FDA) is alteplase, as a 15-mg IV bolus then 85 mg IV over 2 hours (heparin infusion is stopped during alteplase administration). Off-label dosing regimens for alteplase have been described, including a 15-mg bolus with a 85-mg infusion over 90 minutes, used in cardiac arrest with return of circulation.[19] Fibrinolytic therapy has been concluded to be appropriate in patients with confirmed PE and shock. Identification of PE as a cause of shock can be aided by a stepwise approach to diagnosis with consideration of other causes of shock. A bedside echocardiogram and close attention to ECG findings as well as BNP and troponin blood levels may provide clues that shock is secondary to PE. If shock exists and no right heart abnormalities are seen on echocardiogram, PE is a very unlikely explanation for the shock.

Disposition

The patient with a new diagnosis of acute PE should be admitted to the hospital for initiation of anticoagulation and serial evaluations of oxygen saturation, blood pressure, and overall functional capacity. Patients with minimal cardiopulmonary comorbidity who have normal oxygen saturation and no evidence of hypotension are typically discharged shortly after starting warfarin anticoagulation, and trends outside the U.S. have described outpatient treatment of low-risk patients with PE. In either case, patients continue home self-treatment with LMWH for several days until outpatient INR measurements exceed 2.0, at which point they may stop LMWH and continue warfarin.

Patients with low oxygen saturation (less than 95%), right heart strain on echocardiography or ECG, elevated BNP (>90 pg/mL), or elevated troponin (>0.1 pg/mL troponin T or >1.0 pg/mL troponin I) should be observed closely for deterioration. Decisions as to assigning them to the intensive care unit should be made on the basis of the level of specialized care patients need (Box 65-4).

Patients with a history of previous PE present several challenges. *Recurrent PE,* defined as acute clot in a new or different anatomic location, should be treated as acute PE, and if patients are no longer taking anticoagulant agents, they need treatment as previously described. In contrast, persistent clot is seen in the same areas of previous PE and may also

BOX 65-4

Indications for Intensive Care Unit Assignment in a Patient with Pulmonary Embolism

- Shock
- Mental status acutely decreased and not improving
- Respiratory effort poor or worsening
- Cardiac ischemia
- Serum troponin elevation
- Worsening electrocardiographic findings
- High oxygen requirement
- Worsening overall clinical course:
  - Pulse increasing
  - Blood pressure decreasing
  - Oxygen saturations decreasing
  - Recurrent syncope

BOX 65-5

Trends for the Future in Diagnosis, Prognosis, Treatment, and Disposition of Patients with Pulmonary Embolism

- Improved understanding of the diagnostic performance of multidetector computed tomography
- Effective risk stratification for short- and long-term adverse events
- Improved understanding of thrombophilic states
- Outpatient or ED observation-based treatment of selected low-risk patients with new pulmonary embolism
- Oral direct thrombin inhibitors as alternatives to warfarin and low-molecular-weight heparin
- Fibrinolytic therapy for patients at high risk for immediate and later adverse events

look radiographically distinct from acute PE on CT. If patients are appropriately anticoagulated and have no other indications for admission, they may be discharged from the ED provided that no other inpatient evaluation for the symptoms is warranted. However, these patients with no visualized new clot on CT may be suffering from chronic venous thromboembolic syndrome, a condition in which pulmonary hypertension and chronic vascular changes in the lung can lead to chronic disabling dyspnea and other symptoms that may prompt ED evaluation. Such patients should be referred for outpatient echocardiogram and pulmonary consultation, but no specific therapy as of yet exists for this condition, which may affect 1% to 3% of all patients with PE (Box 65-5).

REFERENCES

1. Goldhaber SZ: Pulmonary embolism. Lancet 2004;363:1295-305.
2. McCaig LL: National Hospital Ambulatory Medical Care Survey: 2000 Emergency Department Summary. Hyattsville, MD, National Center for Health Statistics, 2002.
3. Courtney DM, Kline JA: Identification of prearrest clinical factors associated with outpatient fatal pulmonary embolism. Acad Emerg Med 2001;8:1136-1142.
4. Wood KE: Major pulmonary embolism: Review of a pathophysiologic approach to the golden hour of hemodynamically significant pulmonary embolism. Chest 2002;121:877-905.
5. Goldhaber SZ, Visani L, De Rosa M: Acute pulmonary embolism: Clinical outcomes in the International Cooperative Pulmonary Embolism Registry (ICOPER). Lancet 1999;353:1386-1389.
6. Kasper W, Konstantinides S, Geibel A, et al: Management strategies and determinants of outcome in acute major pulmonary embolism: Results of a multicenter registry. J Am Coll Cardiol 1997;30:1165-1171.
7. Kline JA, Hernandez-Nino J, Newgard CD, et al: Use of pulse oximetry to predict in-hospital complications in normotensive patients with pulmonary embolism. Am J Med 2003;115:203-208.
8. Alpert JS, Smith R, Carlson J, et al: Mortality in patients treated for pulmonary embolism. JAMA 1976;236:1477-1480.
9. The Urokinase Pulmonary Embolism Trial: A national cooperative study. Circulation 1973;47(Suppl):II1-II108.
10. Randomised trial of intravenous streptokinase, oral aspirin, both, or neither among 17,187 cases of suspected acute myocardial infarction: ISIS-2. ISIS-2 (Second International Study of Infarct Survival) Collaborative Group. Lancet 1988;2:349-360.
11. American College of Emergency Physicians Clinical Policies Committee; Clinical Policies Committee Subcommittee on Suspected Pulmonary Embolism: Clinical policy: Critical issues in the evaluation and management of adult patients presenting with suspected pulmonary embolism. Ann Emerg Med 2003;41:257-270.
12. Wells PS, Anderson DR, Rodger M, et al: Derivation of a simple clinical model to categorize patients' probability of pulmonary embolism: Increasing the model's utility with the SimpliRED D-dimer. Thromb Haemost 2000;83:416-420.
13. Kline JA, Nelson RD, Jackson RE, Courtney DM: Criteria for the safe use of D-dimer testing in emergency department patients with suspected pulmonary embolism: A multicenter use study. Ann Emerg Med 2002;39:144-152.
14. Kline JA, Mitchell AM, Kabrhel C, et al: Clinical criteria to prevent unnecessary diagnostic testing in emergency department patients with suspected pulmonary embolism. J Thromb Haemost 2004;2:1247-1255.
15. Wells PS: Advances in the diagnosis of venous thromboembolism. J Thromb Thrombolysis 2006;21:31-40.
16. Quiroz R, Kucher N, Zou KH, et al: Clinical validity of a negative computed tomography scan in patients with suspected pulmonary embolism: A systematic review. JAMA 2005;293:2012-2017.
17. Breddin HK, Hach-Wunderle V, Nakov R, Kakkar VV: Effects of a low-molecular-weight heparin on thrombus regression and recurrent thromboembolism in patients with deep-vein thrombosis. N Engl J Med 2001;344:626-631.
18. Konstantinides S, Geibel A, Heusel G, et al: Heparin plus alteplase compared with heparin alone in patients with submassive pulmonary embolism [comment]. N Engl J Med 2002;347:1143-1150.
19. Goldhaber SZ, Nadel ES, King ME, Sharma A: Case records of the Massachusetts General Hospital. Weekly clinicopathological exercises. Case 17-2004: A 42-year-old woman with cardiac arrest several weeks after an ankle fracture. N Engl J Med 2004;350:2281-2290.

Chapter **66**

Venous Thrombosis and Venous Disorders

James V. Ritchie

KEY POINTS

- Deep vein thrombosis (DVT) is difficult to diagnose. Twenty-five percent to 50% of patients do not have known risk factors.
- Known risk factors for DVT are Virchow's triad, blood stasis, vessel wall injury, and hypercoagulable state.
- A patient with a negative evidence-based evaluation has a less than 2% chance of having DVT.
- Ultrasonography is a magnificent tool in diagnosing DVT. However, different ultrasound protocols carry significantly different prognostic values.
- Post-phlebitic syndrome is common and potentially disabling.
- No clear consensus exists as to whether or not to treat for an isolated calf DVT.

Scope and Outline

Venous thrombotic disease is a ubiquitous threat to young and old, causing acute and chronic morbidity. This morbidity may be acute and life-threatening (pulmonary embolus), limb-threatening (phlegmasia cerulea dolens), or chronic and debilitating (post-phlebitic syndrome, venous ulceration, recurrent deep vein thrombosis [DVT]).

Most patients with DVT have well-established risk factors, which are summarized by Virchow's triad. However, 25% to 50% have no identifiable risk factors at the time of evaluation (Table 66-1). Patients without apparent risk factors may have an unrecognized condition, such as cancer, systemic lupus erythematosus, or protein C deficiency.

Symptoms of DVT, when present, are nonspecific and may go unrecognized by both patients and physicians. Although the diagnosis of DVT from simple history and physical findings is unreliable, an evidence-based diagnostic approach using carefully chosen testing is accurate, efficient, and safe.

Low-molecular-weight heparins and warfarin are generally effective in treatment of DVT and prevention of recurrence. Administration of thrombolytic agents is indicated only for extensive limb-threatening thrombosis that is not amenable to vascular surgery.

Post-phlebitic syndrome is a common consequence of DVT, even when the DVT has been properly treated. This syndrome may be permanently disabling.

Perspective

The major manifestations of venous thromboembolic disease are DVT, pulmonary embolism, phlegmasia cerulea dolens, and post-phlebitic syndrome. Minor manifestations include simple thrombophlebitis and pain.

Table 66-1 KNOWN RISK FACTORS FOR DEEP VEIN THROMBOSIS

Damage to the vessel wall	Trauma Vascular surgery Intravenous line
Alterations to flow	Immobility Hospitalization Myocardial infarction Heart failure Pregnancy
Hypercoagulability	Cancer Lupus anticoagulant Anticardiolipin antibody Antiphospholipid antibody Factor V Leiden mutation Factor II G20210A Antithrombin deficiency Protein C deficiency Protein S deficiency Increased concentration of factor VII, IX, or XI Hyperhomocysteinemia Surgery Pregnancy Oral contraceptives and hormone replacement

BOX 66-1

The 25% List for Deep Vein Thrombosis (DVT)*

- 25%-50% of cases of DVT are idiopathic (no commonly recognized risk factors).[2]
- 25% of patients with DVT have some degree of post-phlebitic syndrome.[3,8]
- 25% of patients with DVT have a recurrence after 5 years.[3]
- 10%-25% of patients with suspicion of DVT from the history and physical findings are found by confirmatory testing to have the disease.
- 25% of patients with known DVT have proximal extension of the thrombosis even with appropriate treatment with warfarin.

*Superscript numbers refer to chapter references.

Thrombosis causes inflammation, which may destroy valves, especially if the inflammation is long-standing. Also, distention of the vessel prevents coaption of valves. If valves are rendered incompetent, especially if a significant obstruction remains from residual organized thrombus, the patient is at risk for post-phlebitic syndrome, which causes persistent, sometimes disabling pain and swelling.

Epidemiology

The incidence of DVT is currently impossible to determine, because thromboses may be present without symptoms. Which thromboses are dangerous and which are innocuous have also not been clearly shown.

■ STRUCTURE AND FUNCTION

The body's thrombotic and fibrinolytic systems maintain a healthy balance under normal conditions. The fibrinolytic system demonstrates a mild predominance until local conditions favor the formation of clot.

Thrombotic disease may be characterized as a normal process that has been inappropriately activated. Clot has formed when it is not needed and subsequently threatens normal circulatory function.

■ VIRCHOW'S TRIAD

Virchow's triad summarizes the risk factors for DVT, which are blood stasis, vessel wall injury, and hypercoagulable state.

Fifty percent to 75% of cases of DVT are associated with known risk factors. As few as 25% are idiopathic[1,2] (Box 66-1). Table 66-1 contains a partial listing of known risk factors for DVT. Surgery increases a patient's risk, but orthopaedic surgery, major vascular surgery, and neurosurgery are especially risky. Clots may form in a location remote from the operative site. The greater likelihood of thrombosis persists for months after the procedure. However, the risk of recurrence is low in this population.[3]

Hospital admission, myocardial infarction, heart failure, and acute infection raise the risk for DVT significantly. Cancer also increases the risk, although not equally among the types of cancer. Polycythemia vera, Hodgkin's lymphoma, and brain, liver (primary), ovarian, and pancreatic carcinomas carry the highest risks.[4,5]

■ ABSENCE OF RISK FACTORS

About 25% of patients with DVT have no known risk factors for inappropriate clotting. However, the majority have a condition known to put them at risk.

A significant percentage of those without identifiable risk factors may have an unrecognized clotting disorder. However, extensive testing to find that disorder is probably not helpful. Patients with a known clotting disorder are no more likely to have a second thrombosis than those whose DVT is idiopathic.

In approximately 10% of patients with idiopathic DVT, cancer may be detected at initial or follow-up evaluation. If DVT recurs without apparent cause, the risk of cancer is significantly higher.[6,7] Risk of discovery of subsequent cancer remains higher (odds ratio of 1.3) even 10 years after the initial DVT.[4]

■ PRE-EXISTING ANTICOAGULANT THERAPY

Anticoagulant therapy decreases the incidence and propagation of thrombosis but does not completely prevent it. In approximately 25% of patients with known proximal DVT who are undergoing a therapeutic warfarin protocol, follow-up ultrasound scan demonstrates proximal extension of thrombus.

Anatomy

Venous blood return from the lower extremities is usually resisted by gravity and therefore depends on a system of intact venous valves, active squeezing from muscular contraction, or external pressure. If that system is disabled, through lack of muscular contraction or valve injury, venous flow becomes much more sluggish, and pressure in the veins may increase dramatically.

The venous system of any limb is widely interconnected to allow collateral flow. Because clot often begets clot, a thrombus in one vein may easily propagate into other veins. Once formed in a deep vessel, a thrombus may recanalize, organize, or embolize. The term *recanalize* often is used to represent any of several outcomes of a thrombosed vein. The clot may lyse, may retract with residual clot remaining, or may persist with development of predominantly collateral flow.

Indwelling thrombus is not innocuous to its host vessel, commonly producing inflammation in the vein wall. This inflammation can permanently damage the valves. It can also produce synechiae in combination with clot organization, predisposing to formation of future clots.

If the thrombus does not completely recanalize or resolve (and many of them do not, even with treatment), chronic venous insufficiency may follow. Even if the clot recanalizes, residual clot lining the walls of the vessel may prevent valve function. Most chronic venous insufficiency is caused by valve incompetence rather than by residual obstruction by clot.

Unfortunate nomenclature occasionally contributes to a treatment error. The "superficial" femoral vein is actually a section of the common femoral vein and so is actually part of the deep venous system. Therefore, if clot is reported in the superficial femoral vein, it should be treated as clot in any other deep vein.

Presenting Signs and Symptoms

■ HISTORICAL

Most patients in whom DVT is suspected present with pain or swelling of the involved extremity or with symptoms from embolization. Except in rare obstruction of the inferior vena cava or simultaneous bilateral DVT, the pain and swelling are unilateral. These symptoms may accompany a skin temperature or color change. Patients with chronic DVT may present with chronic skin stasis changes or even venous insufficiency ulcerations. Deep venous thrombi may embolize prior to detection in the legs. Therefore, the presenting symptoms may be those of pulmonary emboli.

■ PHYSICAL EXAMINATION

As expected from the most common complaints, the most common physical findings in DVT are tenderness and swelling. The tenderness may be localized, and the clot may be palpable. However, tenderness may also be regionally generalized owing to distended vessels, inflammation, low-flow ischemia, or other mechanisms.

Pain is a very common, nonspecific symptom. Many DVTs are painless. Therefore, presence or absence of pain is of little utility in diagnosing DVT. The Wells diagnostic criteria award 1 point for pain along the deep venous system only.[9]

Swelling may be minimal or extensive, involving the entire extremity. Pitting edema is more characteristic of an acute thrombus. Chronically involved extremities often demonstrate a dense induration.

Of course, swelling is found in many conditions not associated with DVT, and many patients with DVT have no swelling. Only swelling with conspicuous characteristics has been found to be predictive of DVT. The Wells criteria award points to swelling in an entire leg, swelling producing a calf circumference more than 3 cm larger than in the unaffected leg, and pitting edema greater in the affected leg.[10]

Absence of tenderness and/or swelling has poor negative predictive value for DVT, because as many as 40% of cases are asymptomatic.

Testing for Homan's sign—calf pain elicited by passive dorsiflexion of the ankle—is a virtually useless maneuver, because the results are neither particularly sensitive nor specific. Many other conditions may produce pain with this maneuver, and many patients with DVT do not demonstrate a positive Homan's sign.

RED FLAGS

- The "superficial femoral vein" is really a deep vein. Treat thromboses there as deep vein thromboses (DVTs).
- Patients taking warfarin may still have DVT or extension of a DVT, despite a therapeutic International Normalized Ratio value.
- Do not "rule out" DVT solely on the basis of absence of risk factors. About 25% of DVTs are idiopathic.
- A patient with "idiopathic" DVT has a 10% chance of having an occult malignancy. Ensure follow-up for screening, and advise your patient of your concern.

VARIATIONS AND SUBTLE FEATURES

Phlegmasia Cerulea Dolens

Extensive iliofemoral thrombosis may rarely produce an enlarged, doughy, painful, blue leg, a condition called phlegmasia cerulea dolens (PCD). This condition is limb-threatening, because the majority of venous outflow is clotted and the limb is ischemic. Greatly increased hydrostatic pressure from occluded venous flow results in impressive edema. Intravascular volume suffers as the fluid enters the third space. The edema elevates tissue pressure, which ultimately impedes arterial flow and produces ischemic conditions. If the obstruction is not relieved, venous gangrene may ensue, with limb loss and an associated mortality of approximately 30%.

Post-Phlebitic Syndrome

Inappropriate venous thrombosis may cause chronic valvular incompetence through inflammatory damage, partial recanalization with presence of residual clot, or simple distention producing loss of coaptation. With loss of these valves, blood return from the lower extremity depends on higher venous pressure. This pressure distends the veins and becomes painful. Depending on the extent of valvular damage, the discomfort may be mild or highly disabling. This post-phlebitic syndrome occurs in 23% to 30% of patients with DVT who receive anticoagulants.[8] Patients with severe forms of this disorder may not be able to stand or walk for significant periods and are unable to exercise. Such disability obviously may be career-changing and may occur in young otherwise healthy individuals.

Superficial Thrombophlebitis

Painful inflammation of superficial veins due to thrombus associated with a "palpable cord" is called *superficial thrombophlebitis*. This condition is often considered innocuous but deserves more thought than a quick clinical diagnosis and discharge. A wide range (approximately 0%-50%) in incidence of concomitant or subsequent DVT has been reported. A diagnosis of superficial thrombophlebitis therefore suggests the significant possibility of concomitant DVT and should prompt consideration of ultrasound evaluation. Risk appears to be higher in patients with proximal thrombophlebitis or with known risk factors for inappropriate thrombosis.

If deep venous involvement is not present, a thrombus in the superficial vein is generally not thought to pose a threat of significant embolization. However, this issue is somewhat controversial, especially if the proximal saphenous vein is involved.

Approximately 5% of hospitalized patients with confirmed solitary superficial thrombophlebitis subsequently have DVT with or without pulmonary embolus, and another 15% experience recurrence of superficial thrombophlebitis or extension in the superficial system.[10]

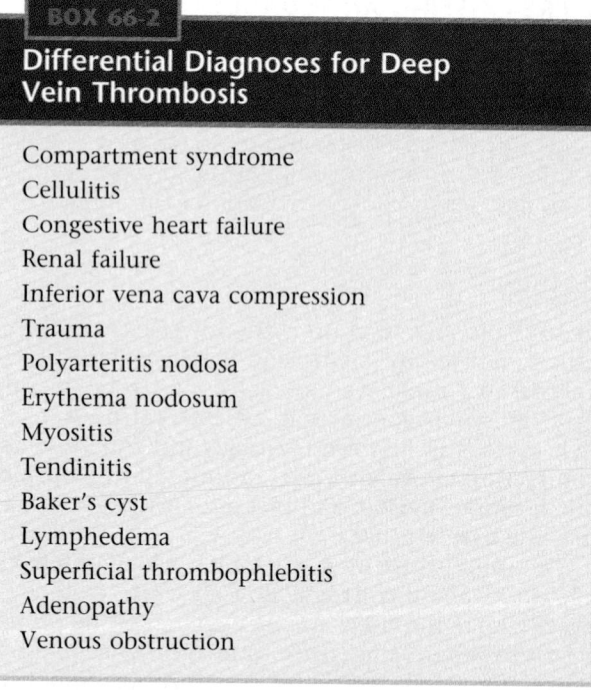

BOX 66-2

Differential Diagnoses for Deep Vein Thrombosis

Compartment syndrome
Cellulitis
Congestive heart failure
Renal failure
Inferior vena cava compression
Trauma
Polyarteritis nodosa
Erythema nodosum
Myositis
Tendinitis
Baker's cyst
Lymphedema
Superficial thrombophlebitis
Adenopathy
Venous obstruction

Differential Diagnosis

Box 66-2 lists the differential diagnosis for DVT. The two most important alternatives are discussed here.

COMPARTMENT SYNDROME

Compartment syndrome is also characterized by pain and swelling. Coolness, diminished pulses, and decreased sensation may be present in advanced cases of either condition. Further, a deep calf compartment syndrome may be present despite a supple superficial compartment. Because compartment syndrome and DVT may coexist, the EP should consider evaluating for both even if one is definitively diagnosed.

CELLULITIS

The pain, swelling, and skin color changes associated with cellulitis may be clinically indistinguishable from the findings in DVT, and the two conditions may also coexist. A site of infection such as an insect bite, fever, clearly demarcated border, and marked increase in skin temperature at the affected site all suggest a diagnosis of cellulitis. However, these findings may also be present in a patient with DVT. The inflammation of thrombophlebitis often causes a fever and local skin temperature increase, as well.

Diagnostic Testing

RISK SCORING

No historical or physical factors are individually dependable in diagnosing DVT, and testing is time-consuming and costly. Such a situation calls for a reliable risk-stratification tool. Wells and colleagues[9] have prospectively validated such a tool, which uses four historical and five physical examination criteria. Such stratification has been shown to be useful and safe in guiding diagnostic testing and is therefore recommended as a first step in the diagnostic evaluation for possible DVT.

RADIOGRAPHY

Ultrasonography

Ultrasound scanning is noninvasive and highly accurate in detection of proximal DVT. Its sensitivity compared with venogram is approximately 97% to 100%, with a specificity of 98% to 99% for proximal thrombosis. The accuracy of ultrasonography is lower for evaluation of the calf because the vessels there are smaller and deeper.[11]

Ultrasound protocols vary widely, even between departments in the same institution or between technicians in the same department. Predictive values for different protocols are not identical. Duplex Doppler imaging studies evaluate vessel filling and pulse waves as well as compressibility.

Comprehensive Ultrasound

A comprehensive ultrasound protocol evaluates compressibility and Doppler assessments at 2-cm intervals from the inguinal ligament to the malleoli. One prospective descriptive trial using experienced vascular technologists evaluated 375 nonpregnant patients suspected to have a first episode of DVT who underwent such a comprehensive ultrasound protocol with negative results. On 3-month follow-up, only approximately 1% of untreated patients had recurrent DVT.[12]

Limited ED Ultrasound Scanning

A limited ultrasound study of the common femoral and popliteal veins performed by EPs appears to have excellent negative predictive value compared with formal, more comprehensive duplex ultrasound studies performed in a radiology department or vascular clinic; several studies have tested this concept.[13-16] Although the amount of operator training and the specific protocols used varied within these studies, reported sensitivity values were high (88.9% to 100%). Specificity values were not as impressive, however (75% to 91.9%). Such a high sensitivity produces a high negative likelihood ratio.

Because reported specificity values for ED ultrasound scanning are lower, the EP should consider obtaining confirmatory studies if the ED ultrasound result is positive or equivocal. False positive scans may occur when a lymph node or chronic clot are mistaken for an acute thrombus

Therefore, according to available data, a clearly negative result of a limited scan performed by a properly trained EP suggests the absence DVT in the proximal leg veins. If results of such a bedside ED study are positive or equivocal, confirmatory studies from the radiology or vascular service should be obtained.

Second Ultrasound Scan

In a patient in whom the results of both a first ultrasound scan (compression only, from femoral vein to trifurcation) and a second scan peformed at 1 week are negative, the risk of symptomatic DVT at 6 months is approximately 1%. Interestingly, only about 1% of patients returning for a scheduled second ultrasound scan are usually found to have DVT.[9,17] The EP should consider arranging for a second scan in 1 week for a patient in whom the initial scan result is negative but the D-dimer result is positive or there is a high risk for DVT.

Venography

Venography remains the historical gold standard for diagnosis of DVT but is now rarely performed. This modality carries potential morbidity, including actually inducing formation of DVT in previously normal vessels, as well as contrast reaction and renal contrast injury. Other less invasive tests are almost as accurate and may be more clinically useful.

Treatment based on venography results may also lead to unnecessary anticoagulation, because the test detects small isolated clots that have low likelihood of causing significant morbidity.

Runoff Venography after Chest Computed Tomography

When computed tomography (CT) of the chest is obtained as part of a pulmonary embolism protocol, many institutions also obtain CT scans through the pelvis and legs to assess for the presence of DVT. A wide variety of protocols have been published. An overall approximate sensitivity of 95% and specificity of 98% are reported, when the protocols are grouped, in comparison with ultrasonography or conventional venography.

LABORATORY TESTS

D-Dimer Test

The D-dimer test alone is an inadequate test to definitively eliminate or establish a diagnosis of DVT.[18] However, a normal D-dimer test result combined

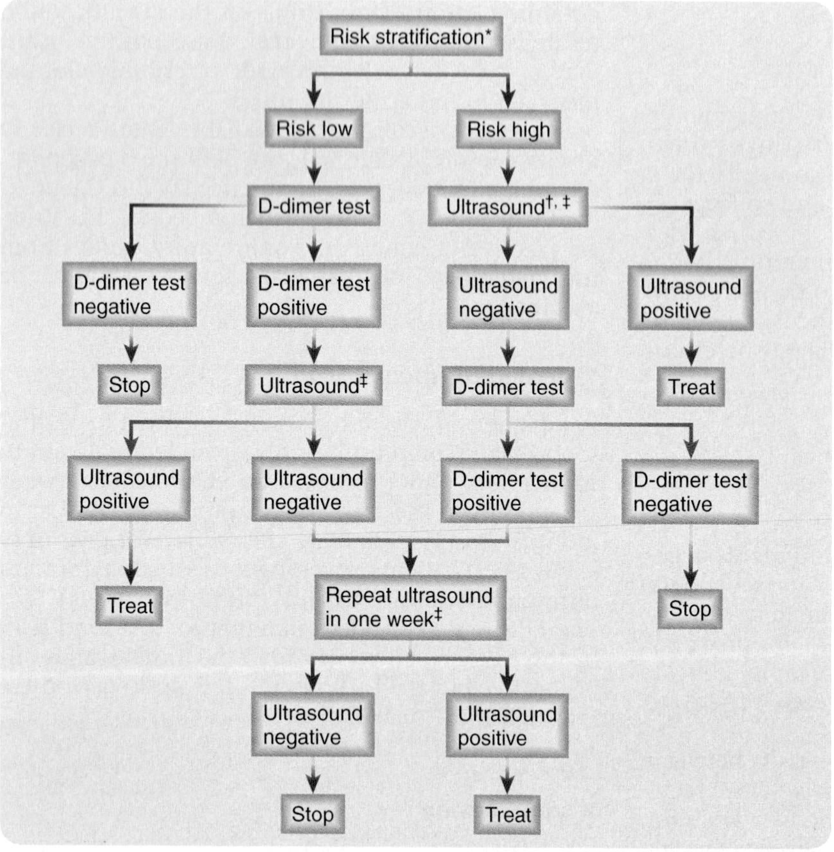
Risk stratification*
Risk low
Risk high
D-dimer test
Ultrasound†, ‡
D-dimer test negative
D-dimer test positive
Ultrasound negative
Ultrasound positive
Stop
Ultrasound‡
D-dimer test
Treat
Ultrasound positive
Ultrasound negative
D-dimer test positive
D-dimer test negative
Treat
Repeat ultrasound in one week‡
Stop
Ultrasound negative
Ultrasound positive
Stop
Treat

FIGURE 66-1 Diagnostic algorithm for a patient with suspicion of deep vein thrombosis in the ED. *Risk stratification is performed using the Wells criteria.[9] †Consider obtaining D-dimer test simultaneously with ultrasound, to speed disposition if results of both are negative. ‡Compression ultrasound scan from femoral vein to top of trifurcation. (Modified from Wells PS, Anderson DR, Rodger M, et al: Evaluation of D-dimer in the diagnosis of suspected deep-vein thrombosis. N Engl J Med 2003;349:1227-1235.)

Tips and Tricks

- Physical examination is unreliable for the diagnosis of DVT, but bedside ultrasound is a highly reliable tool.
- In "low-risk" patients, DVT may be essentially ruled out by a negative D-dimer test result.
- In "high-risk" patients, DVT may be essentially ruled out by negative findings of ultrasound and D-dimer test.

with a low clinical risk effectively rules out DVT.[9,19,20]

■ Testing for Procoagulant Factors

Although many prothrombotic conditions, such as hyperfibrinogenemia, protein C deficiency, and factor V Leiden mutation, may increase the likelihood of development of recurrent DVT, testing for them may not be clinically helpful in predicting future thrombosis. The overall risk for recurrence in patients with these factors is similar to that in patients with idiopathic DVT.[21] Nonetheless, such testing may guide future decisions, such as duration of warfarin treatment. Such testing is usually conducted by the primary care provider.

■ COMBINING LABORATORY AND ULTRASOUND LIKELIHOOD RATIOS

If the result of the ultrasound compression scan from femoral vein to calf trifurcation is negative and a high- or moderate-sensitivity D-dimer test result is also negative, the patient's risk of symptomatic DVT at 6 months with no treatment is approximately 1% to 2%.[17] The safety of this approach is similar to that of repeating the ultrasound scan at 1 week and is valid in all risk groups. Patients found to be at low risk for DVT in a clinical model who also have a negative D-dimer result have a risk of less than 1% of having DVT.

Figure 66-1 provides an evidence-based algorithm for diagnosing lower-extremity DVT using these concepts.

Treatment and Disposition

■ SUPERFICIAL THROMBOPHLEBITIS

Far less is known about the optimal treatment of superficial thrombophlebitis without deep vein involvement. If DVT is not present, superficial thrombophlebitis is usually treated with nonsteroidal anti-inflammatory medications, heat, and compression. The pain may persist for weeks, and the condition may recur. Further, superficial thrombosis may propagate into the deep venous system. The EP should inform the patient about the risks and the need for follow-up.

ISOLATED CALF DEEP VEIN THROMBOSIS

Anticoagulant Therapy Controversial

Treatment of isolated calf DVT with anticoagulants is controversial. Advocates of treatment cite the higher risk of proximal propagation with concomitant risk of clinically significant pulmonary embolus. Post-phlebitic syndrome and recurrent DVT are more prevalent in untreated patients. Opponents argue that isolated calf DVT may embolize but rarely produces clinically significant pulmonary embolus, and that a strategy using a second ultrasound scan in 1 week in untreated patients has been shown to be safe. Further, the risk of bleeding is obviously higher in treated patients.

Follow-up Crucial

The future of a DVT is impossible to predict, even with use of anticoagulants. Some DVTs recanalize, some extend, and some embolize. Especially if no treatment is begun, the EP should arrange for the patient to have a follow-up ultrasound scan in 1 week.

DEEP VEIN THROMBOSIS PROXIMAL TO THE CALF

Anticoagulant Agents

Proximal DVT should be treated in the ED with a low-molecular-weight heparin (LMWH). These agents are as effective as unfractionated heparin at preventing recurrent venous thromboembolism and may reduce overall mortality. Further, they are at least as safe and are associted with a lower incidence of bleeding.[22-24] In the initial treatment of DVT, once-daily dosing appears to be as effective and as safe as twice-daily dosing.[25]

Warfarin therapy is usually begun concurrently and is continued for 3 months after the first episode of DVT. The longer the patient maintains a therapeutic International Normalized Ratio (INR) value (2.0 to 3.0) during the treatment period, the lower the risk of post-phlebitic syndrome.[26] Also, the risk of recurrent venous thromboembolism is reduced for as long as warfarin is used, although the risk of major bleeding remains.[27]

Many physicians are using LMWH rather than warfarin throughout the treatment course. LMWH may be as effective in decreasing the likelihood of recurrent DVT and is safer than warfarin.[28] Administration of LMWH requires more education and involvement of the patient, and higher administration costs, although these costs are offset by the reduction in specific laboratory testing.

Other anticoagulants, such as fondaparinux, a factor Xa inhibitor, and ximelagatran, an oral thrombin inhibitor, appear to be as effective and safe as current regimens and are undergoing further testing.[29,30]

Thrombolytic Agents

Thrombolytic agents are not recommended for treatment of uncomplicated DVT. Standard treatment is effective, and the risk of significant bleeding from thrombolytics outweighs potential benefit. The only present indication for use of thrombolytics is PCD, but only in selected patients.

Thrombolytics may be used systemically or locally, via directed catheter. No one has demonstrated a significant patient-oriented outcome improvement with thrombolysis of DVT unless PCD is present.[31]

Thrombolysis definitely increases clot resolution and diminishes incidence of post-phlebitic syndrome but increases the incidence of bleeding, including hemorrhagic stroke. These risks may diminish with careful patient selection. Improved survival has not been demonstrated, however.[32]

Compression Stockings

Use of elastic compression stockings significantly reduces the incidence and severity of post-phlebitic syndrome in patients with DVT.[33,34]

Surgical Removal

Excision of senechiae and residual obstruction may improve the lot of patients with post-phlebitic syndrome.[35]

Disposition

Recently, some centers have begun treating patients with DVT and even hemodynamically stable pulmonary embolus as outpatients.[36] However, patients with large or physiologically threatening DVT should be hospitalized for initiation of treatment.

PHLEGMASIA CERULEA DOLENS

A diagnosis of PCD should prompt immediate anticoagulation and fluid resuscitation. Unless contraindicated, full-dose heparin should be used. The involved limb should be elevated well above the level of the heart. Because the patient's intravascular volume is probably depleted due to third spacing, fluid resuscitation should also be administered.

The EP should consult with the admission team regarding consideration of thrombolytic therapy or vascular surgery. The two approaches appear to be equally effective in limb salvage. Bleeding complications are more common with thrombolysis, but this risk must be weighed against those of surgery.[37]

Some authorities advocate placement of an inferior vena cava filter prior to thrombolytic therapy of

PATIENT TEACHING TIPS

- Follow up with your primary care manager for ongoing treatment.
- Most people have resolution of the clot within 3 months, if they use their anticoagulants.
- You are at risk for post-phlebitic syndrome, which may leave you with permanent pain and swelling in your leg.
- *When appropriate:* You should have a repeat ultrasound scan in a week.
- *If idiopathic DVT is diagnosed:* You may have a disorder that makes you more likely to form inappropriate clots, and you have a higher risk of forming similar clots in the future. You also have an approximate 10% chance of having cancer. You should follow up with your doctor to consider screening tests.
- *Return precautions:* You should come back to the ED immediately if you have chest pain, difficulty breathing, worsening pain, or swelling in your leg.

PCD, although a clear benefit has not been demonstrated experimentally.

REFERENCES

1. Cushman M, Tsai AW, White RH, et al: Deep vein thrombosis and pulmonary embolism in two cohorts: The longitudinal investigation of thromboembolism etiology. Am J Med 2004;117:19-25.
2. Heit JA, O'Fallon WM, Petterson TM, et al: Relative impact of risk factors for deep vein thrombosis and pulmonary embolism: A population-based study. Arch Intern Med 2002;162:1245-1248.
3. Prandoni P, Lensing AW, Cogo A, et al: The long-term clinical course of acute deep venous thrombosis [see comment]. Ann Intern Med 1996;125:1-7.
4. Baron JA, Gridley G, Weiderpass E, et al: Venous thromboembolism and cancer [erratum appears in Lancet 2000;355:758]. Lancet 1998;351:1077-1080.
5. Sorensen HT, Mellemkjaer L, Steffensen FH, et al: The risk of a diagnosis of cancer after primary deep venous thrombosis or pulmonary embolism [see comment]. N Engl J Med 1998;338:1169-1173.
6. Piccioli A, Lensing AW, Prins MH, et al: Extensive screening for occult malignant disease in idiopathic venous thromboembolism: A prospective randomized clinical trial. J Thromb Haemost 2004;2:884-889.
7. Prandoni P, Lensing AW, Buller HR, et al: Deep-vein thrombosis and the incidence of subsequent symptomatic cancer [see comment]. N Engl J Med 1992;327:1128-1133.
8. Killewich LA, Bedford GR, Beach KW, et al: Spontaneous lysis of deep venous thrombi: Rate and outcome. J Vasc Surg 1989;9:89-97.
9. Wells PS, Anderson DR, Rodger M, et al: Evaluation of D-dimer in the diagnosis of suspected deep-vein thrombosis [see comment]. N Engl J Med 2003;349:1227-1235.
10. Quenet S, Laporte S, Decousus H, et al: Factors predictive of venous thrombotic complications in patients with isolated superficial vein thrombosis. J Vasc Surg 2003;38:944-949.
11. Kyrle PA, Eichinger S: Deep vein thrombosis. Lancet 2005;365:1163-1174.
12. Stevens SM, Elliott CG, Chan KJ, et al: Withholding anticoagulation after a negative result on duplex ultrasonography for suspected symptomatic deep venous thrombosis. Ann Intern Med 2004;140:985-991.
13. Blaivas M, Lambert MJ, Harwood RA, et al: Lower-extremity Doppler for deep venous thrombosis—can emergency physicians be accurate and fast? Acad Emerg Med 2000;7:120-126.
14. Frazee BW, Snoey ER, Levitt A: Emergency department compression ultrasound to diagnose proximal deep vein thrombosis. J Emerg Med 2001;20:107-112.
15. Jang T, Docherty M, Aubin C, et al: Resident-performed compression ultrasonography for the detection of proximal deep vein thrombosis: Fast and accurate. Acad Emerg Med 2004;11:319-322.
16. Jolly BT, Massarin E, Pigman EC: Color Doppler ultrasonography by emergency physicians for the diagnosis of acute deep venous thrombosis. Acad Emerg Med 1997;4:129-132.
17. Kearon C, Ginsberg JS, Douketis J, et al: A randomized trial of diagnostic strategies after normal proximal vein ultrasonography for suspected deep venous thrombosis: D-dimer testing compared with repeated ultrasonography. Ann Intern Med 2005;142:490-496.
18. Heim SW, Schectman JM, Siadaty MS, et al: D-dimer testing for deep venous thrombosis: A metaanalysis. Clin Chem 2004;50:1136-1147.
19. Bates SM, Kearon C, Crowther M, et al: A diagnostic strategy involving a quantitative latex D-dimer assay reliably excludes deep venous thrombosis. Ann Intern Med 2003;138:787-794.
20. Wells PS, Owen C, Doucette S, et al: Does this patient have deep vein thrombosis? JAMA 2006;295:199-207.
21. Christiansen SC, Cannegieter SC, Koster T, et al: Thrombophilia, clinical factors, and recurrent venous thrombotic events. JAMA 2005;293:2352-2361.
22. Dolovich LR, Ginsberg JS, Douketis JD, et al: A meta-analysis comparing low-molecular-weight heparins with unfractionated heparin in the treatment of venous thromboembolism: Examining some unanswered questions regarding location of treatment, product type, and dosing frequency. Arch Intern Med 160;2000:181-188.
23. Gould MK, Dembitzer AD, Doyle RL, et al: Low-molecular-weight heparins compared with unfractionated heparin for treatment of acute deep venous thrombosis: A meta-analysis of randomized, controlled trials. Ann Intern Med 1999;130:800-809.
24. Prandoni P, Carnovali M, Marchiori A; Galilei Investigators: Subcutaneous adjusted-dose unfractionated heparin vs fixed-dose low-molecular-weight heparin in the initial treatment of venous thromboembolism. Arch Intern Med 2004;164:1077-1083.
25. van Dongen CJ, MacGillavry MR, Prins MH: Once versus twice daily LMWH for the initial treatment of venous thromboembolism. Cochrane Database Syst Rev 2005;(3):CD003074.
26. van Dongen CJ, Prandoni P, Frulla M, et al: Relation between quality of anticoagulant treatment and the development of the postthrombotic syndrome. J Thromb Haemost 2005;3:939-942.
27. Hutten B, Prins M: Duration of treatment with vitamin K antagonists in symptomatic venous thromboembolism. Cochrane Database Syst Rev 2006;(1):CD001367.
28. van der Heijden JF, Hutten BA, Büller HR, Prins MH: Vitamin K antagonists or low-molecular-weight heparin for the long term treatment of symptomatic venous thromboembolism. Cochrane Database Syst Rev 2007;4:CD002001.
29. Büller HR, Davidson BL, Decousus H, et al: Fondaparinux or enoxaparin for the initial treatment of symptomatic deep venous thrombosis: A randomized trial. Ann Intern Med 2004;140:867-873.
30. Fiessinger JN, Huisman MV, Davidson BL, et al; THRIVE Treatment Study Investigators: Ximelagatran vs low-molecular-weight heparin and warfarin for the treatment

of deep vein thrombosis: A randomized trial. JAMA 2005;293:681-689.

31. Arcasoy SM, Vachani A: Local and systemic thrombolytic therapy for acute venous thromboembolism. Clin Chest Med 2003;24:73-91.
32. Watson LI Armon MP: Thrombolysis for acute deep vein thrombosis (Cochrane review). Cochrane Database Syst Rev 2007;(4):CD002783.
33. Kolbach DN, Sandbrink MW, Hamulyak K, et al: Non-pharmaceutical measures for prevention of post-thrombotic syndrome. Cochrane Database Syst Rev 2007;(4): CD004174.
34. Prandoni P, Lensing AW, Prins MH, et al: Below-knee elastic compression stockings to prevent the post-thrombotic syndrome: A randomized, controlled trial [see comment]. Ann Intern Med 2004; 141:249-256.
35. Puggioni A, Kistner RL, Eklof B, et al: Surgical disobliteration of postthrombotic deep veins—endophlebectomy—is feasible. J Vasc Surg 2004;39:1048-1052.
36. Wells PS, Anderson DR, Rodger MA, et al: A randomized trial comparing 2 low-molecular-weight heparins for the outpatient treatment of deep vein thrombosis and pulmonary embolism. Arch Intern Med 2005;165:733-738.
37. Berridge DC, Kessel D, Robertson I: Surgery versus thrombolysis for acute limb ischaemia: Initial management [update of Cochrane Database Syst Rev 2000;(4):CD002784]. Cochrane Database Syst Revi 2002;(3):CD002784.

Chapter **67**

Emergency Lower Extremity Venous Ultrasonography for Deep Vein Thrombosis

Emily Baran

KEY POINTS

Emergency ultrasound scanning for deep vein thrombosis is a real-time compression evaluation focusing on the lengths of the common femoral and popliteal veins.

The indication for this examination is clinical suspicion for deep vein thrombosis or pulmonary embolism, and it is performed to answer the question "Is there evidence of deep vein thrombosis?"

A 5- to 10-MHz linear vascular probe is used.

The patient is placed either in the supine position with the head of the bed slightly elevated or in the reverse Trendelenburg position.

The patient's leg should be slightly bent at knee and externally rotated.

Having the patient sit with the legs dangling off the bed or in the prone or decubitus position can be helpful for evaluation of the popliteal vein.

Background

Traditional venous duplex ultrasonography studies are comprehensive and time-consuming because they evaluate all the venous structures along their entire length with both compression and Doppler techniques. Emergency ultrasound for the evaluation of deep vein thrombosis (DVT) is different from duplex studies because its focus is limited to two areas of the proximal lower extremity and it relies primarily on real-time evaluation of vein compression for diagnosis of DVT. Studies have found that limited-compression ultrasonography for DVT has similar results to those of duplex studies for the diagnosis of DVT and can be performed by EPs rapidly at the bedside.[1-4]

Indication

The indication for venous emergency ultrasound of the lower extremity is clinical suspicion for DVT or pulmonary embolus. It is performed to answer the clinical question "Is there evidence of DVT?"

Anatomy and Approach

The patient is most easily imaged either in the supine position with the head of the bed elevated to 30 to

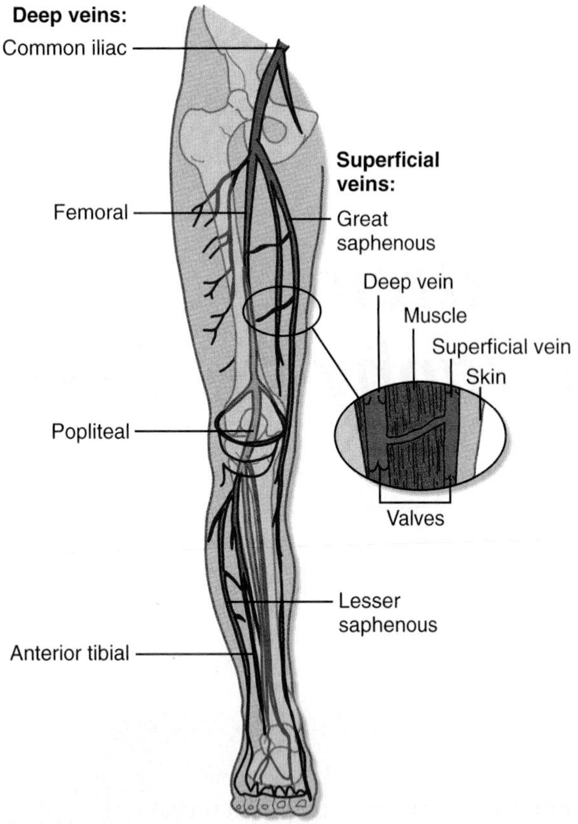
Deep veins:
Common iliac
Femoral
Popliteal
Anterior tibial
Superficial veins:
Great saphenous
Deep vein
Muscle
Superficial vein
Skin
Valves
Lesser saphenous

FIGURE 67-1 Lower extremity venous anatomy. Note that the femoral vein, which is often called the superficial femoral vein, is not actually superficial but instead is a large vein and a common site for deep vein thrombosis in the leg.

45 degrees or in reverse Trendelenburg position to allow venous pooling in the lower extremities. The patient's leg should be slightly bent at knee and externally rotated. The patient can be also be imaged in the sitting position with the legs dangling dependently or changed to a prone or decubitus position for better evaluation of the popliteal vein. A 5- to 10-MHz linear vascular probe is used (see Fig. 5-1).

Representative images of this procedure should include the following views:

- Common femoral vein (before branching) before and with compression
- Proximal femoral vein (after branching) before and with compression
- Distal femoral vein before and with compression (optional)
- Popliteal vein before and with compression

The deep venous anatomy of the lower extremity above the knee is simple, essentially a continuous vascular tube that changes name from knee to groin (Fig. 67-1). The popliteal vein is formed by the joining of anterior and posterior tibial veins with the peroneal vein just below the popliteal crease. The popliteal vein continues through the popliteal fossa, becoming the femoral vein in the distal thigh. The femoral vein joins the deep femoral branch and becomes the common femoral vein, which then becomes the external iliac vein at the level of the inguinal ligament. At this level, the greater saphenous vein (a superficial vein) joins the common femoral vein. The deep femoral branch is short, small, and not regularly imaged because it is not considered a source for significant thrombus. The femoral vein, on the other hand, is often referred to as the superficial femoral vein although it is not a superficial vein but instead a common site for DVT. To avoid confusion, the superficial femoral vein should simply be called the femoral vein.

Below the knee, venous anatomy is variable. Even comprehensive duplex ultrasonography studies can be insensitive for thrombosis below the popliteal vein. This is the biggest limitation of both limited emergency ultrasound and some duplex studies. Patients in whom there is moderate to high clinical suspicion for calf vein thrombosis but in whom findings are normal must undergo a second study in 5 to 7 days to rule out progression of an undiagnosed small clot to the deeper, more proximal veins.

The emergency ultrasound examination for DVT should begin with the probe in transverse orientation high in the inguinal crease to examine the common femoral vein before any branching occurs (Fig. 67-2). The common femoral vein is often next to the artery but then quickly becomes posterior just distal to the inguinal canal. Color flow or pulsed-wave Doppler imaging can be used to help distinguish vein from artery if any variation is present (Fig. 67-3). Interval compression of the vein should then be demonstrated along its length. At a minimum, the common femoral vein should be followed distally beyond branching to the proximal thigh. The femoral vein then can be followed to the distal thigh into the adductor canal. The popliteal vein should then be imaged from posterior to the knee. On the ultrasound screen, the popliteal vein appears anterior to the artery. Anatomically, the vein is actually posterior to the artery, but it is being imaged from the opposite direction, posterior to anterior (Fig. 67-4A). The popliteal vein should be imaged above the popliteal crease and followed distally until it branches.

At each level, the vein should easily and completely compress closed with direct pressure from the ultrasound probe. Enough pressure to slightly deform the artery should be used, and in certain positions, the operator may have to place the other hand posterior to the leg to provide a posterior surface to compress against. Figures 67-4B and C demonstrate the popliteal vein before and with compression.

Interpretation and Limitations

At any site, incompleteness of vein compression when pressure is applied with the probe should be considered a positive result. Figure 67-5 demonstrates a positive study result. In all three areas, the veins do not compress with compression. Intraluminal thrombus may be seen, but its presence is not required for the diagnosis of DVT. All results should be interpreted in the context of the clinical picture (Box 67-1).

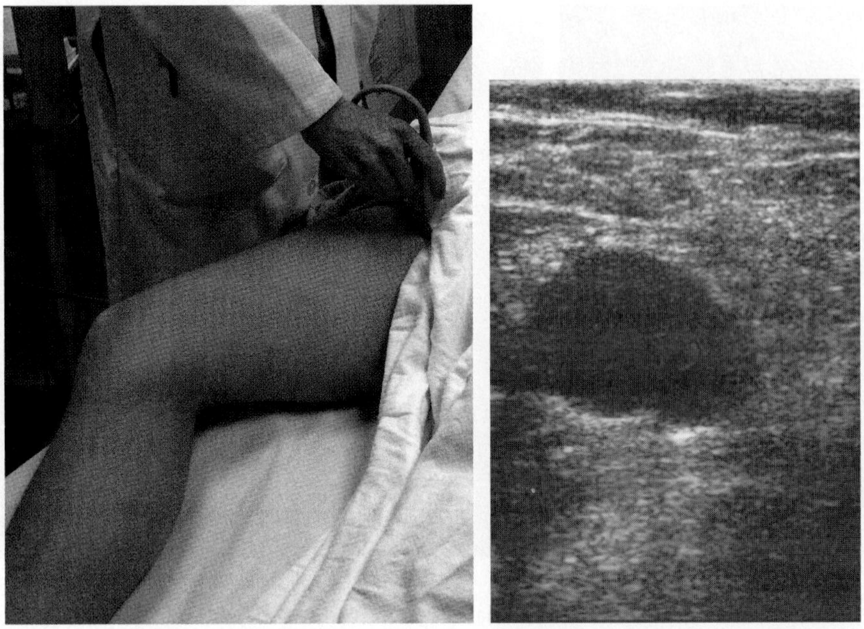

A B

FIGURE 67-2 Probe position for (**A**) and representative normal image of (**B**) emergency ultrasound scanning of the common femoral vein.

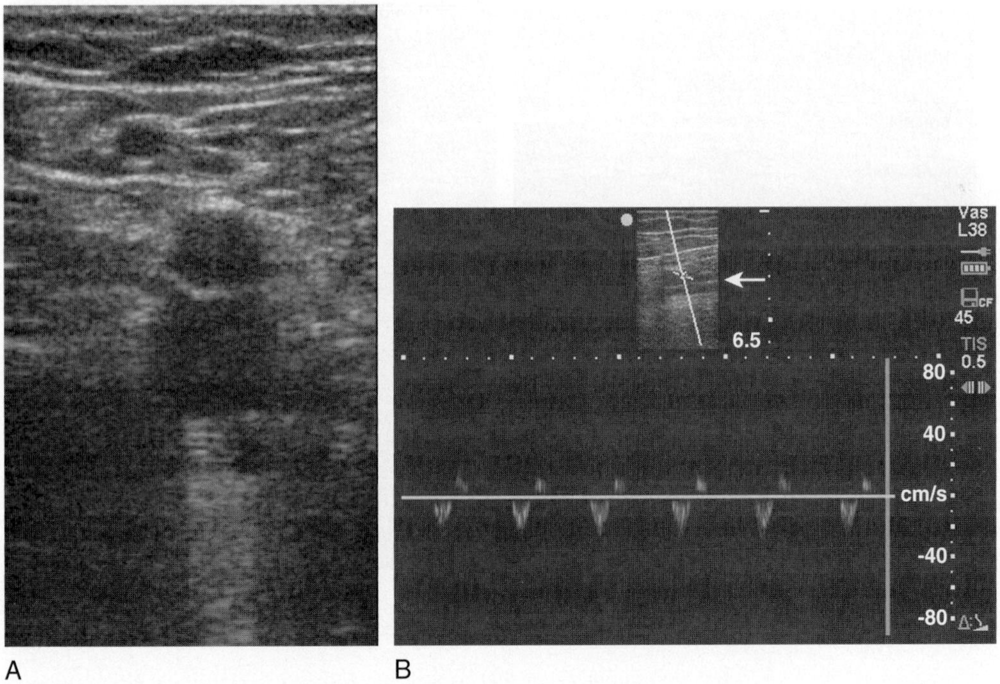
Vas
L38
45
TIS
0.5
6.5
80
40
cm/s
-40
-80

A B

FIGURE 67-3 Normal appearance of femoral vessels in transverse (**A**) and longitudinal (**B**) views. Note that the vein is the posterior tubular structure (*arrow* in **B**) and that the tubular structure lying on top of it has spectral Doppler consistent with an artery.

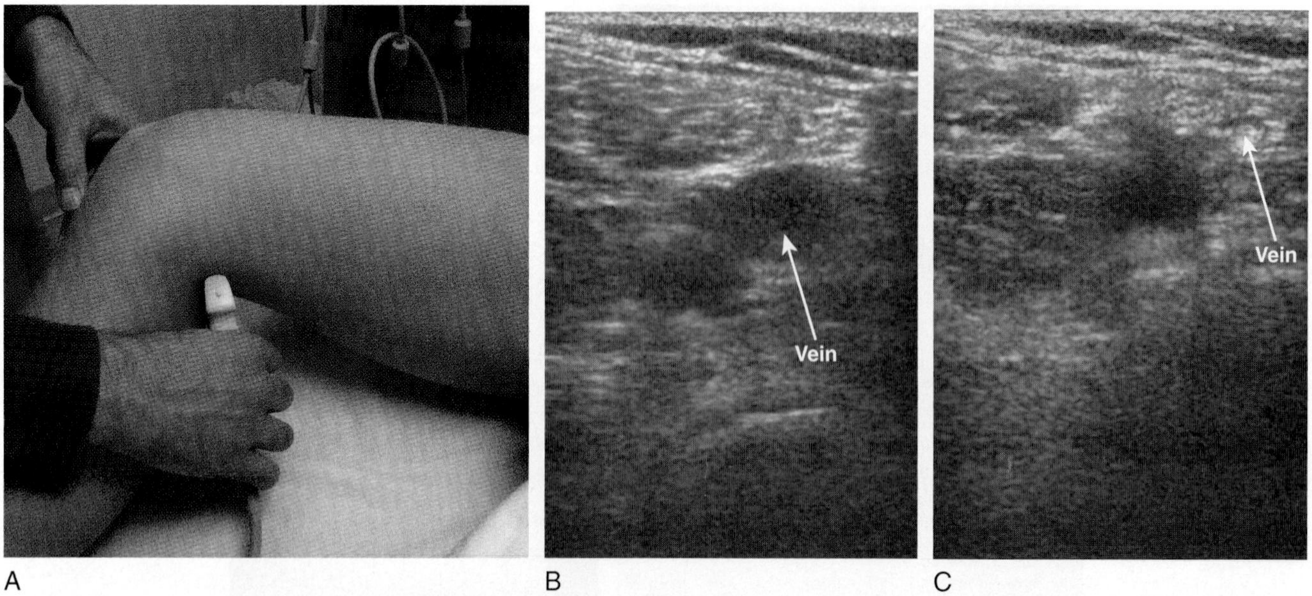
Vein
Vein
A
B
C

FIGURE 67-4 Probe position for (**A**) and representative normal image of (**B**) emergency ultrasound scanning of the popliteal vein. Note that the vein appears on top because the anatomy is being imaged from behind the knee (posterior to anterior). **C,** Image with compression, showing complete closure of the vein and slight deformity of the artery.

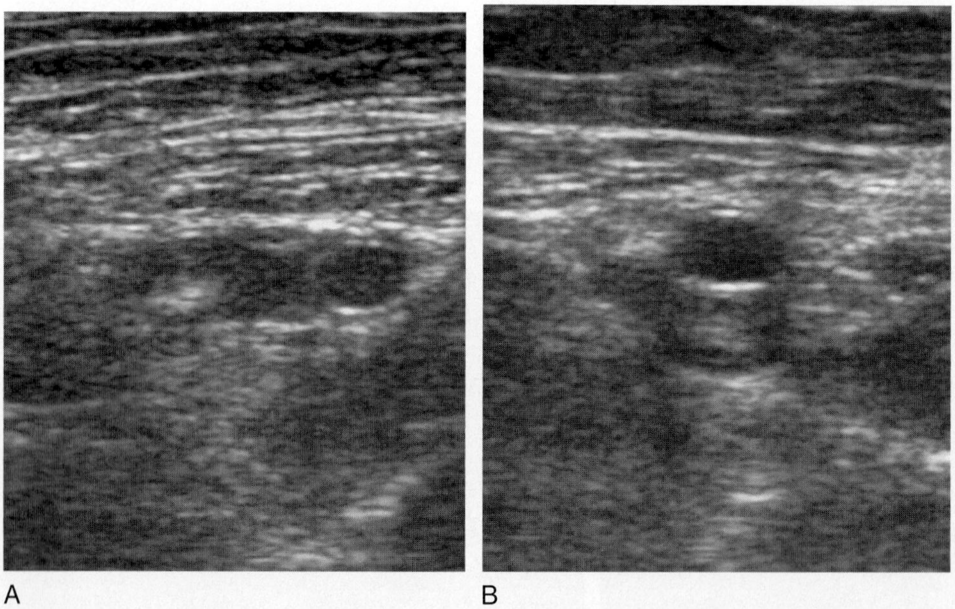
A
B

FIGURE 67-5 **A** to **C,** Images of a positive ultrasound result, in which veins filled with thrombus do not compress when pressure is applied.

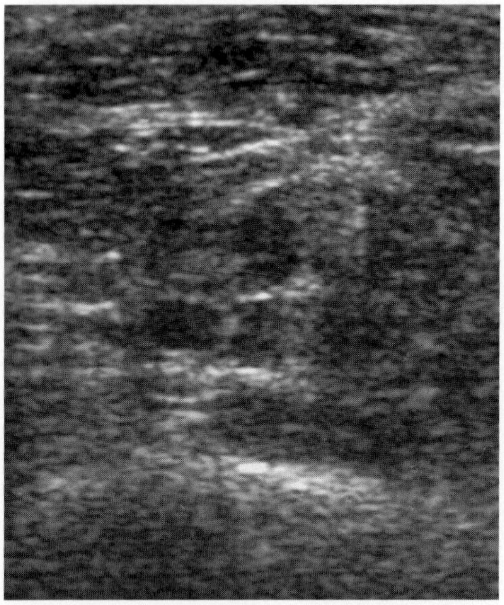

C

FIGURE 67-5, cont'd

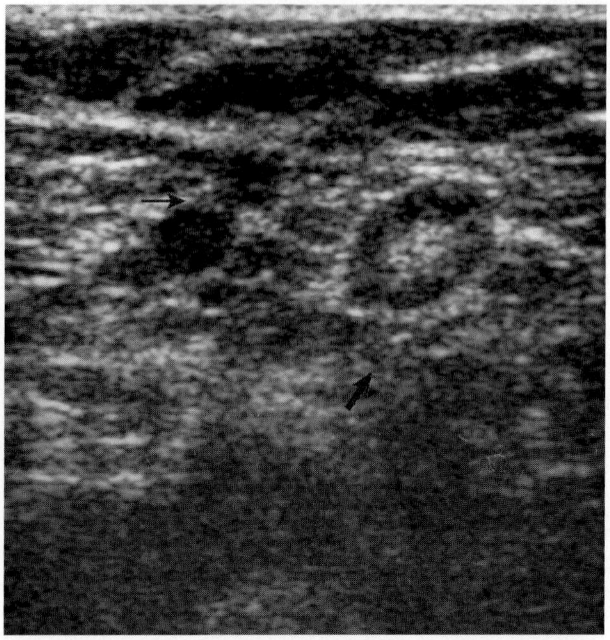

FIGURE 67-6 Inguinal lymph node with appearance similar to that of a transverse image of vein with clot (*large arrow*). Note the actual vascular structures at left (*small arrow*).

BOX 67-1

Pearls and Pitfalls for Emergency Ultrasound for Deep Vein Thrombosis

- Real-time imaging must show complete unequivocal compression in order to rule out deep vein thrombosis.
- If anatomy or compression is questionable, comparison with the other extremity may be helpful.
- Duplication of the popliteal vein can be seen and requires examination of both veins for compression.
- The EP should not be confused by superficial femoral vein terminology. The superficial femoral vein is *the only* femoral vein and should be recognized as part of the deep venous system.
- If there is moderate to high clinical suspicion for venous thrombosis, a second examination should be performed 5 to 7 days later to try to rule out progression of calf thrombus to the deep venous system.

Emergency ultrasound images for DVT can be technically limited in obese patients or because of local tenderness. Indeterminate study results should be followed up with confirmatory testing. For negative scan results in patients with a moderate to high clinical suspicion of DVT, ultrasound should be repeated in 5 to 7 days to rule out progression of potential calf-vein thrombosis.

Inguinal lymph nodes can often look like thrombus-filled femoral vein (Fig. 67-6). The EP can use longitudinal imaging to distinguish between the two, because lymph nodes do not look like tubular vascular structures but have a similar appearance in both transverse and longitudinal imaging planes.

Limited emergency ultrasound for DVT is a focused examination that does not include evaluation of veins below the knee or identify all abnormalities of lower extremity veins.

REFERENCES

1. Pezzullo JA, Perkins AB, Cronan JJ: Symptomatic deep vein thrombosis: Diagnosis with limited compression US. Radiology 1996;198:67-70.
2. Jang T, Docherty M, Aubin C, Polites G: Resident-performed compression ultrasonography for the detection of proximal deep vein thrombosis: Fast and accurate. Acad Emerg Med 2004;11:319-322.
3. Frazee BW, Snoey ER, Levitt A: Emergency department compression ultrasound to diagnose proximal deep vein thrombosis. J Emerg Med 2001;20:107-112.
4. Blaivas M, Lambert MJ, Harwood RA, et al: Lower-extremity Doppler for deep venous thrombosis—can emergency physicians be accurate and fast? Acad Emerg Med 2000;7:120-126.

SECTION **VIII**

Injuries to Bones and Organs

Chapter 68

Traumatic Brain Injury

Daniel Davis

KEY POINTS

Emergency treatment of traumatic brain injury is aimed at both preventing of secondary insults, such as hypoxemia and hypotension, and rapidly identifying of surgically correctable lesions.

Triage to a neurosurgical trauma center is recommended for patients with intracerebral hemorrhage or persistent altered mental status.

Osmotic agents such as mannitol or hypertonic saline are important first-line therapies for patients with elevated intracranial pressure.

Hyperventilation should be avoided but may be needed when a patient has markedly elevated increased intracranial pressure that does not respond to medical therapy.

Early computed tomography (CT) is used to identify intracranial hemorrhage in patients with a significant mechanism of injury, history of altered mental status, or risk factors such as anticoagulant therapy.

Scope

Traumatic brain injury is one of the leading causes of morbidity and mortality, with over 100,000 annual deaths in the United States alone. In addition, an estimated 2 million individuals suffer permanent, life-altering disabilities each year from these injuries. The preponderance of traumatic brain injury among young people has resulted in a greater number of years-of-productive-life lost than either heart disease or stroke. Despite the magnitude of the problem and the enormity of the public health impact, medical science has made little progress in the management of traumatic brain injury and its complications.

Devastating neurologic damage from traumatic brain injury has been implicated as the primary cause of early traumatic death. Traumatic death has been described as occurring in three phases. In the first phase, more than half of all deaths occur in the prehospital environment, even though emergency medical services systems are designed to impact these patients through advanced resuscitation skills, including airway and ventilatory management.[1] The second phase occurs within the first 24 to 48 hours of hospitalization, although hospital trauma systems are designed to deliver emergent, life-saving interventions to this group.[2,3] The final phase of traumatic deaths occurs several days to weeks following hospitalization, typically as a result of multiple organ dysfunction syndrome, acute respiratory distress syndrome, overwhelming sepsis, or other complications of severe trauma.

Modern emergency medical services and organized trauma systems appear to have impacted mortality from nontraumatic brain injury, but there has been little change in traumatic brain injury outcomes over this same period of time. However, evidence suggests that the earliest clinical management and resuscitative maneuvers can lessen later complications.[2,4] Optimal strategies continue to improve as knowledge about the pathophysiology of traumatic brain injury grows. Most important, the impact of early insults such as hypoxia and hypotension on outcome and the optimization of long-term outcome through prompt resuscitation underscore the importance of early clinical maneuvers.

Pathophysiology

Insight into the complex cellular responses to brain injury helps optimize early resuscitative decisions and guide the search for future therapies (Fig. 68-1). For the purposes of this chapter, these responses are separated into macroscopic and microscopic events. This is clearly an artificial construct, however, because the responses to traumatic brain injury are integrated and interrelated. Furthermore, the interactions between events in the brain and the remainder of the body are currently being elucidated and appear to be equally important.

■ MACROSCOPIC EVENTS

The skull represents a rigid compartment containing brain tissue, blood, and cerebrospinal fluid. This is an unforgiving injury model, because hemorrhage or edema following traumatic brain injury leads to rapid increases in intracranial pressure. Initially, cerebrospinal fluid can be shunted out of the skull via the ventricles and cisterns. However, this capacity is quickly overcome by severe traumatic brain injury, leading to a rapid rise in intracranial pressure and a compromise in cerebral blood flow with cerebral ischemia. Ultimately, the brain tissue itself may be forced downward across the rigid tentorium or out of the base of the skull itself, resulting in a herniation syndrome and rapid death. Therapies are designed to decrease intracranial pressure, either through evacuation of intracranial hematomas, decompressive craniectomy, ventricular drainage, controlled hyperventilation, or reduction of cerebral edema via osmotic therapy. These are discussed later in further detail.

Other macroscopic events affect outcome from traumatic brain injury, including systemic hypoxia and hypotension, both of which occur with high frequency. Many investigators have documented an association between these insults and increased mortality in patients with traumatic brain injury. The exact mechanisms are unknown, but hypoxia and hypotension likely exacerbate cellular injury. Although much of our approach to traumatic brain injury resuscitation is driven by the association between secondary insults and outcome, there is little evidence demonstrating that correction of existing physiologic derangements can prevent or reverse neuronal damage. Nevertheless, current practice aims at correction of secondary insults, providing fluid resuscitation in the presence of hypotension, and administration of supplemental oxygen, either invasively or noninvasively, in the presence of hypoxemia.

■ MICROSCOPIC EVENTS

The last decade has led to a dramatic increase in the understanding of the microscopic events that accompany traumatic brain injury. These can be subdivided into cerebrovascular, neurochemical, inflammatory, and intracellular events. Posttraumatic cerebral ischemia appears to be an important mediator of injury. Normal cerebral perfusion is tightly regulated by metabolic byproducts and tissue acid-base status. Disruption of cerebrovascular autoregulatory mechanisms appears to occur rapidly following traumatic brain injury, which may result in either global hypoperfusion and cerebral ischemia or global hyperemia with a subsequent rise in intracranial pressure. These disruptions may occur at different time intervals following injury, even in the same patient. In addition, regional or local hypo- or hyperperfusion may occur, leading to inconsistencies in ischemic injury patterns in individual patients. The individual spatial and

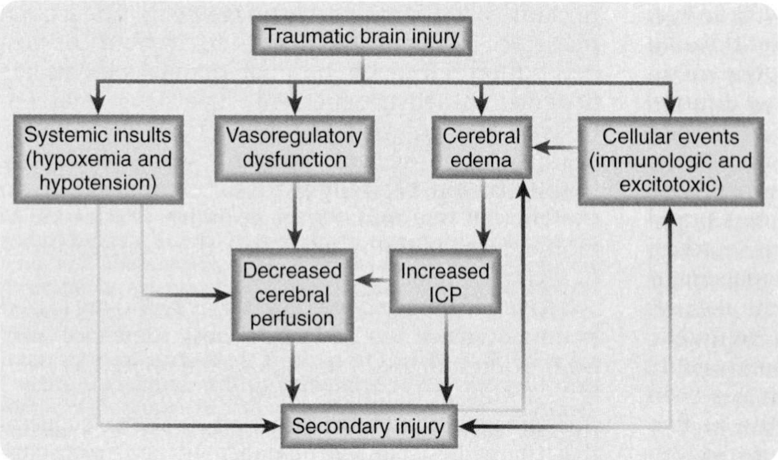
Traumatic brain injury
Systemic insults (hypoxemia and hypotension)
Vasoregulatory dysfunction
Cerebral edema
Cellular events (immunologic and excitotoxic)
Decreased cerebral perfusion
Increased ICP
Secondary injury

FIGURE 68-1 Algorithm showing the pathophysiological mechanisms of traumatic brain injury. ICP, intracranial pressure.

temporal variability with regard to cerebral perfusion, along with the macroscopic intracranial changes that can result in elevated intracranial pressure and a compromise in cerebral blood flow, make cerebral perfusion an attractive target for therapeutic interventions.

Brain tissue is unique in its neurochemical response to injury. Much of the eventual brain injury following traumatic brain injury occurs as the result of excitotoxicity, which involves widespread neuronal depolarization in response to glutamate release. This leads to excitatory receptor activation, with the *N*-methyl-D-aspartate receptor as the best-understood glutamate receptor type. The resultant influx of calcium leads to cellular swelling and rupture as well as intracellular enzyme activation and autolysis. Excitotoxicity may also mediate part of the subsequent inflammatory response to injury as well as initiate a series of intracellular events that result in a delayed cell death via apoptosis.

The inflammatory response to traumatic brain injury also appears an important mediator of outcome. This involves intracerebral inflammatory events as well as the systemic inflammatory response to injury that can affect neurologic outcome directly via circulating cytokines or indirection through such secondary conditions such as multiple organ dysfunction syndrome and acute respiratory distress syndrome. Ultimately, the inflammation-mediated damage appears to occur via direct activation of cell death cascades, indirect effects on cerebral perfusion, and disruption of normal neurotrophoblastic support mechanisms.

Although inflammatory mechanisms of traumatic brain injury were identified several decades ago, specific immunomodulatory therapies have thus far been unsuccessful in improving outcomes. Ironically, hypertonic solutions, originally conceived as a form of osmotic therapy, have demonstrated benefit in traumatic brain injury patients, possibly via their role as immunomodulatory agents.

The least understood pathophysiologic mechanism involves a complex series of intracellular events, including gene transcription and translation, that occurs in response to traumatic brain injury. Each of the other mechanisms discussed previously ultimately produces an intracellular response that can mediate various intercellular and intracellular responses. That response may affect other surrounding cells by undergoing necrosis and perpetuating the local inflammatory response or by releasing neurotransmitters such as glutamate or inflammatory mediators such as tumor necrosis factor. In addition, enzyme activation may occur, resulting in autodigestion via proteolysis or lipolysis. The variability in global and regional cerebral perfusion as well as the potential for secondary insults such as hypoxia and hypotension may also initiate injury mechanisms that mimic the ischemia-reperfusion observed with stroke and cardiac arrest. More recently, a transcriptional response to injury has been identified that may regulate both intracellular and extracellular events and ultimately determine the fate of an individual neuron.

Clinical Evaluation

■ GENERAL

At the present time, no therapies are available to correct the primary brain injury sustained with the initial traumatic insult. Thus, the approach to patients with suspected traumatic brain injury is directed toward reversal of physiologic derangements and avoidance of secondary insults, early triage to a facility with appropriate resources, and expedited neurosurgical care.[1,3,4] It is significant that preventive measures, such as the use of restraint devices or helmets, have been the most effective "therapy" for traumatic brain injury.

■ TRIAGE

An altered level of consciousness in the setting of trauma has been the primary prehospital indicator of traumatic brain injury requiring an advanced level of care. The Glasgow Coma Scale (GCS) score is the method most commonly used to quantify level of consciousness. While the GCS clearly has predictive value, the optimal decision guideline for prehospital triage of potential traumatic brain injury patients has not yet been developed. Furthermore, the GCS has from poor interobserver reliability, and the relationship between the GCS score and outcome is inconsistent at lower values and is nonlinear throughout. However, any change in the GCS is highly predictive of outcome, mandating repeated assessments both in the field and in the ED. In addition, an aging population and increasing use of anticoagulant therapy may lead to more "occult" presentation of traumatic brain injury, such as ataxia, headache, vomiting, and altered mental status remote from the actual traumatic event. The emergence of new technologies to assess traumatic brain injury severity offers hope for more accurate prehospital triage in the future. The ED triage of patients with potential traumatic brain injury includes clinical examination, focusing on the level of consciousness using the GCS score, and radiography using computed tomography (CT). The combination of these assessments can accurately determine which patients require admission for observation or immediate neurosurgical intervention. In addition, the ED assessment should focus on the identification of patients requiring immediate airway intervention or osmotic therapy.

■ CLINICAL FINDINGS

Other clinical findings include pupil reactivity and symmetry, focal sensorimotor deficits, and cerebellar abnormalities. These must be interpreted in combination with mental status to determine whether these lateralizing findings suggest impending herniation or a focal brain injury. For example, an abnormal pupillary examination does not indicate impending herniation in an awake, alert patient. In addition, a thorough cranial examination should be performed to identify external evidence of trauma, potential skull fracture, or evidence of basilar skull fracture. Although the diagnosis of basal skull fracture is largely clinical, classically characterized by periorbital (raccoon's eyes) or retroauricular (Battle's sign) ecchymosis, the significance of this diagnosis is largely related to the potential for associated intracranial hemorrhage diagnosed on CT scanning or because of cerebrospinal fluid leak. With regard to this latter finding, any fluid leaking from the nose or ears should be suspected to be cerebrospinal fluid. It may be useful to test for the presence of glucose, which indicates cerebrospinal fluid rather than other secretions or water.

■ IMAGING

The emergence of CT has revolutionized the management of traumatic brain injury, providing a rapid, accurate imaging modality available in most EDs. Information that can be determined with excellent sensitivity using noncontrast CT includes the presence of intracranial hemorrhage, assessments of mass effect such as ventricular compression or midline shift, and the presence of significant cerebral edema. Acute hemorrhage appears hyperdense on CT scans, with the shape and location of hemorrhage suggesting the underlying pathology.

Epidural hematomas classically are lentiform or "lens-shaped" due to their association with arterial injury, with the higher pressure involuting the brain parenchyma (Fig. 68-2). Subdural hematomas are more commonly crescent-shaped, with blood from torn veins tracking along the surface of the brain beneath the dura mater (Fig. 68-3). Intraparenchymal hemorrhage can exist as a discrete hematoma or as multiple smaller foci throughout a contused area of brain (Fig. 68-4). In addition to focal areas of hemorrhage, cerebral contusions typically involve cerebral edema, which may progress markedly over several days. Skull fractures may be seen on plain radiographs, but more important is the potential for injury to the underlying brain parenchyma or existence of intracranial hemorrhage (Fig. 68-5). Subarachnoid hemorrhage appears as hyperdensities that appear within the ventricles, along the falx and tentorium, and around the circle of Willis (Fig. 68-6). One of the most elusive diagnoses is diffuse axonal injury, in which the CT results are often much less impressive than the degree of obtundation. Small, punctate hemorrhages along the gray-white interface at the cortical periphery suggest this diagnosis, although the initial scan may be completely normal.

Other modalities used to diagnose traumatic brain injury include magnetic resonance imaging, brain acoustic monitoring, and bispectral electroencephalography. The ability of magnetic resonance imaging to identify cerebral edema and diffuse axonal injury is far superior to that of CT. In addition, newer analysis sequences allow appropriately sensitive detection of acute hemorrhage. However, applications of magnetic resonance imaging in the management of traumatic brain injury have been limited due to the lack of availability of this modality and the absence of treatment algorithms guided by magnetic resonance imaging findings. Newer modalities such as brain acoustic monitoring and bispectral electroencephalography appear to be highly sensitive and specific for the presence of traumatic brain injury, with

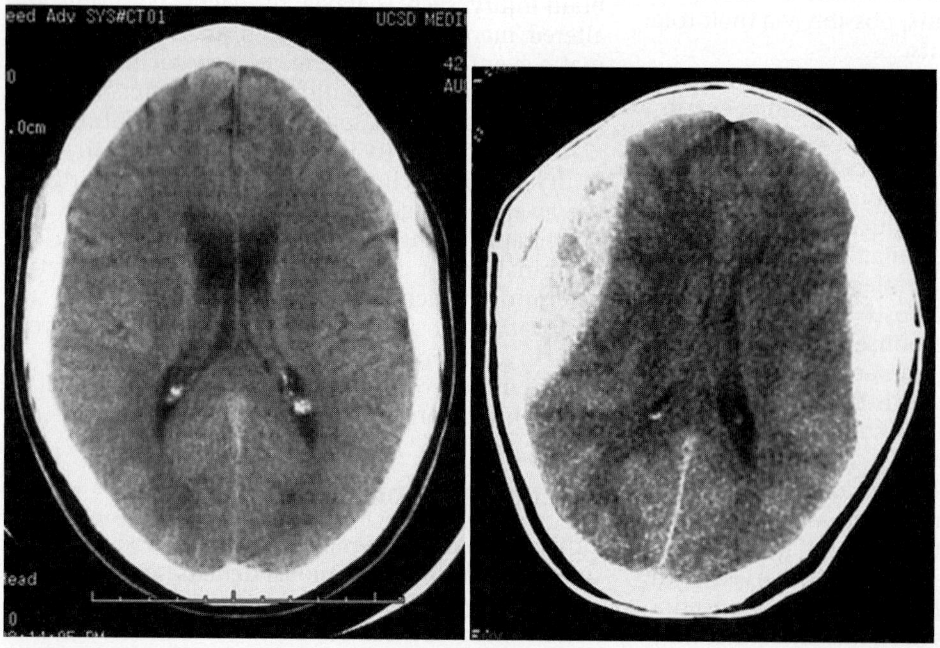
eed Adv SYS#CT01
UCSD MEDI

A B

FIGURE 68-2 **A,** Normal head computed tomography (CT) scan made at the same level as **B. B,** Bilateral epidural hematomas on head CT scan.

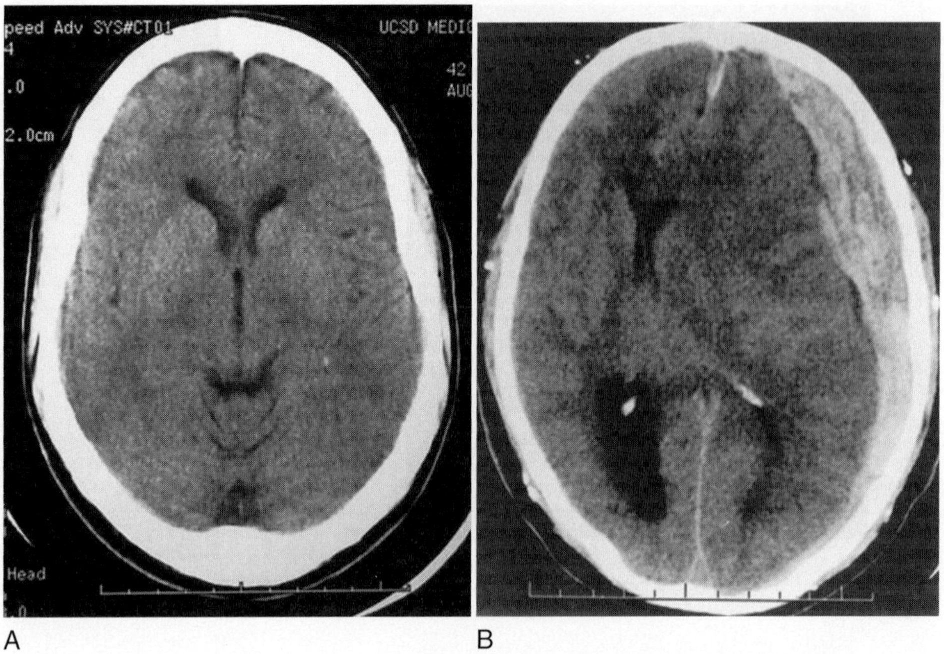
A
B

FIGURE 68-3 **A,** Normal head CT scan made at the same level as **B. B,** Large subdural hematoma with midline shift and compression of ventricles on head CT scan.

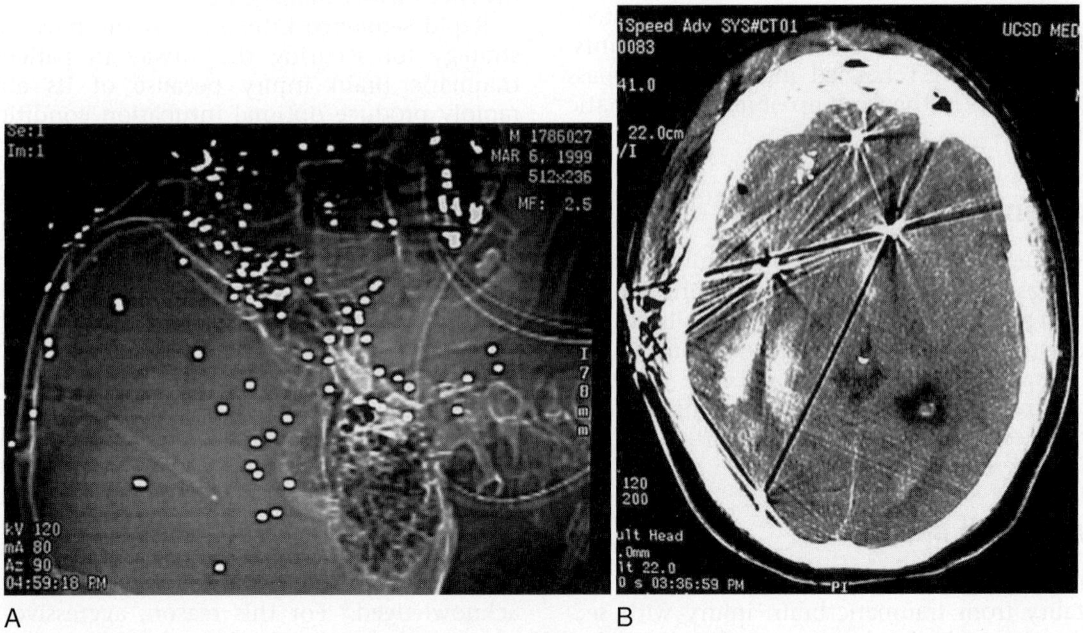
A
B

FIGURE 68-4 **A,** Plain film showing multiple metallic fragments from shotgun blast to eye socket. **B,** Head CT scan of same patient showing intracerebral hemorrhage.

prognostic ability that rivals or exceeds that of CT and with the ability to provide continuous data. Future investigations should focus on the use of these to guide therapy and initiate a more aggressive diagnostic work-up. It is also worth noting that a high coincidence of cervical spine fractures exists with severe traumatic brain injury. For this reason, routine cervical spine radiography should be performed for any traumatic brain injury patient with altered mental status or significant findings on head CT.

Minor Traumatic Brain Injury

The diagnostic and therapeutic decisions surrounding minor traumatic brain injury are somewhat less complex than those of severe injury, but equally controversial. The role of CT in the work-up of minor traumatic brain injury has been much studied, but no census has been achieved with regard to absolute criteria for performing head CT. Important considerations that should suggest head CT scanning include altered mental status at presentation, focal neuro-

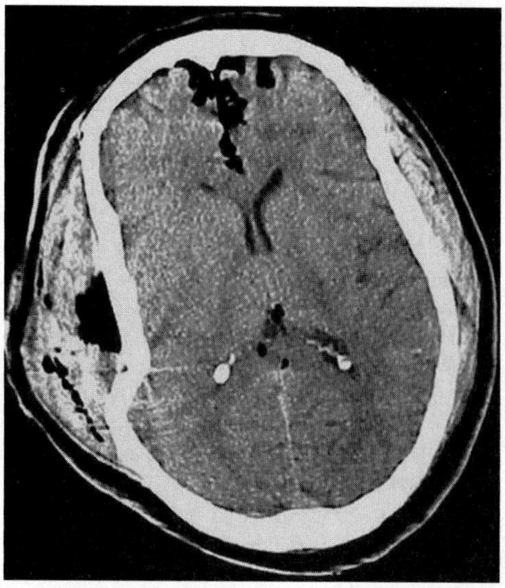

FIGURE 68-5 Depressed skull fracture with intracerebral air on head CT scan.

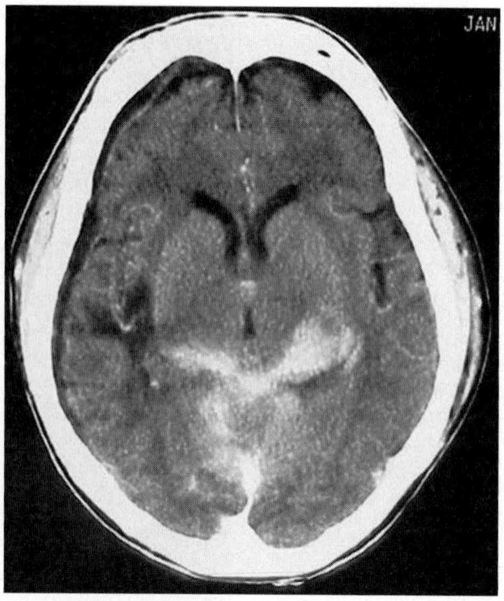
JAN

FIGURE 68-6 Traumatic subarachnoid hemorrhage on head CT scan.

logic deficits, loss of consciousness or amnesia related to the event, seizure, repeated emesis, persistent headache, extremes of age, and use of anticoagulants. The availability of CT has led most EPs to bypass plain radiographs in the work-up of minor traumatic brain injury.

Treatment

The ED management of traumatic brain injury focuses on avoiding secondary insults and reversing physiologic derangement (Fig. 68-7). Conceptually, this is best understood by focusing on oxygenation and perfusion. However, it should be noted that there are important trade-offs with regard to current attempts to reverse these secondary insults and little evidence to support these attempts.

■ AIRWAY AND BREATHING

Many investigators have documented an increase in mortality from traumatic brain injury with secondary insults, including hypoxemia. This has led to an aggressive approach to airway management in patients with severe traumatic brain injury, including early intubation and ventilation with 100% oxygen. The use of pulse oximetry and administration of supplemental oxygen to correct hypoxemia (oxygen saturation <90%) is important in the treatment of all patients with suspected traumatic brain injury.

For patients with severe traumatic brain injury, endotracheal intubation is a critical treatment. The benefits include reversal of hypoxia and prevention of aspiration. Although the axiom "GCS 8, intubate" is ubiquitous in emergency care, the use of the GCS alone may be insufficient because it considers neither oxygenation nor the integrity of airway protective reflexes. Nevertheless, the GCS remains the most commonly used guide to determine the need for invasive airway management.[4]

Rapid sequence intubation is the most common strategy for securing the airway in patients with traumatic brain injury because of its ability to rapidly produce optimal intubation conditions and minimize the adverse effects of laryngoscopy on the injured brain.[1,5-11] Pre-administration of lidocaine may blunt the rise in intracranial pressure associated with laryngoscopy and intubation. Succinylcholine is still the most commonly used neuromuscular blocking agent, due to its rapid onset and short half-life.[1] Recent experimental data suggest that use of succinylcholine during rapid sequence intubation raises intracranial pressure, and the possibility of hyperkalemia with co-existing medical conditions is important to consider; however, succinylcholine remains a first-line paralytic agent because of its ability to rapidly facilitate intubation. The most serious risk associated with rapid sequence intubation is the potential for hypoxia during paralysis and apnea, which is often present but might not be acknowledged.[6] For this reason, aggressive preoxygenation and early use of airway adjunctive measures can minimize hypoxic insults.

Recent data suggest that postintubation ventilation strategies significantly influence outcomes of traumatic brain injury.[7,10] This may reflect the adverse effects of positive-pressure ventilation on cardiac output, hypocapneic cerebral vasoconstriction, or retrograde cerebral transmission of intrathoracic pressure via the jugular venous system, all of which can lead to cerebral hypoperfusion and ischemia. In addition, the use of injurious ventilation strategies in the early resuscitation of critically ill patients appears to result in activation of detrimental inflammatory mechanisms.

Future ventilation strategies should incorporate end-tidal carbon dioxide monitoring to avoid hyper-

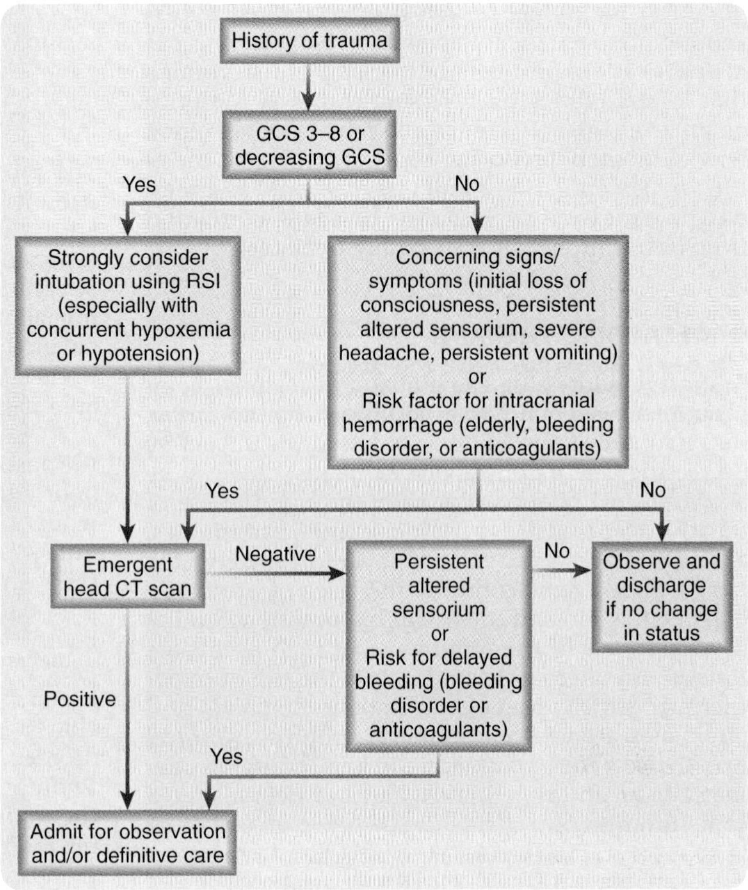

History of trauma
GCS 3–8 or decreasing GCS
Yes
No
Strongly consider intubation using RSI (especially with concurrent hypoxemia or hypotension)
Concerning signs/ symptoms (initial loss of consciousness, persistent altered sensorium, severe headache, persistent vomiting) or Risk factor for intracranial hemorrhage (elderly, bleeding disorder, or anticoagulants)
Yes
No
Emergent head CT scan
Negative
Persistent altered sensorium or Risk for delayed bleeding (bleeding disorder or anticoagulants)
No
Observe and discharge if no change in status
Positive
Yes
Admit for observation and/or definitive care

FIGURE 68-7 Algorithm depicting the differential diagnosis of traumatic brain injury. CT, computed tomography; GCS, Glasgow Coma Scale; RSI, rapid sequence intubation.

ventilation or hypoventilation.[7] These strategies may include the use of positive end-expiration pressure in hemodynamically stable patients with traumatic brain injury.

■ CIRCULATION

Hypoperfusion in the setting of traumatic brain injury is harmful, and every effort should be made to correct and avoid secondary hemodynamic insults.[11] Systemic hypotension has been associated with increased mortality in studies of traumatic brain injury. Although the normal brain can maintain cerebral blood flow despite a range of mean arterial pressures, this ability appears to break down following traumatic brain injury or when there is severe hypotension. In addition, intracranial hypertension requires a high mean arterial pressure to maintain adequate cerebral perfusion pressure. This creates a therapeutic challenge in the treatment of the hypotensive patient with traumatic brain injury.

The use of pressors is generally discouraged in the multiple trauma victim. Thus, the main focus of therapy is volume replacement with blood and IV fluids.[4,11] However, overly aggressive hydration with isotonic fluids may exacerbate cerebral edema. Hypertonic saline solutions appear to have osmotic properties and can lower intracranial pressure and decrease cerebral edema without subsequent diuresis. In addition, hypertonic saline solutions have immunomodulatory effects that may be equally important in mediating outcome from major trauma.

■ CEREBRAL HERNIATION

Cerebral herniation may be central, uncal, or tonsillar. *Uncal herniation* can be caused by a lateral mass of blood that displaces the temporal lobe and compresses the brainstem. Classically, this results in a rapid loss of consciousness, a dilated unilateral pupil, and contralateral hemiparesis.

Central herniation is caused by slowly expanding lesions that create downward pressure, causing altered consciousness but without any localizing signs. Consciousness decreases slowly, eventually leading to small, reactive pupils and Cheyne-Stokes respirations.

Tonsillar herniation occurs when a mass in the posterior fossa pushes cerebellar tonsils through the foramen magnum. The patient experiences occipital headache, posterior neck pain, nausea, vomiting, hypertension, and, sometimes, dizziness and hiccups, followed by a rapid loss of consciousness. The patient may abruptly stop breathing.

Patients with cerebral herniation should receive mannitol, 1 g/kg, repeated every 4 to 6 hours. Hyperventilation to a P_{CO_2} of 25 to 30 temporarily lowers intracranial pressure due to cerebral vasoconstriction. The traditional approach of controlled hyperventilation to reverse intracranial hypertension is out of favor, as the decrease in cerebral blood volume that lowers intracranial pressure comes at the price of an even greater compromise in cerebral blood flow, ultimately producing cerebral ischemia. Therefore, hyperventilation should be used only as a temporizing measure in response to acute herniation from a condition that is surgically treatable.[4,11-15]

■ METABOLIC THERAPY

A strategy addressing the global and regional compromise to cerebral tissue perfusion that accompanies traumatic brain injury is to lessen the impact by decreasing cerebral metabolic demands. This can be accomplished pharmacologically through the use of sedative agents such as benzodiazepines, barbiturates, anticonvulsants, and propofol. Unfortunately, the use of these agents comes at the price of cardiovascular depression and the risk of hypotension. Studies of the efficacy of the routine use of such agents are limited. An alternative approach is the use of hypothermia, which decreases metabolic demands and attenuates delayed cell death via apoptosis. Clinical experience with hypothermia in the setting of traumatic brain injury is limited but has demonstrated some promise.

■ DEFINITIVE CARE

Surgical therapies include evacuation of intracerebral hematomas and decompressive craniectomy. In addition, insertion of intracranial pressure monitors and ventriculostomies allow continuous intracranial pressure measurement to guide clinical decision making.[4,11,12,15] The latter also allows cerebrospinal fluid drainage to reverse intracranial hypertension. Expert trauma and ICU caregivers are necessary to integrate decisions using all available information, provide cardiopulmonary support as needed, and address infectious and inflammatory complications that often accompany critically injured patients.[11,12]

Disposition

The disposition of patients with minor traumatic brain injury is the main consideration for EPs.[13] Intracranial hemorrhage, persistent altered mental status or focal neurologic deficits, or concern about the social situation warrant admission for observation and definitive treatment. A single head CT scan is considered adequate to exclude intracranial hemorrhage in most patients. However, delayed hemorrhage has been reported in patients with a bleeding diathesis or those on anticoagulation, justifying admission for observation and repeat CT after 6 to 12 hours in these patients. Patients with moderate to severe traumatic brain injury, as defined by positive findings on CT scan or persistent altered mental status, should undergo admission and emergent neurosurgical consultation.[11,15]

■ PATIENT TEACHING

The most important considerations when teaching patients sent home from the ED concern the signs and symptoms of an evolving intracranial process, especially in patients how have not had CT imaging. These include increasing headache, persistent vomiting, altered sensorium, confusion, photophobia, and balance problems. Any of these should prompt return to the ED for continued work-up, including appropriate imaging studies.

It is also important to address with patients the possibility of postconcussive syndrome. Although poorly understood, postconcussive syndrome affects many patients with even minor traumatic brain injury. Symptoms may presents weeks to months following the traumatic incident and can include poor concentration, depression, sleep problems, difficulty with relationships, and poor work performance, as well as somatic complaints such as headaches, dizziness, and nausea. There are no specific treatments available for postconcussive syndrome. However, awareness can help validate symptoms that otherwise might not be attributed to the traumatic incident, leading to referrel for neurorehabilitation or psychological services or support groups.

REFERENCES

1. Walls RL: Rapid-sequence intubation in head trauma. Ann Emerg Med 1993;22:1008-1013.
2. Davis DP, Kene M, Vilke GM, et al: Head-injured patients who "talk and die": The San Diego perspective. J Trauma 2007;62:277-281.
3. Fakhry SM, Trask AL, Waller MA, Watts DD. Management of brain-injured patients by an evidence-based medicine protocol improves outcomes and decreases hospital charges. J Trauma 2004;56:492-499.
4. Brain Trauma Foundation: Guidelines for the management of severe head injury. J Neurotrauma 2000;17:457-627.
5. Wang HE, Davis DP, Wayne MA, Delbridge T: Prehospital rapid sequence intubation: What does the evidence show? Prehosp Emerg Car 2004;8:366-377.
6. Wang HE, Peitzman AD, Cassidy LD, et al: Out-of-hospital endotracheal intubation and outcome after traumatic brain injury. Ann Emerg Med 2004;44:439-450.
7. Davis DP, Dunford JV, Ochs M, et al: The use of quantitative end-tidal capnometry to avoid inadvertent severe hyperventilation in patients with head injury after paramedic rapid sequence intubation. J Trauma 2004; 56:808-814.
8. Davis DP, Peay J, Serrano JA, et al: The impact of prehospital endotracheal intubation on outcome in moderate-to-severe traumatic brain injury. J Trauma 2005;59(3):794-801.
9. Davis DP, Hoyt DB, Ochs M, et al: The effect of paramedic rapid sequence intubation on outcome in patients with severe traumatic brain injury. J Trauma 2003;54:444-453.
10. Davis DP, Fakhry SM, Wang HE, et al: Paramedic rapid sequence intubation for severe traumatic brain injury: Perspectives from an expert panel. Prehosp Emerg Care 2007;11:1-8.
11. Advanced Trauma Life Support Course Instructor Manual. Chicago, American College of Surgeons, 7th ed. Chicago, American College of Surgeons, 2004.

12. Bulger EM, Nathens AB, Rivara FP, et al: Management of severe head injury: Institutional variations in care and effect on outcome. Crit Care Med 2002;30:1870-1876.
13. Huizenga JE, Zink BJ, Maio RF, Hill EM: Guidelines for the management of severe head injury: Are emergency physicians following them? Acad Emerg Med 2002;9: 806-812.
14. Marion DW, Spiegel TP: Changes in the management of severe traumatic brain injury: 1991-1997. Crit Care Med 2000;28:16-18.
15. Vukic M, Negovetic L, Kovac D, et al: The effect of implementation of guidelines for the management of severe head injury on patient treatment and outcome. Acta Neurochir (Wien) 1999;141:1203-1208.

Chapter **69**

How to Read a Head CT Scan

Andrew D. Perron

KEY POINTS

Cranial computed tomography (CT) is an extremely useful diagnostic tool used routinely in the care of ED patients.

The EP needs to be able to accurately interpret and act upon certain CT findings without specialist (e.g., radiologist) assistance, because many disease processes are time-dependent and require immediate action.

It has been shown that even a brief educational intervention can significantly improve the EP's ability to interpret cranial CT scans.

Using the mnemonic "blood can be very bad" (where *blood* = blood, *can* = cisterns, *be* = brain, *very* = ventricles, and *bad* = bone) the EP can quickly but thoroughly review a cranial CT scan for significant pathology that demands immediate action.

Cranial CT has assumed a critical role in the practice of emergency medicine for the evaluation of intracranial emergencies, both traumatic and atraumatic. A number of published studies have revealed a deficiency in the ability of EPs to interpret head CTs.[1-6] Significantly, a number of these same studies do show that with even a brief educational effort, EPs can gain considerable proficiency in cranial CT scan interpretation.[2,3] This is important because there are many situations where the EP must interpret and act upon head CT results in real time without assistance from other specialists such as neurologists, radiologists, or neuroradiologists.[7,8] The advantages of CT scanning for CNS pathology in the ED are well known, and include widespread availability at most institutions, speed of imaging, patient accessibility, and sensitivity for a detection of many pathologic processes (particularly acute hemorrhage).

Basic Principles of CT

The fundamental principle behind radiography is the following statement: *X-rays are absorbed to different degrees by different tissues.* Dense tissues such as bone absorb the most x-rays, and hence allow the fewest passing through the body part being studied to reach the film or detector opposite. Conversely, tissues with low density (e.g., air and fat) absorb almost none of the x-rays, allowing most to pass through to the film or detector opposite. Conventional radiographs are two-dimensional images of three-dimensional structures; they rely on a summation of tissue densities penetrated by x-rays as they pass through the body. It should be noted that in plain radiographs, denser objects, because they tend to absorb more x-rays, can obscure or attenuate less dense objects.

As opposed to conventional radiographs, with CT scanning an x-ray source and detector, situated 180 degrees across from each other, move 360 degrees around the patient, continuously detecting and sending information about the attenuation of x-rays as they pass through the body. Very thin x-ray beams are utilized, which minimizes the degree of scatter or blurring that limits conventional radiographs. In CT, a computer manipulates and integrates the acquired data and assigns numerical values based on the subtle differences in x-ray attenuation. Based on these values, a gray-scale axial image is generated that can distinguish between objects with even small differences in density.

ATTENUATION COEFFICIENT

The tissue contained within each image unit (called a pixel) absorbs a certain proportion of the x-rays that pass through it (e.g., bone absorbs a lot, air almost none). This ability to block x-rays as they pass through a substance is known as *attenuation.* For a given body tissue, the amount of attenuation is relatively constant and is known as that tissue's *attenuation coefficient.* In CT, these attenuation coefficients are mapped to an arbitrary scale between −1000 hounsfield units [HU] (air) and +1000 HU (bone) (Box 69-1). This scale is the Hounsfield scale (in honor of Sir Jeffrey Hounsfield, who received a Nobel prize for his pioneering work with this technology).

WINDOWING

Windowing allows the CT scan reader to focus on certain tissues within a CT scan that fall within set parameters. Tissues of interest can be assigned the full range of blacks and whites, rather than a narrow portion of the gray scale. With this technique, subtle differences in tissue densities can be maximized. The image displayed will depend on both the centering of the viewing window and the width of the window. Most CT imaging includes windows that are optimized for brain, blood, and bone (Fig. 69-1).

ARTIFACT

CT of the brain is subject to a few predictable artifactual effects that can potentially inhibit the ability to accurately interpret the images. Besides motion and metal artifact (self-explanatory), the two most common effects are called *beam hardening* and *volume averaging.* It is important to understand these effects and to be able to identify them, because they can mimic pathology as well as obscure actual significant findings.

Beam hardening is a phenomenon that causes an abnormal signal when a relatively small amount of hypodense brain tissue is immediately adjacent to dense bone. The posterior fossa, where there is extremely dense bone surrounding the brain, is particularly subject to this phenomenon. It appears as either linear hyper- or hypodensities that can partially obscure the brainstem and cerebellum. Although beam hardening can be reduced with appropriate filtering, it cannot be eliminated.

Volume averaging (also called partial volume artifact) arises when the imaged area contains different types of tissues (e.g., bone and brain). For that particular image unit, the CT pixel produced will represent an average density for all the contained structures. In the above instance of brain and bone, an intermediate density will be represented that may have the appearance of blood. As with beam hardening, certain techniques can minimize this type of artifact (e.g., thinner slice thickness, computer algorithms), but it cannot be eliminated, particularly in the posterior fossa.

BOX 69-1

Appearance and Density of Tissues on Cranial CT

Appearance

- Black →→ →→ →→ →→ →→ White
- −1000 HU →→ →→ →→ →→ +1000 HU
- Air, fat, CSF, white matter, gray matter, acute hemorrhage, bone

Important Densities

- Air = −1000 HU
- Water = 0 HU
- Bone = +1000 HU

CSF, cerebrospinal fluid; HU, Hounsfield units.

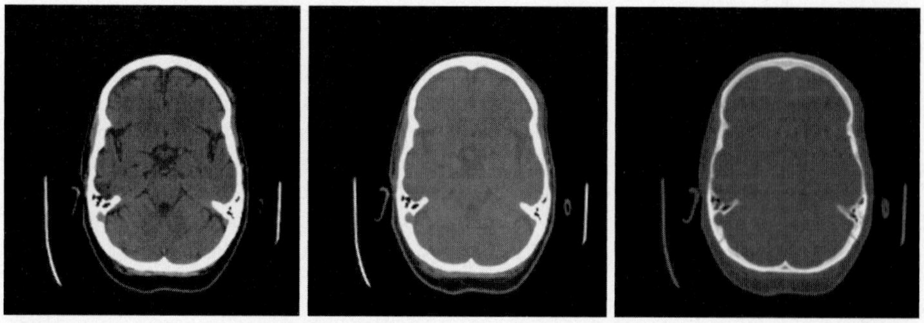

A B C

FIGURE 69-1 CT scan windowing: **A,** brain. **B,** blood. **C,** bone.

Normal Neuroanatomy As Seen on Head CT Scans

As with radiologic interpretation of any body part, a working knowledge of normal anatomic structures and location is fundamental to the clinician's ability to detect pathologic variants. Cranial CT interpretation is no exception. Paramount in head CT interpretation is familiarity with the various structures, ranging from parenchymal areas such as basal ganglia to vasculature, cisterns, and ventricles. Finally, knowing neurologic functional regions of the brain helps when correlating CT results with physical examination findings.

Although a detailed knowledge of cranial neuroanatomy and its CT appearance is clearly in the realm of the neuroradiologist, familiarity with a relatively few structures, regions, and expected findings allows sufficient interpretation of most head CT scans by the EP. Figures 69-2 through 69-5 demonstrate key structures of a normal head CT scan.

▪ IDENTIFYING CNS PATHOLOGY ON CRANIAL CT SCANS

As long as one is systematic in the search for pathology, any number of techniques can be utilized in the review of head CT images. Some recommend a "center-out" technique, in which the examiner starts from the middle of the brain and works outward. Others advocate a problem-oriented approach, in which the clinical history directs the examiner to a particular portion of the scan. In the author's experience, both of these are of limited utility to the clinician who does not frequently review scans. A preferred method, one that has been demonstrated to work in the ED,[2] is to use the mnemonic "*b*lood *c*an *b*e *v*ery *b*ad" (Box 69-2). In this mnemonic, the first letter of each word prompts the clinician to search a certain portion of the cranial CT scan for pathology. The clinician is urged to use the entire mnemonic when examining a cranial CT scan because the presence of one pathologic state does not rule out the presence

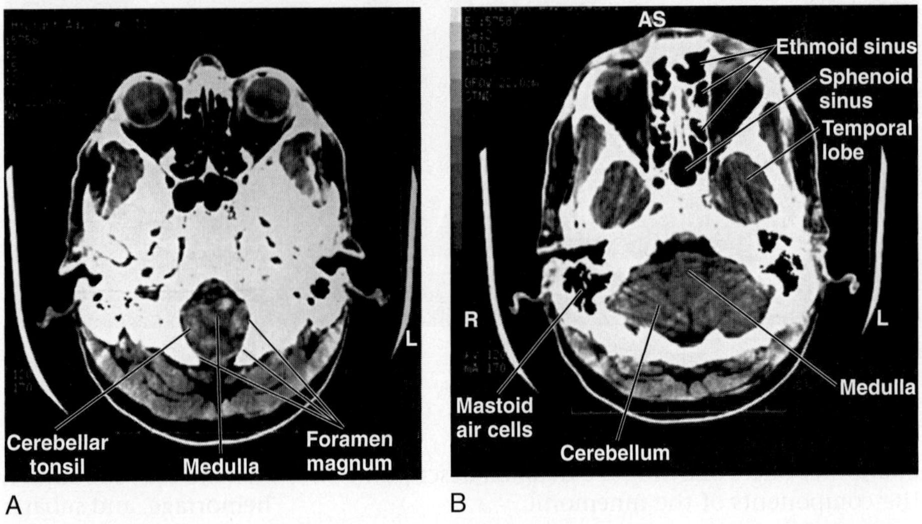
Cerebellar tonsil
Medulla
Foramen magnum
L
A
AS
Ethmoid sinus
Sphenoid sinus
Temporal lobe
R
L
Mastoid air cells
Cerebellum
Medulla
B

FIGURE 69-2 Head CT—Normal anatomy: **A,** posterior fossa; **B,** low cerebellum.

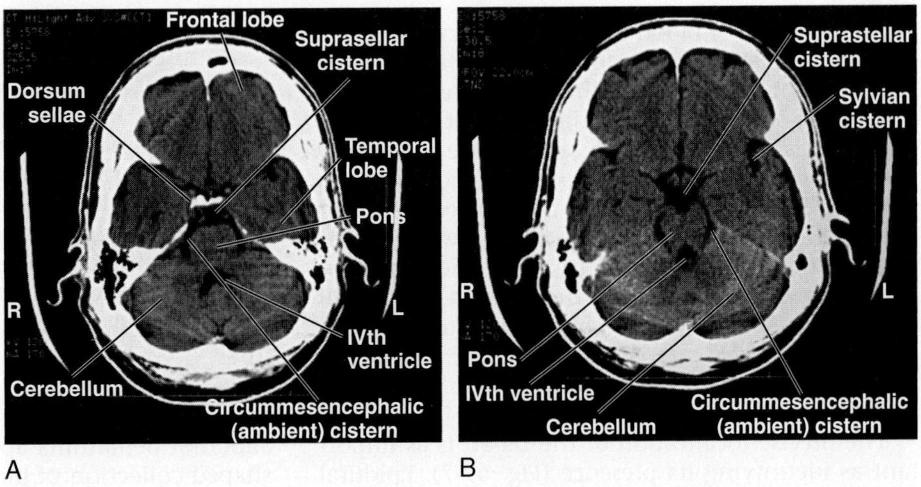
Frontal lobe
Suprasellar cistern
Dorsum sellae
Temporal lobe
Pons
R
L
IVth ventricle
Cerebellum
Circummesencephalic (ambient) cistern
A
Suprastellar cistern
Sylvian cistern
R
L
Pons
IVth ventricle
Cerebellum
Circummesencephalic (ambient) cistern
B

FIGURE 69-3 Head CT—Normal anatomy: **A,** high pons; **B,** cerebral peduncles.

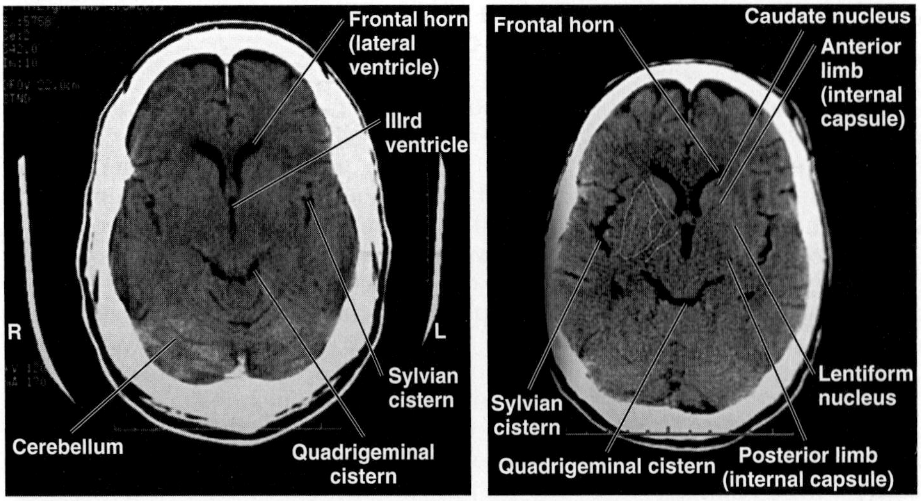
Frontal horn
(lateral
ventricle)
IIIrd
ventricle
Sylvian
cistern
Cerebellum
Quadrigeminal
cistern
R
L
Frontal horn
Caudate nucleus
Anterior
limb
(internal
capsule)
Lentiform
nucleus
Sylvian
cistern
Quadrigeminal cistern
Posterior limb
(internal capsule)

A B

FIGURE 69-4 Head CT—Normal anatomy: **A,** high midbrain level; **B,** basal ganglia region.

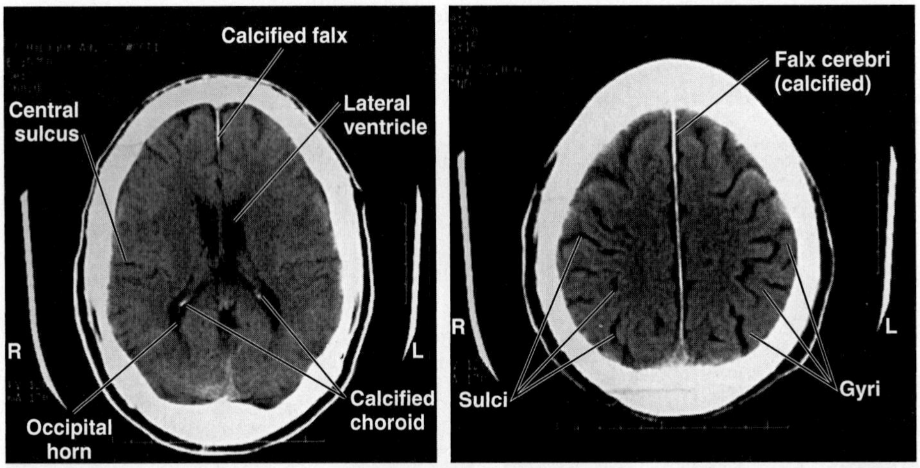
Calcified falx
Central
sulcus
Lateral
ventricle
R
L
Occipital
horn
Calcified
choroid
Falx cerebri
(calcified)
R
L
Sulci
Gyri

A B

FIGURE 69-5 Head CT—Normal anatomy: **A,** lateral ventricles; **B,** upper cortex.

of another one. Following is a detailed description of the components of the mnemonic.

▪ Blood

The appearance of blood on a head CT scan depends primarily on its location and size. Acute hemorrhage will appear hyperdense (bright white) on cranial CT images. This is attributed to the fact that the globin molecule is relatively dense, and hence effectively absorbs x-ray beams. Acute blood is typically in the range of 50 to 100 HU. As the blood becomes older and the globin molecule breaks down, it will lose this hyperdense appearance, beginning at the periphery and working in centrally. On the CT scan, blood will become isodense with the brain at 1 to 2 weeks, depending on clot size, and will become hypodense with the brain at approximately 2 to 3 weeks (Fig. 69-6).

The precise localization of the blood is as important as identifying its presence (Fig. 69-7). Epidural hematomas, subdural hematomas, intraparenchymal hemorrage, and subarachnoid hemorrhage each have a distinct appearance on the CT scan, as well as differing etiologies, complications, and associated conditions.

▪ *Epidural Hematoma*

Epidural hematoma most frequently appears as a lens-shaped (biconvex) collection of blood, usually over the brain convexity. An epidural hematoma will not cross a suture line, as the dura is tacked down in these areas. Epidural hematomas arise primarily (85%) from arterial laceration due to a direct blow, with the middle meningeal artery the most common source. A small proportion, however, come from other injured arteries and can even be venous in origin.

▪ *Subdural Hematoma*

Subdural hematoma appears as a sickle- or crescent-shaped collection of blood, usually over the cerebral

BOX 69-2

The "Blood Can Be Very Bad" Mnemonic*

- *B*lood—Acute hemorrhage appears hyperdense (bright white) on CT. This is due to the fact that the globin molecule is relatively dense and hence effectively absorbs x-ray beams. As the blood becomes older and the globin breaks down, it loses this hyperdense appearance, beginning at the periphery. The precise localization of the blood is as important as identifying its presence.
- Cisterns—Cerebrospinal fluid collections jacketing the brain; the following four key cisterns must be examined for blood, asymmetry, and effacement (representing increased intracranial pressure):
  - *Circummesencephalic*—Cerebrospinal fluid ring around the midbrain; first to be effaced with increased intracranial pressure
  - *Suprasellar* (star-shaped)—Location of the circle of Willis; frequent site of aneurysmal subarachnoid hemorrhage
  - *Quadrigeminal*—W-shaped cistern at top of midbrain; effaced early by rostrocaudal herniation
  - *Sylvian*—Between temporal and frontal lobes; site of traumatic and distal mid-cerebral aneurysm and subarachnoid hemorrhage
- *B*rain—Examine for:
  - *Symmetry*—Sulcal pattern (gyri) well differentiated in adults and symmetric side-to-side.
  - *Gray-white differentiation*—Earliest sign of cerebrovascular aneurysm is loss of gray-white differentiation; metastatic lesions often found at gray-white border
  - *Shift*—Falx should be midline, with ventricles evenly spaced to the sides; can also have rostrocaudal shift, evidenced by loss of cisternal space; unilateral effacement of sulci signals increased pressure in one compartment; bilateral effacement signals global increased pressure
  - *Hyper-/hypodensity*—Increased density with blood, calcification, intravenous contrast media; decreased density with air/gas (pneumocephalus), fat, ischemia (cerebrovascular aneurysm), tumor
- *V*entricles—Pathologic processes cause dilation (hydrocephalus) or compression/shift; hydrocephalus usually first evident in dilation of the temporal horns (normally small and slit-like); examiner must take in the "whole picture" to determine if the ventricles are enlarged due to lack of brain tissue or to increased cerebrospinal fluid pressure
- *B*one—Highest density on CT scan; diagnosis of skull fracture can be confusing due to the presence of sutures in the skull; compare other side of skull for symmetry (suture) versus asymmetry (fracture); basilar skull fractures commonly found in petrous ridge (look for blood in mastoid air cells)

**Blood* = blood, *Can* = cisterns, *Be* = brain, *Very* = ventricles, *Bad* = bone.

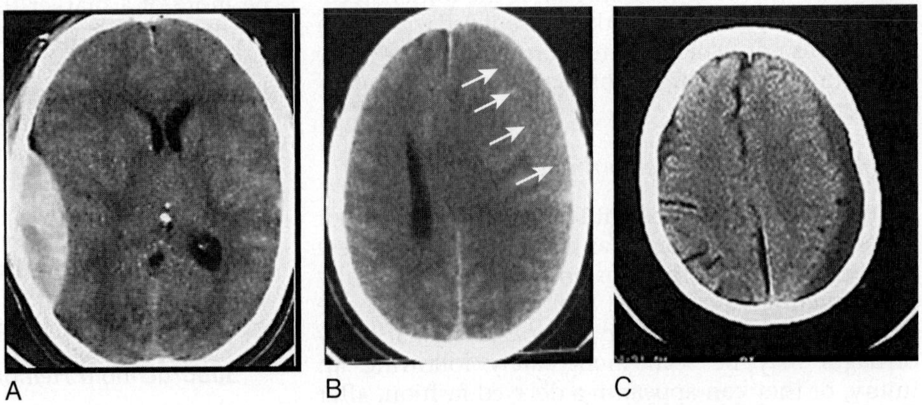
A
B
C

FIGURE 69-6 CT scan appearance of central nervous system hemorrhage: **A,** acute; **B,** subacute; **C,** chronic.

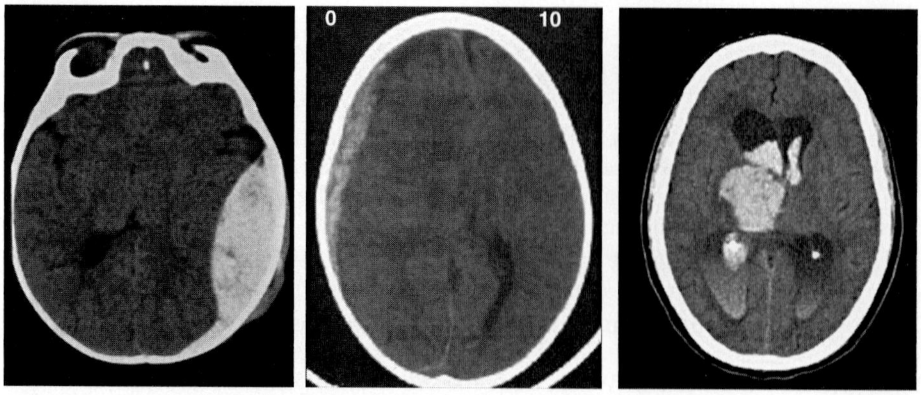
0
10

A B C

FIGURE 69-7 CT appearance of blood of differing etiologies: **A,** epidural hematoma; **B,** subdural hematoma; **C,** intraparenchymal and intraventricular hematomas.

convexity. Subdural hematomas can also be seen as isolated collections that appear in the interhemispheric fissures or along the tentorium. As opposed to epidural hematomas, subdural hematomas will cross suture lines, as there is no anatomic limitation to blood flow below the dura. A subdural hematoma can be either an acute lesion or a chronic one. While both occur primarily from disruption of surface and/or bridging vessels, the magnitude of impact damage is usually much higher in acute lesions. As such, they are frequently accompanied by severe brain injury, contributing to a much poorer overall prognosis than epidural hematoma.

Chronic subdural hematoma, in contrast with acute subdural hematoma, usually follows a more benign course than acute subdural hematoma. Attributed to slow venous oozing after even a minor closed head injury, the clot can gradually accumulate, allowing the patient to compensate. As the clot is frequently encased in a fragile vascular membrane, however, these patients are at significant risk for rebleeding as the result of additional minor trauma. The CT appearance of a chronic subdural hematoma depends on the length of time since the initial bleeding. A subdural hematoma that is isodense with brain can be very difficult to detect on CT, and in these cases contrast may highlight the surrounding vascular membrane.

Intraparenchymal Hemorrhage

Cranial CT can reliably identify intraparenchymal (or intracerebral) hematomas as small as 5 mm. These appear as high-density areas on the CT scan, usually with much less mass effect than their apparent size would indictate. Traumatic intraparenchymal hemorrhages may be seen immediately following an injury, or they can appear in a delayed fashion, after there has been time for swelling. Additionally, contusions may enlarge and coalesce over first 2 to 4 days. Traumatic contusions most commonly occur in areas where sudden deceleration of the head causes the brain to impact on bony prominences (e.g., temporal, frontal, occipital poles).

In distinction to traumatic lesions, nontraumatic hemorrhagic lesions due to hypertensive disease are typically seen in elderly patients and occur most frequently in the basal ganglia region. Hemorrhage from such lesions may rupture into the ventricular space, with the additional finding of intraventricular hemorrhage on CT. Posterior fossa bleeding (e.g., cerebellar) may dissect into the brainstem (pons, cerebellar peduncles) or rupture into the fourth ventricle. Besides hypertensive etiologies, intraparenchymal hemorrhages can be caused by arteriovenous malformations, bleeding from or into a tumor, amyloid angiopathy, or aneurysms that happen to rupture into the substance of the brain rather than into the subarachnoid space.

Intraventricular Hemorrhage

Intraventricular hemorrhage can be traumatic or secondary to intraparenchymal hemorrhage or subarachnoid hemorrhage with ventricular rupture. Identified as a white density in the normally black ventricular spaces, it is associated with a particularly poor outcome in cases of trauma (although this may be more of a marker than a causative issue). Hydrocephalus can be the end result regardless of the etiology. Cerebrospinal fluid (CSF) is produced in the lateral ventricles at a rate of 0.5 to 1 mL per minute, and this will occur regardless of the intraventricular pressure. A block at any point in the CSF pathway (lateral ventricles → foramen of Monro → 3rd ventricle → aqueduct of Sylvius → 4th ventricle → foramina of Luschka and Magendie → cisterns → arachnoid granulations) will result in hydrocephalus, with associated increased intracranial pressure and the ultimate potential for herniation.

Subarachnoid Hemorrhage

Subarachnoid hemorrhage is defined as hemorrhage into any subarachnoid space that is normally filled with CSF (e.g., cistern, brain convexity). The hyperdensity of blood in the subarachnoid space is frequently visible on CT imaging within minutes of the onset of hemorrhage (Fig. 69-8). Subarachnoid

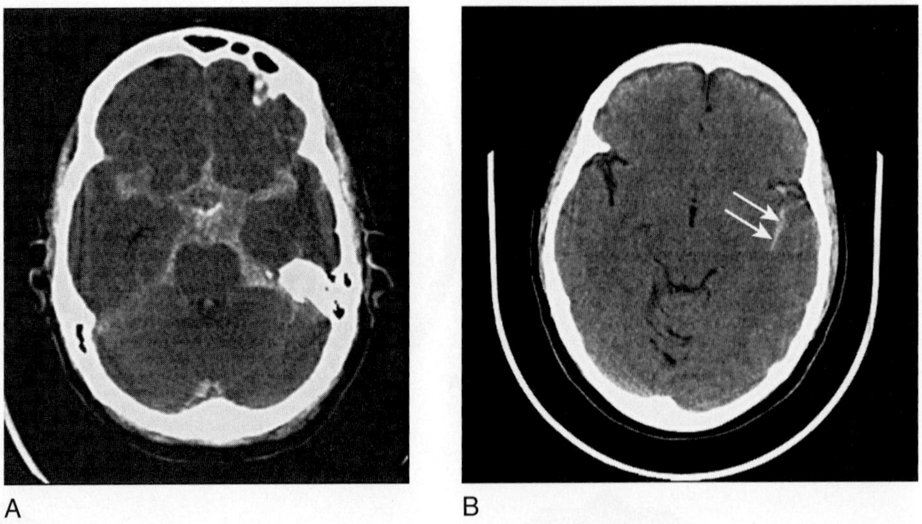
A
B

FIGURE 69-8 CT appearance of subarachnoid hemorrhage: **A,** blood filling the suprasellar cistern; **B,** blood filling the sylvian cistern.

hemorrhage is most commonly aneurysmal (75%-80%), but it can also occur with trauma, tumor, arteriovenous malformations and dural malformations. As a result of arachnoid granulations becoming plugged with red blood cells or their degradation products, hydrocephalus complicates approximately 20% of cases of subarachnoid hemorrhage.

The ability of a CT scanner to demonstrate subarachnoid hemorrhage depends on a number of factors, including the generation of scanner, the time since the initial bleeding, and the skill of the examiner. According to some studies, the CT scan is 95% to 98% sensitive for subarachnoid hemorrhage in the first 12 hours after the ictus.[9-11] This sensitivity is reported to decrease as follows:

90%-95% at 24 hours
80% at 3 days
50% at 1 week
30% at 2 weeks

Extracranial Hemorrhage

The presence and significance of extracranial blood and soft-tissue swelling on CT imaging is often overlooked. The examiner should use this finding to lead to subtle fractures that can be identified in areas of maximal impact (and hence maximal soft-tissue swelling). This will also direct the examiner to search the underlying brain parenchyma in these areas for parenchymal contusions, as well as to areas opposite maximal impact to search for contrecoup injuries.

Cisterns

Cisterns are potential spaces formed where there is a collection of CSF that is pooled as it works its way up to the superior sagittal sinus from the 4th ventricle. Of the numerous named cisterns (and some with multiple names), there are four key cisterns that the EP needs to be familiar with in order to identify increased intracranial pressure as well as the presence of blood in the subarachnoid space (Fig. 69-9). These cisterns are:

- *Circummesencephalic*—Hypodense CSF ring around the midbrain; most sensitive marker for increased intracranial pressure; will become effaced first with increased pressure and herniation syndromes.
- *Suprasellar*—Star-shaped hypodense space above the sella and pituitary; location of the circle of Willis, hence an excellent location for identifying aneurysmal subarachnoid hemorrhage.
- *Quadrigeminal*—W-shaped cistern at the top of the midbrain; can be a location for identifying traumatic subarachnoid hemorrhage, as well as an early marker of increased intracranial pressure and rostrocaudal herniation (Fig. 69-10).
- *Sylvian*—Bilateral CSF space located between the temporal and frontal lobes of the brain; another good location to identify subarachnoid hemorrhage, whether caused by trauma or aneurysm leak (particularly distal middle cerebral artery aneurysms).

Brain

Normal brain parenchyma has an inhomogeneous appearance where the gray and white matter interface. Cortical gray matter is denser than subcortical white matter; therefore the cortex will appear lighter on CT imaging. Given that many disease processes we are looking for in the ED are unilateral (e.g., cerebrovascular aneurysm, tumor, abscess), the clinician should be aware that there will normally be side-to-side symmetry on the scan. Similarly, the cortical gyral and sulcal pattern should be symmetric (Fig. 69-11). Besides symmetry, it is important to examine the brain parenchyma for:

- *Gray-white differentiation*—The earliest sign of an ischemic cerebrovascular aneurysm will be loss of gray-white differentiation. Tumors can also obscure this interface, particularly when there is associated edema (hypodensity).
- *Shift*—The falx should be midline, with ventricles evenly spaced to the sides. With rostrocaudal herniation the midline will be preserved, but this

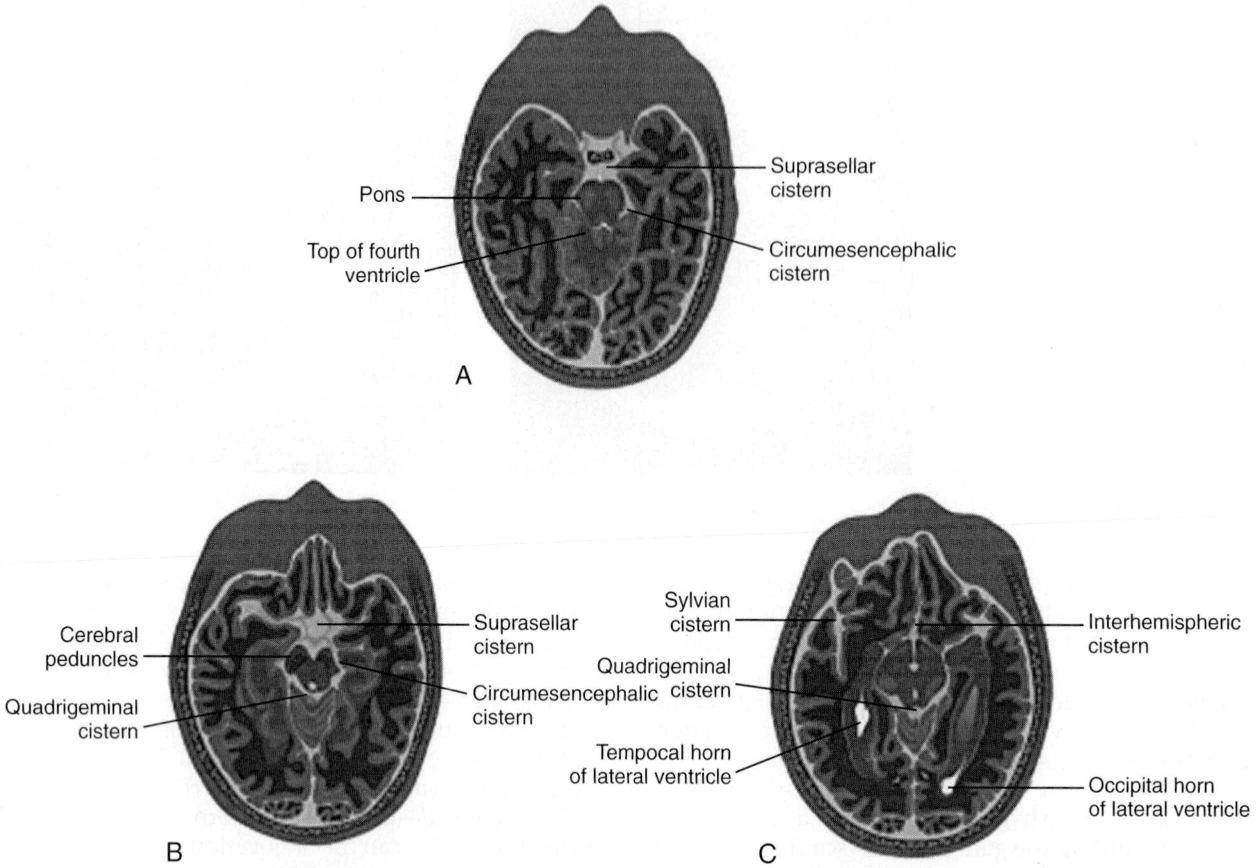
Suprasellar
cistern
Pons
Top of fourth
ventricle
Circumesencephalic
cistern
A
Cerebral
peduncles
Quadrigeminal
cistern
Suprasellar
cistern
Circumesencephalic
cistern
B
Sylvian
cistern
Quadrigeminal
cistern
Tempocal horn
of lateral ventricle
Interhemispheric
cistern
Occipital horn
of lateral ventricle
C

FIGURE 69-9 Three important cerebrospinal fluid cisterns: **A,** cisterns viewed at high pontine level; **B,** cisterns viewed at level of cerebral peduncles; **C,** cisterns viewed at high midbrain level.

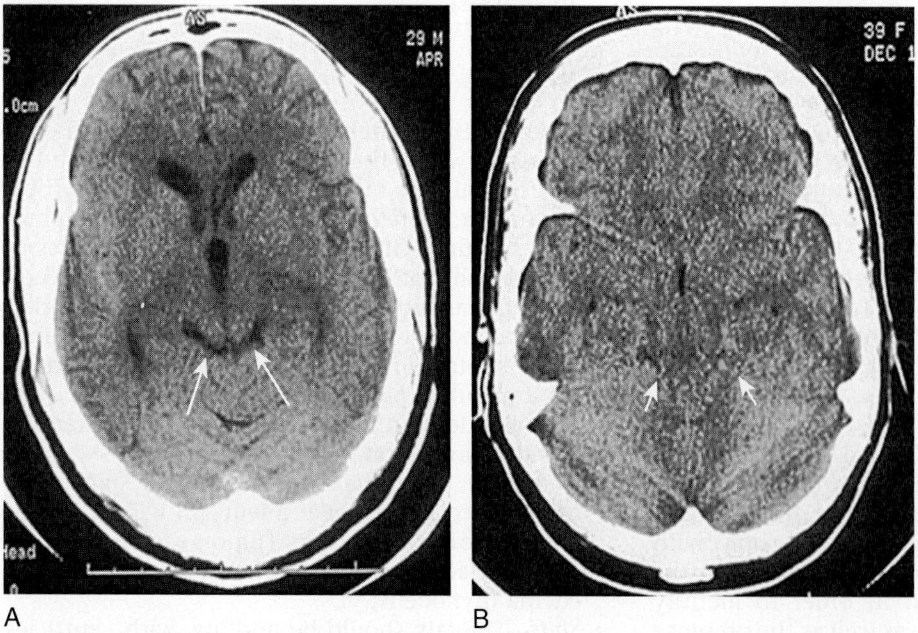
29 M
APR
39 F
DEC
A
B

FIGURE 69-10 CT appearance of increased intracranial pressure: **A,** normal intracranial pressure; **B,** elevated intracranial pressure.

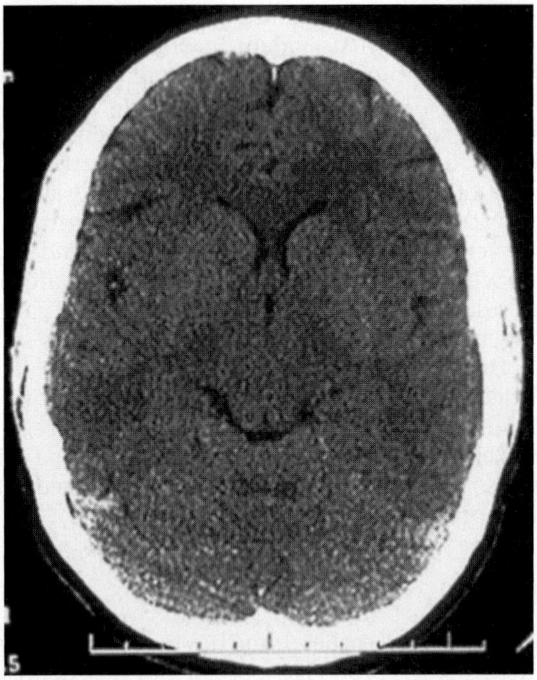

FIGURE 69-11 CT appearance of normal brain.

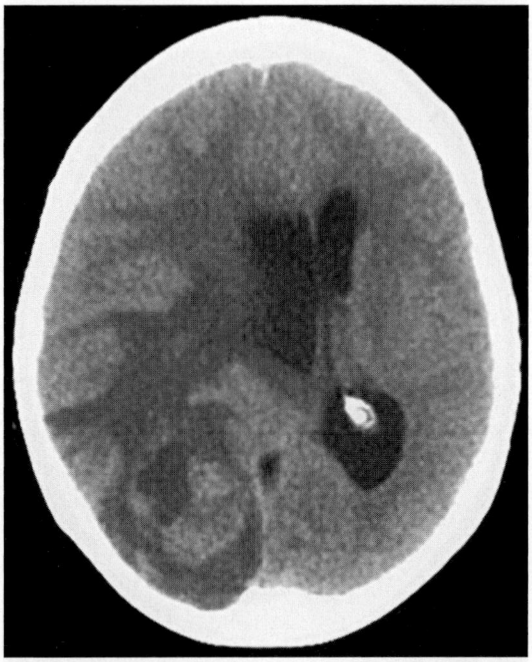

FIGURE 69-12 CT scan appearance of tumor with edema and midline shift.

will usually be evidenced by loss of cisternal spaces. A unilateral effacement of sulci signals increased pressure in one compartment. Bilateral effacement signals global increased pressure.

- *Hyper/hypodensity*—Brain will take on increased density with blood, calcification, and intravenous contrast media. It will take on decreased density with air (pneumocephalus), water, fat, and ischemia (cerebrovascular accident). Tumor may result in either increased or decreased density on CT imaging, depending on tumor type and amount of associated water density (edema).

Specific Brain Parenchymal Lesions

Tumor. Brain tumors usually appear as hypodense, poorly defined lesions on noncontrast CT scans. It is estimated that 70% to 80% of brain tumors will be apparent on plain scans without the use of an intravenous contrast agent. Calcification and hemorrhage associated with a tumor can cause it to have a hyperdense appearance. Tumors should be suspected on a noncontrast CT scan when significant edema is associated with an ill-defined mass. This vasogenic edema occurs because of a loss of integrity of the blood-brain barrier, allowing fluid to pass into the extracellular space. Edema, because of the increased water content, appears hypodense on the CT scan (Fig. 69-12).

Intravenous contrast material can help define brain tumors. Contrast media will leak through the incompetent blood-brain barrier into the extracellular space surrounding the mass lesion, resulting in a contrast-enhancing ring. Once a tumor is identified, the clinician should make some determination of the following information: location and size—intraaxial (within the brain parenchyma) or extraaxial; degree of edema and mass effect—for example, herniation may be impending due to swelling.

Abscess. Brain abscess will appear as an ill-defined hypodensity on non-contrast CT scan. A variable amount of edema is usually associated with such lesions and, like tumors, they will frequently demonstrate ring-enhancement with the addition of an intravenous contrast agent.

Ischemic Infarction. Strokes are classified as either hemorrhagic or nonhemorrhagic. Nonhemorrhagic infarctions can be seen as early as 2 to 3 hours following ictus, but most will not begin to be clearly evident on the CT scan for 12 to 24 hours. The earliest change seen in areas of ischemia is loss of gray-white differentiation, due to influx of water into the metabolically active gray matter. With the loss of blood flow, the energy-dependent cellular ion pumps fail, and the movement of ions such as sodium and potassium is no longer regulated. By osmotic forces, water follows the ions into the cells, where they cease metabolic activity. Because gray matter is metabolically more active than white matter, the gray cells are affected first, become water-filled, and take on the CT appearance of white matter. This loss of gray-white differentiation can initially be a subtle finding but ultimately will become evident and will usually be maximal between days 3 and 5 (Fig. 69-13).

Any vascular distribution can be affected by ischemic lesions (e.g., middle cerebral artery aneurysm, posterior inferior cerebellar artery). One specialized type of stroke frequently identified on CT imaging is

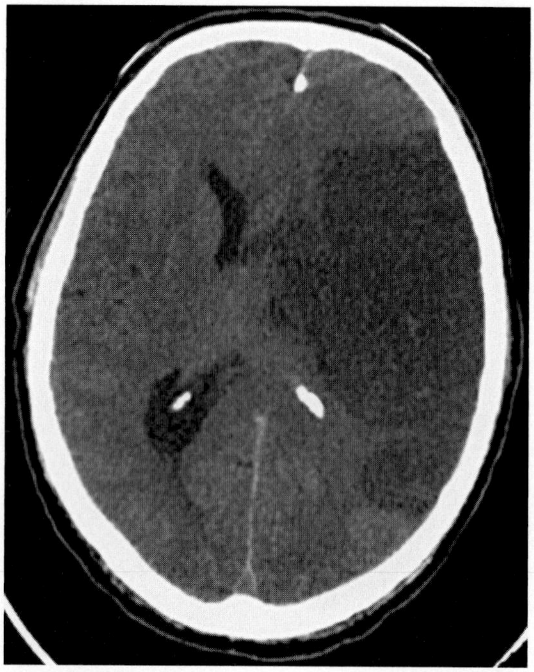

FIGURE 69-13 CT scan appearance of a large left middle cerebral artery stroke. The hypodense brain is the infarcted region. Note midline shift from left to right.

a lacunar infarction, which are small, discrete nonhemorrhagic lesions usually secondary to hypertension and found in the basal ganglia region. They frequently are clinically silent.

▪ Ventricles

Pathologic processes can cause either dilation (hydrocephalus) or compression/shift of the ventricular system (Fig. 69-14). Additionally, hemorrhage can occur into any of the ventricles, resulting in the potential for obstruction of flow and resulting hydrocephalus. The term "communicating hydrocephalus" is used when there is free CSF egress from the ventricular system, with a blockage at the level of the arachnoid granulations. The term *noncommunicating hydrocephalus* is used if there is obstruction anywhere along the course of flow from the lateral ventricles through egress from the 4th ventricle. Hydrocephalus frequently is first evident in dilation of the temporal horns, which are normally small with a slit-like morphology.

When examining the ventricular system for hydrocephalus, the clinician needs to take in the entire picture of the brain, as ventricles can be large for reasons other than increased pressure (e.g., atrophy). If the ventricles are large, the clinician should investigate whether other CSF spaces in the brain are large (e.g., sulci, cisterns). In this case, it is likely that this enlargement is the result of brain volume loss rather than the increased ventricle size. Conversely, if the ventricles are large, but the brain appears "tight" with sulcal effacement and loss of sulcal space, then the likelihood of hydrocephalus is high. The clinician also should look for evidence of increased intracranial pressure (e.g., cisternal effacement).

▪ Bone

As demonstrated earlier, bone has the highest density on the CT scan (+1000 HU). Because of this, depressed or comminuted skull fractures can usually be easily identified on the CT scan; however, small linear (nondepressed) skull fractures and fractures of the skull base may be more difficult to find (Fig. 69-15). Also, making the diagnosis of a skull fracture can be confusing due to the presence of sutures in the skull.

Fractures may occur at any portion of the bony skull. The presence of a skull fracture should increase the index of suspicion for intracranial injury. If intracranial air is seen on a CT scan, this indicates that the skull and dura have been violated at some point (Fig. 69-16). Basilar skull fractures are most commonly found in the petrous ridge (the dense pyramidal-shaped portion of the temporal bone). Due to the density of this bone, the fracture line may not be easily identified in this area. The clinician should not only search for such a fracture line but should also pay close attention to the normally aerated mastoid air cells that are contained within this bone. Any blood in the mastoid air cells means that a skull base fracture is likely. Analogous to the mastoid air cells, the maxillary, ethmoid, and sphenoid sinuses should

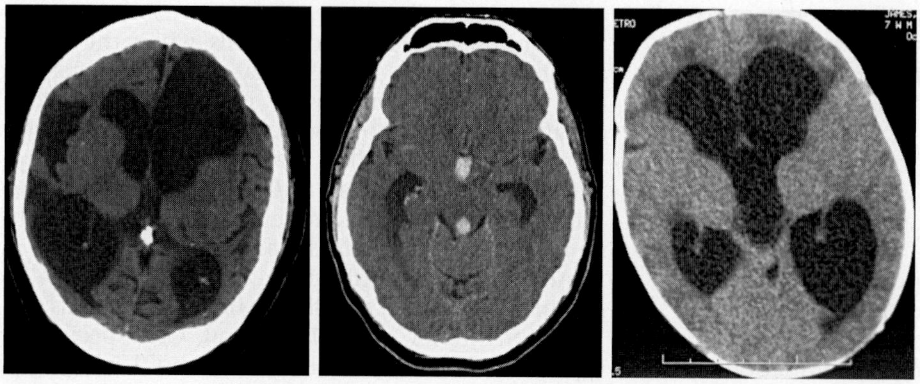

FIGURE 69-14 CT appearance of abnormal ventricles.

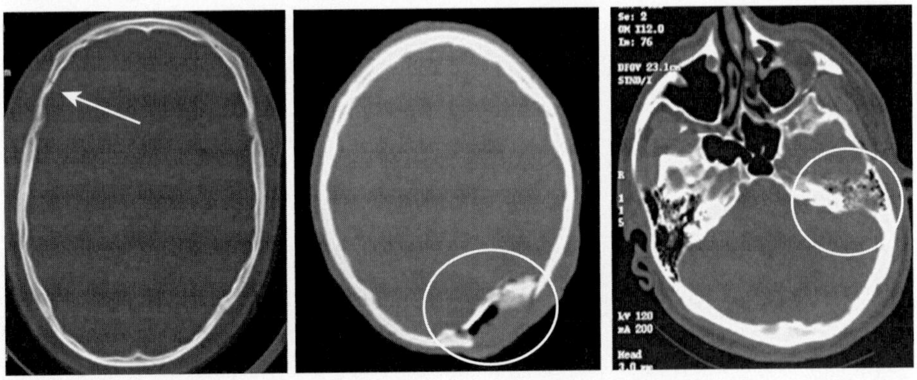

A B C

FIGURE 69-15 CT appearance in bone pathology: **A,** linear skull fracture; **B,** depressed, comminuted skull fracture; **C,** basilar skull fracture.

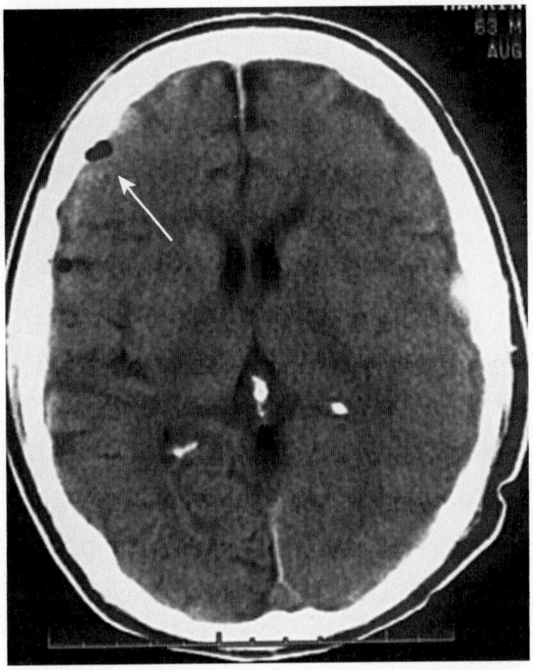

FIGURE 69-16 CT scan appearance of intracranial air.

be visible and aerated; the presence of fluid in any of these sinuses in the setting of trauma should raise suspicion of a skull fracture. In nontraumatic cases, fluid in the mastoids may indicate mastoiditis, and fluid in the sinuses may indicate sinusitis.

Summary

Cranial CT is integral to the practice of emergency medicine and is used on a daily basis to make important, time-critical decisions that directly impact the care of ED patients. An important tenet in the use of cranial CT is that accurate interpretation is required to make good clinical decisions. Cranial CT interpretation is a skill, like ECG interpretation, that can be learned through education, practice, and repetition.

REFERENCES

1. Schreiger DL, Kalafut M, Starkman S, et al: Cranial computed tomography interpretation in acute stroke. JAMA 1998;279:1293-1297.
2. Perron AD, Huff JS, Ullrich CG, et al: A multicenter study to improve emergency medicine residents' recognition of intracranial emergencies on computed tomography. Ann Emerg Med 1998;32:554-562.
3. Leavitt MA, Dawkins R, Williams V, et al: Abbreviated educational session improves cranial computed tomography scan interpretations by EPs. Ann Emerg Med 1997; 30:616-621.
4. Alfaro DA, Levitt MA, English DK, et al: Accuracy of interpretation of cranial computed tomography in an emergency medicine residency program. Ann Emerg Med 1995; 25:169-174.
5. Roszler MH, McCarroll KA, Donovan RT, et al: Resident interpretation of emergency computed tomographic scans. Invest Radiol 1991;26:374-376.
6. Arendts G, Manovel A, Chai A: Cranial CT interpretation by senior emergency departments staff. Australas Radiol 2003;47:368-374.
7. Saketkhoo DD, Bhargavan M, Sunshine JH, et al: Emergency department image interpretation services at private community hospitals. Radiology 2004;231:190-197.
8. Lowe RA, Abbuhl SB, Baumritter A, et al: Radiology services in emergency medicine residency programs: A national survey. Acad Emerg Med 2002;9:587-594.
9. Boesiger BM. Shiber JR: Subarachnoid hemorrhage diagnosis by computed tomography and lumbar puncture: Are fifth generation CT scanners better at identifying subarachnoid hemorrhage? J Emerg Med 2005;29:23-27.
10. Van der Wee N, Rinkel GJE, van Gijn J: Detection of subarachnoid hemorrhage on early CT: Is lumbar puncture still needed after a negative scan? J Neurol Neurosug Psychiatry 1995;58:357-359.
11. Morgenstern LB: Worst headache and subarachnoid hemorrhage prospective, modern computed tomography and spinal fluid analysis. Ann Emerg Med 1998;32:297-304.

Chapter **70**

Spine Trauma and Spinal Cord Injury

Michelle Lin and Swaminatha V. Mahadevan

KEY POINTS

Patients with spinal pain and spine fractures should recive a thorough neurologic examination to look for spinal cord injury.

Patients with spine fractures should be re-examined because of the high incidence of secondary noncontiguous spine fractures and concurrent injuries (abdominal injuries with lumbar fractures and chest injuries with thoracic fractures).

The National Emergency X-radiography Utilization Study (NEXUS) and/or the Canadian Cervical-Spine Rule (CRR) criteria can be used to clinically clear the cervical spine of low-risk patients without the need for radiographic imaging.

Because plain films are significantly less sensitive than computed tomography (CT) scans of the cervical spine for visualizing fractures, radiography should be reserved for low-risk patients with traumatic neck pain.

Spinal shock, which is the transient physiologic transection of the spinal cord from trauma, is different from neurogenic shock, which is the physiologic sympathectomy of the descending pathways in the upper spinal cord, leading to peripheral vasodilation.

Patients with a spinal cord injury caused by blunt trauma are often given high-dose corticosteroids within 8 hours of injury. However, the EP should be aware that high-dose corticosteroid therapy may result in an increased rate of gastrointestinal bleeding and infectious complications.

Scope

The estimated annual costs of spine injuries, including inability to work and health care costs, exceed $5 billion in the United States.[1]

In the ED, all trauma victims are screened for vertebral fractures and spinal cord injuries because of the potentially devastating neurologic consequences of overlooking a spinal fracture. Patients with delayed diagnosis of a spinal fracture are 7.5 times more likely to sustain secondary neurologic deficits.[2] Neurologic deficits from spinal cord injury can be subtle and easily missed if not specifically evaluated. Augmenting these difficulties, plain film radiographs of the spine, although an adequate screening tool for other fractures, can miss 23% to 42% of cervical spinal fractures[3,4] and 13% to 50% of lumbar fractures.[5,6]

Anatomy

Anatomically, the vertebral spine can be divided into structural columns. The cervical spine traditionally is divided into two columns—anterior and posterior. The *anterior column* consists of the load-bearing vertebral bodies, intervertebral disks, anterior longitudi-

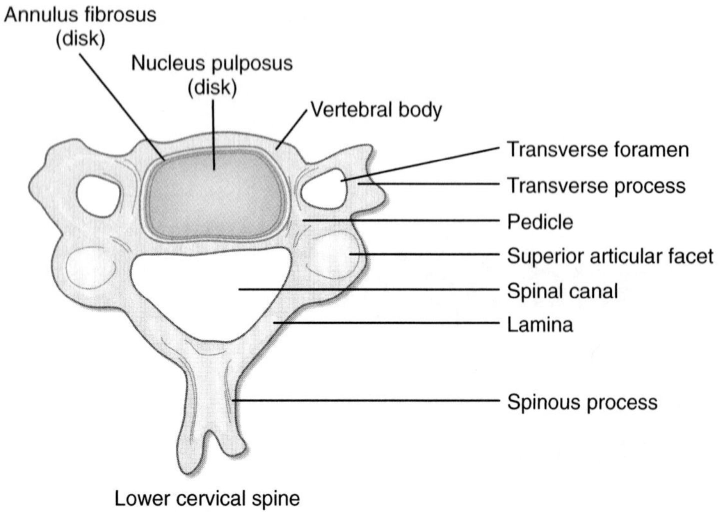
Annulus fibrosus
(disk)
Nucleus pulposus
(disk)
Vertebral body
Transverse foramen
Transverse process
Pedicle
Superior articular facet
Spinal canal
Lamina
Spinous process
Lower cervical spine

FIGURE 70-1 Bony anatomy of a typical lower cervical vertebra (C3-C7): superior axial view with anterior oriented up and posterior oriented down.

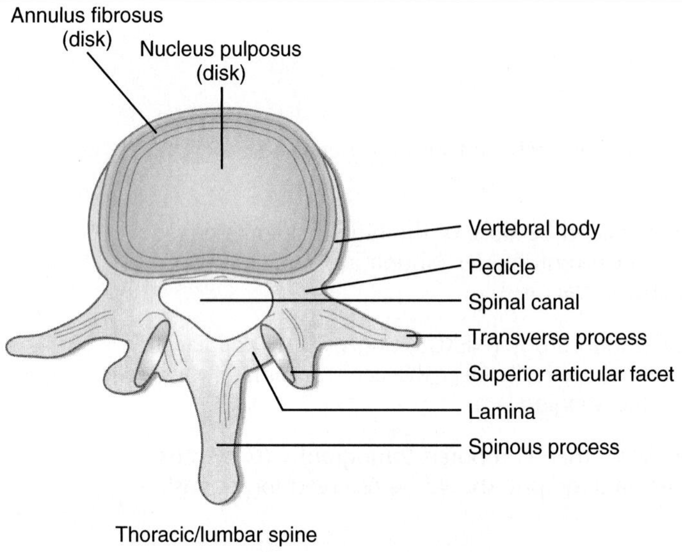
Annulus fibrosus
(disk)
Nucleus pulposus
(disk)
Vertebral body
Pedicle
Spinal canal
Transverse process
Superior articular facet
Lamina
Spinous process
Thoracic/lumbar spine

FIGURE 70-2 Bony anatomy of a typical thoracic and lumbar vertebra (T1-L5): superior axial view with anterior oriented up and posterior oriented down.

nal ligament, and posterior longitudinal ligament (Fig. 70-1). The *posterior column* consists of the more posterior structures, such as the pedicles, laminae, and transverse and spinous processes (Fig. 70-2).

In contrast, the thoracic and lumbar vertebral spines are divided into three columns, based on the modified Denis model—anterior, middle, and posterior (Fig. 70-3). The *anterior column* consists of the anterior longitudinal ligament and anterior two thirds of the vertebral body and intervertebral disk. The *middle column* consists of the posterior longitudinal ligament and posterior one third of the vertebral body and intervertebral disk. Of significance, any disruption in this middle column predisposes a patient to significant spinal cord injury, because the middle column abuts the spinal canal. Note that the anterior and middle columns collectively comprise the same anatomic area defined as the "anterior column" in the cervical spine. The *posterior column* consists of the remaining posterior structures.

The C1 and C2 vertebrae are anatomically unique (Fig. 70-4). C1 (atlas) is a ring-link structure without a vertebral body. It articulates superiorly with the occipital condyles. This articulation allows 50% of normal neck flexion and extension. C2 (axis) projects the dens superiorly to articulate with C1. The transverse ligament tethers the dens to the anterior arch of C1. This atlantoaxial articulation allows 50% of normal neck rotation left and right.

■ VERTEBRAL ARTERY CIRCULATION

The vertebral arteries branch off from the subclavian arteries and course superiorly within the transverse foramina of C2-C6. These arteries then merge to form the basilar artery.

■ THE SPINAL CORD

The spinal cord spans from the foramen magnum to the L1 level, whereupon the spinal cord tapers into the conus medullaris and cauda equina, a collection of peripheral lower lumbar and sacral spinal nerve

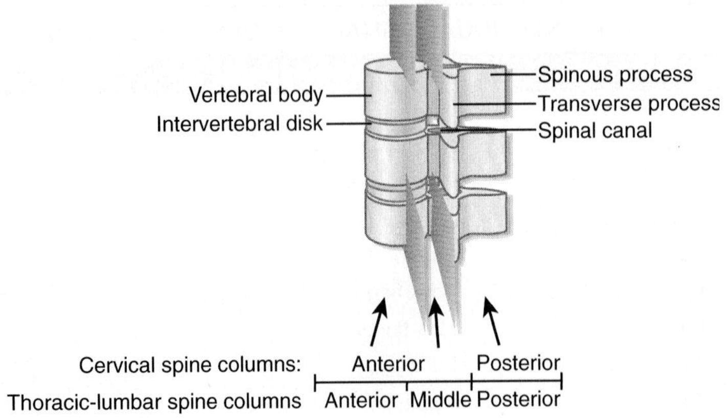
Vertebral body
Intervertebral disk
Spinous process
Transverse process
Spinal canal
Cervical spine columns:
Anterior
Posterior
Thoracic-lumbar spine columns
Anterior
Middle
Posterior

FIGURE 70-3 Schematic diagram illustrating lateral view of the anatomic columns of the cervical and thoracic/lumbar spine. Note that the cervical spine's anterior column is composed of the same structures as the thoracic/lumbar spine's anterior and middle columns.

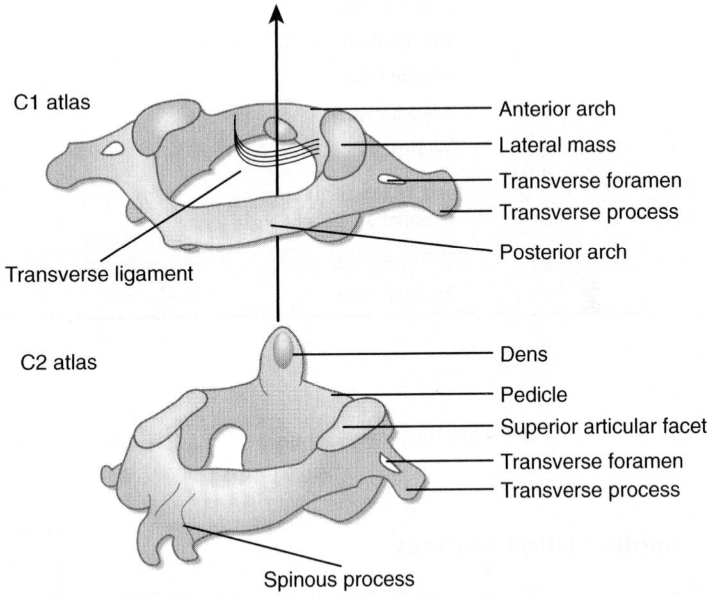
C1 atlas
Anterior arch
Lateral mass
Transverse foramen
Transverse process
Posterior arch
Transverse ligament
C2 atlas
Dens
Pedicle
Superior articular facet
Transverse foramen
Transverse process
Spinous process

FIGURE 70-4 Bony anatomy of the upper cervical spine (C1 and C2): posterolateral view. The C1 lateral masses articulate with the occipital condyles. The C2 dens projects cephalad, articulates with the C1 anterior arch, and is stabilized by the C1 transverse ligament.

roots. Because the spinal cord is thickest in the cervical spine, there is relatively less spinal canal space in the cervical levels compared with the thoracic or lumbar spine. Thus spinal cord injuries occur more frequently in cervical spine trauma than in thoracic or lumbar spine trauma. The neurologic dermatomes can help localize the injury (Table 70-1).

Vertebral Column Fractures

Vertebral column fractures usually are associated with significant midline spinal tenderness on palpation. The likelihood of a fracture is greatest in the cervical spine, followed by thoracolumbar, lumbar, and thoracic regions, in order of frequency.

The thoracolumbar spine, defined as encompassing the T10-L2 vertebral levels, is commonly injured because the spine curvature changes from a kyphotic thoracic spine to a lordotic lumbar spine at this juncture. Thoracic spine fractures are uncommon because the articulating ribs provide spinal column stability.

■ CLINICAL EVALUATION

■ Abdominal Examination

Thoracolumbar and lumbar spine fractures are associated with intra-abdominal injuries. For instance, up to 50% of patients with transverse process fractures[7] and 33% of patients with Chance fractures[8] have concurrent intra-abdominal pathology. These injuries can involve both the hollow viscus and the solid organs. High-risk abdominal signs associated with spinal injuries include significant abdominal tenderness and a transverse ecchymotic finding on the lower abdomen ("seat belt sign").

■ Extremity Examination

Tenderness or ecchymosis of the heel suggests a calcaneal fracture. Ten percent of patients with calcaneal fractures have an associated lower thoracic or lumbar fracture. Because the calcaneus classically is fractured as a result of axial loading, usually from a fall onto the heels, the axial thoracic and

Table 70-1 INDIVIDUAL SPINAL SENSORY DERMATOMES, MOTOR FUNCTION, AND REFLEX ARCS

Spinal Level	Sensory Distribution	Motor Function	Reflex
C2	Occiput		
C3	Thyroid cartilage		
C4	Suprasternal notch	Spontaneous respiration	
C5	Infraclavicular area	Shoulder shrugging	Biceps
C6	Thumb	Elbow flexion	Triceps
C7	Index finger	Elbow extension	
C8	Little finger	Finger flexion (with T1)	
T1		Finger flexion	
T4	Nipple line		
T10	Umbilicus		
L1	Inguinal ligament	Hip flexion (with L2)	
L2	Medial thigh	Hip flexion	
L3	Medial thigh	Hip adduction	
L4	Medial foot	Hip abduction	Patellar
L5	Webspace between big toe and second toe	Foot dorsiflexion	
S1	Lateral foot	Foot plantar flexion (with S2)	Achilles
S2	Perianal area (with S3, S4)	Foot plantar flexion	
S3	Perianal area	Rectal sphincter tone (with S4)	
S4	Perianal area	Rectal sphincter tone	

lumbar spines are mechanistically also at risk for a fracture.

Subtle Clinical Features

The severity and location of spinal pain in vertebral fractures varies depending on (1) the patient's bone density and (2) the fracture location.

Patients older than 65 years and those on chronic corticosteroid therapy are likely osteopenic. They can sustain spinal fractures with mild trauma, such as a fall from a standing position, and often exhibit minimal associated pain. Specifically, patients older than 65 years have an increased risk of cervical spine fractures (relative risk, 2.09).[9] Also, acute back pain in chronic corticosteroid users is correlated with a 99% specificity for a spinal compression fracture.[10] Thus imaging should be obtained to evaluate these potentially osteopenic patients in the setting of neck or back pain.

Not all patients with spinal fractures have midline spinal pain. Transverse process fractures, for instance, may result in pain of varying severity along the paraspinous muscles rather than along the midline spine.

ED INTERVENTIONS AND PROCEDURES

ED management should include protection of the spine and spinal cord until fractures can be identified or excluded. A rigid backboard typically can be promptly removed from cooperative patients because it is unnecessary to maintain spinal column neutrality in a calm person. Extended use of the rigid backboard is associated with complications such as back pain, respiratory impairment, aspiration, and decubitus ulcers.

DIAGNOSIS AND TREATMENT

Diagnosis and treatment of vertebral column fractures are discussed in detail in the following sections on cervical spine injuries and thoracic/lumbar spine injuries.

DISPOSITION

Admission

Most patients with traumatic vertebral column fractures are admitted to the hospital because they fulfill at least one of four admission criteria: (1) intractable pain, (2) fracture involvement of more than one column, (3) a functionally unstable fracture pattern, and (4) the presence or potential for development of a spinal cord injury.

Typical patients who can be discharged home include those with normal neurologic function and (1) an isolated, stable posterior column fracture (spinous process, transverse process) in the cervical, thoracic, or lumbar spine, or (2) a stable wedge fracture in the thoracic or lumbar spine.

Discharge Instructions

Discharged patients without a fracture or spinal cord injury require only conservative management. Discharged patients with a stable spinal fracture require only conservative management with or without an immobilization device, such as a cervical collar or thoracolumbar sacral orthosis (TLSO) back brace. Soft collars and back braces are not recommended because they predispose patients to stiffness of the neck and back, respectively.

Discharged patients with persistent neck pain still at risk for an unstable ligamentous injury, should wear a semi-rigid cervical collar (e.g., Philadelphia or Miami J collar) 7 to 10 days until adequate flexion-extension plain films can be obtained. Discharge instructions should include information about warning signs of spinal cord injury.

Cervical Spine Injuries

IN-LINE CERVICAL SPINE IMMOBILIZATION

During the initial resuscitation phase of trauma victims, patients with a potential cervical spinal injury may require endotracheal intubation before a definitive diagnosis is available. By preventing neck hyperextension during direct laryngoscopy, in-line cervical spine immobilization during intubation maintains cervical spine neutrality (Fig. 70-5).

CLINICAL CLEARANCE

Procedure

Once a cooperative patient is considered to be a candidate for clinical clearance of the cervical spine, the patient's neck should be reevaluated for tenderness. First, unfasten the cervical collar. Next, palpate the patient's posterior neck while applying the other hand to the patient's forehead to prevent spontaneous and reflexive head-lifting. In the absence of significant midline tenderness, remove your hands and instruct the patient to actively lift the head off the gurney and range the neck by looking right, left, caudad, and cephalad. Do not assist the patient.

If the patient is able to move spontaneously and easily, without pain or neurologic symptoms, the patient's neck is considered "clinically cleared" and the collar may be removed.

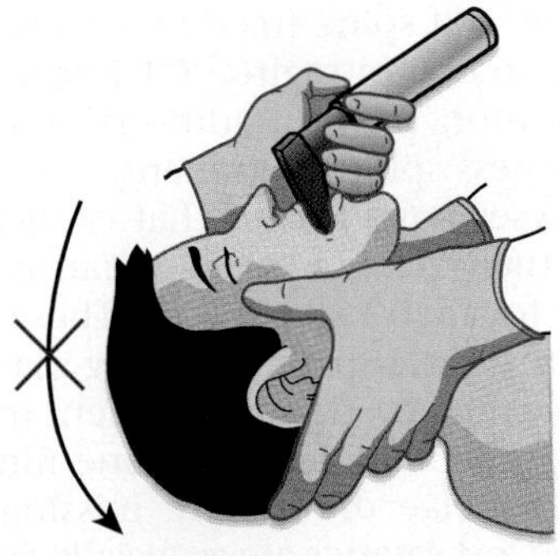

FIGURE 70-5 In-line cervical spine immobilization during endotracheal intubation. Standing to the patient's side, the assistant uses both hands to stabilize the neck to prevent hyperextension.

Is Imaging Necessary?

In 2000, in the hopes of reducing the number of low-risk patients undergoing cervical spine plain film radiography of the cervical spine, a multicenter study by the National Emergency X-radiography Utilization Study (NEXUS) group validated a set of five low-risk criteria, which determined which patients could be "clinically cleared" without radiographic imaging, if all criteria were met (Box 70-1). This clinical decision tool demonstrated a sensitivity of 99.6% and a specificity of 12.9% for detecting clinically significant cervical spine fractures. It was thus extrapolated that 4309 (12.6%) of the enrolled 34,069 patients could have avoided plain film radiography.[15]

Following the development of the NEXUS criteria, the Canadian Cervical-Spine Rule (CCR) was developed (Fig. 70-6). The validated sensitivity and specificity for this decision rule were 99.4% and 45.1%, respectively.[16]

The CCR study excluded the following patients: patients aged less than 16 years; patients with abnormal Glasgow Coma Scale score, abnormal vital signs, injuries more than 48 hours old, penetrating trauma,

BOX 70-1

NEXUS* Low-Risk Criteria for a Cervical Spine Injury

A patient's neck can be clinically cleared safely without radiographic imaging if all five low-risk conditions are met:

1. No posterior midline neck pain or tenderness
2. No focal neurologic deficit
3. Normal level of alertness
4. No evidence of intoxication
5. No clinically apparent, painful distracting injury†

*National Emergency X-radiography Utilization Study.
†Defined as "a condition thought by the clinician to be producing pain sufficient to distract the patients from a second (neck) injury. Examples may include, but are not limited to, the following: (1) a long bone fracture, (2) a visceral injury requiring surgical consultation, (3) a large laceration, degloving injury, or crush injury, (4) large burns, (5) and any other injury producing acute functional impairment. Physicians may also classify any injury as distracting if it is thought to have the potential to impair the patient's ability to appreciate other injuries."
From Hoffman JR, Mower WR, Wolfson AB, et al: Validity of a set of clinical criteria to rule out injury to the cervical spine in patients with blunt trauma. N Engl J Med 2000;343:94-99.

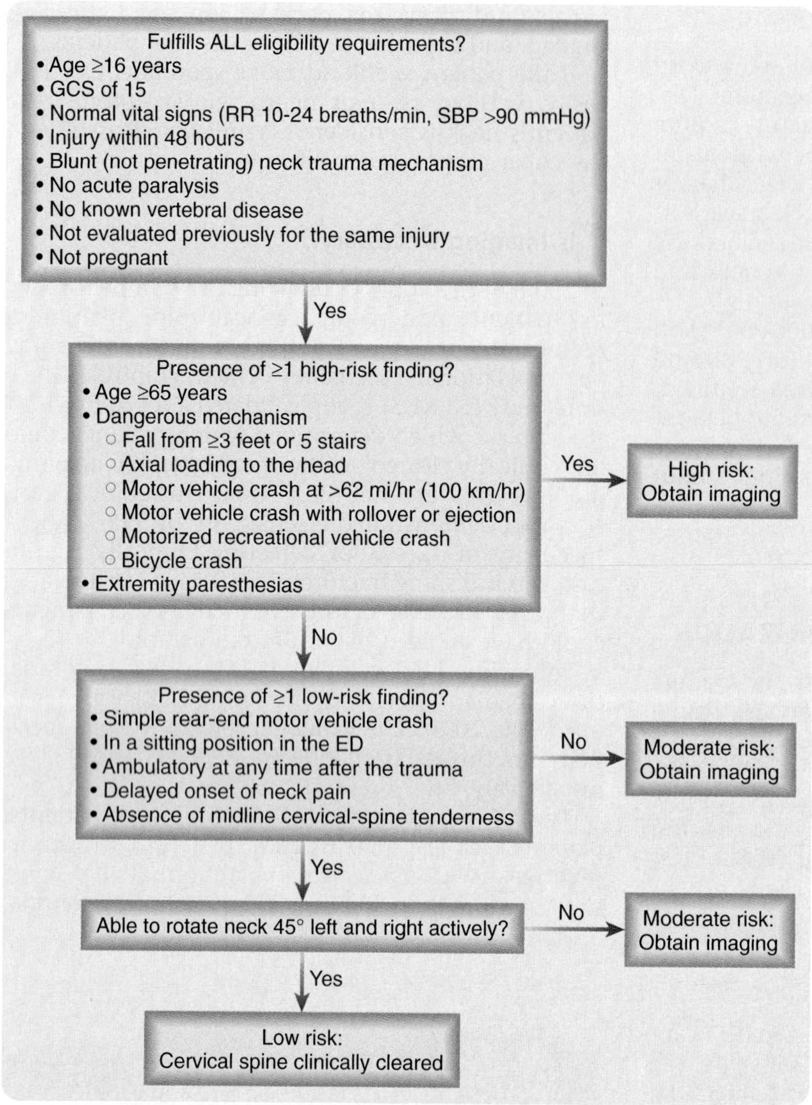
Fulfills ALL eligibility requirements?
• Age ≥16 years
• GCS of 15
• Normal vital signs (RR 10-24 breaths/min, SBP >90 mmHg)
• Injury within 48 hours
• Blunt (not penetrating) neck trauma mechanism
• No acute paralysis
• No known vertebral disease
• Not evaluated previously for the same injury
• Not pregnant
Yes
Presence of ≥1 high-risk finding?
• Age ≥65 years
• Dangerous mechanism
○ Fall from ≥3 feet or 5 stairs
○ Axial loading to the head
○ Motor vehicle crash at >62 mi/hr (100 km/hr)
○ Motor vehicle crash with rollover or ejection
○ Motorized recreational vehicle crash
○ Bicycle crash
• Extremity paresthesias
Yes
High risk: Obtain imaging
No
Presence of ≥1 low-risk finding?
• Simple rear-end motor vehicle crash
• In a sitting position in the ED
• Ambulatory at any time after the trauma
• Delayed onset of neck pain
• Absence of midline cervical-spine tenderness
No
Moderate risk: Obtain imaging
Yes
Able to rotate neck 45° left and right actively?
No
Moderate risk: Obtain imaging
Yes
Low risk: Cervical spine clinically cleared

FIGURE 70-6 Canadian Cervical-Spine Rule (CCR) algorithm for clinical clearance of the cervical spine. The green box signifies a low-risk, negative work-up and clinical cervical spine clearance. Yellow boxes signify a moderate-risk condition, and the red box signifies a high-risk condition, both of which require plain film radiography. GCS, Glasgow Coma Scale; RR, respiratory rate; SBP, systolic blood pressure. (Data from Stiell IG, Clement CM, McKnight RD, et al: The Canadian C-Spine Rule versus the NEXUS low-risk criteria in patients with trauma. N Engl J Med 2003;349: 2510-2518.)

paralysis, history of vertebral disease; patients seen previously for the same injury; and pregnant patients. Because these cases were not studied, the CCR guidelines should not be applied in such patients.

■ Choosing the Imaging Modality for Fracture Evaluation (Fig. 70-7)

When patients require cervical spine imaging because they have at least one high-risk criterion for a spinal fracture, imaging begins with either plain films or CT scans. This decision should take into account the pros and cons of both imaging approaches (Table 70-2).

■ *Computed Tomography (CT)*

With increasing evidence in the literature showing that CT is much more sensitive (98%) than plain film radiography (53%) in detecting cervical spine fractures, future recommendations will likely advocate cervical spine CT imaging as the first-line diagnostic approach for most patients because of the neurologic significance of a missed cervical spine injury.[17] Conventional radiography is especially difficult to interpret in the high (occiput, C1, and C2) and low (C6, C7, T1) cervicothoracic junctions, where coincidentally most cervical spine fractures can be found.[18] It is important to obtain sagittal CT image reconstructions, in addition to the traditional axial views, to adequately assess spinal alignment.

Cost analyses have shown that cervical spine CT scans are actually less expensive than conventional radiography for high-risk patients. These studies factored personnel time spent repeating plain films secondary to inadequacy, delays in patient management while trying to obtain cervical spine films, and the neurologic sequelae of initially missing a cervical spine injury. Cost savings are especially evident if the patient is already undergoing CT imaging of other body parts, such as a head scanning for a closed head injury. With multidetector scanners more readily

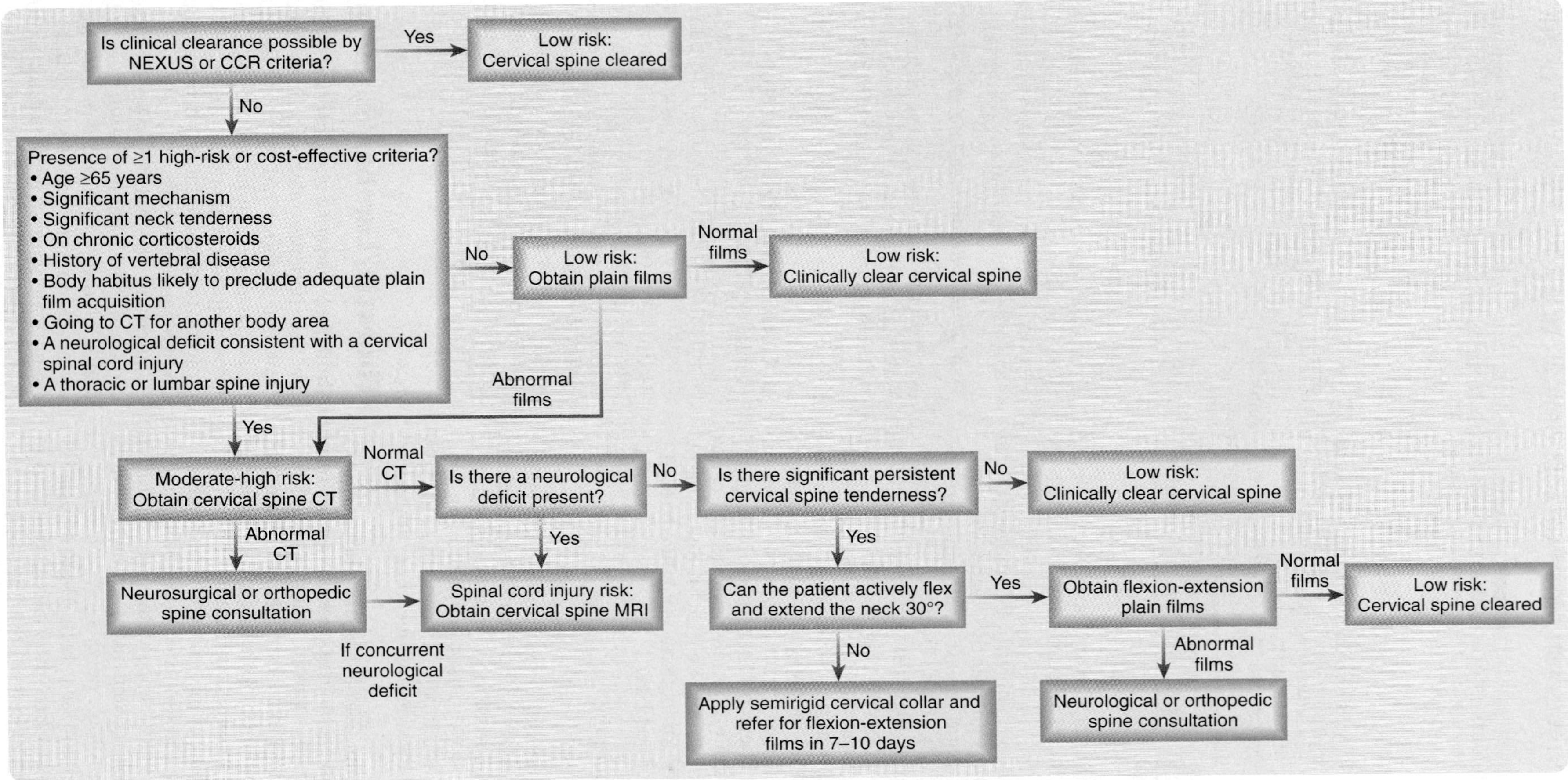
Is clinical clearance possible by NEXUS or CCR criteria?
Yes
Low risk: Cervical spine cleared
No
Presence of ≥1 high-risk or cost-effective criteria?
• Age ≥65 years
• Significant mechanism
• Significant neck tenderness
• On chronic corticosteroids
• History of vertebral disease
• Body habitus likely to preclude adequate plain film acquisition
• Going to CT for another body area
• A neurological deficit consistent with a cervical spinal cord injury
• A thoracic or lumbar spine injury
No
Low risk: Obtain plain films
Normal films
Low risk: Clinically clear cervical spine
Abnormal films
Yes
Moderate-high risk: Obtain cervical spine CT
Normal CT
Is there a neurological deficit present?
No
Is there significant persistent cervical spine tenderness?
No
Low risk: Clinically clear cervical spine
Abnormal CT
Neurosurgical or orthopedic spine consultation
Yes
Spinal cord injury risk: Obtain cervical spine MRI
If concurrent neurological deficit
Yes
Can the patient actively flex and extend the neck 30°?
Yes
Obtain flexion-extension plain films
Normal films
Low risk: Cervical spine cleared
No
Apply semirigid cervical collar and refer for flexion-extension films in 7–10 days
Abnormal films
Neurological or orthopedic spine consultation

FIGURE 70-7 Diagnostic algorithm for a patient with neck pain resulting from blunt trauma. NEXUS, National Emergency X-radiography Utilization Study; CCR, Canadian Cervical-Spine Rule; CT, computed tomography; MRI, magnetic resonance imaging.

Table 70-2 ADVANTAGES AND DISADVANTAGES OF PLAIN FILM AND CT IMAGING OF THE CERVICAL SPINE

	Plain Film Radiography	CT Radiography
Advantages	Less irradiation to the thyroid, breast, and lens Can be performed at the bedside	98% sensitivity in detecting fractures More cost-effective than plain films Less delay in patient management, especially if the patient is already scheduled for CT of another body part
Disadvantages	Only 53% sensitivity for detecting fractures Three-view films are inadequate >50% of the time, especially of the cervicocranial and cervicothoracic junction Inefficient use of radiology personnel, who often must repeat films because of image inadequacy A suspicious or detected fracture on plain films requires additional evaluation by CT for confirmation and further delineation	More irradiation to the thyroid, breast, and lens Requires patient to be hemodynamically stable when being transported from the ED to CT scanner site

CT, computed tomography.

available, an additional cervical spine scan would add less than 5 minutes of scan time at a relatively small cost.[19]

A major deterrent for universal CT imaging of the cervical spine is the significantly greater irradiation dose. The thyroid gland, breast tissue, and lens are exposed to especially high levels of irradiation, placing the patient at high risk for development of thyroid cancers, breast cancers, and cataracts.

Because of high-radiation exposure and overutilization of the CT scanner, low-risk patients should undergo conventional radiography. Only if there is radiographic evidence of a fracture or dislocation on plain films should these patients then undergo CT scanning. For moderate- to high-risk patients, cervical spine CT imaging should be the first-line imaging modality, especially for patients scheduled for CT scanning of another body part.

Plain Film Radiography

A normal cervical CT image adequately excludes a cervical spine fracture but cannot sufficiently evaluate ligamentous instability. In patients who sustained significant flexion, extension, or rotational injury to the neck and who have persistent neck pain, ligamentous stability should be assessed within 10 days either in the ED or by a neurosurgeon or orthopedic spine specialist.

In the ED, patients who are awake and alert and can actively flex and extend the neck 30 degrees may undergo flexion-extension plain film radiography to be evaluated for vertebral column stability. Vertebral body subluxation or focal widening of the spinous processes suggests an unstable ligamentous injury. Manual manipulation of the patient's neck should be avoided during flexion-extension radiography; however, no serious adverse outcomes have resulted from voluntary neck movement by an awake, alert patient without neurologic deficits.

Most of these patient have such severe associated cervical muscle spasms that they have limited neck mobility. As a result, flexion-extension films are often inadequate, and these patients should be immobilized in a semi-rigid cervical collar (e.g., a Philadelphia or Miami J collar) and undergo delayed flexion-extension plain film radiography 7 to 10 days, after the cervical muscle spasms diminish.

Magnetic Resonance Imaging (MRI)

For patients with neurologic deficits, including paresthesias in the arms or legs, emergent cervical spine MRI is warranted to evaluate for potential spinal cord injury.

CLASSIC INJURY PATTERNS

(Tables 70-3, 70-4, and 70-5)

Based on the NEXUS study of 818 patients with cervical spine injury, fractures occurred most commonly at the level of C2 (24% of all fractures), C6 (20%), and C7 (19%). Anatomically, the most commonly fractured part of the cervical spine was the vertebral body, comprising 30% of fractures at the C3-C7 levels. This was more common than fractures of the spinous process (21%), lamina (16%), and articular process (15%). Subluxations occurred most commonly at the C5-C6 (25%) and C6-C7 (23%) levels.[20]

Thoracic/Lumbar Spine Injuries

Similar to patients with cervical spine assessment, low-risk patients may selectively undergo clinical clearance without radiographic imaging. Although there have been no large studies of thoracic/lumbar spine injuries equivalent to the NEXUS and CCR projects, recommendations can be extrapolated from the relevant literature.

Based on the NEXUS criteria, patients with (1) significant back pain or tenderness, (2) clinical evidence of drug- or alcohol-related intoxication, (3) lower extremity neurologic deficits, (4) Glasgow Coma Scale score of less than 15, or (5) a distracting injury cannot be clinically cleared for a thoracic or lumbar fracture. Patients with alcohol intoxication,

Table 70-3 CLASSIC UPPER CERVICAL SPINE INJURY PATTERNS (C1-C2)*

Injury	Mechanism	Stability	Comments
Atlanto-occipital dislocation (Fig. 70-8A)	Flexion	Unstable	Often instantly fatal More common in children because of small, horizontally-oriented occipital condyles Dislocation can be anterior (most common), superiorly distracted, or posterior
Anterior atlantoaxial dislocation (Fig. 70-8B)	Flexion	Unstable	Associated with transverse ligament rupture Most commonly occurs in patients with rheumatoid arthritis and ankylosing spondylitis from ligament laxity Widening of predental space seen on lateral plain films
Jefferson (C1) burst fracture (Fig. 70-8C)	Axial compression	Unstable	33% with associated C2 fracture Low incidence of neurologic injury because of wide C1 spinal canal Usually involves fractures of both the anterior and posterior C1 arches, often with three or four 4 fracture fragments *Complications:* transverse ligament rupture, especially if C1 lateral masses are ≥7 mm wider than expected (MRI recommended); vertebral artery injury (CT angiography recommended)
C1 posterior arch fracture (Fig. 70-8C)	Extension	Stable	An associated C2 fracture (occurs 50% of time) makes the posterior arch fracture unstable On plain films, no displacement of lateral masses on the odontoid view and no prevertebral soft tissue swelling, unlike Jefferson burst fracture
C2 dens fracture (Fig. 70-8D)	Flexion	Variable	*Type I (stable):* Avulsion of dens with intact transverse ligament *Type II (unstable):* Fracture at base of dens; 10% have an associated rupture of the transverse ligament— MRI provides definitive diagnosis of ligament rupture *Type III (stable):* Fracture of dens extending into vertebral body
Hangman's fracture (C2 spondylolisthesis) (Fig. 70-8E)	Extension	Unstable	Bilateral C2 pedicle fractures at risk for disruption of the, C2 anterior subluxation, and C2-C3 disk rupture Low risk for spinal cord injury because of C2 anterior subluxation, which widens spinal canal
Extension teardrop fracture (Fig. 70-8F)	Extension	Unstable	Small triangular avulsion of anteroinferior vertebral body, at insertion point of the ALL Occurs most frequently at C2 level, but can occur in lower cervical spine *Complication:* central cord syndrome due to ligamentum flavum buckling during hyperextension Requires CT differentiation from very unstable *flexion* teardrop fracture (see Table 70-4)

*Listed in progressive order from occipital, C1, to C2.
ALL, anterior longitudinal ligament; CT, computed tomography; MRI, magnetic resonance imaging; PLL, posterior longitudinal ligament.

for example, should be immobilized with full-spinal precautions until they are sober, whereupon they may be cleared clinically if they fulfill no other high-risk criteria.

Furthermore, based on the CCR criteria and the American Healthcare Research and Quality (AHRQ) "red flag" indications for imaging, patients older than 65 years with any degree of back pain or tenderness receiving chronic corticosteroid therapy or with a history of vertebral disease should undergo radiography.

Classic patterns of thoracic/lumbar spine injuries are shown in Table 70-5.

Spinal Cord Injuries

■ PRESENTING SIGNS AND SYMPTOMS

Patients with spinal cord injuries may present with a spectrum of findings ranging from subtle neurologic deficits to grossly obvious paralysis. Spinal cord injuries should be suspected in any trauma victim who complains of neck or back pain, especially pain exacerbated by movement. Neurologic symptoms suggesting spinal cord injury include numbness, tingling, paresthesias, focal weakness, and paralysis. Other worrisome symptoms include urinary or fecal incontinence and urinary retention. Unconscious patients and those with impaired consciousness secondary to intoxication may harbor occult spinal cord injuries.

■ ED EVALUATION

The physical examination is focused on identifying any signs of vertebral fracture, ligamentous instability, and spinal cord injury. The mainstay of diagnosis of a spinal cord injury is a careful, focused neurologic and anogenital examination. Note that in patients

Table 70-4 **CLASSIC LOWER CERVICAL SPINE INJURY PATTERNS (C3-C7)**

Injury	Mechanism	Stability	Comments
Articular mass fracture (Fig. 70-9A)	Flexion-rotation	Stable	Associated with transverse process and vertebral body fractures Uncommon
Burst fracture (Fig. 70-9B)	Axial compression	Stable	Compressive fracture of the anterior and posterior vertebral body Intact ALL and PLL *Complication:* spinal cord injury because of retropulsed vertebral body fragment (especially anterior cord syndrome)
Clay shoveler's (spinous process) fracture (Fig. 70-9B)	Flexion	Stable	Spinous process fracture from forceful neck flexion Most commonly occurs in lower cervical levels, usually C7 Not associated with neurologic injury
Extension teardrop fracture (Fig. 70-8F)	Extension	Unstable	Most commonly occurs at C2 (see Table 70-4)
Facet dislocation, bilateral (Fig. 70-9C)	Flexion	Unstable	Significant anterior displacement (>50%) of spine when bilateral inferior facets displace anterior to the superior facets below At risk for injuring disk, vertebral arteries, and spinal cord
Facet dislocation, unilateral (Fig. 70-9D)	Flexion-rotation	Stable	Usually causes 25-50% anterior displacement of spine *Complication:* vertebral artery injury (CT angiography recommended)
Flexion teardrop fracture (Fig. 70-9E)	Flexion and axial loading	Unstable	One of the most unstable fractures in the lower cervical spine, because it involves both columns Fracture and anterior displacement of anteroinferior vertebral body (appears similar to extension teardrop fracture, except much more unstable) Unique findings for flexion (versus extension) teardrop fractures include same-level fractures and displacement of posterior structures Rupture of both anterior and posterior ligamentous complexes Usually occurs at C5 or C6 Can result from diving into shallow water or football tackling injury Often associated with spinal cord injury and quadriplegia
Subluxation, anterior (Fig. 70-9F)	Flexion	Unstable	Anterior slipping of one vertebra over another Ruptured posterior ligamentous complex, such that anterior and posterior vertebral lines are disrupted *Complication:* vertebral artery dissection (CT angiography recommended) May only be evident on flexion views by conventional radiography when the interspinous distance widens and the vertebral body subluxes anteriorly
Transverse process fracture (Fig. 70-9A)	Lateral flexion	Stable	*Complications:* vertebral artery injury, because the artery travels within the C1-C6 transverse foramina (CT angiography recommended); associated cervical radiculopathy and brachial plexus injuries in 10% of cases
Wedge fracture (Fig. 70-9G)	Flexion	Stable	Compression fracture of only the anterosuperior vertebral body endplate Disruption of anterior vertebral line Intact posterior vertebral body and posterior vertebral line

ALL, anterior longitudinal ligament; CT, computed tomography; PLL, posterior longitudinal ligament.

with neurogenic shock, the extremities may appear warm from peripheral vasodilation.

■ Spinal versus Neurogenic Shock

Spinal shock is a neurologic phenomenon resulting from physiologic transection of the spinal cord. This results in flaccid paralysis and loss of reflexes below the level of the spinal cord lesion. Spinal shock is temporary, most cases commonly lasting 24 to 48 hours, although they can last for weeks. Patients suffering from spinal shock may appear clinically to have a complete spinal cord injury only to "miraculously" recover once the spinal shock has passed. Termination of spinal shock is identified by a return of segmental reflexes; anogenital reflexes are the earliest to return.

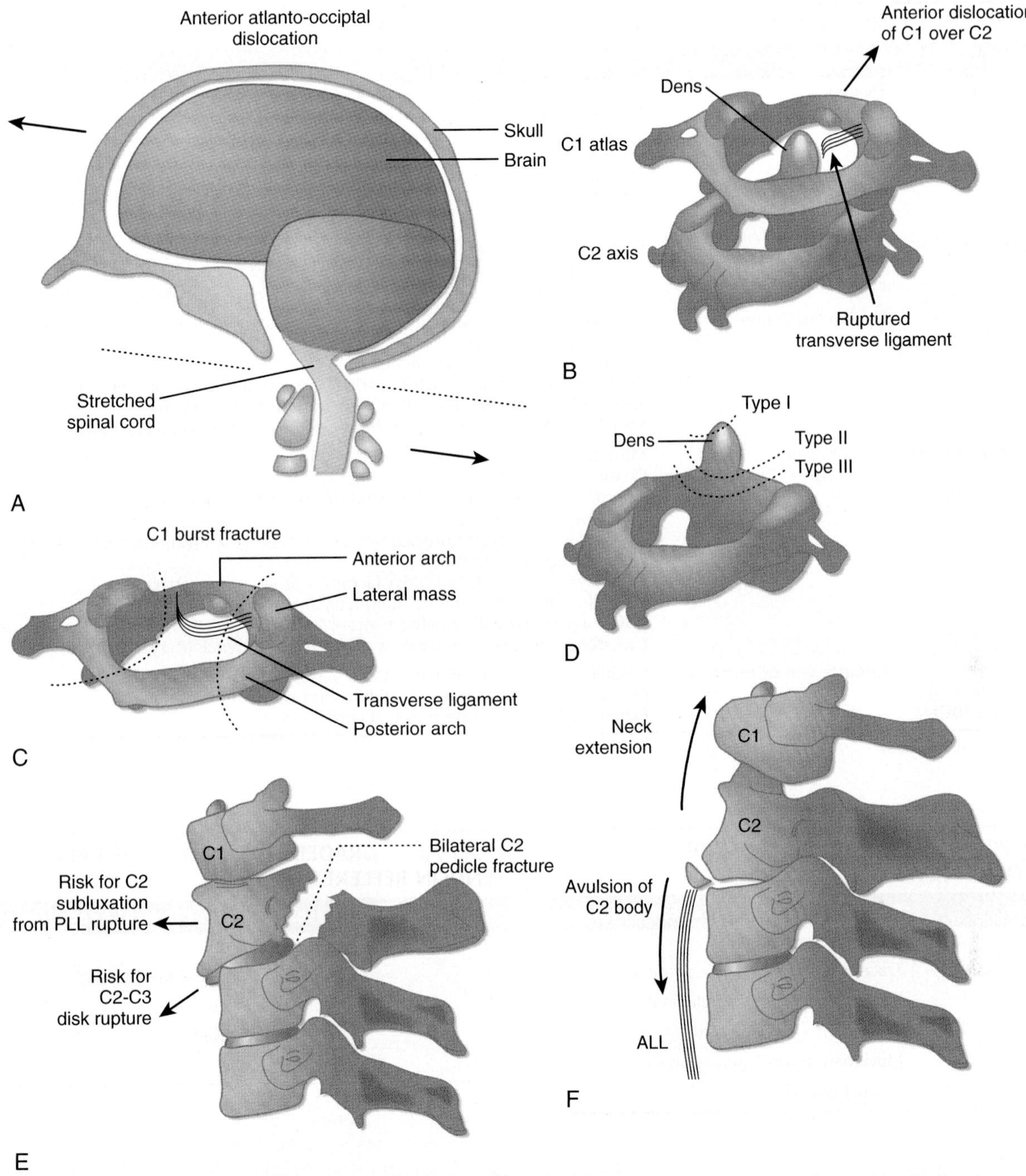
Anterior atlanto-occiptal dislocation
Skull
Brain
Stretched spinal cord
A
Anterior dislocation of C1 over C2
Dens
C1 atlas
C2 axis
Ruptured transverse ligament
B
C1 burst fracture
Anterior arch
Lateral mass
Transverse ligament
Posterior arch
C
Type I
Dens
Type II
Type III
D
C1
C2
Bilateral C2 pedicle fracture
Risk for C2 subluxation from PLL rupture
Risk for C2-C3 disk rupture
E
Neck extension
C1
C2
Avulsion of C2 body
ALL
F

FIGURE 70-8 **A,** Cross-sectional sagittal view of an anterior atlanto-occipital dislocation with associated spinal cord injury. **B,** Posterolateral view of anterior atlantoaxial dislocation from transverse ligament rupture. **C,** Posterolateral view of a C1 Jefferson burst fracture through the anterior and posterior arch, and an isolated C1 posterior arch fracture. **D,** Posterolateral view of the three types of C2 dens fractures. **E,** Sagittal view of a hangman's fracture with bilateral C2 pedicle fracture. PLL, posterior longitudinal ligament. **F,** Sagittal view of C2 extension teardrop fracture. ALL, anterior longitudinal ligament.

Neurogenic shock is a neurocardiovascular phenomenon resulting from impairment of the descending sympathetic pathways in the spinal cord. As a result, there is a loss of vasomotor tone that leads to visceral and peripheral vasodilation and ensuing hypotension. There is also diminished sympathetic innervation to the heart, resulting in relative bradycardia despite hypotension. Neurogenic shock may occur in patients with cervical or high thoracic spinal cord injuries.

■ Neurologic Examination

The neurologic examination includes assessment of the anterior column (motor), lateral spinothalamic tract (sensory), and dorsal column (sensory). The *neurologic level* refers to the most caudal level of the spinal cord with normal sensory and motor function on both sides of the body. Alteration in mental status or intoxication may interfere with accurate determination of the level of injury.

Table 70-5 CLASSIC THORACIC AND LUMBAR SPINE INJURY PATTERNS

Injury	Mechanism	Comments
Wedge fracture (Fig. 70-9G)	Flexion	Most common fracture in the thoracic spine An isolated anterior column fracture Disruption of anterior vertebral line with an intact posterior vertebral line (classic finding) Maintain a low threshold to obtain spine CT to differentiate wedge from burst fracture (up to 22% of burst fractures appear to have an intact posterior vertebral line)
Burst fracture (Fig. 70-9B)	Axial loading	* A fracture of the anterior and middle columns * Disruption of the anterior and posterior vertebral line (classic) * 65% have associated spinal cord injury, because of middle column compromise
Chance fracture (Fig. 70-10A)	Flexion-distraction	Fracture through the anterior, middle, and posterior columns, progressing from posterior to anterior Usually located at T12-L2 junction Classically caused by lap-belt hyperflexion mechanism in motor vehicle collision 33%-89% of fractures associated with intra-abdominal injury Spinal cord injury is uncommon because of the distraction mechanism
Transverse process fracture (Fig. 70-10B)		Most common fracture of the lumbar spine Classically has a vertical fracture orientation Horizontal transverse process fracture orientation suggests a distraction injury (Chance fracture) Over 50% of transverse process fractures missed by conventional radiography, and detected on spine CT Clinically insignificant, but a risk factor for other injury patterns 50% associated with an intra-abdominal injury[7] * 30% associated with a pelvic fracture (especially L5 transverse process fracture) * L2 transverse process fracture is associated with renal artery thrombosis
Fracture-dislocation (Fig. 70-10C)	Compression or distraction	* Significant spinal misalignment and vertebral column discontinuity Fracture through the anterior, middle, and posterior columns Extremely high incidence of spinal cord injury

CT, computed tomography.

Table 70-6 GRADED ASSESSMENT OF MOTOR FUNCTION

Grade	Assessment on Physical Examination
0	No active contraction
1	Trace visible or palpable contraction
2	Movement with gravity eliminated
3	Movement against gravity
4	Movement against gravity and resistance
5	Normal power

Table 70-7 GRADED ASSESSMENT OF DEEP TENDON REFLEXES

Grade	Assessment on Physical Examination
0	Reflexes absent
1	Reflexes diminished but present
2	Normal reflexes
3	Reflexes increased
4	Clonus present

Motor Level

Motor function should be tested and recorded on a scale of 0 to 5 (Table 70-6). The *motor level* is defined as the most caudal segment with at least three fifths of motor function. Injuries of the first eight cervical segments result in tetraplegia (previously known as quadriplegia); lesions below the T1 level result in paraplegia.

Sensory Level

The *sensory level* is defined as the most caudal segment of the spinal cord with normal sensory function. The highest intact sensory level should be marked on the patient's spine to monitor spinal cord injury progression.

Spinothalamic tract sensory function is first evaluated by testing pinprick and light touch bilaterally for each dermatome, starting at insensate levels and moving cephalad. Sensory function is graded as follows: 0 = absent; 1 = impaired; 2 = normal. Posterior column function is assessed by testing vibratory sense with a tuning fork (placed over the bony prominences) and by testing position sense (proprioception) by flexing and extending the great toe.

Deep Tendon Reflexes

On a scale of 0 to 4, the deep tendon reflexes are assessed in the upper (biceps, triceps) and lower (patellar, Achilles) extremities (Table 70-7).

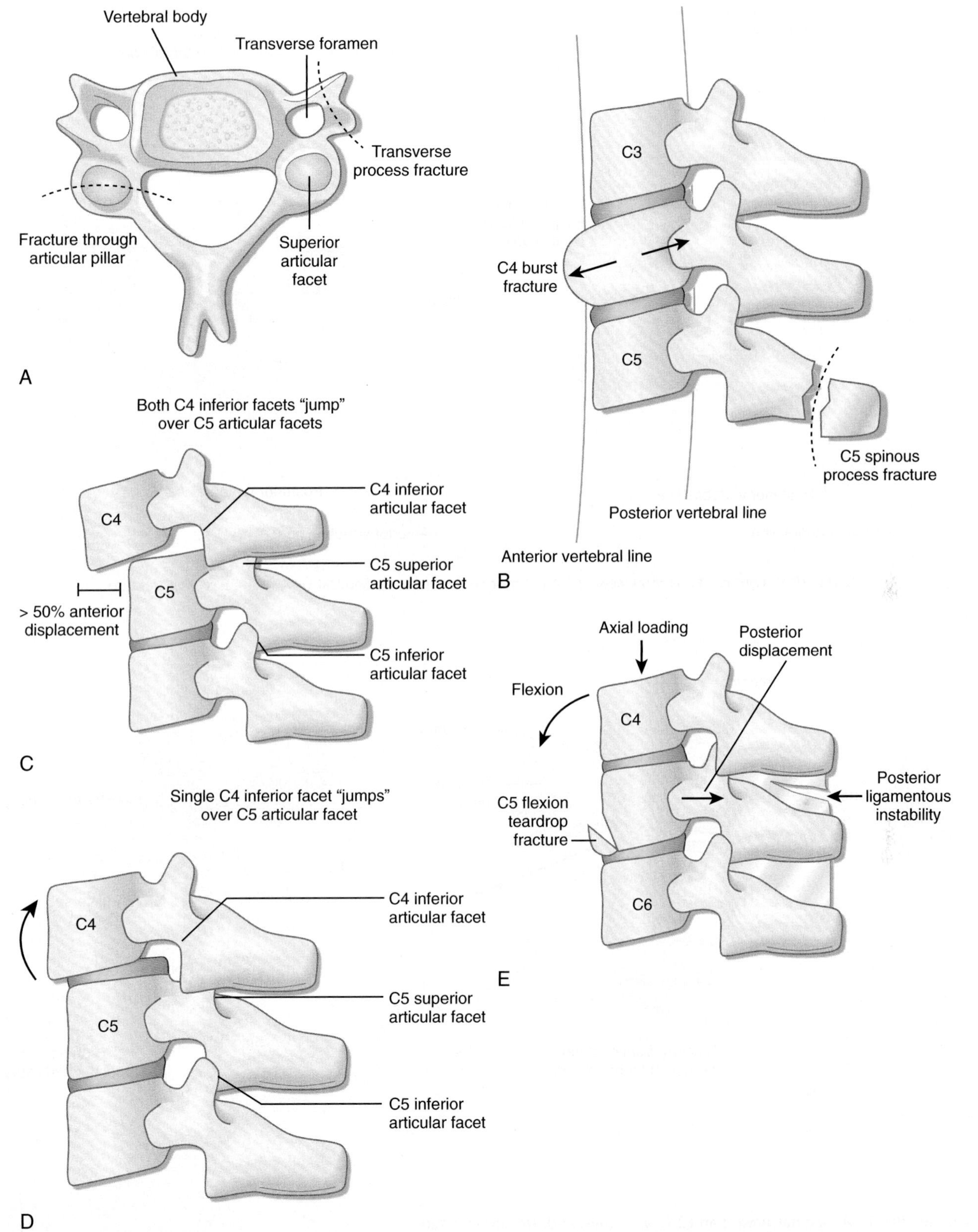
Vertebral body
Transverse foramen
Transverse process fracture
Fracture through articular pillar
Superior articular facet
A
Both C4 inferior facets "jump" over C5 articular facets
C4
C5
C4 inferior articular facet
C5 superior articular facet
> 50% anterior displacement
C5 inferior articular facet
C
Single C4 inferior facet "jumps" over C5 articular facet
C4
C5
C4 inferior articular facet
C5 superior articular facet
C5 inferior articular facet
D
C3
C4 burst fracture
C5
C5 spinous process fracture
Posterior vertebral line
Anterior vertebral line
B
Axial loading
Posterior displacement
Flexion
C4
C5 flexion teardrop fracture
Posterior ligamentous instability
C6
E

FIGURE 70-9 **A,** Superior axial view of articular pillar fracture and transverse process fracture. **B,** Sagittal view of C4 burst fracture and C5 clay shoveler's (spinous process) fracture. **C,** Sagittal view of a C4 bilateral facet dislocation. **D,** Sagittal view of a C4 unilateral facet dislocation. **E,** Sagittal view of a C5 teardrop fracture.

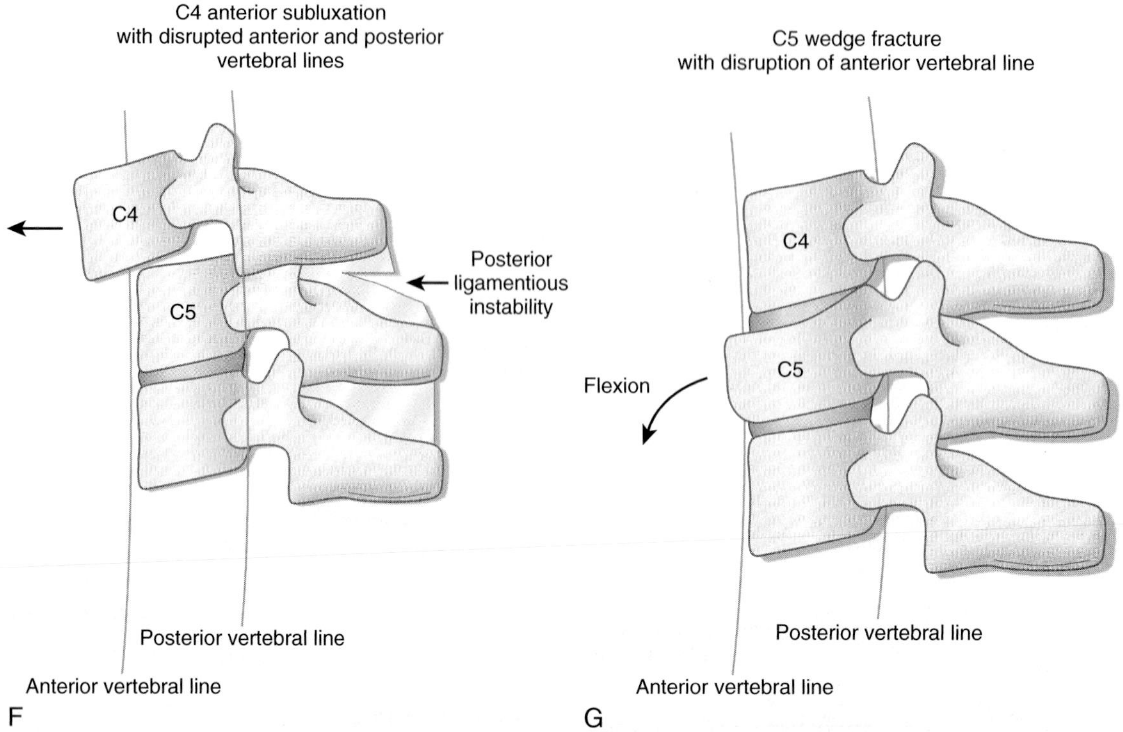
C4 anterior subluxation
with disrupted anterior and posterior
vertebral lines
C4
C5
Posterior
ligamentious
instability
Posterior vertebral line
Anterior vertebral line
F
C5 wedge fracture
with disruption of anterior vertebral line
C4
C5
Flexion
Posterior vertebral line
Anterior vertebral line
G

FIGURE 70-9, cont'd F, Sagittal view of C4 anterior subluxation. G, Sagittal view of a C5 wedge fracture.

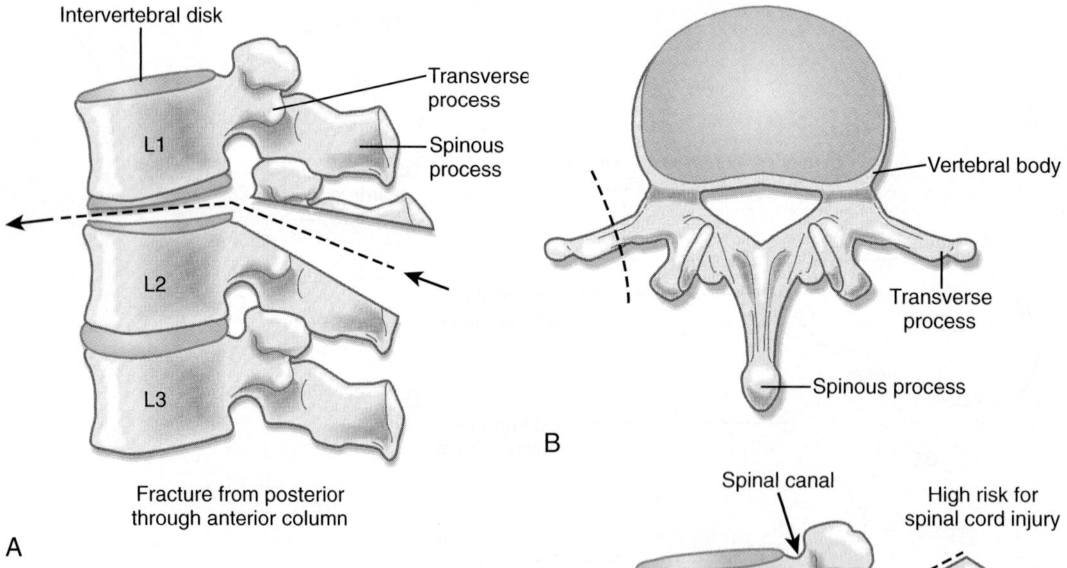
Intervertebral disk
Transverse
process
Spinous
process
L1
L2
L3
Fracture from posterior
through anterior column
A
Vertebral body
Transverse
process
Spinous process
B

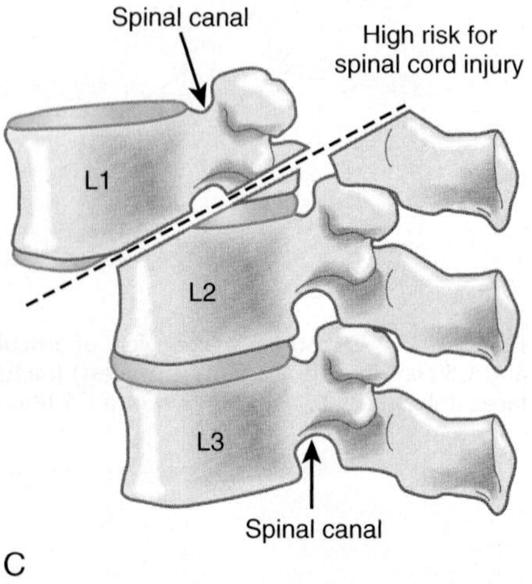
Spinal canal
High risk for
spinal cord injury
L1
L2
L3
Spinal canal
C

FIGURE 70-10 A, Sagittal view of an L2 Chance (flexion-distraction) fracture. **B,** Superior axial view of a transverse process fracture in a typical lumbar spine. **C,** Sagittal view of L1-L2 fracture-dislocation injury, at high risk for a spinal cord injury because of the spinal canal discontinuity.

Anogenital Examination

In the anogenital examination, rectal tone and anogenital reflexes should be assessed, as well as signs of urinary or fecal retention or incontinence, and sacral sensation. The finding of priapism, an abnormal penile erection, may be seen in men with spinal cord injuries.

Anogenital reflexes include the anal wink and bulbocavernosus reflex. An *anal wink* (S2-S4) is present if the anal sphincter contracts in response to stroking the skin of the perianal area. The *bulbocavernosus reflex* (S3-S4) is elicited by squeezing the glans penis/clitoris (or pulling on an inserted Foley catheter), which results in reflexive contraction of the anal sphincter.

Head-to-Toe Physical Examination

After immediate life-threatening concerns have been addressed, a thorough head-to-toe physical examination should be performed. The patient's inability to perceive pain as a result of a spinal cord injury may mask potentially serious injuries elsewhere in the body. Imaging of high-risk regions, such as the abdomen, and of areas of bruising or swelling may be required to exclude occult injuries.

CLASSIFICATION OF SPINAL CORD INJURY

Complete Injury

A spinal cord injury is classified as physiologically complete if the patient has no demonstrable motor or sensory function below the level of injury. During the first few days following injury, this diagnosis cannot be made with certainty because of the possibility of concurrent spinal shock.

Incomplete Injury

A spinal cord injury is incomplete if motor function or sensation or both are partially present below the level of the injury. Signs of an incomplete injury may include (1) the presence of any sensation or voluntary movement in the lower extremities and/or (2) evidence of sacral sparing. Signs of sacral sparing include perianal sensation, voluntary anal sphincter contraction, and voluntary great toe flexion.

Specific incomplete spinal cord injuries include central and anterior cord syndromes, Brown-Séquard syndrome, and conus medullaris syndrome. Patients with these syndromes present with certain characteristic patterns of neurologic injury with distinct physical examination findings.

Central Cord Syndrome

Central cord syndrome is the most common of the spinal cord syndromes, usually resulting from neck hyperextension. Trauma to the central portion of the cord results in injury to the medially located corticospinal motor tracts of the upper extremities. As a result, the upper extremities are predictably and disproportionately weaker than the lower extremities. Many patients exhibit bladder dysfunction (e.g., urinary retention) and varying degrees of sensory loss. Elderly patients are more at risk for central cord syndrome because of underlying cervical spondylosis and/or a thickened ligamentum flavum.

Anterior Cord Syndrome

Anterior cord syndrome results from blunt or ischemic injury to the anterior spinal cord. These patients present with a complete and usually bilateral motor deficit below the level of the injury with loss of pain and temperature sensation a few levels below the lesion. Typically, posterior column function is preserved.

Brown-Séquard Syndrome

Brown-Séquard syndrome is a rare hemicord injury usually associated with penetrating trauma. Patients present with crossed sensory and motor deficits: ipsilateral loss of motor function and position sense below the level of the lesion and contralateral loss of pain and temperature sensation one to two levels below the injury.

Conus Medullaris Syndrome

Conus medullaris syndrome results from injury to the sacral cord with occasional involvement of the lumbar nerve roots. This results in areflexia of the bladder, bowel, and lower extremities. Patients may have perianal numbness. Motor and sensory deficits in the lower limbs vary.

DIAGNOSTIC TESTING

Plain Radiography and Computed Tomography (CT) Imaging

Trauma patients with symptoms suggesting of a spinal cord injury should undergo CT imaging of suspicious areas of the spine. Although plain films and CT imaging do not directly reveal spinal cord injuries, they may supply indirect evidence of such injuries. Spinal cord injury without radiographic abnormality (SCIWORA) is a traumatic myelopathy that presents without identifiable abnormalities on plain films or CT.

Magnetic Resonance Imaging (MRI)

MRI is the best available modality for detection and characterization of spinal cord injury but is less sensitive than CT for cervical spine fractures. Abnormal MRI findings may include the presence of spinal canal compromise, disc herniation, and spinal cord edema or hemorrhage. In the acute trauma patient with potential spine injury, the indications for an emergent MRI include (1) complete or incomplete neurologic deficits suspicious for a spinal cord injury, (2) deterioration of spinal cord neurologic function, and (3) signs of unstable ligamentous injury.

TREATMENT

Management of Neurogenic Shock

Neurogenic shock results from a sympathectomy-induced reduction in blood pressure, heart rate, cardiac contractility, and cardiac output. Overly vigorous fluid resuscitation can be hazardous because of compromised cardiac output. Judicious use of vasopressors such as phenylephrine hydrochloride, dopamine, and norepinephrine is often indicated. Significant bradycardia should be treated hemodynamically with atropine.

A systolic blood pressure greater than 80 mm Hg is rarely due to spinal cord injury alone, and other causes of shock, primarily from hemorrhage, must be excluded. It should never be assumed that hypotension is due to spinal shock until hemorrhage is excluded.

Corticosteroid Therapy

Although controversial, treatment of blunt spinal cord injury with high-dose methylprednisolone is common. This therapeutic recommendation is based on the findings of the National Acute Spinal Cord Injury Study (NASCIS), which demonstrated improved neurologic function in patients receiving high-dose corticosteroids within 8 hours of injury. Improved neurologic function, however, was defined as a modest gain in motor scores but not in functional improvement. In the NASCIS, a loading dose of 30 mg/kg methylprednisolone over 15 minutes is followed by an infusion of 5.4 mg/kg/hour and continued for 24 hours (in patients treated within 3 hours of injury) or 48 hours (in patients treated 3 to 8 hours after injury).[24,25] There was no benefit to steroids administered more than 8 hours of injury.

Steroid therapy is not indicated for penetrating injuries and has not been adequately studied in children less than 13 years old or in patients with cauda equina or spinal root injury.

Finally, systemic corticosteroid therapy is not benign. Complications of steroid therapy include gastrointestinal hemorrhage and wound infections in patients treated with corticosteroid infusions for 24 hours, and higher rates of severe sepsis and severe pneumonia in those treated for 48 hours. The use of steroids for blunt traumatic spinal cord injury is far from the standard of care.[26] More research is needed to verify or refute this controversial therapy.

Surgical Management

Timely reduction of the displaced spinal column and decompression of the spinal cord has been associated with recovery from otherwise devastating spinal cord injuries.[27] The optimal timing of surgery following a spinal injury remains controversial. Some argue for immediate surgery, whereas others advocate delayed surgery because of initial post-traumatic swelling. The sole absolute indication for immediate surgery is a progressively worsening neurologic status in patients with spinal fracture-dislocations who initially present with incomplete or absent neurologic deficits.[28]

In a series of patients with traumatic central cord syndrome, those who underwent early surgery (<24 hours after injury) and had an underlying disk herniation or fracture dislocation had significantly greater overall motor improvement than those who underwent late surgery (>24 hours after injury).[29] Unfortunately, early decompressive surgery does not uniformly improve outcome following spinal cord injury.

DISPOSITION

Admission Criteria

Patients with confirmed or suspected spinal cord injury should be scheduled for early consultation with a neurosurgeon or orthopedist. This may require patient transfer to a spine specialty center.

The level of spinal cord injury, associated neurologic deficits, and other traumatic injuries will determine whether the patient should be admitted to the intensive care unit, neurosurgical observation unit, or general ward. Circular beds, rotating frames, and serial inflation devices are used to protect from pressure sores.

FACTS AND FORMULAS $SI = \frac{SV}{BSA}$

- 10% of spinal fractures have a second noncontiguous fracture along the vertebral spine.
- 10% of patients with a calcaneal fracture have an associated thoracic or lumbar fracture.
- The most commonly fractured cervical spine level is C2, especially in the elderly.
- Approximately 20% of computed tomography–confirmed burst fractures in the thoracic and lumbar spine appear as wedge fractures on plain film radiography.
- High-dose methylprednisolone is administered as a 30 mg/kg bolus and then as a 5.4 mg/kg/hour infusion for 24 hours (if started within 3 hours of injury) or for 48 hours (if started within 8 hours of injury).
- Consider early endotracheal intubation in spinal cord injury patients with a negative inspiratory force (NIF) of less than –25 cm H_2O or vital capacity (VC) of less than 15 mL/kg.

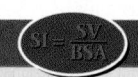

REFERENCES

1. Berkowitz M: Assessing the socioeconomic impact of improved treatment of head and spinal cord injuries. J Emerg Med 1993;11:63-57.
2. Reid DC, Henderson R, Saboe L, et al: Etiology and clinical course of missed spine fractures. J Trauma 1987; 27:980-986.
3. Nunez DB Jr, Zuluaga A, Fuentes-Bernardo DA, et al: Cervical spine trauma: How much more do we learn by routinely using helical CT? Radiographics 1996;16:1307-1318.
4. Woodring JH, Lee C: Limitations of cervical radiography in the evaluation of acute cervical trauma. J Trauma 1993; 34:32-39.
5. Hauser CJ, Visvikis G, Hinrichs C, et al: Prospective validation of computed tomographic screening of the thoracolumbar spine in trauma. J Trauma 2003;55:228-234.
6. Lucey BC, Stuhlfaut JW, Hochberg AR, et al: Evaluation of blunt abdominal trauma using PACS-based 2D and 3D MDCT reformations of the lumbar spine and pelvis.AJR Am J Roentgenol 2005;185:1435-1440.
7. Patten RM, Gunberg SR, Brandenburger DK: Frequency and importance of transverse process fractures in the lumbar vertebrae at helical abdominal CT in patients with trauma. Radiology 2000;215:831-834.
8. Tyroch AH, McGuire EL, McLean SF, et al: The association between Chance fractures and intra-abdominal injuries revisited: A multicenter review. Am Surg 2005;71: 434-438.
9. Lowery DW, Wald MM, Browne BJ, et al: Epidemiology of cervical spine injury victims. Ann Emerg Med 2001; 38:12.
10. Deyo RA, Rainville J, Kent DL: What can the history and physical examination tell us about low back pain? JAMA 1992;268: 760-765.
11. Chiu WC, Haan JM, Cushing BM, et al: Ligamentous injuries of the cervical spine in unreliable blunt trauma patients: Incidence, evaluation, and outcome. J Trauma 2001; 50:457-464.
12. Demetriades D, Charalambides K, Chahwan S, et al: Nonskeletal cervical spine injuries: Epidemiology and diagnostic pitfalls. J Trauma 2000;48:724-727.
13. Domeier RM, Frederiksen SM, Welch K: Prospective performance assessment of an out-of-hospital protocol for selective spine immobilization using clinical spine clearance criteria. Ann Emerg Med 2005;46:123-131.
14. Stroh G, Braude D: Can an out-of-hospital cervical spine clearance protocol identify all patients with injuries? An argument for selective immobilization. Ann Emerg Med 2001;37:609-615.
15. Hoffman JR, Mower WR, Wolfson AB, et al: Validity of a set of clinical criteria to rule out injury to the cervical spine in patients with blunt trauma. N Engl J Med 2000; 343:94-99.
16. Stiell IG, Clement CM, McKnight RD, et al: The Canadian C-Spine Rule versus the NEXUS low-risk criteria in patients with trauma. N Engl J Med 2003;349:2510-2518.
17. Mahadevan SV, Navarro M: The evaluation and clearance of the cervical spine in adult trauma patients: Clinical concepts, controversies, and advances. Trauma Reports 2004;5:1-12.
18. Velmahos GC, Theodorou D, Tatevossian R, et al: Radiographic cervical spine evaluation in the alert asymptomatic blunt trauma victim: Much ado about nothing? J Trauma Injury 1994;40:768-774.
19. Blackmore CC, Ramsey SD, Mann, et al: Cervical spine screening with CT in trauma patients: A cost-effective analysis. Radiology 1999;212:117-125.
20. Goldberg W, Mueller C, Panacek E, et al: Distribution and patterns of blunt traumatic cervical spine injury. Ann Emerg Med 2001;38:17-21.
21. Ballock RT, Mackersie R, Abitbol JJ, et al: Can burst fractures be predicted from plain radiographs? J Bone Joint Surg Br 1992;74:147-150.
22. Dai LY: Imaging diagnosis of thoracolumbar burst fractures. Chin Med Sci J 2004;19:142-144.
23. Blood pressure management after acute spinal cord injury. Neurosurgery. 2002;50(3 Suppl):S58-S2.
24. Bracken MB, Holford TR: Effects of timing of methylprednisolone or naloxone administration on recovery of segmental and long-tract neurological function in NASCIS 2. J Neurosurg 1993;79:500-507.
25. Bracken MB, Shepard MJ, Holford TR, et al: Administration of methylprednisolone for 24 or 48 hours or tirilazad mesylate for 48 hours in the treatment of acute spinal cord injury. Results of the Third National Acute Spinal Cord Injury Randomized Controlled Trial. National Acute Spinal Cord Injury Study. JAMA. 1997;277:1597-1604.
26. Spencer MT, Bazarian JJ: Evidence-based emergency medicine/systematic review abstract. Are corticosteroids effective in traumatic spinal cord injury? Ann Emerg Med. 2003;41:410-413.
27. Brunette DD, Rockswold GL: Neurologic recovery following rapid spinal realignment for complete cervical spinal cord injury. J Trauma 1987;27:445-447.
28. Lindsey RW, Pneumaticos SG, Gugala ZG: Management techniques in spinal injuries. In Browner BD, Jupiter JB, Levine AM, Trafton PG (eds): Skeletal Trauma: Basic Science, Management, and Reconstruction, 3rd ed. Philadelphia, WB Saunders, 2003, pp 746-747.
29. Guest J, Eleraky MA, Apostolides PJ, et al: Traumatic central cord syndrome: Results of surgical management. J Neurosurg 2002;97:25-32.

Chapter 71

Facial Trauma

John H. Burton and Nicholas Armellino

KEY POINTS

Treatment of all facial injuries should be directed initially to maintenance of the airway and ventilation and to stabilization of other life-threatening injuries.

A surgical airway may be required when facial injuries result in impaired function or visualization of oral intubation landmarks.

It should be assumed that a cervical spine injury is present until the spine is clinically and/or radiographically determined to have no injury.

Trauma to the eye is common in facial trauma patients; a complete ocular evaluation should be considered a routine component of the facial examination.

Facial computed tomography imaging is routine for visualization of facial fractures; however, a Water's view plain radiograph may be sufficient in patients with isolated facial injury and a low index of suspicion for a midface fracture.

Scope

The emphasis of this chapter is to provide the reader with fundamental knowledge in the assessment and treatment of patients with facial trauma and to underscore the priority actions needed to ensure patient safety with preservation of an acceptable cosmetic result.

A person's face is the focal point of conversation and social interaction. Within the face is embodied each person's mode of expression and communication. The face also has a receptive importance because of all the special sensory functions of the body located within the facial structures. Thus it is not surprising that facial disfigurement harbors the potential for both physical impairment as well as long-term psychological sequelae.

Death from facial trauma is rare, and the severity of facial injuries is often perceived by the patient to be out of proportion to the actual injury. The goal of the EP is to secure the airway, identify the injury, preserve appearance, and consult with the appropriate surgeon to determine further treatment and follow-up.

General Anatomy

The major bones of the face create its defining features and include the frontal, nasal, zygoma, maxilla, mandible, and temporal bones. The orbit consists of the maxilla, zygoma, frontal, sphenoid, orbital and lacrimal bones (Fig. 71-1).

The face conventionally is divided into thirds: upper, middle, and lower. The borders of each third are loosely defined by the branches of the trigeminal nerve, which provides the sensory innervation to the face. Identification of the exiting foramen for the distributing branches of the trigeminal nerve (cranial

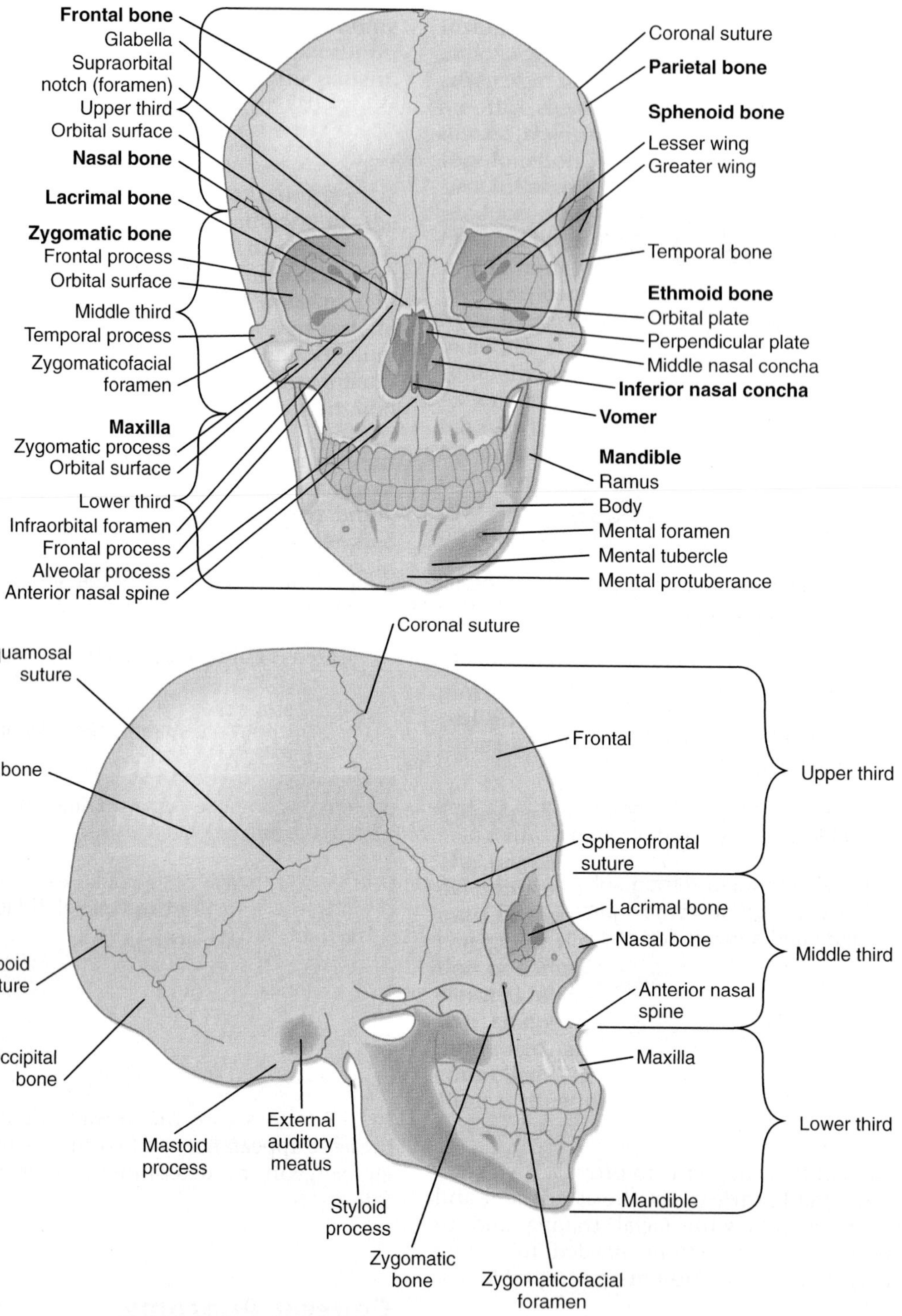

Frontal bone
Glabella
Supraorbital notch (foramen)
Upper third
Orbital surface
Nasal bone
Lacrimal bone
Zygomatic bone
Frontal process
Orbital surface
Middle third
Temporal process
Zygomaticofacial foramen
Maxilla
Zygomatic process
Orbital surface
Lower third
Infraorbital foramen
Frontal process
Alveolar process
Anterior nasal spine
Coronal suture
Parietal bone
Sphenoid bone
Lesser wing
Greater wing
Temporal bone
Ethmoid bone
Orbital plate
Perpendicular plate
Middle nasal concha
Inferior nasal concha
Vomer
Mandible
Ramus
Body
Mental foramen
Mental tubercle
Mental protuberance
Coronal suture
Squamosal suture
Parietal bone
Frontal
Upper third
Sphenofrontal suture
Lacrimal bone
Nasal bone
Middle third
Lamboid suture
Anterior nasal spine
Occipital bone
Maxilla
Lower third
External auditory meatus
Mastoid process
Styloid process
Mandible
Zygomatic bone
Zygomaticofacial foramen

FIGURE 71-1 Facial bones and essential structures of facial anatomy.

nerve V) is crucial when providing local nerve anesthesia (Fig. 71-2).

The facial nerve (cranial nerve VII) intricately courses through the parotid duct, providing parasympathetic innervation, special sensory function to the tongue and soft palate, and general motor function to the 44 muscles of facial expression. Deep facial lacerations between the tragus and lateral canthus may jeopardize the integrity of the facial nerve. Any damage to the facial nerve distal to the stylomastoid foramen can result in facial nerve dysfunction, commonly referred to as Bell's palsy.

The parotid duct lies in a plane with the tragus and inferior corner of the nasal vestibule. Competency of the parotid duct must be considered when there are deep lacerations to this region of the face (Fig. 71-3).

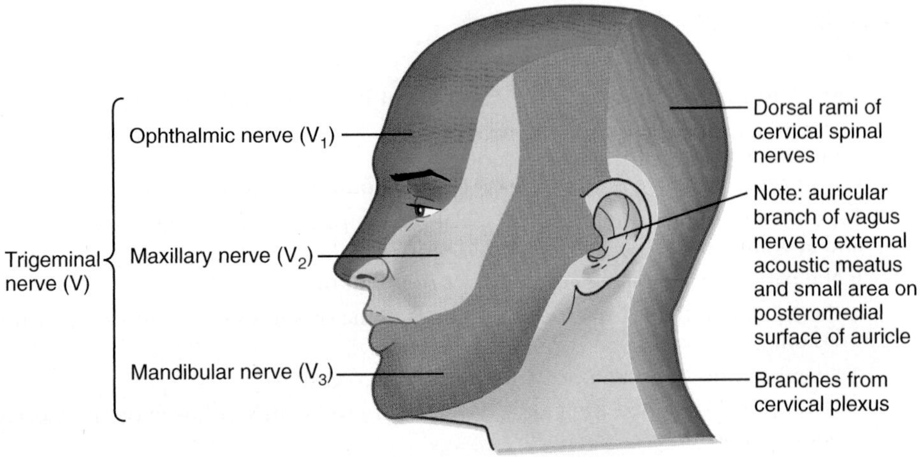
Trigeminal nerve (V)
Ophthalmic nerve (V_1)
Maxillary nerve (V_2)
Mandibular nerve (V_3)
Dorsal rami of cervical spinal nerves
Note: auricular branch of vagus nerve to external acoustic meatus and small area on posteromedial surface of auricle
Branches from cervical plexus

FIGURE 71-2 Anatomic location and distribution of the trigeminal nerve.

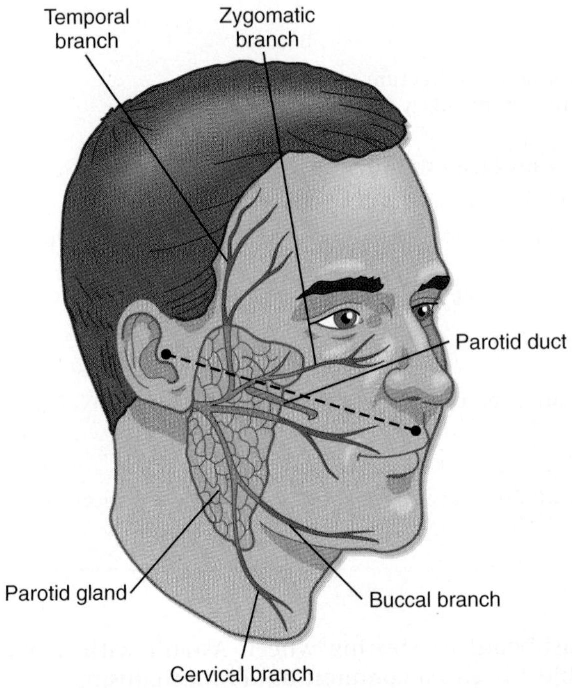
Temporal branch
Zygomatic branch
Parotid duct
Parotid gland
Buccal branch
Cervical branch

FIGURE 71-3 Location of the parotid duct complex.

The external carotid artery is the major vascular supply to the face. There is extensive collateral supply by this vessel to midline tissues through anastomosis (Fig. 71-4).

Approach to the Multitrauma Patient with Facial Injuries

The degree of tissue distortion following facial trauma should not dissuade the initial treatment priorities of the patient. Although rare, facial trauma can be a life-threatening insult, and the EP must address life-threatening injuries before evaluating the obvious facial injury.

The mere presence of a facial fracture, particularly to the midface, greatly increases the risk of traumatic brain injury. The energy required to fracture the midface is often transmitted to the neurocranium and results in an association with a high incidence of brain death. In general, non-surviving patients with facial fractures have higher injury severity scores and lower Glascow Coma Scores and are an older population. Other typical concomitant injuries include pulmonary contusions, abdominal injuries, and cervical spine injuries.

The blood supply to the face consists of a complex system from branches of the internal and external carotid arteries with several anastomoses between them. However, the majority of the vascular supply is via the internal maxillary artery, originating from the external carotid. The internal maxillary artery passes between the Le Fort fracture lines and can be dissected with severe midface trauma.

The treatment of bleeding must begin with inspection of the airway and maintenance of its patency. Local hemorrhage may be controlled with posterior nasal packing or insertion of a Foley catheter advanced into the nasopharynx and inflated with air. The catheter should be gently pulled anterior in an attempt to close the posterior choana. Temporary external reduction of fractures may also provide stabilization of arterial injuries. Finally, surgical ligation of the external carotid artery or transcatheter arterial embolization of the maxillary artery can be performed to effect hemostasis.

Frontal Skull Injuries

■ SCOPE

Fracture of the frontal bone is an unusual isolated fracture and typically is associated with other facial injuries. The force required to fracture the frontal bone is greater than that for other facial structures and should raise the clinician's suspicion of intracranial and/or cervical spine pathology.

PRIORITY ACTIONS

- Suspicious mechanism of injury? Is the patient being physically abused?
  - Obtain a history with only the patient in the room, and ask directed questions concerning the injury mechanism and patient circumstances.
  - Contact appropriate resources if the patient confirms a history of physical abuse.
- Typical concomitant injuries in the facial trauma patient include pulmonary contusions, intracranial pathology, and abdominal and cervical spine injuries.
- Is the patient experiencing a sudden loss of vision or eye pain?
  - Increased retrobulbar pressure from a hematoma or emphysema can lead to acute and permanent loss of vision.
- A lateral canthotomy can be a vision-saving intervention.
  - Loss of the perception of light or of the ability to identify colors without associated eye pain is indicative of optic neuropathy.
- Emergent consultation with an ophthalmologist and computed tomography of the orbits and globes are required when considerating optic nerve impingement.
- Pain with eye movement? Does the patient have muscle entrapment?
  - Obtain computed tomography imaging of the maxilla and orbit when considering a "blowout" injury fracture to the orbit.
- Loss of sensation in distribution of the
  - Superior orbital nerve—consider superior orbital rim or frontal bone fracture.
  - Inferior orbital nerve—consider zygoma, inferior orbital rim, or maxillary fracture.
  - Mandibular nerve—consider mandibular fracture.
- Does the patient have malocclusion? Consider mandibular or maxillary fracture.
- The tongue blade test is useful as a clinical screening examination for mandible fractures.
- Lacerations through the vermilion border require extra attention to detail—slight malalignment may result in substantial cosmetic implications.
- Competency of the parotid duct must be considered for all deep cheek lacerations.
- Do not attempt to realign a fractured nose in the ED.
- Does the patient have a septal hematoma?
  - A septal hematoma requires immediate evacuation, application of a wound dressing, prophylactic antibiotics, and close follow-up for wound care.
- Does the patient have an otohematoma?
  - Otohematomas should be drained with an adherent pressure dressing applied to prevent reaccumulation.
- Is the patient's tetanus immunization up to date?

Documentation

- A detailed cranial nerve examination, with special attention to:
  - Ocular movements
  - Sensory examination of the face
  - Visual acuity
  - Cervical spine "cleared" clinical or radiographic criteria
  - Absence of septal hematoma with a history of nasal trauma

■ PATHOPHYSIOLOGY

The force necessary to fracture the frontal bone is commonly the result of a motor vehicle accident, when the passenger strikes the forehead against the dashboard or steering wheel. Assault with a blunt object is also a common injury mechanism.

■ ANATOMY

The frontal bone is the only constituent of the forehead; the prominent protuberance is called the glabella. Within the frontal bone resides the frontal sinus with communication with the nasopharynx via the frontonasal canal. The anterior bone of the frontal sinus is thicker than the posterior aspect. The intracranial dura mater is adherent to the posterior frontal sinus wall. The cutaneous innervation of the frontal bone is supplied by the superior orbital nerve, a branch of the trigeminal nerve.

■ TREATMENT AND DISPOSITION

Anterior frontal sinus fractures without any concomitant injuries are non–life-threatening; the patient

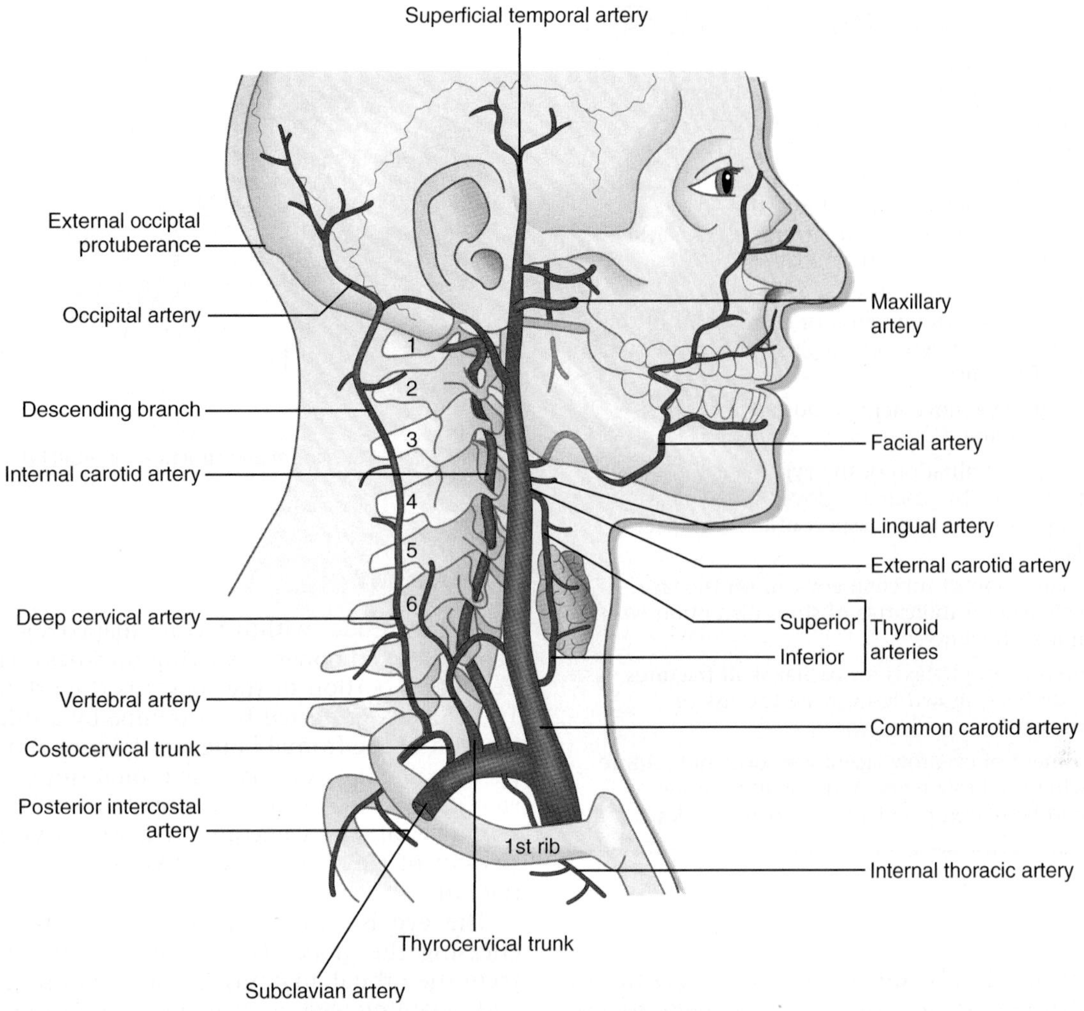
Superficial temporal artery
External occipital protuberance
Occipital artery
Descending branch
Internal carotid artery
Deep cervical artery
Vertebral artery
Costocervical trunk
Posterior intercostal artery
Maxillary artery
Facial artery
Lingual artery
External carotid artery
Superior
Inferior
Thyroid arteries
Common carotid artery
Internal thoracic artery
1st rib
Thyrocervical trunk
Subclavian artery
1
2
3
4
5
6

FIGURE 71-4 Vascular supply to the face and skull.

can be discharged with close consultant follow-up in order to maintain an adequate cosmetic result.

Conversely, frontal bone fractures that involve the posterior wall of the sinus or fractures are associated with cerebrospinal fluid rhinorrhea; the patient will require urgent consultation with a neurosurgeon and admission to the hospital. Although antibiotics have not been shown to decrease the incidence of meningitis associated with a cerebrospinal fluid leak and frontal bone fracture, antibiotic therapy should be based on the consultant's preference after review of the specific injury.

Ocular trauma or sudden loss of vision associated with a frontal bone injury requires immediate ophthalmologic consultation.

Blunt Ophthalmic and Orbital Trauma

■ SCOPE

Trauma to the eye is the second leading cause of blindness in the United States. Traumatic eye injuries may present as a solitary injury to the eye or part of a multitrauma presentation. Immediately after stabilization of the facial trauma patient, the EP must direct attention to evaluation of the eye, as time is of critical importance for saving this organ.

■ PATHOPHYSIOLOGY

Trauma to the eye can result from falls, motor vehicle accidents, and direct blows from an assault or a projectile object (hockey puck, baseball). Serious eye injury has been shown to be most commonly associated with midface fractures.

Ocular trauma can be divided into two broad categories: direct trauma to the globe and trauma to the orbit. Direct globe trauma ranges in severity from a benign corneal abrasion to globe rupture. Orbit trauma involves injuries such as benign contusions and fractures with complications to surrounding structures, including the globe and extraocular muscles.

Orbital fractures are classified as "impure," when the fracture line involves the orbital rim, or as "pure," a fracture with no rim involvement. Compression of the optic nerve (ocular neuropathy) can be caused by

Tips and Tricks

- Identification of the exiting foramen for the distributing branches of the trigeminal nerve is crucial for providing regional anesthesia.
- Severe epistaxis may be controlled with insertion of a Foley catheter advanced into the nasopharynx, inflated, and retracted against the nasopharynx as a posterior nasal pack.
- Upward gaze palsy with vertical diplopia is consistent with dysfunction or entrapment of the inferior rectus muscle and suggestive of an orbital blowout fracture.
- Pain with eye movement is indicative of an orbital fracture.
- Intraoral examination of the zygoma is accomplished by placing a gloved finger along the superior and lateral aspect of the maxillary molars.
- Any palpation of subcutaneous air on the face examination is indicative of sinus disruption with a midface fracture
- Antibiotic prophylaxis for basilar skull fractures has not been shown to decrease the risk of meningitis.
- Treatment of eyebrow lacerations does not require shaving the brow hairs. Additionally, sutures should be placed parallel to the hair follicles.

displacement of a fracture, increased pressure from a retrobulbar hemorrhage, or optic nerve hemorrhage. Each of these processes has the potential to lead to rapidly progressive vision loss and is an ophthalmologic emergency.

The mechanism of orbital "blowout" fractures has been investigated by Waterhouse and colleagues[1] using the same principles as Le Fort a century earlier (see later). Waterhouse investigated the two possible mechanisms for an orbital blowout fracture, the hydraulic and buckling theories. The hydraulic mechanism occurs when the vector of the force directed on an uninjured globe is transmitted to the fixed orbital walls, resulting in a large fracture of the inferior and/or medial orbital wall (Fig. 71-5). This mechanism commonly is associated with herniation of orbital contents through the fractured orbital wall, hence the term "blowout." The buckling mechanism, in contrast, occurs when a traumatic force is directed to the inferior orbital rim causing only the inferior floor of the orbit to buckle, or fracture, with no associated herniation of orbital contents.

Herniation of orbital contents—fatty connective tissue, inferior rectus, and inferior oblique muscles—occurs at the weakest portions of the orbit, specifically the orbital floor and anteromedial wall. With increased pressure to the globe, any defect of these bony structures may lead to herniation of the orbital contents and resultant muscular entrapment.

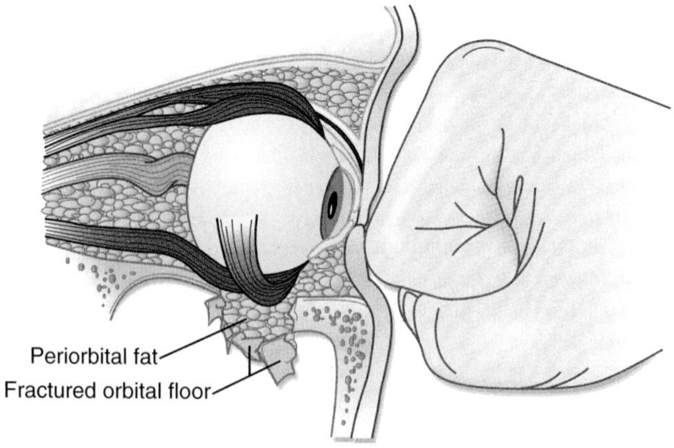
Periorbital fat
Fractured orbital floor

FIGURE 71-5 Mechanism and structures of orbital blowout fracture.

■ ANATOMY

The globe resides within a cone-shaped socket composed of seven bones of varying thickness. The thinnest bony portion of the socket is the orbital floor. The globe is protected from trauma by a thick superior rim of the frontal bone and inferior rim of both the maxilla and zygoma. The orbital rim possesses a smooth contour with occasional notching that is symmetrical when encountered. Any asymmetrical step-off of this rim is indicative of a potential rim fracture.

The eye is cushioned by a retrobulbar fat pad encasing the globe. The extraocular muscles complete the orbital anatomy by surrounding the globe and enabling eye movement. Herniation of any orbital contents through the inferior or medial walls will result in protrusion of these structures, in whole or in part, into the maxillary or ethmoidal sinus, respectively. The inferior rectus and inferior oblique muscles, both innervated by cranial nerve III, lie adjacent to the inferior and medial orbital floors and are therefore the most commonly affected extraocular muscles by a blowout injury.

■ PRESENTING SIGNS AND SYMPTOMS

Patients with a history of facial trauma should undergo a full evaluation of the eye and the encasing orbit. Initial inspection may reveal periorbital ecchymosis and edema, discrepancy of eye level, or enophthalmos. Enophthalmos is consistent with an orbital blowout fracture injury. Anesthesia of the ipsilateral cheek and upper lip is indicative of inferior orbital nerve impingement. Patients should be thoroughly examined for an accurate assessment of visual acuity.

Key points in the patient history include:

- Binocular diplopia (blurring of vision when both eyes are open) is indicative of an ocular muscle imbalance between the two eyes as a consequence of muscle entrapment, contusion, or displacement of the globe secondary to edema from surrounding structures.

- Monocular diplopia (blurring of vision when only one eye is open) often is indicative of a lens dislocation, hyphema, or partial globe rupture.
- Flashing lights, or floaters, can be consistent with a retinal tear, retinal detachment, or vitreous hemorrhage injury.
- Any loss of the perception of light, identification of colors, or central scotomata without association of pain is indicative of optic neuropathy. The absence of light perception following orbital fracture is a poor prognostic indicator for recovery of vision.
- Rapid loss of vision in one eye associated with edema, proptosis, and tension on palpation should heighten suspicion for the presence of a retrobulbar hematoma.
- Pain with eye movement commonly is associated with an orbital fracture.

The examination of the eye should begin with palpation of the orbital rims. The rims should be evaluated for crepitus, a "step-off deformity," subcutaneous emphysema, and/or decreased sensation in the distribution of the inferior and superior orbital nerves.

Examination of pupil size, shape, and light reflex must be observed in consideration of optic nerve status. Full ocular muscle function is evaluated by slow, directed passive range of motion. Upward gaze palsy with vertical diplopia is consistent with dysfunction of the inferior rectus muscle and suggests entrapment from an orbital blowout fracture. Enophthalmos is common when a large amount of tissue herniates through an orbital floor defect and into the adjacent maxillary sinus.

The EP must evaluate both eyes for visual acuity. This examination may be facilitated by using a Snellen eye chart or pocket card or by asking the patient to read the text of a newspaper or other print. Visual impairment should prompt immediate consultation for the suspected injury. If the patient's injury allows proper positioning and cooperation, a slit-lamp examination is warranted to fully evaluate the conjunctiva, lens, iris, sclera, cornea, and anterior chamber of the globe. Intraocular pressures can be measured. However, if there is a question of globe rupture, intraocular pressure assessment should be deferred to an ophthalmologist.

■ DIAGNOSTIC CRITERIA AND TESTING

If there is a low pretest probability of orbital or ocular damage, a Water's view radiograph of the midface is an excellent screening tool for fracture and/or resultant blood in the maxillary sinus. Evidence of a fracture includes clouding of the maxillary sinus, subcutaneous emphysema, depression of bony fragments, or the "hanging teardrop" sign whereby herniated globe structures may be visualized in the maxillary sinus roof.

If there is a high index of suspicion for orbital or ocular injury, computed tomography is the required radiographic study to elucidate the extent of identified injury. This examination should include views of the head as well as axial and coronal cuts of the midface and orbits.

■ TREATMENT

The management of blowout fractures is complicated. There is a great deal of controversy about the care of these injuries, with treatment options ranging from a conservative, nonoperative approach to immediate surgical intervention. Therefore the presence of an orbital fracture with herniation findings on clinical or radiographic examination requires immediate surgical consultation to guide the treatment plan. Immediate indications for surgical intervention include muscular entrapment with gaze restriction and/or acute enophthalmos.

Contraindications for surgery include globe rupture, hyphema, and retinal tears. These injuries should prompt emergent ophthalmologic consultation. An ophthalmologist should also be contacted if there is evidence of lens dislocation, corneal-sclera laceration, or rapid loss of visual acuity.

An increase in retrobulbar pressure from a hematoma or emphysema can lead to acute and permanent loss of vision. A lateral canthotomy can be a vision-saving intervention in this context. This simple procedure is intended to relieve the pressure on the optic nerve and, ultimately, preserve the patient's vision through resolution of optic nerve traction and ischemia.

Immediate ophthalmologic consultation should be obtained to perform the lateral canthotomy; when a consultant is unavailable or if a lengthy response time is anticipated, the procedure should be undertaken by the EP. The following proper anesthetic preparation is necessary.

Local anesthetic without epinephrine is injected to the lateral canthus. An incision is made in the canthus with a pair of fine, sharp scissors. The incision is made in the canthus at the juncture of the upper and lower eyelids between the globe and the orbital rim. Expulsion and drainage of the hematoma should ensue through the incision site.

Patient pain should be controlled as deemed appropriate with prophylactic antibiotics initiated if there is disruption of sinus integrity evident by subcutaneous emphysema or radiographic findings. The use of prophylactic antibiotics generally is recommended, despite the lack of evidence for efficacy in this setting.

■ DISPOSITION

Injury to the globe, acute loss of vision, or globe dysfunction as a result of a blowout injury requires immediate ophthalmologic evaluation. Patients with other types of injuries, including the majority of iso-

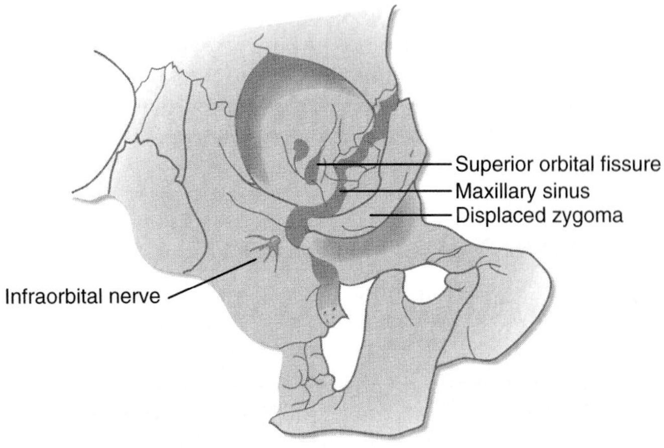
Superior orbital fissure
Maxillary sinus
Displaced zygoma
Infraorbital nerve

FIGURE 71-6 Zygomaticomaxillary complex fracture, also known as a tripod or malar fracture.

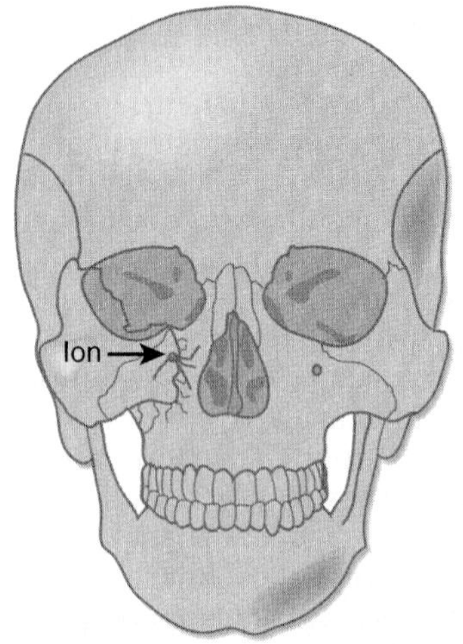
Ion

FIGURE 71-7 Relationship of infraorbital nerve (ION) and foramen to zygomaticomaxillary complex fracture.

lated fractures, will be able to be discharged with planned consultant follow-up.

Zygoma Injury

■ SCOPE

The zygoma, due to its facial prominence, is the second most common facial fracture following fracture of the nasal bone. The zygoma forms the lateral buttress of the face, the inferolateral portion of the orbit, and the roof of the maxillary sinus. Proper diagnosis and recognition of zygoma pathology is essential for maintenance of adequate cosmetic and physiologic function.

■ PATHOPHYSIOLOGY

Zygoma fractures are the result of an anterolateral force to the midface by falls, deceleration injuries, or assault by blunt objects, including a fist. An isolated zygoma fracture, the zygomatic arch fracture, is often due to an assault, whereas more complex fractures are seen with deceleration injuries.

The zygoma is a thick bone, and a direct blow may not necessarily result in fracture, but rather transmit the force to adjacent weaker areas of the orbit and maxilla, causing a complex fracture. An inward/downward displacement of the zygoma in relation to its articulating surfaces results in the classic zygomaticoaxillary complex fracture, also called a tripod or malar fracture (Fig. 71-6). Comminuted fractures of the zygoma are associated with high penetrating trauma as in gunshot wounds.

■ ANATOMY

The term *zygoma* is derived from the Greek word "zygon," meaning a yoke or crossbar by which two draft animals are hitched to a plow. The zygoma forms the lateral buttress of the face, inferior and lateral orbital rim, and a portion of the orbital floor. Thus a zygoma fracture, by definition, is an orbital floor fracture.

The zygoma articulates with four bones: the maxilla, temporal bone, frontal bone, and greater wing of the sphenoid. For this reason, a zygomaticoaxillary complex fracture—typically referred to as a tripod fracture, is technically a misnomer.

The zygoma forms part of the superior and lateral aspect of the maxillary sinus, and disruption may lead to subcutaneous air. Numerous muscles attach to the zygoma, the most prominent being the masseter, which consequently results in the inward/downward displacement of the zygomaticoaxillary complex fracture and trismus.

■ PRESENTING SIGNS AND SYMPTOMS

Common presenting symptoms for a zygoma fracture include:

- Pain over the affected area
- Difficulty opening the jaw secondary to the origin of the masseter (trismus)
- Paresthesia in the distribution of the inferior orbital nerve (Fig. 71-7).
- Binocular diplopia due to entrapment of intraocular muscles

The initial physical examination typically reveals severe edema of the zygoma area with possible inferior displacement of the lateral canthus, periorbital edema, and subconjunctival hemorrhage. The face should be evaluated from the superior and inferior aspect to discern any flattening of the cheek relative to the contralateral side. The zygoma should be palpated for evidence of a step-off of the inferior orbital rim, crepitus of the zygoma, or subcutaneous emphysema.

Intraoral examination of the zygoma is accomplished by placing a gloved finger along the superior and lateral aspect of the maxillary molars. If this area is tender or if the finger is unable to pass under the arch, a fracture of the zygoma is likely.

Finally, a complete ocular examination should be performed to evaluate for entrapment of muscles and possible orbital fracture, because 10% to 20% of zygoma injuries are associated with ocular injury.

■ DIAGNOSTIC CRITERIA AND TESTING

If a nondisplaced, isolated zygoma fracture is suspected, a "jug-handle," submentovertex view on a plain radiograph may be sufficient for diagnosis. Otherwise, a Water's view constitutes an adequate screening radiographic study for a more complicated fracture. If the Water's view reveals a zygomaticoaxillary complex fracture or there is suspicion of ocular muscle entrapment, facial computed tomography scans are required for a more complete injury evaluation.

■ TREATMENT

Initial management of patients with zygomaticoaxillary complex fractures should include prompt diagnosis and exclusion of ocular muscle entrapment or intracranial injuries. If subcutaneous emphysema is present, antibiotics should be initiated immediately; amoxicillin is an effective first-line agent. Analgesia should be achieved with nonsteroidal antiinflammatory drugs (NSAIDs) or narcotic agents.

■ DISPOSITION

Patients with an isolated arch fracture can be discharged with appropriate follow-up. In contrast, patients with a zygomaticoaxillary complex fracture, any injury with impairment of vision, or substantial concomitant injuries require admission to the hospital with surgical consultation for consideration of open reduction and internal fixation.

Maxillary/Midface Contusions

■ SCOPE

Maxillary fractures are the result of high force injuries to the face, the majority secondary to motor vehicle crashes and assault. Due to the high force of impact required to fracture the maxilla, these injuries are uncommonly isolated and often associated with other facial fractures and injuries.

The goal of the approach to suspected and identified maxillary fractures in the ED is to secure the airway, identify the injury, and consult the appropriate surgeon for determination of the need for open reduction and internal fixation.

■ PATHOPHYSIOLOGY

■ Le Fort Classification

Maxillary fractures resulting from severe blows to the head traditionally have been classified based upon the Le Fort classification scheme established by René Le Fort in 1901. Le Fort was a French surgeon who induced trauma to 35 cadaveric heads by striking them with a bat or smashing them against a table edge. Next, Le Fort boiled the heads to remove the soft tissue and documented the fracture lines. In his classic treatise on the subject, Le Fort illustrated three predictable midface fracture lines. These injuries rarely occur in isolation, but they are often used as a reference to describe maxillary trauma (Fig. 71-8).

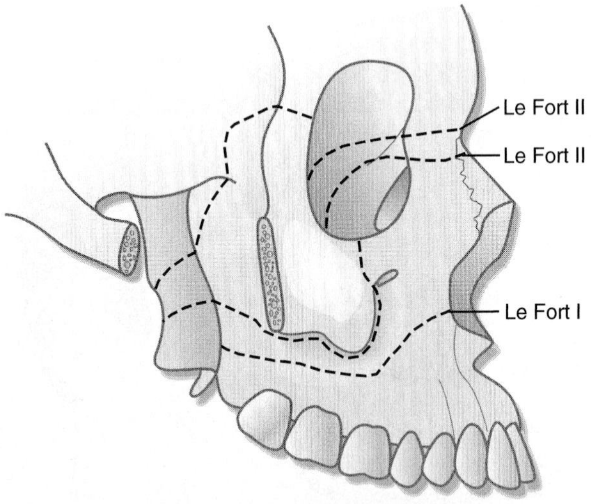
Le Fort II
Le Fort II
Le Fort I

FIGURE 71-8 Fracture lines of the midface as described by Le Fort.

■ *Le Fort I (Transverse)*

This midface fracture is the result of lateral forces to the face. The Le Fort I fracture line extends horizontally above the roots of the teeth, involving only the maxilla. There will be a step-off deformity of the upper palate (if not complete). Rocking of the teeth will lead to motion of the midface, with a sensation similar to that of a loose denture.

■ *Le Fort II (Pyramidal)*

This injury is the result of extreme force to the nose and midface, resulting in separation of the midface from articulating structures. The Le Fort II fracture line extends through the inferior orbital rim and over the nasal ridge separating the upper palate and nose from the remainder of the face.

■ *Le Fort III (Craniofacial Disjunction)*

A Le Fort III is the most severe type of facial fracture whereby the facial fracture line is horizontal, extending through the nasal bone and laterally through the orbits. This injury results in separation of the facial bones from the base of the skull.

■ ANATOMY

The maxilla is primarily innervated by the inferior alveolar nerve, emerging from the inferior orbital

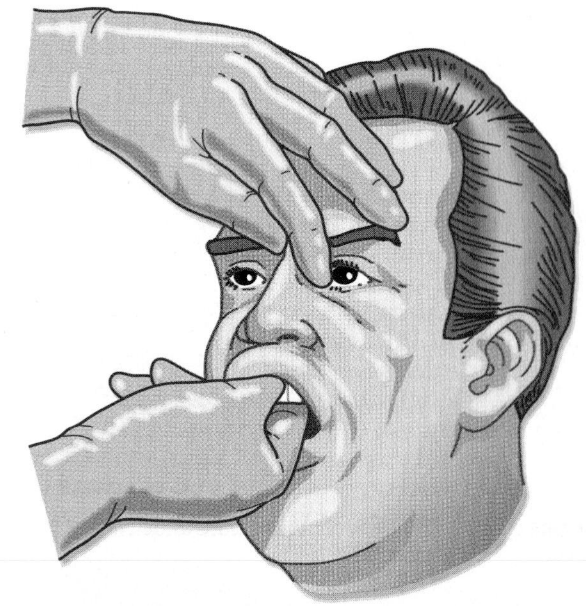

FIGURE 71-9 Examination of the midface for instability.

foramen. Clues to evidence of midface fracture may include parasthesias in the region of the inferior alveolar nerve.

The nose is a highly vascularized structure within the maxilla. Severe epistaxis associated with a maxilla injury can lead to airway obstruction. Therefore, hemostasis is essential in the approach to maxilla injuries.

■ PRESENTING SIGNS AND SYMPTOMS

Initial evaluation of a patient with a maxilla injury varies depending on severity and includes severe edema, malocclusion, periorbital ecchymosis, facial asymmetry, a long or "donkey" face, and enophthalmos. Palpation of maxilla structures may reveal crepitus and abnormal mobility of structures. Anesthesia over the cheek implies disruption of the inferior orbital nerve.

The EP should place one hand on the patient's forehead to stabilize the head, grasping the upper palate by the anterior teeth with the other hand. Gentle, back-and-forth pressure should be applied while palpating the midface for movement (Fig. 71-9). If motion of midface structures is detected with this technique, further classification of the extent of the injury should be performed by localization with the other hand of the nasal ridge or inferior orbital rims. If cerebrospinal fluid rhinorrhea is suspected, testing the fluid for glucose or the "halo sign" may be undertaken; however, both of these assessments have a false-positive rate and are considered unreliable.

■ DIAGNOSTIC CRITERIA AND TESTING

In patients with a high index of suspicion for facial fracture, neurological deficit, or severe facial distortion or in those who are undergoing computed tomography evaluation for any reason other than midface trauma, computed tomography of the facial bones with fine axial and coronal cuts should be the initial imaging study.

If there are no other significant injuries and the clinical examination is ambiguous for facial fracture, a Water's plain radiograph facial view is an excellent screening examination. If plain radiography reveals obvious fracture or opacification of a maxillary sinus, computed tomography is warranted and should be performed in follow-up or at the time of the initial encounter, as dictated by patient needs and surgical consultant preference.

■ TREATMENT

Before a thorough evaluation of the maxilla is undertaken, the EP must first stabilize the patient and assure that the airway is preserved. Airway compromise is more common with Le Forte II and III fractures but also may be seen in a Le Forte I injuries.

Airway obstruction is often secondary to uncontrolled bleeding. Therefore, attempts at hemostasis should be undertaken early in the evaluation. Nasopharyngeal intubation should be avoided with midface injuries. A surgical airway (e.g. cricothyrotomy) may be necessary due to anatomical damage or excessive bleeding.

If hemostasis of the nares cannot be achieved, a Foley catheter should be carefully advanced into the nasopharynx and inflated with air (overinflation may result in septal necrosis). The catheter should be gently pulled anteriorly in an attempt to close the posterior choana. Once this catheter is in place, the nasal cavity can be packed with gauze for anterior epistaxis control. The physician must be careful when advancing any tube through the nares because violation of the anterior cranial base can allow the passage of the catheter into the cranium.

Antibiotic prophylaxis for basilar skull fractures has not been shown to decrease the risk of meningitis; however, prophylactic antibiotic regimens are still commonly utilized, in an effort to prevent translocation of mouth and sinus flora, if there is violation of the sinus mucosa.

■ DISPOSITION

Evidence of a basilar skull fracture or pneumocephalus requires prompt neurosurgical consultation. Maxillary fractures often require surgical repair to restore normal occlusion and facial stabilization; thus consultation and follow-up with an oromaxillofacial or plastic surgeon is important. Patients with demonstrated or suspected Le Fort II or Le Fort III injuries require hospital admission for stabilization and management.

Nasal Contusions

■ SCOPE

Diagnosis of nasal fractures is critical due to the difficulty of reconstruction and detrimental outcomes associated with delayed healing. The nose is the most frequently fractured facial bone and is one of the most commonly fractured structures of the human body. The nose typically is fractured in isolation, and often the fracutre will not be diagnosed; however, a nasal fracture may be associated with the more severe nasoorbitoethmoid fracture.

Because of the common occurrence of nasal fractures, proper attention is required in order to prevent adverse events ranging from unacceptable cosmetic results, including deviation of the septum and saddle nose deformity, to breach of the cribriform plate with cerebrospinal fluid rhinorrhea.

■ PATHOPHYSIOLOGY

Nasal bone fractures are commonly the result of sports-related trauma, assault, and motor vehicle crashes. The force required to fracture the nasal bone ranges from 16 to 66 kPA, the least of any facial bone.

Simple deviated nasal fractures are the result of a lateral force against the nasal prominence. Whereas nasoorbitoethmoid fractures are due to a stronger force directed toward the bridge of the nose and displacing the segments posteriorly, this type of fracture often is associated with other facial and brain injuries.

■ ANATOMY

The nasal bone consists of two small wedged-shaped bones that are fused midline and protrude from the frontal process of the maxilla laterally and frontal bone superiorly. The upper portion of this paired structure is significantly thicker than the lower segments, leading to fractures more commonly of the latter. The external nose is composed of cartilaginous and fatty tissue and has an intricate blood supply from distal branches of the internal and external carotid arteries.

■ PRESENTING SIGNS AND SYMPTOMS

Patients with nasal trauma present for evaluation with complaints of tenderness, edema, epistaxis, and periorbital ecchymosis. Palpation of the area can reveal crepitus, hypermobility, and deformity of the nasal septum.

Each naris must be carefully inspected with a nasal speculum to evaluate for a septal hematoma, which is a collection of blood between the mucoperichondrium or mucoperiosteum of the nasal septum and the septal cartilage. A septal hematoma appears as a purple, bulging, oval structure on the nasal septum that invades the midline (Fig. 71-10). Failure to promptly identify and treat a septal hematoma can lead to necrosis of the septum and, potentially, a "saddle-nose" deformity.

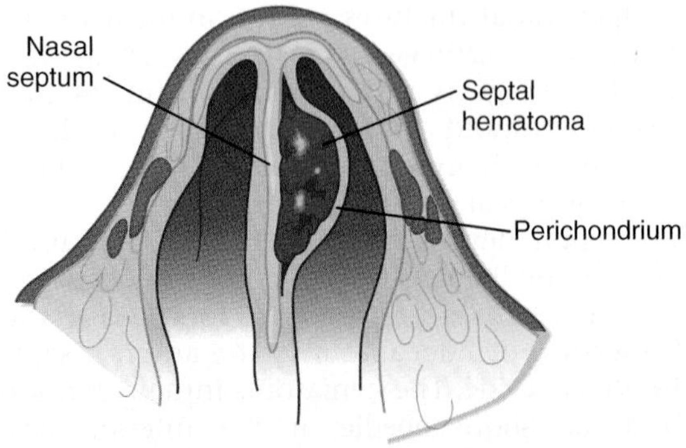
Nasal septum
Septal hematoma
Perichondrium

FIGURE 71-10 Septal hematoma.

A nasoorbitoethmoid fracture should be suspected when there is flattening of the bridge of the nose or telecanthus (an increase in the distance between the medial portions of the eye). Patients may have evidence of ocular injury and cerebrospinal fluid rhinorrhea. Additionally, disruption of the lacrimal apparatus is not uncommon with more severe nasal injuries.

■ DIAGNOSTIC CRITERIA AND TESTING

The use of plain radiographs in simple nasal trauma is of limited value and has no clinical implication in management. If the physician is concerned that a nasoorbitoethmoid fracture is present, axial and coronal computed tomography imaging of the face is required.

■ TREATMENT AND DISPOSITION

Reduction of closed nasal fractures should not be attempted by the EP. Given the extensive edema that generally ensues prior to patient arrival in the ED, the EP will be unable to approximate realignment of the nasal septum. Epistaxis should be addressed during the clinical evaluation. Analgesia should be adequately addressed during the patient visit and in follow-up.

Patients with known or suspected nasal fractures or septal displacement should be referred to an otolaryngologist or plastic surgeon within 1 week of their injury for reevaluation and management planning. Children with nasal fractures should be seen in follow-up within 4 days due to rapid bone healing. Patients should be instructed to avoid blowing the nose, because subcutaneous emphysema may ensue due to air displacement across the injured nasal structures.

Emergent consultation for consideration of nasal reduction is indicated if there is deviation of the nasal pyramid greater than one half the width of the nasal bridge or in patients with an open septal fracture. Open nasal fractures require immediate attention, because cartilage necrosis may ensue if the exposed cartilage is not covered within 24 hours. Nasoorbitoethmoid fractures require a multidisciplinary approach, including oromaxillofacial, plastic, and neurosurgical consultation.

If a septal hematoma is identified, this finding requires immediate evacuation. The nasal passage of the affected side is prepared via topical anesthesia and injection of lidocaine into the anterior septum of the affected side. The hematoma initially is drained with a large-bore needle at the inferior aspect. The needle track is then enlarged with a #15 surgical blade. Next, the anterior nares are tightly packed bilaterally in an attempt to reappose the septal mucosa. Septal hematoma patients should routinely be prescribed a course of antibiotics with otolaryngology follow-up arranged within 4 days to assess the injury for evidence of hematoma reaccumulation.

Lower Face Injuries

■ SCOPE

The mandible is the only mobile bone of the face and, despite its mobility, is the strongest facial bone. The primary function of the mandible is mastication and speech. Trauma to the mandible may result in fracture or dislocation. Fifty percent of mandibular fractures occur at two or more locations due to its psuedo-ring shape. Thus the finding of one fracture site should always prompt a search for a second fracture.

■ PATHOPHYSIOLOGY

Location of mandible fractures have some correlation to the insult received. High-velocity forces to the chin result in symphysis and/or condylar fractures, with a high proportion of these injuries resulting in comminuted fractures. In contrast, assault-related injuries are more commonly associated with fractures of the angle and ramus. The location of trauma impact does not necessarily correlate with the location of the fracture site because force of impact can be transmitted to a distant area.

Dislocations of the mandible can be due to trauma, excessive mouth opening (yawning), seizure, or a dystonic reaction from medication. The mandible dislocates anteriorly and then superiorly, with spasm of the jaw muscles preventing realignment. A unilateral dislocation will cause deviation of the mandible away from the affected side. Bilateral dislocations will result in the patient presenting with an open jaw and underbite appearance.

■ ANATOMY

The mandible is a horseshoe-shaped bone and appears similar to the letter L from a lateral view (Fig. 71-11). The mandible has 16 tooth sockets innervated by the inferior alveolar nerve. The bone articulates with the temporal bone bilaterally via a ginglymoarthrodial (hinge and sliding) joint, forming the temporomandibular joint. Arterial supply to the mandible is via branches of the maxillary artery.

The temporomandibular joint consists of the mandibular condyle process and the mandibular fossa of

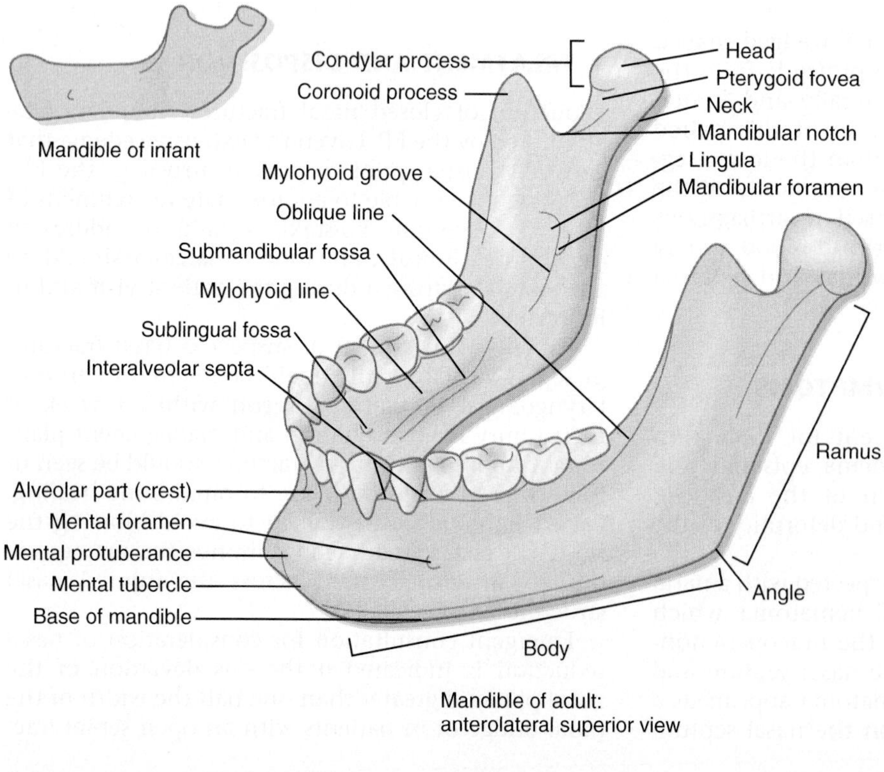

Mandible of infant
Condylar process
Coronoid process
Head
Pterygoid fovea
Neck
Mandibular notch
Lingula
Mandibular foramen
Mylohyoid groove
Oblique line
Submandibular fossa
Mylohyoid line
Sublingual fossa
Interalveolar septa
Alveolar part (crest)
Mental foramen
Mental protuberance
Mental tubercle
Base of mandible
Ramus
Angle
Body
Mandible of adult:
anterolateral superior view

FIGURE 71-11 Anatomy of the mandible.

the temporal bone interspaced with a cartilaginous disc and surrounded by a joint capsule. If the jaw is opened slightly, the hinge action predominates as the condylar process rotates within the socket. However, as the jaw is opened wider, the mandibular condyles glide forward to the articular tubercle of the temporal bone. Overextension of the joint results in anterior dislocation of the mandibular condyle process and subsequent spasm in the masseter and pterygoid muscles, preventing normal mouth closure.

■ PRESENTING SIGNS AND SYMPTOMS

Typical presenting symptoms include mandibular pain, abnormal jaw motion, malocclusion, and paresthesia of the ipsilateral lower lip secondary to disruption of the mandibular nerve. Patients will often state that their "bite is off," a sign of displacement/malocclusion of the mandible or maxilla. If the patient reports pain in the preauricular area, a fracture of the condyle is often present.

The mandible examination should begin with visual inspection for edema, deviation with passive range of motion, and a "widened face," an indication of a bilateral condyle fracture. The EP should palpate the outside of the face to ensure preservation of the smooth contour of the mandible. During the intraoral examination, clues to mandible fracture include ecchymosis of the floor of the mouth and mucosal tears. Any obvious separation of the lower teeth, or step-deformity, is pathognomonic for fracture.

The EP inspects the temporomandibular joint by first performing an otoscopic examination for signs of perforation of the external ear canal or hemotympanum. A "battle axe" sign is indicative of perforation of the glenoid fossa by a fractured condyle. Next, the examiner's fingers are placed in the external canal, and the patient is instructed to open and close the mouth. Tenderness or crepitus elicited with this examination is indicative of a condylar fracture.

If clinical findings are misleading, one can perform the "tongue blade test," demonstrated by Alonso and Purcell to have a high sensitivity in screening for mandible fractures. The test is performed by placing a wooden tongue blade between the molars (Fig. 71-12). The patient is instructed to bite down, and the examiner exerts a twisting motion in an effort to crack the wooden blade between the patient's teeth. If the patient is unable to crack the blade between the teeth during the twisting motion—due to pain or malocclusion—a positive test is confirmed with subsequent enhanced suspicion for a mandible fracture.

■ DIAGNOSTIC CRITERIA AND TESTING

Diagnosis of a mandibular fracture can be made with a dental panoramic radiograph (Panorex). If a Panorex view is unavailable, initial radiographs should include lateral and posteroanterior views and a Towne's view of the mandible. If the index of suspicion for condyle fracture is high despite a normal radiograph, computed tomography with fine cuts of the condyle will be necessary to definitively rule out a fracture. If evidence of an avulsed tooth is present on clinical examination, a chest radiograph should be obtained to evaluate for aspiration.

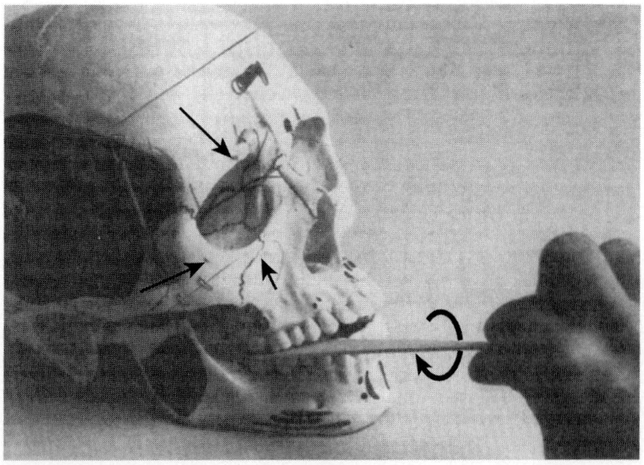

FIGURE 71-12 Performance of the tongue blade test to assess for mandible fracture.

■ TREATMENT

Initial management of a mandible fracture should ensure that the patient can maintain a patent airway without difficulty. Pain relief may then be obtained with NSAIDs and narcotic agents. Due to the potential for wound infection via mouth flora, mandible fracture patients should be started on oral or IV penicillin. Clindamycin is an excellent choice for the penicillin-allergic patient. Stabilization of a displaced mandibular fracture can be achieved with a Barton's bandage.

When a traumatic temporomandibular joint dislocation is encountered, the EP must obtain a dental panoramic study to consider the presence of a concomitant condylar fracture. If no indication of fracture is present, an attempt at reduction of the mandible in the ED may be undertaken with provision of IV benzodiazepines, and occasionally procedural sedation and analgesia, to relax the muscles of mastication and provide an anxiolytic affect for the patient.

To perform reduction, the EP's thumbs are wrapped in gauze (to prevent injury). The EP faces the patient and places the thumbs on the posterior molars of the patient's mandible; the remaining fingers are wrapped around the inferior border of the mandible. Force is directed downward on the thumbs as the symphyseal area is raised toward the EP.

If reduction is unsuccessful, the patient may require general anesthesia. After reduction of an acute dislocation, the patient should be placed on soft diet and instructed not to open the mouth wide for 7 days.

PATIENT TEACHING TIPS

- If the patient begins to lose visual acuity or develops pain with eye movement, medical attention must be sought immediately.
- After sustaining a laceration, any patient who develops a sign of local or systemic infection warrants a prompt medical evaluation.
- If a septal hematoma or otohematoma begins to reaccumulate, the hematoma should be reevacuated.
- Patients with a nasal or midface fracture should refrain from blowing the nose.
- A follow-up appointment with the consulting physician should be arranged at the time of patient discharge.

■ DISPOSITION

Most patients with mandibular fractures require admission for occlusion fixation or mandibular wiring. Prompt consultation with an oromaxillofacial or plastic surgeon is essential to formulate an appropriate treatment plan.

REFERENCES

1. Alvi A, Doherty T, Lewen G: Facial fractures and concomitant injuries in trauma patients. Laryngoscope 2003;113: 102-106.
2. Ardekian L, Rosen D, Klein Y, et al: Life-threatening complications and irreversible damage following maxillofacial trauma. Injury 1998;29:253-256.
3. Howes DS, Dowling PJ: Oral facial emergencies: Triage and initial evaluation of the oral facial emergency. Emerg Med Clin North Am 2000;18:371-378.
4. Hackl W, Fink C, Hausberger K, et al: The incidence of combined facial and cervical spine injuries. J Trauma 2001;50:41-45.
5. Bisson JI, Shepherd JP, Dhutia M: Psychological sequelae of facial trauma. J Trauma 1997;43:496-500.
6. Bynoe RP, Kerwin AJ, Parker HH 3rd, et al: Maxillofacial injuries and life-threatening hemorrhage: Treatment with transcatheter arterial embolization. J Trauma 2003;55: 74-79.
7. Kraus JF, Rice TM, Peek-Asa C, McArthur DL: Facial trauma and the risk of intracranial injury in motorcycle riders. Ann Emerg Med 2003;41:18-26.
8. Nakhgevany KB, LiBassi M, Esposito B: Facial trauma in motor vehicle accidents: Etiologic factors. Am J Emerg Med 1994;12:160-163.
9. Plaisier BR, Punjabi AP, Super DM, Haug RH. The relationship between facial fractures and death from neurologic injury. J Oral Maxillofac Surg 2000;58:708-712.
10. Shaikh ZS, Worrall SF: Epidemiology of facial trauma in a sample of patients aged 1-18 years. Injury 2002;33: 669-671.
11. Shepherd SM, Lippe MS. Maxillofacial trauma: Evaluation and management by the emergency physician. Emerg Med Clin North Am 1987;5:371-392.
12. Villalobos T, Arango C, Kubilis P, Rathore M: Antibiotic prophylaxis after basilar skull fractures: A meta-analysis. Clin Infec Dis 1998;27:364-369.
13. Joondeph BC: Blunt ocular trauma. Emerg Med Clin North Am 1988;6:147-167.
14. Larian B, Wong B, Crumley RL, et al: Facial trauma and ocular/orbital injury. J Craniomaxillofac Trauma 1999;5(4):15-24.
15. Mathog RH: Management of orbital blowout fractures. Otolaryngol Clin North Am 1991;24:79-91.
16. Wang BH, Robertson BC, Girotto JA, et al: Traumatic optic neuropathy: a review of 61 patients. Plast Reconstr Surg 2001;107(7):1655-1664.
17. Waterhouse N, Lyne J, Urdang M, Garey L: An investigation into the mechanism of orbital blowout fractures. Br J Plast Surg 1999;52:607-612.
18. Zingg M, Laedrach K: Classification and treatment of zygomatic fractures: A review of 1025 Cases. J Oral Maxillofac Surg 1992;50:778-790.
19. Greene D, Raven R, Carvalho G, Maas SC: Epidemiology of facial injury in blunt assault. Determinants of incidence and outcome in 802 patients. Arch Otolaryng Head Neck Surg 1997;123:923-918.
20. Bagheri SC, Holmgren E, Katemani D, et al: Comparison of the severity of bilateral Le Fort injuries in isolated midface trauma. J Oral Maxillofac Surg 2005;63:1123-1129.
21. Tessier P: The classic reprint: Experimental study of fractures of the upper jaw. 3. René Le Fort, M.D., Lille, France. Plast Reconstr Surg 1972;50:600-607.
22. Holt GR: Biomechanics of nasal septal trauma. Otolaryngol Clin North Am 1999;32:615-619.
23. Mondin V, Rinaldo A, Ferlito A: Management of nasal bone fractures. Am J Otolaryng 2005;26:181-185.
24. Hallock GG: Microsurgical repair of the parotid duct. Microsurgery 1992;13:243-246.
25. Kerwin AJ, Bynoe RP, Murray AJ, et al: Liberalized screening for blunt carotid and vertebral artery injuries is justified. J Trauma 2001;51:308-314.
26. Alonso LL, Purcell TB: Accuracy of the tongue blade test in patients with suspected mandibular fracture. J Emerg Med 1995;13:297-304.

Chapter **72**

Penetrating Neck Trauma

Niels K. Rathlev, Mark E. Bracken, and Ron Medzon

KEY POINTS

Because patients who appear to have a minor neck wound may have a major injury, thorough vascular and esophageal evaluation is required if any abnormalities are evident on the physical examination or on chest and neck radiographs. However, radiographs do not rule out esophageal injury.

Early airway management is crucial. Orotracheal intubation is the initial method of choice.

A thorough neurologic examination is essential in all patients with neck trauma.

"Hard signs" of vascular injury include bruit, thrill, expanding or pulsatile hematoma, pulsatile or severe hemorrhage, pulse deficit, and central nervous system ischemia.

The gold standard for diagnosis of vascular injury is conventional angiography. Multidetector CT angiography is a noninvasive, relatively expensive, and convenient option.

Admission criteria include signs and symptoms of organ damage and penetration of the platysma muscles.

Perspective

The first account of successful surgical intervention in cases of penetrating neck trauma was documented in 1552. Ambroise Paré, a surgeon in the French army, ligated both common carotid arteries and jugular veins of a soldier with an exsanguinating, traumatic neck injury. The patient survived with aphasia and hemiplegia. In 1803, David Fleming, a young British naval surgeon, ligated a lacerated common carotid artery and reported a successful outcome 5 months following the surgery.

In the Vietnam War, the mortality from penetrating neck injuries was 4% to 7%. The current mortality rate in civilians is approximately 2% to 6%. Patients with zone 1 injuries (see Fig. 72-1) at the base of the neck are at highest risk. Currently, spinal cord injuries and thrombosis of the common and internal carotid arteries account for 50% of all deaths from penetrating neck injuries.

Pathophysiology

The incidence of injuries to the critical airway and the vascular, gastrointestinal, skeletal, and neurologic organs depend on the location and mechanism of injury. In the case of interpersonal violence, the distance between the assailant and victim and the type of weapon must be established. In total, 44% of injuries to critical organs involve vascular structures. This is a major source of morbidity and mortality (Table 72-1).[1]

Unstable cervical-spine fractures and spinal cord injuries are extremely unlikely in the presence of low-risk National Emergency X-radiography Utiliza-

Table 72-1 **INCIDENCE OF NECK INJURIES**

Vascular	%	Aerodigestive	%	Neurologic	%
Subclavian artery	2.6	Trachea	6.0	Spinal cord	1.9
External carotid artery	2.5	Pharynx	5.0	Brachial plexus	2.1
Internal carotid artery	1.3	Esophagus	5.0	Cranial nerves VII, X, XI, XII	1.9
Common carotid artery	0.6	Larynx	2.4	Sympathetic chain	0.2

From Carducci B, Lowe RA, Dalsey W: Penetrating neck trauma: Consensus and controversies. Ann Emerg Med 1986;15:208-215.

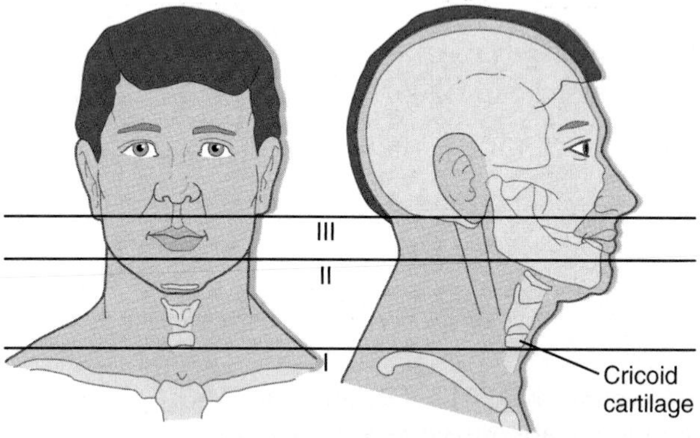
III
II
I
Cricoid cartilage

FIGURE 72-1 Zones of the neck.

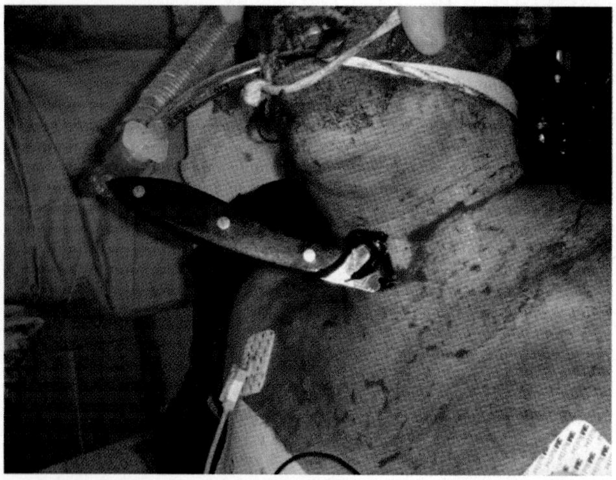

FIGURE 72-2 Stab wound in zone I of the neck.

tion Study I (NEXUS I) criteria—that is, the patient
1. Is alert and awake
2. Is not intoxicated
3. Has no signs or symptoms of neurologic injury
4. Has no spinous process tenderness

Anatomy

The neck consists of three anatomic zones (Fig. 72-1):

- Zone I—base of neck to cricoid cartilage (Fig. 72-2)
- Zone II—cricoid cartilage to the angle of the mandible
- Zone III—above the angle of mandible (Fig. 72-3)

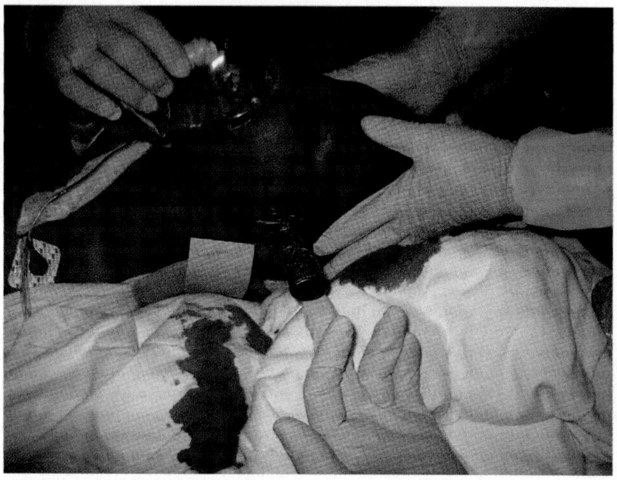

FIGURE 72-3 Injury in zone III of the neck.

The major muscles of the neck are the platysma muscles, extending from the lower jaw to the clavicle (Fig. 72-4). Other critical structures are shown in Figures 72-5 through 72-7.

Presenting Signs and Symptoms

■ AIRWAY INJURY

Symptoms of airway injury include dyspnea, hemoptysis, subcutaneous air, stridor, hoarseness, and dysphonia (Fig. 72-8).

■ VASCULAR INJURY

"Hard signs" that indicate severe vascular injury include the following:

- Bruit or thrill suggestive of a traumatic arteriovenous fistula
- Expanding or pulsatile hematoma
- Pulsatile or severe hemorrhage
- Pulse deficit—pulses may be normal in patients with nonocclusive injuries that require surgical repair such as intimal flaps or pseudoaneurysms.

"Soft signs," which are less predictive of severe vascular injury, include the following:

- Hypotension and shock
- Stable, non-pulsatile hematoma

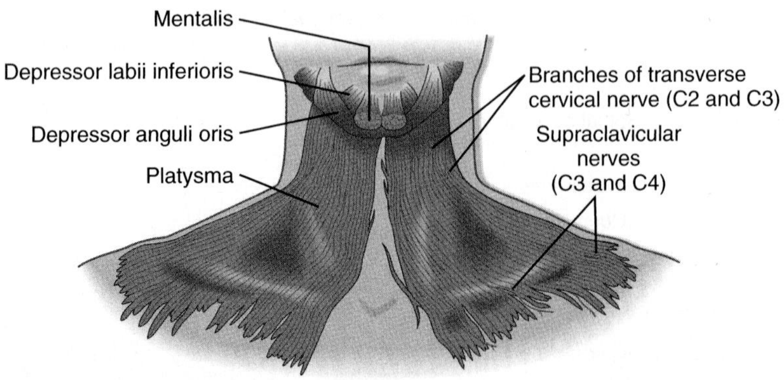
Mentalis
Depressor labii inferioris
Depressor anguli oris
Platysma
Branches of transverse cervical nerve (C2 and C3)
Supraclavicular nerves (C3 and C4)

FIGURE 72-4 Surface anatomy: The platysma. (From Agur AMR, Dalley AF [eds]: Grant's Atlas of Anatomy, 9th ed. Baltimore, Williams & Wilkins, 1991.)

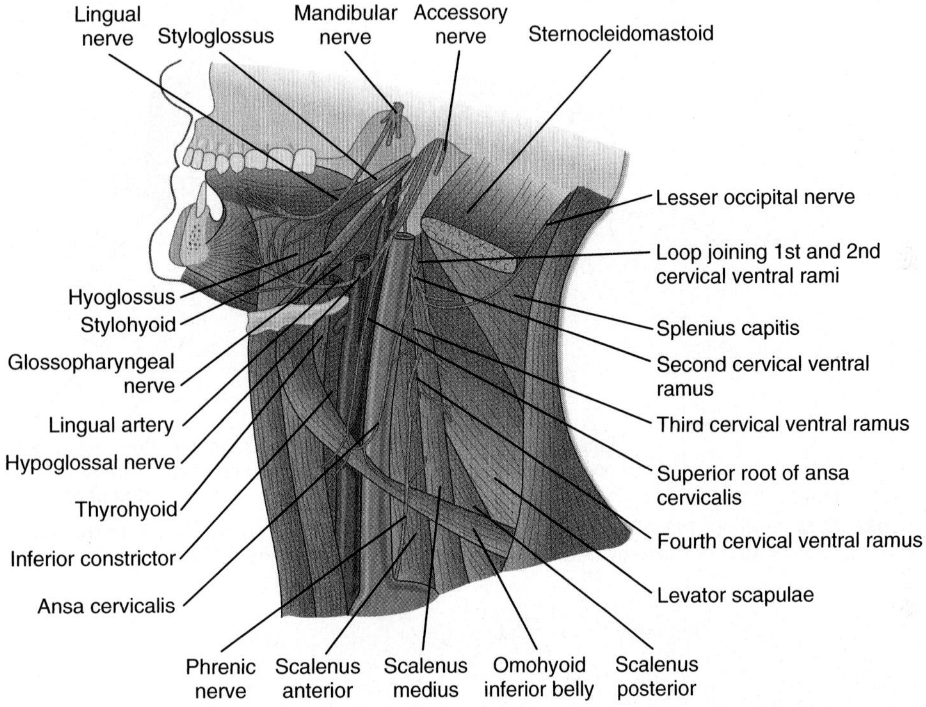
Lingual nerve
Styloglossus
Mandibular nerve
Accessory nerve
Sternocleidomastoid
Lesser occipital nerve
Loop joining 1st and 2nd cervical ventral rami
Splenius capitis
Second cervical ventral ramus
Third cervical ventral ramus
Superior root of ansa cervicalis
Fourth cervical ventral ramus
Levator scapulae
Hyoglossus
Stylohyoid
Glossopharyngeal nerve
Lingual artery
Hypoglossal nerve
Thyrohyoid
Inferior constrictor
Ansa cervicalis
Phrenic nerve
Scalenus anterior
Scalenus medius
Omohyoid inferior belly
Scalenus posterior

FIGURE 72-5 Anterior triangle—anterior border of the sternocleidomastoid muscle to the midline. (From Agur AMR, Dalley AF [eds]: Grant's Atlas of Anatomy, 9th ed. Baltimore, Williams & Wilkins, 1991.)

- Central nervous system ischemia—a neurologic deficit that develops over the course of 1 to 2 hours after injury is consistent with ischemic neurologic injury; an immediate deficit is more likely due to a primary neurologic injury.
- Proximity to a major vascular structure is not considered a high-risk feature in the absence of the preceding criteria (Fig. 72-9).

■ DIGESTIVE TRACT

The pharynx must be examined by visual inspection. Under normal conditions, the esophagus is mobile and collapsed. Symptoms and signs of esophageal injury include subcutaneous air, crepitus, dysphagia, odynophagia, drooling, and hematemesis.

Diagnostic Testing

■ VASCULAR INJURY

■ Conventional Angiography

The gold standard of diagnostic modalities is four-vessel angiography with venous phase imaging (sensitivity >99%) (Fig. 72-10). Very rarely do injuries missed by angiography require repair. A normal study is highly predictive of survival from vessel injury.[2]

■ Duplex Ultrasonography

Duplex ultrasonography is noninvasive, convenient, and relatively inexpensive, but sensitivity for vascular injury is highly operator-dependent. However,

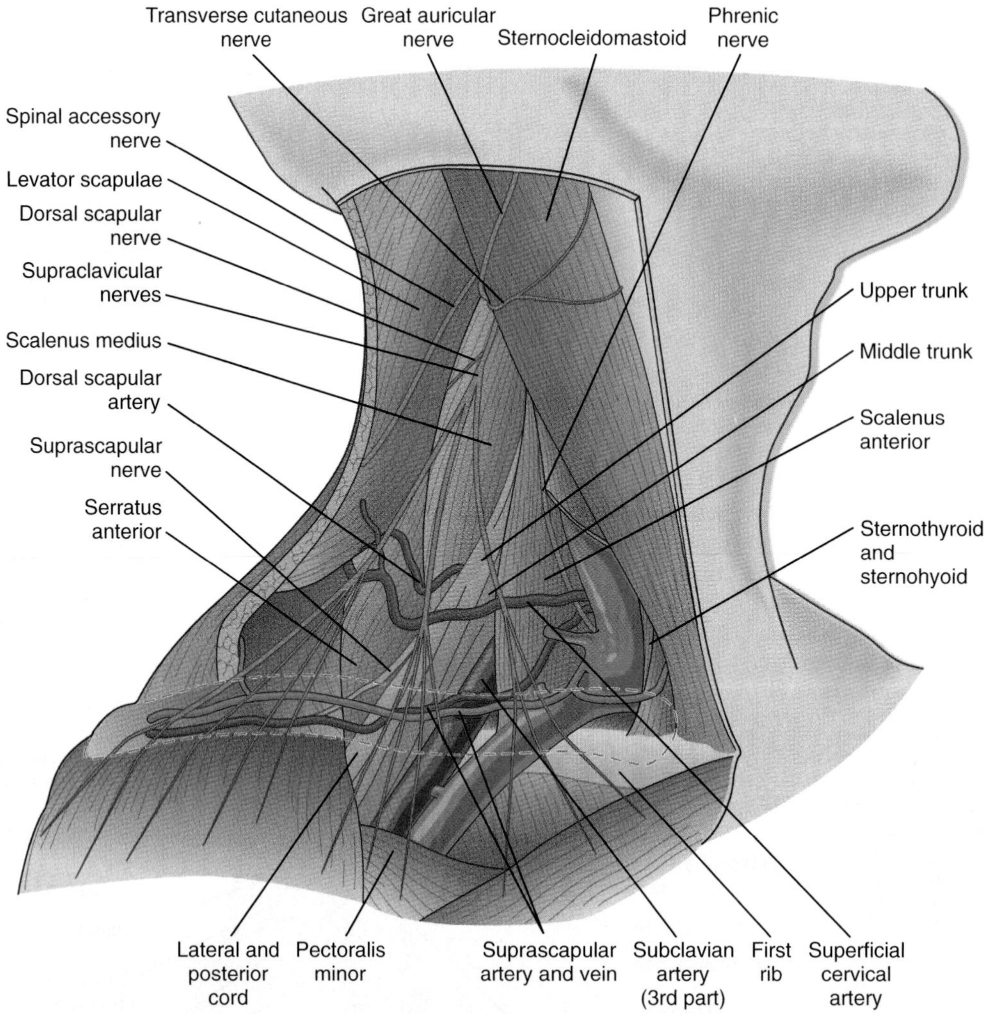
Transverse cutaneous nerve
Great auricular nerve
Sternocleidomastoid
Phrenic nerve
Spinal accessory nerve
Levator scapulae
Dorsal scapular nerve
Supraclavicular nerves
Scalenus medius
Dorsal scapular artery
Suprascapular nerve
Serratus anterior
Upper trunk
Middle trunk
Scalenus anterior
Sternothyroid and sternohyoid
Lateral and posterior cord
Pectoralis minor
Suprascapular artery and vein
Subclavian artery (3rd part)
First rib
Superficial cervical artery

FIGURE 72-6 Posterior triangle—posterior border of the sternocleidomastoid muscle to the trapezius muscle. (From Agur AMR, Dalley AF [eds]: Grant's Atlas of Anatomy, 9th ed. Baltimore, Williams & Wilkins, 1991.)

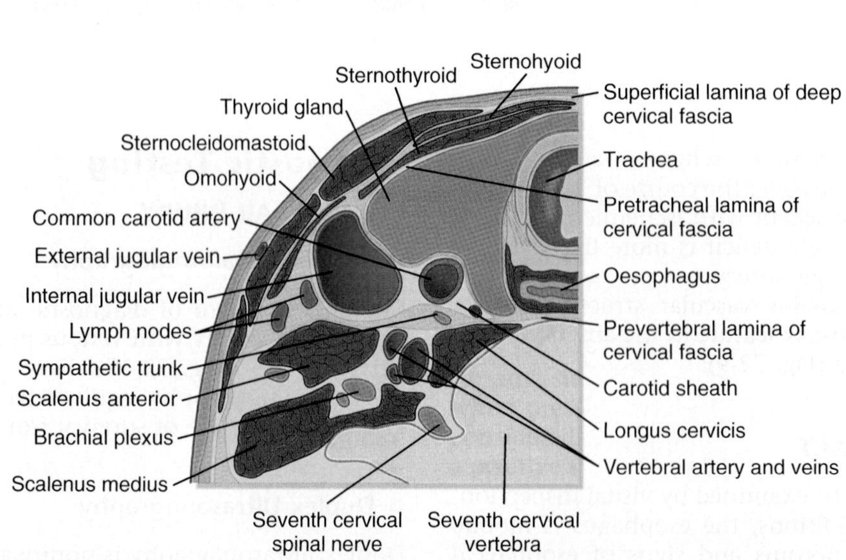
Sternohyoid
Sternothyroid
Thyroid gland
Sternocleidomastoid
Omohyoid
Common carotid artery
External jugular vein
Internal jugular vein
Lymph nodes
Sympathetic trunk
Scalenus anterior
Brachial plexus
Scalenus medius
Superficial lamina of deep cervical fascia
Trachea
Pretracheal lamina of cervical fascia
Oesophagus
Prevertebral lamina of cervical fascia
Carotid sheath
Longus cervicis
Vertebral artery and veins
Seventh cervical spinal nerve
Seventh cervical vertebra

FIGURE 72-7 Transverse section of the neck at level of C7. (From Agur AMR, Dalley AF [eds]: Grant's Atlas of Anatomy, 9th ed. Baltimore, Williams & Wilkins, 1991.)

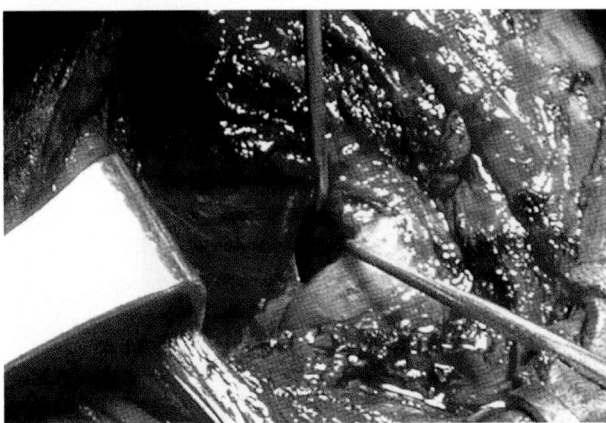

FIGURE 72-8 Tracheal injury.

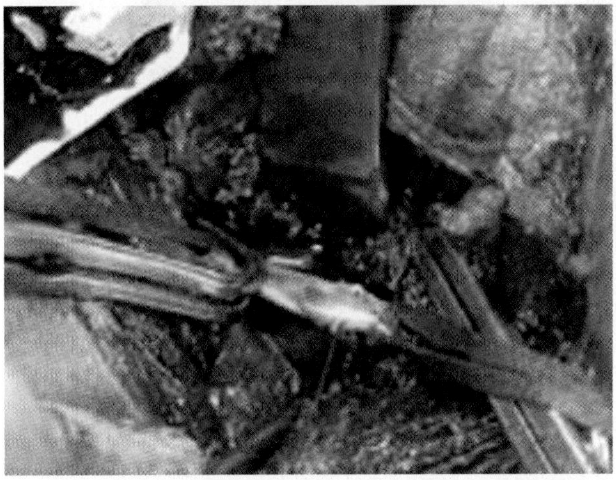

FIGURE 72-9 Common carotid artery injury.

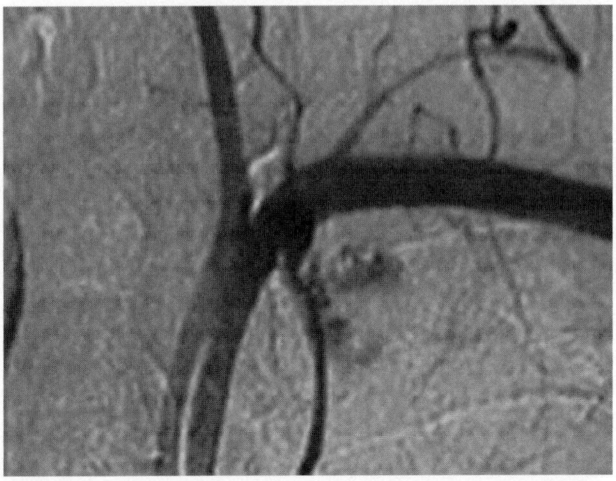

FIGURE 72-10 Angiogram revealing extravasation of contrast caused by a stab wound to the subclavian artery.

sensitivity compared to conventional angiography is 90% to 100% for injuries requiring intervention.[3] Duplex ultrasonography can miss nonocclusive injuries with preserved flow, such as intimal flaps and pseudoaneurysms.

Table 72-2 SENSITIVITIES OF DIAGNOSTIC MODALITIES FOR ESOPHAGEAL INJURY

Diagnostic Test	Sensitivity
Physical examination	80%
Contrast study	89%
Rigid esophagoscopy	89%
Contrast study+esophagoscopy	100%

From Weigelt JA, Thal ER, Snyder WH 3rd, et al: Diagnosis of penetrating cervical esophageal injuries. Am J Surg 1987;154:619-622.

Multi-Detector Helical Computed Tomography (MDCT) Angiography

This diagnostic modality has largely supplanted duplex ultrasonography for patients without obvious indications for immediate operative intervention (Fig. 72-11). The sensitivity of MDCT angiography is 90% with 100% compared with conventional angiography and surgical exploration.[4,5]

Sensitivity is further improved further with high-resolution CT scanning, such as 64-row technology, and increased technical experience using this modality. Compared with conventional angiography, MDCT angiography is faster, less expensive, noninvasive, and does not involve interventional radiology.

ESOPHAGEAL INJURY

Esophageal injuries may be clinically silent initially. Radiographs do not exclude esophageal injury. Contrast studies have a sensitivity of 50% to 90%. Esophagoscopy has a sensitivity of 43% to 100% (Table 72-2).

Rigid endoscopy has a higher diagnostic yield than flexible endoscopy; however, it is associated with a higher incidence of complications, including iatrogenic rupture. A combined approach that includes both contrast studies and esophagoscopy has a sensitivity of 100%.[6]

SELECTIVE EVALUATION

Selective surgical exploration is recommended for patients without obvious indications for surgical repair.[7-9] Nonoperative techniques (Fig. 72-12) are sufficiently sensitive to safely rule out injuries that require an operation. Esophageal and arterial injuries have reportedly been missed during exploration. A selective approach is more cost-effective than mandatory exploration.

NEUROLOGIC INJURY

Fortunately, injuries to the brain, spinal cord, and peripheral nerves are uncommon (Fig. 72-13; see Table 72-1). Patients with primary neurologic injuries present initially with focal deficits or mental status alteration.

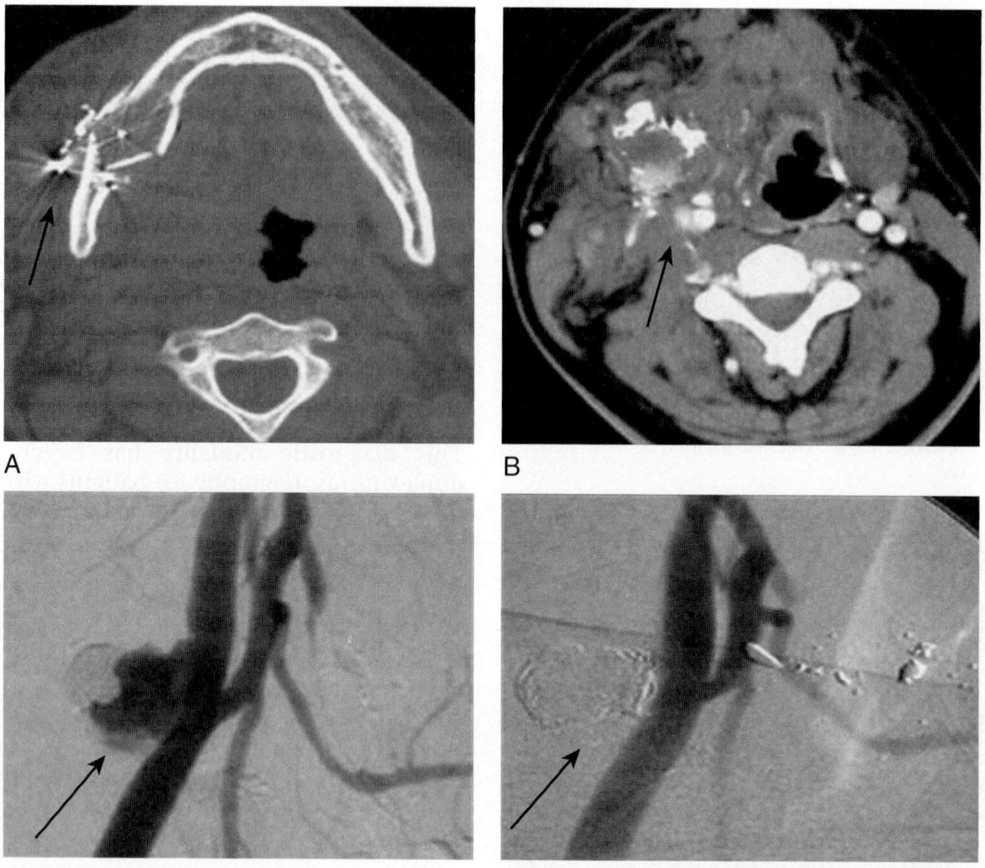

FIGURE 72-11 Gunshot wound to the mandible. **A** and **B,** Helical CT angiography reveals diminished flow through the right common carotid artery (*arrow*). **C** and **D,** Conventional angiography demonstrates a pseudoaneurysm (*arrow*) of the vessel proximal to its bifurcation.

Interventions and Procedures

■ AIRWAY INTERVENTIONS

Direct visualization of the airway is optimal: Orotracheal intubation is the initial method of choice because the procedure is frequently performed and rarely associated with complications.[10,11] Fiberoptic intubation is reserved for semi-elective airway management unless an experienced operator and the necessary equipment are immediately available. Visualization may be impaired due to extensive hemorrhage and secretions.

Cricothyrotomy or tracheostomy is necessary if orotracheal or fiberoptic intubation is unsuccessful. A surgical airway should not be delayed because hematoma or distorted anatomy can develop quickly, resulting in complications. Intubation through an accessible neck wound has a very high success rate (Fig. 72-14).

Nasotracheal intubation is NOT a preferred airway technique. Its success rate varies from 0% to 75%. It is potentially associated with complications, due to the "blind" nature of the procedure. A more direct, visualized approach is suggested (Fig. 72-15).

Treatment

■ WOUND CARE AND EVALUATION

The EP may gently spread wound edges without probing. The patient should be placed in the Trendelenburg position if there is any concern about internal jugular vein injury and possible air embolus. Wounds should be closed only if the depth is clearly visualized; caution is urged because assessment of depth is deceptive. The EP must suspect deep penetration and ensure complete diagnostic evaluation.

■ Vascular Injury

Direct pressure should be used; "blindly" clamping structures with poor visualization should be avoided. Pharyngeal packing of severe oral bleeding may be necessary. Subclavian vein injury should be suspected in patients with zone I injuries. IV access should be placed on the opposite side of the injury to avoid potential extravasation of fluids.

ED thoracotomy is indicated for patients with zone I injuries and refractory shock. Subclavian artery

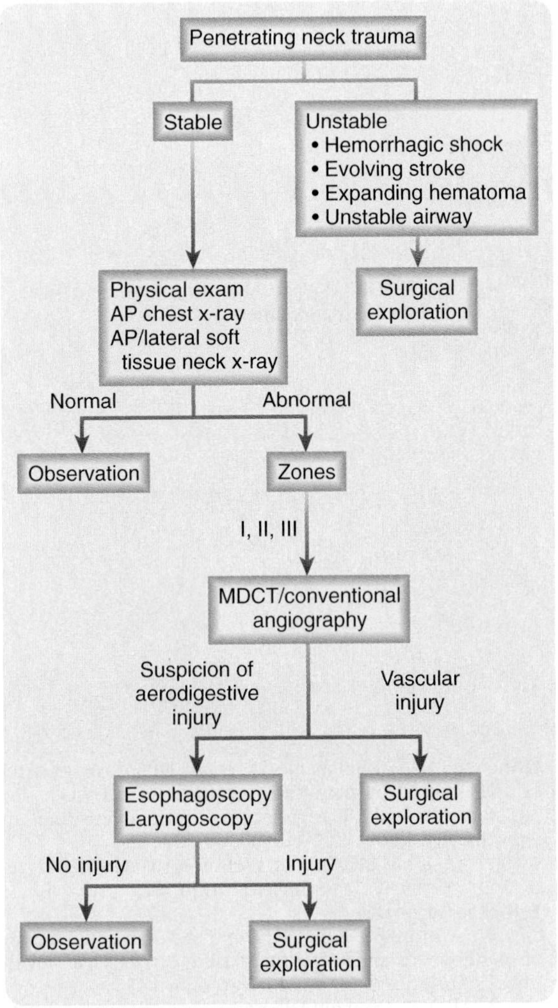
Penetrating neck trauma
Stable
Unstable
• Hemorrhagic shock
• Evolving stroke
• Expanding hematoma
• Unstable airway
Physical exam
AP chest x-ray
AP/lateral soft tissue neck x-ray
Surgical exploration
Normal
Abnormal
Observation
Zones
I, II, III
MDCT/conventional angiography
Suspicion of aerodigestive injury
Vascular injury
Esophagoscopy
Laryngoscopy
Surgical exploration
No injury
Injury
Observation
Surgical exploration

FIGURE 72-12 Algorithm for diagnosis of penetrating neck injuries.

injury should be suspected in these cases. Treatment is determined by angiographic grading of vascular injuries. Primary repair is preferred over graft placement when possible.

Surgical repair is preferred over ligation *except* in the following cases:

- Coma without antegrade flow—high risk of converting an ischemic to a hemorrhagic brain injury
- Uncontrollable hemorrhage
- Inability to place temporary shunt

■ Esophageal Injury

Delayed diagnosis and repair of esophageal injuries is associated with increased morbidity and mortality because of the postential for mediastinitis. When surgery is performed less than 24 hours after the injury, the survival rate is greater than 90%; when surgery is performed more than 24 hours after the injury, it is only 65%.

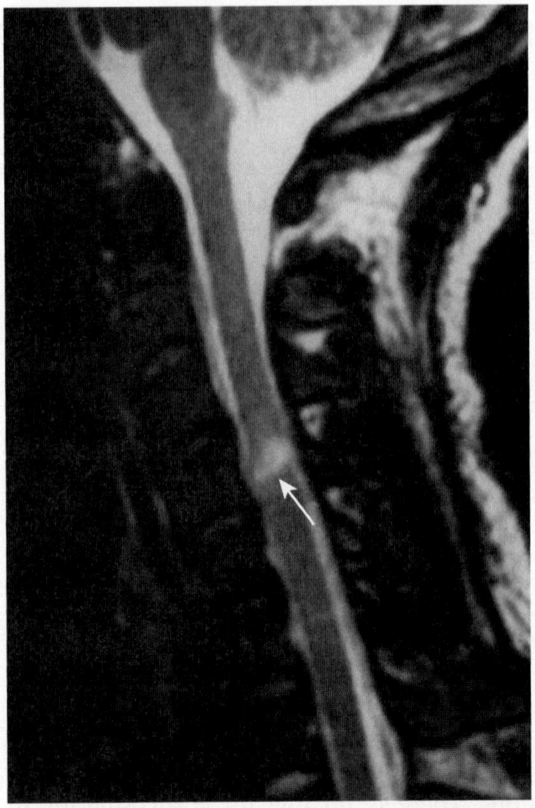

FIGURE 72-13 Magnetic resonance image showing hemisection of the spinal cord at C4 (*arrow*) due to a zone III stab wound. (Firlik AD, Welch WC: Images in clinical medicine: Brown-Séquard syndrome. From N Engl J Med 1999;340:285.)

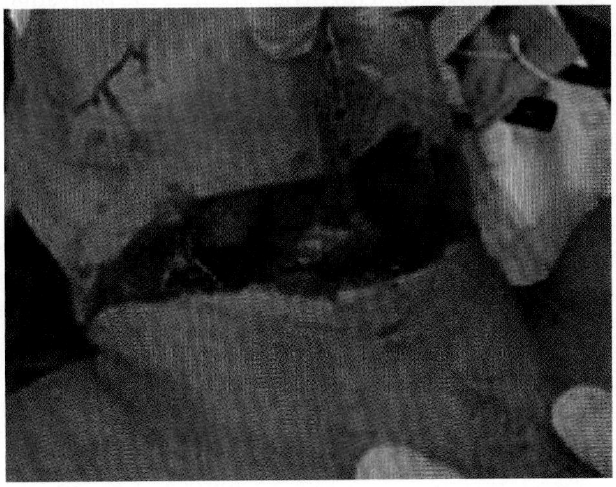

FIGURE 72-14 Emergency airway through accessible wound.

■ Cervical Spine Injury

Rigorous spinal precautions should not be maintained at the expense of managing life-threatening airway or vascular injuries in patients who are awake and neurologically intact without focal deficits.[12,13] Unstable spine fractures almost invariably are associated with focal neurologic deficits or altered mental

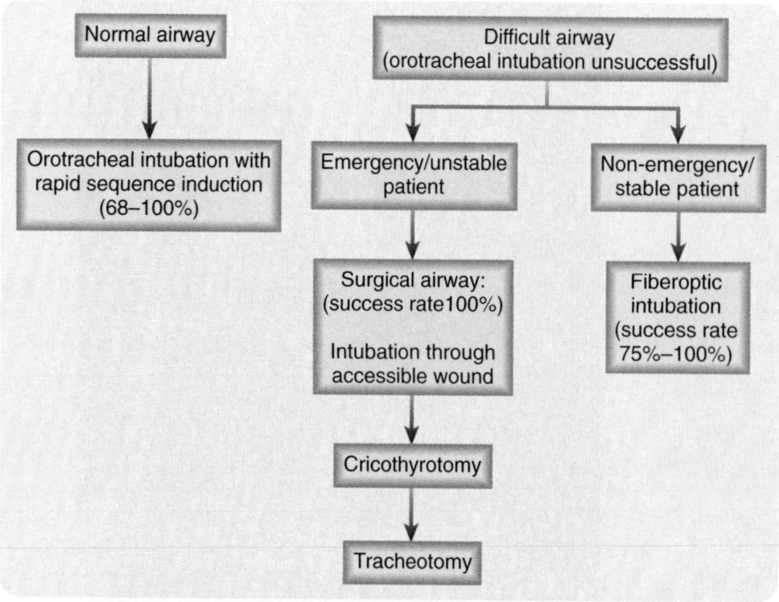
Normal airway
Difficult airway
(orotracheal intubation unsuccessful)
Orotracheal intubation with rapid sequence induction (68–100%)
Emergency/unstable patient
Non-emergency/ stable patient
Surgical airway: (success rate100%)
Intubation through accessible wound
Fiberoptic intubation (success rate 75%–100%)
Cricothyrotomy
Tracheotomy

FIGURE 72-15 Algorithm for emergency airway management.

status. Early fracture stabilization and fixation are mandatory. There is no role for corticosteroids in spinal cord injury due to penetrating trauma.

Disposition

Admission criteria include (1) any signs or symptoms of organ damage and (2) penetration of the platysma, which is only 2 to 3 mm in depth.

REFERENCES

1. Carducci B, Lowe RA, Dalsey W: Penetrating neck trauma: Consensus and controversies. Ann Emerg Med 1986;15:208-215.
2. Snyder WH, Thal ER, Bridges RA, et al: The validity of normal arteriograms in penetrating trauma. Arch Surg 1978;113:424.
3. Kuzniec S, Kauffman P, Molnar LJ, et al: Diagnosis of limb and neck arterial trauma using duplex ultrasonography. Cardiovasc Surg 1998;6:358-366.
4. LeBlang SD, Nunez DB, Rivas LA, et al: Helical computed tomographic angiography in penetrating neck trauma. Emerg Radiol 1997;4:200-2006.
5. Munera F, Soto JA, Palacio D, et al: Diagnosis of arterial injuries caused by penetrating trauma to the neck: Comparison of helical CT angiography and conventional angiography. Radiology 2000;216:356-362.
6. Weigelt JA, Thal ER, Snyder WH, et al: Diagnosis of penetrating cervical esophageal injuries. Am J Surg 1987;154:619-622.
7. Biffl WL, Moore EE, Rehse DH, et al: Selective management of penetrating neck trauma based on cervical level of injury. Am J Surg 1997;174:678-682.
8. Van As AB, Van Deurzen DF, Verleisdonk EJ, et al: Gunshots to the neck: Selective angiography as part of conservative management. Injury 2002;33:453-456.
9. Rathlev NK: Penetrating neck trauma: Mandatory versus selective exploration. J Emerg Med 1990;8:75-78.
10. Shearer VE, Giesecke AH: Airway management for patients with penetrating neck trauma: A retrospective study. Anesth Analg 1993;77:1135-1138.
11. Eggen JT, Jorden RC: Airway management, penetrating neck trauma. J Emerg Med 1993;11:381-385.
12. Medzon R, Rothenhaus T, Bono CM, et al: Stability of the cervical spine after gunshot wounds to the head and neck. Spine 2005;30:2274-2279.
13. Connell RA, Graham CA, Munro PT: Is spinal immobilization necessary for all patients sustaining isolated penetrating trauma? Injury 2003;34:912-914.

Chapter **73**

Thoracic Trauma

John Bailitz

KEY POINTS

All victims of thoracic trauma require meticulous evaluation, but life-saving management begins with prompt interventions such as endotracheal intubation, tube thoracostomy, and proper fluid resuscitation.

Thoracic cage/rib injuries are not always associated with serious injury, but some patients, especially pediatric and elderly patients, may require admission for associated injuries and respiratory therapy.

Pulmonary contusion and flail chest require positive airway pressure and judicious fluid management. Steroids and empirical antibiotics are not effective.

When blunt cardiac injury is suspected, a normal electrocardiogram (ECG) and normal vital signs rule out significant complications and complete the work-up. When a patient has abnormalities, cardiac ultrasonography is needed.

Evaluate patients for traumatic aortic injury when there has been a high-velocity, sudden deceleration mechanism of injury, even with lateral impact and seatbelt use. A normal helical computed tomography (CT) angiogram effectively rules out traumatic aortic injury and often provides valuable information about other injuries.

Suspect a cardiac injury when there has been any penetration of the chest wall medial to the midclavicular lines. Ultrasonographic evidence of cardiac tamponade is the presence of pericardial fluid with diastolic collapse of the right ventricle or atrium.

Scope

Head and thoracic injuries from moving vehicle collisions (MVCs) and firearms account for the majority of the over 160,000 injury-related deaths in the United States each year. Most fatalities occur immediately due to massive cardiac or vascular injury. Although MVCs and firearms account for most deaths, falls and other mechanisms are also common causes of injury. When a patient is transported to the ED by ambulance or private vehicle, whether to a trauma center or a general hospital, prompt injury recognition and intervention is required by the EP. The means of transport is not necessarily an indicator of severity, and some patients who arrive by private vehicle will have life-threatening injuries. It is the mechanism of injury and patient characteristics that are most important.

Anatomy and Pathophysiology

The most common mechanism of blunt thoracic trauma is the MVC, followed by falls, assaults, and crush injuries. Compressive forces directly injure the thoracic cage and underlying viscera, resulting in rib fractures and pulmonary contusion. Deceleration produces traction on fixed structures such as the isthmus of the aorta and the carina resulting in traumatic aortic and tracheobronchial injuries. Blunt thoracic trauma results in penetrating thoracic trauma when rib or clavicle fractures impale thoracic or abdominal viscera.

Gunshot wounds and stab wounds are the most common mechanisms of penetrating thoracic trauma. Low-velocity stab wounds disrupt only the structures penetrated. Medium-velocity handguns and high-velocity military assault rifles produce a permanent and temporary cavity of tissue damage. Missile injuries to the thorax often involve multiple anatomic regions including the neck, diaphragm, abdomen, and retroperitoneum.

Initial Assessment and Management

An organized team approach to trauma improves outcomes. During the primary survey, the EP detects and treats life-threatening emergencies including airway obstruction, tension pneumothorax, open pneumothorax, massive hemothorax, flail chest, and pericardial tamponade (Table 73-1). Methodically thinking about each injury is the first step in recognition and treatment. For all patients with significant mechanism, ill general appearance, altered mental status, or abnormal vital signs, the ED nurse and support staff simultaneously start two large-bore IV intubations in the antecubital fossae while drawing initial laboratory specimens, attaching the patient to the cardiac and pulse oximetry monitor, and obtaining portable chest radiographs and ECGs.

■ BASICS OF EVALUATION: PRIMARY SURVEY

The primary survey begins with a rapid airway assessment.

■ Procedure

First, rule out airway obstruction by first asking patients to state their names while you are inspecting the mouth and neck. A clear voice indicates an intact airway. A hoarse voice indicates injury to the upper airway. Labored speech suggests thoracic injury. No reply indicates loss of the airway secondary to shock, altered mental status, or cardiopulmonary arrest.

Next, inspect the oropharynx for obvious injury and pooling of secretions. Suction secretions if present and check for a gag reflex. Remove the cervical collar if present and inspect the neck for tracheal deviation, jugular venous distention, hematoma, ecchymosis, penetrating injuries, and deformity of the sternoclavicular joint. Quickly listen for breath sounds over the neck and chest. Stridor confirms upper airway injury. The unilateral absence of breath sounds with tracheal deviation in a patient in extremis indicates tension pneumothorax requiring immediate needle thoracostomy prior to intubation.

Apply 100% oxygen by non-rebreather mask to patients with a clear voice and absent to mild respiratory distress. Patients in significant distress require maximal preoxygenation, rapid sequence induction, and endotracheal intubation.

Assess and manage patients' breathing. Evaluate the mental status, color, respiratory rate and pattern, work of breathing, and symmetry of chest rise and fall in patients who are not intubated. In intubated

Table 73-1 LIFE-THREATENING EMERGENCIES IN THE PRIMARY SURVEY

Emergency	Classic Findings	Initial Testing	Further Management
Airway obstruction due to retrosternal clavicular dislocation	Deformity over clavicle and stridor; depressed medial clavicle on chest radiograph	Clinical Dx	Immediate reduction if unable to intubate
Tension pneumothorax	JVD, tracheal deviation, and unilateral absent breath sounds	Clinical Dx	Needle decompression followed immediately by tube thoracostomy
Open pneumothorax	Respiratory distress due to sucking chest wound	Clinical Dx	Three-sided tape over wound and tube thoracostomy
Flail chest	Respiratory distress, tenderness, crepitus, and paradoxical movement	Three or more ribs fractured in two or more places on chest radiograph	Early CPAP and close attention to pain control and fluid status
Cardiac tamponade	Hypotension and tachycardia, JVD, and Beck's triad late	Ultrasound scan confirms diagnosis; chest radiograph; ECG insensitive	IV fluids, pericardiocentesis, and thoracotomy
Massive hemothorax	Respiratory distress, chest wall injury, diminished breath sounds, and dullness to percussion	Ultrasound confirms diagnosis; chest radiograph with fluid collection	Initial chest tube output of 1.5-2 L is indication for surgical intervention

CPAP, continuous positive airway pressure; Dx, diagnostic testing; ECG, electrocardiogram; JVD, jugular venous distention.

patiens, listen for breath sounds high in the axillae and over the epigastrium to assess lung expansion and reconfirm endotracheal tube placement. Quickly percuss areas of diminished breath sounds for dullness suggesting hemothorax or hyperresonance suggesting pneumothorax. Palpate the neck and chest for crepitus, tenderness, and deformity. Life-threatening emergencies that must be recognized and treated during the breathing assessment include tension pneumothorax, open pneumothorax, and flail chest.

Begin the assessment of circulation by again noting patients' mental status, if they are not chemically sedated and paralyzed. A young trauma patient in hypovolemic shock often rapidly progresses from agitation and diaphoresis to obtundation. Life-threatening emergencies to recognize and treat during the circulation assessment include massive hemothorax and cardiac tamponade.

Note the heart rate and blood pressure and ask the nurse to notify the team of new vital signs after administration of each liter of fluid. Assess the strength and symmetry of central and peripheral pulses. Volume-resuscitate young, otherwise healthy patients with unstable vital signs with 2 to 3 liters of normal saline. In patiens who remain hypotensive, further resuscitation will require red blood cell transfusion. In such cases, chest tubes should be prepared to enable autotransfusion.

Permissive hypotension up to a systolic blood pressure of 80 to 100 mm Hg with rapid operative control is the ideal fluid strategy in patients with penetrating trauma and cardiovascular injury. Patients with blunt trauma, especially those with head trauma, require more aggressive fluid resuscitation to a systolic blood pressure above 100 mm Hg.[1] When patients are older than 50 years and are not hemodynamically unstable, use repetitive 500-mL boluses to avoid iatrogenic fluid overload.

For hypotensive patients, focused, bedside ultrasonography can identify pericardial tamponade, pseudo–pulseless electrical activity (secondary to cardiac injury or hypovolemia), hemothorax, and concurrent intraabdominal bleeding. Pulseless electrical activity indicates profound hypovolemia, tension pneumothorax, or cardiac tamponade requiring immediate corrective action.

■ BASICS OF RESUSCITATION: SECONDARY SURVEY

The secondary survey is a complete head-to-toe physical examination of the trauma patient. During the secondary survey, the EP must detect and treat urgent life-threatening conditions such as simple pneumothorax, hemothorax, pulmonary contusion, tracheobronchial injury, blunt cardiac injury, traumatic aortic injury, diaphragmatic injury, and esophageal injuries.

■ Procedure

Meticulously re-inspect the entire patient for all wounds and injuries (see Red Flags box).

Obtain an *ample* history from the patient, paramedics, and/or any witnesses. Ask about allergies, current medications, past medical history, last meal,

RED FLAGS

Subtle Life-Threatening Emergencies in the Secondary Survey

Traumatic Aortic Injury

In patients with injury from any mechanism greater than 30 miles per hour and with chest wall tenderness or positive chest radiograph findings, obtain a computed tomography scan of the chest.

Caution: Patients may have no external sign of trauma. Never say, "she looks too good to have a traumatic aortic injury," or "it was only a lateral impact," or "he was wearing a belt and the airbag went off." The patient will look good until the aorta ruptures; when there is lateral impact in a moving vehicle collision, there may be an increased risk of traumatic aortic injury; and restraints alone do not reduce the risk of traumatic aortic injury.

Esophageal Injury

For any injury near the esophagus, perform esophagography and esophagoscopy.

Caution: Injuries are often subtle until fatal mediastinitis develops.

Diaphragmatic Injury

Penetrating injury anywhere near the diaphragm requires chest radiography, computed tomography scanning, and in some cases, diagnostic peritoneal lavage.

Caution: Small stab wounds may create a diaphragmatic injury that is difficult to detect. However, small wounds can result in incarceration, ischemia, and necrosis of bowel days to years later.

Tracheobronchial Injury

Persistent air leaks despite a functioning chest tube indicate a tracheobronchial injury until proved otherwise. Bronchoscopy must be performed in order to prevent delayed atelectasis and loss of lung function.

Caution: Some patients will have no external sign of injury, although hoarseness or respiratory symptoms will likely be present.

Liver and Splenic Injuries

Three or more rib fractures or any fracture or tenderness of the 6th rib or below is an indication for abdominal computed tomography scanning to rule out liver and splenic injury.

Caution: Point tenderness over the lower ribs indicates a clinical rib fracture and requires abdominal computed tomotraphy scanning to rule out blunt injury to the liver and spleen.

Documentation

- Careful documentation helps to ensure identification and work-up of all significant injuries.
- The documentation chart should reflect the following thought processes and actions:
  - Primary survey assessment and management
  - Secondary survey findings: Use figure or drawing of patient to describe injuries
  - *Ample* history
  - Initial lab and imaging findings
  - Definitive testing
  - Results of consultations
  - Main assessment and plan: Patient, mechanism, and list of injuries with plan for each.
  - Tertiary survey/reassessment prior to discharge:
    - Follow-up provided
    - Patient education provided

and events at the time of the trauma. In case of blunt trauma, specifically ask about vehicle damage severity, intrusion, extrication, ejection, and deaths at the scene.

Note initial symptoms and trends in vital signs, blood loss, and Glascow Coma Scale scores.

Presume the presence of significant injury in pediatric patients, the elderly, and frail patients, including injuries from low-energy mechanisms and even if major injury is not easily apparent.

In patients with penetrating trauma, obtain a detailed history of weapons used and trajectory. Ask about and record the size and angle of the knife or other weapon, type of firearm, number of shots heard, patient position, and distance relative to the shooter. Do not make presumptions or guesses, such as caliber of a bullet. It is best to document known facts and clear, consistent reports of information (see Documentation box).

Initial Laboratory and Imaging Studies

Decisions about initial evaluation and treatment are based on the mechanism of injury, findings on the primary and secondary survey, hemodynamic stability, and prior health of the patient. Blood bank types and crossmatch of packed red blood cells should be carried out, and the baseline complete blood count and chemistry should be assessed in patients with major injury. In all women of childbearing potential, a pregnancy test should be performed. A toxicology screen is commonly sent but is rarely beneficial. A base deficit indicates shock and a higher likelihood of death.

Unstable patients who fail to improve after initial management of life-threatening emergencies and fluid resuscitation require immediate transport to the operating room for exploration and definitive management.

Stable patients require systematic, detailed evaluation. Evidence-based algorithms, discussed later in the chapter, guide evaluation and management based on the mechanism of injury.

Mechanisms of Injury

The otherwise healthy patient with a low-energy mechanism type of injury, normal primary and secondary survey findings, and normal vital signs often requires no further work-up.[2] Older patients, pediatric patients, and those with underlying illness require thorough evaluation because significant injuries are common. Moderate trauma, such as falls, can cause injury, but signs are often not apparent. Systematic, prompt physical evaluation and imaging are prudent.

Patients with blunt thoracic trauma require evaluation for thoracic wall injuries, pneumothorax, hemothorax, pulmonary contusion, blunt cardiac injury, great vessel injury, and esophageal and diaphragmatic injuries. Associated injuries to the head, neck, abdomen, spine, and extremities are also likely.

High-energy mechanisms such as falls from greater than 30 feet or MVCs at greater than 30 miles per hour require more systematic evaluations to exclude life-threatening but clinically inapparent injuries. Patients with high-energy mechanism injuries with chest wall tenderness or with radiographic evidence of a mediastinal hematoma require helical CT angiography to rule out traumatic aortic injury. Abnormal findings on an ECG, hypotension, or dysrhythmia suggesting blunt cardiac injury (blunt cardiac injury) requires cardiac monitoring and hospitalization for 24 hours with repeat electrocardiography every 8 hours.

Penetrating Injury

Patients with penetrating thoracic trauma require evaluation for injury to the lung, mediastinum, and other anatomic structures in the path of the impalement or missile. These patients also require pulse oximetry and posteroanterior (PA) and lateral chest radiographs at 0 and 4 hours to evaluate for pneumothorax and hemothorax.

The thorax is divided into anatomic areas to guide further evaluation. The anterior box is the area between the nipples, clavicles superiorly, and costal margins inferiorly. Injuries potentially involving the anterior box require an emergent FAST (focused assessment with sononography for trauma) to evaluate for pericardial fluid.

The posterior box extends from the shoulders to the inferior costal margins, between the scapulae. Posterior box and transmediastinal gunshot wounds require emergent FAST examination, angiography of the great vessels, esophagogram/esophagoscopy, and bronchoscopy. The initial chest radiograph guides further evaluation of stab wounds to the posterior box. With an abnormal mediastinum and signs and symptoms of injury, perform angiography, esophagogram/esophagoscopy, and bronchoscopy.

The thoracoabdominal area is the area below the nipples and scapulae and above the costal margin. Penetrating injuries potentially involving the thoracoabdominal area require evaluation for thoracic, diaphragmatic, and abdominal injury. Diaphragmatic penetration is evaluated with diagnostic peritoneal lavage; patients with red blood cell counts of 10,000/μL require laparotomy (Box 73-1).

BOX 73-1

Approach to Thoracic Trauma*

Blunt Trauma

- High-energy mechanisms: Falls greater than 30 feet or motor vehicle collisions at more than 30 miles per hour
- All injuries: CXR and pulse oximetery. If pneumothorax or hemothorax, insert chest tube
- Traumatic aortic injury: Mechanism with chest wall tenderness or abnormal CXR evidence requires helical CT angiography; if negative, evaluate for traumatic aortic injury; if findings indeterminate, obtain aortogram; if positive, transfer patient to operating room
- Blunt cardiac injury: Abnormal ECG, hypotension, or dysrhythmia, cardiac monitoring and hospitalization for 24 hours with repeat ECGs every 8 hours; hypotension or symptomatic dysrhythmia, formal echocardiography

Penetrating Injuries

- All injuries: continuous pulse oximetry and PA and lateral CXR at 0 and 6 hours
- Anterior cardiac box: FAST examination to evaluate for pericardial fluid
- Posterior box and transmediastinal gunshot wounds: Angiography for great vessel injury; when there are signs and symptoms of injury, esophagography/esophagoscopy, and bronchoscopy
- Posterior box stab wounds: If abnormal mediastinum on CXR, then angiography for great vessel injury; when there are signs and symptoms of injury, esophagogram/esophagoscopy, and bronchoscopy.
- Thoracoabdominal: DPL with red blood cell count of 10,000 cells/μL, laparoscopy/thoracoscopy or laparotomy to evaluate for diaphragmatic injury

*Protocols and approach may vary based on institutional experience and availability.

CT, computed tomography; CXR, chest radiograph; DPL, diagnostic peritoneal lavage; ECG, electrocardiogram; FAST, focused assessment with sonography for trauma; PA, posteroanterior.

Thoracic Cage Injuries: Rib, Sternum, and Scapula Fractures

■ SCOPE

Rib fractures are the most common thoracic cage injury after blunt thoracic trauma. Isolated first and second rib, sternum, and scapula fractures are no longer considered markers of traumatic aortic injury.[3] However, rib fractures must still be considered markers of significant injury. Most patients presenting to trauma centers with rib fractures will have a hemothorax, pneumothorax, or pulmonary contusion. Three or more rib fractures at any anatomic site dramatically increases the risk of splenic and liver injury. Likewise, scapula fractures are uncommon, yet signify a high-energy mechanism injury, almost always with important associated injuries.

Seat belts have increased the incidence of sternum fractures while reducing the number of lives lost in MVCs. Isolated nondisplaced sternum fractures are no longer considered markers of blunt cardiac injury.[4] More complicated fracture patterns predict associated injuries. Fractures of the manubrium, manubrium-sternal syndochondrosis and proximal sternum, and severely displaced sternum fractures are associated with an increased incidence of spinal fractures. Displaced fractures of the body of the sternum are associated with a higher incidence of intrapulmonary and cardiac injuries.[5]

■ PATHOPHYSIOLOGY

MVCs are the most common cause of rib and sternum fractures. Other mechanisms include pedestrian injury by a moving vehicle, falls, contact sports, and altercations. Fractures occur at the site of direct blows or at their posterior weak point from compressive forces. Ribs 4 to 9 are the most commonly fractured.

All thoracic cage injuries result in significant pain, splinting, and atelectasis and an increased risk of pneumonia. Multiple rib fractures interfere directly with the mechanics of ventilation. Fracture fragments may penetrate the pleura and lungs, resulting in pneumothorax and hemothorax. Traditionally, fractures of the 6th to 12th rib on the right suggest liver injury and on the left suggest splenic injury. However, any fracture, especially multiple fractures, increases the risk of liver and splenic injuries.[6]

Children have more elastic chest walls, transmitting more energy to the underlying lung and requiring a greater force to fracture. Rib fractures in children under 2 years of age suggest child abuse.

■ PRESENTING SIGNS AND SYMPTOMS

Classically, rib fractures present with localized tenderness and pleuritic chest pain, accompanied by splinting, crepitus, and ecchymosis. The patient with a classic sternum fracture presents with localized pain and tenderness with ventral compression, ecchymosis, and deformity. Pain at the site of thoracic cage injuries increases with cough and deep inspiration. Patients with scapular fractures typically present with rib and extremity fractures that often mask the diagnosis of scapula fracture. The upper body of all patients should be exposed completely and examined carefully to avoid missing subtle but serious injuries, especially in patients with multiple injuries and altered mental status.

■ DIAGNOSTIC TESTING

The initial portable anteroposterior (AP) chest radiograph should be inspected to confirm the diagnosis of rib fracture and underlying pleura or lung injury. An upright PA and lateral radiograph should be obtained if high clinical index of suspicion remains for fracture or underlying injury. Both views should be examined carefully for evidence of other fractures and injury to underlying structures. The presence of an occult "clinical rib fracture" with tenderness over the rib should be assumed even in the absence of radiographic findings. Rib radiographs seldom add to the clinical evaluation and are not routinely indicated.

Sternum fractures are best detected on the lateral chest radiograph, which should be carefully inspected for displacement and to identify the location of the injury. Associated rib fractures and mediastinal abnormalities may be evident on the PA view. The ECG should be examined for evidence of cardiac injury. Scapula fractures are often missed on the initial chest radiograph unless the scapulae outline is specifically inspected. Shoulder radiographs can confirm suspected fractures (Fig. 73-1).

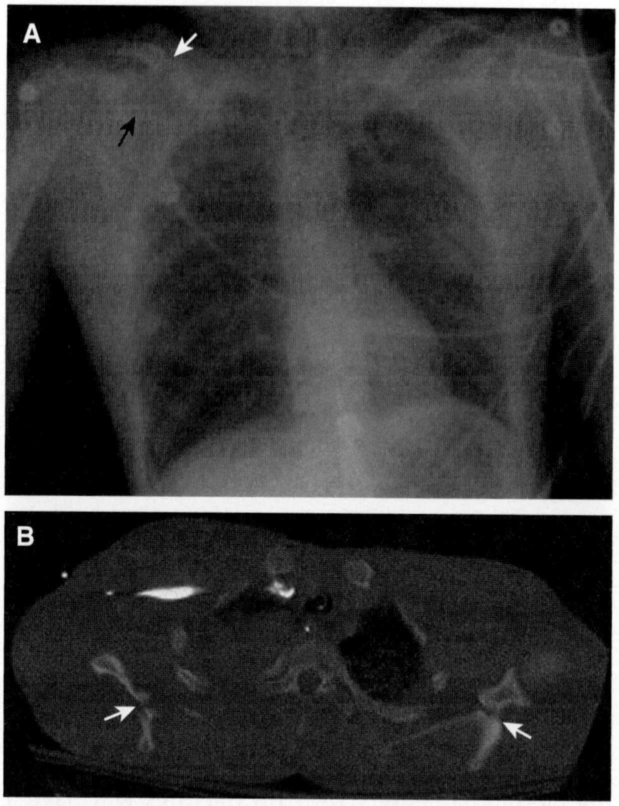
A
B

FIGURE 73-1 **A,** Chest radiograph showing fractures of clavicle (*white arrow*) and scapula (*black arrow*). **B,** Lateral scapula fractures (*arrows*) visible on computed tomography scan. (From Westra SJ, Wallace EC: Imaging of pediatric chest trauma. Radiol Clin North Am 2005; 43:267-281.)

Helical CT angiography should be performed on hemodynamically stable patients when clinically significant underlying injury is suspected.[7] An abdominal CT scan can rule out intraabdominal injury in patients with tenderness or fracture of the 6th rib or below, three or more rib fractures, field or ED hypotension, abdominal or flank tenderness, pelvic or femur fractures, or gross hematuria.[8]

■ TREATMENT AND DISPOSITION

Adequate pain control should be provided to prevent atelectatis in patients with simple acute rib fractures. Patients should be instructed to perform incentive spirometry or take 10 deep breaths every hour.

Binders and belts are not recommended because such devices promote hypoventilation, resulting in atelectasis and pneumonia. Shoulder slings and pendular exercise should be prescribed for most scapular fractures. Displaced fractures, especially those involving the scapular spine and neck, often require consultation with an orthopedic surgeon for repair.

Otherwise healthy patients with isolated rib fractures or sternum or scapula fractures may be discharged home. Elderly patients and patients with multiple comorbidities may require admission for pain control and pulmonary therapy. Intercostal nerve block can be of marked benefit.

Discharged patients should be informed that pain will diminish after 2 weeks but may persist for up to 6 weeks (see Patient Teaching Tips box). Follow-up with a trauma surgeon should be scheduled if pain persists beyond 4 weeks in order to detect delayed rib fracture complications. Patients with isolated scapular fractures should be referred to an orthopedic surgeon.

Flail Chest

■ SCOPE

Flail chest occurs when three or more ribs are fractured in two or more places, producing a discontinuous segment of the thoracic wall that moves paradoxically with respiration. Flail chest occurs in approximately 5% of thoracic trauma patients pre-

PATIENT TEACHING TIPS

RIB FRACTURES/CONTUSIONS

- Take all medicine as directed to ensure that you will be able to breathe deep enough to prevent lung complications.
- Take 10 deep breaths every hour or use incentive spirometer 10 times an hour.
- Binders and belts are not recommended because they prevent effective breathing.
- Pain should diminish after 2 weeks but may persist for up to 6 weeks.
- Return to the ED immediately if you have a fever, worsening shortness of breath, lightheadedness, or other concerns.
- Proper care and follow-up will help to ensure the best possible recovery. However, complications are often unavoidable, so be sure to return to ED if any problems develop.
- If pain persists beyond 4 weeks, return to the ED for follow-up to detect delayed rib fracture complications.

senting to level I trauma centers, typically in the setting of multisystem trauma.

ANATOMY AND PATHOPHYSIOLOGY

Mechanisms include MVCs, crush injuries, assault, falls, and even minimal trauma in elderly patients. Respiratory insufficiency results primarily from underlying pulmonary contusion. Pneumothorax occurs in 50% of cases and pulmonary contusion in 75%.[9]

PRESENTING SIGNS AND SYMPTOMS

The patient may present with the classic signs and sympoms of respiratory distress, tenderness, crepitus, deformity, and paradoxical motion of the affected thoracic wall. Affected segments will move in during inspiration and out during expiration. More commonly, splinting secondary to severe pain or mechanical ventilation masks the diagnosis. Forced expiration and coughing accent the paradox.

DIAGNOSTIC TESTING

A chest radiograph can confirm the diagnosis and detect complications such as pneumothorax and hemothorax. A chest CT scan can further evaluate underlying pulmonary contusion and assess other underlying injuries such as traumatic aortic injury.

TREATMENT

Assessment and management of other injuries including pneumothorax and hemothorax includes immediate chest tube placement. Continuous positive airway pressure is the first-line treatment in the awake and cooperative patient with worsening oxygenation or ventilation.[10] Criteria for intubation include airway obstruction, respiratory distress, shock, closed head injury, and need for surgery. Endotracheal intubation should only be performed when it is necessary to avoid associated nosocomial pneumonia and increased mortality.

Fluid replacement should be managed carefully to avoid over hydration and worsening of lung injury. Analgesia is titrated so that the patient is more willing to make sufficient inspiratory efforts, but excessive sedation should be avoided. Intercostal nerve blocks, epidural anesthesia, or even surgical fixation of the flail segment may be beneficial. Stabilizing the flail segment in the ED or prehospital setting has not been shown to be helpful, and aggressive stabilization efforts impede overall thoracic mechanics.

DISPOSITION

Consultation and admission for trauma or cardiothoracic surgery is advised when flail chest is suspected. Overall mortality from flail chest, while dependent on other injuries, ranges up to 35%. All patients with flail chest should be admitted to the intensive care unit, preferably at a level I trauma center for close observation of respiratory mechanics and worsening of pulmonary contusion.

Retrosternal Clavicular Dislocations

SCOPE

The uncommon retrosternal clavicular dislocation causing airway obstruction must be recognized and appropriately managed as part of the airway assessment. Inability to pass the endotracheal tube requires reduction prior to intubation. Only 100 cases have been described in the past 65 years, with 30% resulting in compression complications.[11]

ANATOMY AND PATHOPHYSIOLOGY

Posterior clavicular dislocations are best described as retrosternal clavicular dislocations because the medial end of the clavicle is actually dislocated medially and posteriorly. The most common mechanism is a blow to the posterior shoulder from a fall or motorcycle crash. A less common but higher-energy mechanism injury occurs with a direct anterior blow to the joint when the chest strikes the dashboard during an MVC. Retrosternal clavicular dislocation may cause compression injuries to any posterior structure, including the trachea, esophagus, great vessels, brachial plexus, and thoracic duct.

■ PRESENTING SIGNS AND SYMPTOMS

In the classic presentation, the patient's neck is flexed toward the side of injury, and the ipsilateral arm is supported by the contralateral arm. Severe pain and tenderness are noted over a depressed and ecchymotic medial clavicle. Symptoms include hoarseness, dypsnea, dysphagia, venous congestion, and ipsilateral neurologic findings. Often the diagnosis is not clinically obvious in the patient with multiple traumatic injuries or altered mental status or in the absence of significant compression of underlying structures.

■ DIFFERENTIAL DIAGNOSIS

Airway obstruction in thoracic trauma more commonly occurs due to associated head and neck injuries. Head injuries often result in loss of protective airway reflexes, inability to handle secretions, and resulting airway obstruction. Injury to the cervical trachea may result from direct strikes from a dashboard or penetrating injury.

Patients with airway obstruction due to head or cervical spine injuries present with loss of consciousness, pooling of secretions, or direct injury to the airway. Patients with retrosternal clavicular dislocations with airway compression have stridorous breath sounds and deformity of the sternoclavicular joint.

■ DIAGNOSTIC TESTING

Clavicular dislocations are often detected on physical examination or initial chest radiograph. When the patient's condition is stable, confirm the diagnosis and assess for injury to underlying structures with chest CT.

■ INTERVENTIONS AND PROCEDURES

Immediate reduction is indicated in patients with airway obstruction. Place a rolled blanket between the scapulae, abduct the arm 90 degrees, and apply longitudinal traction to the affected arm in line with the clavicle. Grasp the depressed medial clavicle with a towel clip and pull forward.

■ TREATMENT AND DISPOSITION

Ideally, reduction is performed in the operating room by an orthopedic specialist with cardiothoracic surgery consultation. Disposition typically is determined by other traumatic injuries. Discharged patients with isolated injuries are instructed to keep the affected arm in a figure-of-eight sling for 4 to 6 weeks and are referred for orthopedic follow-up.

Pneumothorax and Hemothorax

■ ANATOMY AND PATHOPHYSIOLOGY

A simple pneumothorax occurs when air accumulates in the pleural space without shifting the mediastinum or communicating with the atmosphere. Mechanisms include laceration of the pleura or lung by a fractured rib, alveolar rupture from compression of the chest against a closed glottis, or penetrating wound to the thorax.

Tension pneumothorax occurs when injury to the chest wall acts as a one-way valve. Outside air enters the pleural space during inspiration but cannot exit during expiration. Accumulating air increases the intrapleural pressure, eventually shifting the mediastinum, compressing the vena cava, decreasing venous return, and ultimately decreasing cardiac output.

Open or communicating pneumothorax occurs when a significant thoracic wall defect causes the lung to collapse on inspiration and expand on expiration, "sucking" air in and out of the chest and preventing effective ventilation. Mechanisms include high-velocity assault rifle injuries and shotgun wounds.

Hemothorax occurs when blood accumulates in the pleural space, typically from minor lacerations in the lung parenchyma. Injuries to the internal mammary, intercostal, and great vessels produce progressively more significant bleeding. Massive hemothorax is defined as greater then 1.5 liters in the initial chest tube drainage and is an indication for immediate operation. Hemopneumothorax occurs when both air and blood fill the pleural space, commonly resulting from rib fractures or penetrating trauma.

■ PRESENTING SIGNS AND SYMPTOMS

The patient with a simple pneumothorax classically presents with chest pain, diminished breath sounds, crepitus, hyperresonance, and mild to moderate respiratory distress. Patients with tension pneumothorax classically present in extremis (e.g., grabbing the bed with air hunger), jugular venous distention, tracheal deviation, unilateral absent breath sounds, and tachycardia followed by hypotension immediately before death.[12]

Patients with open pneumothorax present with chest wall wounds that produce sonorous sounds and with severe respiratory distress. Typical symptoms of hemothorax are respiratory distress, chest pain, and diminished breath sounds with dullness to percussion.

Atypical presentations are more common than classic. Respiratory distress may occur due to multiple other causes. Patients can have severe pain from distracting injuries. Breath sounds can be difficult to hear in a noisy environment. The physical examination in patients with penetrating thoracic trauma is unreliable for the detection of pneumothorax or hemothorax.[13] Patients with simple pneumothorax may be minimally symptomatic or may be cyanotic and in severe respiratory distress. Tension pneumothorax most commonly occurs in the intubated patient from positive-pressure ventilations, sometimes after overzealous bagging.

Clinical reassessment of the ventilated patient with decreasing oxygen saturation and hypotension may allow faster detection and treatment, even before chest radiograph diagnosis. Open pneumothorax may be missed if the patient is not completely exposed and rolled during the primary survey

■ DIFFERENTIAL DIAGNOSIS AND DISTINGUISHING FEATURES

The differential diagnosis of tension pneumothorax includes cardiac tamponade, massive hemothorax, and right mainstem intubation with left lung collapse. All will produce respiratory distress, hypotension, and tachycardia. Cardiac tamponade results in diminished heart sounds, with normal breath sounds and a midline trachea. Massive hemothorax produces decreased or absent unilateral breath sounds and dullness to percussion. Chest tube insertion confirms the diagnosis. Right mainstem intubation produces jugular venous distention, tracheal deviation to the left, normal resonance, and diminished breath sounds on the left versus the right. In the intubated patient, the endotracheal tube should be checked and pulled back. In the field or resuscitation bay, bilateral needle thoracostomy should be performed when the patient is in distress, even if the diagnosis is uncertain. A rush of air confirms the diagnosis of tension pneumothorax. Chest tubes must be placed after needle decompression, followed by ultrasonographic evaluation to assess for pericardial tamponade or massive hemothorax.

■ DIAGNOSTIC TESTING

A chest radiograph can confirm the diagnosis of a simple pneumothorax and hemothorax. A simple pneumothorax is diagnosed when the thin visceral pleura line is visualized near the lung apex without lung markings beyond. A distance of 1 cm or one fingerbreadth between the chest wall and visceral pleural line correlates with a small, 10% to 15% pneumothorax. Anything larger requires immediate chest tube insertion. On the supine portable AP chest radiograph, a deep sulcus sign suggests a pneumothorax. The affected costophrenic angle appears clearer and deep with depression of the hemidiaphragm due to localized air collection in the supine patient. When there is a high index of clinical suspicion based on symptoms or penetrating injuries, some authorities advocate expiratory upright PA and lateral chest radiographs to make the lung volume smaller and the pneumothorax volume relatively larger and easier to visualize. Clinically significant pneumothoraces should be evident on standard chest radiographs. The chest CT scan is more sensitive for visualizing pneumothorax. Helical border instead of the CT angiogram of the chest often detects small occult pneumothoraces requiring close monitoring.

In the upright patient, the hemothorax appears as a fluid layer in the affected hemithorax. Early collections are noted to blunt the costophrenic angles on the AP and lateral radiograph views. Decubitus views better demonstrate a small hemothorax. The extended FAST scan can diagnose pneumothorax and hemothorax with a higher sensitivity than a portable chest radiograph in experienced hands. The extended FAST scan is especially helpful when chest radiography is not immediately available and in mass casualty situations.[14]

A hemothorax often appears as only a diffuse hazy infiltrate in the supine trauma patient. A hemopneumothorax has a fluid layer with a flat superior fluid meniscus seen with an isolated hemothorax (Figs. 73-2 and 73-3).

■ INTERVENTIONS AND PROCEDURES

Tension pneumothorax and open pneumothorax are both clinical diagnoses requiring immediate treatment, even when based on clinical evaluation, prior to radiographic confirmation.

■ Procedure

Insert a 16-gauge, 2-inch catheter over the needle into the 2nd intercostal space in the midclavicular line immediately over the 3rd rib. The artery and vein course along the inferior rib, so needle placement is superior to the rib. In the out-of-hospital

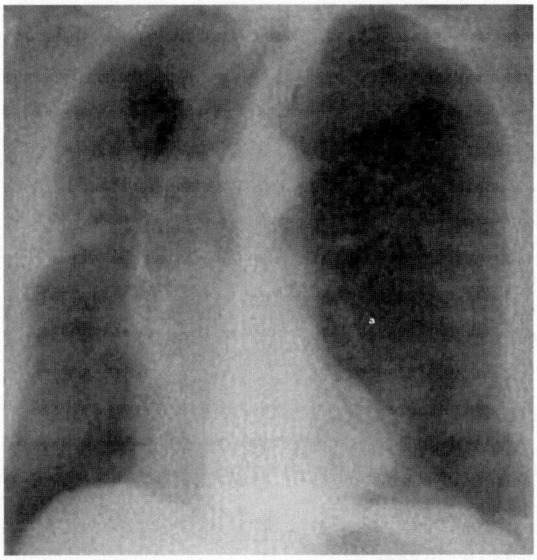

FIGURE 73-2 Chest radiograph showing obvious left-sided tension pneumothorax with mediastinal shift. (From Ullman EA, Donley LP, Brady WJ: Pulmonary trauma emergency department evaluation and management. Emerg Med Clin North Am 2003;21:291-313.)

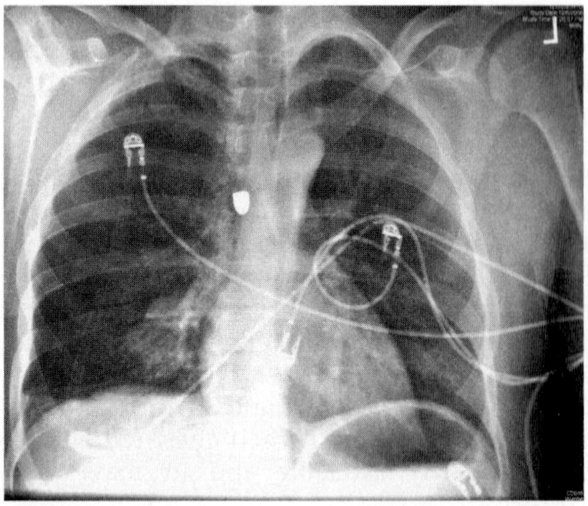

FIGURE 73-3 Chest radiograph showing right hemopneumothorax with bullet. (Image courtesy of Dave Andreski, MD.)

setting, an unpowdered latex glove, with the needle inserted through a fingertip, can act as a one-way valve. If there is no rush of air, a longer needle may be required for patients with a thick thoracic wall. Pulmonary injury should be avoided in lean patients.

Cover all suspicious open chest wounds with petroleum gauze secured on three sides to prevent the entry of air during inspiration and allow the exit of air during expiration.

An immediate tube thoracostomy is indicated if needle decompression has been performed and if there is a clinical suspicion for pneumothorax, even without needle decompression. Insert a chest tube away from the site of the wound to minimize the risk of infection.

Place a 36-40 French chest tube in the 4th to 5th intercostal space in the anterior axillary line and direct the tube apically and posteriorly to remove both blood and air. Be sure that all chest tube holes are within the chest cavity. Prophylactic antibiotics with chest tube insertion do not reduce the risk of empyema or pneumonia.[15] Connect all chest tubes initially to suction using a three-chamber collection system. Observe carefully the initial and subsequent chest tube drainage and check for the presence of air leaks.

Obtain postprocedure radiographs to confirm placement, drainage of air and blood, and re-expansion of lung. Be vigilant to avoid accidental chest tube disconnection or removal.

■ Thoracotomy

Operating room thoracotomy is indicated for patients with the following:

- Massive hemothorax (initial drainage of 1.5 to 2 liters of blood)
- Persistent bleeding of more than 200 mL per hour for 4 hours
- Persistent hypotension or instability despite blood replacement

■ Autotransfusion

Perform autotransfusion when there is massive hemothorax or persistent significant bleeding. It is prudent to prepare for autotransfusion early because most blood loss occurs at the time of initial chest tube insertion.

■ TREATMENT AND DISPOSITION

Traumatic pneumothoraces and hemothoraces generally require tube thoracostomy. The exception is a small stable pneumothorax in an otherwise healthy and symptom-free patient, which may be managed with observation.

Occult traumatic pneumothorax detected on CT scan requires only close observation for respiratory distress, progression, and the development of complications. Tube throracostomy must be immediately available but is not required even with positive-pressure ventilation.[16] Any prolonged operation, diagnostic testing, or transport preventing immediate tube throracostomy requires prophylactic placement.

Chest radiographs are obtained to determine occult pneumothorax resolution without the need for repeat CT scanning. In patients with penetrating injuries and a negative initial chest radiograph, repeat upright PA and lateral chest radiographs should be obtained in 4 hours. Patients with normal repeat radiographs without significant associated injuries are discharged with wound care instructions and follow-up. Patients with asymptomatic blunt chest trauma and normal initial chest radiographs do not require repeat films prior to discharge.

All patients with chest tubes are admitted to the trauma, cardiothoracic, or general surgery service by a unit experienced in managing chest tube equipment.

Pulmonary Contusion

■ SCOPE

Pulmonary contusion is the most common parenchymal lung injury in victims of blunt chest trauma. Although typically described in the setting of flail chest, pulmonary contusion occurs with less significant chest wall fractures and occasionally even in the absence of overlying injury.

■ PATHOPHYSIOLOGY

Pulmonary contusion occurs with blunt, blast, or high-energy penetrating injuries. MVCs and falls are the most commonly reported mechanisms. Injury to the lung parenchyma causes hemorrhage and edema of the alveoli and interstitium, resulting in $\dot{V}/\dot{Q}$ mismatching and ultimately hypoxia and hypercarbia. Hemorrhage worsens over the first 24 to 48 hours and then typically resolves over the next 7 days.

Acute respiratory distress syndrome and pneumonia are the most frequent complications, both with significant morbidity and mortality.

■ PRESENTING SIGNS AND SYMPTOMS

Patients with pulmonary contusion typically present with significant chest wall injury accompanied by dypsnea and tachypnea progressing to hemoptysis, cyanosis, and hypotension. Inspection often reveals obvious flail chest or ecchymosis overlying rib fractures. Auscultation reveals rhonchi, wheezes, rales, or minimal breath sounds. Compliant chest walls result in minimal overlying damage with diffuse pulmonary contusion in children. Blast injuries may also result in significant pulmonary contusion with minimal chest wall injury. Delayed presentations of pulmonary contusion can occur in initially well-appearing patients. Because hemorrhage and edema will worsen, patients with even mild initial symptoms must be observed closely, with continuous monitoring. Clinical findings usually progress over the initial hours, through the first 2 days.

■ DIFFERENTIAL DIAGNOSIS AND DISTINGUISHING FEATURES

The differential diagnosis for the trauma patient with respiratory distress and infiltrates on initial chest radiographs includes pulmonary contusion, congestive heart failure, aspiration pneumonia, and acute respiratory distress syndrome. Symptomatic congestive heart failure may predispose to blunt trauma, result from blunt myocardial injury, or develop during fluid resuscitation. Enlarged heart size, cephalization, and bilateral infiltrates on chest radiograpy confirm the diagnosis of congestive heart failure. Aspiration pneumonia leads to lobar opacification. Acute respiratory distress syndrome typically occurs 24 to 48 hours after the injury, often with diffuse bilateral infiltrates and a normal heart size.

■ DIAGNOSTIC TESTING

The patchy or diffuse air space opacification above the site of injury in pulmonary contusion is often present on the initial chest radiograph and typically progresses over the first 6 hours (Fig. 73-4). Initial CT scanning is more sensitive than chest radiograpy but seldom changes the initial management of pulmonary contusion. Pulse oximetry is essential to detect early clinical deterioration.

■ INTERVENTIONS AND PROCEDURES

Prophylactic intubation is not recommended for patients with minimal symptoms, but its use is prudent for patients with moderate or worsening symptoms. Indications for intubation in adult patients with pulmonary contusion include airway compromise, moderate to severe respiratory distress, hypoxia, hypercarbia, the need for general anesthesia, and as part of care for other injuries.

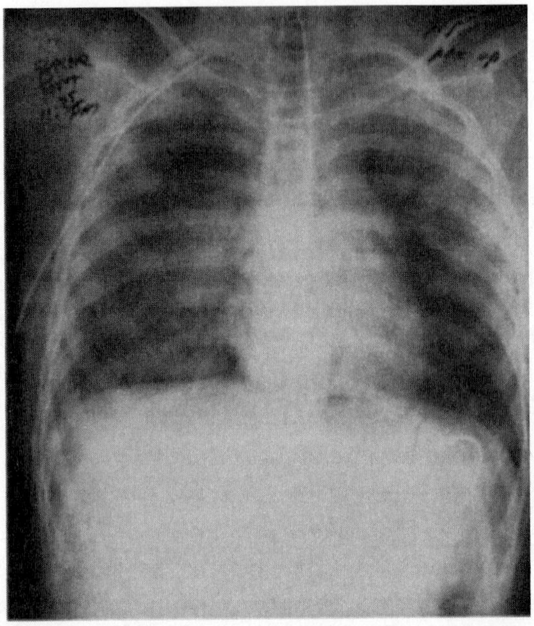

FIGURE 73-4 Chest radiograph showing right pulmonary contusion with pneumomediastinum and pneumopericardium. (From Marx J, Hockberger R, Walls R [eds]: Rosen's Emergency Medicine: Concepts and Clinical Practice, 6th ed. St. Louis, Mosby, 2006.)

■ TREATMENT AND DISPOSITION

Patients with pulmonary contusion require admission to the intensive care unit for oxygen and chest physical therapy for incentive spirometry, suctioning, analgesia, and close monitoring. Overhydration must be avoided to prevent iatrogenic worsening of capillary leak and lung function. Prophylactic steroids and antibiotics are not recommended.[17] Isolated pulmonary contusions typically resolve within 14 days without long-term complications. Disability and mortality is higher in patients with larger areas of contusion, flail chest, acute respiratory distress syndrome, and pneumonia.

Tracheobronchial Injury

■ SCOPE

Tracheobronchial injuries are infrequent but present unique challenges to the EP. Emergent airway management is often both required and complicated by these devastating injuries.

■ ANATOMY AND PATHOPHYSIOLOGY

Penetrating tracheobronchial injuries are more common than blunt injuries. Penetrating injuries to the relatively exposed cervical trachea occur more frequently than injuries to the protected thoracic trachea. Gunshot wounds in the thoracic trachea occur more often than stab wounds. Blunt injuries to the cervical trachea occur with rapid deceleration, resulting in shear stress at the junction of the larynx and trachea; examples of these types of injury include hyperextension injury, direct dashboard strikes, and "clothesline" injuries in snowmobile and motorcycle accidents. Blunt injuries to the thoracic trachea typically occur due to high-energy MVCs crush injuries and falls. Rapid deceleration produces a shearing force with injury typically within 2 cm of the fixed carina.[20] Injuries to the esophagus and spine are the most common associated injuries. Head, vascular, nerve, and intra-thoracic injury also occur frequently in both blunt and penetrating tracheobronchial injuries

■ PRESENTING SIGNS AND SYMPTOMS

Patients with tracheobronchial injuries typically present with dramatic but nonspecific symptoms, including hoarseness, dysphagia, hemoptysis, and dyspnea. Careful inspection for penetrating wounds should be made, and the trajectory and proximity to the trachea of the injury should be estimated. Physical examination findings include air escape from wounds, subcutaneous emphysema in the neck and supraclavicular region, hypoxia, stridor, pneumothorax, and pneumomediastinum. Patients with blunt trauma often have few signs of external injury. Persistent air leaks despite a functioning chest tube suggests tracheobronchial injury. Rarely, patients with tracheobronchial injuries without communication with the pleural space maintain respiration with minimal symptoms until granulation tissue obstructs the airway, resulting in delayed lobar atelectasis.

■ DIAGNOSTIC TESTING

Chest radiographs may have subtle evidence of tracheobronchial injuries such as high rib fractures, "fallen lung" sign, pneumomediastinum, deep cervical emphysema, peribronchial air, and abnormal location of the endotracheal tube. The fallen lung sign occurs when the apical segments of the lung have collapsed and fallen to the level of the hilum. Flexible fiberoptic bronchoscopy usually confirms the injury. Helical CT angiography is particularly effective in the diagnosis of blunt laryngeal injury and often provides additional information in the evaluation of penetrating and thoracic tracheobronchial injuries.

■ INTERVENTIONS AND PROCEDURES

Patients with tracheobronchial injuries who are in respiratory distress require immediate intubation and mechanical ventilation. This is best peformed with flexible fiberoptic bronchoscopy in the operating room if possible. Fiberoptic bronchoscopy is the best diagnostic and management option for cervical and intrathoracic tracheal injuries. When it is not available and immediate airway intervention is required, some authorities recommend orotracheal intubation without paralysis to prevent loss of paratracheal muscle support of the injured trachea. The benefits must be weighed against the suboptimal intubating conditions in a nonparalyzed patient. If paralysis is required, prior preparation for a surgical airway and right-sided thoracotomy is necessary. Skilled specialist support is optimal.

During orotracheal intubation, a smaller-size endotracheal tube should be inserted, placing it past the injury if possible. To prevent worsening of the injury, force should be avoided (e.g., do not attempt to push through resistance) during endotracheal tube placement.

■ PROCEDURE

When orotracheal intubation is not possible, place the endotracheal tube through the anterior neck wound, into the trachea. Be careful to avoid pushing a transected trachea deeper into the thorax.

If there is complete transection and retraction of the trachea, major intervention is required. Perform a right-sided thoracotomy (to avoid the aortic arch on the left), and attempt to visualize the injured trachea, support it, and establish an airway. Extension to a left sided thoracotomy may be needed for complex distal injuries.[18]

Tube thoracostomy is required, often with multiple tubes to drain resulting pneumothorax and re-expand the affected lung.

■ TREATMENT AND DISPOSITION

Stable patients with tracheobronchial injuries and maintained airway are best transported to the operating room immediately for fiberoptic bronchoscopy, intubation, and possible thoracotomy. Definitive surgical repair is necessary to prevent acute and late complications. Acute complications include persistent air leak, pneumothorax, empyema, and mediastinitis. Delayed complications include granulation of partial injuries, resultant atelectasis, and significant loss of pulmonary function. Penetrating and blunt injuries typically are managed early with exploration and repair.

Blunt Cardiac Injury

■ SCOPE

The pathologic spectrum of blunt cardiac injury begins with cardiac concussion; includes myocardial contusion, coronary artery injury, valve and septal injury; and ends with myocardial rupture. Myocardial contusion remains the most common clinical challenge to the EP. Definitive diagnosis can only be made on autopsy, and complications are rare but life-threatening.

■ ANATOMY AND PATHOPHYSIOLOGY

Blunt cardiac injury typically results from MVCs but may occur after falls, crush injuries, blast injuries, direct blows, and chest compression. Low-speed deceleration injuries occasionally result in significant injury. Proposed mechanisms include compression of the heart between the sternum and vertebral bodies and sudden striking of the heart against the sternum in deceleration injuries.

Cardiac concussion, or *commotio cordis,* occurs when a blow to the chest briefly "stuns" the heart, resulting in dysrhythmia, hypotension, syncope, and often sudden death but without permanent cellular damage. Commotio cordis may result from an anterior chest wall impact at a moment when the myocardium is refractory to depolarization, resulting in fatal arrhythmia.

Myocardial contusion occurs when injury to the anterior wall, formed by the right ventricle, results in well-defined areas of red blood cell extravasation and eventually in subendocardial and transmural necrosis. Infrequent delayed complications include mural thrombus, pericardial effusions, constrictive pericarditis, and ventricular aneurysms. Direct injury to already atherosclerotic coronary arteries or severely contused myocardium can result in myocardial infarction. Rare blunt cardiac rupture typically is immediately fatal except when limited to the low-pressure right heart or to small, self-sealing ventricular injuries. Early survival depends on the ability of an intact pericardium to prevent immediate exsanguination. Later survival depends on recognition and treatment of cardiac tamponade and repair of the primary cardiac injury. Other rare but salvageable injuries include injury to the valves and septum.[19]

■ PRESENTING SIGNS AND SYMPTOMS

Blunt cardiac injury typically occurs in patients with multiple blunt trauma injuries. Patients with myocardial contusion typically complain of angina-type chest pain unrelieved by nitroglycerin, pleuritic pain, or pain from associated injuries. Evidence of external trauma is typically but not always present. Information about the scene of the injury often provides the only evidence of blunt cardiac injury in patients who are unconscious or with altered mental status.

Initial and vital sign trends should be carefully noted, including mental status, color, jugular venous distention, and the presence of chest wall ecchymosis or tenderness, gallop rhythms, and friction rubs. Persistent unexplained tachycardia, hypotension, or dysrhythmia suggests blunt cardiac injury. Patients with valve dysfunction typically present with a loud murmur, acute heart failure, and jugular venous distention. The rare patient with cardiac rupture who survives to the ED typically has signs of cardiac tamponade or overt cardiogenic shock.

■ DIAGNOSTIC TESTING

An ECG should be recorded in all patients with suspected blunt cardiac injury. Stable patients with normal initial ECG results are not at risk for complications of blunt cardiac injuries. New ECG findings suggestive of myocardial contusion include unexplained tachycardia, ST- and T-wave changes, conduction abnormalities, and dysrhythmias.

Cardiac markers are not routinely indicated in the evaluation of blunt cardiac injury. The exception is serial troponin I measurement in patients with an ischemic pattern on the initial ECG and in patients in whom cardiac ischemia may have precipitated the trauma. Recent meta-analysis supports the use of troponin I as a sensitive test for myocardial contusion when drawn at admission and 4 to 6 hours later.[22] However, other earlier studies demonstrated that troponin I was not useful in predicting complications in hemodynamically stable patients nor did results affect management of the unstable patient.[23]

Emergent bedside echocardiography is recommended in unstable patients with suspected blunt cardiac injury or with evidence on an ECG of myocardial infarction. Pericardial effusions are easily identified on the initial subxyphoid view of the FAST scan. Formal echocardiography with parasternal and apical views will better identify small effusions, valve dysfunction, and wall motion abnormalities. Transesophageal echocardiography is more sensitive than transthoracic echocardiography and provides additional imaging of the aorta in unstable patients. Routine echocardiography does not predict complications in stable patients with suspected blunt cardiac injury.

■ INTERVENTIONS AND PROCEDURES

Unstable blunt cardiac injury patients require definitive airway control to ensure optimal oxygenation and ventilation. A large-bore internal jugular catheter should be inserted for fluid resuscitation, central venous pressure monitoring, and Swan Ganz catheter placement. Cardiogenic shock secondary to myocardial contusion or cardiac rupture typically requires careful fluid replacement and inotropic support. Refractory cases may require temporary stabilization with an aortic balloon pump after an aortic injury has been ruled out. Cardiac catheterization is necessary in patients with myocardial infarction because antithrombotic therapy is contraindicated after trauma.

■ TREATMENT AND DISPOSITION

Stable patients with a normal initial ECG and without significant associated injuries are safely discharged from the ED. Stable patients with ECG changes suggestive of myocardial contusion require observation for 24 hours with repeat electroencephalography every 8 hours for 24 hours. Oxygen, analgesia, and continuous cardiac monitoring should be provided.

Brief dysrhythmias seldom require treatment and prophylactic antidysrhythmic therapy is not indicated.

Unstable patients with ventricular dysrhythmias, atrial fibrillation, sinus bradycardia, and bundle branch block require intensive care unit admission. In patients with abnormal initial ECGs, the complication rate is low, predominantly occurring in older patients with multiple injuries. Wall motion abnormalities and rhythm disturbances typically resolve within hours. Most patients with myocardial contusion require only supportive care and aggressive management of complicating injuries. Morbidity and mortality are directly related to the presence of other injuries.

Penetrating Cardiac Injury, Cardiac Tamponade, and ED Thoracotomy

■ SCOPE

Penetrating cardiac wounds most commonly result from gunshot wounds, followed by stab wounds. Any gunshot wound to the torso can result in penetrating cardiac injury. Survival is better in patients with stab wounds, single-chamber involvement, and low-pressure right heart injuries. Cardiac tamponade most commonly results from stab wounds to the chest or upper abdomen, followed by gunshot wounds and infrequently by blunt chest trauma.

■ ANATOMY AND PATHOPHYSIOLOGY

Penetrating injuries to the heart result in either death at the scene or tamponade, which allows transport to the ED. Tamponade is more likely to occur with smaller injuries from stab wounds. The tough fibrous sac surrounding the heart prevents immediate exsanguination. As blood accumulates, cardiac filling and eventually output are impaired, often resulting in rapid decompensation after arrival at the ED. Even small amouns of rapidly accumulating pericardial blood can result in pericardial tamponade in the noncompliant pericardial sac. Acutely accumulated pericardial blood may be difficult to visualize on cardiac ultrasonography. The right ventricle is the most commonly injured structure, followed by the left ventricle. Approximately three of four patients will die of the injury.

■ PRESENTING SIGNS AND SYMPTOMS

Patients with pericardial tamponade classically but uncommonly present with Beck's triad of hypotension, jugular venous distention, and muffled heart sounds. Most patients will have at least one of these signs, with all three appearing only briefly before cardiac arrest. More frequently, patients present either relatively stable-appearing or in extremis. Stable-appearing patients have small wounds to the pericardium that allow intermittent decompression of the accumulated blood. Patients with more rapid accumulation are panic-stricken, appear to be in severe respiratory distress, and often have needle thoracostomy performed for presumed tension pneumothorax. In these patients, agitation, tachycardia, and hypotension predominate before progressing to obtundation, bradycardia, and pulseless electrical activity.

■ DIAGNOSTIC TESTING

An ultrasonographic subxyphoid view (Fig. 73-5) may detect pericardial fluid in patients with suspected cardiac injury. Pericardial fluid with diastolic collapse of the right atrium and ventricle are diagnostic of pericardial tamponade. Any pericardial effusion in unstable trauma patients with equal bilateral breath sounds signals tamponade requiring immediate operative intervention.

An initial ECG should be obtained to evaluate for ECG findings suggestive of pericardial tamponade and other cardiac injury. Electrical alternans, low voltage and PR-segment depression are specific but not sensitive for diagnosis of pericardial effusion.[22] A chronic pericardial effusion is more likely to reveal such findings. Acute traumatic pericardial effusion resulting in tamponade does not change the size of the heart on the chest radiograph. However, a chest radiograph can be useful in identifying other injuries and the presence of retained foreign bodies. It is important to remember that normal ECG and chest radograph findings do not rule out traumatic pericardial effusion or tamponade.

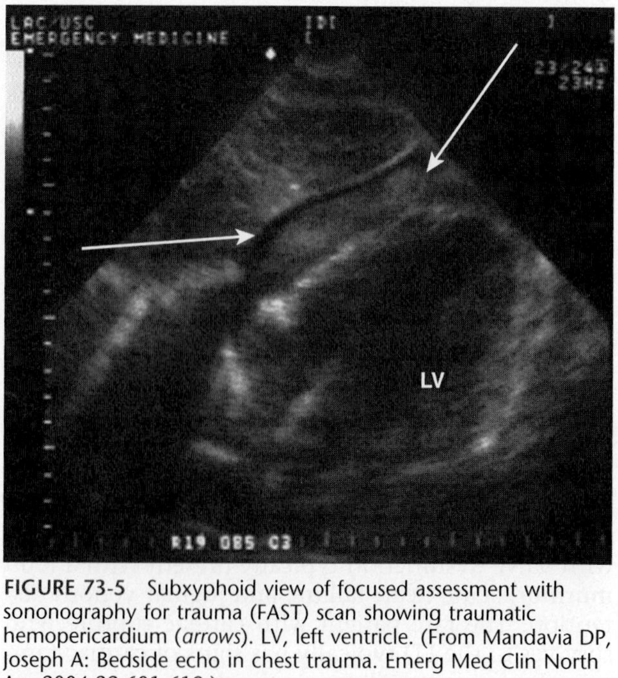
LAC/USC
EMERGENCY MEDICINE
LV

FIGURE 73-5 Subxyphoid view of focused assessment with sononography for trauma (FAST) scan showing traumatic hemopericardium (*arrows*). LV, left ventricle. (From Mandavia DP, Joseph A: Bedside echo in chest trauma. Emerg Med Clin North Am 2004;22:601-619.)

INTERVENTIONS AND PROCEDURES

A central venous line should be placed for volume infusion and central venous pressure monitoring. The injured hemithorax is preferred for central line placement to avoid iatrogenic complications in the uninjured side. The exception is the patient with obvious injury to the clavicle and suspected injury to the subclavian vein. Aggressive fluid resuscitation is mandatory for patients with suspected pericardial tamponade to maximize cardiac filling pressures and cardiac output. Elevated central venous pressure in persistently hypotensive and tachycardic trauma patients suggests impending tamponade.

Pericardiocentesis with catheter placement should be performed in patients with deteriorating vital signs. Pericardiocentesis may serve as a diagnostic and temporizing measure but is never a replacement for thoracotomy and definitive injury repair. Ultrasonography or ECG-guided pericardiocentesis is preferred, if available.

Nonclotting blood traditionally signifies pericardial blood, but aspiration may be unsuccessful because of needle placement, continuous brisk pericardial bleeding, or other reasons. However, the removal of even a small amount of pericardial blood can restore vital signs and aid survival until surgical intervention is available. Thoracotomy is reserved for patients with cardiac tamponade in cardiac arrest or impending arrest.

ED THORACOTOMY

The decision to perform ED thoracotomy requires careful yet rapid answers to two key questions.

First, do the patients have a reasonable chance of functional survival after ED thoracotomy? In 2000, a meta-analysis of 24 studies was published that included 4600 patients and examined survival after ED thoracotomy.[24] The overall survival rate was 7%. Of the survivors, 92% retained neurologic functioning and returned to normal activities of daily living. The authors recommended that careful consideration be given to mechanism of injury, location of major injury, and signs of life.

In another study, blunt trauma patients with arrest in the field had no chance of survival, whereas patients with arrest in the ED had a chance of survival of 0% to 2%.[25] Survival rates were 9% overall, but 4% for those with gunshot wounds and 17% for those with stab wounds. Patients with predominantly cardiac injuries had a 19% survival rate versus 11% for all thoracic injuries, 5% for abdominal injuries, and 1% for multiple locations of injury. Patients with signs of life on arrival had a 12% survival rate versus 9% in patients with signs of life in transport and 1% in patients with no signs in the field. These results were confirmed in a larger review of 7000 patients published as practice management guidelines in 2001.[26]

To summarize, the likelihood of functional survival is greatest for victims of stab wounds with isolated cardiac injury who have signs of life on ED arrival.

Second, is the setting sufficient? Studies have only been done at trauma centers with thoracotomy performed by trauma surgeons. Rural and many small urban community EDs do not have the necessary personnel, training, and equipment to reasonably approximate such outcomes. Physicians must often accompany open chest survivors requiring transport. However, heroic intervention can be justified for selected patients who have no other hope of survival and a potentially treatable cause. Ideally, each ED will have a practical plan, good teamwork, surgical support, and plans for postresuscitation management.

At the trauma center, thoracotomy is performed on victims of penetrating trauma who experienced cardiac arrest in the ED, or within 10 minutes of arrival at the ED, and on blunt trauma patients who experienced cardiac arrest in the ED. In the ED without surgical support, thoracotomy is best performed by a skilled EP only on patients with thoracic stab wounds or isolated gunshot wounds who lost signs of life in the ED or within 10 minutes of arrival in the ED. In all other cases, ED thoracotomy should be performed only if a qualified surgeon is present or immediately available (Table 73-2).

ED Thoracotomy Procedure

All steps in the procedure are derived from the indications. Visualize the pericardium and incise to relieve tamponade. This is the primary goal of ED thoracotomy.[27]

Perform a left lateral incision from the sternum to the bed to best visualize the pericardium and repair the heart. Place and open rib spreaders on the bed to allow sternotomy and right-sided incisions if needed.[26] Deliver the heart from the pericardium and repair cardiac wounds.

Table 73-2 INDICATIONS FOR ED THORACOTOMY

Setting	Penetrating Injuries	Blunt Trauma
Trauma center	Cardiac arrest in the ED or within 10 minutes of ED arrival	Cardiac arrest in the ED
Community ED without emergent surgical backup	Patients with thoracic stab wounds or isolated gunshot wounds who lose signs of life in the ED or within 10 minutes of ED arrival	All other ED thoracotomies should be performed only when a surgeon is available within 10 minutes

Staple linear wounds to temporarily control hemorrhage. Place Foley catheter, and use purse-string sutures for larger wounds.

Perform cardiac compression in patients with cardiac arrest. Defibrillation at 20 J with internal paddles may be needed to treat ventricular fibrillation.

Cross-clamp the aorta to preserve blood flow to the heart and the brain if the patient is unresponsive to other measures or if there is major hemorrhage below the diaphragm.

■ TREATMENT AND DISPOSITION

Immediate operative repair is indicated for all penetrating injuries of the heart to relieve tamponade and repair the initial injury. Identification and initial management of all associated injuries ensure optimal outcomes, but operative intervention must not be delayed. Diagnostic peritoneal lavage should be performed in the operating room to identify intraperitoneal bleeding and assess the need for laparotomy.

Great Vessel Injury

■ SCOPE

Great vessel injury is a significant cause of morbidity and mortality in both blunt and penetrating thoracic trauma. Traumatic aortic injury is the second most common cause of blunt traumatic death. 85% of victims of traumatic aortic injury die immediately. Patients that survive to the ED have incomplete rupture with containment of hemorrhage within the adventitia. The majority of these survivors can be saved with prompt ED diagnosis, blood pressure control, and operative repair. When the injury is not detected, 30% of survivors will die within 24 hours, 50% within 1 week, and 90% within 4 months.[28] Infrequent life-threatening blunt and penetrating injuries occur in the aorta and other great vessels, including the brachiocephalic branches, pulmonary arteries and veins, vena cava, and innominate artery and vein.

■ ANATOMY AND PATHOPHYSIOLOGY

The descending aorta is fixed within the thorax by the ligamentum arteriosum and the intercostal arteries. Sudden deceleration causes the aortic arch to swing forward, producing a shearing force with resultant injury just distal to the take-off of the left subclavian artery. Traditionally, traumatic aortic injuries have only been considered with "major mechanisms of injury," including high-speed MVCs with frontal or side impact and motorcycle crashes. However, the injury has been reported with less impressive mechanisms such as pedestrian-versus-auto collisions, falls, and crush injuries. The use of restraint systems does not protect persons from traumatic aortic injuries.[29,30]

Penetrating wounds to the great vessels typically result from both gunshot penetration and stabbing. Venous injuries result in less severe bleeding than arterial injuries, although the muscular arterial wall may spasm and the advential layer may further help contain very small injuries from stab wounds.

■ PRESENTING SIGNS AND SYMPTOMS

Signs and symptoms of traumatic aortic injury often are not present or are masked by other injuries. Up to one half of all patients have no signs of chest wall injury. Common signs and symptoms include interscapular or retrosternal pain, decreased blood pressure in the left arm, upper extremity hypertension with absent femoral pulses, bruit, and a harsh systolic murmur heard over the precordium or interscapular area. Uncommon findings include extremity pain from distal ischemia, dysphagia from concomitant esophageal injury, and hoarseness due to compression of the laryngeal nerve.

Evidence of penetrating injury to the great vessels depends on the mechanism and location of the injury. High-energy proximal arterial injury typically results in immediate exsanguination or hemorrhagic shock with massive hemothorax. Contained mediastinal hematoma can occasionally impair superior vena cava return, producing engorgement of the soft tissues of the neck, face, and airway. Distal injuries may result in diminished pulses, expanding hematomas, and limb ischemia. Careful palpation for pulse symmetry and blood pressure measurement in both arms are advisable.

Stab wounds should be closely inspected to help determine general trajectory. Deep probing of wounds should be avoided to prevent iatrogenic worsening of the initial injury, dislodgment of clot and massive hemorrhage, and infection. Chest tube output should be closely monitored. The chest tube should be clamped when the patient is being transported to the operating room; when there is massive hemothorax and heavy, continuous bleeding, temporary tamponade within the pleural cavity may be required for this short time.

■ DIAGNOSTIC TESTING

The initial chest radiograph should show evidence of traumatic aortic injury (Fig. 73-6A). The most sensitive criterion is mediastinal widening, usually larger than 8 cm on an AP view; however, a subjective interpretation of mediastinal widening is more reliable. Other mediastinal abnormalities suggesting mediastinal hematoma secondary to traumatic aortic injury are an obscured aortic knob, loss of the AP window, a displaced nasogastric tube, widened paratracheal stripe, widened paraspinal interface, depression of the left mainstem bronchus, left hemothorax, left apical pleural cap, deviation of the trachea to the right, and multiple rib fractures. A normal chest radiograph, however, does not rule out the traumatic aortic injury.

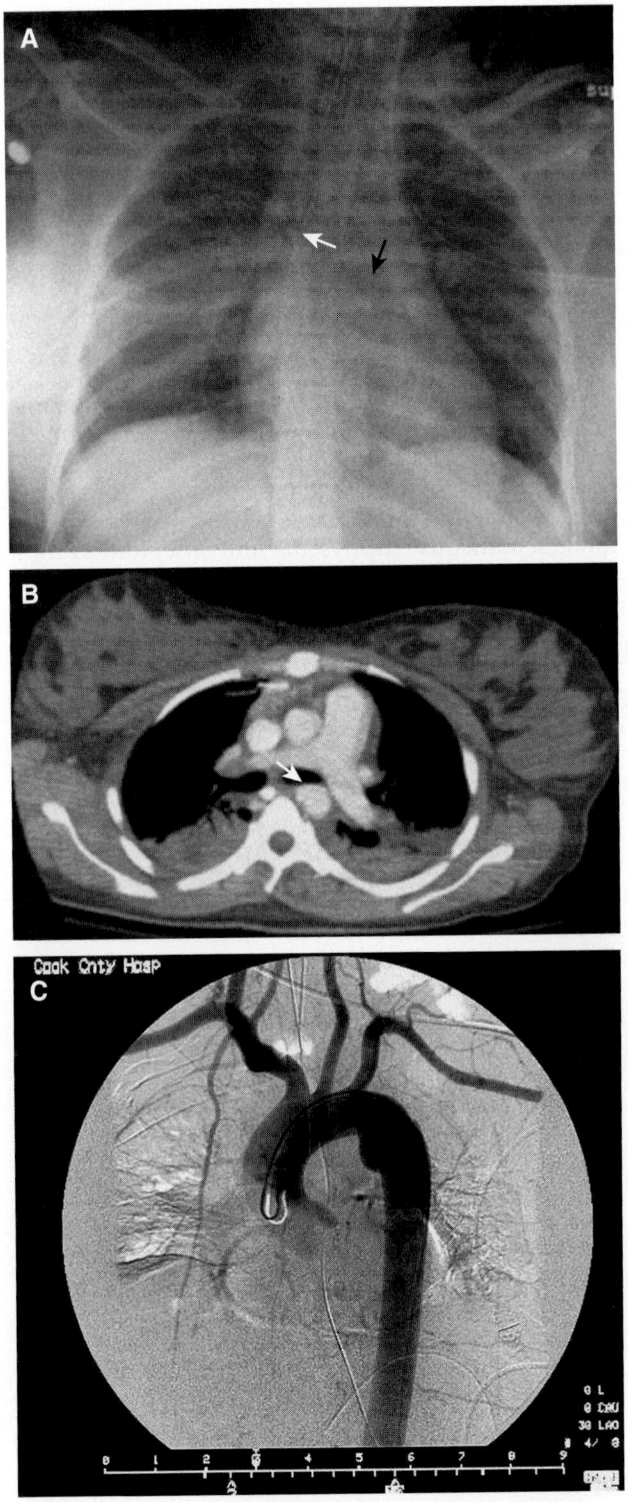
A
B
Cook Cnty Hosp
C

FIGURE 73-6 Chest radiographs showing traumatic aortic injury: **A,** Widened mediastinum, loss of mediastinal contours, depression of left mainstem bronchus (*black arrow*), and deviation of nasogastric tube (*white arrow*). **B,** Traumatic pseudoaneurysm in proximal descending aorta (*arrow*). (From Westra SJ, Wallace EC: Imaging of pediatric chest trauma. Radiol Clin North Am 2005;43:267-281.) **C,** Traumatic pseudoaneurysm seen on aortogram. (Image courtesy of Scott Sherman, MD).

A helical CT angiographic scan can rule out traumatic aortic injury in stable patients with either chest wall tenderness or an abnormal chest radiograph. A normal CT scan rules out traumatic aortic injury[31]; if results are indeterminate, aortography should be performed. Rarely, a positive helical CT angiogram in a stable patient is followed by aortography for further localization of injury and identification of other injuries, such as a pseudoaneurysm (see Fig. 73-6B).

Advantages of helical CT angiography over aortography are that it is faster, noninvasive, requires a smaller volume of contrast, and provides information about other thoracic injuries. A high index of suspicion and low threshold for performing screening helical CT angiography is required to save traumatic aortic injury patients who survive to the ED.

Transesophageal echocardiography should be performed in unstable patients with suspected traumatic aortic injury. Advantages include bedside testing, no contrast, assessment of cardiac function and intimal and medial aortic injuries. Disadvantages include the need for sedation and perhaps intubation, as well as inability to visualize proximal aorta branches. Transesophageal echocardiography is contraindicated in patients with esophageal injuries. Very high sensitivity and specificity have been reported, but these vary widely depending on operator experience.

Aortography remains the gold standard for diagnosis of traumatic aortic injury. False-positive and false-negative results are rare but do occur. Better sensitivity with helical CT angiography has been reported. Aortography offers improved localization of injury prior to surgical repair. Newer techniques such as intravenous digital subtraction angiography have improved the speed while reducing the cost of aortography (see Fig. 73-6C).

A chest radiograph should be obtained in all patients with suspected penetrating great vessel injuries, and all wounds should be noted and marked. The examination should be focused specifically on evidence of mediastinal hematoma, hemothorax, foreign bodies near vessels or in the trajectory of a missile, "fuzzy" missiles created by arterial pulsations, and the absence of a missile in patients with a gunshot wound to the chest, which suggests distal embolization. An angiogram should be obtained to further assess injuries and plan an operative approach in the rare stable patient. With the added benefit of evaluating nearby structures, helical CT angiography will likely replace aortography in the work-up of stable patients with transmediastinal penetrating injury.[32]

■ INTERVENTIONS AND PROCEDURES

Early orotracheal intubation is required because during a period of observation a hematoma can expand and make both orotracheal intubation and a creation of a surgical airway impossible. Tracheostomy is contraindicated in patients with great vessel injury to the upper mediastinum or zone I of the neck because major bleeding can result.

Patients with penetrating great vessel injuries often require ED thoracotomy or immediate thoracotomy in the operating room. In patients with penetrating wounds to the subclavian vessels, traditional left lateral thoracotomy often will not provide adequate exposure.

■ TREATMENT AND DISPOSITION

Before operative repair of traumatic aortic injuries, blood pressure must be controlled, maintaining a systolic pressure of 100 to 120 mm Hg to decrease shear stress and progression of injury. Patients with isolated aortic injuries may be hypertensive and will require short-acting titratable agents such as nitroprusside and esmolol. Surgical repair of traumatic aortic injury is performed after stabilization of other life-threatening intracranial or intraabdominal injuries. Delayed surgical repair is often indicated in elderly patient with multiple comorbidities. The mortality rate during surgery is approximately 10% and is primarily related to the extent of the injury and condition of the patient.

Esophageal Injury

■ SCOPE

Esophageal injuries occur infrequently in both blunt and penetrating trauma. More immediate life-threatening injuries often mask clinical findings, and esophageal leakage can progress to fatal mediastinitis. Esophageal evaluation is indicated when there is a significant penetrating injury to the neck. The majority of esophageal perforations result from medical endoscopic procedures, not from traumatic injuries.

■ ANATOMY AND PATHOPHYSIOLOGY

The lack of an esophageal serosal layer allows gastrointestinal contents direct access to the mediastinum. Penetrating esophageal injury must be considered in any patient with injury near or trajectory through the esophagus. Common mechanisms of penetrating injury include laceration, missile penetration, iatrogenic perforation, and ingested foreign body. Stab wounds to the neck often directly injure the esophagus. High-velocity gunshots result in direct esophageal perforation as well as delayed necrosis. The majority of penetrating injuries occur during routine endoscopy at the proximal or distal esophagus. Rigid endoscopy for foreign body removal and biopsy results in a higher rate of perforation than flexible fiberoptic endoscopy.

Blunt esophageal injuries are much less common than penetrating injuries. Common mechanisms include crush injuries to the cervical esophagus and barotrauma. Blunt laryngotracheal trauma and cervical spine fractures are associated with injuries to the upper esophagus. Blunt injuries to the lower third of the esophagus occur with sudden increases in intraabdominal pressure against a closed upper esophageal sphincter analogous to Boerhaave's syndrome. Both cardiopulmonary resuscitation and the Heimlich maneuver have been associated with perforation of the thoracic esophagus. Blast injury can result in esophageal injury from the primary injury caused by the pressure wave, secondary injury from the impact of the patient against fixed structures, and tertiary injury from blast projectiles.

■ PRESENTING SIGNS AND SYMPTOMS

Typical symptoms of esophageal injury include pleuritic chest pain anywhere along the course of the esophagus, dyspnea, odynophagia, dysphagia, hoarseness, and pain with flexion or extension of the neck. The physical examination should include palpation for subcutaneous emphysema and auscultation for a systolic Hamman's crunch produced by mediastinal air.

Commonly, patients present with emergent life-threatening injuries that obscure the clinical presentation, leading to delayed recognition and management. Fever, tachycardia, hypotension, and progressive dyspnea are noted as mediastinitis develops.

■ DIAGNOSTIC TESTING

AP or PA chest radiographs should be examined for evidence of mediastinal air, subcutaneous emphysema, left-sided pleural effusion, pneumothorax, and a widened mediastinum. A lateral neck radiograph may reveal prevertebral air displacing the tracheal air column forward. Early in the course of a perforation, radiographic evidence is often minimal. Later CT scans of the chest may demonstrate collections of air or fluid as infection develops, but CT usually is not performed for esophageal injury.

Esophagography and esophagoscopy should be performed in all patients with suspected esophageal injury, although neither test alone is sensitive enough to rule out esophageal injury. Initial esophagography is made with gastrograffin to avoid mediastinal irritation from barium leakage. Incidentally, a CT scan after barium ingestion may detect small esophageal perforations and small metallic foreign bodies better than plain radiographs. Negative findings on the esophagogram made with gastrograffin should be followed by the more sensitive barium esophagography. Neither contrast agent prevents the use of endoscopy. If findings in both esophagograms are negative, flexible endoscopy can be used to exclude subtle injuries.

■ INTERVENTIONS AND PROCEDURES

Chest tube drainage is often necessary for associated pneumothorax. Persistent air leak is suggestive of esophageal injury. Food particles in the chest tube confirm major injury.

Keep patients on nothing-by-mouth status. Fluid resuscitation is mandatory. Administer broad-spectrum antibiotics to cover oral anaerobes. Gently place a nasogastric tube to decompress and empty remaining stomach contents.

Consultation with trauma or general surgery specialists for immediate surgical repair dramatically improves outcomes.

Diaphragmatic Injuries

■ SCOPE

Diaphragmatic injuries are a diagnostic challenge and have significant delayed complications. Complications often present weeks to years after the initial trauma with symptoms of visceral herniation. Both blunt and penetrating trauma cause diaphragmatic injuries, but with very different injury patterns. When detected initially, diaphragmatic injury signals that other severe injuries are likely present.

■ ANATOMY AND PATHOPHYSIOLOGY

Gunshot and stab wounds result in diaphragm injuries with nearly equal incidence. Stab wounds with a trajectory reaching the 4th intercostal space superiorly or the 12th intercostal space inferiorly must be considered to have perforated the diaphragm and require prudent evaluation. Stab wounds outside this area may also penetrate the diaphragm, depending on the length and angle of the blade. Gunshot wounds anywhere in the neck, chest, abdomen, or pelvis can penetrate the diaphragm. Blunt forces to the chest or abdomen often result in large tears of the diaphragm. The most common mechanisms are MVCs and falls, followed by pedestrian-versus-vehicle collisions, motorcycle accidents, and crush injuries. Left-sided injuries are more common in survivors,whereas an equal incidence of right- and left-sided injuries is noted at autopsy.[33]

The negative pressure of inspiration prevents closure and promotes herniation through the wound into the chest cavity. If not detected initially, diaphragm injuries often result in visceral herniation months to years later.

Three phases of injury have been described. The acute phase begins with the injury and ends with the initial recovery. In the second, or latent, phase, intermittent herniation of abdominal viscera results in mild and vague symptoms suggesting biliary, gastric, coronary artery, or pulmonary disease. In the last, or obstructive, phase, incarceration, strangulation, and ischemia develop.[34]

■ PRESENTING SIGNS AND SYMPTOMS

The patient with acute diaphragmatic rupture typically will complain of chest pain, abdominal pain, and dypsnea. Physical examination findings include diminished breath sounds in the lung bases, respiratory distress, bowel sounds in the chest, peritoneal signs, and palpation of viscera during chest tube placement. Large left-sided blunt injuries are more obvious than smaller penetrating and right-sided injuries. Acute diaphragmatic injuries are frequently overshadowed by other injuries. Often no abdominal tenderness is noted.

Patients with latent presentations often appear to have other gastrointestinal or cardiovascular diseases and present with vague abdominal pain relieved when upright, or cough and vague chest pain. In the obstructive phase of injury, symptoms of visceral obstruction, ischemia, and ultimately visceral infarction develop. Rarely, tension viscerothorax also develops. Herniation should be considered in any patient with vague complaints of chest or abdominal pain and a history of thoracoabdominal trauma.

■ DIAGNOSTIC TESTING

Inspect the initial chest radiograph for the classic diagnostic finding, which is a nasogastric tube or viscera in the left hemithorax. Other important but more subtle signs include an indistinct or elevated left hemidiaphragm and left lower lobe atelectasis. Hemopneumothorax is present in 50% of patients with penetrating injury. Up to 25% of patients with penetrating diaphragmatic injuries have a normal chest radiograph and no abdominal tenderness.[35] CT scanning is 100% specific but only 66% sensitive for the diagnosis of blunt diaphragmatic injury.[36]

In the latent phase of injury, the chest radiograph typically is abnormal. Findings can be subtle, such as a unilaterally elevated hemidiaphragm, unilateral pleural thickening, basilar atelectasis, or can be significant, such as a shift of the mediastinum or viscera evident above the diaphragm. In cases of delayed herniation, upper or lower gastrointestinal contrast studies may be needed to demonstrate herniation (Fig. 73-7).

Customarily, a diagnostic peritoneal lavage count of less than 10,000 red blood cells/μL is used to rule out a diaphragmatic injury in patients with penetrating thoracoabdominal trauma. Lavage fluid draining from the chest tube is diagnostic. However, diagnostic peritoneal lavage may miss small injuries that bleed into the chest. Laparoscopy or thoracoscopy is the diagnostic study of choice in patients with a high clinical suspicion for diaphragmatic injury not otherwise needing surgery.[37]

■ INTERVENTIONS AND PROCEDURES

Carefully place a nasogastric tube in obstructed patients to avoid further trauma to a herniated gastroesophageal junction. In cases of a tension viscerothorax, place a chest tube into the thoracic cavity but be careful to avoid the viscera. Palpate for viscera and diaphragmatic injuries before chest tube insertion.

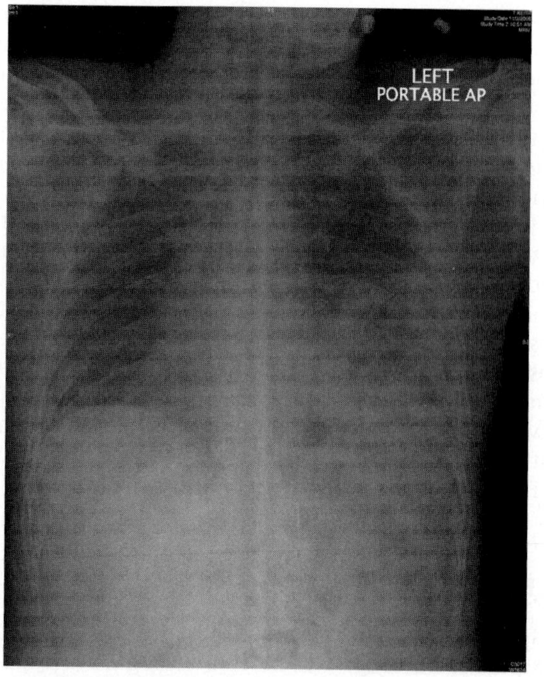
LEFT
PORTABLE AP

FIGURE 73-7 Chest radiograph showing obvious left-sided viscerothorax secondary to stab wound in the diaphragm 3 years earlier. (Image courtesy of Dave Andreski, MD.)

■ TREATMENT AND DISPOSITION

Consultation and admission to trauma or general surgery services is recommended for early surgical repair to prevent delayed complications. Patients with suspected diaphragmatic injuries typically have multiple injuries requiring treatment and hospitalization. The asymptomatic patient with a mechanism for diaphragmatic injury but a negative work-up should be instructed about the need for immediate evaluation if signs of delayed herniation and obstruction develop, such as abdominal discomfort, chest discomfort, shortness of breath, or vomiting.

REFERENCES

1. Soreide E, Deakin CD: Pre-hospital fluid therapy in the critically injured patient—a clinical update. Injury 2005;36:1001-1010.
2. Bokhari F, Brakenridge S, Nagy K, et al: Prospective evaluation of the sensitivity of physical examination in chest trauma. J Trauma 2002;53:1135-1138.
3. Lee J, Harris JH Jr, Duke JH Jr, Williams JS: Noncorrelation between thoracic skeletal injuries and acute traumatic aortic tear. J Trauma 1997;43:400-404.
4. Gouldman JW, Miller RS: Sternal fracture: A benign entity? Am Surg 1997;63:17-19.
5. von Garrel T, Ince A, Junge A, et al: The sternal fracture: Radiographic analysis of 200 fractures with special reference to concomitant injuries. J Trauma 2004;57:837-844.
6. Shweiki E, Klena J, Wood GC, Indeck M: Assessing the true risk of abdominal solid organ injury in hospitalized rib fracture patients. J Trauma 2001;50:684-688.
7. Greenberg MD, Rosen CL: Evaluation of the patient with blunt chest trauma: An evidence based approach. Emerg Med Clin North Am 1999;17:41-62, viii.
8. Holmes JF, Ngyuen H, Jacoby RC, et al: Do all patients with left costal margin injuries require radiographic evaluation for intraabdominal injury? Ann Emerg Med 2005;46:232-236.
9. Ullman EA, Donley LP, Brady WJ: Pulmonary trauma emergency department evaluation and management. Emerg Med Clin North Am 2003;21:291-313.
10. Gunduz M, Unlugenc H, Ozalevli M, et al: A comparative study of continuous positive airway pressure (CPAP) and intermittent positive pressure ventilation (IPPV) in patients with flail chest. Emerg Med J 2005;22:325-329.
11. Ono K, Inagawa H, Kiyota K, et al: Posterior dislocation of the sternoclavicular joint with obstruction of the innominate vein: Case report. J Trauma 1998;44:381-383.
12. Barton ED: Tension pneumothorax: Curr Opin Pulm Med 1999;5:269-274.
13. Bokhari F, Brakenridge S, Nagy K, et al: Prospective evaluation of the sensitivity of physical examination in chest trauma. J Trauma 2002;53:1135-1138.
14. Kirkpatrick AW, Sirois M, Laupland KB, et al: Hand-held thoracic sonography for detecting post-traumatic pneumothoraces: The Extended Focused Assessment with Sonography for Trauma (EFAST). J Trauma 2004;57:288-295.
15. Maxwell RA, Campbell DJ, Fabian TC, et al: Use of presumptive antibiotics following tube thoracostomy for traumatic hemopneumothorax in the prevention of empyema and pneumonia—a multi-center trial. J Trauma 2004;57:742-748.
16. Brasel KJ, Stafford RE, Weigelt JA, et al: Treatment of occult pneumothoraces from blunt trauma. J Trauma 1999;46:987-990.
17. Wanek S, Mayberry JC: Blunt thoracic trauma: Flail chest, pulmonary contusion, and blast injury. Crit Care Clin 2004;20:71-81.
18. Shrager JB: Tracheal trauma. Chest Surg Clin N Am 2003;13:291-304.
19. Huh J, Milliken JC, Chen JC: Management of tracheobronchial injuries following blunt and penetrating trauma. Am Surg 1997;63:896-899.
20. Bansal MK, Maraj S, Chewaproug D, Amanullah A: Myocardial contusion injury: Redefining the diagnostic algorithm. Emerg Med J 2005;22:465-469.
21. Jackson L, Stewart A: Best evidence topic report. Use of troponin for the diagnosis of myocardial contusion after blunt chest trauma. Emerg Med J 2005;22:193-195.
22. Bertinchant JP, Polge A, Mohty D, et al: Evaluation of incidence, clinical significance, and prognostic value of circulating cardiac troponin I and T elevation in hemodynamically stable patients with suspected myocardial contusion after blunt chest trauma. J Trauma 2000;48:924-931.
23. Eisenberg MJ, de Romeral LM, Heidenreich PA, et al: The diagnosis of pericardial effusion and cardiac tamponade by 12-lead ECG. A technology assessment. Chest 1996;110:318-324.
24. Rhee PM, Acosta J, Bridgeman A, et al: Survival after emergency department thoracotomy: Review of published data from the past 25 years. J Am Coll Surg 2000;190:288-298.
25. Branney SW, Moore EE, Feldhaus KM, Wolfe RE: Critical analysis of two decades of experience with postinjury emergency department thoracotomy in a regional trauma center. J Trauma 1998;45:87-94.
26. Practice management guidelines for emergency department thoracotomy: Working Group, Ad Hoc Subcommittee on Outcomes, American College of Surgeons-Committee on Trauma. J Am Coll Surg 2001;193:303-309.
27. Wise D, Davies G, Coats T, et al: Emergency thoracotomy: "How to do it." Emerg Med J 2005;22:22-24.
28. Pretre R, Chilcott M: Blunt trauma to the heart and great vessels. N Engl J Med 1997;336:626-632.
29. Horton TG, Cohn SM, Heid MP, et al: Identification of trauma patients at risk of thoracic aortic tear by mechanism of injury. J Trauma 2000;48:1008-1013.
30. Nagy K, Fabian T, Rodman G, et al: Guidelines for the diagnosis and management of blunt aortic injury: an EAST Practice Management Guidelines Work Group. J Trauma 2000;48:1128-1143.
31. Dyer DS, Moore EE, Ilke DN, et al: Thoracic aortic injury: How predictive is mechanism and is chest computed

tomography a reliable screening tool? A prospective study of 1,561 patients. J Trauma 2000;48:673-682.
32. Stassen NA, Lukan JK, Spain D, et al: Reevaluation of diagnostic procedures for transmediastinal gunshot wounds. J Trauma 2002;53:635-638.
33. Rosati C: Acute traumatic injury of the diaphragm. Chest Surg Clin N Am 1998;8:371-379.
33. Reber PU, Schmied B, Seiler CA, et al: Missed diaphragmatic injuries and their long-term sequelae. J Trauma 1998; 44:183-188.
34. Murray JA, Demetriades D, Cornwell EE III, et al: Penetrating left thoracoabdominal trauma: The incidence and clinical presentation of diaphragm injuries. J Trauma 1997;43:624-626.
35. Allen TL, Cummins BF, Bonk RT, et al: Computed tomography without oral contrast solution for blunt diaphragmatic injuries in abdominal trauma. Am J Emerg Med 2005;23:253-258.

Chapter 74

Blunt Abdominal Trauma

Carlo L. Rosen, Eric L. Legome, and Richard E. Wolfe

KEY POINTS

Intraperitoneal bleeding is an immediate life-threatening injury after blunt trauma.
The management of intraperitoneal bleeding takes priority over many other system injuries (Box 74-1).
The physical examination is unreliable for predicting the presence or absence of injury, except for certain high-risk findings such as the seat belt sign and Kehr's sign.
Bedside ultrasonography is an excellent initial screening tool that facilitates the early triage of patients for either laparotomy or transfer to the radiology suite for computed tomography (CT) scanning.
Helical CT images provide excellent, accurate details of intraperitoneal injuries. CT is highly sensitive for solid organ injuries but has a lower sensitivity for detecting pancreatic, small bowel, and diaphragmatic injuries.
Detailed CT images allow grading of organ injuries and nonoperative management of solid organ trauma in stable patients and the use of angiographic embolization in patients with liver, spleen, and renal injuries.
Early detection of intraperitoneal injuries after blunt trauma and a team approach to management of these injuries significantly improve mortality rates.

Scope and Outline

ED visits by patients with blunt abdominal trauma are commonplace and are a source of frequent mortality and morbidity even when successfully treated. The margin for error when caring for these patients is narrow, and mistakes, errors, and delays are common. Only aggressive and compulsive management can ensure an optimal outcome. Diagnostic and therapeutic decisions are often difficult to make in the ED because underlying injuries can have a wide range of presentations. A patient with blunt abdominal trauma may have an underlying critical injury that can initially present with little or no symptoms. A benign appearance may mask serious, occult injuries that may be life-threatening if not rapidly detected. For these reasons and because abdominal injuries are correctable if rapidly addressed, evaluation of the abdomen is prioritized in trauma patients over other nonabdominal injuries. In particular, abdominal assessment takes priority over lethal injuries such as aortic tears and intracranial hemorrhage.

BOX 74-1

Management of Intraperitoneal Injuries

- Intraperitoneal bleeding is an immediate life-threatening injury after blunt trauma.
- Management of intraperitoneal bleeding takes priority over other system injuries.
- The physical examination is unreliable for predicting the presence or absence of injury, except for certain high-risk findings such as a seat belt sign and Kehr's sign.
- Bedside ultrasonography is an excellent initial screening tool that facilitates the early triage of patients to either laparotomy or the radiology suite for computed tomography (CT) scanning.
- Helical CT images provide excellent, accurate details of intraperitoneal injuries. CT is highly sensitive for detecting solid organ injuries but has a lower sensitivity for detecting pancreatic, small bowel, and diaphragmatic injuries.
- Detailed CT images allow for grading of organ injuries and nonoperative management of solid organ trauma in stable patients and the use of angiographic embolization in patients with liver, spleen, and renal injuries.
- Early detection of intraperitoneal injuries after blunt trauma and a team approach to management of these injuries significantly improve mortality rates.

In the United States, trauma is a serious health problem, both as a cause of mortality as well as significant financial burden. Approximately 25% of all major trauma victims are reported to require an abdominal exploration.[1] In recent years, management of blunt abdominal trauma has started to change because limited health care resources have compelled physicians to find ways to avoid surgical intervention. This has led to an increasingly selective approach to explorative laparotomy.

Abdominal injuries occur in approximately 1% of all trauma patients.[2] Blunt trauma is far more common than penetrating trauma in the United States and carries a greater mortality because of multiple associated injuries and greater diagnostic and therapeutic challenges. The mechanism of blunt trauma may range from high-speed injuries to minor falls or direct blows to the abdomen. Motor vehicle collisions are responsible for approximately 75%, blows to the abdomen for approximately 15%, and falls for approximately 9% of injuries.[3] Evaluation is further complicated by extraabdominal trauma, as well as by altered mental status from head trauma, alcohol intoxication, or recreational drugs.

Structure and Function

Blunt trauma leads to injury when the elastic limit or breaking point of an organ is exceeded by the impact force applied. Exceeding this breaking point causes skin to lacerate, bones to fracture, and organs to tear and rupture. Impact force is defined by the amount of energy involved (e.g., the speed of a vehicle or the height of a fall), the location and surface of the blow to the body, and the duration of the impact. Understanding the mechanism of injury is imperative in assessing the initial risk and subsequent work-up.

The risk of injury may vary slightly according to predisposing factors such as age and gender. Because men are more commonly engaged in dangerous activities, they are more frequently injured than are women. A gravid uterus in a pregnant woman may offer some degree of protection to intraperitoneal structures but adds the unique threat of placental abruption or uterine rupture.

A child's abdomen is less well protected than an adult's because of the thinner musculature, and it is far easier to injure abdominal organs such as the duodenum through compression against the posterior vertebrae. The elastic pediatric rib cage also provides less protection to the spleen and liver.

The risk of specific organ injury is linked to its structure and size. In particular, injuries to the spleen are far more common than injuries to other abdominal organs because of its poor elasticity. This is particularly true of abnormal spleens (e.g., patients with mononucleosis), which are injured with far less force because of their larger size, which favors a greater mass effect, and their thinner capsule, which lacerates more easily. A spleen can be injured by a minor mechanism such as falling over a chair or being hit by a strong ocean wave.

Blunt trauma can lead to injury of any abdominal structure. Direct, focused blows to the epigastrium may lead to contusions and even perforation of the duodenum as well as pancreatic injuries. Deceleration injuries may cause vascular sheering, leading to thrombosis or tears of the renal artery (grade IV renal injury). The incidence and mortality of injuries from blunt abdominal trauma to specific organs are listed in Table 74-1.

Table 74-1 FREQUENCY OF ORGAN INJURY IN BLUNT ABDOMINAL TRAUMA

Organ	Occurrence (%)	Mortality (%)
Spleen	27	14
Kidney	27	8
Liver	15	27
Small bowel	6	10
Duodenum	3	15
Colon	2	20
Pancreas	2	30
Other	17	

BOX 74-2

Splenic Injury Scale

Grade I*

- Subcapsular hematoma with <10% surface area involved
- Capsular tear <1 cm in parenchymal depth

Grade II

- Subcapsular hematoma with 10%-50% surface area
- Intraparenchymal hematoma <5 cm in diameter
- Splenic laceration 1-3 cm in parenchymal depth not involving a parenchymal vessel

Grade III

- Subcapsular hematoma with >50% surface area or expanding
- Ruptured subcapsular or intraparenchymal hematoma
- Intraparenchymal hematoma >5 cm in diameter
- Splenic laceration >3 cm in parenchymal depth or involving trabecular vessels

Grade IV

- Laceration of segmental or hilar vessels producing major devascularization (>25% of spleen)

Grade V

- Completely shattered spleen
- Hilar vascular injury that devascularizes the spleen

*Advance one grade for multiple injuries to same organ up to grade III.
From Moore EE, Cogbill TH, Jurkovich GJ, et al: Organ injury scaling: Spleen and liver (1994 revision). J Trauma 1995;38(3): 323-324

BOX 74-3

Liver Injury Scale

Grade I

- Subcapsular hematoma with <10% surface area involved
- Capsular tear <1 cm in parenchymal depth

Grade II

- Subcapsular hematoma with 10%-50% surface area
- Intraparenchymal hematoma <5 cm in diameter
- Hepatic laceration 1-3 cm in parenchymal depth

Grade III

- Subcapsular hematoma with >50% surface area or expanding
- Ruptured subcapsular or intraparenchymal hematoma
- Intraparenchymal hematoma >5 cm in diameter
- Hepatic laceration >3 cm in parenchymal depth or involving trabecular vessels

Grade IV

- Parenchymal disruption involving 25%-75% of the hepatic lobe or 1-3 Couninaud's segments within a single lobe

Grade V

- Parenchymal disruption involving >75% of a hepatic lobe or >3 Couninaud's segments within a single lobe
- Juxtahepatic venous injuries (e.g., retrohepatic vena cava/central major hepatic veins)

Grade VI

- Hepatic avulsion

From Moore EE, Cogbill TH, Jurkovich GJ, et al: Organ injury scaling: Spleen and liver (1994 revision). J Trauma 1995;38(3): 323-324.

The degree of injury to specific abdominal organs has been classified by the Organ Injury Scaling Committee of the American Association for the Surgery of Trauma (Box 74-2 and Box 74-3). This grading system fosters better communication for outcomes research and allows careful selection of patients for surgical repair.

Anatomy

The abdominal compartment is bounded by the diaphragm, pelvis, and abdominal wall. The boundaries include the vertebral column and the muscles of the abdomen, the most important being the external oblique and the rectus. The rib cage below the 4th intercostal space is considered part of the abdominal wall, as the abdominal compartment extends up into the chest.

The abdominal compartment is subdivided by the peritoneum into an anterior intraperitoneal cavity and the retroperitoneum. The lack of skeletal protection of the muscular anterior abdominal wall leads to a greater risk of injury to intraperitoneal organs, notably the spleen, liver, and small bowel. Ultrasonography and diagnostic peritoneal lavage are excellent for detecting intraperitoneal bleeding; however, they do not evaluate the retroperitoneal cavity, where injuries to structures such as the pancreas, the genitourinary tract, and the rectum are often occult. Organ injuries in the intraperitoneal cavity may bleed freely because of the substantial fluid capacity of this cavity, whereas brisk bleeding will be more contained by the limited space in the retroperitoneum. This risk of exsanguination into the intraperitoneal cavity explains why detection and repair of these injuries receive the highest priority in the management of the trauma patient.

Presenting Signs and Symptoms

Certain presenting signs and symptoms suggest the presence of intraperitoneal injury. Blood pressure and heart rate are the most important vital signs when assessing for significant intraabodminal injury. Isolated pre-hospital hypotension has been shown to be a predictor of mortality and of chest or abdominal injury requiring operative intervention. Prehospital abnormal vital signs should not be discounted even if the patient arrives with "stable" vital signs. Normal vital signs, however, do not rule out intraperitoneal injury. Significant complaints and findings include abdominal pain or tenderness, ecchymoses and abrasions to the abdominal wall, and hematemesis. Peritonitis, even in the absence of hypotension, is a strong predictor of intraabdominal injury.

The physical examination is limited in its ability to identify the presence or absence of intraabdominal injury. Therefore, further diagnostic testing should be performed, despite minimal clinical findings, if there was significant direct trauma to the abdomen such as a baseball bat or handlebar injury. Other significant mechanisms, such as a rollover motor vehicle collision, a motor vehicle collision with ejection or significant intrusion, or a significant fall should be evaluated in light of the patient's clinical picture. A motor vehicle collision with steering wheel deformity is associated with serious abdominal injury in front-seat passengers but not in drivers; direct impact from a bicycle handlebar suggests an increased likelihood of abdominal injury requiring laparotomy. Intraperitoneal injury can also result from minor mechanisms, such as a fall from the standing position onto the abdomen.

Several useful but insensitive clinical signs suggest specific injuries in the blunt trauma patient. Kehr's sign, which is left shoulder pain, suggests splenic rupture. Cullen's sign is ecchymosis around the umbilicus, and Turner's sign is ecchymosis in the flank area. Although rare in the trauma patient, these signs suggest retroperitoneal hemorrhage.

The presence of the "seat belt" sign (erythema, ecchymosis, or abrasions in the pattern of a seat belt) is associated with intraperitoneal injuries—specifically pancreatic, hollow viscous, and mesenteric injuries. Multiple studies have shown a significantly higher incidence of intraabdominal operative pathology in patients with the seat belt sign compared with those lacking one after motor vehicle trauma. The seat belt sign usually results from incorrect use or improper placement of a seat belt restraint. It should be used as a predictor of intraperitoneal injury and therefore as an indication to perform diagnostic imaging in patients with blunt abdominal trauma. A negative CT scan in a patient with abdominal tenderness and the seat belt sign should be followed by observation, diagnostic peritoneal lavage, or laparotomy, depending on findings and clinical suspicion. Although evisceration and clear-cut peritonitis are diagnostic for intraabdominal pathology, neither is a common finding.

Abdominal tenderness is common in many types of abdominal injury; however, often it is absent, even in patients with significant intraperitoneal injury. Drugs, alcohol, hypotension, and the presence of head injury reduce the patient's ability to sense pain or tenderness. Additionally, other significant injuries such as fractures or large lacerations may distract the patient from feeling the pain associated with abdominal injury. In a recent large prospective study, 19% of patients with a positive CT scan for intraabdominal injury did not have abdominal tenderness.[3] Other studies found that only 42% to 75% of patients with small bowel or mesenteric injury had abdominal tenderness.[4,5] The sensitivity, specificity, and negative and positive predictive values of abdominal pain or tenderness in predicting intraabdominal injuries are reported to be 82%, 45%, 93%, and 21% respectively.[6] Furthermore, patients with chest wall injuries and pneumothoraces are at risk for injury and may not have abdominal pain or tenderness. Thus, it is important to avoid relying solely on the physical examination, especially in the multi-trauma patient or patient with altered mental status, when deciding whether to perform diagnostic testing on the blunt abdominal trauma patient.

Stable patients with mild to moderate mechanisms of injury, a normal mental status, a normal abdominal examination, and without other major associated injuries may not need further imaging or work-up to exclude intraperitoneal injury. This approach is obviously based on clinical judgment and the absence of distracting injuries.

Evaluation

The physical examination of the abdomen following trauma consists of observation and palpation. The abdomen should be observed for signs of disruption, evisceration, ecchymoses, abrasions, and distention. Although it is important to perform a rectal examina-

RED FLAGS

- Pre-hospital hypotension indicates the need for diagnostic imaging of the abdomen.
- Abdominal ecchymosis is predictive of intraperitoneal injury.
- The presence of a Chance fracture is predictive of intraperitoneal injury.
- Left shoulder pain suggests splenic injury.
- Low rib fractures are associated with liver and spleen injuries.

tion to assess rectal tone and the prostate for possible urethral injury, a positive stool guaiac test is not predictive of injury. If gross blood is present on the rectal examination, large bowel or rectal injury should be suspected.

The initial physical examination includes assessment of the pelvis for stability and of the urethral meatus for blood as an indicator of an associated urethral injury. These aspects of the examination will help the EP plan the subsequent workup. Patients with pelvic instability may need pelvic fracture stabilization and embolization, whereas those with a urethral injury may need retrograde urethrography and suprapubic Foley catheter placement.

■ INJURY PATTERNS

The specific injuries to be concerned with after blunt abdominal trauma can be broken down into several categories: solid organ (liver and spleen), hollow viscous, mesenteric, vascular (inferior vena cava and aorta), diaphragmatic, and retroperitoneal (renal, bladder, pelvic fractures, and vascular). Other less common injuries are gallbladder, pancreas, and rectus sheath hematomas.

■ Chance Fractures

A single lap belt restraint can result in Chance fractures of the lumbar spine. In a recent report, 33% of patients with Chance fractures had associated intraabdominal injury; of these patients, 22% had hollow viscous injuries.[7] In other studies, up to 89% of patients with Chance fractures had small bowel injuries.[4,8] Some centers consider the presence of Chance fractures and the seat belt sign an indication for exploratory laparotomy.

■ Upper Abdominal Injuries

Low rib injuries may be associated with splenic or liver trauma, as well as kidney injuries. The incidence of splenic injury in patients with "isolated" low rib pain or tenderness (no abdominal tenderness) was 3% in a recent report. Although the only prospective study on the subject is not definitive, it suggests that patients with pleuritic pain and isolated low left rib pain or tenderness, regardless of abdominal tenderness, should undergo imaging.[9] Patients with abdominal tenderness following low chest trauma should undergo diagnostic imaging (e.g., CT scanning).

■ Low Abdominal Injuries

Blunt abdominal trauma may result in retroperitoneal injuries to the kidney or ureters. Intraperitoneal or extraperitoneal bladder ruptures may also occur. Major pelvic fractures are associated with abdominal injuries in 30% of patients.[10] Injury to the abdominal aorta is a rare injury after blunt abdominal trauma. Other less serious injuries are abdominal wall hematomas. These usually do not require operative intervention, but can result in significant blood loss.

■ Injuries with Delayed Presentation

Several injuries notoriously present either in a delayed fashion or with subtle clinical findings. Pancreatic injuries may present in a delayed fashion with abdominal pain and tenderness several hours after trauma. Duodenal hematomas typically present 5 to 7 days after the trauma with vague abdominal pain and vomiting. This is in contrast to patients with duodenal perforations, who have acute pain and tenderness right after the trauma.

Traumatic diaphragmatic hernia can also present in a delayed fashion. These injuries are frequently missed because the sensitivity of CT for diaphragmatic injuries is low and the majority of patients have associated injuries.[11] Most of these injuries result from a vehicular collision. Because the right hemidiaphragm is protected by the liver, the left hemidiaphragm is more commonly involved.

Diaphragmatic injuries present in three phases. In the *acute phase,* immediately after the injury, patients may have decreased or absent breath signs on one side of the chest or bowel sounds in the chest. If the injury is not detected, patients may go through a *latent* phase in which there is intermittent visceral hernation into the chest through the diaphragmatic rupture. These patients may present with vague postprandial abdominal pain (which improves with standing, as the herniated bowel is reduced), nausea, vomiting, and belching. During this phase, the injury can go undetected for months to years. With time, disorder eventually will enter the *obstructive* phase in which there is herniation with incarceration of bowel, intestinal obstruction, and ischemia. These patients present with abdominal pain, distention, and vomiting.

In the acute setting, patients with a diaphragmatic injury can also present with a tension viscerothorax-herniation of bowel into the chest, resulting in increased intrathoracic pressure and mediastinal shift with compression of the superior vena cava. These patients have hypotension and decreased breath sounds on the affected side of the chest.

■ Solid Organ Injuries

The most common type of injury is solid organ injury. More than 90% of injuries in blunt trauma are isolated to the liver and spleen. Patients who present with hypotension from blunt trauma usually have free rupture of a solid organ. Delayed onset of symptoms or pain without hypotension should raise concern about encapsulated hepatic or splenic trauma or hollow viscous injury. Although most intraperitoneal injuries today are managed nonoperatively, delayed diagnosis in some cases can lead to severe

PRIORITY ACTIONS

1. Follow ATLS protocols for initial resuscitation.
2. Determine stability of the patient.
3. Perform chest and pelvic radiography on all major trauma patients.
4. Perform ultrasound examination on all major trauma patients.
5. Arrange transfer immediately for all patients with multi-system trauma or with the potential for intraperitoneal injury if a trauma surgeon is not available.
6. Triage the patient to either CT scan, laparotomy, the angiography suite (pelvic fractures or for embolization of abdominal injuries), intensive care unit, admission for observation, or discharge.

morbidity or mortality. Free intraperitoneal bleeding is the most urgent diagnosis in patients with blunt abdominal trauma. This immediate life-threatening condition may require interventions including transfusion, exploratory laparotomy, and angiography with embolization.

Other less common but important diagnoses of solid organ injuries include diaphragmatic injuries and bowel perforations that require operative repair but are not necessarily associated with significant bleeding.

The Unstable Patient: Interventions and Procedures

■ THE ABCS OF TRAUMA

The initial therapeutic intervention in patients with presumed intraperitoneal injury is to address the ABCs of trauma (airway, breathing, and circulation). Initially all patients should receive high-flow oxygen. Intubation should be performed on very unstable or severely injured multitrauma patients or those with the potential for rapid decline. After breathing is attended to, circulatory status is addressed. Antecubital venous or central line access should be obtained.

■ FLUID AND BLOOD RESUSCITATION

IV fluid resuscitation with normal saline or Ringer's lactate is indicated for patients who are hemodynamically unstable (tachycardia or hypotension). The optimal amount and goal of resuscitation is controversial. Although the standard has been to immediately infuse 2 liters of crystalloid followed by blood transfusion if there is continued instability, many institutions move rapidly to blood transfusion and limit resuscitation to keep the patient "underresuscitated" with a systolic blood pressure of approximately 90 mm Hg.[12,13] Usually this can be accomplished with type O-negative blood in women of childbearing age and type O-positive in all others. Once definitive control of the bleeding lesion is identified and controlled, full resuscitation is instituted. However, this practice is not recommended for patients with possible traumatic brain injury, because hypotension increases the risk of mortality in this population.

The presence of an unstable pelvis on physical examination or on the initial pelvic radiograph is another indication for early blood transfusion, because patients with this condition will bleed profusely. EPs should place a pelvic stabilization binder or simply wrap a sheet tightly around the pelvis to stabilize the fractures. This is a simple but life-saving maneuver that can help stabilize the patient with major pelvic trauma.

■ IMMEDIATE OPERATIVE INTERVENTION

There are several indications to proceed immediately to the operating room without further diagnostic testing. These include evisceration, gross blood per rectum, blood per nasogastric tube or hematemesis, evidence of diaphragmatic injury, and hemodynamic instability with evidence of intraperitoneal injury (e.g., a positive ultrasound examination).

■ Focused Abdominal Sonography in Trauma (FAST) Examination

Once an immediate indication for laparotomy has been ruled out, further evaluation varies, depending on the hemodynamic stability of the patient. In the unstable patient, the next step is to perform a FAST examination to determine whether hemoperitoneum is present.

Bedside ultrasonography has many advantages as an initial triage tool in the unstable trauma patient. It is readily accessible at most Level I trauma centers and in the hands of trained EPs is accurate for the detection of hemoperitoneum.[14] The examination can be performed in less than 2 minutes and can triage patients to the operating room or further diagnostic testing depending on the patient's stability. In trauma patients, the incidence of an indeterminate sonogram result is low (less than 7%),[15] and the reported sensitivity and negative predictive values in unstable patients approach 100%.[16] The presence of hemoperitoneum in the unstable patient is an indication for operative intervention. If the sonogram findings are negative, other sources of bleeding should be addressed, such as pelvic fractures and retroperitoneal bleeding.

■ Diagnostic Peritoneal Lavage

Some authors take a conservative approach and recommend confirming the results of negative ultrasonography with diagnostic peritoneal lavage (DPL) in the hypotensive patient. If ultrasonography is unavailable or if the results are indeterminate, then DPL is required to determine the presence of intraperitoneal bleeding as an indication for immediate laparotomy. Before performing DPL, the EP should place a nasogastric tube and Foley catheter to decompress the stomach and drain the bladder.

DPL involves placing a catheter into the peritoneal space and aspirating with a 10-mL syringe to see if blood is present. In the unstable patient, an initial aspirate of 10 mL of blood is an indication for laparotomy. If the aspirate is negative, other sources of bleeding should be addressed (e.g., pelvic fractures). A liter of normal saline should be instilled into the abdomen if the initial aspirate is negative, and then drained from the abdomen and sent to the laboratory for analysis.

Once the patient has been stabilized or if there is no immediate indication to operate based on the initial FAST examination or DPL aspirate results, further diagnostic testing is indicated.

The Stable Patient: Secondary Survey, Interventions, and Procedures

■ LABORATORY TESTING

Laboratory tests are rarely helpful in the initial resuscitation of the blunt abdominal trauma patient. The utility of ordering individual laboratory tests when there is a specific clinical need versus routinely ordering a standard "trauma panel" has been studied. A significant cost savings, without adverse events, occurs if this practice is followed.[17,18]

Several laboratory tests are useful in the initial evaluation of the blunt trauma patient. A hematocrit should be obtained to be used as a baseline, and may be helpful as an indicator of bleeding if it is very low. Patients with a high likelihood of requiring an operation should have their blood typed and cross-matched in case a transfusion is required. A bedside glucose test should be performed on patients in a single car accident and in patients with altered mental status after trauma.

All women of childbearing age should undergo a pregnancy test and should be questioned about whether they are pregnant. The work-up for a pregnant trauma patient may be slightly different. Serial ultrasonography can be used as the initial and often definitive modality, and CT should be used sparingly in the first 20 weeks of gestation to avoid unnecessary radiation exposure.[19]

Coagulation profiles should be performed in patients with significant mechanism trauma and those who will likely require an operation. Although this does not alter the management of patients, it is helpful to the surgeon to know if a coagulopathy is present. In addition, any patient on coumadin therapy should have a coagulation profile performed.

Lactate levels and base excess are two laboratory tests that have been shown to predict bleeding.[20] In one recent study of stable trauma patients, an increased lactate level (>2.5 mmol/L in ethanol-negative patients and >3 mmol/L in ethanol-positive patients) and an increased base deficit (<0.0 in ethanol-negative patients and ≤3.0 in ethanol-positive patients) were associated with a significant risk of torso injury, whereas patients with a normal base deficit were unlikely to have injury.[21] Other authors consider a base deficit cut-off value of less than or equal to −6 predictive of intraabdominal injury and an indication for diagnostic imaging or DPL.[22] Although these criteria have been strongly advocated by a number of authors, they have not been universally adopted as a standard tool of evaluation at all centers.

Urinalysis should be performed in all blunt trauma patients with a significant mechanism of injury. The presence of gross hematuria is an indication for evaluation of the genitourinary tract. Microscopic hematuria indicates mild renal injuries that do not require treatment; its presence in a stable patient without a significant deceleration injury (associated with renal pedicle injury) does not indicate additional diagnostic imaging.

Amylase and lipase levels do not predict pancreatic injury in the acute setting. However, they may be helpful for detecting traumatic pancreatitis in patients presenting hours after trauma.

In addition to these laboratory tests, the diagnostic modalities available for patients with suspected blunt abdominal injuries include plain chest and pelvis radiographs, the FAST exam, diagnostic peritoneal lavage, computed tomography, and more recently, angiography. The indications for these different studies depend on the stability of the patient.

■ PLAIN RADIOGRAPHS

Plain radiographs cannot rule out intraperitoneal injury after blunt trauma. Chest radiography may diagnose a diaphragmatic rupture (Fig. 74-1). However, plain radiographs of the chest are diagnostic of diaphragmatic rupture in only 50% of patients with left-sided rupture and in only 17% of patients with right-sided rupture.[23,24] Free air is a rare finding on an upright chest radiograph indicating hollow viscous rupture (stomach or small bowel), and upright chest radiography usually is not feasible after blunt trauma. Thus, plain radiographs should not be used to rule out intraperitoneal injury.

Plain chest radiography should be performed in all patients with multisystem trauma to identify rib fractures, flail chest, pulmonary contusions, pneumothorax, and hemothorax and to evaluate the mediastinum. Radiography also is useful for detecting pelvic fractures as a cause of hypotension after blunt trauma and can help guide the work-up for management of associated genitourinary injuries. Although pelvic

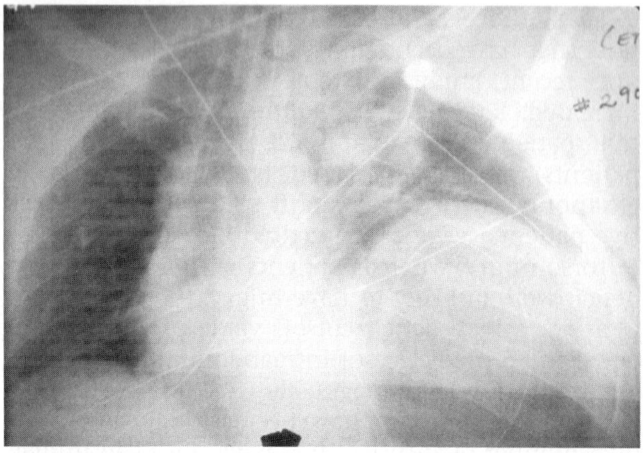

FIGURE 74-1 Chest radiograph of left diaphragmatic rupture.

radiography is not necessary in patients with a normal mental status without pain or tenderness, it should be performed in unstable or seriously injured patients with an appropriate mechanism of injury.

■ ULTRASONOGRAPHY

FAST is recommended for all blunt trauma patients as an initial screening test regardless of patient stability. Ultrasonography, which has its roots in Germany and Japan, has become integrated into the practice in trauma care over the past 15 years in the United States; it is now listed in the Advanced Trauma Life Support algorithm for abdominal trauma used in the majority of Level I trauma centers.[25] In the blunt trauma setting, ultrasonography has become part of the secondary survey to detect hemoperitonum as an indicator of intraperitoneal injury. It can help guide resuscitation and triage of the patient.

If the sonogram shows free fluid and the patient is hemodynamically unstable, exploratory laparotomy is indicated. The stable patient with free fluid should immediately undergo CT to identify the type of injury and determine the need for laparotomy. If the patient becomes unstable at any time during the ED management, laparotomy is indicated. A clinical algorithm that incorporates the FAST examination is shown in Figure 74-2.

The FAST examation also is used for rapid detection of pericardial fluid, hemothorax, and pneumothorax. The test does not replace chest radiography for hemothorax and pneumothorax but may be obtained faster, and can be used to expedite thoracostomy tube placement.

Ultrasonography's major limitation is its inability to identify solid organ injury. The sensitivity for detecting hemoperitoneum as an indicator of intraperitoneal injury ranges from 76% to 90% and the specificities range from 95% to 100%.[14] However, the sensitivity is as low as 33% for splenic injuries and 12% for hepatic injuries for identifying encapsulated solid organ bleeding.[14,26] Ultrasonography is also limited in assessing injuries that are not associated with a large amount of hemoperitoneum, such as retroperitoneal bleeding and injuries of the small bowel or diaphragm. Up to one third of patients with intraperitoneal injury will have a negative FAST examination, including up to 10% of patients who require operation.[27]

Thus, the FAST examination does not replace more definitive tests such as CT, but it can be a triage tool to expedite the work-up and management of patients with blunt abdominal trauma. The amount of intraperitoneal fluid that must be present in order to have an abnormal FAST examination is at least 150 mL and may be as much as 1 liter.[28,29]

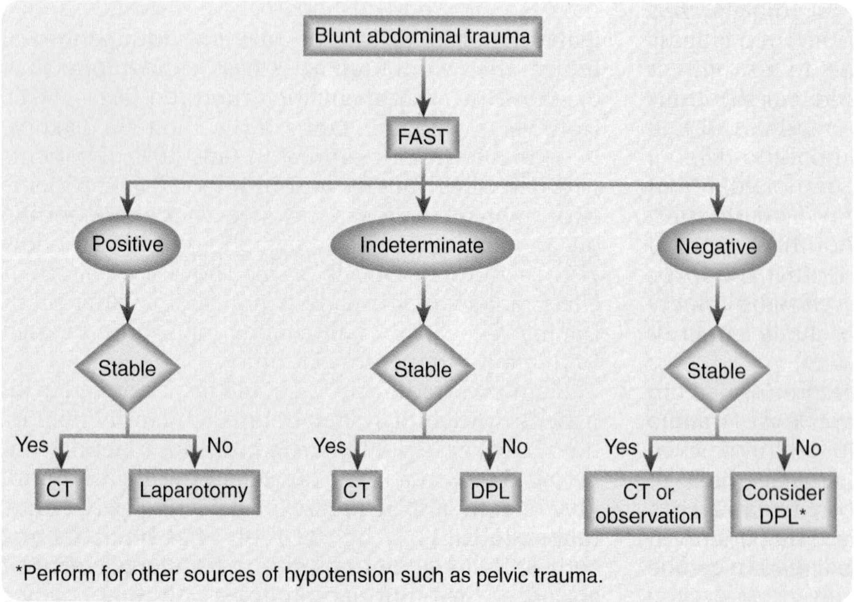
Blunt abdominal trauma
FAST
Positive
Indeterminate
Negative
Stable
Stable
Stable
Yes
No
Yes
No
Yes
No
CT
Laparotomy
CT
DPL
CT or observation
Consider DPL*
*Perform for other sources of hypotension such as pelvic trauma.

FIGURE 74-2 Algorithm for management of blunt abdominal trauma. CT, computed tomography; DPL, diagnostic peritoneal lavage; FAST, focused abdominal sonography in trauma. (From Rosen CL, Promes SB: Use of ultrasound in emergency medicine. Clinical bulletin: State of the Art Emergency Medicine 2003;7[2]:1. Reprinted with permission from Sterling Healthcare. All rights reserved.)

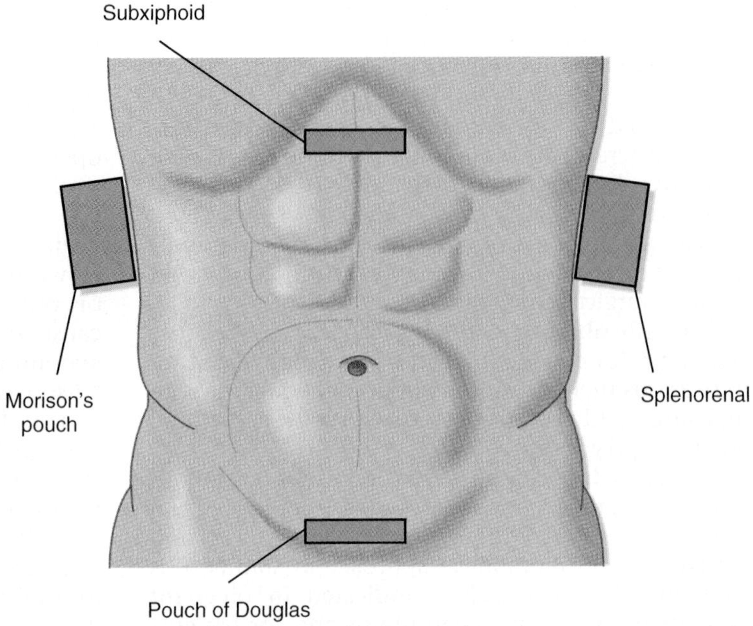

Subxiphoid
Morison's pouch
Splenorenal
Pouch of Douglas

FIGURE 74-3 Focused abdominal sonography for trauma (FAST) examination: Four views.

The technique of bedside ultrasonography in trauma patients is performed using four standard views (Fig. 74-3): right-upper quadrant (Morison's pouch), subxiphoid, left-upper quadrant, and suprapubic (pouch of Douglas). Although there is no standard sequence to this examination, the suprapubic view takes advantage of the full bladder as a sonographic window and should therefore be obtained before Foley catheter placement. Most operators start with the Morison's pouch view because it is technically the easiest.

Obtaining all of the views rather than one single view increases the sensitivity of the test.[30] Performing serial examinations 30 minutes into the resuscitation or if there is a change in the clinical status increases the sensitivity further. Trendelenburg positioning may improve the sensitivity by causing the hemoperitoneum to pool in dependent spaces. However, this is often not practical in blunt trauma patients. Previous abdominal surgery may result in adhesions and pockets of fluid within the abdomen that prevent fluid from accumulating in Morison's pouch or the splenorenal space. A false-positive result may be due to perinephric fat.

The differential diagnosis for fluid seen on ultrasonography includes ascites, as well as urine from an intraperitoneal bladder rupture. All fluid will result in the same black stripe seen on the sonogram.

The finding suggestive of injury is hemoperitoneum, which appears as a black (anechoic) stripe between the kidney and the liver (Fig. 74-4), between the kidney and the spleen, or posterior to the bladder. Because ultrasonography is insensitive for detecting actual parenchymal injuries, the operator should not waste time evaluating the spleen and liver for evidence of injury.

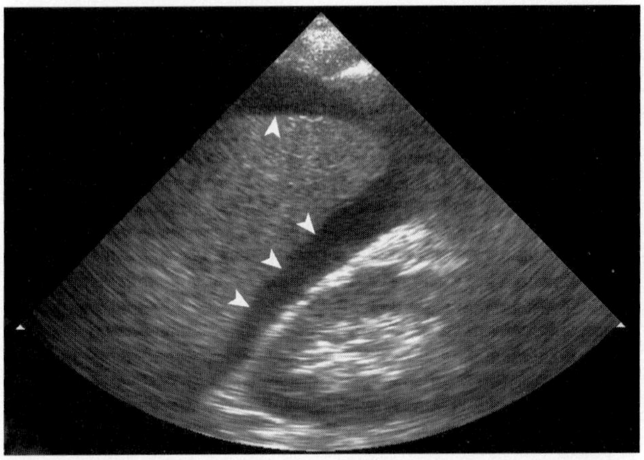

FIGURE 74-4 Morison's pouch, showing fluid (*arrowheads*) in the space between the liver and the right kidney.

■ DIAGNOSTIC PERITONEAL LAVAGE

Diagnostic peritoneal lavage (DPL) was formerly the primary method for evaluating patients with unstable blunt abdominal trauma, but its use has markedly decreased with the widespread use of bedside ultrasonography. Currently, DPL is indicated when ultrasonography is unavailable or if the results are indeterminate in an unstable patient. Some authors recommend DPL to confirm the absence of hemoperitoneum in unstable patients with negative ultrasonography results.[14]

DPL is very sensitive for detecting intraperitoneal bleeding, is rapidly performed, and is inexpensive. It can detect small amounts of intraperitoneal blood (as little as 20 mL).[31] The accuracy of DPL for predicting or ruling out intraperitoneal bleeding is close to 98%.[32,33]

The disadvantages of DPL are that it is invasive, does not identify the specific organ that is injured, and does not sample the retroperitoneal space. It will also detect small amounts of bleeding associated with injuries that do not require operative intervention. The nontherapeutic laparotomy rate for patients with a positive DPL is reported to be as high as 35%.[34] Thus, in stable patients, a positive DPL is not an indication for laparotomy. In unstable patients, however, it is highly predictive of an injury that requires surgical correction.

The only absolute contraindication to DPL is the clear need for emergent laparotomy. Relative contraindications include morbid obesity, previous abdominal surgery (due to the presence of adhesions), and late-term pregnancy.

The procedure can be performed using several different anatomic approaches (supraumbilical, infraumbilical) and techniques (open, semi-open, and closed). The infraumbilical approach is standard. A supraumbilical approach is indicated in pregnant patients to avoid the gravid uterus and for patients with pelvic fractures to avoid placing the catheter through blood that potentially has dissected anteriorly from the retroperitoneal hematoma, yielding a false positive results. The type of DPL performed (open versus closed) varies by institution and also depends on the clinical situation. The open technique is used for pregnant patients or those with pelvic fractures.

DPL findings that predict the presence of intraperitoneal injury after blunt trauma are the presence of greater than 100,000 red blood cells/mm^3, a white blood cell count greater than 500/mm^3, amylase level greater than 10 IU/L, and alkaline phosphatase level greater than or equal to 3 IU/L.

The complication rate for DPL is less than 1%. The most serious complication is bowel perforation; other complications include wound infection and bleeding.

■ COMPUTED TOMOGRAPHY

Abdominal and pelvic computed tomography (CT) is the standard diagnostic imaging modality for the stable patient with possible intraabdominal injury. CT provides excellent detail of solid organ and retroperitoneal injuries. Its performance continues to improve in diagnosing hollow viscous injuries. Multidetector CT has become a rapid and accurate method for evaluating the abdomen and pelvis after blunt trauma. Because of the accuracy and detail of the CT images, nonoperative management of solid organ injury can now be performed safely. Using 3D reconstructions, radiologists can also image the lumbar spine and pelvis to evaluate fractures.

The disadvantages of CT are that it is difficult to monitor and resuscitate a patient in the radiology suite, and there are risks of contrast allergy and renal failure from dye administration. The complication rate is 3%, which includes aspiration of oral contrast material.

CT is indicated in stable patients when there is clinical concern for intraabdominal injury because of abdominal wall findings, traumatic distracting injuries, and significant mechanism of injury. The presence of distracting injury or the need for operative intervention for other injuries (e.g., orthopedic injuries) also are indications for performing CT. The definition of distracting injury has not been well-studied, and remains controversial. However, long bone fractures, pelvic fractures, or other injuries that are judged by the EP to cause enough pain to distract the patient from abdominal pain or tenderness should be considered "distracting."

The determination of when the patient is stable enough to undergo CT remains a point of controversy. An unstable patient should not be sent to the radiography suite, where it is difficult to monitor and resuscitate a sick patient. Most centers use the response to fluid resuscitation and transfusion as an indicator of whether the patient is stable enough to be transferred to the radiography suite for CT. This decision may also be influenced by the proximity and type of CT scanner. A rapid multidetector scanner adjacent to the ED may offer a safer environment than a slower-generation scanner two hospital floors away. Patients whose vital signs normalize after 2 liters of fluid resuscitation are "stable" for CT.

CT is very accurate for diagnosing intraperitoneal injury, especially for detecting solid organ injury. The sensitivity and specificity of CT for intraperitoneal injury is 97% and 95%, respectively.[33] Of even greater importance, the overall negative predictive value of CT for intraperitoneal injury is 99.6%.[3] This means that a normal CT in the patient without other injuries can often lead to discharge.

The limitations of CT lie in its low sensitivity for diaphragm, mesenteric, hollow viscous, and pancreatic injuries. Although the newer-generation multidetector CT scanners appear to have a better resolution and sensitivity for these rare injuries, they are still not highly accurate. The sensitivity for diaphragmatic injury is between 67% and 84%, with specificities reported between 77% and 100%.[11,35-38]

The sensitivity of CT for hollow viscous injury is reported to range from 83% to 94%.[9,11,38-41] However, others report a sensitivity as low as 64%.[42] CT has a reported sensitivity of 96% for identifying mesenteric injury.[38] The reported sensitivity of CT for detecting pancreatic injuries after blunt trauma is 68%, even with spiral CT technology.[43]

In summary, CT is a very sensitive test for excluding solid organ injury. However, its sensitivity is much lower for diaphragmatic, pancreatic, and small bowel injuries. Thus, patients with significant abdominal ecchymosis (an indicator of hollow viscous injury) or those with plain radiographic evidence of diaphragmatic injury should undergo exploratory laparotomy or at least surgical consultation and observation.

■ Oral Contrast or No Oral Contrast?

An ongoing controversy on the use of CT scanning for blunt abdominal trauma is the utility of oral contrast versus IV contrast alone. Oral contrast is associated with increased time and the potential for vomiting and aspiration and other complications, as well as discomfort from nasogastric tube placement (if necessary). Some authors advocate its use to help delineate bowel and mesenteric injury that may not be visualized without contrast extravasation and enhancement. Other authors point to several studies showing that oral contrast is not essential for identifying solid organ, mesenteric, or bowel injuries.[44-47] In one prospective randomized study, the sensitivity of CT without oral contrast for identifying solid organ injury was actually higher than the sensitivity of CT with oral contrast (89% vs. 84%), as well as for small bowel injury (100% vs. 86%).[47]

One small study found that oral contrast may be helpful for detecting pancreatic injuries but not for detecting solid organ or intestinal injuries. Furthermore, this study reported that the use of oral contrast was associated with a significant risk of vomiting and aspiration.[44] Thus, the literature does not seem to support the routine use of oral contrast.

■ Findings in Patients with Blunt Abdominal Trauma

CT findings suggesting solid organ injury are disruption of the parenchyma, contrast extravasation, and hemoperitoneum. Patients with blunt intestinal or mesenteric injuries may have more subtle findings such as free fluid without obvious organ injury, mesenteric stranding or edema, and bowel wall hematoma. Other indicators of bowel and mesenteric injuries are pneumoperitoneum, tears in the bowel wall, and bowel wall thickening.

Isolated intraperitoneal fluid in patients without solid organ injury is associated with a high incidence of bowel or mesenteric injury. In patients without solid organ injury and with more than trace amounts of isolated free fluid, the therapeutic laparotomy rate is 54% to 94%.[48] At operation, small bowel, mesenteric, and diaphragm injuries are usually found. In a large study, Fakhry reported that 84% of patients without obvious solid organ injury and with free intraperitoneal fluid on CT had small bowel injuries.[4]

■ ANGIOGRAPHY

Angiography, when combined with embolization, is both a diagnostic and therapeutic modality. While classically used in blunt trauma for treatment of pelvic fractures, it has been found to be especially useful in the nonoperative treatment of active bleeding from solid organ injuries. High-grade spleen and liver injuries (see Box 74-2 and Box 74-3), as well as renal lacerations, are amenable to this technique. Patients selected for this procedure must be stable and have solid organ injuries with active extravasation (contrast blush) on abdominopelvic CT scans.

Treatment and Disposition

■ TREATMENT

The initial treatment of blunt abdominal trauma patients includes fluid resuscitation, transfusion, and simultaneous consultation with the trauma surgery facility for operative intervention, angiography, or admission for observation. Early involvement of a trauma surgeon in the management of patients with instability or concerning examination is recommended to help guide management and ensure timely operative intervention.

Indications for operative intervention include hemodynamic instability, diaphragmatic injury, and hollow viscous injury. While high-grade splenic and liver injuries once were routinely operated on, the use of angiography with embolization has become more common. Other CT findings that trauma surgeons may consider indications for operative intervention include the presence of intraperitoneal fluid without obvious organ injury as well as evidence of active extravasation.

Because of the high incidence of associated small bowel injury, many institutions consider the presence of a Chance fracture in conjunction with abdominal wall ecchymosis an indication for laparotomy. For similar reasons, the presence of significant amounts of intraperitoneal fluid without solid organ injury indicates the presence of intraperitoneal injury and should be used as an indication for laparotomy.

■ Prioritizing Management of Injuries

ED management of unstable blunt abdominal trauma patients becomes challenging when there are associated injuries. In general, intraperitoneal bleeding trumps other injuries in terms of the immediate need for operative management. An unstable patient with known intraperitoneal hemorrhage and associated pelvic trauma should undergo laparotomy first, followed by management of pelvic injuries (e.g., angiographic embolization of pelvic vessels). In unstable patients with evidence of associated traumatic brain injury, neurosurgical consultation should be obtained for intracranial bolt placement in the operating room while the intraperitoneal injuries are being addressed.

There may not be time for a head CT if the patient is hemodynamically unstable. Suspicion of aortic injuries presents an added challenge in management. The aortic injury is usually not the cause of hemodynamic instability, and the intraperitoneal bleeding should be the presumed source of hypotension. Thus, in patients with concomitant aortic and abdominal

Documentation

- Mechanism and timing of the injury
- Physical examination findings
- Timing and ordering of tests and consultations
- Emergency department procedures
- Changes in clinical status

injuries, laparotomy should be performed first. Abdominal bleeding takes priority over orthopedic injuries; frequently, however, the trauma surgeon can perform a laparotomy at the same time that the orthopedic surgeon is repairing an open fracture.

Nonoperative Treatment

Many reports in the surgical literature document success with nonoperative management of patients with spleen and liver lacerations.[49]

Most centers consider the presence of hemodynamic instability or transfusion requirements indications to operate on patients with solid organ injuries. Age may also be used as an indication for operation; children do well with nonoperative management, whereas elderly patients may have lower success rates for nonoperative care. Nonoperative salvage rates for splenic lacerations are 94%, and up to 80% of grade 4 and 5 splenic injuries can be successfully managed without operative intervention.[50]

In one prospective study, the failure rate of nonoperative management of kidney, liver, and splenic lacerations was 22%; the failure rate was higher for splenic injury than for liver or kidney injuries.[51] Independent predictors of failure of nonoperative management were fluid identified on screening ultrasonography examination, significant blood on CT (>300 mL), and the need for blood transfusion.[51]

Interventional Radiology

In major trauma centers, interventional radiologists in conjunction with trauma surgeons are performing angiography with embolization instead of operative management. The nonoperative salvage rate for patients with splenic lacerations who undergo embolization is 90%.[50] Factors that did not correlate with the need for operative management as opposed to angiographic embolization are age and heart rate. A higher injury severity score, lower blood pressure, lower pH, and the need for transfusion correlate with the need for operative intervention.[52]

Decisions about nonoperative versus operative management or angiographic embolization of blunt solid organ injures are made by the consulting trauma surgeon. Early and accurate detection of intraperitoneal injuries with CT can help the surgeon decide which management strategy to use.

DISPOSITION

Patient Transfer

If the patient is initially transported to a hospital that is not a designated trauma center, then the EP must decide when to transfer to the trauma center and what tests to perform before transfer. If the trauma is isolated to the abdomen and a general surgeon is available to admit the patient or perform a therapeutic laparotomy, then transfer may not be necessary. The decision to keep a trauma patient at a non-trauma center should be based on institutional guidelines. Patients with multi-system trauma or hemodynamic instability require transfer to a trauma center.

It is recommended to only perform a diagnostic test when the results will be acted upon at the first institution, and when the test will not delay life- or limb-threatening intervention. In these cases, performing some diagnostic tests prior to transfer can cause life-threatening delays.

PATIENT TEACHING TIPS

- For patients with nonoperative splenic injuries, avoid contact sports until follow-up and for several weeks.
- Return to the emergency department if experiencing abdominal pain, lightheadedness, vomiting, or blood per rectum.

Tips and Tricks

- Do not underestimate the mechanism of injury. A significant mechanism of injury requires a work-up for intraperitoneal injury even if the patient is stable and the physical examination is normal.
- The presence or absence of abdominal tenderness does not predict intraperitoneal injury.
- Alcohol and distracting injuries can make the physical examination unreliable.
- All blunt abdominal trauma patients should undergo a FAST examination.
- Before performing a DPL, place a nasogastric tube and Foley catheter and obtain a pelvic radiograph.
- A positive FAST examination or DPL aspirate in an unstable patient is an indication for laparotomy.
- Unstable patients should not be transferred to the radiology suite for CT.
- Significant intraperitoneal fluid without solid organ injury on a CT scan suggests the presence of small bowel injury.
- CT can fail to identify injuries of the pancreas, diaphragm, small bowel, and mesenterium.

CT, computed tomography; DPL, diagnostic peritoneal lavage; FAST, focused abdominal sonography in trauma.

REFERENCES

1. Hoyt DB, Coimbra R, Potenza B: Management of acute trauma. In Townsend CM, Beauchamp RD, Evers BM, et al (eds): Sabiston Textbook of Surgery, 17th ed. Philadelphia, WB Saunders, 2004, pp 483-529.
2. Rutledge R, Hunt JP, Lentz CW, et al: A statewide, population-based time-series analysis of the increasing frequency of nonoperative management of abdominal solid organ injury. Ann Surg 1995;222:311-322.
3. Livingston DH, Lavery RF, Passannante MR, et al: Admission for observation is not necessary after a negative abdominal computed tomographic scan in patients with suspected blunt abdominal trauma: Results of a prospective, multi-institutional trial. J Trauma 1998;44:273-280.
4. Fakhry SM, Watts DD, Luchette FA: Current diagnostic approaches lack sensitivity in the diagnosis of perforated blunt small bowel injury: Analysis of 275,557 trauma admissions from the EAST multi-institutional HVI trial. J Trauma 2003;54:295-306.
5. Pikoulis E, Delis S, Psalidas N, et al: Presentation of blunt small intestinal and mesenteric injuries. Ann R Coll Surg Engl 2000;82(2):103-106.
6. Ferrera PC, Verdile VP, Bartfield JM, et al: Injuries distracting from intraabdominal injuries after blunt trauma. Am J Emerg Med 1998;16:145-149.
7. Tyroch AH, McGuire EL, McLean SF, et al: The association between Chance fractures and intra-abdominal injuries revisited: A multicenter review. Am Surg 2005;71: 434-438.
8. Anderson PA, Rivara FP, Maier RV, Drake C: The epidemiology of seatbelt-associated injuries. J Trauma 1991;31: 60-67.
9. Holmes JF, Ngyven H, Jacoby RC, et al: Do all patients with left costal margin injuries require radiographic evaluation of intraabdominal injury? Ann Emerg Med 2005;46: 232-236.
10. Demetriades D, Karaiskakis M, Toutouzas K, et al: Pelvic fractures: Epidemiology and predictors of associated abdominal injuries and outcomes. J Am Coll Surg 2002;195:1-10.
11. Iochum S, Ludig T, Walter F, et al: Imaging of diaphragmatic injury: A diagnostic challenge? Radiographics 2002;22(Spec No):S103-S116.
12. Dutton RP, Mackenzie CF, Scalea TM: Hypotensive resuscitation during active hemorrhage: Impact on in-hospital mortality. J Trauma 2002;52:1141-1146.
13. Pepe PE, Mosesso VN, Falk JL: Prehospital fluid resuscitation of the patient with minor trauma. Prehosp Emerg Care 2002;6:81-91.
14. Rosen CL, Tibbles CD, Tracy JA: The use of ultrasound in trauma. In Ernst A, Feller-Kopman DJ (eds): Ultrasound-Guided Procedures and Investigations: A Manual for the Clinician. New York, Taylor & Francis Group, LLC, 2006, p 75.
15. Boulanger BR, Brenneman FD, Kirkpatrick AW, et al: The indeterminate abdominal sonogram in multisystem blunt trauma. J Trauma 1998;45:52-56.
16. Rozycki GS, Ballard RB, Feliciano DV, et al: Surgeon-performed ultrasound for the assessment of truncal injuries: Lessons learned from 1540 patients. Ann Surg 1998;228: 557-567.
17. Chu UB, Clevenger FW, Imami ER, et al: The impact of selective laboratory evaluation on utilization of laboratory resources and patient care in a level-I trauma center. Am J Surg 1996;172:558-563.
18. Keller MS, Coln CE, Trimble JA, et al: The utility of routine trauma laboratories in pediatric trauma resuscitations. Am J Surg 2004;188:671-678.
19. Brown MA, Sirlin CB, Farahmand N, et al: Screening sonography in pregnant patients with blunt abdominal trauma. J Ultrasound Med 2005;24:175-181.
20. Mackersie RC, Tiwary AD, Shackford SR, Hoyt DB: Intra-abdominal injury following blunt trauma. Identifying the high-risk patient using objective risk factors. Arch Surg 1989;124:809-813.
21. Dunham CM, Sipe EK, Peluso L: Emergency department spirometric volume and base deficit delineate risk for torso injury in stable patients. BMC Surg 2004;4:3.
22. Davis JW, Mackersie RC, Holbrook TL, Hoyt DB: Base deficit as an indicator of significant abdominal injury. Ann Emerg Med 1991;20:842-844.
23. Gelman R, Mirvis SE, Gens D: Diaphragmatic rupture due to blunt trauma: Sensitivity of plain chest radiographs. AJR Am J Roentgenol 1991;156:51-57.
24. Shapiro MJ, Heiberg E, Durham RM, et al: The unreliability of CT scans and initial chest radiographs in evaluating blunt trauma induced diaphragmatic rupture. Clin Radiol 1996;51:27-30.
25. Advanced Trauma Life Support Student Course Manual, 7th Ed. Chicago, American College of Surgeons, 2004.
26. Richards JR, McGahan JP, Pali MJ, et al: Sonographic detection of blunt hepatic trauma: Hemoperitoneum and parenchymal patterns of injury. J Trauma 1999;47:1092.
27. Poletti PA, Kinkel K, Vermeulen B, et al: Blunt abdominal trauma: Should US be used to detect both free fluid and organ injuries? Radiology 2003;227:95-103.
28. Von Kuenssberg Jehle D, Stiller G, Wagner D: Sensitivity in detecting free intraperitoneal fluid with the pelvic views of the FAST exam. Am J Emerg Med 2003;21:476-478.
29. Branney SW, Wolfe RE, Moore EE, et al: Quantitative sensitivity of ultrasound in detecting free intraperitoneal fluid. J Trauma 1995;39:375-380.
30. Ma OJ, Kefer MP, Mateer JR, Thoma B: Evaluation of hemoperitoneum using single- vs multiple-view ultrasonographic examination. Acad Emerg Med 1995;2:581-586.
31. Otomo Y, Henmi H, Mashiko K, et al: New diagnostic peritoneal lavage criteria for diagnosis of intestinal injury. J Trauma 1998;44:991-997.
32. Bilge A, Sahin M: Diagnostic peritoneal lavage in blunt abdominal trauma. Eur J Surg 1991;157:449-451.
33. Liu M, Lee C-H, P'eng F-K: Prospective comparison of diagnostic peritoneal lavage, computed tomography scanning, and ultrasonography for the diagnosis of blunt abdominal trauma. J Trauma 1993;35:267-270.
34. Fryer JP, Graham TL, Fong HM, et al: Diagnostic peritoneal lavage as an indicator for therapeutic surgery. Can J Surg 1991;34:471-476.
35. Shanmuganathan K: Multi-detector row CT imaging of blunt abdominal trauma. Semin Ultrasound CT MR 2004;25:180-204.
36. Larici AR, Gotway MB, Litt HI, et al: Helical CT with sagittal and coronal reconstructions: Accuracy for detection of diaphragmatic injury. AJR Am J Roentgenol 2002;179: 451-457.
37. Allen TL, Cummins BF, Bonk RT, et al: Computed tomography without oral contrast solution for blunt diaphragmatic injuries in abdominal trauma. Am J Emerg Med 2005;23:253-258.
38. Killeen KL, Shanmuganathan K, Poletti PA, et al: Helical computed tomography of bowel and mesenteric injuries. J Trauma 2001;51:26-36.
39. Janzen DL, Zwirewich CV, Breen DJ, Nagy A: Diagnostic accuracy of helical CT for detection of blunt bowel and mesenteric injuries. Clin Radiol 1998;53:193-197.
40. Malhotra AK, Fabian TC, Katsis SB, et al: Blunt bowel and mesenteric injuries: The role of screening computed tomography. J Trauma 2000;48:991-998.
41. Sherck J, Shatney C, Sensaki K, Selivanov V: The accuracy of computed tomography in the diagnosis of blunt small-bowel perforation. Am J Surg 1994;168:670-675.
42. Butela ST, Federle MP, Chang PJ, et al: Performance of CT in detection of bowel injury. AJR Am J Roentgenol 2001;176:129-135.
43. Ilahi O, Bochicchio GV, Scalea TM: Efficacy of computed tomography in the diagnosis of pancreatic injury in adult blunt trauma patients: A single-institutional study. Am Surg 2002;68:704-707.
44. Tsang BD, Panacek EA, Brant WE, et al: Effect of oral contrast administration for abdominal computed tomography in the evaluation of acute blunt trauma. Ann Emerg Med 1997;30:7-13.

45. Clancy TV, Ragozzino MW, Ramshaw D, et al: Oral contrast is not necessary in the evaluation of blunt abdominal trauma by computed tomography. Am J Surg 1993;166: 680-684.
46. ACEP Clinical Policies Committee: Clinical Policies Subcommittee on Acute Blunt Abdominal Trauma: Clinical policy: Critical issues in the evaluation of adult patients presenting to the emergency department with acute blunt abdominal trauma. Ann Emerg Med. 2004;43:278-290.
47. Stafford RE, McGonigal MD, Weigelt JA, Johnson TJ: Oral contrast solution and computed tomography for blunt abdominal trauma. Arch Surg 1999;134:622-626.
48. Cunningham MA, Tyroch AH, Kaups KL, Davis JW: Does free fluid on abdominal computed tomographic scan after blunt trauma require laparotomy? J Trauma 1998;4: 599-602.
49. Ozturk H, Dokucu AI, Onen A, et al: Non-operative management of isolated solid organ injuries due to blunt abdominal trauma in children: A fifteen-year experience. Eur J Pediatr Surg 2004;14:29-34.
50. Haan JM, Bochicchio GV, Kramer N, et al: Non-operative management of blunt splenic injury: A 5-year experience. J Trauma 2005;58:492-498.
51. Velmahos GC, Toutouzas KG, Radin R, et al: Non-operative treatment of blunt injury to solid abdominal organs: A prospective study. Arch Surg 2003;138:844-851.
52. Wahl WL, Ahrns KS, Chen S, et al: Blunt splenic injury: Operation versus angiographic embolization. Surgery 2004;136:891-899.

Chapter **75**

Penetrating Abdominal Trauma

Eric L. Legome and Carlo L. Rosen

KEY POINTS

Patients with diffuse peritonitis after penetrating abdominal trauma require operative intervention.

The evaluation of the patient with stable penetrating trauma depends on resources, local customs, anatomic site of the injury, and the weapon causing the injury.

In injuries of the low chest, back or upper abdomen, It is important to know the anatomic boundaries of the abdomen and to evaluate for potential thoracoabdominal injury.

Rule out concomitant cardiac or pulmonary injury after a stab wound or any gun shot wound to the thoracoabdominal area.

If cardiac or pulmonary injuries are excluded, a hypotensive patient with penetrating abdominal trauma requires laparotomy.

Ultrasonography is useful in the evaluation of penetrating abdominal trauma when results are positive. A negative result can never rule out an intrabdominal injury.

Laparoscopy is the test of choice to evaluate the diaphragm in left-sided low chest, upper abdominal, or lumbosacral wounds.

Scope and Outline

■ PERSPECTIVE

Prior to World War I, penetrating abdominal trauma was treated expectantly. It had high associated morbidity and essentially uniform mortality if a hollow viscus or vascular injury occurred.

Although there were early proponents of surgical intervention, standards of nonoperative management prevailed because of poor success and the desire not to operate under war conditions. World War I, along with the development of antiseptic techniques and anesthesia, heralded the era of mandatory laparotomy, which significantly decreased mortality to about 50%. During World War II, advances in surgical techniques along with antibiotics markedly lowered the death rate to about 25%. Advances during the Vietnam and Korean wars, many spurred by improved surgical management and more rapid evacuation, further improved outcomes.[1,2]

Management of penetrating abdominal trauma has undergone many changes over the last 20 years. Major transformations include rapid transport to trauma centers, "scoop and run" protocols in the field, damage control surgery, increased use of interventional radiologic techniques, and recognition and treatment of abdominal compartment syndrome. Better diagnostic studies, including rational use of computed tomography (CT) and ultrasonography as well as expanded use of laparoscopy, have also improved morbidity rates, although there has not been a marked change in mortality.[3]

Although the management of patients with obvious peritonitis or shock remains essentially unchanged from the perspective of the EP, the patient without obvious intra-peritoneal injury still presents a diagnostic dilemma, with several avenues of diagnostic strategies from which to choose.

■ EPIDEMIOLOGY

World-wide, most penetrating trauma is the result of war or ongoing civil insurrections, although because of the lack of any common reporting scheme, actual numbers are impossible obtain. In the United States, penetrating abdominal trauma is mainly a young urban male phenomenon. Penetrating trauma is a significant public health problem. Unfortunately, while violent crime in the United States has progressively decreased over the last half decade, in 2005 it rebounded with an increase of several percent.[4] There is a high rate of penetrating trauma in low income inner city communities. Illicit drug and alcohol use is strongly associated with victims of penetrating trauma, reaching over 50% in one study of victims who died and even higher in some studies evaluating all patients with penetrating trauma.

Penetrating trauma is overwhelmingly a male disease, as high as 90% in some studies.[5,6] Mortality in the United States due to firearms is almost tenfold higher in men than in women. The highest rate of firearm mortality is in young black males less than 35 years old, followed by young hispanic males and then white males. The largest cause of violent deaths in the age group of 15 to 34 years is due to firearms, comprising approximately 45%. About 5% of deaths are due to piercing or stab wound injuries. In 2003, the Centers for Disease Control calculated that over 275 years of life lost per 100,000 male U.S. populations were due to homicide.[7]

In addition to the tremendous resources needed to care for victims of penetrating trauma, these injuries and deaths impact not only current productivity but also future economic yields of our society.

Since the 1960s, U.S. mortality rates of 9.5% to 12.7% for civilian gunshot wounds and up to 3.6% for stab wounds have been reported. Most deaths due to penetrating trauma occur in the first 24 hours; about 70% occur in the first 6 hours of the patient's course, most commonly in the ED, followed by the operating room. Most of these patients tend to have vascular injuries and succumb to exsanguination or refractory hemorrhagic shock.[3] If patients survive the first 24 hours, later deaths tend to cluster after 72 hours and are mainly related to acute systemic complications such as multiple system organ failure, acute respiratory distress syndrome, pulmonary embolism, and pneumonia.

■ PATHOPHYSIOLOGY

Physiologic evaluation of the patient with penetrating abdominal trauma concentrates on two major findings related to the pathophysiologic basis of the injury—peritonitis and hemodynamic instability. Peritonitis, or inflammation of the peritoneum, develops when the peritoneal envelope and the posterior aspect of the anterior abdominal wall are inflamed by enteric contents. Intra- or retroperitoneal blood and organ contents inflame deeper nerve endings (visceral afferent pain fibers) and result in poorly defined and localized pain. The pain is dull and usually perceived in the epigastrium or periumbilical or hypogastric regions, depending on the developmental origin of the organ injured.

The parietal peritoneum is the innermost layer of the abdominal wall. Direct contact with blood or with organ and bowel contents can cause inflammation. Irritation of somatic pain fibers may present as tenderness to palpation of the abdomen as well as involuntary guarding of the abdominal wall musculature. Due to the unilateral distribution and greater number of somatic pain fibers than visceral fibers in this area, the pain tends to be more localized. However, in many cases of penetrating injury, the dissemination of spillage into the intestinal cavity can lead to a diffusely tender and rigid abdomen.

Patients may also have referred pain. Because of the afferent embryologically related pain fibers that ascend during development, back or shoulder distribution of pain may provide a clue to the damaged organ (e.g., left shoulder pain from a spleen rupture with subphrenic blood). Hemodynamically stable patients with penetrating abdominal trauma and peritonitis can be assumed to have a hollow visceral perforation. They may also have significant intraabdominal hemorrhage but are currently hemodynamically compensated. Thus, peritonitis on physical examination is a trigger for emergent intervention regardless of vital signs. Hypotension, narrow pulse pressure, and tachycardia or other signs of inadequate end organ perfusion in the setting of penetrating abdominal trauma provide evidence of significant intraabdominal injury warranting immediate surgical exploration. Confounding injuries, such as tension pneumothorax or pericardial tamponade that can lead to decompensated shock, need to be excluded as well.

Mortality and morbidity are related to multiple factors. These include mechanism, patient age, underlying pre-morbid state and hemodynamic status, and area of injury.

Although there are multiple specific mechanisms of penetrating trauma, for most purposes it is divided into low- and high-energy injury; in general, these correlate with stab wounds or gunshot wounds. Gunshot wounds may be further divided into low- and high-velocity injuries, although both have the ability to cause secondary injury by energy transfer, fragmentation, and secondary missiles such as bone fragments. Handguns and lower-caliber rifles such as

Table 75-1 APPROXIMATE PERCENTAGE OF INJURED ORGANS IN PENETRATING TRAUMA

Stab Wounds	Gunshot Wounds
Liver (40%)	Small bowel (50%)
Small bowel (30%)	Colon (40%)
Diaphragm (20%)	Liver (30%)
Colon (15%)	Abdominal vasculature (25%)

.22 gauge tend to have lower energy transfer than military rifles and hunting rifles. Shotgun injuries, although having lower velocity, often cause massive tissue damage if the wound is sustained at close range (i.e., less than 3 feet).

Classic teaching is that the majority (about 90%) of gunshot wounds to the abdomen penetrate the peritoneum.[8] However, recent studies looking at nonoperative management show that a larger number of nontangential wounds do not penetrate. If a patient is initially stable and without peritoneal signs, it is probably closer to about 40%; however, abdominal gunshot wounds with peritonitis or instability have clearly penetrated the peritoneum.[9] The majority of wounds that penetrate the peritoneum require a laparotomy for repair. The most commonly injured organs are the small bowel, colon, and liver, followed by vascular structures, stomach, and kidneys (Table 75-1).

Stab wounds, as opposed to gunshot wounds, tend to follow the tract of the wound and have more predictability. Approximately one fourth to one third of anterior abdominal stab wounds penetrate the peritoneum. Of those that penetrate, about one third cause intraabdominal injury that requires operative repair.

Structure and Function

■ ANATOMY

The *anterior abdomen* is the region between the anterior axillary lines from the anterior costal margins to the groin. The thoracoabdominal area is the region in which an injury can enter the chest or abdomen or both. In addition to the boundaries of the anterior abdomen, it includes the low chest bordered by the nipple line or fourth intercostal space anteriorly, the sixth intercostal space laterally, and the inferior scapular tip posteriorly. This is because the diaphragm may extend to this level with expiration. The flank is the area between the anterior and posterior axillary lines bilaterally ranging from the sixth intercostal space to the iliac crest. The back is bordered by the posterior axillary lines, with the inferior scapular tip superiorly and the iliac crest inferiorly. In addition, depending on the type of penetrating object, there may be simultaneous abdominal and thoracic penetration. Within the abdominal cavity, there may be injury to both intraperitoneal and retroperitoneal organs. Intraperitoneal organs include the liver, spleen, small bowel, transverse colon, gallbladder, and bladder. Retroperitoneal structures include the duodenum, pancreas, kidneys, ureters, bladder, ascending and descending colon, aorta and branching vessels, and rectum.[10]

Presenting Signs and Symptoms

■ TYPICAL FINDINGS

Patients may present with peritonitis and hypotension after a penetrating injury. They may have a rigid abdomen with both voluntary and involuntary guarding and generalized tenderness. There may be obvious signs of shock or hypoperfusion of vital organs including tachycardia, tachypnea, diaphoresis, confusion, and decreased urine output. Hypotension early after a penetrating injury is usually due an injury to a vascular structure or to an intraperitoneal solid viscous injury such as a liver or spleen laceration.

■ VARIATIONS

■ Isolated Bowel Injuries

The patient with bowel injury alone or injury to the liver or spleen without significant bleeding may present with minimal symptoms initially. Given that bowel or hollow viscus injury is much more common in penetrating trauma than blunt, the emergency physician must be careful to search for these sometimes subtle or delayed findings. Tenderness at the wound site is normal, but peritoneal findings such as diffuse tenderness and muscular rigidity, regardless of stability, are usually indicative of the need for operative intervention.[11] These findings often will present several hours into a patient's course if injury is due to rupture of hollow viscus. Over time, intraperitoneal inflammation increases, stimulates somatic pain fibers, and manifests clinically.

■ Diaphragmatic Injuries

Diaphragmatic injuries can be diagnostic conundrums, as they may initially present dramatically but also can be occult and present with symptoms or even fatal complications years after the initial injury. Any patient with a thoracoabdominal injury may have a potential diaphragmatic injury. The occurrence of diaphragmatic injury varies from 7% to 42% in patients with penetrating thoracoabdominal trauma. The rate varies with the aggressiveness of evaluation; if it is not looked for, many diaphragmatic injuries will be missed. It tends to be highest in patients with left costal penetration.[12-14] Most left-sided tears, which are much more prevalent than right-sided tears, can be repaired surgically. A small right-sided tear may not need to be repaired because herniation is much less likely on this side due to the protection of the liver.

Table 75-2 OPTIONS FOR EVALUATION

Diagnostic Modalities	Advantages	Disadvantages
Local wound exploration	Inexpensive, bedside test; if negative, can discharge patient	Operator-dependent; may be inconclusive; not good for gunshot wound or impalements
Ultrasonography	Inexpensive, bedside test; high positive predictive value (90%) for therapeutic laparotomy	Operator-dependent; poor sensitivity for bowel injury; if negative, cannot exclude injury
Diagnostic peritoneal lavage	Highly sensitive, inexpensive; can diagnose small bowel and diaphragm injuries	Poor specificity; up to 25% negative laparotomies using lower limits of red blood cell counts
Computed tomography	Excellent for solid organ injuries; can often show lack of peritoneal penetration and obviate need for observation; test of choice for flank/back injuries, as it shows retroperitoneal structures	Expensive; requires radiation; variable sensitivity for bowel and diaphragm injuries; unless penetration of the peritoneum is clearly excluded, observation is required afterward
Laparoscopy	Test of choice for left-sided thoracoabdominal wounds; can exclude peritoneal penetration and also screen for more serious injury; can be used for repair in selected cases	Expensive; associated complications; requires operating room

In addition to wounds involving the abdominal cavity, injuries to the thoracic cavity must also be considered in patients with thoracoabdominal stab wounds or any gunshot wound. It is also useful to take a thorough history to exclude additional blunt trauma or injury due to domestic violence.

Interventions and Procedures

Most interventions and procedures in penetrating trauma (Table 75-2) are aimed at first distinguishing if there was intraabdominal penetration and, if so, then deciding if the patient can avoid a nontherapeutic laparotomy. Although mandatory exploration was once the paradigm for penetrating injuries, knowledge of significant morbidity from negative laparotomy has pushed surgeons toward a much more conservative approach in management.[15,16]

■ LOCAL WOUND EXPLORATION

For the patient with an anterior stab wound, local wound exploration can be a valuable diagnostic aid and should shorten a prolonged evaluation or observation if results are negative. Its utility is dependent on the wound's mechanism and location. Stab wounds to the anterior abdomen are well suited for local wound exploration, because many do not penetrate the fascia. Back, flank, and thoracoabdominal wounds do not allow a clear delineation of the wound tract and extent and are not candidates for this procedure. Likewise, this is a poor option for gunshot wounds or wounds from a sharp pinpoint instrument (e.g., ice pick).

Exploration requires aseptic technique, good overhead lighting, and local lidocaine and epinephrine anesthesia. Inserting a digit into the wound is not acceptable. Obese or noncooperative patients and patients with abdominal scarring from previous operations are not optimal candidates. Paralleling natural skin lines, the wound is enlarged as necessary so that the posterior fascia may be evaluated. If penetration of the anterior fascia has occurred or if the wound exploration is inconclusive, the wound is considered intraperitoneal and must be evaluated further by more invasive methods or by observation and serial examinations. If the fascia is clearly intact, the wound can be irrigated, closed by primary intention if clean, and the patient discharged. Alternatively, the initial wound closed by secondary intention or delayed primary closure.[17]

PRIORITY ACTIONS

- Immediate attention to the ABCs (airway, breathing, and circulation)
- Immediate transport to operating room for diffuse peritonitis or hemodynamic stability
- Evaluation of stable patient to exclude peritoneal penetration
- Admission if there is penetration or evaluation is unclear
- Antibiotics if operation is planned
- Documentation of the location and appearance of all wounds
- Consultation with trauma practitioner or general surgeon
- Exclusion of pulmonary, diaphragm, or cardiac injury

■ DIAGNOSTIC PERITONEAL LAVAGE

Although not practiced as commonly as in the past, diagnostic peritoneal lavage is still a useful and acceptable screening tool for penetrating abdominal trauma. In the patient with unstable blunt trauma, it has been supplanted by ultrasonography. With penetrating trauma, its major benefit is its high sensitivity in screening for intraabdominal penetration and injury to abdominal structures. The main drawback, in addition to a small but real number of complications, is the lack of specificity. That is, it tends to diagnose injuries that may be treated by observation alone. For this reason, diagnostic peritoneal lavage is sometimes used in patients with penetrating trauma in conjunction with less invasive procedures such as laparoscopy. For patients with penetrating trauma who are hemodynamically unstable, it usually is not required to confirm what is already a high pretest probability that they require surgery. It can be of use, however, it there are other possible causes of instability, especially in patients with thoracoabdominal trauma.

A grossly bloody lavage effluent (10 mL of blood on initial aspiration) is always considered positive, although even with this finding, some trauma centers will not immediately operate. If the effluent is not bloody on initial aspiration, a liter of normal saline is instilled and then returned, and the effluent is sent to the lab for analysis. In patients with penetrating anterior abdominal wounds, lavage is always considered positive if the aspirate contains food particles, bile, or urine.

Cell counts tend to be a bit more controversial. There is no universally accepted number for a positive lavage result by cell count. If one is looking for penetration only, which may be useful when assessing gunshot wounds or diaphragm injuries, some institutions use as little as $1000/mm^3$; a more common and specific number, however, is $10,000/mm^3$. Although some centers use the cell count as an indication for laparotomy, others consider it complementary to observation or use CT or laparoscopy, depending on the wound.

When assessing anterior abdominal wounds for injury and not just penetration, many institutions consider a cell count between $50,000/mm^3$ and $100,000/mm^3$ positive; a white blood cell count greater than $500/mm^3$ also has been used. However, these do not seem to be particularly sensitive or specific.[18] Lavage alkaline phosphatase and amylase levels have been advocated; however, it is not clear that they add much to standard criteria.[19]

Although not universally practiced, Otomo's criteria have been shown to be highly accurate in small studies.[20] His criteria for positive results include the following: (1) a lavage white blood cell count greater than a lavage red blood cell count divided by 150 (i.e., L-WBC > [L-RBC/150]); and (2) a lavage white blood cell count greater than or equal to $500/mm^3$ (i.e., L-WBC ≥ $500/mm^3$) combined with a ratio of lavage white blood cell count to red blood cell count divided by a ratio of peripheral white blood cell count to red blood cell count greater than or equal to 1 (i.e., [L-WBC/L-RBC]/[P-WBC/P-RBC] ≥ 1).

Documentation

History

- Time of injury, number of assailants, gunshots, and so on, if known.
- Field interventions.

Physical Examination

- Document all wounds. Do not document as "entrance and exit" but as specific areas. Draw simple picture of wounds.
- Consider having police or security in hospital take photographs of injuries.
- Document that patient was completely examined, including groin, back, and perineal and axillary region.

Treatment

- Document all interventions and response to treatment. If patient is to be transferred, document reason(s) for decision as well as name of accepting physician. Document if surgical service is involved and time of call and arrival.
- Document all radiologic tests and results.
- Document procedure notes for all significant interventions (e.g., wound exploration, chest thoracostomy, diagnostic peritoneal lavage).
- Save and bag all clothing removed from patient.

LAPAROSCOPY

Minimally invasive laparoscopic surgery has gained general acceptance as a diagnostic and therapeutic modality in several circumstances. Although the specific injury may not always be identified, laparoscopy appears highly specific in identifying the need for a therapeutic laparotomy. More important, in many instances it can rule out the need for laparotomy completely with a high degree of sensitivity. Its most accepted use is for low-velocity wounds when there is a possibility of diaphragmatic injury. It is also an excellent tool to use for stable patients with possible or definite anterior abdominal wounds to screen for peritoneal penetration and the need for laparotomy. It may be used in the operating room as an initial intervention in the stable patient with penetrating abdominal trauma and an equivocal physical examination. It allows a survey of the abdominal contents, repair of minor injuries, and possible avoidance of laparotomy with its associated complications. Furthermore, laparoscopy may reduce costs and length of hospital stays when used for evaluating a population of stable patients.[12,14,21]

MEDICATION

Antibiotics

Administer antibiotics to any patient with a penetrating injury who will undergo operative intervention.

Perioperative antimicrobial coverage directed against skin and enteric flora will decrease postoperative wound infections. A single agent with broad-spectrum aerobic and anerobic coverage is recommended. Alternatively, combination therapy with clindamycin or cefazolin and an aminoglycoside is appropriate. Patients allergic to cephalosporin or penicillin may receive vancomycin instead for gram-positive coverage.

There are no clear guidelines for patients with wounds that have not penetrated the peritoneum and who will not undergo operation. Essential to decreasing wound infection is high-pressure irrigation. It may be reasonable to offer a 5-day course of prophylactic antibiotics to patients who have significant devitalized tissue or irretrievable foreign bodies. It is more judicious to allow closure by secondary or delayed primary intention of these wounds.

■ Tetanus Prophylaxis

Due the rarity of the disease and successful public health measures, clinical tetanus is exceedingly rare in the United States. Only one case of a traumatic gunshot wound was reported to cause tetanus in the United States between 1998 and 2000. Penetrating trauma may carry *Clostridium tetani* into the wound, but most U.S.-born patients are properly immunized. A prospective observational case series in 2004 found seroprevalence of tetanus immunity of 90.2% in 1988 patients presenting to five U.S. urban emergency departments with acute wounds. Patients at higher risk are those who are elderly and are from outside North America or western Europe. There appears to be a higher risk in Mexican-Americans between 20 and 44 years of age who were born outside of the United States. Most cases worldwide are due to neonatal tetanus.[22]

If they have not received a tetanus shot within the previous 10 years, patients with stab or gunshot wounds should be treated with tetanus toxoid. All patients not previously fully immunized or with an unclear status should be given both tetanus toxoid and tetanus immunoglobulin. It is not always necessary to give the booster in the ED, as it may be given up to several days after the injury. However, this is often preferable because tetanus immunization may not be part of the usual care in the hospital or outpatient setting.

■ Pain Control

This continues to be a source of controversy and discussion among and within the specialties of emergency medicine, surgery, and anesthesia. Although pain control generally is felt to be appropriate and safe in patients with nontraumatic abdominal pain, there is little scientific literature to guide treatment of patients with traumatic injury when observation is planned.

It seems clear that in a patient who will require operative intervention, withholding pain control offers no diagnostic benefit. Care should be taken, however, before giving large doses of pain medication that may decrease the blood pressure or when treating patients with preexisting shock. Fentanyl, titrated appropriately, due to its better hemodynamic profile, may be a better choice than morphine sulfate in these patients.

Diagnostic Testing

■ PHYSICAL EXAMINATION

Unlike cases of blunt trauma, physical examination clearly plays a role in the management of patients with penetrating abdominal trauma. Serial examinations are a common and time-tested management strategy for low-velocity wounds. Studies show that this is an effective approach and that delay in diagnosis, if less than 24 hours, does not lead to a significant increase in complications. Furthermore, the decrease in morbidity and costs of nontherapeutic laparotomies is considerable.[23-25] In fact, in some centers, even patients with evisceration without peritonitis are observed successfully after replacement of the eviscerated peritoneal contents, although this remains highly controversial.[26-28]

Examination may be used as a sole modality or in conjunction with other modalities. Over the last decade, patients with gunshot wounds have also been managed with serial observation, although usually in conjunction with some other modality, usually a CT scan. The length of time of observation varies by institution. Standard practice is usually a 23-hour observation period, but recent data suggest that all important injuries will manifest within a 12-hour period.[29] Until more data are available, or there is a clear institutional protocol, a 23-hour observation period is appropriate.

■ PLAIN RADIOGRAPHY

Although plain abdominal radiography rarely adds to the evaluation of blunt abdominal trauma, in cases of penetrating trauma with projectiles or retained foreign bodies it allows one to account for bullets, shrapnel, and foreign bodies. If all foreign bodies are not accounted for, one must consider the possibility that the foreign body is intraluminal or intravascular and a potential source of emboli. In patients with stab wounds or injuries without a foreign body, radiography's utility lies in ruling out a broken instrument in the abdomen or in evaluating a large amount of free air consistent with a hollow viscus injury.

In thoracoabdominal trauma, chest radiography can identify the presence of a hemothorax, pneumothorax, and possibly a diaphragmatic injury. Unfortunately, the sensitivity for pneumothorax is variable, and at least two separate radiographs 4 to 6 hours apart must be taken to exclude a clinically significant pneumothorax. Diaphragmatic injuries are seen clearly on plain radiographs only about 30% of the time. They cannot be excluded based on a normal radiograph.

ULTRASONOGRAPHY

Focused assessment by sonography in trauma (FAST) is a useful test if positive (i.e., free fluid is found on the examination). Several authors have shown specificity and positive predictive values in the low 90th percentile for therapeutic laparotomy if the ultrasound reveals free fluid. A positive ultrasound after penetrating abdominal trauma should lead to an exploration, either by laparotomy or laparoscopy. Unfortunately, while the specificity is very high, sensitivity is only 40% to 70%, which is not acceptable to rule out an injury requiring laparotomy.[30-32] Therefore, a FAST test negative for free fluid should be considered an indeterminate test with the need for further observation or testing. The FAST test should be able, in trained hands, to rule out a significant pericardial effusion in thoracoabdominal trauma.

COMPUTED TOMOGRAPHY SCANNING

The use of CT represents a major change in the initial evaluation of penetrating trauma in the past decade. As the technology improves and multidetector CT scans become commonplace, its use in penetrating trauma will continue to broaden and evolve. In the past, CT has been limited in penetrating abdominal trauma because of the high incidence of bowel injuries. Historically, it has been relatively insensitive in diagnosing bowel and mesenteric injuries as well as rents in the diaphragm. The newest-generation CT scanners (i.e., multidetector scanners) have markedly improved resolution and diagnostic capabilities. They may reveal the path of a bullet or knife as well as identify or rule out peritoneal violation and may show with increasing sensitivity signs of hollow viscus perforation (free intraperitoneal air, unexplained free fluid, or bowel edema). They remain excellent in diagnosing solid organ injury. In addition, CT scans may show a "contrast blush," a sign of active bleeding or false aneurysms in solid-organ injuries, and may establish whether early laparotomy or angiographic intervention is warranted.[16]

Although it has not been shown to have high enough sensitivity to rule out diaphragmatic injuries, CT imaging has improved and may one day be useful for this role.[33] CT imaging now has an accepted use in stable patients with penetrating flank trauma. The "triple contrast" (intravenous/oral/rectal) CT can has been found to be highly sensitive in diagnosing injuries to the retroperitoneal structures, including bowel and renal injuries. At this time, however, the sensitivity is too low to fully exclude a bowel injury, and a negative CT scan should be followed by a period of observation, usually 23 hours. The one caveat to this is that it should be clear on CT that the wound tract is superficial and that there was no intra- or retroperitoneal penetration.

Over the past decade, many trauma centers, led by an active group at University of Southern California, have explored the role of CT scanning in nontangential gunshot wounds. They have found that in the stable patient without peritonitis, approximately 25% of those who undergo CT scanning will need laparotomy, and the CT scan has 90% sensitivity and 95% specificity for identifying intraperitoneal injury. There does not appear to be a major increase in morbidity in the few patients who have a delayed operation.[9,16]

Tips and Tricks

- Always fully undress patient and examine back, axilla, and groin areas for occult penetrating trauma.
- Always account for all bullets in cases of penetrating trauma (e.g., if there is only one wound, the bullet should still be inside the body).
- In general, the number of bullets and the number of entrance/exit wounds should add to an even number. For example, a single wound would suggest that there is still a bullet in the body (1 bullet + 1 wound = 2). Three wounds suggests either one or three bullets in the body (2 entrance wounds + 1 exit wound + 1 bullet = 4; 3 entrance wounds + 3 bullets = 6).
- You can use ultrasonography to rapidly distinguish hypovolemic shock from distributive shock by looking for collapse of the inferior vena cava with inspiration.
- Penetrating trauma is a reportable injury in most of the United States. Make sure your ED is in compliance with local laws.
- A single chest radiograph cannot exclude a pneumothorax with a thoracoabdominal wound.
- Negative ultrasonography results have no predictive value with penetrating abdominal trauma; however, positive ultrasonography findings have a high predictive value for a therapeutic laparotomy.

Admission

All patients who have a wound that penetrated the peritoneum should be admitted. Although several trauma centers are attempting early discharge, either in 12 hours or directly from the ED, this is not standard and should be performed only in institutions with well-developed guidelines.

Treatment and Disposition

Final disposition is usually based on injury location, implement used, hemodynamic status, and the EP's and surgeon's preferred evaluation methods. As discussed previously, several different approaches can be taken, with a spectrum of conservative observation to aggressive operative approaches. As is true with all trauma, the ABCs (airway, breathing, and circulation) are the first line in management In general, patients who evidence signs of shock or diffuse peritoneal findings should be taken to the operating room. The one caveat is that patients who may have concomitant cardiac or pulmonary injuries should have them ruled out as a source of hypotension.

Resuscitation of hypotensive patients remains a widely discussed and controversial area of treatment. The Advanced Trauma Life Support (ATLS) standard treatment is to administer two liters of intravenous fluid followed by blood transfusion; however, some ED clinicians prefer to limit resuscitation until definitive control is obtained,[34] because of concerns that elevation in blood pressure through aggressive administration of fluids may disrupt clots and clotting factors, as well as evidence in multiple animal studies that less aggressive resuscitation or "permissive hypotension" leads to improved outcomes.

Only two large prospective trials have been carried out in humans, a study of penetrating torso injuries by Bickell and colleagues[36] and a study of a combination of blunt and penetrating injuries by Dutton and co-workers. The Bickell trial enrolled 598 patients with penetrating trauma and a systolic blood pressure of less than or equal to 90 mm Hg. The authors found a trend toward lower mortality and morbidity in the minimally resuscitated patients, although the "appropriately resuscitated" patients, or those with standard high fluid volume, had blood pressures that were significantly higher after resuscitation, but before surgery. The Dutton study[35] of approximately 100 patients compared outcomes of actively bleeding patients treated with the standard resusciation protocol with patients treated with a "hypotensive resuscitation" protocol, with a target systolic blood pressure of 70 mm Hg. Neither the standard group nor the hypotensive group showed improvements in mortality or worse outcomes; however, there was difficulty reaching target blood pressures. In the authors' judgment, limiting resuscitation with normal saline and blood to reach a target systolic blood pressure of around 90 mm Hg appears reasonable. It may not be feasible, appropriate, or beneficial to allow the blood pressure to decrease much lower.

Disposition and treatment of patients' specific injuries are described in the following sections.

■ ANTERIOR STAB WOUNDS

In patients with anterior stab wounds, the first step is to decide if there was peritoneal penetration. This may be accomplished by local wound exploration, diagnostic peritoneal lavage, or CT scan. If the lavage or local exploration is clearly negative, no further management other than local wound care is indicated. If lavage or CT scanning shows peritoneal penetration but no indication for emergent surgery, options include laparoscopy, laparotomy, and serial observation. Depending on the center, all may be appropriate, although laparoscopy or serial observation provides the best risk/benefit balance. In order for observation to be successful, patients must be able to cooperate with serial examinations, must evidence continued hemodynamic stability, and should not develop peritonitis. Prolonged observation is rarely possible in the ED, and these patients are generally admitted to a surgical service where serial examinations are possible.

■ FLANK WOUNDS

Flank wounds require triple contrast CT scanning. If results are negative, a period of observation is standard. If there is a left-sided thoracoabdominal wound, a negative ED workup is often followed by laparoscopy to exclude an occult diaphragmatic injury. Patients who have stab wounds to the flank or back and are stable and without obvious signs of bowel injury (peritonitis, hypotension) should undergo triple contrast CT scanning of the abdomen and pelvis. If results are negative, such patients should be admitted for 23-hour observation, as previously described.

■ GUNSHOT WOUNDS

It is common and acceptable to explore all gunshot wounds that penetrate the peritoneum. If it is unclear whether penetration has taken place a plain film radiograph may show an intraperitoneal bullet. Alternatively, diagnostic peritoneal lavage with appropriate cell counts is sensitive for intraperitoneal injury. A positive FAST test with free fluid in the abdomen should prompt operative exploration. Although physical examination has been advocated, this usually is performed in conjunction with an intravenous and/or oral contrast CT scan of the abdomen and pelvis. If it is clear that penetration of the peritoneum did not occur, the patient may be discharged. If penetration occurred, the patient may remain under observation or may undergo laparotomy or possibly laparoscopy or angiography, depending on the injury complex.

REFERENCES

1. Bamberger PK: The adoption of laparotomy for the treatment of penetrating abdominal wounds in war. Mil Med 1996;161:189-196.
2. Bennett JD: Abdominal surgery in war—the early story. J R Soc Med 1991;84:554-557.
3. Nicholas JM, Rix EP, Easley KA, et al: Changing patterns in the management of penetrating abdominal trauma: The more things change, the more they stay the same. J Trauma 2003;55:1095-1108; discussion, 1108-1110.
4. Mueller RS III: Federal Bureau of Investigation. Preliminary Annual Uniform Crime Report, 2005. Available at www.fbi.gov/vcr/2005preliminary/index.htm.
5. Zautck JL, Morris RW, Koenigsberg M, et al: Assaults from penetrating trauma in the State of Illinois. Am J Emerg Med 1998;16:553-556.

6. Demetriades, Gkiokas G, Velmahos GC, et al: Alcohol and illicit drugs in traumatic deaths: Prevalence and association with type and severity of injuries. J Am Coll Surg 2004;199:687-692.
7. Centers for Disease Control and Prevention, National Center for Injury Prevention and Control: Web-based Injury Statistics Query and Reporting System. Available at www.cdc.gov/ncipc/wisqars.
8. Moore EE, Moore JB, Van Duzer-Moore S, et al: Mandatory laparotomy for gunshot wounds penetrating the abdomen. Am J Surg 1980;140:847-851.
9. Velmahos GC, Constantinou C, Tillou A, et al: Abdominal computed tomographic scan for patients with gunshot wounds to the abdomen selected for nonoperative management. J Trauma 2005;59:1155-1160; discussion, 1160-1161.
10. Courtney M Jr, Townsend DR, Beauchamp MB, et al (eds): Sabiston Textbook of Surgery, 17th ed. Philadelphia, WB Saunders, 2004.
11. Brown CV, Velmahos GC, Neville AL, et al: Hemodynamically "stable" patients with peritonitis after penetrating abdominal trauma: Identifying those who are bleeding. Arch Surg 2005;140:767-772.
12. Leppaniemi A, Haapiainen R: Occult diaphragmatic injuries caused by stab wounds. J Trauma 2003;55:646-650.
13. Stylianos S, King TC: Occult diaphragm injuries at celiotomy for left chest stab wounds. Am Surg 1992;58: 364-368.
14. Madden MR, Paull DE, Finkelstein JL, et al: Occult diaphragmatic injury from stab wounds to the lower chest and abdomen. J Trauma 1989;29:292-298.
15. Renz BM, Feliciano DV: Unnecessary laparotomies for trauma: A prospective study of morbidity. J Trauma 1995;38:350-356.
16. Demetriades D, Velmahos G: Technology-driven triage of abdominal trauma: The emerging era of nonoperative management. Annu Rev Med 2003;54:1-15.
17. Markovchick VJ, Moore EE, Moore J, et al: Local wound exploration of anterior abdominal stab wounds. J Emerg Med 1985;2:287-291.
18. Soyka JM, Martin M, Sloan EP, et al: Diagnostic peritoneal lavage: Is an isolated WBC count greater than or equal to 500/mm^3 predictive of intra-abdominal injury requiring celiotomy in blunt trauma patients? J Trauma 1990;30:874-879.
19. Megison SM, Weigelt JA: The value of alkaline phosphatase in peritoneal lavage. Ann Emerg Med 1990;19:503-505.
20. Sato T, Hirose Y, Saito H, et al: Diagnostic peritoneal lavage for diagnosing blunt hollow visceral injury: The accuracy of two different criteria and their combination. Surg Today 2005;35:935-939.
21. Ahmed N, Whelan J, Brownlee J, et al: The contribution of laparoscopy in evaluation of penetrating abdominal wounds. J Am Coll Surg 2005;201:213-216.
22. Rhee P, Nunley MK, Demetriades D, et al: Tetanus and trauma: A review and recommendations. J Trauma 2005;58:1082-1088.
23. Ertekin C, Yanar H, Taviloglu K, et al: Unnecessary laparotomy by using physical examination and different diagnostic modalities for penetrating abdominal stab wounds. Emerg Med J 2005;22:790-794.
24. van Haarst EP, van Bezooijen BP, Coene PP, et al: The efficacy of serial physical examination in penetrating abdominal trauma. Injury 1999;30:599-604.
25. Zubowski R, Nallathambi M, Ivatury R, et al: Selective conservatism in abdominal stab wounds: The efficacy of serial physical examination. J Trauma 1988;28:1665-1668.
26. Huizinga WK, Baker WL, Mtshali ZW: Selective management of abdominal and thoracic stab wounds with established peritoneal penetration: The eviscerated omentum. Am J Surg 1987;153:564-568.
27. Nagy K, Roberts R, Joseph K, et al: Evisceration after abdominal stab wounds: Is laparotomy required? J Trauma 1999;47:622-624; discussion, 624-626.
28. Arikan S, Kocakusak A, Yucel AF, et al: A prospective comparison of the selective observation and routine exploration methods for penetrating abdominal stab wounds with organ or omentum evisceration. J Trauma 2005;58: 526-532.
29. Alzamel HA, Cohn SM: When is it safe to discharge asymptomatic patients with abdominal stab wounds? J Trauma 2005;58:523-525.
30. Soffer D, McKenney MG, Cohn S, et al: A prospective evaluation of ultrasonography for the diagnosis of penetrating torso injury. J Trauma 2004;56:953-957; discussion, 957-959.
31. Udobi KF, Rodriguez A, Chiu WC, et al: Role of ultrasonography in penetrating abdominal trauma: A prospective clinical study. J Trauma 2001;50:475-479.
32. Boulanger BR, Kearney PA, Tsuei B, et al: The routine use of sonography in penetrating torso injury is beneficial. J Trauma 2001;51:320-325.
33. Sliker CW: Imaging of diaphragm injuries. Radiol Clin North Am 2006;44:199-211, vii.
34. Salomone JP, Ustin JS, McSwain NE Jr, et al: Opinions of trauma practitioners regarding prehospital interventions for critically injured patients. J Trauma 2005;58:509-515; discussion, 515-517.
35. Dutton RP, Mackenzie CF, Scalea TM: Hypotensive resuscitation during active hemorrhage: Impact on in-hospital mortality. J Trauma 2002;52:1141-1146.
36. Bickell WH, Wall MJ Jr, Pepe PE, et al: Immediate versus delayed fluid resuscitation for hypotensive patients with penetrating torso injuries. N Engl J Med 1994;331: 1105-1109.

Chapter **76**

Pelvic Fractures

Leigh A. Patterson

KEY POINTS

If a patient has displacement of 0.5 cm at any fracture site in the pelvis or has an "open book" pelvic fracture, massive transfusion may be needed.

About 70% of patients with a traumatically disrupted pelvic ring will have major associated injury.

Blood loss from open book pelvic fractures and vertical shear injuries can be life-threatening. Emergent binding of the pelvis can help reduce the pelvic volume and tamponade bleeding. Interventional radiology can embolize the vessels.

Binding the fractured pelvis too tightly should be avoided. Overcorrection may force sharp bony fragments into the pelvic vasculature and organs.

Epidemiology

Fractures of the bony pelvis account for 3% of all fractures; however, the overall mortality from pelvic ring injuries is 10% to 15%. Motor vehicle collisions involving cars or cars and pedestrians cause approximately 60% of pelvic fractures.[1] Side-impact car collisions more commonly cause pelvic fractures than do head-on car collisions.[2] Falls and motorcycle accidents are also significant causes of pelvic ring injuries.

Blood supply and innervation to the pelvic organs and lower extremities are intimately linked to the pelvic architecture. Major disruptions lead to life-threatening blood loss, damage to urogenital organs, and neurologic deficits. The EP must identify patients at risk for pelvic ring disruptions and aggressively work to control bleeding.

Structure and Function

■ BONY ANATOMY

The pelvis provides support for upright mobility by connecting the spine to the lower extremities. When viewed as a whole, the pelvis contains a major ring and two inferior rings. The triangular sacrum and two innominate bones form the major pelvic ring (Fig. 76-1).

The sacrum is a fusion of the five sacral vertebrae and distributes the weight of the upper body to the innominate bones. The sacrum also conducts the sacral nerve roots to the pelvic organs. Each innominate bone is a fusion of the ilium, ischium, and pubic bones, and the intersection of the fusion forms the acetabulum, which articulates with the femur.

Posteriorly, the innominates are anchored to the sacrum by the anterior and posterior iliac ligaments, two of the body's strongest ligaments. The sacrotuberous and sacrospinous ligaments attach the sacrum to the ischial tuberosity and ischial spines bilaterally, further reinforcing the posterior arch of the pelvic ring.

Anteriorly, the innominates are anchored to each other at the cartilaginous pubic symphisis. Because the innominates and sacrum are dense bone anchored together with equally dense connective tissue, disruption of the architecture of the major pelvic ring requires tremendous force and usually results in bony

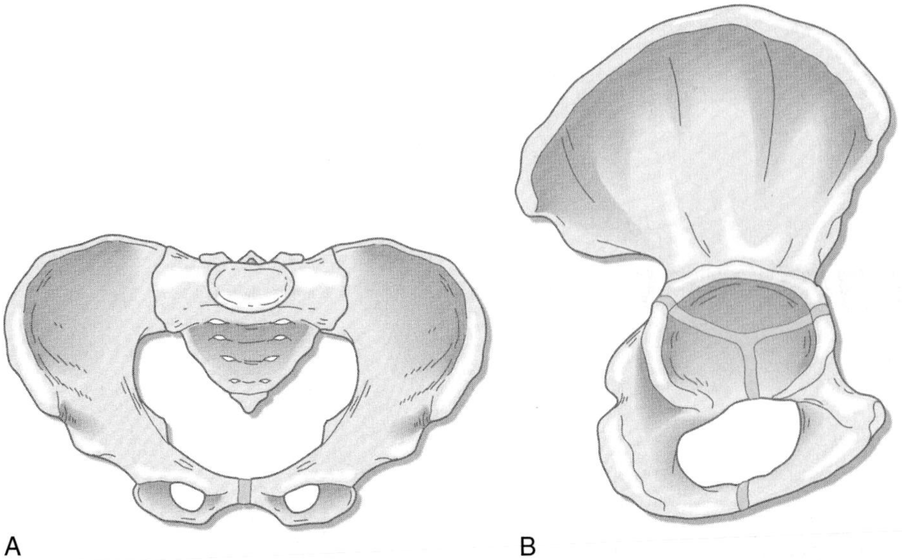
A
B

FIGURE 76-1 Bony pelvis. **A,** anteroposterior view. **B,** Innominate bone (lateral view).

fractures or ligamentous disruptions at two or more sites in the ring.

The inferior rings are formed by the pubic and ischial rami. They serve as attachments for muscles of the thighs and do not bear weight from the upper body. Low-force mechanisms such as straddle injuries and falls onto the buttocks can fracture the rings, usually an isolated pubic ramus.

■ VASCULAR ANATOMY

The left and right internal iliac arteries course in the region of the sacroiliac joints, branching and forming a network of vessels in the posterior pelvic arch. Posteriorly, the superior gluteal artery is commonly injured. Throughout the pelvis, arteries and veins are easily injured during the impact that causes the pelvic fracture, and the bleeding collects in the retroperitoneal space.

Pathophysiology

Lateral compression, from injuries to the side, crushes the pelvis inward; therefore massive pelvic bleeding is uncommon in these types of injury. Sacral crush fractures and horizontal pubic rami fractures can be diagnosed radiographically. Sacroiliac diastasis may also occur.

Anteroposterior compression forces the iliac wings outward, as when a pedestrian is struck directly anteriorly or posteriorly by a car. Pelvic volume increases, the fractures are unstable, and massive pelvic bleeding often occurs. Diastasis of the anterior pelvic ring may be evident, which is often termed an "open book" pelvic fracture. The posterior ligaments (as a guiding principle) can withstand about 2.5 cm of symphyseal diastasis before the sacral ligaments are disrupted. Associated acetabular fractures are common, present in about half of cases.

Vertical shear injuries are less common, resulting from axial force through the legs or spine to the pelvis. The anterior and posterior rings are both disrupted. As the hemipelvis is forcibly sheared, the pelvic volume increases, resulting in massive bleeding.

There are several classification schemes for pelvic ring disruptions that involve the direction of force applied to the pelvis, the bones injured, the degree of instability to the ring, and any associated injuries. Fracture stability and increases in pelvic volume determine the magnitude of blood loss and potential mortality.

■ TILE CLASSIFICATION OF PELVIC FRACTURES

The Tile classification adopted by the Orthopedic Trauma Association[3] describes pelvic fractures by degree of stability. The type and degree of stability predict outcome and associated injuries (Box 76-1). Type A fractures are stable and include avulsion fractures and isolated fractures of an inferior pubic ramus, iliac wing, or distal sacrum. These fractures cause local pain but do involve the major pelvic ring.

Type B and C fractures are unstable fractures resulting from high-energy forces. In both type B and C classes, the pelvic ring is disrupted in two or more places. These disruptions can be any combination of fractures and ligament tears. Disruptions may be unilateral, involving only one hemipelvis, or bilateral, with one or more disruptions to both hemipelves.

Type B fractures are vertically stable but rotationally unstable. These ring disruptions usually involve the anterior structures, the superior pubic rami and pubic symphisis, and the anterior iliac ligaments. The sacrum and the posterior iliac ligaments are spared. Lateral trauma from a side impact MVC or anteroposterior (AP) trauma from a front impact MVC can

Table 76-1 AVULSION PELVIC FRACTURES

Fracture Site	Muscle Involved	Type of Sport	Hip Movement	Initial Treatment	Healing Time
ASIS	Sartorius	Soccer	Flexion/abduction	Limit weight bearing with crutches	10 weeks
AIIS	Rectus femoris	Sprint runner Kicking	Forced flexion in starting block Hyperextension of hip with knee flexion	Bed rest with rectus femoris relaxed (hip and knee flexed)	6 weeks
Ischial tuberosity	Hamstring	Hurdler, long jumper, gymnast	Forced extension at hip	Bed rest	12 weeks

AIIS, anterior inferior iliac spine; ASIS, anterior superior iliac spine.

BOX 76-1

Most Common and Most Threatening Pelvic Fractures*

Most Common

- Inferior pubic ramus fractures (type A)
- Avulsion fractures (type A)
- Lateral compression fractures (type B)

Most Threatening

- Open book pelvic fractures (type B)
- Type C fractures

*See Tile Classification of Pelvic Fractures in text for discussion of types of fractures.

cause fractures in this class. The axis of a bony fracture is determined by the orientation of the force applied to the pelvis.

Type C fractures are both vertically and rotationally unstable because the posterior elements of the major pelvic ring are disrupted by a fracture through the sacroiliac joint, which is a complete tear. In addition to lateral and anteroposterior forces, vertical shear mechanisms, including falls, can cause type C fractures.

Clinical Presentation

■ CLASSIC SIGNS AND SYMPTOMS

The classic presentation of patient with a major pelvic ring disruption includes a chief complaint of pelvic pain or pain with movement at the hips.[4] However, nearly 70% of patients with a disruption of the major pelvic ring have associated injuries such as closed head trauma, blunt chest and abdomen trauma, and long bone fractures[1] that may mask the symptoms of pelvic pain.

The EP should first suspect a pelvic fracture based on the mechanism of injury and then search for additional signs of fracture during the physical examination. Uneven leg length or asymmetry of the iliac wings may indicate a pelvic fracture. The perineum is carefully exposed to visualize any flank ecchymoses, scrotal or labial hematomas, and blood at the urethral meatus. When examining the pelvis, the EP should assume that it is fractured and avoid actions that may distract or displace a fracture. The iliac wings are gently palpated and compressed medially. The pubic symphisis is palpated anteriorly, and the sacrum and sacroiliac joints are palpated posteriorly. The rectum is examined for tone; in females, a manual vaginal examination is performed to check for bone protruding into the vagina.

If there are no obvious fractures of the lower extremities, the femurs are rotated at the hips to assess for pain in the acetabulae. Pain elicited by physical examination is 98% sensitive and 94% specific in predicting pelvic fracture of the posterior aspect of the pelvic ring.[5]

■ VARIATIONS—AVULSION FRACTURES

Avulsion fractures of the pelvis at muscle insertion sites are caused by forced contraction of thigh muscles when moving the hip.[6] The apophyses at the anterior superior iliac spine, the anterior inferior iliac spine, and the ischial tuberosity fuse between the ages of 16 and 25. Adolescent athletes involved in strenuous sports are vulnerable to these injuries. The EP should suspect these injuries based on the mechanism of the injury (Table 76-1).

Differential Diagnosis

The differential diagnosis for major pelvic ring disruption includes fractures of the pelvis, acetabulum, hip, and femur. In a patient who has suffered a simple fall and who is hemodynamically stable and neurologically intact, a non-tender pelvis and leg length asymmetry suggests a hip fracture. However, in the patient who has suffered a major fall or who was injured in a motor vehicle collision, the fracture site may be difficult to differentiate clinically. All can cause leg length asymmetry and significant blood loss, and multiple fractures may exist simultaneously. Perineal hematomas, iliac crest asymmetry, and a palpably unstable pelvis all suggest a pelvic fracture, but this does not rule out a concomitant femur fracture. The patient with a significant traumatic fracture will require additional imaging.

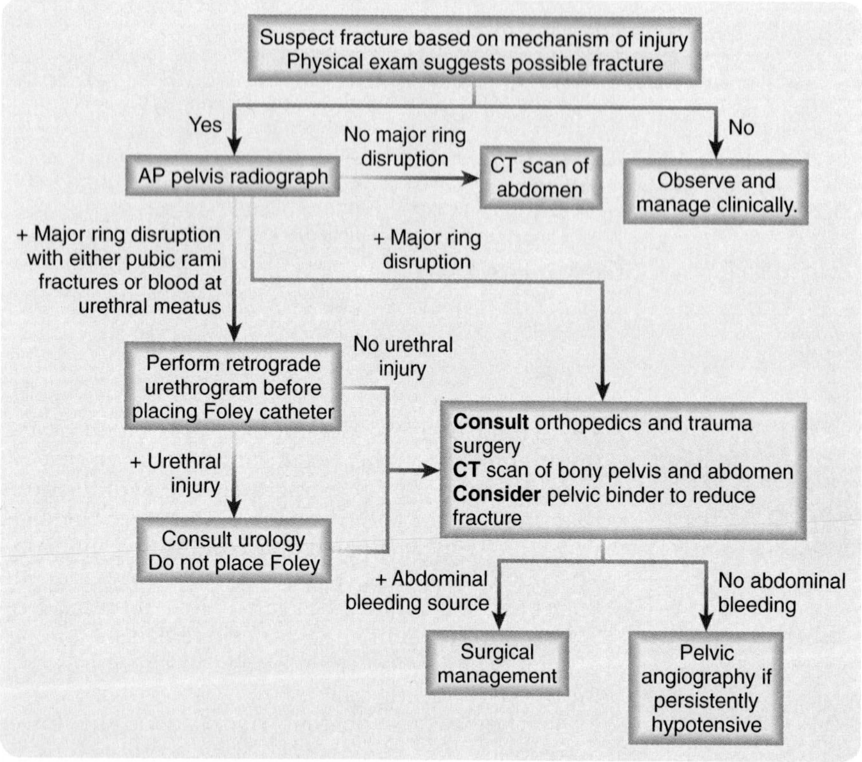
Suspect fracture based on mechanism of injury
Physical exam suggests possible fracture
Yes
No
AP pelvis radiograph
No major ring disruption
CT scan of abdomen
Observe and manage clinically.
+ Major ring disruption with either pubic rami fractures or blood at urethral meatus
+ Major ring disruption
Perform retrograde urethrogram before placing Foley catheter
No urethral injury
Consult orthopedics and trauma surgery
CT scan of bony pelvis and abdomen
Consider pelvic binder to reduce fracture
+ Urethral injury
Consult urology
Do not place Foley
+ Abdominal bleeding source
No abdominal bleeding
Surgical management
Pelvic angiography if persistently hypotensive

FIGURE 76-2 Diagnostic and treatment approach to patient with suspected disruption of major pelvic ring. AP, anteroposterior; CT, computed tomography.

Diagnostic Testing

Figure 76-2 outlines a diagnostic and treatment approach to patients with suspected pelvic ring disruption.

Interventions and Procedures

Pelvic fractures need to be rapidly reduced and fixated to prevent ongoing blood loss and promote healing. Reducing a major pelvic ring disruption should increase the interstitial pressure in the pelvis and at the bony surfaces of a fracture to tamponade venous bleeding. Pelvic volume is also directly related to diastasis at sites of ligamentous disruption, namely the pubic symphisis and sacroiliac joints. A 1-cm widening of the pubic symphisis allows the pelvic volume to expand 4.6%. A combined 8-cm widening of the pubic symphisis and sacroiliac joints would allow potentially 500 mL of blood to accumulate in the pelvis before the soft tissues even begin to tamponade the bleeding.[7]

Treatment and Disposition

Initially, the EP can reduce the fracture by applying a sheet circumferentially around the pelvis and tying it so that the pelvic volume is reduced. Commercial binders can be applied in the same manner. This reduction works best for fractures with external rotation of one or both hemipelves, such as the open book pelvic fracture.[8] The EP should be careful not to overcorrect the external rotation by binding the pelvis too tightly. Overcorrection could force sharp bony fragments into pelvic vasculature and organs.

Orthopedic surgery should be consulted early for reduction of pelvic ring disruptions. Circumferential binding is a temporary reduction and will not stabi-

PRIORITY ACTIONS

RESCUE Pelvis Mnemonic for Treatment of Patients with Pelvic Fractures

Resuscitate Patient

- ATLS protocols, IV fluids, pain control

Examine and Obtain Radiographs of Pelvis and Perineum

- Signs of pelvic fracture/instability, urethral injury, neurologic injury

Stabilize the Pelvic Ring

- Circumferential sheet, commercial pelvic binder

Consult Trauma, Orthopedics, and Urology

- Consult early

Evaluate for Nonpelvic Sources of Bleeding

- FAST, DPL, CT of abdomen

Pelvis Angiography

- Persistent hypotension despite stabilization efforts.

ATLS, advanced trauma life support; CT, computed tomography; DPL, diagnostic peritoneal lavage; FAST, focused assessment with sonography for trauma.

lize a vertically unstable fracture. Patients with ongoing blood loss may need external fixators to stabilize the ring.

Bleeding can be life-threatening. Mortality of patients with hemorrhagic shock from a pelvic fracture is about 50%. Early transfusion, particularly for patients with vertical shear or anteroposterior compression fractures, is indicated. If a patient has an 0.5-cm displacement at any fracture site in the pelvis or has an open book pelvic fracture, massive transfusion will likely be needed. Interventional radiology, for embolization of the bleeding vessels, can be life-saving.

Patients with unstable pelvic fractures will need to be admitted to a surgical intensive care unit for close hemodynamic and neurologic monitoring. Because many of these patients will have additional head, chest, abdomen, and limb injuries, they are best managed primarily by a trauma surgeon. If trauma surgery is not available, the EP must arrange critical care transport for these patients to a designated trauma center.

AVULSION FRACTURES

Initial treatment is supportive, and physical activity is resumed slowly over weeks to prevent repeat avulsion.[5] After pain control has been achieved, these patients can be discharged home with follow-up by the primary care physician. Follow-up should also be scheduled with a sports medicine specialist or orthopedic surgeon who will monitor healing and guide the patient's return to athletic activity.

REFERENCES

1. Gänsslen A, Pohlemann T, Paul C, et al: Epidemiology of pelvic ring injuries. Injury 1996;27(Suppl 1):S-A13-A20.
2. Rowe SA, Sochor MS, Staples KS, et al: Pelvic ring fractures: Implications of vehicle design, crash type, and occupant characteristics. Surgery 2004;136:842-847.
3. Fracture and dislocation compendium. Orthopedic Trauma Association Committee for Coding and Classification. J Orthop Trauma 1996;10 Suppl 1:66-75.
4. Gonzalez RP, Fried PQ, Bukhalo M: The utility of clinical examination in screening for pelvic fractures in blunt trauma. J Am Coll Surg 2002;194:121-125.
5. McCormick JP, Morgan SJ, Smith WR: Clinical effectiveness of the physical examination in diagnosis of posterior pelvic ring injuries. J Orthoped Trauma 2003;17:257-261.
6. Scopp JM, Moorman CT: Acute athletic trauma to the hip and pelvis. Orthoped Clin North Am 200;33:555-563.
7. Moss MC, Bircher MD: Volume changes within the true pelvis during disruption of the pelvic ring—where does the haemorrhage go? Injury 1996;27(Suppl 1):S-A21-A23.
8. Krieg JC, Mohr M, Ellis TJ, et al: Emergent stabilization of pelvic ring injuries by controlled circumferential compression: A clinical trial. J Trauma 2005;59:659-664.

Chapter 77

Genitourinary Trauma

Michael S. Runyon and Michael A. Gibbs

KEY POINTS

Evaluate suspected genitourinary tract injuries in a retrograde fashion; evaluate for urethral disruption before bladder rupture before kidney or ureteral injury.

Suspect urethral injury and ensure integrity with retrograde urethrography prior to Foley catheter placement in blunt trauma patients with a significant pelvic fracture, blood at the urethral meatus, gross hematuria, an absent or abnormally positioned prostate on digital rectal examination, or ecchymosis or hematoma involving the penis, scrotum, or perineum.

Suspect bladder rupture and perform retrograde cystography or retrograde computed tomography (CT) cystography in blunt trauma patients with pelvic trauma and gross hematuria.

Suspect upper tract (kidney or ureter) injury and perform CT scanning with IV contrast, in blunt trauma patients with gross hematuria or microscopic hematuria with shock.

Suspect genitourinary involvement when a penetrating injury is inflicted in proximity to the genitourinary system; investigate accordingly, even in the absence of hematuria.

Scope

Approximately 10% of trauma patients sustain injury to the genitourinary system. The majority of these injuries (approximately 80%) are the result of a blunt trauma mechanism.

Timely identification and management of genitourinary injuries minimizes the associated morbidity, which may include impairment of urinary continence and sexual function. Injury identification depends on a step-wise evaluation with consideration of the mechanism of injury, pertinent physical examination findings, urinalysis, and appropriate diagnostic imaging performed in the correct sequence.

Anatomically, the genitourinary system is divided into the upper and lower tracts. The former consists of the kidneys and ureters; the latter includes the bladder, urethra, and the external genitalia. This division is clinically important as specific mechanisms tend to injure different parts of the genitourinary system.

Initial Assessment

■ HEMATURIA

Hematuria is a marker for potential injury to the genitourinary tract. It is important to inspect the initial urine output to avoid missing transient hematuria that may clear with ongoing fluid resuscitation. A spontaneously voided specimen is ideal but is frequently impractical in the multiply injured patient.

Gross hematuria is defined as urine that is any color other than clear or yellow. This is a necessarily con-

Documentation

- Note the presence or absence of any abnormalities that suggest genitourinary injury. In blunt trauma patients, these include:
  - Flank tenderness, bruising, or swelling
  - Significant pelvic fracture
  - Blood at the urethral meatus
  - An absent or abnormally positioned prostate on digital rectal examination
  - Ecchymosis or hematoma involving the penis, scrotum, or perineum
- In patients with penetrating trauma, note whether the injury trajectory occurs in proximity to the genitourinary tract.
- Document the presence or absence of hematuria in the *initial* urine specimen.

PRIORITY ACTIONS

- Because genitourinary injuries are rarely life-threatening, the initial assessment of the multiply injured patient is focused on the rapid identification of potentially life-threatening injuries with prompt intervention to preserve life.
- During the initial resuscitation, note any findings, such as gross hematuria or unstable pelvic fracture, that may herald genitourinary injury, so that the appropriate investigation may be undertaken once the patient has been stabilized.

servative definition because the degree of gross hematuria does not correlate with the severity of injury; a relatively minor urethral injury may result in impressive hemorrhage whereas major vascular disruption may present with only slightly discolored urine. False-positive results may be caused by many factors, including ingestion of certain food products or dyes, various medications, or the presence of free myoglobin due to rhabdomyolysis.

Microscopic hematuria is defined as more than 5 red blood cells per high-powered field (RBCs/hpf), or a positive dipstick evaluation.

The significance of gross versus microscopic hematuria varies with the mechanism of injury (blunt versus penetrating) and is discussed in more detail later in the chapter.

■ DIAGNOSTIC PRIORITIES AND INJURY STAGING

Ideally, investigation for genitourinary injury is conducted in a retrograde fashion beginning with evaluation of the external genitalia and urethra prior to that of the bladder. The ureters and kidneys are evaluated after lower tract injury is excluded, or after appropriate emergency management of an identified lower tract injury is initiated.

■ GENITOURINARY INJURIES IN THE PATIENT WITH MULTISYSTEM TRAUMA

Except in the rare instance of a shattered kidney or major renal vascular laceration with significant hemorrhage, genitourinary injuries seldom pose a life threat. As such, in the multiply injured patient, evaluation for genitourinary injury is deferred until other, potentially life-threatening injuries are excluded and the patient's condition is stabilized. During the initial evaluation and stabilization, the EP should note any findings that may herald genitourinary injury, so that the appropriate investigation may be undertaken once the immediate life-threatening conditions have been addressed. The patient should not receive any oral fluids until the need for operative intervention has been excluded. IV fluids and analgesics may be administered as needed.

■ Digital Rectal Examination

Although often delegated to the junior-most member of the examining team at teaching institutions, a careful digital rectal examination provides useful clinical information.

First, insert a well-lubricated gloved finger to assess the rectal tone. Decreased tone may be seen in patients with spinal cord injuries or those who have received neuromuscular blocking agents. Next, palpate anteriorly to identify the midline and two lobes of the prostate. An absent or "high-riding" prostate indicates a posterior urethral disruption until proved otherwise. Next, sweep the finger around the entire circumference of the rectal vault, feeling for lacerations and bone fragments. Finally, remove the finger and examine it for the presence of gross blood. To prevent false-positive results during this last step, ensure that the glove is free of blood prior to insertion.

■ Vaginal Examination

Although most multiply injured patients receive a digital rectal examination, the vaginal examination is often omitted in error. To avoid missing occult injuries that may result in significant and potentially life-threatening hemorrhage and infection, a careful vaginal examination should be performed to identify any lacerations or bone fragments in all women with pelvic fractures. This is especially critical in patients with fractures of the anterior pelvic ring.

Lower Genitourinary Tract Injuries

■ ANATOMY

The lower genitourinary tract consists of the external genitalia, urethra, and bladder (Figs. 77-1 and 77-2).

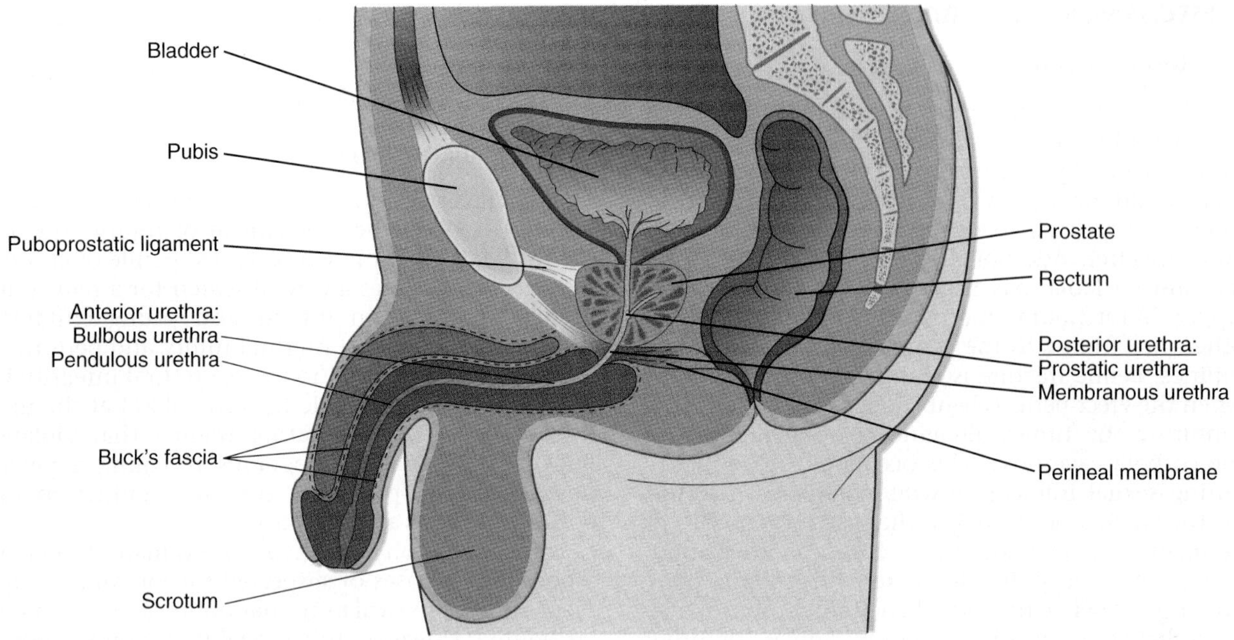
Bladder
Pubis
Puboprostatic ligament
Anterior urethra:
Bulbous urethra
Pendulous urethra
Buck's fascia
Scrotum
Prostate
Rectum
Posterior urethra:
Prostatic urethra
Membranous urethra
Perineal membrane

FIGURE 77-1 Sagittal view of the normal male pelvis.

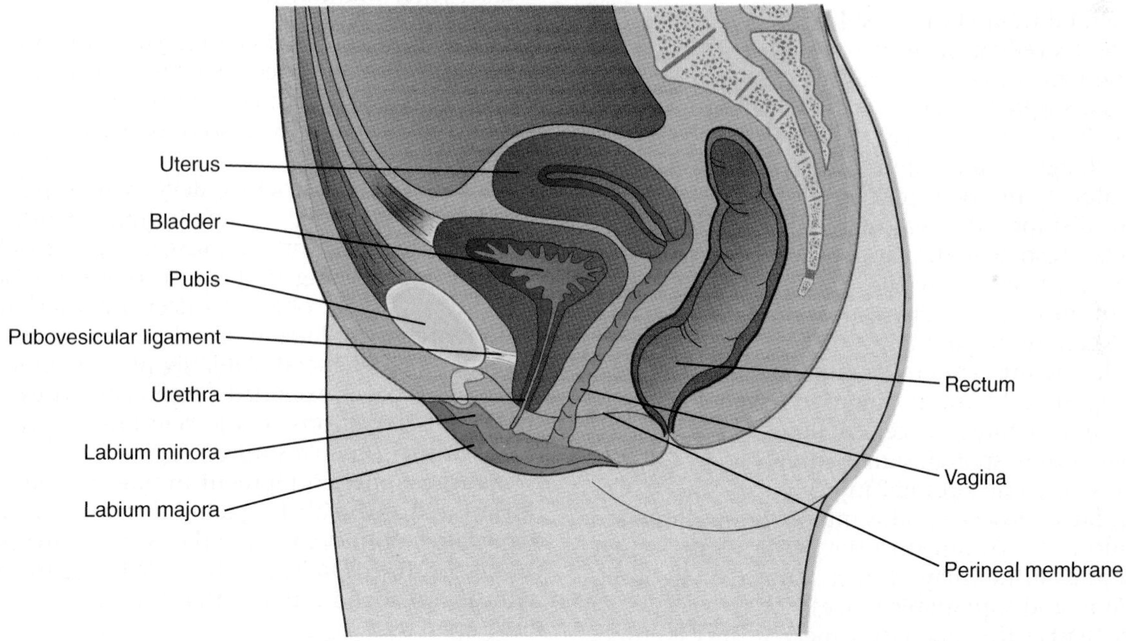
Uterus
Bladder
Pubis
Pubovesicular ligament
Urethra
Labium minora
Labium majora
Rectum
Vagina
Perineal membrane

FIGURE 77-2 Sagittal view of the normal female pelvis.

The male external genitalia consist of the penis, scrotum, testicles, and ejaculatory complex. The female external genitalia consist of the vagina and vulva; the latter includes the labia majora, labia minora, and clitoris. The male urethra is divided into the anterior (bulbous and pendulous) and posterior (prostatic and membranous) urethra. Traditionally, this division has been described at the level of the urogenital diaphragm; however, recent work has questioned the existence of this structure, as classically taught.[1-3] Regardless, the weakest point of the posterior urethra is the bulbomembranous junction and is the area where the majority of posterior urethral disruptions occur.[1]

When empty, the bladder lies along the floor of the pelvis, where it is relatively protected unless the force of an injury fractures the bony pelvis. When distended by urine, the bladder may extend up to the level of the umbilicus, where it is vulnerable to blunt force trauma inflicted on the lower abdomen. The weakest and most mobile area of the bladder is at the peritoneal surface of the dome.

MECHANISMS OF INJURY

External Genitalia

Injuries to the external genitalia may occur by blunt or penetrating mechanisms or by circulatory compromise induced by constricting devices applied either accidentally (as in the case of a hair tourniquet) or intentionally (e.g., to enhance sexual performance and pleasure). Additionally, the skin of the penis, scrotum, or labia may become ensnared by a metal zipper. Blunt trauma mechanisms include a kick or other direct blow to the genitals, falls, and straddle injuries. Penile fracture is a blunt injury that occurs when the erect penis is bent suddenly and forcefully, rupturing the tunica albuginea of one or both of the corpora cavernosa. This occurs most commonly during sexual intercourse when the penis slips out of the vagina and strikes the partner's pubis or perineum, but may also occur during masturbation. Significant injury to the external genitalia may accompany pelvic fractures. Penetrating injuries may be inflicted by gunshot wounds, knives, or other sharp objects.

Clinical Presentation

Blunt scrotal trauma may result in superficial ecchymosis and swelling or testicular rupture, torsion, or displacement. In testicular rupture, the tunica albuginea is disrupted. Even in the absence of testicular rupture, blood or fluid may accumulate between the tunica albuginea and tunica vaginalis, resulting in a hematocele or hydrocele, respectively. Testicular torsion disrupts the vascular supply and causes ischemia. Testicular displacement occurs when the testicle is forced from the scrotum, usually into the peritoneal cavity. Physical examination may be limited because of pain and swelling.

Penile fracture is often accompanied by an audible snapping sound and is followed immediately by severe pain, detumescence, swelling, and ecchymosis. The corpus spongiosum is involved in 20% to 30% of cases, and urethral injury occurs in 10% to 20%. If Buck's fascia remains intact, the swelling and ecchymosis are confined to the penile shaft. If not, blood and urine may dissect into the scrotum, perineum, and suprapubic spaces.[10-11]

In patients with penetrating mechanisms, conduct a careful and complete physical examination for associated or additional occult injuries. In one series, gunshot wounds to the penis were associated with injury to other organ structures in 80% of cases.[12] Violation of the corpora cavernosa requires operative intervention and is heralded by an expanding penile hematoma, significant bleeding from a wound to the penile shaft, or a palpable corporal defect.

Injuries to the female genitalia are often associated with pelvic fractures. Important mechanisms include physical or sexual assault, consensual intercourse, and penetrating injuries. In the presence of a pelvic fracture or blood at the introitus, a meticulous vaginal examination is mandated. The complications of missed vaginal injuries include infection, fistula formation, and significant hemorrhage.[13,14] In one series 25% of women sustaining injury of the external genitalia required red blood cell transfusion because of blood loss from genital injury alone.[13]

Diagnostic Strategies

The diagnosis of injuries to the external genitalia is largely based on the mechanism of injury and the physical examination. Unexplained penile or clitoral swelling necessitates a careful search for a hair tourniquet, especially in infants and young children. Consider concomitant urethral injury and perform a retrograde urethrogram to assess urethral integrity in any patient with a penile fracture, blood at the urethral meatus, or penetrating trauma that violates Buck's fascia. Plain radiographs revealing a pelvic fracture should prompt a careful examination for occult rectal or vaginal injury.

Ultrasonography is used to evaluate testicular blood flow in cases of suspected torsion and to supplement the physical examination in cases of testicular trauma. However, this modality has only modest sensitivity and specificity for detecting testicular rupture and is quite operator-dependent.[11,15]

Emergency Management

Control bleeding with direct pressure. An amputated penis should be wrapped in saline-moistened gauze and placed in a sealed plastic bag, which is then placed on ice in a second plastic bag until reimplantation.

Remove any constricting devices promptly. This may be accomplished by unwinding a hair tourniquet, cutting a tight-fitting constricting ring or band, or wrapping a string or Penrose drain around the penis distal to the object to decrease swelling and facilitate removal. Liberal use of a water-based lubricant may be beneficial. After significant underlying injury has been excluded, copiously irrigate any superficial lacerations to the scrotum or penis and close with absorbable suture.

Manage zipper entrapment injuries by infiltrating the affected area with 1% plain lidocaine followed by application of mineral oil and carefully "unzipping" the zipper. If this fails, cut the slide bar of the zipper with an orthopedic pin cutter and gently pull the teeth apart.

Definitive Management

Traumatic testicular torsion and displacement are treated surgically. All but the most superficial penetrating injuries to the external genitalia require operative exploration, especially those that violate the corpora cavernosa. Prompt surgical exploration and repair of penile fractures minimizes the late complications of penile curvature, erectile dysfunction, and dyspareunia.[10,11] Likewise, in patients with testicular rupture, early operative intervention maximizes the rate of testicular salvage.[11] Reimplantation of an amputated penis should be performed as expeditiously as possible, but has been successful after 16 hours of cold ischemia.[15] The majority of women with vaginal

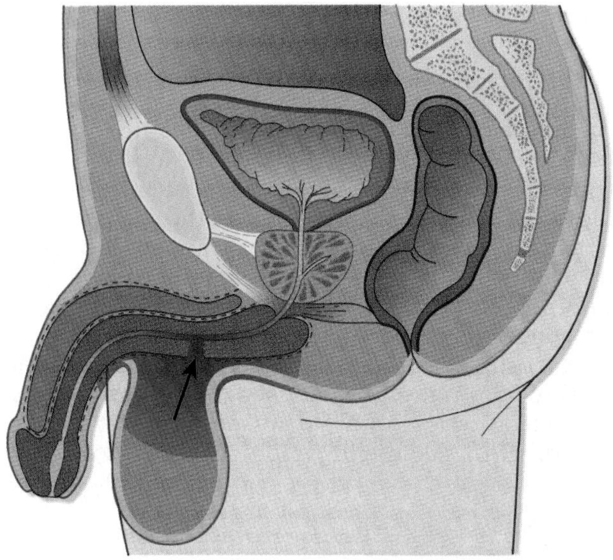

FIGURE 77-3 Anterior urethral injury. Note the extravasation of blood at the injury site with dissection into the tissues of the scrotum and perineum.

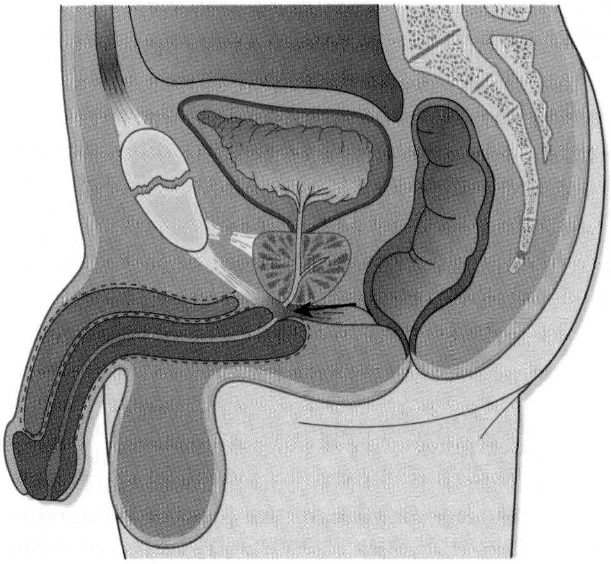

FIGURE 77-4 Posterior urethral injury. Note the displacement of the prostate by the hematoma at the site of injury.

injuries will require operative repair or washout to prevent significant morbidity and mortality.[13]

Urethra

Injuries to the anterior urethra occur from direct blows, straddle injuries, or instrumentation or in conjunction with a penile fracture (Fig. 77-3). By contrast, posterior urethral injuries usually occur in the setting of significant pelvic fractures, often caused by motor vehicle collisions (Fig. 77-4). Penetrating injuries may be inflicted by gunshot wounds, knives, or other sharp objects. Urethral injuries are much less common in women because the female urethra is short, is relatively mobile, and lacks significant attachment to the pubis.

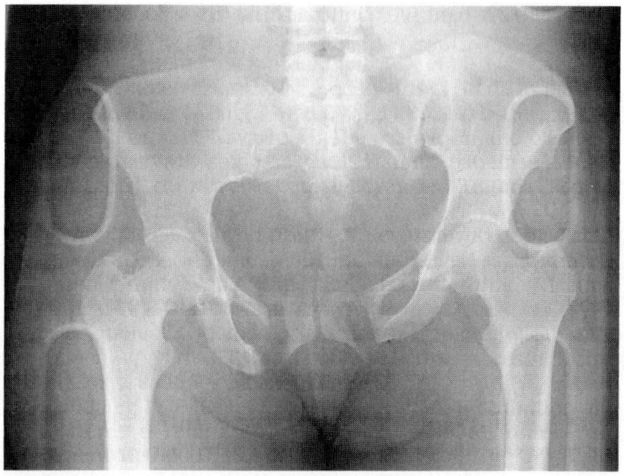

FIGURE 77-5 Straddle pelvic fracture. Note the concomitant fractures of all four pubic rami. This injury confers a high risk of urethral disruption.

Overall, urethral disruption accompanies pelvic fracture in approximately 5% of cases in women and up to 25% of cases in men.[1,4] However, the risk of urethral injury varies with pelvic fracture type. High-risk fractures include concomitant fractures of all four pubic rami (straddle fractures; Fig. 77-5) or when fractures of both ipsilateral rami are accompanied by massive posterior disruption through the sacrum, sacroiliac joint, or ilium.

Low-risk injuries include single ramus fractures and ipsilateral rami fractures without posterior ring disruption. The risk of urethral injury approaches zero with isolated fractures of the acetabulum, ilium, and sacrum.[1] Posterior urethral disruption occurs when a significant pelvic fracture causes upward displacement of the bladder and prostate. Avulsion of the puboprostatic ligament is followed by stretching of the membranous urethra, resulting in a partial or complete disruption at the anatomic weak point, the bulbomembranous junction.[1]

Clinical Presentation

In blunt trauma, the signs and symptoms of urethral injury include blood at the urethral meatus, gross hematuria, inability to void, an absent or abnormally positioned prostate on digital rectal examination, or ecchymosis or hematoma involving the penis, scrotum, or perineum. In penetrating trauma, urethral disruption should be suspected when the injury trajectory occurs in proximity to the course of the urethra.

Diagnostic Strategies

After the initial examination, an anteroposterior (AP) pelvis radiograph should be obtained to assess for fracture. In cases of suspected urethral injury it is imperative to evaluate the integrity of the urethra prior to attempting placement of a Foley catheter. This is accomplished by performance of a retrograde urethrogram. This procedure should be deferred if pelvic angiography is indicated, because extravasated contrast material from a urethral injury may obscure angiography images and complicate attempts to control significant pelvic hemorrhage by vascular embolization.

Retrograde Urethrography Procedure. Keep the patient supine to avoid potentially disrupting a stable pelvic hematoma. Obtain a baseline kidneys, ureter, and bladder (KUB) radiograph and ensure that the film captures the entire course of the urethra and bladder. Retract the foreskin, if present, and control the shaft of the penis with a 4-×4-inch gauze pad to prevent slippage. Stretch the penis obliquely over the thigh to promote unfolding and visualization of the entire urethra. Fill a 60-mL syringe with 10% water-soluble contrast (diluted in sterile saline) and attach a Christmas tree adaptor. Insert the adaptor snugly into the urethral meatus, ensuring a tight fit, because leaking contrast will result in a spurious study.

Alternatively, insert a Foley catheter a few centimeters into the urethra and inflate the balloon to ensure a snug fit within the fossa navicularis; next, attach a catheter-tip syringe filled with contrast as described previously. Inject 50 to 60 mL (0.6 mL/kg in children) of contrast and obtain a KUB radiograph simultaneously with infusion of the final 10 mL. Lack of urethral extravasation with filling of the bladder indicates a normal study. A partial disruption is indicated by urethral extravasation accompanied by partial filling of the bladder. A complete disruption results in urethral extravasation with no filling of the bladder (Fig 77-6).

Emergency Management

In patients with a low-risk pelvic fracture (as defined previously) and no evidence of urethral injury on physical examination, it is reasonable to make a gentle attempt at passage of a Foley catheter. If any significant resistance is met, remove the catheter and obtain a retrograde urethrogram. If the retrograde urethrogram is normal, insert the catheter and inspect the initial output for evidence of hematuria.

If a urethral injury is suspected subsequent to successful placement of a Foley catheter, do not remove the catheter! A retrograde urethrogram may be obtained by inserting a small feeding tube alongside the catheter and proceeding as described previously. Consult a urologist for management of patients with an abnormal retrograde urethrogram results, or in cases of suspected urethral injury when a retrograde urethrogram cannot be obtained. In female patients, suspected urethral injury mandates urologic consultation; retrograde urethrography is not indicated.

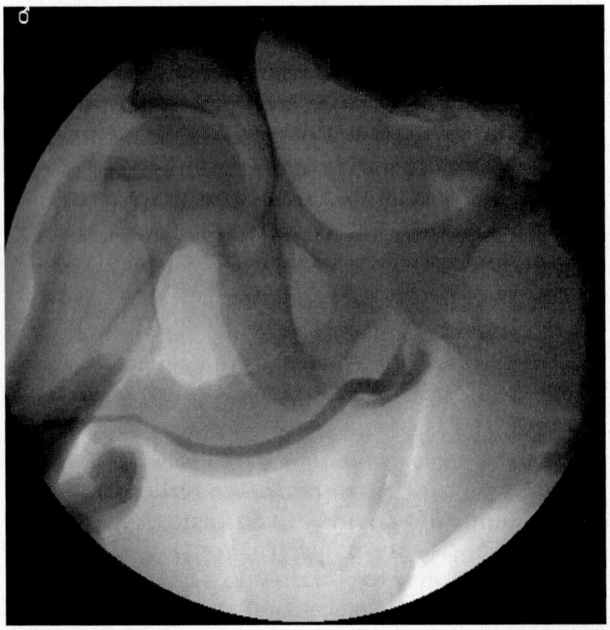

FIGURE 77-6 Retrograde urethrogram with complete urethral rupture at the level of the membranous urethra. Note that no contrast reaches the bladder.

Definitive Management

The optimal definitive management of urethral injuries depends on several factors, including the location (anterior or posterior) and severity (partial or complete) of the injury and the preference and expertise of the consulting urologist. Options vary from simple placement of a Foley catheter to allow a partial anterior urethral injury to heal by secondary intention, to early endoscopic realignment or delayed urethroplasty of posterior urethral injuries. Often, placement of a suprapubic cystostomy tube is required to promote decompression of the bladder and divert urine from the healing urethral injury or anastomosis. Regardless of the approach, the ultimate goal is the maintenance of urinary continence and sexual function.

Bladder

Blunt force bladder injuries are seen with lower abdominal trauma and in conjunction with pelvic fractures, often resulting from a motor vehicle collision. They are classified as contusions, intraperitoneal rupture, or extraperitoneal rupture. *Contusions* are partial thickness injuries to the bladder wall without rupture. *Intraperitoneal rupture* occurs from a blunt force injury to the lower abdomen in a patient with a full bladder, resulting in rupture at the bladder dome followed by extravasation of urine into the peritoneal cavity. *Extraperitoneal rupture* occurs most often in association with a pelvic fracture, in which the injuring force causes extraperitoneal rupture at the anterior or anterolateral wall. In other cases, bony fragments from the pelvic fracture impale the bladder, causing extraperitoneal rupture. Penetrating injuries may be inflicted by gunshot wounds, knives, or other sharp objects.

Clinical Presentation

The vast majority of blunt bladder injuries present with gross hematuria, pelvic fracture, or both. In general, the diagnosis may be excluded clinically when both are absent. Bladder injury may occur with any pelvic fracture but is more likely with fractures of the anterior arch or when all four pubic rami are fractured. A minority of patients will present with pelvic fracture with microscopic hematuria. Additional signs and symptoms include lower abdominal pain or tenderness and inability to void. In patients with penetrating trauma, evaluate for bladder rupture when the injury trajectory occurs in proximity to the bladder.

Diagnostic Strategies

After the initial examination, obtain an AP pelvis radiograph to assess for fracture. Evaluate the initial urine output for gross hematuria. If urethral injury is suspected, obtain a retrograde urethrogram first to ensure urethral integrity prior to placement of a Foley catheter. Once urethral injury is excluded and a Foley catheter has been placed, evaluate for bladder rupture in all patients with gross hematuria and pelvic fracture. This is accomplished by retrograde cystography or retrograde CT cystography. Additional, relative indications for bladder imaging include gross hematuria without pelvic fracture and microscopic hematuria with pelvic fracture.[16]

Retrograde Cystography Procedure. As with the procedure for retrograde urethrography, keep the patient supine to avoid potentially disrupting a stable pelvic hematoma, and take care to avoid contrast spillage, which will result in a spurious study. Obtain a baseline KUB radiograph. Remove the central piston from a 60-mL catheter-tip syringe and attach it to the Foley catheter. Hold the syringe upright above the level of the bladder and instill 400 mL of 10% water-soluble contrast (diluted in sterile saline) by gravity. In patients younger than 11 years, calculate the appropriate amount of contrast in milliliters using the formula "(age in years + 2) × 30." If a bladder contraction occurs prior to instillation of 400 mL of contrast (as evidenced by the contrast level rising in the syringe), wait for the contraction to pass, refill the bladder to the point of contraction, and then forcefully inject another 50 mL of contrast. The goal is to adequately distend the bladder to avoid missing injuries.

The most common reason for false-negative cystography is failure to instill enough contrast. After filling the bladder, clamp the catheter and obtain a KUB radiograph (Fig. 77-7). After ensuring adequacy of the contrast film, unclamp the catheter, allow the bladder to drain, and obtain a post-evacuation film. Extraperitoneal rupture appears as a flame-like area of contrast confined to the pelvis, often extending lateral to the bladder (Fig. 77-8). In cases of intraperitoneal rupture, contrast outlines the bowel and other structures in the peritoneal cavity (Fig. 77-9). Using the baseline film for comparison, carefully scrutinize the post-evacuation film for any subtle areas of extravasation not seen on the contrast-distended view.

For retrograde CT cystography, the bladder is filled in an identical manner. Do not simply clamp the Foley catheter and rely on passive filling of the bladder by intravenously administered contrast for CT cystography. Multiple studies have demonstrated missed injuries with this approach.[6-9] A post-evacuation film is not necessary with retrograde CT cystography.

Emergency Management

Irrigate the Foley catheter as needed to clear any clots and ensure adequate drainage; the primary goal is to keep the bladder completely decompressed. Because bladder injuries are often associated with intra-abdominal trauma, a diligent search for the latter should be undertaken in all patients with positive cystography.

Definitive Management

Operative repair is the rule for most intraperitoneal bladder ruptures. By contrast, the majority of extra-

FACTS AND FORMULAS

PEDIATRIC CONTRAST DOSAGE

- The pediatric dose of contrast for a retrograde urethrogram is 0.6 mL/kg to a maximum of 60 mL.
- In patients younger than 11 years old, calculate the appropriate amount of contrast in milliliters for retrograde cystography using the formula "(age in years+2)×30" to a maximun of 400 mL.

Tips and Tricks

- If a urethral injury is suspected subsequent to successful placement of a Foley catheter, a retrograde urethrogram may be obtained by injecting the contrast through a small feeding tube inserted alongside the catheter.
- Cautions for the EP
  - To avoid the risk of completing a partial urethral disruption, defer Foley catheter placement in a patient with a suspected urethral injury until urethral integrity is assured by the retrograde urethrogram.
  - Perform a careful rectal examination in all patients, and a vaginal examination in women, with a pelvic fracture to evaluate for rectal or vaginal lacerations.
  - For CT cystography, do not simply clamp the Foley catheter and rely on passive filling of the bladder by intravenously administered contrast. Multiple studies have demonstrated missed injuries with this approach.[6-9]
  - In the setting of penetrating trauma, significant renal vascular injury may exist in the absence of hematuria.

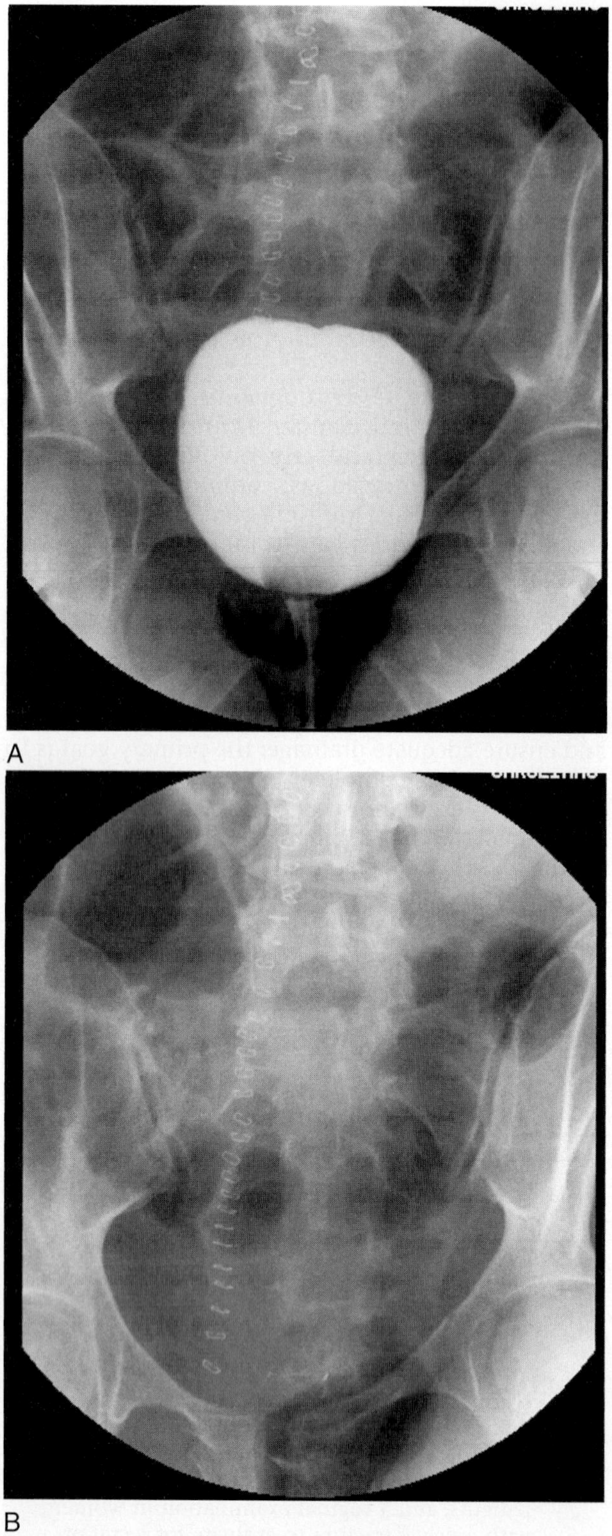
A
B

FIGURE 77-7 **A,** Normal retrograde cystogram. Note the complete retrograde filling of the bladder via a Foley catheter. **B,** Normal retrograde cystogram. Note the complete evacuation of contrast on the post-void film.

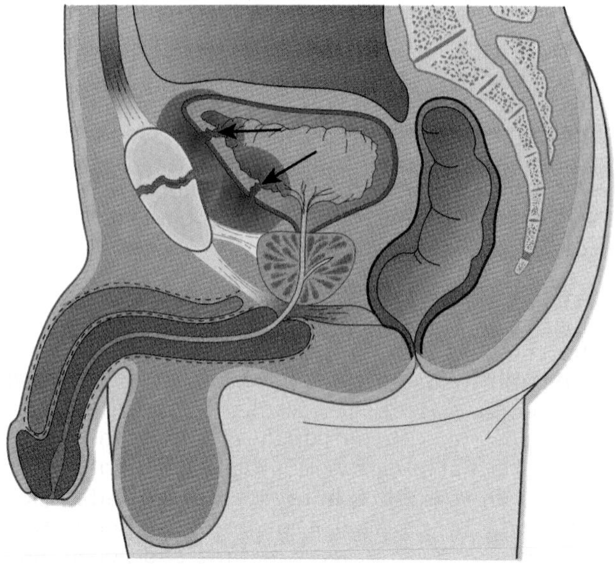

FIGURE 77-8 Extraperitoneal rupture.

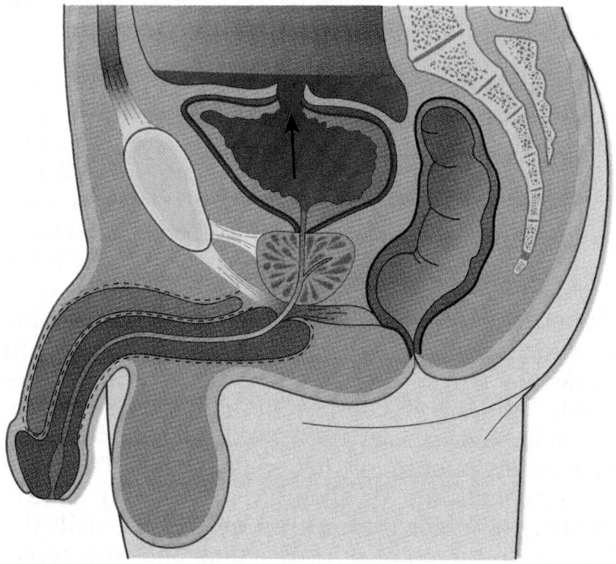

FIGURE 77-9 Intraperitoneal rupture.

peritoneal ruptures can be managed nonoperatively with catheter drainage alone. Exceptions include injuries involving the bladder neck, associated rectal or vaginal injuries, and patients requiring laparotomy for other indications.

Upper Genitourinary Tract Injuries

■ ANATOMY

The upper genitourinary tract consists of the ureters and the kidneys. The kidneys lie in the retroperitoneal space and are protected by the lower ribs, the back musculature, and the perinephric fat. The right kidney extends lower than the left owing to the presence of the liver. The ureters course distally along the psoas muscles and enter the bladder posteriorly and inferiorly at the trigone.

MECHANISM OF INJURY

Ureter

Ureteral injury is rare, consisting of less than 1% of all genitourinary injuries. In adults, penetrating injuries account for approximately 90% of cases, most commonly inflicted by gunshot wounds.[17] In children, the most common mechanism is blunt avulsion at the ureteropelvic junction resulting from a motor vehicle collision or fall from height. This injury pattern is thought to be due to the increased mobility of the pediatric vertebral column, which allows extreme hyperextension resulting in upward displacement of the kidney, separating it from the relatively immobile ureter.

Clinical Presentation

Hematuria (gross or microscopic) is not a reliable predictor of ureteral injury because the urinalysis is normal approximately 25% of the time.[18,19] The diagnosis is frequently missed on the initial evaluation because the signs and symptoms are minimal and nonspecific. Delayed findings include fever, flank pain, and a palpable flank mass (urinoma). Consider this injury in any penetrating injury with a trajectory in proximity to the ureter.

Diagnostic Strategies

The diagnosis of ureteral injury is elusive. Intravenous pyelography has long been the test of choice, although the reported sensitivity is highly variable.[17,19,20] CT imaging has gained popularity of late and is often indicated for identification of related injuries. Delayed CT images are required to allow time for the IV contrast to be excreted by the kidneys (Fig. 77-10). If operative exploration is indicated, the ureters may be directly evaluated in the surgical suite. When the diagnosis remains in doubt, retrograde pyelography may be useful.

Emergency Management

Identification and urologic consultation are the main priorities in the emergency management of ureteral injuries.

Definitive Management

Depending on the degree and location of the ureteral disruption, management options include cystoscopic stent placement or surgically repair over a stent. Urinary diversion may be required.

Kidney

Significant force is required to injure the kidney. Motor vehicle collisions, falls, direct blows, and lower rib fractures are common mechanisms. Significant decelerating forces may cause avulsion of the renal pedicle. In children, bicycle accidents represent a prominent mechanism of renal injury.[18] Penetrating injuries may be inflicted by gunshot wounds, knives, or other sharp objects.

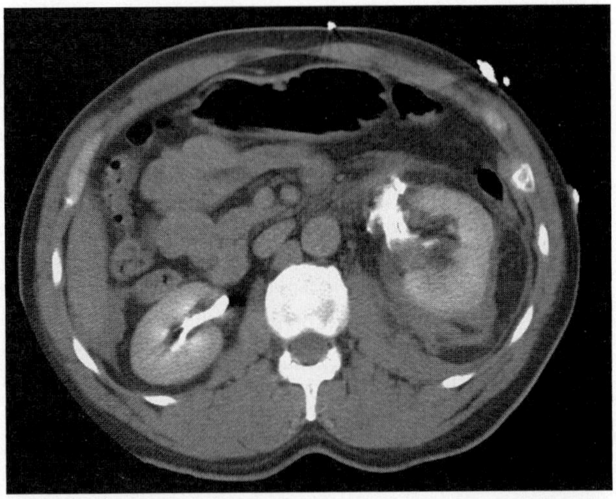

FIGURE 77-10 Injury to the collecting system of the left kidney. This delayed image demonstrates contrast extravasation from the renal pelvis.

Clinical Presentation

Clinical clues to a potential renal injury include bruising, pain, or tenderness to the flank or abdomen; rib or spine fractures; and hematuria, other organ injury, and shock. In patients with penetrating trauma, suspect renal involvement when the injury trajectory occurs in proximity to the kidney.

Diagnostic Strategies

Renal imaging is indicated in all cases of penetrating trauma proximate to the kidneys and in blunt injuries in the presence of gross hematuria or microscopic hematuria with shock (defined as systolic blood pressure <90 mm Hg). Additional, relative indications include a significant decelerating mechanism, such as a high-speed motor vehicle collision or a fall from height.[21,22] The imaging study of choice is CT scanning with IV contrast. If injury to the collecting system is suspected, additional cuts should be obtained 10 minutes after contrast injection. IVP has been used extensively in the past, but has largely been supplanted by CT.

In the unstable patient requiring immediate laparotomy, a "one-shot" intravenous pyelogram obtained in the operating room has some utility. Although this limited study does not provide sufficient sensitivity to exclude all clinically important renal injuries, it will demonstrate major renal disruption and confirm the presence of a functioning contralateral kidney. This study is accomplished by obtaining a KUB radiograph 10 minutes after the rapid bolus injection of IV contrast (2 mL/kg).[5,22] Emergent angiography can be both diagnostic and therapeutic, but it is time-

Table 77-1 AAST ORGAN INJURY SEVERITY SCALE FOR THE KIDNEY*

Grade†	Type	Description
I	Contusion	Microscopic gross hematuria, urologic studies normal
	Hematoma	Subcapsular, nonexpanding without parenchymal laceration
II	Hematoma	Nonexpanding perirenal hematoma confined to renal retroperitoneum
	Laceration	<0.1 cm parenchymal depth of renal cortex without urinary extravasation
III	Laceration	<0.1 cm parenchymal depth of renal cortex without collecting system ruptures or urinary extravasation
IV	Laceration	Parenchymal laceration extending through renal cortex, medulla, and collecting systems
	Vascular	Main renal artery or vein injury with contained hemorrhage
V	Laceration	Completely shattered kidney
	Vascular	Avulsion of renal hilum, devascularizing the kidney

*Appears online at http://www.aast.org/injury/injury.html.
†Advance one grade for bilateral injuries up to grade III.
AAST, American Association for the Surgery of Trauma.

consuming and impractical in many centers. Ultrasonography lacks sensitivity visualizing renal trauma and should not be relied on to exclude significant injury.

Emergency Management

Identification and urologic consultation are the main priorities in the emergency management of ureteral injuries.

Definitive Management

The need for operative intervention correlates with the severity of injury as classified by the American Association for the Surgery of Trauma (AAST) organ injury severity scale for the kidney (Fig. 77-11 and Table 77-1). Most grade I and II injuries can be managed nonoperatively; nearly all grade V injuries (Fig. 77-12) require nephrectomy, which may be lifesaving in the rare case of exsanguinating hemorrhage from a renal vascular injury. Delayed nephrectomy may be indicated in the small subset of patients who develop hypertension or symptomatic renal infarction.[22]

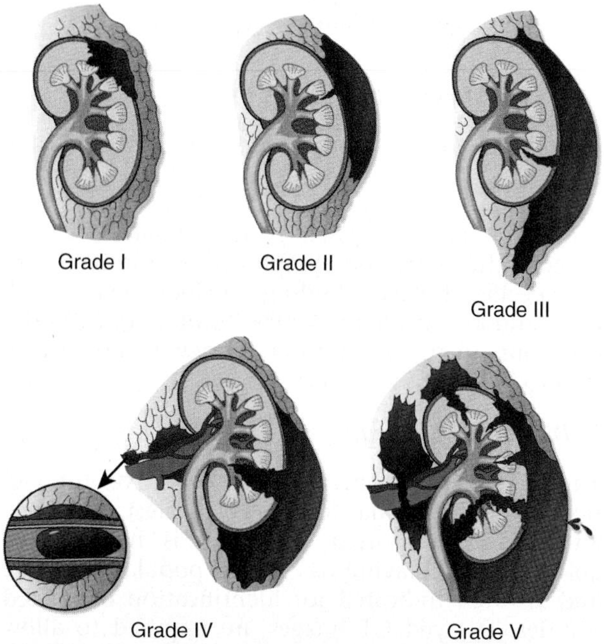
Grade I
Grade II
Grade III
Grade IV
Grade V

FIGURE 77-11 American Association for the Surgery of Trauma (AAST) organ injury severity scale for the kidney.

Pediatric Considerations

There is some controversy as to whether the criteria used to determine the need for renal imaging after blunt trauma in adults may be applied to children. One issue is whether the presence of microscopic hematuria in children warrants imaging even in the absence of shock. Some authors have recommended imaging children when urine microscopy reveals ≥50 RBCs/hpf.[23,24]

Certainly, the criterion of shock as defined by systolic blood pressure less than 90 mm Hg is unhelpful in the pediatric population. Even age-specific definitions of hypotension are of little utility because children manifest shock differently than do adults. A recent study reviewing 720 consecutive pediatric patients with suspected renal trauma concluded that using the criteria of gross hematuria, shock, and significant deceleration injury can identify all cases of renal injury.[25] However, like the definition of shock,

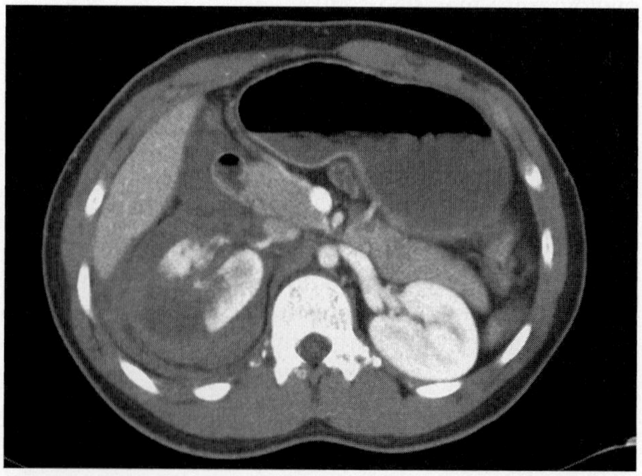

FIGURE 77-12 American Association for the Surgery of Trauma (AAST) grade V renal laceration (*right*) with significant perinephric hematoma due to renal artery disruption with devascularization of the lower pole of the kidney.

"significant deceleration injury" was not well defined in this study.

For now, consensus guidelines recommend that hemodynamically stable children with blunt trauma should be imaged if they have gross hematuria (i.e., ≥50 RBCs/hpf) on urine microscopy.[25] All children with penetrating trauma in proximity to the kidneys warrant imaging.

Disposition

Most patients with significant genitourinary injuries require urgent or emergent urologic consultation in the ED. Additionally, many patients will have associated, nonurologic injuries that mandate trauma surgery or general surgery consultation. In the event that the appropriate specialists are unavailable, expeditious transfer to an appropriate referral center is indicated after the initial evaluation and stabilization.

A minority of hemodynamically stable patients with no other indications for admission may be considered for discharge from the ED after telephone consultation with the urologist who will see the patient for follow-up care. Such cases include minor lacerations and zipper injuries and isolated partial anterior urethral injuries in the presence of a functioning Foley catheter. Counsel these patients on the signs and symptoms of infection and Foley catheter dysfunction, and ask them to return to the ED if they develop these or any other concerning symptoms. Finally, make sure that they understand the importance of complying with the scheduled follow-up plan.

REFERENCES

1. Koraitim MM: Pelvic fracture urethral injuries: The unresolved controversy. J Urol 1999;161:1433-1441.
2. Andrich DE, Mundy AR: The nature of urethral injury in cases of pelvic fracture urethral trauma. J Urol 2001;165: 1492-1495.
3. Dorschner W, Biesold M, Schmidt F, Stolzenburg JU: The dispute about the external sphincter and the urogenital diaphragm. J Urol 1999;162:1942-1945.
4. Chapple CR, Png D: Contemporary management of urethral trauma and the post-traumatic stricture. Curr Opin Urol 1999;9:253-260.
5. Morey AF, McAninch JW, Tiller BK, et al: Single shot intraoperative excretory urography for the immediate evaluation of renal trauma. J Urol 1999;161:1088-1092.
6. Gomez RG, Ceballos L, Coburn M, et al: Consensus statement on bladder injuries. BJU Int 2004;94:27-32.
7. Hsieh CH, Chen RJ, Fang JF, et al: Diagnosis and management of bladder injury by trauma surgeons. Am J Surg 2002;184:143-147.
8. Haas CA, Brown SL, Spirnak JP: Limitations of routine spiral computerized tomography in the evaluation of bladder trauma. J Urol 1999;162:51-52.
9. Vaccaro JP, Brody JM: CT cystography in the evaluation of major bladder trauma. Radiographics 2000;20:1373-1381.
10. Gottenger EE, Wagner JR: Penile fracture with complete urethral disruption. J Trauma 2000;49:339-331.
11. Morey AF, MetroMJ, Carney KJ, et al: Consensus on genitourinary trauma: External genitalia. BJU Int 2004;94: 507-515.
12. Hall SJ, Wagner JR, Edelstein RA, Carpinito GA: Management of gunshot injuries to the penis and anterior urethra. J Trauma 1995;38:439-443.
13. Goldman HB, Idom CB Jr, Dmochowski RR: Traumatic injuries of the female external genitalia and their association with urological injuries. J Urol 1998;159:956-959. [erratum appears in J Urol 1998;159:1650].
14. Lev RY, Mor Y, Golomb J, et al: Missed female urethral injury complicated by myonecrosis of the thigh. J Urol 2001;165:1216.
15. Bandi G, Santucci RA: Controversies in the management of male external genitourinary trauma. J Trauma 2004;56: 1362-1370.
16. Morey AF, Iverson AJ, Swan A, et al: Bladder rupture after blunt trauma: Guidelines for diagnostic imaging. J Trauma 2001;51:683-686.
17. Elliott SP, McAninch JW: Ureteral injuries from external violence: The 25-year experience at San Francisco General Hospital. J Urol 2003;170:1213-1216.
18. Gerstenbluth RE, Spirnak, JP, Elder JS: Sports participation and high grade renal injuries in children. J Urol 2002;168:2575-2578.
19. Carver BS, Bozeman CB, Venable DD: Ureteral injury due to penetrating trauma. South Med J 2004;97:462-464.
20. Perez-Brayfield MR, Keane TE, Krishnan A, et al: Gunshot wounds to the ureter: A 40-year experience at Grady Memorial Hospital. J Urol 2001;166:119-121.
21. Mee SL, McAninch JW, Robinson AL, et al: Radiographic assessment of renal trauma: A 10-year prospective study of patient selection. J Urol 1989;141:1095-1098.
22. Santucci RA, Wessells H, Bartsch G, et al: Evaluation and management of renal injuries: Consensus statement of the renal trauma subcommittee. BJU Int 2004;93: 937-954.
23. Morey AF, Bruce JE, McAninch JW: Efficacy of radiographic imaging in pediatric blunt renal trauma. J Urol 1996;156: 2014-2018.
24. Perez-Brayfield MR, Gatti JM, Smith EA, et al: Blunt traumatic hematuria in children. Is a simplified algorithm justified? J Urol 2002;167:2543-2546.
25. Santucci RA, Langenburg SE, Zachareas MJ: Traumatic hematuria in children can be evaluated as in adults. J Urol 2004;171:822-825.

Chapter **78**

Hip and Femur Injuries

Philip Bossart

KEY POINTS

Isolated hip fractures in the elderly are common injuries seen in the ED. Most of these injuries are secondary to ground-level falls in patients with osteoporosis.

Hip dislocations and femur fractures often are caused by high-energy trauma such as motor vehicle collisions and falls from heights; thus associated injuries are common and should always be looked for.

EPs may relocate hip dislocations in the ED; however, most hip fractures and femur fractures require orthopedic consultation and operative repair.

Scope

Approximately 250,000 hip fractures occur each year in the United States. This number is projected to increase significantly as the population ages. The major causes of hip fractures are ground-level falls in elderly patients with osteoporosis. Hip injuries are a major cause of morbidity and mortality, especially in the elderly, in whom the 1-year mortality after a hip fracture is about 25%.

Femur shaft and distal femur fractures usually are the result of high-energy trauma such as motor vehicle collisions and falls from heights; thus open wounds and associated traumatic injuries are common.

The leading cause of hip fractures are falls in elderly people with underlying osteoporosis. There are about 300,000 hip fractures each year in the United States secondary to osteoporosis.[1] Osteoporosis is a common condition in the elderly, and its incidence increases with advancing age. After about age 30, bone resorption slowly begins to exceed bone formation, and as a result bone mass and bone strength lessens. Approximately 50% of women and 25% of men over the age of 50 will have an osteoporosis-related fracture in their lifetime.[1]

The major cause of hip dislocations is motor vehicle collisions. A great deal of force is required to dislocate a hip; thus associated injuries are common. Patients with hip dislocations have about a 25% risk for osteoarthritis and 20% risk for avascular necrosis. These risks may be decreased by prompt diagnosis and treatment in the ED.

Osteonecrosis (also known as aseptic necrosis, ischemic necrosis, and avascular necrosis) may be caused by acute disruption in the blood supply to the femoral head as a result of a hip fracture or dislocation. Fractures of the femoral neck also can disrupt the blood supply and result in osteonecrosis. Other causes are sickle cell disease, barotrauma, radiation therapy, chemotherapy, atherosclerosis, and Gaucher's disease. Associated conditions include steroid use, excessive alcohol consumption, smoking, connective tissue diseases, pancreatitis, and chronic liver and renal diseases.[2]

The incidence of osteonecrosis after hip dislocation depends on the degree of trauma involved and the duration of the dislocation. Some data suggest that reduction of the hip within 6 hours after dislocation decreases the incidence of osteonecrosis.[3] Therefore, every effort must be made to relocate these as soon as possible. Femoral neck fractures also are associated with a high incidence of osteonecrosis. It is thought that the synovial fluid around the fracture site interferes with normal bone healing. Intertrochanteric fractures and other more distal fractures of the femur are rarely complicated by osteonecrosis.

Anatomy

The hip joint is a ball-and-socket articulation between the femoral head and the acetabulum. The ligamentum teres, the capsular ligaments, and the proximal muscles of the leg make the hip a stable joint requiring very strong forces to dislocate. The femur is the largest and strongest bone in the body. The femoral neck is about 8 to 10 cm in length. The intertrochanteric line is an oblique line that connects the greater trochanter and the lesser trochanter and marks the junction of the femoral neck and the shaft.

The muscles of abduction (gluteus medius and gluteus minimus) insert on the laterally located greater trochanter, and the muscles of flexion (iliopsoas) insert on the medially located lesser trochanter. The major blood supply to the head and neck of the femur is the medial and lateral circumflex arteries, which are branches of the femoral artery.

There are approximately 18 bursae in the hip region. The most common source of hip pain and inflammation is the deep trochanteric bursa, which lies between the gluteus maximus and the greater trochanter.

Presenting Signs and Symptoms

Pain is the most common complaint in patients with hip problems.[4] The location and character of the pain are very helpful in making a diagnosis. Increased pain during and after weight bearing and improvement with rest suggests a structural joint problem such as osteoarthritis. Constant pain, unrelated to use, suggests an infectious, inflammatory, or neoplastic process

Lateral hip pain, especially with tenderness over the greater trochanter, suggests trochanteric bursitis. Lateral hip pain with paresthesias suggests meralgia paresthetica—lateral femoral cutaneous nerve entrapment. This is characterized by a local area of pain (often burning or dysesthesia) that is not influenced by direct pressure of hip or back movement.

Anterior hip or groin pain made worse by joint motion suggests a problem with the hip joint, such as osteonecrosis, occult fracture, synovitis, and septic joint. Anterior hip pain that is not made worse by hip motion or weight bearing suggests inguinal hernia, lower abdominal pathology, or referred lumber nerve root pain. Posterior hip pain suggests sacroiliac joint inflammation, lumbar radiculopathy, or herpes zoster. Anterior thigh pain may be secondary to injury to the hip joint or femur, stress fracture of the femoral neck, or lumbar radiculopathy.

Differential Diagnosis

See Box 78-1.

Diagnostic Testing

Anteroposterior (AP) and lateral radiographs of the hip are usually sufficient to diagnose hip dislocations and fractures. For the AP view, the patient is supine with about 15 degrees of internal rotation of the feet. For the lateral view, the patient is supine with the uninvolved hip flexed and abducted. The radiograph cassette is placed against the lateral aspect of the affected leg, and the x-ray beam is directed horizontanly toward the groin, with 20 degrees of cephalic tilt.

Frog-leg views of the pelvis should not be ordered if there is a possibility of a hip fracture or hip dislocation.

Interventions and Procedures

HIP DISLOCATIONS

In approximately 90% of hip dislocations, the femoral head is posterior to the acetabulum. Typically posterior hip dislocations occur when the knee hits the dashboard during an motor vehicle collision. In pos-

BOX 78-1

Differential Diagnosis of Hip Pain

- Bursitis
- Osteoarthritis
- Hip dislocation
- Hip fracture
- Meralgia paresthetica
- Lumbar radiculopathy
- Osteonecrosis
- Acute synovitis
- Septic arthritis
- Herpes zoster
- Stress fracture of femoral neck
- Aortoiliac occlusive disease
- Sacroiliac joint disease

PRIORITY ACTIONS

- Hip dislocations are true orthopedic emergencies. Reduction should be done as soon as possible. Reduction within 6 hours reduces the incidence of avascular necrosis.
- Significant blood loss is common with hip fractures and femur fractures, especially fractures in young people that usually involve a high-energy force. Good IV access, fluid resuscitation, and monitoring for blood loss are mandatory.

Tips and Tricks

- Consider avascular necrosis in all patients with nontraumatic hip, thigh, or knee pain.
- If hip pain prevents weight bearing, and plain films do not reveal a fracture, obtain a computed tomography or magnetic resonance image scan to confirm the diagnosis.

Documentation

- Always carefully record neurovascular examination findings in patients with an extremity fracture.
- If hip reduction is delayed, record reason for delay.

RED FLAGS

- It is important to look for acetabular fractures before performing closed reduction of a hip dislocation.
- On average, patients with femur shaft fractures lose about two to three units of blood at the fracture site, and about half of these patients will require blood transfusions.
- A hip dislocation or fracture in a young person is strong evidence of serious multisystem trauma.

terior hip dislocations, the leg is flexed, adducted, and internally rotated, with limb shortening. In anterior dislocations the leg is flexed, abducted, and externally rotated.

Because high energy usually is required to dislocate a hip, associated injuries are common.[5] Ligamentous knee injuries, acetabular and femur fractures, and sciatic nerve palsies should be considered. If an associated fracture is not clearly seen on plain films, a computed tomography scan should be ordered.

Posterior dislocations are likely to cause a fracture of the inferior aspect of the femoral head and may cause injury to the sciatic nerve.[6] Anterior dislocations are associated with fractures of the anterior femoral head and also with vascular injuries.

Hip dislocations are orthopedic emergencies. Reduction should be performed as soon as possible; the incidence of avascular necrosis, traumatic arthritis, and joint instability increases with the length of time the hip is dislocated. In addition, orthopedic consultation should be obtained.

Hip relocations require conscious sedation in the ED and general anesthesia in the operating room.

Posterior hip dislocations can be reduced by having an assistant apply pressure to the patient's anterior superior iliac spine while the physician flexes the hip and applies traction to the leg. Initial internal rotation of the leg may be followed by external rotation after the femoral head has cleared the acetabulum. For anterior dislocations, initial traction is followed by external rotation and then internal rotation.

HIP FRACTURES

Hip fractures are classified as intracapsular or extracapsular. Intracapsular fractures include femoral head and femoral neck fractures (Fig. 78-1). These are further categorized as either displaced or nondisplaced. Extracapsular fractures include intertrochanteric and subtrochanteric fractures as well as the less common greater and lesser trochanteric fractures. These can be further categorized by the degree of comminution.

Femoral Head Fractures

These relatively uncommon fractures usually occur in young people involved in motor vehicle collisions, in conjunction with hip dislocations. Because these fractures may not be visualized on plain radiographs, computed tomography or magnetic resonance imaging may be necessary for diagnosis.

Femoral Neck Fractures

Fractures of the femoral neck, which is located between the femoral head and the trochanters, occur within the joint capsule and include susbcapital fractures (fractures through the fused epiphyseal plate). These are common fractures and usually occur secondary to ground-level falls in older patients with osteoporosis and in young people involved in motor vehicle collisions.

This area of the femur has relatively little cancellous bone and very thin or absent periosteum; in addition, blood supply to the femoral head may be disrupted. As a result, degenerative changes to the femoral head and frank avascular necrosis are common after these fractures.[7]

Patients may be able to bear weight with some of these fractures so radiologic examination is impor-

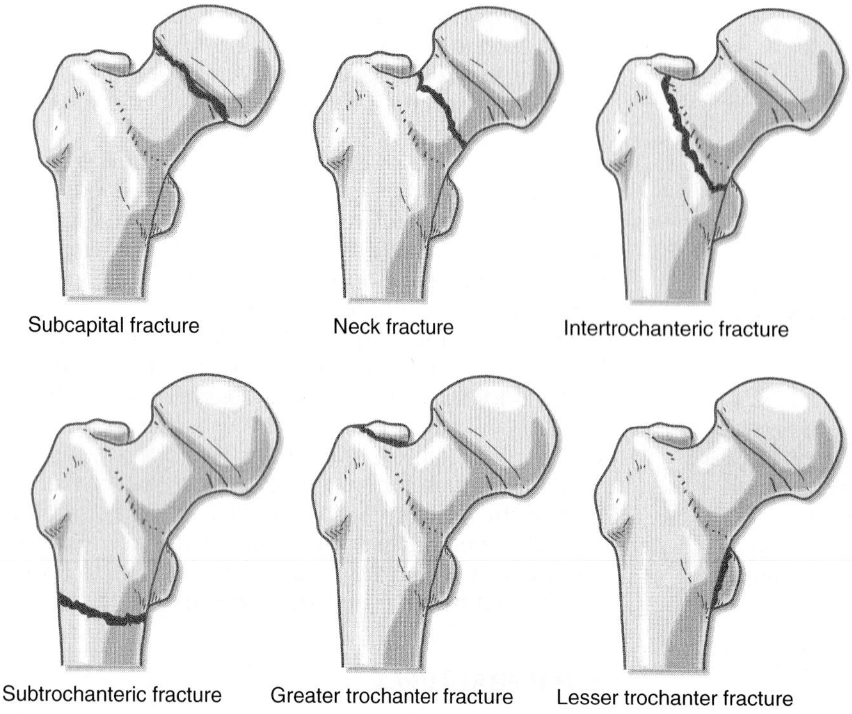
Subcapital fracture
Neck fracture
Intertrochanteric fracture
Subtrochanteric fracture
Greater trochanter fracture
Lesser trochanter fracture

FIGURE 78-1 Types of hip fractures.

tant even if the patient is able to walk. Most femoral neck fractures can be treated with open reduction and internal fixation. Early surgical correction, usually within 12 hours, reduces the incidence of aseptic necrosis.

■ Intertrochanteric Fractures

Intertrochanteric fractures are extracapsular injuries and are the most common type of hip fracture. The majority occur in elderly patients with osteoporosis as a result of ground-level falls. About 80% are comminuted fractures. Patients cannot bear weight; thus the diagnosis is obvious clinically and usually easily confirmed with an AP radiographis view of the hip.

Because patients may lose a much as 1 to 2 liters of blood, IV crystalloid infusion or blood transfusion may be necessary. These are typically elderly, frail patients; ED evaluation includes determining the reason for the fall (e.g., syncope, near-syncope, transient ischemic attack) as well as evaluation of other significant medical problems. The treatment of choice is surgical repair; however, because avascular necrosis is uncommon, surgery does not have to be performed immediately. Medical and postoperative complications are common, and about one third of these patient die within a year of injury.

■ Greater Trochanteric Fractures

Fractures of the greater trochanter are uncommon. In adults they are usually the result of direct trauma; in children they are usually secondary to muscle avulsion. They may be difficult to vizualize on radiographs. Fractures due to direct trauma are usually comminuted but not displaced; those due to avulsion are usually displaced but not comminuted.

If displacement is greater than 1 cm, open reduction and internal fixation are often recommended. However, most of these fractures are usually minimally displaced and do not need surgery. If plain radiographs are uninformative, computed tomography scanning or magnetic resonance imaging may be needed to make the diagnosis.

■ Lesser Trochanteric Fractures

Fractures of the lesser trochanter usually occur in people under age 20 years. If they occur in adults, a pathologic fracture should be suspected. The usual mechanism is a forceful contraction of the iliopsoas muscle during strenuous activity. Patients are unable to lift the affected leg when in the sitting position. Treatment usually is bed rest.

■ Subtrochanteric Fractures

Fractures of the subtrochanter are defined as fractures between the lesser trochanter and a point 5 cm distally. They are associated with severe trauma in young people or mild trauma in people with pathologic bone disease. Like intertrochanteric and midshaft femur fractures, these fractures can be associated with significant blood loss. In addition, associated neurovascular injury to the profunda femoris artery, branches of the lateral circumflex artery, the lateral femoral cutaneous nerve, and the femoral nerve is possible. If the patient has severe swelling in the proximal thigh, then angiography or duplex scanning should be done to look for a vascular injury.

Treatment consists of open reduction and internal fixation. Because of the large stress forces in this area, nonunion is a relatively common complication.

■ FEMORAL SHAFT FRACTURES

The diagnosis of femoral shaft fractures is usually obvious on physical examination, with marked deformity and tenderness. These fractures most commonly occur after high-energy injuries such as motor vehicle collisions and falls; thus associated injuries are common and must be carefully searched for.

If the fracture is associated with an open wound, the wound should be irrigated and covered with moist sterile dressings. Treatment of small, relatively clean wounds includes administration of a first-generation cephalosporin. An aminoglycoside should be given if there is more extensive soft tissue injury. Penicillin is recommended if there are extensive crush injuries or wounds with significant dirt.

Because associated fractures in the hip and knee are common, radiographs should be obtained. About 50% of patient have associated ligamentous injuries of the knee. Blood loss can be significant, but associated neurovascular injuries are rare. On average, these patients lose about two to three units of blood, and about 50% will require blood transfusions.

Traction devices should be removed when the patients present to the ER, but limb immobilization should be maintained.

Treatment includes internal fixation with intramedullary rods. Severely comminuted fractures may be treated with closed reduction. In general, patients do better if the fractures are stabilized within 24 hours of injury. Early stabilization is associated with early patient mobilization and therefore less risk for deep venous thrombosis, pressure ulcers, and pneumonia. Fat embolism syndrome is a possible complication that generally this condition is manifested with signs of pulmonary or central nervous system dysfunction, fever, and rash starting about 12 to 72 hours following injury. In almost all cases, the fractures will have healed and the patients will be functional in 6 months. Nonunion is rare.

■ DISTAL FEMUR FRACTURES

Fractures of the distal femur tend to occur in older patients with severe osteoporosis or in young people with multiple trauma. Supracondylar and intercondylar fractures of the femur are difficult to treat. They are usually unstable and often comminuted. Most are treated operatively. However, malunion, nonunion, and infections are relatively common.

■ STRESS FRACTURES

Stress fractures occur when normal bone is subjected to repeated stress. The bone fails because osteoblasts are unable to lay down new bone fast enough. Symptoms of a femoral neck stress fracture can be very mild pain only. As such, the injury may be mistaken for a muscle strain or arthritis. Pain is typically felt in the groin and medial thigh, is worse with use, and may make weight bearing very painful or impossible.

The physical examination usually is normal, except perhaps some pain at the extremes of hip flexion and internal rotation. Because plain films usually are unrevealing until 14 days after the injury, computed tomography scanning or magnetic resonance imaging may be needed to make the diagnosis. This condition is often bilateral, so any pain in the other hip needs evaluation also.

REFERENCES

1. National Institute of Arthritis and Musculoskeletal and Skin Diseases: Osteoporosis. Available at www.niams.nih.gov/Health_Info/Bone/Osteoporosis/default.asp.
2. National Osteonecrosis Foundation: Osteonecrosis. Available at www.nonf.org/nofbrochure/nonf-brochure.htm.
3. Gurr DE, Gibbs MA: Femur and hip. In Marks JA, Hockberger RS, Walls RM (eds): Rosen's Textbook of Emergency Medicine: Concepts and Clinical Practice, 5th ed. St. Louis, Mosby, 2002, pp 643-672.
4. Anderson BC: Evaluation of the Adult with Hip Pain. Available at www.uptodate.com.
5. Mirza A, Ellis T: Initial management of pelvic and femoral fractures in the multiply injured patient. Crit Care Clin 2004;20:159-170.
6. Fracture dislocations of the hip. In Wheeless' Textbook of Orthopedics (online). Available at www.wheelessonline.com/ostho/fracture_dislocations_of_the_hip.
7. LaVelle DG: Fractures of hip. In Canale ST (ed): Campbell's Operative Orthopaedics, 10th ed. St. Louis, Mosby, 2003, pp 2874-2878.

Chapter 79

Knee and Lower Leg Injuries

Christy McCowen

KEY POINTS

Knee dislocations are associated with a high risk of neurovascular injury and constitute an orthopedic emergency.

A grossly unstable knee should be assumed to be dislocated until proven otherwise.

Patients presenting with fractures and/or dislocations of the knee and lower extremity AND neurovascular compromise should undergo emergency reduction or realignment prior to any radiographic evaluation.

Patients discharged home in knee immobilizers with stable injuries should be instructed to remove the device several times a day and perform range-of-motion and quadriceps-strengthening exercises.

For any person presenting with increasing pain after a lower leg fracture, the cast or splint should be removed, and a careful assessment should be made of the lower leg compartments and neurovascular status.

Scope

Knee and lower leg injuries are both common orthopedic problems that present to the ED. This chapter divides such injuries into discussions of traumatic injuries (soft tissue and cartilaginous injuries, dislocations, and fractures), overuse injuries, and other disorders of the knee and lower leg.

Anatomy

■ KNEE

The knee is the largest and most complex joint in the body. Injuries to this joint are common, so a clear understanding of the anatomy and pathophysiology of the knee are essential to appropriate evaluation, diagnosis, and treatment of disorders in this area.

The knee has a wide range of motion, including flexion, extension, abduction, adduction, and internal and external rotation. Three different articulations occur in this joint: the patellofemoral articulation (anterior) and the articulations between the lateral and medial tibial and femoral condyles. In full extension, the stabilizing ligaments of the knee are tight and prevent rotary motion of the knee. Beyond 20 degrees of flexion, the ligaments are relaxed and allow axial rotation of the joint.

Knee stability is provided solely by ligaments and tendons in and around the joint. These stabilizing structures of the knee can be divided into the static stabilizers (ligaments) and dynamic stabilizers (muscle) (Fig. 79-1; Table 79-1). The knee joint is encapsulated by a fibrous connective tissue lined by a synovial membrane. The knee capsule is continu-

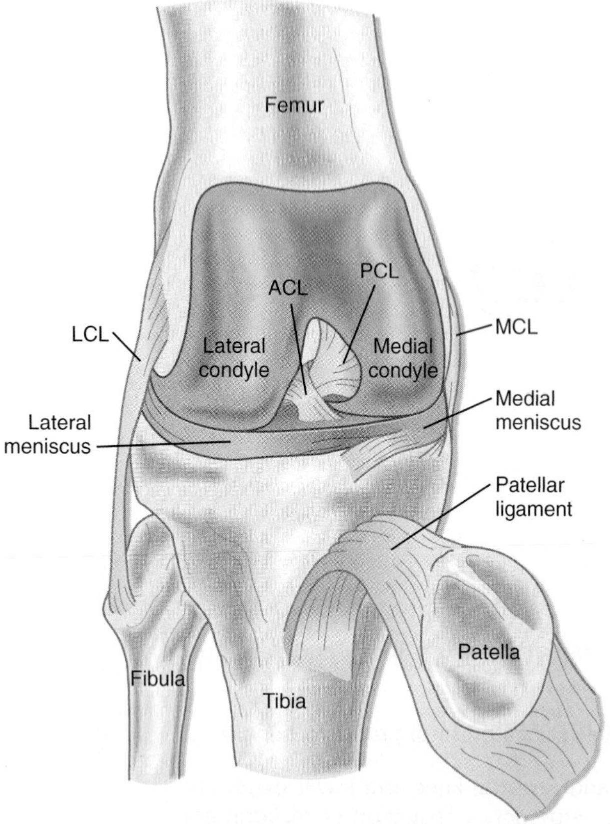
Femur
PCL
ACL
LCL
Lateral condyle
Medial condyle
MCL
Lateral meniscus
Medial meniscus
Patellar ligament
Patella
Fibula
Tibia

FIGURE 79-1 Knee anatomy. ACL, anterior cruciate ligament; LCL, lateral collateral ligament; MCL, medial collateral ligament; PCL, posterior cruciate ligament. (From Brown JR, Trojian TH: Anterior and posterior cruciate ligament injuries. Prim Care 2004;31:925-956.)

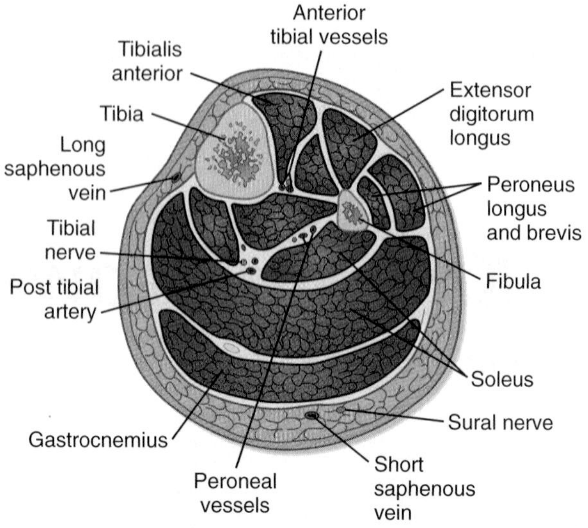
Anterior tibial vessels
Tibialis anterior
Extensor digitorum longus
Tibia
Long saphenous vein
Peroneus longus and brevis
Tibial nerve
Fibula
Post tibial artery
Soleus
Sural nerve
Gastrocnemius
Short saphenous vein
Peroneal vessels

FIGURE 79-2 Cross-section of the lower extremity at the level of the calf. (From Khatri VP, Asensio JA: Operative Surgery Manual. Philadelphia, Saunders, 2003.)

ous with the suprapatellar bursa, which expands when there is a joint effusion.

The popliteal fossa contains the popliteal artery and vein and the peroneal and tibial nerves. The popliteal fossa is delineated laterally by the biceps femoris muscle, medially by the semimembranosus and semitendinosus muscles, and inferiorly by the gastrocnemius muscle.

The popliteal artery is a continuation of the femoral artery after it leaves the adductor hiatus. It gives rise to the geniculate arteries, which form a rich vascular anastomosis around the knee. The popliteal artery divides to form the anterior and posterior tibial arteries at the level of the tibial tubercle. The popliteal artery is immobilized proximally and distally within the popliteal fossa, predisposing it to vascular injury in the setting of traumatic knee injuries.

The tibial nerve and common peroneal nerve (a branch of the tibial nerve) innervate the knee. Because the tibial nerve is not immobilized proximally, it is less likely than the popliteal artery to be injured in the setting of joint disruption. The common peroneal nerve travels around the head of the fibula and divides into the deep and superficial peroneal nerves.

■ LOWER LEG

The lower leg contains the tibia and fibula. The tibia is both the only weight-bearing bone in the lower leg and the most commonly fractured long bone in the body. Its superficial course predisposes it to a higher incidence of open fractures. The two bones are bound together by the superior and inferior tibiofibular joint along with an interosseous membrane. The interosseous membrane aids in the stability of the ankle mortise.

The thigh muscles attach to the upper part of the tibia and lend stability to the knee joint. The muscles of the lower leg, which are enclosed by fascia, can be divided into four compartments: anterior, posterior, deep posterior, and lateral (Fig. 79-2). The *anterior* compartment contains the dorsiflexors of the ankle and foot, the anterior tibial artery, and the deep peroneal nerve. The deep peroneal nerve supplies sensation to the first web space of the foot. The posterior compartment contains the plantar flexors and is divided into a superficial compartment and a deep compartment. The *deep posterior* compartment contains the posterior tibial and peroneal arteries and the tibial nerve, which supplies sensory innervation to the plantar aspect of the foot. The sural nerve travels in the *superficial posterior* compartment and supplies sensory innervation to the lateral aspect of the distal leg and foot. The *lateral* compartment contains the foot everters and the superficial peroneal nerve, which provides sensory innervation to the dorsal aspect of the foot.

Evaluation

■ KNEE

Key aspects of the evaluation of knee are listed in Box 79-1. In general, evaluation of knee complaints should also include examination of the hip and back

Table 79-1 STATIC AND DYNAMIC STABILIZERS OF THE KNEE

Knee Stabilizers	Location	Joint Action	Anatomic Insertions
Static Stabilizers			
Tibial (medial) collateral ligament	Medial	Prevents rotary or valgus stress	Medial femoral/tibial condyles and the medial meniscus
Lateral collateral ligament	Lateral	Offers weak lateral stability to the knee	Lateral femoral epicondyle/fibular head
Posterior capsule	Posterior	Prevents anteromedial/anterolateral rotary instability	Continuation of the deep medial collateral ligament
Anterior cruciate	Noncapsular stabilizer	Prevents anterior displacement of the tibia, excessive lateral mobility in flexion and extension, and tibial rotation	Intercondylar fossa/anterior tibial eminence
Posterior cruciate	Noncapsular stabilizer	Prevents anteroposterior and mediolateral rotation	Intercondylar fossa/posterior tibial eminence
Dynamic Stabilizers			
Quadriceps tendon	Anterior	Primary dynamic stabilizer of the knee	Tendons of the vastus medialis, lateralis, intermedius, and rectus femoris combine to make the patellar tendon Inserts on tibial tubercle
Pes anserinus	Medial	Prevents excessive rotary and valgus stress	Conjoined tendons of the gracilis, sartorius, and semitendinosus
Semimembranosus	Medial/posterior	Three heads stabilize the posterior capsule, flex and internally rotate the knee, and pull the medial meniscus posteriorly during flexion	Semimembranosus inserts on the posterior capsule, posterior horn or medial meniscus, and medial tibial condyle
Iliotibial band	Lateral	Stabilizes lateral knee	Originates from iliac crest, inserts on lateral tibial condyle (Gerdy's tubercle)
Biceps femoris	Lateral	Lateral stability; aids in flexion and external rotation	Inserts on the fibular head
Popliteus	Lateral	Provides posterior motion of lateral meniscus during flexion	Y-shaped tendon (arcuate ligament) inserts on the lateral femoral condyle and on the fibular head

to prevent overlooking a source of pain referred to the lower extremity.

During evaluation, the point of maximal tenderness should be assessed last. Specific tests for evaluating ligamentous and meniscal injuries are detailed in Table 79-2. Comparison with the uninjured or normal knee is helpful, especially for evaluation of ligamentous laxity.

Joint pain or swelling may limit a full evaluation of the knee in the acute setting. Patients with limited evaluations should undergo immobilization and follow-up examination within 7 days. Key physical findings are listed in discussions of specific disorders later in the chapter.

■ LOWER LEG

A directed history of traumatic events, symptom duration, and exacerbating events or activities is necessary to assess lower leg injuries. Examination of lower leg complaints should include an assessment of the back, hips, knee, and ankle to assess for referred pain to the lower leg or associated injuries.

A thorough assessment of the skin integrity, neurovascular status, and leg compartments is essential in the evaluation of any traumatic lower leg injury. The point of maximal tenderness should be evaluated last. Specific tests for neurologic function are listed in Table 79-3.

Diagnostic Testing

■ KNEE

Acute injuries to the knee commonly involve soft tissue injuries, thus plain radiographic examination is not always indicated. The Ottawa knee rules[1] (Box 79-2) and Pittsburgh knee rules[2] (Box 79-3) are useful guides to aid in the decision whether to order plain radiographs. Both criteria are sensitive for fractures, but the Pittsburgh criteria are more specific and can be applied in both children and adults.

BOX 79-1

Evaluation of the Knee

History

- Mechanism of injury:
  - Direction and type of force (high- or low-energy)
  - Position of extremity at time of injury
- Nature and duration of symptoms
- Previous injuries
- Previous surgical procedures
- Associated complaints
- Joint effusion
- Locking of joint
- Ability to ambulate
- Associated injuries

Physical Examination

- Inspection of entire limb with patient sitting or lying and walking (if possible):
  - Deformity, ecchymosis, edema, cutaneous lesions
  - Joint effusions
  - Previous scars
  - Gait and functional range of motion
  - Neurovascular status
- Palpation:
  - Extensor mechanism: quadriceps tendon, patella, patellar tendon, tibial tubercle (tendinitis, prepatellar bursitis, knee effusion, Osgood-Schlatter disease)
  - Femoral or tibial epiphysis in adolescents (physeal fractures)
  - Joint line (meniscal and/or collateral ligament injuries)
  - Posterior aspect of knee (popliteal cyst or pseudoaneurysm)
  - Neurovascular status
- Range of motion:
  - Flexion or extension
  - Internal or external rotation
  - Active straight-leg raise
- Stability testing:
  - Anterior or posterior stability (cruciate ligaments)
  - Medial or lateral stability (collateral ligaments)

If plain radiographs are indicated, a minimum of an anteroposterior (AP) and lateral view should be obtained. Oblique radiographs are helpful for detecting subtle tibial plateau fractures. The intercondylar or tunnel view is helpful to evaluate for tibial spine fractures and osteochondral defects (Fig. 79-3). The patellofemoral joint and patellar tilt (increased propensity for patellar subluxation or dislocation) can be assessed with the Merchant or sunrise view (Fig. 79-4). Comparison radiographs of the unaffected

BOX 79-2

Ottawa Knee Rules

Radiographs indicated if any ONE of the following is present:

- Age ≥55 years
- Tenderness at the head of the fibula
- Isolated tenderness of the patella
- Inability to flex the knee to 90 degrees
- Inability to bear weight for 4 steps both immediately after the injury and in the ED

Data from Stiell IG, Wells GA, McDowell I, et al: Use of radiography in acute knee injuries: Need for clinical decision rules. Acad Emerg Med 1995;2:966-973.

BOX 79-3

Pittsburgh Knee Rules

Radiographs are indicated if the patient sustained a fall or blunt-trauma mechanism *and* one of the following two conditions is present:

- The patient is <12 or >50 years old.
- The patient is unable to walk 4 weight-bearing steps in the ED.

Data from Seaberg DC, Yealy DM, Lukens T, et al: Multicenter comparison of two clinical decision rules for the use of radiography in acute, high-risk knee injuries. Ann Emerg Med 1998;32:8-13.

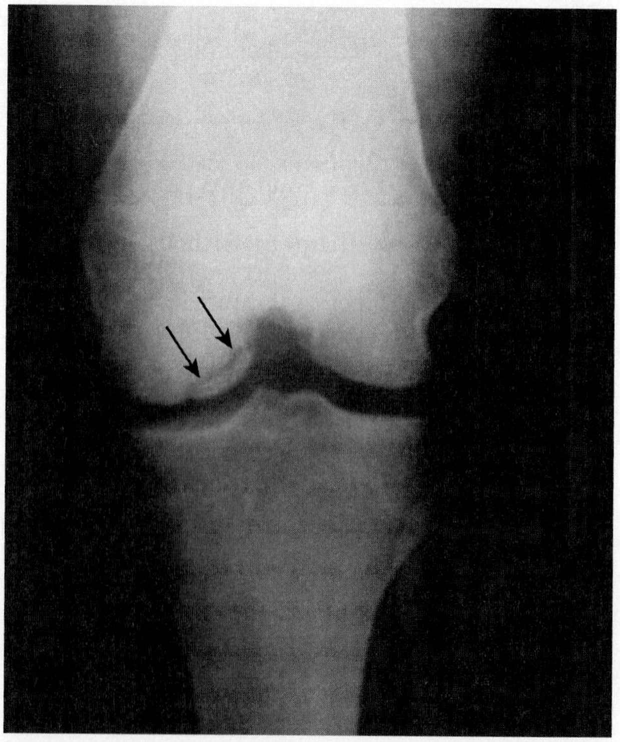

FIGURE 79-3 Knee radiograph, tunnel or intercondylar view, showing osteochondritis dissecans lesion (*arrows*).

Table 79-2 STABILITY TESTING

Test	How Performed	Definition of Positive Result	Comments
Of Anterior Cruciate Ligament (ACL) Stability			
Lachman's test (see Fig. 79-8)	1. Hold knee in 15-30 degrees of flexion. 2. Attempt to pull tibia forward with one hand while holding the femur stationary with the other hand.	Anterior laxity in conjunction with the lack of a firm endpoint (displacement >5 mm compared with opposite side)	Most sensitive test for ACL injury[8]
Anterior drawer test (see Fig. 79-9)	1. Flex hip to 45 degrees and knee to 90 degrees. 2. Stabilize foot with pressure directed toward examination table. 3. Grasp the proximal tibia and pull forward. 4. Perform this maneuver with knee in neutral and internal and external rotation positions.	Increased laxity in neutral position suggests ACL injury (displacement >6 mm compared with opposite side) Increased displacement with external rotation suggests injury to the posteromedial capsule Increased displacement with internal rotation suggests injury to the posterolateral capsule	Not a reliable test for acute ACL injuries
Pivotal shift test (see Fig. 79-10)	1. Flex the hip to 45 degrees, then fully extend knee while holding the heel of the foot. 2. With other hand, hold the knee with the thumb behind the fibular head. 3. Internally rotate the ankle and knee. 4. Apply valgus stress to the knee, then flex the knee while maintaining an internal and valgus stress.	If anterior subluxation of knee is present, reduction of the subluxation occurs at 20-40 degrees of flexion	Maneuvers of this test may be painful Highest positive predictive value for ACL rupture[8]
Of Posterior Cruciate Ligament (PCL)			
Posterior drawer test (see Fig. 79-11)	1. Flex the hip to 45 degrees and the knee to 90 degrees. 2. Stabilize the foot with pressure directed toward the examination table. 3. Apply backward force to the tibia.	>5 mm posterior displacement of tibia or a soft endpoint	Best test for evaluation of a PCL injury
Posterior sag test	1. Put a pillow under the patient's thigh so the knee is flexed to 45-90 degrees. 2. The patient's heel should be resting on the examination table.	Posterior tibial sag with regard to femur Tibia usually sits 10 mm anterior to femoral condyles in this position	Assess prior to posterior drawer test to avoid misinterpretation of posterior drawer test result
Of Lateral and Medial Collateral Ligaments			
Collateral ligament	1. Apply varus and valgus stress to knee in full extension and at 30 degrees. 2. Assess the joint line opening between the tibia and femur.	Laxity in full extension suggests complete collateral ligament tear in addition to injury to secondary stabilizers (ACL, PCL) Laxity at 30 degrees (but not in full extension) isolates injury to the collateral ligament undergoing testing	
For Meniscal Tears			
McMurray's test	1. Hyperflex the knee with patient in a supine position. 2. Hold the lower leg and flex/extend the knee while simultaneously internally and externally rotating the tibia with relation to the femur.	Either (1) examiner feels clicking sensation along the joint line with internal/external rotation or (2) patient experiences pain Internal rotation tests lateral meniscus External rotation tests medial meniscus	Hyperflexion may not be possible in acutely injured knee Poor sensitivity and specificity[10]
Apley's test	1. Have the patient lie in prone position. 2. Flex the knee to 90 degrees. 3. Internally and externally rotate the leg with pressure on the heel.	Pain during application of downward pressure suggests meniscal injury	

Table 79-3 TESTS FOR ASSESSMENT OF PERIPHERAL NERVES AND COMPARTMENTS OF THE LEG

Nerve	Compartment	Motor Function	Sensory Function
Deep peroneal	Anterior	Toe dorsiflexion	Dorsal I-II web space
Superficial peroneal	Lateral	Foot eversion	Lateral dorsum of foot
Tibial	Deep posterior	Toe plantar flexion	Sole of foot
Sural	Superficial posterior	Gastrosoleus	Lateral heel

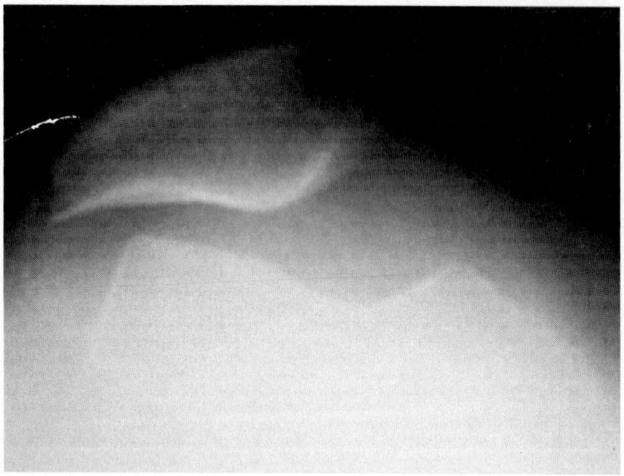

FIGURE 79-4 Merchant's view of knee showing patellar tilt and subluxation.

extremity are helpful in discerning problems in skeletally immature patients.

When describing the knee radiograph, the examiner should note the alignment and joint spacing of the femoral condyles in relation to the tibial plateau. Narrowing of the joint space (particularly in weight-bearing views) indicates articular cartilaginous and meniscal degeneration. Significant joint effusions are evident as water-density lucency on the lateral view, anterior to the distal femur. The patella should be examined for possible fractures (in the event of a direct blow to the anterior knee) and the presence of a bipartite or tripartite patella.[3]

In the setting of acute injuries, radiographs should be observed for the presence of fractures involving the tibial plateau (depression fracture) or tibial spine (suggesting rupture of the anterior cruciate ligament [ACL]). Segond's fractures are avulsion fractures of the lateral tibial plateau at the site of attachment of the lateral capsular ligament. These fractures are associated with ACL and meniscal injuries. The presence of posterior opaque bodies should be noted. These may be fabellae (congenital sesamoids) or loose bodies. More than 75% of loose bodies originate from osteochondral lesions.[3]

Suspected meniscal injuries, ligamentous disruptions, osteochondral lesions, and occult fractures can be confirmed with magnetic resonance imaging (MRI). Computerized tomography (CT) is helpful for establishing the extent of certain fractures (like tibial plateau fractures) and is often more readily available than MRI. Occult fractures that are commonly missed on plain radiographs include patellar, tibial plateau, fibular head, and Segond's fractures.[4]

■ LOWER LEG

Imaging of the lower leg should include the joint above and the joint below the injury. Oblique views are useful for detecting tibial plateau fractures, which may not be seen on routine views.

Traumatic Injuries

■ SOFT TISSUE AND CARTILAGINOUS INJURIES

■ Extensor Mechanism Injuries

The extensor mechanism of the knee is composed of the quadriceps muscles and tendon, patella, patellar tendon, and the tibial tubercle. Injuries can result from direct trauma (direct blow or laceration) or an indirect force (forced flexion of the knee).[5] Rupture of the extensor mechanism is relatively uncommon compared with other injuries to the knee joint.

■ *Quadriceps and Patellar Tendon Injuries*

The quadriceps tendon represents the convergence of the rectus femoris, vastus intermedius, vastus lateralis, and vastus medialis muscles. It inserts on the superior pole of the patella. The patellar tendon travels from the inferior pole of the patella to the tibial tubercle.

Quadriceps ruptures typically occur in patients older than 40 years. Rupture is usually the result of an indirect force causing forced flexion to the knee, which loads the tendon. Direct blows and lacerations can also cause disruptions of the tendon. The most common site of rupture is at or near its insertion on the patella. Predisposing factors are listed in Box 79-4.

Patellar tendon ruptures are less common. Risk factors for patellar tendon rupture are similar to those for quadriceps rupture, with the exception that they usually occur in patients younger than 40 years. Most patellar tendon ruptures occur along the inferior pole of the patella.

Pain, swelling, and ecchymosis are usually localized to the superior pole (quadriceps tendon) or inferior pole (patellar tendon) of the patella. A defect of the patella or quadriceps tendon may be palpable on physical examination. Other physical findings

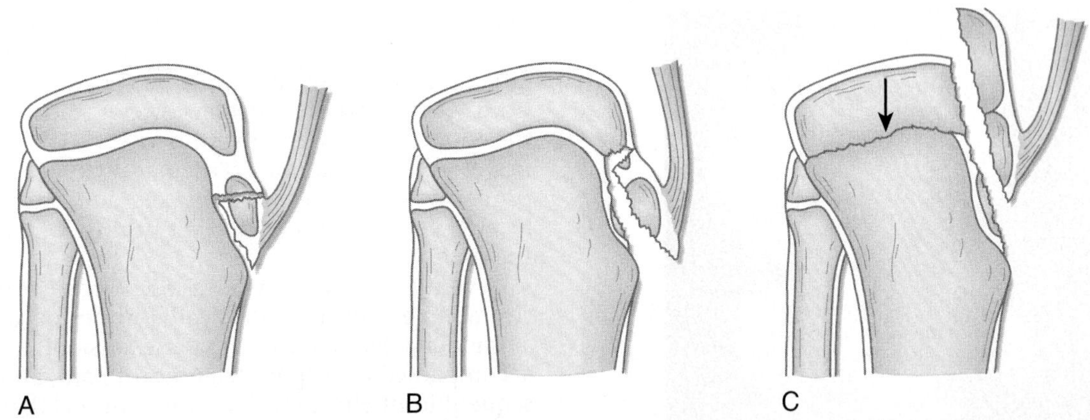

FIGURE 79-5 Avulsion fractures of the tibial tubercle. **A,** Type I fracture. The fracture line is through the secondary ossification center. **B,** Type II fracture. The fracture occurs through the junction of the ossification centers of the proximal end of the tibia and the tuberosity. **C,** A type III fracture is a true Salter-Harris type III injury that is intra-articular. (From Green NE, Swiontkowski MF: Skeletal Trauma in Children, 3rd ed, vol 3. Philadelphia, Saunders, 2003.)

BOX 79-4

Risk Factors for Quadriceps Tendon Rupture

- Age >40 years
- Steroid use
- Insertional tendinopathy
- Chronic metabolic disorders
- Chronic systemic conditions (rheumatoid arthritis, systemic lupus erythematosus, gout)

Data from Perryman JR, Hershman EB: The acute management of soft tissue injuries of the knee. Orthop Clin North Am 2002;33:575-585.

include a low-riding patella (patella baja) with inferior retraction of the patella (quadriceps tendon rupture), high-riding patella (patella alta) with superior retraction of the patella (patellar tendon rupture), inability to perform a straight-leg test, and extension lag.[5]

Extension lag is difficult or halting extension of the leg with the last 10 degrees of extension. Patients with partial tears may be difficult to diagnose on clinical examination, exhibiting weakness or pain only with resisted-leg extension.[5]

AP and lateral radiographs help define the patellar position (alta or baja) and rule out associated fractures. MRI is a helpful in the diagnosis of partial tears. Orthopedic consultation in the ED is indicated for suspected injuries and complete ruptures.

Initial treatment consists of ice, elevation, and immobilization of the leg in an extended position. Partial tears are treated with immobilization for 4 to 6 weeks, whereas complete tears are treated surgically. Diagnosis is essential, given the better outcomes with prompt referral and repair.[5]

Tibial Tuberosity Fractures

The tibial tubercle is a bony prominence that is found approximately 3 cm distal to the proximal articular surface of the tibia and in line with the medial half of the patella. It is the insertion point of the extensor mechanism; thus, accurate reduction and healing of a fracture of this structure is essential. The classifications of tibial tuberosity fractures are shown in Figure 79-5.[6]

Tibial tubercle avulsion fractures are rare injuries. Although they can occur in adults, they are more commonly seen in adolescents undergoing a growth spurt. Most fractures are the result of an indirect force delivered by an eccentric load.[5] A sudden flexion force is applied while the knee is in flexion and the quadriceps is tightly contracted. The quadriceps resists the force, causing an avulsion of the tibial tubercle.

The physical findings depend on the extent of the injury. Swelling and tenderness are present over the anterior aspect of the tibia. A joint effusion may result from associated intra-articular injuries. The injured knee is usually held in 20 to 40 degrees of flexion secondary to hamstring spasm. In addition, the patient may not be able to extend the knee because of either pain or the loss of the extensor mechanism.[7]

Routine AP and lateral radiographs are useful for ruling out associated fractures (Fig. 79-6). Initial treatment is similar to that for both quadriceps and patellar tendon injuries. Minimally displaced fractures are treated conservatively. Displaced fractures frequently require open reduction and internal fixation.[5]

Ligamentous and Meniscal Injuries

Knee stability depends on the static stability of the ligaments and the dynamic stability of the muscles. Injuries to the knee involve the following six common

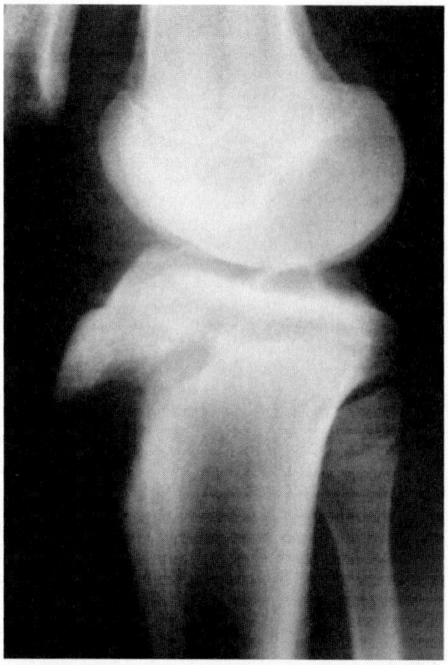

FIGURE 79-6 Lateral knee radiograph of a 14-year-old boy with a displaced fracture of the tibial tubercle. (From Green NE, Swiontkowski MF: Skeletal Trauma in Children, 3rd ed, vol 3. Philadelphia, Saunders, 2003.)

mechanisms: (1) valgus stress (laterally directed), (2) varus stress (medially directed), (3) hyperextension, (4) rotational stress, (5) direct anterior stress, and (6) direct posterior stress. The result of these stressors working in isolation or combination is a myriad of ligamentous, meniscal, or chondral injuries.[5] Common mechanisms of ligamentous knee injuries are shown in Figure 79-7. Ligamentous laxity is graded using the American Medical Association classification system (Table 79-4).

Cruciate Ligament Injuries

Anterior Cruciate Ligament. The ACL prevents the forward displacement of the tibia upon the femur. The ACL travels from the lateral femoral condyle to the medial tibia in anterior, medial, and distal directions. The vascular supply for the ACL originates from the middle genicular artery, a branch of the popliteal artery. Innervation for the ACL is derived from the posterior articular nerve, which primarily innervates the stretch and nociceptors located in the subsynovial layer near the insertion of the ACL.

Seventy percent of ACL injuries occur from noncontact mechanisms. Classically, injury occurs with a sudden deceleration, hyperextension, or twist accompanied by a "pop," significant pain, and a subsequent joint effusion. Common motions that injure the ACL are a plant-and-cut maneuver, a straight-leg landing, and a one-step stop and jump.[8]

ACL-deficient knees rely on the menisci (primarily the medial menisci), soleus, and hamstring muscles as the primary stabilizers of anterior translation. Meniscal tears occur in more than 50% of acute ACL injuries and more than 80% of chronic injuries. Studies have shown that up to 71% of patients who do not sustain a meniscal tear at the time of ACL injury go on to have a meniscal tear.[8]

The formation of a joint effusion within 4 to 6 hours of injury suggests the presence of an intra-articular injury (ACL or meniscal injury) or osteochondral fracture.[8] Lachman's test is the most sensitive test for ACL injury or disruption (see Table 79-2).[5] Stability tests for ACL injury (Lachman's, anterior drawer, and pivot-shift tests) are depicted in Figures 79-8 through 79-10.

Plain radiographs may show findings suggestive of ACL injury, such as an avulsion of the lateral capsule (Segond's fracture) or a tibial spine avulsion, which is seen more commonly in younger patients. Plain radiographs may also show nonspecific findings that can be related to an ACL injury, such as a joint effusion, subtle fractures of the posterior tibial plateau, and impaction of the lateral sulcus.[8] MRI offers a direct, noninvasive view of all of the knee ligaments,

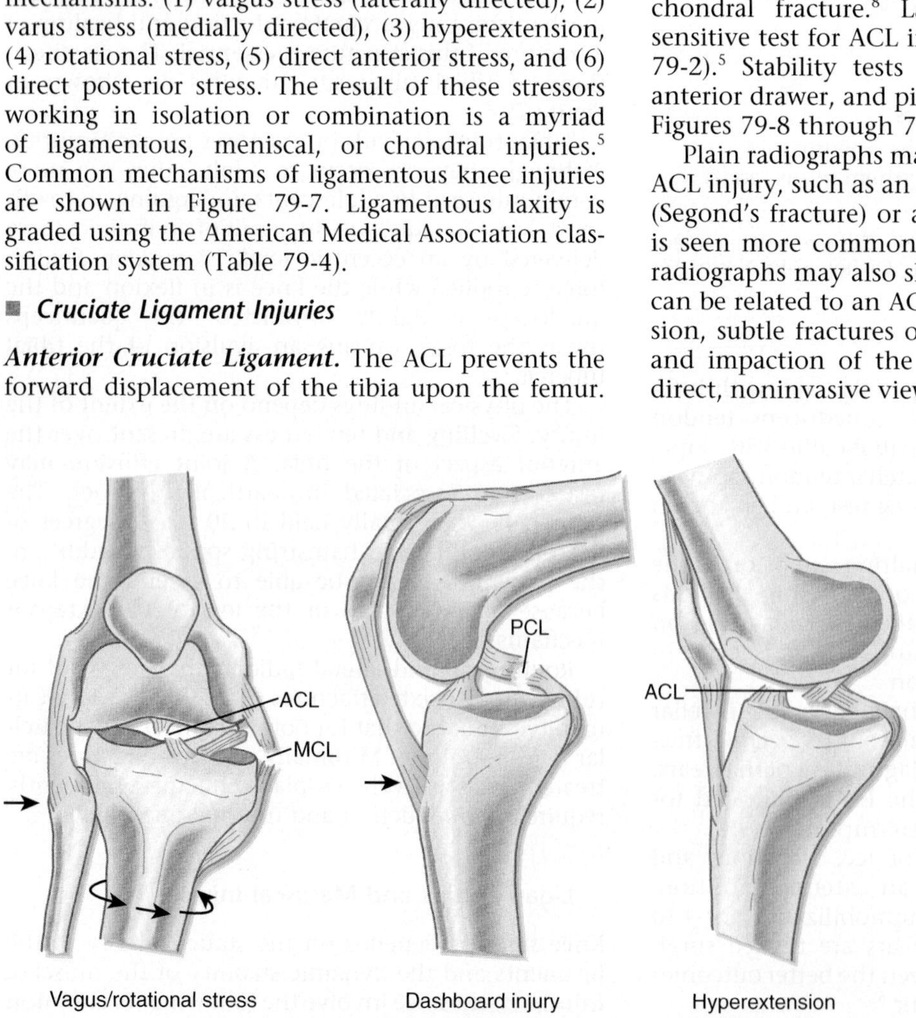
ACL
MCL
PCL
ACL
Vagus/rotational stress
Dashboard injury
Hyperextension

FIGURE 79-7 Common mechanisms of knee injuries. ACL, anterior cruciate ligament; LCL, lateral collateral ligament; MCL, medial collateral ligament; PCL, posterior cruciate ligament. (From Browner BD, Jupiter JB, Levine AM, et al: Skeletal Trauma; Basic Science, Management, and Reconstruction, 3rd ed. Philadelphia, Saunders, 2003.)

Table 79-4 AMERICAN MEDICAL ASSOCIATION CLASSIFICATION OF LIGAMENTOUS LAXITY

Grade	Anatomic Changes	Physical Findings
1	Stretching of ligamentous fibers	No ligamentous laxity on stress testing Firm endpoint
2	Incomplete tear of ligament	Firm endpoint Ligamentous laxity
3	Complete tear of ligament	No endpoint Varying degrees of ligamentous laxity

From Committee on the Medical Aspects of Sports: Standard Nomenclature of Athletic Injuries. Chicago, American Medical Association, 1968.

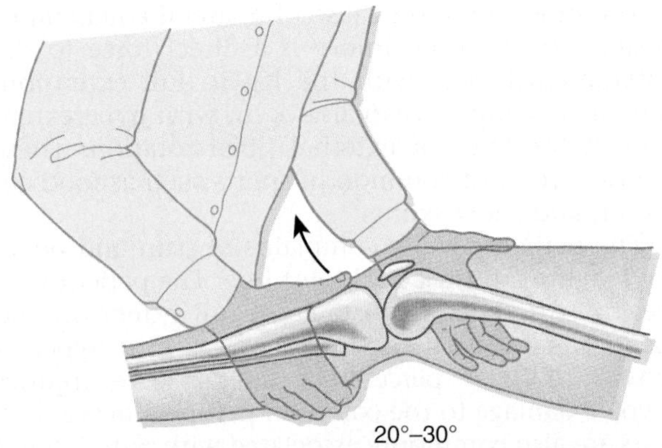
20°–30°

FIGURE 79-8 Lachman's test for anterior drawer instability. The test is done at 20 to 30 degrees of flexion. The examiner stabilizes the femur with one hand and draws the tibia anteriorly with the other hand. (From Browner BD, Jupiter JB, Levine AM, et al: Skeletal Trauma; Basic Science, Management, and Reconstruction, 3rd ed. Philadelphia, Saunders, 2003.)

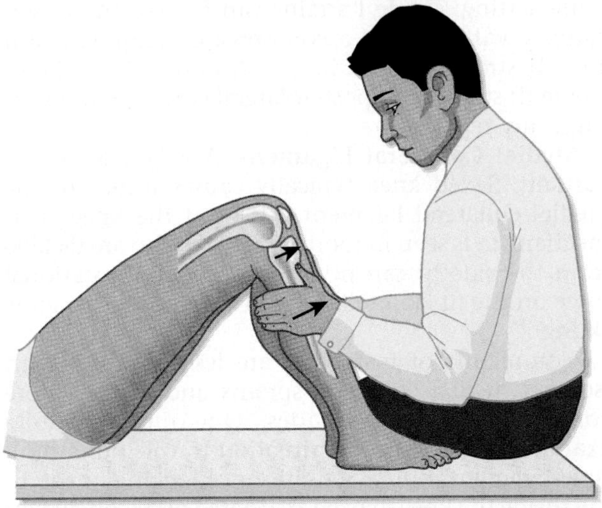

FIGURE 79-9 Anterior drawer test. The knee is placed in 90 degrees of flexion, the foot is stabilized with pressure toward the examination table, and the proximal tibia is grasped and pulled forward. (From Brown JR, Trojian TH: Anterior and posterior cruciate ligament injuries. Prim Care 2004;31:925-956.)

the menisci, and the soft tissue structures; however, it is rarely indicated in the ED.

Initial treatment consists of ice, elevation, pain control, and knee immobilization. Patients should be instructed to perform gentle range-of-motion exercises (flexion or extension) of the knee two or three times a day to maintain joint mobility. Ambulation can resume when the patient is more comfortable. Follow-up and re-examination within a week should be arranged.

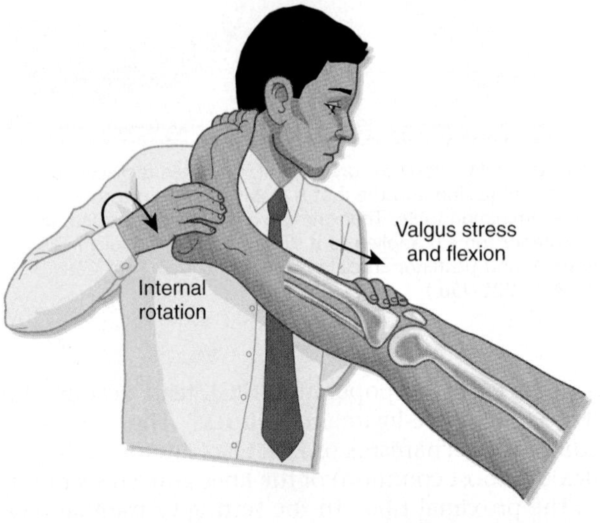
Valgus stress
and flexion
Internal
rotation

FIGURE 79-10 Pivot shift test. With one hand, the examiner flexes the hip to 45 degrees, extends the knee, and holds the heel. With the other hand, the examiner holds the knee with the thumb behind the fibular head. The examiner then internally rotates the leg at the heel and applies valgus stress and flexion at the knee. (From Brown JR, Trojian TH: Anterior and posterior cruciate ligament injuries. Prim Care 2004;31:925-956.)

Posterior Cruciate Ligament. The posterior cruciate ligament (PCL) originates along the lateral border of the medial femoral condyle at the junction of the medial wall and the roof of the intercondylar notch. The PCL lies in proximity to the posterolateral corner, which acts collectively as a secondary stabilizer of posterior tibial translation. The PCL receives its blood supply from branches of the middle geniculate artery, and its nerve supply from the posterior articular branch of the posterior tibial nerve, which provides innervation to pressure, velocity, and pain receptors.[8]

The PCL forms the central pivot about which the knee rotates. It is the primary restraint against posterior tibial displacement. The PCL resists 85% to 100% of posteriorly directed knee forces between 30 degrees and 90 degrees of knee flexion. It is a secondary restraint to external tibial rotation and also prevents hyperextension of the knee.[8]

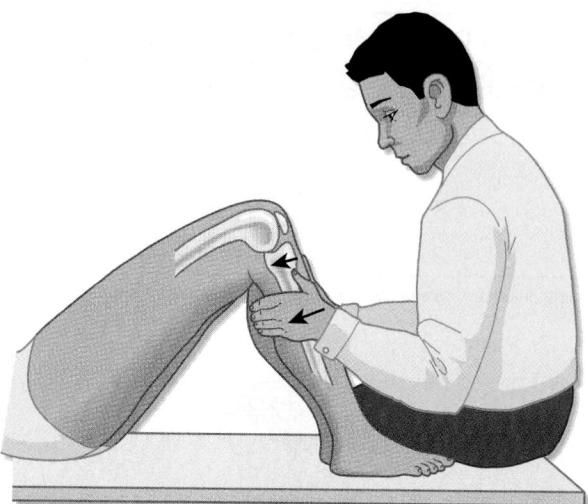

FIGURE 79-11 Posterior drawer test. The knee is placed in 90 degrees of flexion and the foot is stabilized with pressure toward the examination table. Then the proximal tibia is grasped, and a posterior force is applied to it. (From Brown JR, Trojian TH: Anterior and posterior cruciate ligament injuries. Prim Care 2004;31:925-956.)

In the general population, PCL tears account for 3% of all knee-ligament injuries.[8] The two most common mechanisms of PCL tears are forced hyperflexion (most common) of the knee and a direct blow to the proximal tibia. In the setting of trauma, 95% of patients with PCL injuries have associated ligamentous injuries to the same knee. PCL injuries occur more commonly in high-contact sports, such as football and rugby, and less frequently in sports that involve less contact and more pivoting and cutting, such as basketball.[8]

Unlike patients with ACL and MCL injuries, patients with PCL injuries do not describe an event in which they felt a pop or tear indicating ligamentous injury. Instead, they usually report vague symptoms, such as unsteadiness and discomfort.[8] The posterior sag sign and the posterior drawer test (Fig. 79-11) are helpful in the evaluation of the PCL (see Table 79-2).

The majority of PCL injuries can be diagnosed from the history and physical examination. Imaging modalities help confirm the diagnosis and enhance the preoperative assessment of internal injury to the knee. Plain radiographs may exhibit posterior sagging on the lateral view, avulsion fractures at the PCL insertion site, and widening of the lateral joint space if the posterolateral corner is involved. MRI is a highly sensitive and specific modality for detecting PCL injuries. MRI is most useful for preoperative planning and is not indicated as an emergency procedure.[8]

Acute treatment includes ice, compression, elevation, and knee immobilization. The patient may bear weight on the affected leg with crutches. Gentle range-of-motion exercises should be started early, followed by quadriceps strengthening exercises once range of motion is restored.[5] Definitive treatment is based on the severity of injury as well as the patient's activity level and expectations.[8]

Collateral Ligament Injury

Lateral Collateral Ligament. The lateral collateral ligament (LCL) originates on the lateral femoral condyle and inserts into the fibular head. This ligament is taut in full extension but becomes lax after flexion past 30 degrees. The biceps tendon has fibers connecting to the LCL that can put tension on the ligament during flexion.[9]

The most common cause of a lateral collateral or posterolateral corner injury is a direct force to the anteromedial knee with the leg in full extension. Lateral knee injuries can also occur with hyperextension of the knee or external tibial rotation. These injuries are most common in sports such as football, soccer, and snow skiing.[9]

The patient usually complains of pain and possibly swelling at the lateral joint line. The patient may feel that the knee is unstable in full extension and may complain that the knee buckles into hyperextension. Fifteen percent of lateral knee injuries involve damage to the common peroneal nerve. LCL tears are also commonly associated with anterior and posterior cruciate tears.

Varus stress testing should be performed with the knee in full extension and with the knee flexed to 30 degrees (see Table 79-2).[9]

Plain radiographs rule out avulsion fractures and other bony abnormalities. MRI is not indicated in the acute setting. Grade I strains can be treated conservatively with ice and a compression wrap. Grade II and III strains require immobilization of the knee. Grade III strains and posterolateral corner injuries are surgically repaired.[9]

Medial Collateral Ligament. A valgus load to a partially flexed knee typically causes injury to the medial collateral ligament (MCL) of the knee. This mechanism is seen in football players who are tackled from the side or can involve an external rotational force on the tibia in relation to the femur (as in snow skiing).[9]

Complaints of instability are less common with isolated medial collateral sprains and are far more common with ACL injuries. One must carefully examine the ACL in this situation to rule out a multiple-ligament injury. Sensations of locking or catching inside the knee may be associated with concurrent meniscal tears, which occur in up to 5% of isolated MCL injuries. A patient with a MCL tear may describe having felt a "pop" in the medial knee during the injury.[9]

Physical examination testing includes valgus stress testing in full extension and at 30 degrees of flexion on both the injured and uninjured knees (see Table 79-2).

Most MCL injuries can be diagnosed clinically. Plain radiographs detect avulsion fractures due to MCL injuries. MRI is not indicated in the acute setting.[9]

Acute management of isolated MCL injuries consists of ice, immobilization, and crutches. Progressive range-of-motion exercises should be started early. Quadriceps strengthening exercises can begin when range of motion is restored.[5]

Meniscal Injuries

Menisci are composed primarily of type I collagen, which represents 60% to 70% of their dry weight. The meniscal blood supply arises from superior, inferior, medial, and lateral geniculate arteries, which form a peripheral perimeniscal synovial vascular plexus.[10]

Menisci serve many functions, such as increasing the contact area and congruency of the femorotibial articulation. The menisci load-share and reduce contact stresses across the joint. It is estimated that menisci transmit up to 50% to 70% of the load in extension and 85% of the load in 90 degrees of flexion.[10] Meniscal injuries in children younger than 10 years are rare unless associated with a discoid meniscus. The incidence of meniscal and other intra-articular disorders increases with age.

Most meniscal tears are noncontact in nature and occur while a person is cutting, decelerating, or landing from a jump. Because degeneration of the menisci increases with age, tears often occur with trivial injury.

The patient is often not aware of a specific injury, only of the symptoms that follow. Although nonspecific, mechanical symptoms of popping, catching, locking, or buckling along with joint line pain are suggestive of a meniscal tear. Most meniscal tears lead to a mild synovitis, with swelling for several days after the injury and recurrence of symptoms with certain activities.[11]

A positive McMurray's or Apley's test is suggestive of a meniscal injury. However, both tests have a poor sensitivity and specificity (see Table 79-2). Plain radiographs may be obtained to look for associated skeletal injury, presence of loose bodies, and degenerative changes.[11]

Patients should be discharged on a partial weight-bearing status until they are seen at follow-up. A patient presenting with a locked knee should undergo conscious sedation and attempted reduction: The knee is allowed to hang over stretcher or is placed in 90 degrees of flexion. Longitudinal traction is applied to the leg while the knee is internally and externally rotated. If the knee cannot be unlocked with this maneuver, orthopedic consultation is necessary.

Surgical treatment is recommended for most meniscal tears except those causing minor symptoms in less active patients. Surgery is urgently indicated for the locked knee.[11]

MUSCLE STRAINS

Gastrocnemius Muscle Strain

The gastrocnemius, soleus, and plantaris muscles form the superficial muscles of the calf. The tendon of the gastrocnemius muscle has two heads, which arise from the posterior surfaces of the medial and lateral femoral condyles. The tendons of the gastrocnemius and soleus muscles form the Achilles tendon, which inserts on the posterior tubercle of the calcaneus. The gastrocnemius muscle primarily acts as a plantar flexor but also gives some passive support to the posterior joint capsule. The most common mechanism of injury of this muscle is hyperextension of the knee. Posterior dislocation of the tibia during knee flexion may also injure it.

Patients may present with a description of sudden calf pain while running or making a sudden stop or cut. Pain and swelling of the calf develops over the next day, and tenderness is typically found at the musculotendinous junction of the medial (more common) or lateral head of the gastrocnemius muscle. A complete rupture of the head of the gastrocnemius muscle is associated with retraction of the muscle belly. Acute posterior compartment syndrome has been associated with rupture of the medial head of the gastrocnemius muscle.[12]

Plain radiographs are not indicated. MRI may be helpful if a soft tissue injury is in doubt. Acute strains of the gastrocnemius muscle are treated with conservative management, consisting of ice, compression wraps, and anti-inflammatory medications. Gentle passive and active stretching exercises are begun early.

Strain or Rupture of the Plantaris Muscle

The plantaris muscle is a pencil-shaped muscle that originates at the lateral condyle of the femur and passes below the soleus to attach to the Achilles tendon. Strain of the proximal plantaris muscle may occur with an injury to the ACL.

Patients with plantaris muscle rupture may experience a deep, disabling pain in the calf followed by a dull, deep ache. On examination, tenderness is greatest just lateral to the midline of the posterior calf. No diagnostic testing is indicated. Plantaris muscle strains and ruptures are treated conservatively.

Shin Splints

Shin splints are also known as the medial tibial stress syndrome. This syndrome characterized by diffuse tenderness over the posteromedial aspect of the distal third of the tibia. This syndrome is believed to represent a periostalgia or tendinopathy along the tibial attachment of the tibialis posterior or soleus muscle. It may be confused with stress fracture.[13]

Common contributing factors are improper shoe wear, rapid transition in training, inadequate warm-up, running on uneven or hard surfaces, running in cold weather, and anatomic considerations such as muscle imbalance, lower extremity length inequality, femoral anteversion, and tibial or forefoot varus.[13] Patients with mild cases of shin splints have pain during exercise, whereas those with more severe cases have pain at rest.

Diagnostic tests are not indicated for shin splints unless there is a question of a tibial stress fracture. The treatment of shin splints involves relative rest, training adjustment, and anti-inflammatory medications. Runners should be instructed to avoid hill running and running on uneven surfaces.[13]

DISLOCATIONS AND FRACTURES

Knee Dislocations

Knee dislocation is associated with a high risk of neurovascular injury and should be considered an orthopedic emergency. Dislocations are classified on the basis of the direction of tibial movement in relation to the femur. Anterior and posterior dislocations account for between 50% and 75% of all knee dislocations. Knee dislocations may also have associated intra-articular fractures involving the tibial plateau or femoral condyles.

The neurovascular bundle (popliteal artery, popliteal vein, and common peroneal nerve) runs posteriorly behind all bony and ligamentous structures in the popliteal fossa. The popliteal artery is fixed in the fibrous tunnel of the adductor magnus hiatus muscle proximally and traverses the fibrous arch of the soleus muscle and interosseous membrane distally. The relative immobility of the neurovascular bundle makes it susceptible to injury. The popliteal artery is injured in 20% to 30% of all knee dislocations.[14] Traction injuries to the peroneal and tibial nerves are also common.[14]

The most common mechanism of injury for knee dislocations is high-energy trauma such as motor vehicle crashes and auto-pedestrian accidents.[14] Approximately 20% to 30% of high-energy dislocations are open injuries. Low-energy traumatic dislocations are caused by falls and sports injuries.[14]

A grossly unstable knee after a traumatic injury should be assumed to be a reduced dislocation until proven otherwise. Any patient who has a suspected knee dislocation should undergo a careful neurovascular examination. Anterior and posterior dislocations have a higher incidence of vascular injury. Vascular compromise in a dislocated knee requires immediate reduction.

A diminished pulse or arterial pressure index (API) value less than 0.9 in a patient with a knee dislocation necessitates a vascular surgery consultation and arteriogram to rule out vascular injury.[15] Partial or complete dysfunction of the common peroneal nerve should be assessed. Partial injuries are associated with a higher rate of full recovery.[5] Peroneal nerve palsy, present in 14% to 35% of knee dislocations, is associated with medial knee dislocations.[5]

Standard AP and lateral radiographs are adequate for initial evaluation of knee dislocations. Significant controversy exists as to whether all patients with knee dislocation should undergo arteriography to rule out vascular injury. Some surgeons advocate arteriograms in all patients despite vascular status, but others urge more selective use of arteriograms in patients with normal physical findings (Fig. 79-12).[5]

After appropriate analgesia and sedation, emergency reduction of the dislocated knee should be attempted. The knee should be reduced by application of longitudinal traction to the leg while the femur is lifted anteriorly. Neurovascular status should be assessed before and after reduction. Reduction should not be delayed for radiographs. After reduction, the knee should be immobilized in 15 degrees of flexion. Prompt diagnosis of vascular injury is essential, given the chance of development of progressive distal ischemia. When popliteal artery injury exists, patient outcome is directly related to the duration of ischemia.

Patellar Dislocation

The annual incidence of patellar dislocations ranges from 7 per 100,000 to 43 per 100,000, depending on the age and patient population. Thirty percent to 72% of dislocations are sports-related, and 28% to 39% of such dislocations have associated osteochondral fractures.[16]

The patella normally articulates in the groove between the femoral condyles. The vastus medialis, medial retinaculum, medial and lateral patellofemoral, and patellotibial ligaments all stabilize the patella (Fig. 79-13).

The most common mechanism of patellar dislocation involves a direct blow to the superior pole of the patella followed by rotation, resulting in a horizontal dislocation. Less commonly, a direct force to the patella with the knee in flexion causes a patellar dislocation.

The patient may report that the knee "gave out," followed by pain and swelling. Patients may not be able to bear weight on or flex the knee. An acute hemarthrosis is most commonly seen if there is an associated osteochondral fracture. Osteochondral fractures, which usually occur along the articular surface of the patella, are seen in less than 5% of patellar dislocations.

A patellar apprehension test may be useful in a patient who reports a dislocation that resolved spontaneously. The test is performed by moving a nondisplaced patella laterally. The result is positive if the patient shows apprehension, feels pain, or feels a sensation of impending dislocation when the patella is moved laterally (Fig. 79-14). AP and lateral radiographs are adequate to evaluate for acute dislocations and associated fractures.

After proper sedation, the ED can reduce a lateral dislocation by flexing the hip and pushing medially on the patella while extending the knee. Postreduction radiographs are mandatory to rule out osteochondral fractures. Intra-articular, horizontal, and superior dislocations typically require open reduction. Dislocations associated with osteochondral fractures are usually treated surgically.

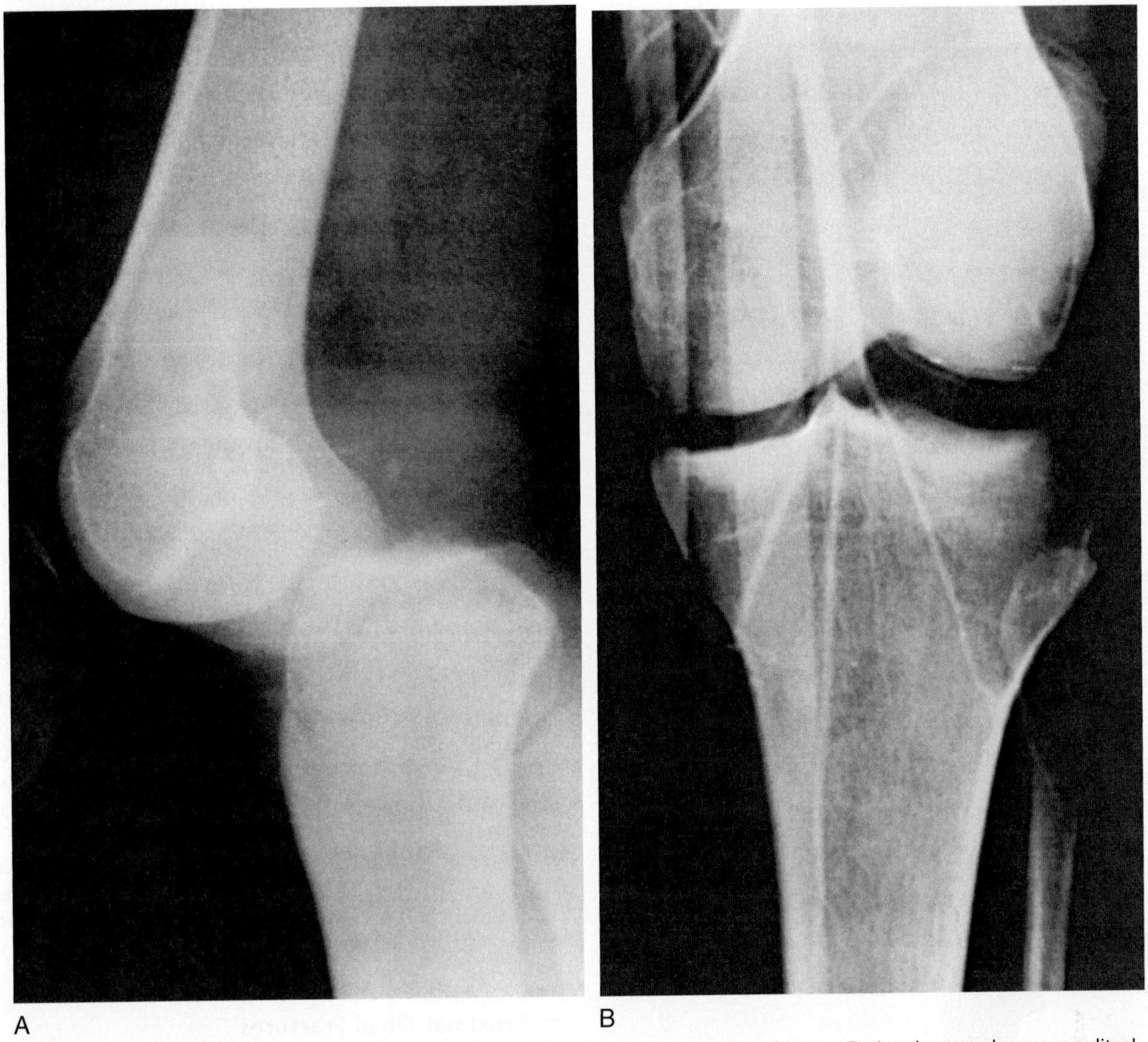

FIGURE 79-12 **A,** Radiograph demonstrates posterior knee dislocation from a dashboard injury. **B,** Arteriogram shows a popliteal artery injury. (From Browner BD, Jupiter JB, Levine AM, et al: Skeletal Trauma; Basic Science, Management, and Reconstruction, 3rd ed. Philadelphia, Saunders, 2003.)

After reduction, the patient should be told to use conservative therapeutic measures, such as ice and elevation, and pain control. The knee should be immobilized, and the patient can start progressive weight bearing when comfortable. Follow-up should be arranged within 1 to 2 weeks.

■ Proximal Tibiofibular Joint Dislocations

A rare injury, proximal tibiofibular dislocation is seen more in adolescents and young adults. It is typically associated with motor vehicle crashes and sports such as sky diving and hang gliding.

The proximal tibiofibular joint is a small joint between the head of the fibula and the inferior aspect of the lateral tibial condyle. It is stabilized by the joint capsule and the anterior and posterior tibiofibular ligaments. Dislocations can be anterior (most common), posterior, or superior.

Pain and tenderness are felt over the proximal tibiofibular joint. On physical examination, the patient has worsening pain with inversion and eversion of the foot or flexion-extension of the ankle. Instability may be present when anterior or posterior pressure is applied to the fibular head. Peroneal nerve injury occurs in approximately 5% of these dislocations.

AP and lateral radiographs are indicated. A comparison view may be helpful to make the diagnosis. Radiographs may demonstrate lateral displacement of the fibular head or diastasis of the proximal tibia and fibula.

Tibiofibular dislocations are reduced by flexing of the knee to 90 degrees while the ankle is everted and dorsiflexed, and application of direct pressure to the head of the fibula. General anesthesia may be necessary. After reduction, the knee should be immobilized in extension or partial flexion. Posterior dis-

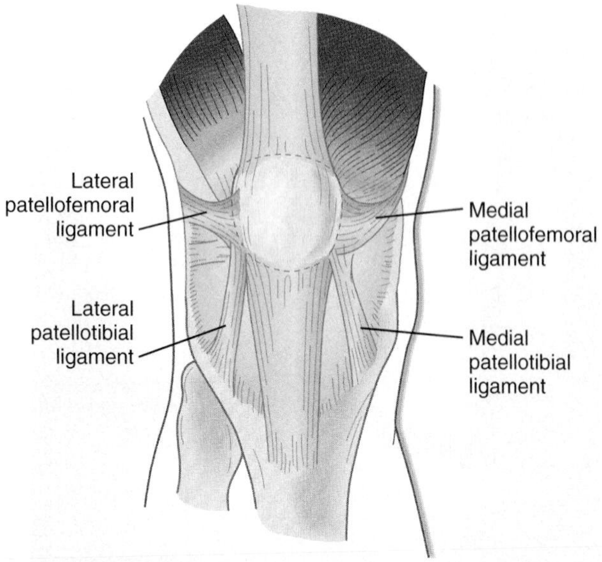
Lateral patellofemoral ligament
Medial patellofemoral ligament
Lateral patellotibial ligament
Medial patellotibial ligament

FIGURE 79-13 Patellofemoral and patellotibial ligaments. These structures act as static stabilizers of the patella. (From DeLee JC, Drez D Jr, Miller MD: DeLee & Drez's Orthopaedic Sports Medicine: Principles and Practice, 2nd ed. Philadelphia, Saunders, 2003.)

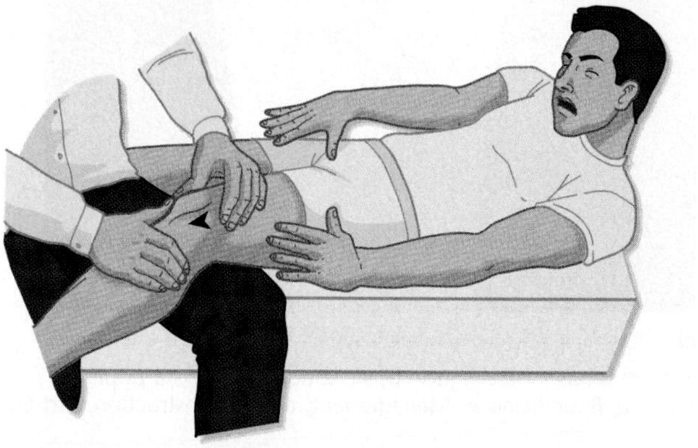

FIGURE 79-14 Positive apprehension test. As the patella is displaced laterally over the lateral femoral condyle, the patient experiences apprehension and discomfort. (From DeLee JC, Drez D Jr, Miller MD: DeLee & Drez's Orthopaedic Sports Medicine: Principles and Practice, 2nd ed. Philadelphia, Saunders, 2003.)

locations may be unstable, and recurrent subluxation may be seen. Degenerative joint disease and arthritis can develop after injury to this joint.

■ Patellar Fracture

The patella, the largest sesamoid bone in the body, is enveloped within the quadriceps tendon and articulates with the trochlear groove of the distal femur. The blood supply of the patella enters via central and distal polar vessels. Disruption of the blood supply can lead to avascular necrosis. The superficial location of the patella makes it more susceptible to injury. Patellar injuries accounts for approximately 1% of all skeletal injuries.

Patellar fractures are the result of either a direct injury or an indirect injury such as violent flexion. Indirect injuries result in an avulsion injury of the patella owing to the pull of the quadriceps muscle against resistance. Transverse patellar fractures are the most common type of fracture and are more likely to be displaced and to manifest as a disrupted extensor mechanism. Comminuted patellar fractures represent one third of all fractures[17] and are common in the elderly population.[18]

The patient usually presents with a swollen, painful knee. Patellar evaluation includes palpation for pain and bony disruption and assessment of extensor weakness.[5]

AP, lateral, and axial (Merchant's) views of the knee should be obtained. A bipartite patella may be difficult to distinguish from patellar fracture, and is most often seen in the superolateral part of the patella. A high-riding patella, or patella alta position, may signify disruption of the distal extensor mechanism; this is best visualized on the AP and lateral views.[17] Acute treatment of patellar fractures consists of ice, elevation, pain control, and knee immobilization in an extended position.[5]

Nonoperative intervention is considered for nondisplaced fractures (<3-4 mm) when the extensor mechanism is intact. Patients discharged from the ED should be referred for follow-up within a few days and can begin progressive weight bearing with crutches.

Surgical management is indicated for displaced fractures and in patients with disruption of the extensor mechanism.[17] Severely comminuted fractures may require patellectomy.[17]

■ Proximal Tibial Fractures

Proximal tibial fractures are those fractures above the tibial tuberosity.

■ *Tibial Plateau Fractures*

The proximal tibia comprises the medial and lateral condyles, which make up approximately three fourths of the proximal tibial surface. The condyles ensure appropriate knee alignment, stability, and motion. Tibial plateau fractures account for about 1% of all fractures of the proximal tibia.[18]

Tibial plateau fractures occur from side loading due to either a varus or a valgus force combined with axial compression, which results in the femoral condyle impacting upon the tibia. Common mechanisms are motor vehicle crashes, falls, and athletic activities such as skiing (Fig. 79-15). Segond's fracture is bony avulsion of the lateral tibial plateau at the site of the attachment of the lateral capsular ligament. This fracture is an important marker for ACL disruption and anterolateral rotary instability.

The Schatzker classification is the most widely accepted classification system for tibial plateau fractures (Fig. 79-16). Types I to III tibial plateau fractures are usually associated with lower-energy mechanisms

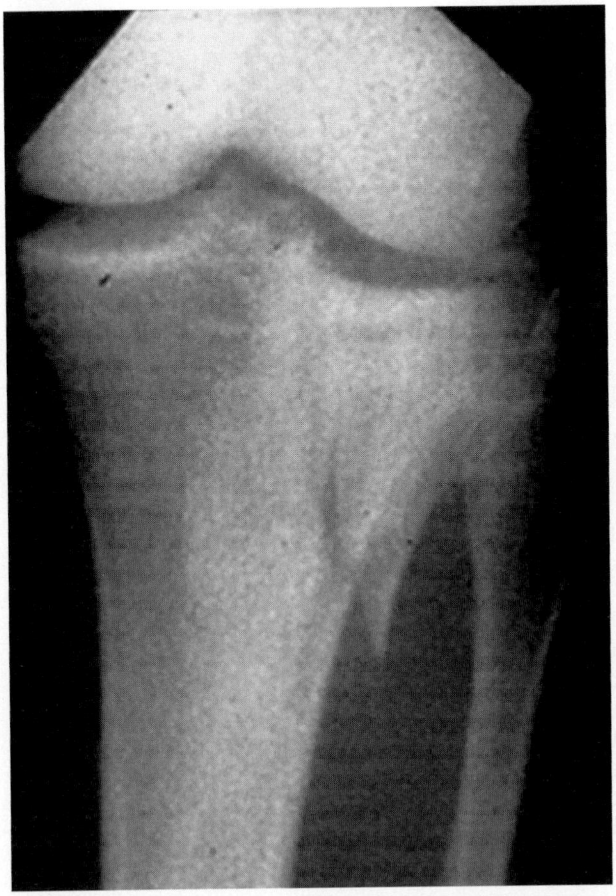

FIGURE 79-15 Lateral tibial plateau fracture. (From Browner BD, Jupiter JB, Levine AM, et al: Skeletal Trauma: Basic Science, Management, and Reconstruction, 3rd ed. Philadelphia, Saunders, 2003.)

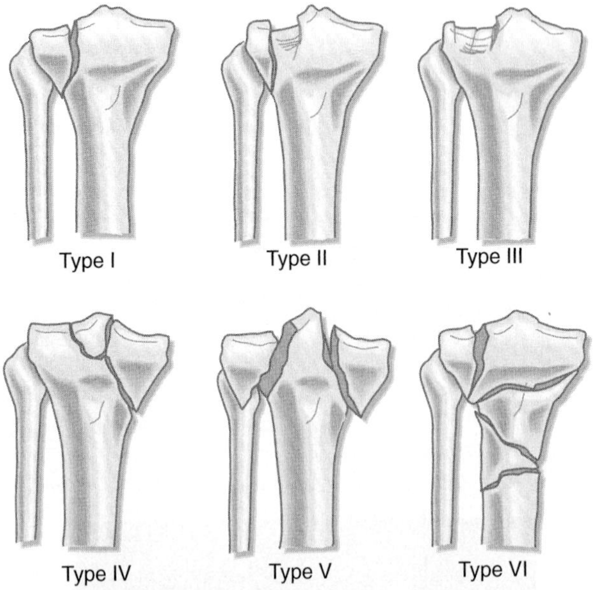
Type I
Type II
Type III
Type IV
Type V
Type VI

FIGURE 79-16 The Schatzker classification. (From Virkus WW, Helfet DL: Tibial plateau fractures. In Insall JN, Scott WN [eds]: Surgery of the Knee, 4th ed. Philadelphia, Churchill Livingstone, 2001.)

than types IV to VI.[19] Associated soft tissue injuries to the collateral ligaments, menisci, and neurovascular structures are common, although low-energy injuries (from athletic activities) usually result in less soft tissue damage.[18]

Patients with tibial plateau fractures exhibit pain and swelling of the knee and present with the knee slightly flexed. A valgus or varus deformity of the knee usually indicates a depressed fracture. Careful assessment of associated ipsilateral bony, soft tissue, and neurovascular injuries is essential, given the high rate of association of such injuries with tibial plateau fractures.[18]

AP, lateral, and oblique radiographs are necessary to evaluate tibial plateau fractures. In addition, a tibial plateau view is also helpful to assess the amount of depression present. Preoperative CT with three-dimensional reconstruction is useful to further evaluate fracture patterns, show the precise extent of articular depression, identify the intact region of the plateau, and assist in planning for optimal operative treatment.[19]

Nonoperative treatment is indicated for minimal or nondisplaced fractures (<3 mm of articular incongruity), peripheral (submeniscal) fractures, and fractures in the elderly, low-demand, or osteoporotic patient. Patients should not bear weight on the affected leg for 4 to 6 weeks.

Absolute indications for surgery are open fractures, arterial injuries, and compartment syndrome. Relative indications for surgery are displaced fractures leading to joint instability and depression of the plateau. The amount of depression that requires operative intervention is controversial, and ranges from 3 to 10 mm in various reports; however, 3 mm is the usual cutoff in athletic patients.[18]

Tibial Spine Fractures

Tibial eminence avulsion fractures occur most often in children 8 to 14 years old but can occur in the skeletally mature patient as well. A fracture of the anterior tibial spine in children is equivalent to an ACL rupture in adults.[20]

The intercondylar eminence, or tibial spine, is the central portion of the proximal tibial surface. Tibial spine injuries usually result from a hyperextension force with or without a valgus or rotational moment about the knee. The fracture also may occur after a direct blow to the distal femur while the knee is flexed. The Meyers and McKeever classification is the most widely accepted classification scheme for these types of fractures (Figs. 79-17 and 79-18).

The patient presents with a suggestive history and a painful, swollen knee. In most cases, the patient is unable to fully extend the knee and exhibits an effusion, and stability test results (Lachman's, anterior drawer) are abnormal. The examiner should carefully evaluate the patient for associated ligamentous injuries.

Routine AP and lateral radiographs are adequate to define these fractures. CT is helpful for looking at

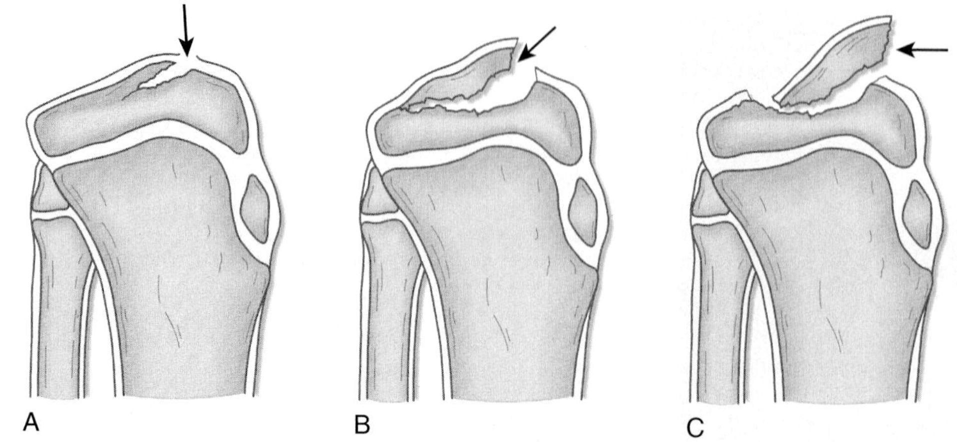
A
B
C

FIGURE 79-17 Meyers and McKeever classification of fractures of the anterior tibial spine. **A,** Type I fracture with no displacement of the fracture. **B,** Type II fracture with elevation of the anterior portion of the anterior tibial spine, but with the fracture posteriorly reduced. **C,** Type III fracture that is totally displaced. (From Green NE, Swiontkowski MF: Skeletal Trauma in Children, 3rd ed, vol 3. Philadelphia, Saunders, 2003.)

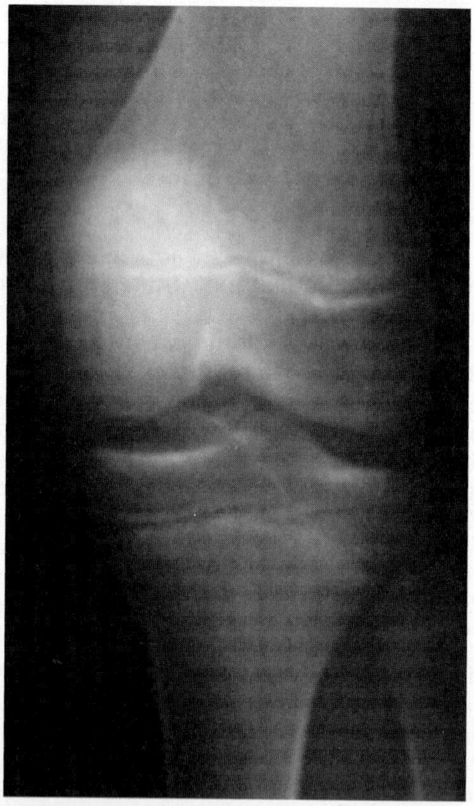

FIGURE 79-18 Type III eminence fracture. Note complete displacement of the avulsed fragment.

displacement, whereas MRI is superior at assessing accompanying soft tissue injuries.

Type I fractures with little or no displacement should be immobilized in a long-leg splint with the knee flexed at approximately 10 to 20 degrees. Type II fractures should undergo closed reduction if there is no ligamentous damage. Most type III fractures should undergo open or arthroscopic reduction with fragment fixation.[20]

Subcondylar Fractures

Subcondylar fractures involve the proximal tibial metaphysis and are usually transverse or oblique. Isolated subcondylar fractures are rare and are usually associated with tibial plateau fractures.[17]

Routine AP and lateral radiographs are adequate for evaluation of subcondylar fractures. The acute management of these injuries involves ice, elevation, and immobilization with a long-leg splint. Stable extra-articular nondisplaced transverse fractures are treated with a long-leg cast for 8 weeks. Fractures that are comminuted or associated with a condylar component require open reduction and internal fixation.[17]

Tibial Shaft Fractures

Tibial shaft fractures are the most common long bone fractures as well as the most common open fracture. They are commonly associated with a fibular fracture or ligamentous injury. The fibula remains intact in only 15% to 25% of tibial shaft fractures. These fractures are associated with a high incidence of infection, delayed union, nonunion, or malunion.

Tibial shaft fractures result from either direct (motor vehicle accidents) or indirect (rotary or compressive forces) trauma. High-energy direct injuries usually cause transverse or comminuted fractures (most common). Indirect trauma commonly results in spiral or oblique fractures (Fig. 79-19).[17]

A good neurovascular examination is essential. Skin integrity should be noted. Documentation of the integrity of the peroneal nerve is mandatory, as is a thorough examination of the knee and ankle. Compartment syndromes may develop 24 to 48 hours after injury; patients who are discharged home from the ED should be educated on the signs of compartment syndrome.

AP and lateral radiographs should be obtained and must include the knee and ankle in both views. Closed tibial shaft fractures are immobilization in a long-leg posterior splint with 10 to 20 degrees of knee flexion. Open fractures should be gently cleansed and dressed. Patients should receive antibiotics and tetanus prophylaxis. Emergency reduction is necessary for injuries in which there is neurovascular com-

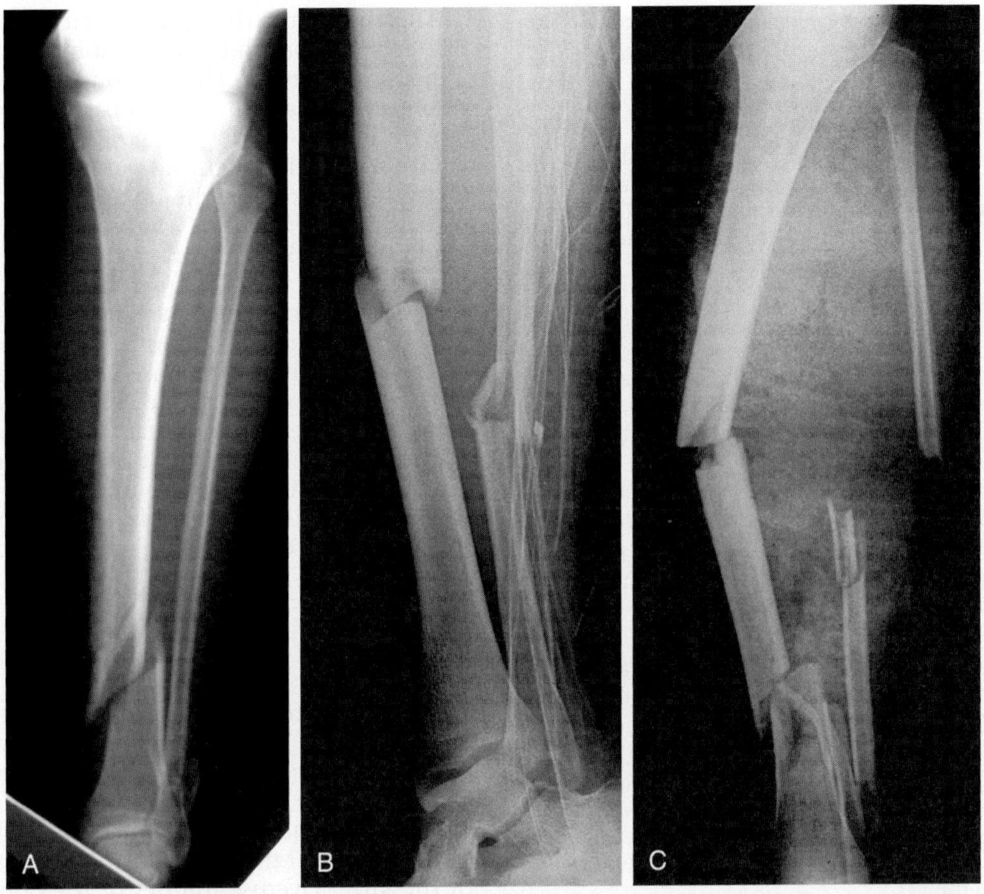
A
B
C

FIGURE 79-19 Radiographic examples of the three grades of tibial fracture severity. **A,** Minor: Spiral fracture caused by a simple slip and fall. **B,** Moderate: Fracture in a pedestrian struck by a slowly moving vehicle. **C,** Major: Fracture caused by a high-velocity motorcycle crash. (From Browner BD, Jupiter JB, Levine AM, et al: Skeletal Trauma: Basic Science, Management, and Reconstruction, 3rd ed. Philadelphia, Saunders, 2003.)

promise. Nonunion or delayed union is more likely in fractures with severe displacement or comminution, in open fractures, and in fractures with severe soft tissue injuries or infections.[17]

■ Proximal Fibular Fractures

Proximal fibular fractures are often seen in conjunction with tibial fractures. Isolated proximal fibular fractures are rare, given that the fibula runs parallel to the tibia and is bound to the tibia via ligaments. Isolated proximal fibular fractures are relatively unimportant because the fibula is not a weight-bearing bone. However, these fractures are often associated with significant knee injuries.[17]

The three main mechanisms of injury are a direct blow over the fibular head, an indirect varus stress to the knee (causing an avulsion fracture to the fibular head), and a valgus strain to the knee (causing a tibial condylar fracture and proximal fibular fracture). Maisonneuve's fracture results from an external rotatory force on the ankle resulting in a proximal fibular fracture and an ankle fracture or deltoid ligament tear with complete or partial syndesmotic disruption.[17]

Isolated fractures of the proximal fibula are treated symptomatically. The EP must rule out other associated injuries, such as LCL injuries, common peroneal nerve injury, arterial injuries, and Maisonneuve's fractures.

Overuse Injuries

■ ILIOTIBIAL BAND SYNDROME

The iliotibial band is a thick band of fascia that is formed proximally by the confluence of fascia from hip flexors, extensors, and abductors. The band originates at the lateral iliac crest and extends distally to the patella, tibia, and biceps femoris tendon. Iliotibial band syndrome is a common knee injury that usually manifests as lateral knee pain due to inflammation of the distal portion of the iliotibial band. Proximal irritation of the band can cause referred hip pain.[21]

The iliotibial band syndrome is caused by excessive friction of the band as it slides over the lateral femoral epicondyle during repetitive flexion and extension of the knee. This disorder is common in

Documentation

The following issues should be clearly documented for a patient with knee or lower leg injury:

- *History:* Mechanism of injury; duration and location of symptoms; associated symptoms; exacerbating or alleviating factors; complaints of weakness, numbness, or instability; complicating medical factors; and prior interventions or imaging or evaluations.
- *Physical examination:* Neurovascular status (before and after splint placement or reduction), compartment assessment, skin integrity, stability assessment, and associated injuries.
- *Radiography:* Anteroposterior or lateral films of the joint above and below the injury. Pre- and post-reduction films are indicated for most reductions (except when there is neurovascular compromise).
- *Medical decision-making:* Any emergency reduction secondary to neurovascular compromise and reasons for emergency or nonemergency consultation or follow-up.
- *Procedures:* Neurovascular status both before and after reduction or splint placement, skin integrity, and post-reduction fracture alignment.
- *Patient instructions:* Discussion with patient regarding splint care, appropriate crutch use, importance of range-of-motion exercises, weight-bearing status, warning signs for neurovascular impairment, and arrangements for follow-up or return to the ED.

athletes who are involved in flexion activities (running, cycling, soccer, tennis, etc.).

The patient with iliotibial band syndrome initially complains of a diffuse pain over the lateral aspect of the knee. The patient usually has no symptoms at rest or after activities, but symptoms become progressive during activity. Maximal tenderness is 2 to 3 cm proximal to the lateral joint line overlying the lateral epicondyle. Strength of the lower extremity should be assessed, especially the knee extensors, knee flexors, and hip abductors, given that muscle weakness can be associated with this disorder.[21]

The clinical diagnosis is based on the history and physical findings. If the diagnosis is in doubt or joint pathology is suspected, MRI is diagnostic. Initial treatment consists of ice, anti-inflammatory medications, and rest or decreased activity. Activities that require repeated knee flexion and extension should be avoided.[21]

■ PATELLAR TENDINITIS

Patellar tendinitis is commonly seen in athletes, especially those involved in some type of repetitive jumping or running activity.[16] The incidence of patellar tendinitis varies by sport, training intensity, and training frequency.[16]

This disorder is thought to occur from the repetitive acceleration and deceleration that occurs with jumping activities. This action can overload the extensor mechanism and lead to microtears in the tendon matrix.[16]

The patient has a chronic pain localized over the quadriceps tendon at the upper pole of the patella, or at the lower pole of the patella in the patellar tendon. The pain can be reproduced by resisted knee extension.[4]

Radiographic changes are rare before symptoms have been present for 6 months and are not indicated in the acute setting.[4] Conservative treatment (ice, rest, anti-inflammatory medications) with activity adjustment is effective in early stages of tendinitis. Advanced-stage injuries that do no respond to conservative treatment may require surgery, although this treatment is rare. Steroid injections may increase the risk of patellar tendon rupture and should be avoided.[16]

■ POPLITEUS TENDINITIS

The popliteus tendon forms part of the floor of the popliteal fossa. The popliteal muscle travels through the popliteal hiatus, traverses the knee joint, and inserts into the lateral femoral condyle.

Popliteus tendinitis is an uncommon disorder that causes pain over the posterior or posterolateral aspect of the knee. Overuse injuries of the popliteus occur with excessive use of the quadriceps muscle, such as running downhill or backpacking. Tenderness is located along the lateral joint line just anterior to the LCL.[22]

Diagnosis is based on history and physical findings. Radiographs are not helpful in establishing the diagnosis. The majority of cases respond to conservative treatment—rest, ice, NSAIDs, and modification of training techniques.[22]

■ OSGOOD-SCHLATTER DISEASE

Osgood-Schlatter disease is an overuse injury that involves traction apophysis at the tibial tubercle. It is often seen in adolescents during a growth spurt, when the apophysis in this region becomes weaker than the surrounding bony and tendinous tissues. The condition is bilateral in 20% to 30% of cases. The cause is unknown.[7]

The patient with Osgood-Schlatter disease complains of pain and swelling over the tibial tuberosity. The patient may describe worsening of the pain with jumping, squatting, or kneeling. The pain may be intermittent and is rarely severe enough to interrupt daily activity. Physical examination demonstrates localized pain and swelling over the tibial tuberosity.[7]

A lateral knee radiograph, the most useful view, shows a separation of the apophyses or fragmentation of a portion of the tibial tubercle. The appearance of tibial tubercle fragmentation may represent

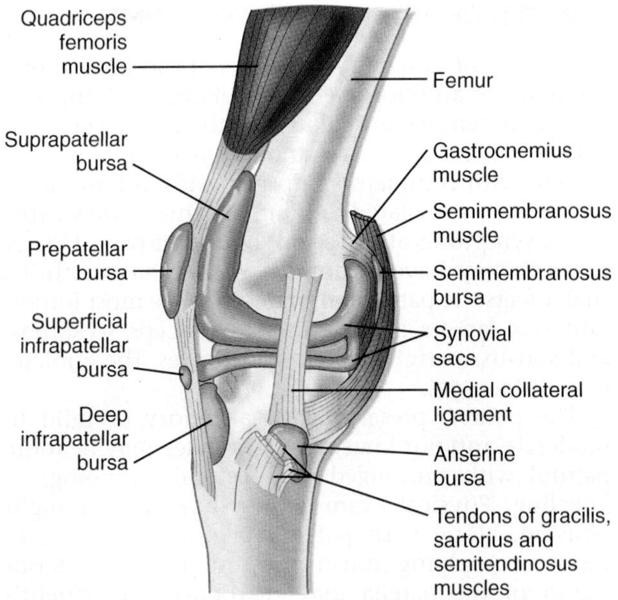
Quadriceps femoris muscle
Femur
Suprapatellar bursa
Gastrocnemius muscle
Semimembranosus muscle
Prepatellar bursa
Semimembranosus bursa
Superficial infrapatellar bursa
Synovial sacs
Medial collateral ligament
Deep infrapatellar bursa
Anserine bursa
Tendons of gracilis, sartorius and semitendinosus muscles

FIGURE 79-20 Multiple bursae around the knee that may become acutely or chronically inflamed. (From Canale ST: Campbells' Operative Orthopaedics, 10th ed. St. Louis, Mosby, 2003; redrawn from O'Donoghue DH: Treatment of Injuries to Athletes. Philadelphia, WB Saunders, 1984.)

a normal variant in the ossification of the tibial tubercle. Radiographic findings without associated clinical symptoms should be interpreted with caution.[7]

Osgood-Schlatter disease is generally a self-limited condition. In most cases, treatment is nonoperative, consisting of activity modification, NSAIDs, and physical therapy. The family of an adolescent with this disorder should be counseled that the symptoms may not resolve for 12 to 18 months.[7]

■ BURSITIS

Several bursae surround the knee (Fig. 79-20). They function to decrease the friction between two structures. Inflammation is commonly caused by direct trauma or chronic repetitive trauma. Other disorders, such as infection and metabolic disorders (gout), can also cause bursitis.

The prepatellar bursa is a common area for inflammation, given its superficial location. Bursitis may occur 1 to 2 weeks after direct trauma or after a repetitive trauma such as kneeling on a hard surface. The patient presents with erythema, warmth, and swelling of the skin over the bursa. Knee range of motion is usually painless except in extreme flexion. Septic bursitis is common in this area. If infection is suspected, the bursa should be aspirated, and the fluid should be sent for a Gram stain, culture and crystal analysis.

Treatment consists of moist heat, rest, anti-inflammatory medications, and protection from further trauma or irritation. Surgical intervention may be needed to drain a septic bursitis or treat resistant cases of bursitis.

■ STRESS FRACTURES

A *stress fracture* is a partial or complete bone fracture that results from repeated stress to a bone. Stress fractures are most common in the lower extremities (tibia, fibula, and metatarsal bones). They occur as a result of a repetitive use injury that exceeds the intrinsic ability of the bone to repair itself. Tibial stress fractures are commonly seen in military recruits as well as track and long distance runners.[13]

Patients present with a localized dull pain of the lower extremity that is not associated with trauma. The pain typically worsens during exercise or weight-bearing. Stress fractures can manifest in a similar fashion to shin splints but have more focal bony tenderness.[13]

Evidence of a stress fracture may not appear on plain radiographs for up to 2 to 10 weeks after symptom onset. The presence of a transverse fracture line across the entire anterior shaft of the tibia on a plain radiograph is considered a poor prognostic sign and is associated with a greater likelihood of nonunion.[17] Radionuclide scintigraphy can confirm the diagnosis as early as 2 to 8 days after the onset of symptoms.[13]

Initial treatment consists of conservative therapy: ice, anti-inflammatory pain medicine, and rest for several weeks or until extremity is pain free. Tibial fractures that do not improve with conservative management may require splinting in a walking boot or air splint. A midshaft tibial fracture is splinted until the extremity is pain free and there is radiographic evidence of healing.[13]

Other Disorders

■ OSTEOCHONDRITIS DISSECANS

Osteochondritis dissecans is a potentially reversible idiopathic lesion of the subchondral bone. It is seen more often in children and adolescents.[25] Osteochondritis dissecans of the knee is seen most commonly on the posterolateral aspect of the medial femoral condyle (70%-80%) (Fig. 79-21). Inflammation, genetics, ischemia, ossification, and repetitive trauma have all been hypothesized as possible causes.[26]

Most children and adolescents with this disorder have a stable lesion and present with nonspecific complaints, such as aches or activity-related knee pain localized to the anterior knee. Both knees should be examined, because the condition is bilateral in 20% to 25% of cases.[26] Initial plain radiographs should include AP, lateral, and tunnel views of the knee.

Stable osteochondritis dissecans lesions have a 50% to 94% healing rate with conservative management (modified activity, NSAIDs, rehabilitative exercises). Patients and their parents should be instructed

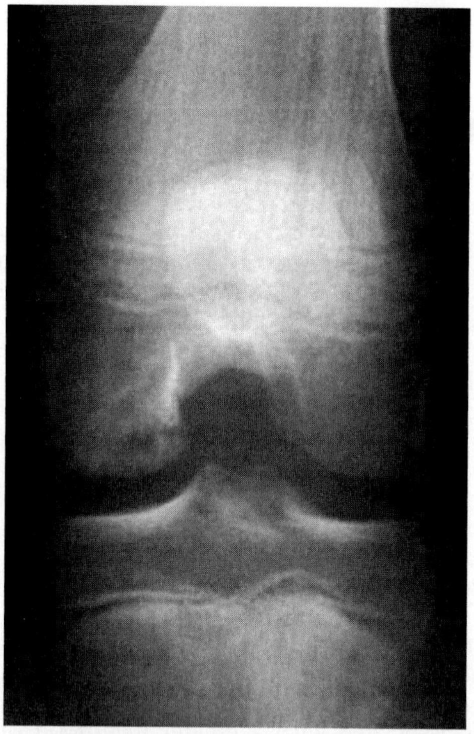

FIGURE 79-21 Tunnel radiographs of a juvenile osteochondritis dissecans lesion of the medial femoral condyle. The lesion can be difficult to see on an anteroposterior radiograph and is often more apparent on the notch view, which images the posterior aspect of the femoral condyle with knee flexion.

that it takes 12 to 18 months for healing to be complete.[26]

■ OSTEONECROSIS

Osteonecrosis of the knee is usually idiopathic and is most commonly located on the medial femoral condyle. It may be associated with steroids, irradiation, and systemic diseases such as sickle cell anemia and the rheumatologic disorders. Osteonecrosis occurs when the blood supply to the bone is disrupted, causing a bone infarction.[25]

The patient presents with a sudden onset of pain over the anteromedial (most common) aspect of the knee. The pain may become worse at night or increase with activity. Idiopathic osteonecrosis is typically seen in women older than 60 years. The patient may have a joint effusion or decreased range of motion of the knee joint.[25]

Radionuclide scintigraphy or CT may be required to detect the disease in early stages. Plain radiographic findings in patients with early disease are usually normal.[25]

Patients with early stages of osteonecrosis are treated conservatively with partial weight-bearing and anti-inflammatory medications. Patients with advanced disease may require surgery to restore the articular surface. Total knee arthroplasty is reserved for disease that has expanded to the lateral compartment.[25]

■ PATELLOFEMORAL PAIN SYNDROME

Patellofemoral pain syndrome refers to the clinical presentation of anterior knee pain related to changes in the patellofemoral articulation. Patients are generally between the ages of 10 and 20 years and usually present with complaints of nonspecific anterior knee pain that is not related to trauma. Athletes may experience symptoms after periods of overactivity. Elderly patients may have symptoms if they have arthritis that affects the patellofemoral joint. The most important risk factors are overuse, quadriceps weakness, and soft-tissue tightness. In most cases, the etiology is multifactorial.[27]

The patient presents with a history of mild to moderate anterior knee pain. The knee may be more painful with prolonged flexion, stair climbing, or kneeling. Physical examination may show a slight effusion, along with patellar crepitus on range of motion. Applying direct pressure to the anterior aspect of the patella may reproduce the patient's pain.[4]

Plain radiographs are not indicated. CT or MRI can detect abnormalities in the articular surface of the patella. In most cases, a physical therapy program that strengthens the quadriceps muscle can successfully reduce symptoms. Surgery may be required for the minority of cases that do not respond to conservative management.[27]

■ OSTEOARTHRITIS

Osteoarthritis results from the loss of hyaline articular cartilage and the replacement of cartilage by bone within the joint. The bone under the cartilage also undergoes extensive remodeling, resulting in denser bone with obliteration of the intratrabecular spaces.

PATIENT TEACHING TIPS

- The patient diagnosed with strain or sprain or stable injury of the knee who is discharged home in a knee immobilizer should be instructed to perform gentle range-of-motion exercises 3 or 4 times a day to prevent joint stiffness.
- The patient with a tibia fracture who is sent home should be educated about compartment syndrome and told to return to the ED if either severe pain or numbness in the foot or leg develops within the first 48 hours.
- The patient with an acute injury should be instructed to:
  - Elevate the injured area above the level of the heart for the first 48 hours after the injury.
  - Apply ice to injured area—avoiding direct contact of ice with bare skin and getting the splint moist.
- For a patient discharged from the ED on crutches:
  - Crutch training should be given.
  - The ability of the patient to safely use crutches should be observed before discharge.

Risk factors for osteoarthritis include the interplay of systemic (age, sex, and genetic) factors with intrinsic joint vulnerabilities (previous damage to the joint, muscle weakness) and extrinsic factors that act on the joint (obesity).[28]

Patients complain of pain that is aggravated by activity and relieved by rest. They may have pain along the joint line, and in severe cases, there may be gross angular deformity of the joint.

Plain radiographs should include weight-bearing, AP, and PA tunnel views. Findings are joint space narrowing, subchondral bony sclerosis, cystic changes, and hypertrophic osteophytes.[4]

Treatment is directed at pain control with anti-inflammatory medications, weight loss, and a rehabilitation program. Surgical treatment with total knee replacement is reserved for advanced cases.

■ POPLITEAL CYST

A popliteal cyst, or Baker's cyst, is an inflammation of the semimembranosus or medial gastrocnemius bursa.[30] A Baker's cyst is produced by herniation of the synovial membrane through the posterior knee capsule (Fig. 79-22). A Baker's cyst is usually the result of synovitis, arthritis, or an internal derangement of the knee that results in excess synovial fluid in the bursa.

Intermittent swelling can develop behind the knee. If the bursa ruptures, the patient may complain of calf pain and the presentation may be similar to that of the patient with thrombophlebitis.

Ultrasonography is helpful to distinguish Baker's cysts from other disorders, such as popliteal artery aneurysms, neoplasms, and thrombophlebitis. Treatment is based on the underlying cause. Asymptomatic cysts found incidentally need no further treatment.[30]

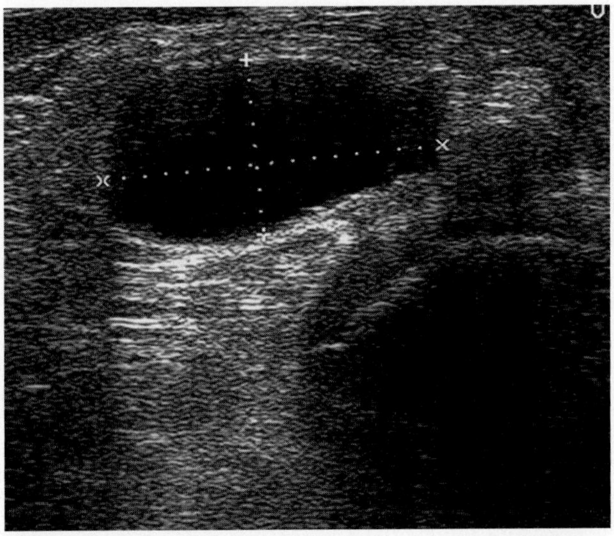

FIGURE 79-22 Ultrasonogram of a Baker's cyst in the popliteal fossa.

REFERENCES

1. Stiell IG, Wells GA, McDowell I, et al: Use of radiography in acute knee injuries: Need for clinical decision rules. Acad Emerg Med 1995;2:966-973.
2. Seaberg DC, Yealy DM, Lukens T, et al: Multicenter comparison of two clinical decision rules for the use of radiography in acute, high-risk knee injuries. Ann Emerg Med 1998;32:8-13.
3. Allen JE, Taylor KS: Physical examination of the knee. Prim Care 2004;31:887-907.
4. Calmbach WL, Hutchens M: Evaluation of patients presenting with knee pain. Part II: Differential diagnosis. Am Fam Physician 2003;68:917-922.
5. Perryman JR, Hershman EB: The acute management of soft tissue injuries of the knee. Orthop Clin North Am 2002;33:575-585.
6. McKoy BE, Stanitski CL: Acute tibial tubercle avulsion fractures. Orthop Clin North Am 2003;34:397-403.
7. Duri ZA, Patel DV, Aichroth PM: The immature athlete. Clin Sports Med 2002;21:461-482, ix.
8. Brown JR, Trojian TH: Anterior and posterior cruciate ligament injuries. Prim Care 2004;31:925-956.
9. Quarles JD, Hosey RG: Medial and lateral collateral injuries: Prognosis and treatment. Prim Care 2004;3:957-975, ix.
10. Kocher MS, Klingele K, Rassman SO: Meniscal disorders: Normal, discoid, and cysts. Orthop Clin North Am 2003;34:329-340.
11. Rath E, Richmond JC: The menisci: Basic science and advances in treatment. Br J Sports Med 2000;34:252-257.
12. El-Dieb A, Yu JS, Huang GS, Farooki S: Pathologic conditions of the ligaments and tendons of the knee. Radiol Clin North Am 2002;40:1061-1079.
13. Wilder RP, Sethi S: Overuse injuries: Tendinopathies, stress fractures, compartment syndrome, and shin splints. Clin Sports Med 2004;23:55-81, vi.
14. Brautigan B, Johnson DL: The epidemiology of knee dislocations. Clin Sports Med 2000;19:387-397.
15. Levy BA, Zlowodzki MP, Graves M, et al: Screening for extremity arterial injury with the arterial pressure index. Am J Emerg Med 2005;23:689-695.
16. Morelli V, Rowe RH: Patellar tendonitis and patellar dislocations. Prim Care 2004;31:909-924, viii-ix.
17. Simon RR, Koenigsknecht SJ: Emergency orthopedics: The Extremities, 4th ed. New York, McGraw-Hill, 2001.
18. Bharam S, Vrahas MS, Fu FH: Knee fractures in the athlete. Orthop Clin North Am 2002;33:565-574.
19. Mills WJ, Nork SE: Open reduction and internal fixation of high-energy tibial plateau fractures. Orthop Clin North Am 2002;33:177-198, ix.
20. Accousti WK, Willis RB.: Tibial eminence fractures. Orthop Clin North Am 2003;34:365-375.
21. Khaund R, Flynn SH: Iliotibial band syndrome: A common source of knee pain. Am Fam Physician 2005;71: 1545-1550.
22. Hunter SC, Poole RM: The chronically inflamed tendon. Clin Sports Med 1987;6:371-388.
25. Soucacos PN, Johnson EO, Soultanis K, et al: Diagnosis and management of the osteonecrotic triad of the knee. Orthop Clin North Am 2004;35:371-381, x.
26. Flynn JM, Kocher MS, Ganley TJ: Osteochondritis dissecans of the knee. J Pediatr Orthop 2004;24:434-443.
27. LaBella C: Patellofemoral pain syndrome: Evaluation and treatment. Prim Care 2004;31:977-1003.
28. Felson DT: An update on the pathogenesis and epidemiology of osteoarthritis. Radiol Clin North Am 2004;42:1-9, v.
30. Handy JR: Popliteal cysts in adults: A review. Semin Arthritis Rheum 2001;31:108-118.

Chapter **80**

Foot and Ankle Injuries

Jorge del Castillo

KEY POINTS

Ankle injuries may at first glance appear common and minor, but a large percentage continue to be symptomatic and develop chronic instability requiring surgical repair.

Most ankle sprains are due to inversion during plantar flexion of the ankle, with 85% involving the lateral ligaments.

Isolated injury to the medial (deltoid) ligament is uncommon and usually involves a medial malleolar fracture.

Uncomfortable approaches to the examination of the ankle result in an incomplete examination and an uncomfortable patient and physician. DO NOT begin the examination at the point of maximal swelling and tenderness.

Stress testing is generally not performed any longer in the acute phase of an ankle injury because magnetic resonance imaging can ascertain the injuries accurately.

Do not mistake subluxing peroneal tendons for an ankle sprain, because the treatment and prognosis are different.

The Thompson test to assess Achilles rupture can be misleading, especially with partial tears.

Dislocations at the level of the tibiotalar joint require prompt anatomic reduction in an effort to diminish cutaneous and neurovascular injury.

Diagnosis of talar dome fractures is missed in 40% to 50% of patients presenting to the ED with an ankle injury. A high index of suspicion is warranted when the patient presents with chronic swelling and/or locking of the ankle 4 to 5 weeks after an injury

Scope and Outline

■ PERSPECTIVE

Injuries to the ankle and foot are the most common orthopedic injuries and the most common of all athletic injuries presenting to the ED. The lateral ligaments are most often involved because of the anatomy of the tibiotalar joint.

The frequency of these injuries often leads the physician to minimize their seriousness and morbidity. It is important to avoid this pitfall and adhere to a methodical physical and radiographic examination. Additionally, one must avoid undertreatment of these injuries and maintain a guarded prognosis, ensuring proper follow-up when necessary.

■ EPIDEMIOLOGY

Inversion injuries occur at a rate of 1 per 10,000 people per day, which is about 28,000 injuries per

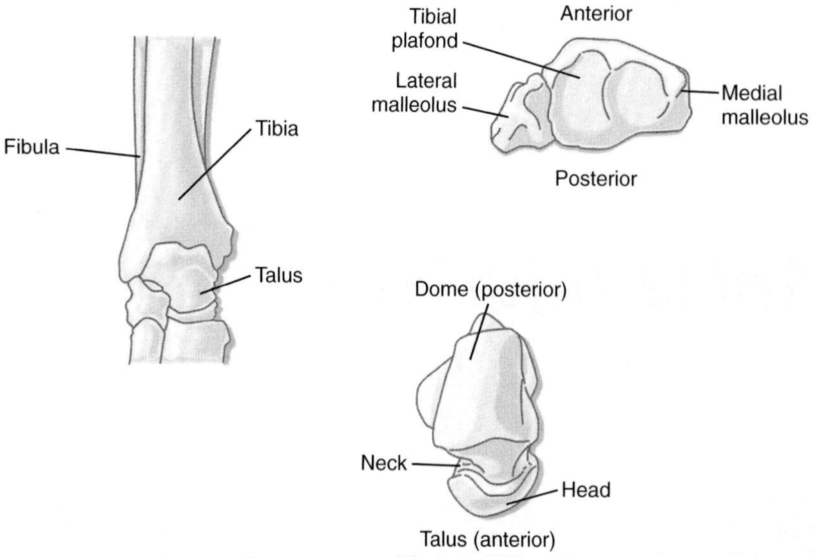
Fibula
Tibia
Talus
Tibial plafond
Anterior
Lateral malleolus
Medial malleolus
Posterior
Dome (posterior)
Neck
Head
Talus (anterior)

FIGURE 80-1 Bony anatomy of the ankle.

day in the United States. Injury to the dominant ankle is more likely than injury to the nondominant ankle. These injuries are common during running recreational sports such as basketball, soccer, baseball, and volleyball.

These injuries may at first glance appear common and minor. A large percentage of these continue to be symptomatic for a year or longer after the injury. Some go on to develop chronic instability and require surgical repair.[1]

Structure and Function

■ ANATOMY

The ankle is composed of two joints: the talar mortise and the subtalar joint. The talar joint is a modified hinge joint similar to a "mortise and tenon," as referred to in carpentry. It is composed of three bones: (Fig. 80-1): the tibia, the mortise, and the talus of the tibula, which forms the tenon. The plafond or "ceiling" of this joint is formed by the tibia with its medial malleolus and its articulation with the fibula.

The dome of the talus has a trapezoidal shape, being wider anteriorly and narrower posteriorly. This anatomic shape confers greater stability in dorsiflexion. However, when the ankle moves into plantar flexion, the narrow part of the talus sits in the mortise. This results in ankle instability and a predisposition to injury.[2,3]

■ Ligaments of the Ankle

The medial side of the ankle is supported by the deltoid ligament (Fig. 80-2). There are five components to the deltoid ligament; one deep and four superficial. The deep ligaments attach to the tibia and the undersurface of the talus. The superficial ligaments are tibionavicualar, anterior talotibial, calcaneotibial, and posterior talotibial.

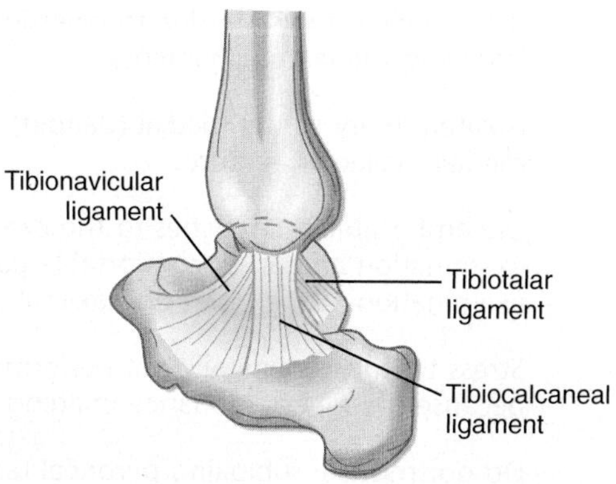
Tibionavicular ligament
Tibiotalar ligament
Tibiocalcaneal ligament

FIGURE 80-2 Medial ligaments of the ankle.

On the lateral aspect of the ankle, there are three supporting ligaments: anterior talofibular, calcaneofibular, and posterior talofibular (Fig. 80-3). Tibiofibular ligaments include the anterior and posterior inferior ligaments, which bind the distal tibia and fibula, and the superior ligaments of the same name, which bind the tibia and fibula at the proximal articulation. Other supporting structures are the inferior transverse ligament and the interosseous ligament. The latter is not part of the ankle but nevertheless provides a strong bond between the tibia and the fibula.[2,3]

Presenting Signs and Symptoms

■ MECHANISM OF INJURY

As previously noted, the ankle is a modified hinge joint; its motion is predominantly executed in a sagittal plane.

Table 80-1 CLASSIFICATION OF ANKLE SPRAINS

Type of Injury	Extent of Injury	Physical Findings
Grade I	Stretch of the ligament with microscopic but not macroscopic tearing	Minor swelling but no joint instability
Grade II	Involves partial tearing of the particular ligament	Minor to moderate swelling and some instability of the affected ankle.
Grade III	Involves the complete rupture of the ligament	Significant swelling, tenderness, and ecchymosis; instability of the joint and inability to bear weight

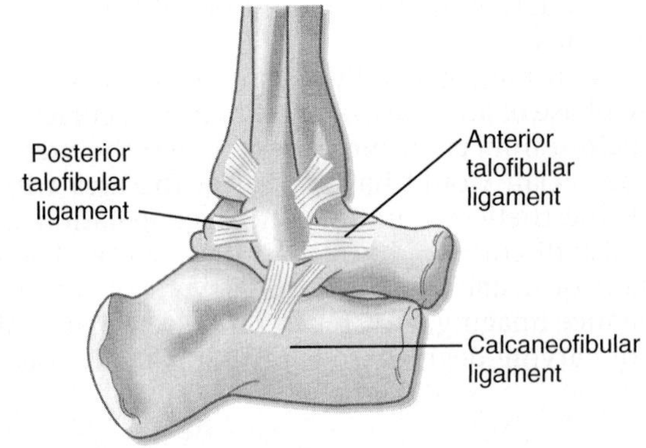
Posterior talofibular ligament
Anterior talofibular ligament
Calcaneofibular ligament

FIGURE 80-3 Lateral ligaments of the ankle.

Most ankle sprains are due to inversion during plantar flexion of the ankle. Thus, approximately 85% of injuries involve the lateral ligaments: the anterior talofibular ligament, calcaneofibular ligament, and posterior talofibular ligament. Of sprains due to inversion, 65% are isolated to the anterior talofibular ligament. In some patients, the subtalar complex may also be injured. The calcaneofibular ligament is rarely injured in isolation. Classification of these injuries and examination findings are noted in Table 80-1.

Isolated injury to the medial (deltoid) ligament is uncommon and usually involves a medial malleolar fracture. Distal tibiofibular syndesmotic rupture is very rare and is associated with forceful dorsiflexion and external rotation.[2,4]

History and Physical Examination

A methodical approach to the history of the injury and the examination of the ankle joint is of paramount importance. Often, the mechanism is unknown due to the sudden and rapid occurrence of the injury. Specific questions about the mechanism, time of injury, ability to bear weight, and prior history of injury to the affected joint are helpful in arriving at a specific diagnosis (Box 80-1).

The physical examination (Box 80-2) should be thorough and orderly with the intent of assessing joint stability and possible neurovascular compromise. Make sure that the patient is in a comfortable position to be examined. Many times we examine patients in hallways and while sitting in chairs, with their feet resting on the floor or wheelchair footrest. Uncomfortable approaches to the examination of the ankle, or of any joint for that matter, are detrimental to the welfare of both the patient and the physician. All that is derived from this approach is an incom-

BOX 80-1

Suggested History for Ankle Injuries

- Has the same ankle been injured before?
- Is there any other relevant medical history?
- What was the mechanism of the injury?
- Where is the point of maximal tenderness?
- Was there a pop or snap?
- Was there immediate swelling?
- Were you able to bear weight?
- Was there any emergent treatment?

BOX 80-2

Sequential Examination of the Injured Ankle

1. Visual inspection
2. Neurovascular assessment
3. Proximal fibula
4. Midshaft tibia and interosseous membrane
5. Medial malleolus and deltoid ligament
6. Lateral malleolus and ligaments
7. Syndesmosis
8. Anterior talofibular ligament
9. Calcaneofibular ligament
10. Posterior talofibular ligament
11. Peroneal tendons
12. Achilles tendon
13. Navicular and bifurcated ligament
14. Base fifth metatarsal
15. Range of motion
16. Other maneuvers (anterior drawer, tilt test, side-to-side)

plete examination and an uncomfortable patient and physician.

Make sure that the seated patient is at a level higher than that of the examiner (e.g., seated on a gurney with the affected limb dependent or seated on the examining table with both extremities on the table). NEVER begin the examination at the point of maximal swelling and tenderness. The examination should begin with visual inspection to assess the degree of swelling and the presence of any deformity and discoloration. Evaluate the neurovascular status of the extremity by testing sensation, capillary refilling, and presence of pulses. Once a preliminary assessment is done proceed in detail from distal to proximal in an orderly fashion as noted in Box 80-2.[5]

■ OTHER MANEUVERS

Other maneuvers sometimes employed in the evaluation of the injured ankle are worth mentioning. The *anterior drawer test* (Fig. 80-4) is used to determine the integrity of the anterior talofibular ligament. It is, unfortunately, not very reliable, especially in acute injuries where there is significant swelling and pain. It is performed by holding the foot at the calcaneus with one hand while the other hand stabilizes the extremity at its middle third. The foot is moved forward while one observes and/or feels for displacement of the foot and ankle anteriorly.

The *side-to-side test* (clunk test) evaluates the integrity of the tibiofibular ligament. The foot is held in a neutral position and then moved from side to side. A "clunk" is heard or felt if the ligament is ruptured.

The *talar tilt test* can be used to assess the deltoid ligament and the calcaneofibular ligament by eversion and inversion stressing, respectively. The calcaneus is held in one hand while the examiner moves the ankle into inversion or eversion (Fig. 80-5). Often it is accompanied by simultaneous radiographic evaluation to determine the amount of "tilt" at the level of the talus.[2]

Stress testing generally is not performed in the acute phase of an injury because of its inaccuracy and the pain it inflicts on the patient. Often the examining physician would have to inject the area with a local anesthetic to attain patient cooperation and diminish discomfort. In the past it was a useful determinant of instability. Since the advent of magnetic resonance imaging, which can reveal soft tissue injuries of varying degrees stress testing is rarely used at all.[2]

Ankle Sprains and Fractures and Other Related Injuries

Ankle sprains result from traumatic rotational forces to the ankle and usually occur in individuals who are involved in sports activities. They have been classi-

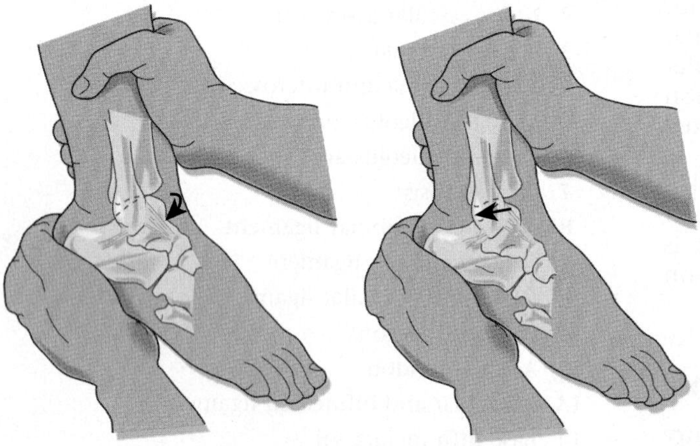

FIGURE 80-4 Anterior drawer test.

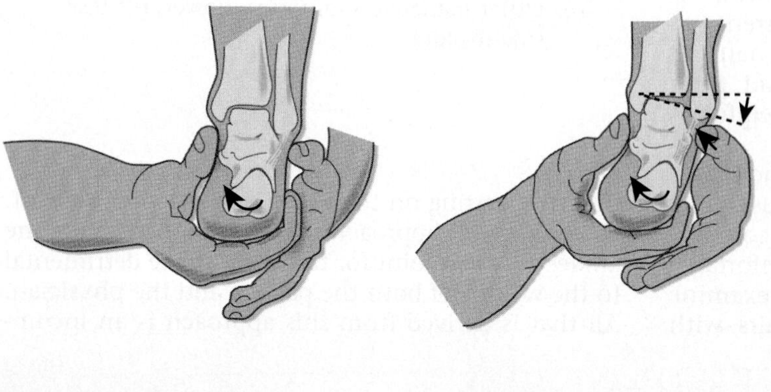

FIGURE 80-5 Talar tilt test.

fied to better understand treatment modalities as well as prognosis.

■ CLASSIFICATION OF ANKLE SPRAINS

■ Subluxation of the Peroneal Tendons

The peroneus longus and brevis tendons lie in a shallow groove immediately posterior to the distal fibula. Rupture of the superior peroneal retinaculum results in the subluxation or dislocation of the peroneal tendons. This injury is often mistaken for a common sprain in the ED. However, it differs due to the location of the pain and swelling along the posterior border of the lateral malleolus. It results from forced dorsiflexion with reflex contraction of the peroneal muscles. Patients complain of pain and a snapping sensation over the posterolateral ankle with weakness of eversion.[6]

In the physical examination, pain is elicited on palpation of the area, and swelling is also noted. Subluxation can be reproduced with dorsiflexion and eversion of the foot.

DO NOT mistake this subluxation of the peroneal tendons for an ankle sprain, because the treatment and prognosis are different.

Treatment is directed at stabilization of the subluxed tendon. A U-shaped felt pad is placed over the lateral ankle with the tip of the fibula lying inside the "U". The ankle is then taped to ensure that the U-shaped pad stays in place. Refer to an orthopedic surgeon for further evaluation in the event corrective surgery is warranted.

■ Achilles Tendon Injuries

The most common conditions affecting the Achilles tendon in patients presenting to the ED range from tendonitis to rupture. Rupture of the Achilles tendon is missed in over 20% of patients presenting with this injury. The rupture may be partial or complete. Occasionally there will be significant swelling and a hematoma over the area, making a discernible defect in the tendon difficult to identify.

History usually includes some form of violent motion around the ankle; the injury is often seen in basketball and tennis players. Weekend athletes in their third or fourth decade are most commonly affected.

Physical examination will reveal swelling and tenderness as well as a partial or complete defect in the tendon. A positive Thompson test is diagnostic. This is performed by having the patient lie prone on a gurney or knee on a chair (Fig. 80-6). The examiner then squeezes the calf muscles. Individuals with normal Achilles tendons will plantar flex as the maneuver is performed.[3]

Note that the Thompson test can be misleading, especially in partial tears, because the accessory ankle flexors are often squeezed together with the contents of the superficial leg compartment.

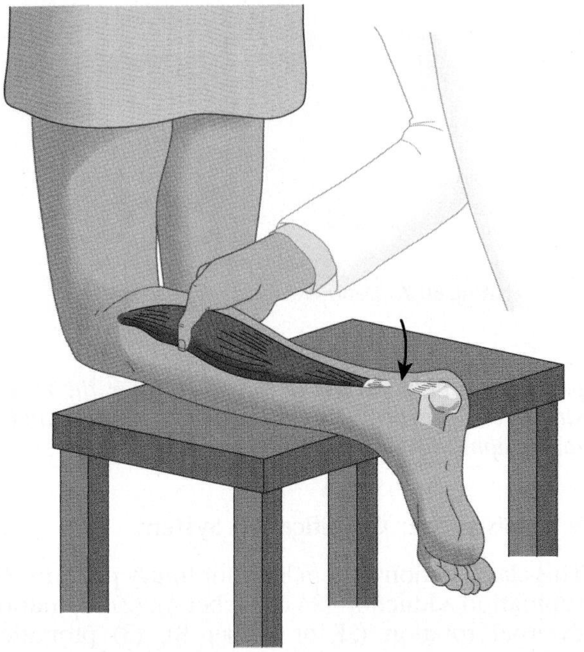

FIGURE 80-6 Thompson test.

Treatment consists of either a compression wrap or a short leg plaster splint with the foot positioned in equinus (plantar flexion). Crutches, non-weight bearing, and analgesics are also indicated. Prompt orthopedic consultation to determine the necessity of surgical repair is advised.

■ CLASSIFICATION OF FRACTURES

Several classifications of ankle fractures have been published over the years in an effort to facilitate accurate description and subsequent treatment. The most comprehensive classification, still in use, was proposed by Lauge-Hansen in 1950 and was based on cadaver experiments using foot position (supination or pronation) and direction of the force exerted on the joint (external rotation, adduction, or abduction) at the time of the injury. The Danis-Weber Arbeitsgemeinschaft für osteosynthesefragen (AO) classification proposes a simpler description based on the location and appearance of the fibular fracture. These fracture lines are A—below the syndesmosis, B—at the level of the syndesmosis, and C—above the syndesmosis (Fig. 80-7).

The Orthopedic Trauma Association (OTA) has since expanded the Danis-Weber classification, keeping the three types (A, B, and C) and adding nine groups (1, 2, and 3 for each type) and 27 subgroups.[3]

In 1987, Tile recommended another classification that identifies ankle fractures by their stability. Because *unstable* fractures require a different treatment approach than *stable* fractures, this is an important clinical distinction. For example, identification of a medial injury will generally determine the stability of the ankle joint. *Therefore, always sus-*

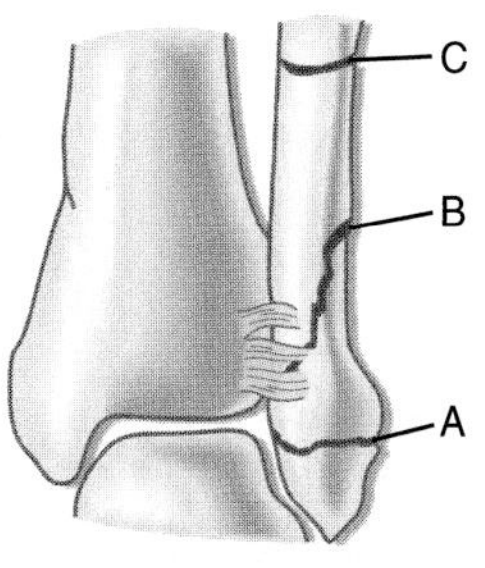
C
B
A

FIGURE 80-7 Danis-Weber classification (see text).

pect an unstable fracture of the ankle when the medial structures are identified as injured clinically and/or radiographically.[4,7]

Danis-Weber Classification System

This classification system has four injury patterns: (1) supination adduction (SA or Weber A), (2) supination external rotation (SE or Weber B), (3) pronation abduction (PA or Weber C1), and (4) pronation external rotation (PE or Weber C2). The names for these injury patterns can be thought of in simple terms as indicating the initial position of the foot (supination or pronation) and the direction of the injuring force acting through the talus (adduction, abduction, external rotation). The location and type of fibula fracture is the key to understanding the classification.[2]

Supination Adduction (SA, Weber A)

The foot is supinated (inverted) and an adducting force is exerted on the talus, resulting in two sequential injuries: transverse fracture of the lateral malleolus below or up to the level of the tibiofibular joint and a ligament tear. (SA I). As the force progresses, the talus impacts the medial malleolus and causes an oblique medial malleolar fracture (SA II) (Fig. 80-8).

Supination External Rotation (SE, Weber B)

This is the most common mechanism of a "twisted ankle" injury. The foot is supinated and an external rotation force acts on the talus, resulting in up to four sequential injuries (Fig. 80-9): tear of the anterior inferior tibiofibular ligament (SE I); short oblique fracture of the fibula (SE II), which is best seen on a lateral radiograph; fracture of the posterior malleolus (SE III); and transverse fracture of the medial malleolus (SE IV) and/or a tear of the deltoid ligament.

Pronation Abduction (Weber C1)

In this injury, the foot is pronated (everted) and an abducting force is exerted on the talus, resulting in up to three sequential injuries (Fig. 80-10). First, transverse fracture of the medial malleolus occurs (PA I); then, as the forces progress, the anterior inferior tibiofibular ligament tears (PA II); finally, further abduction of the talus results in oblique fracture of the distal fibula (PA III). This fibula fracture ends just above the level of the joint line and is best seen on the anteroposterior (AP) or mortise view.

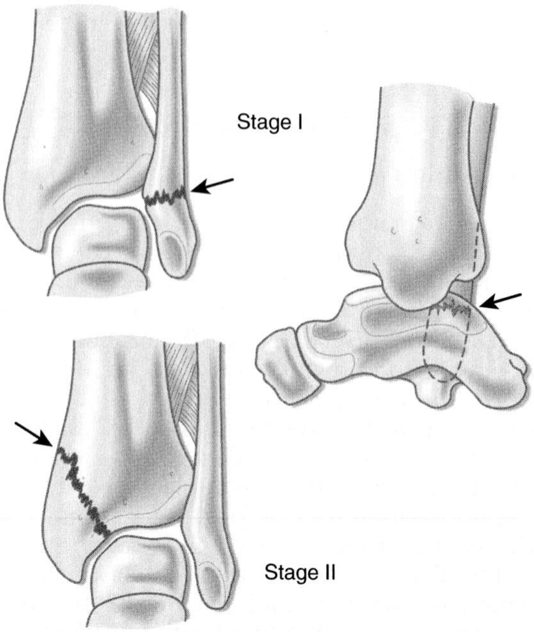
Stage I
Stage II

FIGURE 80-8 Supination adduction (SA, Weber A).

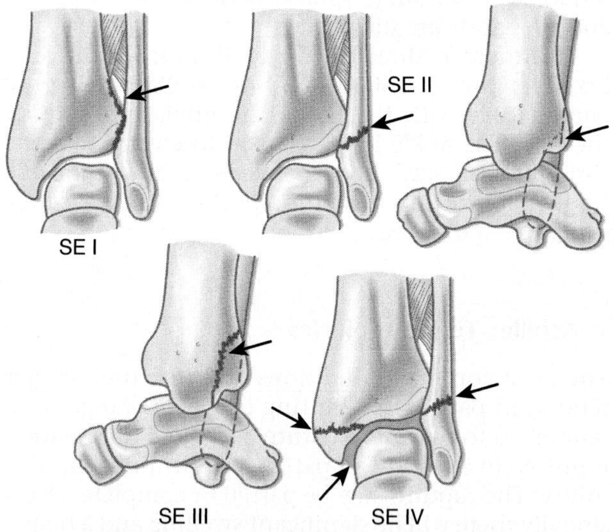
SE I
SE II
SE III
SE IV

FIGURE 80-9 Supination external rotation (SE, Weber B).

Pronation External Rotation (PE, Weber C2)

In pronation external rotation, the foot is pronated (everted) and an external rotation force acts through the talus, resulting in up to four sequential injuries (Fig. 80-11). Similar to the pronation-abduction mechanism, the first two injuries are the same: transverse fracture of the medial malleolus occurs (PE I), followed by a tear of the anterior inferior tibiofibular ligament (PE II). The third injury is a short spiral or oblique fracture usually 6 to 8 cm above the syndesmosis but may be as high as the midshaft level (PE III). The fourth injury is fracture of the posterior malleolus (PE IV).

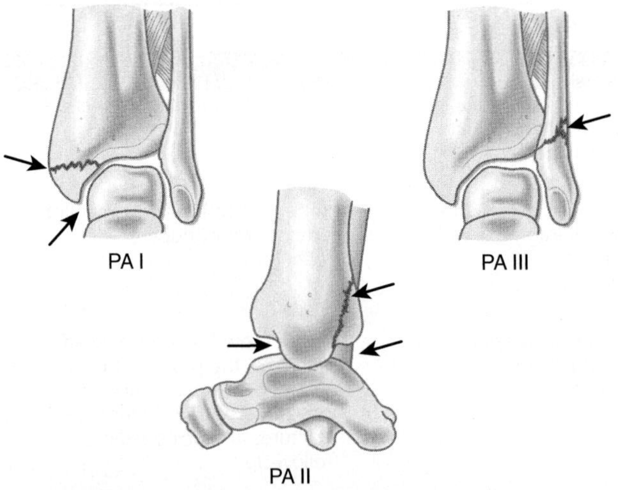
PA I
PA III
PA II

FIGURE 80-10 The foot is pronated (everted) and an abducting force is exerted on the talus, resulting in up to 3 sequential injuries

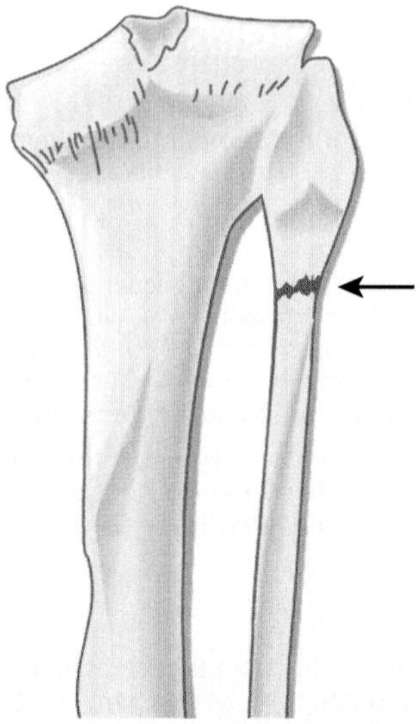

FIGURE 80-12 Maisonneuve fracture.

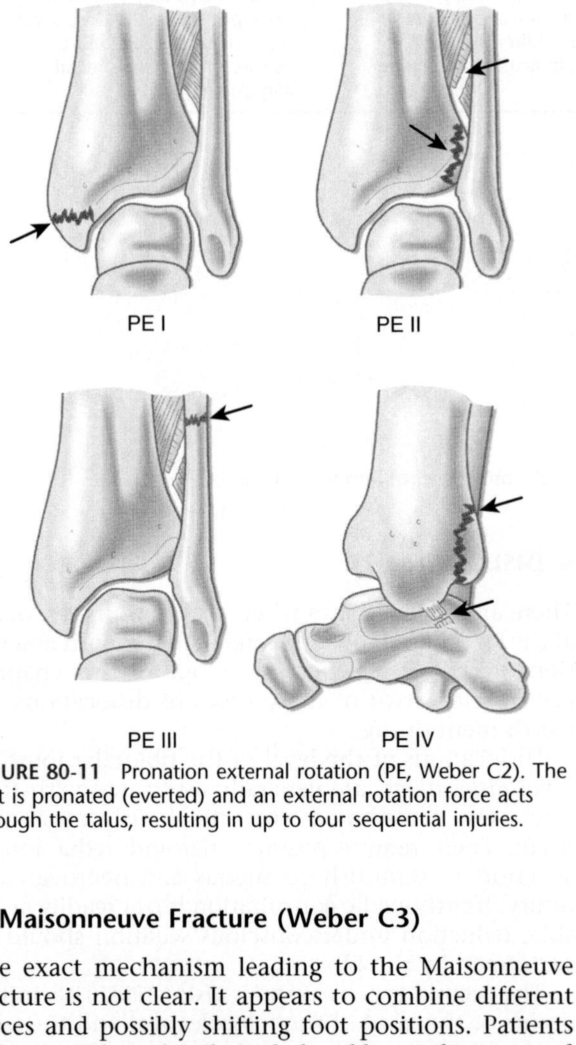
PE I
PE II
PE III
PE IV

FIGURE 80-11 Pronation external rotation (PE, Weber C2). The foot is pronated (everted) and an external rotation force acts through the talus, resulting in up to four sequential injuries.

■ Maisonneuve Fracture (Weber C3)

The exact mechanism leading to the Maisonneuve fracture is not clear. It appears to combine different forces and possibly shifting foot positions. Patients present with isolated medial ankle tenderness and swelling. On further examination, tenderness at the level of the proximal fibula is also identified. *This is an unstable fracture that warrants clinical and radiographic evaluation of the entire lower extremity below the knee.* It often goes unrecognized and is identified merely as "just another ankle sprain." *Therefore, vigilance must be exercised when a medial ankle injury is identified in any patient.* These medial ankle injuries could be limited to the deltoid ligament, an isolated fracture of the posterior tibial tubercle, or a medial malleolar fracture in the absence of a lateral malleolar fracture. The classic appearance of the injury is a fracture of the neck of the fibula—either linear or comminuted (Fig. 80-12). Emergent orthopedic consultation is necessary.[4]

■ Salter-Harris Classification System

The Salter-Harris classification system describes injuries that occur only around growth plates. Hence, only children have Salter-Harris fractures.

Injuries to the ankle in the pediatric population generally occur at the level of the bone physis. The Salter-Harris classification system enables definition of the type and severity of the fracture. Salter-Harris fractures are generally broken down into five categories shown in Figure 80-13 and Table 80-2.[5]

■ Triplane Fractures

This type of fracture is generally seen in older children with partially closed epiphyses and resembles the Salter-Harris type IV fracture. The mechanism is usually external rotation. Even with proper care and reduction, this fracture can result in epiphyseal growth arrest and deformity. If unsure of the fracture lines on plain film radiographs, computed tomography scanning is recommended to ascertain the position of the fracture fragments (Fig. 80-14).

Treatment consists of reduction and immobilization with a long leg cast for 4 weeks followed by a short leg cast for an additional 2 weeks. Displaced fractures that are not easily or anatomically reduced will require open reduction and internal fixation.

Table 80-2 SALTER-HARRIS CLASSIFICATION OF FRACTURES

Type	Description	Radiographic Findings	Treatment
I	Separation of the two portions of bone, with the growth plate being the area of weakest link	No changes seen on radiograph although the growth plate may look wider than that of the other limb	Immobilization for a short period
II	Most common fracture; occurs partially through the growth plate, with the rest of the fracture extending back into the shaft of the bone; that fragment of bone is known as the Thurston-Holland sign	Separation of the physis and metaphyseal fragment with varying degrees of displacement	Immobilization in short leg splint or cast and orthopedic follow-up
III	Fracture occurs partially across the growth plate and then extending out through the epiphysis and into the joint space	Fracture fragment is epiphyseal, with varying degrees of displacement	Because these fractures may affect the joint, the prognosis is more guarded; immobilization as described previously for type II fractures and orthopedic follow-up
IV	Fracture extends from the metaphysis, across the growth plate, and into the joint through the epiphysis; premature arrest of normal growth is common	Combination of types II and III, with varying degrees of displacement	Immobilization and prompt orthopedic follow-up; surgical repair is usually needed to restore proper anatomical alignment.
V	Fracture involves compression of the growth plate; prognosis is variable, with premature arrest of normal growth being the biggest risk	Radiography is generally of little help in diagnosing this fracture; however, obliteration of the physis is indication of severity	Immobilization and emergent orthopedic consultation; surgical repair is usually needed to restore proper anatomical alignment

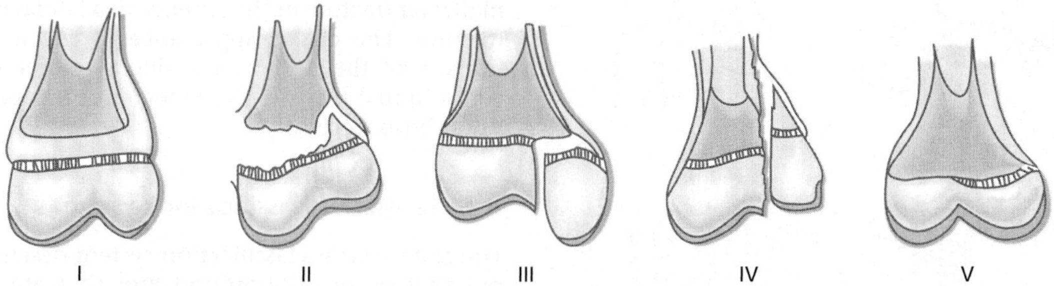
I
II
III
IV
V

FIGURE 80-13 Salter-Harris fractures are generally broken down into five categories.

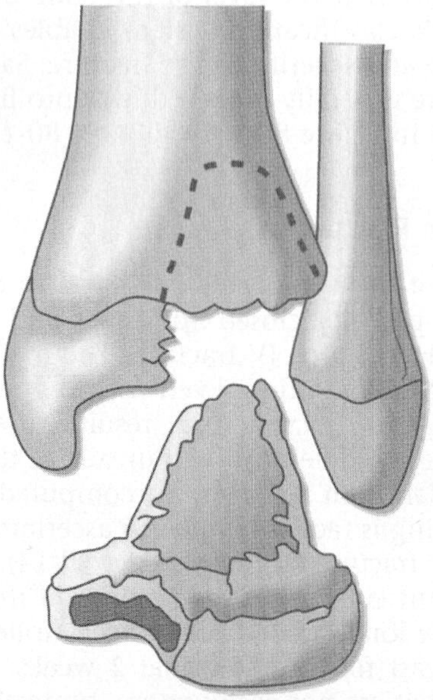

FIGURE 80-14 Triplane fracture.

■ DISLOCATIONS

There are multiple sites where dislocations can occur at the level of the foot and ankle. An in-depth description of these is beyond the scope of this chapter. Nevertheless, two of these types of dislocations are worth mentioning.

Dislocations at the level of the tibiotalar joint, or *tibial dislocations,* are generally associated with fractures. On occasion, a pure tibial dislocation will occur. These require prompt anatomic reduction in an effort to diminish cutaneous and neurovascular injury. If orthopedic consultation is not readily available, reduction under conscious sedation should be performed by the EP.

The second type is *subtalar dislocation.* This injury occurs at the level of the talocalcaneal and the talonavicular joints. Subtalar dislocations can be medial or lateral, depending on the direction of the foot and effecting forces. These are high-energy injuries that result from sports (basketball and baseball) as well as motor vehicle accidents and falls from heights.[6]

The clinical presentation of subtalar dislocations shows significant and obvious deformity. Skin tenting and neurovascular compromise should be promptly assessed and remediated by reduction. Standard lateral radiographs sometimes are not diagnostic, and the AP view of the foot may be the only one that depicts the actual talonavicular dislocation. Computed tomography scanning is recommended to further assess for associated fractures and the integrity of the reduction. Open subtalar dislocations carry significant morbidity and require emergent orthopedic intervention.

FOOT INJURIES

Talar Fractures

Injuries to the talus result from high-energy trauma such as falls from heights or motor vehicle accidents. These injuries may occur at the neck or the body of the talus. Avascular necrosis is common when the injury occurs to the neck of the talus due to the limited blood supply to this area of the bone. Most of these injuries are significant and all warrant orthopedic consultation. In-depth classification is beyond the scope of this chapter; however, a brief summary of the different types of talar fractures is presented in Table 80-3.[3]

Osteochondritis Dissecans (Osteochondral Fracture)

These fractures result from a mechanism similar to that of ankle sprains. When there is forcible inversion of the ankle while it is in plantar flexion or dorsiflexion, the dome of the talus is compressed against the fibula or the tibial plafond. This results in several degrees or "stages" of lesions (Fig. 80-15). More often than not, the initial radiographs are negative, and diagnosis will require computed tomography scanning or magnetic resonance imaging. The diagnosis is missed in 40% to 50% of patients presenting to the ED with an ankle injury. Therefore, a high index of suspicion is warranted in these injuries, especially if the patient presents with a re-injury, chronic swelling, and/or locking of the ankle 4 to 5 weeks after an injury.[2]

Table 80-3 CLASSIFICATION OF FRACTURES OF THE TALUS

Type of Fracture	Classification*
Talar neck fractures	Types I-IV
Talar body fractures	Types I-V
Talar head fractures	
Subtalar dislocations	Medial or lateral
Complete talar dislocation	

*For complete classification details, see Fracture and dislocation compendium: Orthopaedic Trauma Association Committee for Coding and Classification. J Orthop Trauma 1996;10(Suppl 1):104-108.

Calcaneal Injuries

The calcaneus is the most frequently fractured tarsal bone, accounting for more than 60% of tarsal fractures. These fractures are frequently work-related injuries in roofers or other individuals working at heights. The majority are intrarticular, with the remainder being classified as extrarticular.

The most common extraarticular fracture is a calcaneal body fracture. In decreasing frequency, other locations for calcaneal fractures are at the anterior process, the superior tuberosity, and the area of the sustentaculum tali; isolated injuries are rarely seen in these sites. Calcaneus fractures are infrequently encountered as open fractures. Open injuries are reported to occur in only 2% of cases. As a result of the accompanying mechanisms and forces related to calcaneal fractures, other pathology such as spinal injuries and extremity fractures are usually associated with injuries to the os calcis. Multiple complications such as gait abnormalities, arthritis and leg length discrepancy are generally the sequelae of calcaneal fractures.[8]

Plain films including AP, lateral, and axial views of the hindfoot provide a good initial assessment. Computed tomography is generally used to ascertain the true extent of these complex fractures.

One method of assessing the integrity of the calcaneus is done by measuring Böhler's angle. This angle is normally 30 to 35 degrees and is obtained by tracing two lines on the lateral view of the radio-

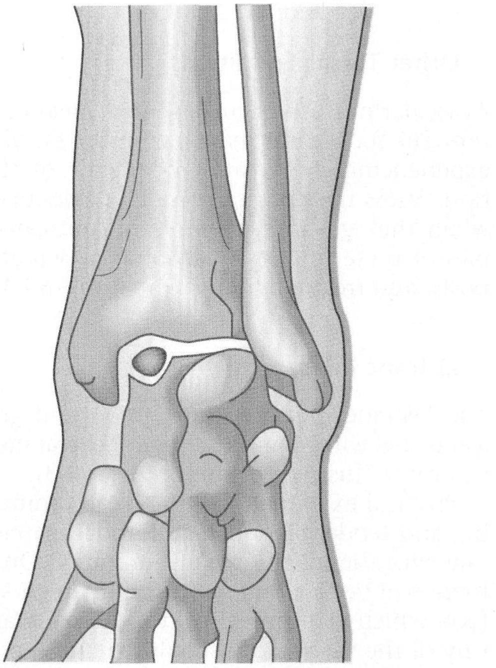

FIGURE 80-15 Osteochondritis dissecans (osteochondral fracture).

Table 80-4 OTHER TARSAL CORDITIONS

	Etiology	History/Physical	Diagnosis	Treatment
Kohler's disease	Self-limited from repetitive trauma; occurs in children ages 3 to 7	Limp and tenderness over the navicular	Radiography of foot	Simple orthotic device; short leg cast for 4 to 6 weeks in recalcitrant cases
Tarsal navicular stress fracture	Occurs in track athletes	Pain in midfoot relieved by rest	Magnetic resonance imaging best; plain film radiography 33% accurate	Immobilization in cast; no weight-bearing for 6 weeks

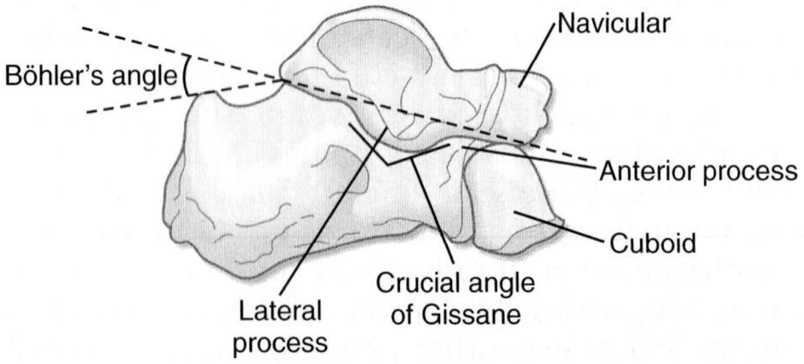
Navicular
Böhler's angle
Anterior process
Cuboid
Crucial angle of Gissane
Lateral process

FIGURE 80-16 Critical angles for evaluating calcaneal fractures.

BOX 80-3

Mechanism of Lisfranc Foot Injuries

Direct Mechanism

Crush injury: e.g., by vehicle running over foot

Indirect Mechanisms

Axial loading: e.g., foot hitting floorboard of car or falling from a height

Severe abduction: e.g., falling off a horse with foot caught in stirrup

graph of the foot (Fig. 80-16). One line is drawn from the posterior tuberosity to the apex of the posterior facet. A second line connects the apex of the posterior facet to the anterior (beak) process. An angle of 20 degrees or less should raise suspicion of a compression fracture of the calcaneus.[3]

Another less frequently used angle measurement is the crucial angle of Gissane. This angle is formed by the downward portion of the posterior facet where it connects to the upward portion. This angle normally measures 100 degrees.[3]

Other Tarsal Conditions

Avascular necrosis occurs in many areas of the skeleton. The foot is not spared, with the tarsal navicular experiencing the greatest frequency of this condition. Stress fractures can result in avascular necrosis when they go unrecognized and untreated.[8] Examples of these injuries, describing preseutation, diagnosis, and treatment, appear in Table 80-4.

Lisfranc Injury

The Lisfranc injury is uncommon and generally is associated with significant force. Several mechanisms can cause this type of injury (Box 80-3).

Physical examination will reveal significant swelling and tenderness of the midfoot area commensurate with the magnitude of the injury. On occasion, there will be ecchymoses of the midarch area of the foot, which is diagnostic of this injury. Careful scrutiny of the vasculature should be made, especially if the intercommunicating arterial branch between the dorsalis pedis artery and the plantar arterial arch is disrupted. This can lead to a compartment syndrome that requires prompt intervention by an orthopedic surgeon.[8]

Metatarsal Injuries

Metatarsal Fractures

Three fracture types commonly occur in the proximal fifth metatarsal (these are from proximal to distal): the tuberosity avulsion fracture, the Jones fracture, and the proximal diaphysial stress fracture. Each has distinct characteristics, and the treatment approach is often controversial. Nevertheless, most of these fractures heal with immobilization over a period of 3 to 8 weeks, depending on location. Treatment of displaced, intraarticular fractures, delayed unions, and nonunions usually requires operative methods. The Jones fracture has a high rate of nonunion and may require surgical intervention. Patients must be warned of this potential problem. Tuberosity fractures and the Jones fracture must not be confused despite their proximity on the fifth metatarsal (Fig. 80-17).[3,9]

Freiberg's Disease

Freiberg's disease is caused by repetitive trauma to the head of the second metatarsal, which deprives the epiphysis of adequate circulation, with consequent necrosis of the metatarsal head and pain in the area of the second metatarsal in the forefoot. Radiography shows flattening of the metatarsal head with a fragmented epiphysis.

Frieberg's disease is most common in adolescent females and is associated with the wearing of high-heel shoes.

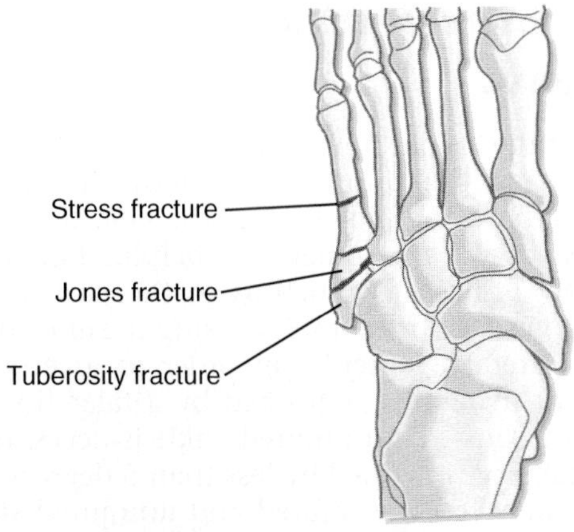
Stress fracture
Jones fracture
Tuberosity fracture

FIGURE 80-17 Metatarsal fracture.

Treatment is directed at prevention of trauma by rest and diminishing of sports activities, as well as wearing flat shoes instead of high heels. Nonsteroidal anti-inflammatory drugs (NSAIDs) may be used as necessary to decrease inflammation.[10]

Sesamoid Bone Fractures

There are many sesamoid bones in the foot. However, those most commonly injured are in the area of the great toe and occasionally in the os trigonum located posterior to the posterior tubercle of the talus. These fractures are infrequent and often go unrecognized. They can occur from direct and indirect trauma. Direct traumatic injuries result from crush-type mechanisms such as falling from a height or direct impact from an external object. Indirectly, the great toe suffers a hyperdorsiflexion-type injury resulting in the fracture. In the case of the os trigonum, plantar flexion is the mechanism. Ballet dancers suffering from these injuries may at some time require removal of the bone due to chronic pain.[3]

Examination reveals localized tenderness over the sesamoid and reproducible pain on dorsiflexion of the great toe. In the case of the os trigonum, the physical examination almost always reveals tenderness anterior to the Achilles tendon and posterior to the tibia, as well as decreased plantar flexion. Pain is reproduced by plantar flexion or resisted plantar flexion of the great toe.

Radiographically, sesamoid fractures appear to have irregular margins as opposed to the smooth contours of a bipartite sesamoid bone. Non-union is frequent due to their poor vascular supply. This can result in chronic pain and swelling as well as disability. It is therefore important to stress the need for orthopedic follow up.

Treatment is directed at protection and immobilization of the affected area in either a walking cast or boot for 4 to 6 weeks.

For fractures of the os trigonum, immobilization in a short leg cast in 15 degrees of plantar flexion for a couple of weeks will suffice.[3]

Toe Fractures

Toe fractures usually are the result of direct trauma such as a heavy object falling on the foot. Occasionally walking or kicking an immobile object will result in a displaced fracture. The eponym "nightwalker" fractures has been given to these injuries that occur at night while navigating in a dark room.

Treatment is directed at anatomic integrity and immobilization. Therefore, reduction of displaced fractures and "buddy tape" immobilization is the standard. All other fractures that are not displaced warrant immobilization in the same fashion; a hard-soled cast shoe is recommended until the pain resolves, at which time an athletic shoe can be worn. In the event of a large intra-articular fracture fragment or a significant displacement of the fragments, orthopedic consultation is emergently required.[8]

Other Conditions of the Foot

Plantar Fasciitis

Plantar fasciitis is a fairly common condition among runners and long-distance walkers. It can have an acute etiology from a sudden excessive loading of the foot; more commonly it becomes symptomatic in a gradual manner from excessive pronation of the foot. These chronic insults result in microtears of the plantar fascia.

Individuals with a high arched foot are more prone to this injury. The patient reports pain in the plantar area of the foot, especially in the morning. Occasionally the pain can be sharp and lancinating, resembling neuropathic pain.

Physical examination reveals tenderness along the plantar area of the hindfoot, near the origin of the plantar fascia. Occasionally swelling may be noted, as well as reproduction of the pain with dorsiflexion of the foot.

Treatment consists of ice massage and gentle stretching of the fascia. The latter is accomplished by Achilles stretching as well rolling the foot back and forth over an object such as a can of soup. An orthotic device is helpful for individuals with excessive pronation on ambulation. Physical therapy in the form of massage and ultrasonography is sometimes necessary. Steroid injections occasionally can be used but should be done judiciously.[5]

Morton's Neuroma

Injury to the third common digital nerve in the third intermetatarsal space of the foot results in perineural fibrosis and pain in this area. Although usually a chronic malady, the presentation also can be acute. It manifests itself in runners or sprinters who experience an electric shock in the forefoot, usually in the early take-off phase of the run.

The history is one of acute or remote trauma during a run or after a fall onto the forefoot. The patient complains of a stabbing or burning pain as well as numbness in the area between the third and

BOX 80-4

Etiologies of Tarsal Tunnel Syndrome

- Trauma
- Medications
- Heavy metals or solvents
- Flat feet (pes planus)
- Tendonitis posterior tibialis
- Varices
- Space-occupying mass
- Medical conditions: diabetes, hypothyroidism
- Alcoholism
- Heel-to-flat shoe transition

fourth toes. Physical examination elicits pain on compression of the interspace. Occasionally a click can be heard when the nerve is pushed from plantar to dorsal and the metatarsals are squeezed together.

Treatment consists of a metatarsal pad in the area of the forefoot to redistribute the weight, thereby relieving pressure on the nerve, and referral to an orthopedist or podiatrist. Custom orthotics, steroid injections, and ultimately surgical excision may be indicated.[10]

Tarsal Tunnel syndrome

Compression of the posterior tibial nerve as it courses through the tarsal tunnel is known as tarsal tunnel syndrome. The tarsal canal is covered by the flexor retinaculum extending posteriorly and distally to the medial malleolus. The floor is formed by the calcaneus, tibia, and talus. The tendons of the flexor hallucis longus, flexor digitorum longus, and tibialis posterior muscles; the posterior tibial nerve; and the posterior tibial artery and vein pass through the tarsal tunnel.

Patients will complain of shooting or radiating pain to the forefoot or the plantar arch. Numbness or a burning or tingling sensation may also be present in the ankle, heel, arch,or toes. Activity will often aggravate the symptoms.

Shooting pain distally may be elicited when the entrapped nerve is percussed (Tinel's sign). Nerve conduction velocity studies are helpful in obtaining a definitive diagnosis. The multiple etiologies are shown in Box 80-4.

There are several treatment options, depending on the etiology. Conservatively, the area can be put at rest by the use of night splints. Orthotics can be used to correct hyperpronation of the foot. Women should stop wearing high-heel shoes.

NSAIDs and occasionally physical therapy may be of benefit. Steroid injections may also be of some help. Ultimately, tarsal tunnel release can be performed to alleviate the condition.

Diagnostic Testing

IMAGING

Views of the ankle should include an AP, lateral, and mortise view. The mortise view allows a fairly good image of both the mortise and the talar dome.

Stress views are sometimes helpful but are not presently utilized as much as in the past. A PA or mortise view is done while stressing the affected ligaments (lateral ligaments) in order to ascertain the degree of instability identified by a talar tilt. Comparison against the uninjured ankle is necessary and joint stability is defined by less than 5 degrees of difference between the injured and uninjured sides. A tilt angle greater than 15 degrees, compared with the uninjured side, often signifies rupture of the anterior talofibular and calcaneofibular ligaments.[2]

Another radiographic method of assessing ankle joint stability is the identification of the medial clear space. This is the distance, as measured on a mortise view, between the lateral border of the medial malleolus and the medial border of the talus. Any measurement greater than 4 mm is considered abnormal and is sign of instability (Fig. 80-18).[3]

Ottawa Ankle rules

In an effort to decrease the number of ankle radiographs used in the diagnosis of acute ankle injuries, Stiell and colleagues from the Ottawa Civic and the Ottawa General Hospitals in Canada conducted a prospective study involving over 750 patients presenting to the ED with acute blunt ankle injuries. They determined that ankle films were necessary only when patients presenting with pain near the malleoli exhibited one or more of the findings shown in Box 80-5.

Likewise, for *injuries to the foot,* radiographs would be necessary only when there is pain in the mid-foot area AND there is bone tenderness at the navicular, the cuboid, or the base of the fifth metatarsal.[11]

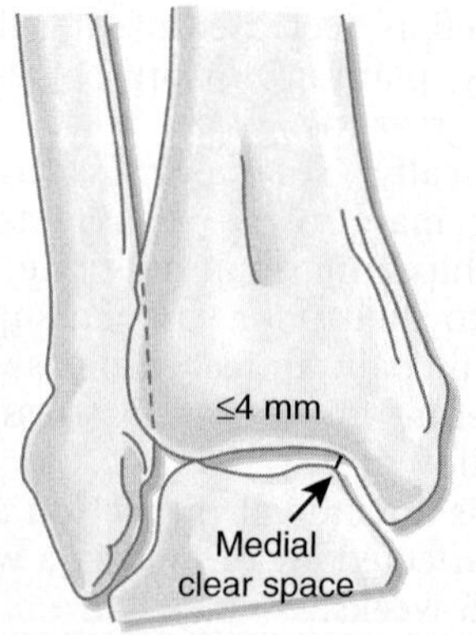
≤4 mm
Medial
clear space

FIGURE 80-18 The distance between the tibial surface and the medial wall of the fibula. Any measurement greater than 4 mm is considered abnormal and a sign of instability.

BOX 80-5

Ottawa Ankle Rules

- Age 55 or greater
- Inability to bear weight immediately and in the ED
- Bone tenderness at the posterior edge or tip of either malleolus

BOX 80-6

ICEMM Mnemonic for Treatment of Fractures of the Foot and Ankle

I**CE:** Every 2 hours or as needed for the first 24 to 48 hours

C**OMPRESSION:** Compression dressing (Webril or Ace) to decrease swelling; ankle stirrup to lend stability, if indicated

E**LEVATION:** To reduce swelling

M**OBILIZATION:** Early, as soon as patient is pain-free

M**EDICATION:** Nonsteroidal anti-inflammatory drugs or narcotics where applicable

Treatment and Disposition

In general, the approach to treatment of foot and ankle injuries is directed at protecting the affected limb from further injury at the same time that other modalities, including early mobilization, are employed. Box 80-6 outlines a brief summary of the standard and basic treatment of these injuries.

An ankle stirrup will protect the joint by preventing lateral motion of the ankle. At the same time, it allows plantar and dorsiflexion, which contribute to early motion and rehabilitation of the affected joint. These devices can be inflated and deflated by the patient, allowing a tolerable degree of compression as well as stability.

BOX 80-7

Guidelines As to When Sports Activities Can Be Safely Resumed

- **Type I injury** (Ligament stretch or minor tear): Return to play in 1 to 10 days.
- **Type II injury** (Partial ligament tear): Return to play in 2 to 4 weeks.
- **Type III injury** (Complete ligament tear): Return to play in 5 to 8 weeks.

The patient can begin exercise when pain subsides (do not use heat) and can return to full activity when full pain-free motion and equal strength are attained in both ankles.

For weekend and other athletes, depending on age and conditioning, Box 80-7 outlines some guidelines as to when sports activities can be safely resumed.

REFERENCES

1. Garrick JG: The frequency of injury, mechanism of injury, and epidemiology of ankle sprains. Am J Sports Med 1977; 56:241-242.
2. Canale TS: Ankle Injuries. In Daugherty K, Jones L (eds): Campbell's Operative Orthopaedics, vol 3, 10th ed. Philadelphia, Mosby, 2003, p 2131.
3. Marsh JL, Saltzman CL: Ankle fractures. In Bucholz RW, Heckman JD (eds): Fractures in Adults, vol 2, 5th ed. Philadelphia, Lippincott Williams & Wilkins, 2001.
4. del Castillo J, Geiderman JM: The Frenchman's fibular fracture (Maisonneuve fracture). JACEP 1979;8:404-406.
5. Trojian TH, McKeag DB: Ankle sprains: Expedient assessment and management. In Howe WB (ed): The Physician and Sports Medicine, vol 26, No. 10. New York, Vendome Group, LLC, 1998.
6. Sammarco GJ: Peroneal tendon injuries. Orthop Clin North Am 1994;25:135-145.
7. Lauge-Hansen N: Fractures of the ankle: Combined experimental-surgical and experimental roentgenologic investigations. Arch Surg 1950;60:957-985.
8. Einhorn TA, Tornetta P III: Foot and ankle. In Thordarson DB (ed): Orthopaedic Surgery Essentials. Philadelphia, Lippincott Williams & Wilkins, 2004, p 243.
9. Lawrence SJ. Botte MJ: Jones' fractures and related fractures of the proximal fifth metatarsal. Foot Ankle 1993;14: 358-365.
10. Simons SM: Foot injuries of the recreational athlete. Phys Sportsmed 1999;27(1).
11. Stiell IG, Greenberg GH, McKnight RD, et al: A study to develop clinical decision rules for the use of radiography in acute ankle injuries. Ann Emerg Med 1992;21:384-390.

Chapter 81

Tendinitis and Bursitis

Erin Lareau and Ted Koutouzis

KEY POINTS

Mechanical overload and repetitive microtrauma are the key to underlying mechanisms in the development of tendon injuries.
Bursitis commonly occurs secondary to overlying tendinosis.
Many bursae are nameless; a new bursa may form anywhere as a result of frequent irritation.
Other emergent medical conditions such as septic arthritis, fractures, and rheumatologic conditions should be excluded in the diagnosis.
The diagnosis is made clinically for both tendinopathy and bursitis; however, magnetic resonance imaging, ultrasonography, and aspiration of bursal fluid can be useful in difficult cases.
Conservative treatment with rest, ice, immobilization, and nonsteroidal anti-inflammatory drugs (NSAIDs) suffices in most cases.
The olecranon bursa and prepatellar bursa are the most commonly infected bursae; thus it is rare to see infection of other bursae.
Depending on the environment in which the injury occurs (workplace, sports), modifying the patient's technique, body position, and repetitive movements can help to prevent fibrous changes and chronic problems.

Scope

Tendinitis and bursitis result from repetitive motion of a patient's arms or legs. The incidence increases with sports activities and occupations that require highly repetitive activities such as baseball, golf, carpentry, and employment as fabricators or operators in some factories. The incidence of tendinitis increases with age as muscles and tendons lose some of their elasticity, and it is highest in the age group of 25 to 54 years. Bursitis affects approximately 1 in 31(3.20%) or 8.7 million people in the United States. According to the Centers for Disease Control and Prevention, in 2001 tendinitis cases involved a median of 10 days away from work, compared with 6 days for all nonfatal injury and illness cases.[1] Most cases involved white, non-hispanic females whose occupations had a highly repetitive component.

Pathophysiology

The primary role of tendons throughout the body is to connect muscle to bone. The activation of muscles creates forces that are transferred through tendons to the human skeleton in order to produce movement. Tendons are composed primarily of type 1 collagen and are arranged in a parallel array of tropocollagen. These structures are in turn grouped together to form larger structures. Through this stacking mechanism, the structural strength of the tendons is increased. Ligaments, functioning more passively to connect bone to bone in the body, do not share this organized arrangement. When viewed under a microscope, tendons appear wavy in the resting state.

As a force is applied, stretching will occur and the tendon will go through different phases of deformation. Initially, microscopic tears occur, followed by complete rupture if the load exceeds the intrinsic strength of the tendon. Tendon injury may occur acutely, and the tendon can be ruptured when an explosive overloading force is applied. These forces are eccentric in nature—for example, when a runner starts a sprint from a standing position. Rupture may be incomplete or complete. Most tendon ruptures occur in the middle of the tendon but may also occur at the bone-tendon insertion, resulting in avulsion fractures.

Most often, tendon injury results from chronic overuse (Fig. 81-1). The term *tendinitis* is somewhat of a misnomer because the disorder is actually a degenerative process with or without inflammatory changes, which may include fibroblastic proliferation. Tendinitis is commonly believed to be caused by repetitive microtrauma to the tendon, causing an early inflammatory response of surrounding tissues and resulting in degenerative changes in the tendon. Because the association between the microscopic degenerative changes and the patient's clinical symptoms is unclear, the term *tendinopathy* often is used to describe chronic tendon pain.[2]

Due to the extensive amount of movement that tendons undergo, overuse injuries are to be expected. Mechanical overload or repetitive microtrauma to the musculotendinous unit may exceed the intrinsic ability of the tendon to repair itself.[3] Although the site and mechanism of injury may vary, the resulting inflammatory response is consistently the same. The classic inflammatory signs of pain, warmth, erythema, and swelling will be experienced, depending on the area injured.

Following this short inflammatory stage, the healing process proceeds through both proliferative and maturation stages. Because much of the process is noninflammatory in nature, some authors question the efficacy of NSAIDs.[4]

In contrast to tendons, bursae are closed, round, flat sacs lined with synovium that may or may not communicate with the synovial cavity. Bursae are most commonly found at sites of friction, between skin, and underlying ligaments and bone. Bursae allow the lubricated movement of soft tissues over areas of potential impingement (e.g., subacromial bursa). Many bursae are nameless, and new bursae may form anywhere as a result of frequent irritation.

During periods of inflammation, synovial bursa cells increase in thickness via villous hyperplasia. With repeated trauma, infection, or systemic disease, this synovial lining may be replaced with granulation tissue prior to fibrous tissue development.

Bursae may become inflamed for many reasons: chronic friction, trauma, crystal deposition, infec-

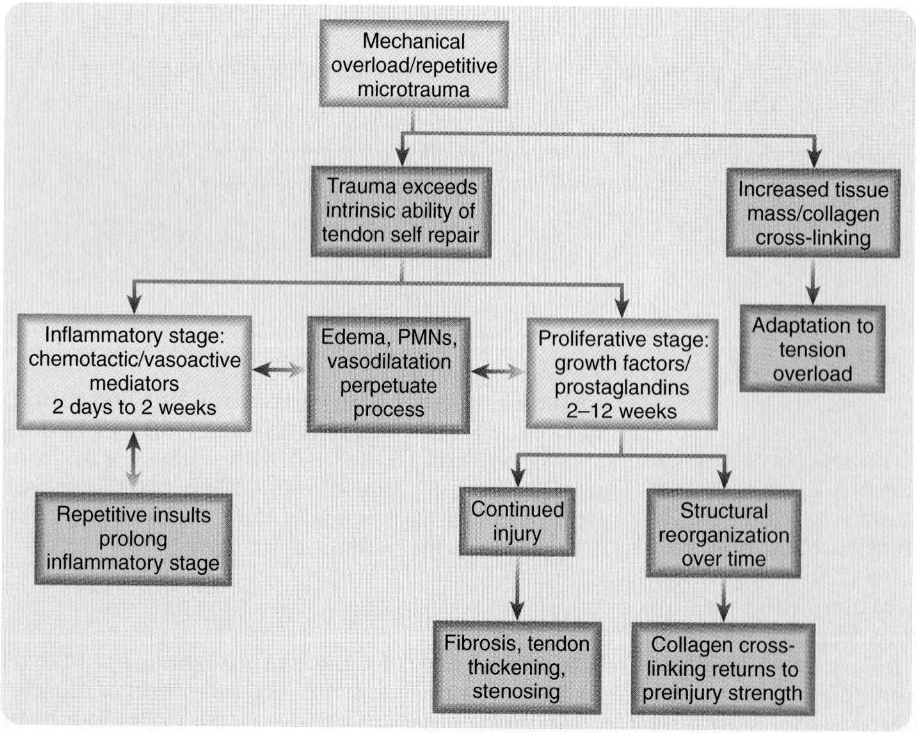
Mechanical overload/repetitive microtrauma
Trauma exceeds intrinsic ability of tendon self repair
Increased tissue mass/collagen cross-linking
Inflammatory stage: chemotactic/vasoactive mediators 2 days to 2 weeks
Edema, PMNs, vasodilatation perpetuate process
Proliferative stage: growth factors/ prostaglandins 2–12 weeks
Adaptation to tension overload
Repetitive insults prolong inflammatory stage
Continued injury
Structural reorganization over time
Fibrosis, tendon thickening, stenosing
Collagen cross-linking returns to preinjury strength

FIGURE 81-1 Algorithm of the pathophysiology of tendon injuries. PMN, polymorphonuclear neutrophil.

Table 81-2 SHOULDER TENDINOPATHIES

Condition	Characteristics	Chief Complaint	Tests	Treatment
Adhesive capsulitis	Fibrosis of joint capsule and restriction of motion due to underlying medical disease or prolonged immobilization	Diffuse, achy pain extending down upper arm	Painful, stiffened "frozen" shoulder with diffuse atrophy; pain reproduced by forcing limits of range of motion (not by palpation)	Pain control; referral to orthopedist, physical therapy
Biceps tendinitis	Inflammation of the long head of the biceps as it passes the biceps groove due to repetitive overhead movements	Acute, intense, localized anterior shoulder pain	Speed's test, Yergason test; pain to palpation along the biceps groove	Analgesics, RICE (*r*est, *i*ce, *c*ompression, *e*levation) if subluxation is present; early mobilization
Calcific tendinitis	Idiopathic deposition of calcium hydroxyapatite crystals in the rotator cuff tendons	Primarily asymptomatic; middle-aged patient with acute attack had pain at rest or at night for 1-2 weeks	Calcium deposits on radiograph; pain on abduction, "catching sensation"	Analgesics, ice; oral/ subacromial steroids controversial
Biceps rupture	Tear of proximal long head of biceps after sudden or prolonged contraction against resistance	Snap or pop; anterior shoulder pain	Swelling, crepitus over bicep groove; "Popeye" deformity (midarm bulge of retracted biceps muscle) with elbow flexion, weak supination	RICE with sling, analgesics; referral to orthopedist for surgical repair

Table 81-3 IMPINGEMENT SYNDROME OF SUPRASPINATUS TENDON

Grade	Characteristics	Tests*	Treatment
Stage 1	Repetitive overhead motion causes reversible edema and hemorrhage with dull, achy, nonspecific pain due to compression of tendons between acromion and humeral head	*Painful arc syndrome:* Flexion and abduction between 70 and 130 degrees elicit pain; no weakness or loss of motion	Rest, activity modification, ice, nonsteroidal antiinflammatory drugs (NSAIDs)
Stage 2	Fibrosis and thickening of tendons and bursa over weeks to months; pain becomes constant and worse at night, localizes to lateral acromion and humeral head	Active motion limited by pain; passive motion preserved. Classic *Neer test:* Raise straight arm in forced forward flexion while preventing scapular rotation	Conservative therapy as in stage 1
Stage 3	Irreversible chronic changes: fibrosis of the tendon bursa, osteophytic bony changes, partial or complete rotator cuff and biceps tendon tears	Muscular atrophy, crepitus, weakness and pain on external rotation, elevation, abduction. *Drop arm test:* patient cannot hold an extended arm at 90 degrees abduction	Conservative therapy and referral to orthopedist for surgical decompression of the subacromial space

*Physical examination maneuvers are considered positive for impingement if they reproduce pain, but usually they are not used for staging.

tendon sheath (A-1 pulley) on the palmar surface over the base of the metacarpal head becomes stenosed and catches as the finger is moved. Typically, symptoms vary from pain to complete locking of the finger in flexion. It is common in middle-aged women.

Conservative treatment with rest, splinting, and antiinflammatory medications may be attempted. Some feel this is inadequate treatment and recommend cortisone injection initially; cure rates from 84% to 91% have been reported with this treatment.[9] Surgical release of the A-1 pulley may also be performed if the conservative treatment fails. For patients with de Quervain's tendinitis, a thumb spica splint is required if cortisone injection provides no improvement.

Table 81-4 ELBOW TENDINOPATHIES

Condition	Characteristics	Tests	Treatment
Lateral epicondylitis (tennis elbow)	Microtrauma due to overuse/inflammation of wrist extensors/supinators: extensor carpi radialis brevis/longus, extensor digitorum communis, extensor carpi ulnaris	Pain with grasping, twisting, or resisted active dorsiflexion of the wrist or middle finger; tenderness at lateral epicondyle	Rest, ice, elevation; compression provides support during activities; banding with or without splint over proximal lateral forearm
Medial epicondylitis (golfer's elbow, pitcher's elbow, bowler's elbow)	Microtrauma due to overuse/inflammation of flexor carpi radialis	Pain with active flexing of the wrist against resistance; tenderness at medial epicondyle	Rest, ice, elevation; circumferential compression band to proximal forearm

Table 81-5 WRIST AND HAND TENDINOPATHIES

Condition	Characteristics	Tests	Treatment	Pearls
De Quervain's tendinitis	Overuse inflammation (repetitive motion) of abductor pollicis longus and extensor pollicis brevis synovia causes radial wrist pain	Thumb held in the palm with ulnar deviation of the wrist (Finkelstein's test) causes pain	Rest, splinting, NSAIDs, referral to orthopedist for cortisone injections; refractory cases require orthopedic consultation for tendon release	Carrying heavy objects (grocery bags) over the wrists can cause symptoms; pregnancy precipitates a flare; differential diagnosis includes SLE, rheumatoid arthritis, CMC joint osteoarthritis, scaphoid fracture/nonunion
Gonococcal tenosynovitis	Hematogenous seeding of CMC joint	Fluid culture, sensitivity	Antibiotics, rest, NSAIDs	Fever, penile or vaginal discharge, skin findings, polyarticular arthritis; differential diagnosis includes Reiter's syndrome and De Quervain's tendinitis
Trigger finger	Overuse tenosynovitis or congenital sheath narrowing causes nodules and A-1 palmar pulley stenosis; "catching" sensation with flexion	Symptoms vary from pain to complete locking of finger in flexion, palpable "pop" during extension	Rest, NSAIDs, splinting; refer to orthopedist for cortisone injections	Differential diagnosis includes infectious flexor tenosynovitis, trisomy 13, rheumatoid arthritis, diabetes mellitus
Dupuytren's contracture	Proliferative disorder of subcutaneous palmar fascia; autosomal dominant with variable penetrance	Place palm down on a flat surface; digits cannot simultaneously lie flat due to contractures (Hueston's table-top test)	No effective presention; observation; refer to orthopedist for fasciotomy	Commonly occurs in older men, patients with alcohol abuse, epilepsy, diabetes, COPD; not symmetric; some patients have Dupuytren's diasthesis, involvement of hands and feet (Letterhose's disease) or penis (Peyronie's disease)

CMC, carpometacarpal; COPD, chronic obstructive pulmonary disease; NSAIDs, nonsteroidal anti-inflammatory drugs; SLE, systemic lupus erythematosus.

■ KNEE (Table 81-6)

■ Iliotibial Band Syndrome

The iliotibial band syndrome, or "runner's knee," is a common tendinopathy occurring in long-distance runners. The etiology is often from chronic overuse through increased volume and intensity of run workouts. Patients report pain in the lateral portion of the knee as the distal iliotibial tract becomes injured, and they may state that the pain resolves after an initial warm up phase, may return at the end of running, and is always prominent the next morning on awakening. On examination, there is point tenderness to palpation, and crepitation may be appreciated.

■ Biceps Femoris and Popliteal Tendinopathy

These two disorders are grouped together because of their commonr anatomic location. The biceps femoris (hamstring) is a large muscle that inserts on the proximal fibula. The popliteal muscle inserts on the lateral aspect of the distal femur. Both tendons cross the knee joint and are subject to acute and overuse injuries, especially in athletes. In acute injuries, radiography should be performed to exclude an avulsion fracture. The diagnosis is made clinically.

Patients report that symptoms occurred while running or playing sports. Tenderness to palpation at the insertions of these muscles is noted.

Table 81-6 KNEE TENDINOPATHIES

Condition	Characteristics	Tests	Pearls
Iliotibial band syndrome (runner's knee)	Tendinopathy of distal iliotibial tract; more common in the morning and at the start or end of workout	Point tenderness and crepitation over lateral knee	Pain is always prominent in the morning on awakening
Biceps femoris (hamstring) tendinopathy	Pain at insertion site during inciting activity (playing sports, running)	Tenderness at proximal fibula	Acute injuries require radiography to exclude avulsion fracture
Popliteal tendinopathy	Pain with activity	Tenderness at lateral aspect of distal femur (over patellar tendon) when under tension	Athletes are particularly subject to knee overuse injury

■ ANKLE

■ Achilles Tendinitis

Achilles tendinitis is a common overuse syndrome that typically affects male athletes. The Achilles tendon arises from the medial and lateral heads of the gastrocnemius muscle and the deep layers of the soleus muscle and inserts on the calcaneal tuberosity. It is the strongest and largest tendon in the body and can withstand tensile loads of up to eight times the body's weight while a person is running.

The Achilles tendon can be injured from direct trauma, overuse, and medication or can become inflamed as part of a systemic disease (ankylosing spondylitis, Reiter's syndrome, gout, pseudogout). However, most causes of Achilles tendinitis are thought to be multifactorial. For instance, an athlete's body mechanics or environmental factors such as uneven terrain may apply valgus or varus stress to the tendon. Thus, techniques, environment, equipment, and body mechanics may underlie the development of Achilles tendinitis. Additionally, the vascular supply creates a watershed area approximately 2 to 6 cm above the calcaneal insertion and is thought to be responsible for the clinical symptoms and pathologic disruption at this site.

Tendinitis progresses through the following series of stages before final rupture occurs. Initially, the tendon sheath becomes inflamed, and tendon inflammation follows. With repeated stress, scar tissue formation and degeneration of the tendon occurs, thereby reducing its strength. Clinically, the patient notes pain, decreased range of motion, and if the tendinitis is chronic, morning stiffness. As with all cases of tendinitis, rest, ice, and NSAIDs are the treatment of choice.

In order to prevent recurrence, correction of limb misalignment with the use of orthotics or heel wedges usually is necessary. Changes in the training environment and in the duration and intensity of exercise should be modified to eliminate undue stress. Achilles injuries and other common injuries in the differential diagnosis are shown in Table 81-7.

Table 81-7 ANKLE TENDINOPATHIES

Condition	Etiology	Examination	Pearls
Achilles tendinopathy (calcaneal paratendinitis)	Multifactorial—direct trauma, overuse (6%-11% of runners), medications, or systemic disease cause inflammation of tendon sheath, resulting in pain, morning stiffness	Tenderness, decreased range of motion; varus or valgus stress exacerbates symptoms	Treatment includes orthotics, heel wedges; never inject steroids
Achilles tendon rupture	Rupture of tendon at watershed area (2-6 cm proximal to calcaneal insertion) due to forced dorsiflexion or direct trauma	Thompson's test; distal calf swelling, palpable tendon defect, weak plantar flexion	Patient describes audible pop or snap; steroids increase risk for rupture
Peroneal tendon subluxation/dislocation	Tear of peroneal retinaculum during forced dorsiflexion; anterior subluxation of peroneus brevis and peroneus longus tendons over lateral malleolus causes "clicking or slipping" over back of ankle	Swelling, tenderness, ecchymosis at posterior aspect of lateral malleolus, anterior subluxation of tendons over malleolus with forced dorsiflexion/eversion	Don't miss avulsion fracture of fibula (50%)
Plantar fasciitis	Overuse, hyperpronation, or improper footwear causes inflammation of fascia at plantar calcaneal insertion	Tenderness to anteromedial aspect of heel; passive dorsiflexion of toes exacerbates pain	Inferior heel pain worst with first steps in the morning; treatment includes arch supports

Bursitis (Table 81-8)

■ TROCHANTERIC BURSITIS

Several bursae in the hip region are common sites of inflammation. The trochanteric bursa has both deep and superficial components. The deep bursa is located between the greater trochanter and the tensor fascia lata. The superficial bursa is the only superficial bursa in the hip and pelvic region and lies between the greater trochanter and skin. Due to its location, it is predisposed to direct trauma.

Patients with trochanteric bursitis generally are middle-aged or older women who complain of acute or chronic pain over the bursal area and lateral thigh.

Trochanteric bursitis can occur as a complication of rheumatoid arthritis. The pain is increased when lying on the hip, walking down or climbing stairs. The pain of superficial bursitis can be reproduced by adduction and that of deep trochanteric bursitis by abduction. Approximately 50% of patients have pain with sequential *f*lexion, *ab*duction, *e*xternal *r*otation, and *e*xtension of the hip while the contralateral knee is held in flexion (Patrick-Fabere test). Internal rotation does not usually provoke symptoms. The hip joint itself appears normal on examination, and no pain is elicited with flexion or extension.

In runners, it is common to see deep trochanteric bursitis as a result of overuse, faulty biomechanics, or extreme mileage. Direct acute trauma can also cause deep trochanteric bursitis.

■ ISCHIAL BURSITIS

Ischial bursitis develops secondary to trauma or from sitting on a hard surface (weaver's bottom). Sometimes the pain radiates down the back of the thigh and mimics sciatic nerve inflammation. The ischial bursa lies adjacent to the ischial tuberosity overlying the sciatic and posterior femoral cutaneous nerves, which can explain these clinical features. This may also explain why this condition is often misdiagnosed as sciatica or disc herniation. The pain can be reproduced by applying pressure over the ischial tuberosity by sitting, standing on tiptoe, or bending forward.

■ PREPATELLAR BURSITIS

Prepatellar bursitis (housemaid's knee, nun's knee) causes swelling over the lower pole of the patella, usually as a result of constant friction, repetitive trauma, rheumatoid arthritis, or localized infection. Repetitive trauma also produces fibrosis and thickened nodules, thereby requiring excision of the bursa. Range of motion may increase the pain associated with prepatellar bursitis as the bursa comes under tension. Examination of the joint usually is normal.

Pyogenic prepatellar bursitis is thought to be more common in children. This condition requires aspiration, immobilization, and antibiotic coverage. If acute episodes are not resolved within 2 days, incision and drainage should be considered.[10]

■ INFRAPATELLAR BURSITIS

The infrapatellar bursa is divided into two parts. Between the patellar ligament and the superior anterior surface of the tibia lies the deep part. The superficial aspect lies between the skin and patellar ligament. Deep infrapatellar bursitis presents with tenderness on both sides of the tendon, which increases with extreme flexion.[11,12]

If signs of infection such as loss of full extension of the knee or resistance to full flexion are present, aspiration of the infrapatellar bursa should be performed along with antibiotic therapy. If infection exists, evaluation for surrounding osteomyelitis is advisable.

Table 81-8 FREQUENTLY INFLAMED BURSAE

Condition	Location
Subacromial	Shoulder: Under acromion and coracoacromial ligament; separates coracoacromial ligament from rotator cuff
Olecranon	Elbow: Superficial olecranon; frequently infected; requires aspiration
Trochanteric	Hip: Deep bursa between greater trochanter and tensor fascia lata Superficial: Between greater trochanter and skin
Ischial (weaver's bottom)	Hip: Adjacent to ischial tuberosity over sciatic and posterior femoral nerves
Iliopsoas	Hip: Between iliopsoas tendon and lesser trochanter
Prepatellar (housemaid's knee or nun's knee)	Swelling over lower pole of patella; frequently infected, requires aspiration
Infrapatellar	Deep: Between patellar ligament and superior tibia Superficial: Between patellar ligament and skin
Anserine	Medial knee 2 inches below joint margin, where medial hamstrings attach
Calcaneal	Deep: Between calcaneus and Achilles tendon Superficial: Between tendon and skin

■ ANSERINE BURSITIS

Anserine bursitis most commonly occurs in obese older women with large legs and a history of osteoarthritis of the knees. Endurance athletes are another group of patients prone to this condition.

Anserine bursitis results from incorrect biomechanics, increased intensity and volume of exercise, or excessive muscle tightness. The mechanism is usually repetitive friction or microtrauma. Pain characteristically increases on climbing stairs and extremes of range of motion and can radiate to the inner thigh and mid-calf. The area of tenderness is localized to the medial aspect of the knee 2 inches below the joint margin, where the medial hamstrings (sartorius, gracilis, and semitendinosus) attach. The area is usually neither swollen nor warm.

■ CALCANEAL BURSITIS

There are two bursa found at the insertion of the Achilles tendon. The superficial bursa lies between the skin and the tendon. It may become inflamed secondarily to Achilles tendinitis or from repetitive friction/overuse. The deep bursa lies between the tendon and calcaneus and is rarely affected. When inflamed though pain with range of motion and tenderness anterior to the Achilles tendon will be noted.

■ SUBACROMIAL BURSITIS

The subacromial bursa lies under the acromion and coracoacromial ligament, to which it is attached. This bursa separates the ligament from the supraspinatus muscle and rotator cuff. The proximity of these anatomic structures contributes to the spread of the inflammatory response. Thus, subacromial bursitis is thought to be an extension of supraspinatus tendinitis and typically follows this disorder's stages of impingement.

Pain and tenderness are localized to the lateral aspect of the shoulder, and signs of impingement are noted on the physical examination. Although not specific to subacromial bursitis, the painful arc of the subacromial space, which is between 70 and 100 degrees of shoulder abduction, is noted. Primary subacromial bursitis rarely may result from rheumatoid arthritis, tuberculosis, gout, and infections.[6]

■ OLECRANON BURSITIS

Due to its superficial location, the olecranon bursa is vulnerable to injury. When traumatized, the resulting bursal hematoma causes pain and swelling mimicking acute bursitis. Systemic conditions such as gout (most common), rheumatoid disease, pseudogout, and uremia and oxalosis induced by dialysis can produce primary bursal inflammation. Infection can occur locally from puncture wounds or lacerations, or systemically from bacteremia. Sometimes microscopic wounds can introduce infection without antecedent trauma. In fact, the olecranon bursa and prepatellar bursa are the most commonly infected bursae. It is thus rare to see infection of other bursae throughout the body.

Symptoms include tenderness to palpation, swelling, fluctuation, and warmth. Early signs of inflammation are limitation of extension and an increase in the normal angle at which the elbow is held at the side. Range of motion should not be affected in aseptic cases. At times in patients with rheumatoid arthritis or gout, nodules or tophi may be appreciated when palpating the bursa. Skin discoloration may also be noted. The diagnosis is based on patient history and clinical examination. If fever is present, septic bursitis must be considered and septic arthritis excluded.

Clinically, the most important question is whether an infection exists. Some distinguishing characteristics of septic bursitis are rapid onset, marked warmth, erythema, and extremely tense and painful bursae. Aspiration of bursal fluid confirms the diagnosis.

Gram stain and culture should be obtained and bursal white blood cell count (WBC) determined. Systemic leukocytosis is neither sensitive nor specific and therefore a routine complete blood count can be omitted. A bursal fluid WBC count higher than $5000/mm^3$ suggests bursal fluid infection; however, but this may not be clear-cut because there is an overlap in the WBC count of bursa fluid in septic versus aseptic cases (synovial fluid analysis is discussed in more detail in Chapter 103). Therefore, if infection is suspected, regardless of Gram stain results, antibiotic treatment should be instituted pending culture results.

The treatment of olecranon bursitis remains controversial. Some experts support aspiration and evaluation of all effusions regardless of physical examination findings; others feel that aspiration only increases the risk of infection and prefer to treat empirically with antibiotics and NSAIDs or antibiotics alone. Staphylococcal infection is most common, and an anti-staphylococcal antibiotic should be chosen if antibiotics are prescribed. Still others view this process as predominantly inflammatory and believe that only NSAIDs need be administered.

These authors believe that unless there is strong evidence of infection, olecranon bursitis should be treated with NSAIDS, compression dressings, and close follow-up. Regardless of which treatment is chosen, intrabursal steroids should not be given if there is the possibility of infection, and close follow-up to assess the patient's response to treatment should be arranged.[9]

Diagnostic Studies

■ PLAIN RADIOGRAPHS

A diagnosis of tendinitis or bursitis is generally made on clinical grounds; however, radiologic studies are sometimes required to confirm the diagnosis by

Documentation

History

- Acute or chronic pain
- Treatments attempted
- Occupation, frequent activities, and aggravating factors
- History of trauma
- Diffuse articular pain or focal periarticular pain
- Is pain monoarticular or polyarticular? Is pain migratory?
- Any systemic complaints

Physical Examination

- Does the patient look ill? Febrile?
- Joint examination: warmth, effusion, deformity, range of motion, pain on motion, tenderness, muscle atrophy
- Systemic signs (e.g., rash)

Studies

- Radiography: Soft tissue swelling, erosions, calcification, osteoporosis, deformity, joint space narrowing/separation, fractures.
- Synovial fluid analysis: cell count, Gram stain, crystals, culture
- Medical decision-making: Document concerns for infection, reasons for starting or not starting antibiotics, alternative diagnoses entertained

Procedures

- Joint fluid aspiration: document indication, approach used, analgesia, and results

Patient Instructions

- Document discussion with patient regarding diagnosis, warning signs and what to do when they occur, follow-up, when to return

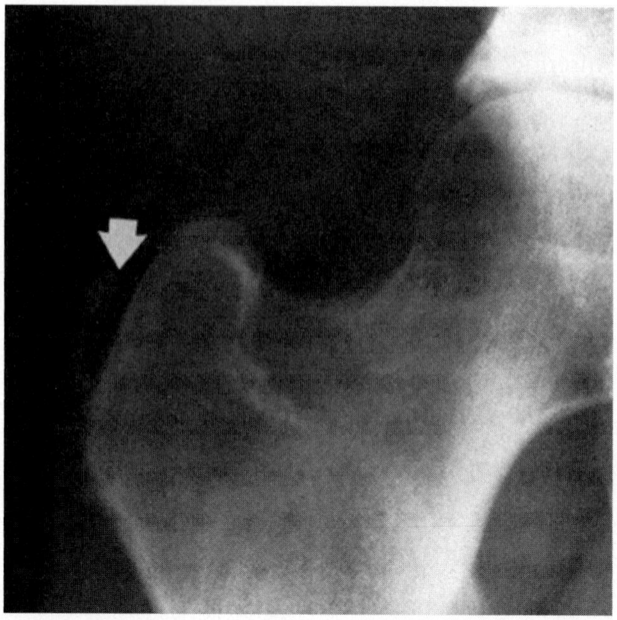

FIGURE 81-3 Calcific trochanteric bursitis. A faint calcification (*arrow*) along the trochanteric bursa is noted along the lateral cortex of the greater trochanter.

RED FLAGS

- Any joint effusion with systemic signs is considered septic arthritis until proved otherwise.
- Any injury in patient with a history of trauma is considered a fracture until proved otherwise.
- Pain with passive motion indicates articular involvement; further investigation is warranted for inflammatory or infectious etiology.
- History of steroid injection into large tendon greatly increases risk for rupture.
- Steroid injections and systemic steroids increase risk for infection.

ruling out other causes of pain. Plain radiographs help distinguish extraarticular from articular sources of pain.[13] In acute injury, radiographs are essential to exclude an avulsion fracture.

The radiograph of a joint should be surveyed using a systematic approach. One such approach is summarized by the mnemonic SECONDS: *S*oft tissue swelling, *E*rosions, *C*alcification, *O*steoporosis, *N*arrowing (joint space), *D*eformity, and *S*eparation (fractures) (Fig. 81-3).

■ ULTRASONOGRAPHY

Ultrasonography is useful in the evaluation of joint effusions and lesions of tendons, ligaments, and skeletal muscles. It is particularly useful in imaging of the shoulder region.[14] It has been shown to be more sensitive than magnetic resonance imaging and is now considered the gold standard for evaluating tendon involvement with concomitant trauma or rheumatic diseases. Ultrasound scanning is especially valuable when other concurrent conditions (e.g., gouty arthritis) obscure the findings of tendinitis. Currently this modality has limited use in the emergency care setting; however, with the increasing presence and practice of ultrasound scanning in the ED, some familiarity will become essential.

In acute or chronic tendinitis, one or more of the following features may be seen on an ultrasound image: loss of fibrillar echotexture, focal tendon-thickening, diffuse thickening, focal hypoechoic areas, extended hypoechogenicity, irregular and ill-defined borders, microruptures, and peritendinous inflammatory edema.[14] Local or diffuse thickening of surrounding soft tissue inflammation and partial and complete tendon tears can also be delineated.

PATIENT TEACHING TIPS

- Instructions should be given regarding proper rest, ice, analgesia, and immobilization.
- If a joint is aspirated, prompt follow-up must be arranged for culture results.
- Septic bursitis requires antistaphylococcal antibiotics and immediate orthopedic consultation. Patients with systemic toxicity require admission for IV antibiotics and operative joint wash-out.
- Patients should call their primary care physician or return to the ED for:
  - Increased pain, swelling, redness around the joint
  - Fever
  - Inability to move the joint due to pain
  - Any other concerning symptoms

BOX 81-1

Management of Tendinopathy and Aseptic Bursitis

- Rest
- Ice for the first 24 to 48 hours post-injury
- Compression of swollen bursa
- Elevation
- Immobilization of involved tendon
- Nonsteroidal anti-inflammatory drugs (NSAIDs)

Treatment and Disposition

Most patients with bursitis and tendinopathy can be managed conservatively with rest and anti-inflammatory medication (Box 81-1). Exceptions to this are olecranon bursitis and prepatellar bursitis, which have a moderate risk of being infected, most likely with *Staphylococcus aureus*. These bursae may require needle aspiration and treatment with antibiotics until culture results are negative. Alternatively, empirical antibiotics may be administered. Most patients can be managed as outpatients as long as close follow-up is assured. Patients with prepatellar bursitis who have systemic symptoms may require admission for intravenous antibiotics.[8]

Patients should rest the involved joint; however, shoulders should not be immobilized for more than a few days because of the risk of adhesive capsulitis. Patients with lateral epicondylitis often benefit from a forearm brace. A Jones-type of compression dressing, with an elastic bandage to prevent recurrent swelling, may be used in olecranon bursitis. De Quervain's tendinitis is immobilized by splinting the wrist and thumb in 20 degrees of dorsiflexion. For patients with Achilles tendinitis, a heel lift or splint in slight plantar flexion is recommended.

Absolute rest can be achieved only with casting, but this should be managed by the consulting orthopedist. The EP can place a splint if indicated.

Reduction of inflammation may be assisted by cold treatment (20 minutes at a time every several hours, for the first 24 to 48 hours), changing to heat treatment for the next several days. NSAIDs provide some pain relief in addition to reducing the inflammatory response. Graduated range-of motion exercises may be useful after immobilization. Tendinopathy and bursitis of the shoulder and rotator cuff tears in older patients are treated initially with gravity pendulum range-of-motion exercises followed by wall climbing with the hand as pain is lessened.

Steroids should not be injected into the Achilles or patellar tendons, which are at risk for spontaneous rupture if already weakened. Steroids should not be instilled in a bursa if there is any suspicion of infection. Complications of intrabursal injections are infection, local subcutaneous atrophy, bleeding, post-injection flare as a result of the release of microcrystals, and tendon rupture.

REFERENCES

1. National Institute for Occupational Safety and Health. Worker Health Chartbook. No. 2004;46:75-80.
2. Sharma P, Maffulli N: Tendon injury and tendinopathy: Healing and repair. J Bone Joint Surg. Am 2005;87: 187-202.
3. Nakama LH, King KB, Abrahamsson S, Rembel DM: Evidence of tendon microtears due to cyclical loading in an in vivo tendinopathy model. J Orthop Res 2005;2: 1199-1205.
4. Marsolais D, Cote CH, Frenette J: Nonsteroidal anti-inflammatory drug reduces neutrophil and macrophage accumulation but does not improve tendon regeneration. Lab Invest 2003;83:991-999.
5. Belzer JP, Durkiu RC: Common disorders of the shoulder. Prim Care 1996;23:365-388.
6. Neviaser RJ: Lesions of the biceps and tendonitis of the shoulder. Orthop Clin North Am 1980;11:343-348.
7. Chop WM: Tennis elbow. Postgrad Med J 1989;36: 307-308.
8. Mitchell M, Howard B, Haller J, et al: Septic arthritis. Radiol Clin North Am 1988;26:1295-1313.
9. Foley B, Christopher TA: Injection therapy of bursitis and tendinitis. In Roberts JR, Hedges JH (eds): Clinical Procedures in Emergency Medicine. Philadelphia, Saunders, 2004.
10. Dlabach JA: Nontraumatic soft tissue disorders. In Canale ST (ed): Campbell's Operative Orthopedics, 10th ed. Philadelphia, Mosby, 2003.
11. Gecha SR, Torg E: Knee injuries in tennis. Clin Sports Med 1988;7:435-452.
12. Safran MR, Fu FH: Uncommon causes of knee pain in the athlete. Orthop Clin North Am 1995;26:547-559.
13. Beachley MC, Franklin JW, Ostlund W, et al: Radiology of arthritis. Prim Care;1993;20:771-794.
14. Grassi W, Filippucci E, Fafina A, et al: Sonographic imaging of tendons. Arthritis Rheum 2000;43:969-976.

Chapter **82**

Injuries to the Shoulder Girdle

M. Scott Linscott

KEY POINTS

- Scapular fractures require high forces and are therefore associated with a high percentage of injuries to the ipsilateral chest wall and lung, resulting in rib fractures, pneumothorax, hemothorax, and pulmonary contusion.
- Posterior dislocation of the sternoclavicular joint may damage vital structures within the superior mediastinum and thorax.
- Most clavicle fractures should be treated with placement of an arm sling. Clavicle fractures requiring urgent open reduction with internal fixation include open fractures and severely displaced type II distal third clavicle fractures.
- The degree of acromioclavicular separation can be diagnosed based on an acromioclavicular-view radiograph taken in the sitting or standing position. Weight-bearing views are of no benefit.
- Axillary lateral shoulder radiographs should be obtained in all suspected glenohumeral dislocations to avoid missing a posterior dislocation.
- Axillary nerve function, both sensory and motor, should be tested in all glenohumeral dislocations.
- Most proximal humerus fractures, especially in older individuals, can be treated conservatively. However, all patients with such fractures should be referred for consultation with an orthopedic surgeon.
- Injuries to the radial nerve are not uncommon in mid-shaft humerus fractures and should always be considered; testing of wrist and finger extension can aid in the diagnosis. Radial nerve palsy following closed reduction of mid-shaft humerus fractures requires immediate surgical intervention.
- Supracondylar fractures in children, especially fractures with significant displacement, may be associated with injuries to the brachial artery and median and radial nerves. Supracondylar fractures in adults are less likely to cause such injuries.
- Rotator cuff tears are the final event in a long history of rotator cuff tendinitis and impingement of rotator cuff tendons.

Scope

This chapter reviews the anatomy of the shoulder girdle (scapula, clavicle, and humerus), followed by a discussion of common injuries and injuries that are potentially limb- and life-threatening. Emphasis is on diagnosis (history, physical examination, and imaging studies), management in the ED, and disposition after discharge.

Anatomy

The shoulder girdle connects the upper extremity to the thorax and axial skeleton. It consists of three bones (scapula, clavicle, and humerus), three joints (sternoclavicular, acromioclavicular, and glenohumeral), and one articulation (scapulothoracic). In addition to ligaments, the shoulder girdle is composed of other soft tissues including muscles, tendons, nerves, arteries, veins, and lymphatics. Injuries to the shoulder girdle include disarticulation (rare), fractures, ligament sprains, joint dislocations, musculotendinous strains, and contusions, as well as injuries to the nerves and vascular structures of the shoulder girdle and humerus.

The scapula and clavicle are attached to the axial skeleton by ligaments at the sternoclavicular joint and by muscles from the blade or body of the scapula to the thorax. The clavicle is attached to scapula by the coracoclavicular ligaments and the acromioclavicular ligaments. The coracoacromial ligament serves as the roof of the coracoacromial arch, beneath which the neurovascular bundle traverses.

Disarticulation of the Shoulder Girdle from the Thorax

This is a rare injury, requiring very high forces and usually seen with falls from a significant height, severe crush injuries, and high-speed motor vehicle crashes. This injury presents with lateral scapular displacement, clavicular disruption, and severe soft tissue injury, often including vascular disruption and avulsion of the brachial plexus. Diagnosis is made clinically and is confirmed by anteroposterior (AP) chest radiographs showing lateral displacement of the scapula. Disarticulation of the shoulder girdle often is associated with other more life-threatening injuries. Emergent orthopedic consultation is required in these cases.

Sternoclavicular Dislocation

■ PATHOPHYSIOLOGY

Anterior dislocations are the most common and usually result from a medial force applied to the shoulder or an indirect force applied to the rolled-back shoulder. *Posterior dislocations* are much less common, but potentially life-threatening because the dislocated medial head of the clavicle may cause a pneumothorax or injuries to the great vessels, esophagus, or trachea (all structures in the superior mediastinum). Posterior dislocations result either from a direct blow or from an indirect force applied to the rolled-forward shoulder.

■ PRESENTING SIGNS AND SYMPTOMS

The patient complains of severe pain in the affected sternoclavicular joint. In anterior dislocations, the protruding medial end of the clavicle is visible, easily palpable, and tender. In posterior dislocations, often there is a cavity where the medial end of the clavicle would normally lie, especially noticeable when compared with the uninjured side. In posterior dislocations, the patient may also have signs and symptoms of pneumothorax, vascular occlusion, and esophageal or tracheal injury.

■ DIAGNOSTIC TESTING

Routine radiographs may not be diagnostic, and computed tomography is usually required to make the diagnosis. This should always be performed with IV contrast media when a posterior sternoclavicular dislocation is suspected to rule out injuries to superior mediastinal vascular structures.

■ TREATMENT, PROCEDURES, COMPLICATIONS, AND DISPOSITION

■ Anterior Sternoclavicular Dislocations

Closed reduction is accomplished with the patient in the supine position and with rolled blankets placed between the shoulder blades. Significant downward pressure on the distal and proximal clavicle usually reduces the dislocation. The patient is discharged with a figure-of-eight clavicle splint with follow-up with an orthopedic surgeon within 1 week. These dislocations often recur when the splint is removed, and open reduction may be necessary.

■ Posterior Sternoclavicular Dislocations

Patients with posterior sternoclavicular dislocations require immediate orthopedic consultation; open reduction usually is necessary. Most reductions should be performed in the operating room with thoracic surgery backup, in case there is injury to superior mediastinal structures. Complications include pneumothorax and vascular, esophageal, and tracheal injuries.

Acromioclavicular Dislocation or Separation

■ PATHOPHYSIOLOGY

Acromioclavicular separations usually are caused by a fall onto the point of the shoulder or acromioclavicular joint with the arm adducted (thus the lay term "shoulder pointer" to describe this injury). It is caused less frequently by a fall onto the outstretched arm in extreme abduction, driving the acromion below the clavicle. Acromioclavicular separations are classified as six types, although only the first three types (I-III) are commonly seen. Types IV to VI are very uncommon and usually require surgical repair.

In type I acromioclavicular separations, the acromioclavicular ligaments are partially torn and the coracoclavicular ligaments are intact, resulting in less than 50% superior dislocation or separation of the clavicle from the acromium. In type II injuries, the acromioclavicular ligaments are completely torn and the coracoclavicular ligaments are stretched or partially torn, resulting in at least 50% superior dislocation or separation of the clavicle from the acromion. In type III injuries, both the acromioclavicular and coracolavicular ligaments are completely torn, resulting in complete superior dislocation or separation of the clavicle from the acromion.

■ PRESENTING SIGNS AND SYMPTOMS

The patient complains of severe pain in the acromioclavicular joint. In type I dislocations, there is tenderness and some swelling over the acromioclavicular joint, with little or no tenderness over the distal clavicle and coracoid process. In type II dislocations, there is tenderness and more swelling over the acromioclavicular joint and some tenderness over the coracoid process. In type III dislocations, the clavicle is obviously dislocated superiorly when the patient is sitting or standing, with less deformity when the patient is supine.

■ DIAGNOSTIC TESTING

Routine shoulder radiographs may miss a type II or type III separation if the radiograph if taken with the patient supine. Acromioclavicular views (a single radiograph that includes both acromioclavicular joints) should be taken in the sitting or standing position, with the arms unsupported. In type I injuries there will be less than 50% cephalad dislocation of the clavicle on the acromion of the affected shoulder. In type II injuries, there will be greater than 50% cephalad displacement of the clavicle on the acromion on the affected side. In type III dislocations, there will be complete dislocation on the sitting or standing film. Using weight-bearing films (the patient holding weights with the affected arm) is of no benefit, because the weight of the shoulder girdle and humerus alone is sufficient to maximize the deformity in the sitting or standing position.[1]

■ TREATMENT, PROCEDURES, COMPLICATIONS, AND DISPOSITION

Types I, II, and III acromioclavicular separations should be initially treated conservatively. In the ED, the patient should be given adequate analgesia and have ice applied to the area of injury. Following diagnosis, the patient should wear a sling or shoulder immobilizer, instructed to ice the injured area for 20 to 30 minutes out of each hour, and given adequate oral analgesia. Types I and II separations have an excellent prognosis, and follow up by the patient's the primary care physician is sufficient. Patients with type III separations should be referred for follow-up consultation with an orthopedic surgeon within 1 to 2 weeks. Most type III fractures should be treated conservatively. Although some orthopedic surgeons may perform an open reduction of these injuries in an athlete who uses the injured arm in overhead activities (e.g., baseball pitcher, football quarterback), recent evidence suggests that conservative therapy is preferable to open reduction even in these patients.[2,3] Types IV, V, and VI fractures are usually severe and patients with these injuries should be referred for consultation with an orthopedic surgeon, because most of these will require open reduction wih internal fixation.

Clavicle Fractures

■ PATHOPHYSIOLOGY

The most common mechanism of injury is a blow to the shoulder. Children will often have a bowing deforming or greenstick fracture, whereas in adults the fracture fragments are often significantly displaced. Clavicle fractures are divided into proximal third, middle third, and lateral third. Lateral third fractures are divided into type I, type II, and type III. Type II fractures are unstable because the coracoclavicular ligament has been disrupted.

■ PRESENTING SIGNS AND SYMPTOMS

Patients present with severe pain at the site of the fracture. They may support the adducted arm of the injured side with the other hand. There is usually an obvious deformity, and the fracture site is tender.

■ DIAGNOSTIC TESTING

The diagnosis is made by radiography of the injured clavicle. If a type II distal clavicle fracture is suspected, both supine and upright films will reveal the degree of instability of the fracture.

■ TREATMENT, PROCEDURES, COMPLICATIONS, AND DISPOSITION

Almost all fractures of the proximal third, middle third, and types I and III distal third heal with conservative treatment (a sling, or a sling and swath for the ipsilateral arm). Even markedly displaced fractures usually heal without surgical intervention. Some attempts at closed reduction may be appropriate if these fractures are markedly displaced or if there is significant skin tenting. Surgical intervention is indicated only if the fracture is open or in cases of a type II distal clavicle fracture. However, even type II distal clavicle fractures may do well with nonoperative therapy, although often there is non-union.[4]

For patients with middle and proximal third fractures, a figure-of-eight clavicle splint may decrease pain and, in an occasional patient, may help keep the fracture reduced. However, this is primarily for the patient's comfort and should not be employed if it increases the pain from the fracture, which it usually does.

The sling should be kept on for 2 to 3 weeks in children and 4 to 6 weeks in adults. Referral to an orthopedic surgeon is only necessary only for patients with severely displaced fractures (>20 mm of shortening), open fractures, fractures associated with neurovascular injury or skin tenting, and type II distal third clavicle fractures.

Complications are uncommon and consist of delayed union or non-union, osteoarthritis of the acromioclavicular joint (in type III distal third clavicle fractures), and malunion (primarily a cosmetic issue).

Scapular Fractures

■ PATHOPHYSIOLOGY

Scapular fractures usually are associated with high-energy forces and thus are often associated with significant life-threatening injuries, especially injuries to the ipsilateral ribs, pleura, and lungs. Most scapular fractures are caused by a direct blow, although fractures of the glenoid and the scapular neck may be from a fall on an outstretched arm.

■ PRESENTING SIGNS AND SYMPTOMS

The patient complains of pain at the site of the fracture. Any movement of the ipsilateral arm will exacerbate the pain, especially with fractures of the glenoid.

■ DIAGNOSTIC TESTING

Fractures of the scapular spine usually are clearly seen on plain films. However, fractures of the neck and the glenoid may not be seen and, if suspected, a computed tomography scan of the scapula should be obtained.

■ TREATMENT, PROCEDURES, COMPLICATIONS, AND DISPOSITION

Most scapular fractures are treated nonsurgically with sling, ice, analgesics, and range-of-motion exercises. Displaced fractures of the glenoid, neck, and coracoid and some acromial fractures may need open reduction with internal fixation; patients with such fractures should be referred for consultation with an orthopedic surgeon.

Glenohumeral Dislocations

■ PATHOPHYSIOLOGY

Dislocations of the glenohumeral joint are divided into anterior, posterior, and inferior (luxatio erecta). More than 95% of dislocations are anterior. Most glenohumeral dislocations are caused by indirect forces such as abduction, extension, and external rotation; however, occasionally they are caused by a direct blow to the proximal humerus.

■ PRESENTING SIGNS AND SYMPTOMS

Patients usually have severe pain in the glenohumeral joint and hold the affected arm in adduction and internal rotation. There is lack of the normal contour, with a depression where the humeral head would normally reside. Patients report extreme pain in the joint with any attempted movement of the arm.

■ DIAGNOSTIC TESTING

AP and axillary or transthoracic lateral radiograph views should be obtained in all patients with suspected dislocations. If displaced fractures of the glenoid or proximal humerus are suggested in plain radiographs, computed tomography scans of the shoulder should be obtained.

■ TREATMENT, PROCEDURES, COMPLICATIONS, AND DISPOSITION

■ Anterior Dislocations

Multiple techniques for closed reduction of glenohumeral dislocations have been recommended. The three main categories are scapular manipulation, traction, and leverage. The hippocratic method (foot in the axilla with traction on the extended arm) and the Kocher maneuver (traction, adduction, internal rotation) should not be employed because of the increased incidence of brachial plexus injuries with the hippocratic method and the increased incidence of proximal humerus fractures with the Kocher maneuver.

For almost all reduction techniques to be successful, adequate sedation/analgesia or anesthesia must be obtained. Conscious sedation with IV fentanyl (50-150 μg) and IV midazolam (1-5 mg) is adequate for most reductions. However, some patients require deep sedation with propofol or etomidate, and occasionally a patient may require general anesthesia to accomplish the reduction. Several commonly used methods used to reduce anterior glenohumeral dislocations are described here.

Scapular Manipulation[5,6]

Ideally, the patient is in the prone position with the dislocated arm hanging over the edge of the stretcher. Traction is applied to the arm, and the operator pushes the tip of the scapula medially while stabilizing the upper scapula. If the patient insists on sitting up, this same technique can be combined with the modified hippocratic method in which one operator applies countertraction superiorly with a sheet-sling in the axilla, another operator puts traction on the arm, and a third operator manipulates the scapula. This is the technique of choice for the author. It requires relatively little sedation/analgesia and is successful in over 90% of cases.

External Rotation[7]

With the patient supine, the affected arm is adducted close to the thorax. The elbow is flexed to 90 degrees and the operator very slowly externally rotates the arm without applying longitudinal traction. This method is safe, easily learned, and relatively atraumatic for the patient.

Snowbird Technique[8]

The patient sits in a chair and supports the affected arm (in 90 degrees of flexion) with the uninjured arm. The operator ties a 3- to 4-foot loop of 4- to 6-inch stockinet around the proximal forearm of the affected arm. The operator places one foot in the other end of the loop and pushes downward. The operator's hands can be used to manipulate the scapula as described previously or to manipulate the humeral head to effect reduction.

Milch Technique[9]

With the patient supine, the operator slowly abducts and externally rotates the arm until the arm is superior to the patient. With the elbow fully extended, traction is applied. Another operator may put pressure on the humeral head superiorly to assist in reduction.

Modified Hippocratic (Traction-Countertraction) Method

With the patient supine, the elbow is abducted slightly and flexed to 90 degrees. The operator ties a sheet around his waist and to the patient's proximal forearm. An assistant slings another sheet around the thorax and under the affected armpit and ties it around the his owns waist. The operator and the assistant pull in opposite directions with their arms and bodies.

Stimson Method

With the patient prone, the affected arm is dangled over the edge of the stretcher and a 10-20 lb. weight is attached to the wrist, producing constant, gentle traction. This method is one of the oldest and has the advantages of not requiring the physician to be present for the reduction and is probably the least traumatic for the patient. The disadvantage is that it often takes 20 or more minutes to affect the reduction and it ties up a nurse for this period of time if the patient has been consciously sedated.

Posterior Dislocations

The most common technique for reduction of posterior dislocation is to apply axial traction in line with the humerus, with an assistant applying countertraction with a sheet slung under the axilla of the affected arm. Gentle pressure is applied by the operator, who also applies slow external rotation to the affected humerus.

Luxatio Erecta (Inferior Dislocations)

An orthopedic consultation should be obtained prior to reduction. The traction-countertraction method is the most effective in reducing this dislocation, although deep sedation or general anesthesia may be required.

DISPOSITION

Although there is debate regarding the ordering of postreduction radiographs, many physicians order them for medicolegal reasons. In uncomplicated cases, following reduction the shoulder should be immobilized with a sling or a sling and swath for 3 to 4 weeks in patients older than 40 years and for 1 to 2 weeks in patients younger than 40 years. The patient should be instructed to avoid significant abduction of the shoulder or overhead activities when the sling is removed for bathing. To prevent adhesive capsulitis, circumduction range-of-motion exercises should be performed at least daily, especially by older patients.

Proximal Humerus Fractures

PATHOPHYSIOLOGY

The two mechanisms that most commonly cause fractures of the proximal humerus are (1) a direct blow to the lateral aspect of the upper arm and (2) indirect forces generated by a fall on an outstretched arm. The position of the humeral shaft in relation to the proximal fragments depends on whether the fall is on the abducted or the adducted arm.

The Neer fracture classification is most commonly used and is based on the position of the articular segment, the greater and lesser tuberosities, and the humeral shaft.[10] According to Neer's classification, a fracture is considered displaced if any major segment is displaced 1 cm or more or is angulated greater than 45 degrees. Fractures are classified as one-part, two-part, three-part, or four-part fractures and are usually differentiated along the classic epiphyseal lines (anatomic neck, surgical neck, greater tuberosity, and lesser tuberosity).

■ PRESENTING SIGNS AND SYMPTOMS

The patient presents with severe pain in the proximal humerus. There may be an obvious deformity, and there is extreme tenderness over the proximal humerus.

■ DIAGNOSTIC TESTING

The trauma radiographic series recommended by Neer, as well as an AP internal rotation view and an axillary lateral view, provide the most complete diagnostic information. A computed tomography scan of the shoulder nay be necessary to better define the extent of injury.

■ TREATMENT, PROCEDURES, COMPLICATIONS, AND DISPOSITION

If the fractures are not displaced (<1 cm of displacement), wearing a sling or a sling and swath may be all the treatment that is required. If significant displacement remains after closed reduction, open reduction with internal fixation will be necessary. Orthopedic consultation should be obtained in almost all of cases.

Successful treatment is most dependent on early mobility. Prolonged immobilization without range-of-motion exercises often results in adhesive capsulitis or marked reduction in mobility of the glenohumeral joint. Patients should be encouraged to perform circumduction range-of-motion exercises after a few days of immobilization, especially elderly patients.

Humerus Shaft Fractures

■ PATHOPHYSIOLOGY

Humerus shaft fractures almost always result from a direct blow to the bone. This usually results in a transverse fracture. Occasionally, a fall onto an outstretched hand or severe twisting forces from supination or pronation or twisting of the entire arm may result in spiral fractures.

■ PRESENTING SIGNS AND SYMPTOMS

Symptoms include pain and deformity at the fracture site. Also, the fracture is usually very unstable. If the radial nerve is injured, the patient will not be able to extend the wrist or fingers.

■ DIAGNOSTIC TESTING

Diagnosis is based on radiographs of the humerus. As in all long bone fractures, the joint above and below the fracture—in this case the shoulder and elbow—should also be radiographed.

■ TREATMENT, PROCEDURES, COMPLICATIONS, AND DISPOSITION

Most humerual shaft fractures can be treated conservatively. If the fracture fragments are minimally displaced, no reduction is necessary. If the fragments are widely separated, reduction may be carried out before splinting.

If the fracture fragments are in reasonable apposition (within 1 to 2 inches) following the reduction, the most commonly employed splinting technique is the coaptation or "sugar tong" splint, whereby a 5-inch plaster or Orthoglass splint is applied over the shoulder, down the lateral side of the upper arm, around the elbow and up the medial side of the upper arm near the axilla. The arm is then placed in a sling, with the sling around the wrist, so that the weight of the splint will bring the fracture fragments together.

If the fracture fragments are separated more than 2 inches after reduction or if there is a spiral fracture, the hanging cast technique may be employed. A lightweight cast is applied 1 to 2 inches proximal to the fracture site up to the palmar crease of the hand. The elbow is flexed at 90 degrees and a loop is placed at the wrist either on the dorsal side to reduce lateral angulation or on the volar side to reduce medial angulation. The hanging cast has the disadvantage of needing gravity for traction; therefore the patient must remain upright at all times, even during sleep. Many patients cannot tolerate this.[11]

The most common and most feared complication of humeral shaft fractures is radial nerve injury. If the nerve function is lost prior to reduction, most authorities treat it expectantly; most of the time nerve function returns because the nerve has been either contused or stretched. After reduction, function of the radial nerve should again be tested. If radial nerve function is compromised but was normal prior to reduction, most authorities recommend open reduction with internal fixation, because the probability is high that the radial nerve is entrapped within the fracture.

All patients with humeral shaft fractures should be referred for consultation with an orthopedic surgeon, preferable within 2 to 3 days.

Distal Humerus (Supracondylar) Fractures

■ PATHOPHYSIOLOGY

Supracondylar fractures are classified as either flexion or extension fractures and occur almost exclusively in children, usually between the ages of 4 to 10 years. More than 95% of these fractures are the extension type and occur when the child falls on the outstretched arm with the elbow in full extension or hyperextension. In the flexion type fracture, the child falls onto the arm with the elbow flexed.

■ PRESENTING SIGNS AND SYMPTOMS

The patient usually presents holding the injured arm in extension with the unaffected hand. There is swelling as well as tenderness to palpation over the distal humerus. There may be an S-shaped deformity if there is significant displacement of the fracture fragments. The patient resists any attempt to flex or extend the elbow.

■ DIAGNOSTIC TESTING

Elbow radiographs (AP and lateral views) should be obtained. The fracture often will be visible only on the lateral view unless there is significant displacement of the fracture fragments. The anterior humeral line should pass through the capitellum. If the capitellum is posterior to the anterior humeral line, this is diagnostic of a subtle supracondylar fracture in a child. Based on radiographic findings, extension fractures are often classified into three types: type I has minimal or no displacement; type II is a displaced fracture with the posterior cortex intact; and type III is a completely displaced fracture, with both the anterior and posterior cortices disrupted.[12]

■ TREATMENT, PROCEDURES, COMPLICATIONS, AND DISPOSITION

Type I supracondylar fractures are treated with a long arm splint with the elbow flexed to 90 degrees. The arm is placed in a sling. Protected active range-of-motion exercises are begun in 3 to 4 weeks.

Type II fractures require reduction even though they're minimally displaced. Following reduction, the long arm splint is applied with the elbow flexed to 100 to 120 degrees. Flexion greater than 90 degrees places tension on the intact posterior periosteum to maintain the reduction. This degree of hyperextension may compromise the neurovascular structures volar to the elbow; thus careful attention should be paid to assure that this complication does not arise, especially in the first 2 to 3 days after the fracture. Orthopedic consultation should be obtained in all cases.

Type III injuries are problematic because they may increase the chance of varus deformity, and they are more likely to cause injury to the neurovascular structures passing through the elbow. Rarely should an attempt be made to reduce these fractures in the ED. The only exception might be the unavailability of immediate orthopedic consultation in a patient who has an obviously occluded brachial artery. The vast majority of these patients should be taken to the operating room immediately and undergo either closed or open reduction. Orthopedic consultation is mandatory in all cases.

The most common complication is the loss of the normal carrying angle, resulting in a cubitus varus deformity. This complication has decreased in incidence as the practice of percutaneous pinning of the fracture has evolved. More serious complications of supracondylar fractures include brachial artery injury and injuries to the radial, median, and ulnar nerves. Most often these are due to contusion or stretching of the nerves, and full recovery is the rule.

Rotator Cuff Tendinitis and Tears and Impingement Syndromes (Subacromial Bursitis)

■ PATHOPHYSIOLOGY

These three disorders have much in common; rotator cuff tears are the end-result of rotator cuff tendinitis and subacromial bursitis. Most rotator cuff tears occur in patients over the age of 40 and result from long-term degeneration and entrapment of the rotator cuff tendons as they pass between the humeral head and the acromion (impingement syndrome). The injury occurs when there is a sudden, powerful elevation of the arm (as in grabbing a tree limb during a fall). Occasionally the injury occurs in weight lifters and in patients who fall onto the shoulder.

In younger patients, these injuries often result in avulsion of bone because their tendons are normal. 30% or more of the tendon must be ruptured to cause a decrease in strength of abduction.

Rotator cuff tendinitis and subacromial bursitis are due to impingement of the tendon between the acromion, the coracoacromial arch, and the humerus. This syndrome occurs more commonly in women between the ages of 35 and 50 years.

■ PRESENTING SIGNS AND SYMPTOMS

The patient complains of pain over the proximal humerus, where the rotator cuff tendons attach to the greater tuberosity. There is significant pain with both active and passive abduction of the shoulder. In other impingement syndromes (supraspinatous tendinitis and subacromial bursitis), the symptoms are similar, with less tenderness over the rotator cuff and greater tenderness proximally.

■ DIAGNOSTIC TESTING

The drop arm test is positive if there has been a significant rotator cuff tear. The patient extends the injured arm at 90 degrees and the operator lightly taps the wrist or forearm. In a positive test, the patient suddenly drops the arm. Also, the patient cannot slowly lower the arm from the abducted position—rather, it drops suddenly to the side. In patients with rotator cuff tendinitis or subacromial bursitis, there is significant pain with abduction, but the drop arm test is negative.

■ TREATMENT, PROCEDURES, COMPLICATIONS, AND DISPOSITION

Treatment depends on the degree of disability (incomplete versus complete tear), the patient's age, and the patient's activity level. In young, active patients with significant tears, arthroscopic repair is indicated. In older patients with a sedentary lifestyle, repairs should rarely be attempted because the outcome is often worse than that with conservative therapy. For evaluation, patients should be referred for consultation with an orthopedist who specializes in shoulder injuries.

Conservative therapy of rotator cuff tears consists of improving the patient's ability to abduct the arm. Having the patient "crawl up the wall" with the affected hand until the pain is unbearable and repeat this exercise daily is beneficial. Also, subacromial injections of a local anesthetic and steroid mixture reduces pain and allows greater range of motion. This should probably be limited to 2 or 3 times a year because of the tendency for steroids to cause tendon rupture. Treatment of subacromial bursitis/supraspinatus tendinitis is similar to that for conservative therapy of rotator cuff tears, with initial treatment consisting of ice and nonsteroidal antiinflammatory drugs (NSAIDs) with subacromial steroid/local anesthetic injections in refractory cases.

Tenosynovitis and Rupture of the Long Head of the Biceps Tendon

■ PATHOPHYSIOLOGY

The long head of the biceps tendon inserts into the glenoid rim and traverses the bicipital groove between the greater and lesser tuberosities. The tendon is irritated by multiple shoulder movements and becomes inflamed. Eventually the tendon becomes weakened and ruptures.

■ PRESENTING SIGNS AND SYMPTOMS

Pain in the anterior shoulder may radiate to the elbow. The pain is made worse with abduction and external rotation. There is tenderness over the biceps tendon in the bicipital groove.

■ DIAGNOSTIC TESTING

Yergason's test is a reliable method for confirming the diagnosis of tenosynovitis of the long head of the biceps tendon. The patient's elbow is flexed to 90 degrees and the patient tries to supinate the forearm against resistance. If this causes increased pain in the bicipital groove, the test is positive.

■ TREATMENT, PROCEDURES, COMPLICATIONS, AND DISPOSITION

Conservative treatment consists of a sling and NSAIDs. If after a week of immobilization the patient continues to have pain, the bicipital canal can be injected with a combined local anesthetic and steroid. Range-of-motion daily exercises should be performed to prevent adhesive tenosynovitis.

Adhesive Capsulitis

■ PATHOPHYSIOLOGY

Adhesive capsulitis is caused by inflammation within the glenohumeral joint capsule. This leads to formation of adhesions within the joint capsule with marked limitation of range of motion of the shoulder. The exact mechanism is unclear; however, this disease usually results from prolonged immobilization of the shoulder joint, particularly when associated with inflammation, such as in rotator cuff tendinitis and subacromial bursitis.

■ PRESENTING SIGNS AND SYMPTOMS

In most cases, the nondominant arm is affected and the patient has pain with minimal activity. The pain is usually worse at night. There is tenderness in the subacromial area and marked limitation of glenohumeral range of motion in all ranges, especially abduction and rotation.

■ DIAGNOSTIC TESTING

The diagnosis is primarily made on the basis of symptoms and signs described previously. Radiographs typically are normal. Arthroscopy or arthrography may be diagnostic, but these modalities are invasive and should be avoided if possible.

■ TREATMENT, PROCEDURES, COMPLICATIONS, AND DISPOSITION

The most important form of therapy should be directed at prevention of this problem. All patients with shoulder injuries or inflammation should be encouraged to perform daily circumduction range-of-motion exercises to prevent adhesive capsulitis. Conservative treatment consists of a gentle exercise program, NSAIDs, and corticosteroid injections. This results in significant improvement in many patients; however, many patients require breaking up of adhesions by putting the shoulder through full range of motion under general anesthesia.

REFERENCES

1. Yap JJ, Curl LA, Kvitne RS, McFarland EG: The value of weighted views of the acromioclavicular joint. Results of a survey. Am J Sports Med 1999;27:806-809.
2. Schlegel TF, Burks RT, Marcus RL, Dunne HK: A prospective evaluation of untreated acute grade III acromioclavicular separations. Am J Sports Med 2001;29:699-703.
3. Press J, Zuckerman JD, Gallagher M, Cuomo F: Treatment of grade III acromioclavicular separations. Operative versus nonoperative management. Bull Hosp Jt Dis 1997;56: 77-83.
4. Deafenbaugh MK, Dugdale TW, Staeheli JW, Nielsen R: Nonoperative treatment of Neer type II distal clavicle fractures: A prospective study. Contemp Orthop 1990;20: 405-413.
5. Kothari RU, Dronen SC: The scapular manipulation technique for the reduction of acute anterior shoulder dislocations. J Emerg Med 1990;8:625-628.

Chapter 83

Forearm Fractures

Trevor J. Mills

KEY POINTS

The goal of Colles' fracture reduction is to restore radial length and correct dorsal angulation, ideally to achieve a normal volar tilt.

A forearm fracture of the ulna may have an associated radial head dislocation (Montaggia fracture); therefore radiographs of joints proximal and distal to the fracture may be required.

Open fractures require early antibiotic therapy and surgical intervention.

Consultation with an orthopedist may be included in ED follow-up or when preparing the patient for surgery.

Scope

Injury is a leading cause of mortality, morbidity, and lost days of work. Traumatic injuries result in over 34 million ED visits each year.[1] The highest rate of injuries occur in persons between the ages of 15 and 24 years old. The annual health care cost of injures is over 9.2 billion dollars. Loss or reduction of function as a result of forearm fractures spans a spectrum of transient annoyance to permanent disability.

Early identification of vascular injury, neurologic compromise, open fractures, and associated dislocations can greatly reduce the complications associated with forearm fractures.

Anatomy

The bones of the forearm are composed of the radius and ulna. These two bones lie in parallel and can be thought of as two cones lying in opposite directions.[2] The bones are connected by joint capsules at the elbow and the wrist, and the shafts are interlocked by a fibrous interosseus membrane. Because of the multiple muscle attachments of the forearm, fractures are often further displaced by muscle contraction.

Pathophysiology

In general, fractures are the result of an external force that exceeds the intrinsic strength of the bone. Most forearm fractures are caused by a sudden force, such as a fall on the outstretched arm. Fractures, and especially forearm fractures, also may occur through smaller repetitive injuries, resulting in a "stress" fracture over time. Any pathophysiologic process that reduces the integrity of the bone, such as osteopenia, osteomyolitis, and bone metastasis, increases the likelihood of fracture, even with "normal" external stress.

External forces that are specific to forearm fractures include direct blows to the forearm, longitudinal compression loads, bending forces, excessive pronation, supination at the wrist, and hyperextension or hyperflexion of the wrist or elbow.

Forearm shaft fractures often undergo a second trauma as the muscles of the forearm contract, leading to further displacement of fractured bone and concurrent dislocation.

Clinical Presentation

Potential symptoms of forearm fractures include pain, forearm edema, forearm ecchymosis, abnormal or reduced mobility from the wrist through the elbow, and complaints of neurovascular compromise. Physical examination findings can include obvious bony deformity, shortening of the forearm, crepitus, tenderness to palpation of the forearm, joint effusions, abnormal mobility of the wrist/forearm/elbow, and neurologic and vascular deficits of the forearm/wrist/hand. Box 83-1 lists signs and symptoms of fractures and complications that indicate serious injury.

In general, forearm fractures are classified by the bone (or bones) involved, anatomic location and alignment of the fracture, and by the presence of angulaton, rotation, comminution, and concurrent dislocations. All fractures should be further described as "open" or "closed," and the presence (or absence) of distal neurologic and vascular function should be noted (Fig. 83-1).

Types of forearm fractures that are frequently mentioned in the medical literature are described in Table 83-1.

Pediatric Fractures

Forearm fractures in the pediatric population include several additional entities, because children have a plastic bone matrix and active growth plates, both of which contribute to unique fractures (Table 83-2). In children, when an external force bends a long bone,

BOX 83-1

Signs and Symptoms of Fractures and Complications That Suggest Serious Injury

Open Fracture
- Open wounds in proximity to fracture, bone fragments protruding from skin
- Skin tenting may indicated high potential for progression to open fracture

Fracture/Dislocation
- In patients with intraarticular fractures and displaced fractures, additional radiographs above and below the injury may reveal concurrent dislocations
- The physical examination should include the joint above and below fracture site

Vascular Compromise
- Loss or reduction of pulse distal to injury
- Reduced capillary refill
- Skin pallor; patient complaints of "cold" extremity or pain out of proportion to injury

Neurologic Compromise
- Loss of strength, sensation, reflexes, two-point discrimination distal to injury
- Complaints of paresthesias or pain distal to injury

Compartment Syndrome
- Tense forearm
- Neurologic or vascular compromise distal to injury

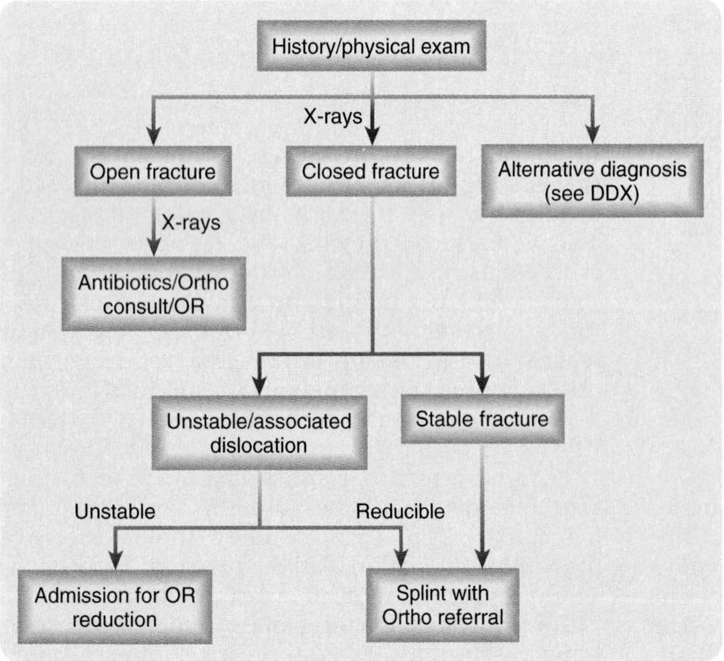
History/physical exam
X-rays
Open fracture
Closed fracture
Alternative diagnosis (see DDX)
X-rays
Antibiotics/Ortho consult/OR
Unstable/associated dislocation
Stable fracture
Unstable
Reducible
Admission for OR reduction
Splint with Ortho referral

FIGURE 83-1 Approach to the patient with a suspected forearm fracture. DDX, differential diagnosis; OR, operating room; Ortho, orthopedics.

Table 83-1 TYPES OF FOREARM FRACTURES

Name	Description
Colles'	Distal radial "extension" fracture (may also include ulna), with dorsal displacement of distal fragment(s)
Smith's	Distal radial "flexion" fracture with volar displacement of distal fragment(s)
Barton's	Intra-articular fracture of the dorsal rim of the distal radius, often associated with carpal dislocation
Hutchinson's	Radial styloid fracture, associated with carpal dislocation
Galeazzi	Distal radial shaft fracture, with concurrent distal radioulnar dislocation
Monteggia	Ular shaft fracture with radial head dislocation

Table 83-2 TYPES OF PEDIATRIC FRACTURES

Name	Description
Torus	Fracture involves compression "buckling" of one or both sides of cortex
Greenstick	Fracture involves distraction of one side of cortex without apparent disruption of the other
Plastic deformity	Bowing of the radius or ulna without obvious fracture lines (multiple microfractures)
Salter-Harris	Fracture involving the growth plates

one side of the cortex may be disrupted while the other side remains intact (greenstick fracture). Alternatively, a deformity of the bone may occur without obvious fracture line (plastic deformity). With compression, buckling of the cortex may be seen (torus fracture). Depending on the age of the child, fractures through the various growth plates of the elbow and wrist also may occur (Salter-Harris fractures).[4]

Differential Diagnosis

The differential diagnosis for forearm fractures includes any soft tissue injury to the forearm, as well as acute skin, soft tissue, and joint infections (Box 83-2). Some clinical aspects of acute arterial occlusion, as well as venous thrombosis, may mimic forearm fractures. Any acute neurologic change, including paresthesias, weakness, and functional loss, should be considered along with forearm fractures. Two normal variants sometimes mistaken for forearm fractures are normal growth plates in children and nutrient vessels.

RED FLAGS

- Open fractures
- Concurrent vascular compromise
- Neurologic deficits
- Symptoms of compartment syndrome
- Concurrent dislocations
- Intra-articular fractures
- Unstable fractures

BOX 83-2

Differerential Diagnosis of Forearm Fractures

Traumatic
- Wrist sprain, elbow sprain
- Ligamentous injuries, forearm contusions, hematomas
- Dislocations of the elbow or wrist (including nursemaid's elbow)

Infectious
- Cellulitis of the forearm, abscesses
- Necrotizing fasciitis

Vascular
- Acute arterial occlusion
- Venous thrombosis

Neurologic
- Neuropraxias, carpal tunnel syndrome
- Systemic neurologic syndromes involving the nerves of the upper extremities

Arthritis
- Septic joint, gonococcal arthritis, rheumatoid arthritis, osteoarthritis
- Pseudogout, gout
- Systemic lupus erythematosus, rheumatic fever, viral syndrome
- Reiter's syndrome, Lyme disease, serum sickness

Other
- Olecranon bursitis, soft tissue masses
- Normal growth plates, nutrient vessels

Diagnostic Testing

The orthopedic literature often recommends radiographs of a suspected fracture and additional films of the joint above and below the injury (Table 83-3; Fig. 83-2). This is true of forearm fractures if they are close to the joint (either elbow or wrist) or have a suspected concurrent dislocation (Fig. 83-3). Additional films usually not necessary in uncomplicated shaft fractures (one bone, nondisplaced). If the fracture is

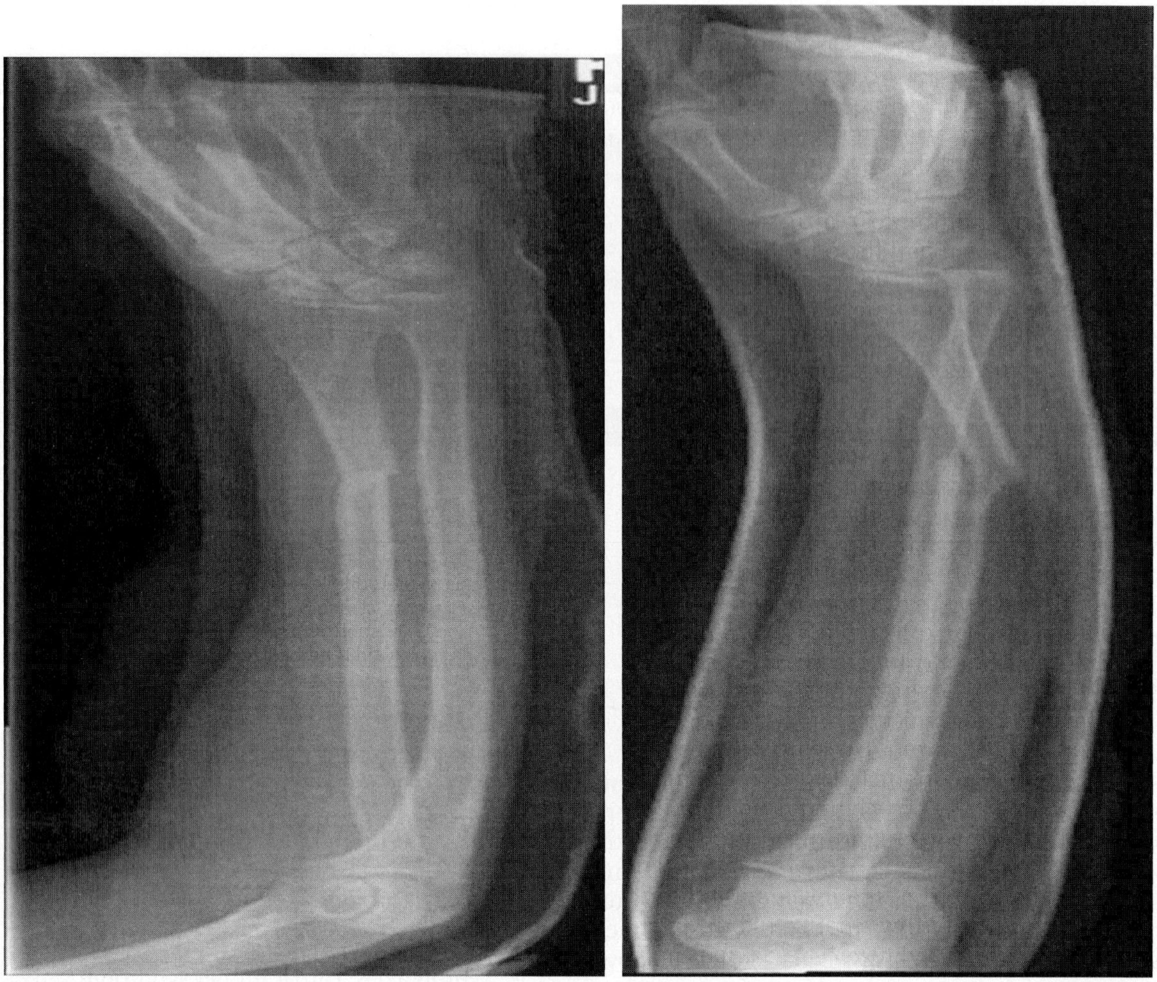

A B

FIGURE 83-2 These radiographs demonstrate the need for at least two views of a fracture. In **A** (anteroposterior view), there appears to be good alignment; in **B** (lateral view), a large amount of displacement is obvious.

PRIORITY ACTIONS

- *History:* Elucidate mechanisms with high potential for open fractures.
- *Physical examination:* Check joints above and below injury; examine skin for open wounds; evaluate and re-evaluate neurovascular status distal to injury.
- *Radiography:* Always look for a second fracture or associated dislocation.
- *Treatment:* Antibiotic therapy for patients with open fractures; early reduction of dislocations and displaced fractures

intra-articular, additional radiographic views or computed tomography or magnetic resonance imaging may be required (Table 83-4).

Although most forearm fractures are evident on plain radiographs, occult fractures of the elbow may be difficult to interpret. One indication of an elbow fracture is the "fat pad" or "sail" sign, indicating a hemarthrosis of the elbow joint and thus a fracture.[3]

Table 83-3 RADIOGRAPHS USEFUL IN DIFFERENTIAL DIAGNOSIS OF FOREARM FRACTURES

Suspected Injury	Views
Proximal forearm fracture	Elbow series (AP and lateral) and forearm servies (AP and lateral forearm)
Shaft fracture	Forearm series
Distal forearm fracture	Wrist series (AP and lateral wrist) and forearm series.

AP, anteroposterior.

Treatment (Intervention and Procedures)

The mainstays of treatment include pain control, reduction of further injury, immobilization, and appropriate disposition.[5] Pain control should include

Chapter **84**

Hand and Wrist Injuries

John C. Southall

KEY POINTS

Tendon, nerve, and bone injuries can sometimes be predicted based on the mechanism of injury.
Anesthesia via radial, ulnar, and median nerve field blocks is easily learned and is often more appropriate than local anesthesia.
Irrigation is the EP's greatest ally in preventing wound infections.
When exploring open hand wounds, the EP should re-create the position of injury when possible.
The final step in the management of almost all hand and wrist injuries is splinting.
All but the most minor hand and wrist injuries merit scheduled follow-up.

Scope

The hand is complicated and injury-prone. The goal of the EP with regard to hand injuries should be to correctly identify the injury via a careful history, a systematic and practiced physical examination, and appropriate radiography. Treatment should then be focused on a return to function, with a bias toward empirical management. Although a significant subset of patients require emergent evaluation by a hand surgeon, the majority can be treated or stabilized in the acute care setting with referral to the surgeon for outpatient follow-up.

Annually, more than 16 million people suffer some form of hand injury, and more than 4.8 million will present to the ED for treatment of these injuries.[1] Traumatic injuries may include lacerations, fractures, and tendon or ligamentous injuries. Fortunately, most injuries are easily identified in the ED by the history, physical examination, and plain film radiography.[2] Because the morbidity from misdiagnosed or mistreated hand injuries can be high, the EP needs to be vigilant when evaluating these injuries.

History

As in all areas of medicine, a careful history is important regarding a chief complaint of injury. Specific questions should focus on the mechanism of the injury, hand position at the time of injury, the direction of the force causing the injury, time elapsed since the injury, and environmental (contamination) considerations. Some mechanisms yield classic injury patterns, such as the "jersey" finger and "mallet" finger, and should increase the EP's index of suspicion. Other injury patterns are known for their poor outcomes, such as "fight bite" or high-pressure injection injuries, and require specific managements. Some wounds are more prone to infection, such as crush injuries and grossly contaminated wounds.

The patient's hand dominance and career should also be ascertained and documented, as well as factors that may compromise healing, such as smoking, drug use, or an immunocompromised state.[2] Although not relevant to the diagnosis of acute injury, the answers to these questions will impact follow-up by affecting the risk/benefit ratios that hand surgeons will use in their discussions with the patient. Also, tetanus immunization status should be ascertained.

Related Anatomy

This chapter assumes that the reader is familiar with the basic bony structures of the hand. The back of the hand is referred to as the dorsal surface; the palm is called either the palmar or volar surface. The lateral borders of the hand are referred to as radial or ulnar. Movement may be in any of these planes. Additionally, fingers may abduct away from, or adduct toward, an imaginary plane bisecting the third finger. The thumb has further planes of movement. These and specific ligaments and tendons of importance are discussed individually.

Physical Examination

Despite its complicated nature, the hand can be adequately examined in a short period of time. Memorizing a rapid, routine hand examination and performing it systematically and regularly will decrease the chances of missing subtle injuries. Box 84-1 lists one technique for performing a rapid but thorough examination.

Assuming that there is no active bleeding requiring immediate attention, the examination of the hand begins with observation. All rings, watches, and other potentially constricting devices should be removed immediately regardless of their proximity to the injury, because soft tissue swelling and edema may spread to uninjured digits.[3] Laceration and other disruptions of the skin integrity usually is easily recognized, but any erythema, soft tissue swelling or ecchymoses should also be noted. It is important to compare the general position of the hand to that of the unaffected side, becauser many fractures or tendon disruptions will alter the outward appearance of the hand. For example, a hand held in flexion may indicate disruption of an extensor tendon, whereas bruising or discoloration at a joint may indicate closed tendon or joint capsule injury.

Vascular integrity can quickly be determined by feeling for ulnar and radial pulses and by documenting intact and symmetric distal capillary refill. Normal capillary refill is less than 2 seconds in a normotensive adult.

Neurologic testing should be performed prior to anesthesia. Radial, median, and ulnar nerves should be individually assessed, and digital nerves interrogated both via light touch and "two-point" testing. Two-point discrimination of 3 to 5 mm is considered normal. Comparison with the unaffected side can be useful, especially in patients with calluses on the hands. Denervated skin will not wrinkle when immersed in water for ten minutes, a fact which can be useful when examining an infant for potential injury.[3]

BOX 84-1

"Two-Minute" Hand Examination

General

- General apperarance
- Obvious deformity

Vascular

- Ulnar, radial pulses
- Capillary refill <2 seconds
- Hemorrhage control

Neurologic

- Ulnar
  - Sensation: light touch distal, volar 5th digit
  - Motor: interosseous—abduction 2nd digit
- Median
  - Sensation: light touch distal, volar 2nd digit
  - Motor: thenar eminence—adduction 1st digit
- Radial
  - Sensation: light touch to dorsal webspace between 2nd and 3rd digit
  - Motor: wrist extension, otherwise sensation only in hand
- Two-point discrimination—2 to 5 mm at finger tip, 7 to 12 mm at palm; measurable difference between digits

Musculoskeletal

- Bony palpation of all digits and joints
- Active range of motion: make fist, fully extend all digits
- Passive range of motion: passively take all digits/joints through all ranges
- Resistance: test all joints, all ranges with resistance to diagnose partial ligament injuries

Ligamentous

- Flexor digitorum profundus tendon—hold proximal interphalangeal joint in extension, flex distal interphalangeal joint against resistance
- Flexor digitorum sublimus tendon—hold metacarpophalangeal joint in extension, flex proximal interphalangeal joint against resistance
- Extensor tendons—place hand palm down, extend digit with resistance at nail bed
- Ulnar collateral—adduct thumb against resistance

To evaluate for radial neuropathy, the dorsal aspect of the second and third webspace are tested for decreased sensation. Proximal limb radial nerve lesions will cause wrist drop. However, the superficial radial nerve, as it courses through the hand, is sensory only.

To test for median neuropathy at the distal, palmar surface of the second digit is assessed for decreased sensation. Placing the hand dorsal side down and abducting the fifth digit toward the ceiling tests motor function. Resistance is applied to the thenar eminence, followed by palpation, to test for contraction of the abductor pollicis brevis muscle.

To test for ulnar neuropathy, distal, palmar surface of the fifth digit is assessed for decreased sensation. Challenging the interosseous muscles best tests ulnar motor function. One method is to ask the patient to place the injured hand on a surface with the fifth digit down and the thumb pointing at the ceiling. The patient then abducts the second finger (spreads the fingers) against resistance; weakness of the first interosseous muscle verifies contraction.

Bone structures should be thoroughly palpated, as should all joints, when looking for signs of pain, laxity, and limited range of motion. Even when a specific injury may be obvious, it is important to examine the entire hand to avoid misdiagnosis of less obvious injuries.

Anesthesia

Multiple techniques exist for anesthetizing the hand and digits; all of which are useful in specific situations. Proper technique is important to limit pain and infection and to ensure proper anesthesia.

Local infiltration is best used for small superficial, nondigital lacerations. Infiltration of anesthetic can be uncomfortable for the patient; however, when anesthesia is done properly, discomfort can be minimal. Pre-mixing one part sodium bicarbonate and nine parts lidocaine decreases the acidity of the solution and lessens initial pain without affecting anesthetic effects.

■ DIGITAL BLOCKS

Digital blocks are preferential for digital lacerations and provide faster anesthesia without disrupting local anatomy. Although digital blocks are safe and effective, contraindications include severe peripheral vascular disease and vasospastic disease (e.g., Raynaud's).[4] Common practice is to use a local anesthetic that does not contain epinephrine. However, a dilute (1:100,000) epinephrine-containing anesthetic may aid repair by decreasing bleeding and prolonging the efficacy of the anesthetic. Historical concerns that utilizing lidocaine with epinephrine for digital blocks will cause necrosis of the digits have been shown to be unfounded.[5] Proper technique is as follows:

1. Inject buffered lidocaine with epinephrine (1:100,000) in small amounts. No more than 2 to 3 mL should be deposited in each digit.
2. Do not inject in a circumferential fashion. This will lead to increased dosage and possible tourniquet effect.
3. Use a small needle (27 gauge) for injection.
4. Avoid the use of postanesthetic hot soaks, excessively tight bandages, and tourniquets when not needed.
5. Inject at the dorsal aspect of the digit; raise a small subcutaneous wheal of anesthetic. Insert the needle, aspirate, and inject 1 mL of anesthetic. Shift the needle to the other side, and repeat. Effect may be seen within 1 to 2 minutes; however, maximum effect will not be seen until after 10 minutes has elapsed.

■ FIELD BLOCKS

Field blocks are a useful technique when treating large or numerous lacerations and are underutilized in many EDs. For example, large palmar lacerations may be best served by field blocks of the ulnar and median nerves.

Perhaps one reason that this technique is underutilized is its perceived failure rate. As practitioners, EPs are most familiar with the almost instant anesthesia induced by local direct injection; however, the goal of the field block is to infiltrate the space around the nerve to avoid damaging the nerves with direct injection. It then takes time for the anesthetic to diffuse and paralyze the nerve. With lidocaine, this process normally takes 10 to 20 minutes; with 0.5% bupivacaine, which is commonly used in the ED, this can take up to 30 minutes.

The effects are longer-lasting than local anesthesia, and one needs to be sure to give the patient appropriate precautions about care of the insensate extremity. It is important to note that field blocks should only be performed once, because reinjection risks damaging an already partially anesthetized nerve. Similarly, a patient complaint of paresthesias or significant pain on injection should prompt immediate withdrawal of the needle.

■ Radial Nerve

The superficial branch of the radial nerve runs along the medial aspect of the brachioradialis muscle before passing between the tendon of the brachioradialis and radius. Dorsal and just proximal to the the radial styloid process, it divides into the digital branches to the dorsal skin of the thumb, index finger, and lateral half of the middle finger. Several branches pass superficially over the anatomic snuff box. Because of these multiple smaller cutaneous branches, 5 mL of local anesthetic should be injected subcutaneously, just dorsal to the radial styloid, aiming medially. The infiltration is then extended laterally, using an additional 5 mL of local anesthetic.

Median Nerve

The median nerve is blocked by inserting the needle between the tendons of the palmaris longus and flexor carpi radialis. The needle is inserted until it pierces the deep fascia, at which point 3 to 5 mL of local anesthetic is injected. After the initial injection, the needle is withdrawn back to the skin level and redirected 30 degrees radially; it is then reinserted, and 2 mL of additional anesthetic is injected. This procedure is then duplicated with ulnar redirection of the needle.

BOX 84-2

Radio-opaque Foreign Bodies

- Metal, bone, teeth
- Pencil graphite, certain plastics, certain glass, gravel, sand
- Some fish bones, some wood, and some aluminum

Ulnar Nerve

The ulnar nerve is anesthetized by inserting the needle under the tendon of the flexor carpi ulnaris muscle close to its distal attachment just above the styloid process of the ulna. The needle is advanced 5 to 10 mm to just past the tendon of the flexor carpi ulnaris, and 3 to 5 mL of local anesthetic solution is injected. Further anesthesia of the hypothenar area can be achieved by injecting 2 to 3 mL of anesthetic subcutaneously, superficial to the flexor carpi ulnaris. This will block the cutaneous branches of the ulnar nerve, which often extend to the hypothenar area.

Open Wounds

CLINICAL PRESENTATION AND EXAMINATION

Open hand and digit wounds are very common in the ED and have the potential to cause great morbidity if not treated properly. Anesthesia and irrigation should follow a complete neurologic and motor examination. Tap water irrigation has proved to be as safe as irrigation with sterile solutions.[6] One effective time-saving technique involves holding the wound under running tap water for 5 to 10 minutes rather than traditional direct irrigation.

When using direct irrigation, a 60-mL syringe and an 18-gauge angiocath or splashguard mechanism will create proper irrigation pressure. The generally agreed-upon pressure goal is 8 to 10 psi and a minimum of 500 mL for clean wounds, with additional irrigation as needed. There are no studies to-date showing benefit of wound soaking or use of antiseptic solution during irrigation.

Exposure is often a problem with open wounds. Finger tourniquets can be helpful in digital injuries. For more proximal injuries a blood pressure cuff applied to the forearm can help to create a bloodless field. All wounds need to be explored for foreign bodies. Plain film radiography is indicated if there is a concern for retained radio-opaque foreign bodies (Box 84-2).

If tendon injury is a concern, it is imperative to manipulate the tendon through its entire range of motion while examining the wound. When possible, an attempt should be made to recreate the specific position of injury. Nonvisualization of the tendon does not rule out tendon injury, because a completely disrupted tendon may retract.[4]

Closed tendon injuries may be difficult to identify, which stresses the need to assess the joints. Every digit and joint should be put through complete active and passive range of motion to assess for pain, weakness, and laxity. Specific tendon function is evaluated by ranging every joint individually. Extensor tendon function is tested by extending all interphalangeal (IP) and metacarpophalangeal (MP) joints against resistance.

Flexor digitorum sublimus tendon injury limits flexion at the PIP joint. This injury is confirmed by holding the MP joint in extension and flexing the PIP joint against resistance. False-negative results occur if all the other digits are not held in complete extension.

Flexor digitorum profundus tendon injury limits flexion at the distal interphalangeal (DIP) joint; its presence is confirmed by holding the PIP and MP joints in extension and flexing the DIP joint against resistance. The uninjured thumb will have complete active range of motion without pain and should be able to appose the fifth digit. Full flexion to a fist and full extension should be normal.

Comparison with the unaffected side may be helpful in patients with chronic conditions such as degenerative joint disease or rheumatoid arthritis. Pain out of proportion to examination may indicate a partial tendon injury.[3]

WOUND REPAIR

Lacerations should be closed with 4.0- to 6.0-mm sutures that are removed in 8 to 10 days. There are no trials comparing absorbable and nonabsorbable suture material in hand injuries. Deep sutures are to be avoided due to the possibility of the development of foreign body reaction. Wounds more than 8 hours in age should be allowed to heal by secondary intention.

A randomized, controlled study of lacerations less than 2 cm in size demonstrated that conservative management decreased pain and anxiety by eliminating suturing and had similar cosmetic and functional outcomes similar to those in the sutured group.[8]

■ RADIOGRAPIC STUDIES

Suspicion of fracture, dislocation, retained foreign body, or high-pressure injection should prompt radiographic evaluation. Anteroposterior (AP), lateral, and oblique views are adequate to visualization of the vast majority of metacarpal and phalangeal joint injuries. Dedicated soft tissue views increase sensitivity in the evaluation of foreign bodies, although not all foreign bodies are identified by this method.

Fractures and Ligament and Tendon Injuries

■ CLASSIC INJURIES

Because of the complexity of the hand and its propensity for injury, the hand enjoys a long list of classic, or "named," injuries. The names themselves are historical and not always intuitive, and therefore warrant special attention. Following is a partial list of these hand injuries.

■ Bennett's/Reverse Bennett's and Rolando Fractures

A Bennett's fracture is a fracture of the proximal thumb metacarpal bone (Fig. 84-1). The classic mechanism is an axial load to a flexed and adducted thumb. For example, a football quarterback strikes the helmet of an opposing player after releasing a throw. In this avulsion injury, the strong abductor pollicis longus muscle fractures the bone at the point of its insertion at the ulnar aspect of the first metacarpal bone. This causes displacement of a bony fragment, which can be seen on plain film. This is usually an unstable fracture, and ED management should consist of referral to a hand surgeon and immobilization in a thumb spica splint. Potential long-term morbidity includes malunion, decreased function, and significant arthritis.

The same injury pattern and mechanism of injury can also occur in the fifth metacarpal joint and is called a reverse Bennett's fracture, which is as unstable as the Bennett's fracture because of the traction exerted by the extensor carpi ulnaris muscle on the distal aspect of the fifth metacarpal. Traction tends to pull the distal segment ulnarly. Closed reduction with ulnar gutter splinting may be attempted, but any articular incongruity must be recognized and referred emergently to a hand surgeon for potential immediate operative repair.

A Rolando fracture is similar to a Bennett's fracture; however, it is comminuted and by definition extends into the joint space. ED management is identical to that for a Bennett's fracture.

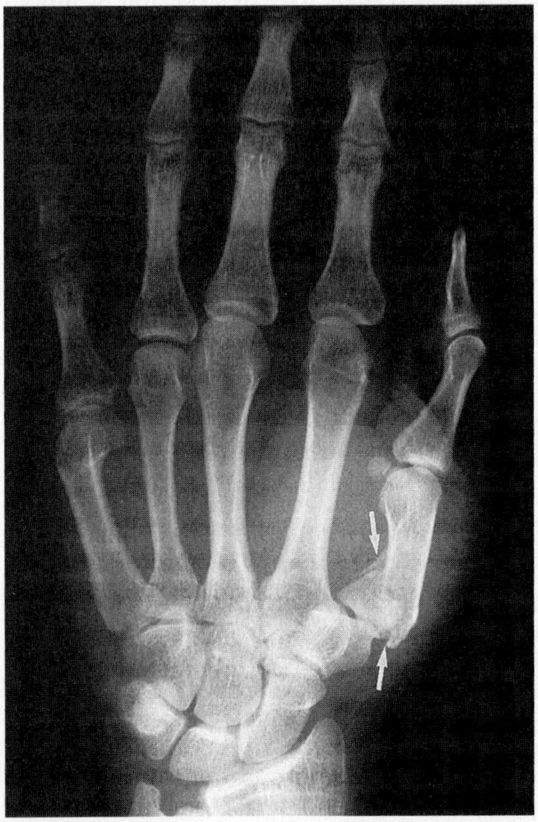

FIGURE 84-1 Bennett's fracture. (From Mettler FA Jr: Essentials of Radiology, 2nd ed. Philadelphia, Elsevier, 2004.)

■ Boutonnière's Deformity

Boutonnière's deformity is not an acute injury. This deformity results from misdiagnosed or inadequately treated central slip rupture. The central slip joins the lateral bands at the dorsal aspect of the PIP joint and is responsible for extension at this joint (Fig. 84-2).

Injury to the PIP joint is common. Acute central slip ruptures occur by one of two mechanisms—the most common is forced flexion of the extended joint. This mechanism is seen in basketball players and martial artists who use hand-blocking techniques. Volar dislocations of the PIP joint are less common but may also cause central slip rupture.

An unreduced volar dislocation will present with obvious deformity of the PIP joint. The middle phalanx is palmar to the proximal phalanx. Patients may present with an acute Boutonnière's deformity,

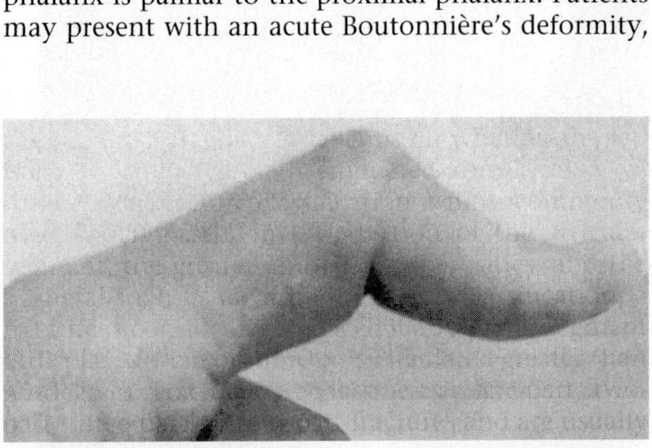

FIGURE 84-2 Boutonnière's deformity. (From Perron AD, Brady WJ: Evaluation and management of the high-risk orthopedic emergency. Emerg Med Clin North Am 2003;21:159-204.)

with flexion of the PIP joint and hyperextension of the DIP and MP joints. In these patients, the PIP joint can be passively brought to full extension, but active extension is not possible. Dislocations may have been relocated in the field, and the EP should have a high index of suspicion for ligament injury.

The physical examination can confirm the diagnosis of central slip injury but may not clarify whether the structure is partially or completely torn. Active extension may still be present, and the patient may be able to fully extend the PIP joint through the action of the lateral bands.

The prudent course is to initially treat all central slip injuries as though they are complete ruptures. The PIP joint should be splinted in extension, leaving the DIP and MP joints free to move. The patient should be instructed to aggressively move the DIP joint to avoid development of an extension contracture. Prompt referral should be made to a hand surgeon.

Boxer's Fracture

Although many people refer to any fracture of the fifth metacarpal joint as a boxer's fracture, the specific injury is a fracture through the neck of the joint (Fig. 84-3). This injury is most frequently seen when a solid object is forcefully struck with a closed fist. True boxer's fractures may carry significant morbidity, because in addition to being an unstable fracture there is often a rotational component to the fracture. If allowed to heal in this position, the hand will be deformed and weakened.

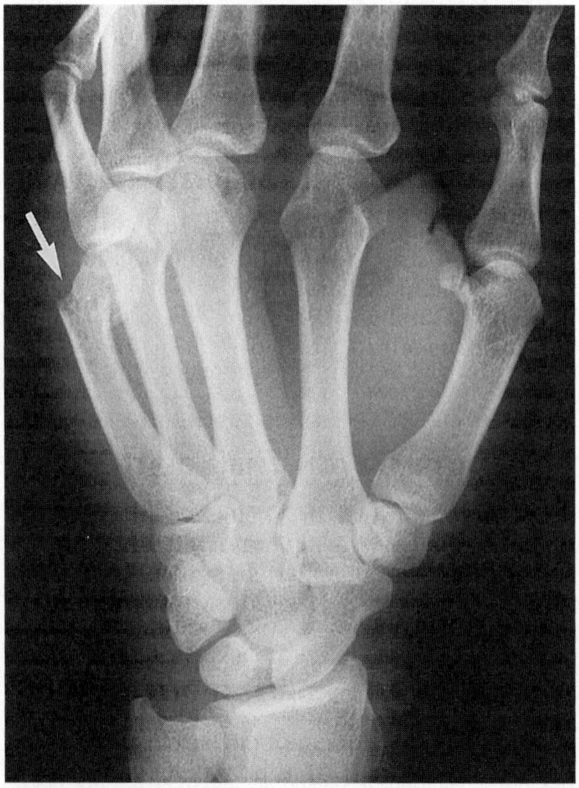

FIGURE 84-3 Boxer's fracture. (From Mettler FA Jr: Essentials of Radiology, 2nd ed. Philadelphia, Elsevier, 2004.)

ED management consists of an attempt at closed reduction and placement of a dorsal-volar splint. Some authors suggest an ulnar-gutter or "cobra" splint. Regardless of the type of splint used, at a minimum the fourth and fifth MP joints should be splinted at 90 degrees of flexion. Because of the instability of this fracture, all patients should be referred to a hand surgeon and warned that there is a significant likelihood that the injury will require operative management.

DeQuervain's Tenosynovitis

DeQuervain's tenosynovitis is an overuse injury of the thumb. The classic example of the mechanism is the fly-fisherman who repetitively collects the line after each cast using the thumb and index finger to grasp the line, resulting in inflammation of the abductor pollicis longus and the extensor pollicis brevis tendons. The diagnosis is made clinically, and a positive Finkelstein's test is said to be pathognomonic. The Finkelstein test is considered positive when pain is elicited with passive ulnar deviation of a closed fist.

It is important to note that patients with this condition may complain of pain upon palpation of the anatomic snuffbox, as the aforementioned tendons form the radial border of that structure. If the history of present illness is suggestive of a possible scaphoid injury, radiography should be performed and a thumb spica splint applied. Treatment for simple DeQuervain's tenosynovitis consists of rest, ice, and nonsteroidal anti-inflammatory drugs (NSAIDs); more severe cases may require splinting to rest the injured joint.

Gamekeeper's/Skier's Thumb

Gamekeeper's thumb is also called skier's thumb (Fig. 84-4). The mechanism is hyperextension of the abducted thumb causing injury to the ulnar collateral ligament and is often associated with an avulsion fracture (Fig. 84-5). Historically old-world "gamekeepers" sustained this injury while dispatching wounded birds during hunts. Today this injury often occurs when a skier falls while grasping the ski pole.

The physical examination will be remarkable because of tenderness at the ulnar collateral ligament, laxity at the MP joint, and inability to actively appose the thumb. Most ulnar collateral ligament ruptures occur at the distal attachment. If the injured joint demonstrates 40 degrees of radial angulation during stressing, a complete ligament rupture should be assumed. There may be an associated avulsion fracture. Treatment is immobilization in a thumb spica splint, NSAIDS, and referral to a hand surgeon for open reduction internal fixation (ORIF). The window of opportunity for ORIF is long (6-8 weeks),

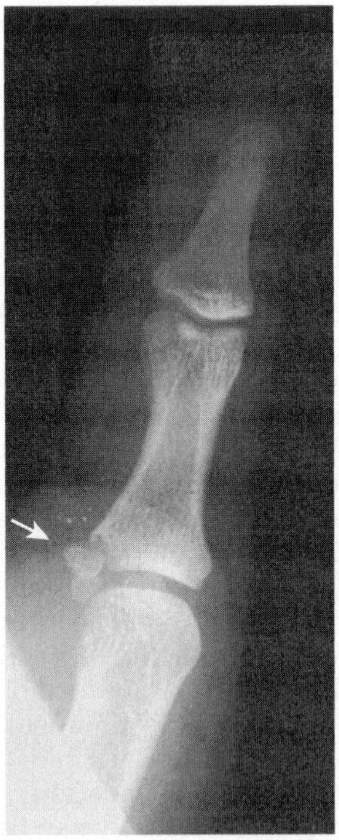

FIGURE 84-4 Gamekeeper's thumb. (From Perron AD, Brady WJ: Evaluation and management of the high-risk orthopedic emergency. Emerg Med Clin North Am 2003;21:159-204.)

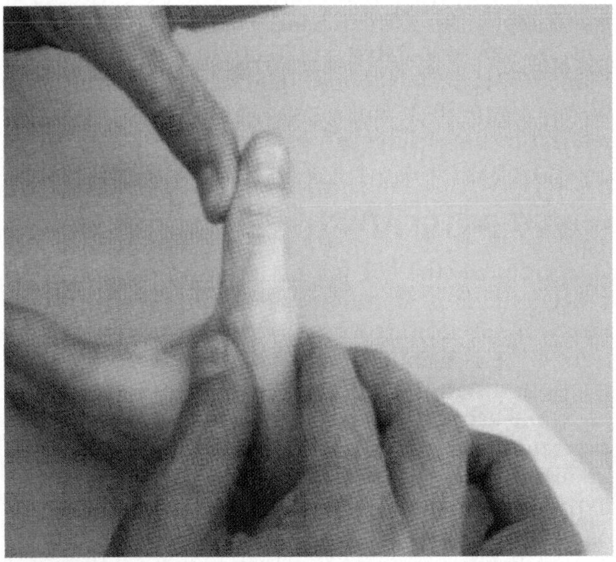

FIGURE 84-5 Testing for ulnar collateral ligament integrity. (From Patel D, Dean C, Baker R: The hand in sports: Update on clinical anatomy and physical examination. Prim Care 2005; 32:71-89.)

and most surgeons will observe the patient for clinical improvement during that time period.

The initial examination may be compromised secondary to pain and spasm. In these cases, the most prudent course of action is immobilization in a thumb-spica splint and referral for reevaluation.

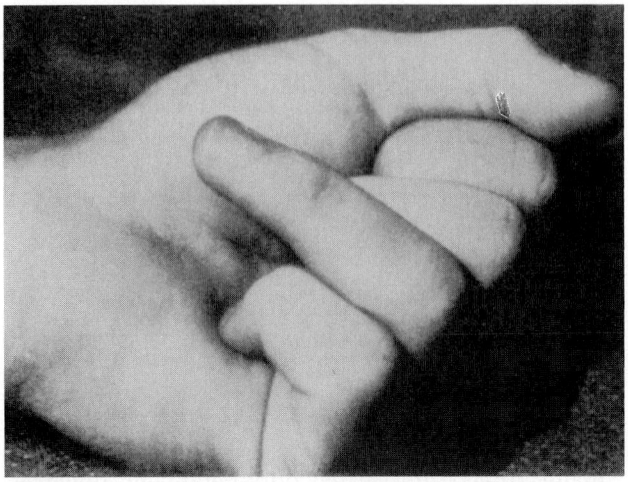

FIGURE 84-6 Jersey finger. (From Perron AD, Brady WJ: Evaluation and management of the high-risk orthopedic emergency. Emerg Med Clin North Am 2003;21:159-204.)

■ Jersey Finger

Jersey finger is an injury often associated with tackling sports (Fig. 84-6). The injury itself is a disruption of the FDP joint, which is responsible for flexion of the digit at the DIP joint. This occurs when a digit (often the 2nd digit) is forced into extension while actively being flexed, as might occur when grabbing an opponent's jersey during a tackle.

On physical examination the injured patient will not be able to flex the digit at the DIP joint when the PIP joint is held (by the examiner) in extension. Examining the DIP joint without holding the PIP joint may result in a false-negative test due to contribution from the lateral bands. The patient may complain of pain more proximally along the flexor tendon sheath, or even in the palm, because the ruptured flexor digitorum profundus tendon will retract. Therefore it is imperative to challenge the distal joint, despite only proximal pain. For full disruption the best outcomes depend on early surgical repair, and all patients should be scheduled for hand surgeon referral.

■ Mallet Finger

Mallet finger is in many ways the functional opposite of jersey finger. In mallet finger, there is a rupture of the distal extensor tendon (Fig. 84-7). This often occurs when the distal phalanx of a finger (or thumb) is forced into flexion while being actively extended. In sports the middle finger is most often affected secondary to length, and this occurs when the finger is jammed, as when attempting to catch a ball.

Because this injury is often painless, it does not always present immediately. The physical examination is remarkable for the inability to extend at the affected DIP joint. Radiographs may demonstrate an avulsion fracture. Treatment is immobilization by splinting the DIP in full extension, which allows full range of motion at the PIP joint. The patient should

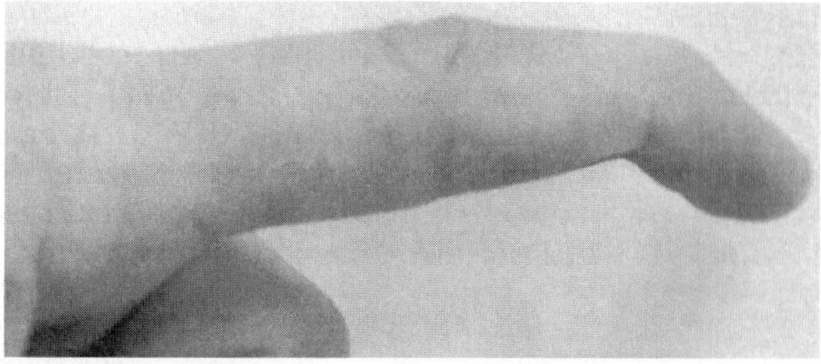

FIGURE 84-7 Mallet finger. (From Perron AD, Brady WJ: Evaluation and management of the high-risk orthopedic emergency. Emerg Med Clin North Am 2003;21:159-204.)

have referral to a hand surgeon follow-up. Most mallet fingers are treated nonoperatively; however, those with large avulsion fracture fragments may require operative management.

■ OTHER FRACTURES

The common characteristic of all phalangeal and metacarpal fractures is intolerance of rotational deformity.[3] Differing degrees of angulations are tolerated in different areas of the hand. Referral depends largely on the necessity for further reduction and the stability of the fracture.

■ Distal Phalanx Fractures

The most common distal phalanx fracture is the tuft fracture, and nail bed injuries are the most common complication of this fracture.[2] There is some controversy regarding the need to repair nail bed injuries; however, most authors recommend performing trephination for nail bed hematomas involving 30% to 50% or greater of the nail bed surface. When there is nail bed involvement, tuft fractures are considered open wound injuries, and although some physicians prescribe empirical antibiotics, evidence suggests that prophylactic antibiotics are not indicated.[9] More proximal distal phalanx fractures are often unstable and require hand surgeon referral for percutaneous wire placement. An attempt to reduce any rotational deformity or angulation should be made prior to splinting. Splinting should isolate the DIP joint alone.

■ Middle and Proximal Phalanx Fractures

Middle and proximal phalanx fractures are managed similarly. The degree of instability depends on the nature of the fracture. Transverse or spiral fractures have greater instability than simple fractures, and are therefore more likely to require percutaneous fixation. It is important to keep in mind that rotational deformity cannot be tolerated. When the hand is held in a relaxed fist, the fingers should all point to the scaphoid region. Visual deviation from this plane suggests a rotational deformity of greater than 10%. Buddy taping is the best management of simple fractures. Rotated, transverse, displaced, or intra-articular fractures should be reduced, splinted in either a dorsal volar or ulnar gutter splint, as indicated, and referred for hand surgery.

■ Metacarpal Bone Fractures

Metacarpal bone fractures cannot be discussed as a group because of the vast differences in both mobility and function between them.

The first metacarpal is very mobile and fractures are relatively uncommon. Management includes proper reduction, thumb spica splint, and follow-up with hand surgery. Bennett's and Rolando fractures are discussed in the section "Classic Injuries."

The second and third metacarpals are the fixed center of the hand, and proper reduction of fractures is crucial for return of function. The fourth and fifth metacarpals, however, are more mobile and have greater ability to compensate for angular deformities. Description of injury and determination of proper reduction are based on angulation and rotational malalignment. Stable fractures may be splinted and referred to a hand surgeon for outpatient follow-up.

All unstable reductions, irreducible, open, or intra-articular fractures, and any fracture with rotational malalignment merit hand surgery consultation.

Metacarpal base fractures are uncommon and usually are of little significance.[2] The exception is at the base of the fifth metacarpal bone, where there can be an associated subluxation of metacarpal-hamate joint. The injured hand should be immobilized in an ulnar gutter splint and scheduled for referral to hand surgery.

■ DIGIT DISLOCATION

Dislocation of the DIP joint is a rare injury, but when it occurs it most commonly dislocates in the dorsal direction after direct force on the finger pad. Relocation is best accomplished after digital block with traction longitudinally and pressure directing the proximal aspect of the distal phalanx back to correct alignment. After relocation, the entire digit is splinted in extension. Some injuries are nonreducible and require operative repair because the volar plate and/or profundus tendon may occupy the joint space. Any indication of joint involvement should prompt referral to a hand surgeon.

PIP joint dislocations result in more complications than DIP joint dislocations. The complex biomechanics of the joint add a degree of intricacy that often results in the need for operative repair. The volar plate may be injured in dorsal dislocations, and the lateral collateral ligaments may be injured in ulnar or radial dislocations. It is important to assess any relocated joint for stability to better rule out the potential for ligament or volar plate injury. Patients with an irreducible or unstable joint should be referred to a hand surgeon for operative repair. If stable, the joint should be splinted in 30 degrees of flexion for 2 to 4 weeks.

MP joint dislocations are seen less commonly than PIP dislocations but have a similar rate of complications. Dislocations may be partial or complete and may involve the volar plate. Care should be taken during the examination not to convert a partial dislocation to a complete dislocation. Injury most commonly occurs as a hyperextension mechanism. With complete dislocations and volar plate involvement, relocation is often impossible because the volar plate may become entrapped in the joint space. For the best chance of relocation, the wrist should be placed in full flexion to relieve all flexor tendon tension and exert longitudinal and volar force. The MP joint should be splinted in full flexion.

■ EXTENSOR TENDON INJURIES

Open wounds on the dorsum of the hand and digits should trigger suspicion of extensor tendon injury. The Verdan extensor tendon injury classification system uses eight anatomic zones to direct treatment (Table 84-1).

Treatment of extensor tendon injuries should usually be coordinated with a hand surgeon. Data concerning suture repair of partial tendon lacerations are lacking, and current treatment is based on flexor tendon treatment. Conservative treatment of injuries of less than 50% of a cross-sectional area has been proposed.

Injuries to zones I and II occur with axial loading to a fully extended DIP, forcing the DIP into flexion and disrupting the distal aspect of the extensor tendon. This creates a mallet injury, as described previously.

Zone III injuries occur either by axial loading and forced flexion of the PIP joint or by direct trauma to the PIP joint. These injuries should be splinted with the joint in extension, and the patient should be referred to a hand surgeon. With complete disruption of the central slip, the lateral bands slide toward the volar surface of the digit, causing the extensor tendons to act as flexors. Untreated injuries lead to a boutonnière deformity, as described previously.

Most zone IV injuries are caused by direct trauma. Open injuries may be treated primarily as in zone IV; by definition, there is no joint involvement. Closed injuries should be splinted with extension of the PIP joint. The extensor tendons of the phalanx are broad and flat, allowing easier primary repair.

"Fight bite" must be considered in all patients with zone V ligament injuries. Patients with open injuries should be referred to a hand surgeon for primary repair. Closed injuries can be treated by splinting the MCP joint in extension while allowing free range of motion of the PIP joint.

Zone VI injuries are usually superficial and easily repaired by the EP. Suture material should be strong, such as braided nylon, and the lacerated tendon completely apposed. After closure, the wrist should be splinted in 30 degrees of extension, the MP joint in 15 degrees of flexion, and the PIP joint should be free. The patient should be referred to a specialist for dynamic splinting.

Zone VII and VIII injuries often involve the extensor retinaculum, and the patient should be scheduled for referral to a hand surgeon for primary closure. The affected tendon often retracts into the forearm, complicating the repair. Due to the density of associated anatomic structures, operative survey of the injury to identify additional injuries is indicated.

■ FLEXOR TENDON INJURIES

All patients with open flexor tendon injuries should be referred to a hand surgeon for emergent evaluation (Table 84-2). However, some knowledge of the nomenclature and prognoses associated with flexor tendon injuries will aid the EP in conversations with both the consultant and the patient.

Repair of complete lacerations is most commonly recommended within 24 hours. Operative repair is usually limited to injuries involving greater than a 50% of a cross-sectional area. Injuries involving less

Table 84-1 VERDAN CLASSIFICATION OF EXTENSOR TENDON INJURIES WITH APPROPRIATE DISPOSITION

Zone	Anatomic Location	Disposition
I	Distal phalange to distal interphalangeal joint	Splint/hand surgeon referral
II	Middle phalanx	Splint/hand surgeon referral
III	Proximal interphalangeal joint	Splint/hand surgeon referral
IV	Proximal phalanx	ED primary repair/splint
V	Metacarpophalangeal joint	Splint/hand surgeon referral
VI	Dorsum of hand/metacarpals	ED primary repair/splint
VII	Dorsum of wrist/carpals	Hand surgeon primary repair
VIII	Distal forearm/proximal wrist	Hand surgeon primary repair

Data from Verdan CE: Primary and secondary repair of flexor and extensor tendon injuries. In Flynn JE (ed): Hand Surgery, 2nd ed. Baltimore, Williams & Wilkins, 1975.

Table 84-2 VERDAN CLASSIFICATION OF FLEXOR TENDON INJURIES WITH APPROPRIATE DISPOSITION

Zone	Anatomic Location	Disposition
I	Distal to insertion of flexor digitorum sublimus tendon	Hand surgeon primary repair
II	Area of flexor sheath with both flexor digitorum sublimus and flexor digitorum profundus tendons	Hand surgeon primary repair
III	Carpal tunnel to the proximal aspect of flexor sheath	Hand surgeon primary repair
IV	Carpal tunnel	Hand surgeon primary repair
V	Forearm proximal to carpal tunnel	Hand surgeon primary repair

Data from Verdan CE: Primary and secondary repair of flexor and extensor tendon injuries. In Flynn JE (ed): Hand Surgery, 2nd ed. Baltimore, Williams & Wilkins, 1975.

than 50% frequently are treated conservatively with splinting. Newer data suggest that conservative management be adequate for injuries of less than 75% of a cross-sectional area; however, this decision should be deferred to the consulting hand surgeon.[1] When splinting flexor tendon injuries, the wrist should be placed in 30 degrees of flexion, MP joint injuries in 70 degrees of flexion, and the DIP/PIP joint injuries in 10 degrees of flexion. Flexor tendon injuries are classified based on anatomic location, treatment, and prognosis. All patients with flexor tendon injuries should be referred to a hand surgeon for operative exploration and repair.

Wrist Injuries

Carpal bone fractures can result in significant long-term morbidity and are easily missed in the physical examination. The two most common carpal fractures are fractures of the scaphoid and triquetrum. Scapholunate, perilunate, and lunate dislocations are the most common dislocations.

■ SCHAPHOID FRACTURES

The scaphoid is the most commonly injured carpal bone. A high index of suspicion is needed when considering this injury, because plain film findings are often subtle or even absent (a dedicated scaphoid view will increase plain film sensitivity). The mechanism of injury is most often a fall onto an outstretched hand.

Morbidity is high with this injury because the bone is anatomically predisposed to avascular necrosis and nonunion. The blood supply to the scaphoid originates from the radial and palmar arteries and flows from distal to proximal. The most proximal aspect of the scaphoid receives blood only from this distal to proximal flow, and if this flow is interrupted by a fracture, the risk of avascular necrosis and nonunion is high. For this reason all patients with a traumatic mechanism and scaphoid tenderness, as assessed by palpation of the anatomic snuff box or pain with axial loading of the thumb, should be treated with a thumb spica splint and referred for follow-up. Roughly 15% of these patients will have a scaphoid fracture, despite unrevealing plain films.[10]

■ TRIQUETRUM FRACTURES

Triquetrum fractures are less common than scaphoid fractures but are often seen with a similar mechanism of hyperextension. Most often the fracture is secondary to an avulsion with an avulsion fragment noted at the dorsal aspect of the triquetrum. This is best seen on a lateral plain film projection. Prognosis is better compared with scaphoid fractures because avascular necrosis is not a common occurrence in these injuries.

Occasionally triquetrum body fractures can be seen; in this case, the EP should look for associated lunate or perilunate dislocations. The wrist should be splinted and the patient referred to a hand surgeon for follow-up.

■ SCAPHOLUNATE, PERILUNATE, AND LUNATE DISLOCATIONS

Scapholunate, perilunate, and lunate dislocations are varying degrees of the same disease process. The mechanism is one of hyperextension. In cadaver work, it was shown that progressive force applied in a hyperextension mechanism to the wrist will reliably re-create these injuries and in a persistent pattern.[11] The reason is anatomically based and the result of progressive ligament injuries.

■ Scapholunate Dislocation

Scapholunate dislocation is the most common of these injuries and occurs with the least amount of force. It can be diagnosed on plain film radiography. Scapholunate dislocation results in a classic radiologic finding—the *Terry-Thomas sign* (Fig 84-8). Terry-Thomas was a 20th-century British comedian who possessed a noticeable gap between his two front teeth reminiscent of the wide space (≥2 mm, when measured on the AP view) seen between the scaphoid and lunate bones when they are dislocated. Stress views accentuate this finding. Additionally, the scaphoid may twist on its access and cause a ringlike shadow known as the "signet ring sign." This is an artifact caused by the x-rays traveling longitudinally down the twisted scaphoid, unlike the normal crosswise orientation. Mayfield and colleagues classified this injury as a stage I injury.[11]

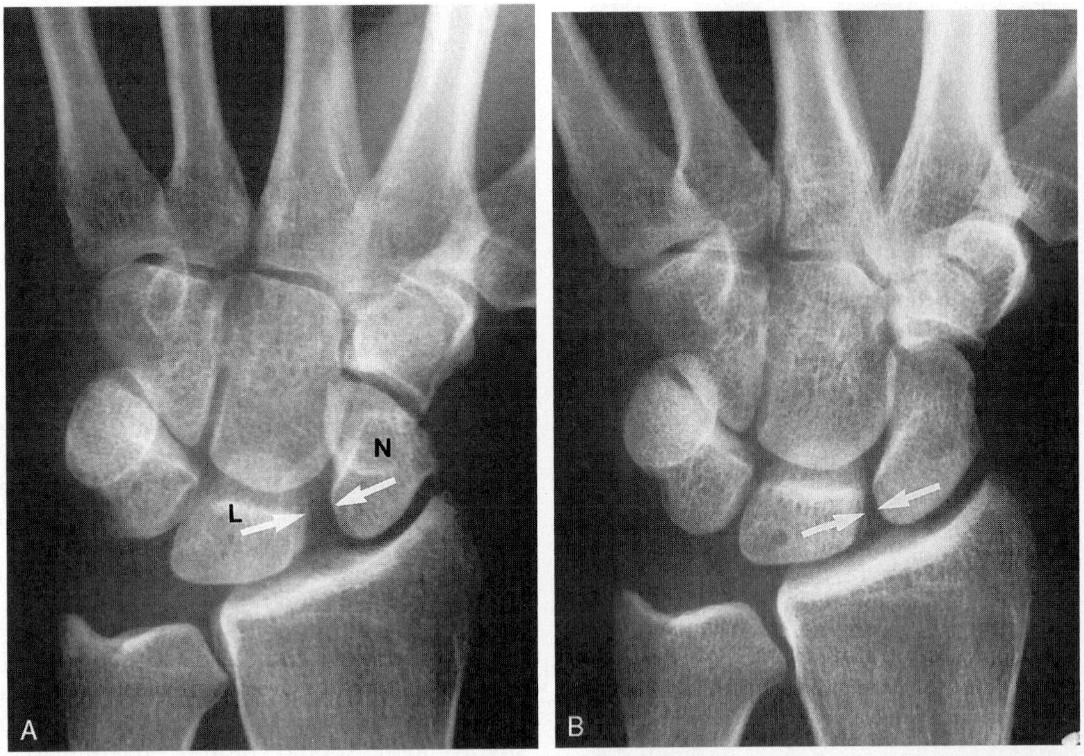
N
L
A
B

FIGURE 84-8 Scapholunate dislocation. **A,** Terry-Thomas sign. **B,** Normal wrist. (From Mettler FA Jr: Essentials of Radiology, 2nd ed. Philadelphia, Elsevier, 2004.)

■ Perilunate Dislocation

Stage II injury is associated with progressively more force (for example, an automobile accident versus a slip and fall) and results in perilunate dislocation (Fig. 84-9). Perilunate dislocations may be a difficult concept because there is no "perilunate" bone. Perilunate dislocation is a disruption of the ligamentous structures around ("peri") the lunate bone. One of these structures is the capitate, which most often dislocates dorsally. Perilunate dislocation may perhaps be better-called capitate dislocation; however, perilunate dislocation is actually a more accurate description of the stepwise disease process as outlined by Mayfield.[11] The dislocation of the capitate can be associated with a scaphoid fracture. The EP should be diligent to assess for one in the setting of the other. Perilunate dislocation is often overlooked despite the classic plain film finding of the capitate and of the remainder of the distal hand lying dorsally to the lunate on the lateral projection.

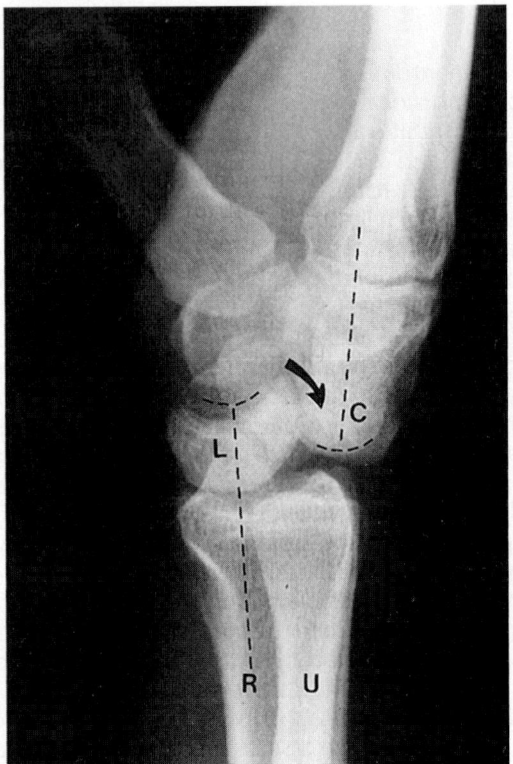
C
L
R
U

FIGURE 84-9 Perilunate dislocation. (From Mettler FA Jr: Essentials of Radiology, 2nd ed. Philadelphia, Elsevier, 2004.)

■ Triquetrum Dislocation

Stage III injury involves dislocation of the triquetrum but is difficult to differentiate radiographically from stage II perilunate dislocation.

Stage IV injury is defined by the presence of a lunate dislocation. This is a complete disruption of

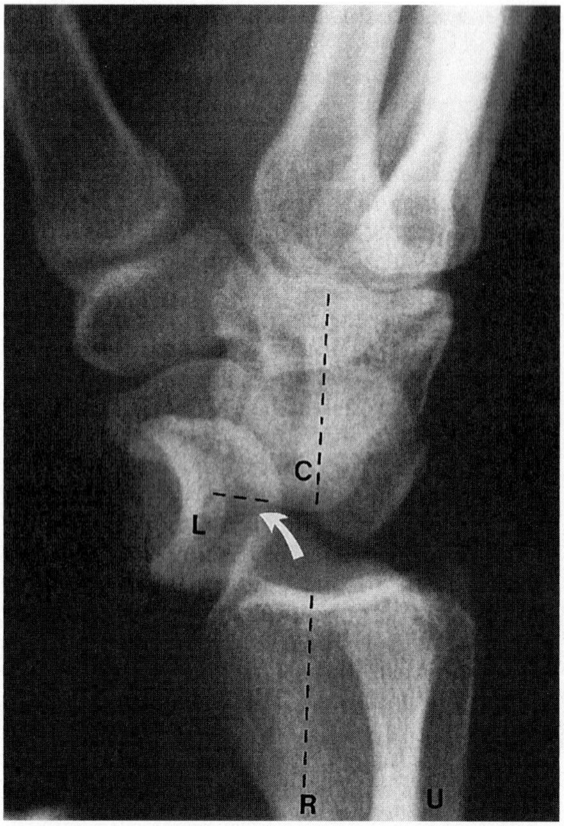
C
L
R
U

FIGURE 84-10 Lunate dislocation: spilled teacup sign. (From Mettler FA Jr: Essentials of Radiology, 2nd ed. Philadelphia, Elsevier, 2004.)

the ligamentous structures of the wrist. In stage I the scaphoid dislocates from the lunate, in stages II and III the capitate and triquetrum dislocate from the lunate, and in stage IV, the lunate dislocates from its articulation with the distal radius. The dislocated capitate, which lies dorsal to the lunate, often will collapse onto the distal radius due to muscular spasm, because the lunate is no longer present to prevent this.

The result is a distal radius and capitate pseudoarticulation, with the lunate lying palmar to the "new" wrist articulation. This is best viewed on a lateral plain film projection, and causes the "spilled teacup" sign (Fig. 84-10). When teaching this concept, the author asked students to imagine a watermelon seed being squeezed between two fingers and then popping forward with force. This is essentially what happens to the lunate as it is "squeezed" by the radius and distal wrist structures, including the capitate, in an extreme hyperextension mechanism. Lunate dislocation often compress the carpal tunnel and can cause median neuropathy.

Plain film radiography is in general adequate to diagnose carpal bone dislocations, although CT scanning can be helpful in ambiguous cases. The EP may attempt closed reduction; however, many of these injuries are unstable. All injuries should be splinted with a long arm splint and patients should be referred to a hand surgeon. Many of these injuries will require internal fixation.

Bite Injuries

Because of the potential for injury and morbidity, all open injuries of the MP joint should be treated as closed fist bite wounds, or "fight bite," until proved otherwise. These often minor-appearing injuries are by definition caused by a clenched fist versus human teeth and are well known for poor outcomes. Potential complications include violation of the joint capsule, extensor tendon injury, and deep fascial space contamination.[12] The potential for infection is great because of the poor vascular supply to the extensor tendon and joint capsule. Treatment of these injuries is threefold: surgical decontamination, antibiotics, and dynamic splinting.[13] These injuries are not limited to fist fights and also commonly occur during sporting events.[10]

Delayed presentation most commonly occurs 2 to 3 days after the inciting event with signs and symptoms of local or significantly advanced infection. Any indication of infection, joint space, or tendon sheath involvement should prompt referral to a hand surgeon for irrigation and débridement. The timing of initiation of IV antibiotics should be made in consultation with the hand surgeon, who may wish to delay antibiotic treatment until after intraoperative cultures have been obtained. Antimicrobial therapy should cover common pathogens found in the human oral and skin flora, including aerobic and anaerobic pathogens. *Staphylococcus aureus* is the most common pathogen, followed by *Streptococcus* species, *Corynebacterium* species, and *Eikenella corrodens*.[14]

If the patient presentation is acute and if there is no indication of fracture, joint space involvement, or extensor tendon injury, then antibiotic therapy and local wound care are sufficient. In this nonoperative patient group, wounds should be treated with high volume irrigation, and they should be left open to heal by secondary intention. The injured hand should be splinted in the position of function, and the patient should be instructed to elevate the affected limb and to return if there is any evidence of infection.

Prophylactic antibiotics for clenched fist bite wounds should be initiated in all but the most superficial injuries. Recommended regimens include amoxicillin/clavulanic acid, a combination of penicillin and dicloxacillin, and a combination of penicillin and a first-generation cephalosporin.[14]

High-Pressure Injection Injuries

Modern technological advances have greatly increased the incidence of high-pressure injection injuries. Many substances are now sprayed under high-pressure, including paint, water, oil and other petroleum-based substances, solvents, and grease. As the incidence continues to grow, the EP should recognize the potential for injury and infection from these injuries.

High-pressure injection injuries can lead to rates of infection, inflammatory reactions, fibrosis, disability, and amputation as high as 50%.[15] An early and aggressive open surgical approach improves the prognosis and the patient's ability to return to previous employment. One report demonstrated 100% amputation rates for patients presenting 6 or more hours after initial injury, thus signifying the importance of early management.[16]

Historical information including the time since injury, material injected, amount injected, temperature of the material, and velocity/pressure of the injection may be helpful in determining the prognosis. For example, the amputation rate is considerably lower with grease injection versus injection of paint or solvent-based material. Thinner and less viscous material is more apt to lead to amputation because of easier spread and subsequent larger extent of injury.

Presentation of a small puncture wound with a history of high-pressure injury is an indication for radiographic imaging. Subcutaneous air and radio-opaque substances may be visualized and can indicate the extent of injury.

The initial pain complaints by patients with high-pressure injection injuries may be significant and large doses of IV narcotic analgesia may be required. Due to the local injury and inflammation, regional anesthesia (digital blocks or infiltration such as Bier blocks), has been shown to worsen outcomes and is contraindicated.[17] Many of the complications from high-pressure injection injuries are related to inflammation; however, there is little data to either support or refute the use of systemic steroids. Similarly, the role of empirical antibiotics is unknown. Tetanus prophylaxis is indicated as with all penetration injuries of the skin.

REFERENCES

1. Amadio P: What's new in hand surgery. J Bone Joint Surg 2005;87A:468-473.
2. Chung KC, Spilson SV: The frequency and epidemiology of hand and forearm fractures in the United States. J Hand Surg 2001;26A:908-915.
3. Harrison B, Holland P: Diagnosis and management of hand injuries in the ED. Emerg Med Pract 2005;7:1-28.
4. Krunic AL, Wang LC, Soltani K, et al: Digital anesthesia with epinephrine: An old myth revisited. J Am Acad Dermatol 2004;51:755-759.
5. Waterbrook, A, Germann C, Southall J: Is epinephrine harmful when used with anesthetics for digital nerve block? Ann Emerg Med 2007;50:472-475.
6. Valente JH, Forti RJ, Freundlich LF, et al: Wound irrigation in children: Saline solution or tap water? Ann Emerg Med 2003;41:609-616.
7. Kotwal PP, Gupta V: Neglected tendon and nerve injuries of the hand. Clin Orthopaed Rel Res 2005;431:66-71.
8. Quinn J, Cummings S, Callaham M, Sellers K: Suturing versus conservative management of lacerations of the hand. BMJ 2002;325:299-300.
9. Sukop A, Kufa R: [Primary surgical treatment of amputated fingers and indications for digital replantation]. Acta Chir Orthop Traumatol Czech 2005;72:129-133.
10. Wackerle JF: A prospective study identifying the sensitivity of radiographic findings and the efficacy of clinical findings in carpal navicular fractures. Ann Emerg Med 1987;16:733-737.
11. Mayfield JK, Johnson RP, Kilcoyne RK: Carpal dislocations: Pathomechanics and progressive perilunar instability. J Hand Surg 1980;5:226-241.
12. Perron AD, Miller MD, Brady WJ: Orthopedic pitfalls in the ED: Fight bite. Am J Emerg Med 2002;20:114-117.
13. Bunzli WF, Wright DH, Hoang AT, et al: Current management of human bites. Pharmacotherapy 1998;18:227-234.
14. Medeiros L, Saconato H: Antibiotic prophylaxis for mammalian bites. Cochrane Database Syst Review. 2003(2):CD001738.
15. Pinto MR, Turkula-Pinto LD, Cooney WP, et al: High-pressure injection injuries of the hand: Review of 25 patients managed by open wound technique. J Hand Surg [Am] 1993;18:125-130.
16. Luber KT, Rehm JP, Freeland AE: High-pressure injection injuries of the hand. Orthopedics 2005;28:129-132.
17. Hayes CW, Pan HC: High-pressure injection injuries to the hand. South Med J 1982;75:1491-1498, 1516.

Chapter **85**

Arterial and Venous Trauma and Great Vessel Injuries

Stephen J. Wolf and Gayle Braunholtz

KEY POINTS

Of patients with great vessel injury who survive until hospital evaluation, 30% die within 6 hours of arrival.

Thirty to fifty percent of patients with blunt aortic injury have no external signs of trauma.

A normal chest radiograph does not exclude great vessel injury when clinical suspicion is high.

Computed tomography angiography (CTA) is the diagnostic test of choice to rule out traumatic aortic injury in hemodynamically stable patients.

For patients too large for a CT scanner, consider transesophageal echocardiographic evaluation of the aorta.

Early definitive operative management should be considered.

Medical management of great vessel injury is used as a bridge to definitive operative care.

Beta adrenergic blockade is instituted before administering nitroprusside in the medical management of great vessel injury in order to avoid the possible reflex tachycardia of vasodilation alone.

Scope and Outline

■ PERSPECTIVE

Few traumatic injuries are more devastating than great vessel injuries. With an average circulating volume of 5 liters and a flow rate up to 4.8 liters per minute in the circulatory system, it is easy to see why great vessel injuries can result in rapid, catastrophic outcomes. In patients surviving an initial injury to the great vessels, rapid diagnosis and treatment is imperative to prevent subsequent exsanguination within the next minutes to hours. This highlights the "golden hour" of trauma resuscitation.

■ EPIDEMIOLOGY

Several contributing factors are important when evaluating great vessel injury (Fig. 85-1). Although the mechanism and the specific vessel injured are the most important of these factors, attention also must be paid to the role of concomitant injuries and comorbid conditions in patients' morbidity and mortality. Unfortunately, on initial evaluation the EP is

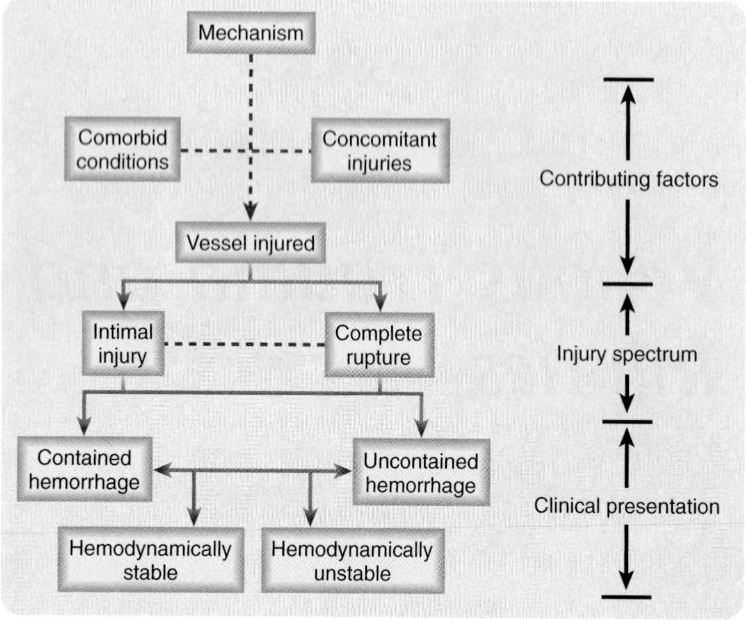
Mechanism
Comorbid conditions
Concomitant injuries
Vessel injured
Intimal injury
Complete rupture
Contained hemorrhage
Uncontained hemorrhage
Hemodynamically stable
Hemodynamically unstable
Contributing factors
Injury spectrum
Clinical presentation

FIGURE 85-1 Algorithm showing contributing factors, injury spectrum, and clinical presentations of great vessel injuries.

often lucky to be aware of one, let alone all, of these factors.

The most important branch point for the likelihood of great vessel injury is a penetrating versus a blunt mechanism. Penetrating mechanisms are associated with greater than 90% of great vessel trauma, and all thoracic vascular structures are at risk.[1] Patients who survive until ED presentation, particularly if they are not in hemorrhagic shock, have a survival rate approaching 50%.[2]

Blunt traumatic injuries to the great vessels most often affect the aorta; the innominate artery, pulmonary hilar vessels, and vena cava are also susceptible. Blunt aortic rupture has an immediate mortality rate of greater than 80% and is responsible for 10% to 15% of motor vehicle accident fatalities.[3] Because of the high association of blunt ascending aortic injury with fatal cardiac injury, the majority of those who survive until hospital evaluation have descending injuries. Of patients who survive until medical evaluation, 30% die within 6 hours and 40% within 24 hours.[3] Because most of these injuries are in young healthy males, their overall survival is much better than expected given the severity of injury.

Although the mechanism is incompletely understood, it has been proposed that blunt aortic injury can result from any combination of shearing forces, rotational forces, increased intraluminal aortic pressures, or a pinching mechanism between the sternum and vertebral column. Thus it is not surprising that motor vehicle collisions cause the majority of blunt aortic injuries. This association increases with the speed of the accident.[4,5] Shearing forces were originally thought to be the highest in front impact accidents, in which deceleration forces are the greatest. However, studies have found that side impact accidents carry the same risk of injury.[4,6] Other attempts to define mechanisms more distinctly have been largely unsuccessful.[4-6] Falls from a height and crushing forces have been known to cause blunt great vessel injury.[6]

Due in part to difficulty isolating the hilum, patients with injuries to the pulmonary arteries and veins and the thoracic vena cava have mortality rates greater than 60%, regardless of whether they are caused by blunt or penetrating forces, although the latter are more common than the former.[7]

Concomitant injuries at presentation clearly play a role in the epidemiology, morbidity, and mortality of great vessel injury. In one study of blunt thoracic trauma, patients with traumatic aortic injury had a mean injury severity score (ISS) of 40, whereas patients without vascular injury had a mean ISS of only 16.[4] In another study, more than half of patients with great vessel injur were diagnosed with closed head injury, with one fourth of those having intracranial hemorrhage.[2]

Comorbid conditions such as underlying vascular disease, cardiopulmonary disease, and renal insufficiency contribute to the morbidity and mortality of great vessel injury. Many disease processes affect a patient's ability to tolerate the initial and delayed physiologic insults associated with severe great vessel injury.

Anatomy

Knowledge of the vascular anatomy of the great vessels and the particular branch points of more distal vasculature is important in potentially preventing morbidity and mortality in the setting of injury. This anatomy can be broken down into arterial, venous, and pulmonary components.

The systemic arterial great vessels include the ascending aorta, aortic arch, and descending thoracic aorta. The innominate artery is the first branch of the aortic arch giving rise to the right subclavian and right common carotid arteries. The left common carotid artery, followed by the left subclavian artery, are the next two branches. These structures course in close approximation to the clavicle, the first and second ribs, and the brachial plexus. Just distal to the left subclavian artery take-off, the descending aorta becomes a more fixed structure in comparison to the arch. The ligamentum arteriosum, a remnant of the ductus arteriosum, and the intercostal arteries tether it to other thoracic structures. This junction, often called the isthmus region, proves to be the most susceptible site of blunt aortic injury, as the arch moves in relation to the relatively fixed descending aorta. Spinal arteries branching off of the descending aorta are of particular importance because they supply the spinal column. Compromised flow to these small branches through direct injury or vascular clamping plays a significant role in patients' risk of paraplegia.

The microanatomy of the artery wall, consisting of intimal, medial, and adventitial layers, is integral in the spectrum of disease (Fig. 85-2). Injuries can range from isolated thrombogenic intimal flaps to full-thickness tears with free hemorrhage.

The venous components of the great vessel system include the confluence of the subclavian and internal jugular veins, which ultimately combine to form the superior vena cava. The inferior vena cava receives blood from the portal system through the hepatic vein in the retrohepatic region. As a whole, this system is characterized by low pressure and resistance and high flow and compliance, unless there is tamponade or heart failure, which results in increased right-sided pressures. These factors can make control of hemorrhage difficult.

The final component of the great vessel system is the pulmonary circulation. As mentioned earlier, the structures of this system reside in the hilum and are deep in the thorax, making them difficult to access. They possess mediastinal and intrathoracic portions, which can result in different clinical presentations, such as mediastinal hematoma and hemothorax.

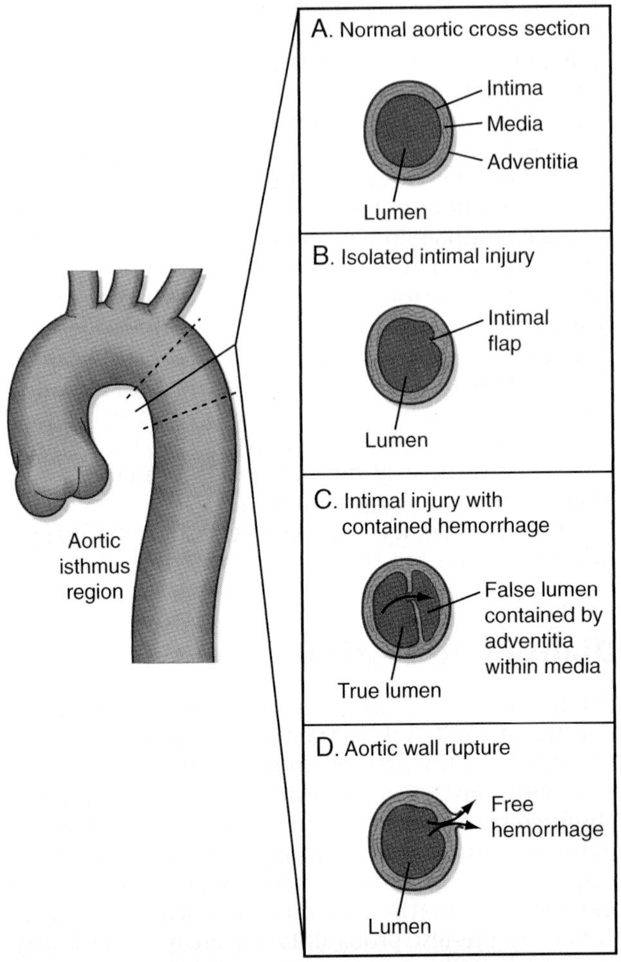
A. Normal aortic cross section
Intima
Media
Adventitia
Lumen
B. Isolated intimal injury
Intimal flap
Lumen
C. Intimal injury with contained hemorrhage
False lumen contained by adventitia within media
True lumen
D. Aortic wall rupture
Free hemorrhage
Lumen
Aortic isthmus region

FIGURE 85-2 Continuum of aortic vessel injury: **A,** normal aortic cross section; **B,** isolated intimal injury; **C,** intimal injury with contained hemorrhage; **D,** complete aortic wall rupture.

Presenting Signs and Symptoms (Box 85-1)

Traditionally, aortic dissection from nontraumatic causes is believed to present with tearing pain radiating through the chest to the interscapular region of the back. This can be accompanied by various associated symptoms, including shortness of breath and vagal complaints. In patients with traumatic injury, this symptom pattern is seen less than 25% of the time; these patients most frequently have either vague, chest-related complaints or no complaints at all, due to distracting injuries. It is remarkable that 30% to 50% of patients with a blunt aortic injury may have no external signs of trauma.[8]

Signs and symptoms of great vessel injury often result from affected blood flow, which can be second-

BOX 85-1

Signs and Symptoms of Great Vessel Injury

Signs	Symptoms
Hemorrhagic shock	Tearing pain
Hypotension	Pain radiating to the back
Tachycardia	Difficulty breathing
Altered mental status	Vagal complaints
Pallor	Vague chest-related complaints
Diaphoresis	Asymptomatic
Hypertension	Neurologic complaints
Dyspnea	
Asymmetric pulse pressures	
Vascular bruits	
Focal neurologic findings	

ary to direct vessel injury, traumatic thrombus formation, or vascular compression from a surrounding hematoma. Of great concern are clinical signs of hemorrhagic shock such as hypotension, tachycardia, altered mental status, pallor, and diaphoresis. Often hypertension occurs as a result of increased stimulation of sympathetic nerve fibers in close proximity to the aortic arch.[9] Additionally, many other signs can be subtle. Dyspnea may result for any number of reasons, including associated pulmonary injury, hemothorax, hypovolemia with poor tissue oxygenation, and tamponade. Neurologic symptoms can be present with arterial injury involving the carotids or spinal arteries.

Extremity findings of altered transmission or diminished intensity of the pulse pressure wave suggest intravascular volume depletion or, if asymmetric, direct vascular injury. Femoral pulses are important to note, particularly with respect to upper extremity pulses, because change can indicate vascular injury in the descending aorta resulting in a pseudocoarctation syndrome. Vascular bruits, resulting from turbulent blood flow in the arterial system, either over the precordium or in the interscapular region, are heard in up to 30% of patients with aortic injury.

Unfortunately, none of the signs and symptoms discussed here are specific for making the diagnosis of great vessel injury.[8]

Differential Diagnosis

Great vessel injury should be considered in the differential diagnosis in all patients who present with thoracoabdominal trauma and an appropriate mechanism of injury. Care must be taken not to exclude the diagnosis based solely on the identification of other injuries that may also be contributing to the clinical presentation.

Great vessel injury is easily misdiagnosed in hemodynamically stable patients, particularly those without external signs of trauma, because of the nonspecific nature of the presenting signs and symptoms. Penetrating injury in proximity to any of the great vessels mandates consideration of great vessel injury. However, a diagnosis of blunt injury requires an assessment of the severity of the causative mechanism (e.g., speed, forces) in combination with the patient's presenting complaints and physical examination findings. This pre-test probability will ultimately be used by the clinician to guide further diagnostic work-up of great vessel injury.

Interventions and Procedures

When great vessel trauma is suspected, adequate vascular access should be obtained immediately. Although two large-bore peripheral intravenous lines are frequently cited as sufficient for trauma patients, the benefits of central venous pressure monitoring and rapid large-volume resuscitation may necessitate central access. Ideally, the suspected vascular injury should not be affected by the site chosen for central venopuncture. For example, when penetrating injury of the descending aorta exists, concomitant venal cava injury is possible; therefore, sole femoral or lower extremity access would not be optimal. Unfortunately, in the setting of undifferentiated thoracic trauma, the options may be limited.

Many of the emergent initial resuscitative efforts needed in patients with great vessel trauma are dictated by hemodynamic instability. Patients in traumatic cardiac arrest or extreme hemodymanic compromise unresponsive to crystalloid and packed red blood cell transfusions are candidates for resuscitative thoracotomy in the ED. This procedure is usually performed without knowledge of the exact injury. As such, it must be executed methodically, such that all potential life-saving interventions are performed. Injuries of the ascending aorta or aortic arch mandate manual pressure for hemorrhage control, whereas injuries of the descending aorta require cross-clamping above the site of injury until stability and repair is achieved. Injuries of the aortic arch branch may be tempered by packing the apex of the injured hemithorax. Suspected injury of the right hemithorax requires extension of the thoracotomy into the right side of the chest. A right-sided thoracotomy could be considered in the rare incidence of an isolated transthoracic right-sided penetrating injury.

Identification of a pulmonary hilar injury or excessive bleeding from deep in the thorax, despite aortic cross-clamping, suggests the need to clamp the affected pulmonary hilum. This is achieved either by manual compression with the hand or a vascular clamp. The goal of ED thoracotomy is to achieve sufficient clinical stabilization to allow definitive operative repair.

In patients who are not in traumatic cardiac arrest or in immediate need of a resuscitative thoracotomy, risk stratification of the likelihood of disease is imperative. This is initially achieved through a combination of assessment of mechanism and interpretation of appropriate diagnostic testing.

Figure 85-3 depicts a diagnostic management algorithm for suspected traumatic aortic injury.

Diagnostic Testing

Often great vessel injury is associated with either significant multisystem trauma or distinct penetrating injury. In the first situation, the presenting signs and symptoms of great vessel injury are frequently obscured by other distracting injuries, altered mental status, or intubation, resulting in the need for a high suspicion and low threshold for diagnostic testing. In the second situation, diagnostic testing is mainly driven by pre-test probability for great vessel injury (i.e., the location and mechanism of the injury).

The chest radiograph is the initial diagnostic screening tool used in patients with history of chest

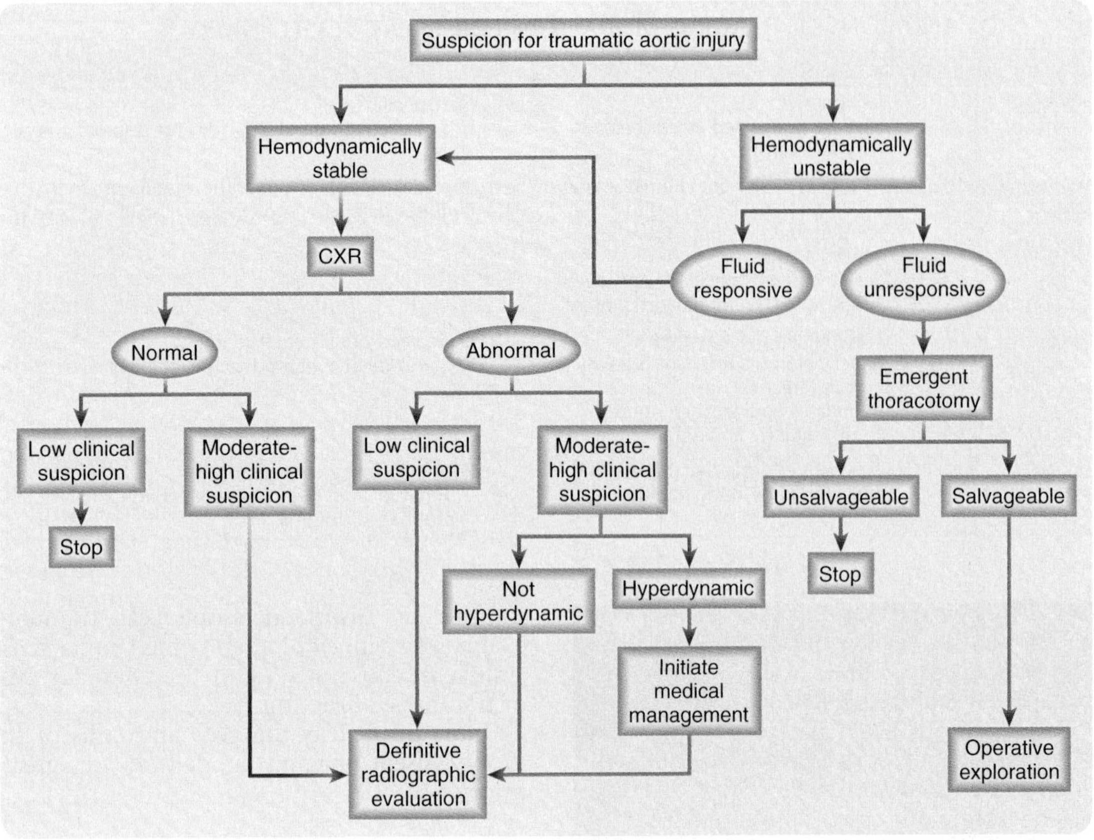
Suspicion for traumatic aortic injury
Hemodynamically stable
Hemodynamically unstable
CXR
Fluid responsive
Fluid unresponsive
Normal
Abnormal
Emergent thoracotomy
Low clinical suspicion
Moderate-high clinical suspicion
Low clinical suspicion
Moderate-high clinical suspicion
Unsalvageable
Salvageable
Stop
Not hyperdynamic
Hyperdynamic
Stop
Initiate medical management
Definitive radiographic evaluation
Operative exploration

FIGURE 85-3 Algorithm for diagnosis and management of suspected traumatic aortic injury.

BOX 85-2

Radiographic Findings Associated with Great Vessel Injuries*

- Superior mediastinal widening
- Indistinct aortic knob
- Left pleural effusion/hemothorax
- Left apical cap
- Deviation of the trachea
- Deviation of nasogastric tube to the right
- Depressed left mainstem bronchus
- Narrowing of carinal angle
- Opacification of aortopulmonary window
- Widening of left or right paraspinous stripe
- Sternal or rib fractures

*Radiographic findings adapted from references 2, 4, and 10.

trauma. An upright, posterior-anterior view provides the best evaluation of the mediastinum. In patients with suspected spinal injury, a portable supine, anterior-posterior view is commonly preferred. Note that in the recumbent position, the mediastinum may appear artificially widened, and a hemothrorax can be obscured.

Chest radiography is not diagnostic for great vessel injury; rather, it is used to identify any of multiple findings suggesting aortic injury. Box 85-2 reviews the classic findings on chest radiographs associated with great vessel injury: a widened superior mediastinum (50%-92%), increased mediastinal width (67%-85%), and indistinct aortic knob (21%-24%) occur with the greatest frequency.[2,10] Figure 85-4 is a chest radiograph demonstrating these three findings.

No single radiograph is sensitive enough to rule out great vessel injury. A normal radiograph is seen in 7% to 10% of injured patients; such a finding should not dissuade the clinician from further testing if the patient's presenting complaint, physical examination, or mechanism of injury indicate a significant pre-test probability.

When great vessel injury is a persistent concern following or despite chest radiography, CTA of the chest should be carried out. This test provides significant information about the patient with thoracic trauma, including identification of mediastinal hematoma and differentiation of the various etiologies. Recent advances in the technology of helical computed tomography have improved the sensitivity and specificity for identifying aortic injury, including isolated intimal tears, such that it approaches 100%.[11,12] Additional benefit exists in its ability to identify concomitant or alternative injuries. The limitations of CTA of the chest for great vessel injury

Table 85-1 PROS AND CONS OF IMAGING MODALITIES FOR GREAT VESSEL INJURY

Modality	Pros	Cons
Chest radiography	Inexpensive May be performed at the bedside Easy to interpret	Nonspecific False-negative rate of 7%-10% for traumatic aortic injury
Computed tomography angiography	Identifies mediastinal hematoma and differentiates its etiologies Identifies aortic injury, including intimal tears Sensitivity and specificity approaches 100% for traumatic aortic injury	Poor delineation of nonaortic vascular injuries Requires relative hemodynamic stability to obtain
Aortography	Traditional gold standard Beneficial in diagnosis of branch vessel injuries Delineates equivocal computed tomography angiograms	Difficult to obtain emergently Requires relative hemodynamic stability
Transesophageal echocardiography	May be performed at the bedside Not limited by body habitus	Poor availability emergently Contraindicated with unstable cervical spine or suspected esophageal trauma

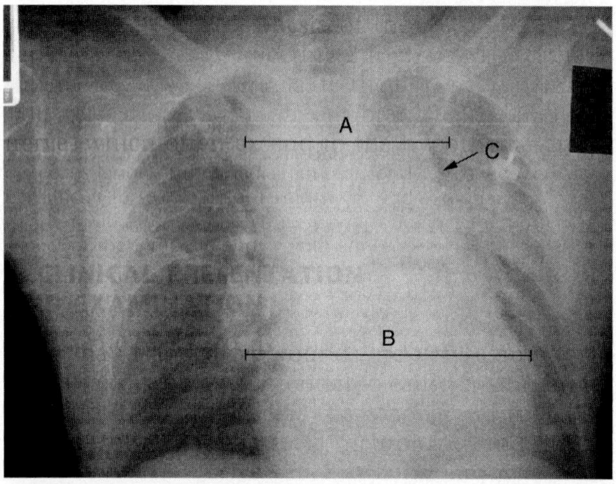
A
B
C

FIGURE 85-4 Chest radiograph demonstrating the three most common findings of traumatic aortic injury: widened superior mediastinum (*A*), increased mediastinal width (*B*), and obscured aortic knob (*C*).

include poor delineation of nonaortic vascular injuries and the need for relative hemodynamic stability in the patient.[4,11]

Because of the ease and accuracy of CTA, use of the traditional gold standard for traumatic aortic injury—aortography—has markedly diminished over the past decade. Its main role now is reserved in the setting of an equivocal CTA finding or to assist in the management of patients requiring delayed management.[4] Arteriography is still used for diagnosis and evaluation of branch vessel injuries when immediate operative intervention is not indicated.

Transesophageal echocardiography is another modality that can be used to evaluate aortic injury. Lack of availability reduces its usefulness in the ED setting, but it should be considered for patients that are too unstable to leave the ED or when body habitus prohibits the use of a CT scanner. Its use is contraindicated in patients with unstable cervical spine injuries or suspected esophageal trauma. Transesophageal echocardiography has similar sensitivities similar to those of CTA of the chest for evaluation of traumatic aortic injury.[12]

Table 85-1 lists the pros and cons of the commonly used imaging modalities for great vessel injury.

Treatment and Disposition

The definitive treatment for great vessel injury usually is surgical repair. With mortality rates associated with these injuries increasing at an estimated rate of 1% per hour over the 48 hours following hospital presentation, expediting the time to operative intervention is imperative.[3] Surgical techniques usually include clamping with aortic reconstruction with or without vascular bypass. Due in part to the need for vascular clamping, paraplegia can be a complication of repair in 4% to 20% of cases.[2,13] Although cross-clamping times are not known to be directly correlated with the incidence of paraplegia, keeping times under 30 minutes is believed to be beneficial.[2,13] More recently, endovascular stenting has become an alternative to open surgical repair.[14,15] Its exact role has yet to be determined, but it may prove most beneficial in patients too unstable for operative repair.

Prior to surgical intervention, medical management is critical and should include pharmacologic reduction of wall tension and shearing forces to prevent propagation of intimal tears and to minimize the risk of subsequent in-hospital catastrophic rupture of a contained hemorrhage. One study demonstrated that starting pharmacologic management as soon as possible, even before a confirmative diagnostic test when suspicion is high, significantly reduced morbidity and mortality.[11]

Beta blockers are first-line medication for reducing wall stress and controlling heart rate. Esmolol is ideal because of its rapid onset of action and its short half-life, making it easy to titrate in a continuous infusion. When further blood pressure control is desired, vasodilators such as nitroprusside can be added after beta-blockade has been established. Because of the potential for reflex tachycardia, which increases shearing forces, caution is advisable when using nitroprusside alone.[16,17]

A second but controversial intervention is permissive hypovolemia, in which blood pressure is controlled by limiting fluid administration. Lower systolic pressures of 60 to 90 mm Hg are believed to decrease the risk of clot rupture and minimize the shear force on traumatized vessels. Patients often have associated pulmonary contusions, which strengthens the rationale for limiting fluid administration prior to operative intervention.[18,19] Animal studies using permissive hypovolemia have shown consistent benefits; human trials have been few with conflicting results.

Two interventions that are often used during global resuscitation require special consideration in the setting of great vessel injury. Central line access provides important information during resuscitative efforts; however, to avoid further vessel damage, it is important to choose a site farthest from the suspected vessel injury. Similar caution must be undertaken when considering chest tube placement to resolve hemothorax. This action may disrupt the containment of a great vessel hemorrhage, with the catastrophic result of patient exsanguination.

Ideally, immediate surgical repair of great vessel injury is recommended. However, delayed repair should be considered in patients with significant associated injuries or hemodynamic instability. Repair of great vessels has been delayed for as long as 6 to 8 months.[20] This approach has yet to be prospectively studied, however, and is not routinely employed.

If a patient survives the first 24 hours without rupture, a stable psuedoaneurysm may develop. In such cases nonoperative management, including close monitoring and pharmacologic control of blood pressure, may be considered.

REFERENCES

1. Campbell NC, Thomason SR, Muckart DJ, et al: Review of 1198 cases of penetrating cardiac trauma. Br J Surg 1997;84:1737-1740.
2. Fabian TC, Richardson JD, Croce MA, et al: Prospective study of blunt aortic injury: Multicenter trial of the American Association of the Surgery of Trauma. J Trauma 1997:42:374-383.
3. Parmley LF, Mattingly TW, Manion WC, et al: Nonpenetrating traumatic injury of the aorta. Circulation 1958;17:1086-1101.
4. Dyer DS, Moore EE, Ilke DN, et al: Thoracic aortic injury: How predictive is mechanism and is chest computed tomography a reliable screening tool? J Trauma 2000; 48:673-683.
5. Ungar TC, Wolf SJ, Haukoos JS, et al: Derivation of a clinical decision rule to exclude thoracic aortic imaging in patients with blunt chest trauma following motor vehicle collisions. J Trauma 2006;61:1150-1155.
6. Horton TG, Cohn SM, Heid MP, et al: Identification of trauma patients at risk of thoracic aortic tear by mechanism of injury. J Trauma 2000;48:1008-1014.
7. Mattox KL, Feliciano DV, Beall AC, et al: Five thousand seven hundred sixty cardiovascular injuries in 4459 patients. Epidemiologic evolution 1958-1988. Ann Surg 1989;209:698-705.
8. Sturm JT, Perry JF Jr, Olson FR, et al: Significance of symptoms and signs in patients with traumatic aortic rupture. Ann Emerg Med 1984;13:876-878.
9. Fox S, Pierce WS, Waldhausen JA: Acute hypertension: Its significance in traumatic aortic rupture. J Thorac Cardiovasc Surg 1979;77:622-625.
10. Mirvis SE, Bidwell JK, Buddemeyer EU, et al: Value of chest radiography in excluding traumatic aortic rupture. Radiology 1987;163:487-493.
11. Fabian TC, Davis, KA, Gavant, ML, et al: Prospective study of blunt aortic injury: Helical CT is diagnostic and antihypertensive therapy reduces rupture. Ann Surg 1998;227: 666-677.
12. Vignon P, Boncoeur MP, Francois B, et al: Comparison of multiplane transesophageal echocardiography and contrast-enhanced helical CT in the diagnosis of blunt traumatic cardiovascular injuries. Anesthesiology 2001;94: 615-622.
13. Razzouk AJ, Gundry SR, Wang N, et al: Repair of traumatic aortic rupture: A 25-year experience. Arch Surg 2000;135: 913-918.
14. Rousseau H, Dambrin C, Marcheix B, et al: Acute traumatic aortic rupture: A comparison of surgical and stent-graft repair. J Thorac Cardiovasc Surg 2005;129:1050-1055.
15. Agostinelli A, Saccani S, Borrello B, et al: Immediate endovascular treatment of blunt aortic injury: Our therapeutic strategy. J Thorac Cardiovasc Surg 2006;131:1053-1057.
16. Walker WA, Pate JW: Medical management of acute traumatic rupture of the aorta. Ann Thorac Surg 1990;50: 965-967.
17. Maggisano R, Nathens A, Alexandrova NA, et al: Traumatic rupture of the thoracic aorta: Should one always operate immediately? Ann Vasc Surg 1995;9:44-52.
18. Bickell WH, Wall MJ Pep P, et al: Immediate versus delayed fluid resuscitation for hypotensive patients with penetrating torso injuries. New Engl J Med 1994;331:1105-1109.
19. Martin RR, Bickell WH, Pep PE, et al: Prospective evaluation of preoperative fluid resuscitation in hypotensive patients with penetrating truncal injury: A preliminary report. J Trauma 1992;33:354-61.
20. Duhaylongsod FG, Glower DD, Wolfe WG: Acute traumatic aortic aneurysm: The Duke experience from 1970-1990. J Vasc Surg 1992;15:331-342.

Chapter **86**

Acute Compartment Syndrome

David A. Peak

KEY POINTS

Pain out of proportion to the clinical situation is the paramount feature of acute compartment syndrome and often is the only early finding.

Acute compartment syndrome can occur in any closed anatomic space, although the most common sites are the lower leg and forearm.

Serial examinations should be performed when acute compartment syndrome is suspected.

Increasing pain, pain refractory to analgesia, and the need for increasing analgesia are common in acute compartment syndrome.

Pain is exacerbated by active or passive movement of the contents of the affected compartment.

In early cases the neurovascular examination often is normal.

Early diagnosis, consultation, and treatment are the keys to a good outcome.

Scope and Outline

Acute compartment syndrome is a condition in which perfusion pressures falls below tissue pressure in a closed anatomic space, with subsequent compromise of circulation and function of tissues. Initially described in the orthopedic and trauma literature in 1872 by Von Volkmann as myofascial compartment syndrome, this concept has been expanded to include the same phenomenon in any circumscribed body cavity. Increased compartment pressure, when exceeding capillary perfusion pressure, leads to a cycle of decreased tissue perfusion, tissue ischemia, and, if not reversed, cell death.[1] Pain out of proportion to the original injury is the paramount feature. Prompt recognition and treatment is required in order to avert devastating results.

The most common anatomic sites are the lower leg and the forearm, but compartment syndrome can occur anywhere in the body where a compartment exists. It has been reported in the hand, forearm, upper arm, abdomen, cranial vault, thorax/mediastinum, buttock, orbit, paraspinal muscles, and entire lower extremity.

Untreated, acute compartment syndrome leads to tissue necrosis, nerve injury, permanent functional impairment, and, in some cases, renal failure and death. Hypoesthesia and painful dysesthesia can result. Little or no return of function can be expected when diagnosis and treatment are delayed. A delayed or missed diagnosis is a potentially devastating occurrence.

Pathophysiology

Tissue perfusion is proportional to the difference between the capillary perfusion pressure (CPP) and the interstitial pressure. This can be stated by the formula LBP = (PA − PV)/R, where LBP is local blood flow, PA is local arterial pressure, PV is venous pressure, and R is local vascular resistance. When fluid is introduced into a fixed volume compartment, tissue pressure increases and venous pressure rises. Some reduction in the local arteriovenous gradient can be compensated for by autoregulatory changes in local vascular resistance. However, once the autoregulatory function is overwhelmed, compartment syndrome is likely to ensue.

When interstitial pressure exceeds CPP (a narrow arteriovenous perfusion gradient), capillaries collapse and muscle and tissue ischemia occurs.[2] Compartment syndrome is characterized by a self-propagating cycle of impaired perfusion resulting in ischemia, edema, and rising interstitial pressures, which further compromise capillary flow.

With myocyte ischemia and necrosis, myofibrillar proteins decompose into osmotically active particles, which attract water from arterial blood, thus further increasing pressure. One milliosmole is estimated to exert a pressure of 19.5 mm Hg; therefore, a relatively small increase in osmotically active particles in a closed space attracts sufficient fluid to cause a further rise in intramuscular pressure.

External pressure-induced functional deficits are likely due to decreased tissue perfusion rather than to a direct mechanical effect. The amount of pressure a limb can tolerate depends on a variety of factors, including blood pressure, limb elevation, hemorrhage, and arterial occlusion. The pathophysiology of acute compartment syndrome with vascular trauma is even more complex secondary to ischemia and reperfusion phenomenon.

Acute compartment syndrome may result from either externally applied compressive forces or internally expanding forces, and many authors make this distinction. Others prefer to separate etiologies into traumatic and atraumatic (so called "well-limb") etiologies (Box 86-1). Myofascial etiologies include long bone fracture, vascular injury, reperfusion after ischemia, crush injury, burns, prolonged positioning from drug overdose or operating procedures, compression from tight casts and dressings (including military antishock trousers [MAST]), overexertion, hemorrhage from coagulopathies, compartment fluid injection, massive IV fluid infusions, envenomations, hypothyroidism, and rhabdomyolysis; it also has been seen with deep vein thrombosis and ruptured Baker's cyst.

The lower leg is the most common site and the anterior component is most frequently affected, followed by the lateral and posterior components. Acute compartment syndrome associated with tibia fracture accounts for as many as 45% of all cases. It is more common in open as compared with closed fractures.[3] Because the incidence of acute compartment syndrome is much higher with an associated vascular damage, many surgeons perform prophylactic fasciotomy at the time of vascular repair in high-risk patients (Fig. 86-1).[4]

BOX 86-1

Etiologies of Acute Compartment Syndrome

Internally Applied Force
- Long bone fractures
- Vascular injury
- Overexertion (including seizures)
- Hemorrhage/coagulopathy
- Compartment fluid injection
- Massive IV infusions
- Envenomations
- Deep venous thrombosis/ruptured Baker's cyst
- Reperfusion after ischemia

Externally Applied Force
- Burns
- Crush injury
- Tight casts, dressings, military antishock trousers (MAST)
- Prolonged awkward positioning
- Closure of fascial defects

Posttraumatic Etiologies
- Long bone fractures
- Vascular injury
- Reperfusion
- Crush injury
- Overexertion
- Compartment fluid injection
- Envenomation

"Well-Limb" Etiologies
- Prolonged awkward positioning
- Hypothyroidism
- Rhabdomyolysis
- Nephrotic syndrome

Presentation

Acute compartment syndrome is a clinical diagnosis. The essential clinical feature in a conscious patient is severe pain out of proportion to the injury, which is aggravated by active or passive stretching of the muscles of the affected compartment. In early cases, pain is the only abnormality. Increasing pain and/or

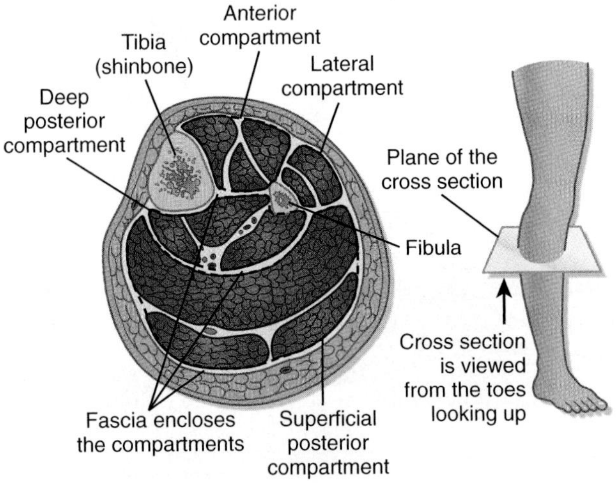
Anterior compartment
Tibia (shinbone)
Lateral compartment
Deep posterior compartment
Plane of the cross section
Fibula
Cross section is viewed from the toes looking up
Fascia encloses the compartments
Superficial posterior compartment

FIGURE 86-1 Compartments of the leg.

pain refractory to analgesics suggests the diagnosis. Severe pain while at rest or without any movement should raise suspicion of acute compartment syndrome.

Increasing need for analgesia or increased dosing of analgesia is common. The diagnosis may be more challenging in unconscious patients, children, and patients with regional nerve blocks or spinal cord injury. Compartment syndromes usually present hours after the inciting event and uncommonly present more than 48 hours of injury.

The EP must remain vigilant and retain a high index of suspicion to avoid missing the diagnosis. Serial examinations are often required.

A high level of suspicion should be maintained when evaluating long bone fractures; penetrating injuries, especially those with vascular injuries due to iatrogenic arterial puncture, extravagated or caustic medications, or repetitive venous sticks; crush injuries; injuries characterized by severe or increasing pain at rest after vigorous muscular activity, after extrinsic compression from casts or dressings, or after prolonged, awkward positioning; injuries due to high-velocity mechanisms; and injuries in patients on anticoagulation therapy or with a coagulopathy. The presence of seizures or tetany also should raise suspicion of compartment syndrome.

The natural progression of untreated acute compartment syndrome is severe pain, decreased sensation, decreased strength, and eventual paralysis of the affected limb. With the exception of pain, the traditional five Ps (pain, paresthesia, pallor, pulselessness, poikilothermia) are NOT clinically reliable. Paresthesia is the earliest objective physical abnormality and represents ongoing ischemia. Severe cases, even those with extensive myonecrosis, can be characterized by palpable pulses and normal capillary refill.

The primary pathology is within the affected compartment, in contradistinction to a vascular injury in which the pathology is downstream to the deficit. Early pulse deficits should raise suspicion

BOX 86-2

Scenarios Suggesting Acute Compartment Syndrome

- Long bone fracture
- High-velocity trauma
- Crush injury
- Reperfusion after ischemia
- Fracture with concomitant vascular injury
- Pain out of proportion to injury/clinical scenario
- Increasing pain/analgesia requirement
- Increasing pain without movement/during rest
- Unconsciousness after significant trauma
- Spinal cord injury/regional nerve block with appropriate precipitant
- Penetrating injury (especially with vascular injury)
- Coagulopathy
- Vascular injury, including iatrogenic arterial puncture
- Extravagated or caustic medications
- Envenomation
- Severe pain after vigorous muscle activity
- Seizures or tetany
- Severe pain after extrinsic compression or prolonged awkward positioning

PRIORITY ACTIONS

1. Suspect acute compartment syndrome when a patient has severe pain, especially with passive movement, but few other objective physical findings.
2. Measure compartment pressures when patient has severe pain.
3. Consult orthopedic or general surgery department.
4. Treat hypotension and anemia, provide oxygen, and reverse coagulopathy if present.

of a vascular injury appearing alone or coexisting with acute compartment syndrome. Scenarios suggesting acute compartment syndrome are listed in Box 86-2.

Special Situations

■ PAINLESS COMPARTMENT SYNDROME

If the diagnosis is significantly delayed, loss of nerve function can result in a "painless" compartment syndrome, but paralysis, weakness, and other physical abnormalities remain. The presentation is normally within hours of the precipitating event, but it is not uncommon for patients, after prolonged awkward positioning (prolonged lithotomy position in the operating room, for example, or a patient with drug or alcohol intoxication), to present up to 12 to 24 hours later.

■ ACUTE ORBITAL COMPARTMENT SYNDROME

Acute orbital compartment syndrome is considered a rare complication of facial trauma (usually blunt) or surgery. The globe and retrobulbar contents are encased in a continuous cone-shaped fascial envelope that is bound on all sides by seven rigid bony walls, except anteriorly, where the orbital septum and eyelids form another, fairly inflexible boundary. The medial and lateral canthal tendons attach the eyelids to the orbit rim and limit the forward movement of the globe.

The orbit may compensate for small increases in orbital volume by forward movement of the globe and prolapse of fat, followed immediately by a rapid rise in orbital tissue pressures. The orbit, therefore, follows pressure-volume dynamics with a pathophysiology akin to other compartment syndromes, in which increased tissue pressures in an enclosed space are associated with decreased perfusion. Ischemia ensues when the orbital pressure exceeds central retinal artery pressure.

Symptoms and signs include eye pain, visual loss, proptosis, reduction of ocular motility, diplopia, increased intraocular pressure, chemosis, and (late) afferent pupillary defect. Diagnosis requires high clinical suspicion and may require serial examinations, including visual acuity tests.

Suspected acute orbital compartment syndrome with a decrease in vision, loss of vision with increasing intraocular pressures, or high suspicion in a comatose patient requires treatment in order to prevent permanent blindness. Computed tomography or magnetic resonance imaging may help identify the etiology of compression, exclude alternative diagnoses, and establish the diagnosis, but these modalities are not necessary in every case. Irreversible optic nerve pathology may occur in as little as 2 hours of ischemia.

Medical therapy and ophthalmologic consultation should proceed promptly, before the diagnosis is established. Osmotic agents and carbonic anhydrase inhibitors are part of established protocols at many centers. Most experts also recommend high-dose steroid therapy. Less agreement exists about the use of topical beta-blockers and multiple osmotic agents.

The emergency procedure of choice for visual acuity loss associated with acute orbital compartment syndrome is lateral canthotomy or cantholysis of the canthal ligaments (Box 86-3; Figs. 86-2 and 86-3; Tips and Tricks box). Primary indications for lateral canthotomy and cantholysis include intraocular pressure greater than 40 mm Hg, as well as proptosis, which may be used as a criterion for unconscious patients whose visual acuity cannot be determined. Secondary criteria include afferent pupillary defect, ophthalmoplegia, cherry-red macula, optic nerve head pallor, and severe pain, but these are all considered less sensitive or very late signs.

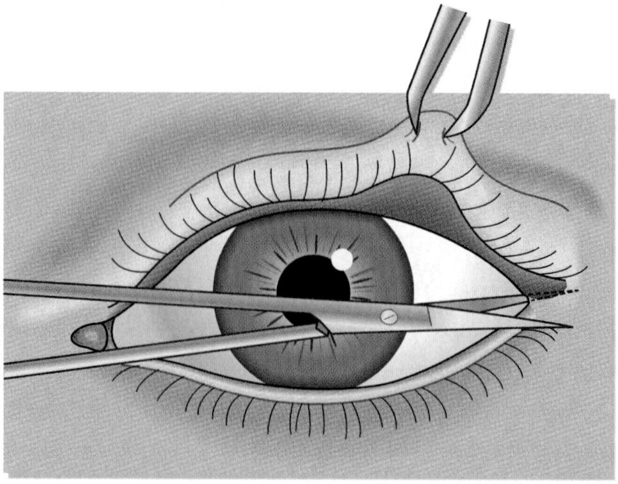

FIGURE 86-2 Lateral canthotomy.

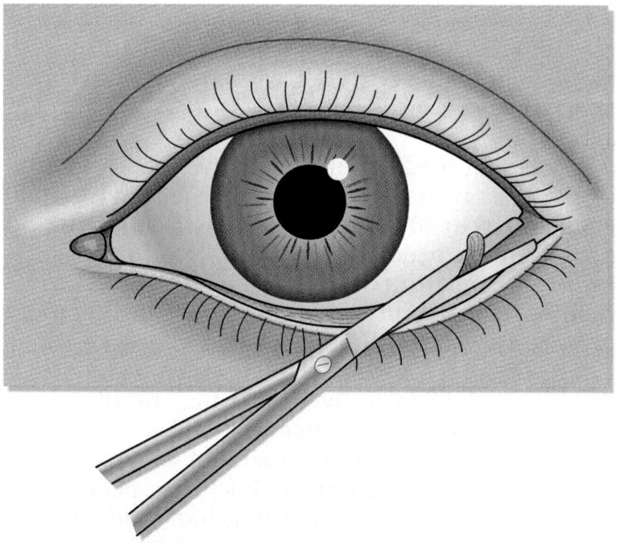

FIGURE 86-3 Canthal ligament cantholysis.

BOX 86-3

Primary Indications for Lateral Canthotomy/Cantholysis

- Suspected orbital compartment syndrome with one or both of the following:
  - Decreasing vision
  - Increasing intraocular pressures
- When vision cannot be assessed (e.g., a comatose patient)

Tips and Tricks

LATERAL CANTHOTOMY/CANTHAL LIGAMENT CANTHOLYSIS PROCEDURE

Lateral Canthotomy

- Stabilize patient's head and lids.
- Anesthesize lateral canthus with lidocaine with or without epinephrine.
- Crush canthus with hemostat for 30 to 60 seconds.
- Incise canthus using straight sharp-edged scissor, making a horizontal incision over crushed canthus and continuing to bony orbital rim (see Fig. 86-2).
- Avoid orbit during incision.

Cantholysis Sweep Technique

- Starting lateral to the midline, carefully sweep the lateral edge of the open faced straight or curved blunt-edged scissors along the palpebral conjunctiva toward the canthotomy incision with care to avoid the orbit/orbital conjunctiva.
- The canthal ligament will be identified as the structure along the orbital rim that prevents a completely smooth sweep to the canthotomy incision.
- Identify and isolate the ligament with the open scissor blade (see Fig. 86-3).
- Carefully maneuver the opposing scissor blade into place avoiding the globe.
- Cut the canthal ligament.
- The lid will now be freely mobile with distraction.
- Repeat for remaining inferior or superior canthal ligaments.

A contraindication for lateral canthotomy is a suspected ruptured globe. In an experimental model, lateral canthotomy produced a mean intraocular pressure decrease of 14.2 mm Hg, isolated disinsertion of 19.2 mm Hg, and combined values of 30.4 mm Hg.[5] EPs should be familiar with and able to perform this procedure in the event that emergent ophthalmology consultation is delayed.

■ ABDOMINAL COMPARTMENT SYNDROME

Abdominal compartment syndrome is a sudden increase in intrabdominal pressure resulting in dysfunction of the respiratory, cardiovascular, and renal systems.[6] Normal intraabdominal pressure is 0 to 5 mm Hg. Acute abdominal compartment syndrome is defined by the 2004 International Abdominal Compartment Syndrome Consensus Definitions Conference Committee as sustained intraabdominal pressure greater than 20 mm Hg that is associated with new organ dysfunction or failure. It is most common after abdominal surgical procedures but can also occur with peritonitis, intraabdominal abscess, intestinal obstructions, ruptured abdominal aneurysms, acute pancreatitis, intra- or retroperitoneal hemorrhage, ascites, ovarian tumors, and massive edema following resuscitation.

Diagnosis depends on a high clinical suspicion combined with the presence of clinical parameters including elevated intraabdominal pressure greater than 20 to 25 mm Hg (most commonly assessed with a device used to measure bladder pressure), distended abdomen, elevated peak airway pressures, large IV fluid requirements, elevated central venous pressure, oliguria or anuria not responding to volume repletion, decreased cardiac output, hypoxemia, hypercapnia, acidosis, and a wide pulse pressure.

Treatment consists of rapid surgical decompression as well as restoration of intravascular volume, maximation of oxygen delivery, and correction of acidosis and/or coagulopathies. Mortality associated with abdominal compartment syndrome can exceed 50%.

■ CHRONIC COMPARTMENT SYNDROME

Chronic compartment syndrome was first described in 1956 and initially thought to be a form of shin splints (anterior tibial enthesitis). Chronic compartment syndrome (also known as exertional or recurrent compartment syndrome) is not a surgical emergency. It is commonly reproducible with a certain specific exercise or exercise distance. Symptoms subside with termination of the exercise and are minimal with normal daily the exercise. When suspected, patients should be advised to rest and be referred to an orthopedic or sports medicine specialist.

Differential Diagnosis

The differential diagnosis includes any disorder that can cause musculoskeletal pain, including fracture, contusions, and hematomas; however, pain due to other etiologies generally dimishes after the inciting event, whereas in acute compartment syndrome, the pain generally increases even while the patient is at rest. The pain will be exacerbated by either active or passive movement of the affected compartment, but movement will exacerbate many types of musculoskeletal pain due to other etiologies.

The increasing need for analgesia is a common finding, and EPs should consider the diagnosis of acute compartment syndrome rather than assume that the patient has a high narcotic tolerance or drug-seeking behavior. The presence of more than one of the traditional five Ps acutely should alert the EP to the possibility of a vascular injury.

Acute compartment syndrome should be on the working list of "worst-case" diagnoses for every patient with musculoskeletal pain.

Physical Examination

The physical examination should focus on evidence of trauma and gross deformity as well as assessment of neurovascular abnormalities. Comparing one extremity to the unaffected side is often very useful.

Excessively vigorous examination may exacerbate the disorder. Sensory nerves are affected before motor nerves, but any abnormal neurologic examination result infers ongoing ischemia. Decreased two-point discrimination is consistently the earliest physical abnormality and can help differentiate which compartments are affected. Correlation has also been reported between decreasing vibratory sense (256 cycles per second) and increasing compartment pressure. On deep palpation, a firm "wooden" feeling is a specific sign when associated with a late diagnosis.

Diagnostic Testing

■ RADIOGRAPHY

The diagnosis cannot be made with radiographic imaging. However, because the differential diagnosis for acute compartment syndrome includes fracture or dislocation, and because the risk of compartment syndrome increases with fracture, radiographic imaging should be useful.

■ COMPUTED TOMOGRAPHY

Computed tomography rarely is indicated but may be helpful in ruling out the diagnosis of orbital and abdominal compartment syndromes.

■ LABORATORY TESTS

A creatine kinase level of 1000 to 5000 U/mL or higher or the presence of myoglobinuria may alert the EP to the presence of compartment syndrome in a muscle. Because the renal threshold for myoglobin is low (about 0.5 mg /100 mL of urine), only approximately 200 g of muscle need to be damaged to cause visible changes in the urine. Serial values may be helpful.

Other laboratory tests that should be checked include blood urea nitrogen/creatinine, potassium (myonecrosis can result in life-threatening hyperkalemia), complete blood count (anemia worsens muscle ischemia), coagulation panel (disseminated intravascular coagulation is a rare occurrence), and urinalysis. It may be prudent to obtain a complete preoperative laboratory test panel.

■ MEASUREMENT OF INTRACOMPARTMENTAL PRESSURES

Measurement of intracompartmental pressures is not necessary if the diagnosis of acute compartment syndrome is clinically apparent.[7] Equivocal cases may require further work-up. Dedicated devices for measuring compartmental pressures are commercially available. Devices that use a side-ported needle or slit catheter are recommended rather than those using a simple needle.

Some EDs use an arterial line set-up. Once calibrated, a needle inserted into the compartment (after local anesthesia) supplies a pressure reading. When formal devices are not available, such a set-up gives a crude indication of the compartment pressure.

Normal intracompartmental pressures are in the range of 0 to 10 mm Hg. Pain and paresthesias are common at 20-30 mmHg, and ischemia generally ensues at pressures greater than 30 mm Hg. Many surgeons traditionally consider a measured compartment pressure of 30 mm Hg or higher as a cutoff indication for fasciotomy,[8] although higher numbers have been used, especially for the thigh. More recently, some authors recommended using a delta-P value (diastolic blood pressure minus the measured intracompartment pressure) of less than 30 to 50 mm Hg as an indication for fasciotomy and have found this more reliable than an absolute compartment pressure.

Treatment

Surgical speciality evaluation is mandatory in suspected cases because the therapy for compartment syndrome is usually surgical decompression. In addition to consultation, the following measures should be considered (Box 86-4).

The affected limb should be placed at the level of the heart. Elevation is contraindicated because it decreases arterial flow, which narrows the arterial venous pressure gradient and thus worsens ischemia. Elevated compartment pressures lead to ischemia pathophysiologically.

Because hypotension potentiates compartment syndrome, it should be corrected with crystalloid or

BOX 86-4

Management of Acute Compartment Syndrome

- Consult surgery department.
- Maintain affected area at level of heart.
- Reverse hypoperfusion/hypotension.
- Maximize oxygenation/employ supplemental oxygen.
- Correct coagulopathy if present.
- Correct anemia if present.
- Modify cast/splint/dressing if this is the precipitant of the syndrome.
- Order antivenoms if envenomation is the cause of the syndrome.

Documentation

- History: Mechanism, timing, paresthesia, weakness, medical conditions that may impair oxygenation or perfusion, coagulopathy or anticoagulation therapy, IV drug use, increasing pain, pain with active or passive movement.
- Physical examination: Neurovascular signs, compartment palpation, discoloration, masses, range of motion.
- Medical decision making: Reasons to pursue or not pursue work-up and/or consultation.
- Procedures: Compartment pressures if measured; canthotomy/cantholysis if performed.
- Patient instructions: Discuss with patient the remote possibility of acute compartment syndrome, warning signs, what to do if symptoms recur, when to return to the ED.

blood products. Routine use of supplemental oxygen should be employed to improve tissue oxygenation.

Pressure from constrictions or casts must be relieved. If a cast is causing pain, the plaster should be cut. Releasing one side of a plaster cast may reduce compartment pressures by 30%, bivalving can produce an additional 35% reduction, and cutting under cast padding may decrease compartment pressures 10% to 20%.

Mannitol is used in some centers. The literature supports its use for rhabdomyolysis but the data are currently insufficient for its effectiveness in compartment syndrome. In renal failure related to myoglobinuria, mannitol decreases blood viscosity and oncotic pressure across the glomerulus, causing an increased glomerlular filtration rate; dilates glomerular capillaries; stimulates prostaglandin release; increases proximal intratubular flow; and possibly reduces tubular cell swelling.

Hyperbaric oxygen promotes hyperoxic vasoconstriction, which reduces swelling and edema and improves local blood flow and oxygenation. Hyperbaric oxygen also increases tissue oxygen tension and improves survival of marginally viable tissue. Compartment syndrome, crush injury, and acute traumatic ischemia are included in the 13 major syndromes amenable to hyperbaric oxygen by the Undersea and Hyperbaric Medical Society Hyperbaric Oxygen Committee, and its use is supported by limited literature.

Treatment of acute compartment syndrome following snake envenomation is extremely controversial. The etiology is multifactorial, and myonecrosis secondary to direct toxic effects plays a key role. These patients should be treated aggressively with antivenoms.

PATIENT TEACHING TIPS

- Inform trauma patient, patient with musculoskeletal pain, and patient leaving with splints/casts/wrappings about the remote possibility of acute compartment syndrome.
- Educate the patient about normal healing of an injury: there should be a consistent, gradual decrease of pain, swelling, and discoloration.
- Instruct the patient to return to the ED if pain increases or if there is numbness or weakness.

Disposition and Referral

- All patients with acute compartment syndrome must be admitted to the hospital. Most will be transferred to the operating room for emergent fasciotomy or surgical decompression.
- Patients with abnormal compartment measurements that do not reach the threshold for emergent surgical decompression should be admitted for observation.
- Patients with suspected impending acute compartment syndrome should be admitted for serial examinations and observation.
- Patients with significant extremity pain, but who do not have clinical evidence of acute compartment syndrome should be counseled to avoid activity, maintain the extremity at the level of the heart, return if there is any increase in pain, and undergo reevaluation, perhaps as soon as the following day.

REFERENCES

1. Whitesides TE, Hanley TC, Morimoto K: Tissue pressure measurements as a determinant for the need of fasciotomy. Clin Orthop Relat Res 1975;113:43-51.
2. Matsen FA III: Compartment syndrome. A unified concept. Clin Orthop Relat Res 1975;113:8-14.
3. DeLee JC, Stiehl JB: Open tibia fracture with compartment syndrome. Clin Orthop Relat Res 1981;160:175-184.
4. Feliciano DV, Cruse PA, Spjut-Patrinely V, et al: Fasciotomy after trauma to the extremities. Am J Surg 1988;156:533-536.
5. Yung CW, Moorthy RS, Lindley D, et al: Efficacy of lateral canthotomy and cantholysis in orbital hemorrhage. Ophthal Plast Reconstr Surg 1994;10:137-141.
6. Schein M, Wittman DH, Aprahamian CC, et al: The abdominal compartment syndrome: The physiological and clinical consequences of elevated intra-abdominal pressure. J Am Coll Surg. 1995;180:745-753.
7. Tiwari A, Haq AI, Myint F, et al: Acute compartment syndromes. Br J Surg 2002;89:397-412.
8. McQueen MM, Court-Brown CM: Compartment monitoring in tibial fractures. The pressure threshold for decompression. J Bone Joint Surg Br 1996;78:99-104.

Chapter **87**

Low Back Pain

Gerard S. Doyle

KEY POINTS

Nonspecific low back pain is usually self-limited and of short duration: about 60% of cases will resolve within 1 week and 90% within 2 to 6 weeks.

Clues pointing to inflammatory, infectious, neurologic, and oncologic disorders as possible causes of low back pain may be subtle and easily missed.

Rather than using broad screening studies, testing should be directed toward specific diagnostic concerns.

The primary treatment option for back pain is nonsteroidal anti-inflammatory drugs (NSAIDs), with opioids used judiciously. Skeletal muscle relaxants have not been shown to improve outcomes and have significant side effects, even though some patients do report relief.

Patients who have pain longer than 2 weeks, or who at any time develop leg weakness, bowel or bladder dysfunction, fever, or new adverse symptoms should be reevaluated.

Scope

Most adults will experience low back pain at some point in their lifetime, and about 30% of adults report having experienced low back pain within a 3-month study period. Yearly direct and total costs due to low back pain are measured in the billions of dollars. Most cases occur without objective evidence of serious pathology, which may lead the physician to complacent evaluation of a benign disorder. Conversely, the pain can be incapacitating, and the patient may perceive the problem as a harbinger of death or disability, regardless of the cause.

Low back pain may be an acute one-time event that responds to treatment and largely resolves within 2 weeks; however, many cases seen in the ED do not fit this category. Low back pain also can be a chronic condition subject to exacerbations, akin to asthma and diabetes mellitus.[1]

Patient expectations of a specific diagnosis of the source of their pain and a complete cure are rarely met and are probably unrealistic. Psychological, social, and economic factors play a role in the natural history of many pain-related conditions, including the progression of low back pain from an acute to a chronic condition. These issues combine to make low back pain a source of frustration for patients and physicians alike.

Pathophysiology

Low back pain is a symptom complex caused by a variety of diseases and anatomic abnormalities. Multiple potential sources of pain both intrinsic and extrinsic to the spinal column have been implicated, including synovial joints (facets and articular processes of the vertebrae and the sacroiliac joint) and cartilaginous joints (intervertebral disk), vertebral bones, periosteum, ligaments, meninges, paraspinous muscles, fascia, blood vessels, and nerves. Additionally, a number of visceral organs may be a source of pain referred to the low back.

Low back pain is often classified as "specific" or "nonspecific," "mechanical" or "nonmechanical," or "primary" or "secondary" or is classified on the basis of presumed etiology (structural, neoplastic, referred pain/visceral, infectious, inflammatory, or metabolic). All these classification systems recognize that in the majority of cases a specific pathoanatomic diagnosis cannot be assigned. Indeed, a clear correlation between a specific anatomic abnormality and pain is rarely established in patients, and proposed mechanisms of pain in the medical literature have been fraught with controversy. For example, in many asymptomatic subjects, magnetic resonance imaging (MRI) studies showed evidence of bulging, prolapsed, or herniated intervertebral disks.[2]

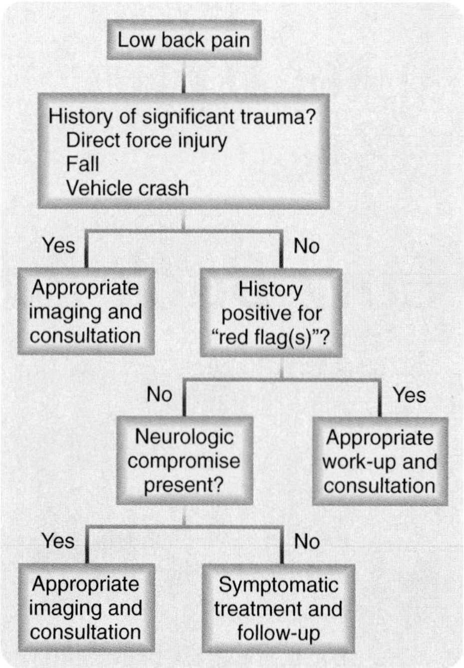
Low back pain
History of significant trauma?
Direct force injury
Fall
Vehicle crash
Yes
No
Appropriate imaging and consultation
History positive for "red flag(s)"?
No
Yes
Neurologic compromise present?
Appropriate work-up and consultation
Yes
No
Appropriate imaging and consultation
Symptomatic treatment and follow-up

FIGURE 87-1 Diagnostic approach to low back pain.

Presenting Signs and Symptoms

■ CLASSIC SYMPTOMS

In general, patients present with pain described as a dull ache that is mild to moderate in intensity. Onset is frequently attributed by patients to lifting or bending or twisting activities and may be abrupt. Movement tends to exacerbate the pain, whereas rest, especially recumbency, minimizes or relieves it. The pain can be midline, unilateral, or bilateral and may radiate to the buttocks or thighs. Due to the recurrent nature of low back pain, many patients have experienced similar pain in the past.

■ TYPICAL VARIATIONS

Pain that is not relieved or that worsens when the patient lies down, as well as pain that awakens the patient from sleep are concerning because they may portend systemic sources of the pain. Pain that is unremitting for more than 4 to 6 weeks or that continues despite adequate analgesia and rest usually has a specific cause.

Low back pain can present alone or as one of a constellation of associated symptoms that frequently are more important than the pain itself in determining an accurate diagnosis and treatment plan. Certain symptoms, comorbid diseases, medication use, and signs are "red flags" in that they point to specific, often serious, diagnoses.

Differential Diagnosis

Nonmechanical causes must be distinguished from mechanical causes of low back pain. The key to this distinction rests on eliminating systemic (infectious, neoplastic, metabolic, or inflammatory) and visceral causes. Figure 87-1 shows one diagnostic approach, and Table 87-1 lists the differential diagnosis of low back pain.

Specific causes of low back pain are shown in Table 87-2, together with signs or symptoms that may suggest these diagnoses. When the history and physical suggest a nonmechanical cause of low back pain, appropriate diagnostic testing and/or specialty consultation is necessary to confirm or rule out the suspected specific cause(s).

Visceral and systemic etiologies of low back pain, although rarely found in most ambulatory care settings, must be addressed. Visceral sources of referred pain that cause low back pain can result from a variety of vascular, pelvic, renal, and gastrointestinal pathology. Pain from aortic dissection, for example, can be referred to the back. Similarly, retroperitoneal pathology of any source, including hematomas and metastatic disease, can cause low back pain. Patients with pain from these sources may or may not have clues to the source of their pain. The diagnostic clues of aortic dissection may include a diminished femoral pulse or mottling of a leg. Because testicular cancer metastasizes to the retroperitoneum, genitourinary examination might identify the pathology.

A retroperitoneal hematoma may be heralded only by tachycardia or, rarely, by hypotension from blood loss. More commonly, warfarin or an antiplatelet agent may be a contributing factor. Any of these clues may be subtle but may also be the only evidence of an important diagnosis.

Systemic causes of low back pain are disease processes that involve the structures of the spinal column, including cancer, infection, inflammation, and degenerative processes. Cancer (with metastatic or primary tumor invasion of the spinal column) typically occurs in those over 50 years of age. Weight

Table 87-1 **DIFFERENTIAL DIAGNOSIS OF LOW BACK PAIN***

Mechanical Lower Back or Leg Pain (97%)†	Nonmechanical Spine Conditions (~1%)‡	Visceral Disease (2%)
Lumbar strain, sprain (70%)§	Neoplasia (0.7%)	Disease of pelvic organs
Degeneration of disks and facets, usually age-related (10%)	Multiple myeloma	Prostatitis
Herniated disk (4%)	Metastatic carcinoma	Endometriosis
Spinal stenosis (3%)	Lymphoma and leukemia	Chronic pelvic inflammatory disease
Osteoporotic compression fracture (4%)	Spinal cord tumors	Renal disease
Spondylolisthesis (2%)	Retroperitoneal tumors	Nephrolithiasis
Traumatic fracture (<1%)	Primary vertebral tumors	Pyelonephritis
Congenital disease (<1%)	Infection (0.01%)	Perinephric abscess
Severe kyphosis	Osteomyelitis	Aortic aneurysm
Severe scoliosis	Septic diskitis	Gastrointestinal disease
Transitional vertebrae	Paraspinous abscess	Pancreatitis
Spondylolysis¶	*Shingles*	Cholecystitis
Internal disk disruption or diskogenic low back pain¶	Inflammatory arthritis (often associated with HLA-B27) (0.3%)	Penetrating ulcer
Presumed instability**	Ankylosing spondylitis Psoriatic spondylitis Reiter's syndrome Inflammatory bowel disease Scheuermann's disease (osteochondrosis) Paget's disease of bone	

*Figures in parentheses indicate the estimated percentages of patients with these conditions among all adult patients with low back pain in primary care. Diagnoses shown in italics often are associated with neurogenic leg pain. Percentages may vary substantially according to demographic characteristics or referral patterns in a practice. For example, spinal stenosis and osteoporosis are more common among geriatric patients, spinal infection among injection-drug users, and so forth.

†The term *mechanical* is used here to designate an anatomic or functional abnormality without underlying malignant, neoplastic, or inflammatory disease. Approximately 2% of cases of mechanical low back pain or leg pain are accounted for by spondylolysis, internal disk disruption or discogenic low back pain, and presumed instability.

‡Scheuermann's disease and Paget's disease of bone probably account for less than 0.01% of nonmechanical spinal conditions.

§"Strain" and "sprain" are nonspecific terms with no pathoanatomic confirmation. "Nonspecific low back pain" or "idiopathic low back pain" may be a preferable term.

¶Spondylolysis is as common among asymptomatic persons as among those with low back pain; thus its role in causing low back pain remains ambiguous.

¶Internal disk disruption is diagnosed by provocative diskography (injection of contrast material into a degenerated disk, with assessment of pain at the time of injection). However, diskography often causes pain in asymptomatic adults, and the condition in many patients with positive diskograms improves spontaneously. Thus the clinical importance and appropriate management of this condition remain unclear. The term "diskogenic lower back pain" is used more or less synonymously with the term "internal disk disruption."

**Presumed instability is loosely defined as greater than 10 degrees of angulation or 4 mm of vertebral displacement on lateral flexion and extension radiograms. However, the diagnostic criteria, natural history, and surgical indications remain controversial.

HLA-B27, human leukocyte antigen B27.

From Jarvik JG, Deyo RA: Diagnostic evaluation of low back pain with emphasis on imaging. Ann Intern Med 2002;137:586-597.

loss, pain with bed rest, and failure of therapy (with pain lasting a month or more) are frequent symptoms. Back pain in any patient with a history of cancer should be considered to be due to a cancerous lesion of the spine until this is ruled out.[3]

Infections involving the spine (osteomyelitis, diskitis, and epidural abscess) are rare and difficult to diagnose but may be detected with careful attention to history and the physical examination. Patients with sickle cell disease are predisposed to *Salmonella* osteomyelitis. Patients with immunosuppression or human immunodeficiency virus, chronic corticosteroid therapy, injection drug use, and recent bacterial infections (cellulitis, pneumonia, urinary tract infection) are at increased risk for abscess, osteomyelitis, and diskitis.

Inflammatory arthridites such as ankylosing spondylitis can cause low back pain but frequently present with other arthritic and systemic symptoms. Patients with these diseases usually report pain that worsens with lying down as well as morning stiffness that gradually improves with activity. Pain is usually chronic, lasting 3 months or more, and is of gradual onset. Ankylosing spondylitis is most common in young men, with symptoms usually appearing before the age of 40.

Once possible visceral and systemic causes of the patient's symptoms have been excluded, the focus should be shifted to determine if there is neurologic compromise. Additionally, diagnoses that may lead to spinal instability (fracture and spondylolisthesis) should be considered.

Table 87-2 "RED FLAGS" IN THE HISTORY AND PHYSICAL EXAMINATION OF PATIENTS WITH LOW BACK PAIN

Disorder	History	Physical Examination
All	Duration of pain >1 month Bed rest with no relief Age: <20 or >50 years*	
Cancer	Age ≥50 years Previous cancer history Unexplained weight loss‡	Neurologic findings† Lymphadenopathy
Compression fracture	Age ≥50 years (≥0 years more specific) Significant trauma§ History of osteoporosis Corticosteroid use Substance abuse¶	
Infection	Fever or chills Recent skin or urinary infection Immunosuppression Injection drug use	Fever (>100°F [38°C]) Tenderness of spinous processes
Inflammatory arthritis	Insidiously presenting pain >3 months Bed rest with no relief Morning stiffness improved with activity	

*Age <20 years is associated with increased risk of spondylolysis, spondylolisthesis, and stress fractures; age >50 years suggests increased risks for cancer and compression fractures.

†Most commonly due to a herniated lumbar disk or lumbar spinal stenosis rather than malignancy.

‡Unexplained weight loss is defined as more than 10 pounds over the preceding 6 months.

§Significant trauma is a fall from height or external trauma such as a motor vehicle accident.

¶Substance abuse can increase the risk for fracture through higher rates of trauma. Alcohol abuse can also increase the risk for fracture through decreasing bone density.

Adapted from Atlas SJ, Deyo RA: Evaluating and managing acute low back pain in the primary care setting. J Gen Int Med 2001;16:120-131.

Table 87-3 NEUROLOGIC EXAMINATION COMPONENTS IN PATIENTS WITH LOW BACK PAIN

Nerve Root	Motor Exam	Functional Test	Sensation*	Reflex
L3	Extend the quadriceps	Squat down and return to standing	Lateral thigh/medial femoral condyle	Patellar tendon
L4	Dorsiflex the ankle	Heel walking	Medial leg/medial ankle	Patellar tendon
L5	Dorsiflex the great toe	Heel walking	Medial leg/medial ankle	N/A
S1	Stand on toes for ≥5 repetitions	Walk on toes	Plantar foot/lateral ankle	Achilles tendon

*Sharp/dull or pinprick.

Low back pain can be associated with leg pain due to radiation, but other causes include radiculopathy and sciatica (pain radiating from the back into the buttock and posterior/lateral aspects of the leg.) Sciatica frequently is caused by lumbar degenerative disk disease. True sciatica usually causes pain below the knee; at least 95% of degenerative disks in the lumbar spine occur at the L4-L5 and L5-S1 vertebral levels. For this reason, the neurologic examination should be focused on the lumbosacral nerve roots for both sensory and motor testing. Table 87-3 details the motor, sensory, and reflex test components of the neurologic examination of patients with low back pain. Note that functional strength testing is more likely to detect subtle muscle weakness than simple motor testing.

Passive straight leg raise (SLR) testing appears to help in the diagnosis of sciatica by stretching the sciatic nerve. A positive ipsilateral SLR, which results in pain below the knee when the leg to which low back pain radiates is raised higher than between 30 and 60 degrees with the patient supine, is sensitive but not specific for sciatica, whereas a positive contralateral SLR (in which pain in the affected leg is provoked or worsened when the opposite leg is raised) is specific but insensitive.[4] A negative SLR may be of greater value, because patients with this finding generally have good long-term outcomes.

Spinal stenosis occurs due to a variety of processes that impinge on the spinal cord (usually hypertrophy of the ligamentum flavum), causing pseudoclaudication—back and leg pain with walking and extension of the spine that improves with sitting and lumbar flexion. Most cases occur in patients 55 year of age or older; they usually report an insidious onset of symptoms.

Cauda equina syndrome results from compression of the conus medullaris of the spinal cord and/or the nerve roots that comprise the cauda equina. It typically is caused by a large central disk herniation but can also occur due to other space-occupying lesions such as spinal stenosis, tumor, abscess, and hematoma.[1] Patients typically have a history of low back pain and present with a triad of new complaints of low extremity weakness, saddle paresthesias, and bowel and bladder dysfunction; central disk herniations may not cause back pain or sciatica, and back pain may be a minor component of the patient's symptoms. The presence of urinary retention has good sensitivity and specificity for cauda equina syndrome.[5]

Expeditious diagnosis and therapy help minimize long-term neurologic deficits in these patients. Most current studies in the literature recommend operative decompression within 48 hours of onset of symptoms,[6] although this remains controversial.

Low back pain without a systemic or visceral cause and without neurologic compromise may nevertheless occur due to a specific mechanical cause, usually involving the spinal column itself. Lumbar fractures usually result from significant trauma (e.g., falls from heights, external trauma) but can occur from minor trauma in older patients, in patients on chronic corticosteroid therapy, and in persons at risk for pathologic fractures (e.g., due to bony metastases or osteoporosis of the spine).

A history of trauma and bony tenderness (to palpation and percussion) suggest fracture as a possible cause of low back pain. Stress fractures of the sacrum and lumbar spine and insufficiency fractures of the sacrum are other causes of low back pain to which athletes (especially young athletes) and older patients (especially women), respectively, are predisposed.

Spondylolisthesis, the slippage of one vertebral body relative to an adjacent vertebral body, is a specific mechanical cause of low back pain that can lead to progressive instability. It occurs due to a defect in the pars interarticularis from either a fracture or spondylolysis, which can be congenital or degenerative in etiology. Spondylolisthesis can also lead to degenerative disk disease and osteophyte development. Instability causes symptoms similar to those of spinal stenosis.

Finally, nonspecific mechanical causes of low back pain may be the root of patients' symptoms when possible systemic and visceral sources have been ruled out and there are no signs of instability or neurologic compromise. Nonspecific low back pain syndromes have been called "lumbago," "lumbar sprain/strain," "idiopathic low back pain," "myofascial strain," and a variety of other names. About 85% to 90% of patients with low back pain in a variety of outpatient settings are considered to have nonspecific low back pain.[7] These patients tend to be most comfortable at rest, and their symptoms worsen with activity and movement. They do not have "red flags" in their history and physical examination that suggest specific musculoskeletal, systemic, or visceral sources of their pain, nor do they have signs or symptoms of neurologic compromise.

Waddell's signs have been promoted as tools to help demonstrate a "nonorganic" cause of patients' symptoms, but they are mainly useful for predicting patients at risk for prolonged recovery from low back pain.[8] Waddell's signs may also point to a diagnosis of depression or other psychoneuroses.

Diagnostic Testing

Plain films of the lumbosacral spine should be limited to patients of age extremes and patients at high risk for specific back pain due to trauma or possible systemic disease; plain films have low sensitivity for tumor and infections, and they have minimal diagnostic utility (although patients frequently expect them).

A rectal examination is performed when evaluation of sacral nerve function is necessary (and to evaluate the male prostate for masses or infection), especially in patients in whom a specific pathologic cause of low back pain is suspected. Postvoid residuals of the bladder should be obtained if cauda equina syndrome is suspected; residuals of more than 100 to 200 mL are highly suggestive of neurogenic bladder as a result of cauda equina syndrome.[5]

Erythrocyte sedimentation rate (ESR) testing should be considered for patients in whom cancer or infection remains part of the differential diagnosis following the history and physical examination; an ESR higher than 20 mm/hour should be viewed with concern in such patients. Patients with an abscess may have back pain as the only symptom, spotty neurologic changes that do not fit a discrete distribution, or pain that mimics sciatica. Prudent suspicion, deliberate consideration, and attention to patient risks are the most important ways to facilitate successful diagnosis.

Urinalysis (and culture as indicated) is recommended for patients in whom urinary tract infection or renal disease are likely. If abdominal aortic aneurysm or dissection is a consideration in the diagnosis, it must be ruled out by an appropriate imaging study, either ultrasonography or computed tomography (CT) scanning.

Advanced imaging such as MRI is reserved for patients who are surgical candidates (e.g., because of cauda equina syndrome or other neurologic compromise). Emergent MRI in patients with a history of low back pain and cancer can be justified if the ESR is 20 mm/hour or higher.[3] Obtain other studies such as myelography (plain or CT), electromyography, and discography are performed at the discretion of consultants.[9]

Interventions and Procedures

Patients with suspected or proven fracture are immobilized until spinal instability has been ruled out. Vascular access is necessary for patients who may need resuscitation and in whom advanced studies or parenteral pain medication therapy is anticipated. Early institution of IV corticosteroids such as dexamethasone (for tumors or disks causing cord or conus

Documentation

Record the Following:

- The presence or absence of historical "red flags" and physical examination finding suggesting specific, systemic, or visceral sources of the patient's signs and symptoms
- The results of a careful, systematic neurologic examination of the lower extremities, including sacral nerve function.
- Assessment of the nature of the patient's symptoms that may require urgent work-up due to possible specific cause, neurologic compromise, or spinal instability
- Discussions with patients and their families or friends, including specific instructions about need for follow-up and warning signs suggesting cauda equina syndrome that requires immediate evaluation

medullaris compression) or IV antibiotics (for osteomyelitis, abscess, and other infectious processes) should be considered if these diagnoses are likely.

Admission to the hospital may be required for further evaluation, testing, and treatment, including obtaining an MRI. The only absolute indications for emergent MRI are suspected cauda equina syndrome, spinal cord compression from any cause, and suspected epidural abscess. MRI is obtained more commonly when the imaging capacity exists at the facility, often facilitating the diagnosis and avoiding unnecessary admissions.

Placement of a Foley catheter may provide improved comfort and convenience in nonambulatory patients, and decompression of the distended bladder in patients with neurogenic bladder may improve later voiding function.

Treatment

Nonspecific low back pain is usually self-limited and of short duration: about 60% of cases will resolve within 1 week and 90% within 2 to 6 weeks. Treatmen is conservative. NSAIDs are first-line analgesics; they usually are prescribed for all patients who don't have contraindications.[10] Patients should be instructed to use NSAIDs routinely because administration only as needed does not seem to be as effective. Narcotic administration is restricted to patients with severe pain and only for short courses; no studies have shown these medications to be more beneficial than other medications for acute or subacute low back pain. Skeletal muscle relaxants can be given and are commonly prescribed but have not been shown to speed functional recovery; a recent clinical trial[11] reported that the addition of cyclobenzaprine to ibuprofen did not improve analgesia in patients with nonspecific low back pain but was associated with a greater prevalence of central nervous system side effects compared with ibuprofen alone.

Corticosteroids (commonly oral methylprednisolone) are frequently given to patients with lumbar degenerative disk disease and sciatica, despite lack of evidence to support their use. Some small studies have shown more rapid return to work, but recent guidelines do not recommend systemic steroids for patients with nonspecific low back pain or sciatica, especially on a chronic basis.

Bed rest has not been shown to improve outcomes in patients with nonspecific low back pain. Patients should be instructed to stay active while avoiding activities that worsen symptoms. If the patient has no contraindications, walking and other routine daily activities are probably as effective as specific stretching and strengthening exercises in patients with acute low back pain.[12,13] Activities that may act as exacerbating factors or precipitants of low back pain—such as bending, twisting, heavy lifting, and prolonged sitting—should be limited.

Patients frequently prefer "alternative" modes of therapy (chiropractic or osteopathic spinal manipulation, acupuncture, massage, magnets) to traditional allopathic approaches. In most cases, there are neither proven benefits nor drawbacks to these therapies[14]; however, patients often will utilize them regardless of physician recommendations. There may be increased risk of cauda equina syndrome following manipulation in patients with disk disease, tumors, or other specific diseases of the spinal column.

Disposition

Patients with nonspecific low back pain can be discharged home in almost all circumstances; there appears to be limited need or utility in admitting patients for pain control. All patients with low back pain who are discharged from the ED should be warned about the risk of cauda equina syndrome and told to return if they experience neurologic or bowel/bladder symptoms.[15]

Inform patients with nonspecific low back pain that the ED work-up has not found any concerning pathology, and that they can expect their pain to get better. Teach them that pain does not necessarily mean danger and that they can safely perform their normal activities of daily living. Finally, advise them to arrange follow-up with a primary care provider, because low back pain can recur frequently and may be better managed with continuity of care.

Patients with specific systemic or visceral sources of their low back pain require specialist consultation.

PATIENT TEACHING TIPS

Low back pain is a common problem, with four out of every five adults having back pain at some time in their lifetime. The most common causes of low back pain are:

Muscle strains and spasm: Poor posture and body mechanics, including improper or excess lifting or twisting, may cause strains or spasms of the muscles that support the back.

Degenerative processes: As people age, the disks between the bones in the spine that provide cushioning and lubrication become dry and hard, and the spine stiffens, leading to pain and discomfort.

Sciatica: Compression or "pinching" of nerves (perhaps from a disc that bulges out from between the backbones) causes pain from the back to travel down the leg.

Treatment for low back pain (what doctors call "conservative therapy") includes:

Over-the-counter pain relievers such as nonsteroidal anti-inflammatory drugs (NSAIDs); examples are ibuprofen (Advil, Motrin, Nuprin), naproxen sodium (Aleve), and aspirin

- Aspirin and other NSAIDs can cause stomach problems and should be taken with food or milk
- If you're taking blood thinners, ask your doctor or pharmacist if it's safe to take NSAIDs or aspirin
- Acetaminophen (Tylenol) is less likely than aspirin and other NSAIDs to bother your stomach

Application of ice in the first 24 hours of symptoms, with moist heat on the following days

Gradual return to normal activities, including walking, without need for special exercises

- "Bed rest" doesn't help and may actually slow the recovery process

Follow-up with your primary care provider to make sure you're getting better and to help minimize recurrence of your symptoms.

If you have back pain plus any of these signs or symptoms, call your doctor!

- Fever above 100.5°F (38° C)
- Past use of steroids, such as prednisone, for more than 1 week
- Losing weight without trying to
- Pain that gets worse or doesn't get better when you stop moving and rest or lie flat in bed
- Pain that wakes you from sleep
- An injury to your back from a fall, a car crash, or an assault
- Bladder or bowel problems
- Weakness in your legs, as opposed to pain
- Severe pain despite use of medications prescribed by your doctor
- A personal history of cancer

REFERENCES

1. Deyo RA, Weinstein JN: Low back pain. N Engl J Med 2001;344:363-370.
2. Jensen MC, Brant-Zawadzki MN, Obuchowski N, et al: Magnetic resonance imaging of the lumbar spine in people without back pain. N Engl J Med 1994;331:69-73.
3. Joines JD, McNutt RA, Carey TS, et al: Finding cancer in primary care outpatients with low back pain: A comparison of diagnostic strategies. J Gen Intern Med 2001;16:14-23.
4. Deyo RA, Rainville J, Kent DL: What can the history and physical examination tell us about low back pain? JAMA 1992;268:760-765.
5. Small SA, Perron AD, Brady WJ: Orthopedic pitfalls: Cauda equina syndrome. Am J Emerg Med 2005;23:159-163.
6. Ahn UM, Ahn NU, Buchowski JM, et al: Cauda equina syndrome secondary to lumbar disc herniation: A meta-analysis of surgical outcomes. Spine 2000;25:1515-1522.
7. Manek NJ, MacGregor AJ: Epidemiology of back disorders: Prevalence, risk factors, and prognosis. Curr Opin Rheumatol 2005;17:134-140.
8. Waddell G, McCulloch JA, Kummel E, Venner RM: Nonorganic physical signs in low-back pain. Spine 1980;5:117-125.
9. Gilbert FJ, Grant AM, Gillan MG, et al: Low back pain: Influence of early MR imaging or CT on treatment and outcome—multicenter randomized trial. Radiology 2004;231:343-351.
10. van Tulder MW, Scholten RJ, Koes BW, Deyo RA: Nonsteroidal anti-inflammatory drugs for low back pain: A systematic review within the framework of the Cochrane Collaboration Back Review Group. Spine 2000;25:2501-2513.
11. Turturro MA, Frater CR, D'Amico FJ: Cyclobenzaprine with ibuprofen versus ibuprofen alone in acute myofascial strain: A randomized, double-blind clinical trial. Ann Emerg Med 2003;41:818-826.
12. Malmivaara A, Hakkinen U, Aro T, et al:. The treatment of acute low back pain—bed rest, exercises, or ordinary activity? N Engl J Med 1995;332:351-355.
13. Vroomen PC, de Krom MC, Wilmink JT, et al: Lack of effectiveness of bed rest for sciatica. N Engl J Med 1999;340:418-423.
14. Assendelft WJ, Morton SC, Yu EI, et al: Spinal manipulative therapy for low back pain. A meta-analysis of effectiveness relative to other therapies. Ann Intern Med 2003;138:871-881.
15. Kostuik JP: Medicolegal consequences of cauda equina syndrome: An overview. Neurosurg Focus 2004;16:e8.

Chapter **88**

Pediatric Orthopedic Emergencies

Russ Horowitz

KEY POINTS

- Ligaments are stronger than bones in young children.
- The history should be consistent with the injury and the developmental stage of the child.
- Children are poor at localizing pain and often refer symptoms to neighboring joints. The pathologic site in knee pain may be the hip.
- Growth plate injuries are subtle but have the potential to lead to growth arrest.
- Radiographs of the contralateral side are useful as comparison views for investigation of subtle fractures.

Radial Head Subluxation

Radial head subluxation, or "nursemaid's elbow," is a common injury affecting children between the ages of 6 months and 5 years. It results from hyperextension with subluxation of the radial head and an acute annular ligament interposition into the radiocapitellar joint. A history of longitudinal traction may not be obtained because the caretaker may not be aware of a particular event or may feel guilty about causing the child's injury. A concern about wrist or shoulder injury may be reported because inadvertent manipulation of the injured elbow caused pain.

■ PRESENTING SIGNS AND SYMPTOMS

Children refuse to use the affected arm and hold it close to the body and in slight flexion. They do not appear in particular distress but may be fearful that examination will elicit pain. There is no bony abnormality or tenderness to palpation. Radiographs are unnecessary unless another particular injury is suspected. Edema and tenderness are present in supracondylar fractures.

A number of reduction techniques are used including the hyperpronation method and the supination-flexion method. The hyperpronation method has proven more effective and appears less traumatic.[1] With the arm held in extension the wrist is hyperpronated. A "click" is sometimes heard. In the supination-flexion approach the examiner places the thumb of one hand over the radial head and provides counter traction. Next, holding the wrist, the elbow is pulled into extension. The final phase is supination and flexion at the elbow. Most children return to full functioning within 15 minutes, and the child should be observed until full range of motion is regained.

In cases in which multiple reductions fail, radiography should be considered. In a child with failed reduction and negative radiographic findings, a sling or posterior splint is necessary with close orthopedic follow-up.

Fractures

Trauma to immature and incompletely ossified bones results in unique pediatric orthopedic injuries including torus, greenstick, bowing, and physeal fractures.

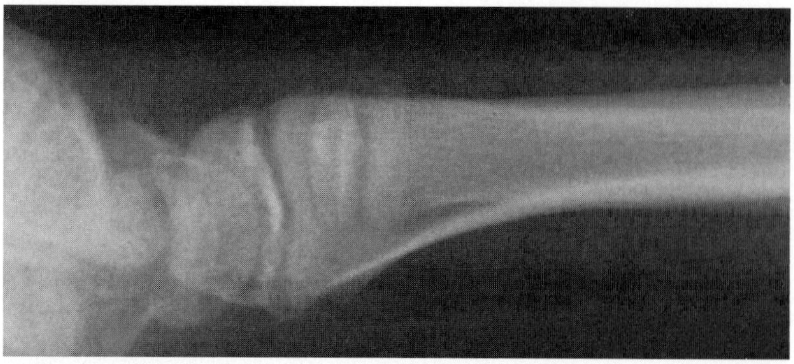

FIGURE 88-1 Torous fracture of the distal radius.

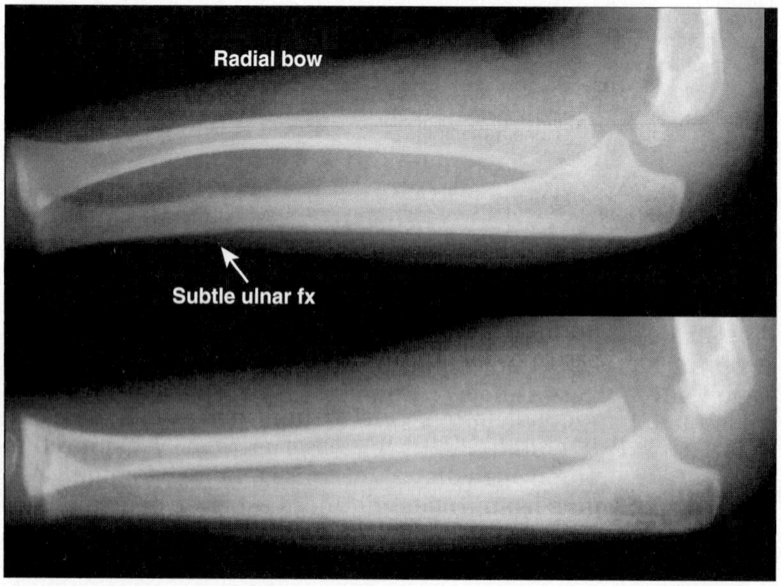
Radial bow
Subtle ulnar fx

FIGURE 88-2 Radial bowing fracture with normal contralateral side shown for comparison.

These patterns do not occur in dense adult bone. Because radiographic findings of some of these abnormalities are incredibly subtle, comparison views are particularly helpful. Trauma that would result in sprains and strains in structurally mature individuals causes the thick periosteum to be ripped from the bony cortex, resulting in avulsion fractures. In children, because ligaments are stronger than neighboring bones, ligamentous tears are uncommon.

Children's bones are apt to bend with a fracture of only one side of the periosteum. Callus formation and remodeling is extensive in pediatric injuries and contributes to the faster healing found in children. The goal of reduction should always be near-perfect alignment; however, growing bones have a dramatic potential for spontaneous correction.

Pediatric bones are less dense and therefore more prone to compression or bending when an axial load is applied. Falls onto an outstretched arm may result in torous or buckle fractures (Fig. 88-1). Greenstick fractures are incomplete, and the the cortex remains intact on one surface. To obtain complete reduction, completion of fracture is necessary. Bowing fractures result when the force is insufficient to cause a complete break but results in deformation of the osseous structure (Fig. 88-2). Cosmetic deformity and functional abnormality will result without complete reduction. Repair is often difficult because both cortices remain intact.

The physis or growth plate is a weak area of cartilage present in developing bone. Trauma that causes strains or joint dislocations in skeletally mature individuals often results in growth plate fractures in children. Anatomic alignment of such fractures is critical for optimal growth.

■ SALTER-HARRIS CLASSIFICATION OF FRACTURES

The most commonly used system to identify physeal injuries is the Salter-Harris classification. Fractures are labeled types I through V, with the higher numbers having the greater risk of growth abnormalities. All such injuries require pediatric orthopedic follow-up.[2]

Type I fractures result from a longitudinal force through the physis that splits the epiphysis from the metaphysis. Radiographs may reveal a widened growth plate. Identification can be difficult, particularly when there is minimal displacement, and a fracture should be suspected in cases of tenderness along

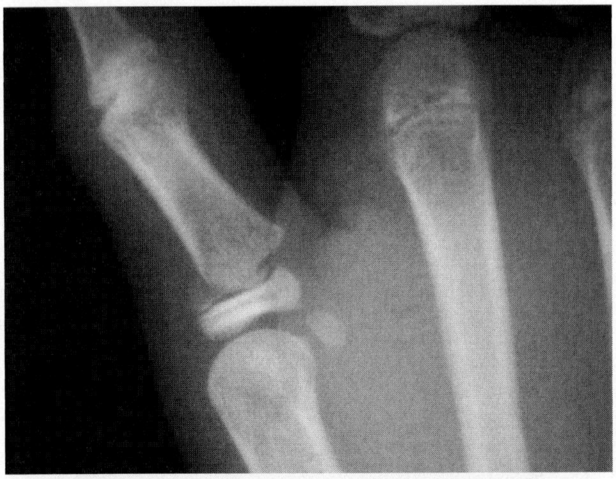

FIGURE 88-3 Type II Salter-Harris fracture at the metacarpal-phalangeal joint of the thumb.

the physis even in the absence of radiologic findings. Type I fractures rarely result in growth disturbances and can be treated effectively with immobilization.

Type II fractures, the most most common type, occur when a piece of the metaphysis remains attached to the epiphysis (Fig. 88-3). They require splinting and generally carry a good prognosis. Types III and IV are intraarticular fractures that also involve the growth plate. In a type III injury, the fracture line extends through the epiphysis into the physis. In type IV, the fracture passes through the epiphysis, physis, and metaphysis. Types III and IV carry risks of growth retardation, altered joint mechanics, and functional impairment and require urgent orthopedic evaluation. Type V fractures are compression injuries and are difficult to visualize on the radiograph. The diagnosis is often made retrospectively following a case of growth arrest.

■ TODDLER'S FRACTURES

Toddler's fractures are nondisplaced oblique or spiral fractures through the distal tibia. Questioning may not reveal any significant injury—simply a refusal to bear weight after a day playing at the park. The examination may reveal mild, diffuse tenderness along the tibial shaft and lack of edema and ecchymosis. Gentle twisting of the lower leg may elicit pain as the fracture plane is opened. Radiographic findings are subtle, and multiple views including anteroposterior, lateral, and oblique images may be necessary. In the case of negative findings, a bone scan may be considered.

If the symptoms persist, one may choose to repeat radiography in 7 to 10 days to look for new subperiosteal bone formation. Immobilization is sufficient to promote healing. When the child limps and radiographic findings are negative, a fracture or injury in another location should be considered. Varied pathology, including appendicitis, toxic synovitis, septic arthritis, foot and ankle fractures, soft tissue injuries, and abuse (Box 88-1) may all present with a limp in a toddler.

BOX 88-1

Fractures Suggesting Abuse*

- Multiple fractures, especially in various stages of healing
- Fracture patterns inconsistent with the history
- Fractures coexistent with soft tissue injuries consistent with abuse
- Corner or bucket-handle fractures
- Lower extremity fractures in nonambulatory children
- Spiral fractures of the humerus
- Multiple depressed skull fractures
- Rib fractures, especially multiple posterior fractures

*A skeletal survey should be done in all cases of suspected abuse.

Data from Belfer RA, Klein BL, Orr L: Use of the skeletal survey in the evaluation of child maltreatment. Am J Emerg Med 2001;19:122-124.

■ SUPRACONDYLAR FRACTURES

Supracondylar fractures are the most common elbow fractures in children and often occur in children 3 to 10 years of age. The most common mechanism is a fall onto an outstretched hand with the elbow hyperextended.

A classification of the types of supracondylar fractures is based on the extent of the injury: type I is nondisplaced (Fig. 88-4), type II is displaced posteriorly with an intact cortex (Fig. 88-5), and type III is completely displaced with no cortical contact (Fig. 88-6). Type I injuries are managed with immobilization for 4 to 6 weeks. Treatment of type II injuries is based on the extent of the damage and an orthopedist should be consulted. The more severe cases require admission, reduction, and internal fixation; milder cases may be treated like type I injuries. All type III fractures require closed reduction with pinning in the operating room.

Radiographic findings may be subtle, particularly in type I injuries (Box 88-2). In cases in which a fracture line cannot be easily visualized, other findings may assist in making the diagnosis. A posterior fat pad or joint effusion located dorsal to the distal humerus at the level of the olecranon fossa is always pathologic and evidence of a fracture. An anterior fat pad is normal unless it is lifted up and squared off inferiorly into a "sail sign." A line drawn along the anterior surface of the humerus should intersect the capitellum in its middle third. Posterior displacement of the distal humerus will cause the line to fall further anteriorly or miss the capitellum entirely.

In cases of more severe injuries, the difficulty is not in making the diagnosis but rather the recognition and reduction of complications. Morbidity includes range of motion abnormalities, neuro-

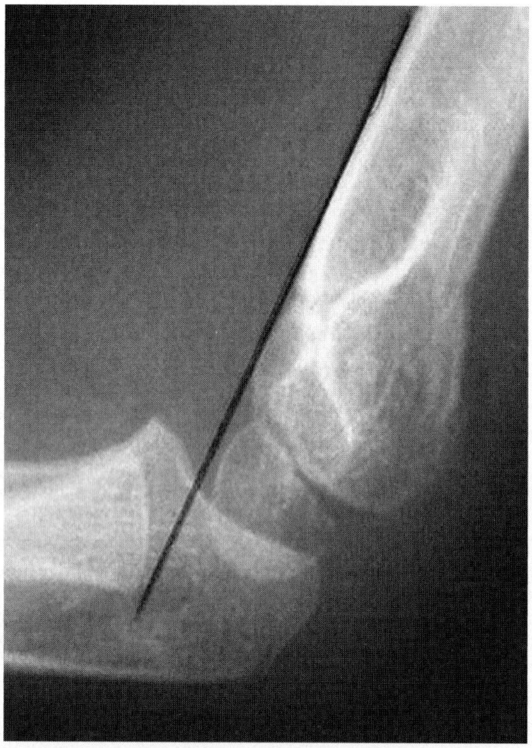

FIGURE 88-4 Type I supracondylar fracture. The anterior humeral line does not intersect with the capitellum. A subtle fracture is visible along the anterior surface of the humerus.

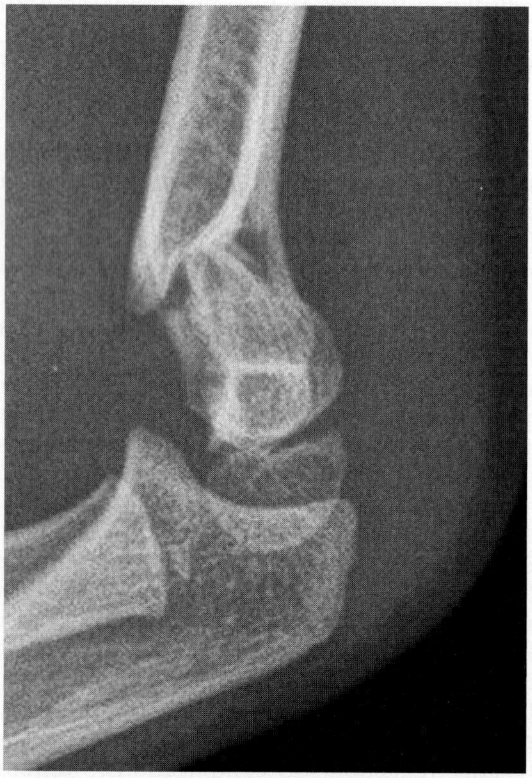

FIGURE 88-5 Type II supracondylar fracture.

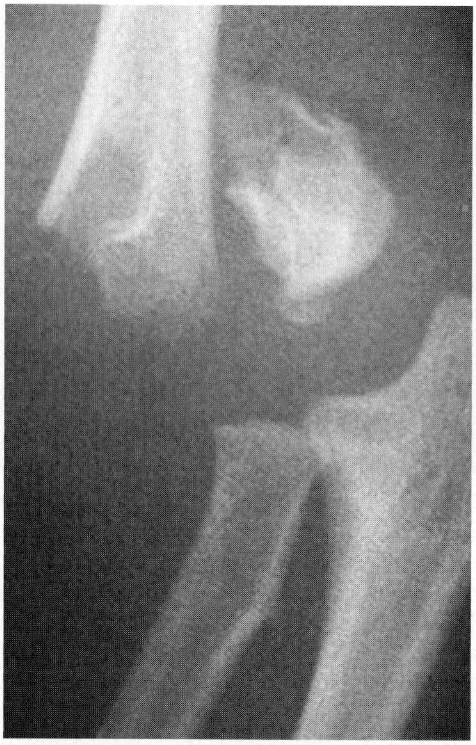

FIGURE 88-6 Type III supracondylar fracture.

BOX 88-2

Radiographic Evidence of Supracondylar Fractures

- Direct fracture visualization
- Posterior fat pad
- Sail sign
- Joint effusion
- Malalignment of anterior humeral line

vascular compromise, and long-term deformities. A thorough examination and documentation of neurovascular status, pain control, and stabilization are mandatory. The limb should be splinted in the deformed position. Motor and sensory function of the median, ulnar, and radial nerves are at risk. Direct vascular injury is uncommon; however, the potential for compartment syndrome does exist, and frequent repeat examinations should be performed and recorded.[3]

Slipped Capital Femoral Epiphysis

Slipped capital femoral epiphysis preferentially affects boys twice as commonly as girls. Most children are diagnosed early in their growth spurt—boys 13 to 15 years of age and girls 11 to 13 years of age (because of girls' earlier onset of pubertal development). Obesity is a risk factor; however, many average-sized children develop slipped capital femoral epiphysis.

■ PRESENTING SIGNS AND SYMPTOMS

Pain and limp are the most common reasons for presentation. Symptoms may have been present for weeks to months. Pain, which can range from dull and intermittent to severe and persistent, may be present in the hip or referred to the knee, groin, or anterior thigh. Sometimes a history of trivial trauma prompts medical evaluation. The physical examination reveals a hip in flexion with mild external rotation. Range of motion is limited, especially full flexion, medial rotation, and internal rotation.

■ DIAGNOSTIC TESTING

Radiographic studies should include both anteroposterior (AP) and frog-leg views, because an AP view alone may miss the diagosis. On the AP view of a normal hip, a line drawn along the superior margin of the femoral neck cortex should transect the epiphysis by a small margin. In slipped capital femoral epiphhysis, the line passes outside the epiphysis or just at the superior edge. Contralateral images or full pelvis views are helpful; however, up to 25% of slipped capital femoral epiphysis are bilateral.

■ TREATMENT

Diagnosis of slipped capital femoral epiphysis necessitates urgent orthopedic evaluation. Management is surgical with screws placed through the femoral neck into the epiphysis. Delay in diagnosis or management may lead to avascular necrosis and long-term disability.

Legg-Calvé-Perthes Disease

Legg-Calvé-Perthes disease is characterized by avascular necrosis and resorption of the femoral head. Its onset occurs in children between 4 and 9 years of age, and it is more common in overweight boys. Although the definitive etiology is unknown, research has focused on clotting abnormalities and increased blood viscosity.

■ PRESENTING SIGNS AND SYMPTOMS

The disease is initially clinically silent and may come to attention incidentally as a result of trauma. The onset of symptoms is usually insidious. Pain may be present in the hip or be referred to the hip, knee, anterior thigh, or groin. Tenderness rarely is present; symptoms include an antalgic gait and decreased hip abduction and medial rotation.

■ DIAGNOSTIC TESTING

AP and frog-leg views of the pelvis allow optimal visualization of the femoral head. Disease findings include widening of the articular cartilage, subcondral fractures, irregularity, and flattening of the epiphysis.

■ TREATMENT AND DISPOSITION

Treatment includes pain management with nonsteroidal anti-inflammatory drugs (NSAIDs) and referral to a pediatric orthopedic surgeon. The majority of children with this disease do well with observation and nonsurgical intervention.[4]

Septic Arthritis

Septic arthritis is a true medical emergency requiring early intervention to prevent permanent joint destruction. There is microbial invasion of the joint space from hematogenous spread, local spread from neighboring infection, or direct inoculation from trauma or surgical infection. Bacterial enzymes cause direct tissue destruction. Synovial edema, increased synovial fluid production, and pus increase the intraarticular pressure, causing damage to vessels and articular cartilage. Commonly involved organisms are *Staphylococcus aureus* and assorted *Streptococcus* species. Group B streptococci and *Escherichia coli* are important causes in neonates, and gonococcal arthritis should be a serious consideration in sexually active adolescents.

■ PRESENTING SIGNS AND SYMPTOMS

Children suffering from septic arthritis are frequently ill-appearing with fever of 104° F (40° C) or higher, limited range of motion of the affected joint, and pain and swelling.[5] The pain is constant and increases with movement. In the case of septic arthritis of the hip, the child lies in a position of comfort with the hip slightly flexed, abducted, and externally rotated. An infected knee will be erythematous, edematous, warm, and tender to palpation.

■ DIAGNOSTIC TESTING

Plain radiographs, complete blood count, erthrocyte sedimentation rate, C-reactive protein, and blood culture are necessary in the evaluation of children with suspected septic arthritis. Radiologic findings include joint space widening, soft tissue swelling, and displacement of adjacent fat pads. Comparison views may be helpful, as a difference of only a few mm from the teardrop of the acetabulum to the medial metaphysis of the femoral neck may be significant. In young children, lack of ossification limits the usefulness of radiographs, and ultrasonography provides more detail.

A convincing clinical and/or laboratory picture justifies joint aspiration for fluid analysis including protein, glucose, Gram stain, and culture. Joint fluid yields a positive culture in approximately 50% to 75% of cases. Blood culture is much less effective and is positive in approximately one third of cases.

■ TREATMENT

Definitive therapy is administration of IV antibiotics and surgical drainage of the purulent material from the joint. Because the potential for joint destruction is great and the yield of Gram stain is low, empirical antibiotic therapy in the emergency department is indicated. Coverage should include an antistaphylococcal agent, either a beta-lactamase resistant penicillin, clindamycin, or a first-generation cephalosporin. Gram-negative coverage should also be considered for neonates.

Toxic Synovitis

Toxic, or transient, synovitis is a benign, self-limited inflammatory condition. A postinfectious inflammatory response has been suggested as the possible cause; however, no definitive etiology has been determined. It affects children 3 to 10 years of age and its presentation mimics that of septic arthritis. Joints most often involved include the hip and knee. Fever is rarely present but when it does occur, is usually low-grade.

■ PRESENTING SIGNS AND SYMPTOMS

Although patients will sit in a position of comfort and will complain with movement of the limb, the affected joint has full range of motion.[5] This is in stark contrast to septic arthritis, in which the child appears systemically ill, is in significant pain, and cannot move the affected join in its full range of motion.[6]

■ DIAGNOSTIC TESTING

White blood cell count, erthrocyte sedimentation rate, and C-reactive protein findings usually are normal or slightly elevated, consistent with an inflammatory process.[5] Radiographs often are normal or may reveal a mild effusion with joint space widening. Sufficient overlap exists in some presentations of septic joint and toxic synovitis that synovial fluid is necessary to make the diagnosis (Table 88-1). When obtained, synovial fluid is sterile.

Table 88-1 SEPTIC ARTHRITIS VERSUS TOXIC SYNOVITIS

Findings	Septic Arthritis	Toxic Synovitis
Fever (°C)	≥38.5	<38.5
Complete blood count (cells/mm^3)	≥12,000	<12,000
C-reative protein (mg/dL)	≥2.0	<2.0
Erythrocyte sedimentation rate (mm/hr)	≥40	<40

Data from reference 6.

■ TREATMENT

Treatment is directed at symptom relief on an outpatient basis with NSAIDs. Pain usually lasts 3 to 4 days but may persist for a few weeks. Children return to full activity and there is no associated morbidity.

REFERENCES

1. Green D, Linares MY, Garcia Pena BM, et al: Randomized comparison of pain perception during radial head subluxation reduction using supination-flexion or forced pronation. Pediatr Emerg Care 2006;22:235-238.
2. Brown JH, DeLuca SA: Growth plate injuries: Salter-Harris classification. Am Fam Physician 1992;46:1180-1184.
3. Campbell CC, Waters PM, Enabs JB: Neurovascular injury and displacement in type III supracondylar fractures. J Pediatr Orthop 1995;15:47-52.
4. Wall EJ: Legg-Calvé-Perthes' disease. Curr Opin Pediatr 1999;11:76-79.
5. Caird MS, Flynn JM, Leung YL, et al: Factors distinguishing septic arthritis from transient synovitis of the hip in children. A prospective study. J Bone Joint Surg 2006; 88A:1251-1257.
6. Kocher MS, Zurakowski D, Kasser JR: Differentiating between septic arthritis and transient synovitis of the hip in children: An evidence-based clinical prediction algorithm. J Bone Joint Surg 1999;81A:1662-1670.

SECTION IX

Neurologic Diseases

Chapter 89

Altered Mental Status and Coma

Jeremy L. Cooke and William G. Barsan

KEY POINTS

The differential diagnosis of coma is broad, requiring a systematic approach to patient evaluation and diagnostic testing.

Patients with altered mental status may have subtle neurologic dysfunction, so careful neurologic examination is helpful.

Once initial stablization of the comatose patient has been addressed, quickly reversible causes should be sought prior to the initiation of a lengthy diagnostic workup. Natoxone, dextrose, and thiamine administration should be considered.

Structural brain lesions that may require operative intervention dictate immediate consultation with a neurosurgical service.

Scope

Altered mental status is a spectrum of disease ranging from sleepiness to confusion to frank coma. Coma is the chief complaint in approximately 3% of patients presenting to the ED. Roughly 85% of cases are caused by metabolic or systemic derangements, whereas 15% are caused by structural lesions. Once the ABCs (airway, breathing, and circulation) have been established and the patient's condition is stable, it is the role of the EP to quickly separate structural from metabolic and systemic etiologies.

Pathophysiology

Consciousness collectively is made up of arousal and cognition. Arousal is defined as the awareness of self and the surroundings. The neuroanatomic structure primarily responsible for arousal is the ascending reticular activating system, which is located in the dorsal part of the brainstem in the paramedian tegmental zone, controls the input of somatic and sensory stimuli to the cerebral cortex, and functions to initiate arousal from sleep. Cognition is the combination of *orientation* (the accurate perception of what is experienced), *judgment* (the ability to process input data to generate more meaningful information), and *memory* (the ability to store and retrieve information). The brain's cognition centers are located primarily in the cerebral cortex.

Coma can be caused by damage to the brainstem (Fig. 89-1), the cerebral cortex, or both. These structures are vulnerable to toxins, metabolic derangements, and mechanical injury. Localized, unilateral lesions in the cerebral cortex usually do not induce altered mental status or coma even as other cognitive functions are impaired. However, if both cerebral hemispheres are affected, altered mental status or coma can occur depending on the size of the insult and its speed of progression. In contrast, a completely intact brainstem is critical for arousal. The ascending reticular activating system can be vulnerable to small, focal lesions in the brainstem. If it is impaired, the cerebral cortex cannot be aroused and coma occurs.[1,2]

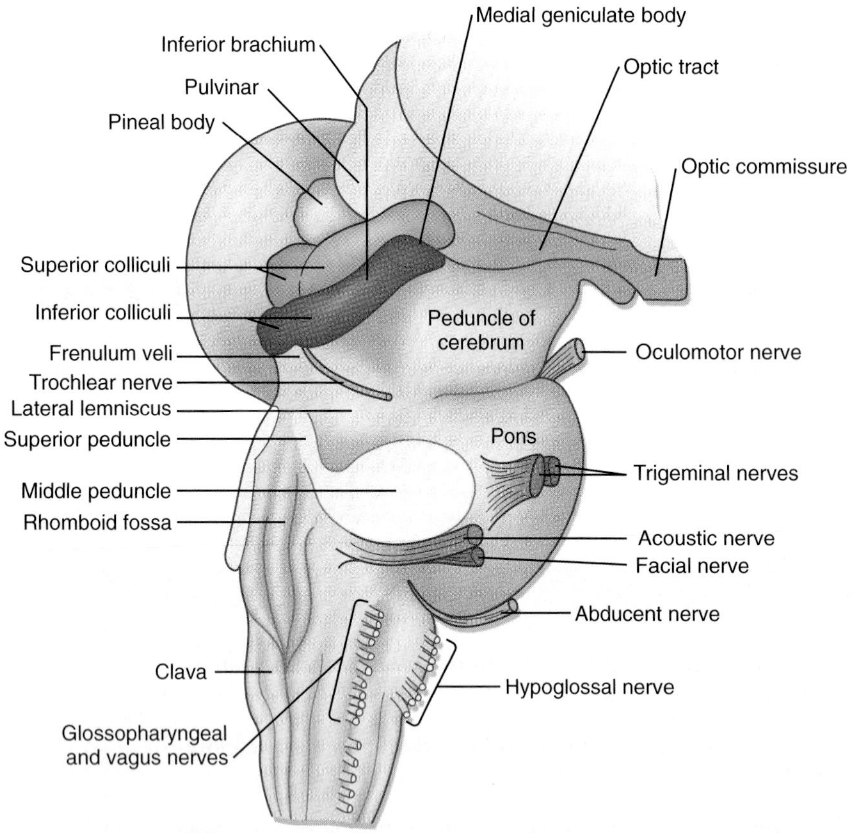
Medial geniculate body
Inferior brachium
Optic tract
Pulvinar
Pineal body
Optic commissure
Superior colliculi
Inferior colliculi
Peduncle of cerebrum
Frenulum veli
Oculomotor nerve
Trochlear nerve
Lateral lemniscus
Superior peduncle
Pons
Trigeminal nerves
Middle peduncle
Rhomboid fossa
Acoustic nerve
Facial nerve
Abducent nerve
Clava
Hypoglossal nerve
Glossopharyngeal and vagus nerves

FIGURE 89-1 Anatomy of the brainstem.

Presenting Signs and Symptoms

The chief complaints by patients and their family members are highly variable along the spectrum of altered mental status. Patients may report increased sleepiness or periods of confusion and disorientation. They may have difficulty concentrating or maintaining focus on tasks that previously gave them no trouble. Family members may describe the patient as less interactive or more difficult to arouse from sleep. Some patients may present to the ED via ambulance after distraught family members are unable to arouse them even with vigorous physical stimuli.

In all of these circumstances, important historical questions must be considered; the family or persons presenting with the patient may be the best source of information. They may know of preceding symptoms about which the patient may have voiced concerns such as headache, nausea, vomiting, or fever. It is important to determine the rate of onset of symptoms or if there was any history of trauma or exposure to drugs or toxins. Family members usually have some knowledge regarding the patient's past medical history, which may include diabetes, liver or renal disease, vascular disease such as hypertension, stroke or transient ischemic attacks, malignancy, seizures, immunocompromised states such as HIV infection, sickle cell disease, organ transplantation, or psychiatric illness.

The age of the patient can be a key historical tool that may focus the physician on the most likely etiology of the patient's presenting complaint (Box 89-1).

> **BOX 89-1**
>
> **Common Age-Related Etiologies**
>
> **Infant**
> - Infection
> - Trauma/abuse
> - Metabolic
>
> **Child**
> - Toxic ingestion
>
> **Adolescent/Young Adult**
> - Toxic ingestion
> - Recreational drug use
> - Trauma
>
> **Elderly**
> - Medication changes
> - Over-the-counter medications
> - Infection
> - Alterations in living environment
> - Stroke

In infants, infectious causes of altered mental status are most common; however, trauma secondary to physical abuse and metabolic derangements from inborn errors of metabolism also are possible causes.[3] Toxic ingestions are commonly seen in young chil-

BOX 89-2

Structural Etiologies of Altered Mental Status and Coma

Trauma
- Subdural hematoma
- Epidural hematoma
- Cerebral concussion/contusion

Stroke Syndromes
- Embolism
  - Cardiac (atrial fibrillation, endocarditis)
  - Paradoxical (fat embolus)
- Thrombosis
  - Cerebral venous sinus thrombosis
  - Hemorrhage
  - Subarachnoid hemorrhage
  - Pontine hemorrhage
  - Cerebellar hemorrhage
  - Intracerebral hemorrhage

Tumor
- Brainstem tumors
- Metastatic disease
- Angiomas
- Pituitary apoplexy
- Acute hydrocephalus

Infection
- Subdural empyema/abscess

dren. Adolescents and young adults often present to the ED after recreational drug use. The elderly are particularly susceptible to infectious etiologies and to disorders related to changes in drug doses, use of over-the-counter medications, and alterations in their living environment.

Differential Diagnosis

The differential diagnosis of altered mental status and coma is extensive and can be daunting for the busy EP (Box 89-2). Fortunately, there are many distinguishing features in the physical examination that, when combined with information gleaned from the patient's history, point to a particular etiology. A systematic approach is best and reduces the likelihood of missing an important clue.[1,2,4]

Patient Evaluation

As with all patients, specific attention should be paid first to assessment of vital signs. Marked hypotension or hypertension should be immediately addressed even if the underlying etiology is unknown. Bradycardia may be the result of increased intracranial pressure as seen in Cushing's response and suggests a state of hypoperfusion. Tachycardia also may result in hypoperfusion and can be the result of toxic/metabolic or primary cardiac causes. Assessment of temperature is crucial because both hypothermia and hyperthermia can cause altered mental status from infectious, structural, or toxic/metabolic etiologies (Box 89-3). Alterations in respiratory patterns such as hyperventilation, Kussmaul's or Cheyne-Stokes breathing, agonal breathing, or apnea should be noted and may suggest toxic/metabolic derangements or primary central nervous system abnormalities.

Signs of trauma should be sought immediately. Scalp lacerations or hematomas, depressed skull fractures, hemotympanum, raccoon eyes, Battle's sign, cerebrospinal fluid rhinorrhea, c-spine stepoffs, and crepitus all suggest a traumatic etiology. Other signs of trauma include lesions on the chest, abdomen, or pelvis; long bone deformities; and gross blood in the rectum or vagina. In the absence of trauma, breath odors may be helpful, including the smell of alcohol, ketones (diabetic/alcoholic ketoacidosis), and bitter almonds (cyanide toxicity). Abdominal findings include ascites, hepatosplenomegaly, ecchymosis, and striae. Lesions on the skin such as rashes, signs of drug use (needle "tracks," medication patches), and embolic phenomena can be telling.

■ NEUROLOGIC EXAMINATION

A systematic neurologic examination is a key tool in determining whether the etiology is structural or systemic or metabolic. The basic examination includes evaluation of the patient's level of altertness, cranial nerves, strength, reflexes, rapid alternating movements, gait, and cerebellar function. Serial measurements of the Glasgow Coma Scale (Table 89-1) are useful in determining whether a patient's mental status is deteriorating or improving over time.

A focal neurologic deficit usually suggests a structural etiology. Pupil findings such as unilateral dilation or a "blown pupil" and loss of reactivity indicate uncal herniation, which is a neurosurgical emergency. Funduscopic examination can demonstrate hemorrhage in the setting of trauma or papilledema, which suggests intracranial pressure.[2]

Testing of eye movements is a hallmark in the neurologic examination of patients with altered mental status or coma. Eye movements are coordinated by ocular centers in the cerebral cortex and the medial longitudinal fasciculus located in the brainstem. Extraocular muscles are innervated primarily by cranial nerves III, IV, and VI. Disconjugate gaze in the horizontal plane is common and can be associated with sedated or drowsy states or alcohol intoxication. Disconjugate gaze in the vertical plane is more ominous and points to pontine or cerebellar lesions. A persistently adducted eye is caused by cranial nerve VI paresis, whereas a persistently abducted eye is caused by cranial nerve III paresis. These are nonlocalizing lesions, however, since

BOX 89-3

Metabolic/Systemic Etiologies of Altered Mental Status and Coma

Hypoxia
- Severe pulmonary disease (hypoventilation)
- Severe anemia
- Environmental/toxin
  - Methemoglobinemia
  - Cyanide
  - Carbon monoxide
  - Decreased atmospheric oxygen (high altitude)
  - Near-drowning

Glucose Disorders
- Hypoglycemia
  - Chronic alcohol abuse and liver disease
  - Excessive doseage of insulin or other hypoglycemic agents
  - Insulinoma
- Hyperglycemia
  - Diabetic ketoacidosis
  - Nonketotic hyperosmolar coma

Decreased Cerebral Blood Flow
- Hypovolemic shock
- Cardiac
  - Vasovagal syncope
  - Arrhythmias
  - Myocardial infarction
  - Valvular disorders
  - Congestive heart failure
  - Pericardial effusion/tamponade
  - Myocarditis
- Infectious
  - Septic shock
  - Bacterial meningitis
- Vascular/hematologic
  - Hypertensive encephalopathy
  - Pseudotumor cerebri
  - Hyperviscosity (sickle cell, polycythemia)
  - Hyperventilation
  - Cerebral vasculitis as a manifestation of systemic lupus erythematosus
  - Thrombotic thrombocytopenic purpura
  - Disseminated intravascular coagulation

Metabolic Cofactor Deficiency
- Thiamine (Wernicke-Korsakoff syndrome)
- Pyridoxine (isoniazid overdose)
- Folic acid (chonic alcohol abuse)
- Cyanocobalamin
- Niacin

Electrolyte/pH Disturbances
- Acidosis/alkalosis
- Hypernatremia/hyponatremia*
- Hypercalcemia/hypocalcemia
- Hypophosphatemia
- Hypermagnesemia/hypomagnesemia

Endocrine Disorders
- Myxedema coma, thyrotoxicosis
- Hypopituitarism
- Addison's disease (primary or secondary)
- Cushing's disease
- Pheochromocytoma
- Hyperparathyroidism/hypoparathyroidism

Endogenous Toxins
- Hyperammonemia (liver failure)
- Uremia (renal disease)
- Carbon dioxide narcosis (pulmonary disease)
- Porphyria

Exogenous Toxins
- Alcohols
  - Ethanol, isopropyl alcohol, methanol, ethylene glycol
- Acid poisons
  - Salicylates
  - Paraldehyde
  - Ammonium chloride
- Antidepressant medications
  - Lithium
  - Tricyclic antidepressants
  - Selective serotonin reuptake inhibitors
  - Monamine oxidase inhibitors
- Stimulants
  - Amphetamines/methamphetamines
  - Cocaine
  - Over-the-counter sympathomimetics
- Narcotics/opiates
  - Morphine
  - Heroin
  - Codeine, oxycodone, meperidine, hydrocodone
  - Methadone
  - Fentanyl
  - Propoxyphene
- Sedative-hypnotics
  - Benzodiazepines
  - Barbiturates
  - Rohypnol
  - Bromide
- Hallucinogens
  - Lysergic acid diethylamide
  - Marijuana

Continued

BOX 89-3

Metabolic/Systemic Etiologies of Altered Mental Status and Coma—cont'd

  - Mescaline, peyote
  - Mushrooms
  - Phencyclidine
- Herbs/plants
  - Aconite
  - Jimsonweed
  - Morning glory
- Volatile substances
  - Hydrocarbons (gasoline, butane, toluene, benzene, choroform)
  - Nitrites
  - Anesthetic agents (nitrous oxide, ether)
- Other
  - Gamma-hydroxybutyrate
  - Ketamine
  - Penicillin
  - Cardiac glycosides
  - Anticonvulsants
  - Steroids
  - Heavy metals
  - Cimetidine
  - Organophosphates

Disorders of Temperature Regulation/ Environmental
- Hypothermia
- Heat stroke
- Malignant hyperthermia
- Neuroleptic malignant syndrome
- High-altitude cerebral edema
- Dysbarism

Primary Glial or Neuronal Disorders
- Adrenoleukodystrophy
- Creutzfeldt-Jakob disease
- Progressive multifocal leukoencephalopathy
- Marchiafava-Bignami disease
- Gliomatosis cerebri
- Central pontine myelinolysis

Other Disorders with Unknown Etiology
- Seizures
- Postictal states
- Reye's syndrome†
- Intussusception†

*Can be associated with dilution of formula in infant feeding.
†Prominent in the pediatric population.

Table 89-1 GLASCOW COMA SCALE

		Score
Eye opening	Spontaneous	4
	To voice	3
	To pain	2
	None	1
Verbal response		
Adult	Oriented	5
	Confused	4
	Inappropriate words	3
	Incomprehensible words	2
	None	1
Pediatric	Appropriate	5
	Cries, consolable	4
	Persistently irritable	3
	Restless, agitated	2
	None	1
Motor response	Obeys commands	6
	Localizes pain	5
	Withdraws to pain	4
	Flexion to pain	3
	Extension to pain	2
	None	1
Maximum score		15

elevated ICP or mass effects from trauma, for example, can compromise cranial nerve functions due to extrinsic compression. In the absence of contraindications, oculocephalic (doll's eyes) or oculovestibular reflex testing can be very helpful. If intact, these reflexes demonstrate functional integrity of a significant majority of the brainstem, making it exceedingly unlikely as the anatomical location for the etiology of the patient's altered mental status.[1,2,4]

Diagnostic Testing

Diagnostic testing in the patient with altered mental status or coma is based on the information gathered from the history and physical examination, which in most cases will point toward a structural versus systemic or metabolic etiology. A general approach to the diagnostic work-up of patients with altered mental status or coma is shown in Fig. 89-2.

■ LABORATORY EVALUATION

Extensive metabolic work-ups should not precede neuroimaging studies in patients with altered mental

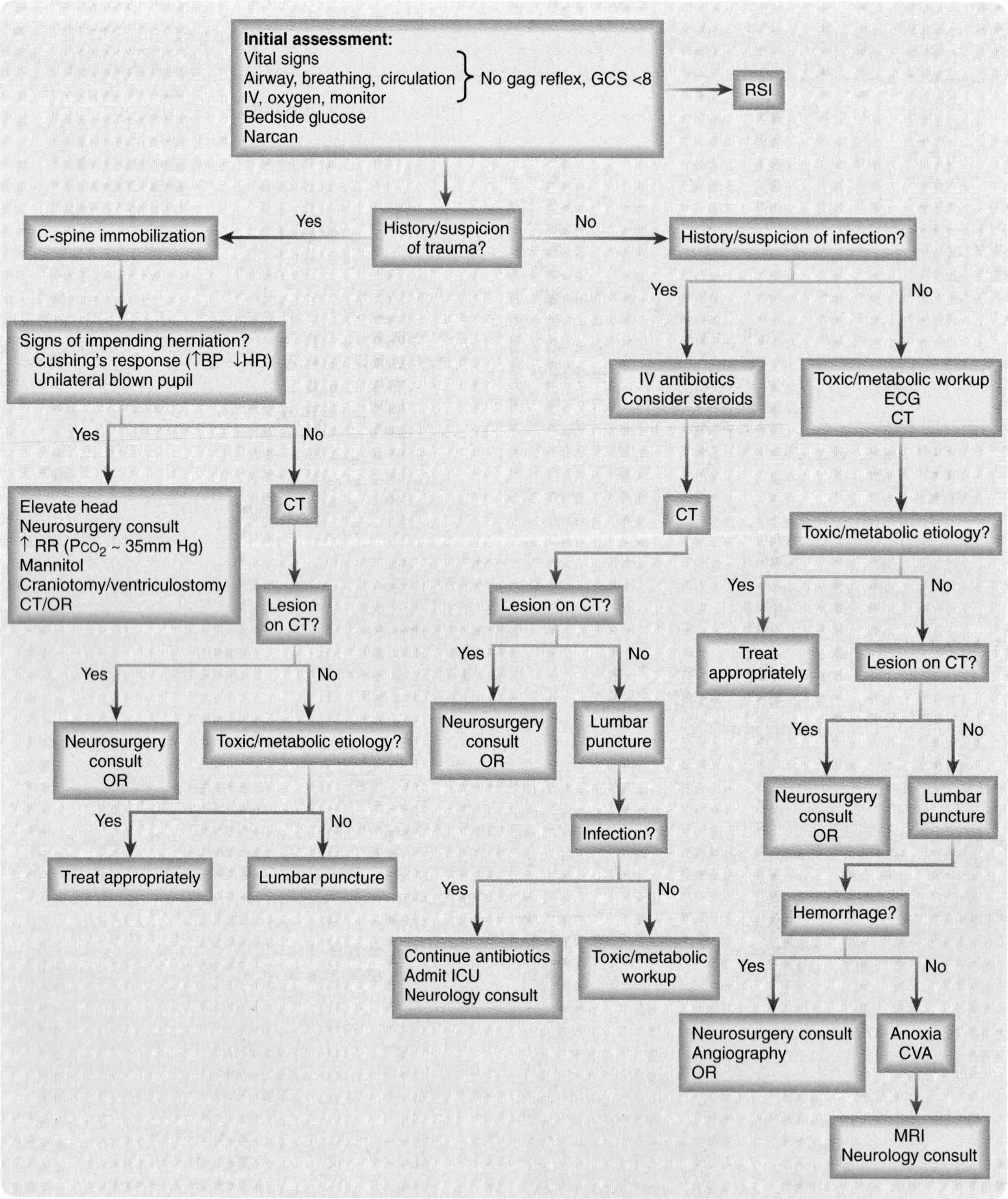
Initial assessment:
Vital signs
Airway, breathing, circulation
IV, oxygen, monitor
Bedside glucose
Narcan
No gag reflex, GCS <8
RSI
History/suspicion of trauma?
Yes
No
C-spine immobilization
History/suspicion of infection?
Signs of impending herniation?
Cushing's response (↑BP ↓HR)
Unilateral blown pupil
Yes
No
Elevate head
Neurosurgery consult
↑ RR (Pco2 ~ 35mm Hg)
Mannitol
Craniotomy/ventriculostomy
CT/OR
CT
Lesion on CT?
Yes
No
Neurosurgery consult OR
Toxic/metabolic etiology?
Yes
No
Treat appropriately
Lumbar puncture
IV antibiotics
Consider steroids
CT
Lesion on CT?
Yes
No
Neurosurgery consult OR
Lumbar puncture
Infection?
Yes
No
Continue antibiotics
Admit ICU
Neurology consult
Toxic/metabolic workup
Toxic/metabolic workup
ECG
CT
Toxic/metabolic etiology?
Yes
No
Treat appropriately
Lesion on CT?
Yes
No
Neurosurgery consult OR
Lumbar puncture
Hemorrhage?
Yes
No
Neurosurgery consult
Angiography
OR
Anoxia
CVA
MRI
Neurology consult

FIGURE 89-2 Diagnostic approach to altered mental status and coma. BP, blood pressure; CT, computed tomography; CVA, cerebrovascular accident; ECG, electrocardiography; GCS, Glasgow Coma Scale; HR, heart rate; ICU, intensive care unit; MRI, magnetic resonance imaging; OR, operating room; RR, respiratory rate; RSI, rapid sequence intubation.

status or coma that may be due to structural causes. Likewise, treatment of suspected narcotic overdose or hypoglycemia should not be delayed in favor of imaging studies.

Laboratory studies are most useful in determining systemic or metabolic causes of altered mental status. Capillary blood glucose measurement—both prehospital and on presentation—can often avoid further extensive metabolic studies, especially in patients with diabetes or alcohol intoxication. Serum electrolytes may demonstrate an anion gap or acidosis. Renal function studies may identify the cause for sodium or potassium imbalance. Serum calcium may be a marker for metastatic disease.

An elevated white blood cell count is rarely helpful in diagnosis of disorders with metabolic or toxic etiologies because it is a nonspecific marker for infection. However, a low count raises concerns for an immunocompromised state. Low platelet levels may indicate sepsis or intracranial bleeding, and the treating physician should exercise caution before performing a lumbar puncture or obtaining central venous access. Serum coagulation studies may be performed to look for bleeding dyscrasias or, when combined with the other liver function studies, may provide evidence of liver dysfunction. Checking the serum ammonia level is controversial; it has not been shown to be a reliable marker for the etiology of altered mental status.

Thyroid function studies are useful in patients with suspected myxedema coma due to hypothyroidism. Arterial blood gas analysis can aid in the classification of acid/base disturbances. In the absence of contraindications, cerebrospinal fluid analysis is mandatory when considering central nervous system infectious etiology or ruling out a subarachnoid hemorrhage after a negative, noncontrast computed tomography scan of the brain.

Urinalysis is a useful tool, providing information about volume status (specific gravity), spilling of glucose as in hyperosmolar coma, and evidence of infection, which is a common cause of altered mental status in the elderly. Urine drug screening for illicit drug use as a cause of altered mental status often is not helpful unless other causes are not forthcoming. Microscopic analysis of urine can reveal calcium oxalate crystals in the setting of ethylene glycol ingestion.

■ IMAGING

The mainstay of diagnostic imaging in the setting of altered mental status is noncontrast computed tomography scanning of the brain. It is fast and readily available in most ED settings, which makes it suitable for the unstable patient. It can reveal the vast majority of intracranial hemorrhages large enough to induce coma. When tumor or infection is suspected, a contrast-enhanced computed tomography scan may be indicated.

A limitation of brain computed tomography scanning is the potential poor view of the posterior fossa due to linear artifacts created by the thick skull base. Magnetic resonance imaging of the brain is more helpful in identifying structural lesions in this area; however, its cost and limited availability make this imaging modality less feasible in most ED settings. In larger tertiary care facilities, angiography may be available for the diagnosis and/or treatment of intracerebral aneurysms or arteriovenous malformations.

Other diagnostic tools include plain radiography, which can reveal specific types of ingestions such as mercury, iron, and lead. This can be particularly helpful in the pediatric population. Electrocardiograms (ECGs) are useful for diagnosing certain ingestions (e.g., tricyclic antidepressants), electrolyte abnormalities (e.g., potassium, calcium), and hypothermia. Although not commonly used in the ED, electroencephalogram monitoring is mandatory for comatose patients with suspected status epilepticus.

Interventions and Treatment

Initial stabilization and quick establishment of the ABCs ares paramount in patients with altered mental status. Patients should be placed immediately on telemetry with concomitant administration of oxygen and initiation of IV access. Definitive airway control with endotracheal intubation is critical in patients without a gag reflex or with a Glascow Coma Scale score of less than 8. Lidocaine should be used for rapid sequence intubation in patients with suspected elevated intracranial pressure. In the setting of trauma, cervical spine immobilization with a backboard in addition to the initiation of IV fluid therapy is mandatory.

Once initial stabilization has been addressed, reversible causes must be sought. A bedside ECG and capillary blood glucose should be obtained immediately. Blood and urine studies should be sent to the laboratory early after the patient's arrival, and the patient should be scheduled for emergent head computed tomography. Empirical administration of a "coma cocktail," which consists of dextrose, thiamine, and naloxone, may bring immediate results and significantly narrows the differential diagnosis.

Physical examination with specific attention to brainstem function dictates further work-up and therapy. Patients whose brainstem function is compromised with evidence of brain herniation require immediate evaluation by neurosurgery. Empirical therapy with mannitol is indicated in this setting. Evidence of brain herniation secondary to a traumatic etiology may necessitate the use of burr holes on the side of the dilated pupil as a last resort. Ventriculostomy and monitoring of intracranial presure often is performed by a neurosurgeon in the ED.

Patients with compromised brainstem function but no evidence of herniation receive supportive care with a concomitant toxic/metabolic work-up. Patients are considered to have unsalvageable brain tissue if they have no brainstem reflexes, have not received neuroactive medications, and are normothermic.

In patients whose brainstem function is intact, supportive care is provided while the work-up proceeds. Lesions discovered on brain computed tomography scans require immediate evaluation by neurosurgery. In general, patients with operable lesions are transferred immediately to the operating room; patients with inoperable lesions continue to receive supportive care. In cases where there is a suspicion for an infectious etiology, empirical antibiotic coverage must not be delayed for lumbar puncture or other diagnostic modalities.

In the setting of suspected toxic ingestion, activated charcoal with or without sorbitol is indicated. Gastric lavage has been used in patients with recent toxic ingestion (less than 1 hour since ingestion) although this intervention is controversial and associated with potential complications, including aspiration and esophageal damage. Specific antidotes, if applicable based on the history and physical examination, should be initiated early. The appropriateness of early hemodialysis should be considered in patients with ingestion of substances amenable to this therapeutic modality.[5]

Disposition

The majority of patients who have significant alterations in mental status require admission for further work-up and treatment. The exception is the patient with an easily reversible cause, such as opiate overdose or hypoglycemia, who may be discharged after a period of observation during which there is a return to baseline mental status. In addition, patients with alcohol intoxication and no other etiology of altered mental status may be discharged once they are deemed clinically sober. Placement in an intensive care unit setting is usually appropriate for patients who require admission.

Immediate consultation with the neurosurgical service is paramount for patients with potentially operable lesions. After definitive airway control, rapid transfer to a center with neurosurgical diagnostic and therapeutic capabilities should be sought if the necessary resources are not available at the site of the patient's initial presentation.

REFERENCES

1. Plum F, Posner J: The Diagnosis of Stupor and Coma, 3rd ed. Philadelphia, FA Davis, 1980.
2. Bateman DE: Neurological assessment of coma. J Neurol Neurosurg Psychiatry 2001;71;13-17.
3. Kirkham FJ: Non-traumatic coma in children. Arch Dis Child 2001;85;303-312.
4. Feske SK: Coma and confusional states: Emergency diagnosis and management. Neurol Clin 1998;16:237-256.
5. Hoffman R, Goldfrank L: The poisoned patient with altered consciousness. JAMA 1995;274:562-569.

Chapter **90**

Cranial Nerve Disorders

Ernest E. Wang

KEY POINTS

The cranial nerves are composed of 12 nerves that supply motor and sensory innervation to the head and neck.

Cranial nerve disorders generally present with visual disturbances, facial weakness, or facial pain or paresthesias, depending on the nerve(s) involved.

Trigeminal neuralgia and Bell's palsy are common cranial nerve disorders.

A thorough history and physical examination should focus on assessing the potential for trauma (skull fracture), tumor, cerebrovascular accidents, vascular derangements (aneurysm, dissection, thrombosis), and infection (meningitis, abscess).

The presence of concomitant focal neurologic or systemic signs should heighten suspicion for a central rather than peripheral cause of the neurologic dysfunction.

Scope

The 12 cranial nerves provide motor and sensory innervation to the head and neck. Some nerves serve purely motor functions (cranial nerves III, IV, VI, XI, and XII), some serve purely sensory functions (cranial nerves I, II, and VIII), and the remainder serve mixed motor and sensory functions (cranial nerves V, VII, IX, and X).

In addition to somatic and visceral sensory components, the cranial nerves provide the *special sensory functions* of sight, smell, hearing, taste, and balance.

Understanding the functions of individual cranial nerves aids in pattern recognition of the clinical syndromes classically associated with disorders of specific cranial nerves.

Cranial Nerve I (Olfactory Nerve)

■ STRUCTURE AND FUNCTION

Cranial nerve I is a special sensory nerve that provides the sense of smell. Inhaled scents are detected by the olfactory *epithelium* lining the nasal cavity and transmitted to the olfactory *bulb,* which lies adjacent to the *cribriform plate* of the *ethmoid bone*. Olfactory sensations are relayed from the olfactory bulb to the brain via the *olfactory tract.*

■ DIFFERENTIAL DIAGNOSIS

The patient should be questioned about a history of head trauma. An anterioposterior *skull fracture* parallel to the sagittal suture or an *anteroposterior shearing injury* can tear olfactory fibers traversing the cribriform plate, leading to disruption of the synapses from the olfactory epithelium to the olfactory bulb.

A *frontal lobe mass* such as a tumor, meningioma, or abscess can compress the olfactory bulb as well, but these presentations tend to be more subacute.

Cranial Nerve II (Optic Nerve)

■ STRUCTURE AND FUNCTION

Visual stimuli are transmitted from the *retina* to the *optic nerve* through the *optic chiasm* to the *lateral geniculate nucleus* in the thalamus, where they synapse. From there, impulses are transmitted along the *optic radiations* (geniculocalcarine tracts, including Meyer's loop) to the primary *visual cortex* in the occipital lobes.

■ PRESENTING SIGNS AND SYMPTOMS

Unilateral loss of vision is most common in injuries of the optic nerve. Patients with bilateral visual loss may not be aware this until an examination is performed. Acute visual loss is often of vascular origin, including arterial or venous occlusion and cerebrovascular disease. Neurologic causes, such as multiple sclerosis, may be suggested by progression of visual loss over hours or days, pain, and a history of additional neurologic complaints with a recurrent waxing and waning pattern. Inflammatory processes such optic neuritis may be the initial symptom of multiple sclerosis.

Neuropathy from temporal arteritis usually occurs in elderly patients and is associated with progressive loss of vision, unilaterally or bilaterally, and constitutional symptoms, jaw claudication, and headache.

Idiopathic intracranial hypertension should be considered in patients with a history of headache, visual scotomata, and visual changes. The typical patient is a young, heavy-set woman who is taking oral contraceptives. The headache and visual changes usually are worsened with cough, bending over, or other maneuvers such as Valsalva.

Orbital compressive tumors or aneurysms cause mass effects that compromise optic nerve function.

■ DIFFERENTIAL DAGNOSIS

The differential patterns of visual loss are described in Box 90-1.

BOX 90-1

Differential Patterns of Visual Loss

- A central retinal etiology of the fovea or optic disc compromises visual acuity or causes a central loss of vision in the affected eye only.
- Unilateral blindness usually is associated with an optic nerve lesion and causes complete visual field loss in affected eye only.
- Unilateral nasal visual field loss can be caused by an internal carotid artery aneurysm compressing the lateral optic chiasm.
- Bitemporal hemianopsia can be caused by a midchiasmatic lesion.
- Homonymous hemianopsia from an optic tract lesion causes full contralateral visual field loss in both eyes.
- Homonymous quadrantanopsia secondary to a Meyer's loop lesion causes contralateral one-quarter visual field loss in both eyes.

Cranial Nerve III (Oculomotor Nerve)

■ STRUCTURE AND FUNCTION

The oculomotor nerve is a pure motor nerve that works in conjunction with the trochlear (cranial nerve IV) and abducens (cranial nerve VI) nerves to coordinate extraocular movements. The oculomotor nerve controls four of the six motor muscles of the globe: superior rectus (globe elevator), medial rectus (globe adductor), inferior rectus (globe depressor), and inferior oblique (globe elevator). It also controls the levator palpebrae superioris (upper eyelid elevator) and the intrinsic visceral motor function of the sphincter pupillae muscles and the ciliary muscles, which perform pupillary constriction and accommodation, respectively.

■ PRESENTING SIGNS AND SYMPTOMS

The patient typically complains of double vision or difficulty seeing out of the affected eye. There may be mild photophobia in bright light. The patient also may complain of inability to raise the eyelid (ptosis).

Cranial nerve III palsy is more common in patients older than 60 years of age and in those with diabetes and/or hypertension (Fig. 90-1).

In patients with herniation syndromes, there will be a history of trauma (Fig. 90-2), tumor, or other neurologic findings.[1]

Pain associated with unilateral mydriasis should alert the EP to look for an aneurysm of the terminal internal carotid artery.

Patients with an abscess or cavernous sinus thrombosis may have headaches, altered mental status, and seizures. Consider this diagnosis in the setting of signs and symptoms in the contralateral eye, prior sinus or midface infection, fever, chemosis, eyelid or periorbital edema, and exophthalmos.

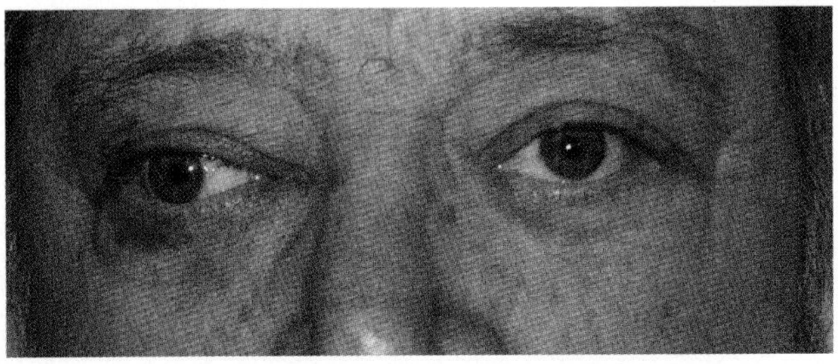

FIGURE 90-1 This 60-year-old man had diabetes mellitus, hypertension, coronary artery disease, chronic renal failure, and multiple myeloma. He presented with double vision (he described the images as "a little side by side but mostly up and down"), diplopia, ptosis, and papillary sparing. Laboratory tests and magnetic resonance imaging/magnetic resonance angiography scans were negative. The patient was evaluated by a neurologist and an ophthalmologist and ultimately was diagnosed with diabetic cranial nerve palsy. He was given an eye patch and scheduled for ophthalmology follow-up.

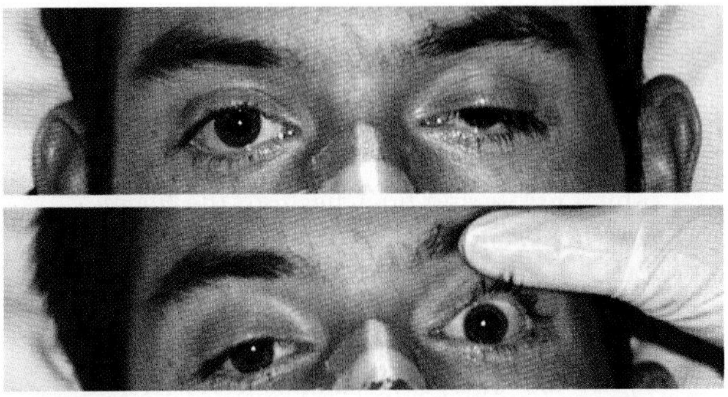

FIGURE 90-2 Ptosis and mydriasis suggest a cranial nerve III palsy. The appearance of these signs after a crush injury indicates that a skull fracture is impinging on the nerve canal. (Reproduced with permission from Baker C, Cannon J: Images in clinical medicine. Traumatic cranial nerve palsy. N Engl J Med 2005;353:1955.)

Cranial Nerve IV (Trochlear Nerve)

■ STRUCTURE AND FUNCTION

The trochlear nerve innervates the superior oblique muscle of the eye and causes inward rotation and downward and lateral movement of the globe. The trochlear nerve nucleus originates in the contralateral midbrain and wraps around the midbrain posteriorly and then anteriorly. It is the smallest cranial nerve and has the longest intracranial course.

■ PRESENTING SIGNS AND SYMPTOMS

Patients with a fourth nerve palsy present with double vision exacerbated by looking downward. The classic complaint is difficulty going down stairs. Most commonly there is a history of trauma. On the physical examination, the patient may unconsciously tilt the head away from the affected side (Fig. 90-3).

Cranial Nerve V (Trigeminal Nerve)

■ STRUCTURE AND FUNCTION

The trigeminal nerve is a mixed motor and sensory nerve. The trigeminal nerve is the primary sensory nerve of the face. It provides motor innervation to the muscles of mastication, as well as sensation from the face, scalp, conjunctiva, globe, mucous membranes of the sinuses, tongue, teeth, and part of the external tympanic membrane.

■ ANATOMY

The motor nucleus is located in the pons. The motor fibers innervate the muscles of mastication: masseter, temporalis, medial and lateral pterygoid, tensor tympani, tensor veli palatini, mylohyoid, and anterior belly of the digastric muscle. These muscles

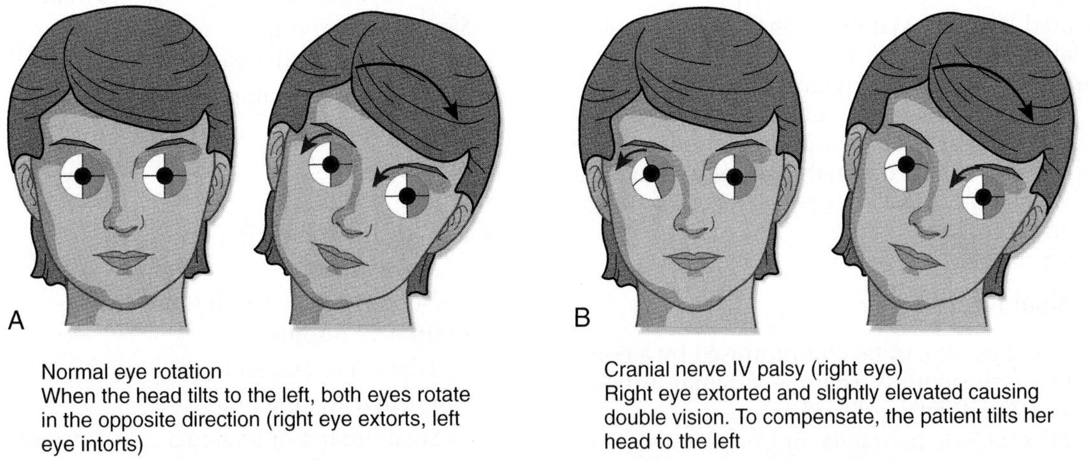
A
B
Normal eye rotation
When the head tilts to the left, both eyes rotate in the opposite direction (right eye extorts, left eye intorts)
Cranial nerve IV palsy (right eye)
Right eye extorted and slightly elevated causing double vision. To compensate, the patient tilts her head to the left

FIGURE 90-3 **A,** Normal eye rotation. When the head tilts, both eyes rotate in the opposite direction. **B,** Cranial nerve IV palsy (right eye). The right eye is extorted and slightly elevated, causing double vision. The patient compensates by tilting the head to the left.

open and close the mouth and move the jaw side to side.

The trigeminal sensory ganglion is located in the mid-cranial fossa and branches into three divisions:

- The *ophthalmic* nerve (V1) exits the superior orbital fissure and branches into the *frontal, nasociliary,* and *lacrimal* nerves. There is also a meningeal branch to the tentorium cerebelli.
- The *maxillary* nerve (V2) exits the foramen rotundum and branches into the *zygomatic, infraorbital,* and *pterygopalatine* nerves. There is also a meningeal branch to the middle and anterior cranial fossae.
- The *mandibular* nerve (V3) exits the foramen ovale and branches into the *buccal, auriculotemporal, lingual,* and *inferior alveolar* nerves. There is also a meningeal branch to the middle and anterior cranial fossae.

PRESENTING SIGNS AND SYMPTOMS

Patients with trigeminal nerve dysfunction present with either sensory or motor deficits. Sensory dysfunctions include paroxysmal pain, paresthesias (abnormal sensations such as burning, pricking, tickling, or tingling), dysesthesias (disagreeable, unpleasant, or painful sensations produced by ordinary stimuli), and anesthesia (loss of sensation). Motor dysfunction usually is described as difficulty chewing and difficulty swallowing.

Peripheral lesions cause loss of sensation or pain in only one division. Positive findings in two or more divisions (e.g., loss of light touch in one division and loss of sensitivity to pain/temperature/pin prick in another division) should raise suspicion of a central cause.

The presence of associated cranial nerve deficits (III, IV, and/or IV) suggests cavernous sinus involvement. In the setting of trauma, if a bruit over the orbit can be detected, a carotid-cavernous sinus fistula may be present. Associated involvement of cranial nerve VII or VIII or gait ataxia should raise suspicion of a cerebellopontine angle or lateral pontine tumor (Table 90-1).

Associated Horner's syndrome may indicate a cervical or lateral brainstem lesion.

The main categories of trigeminal nerve dysfunction are trigeminal neuralgia and trigeminal neuropathy. Sudden onset of symptoms should raise suspicion of a vascular, traumatic, or demyelinating cause, whereas a more indolent course suggests tumor or inflammation (Table 90-2).

Trigeminal Neuropathy

The trigeminal nerve can be compromised by a compression by extrinsic mass, trauma, vascular, inflammatory, or demyelinating disorders.

Symptoms include neuralgia and/or paresthesia to one half of the face. In contradistinction to trigeminal neuralgia, where the pain is more paroxysmal and episodic, the pain in trigeminal neuropathy is more constant. Loss of the corneal reflex is present. The patient's mouth may become more oval and oblique in appearance and, because of loss of masseter muscle strength, the chin may be deviated toward the affected side.

Until proved otherwise, neuropathies of cranial nerve V, of the chin (numb chin; V3), and of the suborbital region (numb cheek) should be presumed to be due to malignancies.[2]

Tic Douloureaux

The term "tic douloureaux" was coined by Nicolaus André, a French surgeon, in 1756. The mechanism is likely due to compression of the trigeminal nerve root within millimeters of entry into the pons.[3] There is a slight predilection in women and increased incidence over age of 60 years.[4] The maxillary and mandibular divisions are most commonly affected, either alone or in combination. The ophthalmic division is least affected. In one longitudinal case series, there were no cases of trigeminal neuralgia affecting both the ophthalmic and mandibular divisions.[4] Causes of tic douloureaux are listed in Box 90-2.

The International Association for the Study of Pain defines tic douloureaux as "a sudden usually unilateral, severe, brief, stabbing, recurrent pain in the distribution of one or more branches of the fifth cranial nerve." The pain is distributed along one or more divisions of the trigeminal nerve and is severe, sudden, intense, sharp, superficial, stabbing, or burning and is precipitated by normal activities such as eating, talking, washing the face, or cleaning the teeth.

A trial of carbamazepine can be therapeutic as well as diagnostic, because failure to improve with carba-

BOX 90-2

Causes of Tic Douloureaux

- Vascular compression by artery or vein
- Saccular aneurysm
- Arterioverous malformation
- Vestibular schwannomas
- Meningioma
- Epidermoid cyst
- Tumor
- Primary demyelinating disorders
  - Multiple sclerosis
  - Charcot-Marie-Tooth (rare)
- Infiltrative disorders
  - Trigeminal amyloidoma
- Nondemyelinating lesions
  - Small infarct or angioma in brainstem
- Familial

Table 90-1 CLINICOANATOMIC CORRELATION OF LOCALIZATION OF LESIONS OF CRANIAL NERVE (CN) V

Anatomic Site of Damage	Clinical Findings	Other Neurologic and Medical Findings	Common Etiologies
Supranuclear			
Sensory cortex	Facial numbness, paresthesias	Neglect, apraxia, aphasia	Stroke, tumor, hemorrhage
Internal capsule	Hemifacial sensory loss	Hemiparesis of arm	Stroke, tumor, hemorrhage, MS
Corona radiata		Central 7th cranial nerve paresis	
VPM thalamus	Facial numbness, paresthesias, pain; cheiro-oral syndrome	Anosmia, hemisensory deficit	Stroke, tumor, hemorrhage
Midbrain	Facial numbness, paresthesias, pain	Ophthalmoparesis	Stroke, MS, tumor, aneurysm
Nuclear			
Pons	Facial numbness and weakness, paresthesias, pain; trigeminal neuralgia	Ophthalmoparesis; CN VI, CN VII, CN VIII palsies; Horner's syndrome	Stroke, tumor, hemorrhage; MS, syringobulbia, abscess, trauma
Medulla	Facial numbness, paresthesias, pain; trigeminal neuralgia	Ataxia, CN X palsy, ophthalmoparesis, nystagmus, Horner's syndrome, Wallenberg's syndrome	Stroke, MS, tumor, aneurysm, abscess, vasculopathy
Preganglionic			
Cerebellopontine angle	Facial numbness	CN VII, CN VIII palsies; headache, cerebellar dysergia	Neuroma, meningioma, meningitis (bacterial, TB, cancer), aneurysm, trauma
Middle cranial fossa			
Gasserian ganglion	Facial numbness and weakness	Gradenigo's syndrome; CN VI, CN VII palsies	Tumor, infection, trauma
Skull base	Facial numbness and weakness	Headache, meningismus	Meningitis (bacterial, TB, cancer, sarcoid)
Trigeminal Nerve Branches			
V1: Cavernous sinus	Facial numbness, pain	Headache, ophthalmoparesis; Horner's syndrome	Tumor, thrombosis, infection, trauma
V1: Carotid-cavernous fistula	Facial numbness	Proptosis, bruit, ophthalmoparesis	Trauma
V2: Maxillary region	Facial numbness; numb cheek syndrome		Tumor, infarct, vasculopathy, trauma
V3: Mandibular region	Weakness of mastication; numb chin syndrome		Tumor, trauma, infarct

MS, multiple sclerosis; TB, tuberculosis; VPM, ventroposteromedial.

mazepine suggests some other cause. Second-line agents include Lioresal and Dilantin.

■ DIAGNOSTIC TESTING

The presence or absence of a corneal reflex should be checked. An intact reflex indicates normal function of the afferent V1 division as well as cranial nerve VII motor efferent function. The absence of a corneal reflex can be caused by posterior fossa and cerebellopontine angle tumors, multiple sclerosis, brainstem strokes (Wallenberg's or lateral medullary syndrome), and Parkinson's disease.

Motor function is evaluated by having the patient open and close the mouth and laterally deviate the jaw against resistance. Loss of muscle bulk or fasciculations in the temporalis or masseter musculature indicate a lower motor neuron lesion.

The jaw jerk reflex test determines the integrity of the V3 division. The examiner places a thumb on the patient's chin; the patient is instructed to relax the jaw completely with the mouth closed, and the examiner then taps the chin, eliciting the jaw jerk reflex. The reflex will be diminished in patients with a lower motor neuron lesion and accentuated in patients with a supranuclear lesion.

Cranial Nerve VI (Abducens Nerve)

■ STRUCTURE AND FUNCTION

The abducens nerve is a pure motor nerve that supplies the ipsilateral lateral rectus muscle of the eye and controls globe abduction. It is the most commonly affected cranial nerve in adults and the second most commonly affected cranial nerve in children

Table 90-2 SELECTED SPECIFIC ETIOLOGIES ASSOCIATED WITH TRIGEMINAL NERVE DISORDERS

Etiology Category	Selected Specific Etiologies
Structural Disorders	
Developmental	Brainstem vascular loop, syringobulbia
Degenerative and compressive	Paget's disease
Hereditary and Degenerative Disorders	
Chromosomal abnormalities, neurocutaneous disorders	Hereditary sensorimotor neuropathy type 1, neurofibromatosis (schwannoma)
Degenerative motor, sensory, and autonomic disorders	Amyotrophic lateral sclerosis
Acquired Metabolic and Nutritional Disorders	
Endogenous metabolic disorders	Diabetes
Exogenous disorders (toxins, illicit drugs)	Trichloroethylene, trichloroacetic acid
Nutritional deficiencies, syndromes associated with alcoholism	Thiamine, folate, vitamin B_{12}, pyridoxine, pantothenic acid, vitamin A deficiencies
Infectious Disorders	
Viral infections	Herpes zoster, unknown
Nonviral infections	Bacteria, tuberculous meningitis, brain abscess, Gradenigo's syndrome, leprosy, cavernous sinus thrombosis
HIV infection, AIDS	Opportunistic infection; abscess, herpes zoster Stroke, hemorrhage, aneurysm
Neurovascular Disorders	
Neoplastic Disorders	
Primary neurologic tumors	Glial tumors, meningioma, schwannoma
Metastatic neoplasms, paraneoplastic syndromes	Lung, breast; lymphoma, carcinomatous meningitis
Demyelinating Disorders	
Central nervous system disorders	Multiple sclerosis, acute demyelinating encephalomyelitis
Peripheral nervous system disorders	Guillain-Barré syndrome, chronic inflammatory demyelinating polyneuropathy Tolosa-Hunt syndrome, sarcoidosis, lupus, orbital pseudotumor
Autoimmune and Inflammatory Disorders	
Traumatic Disorders	
	Carotid-cavernous fistula, cavernous sinus thrombosis, maxillary/mandibular injury
Epilepsy	
	Focal seizures
Headache and Facial Pain	
	Raeder's neuralgia, cluster headache
Drug-Induced and Iatrogenic Neurologic Disorders	
	Orbital, facial, dental surgery

AIDS, acquired immunodeficiency syndrome; HIV, human immunodeficiency virus.
From Goetz CG (ed): Textbook of Clinical Neurology, 2nd ed. Philadelphia, WB Saunders, 2003.

(after cranial nerve IV). Incidence is 2.5 cases per 100,000 population in the United States.

ANATOMY

The motor nucleus lies in the pons. The nerve runs anteriorly toward the globe, crossing the basilar artery, the petrous temporal bone, and the internal carotid artery. It then enters the cavernous sinus and terminates in the lateral rectus. It is the most medial nerve in the cavernous sinus.

PRESENTING SIGNS AND SYMPTOMS

Patients with an abducens nerve palsy usually present with double vision. The head may be turned away from the affected side to maintain binocularity. Ask about a history of diabetes or hypertension, which

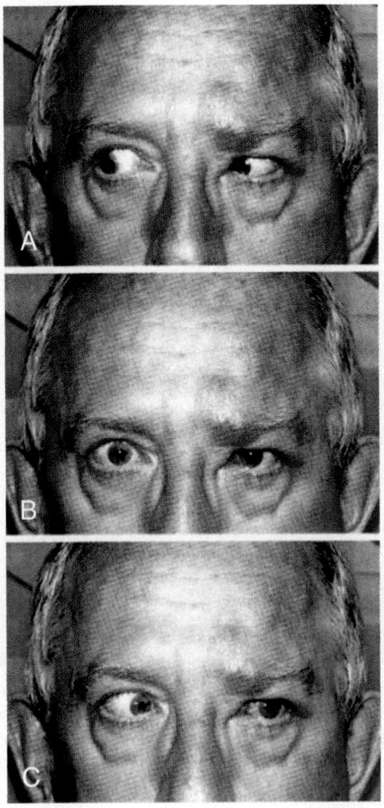
A
B
C

FIGURE 90-4 This 62-year-old man reported acute left retro-orbital pain of 1 week's duration. Double vision developed, a rash appeared on the forehead, and there was restricted abduction of the left eye; this is diagnostic of a left sixth cranial nerve palsy (right, center, and left gaze seen in panels A, B, and C, respectively) and binocular horizontal diplopia. A diagnosis of herpes zoster ophthalmicus was made. The patient was treated with gabapentin and acyclovir for 1 week. Six weeks later, he had minimal residual diplopia, with no postherpetic neuralgia. (Reproduced with permission from Jude E, Chakraborty A: Images in clinical medicine. Left sixth cranial nerve palsy with herpes zoster ophthalmicus. N Engl J Med 2005; 353:e14.)

are common risk factors. Another common sign is "crossed eyes" (esotropia or strabismus) (Fig. 90-4).[5]

■ DIFFERENTIAL DIAGNOSIS

Children are more likely to have a tumor as the principal cause, older individuals are more likely to have an ischemic cause such as temporal arteritis.

An abducens nerve palsy occurring in isolation is rare. In the United States, 8% to 30% are idiopathic, 3% to 30% trauma-related, up to 6% aneurysm-related, up to 36% ischemic, and 10% to 30% due to miscellaneous causes. Usually the seventh and eighth cranial nerves are also involved, signaling a central cause. Causes of abducens nerve palsy are listed in Box 90-3.

Truly isolated sixth nerve palsies are often caused by microvascular ischemia secondary to hypertension or diabetes. A thorough work-up must be performed to rule out a central, inflammatory, infectious, or neoplastic cause. Close follow-up by a neurologist over a 6-month period is indicated; most cases resolve within 3 to 6 months.

BOX 90-3

Causes of Abducens Nerve Palsy

- Trauma—blowout fracture of the orbit may result in trapped medial rectus and mimic a sixth nerve palsy.
- Subarachnoid disorders—hemorrhage, infection (meningitis), tumor
- Vascular—intracavernous aneurysms; sixth nerve palsies are almost always the first clinical feature due to this nerve's close relationship to the carotid artery and the fact that it is unsupported by afibrous covering.
- Giant cell arteritis
- Pontine glioma (in children)
- Pseudotumor cerebri may present with an isolated abducens nerve palsy in 30% of cases.
- Inflammatory (postviral or demyelinating) leptomeningeal involvement secondary to carcinomatous meningitis; inflammatory or infiltrating lesions of the cavernous sinus
- Metabolic—vitamin B deficiency, Wernicke-Korsakoff syndrome
- Congenital absence of cranial nerve VI (Duane syndrome)

Cranial Nerve VII (Facial Nerve)—Bell's Palsy

Bell's palsy is the most common cause of acute facial paralysis worldwide. The peak ages of incidence have been reported as between the ages of 15 and 45 years,[6] but other investigators have noted an increased incidence above the age of 70.[7,8] The mean age of onset is 40 years.[7] There is an associated increased incidence of the disease in pregnant patients and in patients with diabetes. Familial association is noted in 4% of cases.[6]

■ PATHOPHYSIOLOGY

The pathophysiology of Bell's palsy is not clearly established. Several theories have been proposed. One theory involves inflammation and edema of the nerve due to infectious processes, leading to nerve compression within the narrow canal as the nerve exits the stylomastoid foramen. A second hypothesis is the development of an ischemic mononeuropathy due to disturbance in the circulation in the vasa nervorum (the arterial branches supplying the nerve), leading to edema from the subsequent ischemic neuritis. Because the nerve is encased in a tight dural sheath within the temporal bone, this edema then causes additional compression of the vascular supply to the nerve.[9]

The most common cause of Bell's palsy is idiopathic, accounting for 66% of cases in one study.[6] Numerous observed associations are described in the literature. The palsy is often preceded by a viral syndrome. A correlation has been noted with the herpes simplex virus. Its association with shingles and the characteristic blistering (from the herpes zoster virus) is given the designation Ramsay Hunt syndrome. Bell's palsy also may be seen in patients with Lyme disease where the disease is endemic.

Diabetes, hypertension, human immunodeficiency virus (HIV) infection, sarcoidosis, Sjögren's syndrome, parotid-nerve tumors, eclampsia, amyloidosis, and recipients of the intranasal influenza vaccine are associated with the development of Bell's palsy.[7,10] Other common triggers include stress, trauma, fever, tooth extraction, and a "chilling" episode from exposure to drafts and cold.

Complete facial weakness, severe non-ear pain (e.g., retroauricular, cheek), late onset of recovery or no recovery by 3 weeks, diabetes, pregnancy, age over 60 years, hypertension, and Ramsay Hunt syndrome are risk factors for incomplete recovery.[11,12]

Electroneurographic studies demonstrate a steady decline in electrical activity on days 4 to 10. When excitability is retained, 90% of patients recover fully, but when excitability diminishes to absence, only 20% of patients recover completely.[7]

■ ANATOMY

Cranial nerve VII is a mixed motor and sensory cranial nerve, which accounts for the varied symptoms. It wraps dorsomedially around the nucleus of cranial nerve VI (abducens). It emerges from the pons at the cerebellopontine angle close to cranial nerves V, VI, and VIII, running through the internal auditory meatus. As it travels through the petrous temporal bone, cranial nerve VII displays a swelling, the geniculate ganglion, which contains the nerve cell bodies of the taste fibers of the tongue.

The parasympathetic greater petrosal nerve branches at this point to synapse at the pterygopalatine ganglion, which ultimately innervates the lacrimal glands as well as the mucous membranes of the nose and the hard and soft palates. The nerve then travels along the facial canal, gives off motor nerves to the stapedius and the chorda tympani, which gives off parasympathetic motor innervation to the submandibular and sublingual glands and afferent taste fibers from the anterior two thirds of the tongue. As the facial nerve exits the stylomastoid foramen, a small branch bisects the parotid gland to supply the muscles of facial expression.[13]

■ PRESENTING SIGNS AND SYMPTOMS

To the patient, the most alarming symptom of Bell's palsy is the abrupt onset of unilateral facial paralysis.

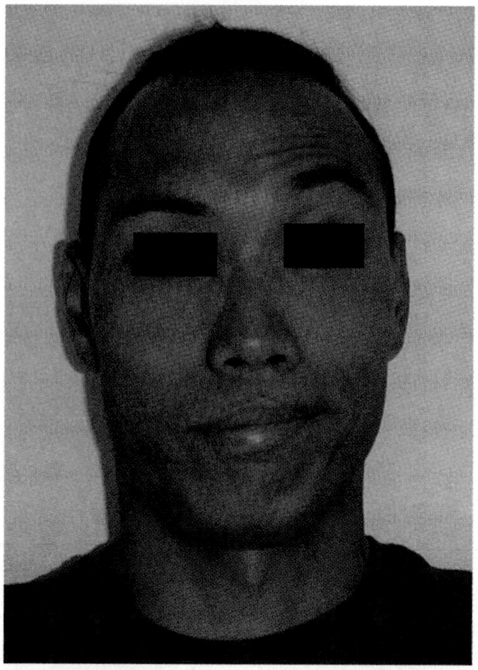

FIGURE 90-5 "Raise your eyebrows." A patient with a peripheral seventh nerve palsy (i.e., Bell's palsy) will have loss of forehead wrinkle at rest and inability to wrinkle the forehead and raise the eyebrow on the affected side (right side in this patient).

Approximately 50% of patients believe that they have suffered a stroke, 25% think they have an intracranial tumor, and the remaining 25% have no clear conception of what is wrong but are extremely anxious.[6]

The EP may note drooping of the eyebrow and/or corner of the mouth and loss of wrinkles on the forehead and/or nasolabial folds. Inability to raise the eyebrow and furrow the forehead is a cardinal sign of Bell's palsy (Fig. 90-5). Preservation of forehead motor neuron innervation should raise suspicion of a central cause.[11] Because the forehead receives bilateral upper motor neuron innervation, a central stroke will spare the forehead, allowing the patient to raise the eyebrow. If the patient can do this, it is not Bell's palsy.

Loss of nasolabial fold and nasal flaring is common. Loss of buccinator strength causes inability to blow out the cheeks. Inability to close the eye on the affected side is a hallmark of Bell's palsy. Speech is affected and may sound slurred or garbled, mimicking dysarthria from a stroke. An asymmetrical smile is often noted on examination (Fig. 90-6).

Signs and symptoms vary depending on the site of the affected nerve. They are listed in Box 90-4.

■ DIAGNOSTIC TESTING AND DIFFERENTIAL DIAGNOSIS

The "blow out your cheeks" test (Fig. 90-7) demonstrates loss of buccinator function. A sensitive variation of this is to ask the patient to hold water in his/her mouth and contract the buccal muscles. The

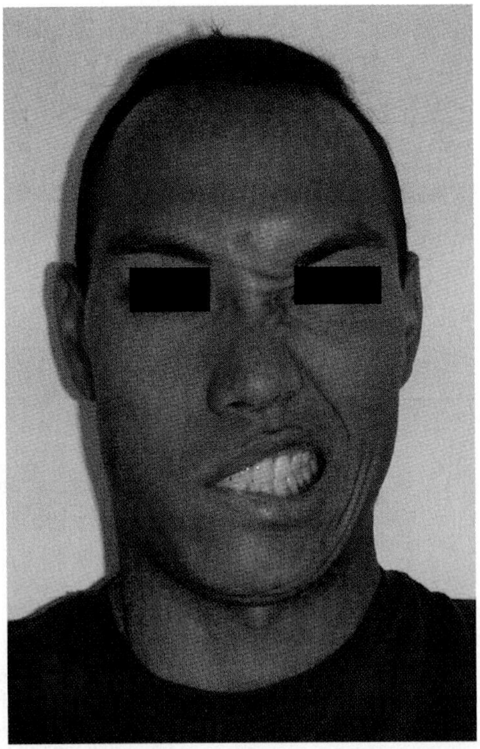

FIGURE 90-6 "Show me your teeth," "wrinkle your nose." Denervation of risorius and orbicularis oris muscles. Notice the inability to corrugate the nose on the affected right side due to loss of nasal and buccal musculature.

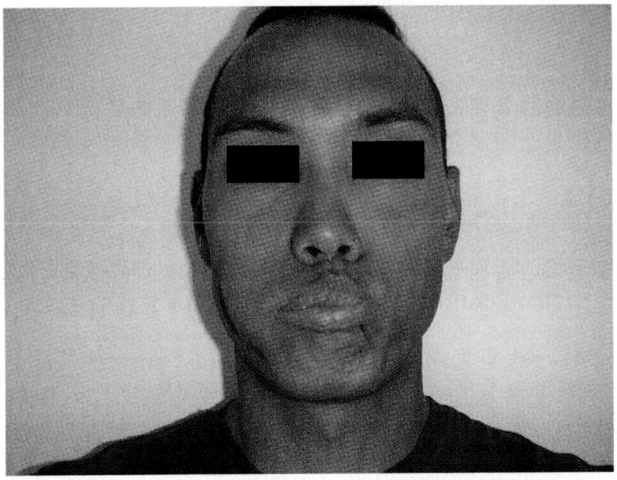

FIGURE 90-7 "Blow out your cheeks." Loss of buccinator function prevents pursing of lips, allowing air (and food and liquids) to escape.

BOX 90-4

Signs and Symptoms of Bell's Palsy

- Ipsilateral tongue numbness
- Loss of taste or dull taste
- Overt paralysis preceded by a sensation of subjective numbness or weakness on the affected side
- Ear pain in the external auditory canal
- Retroauricular pain
- Occipital headache
- Hyperacousis
- Fullness or snapping sound in affected ear
- Tinnitus
- Drooling
- Inability to keep liquids in mouth or chew
- Noticeable dryness of the oral and nasal mucous membranes on the affected side
- Anxiety

water will either dribble out of the corner of the mouth or shoot across the room.

Upon testing of hearing, hyperacousis may be observed on the affected side due to denervation of the stapedius. There should be no hearing loss.

To evaluate taste sensation, a few granules of sugar are placed on the tip of the patient's tongue on the affected side. Decreased taste sensation may be noted.

Other cranial nerves should be normal. The abducens nucleus lies at the level of the genu of cranial nerve VII; infarction in the area can cause concomitant palsy of cranial nerve VI, which signals an upper motor neuron lesion rather than Bell's palsy. There should be no evidence of expressive or receptive aphasia.

The presence of vesicles on the tympanic membrane or in the oropharynx (Fig. 90-8) or the presence of grouped vesicular lesions on the face or around the ear (Fig. 90-9) suggests a diagnosis of Ramsay Hunt syndrome.

Residual synkinesis can result from abnormal regeneration of nerve fibers. This can be manifested as abnormal motor function (e.g., blinking causes involuntary contracture of the risorius), abnormal parasympathetic function classically manifested by "crocodile tears"—lacrimation after a salivary stimulus, or as hemifacial spasm, which can be bothersome especially when the patient is tired.

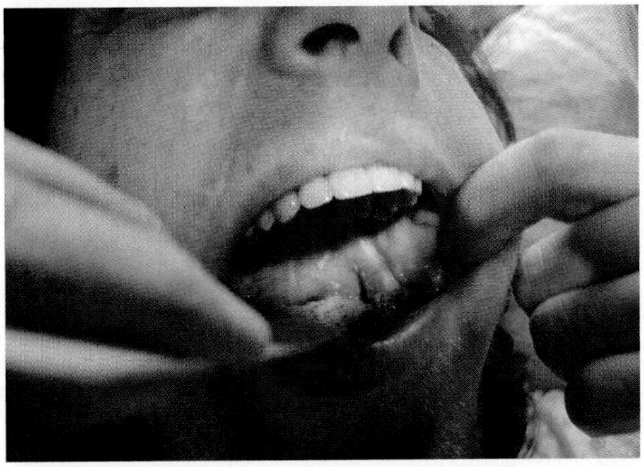

FIGURE 90-8 Buccal herpetic lesions of Ramsay Hunt syndrome.

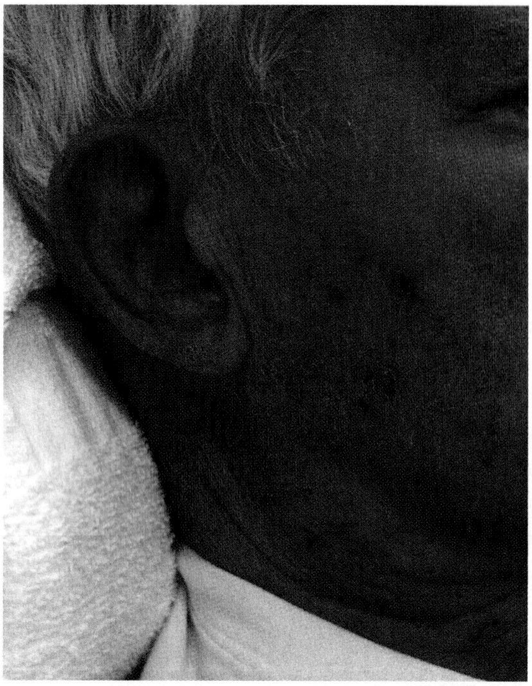

FIGURE 90-9 Characteristic auricular rash of Ramsay Hunt syndrome.

■ TREATMENT AND DISPOSITION

The algorithm shown in Figure 90-10 outlines treatment of patients with Bell's palsy.

Patients can be discharged home with oral medication, instructions for eye care, and expedited follow-up by a neurologist. Additional investigation for Lyme disease may be indicated for patients at risk.

Available evidence indicates that steroids are safe and effective in improving facial function.[7] Patients receiving steroid therapy are up with 1.2 times more likely to attain good functional outcomes compared with untreated patients.[14] No studies demonstrated significantly worse facial functional outcomes in patients treated with steroids.[14]

The most commonly reported treatment regimen is oral prednisone, 1 mg/kg, up to 70 mg per day, split into twice-daily dosing. The starting dose is continued for 6 days and tapered over the next 4 days.[14] Alternatively, prednisone 1 mg/kg/day, may be given for 7 days without a taper. Valacyclovir, 1 g twice a day, or famvir, 750 mg three times a day for 7 days, should also be prescribed.[7]

An eye shield or an eye patch should be worn during the night to prevent drying of the cornea. Commercially available eye patches are available over the counter or via specialty order such as NitEye from Solan Ophthalmic Products (http://www.solan.com). Liberal use of artificial tears during the day and an ophthalmic ointment such as Lacrilube at night should be prescribed to prevent drying of the cornea.

Pain medication should be prescribed because the otalgia and cephalgia can be debilitatingly painful.

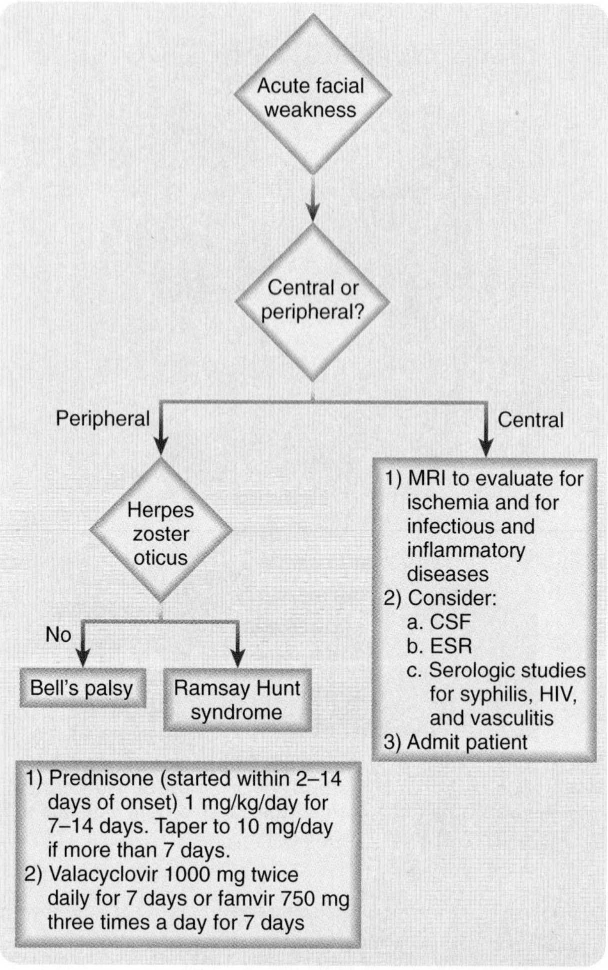
Acute facial weakness
Central or peripheral?
Peripheral
Central
Herpes zoster oticus
No
Bell's palsy
Ramsay Hunt syndrome
1) MRI to evaluate for ischemia and for infectious and inflammatory diseases
2) Consider:
a. CSF
b. ESR
c. Serologic studies for syphilis, HIV, and vasculitis
3) Admit patient
1) Prednisone (started within 2–14 days of onset) 1 mg/kg/day for 7–14 days. Taper to 10 mg/day if more than 7 days.
2) Valacyclovir 1000 mg twice daily for 7 days or famvir 750 mg three times a day for 7 days

FIGURE 90-10 Algorithm outlining treatment of patients with Bell's palsy. CSF, cerebrospinal fluid; ESR, erythrocyte sedimentation rate; HIV, human immunodeficiency virus; MRI, magnetic resonance imaging.

■ Prognosis

In a prospective study describing the spontaneous untreated course of idiopathic peripheral nerve palsy in patients with diabetes, 38% of patients had complete palsies, and only 25% regained normal facial muscle function.[10] This is significantly worse than the observed rate of spontaneous full recovery (94% for incomplete palsies and 61% for complete palsies) at 1 year in nondiabetic patients.[11]

Recurrence is rare (6.3%)[11] and should prompt a work-up for other causes such as myasthenia gravis, lymphoma, sarcoidosis, Lyme disease, and rarely, Guillain-Barré syndrome.[7,15] However, there is a case report of a 22-year-old woman with four left-sided episodes of Bell's palsy without obvious cause.[16] Bilateral seventh nerve palsy has been described, but only 50% are due to a benign, self-limited cause, and thus other causes should be considered.[16]

■ Aftercare

Although the prognosis for recovery is good, the psychological consequences can be long-lasting and are perhaps more significant than the physical disability. Patients report self-consciousness about the facial disfigurement, fear of permanent disfigurement, loss of self-esteem, and social ostracization. Return to work is difficult especially if one's work involves extensive contact with others.

Social embarrassment often occurs due to inadvertent loss of liquids from the mouth and significant difficulty chewing food. Men have difficulty with shaving due to loss of platysma function.

Cranial Nerve VIII (Vestibulocochlear Nerve)

■ STRUCTURE AND FUNCTION

The vestibulocochlear nerve is a special sensory nerve that transmits auditory signals from the cochlea (hearing) and signals from the semicircular canals (balance).

■ ANATOMY

The cochlea sits in the petrous temporal bone. Sound entering the external auditory canal vibrates the tympanic membrane, activates the ossicles, and transmits the sound wave through the cochlea. The cell bodies of the sensory neurons are located in the cochlea and combine to form the spiral ganglion. These neurons leave the cochlea, combine with the vestibular component, enter the posterior cranial fossa via the internal acoustic meatus, and terminate in the pons.

The vestibular apparatus also sits in the petrous temporal bone and is composed of a body consisting of the saccule and utricle and three semicircular canals aligned in three different planes. Hair cells within the endolymph of the canals detect angular movement and transmit the impulses to the vestibular nuclear complex in the floor of the fourth ventricle. The hair cells collectively combine to form the vestibular ganglion.

■ PRESENTING SIGNS AND SYMPTOMS

Patients with vestibulocochlear nerve dysfunction usually present with various degrees of hearing loss, tinnitus, vertigo (a false sensation of movement), falling, and imbalance. The mechanism is the result of asymmetrical integration of vestibular input to the central nervous system or asymmetrical disruption of sensory input from the vestibular organs.[17] If the vertigo is severe, nausea and vomiting also occur.

Symptoms may be constant or episodic; for example, benign paroxysmal positional vertigo can last 10 seconds, whereas vertigo attacks from Ménière's disease typically last 2 hours. Vestibular neuronitis causes vertigo that lasts for weeks, and central vertigo may persist for years.[18]

Patients should be asked about triggers, particularly positional triggers because this may indicate benign paroxysmal positional vertigo. Recent viral and upper respiratory tract infections may be significant because they predispose to vestibular neuronitis. The history should also include use of medications such as anticonvulsants, antihypertensives, sedatives, and ototoxic drugs.

The examination should be focused on determining reproducibility of symptoms, gait, balance, and ataxia; on evaluation of possible acute stroke symptoms; and on the character of the nystagmus and severity of ataxia. The presence or absence of associated cerebellar signs such as lateralizing dysmetria, motor weakness, sensory loss, and abnormal reflexes should be noted, as well as the Babinski reflex and cranial nerve abnormalities such as ophthalmoplegia, dysarthria, and Horner's syndrome.[17] Abnormalities of cerebellar function should prompt consideration of a central cause.

Patients should be examined for vertical and rotatory nystagmus, which are not typically present in patients with peripheral vertigo; their presence warrants imaging and neurologic evaluation.

■ DIAGNOSTIC TESTING AND DIFFERENTIAL DIAGNOSIS

The Dix-Hallpike maneuver commonly is used to elicit positional nystagmus (see Figure 91-1), which is associated with benign paroxysmal positional vertigo and usually lasts 5 to 60 seconds. Prolonged nystagmus is unlikely to be a result of this disorder.

Gait and balance can be assessed with tandem walking and the Romberg test. Ataxia and lateralizing dysmetria can be assessed with finger-to-nose and heel-knee-shin testing.

Hearing can be assessed with the finger rub or finger snap, Weber's test, and Rinne's test. The ear and external auditory canal should be examined for evidence of cerumen, otitis media, tympanic membrane perforation, and mass lesions.

Computed tomography (CT) lacks sensitivity in the evaluation of cranial nerve VIII disorders but may be useful in evaluating the bony temporal region. Magnetic resonance imaging with gadolinium is useful in identifying acoustic neuroma.

When a central cause is suspected, because of abnormalities on cerebellar testing or clinical suspicion, magnetic resonance imaging and/or magnetic resonance angiography should be performed to rule out posterior circulation stroke as a central cause of vertigo.

The differential diagnosis should include other cranial nerve deficits that typically are not present in benign causes of cranial nerve VIII dysfunction. Cranial nerve VII is the most commonly affected nerve because it travels with cranial nerve VIII in the internal auditory canal and is affected earlier by lesions compressing the eighth nerve. Acoustic neuromas may compress the trigeminal nerve when they reach 3 cm or greater; thus patients with complaints of facial numbness should be evaluated for trigeminal neuropathy as well for a mass lesion. Because large tumors can affect cranial nerves IX, X, and XI, these nerves should also be tested.

■ TREATMENT AND DISPOSITION

Some patients who present to the ED with sudden or severe symptoms may not be able to comply with testing because the severity of symptoms limits the ability to open the eyes and turn the head without experiencing nausea and vomiting or exacerbating symptoms. In these cases, it is appropriate to treat the patient symptomatically, initiate a work-up, and reassess clinically for improvement before attempting to move the patient or perform provocative testing.

Cranial Nerve IX (Glossopharyngeal Nerve)

■ STRUCTURE AND FUNCTION

The glossopharyngeal nerve provides branchial motor function to the stylopharyngeus muscle; visceral motor function to the otic ganglion and parotid gland; visceral sensory function from the carotid body; somatic sensory function to the posterior one third of the tongue, the skin of the external ear, and the internal surface of the tympanic membrane; and special sensory function of taste sensation from the posterior one third of the tongue.

■ ANATOMY

Cranial nerve IX originates in various nuclei in the medulla of the brainstem, converges and passes through the jugular foramen, and then branches out again to its terminal innervation.

■ PRESENTING SIGNS AND SYMPTOMS

Patients with a glossopharyngeal nerve palsy usually have associated symptoms involving other cranial nerves, most commonly cranial nerves X and XI.

The most common presenting symptoms are dysphagia and choking. If the vagus nerve is involved, the patient complains of hoarseness and demonstrates ipsilateral paralysis of the soft palate, which is secondary to ipsilateral paralysis of the soft palate, pharynx, and larynx. Head, neck, and oral trauma and surgery can cause acute dysfunction of cranial nerve IX.

Glossopharyngeal neuralgia is a rare disorder consisting of paroxysms of pain in the back of the throat and tongue. The pain is similar to that of trigeminal neuralgia in that attacks are brief, lasting seconds to minutes. It is unilateral and usually triggered by chewing, swallowing, coughing, or sneezing.

■ TREATMENT AND DISPOSITION

CT is warranted to evaluate for a cerebrovascular event or tumor. Rarely, vasovagal syncope can result from bradycardia or asystole caused by vagus nerve cardioinhibitory input. Medical management is similar to that for trigeminal neuralgia, including medications such as carbamazepin and phenytoin. If involvement of other cranial nerves is evident on examination, admit the patient for further evaluation and neurologic consultation.

Cranial Nerve X (Vagus Nerve)

■ STRUCTURE AND FUNCTION

The vagus nerve is a mixed motor and sensory nerve that provides motor function to striated muscle of the pharynx, tongue, larynx, and tensor veli palatine, as well as motor function to smooth muscle and glands of the pharynx, larynx, and thoracic and abdominal viscera

Cranial nerve X provides general sensation from the skin at the back of the ear, the external auditory meatus, the pharynx, and part of the external surface of the tympanic membrane, as well as visceral sensation from the larynx, trachea, esophagus, thoracic and abdominal viscera, chemoreceptors in aortic bodies, and stretch receptors in the walls of the aortic arch.

■ ANATOMY

The vagus nerve originates from brainstem nuclei in the medulla and exits the jugular foramen, giving off motor and sensory branches to the pharynx and the larynx as well as the auricular nerve, which provides sensory function to the skin of the ear, external auditory canal, and tympanic membrane. The remainder of the nerve runs adjacent to the carotid artery and internal jugular vein in the carotid sheath and gives off the recurrent laryngeal nerve at the level of the aortic arch on the left and the subclavian on the right. The remainder of the nerve then continues caudally to its end points in the heart, lungs, and gut.

■ PRESENTING SIGNS AND SYMPTOMS

Patients with palsies of the vagus nerve generally present with hoarseness or difficulty swallowing. A history of recent carotid or thyroid surgery should prompt suspicion for a recurrent laryngeal nerve injury. The patient may also complain about regurgitation of food and liquid into the nose.

The oropharyngeal examination usually reveals a drooped arch of the soft palate and uvular deviation away from the affected side.

■ TREATMENT AND DISPOSITION

A CT scan of the head without contrast should be performed to evaluate for cerebrovascular accident (hemorrhagic or ischemic) or skull-based lesions. Further inpatient evaluation may include magnetic resonance imaging of the head and neck and/or work-ups for metabolic, infectious, or inflammatory disorders as warranted.

Cranial Nerve XI (Accessory Nerve)

■ STRUCTURE AND FUNCTION

The accessory nerve provides motor function to the sternocleidomastoid and trapezius muscles.

■ ANATOMY

Cranial nerve XI arises from the accessory nucleus, passes through the foramen magnum, out of the jugular foramen with cranial nerves IX and X to the sternocleidomastoid and trapezius muscles.

■ PRESENTING SIGNS AND SYMPTOMS

Patients with accessory nerve palsies present with neck and shoulder weakness on the affected side. Inspection may reveal a "dropped" shoulder—that is, the affected shoulder lying downward and in lateral rotation. Testing of the sternocleidomastoid reveals weakness when turning the head against resistance to the contralateral side.

Due to the proximity of cranial nerves IX and X, particular attention should be paid to these nerve functions on examination. The most common etiologies are postoperative trauma (e.g., from cervical lymph node dissection) and cerebrovascular accident.

Treatment and disposition are similar to those for cranial nerves IX and X.

Cranial Nerve XII (Hypoglossal Nerve)

■ STRUCTURE AND FUNCTION

The hypoglossal nerve provides motor function to all of the intrinsic tongue muscles and three of the four extrinsic tongue muscles: the genioglossus, styloglossus, and hypoglossus.

■ ANATOMY

Cranial nerve XII originates in the medulla in the hypoglossal nucleus and exits the skull through the hypoglossal foramina. The relevant structures it courses along with include the internal jugular vein and internal carotid artery. The nerve crosses laterally at the bifurcation of the common carotid artery prior to terminating in the tongue muscles.

■ PRESENTING SIGNS AND SYMPTOMS

Patients with hypoglossal nerve palsies usually present with unilateral tongue weakness.

■ DIFFERENTIAL DIAGNOSIS

The primary diagnostic consideration is distinguishing an upper from a lower motor neuron lesion. An upper motor neuron lesion causes contralateral tongue deviation and fasciculations, and tongue atrophy is absent. A lower motor neuron lesion causes ipsilateral tongue deviation and fasciculations, and tongue atrophy is present. A 26-year review of 100 cases of hypoglossal nerve palsies revealed that tumors, predominantly malignant, produced nearly half of the palsies. Only 15% of patients made complete or near complete recovery.[19]

External lesions that cause compression or stretching of the nerve include internal carotid artery dissection or aneurysm, intracranial tumor, abscess, and other pharyngeal space tumors.

■ TREATMENT AND DISPOSITION

Treatment and disposition are similar to those for cranial nerves IX, X, and XI. If this is concern for cerbrovascular accident or space-occupying lesion, the patient should be admitted for evaluation.

Tips and Tricks

- Patients with palsies of the 12 cranial nerves present with heterogeneous symptoms reflecting the intrinsic function of each nerve.
- Patients with cranial nerve disorders generally present with visual disturbances, facial weakness or facial pain, or paresthesias, depending on the nerve(s) involved.
- Knowledge of the function of each of the cranial nerves helps the EP recognize the classic presentations of cranial nerve palsies.
- Trigeminal neuralgia and Bell's palsy are common cranial nerve disorders encountered in the ED.
- The majority of patients who present with acute onset of facial weakness are concerned about a stroke.
- A thorough history and physical examination should be focused on assessing the potential for trauma (skull fracture), tumor, cerebrovascular accident, vascular derangements (aneurysm, dissection, thrombosis), and infection (meningitis, abscess). Morbidity primary results from these entities.
- The diagnostic work-up and disposition depends on the clinical findings.
- The presence of concomitant focal neurologic or systemic signs should heighten suspicion for a central rather than a peripheral cause of the neurologic dysfunction.

REFERENCES

1. Baker C, Cannon J: Images in clinical medicine. Traumatic cranial nerve palsy. N Engl J Med 2005;353:1955.
2. Vahedi K, Bousser MG: Clinical examination of paralysis of the cranial nerves and principal etiologies. In Doyon D, Marsot-Dupuch K, Francke JP (eds): The Cranial Nerves. Teterboro, NJ, Icon Learning Systems, 2004, pp 1-6.
3. Love S, Coakham HB: Trigeminal neuralgia: Pathology and pathogenesis. Brain 2001;124(Pt 12):2347-2360.
4. Katusic S, Beard CM, Bergstralh E, Kurland LT: Incidence and clinical features of trigeminal neuralgia, Rochester, Minnesota, 1945-1984. Ann Neurol 1990;27: 89-95.
5. Jude E, Chakraborty A: Images in clinical medicine. Left sixth cranial nerve palsy with herpes zoster ophthalmicus. N Engl J Med 2005;353:e14.
6. Peitersen E: Bell's palsy: The spontaneous course of 2500 peripheral facial nerve palsies of different etiologies. Acta Otolaryngol Suppl 2002;549:4-30.
7. Gilden DH: Clinical practice. Bell's palsy. N Engl J Med 2004;351:1323-1331.
8. Katusic SK, Beard CM, Wiederholt WC, et al: Incidence, clinical features, and prognosis in Bell's palsy, Rochester, Minnesota, 1968-1982. Ann Neurol 1986;20:622-627.
9. Gacek RR: Hilger: The nature of Bell's palsy (Laryngoscope 1949;59:228-235). Laryngoscope 1996;106(12 Pt 1): 1465-1458.
10. Mutsch M, Zhou W, Rhodes P, et al: Use of the inactivated intranasal influenza vaccine and the risk of Bell's palsy in Switzerland. N Engl J Med 2004;350:896-903.
11. Allen D, Dunn L: Aciclovir or valaciclovir for Bell's palsy (idiopathic facial paralysis). Cochrane Database Syst Rev 2004(3):CD001869.
12. Holland NJ, Weiner GM: Recent developments in Bell's palsy. BMJ 2004;329(7465):553-557.
13. Wilson-Pauwels L, Akesson EJ (eds): Cranial Nerves—Anatomy and Clinical Comments. Toronto, Philadelphia, BC Decker, 1988, p 177.
14. Grogan PM, Gronseth GS: Practice parameter: Steroids, acyclovir, and surgery for Bell's palsy (an evidence-based review): Report of the Quality Standards Subcommittee of the American Academy of Neurology. Neurology 2001;56:830-836.
15. Keane JR: Bilateral seventh nerve palsy: Analysis of 43 cases and review of the literature. Neurology 1994;44:1198-1202.
16. English JB, Stommel EW, Bernat JL: Recurrent Bell's palsy. Neurology 1996;47:604-605.
17. Delaney, KA: Bedside diagnosis of vertigo: Value of the history and neurological examination. Acad Emerg Med 2003;10:1388-1395.
18. Hain TC: Cranial nerve VIII: Vestibulocochlear system. In Goetz CG (ed): Textbook of Clinical Neurology, 2nd ed. Philadelphia, WB Saunders, 2003, pp 195-210.
19. Keane JR: Twelfth-nerve palsy. Analysis of 100 cases. Arch Neurol 1996;53:561-566.

Chapter 91

Vertigo

Gretchen S. Lent and Andrew K. Chang

KEY POINTS

Not all dizziness is vertigo.
Vertigo is classified as peripheral or central, based on the anatomic location of the cause.
The majority of cases of vertigo arise from a peripheral source (e.g., cranial nerve VIII or vestibular structures).
The patient's description of symptoms, the type of nystagmus, and the physical examination findings help to determine the cause of the vertigo.
Benign paroxysmal positional vertigo (BPPV) is the most common type of vertigo.
The Dix-Hallpike test can be used to confirm the diagnosis of BPPV, and the Epley maneuver can be used at the patient's bedside to treat this disorder.
Central vertigo is less common than peripheral vertigo and results from a lesion affecting the cerebellum or vestibular pathways in the central nervous system.
Central vertigo should be suspected if there are any abnormalities in the neurologic examination.
Because the signs and symptoms of central vertigo can mimic those of peripheral vertigo, it is prudent to always consider a serious etiology.
Vestibular migraine is the most common cause of central vertigo.

Scope

Dizziness is the chief complaint in 7% of emergency department visits.[1] This symptom is more common in elderly patients.[2] Patients use the word *dizzy* to describe many different symptoms, including fatigue, lightheadedness, unsteadiness, headache, confusion, vision changes, and the illusion of motion.

Dizziness is traditionally categorized into four subtypes: vertigo, near-syncope, disequilibrium, and psychophysiologic dizziness.[3] The etiology of dizziness can be determined based on history alone in the majority of patients (Table 91-1).

Roughly half of patients reporting dizziness are diagnosed with vertigo.[4] Vertigo is defined as the sensation of movement when none exists.

Pathophysiology

The visual, proprioceptive, and vestibular systems inform the brain about movement and location of

Table 91-1 CAUSES OF DIZZINESS

	Vertigo	Syncope or Near-Syncope	Disequilibrium	Psycho-physiologic
Description	Spinning Tilting Weaving Rocking Rolling Somersaulting	Passing out Light-headed Fainting Blacking out Falling out	Tilting Feeling of falling Loss of balance Unsteady Staggering	Out-of-body sensation Swimming Dissociation Floating Spinning in head
Exacerbating factors	Turning head Rolling over Lying down	Standing from recumbent position Micturation Stressful event	Walking Turning Poor lighting	Stress Hyperventilation
Associated symptoms	Nausea Vomiting Tinnitus Hearing loss Central neurologic symptoms	Nausea Pallor Sweating Constriction of visual fields	Specific disorientation	Tingling of hands and face Anxiety
Associated signs	Nystagmus Central neurologic signs	Hypotension Irregular heart rate Bradycardia	Unsteady gait	None
Pathophysiology	Peripheral or central vestibular pathology	Loss of postural tone from insufficient blood flow to the brain	Imbalance between sensory inputs and motor outputs	Hypervigilance regarding symptoms, causing great psychological stress

Table 91-2 SENSORY SYSTEMS FOR BODY MOVEMENT AND POSITION

System	Organs	Information
Visual	Retina Occipital cortex	Spatial orientation
Proprioceptive	Proprioceptive sensors in skin, muscles, and joints	Body's location in space
Vestibular	Semicircular canals Otoliths Saccule Utricle	Body's relation to gravity

the body (Table 91-2). Input from these systems is integrated by the central nervous system. Overlapping of these systems allows two of them to compensate when one is deficient.

Vertigo is classified as peripheral or central, based on the anatomic location of the cause. Because peripheral vertigo is generally benign and central vertigo is more serious, it is important to make this distinction. Peripheral vertigo results from pathology to the vestibular system; central vertigo results from interruption of information being processed by the central nervous system.

Presenting Signs and Symptoms

Generalizations exist regarding what symptoms and signs correlate with specific types of vertigo. While these relationships hold true in the majority of cases, there are many exceptions.

The sensation of vertigo often is vague and difficult to describe. As a consequence, patients with dizziness are often very suggestible. Therefore, the EP should use open-ended questions (What do you mean by "dizzy"?) when interviewing vertiginous patients. Other helpful questions are shown in Box 91-1.

A thorough physical and neurologic examination is crucial in the vertiginous patient (Table 91-3).

■ NYSTAGMUS

Nystagmus is an involuntary rhythmic movement of the eyes to and fro that is often seen in patients with vertigo. The factors listed in Table 91-4 should be noted in all patients with nystagmus. It should be kept in mind that on extremes of lateral gaze, several-beat nystagmus is a normal finding in 60% of patients.

The following terms are commonly used to describe nystagmus:

- *Jerk nystagmus*—has a quick and slow component. The slow phase is the pathologic component; the fast phase is the correction mediated by the cortex. The direction of nystagmus is described by the fast phase.
- *Geotropic*—the fast phase beats downward toward the ground.
- *Apogeotropic*—fast phase beats upwards, away from the ground.
- *Torsional*—turning or twisting rotation of the eyes

BOX 91-1

Historical Features Relevant to the Dizzy Patient

Past Medical History
- Diabetes, heart disease, seizures, migraine headaches, cerebrovascular or cardiovascular disease

Psychiatric History
- Anxiety, panic attacks, hyperventilation

Social History
- Drug or alcohol abuse

Family History
- Cancer, atherosclerotic disease, migraines

Medication History
- Aspirin, aminoglycosides, diuretics, chemotherapeutics

- *Spontaneous nystagmus*—occurs when the patient is upright and the eyes are mid-position, may be present when the patient is asymptomatic.
- *Positioning nystagmus*—produced by a sudden change in head position

Differential Diagnosis

Details of the patient's history can narrow the differential diagnosis (Box 91-2). Findings on the physical examination also aid in making the diagnosis.

The major causes of vertigo are listed in Box 91-3 and are discussed in detail throughout the chapter.

Diagnostic Testing

■ BEDSIDE TESTS

■ Head Thrust or Head Impulse Test

The procedure begins by directing patient to look straight ahead and then thrust his or her head rapidly

BOX 91-2

Evaluation of the Vertiginous Patient

Consider the following factors when questioning patients in the ED evaluation:

General
- Sensation
- Length of episode
- Frequency of episodes
- Intermittent or constant
- Whether symptoms are mild, moderate, or severe

Precipitating Factors
- Noise
- Stress
- Head position
- Ameliorating circumstances
- Head or neck trauma
- Barotrauma (airplane flight, scuba diving)
- Ototoxic drugs (aspirin, aminoglycoside, loop diuretic)

Symptoms
- Do you tend to fall? Which side do you fall to?
- Any nausea or vomiting?
- Sensation of linear movement?

Symptoms Associated with Central Vertigo
- Diplopia
- Blurred vision
- Weakness of arms or legs
- Numbness in face or extremities
- Confusion or decreased consciousness
- Slurring of speech
- Clumsiness of arms or legs
- Difficulty swallowing
- Associated headache
- Gait ataxia

Symptoms Associated with Migraine
- Photophobia
- Phonophobia
- Preceding aura

Associated Auditory Symptoms
- Hearing impaired in one or both ears
- Pressure in ears
- History of ear infections
- Ear drainage
- Recent viral illness
- Tinnitus (constant or pulsatile)

Associated Cardiac Symptoms
- Chest pain
- Shortness of breath
- Palpitations

Table 91-3 **PHYSICAL EXAMINATION FINDINGS AND THEIR RELATION TO VERTIGO**

Finding	Result	Possible Etiology and/or Effect
Vital Signs		
Blood pressure	Elevated	Ischemic stroke Hemorrhagic stroke
	Decreased	Syncope/near-syncope Basilar ischemia
	Orthostatic	Syncope/near-syncope Basilar ischemia
	Dissimilar between arms (20 mm Hg difference)	Subclavian steal syndrome Aortic dissection
Heart rate	Elevated Decreased	Syncope/near-syncope Syncope/near-syncope
Respiratory rate	Elevated	Anxiety Hyperventilation syndrome
Temperature	Elevated	Dizziness
Ear		
External auditory canal	Infection Vesicles Cerumen impaction	Peripheral vestibulopathy Ramsey Hunt syndrome Peripheral vertigo
Tympanic membrane	Otitis media Perforation Scarring Cholesteatoma	Peripheral vestibulopathy Peripheral vertigo Peripheral vertigo Perilymph fistula, peripheral vestibulopathy
Mastoid	Tenderness or swelling	Peripheral or central vertigo
Temporal bone	Hematoma, step-off, crepitus	Post-traumatic vertigo or central vertigo
Posterior auricular area	Bruising (Battle's sign)	Post-traumatic vertigo or central vertigo
Hearing	Decreased	Labyrinthitis
Weber's and Rinne tests	Conductive or sensorineural hearing loss	Ménière's disease
Eye		
Ocular examination	Vertical misalignment	Central abnormality
Visual acuity:		
In all extraocular movements	Decreased	Cranial neuropathy or central vertigo
While head is moving	Decreased (oscillopsia)	Vestibulotoxicity
Nystagmus	Suppressed with visual fixation Purely vertical	Peripheral vertigo Central vertigo
Neurologic		
Cranial nerves	Deficit	Central vertigo
Cerebellar testing:		
Hemispheric function	Finger-to-nose deficit (dysmetria)	Central vertigo
	Poor rapid alternating movement (dysdiadochokinesis)	Central vertigo
Midline function	Deficient tandem walk	Central vertigo
	Deficient heel-shin test	Central vertigo
Gait (tandem, heel-toe)	Abnormal posture	Central vertigo
	Decreased length of step	Central vertigo
	Limb or truncal ataxia	Central vertigo
Romberg's test	Patient stands with feet together; steady with eyes open, falls when eyes are closed	Deficit in peripheral sensation, midline cerebellum, or dorsal columns
Standing	Veers toward one side	Peripheral lesion is on side patient veers toward
	Unable to stand	Central vertigo
Motor	Deficit	Central vertigo
Sensory	Deficit	Central vertigo

Table 91-3 PHYSICAL EXAMINATION FINDINGS AND THEIR RELATION TO VERTIGO—cont'd

Finding	Result	Possible Etiology and/or Effect
Proprioception	Deficit	Central vertigo
Vibration	Deficit	Central vertigo
Cardiovascular		
Heart sounds	Dysrhythmia	Syncope/near-syncope Embolic source
	Murmurs (hypertrophic obstructive cardiomyopathy, aortic stenosis)	Syncope/near syncope Embolic source
Carotid artery	Bruit	Embolic source

Table 91-4 CHARACTERISTICS OF NYSTAGMUS

Direction	Axis	Nature	Duration	Associated Factors
Left or right	Vertical or horizontal	Rotary or torsional	Seconds, minutes, or persistent	Spontaneous or positional Effect of visual fixation

to one side approximately 10 degrees; the EP should watch for rapid eye movements (saccades) toward the midline. Normally, no saccades will be seen. In patients with unilateral peripheral vestibular loss, when the head is moved toward the side with the lesion, their eyes cannot maintain focus, and saccades correctively bring the eyes back to midline. Both sides should be tested.

■ Hennebert's Test

Hennebert's test is performed on an intact tympanic membrane. Using a pneumatic otoscope, the EP applies negative and positive pressure to the external auditory canal. A test is positive when this pressure causes vertigo, nausea, and nystagmus. This test can also be performed by Valsalva maneuver or by pressing the tragus against the external auditory canal.

■ IMAGING

Any patient with focal neurologic findings on examination needs urgent brain imaging. Although imaging of the inner ear has dramatically improved, several peripheral causes of vertigo (e.g., benign paroxysmal positional vertigo [BPPV], perilymphatic fistula, Ménière's disease, and vestibular neuritis) cannot be visualized using current modalities.

■ Computed Tomography

High-resolution computed tomography is commonly available. Because skull-related artifacts are common with this modality, it has limited utility for evaluating the posterior fossa. If a patient has a focal neurologic finding and a normal computed tomography scan, further imaging is necessary.

■ Magnetic Resonance Imaging

For assessment of pathologic causes of vertigo, magnetic resonance imaging (MRI) is the modality of choice because it allows visualization of anatomic details in the vestibulocochlear and cerebellar regions and brainstem. However, magnetic resonance imaging is more costly and time-consuming and less readily available than computed tomography.

■ Magnetic Resonance Angiography

Magnetic resonance angiography is a noninvasive technique for visualizing the vessels of the posterior circulation. It detects aneurysms, atherosclerosis, dissections, vasculitis, thrombosis, and other processes.

■ LABORATORY TESTING

Laboratory testing is rarely useful in the initial evaluation of the vertiginous patient. Screening tests include hematocrit, glucose, and electrolyte levels. Thyroid function tests, antinuclear antibody levels, erythrocyte sedimentation rate, and vitamin B_{12} and E assays may be performed when indicated.

■ ELECTROCARDIOGRAPHY

An electrocardiogram is useful to evaluate for signs of ischemia or dysrhythmia.

■ ANCILLARY VERTIGO TESTING

Numerous specialized tests are available to evaluate vestibular function and hearing (Tables 91-5 and 91-6).

BOX 91-3

Major Causes of Vertigo

Peripheral Vertigo

- Autoimmune ear disease
  - Cogan's syndrome
  - Neurosarcoidosis
  - Rheumatoid arthritis
  - Systemic lupus erythematosus
  - Vasculitis
- Benign paroxysmal positional vertigo
  - Posterior canal
  - Lateral canal
  - Anterior canal
- Cerebellopontine angle lesion
  - Compression
  - Acoustic neuroma
- Endolymphatic hydrops (Ménière's disease)
- Focal peripheral diseases
  - Otitis media (acute or chronic)
  - Cholesteatoma
  - Tumor
  - Fistula
  - Genetic anomalies
  - Focal ischemia
- Inflammatory labyrinthitis
  - Otosyphilis
  - Lyme neuroborreliosis
- Ototoxic and vestibulotoxic chemicals
  - Aminoglycosides
  - Loop diuretics
  - Cis-platinum
  - Salicylates
- Perilymph fistula
- Peripheral vestibulopathy
  - Labyrinthitis
  - Vestibular neuronitis
- Post-traumatic vertigo
  - Immediate
  - Delayed onset
  - Ménière's disease–like
  - Post-concussive migraine–like
- Superior semicircular canal
  - Dehiscence syndrome
- Vestibular ganglionitis
- Vestibular paroxysmia
- Vestibulocochlear cranial neuropathy
  - Cerebellopontine angle compression
    - Acoustic neuroma
    - Cholesteatoma
    - Dermoid
    - Lipoma
    - Meningiomas
    - Metastasis
  - Vestibular paroxysmia

Central Vertigo

- Demyelination
  - Acquired
  - Leukodystrophies
  - Multiple sclerosis
- Familial disorders
  - Freiedreich's ataxia
  - Spinocerebellar ataxia
  - Familial episodic ataxia (type 1 and type 2)
  - Olivopontocerebellar atrophy
- Central nervous system infections
  - Lyme neuroborreliosis
  - Meningitis
  - Tuberculosis
- Intrinsic brainstem lesion
  - Tumor
  - Arteriovenous malformation
  - Trauma
- Migraine
  - Basilar
  - Benign paroxysmal positional vertigo of childhood
- Toxins
  - Drugs/alcohol
  - Analgesics
  - Anticonvulsants
  - Antihypertensives
  - Hypnotics
  - Tranquilizers
- Metabolic and endocrine disorders
  - Hyperinsulinism
  - Impaired glucose tolerance
  - Diabetes mellitus
  - Hypertriglyceridemia
  - Hypothyroidism
- Systemic conditions
  - Paget's disease
- Stroke/Ischemia
  - Vertebrobasilar
  - Cerebellar
  - Posterior inferior cerebellar artery syndrome
  - Lateral medullary syndrome
  - Medial medullary infarct
  - Basilar artery syndrome
  - Anterior inferior cerebellar artery
- Other causes of posterior ischemia
  - Subclavian steal syndrome
  - Rotational vertebral artery occlusion syndrome
  - Vertebral artery dissection
  - Vertebral or basilar artery dolichoectasia
  - Neoplasm of the fourth ventricle
  - Chiari malformation
- Superficial siderosis of the central nervous system
- Vestibular epilepsy

Table 91-5 ANCILLARY VERTIGO TESTING

Area Tested	Test	Description	Evaluation
Vestibular function	Electronystagmography	Records changes in the electrical potentials between the cornea and retina and the differences between ears; parts of test include calibration, tracking, and positional and caloric testing	Central versus peripheral vertigo
	Rotary chair testing	Electrodes record reflexive eye movements as the patient is rotated in the dark	Horizontal semicircular canal
	Posturography	Dynamic platform evaluates patient's balance while patient is blindfolded	Vestibular, visual, and somatosensory systems
	Fistula test	Infrared sensors record eye movements while pressure is applied to the ear	Perilymph fistula
	Dynamic visual acuity	Patient's vision is tested while the head is moving	Vestibular-ocular reflex
	Three-dimensional eye movement recording	Scleral search coils record nystagmus; vector analysis is performed	Ewald's first law
	Optokinetic testing	Patient looks at an optokinetic drum	Oculomotor response
Hearing pathway	Audiometry	Formal hearing testing; pure tone and speech are evaluated as well as tone decay and impedance audiometry	Cochlear or central pathology
	Auditory brainstem evoked response	Measures small electrical potentials from the brain in response to auditory stimulus	Auditory brainstem
	Electrocochleography	Measures electrical potentials generated in the inner ear in response to sound	Endolymphatic hydrops
	Click-evoked myogenic potentials	Electrodes on the sternocleidomastoid record the electrical potential generated in response to clicks; electromyograms are generated	Vestibulocollic reflex

Table 91-6 AUDIOMETRY RESULTS FOR VARIOUS CAUSES OF VERTIGO

Cause of Vertigo	Audiometry Results
BPPV	Normal
Labyrinthitis	Normal
Vestibular neuronitis	Normal
Ménière's disease	Low-frequency hearing loss
Acoustic neuroma	High-frequency hearing loss with poor discrimination
Middle ear disorders	Conductive hearing loss

BPPV, benign paroxysmal positional vertigo.

Treatment

■ ANTIVERTIGO MEDICATIONS

Short-term treatment with medications is useful in the management of peripheral vertigo (Table 91-7). It is important to avoid prolonging treatment because this may actually exacerbate symptoms. Therapy is based on the *sensory conflict theory,* which states that a mismatch of information from the vestibular, visual, or proprioceptive inputs will temporarily result in nausea but will resolve as habituation occurs. This mechanism occurs via gamma aminobutyric acid (GABA), acetylcholine, serotonin, and histamine receptors.

■ Benzodiazepines

Benzodiazepines prevent mismatched information from being compared to prior learned stimuli. They bind to GABA brainstem receptors and centrally suppress a labyrinthine response. These medications are helpful in patients whose vertigo is accompanied by anxiety.

■ Anticholinergics

Centrally acting anticholinergic medications are effective in the treatment of vertigo. They work by decreasing the signal-size conflict and are considered by some experts to be the most useful agents in the treatment of vertigo. Atropine generally is not used

Table 91-7 **MEDICATIONS TO TREAT VERTIGO**

Category	Drug	Dosage
Anticholinergic	Scopolamine	0.5-1.5 mg transdermal q3-4d
Antihistamine	Dimenhydrinate Diphenhydramine Meclizine Promethazine	50-100 mg IM, IV, or PO q4-6hr 25-50 mg IM, IV, or PO q4-6hr 25-50 mg PO q6-12hr 12.5-25 mg IM, IV, PO, or PR q6-8hr
Antiemetic	Hydroxyzine Metoclopramide Promethazine Prochlorperazine	25-50 mg PO q6hr 5-10 mg IM, IV, or PO q6-8hr 12.5-25 mg IM, IV, or PO q6-12hr 10-25 mg PR q6-12hr 5-10 mg PO q6-8hr
Benzodiazepine	Diazepam Clonazepam	2-5 mg PO qd-tid 0.25-0.5 mg PO bid-tid
Calcium antagonist	Nimodipine	30 mg PO q4-8hr

due to its serious side effects; scopolamine typically has too long an onset to be useful acutely in the ED.

■ Antiemetics/Antihistamines

These labyrinthine suppressants are the most commonly used medications for the symptomatic treatment of vertigo. H_1 antihistamines are effective, whereas H_2 antihistamines are not. Most of these agents also have anticholinergic properties but are believed to have an additional central action that is helpful. These medications also block the emesis response. Antihistamines suppress the vestibular end-organ receptors and inhibit activation of a vagal response. Side effects include dry mouth and sedation. IV promethazine is considered the best medication for acutely symptomatic patients with vertigo.[3]

■ Calcium Channel Blockers

These agents have antidopaminergic and antihistaminic properties that aid in the treatment of vertigo. These medications also suppress the sensory input of the vestibular apparatus. Calcium channel blockers are used when a patient is unable to take or did not respond to antihistamines or anticholinergics. Such medications are also helpful in treatment of patients with vertiginous migraine.

■ Neuroleptic Drugs

These antidopaminergic medications are second-line agents for patients who fail to respond to the drugs previously discussed. In addition to their anticholinergic and antihistamine properties, they block the dopaminergic receptors in the brainstem, thereby decreasing nausea and vomiting. Promethazine and metoclopramide are the drugs of choice. Other neuroleptics should not be used because they cause orthostatic hypotension, which exacerbates symptoms. Side effects include dystonia and somnolence.

■ Steroids

Steroids are important in the treatment of patients with autoimmune diseases of the inner ear. Intratympanic application allows better penetration than does IV or oral administration.

■ Seritonergic Agents

Seritonergic agents occasionally are used to block the emesis response.

■ PRECAUTIONS

The combination of antihistaminic, anticholinergic, and antidopaminergic medications should be avoided because of overlapping side effects. Patients with chronic vertigo adjust to their condition by enhanced sensory input from their intact senses of proprioception and vision. Certain antivertigo medications may worsen preexisting vertigo by inhibiting this compensation. Therefore, medications such as benzodiazepines, barbiturates, and neuroleptics, as well as alcohol, are to be avoided in patients with chronic vertigo. Antivertigo medications are not recommended for long-term use.

■ REHABILITATION EXERCISES

Vestibular exercises, such as Brandt-Daroff exercises, may be helpful for BPPV, poorly compensated vestibular neuritis, end-stage Ménière's disease, and chronic and psychiatric vertigo.[5] These exercises, which can be performed in the physical therapy unit or at home, give patients control over their symptoms. Rehabilitation exercises are based on the concept of fatigue and facilitation of central compensatory mechanisms.

Disposition

All vertiginous patients should be scheduled for follow-up, even if diagnosed as having peripheral vertigo, because there is an overlap between the signs and symptoms of peripheral and central vertigo. Patients with unrelenting or disabling vertigo need prompt referral to a specialist. Tests for vestibular and audiologic function can be used in consultation with an otolaryngologist, audiologist, neurologist, or neuro-otologist.

■ PSYCHOSOCIAL SUPPORT

It is important to be aware of the psychological facets of vertigo. Anxiety often accompanies vestibular disorders due to a primary psychiatric problem or secondary to the major intrusion the symptoms have on the patient's life. For these reasons, vertigo is associated with serious morbidity, although it is often a benign disease. Early counseling and intervention are especially helpful in treatment of vertiginous patients.

PERIPHERAL VERTIGO

About 80% of cases of vertigo are due to a peripheral lesion. Various types of peripheral vertigo and its causes are discussed in detail throughout the chapter.

Pathophysiology

Peripheral vertigo results from pathology of the vestibular structures or cranial nerve VIII. Because these structures are not vital, peripheral vertigo is considered benign. However, it is important to remember that even though the disorder is not life-threatening, it may cause significant disability.

Anatomy

The inner ear is housed in a chamber inside the petrous portion of the temporal bone, or bony labyrinth. The membranous labyrinth, bathed in perilymph, is suspended inside this chamber where it protects the auditory and vestibular systems. The vestibule is a chamber in the inner ear where the vestibular organs and cochlea converge. The vestibular organs are responsible for equilibrium, whereas the cochlea is responsible for the transmission of sound.

The vestibular system consists of two components—the three semicircular canals and the two otolith organs. Together, these five organs are responsible for balance; the semicircular canals sense rotational movement (angular acceleration) and the otoliths recognize linear movement. The three semicircular canals—anterior (superior/vertical/dorsal), posterior (inferior), and horizontal (lateral)—each contain a dilated area called the ampulla. Inside the ampulla lie the three end-organs, called the cristae ampullaris, attached to a cupulae. Embedded particles on the cupulae allow these sensors to recognize gravity and rotation. The canals are arranged at right angles to one another to allow each canal to sense specific direction and rotation.

The otoliths are found in the sac-like saccule and utricle. Horizontal motion is sensed by the utricle, whereas sagittal movement is sensed by the saccule. The utricle, saccule, semicircular canals, and cochlear duct are filled with endolymph that is absorbed by the endolymphatic sac. Information from these vestibular organs is transmitted by cranial nerve VIII to the vestibular nuclei in the brainstem.

When there is no disease and the head is held motionless, the bilateral vestibular systems fire at a tonic resting frequency. When the head rotates, there is increased firing from one semicircular canal and decreased firing from the others. The cerebral cortex interprets this information, synthesizes it with signals from the visual and proprioceptive systems, and translates it into the consciousness of movement.

Vertigo results when the end organs fire inappropriately at different frequencies, causing unequal input to the brainstem and cerebral cortex.

Presenting Signs and Symptoms

Peripheral vertigo typically is explosive in onset, with intense sensations of spinning or falling. Peripheral lesions are often worsened with rapid head movement and are associated with nausea and vomiting. The hallucination of movement is directed away from the side of the lesion.

By definition, there are no central neurologic findings in peripheral vertigo. In extreme cases patients may have vagally mediated diaphoresis, bradycardia, and hypotension. Other physical findings in peripheral vertigo include nystagmus and a tendency to veer toward the affected side during ambulation.

■ PERIPHERAL NYSTAGMUS

Peripheral vertigo is often diagnosed by the quality of the accompanying nystagmus (Table 91-8). Peripheral nystagmus may be spontaneous or positional.

Signs and symptoms of peripheral nystagmus include the following:

- Alexander's law—spontaneous nystagmus increases in amplitude as the gaze moves towards the direction of the quick phase. Conversely, the amplitude of nystagmus diminishes when the gaze moves in the direction of the slow phase.
- Visual fixation or suppression—when patients fixate their eyes on an object, the spontaneous nystagmus will decrease or disappear. If no nystagmus is present on examination, patients are instructed to close their eyes to eliminate visual fixation; the EP then looks for nystagmus through their eyelids. Visual fixation can also be impaired by the use of high-diopter goggles called Frenzel lenses to distort vision.

Table 91-8 CHARACTERISTICS OF PERIPHERAL NYSTAGMUS THAT INDICATE PERIPHERAL VERTIGO

Sign	Characteristic
Direction of nystagmus	Unidirectional, horizontal-rotary
Purely vertical nystagmus	Never (may be combined vertical and rotational)
Purely horizontal nystagmus	Uncommon
Direction of fast component	Away from side with disease
Effect of visual fixation	Suppressed nystagmus
Anatomic location of the problem	Labyrinth or vestibular nerve
Effect of change in direction of gaze	Unchanged nystagmus
Severity of symptoms	Marked
Tinnitus or hearing loss	May be present
Direction of the fall	Toward slow phase/lesion
Direction of the spin	Toward fast phase/away from lesion
Duration of symptoms	Finite; may be recurrent
Associated central abnormalities	None

- The fast component points away from the side of disease.
- Nystagmus is provoked by having the patient lie with the affected ear dependently.
- Fatigability—symptoms and nystagmus decrease with repeated testing.
- Ewald's first law: the axis of nystagmus matches the axis of the affected semicircular canal (anterior, posterior, and horizontal).
- Ewald's second law: in complete unilateral vestibular lesions, rotation in the direction that excites the vestibular nerve results in more nystagmus than rotation that inhibits the vestibular nerve.

Treatment and Disposition

Peripheral vertigo typically is self-limited. The duration of the vertigo depends on the duration of the cause. Fixed unilateral lesions may have steady symptoms that eventually diminish due to habituation and compensatory mechanisms by the central nervous system.

Once symptoms are controlled, patients with peripheral vertigo can be discharged from the ED with arrangements for follow-up by the primary care physician and, if needed, specialist follow-up.

Types of Peripheral Vertigo

■ BENIGN PAROXYSMAL POSITIONAL VERTIGO (BPPV)

BBBV is the most common type of vertigo.[4] It occurs in all age groups but is most common in the fourth decade. Women are affected twice as often as men. BPPV is underdiagnosed, and patients rarely receive useful treatment.[6]

■ Pathophysiology

BPPV results from a mechanical defect to the inner ear. *Canalolithiasis* is the most accepted hypothesis. According to this premise, the culprits are free-floating calcium carbonate particles called otoconia that form in the macula and saccule. With trauma, labyrinthine disease, inflammation, or aging, the otoconia are displaced from the utricular matrix and inappropriately activate the semicircular canals.[7] With certain head movements, a clump of otoconia move, causing a drag of the endolymph with resultant cupula displacement. Cupula movement triggers neural firing, with consequential vertigo and nystagmus. Free-floating otoconia in the endolymph are referred to as canalolithiasis. When the otoconia adhere to the cupula, this condition is called *cupulolithiasis*.

■ Anatomy

For BPPV to occur, any semicircular canal can be affected; however, the posterior (inferior) canal is involved 95% of the time. This is because the heavy otoliths sink through the endolymph into the most dependent part of the system—the long arm of the posterior canal. The disorder is most often unilateral, and the right labyrinth is affected more often than the left.[8] This may be because patients tend to sleep on the right side (see later).

■ Presenting Signs and Symptoms

In BPPV, sudden transient vertigo is brought on by a change in head position relative to gravity. After movement, there is a delay of a few seconds. Then the room starts to spin, accompanied by nausea. If

Table 91-9 SYMPTOMS OF CENTRAL PERIPHERAL VERTIGO (CPV) VERSUS BENIGN PAROXYSMAL POSITIONAL VERTIGO (BPPV)

Symptoms	BPPV	CPV
Latency	3-10 seconds	None
Intensity of vertigo	Marked	None or mild
Duration	<1 minute	>1 minute
Reproducibility	Variable	Present
Fatigability	Yes	No
Habituation	Yes	No

the head is kept motionless, these symptoms typically resolve within 10 to 60 seconds. Symptoms are worse in the morning; possibly because otoliths have clumped together during sleep. The vertigo will lessen as the day goes on, a process termed "fatigability."

Spontaneous nystagmus is not present but can be induced with head movements. The patient should have a Dix-Hallpike test (see later).

Differential Diagnosis

It is important to distinguish between BPPV and causes of central positional vertigo. This can be done based on the patient's symptoms and nystagmus (Table 91-9).

Diagnostic Testing

Dix-Hallpike Test

The Dix-Hallpike test (also called the Nylan-Bárány test) is used to evaluate for otoliths in the posterior semicircular canal (Fig. 91-1; Box 91-4). Have the patient sit in a position on one end of the examination table so that his or her head will hang over the opposite edge when lying down down. The patient must keep the eyes open during the test. Turn the patient's head 45 degrees to one side and have the patient lie down.[9] The posterior semicircular canal on the dependent side is now aligned with the direction of the turned and recumbent head. If there are otoliths in the canal, they will move, resulting in transient reproduction of the patient's symptoms and transient torsional nystagmus.

Repeat the test with the head rotated 45 degrees to the opposite side.

It is important to note the direction of the fast phase of nystagmus. Symptoms and nystagmus generally resolve as the otoliths settle down in the most dependent part of the canal.

BOX 91-4

Findings on Dix-Hallpike Test in Patients with Benign Paroxysmal Positional Vertigo

- Latency of 3-10 seconds
- Significant subjective vertigo
- Intensity of vertigo escalates, then slowly resolves
- Vertigo and nystagmus last for 5-40 seconds
- Nystagmus is upbeat (toward the forehead) and torsional toward the abnormal ear
- Nystagmus reverses direction when the patient returns to seated position
- Fatigability—the vertigo and nystagmus decrease and eventually subside with repeated positioning

Interventions and Procedures

Repositioning Maneuvers

In patients with BPPV and a positive Dix-Hallpike test, these maneuvers are used to return displaced otoconia from the semicircular canals back to the utricle. The success rate is approximately 80%.

Epley Maneuver/Particle Repositioning Maneuver This maneuver takes approximately 3 minutes and has been shown to be safe and effective.[10] Gravity is used to move the otoconia out of the semicircular canals into the utricle where they will no longer cause vertigo.

As in the Hallpike test, the patient is placed in the supine position and far enough back on the examining table such that the head overhangs the edge when the patient is in the supine position. The head is turned 45 degrees to the affected side.

Next, the patient lies down with the head overhanging the edge of examining table, and the head is rotated 90 degrees to the opposite side. The patient now rolls over to the unaffected side and the head is turned so that the patient is looking toward the ground. The patient is then brought up to the sitting position and the head is brought forward slightly.

Each position is held approximately 30 seconds or until symptoms and nystagmus resolve. It is currently recommended that the patient remain upright only 20 minutes after the maneuver, which may be sufficient time for the otoconia to reattach to hair cells in the utricle.

Semont's Liberatory Maneuver The patient sits upright in the middle of the examining table. The head is turned 45 degrees to the side that is opposite

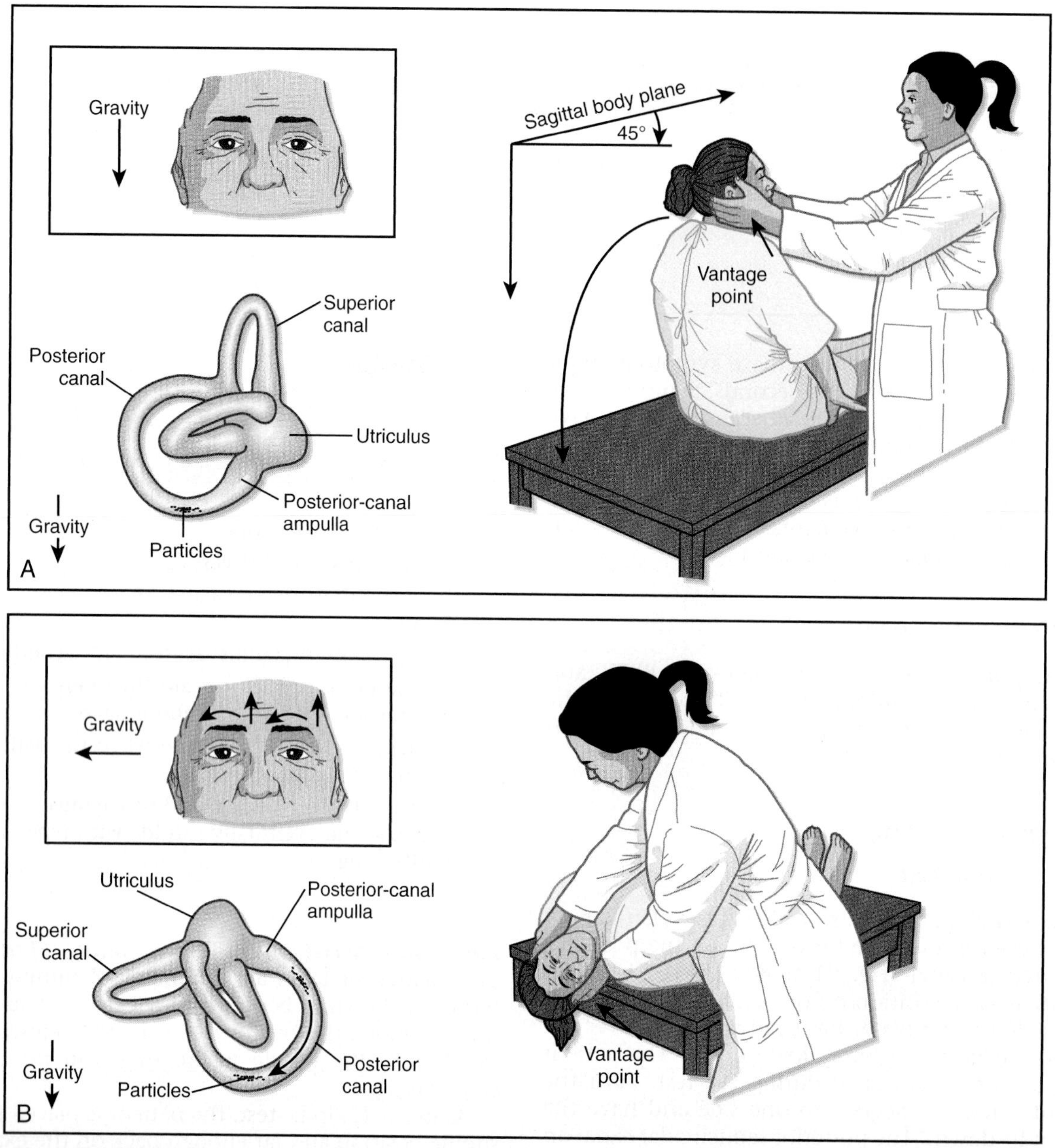
Gravity
Sagittal body plane
45°
Vantage point
Superior canal
Posterior canal
Utriculus
Posterior-canal ampulla
Gravity
Particles
A
Gravity
Utriculus
Posterior-canal ampulla
Superior canal
Posterior canal
Gravity
Particles
Vantage point
B

FIGURE 91-1 The Dix-Hallpike test of a patient with benign paroxysmal positional vertigo affecting the right ear. In **A,** the examiner stands at the patient's right side and rotates the patient's head 45 degrees to the right to align the right posterior semicircular canal with the sagittal plane of the body. In **B,** the examiner moves the patient, whose eyes are open, from the seated to the supine right-ear-down position and then extends the patient's neck slightly so that the chin is pointed slightly upward. The latency, duration, and direction of nystagmus, if present, and the latency and duration of vertigo, if present, should be noted. The *red arrows* in the inset depict the direction of nystagmus in patients with typical benign paroxysmal positional vertigo. The presumed location in the labyrinth of the free-floating debris thought to cause the disorder is also shown. (From Furman JM, Cass SP: Benign paroxysmal positional vertigo. N Engl J Med 1999; 341:1590-1596.)

that of the involved canal. The patient is placed supine very quickly on the side of the involved canal and then rapidly reurned to the other side. The patient then returns to the sitting position.

The rapid movements of this maneuver often are not tolerated, especially by elderly patients.

Brandt-Daroff/Positional Exercises These exercises can be done by the patient at home. The patient sits at the edge of the bed and then lies down quickly on one side with the symptomatic ear down.[11] After the vertigo resolves, the patient sits up. This exercise is repeated multiple times until vertigo is no longer elicited. The patient repeats these exercises three times a day until there are two consecutive days without symptoms.

■ Treatment and Disposition

BPPV typically is self-limited to 2 weeks and recurs up to 50% of the time.[12] Persistent or recurrent vertigo is managed using the maneuvers described previously. Symptomatic treatment can be provided by vestibular suppressants.

Patients who work at heights (builders, roofers) should curtail activities until their symptoms have resolved. All patients can benefit from specialist referral. Outpatient magnetic resonance imaging with contrast may be used to look for an acoustic neuroma or other pathology that can mimic BPPV.

In some intractable incapacitating cases, patients may benefit from neurectomy or non-ampullary plugging of the superior semicircular canal.

HORIZONTAL CANAL BPPV

Horizontal canal BPPV is much less common than posterior canal BPPV.

Pathophysiology

Misplaced otoconia activate the horizontal semicircular canal. Particles can actually shift into the horizontal canal as a consequence of the positional maneuvers discussed previously.

Presenting Signs and Symptoms

The definitive symptom of horizontal canal BPPV is positional vertigo and nystagmus, which occur when the head is turned in either direction.

Diagnostic Testing

The Roll Test

In the roll test, the patient lies supine and then turns the head 90 degrees in either direction. Reproduction of symptoms and nystagmus should occur, with the fast phase of the nystagmus beating toward the ears. The side that is involved is the one that has the more acute symptoms and nystagmus.

Treatment and Disposition

Patients can be treated with the bar-b-que roll maneuver, in which the patient is placed in the supine position with the head turned 90 degrees to the affected side as determined by the roll test. The head is then turned in 90-degree intervals in the opposite direction back to the original starting position. This requires the patient to eventually turn onto the abdomen. Each position is held for 30 seconds or until resolution of the vertigo and nystagmus occurs.

ANTERIOR CANAL BPPV

Less than 2% cases of BPPV arise in the anterior canal, because dislodged otoliths have to be displaced against gravity for this to occur.[12]

Pathophysiology

See pathophysiology of BPPV.

Presenting Signs and Symptoms

The primary symptom is positional vertigo. Positional torsional downbeat nystagmus is also seen.

Treatment and Disposition

The Epley maneuver (see earlier) may be used to treat anterior canal BPPV. However, because downbeat nystagmus can be due to central vertigo, the authors recommend neuroimaging and neurology consultation.

POST-TRAUMATIC VERTIGO

Vertigo is common after injury to the head.[13]

Pathophysiology

Post-traumatic vertigo usually results from trauma to the occiput or temporal area housing the vestibular structures. Vertigo resulting from direct injury to the vestibular structures occurs by the following mechanisms:

- Dislodgment of otoconia from the macula causing BPPV
- Damage to cranial nerve VIII
  - Hemorrhage into the endolymph
  - Fracture of the temporal bone
- Injury to the labyrinth
  - Membranous damage
  - Bony fractures causing perilymphatic fistula

Presenting Signs and Symptoms

These patients may have lost consciousness. Vertigo is accompanied by nausea, vomiting, and possible hearing loss. Spontaneous nystagmus beats away from the side of the injury.

The ED examination may also demonstrate hemotympanum, bleeding from the external auditory canal, or postauricular ecchymosis (Battle's sign). Other details are specific to the injury (Table 91-10).

Diagnostic Testing

Clinically it is difficult to determine the mechanisms causing vertigo in these patients. Temporal bone computed tomography scans should be obtained to detect fractures; neuroimaging may be necessary to detect intracranial injury.

Interventions and Procedures

Immediate consultation with an otolaryngologist and neurosurgeon is mandatory in cases of surgically correctable injuries.

Table 91-10 DIFFERENTIAL DIAGNOSIS, SYMPTOMS, AND TREATMENT OF POST-TRAUMATIC VERTIGO

Type of Vertigo	Symptoms	Treatment
Immediate nonspecific post-traumatic vertigo	Immediate onset of vertigo Improves over days No extensive injury	Symptomatic
Delayed-onset post-traumatic BPPV	Onset days to weeks after minor trauma Identical to BPPV	Same as BPPV
Post-traumatic Ménière's syndrome	Spontaneous vertigo Audiologic symptoms Occur weeks after trauma	Same as Ménière's
Post-concussive migraine–like phenomenon	Typically associated with loss of consciousness	Same as migraine

Treatment and Disposition

Treatment and disposition depend on the diagnosis. Labyrinthine injuries heal over several weeks, and vertigo will resolve over this time.

MÉNIÈRE'S DISEASE (ENDOLYMPHATIC HYDROPS)

Ménière's disease is a form of recurrent unilateral labyrinthine dysfunction. Men and women are affected equally. The first episode typically occurs in persons over the age of 65; however, rare cases occur in childhood.

Pathophysiology

This disorder is associated with an excessive amount of endolymph in the vestibule. Autoimmune migraine-induced vasospasm with ischemia to endolymphatic structures and infectious and genetic causes have been proposed. Progressive hearing loss, which may be permanent, results from damage to the cochlear hair cells.

Anatomy

Both auditory and vestibular structures are affected because they are all filled with endolymph. The excessive fluid damages the cochlea, causing auditory symptoms, and the vestibular labyrinth, resulting in vertigo. The disease begins unilaterally and typically becomes bilateral with time.

Presenting Signs and Symptoms

Symptoms include acute attacks of fluctuating hearing loss, aural fullness, ear discomfort, roaring tinnitus, and peripheral-type vertigo. Nausea and vomiting may occur as well. Attacks usually last for several hours and may occur several times a week. Tinnitus and sensorineural hearing loss are progressive and persist between attacks.

During an attack, nystagmus will be present. The nystagmus of Ménière's disease has a variable fast-phase direction and may point toward or away from the affected side. Patients may also exhibit Tulio's phenomenon (nystagmus and vertigo induced by a loud noise [500 Hz] and a positive Hennenbert sign.

Differential Diagnosis

Ménière's disease may be confused with vestibular migraines.[14] Quantitative vestibular testing helps to make the discrimination. Ménière's disease may coexist with BPPV.

Diagnostic Testing

Glycerol injections into the inner ear have been used for diagnosis. This osmotic agent temporarily decreases vertigo and improves postural control.[15] Electrocochleography and audiologic testing may also assist in the diagnosis.[16,17] Unfortunately, these are not sensitive or specific tests. Currently the only way to diagnose Ménière's disease with certainty is an autopsy.

Treatment and Disposition

Table 91-11 lists medications used to treat patients with Ménière's disease. In addition, a salt restriction diet is recommended. In severe cases intratympanic gentamycin, steroids, or surgical procedures may be necessary. Associated hearing loss cannot be corrected.

Approximately 80% of cases resolve spontaneously within 5 to 10 years. Patients with end-stage disease refractory to medications should be referred to an otolaryngologist for confirmation and treatment. Vestibular rehabilitation may be valuable in these patients.

PERIPHERAL VESTIBULOPATHY

This is a collective term for the benign conditions labyrinthitis and vestibular neuronitis, characterized by inflammation. These disorders most commonly occur in patients in the third to fifth decade of life. Peripheral vestibulopathies typically follow viral gastrointestinal or upper respiratory infections.

Table 91-11 MEDICATIONS TO TREAT MÉNIÈRE'S DISEASE

Medication Class	Specific Medication	Dosage
Diuretics	Hydrochlorothiazide Triamterene Acetazolamide	25-50 mg daily 50-200 mg daily 250 mg daily
Antiemetics	Prochlorperazine	5-10 mg PO qid or 25 mg suppository bid
Antihistamines	Meclizine	25 mg tid to qid

Labyrinthitis

Labyrinthitis is caused by an infectious inflammation of the labyrinth. Viral etiologies are most common, though labyrinthitis also may occur as a result of Lyme neuroborreliosis or otosyphilic infections. Disruption to the round window by otitis media or cholesteatoma gives pathogens access to the labyrinth. Tumors, fistulas, meningitis, or mastoiditis may also create a portal of entry. Unilateral hearing loss and tinnitus are the distinguishing factors of labyrinthitis.

Presenting Signs and Symptoms

Spontaneous, severe, rotary vertigo develops over hours. Nausea and vomiting may occur. Symptoms that accompany a viral illness may also be present. The vertigo is initially severe, requiring 1 or 2 days of bed rest, and then gradually resolves over a few weeks.

Spontaneous nystagmus with peripheral features is seen on examination (see Table 91-10). A third of patients may have positional nystagmus directed away from the affected ear. Postural imbalance with a tendency to fall toward the side of the lesion is also seen. Middle-ear infection or serous fluid may be present. Patients have a positive head thrust test.

Differential Diagnosis

It is important to remember that central lesions may mimic peripheral vestibulopathies.[18,19]

Vestibular Neuritis

Sometimes referred to as vestibular neuronitis, vestibular neuritis occurs as a result of viral inflammation of the vestibular nerve. There are no auditory symptoms.

Diagnostic Testing

Because this syndrome has a benign course and spontaneously resolves, extensive studies and imaging usually are not necessary. The diagnosis is based on clinical features. The hallmark of vestibular neuritis is unilateral hyporesponsiveness of the affected canal detected with a simple head thrust test.

Treatment and Disposition

Although nystagmus may be present for several months, the symptoms of vertigo resolve in approximately 6 weeks. This occurs by vestibular restoration and central compensation. No specific treatment is available; symptomatic therapy is used as needed. Vestibular exercises may improve postural stability.[20] Bacterial infections are managed with antibiotics.

Patients with severe cases or those without resolution may benefit from electronystagmography or neurologic consultation.

PERILYMPH FISTULA

A perilymph fistula is an abnormal opening between the air-filled middle ear and the fluid-filled inner ear.

Pathophysiology

In most instances the fistula is a tear or defect in one or both of the small, thin membranes (i.e., the oval window and the round window) between the middle and inner ears. Head trauma, infections, cholesteatoma, or sudden barotraumas may cause the tear. Through this fistula, middle ear pneumatic changes are inappropriately transmitted to the labyrinth, resulting in vertigo.[21]

Presenting Signs and Symptoms

Symptoms include sensorineural hearing loss and episodic vertigo worsened with Valsalva manerver or changes in barometric pressure. Patients may also describe hearing a popping sound.

Diagnostic Testing

Patient's may exhibit a positive Hennenbert sign and Tulio's phenomenon.

Treatment and Disposition

Because most fistulas heal spontaneously, symptomatic therapy is sufficient.

SUPERIOR SEMICIRCULAR CANAL DEHISCENCE SYNDROME

Superior semicircular canal dehiscence syndrome, a rare variant of perilymph fistula, is also called *inner perilymph fistula.*[22]

Pathophysiology

Abnormal breakdown (dehiscence) of the bone overlying the superior semicircular canals results in a mobile window that inappropriately transduces information to the superior canal. The dehiscence may be a developmental abnormality or may be an acquired defect.

Anatomy

One or both canals may be affected.

Presenting Signs and Symptoms

Recurrent attacks of vertigo are induced by sound and pressure and worsened by positive pressure or Valsalva maneuver. Patients exhibit *autophony,* a condition in which one's own voice, pulse, and eye movements, or self-generated noise, sound louder than normal due to conductive hyperacusis.[23] Low-frequency conductive hearing loss is also present. The sensation of vertigo may be in the vertical plane.

In addition to Hennebert's sign and Tullio's phenomenon, patients can have spontaneous oscillating eye movements that are synchronous with their pulse.[24]

Diagnostic Testing

High-resolution temporal bone computed tomography with 0.1 mm cuts parallel to the superior semicircular canal reveal the dehiscence.

Treatment and Disposition

Conservative measures with symptomatic treatment and trigger avoidance are attempted first. If symptoms worsen, surgical resurfacing or plugging of the affected superior central canal usually is successful.[22]

VESTIBULAR GANGLIONITIS

Vestibular ganglionitis may be a unifying cause of Ménière's disease and vestibular neuronitis.

Pathophysiology

Histopathologic changes in the vestibular ganglion consistent with viral inflammation are seen. It is believed that viruses such as herpes remain dormant in the vestibular ganglion and are reactivated years later, causing a neuropathy.[25] Vestibular ganglionitis is likely associated with the neuropathic disorder Ramsay Hunt syndrome.

Anatomy

Multiple ganglia may be infected.

Presenting Signs and Symptoms

In addition to vertigo, patients may experience sudden ipsilateral deafness and facial paralysis. Peripheral facial nerve palsy may be noted on cranial nerve examination. The external auditory canal should be inspected for the presence of vesicles on a red base.

Differential Diagnosis

This disease is often misdiagnosed as Ménière's disease, peripheral vestibulopathy, or BPPV.

Diagnostic Testing

At this time, vestibular ganglionitis is a clinical diagnosis.

Treatment and Disposition

Within 72 hours of symptom onset, antiviral therapy may be instituted. Patients should be treated symptomatically as well.

VESTIBULOCOCHLEAR CRANIAL NEUROPATHY

Neuropathy of cranial nerve VIII results from infections, toxins, and autoimmune diseases. The gradual onset of vertigo can be positional or spontaneous.[26] Hearing loss is often the most noticeable symptom because central compensation occurs, which minimizes the vertigo the patient might experience.

CEREBELLOPONTINE ANGLE COMPRESSION

Acoustic neuromas, meningiomas, lipomas, cholesteatomas, and tumors (metastasis and dermoid) may disrupt blood flow to the labyrinth, resulting in vertigo.

ACOUSTIC NEUROMA

Also known as a schwannoma, this is a rare slow-growing benign tumor of the cerebellar angle.

Pathophysiology

This tumor slowly expands within the internal auditory meatus until it extends into the posterior fossa and compresses adjacent structures, such as cranial nerve VIII. Because the gradual reduction of the vestibular output may be compensated for by central mechanisms, symptoms may be mild. Acoustic neuroma may occur sporadically or as a part of neurofibromatosis.

Anatomy

Neuromas arise from the vestibular fibers of cranial nerve VIII.

Presenting Signs and Symptoms

Symptoms are gradual and relentless and include mild positional vertigo, ipsilateral sensorineural hearing loss, ear fullness, nausea, vomiting, and tinnitus. Patients often complain of unsteadiness, difficulty understanding speech in ther affected ear, and headache. Because of central compensatory mechanisms, the vertigo may be minimized and the patient may have only auditory symptoms.

Cranial nerves V, VII, and VI are affected progressively as the tumor enlarges. Because cerebellar involvement is common, patients often have ataxia and a tendency to fall toward the side of the lesion. Patients occasionally have nystagmus.

Differential Diagnosis

The diagnosis of acoustic neuroma should be considered in patients with BPPV refractive to treatment.

Diagnostic Testing

Outpatient tests include audiometry and magnetic resonance imaging with gadolinium.

Treatment and Disposition

The patient should be referred to an otolaryngologist and neurologist for evaluation and treatment options including radiotherapy and resection.

VESTIBULAR PAROXYSMIA

This newly described syndrome results from neurovascular compression.[27]

Pathophysiology

Vertigo from vestibular paroxysmia is believed to result from the pathologic excitation of vestibular structures similar to that of trigeminal neuralgia and hemifacial spasm.[28] Compression of cranial nerve VIII occurs from impinging vasculature (pulsating arterial loops) or neurologic structures (arachnoid cysts, tumors).

Anatomy

Loops of the anterior inferior cerebellar artery in the internal auditory canal compress cranial nerve VIII near the cerebellopontine angle. The degree of compression is divided into four types (Box 91-5).

Presenting Signs and Symptoms

Patients report symptoms of rotational vertigo, disequilibrium and motion intolerance. Patients may also complain of hearing loss, tinnitus, aural pressure, and hyperacusis.[28]

BOX 91-5

Types of Vestibular Paroxysma

- Type I Point compression—limited contact
- Type II Longitudinal compression—both run parallel to one another
- Type III Loop compression—a vascular loop encircles the nerve
- Type VI Indentation—the vasculature indents the nerve

Diagnostic Testing

Magnetic resonance imaging demonstrates compression of the vestibulocochlear nerve.

Treatment and Disposition

Patients should be referred to a specialist, such as a neurootologist, for confirmation of the diagnosis. Medical treatment with carbamazepine and surgical options including craniotomy with microvascular decompression are available.

OTHER CAUSES OF PERIPHERAL VERTIGO

Otitis media, cholesteatomas, granulomas of the petrous apex, arachnoiditis, genetic abnormalities, postsurgical complications, and tumors can manifest as peripheral vertigo.

CENTRAL VERTIGO

Sometimes called cortical vertigo, central vertigo occurs as a result of disorders of the central nervous system. Various types and causes of central vertigo are discussed in detail in the following sections.

Pathophysiology

Central vertigo can result from ischemia (stroke, dissection), mass effect (hemorrhage, abscess, neoplasm, metastasis, arteriovenous malformation, granuloma), trauma, demyelination, or inflammation of any of the central structures discussed in the following sections.

Anatomy

The central nervous system integrates information from the visual, proprioceptive, and vestibular systems regarding the body's location in space. The cerebellum, brainstem, and cerebral cortex are the key players in this process.

Afferent fibers relay information from the inner ear vestibule and terminate in the floor of the fourth ventricle in the vestibular nuclei. The vestibular nuclei send this information to the cerebellum, brainstem, vestibulospinal tract, and cranial nerves. The vestibular cerebral cortex is located near the auditory cortex in the temporal lobe.

Because of this extensive distribution of vestibular pathways, lesions in many areas of the central nervous system can result in vertigo.

Presenting Signs and Symptoms

The most important clue to the diagnosis of central vertigo is the presence of associated neurologic signs and symptoms. Symptoms may occur insidiously with a slow-growing lesion such as a tumor, or rapidly from a stroke, intracranial hemorrhage, or trauma. In general, central vertigo is not positional, its intensity is mild, and there is no associated diaphoresis, nausea, vomiting, tinnitus, or hearing abnormality. It is important to note that these clues are generalizations and there are many published exceptions.

■ NYSTAGMUS

Nystagmus in central vertigo is purely vertical or horizontal and changes direction with altered path of gaze (Table 91-12). Downbeat nystagmus, such as might be seen during a Hallpike test, suggests the presence of central vertigo.

Differential Diagnosis

The physical examination can help differentiate central from peripheral vertigo and further localize the defect.

Diagnostic Testing

Emergent neuroimaging is required.

Treatment and Disposition

Causes of central vertigo are serious, and appropriate consultation should be obtained. Although compensation may occur in peripheral lesions, the central nervous system has relatively less plasticity and diminished capacity for compensation over time.

Types of Central Vertigo

■ MIGRAINOUS VERTIGO

Vestibular migraines are the most common cause of central vertigo and occur in 25% of migraine patients.[29] Vestibular migraines tend to occur in females between the third and fifth decades of life.

■ Pathophysiology

It has been theorized that the increased sensitivity to vestibular inputs in patients with vestibular migraine is analogous to the increased sensitivity causing photophobia and phonophobia in seen in typical migraines. There is copious evidence linking vertigo and migraine headaches in general.[29-32] This will be an important topic to watch as research sheds light on this association and its implications.

■ Presenting Signs and Symptoms

If there is a preceding aura, the migraine will develop over minutes and subside within an hour. This is followed by the acute onset of vertigo. Patients usually have an associated headache; however, vertigo may be the headache equivalent.[31] Fluctuating low-

Table 91-12 CHARACTERISTICS OF CENTRAL NYSTAGMUS THAT INDICATE CENTRAL VERTIGO

Sign	Characteristic
Direction of nystagmus	Any direction; may be bidirectional
Purely vertical nystagmus	Occasional
Purely horizontal nystagmus	Common
Direction of fast component	Toward the side with disease
Effect of visual fixation	Unchanged or enhanced
Anatomic location of the problem	Brainstem or cerebellum
Effect of change in direction of gaze	Change in direction of nystagmus
Severity of symptoms	Usually mild
Tinnitus or hearing loss	Usually absent
Direction of the fall	Variable
Direction of the spin	Variable
Duration of symptoms	Chronic
Associated central abnormalities	Extremely common

BOX 91-6

Findings Associated with Migrainous Etiology

- Onset early in life
- Female gender
  - Occurs during menses
- Episodic vertigo
- Spontaneous or positional vertigo
- Episodes last no more than a few days
- Frequent recurrences within a year
- Interferes with daily activities
- History of motion sickness as a child
- Hearing loss
- Symptoms associated with the vertigo
  - Migrainous headache
  - Photophobia
  - Aura (visual, vertiginous)
  - Phonophobia
- Migraine history according to International Headache Society criteria
- Migraine-specific precipitants of vertigo
- Personal history of migraines
- Atypical positional nystagmus
- Migraine medications terminate symptoms
- Other causes of vertigo ruled out
- At least two attacks

frequency hearing loss and tinnitus also can occur (Box 91-6).

When asymptomatic, two thirds of patients will have nystagmus. The neurologic examination usually is normal.

Differential Diagnosis

The differential diagnosis should include all causes of episodic vertigo, including BPPV, Ménière's disease, transient ischemic attack, lesions of cranial nerve VIII, inner-ear diseases, and epileptic vertigo.

Diagnostic Testing

The 2004 International Headache Society (IHS) classification does not include vestibular migraines. Therefore, the diagnosis is made by assumption.[33,34] Magnetic resonance imaging may be performed to evaluate for a cerebellar or brainstem lesion.

Treatment and Disposition

Information concerning specific treatment for vertiginous migraines is limited (e.g., patients should avoid migraine triggers) and is not based on controlled studies. Treatment is divided into symptomatic and prophylactic therapy (Table 91-13).[35] Patients should be referred to a neurologist for follow-up.

Table 91-13 TREATMENT OF MIGRAINOUS VERTIGO

Phase	Therapy
Acute attack	Triptan Vestibular suppressant Antiemetics Metoclopramide Promethazine
Chronic, prophylaxis	Tricyclic amines Calcium channel blockers Flunarizine Beta-blockers Propranolol Antihistamine/serotonin antagonist Pizotifen
Other remedies	Dietary manipulation Physical therapy Lifestyle adaptation Vestibular rehabilitation Biofeedback Acupuncture
Future prospects	Acetazolamide

Basilar Migraines

Basilar migraines tend to occur in young women with a family history of migraines. Symptoms result from vasospasm in the distribution of the basilar artery. Consequently, symptoms are similar to those seen in vertebrobasilar insufficiency (discussed later). Symptoms include recurrent vertigo, occipital headaches, nausea, and vomiting (Box 91-7). Unlike typical migraines, symptoms are bilateral.

BOX 91-7

International Headache Society's Diagnostic Criteria for Basilar Migraine

- Ataxia
- Bilateral paresis
- Bilateral paresthesias
- Bilateral visual symptoms in both the nasal and temporal fields
- Decreased hearing
- Decreased level of consciousness
- Diplopia
- Dysarthria
- Tinnitus
- Vertigo

Table 91-14 SYMPTOMS OF STROKE AND CENTRAL NERVOUS SYSTEM LESIONS BASED ON AFFECTED ANATOMY AND VASCULATURE

Symptom	PICA	AICA	SCA	MMI	VBAT
Vertigo	+	+	+		+
Nystagmus	+			+ (upbeat)	+
Dysarthria	+		+		+
Dysphagia	+				+
Nausea and vomiting	+		+		+
Slurred speech			+		
Paresis	–	C body		C body	U/B
Sensory loss	I—face; C—body	C	–	C	B
Horner's syndrome	I		I		U
Dysmetria	+				+
Hearing loss		I, U	+		+
Ataxia	I, U	+	I		+
Facial weakness		I	–	–	+
Pain and temperature loss	I—face; C—body		C		
Respiratory failure					+
Headache	+		+		+
Diplopia	+				+
Visual loss	–				+
Hoarseness	+				
Babinski sign	–				+
Position and vibration loss				C	
Altered consciousness					+
Crossed findings	+	+	+	+	+
Tinnitus		+	+		+
Autonomic instability	+				+
Other	Hiccups; facial pain			I—tongue weakness	Locked-in syndrome

AICA, anterior inferior cerebellar artery territory; B, bilateral; C, contralateral; I, ipsilateral; MMI, medial medullary infarction; PICA, posterior cerebellar artery territory (Wallenberg, lateral medullary); SCA, superior cerebellar artery territory; U, unilateral; VBAT, vertebral basilar artery thrombosis; VBI, vertebrobasilar insufficiency.

■ STROKE

The central nervous system obtains its blood supply from the carotid and vertebral arteries. The carotid arteries are referred to as the anterior circulation and the vertebral arteries as the posterior. These two arterial systems join at the base of the brain in the vascular circle of Willis. Smaller arteries branch off from this anastomosis to supply specific areas of the brain. A blockage to one of these arteries results in a recognizable pattern of signs and symptoms consistent with the brain territory affected. A stroke is caused by a thrombosis, hemorrhage, or embolism in one of the cerebral arteries.

Twenty percent of strokes involve the posterior circulation, which can affect the vestibular structures or pathways leading to vertigo.

Symptoms of stroke vary based on the affected anatomy and vasculature (Table 91-14). The vascular structures most commonly affected by stroke and other lesions can be divided into anatomic territories, including the vertebrobasilar artery (VBA) territory, the superior cerebellar artery (SCA) territory, and the posterior inferior cerebellar artery (PICA) territory, which are discussed in detail in the following sections.

■ Vertebrobasilar Artery (VBA) Territory

The vertebrobasilar arterial system provides the posterior circulation to the brain. The structures supplied by this blood flow are the brainstem, cerebellum, occipital cortex, and peripheral labyrinths.

■ *Pathophysiology*

Any disease process that decreases the arterial supply to the structures in the posterior fossa will result in vertebrobasilar ischemia. Embolism, thrombosis of penetrating arteries, and dissection are most common.

Other causes include fibromuscular dysplasia, coagulopathies, rotational occlusion, aneurysms, migraines, and drug abuse.[36] A transient ischemic attack in the posterior circulation is referred to as *vertebrobasilar insufficiency*.

Anatomy

The basilar artery is formed from the joining of the two vertebral arteries within the cranium at the level of the medulla. The vertebrobasilar artery has three branches on each side that supply the cerebellum. The posterior inferior cerebellar artery branches from the vertebral artery, whereas the anterior inferior cerebellar artery and the superior cerebellar artery branch from the basilar artery. The anterior inferior cerebellar artery supplies the peripheral labyrinth by the internal auditory end artery.

Presenting Signs and Symptoms

Vertigo is sudden in onset and may be positional. Although other symptoms typically occur (see Table 91-14), vertigo may be the only sign of vertebrobasilar ischemia.[37] This is important because it mimics a peripheral cause but is much more serious. Sixty percent of patients with transient vertigo due to vertebrobasilar insufficiency later develop basilar artery occlusion.[38]

The hallmark of many brainstem strokes is crossed signs (e.g., contralateral sensory and motor findings). Vertigo and nystagmus present early in the progression of ischemia. Dysarthria and oculomotor deficits occur later in the course and portend major neurologic catastrophe.[39]

Patients are often hypertensive. Nystagmus is seen along with limb and truncal ataxia. The neurologic examination may reveal contralateral deficits in pain and temperature sensation, ipsilateral limb and trunk numbness, ipsilateral loss of taste, and visual field defects.

Diagnostic Testing

Acute posterior circulation infarcts are best seen on diffusion-weighted MRI. Magnetic resonance angiography is used to additionally assess vertebral arteries. Patients with contraindications for MRI should undergo computed tomography and computed tomography angiography. Carotid ultrasound scanning is not helpful in patients with posterior ischemia. Electrocardiography, echocardiography, and rhythm monitoring are important in evaluating cardiac and aortic sources of embolism.

Interventions and Procedures

IV tissue plasminogen activator (TPA) may enhance recovery if given within 3 hours of onset of stroke.[40] Mixed results are found when TPA is used for vertebrobasilar disease.[41]

Treatment and Disposition

Hypotension should be corrected because it worsens symptoms and outcome. IV fluids, blood, and pressors should be administered as needed. Neurologic consultation may be useful to guide treatment.

Superior Cerebellar Artery (SCA) Territory

The SCA originates at the base of basilar artery and supplies parts of the midbrain and cerebellum.

Pathophysiology

Stroke, mass, tumors, arteriovenous malformations, compression, hemorrhage or infarction to the SCA territory may cause central vertigo.

Presenting Signs and Symptoms

Although small infarctions to the cerebellum may cause vertigo without other symptoms, patients typically also experience headache, nausea, and vomiting.

On neurological examination, patients with a cerebellar lesion may have truncal or limb ataxia with Romberg's sign and altered tandem gait. Patients may even require assistance to sit upright. There may be a palsy of the cranial nerve VI or eye deviation away from the lesion. Patients with large lesions may have altered consciousness and coma.

Diagnostic Testing

Although computed tomography may show large bleeds, magnetic resonance is best for imaging the posterior fossa.

Interventions and Procedures

Ventriculostomy and occipital craniotomy are often performed to relieve pressure within the posterior fossa associated with hemorrhage or mass effect.

Treatment and Disposition

A neurologist and neurosurgeon should be consulted immediately. Patients with minimal symptoms (Glasgow Coma Scale score >14) may be treated supportively. The prognosis is dismal for comatose patients without brainstem reflexes. Mannitol administration (0.25-2 g/kg IV) should be considered for patients with signs of herniation.

Posterior Inferior Cerebellar Artery (PICA) Territory

Anatomy

The posterior inferior cerebellar artery supplies the posterior medulla and inferior cerebellum.

Presenting Signs and Symptoms

Compromise to this artery may cause orthostasis, diplopia, nausea, vomiting, and positional vertigo that is easily confused with a peripheral cause. Central nystagmus is seen.

Diagnostic Testing

Diagnosis is confirmed by angiography.

Treatment and Disposition

It is important to prevent hypotension in these patients.

LATERAL MEDULLARY SYNDROME

Lateral medullary syndrome is also referred to as Wallenberg syndrome.[42]

Pathophysiology

This syndrome results from ipsilateral ischemia or rarely from demyelination of the lower brainstem.

Anatomy

The PICA or one of its branches supplying the posterior lateral medulla is involved. Cranial nerves IX and X are most commonly affected.

Presenting Signs and Symptoms

Symptoms are complex and variable. Onset typically is acute. Sensory complaints include ipsilateral loss of pain and temperature sensation to the face with contralateral pain and temperature loss to the body, ipsilateral loss of taste, and diplopia.

Motor deficits include dysphagia, dysarthria, dysphonia, and hoarseness. Uncontrollable hiccups, nausea and vomiting, and headache may occur. Vertigo is severe. It is possible for small infarcts in the lateral medulla to present with no other symptoms than vertigo.[43]

Ipsilateral ataxia is seen along with nystagmus. An ipsilateral Horner syndrome often is present. Evaluation and testing may demonstrate loss of the corneal reflex; facial numbness; paralysis of the soft palate, pharynx, and larynx; and contralateral loss of pain and temperature sensation to the limbs and trunk.

Diagnostic Testing

Immediate diagnostic imaging is warranted.

Treatment and Disposition

Urgent neurology consultation is necessary. Treatment is primarily symptomatic.

SUBCLAVIAN STEAL SYNDROME

Subclavian steal syndrome, another cause of posterior circulation ischemia, occurs when blood is siphoned away from the central circulation to the left upper extremity. When the left subclavian artery is stenotic proximal to the origin of the vertebral artery, blood will flow retrograde down the vertebral artery to supply the left arm. In addition to symptoms of vertebrobasilar insufficiency, patients complain of headaches and claudication to their arm, especially when exercised.

ROTATIONAL VERTEBRAL ARTERY OCCLUSION SYNDROME

This syndrome is also known as bow hunter's stroke and may be a cause of posterior circulation ischemia. Simple turning of the head causes vertebral artery occlusion at the C1-C2 level. Patients tend to have stenosis or vascular malformation in the site of occlusion. Symptoms include recurrent attacks of vertigo, nystagmus, ataxia, and other vertebrobasilar manifestations. The diagnosis is confirmed by dynamic angiography during progressive head rotation.[44]

VERTEBRAL ARTERY DISSECTION

Dissetions of the vertebral arteries can cause posterior circulation ischemia. Men and women are equally affected, with a mean age of 48 years. Patients with connective tissue disease are more prone to dissections.

Pathophysiology

Sudden strain to the neck and even trivial injuries can cause dissections. Blood penetrates the arterial wall and compresses the lumen or forms aneurismal dilation. Small emboli and subarachnoid hemorrhages may also occur.

Anatomy

The dissection originates in the most moveable portions of the extracranial vertebral arteries. Maximal distension occurs at the C1 and C2 vertebral levels. Here there is a close relationship between the vertebral artery, carotid artery, sympathetic trunk, and cranial nerves IX to XII. Therefore, these structures are all potentially affected by aneurismal dilation of the vertebral artery.

Presenting Signs and Symptoms

The cardinal symptom for a vertebral artery dissection is pain occurring in the ipsilateral posterior neck and occiput and possibly extending to the shoulder. Sudden unilateral vertigo and deafness may occur along with diplopia and unilateral facial paresthesias and pain. The vertigo may be positional. Other symptoms consistent with basilar and vertebral ischemia may be present. If emboli form, a multitude of other symptoms can occur.

Unilateral Horner's syndrome may be evident along with other cranial nerve palsies.

Differential Diagnosis

Stroke and space-occupying lesions should be included in the differential diagnosis.

Diagnostic Testing

Patients with symptoms of dissection require urgent diagnostic imaging. A computed tomography scan should be obtained to evaluate for subarachnoid hemorrhage. Cerebral angiography was once the standard diagnostic test; however, noninvasive MRI, magnetic resonance angiography, and Doppler ultrasonography are more commonly used today. Patients with spontaneous dissections should be evaluated for vasculitis and arteriopathy.

Interventions and Procedures

Patients with normal computed tomography scans in whom subarachnoid hemorrhage is suspected require lumbar puncture.

Treatment and Disposition

Patients with vertebral dissection require referral to a neurosurgeon. Once subarachnoid hemorrhage is ruled out, patients are treated with anticoagulation and antiplatelet therapy.

VERTEBRAL AND BASILAR ARTERY DOLICHOECTASIA

Vertebral and basilar artery dolichoectasia are rare disorders of the posterior circulation caused by elongation and distension of the affected artery. Dolichoectasia may lead to embolism, thrombosis, compression, or even rupture of the artery.

Clinical Signs and Symptoms

Many symptoms may occur, often including recurrent attacks of vertigo that last hours to days. On examination, nystagmus is immediate without latency, fatigability, or habituation. Symptoms including nystagmus are reproducible with positioning.

Treatment and Disposition

Carbamazepine and oxcarbazepine have been used for treatment.[45] Patients require emergent diagnostic imaging and neurosurgical evaluation.

DRUGS

Many medications and chemicals have been implicated as causes of central vertigo (Box 91-8).

BOX 91-8

Ototoxic and Vestibulotoxic Chemicals

- Phenytoin
- Tricyclic antidepressants
- Neuroleptics
- Opiates
- Alcohol
- Phencyclidine
- Toluene
- Propylene glycol
- Mercury
- Hydrocarbons
- Aminoglycosides
- Quinine derivatives
- Loop diuretics
- Fluroquinolones
- Erythromycin
- Minocycline
- Salicylates
- Nonsteroidal antiinflammatory drugs (NSAIDs)
- Cytotoxic agents
- Vancomycin

METABOLIC AND ENDOCRINE DISORDERS

Hyperinsulinism, impaired glucose tolerance, diabetes, hypertriglyceridemia, and hypothyroidism have all been identified as reversible causes of central vertigo.

SYSTEMIC CONDITIONS

Central vertigo may be caused by Paget's disease.

REFERENCES

1. Kroenke K, Mangelsdorff AD: Common symptoms in ambulatory care: Incidence, evaluation, therapy and outcome. Am J Med 1989;86:262.
2. Oghalai JS, Manolidis S, Barth JL, et al: Unrecognized benign paroxysmal positional vertigo in elderly patients. Otolaryngol Head Neck Surg 2000;122:630-634.
3. Chang AK: Dizziness and vertigo. In Mahadevan SV, Garmel GM (eds): An Introduction to Clinical Emergency Medicine. New York, Cambridge University Press, 2005, pp 241-252.
4. Lempert T, Von Brevern M: Episodic vertigo. Curr Opin Neurol 2005;18:5-9.
5. Beyon GJ: A review of management of benign paroxysmal positional vertigo by exercise therapy and by repositioning maneuvers. Br J Audiol 1997;31:11.
6. Von Brevern M, Lezius F, Tiel-Wilck K, et al: Benign paroxysmal positional vertigo: Current status of medical management. Otolaryngol Head Neck Surg 2004;130:381-382.
7. Parnes LS, McCleure J: Free-floating endolymph particles: A new operative finding during posterior semicircular canal occlusion. Laryngoscope 1992;102:988.

8. Von Brevern M, Seelig T, Neuhauser H, et al: Benign paroxysmal positional vertigo predominantly affects the right labyrinth. J Neurol Neurosurg Psychiatry 2004;75:1487-1488.
9. Dix MR, Hallpike CS: The pathology, symptomatology and diagnosis of certain common disorders of the vestibular system. Ann Otol Rhinol Laryngol 1952;61:987-1016.
10. Hilton M, Pinder D: The Epley (canalith repositioning) maneuver for benign paroxysmal positional vertigo. Cochrane Database Syst Rev 2002;(1):CD003162.
11. Brandt T, Daroff RB: Physical therapy for benign paroxysmal positional vertigo. Arch Otolaryngol 1980;106:484.
12. Honrubia B, Baloh RW, Harris MR, et al: Paroxysmal positional vertigo syndrome. Am J Otol 1999;20:465-470.
13. Hart CW: Evaluation of post-traumatic vertigo. Otolaryngol Clin North Am 1973;6:157.
14. Boyev KP: Ménière's disease or migraine? The clinical significance of fluctuant hearing loss with vertigo. Arch Otolaryngol Head Neck Surg 2005;131:457-459.
15. Di Girolamo S, Picciotti P, Sergi B, et al: Postural control and glycerol test in Ménière's disease. Acta Otolaryngol 2001;121:813.
16. Pappas DG Jr, Pappas DG Sr, Carmichael L, et al: Extratympanic electrocochleography: Diagnostic and predictive value. Am J Otol 2000;21:81-87.
17. Committee on Hearing and Equilibrium: Guidelines for the diagnosis and evaluation of therapy in Ménière's disease. Otolaryngol Head Neck Surg 1995;113:181-185.
18. Hoston JR, Baloh RW: Acute vestibular syndrome. N Engl J Med 1998;339:680-685.
19. Lee H, Cho YM: A case of isolated nodulus infarction presenting as a vestibular neuritis. J Neurol Sci 2004;221:117-119.
20. Strupp M, Arbusow V, Maag KP, et al: Vestibular exercises improve central vestibulospinal compensation after vestibular neuritis. Neurology 1998;51:838-844.
21. Nomura Y, Okuno T, Hara M, et al: "Floating" labyrinth. Pathophysiology and treatment of perilymph fistula. Acta Otolaryngol (Stockh) 1992;112:186-191.
22. Minor LB: Superior canal dehiscence syndrome. Am J Otol 2000;21:9-19.
23. Albuquerque W, Bronstein AM: "Doctor, I can hear my eyes": Report of two cases with different mechanisms. J Neurol Neurosurg Psychiatry 2004;75:1363-1364.
24. Tilikete C, Krolak-Salmon P, Truy E, et al: Pulse-synchronous eye oscillations revealing bone superior canal dehiscence. Ann Neurol 2004;56:556-560.
25. Gacek RR, Gacek MR: Neuritis vestibularis. Ann Otol Rhinol Laryngol 2002;111:103-114.
26. Magnusson M, Karlberg M: Peripheral vestibular disorders with acute onset of vertigo. Curr Opin Neurol 2002;15:5-10.
27. Strupp M, Arbusow V: Acute vestibulopathy. Curr Opin Neurol 2001;14:11-20.
28. Brandt T, Dieterich M: Vestibular paroxysmia: Vascular compression of the eighth nerve? Lancet 1994;343:798-799.
29. Baloh RW: Neurotology of migraine. Headache 1997;37:615-621.
30. Ishiyama A, Jacobson KM, Baloh RW: Migraine and benign positional vertigo. Ann Otol Rhinol Laryngol 2000;109:377-380.
31. Harno H, Hirvonen T, Kaunisto MA, et al: Subclinical vestibulocerebellar dysfunction in migraine with and without aura. Neurology 61:2003;1748-1752.
32. Nauhauser H, Leopold M, von Brevern M, et al: The interrelation of migraine, vertigo, and migrainous vertigo. Neurology 2001;56:436-441.
33. Headache Classification Committee of the International Headache Society. The international classification of headache disorders. Cephalalgia 2004;24:(Suppl.1)1-160.
34. Neuhauser H, Lempert T: Vertigo and dizziness related to migraine: A diagnostic challenge. Cephalalgia 2004;24:83-91.
35. Crevits L, Bosman T: Migraine-related vertigo: Towards a distinctive entity. Clin Neurol Neurosurg 2005;107:82-87.
36. Savitz S, Caplan L: Current concepts in vertebrobasilar disease. N Engl J Med 2005;352:2618-2626.
37. Tang RA: Vascular inner ear partition: A concept for some forms of sensorineural hearing loss and vertigo. ORL Otorhinolargngol Relat Spec 1998;60:78-84.
38. Brandt T, Pessin MS, Kwan ES, et al: Survival with basilar artery occlusion. Cerebrovasc Dis 1995;5:182-187.
39. Devuyst G, Bogousslavsky J, Meuli R, et al: Stroke or transient ischemic attacks with basilar artery stenosis or occlusion: Clinical patterns and outcome. Arch Neurol 2002;59:567-573.
40. The National Institute of Neurological Disorders and Stroke rt-PA Study Group: Tissue plasminogen activator for acute ischemic stroke. N Engl J Med 1995;333:1581-1587.
41. Montavont A, Nighoghossian N, Derex L, et al: Intravenous r-tPA in vertebrobasilar acute infarcts. Neurology 2004;62:1854-1856.
42. Butler K, Humphriss R, Lennox G: Vestibular assessment in a patient with confirmed lateral medullary syndrome. J Laryngol Otol 2006;120;135-137.
43. Kim JS: Vertigo and gait ataxia without usual signs of lateral medullary infarction: A clinical variant related to rostral-dorsolateral lesions. Cerebrovasc Dis 2000;10:471-474.
44. Kuether TA, Nesbit GM, Clark WM, et al: Rotational vertebral artery occlusion: A mechanism of vertebrobasilar insufficiency. Neurosurgery 1997;41:427-432.
45. Carmona S, Nicenboim L, Castagnino D: Recurrent vertigo in extrinsic compression of the brain stem. Ann N Y Acad Sci 2005;1039:513-516.

Chapter **92**

Peripheral Nerve Disorders

Phillip Andrus and Andy Jagoda

KEY POINTS

Peripheral nerve disorders occur in 10% of the population.

Diabetes mellitus is the most common etiology of peripheral nerve disorders.

Central nervous system and life-threatening causes of weakness must be excluded first.

Guillain-Barré syndrome requires prompt intervention; respiratory function is evaluated as soon as the diagnosis is considered and intubation performed before respiratory failure occurs.

Patients with acute myasthenic crisis or botulism require close monitoring of respiratory function.

Most peripheral nerve disorders require formal electrodiagnostic testing before a conclusive diagnosis can be made.

Scope

Peripheral nerve disorders may cause proximal or distal weakness as well as symmetrical or asymmetrical symptoms and may be acute or chronic. Symptoms range from weakness to paralysis, numbness to pain.

Although these disorders are often benign, the role of the EP is to assess each case for serious etiologies including Guillain-Barré syndrome, myasthenia gravis, and botulism. These are acute emergencies associated with respiratory failure and significant mortality and disability when they are not recognized and treated appropriately.

Anatomy

Understanding the anatomy of the spinal cord in general (Fig. 92-1) and of the peripheral nervous system in particular is an important part of evaluating peripheral nerve disorders. The peripheral nervous system is composed of 12 cranial nerves and 31 spinal nerves. The spinal nerves are formed from motor fibers whose cell bodies reside in the ventral horn of the spinal cord and from sensory fibers whose cell bodies are found in the dorsal root ganglion. Motor and sensory fibers join to form one nerve as it exits the spinal canal. Many of these spinal nerves merge with others from several spinal levels at the cervical, brachial, lumbar, and sacral plexuses. The peripheral nerves originate either at these plexuses or, if they are formed from nerves of only one spinal level, as they exit the vertebral foramina.

Peripheral nerves consist of mixed fibers including variable amounts of motor, sensory, and autonomic; small and large; and myelinated and unmyelinated fibers. These fibers, surrounded by endoneurial fluid and covered in perineurium, form a fascicle. Peripheral nerves are made up of fascicles bundled together

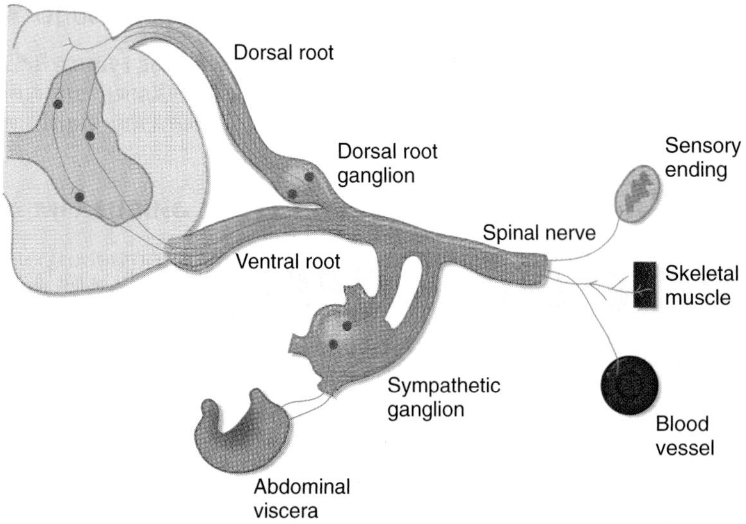
Dorsal root
Dorsal root ganglion
Sensory ending
Spinal nerve
Ventral root
Skeletal muscle
Sympathetic ganglion
Blood vessel
Abdominal viscera

FIGURE 92-1 Cross-section of the spine showing relationship between ventral and dorsal roots, dorsal root ganglion, spinal cord, vertebrae, and peripheral nerve.

Table 92-1 PERIPHERAL NERVE DISORDERS

Process	Definition
Neuropathy	A disturbance of function or pathologic change in one or more peripheral nerves. The injury to the nerve may be at the level of the myelin sheath (myelinopathy), the axon (distal axonopathy, wallerian degeneration) or the nerve cell body (neuronopathy).
Myelinopathy	Segmental demyelination of a myelinopathy involves loss of the protective myelin sheath with sparing of the axon itself and is seen as slowing or conduction block on electrodiagnostic testing. This process is commonly due to inflammatory, autoimmune, or hereditary factors.
Distal axonopathy	Insult at the axonal level, frequently due to diabetes, nutritional deficiency, or toxins, resulting in the "dying-back" phenomenon, as the most distal portion of the axon degenerates with concomitant breakdown of the proximal myelin sheath.
Wallerian degeneration	Initial insult at the axonal level, usually due to direct trauma, results in degeneration of the axons and myelin sheaths distal to the site of injury.
Neuronopathy	Neuropathy that first affects the anterior horn cell or dorsal root ganglion with axonal demyelination extending distally. The prognosis is poor, and recovery often is incomplete, because the initial injury is to the cell body itself.

by the epineurial sheath. This sheath forms a protective barrier akin to the blood-brain barrier in the central nervous system.[1]

Peripheral nerves may be injured by trauma, inflammatory, metabolic, toxic, genetic, or neoplastic processes (Table 92-1). The response of a peripheral nerve to these injuries depends on the insult, and the prognosis is not universally dire. In contrast to the nerves of the central nervous system, injured peripheral nerves regenerate. They do so by following an intact nerve sheath as a guide. This process takes place at a rate of 1 to 3 mm per day. In chronic disease processes, such as diabetic neuropathy and chronic inflammatory demyelinating polyneuropathy, this regeneration occurs repeatedly and may lead to nerve hypertrophy (onion-bulb formation), in which an excess of Schwann cells accumulates.

The differential diagnosis of peripheral nerve disorders is outlined in Box 92-1. A discussion of the most important of these disorders follows.

Guillain-Barré Syndrome

Guillain-Barré syndrome is also known as acute idiopathic polyneuritis, postinfectious polyneuritis, and Landry-Guillain-Barré syndrome.

■ PATHOPHYSIOLOGY

Guillain-Barré syndrome is the prototypical acute inflammatory demyelinating polyneuropathy. It is characterized by immune-mediated peripheral nerve myelin sheath destruction. Biopsy of the affected peripheral nerve frequently reveals a mononuclear inflammatory infiltrate. Although the exact etiology remains unknown, there is a clear association with preceding triggering events such as viral or febrile illness, *Campylobacter jejuni* infection, and vaccination.

Guillain-Barré syndrome is a monophasic illness with symptoms at their worst in 2 weeks in 50% of

BOX 92-1

Differential Diagnosis of Peripheral Nerve Disorders

Central Nervous System
- Cerebrovascular accident (stroke)
- Spinal cord compression
- Brown-Séquard syndrome
- Amyotrophic lateral sclerosis

Autoimmune
- Myasthenia gravis
- Lambert-Eaton myasthenic syndrome

Demyelination
- Guillain-Barré syndrome
- Multifocal motor neuropathy
- Critical illness polyneuropathy

Drug- and Toxin-Related
- Reactions to:
  - Amiodarone, isoniazid
  - Gold, arsenic, lead
- Diphtheria
- Botulism
- Tick paralysis

Hereditary
- Charcot-Marie-Tooth disease
- Acute intermittent porphyria
- Infections

Human Immunodeficiency Virus (HIV) Neuropathy
- Chronic hepatitis
- Acute infectious mononucleosis (Epstein-Barr virus)

Inflammatory
- POEMS (*p*olyneuropathy, *e*ndocrinopathy, *M*-protein production, *s*kin changes)

Metabolic
- Alcoholic neuropathy
- Vitamin B_{12} deficiency
- Hypokalemia

patients, and 4 weeks in over 90% of patients. Recovery can vary from weeks up to a year. Mortality has been reported in 2% to 5% of cases.[2]

PRESENTING SIGNS AND SYMPTOMS

Classic Guillain-Barré Syndrome

Guillain-Barré syndrome generally is preceded by a viral prodrome, followed by acute or subacutely ascending symmetrical weakness or paralysis and loss of deep tendon reflexes. Paralysis may ascend to the diaphragm, compromising respiratory function and requiring mechanical ventilation. One third of patients will require intubation. The diagnosis is strongly suggested by the findings listed in Box 92-2.

BOX 92-2

Findings Suggesting Guillain-Barré Syndrome

- Relative symmetry of symptoms
- Mild sensory signs and symptoms
- Cranial nerve involvement
- Autonomic dysfunction
- Absence of fever at onset
- Cytoalbuminologic dissociation of cerebrospinal fluid
- Typical electrodiagnostic findings
- Progression over days to weeks
- Recovery beginning 2 to 4 weeks after cessation of progression

Variants of Guillain-Barré Syndrome

Acute Motor Axonal Neuropathy

This purely motor form of Guillain-Barré syndrome is associated with *Campylobacter jejuni* infection. It is more likely to be preceded by diarrhea than a viral prodrome. It results in axonal injury rather than demyelination.

Acute Motor and Sensory Axonal Neuropathy

This variant involves loss of both motor and sensory function. As in acute motor axonal neuropathy, electrodiagnostic testing reveals axonal degeneration.

Miller-Fisher Syndrome

Identified in 1956, Miller-Fisher syndrome is characterized by ophthalmoplegia, ataxia, and decreased or absent reflexes. It is differentiated from Guillain-Barré syndrome by significantly decreased weakness and a milder course.

DIAGNOSTIC TESTING

It is critical to assess respiratory function early and often because airway protection given well in advance of respiratory compromise decreases the incidence of aspiration and other complications of emergent intubation. The most well-studied monitoring parameter is vital capacity (VC), in which the normal values range from 60 to 70 mL/kg. However, a simple bedside assessment of ventilatory status is obtained by having the patient count from 1 to 25 with a single breath and trending the values that he or she reaches.

Indications for intubation include:

- Rapid progression of respiratory compromise
- VC < 20 mL/kg
- Negative inspiratory force (NIF) < –30 cm H_2O
- Decrease of >30% of either VC or NIF in the first 24 hours
- Autonomic instability

If the patient's condition does not initially meet the criteria for intubation, the VC should be monitored closely—every hour for the first 4 hours and then every 4 hours.[3]

Lumbar puncture reveals the classic "cytoalbuminologic dissociation," in which CSF protein is high without pleocytosis. The protein level is greater than 45 mg/dL. Cell counts are typically below 10 cells/mL, usually predominantly mononuclear cells. When there are more than 100 cells/mL, other etiologies should be considered including human immunodeficiency virus (HIV) infection, Lyme disease, syphilis, sarcoid, tuberculosis, bacterial meningitis, leukemic infiltration, and central nervous system vasculitis.

Electrodiagnostic testing confirms demyelination typical of Guillain-Barré syndrome. In patients with the acute motor axonal neuropathy or acute motor and sensory axonal neuropathy variants, electromyogram and nerve conduction studies reveal axonal injury rather than demyelination.

■ TREATMENT

The first priority in the treatment of patients with Guillain-Barré syndrome is airway management. Along with frequent assessment of the need for intubation, early consultation with neurology and/or critical care specialists will ensure a coordinated management strategy.

Corticosteroids have shown no benefit in the management of Guillain-Barré syndrome, and may be harmful. The two modalities that have clearly proven beneficial are intravenous immunoglobulin (IVIg) and plasmapheresis. IVIg and plasmapheresis provide equivalent but not additive reduction in duration of symptoms if given within 2 weeks of onset to ambulatory patients and within 4 weeks to nonambulatory patients. Adverse effects may occur with both modalities of treatment. Plasmapheresis has been associated with greater hemodynamic instability, but a lower rate of relapse; IVIg has been associated with thromboembolism and aseptic meningitis.[4]

■ DISPOSITION

The decision to admit the patient to the hospital should be made in consultation with a neurologist and may be based on clinical criteria alone, or with the confirmation of cerebrospinal fluid analysis and nerve conduction studies. Patients who require or may require intubation, are unable to ambulate, or are being considered for plasmapheresis should be admitted to the intensive care unit.

Chronic Inflammatory Demyelinating Polyneuropathy

■ PATHOPHYSIOLOGY

Chronic inflammatory demyelinating polyneuropathy has a much more insidious onset and chronic course than Guillain-Barré syndrome. It is rare and although its etiology remains unclear, it is thought to be the result of an autoimmune process.

This disorder begins with inflammation at the root and peripheral nerve levels, resulting in myelin damage. The ensuing repair of the myelin sheath can take weeks to months. In some cases, the axons themselves may be damaged, leading to a concurrent axonopathy.[5]

■ PRESENTING SIGNS AND SYMPTOMS

■ Classic Inflammatory Demyelinating Polyneuropathy

Symptoms typically progress over the course of weeks to months. Weakness is seen more frequently than sensory symptoms. There is symmetrical involvement of the arms and legs, proximal and distal weakness, and reduced or absent deep tendon reflexes. Lumbar puncture reveals cytoalbuminologic dissociation as seen in Guillain-Barré syndrome. Electrodiagnostic testing results are consistent with demyelination. The progression of symptoms is more gradual than in Guillain-Barré Syndrome, and respiratory failure is rare.[6]

■ Lewis Sumner Syndrome (Multifocal Inflammatory Demyelinating Polyneuropathy)

Lewis Sumner syndrome is far less common than classic inflammatory demyelinating polyneuropathy. These patients usually have asymmetrical involvement in the upper rather than the lower extremities.

■ Sensory Inflammatory Demyelinating Polyneuropathy

Patients with inflammatory demyelinating polyneuropathy have distal sensory loss and pain. Nonetheless, on electrodiagnostic testing some motor slowing will be evident.

■ Inflammatory Demyelinating Polyneuropathy in Diabetes

Compared with diabetic neuropathy, this disorder is more likely to have a rapidly aggressive course, greater motor involvement, proximal muscle involvement, generalized hyporeflexia, and protein cerebrospinal fluid levels of less than 150 mg/dL.

■ DIAGNOSTIC TESTING

Confirming a diagnosis of inflammatory demyelinating polyneuropathy is difficult. No conclusive test is available, and there is considerable disagreement among experts on clinical criteria. The diagnosis may be made on the basis of clinical findings and electrodiagnostic testing, but confirmation with cerebrospinal fluid studies and nerve biopsy may be required. Consultation with a neurologist may be required for electrodiagnostic testing in patients with distal symmetrical polyneuropathy with significant motor involvement.[7,8]

■ TREATMENT AND DISPOSITION

As in Guillain-Barré syndrome, treatment consists of immunomodulatory therapy. However, unlike in Guillain-Barré syndrome, corticosteroids have proven equivalent in efficacy to IVIg and plasmapheresis. Combination therapy does not provide additional benefit. If the response to these therapies is inadequate, other nonstandard immunomodulatory therapies such as antineoplastics may be considered.[9]

Patients who require IVIg or plasmapheresis, whose illness cannot be managed at home due to pain or weakness, or who have comorbid illness requiring admission should be hospitalized.

Diabetic Peripheral Neuropathy

■ PATHOPHYSIOLOGY

Diabetic peripheral neuropathy encompasses any neuropathy in a diabetic patient not attributable to other causes. The most common manifestation is a distal symmetrical polyneuropathy. The converse relationship also exists, because the classic example of distal symmetrical polyneuropathy is diabetic neuropathy. This is not an absolute relationship, however; diabetes also leads to focal neuropathies, and mononeuropathy multiplex neuropathy develops in about 50% of diabetic patients. It is seen in patients with type 1 diabetes after 5 years and early in the course of type 2 diabetes. It is associated with significant morbidity. The most common cause of nontraumatic amputation is injury resulting from impaired sensation due to diabetic peripheral neuropathy that fails to heal due to the impaired blood flow of diabetic vasculopathy.

Hyperglycemia affects peripheral nerves by several proposed mechanisms:

- Oxidative stress
- Glycosylation of nerve proteins
- Changes in diabetic vasculature resulting in increased resistance and decreased flow to peripheral nerves

Motor, sensory, and small and large fibers can be involved. Diabetic peripheral neuropathy is an example of a distal axonopathy resulting in length-dependent "dying back" of the affected nerves. This dying back phenomenon produces the typical stocking-and-glove distribution of diabetic neuropathy.[10]

■ PRESENTING SIGNS AND SYMPTOMS

■ Classic Diabetic Peripheral Neuropathy

Signs and symptoms are many and varied. Motor findings include muscle weakness, atrophy, imbalance, and ataxic gait. Sensory findings consist of pain, paresthesias, numbness, cramping, and antalgic gait.

■ Painful Diabetic Neuropathy

This chronically painful neuropathy is seen in 10% of diabetics. It is usually intermittent, worse when attentive, and occurs at night. It can be experienced variably as pins and needles, throbbing, burning, aching, cramping, and/or a cold sensation. Duration is less than 6 months. When the duration is more than 6 months, the same process is termed *chronic painful diabetic neuropathy.*

■ Insulin Neuritis

Insulin neuritis is a small-fiber neuropathy characterized by pain and paresthesias associated with insulin therapy.

■ Diabetic Neuropathic Cachexia

This rare syndrome causes weight loss and painful dysesthesias of the limbs and trunk.

■ Hyperglycemic Neuropathy

Hyperglycemic neuropathy is seen in newly diagnosed diabetics; this condition normally improves with glycemic control.

■ Asymmetrical Proximal Diabetic Neuropathy (Diabetic Amyotrophy)

Patients with diabetic amyotrophy have pain in the low back, hip, and anterior thigh, which may be bilateral. The disorder may progress to weakness and weight loss. Symptoms may improve after months.

■ TREATMENT AND DISPOSITION

Disease modification is likely to have the greatest effect on progression of diabetic neuropathy. The etiology of this disorder may be multifactorial, but

Table 92-2 **INITIAL THERAPY FOR DIABETIC PERIPHERAL NEUROPATHY**

Type of Therapy	Medication*
Tricyclic antidepressants	Amitriptyline, 50 mg daily Nortriptyline, 50 mg daily
Anticonvulsants	Gabapentin, 300 mg three times daily Valproate, 500 mg twice daily
Topical	Capsaicin, 0.075% up to four times daily Lidocaine 5% patch, 1 patch daily

*All doses are estimated for a 70-kg adult.

there is a clear relationship between glycemic control and neuropathy. The Diabetes Control and Complications Trial showed a 60% reduction in the risk of developing neuropathy when there is tight glycemic control.[11]

Foot care should be stressed to the patient who has already developed neuropathy. Neuropathy-associated anesthesia may result in inadvertent trauma. These injuries, in the setting of impaired healing due to diabetic vasculopathy, can lead to the development of ulcers, cellulitis, and eventually amputation.

Symptomatic management is the patient's most immediate concern. Nonsteroidal antiinflammatory drugs (NSAIDs) may alleviate discomfort but are relatively contraindicated in diabetic patients. Narcotics carry addictive potential. Tricyclic antidepressants, anticonvulsants, and topical capsaicin all have proved beneficial (Table 92-2).[12,13]

Isolated Mononeuropathies

Mononeuropathies, unlike the processes previously discussed, are more likely due to focal compression of a nerve, although systemic processes certainly lead to mononeuropathy. In fact, diabetes, due to its associated microvasculopathy, remains the most common cause of noncompressive focal neuropathy. Focal mononeuropathy can occur at any point of compression along the course of a peripheral nerve. It is seen most commonly along the ulnar, median, radial, and peroneal nerves.

The key to diagnosis of a focal mononeuropathy is careful examination and localization of the affected nerve. Beware, however, that anatomic variations can make localization difficult. Some of these variations are more common and easily recognized, but in other cases they may be unique to the patient.

■ MEDIAN MONONEUROPATHY (CARPAL TUNNEL SYNDROME)

■ Pathophysiology

Median mononeuropathy is virtually synonymous with carpal tunnel syndrome. Compression of the median nerve proximal to the carpal tunnel is rare. Most commonly, it occurs at the wrist where the median nerve passes through the carpal tunnel, bounded superiorly by the carpal bones and inferiorly by the flexor retinaculum (Fig. 92-2). The most common etiology is a repetitive use injury. Other causes include diabetes mellitus, amyloidosis, and trauma. Edema associated with pregnancy and other conditions may result in carpal tunnel syndrome.[14]

■ Presenting Signs and Symptoms

The classic signs of carpal tunnel syndrome are burning, numbness, or pain in the distribution of the median nerve—the palmar aspect of the thumb, index finger, middle and radial aspect of the fourth finger. Patients may report symptoms in the complete hand, but on examination, sensation is preserved in the fifth and ulnar fourth digits.

■ Diagnostic Testing

Provocative testing such as Tinel's and Phalen's signs can confirm the diagnosis. Tinel's sign is elicited by tapping on the palmar aspect of the wrist. Tingling, numbness, or an electric shock sensation shooting into the hand implies compression of the median nerve. In testing for Phalen's sign, the wrists are held in flexion for 60 seconds. Phalen's sign is positive if symptoms of tingling, numbness, or pain are evoked or worsen.

Electrodiagnostic testing may be performed on an outpatient basis to confirm the diagnosis and to aid in deciding whether operative repair is necessary. Results of nerve conduction studies may demonstrate slowing of nerve conduction across the carpal tunnel.[15]

■ Treatment

The initial treatment of carpal tunnel syndrome is conservative. In patients with newly diagnosed carpal tunnel syndrome, behavioral modification is recommended, including weight loss and avoidance of caffeine, nicotine, and alcohol. Patients should be instructed about a reduction in possible repetitive use injury by making changes in workplace ergonomics and by wearing a wrist splint. Antinflammatory medications may provide some relief, but neither NSAIDs nor oral corticosteroid therapy will permanently resolve symptoms. Diuretics may be given if edema is believed to contribute significantly to the patient's symptoms.

■ Disposition

Although carpal tunnel syndrome is not an acute surgical emergency, in the long term patients with this disorder are at risk for impairment and disability. These patients may be safely discharged from the ED

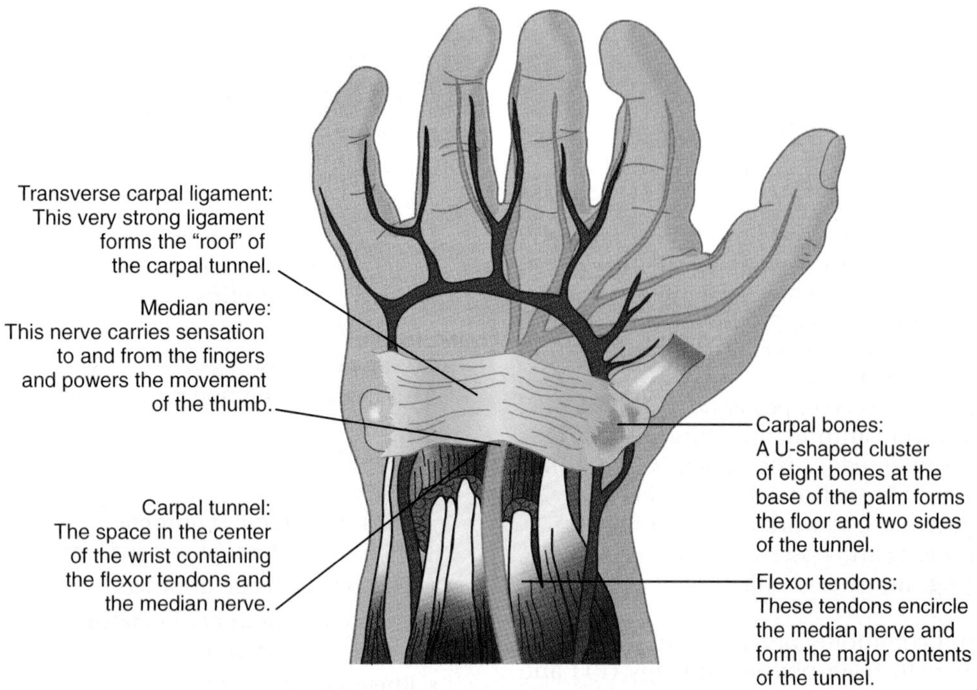
Transverse carpal ligament:
This very strong ligament
forms the "roof" of
the carpal tunnel.
Median nerve:
This nerve carries sensation
to and from the fingers
and powers the movement
of the thumb.
Carpal tunnel:
The space in the center
of the wrist containing
the flexor tendons and
the median nerve.
Carpal bones:
A U-shaped cluster
of eight bones at the
base of the palm forms
the floor and two sides
of the tunnel.
Flexor tendons:
These tendons encircle
the median nerve and
form the major contents
of the tunnel.

FIGURE 92-2 Anatomy of carpal tunnel.

but require close follow-up by their primary care physician or a hand specialist. If conservative treatment fails, the hand specialist may recommentd corticosteroid injection and surgical release of the flexor retinaculum.

■ ULNAR MONONEUROPATHY (CUBITAL TUNNEL SYNDROME)

■ Pathophysiology

Cubital tunnel syndrome is the second most common compressive mononeuropathy. The ulnar nerve extends from the medial cord of the brachial plexus and courses through the cubital tunnel behind the medial epicondyle at the elbow before entering the forearm. At the wrist, it passes through Guyon's canal, bounded by the hamate and pisiform bones and the ligament connecting them. It supplies cutaneous innervation to the medial palm via the superficial terminal branch and to the fifth and medial fourth fingers via the deep terminal branch and innervates the palmaris brevis. The median nerve is most vulnerable to repetitive stress inflammation and trauma as it passes through these two canals.[16]

■ Presenting Signs and Symptoms

Cubital Tunnel Syndrome

Classic symptoms include tingling in the fifth and lateral fourth fingers, the distribution of the ulnar nerve. With time this may progress to numbness and weakness of the intrinsic muscles of the hand. In severe cases, paralysis and wasting of the intrinsics may occur.

Provocative testing as for carpal tunnel syndrome is useful. Tinel's sign is elicited by tapping on the cubital tunnel at the elbow. A positive elbow flexion sign is occurs when symptoms recur within 3 minutes when the elbow is held in flexion with the wrist in extension. Froment's sign may be noted during resistance testing when the thumb intraphalangeal joint flexes to compensate for weakness of the adductor pollicis brevis.

Guyon's Canal Syndrome (Handlebar Palsy)

Compression of the ulnar nerve in this canal bounded by the pisiform and hamate bones is more likely to spare the sensory fibers and present as intrinsic weakness only.

■ Differential Diagnosis

If the diagnosis of cubital tunnel syndrome is suspected, consider cranial nerve VIII (C-VIII) entrapment and thoracic outlet syndrome. C-VIII entrapment can be differentiated by the presence of neck pain and worsening symptoms with neck flexion. Thoracic outlet syndrome worsens with shoulder abduction.

■ Diagnostic Testing

Electrodiagnostic testing demonstrates nerve conduction slowing and serves to precisely localize the lesion. Tests may be ordered by a consulting neurologist or by a surgeon to aid in the decision regarding surgical decompression of the affected nerve.

Treatment and Disposition

In most cases, the goal of treatment in the ED is to initiate conservative treatment and to ensure appropriate follow-up. In cases in which the nerve compression is acute and is possibly due to fracture or hematoma, immediate surgical consultation is mandatory. If this is not the case, prompt surgical referral remains important for either corticosteroid injection or surgical management.

Pain is not a common component of cubital tunnel syndrome; however, antiinflammatory medications such as NSAIDs may reduce the patient's symptoms. The patient should be instructed to rest the elbow by reducing repetitive use at work and/or home and by splinting with a long arm posterior splint. For chronic or longstanding injuries, a sling may suffice for support.

Although not commonly ordered from the ED, the patient may benefit from physical therapy (PT) and occupational therapy (OT) referrals. If the patient's symptoms persist beyond 3 to 6 weeks despite conservative treatment, PT/OT, surgical treatment with nerve decompression, transposition, or medial epicondylectomy is usually required.

MONONEUROPATHY MULTIPLEX

Pathophysiology

Mononeuropathy multiplex consists of a group of disorders that have in common the dysfunction of multiple peripheral nerves separated both temporally and in anatomic location. Early in the progression of these disorders, the affected nerves identified by a careful history and physical examination. As the disorder progresses, signs and symptoms become confluent and more symmetrical. These symptoms may progress over minutes to days and resolve over weeks to months after onset.

Presenting Signs and Symptoms

Patients with mononeuropathy multiplex present with signs and symptoms similar to those of isolated mononeuropathy, including weakness, paresthesias, numbness, aches, and spasms of sharp pain. As the name suggests, however, these symptoms will be present concurrently in several anatomically distinct nerves. The many etiologies of mononeuropathy multiplex suggest the important features that differentiates them (Box 92-3).

Diagnostic Testing

The diagnosis is made based on a careful history and physical examination. Diagnostic testing is based on management of the causative etiology.

BOX 92-3

Etiologies of Mononeuropathy Multiplex

- Diabetes mellitus
- Vasculitides
  - Polyarteritis nodosa
  - Wegener's granulomatosis
  - Temporal arteritis
- Infectious
  - Lyme disease
  - Human immunodeficiency virus (HIV)
  - Leprosy
  - Hepatitis
- Neoplasms
  - Paraneoplastic syndrome
  - Intraneural neoplastic infiltration
- Connective tissue disorders
  - Systemic lupus erythematosus
  - Sjögren's syndrome
- Rheumatoid arthritis
- Sarcoidosis
- Lead poisoning
- Polycythemia vera
- Cryoglobulinemia

Treatment and Disposition

Management depends primarily on the associated etiology and the severity of any concurrent illness.

Along with treatment of underlying disorders, appropriate specialty referral and electrodiagnostic testing should be arranged. Physical and occupational therapy are important components of a management strategy for these patients and help to decrease pain and preserve functional independence.

Disorders of the Neuromuscular Junction—Myasthenia Gravis

PATHOPHYSIOLOGY

Myasthenia gravis has a prevalence of 50 to 125 per million population. The age of onset is bimodal, initially peaking when patients are in their 20s to 30s, affecting women more than men; a second peak occurs during the 6th and 7th decades and affects men more than women.

There are many etiologies, but they all lead to the formation of autoantibodies directed against nicotinic acetylcholine receptors (AChRs) at the neuromuscular junction (Fig. 92-3). This results in autoimmune destruction of AChRs through complement-mediated destruction as well as increased endocytosis by the muscle cells. The culprit autoantibodies further compete with acetylcholine for binding at

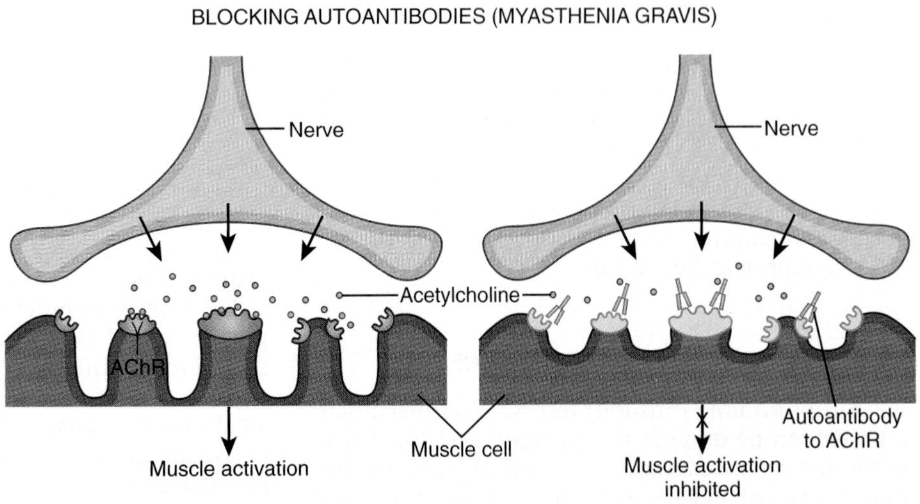
BLOCKING AUTOANTIBODIES (MYASTHENIA GRAVIS)
Nerve
Nerve
Acetylcholine
AChR
Muscle activation
Muscle cell
Autoantibody to AChR
Muscle activation inhibited

FIGURE 92-3 Diagram of motor end plate illustrating the blocking of autoantibodies to acetylcholine receptors (AChRs).

remaining receptors. Thus, with repeated stimulation of the same muscle, fewer and fewer sites are available and fatigue develops.[17]

PRESENTING SIGNS AND SYMPTOMS

New Onset Myasthenia Gravis

Muscular weakness and fatigability are the hallmarks of myasthenia gravis. When patients present to the ED with an initial manifestation of the disease, their symptoms usually consist of mononeuropathy involving the ocular or bulbar muscles. Ocular muscle weakness may be the first sign in up to 40% of patients, although 85% of patients will eventually have ocular involvement. The typical presentation is ptosis, diplopia, or blurred vision. When present, ptosis is often worse toward the end of the day. When bulbar muscles are involved, dysarthria or dysphagia is seen. Respiratory failure is a rare initial presentation. Nevertheless, up to 17% of patients may have weakness of the muscles of respiration.

Acute Myasthenic Crisis

Acute myasthenic crisis is defined as respiratory failure eventually requiring mechanical ventilation. It occurs in 15% to 20% of patients, generally within the first 2 years of disease. With the use of better and more aggressive techniques in the intensive care unit, mortality has declined tremendously.

Underlying infection, aspiration, and changes in medications most often trigger myasthenic crisis, but the precipitant may not be found in up to 30% of cases. Some patients experience an increase in weakness when starting chronic steroid therapy. Other precipitants include surgery and pregnancy.

As in Guillain-Barré syndrome, the initial step in managing the patient in myasthenic crisis is assessing respiratory status and securing the airway, if necessary. A patient who is not yet intubated but is complaining of shortness of breath or difficulty breathing should have frequent vital capacity measurements. In contrast with the steady worsening of Guillain-Barré syndrome, patients in myasthenic crisis may have fluctuating weakness. For these patients, a lower VC of 15 mL/kg is considered an indication for intubation, but the trend of their respiratory function is more useful than a single measurement.

Congenital Myasthenia Gravis

Approximately 12% of pregnant women with myasthenia gravis will give birth to symptomatic infants, bcause of placental transfer of autoantibodies. Infants develop symptoms including impaired sucking, weak cry, limp limbs, and rarely respiratory insufficiency within the first 2 days after birth. Symptoms disappear as antibody titers in the infant decline within days or weeks. In severe cases of respiratory failure, intubation is necessary, and exchange transfusion should be considered.

Lambert-Eaton Myasthenic Syndrome

Lambert-Eaton myasthenic syndrome is a rare disease associated with small-cell carcinoma of the lung in 60% of cases. Autoantibodies formed in patients with this disorder result in an inadequate release of acetylcholine from nerve terminals, affecting both nicotinic and muscarinic receptors. With repeated stimulation, the amount of acetylcholine in the synaptic cleft increases, leading to an increase in strength—the opposite of symptoms seen in patients with myasthenia gravis.

The classic presentation includes weakness that increases with use of muscles, hyporeflexia, and autonomic dysregulation. Management primarily is focused on treating the underlying neoplastic disorder, although plasmapheresis and IgG have been reported to be beneficial.

DIAGNOSTIC TESTING

The diagnosis is based on clinical findings and a combination of serologic testing, the edrophonium test, and electromyography. Receptor-antibody testing is positive in 80% to 90% of patients. Many patients found to be seronegative nonetheless respond to traditional therapy aimed at lowering levels of circulating antibodies, suggesting that antibodies are present but not detected.

INTERVENTIONS AND PROCEDURES

The edrophonium (Tensilon) test is a pharmacologic test that can be done at the patient's bedside.[18] It is performed by measuring the distance between the upper and lower eyelids in the most affected eye, and then measuring again following IV administration of edrophonium, a short-acting acetylcholinesterase (AchE)-blocking agent. Because some patients have a severe reaction to edrophonium, an IV test dose of 1 mg is given initially. If there is no adverse reaction and the patient's symptoms of ptosis, medial rectus weakness, or dysphonia do not dramatically improve in 30 to 90 seconds, a second dose of 3 mg is given. Give another 3 mg dose of edvophonium if there is no response after 30 to 60 seconds. If there is still no response, a final dose of 3 mg is given, for a total maximum dosage of 10 mg.

Adverse reactions to edrophonium include oropharyngeal weakness, cholingeric weakness, abdominal cramps, diarrhea, and bradycardia. Because of the potential for bradycardia, atropine should be available at the bedside during edrophonium testing. Also, due to the potential cholinergic effect of increased airway secretions, this test should be used with caution in asthmatic patients and patients with congestive obstructive pulmonary disease.

The ice test is another bedside test that can be used to quickly confirm the diagnosis. This test is based on the observation that cooling decreases symptoms of myasthenia gravis, and heat exacerbates the symptoms. As in the edrophonium test, the distance between the upper and lower lids is measured before and after the procedure, which in this case consists of application of an ice pack for 2 to 3 minutes to the most severely affected eye.

TREATMENT

Cholinesterase Inhibitors

Cholinesterase inhibitors such as pyridostigmine and neostigmine are the backbone of outpatient chronic therapy and provide symptomatic improvement, although the treatment is not directed at the underlying immunologic basis of the disease.[19] This class of drugs inhibits the hydrolysis of acetylcholine, leading to an increased circulating concentration that stimulates the decreased number of AChRs to compete with the antibody for binding sites.

The most common side effects are those of excessive cholinergic stimulation such as increased airway secretion and increased bowel motility. Other side effects include bradycardia and worsening of weakness, simulating a myasthenic crisis. These drugs are often used as adjunctive therapy to control symptoms while allowing time for other therapy to take effect, after which they are discontinued.

The use of IV pyridostigmine in the setting of acute exacerbation of myasthenia gravis is controversial. There is some evidence that its use may complicate ventilation due to worsening pulmonary secretions.[20] Thus cholinergic drug therapy should be discontinued during a myasthenic crisis. In addition, a "cholinergic crisis," characterized by acute decompensation and excessive muscarinic stimulation, may be caused by excessive medication with acetylcholinesterase (AChE) inhibitors. Cholinergic crisis should be distinguished from an exacerbation of the disease by muscarinic physical examination findings. Muscarinic effects of AChE inhibition include excessive sweating, salivation, lacrimation, miosis, tachycardia, and gastrointestinal hyperactivity.

Immunosuppressant Drugs

Immunosuppressant drugs often are used for the chronic control of the symptoms of myasthenia gravis. They have no role in the acute management of myasthenic crisis, although they may be started prior to extubation of patients recovering from a crisis. Corticosteroids, azathioprine, and cyclosporine have all been used.

Thymectomy

Thymectomy in otherwise well patients between adolescence and 60 years of age results in remission or improvement in up to 50% of cases. However, onset of improvement after thymectomy is often delayed for 2 to 5 years.

Immunomodulatory Therapy

Plasmapheresis and IVIg are reserved for patients with severe exacerbations or are administered preoperatively in patients with stable myasthenia gravis. From 50% to 90% of patients treated with IVIg have some improvement following infusion. Current consensus recommends a dose of 0.4 g/kg/day for 5 days in patients with uncontrolled acute exacerbations.[21]

DISPOSITION

Considering the slow clinical progression of myasthenia gravis and the very low likelihood of complications due to its progression, confirmation of the diagnosis is mainly important in order to facilitate proper discharge referral. It also is important, however, to look for signs of myasthenic crisis in any

BOX 92-4
Drugs That May Exacerbate Myasthenia Gravis

Cardiovascular Drugs
- Calcium channel blockers
- Quinidine
- Lidocaine
- Procainamide

Antibiotics
- Aminoglycosides
- Tetracycline
- Clindamycin
- Lincomycin
- Polymixin B
- Colistin

Other Drugs
- Phenytoin
- Neuromuscular blockers
- Corticosteroids
- Thyroid replacement drugs

patient with myasthenia gravis who presents to the ED. Because a number of medications can exacerbate underlying disease (notably aminoglycosides and immunosuppressants including prednisone) (Box 92-4), medication interactions should be considered when changing or initiating pharmacologic therapy in patients with myasthenia gravis.

Botulism

■ PATHOPHYSIOLOGY

Botulism is a toxin-mediated illness that can cause acute weakness leading to respiratory failure. In 2005, the Centers for Disease Control reported 145 cases of botulism, 96 of which were categorized as infantile botulism.[22] *Clostridium botulinum,* the causative organism, is an anaerobic spore-forming bacterium. Three of eight known toxins produced by *C. botulinum* cause human disease: toxin types A, B, and E. Most cases of botulism are isolated events associated with improperly preserved canned foods, although recently there has been an increased incidence of botulism from wound infections. In 2005, 28 cases of wound botulism were reported in heroin users who injected the drug subcutaneously.[22,23]

Toxin type E is associated with preserved or fermented fish and marine mammals. These are the most important sources of botulism in Alaska, Japan, Russia, and Scandinavia.

The botulinum toxin works by binding irreversibly to the presynaptic membrane of peripheral and cranial nerves inhibiting the release of ACh at the peripheral nerve synapse. As new receptors are generated, patients improve.

■ PRESENTING SIGNS AND SYMPTOMS

■ Classic Botulism

Because the disorder occurs at the neuromuscular junction, there is neither sensory deficit nor pain. Onset of symptoms occurs 6 to 48 hours after the ingestion of tainted food. There may or may not be accompanied signs and symptoms consistent with gastroenteritis, nausea, vomiting, abdominal cramps, diarrhea, or constipation. The classic presentation is a descending, symmetrical paralysis. The nerves and muscles often affected first are the cranial nerves and bulbar muscles, and the patient presents with diplopia, dysarthria, and dysphagia. There may be associated blurring of the vision. Deep tendon reflexes are normal or diminished.

Because the toxins cause decreased cholinergic output, anticholinergic signs may be seen in the form of constipation, urinary retention, dry skin and eyes, and increased temperature. Pupils are often dilated and not reactive to light. This is an important point of differentiation from myasthenia gravis.

■ Infantile Botulism

Infantile botulism occurs as a result of ingestion of *C. botulinum* spores that are able to germinate and produce toxin in the high pH of the gastrointestinal tract of infants (the same spores are not active in the gut of adults due to the lower pH). It occurs in infants between the age of 1 week and 11 months and has been implicated as a cause of sudden infant death syndrome. Clinical presentation includes constipation, poor feeding, lethargy, and weak cry; consequently, this diagnosis must be included in the differential diagnosis of the "floppy" infant.

■ DIAGNOSTIC TESTING

The diagnosis is made on clinical findings and exclusion of other processes. The toxin can be identified in both serum and stool, but the assay is not commonly available in most hospitals and thus requires a prolonged turn-around time. If the suspected food source is available, it also should be tested for the toxin.

■ TREATMENT

Treatment is initially focused on evaluating respiratory effort and securing an airway if there is respiratory compromise. The course of the disease can be shortened by giving botulinum antitoxin. The Centers for Disease Control recommend giving one vial (10 mL) of trivalent equine antitoxin as soon as the diagnosis is made. Skin testing to assess for horse serum sensitivity should be carried out prior to administration.

■ DISPOSITION

Patients diagnosed with botulism require hospitalization and intubation; patients with any signs of respiratory failure should be transferred to the intensive care unit. Suspected cases of botulism should be reported to the Health Department so that other exposures can be prevented.

REFERENCES

1. Kumar V, Abbas A, Fausto N (eds): Robbins and Cotran Pathologic Basis of Disease, 7th ed. Philadelphia, Saunders, 2005, pp 1325-1335.
2. Ropper AH: The Guillain-Barré syndrome. N Engl J Med 1992;326:1130-1136.
3. Lawn ND, Fletcher DD, Henderson RD, et al: Anticipating mechanical ventilation in Guillain-Barré syndrome. Arch Neurol 2001;58:893-898.
4. Shahar E: Current therapeutic options in severe Guillain-Barré syndrome. Clin Neuropharmacol 2006;29:45-51.
5. Lewis RA: Chronic inflammatory demyelinating polyneuropathy and other immune-mediated demyelinating neuropathies. Semin Neurol 2005;25:21-228.
6. Henderson RD, Sandroni P, Wijdicks EF: Chronic inflammatory demyelinating polyneuropathy and respiratory failure. J Neurol 2005;252:1235-1237.
7. Sander HW, Latov N: Research criteria for defining patients with CIDP. Neurology 2003;60(8 suppl 3):S8-S15.
8. Joint Task Force of the EFNS and the PNS: European Federation of Neurological Societies/Peripheral Nerve Society guideline on management of chronic inflammatory demyelinating polyradiculoneuropathy. Report of a joint task force of the European Federation of Neurological Societies and the Peripheral Nerve Society. J Peripher Nerv Syst 2005;10:220-228.
9. Ropper AH: Current treatments for CIDP. Neurology 2003;60(8 Suppl 3):S16-S22.
10. Kelkar P: Diabetic neuropathy. Semin Neurol 2005;25: 168-173.
11. The effect of intensive treatment of diabetes on the development and progression of long-term complications in insulin-dependent diabetes mellitus. The Diabetes Control and Complications Trial Research Group. N Engl J Med 1993;329:977-986.
12. Sindrup SH, Otto M, Finnerup NB, Jensen TB: Antidepressants in the treatment of neuropathic pain. Basic Clin Pharmacol Toxicol 2005;96:399-409.
13. Argoff CE, Backonja MM, Belgrade MJ, et al: Consensus guidelines: Treatment planning and options. Diabetic peripheral neuropathic pain. Mayo Clin Proc 2006;81(4 Suppl):S12-S25.
14. Katz JN, Simmons BP: Clinical practice: Carpal tunnel syndrome. N Engl J Med 2002;346:1807-1812.
15. Jillapalli D, Shefner JM: Electrodiagnosis in common mononeuropathies and plexopathies. Semin Neurol 2005;25:196-203.
16. Robertson C, Saratsiotis J: A review of compressive ulnar neuropathy at the elbow. J Manipulative Physiol Ther 2005;28:345.
17. Drachman DB: Myasthenia gravis. New Engl J Med 1994;330:1797-1810.
18. Pascuzzi RM: The edrophonium test. Semin Neurol 2003; 23:83-88.
19. Massey JM: Acquired myasthenia gravis. Neurol Clin 1997; 15:577-596.
20. Jani-Acsadi A, Lisak RP: Myasthenic crisis: Guidelines for prevention and treatment. J Neurol Sci 2007;261: 127-133.
21. Dalakas MC: Intravenous immunoglobulin in autoimmune neuromuscular diseases. JAMA 2004;291:2367-2375.
22. CDC Division of Bacterial and Mycotic Diseases: Surveillance for botulism summary of 2005 data. Available at www.cdc.gov/ncidod/dbmd/diseaseinfo/files/BOTCSTE2005.pdf.
23. Shapiro RL, Hatheway C, Swerdlow DL: Botulism in the United States: A clinical and epidemiologic review. Ann Int Med 1998;129:221-228.

Chapter 93

Demyelinating Disorders

Scott E. Rudkin

KEY POINTS

Monocular vision loss from optic neuritis is a characteristic presentation of multiple sclerosis.

Elevated body temperature worsens symptoms of multiple sclerosis.

Transverse myelitis usually presents with flaccid paraparesis, which later becomes spastic; there also is loss of sensation and bowel and bladder dysfunction.

Back pain may precede the neurologic symptoms and can be present in patients with multiple sclerosis and Guillain-Barré syndrome.

Patients with Guillain-Barré syndrome may initially present with paresthesias followed by ascending weakness.

Treatment for multiple sclerosis requires thorough supportive care, evaluation for infections, treatment of fevers, and often the administration of steroids to decrease inflammatory consequences of the autoimmune attack that damages the myelin.

Guillain-Barré syndrome patients should have respiratory evaluation of forced vital capacity (FVC) and should be admitted to the intensive care unit if their FVC is less than 20 mL/kg or intubated if it is less than 15 mL/kg. Avoid succinylcholine because it can cause hyperkalemia. Plasmapheresis and IV immunoglobin can reduce recovery time by 50%.

Scope and Outline

■ PERSPECTIVE

Second only to trauma, demyelinating diseases are a major cause of neurologic disability. Nerve conduction relies on the insulation that myelin provides the axon for impulse transmission; demyelination disrupts this insulation and results in abnormal signal propagation. This disruption results in sensory abnormalities, visual dysfunction, and muscle weakness.

Of the demyelinating conditions encountered by the EP, multiple sclerosis is by far the most common. Other demyelinating conditions include optic neuritis, transverse myelitis, and acute inflammatory polyneuropathy (Guillain-Barré syndrome).

■ EPIDEMIOLOGY

Approximately 250,000 to 350,000 people in the United States have multiple sclerosis. It is more than twice as common in women than in men and more frequently afflicts Caucasian patients, but all races can be affected. The onset of disease usually occurs in people between 20 and 50 years of age, with a peak occurring in those 30 years of age. The prevalence of multiple sclerosis varies widely with location; the highest prevalence is found at higher latitudes. The geographic variation suggests that multiple sclerosis may in part be caused by the action of some environmental factor that are more common at high latitudes.

Guillain-Barré syndrome has an incidence of 3 per 100,000, making it the most common cause of flaccid paralysis. There is a slight male predominance. The age of onset is bimodal, afflicting the elderly and young adults most commonly. There does not appear to be a geographic effect.

■ PATHOPHYSIOLOGY

The exact etiology of demyelinating conditions is unknown, but an autoimmune or immune-mediated etiology is most likely. A molecular mimicry model postulates that an autoimmune attack on myelin is precipitated by an infectious organism that contains a protein similar to a myelin protein. The infection elicits a vigorous immune response by lymphocytes that recognize the cross-reactive protein; in the process of eliminating the infectious organism, the activated lymphocytes damage myelin.

Myelin insulates nerves and aids in the transmission of nerve impulses. If the myelin sheath is disrupted through demyelination, normal transmission is disrupted. This slows conduction and creates aberrant signals, with resultant loss of coordinated motor activity and interpretation of sensory information. The majority of the demyelinating disorders cause demyelination of the myelin sheath with relative sparing of the axon.

Multiple sclerosis, transverse myelitis, and optic neuritis all affect the central nervous system. Guillain-Barré syndrome, which primarily afflicts the peripheral nervous system, is now believed to cause both demyelination of the myelin sheath and axonal loss. Inflammatory lesions in peripheral nerve fibers cause focal demyelination with resultant slowing of conduction. Cranial nerves can also be affected.

Clinical Presentation

In general, all of the demyelinating disorders present with an abrupt episode of loss of function. Depending on which area of the brain or nervous system is affected, the patient may have sensory, motor, or autonomic symptoms.

■ MULTIPLE SCLEROSIS

In multiple sclerosis, the initial attack presents abruptly (minutes to hours) from a single lesion. These attacks last between 6 and 8 weeks. Recovery between bouts of demyelination can be incomplete or complete, depending on the amount of remyelination that occurs. Any part of the central nervous system can be affected, but some areas are more common. In decreasing order of frequency, the patient may present with optic neuritis, paresthesias in a limb, diplopia, trigeminal neuralgia, urinary retention, vertigo, or transverse myelitis. Depending on the spinal cord level, the transverse myelitis can also cause loss of bladder or bowel function.

Ocular findings are the most common initial symptom. Optic neuritis presents with subacute monocular vision loss, although it can affect both eyes, and pain exacerbated with eye movement. It is the presenting symptom in 25% and ultimately affects 50% of patients.[1,2] The course usually progresses over 2 weeks and may be associated with headache, retroorbital or periocular pain, and alteration of color vision and visual fields. Slit lamp examination may demonstrate cell and flare in the anterior chamber. The optic disk is frequently swollen on initial presentation. In addition to optic neuritis, the patient may present with an afferent pupillary defect (Marcus-Gunn pupil, decreased pupil constriction on direct light confrontation, but normal consensual response) or intranuclear ophthalmoplegia, which is characterized by a dysconjugate gaze with limited adduction of one eye and nystagmus in the abducting eye on lateral gaze, resulting from a lesion of the medial longitudinal fasciculus.

Sensory symptoms in patients with multiple sclerosis usually include numbness, tingling, pins and needles, and tightness and coldness of the limbs and trunk. Radicular pain and itching may also occur. Symptoms result from involvement of the spinothalamic, posterior column, and dorsal nerve roots. The loss of vibration sense is often most prominent. Ataxia is uncommon at the onset of multiple sclerosis, but it occurs to some degree in most patients. Exacerbation of sensory symptoms can occur frequently and in different patterns with a patchy distribution. Patients may note either paresthesias or loss of sensation.

Sensitivity to heat is a characteristic complaint. Exercise, fever, a hot bath, or other activities that raise body temperature may cause the appearance of new symptoms or the recurrence of old symptoms. These events occur as a result of temperature-induced conduction block across partially demyelinated fibers. The symptoms resolve when body temperature returns to normal.

In addition to loss of sensation, patients may also report "positive" symptoms. In addition to causing a slowing of conduction, demyelination may result in ectopic impulses with resultant abnormal signal transmission and abnormal mechanical sensitivity. These aberrant signals can product Lhermitte's sign—an electric-like tingling or vibrating sensation in the torso or extremities that is produced by neck flexion. The patient may also report flashes of light (phosphenes) and paroxysmal symptom including trigeminal neuralgia, ataxia, and dysarthria or painful tetanic posturing of the limbs triggered by touch or movement.

Motor weakness may occur in any pattern, including paraparesis, hemiparesis, and monoparesis; the lower extremities are usually more affected than the upper extremities. Upper motor neuron dysfunction may also be present, accompanied by spasticity and increased reflexes. Transverse myelitis can occur as initial symptom, with ascending weakness and numbness below the level of the lesion.

Autonomic symptoms are a frequent finding. Patients have difficulty with bladder function, including frequency and urgency, and may experience urge incontinence from bladder spasticity or hesitancy, retention, and overflow incontinence from poor signal conduction. Constipation is the most common bowel complaint. This autonomic dysfunction is frequently very embarrassing and distressful.

The normal disease progression includes variable symptoms. Some may remain indolent or may occur in a progressive manner, with steady accumulation of neurologic deficits in the absence of clearly defined exacerbations. Typically, acute exacerbations are followed by partial or complete resolution. New neurologic deficits develop over the course of several hours or days, remain stable for a period of a few days to a few weeks, and then gradually improve.

With repeated exacerbations, permanent neurologic deficits tend to develop. Patients usually have symptom-free intervals of months or years between attacks. Patients who initially have relapsing-remitting disease (two or more episodes lasting ≥24 hours separated by ≥1 month) and who then enter a progressive phase are said to have *secondary progressive disease* (initial exacerbations and remissions followed by slow progression over at least 6 months), whereas those whose symptoms are progressive from onset are said to have *primary progressive disease* (slow or stepwise progression over at least 6 months). About 15% of patients have primary progressive disease; of those who initially have relapsing-remitting disease, 30% to 50% will experience progressive symptoms during the first 10 years.

■ OPTIC NEURITIS

Optic neuritis may present by itself or may be the presenting symptom of multiple sclerosis. The relation of optic neuritis to multiple sclerosis is controversial. Some regard optic neuritis as a distinct entity, but others consider it part of the clinical continuum of multiple sclerosis. More than half of all patients with multiple sclerosis have optic neuritis at some time during the disease. Patients with completely normal results on magnetic resonance imaging (MRI) and comprehensive cerebrospinal fluid (CSF) evaluation seldom progress to multiple sclerosis. Optic neurits usually presents with unilateral vision loss and retrobulbar pain with eye movement.

■ TRANSVERSE MYELITIS

Like optic neuritis, transverse myelitis may present by itself or be part of the symptomatology of multiple sclerosis. It usually presents with paraparesis, which is initially flaccid and then spastic; loss of sensation with a sensory level on the trunk; and bowel and bladder dysfunction. Back pain precedes the neurologic symptoms, and the sensory symptoms may begin distally and ascend. The thoracic cord is most often affected.

■ GUILLAIN-BARRÉ SYNDROME

Patients with Guillain-Barré syndrome present with weakness, paresthesias, and decreased or absent deep tendon reflexes. The distribution typically includes distal involvement with symmetric paresthesias (pins and needles). It spreads proximally, with weakness presenting a few days later; weakness also progresses to involve the upper extremities. Weakness is most prominent in the lower extremities and tends to involve the proximal muscles. It usually first presents as difficulty rising from a chair. The disease progresses from a few days to 3 to 4 weeks (*progressive phase*), followed by a *plateau phase* (days to weeks), and then by a *recovery phase* lasting from weeks to months. Weakness is varied but can be profound and involve the face and respiratory muscles. A loss or decrease in deep tendon reflexes is frequently the initial finding and should be tested if Guillain-Barré syndrome is suspected. Variants include the acute axonal form, which has a poor prognosis, and the Miller-Fisher syndrome, which presents with ataxia, ophthalmoplegia, and areflexia.

Differential Diagnosis

The differential diagnosis of demyelinating diseases includes conditions that cause progressive weakness. Over time, the diagnosis of a demyelinating disorder becomes clear, because few disorders relapse and remit over time. The role of the EP is to exclude other diseases that need immediate treatment.

■ MULTIPLE SCLEROSIS

Clinical factors that suggest an alternative diagnosis of multiple sclerosis (Table 93-1) include a normal neurologic examination findings, aphasia, pain predominance, abrupt hemiparesis, quick (seconds or minutes) symptom resolution, and ages less than 10 or over 50 years of age.

The diagnosis is usually made by clinical signs and symptoms; MRI and other laboratory tests play a supporting role. The diagnosis requires evidence of the dissemination of lesions in time and space and the careful exclusion of other causes. The patient should have had more than one episode of neurologic dysfunction and should have evidence of white matter lesions in more than one part of the central nervous system.

The diagnosis cannot be confirmed clinically in the ED, because two distinct episodes are required. However, the EP should consider the diagnosis in a young adult with a history of two or more clinically distinct episodes of central nervous system dysfunction or the presence of highly suggestive lesions (optic neuritis or intranuclear ophthalmoplegia).

Table 93-1 DIFFERENTIAL DIAGNOSIS FOR MULTIPLE SCLEROSIS (MS)

Disease/System	Important Factors
Seizures, syncope, or dementia	Present diffusely/globally; MS is usually focal; consider Todd's paralysis in seizure patients
Systemic lupus erythematosus (SLE)	Neurologic findings normally occur in patient with known diagnosis of SLE
Sarcoid	CNS and pulmonary involvement normally occurs in known disease
Lyme disease	Can mimic MS; look for tick exposure, travel history, and Lyme disease titers
CNS infection	Intracranial abscess, meningitis/encephalitis, or epidural abscess can produce focal findings
Bleeding (CNS)	Subdural, subarachnoid, intraparenchymal, or epidural hemorrhage can produce focal findings
Neoplasm	Usually progressive course with more insidious onset
Vascular	Thrombosis, embolism, or vasculitic conditions usually do not have resolution of symptoms
Metabolic	Vitamin B_{12} deficiency, hypoglycemia, hyperglycemia (hyperosmolar)
Neurologic	Migraine headache, postictal state, Bell's palsy
Psychiatric	Diagnosis of exclusion; includes conversion reaction

CNS, central nervous system.

Several sets of established diagnostic criteria for multiple sclerosis are available. The clinically definite category requires the presence of two clinical episodes and two clinically determined central nervous system lesions; less certain cases are classified as probable or possible. All categories require the exclusion of other diagnoses.

Revised criteria that better incorporate MRI into the diagnostic algorithm and that can be used for all disease phenotypes are under review by an international panel of experts and should soon be available. A relatively newer classification of "definite" multiple sclerosis incorporates laboratory testing. This criteria requires the presence of oligoclonal bands or increased synthesis of immunoglobulin G in the CSF along with two attacks or lesions. Although it is possible for a neurologist to diagnosis multiple sclerosis during an initial attack, provided that two clinical lesions are present and with corroborating laboratory testing, it is prudent for the EP to use a more conservative approach that requires two distinct attacks. Table 93-2 lists characteristic differentiating factors of demyelinating disorders.

■ OPTIC NEURITIS

Differential diagnoses for optic neuritis include anterior ischemic optic neuropathy, which is usually painless and found in patients older than 50 years; hereditary diseases such as Leber hereditary optic neuropathy; and toxic or nutritional optic neuropathies.

■ TRANSVERSE MYELITIS

Transverse myelitis may superficially resemble Guillain-Barré syndrome, but its asymmetric involvement, definite sensory level, complete lack of upper extremity involvement, urinary incontinence symptoms, and CSF pleocytosis make the diagnosis of Guillain-Barré syndrome less likely. The differential diagnosis includes other causes of acute myelopathy such as compression of the cord by an extradural structural lesion, spinal cord neoplasms, ischemia, and systemic lupus erythematosus.

■ GUILLAIN-BARRÉ SYNDROME

Heavy metal poisoning can mimic Guillain-Barré syndrome, but it is usually preceded by a gastrointestinal phase with vomiting and diarrhea. As discussed previously, transverse myelitis can superficially resemble this syndrome.

Diagnostic Testing

Routine laboratory tests are usually normal in myelinating disorders, including multiple sclerosis, transverse myelitis, and Guillain-Barré syndrome. Because respiratory muscles are frequently affected in Guillain-Barré syndrome, FVC is essential to determine disposition.

Most cases of optic neuritis are diagnosed clinically. In questionable cases of optic neuritis, serum testing (erythrocyte sedimentation rate, angiotensin-converting enzyme, rapid plasma reagin, thyroid function testing, and antinuclear antibody studies) can be ordered to exclude other causes of optic neuropathy.

■ CEREBROSPINAL FLUID ANALYSIS

■ Multiple Sclerosis

CSF analysis (with electrophoresis) frequently demonstrates albuminocytologic dissociation with increased protein (usually less than 100 mg/dL) and a normal cell count. However, 10% of patients will have a normal CSF protein level.

A mild mononuclear cell pleocytosis can be found during acute relapses, but total cell counts greater

Table 93-2 DIFFERENTIATING BETWEEN THE DEMYELINATING DISORDERS

	Multiple Sclerosis	Optic Neuritis	Transverse Myelitis	Guillain-Barré Syndrome
Diagnostic Findings				
Epidemiology	2:1 female to male ratio; usually northern European descent; peaks at 30 years of age	Patients usually 15 to 45 years of age; usually idiopathic	Peak incidence between 10 and 19 years and 30 to 39 years of age	Annual incidence 1 to 2/100,000; equal male:female incidence
Onset	Abrupt (minutes to hours); lasts 6-8 weeks	Visual loss over days (rarely over hours)	Hours to weeks; 45% within 24 hours	3 days to 3 weeks; usually 1-3 weeks after respiratory infection
Duration	6-8 weeks	4-12 weeks	1-3 months	Weeks to months
Symptoms	Motor weakness; paresthesias; ocular symptoms common (optic neuritis, intranuclear ophthalmoplegia)	Unilateral vision loss and retrobulbar pain with eye movement; loss of light, color, and depth perception more pronounced; bilateral vision loss possible; more common in children	Flaccid,then spastic paresis; loss of sensation and motor function at a specific cord level; bowel and bladder dysfunction common	Rapidly ascending, symmetric paralysis with paresthesias and decreased deep tendon reflexes; autonomic dysfunction common
Diagnosis/testing	MRI (white matter lesions); lumbar puncture (oligoclonal bands); diagnosis largely clinical	MRI with gadolinium may show enhancement of optic nerves; visual field testing; diagnosis largely clinical	MRI (intramedullary lesion at level of symptoms); hyperintense on T_2-weighted imaging; CSF may show elevated protein and leukocytes	CSF analysis (albuminocytologic dissociation); MRI with gadolinium enhancement may show abnormal enhancement of nerve roots in region of conus medullaris and cauda equina; electrodiagnostic testing shows abnormal motor and sensory conduction
Treatment	High-dose, pulsed steroid therapy for exacerbations; interferon and glatiramer acetate for relapse prevention; treat fevers aggressively	IV methylprednisolone (1 g/day for 3 days), followed by oral taper for 11 days	Largely supportive; test FVC to determine respiratory function (intubate if FVC <20 mL/kg) for high-cord lesions; steroids may be helpful to reduce inflammation, and plasmapheresis can be attempted for refractory cases	Largely supportive; test FVC to determine disposition (intubate if FVC<15 mL/kg; admit to ICU if FVC<20 mL/kg); plasmapheresis or intravenous immunoglobulin
Disposition	Acute exacerbations require IV therapy and admission; oral, high-dose outpatient steroid therapy possible	Admit for IV methylprednisolone therapy if known flare; outpatient therapy possible if unilateral vision loss and good follow-up arranged	Admit for respiratory function testing and observation; early mobility therapy for paralyzed limbs can help reduce the risk of muscle atrophy and pressure sores	Admit for respiratory function testing and observation

CSF, cerebrospinal fluid; FVC, forced vital capacity; ICU, intensive care unit; IV, intravenous; MRI, magnetic resonance imaging.

than 50 cells/ mm^3 are uncommon. During acute attacks, especially those involving the spinal cord and brainstem, the CSF may contain measurable amounts of myelin basic protein. Oligoclonal bands or abnormal immunoglobulin synthesis is found in about 90% of patients with clinically definite multiple sclerosis. Although not specific to multiple sclerosis, these findings support the diagnosis of multiple sclerosis in equivocal cases.

■ Transverse Myelitis

CSF studies may demonstrate elevated protein levels and leukocytes.

Optic Neuritis

CSF studies are not usually required for optic neuritis, but are usually obtained to help with diagnosis of multiple sclerosis.

MEASURING NERVE CONDUCTION

Electrodiagnostic testing may demonstrate conduction blocks, differential slowing, or focal slowing. Slowing of conduction over demyelinated segments of axons or over incompletely remyelinated pathways provides a useful marker for identifying additional subclinical lesions in sensory pathways. Conduction can be measured along visual, auditory, and somatosensory pathways by use of summated cortical evoked responses. In these tests, a time-locked recording of the electroencephalogram over the afferent cortex of interest is obtained after repeated visual, auditory, or sensory stimulation. If demyelination is significant, conduction over central pathways will be delayed.

Electrodiagnostic testing may demonstrate abnormal motor and sensory conduction, but these can take a few weeks to develop.

MAGNETIC RESONANCE IMAGING (MRI)

Multiple Sclerosis

MRI permits the exclusion of many diseases that mimic multiple sclerosis and identifies certain lesions, which are hyperintense on T_2-weighted or proton density imaging and are hypointense or isointense on T_1-weighted imaging. Typical lesions are ovoid and periventricular, with the long axis perpendicular to the ventricle, but lesions may appear anywhere in the white matter.

Although MRI is extremely sensitive in detecting white matter lesions in patients with multiple sclerosis, it is not very specific because many other diseases produce multiple white matter lesions. Useful features for increasing the predictive value of MRI for diagnosis of multiple sclerosis include the presence of three or more white matter lesions, lesions that abut the body of the lateral ventricles, infratentorial lesions, lesions greater than 5 mm in diameter, and lesions that demonstrate gadolinium enhancement.

Transverse Myelitis

MRI is extremely useful for excluding structural lesions and for confirming the presence of an intramedullary lesion at the level in the spinal cord commensurate with the symptoms of transverse myelitis. The lesions typically are hyperintense on T_2-weighted imaging; they involve the majority of the cross-sectional area of the cord over several segments and may be enhanced with contrast agents. The lesions may cause swelling of the spinal cord. MRI with gadolinium enhancement may show abnormal enhancement of the nerve roots in the region of the conus medullaris and cauda equina.[3]

Optic Neuritis

MRI is useful both for diagnosing optic neuritis and evaluating multiple sclerosis. Gadolinium enhancement may demonstrate enhancement of the optic nerve. In questionable cases, visually-evoked potentials may demonstrate prolonged latency.

Treatment

For all demyelinating conditions, the EP's goal is to reduce the current demyelinating episode while ensuring that the ABCs (airway, breathing, and circulation) are maintained. Because inflammation is a central component of demyelination, corticosteroids are frequently used; their effectiveness in Guillain-Barré syndrome and optic neuritis is questionable. Preventing and aggressively treating fevers is important because an increased core temperature can worsen the demyelination.

MULTIPLE SCLEROSIS

The treatment of multiple sclerosis can be discussed in terms of the management of acute relapses, the prevention of relapses as a modification of the disease process, and the management of symptoms and fixed neurologic deficits. High-dose pulsed corticosteroid therapy is indicated for exacerbations of acute relapses that adversely affect the patient's function. Intravenous methylprednisolone in doses of 0.5 to 1 g daily for 5 days reduces the maximal neurologic signs and hastens the resolution of associated fatigue. A controversial study by Sellebjerg and colleagues[4] supports the use of oral methylprednisolone (500 mg daily for 5 days, with a 10-day tapering period). Although corticosteroids have a short-term beneficial effect when used for acute exacerbations, their long-term effect on the course of multiple sclerosis is unknown.

In patients with relapsing-remitting multiple sclerosis, disease-modulating drugs reduce the frequency of attacks, the rate of lesion accumulation seen on MRI, and the accumulation of disability. In patients with relapsing disease of mild to moderate severity, interferon beta-1b, given subcutaneously every other day, reduced the year-on-year relapse rate by one third and severe attacks by one half. The effect was maintained for up to 5 years.[5,6] In another study, interferon beta 1-b reduced MRI contrast-enhanced lesions by 1.6%, compared with an increase of 15% in those receiving a placebo. The number of enlarging or new lesions was also significantly reduced.[7] Thirty-five percent of patients taking interferon beta-1b developed antibodies, but there is a lack of consistent effect of antibodies on clinical outcome. Additionally, these antibody levels were found to have disappeared in the majority of patients after 8 years of treatment.[8,9]

Table 93-3 SYMPTOMATIC TREATMENT FOR MULTIPLE SCLEROSIS

Symptom	Treatment Options
Fatigue	Amantadine, pemoline, methylphenidate, modafinil, or SSRI (serotonin selective reuptake inhibitor)
Weakness	Steroids, potassium channel blockers
Loss of balance, coordination, tremor, or ataxia	Clonazepam for tremor, steroids for balance
Sexual dysfunction	Sildenafil, intracavernosal prostaglandins (for erectile dysfunction)
Vertigo	Meclizine, prochlorperazine, diazepam, metoclopramide
Paroxysmal symptoms (itching, burning, twitching, Lhermitte's sign)	Carbamazepine, phenytoin, tricyclic antidepressants, low dose antipsychotics, gabapentin
Bladder urgency	Oxybutynin, tolterodine, imipramine, hyoscyamine, propantheline
Bladder dyssynergia	Phenoxybenzamine, clonidine, terazosin
Bladder retention	Intermittent catheterization, bethanechol
Spasticity (common increased tone in lower extremities)	Baclofen, diazepam, tizanidine, clonazepam, clonidine (adjunctive to baclofen), dantrolene
Paresthesias	Amitriptyline, carbamazepine, gabapentin, corticosteroids if disabling
Optic atrophy, blurred vision, central scotomata	Intravenous methylprednisolone for acute optic neuritis
Intranuclear ophthalmoplegia	Corticosteroids
Ataxia	Clonazepam, gabapentin
Paroxysmal pain	Carbamazepine, phenytoin, misoprostol (trigeminal neuralgia)
Dysesthetic pain	Amitriptyline, phenytoin, gabapentin, valproic acid, carbamazepine, baclofen

Interferon beta-1a produced similar benefits when given intramuscularly three times a week, reducing the relapse rate by 17%. Compared with weekly, low-dose interferon beta-1a, high-dose, given three-times a week, demonstrated a 32% relative reduction in steroid use to treat relapses.[10]

Glatiramer, a synthetic random compound composed of four amino acids, is found in myelin. Its exact mechanism of action is unknown, but it is believed that glatiramer acetate binds to MHC class II antigen and induces organ-specific T helper type 2 cell responses, thus converting pro-inflammatory T cells into anti-inflammatory agents.[11] Treatment with glatiramer acetate reduces the relapse rate by 30% and may delay disease progression.[12]

Specific therapies for symptomatic relief of symptoms are provided in Table 93-3.

■ Transverse Myelitis

Corticosteroids and plasma exchange may be beneficial in the treatment of transverse myelitis.[13] In a small case series, patients treated with steroids were able to walk after a median time of 23 days versus 97 days for historical controls.[14] Plasma exchange is often used for those with more severe disease (e.g., unable to walk) who fail to improve on IV steroid therapy.[15] The prognosis for transverse myelitis is variable.

■ Optic Neuritis

IV methylprednisolone (1 g/day for 3 days) followed by oral prednisone (1 mg/kg/day for 11 days with a 4-day taper) and interferon beta-1a (30 μg intramuscularly once a week) for patients at high risk for multiple sclerosis based on MRI has been shown to hasten vision recovery in patients with optic neuritis.[16] However, this therapy shows little residual benefit at 1 year. Additionally, oral prednisone therapy alone was found to actually increase the recurrence rate.[17] Regardless of therapy, most patients recover their vision within a month.

■ GUILLAIN-BARRÉ SYNDROME

Therapy is largely supportive. Most patients recover function if they survive the acute phase. The key therapeutic measure is ventilatory support. FVC should be measured in all patients in whom Guillain-Barré syndrome is suspected. Patients with an FVC of less than 20 mL/kg should be admitted to the intensive care unit because of the high risk of ventilatory insufficiency. For those with an FVC < 15 mL/kg, intubation is indicated. If intubation is necessary, avoid succinylcholine, which can cause hyperkalemia with resultant arrhythmia and hypotension. Dysautonomia can cause severe paroxysmal hypertension, orthostatic hypotension, arrhythmias. Monitor cardiovascular function carefully. Plasmapheresis and IV gammaglobulin therapy have both been shown to reduce recovery time by 50%. IV gammaglobulin is less expensive and easier to administer, but the risk of viral transmission is greater. IV steroids frequently are administered, but their actual benefit is questionable.

Disposition

All patients with a first episode of demyelination should have neurology consultation. Although outpatient therapy is possible for a subset of these patients, this decision is best left to the neurologist who will be caring for the patient.

■ MULTIPLE SCLEROSIS

As discussed previously, the typical course is a relapsing-remitting pattern. During an acute exacerbation, the patient is frequently admitted for IV steroid therapy, but oral treatment is possible.

■ GUILLAIN-BARRÉ SYNDROME

Hospital admission is required, where FVC measurement guides selection of the appropriate level of care. The majority of patients are hospitalized for a month or longer, and, with careful attention to respiratory function, mortality is now less than 5%.

■ OPTIC NEURITIS

Patients should receive ophthalmology and neurology evaluation. If steroid therapy is necessary, hospital admission is necessary, because steroids may worsen the clinical outcome.

PATIENT TEACHING TIPS

- The National Multiple Sclerosis Society (www.nmss.org), Guillain-Barré Foundation (http://www.gbsfi.com/), and Transverse Myelitis Foundation (http://www.myelitis.org/) provide excellent patient resources and offer support groups for both the family and patients.
- Patients are at risk for symptom exacerbation and disease progression from an elevated core temperature. Aggressive fever control and determination of its etiology is important. Seek medical care quickly whenever a fever develops.
- There is no cure for demyelinating disorders, but current therapies can reduce their frequency and severity. Seek medical care for any new neurologic symptoms.
- Patients with optic neuritis have a worse prognosis with oral steroid therapy. If steroids are used, they must be given intravenously.
- Patients with symptoms of progressive weakness and sensory symptoms must be rapidly assessed for Guillain-Barré syndrome. With aggressive therapy, respiratory failure can be avoided.

REFERENCES

1. Frohman EM: Multiple sclerosis. Med Clin North Am 2003;87:867-897.
2. Miller D, Barkhof F, Montalban X, et al: Clinically isolated syndromes suggestive of multiple sclerosis, part I: Natural history, pathogenesis, diagnosis, and prognosis. Lancet Neurol 2005;4:281-288.
3. Patel H, Garg BP, Edwards MK: MRI of Guillain-Barré syndrome. J Comput Assist Tomogr 1993;17:651-652.
4. Sellebjerg F, Frederiksen JL, Nielsen PM, et al: Double-blind, randomized, placebo-controlled study of oral, high-dose methylprednisolone in attacks of MS. Neurology 1998;51:529-534.
5. Interferon beta-1b in the treatment of multiple sclerosis: Final outcome of the randomized controlled trial. IFNB Multiple Sclerosis Study Group and the University of British Columbia MS/MRI Analysis Group. Neurology 1995;45:1277-1285.
6. Arnason BG: Long-term experience with interferon beta-1b (Betaferon) in multiple sclerosis. J Neurol 2005;252 (Suppl 3):iii28-iii33.
7. Miller DH, Molyneux PD, Barker GJ, et al: Effect of interferon 1-b on magnetic resonance imaging outcomes in secondary progressive multiple sclerosis: Results of a European multi-center, randomized, double-blind, placebo-controlled trial. European Study Group on Interferon-beta 1b in secondary progressive multiple sclerosis. Ann Neurol 1999;46:850-859.
8. Polman C, Kappos L, White R, et al: European Study Group in Interferon Beta-1b in Secondary Progressive MS. Neutralizing antibodies during treatment of secondary progressive MS with interferon beta-1b. Neurology 2003;60:37-43.
9. Rice GP, Paszner B, Oger J, et al: The evolution of neutralizing antibodies in multiple sclerosis patients treated with interferon beta 1-b. Neurology 1999;52:1277-1279.
10. Panitch H, Goodin D, Francis G, et al: EVIDENCE (Evidence of Interferon Dose-response: European North American Comparative Efficacy) Study Group and the University of British Columbia MS/MRI Research Group. Benefits of high-dose, high-frequency interferon beta-1a in relapsing-remitting multiple sclerosis are sustained to 16 months: Final comparative results of the EVIDENCE trial. J Neurol Sci 2005;239:67-74.
11. Arnon R and Aharoni R: Mechanism of action of glatiramer acetate in multiple sclerosis and its potential for the development of new applications. Proc Natl Acad Sci U S A 2004;101(Suppl 2):14593-14598.
12. Johnson KP, Brooks BR, Cohen JA, et al: Copolymer 1 reduces relapse rate and improves disability in relapsing-remitting multiple sclerosis: Results of a phase III multicenter, double-blind placebo-controlled trial. The Copolymer 1 Multiple Sclerosis Study Group. Neurology 1995;45:1268-1276.
13. Krishnan C, Kaplin A, Deshpande D, et al: Tranverse myelitis: Pathogenesis, diagnosis and treatment. Front Biosci 2004;9:1483-1499.
14. Kennedy PG and Weir AI: Rapid recovery of acute transverse myelitis treated with steroids. Postgrad Med J 1988;64:384-385.
15. Weinshenker BG: Plasma exchange for severe attacks of inflammatory demyelinating diseases of the central nervous system. J Clin Apheresis 2001;16:39-42.
16. Balcer LJ, Galetta SL: Treatment of acute demyelinating optic neuritis. Semin Ophthalmol 2002;17:4-10.
17. Visual function 5 years after optic neuritis: Experience of the Optic Neuritis Treatment Trial. The Optic Neuritis Study Group. Arch Ophthalmol 1997;115:1545-1552.

Chapter 94

Seizures

Asim F. Tarabar, Andrew S. Ulrich, and Gail D'Onofrio

KEY POINTS

Intravenous lorazepam is the initial treatment of choice for most seizures because it stimulates the production of gamma-aminobutyric acid (GABA), the main inhibitory neurotransmitter.

Serum glucose levels should be checked in seizure patients as promptly as possible.

Overdose of isoniazid can cause intractable seizures; the antidote is pyridoxine.

Eclamptic seizures, most common in the third trimester of pregnancy, can also occur post partum.

Morbidity and mortality are the result of inadequate cerebral perfusion and consequent insufficient oxygen and glucose supply to the brain.

ED treatment is directed at cessation of ongoing seizures and prevention of further activity.

Scope and Outline

Seizures are a common presenting complaint in the ED. According to some estimates, seizures account for 1% to 2% of ED visits.[1,2]

Epilepsy, a condition resulting in recurrent, unprovoked seizures, affects up to 4 million people in the United States, and 10% of the U.S. population will have at least one seizure during their lifetime.[3,4]

Seizures that occur as a result of pathologic, toxic, or metabolic abnormalities are referred to as *secondary* or *reactive seizures*. One of the primary goals of ED management of seizures is the identification and treatment of reversible causes of secondary seizures. For the majority of these patients, presentation will occur after resolution of seizure activity, often in the postictal phase, which is characterized by confusion and depressed mentation. Very few will have recurrent seizure activity, and even a smaller proportion will continue to have seizures after adequate initial medical treatment.

Patients with active seizures can present in the ED dramatically and unexpectedly. Rapid diagnosis and initiation of treatment is critical in order to limit or prevent end organ damage or permanent neuronal injury, which can result from prolonged uncontrolled seizure activity. Approach to the patients with a first-onset seizure may differ from that for the population who has an established diagnosis of epilepsy or seizure disorder.

Seizures are classified by the resultant clinical presentation of abnormal electrical impulses within the cerebral cortex (Box 94-1). The specific seizure activity is determined by the area in the brain that is involved. Some of these abnormal electrical discharges may remain localized; others may involve larger areas of the brain. The resultant clinical spectrum includes isolated focal motor activity as well as generalized motor and sensory abnormalities, including altered mental status and behavioral changes.

■ PRESENTATION AND EVALUATION

The most common serious condition that can be misinterpreted as a seizure is syncope.[5] Seizures are the result of inappropriate electrical activity in the brain, whereas syncope occurs primarily due to transient hypoperfusion of the brain. It is essential to appropriately identify syncope, as it carries a high risk for significant morbidity and mortality if unrecognized and misdiagnosed as seizure activity. Important clinical signs or preceding events that help differentiate these two entities are listed in Table 94-1.

In many circumstances, patients are unable to provide critical information; thus it is important to obtain an accurate description from anyone who witnessed the event (e.g., family members, co-workers, and emergency medical personnel). Aside from syncope, several other medical conditions that should be included in the differential diagnosis are listed in Box 94-2. Table 94-2 outlines diagnostic tests useful in the evaluation of patients with seizures.

If available, the medical history may reveal risk factors associated with development of seizures

BOX 94-1

Classification of Seizures

Partial Seizures
- Simple (awareness retained)
- Motor
- Somatosensory
- Autonomic
- Psychogenic
- Complex (altered awareness and behavior)

Generalized Seizures (seizures involving whole brain with the alteration of consciousness)
- Tonic-clonic seizures
- "Grand-mal"/convulsions
- Seizures with loss of consciousness (stiffening of body with the jerking movements of limbs)

Secondary Seizures
- Secondary generalized seizures (spreading from one area to the whole brain)
  - Toxin-induced
  - Substance withdrawal–induced
  - Metabolic

Absence Seizures
- "Petit-mal"
  - "Staring fit"or trance-like state
- Tonic or atonic
  - "Drop attack": abrupt fall, with either stiffening (tonic) or loss of muscle tone (atonic)
- Myoclonic
  - Sudden muscle jerks

BOX 94-2

Differential Diagnosis of Conditions with Seizure-like Symptoms

- Breath-holding spells
- Episodic dyscontrol syndrome/rage attacks
- Fugue states
- Hyperventilation
- Hypoglycemia
- Migraine narcolepsy/cataplexy
- Movement disorders
- Night terrors
- Nonepileptic seizures
- Panic attacks
- Paroxysmal vertigo
- Psychogenic seizures
- Syncope
- Transient global amnesia
- Transient ischemic attack/stroke

Table 94-1 SYMPTOMS OF SEIZURE DISORDERS VERSUS SYNCOPE

Seizures (Specific)	Nonspecific*	Syncope (Specific)
Prodromal symptoms	Incontinence	Lightheadedness
Déjà vu	Loss of consciousness	Sweating
Rising abdominal/epigastric sensation		Prolonged standing
Stereotyped tastes or smells		Chest pain
Postictal confusion		Palpitations
Tongue biting		Bradycardia
		Neck turning (carotid sinus)
		Rapid recovery of awareness
		Myoclonus
		Pallor
		Sweating

*Can occur in seizure disorders and in syncope.

Table 94-2 EVALUATION OF PATIENTS WITH SEIZURES

Diagnostic Test	Comment
CBC	May reveal anemia or infectious process
Electrolytes (including Ca/Mg)	Hypocalcemia/hypomagnesemia may be associated with seizures and should be corrected
Pregnancy test	Rule out eclamptic seizures
Serum glucose	Should be ordered immediately and corrected prior to further management
CT of the brain	Useful in first-onset seizures and in patients with new focal neurological deficit or with history of trauma or blood thinner use
Spinal tap	Recommended for patients with suspected CNS infection or HIV/AIDS population
EEG	Use only in patients intubated in the ED or in patients with persistent unconsciousness with identifiable cause (rule out non–tonic-clonic seizure)
MRI	May reveal additional CNS diagnosis

CBC, complete blood count; CNS, central nervous system; CT, computed tomography; EEG, electroencephalography; HIV/AIDS, human immunodeficiency virus/acquired immunodeficiency syndrome; MRI, magnetic resonance imaging.

BOX 94-3

Independent Risks for Development of Seizures

- Depression, suicide attempts
- Family history of epilepsy
- History of cerebrovascular accident (CVA)—particularly after cortical involvement
- History of preeclampsia/eclampsia
- History of traumatic brain injury

(Box 94-3). This can be obtained from the patient (upon normalization of mental status), family, primary care physicians, old medical records, or emergency medical service (EMS) personnel. It should be obtained simultaneously while seizures are being controlled, because certain information can redirect treatment (e.g., exposure to isoniazid [INH], head trauma, central nervous system infection).

First-onset seizures account for about 0.3% of all ED visits. Patients who present with active seizures are often easily identifiable; however, some patients may present after events that are more difficult to categorize as seizures (sudden loss of consciousness, myoclonic movements, incontinence.) In these circumstances, other conditions should be ruled out before making a diagnosis of first-onset seizure.

■ PRE-HOSPITAL AND INITIAL ED MANAGEMENT

If the patient is transported by the EMS, multiple steps of treatment protocol can be initiated and completed by EMS personnel, including administration of anticonvulsants, airway protection, measurement and correction of glucose levels, and an initial history, including drug exposure. Radio notification can improve the level of preparedness of the ED staff. Unlike many other conditions, it is essential to attempt to control seizure activity immediately upon presentation; therefore discussion of treatment should occur simultaneously with discussion of diagnostic approach.

Maintenance of adequate cerebral perfusion and consequent oxygen and glucose supply to the brain is the goal of initial treatment. Rapid control of seizures reduces cerebral metabolic needs and prevents permanent neuronal injuries.

Conceptually, multiple processes are occurring simultaneously during the initial approach to patients with seizure. Airway management, seizure control (administration of anticonvulsants), correction of hypoglycemia, IV line placement, and administration of oxygen can be addressed together with coordinated team care. If there is a question of trauma preceding or secondary to the seizure, cervical spine precautions should be initiated. Work-up of possible cervical spine trauma can be postponed and completed after seizures are treated and controlled.

Interventions and Procedures

■ AIRWAY MANAGEMENT

Most seizures will stop spontaneously or soon after initiation of appropriate treatment. One of the primary goals during the evaluation and treatment of seizures is to preserve patent airway and oxygenation, as well as to prevent aspiration in patients in the postictal phase. This can be achieved with simple maneuvers, including administration of supplemental oxygen and perhaps providing a jaw trust/chin lift, cautiously inserting an oropharyngeal airway, and repositioning the patient's head.

In spite of a very dramatic presentation, including cyanosis, very few patients who are actively seizing require endotracheal intubation. In these instances, the protocol for rapid sequence intubation (see Chapters 1 and 2) should be followed. Patients with suspected increased intracranial pressure from trauma or intracranial bleed should be pretreated with lidocaine (1.5 mg/kg) and a low dose (defasciculating dose) of a nondepolarizing paralytic agent (e.g., vecuronium, 0.01 mg/kg). Cessation of motor seizure activity as a result of chemical paralysis does not indicate cessation of neuronal seizure activity. It is essential to continue to closely monitor for seizures in the intubated patient, including, eventually, electroencephalography (EEG).

■ ELECTROENCEPHALOGRAPHY MONITORING

Patients who have unexplained altered consciousness that may be due to persistent non–tonic-clonic seizure activity, intubated patients, and patients who are paralyzed or have had induction of phenobarbital coma and general anesthesia should be continuously monitored with EEG to exclude seizure activity, because they may not manifest seizure activity due to neuromuscular paralysis.

■ SERUM GLUCOSE TESTING

Patients with possible seizure activity should have a rapid bedside/field finger-stick test performed to evaluate serum glucose levels. One ampule of 50% dextrose should be administered intravenously to the hypoglycemic patient; the dose should be repeated if the patient remains hypoglycemic. As a temporizing measure, glucagon, 1 mg intramuscularly or subcutaneously, should be given to hypoglycemic patients without IV access. However, glucagon can cause vomiting, increasing the risk for aspiration in an unresponsive or seizing patient.

■ OTHER BLOOD TESTS

Although rare, various disturbances in electrolytes may precipitate seizures, including hyponatremia, uremia, and hypocalcemia. It is recommended that serum electrolytes be assayed in patients with new-onset seizures. Between 2.4% and 8% of patients who present with seizures have electrolyte abnormalities. In spite of the fact that the majority of these abnormalities are clinically insignificant, they should be identified and often can be easily corrected in the ED.

If drug overdose is suspected, both blood and urine toxicological screens should be obtained.

Measurement of serum prolactin levels has no clinical utility in the ED because the results cannot be obtained in a timely manner. However, it may be useful for the consulting service that will conduct further work-up to help differentiate between epileptic (generalized tonic-clonic or complex partial) and psychogenic nonepileptic seizures. Prolactin levels should be measured within 10 to 20 minutes after a suspected seizure. Levels of at least twice baseline are considered abnormal (positive). The prudent clinician may decide to order this test, especially if the patient presents with symptoms suggesting nonepileptic or psychogenic seizures.[6]

Diagnostic Testing

■ ELECTROENCEPHALOGRAPHY

EEG records brain electrical activity and is used for definitive diagnosis of epilepsy and related conditions. The need for EEG in the emergent setting is limited, usually for those patients where seizure activity is uncontrollable despite aggressive treatment, or those patients where seizure activity is more difficulty to diagnose.

■ ELECTROCARDIOGRAPHY

An electrocardiogram (ECG) should be obtained in every patient with the first onset of seizures, or with the suspicion of cardiac cause of decreased CNS perfusion. In addition to ischemia, the most important disorders that have to be excluded are related to conduction abnormalities and consequent dysrhythmias (Box 94-4).

Electrocardiography evaluates widening of the QRS complex due to sodium channel blockade after overdose of certain drugs, particularly cyclic antidepressants. More specific ECG changes, such as a terminal 40-millisecond R wave in the AVR lead, can assist in identifying cyclic antidepressant toxicity. A prolonged QTc interval can be found in citalopram (a selective serotonin reuptake inhibitor with proconvulsive properties) overdose. Tachyarrhythmias are often seen in the setting of cocaine and methylxanthine (theophylline, caffeine) toxicity

■ COMPUTED TOMOGRAPHY OF THE BRAIN

Computed tomography (CT) scans of the brain should be obtained in all patients with first-onset seizures or with persistent change of mental status, focal neurologic deficit, or suspicion of organic intracerebral lesion (Box 94-5). Early CT scanning is essential for

BOX 94-4

Conduction Disorders That Should Be Considered a Cause of Seizure-like Activity

- Brugada syndrome: right bundle branch block with ST segment elevation in leads V1-V3
- Short QTc interval
- Long QTc interval
- Wolff-Parkinson-White syndrome
- Torsades de pointes
- Widening of QRS complex
  - Sodium channel blockade with cyclic antidepressants, lidocaine, anticholinergics

BOX 94-5

Indications for Computed Tomography Scanning of the Brain

- Advanced age
- Human immunodeficiency virus/acquired immunodeficiency syndrome (HIV/AIDS)
- Suspicion of parasitic central nervous system infection (neurocysticercosis)
- Persistent change in mental status
- New focal neurological deficit
- History/clinical evidence of trauma

identifying surgically correctable causes. The clinician must ensure that the patient is hemodynamically stable, the airway is protected, and seizure activity has been controlled, prior to transferring the patient to the CT facility. If there is a concern that trauma occurred, CT scanning can be used to rule out cervical spine and intracerebral injury.

■ MAGNETIC RESONANCE IMAGING OF THE BRAIN

In comparison to CT, magnetic resonance imaging (MRI) is more sensitive and can be effective in diagnosing additional lesions, namely, temporal sclerosis, cortical dysplasia, vascular malformations (e.g. AV aneurisms), and some tumors. Its use will depend on availability and time constraints, but it is not typically done on an emergent basis. The majority of patients will be able to complete MRI on the outpatient basis. Also, patients who are intubated or have metal devices implanted may not be candidates for urgent MRI.

Treatment

■ ANTICONVULSANT THERAPY

Tables 94-3 and 94-4 list medications commonly used for the treatment of acute and chronic seizures.

■ Benzodiazepines

Benzodiazepines should be administered immediately because they have been shown to control the majority of seizures regardless of cause, through

Table 94-3 MEDICATIONS USED FOR THE TREATMENT OF SEIZURES

Medication	Dose (Load)	Dose (Maintenance)	Comments
Diazepam	10 mg over 2 min IV	Repeat q 5-10 min	Can cause respiratory depression, hypotension
Lorazepam	2-4 mg IV @ 2 mg/min	Repeat once in 10-15 min if seizure persists	Can cause respiratory depression, hypotension
Midazolam	0.1-0.2 mg/kg or 2.25-15 mg IV	0.001 mg/kg/min	Can cause respiratory depression, hypotension
Phenytoin	18-20 mg/kg @ max rate of 50 mg/min IV	100 mg IV/PO q 6-8 h	Can cause hypotension, ataxia
Fosphenytoin	15-20 mg/kg PE @ max rate of 150 mg/min		Faster loading time; needs to be metabolized to be effective; use PE for dosing
Pentobarbital	5-20 mg/kg IV @ 25 mg/min; 5 mg/kg is usually effective for induction anesthesia	1-3 mg/kg/h	Severe respiratory depression; faster effect than phenobarbital
Phenobarbital	10-30 mg/kg IV @ max rates of 60 mg/min or 2 mg/kg/min	120-240 mg q 20 min	Can cause severe respiratory depression, hypotension
Propofol	1-2 mg/kg IV over 5 min	2-4 mg/kg/h up to 15 mg/kg/h	Can cause severe respiratory depression, acidosis (in children)
Valproic acid	20 mg/kg at 20 mg/min IV	Repeat if needed	Use only as last resort; may be beneficial for patients who are already taking valproic acid in subtherapeutic dosages
Isoflurane	Doses at 1.5 times MAC (approximately 1.8%) produce seizure suppression		Can cause severe respiratory depression
Magnesium sulfate (eclampsia)	4-6 g over 15 min	2 g/h	Can cause respiratory depression with rapid administration; monitor deep tendon reflexes

MAC, minimun alveolar concentration; PE, phenytoin equivalents.

Table 94-4 ADJUVANT MEDICATIONS USED FOR THE TREATMENT OF ACUTE SEIZURES

Medication	Indication	Dose	Comment
Calcium gluconate; calcium chloride	Hypocalcemia	10 mL of 10% calcium gluconate in 50-100 mL of D_5W over 5-10 min; repeat as needed	Watch for hypercalcemia; calcium chloride has three times more calcium than calcium and is more caustic (requires administration through central line)
Magnesium sulfate	Hypomagnesemia	2-4 g of 50% magnesium sulfate diluted in saline or dextrose given IV over 30-60 min; use IV push if severe symptoms	Watch for respiratory arrest and hyporeflexia
3% NaCl (normal saline solution)	Hyponatremia with persistent seizures and neurologic findings	300-500 mL of 3% NaCl over 1-2 h until resolution of seizures	Calculate total sodium deficit; avoid too rapid correction
Baclofen	Baclofen withdrawal symptoms	Same dose that patient was already receiving (PO or IV); consult toxicologist prior to administration	May require restoration of intrathecal pump
Pyridoxine	Persistent status epilepticus; isoniazid overdose	5 g empirically	Requires 50 ampoules of 100 mg of vitamin B_6

D_5W, dextrose 5% in water.

increase of GABA, an inhibitory neurotransmitter. Studies have shown that lorazepam (Ativan) (0.05 to 0.1 mg/kg up to a maximum total dose of 4 mg) was more effective than diazepam (Valium) (0.2 mg/kg up to 20 mg) for the initial control of seizures, although both agents were effective.[2,4] If IV access is difficult, intramuscular (IM) or rectal administration of the rectal form of diazepam (Diastat) (0.2 mg/kg up to 20 mg) or lorazepam (0.1 to 0.2 mg/kg IM) is an alternative. Continued seizure activity should be treated with a second dose of benzodiazepines, along with the addition of a second agent (e.g., barbiturates, propofol, pyridoxine/vitamin B_6), and attention to disorders inciting the seizure (e.g., increased intracranial pressure, central nervous system infection, eclampsia, drug overdose).

■ Phenytoin and Related Drugs

Phenytoin (Dilantin) is the second drug of choice but requires patient monitoring when given intravenously. A loading dose of 18 to 20 mg/kg should be administered simultaneously with benzodiazepines to patients with elevated intracranial pressure (e.g., tumor, bleeding, hydrocephalus) and patients who are noncompliant with prescribed phenytoin. Early initiation of phenytoin helps achieve a therapeutic level in a timely manner because delivery is rate-limited (no faster than 50 mg/min) in order to avoid hypotension. Phenytoin has poor water solubility, which means that the drug must be formulated with propylene glycol, which is responsible for the hypotension.

Fosphenytoin (Cerebryx) is a prodrug of phenytoin. Plasma phosphatase enzymes cleave phenytoin from phosphenytoin. IV administration takes 8 to 15 minutes; IM administration takes approximately 30 minutes for therapeutic levels to be achieved. The dosage of fosphenytoin is expressed in terms of phenytoin equivalents (PE), and its loading dose should be 15 to 20 PE mg/kg at a rate of 100 to 150 PE mg/kg/min. Fosphenytoin is as cardiotoxic as phenytoin; however, it is water-soluble and has far less tissue toxicity at the infusion site. Its use should be reserved for short-term parenteral administration when other means of phenytoin administration are unavailable

If the EP suspects that seizures are drug-related (e.g., withdrawal, alcohol, sedative-hypnotics, baclofen), phenytoin should not be used because mechanistically it will not work (sodium channel blockade) and because of other disadvantages (e.g., negative inotropic and proarrhythmogenic properties). Barbiturates, propofol, or pyridoxine should be considered for drug-related seizures resistant to benzodiazepines.

Patients without intravenous access whose seizure activity has ceased prior to ED arrival may be candidates for oral loading of antiepileptic medications. For the patient with no detectable serum level of phenytoin, the manufacturer recommends 1 g of phenytoin divided into 3 doses (400 mg, 300 mg, and 300 mg) administered orally every two hours. Total administered dose should not exceed 20 mg/kg.

Important caveats to remember in regard to oral loading of dilantin is that a therapeutic level will not be achieved in a substantial proportion of patients and that this regimen should be reserved for patients in a clinic or hospital setting with capabilities for close monitoring of serum levels. Adverse reactions to phenytoin, such as ataxia, somnolence, and confusion, are decreased with a slower loading rate.

A usual outpatient dose is 100 mg three times a day, though doses of 200 mg three times a day may be required. Because the half-life of phenytoin is about 24 hours, some patients may take 300 mg once

Table 94-5 DRUGS WITH MEASURABLE SERUM ANTICONVULSANT LEVELS

Medication (Brand Name)	Daily Dosage	Therapeutic Level	Side Effects
Carbamazepine (Tegretol, Carbatrol)	200 mg bid; can titrate to maximum of 500 mg bid	8-12 mg/L	Anemia, neutropenia, ataxia, drowsiness, nausea
Phenytoin (Dilantin) Fosphenytoin (Cerebryx)	100 mg tid	10-20 mg/L	Anemia, ataxia, gingival hyperplasia
Phenobarbital	150-300 mg daily, divided bid-tid	15-40 mg/L	Respiratory depression, constipation
Valproic acid (Depakote, Depakene)	Start at 10-15 mg/kg/day (250-1250 mg/day); titrate up to 60 mg/kg/day	50-100 mg/L	Hepatotoxicity, hyperammonemia, nausea, weight gain, alopecia, tremor

a day. The therapeutic serum level is 10 to 20 mg/L. Even at this level, some patients will experience mild sedation and cognitive effects (described by some patients as "not feeling as sharp.") With long-term use, thickening of the gums and skin may occur, which may not be reversible. Because phenytoin can cause folate deficiency, leading to anemia and bone problems, daily multivitamins are recommended. One in ten thousand patients experience Stevens-Johnson syndrome.

Patients who are receiving chronic anticonvulsant treatment with carbamazepine, phenobarbital, and/or valproic acid (drugs with real-time measurable serum levels) should receive an additional oral dose prior to discharge if serum levels are subtherapeuti (Table 94-5).

Barbiturates

Because barbiturates are potent respiratory depressants (much more significantly than benzodiazepines), the clinician should be concerned about the potential need for endotracheal intubation. Traditionally, phenobarbital (10-30 mg/kg intravenously, maximum 60 mg/min or 2 mg/kg/min) is the drug of choice, but because of rate-limited administration, pentobarbital (Nembutal, a short-acting barbiturate) (5 mg/kg intravenously at 25 mg/min then 1-3 mg/kg/hr continuous infusion) can be used for the initial control of benzodiazepine-resistant seizures.

Newer Anticonvulsant Agents

In addition to classic/traditional anticonvulsants (e.g., phenytoin, carbamazepine, phenobarbital), the EP may encounter many new anticonvulsants. The majority of new drugs do not have measurable serum levels. It is reasonable to give an additional dose of new anticonvulsants to patients who are noncompliant with treatment (Table 94-6).

TREATMENT OF CHRONIC SEIZURES

Patients with chronic seizures who present with a typical event may require only evaluation of the antiepileptic level and evaluation of triggering factors. However, recent organic pathology that may lower the seizure threshold (e.g., infection, electrolyte abnormality, trauma) should be excluded. More commonly, subtherapeutic levels of anticonvulsants will be the cause (e.g., noncompliance, change of medication, drug interaction). Any precipitating factors that may unmask a chronic seizure disorder or explain an increase in seizure recurrence in patients with therapeutic anticonvulsant levels should be identified (Box 94-6).

BOX 94-6

Factors Precipitating Seizures

- Flashing lights (strobe light–induced seizures/Pokemon seizures)
- Menstrual period (catamenial seizures)
- Recent head trauma
- Metabolic
  - Hypoglycemia/hyperglycemia
  - Hypomagnesemia
  - Hyponatremia/hypernatremia
- New medications (interfering with metabolism of anticonvulsants)
- Sleep deprivation
- Toxins/drug abuse
- Substance abuse/withdrawal (e.g., alcohol)
- Cocaine/sympathomimetics
- Medication noncompliance
- Lack of insurance (unable to refill medications)
- Change of dose/generic vs. brand medications

TREATMENT OF DRUG- AND TOXIN-INDUCED SEIZURES

GABA is the chief inhibitory transmitter in the brain. Every drug that can decrease GABA activity in the central nervous system can cause seizures. Unlike seizures in which there is a focus in the brain (e.g., scar, tumor, bleeding) that initiates excessive distri-

Table 94-6 NEWER ANTICONVULSANT MEDICATIONS

Medication (Brand Name)	Typical Dosage	Indications	Side Effects
Gabapentin (Neurontin)	300-1800 mg/day tid	Adjunctive therapy for partial seizures	Fatigue, dizziness, imbalance
Lamotrigine (Lamictal)	300-500 mg/day bid	Adjunctive therapy for partial seizures	Headache, nausea, dizziness; potentially life-threatening skin rash (when given with valproate)
Levetiracetam (Keppra)	500-3000 mg/day bid	Adjunctive therapy for partial seizures	Fatigue, imbalance, behavioral changes
Oxcarbazepine (Trileptal)	600-1200 mg/day bid	Monotherapy or Adjunctive therapy for partial seizures	Abdominal pain, nausea/vomiting, dizziness, diplopia, drowsiness, fatigue, loss of coordination
Pregabalin (Lyrica)	150-600 mg/day bid	Adjunctive therapy for partial seizures	Blurred vision, difficulty concentrating, dizziness, dry mouth, peripheral edema, somnolence
Primidone (Mysoline) (contains phenobarbital with therapeutic level of 5-12 μg/mL)	250 mg tid-qid	Therapy for grand mal and partial seizures	Blurred vision, fatigue, incoordination, nausea/vomiting, erectile dysfunction, vertigo, weight loss
Tiagabine hydrochloride (Gabitril)	Start at 4 mg/day bid-qid; titrate up to 56 mg/day	Adjunctive therapy for partial seizures	Dizziness, somnolence
Topiramate (Topamax)	50-400 mg/day bid	Therapy for partial and generalized tonic-clonic seizures	Drowsiness, nausea, dizziness, and coordination problems; caveat: acute glaucoma
Zonisamide	100-600 mg qid	Adjunctive therapy for partial seizures	Dizziness, imbalance, fatigue; cross-allergy with sulfonamides

Table 94-7 DRUGS COMMONLY ASSOCIATED WITH SEIZURES

Drug	Comments
Camphor	Causes brief, tonic-clonic seizures; usually self-limited
Cocaine Amphetamines	Presentation includes increased heart rate and blood pressure, high fever, agitation, and history of substance abuse; treat with benzodiazepines and aggressive cooling
Phencyclidine	Presentation includes rotary nystagmus, hallucinations; treat with benzodiazepines and place patient in a quiet room
Cyclic antidepressants	Severe toxicity can cause cardiac dysrhythmias; treatment with bicarbonate will control changes shown on electrocardiogram, but not the seizures; benzodiazepines are drug of choice
Isoniazid (INH)	Treatment is vitamin B_6
Lindane	Topical preparation usually ingested
MDMA (Ecstasy)	Patient typically presents the morning after a "rave" party; usually associated with hyponatremia; fluid restriction is usually sufficient treatment
Strychnine	Usually from ingestion of rat poison; not true seizures; presentation includes agitation, apprehension, painful muscle spasms
Theophylline	Wide pulse pressure; tachycardia, hypokalemia, hyperglycemia

bution of the impulses, in drug-related seizures every cell is excited due to overstimulation (glutamate) or lack of inhibition (GABA withdrawal). Treatment generally is directed at providing GABA stimulus with benzodiazepines. However, certain drugs are associated with particular types of toxicities and may require a specific treatment/antidote (Tables 94-7 and 94-8).

Removal of the toxin or drug and secondary decontamination is the hallmark of treatment for drug/toxin-induced seizures. Decontamination in the ED typically involves administration of charcoal; however, the clinician should be very cautious when treating patients who are postictal or who may develop recurrent seizures, because airway protection is a higher priority.

Drugs of Abuse

Cocaine

The most commonly abused substance that causes seizures is cocaine. Benzodiazepines can help control seizures, agitation, and hyperthermia. In the case of

Table 94-8 CLASSES OF DRUGS/TOXINS ASSOCIATED WITH SEIZURES

Class	Representative Agent(s)
Anesthetics	General: enflurane Local: lidocaine, bupivacaine
Analgesics	Tramadol Propoxyphene Meperidine
Antiasthmatics	Terbutaline Theophylline
Antibacterials	Erythromycin Fluoroquinolones
Anticholinergics	Scopolamine
Anticholinesterases	Physostigmine
Antidepressants	Cyclic antidepressants Citalopram Wellbutrin
Antimalarials	Quinine
Antifungals	Amphotericin B
Antihistamines	Diphenhydramine
Antihelmintics	Albendazole
Antipsychotics	Haloperidol
Antivirals	Amantadine
Contrast agents	Iohexol
Hypoglycemics	Chlorpropamide
Immunosuppressives	Azathioprine
Miscellaneous	Baclofen Flumazenil Nicotine
NSAIDs	Mefenamic acid
Sympathomimetics	Amphetamines Ephedrine
Vaccines	DTP

DTP, diphtheria and tetanus toxoids and pertussis; NSAIDs, nonsteroidal anti-inflammatory drugs.

prolonged, poorly controlled seizures, focal neurologic findings, or persistent change of mental status, CT of the brain should be used to exclude intracerebral bleeding. In is important to maintain adequate fluid resuscitation to protect against renal damage from potential rhabdomyolysis. If the patient is hyperthermic, cooling measures including IV fluids and ice packs, and even ice baths in the case of refractory hyperthermia, should be applied to avoid irreversible enzymatic changes and consequent multiorgan failure and death.

Alcohol

Alcohol-related seizures (ARS) are defined as adult-onset seizures, generally occuring after the age of 25 in the setting of chronic alcohol dependence. ARS typically are brief, generalized tonic-clonic seizures that occur 6 to 8 hours after the last drink. Often they are caused by alcohol withdrawal, but concurrent risk factors such as preexisting epilepsy, structural brain lesions, use of illicit drugs, and metabolic disorders may contribute to seizures in patients who drink heavily. Sixty percent of patients have multiple seizures without treatment, and the interval between the first and the last seizure is typically less than 6 hours.

Lorazepam (Ativan) (2-4 mg intravenously, 2 mg/min, administered immediately on presentation) has been shown to prevent subsequent seizures. In a randomized controlled trial of patients presenting with ARS, only 3% had a subsequent seizure during a 6-hour observation period, compared with 24% in the placebo group.

The diagnosis of ARS is made only after exclusion of other potential causes. New-onset seizures in an alcohol-dependent patient should prompt a thorough evaluation similar to that described for any patient presenting with a new-onset seizure. CT scan of the brain should be performed in all patients with a new-onset seizure, partial seizure, status epilepticus, or prolonged postictal state or if there is evidence of head trauma. A finger-stick test for serum glucose determination is important.

All patients should be offered referral to a specialized alcohol treatment facility, where they can be treated with longer-acting benzodiazepines. If patients refuse referral, they should be kept under observation for a minimum of 3 hours.

Opioids

Opioids generally are not associated with seizures, but there are several exceptions, including meperidine (Demerol), propoxyphene (Darvon), and tramadol (Ultram). Patients taking these drugs may present with an opioid toxidrome and seizure activity. It is interesting that administration of naloxone can actually precipitate and worsen meperidine-associated seizures.

MDMA (Ecstasy)

MDMA (3,4-methylenedioxymethamphetamine) is an amphetamine-related drug associated with seizure activity. Typically, patients who are consuming MDMA during "rave parties" present with brief tonic-clonic seizures due to hyponatremia. MDMA can cause a transient syndrome of inappropriate antidiuretic hormone secretion (SIADH) in addition to dilutional hyponatremia secondary to excessive free water consumption. Most of the these patients can be treated with fluid restriction and observation.

SPECIAL PRESENTATIONS AND POPULATIONS

Status Epilepticus

Status epilepticus is defined as continuous seizure activity in excess of 30 minutes, or consequent seizure activity without return to consciousness. Diagnostic assessment of the patient with status epilepticus should be performed in parallel with treatment;

usually the diagnosis can be made based on the clinical presentation.

Early, aggressive administration of intravenous anticonvulsants is the keystone of successful treatment of status epilepticus. Benzodiazepines and barbiturates will control seizure activity through increased activity of GABA. Patients with seizures of longer duration experience worsening outcomes, as well as theoretical time-dependent loss of synaptic GABA receptors, resulting in loss of responsiveness to gabanergic medications.

The treatment of status epilepticus should include simultaneous administration of additional anticonvulsants without waiting to assess the effects of initial therapy. To avoid delays, it is useful to have a treatment protocol in place that can be activated on patient presentation or after EMS dispatch.

General anesthesia is reserved for patients in status epilepticus who are unresponsive to all other therapeutic measures. For patients who fail to respond to anticonvulsant therapy, especially if isoniazid exposure is suspected (positive chest radiograph result, history of positive purified protein derivative (PPD), family history of tuberculosis), 5 g at 0.5 g/min of vitamin B_6 should be administered intravenously.

■ Pregnancy

Pregnancy per se can precipitate seizure episodes in patients with underlying seizure disorders. Women with epilepsy can experience seizures during and after abortion. During cervical dilation, women may experience "cervical shock," a type of vasovagal syncope resulting in bradycardia, relative central nervous system hypoperfusion, and occasionally tonic-clonic seizures, but it is much shorter in duration and lacks any postictal phase.

■ *Eclampsia*

The incidence of eclampsia in the Western world ranges from 1 in 2000 to 1 in 3000. The incidence of seizures in women with preeclampsia is 1 out of 300. Eclamptic seizures can occur from the 20th week of gestation up to 7 to 26 days after delivery. During this period every new-onset seizure should be initially treated as eclamptic until proved otherwise. The clinician should be aware that up to 30% of eclamptic patients do not necessarily present with the classic symptoms of hypertension, proteinuria, and edema. Recent data show an increase in the proportion of women in whom eclampsia develops beyond 48 hours after delivery.

Other than early detection of preeclampsia, there are no reliable tests for predicting the development of eclampsia. All female patients of childbearing age who present following seizure activity should be tested for pregnancy. Pregnant women who have hypertension, proteinuria, headache, visual disturbances, abdominal pain with nausea, and/or edema should be presumed to have eclampsia until proved otherwise. Cerebral abnormalities in eclampsia (mostly vasogenic edema) are similar to those found in hypertensive encephalopathy.

The treatment of choice is IV administration of magnesium sulfate (which prevents recurrent convulsions in eclampsia) with concomitant delivery of the fetus. A dose of 4 to 6 g of magnesium sulfate is administered intravenously over 15 minutes, followed by a maintenance infusion of 2 g of $MgSO_4$ per hour. An important caveat is to recognize that eclamptic seizures can occur post partum (in 11%-44% of cases). Magnesium is not an anticonvulsant and the mechanism of its activity is unclear.

Following drug administration, the patient's deep tendon reflexes should be monitored because hyporeflexia precedes respiratory insufficiency, a potential complication of hypermagnesemia. Adjunctive administration of hydralazine is usually indicated to manage blood pressure. Benzodiazepines and phenytoin, although not typical first-line agents for the treatment of eclamptic seizures, may have some short-term benefit.

■ Central Nervous System Pathology

Patients with underlying intracranial hemorrhage who are anticoagulated or have elevated isoniazid levels may require administration of fresh frozen plasma and vitamin K to prevent further bleeding. Patients with brain tumors, evidence of increased intracranial pressure, or hydrocephalus need the immediate attention of the neurosurgical service. Administration of steroids may be prudent to reduce mass effect of intracranial tumors.

■ *Neurocysticercosis (NCC)*

Worldwide, NCC is the most common parasitic infection of the central nervous system and has been increasing in the United States since 1980.[7] In endemic areas (Latin America, Asia, Africa) NCC is considered to be main cause of late-onset epilepsy, and seizures are reported to be the most common symptom, occurring in 70% to 90% of patients. The majority of these seizures respond to phenytoin or carbamazepine therapy.

Albendazole is the mainstay of antiparasitic treatment for the treatment of NCC (15 to 30 mg/kg/day divided in two doses bid for 8 days). Patients diagnosed with NCC may require treatment with steroids to control inflammation and treat meningitis, cysticercal encephalitis, or angiitis. Initial treatment is usually started with dexamethasone (4-12 mg/day), which can be replaced with prednisone (1 mg/kg) for long-term treatment.

Patients at high risk for meningitis/encephalitis should be treated with IV administration of ceftriaxone (2 g), vancomycin (1 g), and acyclovir (10 mg/kg), even before results of a spinal tap. In addition, patients should be placed in an isolation room with droplet precaution

Human Immunodeficiency Virus (HIV) Infection

People with HIV infection may have a central nervous system mass or infection as the cause of seizure. This can be the first manifestation of acquired immunodeficiency syndrome (AIDS). HIV-positive patients who have a seizure require CT scanning and, if results are negative, a lumbar puncture. HIV encephalopathy or meningitis must be considered (Box 94-7).

MEDICATIONS TYPICALLY ASSOCIATED WITH SEIZURES

Cyclic Antidepressants

Cyclic antidepressants are notorious for their propensity to cause seizures, due to GABA inhibition. Seizures are a manifestation of severe toxicity; therefore it is important to protect the airway, perform complete gastrointestinal decontamination (charcoal, lavage if indicated) and administer IV benzodiazepines. Bicarbonates are the a primary treatment of cyclic antidepressant overdose and are effective in treating cardiac conduction abnormalities, but they do not affect seizure activity

BOX 94-7

Causes of Seizures In HIV-Positive Patients

- Focal CNS lesions
  - Cerebral toxoplasmosis
  - Primary CNS lymphoma
  - Progressive multifocal leukoencephalopathy (PML)
- Focal viral encephalitis
  - Cytomegalovirus
  - Varicella zoster virus
  - Herpes simplex virus
- Bacterial abscess
- Cryptococcoma
- Tubercular abscess
- Mass lesion
  - Toxoplasmosis
  - Lymphoma
- Meningitis/encephalitis
  - Cryptococcal
  - Bacterial/aseptic
  - Herpes zoster
  - Cytomegalovirus
- HIV encephalopathy/AIDS dementia complex (ADC)
- Progressive multifocal leukoencephalopathy
- CNS tuberculosis
- Neurosyphilis

AIDS, acquired immunodeficiency syndrome; CNS, central nervous system; HIV, human immunodeficiency virus.

Isoniazid (INH)

The typical presentation of isoniazid-induced seizures is status epilepticus that does not respond to conventional treatment, including gabanergic drugs (e.g., benzodiazepines, barbiturates) and dilantin. Isoniazid prevents GABA synthesis. The treatment is administration of vitamin B_6 (pyridoxine), diluted to a concentration of 50 mL/g and administered intravenously over 5 to 10 minutes. If the dose of ingested isoniazid is known, antidote treatment is 1 g of vitamin B_6 for each gram of isoniazid. If the dose is not known, empiric administration of 5 g is recommended. The dose should be repeated if seizures continue or if the patient remains lethargic

Methylxanthines (Caffeine, Theophylline)

Caffeine and theophylline in overdose are notorious for causing seizures, through the antagonism of adenosine (an inhibitory neurotransmitter). Usually the seizures are short and can be controlled with benzodiazepines. However, in severely toxic patients, hemodialysis is necessary. If a markedly elevated theophylline level is identified in a seizing patient, a nephrologist should be consulted, because theophylline is a cause of intractable seizures.

Disposition

Prior to discharge, patients may inquire about their prognosis, which depends on the underlying cause of seizures and most likely is not established in the ED. In the absence of precipitating factors, secondary seizures may be avoidable in the future, but patients usually will be at some risk for recurrent seizures if depending on their underlying condition and lifestyle. Patients should avoid sleeplessness, heavy alcohol use, and other physiologic stresses that can alter the seizure threshold.

Unfortunately, without a complete neurologic work-up, it is impossible to predict recurrence of primary seizures. The natural history of untreated epilepsy is essentially unknown. Based on retrospective data, it was found that in 32% of persons with a first-onset seizure, a second attack occured in 1 month; in 51% it occured in 3 months; and in 87% it occured in 1 year. Some strong predictors for seizure recurrence include history of a previous neurologic insult, abnormal neurologic examination, and an EEG with epileptiform abnormalities and circadian timing. However, about 50% patients diagnosed with epilepsy remain seizure-free with only single drug treatment. Addition of a second and/or third drug controls recurrence in another 20%. About 30% of patients may develop intractable seizures that are poorly responsive to standard medical treatment.

DISPOSITION OF SPECIFIC CASES

- Patients with persistent seizures, change of mental status, or underlying medical condition that

BOX 94-8

Admission Criteria for Seizure Patients

- Change in mental status (e.g., drowsiness, coma)
- Neurologic deficit
- Tumor, bleeding
- Central nervous system infection
- Underlying structural condition
- Underlying treatable medical condition
- Elderly
- Unable to ambulate
- Follow-up as outpatient not possible
- Lack of social support
- Need for placement in facility with higher level of care

BOX 94-9

Discharge Criteria for Seizure Patients

- Normal neurological examination
- Syncope or cardiogenic cause of loss of consciousness ruled out
- Patient has chronic seizures
- Correction of subtherapeutic serum drug levels
- Established workable plan for follow-up with neurology service/consultant

requires hospital treatment (e.g. sepsis, overdose, trauma) should be admitted to the hospital.
- Patients with status epilepticus seizures should be transferred to the intensive care unit.
- Patients with chronic seizures can be discharged after a return to the normal baseline neurologic levels.
- Patients with subtherapeutic drug levels should receive an additional dose of antiepileptics prior to discharge.
- Patients who present with first-onset seizures should have follow-up arranged with the neurology service/consultant for further work-up and eventual treatment if warranted (Boxes 94-8 and 94-9).

■ DISCHARGE INSTRUCTIONS

Patients should be advised to avoid factors precipitating seizure (see Box 94-6), educated about the importance of adherence to anticonvulsant regimens, and given written instructions cautioning about driving motor vehicles or engaging in activities in which unexpected seizures with transient loss of consciousness can lead to injury or death (e.g., diving, rock-climbing).

Pitfalls

- Patients with status epilepticus should be treated aggressively with concurrent administration of multiple medications. The clinician should be aware that administration of phenytoin and phenobarbital is rate-dependent and that patients may continue to seize for 30 minutes before effective serum levels are reached.
- Patients with cocaine abuse with persistent seizures and a recent history of travel abroad should be evaluated for body packing and decontaminated with whole bowel irrigation.
- Not recognizing that a patient is pregnant (or post partum) may cause a serious delay in treatment and obstetrics consultation.
- Patients with seizures should be counseled not to drive and should be accompanied at all times because a recurrent seizure is possible.
- Timely administration of antibiotics and antiviral medication in patients with central nervous sytem infection can improve survival and reduce morbidity.

REFERENCES

1. ACEP Clinical Policies Committee; Clinical Policies Subcommittee on Seizures. Clinical policy: Critical issues in the evaluation and management of adult patients presenting to the emergency department with seizures. Ann Emerg Med 2004;43(5):605-625.
2. Engel J Jr, Starkman S: Overview of seizures. Emerg Med Clin North Am 1994;12:895-923.
3. Walker, MC: The epidemiology and management of status epilepticus (seizure disorders). Curr Opin Neurol 1998;11: 149-154.
4. Dunn MJ, Breen DP, Davenport RJ, Gray A: Early management of adults with an uncomplicated first generalised seizure. Emerg Med J 2005;22:237-242.
5. McKean A, Vaughan C, Delanty N: Seizure versus syncope. Lancet Neurol 2006;5:171-180.
6. Chen DK, So YT, Fisher RS: Therapeutics and Technology Assessment Subcommittee of the American Academy of Neurology. Use of serum prolactin in diagnosing epileptic seizures: Report of the Therapeutics and Technology Assessment Subcommittee of the American Academy of Neurology. Neurology 2005;65:668-675.
7. Takayanagui OM, Odashima NS: Clinical aspects of neurocysticercosis. Parasitol Int 2006;55(Suppl):S111-S115. Epub 2005 Dec 5.

Chapter **95**

Transient Ischemic Attack and Acute Ischemic Stroke

Scott Jolley and Todd L. Allen

TRANSIENT ISCHEMIC ATTACK

KEY POINTS

A new definition of transient ischemic attack (TIA) has been proposed as "a brief episode of neurologic dysfunction caused by focal brain or retina ischemia with clinical symptoms lasting less than 1 hour and without evidence of brain infarction."[1]

TIA is a sudden event that is associated with *negative* symptoms: hemiparesis, hemiparesthesia, dysarthria, aphasia, diplopia, monocular blindness, and imbalance.

TIA is a high-risk warning sign for stroke occurring within 90 days.

TIA commonly is caused by large-artery atherosclerosis, cardioembolism, or small-vessel disease (lacunae).

Patients with a true TIA rarely have symptoms lasting longer than 1 hour.

Patients with TIA can be accurately stratified as at high risk or low risk for recurrent stroke, based on validated clinical scoring systems.

Cerebral and vascular imaging using techniques such as magnetic resonance imaging and magnetic resonance angiography are valuable in differentiating TIA from acute ischemic stroke and in determining the cause of the event.

The goal of management of patients with TIA is to prevent a life-threatening or disabling cardiovascular event or stroke using antiplatelet, anticoagulation, or surgical therapy.

Scope

During the last decade, our understanding of the definition, etiology, and short-term risk of stroke after a transient ischemic attack (TIA) has become clearer. In addition, modern imaging tools for visualizing the brain and vascular system allow differentiation between TIA and stroke. The current definition of TIA as an acute neurological event lasting less than 24 hours is no longer acceptable in an era in which thrombolysis for acute ischemic stroke must occur within 3 hours of the onset of symptoms. In 2002, the TIA working group proposed a new definition of TIA as "a brief episode of neurologic dysfunction caused by focal brain or retinal ischemia, with clinical symptoms lasting less than 1 hour and without evidence of brain infarction."[1] The study concluded that based on this definition, "the distinction between TIA and stroke becomes similar to the distinction between angina and myocardial infarction."[1]

TIA is a symptom of interrupted cerebral blood flow that most commonly is caused by large-artery atherosclerosis, cardioembolism, or small-vessel (lacunae) disease. Recent studies have shown that some patients with TIA have a significant short-term risk of recurrent stroke, myocardial infarction, and death.

In 2000, a group of investigators in California developed a short-term risk stratification method applicable to TIA patients in the ED.[2] In 2005, investigators in the United Kingdom validated a simple scoring system for risk-stratifying patients with TIA.[3] Both groups found that distinct populations are at high risk for stroke in the 7 to 90 days after a TIA (Table 95-1), and that 50% of strokes following a TIA occur in the 48 hours after the TIA.[2,3]

Modern techniques such as diffusion-weighted magnetic resonance imaging (DWI) and magnetic resonance angiography (MRA) assist clinicians in making a clear distinction between TIA and acute ischemic stroke, with more precise localization of the affected area and the source of the event. Although the current literature does not clearly define who should be admitted to the hospital and who can be safely discharged to outpatient follow-up after having a TIA, EPs armed with the new definition of TIA, methods for accurate risk stratification, and modern imaging techniques, can now rapidly determine populations who are at high risk for recurrent events and determine the cause of the TIA in some cases. EPs can institute antiplatelet and/or anticoagulation therapy or schedule early disposition for surgical and endovascular procedures that can prevent acute stroke, death, and disability.

Epidemiology

The yearly incidence of TIA in the Unites States has been estimated as 120,000 to 240,000; however, a more accurate figure may be 500,000 or more because of the high frequency of underreporting these events by medical professionals.[4-6] Some authors have concluded that the annual incidence of TIA would be less and the annual incidence of stroke would be higher if the tissue-based definition were applied to all patients evaluated for TIA.[5] The incidence of TIA in the U.S. population increases with age from 0.1/1000 for patients less than 50 years of age to 11.7/1000 for patients older than 80 years.[4]

The incidence of TIA is significantly higher in blacks than whites and is significantly higher in men than women. TIA is associated with a significantly higher short-term risk (25% in the next 90 days) of recurrent TIA, stroke, and death.[4]

TIAs account for 0.3% of all ED visits. Only 28% of TIA patients arrive at the ED via ambulance, and 36% of patients arrive during daylight hours. EPs obtain CT scans on 56% to 70% of all TIA patients, and MRI scans on 7% of patients. Nearly half of all TIA patients are admitted to the hospital, although there is geographic variability in this practice; another 20% of patients are referred for follow-up. Finally, TIA patients in the ED receive preventive aspirin therapy in 18% of cases, antiplatelet therapy in 7%, and no preventive therapy in an estimated 42%.[7]

Clearly defined risk factors for stroke and adverse events following a TIA are now well described in the literature. In 2000, the California group studied 1707 ED patients who presented with TIA.[2] The study found five risk factors independently associated with stroke:

1. Age greater than 60 years
2. Diabetes
3. Duration of symptoms longer than 10 minutes
4. Weakness
5. Speech impairment

These investigators reported a 10.5% rate of stroke in the 90 days following the TIA, with 50% of these strokes occurring in the immediate 48 hours after the TIA.

In 2005, the Oxfordshire Community Stroke Project in the United Kingdom described a validated 6-point scoring system used to predict a group of TIA patients who were at high risk for stroke in the 7 days following TIA.[3] The system, called the *ABCD*, consisted of the following contributing risk factors:

- ***A***ge >60
- ***B***lood pressure greater than 140 mm Hg systolic and/or greater than 90 mm Hg diastolic
- ***C***linical features such as unilateral weakness or speech disturbance
- ***D***uration of symptoms of the TIA

Patients in the California cohort with a score of 2 or greater had a 7% 90-day risk of stroke (Tables 95-2 and 95-3); patients in the ABCD population–based cohort with a score of 5 or greater had a high-risk (16.3%) for early recurrent stroke (Tables 95-4 and 95-5).[3] These scoring systems are now used in clinical practice to determine high-risk populations that benefit from emergent investigation and therapy to prevent short-term adverse events.

Recent advances in neuroimaging have refuted the old belief that in patients with TIA, complete

Table 95-1 HIGH-RISK FACTORS FOR RECURRENT STROKE

Stroke in 7 Days	Stroke in 90 Days
Age >65 yr	Age >60 yr
High blood pressure	Speech disturbance
Motor weakness	Motor weakness
Speech disturbance	Diabetes
Duration >10 min	Duration >10 min
CHADS2 score ≥4	CHADS2 score >2

CHADS2, **c**ongestive heart failure, **h**ypertension, **a**ge, **d**iabetes, prior transient ischemic attack or **s**troke.

Table 95-2 INDEPENDENT RISK FACTORS FOR STROKE WITHIN 90 DAYS*

Risk Factor	Odds Ratio (95% CI)	*P* Value
Age >60 yr	1.8 (1.1-2.7)	.01
Diabetes mellitus	2.0 (1.4-2.9)	<.001
Duration of episode >10 min	2.3 (1.3-4.2)	.005
Weakness with episode	1.9 (1.4-2.6)	<.001
Speech impairment with episode	1.5 (1.1-2.1)	.01

*Number of patients=1707.
CI, confidence interval.
From Johnston SC, Gress DR, Browner WS, Sidney S: Short-term prognosis after emergency department diagnosis of TIA. JAMA. 2000;284:2901-2906.

Table 95-3 NUMBER OF RISK FACTORS FOR STROKE WITHIN 90 DAYS

Number of Risk Factors	NUMBER (%) Patients	NUMBER (%) Stroke Within 90 Days
0	22 (1)	0 (0)
1	179 (10)	5 (3)
2	509 (30)	35 (7)
3	584 (34)	63 (11)
4	337 (20)	51 (15)
5	76 (4)	26 (34)

From Johnston SC, Gress DR, Browner WS, Sidney S: Short-term prognosis after emergency department diagnosis of TIA. JAMA 2000;284: 2901-2906.

Table 95-4 7-DAY RISK OF STROKE STRATIFIED ACCORDING TO THE ABCD SCORE*

ABCD Score	Patients (%)	Strokes (%)	% Risk (95% CI)
1	2 (1)	0	0
2	28 (15)	0	0
3	32 (17)	0	0
4	46 (24)	1 (5)	2-2 (0-6.4)
5	49 (24)	8 (40)	16.3 (6.0-26.7)
6	31 (16)	11 (55)	35.5 (18.6-52.3)
Total	188 (100)	20 (100)	10.5 (6.2-14.9)

*Data from first assessment in the Oxford Vascular study (OXVASC) validation cohort of patients with probable or definite transient ischemic attack.
ABCD, *A*ge, *B*lood pressure, *C*linical features, and *D*uration of TIA; CI, confidence interval.
From Rothwell PM, Giles MF, Flossmann E, et al: A simple score (ABCD) to identify individuals at high early risk of stroke after transient ischaemic attack. Lancet 2005;366:29-36

Table 95-5 RISK OF STROKE AFTER TRANSIENT ISCHEMIC ATTACK

	Odds Ratio (95% CI)	*P*
Risk Factors		
Age ≥60 yr	2.5 (0.75-8.81)	.133
SBP >140 or DBP ≤ 90 mm Hg	9-67 (2-23-41.94)	.002
Diabetes	4.39 (1.36-14.22)	.014
Clinical Features		
Unilateral weakness	6.61 (1.53-28.50)	.016
Speech disturbance without weakness	2.59 (0.50-13.56)	
Other	1.0	
Duration of Symptoms		
≥60 min	6.17 (1.43-26-62)	.019
10-59 min	3.08 (0.64-14.77)	
<10 min	1.0	

CI, confidence interval; DBP, diastolic blood pressure; SBP, systolic blood pressure.
From Rothwell PM, Giles MF, Flossmann E, et al: A simple score (ABCD) to identify individuals at high early risk of stroke after transient ischaemic attack. Lancet 2005;366:29-36

symptom resolution left no permanent brain injury.[8] In addition, further studies have shown that the cerebral ischemia experienced by patients with TIA is smaller in volume and lesser in severity than that in patients with completed stroke syndromes.[9]

Pathophysiology

An ischemic injury to the central nervous system disrupts the normal cerebral blood flow to the brain (40-60 mL/100 g brain/minute). The extent of injury is based on three principles: the duration of disrupted flow, the flow rate, and collateral circulation. Loss of consciousness occurs within 10 seconds and cell death occurs within minutes of disrupted cerebral circulation.

Cerebral tissues with blood flow between 12 and 20 mL/100 g brain/minute are termed the *ischemic penumbra*. These cells are at risk for permanent injury, but have the ability to recover if flow is reestablished. When cerebral blood flow falls below 10 mL/100 g brain/minute, cell electrical activity ceases and cell death occurs secondary to cytotoxic edema from the disruption of ion-mediated channels, depriving the cells of their energy source (oxygen and glucose).

Many areas of the brain may be protected by the collateral circulation between the anterior and posterior circulation through vessels that comprise the circle of Willis.

Structure and Function

Transient ischemic events and acute ischemic strokes are separate points on a continuum of cerebral vascular disease and share a relationship similar to unstable angina and acute myocardial ischemia. A TIA is a neurologic manifestation of three basic pathophysiologic processes that include atherothromboembolism, causing low flow rates in large arteries; cardioembolism from artery to artery; and cardiac source and small vessel disease of the penetrating arteries that supply the basal ganglia, internal capsule, and pons.

It is estimated that 15% to 30% of patients will have a TIA prior to stroke, and that stroke will occur on the same day of TIA in 17% of patients, on the next day in 9% of patients, and in the first 7 days in 43% of patients.[10] Thus it is important that EPs understand the classification of causes of TIAs, as well as the short-term risk of recurrence.

Classification of a TIA is important because the pathophysiology and risk for recurrent stroke differ among the subtypes. The most commonly used stroke/TIA mechanism classification scheme was derived in the Trial of ORG 10172 in Acute Stroke (TOAST), commonly referred to as the TOAST criteria. The five mechanisms described are large-artery atherosclerosis, cardioembolism, small-vessel disease, other rare determined cause, and undetermined cause.[10,11]

Low-flow transient ischemic events that are uncompensated for by collateral blood flow are brief, recurrent, and similar in character and vascular distribution. Large-artery atherosclerosis is the most common cause of low-flow TIA. Other, less common causes include hypotension, cardiac rhythm disturbance, and arterial dissection. The most commonly affected vascular territories are the origin of the internal carotid and the intracranial portion of the internal carotid (siphon), the middle cerebral artery stem, and the junction of the vertebral and basilar arteries. Patients with large-artery atherosclerosis represent approximately 15% of all cases and have the highest recurrence rates of 4%, 12.6%, and 19.2% at 7, 30, and 90 days, respectively.[12]

Embolic transient ischemic events usually are isolated nonrecurrent events with prolonged duration. Emboli most commonly originate from thrombus in the left atrial appendage (atrial fibrillation) and left ventricle (acute myocardial infarction and dilated cardiomyopathy). Other sources of emboli include mechanical prosthetic heart valves, atrial myxoma, infective endocarditis, patent foramen ovale, and atrial septal aneurysm. Embolic events commonly are found in patients with congestive heart failure or sick sinus syndrome and the period following myocardial infarction. Emboli most commonly affect the middle cerebral artery stem and branches. Patients with embolic TIA represent 25% of cases and have a lower recurrence rate of 2.5%, 4.6%, 11.9% at 7, 30, and 90 days, respectively.

Small-vessel disease (lacunae) events are brief repetitive events that are gradual in onset and stereotyped in presentation. The pathologic basis of these events is disease affecting small penetrating vessels (usually smaller than 300 μm) in the thalamus, basal ganglia, internal capsule and brainstem. Lipohyalinosis is the most common cause of small vessel pathology, followed by atherosclerosis in the branch points of small vessels, and only rarely by small embolic events. Patients with lacunar TIA commonly have hypertension and diabetes and represent 20% of cases. These patients have a favorable prognosis with low, short-term recurrence rates of 0%, 2%, and 3.4% at 7, 30, and 90 days, respectively.

Presenting Signs and Symptoms

Patients who have had a TIA often present without physical findings but with a variety of historical clinical symptoms. Several studies have demonstrated that interobserver disagreement is high when making the diagnosis of TIA.[13,14]

A few basic principles can guide the accurate diagnosis of a TIA. The symptoms are sudden in onset and vascular in nature. True TIA is commonly brief, lasting less than 10 to 15 minutes; the diagnosis of acute stroke should be considered in patients with persistent symptoms. Symptoms are *negative* or associated with function loss. Patients with true TIA report hemiparesis, hemiparesthesia, dysarthria, aphasia, monocular vision loss, diplopia, and gait and balance disturbances. Positive symptoms such as shaking and scotomata or marching of symptoms to other body parts is more consistent with migraine or seizure.[15]

Posterior circulation (vertebrobasilar) TIA is associated with multiple symptoms including vertigo with imbalance, nausea, and vomiting. Patients may present with crossed symptoms associated with cranial nerve deficits and contralateral motor or sensory deficits.

■ OPHTHALMIC ARTERY

Transient monocular blindness, known as amaurosis fugax, is caused by transient occlusion of the ophthalmic artery. It is commonly associated with internal carotid artery stenosis and carries a better prognosis than carotid disease associated with hemispheric TIA.[16]

■ MIDDLE CEREBRAL ARTERY

Patients with middle cerebral artery TIA often complain of hemiparesis and hemiparesthesia involving the face and arm rather than the lower extremity.

These patients often have aphasia (receptive or expressive) that may be accompanied by homonymous hemianopsia. Family members may report cognitive, speech, and spatial orientation deficits.

■ ANTERIOR CEREBRAL ARTERY

The typical patient with anterior cereral artery TIA presents with a history of isolated weakness and numbness of the lower extremity. Some patients may complain of symptoms indicating small branch occlusion, such as memory loss, apathy, dysarthria, and difficulty understanding the written language.

■ VERTEBROBASILAR ARTERIES

TIA in this vascular distribution affects the brainstem, cerebellum, and occipital lobes. Typical patients present with a group of symptoms affecting cranial nerves and the three major long tracts: the spinal thalamic tract, the pyramidal tract, and the posterior column–medial lemniscal tract. Classic crossed symptoms are ipsilateral cranial nerve palsies accompanied by contralateral hemiparesis or hemiparesthesia. Vertigo, ataxia, nausea, and vomiting are commonly reported, as well as visual loss and impaired articulation of speech and swallowing.

■ SMALL-VESSEL DISEASE (LACUNAE)

Patients with lacunar TIA are commonly hypertensive and/or diabetic, and they do not have associated cortical dysfunction (speech, calculation, and spatial orientation deficits). The affected vessels are found mainly in the basal ganglia, pons, and thalamus. The classic presentations are pure motor hemiparesis, pure sensory syndrome, and dysarthria–clumsy hand syndrome.

Diagnosis

The differential diagnosis of TIA is shown in the "Priority Actions" box in the Acute Ischemic Stroke section.

Evaluation, Differential Diagnosis, and Diagnostic Testing

Evaluation of all TIA patients should include a thorough history and physical examination, cerebral imaging, laboratory studies, and electrocardiography (Box 95-1). The results of these fundamental tests combined with risk stratification can guide the EP in determining whether there has been cerebral injury, as well as the cause of the TIA (Fig. 95-1).

A set of key historical facts should be documented in patients presenting with TIAs. The acute nature of the onset, duration, and time of symptoms helps make the distinction between TIA and stroke. Patients presenting with persistent symptoms lasting longer than 1 hour should be presumed to have had an acute stroke. A determination should be made whether this was a single event or the most recent of multiple events and whether the symptoms described can be mapped to a single or multiple vascular territories. Patients should be questioned regarding their history, including risk factors for stroke and use of medications such as antiplatelet and anticoagulation agents.

The physical examination should pay particular attention to the patient's blood pressure. Often it is elevated in patients with transient or permanent ischemic events. The cardiovascular examination should be directed toward examination for the presence or absence of bruits, murmurs, and disturbance of cardiac rhythm. The neurologic examination can be performed in a standard fashion using the National Institutes of Health Stroke Scale (NIHSS) (see Differ-

BOX 95-1

Diagnostic Evaluation for TIA

- History
- Physical examination—blood pressure, cardiac/vascular/neurologic evaluation, NIHSS
- Laboratory tests—chemistry, coagulation, complete blood count, platelets, ESR
- Electrocardiogram
- Cerebral imaging
- Vascular and cardiac imaging

ESR, erythrocyte sedimentation rate; NIHSS, National Institutes of Health Stroke Scale; TIA, transient ischemic attack.

Documentation

PATIENTS WITH TIA

- Time last seen as normal
- Resolution of symptoms and NIHSS score of 0
- Single or multiple events
- History, risk factors, medications
- No evidence of injury on cerebral imaging
- Risk stratification score (California Model/ABCD scores)
- Etiology of the TIA and initiation of preventive therapy
- Specialist consultation and early (within 48 hours) follow-up for low-risk patients discharged from the ED

ABCD, *A*ge, *B*lood pressure, *C*linical features, and *D*uration of TIA; NIHSS, National Institutes of Health Stroke Scale; TIA, transient ischemic attack.

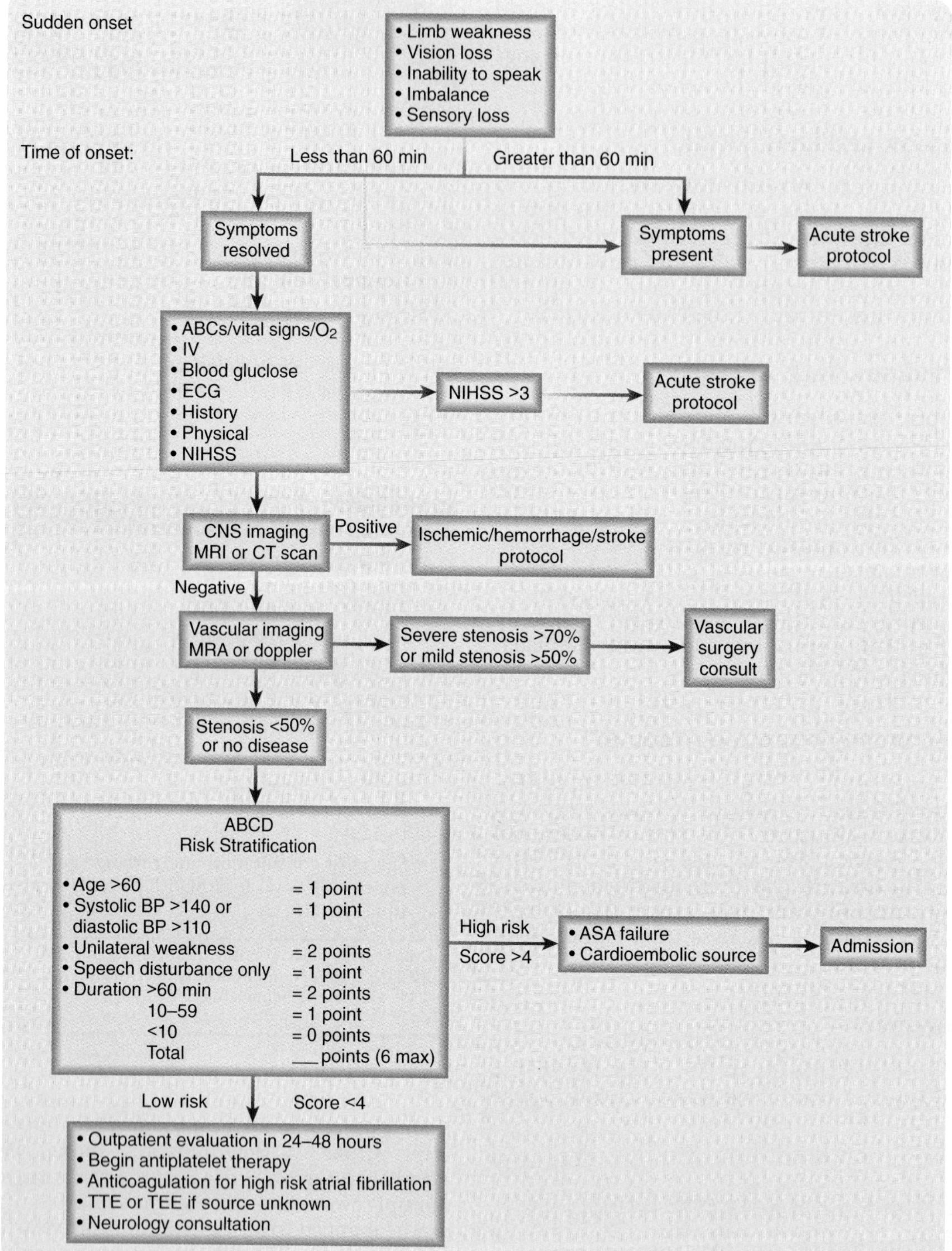
Sudden onset
• Limb weakness
• Vision loss
• Inability to speak
• Imbalance
• Sensory loss
Time of onset:
Less than 60 min
Greater than 60 min
Symptoms resolved
Symptoms present
Acute stroke protocol
• ABCs/vital signs/O2
• IV
• Blood gluclose
• ECG
• History
• Physical
• NIHSS
NIHSS >3
Acute stroke protocol
CNS imaging MRI or CT scan
Positive
Ischemic/hemorrhage/stroke protocol
Negative
Vascular imaging MRA or doppler
Severe stenosis >70% or mild stenosis >50%
Vascular surgery consult
Stenosis <50% or no disease
ABCD
Risk Stratification
• Age >60 = 1 point
• Systolic BP >140 or diastolic BP >110 = 1 point
• Unilateral weakness = 2 points
• Speech disturbance only = 1 point
• Duration >60 min = 2 points
10–59 = 1 point
<10 = 0 points
Total ___ points (6 max)
High risk
Score >4
• ASA failure
• Cardioembolic source
Admission
Low risk
Score <4
• Outpatient evaluation in 24–48 hours
• Begin antiplatelet therapy
• Anticoagulation for high risk atrial fibrillation
• TTE or TEE if source unknown
• Neurology consultation

FIGURE 95-1 Algorithm for management of suspected transient ischemic attack (TIA). ABCs, airway, breathing, and circulation; ASA, American Stroke Association; BP, blood pressure; CNS, central nervous system; CT, computed tomography; ECG, electrocardiogram; IV, intravenous; MRA, magnetic resonance angiography; NIHSS, National Institutes of Health Stroke Scale; US, ultrasonograpy.

ential Diagnosis and Diagnostic Testing in the section "Acute Ischemic Attack" later in this chapter). The NIHSS is a rapidly performed and reproducible tool that provides a universal language when speaking to consultants.

■ LABORATORY TESTS

The American Heart Association (AHA) guidelines recommend the following basic laboratory evaluation in patients presenting with TIA: complete blood

FACTS AND FORMULAS

- 15%-30% of stroke patients have a TIA prior to the stroke.
- 10% of TIA patients have a stroke in the next 90 days.
- 33% of TIA patients will have infarct shown on diffusion-weighted magnetic resonance imaging.
- 50% of TIA patients never report symptoms to a physician.
- 25% of TIA patients will die within 1 year.
- 19.2 % of patients with untreated symptomatic carotid stenosis >70% will have a stroke in the next 90 days.

count with platelets, chemistry (electrolytes, glucose, and lipid) profile, coagulation (prothrombin and international normalized ratio [INR]) studies, and erythrocyte sedimentation rate.

ELECTOCARDIOGRAPHY

An electrocardiogram (ECG) should be obtained for all TIA patients. New-onset atrial fibrillation and myocardial infarction found on the ECG are helpful in determining a cardioembolic cause of the event.

CEREBRAL AND CARDIOVASCULAR IMAGING

The AHA guidelines recommend cerebral imaging for evaluation of patients who present with a TIA, with CT scanning as a first-line choice; however, diffusion-weighted MRI has been proved superior in distinguishing true TIA from cerebral infarct with transient symptoms.[8,9]

Computed Tomography (CT)

CT is available the majority of U.S. hospitals. Image acquisition is rapid and highly sensitive in detecting acute cerebral hemorrhage. CT has been shown to provide an alternative diagnosis in 1% of all cases, and a new infarct has been found within 48 hours in 4% of patients with TIA. In patients with TIA and new infarcts found on CT scanning, 38% went on to have a new ischemic stroke in the next 90 days. CT findings not associated with increased short-term risk for stroke include old infarction, periventricular white matter disease, cerebral atrophy, and vascular calcification.[17] Limitations of CT include the time required to identify an infarct, poor visualization of the cerebellum and brainstem, inability to differentiate infarct from penumbra, and limited visualization of the intracerebral and extracerebral vessels.

Magnetic Resonance Imaging (MRI)

Multimodal MRI (diffusion-weighted MRI, perfusion MRI, and T_2 imaging) has revolutionized our understanding of the pathophysiology of TIA. Multimodal MRI provides physiologic data and a distinction between cytotoxic edema (diffusion-weighted MRI), reduced cerebral blood flow (perfusion MRI), and increased water content, which is a marker of permanent brain injury (T_2 imaging). On average, 42% of TIA patients will have abnormalites on diffusion-weighted MRI, and in up to a third of cases, diffusion-weighted MRI results change the clinically suspected vascular location and etiology of the TIA.[9,18] Clinical predictors of positive findings on diffusion-weighted MRI include symptom duration longer than 1 hour, motor deficits, and aphasia.[19]

Multimodal MRI allows earlier detection of acute or small infarcts, improves diagnostic accuracy, provides better imaging of the brainstem and posterior fossa, and recently has been found to be effective at detecting acute hemorrhage.[20]

Drawbacks of this modality include limited availability, time required to acquire images, relatively high cost, incompatibility with implantable devices, and scarcity of local interpretive expertise. However, if available, multimodal MRI is a first-line imaging modality for patients presenting with transient neurologic symptoms.

Cardiovascular Imaging

Magnetic resonance angiography (MRA), carotid duplex ultrasonography, transcranial Doppler ultrasonography, CT angiography, and echocardiography (transthoracic and transesophageal) are adjunctive imaging modalities for determining the cause of TIAs. In patients with suspected extracranial vascular disease, MRA and carotid Doppler ultrasonography have nearly equal sensitivities (83% and 86%, respectively) for detecting critical stenosis.

Transcranial Doppler ultrasonography is noninvasive method for detecting significant stenosis in the vertebral and basilar arteries. Transthoracic echocardiography is effective for detecting wall motion abnormalities, valvular pathology, and mural thrombus. Transesophageal echocardiography is more sensitive at detecting atrial appendage thrombus, patent foramen ovale, atrial septal aneurysm, and aortic atherosclerotic disease.

Treatment

The goal of management of TIA patients is the introduction of therapy that will prevent stroke and thus avoid permanent disability and untimely death. Three available types of therapy achieve this goal: antiplatelet therapy, anticoagulation therapy, and surgical/endovascular therapy treat atherothrombotic, cardioembolic, and critically stenotic carotid diseases, respectively. In addition, patients should be instructed about measures that modify risk factors for stroke.

■ ANTIPLATELET THERAPY

Antiplatelet agents are the treatment of choice for the prevention of stroke in patients who present with TIA secondary to atherothrombotic disease.[21] Aspirin is the most widely used and the most economical drug available for stroke prevention. Currently, clopidogrel, ticlopidine, and combined dipyridamole-aspirin are antiplatelet agents that have been shown to be effective alternatives to aspirin in the prevention of stroke in patients with cerebral vascular disease. Unfortunately, despite being standard of care in the AHA guidelines, these agents are often underutilized, with only 18% of TIA patients in the ED receiving aspirin, 7% receiving other antiplatelet agents, and 42% receiving no treatment.[7]

Aspirin is the drug of choice for prevention of atherothrombotic stroke in TIA patients. It achieves this benefit though irreversible block of the enzyme cyclooxygenase, which in turn prevents the metabolism of arachidonic acid to the potent vasoconstrictor/platelet aggregator thromboxane A2. The effective dose of aspirin is 50 to 325 mg. Aspirin is associated with an overall reduction rate of 15% to 18% in the combined end points of stroke, myocardial infarction, and death.[22] Aspirin is well tolerated and inexpensive; however, gastrointestinal bleeding is a documented major side effect.

Clopidogrel (75 mg daily) and ticlopidine (250 mg twice daily) are adenosine diphosphate–receptor antagonists that prevent platelet aggregation. Clopidogrel is the preferred agent because of the advantages of once-daily dosing, less neutropenia, and fewer gastrointestinal side effects. It must be noted that clopidogrel has been reported to induce thrombotic thrombocytopenic purpura in a very small percentage of patients.

Large, multicenter randomized control trials have compared clopidogrel to aspirin[23] or combined clopidogrel-aspirin to clopidogrel alone in the prevention of stroke, myocardial infarction, and death.[24] Subgroup analysis failed to find a statistically significant reduction in ischemic stroke in favor of clopidogrel or the combined drugs. In addition, a recent study found no increase in stroke risk reduction by giving aspirin to symptomatic patients currently taking clopidogrel; in fact, major bleeding increased with the combination of the two drugs.[25] Clopidogrel remains a viable option for patients who are aspirin-sensitive and has been shown to be beneficial in patients who have concomitant cerebral vascular and coronary disease.

Dipyridamole is a cyclic nucleotide phosphodiesterase inhibitor with the intended function of inhibiting platelet aggregation by increasing levels of cyclic adenosine monophosphate (cAMP). Extended-release dipyridamole in combination with aspirin has been shown to reduce stroke risk by 37% compared with placebo and to reduce stroke risk by 23% compared with aspirin alone.[26] Current AHA guidelines report that combined dipyridamole-aspirin therapy may be more effective than clopidogrel for patients who have had a TIA while on aspirin therapy.[27] Common side effects include headache and gastrointestinal disturbances.

BOX 95-2

Carotid Endarterectomy (CEA) Recommendations*

- CEA for symptomatic stenosis >70%-99%
- CEA for symptomatic stenosis >50%-69% in men; medical management for women
- CEA best performed within 2 weeks of symptomatic event
- No benefit with CEA for stenosis >30%-49%
- CEA harmful for stenosis <30%
- Antiplatelet therapy should be initiated prior to CEA.

*Assumes that perioperative risk for stroke/death is less than 6% for surgeon or center.

■ ANTICOAGULATION

Atrial fibrillation is responsible for 50% of all cardiogenic embolic events. Patients with a high risk for recurrent stroke and atrial fibrillation who have had TIAs should receive warfarin as the therapy of choice for the prevention of stroke.[28] Risk factors for stroke in patients with atrial fibrillation include congestive heart failure, hypertension, age older than 75 years, diabetes, and previous stroke or TIA.[29] These patients have a target INR of 2.5 (range 2.0-3.0). Warfarin has not been shown to be superior to aspirin in the prevention of noncardioembolic forms of stroke.[30]

■ SURGICAL MANAGEMENT

The North American Symptomatic Carotid Endarterectomy Trial (NASCET) and the European Carotid Surgery Trial (ECST) found that carotid endarterectomy performed in patients with symptomatic severe carotid stenosis greater than 70% to 99% resulted in long-term benefit in stroke prevention.[31,32] Patients with symptomatic stenosis of 50% to 69% also showed benefit if the operation was performed in the 2 weeks following a TIA or minor stroke. The studies also showed that women with symptomatic carotid disease did not obtain stroke reduction benefit if carotid endarterectomy was performed later than 2 weeks following TIA or minor stroke. Finally, carotid endarterectomy showed no benefit in symptomatic patients with stenosis of 30% to 49% and was harmful in symptomatic patients with stenosis of less than 30% (Box 95-2).[33-35]

Other key factors that are part of the decision to operate include risk for stroke, patient co-morbidity, and local surgical expertise. Recently carotid stenting has been found to be a possible alternative to surgical carotid therapy. This therapy should be considered experimental until larger studies are available that show clear benefits over conventional therapy.

Disposition

Although the current guidelines for management of TIA do not specifically state criteria for hospital admission and discharge from the ED, a logical approach can be applied to this population based on several key points obtained from the ED evaluation. The areas that should be emphasized when making decisions regarding admission or discharge are the completeness of the evaluation, the source of the event, and the resolution of symptoms. These issues, coupled with proper risk stratification and cerebral vascular imaging, comprise a logical approach to achieving safe and proper disposition of the patient.

A thorough diagnostic evaluation that determines the cause of the TIA plays a crucial role in the decision to hospitalize or discharge patients from the ED. The evaluation often is limited by time and access to resources such as cerebral and vascular imaging. Patients who are at high risk for recurrent events and who are unable to have appropriate cerebral and vascular imaging should be hopitalized to expedite the evaluation and to allow observation for recurrent events in the period of vulnerability (hours or days) after the event.[10] Diagnostic benefits of hospital admission include rapid evaluation, monitoring for acute neurologic deterioration, and cardiac telemetry monitoring. Therapeutic benefits include the ability to deliver thrombolytic therapy, rapid institution of antiplatelet and anticoagulation therapy, and early consideration for carotid surgery.[36]

Patients who are at high risk for stroke should be admitted to the hospital to investigate the source of the TIA or begin therapy that prevents stroke (see Table 95-5). High-risk populations include patients with a California model score of 2 or higher or an ABCD score of 4 or higher, patients with symptomatic carotid disease and hemispheric symptoms, and patients with cardioembolic TIA.

Patients who are at low risk after a complete evaluation and those who have a clear etiology and who are on preventive therapy can be discharged after appropriate consultation with a neurologist, cardiologist, or vascular surgeon. It should be emphazised to all patients that a TIA is a high-risk event and that the risk of stroke is highest in the next 2 to 90 days. All patients discharged from the ED should be scheduled for follow-up during the next 2 days, which is the most critical period for recurrent events. Preventive therapy, especially antiplatelet therapy, should be initiated prior to discharge.

PATIENT TEACHING TIPS

PATIENTS WHO HAVE HAD TIA

- A TIA is a serious warning sign for stroke, myocardial infarction, and death in the next 2 to 90 days.
- Patients should understand the warning signs of stroke and should be instructed to return to the ED if symptoms recur.
- Patients with significant carotid disease should be evaluated promptly for surgery within the next 2 weeks and should be treated with antiplatelet agents.
- Patients who are discharged should have early outpatient follow-up and evaluation in the following 2 to 7 days.
- Patients should control modifiable risk factors and adhere to antiplatelet, anticoagulation, and antihypertensive therapy.

TIA, transient ischemic attack.

ACUTE ISCHEMIC STROKE

KEY POINTS

Acute ischemic stroke accounts for 80% to 88% of total stokes occurring annually in the United States.

Large-artery atherosclerosis, cardioembolism, and small-vessel disease are the leading causes of ischemic stroke.

The anterior circulation and the middle cerebral artery territories are most commonly affected by ischemic stroke.

The classic ischemic stroke presentation is found in elderly patients with sudden-onset speech disturbances associated with hemiparesis, hemiparesthesia, and homonymous hemianopia in the face and arm rather than in the leg.

Rapid emergency medical services transport and prompt ED evaluation combined with early institution of treatment is mandatory.

Thrombolysis is a controversial therapy that should be given only according to defined protocols. Best outcomes are found with early delivery of recombinant tissue plasminogen activator (rtPA) within established guidelines.

Aggressive treatment of hypoxia, dehydration, fever, and hyperglycemia and administration of antiplatelet agents improve outcome for ischemic stroke patients.

Stroke units and stroke teams, which provide comprehensive stroke care that improves patient outcome, can be established at both academic and community hospitals.

Scope

Ischemic stroke is a general term representing a spectrum of pathologic processes that permanently injure brain tissue and adversely affect or destroy an individual's ability to experience the world through mobility, independence, and the senses. Ischemic stroke is defined as a permanent cerebral injury secondary to prolonged disruption of cerebral blood flow (typically <10 mL/100 g brain/minute).[37]

Common causes of ischemic stroke are similar to those of TIA and include large-artery atherosclerosis (intracranial and extracranial), cardioembolic events, and small-vessel disease. Rare known causes of ischemic stroke include hypercoagulable conditions, vasculitis, arterial dissection, lupus erythematosus, and sickle cell disease. A high percentage of ischemic strokes are classified as unknown or cryptogenic. The early recurrence rate is highest for large artery atherosclerotic disease, and the mortality and disability rates are highest for cardioembolic disease. Recurrence rates and mortality are lowest for ischemic stroke caused by small-vessel disease. Modifiable risk factors include hypertension, diabetes, hypercholesterolemia, hyperlipidemia, cigarette smoking, heavy alcohol consumption, and physical inactivity. Nonmodifiable risks include age, race, sex, and genetic predisposition.

Epidemiology

Ischemic stroke accounts for 80% to 88% of the total strokes occurring annually in the United States and has been estimated to be the cause of approximately 61,000 deaths annually.[38]

Approximately 8% to 12% of all ischemic stroke patients die within 30 days from the initial stroke. Ischemic stroke disproportionately affects the elderly with a mean age of onset at 70.5 years. Ischemic stroke affects black and Hispanic populations more frequently than white populations. The age-adjusted incidence of first ischemic stroke per 100,000 population is 88 in whites, 149 in Hispanics, and 191 in blacks.[39] Ischemic stroke is an enormous economic burden, with an average 30-day cost of $20,346 for a severe stroke and mean lifetime cost of $140,048.[40,41]

The United States spends approximately 56 billion dollars yearly on the direct and indirect cost of stroke care.

Pathophysiology

Large-artery atherosclerosis is defined as greater than 50% narrowing of intra- or extracranial vessel caliber. It accounts for 15% of all ischemic strokes. Symptoms are the result of thrombus formation in a ruptured atherosclerotic plaque or artery-to-artery embolism. It is found more commonly in men than in women and has a greater incidence in African and Hispanic populations. Patients with large-artery atherosclerosis have a higher recurrence rate than patients with other stroke subtypes, and less severe stroke and disability compared with patients with cardioembolic stroke. These patients present with transient or stuttering symptoms in the same vascular territory. There may be a history of vascular disease, and the presence of bruits or decrease pulses may provide clinical support to the diagnosis.

Cardioembolic disease represents 25% of ischemic cerebral vascular events. The most common sources are abnormal cardiac rhythm (49%), abnormal left ventricular wall motion (31.4%), and aortic and mitral valve disease (27%). Clinical features are abrupt in onset, with nonprogressive symptoms; and patients report neurologic deficits in multiple vascular territories. Cardioemboli affect the anterior circulation in 70% of patients and the posterior circulation in 22% of patients. These patients tend to have more severe symptoms and higher mortality rates; disability is more severe in survivors.

Lacunar strokes represent 20% of all ischemic strokes and are caused by small-vessel disease. Symptoms result from small artery obstruction focused in the vessels that penetrate the brain parenchyma at right angles to major parent arteries and supply the basal ganglia, internal capsule, thalamus, and pons. The vessels most commonly involved are small branches of the middle cerebral and basilar arteries.[42] The most common causes of small vessel disease are microatheroma, lipohyalinosis, and Charcout-Bouchard Miliary aneurysms.

Ischemic stroke caused by small-vessel disease can be classified into five major syndromes: pure motor hemiparesis, ataxic hemiparesis, pure sensory syndrome, mixed sensorimotor syndrome, and dysarthria–clumsy hand syndrome.[42] African populations are more affected than white populations, and there does not seem to be a gender preference in patients with lacunar infarcts. This patient population has a better prognosis, with a 30-day recurrence rate of 1.4% and an approximately 2% annual mortality.

Rare causes of stroke account for approximately 2% to 3% of annual cases. Common causes are nonatherosclerotic vasculopathies (acute arterial dissection, polyarteritis, giant cell arteritis, infectious arteritis), hypercoagulable conditions (deficiencies in protein C and S, antithrombin III, antiphospholipid antibody syndrome), and hematologic disorders (sickle cell disease, polycythemia, myeloproliferative disorders).

Patients who present with fever and stroke should be evaluated for the risk of endocarditis and septic emboli as the cause of the stroke.

Cryptogenic stroke is a term used for stroke without a well-defined etiology despite an extensive evaluation. Cryptogenic stroke accounts for 30% to 40% of all strokes in some stroke databases. Conditions commonly considered in this category include patent foramen ovale, atrial septal aneurysm, aortic arch atheromata, mitral valve prolapse, and mitral valve strands. Patients with cryptogenic stroke have a better one-year prognosis than those with other subtypes; the 2-year recurrence risk is 14% to 20%.

Systemic hypoperfusion is an uncommon cause of cerebral ischemia that represents a global decrease in cerebral blood flow. Causes include cardiac pump failure caused by arrest or arrhythmia or due to reduced cardiac output from cardiac ischemia, pericardial effusion, pulmonary emboli, hemorrhage, and medications. Symptoms consist of diffuse brain dysfunction and abnormalities in vital signs accompanied by pallor, diaphoresis, and hypotension. Other symptoms include cerebral blindness, visual disorientation, sensorimotor impairment, disturbance of saccadic eye movement, dyslexia, dysgraphia, and memory deficits.

Structure and Function

The cerebral blood supply is divided into the anterior and posterior circulation. The brain has no capacity for storing its own energy and thus has a constant craving for oxygenated blood and glucose. Although brain tissue represents only 2% of total body weight, it receives 15% of total cardiac output and consumes 20% to 25% of total body oxygen. Autoregulation—the brain's ability to maintain a constant cerebral blood flow despite fluctuations in mean arterial pressure and intracranial pressure—is a neuromyogenic-regulated process that modifies the diameter of the precapillary arterioles to maintain an average cerebral blood flow of 50 mL/100 g brain/minute over a range of cerebral perfusion pressure (50-150 mm Hg).[43,44]

The anterior circulation receives 80% of the total cerebral circulation. It originates as paired carotid arteries that course through the neck, petrous temporal bone, and cavernous sinus, and finally to the subarachnoid space. The internal carotid branches first into the ophthalmic artery, then gives off two smaller branches (the anterior choroidal and the posterior communicating arteries). It then branches into the larger anterior cerebral and middle cerebral arteries. The circle of Willis is completed via the posterior communicating artery linked with the posterior cerebral artery.

The anterior cerebral artery passes above the optic chiasm and divides into A1 (anterior communicating arteries, recurrent artery of Hebner) and A2 (callosomarginal and pericallosal arteries). The larger segments supply the anterior three fourths of the medial aspect of the cerebral cortex. The smaller perforating branches (medial lenticulostriate arteries, recurrent artery of Hebner) supply the anterior limb of the internal capsule, the inferior portions of the head of the caudate nucleus, and the anterior globus pallidus.

The middle cerebral artery is the most commonly affected and the largest branch of the internal carotid artery. It supplies most of the temporal lobe, the anterolateral frontal lobe, and the parietal lobe. In addition, it has small perforating branches that supply the posterior limb of the internal capsule and part of the head and body of the caudate and globus pallidus. The four major segments of the middle cerebral artery are the M1 (sphenoidal), M2 (insular), M3 (opercular), and M4 (cortical). The perforators of the middle cerebral artery generally are referred to as the lateral lenticulostriate arteries.

The posterior cerebral artery is a terminal branch of the basilar artery. Its lateral cortical branches (anterior temporal, posterior temporal, and occipital temporal) supply the anterior temporal cortex, posterior temporal cortex, and occipital cortex, respectively. The medial branches of the posterior cerebral artery supply the calcarine cortex and the splenium of the corpus callosum. Penetrating branches participate in supplying the diencephalon, including the thalamus, subthalamic nucleus, and hypothalamus. Midbrain supply includes the cerebral peduncle, third nerve, and red nucleus.

The vertebral arteries arise from right and left subclavian arteries and ascend through the neck and the upper six cervical vertebrae to enter the skull via the foramen magnum. The two arteries then join at the lower border of one to form the basilar artery. Branches of the vertebral and basilar arteries supply the brainstem, cerebellum, and portions of the spinal cord.

Presenting Signs and Symptoms

Stroke symptoms represent a spectrum of clinical manifestations related to the major artery involved and the cerebral territories it supplies. Symptoms at times are transient or stuttering warning signs, or they may be sudden and completely permanent injuries. The key distinguishing feature of an ischemic stroke is sudden loss of cerebral function or negative symptoms.

Approximately 80% of ischemic strokes occur in the distribution of the intracerebral artery, middle cerebral artery, and anterior cerebral artery; these vessels are known collectively as the *anterior circulation* and give rise to functioning behavior, sensation, movement, and speech and contribute to parts of visual awareness. The minority of strokes occur in the distribution of the vertebral, basilar, and posterior cerebral and cerebellar arteries, which are called collectively the *posterior circulation*. These vessels supply the brainstem, cerebellum, occipital lobes, posterior temporal lobes, and thalamus.

Common posterior circulation symptoms are limb weakness, gait and limb ataxia, oculomotor palsies, and oropharyngeal dysfunction. Patients with posterior circulation ischemia often present with more than one symptom and may have crossed clinical symptoms, often with ipsilateral cranial nerve deficits and contralateral motor and sensory deficits. In addition, they often present with nausea and vomiting due to brainstem involvement, and vertigo and balance disorders related to cerebellar and brainstem injury.

■ MIDDLE CEREBRAL ARTERY

Patients with proximal-stem middle cerebral artery occlusion typically present with sensory loss hemiplegia, severe contralateral sensory loss, and contralateral homonymous hemianopia. Patients with dominant hemispheric lesions have motor or construction aphasia; those with nondominant hemispheric lesions present with contralateral hemisensory neglect. Subtle findings include gaze preference toward the side of the lesion and contralateral gaze weakness.

■ ANTERIOR CEREBRAL ARTERY

Stem lesions in the anterior cerebral artery are rare and secondary to collateral flow from the contralateral anterior cerebral artery through the anterior communicating artery. Branch occlusions are more common and have well-recognized clinical presentations. Patients with anterior cerebral artery lesions typically present with contralateral motor weakness and contralateral sensory deficit in the lower extremity. They complain of urinary incontinence secondary to contralateral weakness in the pelvic floor musculature. Other symptoms include memory loss or apathy secondary to occlusion of the orbital or frontopolar branch, dysarthria secondary to compromise of the medial striate artery, and ideomotor apraxia (inability to perform skilled movements) secondary to occlusion of the pericallosal branch.

■ LACUNAR INFARCTS

Lacunar infarcts result from ischemic events located in the small penetrating branches of the middle cerebral, anterior cerebral, posterior cerebral arteries, and basilar and anterior choroidal arteries. These lesions affect the basal ganglia, internal capsule, thalamus, putamen, and internal capsule. There are five major lacunar syndromes: pure motor hemiparesis, ataxic hemiparesis pure sensory syndrome, mixed sensorimotor syndrome, and dysarthria–clumsy hand syndrome.

■ Pure Motor Hemiparesis Syndrome

This is the most common lacunar syndrome and occurs in 50% of patients with lacunar syndromes. Patients present with stuttering symptoms that develop over hours and with contralateral facial and arm weakness but do not have sensory or higher cortical dysfunction. Injury is located in the corona radiata or internal capsule.[42]

■ Ataxic Hemiparesis Syndrome

Patients present with weakness and dysmetria (inability to fix the range of movement) on the same side. The lower extremity is more often affected than the arm and the face is least affected. The injury is located in the internal capsule, basis pontis, or corona radiate.

■ Pure Sensory Syndrome

Patients with pure sensory syndrome present with contralateral sensory loss in the face, arm, and leg. Symptoms include sensory ataxia, which is a movement disorder secondary to sensory impairment; a wide-stance gait with the gaze directed to the feet; and a walking pattern characterized by a stamping action that maximizes any remaining proprioception in order to move. The injury is located in the ventral posterior nucleus of the thalamus.[42]

■ Mixed Sensorimotor Syndrome

Patients present with hemiparesis or hemiplegia associated with sensory loss on the same side. This syndrome is distinguished from other syndromes by the lack of associated cortical symptoms. The site of injury is located in the posterolateral thalamus and the posterior limb of the internal capsule.[45]

■ Dysarthria–Clumsy Hand Syndrome

This syndrome is the least common of the lacunar syndromes and affects 6% of patients with lacunar stroke. Patients typically are dysarthric secondary to paresis of the lip, tongue, and jaw musculature and report clumsiness of hand movement. The injury site is located in the fibers descending through the genu of the internal capsule.[43]

■ POSTERIOR CIRCULATION ISCHEMIA (VERTEBRAL BASILAR DISEASE)

Twenty percent of ischemic events affect brain tissue supplied by the posterior circulation. Patients who present with posterior circulation ischemia rarely have a single presenting sign or symptom. Typical symptoms are dizziness, vertigo, headache, vomiting, double vision, loss of vision, transient interruption of consciousness, numbness, weakness, and ataxia. These patients often have crossed signs that include ipsilateral cranial nerve deficits associated with contralateral motor deficits. The most common signs include contralateral limb weakness, gait and limb ataxia, oculomotor palsies, and oropharyngeal dysfunction.

■ POSTERIOR CEREBRAL ARTERY

Occlusion of the posterior cerebral artery and its branches leads to a variety of defects in the cerebral cortex, midbrain, thalamus, subthalamic nuclei, and corpus callosum. Stem lesions in the posterior cerebral artery cause isolated contralateral homonymous hemianopia. Midbrain lesions cause crossed symptoms with ipsilateral third nerve palsy accompanied by contralateral motor hemiplegia. Thalamic branch lesions result in contralateral sensory loss accompanied by hemianopia. Subthalamic nuclei injury results in ballism of the contralateral arm. Finally, corpus callosum injury results in the inability to transfer written information from right to left and results in alexia (inability to read written material).[43,46]

■ CEREBELLAR INFARCT

The most common cause of an ischemic injury to the cerebellum is an embolic infarct in the upper cerebellum. Symptoms include dizziness, vertigo, vomiting, blurred vision, and difficulty walking. Patients may report that they veer to a specific side, and family members may report that patients are unable to sit upright or to sit erect without assistance.

Examination of the upper extremities may reveal the side of the lesion. Hypotonia may be present in the arm on the affected side. This sign is best elicited by having patients hold their arms straight out at 90 degrees from the trunk, quickly lower and then abruptly stop the lowering motion. The affected side is detected because the hypotonic arm will overshoot the rapid descent.

Cerebellar infarcts are distinguished from infarcts in other anatomic locations by the lack of hemiparesis or hemisensory deficits.[43,47]

■ LATERAL MEDULLARY SYNDROME (WALLENBERG'S SYNDROME)

Occlusion or narrowing of the intracranial vertebral artery causes signs and symptoms related to ischemic injury of the lateral medullary tegmentum. Symptoms include facial ipsilateral sensory loss, ataxia, and nystagmus. Patients may also present with Horner's syndrome, hoarseness, difficulty swallowing, and contralateral hemisensory loss of pain and temperature sense.

Differential Diagnosis and Diagnostic Testing

Patients with ischemic stroke require a rapid and accurate diagnosis to determine the etiology and location of the event and the extent of the damage. This knowledge allows the EP to estimate the risk and benefit of therapies that will reestablish cerebral blood flow and preserve viable brain tissue.[48]

Rapid diagnosis of acute ischemic stroke begins with public education about the recognition of the major warning signs of stroke. These symptoms include sudden weakness or numbness of the face, arm, or leg on one side of the body; sudden confusion, trouble speaking or understanding; sudden trouble seeing in one or both eyes; sudden trouble walking or dizziness; loss of balance or coordination; or sudden severe headache with no known cause.

Prehospital personnel play a crucial role in early diagnosis and rapid transport of stroke patients to treatment facilities. Tools such as the Cincinnati Prehospital Stroke Scale (CPSS) and the Los Angeles Prehospital Stroke Screen (LAPSS) are used to evaluate facial droop, arm weakness, and speech abnormalities in patients with suspected stroke. In addition, the LAPSS screens for mimics of stroke such as hypoglycemia, hyperglycemia, and seizure and has a high sensitivity (93%) and specificity (97%) for diagnosis of acute stroke.[49,50]

EPs caring for patients with acute ischemic stroke often are under enormous time constraints to accurately determine symptoms, exclude hemorrhage with timely cerebral imaging, and safely deliver therapy using defined protocols. A systematic method is necessary to distinguish patients with stroke from those with conditions that mimic stroke, such as seizures, confusional states, syncope, neoplasm, and subdural hematoma.[51] In addition, the EP must determine the vascular distribution and severity of the stroke and combine these historical and physical data with neurologic imaging results to exclude hemorrhage and determine the extent of injury. These elements, coupled with basic laboratory tests and an ECG, as recommended by the AHA, are the foundation for an accurate diagnosis of an acute ischemic stroke.

The history is the cornerstone of accurate stroke diagnosis. Historical evidence that has been identified as predictive for a patient having a stroke includes persistent focal neurologic deficits, acute onset during the previous week, and no history of head trauma.[52] Clinical symptoms such as arm and leg weakness and speech impairment are more reliable indicators than subjective isolated sensory symptoms. Other key historical factors include the time the patient was last seen as neurologically normal, contraindications to thrombolytic therapy, medications being taken by the patient, heart disease, previous stroke, TIA, and seizures, vomiting, or headache occurring at the beginning of the patient's acute symptoms (see "Priority Actions" box).

EPs must use a reproducible standardized physical examination to assess the severity of injury to the stroke patient. Three key physical findings—facial paresis, arm drift, and abnormal speech—are highly predictive of an acute stroke.

The National Institutes of Health Stroke Scale (NIHSS) (see "Documentation" box) is a valid, standardized tool that records clinical findings and provides information that is helpful in determining the prognosis and therapeutic options. This 42-point scale evaluates level of consciousness, cranial nerves, motor function, ataxia, sensation, speech, and neglect. It can be used for serial examinations and is a predictor of patient outcome and risk of therapy that can be useful when discussing treatment options with specialists, patients, and family members.

Patients with an NIHSS score less than 6 have a predicted excellent outcome at 6 months, and 81% are discharged home. Nearly half the patients with an NIHSS score higher than 15 will require transfer to a nursing facility. Patients with an NIHSS score higher than 20 have a 17% risk of intracerebral hemorrhage when treated with rtPA. Lastly, each additional point on the NIHSS decreases the likelihood of excellent outcome by 17%.[53-55]

Although the history and physical examination are important elements in the accurate diagnosis of patients with acute neurovascular events, neuroimaging is the key diagnostic tool for excluding acute hemorrhage and determining the therapy for each individual ischemic subtype. Currently, EPs have a multitude of imaging options (CT, perfusion CT, MRI) that are based on availability of the imaging modality and local expertise in interpretation of the images. In addition, specific facilities may incorporate simultaneous vascular imaging with CT angiography and MRA.

Noncontrast CT remains the standard imaging technique for evaluating acute stroke patients. It is found in the majority of hospitals, images are rapidly acquired, and it is useful for detecting acute hemorrhage. Unfortunately, CT scans frequently are negative in the first hours after ischemic stroke occurs and are limited in defining posterior fossa structures. Furthermore, non-contrast CT is unable to discriminate between infarct and viable at-risk tissue (penumbra) and provides no information on the presence or location of vascular pathology.

Subtle clues found on CT scanning are cortical hypodensity, hyperdense middle cerebral artery, middle cerebral artery dot sign, sulcal effacement, hypoattenuation of insular ribbon, and obscuration of the lentiform nucleus. The Alberta Stroke Program Early CT Score (ASPECTS) organized these early subtle clues into a semiquantitative 10-point grading system for early ischemic changes in the middle cerebral artery territory found on CT scans. Patients with an ASPECTS over 7 were found to have a much higher incidence of parenchyma hematoma after receiving rtPA therapy.[56]

Perfusion CT is an advanced neuroimaging technique that uses IV contrast in conjunction with helical CT to provide semiquantitative information on cerebral blood flow (CBF) and cerebral blood volume (CBV). Other useful calculations include the mean transit time (MTT) of contrast from arterial to venous circulation and time to peak (TTP), which

PRIORITY ACTIONS

Differential Diagnosis of TIA and Acute Ischemic Stroke

Persistent Focal Neurologic Deficits, Altered Mental Status, Headache

- Does the patient have intracerebral hemorrhage, aneurysm, arterial venous malformation, complicated migraine, venous thrombosis, hypertensive urgency, or brain abscess?
- Exclude hemorrhage and mass with emergent CNS imaging.
- Examine vital signs; if neurologic deficits persist for more than 1 hour, treat as ischemic stroke; exclude aneurysm with CT/LP.

Recurrent Neurologic Symptoms in Multiple Vascular Distributions

- Does the patient have a cardiac rhythm disorder, mechanical heart valve, valvular heat disease, large-artery atheroma, or congenital heart defects?
- Does the patient have a hypercoagulable disease, sickle cell disease, vasculitis, or lupus erythematosus?
- Is the patient on Coumadin therapy and taking the medication?
- Does the patient use IV drugs or is the patient at risk for septic emboli/endocarditis?
- If the presence and/or cause of TIA is undetermined, obtain an echocardiogram and schedule hematologic/coagulation testing.

Acute Onset of Vertigo or Dizziness

- Does the patient have labyrinth disease or Ménière's disease?
- Exclude vertebrobasilar and cerebellar ischemia/hemorrhage with CNS and vascular imaging.

Acute Change in Vision

- Does the patient have multiple sclerosis, retinal detachment, or temporal arteritis?
- Examine the eyes for afferent papillary defect, cranial nerve palsy, and retinal detachment. Palpate for tenderness of the temporal artery and check blood for elevation of ESR.
- If the previous findings are negative, consider amaurosis fugax and look for signs of carotid artery disease using MRI and carotid duplex ultrasonography.

Seizure

- Does the patient have epilepsy or Todd's paralysis?
- Does the patient take seizure medication?
- Does the patient use alcohol, cocaine, benzodiazepines, or amphetamines?

Syncope

- Does the patient have cardiac disease, atrial fibrillation, or valvular heart disease?
- Does the patient have congestive heart failure or take cardiac medications?
- Does the patient have hypotension, shortness of breath, or hematocrit less than 30?
- Obtain ECG and check vital signs; consider cardioembolic disease or border zone ischemia caused by hypotension.

CNS, central nervous system; CT, computed tomography; ECG, electrocardiogram; ESR, erythrocyte sedimentation rate; LP, lumbar puncture; TIA, transient ischemic attack.

measures the time between the first arrival of contrast in the artery and the peak of the bolus within the brain tissue.[57] Baseline values for these measurements in unaffected tissue include:

CBF = 50 mL/100 g brain/minute
CBV = 4 mL/100 g brain
MTT = less than 6 seconds (average: 3.6 seconds)
TTP = less than 8 seconds

Benefits include more rapid identification of ischemic location and the presence of viable tissue. Disadvantages include the need for intravenous contrast and normal renal function, limited imaging of the posterior fossa, and lack of local expertise in interpretation of findings.

MRI with diffusion-weighted imaging is very accurate in early detection of hyperacute stroke and the determination of stroke subtype.[58] MRI coupled with perfusion-weighted imaging and MRA increases diagnostic certainty, allowing detection of ischemic injury, determination of tissue viability, and localization of vascular clot, stenosis, and dissection. MRI provides better imaging the brainstem and posterior fossa than CT. Furthermore, MRI is as accurate as CT in detecting acute hemorrhagic transformation and is more accurate in determining acute hemorrhage from chronic hemorrhage.[20] Limitations include cost, availability, incompability with implantable devices, and requirement for patient tolerance and stability.

Tips and Tricks

- Use diffusion-weighted MRI (DWI) to separate true TIA from acute ischemic stroke.
- Use risk stratification criteria to determine the need for hospitalization.
- Be very concerned about recurrent stroke in patients with LAA.
- Patients with motor and speech deficits and prolonged symptoms are more likely to have positive DWI findings
- Prescribe combined dipyridamole-aspirin for patients with TIA taking aspirin.

LAA, large-artery atherosclerosis; MRI, magnetic resonance imaging; TIA, transient ischemic attack.

Diagnostic testing is completed with laboratory and ancillary tests. Laboratory tests recommended by the AHA include complete blood count, platelets, prothrombin time, partial thromboplastin time, INR, and assays of glucose, cardiac enzymes, and lipids. Other options are pregnancy testing, drug toxicology, and urinalysis. An ECG should obtained to look for atrial fibrillation, acute myocardial infarction, rhythm disturbance, and atrial septal defects. Ancillary testing includes a chest radiograph if pulmonary pathology, aspiration, or congestive heart failure is suspected. Echocardiography and carotid and transcranial Doppler ultrasonography also play limited roles in the diagnostic evaluation.

Treatment

ED management of patients with acute ischemic stroke requires a team approach that is organized, time-sensitive, and goal-directed. The goal is to ensure medical stability, identify the cause of the ischemic event, determine the extent of the injury, and create a therapeutic plan that reestablishes cerebral function and prevents or limits further injury. Four time goals for therapy have been established.

The immediate assessment is completed within 10 minutes of the patient's arrival in the ED. This process includes securing the ABC (airway, breathing, and circulation) and vital signs, providing supplemental oxygen, and cardiac monitoring, establishing IV access, and bedside glucose measurement. Neurologic deficits are assessed, and NIHSS is calculated. Patients with confirmed clinical symptoms of stroke are then transferred for CT scannning, and a stroke team or neurologist is consulted.

The second time goal is 25 minutes from arrival. The CT scan has been completed and time of symptoms onset established. With the neurologist or stroke team present, the patient's history is reviewed.

The third time goal is at 45 minutes from arrival. The CT scan is reviewed and interpreted; the presence of hemorrhage is excluded, and extent of injury and the involved vascular supply are determined. The patient and the family are questioned and laboratory test results are reviewed to determine if there are any contraindications to thrombolysis. During this period the patient is reexamined to determine improving or worsening clinical status. In addition, hypertension (blood pressure >185 mm Hg systolic or >110 mm Hg diastolic), hyperglycemia (glucose >120 mg/dL), and fever (>37.5°C [>99.5°F]) should be treated with the appropriate medications.

After 60 minutes in the ED, the plan for therapy and the risk and benefits are reviewed with the patient and family. Patients who are candidates for thrombolysis are admitted to the intensive care unit, Patients who are not candidates and who do not have central nervous system hemorrhage are screened for aspiration, given aspirin orally or rectally, and admitted for further investigation and therapy.

■ rtPA THERAPY

The only treatment for acute ischemic stroke approved by the Food and Drug Administration (FDA) is IV rtPA therapy, which is recommended for carefully selected patients over the age of 18 years who present within 3 hours of onset of an acute ischemic stroke. Bridging therapies (not FDA-approved) include intra-arterial catheter–based thrombolysis in candidates who present later than 3 hours but less than 6 hours.[59]

Adjuncts to intra-arterial thrombolysis include angioplasty, stenting, and clot retrieval devices. Other therapies include prevention of hypoxemia and dehydration, antiplatelets, anticoagulation, glucose, and temperature control. Areas of future investigation include multimodal therapy for reestablishment of blood flow, cerebral neuroprotective agents, and hypothermia.

■ THROMBOLYSIS

The era of emergent intravenous thrombolysis for acute ischemic stroke began in 1995 based upon Parts 1 and 2 of the National Institute of Neurological Disorders and Stroke (NINDS) rtPA trial. This study was a single, randomized controlled trial that compared patients with ischemic stroke treated with IV rtPA versus placebo (given at 0-90 minutes, 90-180, and 0-180 minutes). The main outcome of the trial was a 30% decrease in disability at 3 months in patients treated with IV rtPA compared with those treated with placebo. Adverse events included a 10-fold increase in intracerebral hemorrhage at 36 hours after treatment with rtPA (6% vs. 0.6%), with 61% of patients with intracerebral hemorrhage not living past 3 months. Additional discoveries in this trial included no difference in NIHSS scores at 24 hours and no difference in mortality between rtPA- and placebo-treated groups at three months after ischemic stroke.[60]

Concerns over data that support the use of thrombolytics for acute ischemic stroke and the external validity in community hospitals have been raised by many EPs.[61] Large randomized trials have investigated the use of thrombolytics, with some using rtPA outside the 3-hour window and only one using modern technology.[62] Three trials using streptokinase were terminated early because of significant mortality in the thrombolysis groups.[63-65] In three other studies, no significant difference in disability and mortality was found at 90 days.[66-68]

The effectiveness of thrombolysis is determined by several variables. Foremost is whether there is an arterial occlusion and the extent of the cerebral infarct. Predictors of poor post-thrombolysis prognosis include patient age, stroke severity (NIHSS), systemic hypertension or hypotension, hyperglycemia, and fever.

Centers that care for stroke patients must develop guidelines for the selection of appropriate patients and develop systems to rapidly deliver thrombolysis therapy to these patients. Large clots in the proximal internal carotid arteries are more resistant to thrombolysis than smaller clots located in the middle cerebral artery. Clots in the basilar artery have been treated successfully with intra-arterial thrombolysis outside the 3-hour window.[69]

Candidates for IV thrombolysis must have a clearly defined time of symptoms and onset less than 180 minutes, must be over age 18, and must have no contraindications for thrombolytic therapy. The dosing regimen is 0.9 mg/kg (maximum 90 mg) of rtPA, with 10% (maximum 9 mg) given as bolus over 1-2 minutes, followed by the remaining dose (maximum 81 mg) infused by pump over 1 hour. The patient's blood pressure should be checked every 15 minutes and should be maintained at less than 180/110 mm Hg. The patient should not receive aspirin or heparin during the first 24 hours after thrombolytic therapy. Furthermore, the patient should have frequent neurologic checks, and the institution must have a protocol for the management of thrombolytic-induced intracerebral hemorrhage.

ENDOVASCULAR PROCEDURES

Endovascular procedures such as intra-arterial thrombolysis, mechanical embolectomy, angioplasty, and carotid stenting are considered experimental therapies that may benefit specific patient groups that present outside the 3-hour window or have contraindications to IV thrombolysis.[70] Benefits of this therapy include lower dose of thrombolytic, direct visualization of the occluded vessel, and higher recanalization rates. Concerns include the following: the number of candidates is extremely limited (3%), the procedure is invasive, and there is a high risk of death due to intracerebral hemorrhage.

ADJUVANT ACUTE ISCHEMIC STROKE THERAPY

Blood Pressure Management

The management of blood pressure in the acute stroke patient is controversial. In an ED study of patients with acute ischemic stroke, a range of systolic and diastolic blood pressure was associated with an increase in 90-day mortality rate. The investigators found that systolic blood pressure outside the range of 155 to 220 mm Hg and diastolic blood pressure outside the range of 71 to 105 mm Hg were associated with increased 90-day mortality. These findings demonstrate the harmful effects of both hypertension and hypotension and indicate that there is an optimal range of blood pressure required to perfuse at-risk tissue in these patients.[71]

Current American Stroke Association (ASA) and European Stroke Initiative (EUSI) guidelines recommend withholding antihypertensive therapy in patients with acute ischemic stroke unless they are thrombolysis candidates or show evidence of end organ dysfunction (acute myocardial infarction, aortic dissection, pulmonary edema, and renal failure). Short-acting IV medications should be used for antihypertensive therapy, with reliable dose response and safety profiles. Medications that meet these requirements include labetolol, nicardipine, and esmolol.[44]

Glucose Management

Hyperglycemia (glucose level >108 mg/dL) is associated with a worsening of clinical and tissue outcome in patients with acute ischemic stroke. Hyperglycemia promotes anaerobic metabolism, lactic acidosis, and free radical production that accelerate the course of ischemic injury and actively convert penumbra to infarcted tissue. Hyperglycemia is a risk factor for hemorrhagic events and poor outcome in patients receiving rtPA therapy.[72] Glycemic control with rapidly acting insulin should be instituted to maintain blood glucose level below 300 mg/dL.[73]

Temperature Management

Hyperpyrexia is defined as a temperature higher than 37.5 to 38.0°C. Elevated temperature is associated with increased morbidity and mortality; the pathologic effects stem from increased neurotransmitter and free radical production and adverse effects on the blood-brain barrier, which seem to be most pronounced at the border zone or penumbra of the infarct, leading to loss of potentially viable tissue. Therefore the source of fever should be actively sought, and the fever treated with acetaminophen.[74]

Anticoagulation

The goal of anticoagulation therapy is to prevent recurrence of another ischemic event. The overall risk of recurrent ischemic stroke in the first 7 to 14 days after an ischemic stroke is 2.2%, but the risk has been estimated to be higher (4.5%-8%) in specific subsets of stroke patients—especially those with atrial fibrillation and other sources of cardioemboli.[75-77] Currently, low-molecular-weight heparin is not recommended in any type of acute ischemic stroke because of the increased risk of secondary hemorrhagic conversion; furthermore, clinical trial data showed no reduction in stroke recurrence or improvement in patient outcome. Unfractionated intravenous heparin is not recommended in the first 48 hours after ischemic stroke because of lack of proven efficacy at preventing recurrence and an increased risk of bleeding complications.[78,79]

Antiplatelet Therapy

The goals of antiplatelet therapy are a reduction in stroke recurrence and a reduction in stroke related morbidity and mortality. Aspirin (50-325 mg/day) therapy resulted in a significant reduction in death and disability when given within 48 hours of ischemic stroke. Aspirin reduces the risk of early recurrent stroke and does not appear to be limited in benefit to any specific stroke subtype. Therefore, patients who are not aspirin-sensitive or at risk for aspiration and are not receiving tPA should receive aspirin within 48 hours of ischemic stroke.

Other antiplatelet agents including clopidogrel, glycoprotein IIB/IIIA inhibitors, and combination drugs such as dipyridamole/aspirin have not been proved to be safer or more cost-effective than aspirin alone, and they play a limited role in stroke prevention therapy. Clopidogrel, with a more favorable side-effect profile than ticlopidine, is recommended for aspirin-sensitive patients who require emergent antiplatelet therapy in the ED. Warfarin has not been shown to be any more effective than aspirin in the prevention of ischemic stroke in populations without atrial fibrillation.

Disposition

All patients with acute ischemic stroke require admission to the hospital to be observed for changes in their condition, to facilitate medical or surgical procedures, to receive preventive therapy, and to recover neurologic function with rehabilitative services. Optimal inter- and intrahospital disposition is dependent on local hospital expertise, severity of the stroke, and intensity of therapy. Following early therapy initiated at a community hospital, patients may be transferred to a stroke center for more comprehensive care. Care of these patients requires a coordinated effort between ED staff, neurologists, and radiologists; stroke teams often coordinate this care in hospitals throughout the United States. Patients receiving thrombolysis should have access to the intensive care unit, neurology and neurosurgery consultation, and blood bank services.

Admission to a stroke unit has been validated in clinical trials as statistically significant in decreasing disability and mortality while increasing the probability that the patient will return home and resume daily living activities.[80] These effects are independent of age, sex, and severity of stroke and are reproducible in a community setting.

Intensive monitoring in a stroke unit allows early detection and treatment of fever, hypoxemia, hyperglycemia, and cardiac rhythm disturbances. Other benefits include early mobilization coupled with physical and occupation therapy. Stroke units have been found to be effective for patients with large artery–associated stroke and more costly but with equal efficacy to medical ward care for patients with small-vessel disease stroke.[81] Hospitals without stroke units should have comprehensive protocols and quality assurance programs that actively manage variables shown to affect outcome and ensure optimal care for all patients.

Patients who require intensive care admission are patients with severe stroke with the potential to compromise breathing and swallowing and patients who are at risk for decompensation from hemorrhage, cerebral swelling, respiratory distress, or medical comorbidities. High-risk populations include patients treated with intravenous or intra-arterial thrombolysis or catheter-based therapies, patients with an NIHSS score greater than 17, and patients with cerebellar or large middle cerebral artery distribution strokes who are at risk for developing cerebral edema.

REFERENCES

1. Albers GW, Caplan LR, Easton JD, et al: Transient ischemic attack—proposal for a new definition. N Engl J Med 2002;347:1713-1716.
2. Johnston SC, Gress DR, Browner WS, Sidney S: Short-term prognosis after emergency department diagnosis of TIA. JAMA 2000;284:2901-2906.
3. Rothwell PM, Giles MF, Flossmann E, et al: A simple score (ABCD) to identify individuals at high early risk of stroke after transient ischaemic attack. Lancet 2005;366:29-36.
4. Kleindorfer D, Panagos P, Pancioli A, et al: Incidence and short-term prognosis of transient ischemic attack in a population-based study. Stroke 2005;36:720-723.
5. Ovbiagele B, Kidwell CS, Saver JL: Epidemiological impact in the United States of a tissue-based definition of transient ischemic attack. Stroke 2003;34:919-924.
6. Johnston SC: Clinical practice. Transient ischemic attack. N Engl J Med 2002;347:1687-1692.
7. Edlow JA, Kim S, Pelletier AJ, Camargo CA Jr: National Study on Emergency Department Visits for Transient Ischemic Attack, 1992-2001. Acad Emerg Med 2006;13: 662-672.
8. Coutts SB, Simon JE, Eliasziw M, et al: Triaging transient ischemic attack and minor stroke patients using acute magnetic resonance imaging. Ann Neurol 2005;57:848-854.
9. Kidwell CS, Alger JR, Di Salle F, et al: Diffusion MRI in patients with transient ischemic attacks. Stroke 1999;30: 1174-1180.

10. Rothwell PM, Warlow CP: Timing of TIAs preceding stroke: Time window for prevention is very short. Neurology 2005;64:817-820.
11. Adams HP Jr, Woolson RF, Clarke WR, et al: Design of the Trial of Org 10172 in Acute Stroke Treatment (TOAST). Control Clin Trials 1997;18:358-377.
12. Lovett JK, Coull AJ, Rothwell PM: Early risk of recurrence by subtype of ischemic stroke in population-based incidence studies. Neurology 2004;62:569-573.
13. Ferro JM, Falcao I, Rodrigues G, et al: Diagnosis of transient ischemic attack by the nonneurologist. A validation study. Stroke 1996;27:2225-2229.
14. Kraaijeveld CL, van Gijn J, Schouten HJ, Staal A: Interobserver agreement for the diagnosis of transient ischemic attacks. Stroke 1984;15:723-725.
15. Shah KH, Edlow JA: Transient ischemic attach: Review for the emergency physician. Ann Emerg Med 2004;43: 592-604.
16. Benavente O, Eliasziw M, Streifler JY, et al: Prognosis after transient monocular blindness associated with carotid-artery stenosis. N Engl J Med 2001;345:1084-1090.
17. Douglas VC, Johnston CM, Elkins J, et al: Head computed tomography findings predict short-term stroke risk after transient ischemic attack. Stroke 2003;34:2894-2898.
18. Saver JL, Kidwell C: Neuroimaging in TIAs. Neurology 2004;62(Suppl6):S22-S25.
19. Crisostomo RA, Garcia MM, Tong DC: Detection of diffusion-weighted MRI abnormalities in patients with transient ischemic attack: Correlation with clinical characteristics. Stroke 2003;34:932-937.
20. Kidwell CS, Chalela JA, Saver JL, et al: Comparison of MRI and CT for detection of acute intracerebral hemorrhage. JAMA 2004;292:1823-1830.
21. Albers GW, Amarenco P, Easton JD, et al: Antithrombotic and thrombolytic therapy for ischemic stroke. Chest 2001;119(1 Suppl):300S-320S.
22. Algra A, De Schryver EL, van Gijn J, et al: Oral anticoagulants versus antiplatelet therapy for preventing further vascular events after transient ischemic attack or minor stroke of presumed arterial origin. Stroke 2003;34:234-235.
23. A randomised, blinded, trial of clopidogrel versus aspirin in patients at risk of ischaemic events (CAPRIE). CAPRIE Steering Committee. Lancet 1996;348:1329-1339.
24. Bhatt DL, Fox KA, Hacke W, et al: Clopidogrel and aspirin versus aspirin alone for the prevention of atherothrombotic events. N Engl J Med 2006;354:1706-1717.
25. Diener HC, Bogousslavsky J, Brass LM, et al: Aspirin and clopidogrel compared with clopidogrel alone after recent ischaemic stroke or transient ischaemic attack in high-risk patients (MATCH): Randomised, double-blind, placebo-controlled trial. Lancet 2004;364:331-337.
26. Diener HC, Cunha L, Forbes C, et al: European Stroke Prevention Study. 2. Dipyridamole and acetylsalicylic acid in the secondary prevention of stroke. J Neurol Sci 1996; 143:1-13.
27. Albers GW, Hart RG, Lutsep HL, et al: AHA Scientific Statement. Supplement to the guidelines for the management of transient ischemic attacks: A statement from the Ad Hoc Committee on Guidelines for the Management of Transient Ischemic Attacks, Stroke Council, American Heart Association. Stroke 1999;30:2502-2511.
28. Secondary prevention in non-rheumatic atrial fibrillation after transient ischaemic attack or minor stroke. EAFT (European Atrial Fibrillation Trial) Study Group. Lancet 1993;342:1255-1262.
29. Gage BF, Waterman AD, Shannon W, et al: Validation of clinical classification schemes for predicting stroke: Results from the National Registry of Atrial Fibrillation. JAMA 2001;285:2864-2870.
30. Mohr JP, Thompson JL, Lazar RM, et al: A comparison of warfarin and aspirin for the prevention of recurrent ischemic stroke. N Engl J Med 2001;345:1444-1451.
31. Barnett HJ, Taylor DW, Eliasziw M, et al: Benefit of carotid endarterectomy in patients with symptomatic moderate or severe stenosis. North American Symptomatic Carotid Endarterectomy Trial Collaborators. N Engl J Med 1998;339: 1415-1425.
32. MRC European Carotid Surgery Trial: Interim results for symptomatic patients with severe (70-99%) or with mild (0-29%) carotid stenosis. European Carotid Surgery Trialists' Collaborative Group. Lancet 1991;337:1235-1243.
33. Chaturvedi S, Bruno A, Feasby T, et al: Carotid endarterectomy—an evidence-based review: report of the Therapeutics and Technology Assessment Subcommittee of the American Academy of Neurology. Neurology 2005;65: 794-801.
34. Rothwell PM, Eliasziw M, Gutnikov SA, et al: Analysis of pooled data from the randomised controlled trials of endarterectomy for symptomatic carotid stenosis. Lancet 2003;361:107-116.
35. Rothwell PM, Eliasziw M, Gutnikov SA, et al: Sex difference in the effect of time from symptoms to surgery on benefit from carotid endarterectomy for transient ischemic attack and nondisabling stroke. Stroke 2004;35:2855-2861.
36. Donnan GA, Davis SM, Hill MD, Gladstone DJ: Patients with transient ischemic attack or minor stroke should be admitted to hospital. Stroke 2006;37:1137-1138.
37. Kucinski T, Koch C, Zeumer H: CT in Acute Stroke. Lincolnshire, IL, Remedica, 2003.
38. Petty GW, Brown RD Jr, Whisnant JP, et al: 1. Ischemic stroke subtypes: A population-based study of functional outcome, survival, and recurrence. Stroke 2000;31: 1062-1068.
39. White H, Boden-Albala B, Wang C, et al: Ischemic stroke subtype incidence among whites, blacks, and Hispanics: The Northern Manhattan Study. Circulation 2005;111: 1327-1331.
40. Leibson CL, Hu T, Brown RD, et al: Utilization of acute care services in the year before and after first stroke: A population-based study. Neurology 1996;46:861-869.
41. Taylor TN, Davis PH, Torner JC, et al: Lifetime cost of stroke in the United States. Stroke 1996;27:1459-1466.
42. Gan R, Sacco RL, Kargman DE, et al: Testing the validity of the lacunar hypothesis: The Northern Manhattan Stroke Study experience. Neurology 1997;48:1204-1211.
43. FitzGerald MJT, Folan-Curan J (eds): Cerebrovascular Disease, 4th ed. Philadelphia, WB Saunders, 2002.
44. Rose JC, Mayer SA: Optimizing blood pressure in neurological emergencies. Neurocrit Care 2004;1:287-289.
45. Fisher CM: Lacunar strokes and infarcts: A review. Neurology 1982;32:871-876.
46. Caplan L: Posterior circulation ischemia: Then, now, and tomorrow. The Thomas Willis Lecture–2000. Stroke 2000;31:2011-2023.
47. Savitz SI, Caplan LR: Vertebrobasilar disease. N Engl J Med 2005;352:2618-2626.
48. Caplan LR: Treatment of acute stroke: Still struggling. JAMA 2004;292:1883-1885.
49. Kidwell CS, Starkman S, Eckstein M, et al: Identifying stroke in the field. Prospective validation of the Los Angeles prehospital stroke screen (LAPSS). Stroke 2000;31:71-76.
50. Kothari RU, Pancioli A, Liu T, et al: Cincinnati Prehospital Stroke Scale: Reproducibility and validity. Ann Emerg Med 1999;33:373-378.
51. Norris JW, Hachinski VC: Misdiagnosis of stroke. Lancet 1982;1:328-331.
52. von Arbin M, Britton M, de Faire U, et al: Validation of admission criteria to a stroke unit. J Chronic Dis 1980;33:215-220.
53. Adams HP Jr, Davis PH, Leira EC, et al: Baseline NIH Stroke Scale score strongly predicts outcome after stroke: A report of the Trial of Org 10172 in Acute Stroke Treatment (TOAST). Neurology 1999;53:126-11.
54. Goldstein LB, Simel DL: Is this patient having a stroke? JAMA 2005;293:2391-202.
55. Schlegel D, Kolb SJ, Luciano JM, et al: Utility of the NIH Stroke Scale as a predictor of hospital disposition. Stroke 2003;34:134-137.
56. Dzialowski I, Hill MD, Coutts SB, et al: Extent of early ischemic changes on computed tomography (CT) before

thrombolysis: Prognostic value of the Alberta Stroke Program Early CT Score in ECASS II. Stroke 2006; 37:973-978.
57. Harrigan MR, Leonardo J, Gibbons KJ, et al: CT perfusion cerebral blood flow imaging in neurological critical care. Neurocrit Care 2005;2:352-336.
58. Kang DW, Chalela JA, Ezzeddine MA, Warach S: Association of ischemic lesion patterns on early diffusion-weighted imaging with TOAST stroke subtypes. Arch Neurol 2003; 60:1730-1734.
59. Adams H, Adams R, Del Zoppo G, Goldstein LB: Guidelines for the early management of patients with ischemic stroke: 2005 guidelines update a scientific statement from the Stroke Council of the American Heart Association/American Stroke Association. Stroke 2005;36:916-923.
60. Tissue plasminogen activator for acute ischemic stroke. The National Institute of Neurological Disorders and Stroke rtPA Stroke Study Group. N Engl J Med 1995;333: 1581-1587.
61. Hoffman JR, Cooper RJ. Stroke thrombolysis: We need new data, not more reviews. Lancet Neurol 2005;4(4):204-205.
62. Hacke W, Albers G, Al-Rawi Y, et al: The Desmoteplase in Acute Ischemic Stroke Trial (DIAS): A phase II MRI-based 9-hour window acute stroke thrombolysis trial with intravenous desmoteplase. Stroke 2005;36:66-73.
63. Randomised controlled trial of streptokinase, aspirin, and combination of both in treatment of acute ischaemic stroke. Multicentre Acute Stroke Trial—Italy (MAST-I) Group. Lancet 1995;346:1509-1514.
64. Thrombolytic therapy with streptokinase in acute ischemic stroke. The Multicenter Acute Stroke Trial—Europe Study Group. N Engl J Med 1996;335:145-150.
65. Donnan GA, Davis SM, Chambers BR, et al: Streptokinase for acute ischemic stroke with relationship to time of administration: Australian Streptokinase (ASK) Trial Study Group. JAMA 1996;276:961-966.
66. Hacke W, Kaste M, Fieschi C, et al: Intravenous thrombolysis with recombinant tissue plasminogen activator for acute hemispheric stroke. The European Cooperative Acute Stroke Study (ECASS). JAMA 1995;274:1017-1025.
67. Hacke W, Kaste M, Fieschi C, et al: Randomised double-blind placebo-controlled trial of thrombolytic therapy with intravenous alteplase in acute ischaemic stroke (ECASS II). Second European-Australasian Acute Stroke Study Investigators. Lancet 1998;352:1245-1251.
68. Clark WM, Wissman S, Albers GW, et al: Recombinant tissue-type plasminogen activator (Alteplase) for ischemic stroke 3 to 5 hours after symptom onset. The ATLANTIS Study: A randomized controlled trial. Alteplase Thrombolysis for Acute Noninterventional Therapy in Ischemic Stroke. JAMA 1999;282:2019-2026.
69. Lindsberg PJ, Soinne L, Tatlisumak T, et al: Long-term outcome after intravenous thrombolysis of basilar artery occlusion. JAMA 2004;292:1862-1866.
70. Choi JH, Bateman BT, Mangla S, et al: Endovascular recanalization therapy in acute ischemic stroke. Stroke 2006; 37:419-424.
71. Stead LG, Gilmore RM, Decker WW, et al: Initial emergency department blood pressure as predictor of survival after acute ischemic stroke. Neurology 2005;65:1179-1183.
72. Lindsberg PJ, Roine RO: Hyperglycemia in acute stroke. Stroke 2004;35:363-364.
73. Klijn CJ, Hankey GJ: Management of acute ischaemic stroke: New guidelines from the American Stroke Association and European Stroke Initiative. Lancet Neurol 2003;2:698-701.
74. Hajat C, Hajat S, Sharma P: Effects of poststroke pyrexia on stroke outcome: A meta-analysis of studies in patients. Stroke 2000;31:410-414.
75. The International Stroke Trial (IST): A randomised trial of aspirin, subcutaneous heparin, both, or neither among 19435 patients with acute ischaemic stroke. International Stroke Trial Collaborative Group. Lancet 1997;349: 1569-1581.
76. Diener HC, Ringelstein EB, von Kummer R, et al: Treatment of acute ischemic stroke with the low-molecular-weight heparin certoparin: Results of the TOPAS trial. Therapy of Patients With Acute Stroke (TOPAS) Investigators. Stroke 2001;32:22-29.
77. Swanson RA: Intravenous heparin for acute stroke: What can we learn from the megatrials? Neurology 1999;52: 1746-1750.
78. Coull BM, Williams LS, Goldstein LB, et al: Anticoagulants and antiplatelet agents in acute ischemic stroke: Report of the Joint Stroke Guideline Development Committee of the American Academy of Neurology and the American Stroke Association (a division of the American Heart Association). Stroke 2002;33:1934-1942.
79. Moonis M, Fisher M: Considering the role of heparin and low-molecular-weight heparins in acute ischemic stroke. Stroke 2002;33:1927-1933.
80. Jorgensen HS, Nakayama H, Raaschou HO, et al: The effect of a stroke unit: Reductions in mortality, discharge rate to nursing home, length of hospital stay, and cost. A community-based study. Stroke 1995;26:1178-1182.
81. Evans A, Harraf F, Donaldson N, Kalra L: Randomized controlled study of stroke unit care versus stroke team care in different stroke subtypes. Stroke 2002;33:449-455.

Chapter **96**

Headache

Joshua N. Goldstein and Jonathan A. Edlow

KEY POINTS

Always inquire about the quality, severity, and associated symptoms of previous headaches. Specifically ask about how the current headache compares with previous headaches; a new headache due to a serious "cannot miss" cause will almost always have a unique quality.

The most frequently missed items on the neurologic examination are visual fields and gait. These cover a large neuroanatomic territory and should be consistently documented.

Any new abnormal neurologic finding must be explored and identified.

When evaluating for a nontraumatic subarachnoid hemorrhage, always follow a negative computed tomography (CT) scan with a lumbar puncture.

When a patient has a "worst-of-life" headache and the maximal intensity is at the onset, CT and lumbar puncture are indicated.

Scope and Outline

Approximately 2% to 4% of all ED visits are for headache.[1] Only a small proportion (as low as 2%) of patients presenting to the ED with a headache suffer a life-, limb-, or vision-threatening illness.[2] However, distinguishing these patients from the much larger group of those with benign headaches is a significant challenge because delayed diagnosis of serious disorders such as meningitis and subarachnoid hemorrhage can lead to catastrophic outcomes.

■ SOURCES OF PAIN

The sensation of headache is rarely due to injury of the brain parenchyma itself. Rather, head pain results from tension, traction, distention, dilation, or inflammation of pain-sensitive structures external to the skull, portions of the dura, and the blood vessels. Each of these mechanisms is likely mediated by a final common biochemical pathway that results in pain; therefore, a favorable response to analgesics should not be used to judge the cause of an individual headache.

■ APPROACH TO PATIENT CARE

EPs should develop a logical, practical, and accurate approach to identification of patients with serious pathology. A comprehensive organizational scheme developed by the International Headache Society has recently been updated (Table 96-1); however, this scheme is cumbersome for the practicing EP. For practical purposes, headaches can be divided into "benign" and "cannot miss" categories, shown in Table 96-2.

Before moving on to the history and physical examination phases of the evaluation, the EP should

Table 96-1 INTERNATIONAL HEADACHE SOCIETY CLASSIFICATION OF HEADACHES

Headache Associated with	Comments
Migraine	Requires five or more attacks of a specific nature, lasting 4 to 72 hours; can be unilateral, pulsating, moderate or severe in intensity, aggravated by physical activity, or associated with nausea, vomiting, photophobia
Tension-type	Requires 10 or more attacks of a specific nature, lasting 30 minutes to 7 days; absence of nausea, vomiting, and photophobia
Cluster type	Requires 5 or more attacks of a specific nature, lasting 15 to 180 minutes; always unilateral; associated with eye, nose, or face symptoms
Other primary headaches	Includes a variety of brief (idiopathic stabbing headache) and situational (cough, exertional, coital) headache syndromes
Head trauma	Includes minor post-injury headaches
Vascular disorders	Includes cerebral ischemia and infarction, all forms of intracranial hemorrhage, venous sinus thromboses, giant cell arteritis, arterial dissections
Nonvascular intracranial disorders	Includes idiopathic intracranial hypertension, post–lumbar puncture headache, and tumor
Substance abuse or their withdrawal	Includes drugs and food additives (e.g., monosodium glutamate headache, or Chinese restaurant syndrome); also includes headache from carbon monoxide poisoning
Infections	Includes headaches due to intracranial (meningitis, abscess) or extracranial infection
Disorders of homeostasis	Includes headaches due to hypercarbia, high-altitude illness, hypertensive encephalopathy, preeclampsia
HEENT (head, eyes, ears, nose, and throat) disorders (includes dental)	Includes narrow angle closure glaucoma, sinusitis, temporomandibular joint disorder
Cranial neuralgias, nerve trunk and deafferentation pain	Most of these are cranial neuropathies or associated with herpes zoster

From Olesen J: International Classification of Headache Disorders, Second Edition (ICHD-2): Current status and future revisions. Cephalalgia 2006;26:1409-1410.

attend immediately to pain management. Appropriate analgesia is all that most patients will require, and comfortable patients are more willing to undergo tests and procedures (such as a lumbar puncture). Immediate pain control results in greater patient satisfaction and more rapid disposition. That said, a given patient's response to analgesics should not alter the diagnostic strategy, and thus there is no diagnostic or therapeutic reason to withhold treatment.

Presenting Signs and Symptoms

The evaluation should focus on those signs and symptoms that can differentiate a benign headache from one requiring emergent work-up and treatment. For example, although headache location is often considered significant, unilateral headache is a hallmark of both primary (migraine, cluster) and secondary (intracerebral hemorrhage, glaucoma) headaches, limiting its usefulness in diagnosis. In contrast, fever and neck stiffness are uncommon in primary headache and are therefore extremely useful.

■ TIMING AND DURATION

Identifying the timing and duration of the headache is critical. Questions such as "What brings you here today, rather than any other day?" can help focus patients on the timing of their symptoms. Worrisome features include a new acute headache or a subacute headache that is increasing in severity. Abrupt or "thunderclap" onset suggests intracranial hemorrhage or cerebral venous sinus thrombosis. If the maximum intensity of the pain was at the onset, sentinel aneurismal bleeding must be considered. Very fleeting headaches, termed "jabs and jolts," that last seconds are typically benign. In abrupt onset headaches, the activity at onset sometimes suggests the etiology, such as in coital headache or benign exertional headache. However, while a history of these activities can be a sensitive indicator for the corresponding diagnoses, specificity is poor. Therefore, subarachnoid hemorrhage cannot be excluded on the basis of pre-headache activity.

■ LOCATION

The location of pain is not very helpful in diagnosis of headache, as there is significant overlap between benign and serious etiologies. Some recommend work-up of patients whose headaches are always on the same side.[3]

■ SEVERITY

Severity of pain also has limitations in differentiating benign from serious headaches. While the "worst-of-life" headache suggests a more serious problem, most severe headaches in the ED have benign causes. That said, patients who have never before sought medical care for a headache should be considered to have a

Table 96-2 "CANNOT MISS" DIAGNOSES

Diagnosis	Suggestive History and Physical Findings	Diagnostic Testing
Meningitis and encephalitis	Fever, stiff neck, jolt accentuation, altered mental status, seizure	LP; if preceded by a CT, give antibiotics before CT
Subarachnoid hemorrhage*	Abrupt onset of severe headache, stiff neck, 3rd nerve palsy	CT scan; LP if CT is non-diagnostic
Stroke (ischemic or hemorrhagic)	Abrupt onset and focal neurologic deficit conforming to an arterial territory	CT scan; MRI if available will give more information (should not delay thrombolytic therapy)
Dissection of craniocervical arteries	Neck pain, abrupt onset, variable presence of neurologic deficit	CT angiography, MRA, or conventional angiography
Hypertensive encephalopathy	Severe (usually chronic) hypertension; often papilledema and other signs of end-organ damage	Careful, titratable lowering of blood pressure by ~25% of the peak blood pressure will decrease the headache
Idiopathic intracranial hypertension	Obese, female patient; papilledema; often 6th nerve palsy	LP (following an imaging study, that by definition will be normal)
Giant cell arteritis	Nearly always age >50 years; symptoms of polymyalgia rheumatica; abnormal scalp vessels	ESR; temporal artery biopsy
Acute angle closure glaucoma	Painful red eye with mid-position pupil and corneal edema	Tonometry
Intracranial mass (tumor, abscess, hematoma)†	Any focal or generalized neurologic finding	CT scan; if available, MRI will provide more information
Cerebral venous sinus thrombosis	Hypercoagulable state of any type	MRI and MRA with venous phase; CT with venous phase
Carbon monoxide poisoning	Cluster of cases, winter season	COHb level
Pituitary apoplexy	Visual acuity or field abnormalities Known pituitary tumor	MRI

*See Figure 96-1.
†See Figure 96-2.
COHb, carboxyhemoglobin; CT, computed tomography; LP, lumbar puncture; MRA, magnetic resonance angiography; MRI, magnetic resonance imaging.

secondary headache until proven otherwise. Even in those with previous visits, a headache of clearly increased severity should lower one's threshold for further diagnostic testing, and most patients with a worst-of-life headache should be evaluated for subarachnoid hemorrhage.

■ QUALITY

The quality of the patient's pain is critical. Most serious headaches are qualitatively unique and unusual. If a patient has chronic headaches that present with new or unusual features, careful evaluation is required.

■ SPECIFIC ASSOCIATED SYMPTOMS

Specific associated symptoms can provide important clues into a dangerous cause of the headache. Fever and neck stiffness are worrisome for meningitis. Syncope, seizure, or any focal neurologic symptoms or new signs associated with a headache should prompt an evaluation. Diplopia suggests a mass, cerebral aneurysm, or elevated intracranial pressure.

Unfortunately, migraine headaches can produce an array of associated symptoms traditionally associated with secondary headaches. Although nausea, vomiting, and photophobia can occur with increased intracranial pressure or infection, they are also associated with migraines. The key differentiating factor in migraineurs is whether they have developed these symptoms for the first time. Visual abnormalities are associated with both migraine headaches and idiopathic intracranial hypertension, temporal arteritis, and pituitary apoplexy.

■ EXACERBATING AND ALLEVIATING FACTORS

Exacerbating and alleviating factors are occasionally helpful. Post–lumbar puncture headache tends to worsen on standing upright, and headache due to sinusitis often worsens on bending forward with the head dependent. In contrast, the classic sign of a headache from brain tumor—that it is worse on awakening—is neither specific nor sensitive, because this also is seen in patients with chronic lung disease and hypercarbia (in which headache worsens during sleep). In terms of alleviating factors, diagnostic significance should not be ascribed to pain relief, even with over-the-counter medications.

BOX 96-1

Critical Features of the History in the ED

Timing
- Abrupt onset, "thunderclap"

Location
- Nonspecific

Severity
- Worst of life, most severe; have never been to an ED before

Quality
- New type, different from previous headaches

Associated Symptoms
- Fever, neck stiffness
- Seizure, syncope
- Focal neurologic complaints
- Visual abnormalities (diplopia)

Exacerbating/Alleviating
- Nonspecific

Past Medical History
- Stroke, vascular disease, cancer
- Immunocompromised
- Coagulopathy or bleeding diasthesis

Family History
- Coagulopathy, bleeding diasthesis, cerebral aneurysm

■ OTHER FACTORS

Age is an important factor because new-onset headache at older ages suggests a secondary cause, such as giant cell arteritis, tumors, subdural hematoma, and side effects of medication.[4] Environmental considerations include winter season and common source clusters, which can indicate carbon monoxide poisoning.

Medical and Family History

The medical history is directed at determining predisposition for a secondary cause of headache. For example, poorly treated hypertension may lead to hypertensive encephalopathy, vascular risk factors can result in stroke, and a medical or family history of cerebral aneurysm increases the likelihood of subarachnoid hemorrhage (Box 96-1).

Hypercoagulability or a history of thromboembolic events should raise the possibility of cerebral venous sinus thrombosis. In contrast, patients with hemophilia are at higher risk of bleeding, and should not only receive a CT scan but should receive factor replacement even before the CT scan. Obesity increases the possibility of idiopathic intracranial hypertension (pseudotumor cerebri), especially in women. A history of metastatic cancer can raise suspicion for brain metastasis, and patients with human immunodeficiency virus (HIV) or taking immunosuppressive medicines are at higher risk of infection.

Physical Examination

The physical examination (Box 96-2) is critical in guiding the differential diagnosis and appropriate work-up.

■ GENERAL APPEARANCE AND VITAL SIGNS

General appearance is in part a function of pain threshold and may be deceiving. For example, shielding one's eyes from the light can be consistent with both migraine and meningeal irritation. Fever is not a symptom of migraine and suggests infection, or a several-day-old subarachnoid hemorrhage. Hypertension suggests hypertensive encephalopathy, stroke, or other secondary causes but also, more commonly, is a result of pain or stress. Early appropriate analgesia can help distinguish these possibilities. The EP should have a low threshold for brain imaging (and possibly lumbar puncture) in patients with headache and persistent hypertension.

■ HEAD AND NECK

The head, eyes, ears, nose, and throat (HEENT) examination may reveal the cause of headache. Vesicles on the scalp, nose, or external ear canal suggest herpes zoster. Temporal artery tenderness, nodularity, or thickening suggests giant cell arteritis. A red eye with an edematous cornea and mid-position pupil suggests narrow angle closure glaucoma. A proptotic eye or chemosis suggests a cavernous sinus thrombosis. Papilledema is specific but poorly sensitive for increased intracranial pressure, whereas venous pulsations in the retina indicate normal intracranial pressure.

Examination of the neck should be directed at signs of meningeal irritation. Meningismus (stiffness on passive flexion of the neck) may be seen in patients with infections (meningitis) or irritation (subarachnoid hemorrhage). However, this finding is not reliably present, and its absence does not exclude these diagnoses. One physical finding that is more reliable in diagnosing meningitis is "jolt accentuation"; when the patient is asked to turn the head horizontally two to three rotations per second, the baseline headache increases in intensity.[5]

Neurologic Examination

A complete neurologic examination should be performed and documented on all patients with the chief complaint of headache. Recognizing that some

BOX 96-2

Critical Features (Potential Diagnoses) of the Physical Examination

Vital Signs

- Fever (meningitis, encephalitis, abscess)
- Elevated blood pressure (ischemic, hemorrhagic stroke)

Head

- Vesicles on scalp (herpes zoster of upper two cervical roots or root of 6th trigeminal nerve)
- Tender temporal artery (giant cell arteritis)
- Tender sinuses (sinusitis)

Eyes

- Red, edematous (acute angle closure glaucoma)
- Proptosis (cavernous sinus thrombosis)
- Papilledema (increased intracranial pressure)

Ears

- Vesicles in external ear canal (Ramsay-Hunt syndrome)

Nose

- Vesicles on tip of nose (herpes zoster of root of 6th trigeminal nerve)

Neck

- Meningismus with positive Kernig's sign; positive Brudzinski's sign (infection; subarachnoid hemorrhage)

Neurologic Examination

- Change in mental status (increased intracranial pressure; infection; toxidrome [carbon monoxide intoxication])
- Decreased visual acuity (giant cell arteritis; acute angle closure glaucoma)
- Visual field cut (mass lesion; pituitary apoplexy)
- Third nerve palsy (subarachnoid hemorrhage; cavernous sinus thrombosis)
- Sixth nerve palsy (increased or decreased intracranial pressure; basilar meningitis)
- Direction-changing nystagmus (cerebellar or brainstem stroke)
- Lower motor neuron 7th nerve palsy (Bell's palsy; Ramsay-Hunt syndrome)
- Eighth nerve palsy (diminished hearing or vertigo; Ramsay-Hunt syndrome)
- Gait ataxia (cerebellar stroke)
- Any focal sensory or motor deficit (mass lesion; stroke)

Documentation

- The history should include timing and severity of headache onset, as well as any neurologic complaints.
- The physical examination should always include an extensive neurologic examination. Any new neurologic findings must be explored.
- Visual fields and gait assessment cover a wide range of neuroanatomic territory and are often either inadequately tested or inadequately documented.
- Be very careful assigning a patient with the diagnosis of "migraine headache" if they do not already have this diagnosis, or if the current headache is quite different from their usual migraines.

Cautions for the Physician

- Just because a patient states that he or she has had "migraine" (or tension, or "sinus") headaches does not mean that the headaches ever formally met these criteria or have ever been evaluated, or that this headache is the same as the previous headaches.
- If head computed tomography (CT) is performed to evaluate for subarachnoid hemorrhage, it should always be followed by lumbar puncture to evaluate for xanthochromia and the presence of blood.
- Response to analgesics has little or no diagnostic significance and should not be used to exclude a secondary cause of headache.

patients with migraine headaches may have neurologic deficits, the presences of new neurologic abnormities should trigger a work-up beyond history and physical examination. Abnormalities may suggest a diagnosis of and the location of a mass lesion or cerebrovascular accident. Abnormal mental status with a new headache suggests increased intracranial pressure, a diffuse process such as meningitis, or carbon monoxide poisoning.

Diagnostic Testing

Following a careful history and physical examination, the physician must determine whether further diagnostic testing is necessary. In patients with new abnormal physical findings, the need for further diagnostic testing is unambiguous. Similarly, patients with a reassuring medical and family history and a normal physical examination may require only appropriate analgesia and follow-up arrangements. Diagnostic dilemmas usually arise with patients who have normal physical examinations but some worrisome aspect of the history. Some decision rules have been published, but for the most part, experience, judgment, careful attention to the history and physi-

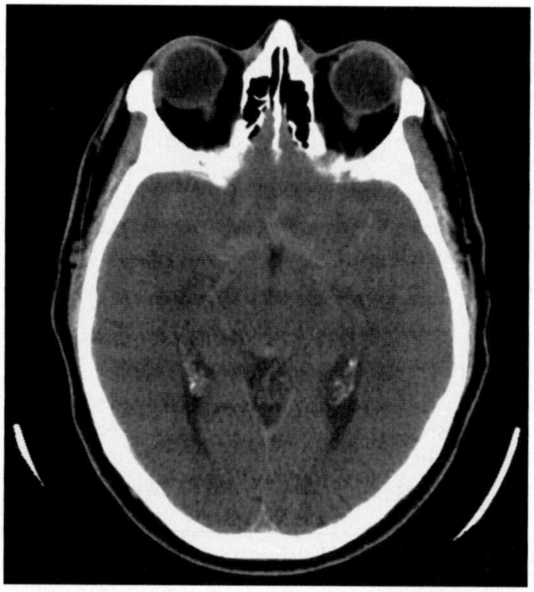

FIGURE 96-1 Subarachnoid hemorrhage.

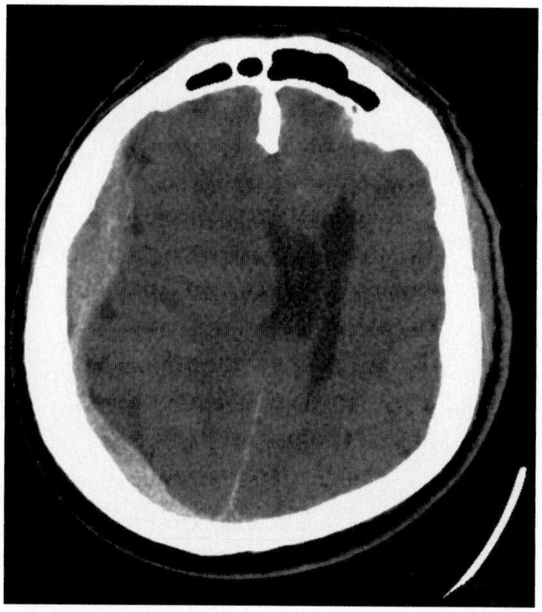

FIGURE 96-2 Subdural hematoma.

cal examination, and the differential diagnosis should guide further testing.

■ COMPUTED TOMOGRAPHY (CT) SCANNING

CT scanning is often the first neuroimaging test, as it is both rapid and widely available. A noncontrast CT scan is extremely sensitive for acute intraparenchymal bleeding and very sensitive for subarachnoid bleeding (Fig. 96-1), but small or less acute subarachnoid bleeding may not be visible. Although some tumors and abscesses are not visible on a scan performed without IV contrast media, most masses large enough to cause a significant headache with focal neurologic findings can be seen on CT even without a contrast agent (Fig. 96-2). It is critical to convey any focal neurologic signs or symptoms to the radiologist reading the CT scan so that appropriate attention can be directed to the anatomic site in question.

Which patients require CT scanning is a matter of some debate.[6] There are no hard and fast rules, but generally, high-risk factors indicate the need for CT (Box 96-3).

The type of CT to perform depends on the specific differential diagnosis under consideration. Imaging of a mass or an abscess can be improved with IV contrast infusion. CT angiography can be performed with a multidetector scanner, and depending on the number of detectors, the software available, and the skill of the neuroradiologist can approach conventional angiography for direct visualization of the cerebral vasculature. For patients in whom an arteriovenous malformation or aneurysm is suspected, this is a useful modality. CT venography can be useful in the diagnosis of cerebral venous sinus thrombosis.

BOX 96-3

Indications for Computed Tomography Scanning

History

- New type of headache
- Hemophilia
- Coagulopathy
- Blunt trauma
- Immunocompromised (human immunodeficency virus infection, chemotherapy)
- Elderly
- Fever with neurologic findings

Physical Examination

- Glascow Coma Scale less than 15 with no clear explanation
- Any focal neurologic finding
- Signs of increased intracranial pressure

■ MAGNETIC RESONANCE IMAGING (MRI)

In general, MRI is superior to CT, especially in evaluating vascular and neoplastic lesions and infections and pathology at the cervicomedullary junction and in the posterior fossa.[3] Brain tumors, abscesses, ischemia and pituitary apoplexy are easily visible. Recent studies suggest that MRI may even identify small cerebral hemorrhages that are not detected by CT scanning.[7] Arterial and venous blood vessels can be evaluated by MR angiography. Carotid and vertebral artery dissections, cerebral aneurysms, and cerebral venous sinus thromboses can be diagnosed using MR angiography and MR venography.

Given the expense and scarcity of this resource, it is critical that the EP carefully evaluate its necessity. For example, a young patient with known coagulopathy, new-onset headache, and signs of cerebellar ischemia, may require MRI evaluation for cerebellar stroke or cerebral venous thrombosis. Similarly, any newly documented neurologic deficit must be explained, and if contrast CT scanning is not sufficient to exclude an emergent cause, patients should be transferred to a facility with available MRI.

■ LUMBAR PUNCTURE

Lumbar puncture has a central role as a diagnostic tool for headache patients. If it is necessary to rule out subarachnoid hemorrhage, the EP must be aware that CT scanning can be nondiagnostic and that a lumbar puncture is the necessary next step.

Lumbar puncture can establish the diagnosis of suspected meningitis with nearly 100% sensitivity. An elevated opening pressure suggests idiopathic intracranial hypertension or cerebral venous sinus thrombosis. However, like all tests in medicine, even the lumbar puncture has limitations. In particular, patients on prednisone therapy who are otherwise immunocompromised may not have the elevated cerebrospinal fluid white blood cell count expected. A lumbar puncture to rule out subarachnoid hemorrhage can be traumatic as well, making interpretation difficult. In such cases an elevated opening pressure may help identify pathology such as subarachnoid hemorrhage.

■ LABORATORY STUDIES

Laboratory studies are rarely helpful in the work-up of headache. The white cell count is too nonspecific for identifying an infectious cause. However, the erythrocyte sedimentation rate (ESR) can be useful in ruling out giant cell arteritis. Although the ESR is not specific, it is highly sensitive. A toxicology screen may show evidence of cocaine or other sympathomimetics, which can raise suspicion of hypertensive intracerebral hemorrhage. Carboxyhemoglobin assay can be useful in patients with other nonspecific symptoms, with a family history of similar symptoms, or with risk factors such as living in an older house or cold weather.

■ TONOMETRY

Tonometry is a critical test in the ED for elderly patients with headache, eye complaints, and risk factors for glaucoma. Acute narrow angle closure glaucoma is an ophthalmologic emergency that can be diagnosed and treated quickly.

■ TEMPORAL ARTERY BIOPSY

Temporal artery biopsy is not a standard ED procedure. However, in a patient in whom there is a strong likelihood of giant cell arteritis, high-dose oral steroid therapy should be initiated emergently, and rapid follow-up arranged to establish the diagnosis.

■ NEUROLOGY CONSULTATON

One final "test" to be considered is a neurology consultation. The timing of a consultation can vary, depending on the differential diagnosis and the duration of the headache. In patients with a new, definite neurologic finding on physical examination and normal results on brain imaging, the physician should consider urgent or emergent neurologic consultation.

Treatment

■ TREATMENT OF EMERGENT CONDITIONS

Airway protection is always paramount in the critically ill patient. If the need does arise, it is usually in patients with impending herniation from a mass lesion or intracranial bleeding. Although a neurologic examination is important in the acute phase of the patient's hospitalization, short-term paralysis for rapid-sequence intubation can and should be used to achieve the optimal intubation conditions.

Once the airway is secure, sedation can be minimized to provide the best possible serial neurologic examination (propofol is a short-acting sedative that is often used for this purpose). Agents such as lidocaine and fentanyl are often advocated to blunt the transient rise in intracranial pressure that accompanies tracheal intubation. If airway management precedes imaging, emergent neuroimaging should rapidly follow intubation.

For patients with signs or symptoms of acute bacterial meningitis, a critical early decision is whether to perform a CT scan or proceed directly to lumbar puncture (Box 96-4).[8] Never delay antibiotic administration in patients who have signs of meningitis. Performing a lumbar puncture directly in an alert

PRIORITY ACTIONS

- Treat pain early. Response to pain should not affect the work-up, so there is no reason to withhold appropriate analgesia.
- Patients with hemophilia and headache require factor repletion emergently, even before head CT, given their high risk for intracranial hemorrhage.
- Patients with signs and symptoms of acute bacterial meningitis require early antibiotics, even if the diagnosis is not yet established.

BOX 96-4

Patient Features That Suggest Performing CT before Lumbar Puncture

History
- Age greater than 60 years
- Immunocompromised
- History of central nervous system disease (such as tumor)
- Recent seizure

Physical Examination
- Altered mental status
- Any new focal neurologic finding
- Papilledema

neurologically intact patient with no medical history usually is safe, especially in those with normal venous pulsations on funduscopy.

BLOOD PRESSURE

Although treatment of elevated blood pressure can be tempting, the EP should avoid this impulse. Elevated blood pressure on arrival in the ED is usually either a nonspecific response to pain or a result of cerebral autoregulation in the face of brain injury or ischemia. Treatment should be undertaken only when the diagnosis is clear.

There are three major indications for blood pressure reduction: hypertensive encephalopathy, ruptured cerebral aneurysm, and intraparenchymal hemorrhage.

Hypertensive Encephalopathy

Reduction of the mean arterial pressure by 25% shculd improve the headache and other signs of end-organ damage.

Ruptured Cerebral Aneurysm

Although high-quality evidence is lacking, it is generally considered prudent to lower the systolic blood pressure to less than 140 or even 120 mm Hg, using labetalol, nitroprusside, or nicardipine. This is in contrast to an ischemic stroke, in which higher blood pressure levels (up to 220/120 mm Hg) are acceptable or even desired.[9]

Intraparenchymal Hemorrhage

In patients with intraparenchymal hemorrhage, the American Heart Association recommends lowering blood pressure to less than 180/105 mm Hg, using labetalol or nitroprusside.[10]

TREATMENT OF URGENT CONDITIONS

Giant Cell Arteritis (Temporal Arteritis)

Giant cell arteritis classically presents with sudden, severe, temporal headache in patients older than 50 years of age. The major differentiating feature of this disease is the presence of ischemic manifestations such as jaw claudication and visual loss.[11] In the ED, this is considered a clinical diagnosis; therefore, the patient should receive immediate empirical administration of prednisone, 40 to 60 mg/day. A temporal artery biopsy should be scheduled within several days to establish a definitive diagnosis, although even a negative biopsy does not definitively rule out this disorder. The decision whether to continue steroid therapy following a negative biopsy should be made by the primary care physician in consultation with appropriate specialists.

Acute Angle Closure Glaucoma

Patients with acute angle closure glaucoma typically present with recurrent unilateral headache behind the eye associated with blurred vision and erythema; often there will be a prolonged course of symptoms before appropriate diagnosis.[12] Although the diagnosis is usually based on clinical findings, tonometry can establish the condition. Intraocular pressure in the affected eye will be elevated up to 40 to 80 mm Hg. In addition to appropriate pain control, any or all of the following therapies may be considered:

1. Acetazolamine: 500 mg intravenously followed by 500 mg orally
2. Timolol: 0.25% to 0.5% applied topically
3. Prednisolone: 1-2 drops to the affected eye
4. Pilocarpine: 2% applied topically
5. Isosorbide: 1.5 g/kg orally or glycerin 1-2 g/kg orally
6. Mannitol: 1.5 to 2 g/kg intravenously
7. Antiemetics and analgesia as needed

The ophthalmology service should be consulted emergently, because peripheral iridectomy or laser iridotomy is the definitive treatment for acute angle closure glaucoma.

Sinusitis-Related Headache

Pain control is the cornerstone of treatment. Nonsteroidal agents and decongestants can be provided. Oxymetazoline nasal spray should be used for no more than 3 days. The Centers for Disease Control and Prevention recommends that the diagnosis of bacterial sinusitis be made only after 7 days of symptoms, and that amoxicillin should be administered as a first-line agent for mild sinusitis with no previous antibiotic use.

Migraine Headache

Migraine headache classically is defined as a throbbing unilateral headache, with a number of associated symptoms including photophobia, pho-

Table 96-3 DIFFERENTIATION OF BENIGN FROM POTENTIALLY PATHOLOGIC HEADACHES

	HEADACHE TYPE		
Finding	Migraine	Tension	Pathologic
History of headaches	Yes	Yes	No
New type of headache	No	No	Yes
Aura	Yes	No	Maybe
Nausea/vomiting	Yes	No	Yes
Focal neurologic finding	Yes	No	Yes
Tender to palpation	No	Yes	No

nophobia, nausea, and vomiting. The headache can be preceded by an "aura," such as scintillating scotomata, jagged lines, or other visual abnormalities. Finally, migraine can be complicated by neurologic abnormalities including hemiparesis, paresthesias, ophthalmoplegia, and aphasia. The patient will usually have a history of headaches of similar quality and often has a family history of migraines.

Of note, migraine is most accurately diagnosed by a history of at least five similar headaches with several specific criteria. New-onset headaches or those of a different or unusual quality, often require further work-up. Table 96-3 lists some of the features that can help differentiate migraine and tension headaches from more serious conditions. One cannot confidently diagnose migraine or tension headache at the initial onset of a new headache.

Pain control is the cornerstone of treatment. The American Academy of Neurology has published a set of evidence-based guidelines for management of acute attacks, some of which are summarized in Box 96-5.[13] Opiates often are used in the ED and are effective; however, they typically should be reserved for rescue therapy in patients who do not respond to initial migraine-specific therapy.

BOX 96-5

Management of Moderate to Severe Acute Migraine Headaches

Triptans
- First-line agents
- Sumatriptan (Imitrex)—nasal spray or subcutaneous
- Zolmitriptan (Zomig)—oral

Ergot Alkaloids and Derivatives
- Can be first-line
- Dihydroergotamine (DHE 45)—nasal spray, subcutaneous, intravenous, or intramuscular
- Ergotamine—oral, rectal (with caffeine)

Antiemetics
- First-line agents
- Prochlorperazine (Compazine)—intravenous; proven statistical and clinical benefit
- Metoclopramide (Reglan)—adjunctive therapy to control nausea, but can be monotherapy
- Serotonin antagonists (Zofran)—less effective for monotherapy but can be adjunctive therapy to control nausea

Nonsteroidal Anti-inflammatory Drugs (NSAIDs)
- Combination agents containing caffeine can be first-line agents
- Acetaminophen, aspirin plus caffeine
- Ibuprofen with or without caffeine

Butalbital-Containing Agents
- Often used but can cause headaches

Opiates
- Parenteral opiates considered for rescue therapy (second-line agents)
- Morphine, dilaudid, methadone

Agents Sometimes Used but of Unclear Efficacy
- Lidocaine—intranasal
- Corticosteroids—rescue therapy for status migrainosus headaches
- Isometheptene

■ CLUSTER HEADACHE

Cluster headache typically presents as a severe unilateral headache that can be accompanied by conjunctival injection, lacrimation, ptosis, miosis, rhinorrhea, and nasal congestion.[14] Attacks can occur up to eight times a day and are severe but short-lived; the autonomic symptoms are typically unilateral and ipsilateral to the pain. Recognition is important because this headache subtype is uniquely sensitive to oxygen. Mainstays of emergency management include oxygen and subcutaneous sumatriptan (Box 96-6).

■ TENSION HEADACHE

Tension headache typically is characterized by throbbing pain that radiates bilaterally from front to back and to the neck muscles. As with migraine headaches, one cannot firmly diagnose tension headache after a single episode, and this diagnosis requires

BOX 96-6

Acute Management of Cluster Headache

- Oxygen (7 L/minute for 15 minutes by face mask)
- Sumatriptan (6 mg subcutaneously or 20 mg nasal spray)
- Dihydroergotamine nasal spray (Note: Do not combine ergotamines with sumatriptan)
- Lidocaine intranasally (1 mL of 4% solution ipsilaterally)

more than nine previous episodes. Pain control consists of nonsteroidal anti-inflammatory drugs (NSAIDs), antiemetics, and perhaps caffeine (Box 96-7). Butalbital-containing agents (as with migraine headaches) may be used with caution, given the risk of dependency and rebound headache.

BOX 96-7

Acute Management of Tension Headache

- Nonsteroidal antiinflammatory drugs (NSAIDs)
- Antihistamines
  - Diphenhydramine (Benadryl)
  - Promethazine (Phenergan)
- Antiemetics
  - Metoclopramide (Reglan)
  - Prochlorperazine (Compazine)
- Butalbital-containing agents
  - Acetaminophen+caffeine+butalbital
  - Aspirin+caffeine+butalbital

REFERENCES

1. Edlow JA: Diagnosis of subarachnoid hemorrhage in the emergency department. Emerg Med Clin North Am 2003;21:73-87.
2. Goldstein JN, Camargo CA Jr, Pelletier AJ, Edlow JA: Headache in United States emergency departments: Demographics, work-up and frequency of pathological diagnoses. Cephalagia 2006;26:684-690.
3. Evans RW: Diagnostic testing for the evaluation of headaches. Neurol Clin 1996;14:1-26.
4. Ramirez-Lassepas M, Espinosa CE, Cicero JJ, et al: Predictors of intracranial pathologic findings in patients who seek emergency care because of headache. Arch Neurol 1997;54:1506-1509.
5. Attia J, Hatala R, Cook DJ, Wong JG: The rational clinical examination. Does this adult patient have acute meningitis? JAMA 1999;282:175-181.
6. Detsky ME, McDonald DR, Baerlocher MO, et al: Does this patient with headache have a migraine or need neuroimaging? JAMA 2006;296:1274-1283.
7. Eliasziw M, Paddock-Eliasziw L: Comparison of MRI and CT for detection of acute intracerebral hemorrhage. JAMA 2005;293:550; author reply, 550-551.
8. Hasbun R, Abrahams J, Jekel J, Quagliarello VJ: Computed tomography of the head before lumbar puncture in adults with suspected meningitis. N Engl J Med 2001;345:1727-1733.
9. Adams H, Adams R, Del Zoppo G, et al: Guidelines for the early management of patients with ischemic stroke: 2005 guidelines update a scientific statement from the Stroke Council of the American Heart Association/American Stroke Association. Stroke 2005;36:916-923.
10. Broderick JP, Adams HP Jr, Barsan W, et al: Guidelines for the management of spontaneous intracerebral hemorrhage: A statement for healthcare professionals from a special writing group of the Stroke Council, American Heart Association. Stroke 1999;30:905-915.
11. Gonzalez-Gay MA, Barros S, Lopez-Diaz MJ, et al: Disease patterns of clinical presentation in a series of 240 patients. Medicine (Balt) 2005;84:269-276.
12. Shindler KS, Sankar PS, Volpe NJ, Piltz-Seymour JR: Intermittent headaches as the presenting sign of subacute angle-closure glaucoma. Neurology 2005;65:757-758.
13. Silberstein SD: Practice parameter: Evidence-based guidelines for migraine headache (an evidence-based review). Report of the Quality Standards Subcommittee of the American Academy of Neurology. Neurology 2000;55:754-762.
14. May A: Cluster headache: Pathogenesis, diagnosis, and management. Lancet 2005;366:843-855.

Chapter 97

Intracranial and Other Central Nervous System Lesions

Steven M. Zahn

KEY POINTS

Subtle neurologic complaints in the patient's history require specific muscle group testing and gait examination in addition to a symptom-focused physical examination.

A thorough neurologic examination based on a complaint of dizziness requires cerebellar testing including finger-nose, heel-shin, dysdiadochokinesia, and gait evaluation.

Fever in the setting of a neurologic complaint requires a thorough neurologic examination and strong consideration of neuroimaging.

Any patient with a first-time seizure warrants a non-contrast head computed tomography (CT) scan regardless of age, due to the possibility of intracranial pathology (Box 97-1).

CT scans reliably demonstrate lesions 1.0 cm or larger; if results are negative but suspicion remains, magnetic resonance imaging (MRI) should be ordered.

Scope

Presenting symptoms and signs in patients with intracranial lesions include headaches, seizures, focal neurologic changes, weakness, and fatigue. Headaches occur in approximately 50% of patients with central nervous system (CNS) tumors; however, brain tumors are uncommon in patients who present with a headache and a normal neurologic examination (<1% of the time).[1] Thus EPs should always consider the presence of a brain tumor in the differential diagnosis but should use neuroimaging judiciously (Table 97-1).[2,3] Focal neurologic changes always warrant further investigation in terms of laboratory tests, radiographic imaging, and neurologic and/or neurosurgical consultation.

Neuroimaging and Neuropathology

Most brain tumors causing clinical symptoms are visible on CT scans, and all are visible using the various contrast-enhanced techniques of CT and MRI. On non-enhanced CT, brain tumors are visualized by mass effect and altered attenuation. Masses may be hypo-, iso-, or hyperdense compared with surrounding structures and can be associated with vasogenic edema, which is visualized by low attenuation in the white matter. Bone-window settings can best appreciate extra-axial lesions because bone erosion or hyperostosis may be present.

Calcification can be useful in isolating brain tumors. Oligodendrogliomas contain calcification in

Table 97-1 GUIDELINES FOR NEUROIMAGING IN PATIENTS WITH A HEADACHE

Clinical Finding	Recommendation
"Thunderclap" headache with abnormal neurologic exam	Emergent neuroimaging recommended
Signs of increased intracranial pressure; fever and nuchal rigidity	Recommended to safely perform lumbar puncture
"Thunderclap" headache Headache radiating to the neck Temporal headache in older individual New onset headache in a patient who is: HIV positive Has a prior diagnosis of cancer In a population at high risk for intracranial disease Accompanied by an abnormal neurologic exam including, but not limited to, papilledema, unilateral loss of sensation, weakness, or hyperreflexia	Neuroimaging should be considered
Migraine and normal neurologic exam	Neuroimaging not usually warranted
Headache worsened by Valsalva maneuver, wakes patient from sleep, or is progressively worsening	No recommendation (some data for increased risk of intracranial abnormality, not sufficient for recommendation)
Tension headache with normal exam	No recommendation (insufficient data)

Adapted from guidelines developed by the U.S. Headache Consortium, American College of Emergency Physicians, and the American College of Radiology (American College of Emergency Physicians: Clinical policy: Critical issues in the evaluation and management of patients presenting to the emergency department with acute headache. Ann Emerg Med 2002;39:108).

BOX 97-1

Indications for CT Brain Scanning in Patients Presenting with First-Time Seizures

- New focal deficit
- Persistent altered mental status
- Fever
- Recent trauma
- Persistent headache
- History of cancer
- Anticoagulant use
- Suspicion or known history of AIDS
- Age older than 40 years
- Partial complex seizure

Adapted from guidelines developed by the U.S. Headache Consortium, American College of Emergency Physicians, and the American College of Radiology (American College of Emergency Physicians: Clinical policy: Critical issues in the evaluation and management of patients presenting to the emergency department with acute headache. Ann Emerg Med 2002; 39:108).

90% of cases. Other tumors with calcification include choroid plexus tumors, ependymoma, central neurocytoma, meningioma, craniopharyngioma, teratoma, and chordoma. Nonmalignant lesions such as neurocysticercosis, toxoplasmosis, and tuberous sclerosis manifest calcific changes on radiographic imaging as well.

The irregular margins of brain lesions tend to favor a diagnosis of metastasis or primary brain lesions over other intracranial pathology. Surrounding edema is often present. When contrast enhancement is used, small or isodense lesions are well visualized and certain tumors will have a large vascular component within the mass. Glioblastoma multiforme (grade 4), oligodendroglioma, and metastases (most commonly breast, lung, and melanoma) typically have a large vascular component within the tumor (Table 97-2).

Clinical Presentation

Brain tumors usually manifest with one of three syndromes: (1) subacute progression of a focal neurologic deficit; (2) seizure; or (3) nonfocal neurologic disorder such as headache (especially with nocturnal features or presentation upon awakening), dementia, personality changes, or gait disorder. The presence of systemic symptoms (malaise, fever, weight loss) suggests a metastatic rather than a primary brain tumor.[4]

■ METASTATIC DISEASE

Autopsy diagnosis reveals that nearly 25% of patients who die of cancer had intracranial metastasis (Fig. 97-1). The lung is the most common origin of brain metastases. Breast cancer (especially ductal carcinoma) has a propensity to metastasize to the cerebellum and the posterior pituitary gland; however, breast cancer that metastasizes to bone tends not to metastasize to the brain.

Other common origins of brain metastases are gastrointestinal malignancies (most commonly colon and rectum), renal carcinoma, and melanoma. In contrast, prostate, esophageal, ovarian cancer, and Hodgkin's disease rarely metastasize to the brain.

Table 97-2 CHARACTERISTIC APPEARANCE OF INTRACRANIAL AND CENTRAL NERVOUS SYSTEM LESIONS

Type of Lesion	Edema	Border	Calcification	Characteristics
Metastatic brain lesion	+	Irregular	±	Present at gray-white matter junction following cerebral blood flow
Central nervous system lymphoma	±	Irregular	–	Dense, homogeneous enhancing periventricular mass; white matter, ring-enhancing mass
Low-grade astrocytoma	+	Irregular	±	Iso- or hypointensity with minimal enhancement
High-grade astrocytomas/ glioblastoma multiforme	+	Irregular	±	Heterogeneous, hypointense, enhancing mass with surrounding edema; can involve both cerebral hemispheres
Ependymoma	±	±	+	Uniformly enhancing mass; well demarcated from adjacent tissue
Meningioma	±	Irregular	+	Extra-axial uniformly enhancing mass
Oligodendroglioma	±	±	+	Well-demarcated frontal-temporal mass with calcific streaks
Medulloblastoma	±	Irregular	±	Contrast-enhancing heterogeneous mass near or involving fourth ventricle
Hemangioblastoma (von Hippel-Lindau disease)	±	Irregular	– (blood may mimic)	Enhancing cerebellar cyst with nodule on wall of cyst; angiography important
Schwannoma	±	Irregular	–	Dense hyperintense mass around eighth cranial nerve; can have mass effect on pons/posterior fossa
Neurocysticercosis	+	Regular	+	Ring-enhancing low-density lesions; often multiple
Toxoplasmosis	+	Regular	+	Ring-enhancing low-density lesions; often multiple
Tuberculoma	–	Irregular	±	Iso- or hypodense lesions that mimic malignancy with contrast
Tuberous sclerosis	–	Irregular	+	Periventricular mass; often multiple
Arteriovenous malformation	–	Irregular	– (blood may mimic)	Heterogeneous hypodense mass with contrast-enhancing rim; lumbar puncture for diagnosis of subarachnoid hemorrhage; angiography required for diagnosis

+, present; –, not present; ±, may or may not be present.

Primary Central Nervous System Lymphoma

Primary CNS lymphoma has increased in prevalence over the last 2 decades due to AIDS and medical immunosuppression. These lesions are high-grade B-cell malignancies occurring in the CNS without evidence of systemic disease and are associated with Epstein-Barr virus.

■ CLINICAL PRESENTATION

Clinical manifestations include behavioral and personality changes, dizziness, confusion, and focal cerebral signs. Signs of increased intracranial pressure, seizures, and headache are less common.

■ DIFFERENTIAL DIAGNOSIS

Contrast-enhanced CT scans and MRI typically show one or more dense homogeneous enhancing lesions that arise in the periventricular matter, as shown in Figure 97-2. Another presentation consisting of a ring-enhancing nodule in the cerebral cortex should also expand the differential diagnosis to include toxoplasmosis, especially in these immunocompromised patients. Multiple sclerosis can be commonly misdiagnosed as primary CNS lymphoma because both may have features of multiple white matter lesions on contrast-enhanced CT or MRI.

■ TREATMENT

In patients less than 60 years of age, current treatment recommendations include chemotherapy with methotrexate and citrovorum or cytosine arabinoside followed by cranial irradiation, with a survival benefit of up to 4 years. Studies have shown that older methods of irradiation and corticosteroids lead to a 90% recurrence of the lymphoma, a median survival of only 10 to 18 months, and even less in immunocompromised patients.

Secondary Central Nervous System Lymphoma

Secondary CNS lymphomas occur in adults who have progressive B-cell lymphoma or B-cell leukemia with involvement of bone, bone marrow, testes, or cranial sinuses.

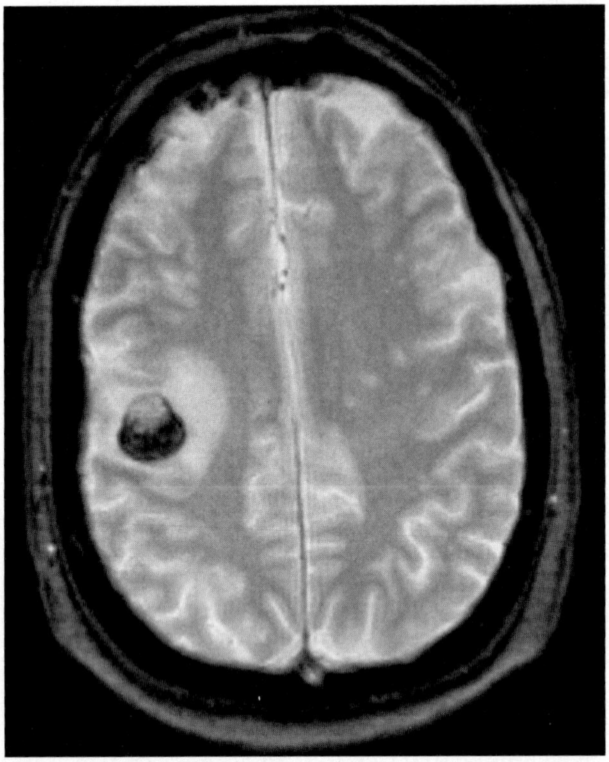

FIGURE 97-1 Axial magnetic resonance image demonstrating a metastatic lesion present at the gray-white matter junction with significant surrounding edema; the hyperintense focus within the lesion likely represents calcification or blood.

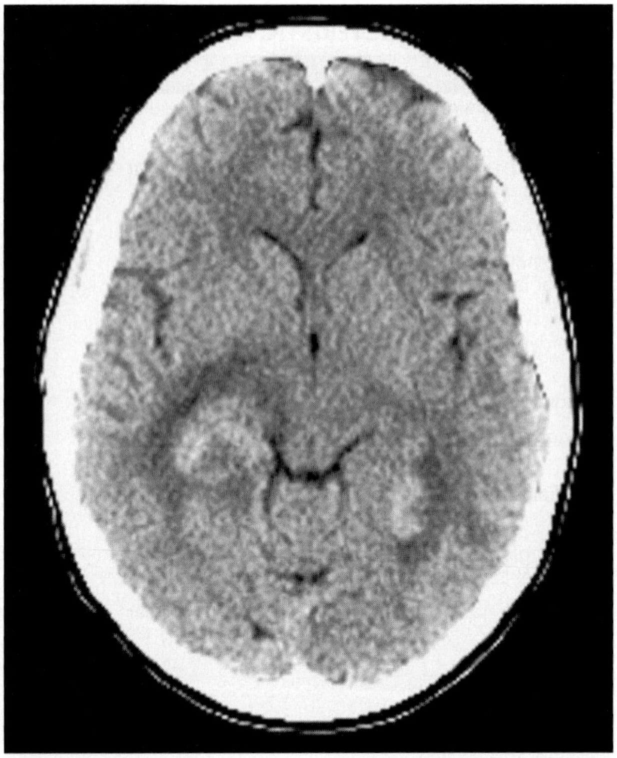

FIGURE 97-2 This computed tomography (CT) image demonstrates the classic periventricular homogeneous lesion of a central nervous system lymphoma; it has a ring-enhancing appearance when viewed with contrast.

■ DIFFERENTIAL DIAGNOSIS AND TREATMENT

Characteristic findings on contrast-enhanced CT scans or gadolinium-enhanced MRI views show leptomeningeal involvement of the lymphoma. Treatment includes systemic and intrathecal chemotherapy as well as irradiation of the brain; however, the overall prognosis is determined by successful treatment of the systemic process.

Astrocytoma

These intracranial lesions are the most common primary brain neoplasm. Astrocytomas of the cerebral hemispheres are diagnosed in adults during the third or fourth decade of life, whereas tumors in other locations of the CNS (most commonly the posterior fossa and the optic nerve) are found in children and adolescents.

■ WHO CLASSIFICATION

Astrocytomas are classified by the World Health Organization (WHO) using a four-tiered grading system based on the tumor's histologic appearance, which determines the patient's prognosis. According to the WHO grading system, grade I pilocytic astrocytomas show dense pilocytic glia cells, no necrosis, and low-grade cellular changes; astrocytic tumors with nuclear atypia alone are grade II; tumors that additionally demonstrate mitotic activity are grade III; and tumors showing atypia, mitoses, endothelial cell proliferation, and/or necrosis are grade IV.[5]

Astrocytomas of the well-differentiated grades (I-II) are much more common in children than in adults and have a better prognosis. These tumors typically are slow-growing and infiltrative and tend to form large cavities or pseudocysts.

Grade I astrocytomas include *juvenile pilocytic astrocytoma, subependymal giant cell astrocytoma* (which occurs in patients with tuberous sclerosis), and *pleomorphic xanthoastrocytoma*. Juvenile pilocytic astrocytomas are the most common primary brain lesion in children.

Grade II astrocytomas (most commonly a low-grade fibrillary type) are tumors with more cellular atypia and varying degrees of cellularity. Surgery is the mainstay of treatment for most low-grade astrocytomas.[6,7]

Grade III (anaplastic astrocytoma) and grade IV (glioblastoma multiforme) astrocytomas show increasing levels of cellularity and atypia, tumor giant cells and cells in mitosis, hyperplasia of endothelial cells of small vessels, necrosis, hemorrhage, and thrombosis of vessels—all leading to the variety of presentations and imaging features of these particular lesions. It is difficult to grade these lesions histologically because often there are foci of undifferentiated cells in a lower-grade tumor that may not be seen without focused pathologic survey of the

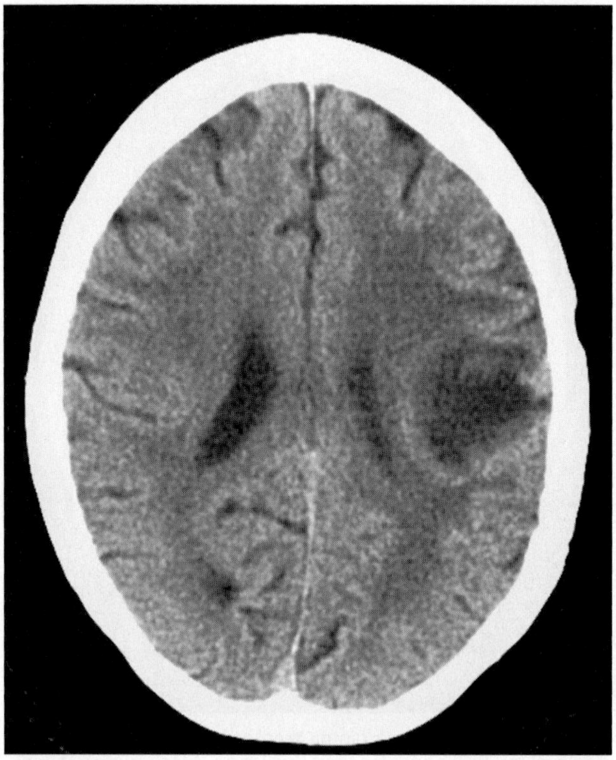

FIGURE 97-3 The lesion in this CT scan illustrates the characteristic features of glioblastoma multiforme: heterogeneous, irregular ring of enhancement, hypointense core, and significant surrounding edema.

biopsy or specimen, thus demonstrating the proliferative nature of this disease.

■ CLINICAL PRESENTATION

The clinical presentation commonly includes seizures or focal neurologic deficits; cognitive changes also can be the presenting sign. These lesions arise deep in the white matter of the brain and can attain a significant size before attracting medical attention. Increased intracranial pressure related to the mass effect is common.

■ DIFFERENTIAL DIAGNOSIS

Radiographic findings in these high-grade tumors are quite irregular and distort the brain matter (Fig. 97-3). The appearance usually is a nonhomogeneous mass, often with a center that is hypointense in comparison to adjacent brain and demonstrating an irregular ring of enhancement surrounded by edema. Part of one lateral ventricle is often distorted, and both lateral and third ventricles may be displaced.

■ TREATMENT

Treatment includes a variety of options, including experimental therapy. The standard regimen currently consists of glucocorticoids, surgery, radiation, and chemotherapy, depending on the involvement and location of the lesion. Dexamethasone (4-10 mg every 6 hours, for a brief period of time) is useful if there are symptoms of mass effect,. This regimen typically is followed by maximal surgical resection with external beam radiation therapy and chemotherapy postoperatively.[8]

Ependymoma

Ependymoma, the most common glioma of the spinal cord, is derived from ependymal cells, which line the ventricles of the brain and central canal of the spinal cord, thus the diagnosis often can be made based on clinical examination and radiographic findings. As expected, these tumors grow into the ventricles or brain matter; the most common location is the fourth ventricle.

■ EPIDEMIOLOGY AND PATHOPHYSIOLOGY

In adults, these lesions typically occur in the spinal canal, especially in the lumbosacral region at the filum terminale (leading to presentations of cauda equina syndrome), whereas in children, these tumors present in the ventricles, most commonly the fourth ventricle. It is important to recognize that although overall this class of brain lesion is fairly uncommon (it accounts for 6% of all intracranial gliomas), 40% of infratentorial ependymomas occur within the first decade of life, making it significant in the pediatric population.

■ CLINICAL PRESENTATION

Clinical symptoms are correlated with the location of the lesion. With infratentorial lesions, most commonly in pediatric patients, signs of hydrocephalus and increased intracranial pressure are frequent. In children, increased intracranial pressure is manifested as nausea, vomiting, papilledema, and lethargy. Cerebral ependymomas present similarly to other gliomas, with seizures seen in about one third of cases.

■ DIFFERENTIAL DIAGNOSIS

Imaging techniques reveal a unique appearance that distinguishes this lesion from other CNS tumors. CT scanning demonstrates uniformally enhancing masses that are well demarcated from adjacent neural tissue, with calcification and cystic changes seen more commonly in supratentorial lesions. On MRI, T_1-weighted images reveal a hypodense lesion, whereas T_2-weighted images show hyperintensity. An intraventricular location visible on CT or MRI views supports the diagnosis of ependymoma; however, meningioma and other lesions cannot be excluded. Metastases from intracranial ependymomas may be seen in the spinal cord; they are termed *drop metastases*.

■ TREATMENT

The most important prognostic factors for patients with ependymomas are histologic grade and tumor resection, making surgical excision the most important factor in the management of these lesions. With neurosurgical intervention, 5-year survival following gross total excision of the lesion is about 80%. Kawabata and colleagues demonstrated that there is no apparent benefit to postoperative radiation, and if relapses do occur, they most often are seen local to the excision site.[9] Rogers and colleagues showed that following gross total resection, adjuvant radiotherapy improved local control of the lesion and increased the 10-year survival rate by 16% compared with those who underwent gross total resection alone.[10] Currently, chemotherapy is not a mainstay of treatment for these lesions.

Meningioma

■ EPIDEMIOLOGY AND PATHOPHYSIOLOGY

Meningiomas are benign and are clearly derived from the meningothelial cells or arachnoidal cells which form the arachnoid villi. These villi most commonly penetrate the dura at the venous sinuses; thus meningiomas are seen at these locations. These lesions are more commonly seen in women (ratio of 2:1) and usually are seen in the sixth to seventh decades of life. There is familial predisposition, with association of the neurofibromatosis 2 gene. Other associations include previous radiation therapy and previous traumatic injury (tumors arising at the site of the fracture line). These lesions contain estrogen and progesterone receptors, which may explain its association with breast cancer, its increased size during pregnancy and its increased overall incidence in women.

■ CLINICAL PRESENTATION

Clinically, these lesions will not present with neurological findings until they have reached a significant size, given their growth along meningothelium. Frequently they invade the skull and less frequently invade the brain. Small meningiomas (2.0 cm or less) often are found at autopsy, as they cause no symptoms. Focal seizures may be seen in patients with tumors overlying the cerebrum, and sylvian fissure lesions are manifested by a variety of motor, sensory and aphasia characteristics depending on their location. Patients with parasaggital, frontoparietal meningiomas may have weakness or numbness of one or both legs and urinary incontinence during later stages of the disease.

■ DIFFERENTIAL DIAGNOSIS

On noncontrast CT scans, lesions typically are isodense or slightly hyperdense, with calcification at the outer surface or heterogeneously within the tumor (Fig. 97-4). The appearance of these lesions on CT and MRI views is characteristically described as a dense contrast-enhancing extra-axial mass. A dural metastasis must be carefully excluded from the differential diagnosis. Angiography is diagnostic as well because all these modalities show the increased vascularity ("tumor blush") and calcifications within the lesion.

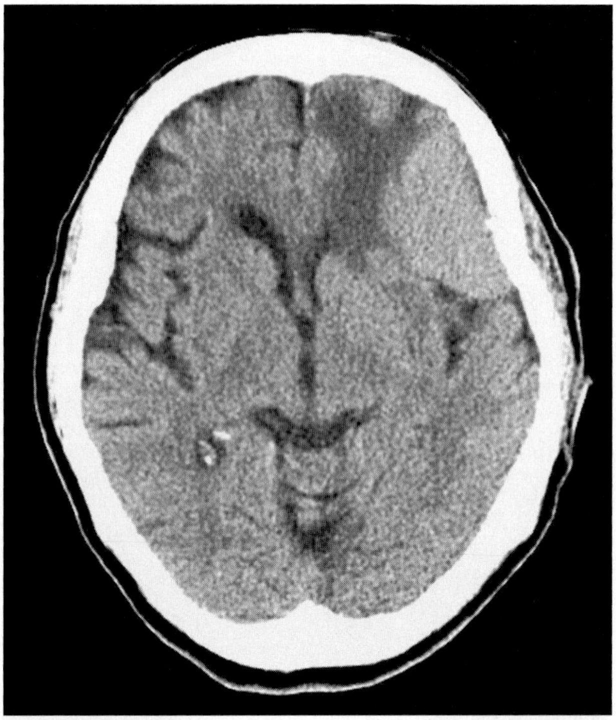

FIGURE 97-4 The meningioma seen on this CT scan has the classic extra-axial appearance of this lesion. Meningiomas often are hyperdense and may demonstrate calcification.

■ TREATMENT

The prognosis is excellent with total surgical resection. Meningiomas along the sphenoid bone or in the parasellar region or anterior to the brainstem are the most difficult to remove. Even if subtotal resection is performed, local external beam radiotherapy reduces the recurrence rate to less than 10%.

Oligodendroglioma

Oligodendrogliomas may be on a spectrum with astrocytomas. Up to half of oligodendrogliomas contain cellular content consistent with astrocytomas—thus the names *mixed glioma* and *oligoastrocytoma*. This is important for prognostication. Oligodendrogliomas account for approximately 5% to 7% of all gliomas in adults and occur more predominantly in males (2:1 ratio).

■ CLINICAL PRESENTATION

The clinical presentation is similar to that of patients with astrocytoma; seizures are the most common symptom. The lesions grow quite slowly, over a period of years. Approximately 15% of patients have signs of increased intracranial pressure, and even fewer have focal neurologic deficits such as hemiparesis.

■ DIFFERENTIAL DIAGNOSIS

Oligodendrogliomas most commonly occur in the frontal and temporal lobes within the white matter, with calcified streaks within the tumor; typically there is little edema surrounding the lesion. This is helpful when interpreting diagnostic images. On noncontrast CT scans, the usual appearance is of a hypodense mass near the cortical surface in the frontal-temporal distribution, with relatively well-defined borders. The presence of calcifications supports the diagnosis, and the presence of an arteriovenous malformation or meningioma may be helpful. An important feature is that the oligodendroglioma will generally not be enhanced with contrast modalities, thereby narrowing the differential diagnosis.

In pathologic analysis of the specimen, the larger the oligodendroglioma component of the lesion, the more benign the clinical course.

■ TREATMENT

Standard treatment for oligodendrogliomas includes adjuvant radiation. Mixed gliomas should also be treated with chemotherapy, given their more malignant features.[11]

Medulloblastoma

Medulloblastomas are rapidly growing embryonic tumors that arise in the posterior part of the cerebellar vermis and neuroepithelial roof of the fourth ventricle in children. Most patients are 4 to 8 years of age, with males being more commonly involved (3:1 incidence). Medulloblastomas of the posterior fossa are the most common malignant brain tumor in children.

■ CLINICAL PRESENTATION

Cinically, these children present similarly to patients with ependymomas because they show features of hydrocephalus and increased intracranial pressure due to obstruction of cerebrospinal fluid at the fourth ventricle.[12] Classic symptoms include vomiting and listlessness, with a morning headache that may mimic an abdominal etiology. A careful neurologic examination may reveal an unstable gait, diplopia, strabismus, and/or oculomotor palsies of the sixth cranial nerve. Dizziness, papilledema, and nystagmus also may be present. Some children may have a sensory loss on one side of the face and a mild facial weakness.

■ DIFFERENTIAL DIAGNOSIS

CT contrast-imaging shows a heterogeneous enhancing mass adjacent to or extending into the fourth ventricle. On MRI scans, the high-signal intensity and heterogeneous appearance with contrast may appear similar to that of gliomas. The classic finding on both CT and MRI studies, however, is that the tumor fills the fourth ventricle and extends into the floor of the ventricle.

■ TREATMENT

Treatment modalities include extensive surgery, radiation, and chemotherapy, which when combined show a 5-year survival rate of about 80%.

Hemangioblastoma

Hemangioblastomas of the cerebellum are commonly associated with von Hippel-Lindau disease. The classic genetic defect is present in a tumor suppressor gene on chromosome 3 and exhibits a dominant pattern of inheritance.

■ CLINICAL PRESENTATION

Patients most often present in the third to fifth decades of life and may have symptoms of hydrocephalus (dizziness, ataxia, and vomiting) due to compression of the mass at the fourth ventricle. Other features of this disease include polycythemia due to an erythropoietic factor expressed by tumor cells, as well as the presence of retinal angiomas. Further work-up may reveal hepatic and/or pancreatic cysts seen on abdominal CT or MRI scans.

■ DIFFERENTIAL DIAGNOSIS

Radiographically, the lesion is demonstrated by a cerebellar cyst with a nodular lesion on the wall of the cyst on contrast-enhanced CT or MRI scans (Fig. 97-5). Further imaging using angiography may reveal a tightly packed cluster of small blood vessels ranging from 1 to 2 cm in diameter. The retinal hemangioma may be seen on CT and MRI studies when searching for the cerebellar lesion.

■ TREATMENT

Ultimately, surgical resection or neurointerventional treatment of the vascular nodule is curative; however, if the entire tumor, including the nodule, is not removed, the tumor will recur.[13]

Schwannoma

These lesions occur occasionally in association with hereditary disorders, such as von Recklinghausen

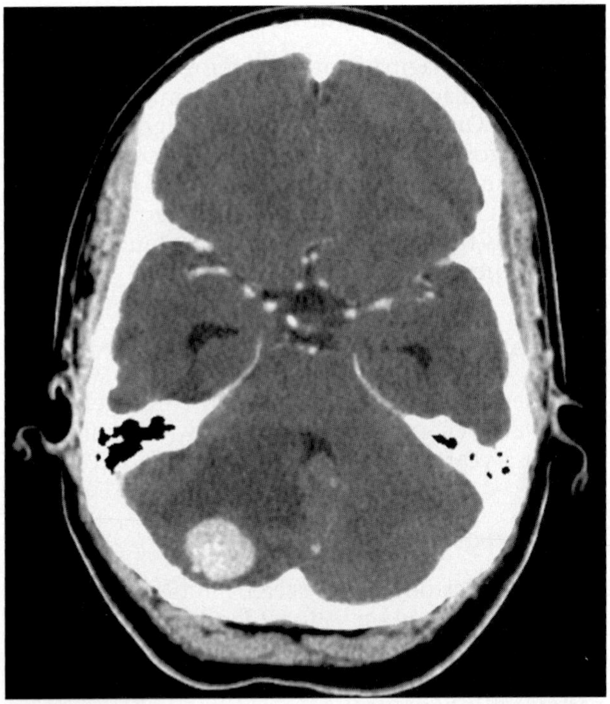

FIGURE 97-5 CT scan with contrast enhancement demonstrates the typical cystic appearanceof a cerebellar hemangioblastoma; a nodular lesion is visible within the wall of the cerebellar cyst.

neurofibromatosis. These lesions, also called neuromas, neurinomas, and neurolemmas, arise from the Schwann cells of nerve roots, most commonly the eighth cranial nerve (also called a vestibular schwannoma or acoustic schwannoma). The fifth cranial nerve is the second most common site, and these lesions can originate from any cranial or spinal nerve root except the optic and olfactory nerves, which are myelinated with oligodendroglia as opposed to the Schwann cells.

■ PATHOPHYSIOLOGY AND CLINICAL PRESENTATION

The position of the lesion affects its clinical presentation. When this tumor arises, it typically begins to grow within the vestibular division of the eighth cranial nerve, just inside the internal auditory canal. As it enlarges, it extends into the posterior fossa between the cerebellum and pons, or cerebellopontine angle. It is at this position that the tumor has the potential to compress the fifth, seventh, ninth, and tenth cranial nerves, leading to potentially diagnostic physical examination findings.

Most commonly, the initial presenting symptom is hearing loss, followed by headaches, gait abnormalities, and vertigo. Other signs and symptoms include eighth nerve impairment of auditory or vestibular distribution, facial weakness, disturbance of taste, and sensory loss over the face, correlating with the cranial nerve dysfunctions discussed previously.

■ DIFFERENTIAL DIAGNOSIS

Unilateral hearing loss without a sufficient cause merits radiographic examination. Contrast-enhanced CT scans demonstrate most lesions larger than 2 cm and lesions extending into the cerebellopontine angle. On contrast-enhanced CT or MRI scans, the lesion appears as an intense dense lesion in the area of the eighth cranial nerve, sometimes showing mass effect on the pons, as the tumor enters the posterior fossa.

■ TREATMENT

With rare exceptions, schwannomas are histologically and clinically benign lesions. If the lesion is small (2.5 cm or less), surgical excision usually can be performed without damage to the patient's hearing.

Neurocysticercosis

■ EPIDEMIOLOGY AND PATHOPHYSIOLOGY

Nonbacterial infections of the CNS include neurocysticercosis, which is the most common parasitic disease of the CNS worldwide. In endemic areas (Latin America, Asia, Africa) neurocysticercosis is considered to be main cause of late-onset epilepsy, and seizures in these areas are reported to be the most common symptom (70%-90% of patients). Because its incidence in the United States has been increasing since 1980, the EP should be aware of this entity.

Humans acquire cysticercosis by ingesting food contaminated with the eggs of the parasite *Taenia solium*. Eggs are contained in undercooked pork and in drinking water and food contaminated with human feces.

■ CLINICAL PRESENTATION

The most common presentation of neurocysticercosis is new-onset partial seizures with or without secondary generalization. When the cyst first appears in the brain, there is little inflammatory response, but subsequent inflammation may manifest as seizure activity. Occasionally, focal neurologic deficits may be present, because the lesion lies in the brain parenchyma, or increased intracranial pressure may result when lesions become lodged in the ventricles and obstruct cerebrospinal fluid outflow.

■ DIFFERENTIAL DIAGNOSIS

Radiographically, lesions appear on CT scans as one or more low-density lesions of variable size, with surrounding edema and ring enhancement, that may show mass effect. Small, eccentric densities may be visualized within the cyst itself. Parenchymal brain calcification is the most common finding and usually is present within the cyst and dense enough to be seen on CT scans. Cysts usually are numerous and can be seen in different phases of development on a single study.

■ TREATMENT

Anticonvulsant therapy is a mandatory for patients who present with seizures and a diagnosis of cysticercosis. The majority of cases respond to treatment with phenytoin or carbamazepine. Albendazole and praziquantel are the mainstays of antiparasitic therapy. Seizure control was shown to be more effective following a course of antiparasitic drugs and glucocorticoids; this combination has been proved to decrease the rate of generalized and recurrent seizures.[14]

Patients diagnosed with neurocysticercosis may require treatment with steroids to control inflammation and treat meningitis, cysticercal encephalitis, and angiitis. Initial treatment is usually started with dexamethasone (4 mg IV every 6 hours for no more than 3 to 4 days), which can be replaced with prednisone (1 mg/kg/day) in the case of long-term treatment.

Serial CT scans are needed to ensure resolution of the lesions, at which point antiepileptic therapy can be stopped unless seizures recur after the resolution of edema and calcification of the degenerating cyst.

Toxoplasmosis

Toxoplasmosis is acquired from the ingestion of undercooked meat and from handling cat feces, which harbor the parasite *Toxoplasma gondii.*

■ CLINICAL PRESENTATION

Primary toxoplasmosis usually is asymptomatic; however, reactivation may occur in the immunocompromised host. The patient at that time may have symptoms including fever, headache, seizures, and/or focal neurologic deficits.

■ DIFFERENTIAL DIAGNOSIS

On neuroimaging, the appearance is very similar to that of neurocysticercosis. Lesions typically have strong ring enhancement, with an area of surrounding edema. Calcification is a finding common to neurocysticercosis and toxoplasmosis. Mass effect may be present, and more than one intracranial lesion may be seen on a single image.

■ TREATMENT

Treatment consists of a combination of sulfadiazine and pyrimethamine with the addition of folinic acid to prevent megaloblastic anemia. Clindamycin can be used in combination with pyrimethamine for patients unable to tolerate sulfadiazine, although this regimen is not as effective. Recent literature has reported resistance of certain toxoplasmosis strains to sulfonamide, in which case clindamycin may have a more prominent role in the treatment of CNS toxoplasmosis.[15]

Tuberculoma

A tuberculoma is a tumor-like mass of tuberculous granulation tissue within the brain parenchyma. It is a manifestation of CNS tuberculosis that may have a different clinical presentation than meningitis. Although rare in the United States, these lesions are common in foreign countries; in some tropical countries, cerebellar tuberculomas are the most common intracranial tumor in children.

■ CLINICAL PRESENTATION

Tuberculomas do not usually manifest with symptoms of focal neurologic disease but can show mass effect if large enough, leading to hydrocephalus and increased intracranial pressure. Tuberculosis can also present with meningitic symptoms of fever, headache, and nuchal rigidity, though it is imperative to rule out these granulomatous lesions on CT.

■ DIFFERENTIAL DIAGNOSIS

Tuberculomas are visible on plain CT scans as rounded lesions that are isodense or slightly denser than the surrounding brain tissue. These lesions produce little if any surrounding edema and can easily be missed on CT studies without IV contrast. On contrast-enhanced CT and MRI views, they may resemble the lesions of a primary malignant brain tumor; thus the clinical setting should be considered carefully.

Small areas of calcification may be present, most likely within the basal cisterns but also seen in the distribution of major cerebral vasculature. CT scans of chronic granulomatous meningitis may show complete obliteration of the basal cisterns with material isodense to the brain.

The general appearance of the tuberculoma can be contrasted with that of metastatic lesions, which have more widespread edema surrounding them.

Tuberous Sclerosis

Tuberous sclerosis is characterized by cutaneous lesions, epilepsy, and mental retardation. Cutaneous lesions include adenoma sebaceum (facial angiofibromas), ash-leaf hypopigmented macules, shagreen patches (yellow thickenings of the skin over the lumbosacral region of the back), and depigmented nevi. Although the disease, autosomal dominant in its inheritance pattern, is apparent within the first few years of life, the intracerebral lesions may manifest clinical signs and symptoms that mandate evaluation in the ED.

■ CLINICAL PRESENTATION

Clinical signs and symptoms of this genetic disorder are evident in patients at a very young age. Slowing of psychomotor development may be the first manifestation of mental retardation. Seizures can sometimes be the presenting symptom and are usually manifested during the first 4 or 5 years of life. Seizure patterns change as these patients mature and are the most reliable index of cerebral lesions; interestingly, focal neurologic lesions typically are not present.

Ultimately, patients have epilepsy and mental retardation resulting from severe involvement of the cortical tubers. Of note, the classic skin lesions—adenoma sebaceum and ash-leaf hypopigmented macules—are seen in patients older than 4 to 5 years.

The tubers of this disease, which are are calcific and tend to lie in a periventricular distribution, are readily seen on CT and MRI views; however, MRI is more sensitive for visualizing giant cell subcortical lesions. Surrounding edema usually is absent. Current research shows that, with increasing numbers of intracranial lesions, there is a proportional relationship with severity of disease.

■ TREATMENT

The prognosis for these patients unfortunately is grim. About 30% of severely affected patients will die before the age of 5 years, and nearly 75% of patients will not live to adulthood. Recent antiepileptic strategies have curtailed deaths due to status epilepticus from this disease, although neoplasms resulting from this disorder have become much more common. Patients inheriting the tuberous sclerosis gene are at increased risk for developing ependymomas and juvenile astrocytomas (of which >90% are subependymal giant cell astrocytomas). These are benign neoplasms that may develop in the retina or along the border of the lateral ventricles; they have been discussed previously in this chapter.

Arteriovenous Malformations

Arteriovenous malformations are congenital vascular malformations that arise from the maldevelopment of the primitive vascular plexus and consist of arteriovenous communications without capillaries. Clinical signs and symptoms may be related to the hemorrhage of the malformation or associated aneurysm or may result from the cerebral ischemia caused by the arteriovenous shunt or venous stagnation. Most lesions are supratentorial, with the majority lying within the territory of middle cerebral artery.

■ CLINICAL PRESENTATION

The most common clinical symptom is hemorrhage, which occurs in over 50% of patients; recurrent seizures and headaches are other common complaints on presentation. Most arteriovenous malformations bleed at some point in the course of the disease—usually in patients younger than 40 years. Small arteriovenous malformations have a stronger propensity for hemorrhage than larger ones.

Focal or generalized seizures are common after hemorrhage or may be the initial presenting complaint, especially in patients with frontal or parietal lesions. Headaches are common if the lesion is in the territory of the external carotid artery, in which case the symptoms may be similar to those of migraine.

■ DIFFERENTIAL DIAGNOSIS

CT scans help immediately determine whether the hemorrhage is subarachnoid or intraparenchymal. Contrast-enhanced CT or MRI scans may identify over 95% of arteriovenous malformations. Lesions appear as a heterogeneous, hypodense mass with hyperintense regions within the mass; an enhancing rim also may be visible (Fig. 97-6). In cases with negative CT findings and a high index of clinical suspicion, lumbar puncture with cerebrospinal fluid analysis is necessary. If there is a high index of clinical suspicion and the diagnosis is suggested by CT scan results, angiography is required to better define the lesion and to develop a management strategy.

■ TREATMENT

Surgery is necessary for patients with increased intracranial pressure and to stop progression of focal neu-

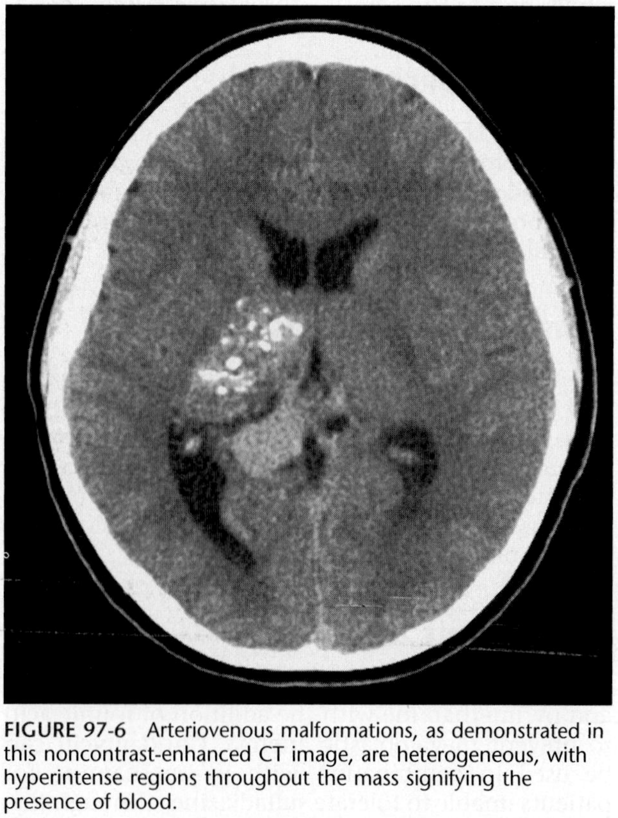

FIGURE 97-6 Arteriovenous malformations, as demonstrated in this noncontrast-enhanced CT image, are heterogeneous, with hyperintense regions throughout the mass signifying the presence of blood.

rologic deficits. Surgery also may be an option if hemorrhage is present, its source is accessible, and the patient has a reasonable life expectancy. Excision of the lesion is definitive therapy when the lesion is accessible. Embolization may be performed not necessarily to reduce the risk of hemorrhage but to potentially stabilize or reverse neurologic deficits.

REFERENCES

1. Evans RW: Diagnostic testing for the evaluation of headaches. Neurol Clin 1996;14:1-26.
2. Schaefer PW, Miller JC, Singhal AB, et al: Headache: When is neuroimaging indicated? J Am Coll Radiol 2007; 4:566-569.
3. Clinical policy for the initial approach to patients with a chief complaint of seizure who are not in status epilepticus. American College of Emergency Physicians. Ann Emerg Med 1993;22:875-883.
4. Engstrom JW: Tumors of the nervous system. In Braunwald E, Fauci AS, Kasper DL, et al (eds): Harrison's Manual of Medicine, 15th ed. New York, McGraw-Hill, 2001, pp 842-844.
5. Doolittle ND: State of the science in brain tumor classification. Semin Oncol Nurs 2004;20:224-230.
6. Peris-Bonet R, Martinez-Garcia C, Lacour B, et al: Childhood CNS tumours—incidence and survival in Europe (1978-1997): Report from Automated Childhood Cancer Information System project. Eur J Cancer 2006;42: 2064-2680.
7. van den Bent MJ, Afra D, de Witte O, et al: Long-term efficacy of early versus delayed radiotherapy for low-grade astrocytoma and oligodendroglioma in adults: The EORTC 22845 randomised trial. Lancet 2005;366(9490):985-990.
8. Nieder C, Adam M, Molls M, Grosu AL: Therapeutic options for recurrent high-grade glioma in adult patients: Recent advances. Crit Rev Oncol Hematol 2006;60:181-193.
9. Kawabata Y, Takahashi JA, Arakawa Y, et al: Long-term outcome in patients harboring intracranial ependymoma. J Neurosurg 2005;103:31-37.
10. Rogers L, Pueschel J, Spetzler R, et al: Is gross-total resection sufficient treatment for posterior fossa ependymomas? J Neurosurg 2005;102:629-636.
11. Lebrun C, Fontaine D, Ramaioli A, et al: Long-term outcome of oligodendrogliomas. Neurology 2004;62:1783-1787.
12. Halperin EC, Watson D, George SL: Duration of symptoms prior to diagnosis is related inversely to presenting disease stage in children with medulloblastoma. Cancer 2001; 91:1444-1450.
13. Zager EL, Shaver EG, Hurst RW, et al: Distal anterior inferior cerebellar artery aneurysms. Report of four cases. J Neurosurg 2002;97:692-696.
14. Del Brutto OH, Roos KL, Coffey CS, et al: Meta-analysis: Cysticidal drugs for neurocysticercosis: Albendazole and praziquantel. Ann Intern Med 2006;145:43-51.
15. Aspinall TV, Joynson DH, Guy E, et al: The molecular basis of sulfonamide resistance in *Toxoplasma gondii* and implications for the clinical management of toxoplasmosis. J Infect Dis 2002;185:1637-1643.

Chapter **98**

Intracranial Hemorrhages

J. Stephen Huff and Chris Ghaemmaghami

KEY POINTS

"Head bleed" is an oversimplified definition of intracranial hemorrhage because different types of hemorrhage have different etiologies, presentations, diagnostic strategies, and therapies.

Cranial computed tomography (CT) without contrast remains the initial diagnostic imaging procedure of choice for detecting intracranial hemorrhage in the ED.

Anatomic description of intracranial hemorrhage should include the anatomic type of hemorrhage, location, estimation of size, presence of midline shift, and whether the hemorrhage is thought to be spontaneous or secondary to another process.

Cranial CT detects more than 95% of acute subarachnoid hemorrhages, but lumbar puncture is recommended in patients whose history strongly suggests subarachnoid hemorrhage.

Recommendations regarding blood pressure management and anticonvulsant administration remain controversial and lack strong evidence-based support.

Scope

Intracranial hemorrhages have different clinical presentations ranging from subtle to catastrophic. The efforts of the EP are directed toward identifying the diagnosis based on clinical information, confirming the diagnosis by cranial computed tomography (CT) or other diagnostic tests, and providing basic supportive care. Strong evidence is lacking of the best course of action concerning basic management issues sush as blood pressure management and use of anticonvulsants. Definitive therapy most often is in the hands of the consultant and admitting physician. Consultation and collaboration with admitting specialists is recommended.

It is tempting to place any intracranial hemorrhage in the diagnostic category *head bleed*. This oversimplification ignores the fact that many different processes may lead to hemorrhage in different intracranial locations. Different types of intracranial hemorrhage may have different etiologies, different natural histories, different diagnostic strategies, different treatments, and often different prognoses. It is important to delineate the various types of intracranial hemorrhage so that correct diagnostic steps and therapeutic interventions are performed. Just as EPs learn fracture terminology to communicate with a consultant, they should know the correct descriptive terminology for intracranial hemorrhages.

For purposes of organization, the following section is divided into discussion of spontaneous intraparenchymal hemorrhages, subarachnoid hemorrhages, traumatic hemorrhages including extra-axial hemorrhages (epidural and subdural), and other causes of intracranial hemorrhage.

Table 98-1 TYPES OF INTRACRANIAL HEMORRHAGES

Type of Hemorrahge	Corresponding Figures in Text	Findings in Figures
Intraparenchmal (synonyms: intracerebral, lobar, hypertensive)	Fig. 98-1	Blood within substance of brain; thalamic hemorrhage
Subarachnoid	Fig. 98-2	Acute hemorrhage with blood in the subarachnoid spaces
Subdural	Fig. 98-3	Blood external to brain; crescent-shaped hemorrhage
Epidural	Fig. 98-4	Blood external to brain; crescent-shaped hemorrhage
Hemorrhagic transformation of ischemic stroke	Fig. 98-5	Hemorrhage within wedge-shaped area of ischemia

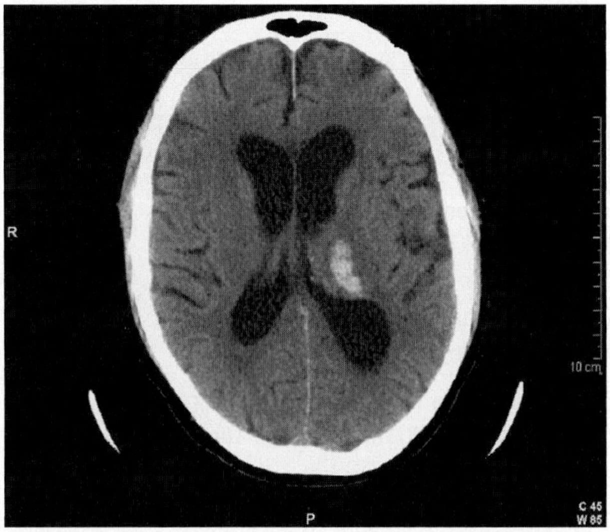
R
10 cm
P
C 45
W 85

FIGURE 98-1 Computed tomography scan: Supratentorial intracerebral hematoma. Note the bright white appearance consistent with an acute hemorrhage. The anatomic location is thalamic.

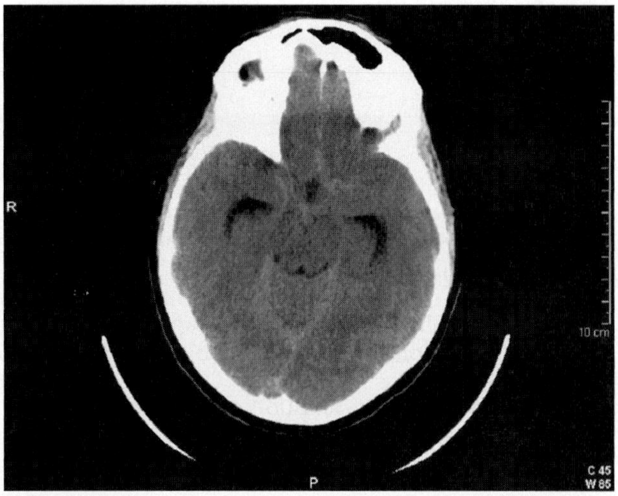
R
10 cm
P
C 45
W 85

FIGURE 98-2 Computed tomography scan: Acute subarachnoid hemorrhage. Blood density is not as dramatic as in Figure 98-13. Hydrocephalus with enlarged temporal horns of lateral ventricle is present.

Pathophysiology and Definitions

Intracranial hemorrhage is the umbrella term used to encompass the many types of bleeding within the cranial vault (Table 98-1; Figs. 98-1 through 98-5). *Intraparenchymal hemorrhage* implies blood within the substance of the brain. When the hemorrhage is spontaneous, this term often is used synonymously with the terms *hypertensive hemorrhage, spontaneous hemorrhage,* and, when anatomically appropriate, *intracerebral hemorrhage.* Intraparenchymal hemorrhages may also occur in the brainstem or cerebellum. *Subarachnoid hemorrhage* (SAH) literally describes blood in the subarachnoid space, but if nontraumatic ("spontaneous") implies a vascular lesion, such as an aneurysm, as the source of the bleeding. Subarachnoid hemorrhage and intraparenchymal hemorrhage frequently co-exist. *Intraventricular hemorrhage* means that blood is visualized within the ventricles by cranial CT and most often is present with other types of intracranial hemorrhage. Intracranial hemorrhages outside of the brain substance are referred to as *extra-axial hemorrhages* and include

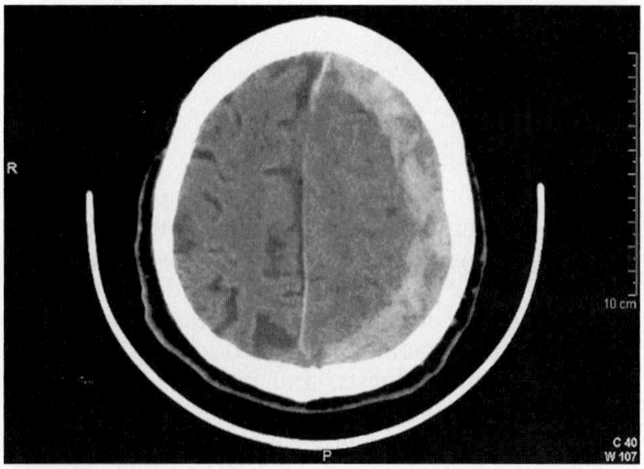
R
10 cm
P
C 40
W 107

FIGURE 98-3 Computed tomography scan: Acute subdural hematoma. Note the crescent-shaped hemorrhage extending the length of the left hemisphere. The mottled appearance is consistent with ongoing bleeding.

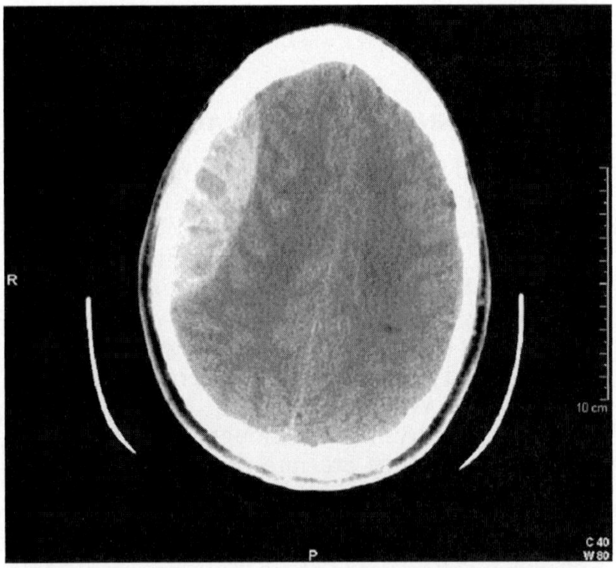
R
10 cm
P
C 40
W 80

FIGURE 98-4 Computed tomography scan: Acute epidural hematoma with "swirl" sign. This is a slice from a repeat CT scan of the patient in Figure 98-10 taken approximately 1 hour later. The marbled density of the clot is consistent with ongoing hemorrhage. Note the lens shape of the hematoma.

both *subdural hemorrhages* and *epidural hemorrhages*. Though uncommon exceptions exist, extra-axial hemorrhages are almost always have a traumatic etiology. The term *hemorrhagic stroke* might literally describe abrupt symptoms with any of the previously mentioned hemorrhages, but is best used in a more restrictive sense to describe hemorrhagic changes in an area of an ischemic stroke to the point of being visible on cranial CT; this is termed *hemorrhagic transformation* of the ischemic stroke.

The pathophysiology of types of intracranial hemorrhages differ, and an understanding of the etiology will help guide therapy. One approach is to consider hemorrhages as traumatic or nontraumatic, or spontaneous or nonspontaneous.

Intracranial bleeding may be of either arterial or venous origin. Because of the closed nature of the cranial vault, any increase in intracranial volume from bleeding may result in increased intracranial pressure and decreased cerebral perfusion pressures. As a mass expands, some initial compensation occurs, with diminished intracranial vascular and cerebrospinal fluid volume. However, at some point compensatory mechanisms fail and the intracranial pressure will dramatically rise with further increase in mass size.

A key concept is cerebral perfusion pressure (CPP), the effective blood pressure presenting to the intracranial contents. CPP is equal to the mean arterial pressure (MAP) minus the intracranial pressure (ICP); that is,

$$CPP = MAP - ICP$$

If intracranial pressure abruptly increases, or if mean arterial pressure falls, CPP falls and central nervous system ischemia follows, which exacerbates neuronal injury.

Hemorrhages cause injury by direct tissue destruction or compression of adjacent structures. Edema formation around a hematoma may further increase mass effect. For example, in cerebellar hemorrhage, tissue damage may cause initial symptoms, but increased intracranial pressure and rapid progression to coma are from compression of the adjacent brainstem.

■ SPONTANEOUS INTRAPARENCHYMAL HEMORRHAGES

Spontaneous intraparenchymal hemorrhages (e.g., intracerebral hemorrhages, lobar hemorrhages, hypertensive hemorrhages) most often are associated with chronic hypertension. Cerebral amyloid angiopathy is increasingly recognized as a contributing process in the elderly. In both hypertension and cerebral amyloid angiopathy, the vessel wall becomes less compliant and the risk of spontaneous rupture increases. Chronic excessive alcohol use is also a risk factor. Hemorrhage usually originates from the rupture of small penetrating branch arteries of the vessels at the base of the brain[1] (Fig. 98-6).

Serial cranial CT demonstrates that many intracerebral hemorrhages are not static but may expand over the course of several hours in some patients.[2] The initial hemorrhage may infiltrate the white matter with little direct destruction, but continued hematoma expansion, white matter edema, additional hemorrhage from surrounding vessels, and hydrocephalus all contribute to increased intracranial pressure and secondary neuronal injury. The frequency of anticoagulant-associated intracerebral hemorrhage is increasing.[3] Warfarin therapy does not appear to increase hematoma volume at presenta-

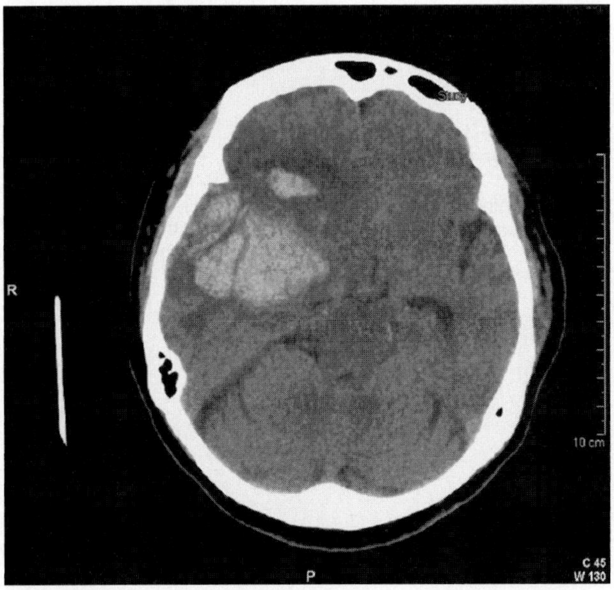
R
10 cm
P
C 45
W 130

FIGURE 98-5 Computed tomography scan: Hemorrhagic transformation of ischemic stroke.

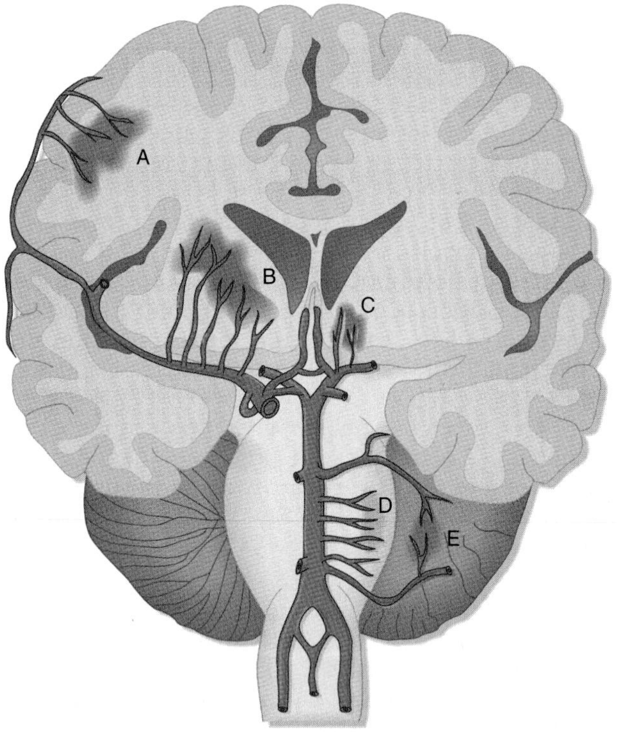
A
B
C
D
E

FIGURE 98-6 Common sites and sources of intracerebral hemorrhage. Intracerebral hemorrhages most commonly involve cerebral lobes, originating from penetrating cortical brances of the anterior, middle, or posterior cerebral arteries **(A)**; basal ganglia, originating from ascending lenticulostriate branches of the middle cerebral artery **(B)**; thalamus, originating from ascending thalamogeniculate branches of the posterior cerebral artery **(C)**; the pons, originating from paramedian branches of the basilar artery **(D)**; and the cerebellum, originating from penetrating branches of the posterior inferior, anterior inferior, or superior cerebellar arteries **(E)**.

tion but does increase risk of later hematoma expansion.[4]

■ SUBARACHNOID HEMORRHAGE

Subarachnoid hemorrhage literally means blood in the subarachnoid space. Trauma is the most common cause. Spontaneous, or nontraumatic, subarachnoid hemorrhage has an entirely different differential diagnosis. About 80% of spontaneous subarachnoid hemorrhages are caused by rupture of saccular (berry) aneurysms of the intracranial vessels, which are commonly located near intracranial arterial bifurcations of the circle of Willis[5,6] (Fig. 98-7).

Saccular aneurysms are thought to be developmental because they are rare in young adults and increase in frequency with age. Vascular flow shear forces are thought to contribute to aneurysm formation, and hypertension predisposes to aneurysm development and rupture. The risk of rupture increases with aneurysm size, consistent with increased tension in the wall of the aneurysm. Aneurysms are often named after the vascular site of origin, such as the anterior communicating artery or middle cerebral artery. Some of the morphologic descriptive terms for these developmental aneurysms are berry, saccular, and fusiform. Aneurysms that develop following vascular infection from endocarditis are termed mycotic aneurysms. Some aneurysms also cause symptoms without rupture from mass effect or from emboli originating within the aneurysm.

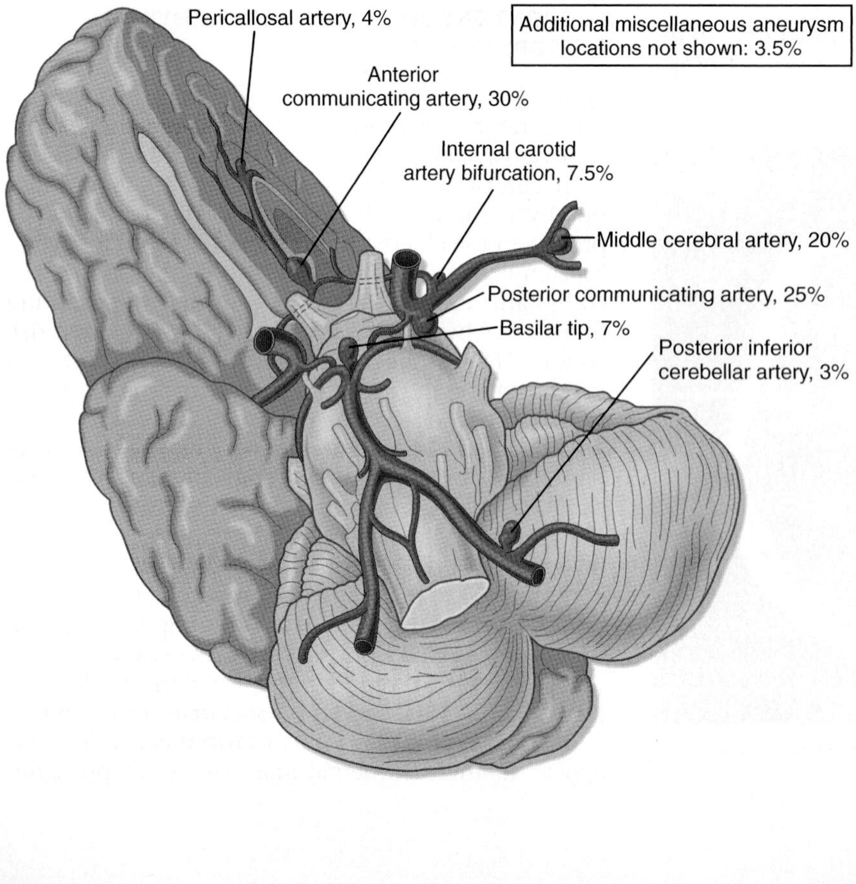
Pericallosal artery, 4%
Additional miscellaneous aneurysm locations not shown: 3.5%
Anterior communicating artery, 30%
Internal carotid artery bifurcation, 7.5%
Middle cerebral artery, 20%
Posterior communicating artery, 25%
Basilar tip, 7%
Posterior inferior cerebellar artery, 3%

FIGURE 98-7 The intracranial vasculature, showing the most frequent locations of intracranial aneurysms.

Rupture of an intracranial aneurysm abruptly raises intracranial pressure with onset of symptoms. The bleeding may be confined to the subarachnoid space or a hematoma may extend into the brain substance, creating an intraparenchymal hemorrhage, which in turn may rupture into the ventricles. Vasospasm of the vascular tree related to the aneurysm typically takes some hours to develop and may worsen regional ischemia.

Arteriovenous malformations are another cause of intracranial hemorrhage, both subarachnoid and intraparenchymal anatomic subtypes. These arteriovenous shunts vary in their anatomy and many patients have saccular aneurysms as well. Lesions with deep venous drainage and high pressure in the feeding vessels are at increased risk for bleeding.[7] Cavernous angiomas are low-pressure vascular lesions associated with small hemorrhages.

■ TRAUMA AND INTRACRANIAL HEMORRHAGE

Diffuse or localized subarachnoid blood is seen in many patients with closed head injuries. Cerebral contusion is a loosely defined term that describes the CT appearance of low density consistent with edema, and there may be some visible hemorrhage within that region.

An epidural hematoma usually reflects arterial bleeding into the epidural space following arterial injury to a meningeal vessel. A common mechanism is skull fracture in the temporal area with associated laceration of the middle meningeal artery. The arterial-pressure hematoma may increase in size until tamponade occurs from resistance of distorted intracranial structures and increased intracranial pressure (at the expense of cerebral perfusion pressure).

Subdural hematomas reflect bleeding from small vessel sources from more diffuse brain injury with hemorrhage accumulating over the surface of the brain. Again, distortion of the cranial contents may occur, as well as increased intracranial pressure. Cortical atrophy that occurs with aging is thought to make the bridging vessels from the cortex to the dura increasingly susceptible to rupture from even trivial trauma in the elderly.

■ OTHER HEMORRHAGES

Other, less common causes of intracranial hemorrhage include dural sinus thrombosis with venous infarction and hemorrhage, intracranial neoplasms, brain abscesses, coagulopathies, vasculitides, and toxins. Cocaine and other sympathomimetic agents are believed to cause transient severe hypertension with resultant hemorrhage.

Anatomy

The anatomic terminology regarding intracranial hemorrhages historically comes from postmortem neuropathology descriptions. In the ED, intracranial hemorrhages are most often diagnosed by cranial CT, which remains the initial diagnostic modality of choice because the appearance of acute hemorrhage usually contrasts vividly with other intracranial contents. As outlined previously, the types of intracranial hemorrhages are anatomically classified primarily by their relationship to the substance of the brain and the meninges.[8] Simplistically, hemorrhages may be thought to be located in the brain substance (intraparenchymal hemorrhage, intracerebral hemorrhage), within the subarachnoid space surrounding the brain, or outside the brain (extra-axial hemorrhages including subdural and epidural hemorrhages) (Fig. 98-8 and Fig. 98-9).

■ SPONTANEOUS INTRACEREBRAL HEMORRHAGE

Intracerebral hemorrhage literally means blood within the substance of the cerebrum, which anatomically is most often defined as the cerebral hemispheres. Jargon often extends the term *intracerebral hemorrhage* to include any well-demarcated hemorrhage within the brain substance. The deep white matter of the cerebrum, basal ganglia, thalamus,

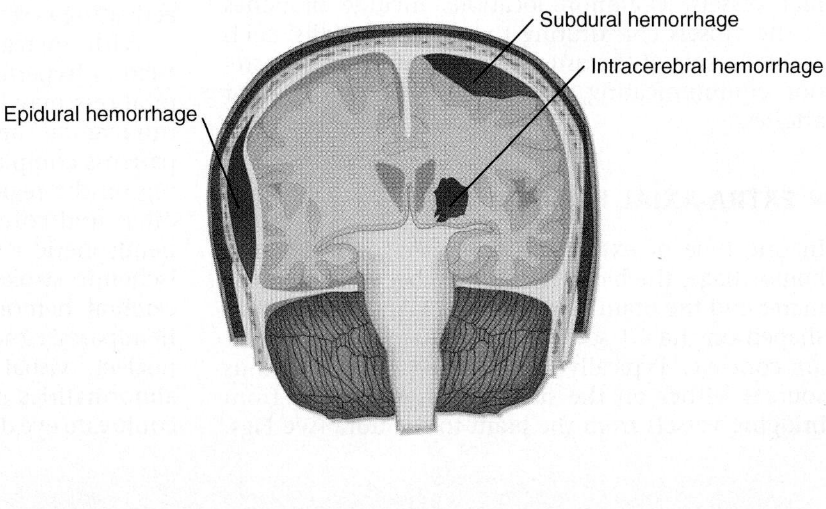
Subdural hemorrhage
Intracerebral hemorrhage
Epidural hemorrhage

FIGURE 98-8 Varieties of intracranial hemorrhage. (From Snell RS, Smith MS: Clinical Anatomy for Emergency Medicine. St. Louis, Elsevier, 1993.)

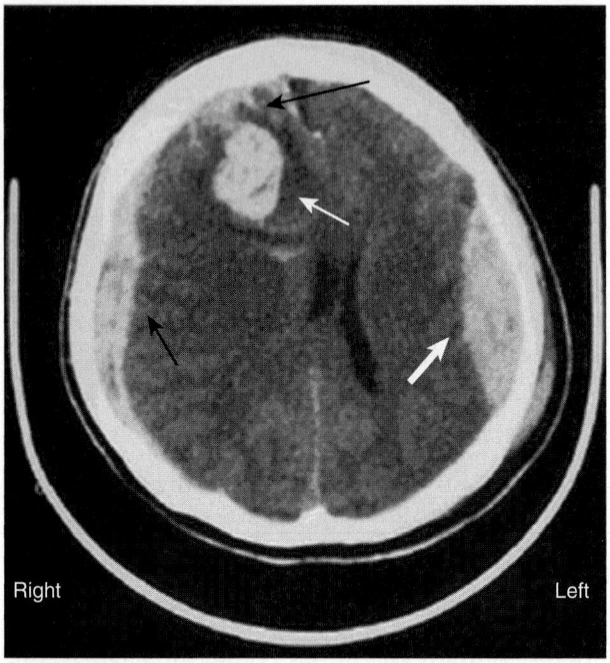
Right
Left

FIGURE 98-9 Axial section of noncontrast computed tomography scan of the head reveals four types of acute posttraumatic intracranial hemorrhage: an epidural hematoma (*short white arrow*) on the left side; a laminated subdural hematoma (*short black arrow*) on the right side; right-sided periventricular and frontal-lobe contusions containing an intraparenchymal hematoma (*long white arrow*); and a subarachnoid hemorrhage (*long black arrow*) in the right frontal region.

brainstem, and cerebellum are the most frequent locations. The hemorrhage is not defined by the relationship with the dura (see Figs. 98-3 and 98-4).

■ SUBARACHNOID HEMORRHAGE

In a subarachnoid hemorrhage, blood is visible by CT or can be identified by lumbar puncture in the subarachnoid space that surrounds the brain and spinal cord. The bleeding is into the cerebrospinal fluid that fills the subarachnoid space and may be visible in the cisterns or in the sulci (see Fig. 98-4). As mentioned in the pathophysiology section, aneurysms are often found intracranially at branch points of the intracranial vessels. Common locations include branches of the vessels constituting the circle of Willis, such as aneurysms of the anterior communicating, posterior communicating, middle cerebral, and basilar arteries.

■ EXTRA-AXIAL HEMORRHAGES

In one type of extra-axial hemorrhage, a subdural hemorrhage, the blood is confined between the dura mater and the brain. These typically appear crescent-shaped on the CT scan, and the margins of the clot are concave. Typically the bleeding is from venous sources, either on the surface of the brain or from bridging vessels from the brain to the dura (see Figs. 98-3 and 98-4). CT scan appearance may vary with the age of the hematoma; acute hemorrhages appear bright white and chronic subdural hematomas have an isodense or hypodense appearance. Subdural hematomas may attain a large size.

An epidural hematoma literally is blood outside the dura, between the dura and the cranium. The dura is tightly adherent to the cranium and the hemorrhage is confined to this epidural space. These hemorrhages often have a distinctive lenticular or lens-shaped configuration (see Fig. 98-3 and 93-4). Typically bleeding is from an arterial source, although often appearing white on CT, acute subdural hematomas may at times have a heterogenous appearance, or "swirl sign," reflecting the rapid bleeding from an arterial source. Often damage to the brain is from external compression with increased intracranial pressure and midline shift.

■ OTHER HEMORRHAGES

In a stroke with hemorrhagic transformation, the hemorrhage occurs into the body of the ischemic tissue so that the underlying wedge-shaped ischemic tissue is seen with hemorrhage into this wedge-shaped bed (see Fig. 98-5).

Presenting Signs and Symptoms

Intracranial hemorrhages of any type may present along a continuum ranging from mild headache, agitation, and confusion to coma, with seizures and stroke symptoms also common presentations.

■ INTRACEREBRAL HEMORRHAGES

Patients with a large intracerebral hemorrhage typically present with a diminished level of consciousness with or without a focal neurologic deficit. Intracerebral hemorrhages account for about 20% of acute strokes. It is not possible to reliably distinguish between an ischemic stroke and an intracerebral hemorrhage at the bedside. Patients with a diminished level of consciousness often have a larger hemorrhage and increased intracranial pressure or distortion of the thalamic and brainstem reticular activating system.[1]

With increased intracranial pressure, Cushing's triad of hypertension, bradycardia, and irregular respirations may be present, but this is not specific for intracranial hemorrhage. If able to speak, many patients complain of headache and nausea. Depending on the region of brain injury, the examiner will often find corresponding neurologic findings. With hemispheric lesions, the picture may be similar to ischemic stroke—that is, patients with a large left cerebral hemorrhage may present with right-sided hemiparesis and aphasia. Other stroke syndromes of neglect, visual field defects, and cortical sensory abnormalities may be present. With frontal lesions, conjugate eye deviation towards the side of the lesion is common. Large hematomas with mass effects may have the clinical picture of uncal herniation with diminished consciousness and third nerve dysfunction, including a large, nonreactive pupil. Third nerve dysfunction usually occurs on the side of the mass lesion but in about 10% of cases is on the opposite side ("falsely localizing third nerve palsy").

Patients with brainstem and posterior-fossa hematomas may show brainstem dysfunction including alteration in consciousness, abnormalities of extraocular motion, other cranial nerve abnormalities, and the so-called crossed signs, with cranial nerve dysfunction on one side and long-tract findings of weakness on the opposite side. One pathognomonic finding on physical examination is in pontine hemorrhage where truly pinpoint pupils (not just small) may be present.

Patients with cerebellar hemorrhages may have profound vegetative signs of diaphoresis and vomiting. A common presentation is acute headache and the inability to ambulate. Smaller cerebellar hemorrhages may demonstrate nystagmus, ataxia, dysmetria, or abnormalities of extraocular motion. If brainstem compression develops, consciousness may abruptly deteriorate.

■ SUBARACHNOID HEMORRHAGE

Subarachnoid hemorrhage typically presents as the "worst headache of my life." Certainly, the abrupt onset of a severe headache that quickly attains maximal intensity is the classic presentation. This presentation—abrupt severe headache reaching maximal intensity within seconds of onset, perhaps occurring with exertion—often leads to the diagnosis. Meningismus may be present. However, initial misdiagnosis of subarachnoid hemorrhage occurs in up to 50% of cases.[9,10]

Patients diagnosed at subsequent visits often have worse outcomes. Because of this, it is important to identify the diagnosis at the time of an initial or "sentinel" hemorrhage or warning leak. The sentinel hemorrhage may present with transient headache or confusional episode. If the patient complains of headache of abrupt onset or that the headache is different from the kind that the patient usually experience, the possibility of subarachnoid hemorrhage exists. If there is accompanying intracerebral hemorrhage there may be additional signs or symptoms.[5]

An expanding unruptured aneurysm may present with cranial nerve abnormalities. Typically this is a third-nerve paresis with asymmetric pupils and impairment of extraocular movement. The pupillary reflex may or may not be impaired.

Cardiac arrhythmias and changes consistent with myocardial ischemia at times confound the diagnosis.[10] Usually these patients have severe symptoms but cases in which the arrhythmia overshadows the clinical presentation are reported as well.

Intracranial hemorrhage is the most common presentation of arteriovenous malformations accounting for roughly half of the presentations. Other presentations include seizures and focal neurologic deficits.[7]

■ TRAUMA

A history of trauma suggests the possibility of an extra-axial hematoma. Progression of symptoms or deterioration in level of consciousness mandates exclusion of an expanding mass lesion from the diagnosis. With epidural hematoma, the classic description (present only in a minority of cases) is that of a transient loss of consciousness followed by an alert or "lucid interval," later followed by progressive decreased level of consciousness. Headache out of proportion to the head blow or the presence of persistent vegetative symptoms such as nausea and vomiting is much more common. As the mass progresses, neurologic findings may progress. Altered mental status following trauma is the typical presentation.

Chronic large subdural hematomas may be found during evaluation of altered mental status or headaches. Occult presentations of intracranial injury are more common in the elderly.

Differential Diagnosis

There is a wide spectrum of presentations of intracranial hemorrhage and diagnostic possibilities. The major differential diagnosis for intracranial hemorrhage presenting with focal neurologic signs or symptoms is ischemic stroke. Both processes may have abrupt onset of symptoms and focal neurologic deficits. Intracranial neoplasms are also in the differential diagnosis. Seizures are not a frequent presenting complaint of intracranial hemorrhage although this does occur with enough frequency to include intracerebral and subarachnoid hemorrhages in the differential diagnosis of seizures. Abnormal decerebrate posturing, which may occur with intracranial hemorrhage, is confused by observers with seizure activity on occasion. Although counter-intuitive, infectious processes such as encephalitis and meningitis at times do have abrupt onset of symptoms as well.

If altered mental status is the presenting complaint, all the causes of altered mental status should be included in the differential diagnosis (see Chapter 100). The expanded differential diagnosis for hemorrhages without focal lesions or altered mental status includes the universe of headache types. Functional headaches or "thunderclap" headaches are at times related to different types of exertions; however, they must be part of a diagnosis of exclusion for the EP.

Diagnostic Testing

■ CRANIAL COMPUTED TOMOGRAPHY

Cranial CT is the current initial imaging test of choice for evaluation of intracranial hemorrhage because of

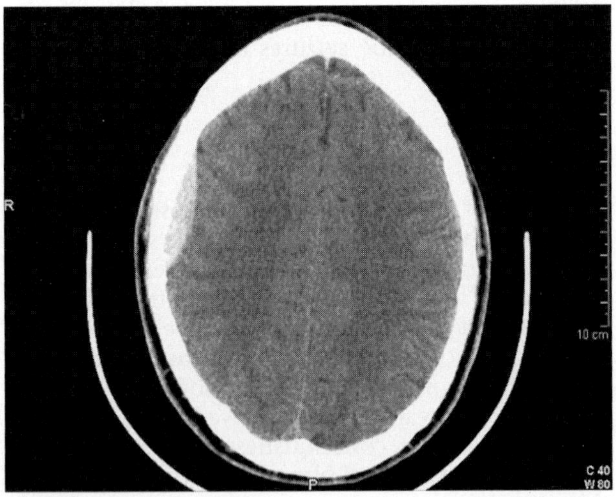
R
10 cm
P
C 40
W 80

FIGURE 98-10 Computed tomography scan: Acute epidural hematoma. Note the high density of the hemorrhage and the lens-shaped clot.

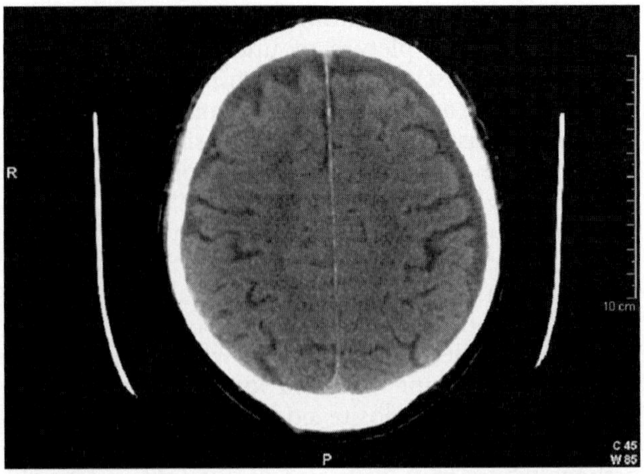
R
10 cm
P
C 45
W 85

FIGURE 98-11 Computed tomography scan: Chronic subdural hematoma (left hemispheric and bifrontal section). Low density is consistent with presence of hemorrage of some days to weeks.

the ability of noncontrast cranial CT to demonstrate the presence of acute hemorrhage. Cranial CT is readily available in most U.S. EDs. Expert interpretation of cranial CT scans unfortunately is often not as readily obtainable, and EPs should be familiar with the basics of CT interpretation as it applies to immediate patient care.

In patients with suspected subarachnoid hemorrhage, CT is very sensitive for detecting acute hemorrhage, to the order of 95% or better.[10,12] The sensitivity starts to diminish as time from the hemorrhage increases, and CT sensitivity is estimated as less than 50% 7 days from the event.

A suggested approach to analyzing CT scans (see Chapter 69) and a useful structure for communicating with consultants is the following series of simple questions:

1. Is there blood present?
2. Where is the hemorrhage?
3. How much blood is present and what is the effect?
4. What is causing the bleeding?

■ Question 1—Is there blood present?

Acute blood appears white or hyperdense on noncontrast CT scans (Fig. 98-10; see Fig. 98-3). Some intracranial structures such as the dura or choroid plexus may calcify and at times simulate hemorrhage. As blood ages, it becomes increasingly low-density or dark (Fig. 98-11). There is a time during this evolution when blood is nearly the same CT density as brain parenchyma and is termed isodense. Clinically, the terms acute, subacute, and chronic are used to reflect the change in appearance on the CT scan. Inhomogeneous density, although usually observed in rapidly bleeding visceral injuries, may be observed on occasions in some cases (see Fig. 98-4). Rarely, the existence of an isodense hematoma must be inferred from cortical sulcus markings that do not reach the cranium.

■ Question 2—Where is the hemorrhage?

If hemorrhage is present, it is then described as external to the brain substance (extra-axial), within the substance of the brain (intraparenchymal), or visible in the subarachnoid or cisternal spaces. Extra-axial hematomas have two basic types of appearance. Subdural hematomas are most often crescentric (see Fig. 98-3), whereas epidural hematomas have a typical lens-shaped pattern (see Fig. 98-10). An intraparenchymal hemorrhage may be in the cerebrum (intracerebral hemorrhage) or in subcortical or brainstem structures. Intracerebral hemorrhages tend to be located in deep white matter or the basal ganglia, or are confined to one lobe of the brain ("lobar") (see Fig. 98-1). These hemorrhages tend to have a stereotypic pattern, and deviation from these patterns may suggest an uncommon etiology of the hemorrhage.

Cerebellar hemorrhages may be hemispheric (Fig. 98-12) or midline and cause brainstem compression. Subarachnoid hemorrhage may be detected by the high density in the suprasellar cistern or perimesencephalic cistern or by blood in the cortical sulci where ordinarily there should be low-density images from the cerebrospinal fluid signal. Depending on the degree of hemorrhage, subarachnoid hemorrhage may be obvious (Fig. 98-13) or relatively subtle (see Fig. 98-2). Intraventricular hemorrhage (literally blood within the ventricles) may result from rupture of an intracerebral hemorrhage into the ventricular system, from trauma, or from a subarachnoid hemorrhage (Fig. 98-14).

■ Question 3—How much blood is present and what is the effect?

Some quantification of the hemorrhage should follow. For extra-axial hemorrhage, the greatest thick-

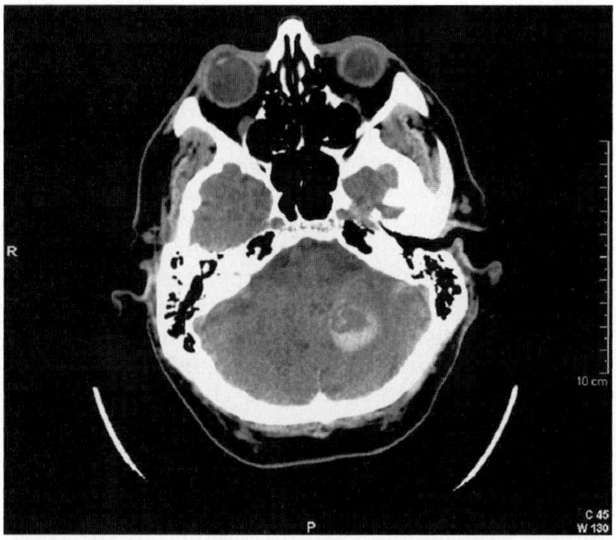
R
10 cm
P
C 45
W 130
FIGURE 98-12 Computed tomography scan: Acute hemispheric cerebellar hemorrhage. The posterior fossa expanding mass places the brainstem at risk for compression.

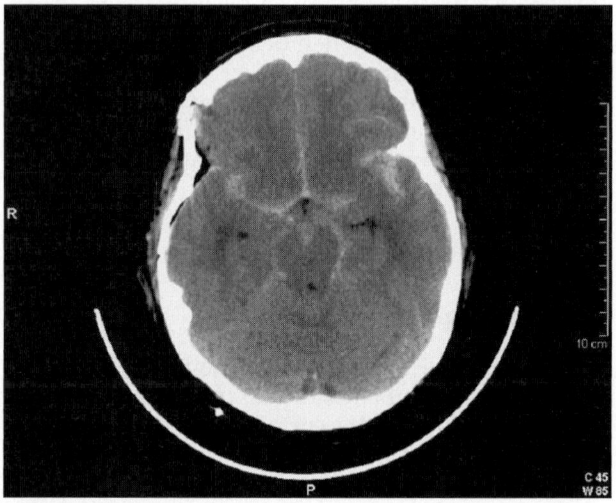
R
10 cm
P
C 45
W 85
FIGURE 98-13 Computed tomography scan: Acute subarachnoid hemorrhage with blood in the suprasellar cistern and over the hemispheres.

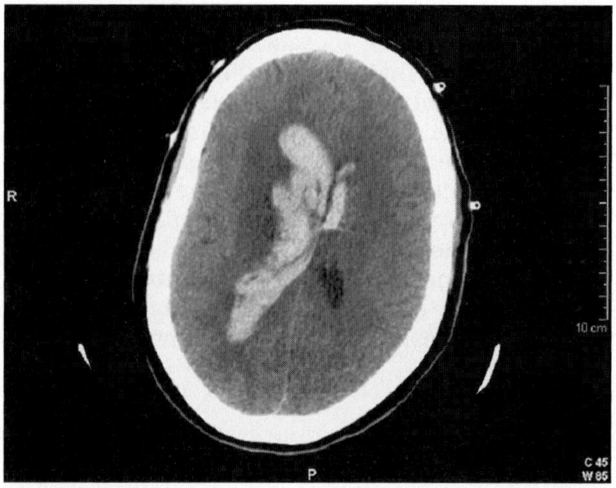
R
10 cm
P
C 45
W 85
FIGURE 98-14 Computed tomography scan: Intraventricular blood from extension of deep intracerebral hemorrhage. The right lateral and third ventricles are filled with blood casts.

ness of the hematoma is easily estimated from the ruler on the CT scan. Volumetric estimation of intraparenchymal hematomas may be estimated from information present on the cranial CT, though this usually is not done frequently by EPs.[11] Of more importance is any effect that the hematoma is having on adjacent structures. This may be estimated qualitatively by noting any compression on the ventricular system and the amount of shift of midline structure.

■ Question 4—What is causing the bleeding?

Some cranial CT scan patterns of hemorrhage are sufficiently typical that an etiologic diagnosis may be suspected. For example, in a middle-aged or elderly patient with a spontaneous intracerebral hemorrhage in the deep white matter, the term *hypertensive hemorrhage* may be used. The same hemorrhage in a much younger patient might suggest a vascular lesion such as an arteriovenous malformation as the cause. One must remember that the specific etiology of a hemorrhage seen on a CT scan is garnered from pattern recognition and is to some degree speculative.

■ ANGIOGRAPHY

Conventional angiography with selective contrast injection traditionally has been used when vascular lesions such as aneurysms or arteriovenous malformations are suspected. CT-angiography with intravenously administered radiographic contrast is being increasingly employed. Selection of direct vascular imaging is directed by a radiologist, neurologist, or neurosurgeon. (Discussion of this modality is outside the scope of this chapter.)

■ MAGNETIC RESONANCE IMAGING

The role of magnetic resonance imaging (MRI) in current emergency medicine practice is evolving. In some centers, MRI-angiography or venography is used, although again this is done in consultation with the admitting physicians or services. The traditional view is that MR is inferior to CT when acute hemorrhage is suspected; however, recent literature suggests that with some technical adaptations MRI may readily detect hemorrhages.

■ LUMBAR PUNCTURE

Lumbar puncture should be performed in patients with suspected subarachnoid hemorrhage and negative or equivocal results on CT scanning. The common procedure is to collect cerebrospinal fluid in four tubes and obtain a cell count in tubes 1 and 4. Findings consistent with subarachnoid hemorrhage include the presence of xanthochromia and a red blood cell count that does not diminish from tube 1 to tube 4. Xanthochromia from red blood cell breakdown may take more than 12 hours to develop and may not be present when lumbar puncture is performed soon after symptom onset. The most common method of determining xanthochromia in the ED is visual inspection, although some studies show that spectrophotometry is superior. Lumbar puncture performed to exclude subarachnoid hemorrhage sometimes reveals unexpected diagnoses such as meningitis.

■ OTHER TESTING

Basic laboratory work should include coagulation studies and platelet counts if hemorrhage is suspected.

ED Interventions and Procedures

■ THE ABCS

Supportive care including appropriate management of ABCs—airway, breathing, and circulation—is of course important. The decision to intubate is based on the judgment of the physician who assesses the patient's ability to protect the airway. It is recommended that certain steps be taken for rapid-sequence induction in patients with intracranial hemorrhage or other conditions with suspected increased intracranial pressure, including use of lidocaine and a defasciculating dose of a paralytic agent, although rigorous proof of efficacy is lacking. In the past, hyperventilation was recommended with the goal of reducing abnormally increased intracranial pressure. Again, evidence is lacking, but the consensus is that hyperventilation beyond that needed to reduce $PaCO_2$ to only a small degree [$PaCO_2$ of 30-35 torr] is not indicated.[13]

■ BLOOD PRESSURE CONTROL CONTROVERSY

Blood pressure management in the setting of intracranial hemorrhage is controversial. In multiple trauma patients with central nervous system injury, hypotension is associated with a poor outcome. In patients with intracerebral hemorrhage, the risk of expanding a hematoma associated with sustained hypertension must be weighed against the risk of impairment of cerebral perfusion if the blood pressure is reduced. In patients with established intracerebral hematoma and hypertension, consensus at this time is to use intravenous agents that can be titrated such as nitroprusside, labetalol, esmolol, or carvedilol, if needed, to maintain blood pressures with an MAP of less than 130 mm Hg. Systolic blood pressure less than 180 mm Hg and diastolic blood pressure greater than 105 mm Hg on two readings taken 5 minutes apart are recommended criteria for intervention.[13]

In patients with subarachnoid hemorrhage, there also is no clear evidence-supported management strategy. Hypertension should be avoided in patients with a ruptured aneurysm, using IV titratable agents, as described previously. Some experts argue that relative hypotension should be induced, based on the theory that the ruptured aneurysm is at risk for rebleeding in the presence of hypertension. Once the aneurysm is secured by interventional techniques, the blood pressure is allowed to return to normal levels. The calcium channel antagonist nimodipine is recommended to reduce the chance of ischemia from vasospasm.[5,6]

Management of intracranial pressure is conjectural if its cause is unknown. However, basic steps such as elevation of the head of the bed, keeping the head midline, and avoiding painful stimulation are clearly indicated. Hyperventilation with the goal of reducing intracranial pressure currently is out of favor. Steroids are of no proven benefit in these conditions. Use of osmotic agents such as mannitol in cases in which a herniation syndrome is present may be useful as a temporizing measure when decompressive neurosurgical therapy is planned.

Intracranial pressure monitoring may be useful in the ED but should be performed under the direction of a neurosurgeon or neurointensivist. Venticulostomy may be performed in the ED by a neurosurgeon.

Treatment

If a patient with intracranial hemorrhage has a seizure, the use of anticonvulsants clearly is indicated. Phenytoin is the current drug of choice. Use of anticonvulsants is common in patients with intracerebral hematomas who have not had seizures, although their efficacy is not evidence-based. Likewise, use of anticonvulsants in patients with subarachnoid hemorrhage who have not had seizures is controversial.

Hyperglycemia and hypothermia are associated with neuronal injury and should be avoided if possible and treated if not. No specific guidelines exist to guide the clinician at this time. If a coagulopathy is present, coagulations studies should be made to detect this.

In cases of intracranial hemorrhage, most activity in the ED is directed at diagnosis. Treatment is governed by the type of hemorrhage, etiology, and any associated medical or surgical conditions. Definitive treatment is under the direction of the consulting and admitting physicians, and the EP works in concert with them. Supportive care is discussed in the preceding rection. In most institutions, subarachnoid hemorrhages and the traumatic hemorrhages will be managed by neurosurgeons. Intracerebral hemorrhages are often managed by neurosurgeons but institutional management patterns will vary.

Intensive care and monitoring will be necessary in many cases.

The condition of the patient may be anywhere in a wide spectrum ranging from deeply comatose to virtually asymptomatic, and obviously the treatment will vary. For deeply comatose patients, intensive supportive care is indicated in the short term. Evidence of the development of hydrocephalus by CT will lead to consideration of placement of a ventriculostomy. Drainage of cerebrospinal fluid and other supportive measures may be guided by continuous measurement of intracranial pressure by a variety of invasive techniques.

Cerebellar hemorrhage is an emergency requiring hematoma removal and relief of brainstem compression that offers the possibility of good recovery in selected cases.[1] Surgery for removal of supratentorial intracerebral hematomas is controversial and generally not recommended.[14] Other inpatient supportive measures for intracerebral hemorrhages might include prophylaxis for thromboembolic events.

Patients with an acute intracerebral hematoma who are taking warfarin should receive fresh frozen plasma (FFP) and vitamin K as soon as possible to correct the coagulopathy. Best dosing regimens are not known, but for patients with a prolonged international ratio, a reasonable recommendation is 10 mg of vitamin K (administered intravenously over 10 minutes) plus 10 mL/kg of fresh frozen plasma administered as soon as possible. Time to treatment of warfarin-coagulopathy in intracerebral hemorrhage has been found to be the most important determinant of 14-hour anticoagulation reversal.[15] Antiplatelet therapy has been noted to be associated with clinical deterioration.

Acute administration of recombinant activated factor VII is currently undergoing study in hopes of limiting expansion of hematomas; early studies indicate some benefit, but thromboembolic complications have been noted.[16,17] A large, multicenter randomized trial is under way at the time of this writing.

■ SUBARACHNOID HEMORRHAGE

In recent years the trend has continued for "early" surgical intervention for subarachnioid hemorrhage—that is, intervention to isolate the aneurysm or occlude it within 1 to 2 days of bleeding.[5,6] Until the aneurysm is secured, the consensus is that blood pressure should be lowered with parenteral medications if necessary. A recent study reported that interventional endovascular coiling may lead to better outcomes in select patients with ruptured aneurysms.[18]

■ ARTERIOVENOUS MALFORMATIONS

Treatment of arteriovenous malformations is complex, controversial, and outside the practice of EPs other than providinge supportive care as outlined previously. Risk of rebleeding is less than for saccular aneurysms. Should seizures occur, anticonvulsant medication should be administered. Additional diagnostic vascular studies besides cranial CT are required and may include angiography, CT-angiography, and MRI studies. Treatment may include radiotherapy, embolization of the arteriovenous malformation, and/or resection.

■ EXTRA-AXIAL HEMORRHAGES

All but the smallest epidural hematomas must be treated with craniotomy and surgical evacuation with investigation of the bleeding site to secure hemostasis. Treatment of subdural hematomas depend on the size and chronicity of the hematoma, the general medical condition of the patient, and signs and symptoms referable to the hematoma. In some patients, chronic subdural hematomas may be of large size with seemingly minimal or no effect on the patient; the problem is underlying atrophy, with the subdural hematoma filling the void. Acute subdural hematomas generally are evacuated if there is any mass effect, but this at times may be difficult to assess because the underlying brain is usually injured and edematous.

In hemorrhages complicating abscesses, tumors, or other conditions, treatment is generally directed at the underlying lesion.

Disposition

If the facility does not have the necessary specialty care, the patient should be transferred after stabilization to an appropriate facility. The urgency of transport corresponds roughly with the clinical condition of the patient; for example, patients with a headache and a chronic subdural hematoma and no other findings may likely be transferred electively. The notable exceptions in which emergency transport is indicated include acute subarachnoid hemorrhages, cerebellar hemorrhages, and epidural hematomas when the natural history includes early clinical deterioration.

REFERENCES

1. Qureshi AI, Tuhrim S, Broderick JP, et al: Spontaneous intracerebral hemorrhage. N Engl J Med 2001;344: 1450-1460.
2. Brott T, Broderick J, Kothari R, et al: Early hemorrhage growth in patients with intracerebral hemorrhage. Stroke 1997;28:1-5.
3. Flaherty ML, Kissela B, Woo D, et al: The increasing incidence of anti-coagulant associated intracerebral hemorrhage. Neurology 2007;68:116-121.
4. Flibotte JJ, et al: Warfarin, hematoma expansion, and outcome of intracerebral hemorrhage. Neurology 2004;63: 1059-1064.
5. Suarez JI, Tarr RW, Selman WR: Aneurysmal subarachnoid hemorrhage. N Engl J Med 2006;354:387-396.
6. Brisman JL, Song JK, Newell DW: Cerebral aneurysms. N Engl J Med 2006;355:928-939.
7. The Arteriovenous Malformation Study Group: Arteriovenous malformations of the brain in adults. N Engl J Med 1999;340:1812-1818.

8. Snell RS, Smith MS: The skull, the meninges, and the blood supply of the brain relative to trauma and intracranial hemorrhage: In Clinical Anatomy for Emergency Medicine. St. Louis, Mosby, 1993, p 284.
9. Kowalski RG, Claasen J, Kreiter KT, et al: Initial misdiagnosis and outcome after subarachnoid hemorrhage. JAMA 2004;291:866-869.
10. Edlow JA, Caplan LR: Avoiding pitfalls in the diagnosis of subarachnoid hemorrhage. N Engl J Med 2000;342:29-36.
11. Kothari RU, Brott T, Broderick JP, et al: The ABC's of measuring intracerebral hemorrhage volumes. Stroke 1996;27: 1304-1305.
12. Mark DG, Pines JM: The detection of nontraumatic subarachnoid hemorrhage: Still a diagnostic challenge. Am J Emerg Med. 2006;24(7):859-863.
13. Broderick JP, Adams HP Jr, Barsan W, et al: Guidelines for the management of spontaneous intracerebral hemorrhage: A statement for healthcare professionals from a special writing group of the Stroke Council, American Heart Association. Stroke 1999;30:905-915.
14. Mendelow AD, Gregson BA, Fernandes HM, et al: Early surgery versus initial conservative treatment in patients with spontaneous supratentorial intracerebral hematomas in the International Surgical Trial in Intracerebral Hemorrhage (STITCH): A randomized trial. Lancet 2005; 365(9457):387-397.
15. Goldstein JN, Thomas SH, Frontiero V, et al: Timing of fresh frozen plasma administration and rapid correction of coagulopathy in warfarin-related intracerebral hemorrhage. Stroke 2006;37:151-155.
16. Mayer SA, Brun NC, Begtrup K, et al: Recombinant activated factor VII for acute intracerebral hemorrhage. N Engl J Med 2005;352:777-785.
17. O'Connell KA, Wood JJ, Wise RP, et al: Thromboembolic adverse events after use of recombinant human coagulation factor VIIa. JAMA 2006;295:293-298.
18. Molyneux AJ, Kerr RS, Yu LM, et al: International subarachnoid aneurysm trial (ISAT) of neurosurgical clipping versus endovascular coiling in 2143 patients with ruptured intracranial aneurysms: A randomised comparison of effects on survival, dependency, seizures, rebleeding, subgroups, and aneurysm occlusion. Lancet 2005;366(9488):809-817.

Chapter **99**

Syncope

James Quinn

KEY POINTS

- Syncope is a symptom, not a diagnosis.
- Patients with cardiac syncope have a 6-month mortality rate of over 10%.
- If the diagnosis can be made, the disposition will be based on that diagnosis.
- When the patient's symptoms have resolved and the cause is unclear, risk stratification can help with disposition decisions.
- Patients with an abnormal electrocardiogram or signs of structural heart disease (especially congestive heart failure), shortness of breath, persistent abnormal vital signs, and a low hematocrit are at higher risk for adverse cardiac outcomes.

Scope and Outline

It is estimated that one in four people will faint during their lifetime and that six of one thousand people per year will suffer from the symptom of syncope. Syncope is responsible for 1% to 2% of all ED visits and the costs of hospitalization for syncope approach 2 billion dollars annually.[1-3]

Syncope is defined as a transient loss of consciousness that does not require resuscitative efforts and results in a return to the patient's baseline neurologic condition. Loss of consciousness associated with neurologic deficits or persistent alteration in level of consciousness is, strictly speaking, not properly described as syncope; although such events are commonly referred to as syncope in the literature, in this chapter they are termed *apparent syncope*.

Pathophysiology

Syncope comes from the Greek word *synkoptein,* meaning "to cut short." Hippocrates was the first to use the term and describe the symptom.[4] Syncope has many causes, but the pathophysiology of the final pathway is the same: hypoperfusion of the cerebral cortex and reticular activating system, which after 8 to 10 seconds of interrupted perfusion causes loss of consciousness; a shorter period results in lightheadedness or dizziness and is referred to as *near syncope*.

Presenting Signs and Symptoms

The symptoms of syncope can be dramatic. Patients may or may not have a warning, or prodrome, and frequently suffer a fall and have associated trauma. Those with prodrome often experience lightheadedness, diaphoretic warmth, and/or nausea and vomiting. Those witnessing the event often conclude that the patient has died or was dead for a short period of time, making it an emotionally charged and anxiety-provoking event.

Classification of Syncope

The American College of Physicians lists four major prognostic categories of syncope: neurally mediated, orthostatic, neurogenic, and cardiac[5]; actually, there is a fifth category ("syncope of unknown cause"), because in most cases the cause of syncope remains unknown even after extensive investigation.

■ NEURALLY MEDIATED SYNCOPE

Neurally mediated syncope is syncope associated with inappropriate vasodilation, bradycardia, or both as a result of inappropriate vagal or sympathetic tone.[6] It is a benign type of cardiovascular syncope that often is associated with a sensation of increased warmth and may be accompanied by preceding lightheadedness (prodrome) with sweating and nausea. A slow, progressive onset suggests the subcategory vasovagal syncope. Sweating and nausea do not occur with orthostatic hypotension, which is another cause of syncope preceded by lightheadedness.

Neurally mediated or vasovagal syncope may occur after exposure to an unexpected or unpleasant sight, sound, or smell; fear or other emotional distress; severe pain; or surgical procedure. It may also occur in association with prolonged standing or kneeling in a crowded or warm place or after exertion. As a result, the vagus nerve is stimulated, causing reflex bradycardia and vasodilation.

Situational syncope occurs during or immediately after coughing, micturition, defecation, or swallowing via a similar mechanism. Carotid sinus syncope can be associated with neck pressure (shaving, tight collar) or head turning resulting in carotid sinus stimulation in the neck.

■ ORTHOSTATIC SYNCOPE

Orthostatic syncope occurs when there is documented postural hypotension associated with syncope or symptoms of pre-syncope.[4] In cases of orthostatic syncope, measurement of blood pressure is recommended, first after the patient is supine for 5 minutes and then after the patient is able to stand for 1 to 3 minutes. A decrease of more than 20 mm Hg in systolic pressure is considered abnormal, as is a drop in pressure below 90 mm Hg independent of the development of symptoms.

Because orthostatic hypotension occurs in asymptomatic individuals, vital signs are neither particularly sensitive nor specific. In fact, positive orthostatic changes have been documented in up to 40% of asymptomatic patients over the age of 70 and in 25% of those younger than 60 years. Similarly, a notable number of children who are asymptomatic have been documented to have orthostatic hypotension.

The most common cause of orthostatic syncope is intravascular volume loss that may be due to dehydration or blood loss. Many serious causes of syncope have orthostatic symptoms.

■ NEUROLOGIC SYNCOPE

Neurologic causes of apparent syncope include seizures, transient ischemic attacks, migraine headaches, subarachnoid hemorrhage, and subclavian steal syndrome. Confusion after apparent syncope that lasts more than 5 minutes, tongue biting, incontinence, and epileptic aura suggest a seizure. A significant differential in the blood pressure in the two arms suggests subclavian steal or dissection. Neurologic causes to be considered as true syncope must by definition be transient in nature and result in a return to baseline neurologic function. Thus loss of consciousness with persistent neurologic deficits or altered mental status is not true syncope. In fact, according to this criterion very few neurologic events (especially strokes or subarachnoid hemorrhage) meet the definition of syncope.[7]

Most cases involving neurologic causes of syncope are easily predicted. In general, when these patients present with symptoms suggesting a specific disease process, the need for intervention based on neurologic symptoms is usually obvious. Most EDs do not recommend routine neurologic work-up of all syncope patients unless the syncopal episode is related to neurologic symptoms. It has been determined that routine neurologic testing and investigation, such as computed tomography (CT) scanning, is not cost-effective in patients without neurologic symptoms.[7]

■ CARDIAC-RELATED SYNCOPE

Cardiac-related syncope is clearly the most dangerous class of syncope, which can be a harbinger of sudden death. Because patients with documented cardiac syncope have a 6-month mortality rate of greater than 10%, timely and thorough evaluation is warranted.[8]

Syncope in this class can be caused by many types of arrhythmias (benign and malignant), valvular and ischemic heart disease, and cardiomyopathies. Although it is clear that patients with known cardiac disease and syncope have a significant increased incidence of cardiac-related death, cardiac disease may not be recognized in many patients with cardiac syncope, and persons with a history of cardiac disease may appear to be very stable. Therefore, depending on the history and age of the patient, a relatively aggressive search for cardiac problems may be necessary. However, the urgency of these investigations is unclear.

■ SYNCOPE OF UNKNOWN CAUSE

Syncope of unknown cause is the largest category of syncope, estimated to be as high as 40%, even with extensive work-up.[2] Some studies have found that after evaluation in the ED, physicians are uncertain as to the cause of syncope more than 50% to 60% of the time.[9] As a result, many serious cases are initially classified in this category, causing a dilemma for EPs who must decide whether to admit or discharge these patients. It is this largest group of patients that present the greatest challenge for EPs.

Recommended Diagnostic Tests

Ongoing or related symptoms associated with syncope should direct the ED investigations. CT scans are not indicated for all patients, but one should not ignore associated symptoms, which should receive a complete work-up[7] (e.g., CT in patients with associated headache or abdominal pain, urine pregnancy tests in females, ultrasonography in pregnant women, troponins and CT angiography in patients with chest pain and dyspnea)

A routine electrocardiogram is almost always indicated, as are rhythm strips and monitoring while the patient is in the ED. Any non-sinus rhythms or new electrocardiographic changes should be a concern. Routine basic laboratory tests in asymptomatic patients are not recommended, and their use should be guided by the history and physical examination.

Prognosis

Perhaps the best data on prognosis for patients with syncope was done by Soteriades and co-workers, using data from the Framingham study.[8] This study assessed the risk of death of a prospective cohort of 7814 patients over a 17-year period. The results were dramatic. Those with documented heart disease and syncope had twice the mortality rate of patients without syncope, and patients with syncope with a neurologic cause were 50% more likely to die. People with syncope of unknown cause also had a significantly increased risk of death of 30%, whereas those with neurally mediated (vasovagal) syncope had a lower risk. The study clearly shows that the increased risk of death in this group requires further scrutiny, as does ED disposition and management.

Other studies suggest that cardiac syncope represents 5% to 40% of the causes of syncope, with a significant increase in mortality. ED management of patients with cardiac symptoms such as chest pain in addition to syncope is obvious; however, of most concern is the asymptomatic patient with syncope.

The absence of cardiac symptoms is not reassuring, because patients can have serious "silent symptoms" (silent myocardial infarction and silent arrhythmia, such as Brugada's syndrome[10]) that may not be obviously associated with syncope on presentation. Such patients may not have a history of cardiac disease, and the presenting syncope may be the first symptom. Patients with cardiac symptoms and syncope clearly require thorough and timely evaluation and thus in most cases require emergent hospitalization.[11]

EPs evaluating patients presenting with syncope who are asymptomatic and without an unclear cause are faced with the following questions:

1. Is the syncope a symptom indicating that known underlying heart disease is active, unstable, and related to the episode?
2. Is the syncope a symptom of occult underlying heart disease?
3. Is the syncope a symptom of an occult noncardiac life-threatening process (e.g., pulmonary embolism, occult bleeding, transient ischemic attack, subarachnoid hemorrhage)?

In order to maximize sensitivity of detecting underlying disease, EPs often properly admit low-risk patients for further evaluation, although such decisions are often questioned.[12] It is this group of asymptomatic syncope patients that are most likely to benefit from risk stratification strategies guiding disposition.

▪ ACUTE RISK STRATIFICATION IN THE EMERGENCY DEPARTMENT

Martin and colleagues developed a risk stratification scheme for patients presenting to the ED with syncope.[13] The stratification was premised on 1-year prognosis of death or cardiac morbidity. Four predictors of death at 1 year were found: age greater than 45 years, history of ventricular dysrhythmias, history of congestive heart failure, and an abnormal electrocardiogram. A similar study found that an abnormal electrocardiogram and history of structural heart disease (primarily congestive heart failure) predicted mortality, but that a much higher age cut-off (age greater than 65 years) could predict death at 1 year.[14]

Sarasin and co-workers developed a risk score for ED patients with syncope.[15] The score was based on three factors associated with increased risk of an arrhythmia: abnormal electrocardiogram, age greater than 65 years, and a history of any cardiac disease (primarily congestive heart failure).

Finally, Quinn and associates derived and validated a decision rule to address short-term risk (7 days) to better address the immediate risk of patients in the ED.[16,17] Again a history of congestive heart failure and an abnormal electrocardiogram were the most important predictors. The decision rule considered all patients with syncope and also determined that shortness of breath, hematocrit greater than 30, and systolic blood pressure greater than 90 mm Hg were important risk factors. Age greater than 75 years was found to be sensitive but nonspecific in this cohort and not useful as a predictor.

Age as a risk factor deserves specific mention beause EPs often admit patients with syncope just because of age. For almost all diseases, older people die sooner than younger people, and health problems in general increase with age. Recommending that all people over 45 years of age (or even those over 65 or 75 years of age) be admitted to the ED because this factor predicts 1-year death is impractical. Age by itself is a poor discriminator; many younger people have significant illness that puts them at even greater risk. This is demonstrated in a study of short-term outcomes of asymptomatic patients with unknown causes presenting with syncope who were older than 50 years; all had benign outcomes.[9]

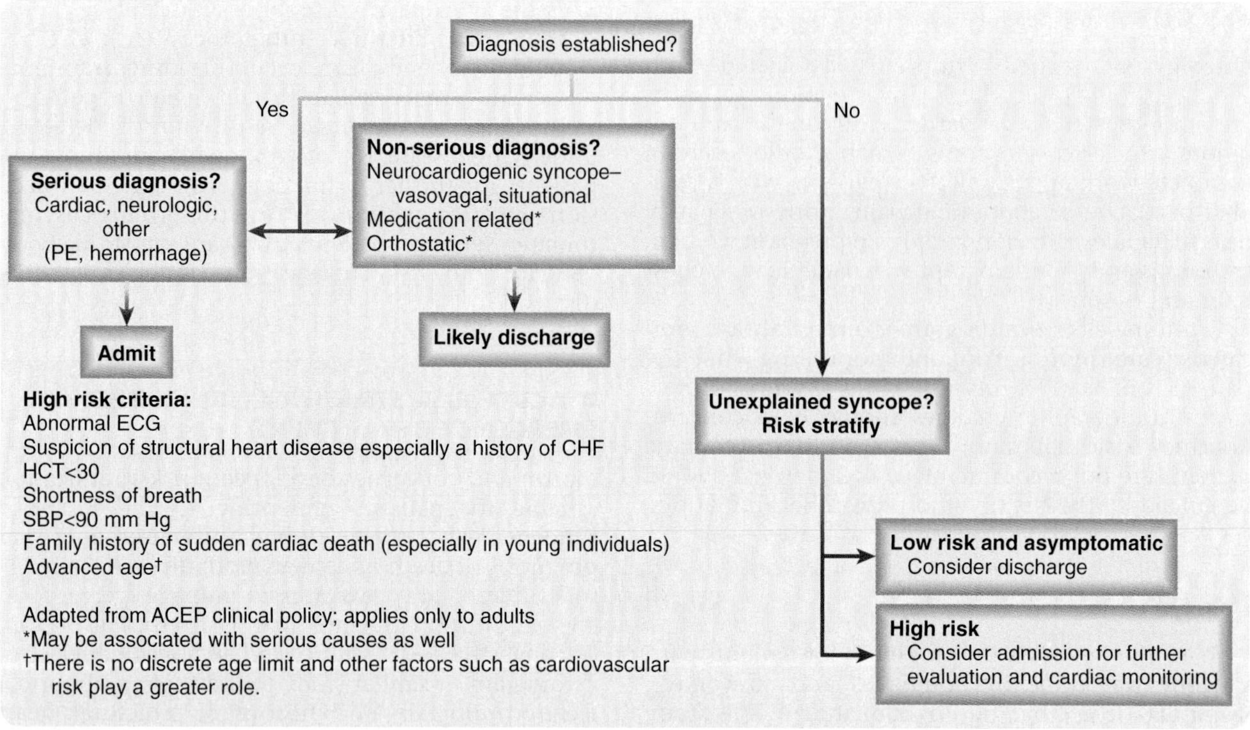
Diagnosis established?
Yes
No
Serious diagnosis?
Cardiac, neurologic, other
(PE, hemorrhage)
Non-serious diagnosis?
Neurocardiogenic syncope–vasovagal, situational
Medication related*
Orthostatic*
Admit
Likely discharge
Unexplained syncope?
Risk stratify
High risk criteria:
Abnormal ECG
Suspicion of structural heart disease especially a history of CHF
HCT<30
Shortness of breath
SBP<90 mm Hg
Family history of sudden cardiac death (especially in young individuals)
Advanced age†
Low risk and asymptomatic
Consider discharge
High risk
Consider admission for further evaluation and cardiac monitoring
Adapted from ACEP clinical policy; applies only to adults
*May be associated with serious causes as well
†There is no discrete age limit and other factors such as cardiovascular risk play a greater role.

FIGURE 99-1 Emergency department evaluation of syncope. ACEP, American College of Emergency Physicians; CHF, congestive heart failure; ECG, electrocardiogram; HCT, hematocrit; PE, pulmonary embolism; SBP, systolic blood pressure.

In summary, advanced age is a risk, but there is no practical age cut-off for risk, and it should be considered only in the presence of other risk factors.

Improved Diagnostic Strategies in the ED

Some investigators reported that diagnosis and prognosis improved with more invasive testing such as echocardiography.[18] This makes sense in that this procedure may identify patients with structural heart disease and a limited ejection fraction; however, another study found that those patients who would benefit from echocardiography could be identified by their history and physical examination, and that this procedure may not be cost-effective.[18] Another group in the United Kingdom found that they could improve risk stratification by implementing a protocol with more aggressive strategies such as tilt-table testing and echocardiography but noted that such strategies may not be cost-effective or practical in the ED.[19] It is unclear whether limited echocardiography has a role in the ED for identifying structural heart disease and increased risk.

Because echocardiography and other invasive tests are not routinely available to the ED 24 hours per day, investigators in the United States have started to utilize observation units with syncope to avoid admission, similar to chest pain units for aggressive work-up in an ED observation unit versus standard inpatient care for a small select group of "intermediate" risk patients who presented to the ED.[20] The study held some promise for syncope observation units, but a formal cost analysis was not done, and although admissions decreased, the safety of the protocol and costs of testing and setting up and maintaining the syncope unit need to be considered in a larger population.

Guidelines for Admission and Disposition

Many specialty societies have devised consensus guidelines for admission to the ED that have focused on the best available data. The American College of Emergency Physicians recently revised its guidelines[21] that recommend that patients with evidence of cardiac and neurologic causes as well as other serious outcomes diagnosed in the ED be admitted. Admission is also recommended for patients with undifferentiated syncope who have risk factors that put them at risk for adverse outcomes (Fig. 99-1).

EPs may consider for discharge asymptomatic, well-appearing patients and patients with a negative work-up for associated symptoms. EPs should remember that many studies show an increased risk for patients with non-sinus rhythms, electrocardiogram abnormalities, a history of congestive heart failure (or other significant heart disease), shortness of breath, anemia, persistent low blood pressure, and advanced age. Patients with these risks, even though they are asymptomatic and well-appearing, have a high risk of adverse outcomes and should be admitted to the hospital.

REFERENCES

1. Wayne NN: Syncope: Physiological considerations and an analysis of the clinical characteristics in 510 patients. Am J Med 1961;30:418-438.
2. Kapoor WN, Karpf M, Wieand S, et al: A prospective evaluation and follow-up of patients with syncope. N Engl J Med 1983;309:197-204.
3. Sun BC, Emond JA, Camargo CA Jr: Direct medical costs of syncope-related hospitalizations in the United States. Am J Cardiol 2005;95:668-671.
4. Grubb BP, Jorge Sdo C: A review of the classification, diagnosis, and management of autonomic dysfunction syndromes associated with orthostatic intolerance. Arq Bras Cardiol 2000;74:537-552.
5. Linzer M, Yang EH, Estes NA 3rd, et al: Diagnosing syncope. Part 2: Unexplained syncope. Clinical efficacy assessment project of the American College of Physicians. Ann Intern Med 1997;127:76-86.
6. Boehm KE, Morris EJ, Kip KT, et al: Diagnosis and management of neurally mediated syncope and related conditions in adolescents. J Adolesc Health 2001;28:2-9.
7. Eagle KA, Black HR: The impact of diagnostic tests in evaluating patients with syncope. Yale J Biol Med 1983;56:1-8.
8. Soteriades ES, Evans JC, Larson MG, et al: Incidence and prognosis of syncope. N Engl J Med 2002;347:878-885.
9. Morag RM, Murdock LF, Khan ZA, et al: Do patients with a negative Emergency Department evaluation for syncope require hospital admission? J Emerg Med 2004;27:339-343.
10. Juang JM, Huang SK: Brugada syndrome—an under-recognized electrical disease in patients with sudden cardiac death. Cardiology 2004;101(4):157-169.
11. Oh JH, Hanusa BH, Kapoor WN: Do symptoms predict cardiac arrhythmias and mortality in patients with syncope? Arch Intern Med 1999;159:375-380.
12. Quinn JV, Stiell IG, McDermott DA, et al: San Francisco Syncope Rule vs. physician judgment and decision making. Am J Emerg Med 2005;23:782-786.
13. Martin TP, Hanusa BH, Kapoor WN: Risk stratification of patients with syncope. Ann Emerg Med 1997;29:459-466.
14. Colivicchi F, Ammirati F, Melina D, et al: Development and prospective validation of a risk stratification system for patients with syncope in the emergency department: The OESIL risk score. Eur Heart J 2003;24:811-819.
15. Sarasin FP, Hanusa BH, Perneger T, et al: A risk score to predict arrhythmias in patients with unexplained syncope. Acad Emerg Med 2003;10:1312-1317.
16. Quinn JV, Stiell IG, McDermott DA, et al: Derivation of the San Francisco Syncope Rule to predict patients with short-term serious outcomes. Ann Emerg Med 2004;43:224-232.
17. Quinn J, Stiell I, McDermott D, et al: Prospective validation of the San Francisco Syncope Rule to predict patients with serious outcomes. 2006;47:448-454.
18. Sarasin FP, Junod AF, Carballo D, et al: Role of echocardiography in the evaluation of syncope: A prospective study. Heart 2002;88:363-367.
19. Crane SD: Risk stratification of patients with syncope in an accident and emergency department. Emerg Med J 2002;19:23-27.
20. Shen WK, Decker WW, Smars PA, et al: Syncope Evaluation in the Emergency Department Study (SEEDS): A multidisciplinary approach to syncope management. Circulation 2004;110:3636-2645.
21. Huff JS, Decker WW, Quinn JV, et al: Clinical policy: Critical issues in the evaluation and management of adult patients presenting to the emergency department with syncope. Ann Emerg Med 2007;49:431-444.

Chapter **100**

Delirium and Dementia

Yasuharu Okuda and Andy Jagoda

KEY POINTS

Delirium is a medical emergency that can occur superimposed on a chronic condition such as dementia.

A high mortality risk is associated with undiagnosed delirium.

A detailed family and medical history, thorough physical examination, and attention to vitals signs are crucial in the diagnosis.

During the ED evaluation it is important to look for easily reversible causes of delirium such as hypoglycemia and hypoxia, to inquire about new medications or changes in dosages as a cause of delirium, and to consider reversible causes of dementia such as vitamin deficiency and endocrine disorders

Early antibiotic therapy for patients with sepsis, which causes delirium, improves outcome.

In cases of suspected chemical exposure, proper decontamination procedures should be initiated to avoid additional exposure to healthcare workers.

Scope and Outline

The word *delirium* is derived from the prefix *de,* meaning "away," and the Latin root *lira,* meaning "furrow in a field," implying that in ancient times going off the furrow was considered madness.

A patient with delirium has impaired consciousness with inability to focus or shift attention and disturbance in cognition such as loss of memory, disruption in speech, and disorientation. The onset of delirium typically is acute and has a fluctuating course. Criteria of *The Diagnostic and Statistical Manual of Mental Disorders, Fourth Edition* (DSM-IV) include early loss of the sleep/wake cycle.

The word *dementia* is derived from the Latin word *mens,* which means "mind"; thus an individual with dementia has drifted away from his mind. Dementia also is associated with a deterioration of cognitive function but occurs insidiously and is characteristically progressive. Patients with dementia have difficulty processing new information and recalling learned information (Table 100-1).

■ PERSPECTIVE

Altered mental status is a presenting complaint in 5% to 10% of ED visits and in up to 30% of visits by the older population.[1-3] Delirium and dementia account for a significant portion of these complaints. Some studies suggest a mortality rate as high as 9% in patients who are admitted to the hospital because of altered mental status. One study found that patients who were discharged home with unrecognized delirium had a mortality of 30.8% at 6 months.[4] The challenge for the EP, who generally has not previously seen the patient, is recognizing delirium—an acute process—when it is superimposed on demen-

Table 100-1 CLINICAL CHARACTERISTICS OF DELIRIUM VERSUS DEMENTIA

Characteristic	Delirium	Dementia
Onset	Acute	Insidious
Course	Fluctuating	Progressive
Orientation	No	Yes
Attention	Impaired	Intact
Cognitive function	Impaired*	Impaired
Speech	Pressured or unintelligible	Normal

*Some of the cognitive impairment reported in delirium may actually be due to inattention.

tia—a chronic process. Therefore, a systematic approach to the ED evaluation is necessary.

Delirium

■ PATHOPHYSIOLOGY

The exact mechanism of delirium is not known, but it is believed to arise from an imbalance of neurotransmitters at the cortical and subcortical levels. The principal neurotransmitters implicated in causing delirium include dopamine, an excitatory neurotransmitter, and acetylcholine and gamma-amniobutyric acid (GABA), inhibiting neurotransmitters.[5] Physiologic stressors such as infection, medications, and metabolic disturbances can alter the balance of the levels of the neurotransmitters, leading to changes in cognition and attention. Inflammatory mediators such as cytokines and histamines are thought to be involved as well.

■ CLINICAL PRESENTATION

■ General Considerations

Delirium is a syndrome and not a specific disease; therefore, identifying the underlying etiology requires a comprehensive approach that includes a medical and family history, physical examination, and diagnostic testing. The Confusion Assessment Method (CAM) is a useful tool to screen for delirium in the medical setting.[6] In an uncooperative or severely confused patient, information obtained from emergency medical service personnel and the patient's family, personal items brought in with the patient, and a detailed physical examination with close attention to vital signs are important. The EP should consider all possible reversible medical causes of delirium so that treatment can be initiated as soon as possible (Box 100-1).

■ Infection

One of the most common causes of delirium in the elderly is infection. A simple urinary tract infection or pneumonia, which is easily handled by the immune system of a healthy adult, can have deleterious effects on the mental balance of an elderly patient who has little physiologic reserve. Progression to sepsis often worsens the delirium and can lead to coma. A history of recent cough, fever, or urinary symptoms can help establish the diagnosis of delerium in elderly patients.

Central nervous system infections range from localized abscess, meningitis, and encephalitis to late manifestations of syphilis. All of these disease forms may present symptoms of delerium ranging from minimal mental status changes to severe confusion. Fever, headache, nuchal rigidity, and photophobia suggest meningitis and encephalitis. A history of IV drug use or presence of a prosthetic heart valve with heart murmur and fever suggests intracerebral abscess as a cause of delirium. Argyll-Robertson pupils seen on the phyical examination plus a history of sexually transmitted diseases including syphilis should prompt a work-up for neurosyphilis.

Human immunodeficiency virus infection can cause delirium in its late stages, but patients with a significantly compromised immune system are more susceptible to delirium due to other central nervous system infections such as cytomegalovirus, herpes simples virus, toxoplasmosis, and cryptococcus.

■ Metabolic, Fluid, and Electrolyte Disturbances

Hypoglycemia is a common cause of delirium seen in the ED and one that is readily treatable. The patient presents with symptoms ranging from mild agitation to coma; the diagnosis may not be suspected if a hypoglycemia-induced focal neurologic deficit is present. Tachycardia and diaphoresis are commonly seen in these patients, but these findings may be absent in patients taking beta-blockers. A history of diabetes, medications, and time of last meal are important; documentation by the emergency medical service of administration of medications such as dextrose, thiamine, and narcan, and the patient's response to the medications, should be obtained.

Diabetic ketoacidosis and hyperosmolar hyperglycemic nonketotic coma can both present with an acute confusional state. Symptoms in patients with diabetic ketoacidosis include polyuria, polydypsia, nausea, vomiting, abdominal pain, the characteristic fruity acetone breath odor, and Kussmaul breathing.

BOX 100-1

Causes of Delirium

Infections

- Systemic
  - Urinary tract infection, pneumonia
- Central nervous system (CNS)
  - Meningitis, seizures, encephalitis, abscess, mass
- Human immunodeficiency virus (HIV)
  - Toxoplasmosis, cytomegalovirus, cryptococcus

Metabolic and Fluid Disorders

- Electrolyte
  - Hypoglycemia, hyperglycemia, hyponatremia, hypercalcemia
- Hypovolemia
  - Dehydration, bleeding
- Other
  - Uremia, hepatic encephalopathy

Drugs

- Withdrawal
  - Alcohol, benzodiazepine
- Illicit and abuse
  - Sympathomimetics, hallucinogen, alcohol
- Prescription medications (see Box 100-2)

Cerebrovascular

- Medical
  - Hypertensive emergency, stroke
- Traumatic
  - Intracerebral bleeding, axonal injury

Hypoxia and Hypercapnia

- Pulmonary
  - Asthma, chronic obstructive pulmonary disease (COPD), pulmonary embolism
- Hematologic
  - Carbon monoxide, methemoglobinemia
- Endocrine
  - Hyperthyroidism, hypothyroidism, Cushing's syndrome, hyperparathyroidism

Environment and Toxicity

- Toxic exposure
  - Pesticides, cyanide, carbon monoxide, methemoglobinemia, lead, mercury
- Temperature
  - Heat stroke, hypothermia
- Other
  - Bites, stings, plants (see Box 100-4)

Vitamin Deficiency

- Vitamin B_1, vitamin B_{12}

Hyperosmolar hyperglycemic nonketotic coma is seen more commonly in elderly patients presenting with no history of diabetes or in patients with adult-onset diabetes with an underlying stressor such as infection. Both have a high risk of morbidity and mortality if untreated and must be aggressively managed.

Hyponatremia can cause delirium but is related to the rate of sodium reduction and not the absolute number. A patient with a slight, sudden decrease in serum sodium can present with delirium, whereas a larger, more gradual reduction (over days) is well tolerated in many patients. Hyponatremia has many causes from underlying medical conditions such as syndrome of inappropriate secretion of antidiuretic hormone (SIADH) to intentional and unintentional water ingestion. SIADH must be included in the differential diagnosis in a delirious patient with a history of lung cancer. In a marathon runner presenting with confusion on a hot summer day, water intoxication must be considered.

Hypercalcemia is one of the few oncologic emergencies that may be associated with delirium. The normal range of total serum calcium is between 8.5 and 10.5 mg/dL. Patients with elevation above this range can present with confusion, depending on the rate of increase. Symptoms such as abdominal pain, vomiting, nausea, kidney stones, joint pain, polyuria, and constipation may be seen in a confused patient with a history of malignancy.

Patients with end-stage kidney and liver disease can present with delirium. The patient's medical history or family members may document dialysis or a history of encephalopathy. The underlying process causing the encephalopathy, such as infection or lack of compliance with treatment, should be investigated.

Drug Withdrawal

Alcohol withdrawal in its severe form can cause delirium and is known as delirium tremens. This patient will come to the ED severely agitated and confused, with visual and/or auditory hallucinations and delusions. Diagnosis of delirium tremens is based on a history of chronic alcohol abuse and symptoms of acute confusion and sympathetic hyperactivity. Typically the last drink of alcohol was greater than 48 hours prior to presentation. Vital signs may show severe hypertension, hyperthermia, and tachycardia. On the physical examination, the patient is often tremulous, diaphoretic, and has mydriasis.

Withdrawal from chronic benzodiazepine abuse can present similarly, but the onset is variable, depending on the time of the last dose and the half-life of the drug.

Drug Toxicity

Alcohol intoxication is a common presenting complaint in the ED. The patient often is agitated, confused, and combative. Information provided by the prehospital provider and family is often useful in the diagnosis. If the patient was found actively consuming alcohol or has a known history of alcoholism, this can help with the diagnosis. This patient population is more susceptible to other causes of delirium including infection, trauma, and co-ingestion; therefore a thorough, unbiased evaluation is important.

Common classes of abused drugs causing delirium include sympathomimetics such as cocaine and amphetamine and hallucinogens such as lysergic acid diethylamide (LSD) and ketamine. Close attention to vital signs and the identification of a toxic syndrome ("toxidrome") is essential in the diagnosis. In patients with sympathomimetic toxicity, there may be significant increases in heart rate, blood pressure, and temperature with associated hyperactivity, agitation, and diaphoresis. Clinical findings associated with ketamine abuse include vertical and rotatory nystagmus, mid-positioned pupils, hallucinations, labile affect, hyperthermia, and muscle rigidity. Mild tachycardia and hypertension may be seen. Investigation of personal belongings for pills and interview of family members may augment the diagnosis.

Many commonly prescribed medications can cause delirium due to improper dosing, change in metabolism, intentional overdose, and drug-drug interactions (Box 100-2).[7,8] Family members or the patient's personal physician may be able to give valuable information about recent changes in medication dosages or additions of new medications.

Digoxin is a medication commonly seen in the ED; toxicity in both chronic and acute forms can cause delirium. Careful attention to symptoms such as nausea and vomiting, headaches, and visual disturbance can aid in making the diagnosis. Bradycardia may be the only initial abnormality in the vital signs. Anticholinergic medications are also commonly used in the ED and outpatient settings. Delirium associated with mydriasis, hyperthermia, anhydrosis, and hyperemia is seen in this toxidrome.

BOX 100-2

Medications Associated with Delirium

Anticholinergics

- H_1 receptor blockers (diphenhydramine, meclizine, hydroxyzine)
- Antiparkinson drugs (benztropine)
- Phenothiazine (promethazine)

Antidepressants

- Tricyclic (amitriptyline, nortriptyline)
- Selective serotonin reuptake inhibitors (SSRIs) (fluoxetine, sertraline)

Sedatives

- Benzodiazepine (alprazolam, diazepam)

Analgesics

- Opioids (codeine, morphine)

Anti-inflammatory Agents

- Nonsteroidal anti-inflammatory drugs (NSAIDs) (aspirin, ibuprofen)
- Corticosteroids (hydrocortisone, prednisone)

Antihypertensives and Antiarrythmics

- Beta-blockers (metoprolol, propranolol)
- Angiotensin-converting enzyme (ACE) inhibitors (lisinopril, captopril)
- Calcium channel blockers (amlodipine, nifedipine)
- Other (digoxin)

Antibiotics

- Quinolones (levofloxacin, ciprofloxacin)
- Macrolides (azithromycin, clarithromycin)

Anticonvulsive Agents

- Barbiturates (phenobarbital)

Cerebrovascular Disorders

With the nationwide advancement of stroke centers, the early recognition of cerebral infarction has increased. Patients with stroke in both its ischemic and hemorrhagic forms can present with delirium. Opthalmoplegia on careful cranial nerve examination suggests a paramedian thalamic infarction. An anterior cerebral artery stroke exclusively involving the frontal lobe can affect cognitive function and attention without other focal neurologic findings. Associated bowel and bladder incontinence as well as the grasp and suck reflexes may be present. Patients with posterior cerebral artery infarction can present with agitation, disorientation, and restlessness without focality.[9] These patients may have cortical blindness from bilateral infarctions of the occipital lobe and may exhibit Anton's syndrome, which is a form of cortical blindness in which the patient denies the problem. For example, the patient may bump into objects while walking but deny that this occured.

Hypertensive emergency is associated with delirium if target organ damage affects the brain, causing hypertensive encephalopathy. Blood pressures are typically significantly elevated. Other signs of end organ damage include heart failure and renal failure.

Patients can present with delirium from a primary traumatic brain injury or secondary to multitude of other causes including hypotension, toxic ingestion, and hypoxia. Aggressive systematic evaluation of the reversible secondary causes of acute confusion is necessary while maintaining optimal cerebral perfusion and oxygenation. Intracerebral bleeding and diffuse axonal injury and edema can cause elevations in intracerebral pressure, resulting in cerebral herniation. The elevation in intracranial pressure can manifest with hypertension, bradyacardia, and irregular breathing, known as the Cushing's triad. Cheyne-Stokes breathing is an example of the irregular breathing characterized by alternating periods of apnea and hyperpnea. A thorough physical examination looking for signs of head injury must be performed.

Hypoxemia and Hypercarbia

Acute elevations in PCO_2 and a low PO_2 can cause alterations in cognition and awareness. Pulmonary disorders such as pneumonia, pulmonary embolism, asthma, and pneumothorax can cause hypoxia. Abnormal chest excursion and rate, depth, and effort of breathing are significant findings in the physical examination. Symptoms important in the history include dyspnea, fever, cough, and pleuritic chest pain as well as recent travel and a family history of connective tissue disease.

Hypercarbia is a normal finding in many patients with chronic obstructive pulmonary disease, but an acute rise in PCO_2 can lead to an alteration in consciousness. Oxygenation in not an adequate measurement of ventilation, and therefore serial monitoring of the patient's mental status should be initiated in the absence of bedside capnography.

Endocrine Disorders

Patients with endocrine disorders such as hyperthyroidism, hypothyroidism, Cushing's syndrome, and hyperparathyroidism may present initially with altered mental status.[10] Delirium is more common in severe manifestations of these disease, as in the cases of thyroid storm and myxedema coma. Abnormalities in vital signs such has tachycardia and fever in thyroid storm and bradycardia and hypotension in myxedema coma may be the only initial clues to the diagnosis.

Chemical Exposure

Delirium can be the presenting symptom in patients exposed to a chemical weapon or contaminated environment. History of exposure is important, but oten the patient presents with confusion and there is no history available. If there is a suspicion of chemical exposure, the patient must be brought to the proper decontamination area immediately. Universal precautions should be practiced as well as use of a proper-level HAZMAT suit. The patient should be stabilized and evaluated for examination findings and vital signs suggesting the cause of the contamination and the antidote (Box 100-3).

BOX 100-3

Chemical Agents Associated with Delirium

- Organophosphates
  - Sarin (isopropyl methylphosphonofluoridate)
  - Diethyl parathion
  - VX (*O*-ethyl *S*-2-[diisopropylamino]ethyl-methylphosphonothioate)
- Carbamates
  - Aldicarb (Tres Pasitos)
  - Propoxur (Baygon)
- Organochlorines
  - DDT (dichlorodiphenyltrichloroethane)
  - Lindane
- Other
  - DEET (diethyltoluamide)
  - Pyrethrins

Environmental Agents

Stroke from heat exposure occurs in the very young and the elderly, but exertional heatstroke can occur acutely in persons of all age. Patients with heatstroke present with confusion, hyperthermia (typically greater than 40°C), tachycardia, tachypnea, and hypotension. Delirium may be the initial presenting complaint because the central nervous system often is the first organ system to be affected by the elevation in temperature.

In contrast to heat illnesses, patients suffering from cold exposure can present with acute confusion. Patients with temperatures below 35°C present with apathy, slurred speech, confusion, forgetfulness, and shivering. As the temperature drops further, symptoms progress from delirium to coma.

Exposure to plants, insect stings, and animal bites may all result in delirium related to the toxin or chemical involved in the exposure. The initial complaint may be related to the cause of injury or rash, but progression to systemic complications can ensue rapidly. A careful history should be obtained, including history of travel; description of the offending plant, insect, or animal; and the time course of symptoms. Evaluation of the wound or rash may be helpful in making the diagnosis (Box 100-4).

Central Nervous System Disease

Depending on the location of the mass, intracerebral tumors can present with delirium without focal motor deficits. Frontal lobe tumors are more commonly associated with acute changes in personality or behavior.

Absence seizures, seen primarily in children 5 to 10 years of age, may be characterized by acute-onset altered mental status without motor activity. The

BOX 100-4

Environmental Agents That May Cause Delirium

Plants and Mushrooms

- Plants
  - Camphor
  - Water hemlock
  - Strychnine
  - Belladonna
  - Angel's trumpet
  - Jimson weed
  - Peyote
  - Nutmeg
  - Morning glory
- Mushrooms
  - *Amanita muscaria*
  - *Amanita pantherina*
  - *Psilocybe cubensis*
  - *Panaeolus foenisecii*

Insects and Animals

- Insects
  - Black widow spider
  - Scorpion
- Animals
  - Portuguese man of war
  - Box jellyfish
  - Scorpionfish

seizure episodes typically last for seconds and resolve without a postictal state.

Patients with nonconvulsive status epilepticus may present with a history of seizure disorder as well as with a new-onset seizure. Symptoms include confusion, personality changes, hallucinations, and delusions without focal motor findings.[11] The diagnosis should be suspected in patients with a prolonged postictal phase or in patients with a history of seizures with atypical change in mental status. Nystagmus and subtle motor activity are possible clues, but emergent electroencephalography confirms the diagnosis.

The postictal state after a generalized seizure is associated with impaired cognition and consciousness. Episodes typically resolve after a few hours. If the postictal state continues for a longer period, other causes of delirium should be considered and electroencephalograpy should be performed to evaluate for nonconvulsive seizure.

Vitamin Deficiency

Deficiency in certain vitamins can cause altered mental status. Patients with Wernicke encephalopathy, which is caused by a deficiency of thiamine (vitamin B_1), present with delirium, ataxia, and ophthalmoplegia. Advanced cases of vitamin B_{12} deficiency can also cause altered mental status, associated with a history of paresthesias, weakness, diarrhea, and loss of appetite.

DIFFERENTIAL DIAGNOSIS

If after a thorough work-up of a patient presenting with confusion, delirium is excluded, other causes of altered cognition should be considered. An elderly patient with newly recognized or worsening dementia may present to the ED with an acute decline in consciousness. Family members may recall changes in memory and function over a longer period of time, suggesting dementia rather than delirium.

First-time presentation of psychiatric disorders or exacerbation of underlying psychiatric disease can often be confused with delirium and present similarly. Because patients with psychiatric illness can present with delirium, medical and reversible causes of the confusion must be excluded before transfer of care to a psychiatrist.[12]

DIAGNOSTIC TESTING

See Priority Actions: Tests Useful in the Diagnosis of Delirium.

TREATMENT AND DISPOSITION

Once the etiology of the delirium is discovered, appropriate treatment should be initiated immediately. Antibiotic therapy should be started for patients with suspected meningitis, hypoglycemia should be corrected with dextrose, and patients with hypoxia should receive oxygen supplementation. Delay of diagnosis and treatment can increase overall morbidity and mortality.

Disposition depends on the cause of the delirium and the patient's response to treatment. If the patient does not improve or if the cause is not found, the patient should be transferred to the appropriate inpatient facility. In some cases, with improvement to baseline vaues, the patient can be discharged home.

Dementia

Alzheimer's dementia is the most common form of dementia in adults (occurring in 50%-60% of patients), followed by vascular dementia (15%-25%), Lewy body dementia (5%), and Parkinson's dementia (5%).[13,14]

PATHOPHYSIOLOGY

At the anatomic level, Alzheimer's dementia is characterized by atrophy at both cortical and subcortical structures, which is seen most prominently in the hippocampus and temporal cortex. Histologic examination reveals an accumulation of extracellular

PRIORITY ACTIONS

Tests Useful in the Diagnosis of Delirium

Infections
- Pneumonia
  - *Chest radiography, blood culture*
- Urinary tract infection
  - *Urinalysis, urine culture*
- HIV
  - *Head and contrast CT; lumbar puncture*

Metabolic Disorders
- Hypoglycemia/hyperglycemia
  - *Glucose finger-stick test; serum chemistry panel*
- Electrolyte abnormalities
  - *Serum chemistry panel; ECG*
- Hypovolemia
  - *Vital signs, hematocrit*
- Uremic encephalopathy
  - *BUN, serum chemistry panel*

Drugs
- Withdrawal
  - *History and vital signs*
- Illicit and abuse
  - *History and vital signs*

Cerebrovascular Disorders
- Hypertensive emergency
  - *ECG; serum chemistry panel*
- Stroke
  - *Head CT and/or head MRI; ECG; radiography*
- Intracerebral bleeding, axonal injury
  - *Head CT*

Hypoxia and Hypercapnia
- Asthma and COPD
  - *Pulse oximetry; capnography*
- Pulmonary embolism
  - *Ventilation-perfusion scan or CT angiography of chest; D-dimer*
- Carbon monoxide
  - *Assay of carboxyhemoglobin level or CO-oximetry*
- Methemoglobinemia
  - *Serum methemoglobin level; CO-oximetry*

Endocrine Disorders
- Thyroid storm
  - *Vital signs*
- Myxedema coma
  - *ECG; serum chemistry panel; glucose finger-stick test*
- Acute adrenal failure
  - *Serum chemistry panel (K↑, Na↓, glucose↓)*

Toxic Exposure
- Pesticides
  - *Toxidrome*

Thermal Disorders
- Heat stroke
  - *Temperature; ECG; liver function test; serum chemistry panel*
- Hypothermia
  - *Temperature; ECG*

Central Nervous System Disorders
- Meningitis and encephalitis
  - *Lumbar puncture*
- Abscess
  - *Head and contrast CT or MRI*
- Mass
  - *Head CT*
- Seizure
  - *Head CT*

Vitamin B_1 and B_{12} Deficiency
  - *Serum vitamin level assays*

BUN, blood urea nitrogen; COPD, chronic obstructive pulmonary disease; CT, computed tomography; ECG, electrocardiography; HIV, human immunodeficiency virus; MRI, magnetic resonance imaging.

amyloid plaques and neurofibrillary tangles that attract inflammatory mediators and impede neurotransmitter delivery along the axons, respectively. Deficiencies in the neurotransmitters acetylcholine and norepinephrine are also thought to be responsible for the dementia in Alzheimer's disease. Pathophysiologic and clinical characteristics of types of dementia are shown in Table 100-2.[15]

■ CLINICAL PRESENTATION

Alzheimer's disease is characterized by a gradual onset of dementia, as defined by the DMS-IV (Box 100-5), with continuous functional decline. The cognitive impairment seen in Alzheimer's disease is not explained by other causes of dementia. Most patients in the ED with Alzheimer's disease will already carry

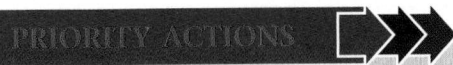

Table 100-2 CLINICAL AND PATHOPHYSIOLOGIC SYMPTOMS AND SIGNS IN TYPES OF DEMENTIA

	SYMPTOMS AND SIGNS	
Disorder	**Clinical**	**Pathophysiologic**
Alzheimer's disease	Gradual and continuing functional decline not explained by another cause of dementia	Amyloid plaques, neurofibrillary tangles, hippocampal and temporal atrophy
Vascular dementia	Sudden onset, focal neurologic findings, stepwise deterioration	Multiple infarcts
Lewy body dementia	Visual hallucinations, fluctuating cognition, mild parkinsonism seen less than 1 year prior to dementia	Lewy bodies, Lewy neuritis
Parkinson's dementia	Extrapyramidal signs, visual hallucinations, fluctuating cognition	Lewy bodies, Lewy neuritis
Frontotemporal dementia (Pick's disease)	Personality changes, restlessness, disinhibition, impulsiveness, ataxia, parkinsonism	Pick bodies, frontal and temporal atrophy
Infectious dementia (Creutzfeldt-Jakob)	Visual disturbances, ataxia, myoclonus, progressive dementia	Prion protein accumulation, spongiform change of brain

BOX 100-5

DSM-IV Criteria for Dementia

1. Memory impairment (inability to learn new information or to recall previously learned information)
2. At least one of the following:
   a. Aphasia (language disturbance)
   b. Apraxia (problems with motor activities despite intact motor function)
   c. Agnosia (problems recognizing or identifying objects despite intact sensory function)
   d. Disturbance in executive functioning (planning, organizing, sequencing, abstracting)
3. The deficits listed above significantly impair social or occupational functioning and are a significant decline from a previous level of functioning.
4. The deficits do not occur exclusively during the course of a delirium.
5. The deficits are not better accounted for by another disorder.

DSM-IV, Diagnostic and Statistical Manual of Mental Disorders, Fourth Edition.

the diagnosis and likely have an associated presenting complication such as infection or exacerbation of their dementia.

Because the clinical presentation of dementia is subtle and gradual, it is important to maintain a high index of suspicion in the evaluation of elderly patients in the ED. Initial symptoms, such as depression, fatigue, insomnia, and irritability, can be nonspecific. Inquiring about missing appointments and increased forgetfulness can be helpful, but patient often deny difficulties in cognitive abilities by changing the subject. Family members or caregivers may bring patients to the ED because they are unable to care for them or because patients are no longer able to care for themselves. It is important to recognize early dementia (mild cognitive impairment) in the ED setting to prevent secondary complications such as injuries from falls and fires, noncompliance with medications, and malnutrition and dehydration. Evaluation for reversible cause of dementia and delirium must be initiated.

Although dementia in less than 5% of these patients has a reversible cause, a thorough history and physical examination must be undertaken to identify this subcategory (see Priority Actions: Tests Useful in the Diagnosis of Reversible Causes of Dementia). Normal pressure hydrocephalus is characterized by ataxia, urinary incontinence, and dementia, all of which are reversible. Diagnosis is made by CT scan of the head and the finding of elevated opening pressure on lumbar puncture. Treatment is insertion of a surgical shunt.

■ DIFFERENTIAL DIAGNOSIS

Pseudodementia is a term used to describe patients who appear demented but actually have severe depression. Differences from genuine dementia can be subtle; patients with pseudodementia usually have a preexisting history of depression with acute onset (often after a specific event), emphasize and appear more distressed about cognitive deficits, and have preserved attention. If the diagnosis of depression is suspected, patients should be asked about thoughts of suicidality and their social support structure. Appropriate consultation and follow-up with a psychiatrist or social worker or hospitalization may be necessary to ensure the patient's safety.

■ TREATMENT AND DISPOSITION

As with the treatment of delirium, the reversible causes of dementia should be addressed and treatment initiated immediately. Frequently the dementia

PRIORITY ACTIONS

Tests Useful in the Diagnosis of Reversible Causes of Dementia

Central Nervous System Disorders

- Normal pressure hydrocephalus
  - *Head CT; lumbar puncture*
- Subdural hematoma
  - *Head CT*

Infections

- Neurosyphilis
  - *VDRL and RPR tests; lumbar puncture*
- AIDS
  - *HIV titers*

Heavy Metal Toxicity

- Lead
  - *Blood lead level assay*
- Mercury
  - *Urine mercury level assay*

Endocrine Abnormalities

- Hypothyroidism
  - *Serum assay for TSH*

Vitamin Deficiency

- Vitamins B_1 and B_{12}
  - *Serum vitamin level assay*

AIDS, acquired immunodeficiency syndrome; CT, computed tomography; HIV, human immunodeficiency virus; RPR, rapid plasma reagin; TSH, thyroid-stimulating hormone; VDRL, Venereal Disease Research Laboratory.

will have no reversible causes; the patient presents with a new diagnosis of dementia or worsening of an underlying condition.

In such cases, disposition is based on the patient's ability to function independently at home or on the family's capacity to care for the patient. If the family is unable to further care for the patient, admission to the hospital for the evaluation of nursing home placement or assisted home care is necessary. If there is adequate support by family and patient safety can be ensured, the work-up of patients with new-onset dementia can be done in an outpatient setting with appropriate coordinated care by the primary physician.

REFERENCES

1. Elie M, Rousseau F, Cole M, et al: Prevalence and detection of delirium in elderly emergency department patients. CMAJ 2000;163:977-981.
2. Hustey F, Meldon S: The prevalence and documentation of impaired mental status in elderly emergency department patients. Ann Emerg Med 2002;39:248-253.
3. Hustey F, Meldon S, Smith M, Lex C: Care of elderly emergency department patients. Ann Emerg Med 2003;41: 678-684.
4. Kakuma R, Galbaud du Fort G, Arsenault L, et al: Delirium in older emergency department patients discharged home: Effect on survival. J Am Geriatr Soc 2003;51:443-450.
5. Pandharipande P, Jackson J, Ely W: Delirium: Acute cognitive dysfunction in the critically ill. Curr Opin Crit Care 2005;11:360-368.
6. Monette J, Galbaud du Fort G, Fung S, et al: Evaluation of the confusion assessment method (CAM) as a screening tool for delirium in the emergency room. Gen Hosp Psychiatry 2001;23:20-25.
7. Alagiakrishnan K, Wiens C: An approach to drug-induced delirium in the elderly. Postgrad Med J 2004;80:388-393.
8. Gray S, Lai K, Larson E: Drug-induced cognition disorders in the elderly. Drug Safety 1999;2:101-122.
9. Vatsavayi V, Malhotra S, Franco K: Agitated delirium with posterior cerebral artery infarction. J Emerg Med 2003; 24:263-266.
10. Bazakis A, Kunzler C: Altered mental status due to metabolic or endocrine disorders. Emerg Med Clin North Am 2005;23:901-908.
11. Treiman D, Walker M: Treatment of seizure emergencies: Convulsive and non-convulsive status epilepticus. Epilepsy Res 2006;68(Suppl 1):S7-S82.
12. Reeves R, Pendarvis E, Kimble R: Unrecognized medical emergencies admitted to psychiatric units. Am J Emerg Med 2000;18:390-393.
13. Dugu M, Neugroschl J, Sewell M, Marin D: Review of dementia. Mt Sinai J Med 2003;70:45-53.
14. Tolosa E, Wenning G, Poewe W: The diagnosis of Parkinson's disease. Lancet Neurol 2006;5:75-86.
15. Love S: Neuropathological investigation of dementia: A guide for neurologists. J Neurol Neurosurg Psychiatry 2005;76:8-14.

Chapter **101**

Neurologic Procedures

Edward C. Jauch and Brian A. Stettler

KEY POINTS

Lumbar puncture with an opening pressure can quickly make or exclude the diagnosis of many central nervous system diseases as a cause of headache or altered mental status.

Liberal administration of lidocaine and small doses of an anxiolytic agent can expedite performance of a lumbar puncture in an anxious patient.

To obtain an accurate opening pressure when performing a lumbar puncture, patients should lie on the side with the head supported by a pillow and the legs straight; also, the fluid should be allowed to equilibrate in the manometer.

A smaller-gauge needle, such as a 22-gauge, will help decrease complications such as post–dural puncture headache.

Scope

The most common neurologic procedure, lumbar puncture, is performed daily by EPs to evaluate a wide range of chief complaints in the ED, including headache, altered mental status, and fever. Lumbar puncture can be performed quickly and successfully at the bedside and can diagnose or eliminate the possibility of life-threatening conditions of the central nervous system. To optimize patient care, it is important for the EP to be knowledgeable about the indications for this procedure as well as proficient in its performance.

Other emergent neurologic procedures, including ventriculostomy for drainage of cerebrospinal fluid, intracranial pressure monitoring, and aspiration of an indwelling ventriculoperitoneal shunt, are used less frequently and should only be performed in consultation with a neurosurgeon.

Lumbar Puncture

Lumbar puncture has been performed for decades to diagnose and treat a variety of complaints. Currently, this procedure is used mainly for assessment of the complaint of headache or altered mental status in the ED. Analysis of cerebrospinal fluid and opening pressure measurements obtained from the lumbar puncture can make or exclude the diagnosis of meningitis, subarachnoid hemorrhage, pseudotumor cerebri, and other morbid diseases.

■ PROCEDURE

After consent is obtained, place the patient on a flat gurney on the side with a pillow under the head. The procedure is typically started with the patient in the fetal position and the person performing the procedure seated, facing the patient's back.

Place an absorbent towel under the patient to capture dripping betadine and then cleanse the patient's back, using at least three swabs or pieces of gauze soaked in betadine. Locate the iliac crest with gloved fingers, and use the thumbs to palpate the spinous processes in the midline of the back. This is roughly the L4-L5 interspace and is an appropriate interspace to use. In adults, the L3-L4 interspace also can be used, because both lie below the termination

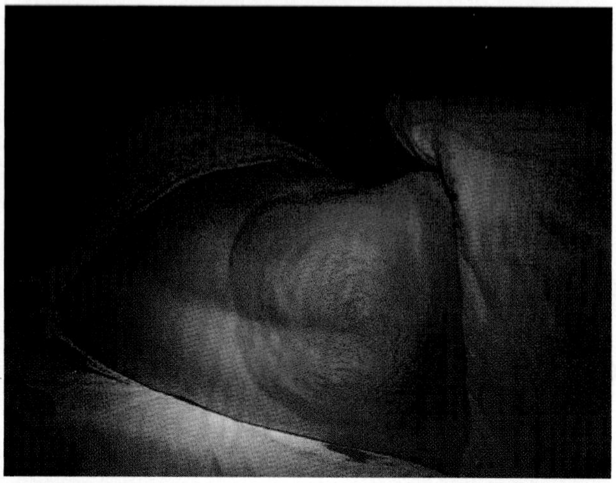

FIGURE 101-1 Lumbar puncture procedure showing patient preparation.

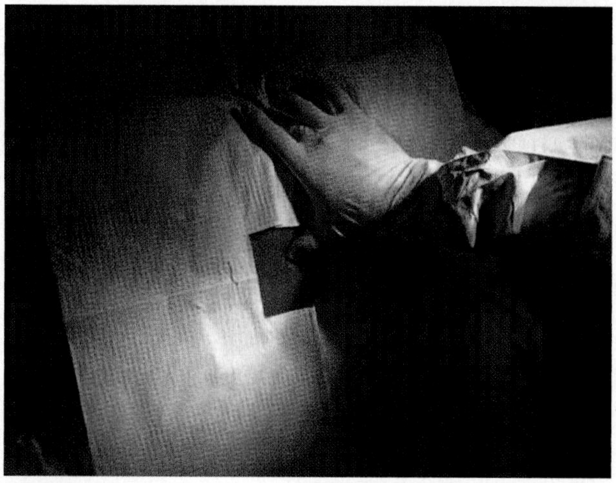

FIGURE 101-2 Lumbar puncture procedure showing identification of space.

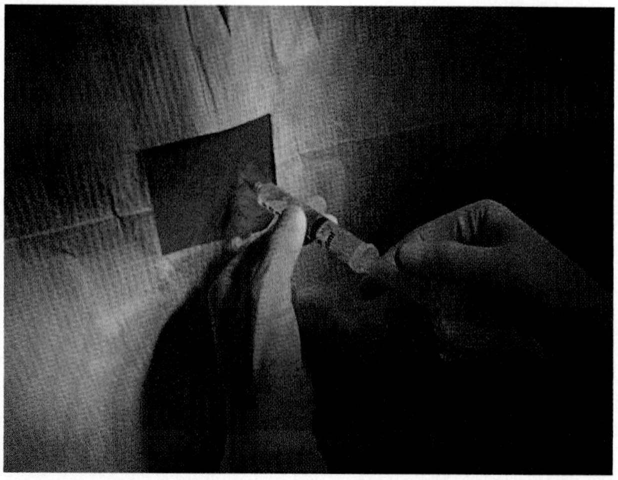

FIGURE 101-3 Lumbar puncture procedure showing placement of local anesthesia.

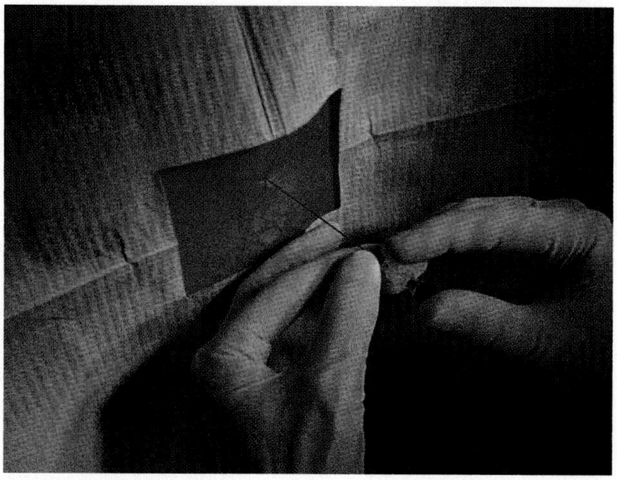

FIGURE 101-4 Lumbar puncture procedure showing insertion of needle.

of the spinal cord within the spinal canal. Use the betadine-soaked gauze to make circular motions to scrub the back in gradually expanding circles, starting at the midline of the L4-L5 interspace. The preparation is complete when the area all the way to the iliac crests and up to the lower thoracic spine is scrubbed (Fig. 101-1). A wider sterile field is always better.

Next, open the lumbar puncture kit and put on sterile gloves. Use the sterile drape to align the hole in the center of the drape overlying the previously identified interspace (Fig. 101-2).

The procedure may be made somewhat easier by having the patient sit up and lean over a bedside table while being stabilized by a helper, but this prevents measurement of the opening pressure, which can be very useful. Consider using this technique, however, in very obese patients with landmarks that are difficult to palpate.

The procedure may be augmented in very anxious patients by the administration of a small dose of a benzodiazepine such as midazolam. Ultrasonography has been described for the identification of landmarks in the difficult patient but is not widely in use at this time.

Reassess landmarks and place 2 mL of sterile lidocaine subdermally with a 27-gauge or 25-gauge needle at the identified interspace to anesthetize the skin (Fig. 101-3). Allow the lidocaine to take effect while setting up the remainder of the kit. After 1 to 2 minutes, using a longer, 22-gauge needle, anesthetize the deeper tissues, aspirating and advancing slowly. Up to 10 mL of lidocaine may be necessary to achieve good anesthesia, and this is a key segment of the procedure.

Next, check landmarks again, including the iliac crests and the midline spinous processes. After the patient is fully anesthetized, use a 22-gauge spinal needle to advance into the previously identified space (Fig. 101-4). Advance slowly while controlling the needle at the skin with the nondominant hand. An angle with the needle directed slightly cephalad may

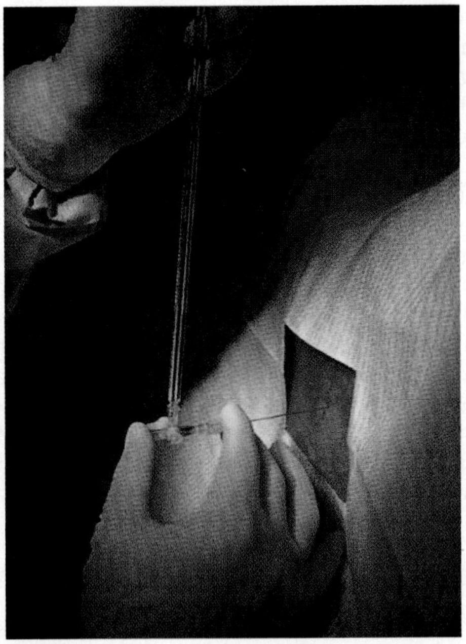

FIGURE 101-5 Lumbar puncture procedure showing measururement of intracranial pressure.

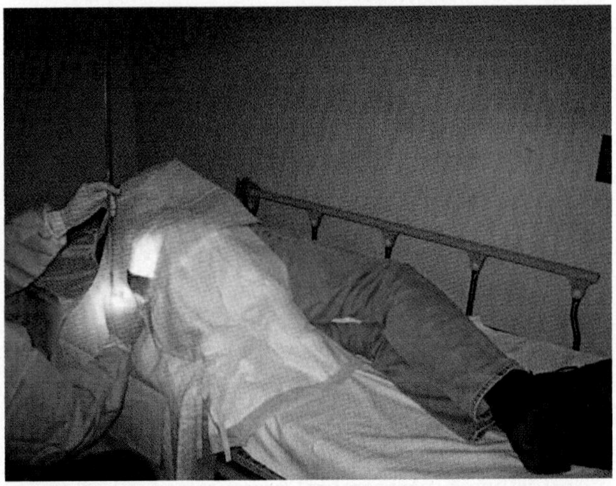

FIGURE 101-6 Lumbar puncture procedure showing measururement of intracranial pressure.

be required, due to the tilt of the spinous processes. The widely discussed "pop" is not always felt, so once you have traversed the ligamentum flavum, you may remove the introducer every few millimeters of advancement to see if fluid has been obtained. It is important to keep the direction of the needle in the midline to avoid nerve roots as they exit the spinal canal. Keep the bevel of the needle parallel to the dural fibers, which run cephalad-caudad, to minimize post–dural puncture headache.

Once fluid is seen in the needle, attach the manometer that comes with the kit to measure the opening pressure (Fig. 101-5). Have an assistant help the patient to straighten the legs and wait for the fluid to equilibrate in the column of the manometer (there will be slight respiratory variation) (Fig. 101-6). Record this as the opening pressure, which, in the absence of obstructive hydrocephalus, is equivalent to the intracranial pressure. The manometer may then be removed or left in place.

After placing 1 to 2 mL of cerebrospinal fluid in each of four tubes, remove the needle from the patient's back, continue to apply pressure briefly with a piece of gauze, and apply a bandage. The patient at this point may be returned to any position of comfort.

■ COMPLICATIONS

■ Post–Dural Puncture Headache

The most common complication associated with lumbar puncture is the development of a "post–dural puncture" headache, which occurs roughly 5% to 40% of the time after lumbar puncture, depending on the technique and type and size of needle used.[2-5] Post–dural puncture headache develops roughly 2 days after the performance of a dural puncture, is worse with standing, and is partially relieved by lying down. The exact cause of this complication is uncertain, but it is thought to result from continued leakage of cerebrospinal fluid through the dural rent created by the needle. The headache is typically self-limited but can last up to a week and be fairly debilitating during that time. This complication can be minimized by use of the smallest-gauge needle possible, because the incidence is directly correlated with needle gauge.[2]

When using a sharp bevel, or "Quincke" needle, the needle bevel should be oriented parallel to the dural fibers to avoid cross-cutting of the fibers. The patient's position following dural puncture does not appear to be associated with the development or prevention of a headache, nor does administration of a periprocedure fluid bolus.

Post–dural puncture headache can be treated with administration of fluids and analgesia or IV caffeine. Severe headache may require the placement of a blood patch, which is curative in 80% to 90% of cases.

■ Other Complications

Other complications of lumbar puncture include development of an epidural hematoma, which is more common in the setting of anticoagulation, platelet disorders, thrombocytopenia, and other causes of hypocoagulation. This can be a surgical emergency, because the hematoma can place pressure on the cauda equina, resulting in neurologic dysfunction.

Infection with resulting vertebral osteomyelitis, meningitis, or abscess is possible but can be avoided by observing strict sterile technique. In procedures performed at the proper level (i.e., L3-L4 or lower in an adult and L4-L5 or lower in a child), paralysis is not a complication in the absence of a significant epidural hematoma.

Cerebrospinal Fluid Analysis

Tests for cerebrospinal fluid analysis vary depending on the indication for the lumbar puncture. If infection is suspected, a Gram stain and bacterial culture should be obtained. This can be performed on any sample, as all fluid should be sterile. Cultures or assays for other organisms should be ordered as needed, including viral and fungal cultures, polymerase chain reaction cryptococcal antigen, testing for acid-fast bacilli, India ink, and testing for other specific pathogens. Some of these assays may require more than 1 to 2 mL of cerebrospinal fluid, so extra fluid should be obtained in immunocompromised patients or when unusual pathogens are suspected.

A protein assay can be helpful in the setting of infection, as many infectious processes increase the protein level beyond the normal range. Glucose levels will sometimes be depressed in the setting of infection, because glucose is consumed by leukocytes in the cerebrospinal fluid; however, this value must be interpreted in the setting of the plasma glucose, because glucose freely crosses the blood-brain barrier. In general, when cerebrospinal fluid analysis reveals high protein and low glucose values relative to the serum glucose, there shoud be a high index of suspicion for infection.

Cell counts must be obtained in setting of infection, primarily to assess the number and type of leukocytes present in the cerebrospinal fluid. If the lumbar puncture is obviously bloody or blood-tinged, counts should be obtained on multiple tubes, correcting the number of leukocytes for the number of erythrocytes present. The standard correction that has been applied in the past has been 1 leukocyte for every 500 erythrocytes in a traumatic tap; however, this number is subject to debate and unreliable in clinical practice and should be used only as a guide.[1] More than 5 leukocytes/high-power field in the cerebrospinal fluid is considered abnormal, although infection typically presents with higher values. Lower leukocyte counts that are still above the cutoff may also signify central nervous system vasculitis, viral infection, or malignancy depending on the cell type present.

In the setting of suspicion of subarachnoid hemorrhage, cell counts obtained on tubes No. 1 and No. 4 should be used for comparison, because the number of erythrocytes is very important in this disease process. A specific value has not been established to determine the number of erythrocytes that differentiate a traumatic tap from subarachnoid hemorrhage; however, the number of cells in the last tube collected should be substantially less than those in the first sample collected in the setting of a traumatic tap.

Cerebrospinal fluid also should be analyzed for the presence of xanthochromia when subarachnoid hemorrhage is suspected, preferably by spectrophotometry for maximum sensitivity. The presence of xanthochromia should cause concern about red blood cell (RBC) lysis and hemoglobin enzymatic degradation in the cerebrospinal fluid, because this indicates that the RBCs were present before the performance of the lumbar puncture, as would be seen in a subarachnoid hemorrhage. Although xanthochromia usually develops more than 12 hours after the initial bleeding event, its absence prior to this does not rule out subarachnoid hemorrhage. Xanthochromia persists for at least 1 week; its presence thereafter suggests repeated bleeding or an alternative explanation, such as jaundice or medications such as rifampin.

Intracranial Pressure Monitoring

Placement of an invasive pressure monitor is typically performed in a head-injured patient with a Glascow Coma Scale (GCS) score of 7 to 8 or less, because a standard neurologic examination may be difficult to perform in these patients. Intracranial hypertension that is sustained at levels greater than 15-20 mm Hg is associated with a worse outcome. In order to assess intracranial pressure in patients with a negative neurologic examination and altered level of consciousness, a monitor can be placed directly in the skull or brain. The procedure is performed in sterile fashion at the bedside but should only be performed after consultation with and under the guidance of the neurosurgeon who will be caring for the patient after admission. Furthermore, placement of an invasive monitor should be reserved for patients with some chance for recovery from their injuries.

Intraventicular catheterization is the gold standard of invasive intracranial pressure monitoring. Ventriculostomy is performed to achieve invasive monitoring of intracerebral pressure as well as drainage of cerebrospinal fluid in the setting of elevated intracranial pressure from any cause, including obstructing or nonobstructing hydrocephalus, diffuse cerebral edema, and hemorrhage.

■ PROCEDURE FOR INTRAVENTRICULAR CATHETERIZATION

A fluid-filled catheter is placed into the lateral ventricle through a burrhole in the skull. The pressure is transmitted through the fluid-filled catheter back to a pressure transducer. Cerebrospinal fluid can be drained from the ventricle through the catheter in the setting of elevated intracranial pressure, particularly in cases of obstructive hydrocephalus, such as is found in subarachnoid hemorrhage, intraventricular hemorrhage, or mass lesion. The goal of drainage of cerebrospinal fluid from the fixed-volume intracranial space is to decrease intracranial pressure to allow a more acceptable range for cerebral perfusion pressure.[6]

■ OTHER METHODS

Other methods of monitoring intracranial pressure include the Camino intraparenchymal monitor (Camino, San Diego, CA) and the Richmond bolt. Both of these methods monitor local tissue pressure but do not extend into the ventricular system. Both are inserted on the ipsilateral side to the lesion to get the most accurate pressure; however, they fail to reflect the global pressure on the brain with the same level of fidelity of an intraventricular catheter. The advantages of the Camino catheter and Richmond bolt include ease of insertion and some decrease in hemorrhagic complications.[7]

■ COMPLICATIONS

Complications associated with the insertion of an intracranial pressure monitor include hemorrhage and infection. Hemorrhage—including subdural, intraparenchymal, and intraventricular hemorrhage—can occur anywhere along the tract of the catheter. Infection—including scalp cellulitis, calvarial osteomyelitis, meningitis, and encephalitis—likewise also can occur. Risk of infection seems to be increased with flushing of the catheter and is prevented only by strict sterile technique when inserting and caring for the catheter. Infectious risk is approximately 10% and is not reproducibly affected by the use of periprocedural antibiotics.[8] Conflicting data show that infectious complications may increase as the duration of monitoring increases; therefore a monitor that is no longer being used to make clinical decisions should be discontinued as soon as possible.

Aspiration of a Ventriculoperitoneal Shunt

Ventriculoperitoneal shunts are placed for persistent hydrocephalus from many causes, including congenital malformations, previous subarachnoid hemorrhage, obstructive processes such as a neoplasms, and normal-pressure hydrocephalus. Aspiration of a ventriculoperitoneal shunt is typically performed when central nervous system infection is suspected in patients who present to the ED with headache, fevers, or altered mental status and who have such hardware in place. It can also be used to aspirate larger volumes of cerebrospinal fluid in the setting of a malfunctioning shunt and acute hydrocephalus.

A standard shunt assembly consists of a catheter tip located in the ventricle, a shunt tubing traversing the cerebrum and exiting the skull, and a cerebrospinal fluid reservoir and check valve placed subcutaneously under the scalp. The shunt is tunneled down the neck and empties into the peritoneum. Aspiration of a ventriculoperitoneal shunt should only be done in consultation with a neurosurgeon; the EP performing the procedure should have some experience in the procedure and its complications. Only shunts that have a reservoir are amenable to aspiration (most shunts installed within recent years have reservoirs).

■ PROCEDURE

Aspiration is a relatively simple procedure, involving palpation of the reservoir under the scalp as a landmark. Once the landmark is identified, the skin is prepped sterilely with betadine. Absolute sterility is imperative because the procedure violates the sterile space of the central nervous system through a retained foreign body (i.e., the shunt), and infection can result in disastrous consequences.

Once sterility is assured, a 23-gauge or 25-gauge butterfly needle is introduced into the reservoir, such that the bevel of the needle is contained with the reservoir and cerebrospinal fluid can be aspirated for standard cerebrospinal fluid analysis (as discussed previously). The location of the reservoir is subcutaneous, so its depth below the skin, and therefore the depth of needle penetration, should only be that of the thickness of the scalp. If desired, a manometer can be connected to the butterfly needle so that pressure within the central nervous system can be assessed. If so, a larger-gauge needle such as the 23-gauge may be needed to produce more accurate results.

■ COMPLICATIONS

The most common complication of ventriculoperitoneal shunt aspiration is infection, potentially resulting in meningitis or encephalitis; thus meticulous sterile technique is mandatory. Other complications include subdural hemorrhage from overly aggressive cerebrospinal fluid decompression, bleeding or persistent cerebrospinal fluid leakage from the site of aspiration, and disruption of the valve by a misplaced aspiration attempt.

One can attempt to avoid creation of a subdural hematoma by gentle aspiration of fluid in as small a volume as is clinically required. Shunt malfunction secondary to mechanical blockage is a known problem with the shunts themselves but is an unlikely complication of aspiration unless blood or clots are irrigated through the catheter.

REFERENCES

1. Novak RW: Lack of validity of standard corrections for white blood cell counts of blood-contaminated cerebrospinal fluid in infants. Am J Clin Pathol 1984;82(1):95-97.
2. Turnbull DK, Shepherd DB: Post–dural puncture headache: Pathogenesis, prevention and treatment. Br J Anaesth 2003;91:718-729.
3. Strupp M, Schueler O, Straube A, et al: "Atraumatic" Sprotte needle reduces the incidence of post–lumbar puncture headaches. Neurology 2001;57:2310-2312.

4. Vallejo MC, Mandell GL, Sabo DP, Ramanathan S: Postdural puncture headache: A randomized comparison of five spinal needles in obstetric patients. Anesth Analg 2000;91: 916-920.
5. Luostarinen L, Heinonen T, Luostarinen M, Salmivaara A: Diagnostic lumbar puncture. Comparative study between 22-gauge pencil point and sharp bevel needle. J Headache Pain 2005;6:400-404.
6. Jordan KG: Neurophysiologic monitoring in the neuroscience intensive care unit. Neurol Clin 1995;13:579-626.
7. Lang EW, Chesnut RM: Intracranial pressure: Monitoring and management. Neurosurg Clin North Am 1994;5: 573-605.
8. Rajshekhar V, Harbaugh RE: Results of routine ventriculostomy with external ventricular drainage for acute hydrocephalus following subarachnoid haemorrhage. Acta Neurochir (Wien) 1992;115:8-14.

SECTION X

Allergic, Inflammatory, and Autoimmune Disorders

Chapter 102

Allergies, Allergic Disease, and Anaphylaxis

T. Paul Tran and Robert L. Muelleman

KEY POINTS

Anaphylaxis is an acute life-threatening multiorgan-allergic syndrome that is precipitated within minutes after exposure to an allergen or drug.

The prevalence of allergic disease has been increasing for the last few decades.

Angioedema caused by angiotensin-converting enyme (ACE) inhibitors or due to C1 esterase inhibitor deficiency (hereditary angioedema) requires special considerations and treatment.

ACE-induced angioedema is not mediated by histamine (non–immunoglobulin E [non-IgE] antibody angioedema); therefore antihistamines and steroids may not be as effective in the treatment of laryngeal swelling and upper airway obstruction in patients with this type of angioedema as in other cases of allergic angioedema.

Foods, antibiotics, therapeutic agents, insect stings, and latex are the most common identifiable etiologic agents of anaphylaxis.

Deaths from anaphylaxis result from acute respiratory failure and cardiovascular collapse.

If mild anaphylaxis is recognized and treated early, most patients can be safely discharged home.

Epinephrine is the primary treatment for anaphylaxis.

Both types of antihistamines (drugs that block the H_1 histamine receptors and those that block the H_2 receptors) should be used in cases of anaphylaxis.

Prevention of anaphylaxis by identifying and avoiding the causative agent is important in long-term management and should be discussed by the EP with the patient and family before discharge.

Scope

For allergic diseases to occur, patients need first to be sensitized—that is, they must have developed specific IgE antibody from previous contacts with the allergen. Some patients who possesses IgE antibody do not develop allergic reactions upon re-exposure; these patients are said to be sensitized but not allergic.

The term *atopy* is used to describe the propensity in affected patients to produce IgE antibody in response to otherwise innocuous environmental allergens. Atopic patients have higher serum levels of IgE antibody and one or more atopic diseases (e.g., allergic asthma, allergic rhino-conjunctivitis, atopic dermatitis [eczema], urticaria, angioedema, drug allergy, anaphylaxis). In contrast, nonatopic allergic disorders include such conditions as contact dermatitis, tuberculin reaction, and hypersensitivity pneumonitis.

Anaphylaxis is a life-threatening multiorgan-allergic syndrome that is precipitated within minutes of exposure to a specific allergen in a sensitized person. The offending agent remains unknown in the majority of cases, followed in incidence by food, medication, exercise, and latex.[1]

Epidemiology

It is estimated that up to 42% of Americans suffer from some form of allergic rhinitis at any one time, and thus it is not uncommon to see patients with a non-emergent allergic disease in the ED.[2] The prevalence of allergy in urbanized and Western societies has been increasing steadily in the last three decades. Features of Western lifestyles such as changes in infant diets, widespread use of antibiotics, smaller family size, and cleaner child care are believed to reduce stimulatory antigenic exposure in an individual's early years, leading to an environment in which the immune system is dominated by a persistent allergy-prone system.[3]

Pathophysiology

Development of allergic disease requires the genetically predisposed patient to be sensitized—that is, exposed to an antigen that provokes an IgE antibody response and then re-exposed to the same allergen at a later time. Some of the more common and important allergens include house dust mite, cat dander, tree allergens, grasses, ragweed, and latex (sap harvested from the rubber tree). Haptens, on the other hand, are small molecules that by themselves are not immunogenic, unless they are attached to a larger molecule (carrier). Benzylpenicillin, semisynthetic penicillins, and cephalosporins are important examples of haptens.

Allergic reactions are mostly mediated by IgE antibodies. Cross-linking of a pair of IgE molecules on the surface of the effector cell by a specific allergen causes secretion and degranulation of preformed and newly formed mediators such as histamine from mast cells (and basophils), formation of lipid mediators and cytokines, and subsequent activation of various inflammatory pathways. These mediators and products of secondary inflammatory pathways cause adherence and chemotaxis of inflammatory cells, increased capillary permeability, vasodilation, smooth muscle contraction, and sensory nerve stimulation. Depending on where the allergen is first introduced into the host's body (skin, eyes, nose, lungs, or intestine), the initial signs and symptoms of an allergic reaction can include sneezing, rhinorrhea and bronchorrhea, nasal congestion, dyspnea, wheezing, urticaria, angioedema, ocular itching and swelling, ocular discharge, nausea, vomiting, diarrhea, or abdominal pain.

Allergic Rhinitis

■ CLINICAL PRESENTATION

A detailed history is crucial in diagnosing allergic rhinitis (AR). Patients usually complain of a history of seasonal allergy ("hay fever"), nasal congestion, itching of the nose, sneezing, rhinorrhea, cough (mild), headache, low-grade fever, malaise, or xerostomia (from mouth breathing). Often, patients report a temporal association with exposure to certain environment allergens (seasonal allergy, pollens, animal danders). On the physical examination, nasal membranes are swollen with enlarged, pale turbinates and clear nasal discharge. Maxillary sinuses may feel full and tender on palpation.

Patients with allergic rhinitis often suffer from symptoms of allergic conjunctivitis such as eye itching, swelling, and discharge (clear or can resemble strings of cheese). In atopic patients, the EP should consider the diagnosis of atopic keratoconjunctivitis (Fig. 102-1) and vernal keratoconjunctivitis (Fig. 102-2)—two types of chronic allergic conjunctivitis with the potential to cause corneal erosions and ulcers leading to vision loss. Patients

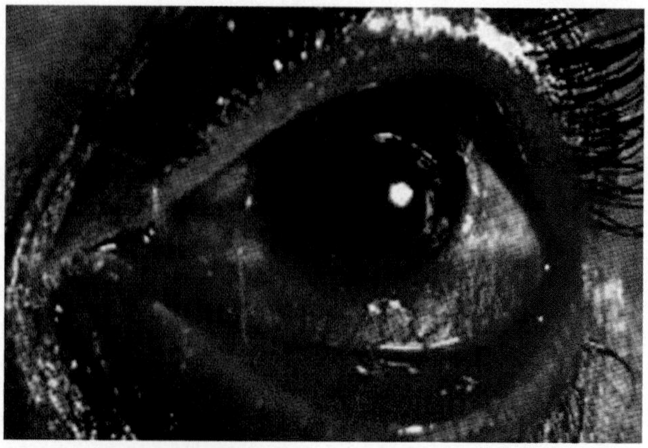

FIGURE 102-1 Atopic keratoconjunctivitis. (From Baba I: Red eye—first aid at the primary level. Commun Eye Health 2005;18:70-72.)

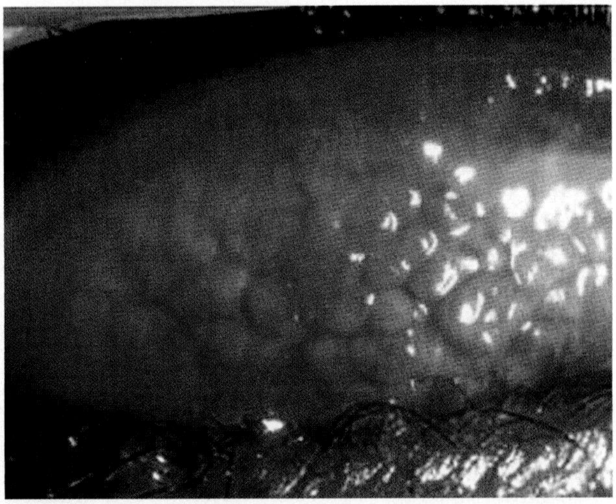

FIGURE 102-2 Vernal keratoconjunctivitis. Notice the lumpy appearance on the conjunctivae. (From Yorston D, Zondervan M: Red eye picture quiz. Community Eye Health 2005;18:72-78.)

with either of these conditions may present with severely inflamed conjunctivae, lids, and periorbital structures, and their treatment should be managed in consultation with an ophthalmologist.

DIFFERENTIAL DIAGNOSIS

Causes of rhinorrhea and nasal congestion are listed in Box 102-1. Because allergic rhinitis is usually first diagnosed in the teenage years, newly diagnosed rhinitis in patients older than 20 years should be investigated for nonallergic causes (such as polyps) either as the primary culprit for the nasal symptoms or as a significant contributor to the underlying allergic rhinitis that patients already have.

DIAGNOSTIC STUDIES

Usually, no diagnostic tests are performed in the ED. Specific IgE serum assays such as the radioallergosorbent test (RAST) and the enzyme-linked immunosorbent assay (ELISA) and the skin prick test and nasal smears usually are performed by an allergy specialist.

TREATMENT

Patients are advised to avoid allergens when practically feasible. Those who are sensitive to pollens should minimize time spent outdoors during periods of high pollen count and lessen the allergen load indoors by keeping windows closed and using HEPA (high-efficiency particulate air) filters, infestation (cockroach) controls, and impermeable covers for mattresses, pillows, quilts, and blankets.

Oral second-generation H_1 blockers (loratadine, fexofenadine), oral HEPA filters (pseudoephedrine), and/or nasal decongestants (oxymetazoline, phenylephrine) can be used for mild, intermittent symptoms. Moderate to severe, intermittent and mild, persistent nasal symptoms are treated similarly with oral H_1 blockers and/or nasal decongestants or with intranasal steroids (fluticasone, triamcinolone, mometasone) or chromone derivatives such as cromoglycate and nedocromil. Intraocular antihistamine (olopatadine), intraocular chromone, or intraocular ketorolac can be used for ocular allergies including conjunctivitis.[4,5]

BOX 102-1

Causes of Rhinorrhea and Nasal Obstruction

Non-Allergic Rhinitis with Eosinophilia Syndrome
- Nasal smears are negative for allergens but have an abundance of eosinophils

Mechanical Obstruction
- Foreign body
- Previous trauma to septum
- Polyps
- Adenoid disease

Infectious Rhinosinusitis
- Primary or secondary bacterial/viral/fungal infections

Vasomotor Rhinitis
- Profuse, clear rhinorrhea and nasal congestion—may be triggered by environmental conditions such as cold air, odors, or atmospheric pressure changes or by ingestion of hot or spicy foods

Drug-Induced
- Includes entities such as rhinitis medicamentosa (rebound from topical decongestant prolonged use)
- May be triggered by aspirin, nonsteroidal antiinflammatory drugs, or oral contraceptive use

Systemic Disease
- Wegener's disease, sarcoidosis
- Head trauma

Modified from Greiner AN: Allergic rhinitis: Impact of the disease and considerations for management. Med Clin North Am 2006;90:17-38.

Urticaria and Angioedema

CLINICAL PRESENTATION

Urticaria, or wheals or hives, is an itchy, erythematous, nonpitting, raised edematous reaction that blanches on palpation (Fig. 102-3) and that can last from hours to a few weeks in response to an aller-

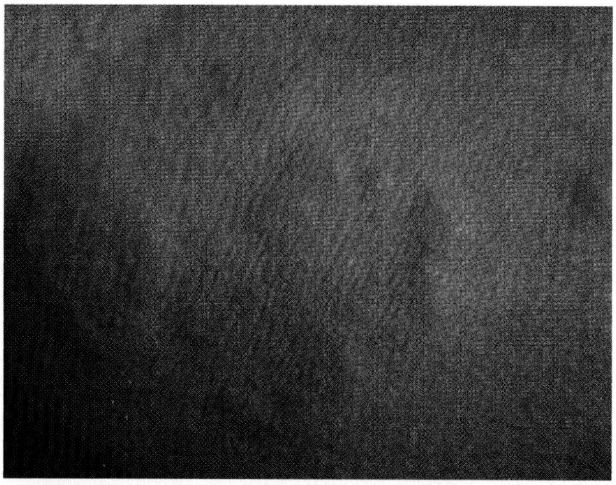

FIGURE 102-3 Acute urticaria. (Copyright 2001-03, Johns Hopkins University School of Medicine. Shahbaz Janjua: Dermatlas; http://www.dermatlas.org, with permission.)

genic exposure. The wheals can be round or oval with serpiginous borders, range in size from millimeters (cholinergic urticaria) to the size of a palm (drug reaction). An urticarial lesion usually first starts with erythema (flare), which is due to capillary vasodilation in the superficial layer of the dermis, and then evolves into raised wheals, which are due to the extravasation of protein-rich fluid from these blood vessels into the surrounding tissue. The lesion can then change from red to white as the edema builds up, and then is slowly absorbed by the body.

When the extravasation and edema occur at subcutaneous layers, the resulting hive-like, brawny edema is called *angioedema*. Itching in angioedema is less than that in urticaria because there are fewer sensory nerve endings in subcutaneous layers than in the superficial dermal layers, which are affected in urticaria. Angioedema tends to involve the face, tongue, mouth, lips, larynx, mucosa of the gastrointestinal tract, extremities, and in men, genitalia. Patients commonly complain of pain or a burning sensation at the affected sites. Involvement of the gastrointestinal tract can cause nausea, vomiting, diarrhea, and abdominal pain.

Recurrent attacks of angioedema and urticaria lasting less than 6 weeks are considered acute (about 90% of cases); those that persist longer than 6 weeks are classified as chronic (about 10% of cases). Acute urticaria and angioedema tend to occur simultaneously in about half of cases. In about 40% of cases, urticaria is the sole presentation.

Attention should be given to cases in which angioedema occurs without urticaria (about 10%), as this may be a presentation of hereditary angioedema, a genetic condition caused by a dysfunctional or absent C1 esterase inhibitor. Hereditary angioedema usually presents in late childhood and teenage years and is characterized by striking swelling of the face, oropharynx, and extremities and mucosal swelling of the gastrointestinal tract. Itching is rare. Upper airway obstruction accounts for up to 30% of deaths associated with hereditary angioedema. Patients with this disease need to be identified and referred to an allergist for further work-up and treatment.

In contrast, onset of recurrent angioedema later in life (e.g., middle age) without urticaria may suggest the presence of acquired angioedema characterized by lack of inheritance and low levels of or nonfunctional C1-esterase inhibitor.

Perhaps the most common form of angioedema seen in the ED is that associated with the use of ACE inhibitors. About 0.1% to 0.2% of patients on ACE-inhibitor therapy develop angioedema. Typically, about 50% of these patients develop symptoms within the first week, whereas others may develop symptoms months or years later.[6] ACE-induced angioedema tends to have a predilection for the lips, tongue, and oropharynx, making this form of angioedema potentially lethal. Because ACE-induced angioedema is mediated by bradykinin and substance P and not histamine (non-IgE), antihistamines and steroids may not be as effective in the treatment of laryngeal swelling and upper airway obstruction caused by ACE as in other cases of allergic angioedema.

■ DIFFERENTIAL DIAGNOSIS

In the majority of cases seen in the ED, a temporal association between a preceding exposure and the onset of symptoms can never be established with complete certainty. The first step in narrowing the differential diagnosis of urticaria is to determine if the urticaria is acute (<6 weeks of symptoms) or chronic (≥6 weeks of symptoms). The differential diagnosis of urticaria is outlined in Box 102-2 and illustrated in Figure 102-4.

When angioedema is suggested by the physical examination, other conditions that can cause swelling should be considered (Box 102-3).

■ DIAGNOSTIC TESTING

The evaluation of urticaria/angioedema is based on a careful history and skin examination; little additional laboratory testing should be needed for acute urticaria.

Patients suspected to have hereditary angioedema should first have their complement-4 (C4) level checked, followed by a CH50 (total complement activity) test, C1-esterase inhibitor test, C1 functional assay, and C2 level measurement, or as recommended by the consultant allergist/internist.

Selected screening tests that can be done in the ED include pelvic examination, sinus films, Panorex, erythrocyte sedimentation rate, thyroid panel, thyroid microsomal antibodies, complete blood count, urinalysis, RPR/MHA-TP (rapid plasma reagin/microhemagglutination assay for antibodies to *Treponema pallidum*) tests for syphilis, and chemistry panel.

BOX 102-2

Differential Diagnosis of Urticaria

Foods/Additives

- Seafood (fish, shellfish, scombroid), tree nuts, eggs, seeds
- Foods containing allergens that are cross-reactive with latex including bananas, avocados, kiwi fruit, chestnuts
- Food preservatives such as tartrazine, benzoates, and sulfites
- Other: cow's milk, pork, strawberries, wheat, chocolate, tomatoes

Medications

- IgE-mediated: penicillins, sulfonamides, cephalosporins
- Nonimmunologic release of histamine: acetylsalicylic acid, nonsteroidal antiinflammatory drugs, indomethacin, angiotensin-converting enzyme inhibitors, morphine, codeine, acetylcholine, iodinated contrast dye, beta-blockers, vancomycin

Infections

- Viral infections: Epstein-Barr virus, hepatitis, coxsackievirus
- Bacterial (occult) infections: sinusitis, dental infections/abscesses, chronic cholecystitis
- Fungal infections: candidiasis, dermatophytosis
- Parasitic infections

Systemic Disease

- Rheumatologic/immunologic: vasculitis, serum sickness, systemic lupus erythematosus, juvenile rheumatoid arthritis
- Endocrinologic: thyroid (both hyper- and hypothyroid) disease, progesterone dermatitis, pruritic urticarial papules and plaques of pregnancy (PUPP), premenstrual flare-up
- Skin disease: mastocytosis, dermatitis herpetiformis, amyloidosis, pemphigoid
- Neoplastic: paraneoplastic syndrome, Hodgkin's disease, leukemia

Inhalants

- Pollen
- Animal danders
- House mite dusts
- Mold spores
- Household chemicals/aerosols

Hymenoptera

- Yellow jackets, honeybees, hornets, wasps most commonly reported; fire ants

Types of Urticaria

- Dermatographism: may begin suddenly after a viral illness or drug therapy
- Pressure/vibratory urticaria: caused by tight clothing around the waist (may be misdiagnosed as scabies)
- Heat urticaria: may be caused by a rise in core temperature after a hot bath, fever, vigorous exercise (also known as cholinergic urticaria because it can be induced by injection of cholinergic agent)
- Cold urticaria: due to exposure to cold temperatures
- Solar urticaria: occurs after exposure to intense sunlight or artificial light (antigens produced in the skin may interact with immunoglobulin E)
- Water urticaria: prickling skin sensation without skin lesions within 15 min of contact with water
- Exercise urticaria: may progress to anaphylaxis
- Household chemicals/aerosols
- Contact urticaria: urticarial wheals/hives develop within 30 to 60 minutes after cutaneous exposure to certain agents including plants (nettles), animals (caterpillars, jellyfish), latex, cosmetics, and various chemicals

Modified from Dibbern DA Jr: Urticaria: Selected highlights and recent advances. Med Clin North Am 2006;90:187-209.

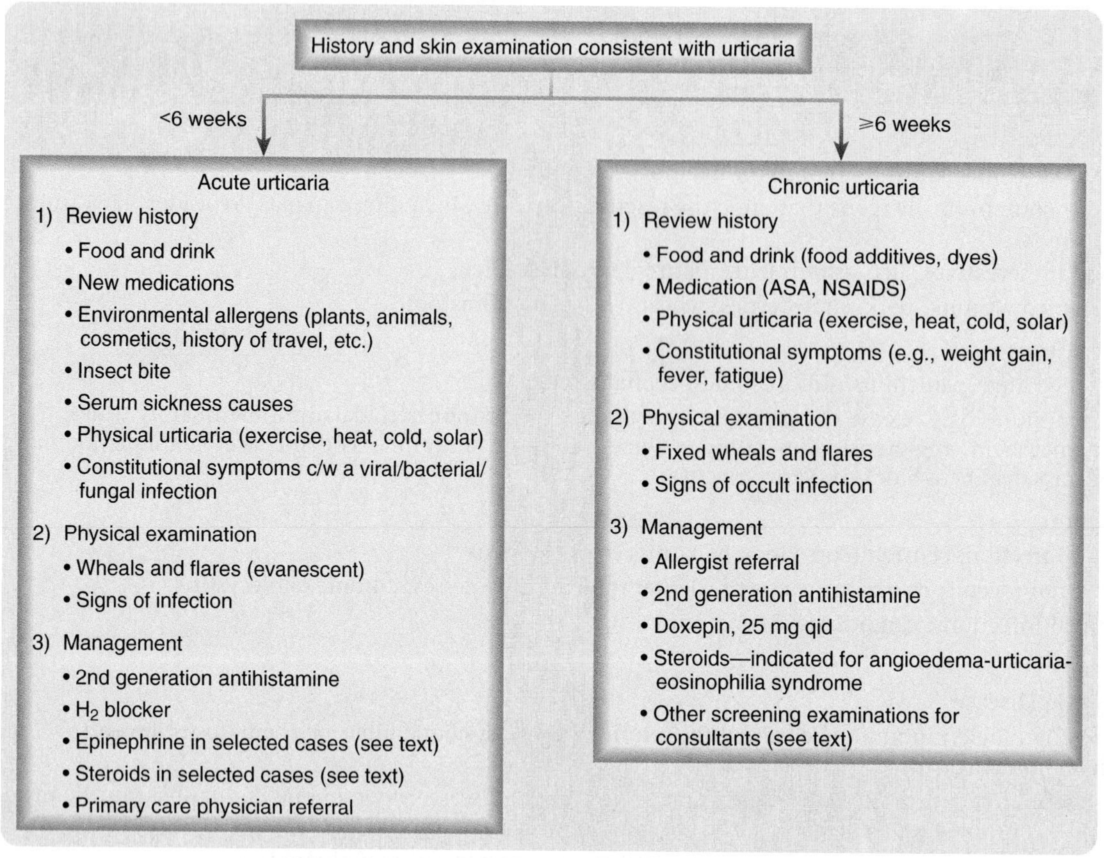
History and skin examination consistent with urticaria
<6 weeks
≥6 weeks
Acute urticaria
1) Review history
• Food and drink
• New medications
• Environmental allergens (plants, animals, cosmetics, history of travel, etc.)
• Insect bite
• Serum sickness causes
• Physical urticaria (exercise, heat, cold, solar)
• Constitutional symptoms c/w a viral/bacterial/ fungal infection
2) Physical examination
• Wheals and flares (evanescent)
• Signs of infection
3) Management
• 2nd generation antihistamine
• H2 blocker
• Epinephrine in selected cases (see text)
• Steroids in selected cases (see text)
• Primary care physician referral
Chronic urticaria
1) Review history
• Food and drink (food additives, dyes)
• Medication (ASA, NSAIDS)
• Physical urticaria (exercise, heat, cold, solar)
• Constitutional symptoms (e.g., weight gain, fever, fatigue)
2) Physical examination
• Fixed wheals and flares
• Signs of occult infection
3) Management
• Allergist referral
• 2nd generation antihistamine
• Doxepin, 25 mg qid
• Steroids—indicated for angioedema-urticaria-eosinophilia syndrome
• Other screening examinations for consultants (see text)

FIGURE 102-4 Algorithm for diagnosis and treatment of urticaria.

BOX 102-3

Differential Diagnosis of Angioedema

- Cellulitis/erysipelas
- Acute contact dermatitis
- Crohn's disease (of mouth and lips)
- Dermatomyositis
- Venous obstructive disease (superior vena cava syndrome)
- Heart failure
- Photodermatitis
- Tumid discoid lupus erythematosus
- Melkersson-Rosenthal syndrome
- Ascher syndrome
- Facial lymphedema
- Renal disease

From Kaplan AP, Greaves MW: Angiodema. J Am Acad Dermatol 2005;53:373-388.

These tests, designed to screen for occult infections, hematology/oncology pathologies, and rheumatologic and inflammatory disorders, may aid the allergist/internist consultant in the subsequent evaluation of these patients.

■ TREATMENT

■ Urticaria

The mainstay of treatment for acute urticaria includes discontinuation of any suspected offending agent and administration of antihistamines (see Fig. 102-4). First-generation antihistamines (diphenhydramine, chlorpheniramine, hydroxyzine) are effective, but they can be sedative with anticholinergic side effects. Second-generation antihistamines (cetirizine, loratadine, fexofenadine, desloratadine) are usually preferred because they are equally effective with significantly less sedation and less psychomotor impairment. Steroids should be avoided if possible.

For urticaria judged difficult to control with antihistamines alone, prednisone (taper: 40 mg PO once a day to 10 mg, tapering over 10 days for an average-sized adult; or pulse: 40-60 mg once a day for 5 days) can be added.[7] If itching is intense and/or the urticarial rash is extensive, epinephrine can be administered (0.3-0.5 mL 1:1000 intramuscularly [IM] or subcutaneously), repeated every 1 to 2 hours as needed. Caution is advised when epinephrine is used in patients older than 40 years of age and is contraindicated in patients with a history of severe cardiovascular disease.

Angioedema

The first priority in the management of patients with the acute allergic syndrome of angioedema is to secure a patent airway. IV access should be established, oxygen applied, and the patient put on a monitor. Because the majority of cases of angioedema are type-I hypersensitivity reactions, combined H_1 and H_2 antihistamine administration remains first-line pharmacotherapy in the ED. H_2 antihistamines are well tolerated and may provide additional, albeit small, benefits to those provided by H_1 antihistamines.[7]

Epinephrine can be administered (0.3-0.5 mL 1:1000 IM), repeated every 1-2 hours as needed for symptoms and signs of airway compromise or hypoxia. Nebulized racemic (or regular) epinephrine (0.5 mL of 2.25% racepinephrine solution; multiple doses are acceptable if there is no IV access) can be a temporizing measure for pharyngeal and laryngeal edema, prior to or in addition to parenteral administration of epinephrine. Parenteral steroids (methylprednisolone, 125 mg intravenously) should be administered for moderately severe disease.

Antihistamines and glucocorticosteroids generally are ineffective in treatment of hereditary angoedema. IV fresh frozen plasma can be given while a search for a C1-esterase inhibitor concentrate is under way. The currently available lyophilized vapor-heated C1-esterase inhibitor concentrate (Immuno, Aventis) can be given (25 plasma U/kg to a total of 1000 U), repeated once as needed. It has been reported to reduce the submucosal swelling within 4 hours, and sometimes within minutes.[6]

DISPOSITION

Urticaria

Most patients with urticaria (acute and chronic) can be managed as outpatients.

Angioedema

Patients with allergic angioedema usually can be managed as outpatients; however, patients with ACE-induced angioedema who were sick enough to be administered epinephrine are candidates for overnight hospital observation, and ACE-inhibitor therapy should be stopped in those who are sent home. These patients should be warned about recurrent symptoms and instructed to return to the ED if they have any respiratory symptoms.

Replacement alternatives for ACE inhibitors include calcium channel blockers and thiazides. Alternatively, an angiotensin-receptor blocker can be used because the risks of angioedema from these agents are acceptably low.[8] Beta-blockers are not advised in the initial setting because of the theoretical risk of exacerbating the angioedema and the potential antagonistic effects to epinephrine. Additionally, these patients should be given second-generation antihistamines and H_2 blockers, Epi-Pens, and prednisone.

Patients with hereditary angioedema should be managed in the ED in consultation with their primary physician and/or allergist. Most of these patients, especially those with faciolaryngeal involvement, usually warrant observation overnight in the hospital.

Insect Stings (Hymenoptera Venom Allergy)

PATHOPHYSIOLOGY AND EPIDEMIOLOGY

The venom from insects in the Hymenoptera order (yellow jackets, hornets, honeybees, wasps, and fire ants) contain histamine, dopamine, kinins, and various peptides and protein enzymes that either are vasoactive or can elicit allergic reactions in the host.

Serious systemic reactions from insect stings are rare, occurring in 0.4% to 3% of individuals and accounting for approximately 50 deaths in the United States per year from anaphylactic reaction.[9] These most serious reactions are type I hypersensitivity (IgE-mediated) reactions (see Box 102-4). There is a 2:1 male:female distribution in the victims; the most vulnerable population is that of adult male agricultural workers.[10]

CLINICAL PRESENTATION

Most stings typically result in self-limited local reactions with itching, pain, swelling, and redness. These reactions usually last for a few hours, are not IgE-mediated, and do not put patients at risk for future systemic reactions.[9] In some patients, the reaction can involve a large part of the body (e.g., an entire limb) and can last for longer than 24 hours.

Caution should be exercised when the sting and subsequent swelling reaction occur near the oropharynx (either cutaneous or swallowed), because airway compromise can result.

DIFFERENTIAL DIAGNOSIS

Considerations include secondary bacterial infection, cellulitis, abscess, urticaria, angioedema, and anaphylactic reaction.

DIAGNOSTIC STUDIES

Screening laboratory examinations for infection (complete blood count, wound culture) should be made if there are signs of infection on physical examination.

■ TREATMENT

The stinger should be removed if present. For minor local reactions, antihistamines and nonsteroidal anti-inflammatory drugs (NSAIDs) (ibuprofen) should be sufficient. Ice can be used to decrease the inflammatory response. Elevation will decrease the swelling. Antibiotics should be prescribed if there are signs of secondary bacterial infection. Coverage for methicillin-resistant *Staphylococcus aureus* should be considered. Management of more systemic reactions is similar to that of anaphylaxis.

Stings by fire ants can cause the formation of a pustule-like lesion that contains mostly necrotic materials, and these should be managed like second-degree burns.

■ DISPOSITION

Patients who have systemic reactions to stings warrant overnight observation in the hospital. Patients with limited or extensive local reactions to stings can be managed as outpatients.

Patients with urticaria or angioedema reactions to insect stings should be referred to an allergist for possible skin testing and venom immunotherapy. These patients should wear a Med-Alert bracelet at all times, be educated about prevention of stings, the early signs of a systemic reaction, how to call for help, and how to self-administer Epi-Pen. At least two Epi-Pens should be prescribed for emergency self-injection.

Patients should be instructed about preventive measures, such as *always* wearing shoes when outdoors and *not* wearing brightly colored clothes or fragrances in high-risk areas.

Drug Allergy and Adverse Drug Reactions

An adverse drug reaction is defined by the World Health Organization (WHO) as a noxious, unintended, or undesired response to a drug taken at a normal dose for the prevention, diagnosis, or treatment of a disease. Adverse drug reactions affect 10% to 20% of hospitalized patients and up to 7% of the general population.[11] The majority of these reactions (80%) are classified as "predictable" or type A, meaning that they are dose-dependent and related to the known pharmacology of the drugs, known side effects (antibiotic-associated diarrhea), toxicity if taken in overdose, and/or drug-drug interactions. The remaining 20% are classified as "unpredictable" or type B and include hypersensitivity reactions, drug idiosyncrasy, and psycho-physiologic responses (hyperventilation, vasovagal).

Although the true frequency is unknown, drug allergy probably accounts for about one third of adverse drug reactions.[11]

■ CLINICAL PRESENTATION

Patients may present with an acute reaction or they may report a history of drug allergy (e.g., penicillin) first occurring in childhood, for example. The most prudent approach in the ED for management of possible drug-allergy related complaints is to discontinue the suspect medication(s), provide supportive care for the presenting symptoms, and prescribe a suitable alternative medication. Before making the diagnosis of drug allergy, the EP may determine from clinical history whether the presenting symptoms represent an adverse drug reaction, the time course and nature of the drug reaction, and whether the reaction is an adverse drug reaction or a true drug allergy. At the end of the ED visit, the EP should educate the patient about the nature of drug allergy vs. adverse drug reaction, because patients often considered drug allergy to be synonymous with adverse drug reaction.[12]

Penicillin is one of the most commonly prescribed antibiotics and most studied drug causing allergic reactions. Table 102-1 shows the incidences of allergic reactions to penicillin.[13] Those rare patients who present with urticaria, angioedema, respiratory insufficiency, or cardiac insufficiency 20 minutes after oral or parenteral administration of penicillin are having an immediate hypersensitivity (type I) reaction (Box 102-4). More commonly, patients who present with maculopapular exanthems and non-urticarial morbilliform rash a few days after taking penicillin are probably having a T-cell mediated hypersensitivity (type IV) reaction. There are a variety of factors that can cause the T cells to falsely identify the penicillin

Table 102-1 ESTIMATED INCIDENCE OF ALLERGIC REACTIONS TO PENICILLIN

Type of Reaction	Manifestation	Time of Occurrence after First Dose	Percentage of Patients Showing Reaction
Late	Skin rash	≥72 hr	1.4
Accelerated	Urticaria	1-72 hr	0.3
Immediate	Generalized urticaria	2-30 min	0.3
	Anaphylaxis	2-30 min	0.04
	Death due to anaphylaxis		0.001

From Asthma and the other allergic diseases. NIAID Task Force Report, NIH publ no. 79-387, 1979.

BOX 102-4

Types of Hypersensitivity

Type I Hypersensitivity

Immediate or immunoglobulin E (IgE)–mediated: Binding of antigens to IgE on the surface of mast cells/basophils leads to release of imflammatory mediators (maximal reaction in 20 minutes). This type of hypersensitivity reaction is seen in allergic diseases, drug reactions, urticaria/angioedema, and anaphylaxis. *Pseudoallergic syndrome* and *anaphylactoid reaction* are terms referring to the direct release of preformed contents of mast cells and the clinical sequelae independent of the IgE mechanism.

Type II Hypersensitivity

Cytotoxic antibody reaction: Binding of antigens to their own cells (or foreign cells with foreign antigens) attracts binding by IgM/IgG antibodies, which subsequently causes injury and lysis of cells via the complement or mononuclear cell system.

Type III Hypersensitivity

Immune complex (IC)-mediated reaction: Binding of antigens to IgE forms soluble ICs, which deposit on vessel walls, causing a local inflammatory reaction (Arthus reaction) by attaching to FγRIII receptors on inflammatory cells (maximum reaction 4-8 hours).

Type IV Hypersensitivity

Cell-mediated delayed hypersensitivity: Sensitized lymphocytes (T_H1 cells) recognize the antigen, recruit additional lymphocytes and mononuclear cells to the site, starting the inflammatory reaction. This type of hypersensitivity reaction is seen in contact dermatitis, erythema multiforme, Stevens-Johnson syndrome, and toxic epidermal necrolysis (maximum reaction 48-72 hours).

epitope as allergic. For example, up to half (50%) of patients with mononucleosis develop a maculopapular rash after taking amoxicillin. These same patients often have no adverse drug reactions on subsequent challenge with amoxicillin at a later time. These patients should not be diagnosed as having penicillin allergy.

Studies of cephalosporins show that 4.4% of patients whose penicillin allergy history was confirmed by a positive skin test have adverse drug reactions to cephalosporins,[14] and only 10% to 20% of patients who report a history of penicillin allergy are truly allergic when assessed by skin testing.[15] Thus the overall risks of a cross-allergic reaction to cephalosporins in patients with a unsubstantiated history of penicillin allergy seem low; however, the use of cephalosporins requires weighing risks versus benefits based on an informed discussion by the patient and treating physician.

■ DIFFERENTIAL DIAGNOSIS

Common entities to consider are infection (viral exanthem, mononucleosis, Rocky Mountain spotted fever, syphilis, cellulitis, sepsis), insect bite, pityriasis rosea, serum sickness, vasculitides, contact dermatitis, fixed drug eruption, and drug hypersensitivity syndrome.

■ DIAGNOSTIC STUDIES

The diagnosis of adverse drug reaction relies on a careful history and thorough skin examination. A complete blood count, chemistry panel, and erythrocyte sedimentation rate may be ordered to evaluate possible infections or vasculitis. Skin testing is only of limited value. RAST and ELISA for serum IgE require known immunogenic epitopes for the drugs, information that is normally unavailable. In cases of hemolytic anemia, the indirect Coombs test can be used to diagnose the immune-mediated destruction of red blood cells.

■ TREATMENT

The standard approach to managing adverse drug reactions includes discontinuation of the possible offending drugs, treatment of allergic symptoms, and provision for suitable alternatives to the discontinued drugs. An antihistamine can be prescribed for itching, flushing, and rash. Steroids are reserved for cases of serious or extensive drug reactions.

Following observation in the ED, patients with more serious symptoms are triaged to home, observation unit, regular hospital floor, or the intensive care unit. Respiratory insufficiency is first corrected with oxygen and nebulized beta-agonists and intubation if necessary. Hypotension from vasodilation and capillary leak syndrome is corrected with crystalloids and pressors (dopamine, 10-20 μg/kg/min and/or norepinephrine 2-8 μg/min). Patients with Stevens-Johnson syndrome and toxic epidermal necrolysis require a multidisciplinary effort from an intensivist, burns surgeon, and endocrinologist/allergist.

■ DISPOSITION

The majority of patients with late (>1 hour to days) reactions to medications who have mild/moderate rash can be safely discharged to home. Those with immediate drug reactions (<1 hour) need to be observed in the ED. If symptoms are completely resolved while patients are in the ED, they can be discharged to home accompanied by a family member, with two Epi-Pens, the treatment medications previously described, and a Med-Alert bracelet.

Patients judged to be at risk for prolonged effects of the drug reaction, with poor social support, with significant comorbid conditions, and/or with moderate to severe allergic syndromes warrant a hospital stay.

Anaphylaxis

Anaphylaxis is an acute life-threatening allergic syndrome caused by sudden systemic release of mediators from mast cells and basophils in response to an allergenic activation in previously sensitized individuals. Symptoms include rapid clinical deterioration—moving from seemingly benign itchy urticarial rash at initial presentation to urgent laryngeal edema, bronchospasm, emergent upper airway obstruction, acute respiratory failure, cardiovascular instability, hypotension, shock, and death.

■ EPIDEMIOLOGY AND PATHOPHYSIOLOGY

The incidence of anaphylaxis is estimated to be about 1% of the population.[16] Risk factors for experiencing anaphylaxis include a history of atopy, male less than 16 years of age, female less than 30 years of age, route of allergen administration, economic status, and time of the year.

Anaphylaxis is commonly a type I immediate hypersensitivity reaction (see Box 102-4), but it can also be type II (cytotoxic) or type III (immune complex). In addition, anaphylaxis can result from agents with the ability to alter arachidonic metabolism (e.g., acetylsalicylic acid, NSAIDs), agents that can cause direct degranulation of mast cells (opiates, radiocontrast media), and physical agents (exercise, heat, cold). Furthermore, anaphylaxis can occur in certain patients without any obvious inciting events (idiopathic). The resulting syndromes of these IgE-independent reactions are clinically indistinguishable from those of classic anaphylaxis; the term *anaphylactoid* has been used to refer to these IgE-independent reactions.

Histamine is the most important mediator and responsible for most of the clinical manifestations of anaphylaxis. Histamine exerts its effects on multiple organs, causing vasodilation and increased vascular permeability, fluid shifts to extravascular space, lowered peripheral vascular resistance, increased rate of force of atrial and ventricular contraction, bronchoconstriction of the lungs, hypermotility of the gastrointestinal tract (causing abdominal pain, nausea, vomiting, and diarrhea), and uterine contractions. Presumably, with the activation of the rest of the inflammatory cascades and mediators, shock ultimately ensues.

As the anaphylaxis progresses, intravascular volume deficit grows due to third spacing, and cardiac output falls as a result of myocardial depression and decreased preload. Even though blood pressure plummets, peripheral vascular resistance is often noted to rise, probably as a response to endogenous vasopressors. Without additional volume infusion, more pressors will only lead to further vasoconstriction at the expense of the heart.

■ CLINICAL PRESENTATION

In general, the sooner the clinical syndrome manifests after allergenic exposure, the more severe the reaction. The clinical expression depends on the degree of hypersensitivity by the host, the quantity, route, and rate of antigen exposure, and the target organ sensitivity and responsiveness. Rapid progression from mild urticaria and bronchospasm to shock and acute respiratory failure may occur in minutes. Most anaphylactic reactions become clinically evident within seconds to minutes (average 5-30 minutes) after parenteral exposure and within hours (average, 2 hours) after ingestion of an anaphylactic allergen.

Most fatalities occur within the first 30 minutes after the allergenic exposure; however, a delay of hours or even days can occur in rare situations. In about 20% of the cases, the anaphylactic reaction follows a biphasic pattern; patients seem to recover from the initial episode and appear asymptomatic, only to have a second phase of the anaphylactic reaction, which usually occurs within the first 8 hours and sometimes up to 72 hours later.

Anaphylaxis is a multiorgan allergic syndrome; the following organs are most often involved: cutaneous, respiratory, gastrointestinal, cardiovascular, and central nervous systems. Cutaneous symptoms are by far the most common, present in more than 90% of cases, and often considered the sine qua non condition of anaphylaxis.

Patients may report generalized warmth and tingling of the face, mouth, upper chest, palms, soles, or the site of the allergenic exposure. This may progress to a flush syndrome or an abrupt eruption of itchy, red, raised wheals that spread rapidly. In the setting of shock, cutaneous symptoms may be absent as a result of compensatory vasoconstriction, and deaths have been reported from acute respiratory failure in the absence of cutaneous findings.

Signs and symptoms of anaphylaxis on physical examination include angioedematous and urticarial rash, tachypnea, nasal obstruction with discharge, ocular tearing with conjunctivitis, wheezing, stridor, tachyarrhythmia, altered mental status, and hypotension. The constellation of laryngeal stridor, hypersalivation, hoarseness, and angioedema indicates upper airway obstruction, whereas coughing, wheezing, rhonchi, and diminished air movement suggest lower airway bronchoconstriction. Tachycardia and hypotension suggest cardiac insufficiency. Electrocardiographic changes include sinus tachycardia, premature atrial and ventricular contractions, nodal rhythm, atrial fibrillation, nonspecific and ischemic ST-T wave changes, right ventricular strain, and intraventricular conduction defects. Any of these clinical patterns may occur independently of, in combina-

BOX 102-5

Differential Diagnosis of Anaphylaxis

Flush Syndromes
- Hereditary angioedema
- Urticaria vasculitis
- Carcinoid syndrome
- Systemic mastocytosis/urticaria pigmentosa
- Vasointestinal polypeptide-secreting tumors
- Medullary carcinoma of the thyroid
- Pheochromocytoma
- Acute alcohol syndrome
- Monosodium glutamate toxicity
- Sulfites
- Scombroidosis

Infections/Respiratory Syndromes
- Epiglottitis/supraglottitis
- Retropharyngeal, peritonsillar abscess
- Laryngeal spasm, foreign body aspiration, tumor
- Acute asthma exacerbation/chronic obstructive pulmonary disease

Shock Syndromes
- Hemorrhagic
- Cardiogenic
- Septic
- Spinal shock

Somatoform/Psychogenic
- Panic attacks
- Munchausen/factitious disorder
- Somatoform idiopathic anaphylaxis

Miscellaneous
- Idiopathic
- Vasodepressor (vasovagal) reactions
- Progesterone anaphylaxis
- Red man syndrome (vancomycin)
- Capillary leak syndrome

tion with, or in association with cramping abdominal pain with nausea, vomiting, diarrhea, tenesmus, incontinence, pelvic pain, headache, or a sense of impending doom.

■ DIFFERENTIAL DIAGNOSIS

Because anaphylaxis involves multiple organs, its clinical spectrum overlaps several other clinical syndromes, especially those involving the skin and respiratory system (Box 102-5).

Vasovagal reaction is the most common differential diagnosis in the patient presenting to the ED with syncope, perhaps as a result of parenteral administration of a medication. Both anaphylaxis and vasovagal reaction are characterized by syncope and nausea and vomiting; patients with vasovagal reaction may have bradycardia, hypotension, diaphoresis, and pallor, as opposed to the tachycardia, hypotension, diaphoresis, and wheals and flares usually associated with anaphylaxis. The absence of any other clinical manifestations of anaphylaxis, along with history of stress, pain, and previous episodes of simple syncope suggests the diagnosis of vasovagal reaction.

Patients who present in anaphylactic shock may appear clinically indistinguishable from patients in septic and spinal shock, because signs in both types of shock include end organ hypoperfusion and vasodilation. The skin is usually moist and warm, suggesting a state of decreased peripheral vascular resistance.

Patients in cardiogenic, restrictive, hypovolemic, or hemorrhagic shock are more likely to be seen with cold, clammy skin as a result of increased peripheral vascular resistance.

Because anaphylactic shock can progress to cardiogenic shock, measurement of central venous pressures may be necessary. A history of atopy, the characteristic angioedematous urticarial rash seen in anaphylaxis, and a history of antecedent allergenic exposure immediately prior to the onset of symptoms may help distinguish anaphylactic shock from the other forms of shock. Ordinary allergic reactions and especially anaphylaxis can precipitate an acute coronary syndrome.[17]

■ DIAGNOSTIC STUDIES

The diagnosis of anaphylaxis is based on the history and physical examination. A starting diagnostic panel includes complete blood count, complete metabolic panel (hypoglycemia), coagulation panel including international normalized ratio and prothrombine time/partial thromboplastin time, cardiac enzyme assays, an electrocardiogram (to rule out an acute coronary syndrome), urinalysis, erythrocyte sedimentation rate, and a chest radiograph.

Serum levels of serotonin and urinary 5-hydroxyindole acetic acid, catecholamines (free plasma metanephrine), and vanillylmandelic acid are useful to rule out carcinoid syndrome and pheochromocytoma. A serum vasointestinal polypeptide hormone panel, if available, can be used to look for vasoactive peptides that can be due to a gastrointestinal tumor or medullary carcinoma of the thyroid. Serum levels of urinary histamine and serum tryptase are helpful to confirm the diagnosis of anaphylaxis after the fact. The optimal time to obtain the serum level of histamine is within 1 hour, of serum tryptase within 1 to 2 hours (but no longer than 6 hours) after the onset of symptoms. A 24-hr urine collection for histamine metabolites (methylhistamines) is another useful confirmatory test for anaphylaxis.

■ TREATMENT

The early administration of epinephrine is the mainstay of treatment for anaphylaxis (Box 102-6). For prophylaxis, 50 mg of oral diphenhydramine hydrochloride can be taken by high-risk patients after possible allergenic exposure. At the first signs of clinical manifestations of anaphylaxis, the patient should self-administer epinephrine if available. Susceptible patients may use aerosolized epinephrine via a metered-dose inhaler, if available. Multiple inhalations (e.g., 10 to 20 doses [0.22 mg/min], resulting in the inhalation of 1.5 to 3 mg of epinephrine) produce therapeutic plasma levels, with the advantages of ease of administration, rapid absorption, and high epinephrine levels in the upper and lower airways.

Local measures to decrease antigen absorption from an extremity include dependent positioning of the extremity, ice for local vasoconstriction, and application of a loose tourniquet to obstruct the venous and lymphatic circulation. The tourniquet should be released for 1 of every 10 minutes. If an insect stinger remains, the wound should not be squeezed because this may inject more venom into the patient. The stinger should be removed gently with instruments, avoiding disturbance of the venom apparatus.

Most cases of morbidity and mortality from anaphylaxis are related to asphyxia from upper respiratory tract obstruction, acute respiratory failure from bronchospasm, or cardiovascular collapse; therefore priority should be given to stabilizing any cardiorespiratory insufficiency (Fig. 102-5).

Epinephrine and antihistamines (H_1 and H_2 blockers) should be administered early. A nebulized beta-agonist can be given simultaneously for wheezing. All patients should have supplemental oxygen administered, large-bore IV lines inserted to infuse crystalloid or colloid solutions (normally not necessary), and continuous cardiac monitoring. A large volume of crystalloid fluid may be required to reverse the hypotension associated with anaphylaxis.

Upper airway obstruction from laryngeal edema or angioedema can progress rapidly. Racemic epineph-

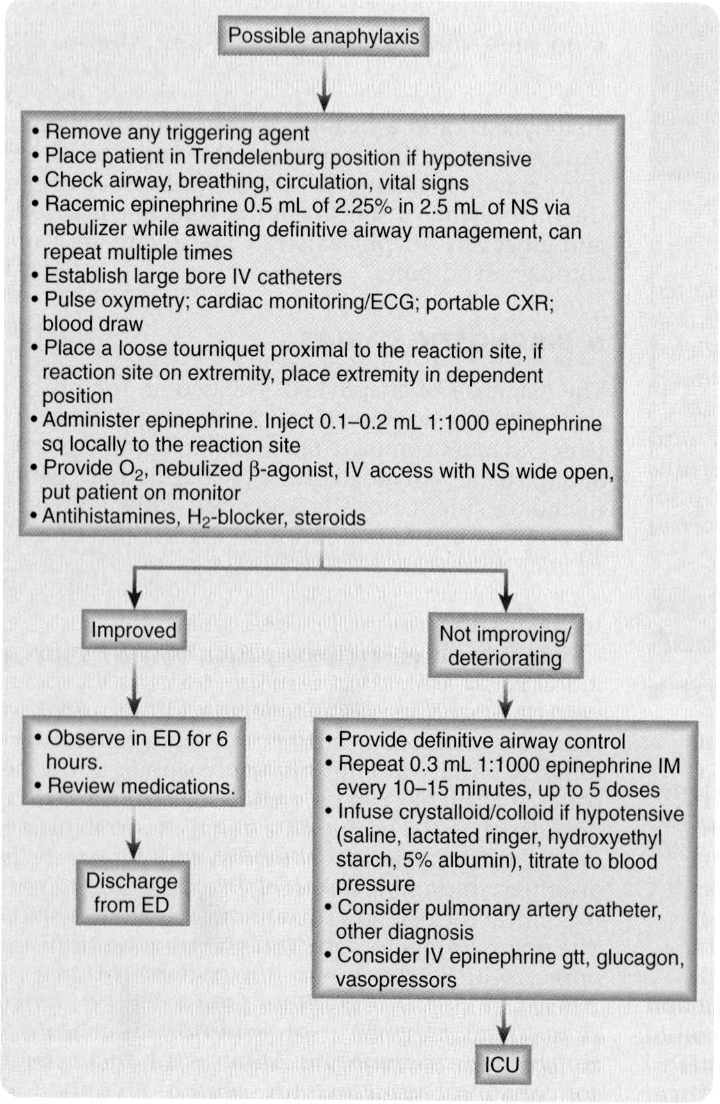
Possible anaphylaxis
• Remove any triggering agent
• Place patient in Trendelenburg position if hypotensive
• Check airway, breathing, circulation, vital signs
• Racemic epinephrine 0.5 mL of 2.25% in 2.5 mL of NS via nebulizer while awaiting definitive airway management, can repeat multiple times
• Establish large bore IV catheters
• Pulse oxymetry; cardiac monitoring/ECG; portable CXR; blood draw
• Place a loose tourniquet proximal to the reaction site, if reaction site on extremity, place extremity in dependent position
• Administer epinephrine. Inject 0.1–0.2 mL 1:1000 epinephrine sq locally to the reaction site
• Provide O_2, nebulized β-agonist, IV access with NS wide open, put patient on monitor
• Antihistamines, H_2-blocker, steroids
Improved
Not improving/ deteriorating
• Observe in ED for 6 hours.
• Review medications.
Discharge from ED
• Provide definitive airway control
• Repeat 0.3 mL 1:1000 epinephrine IM every 10–15 minutes, up to 5 doses
• Infuse crystalloid/colloid if hypotensive (saline, lactated ringer, hydroxyethyl starch, 5% albumin), titrate to blood pressure
• Consider pulmonary artery catheter, other diagnosis
• Consider IV epinephrine gtt, glucagon, vasopressors
ICU

FIGURE 102-5 Treatment algorithm for anaphylaxis (see Box 102-6 for drug dosages and indications). CXR, chest radiograph; ECG, electrocardiogram; ICU, intensive care unit; IM, intramuscularly; IV, intravenous; NS, normal saline.

BOX 102-6

Treatment Options for Anaphylaxis

Epinephrine

- Intramuscular (subcutaneous acceptable)—1:1000; adult: 0.3-0.5 mL, every 10-15 min as necessary, titrated to effects; pediatric: 0.01 mL/kg, every 5 min as necessary, titrated to effects)
- Alternatively, EpiPen (0.3 mL) or EpiPen Jr (0.15 mL) can be administered into anterolateral thigh; removal of clothing unnecessary
- IV infusion—1:100,000; 0.1 mL of 1:1000 in 10 mL of normal saline (NS), 100 μg, over 10 minutes; equivalent to 10 μg/min for 10-min period, titrated to effects; repeat as necessary; continuous hemodynamic monitoring required
- Continuous infusion—1 mL of 1:1000 dilution of epinephrine in 250 mL of D_5/W results in concentration of 4 μg/mL; can be started at 1 μg/min and increased to 4 μg/min if needed
- Pediatric continuous infusion—rate of 0.1 μg/kg/min (up to 30 kg) advised, increasing in increments of 0.1 μg/kg/min to a maximum of 1.5 μg/kg/min.

Antihistamines

- Diphenhydramine (IV or PO)—adult: 50-100 mg, up to 400 mg/24 hr, titrated to effects; pediatric: 0.02 mg/kg, up to 300 mg/24 hours, titrated to effects
- Ranitidine or other H_2 blocker (IV or PO)—adult: 50 mg IV, 300 mg PO (4 mg/kg); pediatric: 1 mg/kg

Aerosolized Beta-Agonists and Others

- Albuterol—adult: 2.5 mg; pediatric: 0.02 mL/kg up to 2.5 mg in 3 mL of NS; may be given continuously
- Ipratropium—adult: 0.5 mg; pediatric: 0.25 mg in 3 mL of NS; repeat as necessary

Methylprednisolone

- IV infusion—adult: 125-250 mg; pediatric: 40-80 mg

Glucagon

- IV infusion—adult: 1-5 mg over 5 min; pediatric: 0.5 mg, followed by 5-15 μg/min gtt; for refractory hypotension or patients on beta-blockade

Dopamine

- IV infusion—5-20 μg/kg/min gtt and/or dobutamine, 5-20 μg/kg/min gtt

Norepinephrine

- IV infusion—8-12 μg/min gtt (2-3 mL/min; 4 mg added to 1000 mL of D_5W provides concentration of 4 μg /mL)

Transcutaneous Pacing for Bradycardia

Atropine for Bradycardia

- IV infusion or subcutaneous—adult: 0.3-0.5 mg, to a maximum of 3 mg; pediatric: 0.02 mg/kg, to a maximum of 2 mg

Isoproterenol

- IV infusion: 0.05- 0.2 μg /kg/min (1-2 mg in 500 mL of D_5W, infused at rate of 0.5 to 2 mL/min)

Aminophylline

- IV infusion—5-6 mg/kg loading dose over 20 min, followed by 0.1-1.1 mg/kg/hr gtt; for refractory bronchospasm

Nitroprusside

- IV infusion—0.3-10 μg/kg/min gtt plus phentolamine, 5-20 mg; for hypertensive crisis due to unopposed alpha-blockade

Lidocaine

- IV infusion—1-2 mg/kg bolus, followed to 2 mg/min gtt; for dysrhythmia rine, delivered as a 2.25% solution, may be a temporizing measure. The success rate of intubation will be improved when it is performed early and before soft tissue swelling has advanced. Oral endotracheal intubation is the route of choice because significant anatomic distortion may be present as a result of edema. Once a patent airway has been obtained and supplemental oxygen delivered, therapy should be focused on relieving the patient's bronchospasm.

Epinephrine usually is administered as an intramuscular injection. A fraction of the total dose (0.1 to 0.2 mL) should be administered at the site of antigenic exposure if it is accessible (e.g., a bee sting or antigen injection in an extremity). If the patient demonstrates severe upper airway obstruction, acute respiratory failure, or shock, intravenous epinephrine can be administered; however, the risk of supraventricular, accelerated idioventricular, and ventricular tachydysrhythmia; accelerated hypertension; and myocardial ischemia is increased by using the IV route. Because of these risks, dilution and slow administration are recommended. If no improvement is seen, a continuous infusion should be set up. If a percutaneous IV line cannot be established, intraosseous or sublingual injection or endotracheal nebulization should be considered. Continuous cardiac monitoring during IV therapy is mandatory at all times.

Diphenhydramine is the H_1 antihistamine most commonly used for anaphylaxis. Commonly used H_2 blockers are ranitidine and cimetidine.

Bronchospasm refractory to epinephrine may respond to a nebulized beta-agonist such as albuterol sulfate, bitolterol, pirbuterol, and metaproterenol. Continuous nebulization may be necessary for persistent bronchospasm. The use of anticholinergic therapy with ipratropium bromide is an additional option in the management of acute bronchospasm.

As second-line therapy for refractory bronchospasm, an aminophylline IV bolus (5.6 mg/kg loading dose over 20 minutes), followed by maintenance infusion (0.1-1.1 mg/kg/hour), can be added. Aminophylline is an old drug with a narrow therapeutic window. Its main purported action is bronchodilation, although it may also act to potentiate the action of catecholamines.

Systemic corticosteroids have an onset of action of approximately 4 to 6 hours after administration and therefore are of limited benefit in the acute treatment of the anaphylactic patient. They are most useful for persistent bronchospasm or hypotension and should be used to prevent the biphasic reaction of anaphylaxis. Rare cases of deterioration after corticosteroid administration may be the result of anaphylactic sensitivity to this medication.

In patients with persistent hypotension despite epinephrine and large volumes of intravenous crystalloid administration, the use of colloid solutions (e.g., 5% albumin) should be considered in addition to crystalloids because of increased vascular permeability in anaphylaxis. If the central venous pressure is less than 12 mm Hg, crystalloid and colloid fluids should first be administered. If the pressure is greater than 12 mm Hg, dopamine (5µg/kg/minute) should be started and titrated to effects. Dobutamine can be added if myocardial depression is judged to be an important cause of the hypotension.

Causes of elevated filling pressures other than vascular volume or myocardial dysfunction should be considered (e.g., vasopressor administration, increased intraperitoneal and intrathoracic pressures, vasoconstriction, pulmonary artery hypertension). If pulmonary hypertension exists, hyperventilation, hyperoxygenation, and large doses of steroids should be considered. The use of pressors with primarily alpha-adrenergic activity, such as norepinephrine, should be considered if all of these measures fail to restore the inadequate hemodynamics. In the rare case that the anaphylactic patient develops a hypertensive crisis secondary to unopposed alpha-adrenergic activity from the treatment, nitroprusside drips or phentolamine may be necessary.

RED FLAGS

Management of Anaphylaxis

- Failure to diagnose anaphylaxis early or to recognize the need to secure the airway early; reluctance to use epinephrine when indicated
- Incorrect administration of IV epinephrine (e.g., not diluting)
- Failure to identify vernal and atopic keratoconjunctivitis—two types of chronic allergic conjunctivitis that can cause corneal erosions and ulcers leading to vision loss

SPECIAL CONSIDERATIONS: PATIENTS ON BETA-BLOCKERS

Glucagon, with positive inotropic and chronotropic cardiac effects mediated independently of beta-1 and beta-2 receptors, may be helpful in patients who are on beta-blockers and who do not respond to epinephrine and antihistamines.[18] Atropine and isoproterenol can be tried as second-line therapy. Atropine is probably more useful for bradycardia. Isoproterenol should only be used as a last resort for the rare patient who is in refractory shock despite receiving the therapy previously described.

DISPOSITION

Guidelines for disposition of patients with anaphylaxis are shown in the Tips and Tricks Box. The majority of patients with mild to moderate anaphylaxis can be treated successfully in the ED and safely discharged to home if symptom resolution was rapid and complete and there was no recurrence during an observation period of 2 to 6 hours in the ED.[19] Oral H_1 antihistamines such as diphenhydramine (50 mg

Tips and Tricks

PREVENTION OF ANAPHYLAXIS AND ANAPHYLACTIC DEATH

- Obtain a thorough drug allergy and atopic history.
- Check all drugs for proper labeling.
- Give drug orally rather than parenterally when possible.
- Give drug in distal extremity if possible when parenteral route is necessary.
- Always have resuscitation equipment available when administering antigenic compounds.
- Ensure that patients remain in the ED for at least 30 minutes after drug administration.
- Use unrelated drugs when feasible in susceptible patients.
- When antiserum is essential, use human type if available.
- If heterologous serum is essential, always perform pretest.
- Instruct predisposed patients to carry warning identification (Medic-Alert, wallet ID).
- Teach predisposed patients technique of self-injection of epinephrine; tell them to carry treatment kit at all times.
- Instruct patients to avoid known antigens (stinging insects, foods, antibiotics).
- Perform skin test and consider hyposensitization immunotherapy.
- Pretreat with antihistamines or steroids when appropriate (see Box 102-7).

every 6 hours for 72 hours) and H_2 blockers such as ranitidine (150 mg every 12 hours for 72 hours) along with oral prednisone may prevent possible relapse. These patients should be instructed to return to the ED if experiencing symptoms such as hoarseness, voice changes, aphonia, dysphagia, dyspnea, wheezing, dizziness, recurrent rash, and/or swelling. Patients with bronchospasm should be continued on metered-dose beta-adrenergic bronchodilator inhalant therapy.

Hospital admission should be considered for patients who, in the course of the ED stay, show slow clinical improvement and have hypotension, upper airway involvement, and/or persistent bronchospasm. Patients who are at risk for a biphasic reaction such as those on chronic beta-blocker therapy also may be candidates for extended observation in the hospital.

Because most anaphylactic reactions that occur following parenteral drug administration begin within 30 minutes, patients should be held for observation in the ED during this period, discharged only if completely asymptomatic, and given a warning to return if there are subsequent symptoms.

BOX 102-7

Standard Pharmacologic Treatment Protocol for Patients with a History of Radiocontrast-Induced Anaphylaxis

- Prednisone, 50 mg PO given 13 hours, 7 hours, and 1 hour before procedure
- Diphenhydramine, 50 mg intramuscularly given 1 hour before procedure.
- Consider giving an H_2 antagonist, such as ranitidine, 300 mg PO gtt, 3 hours before procedure

Modified from Lieberman P: Anaphylaxis. Med Clin North Am 2006;90:77-95.

Human antiserum is now available for rabies, tetanus, and diphtheria; however, heterologous equine antisera is still used (e.g., for snake bites). Intradermal pretesting should be performed before treatment if time permits, following the instructions in the product monograph. It should be kept in mind that even pretesting solution can precipitate an anaphylactic reaction. Furthermore, unnecessary pretesting sensitizes predisposed patients to future hypersensitivity reactions to antiserum.

Predisposed patients who have experienced a moderate or severe anaphylactic reaction should be taught self-administration of an oral antihistamine (e.g., diphenhydramine) on known exposure, and self-injection of epinephrine (Epi-Pen Ana-Kit) at the first symptom or sign of an anaphylactic reaction. Epinephrine injection kits have a limited shelf life that is prolonged by refrigeration. These kits should be readily available to the patient at all times; preferably one kit available at home, one at work or school, one in patient's purse or briefcase, and one in the patient's automobile. Predisposed patients should be encouraged to wear a Medic-Alert bracelet or carry a wallet card identifying their hypersensitivity.

Pretreatment with antihistamines and steroids significantly decreases the frequency and severity of anaphylactoid reactions in patients who have sustained a previous reaction after injection of radiocontrast media. Each hospital has its own pre-treatment protocols for clinical procedures; Box 102-7 reproduces one such protocol.[20]

Skin testing and hyposensitization immunotherapy by an allergist are recommended to minimize the frequency and severity of subsequent anaphylactic reactions from bee stings in an appropriately sensitive population.

REFERENCES

1. Webb LM, Lieberman P: Anaphylaxis: A review of 601 cases. Ann Allergy Asthma Immunol 2006;97:39-43.
2. Settipane RA: Demographics and epidemiology of allergic and nonallergic rhinitis. Allergy Asthma Proc 2001;22: 185-189.

3. Weiss ST: Eat dirt—the hygiene hypothesis and allergic diseases. N Engl J Med 2002;347:930-931.
4. Bachert C, van Cauwenberge P, Khaltaev N: Allergic rhinitis and its impact on asthma. In collaboration with the World Health Organization. Executive summary of the workshop report. 7-10 December 1999, Geneva, Switzerland. Allergy 2002;57:841-855.
5. Owen CG, Shah A, Henshaw K, et al: Topical treatments for seasonal allergic conjunctivitis: Systematic review and meta-analysis of efficacy and effectiveness. Br J Gen Pract 2004;54:451-456.
6. Kaplan AP, Greaves MW: Angioedema. J Am Acad Dermatol 2005;53:373-388.
7. Dibbern DA Jr: Urticaria: Selected highlights and recent advances. Med Clin North Am 2006;90:187-209.
8. Malde B, Regalado J, Greenberger PA: Investigation of angioedema associated with the use of angiotensin-converting enzyme inhibitors and angiotensin receptor blockers. Ann Allergy Asthma Immunol 2007;98:57-63.
9. Ellis AK, Day JH: Clinical reactivity to insect stings. Curr Opin Allergy Clin Immunol 2005;5:349-354.
10. Fernandez J, Soriano V, Mayorga L, Mayor M: Natural history of Hymenoptera venom allergy in Eastern Spain. Clin Exp Allergy 2005;35:179-185.
11. Gomes ER, Demoly P: Epidemiology of hypersensitivity drug reactions. Curr Opin Allergy Clin Immunol 2005;5:309-316.
12. Bowrey DJ, Morris-Stiff GJ: Drug allergy: Fact or fiction? Int J Clin Pract 1998;52:20-21.
13. Asthma and the other allergic diseases. NIAID Task Force Report, NIH publ no. 79-387, 1979.
14. Kelkar PS, Li JTC: Cephalosporin allergy. N Engl J Med 2001;345:804-809.
15. Salkind AR, Cuddy PG, Foxworth JW: The rational clinical examination. Is this patient allergic to penicillin? An evidence-based analysis of the likelihood of penicillin allergy. JAMA 2001;285:2498-2505.
16. Simons FE, Peterson S, Black CD: Epinephrine dispensing patterns for an out-of-hospital population: A novel approach to studying the epidemiology of anaphylaxis. J Allergy Clin Immunol 2002;110:647-651.
17. Constantinides P: Infiltrates of activated mast cells at the site of coronary atheromatous erosion or rupture in myocardial infarction. Circulation 1995;92:1083.
18. Javeed N, Javeed H, Javeed S, et al: Refractory anaphylactoid shock potentiated by beta-blockers. Cathet Cardiovasc Diagn 1996;39:383-384.
19. Yocum MW, Klein JS: Emergency room incidence of community onset anaphylaxis. J Allergy Clin Immunol 1994;93:302.
20. Lieberman P: Anaphylaxis. Med Clin North Am 2006;90:77-95.

Chapter **103**

Arthritis and Inflammatory Joint and Synovial Disorders

Kathleen Schrank and Amy Zosel

KEY POINTS

Septic arthritis is an emergency and must be treated with parenteral antibiotics and possible surgical intervention.

Artificial joint, immunosuppression, fevers/chills, and recent infection are risk factors for septic joint.

Analysis of joint fluid may diagnose septic joint, crystalline disease, or hemorrhage. A white blood cell count higher than 50,000 mm^3 is suggestive of septic joint; however, lower counts do not rule out this diagnosis. If there is a high index of clinical suspicion for septic joint but nondiagnostic test results, the disorder should be treated as an infection.

Gout and pseudogout are crystal-induced arthritides that, although benign, may cause significant pain and morbidity. The patient's pain can be significantly improved with anesthetic and steroid injection after arthrocentesis.

A sexually active young adult with an inflamed, painful joint is considered to have gonococcal arthritis until proved otherwise and should be treated accordingly.

Early pain relief (medications, joint support, ice) should be provided in the ED, followed by more thorough reexamination of the joint after analgesia.

The whole patient, not just the joint, must be considered to better determine diagnosis and treatment.

It is important to distinguish whether joint pain is inflammatory (infection, chronic arthritides, crystalline disease) or noninflammatory (mechanical, traumatic) and to narrow the differential diagnosis as much as possible—a specific diagnosis may be impossible in only a single ED visit.

Scope

Arthritis afflicts hundreds of millions of persons worldwide—an estimated 20 million people in the United States have osteoarthritis, and 2 to 3 million have rheumatoid arthritis. The total cost of medical care, lost work time, and disability for osteoarthritis alone is estimated to run 2% of the gross national product.

Pathophysiology

In addition to bone, muscles, and joints, musculoskeletal pain may come from nerves, skin, or periarticular structures (ligaments, tendons, bursae). Diarthrodial joints are the most common type of joint, including all extremity and most axial joints. Their structure includes: synovium, synovial fluid, articular cartilage, intraarticular ligaments, joint capsule, and juxtaarticular subchondral bone (on both sides).

Arthrosis is a mechanical insult, whereas arthritis is synovial inflammation. Mechanical or metabolic disturbances may lead to an inflammatory response that can involve adjacent or contiguous structures, or an inflamed structure (such as a tendon) may rupture (Box 103-1). Inflammation consists of white blood cell infiltration, release of cytokines (e.g., tumor necrosis factor-alpha and interleukins) and other inflammatory mediators, and proliferation of cells or tissue. Edema collects around the joint, causing stiffness. With prolonged inflammation, eventually bony erosion and destruction of the joint may produce deformity and chronic disability.

BOX 103-1

Initial Causes of Joint Disorders

Mechanical
- Loss of articular surface
- Trauma
- Microfractures/remodeling/arthrosis
- Congenital dysplasias

Metabolic
- Crystal deposition
- Osteoporosis
- Inherited storage diseases (e.g., Gaucher's)
- Endocrinopathies (e.g., acromegaly, hyperparathyroidism)
- Metabolic bone disease (e.g., osteoporosis, Paget's)

Inflammatory
- Infection
- Immunologic response

Clinical Presentation

Clinical features of arthritides are listed in Table 103-1. Musculoskeletal pain is a common chief complaint among ED patients of all ages. Patients may also present with serious nonarticular complications of their disease or its treatment.The initial assessment

Table 103-1 CLINICAL FEATURES OF THE ARTHRITIDES

	Pain	Mono vs. Poly	Effusion	Skin	Fever	Other
Osteoarthritis	Long onset	Usually mono at first; often DIP or first CMC	Possibly	Possible swelling, no redness	No	Presence of osteophytes, morning stiffness (<1 hr)
Rheumatoid arthritis	Long onset (weeks to months)	Mono or poly; symmetric; often MCP, PIP, or wrist	Often	Swelling and redness	Possibly; low-grade	Rheumatoid nodules; possible friction rub or pleuritic rub; morning stiffness (>1 hr)
Septic joint	Quick onset	Mono; often knee		Swelling and redness	Yes; often high	May be toxic-appearing
Gout/crystalline-induced	Quick onset	Mono or oligo; often first MTP (podagra), knee	Often	Swelling +/− redness	Possibly; low-grade	Tophi
Systemic lupus erythematosus	Variable	Poly	Often	Swelling +/− redness	Possibly; low-grade	Butterfly/malar rash and oral lesions
Meniscal tear and/or ligament injury	Quick onset	Mono		Swelling	No	
Gonococcal arthritis	Migratory polyarthritis in acute phase (2-3 d); localizing phase (3-6 d)	Often migratory; mono symptoms in 25% of cases; poly symptoms in >60% of cases; wrists, hands, knees, elbows, shoulders, but any joint may be affected		Cervicitis and pustular lesions of skin Swelling +/− redness	Possibly; low-grade	Arthritis-dermatitis syndrome (60%); localized septic arthritis (40%)

CMC, carpometacarpal; DIP, distal interphalangeal joint; oligo, oligoarticular; mono, monoarticular; MTP, metatarsophalangeal joint; PIP, proximal interphalangeal; poly, polyarticular.

BOX 103-2

Key Historical Points

- What is the source and type of pain?
  - Muscle, nerve, skin, periarticular/articular structures, or joint?
  - Acute, chronic, or chronic with acute complication?
  - Monoarticular, oligoarticular (two or three joints), or polyarticular (more than three joints)?
- If polyarticular, is there a symmetric and/or migratory pattern?
- Exacerbating or alleviating factors? Limit activity?
- Fever/chills/recent infections?
- Evidence of inflammation?
- Prior diagnosis of arthritis or other diseases? How does this compare?
- Medications, especially thiazides (can increase serum uric acid), isoniazid, procainamide, and hydralazine (can precipitate lupus)?
- Personal history
  - Trauma?
  - Joint surgery? Prosthesis?
  - Joint instability or locking?
  - Repetitive use?
  - IV drug use?
  - What is the PQRST (*p*alliation/aggravation, *q*uality, *r*adiation, *s*everity, and *t*iming) of the pain?
- Family history of arthritis?
- Associated systemic symptoms (rash, eye complaints, fatigue, weight loss)?
- Brief or prolonged morning stiffness?
- Prior treatments? Results?
- Use of nontraditional remedies?

Documentation

- Document the presence/absence of:
  - Cardinal signs of inflammation (pain/tenderness, heat, erythema, swelling)
  - Functional impairment and ability to bear weight
  - Constitutional and systemic symptoms
  - Traumatic injury
  - Risk factors for joint space infection
  - Risk factors for adverse effect of planned treatment regimen
- Clearly identify specific anatomic site(s) of tenderness, swelling, erythema
- Assess and document:
  - Characteristics of pain (PQRST mnemonic*)
  - Full set of vital signs
  - Approximate range of motion of affected joint(s); level of activity
  - Witnessed functional impairment, weight bearing, and gait
  - Distal neurovascular status
  - Patient consent and procedure; note if arthrocentesis is performed
- Document specific discharge instructions:
  - Medications and potential serious side effects and/or drug interactions
  - Adjunctive measures as indicated (splinting, rest, ice, elevation)
  - Follow-up plan for any pending test results
  - Recommended follow-up visits
  - Need to bring all medications to follow-up visits
  - Potential reasons to return to ED for reassessment

*PQRST=*p*alliation/aggravation, *q*uality, *r*adiation, *s*everity, and *t*iming.

must first determine the anatomic site of the problem and then the general category of disease (e.g., inflammatory, noninflammatory, septic) (Box 103-2).

Mechanical pain is worse with use, relieved rapidly with rest, and often least severe in the morning. Inflammatory pain also is often worse with use but is not so quickly relieved with rest and may be associated with prolonged morning stiffness (longer than an hour). Stiffness in the morning is common in all patients with arthritis. This stiffness tends to be brief in patients with osteoarthritis and significant and prolonged in patients with rheumatoid arthritis. Widespread pain with morning stiffness typically is due to inflammatory arthritis or fibromyalgia. Subjective pain without joint findings on examination is arthralgia. "Gelling" (stiffness and immobility) after sitting in one position can have both inflammatory and noninflammatory causes. Rapid onset over minutes suggests trauma, internal derangement, or a loose fragment in the joint. If patients have tried medications without relief, how much they took, how often, and for how long should be determined (inadequate dosing is common).

The musculoskeletal examination attempts to identify the exact site of the problem—joint versus bone, muscle, periarticular, or superficial skin pain. True joint pain is diffuse with joint palpation and increases with active and passive motion. Periarticular inflammation (tendinitis, bursitis, cellulitis) usually is more focal, with pain being produced by only certain movements—most often resisted active contraction or passive stretching of involved muscles or tendons, and usually only toward one side.

During the examination:

- Look for erythema, wounds, and differences from the nonaffected side.
- Palpate for warmth, tenderness, crepitus, swelling, joint effusion, nodules, and synovial thickening.
- Check for limitation of range of motion (compare with nonaffected side or with examiner's range).

Table 103-2 **DIFFERENTIAL DIAGNOSES FOR ACUTE ARTHRITIS**

Nonarticular Disorders	Noninflammatory Joint Disorders	Inflammatory Joint Disorders
Abscess	Avascular necrosis of the hip	Amyloidosis
Bone tumor	Charcot/neuropathic arthropathy	Connective tissue diseases: systemic lupus erythematosus, scleroderma, Sjögren's syndrome, mixed connective tissue disease
Bursitis	Congenital hip dysplasia	Crystal deposition: gout, pseudogout
Cellulitis	Decompression sickness/bends	Drug reaction/serum sickness
Compartment syndrome	Hemarthrosis/hemophilic arthropathy	Erythema nodosum
Fibromyalgia/myofascial pain syndromes	Hemoglobinopathies	Familial Mediterranean fever
Inflammatory myopathies	Hypertrophic pulmonary osteoarthropathy	Foreign body reaction
Myalgia/myositis	Inherited storage diseases (e.g., Gaucher's)	Infection-related
Neuropathic pain	Liquid lipid microsphere disease	Juvenile rheumatoid arthritis and subtypes
Osteomyelitis	Malignancy	Multicentric histiocytosis
Polychondritis	Osteoarthrosis	Osteoarthritis/degenerative joint disease
Polymyalgia rheumatica	Osteochondritis dessicans	Palindromic rheumatism
Reflex sympathetic dystrophy	Osteochondroma	Polymyalgia rheumatica with joint involvement
Shoulder capsulitis	Osteonecrosis	Rheumatoid arthritis
Temporal arteritis	Pigmented villonodular synovitis	Sarcoidosis
Tendinitis/tenosynovitis	Slipped capital femoral epiphysis	Seronegative spondyloarthropathies
Trauma (ligament, tendon, muscle, bone)	Trauma	Vasculitides

- For lower extremity problems, check ability to rise from a chair and walk.
- If inflammation is present, look for other involved joints—a quick range of motion of major joints and palpation of finger joints only takes a minute, and identification of polyarticular arthritis is especially helpful in the differential diagnosis (Box 103-3).

Although pain usually is the main concern of patients with joint disease, it is important to determine if there are other associated symptoms that can aid in narrowing the differential diagnosis (Table 103-2).

Rheumatoid Arthritis

■ SCOPE

Rheumatoid arthritis is the most common inflammatory arthritis, afflicting about 0.8% of the world's population, and generally lacking ethnic or racial prevalence but with a 3:1 female predominance. It can begin at any age, but most commonly starts in the 40s.

Onset is typically insidious, although it sometimes can be abrupt. The usual time from onset to diagnosis is 6 to 12 months. Multiple joints are affected, usually with a symmetric pattern. Joint damage occurs early, with 30% of patients having bony erosions at the time of diagnosis. The inflammatory process usually responds well to disease-modifying treatment, but the damage already done is not reversible. The course is highly variable, with about 70% of patients experiencing chronic remitting disease, 10% to 20% developing disease with an aggressive, destructive pattern and severe disability, and a small group undergoing spontaneous and long-lasting remission.

BOX 103-3

Articular Diseases Associated with Joint Location

Monarticular
- Osteoarthritis
- Septic arthritis
- Gout
- Pseudogout
- Trauma
- Hemarthrosis

Polyarticular
- Rheumatoid arthritis
- Systemic lupus erythematosus
- Viral arthritis
- Rheumatic fever
- Reiter's syndrome
- Lyme disease
- Serum sickness
- Drug-induced

Periarticular
- Bursitis
- Tendinitis
- Cellulitis

■ PATHOPHYSIOLOGY

Rheumatoid arthritis is a systemic inflammatory autoimmune disease that primarily targets the synovium, transforming it into hyperplastic inflamed and thickened tissue that proliferates into a pannus.

BOX 103-4

1987 American College of Rheumatology Revised Criteria for the Classification of Rheumatoid Arthritis

A diagnosis of rheumatoid arthritis requires at least four of the following criteria:

- Morning stiffness in and around joints, lasting longer than 1 hour before maximal improvement*
- Arthritis of three or more joint areas at same time, with soft tissue swelling or joint fluid observed by physician*
- Arthritis of hand joints (at least one joint of wrist or metacarpophalangeal or distal phalangeal joint)*
- Symmetric arthritis*
- Rheumatoid nodules
- Serum rheumatoid factor
- Radiographic changes typical of rheumatoid arthritis on hand and wrist radiographs

*Must have been present for at least 6 weeks.

The pannus is unique to rheumatoid arthritis—the leading edge of synovium grows over the articular cartilage and erodes into bone, causing destruction and deformity.

The etiology remains unknown, although there is likely a combination of environmental factors plus genetic susceptibility, with several contributing genes, particularly the Class II major histocompatibility complex. An ongoing and uncontrollable immune response is elicited, perhaps against an autoantigen. Rheumatoid factors include immunoglobulin M (IgM) or IgG antibodies synthesized in the synovium that form immune complexes with IgG in the blood or joints.

■ CLINICAL PRESENTATION

Rheumatoid arthritis is characterized by symmetric polyarthritis persisting for more than 6 weeks, prolonged morning stiffness (>30 minutes), and systemic symptoms of fatigue, malaise, and weight loss. Diagnostic criteria are listed in Box 103-4.[1] Arthritis typically starts in the small joints of the hands (metacarpophalangeal and proximal interphalangeal) and feet and later affects larger extremity joints. Migratory polyarthralgias occur, and symptoms may wax and wane. Cervical spine involvement is prevalent, but the rest of the spine is usually spared. Rheumatoid arthritis increases the risk of a septic joint or tendon rupture. Temporomandibular joint problems are common.

In the early stages of the disease, there is usually tenderness, swelling, and limited range of motion of at least three joints, especially in the hands and feet. Warmth and erythema are uncommon. Distal interphalangeal joint involvement is very mild or absent. Palpation may reveal loss of normal contour across the joints (especially the metacarpophalangeals) from pannus.

Rheumatoid nodules are found in 20% of patients, appearing anywhere, but especially over bony prominences, pressure points, and tendon sheaths. The nodules may be fixed or mobile with a rubbery or granular texture; they may be indistinguishable from gouty tophi. They are not serious problems, unless they occur in the vocal cords or cardiac conduction tissue.

Typical later joint deformities are radial deviation at the wrist (usually the earliest deformity), ulnar deviation at the metacarpophalangeals (the most characteristic deformity of rheumatoid arthritis), swan neck or boutonniere deformities of the fingers, cock-up toes, loss of arches, and hallux valgus. There are many extraarticular manifestations. Acutely life-threatening complications, including complications of chronic treatment, are rare but disastrous (Box 103-5).

■ DIFFERENTIAL DIAGNOSIS

It is important to determine whether the patient's complaints are actually due to arthritis versus other musculoskeletal problems. Mechanical, inflammatory, or metabolic causes of arthritis must be considered (see Box 103-1). A new diagnosis of a specific type of inflammatory arthritis may not be possible in a single ED visit, but recognition that the case is inflammatory with findings suggestive of rheumatoid arthritis is important for interim care.

Identification of septic arthritis is the top priority, given its risk of rapid joint destruction or systemic infection. An infected joint is especially likely in patients with severely painful acute monoarticular arthritis, with or without fever. Patients with known rheumatoid arthritis are at significantly increased risk, and clinical findings may be subtle due to their drug regimens.

Signs and symptoms may overlap, but crystals found on arthrocentesis are diagnostic of crystal-induced arthritis. The recent addition of a medication that can cause hyperuricemia may be a clue, but serum uric acid levels alone do not make or rule out the diagnosis of gout. Often the patient has had multiple bouts of pain in the same joint, most commonly the great toe in gout.

Self-limited arthritic syndromes (e.g., viral infections or Lyme disease) can be difficult to distinguish clinically from the initial presentation of rheumatoid arthritis; thus the rheumatoid arthritis criteria include persistence of joint symptoms for longer than 6 weeks. The list of known inflammatory arthritides is long. Systemic vasculitides and lupus are the greatest threats, since they may rapidly cause multiorgan damage.

Careful history and examination, pattern of joint involvement, clinical course, associated signs and

BOX 103-5

Rheumatoid Arthritis: Extraarticular Manifestations and Complications*

- Anemia of chronic disease
- Cardiac
  - **Heart block** (rheumatoid nodules in or around atrioventricular node) and syncope
  - Myocarditis
  - Pericardial effusion (ranging from asymptomatic to **tamponade**)
  - Pericarditis (may be constrictive)
  - Premature atherosclerosis
  - Valvular insufficiency (any valve due to nodules; aortic insufficiency due to aortic root dilation)
- Cervical spine disease—atlantooccipital subluxation with myelopathy (major caution with endotracheal intubation!)
- Compression neuropathies (carpal tunnel, tarsal tunnel syndromes)
- Ear, nose, and throat
  - Episcleritis (mild irritation; not serious)
  - Scleritis (severe pain; if serious, may lead to perforation)
  - Sicca syndrome (corneal erosion or ulceration, oral thrush, dental caries)
  - Felty's syndrome (neutropenia and splenomegaly)
  - Osteopenia
- Pulmonary
  - Bronchiolitis obliterans
  - **Cricoarytenoid arthritis** (ranging from hoarseness to emergent airway compromise)
  - Interstitial lung disease
  - Parenchymal rheumatoid nodules
  - Pleural effusions (typically exudative with low glucose and complement)
  - Pleural inflammation or rheumatoid nodules
  - **Vocal cord nodules with airway compromise**
  - Raynaud's phenomenon
  - Rheumatoid nodules
  - Synovial cysts (popliteal Baker's cyst may rupture or occlude popliteal vein)
  - **Systemic vasculitis** (much more common in men than in women; mononeuritis multiplex with wrist or foot drop; sensory deficit; palpable purpura)
  - Septic joint
  - Temporomandibular joint subluxation
  - Tendon rupture

*Items shown in bold type may be imminently life-threatening.

symptoms, and judicious serologic testing combine to establish the exact diagnosis, generally in the outpatient follow-up setting.

Osteoarthritis is the most common diagnostic consideration; however, its pattern of joint involvement (especially in the hands) and minimal-to-absent systemic symptoms distinguish it from rheumatoid arthritis.

■ DIAGNOSTIC STUDIES

Blood tests are rarely diagnostic in synovial disorders but may be ordered to assist in management decisions. Useful studies include a complete blood count and basic chemistry profile to look for anemia, white blood cell count, and renal dysfunction (may affect use of nonsteroidal antiinflammatory drugs [NSAIDs]). Erythrocyte sedimentation rate (ESR) and C-reactive protein (CRP) are nonspecific but useful markers of inflammation. If clinical assessment raises concern about other autoimmune diseases, screening for multiorgan involvement with a urinalysis and liver enzymes should be performed. Coagulation studies are made prior to arthrocentesis only if a bleeding disorder is suspected. Rheumatoid arthritis typically produces a mild normochromic normocytic anemia and thrombocytosis, with normal white blood cells (unless there is infection or Felty's syndrome), an ESR of 30 to 60 mm/hour, and elevated CRP levels.

Plain radiographs are obtained if there is a high index of suspicion of fracture, foreign body, septic joint, or tumor. Radiograpy is useful in the diagnosis of rheumatoid diseases (Box 103-6), although findings may be negative early in the course of disease.

Rheumatoid arthritis characteristically produces joint space narrowing (especially in the metacarpophalangeals, proximal interphalangeals, and wrist), marginal bony erosions, periarticular osteopenia, and soft tissue swelling (Fig. 103-1). Late, progressive disease shows joint destruction (e.g., femoral head can protrude through the acetabulum).

Arthrocentesis is essential in cases of acute monoarthritis to identify joint infection, crystals, and hemarthrosis (indications and methods for arthrocentesis are discussed later in the section on septic arthritis, gout, and pseudogout). Rheumatoid arthritis fluid is inflammatory—cloudy yellow with low viscosity; 5 to 50,000 white blood cells per mm^3, with 50% to 75% polymorphonuclear leukocytes; glucose normal or mildly reduced. The white blood cell count may be elevated with no infection or low with infection (see later discussion).

Serologic testing (rheumatoid factor, possibly antinuclear antibody, other tests such as Lyme serology, depending on clinical suspicion) for new presentations is generally best done in the follow-up setting and is not needed in the ED for known cases. False-positive and false-negative results do occur, so results must always be interpreted in clinical context. Although 85% of patients develop positive rheumatoid factor titers (≥1:80) in the first year of their

BOX 103-6

SECONDS Mnemonic for Radiographic Evaluation of Arthritis[2]

Soft tissue swelling—Often seen in acute arthritides such as gout, pseudogout, and septic arthritis, as well as tubercular arthritis; also present in trauma.

Erosions—May be present in late rheumatoid arthritis; proliferating cells form a pannus and erode into the articular cartilage and bone.

Calcification—In late pseudogout; may be linear calcification in cartilage.

Osteoporosis—Sometimes present in late septic arthritis. Note that it takes about 8-10 days of septic arthritis before changes are evident on plain films. By this point, there has likely been severe joint destruction. Osteoporosis or periarticular bone may be seen in late rheumatoid arthritis but in NOT seen in pseudogout or osteoarthritis.

Narrowing of joint space—Present in late septic arthritis; asymmetric joint space narrowing is consistent with late pseudogout and osteoarthritis; symmetric joint space narrowing is consistent with late rheumatoid arthritis. Joint space typically is preserved in tubercular arthritis.

Deformity—In late septic arthritis, subchondral bone destruction and periosteal new bone may be visualized; in late pseudogout and osteoarthritis, changes may include sclerosis, osteophyte formation, and subchondral cyst formation.

Separation from fracture.

disease, unfortunately half are negative for the first 6 months, just when early intervention is most effective. Rheumatoid factor frequently is positive in other settings, such as subacute bacterial endocarditis and rheumatic fever, and is present in low titers in 20% of elderly patients without disease.

▪ TREATMENT AND DISPOSITION

ED care is focused on early relief of pain, typically with NSAIDs (e.g., ibuprofen, 800 mg orally), ice, and limb support in a position of comfort (usually partial flexion). If pain is severe or unrelieved by NSAIDs, tramadol or narcotic analgesics and immobilization of the joint may be effective.

The majority of patients are discharged home from the ED, unless they have a septic joint (requiring antibiotics and orthopedic consultation), other serious infection, or a significant complication (e.g., new vasculitis, myelopathy, heart block, hypoxic lung involvement). Immunosuppressed patients

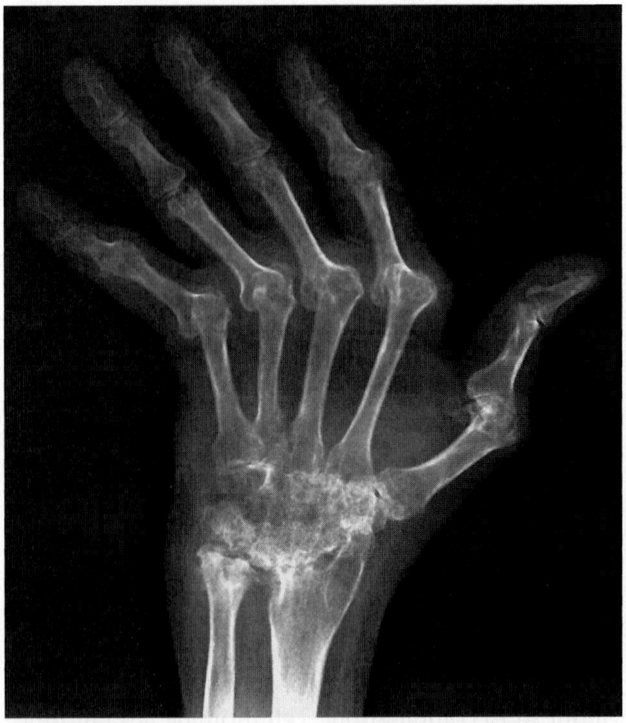

FIGURE 103-1 Ulnar deviation in rheumatoid arthritis. Severe ulnar deviation with extensive erosions is present at the metacarpophalangeal joints. Pancompartmental bony ankylosis and erosion are also seen in the wrist. (From Harris E [ed]: Kelley's Textbook of Rheumatology, 7th ed. Philadelphia, Saunders, 2005.)

warrant a high index of suspicion for infection. Follow-up visits with either a primary care physician or rheumatologist (if new diagnosis or if chronic rheumatoid arthritis is not responding to treatment) are essential. Chronic severe joint dysfunction merits orthopedic referral for potential surgical intervention. Joint replacement of hips or knees has been very effective in reducing pain and disability, and so have artificial joints or arthrodesis in the hands and synovectomy in the knees and wrists.

NSAIDs are the mainstay of initial symptomatic treatment, although these drugs do not modify the course of the disease. Choice of NSAID is based on low cost and safety profile; a high dose (e.g., ibuprofen 800 mg, three times a day) is administered for a minimum 2-week trial. Nonresponders may be switched to a different NSAID, often with good results. The patient should be instructed to take the medication with food, especially if there is any stomach upset; an alternative is co-treatment with an H_2 blocker or a proton pump inhibitor. Celecoxib has less risk of gastrointestinal bleeding, but concern regarding cardiovascular complications has limited its prolonged use. Concomitant use of acetaminophen or tramadol is often helpful, or these may be used when NSAIDs are contraindicated (gastrointestinal bleeding, renal failure). Judicious use of narcotic analgesics is also appropriate.

Low-dose corticosteroids (prednisone, 5-10 mg daily) are often helpful for rapid symptom relief, but usually are initiated by the primary care physician, and they can be very difficult to taper off in the future. In patients with rheumatoid arthritis, corticosteroids are usually superimposed on other treatment regimens. Prednisone may be considered for patients who have had an adequate trial with more than one NSAID and other general measures, but who remain unable to handle self-care, activities of daily living, or a normal work schedule. If the patient has only one or two very problematic joints that are clearly NOT infected, intraarticular corticosteroids (triamcinolone hexacetonide, ranging from 5 mg in a finger joint to 40 mg in large joint) can produce rapid improvement lasting for several months; they usually are prescribed by the physician providing ongoing care, but they may be given in the ED.

Disease-modifying anti-rheumatic drugs (DMARDs) are essential to prevent joint damage, and combinations are now initiated as early as possible after diagnosis. However, these are appropriately started in a continuity care setting, not in the ED. Many DMARDs with varying efficacy and safety profiles are available, and new agents have dramatically improved care in recent years. The mainstay remains methotrexate, alone or in combination.[3] Leflunomide (an immunomodulatory drug) and sulfasalazine are alternatives. Exciting new and effective agents include the tumor necrosis factor antagonists (e.g., etanercept) and an interleukin-1 receptor antagonist (anakinra). The latter have a rapid onset of action and appear to particularly helpful in stopping early disease progression.[4] Abatacept, an inhibitor of T cell stimulation, is another option.

General treatment measures (ice and/or heat, temporary support with elastic bandage or brace, cane or walker) should be considered, but unnecessary immobilization should be avoided. Appropriate life style recommendations for patients with rheumatoid arthritis are to stay as active as possible with daily activities and exercise programs. Physical and occupational therapy may contribute greatly to improved quality of life and ability to maintain independence in self-care. Initial range of motion and later strengthening and aerobic exercise regimens are recommended; swimming pool exercise programs are quite helpful (Box 103-7).

RED FLAGS

- Severely painful acute monoarticular arthritis, with or without fever, is highly likely to be a septic joint.
- Acute monoarticular arthritis in a sexually active young adult is considered gonococcal arthritis until proved otherwise.
- Overlying soft tissue infection may preclude arthrocentesis, or warrant a different approach.
- Acute problems in a prosthetic joint merit immediate discussion with an orthopedic surgeon.
- Syncope may be a warning of high risk of sudden cardiac death in patients with systemic inflammatory diseases.
- Cervical spine disease is common with rheumatoid arthritis and osteoarthritis, and must be considered prior to any endotracheal intubation attempt using forced flexion.
- Serious complications of arthritides are rare, but may be life- or limb-threatening:
    - Acute airway compromise may occur with rheumatoid arthritis—this represents a difficult airway!
    - Cervical spine subluxation and myelopathy
    - Vasculitis
    - Syncope and heart block
    - Hypoxic lung disease
    - Septic joint
- Patients may present with serious complications from their chronic treatment:
    - Gastrointestinal bleeding from nonsteroidal antiinflammatory drugs (NSAIDs)
    - Hyperglycemia/hyperosmolar states from corticosteroid-induced hyperglycemia
    - Bacterial or tubercular infections from immunosuppressive therapy

Osteoarthritis

SCOPE

Osteoarthritis is the most common cause of joint pain worldwide and frequently leads to chronic pain and disability. In the United States, symptomatic knee osteoarthritis occurs in 6% of persons over age 30, and hip osteoarthritis in 3%. About one third of adults aged 25 to 74 years have radiographic evidence of osteoarthritis in at least one joint group, most commonly the hands, followed by the feet and knees.

Prevalence increases considerably with age, and osteoarthritis is a major cause of disability, lost work time, and early retirement. Before age 50, prevalence in most joints is higher in men, but at older ages, women are more often affected by osteoarthritis in the hands, feet, and knees. Hip osteoarthritis is more prevalent in men than in women at all ages. Although there appear to be some ethnic differences, data are conflicting.[5]

Other risk factors include obesity, trauma, family history of osteoarthritis, and occupations requiring repetitive knee/hip bending and lifting (e.g., farmers, dockworkers, some athletes). The role of aggressive avocational exercise remains unclear, although moderate running appears to be a low-risk activity. High-intensity contact sports and those with repetitive joint impact and twisting are higher-risk categories.

PATHOPHYSIOLOGY

Osteoarthritis is a disease of articular cartilage and subchondral bone, characterized by patchy loss of

BOX 103-7

General Treatment Measures for Chronic Arthritis

Patient Education
- Nature and usual course of disease
- Exacerbating and relieving factors
- Avoidance of repetitive injuries/impacts
- Arthritis self-help course available from the Arthritis Foundation (www.arthritis.org)

Painful Joint
- Analgesics (take bedtime dose if early morning pain)
- Acute exacerbations:
  - Rest, ice, compression, elevation
  - Temporary limitation of range of motion and forceful use
- Correction of misalignment—joint sleeve or brace, orthotics
- Chronic pain—trials with ice, heat, in-water therapy
- Unloading joint stress with cane or crutch (contralateral to affected leg)

Physical Therapy
- Relief of pain and muscle spasm (massage, heat, ultrasonography, electrical stimulation therapy, physical maneuvers)
- Improvement in and preservation of range of motion
- Strengthening (general or surrounding specific joint)
- Progressive individualized exercise regimen
- General conditioning

Occupational Therapy
- Improved activities of daily living
- Assist devices
- Temporary splinting
- Protective techniques
- Energy conservation skills

Life Style
- Weight loss program
- Adequate nutrition and calcium intake
- Range of motion preservation
- Exercise program with low impact aerobic conditioning
- Evaluation of home for fall prevention, improved functionality
- Well-cushioned shoes or orthotics

Acupuncture
- Role unclear; efficacy not well supported by available evidence; appears beneficial for knee pain

Glucosamine/Chondroitin
- Role unclear; efficacy not well-supported by available evidence

cartilage, overgrowth of bone at the joint margins (osteophytes are hallmarks of osteoarthritis), hypertrophy of subchondral bone, fibrosis in the joint capsule, loss of joint space, and mild inflammation of the synovium. Loss of cartilage allows the underlying bones to rub together, producing pain, swelling, and limited range of motion. The primary process is mechanical, not inflammatory, but past views of osteoarthritis as being entirely mechanical (hence names used in the past such as degenerative joint disease and osteoarthrosis) are inaccurate. Recent evidence has found considerably more synovial inflammation than was previously considered. Local mechanical factors (malalignment, laxity, proprioception) do contribute to development and progression of osteoarthritis, but the pathogenesis likely involves not only chronic mechanical microdamage but also disturbed chondrocyte regulation of the the synthesis and degradation of matrix, genetic factors, and inflammatory pathways.

Most cases of osteoarthritis are classified as idiopathic or primary. Secondary osteoarthritis may result from congenital or developmental diseases, trauma, deposition disorders (calcium, hemochromatosis), neuropathic arthropathy, or endocrinopathies (acromegaly, hyperparathyroidism).

■ CLINICAL PRESENTATION

Osteoarthritis most commonly affects the knees, hips, spine, fingers (especially the distal interphalangeal joints and first carpometacarpal joint) and toes (especially the metatarsophalangeal joints). Patients typically complain of gradual onset of pain and stiffness in one or a few joints, with limited range of motion. Locking or instability of the knee is common. Pain is usually moderate, worse with use, and rapidly better with rest. Commonly, symptoms are worse in damp, cool weather. Systemic symptoms are minimal or absent.

On examination, disease is limited to the symptomatic joints. Joint tenderness, bony enlargement, and crepitus on joint motion are common findings. Heberden's nodes, which are hard nodules on the dorsal aspects of distal interphalangeal joints, are commonly found in older women with osteoarthritis. Malalignment is found in about half of knees with osteoarthritis, typically with a varus (bow leg) deformity and often with instability upon excess range of motion. Patients are prone to coexisting pseudogout in the knee, or they may develop gout. Joints may be mildly warm, especially if there is an effusion, but not dramatically inflamed. Late in the disease course, significant joint disability is evident.

■ DIAGNOSTIC STUDIES

Laboratory studies are not generally needed, but if ordered, results usually are normal. Joint fluid is usually noninflammatory, with white blood cell counts greater than 2000 per mm^3; inflammatory joint fluid suggests gout or infection.

Radiologic results must be applied in context with the clinical picture. In asymptomatic patients over age 40, radiographic studies often show degenerative changes in the joints; thus a label of osteoarthritis would be misapplied in those patients. Classic changes from osteoarthritis are degenerative, with marginal osteophyte formation, subchondral bony sclerosis, and asymmetric joint space narrowing (Fig. 103-2). Later, subchondral cysts form with sclerotic walls, and bone remodeling distorts the bone ends. Bony demineralization and marginal erosions suggest an inflammatory arthritis, such as rheumatoid arthritis.

■ TREATMENT AND DISPOSITION

Initiate pain relief in the ED with analgesics, ice pack, and support in a position of comfort. Acetaminophen (1 g orally) or ibuprofen (600-800 mg orally) may be adequate. If the patient has already adequately tried and failed to get relief with these medications, consider tramadol or narcotic analgesics.

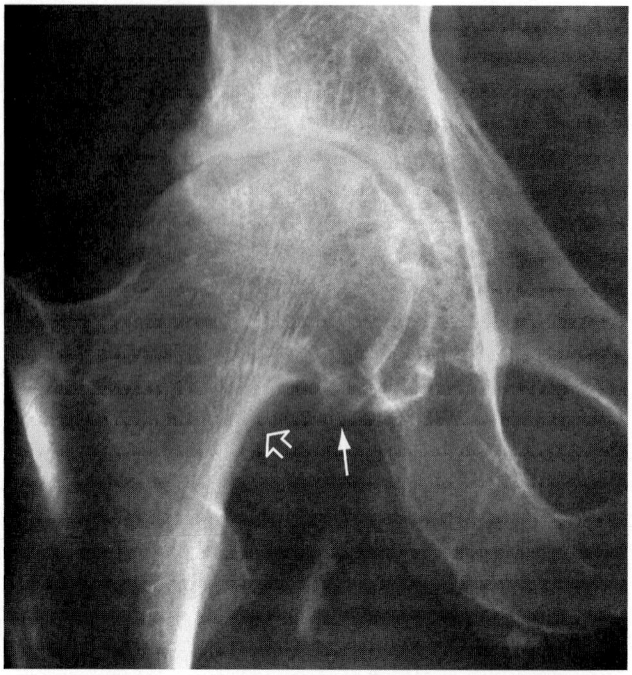

FIGURE 103-2 Osteoarthritis of the hip. This anteroposterior view of the hip shows complete cartilage space loss superiorly. There is osteophytic lipping from the femoral head, especially medially *(arrow)*, and buttressing bone *(open arrow)* is present along the femoral neck. (From Harris E [ed]: Kelley's Textbook of Rheumatology, 7th ed. Philadelphia, Saunders, 2005.)

The vast majority of patients are discharged home from the ED with primary care follow-up recommendations. Those with known or strongly suspected joint infection need admission. Chronic severe joint pain with disability merits orthopedic referral.

Several options are available for discharge analgesia, although patients with mild osteoarthritis may need only general care measures. Acetaminophen (650 mg to 1 g four times a day) or NSAIDs (e.g., ibuprofen, 600-800 mg three times a day) are first-line choices. In some studies, both were effective in reducing pain, although NSAIDs or celecoxib were modestly better. However, acetaminophen has less risk of side effects, so is usually the first choice. Topical capsaicin (thin film of 0.025% cream applied four times a day) or NSAIDs were also helpful, although not as effective as oral agents; maximal benefit took 3 to 4 weeks.[6] Effective additions or alternatives included tramadol or short-term use of oxycodone. Glucosamine sulfate (1500 mg/day) and chondroitin sulfate (1200 mg/day) were reported to shift cartilage metabolism toward a positive balance and are widely used, but overall evidence to date shows limited efficacy[7,8]; these are over-the-counter preparations that may vary considerably in composition. Of note, placebo arms of several trials showed high response rates.

Intraarticular corticosteroids are also effective, especially in the knee and the thumb metacarpophalangeal joint, with pain relief lasting 1 to 4 weeks in some studies. Because repeated use raises concern over cartilage damage, use in same joint is limited to every 3 to 4 months. Intraarticular hyaluronic acid injections have been used in the knee, but efficacy was limited.[9]

General care measures and patient education are important.[10] Evidence supports the benefit of exercise regimens and weight loss in knee arthritis. Correction of malignment of the knee with a neoprene sleeve, valgus brace, and/or orthotics is beneficial. Evidence of the benefits of acupuncture is limited and mixed. Physical and occupation therapy are helpful in patients with limiting disability.

Surgical interventions are useful in selected situations: Knee arthroscopy is beneficial if cartilage flaps, loose bodies, or meniscal disruption cause mechanical locking or instability or if recurrent pseudogout occurs. Total joint replacement for knee or hip osteoarthritis often dramatically improves severe refractory pain and disability, particularly if the patient has a relatively low body mass index. Chondrocyte transplantation is a promising intervention for future care.

Reiter's Syndrome and Reactive Arthritis

■ SCOPE

Reiter's syndrome and reactive arthritis are seronegative spondyloarthropathies that are much less common than osteoarthritis and rheumatoid arthritis; however, identification is important to guide management. Most are self-limited illnesses, but a minority of patients (particularly those with AIDS), develop persistent and severe disease. Prevalence parallels that of human leukocyte antigen (HLA) B27 genes in different populations. In the United States, 6% to 14% of Caucasians have HLA B27, as do 2% to 3% of blacks. The peak onset of Reiter's syndrome is during the third decade of life, but cases have occurred in children and in octogenarians. There is a 5:1 to 6:1 male predominance, but cases in women may be underdiagnosed—women tend to have milder symptoms, and the genitourinary manifestations may be occult. Incidence is estimated at 3 to 6 cases per year per 100,000 males less than age 50 years.

Inflammation of the entheses, eyes, and mucosal surfaces are distinctive features of reactive arthritis. The illness tends to be self-limited over several months, but relapses occur in about one third of patients. Persistent symptoms develop in 10% to 20% of patients with Reiter's syndrome.

■ PATHOPHYSIOLOGY

Reiter's syndrome consists of the classic triad of acute peripheral arthritis (asymmetric, oligoarticular, additive), conjunctivitis (mild, usually several days before joint pain), and nongonococcal urethritis and/or cervicitis (usually mild, precedes joint pain). It is a subset of the larger group of reactive arthritides, in which a sterile inflammatory arthropathy arises within a month of a primary infection elsewhere in the body. Most patients with reactive arthritis do not manifest the full Reiter's syndrome triad, but the pathophysiology is the same. Other seronegative spondyloarthropathies have a more severe axial component, such as sacroiliitis in ankylosing spondylitis.[11]

Onset typically occurs 1 to 4 weeks after the triggering infectious illness, such as a gastrointestinal or genitourinary infection, is resolved. Enteric pathogens include *Shigella, Yersinia, Salmonella,* and *Campylobacter* (e.g., *C. difficile*). Sexually transmitted pathogens include *Chlamydia* (mainly *C. trachomata*), *Ureaplasma urealyticum,* and human immunodeficiency virus (HIV). Presumably, microbial material or products are disseminated to the joints and extraarticular structures, triggering an inflammatory response with mononuclear infiltration (helper T cells and macrophages) into the joints and entheses, synovial effusions, and inflammatory mediators. Most patients carry HLA B27. In many, the inciting infection is not identifiable. HIV-associated reactive arthritis does not usually manifest as the full Reiter's syndrome but tends to be a more aggressive, severe joint disease with poor response to anti-inflammatory drugs.

■ CLINICAL PRESENTATION

ED presentations of reactive arthritis are likely to be new diagnoses. Typically, the patient reports one or several sites of acute joint pain, often asymmetric and with sequential onset (Box 103-8). Common sites include large joints (one or both ankles, wrists, knees) and small joints in the feet; upper extremities may be involved later. Fever (up to 102.2°F [39°C]), constitutional symptoms (fatigue, malaise, weight loss), and eye problems are common symptoms. Recent diarrhea or genitourinary infections may have been the inciting event, as well as more recent conjunctivitis and genitourinary symptoms from the immune response. Low back pain, back stiffness, or sacroiliac joint pain occurs in half the patients.

Later complications can include uveitis, cardiac involvement (in about 10% of patients) with conduction blocks, nonspecific ST-segment changes, Q waves, and aortic regurgitation.

■ DIFFERENTIAL DIAGNOSIS

With an acute hot joint, infection (especially gonococcal) must be ruled out. Active infection elsewhere (especially the gastrointestinal and genitourinary tracts) must also be considered. Reactive arthritis and Reiter's syndrome should be distinguished from seronegative rheumatoid arthritis, crystal-induced arthritis, sarcoidosis, acute rheumatic fever, psoriatic arthritis, and erythema nodosum. A carefully constructed clinical picture will usually distinguish reac-

BOX 103-8

Classic Signs of Reiter's Syndrome

- Enthesitis—periarticular, classically Achilles or plantar tendinitis
- Peripheral arthritis pattern—may be a hot erythematous joint when active infection must be ruled out; often asymmetric oligoarthritis
- Dactylitis—"sausage digits"
- Conjunctivitis—bilateral or unilateral, usually painful
- Urethritis/cervicitis
- Circinate balanitis on shaft or glans of penis; vulvitis in women—ranging from vesicles to ulcerations
- Keratoderma blenorrhagicum—painless papulosquamous rash on palms and soles, similar to pustular psoriasis
- Oral ulcerations—painless

Tips and Tricks

ED EVALUATION AND MANAGEMENT

- Improve assessment by:
  - Careful examination to distinguish joint involvement from periarticular or other sources
  - Determination of both active and passive range of motion
  - Repeat, more aggressive examination of joint after analgesia and review of radiographs
- Improve acute pain relief by:
  - Starting with maximal dose of selected analgesic drug
  - Supporting joint in position of comfort (usually partial flexion)
  - Ice pack application
  - Reassessing patient for adequacy of response to analgesic
  - Assuring timely continuing doses of analgesics as needed
- Although short-term (1-2 days) immobilization of an acutely painful joint is often beneficial in chronic arthritis, longer immobilization should be avoided; progressive exercise optimizes functional recovery.
- If there is a high index of clinical suspicion of joint infection, treat as infection even if fluid results are nondiagnostic

tive arthritis, but this may not be easily done on a single ED visit.

■ DIAGNOSTIC STUDIES

Given the frequent presentation with fever, acute arthritis, and involvement of mucosal surfaces, laboratory studies are appropriate (complete blood count and chemistries, liver enzymes, urinalysis, ESR, arthrocentesis, joint fluid cultures, and usually blood cultures). In Reiter's syndrome, there usually is a modest increase in white blood cells, platelets, and ESR. Mild anemia is common. Active urethral or gastrointestinal infection should be considered and tests for *Chlamydia* and gonorrhea are appropriate if there are recent genitourinary symptoms. If the precipitating infection was dysenteric, stool cultures should be obtained. Serologic testing and HLA typing are not needed in the ED.

■ TREATMENT AND DISPOSITION

Full-dose NSAIDs are the mainstay of therapy in reactive arthritis—a good response is typical. General care measures are also appropriate (see the section on osteoarthritis), especially encouragement of continuing exercise. Systemic corticosteroid therapy generally is not indicated, but intraarticular glucocorticoids may help in cases with persistently problematic joints after ruling out infection. Second-line medications for nonresponders include sulfasalazine and methotrexate. Experience with anti–tumor necrosis factor agents is limited but promising.

Antibiotic treatment for *Chlamydia* infection is appropriate if the initial infection was untreated or is found on testing. An empirical antibiotic for patients with a prior history of gastrointestinal infection is not useful unless current stool cultures show persistence of a pathogenic trigger for Reiter's syndrome.

Many of these patients can be discharged home from the ED with primary care follow-up, but admission is indicated if the patient is febrile or if active joint infection is likely. Referral to ophthalmology services is advised if uveitis is suspected.

Septic Arthritis, Gout, And Pseudogout

■ SCOPE

The incidence of septic arthritis varies between 2 and 5 per 100,000 per year in the general population, 5 and 12 per 100,000 per year in children, 28 and 38 per 100,000 per year in patients with rheumatoid arthritis, and 40 and 68 per 100,000 per year in patients with joint prostheses. Septic arthritis occurs in all age groups but is more common in children than in adults. Males are usually affected more commonly than females, although in patients with underlying rheumatoid arthritis, females are affected more often.

The organisms causing bacterial arthritis depend on the epidemiologic circumstances. For example, monoarthritis of a prosthetic joint in an elderly man is likely due to *Staphylococcus* species, whereas a migratory arthritis in a sexually active woman with skin lesions is likely due to disseminated gonococcal infection.

Risk factors for the development of septic arthritis include age older than 60 years, diabetes mellitus, immunodeficiency states, preexistent joint damage (particularly rheumatoid arthritis), skin infection, intravenous drug use, debilitating conditions, hemoglobinopathy, and joint prostheses.

Risk factors for septic arthritis include older age, diabetes mellitus, rheumatoid arthritis, immunodeficiency, and preexisting joint disease.[12] The most common site is the knee, followed by the hip and shoulder, with more than 10% having polyarticular involvement (>50% of polyarticular forms occur in patients with rheumatoid arthritis).

The incidence of gout ranges from 1% to 15% of the general population. The incidence increases with age and with increases in serum urate. In adults, serum urate levels correlate strongly with serum creatinine and urea nitrogen levels, body weight, height, age, blood pressure, and alcohol intake. In epidemiologic studies, body bulk has proved to be one of the most important predictors of hyperuricemia in people of widely differing races and cultures, with rare exceptions. Radiography and autopsy studies have found the incidence of pseudogout to be 15% at age 65 and 50% at age 85.

■ PATHOPHYSIOLOGY

Bacteria can cause infection in the joint via hematogenous spread and direct inoculation (arthrocentesis, trauma, surgery) or through contiguous contact (cellulitis, bursitis, tenosynovitis). Any microorganisms, including bacteria, fungi, viruses, and protozoa, may invade joints; however, the overwhelming majority of cases (90%) are caused by the pyogenic bacteria *Staphylococcus* and *Streptococcus*.[13] Once the microbial agent penetrates the joint space, it initiates a series of inflammatory reactions that may lead to joint destruction and permanent joint damage. Microorganisms and/or their products activate the release of proinflammatory cytokines, such as tumor necrosis factor-alpha and interleukin-1, and proteolytic enzymes, such as metalloproteinases and other collagen-degrading enzymes. These substances may induce synovial membrane proliferation, granulation tissue, neovascularization, and infiltration by polymorphonuclear cells and may result, if untreated, in cartilage and bone destruction. The articular damage may progress even after eradication of microorganisms by antibiotic therapy because persistence of bacterial antigens and metalloproteinases within the joint will continue to promote an inflammatory response.

Tophi commonly develop in osteoarthritic interphalangeal joints, suggesting roles of connective tissue matrix structure and turnover in urate crystal deposition. The predilection for marked urate crystal deposition in the first metatarsophalangeal joint may be related to repetitive minor trauma at that site. Microscopic tophaceous deposits of urate crystals are often present in the synovial membrane at the time of the first gouty attack and may also be detected within cartilage. Abrupt increases and decreases in serum urate levels—as stimulated by diuretics or alcohol use and with initiation of therapy with antihyperuricemic drugs—may promote release of urate crystals from tophi via changes in packing of crystals in tophaceous deposits. Free urate crystals have considerable proinflammatory potential because of their ability to activate synovial lining cells and leukocytes and to trigger multiple inflammatory cascades. In some individuals with gout, urate crystals can be found in asymptomatic metatarsophalangeal and knee joints that have never been involved in an acute attack or are present in noninflamed joints between acute attacks of gout at those sites. These findings reinforce the theory that urate deposition in tissues is asymptomatic.

The ingress of neutrophils into the joint is central in triggering acute gouty arthritis, and effects on neutrophil-endothelial cell interactions likely represent a major locus for the prophylactic and therapeutic effects of colchicine. IL-8 (interleukin-8) and closely related chemokines that bind the IL-8 receptor CXCR2 (including GRO-alpha) appear to be critical in initiating and perpetuating neutrophil ingress in acute gouty inflammation.

The acute gouty attack often is spontaneously self-limited to 7 to 10 days, likely mediated by an altered balance between proinflammatory and antiinflammatory mediators in the joint. Low-grade synovitis may persist in affected joints. Inflammatory mechanisms in gout, especially in untreated disease, can lead to chronic synovial proliferation, cartilage loss, and bone erosion.

Calcium-containing crystals deposited in the pericellular matrix of cartilage are often in the form of calcium pyrophosphate dihydrate, a disorder termed *chondrocalcinosis pyrophosphate arthropathy* and, when associated with acute arthritis, *pseudogout*.

■ CLINICAL PRESENTATION

Septic arthritis, gout, and pseudogout are forms of arthritis that often present acutely. Symptoms include joint pain, swelling, erythema, pain, and tenderness. In general, a septic joint will be redder and warmer and a gouty joint will have more fluid. Septic arthritis is usually monoarticular, but some patients can have polyarticular involvement. Classically, gout affects the first metatarsophalangeal joints. The knee is commonly the joint affected in septic arthritis, gout, and pseudogout. Severe pain with range of motion of the joint is common in septic arthritis, although pain with range of motion is also common with gout and pseudogout. Whereas low-grade fever is common with many types of inflammatory arthritis, high

Table 103-3 ADVANTAGES AND DISADVANTAGES OF LABORATORY STUDIES IN JOINT DISEASE

Lab Test	Advantage	Disadvantage
Complete blood count	Fast; white blood cell count may be elevated due to infection (only 48% in septic arthritis); patients with chronic rheumatic diseases may have associated anemia	Not specific
Erythrocyte sedimentation rate (ESR)	Inexpensive; monitoring ESR reported to be diagnostic and useful for monitoring of temporal arteritis and polymyalgia rheumatica[17]	Not specific; must be run within 2 hr of collection; increased in infections, inflammatory diseases, neoplasms, and anemias; by itself is not diagnostic of any particular disease[17]
C-reactive protein	Inexpensive; marker of inflammation	Not specific
Others (rheumatoid factor, complement levels, antinuclear antibody, Lyme serologies)	May be helpful in making final diagnosis	Unlikely to be completed during single ED visit

BOX 103-9

Classic Joint Involvement in Arthritides

- First metatarsophalangeal joint: Gout
- Metatarsophalangeal, metacarpophalangeal, proximal interphalangeal, and tarsometatarsal joints; cervical spine: Rheumatoid arthritis
- Distal interphalangeal, proximal interphalangeal, and first carpometacarpal joints; knee, hip, cervical spine, and umbosacral spine: Osteoarthritis
- Knee: Septic arthritis, pseudogout, gout, osteoarthritis

fevers and chills are more commonly associated with a septic joint. As presentations for these entities are very similar, it is necessary to rule out a septic joint with joint fluid analysis.

■ DIFFERENTIAL DIAGNOSIS

The differential diagnosis for septic arthritis, gout, and pseudogout is broad (Box 103-9). Because septic arthritis has the most serious potential for morbidity and mortality, it is important to keep the possibility in the forefront of one's mind when doing a working-up of acute arthritis. A history of gout makes a recurrent gout attack more likely. However, patients with gout are more susceptible to septic arthritis. Gouty arthritis may present in a polyarticular fashion, whereas septic arthritis is usually limited to a single joint. The differential diagnosis is similar that for rheumatoid arthritis and osteoarthritis.

■ DIAGNOSTIC STUDIES

Laboratory studies commonly used in the diagnosis of joint disorders are compared in Table 103-3. Arthrocentesis is an important diagnostic methodology for joint disease, and it can be therapeutic. It is the only reliable means to rule out a septic joint. (Table 103-4; also see Tips and Tricks: Joint Fluid Collection box). Possible complications of arthrocentesis include introducing infection into the joint space, causing hemarthrosis, and allergic or adverse reactions to medications injected (Box 103-10).

Normal synovial fluid is clear in appearance. In degenerative joint disease, the fluid itself is normal and thus remains clear. Bloody fluid suggests hemarthrosis. Fat droplets may suggest traumatic arthritis. Turbid fluid is observed in gout, pseudogout, and septic arthritis, as well as in rheumatoid and seronegative arthritides.

Crystal analysis is performed under polarizing microscopy. In patients with gout, monosodium urate crystals are present in the joint fluid of the affected joint. Crystals typically are needle-shaped, appearing yellow when parallel to the compensator. They are considered to be negatively birefringent. In pseudogout, on the other had, the crystals are positively birefringent, blue when parallel to the compensator, and usually rhomboid-shaped.

Glucose may be decreased compared with serum glucose in severe inflammatory disorders, including both septic joint and other inflammatory arthritides. Joint fluid glucose may be less than 50% of the serum glucose in septic arthritis and 50% to 75% of the serum glucose in rheumatoid and seronegative arthritides. However, evidence suggests that chemistry studies of synovial fluid should be discouraged because they are likely to provide misleading or redundant information.[15]

Viscosity can be measured grossly in the laboratory or by the person collecting the sample. Inflammation of the joint causes a decrease in the hyaluronate portion of the synovial fluid; thus viscosity decreases. Normal synovial fluid when dropped from a syringe makes a 5- to 10-cm string of fluid before dropping. If viscosity is decreased in the setting of inflammation, the string of fluid will be shorter or the fluid may simply form droplets.

According to a published study, although several emergency medicine texts indicate that a joint white blood cell count greater than 50,000 cells/mm^3 is

Table 103-4 JOINT FLUID ANALYSIS OF THE VARIOUS ARTHRITIDES[19]

Diagnosis	Appearance	WBCs/mm³	PMN Leukocytes	Glucose (% Blood Level)	Crystals under Polarized Light	Culture
Normal	Clear	<200	<25	95-100	None	Negative
Degenerative joint disease	Clear	<4000	<25	95-100	None	Negative
Traumatic arthritis	Straw-colored, bloody, xanthochomic, occasionally with fat droplets	<4000	<25	95-100	None	Negative
Acute gout	Turbid	2000-50,000	>75	80-100	Negative birefringence; needle-like crystals	Negative
Pseudogout	Turbid	2000-50,000	>75	80-100	Positive birefringence; rhomboid crystals	Negative
Septic arthritis	Turbid/purulent	5000 to >50,000	>75	<50	None	Usually positive
Rheumatoid arthritis/ seronegative arthritis	Turbid	2000-50,000	50-75	≈75	None	Negative

PMN, polymorphonuclear; WBCs, white blood cells.

BOX 103-10

Arthrocentesis: Indications and Contraindications

Indications

- Suspected septic arthritis
- Diagnosis of nontraumatic joint disease by synovial fluid analysis
- Diagnosis of ligamentous or bony injury by confirmation of blood in the joint
- Establishment of the existence of an intraarticular fracture by the presence of blood with fat globules in the joint
- Relief of pain of an acute hemarthrosis or a tense effusion.
- Local instillation of medications in acute and chronic inflammatory arthritides
- Obtaining fluid for analysis (culture, cell count, crystal studies)

Contraindications (Relative)

- Infection in tissue overlying the site to be punctured.
- Presence of bacteremia
- Coagulopathy
- Joint prosthesis
- Uncooperative patient

"positive," it is known that septic arthritis can occur in patients with low joint white blood cell counts, especially early in infection (36% of patients with septic arthritis had joint white blood cell counts <50,000 mm³).[16] Also, patients with inflammatory arthritides such as rheumatoid arthritis, gout, and pseudogout may have very high joint white blood cell counts. The overall white blood cell count, ESR, and joint white blood cell count are extremely variable in adults with septic arthritis.[17]

Laboratory tests do not rule out septic arthritis with accuracy. Therefore if suspicion for septic arthritis is high in the setting of negative testing, the EP should not hesitate to treat for infection while awaiting bacterial culture results. Hospital admission or extremely close follow-up and perhaps repeat arthrocentesis may be indicated. Adequate treatment involves drainage of purulent fluid as well as antimicrobial therapy. Empirical therapy should be initiated after cultures are drawn.

According to *Guidelines for the Initial Evaluation of the Adult Patient with Acute Musculoskeletal Symptoms* published by the American College of Rheumatology,[18] routine blood or urine tests including a complete blood count, urinalysis, basic metabolic panel, and liver function tests should be ordered if a systemic illness is suspected. If liver function tests are elevated, measurement of hepatitis serologies should be considered. A creatine phospokinase analysis should be performed if muscle pain or weakness is detected.

Imaging studies are indicated when the physical examination and laboratory tests cannot localize the anatomic structure that is causing symptoms, espe-

Table 103-5 MOST COMMON ORGANISMS AND SUGGESTED ANTIBIOTICS FOR VARIOUS PATIENT GROUPS WITH ARTHRITIS

Age/Group	Most Common Organisms	Suggested Empirical Antibiotics
Overall	*Staphylococcus aureus* most common; also streptococci, gram-negative organisms, anaerobes, *Neisseria gonorrhoeae*	At risk for STD—ceftriaxone; not at risk for STD—oxacillin/nafcillin+ceftriaxone
Infants (<6 months)	*Escherichia coli,* group B streptococci	Oxacillin/nafcillin+cefotax/ceftriaxone
Children 6-24 months	Staphylococci, *Kingella kingae* (no longer *Haemophilus influenzae)*	Oxacillin/nafcillin+cefotax/ceftriaxone
Pediatric group in general	*N. gonorrhoeae,* pneumococci	Oxacillin/nafcillin+cefotax/ceftriaxone
IV drug abusers	*Staphylococcus aureus,* gram-negative organisms	Oxacillin/nafcillin+ceftriaxone
Prosthetic joint	MSSA/MRSA, MSSE/MRSE, *Enterobacteriaceae, Pseudomonas*	Vancomycin+ciprotlaxin

MSSA/MRSA, methicillin-sensitive/resistant *Staphyloccous aureus*; MSSE/MRSE, methicillin-sensitive/resistant *Staphylococcus epidermidis*; STD, sexually transmitlerd disease.

Tips and Tricks

JOINT FLUID COLLECTION

- Prior to the procedure, educate the patient about its risks and benefits.
- If local anesthesia is planned, identify and mark landmarks before infiltration.
- Pre-procedure ice pack use will decrease procedural pain.
- Support the joint in a position of comfort during and after procedure.
- If there is possible overlying soft tissue infection, use an alternative approach if available.
- Utilize sonographic localization of joint fluid if uncertain about effusion.
- Have the patient rest the joint for 12 to 24 hours after injection of corticosteroids.
- Prepare the area thoroughly with antiseptic of choice to prevent seeding of the joint with skin flora. Use sterile gloves and equipment.
- Use an 18- to 22-gauge needle depending on size of the joint; smaller needles may not be sufficient to collect joint fluid.
- Fluid may be sent to the laboratory for cell count and differential, Gram stain and culture, presence of crystals, and glucose and viscosity testing.
- Familiarize yourself with the appropriate tubes for collection before sending specimen to the laboratory. It may be helpful to contact the laboratory technicians before collecting the fluid to ensure that the correct tubes are readily available; for example, the specimen for crystal analysis must be sent with liquid heparin in the tube.
- Know ahead of time where the fluid is to be sent (e.g., cell count to hematology lab, Gram stain to microbiology lab).
- Attaching a piece of extension tubing between the needle hub and collection syringe is helpful because it decreases movement of the needle in the joint space and eases changing of syringes in large-volume arthrocentesis. It also makes injection of anesthetics and steroids into the joint space easier. Make sure that you flush the tubing when injecting steroids, so the dose actually enters the joint space.
- Collect enough fluid for appropriate testing (this is not an easily repeated procedure). According to one study, seeding the fluid on blood culture flasks immediately after aspiration increases the yield.

cially after significant trauma and when there is loss of joint function, pain continues despite conservative management, a fracture or bone infection is suspected, or there is a history of malignancy.

Radiographs can confirm the diagnosis of osteoarthritis and assess its severity, but normally findings do not rule out osteoarthritis. The earliest changes in rheumatoid arthritis are nonspecific and include soft tissue swelling and periarticular osteoporosis, but these features are often abscent at the initial presentation. Calcification of fibrocartilage is often found in calcium pyrophosphate disease but is frequently an asymptomatic finding in elderly patients. Repeat films in 7 to 10 days may be appropriate when a fracture is suspected despite an unrevealing initial evaluation. Callus formation or abnormal alignment may be present.

Magnetic resonance imaging, which is suitable for soft tissue imaging, may be useful for diagnosing such problems as rotator cuff tear, spinal stenosis, and avascular necrosis of bone. Bone scans are best for assessing bone turnover and can be helpful in evaluation of osteomyelitis, stress fracture, and bony metastasis.

BOX 103-11

ED Disposition[23]

Rheumatology or Orthopedic Outpatient Follow-Up Is Indicated for:

- Diagnostic uncertainty
- Uncontrolled symptoms
- Increasing disability or deformity
- Disease complications
- Management uncertain
- Consideration of immunosuppressive therapy
- Proposed surgical intervention
- Medication complications
- Patient request for specialist opinion

Time Line for Follow-Up:

- **In 2-3 days:** EP unsure of diagnosis, but no indication for admission
- **Within 1 week:** Lupus flare (no central nervous system or renal involvement; complete blood count OK); consult with rheumatologist and possibly increase steroids.
- **In 1-2 weeks:** Patient with known rheumatology sick enough to come to ED but not severely ill; if joint was injected with steroids (tell patients that maximum effect will be in 1 week, although they should feel better by the next morning); hot joint, otherwise negative (not septic)
- **In 1 month:** Chronic complaints

When to Admit:

- Inability to control pain
- Inability to ambulate
- Inability to care for self at home (physical and occupational therapy; social/placement issues)
- Need urgent operative intervention
- Need parenteral antibiotics (septic joint)
- Acute symptoms in prosthetic joint
- Rare but high-risk complications (systemic vasculitis, cardiac involvement, hypoxic lung disease)

PATIENT TEACHING TIPS

ED DISPOSITION

- Instruct patients to return to the ED immediately if they have a temperature higher than 101° F, spread of redness or swelling, or any other urgent problems or concerns; also specify specific problems to watch out for—for example, tell patients taking nonsteroidal antiinflammatory drugs (NSAIDs) to "stop your medicine and come to the ED if you have black or bloody stools."
- Educate patients about their condition. Tell them that osteoarthritis is a chronic condition that is treated with NSAIDs, general measures, physical and occupational therapy, and in some cases surgical intervention (joint replacement).
- Warn patients that gout and pseudogout often recur and advise them to maintain hydration, avoid meat and alcohol in excess, and avoid certain medications.
- Remind patients with gonococcal arthritis that all sexual partners must be treated and educate them about protected sex and the need for follow-up testing for other sexually transmitted diseases, including human immunodeficiency virus, hepatitis B and C, and syphilis.
- Patients with inflammatory arthritis must understand that antiinflammatory medicines need to be continued as directed, even after pain improves.
- Patients should be aware that many rheumatologic diseases are chronic, or cannot be diagnosed in a single ED visit, or need specialized treatments not normally done in the ED; and many patients will need follow-up with rheumatology consultation and primary care.
- Patients must inform their caregivers about all the medications they are taking, including over-the-counter and herbal/alternative preparations.
- Patients must understand and comply with recommended medication doses and directions for treatment.
- Results of the ED visit and discharge recommendations need to be discussed in language understood by the patient; if the patient agrees, discuss recommendations with a family member also.
- Preprinted discharge instructions and disease education pamphlets are helpful, especially if notes are added to adapt them to the specific needs of individual patients.

■ TREATMENT AND DISPOSITION

Offending organisms and recommendations for treatment of septic arthritis are listed in Table 103-5 for some common etiologies. Although colchicine traditionally has been used in the acute treatment of gout, rheumatologists prefer NSAIDs, oral prednisone (40 mg/day for 1 week; no need to taper if less than 2-3 weeks), or intraarticular steroids. Allopurinol may be used as preventive therapy. Colchicine is seldom used in the acute setting but can be given prophylactically with allopurinol.

Pseudogout can be treated with NSAIDS such as indomethacin. For patients who cannot tolerate NSAIDs, an alternative option is cortisone injection in the affected joint. Effective prevention may be obtained with low doses of colchicine or NSAIDs.

All patients with rheumatologic complaints need primary care follow-up (Box 103-11). Many of these patients presenting with joint complaints have had past studies. It may be helpful to discuss prior work-up with their primary care physician to avoid redundancy.

REFERENCES

1. O'Dell J: Rheumatoid arthritis: clinical aspects. In Koopman W, Boulware D, Heudebert G (eds): Clinical Primer of Rheumatology. Philadelphia, Lippincott Williams and Wilkins, 2004, p 97.
2. Beachley MC, Franklin JW, Ostlund W, et al: Radiology of arthritis. Prim Care 1993;20:771-794.
3. Goekoop-Ruiterman YP, DeVries-Bouwstra JK, Allaart CF, et al: Comparison of treatment strategies in early rheumatoid arthritis: A randomized trial. Ann Intern Med 2007;146:406-415.
4. Scott DL, Kingsley JW: Tumor necrosis factor inhibitors for rheumatoid arthritis. N Engl J Med 2006;355:704-712.
5. Felson DT, Lawrence RC, Dieppe PA, et al: Osteoarthritis: New insights. Part 1: The disease and its risk factors. Ann Intern Med 2000;133:635-646.
6. Dieppe P, Brandt KD: What is important in treating osteoarthritis? Whom should we treat and how should we treat them? Rheum Dis Clin North Am 2003;29:687-716.
7. Clegg DO, Reda DJ, Harris CL, et al: Glucosamine, chondroitin sulfate, and the two in combination for painful knee osteoarthritis. N Engl J Med 2006;354:795-808.
8. Reichenbach S, Sterchi R, Scherer M: Meta-analysis: Chondroitin for osteoarthritis of the knee or hip. Ann Intern Med 2007;146:580-590.
9. Felson DT: Clinical practice. Osteoarthritis of the knee. N Engl J Med 2006;354:841-848.
10. Glass GG: Osteoarthritis. Clin Fam Practice 2005: 7:161-179.
11. Khan MA: Update on spondyloarthropathies. Ann Intern Med 2002;136:896-907.
12. Dubost JJ, Soubrier M, Sauvezie B: Pyogenic arthritis in adults. Joint Bone Spine 2000;67:11-21.
13. Ho G, Jue SJ, Cook PP: Arthritis caused by bacteria and their components. In Harris ED Jr, Budd RC, Genovese MC, et al (eds): Kelley's Textbook of Rheumatology. Philadelphia, Saunders, 2005.
14. Parillo S, Fisher J: Arthrocentesis. In Roberts JE, Hedges JR, Chanmugam AS, et al (eds): Clinical Procedures in Emergency Medicine, 4th ed. Philadelphia, Saunders, 2004.
15. Shmerling RH, Delbanco TL, Tosteson AN, Trentham DE: Synovial fluid tests. What should be ordered? JAMA 1990;264:1009-1014.
16. Li SF, Henderson J, Dickman E, Darzynkiewicz R: Laboratory tests in adults with monoarticular arthritis: Can they rule out a septic joint? Acad Emerg Med 2004;11: 276-280.
17. Sox HC, Liang MH. The erythrocyte sedimentation rate: Guidelines for rational use. Ann Intern Med 1986;104:515-523.
18. Dore RK, MD, Clements PJ, Fox RI, et al: Guidelines for Rheumatology Referral. American College of Rheumatology, revised Sept 25, 1996.

Chapter 104

Systemic Lupus Erythematosus

James G. Adams and Clare Sercombe

KEY POINTS

Systemic lupus erythematosus (SLE) is an autoimmune disease that damages skin, kidneys, bones, lungs, brain, and nearly every other body organ.
The damage is due to inflammation from direct antibody reaction to body tissues, from the deposits of immune complexes, and from secondary thrombosis.
A characteristic presentation is fever, malar rash, and joint pain in a young, premenopausal woman.
Sunlight and certain viruses and drugs can induce an autoimmune response in the genetically susceptible host.
Basic treatment is nonsteroidal anti-inflammatory medications or steroids. Many patients additionally require immunosuppressants, antimalarial drugs, and other therapies prescribed by a rheumatologist.
Patients with SLE have an increased risk for serious infection, often because of the steroids and immunosuppressants required to treat the disease.
Morbidity is due to organ failure, primarily of the kidney and brain.

Scope

Systemic lupus erythematosus (SLE) is a chronic autoimmune disease with widespread physical effects due to the production of autoantibodies to components of cellular nuclei.[1] The term *lupus* (Latin for wolf) is attributed to the thirteenth-century physician Rogerius who used it to describe the characteristic facial lesions that were reminiscent of a wolf's bite.

In some patients the illness is mild. Other patients suffer early, catastrophic organ damage. Early deaths are often due to injury to the kidney and brain. Later deaths often occur as the result of acute myocardial infarction, stroke, or infection. Steroids used for treatment may cause or worsen complications.

Epidemiology

SLE is more common by a ratio of 12:1 in women ages 15 to 45 years of age and by a ratio of 2:1 ratio in younger and older women. Overall prevalence of this disease is about 1 in 1000.[2]

In most studies of SLE, about 90% of enrollees are women. In the United States, the disease is three times more common among black women than white women. In addition to genetic factors, age, sex, race, and socioeconomic status impact disease expression and prognosis.

With optimal management, the 20-year survival approaches 70% and the 1-year survival is about 90%.

Pathophysiology

SLE is a prototypical autoimmune disease, characterized by tissue damage from excess antibody production and immune complex deposition. The chronic inflammation characteristic of the disease originates from overproduction of autoantibodies and a failure of the body to suppress them.

Nearly every tissue of the body can be affected. Autoantibodies directly react to human antigens, immune complexes deposit in tissue and blood vessels, and the complement cascade is activated, resulting in inflammation and organ damage.

The exact cause is unknown, but genetic predisposition, viruses, ultraviolet light (including sunlight), and medications such as hydralazine, isoniazid, and procainamide are known to be involved in certain patients. There is a relationship to specific human leukocyte antigen (HLA) genotypes.

Autoantibodies to lupus erythematosus are found in laboratory workers who handle lupus sera. Exposure to certain drugs can produce a SLE–like syndrome. Hormonal factors include an association to estrogens, which may explain the higher prevalence in women.

Clinical Presentation and ED Evaluation and Management

■ CLASSIC SIGNS AND SYMPTOMS

The triad of fever, joint pain, and rash in a woman of childbearing age suggests SLE. The most well-recognized cutaneous finding is the red, raised "butterfly rash" (Fig. 104-1), but malaise, fatigue, aches, fever, and weight loss are the most common symptoms. The rash, which does not cross the nasolabial fold, may be painful or pruritic. It may be precipitated by sunlight and may last from days to weeks.

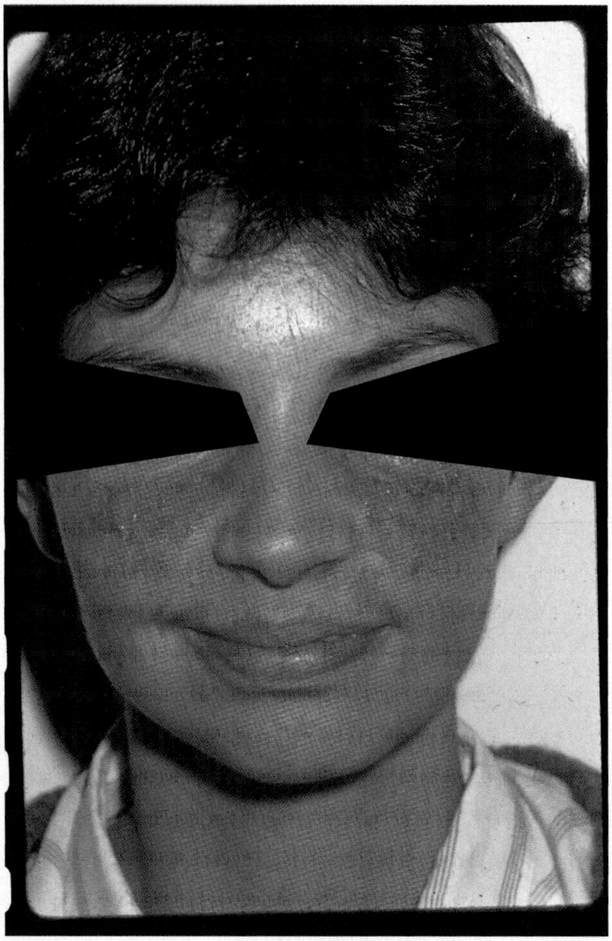

FIGURE 104-1 Erythematous malar rash of sytemic lupus erythematosus. Note that the rash does not cross the nasolabial fold. (From Gladman DD, Urowitz MB: Clinical features. In Hochberg MC, Silman AJ, Smolen JS: Rheumatology. Philadelphia, Mosby, 2003, pp 1359-1379.)

More than two thirds of patients have vague constitutional symptoms. A thorough evaluation is required before attributing such symptoms to lupus alone. Patients can have kidney failure, infections, adrenal failure, and other complications with similar symptoms.

Clinical presentations range widely, from mild to life-threatening. About half of patients have severe disease, defined as complications that threaten life or organ function. The most common and most severe manifestations are listed in Table 104-1. This disease activity index allows systematic tracking, especially useful in research.[3]

A substantial majority of patients develop some rash and/or arthritis. At least half of patients have Reynaud's phenomenon, mucous membrane involvement, and renal or central nervous system involvement. About half of patients report photosensitivity. A quarter to a third of patients will develop pleurisy, vasculitis, or gastrointestinal involvement. Less common but important manifestations include pancreatitis, myositis, and myocarditis.

■ ORGAN-SPECIFIC CLINICAL FINDINGS

■ Arthritis, Arthralgia, Myalgia, and Osteonecrosis

Almost all patients occasionally have arthralgias and myalgias. Hand inflammation is symmetrical, as in rheumatoid arthritis, but joint deformities are less common. Thirty percent of patients develop "hitchhiker's thumb" (hyperextension of the interphalangeal joint of the thumb). Tenosynovitis and tendon rupture also may occur, especially in patients taking corticosteroids. Avascular necrosis of the large joints, especially the femoral heads, also may be seen, due to ischemia caused by the vasculitis or as a complication of corticosteroid therapy.

■ Skin

The malar or butterfly facial rash of acute cutaneous SLE is a hallmark of the disease. Notably, it does not cross the nasolabial folds of the face, although it may involve the chin and ears. This facial eruption, seen

Table 104-1 SYSTEMIC LUPUS ERYTHEMATOSUS DISEASE ACTIVITY INDEX

Symptom	Score (Points)*
Seizure	8
Altered mentation	8
Retinal changes	8
Cranial nerve neuropathy	8
Lupus headache	8
Cerebrovascular accident	8
Vasculitis	8
Arthritis	4
Myositis	4
Urine casts	4
Hematuria	4
Proteinuria	4
Pyuria	4
New malar rash	2
Alopecia	2
Oral/nasal ulceration	2
Pleurisy	2
Pericarditis	2
Low complement	2
Increased DNA binding	2
Fever	1
Thrombocytopenia	1
Leukopenia (<3000 mm^3)	1

*Weighted score based on the presence of the symptom at the time of the visit or within the preceding 10 days.

in up to 40% of patients, may be the first sign or may accompany flares of the disease. It can be exacerbated by exposure to ultraviolet light.

Discoid lupus erythematosus, which is primarily a cutaneous disease, is characterized by raised plaques with scales, usually on the face, head, or neck. This can be associated with alopecia. Only 10% of these patients have SLE, but up to 25% of patients with SLE develop skin lesions consistent with discoid lupus erythematosus.

Kidneys

Clinical nephritis, defined as persistent proteinuria, is seen in approximately 50% of patients with SLE, although mesangial and glomerular immunoglobulin deposition is seen in almost all patients.[4] Usually there are no symptoms from the nephritis until it progresses to an advanced stage. Serum creatinine is an important but insensitive indicator of early renal disease, because many nephrons must be damaged before the creatinine level is elevated. Renal complications are recognized by hematuria, proteinuria, and red blood cell casts. Active urine sediment with excretion of red blood cell casts and increasing proteinuria is cause for concern.

Patients with active urine sediment may benefit from aggressive steroid or other immunosuppressive therapy. Indications for treatment include worsening renal failure, decreasing serum complement levels, increasing anti–double-stranded DNA (dsDNA) levels, and nephritic urinary sediment, especially when accompanied by increasing or nephrotic-range proteinuria. Renal biopsy can be useful in making treatment decisions. High-dose corticosteroids with immunosuppressive agents as therapy for renal disease are conventional but controversial. Patients who have end-stage SLE renal disease have survival rates similar to other patients on dialysis, approaching 85% at 5 years. Although patients on dialysis experience an improvement of their nonrenal SLE manifestations, they run a high risk of dying from severe SLE or infection in their first year of dialysis. Renal transplantation has been successful in these patients, and recurrent nephritis in the allograft is rare.

Central Nervous System

Seizures, stroke, migraines, peripheral neuropathies, and psychosis are common. These symptoms may appear early but are rarely the initial sign of SLE. Central nervous system involvement occurs in approximately 50% of patients with SLE. Full recovery from neuropsychiatric manifestations is approximately 70% to 85%, although the mortality from such events is 10% to 15%.

Seizures are the most frequent central nervous system manifestation. Strokes as a result of vascular inflammation and thrombosis also are common, especially in association with antiphospholipid syndrome.

Cerebritis should be considered in any patient with SLE who exhibits a change in behavior or altered mental status. Infection should also be considered, especially in patients on immunosuppressive therapy. These patients are at risk for bacterial, fungal, and tuberculous infections, in addition to brain abscesses. A head computed tomography scan and lumbar puncture usually are required to confirm the diagnosis. Subtle behavior changes and frank psychosis can be seen. Again, either the SLE or corticosteroid use may be the cause. In general, steroids are an important therapy modality for patients with lupus-associated cerebritis.

Cardiovascular System

Pericarditis

Pericarditis is the most common heart-related problem, reported to occur in 20% to 30% of patients, but present in up to 60% at autopsy. Electrocardiogram (ECG) findings alone may lead to the diagnosis, because the pericarditis can be clinically inapparent. Alternatively, some patients will have fever, tachycardia, chest pain, and a cardiac rub. The pericarditis usually is fairly benign and responds well to ibuprofen or corticosteroids. Pericardial effusion, typically a transudative serous fluid, occurs in about 20% of patients. Tamponade is rare but has been noted.

An uncommon but dangerous complication is purulent pericarditis, which should be suspected in patients who appear especially ill. Typical causes are *Staphylococcus aureus* and tuberculosis. Purulent pericarditis is exudative with a high C-reactive protein level and white blood count.

Myocarditis

Myocarditis is rarely diagnosed clinically but is found on autopsy in about 40% of patients. The 10% of patients in whom the diagnosis is made typically present with symptoms that resemble a cardiomyopathy, including congestive heart failure, ventricular dysrhythmia, tachycardia, and nonspecific ECG changes. Severe myocarditis should be treated with large doses of systemic corticosteroids, control of hypertension, and correction of volume overload.

Endocarditis

Libman-Sachs vegetations, present in up to 10% of patients with SLE, are growths on heart valves that usually cause no symptoms. Occasionally, these vegetations may be complicated by infection, valvular dysfunction, and rarely thromboembolism. The mitral valve is most commonly involved, although all four valves may have vegetations. Valvular dysfunction may occur independent of vegetations secondary to valvulitis, mucoid degeneration, or aortic dissection. The aortic valve has the highest incidence of hemodynamically significant regurgitation, followed by the mitral valve.

Coronary Artery Disease and Coronary Vasculitis

Accelerated atherosclerosis due to corticosteroid use may cause coronary ischemia. Mortality due to coronary artery disease is seen in up to 30% of patients with SLE despite improved survival of patients with renal and cerebral SLE. Hypertension, smoking, and hypercholesterolemia significantly increase the mortality risk in these patients. Patients who present with acute cardiac ischemia should be treated with standard interventions.

Coronary vasculitis is rare and best treated with steroids. Treatment differences make the distinction between the coronary vasculitis and coronary artery disease important. The diagnosis can be made by coronary angiography. Evidence of aneurysmal dilation of the coronary arteries is seen in patients with coronary vasculitis.

Pulmonary System

Hypertension

Patients with SLE often have systemic hypertension secondary to lupus nephritis and steroid use. The incidence has been reported in 25% to 50% of patients with SLE. Hypertension is particularly noted in patients who take high, long-term doses of corticosteroids.

Pleuritis

Pleurisy and pleural effusions are common, occurring in more than half of patients with SLE.[5] Pleural effusions usually are small and bilateral but occasionally can be very large. Pleural fluid usually is exudative, with glucose levels similar to serum glucose levels. In contrast, pleural fluid of patients with rheumatoid arthritis has very low glucose levels.

Pneumonitis

Pneumonitis in patients with SLE causes diffuse interstitial infiltrates, although patients have usually had the disease for several years before they suffer from pneumonitis. Bacterial, fungal, and opportunistic infections must be considered, especially in patients taking immunosuppressive agents, before confirming the diagnosi. Patients with SLE are particularly at risk for pneumococcal disease, in part due to autosplenectomy or splenic dysfunction.

Pulmonary Fibrosis

Patients with SLE may also develop chronic interstitial infiltrates leading to pulmonary fibrosis. These patients need inpatient treatment, and their conditions may progress to chronic hypoxia, pulmonary hypertension, and right-sided heart failure.

Shrinking Lung Syndrome

When a patient has shortness of breath, low lung volumes seen on a chest radiogram, and no other identifiable etiology, shrinking lung syndrome is signaled. Elevated diaphragm, but clear lung fields, are characteristic. This syndrome may be chronic, the result of impaired respiratory mechanics, weak muscles, and poor diaphragmatic function. If the presentation is acute, the patient may have a good response to steroids.

Gastrointestinal System

Mucous membrane lesions (small, shallow ulcerations in the mouth) are seen in up to 19% of patients. Oral ulcerations usually accompany disease flares. Esophageal dysmotility is occasionally seen; however, it is much less common in patients with SLE than in patients with scleroderma.

Patients with intestinal pseudo-obstruction may have crampy abdominal pain, and a clinical and radiographic picture consistent with obstruction. They should be observed for resolution.[6] Pancreatitis can be seen as a result of a disease flare or corticosteroid therapy and has been reported in up to 8% of patients. Spontaneous bacterial peritonitis also has been reported. Elevated liver function tests are common, usually the result of the medications given to treat SLE, such as azathioprine. Cytomegalovirus infection while the patient is on immunosuppressive therapy also may occur. Portal hypertension caused by scarring and fibrosis is seen in 4% of patients.

Mesenteric vasculitis is the most serious gastrointestinal complication. The patient has abdominal pain and, typically, bloody diarrhea along with evidence of vasculitis elsewhere. Bowel vasculitis may progress to perforation, gangrene, and peritonitis.

Hematologic Disorders

Anemia, affecting up to 40% of patients, may result from hemolysis, drugs, renal disease, blood loss, or chronic disease. The most important etiology is autoimmune hemolytic anemia. The Coombs test, which detects the hemolysis caused by antibodies directed against red blood cell antigens, usually is positive.

Thrombocytopenia occurs in 25% of patients. Antiplatelet antibodies may cause the low platelet count seen in patients with active SLE. Treatment for severe lupus-related thrombocytopenia is controversial; some authors advocate the use of vinca alkaloids and intravenous gammaglobulin.

An important cause of thrombocytopenia is thrombotic thrombocytopenic purpura. This may be difficult to distinguish from acute autoimmune hemolysis. Patients with thrombotic thrombocytopenic purpura typically present with low platelets, hemolytic anemia, central nervous system dysfunction, renal insufficiency, and fever. Symptoms can appear similar to those of a lupus flare. Treatment requires plasma exchange, so it is important to either clinically distinguish or empirically initiate the plasma exchange. Thrombotic thrombocytopenic purpura should be considered when a patient presents with a combination of microangiopathy, seizures, coma or altered mental status, and renal failure.

DRUG-INDUCED LUPUS ERYTHEMATOSUS

Procainamide has been known to induce a lupus reaction for over 40 years. Since then, a large number of agents have been implicated, with hydralazine and procainamide being the most common (Table 104-2). The clinical manifestations vary, with most patients experiencing arthralgias and occasional pleuropericardial pain. The full manifestations are present in less than 1% of patients taking high-risk drugs, although a positive antinuclear antibody (ANA) titer can be found in more than 50%. Patients usually are women, middle-aged or older, and rarely African-American, but this may be representative of the group of patients. The condition usually is reversible when drug therapy is stopped, with resolution within days or weeks. Manifestations lasting for years have been reported. In patients with significant pleuropericardial disease, a short course of tapered steroids has been used successfully once the implicated medication has been discontinued.

Differential Diagnosis and Diagnostic Testing

The American Rheumatism Association Revised Criteria for the Classification of Lupus was published in 1982. These criteria consist of 11 conditions associated with SLE (Box 104-1). Patients must have four criteria present, serially or simultaneously, to be given the diagnosis of SLE.

The diagnosis often can be confirmed by ANA testing. Positive titers are found in more than 95% of patients. The degree of positivity of the test is important, with higher titers having a positive predictive value. ANA titers may be positive in elderly patients taking certain medications such as hydralazine and procainamide and in patients with subacute bacterial endocarditis, infectious hepatitis, and primary biliary cirrhosis and other immune disorders. From 5% to 7% of healthy people may have a positive ANA titers.

Antibodies to dsDNA and anti-Smith (anti-Sm) antibodies are most specific titers for diagnosis of SLE. Patients with disease flares may show an increase in ANA or dsDNA titers. Decreases in complement levels of C3 and C4 also correlate with disease flares in certain patients.

The erythrocyte sedimentation rate (ESR) is a very poor index of disease activity. Patients who have an ESR of 50 to 100 mm/hour often show minimal disease activity. C-reactive protein levels often remain low except in patients with concurrent infection.

Table 104-2 DRUGS IMPLICATED IN LUPUS-LIKE SYNDROMES

System	Drug	Risk
Cardiovascular	Procainamide, quinidine, practolol*	High
Antihypertensive	Hydralazine, methyldopa, reserpine	High
Antimicrobial	Isoniazid, nitrofurantoin, penicillin, sulfonamides, streptomycin, tetracycline	Moderate
Anticonvulsant	Ethosuximide, mephenytoin, phenytoin, primidone	Moderate
Antithyroid	Methylthiouracil, propylthiouracil	Low
Psychotropic	Chlorpromazine, lithium carbonate	Low
Miscellaneous	Allopurinol	High
	Aminoglutethimide, gold salts, D-penicillamine, phenylbutazone, methysergide	Low

*Removed from market because of lupus-like syndrome.

Adapted from Rosen's Emergency Medicine: Concepts and Clinical Practice, 5th ed. St. Louis, Mosby, 2001.

BOX 104-1

Criteria for the Classification of Systemic Lupus Erythematosus*

Malar rash
- Fixed erythema, flat or raised, over the malar eminences, sparing the nasolabial folds

Discoid rash
- Erythematous raised patches with adherent keratotic scaling and follicular plugging; atrophic scarring may occur in older lesions

Photosensitivity
- Skin rash as a result of unusual reaction to sunlight, as determined by patient history or physician observation

Oral Ulcers
- Oral or nasopharyngeal ulceration, usually painless, observed by physician

Nonerosive Arthritis
- Involving two or more peripheral joints and characterized by tenderness, swelling, or effusion

Pleuritis or Pericarditis
- Pleuritis
  - Convincing history of pleuritic pain or rub heard by physician, or evidence of pleural effusion
- Pericarditis
  - Documented by electrocardiogram or rub, or evidence of pericardial effusion

Renal Disorder
- Persistent proteinuria >0.5 g/day or >3+ if quantitative assay is not performed
- Cellular casts—may be red blood cell, hemoglobin, granular, tubular, or mixed

Seizures or Psychosis
- Seizures
  - In the absence of offending drugs or known metabolic derangement (e.g., uremia, ketoacidosis, electrolyte imbalance)
- Psychosis
  - In the absence of offending drugs or known metabolic derangement (e.g., uremia, ketoacidosis, electrolyte imbalance)

Hematologic Disorder
- Hemolytic anemia with reticulocytosis
- Leukopenia—<4000/mm^3 on two occasions
- Lymphopenia—<1500/mm^3 on two occasions
- Thrombocytopenia—<10,000/mm^3 in the absence of offending drugs

Immunologic Disorder
- Anti-DNA—antibody to native DNA in abnormal titers
- Anti-Sm—presence of antibody to Sm nuclear antigen
- Positive finding of antiphospholipid antibodies based on:
  - Abnormal serum concentration of IgG or IgM anticardiolipin antibodies
  - Positive test for lupus anticoagulant using a standard method
  - False-positive test for at least 6 months and confirmed by *Treponema pallidum* immobilization or fluorescent treponemal antibody absorption test

Positive ANA Test
- Abnormal ANA titers by immunofluorescence or an equivalent assay at any time in the absence of drugs

*Based on The American Rheumatism Association Revised Criteria for the Classification of Lupus. The criteria consist of conditions associated with systemic lupus erythematosus including clinical symptoms, systemic complications, and diagnostic and laboratory test findings (see text for discussion).

Modified from Hochberg MC, Silman AJ, Smolen JS (eds): Rheumatology, vol 2, 3rd ed. London, Mosby, 2003, Ch 122.

ANA, antinuclear antibody; anti-Sm, anti-Smith; IgG, immunoglobulin G; IgM, immunoglobulin M.

Patients may have false-positive VDRL (Venereal Disease Research Laboratory) or RPR (rapid plasma reagin) test results.

Medical Therapy

Medical therapy attempts to reduce inflammation, suppress the immune system, and control pain. Mild symptoms might be controlled with acetominophen, but nonsteroidal antiinflammatory drugs (NSAIDs), corticosteroids, and immunosuppressive agents are the mainstays of treatment.

Aspirin and other NSAIDs are the primary treatment for arthralgias, pleurisy, and pericarditis. The maximum standard recommended doses of these agents usually are needed. These agents should be avoided in patients with severe gastrointestinal complications, renal insufficiency, nephritis, or thrombocytopenia. Treatment with NSAIDs can worsen lupus nephritis, either by causing interstitial nephritis or by inhibiting prostaglandins.

Topical corticosteroids control most rashes. Minor disease (arthralgias, fatigue, pleurisy) is usually controlled with *low-dose steroids* such as prednisone (0.5 mg/kg or less) in a single daily dose. However, anti-inflammatory and antimalarial drugs have been advocated for patients with minor symptoms to avoid the long-term complications of corticosteroid therapy.[6]

High-dose steroids (e.g., 1 mg/kg/day of prednisone or 1 g of IV methylprednisolone) is used when major organs are involved and also for hemolytic anemia and severe thrombocytopenia. For example, in patients with lupus-related cerebritis or acute worsening of lupus nephritis, 1 g/day of IV methylprednisolone may be given for several days. Treatment of glomerulonephritis with long-term steroids has not been proved to alter the outcome or course in patients with SLE, and their long-term use remains controversial.[6]

Corticosteroids have well-known long-term complications including steroid-induced diabetes, osteoporosis, weight gain, pancreatitis, osteonecrosis, accelerated atherosclerosis, and—most important—immunosuppression. Patients receiving steroid therapy should be monitored for evidence of infection and should be evaluated for any episode of fever.

When patients who are taking corticosteroids present with an acute serious illness or other physiologic stress (e.g., surgery, childbirth) the patient should also be given IV hydrocortisone (100 mg IV every 8 hours). Patients with overwhelming sepsis or shock should be given stress-dose steroids (e.g., 100 mg of IV hydrocortisone) in addition to the usual treatment with broad-spectrum antibiotics and IV resuscitation fluid.

Antimalarial drugs are effective for the cutaneous and musculoskeletal manifestations of SLE. Hydroxychloroquine and chloroquine are given on an outpatient basis in a loading dose for 4 weeks, followed by maintenance dosing once symptoms are under control. Withdrawal of the drug may result in disease flare.

Immunosuppressive agents (azathioprine, methotrexate, cyclophosphamide) are reserved for patients with severe renal or cerebral disease in whom other therapies have failed and for patients who cannot tolerate corticosteroids. Studies of the use of immunosuppressants have shown decreased chronic renal scarring and reduced likelihood of end-stage renal disease, without an increase in mortality. The toxicities of such drugs are numerous and include myelosuppression, risk of neoplasms, and infections,[6] especially gram-negative organisms, encapsulated gram-positive organisms, herpes zoster, and opportunistic organisms. Febrile patients who are on azathioprine, methotrexate, or cyclophosphamide should be admitted whether a source is evident or not, because gram-negative or streptococcal sepsis occurs in this population. Patients with localized herpes zoster should be admitted for intravenous acyclovir administration to prevent viral dissemination.

Specialized treatments include rituximab, new anti–B cell drugs, IV immunoglobulins, mycophenolate mofeti (an inhibitor of purine synthesis), and autologous marrow stem-cell transplantation.

Disposition

Patients with known SLE may come to the ED because of a flare of their disease, new systemic complaints, fevers, or illnesses not directly caused by the disease. Patients with known disease usually are able to tell the EP if the problem is typical.

Patients with known disease and increasing arthritic pain or with a mild flare without fever may be treated with NSAIDs or corticosteroids as an outpatient. Pleuritis and arthralgias can be treated on an outpatient basis. It may be prudent to perform urinalysis to ensure that there is no evidence of renal involvement, which might signal significant disease activity. If there is no major organ involvement, the patient can be scheduled for prompt follow-up with a rheumatologist.

Patients with a new diagnosis of pericarditis, myocarditis, pleural effusion or infiltrates or with evidence of vasculitis or renal insufficiency should almost always be admitted to the hospital. If there is uncertainty regarding diagnosis or severity of any circumstance, patients should be admitted for observation, testing, and treatment. Patients with worsening disease who are taking large doses of steroids or immunosuppressive agents should be admitted for aggressive treatment.

Patients with evidence of lupus nephritis and worsening renal failure should be admitted for therapy with steroids and, often, immunosuppressive agents.[7] The serum creatinine level may be elevated, but serious disease may be present even with normal creatinine levels. Proteinuria may be present, or red blood cell casts in the urine may be the only sign of severe renal involvement.

Patients with SLE have a higher risk of coronary artery disease, so the complaint of chest pain should prompt evaluation for cardiac ischemia. If pericarditis is suspected, evaluation of pericardial effusion may be necessary, although tamponade is rare. Patients with myocarditis should be observed for evidence of congestive heart failure and dysrhythmias.

Shortness of breath suggests lung infection from typical or atypical organisms. Opportunistic infection, tuberculosis, and lupus pneumonitis need to be considered. In the hypoxic patient, it is prudent to consider the possibility of pulmonary embolism due to antiphospholipid antibody with thrombosis. Patients with significant pleural effusions should be admitted for consideration of diagnostic thoracentesis and treatment. Pleural effusions may be complicated by infection, tuberculosis, or malignancy.

SLE predisposes patients to anemia and thrombocytopenia. Patients should be admitted if there is evidence of active hemolysis with decreased hematocrit levels or hemolysis that is evident on the blood smear. Patients with thrombocytopenia should be admitted if there is evidence of bleeding or if platelet counts are severely decreased ($<50,000/mm^3$). If the patient is actively bleeding, platelet transfusion is appropriate; however, rapid destruction of the platelets may occur. Simultaneous administration of IV corticosteroids and IV gammaglobulin will aid in increasing the platelet count and decreasing the amount of platelet destruction.

Patients with evidence of arterial or venous thrombosis should be admitted for anticoagulation and possible embolectomy. Anticoagulation can be achieved acutely with heparin, although large doses occasionally are needed to overcome the antibody effect. The partial thromboplastin time (PTT), if not elevated, can be followed to assess evidence of adequate anticoagulation, with careful observation for bleeding in patients who also are thrombocytopenic. Otherwise, patients with prolonged PTT and evidence of lupus anticoagulant can be followed with thrombin times if necessary. Patients with an INR less than 2.5 should nevertheless be considered to have a possible thrombus if they have a history of antiphospholipid syndrome.

Pregnant patients should have early follow-up with a high-risk obstetrician. Emergency delivery for the pregnant patient with SLE should include stress-dose steroid administration and close observation of the neonate for congenital complete heart block (i.e., neonatal lupus). Emergent cardiac pacing may be necessary for the infant.

REFERENCES

1. Moldovan I: Systemic lupus erythematosus: Current state of diagnosis and treatment. Compr Ther 2006;32:158-162.
2. Ward MM: Prevalence of physician-diagnosed systemic lupus erythematosus in the United States: Results from the third national health and nutrition examination survey. J Womens Health 2004:13:713-718.
3. Gordon C: Assessing disease activity and outcome in systemic lupus erythematosus. In Hochberg MC, Silman A, Smolen JS, et al (eds): Rheumatology. Philadelphia, Mosby, 2003, pp 1390-1391.
4. O'Callaghan CA: Renal manifestations of systemic lupus erythematosus. Nephrol Ther 2006:2;140-151.
5. Ion DA, Chivu RD, Chivu LI: Aspects of pleural/pulmonary involvement in systemic lupus erythematosus. Pneumologia 2006;55:151-155.
6. Sercombe CT: Systemic lupus erythematosus and the vasculidites. In Marx J, Hockberger R, Walls R (eds): Rosen's Emergency Medicine: Concepts and Practice, 6th ed. Philadelphia, Mosby, 2006, pp 1805-1818.
7. Boumpas DT, Sidiropoulos P, Bertsias G: Optimum therapeutic approaches for lupus nephritis: What therapy and for whom? Nat Clin Pract Rheumatol 2005;1:22-30.

Chapter **105**

Connective Tissue and Inflammatory Disorders

Raveendra S. Morchi

KEY POINTS

In this chapter, the specific connective tissue diseases Sjögren's syndrome, systemic sclerosis, sarcoidosis, and Raynaud's phenomenon are discussed.

Dry eyes and dry mouth unrelated to a medication side effect suggest primary Sjögren's syndrome.

Loss of sensation, paresthesias, and pain in the digits upon exposure to cold or emotional stress are characteristics are of Raynaud's phenomenon.

Many patients who eventually go on to develop systemic sclerosis initially have only symptoms of Raynaud's phenomenon and symmetric, nonpitting digital edema (without any fibrosis).

Gastrointestinal symptoms in the presence of symmetric, digital edema or fibrosis suggest systemic sclerosis.

Symptoms of edema and fibrosis proximal to the elbows or knees can represent an aggressive, diffuse form of systemic sclerosis, diffuse scleroderma, with a high likelihood of internal organ involvement.

An angiotensin-converting enzyme inhibitor should be considered for the hypertensive patient with a presumed or definitive diagnosis of systemic sclerosis

In patients with only bilateral hilar lymphadenopathy by chest radiography, especially if they have longstanding pulmonary complaints, the diagnosis of sarcoidosis should be suspected.

Early, vague subjective symptoms of fatigue, joint pain, or muscle discomfort may herald autoimmune disease. Patients who present later in the clinical course of their disease may have characteristic findings that can pinpoint the diagnosis.

SJÖGREN'S SYNDROME

Scope

Sjögren's syndrome is a slowly progressive, autoimmune destruction of the lacrimal and salivary glands. The resulting exocrine dysfunction produces the characteristic clinical presentation of dry eyes and dry mouth. An incidence of 4 per 100,000 per year has been noted. Ninety percent of cases are in women, and the incidence increases with age. Patients may be anywhere from the fourth to eighth decade of life. If dry eyes and dry mouth dominate the clinical picture, the patient may have primary Sjögren's syndrome. However, these symptoms can be associated with a number of other underlying autoimmune disorders that more accurately characterize the clinical presentation (rheumatoid arthritis, systemic lupus erythematosus, scleroderma); these patients probably have secondary Sjögren's syndrome.

Pathophysiology

Infiltration of the salivary or lacrimal gland by periductal and periacinar foci of aggressive T lymphocytes produces the destruction that eventually leads to loss of exocrine function. Polyclonal activation of B cells within, and at the border of, foci can result in hypergammaglobulinemia and a characteristic serum antibody profile. There are many other exocrine glands in the body (e.g., those lining the respiratory tree, integument, and vagina) and they too can be destroyed in Sjögren's syndrome, producing symptoms of a dry cough, dry skin, dysuria, or dyspareunia.

Because gland dysfunction is only an expression of the real problem in Sjögren's syndrome—an underlying systemic lymphocyte disorder—many other organs may be affected, resulting in less common "extraglandular" symptoms. This level of immune activation may be responsible for the increased risk of lymphoproliferative disorders and autoimmune endocrinopathies that have been noted in Sjögren's syndrome patients.

Clinical Presentation

■ GLANDULAR

Dry eyes, foreign body sensation, ocular grittiness, fatigue, and easy irritation are common complaints related to the lacrimal system. The patient may also have blurred vision, trouble with bright lights, or red eye. Signs include keratitis, conjunctivitis, mucous filaments at the inner canthus, blepharitis from meibomian gland dysfunction, and lacrimal enlargement.

Dry mouth and lips, an unpleasant taste in the mouth, difficulty chewing and swallowing dry food, and possibly a clicking quality to speech from the tongue sticking to the hard palate are all symptoms of diminished saliva production. Signs of poor salivary flow include secondary dental caries, gingivitis, irritation of oral mucosa, oral candidiasis, parotid gland enlargement, and diminished pooling of sublingual saliva upon direct inspection.

■ EXTRAGLANDULAR

The T- and B-lymphocyte activity that infiltrates and destroys exocrine glands can also affect other nonglandular organs. These extraglandular manifestations may portend a worse prognosis. Fatigue, myalgias, arthralgias, arthritis, and subjective fever are nonspecific and will not help distinguish Sjögren's syndrome. Most renal disease will be tubular in origin and related to invading lymphocytes. Signs may be minimal, but urinary sediment consisting of small amounts of protein or evidence of tubular malabsorption with or without systemic acidosis (renal tubular acidosis) may be seen.

Patients may have abdominal pain or nausea and vomiting consistent with gastritis or hepatitis. There may be an association between Sjögren's syndrome and hepatitis C, especially in patients with cryoglobulinemia. Celiac disease, another condition characterized by aggressive lymphocytes, may be associated with Sjögren's syndrome.

Patients may have symptoms of Raynaud's phenomenon because of abnormal regulation of vascular caliber. Purpuric, maculopapular, or urticarial rash from hypergammaglobulinemia or cryoglobulinemia results from polyclonal B cell activation and immunoglobin production.

Peripheral (median or peroneal) and cranial (V, VII, VIII) neuropathies may be secondary to autoimmune mediated vasculitis. Central nervous system involvement is less common and may consist of focal lesions mimicking multiple sclerosis, diffuse encephalopathy, or aseptic meningitis.

Differential Diagnosis

See Box 105-1.

Diagnostic Studies

The cracker test, in which the patient tries to chew and swallow a dry cracker, is probably the most useful bedside diagnostic maneuver. Patients with Sjögren's syndrome will have a difficult time completing this task, with adherence of food to the buccal mucosa. Slit lamp testing with fluorescein may show epithelial defects over the cornea consistent with keratitis secondary to dryness. Rose bengal staining (Fig. 105-1) generally is regarded as a more sensitive way of depicting these defects but usually is performed by an ophthalmologist. Schirmer's test involves placing standardized tear testing strips between the unanesthetized eyeball and the lateral margin of the lower lid and noting the advancement of a tear film over a

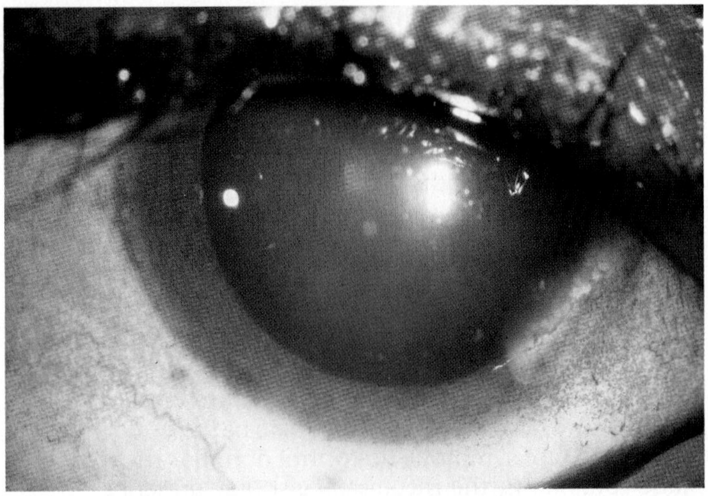

FIGURE 105-1 Keratitis by rose bengal stain. (From Yanoff M, Duker JS [eds]: Ophthalmology, 2nd ed. St. Louis, Mosby, 2004.)

BOX 105-1

Differential Diagnosis of Sjögren's Syndrome

Most Common

- Medication effects (anti-hypertensives, antipsychotics, antihistamines, antidepressants)
- Viral sialadenitis, human immunodeficiency virus, human T-lymphotropic virus 1
- Lacrimal gland infiltration in sarcoidosis or amyloidosis
- Chronic sialadenitis/conjunctivitis/blepharitis
- Prior radiation treatment
- Malnutrition (alcoholism, bulimia)
- Diabetes

Most Threatening

- Bacterial sialadenitis or parotitis
- Lymphoproliferative disorders
- Graft-versus-host disease
- Thyroiditis
- Salivary gland tumor

period of 5 minutes. Anything less than 5 mm is considered abnormal.

Treatment

There are two objectives to the treatment of Sjögren's syndrome: improve symptoms of exocrine gland dysfunction and attempt to control the underlying autoimmune lymphocyte activity. The former has had more success than the latter.

■ IMPROVING SYMPTOMS OF EXOCRINE GLAND DYSFUNCTION

■ Xerophthalmia

Artificial tears with or without preservatives may be used throughout the day, and lubricating ointments can be used at night. Oral pilocarpine, 5 mg four times a day, will stimulate muscarinic gland receptors, increase lacrimal flow, and provide subjective improvement.[1,2] More severely affected patients with keratoconjunctivitis sicca taking cevemiline, 30 mg three times a day, have reported a reduction in severity of symptoms.[3] Occlusion of the nasolacrimal duct temporarily with plugs or permanently by surgical intervention are last-line therapies. Topical ocular steroid preparations may be used for a short term and should be prescribed by an ophthalmologist.

■ Xerostomia

Although available, artificial salivas tend to be short-lived and less well accepted by patients. Meticulous oral hygiene is necessary to prevent dental caries, gingivitis, or periodontitis secondary to dryness. Sugarless sialogogues (lemon drops) stimulate flow. Lifestyle modifications like the use of a humidifier or avoidance of dry environments or excessive air conditioning help retain moisture. Mycostatin oral suspension, mycostatin vaginal tablets (also dissolve orally), or clotrimazole troches should be considered as alternatives to nystatin for treatment of oral candidiasis in the Sjögren's syndrome patient. Oral pilocarpine 5 mg four times a day or cevemiline 30-60 mg three times a day can stimulate muscarinic receptors and improve salivary flow in those with more significant symptoms.[4,5,6] Beware of side effects related to systemic muscarinic activation including bradycardia, bronchospasm, gastrointestinal symptoms, or impaired mydriasis and trouble with night vision.

■ Other Types of Xerosis

Humidified air and guaifenesin are useful for a dry respiratory tree. Avoidance of tight or restrictive clothing and the use of moisturizing creams, lotions, and bathing products can help dry skin. Mild corticosteroid cream may be added for pruritis. Proprionic acid gel is an effective vaginal lubricant.

■ ATTEMPTING TO CONTROL THE UNDERLYING AUTOIMMUNE LYMPHOCYTE ACTIVITY

Although non-steroidal anti-inflammatory drugs (NSAIDs) and hydroxycholoroquine can be prescribed from the ED for symptomatic control of minor rheumatic complaints, the rheumatologist may prescribe prednisone, cyclosporine, methotrexate, and azathioprine to control the lymphocyte activity.

Disposition

Patients with suspected primary or secondary Sjögren's syndrome should have outpatient primary care and rheumatology follow-up for further work-up within two to four weeks. Outpatient ophthalmology or dental evaluation is advisable. Patients should be advised to return to the ED for significant ocular pain or visual disturbance, which may signify keratitis. Severe keratitis may be complicated by globe perforation.

BOX 105-2

Types of Systemic Sclerosis

- *Localized scleroderma* consists of fibrosis in scattered, circular patches of skin (morphea), linear streaks (linear scleroderma), or nodules and is seen primarily in children. There is no systemic or internal organ involvement, and sequelae are cosmetic and sometimes functional.
- *Limited scleroderma* implies that fibrosis occurs distal to the elbows or knees and above the clavicles only.
- *CREST syndrome* refers to a type of limited scleroderma with evidence of three of the following symptoms: *c*alcinosis cutis, *R*aynaud's phenomenon, *e*sophageal dysfunction, *s*clerodactyly, and *t*elangiectasia. The inflammatory and fibrotic involvement of the esophageal wall results in poor motility with symptoms of dysphagia, reflux, and secondary esophagitis.
- *Diffuse scleroderma* is characterized by fibrosis extending proximal to the elbows and knees. It may be rapidly progressive and can be associated with significant internal organ fibrosis.

SYSTEMIC SCLEROSIS (SCLERODERMA)

Scope

Systemic sclerosis is a generalized thickening and fibrosis of skin and internal organs. Patients may present with localized patches of skin fibrosis (morphea or linear scleroderma), or the disorder may progress to diffuse skin involvement with internal organ fibrosis and dysfunction. The incidence is about 20 cases per million per year. Women are more likely to be affected than men, with the onset of disease peaking between 30 and 50 years of age.

Pathophysiology

Although the precise etiology is unknown, an underlying functional and microstructural vascular abnormality is believed to play a central role. Endothelial dysfunction, intimal and adventitial changes, and vascular smooth muscle reactivity incite a *secondary* inflammatory response composed of lymphocytes and fibroblasts that lay down increasing amounts of extracellular matrix, including collagen. Evolution of this inflammation results in the progression from edema to fibrosis, producing the characteristic clinical signs and symptoms of scleroderma.

If the primary vascular and secondary inflammatory abnormalities occur in scattered patches of skin only, the patient may have localized scleroderma (morphea or linear). If there is involvement of fingers (sclerodactyly) and the esophageal wall, patients may be classified as having the CREST (*c*alcinosis cutis, *R*aynaud's phenomenon, *e*sophageal dysfunction, *s*clerodactyly, and *t*elangiectasia) syndrome. However, if a patient has extensive, symmetric skin involvement with one or more internal organs affected (beyond that of the esophagus), the term *diffuse scleroderma* is applicable (Box 105-2).

Clinical Presentation

Raynaud's phenomenon is the initial complaint in the majority of patients and precedes clinically detectable skin fibrosis. Vascular malfunction antedates inflammation, edema, and collagen deposition. Notably, most patients with Raynaud's phenomenon will never develop systemic sclerosis. In patients with systemic sclerosis, the skin blanching of Raynaud's phenomenon may not be present, but paresthesias or sensory deficits followed by throbbing pain in the fingers, toes, and sometimes cheeks, nose, or tongue upon exposure to cold are more consistent findings.

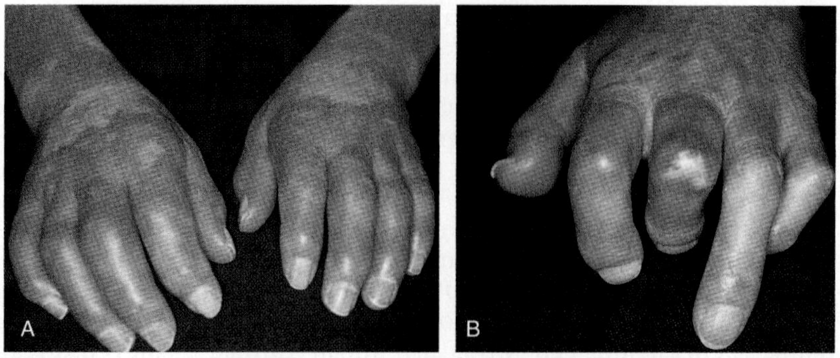
A
B

FIGURE 105-2 Hand changes associated with connective tissue diseases. **A,** Edematous phase; **B,** atrophic phase with contractures and skin thickening (sclerodactyly). (From Goldman L, Ausiello D [eds]: Cecil Textbook of Medicine, 22nd ed. Philadelphia, Saunders, 2004.)

Musculoskeletal complaints consisting of arthralgias, myalgias, and generalized weakness are nearly universal in patients with systemic sclerosis and other connective tissue disorders. Sometimes patients will have palpable or audible tendon friction rubs. Musculoskeletal problems are often some of the first symptoms and may be refractory to standard therapy with NSAIDs.

Skin findings are the most useful findings in the ED. Edema is a hallmark of early scleroderma as well as of rheumatoid arthritis, systemic lupus erythematosus, and other connective tissue disorders. Painless swelling of the fingers and hands also is common in these disorders (Fig. 105-2). Erythema and pruritus are associated findings due to microvascular abnormalities, an early inflammatory response, and deposition of components of the extracellular matrix. Non-pitting edema of this sort need not be limited to the distal extremities but may spread proximally or to the face and neck over the course of weeks.

Fibrosis may ensue over the course of months. Gradually collagen is deposited and the edematous areas are replaced by firm, thick, taut skin that may become bound to underlying tissue. In the fingers, tight skin can produce joint flexion contractures plus breaks or ulcerations as it is stretched over bony prominences (knuckles) in the condition termed *sclerodactyly* (see Fig. 105-2). Digital ulcerations, pitting scars, and loss of the finger pad can result from poor distal perfusion through intervening fibrotic tissue. This may be followed by calcium deposition (calcinosis).

A mask-like appearance to the face (Fig. 105-3) with a loss of natural skin creases and diminished hair growth is characteristic. "Salt and pepper" alterations in pigmentation and disorganized arrays of blood vessels (telangiectasias) scattered over the extremities, face, and mucous membranes are sequelae of this chronic, fibrotic inflammatory response.

Gastrointestinal symptoms are very common and related to intestinal wall edema and fibrosis that may occur anywhere from the esophagus to the rectum. In the esophagus, reflux esophagitis, strictures, and even Barrett's esophagus can occur. Throughout the rest of the bowel, complications include smooth muscle dysfunction, dysmotility, ileus, development of diverticuli due to uncoordinated peristaltic activity, bacterial overgrowth, and malabsorption. Nausea, anorexia, bloating, constipation, and diarrhea are potential complaints in these patients.

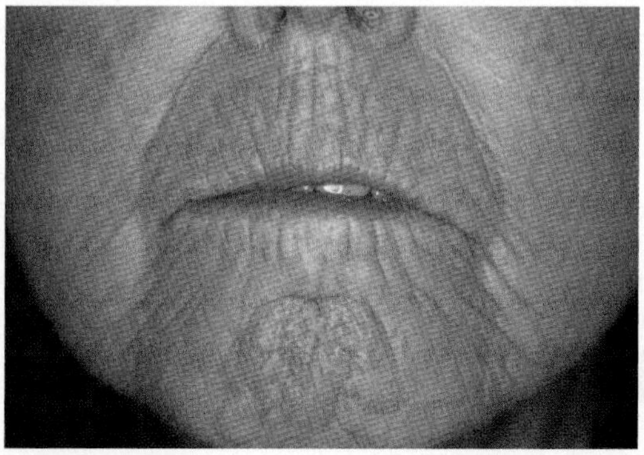

FIGURE 105-3 Facial features in scleroderma. Note the vertical lines or furrowing around the mouth in this patient with diffuse scleroderma. (From Goldman L, Ausiello D [eds]: Cecil Textbook of Medicine, 22nd ed. Philadelphia, Saunders, 2004.)

Pulmonary involvement is the leading cause of mortality in systemic sclerosis. Symptoms generally include dyspnea on exertion and a nonproductive cough. Interstitial fibrosis is more common in the diffuse form of scleroderma, and scattered rales may be heard. Like other fibrotic conditions, systemic sclerosis is a restrictive lung disease. Pulmonary hypertension from an obliteration of pulmonary vasculature associated with intimal and medial vessel wall changes can occur in the absence of significant interstitial fibrosis and is seen in a subset of patients with the limited form of scleroderma.

Renal vascular involvement can parallel that of other organs. The main difference is that when flow through arcuate and interlobular renal arterioles is diminished secondary to the microvasculopathy and spasm characteristic of systemic sclerosis, the distal glomerulus and juxta-glomerular apparatus will respond to this decrease in perfusion by producing renin and beginning a cycle of fluid retention and vascular constriction via angiotensin II and aldosterone. The result is hypertension with systemic vasoconstriction that can cause further damage to blood vessels and even hemolysis of red cells as they pass through damaged vasculature. In this sense, patients with renal involvement can present anywhere on a spectrum between asymptomatic hypertension, to malignant hypertension with characterisitic funduscopic changes, to hypertensive emergency.

Cardiac inflammation results in pericarditis with effusion. Pericardial disease may be asymptomatic or present with classic pain. In the myocardium, patchy areas of fibrosis may be a secondary event to coronary artery vasospasm and vasculopathy (in the same manner as other areas of the body affected by systemic sclerosis) and can physically impair cardiac conduction tissue or provide scar tissue that serves as points of re-entry. Secondary conduction deficits and supraventricular or ventricular arrhythmias will follow. Myocardial involvement and arrhythmias are asymptomatic in most, but dyspnea on exertion, CHF, syncope, or sudden death can occur.

Other features include thyroid, salivary, and lacrimal gland dysfunction secondary to fibrosis. Fibrosis in soft tissue can result in an entrapment neuropathy of susceptible peripheral nerves including the median, lateral femoral cutaneous, trigeminal, and facial nerves. Many men have erectile dysfunction from impaired blood flow secondary to vasculopathy and fibrosis.

Differential Diagnosis

See Box 105-3.

Diagnostic Studies

The skin examination is by far the most important diagnostic tool for the EP suspecting systemic sclerosis. Nailfold capillary examination may be useful for the patient with Raynaud's phenomenon who does not yet have skin changes indicative of sclerosis. Using an ophthalmoscope and immersion oil applied to the skin, dilated and tortuous capillaries mixed with areas of capillary loss may be seen in patients with secondary Raynaud's phenomenon as a result of a burgeoning connective tissue disease.

Serum electrolytes and urinalysis should be obtained to evaluate renal function. Because the disease does not usually involve the glomerulus or nephron tubular cells directly, but rather the arterioles upstream, urinalysis findings are frequently normal or limited to mild proteinuria with few cells or casts. Therefore, elevations in serum creatinine alone in a patient with other clinical evidence of systemic sclerosis should raise the possibility of scleroderma renal disease.

A complete blood count and smear should be obtained for those patients with suspected microangiopathic hemolysis from malignant hypertension. An electrocardiogram and rhythm strip should be evaluated for suspected conduction deficits or arrhythmia secondary to myocardial fibrosis.

Non-emergent work-up includes specific autoantibody profiling, gastrointestinal contrast studies for dysmotility, testing for suspected pulmonary fibrosis, echocardiography to evaluate myocardial contractile function or pulmonary hypertension, and biopsy to reveal characteristic fibrotic skin or gland changes.

BOX 105-3

Differential Diagnosis of Systemic Sclerosis

Most Common

- Primary Raynaud's phenomenon
- Localized scleroderma (linear or morphea)
- Other connective tissue disorders
- Scleredema and scleromyxedema
- Eosinophilic fasciitis and eosinophilia-myalgia
- Amyloidosis
- Reflex sympathetic dystrophy
- Diabetic sclerodactyly
- Myxedema

Most Threatening

- Chronic graft-versus-host disease
- Bleomycin
- Mycosis fungoides

Treatment

Because the mechanics and primary inciting events of systemic sclerosis are not yet well understood, therapy generally is aimed at improving symptoms and curbing end-organ dysfunction. Treatment for Raynaud's phenomenon includes lifestyle changes, calcium channel blockers, alpha blockers, antiplatelet agents, and sympathectomy. These are discussed later in the chapter.

Musculoskeletal symptoms may respond to ibuprofen or another NSAID in standard doses combined with physical and occupational therapy. More aggressive treatment with glucocorticoids or methotrexate should be left to a specialist, as benefit may be unclear.

Skin therapy includes moisturizers, topical glucocorticoid or antihistamine cream for pruritus, and local wound care with topical antibiotics for ulceration. High- or low-dose D-penicillamine cannot be recommended as an effective treatment at this time.[7]

Gastroesophageal reflux responds to standard changes in dietary habits and daily oral administration of omeprazole, 10 to 20 mg. Refractory cases may require surgical intervention, and reflux esophagitis–induced strictures may need periodic dilation.

Asymptomatic hypertension in a patient with known or suspected systemic sclerosis is presumed to be hyper-reninemic in origin from renal arteriolar disease and should be treated as such with an angiotensin-converting enzyme inhibitor. Oral administration of captopril, 6.25-12.5 mg three times a day, is a recommended starting point.[8,9] These patients require close outpatient monitoring of renal function. Patients with a hypertensive emergency or malignant hypertension may require intravenous enalaprilat or tighter control of systemic vascular resistance and heart rate via short-acting agents. Dialysis and renal transplantation remain last-line treatments for patients whose condition progresses to end-stage renal disease despite medical management.

SARCOIDOSIS

Scope

Sarcoidosis is characterized by the presence of noncaseating granulomas in multiple organ systems. Granulomas are composed of macrophages and other antigen-presenting cells as well as T lymphocytes helping to organize the response. They represent the immunologic response to organisms or antigens that cannot be properly disposed of, so instead are simply contained and walled off. Sometimes the contents of the granuloma undergo what is described pathologically as caseous necrosis (i.e., the granulomatous response to tuberculosis). At other times there is no necrosis, and the granulomas are termed noncaseating. In sarcoidosis these noncaseating granulomas can be found anywhere in the body but are primarily situated in the mediastinal and hilar lymphatic tissue, airways, and pulmonary parenchyma. Pulmonary or not, nearly every clinical manifestation of sarcoidosis can be traced to the physical presence of granulomas within the organ.

Because there are many causes of granulomatous inflammation, the exact worldwide prevalence and incidence of sarcoidosis are not known. Most patients with the disease are below age 40 years. Women are affected slightly more often than men. Worldwide, the majority of cases are in white persons, but within the U.S. the disease is more frequent in African-Americans.

Pathophysiology

Although the exact cause of sarcoidosis is unknown, there is evidence that an environmental, chemical, or infectious agent provides the antigenic stimulus to macrophages. Once processed and presented, these antigens trigger a CD4 T cell–mediated hypersensitivity reaction that subsequently incites increasing numbers of macrophages and neighboring epithelial cells to partake in the formation of noncaseating granulomas and produce the clinical signs and symptoms of sarcoidosis.

In addition to the environmental trigger, a genetic component mediating the T cell hypersensitivity may need to be present. In this way, only a genetically susceptible individual exposed to the unidentified antigen may develop clinical sarcoidosis.

Clinical Presentation

Pulmonary disease is the hallmark of sarcoidosis. Granulomas are spread throughout mediastinal and hilar lymph nodes, in the lining of bronchi, and within the pulmonary parenchyma. Dyspnea on exertion, nonproductive cough, and nonspecific retrosternal chest pain are the most common symptoms. Depending on the location and extent of granulomatous tissue, patients may have primarily wheezing and a prolonged expiratory phase from endobronchial lesions, or rales from parenchymal involvement. Alternatively, many patients have no symptoms or a clear lung examination despite radiographic evidence of disease.

Skin findings are present in up to 25% of patients (Fig. 105-4). Most are chronic and due to direct granulomatous involvement of the dermis. Unfortunately, they may take the form of papules, plaques, nodules, keloids at the site of surgical scars, or even lupus pernio (a violaceous discoloration over the nose, cheeks, chin, and ears). It is difficult for the EP to make the diagnosis of sarcoidosis based on the presence of skin lesions alone due to the variety of presentations. Erythema nodosum may be one exception. Unlike other lesions, it is acute in onset and does not consist of granulomas, but rather of cellular inflammation and edema to the dermis and subcutaneous tissue that produces the characteristic raised, red, tender, nodular lesions most often seen on the ante-

RED FLAGS

- Many connective tissue diseases have associated severe keratitis that may be complicated by globe perforation.
- Sarcoid granulomas can block the normal conduction syst, with complete heart block as the most common manifestation.
- Consider sarcoidosis in patients with *only* bilateral hilar lymphadenopathy shown on a chest radiograph, especially if they have longstanding pulmonary complaints.
- Before diagnosing sarcoidosis in patients, consider tuberculosis, histoplasmosis, community-acquired pneumonia, and lymphoma. Some of these patients will have to be admitted or empirically treated for an infectious process before a diagnosis can be secured via more extensive work-up.
- Patients who have functional impairment and no known history of sarcoidosis will need to be admitted for evaluation for the other infectious and neoplastic processes before a definitive diagnosis can be made and treatment started.

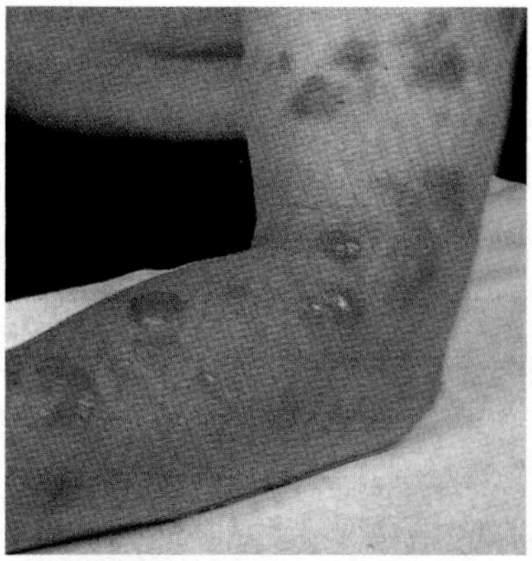

A

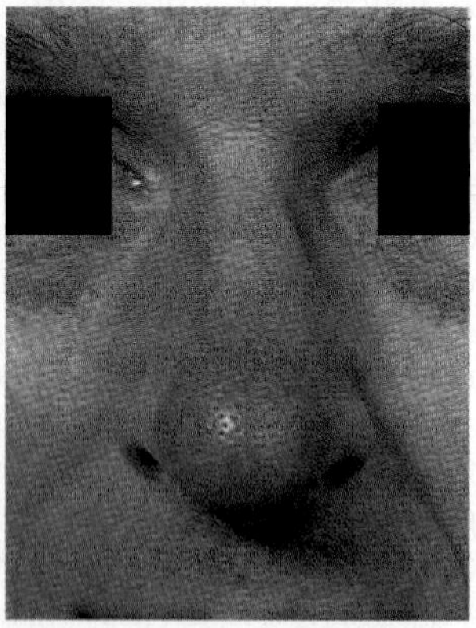

B

FIGURE 105-4 Skin lesions of sarcoidosis. **A,** Sarcoid lesions may occur at any site, and they may take nodular, papular, or plaque forms. Biopsy is often necessary for diagnosis. **B,** *Lupus pernio* is the term used to describe a dusky-purple infiltration of the skin of the nose, cheeks, or ears in chronic sarcoidosis. (From Goldman L, Ausiello D [eds]: Cecil Textbook of Medicine, 22nd ed. Philadelphia, Saunders, 2004.)

rior tibial surface. Also unlike other skin lesions, erythema nodusum can be used to confirm the diagnosis of sarcoidosis in patients who have bilateral hilar lymphadenopathy on chest radiography.

This combination of findings describes a subset of sarcoidosis patients said to have Löfgren's syndrome. Note that erythema nodosum without bilateral hilar adenopathy may be present in a number of other infectious or neoplastic conditions and should not be considered diagnostic for sarcoidosis.

Ocular sarcoidosis most frequently takes the form of anterior uveitis with symptoms of eye pain, irritation, visual disturbances, including red eye and photophobia. Cell and flare or even hypopyon may be seen on slit lamp examination. Posterior uveal tissue can also be involved with signs of chorioretinitis seen by fundoscopy. Keratitis and globe perforation are sequelae of corneal involvement, and nodules representative of granulomatous tissue can be seen on the conjunctiva of affected patients.

Cardiac disease, although less common, can be life-threatening. Appropriately placed septal granulomas can block the normal conduction system, with complete heart block as the most common manifestation. They can also serve as foci for reentry or automaticity and thereby predispose to arrhythmias. Within papillary tissue, granulomas can result in muscle dysfunction and secondary valvular incompetence. Extensive ventricular muscle involvement or valvular insufficiency can result in congestive heart failure.

Musculoskeletal manifestations consist of symmetric arthralgias or inflammatory arthritis of the ankles, knees, wrists, and elbows. Most patients do not have chronic arthritis or joint destruction. Lytic or sclerotic bony lesions are noted in the hands and feet, and many patients are asymptomatic. Granulomatous muscle involvement is often subclinical.

Neurologic complications develop in up to 10% of patients and can involve any part of the central or peripheral nervous system. Aseptic (predominantly basal) meningitis, encephalopathy, seizures, hypothalamic and pituitary disturbances (with diabetes insipidus or secondary thyroid or adrenal dysfunction), cranial neuropathies (especially unilateral or bilateral nerve VII palsies), or communicating/noncommunicating hydrocephalus from granulomatous impairment of ventricular drainage are all potential intracranial presentations. Peripheral neuropathies and spinal cord dysfunction are secondary to extracranial granulomatous inflammation.

Glandular exocrine insufficiency from granulomatous invasion can result in swollen lacrimal, parotid, and salivary glands, with symptoms of dry eyes and mouth. Other signs and symptoms related to systemic T-cell activation and granuloma formation include nonthoracic lymphadenopathy, splenomegaly, fever, and malaise. Increased granulomatous calcitriol production with longstanding hypercalcemia and hypercalciuria can result in renal calcium deposition and renal dysfunction.

Differential Diagnosis

Pulmonary symptoms and typical radiographic signs in a young or middle-aged patient with erythema nodosum, iritis, or nonspecific, symmetric musculoskeletal complaints can help the EP distinguish sarcoidosis from other infectious or autoimmune processes (Table 105-1). Even then a definitive bedside diagnosis may be difficult to make, and the EP may need to consider tuberculosis, histoplasmosis, community-acquired pneumonia, and lymphoma before diagnosing sarcoidosis (Box 105-4). Some of these patients will have to be admitted or empirically treated for an infectious process before a diagnosis can be secured via more extensive work-up. Given the array of organ systems affected and the lack of pulmonary symptoms in many patients, sarcoidosis may go unrecognized in the ED.

Diagnostic Studies

A chest radiograph is the most useful tool for patients with cough, dyspnea, or chest pain. Patients in whom

Table 105-1 SUMMARY OF CONNECTIVE TISSUE DISEASES

Syndrome	Testing	Treatment	Tips
Sjögren's syndrome	Cracker test Slit-lamp examination Schirmer's test	Artificial tears Sialogogues Pilocarpine Nasolacrimul duct occlusion	Use humidifier and moisturizers Avoid dry environments
Systemic sclerosis and Raynaud's phenomenon	Skin exam Serum creatinine Urinalysis	Omeprazole Captopril	GERD precautions Regular BP checks Patients should be advised of the chronic and progressive nature of systemic sclerosis
Sarcoidosis	Chest radiograph ECG Slit-lamp examination	Prednisone NSAIDs Cycloplegics	Most cases abate within 2 years
Raynaud's phenomenon	Normal nailfold capillary examination	Nifedipine	Avoid cold Avoid tobacco Wear warm clothing

BP, blood pressure; ECG, electrocardiogram; GERD, gastroesophageal reflux disease; NSAIDs, nonsteroidal anti-inflammatory drugs.

BOX 105-4

Differential Diagnosis of Sarcoidosis

Most Common

- Other granulomatous disease (tuberculosis, fungal, spirochetes, viral, parasitic)
- Environmental antigens
- Chemical antigens (silica, beryllium)
- Other autoimmune conditions (Sjögren's syndrome)
- Human immunodeficiendy virus

Most Threatening

- Primary cardiac arrhythmia, conduction deficit, cardiomyopathy
- Neoplasm (pulmonary or lymphoma)
- Globe perforation
- Bacterial or aseptic meningitis

BOX 105-5

Stages of Sarcoidosis

Stage I	Bilateral hilar lymphadenopathy (Fig. 105-5)
Stage II	Bilateral hilar lymphadenopathy plus parenchymal infiltrate
Stage III	Parenchymal infiltrate without hilar adenopathy (see Fig. 105-5)
Stage IV	Parenchymal fibrosis

the diagnosis of sarcoidosis is considered because of erythema nodusum, iritis, or cranial neuropathy should also have chest radiography, even in the absence of pulmonary signs or symptoms. Four stages of sarcoidosis are described in Box 105-5, but patients normally do not progress from one stage to the next. The higher stages indicate a lower likelihood of spontaneous resolution.

An ECG should be obtained for any patient with syncope, dyspnea, or rhythm abnormalities. Cardiac granulomas can produce first- through third-degree atrioventricular block, fascicular block, or bundle branch blocks.

Patients should have a slit-lamp examination for evaluation of the red eye. Consensual photophobia, pain at a given distance of accommodation, and cell and flare are indicative of iritis. The funduscopic examination may provide evidence of posterior uveitis (vitreous, retinal, or choroid disease). Corneal staining and Seidel's test are useful for the diagnosis of keratitis and corneal perforation.

Arthrocentesis will be consistent with nonseptic, inflammatory arthritis. A head computed tomography or lumbar puncture should be obtained for patients with suspected focal intracranial or diffuse meningeal neurologic involvement. Two thirds of patients will have an elevated cerebrospinal fluid protein, and one half may have a predominantly mononuclear pleocytosis. These findings in some patients with extraneural sarcoid features may suggest the diagnosis of neurosarcoidosis.

Laboratory work will likely not help the EP make a diagnosis, but findings may include anemia of chronic disease, thrombocytopenia from splenomegaly, elevated serum calcium levels from granuloma-related abnormalities in calcitriol production, and nonspecific transaminitis from asymptomatic hepatic granulomas.

Further work-up with a tuberculin skin test, chest computed tomography scan, pulmonary function tests, echocardiography, angiotensin-converting enzyme levels, radionuclide imaging, endomyocardial biopsy for myocardial involvement, or endobronchial/transbronchial/mediastinal/thoracoscopic biopsies may be considered for patients on an

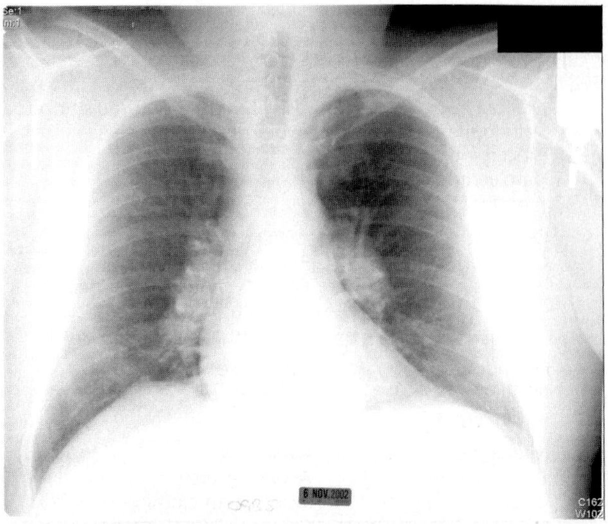

A

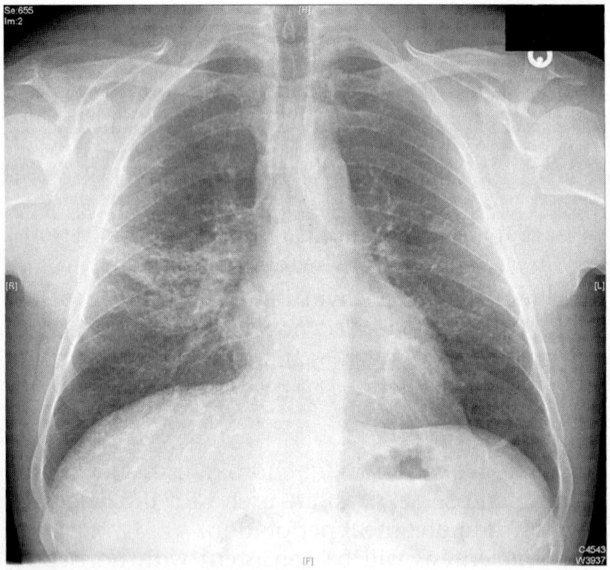

B

FIGURE 105-5 **A,** Stage I sarcoidosis: Prominent hilar lymphadenopathy and normal lungs. **B,** Stage III sarcoidosis: Interstitial infiltrate without hilar lymphadenopathy. (From Mason RJ, Broaddus VC, Murray JF, Nadel JA: Murray and Nadel's Textbook of Respiratory Medicine, 4th ed. Philadelphia, Saunders, 2004.)

inpatient or outpatient basis with specialist consultation.

Treatment

Two thirds of cases of sarcoidosis will spontaneously resolve within 2 years, and many patients can be managed with observation alone. Treatment focuses on suppression of granuloma formation with glucocorticoids and is reserved for individuals with functional impairment or chronic disease.

Many patients with pulmonary involvement will not require ED treatment. Simple observation by a primary care physician on an outpatient basis for development of treatable symptoms or abnormal pulmonary function tests will suffice. Patients who present to the ED with significant dyspnea, functional impairment, and parenchymal disease on radiography are candidates for therapy with prednisone, 0.5 to 1 mg/kg/day if bacterial, mycobacterial, fungal and neoplastic processes can be excluded. Patients may need specialist consultation, hospital admission, or (at the very least) close outpatient follow-up. Doses may be tapered over a 6- to 12-month period by the patient's primary physician, depending on symptomatic response.

Musculoskeletal complaints and erythema nodusum are best treated with standard doses of nonsteroidal anti-inflammatories. Patients presenting with cardiac or neurologic involvement should first have standard ED management, then specialist consultation and consideration given to systemic glucocorticoids. Invasive interventions like transvenous cardiac pacing or an intraventricular drain for obstructive hydrocephalus may be required. Ocular manifestations can be treated with topical cycloplegics and, after consultation with an ophthalmologist, topical corticosteroids. Suspected globe perforation from severe keratitis warrants an ophthalmologic evaluation in the ED.

Weekly methotrexate and daily azathioprine are corticosteroid-sparing agents that may be prescribed by a pulmonologist or rheumatologist for steroid-dependent or refractory cases. Antitumor necrosis factor medication may also be considered in refractory cases. Radiation therapy and surgical intervention have been used for focal intracranial disease refractory to multiple agents.

Disposition

The EP should give first consideration to bacterial, mycobacterial, or fungal causes of the patient's presentation. Lymphoma and other neoplastic processes are also potential diagnoses. If these entities can be excluded or if patients have known sarcoidosis, they may be discharged with oral prednisone prescribed to be taken if needed for symptomatic control; however, close outpatient primary care follow-up is mandatory.

Most patients who have functional impairment and no known history of sarcoidosis will need to be admitted for evaluation of the other infectious and neoplastic processes before a definitive diagnosis can be made and treatment started.

PRIMARY RAYNAUD'S PHENOMENON

Scope

Raynaud's phenomenon is a vasospastic disorder marked by minute- to hour-long episodes of digital ischemia on exposure to cold or emotional stress. Up to 20% of the population may suffer from Raynaud's phenomenon. Cases commonly involve women and occur in cooler environments.

Clinical Presentation

Intense vasoconstriction results in decreased perfusion, well-demarcated pallor, and loss of sensation to fingers and toes, and rarely the nose and ears. With the return of sluggish flow, the extremity turns from white to blue. Parasthesias may be present. Then, with increased flow, digits become bright red in a phase termed *reactive hyperemia*. It is during this time of reperfusion that patients will have throbbing pain. Although the triphasic color changes are not always present, it is a predictable response to cold or stress that defines Raynaud's phenomenon.

In primary Raynaud's phenomenon, the microstructure of distal vessels is entirely normal and symptoms are due to an intrinsic hyperreactivity of these vessels when exposed to cold or emotional stress. The appearance of the vasculature and the patient's digits between attacks is normal.

In secondary Raynaud's phenomenon, the symptoms occur because of arterial luminal occlusion or stasis to flow, external compression, fibrosis, or abnormal neural innervation. Given this, symptoms in secondary disease are not always symmetric. Over time, there may be structural changes to distal vessels and permanent changes to the clinical appearance of the patient's digits.

Differential Diagnosis

The cardinal stigmata of autoimmune diseases (sclerodermatous skin changes, muscle weakness, rash) may not be present at the time a patient has Raynaud's phenomenon symptoms (Box 105-6). On an initial visit, a diagnosis of primary Raynaud's phenomenon may be made when, in actuality, the patient's symptomatology indicates secondary Raynaud's phenomenon due to an underlying disease yet to become manifest.

Diagnostic Studies

A well-demarcated symmetric color change occurs during an attack or can be precipitated by placement of the extremity in ice water. Fibrosis, pitting, or ulceration of the fingertips is indicative of structural vascular and dermal changes in secondary Raynaud's phenomenon. In the nailfold capillary examination, immersion oil is placed over the skin at the proximal nail and an ophthalmoscope used to denote normal-appearing capillaries. Abnormally tortuous, enlarged capillaries or a heterogeneous appearance may be indicative of Raynaud's phenomenon secondary to scleroderma, idiopathic inflammatory myopathy, or another vascular disease.

BOX 105-6

Differential Diagnosis of Raynaud's Phenomenon

Most Common

- Scleroderma
- Systemic lupus erythematosus
- Other connective tissue diseases
- Occupational arterial injury (hypothenar hammer syndrome)
- Medications (beta-blockers, ergotamines)
- Thoracic outlet syndrome
- Carpal tunnel syndrome
- Cryoglobulinemia

Most Threatening

- Arterial occlusion
- Thromboangiitis obliterans

Autoantibodies, cryoglobulins, and serum or urine protein electrophoresis to determine secondary causes of Raynaud's phenomenon are not standard in the ED work-up.

Treatment

Patients should be instructed to avoid cold and stress, cease tobacco consumption, and wear warm clothing. Oral administration of nifedipine, 10 to 20 mg, taken 30 minutes prior to cold exposure can minimize attacks.[10] Alternatively, patients may take up to 60 mg/day divided into three doses. Once-a-day extended-release tablets are also available. Caution should be used in the elderly and those with cardiac and vascular disease. Prazosin and topical nitrates are second-line agents.[11] Intravenous infusions of the prostacyclin analogue iloprost and surgical palmar sympathectomy or arteriolysis (release of fibrotic adventitia) are last-line treatments.

Disposition

Most patients with primary or secondary Raynaud's phenomenon can be discharged home for primary care follow-up in the following 2 to 4 weeks.

In addition to digital artery spasms, chest pain from coronary artery vasospasms may occur in a subset of patients who may require admission.

REFERENCES

1. Vivino FB, Al-Hashimi I, Khan Z, et al: Pilocarpine tablets for the treatment of dry mouth and dry eye symptoms in patients with Sjögren syndrome: A randomized, placebo-controlled, fixed-dose, multicenter trial. P92–01 Study Group. Arch Intern Med 1999;159:174-181.

2. Tsifetaki N, Kitsos G, Paschides CA, et al: Oral pilocarpine for the treatment of ocular symptoms in patients with Sjögren's syndrome: A randomised 12 week controlled study. Ann Rheum Dis 2003;62:1204-1207.
3. Petrone D, Condemi JJ, Fife R, et al: A double-blind, placebo-controlled study of cevimeline in Sjögren's syndrome patients with xerostomia and keratoconjunctivitis sicca. Arthritis Rheum. 2002;46:748-754.
4. Vivino FB: The treatment of Sjögren's syndrome patients with pilocarpine-tablets. Scand J Rheumatol Suppl 2001; 115:1-9.
5. Moutsopoulos NM, Moutsopoulos HM: Therapy of Sjögren's syndrome. Springer Semin Immunopathol 2001;23:131-145.
6. Fox RI, Petrone D, Condemi J, et al: Randomized, placebo-controlled trial of SNI-2011, a novel M3 muscarinic receptor agonist, for treatment of Sjögren's syndrome [abstract]. Arthritis Rheum 1998;41:S80.
7. Clements PJ, Furst DE, Wong WK, et al: High-dose versus low-dose D-penicillamine in early diffuse systemic sclerosis: Analysis of a two-year, double-blind, randomized, controlled clinical trial. Arthritis Rheum 1999;42:1194-1203.
8. Whitman HH, Case DB, Laragh JH, et al: Variable response to oral angiotensin-converting-enzyme blockade in hypertensive scleroderma patients. Arthritis Rheum 1982;25:241.
9. Beckett, VL, Donadio JV, Brennan LA Jr, et al: Use of captopril as early therapy for renal scleroderma: A prospective study. Mayo Clin Proc 1985 60:763.
10. Thompson AE, Pope JE: Calcium channel blockers for primary Raynaud's phenomenon: A meta-analysis. Rheumatology (Oxf) 2005;44:145-150.
11. Russell IJ, Lessard JA: Prazosin treatment of Raynaud's phenomenon: A double-blind single crossover study. J Rheumatol 1985;12:94.

Chapter **106**

Vasculitis Syndromes

Paul J. Allegretti

KEY POINTS

A patient's combined genetic predisposition and regulatory mechanisms control expression of an immune response to antigens.
Negative test results for antineutrophil cytoplasmic antibodies (ANCA) do not exclude disease nor do positive results indicate a specific syndrome.
The combination of clinical, laboratory, biopsy, and radiographic findings usually points to a specific vasculitis syndrome.
The definitive diagnosis of a vasculitic syndrome depends on demonstration of vascular involvement and may be accomplished by biopsy or angiography.
Differentiation of primary and secondary vasculitis is essential because the pathophysiologic, prognostic, and therapeutic aspects differ.
The diagnosis of vasculitis should be considered in any patient with febrile illness and organ ischemia without other explanation.

Scope

The first account of a vasculitic syndrome was documented in 1866 by Kussmaul and Maier. Descriptions of other vasculitides followed, and in 1952 Zeek developed the first classification system. The American College of Rheumatology introduced classification criteria for seven forms of vasculitis in 1990. Finally in 1994, the Chapel Hill Consensus Conference named and defined the ten most common forms of vasculitides based on vessel size (Box 106-1). This system is based on the fact that different forms of vasculitis attack different vessels.[1,2] These criteria were established to differentiate specific types of vasculitis, but they are often used as diagnostic criteria. The vasculitic syndromes feature a great deal of heterogeneity and overlap, leading to difficulty with regard to categorization.[3] In addition, many patients display incomplete presentations, adding to the confusion. EPs should keep in mind the fact that nature does not always follow the patterns and artificial boundaries drawn by classification systems.[4]

Pathophysiology

Vasculitis, also known as the vasculitides or the vasculitis syndromes, is a clinicopathologic process that results in inflammation and damage to blood vessels.[3] Cell infiltration with inflammatory modulators causes swelling and changes in the function of the vessel walls. This compromises vessel patency and integrity, leading to tissue ischemia, necrosis, and bleeding. Because most forms of vasculitis are not restricted to a certain vessel type or organ, the syndromes are broad and heterogeneous. Because vasculitis is a

BOX 106-1

The Chapel Hill Consensus Conference Classification of Primary Vasculitides

Large Vessel
- Giant cell (temporal) arteritis
- Takayasu's arteritis

Medium Vessel
- Polyarteritis nodosa
- Kawasaki disease

Small Vessel
- Wegener's granulomatosis
- Churg-Strauss syndrome
- Microscopic polyangiitis
- Henoch-Schönlein purpura
- Cryoglobulinemic vasculitis
- Cutaneous leukocytoclastic vasculitis

From Kallenberg CG: Vasculitis: Clinical approach, pathophysiology, and treatment. Wien Klin Wochenschr 2000; 112:656-659.

systemic multiorgan disease; the presentation may be dominated by a single or a few clinical organ manifestations.[4]

Vasculitis can be separated into two broad categories. It may present de novo as a primary manifestation of vessel inflammation without a known cause. Alternatively, it may present as a secondary manifestation of an underlying disease or exposure to a drug. Distinction between primary and secondary vasculitis is essential because the pathophysiologic, prognostic, and therapeutic aspects differ.

Management of patients with the secondary forms of vasculitis needs to be directed toward the underlying disease process. The primary vasculitides, once thought to be uncommon, have proved to be much less rare than previously estimated, and there has been a recent increased awareness of the incidence and prevalence of all forms of vasculitis.[5] This chapter focuses on the primary or de novo vasculitides.

The pathophysiology of the vasculitis syndromes remains poorly understood. Variation between disease states contributes to the difficulty. It also is not clear why certain patients develop vasculitis in response to antigenic stimuli and others do not; however, in each disease state, immunologic mechanisms play an active role in mediating blood vessel inflammation.[1] There are three potential mechanisms of blood vessel damage (Box 106-2).[6]

Immune complex deposition in vessel walls is the most well known pathogenic mechanism of vasculitis, and results in tissue damage from that deposition. Complement components are then activated and infiltrate the vessel walls. The immune complexes are phagocytosed and release damaging enzymes. As the condition progresses and becomes subacute, the vessel lumen may become compromised leading to tissue ischemia.

BOX 106-2

Three Potential Mechanisms of Blood Vessel Damage in Vasculitis with Corresponding Diseases

Pathogenic Immune Complex Formation
- Henoch-Schönlein purpura
- Vasculitis associated with collagen vascular diseases
- Serum sickness
- Cutaneous vasculitic syndromes
- Hepatitis C/cryoglobulinemia
- Hepatitis B/polyarteritis nodosa

Antineutrophilic Cytoplasmic Antibodies
- Wegener's granulomatosis
- Churg-Strauss syndrome
- Microscopic polyangiitis

Pathogenic T-Lymphocyte Responses and Granuloma Formation
- Temporal arteritis
- Takayasu's arteritis
- Wegener's granulomatosis
- Churg-Strauss syndrome
- Kawasaki disease

From Fauci AS, Sneller MC: Pathogenesis of vasculitis syndromes. Med Clin North Am 1997;81:221-242.

Antineutrophil cytoplasmic antibodies (ANCA) develop in a large number of patients with systemic vasculitis, especially Wegener's granulomatosis. These antibodies attack proteins in the cytoplasm of neutrophils. Two main types of ANCA are differentiated by the different targets of the antibodies: *perinuclear ANCA,* or *p-ANCA,* attacks the enzyme myeloperoxidase; *cytoplasmic ANCA,* or *c-ANCA,* attacks the proteinase-3 enzyme.

The exact role of ANCA in the pathogenesis of vasculitis is unclear. Althugh a number of mechanisms have been proposed, confusion remains because many patients develop vasculitis without ANCA, there is a lack of correlation with the quantitative value of ANCA and disease activity, and many patients in remission continue to exhibit high ANCA titers.

Pathogenic T lymphocyte responses and granuloma formation may also be involved in damaging blood vessels. Delayed hypersensitivity and cell-mediated immune injury are the most common mechanisms in this category. Direct cellular toxicity or antibody-dependent cellular toxicity may also occur.

Two main factors are involved in the expression of a vasculitic syndrome: genetic predisposition and regulatory mechanisms associated with the immune response to antigens. Only certain types of immune complexes cause vasculitis, and the process may be selective for only certain vessel types. Other factors also are involved—for example, the reticuloendothelial system's ability to clear the immune complex, the size and properties of the complex, blood flow turbulence, intravascular hydrostatic pressure, and the preexisting integrity of the vessel endothelium.[3]

Clinical Presentation

The diagnosis of many vasculitic syndromes is based more on clinical presentation rather than laboratory results; therefore a detailed history and physical examination is an essential first step in the diagnosis.[7] A high index of suspicion is necessary. The diagnosis should be considered in any patient with systemic febrile illness with signs of organ ischemia without a direct explanation. Nonspecific symptoms such as weight loss, night sweats, and malaise are common. The vessels involved may correlate with specific symptoms displayed.[8]

Diagnostic Studies

▪ LABORATORY TESTS

The complete blood count may reveal leukocytosis, normocytic/normochromic anemia, and thrombocytosis. The C-reactive protein (CRP) and erythrocyte sedimentation rate (ESR) may be elevated. Complement levels may be low. Because of renal involvement, urinalysis may reveal proteinuria or active sediment. Cerebral spinal fluid findings in central nervous system vasculitis reveal an elevated protein.

▪ ANCA Testing

ANCA associated with Wegener's granulomatosis, first reported in 1985, is now an established entity in the evaluation of patients with suspected vasculitis. As with any diagnostic test, the predictive value of ANCA depends on the pretest probability of the disease. A negative test does not exclude the disease nor should the diagnosis of a vasculitic syndrome be made or treatment initiated based on a positive ANCA titer alone. There have been reports of positive titers of ANCA in patients with chronic infections and clinical features similar to systemic vasculitis. Therefore, caution is advised and testing for c-ANCA should not replace a tissue biopsy.

▪ BIOPSY AND ANGIOGRAPHY

The definitive diagnosis is dependent on demonstration of vascular involvement and may be accomplished by biopsy or angiography. A biopsy is preferred and should be directed toward tissue showing evidence of clinical involvement. The biopsy provides the distinct advantage of differentiating active versus chronic disease. This differentiation allows for appropriate treatment.

Angiography is an excellent diagnostic modality when medium and large vessels are involved and when visceral organ involvement is likely. This modality is the gold standard in the work-up of Takayasu's arteritis, for which a full evaluation of the aorta is recommended. Angiography demonstrates luminal patency but provides no information about cellular or tissue status. Early vessel inflammation may still be present in a fully patent vessel. On the other hand, vessel narrowing may also be due to fibrosis, not active disease.[8] Therefore, clinical correlation is advised with each angiographic finding.

▪ NONINVASIVE IMAGING

Noninvasive imaging modalities are useful in evaluating vessel wall changes not evident on angiography. They are associated with less morbidity than angiography and biopsy and have recently gained popularity in the serial evaluation and detection of early disease in vasculitis.

High-resolution ultrasonography is an efficient, noninvasive, and inexpensive method of following known cases of vasculitis. An example of clinical application is the evaluation of stenotic vessels of the carotid arteries. The progression, or hopefully resolution, with treatment of this pathology can also be followed with ultrasonography. This modality is limited by the fact that it cannot detect disease in all vessels, particularly the pulmonary, thoracic, and abdominal visceral vessels.

Computerized tomography (CT) can be useful to detect vessel wall thickening especially in early Takayasu's arteritis. CT angiography, high-resolution CT, and electron beam CT have all improved diagnostic outcomes. CT may also be used to evaluate sinus pathology or pulmonary lesions in Wegener's granulomatosis. To exclude infection, sarcoidosis, and malignancy, biopsies should follow CT when evaluating these lesions.

Magnetic resonance imaging (MRI) can be used to assess vessel wall thickening and has the advantage of axial, sagittal, and coronal plane views. Magnetic resonance angiography (MRA) correlates well with CT angiographic findings when evaluating the aorta or renal arteries. Further studies are needed before MRI/MRA can be considered first-choice diagnostic tools.

Positron emission tomography (PET) measures glucose metabolism in tissues. Increased glycolysis is seen in inactivated leukocytes and macrophages and is a hallmark of inflammation in certain vasculitides, especially giant cell artertitis.

Single-photon emission computed tomography (SPECT) uses multiplanar nuclear imaging to investigate perfusion abnormalities, especially when evaluating central nervous sytem vasculitis. Clinical correlation is necessary because perfusion defects may not distinguish vasculitis from entities such as vasospasm, thromboembolism, atherosclerosis, and malignant hypertension. SPECT may also be useful in evaluating the coronary arteries in Kawasaki disease.[8]

Treatment

The combination of clinical, laboratory, biopsy, and radiographic findings usually points to a specific syndrome (Table 106-1). Therapy should then be initiated as appropriate. If the vasculitis is associated with a specific disease such as neoplasm, infection, or connective tissue disease, the underlying disease should be treated. If the syndrome resolves, no further treatment is needed. If the syndrome persists, treatment for vasculitis should be initiated. Likewise, if an offending antigen is recognized, it should be removed if possible. No further treatment is needed if the syndrome resolves; however, if the syndrome continues, treatment must be initiated. Treatment initiated for a primary vasculitis syndrome should focus on using the most effective and least toxic options based on published experience.[9]

Individual vasculitis disorders are discussed in detail in the following section.

Temporal (Giant Cell) Arteritis

▪ DEFINITION, EPIDEMIOLOGY, AND PATHOPHYSIOLOGY

Temporal, or cranial or giant cell, arteritis is a granulomatous large-vessel vasculitis affecting the extracra-

Table 106-1 COMPARING THE VASCULITIDES

Vasculitides	Pathophysiology	Classic Features	Testing	Treatment
Temporal arteritis	Mononuclear cell infiltration and giant cell formation	Headache Scalp tenderness Visual disturbance	ESR CRP Biopsy	Prednisone
Takayasu's arteritis	Mononuclear cell infiltration and giant cell formation	Visual disturbance, chest pain, abdominal pain, differences in extremity blood pressure and pulses	Angiography	Prednisone Surgical or angiographic intervention
Polyarteritis nodosa	Polymorphonuclear infiltration	Fever, hypertension, myalgias, abdominal pain, hematuria, CHF, GI bleeding, orchitis	ESR, CRP Biopsy Angiography	Prednisone plus cyclophosphamide
Kawasaki disease	Polymorphonuclear infiltration	5-day fever, conjunctivitis, oral lesions, rash, red palms and soles, edema, cervical lymphadenopathy	ESR, CRP Leukocytosis Thrombocytosis Echocardiography	Aspirin plus IV gamma globulin
Wegener's granulomatosis	Granuloma formation secondary to aggregating neutrophils	Upper and lower respiratory symptoms, renal insufficiency, skin lesions, visual disturbance	ESR CRP c-ANCA	Cyclophosphamide plus prednisone
Churg-Strauss syndrome	Eosinophilic infiltration Allergic granulomas	Allergic rhinitis Nasal polyps Asthma	Leukocytosis Eosinophilia ESR, CRP Biopsy	Prednisone plus or minus cyclophosphamide
Henoch-Schönlein purpura	IgA complex deposition	Palpable purpura, arthralgias, GI disturbances, glomerulonephritis	Leukocytosis Eosinophilia IgA elevation Skin biopsy	Usually self-limited Prednisone if necessary
Cryoglobulinemic vasculitis	Cold precipitable monoclonal or polyclonal immunoglobulins	Palpable purpura, glomerulonephritis, myalgias, weakness, peripheral neuropathy	Low complement levels Hepatitis C Renal biopsy	Interferon-alpha plus ribaviron
Cuntaneous leukocytoclastic vasculitis	Neutrophilic infiltration Mononuclear and eosinophilic infiltration	Palpable purpura, macules, vesicles, bullae, urticaria	Skin biopsy	Prednisone
Behçet's syndrome	Polymorphonuclear infiltration	Recurrent oral aphthous ulcers, genital ulcers, skin lesions, visual disturbance	ESR, CRP Leukocytosis Oral mucosa auto antibodies	Topical glucocorticoids Prednisone

c-ANCA, cytoplasmic antineutrophil cytoplasmic antibodies; CHF, congestive heart failure; CRP, C-reactive protein; ESR, erythrocyte sedimentation rate; GI, gastrointestinal; IgA, immunoglobulin A; IV, intravenous.

nial branches of the carotid artery, particularly the temporal artery. Females are affected two to four times more often than males; the disorder usually occurs in patients older than 55 years. Its incidence is estimated to be 1 per 3000 patients over 50 years. Up to 59% of the time it is associated with polymyalgia rheumatica, which is characterized by pain and stiffness in the shoulders, neck, and pelvis along with an elevated ESR.

Giant cell arteritis is a panarteritis with inflammatory mononuclear cell infiltrates and giant cell formation in vessel walls. The intima proliferates and the internal elastic lamina fragments. Organ pathology results from ischemia related to the involved vessel derangement.[3]

▪ CLINICAL PRESENTATION

Patients present with local symptoms related to the arteries involved. Headache, scalp tenderness associated with the inflamed temporal artery (Fig. 106-1), jaw claudication, and visual disturbances are typical. Symptoms associated with polymyalgia rheumatica are frequently displayed. Constitutional symptoms such as fever, malaise, fatigue, anorexia, weight loss, arthralgias, and night sweats are also common.

The most serious complication is ocular involvement due to ischemic optic neuropathy. This may lead to blindness; however, vision loss usually is avoided with proper treatment. A later complication may be an aortic aneurysm.[10-12]

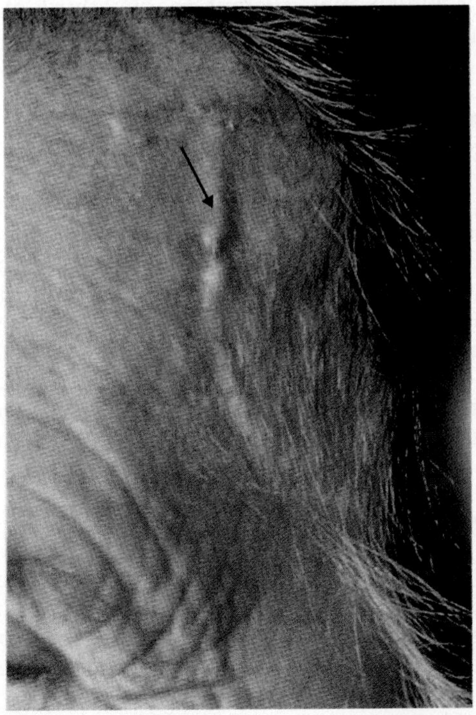

FIGURE 106-1 Temporal artery inflammation. (From Kumar V [ed]: Robbins and Cotran Pathologic Basis of Disease, 7th ed. Philadelphia, Saunders, 2005.)

▪ DIAGNOSTIC STUDIES AND DIFFERENTIAL DIAGNOSIS

Classic laboratory manifestations include elevated ESR and CRP. Normochromic anemia and thrombocytosis due to the chronic inflammation are common. Liver function abnormalities, particularly an elevated alkaline phosphatase, are common.

The diagnosis can be determined clinically because of the classic scenario of headache, fever, anemia, and an elevated ESR. A temporal artery biopsy is confirmatory. Because involvement of the vessel may not be contiguous, several separate biopsies may be needed. Color duplex ultrasonography, angiography, or magnetic resonance imaging may play a role in making the diagnosis. A rapid clinical response to treatment also confirms the diagnosis.

▪ TREATMENT AND DISPOSITION

Treatment should commence immediately and not be delayed by diagnostic procedures. Administration of 40 to 60 mg of prednisone daily for 1 month is followed by a taper to 7.5 to to 10 mg daily. This should be continued for 1 to 2 years to prevent relapse. Disease activity is monitored by clinical symptoms and ESR.

Prognosis is good; the majority of cases go into remission and remain in remission after discontinuation of steroids. Patients with severe disease or impending vision loss should be hospitalized and given high dose intravenous steroids.

Takayasu's Arteritis

▪ DEFINITION, EPIDEMIOLOGY, AND PATHOPHYSIOLOGY

Takayasu's arteritis (also referred to as aortic arch syndrome) is a granulomatous large-vessel vasculitis primarily affecting the aorta, its branches, and pulmonary and coronary arteries.[1] This is a rare disease that predominantly affects females in the 20- to 30-year age group and is more common in Asian and South American patients. The inflammation involves all vessel wall layers of medium- and large-sized vessels, especially the aorta and its branches. Panarteritis with inflammatory mononuclear cell infiltrates and giant cells predominates. This results in scarring and fibrosis with disruption and degeneration of the elastic lamina. Narrowing of the vessel lumen (Fig. 106-2) follows with frequent thrombosis.[3] Vessel dilation and formation of aneurysms may also occur. Organ pathology results from ischemia.

▪ CLINICAL PRESENTATION

Patients present with ischemic symptoms of the involved vessels, including visual problems, faint or absent pulses in the upper extremities, and myocardial, abdominal, and lower extremity ischemia. Dif-

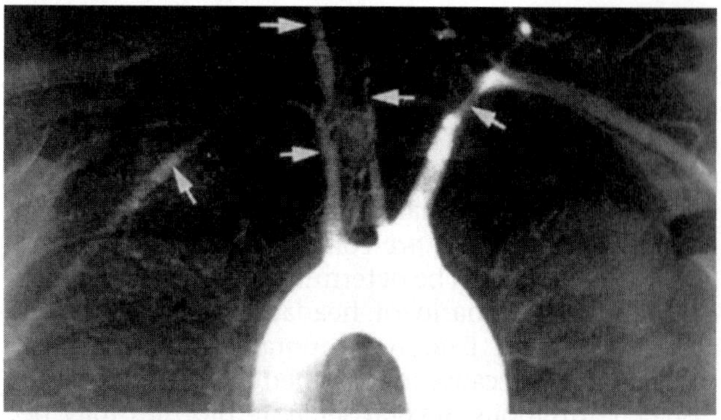

FIGURE 106-2 Aortic arch angiogram of aortic arch showing narrowing of brachiocephalic, carotid, and subclavian arteries (*arrows*). (From Kumar V [ed]: Robbins and Cotran Pathologic Basis of Disease, 7th ed. Philadelphia, Saunders, 2005.)

ferences in extremity blood pressures and bruits may also be present. Up to 40% of patients may experience systemic symptoms such as fever, malaise, night sweats, arthralgias, myalgias, weight loss, and anorexia. Death usually occurs from congestive heart failure or stoke. The course may be progressive and unremitting and become fulminant or may stabilize into remission.[3] Mortality ranges from 10% to 75%.

▪ DIAGNOSTIC STUDIES AND DIFFERENTIAL DIAGNOSIS

Laboratory findings during active disease include elevated ESR and CRP Levels.[4] Angiography demonstrates stenosis, occlusion, dilation, and aneurysms of the aorta and its branches. The entire aorta should be visualized to fully appreciate the spectrum of this disease.[3] Spiral computed tomography/angiography and magnetic resonance angiography have been shown to be useful.

The diagnosis should be suspected in any young woman with the systemic signs and symptoms previously described and with any blood pressure or pulse discrepancies or bruits. Establishment of the diagnosis must then be obtained by radiologic procedures.

▪ TREATMENT AND DISPOSITION

Treatment consists of the combination of 40 to 60 mg per day of prednisone with aggressive surgical or angiographic procedures directed toward stenotic vessels. This approach corrects hypertension due to renal artery stenosis, improves blood flow in ischemic vessels, and decreases stroke risk,[3] resulting in decreased morbidity and improved survival. It is the best practice but not always possible to control vascular inflammation with prednisone prior to any surgical procedures. Hospital admission for diagnostic testing and treatment should be considered for suspected cases.

Polyarteritis Nodosa

▪ DEFINITION, EPIDEMIOLOGY, AND PATHOPHYSIOLOGY

Polyarteritis nodosa is a multisystem necrotizing vasculitis of small- and medium-sized muscular arteries. Visceral and renal artery involvement is characteristic.[3] The mean age of onset is 50 years, although it can occur at any age. Men, women, and racial groups are all affected equally. This rare disease affects less than 10 per 1 million persons worldwide.

The inflammatory lesions are segmental and involve the bifurcations and branches of the arteries. Polymorphonuclear neutrophils infiltrate all layers of the vessel wall. This results in intimal proliferation with degeneration of the vessel wal, leading to vascular necrosis, which in turn results in thrombosis, compromised blood flow, and infarction of the involved tissues and organs. Characteristic aneurismal dilations of up to 1 centimeter are common. Multiple organ systems are involved.[3]

▪ CLINICAL PRESENTATION

The most common symptoms are fever, hypertension, myalgias, arthralgias, weight loss, malaise, and headache. Renal involvement evolves as flank pain, hematuria, renovascular hypertension, and renal failure. Skin lesions range from subcutaneous nodules to distal ischemia. Gastrointestinal manifestations include pain, malabsorption, bleeding, and perforation. Congestive heart failure secondary to coronary artery vasculitis may occur. A classic symptom is orchitis which may present in one third of male patients.[4]

▪ DIAGNOSTIC STUDIES AND DIFFERENTIAL DIAGNOSIS

There are no diagnostic serologic tests for polyarteritis nodosa, and laboratory findings are nonspecific; ESR, CRP, and leukocytes are elevated. Normochromic anemia is present, indicating chronic disease. The diagnosis may be achieved via biopsy demonstrating histologic necrotizing inflammation in the arteries. If a biopsy is not possible, angiography demonstrating microaneurysms, stenosis, or sequential narrowing and dilation suggests the diagnosis.

▪ TREATMENT AND DISPOSITION

Combination therapy of prednisone (1 mg/kg/day) and cyclophosphamide (2 mg/kg/day) has resulted in a long-term remission rate of 90% after therapy has been discontinued. Glucocorticoids alone may be used alone in mild cases. Discharge home with follow-up is appropriate unless there is evidence of end-organ failure.

Kawasaki Disease

▪ DEFINITION AND EPIDEMIOLOGY

Kawasaki disease, also referred to as mucocutaneous lymph node syndrome, primarily affects children less than 5 years of age. This acute systemic vasculitis is a febrile multisystem disease that is the leading cause of acquired heart disease in children in the United States.[1] The disease occurs worldwide but predominates in Japan, Asia, and the United States.

▪ CLINICAL PRESENTATION

The characteristic clinical features of Kawasaki disease are a fever for at least 5 days, conjunctivitis, oral mucosa changes, a generalized rash, red palms and soles, indurative edema with subsequent skin desquamation, and cervical lymph adenopathy.[4] The presence of five of these symptoms confirms the diagnosis. Of course, atypical cases with fewer symptoms occur.

▪ DIAGNOSTIC STUDIES AND DIFFERENTIAL DIAGNOSIS

Echocardiography and angiography confirm the cardiac complications and vasculitis. Laboratory findings include elevated leukocytes, platelets, ESR, and CRP.

Although the disease is generally benign and self-limited, coronary artery aneurysms occur in 20% to 30% of cases, usually during the 3rd or 4th week as convalescence ensues. Four symptoms along with coronary artery aneurysms are diagnostic. Case fatality rate secondary to coronary artery aneurysm is 0.5% to 2.8%. As in other vasculitides, there is typical intimal proliferation and infiltration of the vessel wall with mononuclear cells, leading to bead-like aneurysms and thrombosis. Although a strong predilection for the coronary arteries is seen, this vasculitis is systemic and may involve medium-sized arteries with corresponding manifestations. Cardiomegaly, pericarditis, myocarditis, myocardial ischemia, and infarction may result.[3]

▪ TREATMENT AND DISPOSITION

Except for rare fatal cardiac complications, prognosis is good, with a typical full recovery.[3] Treatment consists of high-dose IV gamma globulin (2 g/kg over 10 hours) concurrently with aspirin (80 to 100 mg/kg/day for 2 weeks followed by 3 to 5 mg/kg/day for several more weeks). Early therapy has proven beneficial in the reduction of coronary artery abnormalities. Children who develop aneurysms require close follow-up after discharge, and some patients with severe disease may need long-term anticoagulation.

Wegener's Granulomatosis

▪ DEFINITION, EPIDEMIOLOGY, AND PATHOPHYSIOLOGY

Wegener's granulomatosis is a vasculitis of the upper and lower respiratory tract and kidneys. A systemic small-vessel vasculitis also is involved. This disease may occur at any age but has a mean onset at 40 years of age. It affects men and women equally and involves whites more commonly than blacks.

The pathology involves a necrotizing vasculitis of small vessels with granuloma formation. The typical necrotizing granulomatous vasculitis in the lungs commonly leads to scarring, atelectasis, and obstruction. Upper airways also become inflamed, with necrosis and granuloma formation. Renal involvement is that of a focal and segmental glomerulonephritis that may become rapidly progressive. Few or no immune complexes are found on biopsy; the involvement of immunopathology is unclear. A large number of these patients develop c-ANCA, but this correlation is not clear.[3] Besides the typical sinus, lung, and kidney involvement, other organs may be affected, because Wegener's granulomatosis is a systemic small-vessel vasculitis.

▪ CLINICAL PRESENTATION

The characteristic presentation involves symptoms in the upper and/or lower airways for a prolonged period before the disease becomes systemic. Up to 90% of patients seek medical attention for sinus or pulmonary problems earlier.[1] Upper respiratory symptoms include pain, purulent or bloody drainage, ulcerations, hoarseness, stridor, and deafness. Pulmonary findings manifest as cough, dyspnea, chest pain, and hemoptysis, which may become severe. Pulmonary nodules, infiltrates, or cavitations may be seen on chest radiographs. Hypoxemia ensues when the lungs become affected.

Other manifestations include ocular inflammation ranging from conjunctivitis, episcleritis, and scleritis to retinal vasculitis and retro-orbital masses. Skin lesions may appear as ulcerations, subcutaneous nodules, or purpura with necrosis. Central nervous system symptoms stem from infarction, cranial nerve neuropathy, and mononeuritis multiplex. Bowel perforation and bleeding may be symptoms of gastrointestinal involvement; pericarditis, coronary ischemia, and cardiomegaly may signal cardiac involvement.[3] Vague symptoms such as malaise, weakness, arthralgia, fever, and anorexia are common.

Glomerulonephritis is present in 20% of patients at the time of diagnosis and develops in 80% at some point as the disease progresses. If not treated properly, renal involvement accounts for most mortality.

▪ DIAGNOSTIC STUDIES AND DIFFERENTIAL DIAGNOSIS

Laboratory findings include an elevated ESR and CRP, anemia with leukocytosis, thrombocytosis, and positive tests for ANCA, which is seen especially when the kidneys are affected.

The diagnosis is made by biopsy demonstrating necrotizing granulomatous vasculitis with an aggregation of neutrophils in nonrenal tissue. The renal biopsy reveals focal, segmental, necrotizing, crescentic glomerulonephritis.[4] Biopsy findings coincide with the characteristic clinical findings of sinus, pulmonary, and renal symptoms. Although the use of ANCA testing is only adjunctive, the specificity is 90% for Wegener's granulomatosis if active glomerulonephritis is present.

▪ TREATMENT AND DISPOSITION

Outpatient management is appropriate except in cases of advanced end-organ involvement. The administration of cyclophosphamide (2 mg/kg/day) combined with prednisone (1mg/kg/day) has proved to be the most successful therapy. Reported results are 75% complete remission, 80% survival, and 91% marked improvement.[1] Although very effective, cyclophosphamide may be associated with severe bone marrow toxicity. Leukocytes must be monitored closely and kept above 3000 U/L.

Full-dose cyclophosphamide therapy should be continued for 1 year after remission and then tapered off. Prednisone therapy may be changed to alternate-day administration after 1 month and then tapered off by 6 months.[3] Methotrexate has shown some success in patients who cannot tolerate cyclophosphamide.

Upon achievement of remission, long term follow-up is essential. Up to 50% of patients have one or more relapses. With close follow-up and immediate reinstitution of therapy, reinduction of remission is almost always a success. Many patients, especially those with multiple relapses, develop some degree of long-term morbidity such as renal insufficiency, tracheal stenosis, hearing loss, or sinus impairment.[3] Aggressive prompt therapy during the initial manifestation of the disease as well as during relapses helps diminish the degree of chronic morbidity.

Churg-Strauss Syndrome

▪ DEFINITION, EPIDEMIOLOGY, AND PATHOPHYSIOLOGY

Churg-Strauss syndrome is a rare small-vessel vasculitis manifested by fever, asthma, and hypereosinophilia.[1] This disease also referred to as allergic angiitis and granulomatosis, particularly when it affects the lungs.

It is estimated that about 3 million people are affected worldwide, with incidence occurring equally between sexes. It is seen in all ages with a mean onset of 44 years of age.

The characteristic histopathologic features include tissue infiltration by eosinophils, necrotizing small vessel vasculitis, and extravascular "allergic" granulomas.[1] The process can occur in any organ, but lung involvement predominates, with a strong association with asthma. The combination of asthma, eosinophilia, granulomas, and vasculitis strongly suggests a hypersensitivity reaction as the triggering factor.[3]

▪ CLINICAL PRESENTATION

Symptoms such as fever, anorexia, malaise, and weight loss suggest a multisystem disease. Churg-Strauss syndrome has three identifiable phases. It begins with a prodrome of allergic rhinitis, nasal polyps, and asthma. The next phase includes a peripheral eosinophilia and eosinophilic tissue infiltrates, especially in the lungs. The third phase consists of a systemic vasculitis involving the lungs, heart, kidneys, central nervous system, and gastrointestinal tract. These phases may not occur in sequence and may not be seen in all patients.

The disease is best known for its severe and frequent exacerbations of asthma and relapsing vasculitis.[1] The asthma associated with Churg-Strauss syndrome is not a classic allergic asthma that begins early in life; rather, it begins later in life around age 35 years. It is severe, and patients frequently becoming steroid-dependent.[4]

▪ DIAGNOSTIC STUDIES AND DIFFERENTIAL DIAGNOSIS

Classic laboratory findings include leukocytosis with notable eosinophilia, anemia, and elevated ESR and CRP. Diagnosis is confirmed via biopsy in a patient with the characteristic clinical manifestations.

▪ TREATMENT AND DISPOSITION

Outpatient management is appropriate except in cases of advanced end-organ involvement. The prognosis for untreated cases is a 25% 5-year survival rate; this improves to 50% with proper treatment.[1] The most effective therapy is prednisone (1 mg/kg/day). The vasculitis usually remits more readily than the asthma, which may remain moderate to severe, making discontinuation of prednisone therapy difficult.[1] Cyclophospamide at 2 mg/kg/day may be added to the prednisone in cases not responsive to prednisone alone.

Henoch-Schönlein Purpura

▪ DEFINITION, EPIDEMIOLOGY, AND PATHOPHYSIOLOGY

Henoch-Schönlein purpura (anaphylactoid purpura) is a small-vessel vasculitis predominately affecting children and characterized by palpable purpura, arthralgia, glomerulonephritis, and gastrointestinal symptoms.[3] Although also seen in adults, 75% of cases occur in children younger than 8 years of age. It is more common than other vasculitides and affects males to females in a 2:1 ratio. It has a peak incidence in winter and spring and usually follows an upper respiratory tract infection.

Henoch-Schönlein purpura is an immune complex disease with deposition of immunoglobulin A (IgA)–containing complexes. Suggested but unproved inciting antigens include upper respiratory infections, foods, drugs, insect bites, and vaccinations.[3]

▪ CLINICAL PRESENTATION

The classic clinical picture includes four cardinal manifestations—palpable purpura, arthralgias, gastrointestinal involvement, and glomerulonephritis. The palpable purpura occurs in nearly all cases and presents most commonly over the buttocks and legs (Fig. 106-3). Most patients also develop polyarthralgias. Gastrointestinal symptoms include abdominal pain with nausea, vomiting, diarrhea, constipation, and occasional gastrointestinal bleeding.

Renal disease is characterized by a mild glomerulonephritis with hematuria and proteinuria. Glomerulonephritis is seen in 20% to 50% of patients, with 2% to 5% progressing to end-stage renal disease.[1]

▪ DIAGNOSTIC STUDIES AND DIFFERENTIAL DIAGNOSIS

Laboratory studies are nonspecific and may reveal a mild leukocytosis and occasional eosinophilia. Serum IgA levels are elevated in 50% of patients.[3] The diagnosis remains a clinical diagnosis based on the characteristic presentation. A skin biopsy occasionally is necessary needed for confirmation and reveals leukocytoclastic vasculitis with IgA immune deposition. Renal biopsy better serves as a prognostic indicator.[1]

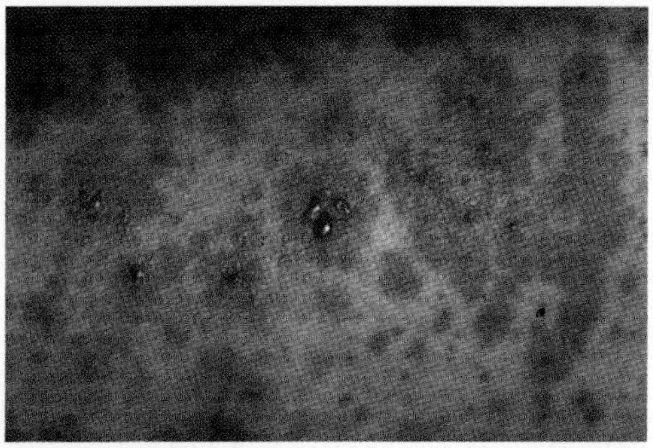

FIGURE 106-3 Palpable purpura in a patient with Henoch-Schönlein purpura. (From Hoffman R, Benz EJ Jr, Shatttil SJ, et al [eds]: Hematology: Basic Principles and Practice, 4th ed. Philadelphia, Saunders, 2005.)

▪ TREATMENT AND DISPOSITION

Although renal failure is the most common cause of death, Henoch-Schönlein purpura usually resolves without therapy. In general, the disease is self-limited with an excellent prognosis for a full recovery in as little as a few weeks.

However, when required, prednisone at 1 mg/kg/day is effective in lessening tissue edema, arthralgias, and abdominal pain. The dose should be tapered as symptoms abate. Glucocorticoids have no proven benefit on skin and renal involvement and have not been shown to shorten the disease or prevent relapse.[3]

All aspects of the disease are more serious when an adult is affected.

Cryoglobulinemic Vasculitis

▪ DEFINITION AND PATHOPHYSIOLOGY

Cryoglobulinemic vasculitis is an entity of cold-precipitable monoclonal or polyclonal immunoglobulins that can induce a general vasculitic or renal injury depending on the rapidity, severity, and site of immunoglobulin deposition. The immune deposits, which affect small vessels, occur in a variety of disease processes including as plasma cell and lymphoid neoplasms, chronic infections, and inflammatory diseases. It has been found that the majority of cases are related to hepatitis C virus infectivity.[1]

▪ CLINICAL PRESENTATION

Clinical features frequently overlap with those of other small-vessel vasculitides. Common findings include palpable purpura, glomerulonephritis, arthralgias, myalgias, weakness, malaise, and peripheral neuropathy. The disorder frequently is evident in the skin as palpable purpura; transitions to chronic ulcerations usually occur in the lower extremities above the malleoli.[13] Another feature suggesting cryoglobulinemic vasculitis is Raynaud's phenomenon.

▪ DIAGNOSTIC STUDIES AND DIFFERENTIAL DIAGNOSIS

Low complement levels and concurrent hepatitis C infection are indicative. A renal biopsy is very useful in making the diagnosis of cryoglobulinemic vasculitis; the specific lesion of a type-1 membranoproliferative glomerulonephritis is often found on renal biopsy.[14]

■ TREATMENT

Treatment consists of combination therapy with interferon alfa and ribavirin. Because a high prevalence of hepatitis C virus is known to be present in cryoglobulinemic vasculitis patients, the primary treatment has moved away from the typical glucocorticoid and cyclophospamide combination because the immunosuppressive effects of this therapy may lead to an increase in hepatitis C viral load. However, immunosuppressive drugs may be needed on a short-term basis in patients with a severe inflammatory reaction to the disease. In addition, short-term plasmapheresis may be necessary in severe, rapidly progressive cases.[1] Hospital admission for diagnostic testing and initiation of therapy may be necessary.

Weaning from the immunosuppressive drugs as soon as possible is advantageous because patients do best when a positive virologic response is obtained. Long-term combination interferon alpha/ribavirin therapy usually is necessary.

Cutaneous Leukocytoclastic Vasculitis

■ DEFINITION, EPIDEMIOLOGY, AND PATHOPHYSIOLOGY

This disorder, also called hypersensitivity vasculitis or predominantly cutaneous vasculitis, involves small vessels of the skin and is the most common vasculitic manifestation seen in clinical practice.[1] It has an incidence of 15 per one million.[4] In about 70% of cases, cutaneous vasculitis occurs along with an underlying process such as infection, malignancy, medication exposure, and connective tissue disease or as a secondary manifestation of a primary systemic vasculitide.

The pathology predominantly involves small vessels, especially postcapillary venules. Acutely, neutrophils infiltrate the vessels causing destruction and resulting in nuclear debris; thus the term *leukocytoclastic*. As the process becomes more chronic, mononuclear cells and eosinophils become involved. Erythrocytes frequently extravasate, causing a classic palpable purpura, which is a hallmark of the disease.[3]

■ CLINICAL PRESENTATION

Clinically, besides purpura, patients may exhibit macules, papules, vesicles, bullae, subcutaneous nodules, or urticaria. The skin usually becomes pruritic and painful and the lesions may progress to ulcers. Although the skin is predominantly involved, patients may exhibit systemic symptoms such as myalgias, fever, anorexia, and malaise.[3] The course of the disease ranges from a brief single episode to multiple prolonged recurrences with infrequent progression to systemic vasculitis.

■ DIAGNOSTIC STUDIES AND DIFFERENTIAL DIAGNOSIS

Laboratory values are usually within normal limits, including ESR and CRP levels. Mild leukocytosis and eosinophilia may be present. Laboratory studies should be used primarily to rule out the presence of systemic vasculitis. Minimal to no signs of inflammation should be found.[4] The diagnosis is made by skin biopsy and by carefully ruling out systemic disease or exogenous reasons for the vasculitis.

The clinical and histopathologic appearance of the lesions is indistinguishable from the cutaneous manifestations of the systemic vasculitides; therefore, the diagnosis should be one of exclusion after other causes have been ruled out.[2] Only then can the disorder be called true cutaneous leukocytoclastic vasculitis or idiopathic cutaneous vasculitis.

■ TREATMENT

If an underlying process is discovered as the cause of the cutaneous symptoms, treatment should be aimed at the underlying process. If an exogenous agent is the culprit, its removal usually results in remission of the skin process. If true cutaneous leukocytoclastic vasculitis is determined to be the etiology, glucocorticoids at 1 mg/kg/day have proved effective.[3]

Often the disease is self-limited; otherwise, it usually responds very rapidly to steroid therapy. Some symptomatic agents may be used on occasion, such as antihistamines, nonsteroidal antiinflammatory drugs, and colchicine. In the rare scenario where glucocorticoids are not effective, cytotoxic agents such as methotrexate, azothioprine, and cyclophosphamide may be used, but these should be reserved for severe cases. This disorder may be managed on an outpatient basis.

Behçet's Syndrome

■ DEFINITION, EPIDEMIOLOGY, AND PATHOPHYSIOLOGY

Behçet's syndrome is a multisystem inflammatory disease that affects vessels of all sizes.[1] It presents with recurrent aphthous oral and genital ulcerations along with ocular involvement. It is most prevalent at ages 20 to 35 years, with males suffering more severe disease. The main pathology is vasculitis with a tendency to form venous thrombi.

■ CLINICAL PRESENTATION

Patients present with painful ulcers that occur as one ulcer or multiple ulcers that last for 1 to 2 weeks and resolve without scars. Besides oral ulcers, patients with Behçet's syndrome may exhibit two or more of the following signs or symptoms: recurrent genital ulcers, skin lesions, eye lesions, and a positive pathergy test.[1]

Tips and Tricks

- Although antineutrophil cytoplasmic antibodies (ANCA) are quite common in vasculitis, their role is not clear. ANCA testing may actually confuse the diagnostic picture when results are negative in a patient with clinical vasculitis, when there is a lack of quantitative correlation with disease activity, and when high titers are found in patients whose disease has fallen into remission.
- Vision loss associated with temporal arteritis may be prevented with immediate and proper treatment. If there are any signs of this complication, do not delay treatment because permanent vision loss may ensue.
- Patients with Wegener's granulomatosis often have prolonged signs and symptoms of upper and/or lower airway dysfunction. 90% of these patients have previous presentations for sinus problems that become chronic. A high index of suspicion is required.
- The asthma of Churg-Strauss syndrome is a severe condition that usually begins when the patient is about 35 years of age. With treatment, the vasculitis commonly subsides much more readily than the asthma.

The genital ulcers resemble the oral ulcers. Skin lesions range from erythema nodosum and folliculitis to a general inflammatory exanthem. The ocular manifestations usually present at onset of the disease but may develop later in the first few years. Iritis, posterior uveitis, retinal artery and vein occlusions, and optic neuritis may be seen. Hypopyon uveitis is rare but is pathognomonic for the disease. The ocular involvement may lead to blindness.

Other symptoms include mild arthritis of the lower extremity joints, gastrointestinal inflammation, and ulcerations. Central nervous system manifestations include meningoencephalitis, benign intracranial hypertension, multiple sclerosis–like symptoms and psychiatric disturbances. Large venous or arterial thrombi or occlusions occur in 25% to 38% of patients.[1,3] Pulmonary emboli are possible.

▪ DIAGNOSTIC STUDIES AND DIFFERENTIAL DIAGNOSIS

Laboratory findings indicate nonspecific inflammation such as leukocytosis and elevated ESR and CRP levels. Half of patients are found to have autoantibodies to human oral mucous membranes. The diagnosis is based on the clinical findings of recurrent aphthous oral ulcerations.

▪ TREATMENT

Treatment is based on disease manifestations. Oral and skin lesions respond well to topical glucocorticoids, dapsone, or colchicine. Thrombophlebitis is treated with aspirin. Ocular and central nervous system manifestations require aggressive treatment with immunosuppression utilizing glucocorticoids, azothioprine, or cyclosporine.[1] Treatment may be managed on an outpatient basis unless ocular or central nervous system manifestations are evident upon presentation.

REFERENCES

1. Fauci AS: The vasculitis syndromes. In Harrison TR: Harrison's Principles of Internal Medicine, 15th ed. New York, McGraw-Hill, 2001, pp 1956-1958.
2. Stegeman CA, Kallenberg CG: Clinical aspects of primary vasculitis. Springer Semin Immunopathol 2001;23: 231-251.
3. Luqmani RA, Robinson H: Introduction to, and classification of, the systemic vasculitides. Best Pract Res Clin Rheumatol 2001;15:187-202.
4. Langford CA: Vasculitis. J Allergy Clin Immunol 2003;111(2 Suppl):S602-S612.
5. Savage OS: The evolving pathogensis of systemic vasculitis. Clin Med 2002;2:458-464.
6. Kallenberg CG: Vasculitis: Clinical approach, pathophysiology and treatment. Wien Klin Wochenschr 2000; 112:656-659.
7. Fauci AS, Sneller MC: Pathogenesis of vasculitis syndromes. Med Clin North Am 1997;81:221-242.
8. McLaren JS, McRorie ER, Luqmani RA: Diagnosis and assessment of systemic vasculitis. Clin Exp Rheumatol 2002;20:854-862.
9. Mohan N, Kerr GS: Diagnosis of vasculitis. Best Res Pract Clin Rheumatol 2001;15:203-223.
10. Langford CA: Management of systemic vasculitis. Best Pract Res Clini Rheumatol 2001;15:281-297.
11. Seo P, Stone JH: Large-vessel vasculitis. Arthritis Rheum 2004;51:128–139.
12. Younger DS: Headaches and vasculitis. Neurol Clin 2004;22:207–228.
13. Younger DS: Vasculitis of the nervous system. Curr Opin Neurol 2004;17:317-336.
14. Sansonno D, Dammacco F: Hepatitis C virus, cryoglobulinaemia, and vasculitis. Immune complex relations. Lancet Infect Dis 2005;5:227-236.
15. Jennette JC, Falk RJ: Overview of the nomenclature and diagnostic categorization of vasculitis. Wien Klin Wochenschr 2000;112:650-655.

SECTION XI

Genitourinary and Renal Diseases

Chapter **107**

Male Genitourinary Emergencies

Jonathan E. Davis

KEY POINTS

There are five major male genitourinary emergencies: testicular torsion, Fournier's disease (necrotizing fasciitis of the perineum), priapism, paraphimosis, and genitourinary tract trauma.

Ultrasound examination is the primary diagnostic tool for differentiation of causes of acute scrotal pain.

Urology services should be consulted immediately after initial patient evaluation when testicular torsion is suspected.

When a patient has pain out of proportion to findings on the physical examination, a necrotic or ischemic cause should be suspected. For example, the appearance of physical findings in Fournier's disease indicates advanced disease, at which point treatment may not mitigate morbidity and mortality.

A trial of terbutaline (a beta-adrenergic agonist) is a first-line ED treatment for priapism.

Successful reduction of paraphimosis can often be performed without specialty consultation.

A urologist should be consulted in all but the most minor cases of genitourinary trauma.

Anatomy and Pathophysiology

The male genitalia is composed of the penis, with paired erectile bodies and penile urethra, and the scrotum, which encases the testis, epididymis, and spermatic cord bilaterally. Beneath the scrotal skin are the dartos muscle and fascia, which is contiguous with the fascia of the abdomen (Scarpa's fascia), perineum (Colles' fascia), and penis (dartos fascia). The spermatic fascia lies beneath the dartos fascia; it has three layers, with the middle layer forming the cremasteric muscle. These anatomic layers may provide a conduit for the rapid spread of infection.

The fibrous capsule of the tunica albuginea surrounds the testes. A break in the integrity of the tunica albuginea represents a "ruptured" testicle, which can be caused by blunt trauma. External to the testicular parenchyma and tunica albuginea is the tunica vaginalis, which envelops each testicle and fastens it to the posterior scrotal wall.

The scrotal ligament (gubernaculum) anchors each testicle inferiorly, providing additional stability. The tunica vaginalis consists of both visceral (contiguous with the tunica albuginea) and parietal leaves, with an interposed potential space. The significance of this potential space is that a lack of firm attachment of the testicle to the posterior scrotal wall makes the testis prone to rotation in a horizontal plane about the spermatic cord within the tunica vaginalis, a condition termed *testicular torsion*.

The testicular artery originates from the aorta, typically just below or directly from the renal artery. The spermatic cord contains both the blood supply to each testicle (via the gonadal vessels) and the vas deferens (described later). Interruption of blood flow to the testis by twisting the spermatic cord can lead to rapid ischemia and subsequent infarction of the affected testicle in cases of testicular torsion.

The appendix testes are embryologic remnants with no known physiologic function, located at the uppermost pole of the testes. These appendages are prone to torsion as well, leading to localized, self-limited necrosis. This results in pain that can be confused with that of testicular torsion.

The epididymis is a fine tubular structure that adheres closely to the posterolateral aspect of each testis. It is involved in promoting sperm maturation and motility. Similar to the appendix testes, the appendix epididymis is an embryologic remnant (with no known function) attached to the head of each epididymis. These too are prone to torsion, similarly leading to localized necrosis of the appendage.

The vas deferens is a tubular structure involved in sperm transit, extending from the epididymis distally to the prostatic portion of the urethra proximally.

The penis consists of the corpora cavernosa (erectile bodies), and the corpus spongiosum, which surrounds the urethra. In uncircumcised males, the retractile penile foreskin covers the glans. The potential constricting effect of proximally retracted foreskin may lead to *paraphimosis*. In paraphimosis, glans venous engorgement and edema resulting from constriction can potentially progress to arterial compromise and gangrene of the distal penis. Each corpus cavernosum is surrounded by a dense connective tissue layer (also termed the tunica albuginea).

Priapism is a pathologic condition defined as the presence of a persistent erection lasting longer than 4 hours in the absence of sexual desire or stimulation. It most frequently results from engorgement of the corpora cavernosa with stagnant blood (termed low-flow priapism). Box 107-1 lists some etiologies of low-flow priapism.

High-flow priapism is rare and results from the development of traumatic arterial-cavernosal fistulae, resulting in the accumulation of oxygen-rich blood in the corpora.

BOX 107-1

Selected Etiologies of Low-Flow Priapism

Medications

- Impotence treatments
  - Intracavernosal therapies (prostaglandin E_1, papaverine, phentolamine)
  - Oral agents (sildenafil)
- Antihypertensives
  - Hydralazine, prazosin, doxazosin
- Antidepressants
  - Trazadone, fluoxetine, sertraline, citalopram
- Antipsychotics
  - Phenothiazines, atypical antipsychotics
- Illicit substances
  - Cocaine, marijuana
- General anesthetics
- Miscellaneous
  - Hydroxyzine, metoclopramide, omeprazole
  - Total parenteral nutrition

Hematologic Disorders

- Sickle cell disease
- Leukemia
- Myeloma

Central Nervous System

- Brain
  - Cerebrovascular accident
- Spinal cord
  - Spinal stenosis, spinal cord injury, lumbar disc herniation

Others

- Infections
  - Malaria, rabies
- Toxins
  - Black widow spider, scorpion
- Carbon monoxide
- Hypertriglyceridemia
- Idiopathic

Clinical Presentation

Genitourinary complaints often are influenced by patient embarrassment and apprehension; this is especially true in children and adolescents. Complaints of abdominal pain, fever, or nausea may be offered by the patient, but information about scrotal or penile issues may be withheld. It is important to speak with the patient alone to maximize patient disclosure, privacy, and confidentiality.

■ ACUTE SCROTAL PAIN

One of the most challenging aspects of male genitourinary complaints is that a wide variety of clinical conditions may all present with acute, unilateral (or bilateral) pain and swelling of the scrotum. Although the differential diagnosis for such presentations is extensive, the vast majority of acute testicular pain can be attributed to one of three diagnostic entities: testicular torsion, epididymitis, or appendage torsion (Table 107-1).

Table 107-1 DIFFERENTIATION OF TESTICULAR TORSION, EPIDIDYMITIS, AND APPENDAGE TORSION

	Testicular Torsion	Epididymitis*	Appendage Torsion
Historical Features			
Age	Incidence peaks in neonatal and adolescent groups but may occur at any age	Primarily adolescents and adults	Prepubescent males
Risk factors	Undescended testicle (neonate), rapid increase in testicular size (adolescent), failure of prior torsion repair	Multiple sexual partners, genitourinary anomalies, genitourinary instrumentation	Predisposing anatomy
Pain onset	Sudden or intermittent	Gradual and progressive	Gradual or sudden
Previous episodes of similar pain	Possible	Unlikely	Occasional
History of trauma	Possible	Possible	Possible
Nausea/vomiting	Common	Rare	Rare
Dysuria	Rare	Common	Rare
Physical Findings			
Fever	Rare	Common in advanced disease (epididymo-orchitis)	Rare
Location of swelling/ tenderness	Testicle, progressing to diffuse hemiscrotal involvement	Epididymis, progressing to diffuse hemiscrotal involvement	Localized to head of affected testicle or epididymis
Cremasteric reflex	Absent	Present	Present
Testicle position	High-riding testicle with transverse alignment	Normal position with vertical alignment	Normal position with vertical alignment
Pyuria	Rare	Common	Rare

*Including epididymo-orchitis.

■ HISTORY

Pain may be due to structures within or adjoining a particular region or may be referred from other areas. Delineation of the source of the pathology is essential. For example, pain from abdominal aortic aneurysms, renal colic, and pyelonephritis can radiate to the testicles.

■ ONSET OF SYMPTOMS

Pain that begins abruptly and severely suggests testicular torsion (intermittent pain can signal intermittent torsion). Twisting of the spermatic cord leads to rapid diminution of blood supply to the affected testicle, causing ischemic pain. This is in contrast to the more indolent pain of epididymitis, a gradually progressive inflammatory process. Patients with long-standing inguinal hernias often present with isolated genital pain of prolonged duration. However, patients with incarcerated hernias (those that cannot be reduced) or strangulated hernias (with ischemic or infracted, herniated bowel) may present with more acute pain.

Testicular torsion often accompanies a report of minor trauma. Testicular torsion can also occur in the absence of such events and may even happen during sleep.

■ CHARACTER OF SYMPTOMS

The distinction between constant/progressive and intermittent/colicky pain is potentially useful in the diagnosis of acute scrotal pain. Constant and progressive pain typically results from progressive inflammatory processes such as epididymitis. Patients may exhibit pain with ambulation and other movements as a result of the inflammation. Intermittent and colicky pain is more consistent with rapid "onset" and "offset" conditions, as occurs with twisting of the spermatic cord, either suddenly or intermittently.

Patients with testicular torsion often complain of severe pain as a consequence of ongoing testicular ischemia, leading to necrosis. Pain resulting from inflammatory processes (epididymitis) may be temporarily relieved by rest and scrotal elevation with a supportive undergarment such as a "jockstrap." Similarly, the inflammatory pain is often exacerbated by movement, leading a patient to remain still. Alternatively, patients exhibiting the colicky symptoms of testicular torsion may writhe in pain as they try (and fail) to find a position of comfort. These symptoms are generalizations and, when considered alone, lack high sensitivity or specificity.

■ ASSOCIATED SYMPTOMS

Patients with nausea or emesis are less likely to have torsion of an appendage or simple, uncomplicated epididymitis. It is more likely that a substantial pathology is present. Patients with abdominal pain, nausea, or constitutional symptoms may have testicular torsion, an incarcerated hernia, or other process. Patients with epididymitis may present with a low-grade fever, nausea, and malaise; those with advanced infection (e.g., epididymo-orchitis) may demonstrate more pronounced constitutional symptoms.

Urinary symptoms such as dysuria and urgency may accompany epididymitis. Inability to void spontaneously may indicate either urethral obstruction or severe volume depletion. Yellow-green penile discharge may provide clues to the diagnosis of urethritis or epididymitis, often caused by gonorrhea or *Chlamydia* infection in sexually active males. Hematospermia may also be present in cases of epididymitis, because the inflammatory process leads to a breach in the integrity of the vascular endothelium and spilling of blood into the seminal fluid.

Physical Examination

■ ABDOMINAL EXAMINATION

Because many intra-abdominal conditions may present with genitourinary pain, abdominal, flank, and back evaluation is useful. It is important to assess for lower abdominal tenderness or mass, potentially signaling acute appendicitis, inguinal hernia, genitourinary malignancy, abdominal trauma, or advanced perineal infection (such as Fournier's disease). Costovertebral angle tenderness may be present in retroperitoneal processes such as pyelonephritis, renal colic, and expanding or ruptured abdominal aortic aneurysm.

■ GENITAL EXAMINATION

The genitalia should be examined both while the patient is standing and lying supine. Caution should be used when examining a standing patient, as some males experience a strong vagal response to scrotal (or prostate) stimulation, leading to presyncope or syncope. Also, examination of the testicles and epididymis may cause significant discomfort even in the absence of pathology. As many patients have unilateral pain, the unaffected side should be examined first. This serves as a control and helps to gain the trust of the patient.

Visual examination of the genitals may reveal cutaneous rashes or lesions, abnormal testicular symmetry or position, edema (evident by loss of scrotal skin folds), and masses. Key visual features of testicular torsion include a high-riding and a transverse lie of the affected testicle, both of which result from twisting of the spermatic cord.

It is important to look for evidence of scrotal and perineal erythema or ecchymoses, particularly in older patients with scrotal pain. This may be the only clue to the presence of Fournier's disease (necrotizing fasciitis of the perineum), which often affects diabetics and other immunocompromised individuals. However, a prominent feature of necrotizing fasciitis is significant pain in the *absence* of pronounced physical findings.

A digital rectal examination provides information regarding the prostate and the prostatic portion of the urethra. Exquisite prostate tenderness may indicate acute infection (prostatitis). Firmness and enlargement of the prostate are signs of benign prostatic hypertrophy; nodularity is concerning for prostate carcinoma. These conditions may present with variable genitourinary symptoms.

■ ACUTE PENILE PAIN

Patients with low-flow priapism often complain of an exquisitely painful and prolonged erection. Stagnant, oxygen-poor, acidic blood accumulates in the corpora, resulting in ischemic pain. Ischemia may lead to irreversible cellular damage, permanent fibrosis, and impotence with prolonged duration of the pathologic erection. Of note, the use of oral erectile dysfunction treatments such as sildenafil (Viagra) have only rarely been associated with priapism.[1] Patients with high-flow priapism often complain of a persistent, yet painless erection as there is a continuous inflow of well-oxygenated blood via traumatic arterial-cavernosal fistulae.

Paraphimosis classically develops in uncircumcised males when the proximally retracted foreskin acts as a constricting band on the mid to distal portion of the penile shaft. Disruption of venous drainage by the constricting foreskin leads to a vicious cycle of progressive glans edema. Progressive glans edema will eventually cause arterial compromise, ischemic pain, and subsequent glans necrosis and gangrene. Penile foreskin should always be replaced after retraction during examination or urethral catheter placement to avoid development of iatrogenic paraphimosis.

Penile constriction analogous to paraphimosis can occur. Objects constricting the mid to distal shaft lead to the same pathophysiologic derangements seen with paraphimosis. These objects may be placed intentionally (e.g., string, metal, or rubber rings) or may occur sporadically, as in the case of a hair tourniquet in infants. Hair tourniquets may be very difficult to diagnose, as the offending hair is nearly invisible within an edematous coronal sulcus. An occult hair tourniquet should be considered along with testicular torsion in a male infant with inconsolable crying. Removal of the offending hair from the coronal sulcus can be difficult. It has been reported that over-the-counter hair removal products (depilatories such as Nair) have been used successfully for the removal of digital (finger, toe) hair tourniquets, suggesting its utility for penile hair tourniquets as well.[2]

■ GENITOURINARY TRAUMA

Trauma to the testicle and its associated structures (epididymis and spermatic cord) occurs infrequently because of testicular mobility and the protective cremasteric reflex. In addition, each testicle is encapsulated by the tunica albuginea, which may protect the testicular parenchyma from injury. Blunt force injury may cause a testicular contusion or, less frequently, rupture of the tunica albuginea. Also, traumatic dislocation of the testicle to a location outside of the scrotal confines is possible with significant blunt force injury.

All but the most superficial penetrating scrotal injuries require specialty consultation for possible exploration.

Patients with blunt or penetrating genitourinary trauma may present with a hematocele, which is a painful, tender ecchymotic scrotal mass resulting from the accumulation of blood in the tunica vaginalis.

Trauma to the penis often presents with distressing pain. A penile fracture is an acute tear or rupture of the tunica albuginea of the corpus cavernosum. Patients often relate a history of a sudden "snapping" sound during intercourse or other sexual activity, or as a result of blunt trauma in the setting of an erect penis. Physical examination reveals a swollen, ecchymotic, detumescent (limp) penis which is tender to palpation at the site of injury.

A penile contusion results from less severe direct blunt force trauma to the penis. In a penile contusion, the tunica albuginea remains intact and the patient presents with localized bruising and tenderness at the trauma site. This may result from a toilet seat injury sustained while "potty-training" in the toddler age group, or as a result of a "straddle" mechanism at any age.

Penetrating penile injuries require specialty consultation in virtually all cases.

■ SEXUALLY TRANSMITTED DISEASES

Genital infections that are likely to cause acute symptoms can generally be divided into diseases characterized by genital ulceration (e.g., herpes) and diseases causing penile discharge (e.g., urethritis).

Among the many infections that can cause genital ulceration, genital herpes, syphilis, and chancroid are most commonly seen in the United States; genital herpes is the most prevalent.

Genital herpes (either primary or recurrent) may present with severe pain, pruritus, or burning localized to the penis, scrotum, rectum, or elsewhere in the perineum. The typical pattern of multiple grouped vesicular or ulcerative lesions may be absent entirely in many acutely infected persons, however, rendering the diagnosis elusive.

Syphilis is a systemic disease caused by *Treponema pallidum.* Patients who have syphilis may seek treatment for signs or symptoms of primary infection, which is often a painless ulcer (or chancre) at the infection site, typically on the head or distal shaft of the penis.

Chancroid is caused by *Haemophilus ducreyi,* and classically presents with the combination of a painful ulcer and tender inguinal adenopathy.

Diagnosis of any of these ulcerative infections based on the history and physical examination alone is frequently inaccurate. Therefore, evaluation of all patients with genital ulcers should include a serologic test for syphilis and a diagnostic evaluation for genital herpes. Testing for *Haemophilus ducreyi* should be performed in settings where chancroid is prevalent.

Findings suggestive of a urinary tract infection (pyuria, bacteruria, nitrites, leukocyte esterase) may be present in cases of urethritis or epididymitis. Urethritis typically is characterized by discharge of mucopurulent or purulent material, with or without accompanying dysuria or urethral pruritus. The principal bacterial pathogens of proven clinical importance in men who have urethritis are *Neisseria gonorrhoeae* and *Chlamydia trachomatis.* Asymptomatic infections are common as well.

Special Signs and Techniques

Several adjuncts to the traditional examination are commonly employed in assessing the male genitourinary tract. Certain signs may aid in the proper identification of particular male genital pathology.

An intact ipsilateral cremasteric reflex is sensitive, although imperfect, for excluding the diagnosis of testicular torsion.[3-5] This reflex is elicited by stroking the ipsilateral inner thigh with a tongue depressor or hand, resulting in a reflexive elevation of the testicle through contraction of the cremasteric muscle. Although the presence of an intact cremasteric reflex is useful in excluding torsion, the absence of this reflex is nonspecific, because some healthy individuals lack the reflex (particularly males in the first few years of life).[6] Of note, there have been several published reports of testicular torsion presenting with an intact cremasteric reflex.[7-9]

Prehn's sign, or relief of pain with scrotal elevation, was previously thought to help in differentiating epididymitis from testicular torsion (no change in symptoms with elevation). However, this sign has been found to be unreliable in distinguishing these two disorders, and its use for this purpose is not recommended.

In cases of suspected appendage torsion, the "blue dot sign" is pathognomonic. Because appendage torsion is most common in the prepubescent age group, visualization of the infarcted appendage (the blue dot) is seen through thin, nonhormonally stimulated prepubertal skin.

Scrotal transillumination may be performed in cases of suspected hydrocele. The scrotal contents will supposedly transilluminate when filled with light-transmitting fluid, as is the case with a hydrocele. However, transillumination is neither sensitive nor specific for the diagnosis of hydrocele, and results should be interpreted with caution.

Diagnostic Testing

Most routine diagnostic aids (such as blood work, urinalysis) add little to distinguish among the common etiologies of acute scrotal pain. Rather, they may actually worsen patient outcome by causing delays in consultation and therapeutic action—"castration through procrastination." If the history and examination suggest the diagnosis of testicular torsion, consult urology (or general surgery) services and plan for immediate surgical exploration without delay. A patient of appropriate age with classic history and examination findings of testicular torsion does not require any diagnostic tests. In low-risk or unclear circumstances, a confirmatory radiologic study (typically ultrasonography) is indicated.

In cases of Fournier's disease, a delay in recognition and surgical débridement can be life-threatening. Early consultation and administration of broad-spectrum antibiotics is indicated in all suspected cases; however, surgical débridement remains the definitive treatment.

■ LABORATORY TESTING

Any patient presenting to the ED with penile discharge should be assumed to have infectious urethritis. The Centers for Disease Control and Prevention (CDC) guidelines recommend testing to determine the specific etiology.[10] Urine polymerase chain reaction testing for gonorrhea and *Chlamydia* infection is available at most institutions. Urine samples for urethritis testing should be collected at the initiation of the urine stream without cleansing of the glans; mid-stream collection and glans cleansing are necessary for urine culture in suspected cystitis or pyelonephritis. If polymerase chain reaction testing is unavailable, swabs of the lining of the distal 1 to 2 cm of the penile urethra are necessary for testing.

An elevated systemic white blood cell count may be present in cases of inflammation as well as infection, but does little to narrow the differential diagnosis, and awaiting results could delay definitive management. Patients with advanced infections (such as scrotal abscess, epididymo-orchitis, and Fournier's disease) may have a markedly elevated white blood cell count or granulocyte predominance, but the test lacks sufficient sensitivity and specificity.

■ ULTRASONOGRAPHY

Ultrasound visulization is the most useful diagnostic modality for the evaluation of genitourinary complaints. A color flow duplex Doppler ultrasound scan generally is helpful in distinguishing potential etiologies of acute scrotal pain. The classic finding suggestive of testicular torsion is diminished intratesticular blood flow. In addition, examination of the spermatic cord with high resolution gray-scale sonography may reveal "kinking" of the cord.[11] In epididymitis, perfusion is normal or increased due to the effects of inflammatory mediators on local vascular beds.

Ultrasonography may also identify an infarcted appendage (resulting from appendage torsion), hydroceles, hematoceles, varicoceles, hernias, tumors, abscesses, and gonadal vasculitis. In patients with testicular trauma, ultrasonography may identify disruption of the tunica albuginea, which signals testicular rupture. Doppler blood flow studies can measure the adequacy of blood flow. Absent blood flow means that traumatic torsion or vascular injury has occurred.

■ COMPUTED TOMOGRAPHY

Computed tomography scanning may be helpful in assessing the extension or depth of genitourinary abscess or Fournier's disease and may aid in the search for coexisting injuries or foreign bodies in the evaluation of a trauma patient.

Treatment and Dispositon

■ ANALGESIA

Analgesia should be administered parenterally in most cases, because of the significant pain associated with most of the conditions. Analgesia should not be withheld pending consultation. If the likelihood of surgical intervention is low, or if the pain is mild on presentation, a trial of oral medications can be offered. The agents most frequently used are narcotic analgesics, nonsteroidal antiinflammatory drugs (NSAIDs), and acetaminophen.

■ MANUAL TESTICULAR DETORSION

In the case of prolonged time to definitive treatment, manual testicular repositioning may be attempted. Because testicular torsion usually occurs in a lateral to medial fashion, detorsion is often accomplished by rotation of the affected testicle from medial to lateral. The end point of the detorsion procedure is relief of pain.

■ EMERGENT SURGERY FOR TESTICULAR TORSION

Testicular salvage rates are time-dependent; 96% of testicles are salvaged if detorsion occurs within 4 hours after onset of symptoms, whereas the salvage rate is 10% when there is delay of greater than 24 hours until treatment.[12] Immediate surgical consultation is important when testicular torsion is likely.

SCROTAL ELEVATION

Elevation of the scrotum may be beneficial in patients with inflammatory conditions such as epididymitis. This is easily accomplished by use of a towel roll or supportive undergarments (such as a "jockstrap"). In addition, ice may reduce edema and provide mild symptomatic relief.

PRIORITY ACTIONS

Testicular Torsion

- Emergent urology consultation in all moderate to high-probability cases
- Consider ultrasound imaging only if diagnosis is equivocal based on history and physical findings

Fournier's Disease

- Emergent surgical consultation for débridement
- Broad-spectrum antibiotics (covering gram-positive, gram-negative, and anaerobic species)
- IV fluids and supportive measures as dictated by clinical picture

Priapism

- Urology consultation
- Consider treatment with terbutaline
- Consider corporal aspiration and irrigation

Paraphimosis

- Attempt reduction in the ED; urology consultation if unsuccessful

Genitourinary Trauma

- Maintain a very low threshold for urology consultation and ultrasound imaging
- Search meticulously for other coexisting injuries

ANTIBIOTIC THERAPY

Antimicrobial agents are indicated in cases of suspected or proven infection. Early broad-spectrum antibiotic therapy (to cover gram-positive, gram-negative, and anaerobic species) is imperative in any case of suspected Fournier's disease. Suggested regimens include extended-spectrum penicillin/beta-lactamase inhibitors (e.g., ampicillin/sulbactam, piperacillin/tazobactam), a third-generation cephalosporin plus clindamycin, or vancomycin plus flagyl plus a quinolone in penicillin-allergic patients.

SEXUALLY TRANSMITTED DISEASES

Timely follow-up counseling and treatment of patients with abnormal test results is impractical in the ED setting. Thus, empirical antimicrobial treatment for likely pathogens should be initiated (Table 107-2), and counseling regarding notification of the patient's sexual contacts should be underscored. Patients should wear a condom during intercourse following treatment until 1 week after symptoms have resolved.

Antibiotics are the cornerstone of therapy for epididymitis. Antimicrobial selection is guided by patient demographics: younger (less than 35 years old), sexually active males are treated presumptively for *Neisseria gonorrhoeae* and *Chlamydia trachomatis* (intramuscular ceftriaxone with oral doxycycline. Broader coverage should be considered for both coliform and fungal species in males who engage in anal insertive intercourse (with presumed gonorrhea and *Chlamydia* co-infection).

Patients older than 35 years are treated with oral fluoroquinolones for the common "urinary" pathogens (*Escherichia coli* and *Klebsiella* species) most frequently encountered in this demographic group.

The distinction between urethritis with or without accompanying epididymitis is critical in the patient presenting with penile discharge, because it has important management implications. When accom-

Table 107-2 MEDICATION DOSAGES FOR SEXUALLY TRANSMITTED DISEASES

Disease	Recommended Treatment	Alternative
Ulcerative Disease		
Genital herpes:		
Primary	Acyclovir 400 mg tid × 7-10 d	Valacyclovir 1 g bid × 7-10 d
Recurrent	Acyclovir 400 mg tid × 5 d	Valacyclovir 1 g once daily × 5 d
Syphilis	Benzathine Penicillin G 2.4 million units IM ×1 dose	Doxycycline 100 mg bid × 14 d
Chancroid	Azithromycin 1 g PO × 1 dose	Ceftriaxone 250 mg IM × 1 dose
Urethritis		
Gonorrhea	Ceftriaxone 125 mg IM × 1 dose	Cefixime 400 mg PO × 1 dose
Chlamydia	Azithromycin 1 g PO ×1 dose	Doxycycline 100 PO bid × 7 d

Data from U.S. Centers for Disease Control and Prevention (CDC): Sexually transmitted diseases treatment guidelines, 2006. MMWR Morb Mortal Wkly Rep 2006;55 (No. RR-11); CDC: Update to CDC's sexually trasmitted diseases treatment guidelines, 2006: Fluoroquinolones no longer recommended for treatment of gonococcal infections. MMWR Morb Mortal Wky Rep 2007;56:332-336.

panying epididymal pain or tenderness is present, both the dosage and duration of antimicrobial treatment must be increased because epididymitis represents a more advanced stage of reproductive tract disease. The typical treatment regimen for isolated urethritis is a single dose of ceftriaxone, 125 mg intramuscularly (IM) (for gonorrhea), plus a single dose of azithromycin, 1 g orally (for *Chlamydia*); typical treatment for epididymitis is a single dose of ceftriaxone, 250 mg IM, plus doxycycline, 100 mg orally given twice a day for 10 days. Based on the degree of epididymal (or testicular) involvement and individual clinical circumstances, a comprehensive evaluation for other causes of acute scrotal disease or abscess may be indicated.

Epididymitis may also occur in prepubescent males due to reflux of sterile urine into the epididymis (often as a result of minor congenital genitourinary anomalies). Treatment of the resulting "chemical" (noninfectious) inflammation is with prophylactic oral trimethoprim/sulfamethoxazole.

■ PRIAPISM

The treatment of priapism usually is managed by a urologist; however, in certain circumstances the EP may have to initiate treatment for low-flow priapism. The classic teaching is that the initial treatment—oral (or subcutaneous) terbutaline—is the same regardless of inciting etiology, although its utility is debated.[13-15] It is thought that terbutaline, a beta-2 adrenergic agonist, increases venous outflow from the engorged corpora by way of relaxation of venous sinusoidal smooth muscle. Terbutaline is of unproved benefit; however, given its limited propensity for adverse effects it is still warranted in select circumstances while awaiting urology consultation.[16]

If terbutaline fails, the next step in the treatment of priapism is corporal blood aspiration, saline irrigation, and injection of an alpha-adrenergic receptor agonist (e.g., phenylephrine, epinephrine, pseudoephedrine).

The goal of treatment for patients with sickle cell disease and priapism is reduction of red blood cell sickling, thereby reducing vascular sludging and vaso-occlusion. Treatments in this setting include oxygen, intravenous hydration, and simple or exchange transfusions.

Regardless of the precipitating etiology of priapism, surgical shunt procedures are used as a last resort in patients with low-flow priapism unresponsive to the aforementioned treatments.

■ PARAPHIMOSIS

Paraphimosis can frequently be managed in the ED without the need for emergent specialty consultation. There are many reported methods of successful paraphimosis reduction; however, the most commonly employed initial maneuver involves manual compression of the distal glans penis to decrease edema, followed by reduction of the glans penis back through the proximal constricting band of foreskin.[17]

■ TESTICULAR TRAUMA

Patients with penetrating injury to the scrotum are generally explored in the operating room. Patients with blunt testicular trauma with ultrasonographic evidence of significant testicular injury also generally undergo surgical exploration for débridement of devitalized tissue, treatment of an acute hematocele larger than 5 cm, and repair of the tunica albuginea. Documented testicular injury requires early repair to minimize the potential for infection, infarction, necrosis, torsion, abscess, infertility, atrophy, and testicular loss.

REFERENCES

1. Goldmeier D, Lamba H: Prolonged erections produced by dihydrocodeine and sildenafil. BMJ 2002;324(7353):1555.
2. Barton DJ, Sloan GM, Nichter LS, et al: Hair-thread tourniquet syndrome. Pediatrics 1998;82:925-928.
3. Rabinowitz R: The importance of the cremasteric reflex in acute scrotal swelling in children. J Urol 1984;132:89-90.
4. Caldamome AA, Valvo JR, Altebarmakian VK, et al: Acute scrotal swelling in children. J Pediatr Surg 1984;19: 581-584.
5. Melekos MD, Asbach HW, Markou SA: Etiology of acute scrotum in 100 boys with regard to age distribution. J Urol 1988;139:1023-1025.
6. Caesar RE, Kaplan GW: The incidence of the cremasteric reflex in normal boys. J Urol 1994;152:779-780.
7. Feldstein MS: Re: The importance of the cremasteric reflex in acute scrotal swelling in children. J Urol 1985;133:488.
8. Hughes ME, Currier SJ, Della-Giustina D: Normal cremasteric reflex in a case of testicular torsion. Am J Emerg Med 2001;19:241-242.
9. Nelson CP, Williams JF, Bloom DA: The cremasteric reflex: A useful but imperfect sign in testicular torsion. J Pediatr Surg 2003;38:1248-1249.
10. United States Centers for Disease Control and Prevention (CDC). Sexually transmitted diseases treatment guidelines, 2006. MMWR Morb Mortal Wkly Rep 2006;55(No. RR-11). Available from: http://www.cdc.gov/std/treatment/default.htm.
11. Kalfa N, Veyrac C, Lopez M, et al: Multicenter assessment of ultrasound of the spermatic cord in children with acute scrotum. J Urol 2007;177:297-301.
12. Knight PJ, Vassy LE: The diagnosis and treatment of the acute scrotum in children and adolescents. Ann Surg 1984; 200:664-673.
13. Lowe JC, Jarow JP: Placebo-controlled study of oral terbutaline and pseudoephedrine in management of prostaglandin E_1-induced prolonged erections. Urology 1993;42: 51-54.
14. Govier FE, Jonsson E, Kramer-Levin D: Oral terbutaline for the treatment of priapism. J Urol 1994;151:878-879.
15. Erectile Dysfunction Guideline Update Panel: The Management of priapism. Baltimore, American Urological Association, 2003.
16. Priyadarshi S: Oral terbutaline in the management of pharmacologically induced prolonged erection. Int J Impot Res 2004;16:424-426.
17. Choe JM: Paraphimosis: Current treatment options. Am Fam Physician 2000;62:2623-2626.

Chapter 108

Nephrolithiasis

Carl R. Menckhoff

KEY POINTS

Ureteral calculi less than 5 mm in diameter spontaneously pass through the urinary tract in 90% of cases, whereas stones larger than 8 mm in diameter cause impaction in 95% of instances.

Impaction most commonly occurs at the ureterovesicular junction, the ureteropelvic junction, or the pelvic brim.

Patients with abdominal aortic aneurysms are commonly misdiagnosed as having renal colic.

Hematuria is absent in 15% of patients with symptomatic nephrolithiasis.

Scope and Outline

Renal colic is defined as severe, spasmodic pain caused by the impaction or passage of a calculus in the renal pelvis or ureter. Approximately 15% of the U.S. population will develop symptomatic nephrolithiasis during their lives[1]; the majority of these patients will present to the ED.

▪ EPIDEMIOLOGY

Most cases of renal colic occur in men between 20 and 50 years of age. The incidence of first-time ureteral stones in men is 0.3% per year, with a recurrence rate of 37% and 50% at 1 and 5 years, respectively.[2,3] The most significant risk factors for renal stone disease are listed in Box 108-1.

▪ PATHOPHYSIOLOGY

Renal stones form when the urine becomes supersaturated with calcium, oxalate, cystine, uric acid, or struvite. Hypercalciuria accounts for the development of 60% of calculi and results from increased intestinal absorption, decreased renal tubular reabsorption, or excessive bone resorption of calcium. Decreased urine output can further promote calculus formation due to reductions in citrate, magnesium pyrophosphate, and other inhibitors of urine crystallization. Table 108-1 describes features of the five main types of renal calculi.

Stone impaction may occur anywhere along the path of the genitourinary tract. Resultant ureteral obstruction can shift hydrostatic pressures and cause blood flow to be redistributed to the opposite renal artery. The overall rate of glomerular filtration decreases as renal excretion becomes a task of the unaffected kidney. A transient increase in serum creatinine follows this decrease.

Although an initial rise in creatinine may quickly resolve, irreversible kidney damage can occur after 7 days of complete obstruction.[3,4] Prolonged obstruction impairs recoverable kidney function over time,[4,5] but case reports show that some recovery may be possible for up to 150 days.[5,6]

Ureteral obstruction is primarily determined by calculus size. Most stones smaller than 5 mm in diameter will pass spontaneously (90%), whereas

Table 108-1 THE FIVE MAIN TYPES OF RENAL CALCULI

Mineral Type	Frequency	Etiologies	Pearls
Calcium oxalate	70%	Hypercalciuria High calcium intake (cheese, milk, antacids) Jejunal hyperabsorption Hyperparathyroidism Hyperoxaluria Dietary (tea, coffee, sodas, plums, rhubarb, cranberries, citrus fruit, green leafy vegetables) Inflammatory bowel disease	Most common
Calcium phosphate	10%	Type 1 renal tubular acidosis	Most dense
Struvite (magnesium-ammonium-phosphate)	10%	Urinary tract infections with urea-splitting bacteria such as *Klebsiella, Serratia, Enterobacter, Pseudomonas, Proteus, Staphylococcus*	Alkaline urine (pH > 7.6); staghorn calculi
Uric acid	10%	Hyperuricosuria (dietary: meat, fish, poultry)	Radiolucent Least dense
Cystine	1%	Inborn error of metabolism causing increased cystine secretion	Rare; radiolucent; staghorn calculi

BOX 108-1

Risk Factors for Renal Calculus Formation

- Family history of nephrolithiasis
- Age (third to sixth decades of life)
- Male gender
- Living in a hot, dry climate
- Low water intake
- Primary hyperparathyroidism
- Type 1 renal tubular acidosis
- Crohn's disease
- Laxative abuse
- Sarcoidosis
- Recurrent urinary tract infections
- Milk-alkali syndrome
- Sedentary lifestyle
- High animal protein diet

passage of stones larger than 8 mm is unlikely (5%). Table 108-2 compares ureteral stone size with percent likelihood of spontaneous passage.

Anatomy

Stone impaction most commonly occurs at the ureterovesicular junction, the narrowest part of the genitourinary tract. Other common areas of impaction include the ureteropelvic junction (where the renal pelvis narrows from 1 cm down to 2 mm) and the pelvic brim (where the ureter arches anteriorly across the iliac vessels) (Fig. 108-1).

Table108-2 RENAL CALCULUS SIZE AND LIKELIHOOD OF SPONTANEOUS PASSAGE

Stone Size (diameter)	Percent Likelihood of Spontaneous Passage
<5 mm	90
5-8 mm	15
>8 mm	5

Clinical Presentation

■ HISTORY

Renal colic classically presents as a *sudden* onset of excruciating, intermittent flank pain that radiates to the groin. This swift presentation often is accompanied by a deeper flank ache and nausea and vomiting. The severe, spasmodic pain of renal colic is caused by hyperperistalsis of smooth muscle from the calices to the ureter. The dull, deep, aching pain reflects ureteral obstruction and distention of the renal capsule.

The location of the ureteral calculus determines the presenting symptoms, as outlined in Table 108-3.

Table 108-3 URETERAL CALCULUS LOCATION AND ASSOCIATED SYMPTOMS

Location of Calculus	Symptoms
Renal pelvis or calyx	Deep flank ache
Proximal or mid-ureter	Severe flank pain radiating to the groin
Distal ureter	Flank discomfort and/or low abdominal pain
Bladder	Dysuria, frequency, urgency, retention, suprapubic discomfort

Table 108-4 PHYSICAL EXAMINATION FINDINGS AND POTENTIAL ALTERNATIVE DIAGNOSES

Finding	Consideration
Vital Signs	
Fever	Infected stone, pyelonephritis, perinephric abscess
Hypotension	Sepsis, abdominal aortic aneurysm
Abdomen	
Bruit	Abdominal aortic aneurysm, renal artery stenosis
Pulsatile mass	Abdominal aortic aneurysm
Pronounced costovertebral angle tenderness	Pyelonephritis
Lower abdominal/pelvic tenderness	Ectopic pregnancy, appendicitis, pelvic inflammatory disease
Genitourinary	
Testicular tenderness	Torsion, epididymitis, orchitis
Mass	Hernia, cancer
Pulmonary	
Focal findings	Lobar pneumonia
Cardiovascular	
Asymmetric lower extremity pulses	Abdominal aortic aneurysm
Skin	
Vesicular rash	Herpes zoster

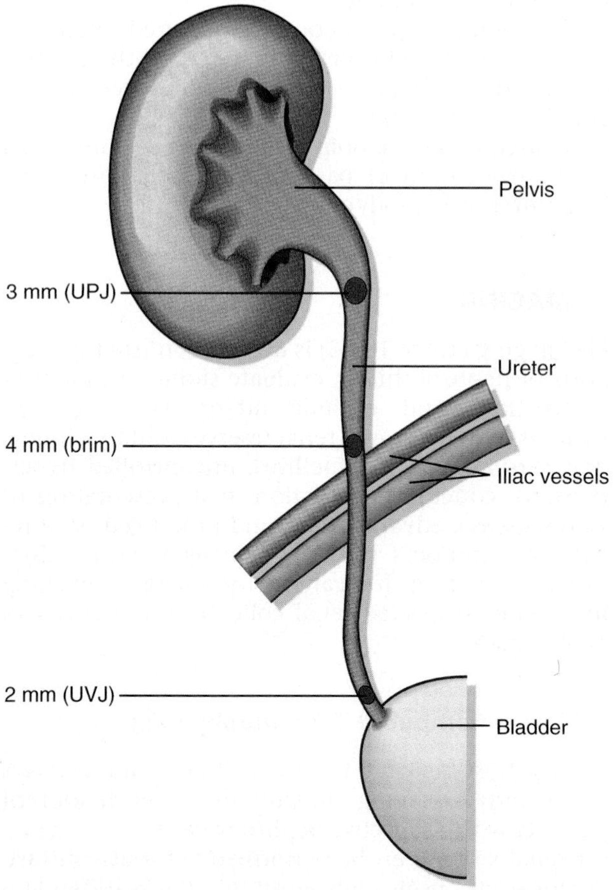
Pelvis
3 mm (UPJ)
Ureter
4 mm (brim)
Iliac vessels
2 mm (UVJ)
Bladder

FIGURE 108-1 Common sites of renal calculus impaction.

■ PHYSICAL EXAMINATION

Patients with renal colic typically appear uncomfortable and are commonly described as "writhing" on the gurney. The abdominal examination generally is unremarkable, though thin patients with distal ureteral stones and obstruction may exhibit some tenderness. Costovertebral angle tenderness can develop as a result of worsening hydronephrosis; this sign is mild or absent early in the presentation. Abnormal physical examination findings should raise suspicion of alternative diagnoses, as reviewed in Table 108-4.

Differential Diagnosis

Many disease processes can mimic symptomatic nephrolithiasis. Abdominal aortic aneurysm, aortic dissection, renal artery dissection, and renal infarction are the most lethal conditions that may present similarly to renal colic. In one study, approximately 20% of patients with an abdominal aortic aneurysm who were older than age 60 years were initially misdiagnosed as having a kidney stone.[7] Box 108-2 lists the differential diagnoses of renal colic.

Diagnostic Testing

■ LABORATORY TESTS

■ Urinalysis

A bedside urine dipstick test or urinalysis should be obtained in all patients with suspected renal colic to evaluate for hematuria and infection. A urine culture

BOX 108-2

Differential Diagnoses of Renal Colic

Vascular
- Abdominal aortic aneurysm
- Aortic dissection
- Renal artery dissection
- Renal artery stenosis
- Renal vein thrombosis
- Renal infarct
- Mesenteric ischemia
- Retroperitoneal hemorrhage

Gastrointestinal
- Incarcerated hernia
- Appendicitis
- Cholecystitis
- Biliary colic
- Pancreatitis
- Bowel obstruction
- Diverticulitis

Genitourinary
- Testicular torsion
- Pyelonephritis
- Perinephric abscess
- Urinary tract tumor
- Renal papillary necrosis
- Upper urinary tract hemorrhage

Gynecologic
- Ectopic pregnancy
- Ovarian torsion
- Tubo-ovarian abscess
- Pelvic inflammatory disease
- Endometriosis

Musculoskeletal
- Lumbar strain
- Radiculopathy
- Disc herniation
- Vertebral compression fracture

Dermatologic
- Herpes zoster

Miscellaneous
- Factitious

should be ordered if leukocytes, nitrites, or bacteria are identified.

Hematuria is a common but inconsistent finding in patients with ureteral stones. The amount of gross or microscopic hematuria does not correlate with stone impaction or the degree of obstruction; rather, hematuria results from direct ureteral trauma caused by the passing stone.[8] Hematuria is absent in 15% of patients with ureteral stones.[9,10]

Alkaline urine (pH > 7.6) may indicate infection with a urea-splitting organism, a common finding in patients with struvite stones. A urine pH less than 5.0 suggests the presence of a uric acid stone.

Uric acid or oxalate crystals may be detectable in the urine with a variety of conditions; this finding does not imply the presence of nephrolithiasis and should be interpreted with caution.

Urine Pregnancy Test

Urine human chorionic gonadotropin levels should be checked in female patients of child-bearing age. Although pregnant patients may present with renal colic, a newly positive result should raise suspicion of ectopic pregnancy.

Blood Tests

Blood urea nitrogen and creatinine can be obtained if symptoms have been prolonged or there is a concern for renal impairment, but these tests are not routinely indicated.

If a complete blood count is obtained, increased leukocytosis should be interpreted with caution because it can indicate either pain-induced demargination or infection.

A baseline hemoglobin level should be considered in the evaluation of patients with persistent gross hematuria or hemodynamic compromise.

IMAGING

ED imaging (Table 108-5) is used to confirm the diagnosis of nephrolithiasis, evaluate stone size, identify obstruction, and exclude alternative diagnoses. Patients with decreased renal reserve (solitary kidney, uncontrolled diabetes mellitus, uncontrolled hypertension), concurrent infection, first presentation of stone disease, advanced age, and prolonged or unrelenting symptoms should be imaged during their initial evaluation. Indications for emergent imaging in cases of suspected renal colic are summarized in Table 108-6.

Helical Computed Tomography (CT)

Noncontrast helical CT of the abdomen and pelvis is the preferred imaging modality for the evaluation of patients with suspected nephrolithiasis. CT imaging for renal stones can be performed without contrast, demonstrates both high sensitivity (94%-100%) and specificity (96%-100%),[11-15] and allows alternative diagnoses to be simultaneously identified.[15,16] Sagittal images are obtained in 5-mm intervals from the top of the kidney to the bottom of the bladder (Figs. 108-2 and 108-3).

Table 108-5 IMAGING MODALITIES FOR THE DETECTION OF NEPHROLITHIASIS

Test	Sensitivity (%)	Specificity (%)	Pros and Cons
Computed tomography	94-100	96-100	Pros: noncontrast, rapid, identifies alternative diagnoses Cons: radiation exposure, cost
Intravenous pyelography	52-85	97-100	Pros: functional study Cons: need for contrast, radiation exposure, duration of imaging
Ultrasonography	66-93	83-100	Pros: noncontrast, no radiation Cons: false-negative results in cases of small, nonobstructing stones
KUB (kidney-ureter-bladder) radiography	58-62	67-69	Pros: quick, readily available Cons: lower sensitivity and specificity

Table 108-6 INDICATIONS FOR DIAGNOSTIC IMAGING OF SUSPECTED RENAL COLIC

Finding	Indication for Diagnostic Imaging
Solitary kidney; uncontrolled diabetes*; uncontrolled hypertension*	To exclude obstruction in a patient with decreased renal reserve
Advanced age	To exclude alternative diagnoses, especially vascular disease
Concurrent infection	If concurrent with obstruction, urologic intervention is indicated
Prolonged symptoms	To exclude renal impairment that is associated with obstruction longer than 1 week in duration
Refractory symptoms; first presentation*	To exclude alternative diagnoses, especially ischemia/infarction

*Relative indication.

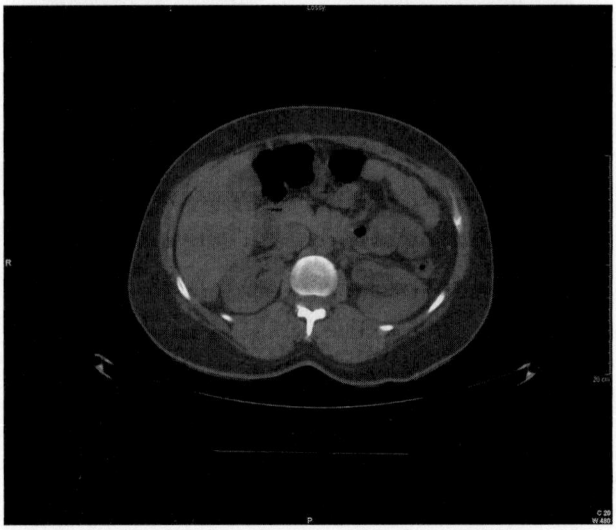

FIGURE 108-2 Noncontrast renal protocol computed tomography scan showing moderate hydronephrosis of the renal pelvis.

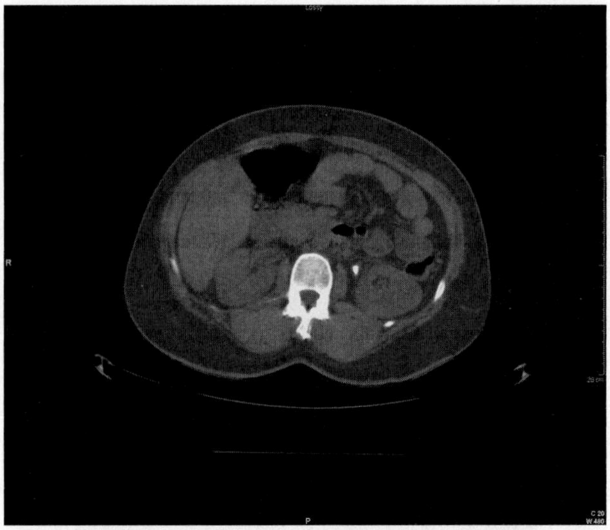

FIGURE 108-3 Noncontrast renal protocol computed tomography scan showing a stone at the left ureteropelvic junction.

■ Intravenous Pyleography

Intravenous pyelography (Fig. 108-4) yields a sensitivity of 52% to 85% and specificity of 97% to 100% for the detection of ureteral calculi.[11,17,18] It provides a visual interpretation of renal function as well as genitourinary anatomy. The earliest sign of ureteral obstruction on an intravenous pyleograph is a delayed nephrogram; other abnormal findings include a "standing column" (the entire ureter seen on one image; Fig. 108-5), hydroureter, hydronephrosis, contrast cutoff at the point of impaction, and extravasation of contrast material. The use of intravenous pyelography is limited by the need for contrast, a decreased sensitivity compared with helical CT, and the length of time required to obtain multiple delayed images.

■ Sonography

Ultrasonography is a useful modality for identifying hydronephrosis caused by ureteral obstruction (Fig. 108-6). Advantages include its ease of use; diagnostic images can be obtained rapidly, at the bedside, without the need for contrast or radiation. It is the

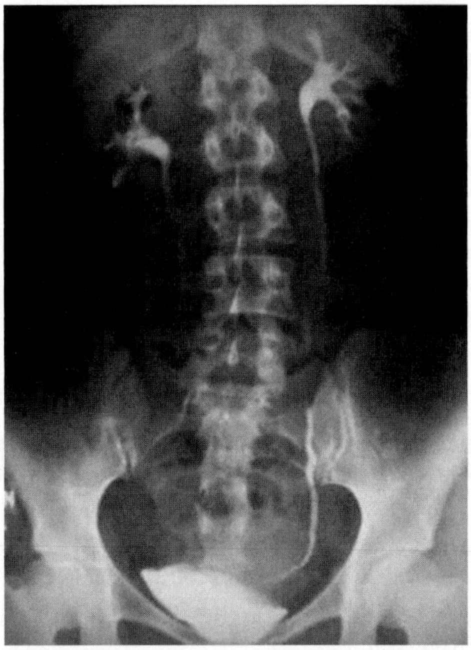

FIGURE 108-4 Normal intravenous pyleograph.

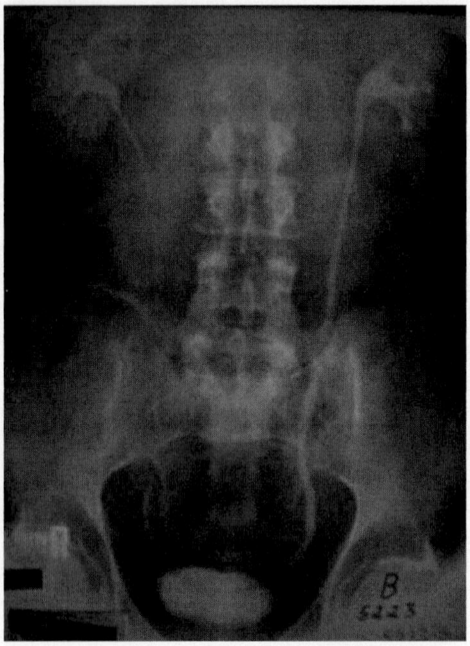

FIGURE 108-5 Intravenous pyleograph showing the entire left ureter in one view. This is known as a standing column and is caused by lack of ureteral peristalsis due to a ureteral stone.

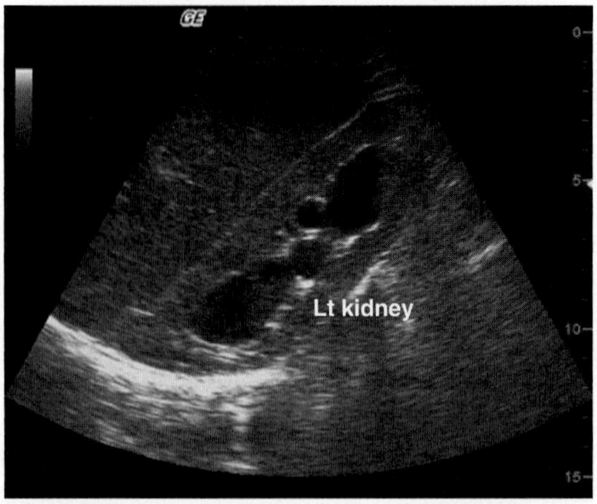
Lt kidney

FIGURE 108-6 Renal ultrasound showing moderate hydronephrosis.

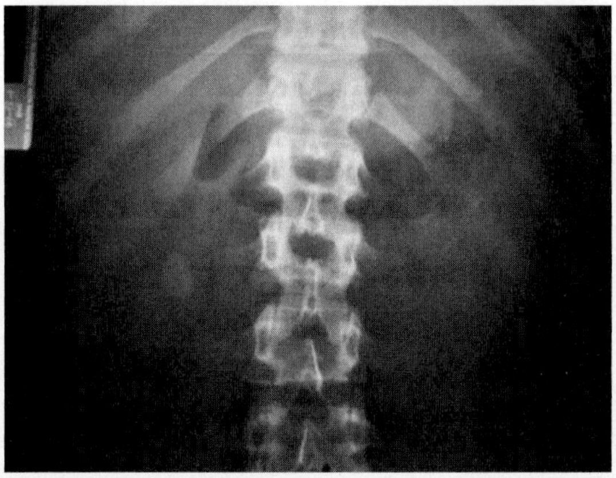

FIGURE 108-7 Kidney-ureter-bladder (KUB) radiograph showing a large kidney stone on the right.

imaging technique of choice for the evaluation of suspected renal colic in pregnancy. Ultrasonography is limited by its false negative rate, which is observed in cases of small calculi that do not cause significant obstruction or hydronephrosis. Sensitivity and specificity of ultrasonography in the diagnosis of urologic stone disease is 66% to 93% and 83% to 100%, respectively.[18-20]

Plain Radiography

The utility of plain radiography ("KUB" [kidney-ureter-bladder] performed in the supine position) is dependent upon the radiodensity of the suspected kidney stone. Although 90% of stones are radiopaque (Fig. 108-7), uric acid and cystine calculi are radiolucent. KUB imaging is limited technically by overlying soft tissue, air, and bone; a low sensitivity (58%-62%) and specificity (67%-69%) are observed in clinical practice.[21,22] The combination of ultrasonography and KUB radiography improves the usefulness of these imaging modalities. Studies that employed both ultrasound and plain radiography for the detection of nephrolithiasis demonstrated a sensitivity and specificity of 89% and 100%, respectively, when both tests were positive[20] and a sensitivity and specificity of 95% and 67%,[23] respectively, when either test was positive.

PRIORITY ACTIONS

- Institute symptom management (NSAIDs, opiates, antiemetics).
- Evaluate need for imaging:
  - Advanced age
  - Signs of infection—treat with antibiotics if present
  - Symptoms for longer than 7 days
  - Symptoms refractory to treatment
  - Known renal impairment
- Determine the need for urgent urology consultation and intervention.

Tips and Tricks

- A young, healthy patient with a typical presentation of renal colic, history of previous nephrolithiasis, no signs of infection, and easily managed symptoms may be discharged with analgesics, antiemetics, and a urine strainer for follow-up within 7 days.
- All other patients require evaluation for likely imaging and possible urology consultation.

RED FLAGS

- Patients older than 60 years: Consider a vascular etiology for their pain.
- Signs of infection: Exclude concurrent obstruction.
- Large calculi: 5-mm stones have 50% chance of passing; stones larger than 8 mm have 5% chance of passing.

Treatment

■ PHARMACOLOGIC MANAGEMENT

Patients with renal colic will likely require immediate pain control. Several options are available for rapid analgesia.

■ Nonsteroidal Anti-inflammatory Drugs (NSAIDs)

NSAIDs decrease ureteral spasm by inhibiting prostaglandin synthesis. Renal blood flow may be reduced when NSAIDs are administered in the setting of ureteral obstruction,[24] thereby improving symptoms through a decrease in urine production and ureteric pressure. Ketorolac (Toradol) (30 mg intravenously or 60 mg intramuscularly) has efficacy equivalent to oral administration of 800 mg of ibuprofen, although the latter may be less well tolerated in patients with concomitant nausea.

Some urologists debate the routine use of NSAIDs for the treatment of nephrolithiasis, because these medications may promote bleeding following the placement of a ureteral stent. Data to support such observations are inconclusive.

■ Opiates

Intravenous narcotics provide adequate symptom relief for most patients with renal colic. Opiates have similar analgesic effects at equivalent dosing. Although meperidine (Demerol) demonstrates smooth muscle relaxation when tested in vitro,[25] this spasmolytic effect does not appear to improve its clinical utility in therapy for renal colic.[26] Given the potential for drug interactions with meperidine, preferred opiates for emergency department use include hydromorphone (0.01-0.02 mg/kg) or morphine (0.1 mg/kg).

Multiple studies have shown that both NSAIDS and opiates are effective and appropriate treatments in renal colic.[24-31] One meta-analysis of 19 studies showed that NSAIDs and opiates are equally effective in the acute management of renal colic symptoms.[28] Many experts recommend the use of NSAIDs followed by opiates for continued pain.

Documentation

- Patient's age
- Onset, location, and duration of pain
- Urinalysis results
- Medical decision-making for imaging
- Medical decision-making for disposition
- Discharge instructions and return precautions
- Follow-up within 7 days

■ OTHER SYMPTOM MANAGEMENT

Tamsulosin (Flomax), an alpha-adrenergic blocker, reduces ureteral spasm. One study suggests that oral tamsulosin (0.4 mg per day) may help promote ureteral passage of juxtavesical stones.[32] Antiemetics should be administered to patients experiencing concomitant nausea or vomiting. IV crystalloid administration was once thought to promote stone migration by stimulating ureteral peristalsis; however, there is no supporting evidence to show that hydration consistently improves symptoms by this mechanism.[33]

Disposition

The patient with uncomplicated renal colic whose symptoms are easily controlled should be discharged with analgesics, a urine strainer, antiemetics, and

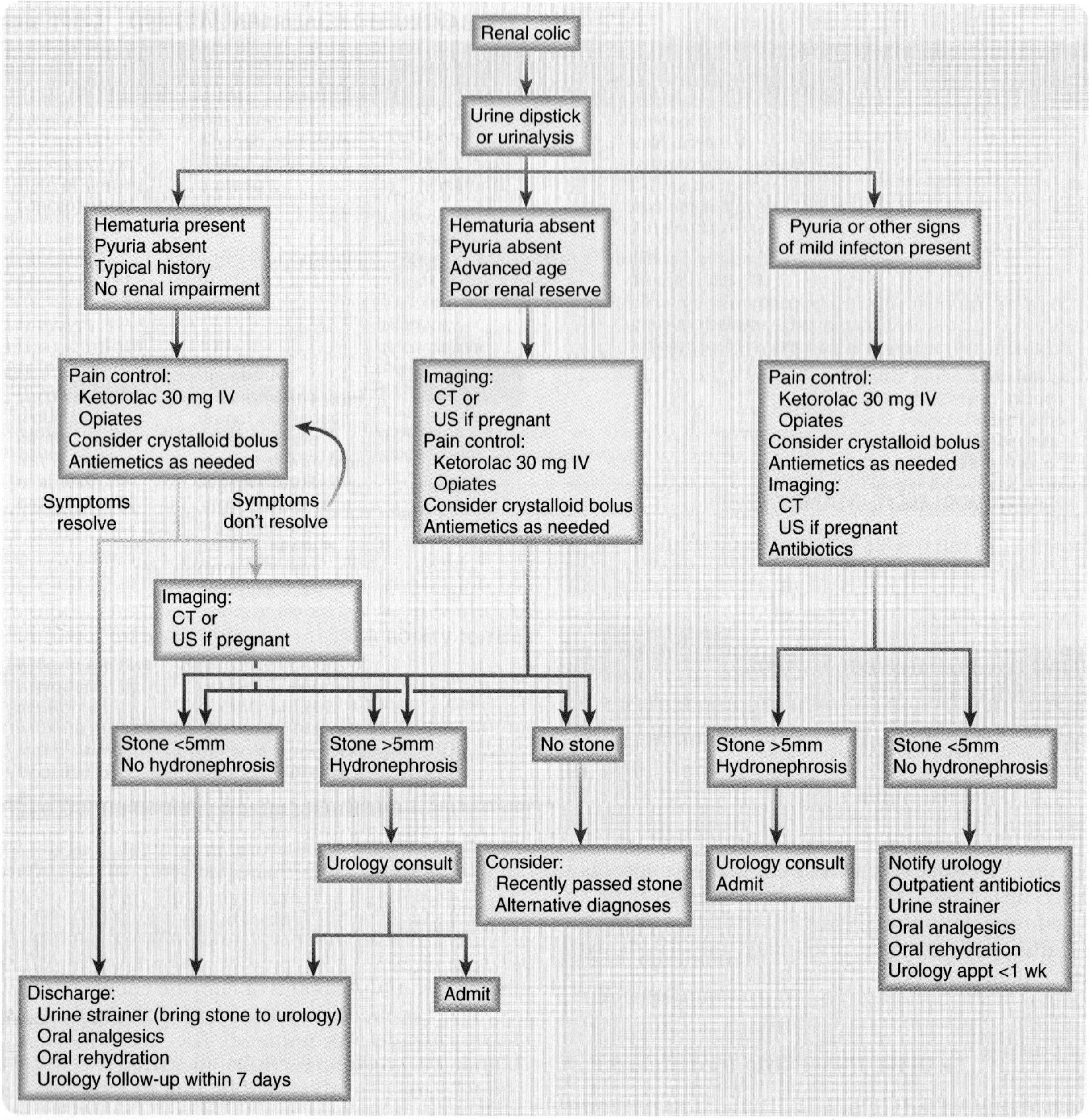
Renal colic
Urine dipstick or urinalysis
Hematuria present
Pyuria absent
Typical history
No renal impairment
Hematuria absent
Pyuria absent
Advanced age
Poor renal reserve
Pyuria or other signs of mild infecton present
Pain control:
Ketorolac 30 mg IV
Opiates
Consider crystalloid bolus
Antiemetics as needed
Imaging:
CT or
US if pregnant
Pain control:
Ketorolac 30 mg IV
Opiates
Consider crystalloid bolus
Antiemetics as needed
Pain control:
Ketorolac 30 mg IV
Opiates
Consider crystalloid bolus
Antiemetics as needed
Imaging:
CT
US if pregnant
Antibiotics
Symptoms resolve
Symptoms don't resolve
Imaging:
CT or
US if pregnant
Stone <5mm
No hydronephrosis
Stone >5mm
Hydronephrosis
No stone
Stone >5mm
Hydronephrosis
Stone <5mm
No hydronephrosis
Urology consult
Consider:
Recently passed stone
Alternative diagnoses
Urology consult
Admit
Notify urology
Outpatient antibiotics
Urine strainer
Oral analgesics
Oral rehydration
Urology appt <1 wk
Discharge:
Urine strainer (bring stone to urology)
Oral analgesics
Oral rehydration
Urology follow-up within 7 days
Admit

FIGURE 108-8 Algorithim for evaluation, treatment, and disposition of the patient with presumed renal colic. CT, computed tomography; IV, intravenously; US, ultrasonography.

follow-up within 7 days. Stones captured by urine straining should be brought to the urologist for evaluation by pathology. Return precautions include uncontrolled pain, protracted vomiting, and fever (Fig. 108-8).

A urologist should be consulted if patients have uncontrollable pain or evidence of infection. The presence of white blood cells in the urine may indicate an infection and warrant urology department consultation for urgent stone removal.

Some patients will have few white blood cells in the urine (e.g., <10) but no clinical signs of infection. These patients will be otherwise asymptomatic following medication for pain (i.e., afebrile). In the absence of concomitant obstruction, urgent stone removal in such cases is not routine. Patients with coexisting, complicating diseases may be treated with antibiotics and observed in the hospital. Patients without underlying disease may be treated with antibiotics as an outpatient and followed carefully. A urine culture should be obtained from any patient with white blood cells in the urine.

Box 108-3 summarizes common indications for admission or urology consultation.

BOX 108-3

Indications for Admission or Consultation with a Urologist

Indications for Admission

- Obstruction with infection
- Solitary kidney with obstruction or a stone unlikely to pass spontaneously
- Refractory pain
- Refractory emesis

Indications for Consultation with a Urologist

- Infection without obstruction
- Stone unlikely to pass spontaneously
- Moderate to severe hydronephrosis
- Solitary kidney
- Intrinsic renal disease

REFERENCES

1. Trivedi B: Nephrolithiasis: How it happens and what to do about it. Nephrolithiasis 1996;100:63-78.
2. Ahlstrand C, Tiselius H: Recurrences during a 10-year follow-up after first renal stone episode. Urol Res 1990; 18:397-399.
3. Kerr WS Jr: Effect of complete ureteral obstruction for one week on kidney function. J Appl Physiol 1954;6:762-772.
4. Vaughan E, Gillenwater J: Recovery following complete chronic unilateral ureteral occlusion: Functional, radiographic and pathologic alterations. J Urol 1971;106: 27-35.
5. Shapiro S, Bennett A: Recovery of renal function after prolonged unilateral ureteral obstruction. J Urol 1976;115: 136-140.
6. Okubo K, Suzuki Y, Ishitoya S, et al: Recovery of renal function after 153 days of complete unilateral ureteral obstruction. J Urol 1998;160:1422-1423.
7. Borrero E, Queral LA: Symptomatic abdominal aortic aneurysm misdiagnosed as nephroureterolithiasis. Ann Vasc Surg 1988;2:45-49.
8. Stewart D, Kowalski R, Wong P, Krome R: Microscopic hematuria and calculus-related ureteral obstruction. J Emerg Med 1990;8:693-695.
9. Luchs J, Katz D, Lane M, et al: Utility of hematuria testing in patients with suspected renal colic: Correlation with unenhanced helical CT results. Urology 2002;59:839-842.
10. Press S, Smith A: Incidence of negative hematuria in patients with acute urinary lithiasis presenting to the emergency room with flank pain. Urology 1995;45:753-757.
11. Yilmaz S, Sindel T, Arslan S, et al: Renal colic: Comparison of spiral CT, US and IVP in the detection of ureteral calculi. Eur Radiol 1998;8:212-217.
12. Fielding J, Steele G, Fox L, et al: Spiral computerized tomography in the evaluation of acute flank pain: A replacement for excretory urography. J Urol 1997;157:2071-2073.
13. Dalrymple N, Verga M, Anderson K, et al: The value of unenhanced helical computerized tomography in management of acute flank pain. J Urol 1998;159:735-740.
14. Boulay I, Holtz P, Foley W, et al: Ureteral calculi: Diagnostic efficacy of helical CT and implications for treatment of patients. AJR Am J Roentgenol 1999;172:1485-1490.
15. Smith R, Verga M, McCarthy S, et al: Diagnosis of acute flank pain: Value of unenhanced helical CT. AJR Am J Roentgenol 1996;166:97-101.
16. Colistro R, Torreggiani W, Lyburn I, et al: Unenhanced helical CT in the investigation of acute flank pain. Clin Radiol 2002;57:435-441.
17. Sourtzis S, Thibeau J, Damry N, et al: Radiologic investigation of renal colic: Unenhanced helical CT compared with excretory urography. AJR Am J Roentgenol 1999;172:1491-1494.
18. Hill M, Rich J, Mardiat J, et al: Sonography vs excretory urography in acute flank pain. AJR Am J Roentgenol 1985;144:1235-1238.
19. Patlas M, Farkas A, Fisher D, et al: Ultrasound vs CT for the detection of ureteric stones in patients with renal colic. Br J Radiol 2001;74:901-904.
20. Gorelik U, Ulish Y, Yagil Y: The use of standard imaging techniques and their diagnostic value in the workup of renal colic in the setting of intractable flank pain. Urology 1996;47:635-642.
21. Mutgi A, Williams J, Nettleman M: Utility of the plain abdominal roentgenogram. Arch Intern Med 1991; 151:1589-1592.
22. Roth C, Bowyer B, Berquist T, et al: Utility of the plain abdominal radiography for diagnosing ureteral calculi. Ann Emerg Med 1985;14:311-315.
23. Palma L, Stacul F, Bazzocchi M, et al: Ultrasonography and plain film versus intravenous urography in ureteric colic. Clin Radiol 1993;47:333-336.
24. Perlmutter A, Miller L, Trimble LA, et al: Toradol, an NSAID used for renal colic, decreases renal perfusion and ureteral pressure in a canine model of unilateral ureteral obstruction. J Urol 1993;149:926-930.
25. Lennon G, Bourke J, Ryan P, et al: Pharmacological options for the treatment of acute ureteric colic. Br J Urol 1993;71:401-407.
26. Jasani NB, O'Conner RE, Bouzoukis JK: Comparison of hydromorphone and meperidine for ureteral colic. Acad Emerg Med 1994;1:539-543.
27. Cordell W, Larson T, Lingeman J, et al: Indomethacin suppositories versus intravenously titrated morphine for the treatment of ureteral colic. Ann Emerg Med 1994; 23:262-269.
28. Labrecque M, Dostaler L, Rousselle R, et al: Efficacy of nonsteroidal anti-inflammatory drugs in the treatment of acute renal colic. Arch Intern Med 1994;154:1381-1387.
29. Lundstam SO, Leissner KH, Wåhlander LA, Kral JG: Prostaglandin-synthetase inhibition with diclofenac sodium in treatment of renal colic: Comparison with use of a narcotic analgesic. Lancet 1982;1(8281):1096-1097.
30. Larkin G, Peacock W, Pearl S, et al: Efficacy of ketorolac tromethamine versus meperidine in the ED treatment of acute renal colic. Am J Emerg Med 1999;17:6-10.
31. Cordell W, Wright S, Wolfson A, et al: Comparison of intravenous ketorolac, meperidine, and both (balanced analgesia) for renal colic. Ann Emerg Med 1996; 28:151-158.
32. Dellabella M, Milanese G, Muzzonigro G: Efficacy of tamsulosin in the medical management of juxtavesical ureteral stones. J Urol 2003;170:2202-2205.
33. Edna T, Hesselberg F: Acute ureteral colic and fluid intake. Scand J Urol Nephrol 1983;17:175-178.

Chapter **109**

Hematuria

Edward John Ward

KEY POINTS

- Hematuria results from the admixture of blood and urine at any point along the genitourinary tract, often due to infection, cancer, structural abnormalities, or unknown cause.
- Hematuria is of variable clinical significance and can be found in up to 10% of the general population at any given time.
- Stable patients with incidental microscopic hematuria should have a repeat urinalysis with their primary care provider 1 week after ED discharge.
- Patients with hematuria may require evaluation for carcinoma.
- Stable patients with large amounts of blood may require Foley catheter irrigation.

Scope and Definitions

Hematuria is the presence of red blood cells in the urine. Screening of asymptomatic individuals suggests that up to 10% of adults may have some degree of hematuria at any given time. Although often there is spontaneous resolution of the transient bleeding, some cases have undiagnosed structural, neoplastic, or infectious causes.[1]

Microscopic hematuria refers to the detection of greater than 2 to 10 red blood cells per high-powered field (hpf) in a spun sample of urine sediment.[1,2] Microscopic hematuria cannot be detected by visual inspection of urine. Hematuria present at microscopic levels is usually asymptomatic but can cause mild dysuria with greater degrees of bleeding.

Macroscopic hematuria (gross hematuria), visualized as red-colored urine, can occur when as little as 1 mL of blood mixes with a liter of urine. Macroscopic hematuria is very disconcerting to most patients, who will often present to the ED for the initial evaluation of this chief complaint. Dysuria is common among patients with macroscopic hematuria, and urinary retention may develop if high-volume bleeding leads to clots that obstruct urethral outflow.[2,3]

Pathophysiology

Hematuria results from the admixture of blood and urine at any point along the urinary tract. Box 109-1 summarizes the sources of genitourinary blood supply. Vascular disruption from any of these sources can result in variable degrees of hematuria. Clinically insignificant causes of minor vascular disruption leading to microscopic hematuria are generally traumatic in nature and resolve spontaneously.[3] Examples of such minor trauma include long-distance running, biking, contusion from low-impact direct blows, or shearing forces associated with motor vehicle collisions. Persistent or high-volume bleeding is generally pathologic in nature and mandates further evaluation.

Clinical Presentation

The ED presentation of hematuria can be divided into two groups: incidental and suspected. Incidental

BOX 109-1

Sources of Genitourinary Blood Supply

- The kidney receives blood from the renal arteries.
- The renal arteries divide multiple times until they form the efferent and afferent arterioles in the juxtamedullary complex within the capsule of the kidney.
- The ureters receive their blood supply from branches of the renal, aortic, iliac, and vesical arteries.
- The bladder is supplied by the vesical arteries and the urethra via the corpus spongiosum.
- Extra urethral tissue is supplied by multiple different sources.

BOX 109-2

Differential Diagnosis of Hematuria

- Infection
  - Cystitis
  - Pyelonephritis
  - Urethritis
  - Epididymitis
  - Sexually transmitted diseases
- Obstruction
  - Renal calculus
  - Cancer
  - Prostate hypertrophy
- Systemic disorders
  - Glomerulonephritis
  - Systemic lupus erythematosus
- Metabolic disorders
  - Hypercalcemia
  - Hyperuricosemia
- Genetic disorders
  - Sickle cell anemia
  - Von Hippel-Lindau disease
  - Polycystic kidney disease
  - Medullary sponge kidney
  - Thin basement membrane disease
  - Alport's syndrome—hereditary nephritis
- Trauma
  - Blunt
  - Penetrating
  - Exercise-related
  - Post-procedure/iatrogenic
- Medications (anticoagulants)

discovery of microscopic hematuria is generally noted in patients who have no abnormal vital signs or complaints attributable to the presence of red blood cells in their urine.[3] Urinalysis is ordered in these patients for unrelated reasons (e.g., suspected ketonuria or proteinuria).

The presentation of patients with suspected hematuria varies greatly depending on the underlying cause. Symptoms that suggest hematuria include dysuria, red-colored urine, suprapubic or flank pain, urinary retention, and urinary tract infection or urethritis. Unexplained anemia or renal insufficiency should also raise suspicion for coincident, undiagnosed hematuria.[2,3]

Differential Diagnosis

Hematuria may be a sign of a large number of diseases (Box 109-2).[1-4] Infection at any location in the genitourinary tract can cause hematuria. Bacterial irritation of the urinary bladder epithelium may result in hematuria, either microscopic or macroscopic (hemorrhagic cystitis). In addition to pyuria and bacturia, pyelonephritis may feature hematuria or casts of red and white blood cells. Sexually transmitted infections of the distal urethral tract irritate the mucosa and may result in bleeding, as well as pyuria and purulent discharge.[1]

Nephrolithiasis usually presents with acute flank pain, nausea, and vomiting as the chief complaints but may include gross hematuria as well. Microscopic hematuria is a common finding in cases of suspected ureteral colic; however hematuria may be absent with complete ureteral obstruction. As the stone descends through the ureter it abrades the mucosal tissue, resulting in hematuria.[1,3]

Benign prostatic hypertrophy is a common cause of microscopic hematuria as men age. Gradual-onset associated symptoms include difficulty initiating urination, increased frequency, and incomplete voiding. An enlarged, firm, smooth prostate will be found on examination.[2]

Glomerulonephritis is caused by an immunologic reaction that triggers inflammation and proliferation of glomerular tissue. Patients usually present with hematuria and back pain, with eventual progression to renal insufficiency or failure. A history of recent upper respiratory tract infection or diagnosed streptococcus infection is helpful in making the diagnosis of poststreptococcal glomerulonephritis. Systemic lupus erythematosus and other chronic inflammatory connective tissue disorders can also cause hematuria by similar mechanisms.[2]

Rare genetic disorders can also present with hematuria. They include von Hippel-Lindau disease and familial disorders such as polycystic kidney disease, medullary sponge kidney, thin basement membrane disease, hereditary nephritis (Alport's syndrome), Fabry's disease, and nail-patella syndrome.[2]

BOX 109-3

Causes of Red-Colored Urine Not Associated with Red Blood Cells

- Myoglobinuria
  - Significant rhabdomyolysis
  - Burns
  - Crush injury
  - Myositis
  - Prolonged generalized seizures
- Hemoglobinuria (hemolytic anemias)
- Contamination
  - Menstrual bleeding
  - Factitious addition of blood to the urine
- Medications (phenazopyridine)
- Ingestion of beets or blackberries

Hematuria can represent an adverse reaction to several medications, including quinine, rifampin, phenytoin, and anticoagulants (e.g., warfarin, aspirin, lovenox, nonsteroidal antiinflammatory drugs, clopidogrel). Additionally, some medications can induce nephritis.[1,4]

Blunt trauma will often result in microscopic hematuria that is generally self-limited. Macroscopic hematuria is most common in the setting of penetrating trauma. Vigorous exercise will elicit hematuria due to minor repetitive trauma to the bladder or prostate, especially in younger athletes who engage in long-distance running or biking.[3]

Box 109-3 lists several causes of red-colored urine that do not involve the presence of red blood cells.

Diagnostic Testing

Two tests to detect hematuria are readily available—the urine dipstick text and standard urinalysis. The rapid and inexpensive urine dipstick test is routinely performed on most urine specimens screened in the ED. This point-of-care test is able to detect the equivalent of 1 to 2 red blood cells/hpf. Although the urine dipstick test is very sensitive, false-positive results can occur with myoglobinuria or hemoglobinuria.[5]

If a urine dipstick test is positive for the detection of blood, standard urinalysis should be performed on a spun urine specimen in the laboratory. This is the optimal means for diagnosing hematuria. Urinalysis is highly sensitive and specific; however, it is more expensive and time-intensive than the urine dipstick test. Urinalysis quantifies the amount of blood present and can differentiate the presence of myoglobin or hemoglobin.[1,3]

Incidental microscopic hematuria without associated symptoms or hemodynamic instability requires no further ED testing but mandates follow-up evaluation as an outpatient.[2] A repeat urinalysis should be checked in a primary care setting 1 week after ED discharge. Persistent microscopic hematuria requires further testing, including imaging, cystoscopy, and renal biopsy. Studies have demonstrated that 19% to 68% of cases of asymptomatic microscopic hematuria will not have an identifiable etiology, even after extensive outpatient testing.[1]

Computed tomography is routinely performed to assess renal anatomy and screen for suspected tumors, infection, or nephrolithiasis in cases of hematuria. Such imaging may be performed as an outpatient in otherwise stable patients, in consultation with the primary care provider or a urologist.

Other outpatient tests that may be performed in the evaluation of hematuria include[2]

- Renal ultrasonography (to assess kidney size, blood flow, and suspected hydronephrosis)
- Renal biopsy (for tumors noted on computed tomography scans or for suspected glomerulonephroses)
- Renal angiography
- Cystoscopy (routinely performed in the outpatient evaluation of lower urinary tract tumors)[1,2,4]

Treatment and Disposition

Treatment varies depending on the underlying diagnosis. Consultation with a nephrologist may be helpful in cases of persistent microscopic hematuria. Urology consultation should be obtained for patients with urinary tract tumors identified by computed tomography or ultrasonography patients with suspected tumors based on evidence of high-volume, noninfectious gross hematuria. Most cases of hematuria can be further managed on an outpatient basis.[3]

Patients with gross hematuria resulting in significant dysuria or obstruction require placement of a Foley catheter. Bladder irrigation with sterile saline may dislodge clots and allow bladder decompression. A multiple-lumen catheter may be advantageous if large-volume, continuous bladder irrigation is required to clear significant bleeding. Stable patients with improved symptoms may be discharged with a leg bag and instructions for urology follow-up in 3 to 5 days. Prophylactic antibiotics should be prescribed to prevent urinary tract infection.

The vast majority of patients with microscopic hematuria are discharged with further care as an outpatient. Incidental cases require repeat urinalysis in 1 week; persistent hematuria mandates further testing. Return precautions include fatigue, dizziness, fever, pain, worsening dysuria, and macroscopic hematuria.[1,3]

Patients with macroscopic hematuria rarely require admission to the hospital. Those with unstable vital signs secondary to significant blood loss or infection should be admitted to a medical or urological service.[3]

REFERENCES

1. Cohen R, Brown R: Microscopic hematuria. N Engl J Med 2003;348:2330-2338.
2. Kincaid-Smith P, Fairley K: The investigation of hematuria. Semin Nephrol 2005;25:127-135.
3. Gordon C, Stapleton F: Hematuria in adolescents. Adolesc Med Clin 2005;16:229-239.
4. Ahmed Z, Lee J: Asymptomatic urinary abnormalities. Med Clin North Am 1997;3:641-652.
5. Liao J, Churchill B: Pediatric urine testing. Pediatr Clin North Am 2001;6:1425-1440.

Chapter 110

Pediatric Genitourinary and Renal Disorders

Ingrid T. Lim and N. Ewen Wang

KEY POINTS

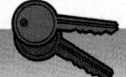

Because children often cannot differentiate between abdominal pain and groin pain, a complete physical examination is necessary.

Nephrotic syndrome is characterized by edema, hypoproteinemia, and marked proteinuria. The most common primary cause in children is minimal change disease.

The most common cause of acute renal failure in children is hemolytic uremic syndrome.

Post-streptococcal glomerulonephritis is the most common cause of acute glomerulonephritis. IgA nephropathy is the most commonly diagnosed cause of glomerulonephritis in adolescents.

One third of patients with Henoch-Schönlein purpura have renal involvement. This disorder is the most common form of vasculitis in childhood, usually presenting with the triad of abdominal pain, arthritis, and purpura.

The most common types of renal tubular acidosis seen in children are type 1 (distal, H^+ transport defect) and type 2 (proximal, bicarbonate-wasting).

Anatomy of the Genitourinary Tract

The genital organs originate within the abdominal cavity and then migrate externally during fetal development. Delays in testicular migration explain much of the pathology of scrotal masses. The testes, attached to their blood supply, drag their peritoneal covering (known as the tunica vaginalis) through the inguinal canal and into the scrotal sac.

The left testicle usually completes migration before the right testicle thus explaining the increased frequency of right-sided inguinal hernias and undescended right testicles. Impediments to migration cause cryptorchidism. Failure of the peritoneal space to close after testicular migration can lead to hydroceles and inguinal hernias. Failure of fixation of the testes within the scrotal sac can cause testicular torsion. Differences in venous return make left-sided varicoceles much more common than right-sided.

Posterior urethral valves (PUV) represent a disturbance of urethral development in males that is the leading cause of lower urinary tract obstruction in neonates. One third of patients progress to end-stage renal disease, and 10% to 15% of children who require renal transplantation have posterior urethral valves.

Anatomy of the Kidneys

The full complement of nephrons is present at birth, although newborn nephrons are heterogeneous in glomerular size and proximal tubule length. Anatomy and function mature postnatally. Although fetal urine is excreted into the bladder by 10 to 11 weeks of gestation, ability to conserve and excrete sodium, concentrate urine, and reabsorb substrates such as glucose evolves to maturity over the first two years of life. In utero, the glomerular filtration rate (GFR) is minimal secondary to placental function; at birth, GFR is 10% of adult values and matures by 12 to 24 months of age. Thus an increase in an infant's creatinine to "normal" adult ranges can indicate pathology.

GENITOURINARY DISORDERS

Cryptorchidism (Undescended Testis)

Usually the testes have descended from the abdominal cavity into the scrotum by birth; only 4% of newborns have an undescended testicle. By 1 year of age, spontaneous descent is unlikely—0.8% of males are still affected at 12 months of age. In a careful physical examination, 80% of undescended testes are palpable, usually in the inguinal canal. Children with undescended testes are at higher risk for torsion, trauma, and malignancy.

■ CLINICAL PRESENTATION AND DIAGNOSIS

Abdominal pain in children with undescended testes should prompt evaluation for intra-abdominal torsion. The differential diagnosis includes retractile testes. Children less than 1 year of age should be examined while they are relaxed in a warm bath, because the testes can be retracted during examination. Children older than 1 year of age should be examined by a urologist. Histologic deterioration of the testes, presumably secondary to increased ambient temperature, begins during the second year of life and is correlated with infertility even in cases of unilateral undescended testes.

■ TREATMENT

The optimal time for surgical intervention is shortly after the first birthday.

Hydrocele

A hydrocele is a collection of fluid that accumulates within the tunica vaginalis. Hydroceles are often present at birth and occur most frequently on the right side secondary to delayed migration of the right testicle.

■ CLINICAL PRESENTATION AND DIAGNOSIS

Hydroceles usually are painless. Physical examination reveals enlargement of the scrotum that may transilluminate. Ultrasonography is necessary to exclude acute pathology if the infant appears to be in pain. The majority of hydroceles not associated with inguinal hernia tend to resolve spontaneously between 12 and 24 months of age.

■ TREATMENT

Hydroceles associated with an inguinal hernia, or those that occur or persist after 2 years of age, require outpatient surgical repair.

Varicocele

A varicocele is a collection of venous varicosities of the spermatic veins in the scrotum caused by incomplete drainage of the pampiniform plexus. They are rare in children younger than 10 years of age. Varicoceles arise between 10 and 15 years of age, with an overall incidence in approximately 15% of males.[1,2]

■ CLINICAL PRESENTATION AND DIAGNOSIS

The majority (85%-95%) of varicoceles are left-sided, the result of spermatic venous incompetence due to drainage of the left spermatic vein into the renal vein at a right angle. Right-sided varicoceles should prompt an evaluation for intra-abdominal pathology such as thrombosis or tumor causing compression of the inferior vena cava.[3] A sudden-onset left-sided varicocele should raise suspicion of renal cell carcinoma with obstruction of the left renal vein. The differential diagnosis of varicoceles and other scrotal masses is outlined in Table 110-1.

Varicoceles can cause mild discomfort and may lead to infertility in adult males. They are usually diagnosed on routine physical examination and are characterized by a full hemiscrotum without skin changes and a classic "bag of worms" finding on palpation.

■ TREATMENT

A varicocele is usually an incidental finding in adolescence and is not an emergency. Referral to outpatient urology is appropriate.

Hernias

An inguinal hernia occurs when a portion of the intestine herniates into a patent processus vaginalis. An incarcerated hernia refers to an intestinal loop that is not reducible. A strangulated hernia results when the blood supply to the intestinal loop is obstructed and bowel ischemia ensues.

■ EPIDEMIOLOGY AND PATHOPHYSIOLOGY

Inguinal hernias occur in 15 out of every 1000 live births and are 6 to 10 times more common in males.

Table 110-1 AGE-BASED DIFFERENTIAL DIAGNOSIS OF PEDIATRIC SCROTAL MASSES AND PAIN

Diagnosis	Age at Onset	Pain	Position of Testes, Tenderness	Systemic Symptoms	Comment
Testicular torsion*	All ages; peak onset 12-18 years	60% sudden onset; diffuse tenderness	High riding horizontal lie	Vomiting common; dysuria and fever uncommon	
Testicular appendix torsion	Pre-puberty; average age 10 years	Acute or gradual; focal tenderness	Normal lie; blue dot	Vomiting, dysuria, and fever uncommon	
Epididymo-orchitis	>16 years	Gradual; posterior tenderness	Normal lie	Vomiting uncommon; dysuria and fever common	Adolescent etiology: STD
Hydrocele	Most common during first year of life	Painless	Normal lie	None	Usually resolves by 12 months of age
Inguinal hernia (incarcerated hernia, strangulated hernia*)	Most common during first year of life	Pain with incarceration/ strangulation	Normal	Vomiting abdominal pain with incarceration/ strangulation	Occurs 10 times more frequently in males than in females; right-sided more common
Varicocele	10-15 years	Painless, mild discomfort, "pressune or fullness"	Normal lie	None	Associated with infertility; right-sided varicocele should prompt evaluation for tumor causing IVC compression
Testicular tumor	Rare; most occur in patients <3 years of age	Painless	Normal lie, nontender mass	None unless advanced tumor	

*Emergent condition.
IVC, inferior vena cava; STD, sexually transmitted disease; UTI, urinary tract infection.

The incidence is highest during the first year of life, with a peak in diagnosis during the first month; one third of cases are diagnosed in children less than 6 months of age. The incidence is higher (30%) in premature infants. Due to improved neonatal care of premature infants, neonatal inguinal hernias and hydroceles are increasingly being identified.

Indirect hernias are more common on the right side (60%) secondary to late testicular descent into the scrotum. If a left-sided hernia exists, there is a strong possibility that an occult right-sided hernia is present. A family history of hernia, prematurity, or undescended testicle is associated with inguinal hernias.

■ CLINICAL PRESENTATION

Incarceration is more common with small hernias and occurs frequently during the first 6 months of life; it is less common after 2 years of age and is relatively rare after age 5. Strangulation and perforation can occur within two hours of decreased blood flow. In females, although incarceration occurs more frequently, strangulation is less common because the ovaries, not the intestines, herniate.

■ TREATMENT

Hernias found on routine examination without symptoms should be referred for surgical repair because incarceration is frequent during the first year of life. Approximately 90% of complications can be avoided if surgery is performed within the first month of diagnosis.

Idiopathic Scrotal Edema

Idiopathic scrotal edema presents as painless erythema and induration of the scrotum. Over 75% of cases occur in boys less than 10 years of age. Two thirds of cases are unilateral.

■ CLINICAL PRESENTATION

Patients may complain of pruritus. Edema and erythema may extend to the phallus, groin, and abdomen. The testes and epididymis have no palpable masses and systemic symptoms are rare.

TREATMENT AND DISPOSITION

If acute pathology has been excluded, patients can be discharged home with outpatient follow-up. Most cases spontaneously resolve within a few days and do not require specific treatment. There is a 21% recurrence rate.

Carcinoma

Testicular and scrotal cancer account for 1% of solid tumors in children. There is an increased incidence in patients with bilateral cryptorchidism. Lymphoma and leukemia can metastasize to the testicles as well.

CLINICAL PRESENTATION AND DIAGNOSIS

On examination, a painless unilateral mass can be palpated separately from the testis; there also may be a sensation of fullness, tugging, or increased weight in the scrotum associated with testicular enlargement. A reactive hydrocele is present in 7% to 25% of patients and may lead to a delay in diagnosis. Further examination reveals a firm mass, either smooth or nodular, that does not transilluminate. Lymphadenopathy, petechiae, abdominal masses, hepatosplenomegaly, or gynecomastica may be present.

A complete blood count, urinalysis, urine test for human chorionic gonadotropin (produced by germ cell tumors), and testicular ultrasound images should be obtained.

TREATMENT

Management consists of prompt urologic and oncologic consultation and biopsy.

Phimosis

Phimosis is a constriction of the penile foreskin resulting in inability to retract the prepuce over the glans. A fully retractable foreskin is present in 4% of newborns, 50% of 1-year-olds, 80% of 2-year-olds, and 90% of 4-year-olds. In the remaining cases, the foreskin may not be retractable until puberty.[4]

CLINICAL PRESENTATION

Symptoms include pain, hematuria, and in severe cases, urinary obstruction. Most cases of phimosis are physiologic. Adolescents may complain of pain on erection secondary to tension on the foreskin from glandular adhesions. Phimosis can also result from trauma, infection, chemical irritation, and poor hygiene or as a complication of circumcision. Severe stenosis or obstructive uropathy can result from chronic symptomatic phimosis.

TREATMENT

Because the ability to retract the foreskin is age-related, parents should not forcefully retract the prepuce. Good hygiene should be taught. If the child has signs of urinary outlet obstruction, dilation of the meatus by gentle use of forceps is warranted.

Steroid preparations (betamethasone cream 0.05-5% two to four times daily or hydrocortisone cream 1% two to three times daily) have been used with varying success.[5]

Balanitis and Balanoposthitis

Balanitis is an infection of the glans penis; *balanoposthitis* is an infection of the foreskin as well as of the glans. Balanitis occurs in approximately 3% of boys, usually between 2 and 5 years of age, especially if they are uncircumcised.[6]

CLINICAL PRESENTATION AND DIAGNOSIS

Balanitis can be caused by trauma, infection, or irritation such as contact dermatitis from urine, soaps, powders, and ointments. Balanoposthitis is often a mixed infection but may be caused by group A beta-hemolytic streptococci. Most children present with a characteristic moist balanoposthitis caused by a nonretractable prepuce.[7] In severe cases, cellulitis can extend down the penile shaft. Palpable inguinal adenopathy is often present.

Signs of group A beta-hemolytic streptococcal infection include pain, intense fiery redness, and a moist, glistening transudate or exudate under the prepuce and over the glans. Streptococcal infection occurs without associated pharyngitis.

The differential diagnosis includes sexually transmitted diseases. Gonorrhea and chlamydia without frank urethral discharge is unusual in preschool children. After puberty, gonorrhea can be isolated in the absence of urethral discharge.[8] Thin, purulent discharge in the preputial glandular sulcus without true urethral discharge may signal a streptococcal infection, which can be diagnosed by rapid antigen detection and culture.

TREATMENT AND DISPOSITION

Patients with urinary retention, fever, or cellulitis of the penile shaft should be treated with oral antibiotics for 7 days (cephalexin, cefadroxil). Warm water sitz baths and topical antibiotics also are helpful. Poor urinary flow, urine dribbling, or severe phimosis may mandate incision of the dorsal inner foreskin by a urologist.

Indications for admission include severe infection and urinary retention.

Meatal Stenosis

Meatal stenosis is a narrowing of the urethral meatus, usually secondary to recurrent episodes of subclinical meatitis. It can be caused by ammonia diaper irritation in circumcised boys and by recurrent balanoposthitis in uncircumcised boys. Acquired meatal stenosis usually only occurs in circumcised boys because the foreskin acts as a protective cover for the meatus. Congenital meatal stenosis is rare.

■ CLINICAL PRESENTATION AND DIAGNOSIS

Obstructive symptoms occasionally occur, including hesitancy, straining, urgency, frequency, and postvoid dribbling. An abnormal urinary stream may be seen, but urinary retention is rare. An erythematous swollen meatus is noted, often with purulent discharge. Radiographic studies are seldom necessary.

■ TREATMENT

Treatment of purulent meatitis includes sitz baths and administration of oral antibiotics (e.g., cephalexin) for 7 days. Urinary retention is an indication for urology consultation and admission; otherwise prompt outpatient follow-up is sufficient.

Urethral Stricture

In the United States, most cases of urethral stricture are acquired by infection and trauma. Infectious causes are usually secondary to gonococcal urethritis or an indwelling Foley catheter. In developing countries, sexually transmitted urethritis is the most common cause. Trauma can result in urethral stricture secondary to pelvic fracture and straddle injury.

■ CLINICAL PRESENTATION AND TREATMENT

Clinically, the patient has difficulty passing urine. There may be slowing, spraying, or dribbling of the urine stream. When patients with this condition present to the ED, outpatient management is appropriate. Patients are usually given prophylactic antibiotics. Urethrography or voiding cystourethrography should be performed before dilation of the stricture if this procedure is necessary.

Urethral Foreign Body

A urethral foreign body in older male children may have been inserted for sexual purposes. Most objects are palpable if they are in the anterior urethra. Retained foreign body should be included in the differential diagnosis of a male with signs and symptoms of recurrent urinary tract infection and no urogenital abnormalities. Most foreign bodies can be removed endoscopically.

Urethral Prolapse

Prolapse of the urethra is most common in young African-American females. The prolapsed mucosa is visible and may be irritated, congested, and hemorrhagic. Although quite alarming on physical examination, it is not associated with sexual abuse. Treatment consists of sitz baths three times a day.

RENAL DISORDERS

Nephrotic Syndrome

Nephrotic syndrome is the clinical manifestation of a variety of primary and secondary glomerular disorders characterized by the following findings:

- Hypoproteinemia (serum albumin <3 g/dL)
- Marked proteinuria (>40 g/m^2/hour in a 24-hour period)
- Edema
- Hyperlipidemia (predominantly triglycerides and cholesterol)

■ PATHOPHYSIOLOGY

Nephrotic syndrome most commonly presents in children as idiopathic nephrotic syndrome (also known as minimal change disease because of the minimal changes seen on renal biopsy). *Primary* nephrotic syndrome refers to diseases limited to the kidney; *secondary* nephrotic syndrome includes systemic disease that involves renal complications. Ninety percent of children with nephrotic syndrome have the primary type.

Idiopathic nephrotic syndrome is classified by its response to corticosteroids: steroid-responsive (90%) and steroid nonresponsive (10%). Lack of response to steroids portends a poor prognosis and a 50% risk of advancement to end-stage renal failure.

■ EPIDEMIOLOGY

Boys are twice as likely to be affected as girls. The incidence and prevalence of nephrotic syndrome in children less than 16 years of age are 2 to 7 per 100,000 per year and 15 cases per 100,000, respectively. Usually sporadic, the disease can be familial, with a polygenic inheritance pattern. The typical age of presentation of primary nephrotic syndrome is 18 months to 6 years. Children older than 5 years are more likely to have the secondary form. If nephrotic syndrome appears in the neonatal period, it is likely the congenital (Finnish) type, which is steroid-resistant and generally fatal. In adolescents, nephrotic syndrome is most often associated with a primary or secondary form of an underlying nephritis.

CLINICAL PRESENTATION

The usual presenting sign in a child with nephrotic syndrome is edema. The edema starts with early-morning periorbital swelling, often misattributed to a cold or allergies. As the edema spreads to the abdomen, trunk, and extremities, children have increasing difficulty fitting into their pants and shoes, and parents often mistake this for weight gain. The child otherwise appears well, although ascites, pleural effusion, or pulmonary edema may be present. Ascites and an edematous intestinal wall can manifest as abdominal pain, nausea, vomiting, and diarrhea.

COMPLICATIONS

Complications include infection, hypercoagulability, hypovolemia, respiratory distress, and acute renal failure.

Infection

The most common infection is peritonitis, although cellulitis, pneumonia, sepsis, and meningitis are also seen. Infection with encapsulated bacteria such as *Escherichia coli, Haemophilus influenzae,* and *Streptococcus pneumoniae* is the main cause of death in children with nephrotic syndrome. Steroid therapy may mask the typical signs of infection.

Hypercoagulability

Hypercoagulability occurs in 3% of patients with nephrotic syndrome; thromboembolic events can involve arteries and veins, particularly renal veins. Sudden onset of gross hematuria or renal failure should prompt investigation for renal vein thrombosis.

Prednisone exerts an anti-heparin effect. For this reason, deep venous punctures should not be attempted in these patients unless no alternative exists.

Respiratory Distress

Pleural effusions, pulmonary edema, and massive ascites can cause respiratory distress.

TREATMENT

The goals of ED management are volume restoration and treatment of symptomatic edema. Patients in shock are treated with isotonic hydration at a 20 mL/kg bolus per hour until they are normotensive. If the patient is clinically dehydrated with hemoconcentration but not in shock, a trial of sodium-deficient fluids administered orally at twice the maintenance dose is preferable to IV hypotonic solutions. Small amounts of oral hydration fluids should be administered frequently to avoid vomiting caused by an edematous gut.

If the patient is well hydrated and exhibits symptomatic edema, diuretics may be warranted but should be used judiciously, as these children are prone to thromboembolic events and have decreased circulating volume. IV or oral administration of furosemide, 1 to 2 mg/kg/24 hours divided into two doses, can be used. Loop diuretics work best, but additional diuretics such as hydrochlorothiazide or spironolactone may be used if there is no response. Diuretics are not effective with albumin concentrations of less than 1.5 g; albumin infusions may be necessary prior to diuretic administration (0.5-1g/kg given as 25% salt-deficient albumin, followed by 0.5-1 mg/kg of furosemide).

The mainstay of treatment for nephrotic syndrome is steroid therapy. Generally, patients are started on prednisone, 2 mg/kg/24 hours (maximum 60 mg/24 hours) divided into two or three doses. Approximately 90% of patients with idiopathic nephrotic syndrome respond to steroid therapy by the end of a 4-week course, with response defined as trace or negative amounts of urine protein for three days. Failure to respond to steroid treatment increases the likelihood that the renal pathology is not due to minimal change disease.

Prophylactic antibiotics are not necessary unless infection is suspected and cultures collected. Any child with nephrotic syndrome and an unexplained fever must considered to have a bacterial infection until proved otherwise. Because persons on steroid therapy may not demonstrate abdominal pain or other signs of peritonitis, diagnostic paracentesis is necessary to confirm the diagnosis in children with fever and ascites or with signs of peritonitis without fever. Treatment with ampicillin and/or gentamicin or cephalosporins is recommended.

DISPOSITION

Admission Criteria

- Any infant with nephrotic syndrome
- Any patient with respiratory distress or shock
- Nephrotic patients with infections, unexplained fever, refractory edema, renal insufficiency, dehydration, abdominal complaints, or hemoconcentration greater than 50%
- Newly diagnosed patients, to complete the evaluation and educate parents about outpatient management

Follow-up for Patients with Non-Nephrotic Proteinuria

Very few patients with dipstick proteinuria have renal disease. In the absence of edema, hypertension, oliguria, or hematuria, a repeat urinalysis in 2 to 4 weeks is recommended.

BOX 110-1

Hallmarks of Hemolytic Uremic Syndrome

- Acute renal failure
- Microangiopathic hemolytic anemia
- Fever
- Thrombocytopenia

Hemolytic Uremic Syndrome

Hemolytic uremic syndrome is the most common cause of acute renal failure in children, with an incidence of 1 to 10 cases per 100,000 during childhood. The mean age at presentation is 3 years, and the diagnosis is less likely after 5 years of age. Caucasian children are more often affected than others and there is no gender preference.

■ PATHOPHYSIOLOGY

Hemolytic uremic syndrome is defined by the presence of the classic triad of microangiopathic hemolytic anemia, thrombocytopenia, and acute renal failure (Box 110-1).

In contrast to the adult form of the disease (thrombotic thrombocytopenic purpura), the microthrombi of hemolytic uremic syndrome are essentially confined to the kidneys. Thrombotic thrombocytopenic purpura has a predominantly neurologic presentation, a higher mortality rate, and a better response to plasmapheresis and fresh-frozen plasma. Renal involvement is the defining feature of hemolytic uremic syndrome.

The usual cause of epidemic hemolytic uremic syndrome is the verotoxin-producing strain of *Escherichia coli* serotype O157:H7, although it can be caused by *Shigella* organisms that produce a similar toxin. Transmission is through person-to-person contact or ingestion of contaminated food, such as unpasteurized dairy products or undercooked beef. The verotoxin binds to and destroys the colonic mucosa, leading to bloody diarrhea.

■ CLINICAL PRESENTATION

The epidemic form begins with a prodrome of nausea, vomiting, watery diarrhea, crampy abdominal pain, and occasionally fever. Patients typically develop bloody stools on the second or third day of symptoms. After the prodromal gastroenteritis, there is a sudden onset of pallor, listlessness, irritability, and oliguria. Symptoms also may include dehydration, edema, hypertension, petechiae, hepatosplenomegaly, jaundice, hemolytic anemia, thrombocytopenia, acute renal insufficiency, and neurologic manifestations (obtundation, hemiparesis, seizures, brainstem dysfunction).

Possible gastrointestinal complications are toxic megacolon, ischemic colitis, intussusception, and perforation. Pancreatic insufficiency from microinfarcts in the pancreas can lead to permanent insulin-dependent diabetes mellitus.

■ DIAGNOSTIC TESTING

Hemolytic uremic syndrome primarily is diagnosed by clinical symptoms coupled with consistent laboratory findings. A complete blood count may show leukocytosis, profound anemia (with hemoglobin levels of 5 to 9 g/dL), and mild to moderate thrombocytopenia (generally platelet counts are around 40,000/mm^3).

The presence of microangiopathic hemolytic anemia is necessary to establish the diagnosis. The peripheral blood smear demonstrates signs of a microangiopathic process: tear drop cells, helmet cells, spherocytes, and burr cells.

C-reactive protein levels may be elevated, and the coagulation profile is usually normal. Serum fibrin split products might be elevated, though fulminant disseminated intravascular coagulation is rare. Chemistry abnormalities include hyponatremia, hyperkalemia, azotemia, metabolic acidosis, hyperbilirubinemia, low total protein from proteinuria, and elevated lactate dehydrogenase. Urinalysis often shows hematuria, proteinuria, and pyuria. Granular and hyaline casts are seen in the urine sediment.

Specific serologic testing for antibodies to the lipopolysacchande of *Escherichia coli* O157:H7 is necessary, since routine stool cultures may not always detect the bacteria or verotoxin.

■ TREATMENT AND DISPOSITION

Indications for dialysis in hemolytic uremic syndrome are similar to those in children with renal failure: signs and symptoms of uremia, azotemia, severe fluid overload, and electrolyte disturbances not responsive to medical therapy. Rehydration should be done slowly to avoid fluid overload. Transfusion of packed red blood cells is necessary if hemoglobin level falls below 6 g/dL; Platelet transfusion is recommended only if there is active bleeding or prior to a required invasive procedure.

Hypertension is usually responsive to administration of calcium-channel blockers, labetalol, captopril, or hydralazine or, in refractory cases, nitroprusside. Seizures will respond to benzodiazepines and phenytoin, but consider hypertonic 3% saline if hyponatremic seizures occur. Plasmapheresis or fresh-frozen plasma infusion has no proven efficacy in diarrhea-associated hemolytic uremic syndrome but may be useful in recurrent, inherited, drug-induced, or idiopathic hemolytic uremic syndrome, especially if there is neurologic involvement.

The role of antibiotics remains controversial—it is theorized that antibiotics may enhance the release of verotoxin from the bacteria, and therefore are generally not recommended. Antimotility agents should be avoided because they may cause toxic megacolon.

Patients require admission and pediatric nephrology consultation. Prognosis is poor in patients who have nondiarrheal forms of the disease, are less than 1 year of age, or have prolonged anuria, hypertension, or severe central nervous system disease. In general, prognosis is excellent, with less than 5% mortality. An additional 5% will have long-term consequences of end stage renal failure or stroke.

Acute Glomerulonephritis

Acute glomerulonephritis refers to a spectrum of inflammatory renal disorders characterized by hematuria and proteinuria.

■ PATHOPHYSIOLOGY

The most common form of acute glomerulonephritis in children occurs following infection with group A beta-hemolytic streptococci. Acute glomerulonephritis also can occur following a pharyngitis or a cutaneous infection approximately 1 to 3 weeks prior to presentation. School-age male children are commonly affected. In warmer climates, pyoderma is the antecedent infection common to younger preschool children. The latency period for both pharyngeal and cutaneous forms can be as long as 6 weeks. Anuria and renal failure occur in 2% of patients.

■ CLINICAL PRESENTATION

Signs and symptoms of acute glomerulonephritis are shown in Box 110-2.

The diagnosis usually is made in the ED based on the patient's history. The typical patient is a 5- or 6-year-old boy who presents to the ED 1 to 2 weeks after a preceding streptococcal infection, or 3 to 6 weeks after onset of pyoderma, with sudden onset of brown, tea-colored, or grossly bloody urine, decreased urine output, and edema, involving the face, periorbital areas, and extremities. On examination, hypertension (both systolic and diastolic) may be found. Some children may be asymptomatic except for the change in urine color. Rarely, patients with advanced disease may present which congestive heart failure, hypertensive encephalopathy, or other life-threatening complications of renal failure.

BOX 110-2

Presenting Signs and Symptoms of Acute Glomerulonephritis

- Hematuria (gross or microscopic)
- Dysmorphic red blood cells and red blood cell casts
- Proteinuria
- Hypertension
- Edema
- Renal insufficiency

■ DIAGNOSTIC TESTING

Urinalysis is the single most important test in categorizing glomerulonephritis. Proteinuria is almost always more than 2^+ on the dipstick, indicating that the measured protein is not merely secondary to hematuria. In 60% of cases, red blood cell casts are seen on microscopic analysis. Hyaline granular casts and pyuria are common. A urine culture should always be obtained.

Serologic testing can confirm streptococcal infection. Antistreptolysin O (ASO) titers are elevated in 90% of cases and peak at 10 to 14 days, returning to normal after 3 to 4 weeks; antihyaluronidase titers peak at 3 to 4 weeks. In patients with skin infections, anti-DNAse-B antibodies can be measured.

■ TREATMENT AND DISPOSITION

The key to a successful outcome is early diagnosis in the ED and treatment of life-threatening emergencies such as hyperkalemia, hypertension, and congestive heart failure. The management of patients with nephritis is primarily supportive, with restricted fluid and sodium intake. Antibiotics are required for ongoing infectious processes.

Any child who is oliguric or hypertensive should be hospitalized and scheduled for nephrology consultation. Otherwise, discharge from the ED is reasonable, with instructions for a low-sodium diet and close follow-up with the pediatrician. Advise the family to monitor the patient's urine output and weight and observe for signs of congestive heart failure or hypertension. In general, the prognosis is excellent—approximately 80% to 90% of these children recover without any persistent renal abnormalities, except for microhematuria, which may persist for up to 18 months.

IgA Nephropathy

IgA nephropathy, also known as *Berger's disease,* is the type of glomerulonephritis most commonly diagnosed in adolescence.[9] This disease accounts for up to 25% of glomerulonephritis cases in Asia and Europe and up to 10% in the United States.

■ CLINICAL PRESENTATION AND DIAGNOSIS

The classic presentation is hematuria or proteinuria with preceding upper respiratory infection. Diagnosis is confirmed by a renal biopsy, showing deposition of 1gA in the mesangium.

TREATMENT AND DISPOSITION

Gross hematuria usually resolves spontaneously within days without serious sequelae in 85% of patients. As the prognosis is good in most cases where there is not significant proteinuria or renal dysfunction, treatment is usually not needed. However, proteinuria, hypertension, or renal insufficiency portend a poor prognosis and should be managed in consultation with nephrology.

Henoch-Schönlein Purpura with Renal Involvement

Henoch-Schönlein purpura is the most common form of small-vessel vasculitis in childhood. Most patients present with the triad of abdominal pain, arthritis, and purpura. A third of the patients have renal involvement, of whom 80% will have asymptomatic hematuria. The populations most affected are school-age children and young adults, and the disorder occurs more commonly in Caucasians and males. One third to three fourths of patients have a preceding respiratory infection.

CLINICAL PRESENTATION

Usually occurring within the first month of illness, renal involvement develops in 20% to 50% of patients, with progression to end-stage renal disease in less than 1%. Predictors of worse prognosis include late onset of renal involvement in older children, and massive proteinuria; 20% of such cases result in end-stage renal failure. Approximately 50% of patients who develop nephritic syndrome with Henoch-Schönlein purpura will develop end-stage renal disease within 10 years.

Diagnosis is clinical and not based on laboratory studies.

TREATMENT

There is no specific treatment other than corticosteroids. Prednisone 1-2 mg/kg/day for 2 weeks, then tapered over 2 weeks, has been shown to improve gastrointestinal and joint symptoms and lessen the severity of nephritis. About one third of affected patients will have a recurrence of at least one symptom. Fortunately most patients recover quickly in several weeks with supportive treatment.

Renal Tubular Acidosis

The normal response to acidemia is to reabsorb all the filtered bicarbonate and to increase excretion of hydrogen, primarily by excreting ammonium ions in the urine.

Renal tubular acidosis occurs when the renal tubules are unable to pertorm these functions. The accumulation and subsequent metabolic acidosis can cause growth retardation, kidney stones, bone disease, and progressive renal failure.

There are four subtypes of renal tubular acidosis:
Type 1—distal (classic form)
Type 2—proximal (bicarbonate-wasting)
Type 3—a combination of types 1 and 2
Type 4—hyperkalemic (rare in children)

Types 1 and 2 are encountered most frequently in children. The diagosis of all types requireses a serum electrolyte panel and urinalysis with urine pH.

TYPE 1 RENAL TUBULAR ACIDOSIS

Distal renal tubular acidosis results from a defect in the tubular transport of hydrogen in the distal nephron. The most common form in children is hereditary, but it can be a complication of systemic diseases seen more commonly in adults such as Sjögren's syndrome, lupus erythematosus, and hyperparathyroidism. Patients present with failure to thrive, anorexia, vomiting, and dehydration. Hyperchloremic metabolic acidosis and hypokalemia may be seen. Hypercalciuria can manifest as rickets, nephrocalcinosis, nephrolithiasis, and renal failure. The urine pH usually exceeds 6.5.

The classic diagnostic test for distal renal tubular acidosis is an acid load from ammonium chloride; however, this is a tedious test that can generate severe acidosis. Distal renal tubular acidosis can be permanent, but children may outgrow it by the time they are school-aged. Treatment is focused on correction of the acidosis with sodium bicarbonate or sodium citrate, which may also prevent kidney stone formation. Target serum HCO_3 levels should be between 20 and 22 mEq/L in infants and between 22 and 26 mEq/L in children.

TYPE 2 RENAL TUBULAR ACIDOSIS

Proximal renal tubular acidosis is the most common form found in children. It is characterized by an alkaline urine (usually pH > 7), loss of bicarbonate in the urine, and mildly reduced serum bicarbonate concentration. Approximately 85% to 90% of bicarbonate reabsorption occurs in the proximal tubules.

Proximal renal tubular acidosis can result from inherited disorders (hereditary fructose intolerance, Wilson's disease, cystinosis, Fanconi's syndrome, Lowe's syndrome), medication exposure (chemotherapy agents, acetazolamide, sulfonamides), anatomic abnormalities (obstructive uropathy, reflux), or heavy metal exposure. Treatment consists of alkaline therapy with citrate solutions (Bicitra, Polycitra) or sodium bicarbonate. Potassium supplements may also be required because the added sodium load may increase potassium loss in the distal tubule.

Urinary Tract Infections

CLINICAL PRESENTATION

Urinary tract infections are common in children; however, children do not always present with typical

Table 110-2 GENERAL APPROACH TO URINALYSIS

Finding	Interpretation: False-negative	Interpretation: False-positive	Significance	Comment
Proteinuria >10 mg/dL; dependent on state of urinary concentration	Dilute urine; non-albumin proteinuria (Bence Jones protein)	Concentrated urine, highly alkaline urine, gross hematunia	Likelihood of significant renal disease in asymptomatic patient is <1%; no further tests needed unless proteinuria persists	
>3 RBCs/high-powered field	Vitamin C or captopril (oxidants)	Presence of hemolysis or myoglobinuria	Likelihood of significant disease is 2%-3%; follow up with repeat urinalysis before performing other tests	
Nitrite—tests bacterial nitrate reduction to nitrite; positive test is evidence of at least 10^5 organisms/mL	Gram-positive organisms and yeast do not not reduce nitrate and are associated with false-negative results if large number of organisms are present; nitrite is converted to ammonia, nitric oxide, or nitrous oxide	Contamination		Dipstick nitrite often has a low sensitivity in infants and young children who void frequently, because urine must be in the bladder for at least 4 hours for bacteria to produce nitrites
Leukocyte esterase is produced by neutrophils within urine and is strong evidence of active inflammation	High concentrations of vitamin C, albumin or other proteins, glucose (>3000 mg/dL) or ketones; Urine with high specific gravity			Used in combination, nitrites and leukocyte esterase assays are very specific for UTI; negative predictive value of both tests is more than 97% in excluding diagnosis of UTI

RBCs, red blood cells; UTI, urinary tract infection.
From Handrigan MT, Thompson I, Foster M: Diagnostic procedures for the urogenital system. Emerg Med Clin North Am 2001;19:745-761.

symptoms reported by adults. The diagnosis should be considered in all children with the classic symptoms of dysuria, urgency, and frequency, as well as in patients with nonspecific symptoms such as fever, nausea, vomiting, and abdominal and flank pain. Urinary tract infections are typically separated into lower tract disease (cystitis and urethritis) and upper tract disease.

Urethritis is an inflammation of the urethral mucosa caused by local irritation (chemical, infection, foreign-body insertion). Infectious etiologies are rare in prepubertal children, whereas sexually transmitted disease is the most common cause in sexually active adolescents.

■ DIAGNOSTIC TESTING

Clean-catch mid-stream urine sampling for urinalysis and culture are difficult to obtain in young children. Catherization is preferable to bag specimens for diagnostic accuracy.

■ TREATMENT AND DISPOSITION

Empirical treatment is similar to that for adults, based on local hospital susceptibilities, except for the exclusion of fluroquinolones and the need for longer durations of therapy. Children treated for pyelonephritis or febrile urinary tract infections should have follow-up within 24 to 48 hours to assure favorable response to antibiotics, to monitor bacterial susceptibility to empirical antibiotics, and to arrange for outpatient imaging if needed.

Urinary Retention

Urinary retention is defined as failure to urinate for more than 12 hours. More than 90% of all newborns void within the first 24 hours of life, and 99% within the first 48 hours. In male children, posterior urethral valves are the most common cause of retention. Other etiologies include urethral polyps, urethral stricture, urethral diverticulum, meatal stenosis, and fecal impaction. In female infants, the differential

RED FLAGS

- Do not attempt deep venous punctures in children with nephrotic syndrome receiving chronic prednisone therapy because they are at increased risk for thromboembolic events.

diagnosis includes prolapsing ureterocele, urethral prolapse, and foreign bodies. Infections, medications, spinal cord abnormalities, and sexual abuse can cause retention in both male and female children. Diagnostic tests in the ED include blood urea nitrogen, creatinine, and urinalysis (Table 110-2).[10]

REFERENCES

1. Niedzielski J, Paduch D, Raczynski P: Assessment of adolescent varicocele. Pediatr Surg Int 1997;12:410-413.
2. Kass EJ: Adolescent varicocele. Pediatr Clin North Am 2001;48:1559-1569.
3. Bomalaski MD, Mills JL, Argueso LR, et al: Iliac vein compression syndrome: An unusual cause of varicocele. J Vasc Surg 1993;18:1064-1068.
4. Brown MR, Cartwright PC, Snow BW: Common office problems in pediatric urology and gynecology. Pediatr Clin North Am 1997;44:1091-1115.
5. Van Howe RS: Cost-effective treatment of phimosis. Pediatrics 1998;102:E43.
6. Winkler A, Kohan A: Genitourinary emergencies: In Crain EF, Gershel JC (eds): Clinical Manual of Emergency Pediatrics. New York, McGraw Hill, 2003, p 257.
7. Waugh MA: Balanitis. Dermatol Clin 1998;16(4):757-797.
8. Schwartz RH, Rushton HG: Acute balanoposthitis in young boys. Pediatr Infect Dis J 1996;15:176-177.
9. Lau KK, Wyatt RJ: Glomerulonephritis. Adolesc Med 2005;16:67-85.
10. Handrigan MT, Thompson I, Foster M: Diagnostic procedures for the urogenital system. Emerg Med Clin North Am 2001;19:745-761.

Chapter **111**

Renal Failure

Troy P. Coon and Michael A. Miller

KEY POINTS
Renal failure is a diagnosis, not a presentation.
Acute renal failure is "an abrupt and sustained decrease in renal function."
Management of renal failure should be aimed at identifying life-threatening abnormalities created by the disorder and preventing further injury to the kidneys.
Supportive care of patients with newly diagnosed or worsening renal failure includes treatment of collecting system obstruction, supplemental oxygen delivery, and avoidance of pharmacologic harm.
Uremia refers to the accumulation of nitrogenous waste products and is characterized not only by renal excretory failure but also by a host of disturbed metabolic and endocrine functions.
Acute pulmonary edema is a potentially life-threatening complication of renal failure that must be managed expeditiously.
One of the most lethal complications of renal failure is severe hyperkalemia.
All patients with renal failure should have an electrocardiogram (ECG) to screen for hyperkalemia.

Scope

Renal failure is a diagnosis that lacks a specific pattern or clinical presentation. It may be the *cause* of a variety of complaints (shortness of breath, edema, altered mental status) or may be the *result* of pathologic processes (diabetes, hypertension, vasculitis). The delineation of renal failure as the cause or effect of a condition is not crucial in the care of patients presenting to the ED; rather, EPs should be able to recognize and manage the most common presentations associated with renal failure and the resultant complications of renal failure and its treatments.

The Acute Dialysis Quality Initiative (ADQI) consensus defines acute renal failure as "an abrupt and sustained decrease in renal function" and has proposed the RIFLE (*r*isk, *i*njury, *f*ailure, *l*oss, and *e*nd-stage kidney disease) classification system to describe severity based on the degree of change in serum creatinine or urine output from a baseline measurement (Table 111-1).[1]

This chapter avoids terminology that further distinguishes between acute and chronic renal failure; rather, reference to patients with renal dysfunction implies the need for some form of renal replacement therapy.

Table 111-1 RIFLE CLASSIFICATION SYSTEM

Parameter	GFR Criteria	Urine Output (UO) Criteria
Risk	Serum creatinine ×1.5	UO<0.5 mL/kg/hr ×6 hr
Injury	Serum creatinine ×2.0	UO<0.5 mL/kg/hr ×12 hr
Failure	Serum creatinine ×3 *or* serum creatinine ≥4 mg/dL with an acute rise >0.5 mg/dL	UO<0.3 mL/kg/hr ×24 hr *or* anuria ×12 hr
Loss	Persistent acute renal failure=complete loss of kidney function for >4 wk	
End-stage kidney disease	Duration >3 months	

GFR, glomerular filtration rate; RIFLE, *r*isk, *i*njury, *f*ailure, *l*oss, and *e*nd-stage kidney disease.

Anatomy and Physiology

The kidneys are located in the retroperitoneal space and are composed of three basic structures: vasculature, parenchyma, and the collecting system. The renal arterial system supplies the kidneys with 20% to 25% of cardiac output, divided into an intricate network of arteries, arterioles, and capillaries that eventually drain into the renal vein. The renal parenchyma is composed of the medulla and cortex, which houses the functional unit of the kidney, the nephron. A single nephron consists of a glomerulus, proximal tubule, thin limbs of Henle, and a distal tubule. The connecting tubule joins the nephron to the collecting system, including the renal pelvis, minor and major calyces, and the ureter, bladder, and urethra (Fig. 111-1).

In a person weighing 70 kg (153 lb), the kidney forms approximately 180 liters of glomerular filtrate each day. Cardiac output in combination with effective intravascular volume generates hydraulic pressure that drives fluid from the capillaries into the urinary space, which comprises the main mechanism of urine formation. The final urinary filtrate is determined by a complex interaction between hydraulic and oncotic pressure, molecular size and charge, absorption, reabsorption, and secretion under hormonal control.

■ DIAGNOSTIC IMPLICATIONS

The diagnosis of renal failure has classically been based on a prerenal, intrarenal, and postrenal classification system. The value of this framework is questionable, however, because many causes of renal failure demonstrate variations in FeNa (fractional excretion of sodium) measurements.[2] A thorough understanding of basic renal anatomy and physiology, combined with elements of the history and physical, is all that is needed to generate a useful differential diagnosis, management strategy, and disposition in the ED.

The measurement of urinary sodium, ratio of blood urea nitrogen to creatinine, and FeNa does not improve the ED management of patients with renal dysfunction and may instead lead to incorrect conclusions regarding cause and effect. Once a diagnosis

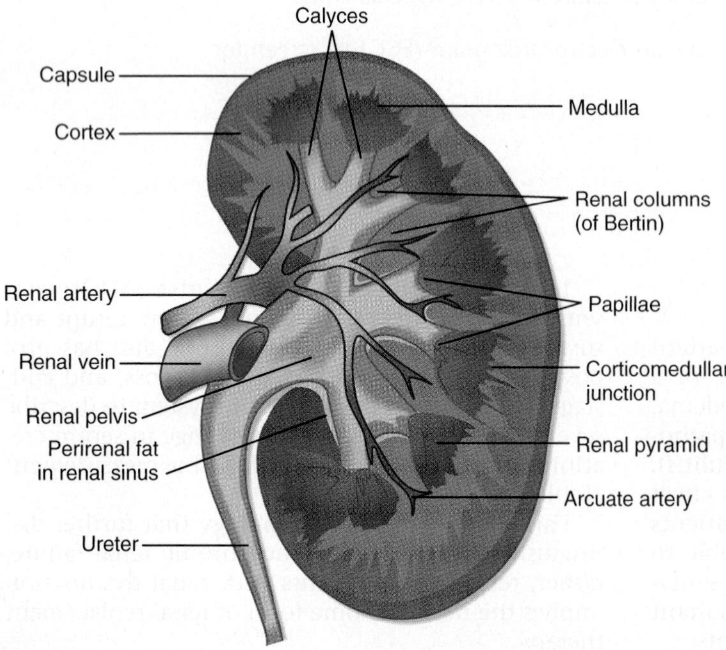
Calyces
Capsule
Cortex
Medulla
Renal columns
(of Bertin)
Renal artery
Papillae
Renal vein
Corticomedullary
junction
Renal pelvis
Perirenal fat
in renal sinus
Renal pyramid
Arcuate artery
Ureter

FIGURE 111-1 Gross anatomy of the kidney.

BOX 111-1

Causes of Renal Failure Secondary to Vessel Injury

Large-Vessel
- Renal artery thrombosis or stenosis
- Renal vein thrombosis
- Atheroembolic disease
- Aortic dissection
- Angiography

Small- and Medium-Vessel
- Scleroderma
- Malignant hypertension
- Hemolytic uremic syndrome
- Thrombotic thrombocytopenic purpura
- Sickle cell nephropathy
- Toxemia of pregnancy
- Trauma

of renal failure is made through creatinine screening, a differential diagnosis is generated of associated conditions or complications by considering potential diseases of the vasculature, parenchyma, and collecting system, as well as the process of urine formation within the context of the patient presentation.

VASCULATURE

Vascular disease of the kidney can be classified according to the size of the artery involved (Box 111-1). Patients may present with a variety of complaints, ranging from the complications of renal failure secondary to vascular insufficiency to sudden onset of back or flank pain due to acute renal artery embolism. Large-vessel injury may occur secondary to trauma, thrombosis, embolization, aortic dissection, or angiography. Renal artery stenosis may produce an indolent renal failure, further exacerbated by the initiation of angiotensin-converting enzyme (ACE) inhibitors to treat associated hypertension. Smaller, intrarenal vessels may be damaged by vasculitis.

PARENCHYMA

The working unit of the kidney is the nephron, which is composed of a variety of cell types that are susceptible to many disease processes (Box 111-2). Exposure to toxins may affect the entire renal parenchema; diseases such as Goodpasture's syndrome may injure only the glomerular basement membrane. Infection may lead to acute interstitial disease presenting as fever, rash, and eosinophilia, whereas severe shock may cause diffuse tissue ischemia.

BOX 111-2

Causes of Renal Failure Secondary to Parenchymal Injury

Systemic Disease
- Systemic lupus erythematosus
- Infective endocarditis
- Systemic vasculitis
- Henoch-Schonlein purpura
- Essential mixed cryogobulinemia
- Goodpasture's syndrome

Primary Renal Disease
- Poststreptococcal glomerulonephritis
- Rapidly progressive glomerulonephritis

Ischemia
- Shock
- Severe volume depletion

Nephrotoxins
- Antibiotics
- Contrast agents
- Pigment-induced (rhabdomyolysis)
- Drugs (nonsteroidal antiinflammatory drugs)
- Toxins
- Multiple myeloma

Hereditary
- Polycystic kidney disease
- Alport's syndrome
- Medullary cystic disease

Infections

Severe Liver Disease

Allergic Reactions

COLLECTING SYSTEM

The collecting system of the kidneys is composed of the calyces, renal pelvis, ureter, bladder, and urethra—obstruction may occur at any level (Box 111-3). Obstruction to urinary flow generally is a reversible cause of renal failure. Alert patients may present with symptoms of urinary retention or nephrolithiasis that are dramatic and obvious. Occult, potentially reversible renal obstruction should always be considered in patients with altered mental status due to acute renal failure.

URINE FORMATION

Urine formation is a complex process regulated by many factors. The hydraulic pressure used to generate flow from the capillaries to the urinary space is dependent on cardiac output and effective intravascular volume. Volume depletion, redistribution, or

BOX 111-3

Causes of Renal Failure Secondary to Collecting System Obstruction

Intrarenal and Ureteral
- Kidney stone
- Sloughed papilla
- Malignancy (obstructive)
- Crystal precipitation
- Retroperitoneal fibrosis

Bladder
- Kidney stone
- Blood clot
- Prostatic hypertrophy
- Bladder carcinoma
- Neurogenic bladder

Urethra
- Phimosis
- Stricture
- Reflux nephropathy

BOX 111-4

Causes of Renal Failure Secondary to Urine Formation Disturbances

Volume Loss
- Vomiting and diarrhea
- Diuresis
- Blood loss
- Insensible losses
- Third spacing
- Peritonitis
- Trauma and burns

Decreased Perfusion
- Congestive heart failure
- Valvular disease
- Septic shock
- Anaphylaxis
- Antihypertensive medications
- Neurogenic shock

Oncotic Pressure
- Hypoalbuminema
- Nephrotic syndrome
- Liver disease

decreased cardiac output may all impair renal perfusion pressure and urine formation. Volume depletion may occur with vomiting, diarrhea, hemorrhage, burns, or increased insensible losses. A decrease in cardiac output (from congestive heart failure or valvular disease), shock states, nephrosis, cirrhosis, hypoalbuminemia, and third spacing can affect the effective intravascular volume, all resulting in poor renal perfusion (Box 111-4).

■ RENAL FUNCTION

The kidney is responsible for maintaining the volume and ionic composition of body fluids, excreting metabolic waste products such as urea, and eliminating exogenous drugs, hormones, and toxins. The kidneys also serve as a major endocrine organ through production of renin, erythropoietin, 1,25-dihydroxycholecalciferol, prostaglandins, and kinins. Metabolic functions of the kidney do not include catabolism of small-molecular-weight proteins and anabolic roles in ammoniagenesis and gluconeogenesis.

Pathophysiology

Renal failure can be divided into two categories: primary disturbances or secondary disturbances. Primary disturbances reflect a direct failure of the kidneys to perform critical functions, such as failure to excrete sodium (leading to volume overload) or a decrease in erythropoietin production (leading to anemia). Secondary disturbances result from an accumulation of metabolic products in other organ systems, as when hyperphosphatemia causes hyperparathyroidism or when nitrogenous waste products promote platelet dysfunction. The combination of primary and secondary disturbances disrupts the homeostatic balance of almost every organ system (Box 111-5).

■ PRIMARY DISTURBANCES

When the kidney can no longer perform excretory functions, the result is volume overload, hyperkalemia, and hyperphosphatemia. As renal endocrine function declines, hypocalcemia and anemia develop. Renal failure can cause an increased circulating concentration of insulin and lower insulin requirements in diabetics. The loss of ammoniagenesis and the ability to excrete phosphate impairs the metabolic acid load cleared by the kidneys and may lead to acidosis. Adverse drug reactions at normal dosages can occur.

■ SECONDARY DISTURBANCES

The accumulation of nitrogenous waste products, generically referred to as *uremia,* is characterized not only by renal excretory failure but also by a host of metabolic and endocrine disease states. Derangements in protein, carbohydrate, and lipid metabolism will ensue, associated with anemia, malnutrition, and metabolic bone disease. Loss of renal catabolism

BOX 111-5

Organ System Effects of Renal Failure

Cardiovascular
- Pulmonary edema
- Arrhythmia
- Hypertension
- Pericarditis
- Pericardial effusion
- Myocardial infarction

Metabolic
- Hyponatremia/hypernatremia
- Hyperkalemia
- Acidosis
- Hypocalcemia
- Hyperphosphatemia
- Hypermagnesemia
- Hyperuricemia

Neurologic
- Asterixis, hiccups, myoclonic twitching
- Sensorimotor neuropathy
- Neuromuscular irritability
- Mental status changes (acute/chronic)
- Lethargy, somnolence, coma
- Encephalopathy
- Dialysis dementia (dementia, altered mental status, movement disorders)
- Seizures

Immune System
- Immunosuppression

Pulmonary
- Pleural effusions
- Uremic pleuritis
- Pulmonary edema
- Pneumonia

Gastrointestinal
- Nausea and vomiting
- Gastritis
- Ulcers
- Bleeding
- Pancreatitis
- Malnutrition

Hematologic
- Anemia
- Platelet dysfunction

Endocrine
- Hyperparathyroidism
- Glucose intolerance

Musculoskeletal
- Renal osteodystrophy
- Arthritis
- Cramps
- Spontaneous tendon rupture
- Myopathy
- Carpal tunnel syndrome
- Amyloid arthropathy

Skin
- Uremic frost
- Diffuse pruritus

and an increase in endocrine secretion affects many hormones, including insulin, glucagon, luteinizing hormone, and prolactin. A normal platelet count may be maintained, although platelet function and bleeding time will likely become abnormal. Poorly understood immune system interactions can lead to immunosuppression, overwhelming infection, septic shock, and death.

Management

Once a differential diagnosis has been established, ED management of patients with renal failure should be aimed at (1) identifying life-threatening abnormalities caused by renal failure, and (2) preventing further injury to the kidneys. Patients receiving renal replacement therapy and those with known renal abnormalities who present with a worsening of renal function ("acute on chronic failure") should be treated the same as patients without a history of renal insufficiency. It is not possible to predict which patients will improve with therapy and experience a return to baseline renal function.

Preventing further injury to the kidneys requires hospital admission and nephrology consultation. The entire list of potential causes of renal failure cannot be reviewed in a single chapter, because most causes are diagnoses unto themselves. In general, supportive care should be provided in the ED while awaiting admission.

Supportive care includes the treatment of collecting system obstruction, supplemental oxygen delivery, and avoidance of iatrogenic (pharmacologic) harm. The use of diuretics to improve urinary flow is controversial, and urine indices should be examined with consultants prior to use.[3]

In cases of parenchymal injury, any obvious toxic exposures (drugs, antibiotics, toxins) should be stopped, proper hydration (for conditions such as rhabdomyolysis, contrast-induced nephropathy) should be provided, and infections or severe shock states should be treated. The use of specific antidotes and pharmacologic treatments (e.g., bicarbonate and mannitol for patients with rhabdomyolysis) is controversial; consultation should be obtained before initiating any therapy (beyond fluid replacement) aimed at maintaining adequate urine output.

Efforts should be made to treat collecting system obstruction. Distal obstructions may be relieved with a Foley catheter, but more proximal obstructions require urology consultation and nephrostomy tubes.

Treatment of vascular compromise in large vessels (embolization, thrombosis, dissection) should focus on return of normal blood flow, and consultation with urology, vascular surgery, and/or interventional radiology may be required. Small-vessel disease may be acute or chronic (e.g., thrombotic thrombocytopenic purpura or scleroderma, respectively), and treatment should be focused on the underlying etiology.

Patients with abnormalities of urine formation due to a decrease in perfusion should receive appropriate hydration. Caution should be taken to avoid volume overload in patients with congestive heart failure, liver disease, or cirrhosis.

Management of Complications of Renal Failure

Patients may present to the ED with a wide range of symptoms reflecting either a primary or secondary disturbance in renal function. Management depends on the patient's presentation and the underlying etiology. Life-threatening complications should be treated expeditiously.

Although there is little variability in treatment of most renal failure complications, certain management considerations should not be overlooked (Box 111-6). In patients with grafts or arteriovenous fistulas, intravenous access and external blood pressure devices should be used in the contralateral extremity. For patients with emergent life-threatening conditions in whom IV access cannot be established, grafts and fistulas may be accessed with caution to avoid puncturing both sides. Fluid and electrolyte administration should be adjusted according to renal function, avoiding volume overload and pulmonary edema. Medication dosages or regimens may need to be reduced or discontinued. Certain procedures carry a high risk of increased bleeding secondary to platelet dysfunction. The ability to excrete radiographic contrast is dependent on adequate renal function—for example, patients on renal replacement therapy without any remaining renal function can tolerate contrast administration, whereas patients with minimal renal function may suffer detrimental renal injury.

BOX 111-6

Management Considerations for Patients with Renal Failure

Intravenous Access
- Avoid the side of grafts and fistulas
- In life-threatening emergencies, grafts and fistulas may be accessed
- Maintain needlestick precautions

External Blood Pressure Measurements
- Avoid the side of grafts and fistulas

Volume and Electrolyte Replacement
- Careful titration of fluid administration may be needed to avoid volume overload and pulmonary edema
- Avoid overzealous electrolyte replacement

Medications
- Dosages may need adjustments
- Antibiotic regimens may change
- Anticoagulants may need to be adjusted (low-molecular-weight heparin)

Radiographic Contrast Agents
- If no renal function remains, contrast dye should be tolerated
- Avoid further injury, if possible, in patients with remaining renal function

Procedures
- Increased risk of bleeding is possible

Disposition
- Inpatient dialysis should be available
- The threshold for intensive care unit admission may be lower in these patients

Resuscitation Wishes
- Ask patients about their wishes for intubation and resuscitation

■ LIFE-THREATENING COMPLICATIONS

■ Volume Overload

Extracellular fluid volume is determined by the balance between sodium and water. Renal failure may promote sodium retention or result in failure to excrete excessive sodium intake, leading to a positive sodium balance and extracellular fluid volume expansion. The most concerning clinical presentation of volume overload is pulmonary edema with respira-

PRIORITY ACTIONS

Volume Overload and Pulmonary Edema

- Assess airway and ventilation
  - Intubation, CPAP, or BiPAP may be necessary
- Provide supplemental oxygen
  - 100% non-rebreather mask should be used if above measures are not employed
- Position patient upright
- Apply cardiac rhythm strip and monitor
  - Look for contributing dysrhythmias
- Obtain IV access
- Obtain ECG
  - Always screen for hyperkalemic changes
- Venodilating agents (when blood pressure allows)
  - Nitroglycerin, sublingual or intravenous infusion may be given in hypotensive patients once inotropes or pressors are employed and blood pressure is stabilized
  - IV nitroprusside
- Diuretics
  - May be effective even when there is no renal function
- Inotropes and vasopressors
  - May be necessary when cardiac function is depressed or hypotension is present
- Schedule dialysis
  - This should be done early, because patients may not respond to standard therapies
- Exclude other causes of pulmonary edema and dyspnea

BiPAP, bi-level positive airway pressure; CPAP, continuous positive airway pressure; ECG, electrocardiogram.

tory distress. The presence or lack of previous renal replacement therapy should not alter the management of acute pulmonary edema. Volume overload remains one of the most common reasons for emergent dialysis—dialysis should be considered as early as possible in patients with renal failure and severe pulmonary edema. Volume overload may manifest as hypertensive encephalopathy or cardiovascular decompensation in patients with renal insufficiency.

Hyperkalemia

One of the most lethal complications of renal failure is hyperkalemia. The presentation of patients with severe hyperkalemia is usually silent until it is fatal—any patient with suspected renal failure or hyperkalemia should have an ECG screen on arrival to the ED. Patients with ECG changes consistent with hyperkalemia should receive immediate treatment without waiting for serum confirmation. However, a normal ECG does not exclude hyperkalemia, and serum confirmation should be made when the suspicion for hyperkalemia remains high. Treatment includes intravenous calcium, insulin and dextrose, bicarbonate, and oral polystyrene sulfonate.

PRIORITY ACTIONS

Severe Hyperkalemia

- Cardiac arrest and known renal failure
  - Calcium chloride and sodium bicarbonate should be given along with usual resuscitative measures
- Suspected hyperkalemia
  - Screening ECG should be performed
  - Normal ECG does not exclude hyperkalemia and serum confirmation should be performed
- ECG changes consistent with hyperkalemia
  - Myocardial stabilization is needed immediately with calcium chloride
- Normal ECG with elevated serum potassium
  - Intracelluar movement and removal should be the focus of treatment
- All patients with hyperkalemia
  - Emergent consultation and admission to hospital with inpatient dialysis
  - Efforts to shift potassium are only temporizing

ECG, electrocardiogram.

Patients with renal failure have abnormal potassium clearance, and changes in diet or medications, new medications (beta-blockers, ACE inhibitors, antibiotics), infections, or dialysis noncompliance may lead to dangerous elevations in serum potassium.

All patients with known renal failure who present in cardiac arrest should receive treatment for hyperkalemia along with usual resuscitative measures. The extremities and upper chest should be checked for dialysis access devices when patients present in cardiac arrest.

Emergent dialysis should be arranged for all patients unresponsive to standard therapies.

Other Electrolyte and Acid-Base Disturbances

Additional metabolic derangements seen in cases of renal failure include hypermagnesemia, hypernatremia, hyponatremia, hypercalcemia, hypocalcemia, hyperglycemia, hypoglycemia, and metabolic acidosis (refer to specific treatment strategies in corresponding chapters). In many instances, severe electrolyte disturbances mandate urgent dialysis.

Chest Pain

The leading cause of death in patients with renal failure is acute coronary syndrome. Precluding illnesses (diabetes, hypertension) compounded with complications of renal failure (dyslipidemia, chronic volume overload, hyperphosphatemia, anemia, hyperparathyroidism) present a host of risk factors for cardiovascular disease. Renal failure does

Table 111-2 SOURCES OF INFECTIONS IN PATIENTS WITH RENAL FAILURE

Source	Comments
Skin and bone: Soft tissue abscesses Osteomyelitis Epidural abscess	Usually *Staphylococcus aureus;* repeated punctures and associated neuropathies increase risk Osteomyelitis most commonly involves ribs and thoracic vertebrae
Access site–associated bacteremias: Endocarditis Epidural abscess Recurrent bacteremias Septic arthritis	*Stapylococcus aureus* most common; enterococci and aerobic gram-negative bacilli make up the remainder Empirical treatment should cover both gram-positive and gram-negative bacteria Catheter removal may be life-saving in patients with fever or positive blood cultures and in unstable patients
Vancomycin-resistant enterococci	Colonization—only standard precautions needed; infection—requires treatment with chloramphenicol, doxycycline, or linezolid
Septicemia	Vascular access most common source; decubitus ulcers, urinary tract infections, and nosocomial pneumonia make up the majority of remainder *Staphylococcus* species common in vascular sites; other organisms are *Pseudomonas* and gram-negative bacteria from contaminated dialysis equipment
Central nervous system: Meningitis	Usual bacteria plus mucormycosis
Pulmonary	Pneumonia no more common than in general population, but diagnostically more difficult secondary to fluctuating volumes and pulmonary edema Increased risk for tuberculosis, particularly in first year of dialysis
Gastrointestinal: Peritonitis Perirectal abscess	90% risk after 3 years of peritoneal dialysis *Staphylococcus epidermidis* and *aureus* account for most causes
Retropharyngeal abscess	Polymicrobial infections increase suspicion for perforated viscus; a rectal exam must be performed to avoid missing any potential abscesses
Urogenital	Same bacteria as in general population Fungal infections are associated with dialysis and extensive use of antibiotics, predominantly *Candida* species Symptomatic patients should be treated the same as other populations; asymptomatic patients should have culture-driven treatment because pyuria correlates poorly with urinary tract infection

From Minnaganti V, Cunha B: Infections associated with uremia and dialysis. Infect Dis Clin North Am 2001;15:385-406.

not change the treatment for acute myocardial infarction.

Other causes of life-threatening chest pain should be considered. Patients with renal failure have abnormalities in platelet adhesion, and they are also prone to thromboembolic disease and pulmonary embolism.

Uremic Pericarditis

Pericarditis secondary to uremia occurs prior to the initiation of dialysis; classic symptoms of fever, chest pain, friction rub, and worsening pain when the patient is supine may not be present. Electrocardiographic changes may be absent as well. If no signs of pericardial tamponade are present, pain control and hospital admission are appropriate. Uremic pericarditis traditionally prompts the initiation of dialysis in patients not receiving renal replacement therapy.

Dialysis-associated pericarditis is not well understood, but large effusions may be present requiring either increased dialysis or surgical correction.[4]

Acute Pericardial Tamponade

Many patients with long-standing renal failure have preexisting pericardial effusions and volume overload that complicates the diagnosis of pericardial tamponade. Chest radiography may not reveal classic abnormalities in heart shape because many patients may have long-standing cardiomegaly. Diagnostic echocardiographic findings may be altered in patients with chronic volume overload, decompensated myocardium, and preexisting pericardial pathology. The lack of diagnostic findings in patients with renal failure and clinically suspected tamponade should not alter standard treatment.[5]

Hemorrhage

Prolongation of bleeding time, decreased activity of platelet factor III, abnormal platelet aggregation, and impaired prothrombin consumption contribute to abnormal hemostasis in patients with renal failure. Patients may present with abnormal bleeding from minor wounds or surgeries, epistaxis, spontaneous gastrointestinal bleeding, or hemorrhages in the liver, pericardial sac, or brain. Gastrointestinal bleeding is both more common and more severe in patients on renal replacement therapy.[4] Patients with renal failure may have pre-existing anemia and small drops in hemoglobin may be detrimental. Blood transfusions that maintain a hematocrit above 30% have been shown to improve platelet dysfunction. Desmopres-

BOX 111-7

Interventions to Reduce Bleeding in Patients with Renal Failure

- Packed red blood cell transfusions
  - Hematocrit goal: ≥30%
- Conjugated estrogens
  - 0.6 mg/kg/d IV for 5 consecutive days or 25 mg orally or 50-100 μg/24 h transdermally q3d
- Intensification of dialysis regimen
- Recombinant erythropoietin
- Desmopressin (DDAVP)
  - 0.3 μg/kg (IV, SC, or intranasal)
- Cryoprecipitate

Data from Dember LM: Critical care issues in the patient with chronic renal failure. Crit Care Clin 2002;18: 421-440.

sin, erythropoietin, cryoprecipitate, and conjugated estrogens may all be of benefit (Box 111-7).

■ Infection

Infections are the second most common cause of mortality in patients on dialysis; most infections are bacterial in origin.[12] Both immunomodulators and cellular components of the immune system are altered in renal failure, leading to a greater risk of infections. Vascular grafts, recurrent needle sticks, and peritoneal ports break down the skin's protective barrier and offer more opportunities for bacteria to enter the circulation (Table 111-2).

■ COMPLICATIONS OF RENAL REPLACEMENT THERAPY

Renal replacement therapy produces its own unique set of complications. Patients with grafts and fistulas may present with infections, bleeding, or thrombosis of their access sites. Peritoneal dialysis patients may develop port malfunction, infection, or peritonitis. Dialysis-related complications include hypotension and disequilibrium syndrome (refer to Chapter 113 for a detailed discussion of dialysis-related emergencies).

Disposition

Stable patients who are compliant with renal replacement therapy may be discharged with appropriate diagnoses. Patients with no known history of renal failure or a worsening of already poor renal function should be admitted to the hospital. Availability of inpatient dialysis should be considered when admitting patients with renal failure. Admission to an intensive care unit is required for all life-threatening complications of renal failure.

REFERENCES

1. Kellum JA, Ronco C, Mehta R, Bellomo R: Consensus development in acute renal failure: The Acute Dialysis Quality Initiative. Curr Opin Crit Care 2005;11:527-532.
2. Pascual J, Fernando L, Ortuno J: The elderly patient with acute renal failure. J Am Soc Nephrol 1995;6:144-153.
3. Albright R: Acute renal failure: A practical update. Mayo Clin Proc 2001;76:67-74.
4. Dember LM: Critical care issues in the patient with chronic renal failure. Crit Care Clin 2002;18:421-440.
5. Klein LW: Diagnosis of cardiac tamponade in the presence of complex medical illness. Crit Care Med 2002;30: 721-723.
6. Minnaganti V, Cunha B: Infections associated with uremia and dialysis. Infect Dis Clin North Am 2001;15:385-406.

Chapter **112**

Emergency Renal Ultrasonography

Emily Baran

KEY POINTS

- Emergency renal ultrasonography is indicated when there is clinical suspicion of hydronephrosis in a patient with acute abdominal pain or a clinical suspicion of urinary retention.
- Both kidneys should be examined in longitudinal and transverse views. The bladder should be examined for evidence of distention or stones.
- A 2- to 5-MHz curvilinear abdominal probe should be used.
- The patient should be supine during the procedure. Right lateral decubitus positioning can help obtain left renal views.
- Evidence of obstruction/hydronephrosis, renal calculi, or bladder distention should be interpreted in the clinical setting.

Background

Flank pain is a common chief complaint in the ED. Computed tomography generally is the preferred modality for the evaluation of patients with flank pain because of its ability to identify the exact size and location of kidney stones as well as its ability to diagnose other etiologies of abdominal pain.[1] Endoscopic ultrasonography can identify hydronephrosis as a marker for kidney stones with reasonable sensitivity and specificity. It is a limited, focused examination that can be performed easily at the bedside.[2] Rapid differentiation of nephrolithiasis from other causes of abdominal pain can help direct patient care, additional evaluation, and disposition. Early ultrasound scanning of the bladder is important in the setting of acute renal failure to detect bilateral renal obstruction and to estimate bladder volumes in cases of urinary retention.

Indication

Emergency ultrasonography is indicated when hydronephrosis is clinically suspected in patients with acute abdominal pain or when there is clinical evidence (e.g., bladder distention) of urinary retention.

Anatomy and Approach

The kidneys are paired, bean-shaped, retroperitoneal structures that lie slightly oblique to the long axis of the body. They are surrounded by Gerota's fascia, which appears as an echogenic (bright) outline and

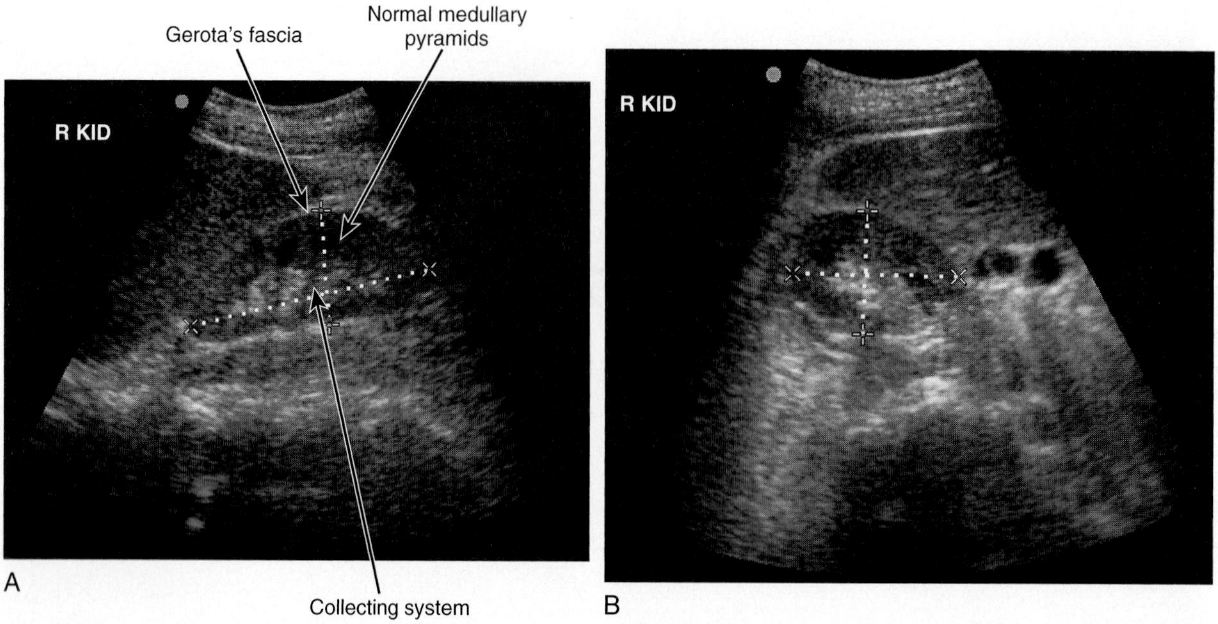
Gerota's fascia
Normal medullary pyramids
R KID
R KID
A
Collecting system
B

FIGURE 112-1 **A,** Normal longitudinal view of the right kidney. Note the central bright collecting system, which appears collapsed (not dilated), normal hypoechoic medullary pyramids in the parenchyma, and bright outline of Gerota's fascia. **B,** Normal transverse view of the right kidney.

is nestled next to the liver and spleen in the right and left upper quadrants, respectively.

The patient usually is imaged in the supine position with the head of the bed as flat as possible. A 2- to 5-MHz abdominal curvilinear probe or similar smaller-footprint probe can be used.

Initial probe positioning begins approximately at the mid-axillary line in both upper quadrants similar to focused assessment with sonography for trauma (FAST) imaging (see Chapter 8). Patient inspiration can help move the kidneys below rib shadowing for better imaging. The left kidney is more difficult to image than the right. Placing the probe more posteriorly, imaging from a transcostal approach, or positioning the patient in a right lateral decubitus position can help obtain better views of the left kidney.

Each kidney is then imaged as completely as possible in two planes. To image the kidney in the longitudinal axis, the probe indicator is aimed at the patient's head and rotated slightly to get between the ribs and to find the kidney in its longest axis. Once the longest axis of the kidney is found, the kidney should be scanned from midline to each side with a fanning or rocking maneuver to ensure visualization of all areas of the kidney.

To image the kidney in the transverse axis, the probe indicator is turned 90 degrees counterclockwise (to the patient's right) from the long axis. Again, the kidney should be scanned from top to bottom with a fanning or rocking maneuver to ensure visualization of all areas of the kidney.

Normal images of the kidney in the longitudinal and transverse axes are illustrated in Figure 112-1. The bladder can be imaged in longitudinal and transverse imaging with probe placement similar to that for FAST pelvic imaging just above the symphysis pubis (see Chapter 8).

Examination Interpretation and Limitations

Dilation of the renal collecting system generally is categorized as mild, moderate, or severe hydronephrosis based on the degree of anechoic (black) distention of the renal collecting system (bright) (Fig. 112-2). Comparison from side to side can help identify mild hydronephrosis. Normal medullary pyramids can often be confused with mild hydronephrosis, but these hypoechoic areas are not surrounded by an echogenic collecting system (bright) but rather blend with the renal parenchyma (see Fig. 112-1A). Renal cysts (Fig. 112-3), solid masses, and anatomic variations are commonly seen with renal imaging. Confirmatory imaging often is necessary in patients with abnormal ultrasound findings. Figure 112-4 shows a full bladder with clot in a patient with hematuria and urinary retention.

Emergency renal ultrasonography may be technically limited by obesity, bowel gas, or significant abdominal tenderness. It is also limited by the fact it only looks for hydronephrosis as a marker for nephrolithiasis. Hyperechoic (bright) stones with shadowing similar to gallstones can be identified, but in general this modality does not have the ability to detect small stones, especially in the ureters. Hydronephrosis should be interpreted in the clinical setting. Failure to identify or adequately image the kidneys should prompt additional imaging studies.

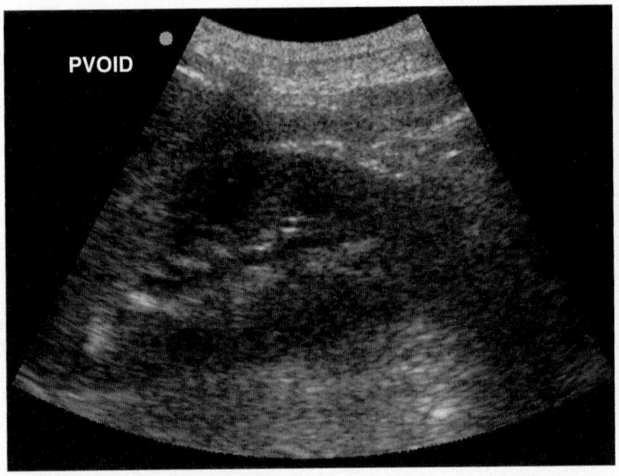
PVOID

A

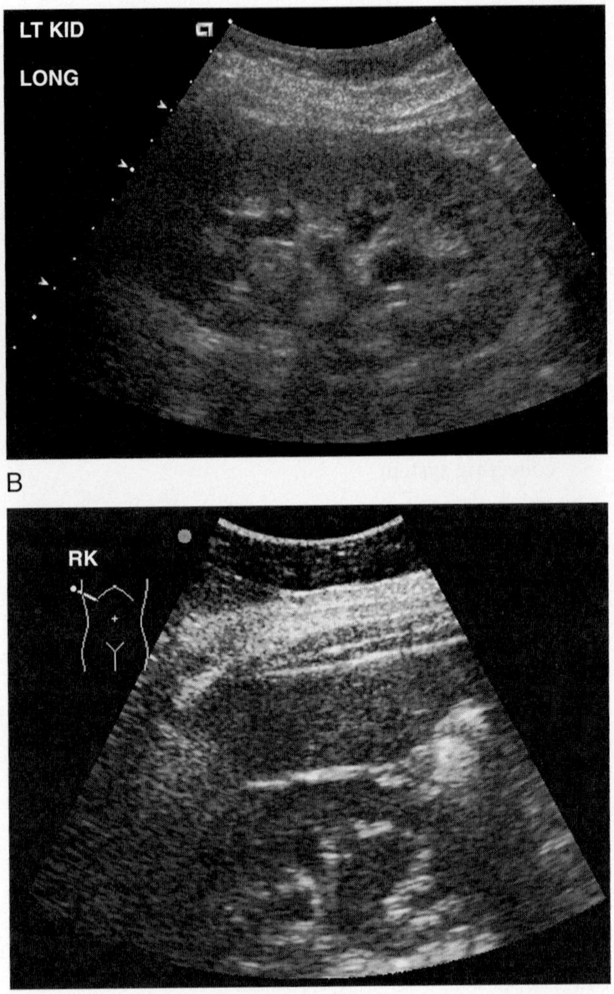
LT KID
LONG
RK

B

C

FIGURE 112-2 A simple grading scale describes a dynamic continuum from minimal distention of the pelvis and calyces to thinning of the renal cortex from an enlarged collecting system. **A,** Mild hydronephrosis; **B,** mild to moderate hydronephrosis; **C,** moderate to severe hydronephrosis.

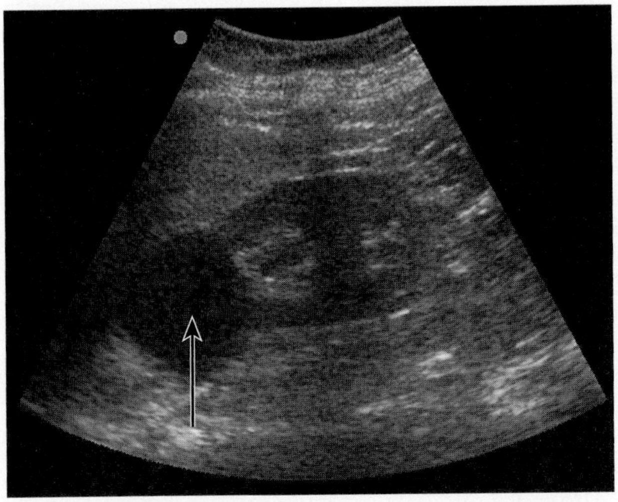

FIGURE 112-3 A simple renal cyst (*arrow*).

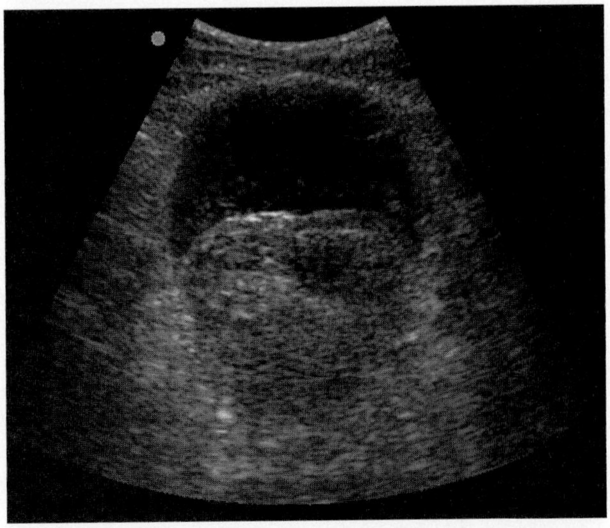

FIGURE 112-4 Transverse image of bladder with clot.

Tips and Tricks

PEARLS AND PITFALLS

- Remember to scan the aorta for aneurysms in clinically appropriate patients with flank pain.
- Hydronephrosis appears as anechoic (black) dilation of the normally hyperechoic (bright) collecting system.
- Absence of hydronephrosis does not rule out nephrolithiasis, because many stones do not cause obstruction.
- Comparison with the other kidney can help identify mild hydronephrosis.
- Larger stones can sometimes be visualized as hyperechoic areas with shadowing in the renal collecting system

The EP should always include a differential diagnosis in the work-up and schedule additional testing as appropriate. Renal endoscopic ultrasonography is a focused examination not intended to accurately identify all renal pathology.

REFERENCES

1. Sheafor DH, Hertzberg BS, Freed KS, et al: Nonenhanced helical CT and US in the emergency evaluation of patients with renal colic: Prospective comparison. Radiology 2000; 217:792-797.
2. Gaspari RJ, Horst K: Emergency ultrasound and urinalysis in the evaluation of flank pain. Acad Emerg Med 2005;12: 1180-1184.

Chapter 113

Dialysis-Related Emergencies

Yi-Mei Chng and Gregory H. Gilbert

KEY POINTS

Infection is a common cause of morbidity and mortality in dialysis patients. Tunneled lines and temporary dialysis catheters are more likely to become infected than grafts and native arteriovenous (AV) fistulas.
Differential diagnosis of hemodynamic instability in the hemodialysis patient is dependent on associated signs or symptoms (such as fever and chest pain), as well as time and speed of onset.
Early vascular surgery consultation is necessary for patients with clotted hemodialysis access.
Peritonitis is a common infection associated with peritoneal dialysis. Turbidity is one of the earliest signs of infection.
Peritoneal effluent should be centrifuged prior to culture to decrease false-negative results.

Scope

In the United States, approximately 300,000 patients with renal failure rely on some form of dialysis as life-sustaining renal replacement therapy. Over 90% of these patients are managed using hemodialysis, whereas just under 5% use peritoneal dialysis.[1] The most common complication associated with either dialysis modality is infection, although many access site malfunctions and dialysis-related emergencies prompt ED presentation in this population.

Hemodialysis

■ STRUCTURE AND FUNCTION

Hemodialysis can be performed through native AV fistulas, prosthetic AV grafts composed of polytetrafluoroethylene (PTFE), tunneled (Permacath) central venous catheters, and non-tunneled (temporary) central venous catheters. The rate of infection is lowest with native AV fistulas.

Native AV fistulas (Fig. 113-1) are created by connecting an artery (usually in the forearm) directly to a vein. Over months, the increased blood flow creates a larger, stronger vein with adequate blood flow for dialysis. Native AV fistulas are less likely to become infected or form clots than other forms of hemodialysis access.

Synthetic AV grafts (Fig. 113-2) are used when forearm veins are unsuitable for native grafts. Synthetic grafts can be used within weeks of placement; however, they are at higher risk for infection and clotting.

Central venous catheters (Fig. 113-3) are used when dialysis access is needed before permanent AV grafts have had time to mature or when fistula or graft surgery fails. Approximately 25% of the hemodialysis patients in the United States use central venous catheters as their primary vascular access. Tunneled, cuffed catheters have a lower infection rate than nontunneled catheters. All these catheters have a double lumen and are at higher risk for infection and clotting than AV fistulas.

■ COMPLICATIONS

■ Infection

Infectious complications are among the foremost causes of morbidity and mortality in hemodialysis patients. The risk of infection results from both impaired immune function related to the renal failure (e.g., altered granulocyte function in uremia) and repetitive access of the vasculature across the protective skin barrier. Vascular access is the source of bacteremia in 48% to 73% of infected hemodialysis patients.[2]

The clinical presentation may include findings of fever, hypotension, altered mental status, skin infection at the access site, and severe sepsis. Patients with diabetes may present with ketoacidosis. The differential diagnosis of various clinical presentations in hemodialysis patients is described in Table 113-1.

Antimicrobial therapy for infections believed to be related to hemodialysis access (whether catheter or graft) should cover gram-positive species including methicillin-resistant *Staphylococcus aureus*. Gram-positive species account for up to two thirds of hemodialysis access–related bacteremia. *Enterococcus* and gram-negative rods also are frequently implicated. Empirical broad-spectrum antibiotic coverage should be initiated until culture results are available, especially in patients who have a history of gram-negative bacteremia or who may be septic from a secondary source. The recommended regimen is 1 g of IV vancomycin (with sequential doses according

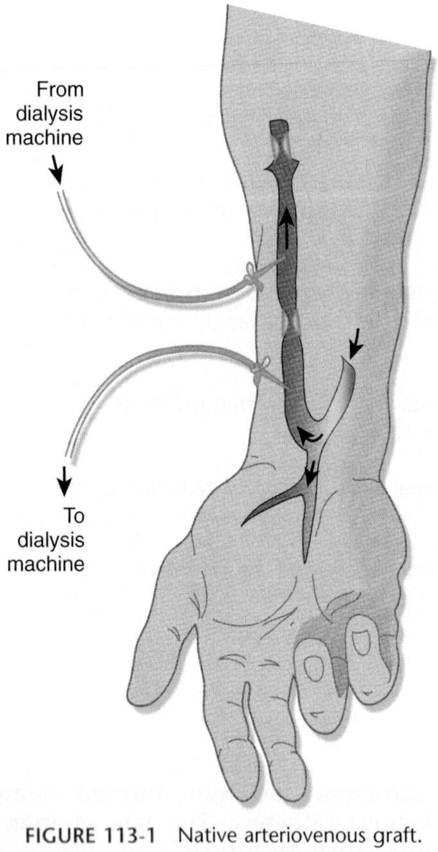
From
dialysis
machine
To
dialysis
machine

FIGURE 113-1 Native arteriovenous graft.

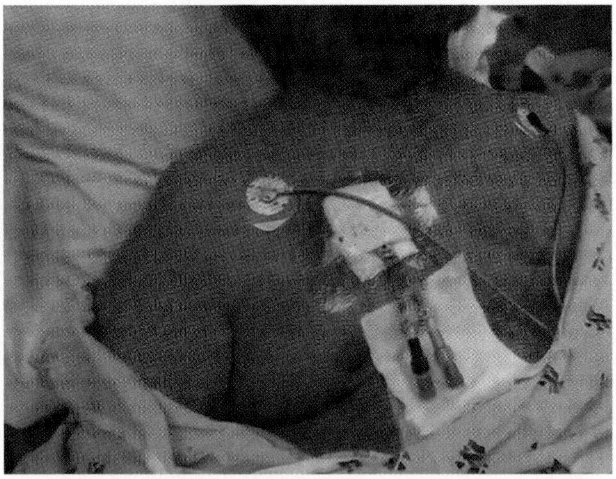

FIGURE 113-3 Tunneled central venous catheter.

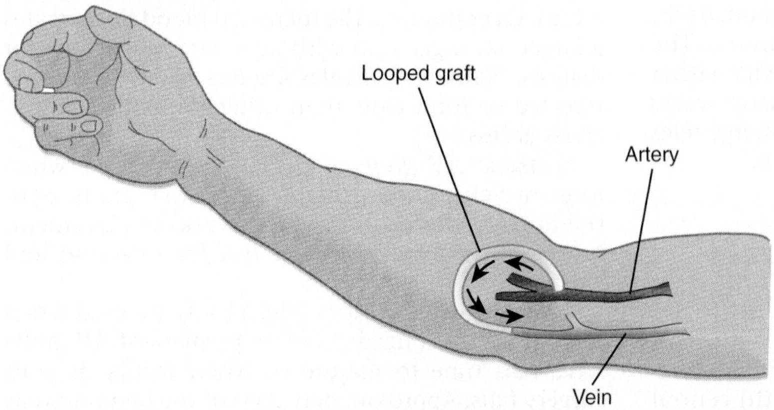
Looped graft
Artery
Vein

FIGURE 113-2 Arteriovenous graft.

Table 113-1 DIFFERENTIAL DIAGNOSIS OF VARIOUS CLINICAL PRESENTATIONS IN HEMODIALYSIS PATIENTS

Clinical Presentation	Differential Diagnosis and Critical Actions
Hypotension	If accompanied by fever—consider sepsis. If sudden onset during dialysis—consider hypovolemia due to excessive ultrafiltration, anaphylaxis/anaphylactoid reaction, or air embolism. If accompanied by chest pain—consider tamponade, arrhythmia, or acute coronary syndrome.
Altered mental status	If onset is immediately after first hemodialysis session, consider dialysis disequilibrium syndrome. If onset is gradual, consider dialysis dementia. Infection is a common cause of altered mental status (delirium) in hemodialysis patients, and the presence of a fever should prompt antibiotic administration and a search for the source. Also consider stroke, hypotension, drug effect, seizure, and/or metabolic derangement (acidosis, hyperkalemia).
Chest pain	Consider acute coronary syndrome, pulmonary embolus, air embolus, uremic pericarditis, and arrythmias due to electrolyte imbalance.
Shortness of breath	Consider fluid overload, cardiac tamponade, acute coronary syndrome, air embolism, and anaphylactoid reactions.
Bleeding	Can be due to excessive anticoagulation during dialysis or uremic coagulopathy.
Fever	Consider line infection if there is warmth or erythema of the skin overlying the dialysis access site. Consider sepsis if the patient is hypotensive or in shock; obtain blood cultures and administer antibiotics. Fever is almost always due to infection, but overheated dialysate is a potential cause.

to level at dialysis) plus gram-negative coverage with either an aminoglycoside or a third-generation cephalosporin.

Removal or exchange of an infected catheter is advisable because a bacterial biofilm can form rapidly in the lumens of most indwelling central vein catheters and serve as a source of continued infection. Systemic antibiotics given alone are relatively ineffective at eradicating infection if the catheter is not removed.[3] Tunneled catheters can be replaced with temporary non-tunneled catheters or can be changed over a guide wire, thus avoiding disruption of the patient's dialysis schedule.

■ Thrombosis

Thrombosis of hemodialysis access grafts and catheters is a significant cause of morbidity. The failure of hemodialysis grafts occurs mainly due to progressive intimal hyperplasia at the venous anastomosis resulting in decreased flow and graft thrombosis.[4]

Signs and symptoms of impending graft thrombosis include loss of thrill or bruit, increased "water-hammer" pulses, increased venous pressure, and poor flow rates.

Success of treatment decreases with time. A vascular surgeon should be consulted immediately for definitive treatment by thrombectomy (percutaneous or surgical) or surgical revision. To avoid rupture or distal embolization, the access site should not be forcibly irrigated or manipulated.

Thrombolytic agents can be initiated in consultation with a vascular surgeon. There are several different thrombolytic regimens. One protocol involves the use of 2 to 4 mg of Alteplase infused through an 18- to 22-gauge IV while waiting for the availability of angiography, with an additional 2 mg given if the wait time is greater than 30 minutes.[5] Care must be taken to confirm that the IV tubing has actually been inserted into the graft pointing toward the occlusion and not into the surrounding tissue or other vessel before the infusion of the thrombolytic agent. The arterial limb of the graft should also be occluded while the thrombolytic agent is being infused.

■ Bleeding

Bleeding from dialysis puncture sites or around tunneled catheters can occur hours after hemodialysis is complete. Bleeding usually can be controlled with firm (but non-occlusive) pressure on the site. A thrill should be documented after bleeding stops in peripheral hemodialysis grafts. Surgicel may be placed around the entry port of a tunneled catheter to promote hemostasis. Patients should be evaluated for significant blood loss and observed in the ED to ensure that bleeding does not occur. If bleeding cannot be controlled, a vascular surgeon should be consulted.

Hemodialysis patients are at risk for hemorrhage from other sites because they receive anticoagulation during the dialysis. Platelet dysfunction due to uremia also contributes to hemorrhage in patients with renal failure, and it is only partially corrected by hemodialysis. Administration of desmopressin (DDAVP) improves the hemostatic function of platelets and is useful in treating hemorrhage in hemodialysis patients.

■ Dialyzer Reactions

Patients undergoing their first hemodialysis or those switching to a new dialyzer may experience anaphy-

Tips and Tricks

USE OF HEMODIALYSIS GRAFT OR CATHETER FOR EMERGENCY VASCULAR ACCESS

Peripheral hemodialysis access sites may be used for IV placement in an emergency when no other access is available:

- Do not use a tourniquet.
- Avoid puncturing the back wall of the vessel.
- Use a small IV catheter if possible.
- Secure all sources of IV access tightly. Infusions may need to be given under pressure because of the relatively high pressures within the peripheral graft.
- Apply firm but non-occlusive pressure for 10 to 15 minutes after removing the IV catheter. Ask a nurse experienced with hemodialysis for assistance with removal if available.
- Document the presence or absence of a thrill before and after the procedure.

Central venous hemodialysis access may also be used in an emergency when no other access is available:

- Either the red or blue port may be used, as both lead to the vein (even though one is used to withdraw blood during hemodialysis and the other to return it). The "arterial" (red) port is proximal to the "venous" (blue) port to avoid recirculation during dialysis.
- Aspirate at least 2 mL from the port being used because it usually contains heparin between hemodialysis sessions.
- After use, contact a nurse experienced with hemodialysis to clear and prepare the catheter according to standard protocols.

laxis or an anaphylactoid reaction to a component of the dialyzer or dialysate. Anaphylactoid reactions have been observed with dialyzers made of cuprophane and with polyacrylonitrile dialysis membranes (particularly in patients receiving angiotensin-converting enzyme inhibitors). Treatment consists of epinephrine, antihistamines, and steroids.[6]

PATIENT TEACHING TIPS

HEMODIALYSIS

- Keep your access site clean and allow use only for dialysis or emergency access.
- Do not allow placement of a blood pressure cuff on your access arm.
- Do not lift heavy objects or put pressure on your access arm.
- Check the pulse (thrill) in your forearm access graft daily.

Air Embolism

Venous air embolism is a rare complication of hemodialysis that can occur during a session or during insertion of (or more rarely during removal of) a tunneled venous catheter. Air enters the systemic venous system and is transported to the right heart and pulmonary arteries, potentially leading to changes in gas exchange, cardiac arrhythmias, and death.

When air embolism is suspected, 100% oxygen is administered and the patient is intubated if necessary. The patient is placed in the Trendelenburg and left lateral decubitus positions to attempt to trap air in the apex of the right ventricle, in an effort to prevent migration to the pulmonary arterial system. Transfer to a hyperbaric chamber should be considered if the patient is stable. If the patient is unstable or suffering arrest, chest compressions may break up the air bubbles—aspiration of intracardiac air should be considered.

Cardiac Tamponade

Many dialysis patients have small pericardial effusions that do not cause clinical symptoms. Symptomatic cardiac tamponade can occur in these patients either as a result of an acute pericardial hemorrhage (possibly after heparin administration during hemodialysis) or as an exacerbation of volume overload in the setting of a preexisting effusion. Hemodynamically compromised patients with significant pericardial effusions confirmed by ultrasonography (particularly if right ventricular collapse in diastole is noted) may be treated with emergency pericardiocentesis if they are not sufficiently stable to be transferred for a pericardial window. Providers should be prepared for complications of hemorrhage in renal failure patients requiring pericardiocentesis.

Dialysis Disequilibrium Syndrome

Dialysis disequilibrium syndrome is characterized by nausea, headache, malaise, vomiting, fatigue, and muscle cramps that occur during or immediately after hemodialysis. In severe cases, patients can present with altered mental status, seizures, or coma (though other likely causes of these altered mentation states should be excluded before attributing such symptoms to dialysis disequilibrium syndrome).

The exact pathogenesis of the syndrome is unclear; it is believed to result from cerebral edema caused by shifts in osmolarity and pH during dialysis. The removal of small solutes such as urea from the serum causes a rapid drop in serum osmolarity in the brain. This leads to the rapid ingress of free water, resulting in cerebral edema.

The mainstay of treatment is prevention by avoiding rapid shifts in serum osmolarity during dialysis. Symptoms usually are self-limited and resolve within a few hours; severe cases can be treated by raising the serum osmolarity with infusions of hyperosmolar solutions such as hypertonic saline or mannitol, in consultation with a nephrologist.[7,8]

Table 113-2 COMPLICATIONS OF PERITONEAL DIALYSIS (IN ORDER OF FREQUENCY)

Mechanical	Infectious	Medical
Catheter dislodgment	Peritonitis	Malnutrition/hypoalbuminemia
Catheter malfunction	Cellulitis/tunnel infection	Bowel obstruction
Leakage/hernias/effusions	Abscess	Hyperglycemia

Data from U.S. Renal Data System, USRDS 2005 Annual Data Report: Atlas of End-Stage Renal Disease in the United States, National Institutes of Health, National Institute of Diabetes and Digestive and Kidney Diseases, Bethesda, MD, 2005.

Dialysis Dementia

Dialysis dementia is a form of dialysis encephalopathy associated with dyspraxia and multifocal seizures. Unlike the dialysis disequilibrium syndrome, dialysis dementia is slowly progressive in onset and generally occurs in patients who have been on hemodialysis for at least 2 years. There are three forms:

1. An epidemic form believed to be due to contamination of dialysate with aluminum, which is usually excreted by the kidneys (the use of deionized water in dialysis has decreased the incidence of this form)
2. A sporadic endemic form whose cause remains unclear
3. A pediatric form that occurs in children with renal failure even when they have not yet been dialyzed (this may be related to exposure to aluminum-containing medications)

Seizures in the ED should be treated with benzodiazepines; a serum aluminum level should be obtained in addition to other standard laboratory tests if dialysis dementia is suspected (Table 113-1).

Peritoneal Dialysis

STRUCTURE AND FUNCTION

Peritoneal dialysis can be performed in a number of different ways; however, the complications associated with these various methods are similar. Typically peritoneal dialysis is performed using a Tenckhoff catheter (it can be straight or curved, single or dual-cuffed) inserted in a median or paramedian line with or without omentectomy. Omentectomy is associated with fewer complications. The dialysate is infused into the abdomen using either a pump or gravity. It remains in the abdomen for a period, known as "dwell time," long enough to allow osmosis and diffusion. The effluent (or dialysate, after dwelling in the abdomen) is then drained (Fig. 113-4).[9]

COMPLICATIONS

In this chapter, complications of peritoneal dialysis are organized into three groups: mechanical, infectious, and medical (Table 113-2).

The most common and life-threatening complication is peritonitis, which causes the effluent to be turbid and cloudier than usual. This symptom should not be ignored. Patients are typically afebrile and otherwise well-appearing. They do not present with a rigid abdomen—instead, the physical examination is usually unimpressive, and the patient may at most complain of mild abdominal pain.

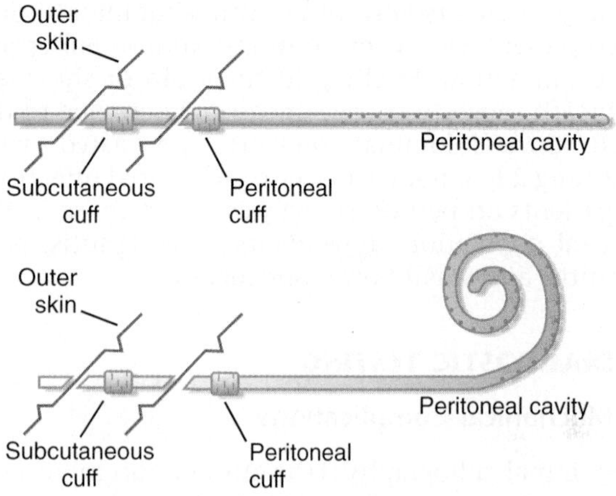
Outer skin
Peritoneal cavity
Subcutaneous cuff
Peritoneal cuff
Outer skin
Peritoneal cavity
Subcutaneous cuff
Peritoneal cuff

FIGURE 113-4 Peritoneal dialysis catheters.

Peritonitis usually is the most common presentation in patients with peritoneal dialysis catheter malfunction, but other problems can arise.[1] Blood in the effluent can suggest solid organ damage (especially if the catheter was recently placed), ruptured or leaking abdominal aortic aneurysm, or coagulopathy.

Mechanical Complications

Mechanical complications are related to the process of dialysis. These include pump malfunction (for patients on continuous cyclic or intermittent dialysis), inability to instill the dialysate or failure of the effluent to drain due to catheter malfunction or dislodgment, or fluid leakage into the groin, across the diaphragm or out of the abdominal wall.

Infectious Complications

Infectious complications include peritonitis, cellulitis at the catheter site, infection in the tunnel site itself, or intra-abdominal abscesses.

Medical Complications

Most frequently, medical complications are related to nutrition. Hypoalbuminemia results from poor dietary intake and a daily loss of 15 g of protein that promotes infection by impairing normal immune function.[10] Hyperglycemia occurs secondary to a large glucose load in the dialysate.[11] Bowel obstruction can occur secondary to abdominal surgery.

Differential Diagnosis

Although peritonitis is associated with few clinical findings, patients with other intra-abdominal infections present with fever, vomiting, and/or tenderness on examination. Swelling in the groin or shortness of breath suggests leakage of the dialysate due to the high intra-abdominal pressures associated with instilling 2 L of fluid. Common abdominal infections in patients on peritoneal dialysis reflect those in the general population: appendicitis, cholecystitis, pancreatitis, and small bowel obstruction.

RED FLAGS

Complications of Peritoneal Dialysis

- Fever
- Vomiting
- Severe abdominal tenderness
- Known or suspected fungal infection

DIAGNOSTIC TESTING

Mechanical Complications

Abdominal radiography is the most important modality. Radiographs confirm that the tube placement is correct in the true pelvis, that there are no kinks, and that the tube has not broken into multiple pieces. Chest radiographs can reveal evidence of pleural effusion; bowel obstruction is apparent on upright and lateral decubitus abdominal views. For suspected leaks, intraperitoneal water-soluble contrast can be instilled to demonstrate communication with noted areas of swelling.

Infectious Complications

Culture is critical when testing for infectious complications. Bacteria in the peritoneal cavity have been diluted significantly by the dialysate and this leads to negative cultures at standard volumes. To improve diagnostic results, 50 mL of effluent should be centrifuged down, and the sediment resuspended in 3 to 5 mL of sterile saline before inoculation of both solid and liquid blood culture media. Alternatively, a minimum of 10 mL of effluent per blood culture bottle can be used. Blood cultures are not helpful unless the patient appears septic. A test result of greater than 50% polymorphonuclear cells in the effluent is highly sensitive for peritonitis regardless of the total white blood cell count.[12]

Medical Complications

A comprehensive metabolic panel and serum lipase should be obtained. Liver function tests and serum lipase levels can differentiate other causes of abdominal pain. Albumin levels are useful markers of malnutrition, which is present in 40% of these patients (25% of whom are severely malnourished). Hypoalbuminemia significantly increases the incidence of morbidity and mortality, especially in patients with peritonitis and those with a serum albumin less than 35 g/L. Hypokalemia causes decreased gut motility and constipation, which is associated with peritonitis; both conditions should be treated. Hyperglycemia, inadequate dialysis, and volume depletion/overload can be evaluated by physical examination and standard laboratory testing.[10]

TREATMENT

Mechanical Complications

Most complications require removal of the peritoneal catheter or some type of surgical repair; patients need to be switched to hemodialysis until the catheter malfunction is resolved.

For a clogged catheter, attempts to empty the bladder and then the bowel (with laxatives) may improve function. If the catheter is clogged with fibrin or clot, heparin (500 units/L) can be added to the dialysate. If this fails, urokinase can be used as a last resort (5000 IU diluted in saline), which has a success rate of 10% to 15%.[9]

For catheter leakage, the amount of the dialysate infused is decreased to lower the intra-abdominal pressure; the patient will likely still need surgical repair for correction.

For catheter migration, kinking, dislodgment, and cuff extrusion, a one-time 2-g dose of IV ampicillin should be given for prophylaxis in the setting of tube manipulation.[9]

Infectious Complications

Gram-positive organisms account for three fourths of peritoneal dialysis–associated infections; one half of these are *Staphylococcus epidermidis*. Concerning organisms observed in infections are *Pseudomonas*, *Staphylococcus aureus* (including methicillin-resistant *Staphylococcus aureus* [MRSA]), and fungal species.[12]

If the patient has had culture-positive results in the past, these results can help guide antibiotic therapy. Otherwise, empirical antibiotic therapy should cover gram-positive and gram-negative organisms based on local hospital sensitivities.

Intermittent or continuous antibiotic therapy can be used with continuous ambulatory peritoneal dial-

Table 113-3 ANTIBIOTIC THERAPY FOR PERITONEAL DIALYSIS

Antibiotic	Intermittent Therapy	Continuous Therapy
Cefazolin	15 mg/kg IP	LD, 500 mg/L; MD, 125 mg/L
Ceftazidime	1000-1500 mg/day IP	LD, 500 mg/L; MD, 125 mg/L
Vancomycin	15-30 mg/kg every 5-7 days IP	LD, 1-2 g/L; MD, 25-50 mg/L
Gentamicin	0.6 mg/kg IP	LD, 8 mg/L; MD, 4 mg/L

IP, intraperitoneally; LD, loading dose; MD, maintenance dose.
Data from Dasgupta MK: Management of patients with type 2 diabetes on peritoneal dialysis. Adv Perit Dial 2005;21:120-122.

ysis. For intermittent treatment, antibiotics are added to only one of the four daily exchanges. For continuous therapy, a loading dose is given in the first exchange and then a maintenance dose is given in each exchange for the remainder of the 2 weeks.[12]

One suggested regimen is cefazolin (15 mg/kg intraperitoneally [IP] daily) for intermittent treatment, or for continuous therapy administer a 500-mg loading dose with 125-mg maintenance doses. For gram-negative organisms, an antibiotic that also treats *Pseudomonas* infection should be given, such as ceftazidime (1000-1500 mg IP daily), or for continuous therapy use a 500-mg loading dose and 125-mg maintenance doses. If MRSA infection is suspected, vancomycin (15 to 30 mg/kg) can be added to the dialysate and should be used in place of cefazolin[12] (Table 113-3).

Doses for renally excreted drugs should be increased by 25% if the patient produces over 100 mL of urine per day.[12]

Fungal infections may occur after antibiotic treatment. These require removal of the catheter and are associated with a mortality of 25%.[12]

Exit site infections should be treated with oral antibiotics. Therapy is guided by the Gram stain of the purulent drainage and by prior treatment regimens. For first-time infections, immediate empirical antibiotic treatment for gram-positive organisms should be initiated (Cephalexin, 500 mg PO qid). Suspected MRSA infections should be treated with vancomycin, Bactrim, or rifampin. Patients with MRSA infections should be given intranasal and local mupirocin twice a day for 5 to 7 days. Suspected pseudomonal infections should be treated with quinolones[12] (Table 113-4).

Table 113-4 ANTIBIOTICS FOR EXIT SITE INFECTIONS

Antibiotic	Dosage (for at least 2 weeks)
Cephalexin	500 mg PO qid
Ciproflaxin	250-500 mg PO bid
Bactrim SS	80-400 mg qd

Data from Dasgupta MK: Management of patients with type 2 diabetes on peritoneal dialysis. Adv Perit Dial 2005;21:120-122.

Medical Complications

Management of most medical complications in peritoneal dialysis patients is similar to that in the general population. Hyperglycemia can be treated with intraperitoneal insulin, but at higher doses.[11] Hypokalemia should be aggressively treated because this leads to constipation and risk for peritonitis. Hypoalbuminemia should be managed with protein supplements and education of the patient. In severe cases, total parenteral nutrition and/or IV albumin may be necessary.[10]

DISPOSITION

Mechanical Complications

The patient can be safely discharged home if dialysate goes in, effluent comes out, and there are no signs of infection. If the patient is unable to use the peritoneal dialysis catheter, hospital admission and scheduling for hemodialysis in consultation with a nephrologist is necessary.

Infectious Complications

The majority of patients with peritonitis are stable and can be treated at home. Those with fever, vomiting, intractable pain, fungal infection, concomitant catheter site infection, and those refractory to outpatient treatment require hospital admission. Discharge and urgent follow-up should be arranged with the team that placed the catheter and with the patient's nephrologist.[1]

Medical Complications

Disposition of patients with medical complications depends on the severity of the specific disease process. Nutritional problems can usually be treated with patient education and close outpatient follow-up.

PATIENT TEACHING TIPS

PERITONEAL DIALYSIS

- Wear loose clothing.
- Do not submerge in unchlorinated water (baths, rivers, lakes).
- Avoid heavy lifting and abdominal exercise.
- Wash hands and peritoneal dialysis site with antibacterial soap.

REFERENCES

1. U.S. Renal Data System, USRDS 2005 Annual Data Report: Atlas of End-Stage Renal Disease in the United States, National Institutes of Health, National Institute of Diabetes and Digestive and Kidney Diseases, Bethesda, MD, 2005.
2. Nassar GM, Ayus JC: Infectious complications of the hemodialysis access. Kidney Int 2001;60:1-13.
3. Allon M: Dialysis catheter–related bacteremia: Treatment and prophylaxis. Am J Kidney Dis 2004;44:779-791.
4. Rotmans JI, Pasterkamp G, Verhagen HJ, et al: Hemodialysis access graft failure: Time to revisit an unmet clinical need? J Nephrol 2005;18:9-20.
5. Sofocleous CT, Hinrichs CR, Weiss SH, et al: Alteplase for hemodialysis access graft thrombolysis. J Vasc Interv Radiol 2002;13:775-784.
6. Ebo DG, Bosmans JL, Couttenye MM, Stevens WJ: Haemodialysis-associated anaphylactic and anaphylactoid reactions. Allergy 2006;61:211-220.
7. Arieff AI: Dialysis disequilibrium syndrome: Current concepts on pathogenesis and prevention. Kidney Int 1994;45:29-35.
8. Himmelfarb J: Hemodialysis complications. Am J Kidney Dis 2005;45:1122-1131.
9. Bhatla B, Khanna R, Twardowski ZJ: Peritoneal access. J Postgrad Med 1994;40:170-178.
10. Gokal R, Mellnick NP: Peritoneal dialysis. Lancet 1999; 353:823-828.
11. Piraino B, Bailie GR, Bernardini J, et al: Peritoneal dialysis related infections recommendations: 2005 update. Perit Dial Int 2005;25:107-131.
12. Dasgupta MK: Management of patients with type 2 diabetes on peritoneal dialysis. Adv Perit Dial 2005;21: 120-122.

Chapter 114

Renal Transplant Complications

Gerald Maloney

KEY POINTS

Renal transplantation has been highly successful. With appropriate immunosuppressive therapy, the rate of acute rejection during the first post-transplant year is less than 25%; 1-year survival now approaches 100%.

Surgical complications that may be seen in the ED include hematoma formation, ureteral anastomotic leak, and ureteral obstruction. Computed tomography imaging is the diagnostic modality of choice for these surgical emergencies.

Surgical infections that are common in the first post-transplant month include pneumonia, line sepsis, and wound infection. Opportunistic infections reach their peak incidence during the remainder of the first post-transplant year. After the first year, community-acquired infections predominate.

Renal transplant patients have a high risk for atherosclerotic disease. Cardiovascular conditions accounts for 30% to 50% of deaths during the first post-transplant year.

Fluoroquinolones and macrolides may increase levels of cyclosporine and tacrolimus; these antibiotic classes should not be used as first-line agents for treatment of patients with post-transplant pneumonia.

Fever and tenderness over the graft site may indicate acute rejection.

Transplant recipients on corticosteroid therapy have functional adrenal insufficiency and require pulse-doses of corticosteroids when they encounter physiologic stress.

Scope

Advances in organ selection, surgical techniques, and postoperative management have led to a significant increase in solid-organ transplantation over the past several decades. The kidney is the most commonly transplanted solid organ. According to the United Network for Organ Sharing, there have been over 221,000 kidney transplants to date.[1] As more patients receive successful transplants, it is increasingly likely that EPs outside of tertiary referral centers will encounter a post-transplant patient and be required to perform initial management and stabilization. It is important for the practicing EP to have a general understanding of the often complex management of post-transplant patients.

Developments in Renal Transplantation

The first successful kidney transplant was performed between twin brothers in 1954.[2] The development of immunosuppressive medication led to more

BOX 114-1

Diseases Leading to Renal Transplantation

- Chronic kidney disease
- Polycystic kidney disease
- Trauma
- Rapidly progressive glomerulonephritis
- Toxic nephropathies

BOX 114-2

Common Immunosuppressive Drugs Used in Renal Transplant Recipients

- Cyclosporine (Sandimmune, Neoral)
- Tacrolimus (Prograf)
- Azathioprine (Imuran)
- Mycophenolate mofetil (Cellcept)
- Prednisone, methylprednisolone
- Sirolimus (Rapamune)
- Polyclonal anti-thymocyte globulin
- Rituximab
- Daclizumab

widespread use of transplant procedures after 1963.

Today, the primary indication for renal transplantation is stage V chronic kidney disease (formerly called end-stage renal disease). Transplantation is recognized as the most effective form of renal replacement therapy for these patients.

Specific disease entities that cause chronic kidney disease are outlined in Box 114-1. Diabetic nephropathy is the most common single disease process leading to renal transplantation.[1]

Most renal grafts now function for longer than 10 years. The 1-year survival rate for renal transplant recipients is 95% to 98%. Renal transplants are more effective than hemodialysis at prolonging the life of patients with chronic kidney disease.[3]

Previously, the highest surgical success rates were with histologically matched donor kidneys from a living recipient. Improvements in immunosuppressive medication regimens have improved the success rate using cadaveric kidneys, which now approaches that using kidneys of living donors.

Preoperative clearance for renal transplantation is extensive. Of specific note for patients with cancer, the suggested disease-free interval before transplantation is 5 years. HIV infection is considered a contraindication to renal transplantation in many institutions, although transplantation has been successful in many patients with well-maintained CD4 counts.

Cholecystectomy was previously performed in all patients undergoing renal transplant. Currently, cholecystectomy is performed only if there is evidence of cholelithiasis or cholecystitis.

The surgical approach to renal transplantation varies depending on the age of the patient and location of the kidney and the anastomosis. The recipient's native kidneys and collecting system are generally left in place unless there is another indication for nephrectomy. The donor kidney is placed in one of the lower abdominal quadrants (more commonly the right) and the ureter is anastomosed to the bladder; arterial and venous anastomoses generally arise from the iliac vessels, aorta, or inferior vena cava. The transplanted kidney usually is palpable on abdominal examination.

Immunosuppression is initiated after transplantation and is divided into two phases: induction and maintenance.[2] Azathioprine and corticosteroids were the first available immunosuppressive agents. The addition of cyclosporine in 1983 improved the success rate for cadaveric kidney transplants. Currently used agents such as tacrolimus and mono- and polyclonal antibodies are included in the induction and maintenance phases of treatment (Box 114-2). With the use of immunosuppressive medications, the one-year incidence of acute rejection is 15% to 25%.

Complications

The complications of renal transplantation can be categorized by etiology as either surgical or medical, and further divided by time of occurrence as either early or delayed.

■ SURGICAL COMPLICATIONS

Surgical complications include graft malfunction, thrombosis and aneurysms of the graft vessels, and stricture or obstruction of the ureter. Some of these complications will be evident shortly after surgery; others may occur years after the procedure, causing symptoms that will likely prompt ED evaluation.

Graft function may be delayed in up to 30% of cadaveric transplants, likely due to prolonged cold ischemia of the kidney during the period between harvesting and transplantation.[4] Delayed graft function is a rare complication in living-donor transplants. Patients may require continued dialysis until adequate post-transplant function is demonstrated.

Acute thrombosis of the arterial or venous anastomoses is usually seen within the first post-transplant week.[2,4] Treatment is surgical exploration in an attempt to salvage the donor kidney.

Renal artery stenosis has been reported in allografts and can cause hypertension in post-transplant patients. This is generally a delayed complication. Aneurysms of the graft vessels are uncommon, delayed events.

Hematomas may develop around the transplanted kidney. Hematoma formation may be an early postoperative complication or rarely may be the result of acute rejection with spontaneous rupture of the kidney.[4] Acute hematomas are surgical emergencies.

Ureteral complications include anastomotic leak (usually within the first post-transplant month), acute ureteral obstruction, and lymphocele. These complications will occur within the first 3 months following transplant. Computed tomography of the abdomen is the preferred imaging modality for ureteral complications. Ureteral obstruction often requires emergent surgical intervention.

■ MEDICAL COMPLICATIONS

Medical complications are numerous and often subtle in presentation. Post-transplant patients are at risk for atypical infections, cardiovascular death, renal failure, and, of course, rejection. Adverse reactions from immunosuppressive medications account for many delayed medical complications in transplant patients.

■ Fever

Management of fever in post-transplant patients should be approached similarly to that of fever in other immunocompromised patients.[5] Due to suppressed immunologic and inflammatory responses, post-transplant patients may not exhibit common findings of acute infection. Fever may or may not be associated with clinically significant infection.

One cause of fever that is present across time frames is acute rejection. Decisions regarding appropriate diagnostic testing and disposition of a post-transplant patient with fever should be made in conjunction with the transplant service.

■ Infections

The incidence of infection in the first post-transplant year has been reported as 25% to 80%. Expected infections vary according to post-transplant time (Box 114-3). Infections in the first post-transplant month are typical postoperative infections—pneumonia, sepsis from central lines or urinary catheters, and wound infections.[2,5] Atypical or opportunistic infections are uncommon.

After the first month through the end of the first post-transplant year, opportunistic infections reach their peak incidence. A variety of atypical bacterial, viral, fungal, protozoal, and parasitic infections may occur. Individual transplant services maintain current information on the opportunistic infections seen at their institution. Cytomegalovirus is one of the most common opportunistic infections, occurring in up to 25% of renal transplant recipients.[5] It can cause systemic or invasive disease and is associated with acute rejection.

BOX 114-3

Infections in the Post-transplant Patient

First Month Post-transplant

- Typical postsurgical infections (pneumonia, urinary tract infection, line sepsis, wound infection)
- Opportunistic infections uncommon

Infections in the First Post-transplant Year

- Opportunistic infections (*Pneumocystis* pneumonia, *Cryptococcus,* fungal infections, viral infections; highest incidence in months 2-6)
- Cytomegalovirus (most common)
- Tuberculosis

Infections >1 Year Post-transplant

- Community-acquired more common than opportunistic infections
- Typical organisms causing cellulitis, pneumonia, urinary tract infections

After the first year, the incidence of opportunistic infections decreases and typical community acquired pathogens predominate.

Leukocytosis is a poorly sensitive and inconsistent indicator of fever source. Peritoneal findings may be minimal or absent in the presence of an acute intra-abdominal catastrophe. Due to the degree of immunosuppression, infections may follow a fulminant course.

■ Cardiovascular Emergencies

Because the majority of renal transplant recipients in the United States have diabetes and/or hypertension, risk for concomitant cardiovascular disease is high. Furthermore, the combination of cyclosporine and corticosteroids worsen dyslipidemias and atherogenesis.[7] Cardiovascular disease accounts for 30% to 50% of deaths in the first post-transplant year, and the incidence of atherosclerotic vascular disease is up to five times greater in transplant recipients than in other hospitalized patients.[6]

The approach to the diagnosis and management of suspected cardiac ischemia is standard in the post-transplant population; however, higher risk-stratification for these patients is critical.

Varying degrees of hypertensive urgencies or emergencies may be seen in post-transplant patients. Likewise, patients may present with acute or chronic dysrhythmias (such as chronic atrial fibrillation) unrelated to the transplant. Although no single antihypertensive or antidysrhythmic agent is contraindicated, care should to be taken to avoid drug interactions (Box 114-4).

BOX 114-4

Drug Interactions in Patients Taking Immunosuppressive Medications

Cyclosporine
- Levels *increased* (potential nephrotoxicity) by diltiazem, verapamil, azole antifungals, macrolides
- Levels *decreased* (potential subtherapeutic levels and risk for rejection) by phenobarbital, phenytoin, carbamazepine, isonicotine hydrazine (INH), rifampin, nafcillin
- Aminoglycosides—can exacerbate nephrotoxicity
- Statins—may predispose to hepatotoxicity/rhabdomyolysis; cyclosporine may increase statin levels

Azathioprine
- Allopurinol—levels of azathioprine *increased,* causing increased risk of myelosuppression

Pulmonary Emergencies

Pneumonia remains the most common pulmonary emergency in transplant recipients.[8] The causative organisms vary depending on timing of presentation. Chest radiograph findings may be nonspecific; immunosuppressive medications blunt the appearance of infiltrates.[2,8] Additionally, sirolimus has been noted to cause an interstitial pneumonitis.[9] Chest computed tomography may be required to help delineate etiologies of an abnormal chest radiograph.

The threshold for hospital admission for post-transplant patients with pneumonia is lower given the potential for rapidly progressive disease and opportunistic infections. Appropriate efforts should be made to obtain sputum for Gram stain and culture, given the potential for unusual organisms. Antimicrobial choices need to be tailored to the most likely organisms, based on the clinical picture and time from transplant.

Fluoroquinolones and macrolides may increase levels of cyclosporine and tacrolimus; these antibiotic classes should not be used as first-line agents in treatment of patients with post-transplant pneumonia.

Gastrointestinal Emergencies

Abdominal pain in renal transplant recipients may be due to a variety of causes. Diagnostic imaging studies should be liberally ordered, given the potential for patients with serious intra-abdominal processes to present with relatively minimal findings on physical examination.[2,10]

Mortality from cholecystitis is high in renal post-transplant patients. Diverticulitis is the most common bacterial gastrointestinal infectious process.[10] Diarrhea may be due to any number of infectious organisms, including *Salmonella, Listeria,* cytomegalovirus, and *Cryptosporidium.*

Abdominal pain in the area of the allograft should prompt consideration of acute rejection.

Opportunistic infections may affect any area of the gastrointestinal tract, from mouth to anus. Common opportunistic infections include candidiasis, cytomegalovirus, and herpes simplex.[10,11] Cytomegalovirus and Epstein-Barr virus can cause acute hepatitis.

Various immunosuppressive drugs can cause stomatitis, ulcerations, or acute hepatitis.[10] There is an increased incidence of acute pancreatitis in renal transplant recipients that may be related to immunosuppressive agents.[10]

Genitourinary and Renal Emergencies

Renal transplant recipients are prone to the same genitourinary and renal disorders as the general population. The one truly unique renal emergency in this population is rejection.

Urinary tract infections are more severe in transplant recipients.[12] Pyelonephritis may follow a fulminant course and patients with this disorder should not be managed as an outpatient. These patients often require two broad-spectrum antibiotics for adequate treatment. Aminoglycosides are nephrotoxic and should be avoided if possible.

Hematuria in renal transplant recipients may be due to infection or obstruction in the allograft or in the native kidneys; imaging studies are recommended. Hemolytic-uremic syndrome, another cause of hematuria and acute renal failure in post-transplant patients, may be related to infection (cytomegalovirus), rejection, or medication toxicity (cyclosporine and tacrolimus).[13]

When evaluating acute renal failure in post-transplant patients, common causes of renal insufficiency seen in non-transplant patients must be considered; rejection is a later consideration, after other more likely causes have been excluded.

If hydronephrosis is present, ultrasound studies should be ordered to look for ureteral obstruction. Arterial Doppler imaging may be needed to evaluate the adequacy of blood flow to a graft. Obstruction of an allograft is a true surgical emergency and generally requires placement of a percutaneous nephrostomy tube.

Rejection can be acute, chronic, or acute-on-chronic. Acute rejection occurs in the early post-transplant period. Chronic rejection is the most common cause of renal allograft dysfunction after the first post-transplant year.

A common cause of acute renal failure in renal transplant patients is nephrotoxicity due to cyclosporine or tacrolimus.[2,14] Rejection may not be distinguished from nephrotoxicity without a biopsy. Fever and tenderness over the graft site suggest the presence of rejection, whereas elevated trough levels of cyclosporine or tacrolimus suggest drug-induced nephrotoxicity.

If acute rejection is the most likely diagnosis, the transplant service should be consulted about inpatient management, and high-dose methylprednisolone therapy should be started at a dose of 500 to 1000 mg daily.

■ Endocrine and Metabolic Emergencies

Transplant recipients on corticosteroid therapy have functional adrenal insufficiency and require pulse doses of corticosteroids when they encounter physiologic stress. Administer stress-dose hydrocortisone to transplant patients with unexplained or refractory hypotension, unless they have been off corticosteroid therapy for more than 6 months.

Electrolyte disorders, especially hyperkalemia, are common in post-transplant patients due to cyclosporine- or tacrolimus-induced impairment of potassium excretion.[15] This impairment may be exacerbated by the use of potassium-sparing diuretics and angiotensin-converting enzyme inhibitors.

Cyclosporine and corticosteroids both contribute to an increased incidence of new-onset diabetes in transplant recipients.[16]

■ Neurologic Emergencies

Cryptococcal meningitis and central nervous system lymphoma are seen with greater frequency in post-transplant patients, due to immunosuppression.[17] Patients presenting with fever of unknown origin, headache, or altered mental status should undergo intracranial imaging and lumbar puncture as appropriate. Computed tomography scanning of the brain with and without contrast is preferable in this population, to more readily identify space-occupying lesions. The risk of contrast-induced nephrotoxicity must be weighed against the benefit of diagnostic accuracy when brain lesions are suspected.

■ Adverse Drug Reactions

Immunosuppressive medications cause illness through the direct toxic effects of these drugs or resulting from interaction with other common medications. Medication reconciliation is critical as new drug regimens become more complex.

Initial post-transplant regimens typically consist of three agents: a corticosteroid, a calcineurin inhibitor (cyclosporine, tacrolimus, sirolimus), and a purine synthesis inhibitor (azathioprine, mycophenolate mofetil).[18] Most patients are weaned off corticosteroid in 6 months, and maintenance is continued with only two drugs.

During the initial induction phase of immunosuppression, other agents such as anti-thymocyte monoclonal and polyclonal antibodies are used. Because these medications generally are reserved for inpatient use, it is unusual for patients to present to the ED with an acute complication from these agents.

Corticosteroid therapy has many well-recognized complications. In addition to functional adrenal suppression, corticosteroids can induce diabetes, steroid psychosis, gastric ulceration, pancreatitis, changes in body habitus, and avascular necrosis.

Azathioprine is one of the oldest agents used to treat rejection. It is an alkylating agent similar to other chemotherapeutic drugs, and thus its primary toxicity is bone marrow suppression (particularly leukopenia). When given with allopurinol, increased levels of azathioprine may result in myelosuppression. Azathioprine and mycophenolate mofetil demonstrate an additive risk of myelosuppression. Hepatotoxicity from azathioprine is less than with other agents.

Cyclosporine interacts with multiple other medications and demonstrates significant nephrotoxicity. Increased serum creatinine levels are observed in up to one third of patients taking cyclosporine.[15] As these levels rise, cyclosporine excretion decreases and renal failure worsens. Trough measurements of cyclosporine (drawn 3 hours prior to the next scheduled dose) differentiate drug-induced nephrotoxicity from other causes of renal insufficiency.

Tacrolimus and sirolimus both carry the risk of multiple drug interactions and worsening nephrotoxicity. Drugs that increase the metabolism of these agents may decrease their effective serum levels, thus resulting in acute rejection due to inadequate immunosuppression.

Disposition

Concerns about chronic immunosuppression, graft rejection, and multiple drug interactions make management of transplant patients among the most difficult challenges encountered in the ED. As a rule, these patients require extensive laboratory and imaging studies; there is no data to predict which of these patients can safely forgo such testing in an emergency setting. Consultation with an experienced transplant team will improve outcomes. The majority of transplant patients with serious chief complaints require hospital admission for observation and further management.

REFERENCES

1. Data from www.unos.org; accessed 3/31/06.
2. Schulak JA: What's new in general surgery: Transplantation. J Am Coll Surg 2005;200:409-417.
3. Djamali A, Kendziorski C, Brazy PC, et al: Disease progression and outcomes in chronic kidney disease and renal transplantation. Kidney Int 2003;64:1800-1807.
4. Denton MD, Magee CM, Sayegh MH: Immunosuppressive strategies in transplantation. Lancet 1999;353:1083-1091.
5. Venkat KK, Venkat A: Care of renal transplant recipients in the emergency department. Ann Emerg Med 2004;44: 330-341.
6. Akbar Sam Jofri SZ, Amendola MA, et al: Complications of renal transplantation. Radiographics 2005;25:1335-1356.
7. Kendrick E: Cardiovascular disease and the renal transplant recipient. Am J Kidney Dis 2001;38:36-43.

8. Rubin RH: Infectious disease complications of renal transplantation. Kidney Int 1993;44:221-236.
9. Pham PT, Pham PC, Danovitch GM, et al: Sirolimus-associated pulmonary toxicity. Transplantation 2004;77:1215-1220.
10. Abou-Saif A, Lewis JH: Gastrointestinal and hepatic disorders in end-stage renal disease and renal transplant recipients. Adv Renal Replace Ther 2000;7:220-230.
11. de Francisco AL: Gastrointestinal disease and the kidney. Eur J Gastroenterol Hepatol 2002;14:11-15.
12. Brown PD: Urinary tract infections in renal transplant recipients. Curr Infect Dis Rep 2002;4:525-528.
13. Agarwal A, Mauer SM, Matas AJ, Nath KA: Recurrent hemolytic uremia syndrome in an adult renal allograft recipient: Current concepts and management. J Am Soc Nephrol 1995;6:1160-1169.
14. Williams D, Haragsim L: Calcineurin nephrotoxicity. Adv Chronic Kidney Dis. 2006;13:56-61.
15. Caliskan Y, Kalayoglu-Besisik S, Sargin D, Ecder T: Cyclosporine-associated hyperkalemia: Report of four allogeneic blood stem-cell transplant cases. Transplantation 2003;75:1069-1072.
16. Marchetti P: New-onset diabetes after transplantation. J Heart Lung Transplant 2004;23:194-201.
17. Palmer CA: Neurologic manifestations of renal disease. Neurol Clin 2002;20:23-34.
18. Halloran PF: Immunosuppressive drugs for kidney transplantation. New Engl J Med 2004;351:2715-2729.

SECTION XII

Women's Health and Gynecologic Diseases

Chapter **115**

The Healthy Pregnancy

Jon D. Van Roo and Matthew Kippenhan

KEY POINTS

The incidence of venous thromboembolism increases by a factor of 5 during pregnancy; pulmonary embolism is a leading cause of maternal mortality in the United States.

Approximately 2% to 10% of gravid and nongravid patients have asymptomatic bacteriuria, which will eventually progress to acute pyelonephritis in as many as 40% of gravid patients.

Acute pyelonephritis during pregnancy increases the risk for preterm labor; these patients should be admitted for IV antibiotic therapy.

One third of patients will have improvement in their asthma symptoms during pregnancy, one third with remain the same, and one third will have worsening of symptoms.

As many as one third of patients with epilepsy will experience an increase in seizure activity during pregnancy.

Migraine headaches are reduced or resolved in 60% to 80% of women during pregnancy.

Treatment of human immunodeficiency virus (HIV) infection during pregnancy with zidovudime can reduce the incidence of perinatal transmission from the mother to the infant by 70%.

Scope

Each year there are 4.1 million live births in the United States resulting from approximately 6.5 million pregnancies.[1,2] These women routinely present to the ED with general medical complaints as well as pregnancy-specific issues. In addition, pregnancy can be an emotionally stressful condition requiring special attention from caregivers. Because diagnostic and management strategies are altered in pregnancy, a thorough understanding of the physiologic changes that accompany pregnancy is mandatory (Box 115-1).

Definitions

Gravidity refers to the total number of pregnancies conceived including the current pregnancy. *Parity* characterizes the outcome of the pregnancy, and it is further subdivided into four categories described by the mnemonic TPAL (number of *t*erm infants, *p*reterm infants, *a*bortions, and *l*iving children (Box 115-2).

A *term pregnancy* lasts from 37 to 42 weeks and is divided into trimesters. The first trimester begins at conception and lasts until the 14th week. The second trimester encompasses weeks 14 to 28, and the third trimester lasts from the 28th to the 42nd week.

BOX 115-1

Physiologic Changes in Pregnancy

Respiratory System
- Reduction of total lung capacity (TLC)
- Reduction of functional residual capacity (FRC)
- Increased tidal volume (TV)
- Increased minute ventilation (Ve)
- Decreased $Pa{CO_2}$

Hematologic/Immunologic System
- Increased blood volume
- Increased plasma volume
- Decreased hemoglobin (dilutional)
- Increased procoagulation factors
- Increased white blood cell count (WBC)

Cardiovascular System
- Increased cardiac output (CO)
- Increased heart rate
- Increased stroke volume
- Decreased systemic vascular resistance (SVR)
- Decreased blood pressure

Gastrointestinal System
- Decreased stomach motility and tone
- Increase in gastroesophageal reflux

Dermatologic System
- Striae gravidarum
- Linea nigra
- Chloasma or melasma
- Spider angioma

Urinary System
- Increased glomerular filtration rate (GFR)
- Dilation of ureters, renal pelvis, and renal calices
- Decrease in creatinine and blood urea nitrogen (BUN)

Musculoskeletal System
- Increased spinal lordosis
- Increased pubic in ligament laxity
- Breast enlargement and tenderness

Endocrine System
- Increased pituitary gland size
- Glucose intolerance

Infants delivered prior to 37 weeks are considered premature, whereas those delivered after 42 weeks are considered post-term. The due date can be estimated using Naegele's rule, applied by subtracting 3 months from the first day of the patient's last menstrual period and adding 7 days to that date. First-trimester ultrasound scans provide more reliable estimates of gestational age.

BOX 115-2

Gestation and Parity Notation

Gestatation (G): Total number of pregnancies

Parity (P): Subdivided into four categories described by the mnemonic TPAL—number of *t*erm infants, *p*reterm infants, *a*bortions, and *l*iving children

Example: G4P3 describes a woman who has had four pregnancies and three deliveries; G4P3 (2-1-1-3), also written as G_4P_{2113}, describes a woman who has had two term deliveries, one preterm delivery, and one abortion (spontaneous or induced) and has three living children.

Clinical Presentation—Anatomic/Physiologic Changes in Pregnancy

EPs should consider the possibility of pregnancy in every female patient of childbearing age regardless of the chief complaint or symptoms. One study documented pregnancy in 7% of ED respondents who indicated that their last menstrual period was on time and normal, and that there was "no chance" they were pregnant.[3] Early signs of pregnancy include missed menses, vaginal bleeding, nausea, vomiting, breast tenderness, urinary frequency, fatigue, near-syncope, and abdominal pain or bloating. Some patients may not have these symptoms or may ignore them, presenting later with an obviously enlarged uterus or in labor.

■ RESPIRATORY SYSTEM

The physiology of breathing in pregnancy is altered by both anatomic and hormonal changes. Anatomic changes include increase in chest diameter and circumference, as well as a rise in the level of the diaphragm. The result is a reduction in total lung capacity by 5%, and functional residual capacity by 20%. In contrast, the vital capacity does not change.[4] The respiratory rate also remains constant, but due to a progesterone-mediated increase in both tidal volume and minute ventilation there is a decrease in $Pa{CO_2}$ to an average of 30 mm Hg. The sensation of dyspnea is increased during pregnancy.

■ HEMATOLOGIC/IMMUNOLOGIC SYSTEM

Blood volume increases during pregnancy by an average of 40% to 50%, secondary to both plasma volume expansion and increased erythrocyte mass. Plasma volume increases approximately 50%, reaching a plateau at 30 weeks of gestation. Erythrocyte mass increases 20% to 30% over prepregnancy levels, peaking near term, with greater increases associated with iron supplementation. The asymmetric expansion of plasma and erythrocyte mass results in a relative anemia, referred to as the *physiologic anemia of pregnancy*. Plasma expansion begins earlier than erythropoiesis but then stabilizes, resulting in a nadir in hemoglobin concentration that occurs between weeks 16 and 28.[5] Hemoglobin levels normally do not drop below 10.5 g/dL during the nadir period and should measure 11 g/dL or more during the remaining pregnancy.

Procoagulation factors are increased during pregnancy, whereas inhibitors of coagulation levels are reduced or unchanged. These changes in the coagulation cascade may serve to protect a mother against peripartum hemorrhage but, when combined with venous stasis and vessel wall injury, predispose a patient to thromboembolic disease.[6]

Pregnancy has been described as a state of immunodeficiency but is more accurately described as a period of modified immune response.[7] The peripheral white blood cell count is elevated during pregnancy, ranging from 5110/mm^3 to 12,200/mm^3 during gestation and rising even higher during labor. Additionally, there are changes in both the chemotaxis and adherence of neutrophils and a shift by the immune system away from the cell-mediated immune response toward antibody-mediated immunity. This altered immune focus allows tolerance of the maternal immune system to paternal antigens, but increases susceptibility to pathogens and variation in activity of autoimmune disease.[8]

■ CARDIOVASCULAR SYSTEM

Changes in diaphragm position and rib cage dimension cause the heart to be displaced to the left and upward and rotated on its long axis. On radiographic studies these changes are manifested as an increase in heart silhouette in the absence of actual cardiomegaly. Likewise, this positional change is responsible for apparent left axis deviation on electrocardiography.

Cardiac output consistently and dramatically increases during pregnancy, rising 37% to 53% over prepregnancy values.[9] This increase is driven by increases in both heart rate and stroke volume. Heart rate increases 15 to 20 beats per minute over pregravid rates, and stroke volume increases by 20% to 30%. In later stages of pregnancy, cardiac output is also dependent on maternal position because of compression of the inferior vena cava. The highest levels of cardiac output occur in the right and left lateral positions; the lowest levels occur in the supine, sitting, and standing positions. A small number of pregnant patients (5%-10%) develop supine hypotension with symptoms such as dizziness, nausea, and syncope.[6] Despite the increase in cardiac output, pregnancy-associated reduction in systemic vascular resistance causes an overall reduction in maternal blood pressure. Blood pressure, like cardiac output, is position-dependent, being highest when sitting and lowest in the lateral recumbent position.

■ DERMATOLOGIC SYSTEM

Striae cutis distensae, also known as *striae gravidarum* ("stretch marks"), occur in 50% to 90% of pregnancies during the late second or third trimester. Formation requires stretching of the skin, but hormonal changes affecting the dermis are also implicated. Hormonal stimulation of melanocyte activity is responsible for the hyperpigmentation seen in as many as 90% of pregnancies

■ GENITOURINARY SYSTEM

Urinary system changes during normal pregnancy include increases in kidney size, glomerular filtration rate, and renal blood flow. Additionally, there is dilation of the ureters, renal pelvis, and renal calices, which is secondary to mechanical compression caused by the expanding uterus and ovarian structures, as well as progesterone-mediated smooth muscle relaxation. The right ureter is more commonly affected than the left, likely secondary to anatomic susceptibility. The glomerular filtration rate increases 50% over non-gravid values by the end of the first trimester and is maintained throughout pregnancy. This increase, and the subsequent increase in filtration fraction, leads to decreases in both creatinine and blood urea nitrogen levels. Dependent edema accumulated during the day is mobilized at night, resulting in increased nocturia during pregnancy. Increased incidence of glycosuria is common during pregnancy and may be unrelated to blood glucose levels or kidney dysfunction, but hematuria or protenuria prior to labor are pathologic.

The weight of the uterus increases from 70 g to 1100 g, and intrauterine volume increases from 10 mL to 5000 mL. The gradual color change of the vaginal walls to a dark blue or black color (Chadwick's sign) is secondary to venous congestion.

■ GASTROINTESTINAL SYSTEM

Changes in the gastrointestinal system during pregnancy include an overall decrease in stomach tone and motility. This is consistent with, and likely related to, a decrease in lower esophageal sphincter tone and esophageal dysmotility caused by altered hormonal levels. This muscle relaxation, coupled with the compression of the stomach by the expanding uterus leads to an increase in gastroesophageal reflux disease (GERD). Paradoxically, there is a concurrent decrease in peptic ulcer disease.

Liver anatomy and function are essentially unchanged. However, serum alkaline phosphatase is elevated during the third trimester secondary to placental production of the isoenzyme. Gallbladder emptying is slower and less efficient during pregnancy. In addition to stasis, chemical composition changes in bile lead to increased formation of cholesterol crystals. The result is an increase in symptomatic cholelithiasis.

■ MUSCULOSKELETAL SYSTEM

In order to counterbalance the expanding uterus and prevent an anterior shift in the center of gravity, there is an increasing degree of lordosis of the lumbar spine throughout pregnancy. This often results in low back pain. Increased laxity of the ligament of the pubic symphysis and sacroiliac joints can also result in pain. Increasing tenderness of the breasts is common in pregnancy.

■ ENDOCRINE SYSTEM

Enlargement of the breasts and nipples is normal, and discharge of colostrum from the nipples during the later stages of pregnancy is not uncommon. Hypothyroidism during pregnancy is associated with fetal neurologic defects such as mental retardation and lower IQ scores.[10,11] Despite histologic changes, women remain euthyroid during pregnancy, and the slight increase in thyroid size that does occur is not clinically detectable. Palpable increase in the thyroid during pregnancy is pathologic and must be further evaluated. Results of laboratory tests commonly used to evaluate thyroid function should be within normal limits.

The pituitary gland increases 136% in size compared with prepregnancy size. This size increase makes the gland more susceptible to infarct with hemorrhage (Sheehan's syndrome) but does not impair the optic chiasm.

Some level of glucose intolerance is associated with pregnancy. Normal pregnancy is marked by hyperglycemia after eating, followed by hypoglycemia when fasting. Postprandial hyperglycemia ensures adequate nutrient delivery to the fetus.

Common Medical Diseases and Pregnancy

■ DIABETES

Diabetes occurs in approximately 3% to 5% of all gestations.[12] Three types of diabetes affect pregnancy: type 1, type 2, and gestational diabetes. Gestational diabetes represents 90% of cases. Fetal risks during pregnancy for women with diabetes include congenital malformation, intrauterine growth retardation, macrosomia, fetal hypoglycemia, fetal respiratory distress syndrome, neonatal hypocalcemia, hyperbilirubinemia, polycythemia, intrauterine demise, and neonatal jaundice. These risks are greatest for women with type 1 diabetes, although type 2 and gestational diabetes are also associated with a significant increase in fetal mortality.

With tight glucose control, the perinatal mortality rate of diabetic pregnancies can approach that of uncomplicated pregnancies. However, maintaining normal blood sugar levels is extremely difficult due to a changing degree of insulin resistance throughout pregnancy.

Patients who are unable to achieve glucose control with diet and exercise require insulin therapy. The effects of oral hypoglycemic agents in pregnant patients has not been studied extensively. Some agents may be associated with an increased rate of congenital malformation, and often they do not provide adequate glucose control.

Diabetic ketoacidosis occurs in as many as 10% of patients with type 1 diabetes. Treatment during pregnancy is the same as for a nongravid patients but should include assessment of fetal status and supportive measures such as oxygen and the use of the left lateral decubitus position to maximize fetal blood flow.

■ URINARY TRACT INFECTIONS

The incidence of acute cystitis or acute pyelonephritis is approximately 1% during pregnancy. Asymptomatic bacteriuria is a related condition in which a urine culture is positive in an asymptomatic patient. The incidence of asymptomatic bacteriuria is similar in both gravid and nongravid populations, affecting 2% to 10% of the population.[13] Gravid patients have a much higher rate of progression to symptomatic infection, with as many as 40% of cases eventually progressing to acute pyelonephritis. All three conditions—chronic cystitis and chronic and acute pyelonephritis—are associated with negative outcomes, and patients should receive antibiotic therapy. Patients with recurrent asymptomatic bacteriuria or urinary tract infection may require daily suppressive therapy or postcoital prophylaxis.

Treatment of asymptomatic bacteriuria and acute cystitis can be accomplished with 3 to 7 days of oral therapy using amoxicillin, a cephalosporin, or nitrofurantoin. Unless sensitivities are known, nitrofurantoin is the preferred agent because of high levels of resistance to other agents. Acute pyelonephritis during pregnancy increases the risk for preterm labor and should be managed aggressively. Patients require admission and IV antibiotic therapy until clinical improvement is demonstrated.

■ ASTHMA

Asthma is a complication in approximately 4% of pregnancies,[14] roughly mirroring its incidence in women of childbearing age. The course of asthma during pregnancy is not uniformly predictable. One third of patients will have improvement of symptoms during pregnancy, one third will experience stable disease, and another third will have worsening of symptoms.[15] Although this finding is somewhat controversial, patients with asthma have been

RED FLAGS

- Most antiepileptic drugs are teratogenic; increased seizure activity may be related to the known higher prevalence during pregnancy, but the increase may also be related to medicine noncompliance.
- New seizure activity during pregnancy merits investigation; eclampsia must always be suspected in the third trimester.
- Hemoglobin levels do not normally drop below 10.5 g/dL during pregnancy and should usually measure 11 g/dL.
- Pregnancy is a state of immunodeficiency, and pregnant women have increased susceptibility to pathogens.

reported to have increased rates of preeclampsia, cesarean delivery, asthma exacerbations, and preterm rupture of membranes. Fetal risks include increased mortality, prematurity, intrauterine growth retardation, and low birth weight.

Monitoring and treatment of asthma in pregnant patients are much the same as for nonpregnant patients. Commonly used measures include the peak expiratory flow rate (PEFR) and the forced expiratory flow in 1 second (FEV_1). Beta-agonists are the initial medication of choice both for acute exacerbation and for maintenance. Inhaled corticosteroids are safe and effective, but during acute exacerbation IV corticosteroids may be required.

■ SEIZURE DISORDERS

Epilepsy is associated with an increased incidence of obstetric and fetal complications. However, over 90% of pregnant women with epilepsy have a normal pregnancy with a good outcome.[16] Seizure disorders affect approximately 1% of the general population and affect a similar percentage of gestations. As many as one third of women with epilepsy experience an increase in seizure activity during pregnancy. Patients who experience a higher pregravid incidence of seizures are at a greater risk for increased seizure activity during pregnancy. The cause of this change in seizure activity may result from decreased compliance with medical therapy, altered pharmacologic distribution, increased elimination of medications, or a combination of factors.

Status epilepticus during pregnancy is a gravely danger for both mother and fetus and should be treated aggressively with early intubation, pharmacologic therapy, and evaluation for eclampsia. Benzodiazepines, phenytoin, and fosphenytoin are all effective in treatment of status epilepticus. New seizure activity during pregnancy merits investigation to determine etiology; eclampsia should be suspected in the third trimester.

■ MIGRAINE

Migraine symptoms are reduced or resolved in 60% to 80% of women during pregnancy. Acceptable pharmacologic agents to treat symptoms include acetaminophen, narcotics, and antiemetics such as prochlorperazine, promethazine, and metoclopramide. Caffeine is sometimes effective and may be used in moderation. Propranolol is generally considered safe for migraine prophylaxis, but may carry a risk of intrauterine growth retardation.

Other commonly used agents should be avoided. Ergotamines may cause birth defects secondary to vascular alteration. Triptans may cause vasospasm resulting in increased incidence of preterm birth and intrauterine growth retardation. As is the case in other conditions, nonsteroidal antiinflammatory drugs (NSAIDs) should be avoided.

■ THROMBOEMBOLIC DISEASE

Thromboembolic disease is a major source of maternal morbidity and mortality during pregnancy. The incidence of venous thromboembolism increases by a factor of 5 during pregnancy, and pulmonary embolism is a leading cause of maternal mortality in the United States.[17] Factors believed to contribute to the increased incidence of venous thromboembolism include alteration of normal clotting factor levels, increased stasis, and vessel damage. These factors may be aggravated by advanced maternal age and inherited or acquired thrombophilias.

Ultrasonography safely and reliably detects lower-extremity deep vein thrombosis. If pelvic or iliac thrombosis is suspected, venography may be required for diagnosis; however, magnetic resonance imaging is increasingly being used. Ventilation-perfusion scans are useful in the assessment for pulmonary embolism; however, spiral computed tomography, available at most institutions, delivers lower fetal radiation exposure than ventilation-perfusion scans. Both heparin and low-molecular-weight heparin are commonly used in the treatment of acute thromboembolism. Warfarin is contraindicated in pregnant patients because of its association with fetal malformation and fetal demise.

■ HYPERTENSION

Pregnant women with elevated blood pressure may have preexisting hypertension, gestational hypertension, preeclampsia, or eclampsia.

There currently is no established consensus regarding initiation of antihypertensive therapy during pregnancy. Most authorities prescribe treatment for patients with blood pressure of 160/105 or higher; others argue that a lower threshold of 150/100 should be the criterion for treatment. In one review of pregnant patients experiencing stroke secondary to preeclampsia, systolic blood pressures recorded before the event were 159 to 198 mm Hg, and diastolic blood pressures were 81 to 113 mm Hg[18]; arterial hemorrhage was the cause of stroke in 93% of those patients who underwent intracranial imaging. Of note, there is not sufficient evidence to recommend bed rest as an effective or practical treatment for hypertension during pregnancy.[19]

■ ALCOHOL AND OTHER RECREATIONAL DRUGS

Alcohol use is reported in 10% to 15% of pregnancies; no safe level of intake has been determined. Alcohol abuse is associated with fetal alcohol syndrome. Common features of this syndrome include low IQ, microcephaly, short palpebral fissures, smooth filtrum, thin upper lip, and ventricular septal defects.

Cigarette smoking increases the risk of spontaneous abortion, prematurity, small-for-gestational age births, abruptio placentae, placenta previa, and prolonged rupture of membranes. The adverse effects of smoking are dose-related and reduced by cessation of smoking even after a pregnancy is diagnosed.

Opiate, cocaine, and methamphetamine are all associated with obstetric complications. Cocaine use during pregnancy is believed to cause increased rates of abruptio placentae, preterm labor, and small-for-gestational age infants. However, these studies are limited in that many of the mothers using cocaine were polysubstance abusers.

EPs should be aware of the reporting requirements of drug abuse in the states in which they practice.

■ HIV/AIDS

Treatment of HIV infection during pregnancy with zidovudine can reduce the incidence of perinatal transmission from mother to infant by 70%. The combination of zidovudine therapy and elective cesarean delivery may reduce perinatal HIV transmission by as much as 85%. In the United States, where safe breast milk replacement is readily available, breastfeeding is discouraged due to the risk of transmission from mother to child. Referral to infectious disease and high risk obstetrics services is mandatory for pregnant women who are known to be HIV-positive.

Medication Use during Pregnancy

Medication use during pregnancy can be a source of apprehension for both patients and physicians due to the paucity of safety data. Pharmaceutical companies have excluded pregnant patients from the testing of new agents for decades, resulting in little knowledge about the teratogenicity of products in humans. Additionally, animal models may not be representative of human risk. EPs prescribing medication for pregnant or lactating women should use resources available in both electronic and text formats.

Fetal toxicity is affected by dose, duration of exposure, and the gestational age when exposure occurs. During the 31-day period following the last menstrual period, teratogens have essentially a binary (all-or-nothing) effect—the conceptus is either aborted or survives without harm. The next stage of development is the crucial period of organogenesis, lasting from 31 to 71 days after the last menstrual period. The effect of exposure to a teratogen is time-dependent during this period. Early exposure may affect the cardiovascular and/or central nervous systems, whereas later exposure may affect the palate and ears.

The United States Food and Drug Administration (FDA) classifies medications into five categories based on potential fetal risk based on animal and human studies (Table 115-1).[20] Medications commonly

Table 115-1 UNITED STATES FDA PHARMACEUTICAL PREGNANCY CATEGORIES

Pregnancy Category	Description
A	Adequate well-controlled studies in pregnant women have not shown an increased risk of fetal abnormalities.
B	Animal studies have revealed no evidence of harm to the fetus; however, there are no adequate and well-controlled studies in pregnant women. *or* Animal studies have shown an adverse effect, but adequate and well-controlled studies in pregnant women have failed to demonstrate a risk to the fetus.
C	Animal studies have shown an adverse effect, and there are no adequate well-controlled studies in pregnant women. *or* No animal studies have been conducted, and there are no adequate well-controlled studies in pregnant women.
D	Adequate well-controlled or observational studies in pregnant women have demonstrated a risk to the fetus. However, the benefits of therapy may outweigh the potential risks.
X	Adequate well-controlled or observational studies in animals or pregnant women have demonstrated positive evidence of fetal abnormalities. The use of the product is contraindicated in women who are or may become pregnant.

FDA, Food and Drug Administration.
Modified from Meadows M: Pregnancy and the drug dilemma. FDA Consum 2001;35:16-20. Available at http://www.fda.gov/fdac/features/2001/301_preg.html.

BOX 115-3

Medications Considered Safe during Pregnancy

- Analgesics
  - Acetaminophen
  - Opiates*
- Antiemetics
  - Dopamine agonists: (phenothiazides, promethazine, chlorpromazine, perphenazine, metoclopramide)
  - Serotonin 5-HT_3 receptor antagonist: (ondansetron)
  - Other (vitamin B_6, ginger)
- Antihypertensives
  - Alpha-methyldopa
  - Hydralazine
  - Beta-blockers (labetolol, metoprolol, propranolol)
  - Calcium channel blockers (nifedipine, diltiazem, verapamil)
  - Diuretics
- Antimicrobials
  - Penicillin and derivatives (ampicillin, nafcillin, ticarcillin, piperacillin)
  - Cephalosporins (1st, 2nd, 3rd, 4th generation)
  - Macrolides (erythromycin,† azithromycin, clarithromycin)
  - Benzodiazepines‡
  - Others (clindamycin, nitrofurantoin)
- Anticoagulants
  - Heparin
  - Low-molecular-weight heparin
- Antiepileptics
  - Benzodiazepines‡
- Asthma medications
  - Beta-agonists
  - Corticosteroids
- Diabetes medications
  - Insulin (lispro, aspart, regular, glargine)
- Prophylaxis
  - Tetanus toxoid
  - Influenza vaccine

*Avoid chronic use of opiates during pregnancy. Also, use caution when giving opiates near time of delivery because of risk of respiratory and central nervous system depression.
†Do not give estolate salt of erythromycin because of risk of maternal hepatic toxicity.
‡Use caution when giving benzodiazepines near time of delivery because of risk of respiratory depression. Early studies showed teratogenicity, uncomfirmed in later studies; however, the drug is still class D and should be used with caution in the first trimester.

used in the ED and generally considered safe are listed in Box 115-3; often-used medications considered unsafe for use during pregnancy are listed in Table 115-2.

■ ANALGESIC AGENTS

There is no evidence implicating acetaminophen as a teratogen; thus it is the preferred agent when a mild analgesic or antipyretic is indicated. The use of NSAIDs such as ibuprofen and naproxen is generally discouraged during pregnancy, although the risk appears to be mostly in the third trimester. Indomethacin has been reported to be associated with oligohydramnios, pulmonary hypertension, and constriction of the ductus arteriosus.

Although there is no conclusive human data indicating that aspirin is a teratogen, its other ill effects limit its use during pregnancy. Aspirin has been linked to delayed onset of labor, protracted labor, and increased risk of prolonged pregnancy. It inhibits prostaglandin synthesis, leading to premature closure of the ductus arteriosus, as well as increases the incidence of hemorrhage due to a decrease in platelet aggregation.

The use of opiates is considered safe throughout pregnancy. However, opiate use shortly before deliv-

Table 115-2 COMMON ED PHARMACEUTICAL AGENTS CONTRAINDICATED IN PREGNANCY

Agent	Contraindication
Analgesics	
Aspirin	Premature closure of the ductus arteriosus and increased incidence of hemorrhage
NSAIDs (ibuprofen, indomethacin, and naproxen)	Oligohydramnios, pulmonary hypertension, and constriction of the ductus arteriosus
Antimicrobials	
Tetracyclines	Discolored teeth, inhibition of bone growth
Fluoroquinolones	Arthropathy in immature animals
Aminoglycosides	Ototoxicity, nephrotoxicity
Anticoagulants	
Warfarin	Nasal bone hypoplasia, bone stippling, ophthalmologic abnormalities, and mental retardation
Antiepileptics	
Phenytoin	Fetal hydantoin syndrome (ossification abnormalities, cleft lip and palate, impaired growth, and cardiac abnormalities)
Carbamazepine, valproic acid	Dysmorphic syndrome, similar to fetal hydantoin syndrome
Antihypertensives	
ACE inhibitors	Renal malformation, oligohydramnios, craniofacial malformations and lung malformations
Angiotensin II receptor blockers	Linked to similar malformations similar to those from ACE inhibitors
Other	
Isotretinoin	Craniofacial, cardiac, thymic, and CNS malformations

ACE, angiotensin-converting enzyme; CNS, central nervous system; NSAIDs, nonsteroidal antiinflammatory drugs.

ery can result in respiratory and central nervous system depression in the newborn. Because long-term opiate use during pregnancy can cause newborn addiction and withdrawal, patients using opiates chronically should be carefully followed by their physician during pregnancy.

■ ANTICOAGULANTS

Warfarin is a known human teratogen, associated with nasal bone hypoplasia, bone stippling, ophthalmologic abnormalities, and mental retardation; therefore, it is contraindicated in pregnancy. Heparin and low-molecular-weight heparin are thought to be safe during pregnancy and can be used when anticoagulation is indicated.

■ ANTIEMETICS

Antiemetic agents commonly are prescribed during early pregnancy. Dopamine agonists such as phenothiazides, promethazine, chlorpromazine, perphenazine, and metoclopramide are all well tolerated and appear to be safe in pregnancy. The serotonin 5-HT_3 receptor antagonist, ondansetron, also appears to be both safe and effective for nausea and vomiting during pregnancy, although less data are available about this agent.

Vitamin B_6 has been reported to be an effective treatment for nausea and vomiting in several randomized, double-blind, placebo-controlled trials.

Tips and Tricks

- EPs should not initiate, cease, or adjust antiepileptic drugs during pregnancy.
- Spiral computed tomography should be used in preference to ventilation-perfusion scanning in pregnancy because of the the lower radiation exposure.
- Some level of glucose intolerance is associated with pregnancy; normal pregnancy is marked by hyperglycemia after eating, followed by hypoglycemia when fasting.
- Lorazepam (Ativan) is preferable to diazepam (Valium) for control of seizures because it crosses the placenta more slowly and has a shorter half-life.

■ ANTIMICROBIAL AGENTS

All antibiotics have been shown to cross the placenta and the fetal circulation.[21] Penicillin and its derivative compounds including nafcillin, dicloxacillin, amoxicillin, and ampicillin have been used extensively in pregnant patients and no ill-effects on fetal development have been reported. Newer derivatives, such as pipericillin and ticarcillin, have not been used as extensively but are believed to be safe in pregnancy. Cephalosporins are routinely prescribed, although there is less experience with use of cephalosporins than with penicillin and ticarcillin.

The macrolides (erythromycin, azithromycin, clarithromycin) are considered safe during pregnancy with the exception of erythromycin estolate, which is contraindicated because of the risk of maternal hepatotoxicity. Clindamycin and nitrofurantoin, antibiotics commonly used during pregnancy, are both considered safe.

Metronidazole has not been shown to be a human teratogen. However, its use is somewhat controversial due to potential mutagenesis and carcinogenicity. Trimethoprim-sulfamethoxazole has two contraindications, one related to each of its constituents—trimethoprim should be avoided during the first trimester because it is a folate antagonist and its use may lead to an increased incidence of neural tube defects; sulfamethoxazole use is discouraged near term due to competitive binding of albumin with bilirubin, leading to a concern for increased risk of kernicterus. Although this concern exists for all sulfonamides, there are no reported cases of kernicterus resulting from prenatal use.[21]

Tetracyclines are contraindicated during pregnancy due to calcium binding, which causes staining of the deciduous teeth, poor development of tooth enamel, and inhibition of skeletal growth in the fetus. Fluoroquinolones have not been shown to increase the rate of fetal malformation in humans but are contraindicated because of the development of arthropathy in immature animals exposed to quinolones.[22,23]

The aminoglycosides streptomycin and kanamycin are associated with ototoxicity and are potentially nephrotoxic. If gentamycin, also an aminoglycoside and potentially ototoxic and nephrotoxic, is to be used, dosing must be adjusted for renal function and it should be used with caution.

▪ ANTIVIRAL AGENTS

Women with disseminated herpes infections or a first genital herpes virus infection occurring during pregnancy should be treated with acyclovir. There is no known incidence of fetal abnormalities caused by acyclovir. A genital herpes outbreak at term necessitates cesarean delivery.

▪ ANTIEPILEPTIC DRUGS

Management of epilepsy during pregnancy is difficult and requires a multidisciplinary approach. The risk of maternal death during pregnancy can be as much as ten times higher than that for patients without epilepsy.[24] In addition, rates of intrauterine fetal demise and malformation are also increased. Many commonly available anticonvulsive medications are known or suspected teratogens, which can make management decisions difficult for both caregivers and patients.

Phenytoin, carbamazepine, valproate, and lamotrigine are associated with an increased incidence of congenital abnormalities. A recent review of data from 25 epilepsy centers recorded the following rates of serious adverse outcomes: valproate (20.3%), phenytoin (10.7%), carbamazepine (8.2%), and lamotrigine (1.0%).[25] Newer antiepileptic drugs including levetiracetam, felbamate, gabapentine, oxcarbazepine, tiagabine, and topiramate seem to be safe for use in pregnancy, although there are less data available for these agents.[26]

Despite these risks, most physicians agree that patients with a well established diagnosis of epilepsy should be continued on medication during pregnancy. Women taking antiepileptic drugs during pregnancy should have folic acid supplementation and frequent monitoring. Seizures occurring during pregnancy or labor may be treated with benzodiazepines. Early studies demonstrated a risk for teratogenesis (mostly cleft abnormalities), but these findings have not been reproduced in more recent studies. Lorazepam (Ativan) does not cross to the placenta at as fast a rate as other benzodiazepines and, except during the first trimester, is considered safe. Sedation of the fetus peridelivery is a minor concern.

▪ ANTIHYPERTENSIVE MEDICATIONS

Several agents for the treatment of hypertension during pregnancy have had good safety data. Commonly used medications include alpha-methyldopa and hydralazine. Hydralazine has been used extensively in pregnancy and is available in both IV and oral formulations.[27,28] Beta-blockers are believed to be safe in pregnancy, although there is some association with lower placental and fetal weights with atenolol.[29] Labetolol is the preferred agent because it does not carry this risk. The combined alpha- and beta-blocking characteristics of labetolol may act to preserve uteroplacental blood flow.

Although there are less data available about calcium channel blockers, they also appear to be safe and effective for use during pregnancy. Short-acting sublingual formulations of nifedipine may cause maternal hypotension and fetal distress and should be avoided. Diuretics are safe but are not often used during pregnancy because preeclampsia may arise from a fluid-depleted state.

Two classes of antihypertensive agents, angiotensin-converting enzyme inhibitors and angiotensin II receptor blockers (ARBs), are contraindicated during pregnancy. Angiotensin-converting enzyme (ACE) inhibitors have been associated with fetal renal malformation, oligohydramnios, craniofacial malformations, and lung malformations. Angiotensin II receptor blockers are associated with similar set of malformations likely due to a similar mechanism.

■ ANTIHYPERGLYCEMIC AGENTS

Insulin is the primary medication for the treatment of diabetes during pregnancy and is proven to be safe and effective. A regimen including multiple daily doses of both short- and long-acting insulin is often required. Data regarding the use of oral hypoglycemic agents in pregnancy are still limited. Glyburide and metformin have been used and appear to be safe, but there is little indication for initiating these agents in the ED setting. Patients are at an increased risk for hypoglycemic episodes associated with oral hypoglycemic use and thus should be monitored closely when using these medications.

■ IMMUNIZATIONS

Indications for vaccines composed of toxoid or inactivated virus are similar to those for the nongravid female. In general, the protection gained by vaccination during pregnancy usually outweighs the risks.[30] Live-virus or attenuated vaccines (measles, mumps, poliomyelitis, rubella, yellow fever, and varicella) may cause infection and/or malformation in the fetus, and are therefore contraindicated.

Influenza is a significant exception, and immunization for influenza is indicated for all women who will be pregnant during the flu season (October-March) and for all women at high risk for pulmonary complications.[31] The EP should be aware that tetanus-diphtheria toxoid is administered as usual for tetanus prone wounds.

■ OVER-THE-COUNTER MEDICATIONS

Most over-the-counter cold medications contain a combination of compounds. Little information is available regarding the affects of these agents alone, and less when they are used in combination. Decongestants act via vasoconstriction, and that mechanism also serves, at least theoretically, as a pathway for increased birth defects. Decongestant use during pregnancy should be avoided. Antihistamines, like diphenhydramine, have been used during pregnancy and are considered safe. However, it should be noted that over-the-counter cold remedies are effective for symptom relief only and do not modify the course of disease; rest, hydration, and time are still the best treatment for the common cold.

REFERENCES

1. Martin JA, Hamilton BE, Sutton PD, et al: Births: Final data for 2004. Natl Vital Stat Rep 2006;55:1-101.
2. Ventura SJ, Abma JC, Mosher WD, Henshaw S: Estimated pregnancy rates for the United States, 1990-2000: An update. Natl Vital Stat Rep 2004;52:1-9.
3. Ramoska EA, Saccetti AD, Nepp M: Reliability of patient history in determining the possibility of pregrency. Ann Emerg Med 1989;18:48-80.
4. Crapo RO: Normal cardiopulmonary physiology during pregnancy. Clin Obstet Gynecol 1996;39:3-16.
5. CDC criteria for anemia in children and childbearing-aged women. MMWR Morb Mortal Wkly Rep 1989;38: 400-404.
6. Gabbe SG, Niebyl JR, Simpson JL: Obstetrics: Normal and Problem Pregnancies, 4th ed. New York, Churchill Livingstone, 2002.
7. Stirrat GM: Pregnancy and immunity. BMJ 1994;308(6941): 1385-1386.
8. Wilder RL: Hormones, pregnancy, and autoimmune diseases. Ann N Y Acad Sci 1998;840:45-50.
9. van Oppen AC, Stigter RH, Bruinse HW: Cardiac output in normal pregnancy: A critical review. Obstet Gynecol 1996;87:310-318.
10. Haddow JE, Palomaki GE, Allan WE, et al: Maternal thyroid deficiency during pregnancy and subsequent neuropsychological development of the child. N Engl J Med 1999;341: 549-555.
11. Utiger RD: Maternal hypothyroidism and fetal development. N Engl J Med 1999;341:601-602.
12. Gabbe SG, Graves CR: Management of diabetes mellitus complicating pregnancy. Obstet Gynecol 2003;102: 857-868.
13. Lucas MJ, Cunningham FG: Urinary infection in pregnancy. Clin Obstet Gynecol 1993;36:855-868.
14. Blaiss MS: Management of rhinitis and asthma in pregnancy. Ann Allergy Asthma Immunol 2003;90(Suppl 3): 16-22.
15. Clark SL: Asthma in pregnancy. National Asthma Education Program Working Group on Asthma and Pregnancy. National Institutes of Health, National Heart, Lung and Blood Institute. Obstet Gynecol 1993;82: 1036-1040.
16. Practice parameter: Management issues for women with epilepsy (summary statement). Report of the Quality Standards Subcommittee of the American Academy of Neurology. Neurology 1998;51:944-948.
17. Berg CJ, Atrash HK, Koonin LM, Tucker M, et al: Pregnancy-related mortality in the United States, 1987-1990. Obstet Gynecol 1996;88:161-167.
18. Martin JN Jr, Thigpen BD, Moore RC, et al: Stroke and severe preeclampsia and eclampsia: A paradigm shift focusing on systolic blood pressure. Obstet Gynecol 2005;105: 246-254.
19. Meher S, Abalos E, Carroli G: Bed rest with or without hospitalisation for hypertension during pregnancy. Cochrane Database Syst Rev 2005;4:CD003514.
20. Meadows M: Pregnancy and the drug dilemma. FDA Consum 2001;35:16-20.
21. ACOG educational bulletin. Antimicrobial therapy for obstetric patients. Number 245, March 1998 (replaces no. 117, June 1988). American College of Obstetricians and Gynecologists. Int J Gynaecol Obstet 1998;6:299-308.
22. Ciprofloxacin. 2004 (cited 2007 03/08/07). Available from http://www.fda.gov/cder/foi/label/2005/019537s057, 020780s019lbl.pdf.
23. Linseman DA, Hampton LA, Branstetter DG: Quinolone-induced arthropathy in the neonatal mouse. Morphological analysis of articular lesions produced by pipemidic acid and ciprofloxacin. Fundam Appl Toxicol 1995;28:59-64.
24. Adab N, Kini U, Vinten J, et al: The longer term outcome of children born to mothers with epilepsy. J Neurol Neurosurg Psychiatry 2004;75:1575-1583.
25. Meador KJ, Baker GA, Finnell RH, et al: In utero antiepileptic drug exposure: Fetal death and malformations. Neurology 2006;67:407-412.
26. Morrell MJ: The new antiepileptic drugs and women: Efficacy, reproductive health, pregnancy, and fetal outcome. Epilepsia 1996;37(Suppl 6):34-44.
27. ACOG Practice Bulletin. Chronic hypertension in pregnancy. ACOG Committee on Practice Bulletins. Obstet Gynecol 2001;98:177-185.
28. Abalos E, Duley L, Steyn DW, Henderson-Smart DJ: Antihypertensive drug therapy for mild to moderate hyperten-

sion during pregnancy. Cochrane Database Syst Rev 2007;1: CD002252.
29. Montan S, Ingemarsson I, Marsal K, Sjoberg NO: Randomised controlled trial of atenolol and pindolol in human pregnancy: Effects on fetal haemodynamics. BMJ 1992; 304(6832):946-949.
30. ACOG Committee Opinion. Immunization during pregnancy. Obstet Gynecol 2003;101:207-212.
31. ACOG Committee Opinion. Influenza vaccination and treatment during pregnancy. Obstet Gynecol 2004;104(5 Pt 1):1125-1126.

Chapter **116**

Disorders of Early Pregnancy

Matthew Kippenhan

KEY POINTS

Complications of early pregnancy include abdominal pain, vaginal bleeding, and vomiting, which can either be benign or represent pathologic conditions such as spontaneous abortion, ectopic pregnancy, hyperemesis gravidarum, and gestational trophoblastic disease.

Increasing use of ultrasonography in the ED gives the EP better diagnostic ability, but also more responsibility. Accuracy and skill with pelvic ultrasonography is becoming essential.

Often, definitive diagnosis of these disorders can be made only after specialized studies and subsequent observation. Some patients will leave the ED with a still uncertain diagnosis. Patients need clear discharge instructions and education to understand the dangers and potential complications of their disorders.

SPONTANEOUS ABORTION

Scope and Outline

Spontaneous abortion, also known as miscarriage, occurs when a pregnancy ends before the fetus has reached viability. This correlates to a fetus larger than 500 g, or approximately the size at 20 to 22 weeks of gestation. Miscarriage is common, occurring in one third of all pregnancies. Eighty percent of miscarriages occur before the 12th week of gestation, and up to 25% occur in pregnancies that are not even recognized clinically, in which human chorionic gonadotropin (HCG) can be detected in the urine but the patient has no missed menses.[1]

Approximately 25% of patients will experience some bleeding in the first trimester of pregnancy, with half of these proceeding to miscarriage. The risks for spontaneous abortion include advanced maternal age, previous spontaneous abortion, and prolonged time from ovulation to implantation. Other risk factors are smoking, alcohol, cocaine, caffeine, and use of nonsteroidal anti-inflammatory drugs.

Structure and Function

The etiology of miscarriage can be classified as either intrinsic or extrinsic to the embryo. Intrinsic factors include genetic abnormalities and congenital conditions. Most cases of spontaneous abortion are due to genetic factors, either anembryonic gestations or chromosomal abnormalities. The majority of these defects arise de novo during fertilization and are not inherited. Genetic factors tend to lead to miscarriage early because of abnormal growth and development.[2] In contrast, later miscarriage is more often from extrinsic factors.

Extrinsic causes of miscarriage include host factors such as such as fibroids, intrauterine adhesions, and septate uterus; teratogen exposure; and trauma. Maternal infection with listeria, toxoplasmosis, parvovirus B19, rubella, herpes simplex virus, cytomegalovirus, or lymphocytic choriomeningitis virus can lead to miscarriage, as can maternal conditions such as hypercoagulable states and endocrine abnormalities. Although blunt trauma to the abdomen is an unlikely cause of miscarriage because of the well-protected placement of the uterus in the pelvis, traumatic procedures such as chorionic villus sampling and amniocentesis may induce miscarriage.

Clinical Presentation

Spontaneous abortion is classified as threatened, inevitable, incomplete, complete, missed, or septic. Table 116-1 lists characteristics of these categories. Symptoms of spontaneous abortion include vaginal bleeding, suprapubic cramping or pain, and passage of tissue. Bleeding can vary from minor spotting to severe hemorrhage.

Threatened abortion is defined by vaginal bleeding with or without mild suprapubic cramping or pain. It is the most common presentation of spontaneous abortion seen in the ED. Examination shows a closed cervix, uterine size that correlates to gestational age, and bleeding varying from scant to heavy. Ultrasound imaging confirms an intrauterine pregnancy and fetal heart tones in appropriate gestational ages. Threatened abortion may resolve with progression to normal pregnancy, or may progress to other forms of miscarriage.

Prior to the 12th week of gestation most spontaneous abortions will progress to completion with few complications. After this time, patients are more likely to have an incomplete abortion and require medical or operative intervention. "Missed abortion" is an outdated term. It is now recognized that most pregnancies are deemed nonviable before bleeding begins, and the current terminology of first or second trimester fetal demise is preferred.

A septic abortion occurs when infection occurs during any stage of the abortion process. Implicated agents include *Staphylococcus aureus*, gram-negative rods, gram-positive cocci, and anaerobes. Risk factors include elective abortion, cytomegalovirus infection, amniocentesis, and incomplete abortion.

Differential Diagnosis

As mentioned previously, bleeding in early pregnancy is common (Fig. 116-1). It may represent benign bleeding from implantation or marginal separation of the placenta. Pathologic processes in the differential diagnosis include ectopic pregnancy, gestational trophoblastic disease, cervicitis, subchorionic hemorrhage, rupture or torsion of a corpus luteum cyst, and cervical or vaginal malignancy. Vaginal lacerations from intercourse or trauma may be to blame. Occasionally, nongynecologic sources such as rectal bleeding or hematuria are mistaken for vaginal bleeding. Finally, some patients will have idiopathic bleeding in a viable pregnancy.

Diagnostic Testing

Pregnancy should be confirmed by positive urine HCG test. A speculum examination should be performed to assess the degree of bleeding and cervical dilation, as well as to inspect for expelled products of conception. Bimanual examination can assess uterine size, cervical opening, and any abnormal masses or tenderness.

Laboratory studies include a complete blood count, quantitative human HCG, and blood type with Rh status. For those with significant bleeding or other medical disease, order coagulation parameters and type and cross-match for blood products. Ultrasonography is essential for a full diagnosis and for guiding further management. Even if it appears that the patient has passed the embryo, she should undergo ultrasound imaging to evaluate for any retained products.

Table 116-1 CLASSIFICATION OF SPONTANEOUS ABORTION

Category	Definition/Clinical Characteristics	Ultrasonographic Findings
Threatened	Bleeding and/or cramping with no passage of tissue; closed os; uterine size appropriate for dates; pregnancy viable	Intrauterine pregnancy (IUP); fetal heart tones (if age appropriate)
Inevitable	Open os without passage of products; pregnancy nonviable	IUP or products in cervical canal
Incomplete	Partial passage of products; open os, uterus not well contracted; variable bleeding; pregnancy nonviable	Persistent gestational tissue in uterus
Complete	Products of pregnancy completely passed; closed os; minimal bleeding; uterus well contracted	Empty uterus
Missed	Intrauterine demise with no spontaneous passage of products; closed os	Absent fetal cardiac activity or anembryonic gestation; absent heart tones with crown rump length >5 mm; absent fetal pole with >18-mm mean sac diameter
Septic	Infection complicating any of the previously described categories	Persistent products of conception or hemorrhage within uterine cavity

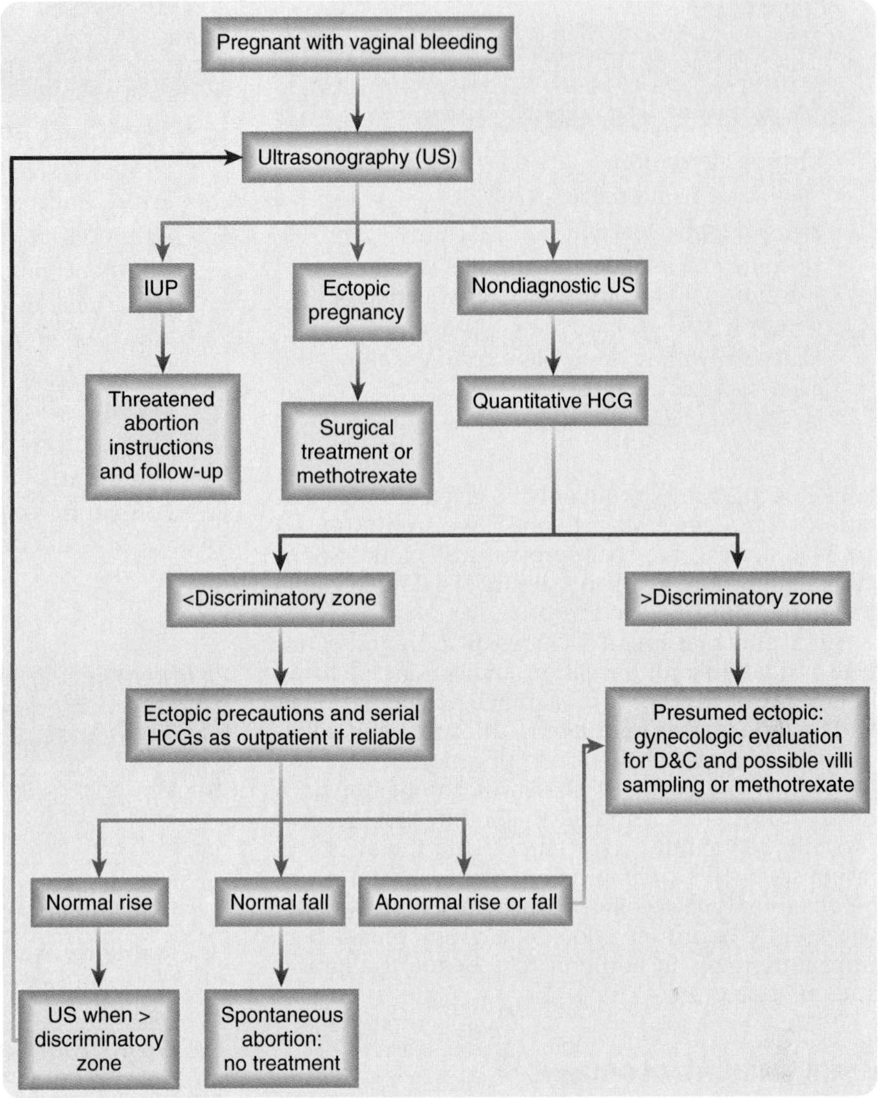
Pregnant with vaginal bleeding
Ultrasonography (US)
IUP
Ectopic pregnancy
Nondiagnostic US
Threatened abortion instructions and follow-up
Surgical treatment or methotrexate
Quantitative HCG
<Discriminatory zone
>Discriminatory zone
Ectopic precautions and serial HCGs as outpatient if reliable
Presumed ectopic: gynecologic evaluation for D&C and possible villi sampling or methotrexate
Normal rise
Normal fall
Abnormal rise or fall
US when > discriminatory zone
Spontaneous abortion: no treatment

FIGURE 116-1 Algorithm for evaluation of vaginal bleeding in the pregnant patient. D&C, dilation and curettage; HCG, human chorionic gonadotropin; IUP, intrauterine pregnancy.

Treatment

Many patients presenting with spontaneous abortion often need little or no intervention following accurate diagnosis and the exclusion of other pathology. Expectant management is the only option for threatened abortion; patient education and ensuring adequate follow-up care are essential. The presence of fetal heart tones in women with symptoms of threatened abortion is reassuring; less than 5% of women less than 36 years old will miscarry, but this risk rises to 29% for those over age 40.[3]

Inevitable abortions may be managed either expectantly or by dilation and curettage. Both methods are generally acceptable. If products of conception are visible in the cervical os, gentle removal with ring forceps may allow the cervix to close and may control bleeding. A complete abortion requires no further treatment as long as ultrasound scanning confirms that there are no retained products. Examine any retrieved tissue for villi, which will have a frond-like appearance.

Incomplete or missed abortions can be managed expectantly as long as there are no signs of shock, fever, or significant ongoing bleeding. The time course for completion of a spontaneous abortion is highly variable, and patients will need education and routine gynecologic care to plan for dilation and curettage if tissue does not pass spontaneously or if bleeding becomes heavy. Patients should attempt to collect the products of conception for examination and should undergo subsequent ultrasonography to assess whether all products of conception have passed. Studies have proved the safety of this practice.[4] Approximately 90% of patients with incomplete and 76% of those with missed abortions required no surgical management when followed expectantly for four weeks. Complications occur in 1%, less than in those managed surgically.[5]

Prostaglandins such as misoprostol can effectively induce abortion for pregnancy failure longer than 12 weeks and may help to control bleeding in patients with inevitable or incomplete abortions. The dose of misoprostol is 800 μg administered vaginally or rec-

BOX 116-1

Indications for Dilation and Curettage in Patients with Spontaneous Abortion

- Incomplete abortion
- Significant hemorrhage
- Signs of septic abortion
- Documented fetal demise or blighted ovum with no spontaneous passage (after period of observation)
- Patient unwilling or unable to comply with expectant management

tally, but this drug should only be given after consultation with a gynecologist. One large study showed an 84% success rate.[6] Misoprostol will induce spontaneous abortion, so any possibility of a desired viable pregnancy must be excluded.

Surgical management includes dilation and curettage or dilation and evacuation. Indications are listed in Box 116-1. Risks of surgical management are small and include uterine perforation, infection, and adhesions, as well as anesthetic complications.

Women presenting with significant hemorrhage or hemodynamic instability should first receive crystalloid volume replacement. If there is no response to this or if bleeding persists, administer blood either type-specific or type O-negative. Patients with septic abortions should be given broad-spectrum antibiotics in addition to scheduling dilation and curettage.

■ RH$_0$ IMMUNE GLOBULIN

Rh$_0$ immune globulin (Rh$_0$ IG) should be administered to any Rh-negative woman with signs of spontaneous abortion, unless the father is also known to be Rh-negative. It is administered in a dose of 50 μg before the 12th week of gestation and in a dose of 300 μg after 12 weeks. It is estimated that 50 μg will neutralize 2.5 mL of fetal blood, and that the 300-μg dose will neutralize 15 mL. A 12-week-old fetus has approximately 4.8 mL of blood, and a 16-week-old fetus has about 30 mL of blood. It is unlikely that significant amounts of fetal blood will transfer to the maternal circulation during first-term miscarriage, so the single, appropriate dose of immune globulin will be fully sufficient to prevent maternal antibody formation against the Rh antigen.

Rh$_0$ IG is effective for up to 12 weeks after administration, so patients presenting with recurrent bleeding who already received immunization within that time frame do not need a repeat dose. If significant hemorrhage occurs later in pregnancy, especially in the setting of trauma, additional doses are necessary. Ideally, Rh$_0$ IG is administered within 72 hours of the event leading to fetal-maternal hemorrhage (Box 116-2).

BOX 116-2

Indications for Rh$_0$ Immunization

- Spontaneous abortion (any phase)
- Elective pregnancy termination
- Ectopic pregnancy
- Amniocentesis
- Chorionic villus sampling
- Gestational trophoblastic disease
- Blunt abdominal trauma
- Placenta previa
- Placental abruption
- Immune thrombocytopenic purpura
- Routine at 28 weeks of gestation
- Postpartum (if Rh-positive infant)

PATIENT TEACHING TIPS

SPONTANEOUS ABORTION

- Miscarriage affects up to one third of pregnancies. Most patients will subsequently have normal pregnancies.
- Reassure the patient that in most cases genetic factors are responsible—not patient behavior.
- In threatened abortion with detectable fetal heartbeat, 95% of cases will progress to normal pregnancy.
- Women with recurrent miscarriage should receive fertility and genetic evaluation.
- Warn that it will take about 6 weeks for next menses.
- Advise 2 weeks pelvic rest and suggest waiting 2 to 3 months before trying to get pregnant again (although there are no studies confirming either recommendation).

Disposition

Emergency gynecologic consultation is needed for patients with significant hemorrhage or signs of infection. Others may be managed expectantly or with close follow-up as long as adequate outpatient care is assured. Patients with missed abortions may ultimately need surgical management if they do not spontaneously pass tissue.

Instruct patients to contact their physician or return to the ED if heavy bleeding, severe pain, or fever develops. Bleeding should resolve over a few weeks, and menses will generally resume within 6 weeks. Pelvic rest (no vaginal intercourse, tampons, or douching) for 2 weeks is often recommended because of the theoretical risk of infection, although no studies support this risk. Patients are often advised not to become pregnant for 2 to 3 months, but again no studies show worse outcomes if another pregnancy is achieved during this interval.

Psychosocial issues surrounding miscarriage are common, including feelings of guilt and sadness. Reassuring women that most miscarriages are due to genetic abnormalities and are not the result of their actions is essential. Women with substance abuse leading to abortion should be counseled appropriately. Referrals for grief counseling may be appropriate. Patients with recurrent miscarriages should be offered referral for fertility treatment and genetics counseling.

ECTOPIC PREGNANCY

Scope and Outline

Ectopic pregnancy, in which the developing embryo implants outside of the uterine cavity, is responsible for the greatest morbidity and mortality of early pregnancy. There has been an increased incidence of ectopic pregnancy in the United States over the past 30 years, now accounting for 19 of every 1000 pregnancies.[7] This increase has been attributed to rising rates of pelvic inflammatory disease, as well as the advent of assisted reproductive technologies.

At the same time, there has been a decrease in the morbidity and mortality of ectopic pregnancy due to better diagnosis (pelvic ultrasonography) earlier in the pregnancy and alternative methods (methotrexate) for terminating an ectopic pregnancy. Despite advances in diagnosis and management, ruptured ectopic pregnancy remains responsible for 10% of pregnancy-related deaths.

Structure and Function

Risk factors for ectopic pregnancy are outlined in Box 116-3. Tubal pathology is the most significant risk factor, leading to abnormal transport and implantation of the embryo. The majority of cases arise in women with a history of pelvic inflammatory disease. Women undergoing in vitro fertilization treatment are also susceptible, doubling their risk from 3% to 6%. Women with a previous ectopic pregnancy have a 15% recurrence rate.

Genetic abnormalities in the embryo have not been found to be a risk factor for abnormal implantation. Although women using an intrauterine device or those who have undergone a sterilization procedure are at decreased risk of pregnancy, there is an increased incidence of ectopic pregnancy among those who do become pregnant. For example, the pregnancy rate after tubal ligation is 0.1% to 0.8%, but as many as one third of these pregnancies are ectopic.

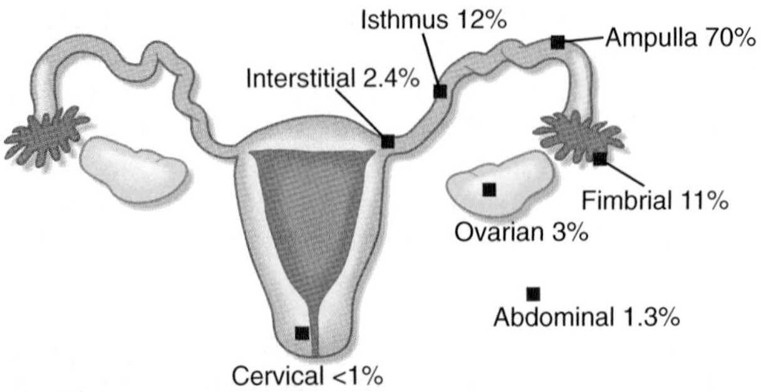
Isthmus 12%
Ampulla 70%
Interstitial 2.4%
Fimbrial 11%
Ovarian 3%
Abdominal 1.3%
Cervical <1%

FIGURE 116-2 Sites and rate of occurrence at each site ectopic implantation.

BOX 116-3

Risk Factors for Ectopic Pregnancy

High Risk
- History of pelvic inflammatory disease
- Tubal surgery
- Previous ectopic pregnancy
- Tumor or congenital tubal abnormality
- In utero diethylstilbestrol exposure

Moderate Risk
- Previous genital infection, especially if recurrent
- Infertility
- More than one lifetime sexual partner

Low Risk
- Smoking
- Douching
- First intercourse when less than 18 years old
- Age older than 35 years
- In vitro fertilization
- Tubal ligation

The most common location for ectopic implantation is the fallopian tube, accounting for 95% of all ectopic pregnancies. The growing blastocyst leads to tubal distention and bleeding into the peritoneal cavity. If the pregnancy continues and is undetected, it can lead to rupture of the tube with subsequent hemorrhage. Less commonly, ectopic pregnancies implant on the ovary, abdominal viscera, or cervix. In these cases, significant hemorrhage or perforation of abdominal structures may occur. See Figure 116-2 for sites of ectopic implantation.

Clinical Presentation

As ultrasonography and HCG assays become more sensitive, the diagnosis of ectopic pregnancy usually is made earlier, leading to a significant decrease in morbidity and mortality. Most ectopic pregnancies present 6 to 8 weeks after missed menses, and significant tubal distention and bleeding usually occur by that point. Up to 50% of women have no identifiable risk for ectopic pregnancy.[8]

Symptoms may mimic the signs of spontaneous abortion. The classic triad consists of abdominal pain, vaginal bleeding, and a missed menstrual period, although these vary with timing of presentation. Patients presenting with early ectopic pregnancies may show no abdominal tenderness or vaginal bleeding, and the ectopic inplantation may be found only incidentally on ultrasonography. In contrast, a woman with a tubal rupture may display hemodynamic instability and signs of surgical abdomen. Approximately one half of patients are asymptomatic before tubal rupture. Of those with rupture, 99% have abdominal pain, 74% amenorrhea, and 56% vaginal bleeding.

BOX 116-4

Differential Diagnoses of Ectopic Pregnancy

- Spontaneous abortion
- Benign bleeding from implantation
- Hemorrhage/rupture/torsion of corpus luteum cyst
- Molar pregnancy
- Pelvic inflammatory disease
- Endometriosis
- Appendicitis
- Diverticulitis
- Urinary tract infection
- Nephrolithiasis

Variations of Ectopic Pregnancies

An interstitial, or corneal, pregnancy occurs when the embryo is implanted in the proximal portion of the tube that is embedded in the muscle of the uterus. The tube at this location is more distensible, so the embryo may grow undetected for a longer period of time. Presentation may not be until 12 weeks or later. Ultrasonography demonstrates an asymmetric uterine thickness surrounding the gestational sac. However, this observation requires a skilled ultrasonographer, and in its early stages a corneal pregnancy may be mistaken for a normal intrauterine pregnancy. Corneal pregnancy has a 2% to 2.5% maternal mortality rate and is more likely than other tubal pregnancies to require hysterectomy.

Ectopic pregnancy implanting outside of the fallopian tube is less common. In ovarian pregnancy, the ectopic embryo may be mistaken for a hemorrhagic cyst. Without treatment, rupture will occur. In abdominal pregnancy, the embryo is implanted on either abdominal viscera or the peritoneal surface, which can lead to hemoperitoneum or rupture of organs such as the bowel. In cervical pregnancy, the growing embryo causes distention of the os and excessive bleeding. More common in patients undergoing in vitro fertilization, a cervical pregnancy may be seen on speculum examination.

Heterotopic pregnancy occurs when an intrauterine pregnancy is present with a simultaneous ectopic gestation. Incidence was at one time estimated at 1/30,000, but the true incidence is unknown. Thus, an ectopic gestation essentially can be excluded if an intrauterine pregnancy is demonstrated by ultrasonography. Patients using assisted reproductive techniques have up to a 1% incidence of ectopic pregnancy, highest in those with patients with transfer of multiple embryos. In these patients, an ectopic gestation should not be excluded solely based on the presence of an intrauterine pregnancy.[9]

Differential Diagnosis

The differential diagnoses of ectopic pregnancy are listed in Box 116-4. Because of the high potential for morbidity, any patient presenting with abnormal vaginal bleeding or abdominal or pelvic pain should be considered to have an ectopic pregnancy until proved otherwise. Urinary HCG testing is essential for any woman of childbearing age with abdominal pain.

Diagnostic Testing

■ QUANTITATIVE HUMAN CHORIONIC GONADOTROPIN (HCG) TESTING

The initial diagnostic maneuver is to obtain urine for HCG testing. Commercially available kits detect as low as 20 mIU/mL, although there have been case reports of ectopic pregnancy with an undetectable urine HCG level.[10] If high clinical suspicion still exists despit a negative UCG, a serum HCG test should be ordered.

In normal pregnancy, HCG production begins shortly after fertilization with a peak of about 100,000 mIU/mL at approximately 41 days gestational age. In the early weeks of normal pregnancy, HCG levels are expected to double roughly every 48 hours, with a range of 1.4 to 2.1 days. In contrast, HCG levels generally rise more slowly in ectopic and nonviable intrauterine pregnancies. However, in some normal pregnancies, HCG levels may increase as little as 66% over 48 hours,[11] and up to 17% of ectopic pregnancies have normal doubling times. Patients should have serial measurements done by the same laboratory, because interassay variability may be as high as 15%.

■ ULTRASONOGRAPHY

Transvaginal ultrasonography is essential for making the diagnosis. The diagnosis of ectopic pregnancy is confirmed by a visible extrauterine gestational sac with yolk sac or embryo, but this is seen in less than half of the cases. Highly suggestive findings include a complex adnexal mass or free fluid in the pelvis, in conjunction with an empty uterus. Color flow Doppler imaging demonstrating increased flow to the tube containing the ectopic pregnancy can be added to increase sensitivity, but this requires a highly skilled ultrasonographer.

■ Ultrasonographic Findings plus HCG

To obtain the full benefit of transvaginal ultrasonography, serum HCG levels must be taken into consideration.

The earliest ultrasonographic confirmation of intrauterine pregnancy is a true gestational sac seen within the uterine cavity. This is routinely visualized when HCG levels reach 1500 to 2000 mIU/mL, but can be detected with levels as low as 800 mIU/mL. The discriminatory zone refers to the level of HCG at which a true gestational sac can be seen. Lack of an intrauterine pregnancy with an HCG above the discriminatory zone raises concern for ectopic pregnancy or a failed intrauterine gestation. The discriminatory zone is generally accepted to be in the range of 1500 mIU/mL but is dependent on equipment quality and operator skill.

Transvaginal sonograms are more likely to be nondiagnostic in women with very low HCG levels, but they may still be useful. In a study by Kaplan and colleagues, 19% of patients with HCG levels greater than 1000 mIU/mL at the time of presentation had transvaginal sonograms diagnostic of ectopic pregnancy. The specificity of ultrasonography findings was 100%. Given its safety, transvaginal ultrasonography should be performed on all women with suspected ectopic pregnancy, even those with HCG levels below the discriminatory zone.[12]

As discussed previously, ectopic pregnancy is visualized by ultrasonography only half of the time; therefore, women with serum HCG levels below the discriminatory zone and nondiagnostic ultrasonography findings present a clinical challenge. These findings may represent an ectopic pregnancy or a nonviable early intrauterine pregnancy. In these cases, HCG testing and ultrasonography should be repeated at 48 to 72 hours. HCG levels increasing normally at 48 to 72 hours should be monitored until the intrauterine pregnancy can be seen on the sonogram. A decreasing HCG level is most consistent with failed pregnancy or spontaneously resolving ectopic pregnancy. In these cases, serial measurements should be followed until HCG reaches non-detectable levels.

Patients with HCG levels that plateau or rise by less than double in 72 hours are likely to have either a nonviable intrauterine or an ectopic pregnancy. Repeat transvaginal ultrasonography may be helpful to distinguish the two. Failure to visualize an intrauterine gestation with HCG levels higher than 2000 mIU/mL excludes the possibility of viable pregnancy.

These patients have a high likelihood of having an ectopic gestation and should be treated accordingly.[13] Patients with HCG levels higher than 1500 mIU/mL may undergo dilation and curettage to obtain tissue for examination. Confirmation of villi in the curettage specimen confirms the diagnosis of a failed intrauterine pregnancy, whereas their absence suggests ectopic pregnancy. Laparoscopy may then be used to provide definitive diagnosis and to guide treatment.

Treatment

Ruptured ectopic pregnancy may present dramatically, with the patient in hemorrhagic shock. Rapid stabilization with IV fluids and packed red blood cells is essential. Type-specific blood is preferable, but unstable patients may require O-negative blood until a full cross-match is performed. Laboratory studies include a complete blood count, quantitative HCG, and coagulation studies. The gynecology department should be consulted about operative management. Rh-negative patients should receive Rh_0 IG.

In stable patients, treatment of confirmed unruptured ectopic pregnancy may be medical, surgical, or expectant.

■ METHOTREXATE THERAPY

The medical treatment of choice is methotrexate, a folate antagonist that inhibits DNA synthesis in rapidly dividing cells such as embryonic tissue. This action leads to medically-induced abortion of the embryo. Although there are limitations, methotrexate use allows for non-invasive management and has proven successful in properly selected patients.

The ideal candidate for methotrexate therapy is relatively asymptomatic with no significant pain or bleeding. Multiple visits and close follow-up care are essential, so this also must be taken into consideration. A minority of patients will fail treatment or progress to rupture, and the patient must be made aware of these possibilities. Criteria predicting success include diameter less than 3.5 cm, absence of cardiac activity on ultrasonography, and HCG level less than 5000 mIU/mL. Patients with lower HCG levels tend to have fewer treatment failures.[14]

Patients should be counseled on the risks and benefits of methotrexate therapy. They must be willing to comply with treatment and have ready access to care. The patient should be aware of the possibility of treatment failure.

Relative contraindications include a high HCG level (>6000-15,000 mIU/mL), visible cardiac activity, and a large ectopic mass. Although visible cardiac activity generally is considered a contraindication,

BOX 116-5

Contraindications for Methotrexate Therapy

- Hypersensitivity to methotrexate
- Breastfeeding
- Immunodeficiency
- Alcoholic or other liver disease
- Blood dyscrasias
- Active pulmonary disease
- Peptic ulcer disease
- Renal dysfunction

BOX 116-6

Side Effects of Methotrexate

- Stomatitis
- Conjunctivitis
- Enteritis
- Dermatitits
- Pleuritis
- Alopecia
- Bone marrow suppression
- Abdominal pain
- Elevated liver function levels

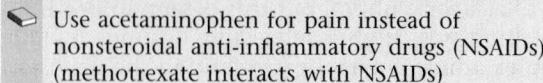

PATIENT TEACHING TIPS

INSTRUCTIONS AFTER RECEIVING METHOTREXATE

- Use acetaminophen for pain instead of nonsteroidal anti-inflammatory drugs (NSAIDs) (methotrexate interacts with NSAIDs)
- No intercourse, no pelvic examination for 7 days or as advsed by gynecologist (theoretically could rupture the ectopic mass)
- No pregnancy for at least one cycle
- Return to ED if there is an increase in pain, especially if acute onset
- Repeat human chorionic gonadotropin (HCG) measurements should be obtained 4 to 7 days post-methotrexate therapy; if the HCG level fails to decrease by 25%, repeated methotrexate therapy may be necessary.
- Success rate of methotrexate therapy is 86% to 94%.

one study showed good results despite this finding.[15] Absolute contraindications to the use of methotrexate include hemodynamic instability, as well as the factors listed in Box 116-5.

Side effects of methotrexate are listed in Box 116-6. Thirty percent of patients are affected, but most symptoms are mild and self-limited. Most patients will experience some abdominal pain, usually 2 to 3 days after methotrexate administration, due to tubal abortion with subsequent hematoma formation. In contrast to the pain from rupture, this pain is milder, and patients do not have hemodynamic instability or signs of a surgical abdomen. Although only 20% of patients with abdominal pain following methotrexate administration will ultimately need laparoscopy to evaluate for rupture, this subset can be difficult to identify. Transvaginal ultrasonography should be performed in these patients to evaluate for rupture.[16]

It is normal for HCG levels to increase for as long as 4 days following methotrexate administration. Patients typically have repeat HCG testing between days 4 and 7. By day 7, if the serum HCG level has not decreased by 25%, a second dose of methotrexate is given (required in 15%-20% of patients), and HCG values are monitored weekly until levels decrease to less than 10 to 15 mIU/mL. Success rates with methotrexate range from 86% to 94%.

Methotrexate protocols vary by institution, but single-dose treatment is widely used, with an intramuscular injection of 50 mg/m^2 of body surface area. Multiple-dose treatment (days 1, 3, 5, and 7) with leucovorin rescue has had good results, but patients suffer more side effects. No studies have directly compared the two methods, but most institutions now use single-dose treatment with second-dose administration as needed. Multiple-dose treatment is used for interstitial or cervical pregnancies.

Surgical Treatment

As mentioned earlier, surgical treatment is the only option for unstable patients with ectopic pregnancy. It is also indicated for patients with large ectopic masses, patients unable or unwilling to comply with the monitoring associated with methotrexate therapy, and patients with poor access to emergency care.

Resection of the ectopic mass with preservation of normal anatomy is ideal. Thus, salpingostomy is preferred over salpingectomy. Laparoscopic resection is the standard approach, although laparotomy is occasionally required. After surgery, patients should be monitored with weekly HCG testing, given the slight possibility of persistent ectopic tissue following resection.

A recent review showed the highest success rates with salpingostomy, although single-dose methotrexate therapy had the lowest financial cost and the least impact on quality of life.[17] Methotrexate therapy was less costly in patients with HCG levels less than 1500 mIU/mL. The cost of medical therapy increases

PATIENT TEACHING TIPS

HYPEREMESIS

- Daily multivitamin at time of conception may decrease severity of nausea and vomiting.
- Avoid triggers such as noxious odors, brushing teeth after eating, and iron supplements.
- Eat small, frequent meals rich in protein and carbohydrates and low in fat. Avoid spicy foods.
- Eat as soon as you feel hungry.
- Drink small amounts of liquids often. Cold, clear, carbonated, and sour liquids are best tolerated.
- Aromatic mint tea and teas with lemon/orange flavoring may be helpful.

safety data. Antihistamines have the best safety profile, whereas phenothiazines and metoclopramide are safe as well. Ondansetron appears to have a good safety profile in pregnancy, although it is much more expensive than traditional therapies. Its use is increasing, in part due to an oral dissolving formulation that is easy to administer to nauseated patients.

Gynecologists may prescribe oral corticosteroids for patients with refractory nausea and vomiting. Studies have shown conflicting results of effectiveness, and there appears to be a slightly increased incidence of cleft palate in infants whose mothers received methylprednisolone in the first trimester of pregnancy. Steroids should thus be reserved as a last resort.[31,32]

Many patients are reluctant to use pharmacotherapy because of perceived fear of birth defects. These patients may be agreeable to adjunctive therapies such as acupuncture, hypnosis, and powdered ginger. Studies of acupuncture and acupressure have yielded conflicting results,[33] whereas hypnosis has been shown to decrease vomiting in patients with hyperemesis. Powdered ginger (250 mg to 1 g/day) is as effective as pyridoxine, but its safety is not well established.[34]

The ultimate goal of treatment is restoration of nutrition. Many patients are able to tolerate feeding after a short course of rehydration along with gut rest. The Patient Teaching Tips (Hyperemesis) box outlines dietary suggestions.

Patients who cannot maintain their weight despite rehydration and antiemetics are candidates for enteral nutrition. Those who cannot tolerate enteral feedings should be given total parenteral nutrition. This regimen carries the usual risks of infectious and metabolic complications.

Disposition

Patients with mild dehydration may be discharged home after fluid and electrolyte repletion. Antiemetics can be prescribed for home use after appropriate discussions with the patient and the primary physician. Many patients present to the ED before they have established prenatal care; ensuring adequate outpatient care is essential. Patients with severe dehydration, significant electrolyte abnormalities, progressive weight loss, and intractable vomiting despite antiemetics should be admitted to the hospital.

Patients should be instructed to return to the ED if vomiting persists or if they experience new symptoms such as abdominal pain and fever. Patients with mild nausea and vomiting are not at increased risk of low-birth-weight infants or birth defects. Although patients with hyperemesis do have a higher incidence of low-birth-weight infants, appropriate weight gain later in pregnancy reduces this risk.[35]

REFERENCES

1. Wilcox AJ, Weinberg CR, O'Connor JF, et al: Incidence of early loss in pregnancy. N Engl J Med 1988;319:189-194.
2. Klein J, Stein Z: Epidemiology of chromosomal anomalies in spontaneous abortion: Prevalence, manifestation and determinants. In Bennett MJ, Edmonds DK (eds): Spontaneous and Recurrent Abortion. Oxford, Blackwell Scientific Publications, 1987, p 29.
3. Deaton JL, Honore GM, Huffman CS, et al: Early transvaginal ultrasound following an accurately dated pregnancy: The importance of finding a yolk sac or fetal heart motion. Hum Reprod 1997;12:2820-2823.
4. Chipchase J, James D: Randomised trial of expectant versus surgical management of spontaneous miscarriage. Br J Obstet Gynaecol 1997;104:840-841.
5. Luise C, Jermy K, May C et al: Outcome of expectant management of spontaneous first trimester miscarriage: Observational study. BMJ 2002;324:873.
6. Zhang J, Gilles JM, Barnhart K, et al: A comparison of medical management with misoprostol and surgical management for early pregnancy failure. N Engl J Med 2005;353:761.
7. Centers for Disease Control and Prevention. Ectopic pregnancy—United States, 1990-1992. MMWR Morb Mortal Wkly Rep 1995;44:46-48.
8. Tulandi T, Sammour A: Evidence-based management of ectopic pregnancy. Curr Opin Obstet Gynecol 2000;12:289-292.
9. Svare J, Norup P, Grove Thomsen S, et al: Heterotopic pregnancies after in-vitro fertilization and embryo transfer—a Danish survey. Hum Reprod 1993;8:116-118.
10. Maccato ML, Estrada R, Faro S: Ectopic pregnancy with undetectable serum and urine beta-hCG levels and detection of beta-hCG in the ectopic trophoblast by immunocytochemical evaluation. Obstet Gynecol 1993;81:878-880.
11. Kadar N, Caldwell BV, Romero R: A method of screening for ectopic pregnancy and its indications. Obstet Gynecol 1981;58:162-166.
12. Kaplan BC, Dart RG, Moskos M, et al: Ectopic pregnancy: Prospective study with improved diagnostic accuracy. Ann Emerg Med 1996;28:10-17.
13. Mol BWJ, Hajenius PJ, Engelsbel S, et al: Serum human chorionic gonadotropin measurement in the diagnosis of ectopic pregnancy when transvaginal ultrasound is inconclusive. Fertil Steril 1998;70:972-981.
14. Lipscomb GH, McCord ML, Stovall TG, et al: Predictors of success of methotrexate treatment in women with tubal ectopic pregnancies. N Engl J Med 1999;341:1974-1978.
15. Lipscomb GH, Bran D, McCord ML, et al: Analysis of three hundred fifteen ectopic pregnancies treated with single dose methotrexate. Am J Obstet Gynecol 1998;178:1354-1358.
16. American College of Obstetricians and Gynecologists: Medical management of tubal pregnancy. ACOG Practice Bulletin 3. Washington, DC, ACOG; 1998.

17. Hajenius PJ, Mol BW, Bossuyt PM, et al: Interventions for tubal ectopic pregnancy. Cochrane Database Syst Rev 2000;CD000324.
18. Yao M, Tulandi T: Current status of surgical and nonsurgical treatment of ectopic pregnancy. Fertil Steril 1997;67:421-433.
19. Smith HO: Gestational trophoblastic disease epidemiology and trends. Clin Obstet Gynecol 2003;46:541.
20. Sclaerth JB, Morrow CP, Montz FJ, et al: Initial management of hydatidiform mole. Am J Obstet Gynecol 1998;158:1299-1306.
21. Tidy JA, Rustin, GJ, Newlands ES, et al: Presentation and management of choriocarcinoma after non-molar pregnancy. Br J Obstet Gynaecol 1995;102:715-179.
22. Montz FJ, Schlaerth JB, Morrow CP: The natural history of theca lutein cysts. Obstet Gynecol 1988;72:247-251.
23. Kohorn EI: The new FIGO 2000 staging and risk factor scoring system for gestational trophoblastic disease: Description and clinical assessment. Int J Gynecol Cancer 2001;11:73-77.
24. Berkowitz RS, Im SS, Bernstein MR, et al: Gestational trophoblastic disease: Subsequent pregnancy outcome, including repeat molar pregnancy. J Reprod Med 1998;43: 81-86.
25. Goodwin TM, Montoro M, Mestman JH: Transient hyperthyroidism and hyperemesis gravidarum: Clinical aspects. Am J Obstet Gynecol 1992;167:648-652.
26. Adams MM, Harlass FE, Sarno AP, et al: Antenatal hospitalization among enlisted servicewomen, 1987-1990. Obstet Gynecol 1994;84:35-39.
27. Depue RH, Bernstein L, Ross RK, et al: Hyperemesis gravidarum in relation to estradiol levels, pregnancy outcome, and other maternal factors: A seroepidemiologic study. Am J Obstet Gynecol 1987;156:1137-1141.
28. Goodwin, TM: Hyperemesis gravidarum. Clin Obstet Gynecol 1998;41:597-605.
29. Vutyavanich T, Wongtra-ngan S, Ruangsri R: Pyridoxine for nausea and vomiting of pregnancy: A randomized, double-blind, placebo-controlled trial. Am J Obstet Gynecol 1995;173:881-884.
30. McKeigue PM, Lamm SH, Linn S, et al: Bendectin and birth defects: I. A meta-analysis of the epidemiologic studies. Teratology 1994;50:27-37.
31. Yost NP, McIntire DD, Wians FH Jr, et al: A randomized, placebo-controlled trial of corticosteroids for hyperemesis due to pregnancy. Obstet Gynecol 2003;102:1250-1254.
32. Carmichael SL, Shaw GM: Maternal corticosteroid use and risk of selected congenital anomalies. Am J Med Genet 1999;86:242-244.
33. Jewell D, Young G: Interventions for nausea and vomiting in early pregnancy. Cochrane Database Syst Rev 2003: CD000145.
34. Vutyavanich T, Kraisarin T, Ruangsri R: Ginger for nausea and vomiting in pregnancy: Randomized, doublemasked, placebo-controlled trial. Obstet Gynecol 2001;97:577-582.
35. Tsang IS, Katz VL, Wells SD: Maternal and fetal outcomes in hyperemesis gravidarum. Int J Gynaecol Obstet 1996;55:231-235.

Chapter **117**

First-Trimester Ultrasonography: Evaluation for Intrauterine Pregnancy

Mary Ann Edens and Emily Baran

KEY POINTS

Ultrasonography is indicated for patients with first-trimester pregnancy complicated by vaginal bleeding, abdominal pain, or other clinical suspicion of ectopic pregnancy.

Ultrasonography during the first trimester primarily is used to determine the presence or absence of intrauterine pregnancy.

Common ultrasound findings in the setting of ectopic pregnancy are an ovarian mass or free fluid in the pelvis.

The patient should have a full bladder when a transabdominal pelvic examination is performed; the bladder should be empty when a transvaginal pelvic examination is performed. Transvaginal ultrasonography ideally should immediately follow the pelvic examinations.

A 2- to 5-MHz curvilinear abdominal probe is used for transabdominal imaging.

A 5- to 8-MHz intracavitary probe is used for transvaginal imaging; the patient should be supine with lithotomy positioning.

Scope

Abdominal pain and vaginal bleeding in the first trimester of pregnancy are common presentations. The incidence of ectopic pregnancy is approximately 2% in the general population and increases to 7% to 13% in symptomatic ED patients.[1,2]

Once a symptomatic pregnancy is recognized, a focused ultrasound examination can be performed as part of the physical examination because 7% to 75% of these patients can be diagnosed with intrauterine or ectopic pregnancy by ultrasonography.[3-5]

Quantitative beta–human chorionic gonadotropin (beta-hCG) levels in the setting of ectopic pregnancy may be low, normal, or elevated; therefore it is important to perform an ultrasound scan on all symptomatic patients regardless of their beta-hCG levels.[6]

First-trimester ultrasonography is a limited, focused test that can be performed rapidly at the bedside in order to direct patient care, additional evaluation, and disposition. First-trimester ultrasonography has shown to decrease length of stay for patients with intrauterine pregnancy and improve morbidity associated with ectopic pregnancy.[7-9]

Indications

The primary indication for first-trimester ultrasonography is first-trimester pregnancy complicated by vaginal bleeding, abdominal pain, or other clinical signs of ectopic pregnancy. The primary goal of first-trimester ultrasonography is to evaluate for an intrauterine pregnancy, and by doing so rule out an ectopic pregnancy. Additionally, depending on the sonographer's level of experience, evaluation for other pelvic pathology such as tubo-ovarian abscess, pelvic mass, or ovarian torsion can be performed.

Anatomy and Approach

The uterus is a pear-shaped organ usually 7 to 9 cm × 4 to 6 cm in size. The ovaries are paired oval structures normally 3 cm × 2 cm in size that should appear posterolateral to the uterus. Ovaries appear relatively hypoechoic to the uterus with small anechoic (black) follicles outlining their periphery (Fig. 117-1). They often can be identified by their position anterior and medial to the internal iliac vessels.

Intrauterine pregnancy is defined as a gestational sac with a circumferential myometrial mantle containing a yolk sac or fetal pole (with or without cardiac activity). An isolated gestational sac regardless of size or location should not be considered an intrauterine pregnancy.

There are two basic approaches to ultrasonography in the first trimester—transabdominal and transvaginal. The transabdominal approach should be performed first as it can identify intrauterine pregnancy with gestation greater than 7 weeks and provide a useful overview of the pelvis, identifying the general position of the uterus and any concerning free intraperitoneal fluid. A full bladder provides a better sonographic window for transabdominal ultrasound. A 2- to 5-MHz curvilinear probe generally is used; the uterus is imaged in both longitudinal and transverse planes.

First-trimester ultrasonography ideally should immediately follow the pelvic examinations. Both approaches should include the features shown in Box 117-1.

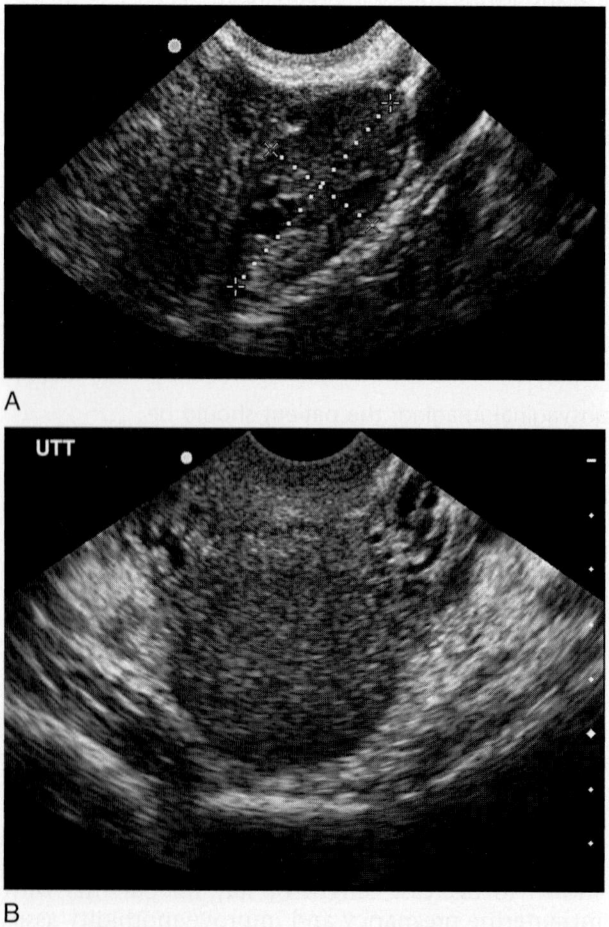
A
UTT
B

FIGURE 117-1 **A,** Ovary. **B,** Uterus with ovaries.

■ TRANSABDOMINAL APPROACH

To image the uterus in the longitudinal or long-axis plane, the transducer is placed in the midline just above the symphysis pubis with the probe indicator pointed toward the patient's head. The ultrasound probe may need to be rocked inferiorly toward the pelvis to locate the uterus, especially during early pregnancy. The EP should be sure that the transducer foot remains in contact with the patient. Once the long axis of the uterus is located (may need to rotate slightly left or right of midline), the transducer should be fanned from left to right to sweep from one side through to the other side of the uterus.

To image the uterus in the transverse or short-axis plane, the transducer should be turned 90 degrees counter-clockwise to the patient's right. In the transverse plane, the transducer should be fanned upward (cephalad) and downward (caudad) to sweep through the entire uterus. The goal is to see the entire uterus through this process.

BOX 117-1

Features of Transabdominal and Transvaginal Pelvic Ultrasound Examinations

- Longitudinal examination of uterus, cervix, and vaginal stripe
- Transverse examination of uterus
- View of right adnexa
- View of left adnexa
- Determination of gestational age by crown rump length, if fetus is present
- M-mode imaging of cardiac activity, if present

■ TRANSVAGINAL APPROACH

The second approach for first-trimester ultrasonography is the transvaginal approach. Unlike the transabdominal approach, a full bladder can be a hindrance, as it may push the uterus out of view; therefore the patient's bladder should be emptied prior to transvaginal imaging. The ultrasound imaging should be done as part of the pelvic examination in the lithotomy position.

The procedure can be described to the patient as similar to the bimanual examination, except that the examiner's bottom hand is replaced by the ultrasound probe. Similar to the bimanual examination, the sonographer's top hand can be used on the abdomen to help visualize the ovaries and determine adnexal tenderness. An assistant to chaperone the procedure is recommended.

A 5- to 8-MHz intracavitary transducer is used. Ultrasound gel is applied directly to the footprint of the transducer, and then a cover (condom, glove, or probe-specific sheath) is placed over the transducer. Water-based lubricant is then applied to the footprint of the probe on the outside of the cover. The transducer is then slowly inserted into the vaginal vault. The normal position of the uterus is at a 90-degree angle to the vaginal vault. This relationship helps to explain why a better examination is obtained with an empty bladder and by not inserting the probe too deeply.

During the transvaginal examination, the uterus is imaged in both sagittal (long-axis) and coronal (short-axis) planes. To image the uterus in the long-axis plane, the indicator on the transducer is pointed anteriorly (up to the ceiling) (Fig. 117-2). Small movements angling or rocking the tip of the transducer up and down should help visualize at the fundus and cervix, respectively. Next, small movements fanning through the uterus from left to right are necessary to sweep through the entire uterus. The ovaries may be visualized along each side of the uterus.

To image the uterus in the short-axis plane, the transducer is turned 90 degrees counterclockwise to the patient's right. Small movements fanning the probe up and down are necessary to scan through the entire uterus. Small movements angling or rocking the transducer to the left and right can visualize each adnexa. The ovaries are often easier to visualize in this plane.

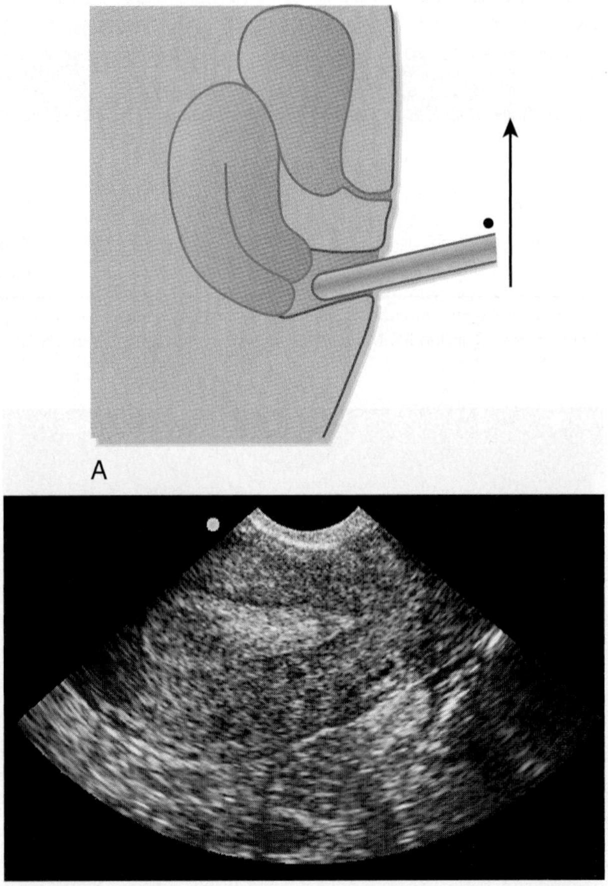

A

B

FIGURE 117-2 **A,** Transducer placement for transvaginal long-axis view (*arrow* shows direction of probe indicator). **B,** Normal transvaginal long-axis image of uterus. Note the thickened endometrial stripe.

Clinical Questions and Examination Interpretation

■ QUESTION #1: IS THERE AN INTRAUTERINE PREGNANCY?

The primary goal of first-trimester ultrasonography is to diagnose an intrauterine pregnancy. The first sonographic indication of pregnancy is a gestational sac. The gestational sac should appear as a dark fluid–filled structure within the uterus. It should be round or oval-shaped with no sharp edges (Fig. 117-3). A gestational sac alone is not sufficient to diagnose an intrauterine pregnancy because in the setting of ectopic pregnancy, hormonal stimulation of the uterus can cause an anechoic area or pseudogestational sac to be present. A gestational sac should be

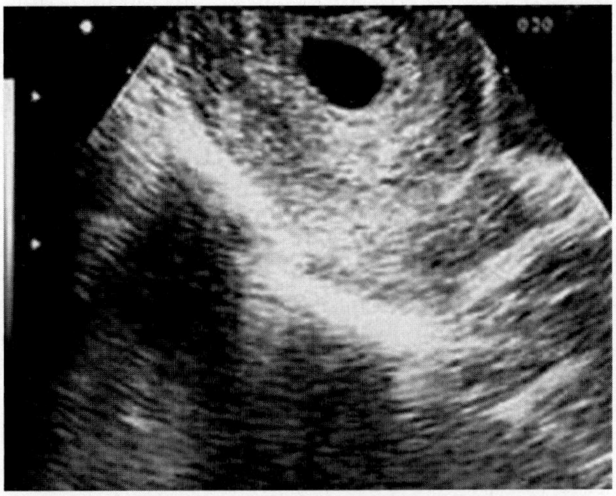

FIGURE 117-3 Gestational sac in the uterus.

Table 117-1 GESTATIONAL AGE (GA) AND BETA-HCG CORRELATION WITH EUS FINDINGS

GA (Weeks)	Beta-hCG (mIU/mL)	EUS Findings	
		Transabdominal Approach	Transvaginal Approach
4-5	<1000	—	—
5	1000-2000	—	Gestational sac
5-6	>2000	Gestational sac	Yolk sac ± fetal pole
6	10,000-20,000	Yolk sac ± fetal pole	Embryo ± cardiac activity
7	>20,000	Embryo ± cardiac activity	Clear torso and head

Beta-hCG, beta–human chorionic gonadotropin; EUS, endoscopic ultrasonography.
Adapted from Reardon RF, Martel M: First trimester pregnancy. In Ma OJ, Mateer JR (eds): Emergency Ultrasound. New York, McGraw-Hill, 2003, p 254.

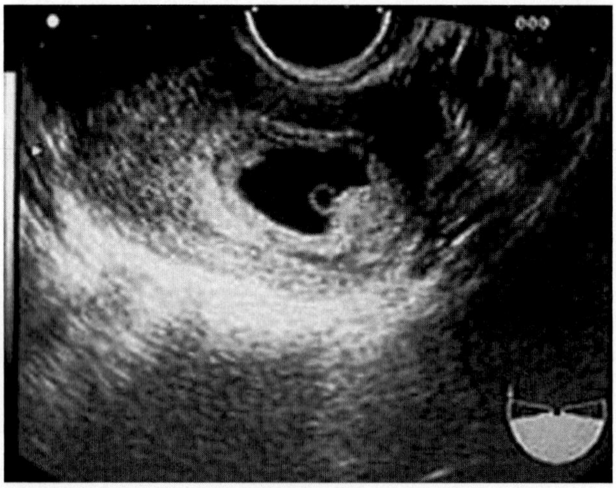

FIGURE 117-4 Bright, ring-like yolk sac within the gestational sac in the uterus.

seen at 5 to 6 weeks of gestation using the transabdominal approach and approximately 1 week earlier using the transvaginal approach. Ultrasound findings at different gestational age and beta-hCG levels are listed in Table 117-1.

Most sonographers agree that the first reliable indication of an intrauterine pregnancy is a yolk sac. A yolk sac appears in the 5th to 6th week of gestation as a small, bright ring-like structure within the gestational sac (Fig. 117-4). A yolk sac should be visible when the mean gestational sac diameter is larger than 8 mm transvaginally and 20 mm transabdominally. A fetal pole becomes visible at 6 to 7 weeks of gestation and resembles a small mass initially seen at the edge of the yolk sac (Fig. 117-5). A fetal pole should be visible when the mean gestational sac diameter is larger than 16 mm transvaginally and 25 mm transabdominally. Fetal cardiac activity usually can be detected by transvaginal scan at 6 weeks of gestation. The fetal heart rate can be measured using M-mode imaging (Fig. 117-6). A measurement of the embryo excluding legs and yolk sac, or crown rump length (CRL), can be used to estimate gestational age (Fig. 117-7). After the 13th week of gestation, other measurements such as head circumference, biparietal diameter, and femur length should be used to determine gestational age.

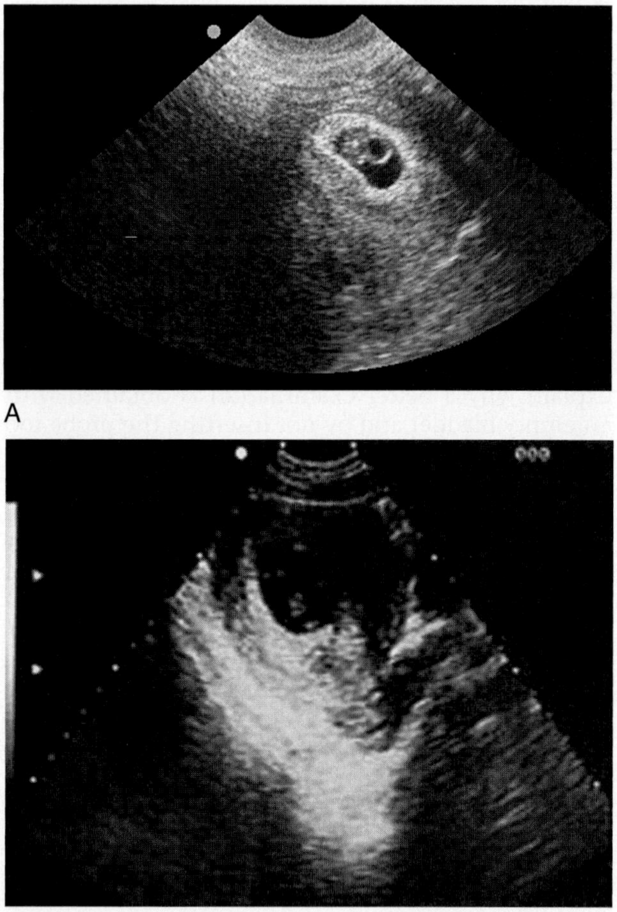

A

B

FIGURE 117-5 Fetal pole within the gestational sac.

The discriminatory zone is the beta-hCG level above which a normal intrauterine pregnancy should be visible on ultrasound evaluation. This level is approximately 6500 mIU/mL for transabdominal scans and 1000-2000 mIU/mL for transvaginal scans.

■ QUESTION #2: IF NO INTRAUTERINE PREGNANCY IS SEEN, ARE THERE INDICATIONS OF AN ECTOPIC OR ABNORMAL PREGNANCY?

The second purpose of first-trimester ultrasonography is to look for signs of ectopic or abnormal pregnancy. A definitive ectopic pregnancy is seen as an

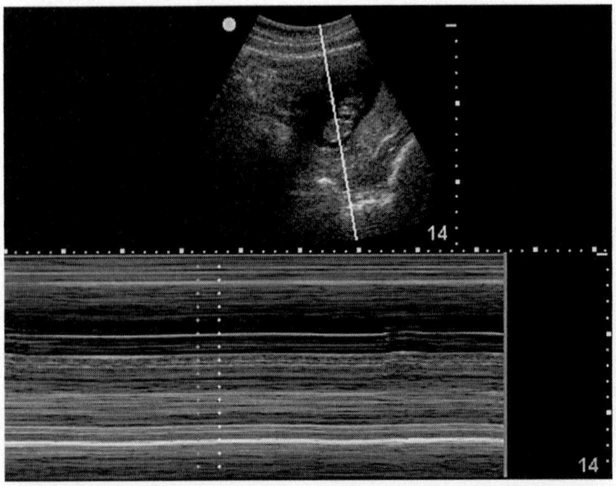
14
14

FIGURE 117-6 Fetal heart beat demonstrated and measured using M-mode imaging.

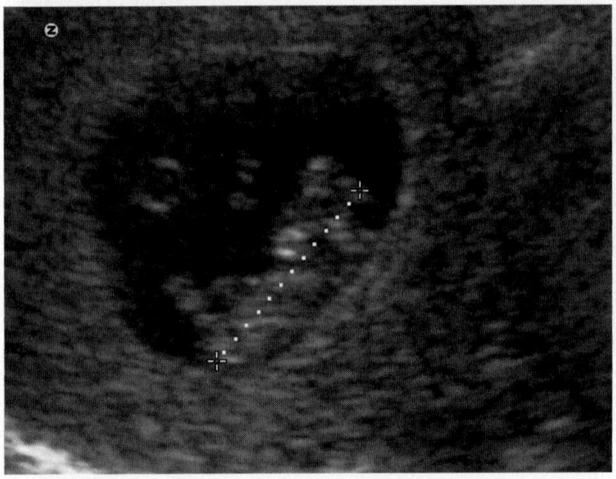

FIGURE 117-7 Measurement of crown rump length (CRL) to estimate gestational age.

extrauterine gestational sac containing either yolk sac or fetal pole (± cardiac activity) in up to 20% of ectopic pregnancies (Fig. 117-8). Other findings suggestive of ectopic pregnancy are listed in Box 117-2. Figure 117-9 shows ultrasound images highly suggestive of ectopic pregnancy.

Patients with an empty uterus and beta-hCG levels above the discriminatory zone or with any suggestive or definitive evidence of ectopic pregnancy on ultrasonography should have immediate obstetric evaluation.

The goal of first-trimester ultrasonography is not just to identify a gestational sac with contents that look like a normal pregnancy but to make sure that the pregnancy is actually within the uterus. The entire uterus and adnexa should be visualized. The importance of making sure that the gestational sac is symmetrically surrounded by the uterus (8-10 mm of myometrium measured on each side) cannot be overemphasized.

BOX 117-2

Findings Suggestive of Ectopic Pregnancy

- Tubal ring in ovary
- Complex ovarian mass
- Free fluid in the pelvis
- Free fluid in Morrison's pouch

Tips and Tricks

PEARLS AND PITFALLS

- Make sure to remove air bubbles from the footprint of the transvaginal transducer, which can cause artifacts in the image.
- In general, pulsed-wave and color Doppler ultrasonography should not be used in early pregnancy because of potential adverse affects on the fetus.
- An ectopic pregnancy is not a normal pregnancy and may be present with a low, normal, or high beta-hCG levels. In up to 40% of ectopic pregnancies, including ruptured ectopic pregnancies, levels are higher than 1000 mIU/mL.
- Make sure the normal-appearing pregnancy is actually within the uterus, with clear symmetrical-appearing myometrium on all sides.
- Heterotopic pregnancy does occur; therefore, maintain a high index of clinical suspicion for this disorder, and ask the patient about fertility treatments.

If there is asymmetry, an interstitial pregnancy may be present. This type of ectopic pregnancy lies on the margin of the uterine wall. Interstitial ectopic pregnancy carries a greater risk of bleeding and higher mortality if ruptured.

First-trimester ultrasonography often can identify other signs of abnormal pregnancy. One sign of abnormal pregnancy is a *blighted ovum*. In this case, the gestational sac will be larger than 16 to 20 mm, but no yolk sac or fetal pole is visualized (Fig. 117-10). Other sonographic findings suggestive of embryonic demise can be seen on endoscopic ultrasonography. In general, all findings of embryonic demise should be interpreted conservatively, and these patients should be referred for confirmatory obstetric tests.

Another type of abnormal pregnancy that can be seen on ultrasound scans is a hydatidiform mole, or *molar pregnancy*. In this condition the uterus appears enlarged, but no intrauterine pregnancy is visualized. Instead, the uterus is filled with abundant cystic placental material (Fig. 117-11). Beta-hCG levels will be abnormally elevated, often >200,000 mIU/mL.

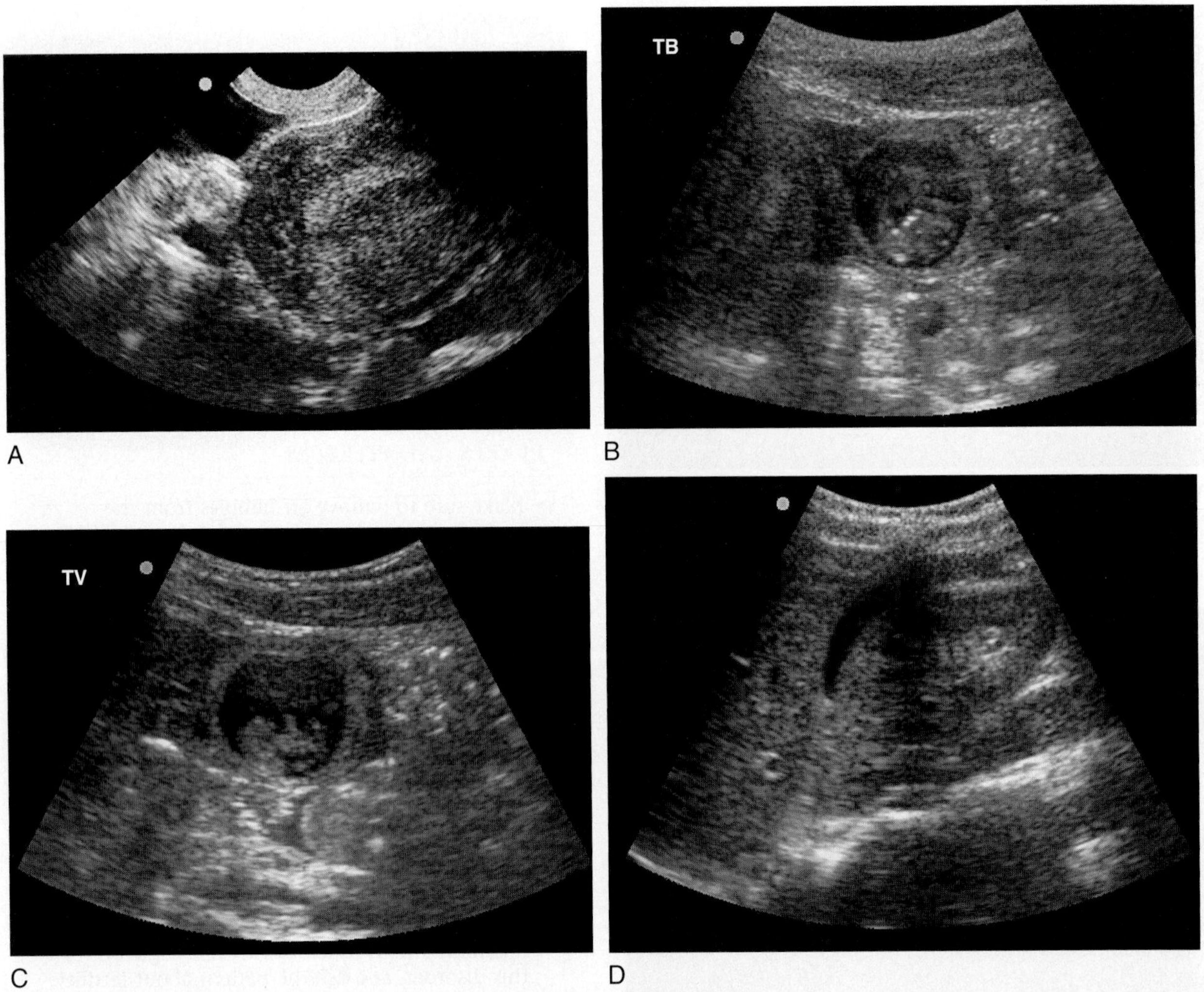
A
TB
B
TV
C
D

FIGURE 117-8 This patient had evidence of an extrauterine embryo (**B and C**) with cardiac activity and fetal movement on real-time ultrasound images. Free fluid is present both in the pelvis (**A**) and in Morrison's pouch (**D**).

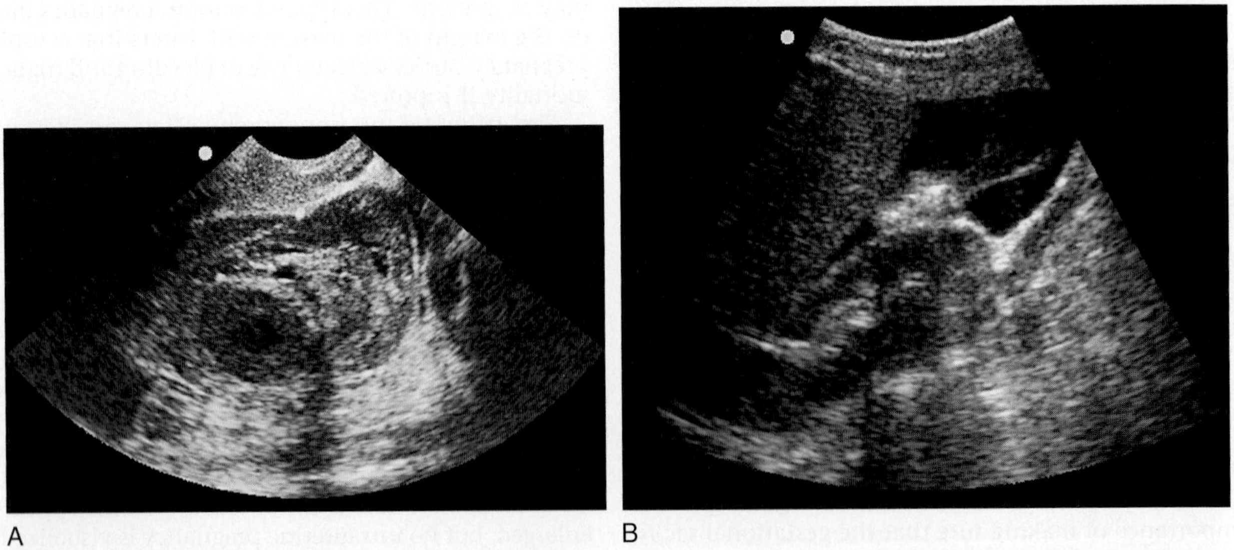
A
B

FIGURE 117-9 These ultrasound images from the same patient demonstrate a complex ovarian mass (**A**), a pseudogestational sac, and a large amount of free intraperitoneal fluid with clot (**B**).

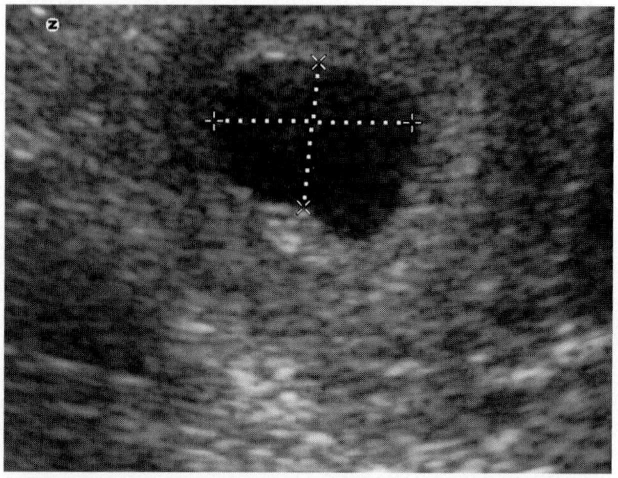

FIGURE 117-10 Large, empty gestational sac constistent with a blighted ovum.

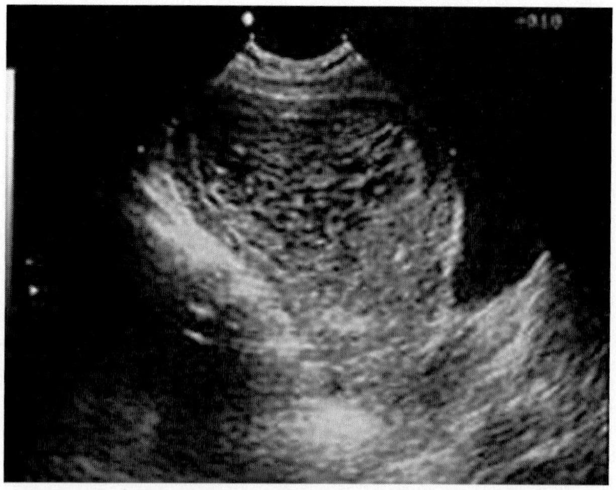

FIGURE 117-11 Enlarged uterus with hyperechoic grape-like clusters consistent with a molar pregnancy.

Limitations

Because beta-hCG urine tests are positive at 20 mIU/mL (1 week post-conception or 3 weeks gestational age) and a normal pregnancy usually is not visualized on ultrasound scans until quantitative beta-hCG levels are higher than 2000 mIU/mL (5-6 weeks gestational age), ultrasonography cannot be used to confirm an intrauterine pregnancy for approximately 3 weeks of early pregnancy. Clinical suspicion for ectopic pregnancy and reliability of dates should be factored into decision making for these patients.

The presence of an intrauterine pregnancy does not rule out an ectopic pregnancy in the setting of fertility treatments, where there is a high risk of heterotopic pregnancy.

REFERENCES

1. Stovall TG, Kellerman AL, Ling FW, Buster JE: Emergency department diagnosis of ectopic pregnancy. Ann Emerg Med 1990;19:1098-1103.
2. Mateer JR, Valley VT, Aiman EJ, et al: Outcome analysis of a protocol including bedside endovaginal sonography in patients at risk for ectopic pregnancy. Ann Emerg Med 1996;27:283-289.
3. Tayal VS, Cohen H, Norton HJ: Outcome of patients with an indeterminate emergency department first-trimester pelvic ultrasound to rule out ectopic pregnancy. Acad Emerg Med 2004;11:912-917.
4. Durham B, Lane B, Burbridge L, Balasubramaniam S: Pelvic ultrasound performed by emergency physicians for the detection of ectopic pregnancy in complicated first-trimester pregnancies. Ann Emerg Med 1997;29:338-347.
5. Kaplan BC, Dart RG, Moskos M, et al: Ectopic pregnancy: Prospective study with improved diagnostic accuracy. Ann Emerg Med 1996;28:10-17.
6. Counselman FL, Shaar GS, Heller RA, King DK: Quantitative β-hCG levels less than 1000 mIU/mL in patients with ectopic pregnancy: Pelvic ultrasound still useful. J Emerg Med 1998;16:699-703.
7. Blaivas M, Sierzenski P, Plecque D, Lambert M: Do emergency physicians save time when locating a live intrauterine pregnancy with bedside ultrasonography? Acad Emerg Med 2000;7:988-993.
8. Shih CH: Effect of emergency physician–performed pelvic sonography on length of stay in the emergency department. Ann Emerg Med 1997;29:348-351.
9. Rodgerson JD, Heegaard WG, Plummer D, et al: Emergency department right upper quadrant ultrasound is associated with a reduced time to diagnosis and treatment of ruptured ectopic pregnancies. Acad Emerg Med 2001;8:331-336.

Chapter **118**

Complications of Third Trimester Pregnancy

Sally A. Santen and Robin R. Hemphill

PREECLAMPSIA AND ECLAMPSIA

KEY POINTS

Preeclampsia is a disease of the third trimester of pregnancy characterized by sustained elevation of blood pressure and proteinuria.

The HELLP syndrome is a particularly severe form of preeclampsia with high maternal morbidity, characterized by *he*molysis, *e*levated *l*iver enzymes, and *l*ow *p*latelets.

Edema is common in preeclampsia but is no longer considered to be necessary for the diagnosis.

Eclampsia is defined by seizures usually in the setting of preeclampsia.

In patients with severe preeclampsia and eclampsia, basic management involves support of maternal vital signs, control of hypertension, prevention and treatment of seizure activity, and consultation with the obstetrics department to determine the need for early delivery.

Perspective

Preeclampsia is a disease of the third trimester of pregnancy characterized by sustained elevation of the blood pressure (>140/90 mm Hg) and proteinuria. Edema is common in preeclampsia but is no longer considered to be necessary for the diagnosis. Eclampsia is defined by seizures, usually in the setting of preeclampsia. Seizures are rare without underlying preeclampsia. Preeclampsia occurs most commonly after the 20th week of pregnancy. It can also present in the postpartum period, usually within the first 24 to 48 hours, although cases with delayed presentation of 2 weeks or more have been reported.

■ EPIDEMIOLOGY

Preeclampsia complicates 5% to 11% of pregnancies in the United States, and has an even higher rate in developing nations. It represents 15% of pregnancy-related deaths. Fetal complications such as prematurity and low birth weight are common, with death occurring in 129 of every 1000 cases. Maternal complications are common in both severe eclampsia and preeclampsia, including HELLP syndrome (11%), placental abruption (10%), disseminated intravascular coagulation (DIC) (6%), neurological deficits (6%), aspiration pneumonia (6%), pulmonary edema (5%), renal failure (4%), and death (1%).

First pregnancies are at the greatest risk. Other risk factors include extremes of reproductive age, more than 10 years between pregnancies, multiple gestations, molar pregnancies, previous or family history of preeclampsia, underlying diseases (hypertension, diabetes, autoimmune or renal diseases, obesity), and thrombophilia (e.g., antiphospholipid syndrome, factor V Leiden deficiency, activated protein C resistance).[1]

Pathophysiology

The etiology of preeclampsia is unclear and is likely multifactorial. The disease is thought to originate within the placenta which, for reasons that remain obscure, has inappropriately decreased perfusion. This decrease in placental perfusion in some cases results in development of preeclampsia. There is ensuing hypoperfusion and multi-organ effects from decreased intravascular volume and endothelial vascular leakage causing increased interstitial volume, interstitial protein leakage, and vasoconstriction.[2]

Preeclampsia affects nearly every organ system. Severe preeclampsia is characterized by hypertension due to severely increased peripheral resistance. However, the profound elevation of blood pressure is the result rather than the cause of the underlying pathophysiology. Effects on the liver include edema, hepatocellular necrosis, and periportal and subcapsular hematomas. Decreased renal flow with high perfusion pressures can cause glomerular and tubular injury resulting in proteinuria or, worse, renal failure. Cerebral vasospasm creates edema, microinfarction, and hemorrhage. Patients experience a variant of chronic DIC with thrombocytopenia and hemolysis that can worsen the organ system dysfunctions already mentioned.

The HELLP syndrome is a particularly severe form of preeclampsia characterized by *he*molysis, *e*levated *l*iver enzymes, and *l*ow *p*latelets. This syndrome is associated with severe maternal morbidity. The risk factors of HELLP syndrome (multiparity, age older than 25 years, and white race) differ from those of preeclampsia.[3]

Preeclampsia has long-term implications for the health of these patients. After delivery, women with preeclampsia are at increased risk for development of chronic hypertension, cardiovascular diseases, and psychosomatic disorders.[4]

Presenting Signs and Symptoms

Classic clinical findings of preeclampsia include proteinuria and an associated blood pressure elevation; when these develop late in the pregnancy of a primigravida, the diagnosis of preeclampsia is clear. However, preeclampsia does not always present in this straightforward manner. For instance, a patient with chronic hypertension complicated by chronic renal disease can be difficult to differentiate from one who has preeclampsia. Likewise, seizures in pregnant patients do not always herald eclampsia, and other structural, toxic, and metabolic causes have to be considered.

Patients may present with the classic symptoms of severe preeclampsia, such as seizures superimposed on hypertension and proteinuria, or may have incidentally noted hypertension, proteinuria, and edema.

Persistent blood pressure elevation is the hallmark of preeclampsia. Hypertension is defined as blood pressure greater than 140/90 mm Hg. Blood pressure readings ideally should be taken more than 6 hours apart; however, for most patients in the ED, therapy should not be delayed. Early in pregnancy the diastolic blood pressure decreases but returns to normal toward the 28th week of gestation. Therefore, a sustained diastolic blood pressure of greater than 90 mm Hg at the midpoint of pregnancy should be considered elevated unless the patient has a clearly documented history of prior hypertension.

If the patient's blood pressure before pregnancy is known, a systolic blood pressure increase of 30 mm Hg or greater and a diastolic blood pressure increase of 15 mm Hg or greater are diagnostic for preeclampsia. In addition to hypertension, the patient will have proteinuria of greater than 1+ on urinalysis.

Patients with severe preeclampsia may present with additional symptoms of organ involvement (Box 118-1),[5] including significant edema, especially facial edema, and documented weight gain greater than 5 pounds per week. Findings ominous for severe preeclampsia include blood pressure greater than or equal to 160 mm Hg systolic and 110 mm Hg diastolic, visual disturbances (blurred vision or scotomata), severe headache, altered mental status, seizures (this defines eclampsia), hyperreflexia with clonus, severe epigastric or right upper quadrant pain on examination, retinal hemorrhage with exudates and papilledema (this is rare and more commonly indicates underlying chronic hypertension), bibasilar rales and evidence of frank pulmonary edema, oliguria, and petechiae and bleeding from puncture sites.

Fetal growth retardation and oligohydramnios may be seen in cases of severe preeclampsia, but this information usually is not available. Sudden onset of abdominal pain with a firm painful uterus suggests placental abruption, which complicates up to 10% of preeclamptic pregnancies.

Differential Diagnosis

The current classification of hypertension in pregnancy is divided into four categories: preeclampsia, gestational or transient hypertension, chronic hypertension, and preeclampsia superimposed on chronic hypertension (Box 118-2).[6] In addition, occult renal disease can be manifest with proteinuria and associated hypertension.

Thrombotic thrombocytopenic purpura and preeclampsia can have identical findings of thrombocytopenia, hemolytic anemia, renal disease, and

BOX 118-1

Clinical Manifestations of Severe Preeclampsia

Cardiovascular

- Increased cardiac output, systemic vasoconstriction, systemic hypertension, increased hydrostatic pressure, generalized edema

Obstetric

- Uteroplacental insufficiency, fetal growth retardation, fetal hypoxemia and distress, decidual ischemia or thrombosis, placental abruption, placental infarcts

Renal

- Decreased renal blood flow and glomerular filtration rate, endothelial damage, proteinuria, elevated creatinine levels and decreased creatinine clearance, oliguria, elevated uric acid levels, renal tubular necrosis, renal failure

Hematologic

- Intravascular hemolysis (schistocytes, burr cells, elevated free hemoglobin and iron, decreased haptoglobin levels), thrombocytopenia, DIC (increased fibrin split products, decreased fibrinogen)

Cerebrovascular

- Ischemia, generalized grand mal seizures (eclampsia), high cerebral perfusion pressure with regional ischemia, cerebral hemorrhage, cerebral edema, coma, central blindness, loss of speech

Hepatic

- Ischemia, hepatic cellular injury, elevated liver enzymes, mitochondrial injury, intracellular fatty deposits

neurologic abnormalities. In patients with preeclampsia, the hypertension, proteinuria, and edema tend to precede the hematologic findings. In patients with thrombotic thrombocytopenic purpura they generally follow, and are a result of, the hematologic abnormalities.

In addition, laboratory test abnormalities seen in HELLP syndrome can be seen in other diseases noted in Box 118-3.

Diagnostic Testing

Laboratory tests may help clarify the diagnosis and determine the severity of the preeclampsia. If proteinuria is 1+ or greater on urinalysis, a hypertensive pregnant woman should be considered to have preeclampsia unless proved otherwise. A 24-hour urine collection is more sensitive for this purpose, but its use is not realistic in the ED.

A complete blood count should be performed with manual differential and haptoglobin to evaluate for hemolysis. The finding of hemoconcentration favors the diagnosis of preeclampsia, although the count may be low if hemolysis accompanies the disease. Decreased platelet counts (less than 100,000/mm^3) are associated with severe disease. Fibrinogen levels, fibrin split products, and prothrombin time/partial thromboplastin time (PT/PTT) tests should be ordered to evaluate for DIC, which may complicate severe preeclampsia.

BOX 118-2

Classification of Hypertension in Pregnancy

Preeclampsia

- Hypertension and proteinuria after the 20th week of gestation

Gestational or Transient Hypertension

- Hypertension without proteinuria after 20th week of gestation

Chronic Hypertension

- Hypertension diagnosed before the 20th week of gestation or before the pregnancy

Preeclampsia Superimposed on Chronic Hypertension

- Development of accelerated hypertension or proteinuria after the 20th week of gestation in a patient with hypertension diagnosed before the 20th week or before the pregnancy

BOX 118-3

Differential Diagnosis of HELLP* Syndrome

- Hemolytic uremic syndrome
- Acute fatty liver of pregnancy
- Thrombotic thrombocytopenic purpura
- Immune thrombocytopenic purpura
- Systemic lupus erythematosus
- Antiphospholipid antibody syndrome
- Cholecystitis
- Fulminant viral hepatitis
- Acute pancreatitis
- Disseminated herpes simplex
- Hemorrhagic or septic shock

*Hemolysis, *e*levated *l*iver enzymes, and *l*ow *p*latelets.

A comprehensive metabolic profile should be obtained because serum creatinine elevation, especially when associated with oliguria, and elevated liver transaminases suggest severe preeclampsia. Uric acid levels should be assayed; the degree of elevation of uric acid has been shown to correlate with the severity of the preeclampsia. Elevated lactate dehydrogenase (LDH) levels indicate hemolysis but can also be a result of liver involvement. Typing and cross-matching of blood is necessary in cases of severe preeclampsia or anticipated delivery.

HELLP syndrome is characterized by peripheral smears showing schistocytes and burr cells, elevated LDH levels (>600 U/L), elevated liver enzymes (bilirubin >1.2 and aspartate aminotransferase [AST] >70 U/L), and low platelet count (<100,000).

Treatment and Disposition

Pregnant women presenting for any complaint should have careful consideration of blood pressure. Mild preeclampsia may progress rapidly to severe preeclampsia with little warning. If a pregnant patient is found to have elevated blood pressure, the initial assessment should include a complete history and physical examination with attempts to determine whether the blood pressure elevation is new or old, and whether there is other evidence of preeclampsia (Fig. 118-1). If there is concern that the blood pressure elevation indicates preeclampsia, the patient will usually need admission for close monitoring and therapy.

Mild preeclampsia, especially with prematurity, may be closely managed without immediate delivery. Therefore it is important to differentiate between mild and severe preeclampsia (Table 118-1).[7]

In patients with severe preeclampsia and eclampsia, basic management involves the following measures: (1) support of maternal vital functions and initiation of laboratory test evaluation, (2) control of severe hypertension, (3) prevention and treatment of seizures, and (4) evaluation for early delivery and obstetric consultation.

The patient should be placed in the left lateral decubitus position with large-bore IV access; however, large amounts of fluid should be avoided. Patients should receive supplemental oxygen and, if the airway is in danger of compromise, should be intubated, with attempts to minimize elevation of intracranial pressure. Vital signs should be continuously monitored. Fever may indicate infection or may be the result of prolonged seizures. After the maternal condition has been stabilized, the fetal heart rate should be monitored.

In the preeclamptic patient, the mainstay of treatment is magnesium administered when the diastolic blood pressure exceeds 100 mm Hg, for seizure prophylaxis. (Magnesium is superior to dilantin or diazepam for prevention of eclamptic seizures, although the mechanism of action is not well understood.)

The recommended dosage is 4 to 6 g of magnesium administered intravenously over 15 minutes, followed by an infusion of 1 to 2 g /hour, with a goal of serum levels of 4 to 6 mEq/L. Magnesium should be used cautiously in patients with renal insufficiency or oliguria.

When systolic blood pressure reaches 160 mm Hg or diastolic pressure reaches 105 mm Hg, most experts recommend the use of an antihypertensive agent. The ideal antihypertensive agent for preeclampsia is one that reduces blood pressure in a controlled manner and has minimal side effect (Table 118-2).[8,9] The exact degree of reduction is controversial, but it is reasonable to maintain diastolic blood pressure between 90 and 110 mm Hg.

Hydralazine hydrochloride (Apresoline) has been the antihypertensive agent of choice for 50 years. The mechanism of action is through direct relaxation of arteriolar smooth muscle. This drug can be given as 5- to 10-mg boluses every 15 to 20 minutes until a response is seen in the blood pressure. Side effects include tachycardia, nausea, vomiting, headache, and epigastric pain.

Labetalol, a combination alpha- and beta-adrenergic blocking agent, is a second-line treatment. The dose is 20 to 40 mg administered as slow IV push every 20 to 30 minutes. This can be followed by 1 to 2 mg/min given by a continuous infusion or by IV dosing every 3 hours after blood pressure has been controlled. Side effects include flushing, orthostatic hypotension, and tremulousness. Labetolol should not be used in patients with asthma or evidence of heart failure.

Antihypertensive agents to use with caution, if at all, include nifedipine and nitroglycerin. Calcium channel blockers such as nifedipine (10 mg PO q30 min) have been used for refractory cases of hypertension. However, there is concern about precipitous blood pressure decrease when magnesium and nifedipine are used together. Nitroglycerin, a venous (predominantly) and arterial vasodilator, also

Table 118-1 COMPARISON OF SYMPTOMS OF SEVERE AND MILD PREECLAMPSIA

	Mild	Severe
Hypertension	140-150/ 90-100 mm Hg	>160/110 mm Hg
Proteinuria	1+	>3+
Oliguria	Absent	Present
Visual disturbances, particularly scotomata	Absent	Present
Epigastric pain	Absent	Present
Headache	Absent	Present
Pulmonary edema or cyanosis	Absent	Present
Seizures (eclampsia)	Absent	Present
Laboratory test abnormalities (elevated creatinine and liver enzymes; thrombocytopenia)	Absent	Present

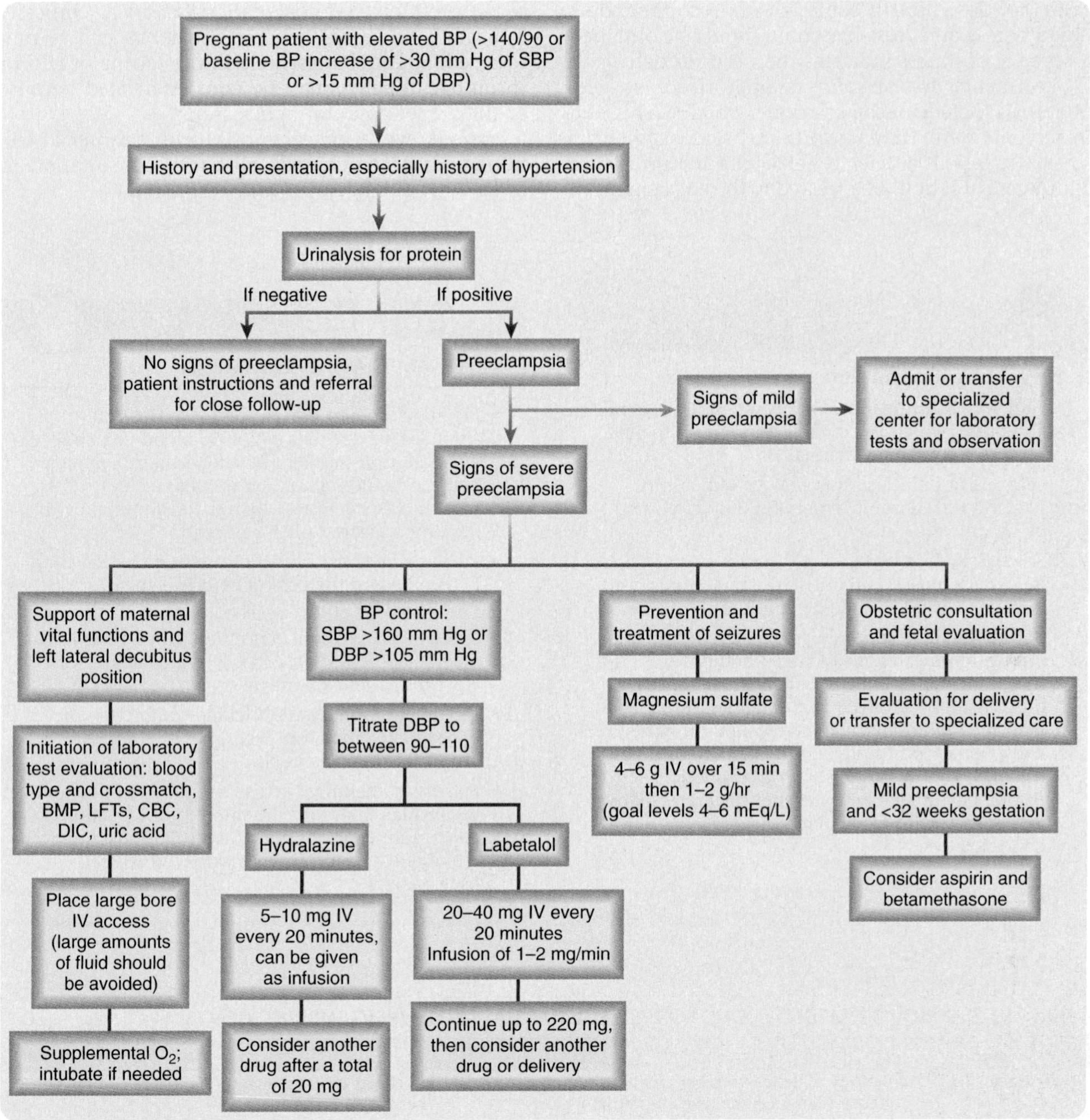
Pregnant patient with elevated BP (>140/90 or baseline BP increase of >30 mm Hg of SBP or >15 mm Hg of DBP)
History and presentation, especially history of hypertension
Urinalysis for protein
If negative
If positive
No signs of preeclampsia, patient instructions and referral for close follow-up
Preeclampsia
Signs of mild preeclampsia
Admit or transfer to specialized center for laboratory tests and observation
Signs of severe preeclampsia
Support of maternal vital functions and left lateral decubitus position
Initiation of laboratory test evaluation: blood type and crossmatch, BMP, LFTs, CBC, DIC, uric acid
Place large bore IV access (large amounts of fluid should be avoided)
Supplemental O2; intubate if needed
BP control: SBP >160 mm Hg or DBP >105 mm Hg
Titrate DBP to between 90–110
Hydralazine
5–10 mg IV every 20 minutes, can be given as infusion
Consider another drug after a total of 20 mg
Labetalol
20–40 mg IV every 20 minutes Infusion of 1–2 mg/min
Continue up to 220 mg, then consider another drug or delivery
Prevention and treatment of seizures
Magnesium sulfate
4–6 g IV over 15 min then 1–2 g/hr (goal levels 4–6 mEq/L)
Obstetric consultation and fetal evaluation
Evaluation for delivery or transfer to specialized care
Mild preeclampsia and <32 weeks gestation
Consider aspirin and betamethasone

FIGURE 118-1 Algorithm for approach to patient with suspected preeclampsia. BMP, basic metabolic profile; BP, blood pressure; CBC, complete blood count; DBP, diastolic blood pressure; DIC, disseminated intravascular coagulation; LFTs, liver function tests; SBP, systolic blood pressure.

has been used for refractory cases of hypertension. However, when high doses are used, the patient should be monitored for the development of methemoglobinemia. These antihypertensive agents should be used with caution, if at all.

Other antihypertensive agents to avoid include sodium nitroprusside and angiotensin-converting enzyme inhibitors. Sodium nitroprusside should only be used as a last resort, because fetal cyanide poisoning has been reported in animal studies.[10] Angiotensin-converting enzyme inhibitors have been shown to cause fetal death in diverse animal species,[11] and possibly renal failure in neonates, and thus should not be used in pregnancy. Clonidine and alphamethyldopa are not administered parenterally and therefore are rarely used in initial management of preeclampsia.

Treatment of eclampsia is delivery. The method of delivery (cesarean or vaginal) depends on gestational age, cervical maturation, and clinical status. In patients with less than 32 weeks' gestation and mild preeclampsia it may be best to delay delivery. In these cases low-dose aspirin sometimes is recommended. Blood typing and cross-matching should be obtained if severity of illness indicates the need for delivery.

Treatments for specific complications of preeclampsia include dexamethasone, which may useful in patients with HELLP syndrome, and betamethasone, which will accelerate fetal lung maturity after 24 hours. DIC should be treated with replacement of blood products and coagulation factors as clinically indicated; however, heparin usually is not recommended. Epidural anesthesia in the setting of DIC or thrombocytopenia may be contraindicated because of the risk of epidural hematoma.

Patients with preeclampsia and eclampsia will need to have emergency obstetrics consultation to assist with management and admission.

RED FLAGS

Preeclampsia and Eclampsia

- Pain with a firm painful uterus suggests placental abruption, which is a complication in up to 10% of preeclamptic pregnancies.
- Diagnosis of preeclampsia may be difficult in patients with chronic hypertension complicated by chronic renal disease.
- Seizures in pregnant patients do not always herald eclampsia, and other structural, toxic, and metabolic causes should be considered.
- Both thrombotic thrombocytopenic purpura and preeclampsia can have identical findings of thrombocytopenia, hemolytic anemia, renal disease, and neurologic abnormalities. In patients with preeclampsia, the hypertension, proteinuria, and edema tend to precede the hematologic findings, and in patients with thrombotic thrombocytopenic purpura, they generally follow, and are a result of, the hematologic abnormalities.

Documentation

PREECLAMPSIA AND ECLAMPSIA

- Pregnant women presenting for evaluation should have documentation of blood pressure; any elevation needs to be addressed. A complete history should include symptomatic clues (e.g., headache, vision changes, abdominal pain) identifying causes of the elevation.
- Review of records may indicate that the elevation is chronic and that the patient is being monitored for this finding.
- If the blood pressure is not dangerously high, it may be addressed by making arrangements for close outpatient follow-up.
- Documentation should include completion of appropriate laboratory testing (e.g., complete blood count, urinalysis).
- Patients presenting with severe preeclampsia and eclampsia require documentation of all actions taken, interventions given, consultations requested, and the time at which all were ordered.

Table 118-2 PRIORITY MEDICATIONS FOR PREECLAMPSIA: ANTIHYPERTENSIVE AGENTS

Drug	Dosage	Comments
Hydralazine	5-10 mg IV q20 min; consider another drug after a total of 20 mg; can be given as infusion	Side effects include tachycardia, nausea, vomiting, headache, epigastric pain
Labetalol	20-40 mg IV q20 min; continue up to 220 mg; give 1-2 mg/min as infusion or repeat IV doses every 3 hr	Second-line treatment; side effects include flushing, orthostatic hypotension, tremulousness; do not use in patients with asthma or heart failure
Nifedipine	10 mg sublingually; response time is 10 min, with maximum effect at 30 min; if no response after 20 mg, consider alternatives	Third-line treatment; avoid in older patients or patients with family or personal history of coronary disease, especially if smokers; may cause precipitous blood pressure decrease, especially when used with magnesium
Clonidine	0.1 mg PO in 30 min, then 0.1 mg every hour	Third-line treatment; no parenteral form; not good for initial management

THIRD TRIMESTER BLEEDING

KEY POINTS

Placental abruption and placenta previa are the most serious causes of vaginal bleeding in late pregnancy.

Painful bleeding in late pregnancy is likely due to placental abruption; however, when the vaginal bleeding is painless, the etiology is more likely placenta previa.

Ultrasound evaluation of third trimester bleeding is useful in cases of placenta previa, but less so for placental abruption (only detects 25%-50%).

Treatment for third trimester bleeding includes stabilization of the patient, assessment of fetal status using ultrasound and fetal monitoring, and consultation with the obstetrics department to determine need for delivery.

Scope and Outline

Vaginal bleeding is found in about 3% to 4% of second and third trimester pregnancies. It can herald catastrophic problems for both mother and fetus.

Placental abruption and placenta previa are the most serious causes of vaginal bleeding in late pregnancy. In 20% of cases it is due to placenta previa, and in 33% to placental abruption. Placental abruption is estimated to occur in about 1% of all pregnancies. Of these pregnancies, 20% to 40% will have perinatal morbidity or mortality of mother or fetus. Maternal death, although diminishing in incidence (0.03% of pregnant women), remains significant.

Ultrasound studies estimate that the incidence of placenta previa is higher (about 5%) in the second trimester. The incidence decreases to about 0.5% of pregnancies at delivery, as the uterus enlarges, pulling the placenta away from the cervical os.

Vaginal bleeding in late pregnancy has causes other than placenta previa or placental abruption (such as cervical and vaginal abrasions or polyps) in about 50% of patients; nonetheless, these women need close follow-up. Investigation of other causes of vaginal bleeding should be delayed until the diagnosis of placenta previa or placental abruption is ruled out.

In some studies the risk of second trimester abortion or perinatal mortality is as high as 30% in this group. Therefore, vaginal bleeding in all patients should receive serious consideration, even if the bleeding appears self-limited.

Pathophysiology

■ PLACENTAL ABRUPTION

Placental abruption, or abruptio placentae in Latin (meaning "the rending asunder of the placenta"), is the premature separation of the normally implanted placenta from the uterine decidual lining. The margin, or a part, or all of the placenta may separate, creating minimal to large amounts of bleeding. The bleeding may be seen vaginally or may be concealed behind the placenta. In placental abruption, there is initial bleeding into the placental decidua basalis, a thin layer adherent to the myometrium, and then bleeding into the abrupted placental tissue. The blood creates a potential space, tracking to the cervix and causing vaginal bleeding. It can also disrupt the placenta, resulting in bloody amniotic fluid.

The vascular placental bed can bleed significantly, causing maternal hypotension, or the loss of placental circulation may cause fetal distress or death. Hematoma between the layers prevents that area of placenta from exchanging nutrients and oxygen for the fetus. In addition, typically there is significant uterine spasm. The combination of spasm and decreased perfusion causes the fetus to become hypoxic. Fetal bleeding can occur but is more likely in traumatic placental abruption. The hallmark of placental abruption is vaginal bleeding and uterine tenderness.

Risk factors for placental abruption include cocaine, hypertension in pregnancy (preeclampsia, gestational or chronic hypertension), previous placental abruption, current placenta previa, twin pregnancies, trauma, and multiparity. Other risk factors associated with placental abruption are fetal malformation, premature rupture of membranes, uterine leiomyomas, advanced maternal age, cigarette smoking, intravenous drug use, malnutrition, low socioeconomic status, and being African American.

Hypertension increases not only the risk for placental abruption but also the risk for more severe placental abruption and increased fetal mortality. Elevations in blood pressure may predispose the placenta to bleeding, but the exact initiating event is still elusive. Major trauma as well as seemingly insignificant trauma are important causes of placental abruption. Because pregnant trauma patients are initially managed in the ED, the EP should be vigilant for signs of placental abruption.

Coagulopathy and progression to DIC may develop as well. The etiology of consumptive coagulopathy is multifactorial. The larger the abruption, the more likely is DIC to develop. The concealed hemorrhage serves as a nidus for activation of the intrinsic and extrinsic pathways of coagulation. Another mechanism for the development of DIC is the loss of endothelial integrity; exposure of thromboplastin stimulates the coagulation cascade.

Other complications of placental abruption include maternal morbidity, massive blood loss, renal failure, fetal mortality, preterm births, and low birth weight.

■ PLACENTA PREVIA

Painful bleeding in late pregnancy is likely due to placental abruption; however, when vaginal bleeding is painless the etiology is more likely placenta previa, in which the placenta is located either partially or completely over the cervical os. In preparation for labor, the softening of the lower uterine segment and effacement of the cervix tear the implanted placenta previa resulting in painless vaginal bleeding. Only 10% of women have contractions or uterine tenderness coincident to the initial vaginal bleeding. Many women have brief painless bleeding initially, which is a warning that placenta previa exists. As the cervix dilates further, the bleeding can become rapid and life-threatening.

Placenta previa can be total, partial, marginal, or low-lying. The etiology of placenta previa also is unclear. Factors that decrease the richness of the vascular bed of the uterus (defective decidual vascularization), or "scar" the uterus, predispose to placental implantation in the lower uterine segment and cervix. The risk of placenta previa is increased with prior cesarean section and advanced maternal age. Other risk factors include multiparity, malpresentation, multiple gestation, previous placenta previa, and smoking. Presumably, the presence of multiple implantation sites of multiparous women and multiple gestations increases the risk. In addition, the placenta often preferentially implants near the scar of a previous cesarean section, but then migrates to cover the cervix as well. It is uncertain whether the lower uterine scar prevents the normal elongation of the lower uterine segment that would normally pull the placenta away from the cervix or if the uterus is not rich enough to support the placenta, causing it to enlarge and cover the cervix. Whatever the cause, the eventual vaginal bleeding is caused by softening of the lower uterine segment, disrupting the placental attachment.

Although placenta previa may be diagnosed in the second trimester, in many women, as the uterus enlarges it pulls the placenta away from the cervix, eliminating the previa; thus 90% of cases of placenta previa diagnosed before the 20th week of gestation resolve. Therefore a definitive diagnosis of placenta previa is made after the 24th week of gestation.

Presenting Signs and Symptoms

The classic presentation of placental abruption is painful vaginal bleeding associated with fetal distress. Most patients have uterine contractions at the time, and in about one third of cases there is uterine hypertonus. Symptoms also may include abdominal and back pain. In the majority cases, the abruption is not due to trauma; however in the ED population, trauma is an important cause. One half of abruptions occur in the period just before labor.

In contrast to placental abruption, the classic presentation of placenta previa is painless bleeding.[12] The onset of bleeding is usually sudden and may be profuse. Placenta previa usually occurs after the 28th week of gestation.

Vaginal bleeding past the first trimester of pregnancy is abnormal and should be taken seriously. The patient's obstetric history as well as social and medical history may contribute to the diagnosis and alert the physician to complicating factors. The onset, duration, and quantity of vaginal bleeding are relevant to determine the patient's stability; trauma and sexual activity may stimulate bleeding. Bleeding after trauma is more likely due to placental abruption, whereas intercourse may provoke bleeding from placenta previa.

The duration of bleeding, estimated volume of blood, and number of pads used can help determine the volume of blood loss. The typical saturated pad holds about 30 mL of blood. Since several liters of blood can remain concealed in the uterus, it is easy to underestimate the volume of blood lost.

During the initial evaluation, patients should be asked if they have felt fetal movements in the past few hours. Lack of movement may indicate fetal death or compromise.

The physical examination should not include speculum or manual pelvic examination as part of the evaluation of patients with third trimester bleeding. In the presence of a placenta previa, cervical manipulation may cause torrential vaginal bleeding. The evaluation should include fundal height measurement and evidence of uterine tenderness, contractions, or a hypertonic uterus. Severe placental abruption causes uterine irritability manifested by frequent contractions with increased baseline tone (high frequency contractions). In patients with placenta previa, the uterus should be soft, although 10% of these patients may be in labor and have contractions that should not be confused with the uterine irritability of placental abruption. The fetal descent into the pelvis should be noted, and the presenting part may be determined using Leopold maneuvers.

In cases of vaginal bleeding caused by trauma, placental abruption is highest on the list of differential diagnoses. However, if the pain is caused by trauma to other organs, the bleeding might be due to placenta previa. In about 10% of cases, abdominal pain occurs with placenta previa. The pain may be due to the bleeding or due to the onset of labor.

Although vaginal bleeding occurs in 80% of cases of placental abruption, some abruptions are con-

Tips and Tricks

THIRD TRIMESTER BLEEDING

- Do not do a speculum examination in patients presenting with third trimester bleeding.
- Major trauma as well as seemingly insignificant trauma are important causes of placental abruption.
- All vaginal bleeding during the third trimester should be considered serious; investigation for other causes of vaginal bleeding should be delayed until the diagnosis of placenta previa or placental abruption is ruled out.
- Focus on maternal stabilization—when mom does well, the fetus has a better chance to do well.
- The diagnosis of placental abruption is based on clinical signs; the diagnosis should always be considered in pregnant women presenting to the ED with significant uterine contractions and fetal distress.

Placental Abruption

- Painful vaginal bleeding
- Concealed abruption is difficult to diagnose
- Uterine contractions
- More likely after trauma

Placenta Previa

- Painless vaginal bleeding
- Usually occurs after 28th week of gestation
- Uterine irritation not present
- Bleeding more likely to start after sexual intercourse

cealed and there is no evidence of overt bleeding, making diagnosis difficult. Thus it is important to realize that abruption may present with symptoms that can be either minor or severe (shock, fetal demise, tetanic contractions).

Differential Diagnosis

Uterine rupture is a rare but catastrophic event that should be considered in the differential diagnosis of placental abruption. It is most commonly seen in women with prior cesarean section or after severe trauma. Fetal mortality is close to 100%, and maternal mortality is significant. There may or may not be bleeding, but usually there is severe abdominal pain and a rigid gravid abdomen. The diagnosis is made operatively or by ultrasonography.

The maternal response to volume depletion is to decrease blood flow to nonvital organs including the uterus, with resultant fetal hypoxia manifesting as bradycardia with a fetal heart rate less than 100 beats/min. Bradycardia and fetal distress may have a variety of causes and may be present in placental abruption without maternal compromise. In addition, it should be noted that up to 20% of cases of placental abruption present with fetal demise.

Following clinical examination, ultrasound imaging may be performed; in 25% to 50% of cases another diagnosis is found (Box 118-4). About 10% of pregnant patients presenting with abdominal pain and bleeding may have preterm labor pains, a heavy bloody show with the onset of labor, or marginal placental or subchorionic bleeding. These patients should be admitted for monitoring.

Other causes of vaginal bleeding are vaginal or cervical polyps, cervical lacerations or erosions, cervical carcinoma, and vulvar injury.

Patients in the second half of pregnancy with abdominal or back pain but without vaginal bleeding should first be considered to have placental abruption, because concealed hemorrhage is present in 10% of placental abruptions. Other causes of abdominal pain should be considered such as pyelonephritis, nephrolithiasis, appendicitis, ovarian torsion, and other abdominal processes. Abnormal laboratory findings such as blood in the urine and an elevated white blood cell count may help in the differential diagnosis.

Diagnostic Testing

In patients with third trimester bleeding, ultrasonography may be performed to rule out placenta previa, to determine fetal age and viability, and to look for placental abruption. However, only 25% to 50% of placental abruptions are identified on ultrasound scans, and the appearance may be unimpressive because the clot looks similar to the placenta. The diagnosis of placental abruption is clinical, and the EP should suspect placental abruption in the pregnant woman presenting with significant uterine contractions and fetal distress. Fetal heart rate and uterine contraction (toco) monitoring should be initiated early. The diagnosis is confirmed by examination of the placenta after delivery.

Laboratory evaluation includes a complete blood count, comprehensive metabolic profile, prothrombin time/partial thromboplastin time (PT/PTT) tests, DIC panel (fibrinogen, fibrin split products), urinalysis, and blood typing and cross-match. Anemia is a concern both in placental abruption and placenta

BOX 118-4

Differential Diagnosis of Third Trimester Bleeding

- Placental abruption
- Placenta previa
- Bloody show (extrusion of cervical mucus)
- Vasa previa
- Disseminated intravascular coagulopathy
- Uterine rupture
- Cervicitis, cervical cancer, or other cervical abnormality
- Vaginal laceration

Documentation

THIRD TRIMESTER BLEEDING

- Vital signs of patient, as well as fetal monitoring
- Size of the gravid uterus and the degree of uterine spasm as determined during the physical examination
- The presence or absence of vaginal bleeding, and its onset, quantity, and duration
- Events prior to the onset of bleeding
- Type and time of interventions as well time when consultation was requested
- Personal and family history, with focus on risks for placental abruption
- Medical (including obstetric) history, especially in regard to cesarean section

RED FLAGS

Third Trimester Bleeding

- Hypertension not only increases the risk of placental abruption; it also predisposes to more severe placental abruption and increased fetal mortality.
- Although vaginal bleeding occurs in 80% of cases of placental abruption, some abruptions are concealed, with no evidence of overt bleeding.
- Placental abruption in patients presenting to the ED may be the result of abuse.
- Many women with vaginal bleeding will have brief painless bleeding initially; this is a sign of placenta previa.

previa. DIC can complicate placental abruption; therefore it is important to perform the relevant tests. The Kleihauer-Betke test, which confirms the presence of fetal blood cells in the maternal circulation, should be performed if fetal-maternal transfusion is suspected.

Treatment and Disposition

Basic management of vaginal bleeding in third trimester pregnancy includes determination of the hemodynamic status of the mother, with resuscitation as needed; assessment of fetal condition and age by fetal monitoring and ultrasonography; and decision-making about optimal timing of delivery.[13] Early consultation with the obstetrics department is critical.

The patient should be placed on her left side to increase venous return. Initial management of significant vaginal bleeding is volume resuscitation and transfusion as needed. Although normal vital signs are optimal, they may be falsely reassuring due to the physiologic increase in maternal volume.[14,15] Fetal heart rate may be a good indicator of maternal status; however, this is not specific.

After stabilization of the mother is assured, the status of the fetus is assessed with continuous monitoring and ultrasound imaging to determine viability and age.

Ultrasonography may diagnose placenta previa. This disease is managed by delaying delivery if the patient is stable and the fetus is premature. If there is heavy bleeding or the pregnancy is near-term, delivery should be by cesarean section, regardless of fetal viability.

Management of placental abruption is contingent on the viability or distress of the fetus. In cases of mild placental abruption without fetal distress and severe placental abruption with fetal mortality, infants are delivered vaginally. In cases of moderate placental abruption with fetal distress, cesarean section is preferred.

Rh-negative women should be given 300 units of Rhogam. This dose is adequate to prevent maternal sensitization to up to 15 mL of fetal blood. A larger dose may be necessary if the fetal-to-maternal transfusion is greater as determined by the Kleihauer-Betke test.

Women with vaginal bleeding late in pregnancy need to be admitted. If the hospital does not have critical obstetrics and neonatal care facilities, transfer to a tertiary hospital is required.

REFERENCES

1. Duckitt K, Harrington D: Risk factors for pre-eclampsia at antenatal booking: Systematic review of controlled studies. BMJ 2005;330(7491):565.
2. Pridjian G, Puschett JB: Preeclampsia. Part 1: Clinical and pathophysiologic considerations. Obstet Gynecol Surv 2002;57:598-618.
3. Baxter JK, Weinstein L: HELLP syndrome: The state of the art. Obstet Gynecol Surv 2004;59:838-845.
4. Van Pampus MG: Long-term outcomes after preeclampsia. Clin Obstet Gynecol 2005;48:489-494.
5. National High Blood Pressure Education Program Working Group Report on High Blood Pressure in Pregnancy. Am J Obstet Gynecol 1990;163:1691-1712.
6. Norwitz ER, Hsu CD, Repke JT: Acute complications of preeclampsia. Clin Obstet Gynecol 2002;45:308-329.
7. O'Brien JM, Barton JR: Controversies with the diagnosis and management of HELLP syndrome. Clin Obstet Gynecol 2005;48:460-477.
8. Roberts JM, Gammill HS: Preeclampsia: Recent insights. Hypertension 2005;46:1243-1249.
9. Vidaeff AC, Carroll MA, Ramin SM: Acute hypertensive emergencies in pregnancy. Crit Care Med 2005;33(10 Suppl):S307-S312.
10. Briggs GG: Drug effects on the fetus and breast-fed infant. Clin Obstet Gynecol 2002;45:6-21.
11. Naulty J, Cefalo RC, Lewis PE: Fetal toxicity of nitroprusside in the pregnant ewe. Am J Obstet Gynecol 1981; 139:708-711.
12. Usta IM, Hobeika EM, Musa AA, et al: Placenta previa-accreta: Risk factors and complications. Am J Obstet Gynecol 2005;193:1045-1049.
13. Chamberlain G, Steer P: ABC of labour care: Obstetric emergencies. BMJ 1999;318(7194):1342-1345.
14. Bhide A, Thilaganathan B: Recent advances in the management of placenta previa. Curr Opin Obstet Gynecol 2004;16:447-451.
15. Neilson JP: Interventions for suspected placenta praevia. Cochrane Database Syst Rev 2003;(2):CD001998.

Chapter 119

Emergency Delivery and Peripartum Emergencies

Rachel Reisner and Jeremy Branzetti

KEY POINTS

Practitioners underestimate blood loss in postpartum hemorrhage by as much as 50%.

Uterine inversion is relatively uncommon (1 in 2500 deliveries) but is associated with significant morbidity if not recognized and treated promptly.

Patients with uterine rupture present without pain in 87% of cases, and without vaginal bleeding in 89%.

Perimortem cesarean delivery is indicated in gravid patients if more than 24 weeks of gestation and if arrest continues after 4 to 5 minutes of cardiopulmonary resuscitation.

Emergency cesarean delivery protocols should be started as soon as the patient has signs of cardiac arrest.

Abnormal vital signs are late indicators of severe hemorrhage.

The clinical examination of term pregnant patients is notoriously unreliable.

Treatment for anaphylactoid syndrome of pregnancy is similar to that for sepsis and disseminated intravascular coagulation and should begin immediately; the diagnosis is one of exclusion and patients must be treated promptly to survive.

Postpartum Hemorrhage

■ SCOPE

Hemorrhage is a significant cause of maternal morbidity and is the second most common cause of pregnancy-related deaths (following amniotic fluid embolism). Hemorrhage was a direct cause of more than 18% of 3201 pregnancy-related maternal deaths in the United States from 1991 to 1997.[1] Worldwide, hemorrhage has been identified as the single most important cause of maternal death, responsible for almost half of all postpartum deaths in developing countries.[2]

Postpartum hemorrhage is the term used to describe excessive blood loss after delivery. Classically, it is defined as more than 500 mL of blood loss in a vaginal delivery or more than 1000 mL of blood loss in a cesarean delivery; however, careful quantitative measures reveal that blood loss in the range of 500 to 1000 mL is actually average for both types of delivery. Of note, practitioners underestimate blood loss by as much as 50%.[3]

Table 119-1 **RISKS FOR POSTPARTUM HEMORRHAGE**

Hypotonic Myometrium (50%)	Anomalies of Uterus or Placenta (20%)	Trauma (20%)	Other
Poor myometrium perfusion	Uterine anomalies/malformation	Ruptured uterus	Coagulopathy
Leiomyomata	Succenturiate lobe	Episiotomy	Preeclampsia
Multiparity	Uterine inversion	Lacerations	Advanced maternal age
Previous atony	Uterine arteriovenous malformations	Instrumental delivery	Previous postpartum hemorrhage
Chorioamnionitis	Retained placental tissue: placenta accreta, increta, percreta	Cesarean delivery	Hypertensive disorders
Dermatomyositis	Placenta previa		
Multiple gestation	Low-lying placenta		
Polyhydramnios			
Macrosomia			
Inhalation anesthesia			
Oxytocin use			
Prolonged 2nd or 3rd stage			
Precipitate labor			
Dysfunctional labor			
Instrumental or cesarean delivery			

■ PATHOPHYSIOLOGY

Separation and delivery of the placenta constitutes the third stage of labor. With separation of the placenta, there is also severance of the numerous uterine arteries and veins that carry 600 mL/min of blood through the intervillous space. The most important factor for hemostasis is contraction and retraction of the myometrium to compress and obliterate the open lumens of the vessels. Uterine atony can lead to catastrophic postpartum hemorrhage, and a majority (50%-80%) of cases are the result of a hypotonic uterus or uterine atony. Factors that lead to uterine overdistention or that interfere with uterine contractility can cause uterine atony and are associated with postpartum hemorrhage (Table 119-1). Although it is important to keep these associations in mind, most cases of postpartum hemorrhage occur without any known predisposing factors.

■ CLINICAL PRESENTATION

The patient may lose a substantial amount of blood before becoming hypotensive or feeling symptomatic. Immediate postpartum hemorrhage should be recognized as a potential complication of a precipitous delivery. The classic clinical presentation is a woman who presents with sudden massive vaginal bleeding and is tachycardic, pale, and possibly diaphoretic or hypotensive. Three factors make this classic presentation flawed. First, it is important to keep in mind that the pulse and blood pressure may remain reasonably normal until large amounts of blood have been lost. Second, many patients will have a steady bleeding that, although moderate-appearing, can lead to very serious blood loss. The condition of these patients may escape notice until serious hypovolemia develops. Third, intrauterine, intravaginal, intraperitoneal, and retroperitoneal accumulation of blood can be overlooked.

■ DIFFERENTIAL DIAGNOSIS

Postpartum hemorrhage is a sign, not a diagnosis; it is important to consider the etiology of the postpartum hemorrhage because it will often direct the treatment.

Abnormal placentation (placenta accreta, increta, or percreta) can contribute to postpartum hemorrhage in different ways: (1) an adherent placenta or large blood clots prevent effective contraction of the myometrium, thereby impairing hemostasis at the implantation site; and (2) significant bleeding from the implantation site is more likely with placental separation of abnormally adherent tissue. Trauma to the genital tract during labor and delivery (lacerations to the perineum, vagina, vulva, or cervix) is the second most common cause of postpartum hemorrhage.

Although congenital coagulation defects may be relatively rare, consumptive, dilutional, and disseminated intravascular coagulopathies are important considerations. A depletion of platelets and soluble clotting factors after blood loss and subsequent crystalloid and packed red blood cell replacement is difficult to distinguish clinically from disseminated intravascular coagulopathy. Placental abruption, amniotic fluid embolism, HELLP syndrome (*h*emolysis, *e*levated *l*iver enzymes, *l*ow *p*latelet count), and intrauterine demise are pregnancy-related risk factors for disseminated intravascular coagulation.

■ DIAGNOSTIC TESTING AND TREATMENT

The most important aspects of managing postpartum hemorrhage are hemostasis and treatment for shock. This includes supplemental oxygen, placement of two large-bore IV lines, hemodynamic monitoring, and volume replacement. In addition, blood should be typed and cross-matched and 4 to 6 units of packed red blood cells should be available. Consultation with the obstetrics service should be arranged.

Table 119-2 MEDICATIONS FOR POSTPARTUM HEMORRHAGE

Drug	Dosage	Class	Commentse
Uterotonic			
Oxytocin (Pitocin)	20-40 units/L IV infusion @10 mL/min, or 10-20 units IM	Ergot	Do not give IV bolus; IV infusion 1st-line choice, IM second choice
Methylergonovine (Methergine or Ergonovine)	0.2 mg IM, may repeat q2h (max 5 doses)		Contraindicated in preeclampsia or hypertension
Carboprost tromethamine (Hemabate)	0.25 mg (250 μg) IM, may repeat q15-90min (max 8 doses)	Prostaglandin (15-methyl prostaglandin $F_{2\alpha}$ analogue)	May cause transient O_2 desaturation; contraindicated in active cardiac, renal, pulmonary, or hepatic disease
Misoprostol (Cytotec)	600-1000 μg SL or PR; single dose	Prostaglandin (prostaglandin E_1 analogue)	May cause bronchospasm
Prostaglandin E_2 (Dinoprostone or Prostin E_2)	20-mg uterine suppository, may repeat q2h	Prostaglandin	May transiently decrease blood pressure
Hemostatic			
Factor VIIa (NovoSeven)	35-200 μg/kg, may repeat q2h until hemostasis achieved	Human recombinant factor VIIa	

IM, intramuscularly; PR, per rectum; SL, sublingually.

Along with the initial resuscitation, bimanual massage and IV oxytocin should be initiated (Fig. 119-1 and Table 119-2).

Initial laboratory studies include a complete blood count, coagulation studies, disseminated intravascular coagulation panel, liver function tests, and basic metabolic panel.

A Foley catheter should be placed. An operator experienced with bedside ultrasonography may be able to identify retained products or clot in the uterus, but manual exploration is still needed. In select circumstances, with stable patients, a computed tomography scan can be useful in the diagnosis in postpartum hemorrhage (retroperitoneal hematoma).

The key to identifying the etiology of postpartum hemorrhage is the physical examination. Because uterine atony is the most common cause of postpartum hemorrhage, accurate assessment of the uterine tone is essential. To assess uterine tone, a hand is placed on the anterior wall of the uterus (over the fundus) and palpated. If a soft, boggy, or very large uterus is felt, the diagnosis of uterine atony is established. At this point, management of uterine atony should be a priority over inspection for secondary causes of bleeding. If a firm, contracted uterus is felt, a search for other causes should be initiated promptly.

If the placenta has been delivered, manual uterine exploration may reveal uterine rupture or retained products or clots (which should be removed manually to improve uterine contraction). If the placenta is still in place and bleeding is ongoing, the placenta should be removed if a distinct cleavage plane is palpated on exploration. If an indistinct cleavage plane is revealed, the diagnosis of placenta accreta is likely. in the case of placenta accreta, the placenta should not be removed in the ED. Bimanual uterine compression should continue, with the goal being to stabilize patients until they can be taken to the operating room.

Trauma to the genital tract can be diagnosed with careful inspection of the labia, vagina, and cervix for laceration or hematoma. Noncomplex (1st- or 2nd-degree), easily accessible lacerations can be repaired with absorbable sutures. Cervical lacerations and 3rd- and 4th-degree lacerations should be repaired by an obstetrician. Temporary hemostasis may be achieved by direct pressure or, in the case of cervical lacerations, by gentle application of ring forceps to the bleeding point.

Retroperitoneal hematoma is a potentially life-threatening condition that may present as hypotension, cardiovascular shock, or flank pain. Once a diagnosis is made, treatment should be supportive until the obstetrician, interventional radiology, or the operating room is available.

First-line interventions for atony are part of the initial management of postpartum hemorrhage—namely, initiation of bimanual uterine compression, IV oxytocin, and clearing products of conception/clots from the uterus. If bleeding persists after initial interventions, additional uterotonic medications should be given (see Table 119-2). The choice of agent may be influenced by the side-effect profile, but the best drug is probably the agent that is the most quickly available in the ED. Interventional radiology may be beneficial, because embolization may control the bleeding. In any case, temporizing measures may be required until definitive intervention (Table 119-3).

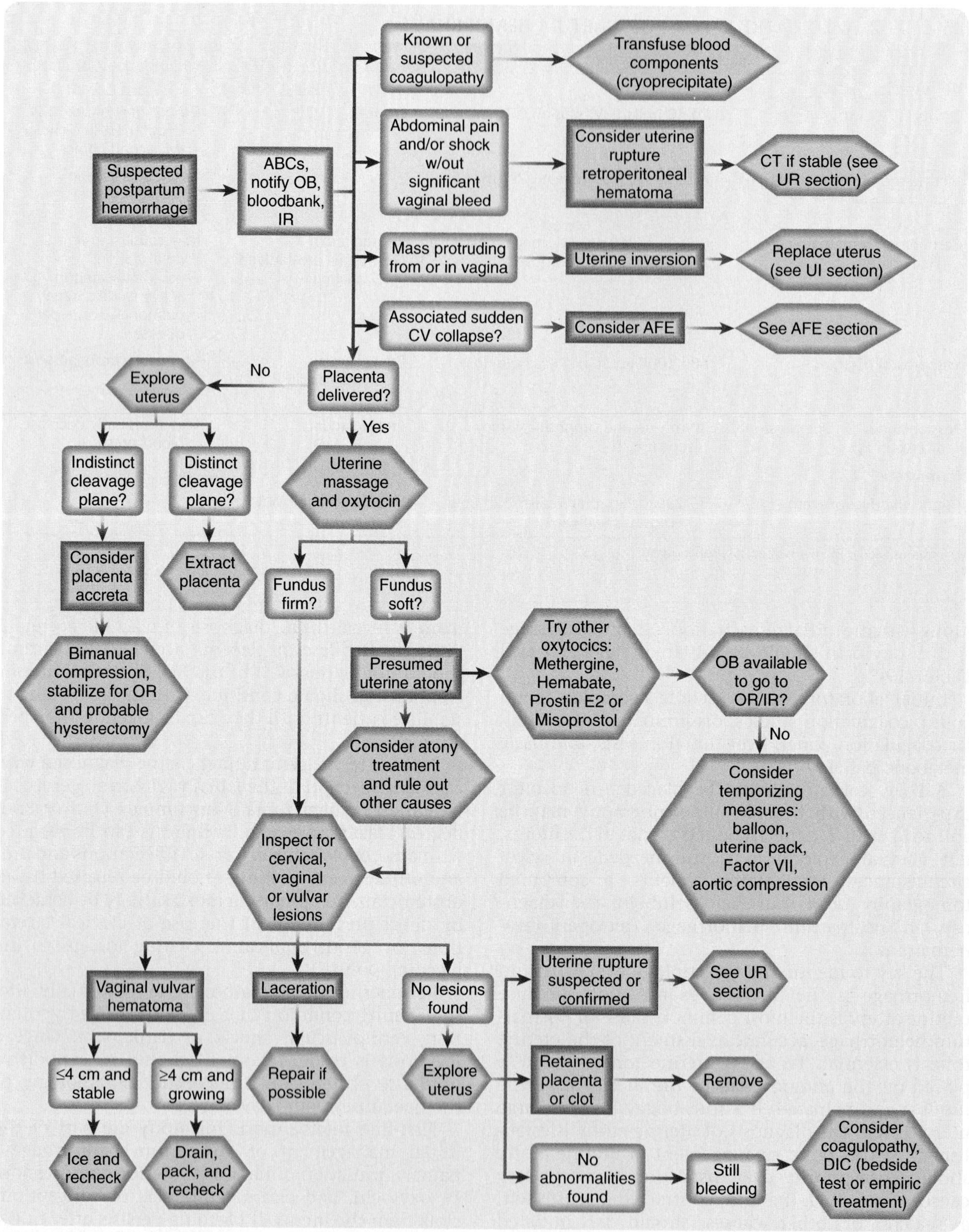
Suspected postpartum hemorrhage
ABCs, notify OB, bloodbank, IR
Known or suspected coagulopathy
Transfuse blood components (cryoprecipitate)
Abdominal pain and/or shock w/out significant vaginal bleed
Consider uterine rupture retroperitoneal hematoma
CT if stable (see UR section)
Mass protruding from or in vagina
Uterine inversion
Replace uterus (see UI section)
Associated sudden CV collapse?
Consider AFE
See AFE section
Placenta delivered?
No
Explore uterus
Yes
Indistinct cleavage plane?
Distinct cleavage plane?
Uterine massage and oxytocin
Consider placenta accreta
Extract placenta
Fundus firm?
Fundus soft?
Bimanual compression, stabilize for OR and probable hysterectomy
Presumed uterine atony
Try other oxytocics: Methergine, Hemabate, Prostin E2 or Misoprostol
OB available to go to OR/IR?
No
Consider atony treatment and rule out other causes
Consider temporizing measures: balloon, uterine pack, Factor VII, aortic compression
Inspect for cervical, vaginal or vulvar lesions
Vaginal vulvar hematoma
Laceration
No lesions found
Uterine rupture suspected or confirmed
See UR section
≤4 cm and stable
≥4 cm and growing
Repair if possible
Explore uterus
Retained placenta or clot
Remove
Ice and recheck
Drain, pack, and recheck
No abnormalities found
Still bleeding
Consider coagulopathy, DIC (bedside test or empiric treatment)

FIGURE 119-1 Algorithm for postpartum hemorrhage management strategies. ABCs, airway, breathing, and circulation; AFE, amniotic fluid embolism; CV, cardiovascular; DIC, disseminated intravascular coagulation; IR, interventional radiology; OB, obstetrics; OR, operating room; UI, uterine inversion; UR, uterine rupture.

Table 119-3 TEMPORIZING MEASURES FOR HEMOSTASIS OF POSTPARTUM HEMORRHAGE

Method	Procedure	Comments
Uterine packing	Layer sterile gauze within uterus, with the distal end going out through the os	May adhere to uterine wall and removal required; does not allow for monitoring of ongoing bleeding; start prophylactic antibiotics
Balloon tamponade		If available and time allows, use bedside ultrasonography to confirm that balloon is beyond the internal os prior to inflation to avoid damage to the cervical canal; give prophylactic antibiotics and continue oxytocin infusion
Foley catheter	Insert large bulb catheter (24F) into uterus Instill with 80-100 mL saline Pack vagina to avoid expulsion of catheter	Multiple catheters may be needed (in sterile overbag), which makes inner lumen difficult to monitor
SOS Bakri balloon	Insert into uterus Instill 300-500 mL of saline through stopcock Pack vagina	Best option if available; allows direct measurement of ongoing bleeding via open inner lumen; developed for postpartum hemorrhage; balloon conforms to shape of uterine cavity
Sengstaken-Blakemore tube	Cut off distal ("stomach") end of tube Insert inside uterine cavity Infuse 75-300 mL of saline Pack vagina to avoid expulsion of tube	Does not conform to shape of uterine cavity; with end cut off, proximal bleeding can be monitored through lumen; may be available from gastrointestinal department lab if not available in ED
Rusch catheter	Using 60-mL bladder syringe, inflate balloon via the drainage port, with 150-500 mL of saline Pack vagina to avoid expulsion of tube	Urologic catheter used for bladder stretching; may be available in urology department
Condom catheter	Slide condom over end of Foley and tie off with string to close end Inflate with 250-500 mL of saline and clamp end Pack vagina to avoid expulsion of tube	Sterile rubber catheter is fitted with a condom
Vaginal packing	Pack vagina with blood pressure cuff placed inside a sterile glove Increase pressure to 10 mm Hg above systolic blood pressure	Various techniques have been described; concern for bleeding proximal to vaginal pack
Noninflatable antishock garment	Begin application at the ankles and progress sequentially up to the abdomen	Adjust panels if any discomfort or dyspnea; contraindicated in women with heart failure or mitral stenosis

Uterine tamponade with sterile gauze and balloon tamponade are commonly used temporizing measures. Uterine balloon tamponade has been described using large Foley catheters, Sengstaken-Blakemore tubes, condom catheters, sterile gloves, and Rusch urologic catheters, as well as catheters specifically designed to be used for uterine tamponade in postpartum hemorrhage (SOS Bakri tamponade balloon).[4]

Uterine Inversion

■ SCOPE

The term *uterine inversion* refers to prolapse of the uterine corpus to or through the cervix (by inverting or turning inside-out). The majority of uterine inversion cases occur in the third stage of labor, with traction on the umbilical cord during placenta removal. Non-puerperal uterine inversion is very rare and is usually associated with uterine tumors. Uterine inversion is relatively uncommon (1 in 2500 deliveries)[3] but is associated with significant morbidity if not recognized and treated without delay. Uterine inversion is a potential cause of postpartum hemorrhage or profound shock.

■ PATHOPHYSIOLOGY

Acute, significant hypotension is common in uterine inversion. The traditional teaching was that patients present with "shock out of proportion" to the blood loss. The added shock was attributed to parasympathetic reflex from stretching of the broad ligament or compression of the ovaries. More conventional teaching is that hypovolemia from hemorrhage is primarily responsible for the observed hypotension, and that the blood loss is regularly underestimated. The estimated average blood loss in uterine inversion is 800 to 1800 mL.[5]

Tips and Tricks

PERIPARTUM HEMORRHAGE

- Use an endotracheal tube 0.5 to 1 mm smaller than you would normally use because airway may be narrowed from edema.
- Use reduced ventilation volumes because of elevated diaphragm.
- Left lateral position, manual uterine displacement, and perimortem cesarean delivery may improve maternal circulation
- Do *not* use femoral vein for central line.
- Perform chest compressions higher on the sternum because the gravid uterus elevates the diaphragm and abdominal contents.
- Follow the standard advanced cardiac life support (ACLS) guidelines for resuscitation, medications, and defibrillation doses (remove any fetal or uterine monitors prior to defibrillation).
- Administer calcium gluconate (1 ampule or 1 g) for arrest from suspected magnesium toxicity.
- Acute cononary syndrome (ACS): Percutaneous coronary intervention is preferred (over fibrinolytics) for ST-elevation myocardial infarction.

■ CLINICAL PRESENTATION AND DIFFERENTIAL DIAGNOSIS

Uterine inversion is classified by the amount of inversion and its duration. If the uterus is inverted but does not go through the cervix, it is called an *incomplete* inversion. In a *complete* inversion, the fundus protrudes through the cervix. In a more extreme version, the entire uterus may prolapse out of the vagina. Most cases are *acute,* occurring immediately after delivery and before the cervical ring constricts. If the inversion occurs or is noted after cervical contraction, the inversion is termed *subacute. Chronic* inversion refers to inversion occurring more than 4 weeks after delivery.

In a reported case series, the most common presenting signs are shock and hemorrhage.[5] Symptoms may include acute lower abdominal pain with a bearing-down sensation. In a complete inversion, the prolapsed uterus may be visible as a large, dark red, polypoid mass within the vagina or protruding through the introitus. If the fundus remains within the vagina, the diagnosis may be suspected because of dimpling, indentation, or absence of the uterine fundus on abdominal examination or because a mass is palpated in the cervix on bimanual examination. Establishing the diagnosis of an incomplete inversion is more difficult, and severe hypotension, postpartum hemorrhage, and subtle abnormalities on abdominal examination may be the only clues.

Without palpation or visualization of the prolapsed uterus, it may be difficult to differentiate uterine inversion from severe atony. Heavy bleeding may make visualization of the cervix impractical. In addition, abdominal palpation for a uterine fundus may be impossible in an obese patient. Depending on the stability of the patient, the uncertainty of the diagnosis, and the resources of the hospital, diagnosis via ultrasonography or laparotomy may be appropriate. In stable cases in which diagnosis is uncertain and resources are available, prompt ultrasound scanning may be helpful.[6] If the accompanying hemorrhage or shock is sufficiently alarming to require immediate exploration, the correct diagnosis may be established only at laparotomy.

■ DIAGNOSTIC TESTING AND TREATMENT

Management of uterine inversion has two important components: the immediate treatment of the hemorrhagic shock and repositioning of the uterus (Fig. 119-2). Resuscitation should be initiated immediately and continued while attempts are made to reposition the uterus manually. If oxytocin is being infused, it should be stopped once uterine inversion is suspected.

A maneuver to reposition the uterus should be attempted simultaneously with resuscitation. The emphasis is on an initial attempt at repositioning without delay because the success of nonsurgical replacement depends on completion before the myometrium regains its tone. If the uterus is flaccid, it may be repositioned easily and without the use of tocolytics. The reported rate of successful immediate reduction is between 40% and 80%.[7] If initial measures are delayed or fail to relieve the condition, the inversion may progress to the point at which operative treatment or even hysterectomy is necessary.

The most common nonsurgical replacement method is a variation of the "Johnson maneuver."[8] The prolapsed uterus is cupped in the operator's palm, and a firm upward pressure is applied to move the uterus up through the cervix, following the natural curve of the pelvis, toward the umbilicus, until it is in place. Usually when the inverted mass is pushed upward, the uterus automatically reverts, with the fundus returning to its anatomic position. If the placenta has not separated, it should not be removed.

If initial repositioning is unsuccessful, myometrial relaxation with pharmacologic agents should be started. Magnesium sulfate, terbutaline, and recently nitroglycerin are the agents most commonly used (Table 119-4).[9]

If the patient's blood pressure is adequate, nitroglycerin has many advantages, including its availability in the ED. Furthermore, nitroglycerin has a rapid onset of 30 to 60 seconds and a short half-life, which enables the uterus to contract again after it has been repositioned, minimizing further blood loss. Hemodynamic monitoring and crystalloid IV infusion should be maintained during administration of nitroglycerin. If significant hypotension follows, it can be reversed with ephedrine (10 mg IV).

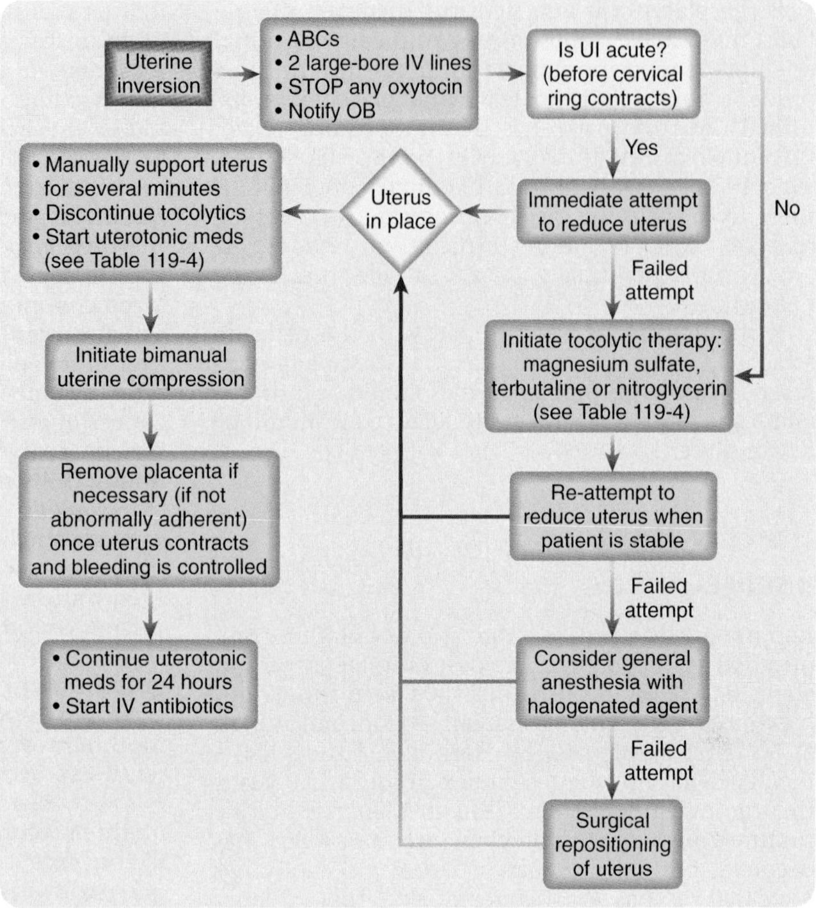
Uterine inversion
• ABCs
• 2 large-bore IV lines
• STOP any oxytocin
• Notify OB
Is UI acute? (before cervical ring contracts)
Yes
No
Immediate attempt to reduce uterus
Uterus in place
• Manually support uterus for several minutes
• Discontinue tocolytics
• Start uterotonic meds (see Table 119-4)
Failed attempt
Initiate tocolytic therapy: magnesium sulfate, terbutaline or nitroglycerin (see Table 119-4)
Initiate bimanual uterine compression
Remove placenta if necessary (if not abnormally adherent) once uterus contracts and bleeding is controlled
Re-attempt to reduce uterus when patient is stable
Failed attempt
• Continue uterotonic meds for 24 hours
• Start IV antibiotics
Consider general anesthesia with halogenated agent
Failed attempt
Surgical repositioning of uterus

FIGURE 119-2 Algorithm for uterine inversion management strategies. ABCs, airway, breathing, and circulation; OB, obstetrics; UI, uterine inversion.

Table 119-4 PRIORITY MEDICATIONS FOR UTERINE INVERSION

Drug	Dosage	Comments
Tocolytic		
Magnesium sulfate	4 g IV over 20 min, then 2-3 g/h infusion	Monitor for side effects; has prolonged effects; calcium gluconate may be needed to reverse tocolysis when uterus in place
Terbutaline	0.25 mg SC, may repeat q20min	May cause hypotension; tachycardia common; hold if heart rate >120 beats/min
Nitroglycerin	50 to 100 μg IV, may repeat as needed	Rapid onset/half-life; transient hypotension; have ephedrine (10 mg IV) available as remedy
Uterotonic		
Oxytocin (Pitocin)	20-40 units in 1 L normal saline/lactated Ringer's solution given as IV infusion @5 mL/min	Do not give an IV bolus; titrate to sustain uterine contractions
Methylergonovine (Methergine or Ergonovine)	0.2 mg IM	Contraindicated in preeclampsia or hypertension

IV, intravenously; IM, intramusculanly; SC, subcutaneously.

Attempts at manual repositioning of the uterus should continue. Eventually, if all other efforts have failed to reposition the inverted uterus, operative intervention may be required. If manual repositioning of the uterus is successful, the uterus should be supported for several minutes to allow the ligaments to return to their original state. Uterine relaxant administration is discontinued, and uterotonics are then administered to firm the myometrium. If magnesium sulfate was administered as a tocolytic, calcium gluconate can be given to reverse the tocolytic effect. Fluid and blood replacement and manual uterine massage should be maintained until the uterus is well contracted and bleeding has stopped. Antibiotics should be started as soon as is practical. Uterotonics are continued for at least 24 hours.

If the placenta is attached, the increased uterine bulk may make repositioning difficult; if initial attempts at repositioning are unsuccessful, the most prudent approach is to leave the placenta undisturbed until the patient is in the operating room. Placenta removal initially will increase blood loss even in cases with normal placental adherence. If there is a placenta accreta, increta, or percreta, removal will be more difficult or impossible and could potentially cause a life-threatening hemorrhage.

If the uterus was repositioned with the placenta attached, manual removal can be attempted once relaxants are stopped. Uterotonics should be initiated and if the placenta is not easily removed it should be left in place.

Uterine Rupture

■ SCOPE

Rupture of the uterus is a rare and devastating complication of pregnancy. The best estimate is rates of about 0.05% of all pregnancies, 0.8% in those with previous lower-segment cesarean section, and as high as 5% after classic cesarean section.[10] Although the incidence has not changed much in the last 20 years, the leading etiologies have. The incidence of uterine rupture cases without previous uterine surgery has declined, but the number of cesarear sections has increased, as has the frequency of a trial of labor post-cesarean, which results in the overall uncharged incidence.[11]

In the United States, uterine rupture is responsible for 5% of maternal deaths.[12] The major primary mechanism for maternal morbidity and mortality with uterine rupture is hemorrhagic shock and infection. The associated fetal outcomes with uterine rupture are worse. Fetal mortality is reported as 60% to 70%, and almost 100% in cases of uterine rupture from blunt trauma.[13]

Uterine rupture complicates about 1% of traumas. The maternal mortality rate in these cases is less than 10%, and most deaths are the result of concurrent injuries. In contrast, the incidence of fetal demise following traumatic uterine rupture approaches 100%.[14] Most penetrating wounds in this patient population are gunshot or stab wounds. In these cases the gravid uterus is protective for the mother while leaving the fetus particularly vulnerable. The fetus may be injured in up to 70% of penetrating trauma cases, whereas the mother suffers visceral injuries in only 19% of such cases. The rate of fetal mortality is as high as 70%, whereas maternal mortality is approximately 5%.[15]

■ PATHOPHYSIOLOGY

Uterine rupture is classified by degree of defect: complete or incomplete; spontaneous or traumatic. An added delineation is often made in uterine rupture in a previously scarred uterus versus uterine rupture in an unscarred uterus.

A *complete* uterine rupture is defined as a full-thickness separation of the uterine wall and overlying serosa; it is associated with life-threatening maternal and fetal compromise. After complete rupture, the uterine contents may escape or partially extrude from the uterus and into the peritoneal cavity.

An *incomplete* uterine rupture is defined as uterine muscle separation with intact visceral peritoneum. Most commonly, an incomplete uterine rupture is actually uterine scar dehiscence. In an incomplete rupture, hemorrhage frequently extends into the broad ligament, which has a tamponading effect. A concerning alternative is a retroperitoneal hematoma which, if large enough, can cause fatal exsanguination with its rupture.

Traumatic uterine rupture ranges from blunt (motor vehicle collisions, abuse, and falls) and penetrating injury (gunshot wounds, stab wounds) to even routine obstetric procedures (external cephalic version or forceps delivery).

Spontaneous rupture can occur prior to the onset of labor, during labor, or at the time of delivery and is usually associated with a scarred uterus.[6] Although rupture most commonly occurs in the third trimester, it can occur even in early pregnancy.

Many factors have been identified as risks for uterine rupture; however, each individual associated factor, except for previous uterine scar, is inconsequential by itself. It is the combination of the associated factors that makes the risk of uterine rupture significant (Box 119-1).

■ CLINICAL PRESENTATION AND DIFFERENTIAL DIAGNOSIS

The presentation of uterine rupture can be nonspecific or subtle. Timely diagnosis and definitive intervention may be impossible if the possibility of rupture is not considered. The classic presentation of uterine rupture is "ripping" or "tearing," suprapubic pain and tenderness, absence of fetal heart sounds, recession of presenting parts, and vaginal hemorrhage. This may be followed by signs and symptoms of hypovolemic shock and hemoperitoneum. The classic presentation actually is rare; uterine rupture presents without pain in 87% of cases and without vaginal bleeding in 89%.

The clinical abdominal examination is notoriously unreliable in term pregnant patients. The stretched abdominal wall significantly alters the normal noxious response to intraperitoneal stimuli. Most reports of uterine rupture describe patients with normal blood pressure or even elevated blood pressure without tachycardia. Abnormal maternal vital signs are late indicators of severe hemorrhage.

On presentation, vague or mild abdominal discomfort is more common than severe abdominal pain. Patients with uterine rupture can present with chest or shoulder pain referred from hemoperito-

BOX 119-1

Risks for Uterine Rupture

Surgery or Procedure

- Previous cesarean delivery (most common by far) (1/125 subsequent pregnancies)
- Previous uterine rupture
- Abortion with instrumentation
- Previous myomectomy incision (1/40 subsequent pregnancies)
- External or internal version
- Forceps delivery
- Breach extraction
- Forceful uterine pressure during delivery
- Complicated manual removal of placenta

Trauma or Environmental

- Trauma*
  - External blunt or penetrating trauma
  - Internal trauma (e.g., uterine pressure catheter)
- Cocaine use

Anomaly

- Congenital uterine anomaly
- Prior invasive molar pregnancy
- Placenta increta or percreta
- Adenomyosis
- Neoplasia
- Fetal anomaly or macrosomia distending lower uterine segment

Pregnancy-Related

- Silent rupture in previous pregnancy
- Persistent, intense contractions (spontaneous or induced)
- High parity (1/100 subsequent pregnancies); grand multiparity (≥7) increases the risk of rupture 20-fold.[16]
- Maternal age
- Uterine wall <2 mm (measured at 38-39 weeks of gestation by ultrasound)
- In vitro fertilization

*Most common cause of uterine rupture in patients without previous uterine surgery.

neum irritating the diaphragm. Fetal distress is the most consistent finding (80%-100%), with fetal bradycardia being the most common finding.[17]

The symptoms of rupture and abruption may be difficult to distinguish on clinical examination, but placental abruption is a more common complication of trauma than is rupture.

■ DIAGNOSTIC TESTING AND TREATMENT

The initial management differs and is based on the stability of the patient and fetus. Because most patients with uterine rupture present with a normal maternal examination, and because fetal distress is the most common finding, the initial management will probably be the same as that for other causes of acute fetal distress—urgent delivery.

The EP should refer the patient for obstetrics consultation, ensure adequate IV access, notify the bloodbank, and alert the neonatal team to be ready for intensive-care newborn resuscitation. If these resources are not available in the hospital, the EP should make arrangements for immediate transfer.

Quick definitive care is necessary for a good fetal outcome. Fetal morbidity invariably occurs because of catastrophic hemorrhage, fetal anoxia, or both. In a study of 99 cases of uterine rupture, best fetal outcomes were noted when surgical delivery was accomplished within 17 minutes from the onset of fetal distress.[17] If there are any signs of or concerns about maternal stability, a solid effort at resuscitation should be initiated, but surgery should not be delayed because of shock. The shock may not be reversible until the hemorrhage is controlled with repair or hysterectomy.

If the patient is stable, there are no signs of fetal distress, and the diagnosis is unclear, ultrasonography can be useful. Ultrasound findings include lack of normal orientation, uncertain placental location, fetal demise, and absence of amniotic fluid.

■ DISPOSITION

Patients with uterine rupture should be admitted to the intensive care unit or obstetric services after leaving the operating room. If the hospital does not have direct access to obstetric services, patients should be transferred to another hospital once it has been determined that their condition is stable enough for transfer. Morbid outcomes of uterine rupture include infection, hysterectomy, damage to ureter, amniotic fluid embolism, disseminated intravascular coagulation, and pituitary failure.

Perimortem Cesarean Delivery

■ SCOPE

Maternal arrest is estimated to occur in 1:4000 to 1:6500 pregnancies in the United States.[18-20] In any maternal arrest that occurs beyond 24 weeks, perimortem cesarean delivery should be considered as a potentially life-saving intervention for the both the mother and the fetus.[21]

Comparing causes of death in the cohort of women undergoing perimortem cesarean delivery to all maternal deaths, the etiologies are the same but trauma accounts for a larger proportion in the former group.[22] Perimortem cesarean delivery is one of the oldest surgical procedures in history, with the first reference to a successful postmortem cesarean section recorded in 237 BCE.[23] Under the emperors of Rome, the Caesars, a law decreeing that a child be excised from the womb of any woman who died late in pregnancy became known as the "lex caesare"—consequently the name *cesarean operation.* The first documented maternal survival from cesarean delivery was that of a Swiss woman sectioned by her husband in 1500.

In the 1980s DePace and Marx, pioneers in the world of perimortem cesarean delivery, published two papers describing unanticipated maternal survivals after postmortem cesarean deliveries.[24,25]

In 1986, Katz and colleagues published a comprehensive review of perimortem cesarean delivery cases between 1900 and 1985.[26] These studies suggested that emptying the uterus as part of early resuscitation would not only improve fetal outcomes but would also improve maternal survival, because cardiopulmonary resuscitation is likely to be ineffective in the third trimester. These workers concluded that "perimortem delivery" should be performed within 4 minutes of maternal arrest if resuscitation was ineffective. An update published in 2005 strongly supported this conclusion.[21]

The 2005 American Heart Association guidelines for cardiac arrest associated with pregnancy include the following statement regarding perimortem cesarean delivery in the secondary survey: "The resuscitation team leader should consider the need for an emergency hysterotomy (cesarean delivery) protocol as soon as a pregnant woman develops cardiac arrest."[27]

Pathophysiology

In the nonpregnant patient, under ideal conditions, chest compressions produce cardiac output less than one third of normal; in a gravid patient, the near-term uterus reduces cardiac output another two thirds (to about 10% of normal). Cardiac output can be improved by displacement of the uterus or tilting the patient (left lateral decubitus position); however, a decrease in effective chest compressions occurs with an increase in the patient's body tilt.[28]

Perimortem cesarean delivery is indicated for gravid patients more than 24 weeks of gestation if arrest continues after 4 to 5 minutes of cardiopulmonary resuscitation. In the recent Katz study,[21] among the cases with available data on maternal hemodynamics during resuscitation, more than one half of the women had "sudden and often profound improvement, including return of pulse and blood pressure at the time the uterus was emptied."

There are no reported cases of perimortem cesarean delivery worsening maternal hemodynamic status. Among women delivered in less than 15 minutes, almost 50% showed return of spontaneous circulation or improved hemodynamic status. In the cohort delivered after 15 minutes, only one in five showed improvement.[22]

Fetal outcomes are most directly related to the time from maternal arrest to delivery. Other important variables are the maturity of the fetus, the performance and effectiveness of maternal cardiopulmonary resuscitation, the etiology of maternal arrest, and the availability of a neonatal intensive care unit. Perimortem cesarean delivery before the point of fetal viability (approximately 24 weeks) is not indicated. Katz advises that if four fingers can be placed between the umbilicus and the top of the fundus, this is the beginning of aortocaval compression and also the time when there is fetal viability.[21]

Neurologic outcome is optimized by early delivery; in one study, 93% of infants delivered within 5 minutes were normal and only 45% of infants delivered within 15 minutes were without neurologic sequelae (Fig. 119-3).[22]

Treatment

See Box 119-2: Procedure for Perimortem Cesarean Delivery.

Amniotic Fluid Embolism

■ SCOPE

Amniotic fluid embolism and the resulting anaphylactoid syndrome of pregnancy occur in late preg-

BOX 119-2

Procedure for Perimortem Cesarean Delivery

- Using a #10 blade, make a midline vertical incision, going through all abdominal layers to the peritoneal cavity, which extends from the umbilicus to the pubic symphysis.
- Separate the rectus muscles in the midline and enter the peritoneum. If available, retractors can be used to expose the anterior surface of the uterus. If the bladder is full, it may be seen inferior to the uterus. A Foley catheter is optimal, but under pressing conditions the bladder can be drained with a small scalpel incision and applied pressure.
- To enter the uterus, start with a vertical incision through the lower uterine segment until amniotic fluid is obtained or until the uterine cavity is clearly entered. Next, lift the uterine wall away from the fetus with two fingers and use blunt scissors to extend the incision vertically to the fundus, allowing for generous exposure. The membranes should be ruptured and the baby delivered.
- Suction the infant's mouth and nose, and clamp and cut the cord. When the mother regains stable vital signs, remove the placenta and repair the uterus, abdomen, and bladder.

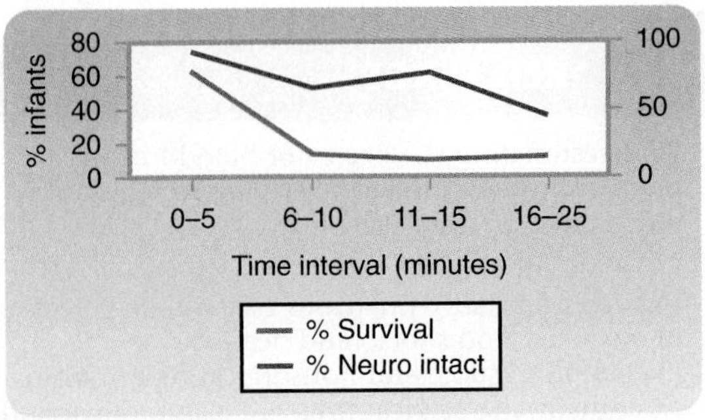
% infants
80
60
40
20
0
100
50
0
0–5
6–10
11–15
16–25
Time interval (minutes)
% Survival
% Neuro intact

FIGURE 119-3 Perimortem cesarean delivery: fetal outcomes in relation to time interval from maternal arrest to delivery.

nancy or immediately postpartum. Amniotic fluid embolism is rare, occurring in roughly 1 in 8000 to 1 in 80,000 pregnancies, but because of its devastating outcomes it is responsible for about 10% of all maternal deaths in the United States and is the most common cause of peripartum death.[29]

The syndrome of amniotic fluid embolism was first described in 1926 and established as a clinical entity in 1941.[30] Despite knowledge of this deadly syndrome for more than 80 years, the etiology and pathophysiology is not fully understood; the criteria to make the diagnosis are still controversial, and there are no management interventions that have been proved to improve the outcomes or prevent the syndrome.[31] The term *anaphylactoid syndrome of pregnancy* is considered more appropriate than the term *amniotic fluid embolism* to avoid misunderstanding the likely pathophysiology because of a lack of evidence supporting a causative embolic event.[32]

■ PATHOPHYSIOLOGY

Anaphylactoid syndrome of pregnancy, from a clinical, hemodynamic, and hematologic standpoint, is similar to anaphylaxis and septic shock and suggests the possibility of a shared pathophysiologic mechanism.[32] The syndrome appears to be initiated after maternal intravascular exposure to fetal tissue. Fetal-maternal tissue transfer is common and probably normal. It is proposed that when fetal antigens breach a maternal immunologic barrier in some women, release of endogenous mediators is triggered, and an anaphylactoid syndrome can occur.[33]

Neurologic damage is seen in as many as 85% of survivors of anaphylactoid syndrome.[32] The mechanism of neurologic injury is thought to be severe hypoxia leading to encephalopathy and seizures. The increased metabolic demand concurrent with seizures (seen in 50%) may worsen the brain injury, especially in the setting of hypoxia.[32] Disseminate intravascular coagulation developed within 4 hours of initial presentation in more than 80% of patients.[32] If diffuse bleeding occurs, hemorrhagic shock can contribute to the hypotension.

Table 119-5 SIGNS AND SYMPTOMS OF ANAPHYLACTOID SYNDROME OF PREGNANCY

Finding	Incidence (%)
Hypotension	100
Fetal distress	100
Pulmonary edema or ARDS	93
Cardiopulmonary arrest	87
Cyanosis	83
Coagulopathy	83
Dyspnea	49
Seizure	48
Atony	23
Bronchospasm	15
Transient hypertension	11
Cough	7
Headache	7
Chest pain	2

ARDS, acute respiratory distress syndrome.

■ CLINICAL PRESENTATION AND DIFFERENTIAL DIAGNOSIS

The classic presentation of anaphylactoid syndrome of pregnancy is acute hypoxia or respiratory arrest with associated cardiovascular failure, altered mental status, seizures, and coagulopathy in the immediate peripartum period (Table 119-5). Rare cases have been diagnosed in the first and second trimester in association with abortions, other procedures, and trauma. In about 10% of patients the diagnosis is made postpartum, and it has been diagnosed as late as 48 hours postpartum.

Anaphylactoid syndrome of pregnancy classically presents abruptly and with catastrophic outcomes, but less severe forms of this syndrome have been described. The National Registry's criteria for diagnosis of amniotic fluid embolism are included in Box 119-3.

■ DIAGNOSTIC TESTING AND TREATMENT

The diagnosis of anaphylactoid syndrome of pregnancy is a diagnosis of exclusion. The dramatic and rapid onset should prompt immediate action; death has been reported in 30 minutes to 7 hours from onset, with most deaths occurring in the first 2 hours. The initial presentation can be difficult to differentiate from that of other serious causes, but management, focusing on cardiopulmonary stabilization, is similar (Box 119-4).

There are no studies showing that targeted intervention improves maternal prognosis. Management includes early definitive airway control with endotracheal intubation, IV fluids, vasopressors, and inotropes as needed. The bloodbank should be notified and packed red blood cells, platelets, fresh frozen

BOX 119-3

National Registry Criteria for Diagnosis of Amniotic Fluid Embolism

- Acute hypotension or cardiac arrest
- Acute hypoxia (defined as dyspnea, cyanosis, or respiratory arrest)
- Coagulopathy (defined as laboratory evidence of intravascular consumption or fibrinolysis or severe clinical hemorrhage in the absence of other explanations)
- Onset during dilation and evacuation, labor, cesarean delivery, or within 30 minutes postpartum
- Absence of other significant, confounding condition or explanation of symptoms and signs listed here

Modified from Clark SL, Hankins GD, Dudley DA, et al: Amniotic fluid enbolism: Analysis of the national registry. Am J Obstet Gyrecol 1995;172:1158-1169.

BOX 119-4

Differential Diagnosis of Anaphylactoid Syndrome of Pregnancy (Amniotic Fluid Embolism)

Cardiovascular Collapse/Hypotension
- Acute coronary syndromes/myocardial infarction
- Cardiomyopathy
- Pulmonary embolism
- Anesthesia complications/transfusion reaction
- Sepsis/systemic inflammatory response syndrome

Respiratory Arrest
- Pulmonary embolism, air embolism
- Anesthesia complications/transfusion reaction
- Aspiration

Altered Mental Status/Seizure
- Eclampsia
- Cerebrovascular accident
- Hypoglycemia

Coagulopathy
- Disseminated intravascular coagulation
- Consumptive coagulopathy from hemorrhage

plasma, cryoprecipitate, and factor replacement should all be used as needed to treat disseminated intravascular coagulation.

If the fetus is still undelivered at the time of arrest, perimortem cesarean delivery should be initiated within 4 to 5 minutes of resuscitation.

RED FLAGS

- Underestimating the degree of blood loss in peripartum hemorrhage or not appreciating moderate-appearing bleeding.
- Delaying uterine inversion replacement, which increases mortality (increases risk and degree of hemorrhage and shock) and decreases the likelihood of successful nonsurgical repositioning (eventually the cervical ring will clamp down and make replacement more difficult, but this takes time).
- Not performing an emergency cesarean delivery in maternal (≥24 weeks of gestation) cardiac arrest not immediately reversed by cardiopulmonary resuscitation.
- Overlooking intrauterine, intravaginal, intraperitoneal, or retroperitoneal accumulation of blood.
- Presuming minimal bleeding or a less severe presentation in patient with normal vital statistics.

DISPOSITION

Patients who survive long enough to be transferred to the intensive care unit have a better prognosis, but the overall mortality is reported as 60%.[32] In one study, only 8% of patients who had cardiac arrest as part of the initial presentation survived neurologically intact. Infant survival was reported as 70%, but almost half of the survivors had neurologic damage. If arrest occurs, a short arrest-to-delivery interval is associated with improved neonatal outcomes.[32]

REFERENCES

1. Berg CJ, Chang J, Callaghan WM, et al: Pregnancy-related mortality in the United States, 1991-1997. Obstet Gynecol 2003;101:289-296.
2. McCormick ML, Sanghvi HC, Kinzie B, McIntosh N: Preventing postpartum hemorrhage in low-resource settings. Int J Gynaecol Obstet 2002;77:267-275.
3. ACOG Practice Bulletin: Clinical Management Guidelines for Obstetrician-Gynecologists, Number 76, October 2006: Postpartum hemorrhage. Obstet Gynecol 2006;108: 1039-1047.
4. Condous GS, Arulkumaran S, Symonds L, et al: The "tamponade test" in the management of massive postpartum hemorrhage. Obstet Gynecol 2003;101:767-772.
5. You WB, Zahn CM: Postpartum hemorrhage: Abnormally adherent placenta, uterine inversion, and puerperal hematomas. Clin Obstet Gynecol 2006;49:184-197.
6. Ripley DL: Uterine emergencies. Atony, inversion, and rupture. Obstet Gynecol Clin North Am 1999;26: 419-434.
7. Brar HS, Greenspoon JS, Platt LD, Paul RH: Acute puerperal uterine inversion. New approaches to management. J Reprod Med 1989;34:173-177.
8. Johnson AB: A new concept in the replacement of the inverted uterus and a report of nine cases. Am J Obstet Gynecol 1949;57:557-562.
9. Morini A, Angelini R, Giardini G: Acute puerperal uterine inversion: A report of 3 cases and an analysis of 358 cases in the literature. Minerva Ginecol 1994;46:115-127.

10. Kieser KE, Baskett TF: A 10-year population-based study of uterine rupture. Obstet Gynecol 2002;100:749-753.
11. Eden RD, Parker RT, Gall SA: Rupture of the pregnant uterus: A 53-year review. Obstet Gynecol 1986;68: 671-674.
12. Sakka M: Rupture of the pregnant uterus: A 21-year review. Int J Gynecol Obstet 1998;63:105-108.
13. Bujold E, Gauthier RJ; Neonatal morbidity associated with uterine rupture: What are the risk factors? Am J Obstet Gynecol 2002;186:311-314.
14. Pearlman MD, Tintinalli JE, Lorenza RP: Blunt trauma during pregnancy. N Engl J Med 1990;323:1609-1613.
15. Connolly AM, Katz VL, Bash KL, et al: Trauma and pregnancy. Am J Perinatol 1997;14:331-336.
16. Fuchs K, Peretz BA, Marcovici R, et al: The "grand multipara"—Is it a problem? A review of 5785 cases. Int J Gynaecol Obstet 1985;23:321-326.
17. Leung AS, Leung EK, Paul RH: Uterine rupture after previous cesarean delivery: Maternal and fetal consequences. Am J Obstet Gynecol 1993;169:945-950.
18. Deneux-Tharaux C, Berg C, Bouvier-Colle MH, et al: Underreporting of pregnancy-related mortality in the United States and Europe. Obstet Gynecol 2005;106:684-692.
19. Horon IL, Cheng D: Underreporting of pregnancy-associated deaths. Am J Public Health 2005;95:1879.
20. Horon IL: Underreporting of maternal deaths on death certificates and the magnitude of the problem of maternal mortality. Am J Public Health 2005;95:478-482.
21. Katz V, Balderston K, DeFreest M: Perimortem cesarean delivery: Were our assumptions correct? Am J Obstet Gyneco. 2005;192:1916-1920.
22. Kloeck W, Cummins RO, Chamberlain D, et al: Special resuscitation situations: An advisory statement from the International Liaison Committee on Resuscitation. Circulation 1997;95:2196-2210.
23. Whitten M, Irvine LM: Postmortem and perimortem caesarean section: What are the indications?. J R Soc Med 2000;93:6-9.
24. DePace NL, Betesh JS, Kotler MN: Postmortem cesarean section with recovery of both mother and offspring. JAMA 1982;248:971.
25. Marx GF: Cardiopulmonary resuscitation of the late pregnant woman. Anesthesiology 1982;56:156.
26. Katz VL, Dotters DJ, Droegemueller W. Perimortem cesarean delivery. Obstet Gynecol 1986;68:571.
27. American Heart Association Guidelines for Cardiopulmonary Resuscitation and Emergency Cardiovascular Care: Part 10.8: Cardiac arrest associated with pregnancy. Circulation 2005;112:IV150-IV153.
28. Rees GA, Willis BA: Resuscitation in late pregnancy. Anaesthesia 1988;43:347-349.
29. Clark SL, Hankins GD, Dudley DA, et al: Amniotic fluid embolism: Analysis of the national registry. Am J Obstet Gynecol 1995;172:1158-1169.
30. Morgan M: Amniotic fluid embolism. Anaesthesia 1979; 34:20-32.
31. Moore J, Baldisseri, MR: Amniotic fluid embolism. Crit Care Med 2005;33(10 Suppl):S279-S285.
32. Locksmith GJ: Amniotic fluid embolism. Obstet Gynecol Clin North Am 1999;26:435-444.
33. Azegami M, Mori N: Amniotic fluid embolism and leukotrienes. Am J Obstet Gynecol 1986;155:1119-1124.

Chapter 120

Postpartum Emergencies

Fiona E. Gallahue

KEY POINTS

The most common cause of infection after childbirth is a genital tract infection.

Because lochia will contaminate a clean-catch specimen between 4 and 8 weeks postpartum, urine should be obtained by catheterization in the postpartum period to rule out a urinary tract infection.

In the immediate postpartum period, an acute abdomen may not manifest with abdominal rigidity on examination due to the laxity of the abdominal wall tissue at this time.

Leukocytosis cannot be used to help differentiate an infection in the first 2 weeks postpartum due to the physiologic leukocytosis that occurs during pregnancy and delivery.

Fever is the most important criterion for the diagnosis of postpartum metritis.

Scope

Despite the fact that the first postpartum visit is generally scheduled at 6 weeks, most life-threatening complications arise within the first 3 weeks following delivery, and thus they are likely to be seen in the ED. These complications are primarily related to infection, hemorrhage, pregnancy-induced hypertension, and embolic events.[1,4] The most common complaints are fatigue (56%), breast problems (20%), backache (20%), depression (17%), hemorrhoids (15%), and headache (15%).[5]

Additionally, there is a high frequency of late maternal morbidity; up to 87% of women note problems in the during the first 6 weeks postpartum, and as many as 76% of these patients contine to have these problems for as long as 18 months following delivery.

The Puerperium

Originally the puerperium was defined as the period of confinement during and just after birth; now it is generally accepted to mean the 6 weeks after delivery. The puerperium has also been referred to as "the fourth trimester." This period is marked by multiple physiologic changes (Table 120-1) as the woman returns to the prepregnant state, including healing physically from any trauma from delivery, and adjusts to the many physiologic and psychological demands involved in caring for a newborn. Just as in pregnancy, when there are so many physiologic changes, the potential exists for the normal healing process to go awry and emergencies to occur.

Puerperal Fever and Infections

Puerperal fever is defined as a temperature of 38°C (100.4°F) or higher that occurs on any 2 of the first 10 days postpartum, exclusive of the first 24 hours, and which is taken orally by a standard technique at least four times daily.[2] The usual cause is a genital tract infection, which can lead to significant morbidity and mortality. Infection is one of the top five causes of mortality, causing approximately 13% of pregnancy-related deaths between 1991 and 1999.[4]

RED FLAGS

- Metritis should improve within 48 to 72 hours; failure to improve suggests complications such as parametrial phlegmon, pelvic or incisional abscess, infected hematoma, septic pelvic thrombitis, retained products of conception, or bacterial resistance.
- Central venous thrombosis, a rare occurrence usually presenting within 1 to 3 weeks postpartum, can be associated with throbbing headache (75%), a feeling of lethargy, subjective numbness, nonspecific weakness, mild elevations of body temperature, dehydration, polycythemia, and increased platelet counts and fibrinogen levels.
- Initial diagnosis of peripartum cardiomyopathy (PPCM) may be difficult to make and often presents with symptoms similar to amniotic fluid or pulmonary thromboembolism. Patients with PPCM are at high risk for thromboembolic events. Severe left ventricular dysfunction from PPCM results in blood stasis and may lead to left ventricular thrombi and subsequent emboli.
- Postpartum thyroiditis is associated with a period of transient hyperthyroidism occurring 2 to 6 months postpartum; symptoms include fatigue, palpitations, irritability, heat intolerance, and nervousness. These symptoms often are attributed to the stress of motherhood, and the correct diagnosis may be missed.
- Sterile pyuria and hematuria may be seen in appendicitis. The uterus is still enlarged for much of the puerperium, displacing the appendix upward toward the right upper quadrant and lifting the abdominal wall away from the inflamed appendix, which minimizes clinically apparent signs of peritoneal irritation.
- Patients with postpartum psychosis may have symptoms such as delusions, hallucinations, rapid mood swings, sleep disturbances, and obsessive thoughts about the baby. These patients require emergent hospitalization because approximately 5% commit suicide and 4% commit infanticide.

A small proportion of women will develop postpartum fever due to breast engorgement, but this rarely exceeds 39° C (102.2° F) in the first few postpartum days and usually lasts less than 24 hours.

The most common source of infection in the postpartum period is genital tract infection, but other sources must be eliminated, especially urinary tract infection and pneumonia. The puerperal bladder is prone to urine retention, especially after instrumental delivery and epidural analgesia; also, the dilation of the ureters and renal pelvis makes them potential sites of infection.

Mild hypoventilation post-delivery due to pain and/or limited ambulation predispose some women to pneumonia. Additionally, minor temperature elevations are occasionally caused by superficial or deep vein thrombosis of the lower extremities (Table 120-2).[1,2]

Tips and Tricks

- Because lochia will contaminate a clean-catch urine specimen during the first 30 to 60 days postpartum, a catheterized urine specimen should be obtained and sent to the laboratory to rule out urinary tract infection.
- The second most common cause of early postpartum bleeding is laceration of the reproductive tract. In some of these cases, areas of bleeding can be concealed, especially if the source is above the pelvic diaphragm; this condition is very uncomfortable and not always obvious on examination.
- Although 75% of deep venous thrombosis events occur antepartum, 66% of pulmonary thromboembolism events occur postpartum.
- Psoas, obturator, and Rovsing's signs are not predictive of appendicitis in pregnant and postpartum patients.

Uterine Infections (Metritis)

In the past, uterine infections had different names based on the assumed location of the infection; however, the accepted terminology is now *metritis* or *metritis with cellulitis,* because uterine infection often involves multiple tissue layers, usually the decidua as well as the myometrial and parametrial tissues.

The single most significant risk factor in the development of metritis is the route of delivery. Women who deliver by cesarean section have a 6% to 18% incidence of metritis compared with 0.9% to 3.9% in vaginal deliveries.[6,7] Other recognized risk factors for developing metritis are chorioamnionitis, anal sphincter laceration, prolonged rupture of membranes, and weight on admission of more than 200 pounds. The rates of metritis are lower now than in the past 2 decades due to the routine use of prophylactic antibiotics in cesarean deliveries.[2,6]

Symptoms of metritis are fever and abdominal pain. Fever (>38° C [100.4° F]) is the most important criterion for the diagnosis of metritis. Lochia may be foul-smelling or have no odor. Leukocytosis is often present but normally is elevated during the first 2 weeks postpartum. Chills may indicate bacteremia, which occurs in 10% to 20% of women with pelvic infection after cesarean delivery. Patients with mild metritis after being sent home following vaginal delivery can be treated with an oral microbial agent such as doxycycline or azithromycin. Patients with moderate to severe metritis as well as those who have delivered by cesarean section should be treated with broad-spectrum intravenous antibiotics to cover mixed flora and should be observed in the hospital (Table 120-3).

Table 120-1 PHYSIOLOGIC CHANGES IN THE PUERPERIUM

Immediately Following Delivery	By Postpartum Time*
Uterus palpable at umbilicus	By 2nd week, uterus has shrunk back into the pelvis; complete involution takes 6-8 weeks
Uterine blood flow via uterine artery = 500 – 600 mL/min	By 2nd week, uterine blood flow = 30-45 mL/min
Cardiac output and blood volume increased by 30% to 50%	By 2nd week, values are normalized to baseline
Breasts produce colostrums	By day 5, mature breast milk produced
Thyroid size and function increase	In 3 months, size of thyroid decreases; by 4th week, biochemical changes resolve (T_3,T_4, TSH are normalized)
Bladder has enlarged capacity and insensitivity to increased intravesicular pressure; renal pelvis and ureters dilated	2-3 months to return to normal
GFR increased	8 weeks to return to prepregnant GFR
Rectus abdominis muscles lengthened	3-4 weeks minimum to shorten; may be altered by exercise and overall baseline tone of mother
Leukocytosis	2 weeks to return to baseline
Fibrinogen level elevated	Increases on days 2-4; returns to normal levels by end of first week
Stretch marks	6-12 months; depigmentation occurs, never fully resolves
Thicker and fuller hair	3-4 months; delayed alopecia
Lower mean velocities of blood flow in the common femoral vein after cesarean section	6 weeks to return to baseline

*Approximate time.
GFR, glomerular filtration rate; T_3, triiodothyronine; T_4, thyroxine; TSH, thyroid-stimulating hormone;

Table 120-2 DIFFERENTIAL DIAGNOSIS OF POSTPARTUM FEVER

Most Common	Most Threatening
Metritis	Toxic shock syndrome
Urinary tract infection	Necrotizing fasciitis
Pneumonia	Pelvic phlegmon
Wound infection	Pelvic abscess
Mastitis	Peritonitis
Superficial or deep venous thrombosis	Septic pelvic thrombosis Breast abscess

Table 120-3 RECOMMENDED TREATMENT REGIMENS FOR METRITIS*

Regimen	Use
Clindamycin+gentamycin +ampicillin	First-line treatment; 90%-95% resolution rate
Clindamycin+aztreonam	Alternative regimen
Beta-lactam antimicrobials, semisynthetic penicillins, broad-spectrum second- and third-generation cephalosporins	Alternative regimen
Metronidazole+ampicillin +aminoglycoside	Alternative regimen
Imipenem+cilastatin	Reserved for the most serious infections

*90% cure rate.[2,7,8]

Most patients should improve within 48 to 72 hours, and failure to improve suggests a complication of metritis such as parametrial phlegmon, pelvic or incisional abscess, infected hematoma, septic pelvic thrombitis, retention of fetal parts, or bacteria resistant to the treatment regimen. Computed tomography or magnetic resonance imaging is recommended to confirm the diagnosis.

Complications of Infections

Toxic shock syndrome (TSS) is a rare but worrisome postpartum infection with a mortality of 10% to 15%. Group A *Streptococcus* and *Staphylococcus aureus* are the predominant causes of TSS. These bacteria colonize the mucosa of the vaginal tract and infect the postpartum uterus, cervix, and vagina, all of which are susceptible due to the trauma that accompanies delivery. Most cases of TSS occur in the first 8 weeks postpartum, but TSS can be seen up to week 10. Symptoms include fever of 39°C (102.2°F) or higher; erythematous diffuse rash; headache, photophobia, myalgias, and altered sensorium; gastrointestinal complaints including nausea, vomiting, and watery diarrhea; and rapid progression to renal failure, hepatic failure, disseminated intravascular coagulation, and circulatory collapse. Treatment includes aggressive fluid management with crystalloids, supportive care, and pressors as needed. Antibiotics do not alter the course of TSS, but they decrease the recurrence rate by 50%. An antistaphylococcal agent such as nafcillin, vancomycin, or cefazolin combined with an aminoglycoside such as gentamicin is appropriate.[8]

Complications of pelvic infections can be quite severe. If a patient with metritis does not respond to antibiotics after 48 to72 hours, there should be high suspicion for complications.

Wound infections are the most common cause of antimicrobial failure in women treated for metritis and are usually associated with fever around the fourth postoperative day in patients who deliver by cesarean section. Wound dehiscence, separation of the fascial layer, is a complication of incisional infections and is associated with fascial infection and tissue necrosis.

One of the most severe complications of a pelvic infection is necrotizing fasciitis. It has a devastatingly high mortality of approximately 50%, even with appropriate treatment, and may be a complication of a cesarean incision or episiotomy or perineal lacerations. Risk factors for necrotizing fasciitis are diabetes, obesity, and hypertension. Treatment includes clindamycin and a beta-lactam antimicrobial along with emergent operative debridement of the area.

Other complications include pelvic phlegmon, which is cellulitis that has extended to the broad ligament. These infections can extend into any blood collections that develop after a cesarean delivery, such as under the bladder flap, and cause an infected hematoma. If left untreated, a phlegmon can suppurate into an abscess. Pelvic abscesses can develop in the broad ligament, ovaries, rectovaginal septum, or psoas muscle. Treatment includes intravenous antibiotics and possible percutaneous drainage.

Peritonitis presents with severe abdominal pain but may be misdiagnosed because abdominal rigidity, guarding, or rebound tenderness often are not present on physical examination due to the laxity of the rectus abdominus muscles. Commonly, an adynamic ileus is the first presenting sign.

Infections can extend into the veins and cause septic pelvic thrombosis, which usually involves one or both ovarian venous plexuses and occurs more predominantly on the right due to the slightly longer vein on the right and dextrotorsion of the puerperal enlarged uterus. In 25% of patients, these clots extend into the inferior vena cava and occasionally into the renal veins. Heparin and intravenous antibiotics are currently the mainstay of therapy despite studies indicating that use of heparin does not alter outcome.

■ MASTITIS

Among women who breastfeed, mastitis is a common problem, usually peaking between the second and sixth postpartum weeks. Most often the mastitis is unilateral and is caused by infant oral bacterial flora and relative obstruction of a milk duct. The most commonly isolated organism is *Staphylococcus aureus*.

The affected breast appears hard and reddened, and the patient complains of severe pain. Ten percent of women with mastitis develop an abscess. Patients with breast abscesses may have constitutional symptoms of fevers, chills, or rigor along with fluctuance of the area. Ultrasonography can be useful in detecting an abscess.

First-line agents for treatment for mastitis are penicillin, cephalosporin, or erythromycin (for penicillin-sensitive patients); all are considered safe in the lactating woman. The infection should show improvement within 48 hours. Lack of improvement over this time period suggests an abscess or resistant organism. Abscesses require incision and drainage with packing or ultrasound-guided needle aspiration, which has a success rate of 80% to 90%.

If resistant organisms are suspected, a culture of the milk from the affected breast should be sent on a swab for testing, and the patient should be started on an antimicrobial agent effective against methicillin-resistant *Staphylococcus aureus* (MRSA) such as vancomycin. Continued breastfeeding on the affected side is important in order to help clear the infection. If the baby is having difficulty latching because of surrounding erythema/induration, the affected breast can be gently pumped. Patients should be referred for a follow-up visit within 72 hours to their primary care physician or gynecologist to ensure that they are responding to the prescribed medication.

Hemorrhagic Complications

Severe bleeding complications usually occur early in the puerperium. The most common cause of early postpartum hemorrhage is uterine atony. Because this complication usually presents immediately after delivery of the placenta, it is not likely to be seen in the ED unless the mother delivered at home or at a birth center without medical backup. Treatment of uterine atony is fundal massage or bimanual uterine elevation and compression, oxytocin (10 IU IV or intramuscularly [IM]) or methergine (0.2 mg IM) to contract the uterus, and emergent obstetrics department consultation. Additionally, 40 IU of oxytocin can be added to 1 liter normal saline and infused based on the severity of hemorrhage and patient response.

The second most common cause of early postpartum bleeding is vaginal or cervical laceration of the reproductive tract. Sometimes these areas of bleeding can be concealed, especially if the source is above the pelvic diaphragm, and can be very uncomfortable and not obvious on examination.

Delayed bleeding is the hemorrhagic complication most likely to be evaluated in the ED. Most cases of delayed postpartum hemorrhages are associated with infected retained placental fragments or membranes. A persistently patent cervix, especially if associated with bright red bleeding, should suggest retained products of conception. Treatment is broad-spectrum antibiotics and emergency obstetric consultation for dilation and curettage. Disseminated intravascular coagulation may occur in these cases and may require aggressive management with platelets, fresh frozen plasma, and packed red blood cells.[1]

A rare cause of hemorrhage (0.2 to 1 case per million) is an acquired hemophilia that usually presents within the first 3 months after delivery, occasionally as early as the first day postpartum. Mortality is 12% to 22% due to hemorrhage. Of these patients, 54% have other previously diagnosed immune system diseases such as rheumatoid arthritis, systemic lupus erythematosus, and inflammatory bowel diseases. A prolonged partial thromboplastin time with a normal prothrombin time localizes the coagulation defect in the intrinsic pathway of the coagulatory cascade, suggesting hemophilia as the cause of hemorrhage. This finding should prompt a hematology consultation. Currently, no universally accepted protocol exists in the care of these patients but immunosuppressive drugs and plasmapheresis have shown benefit. In most of these cases, there is spontaneous remission of the acquired hemophilia within months of delivery.[9]

Thromboembolic Complications

Certain significant changes in the physiology of the coagulation system during pregnancy persist past delivery and into the puerperium. These include major changes in the coagulation and fibrinolytic system as well as a reduction in venous blood flow in the deep venous system. Combined, these alterations increase the thrombotic potential in near-term and immediate postpartum patients.

In the general population, the incidence of pregnancy-induced venous thromboembolism is approximately 1 in 1500 deliveries. The risk of venous thromboembolism is five times higher in a pregnant than in a nonpregnant patient. Although 75% of deep venous thrombosis cases occur antepartum, 66% of cases of pulmonary thromboembolism occur postpartum.[10,11] The majority of deaths due to venous thromboembolism occur during the first 2 weeks of the puerperium, but a significant number of these events occur 2 to 6 weeks after delivery.[10]

The pregnant patient around term and immediately postpartum has significant increases in factors I, V, VII, IX, X, and XII, von Willebrand factor antigen, and ristocetin co-factor activity. The endogenous anticoagulants protein C and antithrombin remain unchanged throughout pregnancy but there is a reduction in protein S. Fibrinolytic activity is impaired during pregnancy due to placentally derived plasminogen activator inhibitor type II, and pregnancy-induced increases (approximately threefold) of endothelial and hepatic-derived inhibitor of plasminogen activator type I. These changes rapidly return to normal following delivery.

During normal pregnancy, there is a significant reduction of blood flow to the deep venous system as well as an increase in diameter of the major leg veins. These changes do not occur evenly in both legs. Studies of patients in the puerperium have reported greater diameter and slower blood flow in the left common femoral vein than the right. These differences are manifested clinically; in nonpregnant patients, the left leg was affected in 55% of cases of deep venous thrombosis, whereas in pregnancy the rate is 85%. Mode of delivery also affects the deep venous system. Women who delivered by cesarean section had lower mean velocities of blood flow in the common femoral vein during the puerperium compared with those who had delivered vaginally. These changes in flow velocity and diameter take 6 weeks to return to baseline. Another significant clinical difference seen in pregnant and immediate postpartum patients is that the majority of deep venous thrombosis events seen during this time occur in the iliofemoral segments, rather than in the calf veins, and therefore are more likely to result in pulmonary thromboembolism. Additional underlying risk factors that increase the likelihood of thrombotic complications are age older than 35 years, delivery by cesarean section, weight greater than 175 lb, and family or personal history of thrombosis and thrombophilia (protein C or S deficiency, factor V Leiden).

The index of suspicion for venous thromboembolism should remain high because although complaints of dyspnea, tachypnea, leg swelling, and leg discomfort are common at term, they may also indicate pulmonary or deep venous thrombosis. One study found that approximately 24% of women who developed deep venous thrombosis during pregnancy or the puerperium were asymptomatic, and 55% complained of isolated leg swelling.[10]

Diagnosis of deep venous thrombosis is best done by duplex ultrasonography, because no radiation is involved; if the diagnosis is still uncertain, ultrasonography can be repeated or venography can be performed. To confirm the diagnosis of pulmonary thromboembolism, ventilation-perfusion lung scan or spiral computed tomography can be performed safely in patients in the puerperium. Treatment for the postpartum patient is unfractionated or low-molecular-weight heparin and transition to coumadin, which is safe in the lactating patient because it does not significantly cross over into breast milk.[10,12]

Neurologic embolic events such as cerebral embolism and cerebral venous thrombosis can also occur in the puerperium. Cerebral embolism usually involves the middle cerebral artery and is commonly associated with a cardiac arrhythmia, especially from atrial fibrillation associated with rheumatic heart disease. However, these emboli may also be associated with rheumatic heart disease without arrhythmia, mitral valve prolapse, and infective endocarditis. Management is supportive care and consideration of anticoagulation.

Central venous thrombosis is a rare occurrence in developed countries, with an incidence of 1 in 11,000 to 45,000 patients. Usually presenting within 1 to 3 weeks postpartum and located in the lateral or superior sagittal venous sinus, it has a high mortality—between 10% and 30%.[13] Central venous thrombosis is associated with preeclampsia, sepsis, thrombophilias, and thyrotoxicosis. Headache, typically described as "throbbing," is the most common presenting symptom, occurring in 73% of cases; 10% of patients will have seizures. Patients may also describe feelings of lethargy, subjective numbness, and nonspecific weakness. There may be mild elevations of body temperature, dehydration, polycythemia, and increased platelet counts and fibrinogen levels. A prior history of prothrombotic conditions, hypertension in pregnancy, or dehydration should raise the index of suspicion for central venous thrombosis. Magnetic resonance imaging or angiography is the test of choice for diagnosis. Management includes anticonvulsants to control seizures, emergent neurology consultation, and antimicrobials if septic thrombosis is suspected. Heparin therapy is controversial because spontaneous bleeding may develop.[2,13]

Cardiac Complications

■ PERIPARTUM CARDIOMYOPATHY

Peripartum cardiomyopathy is a rare disorder that occurs in 1 of every 3000 to 4000 pregnancies in the United States, but it is a potentially fatal complication in the puerperium. The diagnostic criteria include onset of heart failure in the last month of pregnancy or in the first 5 months postpartum; absence of determinable cause for cardiac failure; absence of a demonstrable heart disease before the last month of pregnancy; and impairment of left ventricular systolic function as demonstrated by echocardiography. The cause of peripartum cardiomyopathy is not known. Multiparity, twin births, advanced maternal age (>30 years), preeclampsia or eclampsia, hypertension, use of tocolytic therapy, and African descent are documented risk factors. The mortality of peripartum cardiomyopathy ranges from 25% to 90%.[16] Survival is largely dependent on recovery of left ventricular function. If recovery does occur, it usually does so within 6 months.

Patients who fail to recover within 6 months may require cardiac transplantation. The patients who undergo transplantation have a 30% higher rate of early rejection than patients with idiopathic cardiomyopathy, but survival at 2 years is 86%.[17,18] Without transplantation, patients with persistent or progressive cardiomyopathy have a 5-year mortality rate approaching 50%.

Clinical signs and symptoms include fatigue, dyspnea, cough, orthopnea, hemoptysis, chest pain, palpitations, abdominal pain, tachycardia, elevated blood pressure, pulmonary rales, third heart sound, mitral regurgitant murmur, and peripheral edema. Symptoms often are similar to those of thromboembolus.

Initial diagnostic evaluation includes electrocardiography, plain chest radiography, serum tests (electrolytes, liver function panel, complete blood count) and urinalysis. The electrocardiogram may be normal or tachycardic, may show nonspecific ST or T-wave changes, atrial or ventricular dysrhythmias, left ventricular hypertrophy, PR or QRS prolongation, and conduction disturbances. Plain chest radiography usually shows cardiomegaly with pulmonary venous congestion and occasionally pleural effusion.

The diagnostic study of choice is echocardiography because it can be performed at the bedside, presents no radiation risks to the pregnant patient, can differentiate between a pulmonary embolism and amniotic embolism, and can provide prognostic information based on the degree of left ventricular dysfunction. The biggest drawback often is lack of availability in the ED.

Patients with peripartum cardiomyopathy are at especially high risk for thromboembolic events because of severe left ventricular dysfunction that results in blood stasis that may lead to left ventricular thrombi and subsequent emboli.

Treatment is the same as that for nonischemic dilated cardiomyopathy unless the well-being of the fetus is an issue. Management should be supportive with sodium (no more than 4 g daily of salt) and fluid (no more than 2 liters daily fluid intake) restriction. Preload and afterload reducing agents plus positive inotropic agents, if the patient is acutely ill, are the cornerstones of treatment. For the antepartum patient, afterload reduction can be accomplished with hydralazine; positive inotropy with digoxin; and preload reduction with diuretics, nitroglycerine, and beta-blockers; however, diuretics can cause dehydration and beta-blockers are associated with low birth weight in infants, so they must be used with caution. Postpartum patients should receive angiotensin-converting enzyme inhibitor therapy, which has been shown to improve survival in patients with dilated cardiomyopathies.[17] The breastfeeding mother should curtail breastfeeding because angiotensin-converting enzyme inhibitors are excreted in breast milk and their safety is unproved.[12,16]

Endocrine Disorders

■ SHEEHAN'S SYNDROME

This syndrome of pituitary ischemia and necrosis associated with obstetric blood loss, first described in 1937, is an extremely rare occurrence in the developed world, now that hemorrhage and shock are managed aggressively.

■ THYROIDITIS

Postpartum thyroiditis is a usually self-limited autoimmune disorder marked by the development of postpartum thyroid dysfunction that occurs up to 9 months following delivery. Classically, a period of transient hyperthyroidism occurs between postpartum months 2 and 6, followed by a transient hypothyroid stage, with a return to the euthyroid state by 1 year postpartum. Incidence ranges from 1.1% to 16.7%.

Risk factors include presence of thyroid antibodies, a previous episode of postpartum thyroiditis, type 1 diabetes mellitus, and a positive family history of thyroid disease. These patients have an increased risk of developing permanent hypothyroidism in the following 5 to 10 years. Diagnosis is based on thyroid-stimulating hormone (TSH) levels and free triiodothyronine (T_3) and thyroxine (T_4) levels.

During the *hyperthyroid* state of postpartum thyroiditis, TSH is suppressed and free T_3 and T_4 levels are elevated. Symptoms include fatigue, palpitations, irritability, heat intolerance, and nervousness. Many of these symptoms are often attributed to the stresses of motherhood, and diagnosis is often missed. During the *hypothyroid* state, TSH is elevated with suppressed levels of free T_3 and T_4. Symptoms include impaired concentration, carelessness, lack of energy, poor memory, dry skin, cold intolerance, and aches and pains.

Most women in the hyperthyroid stage need no treatment or intervention. Symptomatic patients in this stage usually can be managed with beta-blockers and referral to an endocrinologist. The hypothyroid stage is multifactorial, and management is more difficult; these patients should also be referred to an endocrinologist for long-term follow-up. Patients with a TSH greater than 10 mU/L or who are symptomatic with a TSH between 4 and 10 mU/L should be treated with levothyroxine. Women who are planning to get pregnant again should be cautioned to wait until they have discussed the issue with an endocrinologist because even subclinical hypothyroidism can cause an increased miscarriage rate and may result in impaired cognitive performance in the child.[19]

Gastrointestinal and Abdominal Pain

Abdominal pain is a common complaint in the puerperium. In fact, one questionnaire given to women 48 hours after vaginal delivery noted that 50% of primiparous and 86% of multiparous women complained of lower abdominal pain.[20]

Abdominal pain can be a difficult complaint to evaluate in the postpartum patient and requires a higher level of suspicion for a surgical emergency or infectious or thrombotic complications. Because patients expect to experience a certain amount of pain and discomfort after delivery, they often present late to the ED with these symptoms. During the preliminary ED evaluation, it may be difficult for the EP to assess these patients, and the proper diagnosis may be further delayed.

■ APPENDICITIS

In puerperal patients with appendicitis, peritoneal tenderness, because of the laxity of the rectus abdominis muscles following pregnancy, may not be present; the uterus is still enlarged for much of the puerperium, displacing the appendix upward toward the right upper quadrant and lifting the abdominal wall away from an inflamed appendix, minimizing clinically apparent signs of peritoneal irritation. Psoas, obturator, and Rovsing's signs are not predictive of appendicitis in pregnant and postpartum women. Other tests have been suggested such as Bryan's sign (pain elicited by movement of the enlarged uterus to the right) for appendicitis and Alder's test (maintaining constant pressure at the area of maximum tenderness while the patient rolls from a supine position to the left side) to differentiate pain of intrauterine origin (which diminishes as the uterus falls away with the maneuver) from pain of extrauterin origin. The sensitivity and specificity of these tests are unknown.

The incidence of appendicitis is not increased during the puerperium, although outcome is poorer due to delayed diagnosis. The incidence of certain pathologies such as obstruction, ileus, acute cholecystitis and perihepatitis, and Fitz-Hugh-Curtis syndrome (often misdiagnosed as acute cholecystitis) *is* increased during this period. Postpartum ileus is usually associated with cesarean section; other obstructions may occur more frequently due to compression of the enlarged uterus. Perihepatitis is often a sequela of latent or asymptomatic infection. Ovarian cysts and torsion need to be ruled out in the differential diagnosis, as well as complications of metritis and urinary tract infections.

Evaluation tools include a careful pelvic examination with appropriate cultures to rule out infection of the genital tract, a catheterized urine specimen to avoid contamination with lochia for urinalysis and culture, and standardized laboratory values such as electrolytes, liver function tests, serum amylase, and a complete blood count. In puerperal patients with appendicitis, urinalysis may show a sterile pyuria of more than 5 white blood cells per high-power field, and 15% to 30% of these patients have hematuria because of the proximity of the inflamed appendix to the ureter. The white blood cell count is difficult to interpret in the puerperal patient because of the leukocytosis that normally occurs during the first 2 weeks of the puerperium.

Radiographic findings typically are nonspecific. Ultrasonography is useful to identify uterine, adnexal, ovarian, pelvic, or hepatobiliary abnormalities and may diagnose appendicitis. Contrast computed tomography is better for identifying appendicitis and complications of metritis such as septic pelvic thrombophlebitis.[3,21]

Genitourinary Complications

■ PERINEAL PAIN

Although some discomfort is to be expected post-delivery due to the disruption and distention of the birth canal soft tissues, painful perineal tissues are a significant issue for many women. In fact, perineal pain was noted by 42% of recently delivered women to be a significant problem in the first 2 weeks following delivery, and as might be expected, this number was higher in patients with assisted vaginal deliveries (84%). By 8 weeks postpartum this number was down to 22%, by 12 weeks to approximately 7%.[5]

Early application of cold compresses or ice packs to soft tissue trauma reduces swelling and discomfort. Sitz baths are also recommended to alleviate discomfort. Acetaminophen or nonsteroidal antiinflammatory drugs (generally considered safe in breastfeeding patients) are initial medications of choice for pain.

Careful examination is required for these patients, especially those with persistent and significant discomfort, to look for evidence of hematoma formation, abscess, or genital tract infections such as cellulitis and necrotizing fasciitis.

■ URINARY TRACT DYSFUNCTION

The puerperal bladder is predisposed to some urinary retention as well as urinary tract infections especially in patients who had instrumentation or prolonged labor in delivery, as well as epidural or spinal analgesia. In the immediate postpartum period, the bladder has an increased capacity and relative insensitivity to increased intravesical pressure. The ureteral and renal pelvic dilation seen in late pregnancy take approximately 2 to 3 months to resolve. These factors, combined with the stasis of urine, create an excellent environment for development of a urinary tract infection.

Any patient with complaint of urinary retention should have a catheterized urinalysis and culture sent the laboratory to rule out urinary tract infection. Most patients with urinary retention will note incomplete voiding and will not require catheterization, but they should be referred to the urology or urogynecology department for urodynamic testing.

Stress urinary incontinence is another complaint that occurs in the postpartum period. The ED usually lacks the facilities to address this complaint, but these patients should be referred to the urology or urogynecology department for work-up and management.

Lactation and Breast Dysfunction

■ BREAST ENGORGEMENT

Milk leakage, engorgement, and breast pain peak at 3 to 5 days postpartum. During the state of engorgement, breast pain can be partially alleviated by a supportive brassiere or breast binder, avoidance of nipple stimulation, ice packs, and oral analgesics.[1,2]

■ GALACTOCELE

A milk duct can be clogged by inspissated secretions or milk. This may form a fluctuant mass and resultant pain. Warm compresses may help the situation resolve spontaneously, but if there is a large amount of pain and fluctuance, needle aspiration may be required.

Neurologic Complications

■ HEADACHES

Headache is a common complaint in the postpartum patient; it has been noted to occur in the first 2 weeks after delivery by about 14% of patients. The differential diagnosis of the cause of headache is extensive, and certain life-threatening complications need to be excluded such as central venous thrombosis, meningitis, and intracranial bleeding from an undiagnosed aneurysm or arteriovenous malformation. The patient's personal and medical history is of the greatest importance to aid in diagnosis, because it may suggest an etiology such as migraine, postdural puncture headache, or pneumocephalus.

The pain from pneumocephalus associated with epidural anesthesia usually is immediately noted as back pain at the level of the needle insertion, spreading to the posterior neck and then to occipital and frontal areas. Generally, this complication, which occurs when the patient is in labor, resolves with supportive care, and the patient has no neurologic deficits.

Postdural puncture headaches also are associated with epidural anesthesia. This is a "nonthrobbing" headache that is worsened on change of posture from a horizontal to an upright position. These headaches are postulated to be caused by a persistent loss of cerebrospinal fluid at a dural puncture site. Up to 90% of these headaches begin within 3 days of the procedure. Auditory and ocular symptoms may occur with prolonged or severe presentation. Hydration and analgesic agents are the first-line agents of choice. If these measures fail, consultation with the anesthesiology department to consider an epidural blood patch is recommended.[13]

Psychiatric Complications

Fatigue is one of the most common complaints during the puerperium. Some fatigue is normal, given the demands of taking care of a newborn infant after

PATIENT TEACHING TIPS

- After starting antibiotics for mastitis, improvement should be seen by 48 to 72 hours; if the condition does not improve or worsens, an abscess or resistant organism may be the cause of the infection, and reevaluation is necessary.
- Patients with mastitis should be instructed to continue breastfeeding on the affected side in order to help clear the infection.
- To avoid complications in a second pregnancy, patients with hypothyroidism should not get pregnant again until management of the disorder is successful and cleared by an endocrinologist.
- Patients with abdominal pain should be counseled on the difficulty of making intraabdominal diagnoses in the puerperium and should have clear follow-up and return visit instructions.
- Patients with postpartum blues should be reassured that this is normal and usually resolves within a few days. If there is no improvement in their symptoms by the end of a week, they should be reevaluated either in the ED or by a psychiatrist.

the physical rigors of labor and delivery; however, this complaint should be taken seriously, because this can be the first symptom of anemia, new-onset diabetes, hypothyroidism, or a psychiatric disorder.

The most common postpartum mood disturbance is the postpartum blues, which affects 50% to 80% of new mothers. Symptoms include mild depression, irritability, confusion, mood instability, anxiety, headache, fatigue, and forgetfulness. Usually the postpartum blues appear in the first 2 weeks after delivery and last from a few hours to a few days. Although this is generally a self-limited and benign condition, patients should be evaluated for personal or family history of depression as well as the strength of their social support structure. Patients with postpartum blues should be referred to their primary care physicians for follow-up. Those with risk factors for a major depressive episode (see the following paragraph) should be educated about signs and symptoms of major depression and encouraged to seek help if they experience these symptoms.

More severe than postpartum blues is postpartum depression. Up to 20% of women with postpartum blues will have a major depressive episode in the first postnatal year. Multiple risk factors have been identified for postpartum depression: personal or family history of depression, prior episode of postpartum depression, depression or anxiety during pregnancy, an unplanned or unwanted pregnancy, recent stressful life events, poor social support, and marital discord. Neonatal infant medical problems or occurrence of postpartum blues also increases the risk for postpartum depression.

Documentation

- Mode of delivery is an important factor in puerperium complications; delivery by cesarean section has higher rates of infection as well as of other disorders. Note method of delivery, pregnancy and delivery complications, and associated risk factors.
- Document social support for patient and infant.
- Give and record instructions about potential complications.
- Patients with abdominal pain are at increased risk for complications; provide clear instructions on where and when follow-up should be carried out, list reasons to return to the ED, and discuss potential causes of abdominal pain.
- In patients with headache in the first 3 postpartum weeks, document timing of headache, worsening on change of position, and quality of headache.

Usually beginning within the first 4 weeks after delivery, postpartum depression is highly variable in severity and duration. It occurs in 5% to 20% of new mothers and is especially prevalent in adolescent mothers. The diagnosis of depression is difficult to make in a postpartum mother because the typical signs and symptoms have significant overlap with normal issues of the puerperium such as disturbances in sleep, weight, and energy. These patients require psychiatric evaluation and follow-up.

The most severe form of psychiatric disease in the postpartum period is postpartum psychosis. Fortunately this is a rare condition occurring in less than 2 of every 1000 deliveries. The onset of postpartum psychosis usually is within the first 3 weeks after delivery, and occasionally within a few days after delivery. Many of these patients have a history of schizophrenia or bipolar disorder. Symptoms include delusions, hallucinations, rapid mood swings, sleep disturbances, and obsessive thoughts about the baby. Patients with postpartum psychosis require emergent hospitalization because 5% of these women patients commit suicide and 4% commit infanticide.[22]

REFERENCES

1. Varner MW: Medical conditions of the puerperium. Clin Perinatol 1998;25:403-416.
2. Cunningham FG, Hauth JC, Leveno KJ, et al (eds): Williams' Obstetrics, 22nd ed. New York, McGraw-Hill, 2005.
3. Brennan DF, Harwood-Nuss AL: Postpartum abdominal pain. Ann Emerg Med 1989;18:83-89.
4. Chang J, Elam-Evans LD, Berg CJ, et al: Pregnancy-related mortality surveillance—United States, 1991-1999. MMWR Surveill Summ 2003;52:1-8.
5. Glazene CM, Abdalla M, Stroud P, et al: Postnatal maternal morbidity: Extent, causes, prevention and treatment. Br J Obstet Gynaecol 1995;102:282-287.
6. Burrows LJ, Meyn LA, Weber AM: Maternal morbidity associated with vaginal versus cesarean delivery. Obstet Gynecol 2004;103:907-912.

7. Normand MC, Damato EG: Postcesarean infection. J Obstet Gynecol Neonatal Nurs 2001;30:642-648.
8. Davis D, Gash-Kim TL, Heffernan EJ: Toxic shock syndrome: Case report of a postpartum female and a literature review. J Emerg Med 1998;16:607-614.
9. Grio R, Smirne C, Leotta E, et al: Acquired post-partum hemophilia. Panminerva Med 2004;46:201-203.
10. Greer IA: The special case of venous thromboembolism in pregnancy. Haemostasis 1998;28(Suppl 3):22-34.
11. Pabinger I, Grafenhofer H: Pregnancy-associated thrombosis. Wien Klin Wochenschr 2003;115:482-484.
12. American Academy of Pediatrics Committee on Drugs: Transfer of drugs and other chemicals into human milk. Pediatrics 2001;108:776-789.
13. Ponder TM: Differential diagnosis of postdural puncture headache in the parturient. CRNA 1999;10:145-154.
14. Felz MW, Barnes DB, Figueroa RE: Late postpartum eclampsia 16 days after delivery: Case report with clinical, radiologic, and pathophysiologic correlations. J Am Board Fam Pract 2000;13:39-46.
15. Sibai BM, Coppage KH: Diagnosis and management of women with stroke during pregnancy/postpartum. Clin Perinatol 2004;31:853-868, viii.
16. Chan L, Hill D: ED echocardiography for peripartum cardiomyopathy. Am J Emerg Med 1999;17:578-580.
17. Mehta NJ, Mehta RN, Khan IA: Peripartum cardiomyopathy: clinical and therapeutic aspects. Angiology 2001; 52:759-762.
18. Cole WC, Mehta JB, Roy TM, et al: Peripartum cardiomyopathy: Echocardiogram to predict prognosis. Tenn Med 2001;94:135-138.
19. Stagnaro-Green A: Postpartum thyroiditis. Best Pract Res Clin Endocrinol Metab 2004;18:303-316.
20. Murray A, Holdcroft A: Incidence and intensity of postpartum lower abdominal pain. BMJ 1989;298(6688):1619.
21. Munro A, Jones PF: Abdominal surgical emergencies in the puerperium. Br Med J 1975;4(5998):691-694.
22. Newport DJ, Hostetter A, Arnold A, et al: The treatment of postpartum depression: Minimizing infant exposures. J Clin Psychiatry 2002;63(Suppl 7):31-44.

Chapter 121

Gynecologic Pain and Vaginal Bleeding

Colleen Roche

KEY POINTS

The possibility of pregnancy must be assessed in every patient with either vaginal bleeding or pelvic pain.

Abnormal vaginal bleeding may be a sign of malignancy, chronic disease, or sexual abuse.

With the exception of physiologic withdrawal bleeding in the neonate, vaginal bleeding is always abnormal in the prepubescent female.

Patients with ovarian torsion may have normal ultrasound findings in up to 50% of cases.

Dysfunctional uterine bleeding is a diagnosis of exclusion.

Postmenopausal women who have new onset vaginal bleeding must be evaluated for cancer.

Ectopic pregnancy, acute appendicitis, and ovarian torsion must be ruled out in every patient with acute pelvic pain.

Scope

Vaginal bleeding and pelvic pain are relatively common complaints in women presenting to the ED. When approaching a patient with vaginal bleeding and/or pelvic pain, it is essential to determine if the patient is pregnant. When caring for any woman of childbearing age, pregnancy and pregnancy-related pathologies must be considered, such as ectopic pregnancy and placental abruption. Vaginal bleeding and pelvic pain in the pregnant patient are discussed in Chapters 116, 118, and 119; this chapter is focused solely on vaginal bleeding and pelvic pain in the nonpregnant female.

Vaginal bleeding may occur in women of all ages, from infancy into the postmenopausal years. The normal menstrual cycle ranges from 21 to 35 days and lasts from 2 to 6 days. The average volume exuded in a normal menstrual cycle is 20 to 60 mL per cycle, although it has been found that patients cannot adequately estimate the amount of their menses. Normal menstrual blood does not clot.

Pelvic pain uncommonly occurs concurrently with vaginal bleeding in the nonpregnant patient. Pelvic pain in nonpregnant women may be indicative of either an acute or a chronic process. Pelvic pain tends to affect women of childbearing age more than women at the extremes of age. Pelvic pain can occur in postmenopausal women but is often a late finding of a more insidious disease process such as cancer. Noninfectious causes of pelvic pain are discussed in this chapter.

Structure and Function

The female reproductive system is controlled by the hypothalamic-pituitary-ovarian axis. The hypothalamus releases gonadotropin-releasing hormone (GnRH), which affects the pituitary gland to release follicle-stimulating hormone (FSH) and luteinizing hormone (LH). Both FSH and LH act on the ovaries in a feedback loop to control the amount of estrogen and progesterone produced by the ovaries themselves. Estrogen and progesterone production are ultimately responsible for the proper functioning of the female reproductive tract.

The normal female reproductive cycle is 28 days, although it ranges from 21 to 35 days. Days 1 to 14 are known as the follicular or proliferative phase. During this time, FSH levels increase, allowing a dominant ovarian follicle to mature and produce estrogen. The initial increase in estrogen halts menstruation from the previous cycle. As estrogen levels increase, the endometrium begins to thicken and stabilize, and gives positive feedback to the pituitary gland to release LH. LH stimulates ovulation on day 14. Days 14 to 28 comprise the luteal or secretory phase. The corpus luteum that remains in the ovaries after ovulation then begin to secrete progesterone, which halts proliferation of the endometrium. If implantation does not occur, the corpus luteum involutes, estrogen and progesterone levels drop markedly, and menstruation occurs.

This highly orchestrated process requires that each individual component functions properly. Any irregularities or pathology of either the hypothalamic-pituitary-ovarian axis or the female reproductive tract can lead to abnormal vaginal bleeding and can contribute to pelvic pain. Table 121-1 lists common terminology and definitions associated with abnormal vaginal bleeding.

Clinical Presentation

In the evaluation of a patient presenting to the ED with vaginal bleeding or pelvic pain, careful history and a complete physical examination can narrow the differential diagnosis significantly and can accurately delineate the diagnosis. Acute trauma, infection, and systemic disorders may be properly diagnosed without further testing. The Documentation box lists important aspects of the history necessary to the proper care of a nonpregnant patient with vaginal bleeding or pelvic pain.

Presenting Signs and Symptoms

PELVIC PAIN

Women may present to the ED with either acute or chronic pelvic pain. Acute pelvic pain may be secondary to life-threatening or organ-threatening processes and requires prompt attention. Chronic pelvic pain is usually indicative of a more indolent process

Documentation

- Age of patient
- Onset and duration of symptoms
- History of prior pregnancies
- Duration and frequency of past periods
- Number of sexual partners
- Contraception methods
- Presence of postcoital bleeding
- History of previous abnormal Papanicolaou (PAP) smears
- History of previous or sexually transmitted diseases or pelvic infections
- History of past or present exogenous hormone utilization
- Recent trauma
- Associated symptoms including fever, breast changes, anorexia, vomiting, weight fluctuation, hirsutism, and bowel or bladder changes
- Past medical and surgical history
- Medication history

Table 121-1 COMMON TERMINOLOGY AND DEFINITIONS

Terminology	Definition
Amenorrhea	Cessation of menses for >6 months
Dysmenorrhea	Pain associated with menses
Hypomenorrhea	Menstrual volumes <20 mL/cycle
Menometrorrhagia	Prolonged or heavy bleeding at irregular intervals
Menorrhagia	Menses >80 mL/cycle or occurring for >6 days
Metrorrhagia	Vaginal bleeding between menstrual cycles; irregular cycles
Oligomenorrhea	Decreased frequency of menstrual cycles; >35 days between cycles
Polymenorrhea	Increased frequency of menstrual cycles; <21 days between cycles
Postmenopausal bleeding	Bleeding occurring 6 to 12 months after menopause

such as abnormal scarring or cancer. This chapter addresses more common causes of pelvic pain in a nonpregnant female. Infectious etiologies of pelvic pain are addressed in Chapter 123.

■ VAGINAL BLEEDING

Vaginal bleeding occasionally can be mistaken for urinary or rectal bleeding, and it is important to make that distinction through the history and physical examination.

Differential Diagnosis

■ VAGINAL BLEEDING

The most common causes of abnormal vaginal bleeding in the nonpregnant patient are uterine leiomyomas and dysfunctional uterine bleeding. Box 121-1 lists the differential diagnoses of vaginal bleeding in the nonpregnant patient.

■ Trauma

Vaginal bleeding can be the result of injuries to the female genitalia by either blunt or penetrating trauma. These injuries occur from childhood through adulthood. Pain of the external genitalia often is pronounced, and patients may even avoid urination because of the associated pain.

Blunt injuries to the external genitalia, such as straddle injuries, commonly result in lacerations of the labia majora and minora. Less common injuries include vulvar hematomas and lacerations of the posterior fourchette. Bleeding is often self-limited, but further intervention may be warranted.

Hymenal and vaginal injuries are not related to blunt trauma and indicate a penetrating mechanism. These injuries are often attributed to consensual sexual practices, but the possibility of sexual abuse should be explored in every patient. Hymenal or vaginal lacerations in a minor should always suggest sexual abuse, and further investigation is paramount.

BOX 121-1

Differential Diagnosis of Vaginal Bleeding in Nonpregnant Females

Trauma
- Direct trauma, foreign bodies

Infection
- Vaginitis, cervicitis, endometritis

Dysfunctional Uterine Bleeding
- Ovulatory, anovulatory

Benign Abnormalities
- Uterine leiomyomas, polyps

Malignancy
- Vulvar, vaginal, cervical, uterine, ovarian

Systemic Disease
- See Table 121-2

Medication Effects
- See Box 121-2

■ Vaginal Foreign Body

Mild vaginal bleeding may be the only presenting sign in a patient with a retained vaginal foreign body. Vaginal foreign bodies can lead to vaginal bleeding due to direct trauma, local irritation, and/or superimposed infections. Females are often aware that they have a retained vaginal foreign body, although some are not, and a thorough speculum examination may be warranted. Previously unrecognized vaginal foreign bodies are often discovered in both minors and adults with psychiatric illnesses. The two most common retained foreign bodies are toilet tissue (minors) and tampons, although a wide range of retained vaginal foreign bodies have been recognized. Despite the fact that children tend to place foreign bodies in novel places, the presence of vaginal foreign bodies in a minor should prompt a serious consideration of sexual abuse.

■ Infection

Although patients with vaginal and pelvic infections may present initially with vaginal bleeding, this symptom rarely exists in isolation. Patients often have a concurrent vaginal discharge and may even have pelvic pain or fever depending on the extent of the infection.

Sexually active women with vaginal infections can have mild vaginal bleeding from the local inflammatory process. This mild bleeding is most often linked to *Trichomonas* infection and is self-limited. Examination often reveals inflammation of the vaginal walls and a friable cervix.

■ Dysfunctional Uterine Bleeding

Dysfunctional uterine bleeding is the most common cause of menorrhagia (excessive uterine bleeding) in menstruating females. It can be ovulatory or anovulatory.

Ovulatory dysfunctional uterine bleeding is less common than anovulatory dysfunctional uterine bleeding and is secondary to abnormalities of uterine hemostasis regulated through cytokine and prostaglandin production. Patients with ovulatory dysfunctional uterine bleeding present with increased menstrual flow, but it occurs at expected intervals.

Anovulatory dysfunctional uterine bleeding occurs when ovulation has failed. This can be due to a disruption in the hypothalamic-pituitary-ovarian axis or to systemic disease. Primary ovarian disorders, most notably polycystic ovarian disease, are associated with anovulation. When ovulation fails to occur, progesterone is not produced, and the uterine lining is exposed to an unopposed estrogen supply. Eventually, the endometrium outgrows its vascular supply and degenerates, leading to irregular menses with flow alternating between heavy and scanty. Blood loss may be extreme and patients may present with signs and symptoms of hypovolemia and anemia.

Anovulatory dysfunctional uterine bleeding is most common in post-pubescent females, secondary to immaturity of hypothalamic function. As the hypothalamic function develops, the menses ultimately are regulated.

Women of reproductive age can experience anovulatory cycles secondary to extreme weight fluctuations, exercise, or stress. Anovulatory cycles can occur in perimenopausal women as well but can be indistinguishable in the ED from more pathologic etiologies such as endometrial cancer.

Benign Uterine Abnormalities

Polyps

Women may present to the ED with vaginal bleeding secondary to benign uterine or cervical polyps. This painless vaginal bleeding is often seen in women of reproductive age shortly after intercourse, secondary to direct trauma. Whereas cervical polyps usually are easily visualized on examination, uterine polyps may not be. Polyps rarely become malignant, and bleeding is self-limited.

Uterine Leiomyomas (Fibroids)

One of the most common causes of menorrhagia is uterine leiomyomas. These benign tumors develop from the myometrium and distort the normal contour of the endometrium. The resulting increase in the surface area of the endometruim results in greater menstrual volumes.

Patients with uterine leiomyomas often have a history of menorrhagia over several months to years. These benign tumors typically are discovered in the fourth decade of life and are most prevalent in black females. Patients may experience pain from uterine cramping or infarction (resulting from the tumor outgrowing its blood supply or twisting and cutting off the blood supply). On examination, these tumors often cannot be palpated and are ultimately discovered by sonography. There may be a significant blood loss from uterine leiomyomas, and secondary signs of anemia, including shock, should be rapidly recognized.

Malignancy

Malignancy of the female reproductive tract can lead to irregular vaginal bleeding. Bleeding can occur secondary to anatomic changes, local inflammation, or hormone production. Primary cancers of the external genitalia and vagina are rare and can be recognized on thorough examination of the genitalia. Postmenopausal women are at greater risk for these malignancies. More common malignancies are discussed in the following sections.

Endometrial Cancer

Patients with endometrial cancer experience perimenopausal and postmenopausal bleeding. This bleeding is often painless but occasionally can be severe. Risk factors for the development of endometrial cancer include age older than 35 years, history of anovulatory cycles, diabetes mellitus, nulliparity, obesity, history of tamoxifen therapy or exogenous estrogen use without progestins. Whereas routine Papanicolaou smears can detect approximately 50% of cases of endometrial cancer, many cases remain undiagnosed, and many patients may present initially to the ED with abnormal vaginal bleeding.

Cervical Cancer

Patients with undiagnosed cervical cancer may present to the ED with painless, abnormal vaginal bleeding. Bleeding is often postcoital or associated with localized inflammation. Physical examination often does not reveal obvious abnormalities. The peak incidence of cervical cancer is in women from 45 to 54 years of age, although it is being diagnosed with increased frequency in women in their 20s and 30s, due to the increased incidence of human papillomavirus. Risk factors include multiple sexual partners, early intercourse, early pregnancy, and history of prior sexually transmitted diseases.

Ovarian Tumors

Patients with ovarian tumors may present with vaginal bleeding from abnormal hormone secretion, but more commonly present with signs and symptoms related to mass effect. Patients typically complain of urinary frequency, constipation or rectal fullness, pelvic pressure, abdominal pain, and bloating. The physical examination may reveal a palpable mass. A palpable ovary in a postmenopausal woman should be considered cancerous until proved otherwise. The peak incidence of ovarian tumors is in women 55 to 65 years of age. Risk factors include frequent ovulation, nulliparity, late menopause, and late childbearing age. Previous use of oral contraceptives is believed to decrease the risk of ovarian cancer.

Systemic Disorders

Multiple systemic illnesses, particularly those that affect hematologic or endocrine homeostasis, can lead to abnormal vaginal bleeding. Table 121-2 lists systemic disorders associated with abnormal vaginal bleeding. Exogenous medications that may contrib-

Table 121-2 SYSTEMIC ETIOLOGIES OF ABNORMAL VAGINAL BLEEDING

Etiology	Mechanism
Hypothalamic suppression	Abnormal production of gonadotropin-releasing hormone (GnRH); can occur secondary to weight loss, stress, or exercise
Hypothyroidism	May cause anovulation
Hyperthyroidism	Changes androgen and estrogen production
Liver failure	Decreased production of vitamin K–dependent clotting factors; decreased metabolism of estrogen leading to unopposed estrogen effects
Renal failure	Platelet dysfunction
Bleeding disorders	Affect normal clotting cascade
Blood dyscrasias	Abnormal platelet production or function
Splenic disease	Thrombocytopenia
Polycystic ovarian disease	Causes anovulatory cycles

BOX 121-2

Medications Associated with Abnormal Vaginal Bleeding

- Anticoagulants
- Antipsychotics
- Corticosteroids
- Hormone therapies
- Contraceptives: intrauterine device with hormones, Norplant, Depo-Provera, oral contraceptives
- Tamoxifen
- Selective serotonin reuptake inhibitors

ute to abnormal vaginal bleeding are shown in Box 121-2.

PELVIC PAIN

The differential diagnosis of pelvic pain in the female is extensive, and includes diseases of the intestinal tract and urinary system. Appendicitis and ectopic pregnancy must be effectively ruled out in any patient presenting with acute pelvic pain. Table 121-3 lists the differential diagnosis of pelvic pain.

Ovarian Torsion

Ovarian torsion occurs when the ovary and fallopian tube twist upon their own vascular supply. Venous congestion and lymphatic obstruction occur initially, leading to edema of the ovary. As the edema progresses there is a decline in arterial flow to the ovary. This process results in necrosis of the ovary, and the viability of the ovary is compromised.

Patients with acute ovarian torsion present with the acute onset of unilateral pelvic pain. The pain is often severe and may be associated with nausea and vomiting. Fever may be present if ovarian necrosis has occurred. Physical examination reveals unilateral adnexal tenderness, and peritoneal signs may be present on abdominal examination.

Ovarian torsion affects women in their reproductive years, with the highest incidence in women in their mid-20s. Enlargement of the ovaries that occurs with cysts or pregnancy predisposes women to

Table 121-3 DIFFERENTIAL DIAGNOSIS OF PELVIC PAIN IN NONPREGNANT FEMALES

Gynecologic Diagnoses	Nongynecologic Diagnoses
Degenerating fibroid	Appendicitis
Mittelschmerz	Mesenteric lymphadenitis
Cervicitis	Diverticulitis
Endometritis	Intraabdominal abscess
Pelvic inflammatory disease	Inflammatory bowel disease
Salpingitis	Bowel obstruction
Tubo-ovarian abscess	Cystitis
Endometriosis	Renal colic
Ovarian torsion Ruptured ovarian cyst Degenerating ovarian tumor	Musculoskeletal injury

ovarian torsion. Ovarian torsion can occur in smaller ovaries, and the absence of any mass does not preclude the diagnosis. The right ovary is more commonly affected than the left. 10% of women with ovarian torsion will experience torsion of the contralateral ovary in their lifetime.

■ Corpus Luteal Cysts (Hemorrhagic Cysts)

As the normal corpus luteum degenerates during the normal reproductive cycle, a small cystic space forms. Thin-walled capillarites invade these cysts and can cause minimal, self-limited bleeding into the cyst. Occasionally, bleeding can be rapid or more extensive. Intracystic pressures can then rise, leading to rupture of the corpus luteum.

Patients with ruptured corpus luteal cysts present with acute onset of unilateral pelvic pain, ranging from mild to severe. Nausea and vomiting frequently are associated symptoms. Rectal pain may occur due to the presence of blood in the cul-de-sac. The amount of bleeding is variable. Hemorrhage may occur into the peritoneal cavity, particularly if the patient has received anticoagulation. Signs of hypovolemia and peritonitis may then be present.

■ Endometriosis

Endometriosis is defined as the presence of endometrial tissue in a location outside of the uterine cavity. This heterotopic tissue is most commonly located near the ovary and in other dependent portions of the pelvis. The tissue is subject to hormonal variations, and pain can ensue from bleeding and the presence of scar tissue.

Endometriosis generally affects women of reproductive age and is most commonly seen in nulliparous women in their mid-30s. Pain is often chronic in nature and poorly localized. A history of cyclical pain is often elicited. Endometriosis can be associated with dysmenorrhea or dyspareunia. Gastrointestinal symptoms and constitutional symptoms, such as fever, may occur but are rare.

Diagnostic Testing

Certain diagnostic tests can enhance the diagnostic ability of the EP and aid in the disposition of the patient (Fig. 121-1). Vaginal wet preparations and cultures can properly identify infectious agents. Complete blood counts can reveal the presence of leukocytosis, anemia, or thrombocytopenia. Coagulation studies and blood urea/creatine and liver function tests can help diagnose systemic disease processes. Urinalysis can reveal cystitis or other infectious processes.

Pelvic sonography should be performed in the ED if there are any signs or symptoms of ovarian torsion or tuboovarian abscess. Doppler flow studies should be performed in any patient with suspected ovarian torsion, although up to 50% of these studies are normal in the setting of acute torsion. If the index of clinical suspicion remains high, the gynecology service should be consulted for intraoperative diagnosis.

Pelvic sonography is sensitive for diagnosis of uterine leiomyomas, polyps, masses, and endometrial cancer, and it can be performed on an outpatient basis.

Diagnostic tests cannot identify dysfunctional uterine bleeding; it is a diagnosis of exclusion, and all other causes of vaginal bleeding must be excluded by the EP before that diagnosis is made.

Treatment

Although vaginal bleeding in the nonpregnant patient rarely leads to significant blood loss, aggressive resuscitation is necessary for patients with symptomatic hypovolemia or anemia. Volume repletion can be enhanced by packed red blood cells and fresh frozen plasma or platelet transfusion if necessary. Dilation and curettage may be necessary to halt ongoing hemorrhage, and early gynecology consultation is of utmost importance.

Pain management is essential. Rapid treatment of pain with narcotic or non-narcotic agents and frequent reassessment of the patient's pain are paramount.

■ TRAUMA

Mild abrasions or non-repairable lacerations should be cleaned and dressed with topical antibiotic ointment. External lacerations requiring repair should be properly anesthetized and cleaned. Absorbable suture material should be used. The gynecology service should be consulted for definitive repair of all vaginal or cervical lacerations.

Tips and Tricks

- All women of childbearing age presenting to the ED are assumed to be pregnant until proved otherwise with a pregnancy test.
- Ovarian torsion presents as acute severe unilateral pain and a gynecologist should evaluate the patient with a history suggestive of torsion even when ultrasound findings are negative.
- Adolescents with abnormal bleeding should be evaluated for potential pregnancy, sexual abuse, and eating disorders. If results are negative, the patient can be discharged with reassurance that the bleeding is likely due to anovulation, which will become more regular with time.
- About 20% to 25% of cases of endometrial cancer occur prior to menopause; all patiens with abnormal uterine bleeding should referred to the gynecology service for endometrial evaluation as an outpatient.
- Hypothyroidism can cause severe menorrhagia.

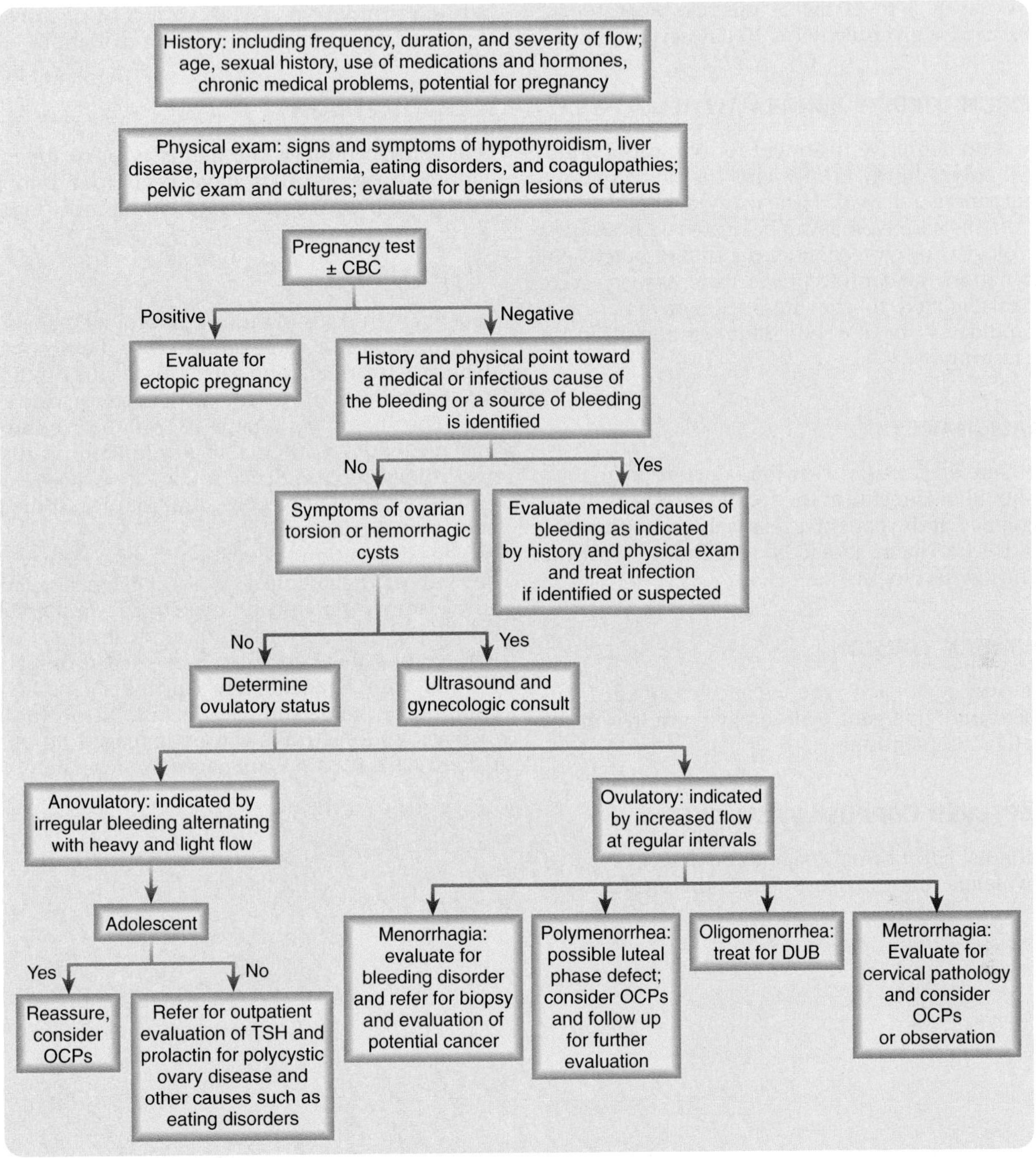
History: including frequency, duration, and severity of flow; age, sexual history, use of medications and hormones, chronic medical problems, potential for pregnancy
Physical exam: signs and symptoms of hypothyroidism, liver disease, hyperprolactinemia, eating disorders, and coagulopathies; pelvic exam and cultures; evaluate for benign lesions of uterus
Pregnancy test ± CBC
Positive
Negative
Evaluate for ectopic pregnancy
History and physical point toward a medical or infectious cause of the bleeding or a source of bleeding is identified
No
Yes
Symptoms of ovarian torsion or hemorrhagic cysts
Evaluate medical causes of bleeding as indicated by history and physical exam and treat infection if identified or suspected
No
Yes
Determine ovulatory status
Ultrasound and gynecologic consult
Anovulatory: indicated by irregular bleeding alternating with heavy and light flow
Ovulatory: indicated by increased flow at regular intervals
Adolescent
Yes
No
Reassure, consider OCPs
Refer for outpatient evaluation of TSH and prolactin for polycystic ovary disease and other causes such as eating disorders
Menorrhagia: evaluate for bleeding disorder and refer for biopsy and evaluation of potential cancer
Polymenorrhea: possible luteal phase defect; consider OCPs and follow up for further evaluation
Oligomenorrhea: treat for DUB
Metrorrhagia: Evaluate for cervical pathology and consider OCPs or observation

FIGURE 121-1 Algorithm outlining an approach to the patient with abnormal vaginal bleeding. CBC, complete blood count; DUB, dysfunctional uterine bleeding; OCPs, oral contraceptive pills; TSH, thyroid-stimulating hormone.

■ FOREIGN BODIES

Vaginal bleeding secondary to foreign bodies is generally resolved once the offending agent has been removed.

■ INFECTION

Once the cause of vaginitis has been adequately diagnosed by examination and wet preparation assay, treatment should be directed at elimination of the offending organism.

■ DYSFUNCTIONAL UTERINE BLEEDING

Gynecologists manage dysfunctional uterine bleeding with nonsteroidal antiinflammatory drugs (NSAIDs), progestins, and estrogens. Because dysfunctional uterine bleeding is a diagnosis of exclusion, it is difficult to prescribe definitive therapy in the ED.

Treatment for acute episodes includes low-dose oral contraceptives two to three times daily for 7 days, 7 days off for withdrawal bleeding, and then once daily for 3 months. Chronic bleeding can be approached by starting oral contraceptives at a regular daily dose, or 5 to 10 mg of medroxyprogesterone acetate can be given daily for 10 days every month.

BENIGN UTERINE ABNORMALITIES

There is no definitive treatment for cervical or endometrial polyps in the ED. Patients should be referred for outpatient removal. Mild to moderate bleeding from uterine leiomyomas can be treated with NSAIDs; gynecologists often recommend a trial of outpatient combination oral contraceptives. Patients with severe problems related to the uterine leiomyomas may be candidates for uterine artery embolization or hysterectomy.

MALIGNANCY

Treatment of patients with reproductive malignancies should be directed at the secondary effects of the malignancy. If the patient is relatively asymptomatic, definitive treatment should be coordinated with the patient's gynecologist.

OVARIAN TORSION

Acute ovarian torsion requires adequate pain management and emergent gynecology consultation for operative intervention.

RUPTURED CORPUS LUTEAL CYST

In patients with normal coagulation and no signs of hypovolemia, pain management is the most important intervention in the ED. Oral contraceptives can be started in ED to prevent future ovulation.

ENDOMETRIOSIS

Oral contraception is the mainstay of treatment for endometriosis. NSAIDs have been found to have minimal efficacy in the treatment of endometriosis.

Disposition

Patients with signs of either symptomatic anemia or hypovolemia should be admitted to the hospital for definitive treatment and care. This occurs in a minority of nonpregnant patients with acute vaginal bleeding. The majority of patients can be treated and managed as outpatients in conjunction with the gynecology service. Strict follow-up is necessary to ensure cessation of bleeding and to rule out the presence of malignancy.

The disposition of patients with pelvic pain depends on their clinical state and diagnosis. Patients with acute ovarian torsion need to be admitted to the gynecology service for definitive treatment. Patients with corpus luteal cysts can be treated as outpatients if their pain is adequately controlled and if their condition is stable and without risk factors for hemorrhage. Endometriosis can be managed on an outpatient basis if pain is managed appropriately.

Chapter **122**

Complications of Gynecologic Procedures, Abortion, and Assisted Reproductive Technology

Christine Yang-Kauh and Tara Khan

KEY POINTS

The most common chief complaints are pain, bleeding, infection, and vomiting.
The EP should maintain suspicion for hemorrhage, severe infections, damage to intra-abdominal structures, and pulmonary embolism.
Ureteral injuries are rare but are the leading cause of legal action against gynecologic surgeons.
Bedside ultrasonography is useful in evaluating the post-procedural patient.
Abortion is one of the most common surgical procedures performed in the United States and overall has very low complication rates.
The most feared complication of assisted reproductive technology (ART) is ovarian hyperstimulation syndrome. There is no cure, so prevention and early intervention are key measures.
Gynecology consultation is important for all but the most minor complications.

Gynecologic procedures run the gamut from minor office procedures to major surgery, diagnostic and therapeutic procedures, and procedures intended to terminate pregnancy or to initiate it. They are among the most common surgical procedures performed in the United States today. Abortions alone account for almost a million reported cases per year (ranking near the top),[1] and almost 100,000 cycles of ART were reported from 383 sites in the year 2000.[2]

With shortened hospital stays and minimally invasive or outpatient surgery, patients with complications that might previously have been diagnosed early during hospitalization are presenting to the ED, often in a delayed fashion.

This chapter is divided into three main sections—complications of gynecologic procedures; complications following medical and surgical abortion; and complications of ART, including procedures for male infertility.

COMPLICATIONS OF GYNECOLOGIC PROCEDURES

Scope

This section focuses on common and threatening complications of diagnostic and therapeutic gynecologic procedures and their evaluation and treatment in the ED (Fig. 122-1). Catastrophic complications usually declare themselves intraoperatively. Complications with slower evolution often go unrecognized before discharge, only to present in a delayed fashion to the ED (Table 122-1). The most critical complications are hemorrhage, septic shock and other severe infections (toxic shock syndrome, necrotizing fasciitis), and thromboembolism.[3]

When a patient with post-procedure complications presents to the ED, the physician who performed the procedure should be contacted; definitive management often requires gynecological intervention.

It is important to avoid narrowing the differential diagnosis to only postoperative complications. Even though the patient has had a surgical procedure, she is still subject to the risks of other conditions (Box 122-1).

Documentation

PATIENTS WITH COMPLICATIONS OF GYNECOLOGIC PROCEDURES

History
- Gravida, para, aborta, current pregnancy status
- Last normal menstrual period or onset of menopause
- Procedure performed, including any prior associated complications
- Time lapse since procedure
- If bleeding, quantify rate and whether symptoms of anemia are present

Physical Examination
- Are the vital signs normal?
- Does the patient look ill? pale? febrile? uncomfortable?
- Abdominal examination—Distention, soft, tender, peritoneal signs
- Speculum examination—Vaginal discharge, bleeding color and quantity
- Bimanual examination—Uterine and ovarian size and texture, tenderness

Diagnostic Studies
- Bedside ultrasound imaging results, if performed, to evaluate for free fluid, hydronephrosis, bladder fullness or uterine contents; other imaging or laboratory study results

Medical Decision Making
- Time and person contacted for gynecology consultation

Patient Instructions
- Document discussion with patient regarding diagnosis, recognizing warning signs, what to do if they occur, follow-up, when to return to the ED.

Diagnostic Testing

Bedside ultrasonography is rapidly becoming an indispensable tool for EPs. For patients presenting with complications after a gynecologic procedure, bedside ultrasonography in the hands of a skillful operator can provide rapid recognition of intraabdominal pathology.

Free fluid in Morrison's pouch (the hepatorenal fossa), in the splenorenal fossa, or behind the bladder suggests a perforated vessel or viscus (Fig. 122-2). Ultrasound-guided paracentesis allows definitive fluid diagnosis.

Urinary Tract Injury

Ureteral injuries occur in only 1% of cases but are the number one cause of legal action against gynecologic surgeons. Although injuries to the bowel or bladder are more common, ureteral injury carries a higher morbidity because it is likely to be discovered later in its course. Unilateral ureteral injury presents postoperatively in more than 70% of cases.

Typical symptoms are fever, flank pain, prolonged ileus, and prolonged abdominal distention. Unexplained hematuria or watery vaginal discharge may be present. Anuria suggests bilateral compromise or renal failure. A full, distended bladder noted on ultrasound images and/or urine output greater than 500 mL on Foley catheter placement differentiates

BOX 122-1

Most Threatening and Most Common Complications of Gynecologic Procedures

Most Threatening
- Vascular injury
- Bowel injury
- Urinary tract injury
- Sepsis/severe infection
- Pulmonary embolism

Most Common
- Pain
- Bleeding
- Fever
- Nausea and vomiting

PRIORITY ACTIONS

Differential Diagnosis: Complications of Gynecologic Procedures

Abnormal Vital Signs?

- Anemic? Consider hemorrhage (vascular injury); resuscitation and exploratory laparotomy required.
- Fever? Consider septic shock, toxic shock syndrome, necrotizing fasciitis; administer broad-spectrum antibiotics and search for source of infection; emergent surgical débridement required for necrotizing fasciitis.
- Abdominal distention? Consider perforated bowel or urinary tract or bowel obstruction.
- Shortness of breath? Consider pulmonary embolism, fluid overload, and aspiration pneumonia.
- If post-laparoscopy, also consider pneumothorax.

Vaginal Bleeding—Is It Cervical or Uterine in Origin?

- For cervical or vaginal lacerations: Controlled by simple measures in the ED?
  - If not, or if post-conization, consult gynecologist about return to the operating room for bleeding control.
- For uterine bleeding: Is retained tissue noted on ultrasound imaging?
  - If not, consider uterine perforation; if uterine perforation is present, maintain high suspicion for perforated viscus.

Abdominal Pain with Distention?

- Ileus or small bowel obstruction on radiograph? Nasogastric tube if excessive vomiting; surgical consultation required.
  - If not, consider intestinal, urinary, or vascular injury.

Unable to Urinate?

- >500 mL of urine output on Foley catheter placement? Substitute a leg bag and treat for UTI, if present; schedule follow-up with urology.
  - If not, consider renal failure due to medications or bilateral ureteral obstruction.

Dysuria?

- Hematuria and abdominal pain? Or persistent/recurrent UTI? Suspect urinary tract injury; obtain imaging to evaluate for ureteral or bladder compromise.
  - If not, treat as UTI with antibiotics, urine culture and close follow-up.

Wound Redness and Drainage?

- Is it localized? If so, check the fascia; if it is intact, treat as superficial wound infection with packing and close follow-up.
  - If fascia is not intact, consider subfascial abscess, early necrotizing fasciitis, or hernia/evisceration; make sure it is not an incarcerated hernia; gynecology consultation and possible surgery evaluation required.
- If wound is widespread, consider cellulitis or fasciitis; administer antibiotics and hospitalize patient unless the cellulitis is mild; then very close follow-up and explicit return instructions are required.

UTI, urinary tract infection.

these cases from urinary retention. Bedside ultrasonography is useful to evaluate for urinary ascites and hydronephrosis.

Laboratory testing includes a complete blood count and differential, electrolytes and kidney function, preoperative blood assays, and urinalysis. If ascites or other fluid is obtained, fluid creatinine levels should be measured to determine if it is urinary in origin. Imaging to evaluate the status of the urinary system is indicated, such as intravenous urography, abdominal/pelvic computed tomography with contrast, and renal ultrasonography with retrograde ureteropyelography.

If ureteral obstruction is suspected, renal ultrasonography to identify hydronephrosis lends further credence to the diagnosis. Urinary retention can also be differentiated from anuria by a full, distended bladder on ultrasound imaging (as well as by urinary catheterization).

Ureteral injury can be repaired urgently on the day of diagnosis, or if the patient is unstable, a percutaneous nephrostomy can be placed to decompress the kidney while awaiting definitive repair.

Complications of ureteral obstruction (due to ligation, stricture, or external compression by another structure) are hydronephrosis and progressive kidney damage, ultimately leading to failure of the ipsilateral kidney. Urinary leakage due to ureteral disruption can cause urinary ascites or an enclosed uroma. Bilateral injury (or unilateral injury of a solitary functioning kidney) may simply present with anuria and subsequent renal failure.

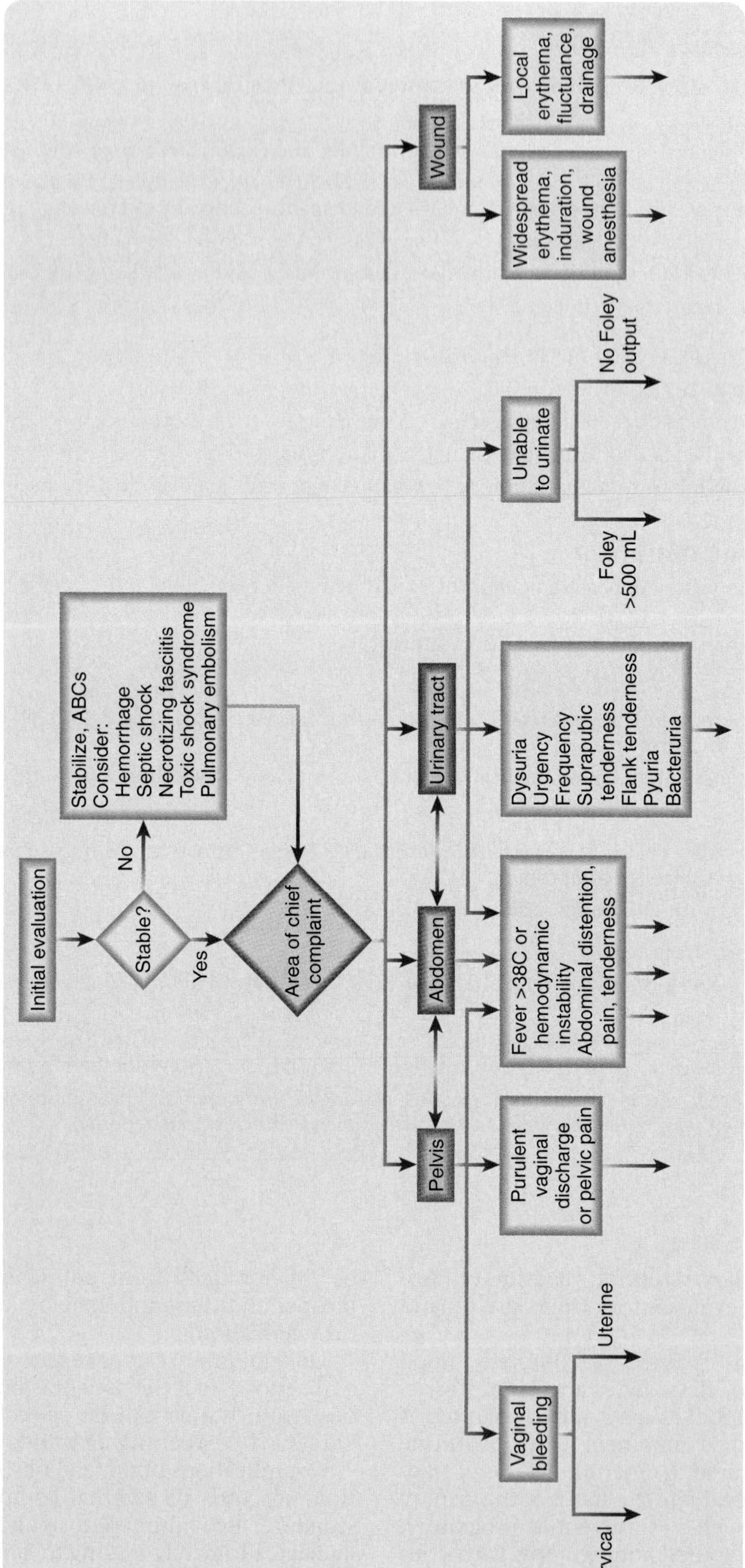
Initial evaluation
Stable?
No
Yes
Stabilize, ABCs
Consider:
Hemorrhage
Septic shock
Necrotizing fasciitis
Toxic shock syndrome
Pulmonary embolism
Area of chief complaint
Pelvis
Abdomen
Urinary tract
Wound
Vaginal bleeding
Cervical
Uterine
Purulent vaginal discharge or pelvic pain
Fever >38C or hemodynamic instability
Abdominal distention, pain, tenderness
Dysuria
Urgency
Frequency
Suprapubic tenderness
Flank tenderness
Pyuria
Bacteruria
Unable to urinate
Foley >500 mL
No Foley output
Widespread erythema, induration, wound anesthesia
Local erythema, fluctuance, drainage

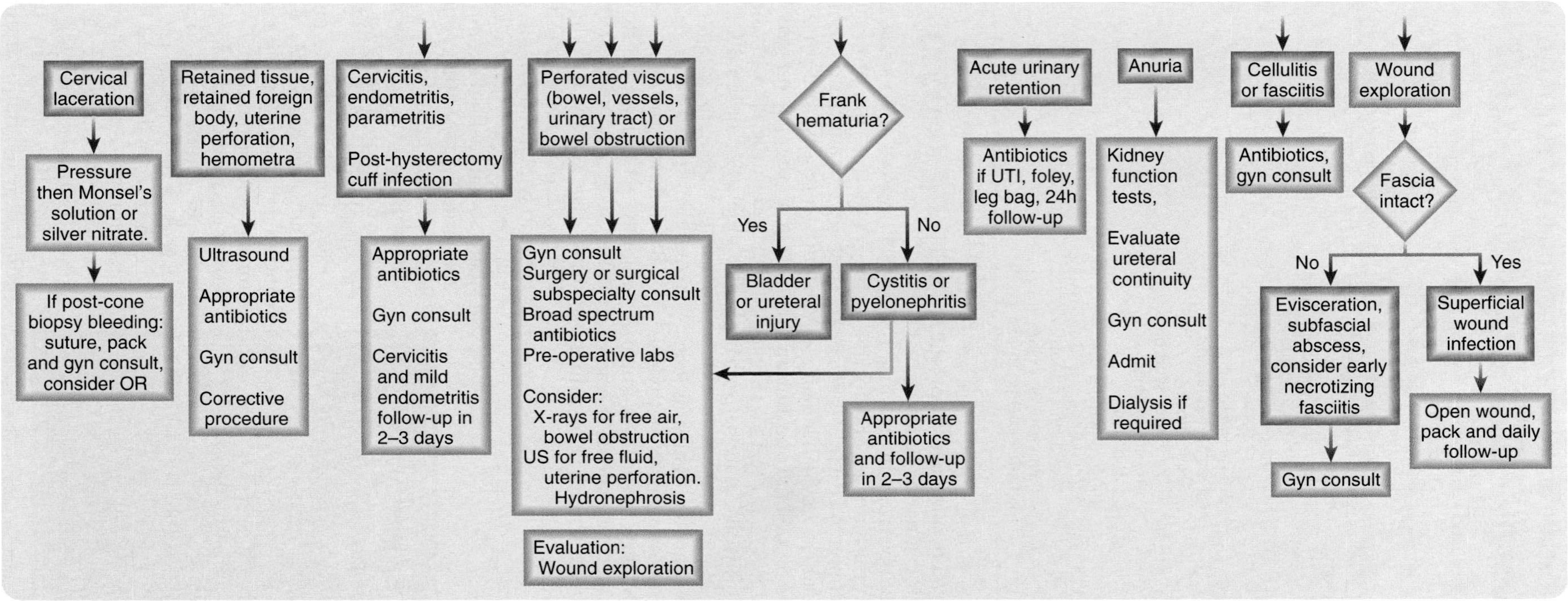
Cervical laceration
Pressure then Monsel's solution or silver nitrate.
If post-cone biopsy bleeding: suture, pack and gyn consult, consider OR
Retained tissue, retained foreign body, uterine perforation, hemometra
Ultrasound
Appropriate antibiotics
Gyn consult
Corrective procedure
Cervicitis, endometritis, parametritis
Post-hysterectomy cuff infection
Appropriate antibiotics
Gyn consult
Cervicitis and mild endometritis follow-up in 2–3 days
Perforated viscus (bowel, vessels, urinary tract) or bowel obstruction
Gyn consult
Surgery or surgical subspecialty consult
Broad spectrum antibiotics
Pre-operative labs
Consider:
X-rays for free air, bowel obstruction
US for free fluid, uterine perforation.
Hydronephrosis
Evaluation:
Wound exploration
Frank hematuria?
Yes
No
Bladder or ureteral injury
Cystitis or pyelonephritis
Appropriate antibiotics and follow-up in 2–3 days
Acute urinary retention
Antibiotics if UTI, foley, leg bag, 24h follow-up
Anuria
Kidney function tests,
Evaluate ureteral continuity
Gyn consult
Admit
Dialysis if required
Cellulitis or fasciitis
Antibiotics, gyn consult
Wound exploration
Fascia intact?
No
Yes
Evisceration, subfascial abscess, consider early necrotizing fasciitis
Gyn consult
Superficial wound infection
Open wound, pack and daily follow-up

FIGURE 122-1 Suggested algorithm for the evaluation and treatment of postoperative gynecologic patients. ABCs, airway, breathing, and circulation; gyn consult, gynecology consultation; US, ultrasonography; UTI, urinary tract infection.

Table 122-1 **COMPLICATIONS OF GYNECOLOGIC PROCEDURES BY ESTIMATED TIMELINE**

Immediate (<24 hr)	Early (1 day-1 wk)	Delayed (1 wk-1 year)	Late (years)

Complications of anesthesia
Emesis:
  Postoperative ileus
  Medication reaction
Fever:
  Atelectasis
  Hematoma
  Pyogenic reaction to tissue trauma
Bleeding:
  Vaginal or cervical
  Laceration
  Uterine perforation
  Visceral perforation
  Vascular injury
  Retained tissue
  Retained foreign body
Laproscopic:
  Visceral injuries
  Fluid overload
  Gas embolization
  Pneumothorax
  Pneumomediastinum
	Bleeding:
	  Laceration
	  Perforation
	  Injury to vasculature
	  Infection
	  Retained tissue
	  Retained foreign body
	Infection:
	  Superficial wound infection
	  Clostridial infections
	  Pelvic cellulitis/abscess
	  Septic pelvic
	  thrombophlebitis
	  Necrotizing fasciitis
	  Septic shock
	  Toxic shock syndrome
	Postoperative ileus
	Constipation
	Urinary retention
	Thrombosis:
	  Venous thrombosis
	  Pulmonary embolism
	Retained foreign bodies
		Wound dehiscence
		Suture sinuses
		Postoperative small bowel obstruction
		Incisional hernia
		Vaginal evisceration
		Fistula formation
		Amenorrhea
			Vaginal eversion
			Postoperative small bowel obstruction
			Fistula formation
			Decreased fertility:
			  Amenorrhea
			  Uterine synechiae
			  Cervical stenosis

On a delayed basis, watery drainage from the vagina may herald a ureterovaginal or vesicovaginal fistula. Bedside diagnosis can be made by first inserting a tampon and then administering an oral dose of phenazopyridine and instilling methylene blue or indigo carmine into the bladder. An orange tampon indicates a ureterovaginal fistula, a blue one indicates a vesicovaginal fistula (Table 122-2). The EP should be aware that both types of fistulae may be present concurrently.

Suspicion of a ureterocutaneous fistula is confirmed if, after administering intravenous methylene blue, the watery wound discharge turns blue. Analogous testing can be performed to evaluate if watery discharge from a suprapubic wound is of urinary origin.

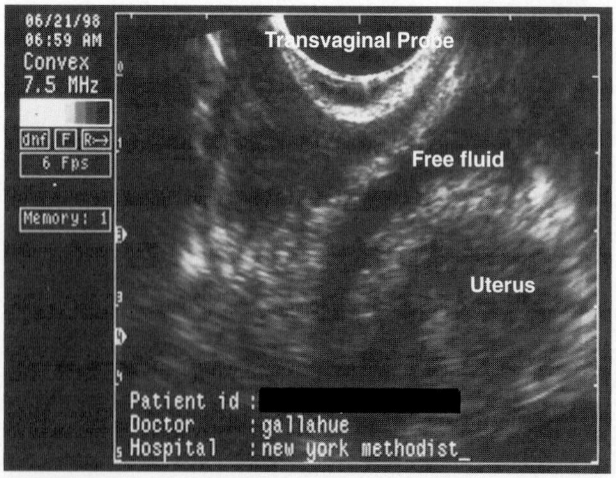
06/21/98
06:59 AM
Convex
7.5 MHz
6 Fps
Memory: 1
Transvaginal Probe
Free fluid
Uterus
Patient id : [redacted]
Doctor : gallahue
Hospital : new york methodist_

FIGURE 122-2 Transvaginal ultrasound image showing free fluid in the cul de sac consistent with hemorrhage.

Vaginal Bleeding

Bleeding from the vagina needs to be evaluated in the context of the procedure performed. A careful speculum examination is key to determining the source, quantity, and persistence of the bleeding.

Minor vaginal or cervical lacerations can be managed in the ED with direct pressure followed by the application of Monsel's solution or silver nitrate. Persistent bleeding in spite of these measures may require sutures or electrocautery.

Blood flowing from the cervical os implies a uterine etiology. This may be from hemometra, retained tissue, retained foreign bodies, infection, or uterine injury. The bimanual examination helps to ascertain the size and tenderness of the uterus. If the patient is hemodynamically stable, a pelvic ultrasound scan can be performed to assess uterine contents. An acute abdominal radiography series (flat and upright abdominal views with an upright chest radiogram) to look for signs of perforation may be obtained, unless laparotomy or laparoscopy was performed within the last 72 hours, in which case residual postsurgical free air may be present.

Symptoms of uterine perforation include pelvic cramping and vaginal bleeding. A high index of suspicion for injury to adjacent bowel or other structures should be maintained. Broad-spectrum antibiotic coverage is indicated. Rapid bedside ultrasonography by the EP can be useful to assess for free pelvic fluid suggesting hemorrhage (see Fig. 122-2).

Definitive management consists of laparoscopy or laparotomy to evaluate the extent of the damage and to stop the bleeding. However, cases in which bleeding is controlled, the patient is stable and comfortable, and the EP is sure that the perforation was inflicted by a blunt instrument (e.g., dilator) can be managed conservatively with close observation.

Table 122-2 CLINICAL PRESENTATION AND BEDSIDE DIAGNOSIS OF PELVIC FISTULAS

Type of Fistula	Presentation	Bedside Diagnosis
Ureterovaginal	Copious, watery vaginal discharge; multiple urinary tract infections	To confirm and differentiate these fistulas: 1) Place a tampon in the vagina 2) Administer phenazopyridine, 200 mg orally 3) Instill normal saline tinted with methylene blue into the bladder. Results: Orange tampon = ureterovaginal fistula Blue tampon = vesicovaginal fistula Please note that BOTH types may be present concurrently
Vesicovaginal	Copious, watery vaginal discharge; multiple urinary tract infections	
Enterovaginal	Vaginal discharge may contain intestinal contents; severe vaginovulvar irritation may be present due to the pH	Acidity can be tested using litmus paper or the pH portion of a urine dipstick. Place a tampon in the vagina and administer oral activated charcoal. A stained tampon is diagnostic.
Colovaginal	Brown, feculent vaginal discharge	Place a tampon in the vagina and instill normal saline tinted with methylene blue into the rectum. A stained tampon is diagnostic of a rectovaginal fistula. Higher colonic lesions may be diagnosed by using orally administered activated charcoal.
Ureterocutaneous	Copious, watery wound drainage	Administer methylene blue intravenously. Blue watery discharge is diagnostic.

Symptoms of acute hemometra (intrauterine hematoma) include severe, progressive, cramping pelvic pain. Vaginal bleeding may be minimal if the os is obstructed by the enlarging hematoma. Blood loss is insufficient to cause hypotension or anemia. Bimanual pelvic examination reveals an extremely distended and tender uterus. Suction evacuation of the uterus provides prompt relief and typically can be performed without anesthesia or cervical dilation. Methylergonovine maleate (0.2 mg intramuscularly [IM]) should then be administered to induce uterine contraction, unless contraindicated by hypertension. In that case, a 1000-mg rectal suppository of misoprostol can be given instead.

In rare cases of persistent bleeding without explanation, an unrecognized bleeding diathesis must be considered. Von Willebrand disease is the most common bleeding disorder in women of childbearing age.

Bright red cervical bleeding post-hysterectomy should prompt a search for bleeding sites at the excised vaginal cuff. Dark blood from the os should prompt suspicion of a cuff hematoma. Purulent drainage indicates infection. Administration of antibiotics appropriate for pelvic imflammatory disease should be initiated.

Endometritis

Patients with endometritis typically present to the ED 3 to 7 days post-instrumentation with fever and pelvic or low abdominal pain and tenderness. Vaginal bleeding also is frequently present. Potential pathogens include those of pelvic inflammatory disease as well as those that may have been introduced during the procedure. Thus risk factors include retained tissue as well as pelvic inflammatory disease and insufficiently aseptic operating conditions.

Management consists of suction curettage preceded by a first dose of IV antibiotics. The procedure should be performed in an operating suite due to the high risk of hemorrhage during instrumentation of infected tissue, and the patient should be hospitalized for IV administration of antibiotics.

Recommended antibiotic regimens for outpatient care are ceftriaxone, 250 mg IM, with doxycycline, 100 mg orally twice a day for 14 days, or amoxicillin/clavanulate and doxycycline. Anaerobic coverage should be included as well. For severe endometritis, inpatient admission is necessary for IV administration of clindamycin, 900 mg every 8 hours, and gentamicin, 1.5 mg/kg every 8 hours. Alternatives are triple IV therapy with ampicillin, 2 g every 6 hours, plus gentamicin, 1.5 mg/kg every 8 hours, and metronidazole, 500 mg every 6 hours; or IV ampicillin/sulbactam, 3.0 g every 8 hours as monotherapy. Doxycycline, 100 mg twice a day for 14 days, should be added if *Chlamydia* is a possible pathogen.

Cuff Infections

Patients with post-hysterectomy cuff infections can present with purulent vaginal discharge, pain, and fever. Induration and tenderness of the vaginal apex are consistent with cuff cellulitis. The presence of abscess is noted on ultrasound imaging.

Necrotizing Fasciitis

Necrotizing fasciitis is a devastating infection with high mortality characterized by extensive necrosis of the superficial fascia that undermines the skin but lacks muscular involvement. It is often accompanied by systemic toxicity out of proportion to the apparent local infection. Necroting fasciitis is difficult to diagnose early. The initial presentation may be nonspecific edema and induration with erythema or duskiness of the skin. As the infection spreads, superficial bullae may develop. Fever and leukocytosis are common, and patients also may present with significant hypotension, tachycardia, and lethargy.

Although it can arise from minor injuries, approximately 50% of cases of necrotizing fasciitis occur in association with surgical incisions. Risk factors include immunosuppression, diabetes, elderly age, peripheral vascular disease, malnutrition, obesity, hypertension, malignancy, radiation therapy, and renal insufficiency.

On evaluation, the lack of fascial resistance to probing in the wound in a toxic-appearing patient is highly suspicious. ED management relies on the immediate administration of broad-spectrum parenteral antibiotics; aggressive repletion of IV fluids, colloids, and calcium; and immediate surgical consultation to arrange for definitive treatment—emergent wide surgical debridement. Hyperbaric therapy should be considered. Central venous monitoring and admission to the intensive care unit are essential for all unstable patients.

Drugs of choice are penicillin G, 18 million units daily in divided doses; clindamycin, 900 mg every 8 hours for streptococcal or clostridial infection; imipenem, 500 g every 6 hours; or meropenem, 1 g every 8 hours for polymicrobial infections.

If toxic shock is present, intravenous administration of IV immunoglobulin, 1 g/kg on day 1 followed by 0.5 g/kg for 2 more days, decreases sepsis-related organ failure. Wound cultures should be sent to the laboratory for testing to guide treatment.

Superficial Wound Infections

Superficial wound infections occur in up to 10% of patients who have undergone gynecologic surgery without perioperative antibiotics. The most common causes are *Staphylococcus aureus* and vaginal or enteric flora. Typically, serosanguinous or seropurulent drainage is noted 5 to 7 days postoperatively. Fever and leukocytosis also may be present. The great majority of these infections are minor, although systemic toxicity or extensive infection may occur if the initial infection is neglected, or in the presence of immunosuppression, diabetes, or obesity.

Thorough evaluation requires opening the wound to drain and to allow examination for deep fascial or muscular involvement. Truly superficial wound infections can be managed without antibiotics, using meticulous wound care, irrigation with diluted hydrogen peroxide or Dakin's solution four times a day, and dry gauze packing. Delayed wound closure can be performed if necessary. Wound cultures have little clinical significance.

Group A beta-hemolytic *Streptococcus* wound infections usually present within 1 to 2 days and are characterized by rapidly advancing erythema, lymphangitis, and lymphadenopathy, with scant, watery drainage. A confirmed diagnosis of uncomplicated Group A beta-hemolytic *Streptococcus* infection can be treated with oral ampicillin/clavulanate, or a first-generation cephalosporin without opening the wound. An initial IV dose of 2 g of nafcillin or oxacillin may be given.

If the diagnosis is uncertain, treatment should include wound care as described previously plus broad-spectrum antibiotics, including coverage for possible community-acquired MRSA (methicillin-resistant *Staphylococcus aureus*).

Wound Dehiscence

Wound dehiscence, or complete fascial disruption, occurs in about 0.5% of gynecologic surgical cases and has a mortality of 10% to 35%. Risk factors include obesity, malnutrition, malignancy, previous surgical incision, infection, abdominal distention, bronchopulmonary disease, corticosteroid therapy, prior radiation therapy, and use of absorbable sutures and layered closure as opposed to mass closure. Severe cases may be accompanied by evisceration (herniation of abdominal contents through the wall).

The patient may note a protruding lump, bloody drainage, pain, or a frankly open incision following a sudden movement or action that increases intraperitoneal pressure, such as a violent cough. Even without other symptoms, bloody drainage from the wound should prompt evaluation. Gentle probing with a sterile gloved finger or sterile cotton swab can evaluate the integrity of the fascial layer. If the skin is still intact, ultrasound imaging may reveal herniated bowel loops just below the surface.

Exposed organs must be covered immediately and protected with a wet sterile dressing, and gastric and bladder decompression performed. Wound infection must be considered and treated if present, ideally after cultures are obtained. Resuscitation and repletion of fluid, electrolyte and nutritional deficits take precedence over wound closure. Once the patient is stable, careful wound evaluation and management in the operating room is recommended, with removal of the old suture material, abscess drainage, wound debridement, and peritoneal cavity lavage before closure of the abdominal wall. Often the skin is left to heal by secondary intent. Complications include sepsis, hernias, and poor cosmetic outcome.

Incisional Hernias

Poor healing of the fascia and muscle in a wound leads to incisional hernias, allowing the peritoneum to abut the superficial tissues. Presentation can be acute, with a tearing sensation during a maneuver with increased intrabdominal pressure, or can be subacute, with a pulling sensation during straining or walking over a long period of time.

The size of the peritoneal bulge may have no relation to the size of the hernia. The smaller the fascial defect, the more likely it is to result in the most serious complication of incarcerated bowel and bowel necrosis.

During the physical examination, it is crucial to confirm that the hernia is reducible. Tenderness over the hernia, inability to reduce it, and obstructive or peritoneal signs require prompt surgical consultation. Reducible hernias can be repaired on an elective basis if desired, or can be managed conservatively with an abdominal binder.

Fistula Formation

Fistulas can occur between almost any two mucosa-covered surfaces after the extensive dissection involved in pelvic surgery, particularly if there is occult injury to hollow viscera.

Vaginal Evisceration

Vaginal evisceration is rare, yet dramatic, and has a mortality of up to 10% due to associated intestinal necrosis, peritonitis, or other underlying or global illness. It occurs with increased intraperitoneal pressure in the setting of a ruptured vaginal enterocele or an unrecognized uterine perforation. The diagnosis is made based on physical examination.

A moist covering must be placed immediately to protect the viscera. Bed rest in the supine or Trendelenburg position is recommended to prevent further outward pressure. Broad-spectrum antibiotics should be administered, and gynecology consultation should be obtained immediately to schedule surgical repair.

Laparoscopy

Laparoscopic procedures usually are characterized by more rapid recovery and lower complication rates than open surgical procedures (Box 122-2). However, unique complications are associated with needle/trocar insertion, induced pneumoperitoneum, and the extensive use of electrocautery.[4]

BOX 122-2

Most Threatening and Most Common Complications of Laparoscopy

Most Threatening

- Vascular injury
- Thermal bowel injury
- Traumatic bowel injury
- Urinary tract injury
- Complications of anesthesia
- Sepsis

Most Common

- Ileus
- Urinary tract infection

■ NEEDLE/TROCAR INSERTION

The introduction of the Veress needle at the start of the laparoscopic procedure is usually performed blindly and can result in traumatic injury to the bowel (particularly in the presence of adhesions) and vasculature. In rare instances, the diaphragm is transversed, creating a pneumothorax. These catastrophic injuries usually are noted and managed intraoperatively.[5]

Less critical is injury to abdominal wall vessels, leading to abdominal wall hematomas. If the injury is extensive or if the size cannot be estimated due to habitus, a complete blood count should be obtained to estimate blood loss. Blood loss usually is not sufficient to require transfusion.

Incisional hernias from trocar sites can occur; due to their small size, they are more likely to incarcerate if abdominal contents protrude into them. These require surgical repair when symptomatic.

■ LAPAROSCOPIC ELECTROCAUTERY

Unlike significant traumatic injuries, thermal injuries such as those caused by laparoscopic electrocautery usually are not recognized intraoperatively. With thermal injury, there is no intraoperative bleeding, but diathermy-induced coagulative necrosis leads to a dry injury that weakens the wall and eventually ruptures.

Thermal bowel injuries are serious and typically present days or even weeks after laparoscopy. Symptoms include abdominal distention, unexpectedly severe lower abdominal pain, and tenderness with fever, often accompanied by nausea, vomiting, and peritoneal signs. Blood tests reveal leukocytosis. Abdominal radiographs may show free air or ileus. The EP should not mistake the free air for residua from induced pneumoperitoneum greater than 24 hours after laparoscopy. Early gynecology consultation should be obtained if thermal injury is suspected.

Thermal ureteral injuries also present in a delayed fashion, usually with peritonitis or, if very late, as a fistula. IV pyelograms reveal urine extravasation or a uroma. If pyelography is unavailable, abdominal/pelvic computed tomography with IV contrast may be used; however, its ability to pinpoint ureteral discontinuity or minor injuries is limited.

Vascular injuries are a major cause of death from laparascopic surgery, with a mortality of 15%. They are almost universally discovered intraoperatively.[6]

■ PNEUMOPERITONEUM

The major complications of pneumoperitoneum (the use of inert gases to distend the abdomen for laparascopic surgery) are associated with a high mortality rate; they will occur intraoperatively if significant. These include pneumothorax, pneumomediastinum, and gas embolism.

Hysteroscopy

Hysteroscopy involves filling the uterus with fluid to distend it and allow fibroscopic evaluation and procedures such as biopsy, endometrial ablation, myomectomy, and resection of uterine septa. In addition to the usual risks of transcervical procedures, absorption of excess amounts of hysteroscopic fluid (30% dextran-70, glycine, sorbitol) may result in electrolyte imbalances, water intoxication, and systemic or pulmonary edema. Patients with complications from hysteroscopy usually are recognized intraoperatively and must be hospitalized for medical management.

Uterine Fibroid Embolization

Uterine fibroid embolization (Box 122-3) typically is performed by an interventional radiologist to treat bleeding fibroids in patients who are poor candidates for major surgery, are not interested in reproduction, or wish to preserve menses for personal or ethnoreligious reasons. The procedure consists of the injection of a mass of microspheres (tris-acryl gelatin) or polyvinyl alcohol directly into the uterine artery in order to occlude it. The goal is to cut off the blood supply to the fibroids so that they will shrink and degenerate.

BOX 122-3

Most Threatening and Most Common Complications of Uterine Fibroid Embolization

Most Threatening

- Sepsis
- Non-target embolization
- Uterine ischemia/rupture
- Endometritis/pyometrium
- Contrast-induced renal failure
- Thromboembolic disease

Most Common

- Post-embolization syndrome
- Severe pain
- Bleeding
- Allergic reactions
- Groin hematoma
- Retained tissue
- Embolization failure
- Iatrogenic menopause*

*Incidence is 1% to 5% in all women, but up to 43% in women over 45 years of age.

A relatively new procedure, it has been rapidly gaining popularity in the United States, increasing from 50 cases in 1996 to more than 10,000 cases in 2000. Early results show a success rate of about 90% and a complication rate of about 5% by American College of Gynecology criteria.[7] These patients are likely to present to the ED with gynecologic complaints.

Post-embolization syndrome (low-grade fever, malaise, pelvic pain, nausea, and vomiting) affects most of these patients to some degree. Only symptomatic treatment is warranted as long as other causes are ruled out.

Severe pain from degenerating fibroids can be treated with nonsteroidal anti-inflammatory drugs and oral opioids (e.g., acetaminophen plus hydrocodone). Infected necrotic tissue or intractable pain may require hysterectomy. Severe bleeding or a sloughed fibroid that does not spontaneously expulse vaginally require evacuation.

Iatrogenic menopause due to inadvertent compromise of ovarian blood supply may occur. Occasionally, the embolization goes awry ("nontarget embolization") and severe tissue ischemia and necrosis occur in undesirable areas such as the buttock, labia, and vaginal vault. Late complications include decreased fertility and fistula formation.

These patients are at risk for angiographic complications such as femoral hematoma, site infection, pseudoaneurysm, arteriovenous fistula formation, thromboembolism, and contrast nephropathy.

Cervical Procedures

Cervical cancer used to be the top cancer killer of women in the United States. Although numbers have declined over the past few decades because of the emphasis on regular PAP (Papanicolaou) tests, in 2003 11,820 women were diagnosed with cervical cancer, and 3919 women died from the disease.[8] Cervical procedures such as cervical conization (laser conization, cold-knife conization, loop electrosurgical excision [LEEP]), colposcopy, and cryotherapy are used in the diagnosis and treatment of early cervical neoplasia.

Cold-knife conization (surgical excision with a scalpel) is always performed in the operating room, usually with general or spinal anesthesia. Because intraoperative and postprocedural bleeding can be profuse, cerclage often is placed prophylactically prior to the procedure as a tourniquet. Postconization bleeding usually presents 1 to 2 weeks after the procedure. Vaginal packing may be attempted, but usually the patient needs to return to the operating room for hemorrhage control.

Laser conization has only slightly lower rates of bleeding. Cervical cryotherapy and LEEP cause only minor bleeding and thus often are performed in the outpatient setting.

Other potential complications of cervical procedures are cervical stenosis, preterm labor in subse-

PATIENT TEACHING TIPS

POST–GYNECOLOGIC PROCEDURE INSTRUCTIONS

- Explain the normal postoperative course to the patient.
- If the patient is not being admitted, schedule follow-up with the patient's physician in the next 1 to 3 days.
- If antibiotics are prescribed, instruct the patient to complete the entire course of therapy as indicated.
- Tell the patient to call her physician or return to the ED if she has:
  - Worsening abdominal or pelvic pain or abdominal distention
  - Intractable vomiting
  - Any evidence of wound infection or discharge
  - Vaginal bleeding soaking more than 1 maxipad an hour for at least 4 hours
  - Foul-smelling, milky, green, or other abnormal vaginal discharge
  - Fever greater than 100.3°F
  - Any other concerning symptom

quent pregnancies, cervical incompetence, and postconization carcinoma.

POST-ABORTION COMPLICATIONS

Scope

The termination of pregnancy can be achieved medically or surgically. The selection of abortion method is largely dictated by gestational age. Medical terminations are limited to pregnancies less than 8 weeks of gestation. Curettage, including dilation and evacuation, accounts for the great majority of all abortions performed. Intrauterine instillation has plummeted in usage due to the high complication rate. Hysterotomy and hysterectomy are extreme measures that are now rarely used for the purposes of induced abortion.

Epidemiology

Since becoming legalized nationwide in 1973, induced abortion has become one of the most frequently performed operative procedures in the United States with about a million cases a year (>850,000 legal abortions reported to the Centers for Disease Control and Prevention [CDC] from 49 sites in 2002). An estimated half of all pregnancies are unplanned, and 40% of unintended pregnancies are terminated. In fact, each year approximately 3% of all women of childbearing age have abortions, accounting for almost one fourth of all pregnancies. Most abortions are performed during the first trimester—60% within the first eight weeks and 88% within the first 13 weeks.[9]

Complications

In addition to the particular risks of the method chosen, general complications of abortion include hemorrhage, infection, retained pregnancy, and retained products of conception. Overall complication rates are low, ranging from 1% to 5% of cases, and associated maternal mortality is extremely rare. In fact, the overall maternal mortality rate of legal abortions was 0.6 per 100,000 in 1997, which is less than one tenth of the U.S. maternal mortality rate of 7.5 per 100,000 for live births. In fact, for every gestational age, mortality is lower for abortion than for pregnancy and childbirth.[10]

Post-abortion infection seems to be the only predictor of decreased fertility. For instance, ectopic pregnancy risk increases only in cases of post-abortion infections. Vacuum aspiration does not increase the subsequent risk incidence of second-trimester spontaneous abortion or preterm delivery. Also, it does not increase the risk of placenta previa, whereas multiple sharp curettage may.

Ovulation can resume as early as two weeks after abortion. Contraception should be initiated soon after abortion.

General complications of abortion include retained pregnancy, hemorrhage, infection, retained products or incomplete evacuation, and intra-abdominal expulsion (Table 122-3); the most threatening and most common complications of abortion are listed in Box 122-4. In the long term, there is an

BOX 122-4

Most Threatening and Most Common Complications of Induced Abortion

Most Threatening
- Uterine perforation
- Vascular injury
- Bowel injury
- Urinary tract injury
- Sepsis
- Uterine rupture

Most Common
- Bleeding
- Pain/cramping
- Medication intolerance (medical abortion)
- Cervical laceration
- Retained products of conception
- Retained pregnancy

Table 122-3 POST-ABORTION COMPLICATIONS

Abortion Method	Gestational Age	Complications: Immediate (<24 hr)	Complications: Early (1 day-4 wk)	Complications: Delayed	Complications: Late
Medical					
Mifepristone (Single 200-mg oral dose) Methotrexate ± misoprostol	<8 weeks	Nausea Bleeding Pain/cramping Ruptured ectopic pregnancy Rh isoimmunization	Bleeding Retained pregnancy Retained products Infection: Endometritis Sepsis Toxic shock syndrome Rh isoimmunization	Psychological trauma Rh isoimmunization	Psychological trauma Rh isoimmunization
Misoprostol/ vaginal prostaglandins	Up to 23 weeks				
Surgical					
Curettage (suction or sharp): Without dilation With dilation Dilation and evacuation	 <7 weeks 7 to 13 weeks >13 weeks	Pain Bleeding Cervical laceration Uterine perforation Inability to complete procedure Combined (intrauterine and tubal) pregnancy	Bleeding Retained products Infection: Endometritis Sepsis Toxic shock syndrome Rh isoimmunization	Post-abortive amenorrhea Rh isoimmunization	Post-abortive amenorrhea Psychological trauma Rh isoimmunization

increased incidence of decreased fertility and amenorrhea.

Surgical abortion carries the risks of anesthesia in addition to those of the procedure. Complications categorized as immediate, delayed, and long-term are listed in Box 122-5 These and other complications related to specific abortion methods are discussed separately.

A review of medical abortion methods follows.

Medical Abortion

■ SCOPE AND EPIDEMIOLOGY

Medical abortion has a success rate of 80% to 97% (higher for gestations <50 days); 2% to 5% of patients with failed abortions require subsequent surgical abortion, with a 5% to 10% rate of incomplete evacuation of products of conception.[11]

The three most commonly used abortion medications are *mifepristone* (an antiprogestin), and *misoprostol* (a prostaglandin), both of which trigger uterine contraction, and *methotrexate,* which is an antimetabolite and interrupts embryonic development. Methotrexate and misoprostol are also teratogenic. Thus their use requires that the termination be completed, even if surgical means are ultimately necessary.

Medical abortion between 13 to 28 weeks of gestation of both live and deceased fetuses is uncommon but can be performed with prostaglandin E_2 suppositories, carboprost tromethamine, misoprostol, or high-dose oxytocin (80%-90% effective). The most feared complication is uterine rupture, especially in women with a scarred uterus (e.g., previous cesarean delivery), grand multiparity, and nulliparity with an insufficiently ripened cervix.

■ COMPLICATIONS

Complications include bleeding, abdominal pain, and uterine cramping that can be severe and prolonged. It is important to distinguish expected heavy bleeding due to the natural course of medical termination from incomplete abortion or uterine rupture. Transfusions are rarely required despite heavy bleeding. Common side effects include nausea, vomiting, and diarrhea. Headache, dizziness, back pain, and fatigue may also occur.

Dilation and Curettage/Evacuation

Dilation and curettage is the most frequently utilized abortion method in the United States (over 90% of abortions).[1] The cervix is manually dilated, and uterine contents scraped out with a curette or aspirated via vacuum extraction. It is typically performed in the first trimester. The overall risk profile is low (0.1%-0.3%), and even lower with regional anesthesia. However, the complication rate does increase with gestational age.

Dilation and evacuation is performed to terminate pregnancies over 16 weeks of gestation. Dilation is achieved via osmotic dilators (i.e., laminaria) or vaginally administered prostaglandins, as opposed to

BOX 122-5

Complications of Surgical Abortion

Immediate Complications (<24 hours)

Minor

- Mild infection
- Incomplete abortion
- Hematometra (uterine distention syndrome)

Major

- Hemorrhage due to
  - Incomplete abortion (retained products of conception)
  - Uterine perforation +/– injury to adjacent structures
  - Cervical laceration
- Severe infection and sepsis
- Injury to adjacent structures
- Missed heterotopic pregnancy

Delayed Complications (1 day-4 wk)

- Infection (e.g., endometritis)
- Hemorrhage
- Retained foreign body or products of conception
- Cervical stenosis

Long-Term Complications

- Future fertility problems
- Post-abortion amenorrhea
- Adhesions
- Uterine synechiae
- Ectopic pregnancy
- Premature labor
- Very-low-birthweight infants

instrumentation, and the uterine contents are removed with forceps and vacuum. This technique also is used in the management of spontaneous abortion, retained products of conception, intrauterine fetal demise, and gestational trophoblastic neoplasia. Its use depends on uterine volume, age of gestation, and operator experience.[12]

Complications include uterine perforation, cervical laceration, hemorrhage, incomplete removal of the fetus and placenta, and infection. Very rarely, a curettage performed in advanced pregnancy results in a severe, fatal, consumptive coagulopathy.

The most common postprocedural complaints are bleeding and pain. The EP must first establish that the patient is stable, resuscitate if necessary, and then determine if the source of bleeding is vaginal, cervical, or uterine.

Lacerations of the vagina or cervix are treated with pressure and Monsel's solution or silver nitrite.

Uterine bleeding may be due to retained products of conception, uterine atony, infection, uterine arteriovenous malformation, placenta accreta, coagulopathy (due to high levels of tissue thromboplastin released during the procedure), or uterine perforation.

Table 122-4 PRESENTATION OF UTERINE PERFORATION

Site	Signs and Symptoms
Any site	Unexpected pain Vaginal bleeding Symptoms of anemia
Any site with bowel injury	Abdominal pain ± distention or peritoneal signs Fever
Fundal	Unexpected pain
Lateral	Diffuse lower abdominal pain Pelvic mass Fever
Anterior	Hematuria

■ UTERINE PERFORATION

Uterine perforation is feared because it carries a high risk of concomitant damage to intraperitoneal structures and severe hemorrhage. Delayed presentation is not uncommon because fundal perforations (accounting for two thirds of all perforations) have scant bleeding. Lateral perforations may have heavy bleeding hidden in the broad ligament, and a lacerated uterine artery may initially spasm. Presentation depends on the site of perforation (Table 122-4).

Resuscitation of the unstable patient is paramount. Management includes rapid diagnosis, placement of two large-bore IV catheters, fluid resuscitation and/or transfusion, and gynecologic consultation. Laboratory tests include a complete blood count, electrolytes, blood urea nitrogen and creatinine, beta–human chorionic gonadotropin (beta-hCG), coagulation profile, and blood type and screen (or blood type and cross if bleeding is profuse). An upright chest radiograph revealing free air is sufficient evidence of perforation and the need for emergent exploratory laparotomy.

In the stable patient, ultrasound imaging is required to evaluate the pelvic structures, followed by a computed tomography scan if the ultrasound image is equivocal. Laparotomy or laparoscopy to examine the abdominal contents is usually indicated, although small perforations may be managed expectantly. In the presence of rapid bleeding, a Foley catheter inserted into the uterus and inflated with 60 mL of saline can serve as a temporizing tamponade (Table 122-5).

Post-Abortion Infection

Post-abortion infection is extremely rare. Usually it is due to retained products of conception or unrecognized preexisting infection. Antibiotic therapy

Table 122-5 TREATMENT OF POST-ABORTION HEMORRHAGE WITHOUT PERFORATION

Cause of Hemorrhage	Treatment
Uterine atony	Methylergonovine maleate (Methergine), 0.2 mg IM Carboprost tromethamine (Hemabate), 250 µg IM q15-90 min (maximum total dose 2 mg) Misoprostol, 1000 mg suppository per rectum Pitocin, 40 U in 1 L of 5% dextrose in normal saline (NS) at IV drip rate titrated to bleeding control
Retained tissue	Dilation and curettage Consider antibiotics if endometritis is suspected
Placenta accreta	Uterine artery embolization
Severe continued bleeding	Temporizing measure: Intrauterine tamponade via uterine packing or transcervical Foley catheter placement with balloon inflation using 30 mL of sterile NS (or 100 mL NS for a 30-mL balloon)

usually is based on the CDC guidelines for treating pelvic inflammatory disease.

Patients with endometritis usually present with fever, prolonged vaginal bleeding, and pelvic pain. A midline boggy mass may be noted on examination. The leading cause is retained products of conception. Laboratory tests include complete blood count, coagulation profile, beta-hCG, and cervical cultures. Transvaginal pelvic ultrasonography should be performed to evaluate for retained tissue. These cases require not only antibiotics but also repeat suction curettage.

Recommended antibiotic regimens include IV clindamycin, 900 mg every 8 hours, plus gentamicin, 1.5 mg/kg every 8 hours; triple coverage with ampicillin, gentamicin, and metronidazole is indicated for sicker patients; and ampicillin/sulbactam as monotherapy in less severe cases.

Although extremely rare and seen mostly in illegal abortions, severe and fatal infections are possible. Severe hemorrhage, sepsis, bacterial shock, and acute renal failure have occurred in association with abortion. Uterine infection is most common but parametritis, endocarditis, peritonitis, and septicemia may be seen. The infecting organisms usually are anaerobic bacteria coliforms.

Diffuse abdominal tenderness with guarding, fever, tachycardia, and hypotension suggest severe sepsis. After rapid stabilization and IV fluid resuscitation, laboratory tests should include complete blood count with differential, electrolytes, kidney and liver function, coagulation profile, lactate studies, beta-hCG, urinalysis, and cervical and urine cultures. Treatment includes prompt IV administration of broad-spectrum antimicrobials followed by evacuation of the products of conception. A severe complication is disseminated intravascular coagulopathy.

PATIENT TEACHING TIPS

POST-ABORTION INSTRUCTIONS

- Instruct the patient about the natural course of recovery, in particular how much bleeding can be anticipated and when to be concerned.
- If antibiotics are prescribed, the patient should complete the entire course as indicated.
- Inquire if the patient wishes to use contraception. Also clarify that only barrier contraception protects against sexually transmitted diseases as well.
- Tell the patient to call her physician or return to the ED if she has:
  - Vaginal bleeding soaking more than 1 maxipad an hour for at least 4 hours
  - Foul-smelling, milky, or green vaginal discharge
  - Increasing abdominal or pelvic pain
  - Any other concerning symptoms

■ RETAINED PRODUCTS OF CONCEPTION

Patients with retained products of conception usually present with bleeding. Endometritis can occur as a result, as described in the previous section. Definitive treatment is repeat dilation and curettage.

Procedures Out of Favor

Intact dilation and extraction (politically termed "partial birth abortion") is a procedure in which the fetus is removed via a modified assisted breech delivery with decompression of the calvarium to deliver the fetus intact. Complication rates are comparable to those of dilation and evacuation. Currently, there is a nonenforced ban on this procedure.

Intrauterine instillation of abortifacients, hysterectomy, and hysterotomy have been largely abandoned for uterine evacuation due to their high rates of associated maternal morbidity and mortality.

COMPLICATIONS OF ASSISTED REPRODUCTIVE TECHNOLOGY

Scope and Epidemiology

On July 25, 1978, Louise Brown, the original "test-tube baby" was born in England. Conceived by in vitro fertilization, her birth was a landmark in the history of assisted reproductive technology (ART).

PRIORITY ACTIONS

Diagnosis: Complications of ART

Induction Phase

- Abdominal pain, distention or ascites? Initiate work-up and symptomatic treatment for OHSS. Obtain US scan and estradiol levels.
- Difficulty breathing and unstable? If signs of third spacing, suspect severe OHSS; symptomatic treatment, possible admission to the ICU required.
- No evidence of third spacing, or only leg edema? Consider pulmonary embolism; obtain chest radiograph to rule out other causes; anticoagulation and lower-extremity vascular Doppler US required to evaluate for deep venous thrombosis.
- Pelvic pain? Consider early OHSS.

Any Time during ART

- Pelvic pain? Doppler US required to evaluate for ovarian torsion versus ovarian cyst ± rupture.

After Oocyte Harvesting

- Fever? Consider infection; administer antibiotics and evaluate, if stable, for discharge.
- Vaginal bleeding from puncture site? Place pressure. If bleeding does not stop, consider Monsel's solution or silver nitrate.
- Abdominal pain or peritoneal signs? Consider intraperitoneal hemorrhage; cardiovascular stabilization and definitive exploratory laparotomy required.

After Implantation or Embryo Transfer

- Pelvic pain or vaginal bleeding? Schedule US and obtain quantitative hCG to evaluate for ectopic/heterotopic pregnancy or threatened spontaneous miscarriage.

ART, assisted reproductive technology; hCG, human chorionic gonadotropin; OHSS, ovarian hyperstimulation syndrome; US, ultrasonography.

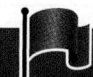

Four years later, the first child conceived by ART in the United States was born. In 1996, 64,724 ART procedures were reported in the United States; since then the numbers have skyrocketed to 115,392 cycles reported in 2002, resulting in 45,751 infants.[13] In spite of the growing popularity of ART, however, there are limited published data on complications.

Literature on complications of in vitro fertilization focuses primarily on outcomes of the pregnancy (multiple-birth gestations, low birthweight babies, cesarean sections, and pre-term delivery), as well as long-term effects on women, and effects on the resultant children.[14] These complications are dealt with only indirectly in the ED.

RED FLAGS

Complications of Assisted Reproduction Technology (ART)

- Increased abdominal girth, abdominal pain, edema, dyspnea during ovulation induction or early post-implantation are suspicious for ovarian hyperstimulation syndrome.
- Unilateral pelvic pain is suspicious for ectopic pregnancy or ovarian torsion.
- Severe pain, fever, brisk bleeding, and peritoneal signs are suspicious for perforation.
- Shortness of breath, possibly with pleuritic chest pain, should prompt evaluation for pulmonary embolism, although pleural effusions due to ovarian hyperstimulation syndrome also are possible.

Structure and Function

Many techniques are used in the course of assisted reproduction, with rapid advances having been made over the last 2 decades. There are five basic stages of ART for women: ovulation (natural or induced), egg harvesting, implantation of the egg and sperm or fertilized zygote, pregnancy, and delivery. For men, risks are mostly limited to procedures for correction of anatomic abnormalities or for sperm acquisition. Complications of the earlier stages are more likely to be related to the specific procedure. The EP must keep in mind that often infertility specialists are very involved in the management of their patients, and thus these patients typically will have very close follow-up.

The subfertility of a couple can be attributed to male factor, female factor, or incompatibility issues. Male factor infertility includes dysfunctional sperm, inadequate sperm concentration, and obstruction. Female factor infertility can be due to ovulatory dysfunction, poor egg quality, anatomic abnormalities, or hormonal imbalance. Compatibility factors include hostile environment.

ART incorporates techniques of controlled ovarian hyperstimulation, egg or sperm retrieval, insemination, and embryo transfer. The choice of ART methods depends on an extensive evaluation of both individuals and compatibility.

Major Complications

Major complications of ART likely to be encountered in the ED include ovarian hyperstimulation syndrome, ectopic/heterotopic pregnancy, miscarriages, ovarian torsion, ovarian rupture, thromboembolism, and post-procedural complications (Table 122-6 and Box 122-6). Infertility specialists typically follow their patients very closely and should be contacted early.

Table 122-6 COMPLICATIONS OF ASSISTED REPRODUCTIVE TECHNOLOGY

	Time of Onset			
Complication	**Immediate**	**Early**	**Delayed**	**Late**
Controlled ovarian hyperstimulation: Clomiphene citrate, gonadotropins (FSH/LH, GnRH, hMG)	Medication side effects	OHSS,* ovarian torsion, ovarian cyst, rupture	Multifetal pregnancy, thromboembolic disease*	Ovarian cancer is NOT supported by trials
Oocyte retrieval	Risks of anesthesia, bleeding from vaginal puncture site, intraperitoneal bleeding	Bleeding from vaginal puncture site, intraperitoneal bleeding, ovarian torsion, infection	Bowel endometriosis	
Embryo transfer	Contractions expelling the embryos	Infection, OHSS	Multifetal pregnancy	
Pregnancy	Early pregnancy, bleeding, placenta previa	OHSS, ectopic/heterotopic pregnancy,* spontaneous abortion, thromboembolic disease*	Multifetal pregnancy, preeclampsia/eclampsia, thromboembolic disease,* placental abruption	Multifetal pregnancy, preeclampsia/eclampsia, thromboembolic disease*
Delivery	Pre-term labor/PROM, preeclampsia/eclampsia, primary inadequate contractions, secondary uterine inertia; increased risk of cesarean section, multifetal delivery; EVLBW/VLBW/LBW infants	Thromboembolic complications, retained placenta; bleeding associated with vaginal delivery; preeclampsia/eclampsia		

*Major complication.
EVLBW, extremely very-low-birthweight; FSH/LH, follicle-stimulating hormone/luteinizing hormone; GnRH, gonadotropin-releasing hormone; hMG, human menopausal gonadotropin; LBW, low-birthweight; OHSS, ovarian hyperstimulation syndrome; PROM, premature rupture of membrane; VLBW, very-low-birthweight.

BOX 122-6

Most Threatening and Most Common Complications of Assisted Reproductive Technology (ART)

Most Threatening
- Ovarian hyperstimulation syndrome
- Ectopic/heterotopic pregnancy
- Ovarian torsion
- Pulmonary embolism/deep venous thrombosis

Most Common
- Medication side effects
- Multiple gestation pregnancies
- Preterm labor
- Bleeding
- Infection
- Miscarriage
- Pain

■ OVULATION INDUCTION

During artificially modulated ovarian stimulation, the majority of complaints arise from medication reactions and pain that is due to ovarian cysts, exacerbation of endometritis, or enlarging fibroids. Pain should be taken seriously as a possible sentinel of diagnoses such as ovarian hyperstimulation syndrome and ovarian torsion.

■ OVARIAN HYPERSTIMULATION SYNDROME

Ovarian hyperstimulation syndrome is the most feared complication of ovulatory stimulation. In its most severe form, it is life-threatening. Severe cases occur in an estimated 0.5% to 5% of ART cycles and also occur rarely in spontaneous pregnancy. The estimated mortality rate is 1/450,000 to 1/50,000 patients.[15]

■ Pathophysiology

Ovarian hyperstimulation syndrome is characterized by increased capillary permeability with third-spacing

BOX 122-7

Risk Factors for Ovarian Hyperstimulation Syndrome

- <35 years of age
- Low body mass index
- Use of gonadotropin-releasing hormone analogues and gonadotropins
- Elevated estradiol levels
- Increased number of stimulated follicles during controlled ovarian hyperstimulation
- Polycystic ovarian disease
- Previous episode of ovarian hyperstimulation syndrome

of protein-rich fluid resulting in hemoconcentration with severe intravascular hypovolemia manifested as edema, ascites, and pleural and pericardial effusions. Multisystem organ failure, renal failure, immunosuppression, pulmonary failure, thromboembolism, and death may result.

The mechanism is unclear, but hCG appears to be a trigger because it usually manifests within a week of exogenous hCG administration and oocyte retrieval, with a second peak noted after implantation, due to endogenous hCG.

Presenting Signs and Symptoms

Patients present with abdominal pain and distention, nausea, and vomiting and may have constipation or diarrhea. Chest discomfort, dyspnea, concentrated oliguria, rapid weight gain, and peripheral edema are symptoms of more severe cases.

Risk Factors

Risk factors include young age, low body mass index, use of gonadotropin-releasing hormone analogues and exogenous hCG (endogenous hCG from pregnancy may rarely also be causative), elevated estradiol levels, increased number of stimulated follicles during controlled ovarian hyperstimulation ("necklace sign" or "string of pearls" appearance on ultrasound images), polycystic ovarian disease, and previous ovarian hyperstimulation syndrome (Box 122-7).

Differential Diagnosis, Diagnostic Criteria, and Diagnostic Testing

Physical examination reveals abdominal distention with tenderness in the bilateral lower quadrants and tender, enlarged ovaries. Increasing evidence of third spacing such as peripheral edema, ascites, dull lung fields consistent with pleural effusion, and distant

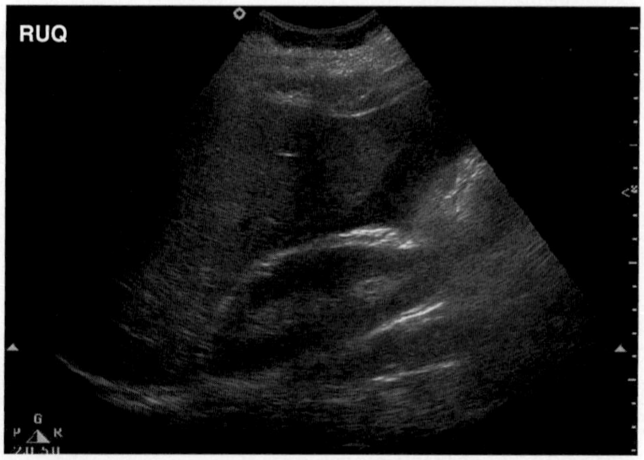
RUQ

FIGURE 122-3 Ascites and pleural effusion in a patient with ovarian hyperstimulation syndrome.

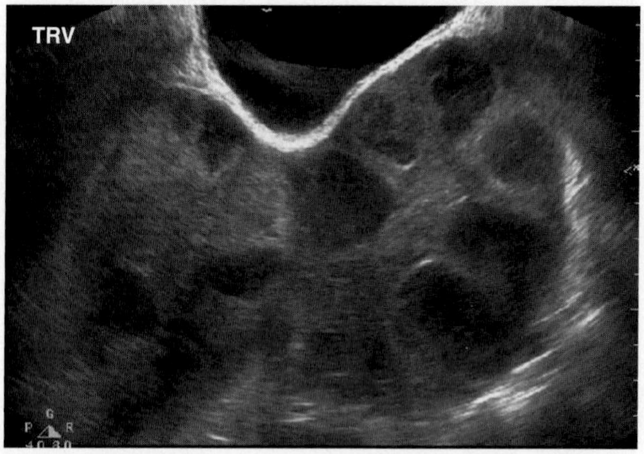
TRV

FIGURE 122-4 Polycystic ovarian syndrome affecting both ovaries in a patient with ovarian hyperstimulation syndrome.

heart sounds are evident in patients with severe disease. Laboratory testing reveals elevated serum estradiol levels greater than 3000 pg/mL, hemoconcentration with hyponatremia and hyperkalemia, and decreased renal function. Pelvic Doppler ultrasonography is essential to evaluate the extent of follicular recruitment (Fig. 122-3) and the presence of ascites (Fig. 122-4). as well as, to rule out alternative diagnoses such as ovarian torsion.

Treatment

There is no specific cure for ovarian hyperstimulation syndrome; treatment is empirical and focused on supportive care until spontaneous resolution occurs (Table 122-7). Usually the syndrome is self-limited.

Early detection and prevention are key. Individuals at risk should receive only low-dose gonadotropins and be closely monitored. The development of symptoms, elevated estradiol levels (>3000 pg/mL), or excessive follicular recruitment (>20) calls for the initiation of preventive treatment strategies such as decreasing hormone dosages, freezing the embryos rather than waiting for fresh embryo transfer, admin-

Table 122-7 MANAGEMENT OF PATIENTS WITH OVARIAN HYPERSTIMULATION SYNDROME

Severity	Signs and symptoms	Management
Mild	Abdominal discomfort, distention, pain Enlarged ovaries (up to 5 cm) Minimal ascites Weight gain of <10 pounds	Outpatient management Analgesia Increased oral fluid intake (high-salt solutions) Close follow-up with regular visits Report if symptoms worsen
Moderate	**AS ABOVE, PLUS:** Enlarged ovaries (5-12 cm) Nausea, vomiting, diarrhea Ultrasonographic evidence of ascites Hemoconcentration (Hct<45%)	Admit to hospital Daily assessment Thromboembolic prophylaxis Monitor lab studies—CBC, electrolytes, blood urea nitrogen, Cr, liver function tests, coagulation profile
Severe	**AS ABOVE, PLUS:** Clinical evidence of ascites Palpable ovaries Hepatic dysfunction Hydrothorax, dyspnea Peripheral edema, anasarca Oliguria Hemoconcentration (Hct>45%, Hg>15 g) Hypotension Renal insufficiency (Cr 1.0-1.5 mg/dL)	Admit to intensive care unit Strict fluid balance with input of 3 L or more 2 large-bore IV catheters Consider central venous pressure line Consider IV albumin Thoracentesis or paracentesis as needed Thromboembolic prophylaxis Terminate ART cycle
Critical	**AS ABOVE, PLUS:** Severely contracted blood volume (Hct>55%, WBC>25,000) Renal failure (Cr>1.6 mg/dL) Thromboembolism Acute respiratory distress syndrome	Admit to intensive care unit Strict fluid balance with input of 3 L or more 2 large-bore IV catheters/central venous pressure line IV albumin Intubation and ventilation Thoracentesis or paracentesis as needed Hemodialysis as needed Anticoagulation or IVC filter as required Terminate ART cycle

ART, assisted reproductive technology; CBC, complete blood count; Cr, creatinine; Hct, hematocrit; IVC, interior vena cava; WBC, white blood cells.

istering albumin during oocyte harvesting, and "coasting" (withholding further gonadotropin administration until estradiol levels decrease, which allows fresh embryo retrieval and transfer). In extreme circumstances, the stimulation protocol should be terminated.

Mild Cases

Mild cases can be managed on an outpatient basis with very close follow-up and daily monitoring of weight, abdominal girth, and urine output. Conservative management focuses on treating pain and maintaining hydration, although some treatment strategies include high-protein diets and high-sodium drinks (e.g., exercise rehydration drinks). Progressive symptoms or weight gain of more than 2 pounds should prompt hospital admission. In the absence of pregnancy, symptoms are expected to resolve about 2 weeks after hCG was administered.

Moderate Cases

Patients with moderate disease require a complete laboratory and ultrasonography work-up, as well as hospitalization for close observation and serial examinations, particularly if the patient has disabling nausea, intractable abdominal pain, tense ascites, abnormal laboratory values, or other indications of a downward trajectory. Pelvic examination is NOT recommended in moderate or severe cases because of the risk for cyst rupture with hemorrhage.[16] There is a low threshold for admission for monitoring, and if discharged, the patient should maintain a record of fluid balance and be seen in 2 to 3 days. Physical activity should be avoided.

Severe Cases

Severe ovarian hyperstimulation syndrome requires inpatient care in the intensive care unit.[17] Strict monitoring of fluid balance and hemodynamics is critical. Two large-bore IV catheters (18 gauge or larger) must be placed, and a subclavian line for central venous pressures is advisable. Aggressive repletion of the intravascular space starts with at least two to three liters of normal saline. If urine output remains inadequate (<50 mL/hour), salt-poor IV albumin (or hydroxyethyl starch) is the next step. Lactated Ringer's solution should be avoided due to elevated potassium levels. If oliguria and renal failure ensue in the face of aggressive volume repletion, elevated intraperitoneal pressure compressing the renal vasculature must be considered, and paracentesis may help.

Ultrasound guidance is recommended to avoid puncturing the enlarged ovaries. Diuretics may deplete the intravascular space and increase the risk of thromboembolism; however, once hemodilution has been achieved, following each 100 mg of albumin

PATIENT TEACHING TIPS

OVARIAN HYPERSTIMULATION SYNDROME

- Clarify details of the anticipated post-procedural course.
- Schedule follow-up with the patient's physician in 1 to 3 days.
- If the procedure is still in the induction phase, instruct the patient to call her physician or return to the ED immediately if she develops symptoms of ovarian hyperstimulation syndrome, including:
  - Chest discomfort, difficulty breathing
  - Abdominal pain and bloating, rapid weight gain
  - Decreased urination
  - Severe or persistent vomiting
- Warn the patient that there can be a second peak in symptoms AFTER implantation triggered by the patient's own hormonal surge.

with 10 to 20 mg of furosemide may be of benefit in patients with recalcitrant prerenal azotemia. Deep venous thrombosis prophylaxis is essential, given the high risk of thromboembolic disease. Syndrome-associated hypoglobulinemia results in a relative immunodepression. Antibiotics should be selected for specific suspected infectious etiologies. Prescription of medications should take into consideration the presence of early pregnancy.

Critical Cases

Critical cases with complications such as renal failure, thromboembolism, or acute respiratory distress syndrome require all of the previously described measures and termination of the pregnancy.

OVARIAN TORSION

Ovarian enlargement predisposes to torsion. ART patients are at particular risk because they are actively seeking to attain hyperovulation and pregnancy. In addition, patients with elevated risk due to preexisting conditions such as polycystic ovarian syndrome are overrepresented in the ART population.

Severe unilateral adnexal or pelvic pain initially may be intermittent as the ovary twists and untwists; the pain then become sustained when the torsion persists and the ovary becomes ischemic. Immediate pelvic Doppler ultrasonography of the ovarian vessels is the key to diagnosis and differentiation from benign etiologies of pelvic pain. Emergent surgical intervention is indicated to avoid permanent damage to the ovary.

THROMBOEMBOLIC DISEASE

ART patients are at high risk for thromboembolism due to the high levels of hormones being maintained. A high index of suspicion must be maintained, but evaluation should take into consideration the ongoing attempts at pregnancy. Before any type of imaging is performed pregnancy status should be established.

If the patient is pregnant, ventilation perfusion scans are not recommended because of the use of radioactive materials. Chest computed tomography can be performed with shielding, but informed consent should be obtained from the patient first, allowing her to weigh the risks and benefits of the procedure. Echocardiography can evaluate for signs of critical pulmonary enbolism. Lower extremity vascular studies should be performed first, although sensitivity is low if there are no leg symptoms; if deep venous thrombosis is present, however, treatment should be instituted without further investigation.

Oocyte Harvesting

Transvaginal ultrasound-guided oocyte aspiration typically is an ambulatory procedure with intravenous analgesia and sedation. Risks include vascular injury with bleeding from the vaginal puncture site, hemoperitoneum, rupture of ovarian cysts, bowel perforation, injury to pelvic organs, and infection.

Bleeding from the vaginal mucosa due to the punctures required for harvesting usually spontaneously resolves by the end of the procedure, or with direct pressure. Persistent or significant bleeding despite these measures or administration of topical hemostatic agents requires suturing. Intraabdominal bleeding should be suspected in the face of post-procedural symptoms of anemia even before peritoneal signs manifest.

If vital signs remain stable and the patient is minimally symptomatic, conservative management is possible; however, if the patient is hemodynamically unstable and does not recover with basic fluid resuscitation, or if the hemoglobin continues to fall and the patient is symptomatic, emergent exploratory laparotomy is required for definitive diagnosis and correction. Typed and crossed blood should be used for transfusion if the patient is sufficiently stable. Uncrossed O-negative blood can be used for immediate transfusion if necessary.

Embryo Transfer

Embryo transfer may be complicated by pelvic infection, ectopic or heterotopic pregnancy, spontaneous expulsion of the embryo, and multiple gestation pregnancy.

PELVIC INFECTION

Patients with post-procedure pelvic infection present with pelvic pain and fever several days after the procedure; vaginal discharge also may be present (Table 122-8). Cultures should be sent to the laboratory. Other laboratory tests may show leukocytosis with a

Table 122-8 POST-PROCEDURAL PELVIC INFECTIONS

Procedure	Complication	Presentation
Minor gynecologic surgery	Cervicitis	Inflammation and cervical discharge
	Endometritis/parametritis	Inflammation, cervical discharge, uterine and/or adnexal tenderness
Hysterectomy	Cuff infection	Malodorous discharge
	Cuff cellulitis	Induration and tenderness of the vaginal apex; fever, leukocytosis
	Cuff abscess	Induration and tenderness of vaginal apex; fever, leukocytosis; discrete mass by palpation or ultrasonography

left shift. Administration of amoxicillin/clavulanate, 875 mg twice daily for 5 days, is usually adequate treatment.

■ ECTOPIC/HETEROTOPIC PREGNANCIES

In spite of the careful placement of embryos into the uterus, approximately 4% of in vitro fertilization pregnancies are ectopic. This incidence is slightly reduced with ultrasound guidance of embryo placement; however, migration of the embryo may occur. Ectopic pregnancies due to ART are usually diagnosed very early because of close ultrasound monitoring by the fertility specialist.

Heterotopic pregnancies (multigestational pregnancies with at least one ectopic and one intrauterine pregnancy) are very rare in spontaneous conception (1:30,000) but occur in up to 1% of assisted conception cycles. This number is expected to decrease as technology continues to improve and the use of single-embryo transfer increases. In the presence of symptoms consistent with a possible ectopic pregnancy, the presence of an intrauterine pregnancy does not rule out a heterotopic ectopic pregnancy, and a full work-up should be performed.

Management of patients who have undergone the psychological, physical, and financial burden of using ART and have a heterotopic pregnancy should be focused on maintaining the intrauterine pregnancy while eliminating the ectopic pregnancy and avoiding excess risk to the mother.

■ MULTIPLE GESTATION PREGNANCIES

In 2003, 51% of infants born as a result of ART were multiple gestation births, in contrast to approximately 3% of births in the general population.[18]

Multiple embryos often are placed in the uterus because of the low implantation rate per embryo (10%-25%). Although this can be welcome news to the expectant parents, these multifetal pregnancies are associated with an increased risk of mortality and morbidity for both mother and fetuses.

Maternal complications include preterm labor, placental abruption and placenta previa, cesarean section, postpartum hemorrhage, gestational diabetes, and preeclampsia. Fetuses are at risk for the secondary effects of maternal complications as well as premature birth, low birth weight, intrauterine demise, and congenital conditions such as cerebral palsy. As new technological developments increase the success of implantation, however, protocols are changing to dictate the transfer of only one or two embryos.

Male Factor Infertility Treatment

Oligospermia is the number one reason for male factor infertility. Fortunately, treatment for this condition entails minimal complications. If more than two million sperm can be obtained via ejaculation, artificial insemination is used to directly place the sperm in a position amenable to fertilizing the ova.

The introduction of intracytoplasmic sperm injection in 1993 has given hope to men with severe oligospermia. In this procedure, sperm is surgically obtained and a single sperm injected directly into the oocyte. The fertilized embryo is then placed in the uterus for implantation. In vitro fertilization success rates using this method are close to those achieved with in vitro fertilization from ejaculated spermatozoa.

Physical complications during in vitro fertilization cycles are therefore limited to those of diagnostic testicular biopsy and of procedures to obtain sperm if ejaculated sperm are inadequate.

Other complications include pain, bleeding, bruising, and, in the long term, scarring from the surgical procedure. Psychological benefits may outweigh physical complications.

REFERENCES

1. Strauss LTT, Herndon J, Chang J, et al: Abortion Surveillance—United States, 2002. MMWR Surveill Summ 2005;54:1-31.
2. ASRM/SART Registry: Assisted Reproductive Technology in the United States: 2000 results generated from the American Society for Reproductive Medicine/Society for Assisted Reproductive Technology Registry. Fertility and Sterility. 2004;81;1207-1220.
3. Waterstone M, Bewley S, Wolfe C: Incidence and predictors of severe obstetrical mortality: A case review. Obstet Gynecol Surv 2002;57:139-140.
4. Magrina JF: Complications of laparoscopic surgery; Clin Obstet Gynecol 2002;45:469-480.

5. Bishoff JT, Allaf ME, Kirkels W, et al: Laparoscopic bowel injury: Incidence and clinical presentation. J Urol 1999;161:887-890.
6. Chapron CM, Pierre F, Lacroix S, et al: Major vascular injuries during gynecologic laparoscopy. J Am Coll Surg 1997;185:461-465.
7. Walker WJ, Pelage JP, Sutton C: Fibroid embolization. Clin Radiol 2002;57:325-331.
8. U.S. Cancer Statistics Working Group: United States Cancer Statistics: 2003 Incidence and Mortality (preliminary data). Atlanta, U.S. Department of Health and Human Services, Centers for Disease Control and Prevention, and National Cancer Institute, 2006.
9. Finer LB, Henshaw SK: Abortion incidence and services in the United States in 2000. Perspect Sex Reprod Health 2003;35:6-15.
10. CDC: Maternal Mortality—United States, 1982-1996; MMWR Morb Mortal Wkly Rep 1998;47;705-707.
11. Christin-Maitre S, Bouchard P, Spitz IM: Medical termination of pregnancy. N Engl J Med 2000;342:946-956.
12. American College of Obstetricians and Gynecologists (ACOG): Methods of midtrimester abortion. ACOG technical bulletin #109. Washington, DC, 1987.
13. CDC: 2002 Assisted Reproductive Technology (ART) Report: Section 5—ART trends, 1996-2002. Oct 17, 2005.
14. Land JA, Evers JL: Risks and complications in assisted reproduction techniques: Report of an ESHRE (European Society of Human Reproduction and Embryology) consensus meeting. Hum Reprod 2003;18:455-457.
15. Budev MM, Arroglia AC, Falcone T: Ovarian hyperstimulation syndrome. Crit Care Med 2005;33(Suppl):S301-S306.
16. Fawzy M, Harrison RF, Walshe J: Ovarian hyperstimulation syndrome: Diagnosis, prevention and management. Ir Med J 1998;91:86-87.
17. Delvigne A, Rozenberg S: Review of clinical course and treatment of ovarian hyperstimulation syndrome (OHSS). Hum Reprod Update 2003;9:77-96.
18. CDC: Assisted Reproductive Technology Surveillance—United States, 2003. MMWR Surveill Summ 2006;55:1-22.

Chapter **123**

Gynecologic Infections

Jamil Bayram and Mamta Malik

KEY POINTS

- Not all gynecologic infections, including pelvic inflammatory disease, are sexually transmitted, although many are. They are often asymptomatic in women and their sex partners.
- Sexually transmitted diseases are common, particularly in young, sexually active women with multiple sex partners.
- Careful history, physical examination, and diagnostic tests are important to differentiate gynecologic infections, because modalities of treatments vary.
- Microscopic diagnosis of yeast infections has a sensitivity of only 50% and fails to diagnosis the disorder in a large percentage of patients with symptomatic vulvovaginal candidiasis.
- Most young, sexually active patients with genital ulcers have a genital herpes infection, syphilis, or chancroid disease, with genital herpes infection being the most common.
- Treatment should be instituted for most gynecologic infections based on presumed diagnosis because many patients with genital infections will not have a laboratory-confirmed diagnosis.

Scope

A large number of microbes are naturally present in the female reproductive tract and can predispose to infectious processes. Many of these infections—but not all—are sexually transmitted. In this chapter, gynecologic infections are grouped according to their anatomic location: namely, vulvar, vaginal, cervical, pelvic, abdominal, genitourinary, and systemic. It should be kept in mind that some infections affect more than one area of the female genital tract. Populations requiring specific consideration (e.g., pregnant patients, human immunodeficiency virus [HIV]-positive patients) are discussed separately.

Diagnosis and management of common gynecologic infections are summarized in Table 123-1.

Vulvar Infections

■ HUMAN PAPILLOMAVIRUS

Human papillomavirus (HPV) infection is a sexually transmitted disease that usually is asymptomatic but can cause disease processes ranging from benign anogenital warts to invasive cancer (Fig. 123-1). Genital warts (*Condylomata acuminata*), most commonly caused by HPV subtype 6 or 11,[1] can occur on the vulva, perianal area, urethra, vaginal walls, or cervix.

Table 123-1 DIAGNOSIS AND TREATMENT OF GYNECOLOGIC INFECTIONS IN WOMEN

Infection	Diagnosis	Treatment	Follow Up or Special Concerns
Human papillomavirus infection	Diagnosis is made by visual inspection and identification of genital warts.	Patient-applied: podofilox 0.5% solution or gel bid for 3 days; or imiquimod 5% cream qhs 3 times per week for 16 weeks Provider-applied: cryotherapy with liquid nitrogen or cryoprobe; podophyllin resin 10%-25% in a compound tincture of benzoin; tricholoracetic acid or bichloracetic acid 80%-90% weekly Surgical excision Intralesional interferon Laser surgery	No treatment is started in ED; patient may schedule follow-up at earliest convenience.
Genital herpes simplex virus infection	The first episode may result in severe local symptoms such as painful bilateral genital ulcers or vesicles, inguinal adenopathy, along with fever, malaise, and myalgia. The classic appearance is vesicles or ulcers in various stages of development. Prodrome of itching or burning is common in patient with recurrent infection.	First clinical episode: Acyclovir, 400 mg PO tid for 7 to 10 days; or famciclovir, 250 mg PO tid for 7 to 10 days; or valacyclovir, 1 g PO bid for 7 to 10 days. Recurrent episodes: Acyclovir, 800 mg PO bid or 400 mg PO tid for 5 days; or famciclovir, 125 mg PO bid for 5 days; or valacyclovir, 500 mg PO bid for 3 days or 1.0 g qd for 5 days. Recommended regimens for daily suppressive therapy: Acyclovir, 400 mg PO bid; or famciclovir, 250 mg PO bid; or valacyclovir, 500 mg qd or 1000 mg qd	Sex partners of patients who have genital herpes infection are likely to benefit from evaluation and counseling. Make sure that patient understands risks of transmission even when she is asymptomatic.
Chancroid	Patient has one or more painful genital ulcers and has no evidence of *Treponema pallidum* infection by dark-field examination of ulcer exudate or by serologic test for syphilis performed at least 7 days after onset of ulcers. Clinical appearance of genital ulcers and regional lymphadenopathy, if present, is typical of chancroid, and test for herpes simplex virus is negative.	Azithromycin, 1 g orally in a single dose; or ceftriaxone, 250 mg IM in a single dose; or ciprofloxacin, 500 mg PO tid for 3 days (contraindicated in pregnant and lactating women and patients <18 years old); or erythromycin base, 500 mg PO tid for 7 days.	Patients should be reexamined 3 to 7 days after initiation of therapy.
Granuloma inguinale	Painless progressive ulcerative lesions without regional lymphadenopathy. Lesions are highly vascular and bleed easily on contact.	Doxycycline, 100 mg PO bid for a minimum of 3 weeks; or TMP-SMZ, one DS tablet PO bid for a minimum of 3 weeks; or ciprofloxacin, 750 mg PO bid for a minimum of 3 weeks; or azithromycin, 1 g PO once a week for at least 3 weeks; or erythromycin base, 500 mg PO qid for a minimum of 3 weeks.	Follow-up within a few days to ensure healing.

Table 123-1 DIAGNOSIS AND TREATMENT OF GYNECOLOGIC INFECTIONS IN WOMEN—cont'd

Infection	Diagnosis	Treatment	Follow Up or Special Concerns
Lymphogranuloma venereum	Women and homosexually active men: proctocolitis or inflammatory involvement of perirectal or perianal lymphatic tissues can result in fistulas and strictures.	Doxycycline, 100 mg PO bid; or erythromycin base, 500 mg PO qid for 21 days.	Surgical excision of scarred areas may be necessary.
Syphilis	Patients with syphilis may seek treatment for signs or symptoms of primary infection (ulcer or chancre at site of infection), of secondary infection (rash, mucocutaneous lesions, adenopathy), or of tertiary infection (cardiac, neurologic, ophthalmic, and auditory, and gummatous lesions).	Benzathine penicillin G, 2.4 million U IM in a single dose; doxycycline, 100 mg PO bid for 2 weeks; or tetracycline, 500 mg orally four times a day for 2 weeks if penicillin-allergic.	All patients should be tested for HIV and, if high risk, retested at 3 months if negative.
Mucopurulent cervicitis: likely *Chlamydia trachomatis* or *Neisseria gonorrhoeae* infection	Many patients are asymptomatic, but a yellow endocervical exudate often is seen. Other symptoms include abnormal vaginal discharge and abnormal vaginal bleeding (e.g., after intercourse). The condition can be caused by *C. trachomatis* or *N. gonorrhoeae,* although often neither organism can be isolated.	Azithromycin, 1 g PO in a single dose; or doxycycline, 100 mg PO bid for 7 days.	Patients should be instructed to refer all individuals who were sex partners within the preceding 60 days for evaluation and treatment. Patients should avoid sexual intercourse until both they and their sex partners are cured. In the absence of a microbiologic test of cure, this means that abstinence should be practiced until therapy is completed and patients and partners are without symptoms.
Gonococcal infections	Asymptomatic carriage may occur in 12%-50% of men and up to 80% of women. Typically in men there is a purulent discharge from the anterior urethra with dysuria appearing 2 to 7 days after the infecting exposure. Women may experience initial urethritis and cervicitis, accompanied by purulent discharge. Fever and abdominal and adnexal tenderness can occur with acute gonococcal pelvic inflammatory disease. Disseminated gonococcal infection results from gonococcal bacteremia. Patients may present with petechial or pustular acral skin lesions, asymmetrical arthralgias, tenosynovitis, and septic arthritis.	Cefixime, 400 mg PO in a single dose; or ceftriaxone, 125 mg IM in a single dose; or ciprofloxacin, 500 mg in a single dose. Disseminated gonococcal infection: Hospitalization is recommended for initial therapy; recommended initial regimen is ceftriaxone, 1 g IM or IV every 24 hours. All regimens should be continued for 24-48 hours after improvement begins, at which time therapy may be switched to one of the following regimens to complete a full week of antimicrobial therapy: cefixime, 400 mg PO bid; or ciprofloxacin, 500 mg PO bid.	Patients infected with *N. gonorrhoeae* often are coinfected with *C. trachomatis;* this finding has led to the recommendation that patients treated for gonococcal infection also be treated routinely with a regimen effective against uncomplicated genital *C. trachomatis* infection. Patients should be instructed to refer for evaluation and treatment all individuals who were sex partners within the preceding 60 days. Patients should be instructed to avoid sexual intercourse until patient and partners are cured. In the absence of a microbiologic test of cure, this means until therapy is completed and patient and partners are without symptoms.

Continued

Table 123-1 DIAGNOSIS AND TREATMENT OF GYNECOLOGIC INFECTIONS IN WOMEN—cont'd

Infection	Diagnosis	Treatment	Follow Up or Special Concerns
Trichomoniasis	*Trichomonas vaginalis* typically causes a diffuse, malodorous, yellow-green discharge with vulvar irritation.	Recommended regimen: metronidazole, 2 g orally in a single dose. Alternative regimen: metronidazole, 500 mg bid for 7 days. Treatment of patients and sex partners results in relief of symptoms, microbiologic cure, and reduction of transmission. Metronidazole gel has been approved for the treatment of bacterial vaginosis, but it is less efficacious than oral preparations of metronidazole and therefore is not recommended.	Persistent discharge after adequate treatment for trichomoniasis should lead to repeat examination for trichomoniasis, candidiasis, and gonorrhea
Bacterial vaginosis	This condition is the most prevalent cause of vaginal discharge or malodor. However, half the women who meet clinical criteria for bacterial vaginosis have no symptoms.	Metronidazole, 500 mg PO bid for 7 days; or metronidazole gel 0.75%, one full applicator (5 g) intravaginally qd for 5 days; or clindamycin cream 2%, one full applicator (5 g) intravaginally at bedtime for 7 days. Alternative regimens: clindamycin, 300 mg PO bid for 7 days or clindamycin ovules, 100 mg intravaginally once daily at bedtime for 3 days.	Treatment of male sex partners has not been found to be beneficial in preventing the recurrence of bacterial vaginosis. Only symptomatic patients should be treated. Patients should be advised to avoid using alcohol during treatment with metronidazole and for 24 hours thereafter. Clindamycin cream is oil-based and may weaken latex condoms and diaphragms.
Vulvovaginal candidiasis	Typical symptoms are pruritus and vaginal discharge. Other symptoms include vaginal soreness, vulvar burning sensation, dyspareunia, and external dysuria. None of these symptoms is specific for vulvovaginal candidiasis.	Fluconazole, one 150-mg oral tablet (single dose); or clotrimazole, 1% cream, 5 g intravaginally for 7-14 days, or clotrimazole, 100 mg vaginal tablet for 7 days; or butoconazole 2% cream, 5 g intravaginally for 3 days; or terconazole 0.8% cream, 5 g intravaginally for 3 days.	Vulvovaginal candidiasis usually is not sexually acquired or transmitted, but about 15% of male sexual partners have symptomatic balanitis and should be treated.

These subtypes also can cause laryngeal or respiratory papillomatosis in infants and children; the route of transmission is not completely understood. The prevalence of HPV is highest in the youngest age group (50% in females 20 to 24 years of age). This prevalence declines substantially after the age of 24 years.[2] However, gross clinical prevalence of HPV is less than 1%.[3]

■ Clinical Presentation

The average incubation period for visible warts is about 3 months. Genital warts may be asymptomatic but can be pruritic. On clinical examination, they usually are papillary, verrucous (wartlike), or macular in character. Fissures may be present at the posterior fourchette. They originally appear as individual lesions, although large confluent growths can develop. Vaginal and cervical warts are more common than labial warts, although most of these are flat lesions visible only by colposcopy.

■ Differential Diagnosis and Diagnostic Testing

Several laboratory methods such as polymerase chain reaction (PCR) have been developed for confirmation of genital human papillomavirus infection, but the ED diagnosis remains primarily clinical. Vulvar warts must be differentiated from the less verrucous, flatter growths of syphilitic *Condyloma latum* and from car-

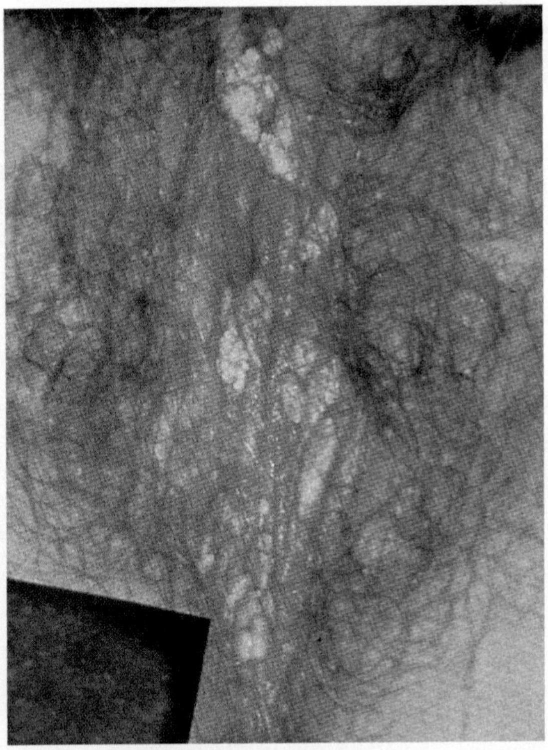

FIGURE 123-1 Vulvovaginal human papillomavirus infection. (From Cohen J, Powderly WG: Infectious Diseases, 2nd ed. Philadelphia Mosby, 2004.)

cinoma in situ of the vulva. Dark field examination or punch biopsies may be required to differentiate these lesions. Vulvar lesions may be obviously wart-like or may be diagnosed only after application of 4% acetic acid (vinegar) and colposcopy, when they appear whitish, with prominent papillae.

Treatment

Although not necessary in the ED, recommended provider-applied treatments for vulvar warts include 10% to 25% podophyllum resin in tincture of benzoin (do not use during pregnancy or on bleeding lesions); 80% to 90% trichloroacetic or bichloroacetic acid; cryotherapy with liquid nitrogen or cryoprobe; or surgical removal. Alternative treatments include interlesional interferon or laser therapy. Patient-applied regimens include 0.5% podofilox solution or gel and 5% imiquimod cream.[1] Vaginal warts may be treated with cryotherapy with liquid nitrogen, trichloroacetic acid, or podophyllum resin. Extensive warts may require treatment with CO_2 laser under local or general anesthesia. Interferon is not recommended for routine use because it is expensive, associated with systemic side effects, and no more effective than other therapies.

Routine examination of sex partners is not necessary for the management of genital warts because the risk of reinfection is minimal and curative therapy to prevent transmission is not available. However, partners may wish to be examined for detection and treatment of genital warts and other sexually transmitted diseases. A vaccine that has been reported to be effective for the prevention of human papillomavirus infection and for the treatment of human papillomavirus–related neoplasms is recommended for adolescent girls because of the possibility of exposure.

Special Considerations

Pregnancy

Although proliferation of genital warts can occur during pregnancy, imiquimod, podophyllin, and podofilox should not be used for treatment because they can be absorbed systemically and cross the placenta to the fetus.

Immunosuppression

Growth of warts is supported when immune response is compromised.

HERPES SIMPLEX VIRUS

Approximately 50 million people in the United States are thought to be infected with herpes simplex virus.[1] It is the most common cause of genital ulcers. Subtype 2 (HSV-2) is the most common variant causing genital infections; subtype 1 (HSV-1) also is implicated, causing up to 10% to 15% of cases.[3] These subtypes are clinically indistinguishable. Transmission via sexual contact is variable but occurs through contact with infectious secretions. The incubation period ranges from 2 to 7 days.[3]

Clinical Presentation

Up to 70% of women infected are asymptomatic.[4] Symptoms usually begin 1 to 4 weeks after exposure and consist of painful lesions often described as burning (Fig. 123-2). These lesions begin as vesicles and then rupture, exposing an ulcerated base that persists for 1 to 2 weeks before crusting over and healing without scars. Vesicles and ulcers contain many highly infectious virus particles, and viral shedding occurs until the lesions disappear. Vulvar lesions may last for 3 or more weeks before complete healing. The cervix and vagina also may be involved, resulting in a gray, necrotic cervix and profuse leukorrhea. External dysuria is common, and bilateral inguinal lymphadenopathy is usual.

The primary episode, defined as genital herpes with the absence of antibodies to HSV-1 and HSV-2, typically is associated with systemic symptoms including headache, fever, malaise, and other flu-like symptoms in about two thirds of the cases. Following primary infection, latent herpes simplex virus usually localizes in the sacral ganglion and perhaps the dermis. Recurrent attacks tend to be subtler in presentation and are the most frequently seen outbreaks

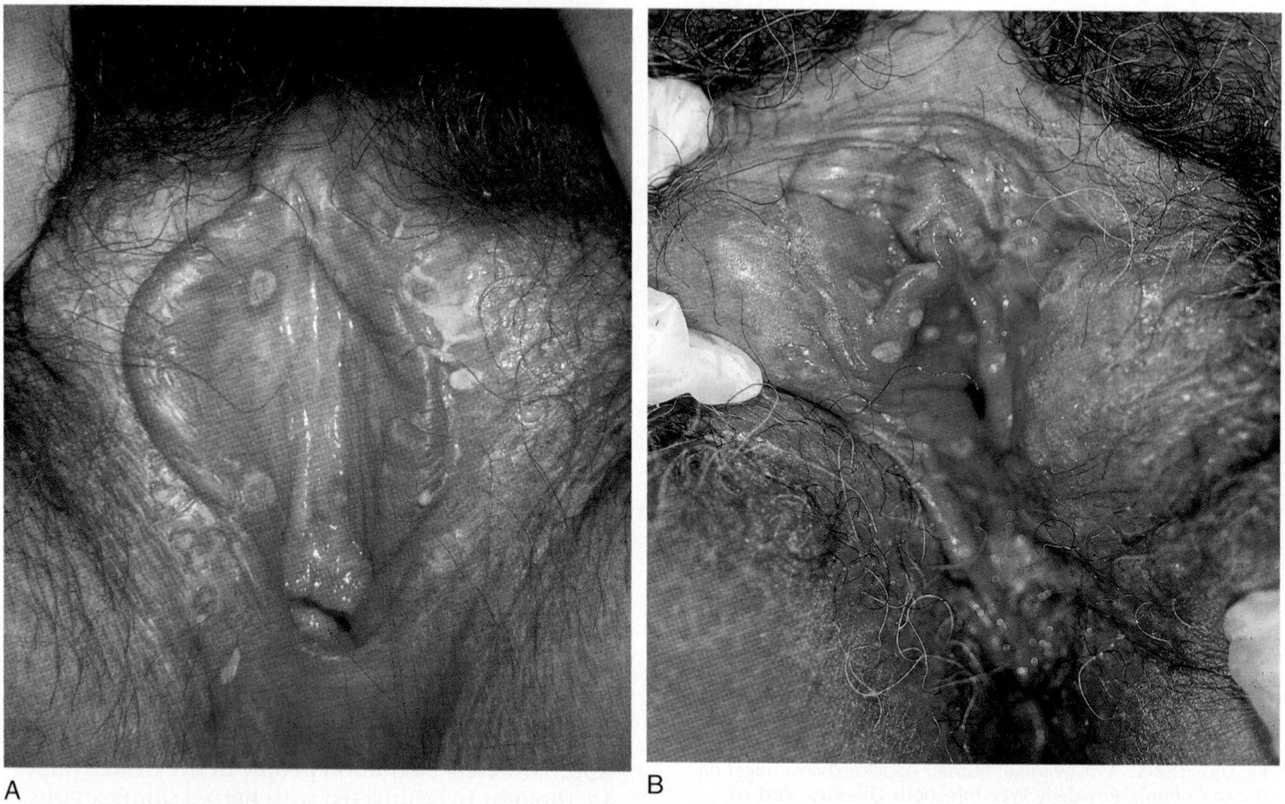

FIGURE 123-2 Primary herpes simplex. **A,** Scattered erosions covered with exudate. **B,** Numerous erosions appeared 4 days after contact with an asymptomatic carrier. (From Habif, TP: Clinical Dermatology, 4th ed. Philadelphia, Mosby, 2004.)

in the ED. Recurrence can be precipitated by immunodeficiency, trauma, fever, or sexual intercourse.

Differential Diagnosis and Diagnostic Testing

Genital ulcers also may be caused by syphilis, chancroid, lymphogranuloma venereum, and granuloma inguinale.

A significant number of patients who present with typical signs and symptoms of herpesvirus infection are later found to have syphilis; therefore, screening for treponemal antibodies is an important part of the ED evaluation.

The diagnosis of herpes simplex virus infection can be made clinically if typical, painful, shallow multiple vulvar ulcers are present. However, many lesions are atypical. Laboratory confirmation of atypical lesions and lesions that appear during pregnancy is best attained by virus isolation (which can usually be achieved within 48 hours) or by PCR testing.

Treatment

Recommended treatment regimens vary based on whether the presentation represents primary infection or recurrence; in both instances treatment is directed at improving lesion healing and reducing symptoms.

Episodic antiviral therapy is used initially, although patients experiencing six or more recurrences a year may require continuous antiviral therapy. Antiviral treatment for initial infection should be given for 7 to 10 days and includes oral acyclovir (400 mg three times a day or 200 mg five times a day), oral famciclovir (250 mg three times a day), or oral valacyclovir (1 g twice a day). The following recurrence regimens for all three drug options are prescribed orally as follows: acyclovir (400 mg three times a day for 5 days or 800 mg twice a day for 5 days or 800 mg three times a day for 2 days), famciclovir (125 mg twice a day for 5 days or 1 g twice a day for 1 day), or valcyclovir (500 mg twice a day for 3 days or 1 g once a day for 5 days).[1]

Special Considerations

Pregnancy

Medications are not contraindicated but should be reserved for patients that are significantly symptomatic and present within 48 hours of symptom onset. Transmission of the virus from mother to fetus occurs with increasing frequency as gestational age at the time of infection advances, and represents the most serious consequence of genital HSV infection. Neonatal infection is caused by contact with infected genital secretions at the time of labor, with a transmission rate of up to 40% to 50%.[3] Referral to obstetrics for potential cesarean section should be immediate if rupture of membranes has occurred in a patient with herpes genital ulcers.

Immunosuppression

Herpes simplex virus serves as a cofactor in the transmission of HIV. Prolonged or severe episodes are more commonly seen in immunocompromised patients. If lesions persist or recur in HIV-positive patients receiving herpes simplex virus antiviral therapy, resistance should be suspected. These patients should be managed in conjunction with infectious disease specialists.

LYMPHOGRANULOMA VENEREUM

Lymphogranuloma venereum is an acute or chronic sexually transmitted disease caused by *Chlamydia trachomatis* types L1-L3. The disease is acquired during intercourse or through contact with contaminated exudate from active lesions.

Clinical Presentation

The initial vesicular or ulcerative lesion (on the external genitalia or anorectal region) is transient and often goes unnoticed. Inguinal buboes appear 1 to 4 weeks after exposure, often are bilateral, and have a tendency to fuse, soften, and break down to form multiple draining sinuses, with extensive scarring. In women, the genital lymph drainage is to the perirectal glands.

Early anorectal manifestations include proctitis with tenesmus and bloody purulent discharge; late manifestations are chronic cicatrizing inflammation of the rectal and perirectal tissue. These changes lead to obstipation and rectal stricture and, occasionally, rectovaginal and perianal fistulas.

Differential Diagnosis and Diagnostic Testing

The early lesion of lymphogranuloma venereum must be differentiated from the lesions of syphilis, genital herpes simplex, chancroid, and granuloma inguinale; lymph node involvement must be distinguished from that due to tularemia, tuberculosis, plague, neoplasm, or pyogenic infection; and rectal stricture must be distinguished from that due to neoplasm and ulcerative colitis. The complement fixation test may be positive, but cross-reaction with other chlamydiae occurs. Although a positive reaction may reflect remote infection, high titers usually indicate active disease. Specific immunofluorescence tests for immunoglobulin M (IgM) are more specific for acute infection.

Treatment

The antibiotic of choice is doxycycline, 100 mg orally twice daily for 21 days.[1] Erythromycin, 500 mg four times a day for 21 days, also is effective. Large lymph nodes should be aspirated to avoid chronic drainage. Surgical excision of scarred areas may be necessary.

Special Considerations

Pregnancy

Doxycycline is contraindicated in pregnant and lactating women. When indicated, they should be treated with erythromycin.

Immunsuppression

Delay in resolution of symptoms may occur in HIV-positive patients, necessitating prolonged therapy.

GRANULOMA INGUINALE

Granuloma inguinale is a chronic, relapsing, granulomatous anogenital infection due to *Calymmatobacterium* (Donovania) *granulomatis*. It is usually considered a sexually transmitted disease, although gastrointestinal transmission can occur.

Clinical Presentation

The incubation period is 3 to 30 days,[5] and onset is insidious. Lesions, which occur on the skin or mucous membranes of the genitalia or perineal area, are relatively painless, infiltrated nodules that soon slough. A shallow, sharply demarcated ulcer forms, with a beefy-red friable base of granulation tissue. The lesions spread by contiguity. The advancing border has a characteristic rolled edge of granulation tissue. Large ulcerations may advance onto the lower abdomen and thighs. Scar formation and healing occur along one border while the opposite border advances. Superinfection with spirochete-fusiform organisms is common. The ulcer then becomes purulent, painful, and foul-smelling.

Differential Diagnosis and Diagnostic Testing

Calymmatobacterium granulomatis is difficult to culture because it is an intracellular parasite. The identification is usually made from scraped material or a biopsy specimen obtained from the periphery of the lesion. Bipolar-staining bacteria are best identified within mononuclear cells (Donovan bodies) by Wright or Giemsa staining.

Genital ulcers also are caused by syphilis, chancroid, or lymphogranuloma venereum.

Treatment

Because of the indolent nature of the disease, duration of therapy is relatively long. Several therapies are available.

The regimen of choice is doxycycline, 100 mg orally twice a day for at least 3 weeks and until all lesions are completely healed. Alternative oral regimens include azithromycin, 1 g per week; ciproflaxin, 750 mg twice a day; erythromycin base, 500 mg four times a day; or trimethoprim-sulfamethoxazole,

160 mg/800 mg (1 tablet) twice a day; all for a duration of at least 3 weeks and until all lesions have completely healed.[1]

Special Considerations

Pregnancy

Doxycycline and ciproflaxin are contraindicated in pregnant and lactating women, and pregnancy is a relative contraindication to the use of sulfonamides. When indicated, treatment should be with erythromycin, and consideration should be give to the addition of a parenteral aminoglycoside (e.g., gentamycin). There is no published data on the efficacy of azithromycin in the treatment of granuloma inguinale during pregnancy.

Immunosuppression

In HIV-positive patients with granuloma inguinale, consider the addition of a parenteral aminoglycoside.

SYPHILIS

Syphilis is a systemic sexually transmitted disease caused by the spirochete *Treponema pallidum*. It can also be acquired congenitally. The risk of transmission following sexual exposure depends on many factors. It is estimated to be about 30%.[6]

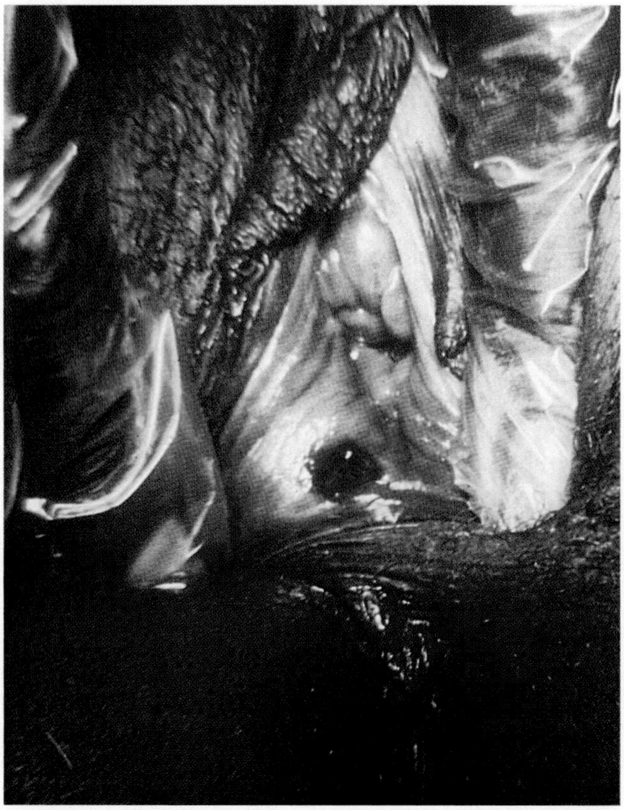

FIGURE 123-3 Primary syphilis with chancre in vagina. Lesions are painless and may never be detected.

Clinical Presentation

ED presentation can occur at any of the four stages through which untreated syphilis can pass. Primary infection manifests as a single, painless ulcer, usually within 3 weeks but sometimes 2 to 3 months after infection[6] (Fig. 123-3). The labia and vaginal walls are most often affected, but lesions can occur on the cervix.

Secondary syphilis is associated with a characteristic maculopapular generalized rash on the palms and soles and may include components of arthralgias, pharyngitis, and lymphadenopathy. This stage typically is seen 4 to 10 weeks after the initial appearance of a chancre. Infectivity can occur in the first two stages (up to 2 to 4 years following infection).

The third stage—the asymptomatic latent phase—may last many years. The fourth stage—tertiary syphilis—has numerous neurologic, cardiovascular, and other systemic effects and develops in about 25% of untreated patients.[6]

Differential Diagnosis and Diagnostic Testing

The diagnosis of syphilis should be considered in any patient with an ulcerative lesion in the genital area, as well as in patients with unexplained rashes, arthralgias, and neurologic or systemic complaints. Screening includes rapid plasma reagin (RPR) and Venereal Disease Research Laboratory (VDRL) tests and must be followed by confirmatory testing when positive. If the serologic results are nonreactive, and spirochetes cannot be demonstrated by dark-field examination, serologic tests should be repeated in 1 month. All patients need to be followed with quantitative serologic tests to monitor treatment results and offered HIV testing. All sex partners need to be contacted and tested for syphilis.

Treatment

Penicillin remains the mainstay of treatment. Patients with primary and secondary infections should receive a single dose (2.4 million units intramuscularly [IM]) of benzathine penicillin G. Several antibiotics may be effective in nonpregnant, penicilin-allergic patients with primary and secondary infection including a 14-day course of oral doxycycline (100 mg twice a day) or oral tetracycline (500 mg four times a day). Some studies recommend IV or intramuscular ceftriaxone (1 g daily for 8 to 10 days) as an alternative.[1]

Benzathine penicilin G is also the recommended treatment in patients with latent and tertiary syphillis, but the doses and duration of treatment need to be adjusted. For example, benzathine penicillin G (2.4 million units IM) should be given every week for three doses (total 7.2 million units). Oral doxycycline (100 mg twice daily) or tetracycline (500 mg four times daily) continue to be alternatives for the penicillin-allergic patient, but also should be given for a longer duration of 28 days.

Patients with neurosyphilis require hospital admission for IV administration of 18 to 24 million units of aqueous crystalline penicillin (3 to 4 million units every 4 hours for 10 to 14 days) or a 14-day course of procaine penicillin (2.4 million units IM once daily) plus oral probenecid (500 mg four times a day).[1] As no proved alternatives to penicillin exist, penicillin-allergic patients should undergo desensitization.

■ Special Considerations

■ *Pregnancy*

Parenteral penicillin is the only documented efficacious treatment in pregnancy. Treatment with penicillin is the same as for the corresponding stage of syphilis among nonpregnant women. For pregnant patients who are allergic to penicillin, tetracycline is not used because of toxicity and erythromycin is not used because of high failure rates to cure the fetus. Penicillin is so superior to other antibiotics for treating syphilis in pregnancy that pregnant, penicillin-allergic patients should be skin-tested and desensitized.

The Jarisch-Herxheimer reaction, caused by massive release of treponemal antigens and manifested by fever, headache, and myalgias, can occur in any patient in the first 24 hours following initiation of therapy and is observed most often in patients with early syphilis (frequently in secondary syphilis).[6] This reaction in pregnant women may precipitate early labor or cause fetal distress; thus these patients should be hospitalized for monitoring. Concern for this reaction should not prevent or delay therapy. Systemic glucocorticoids administered 12 hours before or concurrent with antibiotics may minimize the effects, and antipyretics have been used for supportive care.

Maternal-fetal transmission may result in fetal death, premature delivery, or congenital syphilis.

■ *Immunosuppression*

All syphilis patients should be tested for HIV infection. Syphilis increases likelihood of HIV transmission six- to sevenfold.

■ *Pediatrics*

Treatment regimen for penicillin in children mimics the duration and route specified for adults at the adjusted dose of 50,000 units/kg up to 2.4 million units per dose.[1]

■ CHANCROID

Chancroid is a sexually transmitted disease caused by the short gram-negative bacillus *Haemophilus ducreyi* and is characterized by painful genital ulcers and painful lymphadenopathy. The incubation period is 4 to 7 days.[7]

■ Clinical Presentation

At the site of inoculation, a vesicopustule develops that breaks down to form a painful, soft ulcer with a necrotic base, surrounding erythema, and undermined edges. There may be multiple lesions due to autoinoculation. The adenitis is usually unilateral and consists of tender, matted nodes of moderate size with overlying erythema. These may become fluctuant and rupture spontaneously. With lymph node involvement, fever, chills, and malaise may develop. Women may have no external signs of infection.

■ Differential Diagnosis and Diagnostic Testing

Chancroid must be differentiated from other genital ulcers. The chancre of syphilis is clean and painless, with a hard base. The diagnosis is established by culturing a swab of the lesion onto a special medium. Mixed sexually transmitted disease is very common (including syphilis, herpes simplex virus infection, and HIV infection), as is infection of the ulcer with fusiforms, spirochetes, and other organisms.

■ Treatment

A single dose of azithromycin (1 g orally) or ceftriaxone (250 mg IM) is effective treatment. Alternative regimens are erythromycin (500 mg orally) three times a day for 7 days and ciprofloxacin (500 mg orally) twice a day for 3 days.[1]

■ Special Considerations

■ *Pregnancy*

No adverse effects of chancroid on pregnancy outcome have been described.

■ *Immunosuppression*

HIV-positive patients are more likely to experience treatment failure or have prolonged ulcer healing times requiring longer courses of medication therapy.

■ BARTHOLIN GLAND ABSCESS

Bartholin glands are bilateral vulvovaginal secretory structures located in the labia minora on the posterolateral aspect of the vestibule. Normally pea-sized, these glands drain fluid through a 2.5-cm duct into a fold between the hymeneal ring and the labium that serves to maintain the moisture of the vaginal mucosa. Duct occlusion can result in cyst and subsequently abscess formation. Isolates from abscess cultures are most commonly anaerobic organisms (*Bacteroides fragilis, Peptostreptococcus*); aerobic *Neisseria gonorrhoeae* is the causative agent in approximately 10% to 15% of cases[8]; and *Chlamydia trachomatis* is found even less frequently. Patients typically are 20 to 30 years old. Occurrence in patients older than 40 years of age is unusual and should raise concern for malignancy as an alternative cause.

Clinical Presentation

Disease onset can occur rapidly over several hours or may progress more gradually over several days. Presenting symptoms are pain, dyspareunia, and sometimes fever. The physical findings demonstrate a unilateral labial mass with tenderness, redness, and swelling in the Bartholin gland area. Elevated temperature is observed in approximately one third of patients.

Microscopically, the Bartholin duct has acute inflammation within the duct as well as within the gland stroma about the duct. The abscess, when fully developed, contains purulent exudate.

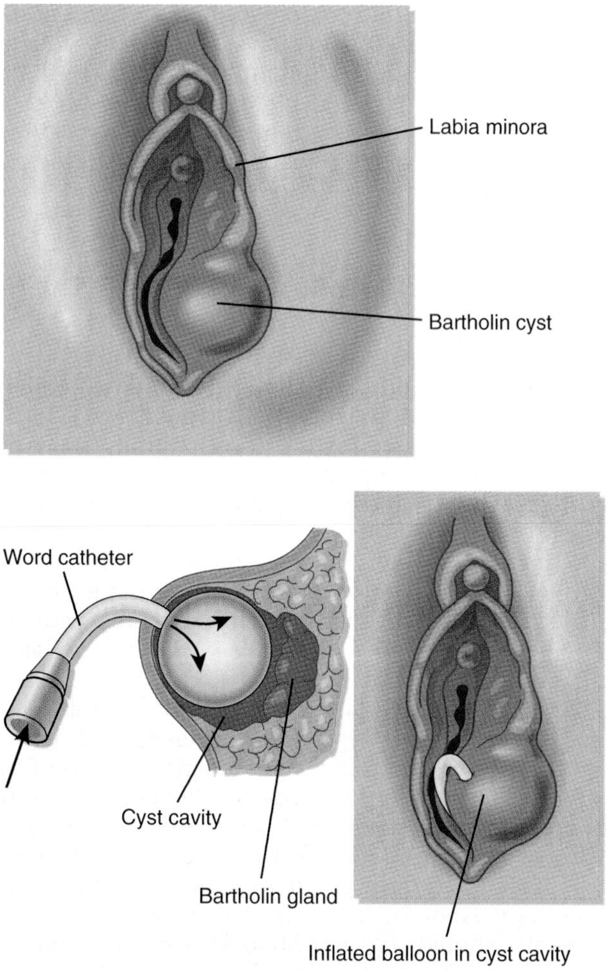
Labia minora
Bartholin cyst
Word catheter
Cyst cavity
Bartholin gland
Inflated balloon in cyst cavity

FIGURE 123-4 **A,** Scalpel incision of Bartholin duct cyst. **B,** Placement of Word catheter in the cyst.

Differential Diagnosis and Diagnostic Testing

Cultures and a Gram stain of material expressed from the duct may identify gonococci. Cervical gonococcal and chlamydial cultures should be obtained, and treated, if present.

Treatment

Management of the abscess consists of simple incision and drainage. Patient comfort will significantly improve the likelihood of successful drainage and therefore local anesthesia should be administered prior to the procedure. Conscious sedation may be required for some patients. After sterile preparation of the area, a scalpel stab incision ideally no more than 1.5 cm long (longer incisions will make it difficult to keep the Word catheter [see later] in place) should be performed deep into the abscess from the inside of the labium. Outside incision can cause permanent fistula formation.

Loculations should be broken manually followed by placement of a Word catheter with its balloon tip inserted into the abscess before inflation with water or lubricating gel (Fig. 123-4). Simple incision and drainage without Word catheter placement may be inadequate and result in recurrence. The catheter is left in place for 2 to 4 weeks, and the patient should scheduled for follow-up with a gynecologist for removal.

Vaginal Infections

Vaginitis may be due to various causes, most of which are infectious (95%).[9] It is the most common reason for a visit to a gynecologist. Symptoms of vaginitis include increased vaginal discharge, vulvar irritation and pruritus, external dysuria, and yellow discharge with a foul odor. However, symptoms are very poor indicators of the specific cause of vaginitis. Women with infectious vaginitis have a sexually transmitted disease (e.g., trichomonads, chlamydia) or a quantitative increase in normal flora (e.g., *Candida, Gardnerella vaginalis,* anaerobes). A specific diagnosis is mandatory to select effective therapy. Every effort should be made to establish the diagnosis of one of these specific infections and to avoid the diagnosis of a nonspecific vaginitis.

Other conditions that may cause excessive vaginal discharge include cervicitis, normal cervical mucus from cervical ectopy, vaginal foreign bodies (most commonly retained tampons), and allergic reactions to douching or vaginal contraceptive agents. Atrophic vaginitis among postmenopausal women can cause burning and dyspareunia, but an infectious cause is not established. A small amount of vaginal discharge may be normal, particularly midcycle, when large amounts of cervical mucus production produce a clear vaginal discharge. A normal vaginal discharge should not have a foul odor or cause irritation or pruritus.

The most common causes of vaginitis in premenopausal women are bacterial vaginosis (prevalence of 40%-50%), vaginal candidiasis (20%-25%), and trichomoniasis (15%-20%).[9] Symptoms alone are inadequate for differentiation of these potential causes but may be useful for exclusion of certain etiologies in the differential diagnosis. Similarly, physical examination signs have limited diagnostic capability. Self-diagnosis has been shown to be a reliable indicator of etiology.

Microscopy is the most reliable way of differentiating between vaginal candidiasis, bacterial vaginosis, and vaginal trichomoniasis. Testing of vaginal pH is also useful, but potential confounders of accurate readings include gel on the speculum, semen, douching, and intravaginal medications. Characteristic pH levels for each etiology are ≤ 4.5 (normal vaginal pH) for candidiasis, 5 to 6 for bacterial vaginosis, and 6 to 7 for *Trichomonas*.[10]

■ CANDIDA VAGINITIS

Candida albicans is a normal vaginal flora that is the primary cause of 25% of cases of vaginitis and approximately 90% of vaginal yeast infections (noncandidal species cause the remaining infections).[9] These saprophytic fungi are isolated from the vagina in 20% to 40% of asymptomatic women.[11] Infection should especially be suspected in women who have been recently been taking antibiotics or high-dose estrogen oral contraceptives and in women who are immunosuppressed (e.g., diabetics, on corticosteroid therapy).

■ Clinical Presentation

Common symptoms include vulvovaginal pruritus, dyspareunia, dysuria, and white, thick, curdlike vaginal discharge. The physical examination typically reveals erythematous or edematous mucosa in addition to the classic discharge described previously.

■ Differential Diagnosis and Diagnostic Testing

Several infections may mimic candida vaginitis; however, diagnosis is based on the characteristic clinical presentation along with microscopy. Microscopic evaluation reveals a normal pH (4-4.5) with hyphae, pseudohyphae, or budding yeast on a saline wet preparation or 10% potassium hydroxide preparation. 50% of women with candidiasis have a negative wet mount, but a positive *Candida* culture.

■ Treatment

Local vaginal therapy is necessary because most antifungal preparations are not absorbed from the intestinal tract. For uncomplicated infection, various intravaginal azole agents administered for 3 to 5 days are equally effective for women with primary and infrequent *Candida* vaginitis. These agents include miconazole, clotrimazole, butoconazole, tioconazole, and terconazole. Azole drugs are not absorbed to any degree from the vagina, and these local regimens can be used safely in pregnancy. The insertion of boric acid powder in capsules into the vagina is also effective. A one-time dose of fluconazole (150 mg orally) is also effective for cases of with uncomplicated infection. Patients with complicated infection from severe symptoms should receive 7 to 14 days of intravaginal azole therapy or 150 mg of fluconazole with the dose repeated in 3 days.[1] About 15% of male sexual contacts of women with candidiasis have symptomatic balanitis; symptomatic males should be identified and treated to prevent recurrent female infection.

■ Special Considerations

■ *Pregnancy*

Because oral fluconazole is contraindicated, only a topical 7-day course of an azole drug should be prescribed in pregnancy.

■ *Immunosuppression*

Long-term prophylactic therapy with oral fluconazole (200 mg given once a week) may be effective in HIV-positive patients with persistent symptomatic vaginal candidal infections.

■ BACTERIAL VAGINOSIS

Polymicrobial anaerobic infection (*Gardnerella vaginalis, Mycoplasma hominis, Mobiluncus curtisii*) resulting from disruption of normal flora. Bacterial vaginitis can be a precursor infection to upper genital tract extension including cervicitis and pelvic inflammatory disease.

■ Clinical Presentation

Clinical signs include a thick, homogeneous, milky vaginal discharge. Prevalence depends on the population studied but ranges from 4% to 40%.[12]

■ Differential Diagnosis and Diagnostic Testing

Clinical diagnosis requires three of the following four criteria:

- Homogeneous, thin vaginal fluid that adheres to vaginal walls
- Vaginal fluid pH>4.5
- Release of amine odor with alkalinization of vaginal fluid ("whiff test")
- Presence of vaginal epithelial cells with borders obscured by adherent small bacteria ("clue cells")

■ Treatment

Benefits of therapy in nonpregnant patients are primarily directed toward relief of symptoms and minimizing the risk of extension of infection after instrumentation during a procedure. All women with symptoms require treatment. Therapeutic options include oral metronidazole (500 mg bid for 7 days), intravaginal metronidazole (5 g of 0.75% gel once daily for 5 days), and 2% clindamycin vaginal cream (5 g once daily at bedtime for 7 days).[1]

Sex partners do not need to be treated. Women's likelihood of recurrence and response to treatment do not seem to be affected by treating the male partner.

Special Considerations

Pregnancy

Bacterial vaginitis occurring during pregnancy is associated with a higher incidence of first trimester miscarriage, premature rupture of membranes, preterm labor, preterm delivery, and postpartum endometritis. Pregnant women should receive treatment regardless of the presence or absence of symptoms. The preferred regimen is oral metronidazole (500 mg twice a day or 250 mg three times a day for 7 days) or oral clindamycin (300 mg twice a day for 7 days). Intravaginal clindamycin cream should not be used in pregnancy because it is associated with an increased risk of preterm delivery.

Immunosuppression

Additional associated morbidity includes increased risk of HIV infection. However, treatment regimens are identical regardless of HIV status.

TRICHOMONAS VAGINITIS

Trichomoniasis affects 2 to 3 million American women annually[13] and is caused by *Trichomonas vaginalis,* an anaerobe protozoan that is transmitted primarily through sexual activity. It is identified in 30% to 40% of male sexual partners of infected women.[9]

Clinical Presentation

Typical symptoms include vulvar irritation, dyspareunia, dysuria, urinary frequency, and a malodorous, profuse, purulent vaginal discharge. The physical examination may reveal an erythematous vaginal mucosa or punctate hemorrhages on the cervix.

Differential Diagnosis and Diagnostic Testing

Although candidiasis and bacterial vaginosis are included in the differential diagnosis of vaginitis, trichomonal infections are less typically associated with pruritus or malodor.[1] Diagnosis is made by identification of motile trichomonads on a saline wet preparation but are seen in only 60% to 70% of confirmed cases when cultures are used.[9]

Treatment

Current recommended therapy is oral metronidazole (2 g as a single dose). Alternative regimens include metronidazole, 500 mg twice a day for 7 days, or tinidazole. Sex partners also should be treated. Persistent discharge after adequate treatment for trichomoniasis should lead to repeat examination for trichomoniasis, candidiasis, and gonorrhea.[1]

Special Considerations

Pregnancy

Vaginal trichomoniasis has been associated with adverse pregnancy outcomes in the form of premature rupture of membranes, preterm delivery, and low birth weight. Single-dose therapy with metronidazole is the preferred regimen, and treatment should be limited to symptomatic women. Treatment of asymptomatic pregnant women should be in consultation with a specialist.

Immunosuppression

Transmission of HIV infection is facilitated by coinfection with *T. vaginalis.*[14] Treatment regimens are identical regardless of HIV status.

Cervical Infections

The most common causes of cervicitis are *C. trachomatis* and *N. gonorrhoeae,* which can be isolated in combination in about 20% to 40% of women with purulent cervicitis.[15] However, 80% to 90% of women infected with these pathogens are asymptomatic.[16] Other potential pathogens include *Actinomycetes* (classically in patients with intrauterine devices), *Mycoplasma hominis, Ureaplasma urealyticum, Cytomegalovirus,* and tuberculosis.

Mucopurulent cervicitis is not a sensitive predictor of infection because most patients with *C. trachomatis* or *N. gonorrhoeae* infection do not have this finding.

Complications of cervical infection include spread to the upper genital tract and increased susceptibility to HIV infection.

GONORRHEA

Gonorrhea is caused by *Neisseria gonorrhoeae,* a gram-negative diplococcus typically found inside polymorphonuclear cells. It is transmitted during sexual activity and has its greatest incidence in the 15- to 24-year-old age group.[17] In 2006, the rate of gonorrhea infection in African Americans was 18 times higher than that of whites.[18] The incubation period is usually 3 to 5 days.[15] Gonococcal infection in women often becomes symptomatic during menses.

Clinical Presentation

Patients may have dysuria, urinary frequency, and urgency, with a purulent urethral discharge. Vaginitis and cervicitis with inflammation of Bartholin's glands are common findings. Infection may be asymptomatic, with only slightly increased vaginal discharge and moderate cervicitis on physical examination. Infection may remain as a chronic cervicitis—an important reservoir of gonococci. It can progress to acute or chronic salpingitis affecting the uterus and tubes, causing scarring of tubes and sterility. Systemic complications follow the dissemination of gonococci from the primary site via the blood stream and include meningitis, endocarditis, and arthritis.

Differential Diagnosis and Diagnostic Testing

Gonococcal urethritis or cervicitis must be differentiated from nongonococcal urethritis; cervicitis or vaginitis due to *C. trachomatis, Gardnerella vaginalis, T. vaginalis, Candida albicans;* and many other pathogens associated with sexually transmitted disease. Gram stains often are negative. In the past, culture has been the gold standard for diagnosis; however, nucleic acid amplification tests that detect both *N. gonorrhoeae* and *C. trachomatis* in cervical and urethral swab specimens and urine. These tests permit rapid diagnosis and have excellent sensitivity and specificity.

Treatment

Therapy typically is administered before antimicrobial susceptibilities are known. Treatment should be based on laboratory confirmation except in cases with a high likelihood of disease or those likely to be lost to follow-up. Empirical therapy should be given in these groups. Sex partners should be identified and treated. Patients should abstain from unprotected intercourse for 7 days after completion of the treatment regimen.

Penicillin is no longer recommended to treat gonorrhea because of growing resistance. Quinolone-resistant *N. gonorrhoeae* (G RNG) is also becoming increasingly common in various parts of the United States. For uncomplicated urethritis or cervicitis, treatment options include cefixime (400 mg orally as a single dose), ceftriaxone (125 mg IM), ciprofloxacin (500 mg orally as a single dose), ofloxacin (400 mg orally as a single dose), and levofloxacin (250 mg orally as a single dose). Spectinomycin (2 g IM in a single dose) may be used for cephalosporin- or quinolone-intolerant patients.[1] Anal gonorrhea in women responds to the same drugs.

Because coexistent chlamydial infection is common, the recommended treatment is azithromax (1 g orally as a single dose) or doxycycline (100 mg twice daily orally for 7 days) if *C. trachomatis* has not been excluded.

Patients with gonorrhea should have serologic tests for syphilis. Specific antibiotic regimens are recommended for patients with complicated gonococcal infections such as bacteremia, endocarditis, arthritis, meningitis, and conjunctivitis.

Special Considerations

Pregnancy

Quinolones and tetracycline should not be used in pregnancy because of potential risk to the developing fetus. Alternatives include a cephalosporin or a single dose of spectinomycin (2 g IM). Pregnant patients should have repeat testing 3 weeks after treatment to demonstrate efficacy.[1]

CHLAMYDIA

Chlamydia trachomatis is a sexually transmitted bacterium that is often associated with gonorrhea. Chlamydiae infect the same tissues and produce the same symptoms and diseases as gonorrhea. Treatment of *C. trachomatis* in pregnancy reduces premature delivery. *C. trachomatis* is three to five times more common than *N. gonorrhoeae* in developed countries because it is not routinely looked for in asymptomatic patients. *C. trachomatis* is associated with serious sequelae, including tubal infertility and ectopic pregnancy, and it appears to produce permanent tissue damage more readily than *N. gonorrhoeae.* Young females aged 15 to 19 years have the highest chlamydia rate, and the rate of infection of African American women was 7 times that of white females in 2006.[18] The incubating period for genital chlamydial infection ranges from 7 to 21 days.[19]

Clinical Presentation

Chlamydial infections usually are asymptomatic and frequently are not identified until overt infection occurs. Clinical signs and symptoms include urethritis, bartholinitis, cervicitis, endometritis, salpingitis, Fitz-Hugh-Curtis syndrome (see later), and lymphogranuloma venereum.

Differential Diagnosis and Diagnostic Testing

Chlamydial infections can be diagnosed by culture, a direct monoclonal antibody slide test, enzyme-linked immunosorbent assay (ELISA), or DNA techniques. New DNA methods using ligase chain reaction or PCR offer both sensitivity and specificity not achieved with older tests. For DNA tests, samples should be taken from the cervix or from urine. As with all sexually transmitted diseases, studies for HIV and syphilis should be performed. Sex partners should be referred for evaluation, testing, and treatment.

Treatment

Recommended first-line treatment for chlamydial cervicitis is azithromycin (1 g orally as single dose) or doxycycline (100 mg orally twice a day for 7 days; contraindicated in pregnancy). Alternative 7-day regimens include erythromycin base (500 mg orally four times a day), erythromycin ethysuccinate (800 mg orally four times a day), ofloxacin (300 mg orally twice a day), and levofloxacin (500 mg orally once a day).

Special Considerations

Pregnancy

Azithromycin and amoxicillin (500 mg orally three times a day for 7 days) are preferred for pregnant patients. Erthyromycin base may be used as well, but the side effects may discourage compliance and thus the alternative regimen of 250 mg four times a day for 14 days may be preferred. Erythromycin estolate is contraindicated in pregnancy because of drug-related hepatotoxicity. Pregnant patients should have repeat testing 3 weeks after treatment to demonstrate efficacy.

BOX 123-1

Findings Suggesting the Diagnosis of Pelvic Inflammatory Disease

- Oral temperature greater than 101°F (38.3°C)
- Abnormal cervical or vaginal discharge with white cells on saline microscopy
- Elevated erythrocyte sedimentation rate
- Elevated C-reactive protein
- Laboratory documentation of cervical infection with *N. gonorrhoeae* or *C. trachomatis*

PELVIC INFLAMMATORY DISEASE

Pelvic inflammatory disease is a polymicrobial infection of the upper genital tract (endometrium, fallopian tubes, ovaries) that is associated most commonly with the sexually transmitted organisms *N. gonorrhoeae* and *C. trachomatis,* and to a lesser extent with some endogenous organisms including anaerobes, *Haemophilus influenzae,* enteric gram-negative rods, and streptococci. Pelvic inflammatory disease is an ascending infection that can cause endometritis, salpingitis, oophoritis, and tubo-ovarian abscess. It is most common in young, nulliparous, sexually active women with multiple sex partners.

Postinfectious tubal factor infertility is the second most common cause of female infertility in the United States. Following pelvic inflammatory disease, infertility occurs in 12% of women; the risk of ectopic pregnancy increases 7- to 10-fold, and approximately 20% of women develop chronic pelvic pain.[20]

Clinical Presentation

Symptoms suggesting pelvic inflammatory disease include abdominal pain, dyspareunia, vaginal discharge, and abnormal vaginal bleeding. Mucopurulent discharge or leukorrhea in the vaginal vault has good sensitivity but low specificity for pelvic inflammatory disease.

Differential Diagnosis and Diagnostic Testing

The ED diagnosis of pelvic inflammatory disease usually is based on clinical findings of lower abdominal tenderness, cervical motion tenderness, and adnexal tenderness for which another cause is not likely. The diagnosis is complicated by the fact that many women may have subtle or mild symptoms that are not readily recognized as pelvic inflammatory disease. Box 123-1 lists certain critera that can enhance the specificity of the diagnosis.

Appendicitis, ectopic pregnancy, septic abortion, hemorrhagic or ruptured ovarian cysts or tumors, twisted ovarian cyst, degeneration of a myoma, and acute enteritis must be considered in the diagnosis. Patients with uterine adnexal or cervical motion tenderness should be considered to have pelvic inflammatory disease and should be treated with antibiotics unless there is a competing diagnosis such as ectopic pregnancy or appendicitis.

Endocervical culture should be performed routinely, but treatment should not be delayed while awaiting results. In selected cases when the diagnosis based on clinical or laboratory evidence is uncertain, the following criteria may be used:

1. Histopathologic evidence of endometritis on endometrial biopsy
2. Transvaginal ultrasonography, computed tomography (Fig. 123-5), or magnetic resonance imaging scan showing thickened, fluid-filled tubes with or without free pelvic fluid and tubo-ovarian complex
3. Laparoscopic abnormalities consistent with pelvic inflammatory disease

A pregnancy test should be obtained to rule out ectopic pregnancy. Pelvic and vaginal ultrasonography is helpful in the differential diagnosis of ectopic pregnancy. Laparoscopy is often used to diagnose pelvic inflammatory disease, and it is imperative if the diagnosis is not certain or if the patient has not responded to antibiotic therapy after 48 hours. The appendix should be visualized at laparoscopy to rule out appendicitis. Cultures obtained at the time of laparoscopy are often specific and helpful.

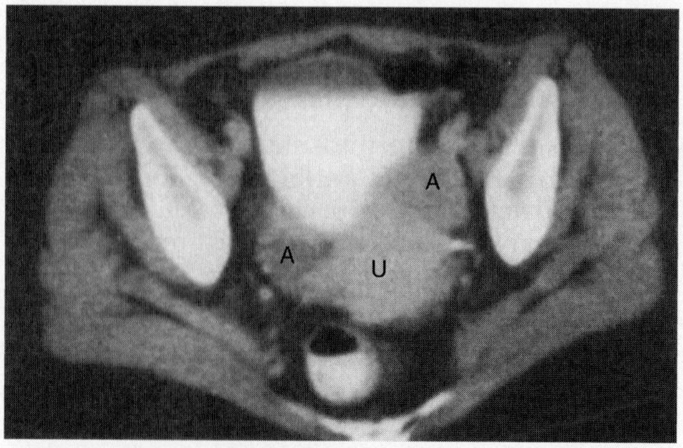
A
A
U

FIGURE 123-5 Computed tomography scan of patient with pelvic inflammatory disease showing bilateral adenexal masses. A, tubo-ovarian abscesses; U, uterus.

BOX 123-2

Pelvic Inflammatory Disease

Definition

- Pelvic inflammatory disease in women comprises a spectrum of inflammatory disorders of the upper genital tract and may include any combination of endometritis, salpingitis, tubo-ovarian abscess, and pelvic peritonitis.

Etiology

- Sexually transmitted organisms, especially *Neisseria gonorrhoeae* and *Chlamydia trachomatis,* are implicated in the majority of cases.
- Microorganisms that are found in the vaginal flora such as anaerobes, *Gardnerella vaginalis, Haemophilus influenzae,* enteric gram-negative rods, and *Streptococcus agalactiae* can cause pelvic inflammatory disease.
- Some experts believe that *Mycoplasma hominis* and *Ureaplasma urealyticum* are causative agents of pelvic inflammatory disease.

Diagnosis

- Acute pelvic inflammatory disease is difficult to diagnose because of the wide variation in the symptoms and signs. Many women have subtle or only mild symptoms.
- No single historical, physical, or laboratory finding is both sensitive and specific for the diagnosis of acute pelvic inflammatory disease.
- Minimal criteria for the diagnosis of pelvic inflammatory disease:
  - Uterine/adnexal tenderness, or
  - Cervical motion tenderness
- Additional criteria:
  - Oral temperature greater >101° F (38.3° C)
  - Abnormal cervical or vaginal mucopurulent discharge
  - Presence of white blood cells on saline microscopy of vaginal secretions
  - Elevated erythrocyte sedimentation rate
  - Elevated C-reactive protein level
  - Laboratory documentation of cervical infection with *N. gonorrhoeae* or *C. trachomatis*
- More specific criteria:
  - Histopathologic evidence of endometritis on endometrial biopsy
  - Transvaginal ultrasonography, computed tomography, or magnetic resonance imaging scans showing thickened, fluid-filled tubes with or without free pelvic fluid or tubo-ovarian complex
  - Laparoscopic abnormalities consistent with pelvic inflammatory disease

Treatment

- Antimicrobial coverage should include *N. gonorrhoeae, C. trachomatis,* gram-negative facultative bacteria, anaerobes, and streptococci. No single therapeutic regimen has been established.
- When selecting a treatment regimen, PEs should consider availability, cost, patient acceptance, and regional differences in antimicrobial susceptibility of likely pathogens.
- Outpatient management is appropriate for most patients; however, follow-up within 72 hours is recommended to assess the patient's response to antimicrobial therapy. (See Box 123-3 for criteria for hospitalization of patients.)
- Outpatient treatment regimens:
  - Ofloxacin, 400 mg PO bid for 14 days; or levofloxacin, 500 mg PO qd for 14 days, with or without metronidazole, 500 mg PO bid for 14 days
  - Ceftriaxone, 250 mg IM once, plus doxycycline, 100 mg PO bid for 14 days, with or without metronidazole, 500 mg PO bid for 14 days
- Inpatient treatment regimens:
  - Cefotetan, 2 g IV q12h, or cefoxitin, 2 g IV q6h, plus doxycycline, 100 mg IV or orally q12h; parenteral therapy may be discontinued 24 hours after the patient improves clinically, and oral therapy with doxycycline, 100 mg orally bid, should be continued for a total of 14 days
  - Clindamycin, 900 mg IV q8h, plus gentamicin, loading dose IV or IM of 2 mg/kg, followed by maintenance dose of 1.5 mg/kg q8h; single daily doses may be substituted; parenteral therapy may be discontinued 24 hours after a patient improves clinically, and oral therapy (doxycycline, 100 mg PO bid, or clindamycin, 450 mg PO qid) should be continued for a total of 14 days

■ Treatment

Recommended outpatient and inpatient treatment regimens are shown in Box 123-2.

Patients with acute pelvic inflammatory disease who meet the criteria for hospital admission require IV antibiotic therapy. Criteria for admission (Box 123-3) include possible appendicitis, pregnancy, lack of response to oral antimicrobial therapy, inability to tolerate outpatient oral regimens, presence of a tubo-ovarian abscess, and severe symptoms such as nausea, vomiting, and high fever.

BOX 123-3

Criteria for Hospitalization of Patients with Pelvic Inflammatory Disease

- Surgical emergencies such as appendicitis cannot be excluded in the diagnosis.
- The patient is pregnant.
- The patient has a tubo-ovarian abscess.
- The patient has severe illness such as nausea and vomiting or high fever.
- The patient is unable to follow or tolerate an outpatient oral regimen.
- The patient does not respond clinically to oral antimicrobial therapy.

Special Considerations

Pregnancy

Pelvic inflammatory disease during pregnancy is uncommon but can occur, most frequently in the first trimester. Hospital admission for parenteral antibiotic therapy is recommended because of the increased risk for preterm delivery, fetal demise, and maternal morbidity.

TUBO-OVARIAN ABSCESS

Tubo-ovarian abscess is a complication of pelvic inflammatory disease; up to one third of patients hospitalized with pelvic inflammatory disease develop this sequela. Rupture rates can be as high as 15% and constitute a surgical emergency.[8] Most cases of arise from oophoritis, which is secondary to salpingitis. The ovary becomes infected when purulent material from the fallopian tube enters it. If tubal fimbriae are adherent to the ovary, the tube and ovary together may form a large, retort-shaped tubo-ovarian abscess, which is the most common intra-abdominal abscess in premenopausal women.

Most tubo-ovarain abscesses consist of polymicrobic anaerobic bacteria, and not all are associated with pelvic inflammatory disease. Disease can be bilateral, although unilateral disease is more common and accounts for 60% of such abscesses.[15]

Clinical Presentation

Patients with a tubo-ovarian abscess typically present with abdominal pain and severe, asymmetrical tenderness, often exhibiting peritoneal signs on palpation. Fever and leukocytosis are usually, but not always, present as well.

Differential Diagnosis and Diagnostic Testing

Definitive diagnosis is made by direct visualization or an imaging study. Pelvic ultrasonography has a reported sensitivity of 93% and specificity of 98%.[8] Computed tomography may be used to define the abscess better or may be appropriate if the ultrasound evaluation is inconclusive.

Treatment

All patients with suspected tubo-ovarian abscess should be hospitalizd. Initial parenteral therapy options are the same as those listed for pelvic inflammatory disease, but continued oral therapy should include clindamycin or metronidazole in addition to doxycycline.

Tubo-ovarian abscesses may require transcutaneous or transvaginal aspiration. Surgical excision is also an option. Unless rupture is suspected, institute high-dose antibiotic therapy should be instituted, and therapy should be monitored with ultrasonography. Ruptured tubo-ovarian abscess is a life-threatening condition and requires immediate medical therapy associated with surgery.

Unilateral adnexectomy is acceptable for unilateral abscess. Hysterectomy and bilateral salpingo-oophorectomy may be necessary for overwhelming infection or in cases of chronic disease with intractable pelvic pain.

Special Considerations

Pregnancy

Although rare in pregnancy, tubo-ovarian abscesses can occur, most commonly in the first trimester.

Immunosuppression

HIV-positive women develop tubo-ovarian abscesses more frequently than HIV-negative women.

Abdominal Gynecologic Infections

FITZ-HUGH-CURTIS SYNDROME

Perihepatitis consisting of liver capsule inflammation without liver parenchymal damage is referred to as Fitz-Hugh-Curtis syndrome. This disorder is an extrapelvic manifestion of pelvic inflammatory disease. Swelling of the liver capsule produces pain with inspiration, usually in the right upper quadrant. A purulent or fibrinous exudate appears on the capsular surface.

Clinical Presentation

Illness consists of two phases. The acute phase is characterized by sharp, right upper quadrant, pleuritic abdominal pain that can radiate to the shoulder; the chronic phase results from the formation of peritoneal adhesions that cause persistent, typically right upper quadrant, abdominal pain. Tubal infections may or may not be concurrently present.

■ Differential Diagnosis and Diagnostic Testing

Perihepatitis was formerly believed to be caused solely by *N. gonorrhoeae,* but *C. trachomatis* is now more often the causative agent. Salpingitis is invariably the source, but the syndrome occasionally follows appendicitis and other causes of peritonitis. Fitz-Hugh-Curtis syndrome is frequently misinterpreted as cholecystitis, pneumonia, perforated peptic ulcer, or renal colic. Liver enzyme levels may be mildly elevated.

Diagnosis is difficult and clinically based. A high index of suspicion should be maintained in women presenting to the ED with upper abdominal pain and normal routine results in gallbladder and liver function tests. Fitz-Hugh-Curtis syndrome is a more likely cause of upper quadrant pleuritic pain than cholecystitis and should be suspected in any woman with pleuritic upper quadrant pain and physical signs of salpingitis. Associated signs and symptoms of fever, leukocytosis, abdominal pain, cervicitis, or pelvic inflammatory disease may be present but their absence does not exclude the diagnosis.

Laparoscopy is useful to identify unclear cases and, in conjunction with positive cervical or abdominal cultures, represents the criterion standard for diagnosis. Negative cervical cultures alone, however, do not rule out the diagnosis. "Violin string" adhesions may be seen on ultrasound or computed tomography scans (Fig. 123-6).

■ Treatment

The goal of treatment is to prevent chronic abdominal pain via bacterial eradication with antibiotics and surgical lysis of adhesions. Complications are uncommon but can include subdiaphragmatic abscess and small bowel obstruction.

Although no formal antibiotic recommendations exist, options include oral doxycycline (100 mg twice a day for 14 days) plus ceftriaxone (250 mg IM once) or ofloxacin (400 mg) and metronidazole (500 mg), both given orally twice a day for 14 days.[8]

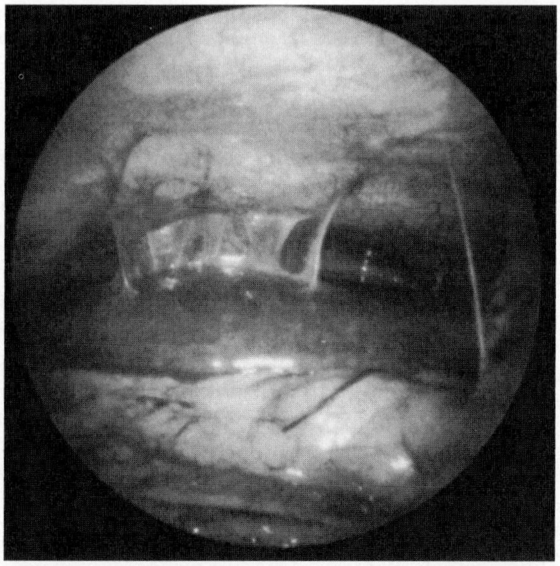

FIGURE 123-6 "Violin string" adhesions are visualized in this scan of a patient with Fitz-Hugh-Curtis syndrome. (From Ferri FF: Ferri's Clinical Advisor 2007: Instant Diagnosis and Treatment, 9th ed. Philadelphia, Mosby, 2007.)

Genitourinary Infections

■ ACUTE URETHRAL SYNDROME

Most women with symptoms of dysuria and urinary frequency have acute cystitis caused by coliform or staphylococcal organisms. The pyuria that occurs with recent onset of dysuria and urinary frequency and negative urine cultures is termed acute urethral syndrome. The infectious agent usually is *C. trachomatis*. Therapy consists of antibiotics directed against the infectious agent (coliform or *Staphylococcus saprophyticus* cystitis, *C. trachomatis* urethritis).

Systemic Gynecologic Infections

■ HUMAN IMMUNODEFICIENCY VIRUS AND HEPATITIS B AND C

HIV and hepatitis B and C can all be sexually transmitted and have systemic but not localized gynecologic manifestations of illness.

■ GENITAL TUBERCULOSIS

Female genital tuberculosis is rare in the United States. The overall incidence of pelvic tuberculosis in patients with pulmonary tuberculosis is approximately 5%.[15] Virtually all genital tuberculosis is secondary to pulmonary infection, which usually spreads by the blood stream from the lungs to the fallopian tubes within 1 year of the primary pulmonary infection. Direct extension occurs from the tube in several directions: to the pelvic peritoneum and ovary, the endometrium, and the cervix. In the latent form, genital tuberculosis appears partially or completely arrested after the initial tubal infection, and patients have few or no pelvic complaints. In the active form, it may cause tuberculous salpingitis or peritonitis and is treated accordingly.

■ TOXIC SHOCK SYNDROME

Toxic shock syndrome is an acute illness caused by toxin-producing *Staphylococcus aureus*. 5% to 10% of women carry *S. aureus* in the vagina, but only 1% carry the toxin producing form.[21] The syndrome is associated with menstruation, and probably with tampon use, but it also can occur as a result of *S. aureus* infection of the breast and endometrium after delivery and from abdominal surgical wounds.

PATIENT TEACHING TIPS

- Patients diagnosed with suspected infection should be instructed on the use of condoms and told to avoid sexual contact for at least 7 days.
- Patients at risk should be advised to schedule follow-up for HIV and syphilis testing as an outpatient.
- Patients should be instructed that all sex partners need treatment.
- Patients diagnosed with herpes simples virus infection should be informed about the course of the disease and the continued risk of transmission to others even when they are asymptomatic.

■ Clinical Presentation

Characteristic features include a high fever (>102° F [38.9° C]), a diffuse rash, hypotension, skin desquamation (usually 1-2 weeks later), and a wide variety of systemic effects, including gastrointestinal (vomiting, diarrhea), muscular (myalgia), mucous membrane (hyperemia), renal (elevated blood urea nitrogen or creatinine level), hepatic (enzyme abnormalities), hematologic (thrombocytopenia), and neurologic (disorientation, coma) symptoms.

■ Differential Diagnosis and Diagnostic Testing

Vaginal or specific-site cultures recover *S. aureus*. Blood, throat, and cerebrospinal fluid cultures, together with serologic tests for Rocky Mountain spotted fever, leptospirosis, and measles, are usually indicated to exclude diseases with similar clinical presentations.

■ Treatment

A vaginal tampon, if present, should be removed. Patients should be hospitalized and, when indicated, given large fluid volumes for blood pressure maintenance. Beta-lactamase–resistant antibiotics are recommended (nafcillin, oxacillin) or vancomycin for pericillin-allergic patients.

Other supportive measures such as intubation, vasopressor administration, steroids, and dialysis may be necessary.

Women with toxic shock syndrome should be warned of recurrent episodes and advised against resuming tampon use.

Although the effectiveness of this measure is uncertain, it is prudent for all women to avoid *prolonged* use of tampons. It is recommended that women do not use tampons for 6 to 8 weeks after delivery.

REFERENCES

1. Sexually transmitted disease treatment guidelines 2006. Centers for Disease Control and Prevention. MMWR Recomm Rep 2006;55(RR-1):1–85.
2. Dunne EF, Unger ER, Sternberg M, et al: Prevalence of HPV infection among females in the United States. JAMA 2007;297:813–819.
3. Mazdisnian F: Benign disorders of the vulva and vagina. In DeCherney AH, Nathan L (eds): Current Obstetric and Gynecologic Diagnosis and Treatment, 10th ed. New York, McGraw-Hill, 2007.
4. Koutsky LA, Ashley RL, Holmes KK, et al: The frequency of unrecognized type 2 herpes simplex virus infection among women. Sex Transm Dis 1990;17:90–94.
5. Mabey L, Peeling RW: Lymphogranuloma venereum. Tropical Medicine Series. Sex Transm Inf 2002;78:90–92.
6. Augenbraun M: Syphilis. In Klausner JD, Hook EW III (eds): Current Diagnosis and Treatment of Sexually Transmitted Diseases. New York, McGraw-Hill, 2007.
7. Taylor SN, Martin DH: Chancroid. In Klausner JD, Hook EW III (eds): Current Diagnosis and Treatment of Sexually Transmitted Diseases. New York, McGraw-Hill, 2007.
8. Zeger W, Holt K: Gynecologic infections. Emerg Med Clin North Am 2003;21:631–648.
9. Sobel JD: Vaginitis. N Engl J Med 1997;337:1896–1903.
10. Schwebke JR: Vaginal discharge. In Klausner JD, Hook EW III (eds): Current Diagnosis and Treatment of Sexually Transmitted Diseases. New York, McGraw-Hill, 2007.
11. Sobel JD: Candida vulvovaginitis-vulvar disorders. Semin Cutan Med Surg 1996;15:17–28.
12. Sobel JD: Bacterial vaginosis. Annu Rev Med 2000;51: 349–356.
13. Lossick JC: Epidemiology of urogenital trichomoniasis. In Honigberg BM (ed): Trichomonads Parasitic in Humans. New York, Springer-Verlag, 1990, pp 311–323.
14. Sorvillo F, Smith L, Kerndt P, et al: Trichomonas vaginalis, HIV, and African-Americans. Emerg Infect Dis 2001; 7(6):927–32.
15. Ainbinder SW, Ramin SM, DeCherney AH: Sexually transmitted diseases and pelvic infections. In DeCherney AH, Nathan L (eds): Current Obstetric and Gynecologic Diagnosis and Treatment, 10th ed. New York, McGraw-Hill, 2007.
16. Marrazzo JM: Cervicitis. In Klausner JD, Hook EW III (eds): Current Diagnosis and Treatment of Sexually Transmitted Diseases. New York, McGraw-Hill, 2007.
17. Weinstock H, et al: Sexually transmitted diseases among American youth: Incidence and prevalence estimates, 2000. Perspect Sex Reprod Health 2004;36(1):6–10.
18. National Surveillance Data for Chlamydia, Gonorrhea, and Syphilis—Trends in Reportable Sexually Transmitted Diseases in the United States, 2006. Centers for Disease Control and Prevention. Available at www.cdc.gov/std/stats/trends2006.htm.
19. Geisler WM, Stamm WE: Genital chlamydial infections. In Klausner JD, Hook EW III (eds): Current Diagnosis and Treatment of Sexually Transmitted Diseases. New York, McGraw-Hill, 2007.
20. Cohen CR: Pelvic inflammatory disease. In Klausner JD, Hook EW III (eds): Current Diagnosis and Treatment of Sexually Transmitted Disease. New York, McGraw-Hill, 2007.
21. Davis D, Gash-Kim T, Hefferman E: Toxic shock syndrome: Case report of postpartum female and a literature review. J Emerg Med 1998;16(4)607–614.

Chapter **124**

Breast Disorders

Karen Jubanyik

KEY POINTS

There are very few true breast emergencies, and immediately life-threatening causes such as traumatic breast rupture or necrotizing fasciitis are exceedingly rare.

Breast pain, particularly if cyclical, is common, and benign causes predominate.

Breast cancer is a possible diagnosis in any patient who presents for medical care with a chief complaint related to the breast, including breast pain or mass, nipple discharge, or skin lesions.

Most patients diagnosed with breast cancer have no risk factors except age older than 50 years and female sex, and eight of nine patients have no family history of breast cancer.

The EP can play a role in the reduction of the risk of lymphedema by early and aggressive treatment of even very minor infections and burns.

Most medications are safe for use while breastfeeding, and the benefits of continuing breastfeeding generally outweigh the potential for harm.

Few maternal infections, other than human immunodeficiency virus (HIV), present a significant risk to the breastfeeding infant.

Scope

It is estimated that one in three women sees a physician for a breast-related complaint in her lifetime. There are very few true breast-related emergencies. Increased public health campaigns to promote breast cancer awareness have led to an overestimation of its prevalence, and many patients worry unduly that any new breast symptom is due to malignancy. Common breast complaints include pain, masses, nipple discharge, and skin changes. In addition, patients may present with acute, subacute, or chronic conditions related to trauma, lactation, cosmetic breast surgery, and breast cancer or its treatment.

Approximately one half of physician visits for breast complaints are for pain. A new, palpable mass is another common breast-related complaint. Although 9 of 10 premenopausal women with a palpable breast mass will be diagnosed with a benign condition, a new mass in a 75-year-old woman is malignant in up to 70% of cases. Breast cancer is the most common cause of cancer-related mortality in women worldwide and second only to lung cancer in women in the United States. In 2006, it accounted for one third of all cancer diagnoses in women in the United States.[1]

Because EPs frequently perform diagnostic studies, diagnose infectious diseases, and initiate drug therapy in women who are nursing, it is important for them to be aware of the impact that these decisions may have on the safe continuation of breastfeeding. It is an explicit goal of the Healthy People 2010 campaign to increase the rate and duration of breastfeeding in the United States; specifically, the goal is for 75% of women to breastfeed in early infancy, 50% through 6 months, and 25% to the end of the first postpartum year.

Breast surgery is relatively common in the United States. In addition to the 90,000 mastectomies performed annually, there are approximately 100,000 cosmetic augmentations and 100,000 reduction mammoplasties. Many patients undergoing breast augmentation, either for reconstruction or cosmesis, experience significant complications and require additional surgeries for correction or explantation; these cases account for tens of thousands of additional procedures.

Men can develop most of the breast conditions seen in women. Although breast cancer in men accounts for fewer than 1% of the total number of breast malignancies diagnosed in the United States, in other areas in the world (e.g., central Africa), male breast cancer is significantly more common.

Normal Anatomy and Physiology of the Adult Breast

The mammary glands arise along milk lines that appear during the fifth week of gestation and extend from the groin to the axilla. By approximately the ninth week, the lower portion of the milk line regresses. Failure of regression can lead to accessory breast tissue or nipples at any point along the milk lines, and abnormal regression may lead to breast hypoplasia or amastia.

Each breast contains approximately 20 glandular units (lobes), each composed of a tubulo-alveolar gland and adipose tissue (Fig. 124-1). Each lobe drains into a lactiferous duct, and multiple lactiferous ducts fuse before exiting the skin. Just below the surface of the nipple, the lactiferous ducts form large dilations called lactiferous sinuses. Lactiferous sinuses store milk during lactation. The lobes and ducts account for approximately 20% of the mass of the breast; 80% of the breast is composed of stromal tissue (fat and fibrous connective tissue), which give the breast its size, shape, and support.

The arterial blood supply to the breast arises from branches of the internal mammary, lateral thoracic, thoracodorsal, and subscapular arteries. A plexus of veins in the subareolar region drains into the intercostal, internal mammary, and axillary veins. Lymphatic drainage is primarily to the axilla, although there is some drainage to the internal mammary lymph nodes. There is additional drainage to the subclavicular and mediastinal nodes. Lymph can flow from any quadrant of the breast to any axillary lymph node or to any of the other channels mentioned.

Between menarche and menopause, cyclic variations in circulating hormonal levels, principally progesterone and estrogen, cause breast swelling, engorgement, and tenderness. Interlobular edema can increase breast size by 15%. These symptoms are most pronounced in the few days prior to the onset of menses and subside substantially by day 7 of the menstrual cycle. Hormonal changes leading up to menopause cause a significant loss of glandular tissue, particularly lobular elements. The postmenopausal breast consists of relatively more fat and connective tissue.

Traumatic Injuries to the Breast

Trauma to the breast is usually due to blunt forces and rarely appears in isolation. Multiple thoracic injuries are typical, including rib fractures, clavicle fractures, lung and cardiac trauma, and injuries to the great vessels. In cases of apparent breast trauma without significant mechanism, the EP should be concerned about potential intimate partner violence or malignancy. Hematomas occasionally occur spontaneously or in the setting of very minor trauma in women with breast cancer, and they may be the first symptom of occult malignancy. Breast trauma normally heals within 4 to 6 weeks. Symptoms that persist require evaluation for possible malignancy.

Mandatory three-point lap-shoulder restraint laws have been effective in decreasing overall mortality from motor vehicle crashes; however, there has been an increase in the incidence of soft tissue injury to the chest wall. The three-point diagonal chest restraint seat belt produces a shearing force on the

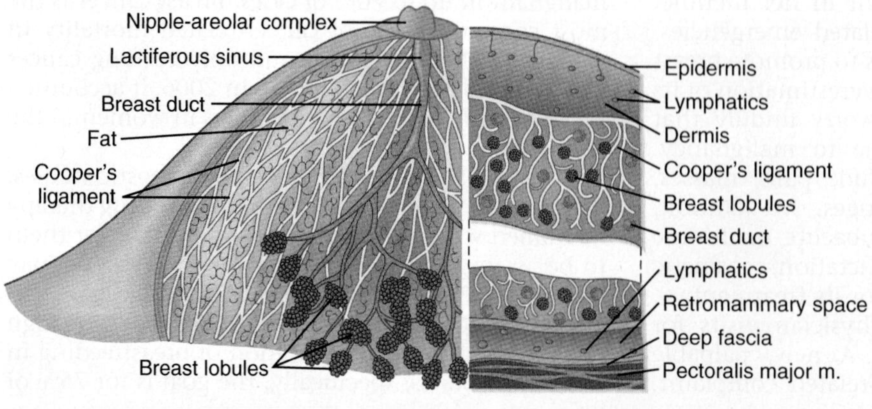
Nipple-areolar complex
Lactiferous sinus
Breast duct
Fat
Cooper's ligament
Breast lobules
Epidermis
Lymphatics
Dermis
Cooper's ligament
Breast lobules
Breast duct
Lymphatics
Retromammary space
Deep fascia
Pectoralis major m.

FIGURE 124-1 The breast contains approximately 20 glandular units (lobes), each composed of a tubulo-alveolar gland and adipose tissue. (From Iglehart JD, Kaelin CM: Diseases of the breast. In Townsend CM, Beauchamp RD, Evers BM, Mattox KL [eds]: Sabiston's Textbook of Surgery, 17th ed. Philadelphia, Elsevier, 2004.)

breast by the diagonal chest strap, as well as a compression injury to the breast tissue between the chest restraint and the bony thorax. Simple hematomas are the most common problem after trauma. Crush injuries to the breast from seat belts have, in rare cases, caused subcutaneous transection of the breast. A permanent furrow deformity may result and is acutely managed surgically. Because the breast is mobile over the pectoral fascia, a sudden forceful movement of the breast can also cause complete avulsion of the breast from the chest wall. This type of injury causes complete rupture of the perforating arteries (which arise from the second, third, and fourth intercostal arteries) to the breast. A transected artery may massively bleed immediately or may retract into the pectoral musculature, resulting in life-threatening hemorrhage after vascular spasm resolves.

Simple hematomas can be managed conservatively with analgesics such as acetaminophen or oxycodone and instructions to the patient to wear a tight-fitting bra. The EP must be alert to patients with an acute injury and an expanding hematoma, particularly patients with coagulopathies or taking anticoagulant medication. The EP must begin anticoagulation reversal promptly with fresh-frozen plasma and vitamin K and immediately consult a surgeon. Patients presenting more than 48 hours after injury rarely have bleeding from a discrete vessel, and the blood is diffusely located within the breast tissue and therefore not amenable to surgery. Aspiration is not effective until clot liquefication occurs.

Posttraumatic hematomas can become infected, even months after injury. Management strategies include both open surgical drainage and packing or ultrasound-guided placement of a drain in combination with oral antibiotics. Appropriate antibiotic options in uncomplicated cases include a first-generation cephalosporin (cephalexin, 500 mg PO qid) or an antistaphylococcal penicillin (dicloxacillin, 250 mg PO qid).

■ FAT NECROSIS

The most common long-term complication after trauma to the breast is fat necrosis.[2] Fat necrosis is an inflammatory condition that can be a sequela of trauma, surgery, infection, or radiation, or it may appear spontaneously, particularly in women with large, pendulous breasts. The pathophysiology of fat necrosis is multifactorial but seems to involve the breakdown of fat cells by blood and tissue lipases. Clinically, mammographically, and sonographically, the condition may mimic carcinoma of the breast. Usually there is a firm, poorly mobile, nontender mass in the superficial subcutaneous tissues. Overlying skin may be erythematous, ecchymotic, or indurated. Axillary lyphadenopathy and nipple retraction may be present. Fat necrosis typically resolves spontaneously, but because it is hard to differentiate from malignancy, tissue sampling often is necessary.

■ MONDOR'S DISEASE

Although often idiopathic, Mondor's disease[3] may be associated with trauma, large breasts, febrile illness, contact dermatitis, or occasionally with breast cancer. Mondor's disease is a superficial phlebitis of the lateral thoracic, thoracoepigastric, or superior epigastic vein. It typically occurs in middle-aged women but can occur in men as well; the condition can be unilateral or bilateral and may be asymptomatic or associated with pain and tenderness. The classic Mondor cord is 2 to 3 mm in diameter, initially red and tender, and tracks from the lateral margin of the breast, across the costal margin and extending to the abdominal wall (Fig. 124-2). The cord is firmly attached to the overlying skin and can extend 2 to 30 cm or more. Any tenderness should resolve within weeks, but the cord may remain palpable for up to six months. There is no risk of systemic embolization.

Discomfort can be managed with warm compresses and antiinflammatory medications such as ibuprofen or naproxen. As with any breast condition seen in the ED, patients with presumed Mondor's disease must have close outpatient follow-up, particularly in light of the rare association with breast cancer.

Breast Pain

Breast pain, especially as an isolated symptom, can be thought of as originating from one of three broad categories: cyclic mastalgia, noncyclic mastalgia, or

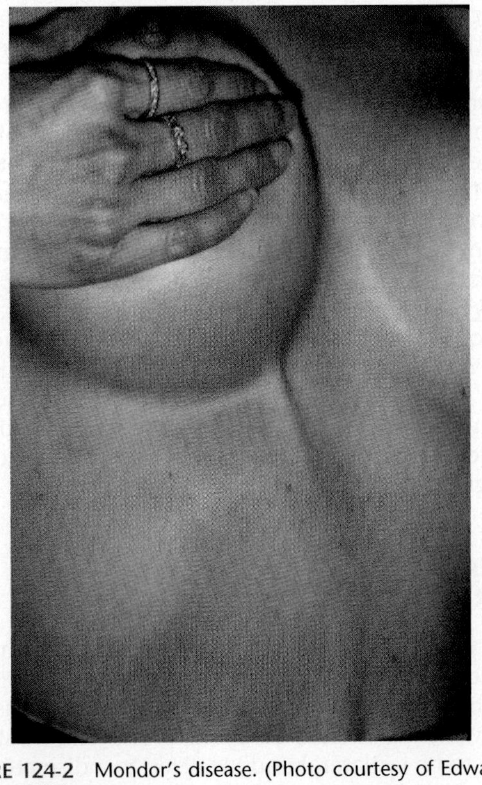

FIGURE 124-2 Mondor's disease. (Photo courtesy of Edward Pechter, MD.)

extramammary. Regardless of suspected etiology, all patients should be referred for follow-up care.

■ CYCLIC MASTALGIA

The term *fibrocystic breast disease* has been replaced by the term *fibrocystic breast condition* to emphasize that this is not considered a disease and represents a spectrum of histologic entities in women. Women with predominantly fibrotic changes may have rubbery areas of fibrosis that are hard and firm. Women with significant cysts often find that these enlarge and become more painful just prior to menstruation, causing cyclic mastalgia.

Cyclic mastalgia occurs in premenopausal women, is associated with worsening symptoms in the late luteal phase of the menstrual cycle, and accounts for two thirds of patients with mastalgia. The typical pain of cyclic mastalgia is:

- Bilateral
- Predominantly in the upper outer quadrants
- Described as achy or heavy
- Resolves with onset of menses

The physical examination may be normal or may reveal tender nodularities. Fibrocystic breast conditions are not associated with axillary lymphadenopathy, skin thickening, edema or discoloration, or nipple abnormalities such as retraction or discharge. The presence of any of these findings raises the probability that the patient has another condition instead of, or in addition to, cyclic mastalgia. The EP should educate patients about symptoms not generally associated with cyclic mastalgia, and encourage women to seek medical attention for any new or worrisome changes.

Although most patients require only mild analgesics, such as acetaminophen or ibuprofen, and referral for outpatient follow-up, a number of alternative potential treatment modalities are available to women with cyclic mastalgia.[5] Many of these therapies have little more than anecdotal evidence to support their use, but because they pose little risk to patients, the EP should be familiar with them and selectively offer options that a given patient may believe are potentiallly beneficial (Box 124-1).

Women with *severe* cyclic mastalgia, defined as pain interfering with work and other activities of daily living for more than 7 days a month, despite treatment with conservative measures, should be referred for specialty care, preferably to an endocrinologist or reproductive endocrinologist.

BOX 124-1

Management Strategies for Cyclic Mastalgia

- Improved mechanical support with a properly fitting bra and use of a sports bra during exercise.
- Application of warm compresses or ice packs
- Decreasing dietary fat to less than 20% of energy intake
- Eliminating caffeine in the diet
- Smoking cessation
- Evening primrose oil (gamma-linolenic acid), 1000 mg PO tid for 6 months*
- Oral contraceptive pills with low estrogen content
- Parenteral medroxyprogesterone acetate (Depo-Provera)
- Micronized progesterone vaginal cream applied to breast
- Vitamin E
- Acupuncture
- Relaxation training

*Caution is urged because this is a nutritional supplement/herb and is not regulated by the U.S. Food and Drug Administration.

■ NONCYCLIC MASTALGIA AND EXTRAMAMMARY PAIN

Noncyclic mastalgia and extramammary pain are caused by a variety of conditions (Table 124-1)[6]; they may be constant or intermittent, but are not associated with the menstrual cycle. Noncyclic mastalgia tends to be unilateral and localized to a discrete area. Women with noncyclic breast pain tend to be older than 40 years, and the cause is likely to be related to an anatomic lesion in the breast. Although breast cancer does not typically present with pain as the sole symptom, breast cancer, particularly inflammatory breast cancer, is diagnosed in a small percentage of patients presenting with pain. A number of medications, many of which also cause galactorrhea or gynecomastia (discussed in detail later in this chapter), are also associated with noncyclic mastalgia.

Table 124-1 DIFFERENTIAL DIAGNOSIS OF NONCYCLIC MASTALGIA

Breast-related	Extramammary
Mastitis	Costochondritis
Breast trauma	Chest wall trauma
Mondor's disease	Acute coronary syndrome/ angina
Breast cancer	Pericarditis
Benign breast mass	Pulmonary embolus
Breast cyst	Pleurisy
Duct ectasia	Biliary disease
Postoperative pain	Peptic ulcer disease
Diabetic fibrous mastopathy	Fibromyalgia
Medication side effects	Arthritis
	Phantom pain (post-mastectomy)

Postoperatively, pain can be prolonged; 30% to 40% of patients report significant pain 1 year after reduction or augmentation mammoplasty, and the number is higher after mastectomy with reconstruction. Phantom breast pain after mastectomy occurs in up to 12% of patients 1 year after surgery.[7] Extramammary breast pain can arise from the chest wall or from other sources. Although most of the conditions that cause isolated breast pain are not immediately life-threatening, the EP must be aware that some emergent conditions, including acute coronary syndrome and pulmonary embolus, can present with pain that appears to be originating from the breast.

Breast Mass

Although breast pain is the most common symptom causing women to seek medical care related to their breasts, a palpable breast mass is associated with significant anxiety and often prompts a visit to a physician. For the woman presenting with a chief complaint of a breast mass, evaluation and treatment will likely be based upon the findings on physical examination, the patient's age, and other risk factors. The EP must make arrangements for prompt surgical referral particularly when the physical examination reveals a mass and any of the following associated findings:

- Axillary or supraclavicular lymphadenopathy
- Skin rash, ulceration, or dimpling
- Nipple retraction, ulceration, or discharge

Women without these worrisome findings still need referral for outpatient evaluation and follow-up, although many can be managed in a primary care setting.

Breast cancer is exceedingly rare in women less than 20 years of age and accounts for only a small fraction of a percent of breast disease in women younger than 30 years. Most women younger than 35 years who present with a solitary painless breast mass will have a fibroadenoma. Typically, outpatient ultrasonography, with or without fine needle aspiration cytology, and referral to a breast surgeon is needed.

The EP should be suspicious of a malignancy in patients younger than 30 years who present with a mass if the patient history is positive for the following:

- Childhood malignancy
- Chest radiation
- Inheritance of the *BRCA1* or *BRCA2* gene
- Multiple family members with early-onset breast cancer, particularly if bilateral or in males

Women over the age of 30 are at increased risk for breast cancer particularly if the history includes the following findings:

- Family history of first-degree relative with breast cancer
- Biopsy-proven atypical hyperplasia
- Increased exposure to endogenous estrogens (nulliparity, delayed childbearing)

All women older than 35 years with dominant masses require triple testing in the outpatient setting, including clinical evaluation, mammography with or without ultrasonography, and biopsy. Biopsy is required regardless of the results of imaging studies; lobular carcinoma is an example of a lesion frequently not visible on mammography. Surgeons disagree about the need for biopsy in women younger than 35 years of age who have a discrete mass consistent with fibroadenoma on both examination and ultrasonography because 99% of these women will be confirmed to have a benign lesion on biopsy. EPs should be aware of the usual approaches for outpatient evaluation of breast masses in order to provide optimal patient education.

Common benign breast masses (Table 124-2) include fibroadenomas, cysts, phylloides tumors (malignant 5% of the time), and intraductal papillomas. Other benign tumors found in breast tissue, but not limited to the breasts, include lipomas, hamartomas, hemangiomas, neurofibromas, granular cell tumors, and fat necrosis. None of these conditions appears to increase the risk for subsequent development of breast cancer.

■ BREAST CANCER

Breast cancer is the most common cancer diagnosed in women in the United States, and the second leading cause of cancer-related death (after lung cancer). Breast cancer can begin in either the ducts or the lobes and can remain *in situ* or invade through the duct or lobule. Eighty percent of all breast cancers are infiltrating (or invasive) ductal carcinomas; less than 10% are of the infiltrating lobular type. Rare variants of infiltrating ductal breast cancer include medullary, colloid, and tubular carcinomas.

A female born in the United States today has a 13% probability of developing breast cancer during her lifetime, which is slightly increased over the past decade.[9] Most women who develop breast cancer have only two risk factors (being female and older than age 50), and it is believed that the growing incidence of breast cancer is due to a number of lifestyle markers of Western industrialized society. The list includes delayed childbirth, lower parity, decreased incidence and duration of lactation, obesity, alcohol, affluence, and probably increased fat in the diet.

Recent reduction in breast cancer mortality in the United States is believed to be due to the following factors:

- Mammography screening programs
- Increased use of ultrasonography as an adjunctive screening tool
- Identification of high-risk patients with *BRCA1* and *BRCA2* gene mutations
- Use of adjuvant hormonal therapy in receptor-positive disease
- Use of adjuvant biologically targeted therapy in patients with *HER2/neu* gene amplification

Table 124-2 BENIGN BREAST TUMORS

Tumor	Tissue	Age	Size	Characteristics	Diagnostic Findings	Follow-Up
Fibroadenoma	Both glandular and stromal tissue elements; typically solitary	Common in women <40 yr; Uncommon >50 years	From microscopic to 5 cm	Tender premenstrually, often asymptomatic; complex fibroadenomas increase risk for malignancy	MF: poor (look the same as surrounding parenchyma); UF: well-circumscribed, homogeneous, hypoechoic lesions with edge-shadowing; diagnosis depends on fine needle, core, or surgical biopsy	Specialist evaluation and follow-up
Cyst	Lobular lesions; obstruction, involution, and aging of ducts produce loculations that enlarge as cysts	Common in women 40-50 yr but rare in post-menopausal women	Microscopic to several cm	Usually round, mobile; can be tender premenstrually	MF: poor; UF: typical simple cyst (well-defined round or oval anechoic lesions)	Ultrasonography for benign cysts; biopsy for atypical cases
Phylloides tumor	Glandular tissue and stromal tissue (mostly stromal)	Any age; median of 50-60 yr	5 cm average size; up to 30 cm seen	Rare; painless, rapid-growing; 5% are malignant	MF and USF similar to findings for fibroadenoma; definitive diagnosis depends on tissue sampling and biopsy	All tumors, including benign growths, are resected;. high mortality at 3 years
Intraductal papilloma	Wartlike growths of glandular and fibrovascular tissue within ducts	Typically 45-50 yr	Usually <1 cm	Single tumors involving large ducts near the nipple; clear or bloody discharge; may be felt as a small lump behind or adjacent to nipple	Ductography is particularly helpful	Surgical treatment generally recommended; involves removal of papilloma and portion of duct

MF, mammography findings; USF, ultrasound findings.

Table 124-3 AMERICAN CANCER SOCIETY BREAST CANCER SCREENING GUIDELINES 2003

Category	Guidelines
Women at average risk	Breast self-exam beginning in 20s and clinical breast examination (CBE) should be performed at least every 3 years. Beginning at age 40 years, CBE and mammography should be performed annually.
Women at increased risk	Earlier initiation of screening, shorter screening intervals, or addition of screening modalities such as ultrasonography and magnetic resonance imaging recommended. Current evidence is insufficient to make specific recommendations.
Older women	Screening decisions are based on health and life expectancy. If woman is in reasonably good health and would be a candidate for treatment, mammography and CBE are warranted.

From Smith RA, Saslow D, Sawyer KA, et al: American Cancer Society guidelines for breast cancer screening: Update 2003. CA Cancer J Clin 2003;53:141-169.

ROUTINE SCREENING RECOMMENDATIONS

Regular screening according to evidence-based guidelines has been shown to decrease mortality in the population by detecting early, asymptomatic breast cancers. Patients diagnosed with stage I disease experience close to 90% overall survival at 10 years, but this falls to less than 5% in patients presenting with stage IV disease. The EP should be familiar with current breast cancer screening guidelines (Table 124-3)[10]. because they are in a unique position to educate women, particularly those who lack adequate access to primary care, about the importance and availability of screening tools. In particular, immigrant and minority women experience a number of barriers when seeking preventive health care, and the special nature of breast cancer adds layers of sociocultural and psychological complexity.[11] The literature on the effectiveness of breast self-examination (BSE) has shown mixed results, and the current version of the guidelines contains no specific recommendations either for or against BSE.

Treatment of Breast Cancer and Associated Complications

Patients undergoing treatment for breast cancer frequently present to the ED with complications related to their disease or treatment.

RED FLAGS

- Most women with breast cancer have no discernible risk factors.
- Missed diagnoses occur more frequently in women younger than age 40 years, those from lower socioeconomic backgrounds, and those with normal mammograms.
- Although 9 of 10 premenopausal women with a palpable breast mass will be diagnosed with a benign condition, a new mass in a 75-year-old woman is malignant in up to 70% of cases.
- Breast trauma normally heals within 4 to 6 weeks; symptoms that persist require evaluation for possible malignancy.
- With complete avulsion of the breast from the chest wall, rupture of the perforating arteries (which arise from the second, third, and fourth intercostal arteries) may occur, and the transected artery may bleed massively immediately or may retract into the pectoral musculature, resulting in life-threatening hemorrhage after the vascular spasm resolves.
- Prompt surgical referral is indicated for a mass and associated axillary or supraclavicular lymphadenopathy, skin rash, ulceration, dimpling, nipple retraction, or discharge.
- All women older than 35 years with a dominant mass require triple testing in the outpatient setting, including clinical evaluation, mammography with or without ultrasonography, and biopsy.
- Given the outward similarity of periductal mastitis and subareolar abscess to some types of breast cancer, all patients in whom these disorders are suspected should be scheduled for outpatient work-up, which typically includes imaging studies and tissue sampling
- Spontaneous nonpuerperal infections other than those associated with periductal mastitis are very rare, and the EP should maintain a high index of suspicion for malignancy, especially inflammatory breast cancer.

COMPLICATIONS OF METASTATIC SPREAD

Common sites of metastases of breast cancer include local and regional as well as distant sites, including lung, pleura, pericardium, bone, and brain. Pleural effusions, generally ipsilateral to the primary tumor, are believed to result from lymphatic spread and are typified by exudates with high glucose concentrations relative to the serum glucose. Breast cancer is the most common extrathoracic primary neoplasm causing metastases to the heart and pericardium; the EP should perform or arrange for emergent echocardiography when managing a patient with a history of breast cancer and symptoms consistent with pericardial effusion.

Radiographically, bone metastases appear as lytic or sclerotic lesions or both. The development of back pain in a woman with a history of breast cancer should prompt initiation of diagnostic studies and treatment for cord compression. The most sensitive imaging study is magnetic resonance imaging, and it should be performed for back pain even when no associated neurologic finding is present (waiting for symptoms can be too late).

■ LYMPHEDEMA

Most patients who are treated for breast cancer undergo surgery with lumpectomy, segmental mastectomy, or mastectomy first. An axillary lymph node dissection or sentinel lymph node biopsy may be performed as well. Lymphedema affects 10% to 30% of women who undergo axillary lymph node dissection; radiation and infection increase the risk. Lymphedema may range from mild to severe, and can develop even years after treatment. It is usually permanent; a few institutions have reported success with autologous lymph node transplantation,[12] but this is not an option for most women.

Those at risk for developing lymphedema are encouraged to have blood drawn and intravenous lines placed in the unaffected arm. Impeccable nail hygiene and aggressive avoidance and treatment of even minor burns, insect bites, and cuts are advised. In addition to avoiding arm compression by blood pressure cuffs, the patient should should avoid any type of squeezing or constriction of the arm, such as that caused by tight clothing, jewelry, bra straps, and purse straps. Patients should be counseled to avoid heavy lifting with the affected arm and to maintain a normal body weight.

■ COMPLICATIONS OF RADIATION THERAPY

Women who choose lumpectomy or partial (segmental) mastectomy usually undergo 6 weeks of external beam radiation. Radiotherapy may also be given in the form of radioactive seeds placed at the tumor site. In another method, called MammoSite, a saline-filled balloon is placed into the lumpectomy site; radioactive material is instilled and drained twice daily for 5 days.

Regardless of the radiation method, the most common complications are radiation-induced dermatitis[13] (90% of patients), which can progress to dry desquamation (50% of patients) in the first few weeks, and moist desquamation (<10% of patients), which appears within 3 to 6 weeks. A corticosteroid cream such as mometasone furoate can be used as prophylaxis or treatment of dry desquamation, preferably in consultation with a medical or radiation oncologist. Wet desquamation, a partial-thickness injury, is best treated with hydrocolloid dressings and should be managed in consultation with a plastic surgeon or radiation oncologist.

Late effects of radiation may develop months or years after radiation therapy. Symptomatic radiation pneumonitis typically presents with cough, fever, and shortness of breath 1 to 10 months after completion of radiation therapy. Radiographic changes, which can present as diffuse haziness and progress to patchy consolidations, are generally confined to the field of radiation. Dermal necrosis is a complication that may present years after treatment. Radiation-induced brachial plexopathy,[14] which may develop up to 30 years after breast cancer therapy, is a permanent debilitating condition that can progress to complete sensory and motor impairment of the ipsilateral upper extremity, with chronic neuropathic pain. The EP must be aware that any woman treated with radiotherapy for breast cancer in the past is at risk for developing secondary malignancies, including lung cancer, acute myeloid leukemia, esophageal cancer, new breast cancer, osteosarcoma, and angiosarcoma. Postradiation angiosarcomas typically involve the dermis, appear on the breast or in a lymphedematous upper extremity, and present with mild skin changes (thickening, edema) that mimic many benign conditions.

PATIENT TEACHING TIPS

- Any new breast symptom requires evaluation by a physician; the patient should seek prompt reevaluation if initial treatment for a diagnosed condition is not effective.
- Although most causes of breast lumps, skin changes, breast pain, and nipple discharge are benign, many conditions appear similar on physical examination and even on imaging studies.
- Making a definitive diagnosis of any breast condition may require several follow-up outpatient visits and tests.
- Patients should be familiar with the American Cancer Society's recommendations for breast cancer screening for their age group.
- Most patients fail to appreciate the significance of the false-negative rate of mammography. Mammograms fail to diagnose breast cancer in up to 15% of cases; therefore a recent "normal" screening mammogram should not falsely reassure a patient with a suspicious complaint. Tissue sampling is indicated in these situations.
- The patient should be informed that cyclical breast pain, frequently synonymous with fibrocystic breast conditions, may be improved by wearing a tight-fitting bra and avoiding caffeine, tobacco, and dietary fat.
- Patients who have had surgery and/or radiation therapy for breast cancer are at high risk for the development of lymphedema. They should be instructed to avoid compression of the ipsilateral arm and should seek immediate medical care for treatment of insect bites, burns, lacerations, and infections, all of which increase the risk for lymphedema.

Table 124-4 DRUGS COMMONLY USED TO TREAT BREAST CANCER

Cytotoxic Drugs	Hormonal Therapy	Other Drugs
Doxorubicin	Tamoxifen	Trastuzumab (monoclonal antibody to *HER-2/neu* receptors)
Cyclophosphamide	Toremifene	Pertuzumab (similar to Trastuzumab)
Epirubicin	Fulvestrant	Bevacizumab (monoclonal antibody to vascular endothelial growth factor)
Paclitaxel	Anastrozole	Pamidronate (biphosphonate)
Vinorelbine	Letrozole	
Docetaxel	Luprolide	
Gemcitabine	Megesterol	
Fluorouracil	Goserelin	
Methotrexate	Raloxifene	

Although adverse reactions to chemotherapy are beyond the scope of this chapter, drugs commonly used to treat breast cancer are listed in Table 124-4. The EP should be aware of specific drugs being used by the patient. In addition, the EP should always query patients about their use of complementary and alternative medicine. Many patients with breast cancer use these treatments but typically do not offer this information unless specifically asked.

Dermatologic Conditions of the Breast and Nipple

Dermatitis of the breast and nipple-areolar complex is common and may be caused by a number of benign and malignant conditions (Table 124-5). Often the clinical history and physical examination will yield the likely diagnosis, but close outpatient follow-up of all patients is mandatory and may include short-term reevaluation of response to treatment initiated in the ED. The EP shouldt refer all patients with concerning skin lesions to a breast clinic or surgeon. Further work-up typically involves triple testing with clinical assessment, imaging studies (mammography or ultrasound), and tissue sampling.

■ NECROTIZING FASCIITIS

Necrotizing fasciitis has been reported in the female breast and has caused fatal and near-fatal illness. Although patients with necrotizing fasciitis usually are quite ill systemically on presentation, examination of the breast may show only mild changes. Signs of inflammation with skin color changes from red to dusky blue along with severe pain disproportionate to the examination findings, particularly in a patient with significant systemic toxicity, should alert the EP to the possibility of necrotizing fasciitis.

Risk factors include advanced age, diabetes mellitus, peripheral vascular disease, AIDS, and use of immunosuppressive medications including steroids, cytotoxic agents, and anti-rejection medications. Many patients have had recent breast trauma or breast surgery, but some cases are idiopathic. These life-threatening, polymicrobial infections are managed by prompt initiation of broad-spectrum antibiotics and early, aggressive surgical debridement.

■ INFLAMMATORY BREAST CANCER

Inflammatory breast cancer is the breast malignancy most likely to present to the ED as an acute illness.

Table 124-5 SKIN CONDITIONS INVOLVING THE BREAST OR NIPPLE

Most Threatening	Most Common
Necrotizing fasciitis	Contact dermatitis (irritant, allergic)
Inflammatory breast carcinoma	Atopic dermatitis (nipple eczema)
Direct spread of invasive carcinoma	Candidiasis
Mammary Paget's disease	Lactational mastitis or abscess
Metastatic disease (from lung, ovary, kidney, stomach, pancreas, bladder)	Periductal mastitis (mammary duct ectasia)
Malignant melanoma	Psoriasis
Lymphomas/sarcomas	Hidradenitis suppurativa
Systemic infections (tuberculosis, syphilis)	Herpes zoster
Manifestation of intimate partner violence (bites, bruises)	Papillary adenoma of the nipple
Warfarin-induced skin necrosis	Post-radiation dermatitis

Data from Whitaker-Worth DL, Carlone V, Susser WS, et al: Dermatologic diseases of the breast and nipple. J Am Acad Dermatol 2000;43:733-751.

It accounts for 4% of invasive breast cancers, usually arising from invasive ductal carcinoma. It is associated with particularly high mortality, because most cases are at least stage III when diagnosed. Although most patients diagnosed with breast cancer do not present with pain, patients with imflammatory breast cancer are an exception. Patients may present with rapid, unilateral breast enlargement because tumor infiltration of dermal and intramammary lymphatics causes an inflammatory response in the stroma. On examination, the breast typically exhibits erythema, edema, warmth, tenderness, and the classic peau d'orange appearance. Nipple retraction and flattening are common. An underlying mass is detectable on physical examination in approximately one half of cases.

Many cases of inflammatory breast cancer are indistinguishable from a number of benign causes (Table 124-5). Patients diagnosed with breast infections who fail to respond to traditional therapy should be referred promptly for evaluation and work-up of possible inflammatory breast cancer. The EP should counsel all patients diagnosed with infections that failure to respond to antibiotic therapy is worrisome and warrants prompt reevaluation.

■ MAMMARY PAGET'S DISEASE

Mammary Paget's disease of the nipple, first described by James Paget in 1874, is a neoplastic condition accounting for 2% to 4% of breast malignancies. The lesion involves the nipple-areolar complex and may spread to the surrounding skin. Usually, malignant cells spread to the skin of the nipple and areola from an underlying invasive carcinoma or ductal carcinoma in situ. Rarely, the malignant cells are limited to the nipple epidermis. Patients with early disease may present with only a burning and itching sensation around the nipple area. Clinically, the disease ranges from a small vesicular eruption on the nipple to a large, disfiguring lesion involving most of the breast (Fig. 124-3). On examination, the lesion is usually demarcated, thickened, eczematoid, and erythematous. Weeping, crusted, or ulcerated lesions with irregular borders are common. There may be spontaneous nipple discharge, and the nipple may be inverted. A central palpable breast mass is present in 60% of cases.[15]

Patients diagnosed with mammary Paget's disease usually undergo mastectomy with either lymph node dissection or sentinal node biopsy, although breast-conserving surgery combined with radiotherapy or radiotherapy alone is an option in selected cases. Men can develop Paget's disease.

■ TUBERCULOSIS OF THE BREAST

The first case of mammary tuberculosis or "scrofulous swelling of the bosom" was documented by Sir Astley Cooper in 1829. Tuberculosis of the breast is rare in the United States but may represent 4% to 5% of

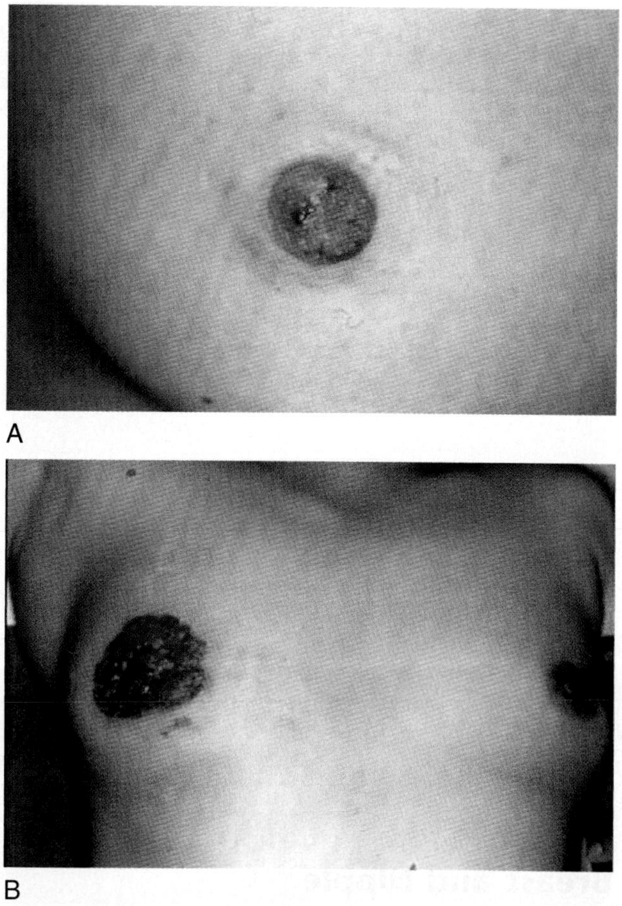

FIGURE 124-3 A and B, Paget's disease of the nipple. (Courtesy of Sehwan Han, MD.)

surgically treated lesions in areas of the world where tuberculosis is endemic.[16] There are reports of primary breast lesions resulting from infection of the breast from abraded skin or through nipple ducts, but most cases of breast tuberculosis have probably spread hematogenously, through lymphatics, or directly from contiguous structures. Cases of primary breast lesions may arise from infection residing in the tonsils of a nursing infant. Patients with mammary tuberculosis complain of a solitary painful mobile lump, either centrally or in the upper, outer quadrants. Nipple retraction and discharge are common. Typically, one third of affected patients have systemic symptoms including fever, weight loss, night sweats, and fatigue, but very few have pulmonary complaints of cough or hemoptysis.

Diagnosis is dependent on tissue sampling that typically shows granulomas with caseating necrosis; diagnostic imaging studies (mammograms, computed tomography, magnetic resonance imaging, and ultrasonography) often mistake the lesions for cancer. Because carcinoma and tuberculosis of the breast occasionally co-exist, a tissue diagnosis is needed for each mass, if multiple lesions are present.

Treatment consists of antitubercular chemotherapy and surgery. Typically, a 6-month course is prescribed: four drugs for 2 months, and then two drugs for 4 months. Medication choices include ethambutol, streptomycin, rifampicin, isoniazid, and pyrazinamide. Surgical options range from excision biopsy to mastectomy, depending on the size of the lesion. Other mycobacterial species associated with breast disease include *Mycobacterium xenopi, M. fortuitum, M. chelonei,* and *M. avium intracellulare. M. avium intracellulare* has been specifically linked to breast implant infections.

■ SKIN NECROSIS[17]

Warfarin-induced skin necrosis is a rare complication of oral anticoagulant therapy, affecting only 0.01% to 0.1% of patients who take the medication. Warfarin-induced skin necrosis has a propensity for fatty areas; it involves one or both breasts in approximately 15% of cases. The typical patient is a middle-aged, obese woman taking coumadin for 3 to 5 days, although cases have been reported occurring well into a year of therapy. High initial doses of greater than 10 mg of warfarin increase the risk for this disorder.

Lesions can be single or multiple and present with intense pain. Initially, erythematous plaques appear, followed by petechiae, ecchymoses, hemorrhagic bullae, necrosis, gangrene, and eschar formation. The diagnosis is made on clinical grounds; prothrombin times are usually in the therapeutic range on presentation. Patients who develop this condition are often subsequently found to have inherited protein C, protein S, or antithrombin III deficiencies.

Initial management includes discontinuation of the drug, and prompt surgical evaluation; more than 50% of cases involving the breast require mastectomy. The EP should administer vitamin K and fresh-frozen plasma immediately and start the patient on heparin if anticoagulation is necessary.

■ INTIMATE PARTNER VIOLENCE AND SEXUAL ASSAULT

The breast is a common site of injuries in cases of intimate partner violence and sexual assault. The EP should recognize abnormalities on the breast examination that suggest these types of injuries, both when evaluating patients presenting with complaints specific to the breast and as part of a comprehensive examination. During sexual assault in which a female victim is bitten, 20% to 30% of the bites are on the breast. Intimate partner violence frequently involves areas of the body that are not outwardly visible when clothed. Recognizing and making appropriate referrals in cases of intimate partner violence could be life-saving both for the victim and for her dependents.

■ ATOPIC, ALLERGIC, AND CONTACT DERMATITIS

Nipple eczema is the most common presentation of atopic dermatitis that involves the breast. It is so common that it is listed as a minor criterion in the diagnosis of atopic dermatitis. The patient typically presents with burning and itching, and examination of the breast may reveal erythema, erosions, weeping, crusting, fissures, or lichenification. The condition is often bilateral.

Management includes topical steroids, lubricants, and avoiding atopic triggers. In breastfeeding women, nipple dermatitis tends to develop after initiating supplemental foods, likely representing an allergy to food residue in the infant's mouth; candidal infections are common causes of erythema and pain.

The presentation of allergic contact dermatitis of the breast is similar to that of atopic dermatitis. Triggers include soaps, shampoos, detergents, or body lotions. Most ointments available for use in lactation contain ingredients that can trigger allergic contact dermatitis. Treatment is dependent on identifying and discontinuing the inciting agent.

Irritant dermatitis of the nipple—"jogger's nipple" —is common in long-distance runners; during a marathon, up to 15% of runners will experience this problem. The repetitive friction between the runner's shirt and nipple can cause painful, erythematous crusted erosions of the nipple and areola. Lesions may crack and fissure, causing bleeding. Prevention strategies include wearing synthetic shirts that wick moisture and applying petroleum jelly, adhesive patches, or tape. Treatment includes petroleum jelly or antibiotic ointment (e.g., Bacitracin).

■ CANDIDAL BREAST INFECTIONS

Candida albicans intertrigo is a common skin condition, especially in the inframammary area. The nipple-areolar complex may be involved as well, particularly in lactating women. Predisposing factors include obesity, diabetes, and excess mammary tissue. The rash is often beefy red with typical satellite lesions. Pruritus and maceration are common. Local treatment is indicated, including topical anticandidal agents and low-potency corticosteroids; the patient should be instructed to keep the affected area dry.

■ NONPUERPERAL MASTITIS AND ABSCESS

Lactational or puerperal mastitis is discussed later in this chapter. Periductal mastitis, sometimes called ductal ectasia, is the classic form of nonpuerperal mastitis. However, recent evidence suggests that ductal ectasia and periductal mastitis are really two distinct inflammatory entities. Ductal ectasia is minimally inflammatory, generally asymptomatic, and characterized by normal aging and dilation of the subareolar ducts. Occasionally, a mass may be palpated.

In contrast, periductal mastitis is a symptomatic inflammatory condition seen especially in middle-aged women smokers that has the following characteristics:

- Unilateral or bilateral fistular or erosive lesions in the periareolar area
- Erythema and peau d'orange skin
- Reactive axillary adenopathy
- Nipple discharge ranging in color from creamy to straw to green or brown

Periductal mastitis may be confused with cellulitis or inflammatory breast cancer. Bacteria have been isolated from the discharge, and although periductal mastitis has not been proved to be infectious in origin, the standard of care is oral broad-spectrum antibiotic therapy. Amoxicillin/clavulanic acid or levofloxacin plus metronidazole are appropriate antibiotic regimens. Combination therapy is often necessary for adequate aerobic and anaerobic coverage.

Virtually 90% of nonpuerperal breast abscesses are subareolar.[18] Chronic fistula formation is common. Because of the outward similarity of periductal mastitis and subareolar abscess to some types of breast cancer, all patients in whom these disorders are suspected should be scheduled for outpatient work-up, which typically includes imaging studies and tissue sampling. In addition to broad-spectrum antibiotic coverage, treatment of subareolar abscesses requires incision and drainage, and often excision of the affected lactiferous duct and surrounding chronically infected tissue. The EP should not attempt surgical treatment of this condition; a breast surgeon should be consulted.

Spontaneous nonpuerperal infections other than those associated with periductal mastitis are very rare and the EP should have a high index of suspicion for malignancy, especially inflammatory breast cancer. Particularly if the infections are resistant to treatment or are recurrent, the EP must also consider unusual diseases such as syphilis, tuberculosis, and actinomycosis.

A new form of nonpuerperal mastitis and abscess has recently emerged with the popularization of nipple-piercing. The generally unregulated nature of the body art industry has led to high local infection rates (mastitis and abscess) and to piercings in individuals with contraindications for minor procedures. Infection within the first year following nipple-piercing is common (as high as 20%) and is of special concern in patients who are immunosuppressed due to HIV infection, diabetes mellitus, or glucocorticoid use. Other high-risk patients are those who have previously undergone breast augmentation or surgery for congenital heart defects. Nipple-piercing, especially in these high-risk patients, can lead to endocarditis or even sepsis.

Common pathogens include *Staphylococcus aureus, Staphylococcus epidermidis,* and *Streptococcus* species. Unusual pathogens, such as *M. fortuitum,* have been reported and are characterized by a "cold" abscess. A cold abscess lacks the usual erythema, tenderness, and fluctuance seen in soft tissue infections. *M. fortuitum* infections is best diagnosed by tissue culture; therapy requires a prolonged antibiotic course with at least two antibiotics (to prevent development of resistance). Appropriate choices include cephalexin, doxycycline, gentamicin, and trimethoprim/sulfamethoxazole. In addition, nipple-piercing carries the risk of blood-borne viral infections, including HIV, hepatitis B, and hepatitis C; the EP should consider these infections in the evaluation of a pierced patient with vague, systemic symptoms.

Nipple Discharge

Discharge from the nipple is a common complaint. Nipple discharge is often categorized based on the following factors:

- Spontaneous or on expression—whether fluid is secreted without pressure or squeezing
- Fluid color (clear, milky, green, brown, or bloody)
- Unilateral or bilateral
- Number of ducts involved (single or multiple)

Any discharge in the presence of a mass dictates prompt outpatient evaluation. In the absence of a mass, most physiologic discharge is yellow, milky, or green; is bilateral from multiple ducts; and occurs only with compression. Other types of physiologic discharge include persistent lactation in women for up to 3 months postpartum or for as long as 2 years after discontinuation of lactation. Galactorrhea may be caused by hyperprolactinemia due to medications or medical conditions including hypothyroidism or pituitary ademoma. Once medications are eliminated as a possible cause, outpatient studies frequently include prolactin and thyrotropin levels as well as magnetic resonance imaging.

Nipple discharge that is spontaneous, unilateral, localized to a single duct, and either clear or bloody is pathologic and requires outpatient follow-up. The most common cause of bloody discharge from a single duct is a benign intraductal papilloma. Other common causes of nipple discharge are listed in Table 124-6. Mammography, ultrasonography, cytologic assessment of nipple fluid, ductography, ductal exploration, and biopsy may be used to evaluate pathologic nipple discharge.

Lactation and Its Complications

Many EPs lack sufficient knowledge about the relative safety of medications, infectious conditions, and radiation exposure in breastfeeding women, and unnecessarily recommend lactation cessation or withhold helpful medications or diagnostic studies in a misguided effort to protect the infant.

■ PUERPERAL MASTITIS

Puerperal mastitis, or mastitis that develops while breastfeeding, is a common cause of premature lactation cessation and results in voluntary discontinuation of breastfeeding in up to 25% of patients.[19] It

Table 124-6 CAUSES OF NIPPLE DISCHARGE

Malignant	Benign	Galactorrhea

Paget's disease
In-situ ductal carcinoma
Invasive breast cancer
Inflammatory breast cancer
	Duct ectasia
	Duct papilloma (usually benign)
	Nipple eczema
		Pregnancy
		Hypothyroid disorders
		Hypercortisolism
		Pituitary adenomas*
		Other neoplasms
		  Lymphoma
		  Bronchogenic carcinoma
		  Renal cell carcinoma
		Drugs
		  Tricyclics
		  MAOIs
		  SSRIs
		  Antipsychotics (phenothiazines)
		  Antihypertensives
		  Illicit drugs

*Often associated with hirsutism, acne, visual field defects, and headaches.
MAOIs, monoamine oxidase inhibitors; SSRIs, selective serotonin reuptake inhibitors.

develops in about one third of nursing mothers, with 80% of cases occuring in the first 3 months, although some cases appear around the time of infant teeth formation. Mastitis can rarely progress to abscess; this is significantly more common in the first 6 weeks after birth. Risk factors for puerperal mastitis include older mothers, primiparity, nipple damage, employment outside the home, ineffective nursing technique, and milk stasis.

Symptoms of puerperal mastitis include a painful, erythematous area or mass on the breast and systemic symptoms of fever, chills, malaise, and myalgia. The most common causative organism is *S. aureus,* though *Eschericia coli, Streptococcus species, Salmonella species, Mycobacteria, Candida,* and *Cryptococcus* have also been identified, and infections may be polymicrobial. If mastitis is suspected, the EP should immediately institute a 10-day course of oral therapy with dicloxacillin (500 mg qid) or cephalexin (500 mg qid); either may be given as 1 g bid for increased compliance. Penicillin-allergic patients can be treated with or clindamycin (300 mg qid) for 10 days.

The patient should be instructed to continue breastfeeding, even on the affected side. If this is painful, she should pump the affected breast frequently. Patients must have close follow-up and should be instructed to return to the ED if there are worsening symptoms at any time or if there is failure to improve within 48 hours. Additional management may include referral to a lactation specialist, if available, for instruction of infant positioning and attachment; this can hasten healing and reduce the chance of recurrent infection.

Indications for possible inpatient admission include failure of outpatient therapy, infections in immunocompromised patients (AIDS, diabetes, therapy with cytotoxic agents or glucocorticoids), and patients with significant signs of systemic toxicity. Rarely, patients can develop sepsis, gangrene, or necrotizing soft tissue infections.

Differentiating between mastitis and abscess is often difficult, and it is possible that the two conditions exist on a continuum. However, it is important to distinguish between the two conditions because the treatment for each is markedly different. Although an abscess usually is associated with significant fluctuance, it may appear as only a focal induration. Ultrasonography of the affected area should be performed to identify a subcutaneous fluid collection, which can be aspirated with a 16-gauge needle.

In contrast to mastitis, when an abscess is diagnosed, the EP should instruct patients who wish to continue breastfeeding to pump and discard all milk until the abscess is healed in order to prevent transmission of the infection to the infant. A surgeon should be consulted immediately about open surgical drainage. Oral or parenteral antibiotics are generally prescribed, depending on the extent of tissue involvement, degree of systemic toxicity, and host factors. Parenteral choices include nafcillin (2 g IV q6h), cefazolin (1 g IV q8h), and vancomycin (1 g IV q8h).

Fungal infection in the lactating breast appears to be more common than was previously thought. *C. albicans* may be the cause of unresolved pain in lactating women and may contribute to premature weaning. The pain is persistent, burning, and severe. Candidal infections can involve the superficial skin or lie deep in the mammary ducts and likely originate from the infant's mouth. Diagnosis is generally made on clinical grounds, although milk can be examined microscopically and cultured. Treating the mother-infant dyad is thought to be most effective. Unfortunately, increasing numbers of *Candida* species are developing resistance to common antifungal medications. Antifungal choices include the following:

- Nystatin cream or ointment applied four times daily to the nipples, nystatin oral drops for the infant, 500,000 U four times daily.

- Clotrimazole cream applied to the nipples four times a day after feedings and wiped off prior to the next feed.
- Oral fluconazole, 200 mg daily for 14 to 28 days for the mother; treatment for the infant should be determined in consultation with a pediatrician.

■ RISKS OF LACTATION IN SPECIAL CIRCUMSTANCES

Breastfeeding has been proved superior to manufactured infant formula for its nutritional, cognitive, emotional, and immunologic benefits and is compatible with a number of maternal infections and medications. Not all medications contraindicated during pregnancy are similarly dangerous to the nursing infant. The inappropriate cross-referencing of drug information in pregnancy to lactation may result in inaccurate information given to patients. Many drugs strongly contraindicated in pregnancy, such as angiotensin-converting enzyme inhibitors, are considered safe during lactation. It is important to have a basic understanding of pharmacokinetics when assessing the safety of a medication to be used during lactation. On average, 1% to 2% of a maternal dose of a drug is delivered to the infant, although this varies depending on the drug. Factors that affect drug concentrations in milk include:

- Molecular weight (high-molecular-weight compounds such as heparin and insulin are not found in milk)
- Lipid solubility (high lipid solubility of drugs such as fluoxetine leads to higher levels in the milk)
- Degree of ionization (weak bases, such as beta-blockers, tend to accumulate in milk)
- Degree of protein binding (highly protein-bound drugs such as warfarin exist in low concentrations in breast milk)
- Bioavailability of medication from infant gastrointestinal tract

Because the milk compartment is bidirectional, a drug that peaks in milk after 30 minutes may leave the milk compartment prior to the next feeding. Therefore it is recommended that when possible, a nursing mother take medications immediately after a feeding to decrease the amount delivered to the infant in the next feeding.

There are some circumstances that can change the risk:benefit ratio in favor of discontinuation of breastfeeding, either transiently or permanently; the EP should be familiar with these circumstances, which include administration of certain drugs, exposure to radioactive agents, and certain infectious conditions. Little evidence-based data are available that determine which drugs are safe to use in lactation. Review of multiple sources reveals that many drugs considered safe by some sources are relatively contraindicated or absolutely contraindicated by others. In most cases, an effective drug can be chosen from the list of drugs considered safe. EPs concerned about the safety of a particular medication in a lactating woman can consult the American Academy of Pediatrics Committee on Drugs,[20] a continuously updated document available on the World Wide Web. Interestingly, in the newest version of the document, nicotine has been moved out of the "drugs to be avoided" category. Although it is always advisable to counsel women to stop smoking, and there are numerous studies documenting the risks of second-hand smoke to infants, the most recent guidelines from the American Academy of Pediatrics state that the benefits of breastfeeding outweigh the risks. Particular concern has also been raised in the case of psychotropic medications, including anti-anxiety, antidepressant, and antipsychotic agents. There are few specific reports of adverse effects, but there is theoretical concern that these drugs, especially when given for extended periods of time, may have long-term consequences by altering neurotransmitter levels in the developing brain (Table 124-7).

Table 124-7 SELECTED LIST OF CONTRAINDICATED DRUGS AND DRUGS TO AVOID DURING LACTATION

Contraindicated Drugs	Reason for Concern	Drugs to Avoid	Reason for Concern
Fluroquinolones	Cartilage effects	Atenolol	Cyanosis, bradycardia
Metronidazole	In vitro mutagen	Pseudoephedrine	Irritability, poor feeding
Combination oral contraceptive pills	May decrease milk supply	Phenobarbital, Primidone	Sedation, withdrawal symptoms
Ergotamine	Vomiting, diarrhea, seizures	Phenytoin	Methemoglobinemia
Lithium	33% therapeutic blood level in infant	Aspirin	One case of metabolic acidosis
Cocaine	Vomiting, diarrhea, seizures, irritability	Antihistamines	May decrease milk supply
Heroin	Tremors, vomiting, restlessness, poor feeding	Sulfisoxazole	Use with caution in ill, premature infants
Phencyclidine	Hallucinogen	Tetracyclines	Staining of decidual teeth
Amphetamines	Irritability, poor sleeping		

Data from American Academy of Pediatrics Committee on Drugs: Transfer of drugs and other chemicals into human milk. Pediatrics 2001;108:776-789.

Administration of radioactive compounds to a lactating mother may require temporary cessation of breastfeeding (Table 124-8). Expressing and discarding milk for the duration of five half-lives is recommended. A nursing mother receiving Iodine-125 (half-life of 60 days) therapy essentially is required to wean the infant.

When ordering a nuclear medicine study for a lactating woman, the EP should speak directly to the nuclear medicine radiologist to determine whether a radionuclide with a shorter half-life could be used. Milk samples can be screened using radiology before resuming breastfeeding.

BREASTFEEDING AND MATERNAL INFECTIONS

Despite the overwhelming evidence that "breast is best," certain maternal infections affect the advisability of breastfeeding (Table 124-9). HIV infection profoundly alters the risk:benefit ratio in women in developed countries. In communities in which replacement feeding is acceptable, affordable, sustainable, and safe, avoidance of breastfeeding is recommended. Modeling exercises have shown, however, that in situations in which infant mortality is more than 40 per 1000 live births, breastfeeding is superior.[21]

The risk of transmission of HIV to an HIV-negative infant is 4% per 6 months of breastfeeding. The risk increases if the mother alternates formula feedings with nursing; therefore it is recommended that HIV-positive breastfeeding mothers attempt exclusive breastfeeding for 6 months and then wean the child. Low CD4 counts and high viral load in the mother are associated with higher rates of infant infection. Avoidance of mastitis and cracked nipples seems to reduce the risk of transmission. If mastitis or abscess develops in an HIV-positive woman, the milk must be expressed and discarded.

Table 124-8 RADIOACTIVE DRUGS THAT REQUIRE TEMPORARY CESSATION OF BREASTFEEDING

Drug	Time for Cessation
Gallium 67	14 days
Iodine 125	12 days
Iodine 131	2-14 days, depending on study
Radioactive sodium	4 days
Copper 64	50 hours
Technetium 99m	15-36 hours
Iodine 123	36 hours
Indium 111	20 hours

Data from American Academy of Pediatrics Committee on Drugs: Transfer of drugs and other chemicals into human milk. Pediatrics 2001;108:776-789.

COMPLICATIONS RELATED TO BREAST SURGERY (MASTECTOMY, AUGMENTATION, REDUCTION MAMMOPLASTY)

More than 2,000,000 women in the United States have undergone breast augmentation and are living with saline or silicone gel–filled implants. Another 100,000 women undergo this surgery per year. A similar number undergo reduction mammoplasty and approximately 80,000 have mastectomies annually.[22] Although 80% of augmentations are performed purely for cosmetic reasons, the 20% representing reconstruction following mastectomy account for a disproportionate percentage of local complications. Over time, nearly a one third will require additional

Table 124-9 BREASTFEEDING RECOMMENDATIONS IN SELECTED MATERNAL INFECTIONS

Infection	Clinical Significance and Impact on Breastfeeding
CMV	Rarely causes illness in full-term infants due to placentally acquired antibodies.
Hepatitis A	Found in breast milk, but unusual mode of transmission; give immunoglobulin to infant and continue breastfeeding.
Hepatitis B	Give infant routine hepatitis B vaccine and immunoglobulin and continue breastfeeding.
Hepatitis C	Not proved to be transmitted by breastfeeding; continue breastfeeding.
VZV	Close contact with a person with acute VZV infection requires VZV immunoglobulin; infant must avoid infected person until lesions crust over; expressed breast milk may be given, unless lesions are present on nipple-areolar complex.
HSV 1 and 2	Breastfeeding can be continued unless lesions are present on breast.
Lyme disease	If organism can be detected by PCR in breast milk, but infant has no signs of clinical illness, continue breastfeeding.
Syphilis	Delay breastfeeding and express breast milk until maternal therapy has been given for 24 hr; treat infant empirically.
TB	Transmission via breast milk seen only in TB mastitis; if no breast lesions, stop breastfeeding for 14 days and give isoniazid to infant; may use expressed breast milk.
Gonorrhea	If mother is treated with ceftriaxone, continue breastfeeding; if other medications are used, delay breastfeeding for 24 hr.

CMV, cytomegalovirus; HSV, herpes simplex virus; PCR, polymerase chain reaction; TB, tuberculosis; VZV, varicella-zoster virus.
Data from Lawrence RM, Lawrence RA: Breast milk and infection. Clin Perinatol 2004;31:501-528.

BOX 124-2

Short- and Long-Term Complications of Breast Surgery

- Pain; up to 30% of patients at 1 year report significant pain
- Seroma
- Hematoma and hemorrhage
- Infection of the wound and around an implant; serious infections, including toxic shock, have been reported
- Galactorrhea
- Implant rupture
- Sensory loss or paresthesia (permanent in approximately 15% of patients)
- Fibrous contracture of the implant capsule ulceration
- Necrosis of the breast, nipple, or mastectomy or reconstruction flap
- Implant extrusion or displacement of contents

surgeries within 5 years to address these complications (Box 124-2).[23] At 5 years following operation, more than 70% of implants will have ruptured.

Analysis of data from multiple studies has not shown a causative relationship between silicone implants and connective tissue disease; nevertheless, the U.S. Food and Drug Administration (FDA) temporarily placed significant restrictions on the use of silicone breast implants in 1992.

Seroma

The most common perioperative complication after any type of breast surgery is a seroma, or collection of serous fluid in a pocket created either by the removal of tissue (e.g., mastectomy) or the insertion of a foreign body (e.g., breast prosthesis). On physical examination, the accumulation presents as a soft, moveable mass with no evidence of infection and a "water-bed" consistency when depressed and released. Seromas typically appear 7 to 10 days after surgery or 1 to 2 days after the removal of a drain; in most cases they will resolve independently as the fluid is absorbed into surrounding tissues. Although a seroma typically is sterile, a persistent, untreated seroma can lead to infection or skin-flap necrosis. An especially large accumulation may also produce deleterious tension on the healing incision and hinder the initiation of adjunctive therapy.

In the case of a persistent or very painful seroma, or one that compromises surrounding tissue or incisions, fine needle aspiration is indicated. Because drainage may result in rupture of the prosthesis, aspiration is best performed by a plastic surgeon. Seromas often will reappear; if after two or three aspirations the seroma persists, insertion of a drain and simultaneous antibiotic administration to prevent infection may be necessary.

Hematoma

Hematomas that present within 48 hours of breast surgery might indicate bleeding from a single vessel and may require additional surgery or drainage. Hematomas that present later than 48 hours after surgery are best managed conservatively with a cold compress or a compressive bra. Patients should avoid aspirin and ibuprofen as these can exacerbate the bleeding. As with seromas, there is a possibility of associated infection, and prophylactic draining of large hematomas should be left to the discretion of the surgeon.

Infection

Many plastic surgeons use perioperative antibiotic prophylaxis. This precaution has decreased the rate of postoperative infections, which otherwise ranges from 2% to 4% within the first month. The highest risk of infection is in patients who choose reconstruction at the time of mastectomy. The most common pathogen is *S. aureus* (75%), followed by *S. epidermidis* (10%), both of which can be treated with first-generation cephalosporins.

Toxic shock syndrome has been reported in some patients after augmentation or explantation; patients present with sudden pyrexia (>102°F), swelling of the infected breast, vomiting, diarrhea, dizziness, and often a sunburn-like rash. Treatment entails immediate surgical removal of the prosthesis, surgical debridement of surrounding tissue, parenteral antibiotics active against polymicrobial infections, and admission to an intensive care unit.

Galactorrhea

In the first days of recovery from surgery, 1% of women will experience galactorrhea (inappropriate lactation); this figure is slightly higher among women who have previously breastfed. Galactorrhea is a benign symptom that should resolve spontaneously after a few days. Bromocriptine can be administered if symptoms are persistent and bothersome.

Capsular Contracture

In capsular contracture, tightly-woven collagen fibers form naturally around all implants and represent the body's attempt to isolate them from endogenous tissue. In 15% of women, this capsule becomes hard and resistant, contracting around the implant and causing pain, deformation, and rupture. The risk is greater among women who experience perioperative seroma, hematoma, or infection, and those who opt for silicone implants or subglandular placement. In cases in which there is notable breast hardness and

Documentation

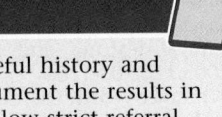

- The EP must perform a careful history and physical examination, document the results in meticulous fashion, and follow strict referral principles when evaluating a patient with a complaint related to the breast or when an abnormality is discovered incidentally.
- Impeccable documentation is required in cases of suspected intimate partner violence or sexual assault because of the possibility of a criminal investigation or a civil lawsuit.
- When treating a lactating patient, all discussions about the advisability and possible risks of continuing breastfeeding should be documented, especially when diagnosing infectious conditions, prescribing medications, and ordering radionuclide imaging.
- The history should include attention to current medications as well as past hormonal therapy, menopausal status, reproductive and breastfeeding history, family history of breast cancer or ovarian cancer (particularly if bilateral or pre-menopausal), radiation exposure, and previous breast problems.
- Documentation of the physical examination should include the appearance of the breasts, including the nipple-areolar complex, with the patient sitting, with arms raised, and supine. Results of palpating the breast with the patient supine with the ipsilateral hand under the head, should be recorded, as well as the results of gentle nipple-squeezing. Axillary, cervical, and supraclavicular areas should be palpated for nodularity.
- All abnormalities should be diagrammed and described in terms of location (position of clock face) and distance from the nipple. Size, mobility, consistency, and symmetry compared with the opposite breast are important to document. Lymph nodes should be noted in terms of number, size, consistency, and mobility.
- An inclusive list of conditions in the differential diagnosis should be documented, specifically listing cancer if it is possible that the complaint is due to malignancy. In these cases, documented discussions with the patient should include mention of the physician's concerns and need for prompt follow-up.
- Written discharge instructions should include follow-up plans and phone numbers for referral physicians. Patients anticipated to have trouble navigating the local healthcare system for follow-up because of a language barrier, lack of insurance, or transportation problems may require short-term reevaluation in the ED, and special arrangements may be necessary to ensure timely specialist care. All such efforts should be documented.

distortion, surgery may br required to remove the implant or to reduce tension by scoring the capsule tissue (open capsulotomy). The patient should be counseled that manual manipulation of the breast to sever resistant fiber-capsules is not advised, as it can lead to rupture.

Rupture

The median lifespan of a silicone gel–filled implant has been approximated as 16 years, and that of a saline implant as 10 years. Although most ruptures do not result from ascertainable trauma, they have been reported following mammography, motor vehicle collisions, gunshots, falls, and surgical procedures in the chest (central venous catheter insertion, thoracostomy). Ruptures are classified either as intracapsular (implant contents remain within the fibrous capsule) or extracapsular (implant contents escape the capsule). Clinical examination alone is unsatisfactory to identify most ruptures and should be supplemented with magnetic resonance imaging (90% accurate) or computed tomography (80% accurate).

Saline implant rupture (even extracapsular rupture) rarely requires emergency intervention, as the saline is quickly absorbed into surrounding tissues. Patients should be referred to a plastic surgeon for removal of the silicone lumen and cosmetic correction of breast deflation. Following rupture of a silicone gel–filled implant, however, extruded silicone may cause localized inflammation or silicone granulomas (siliconomas) that can migrate as far as the lower back, groin, abdomen, and upper extremities.

Breast Disease in Men

Virtually all breast conditions seen in women are seen in men as well. This includes benign conditions such as fat necrosis, allergic and irritant dermatitis, mastitis and abscess, and mammary tuberculosis. Malignant entities such as adenocarcinoma of the breast, Paget's disease of the nipple, and lymphomas are seen less frequently than in women. However, possibly due to sun exposure, men are at higher risk for developing malignant melanoma and basal cell carcinoma of the breast. One condition, gynecomastia, occurs exclusively in men.

REFERENCES

1. American Cancer Society: Estimated new cancer cases and deaths by sex for all sites. United States, 2006. American Cancer Society Surveillance Research, 2006.
2. Haj M, Loberant N, Salamon V, Cohen I: Membranous fat necrosis of the breast: Diagnosis by minimally invasive technique. Breast J 2004;10:504-508.
3. Dirschka T, Winter K, Bierhoff E: Mondor's disease: A rare cause of anterior chest pain. J Am Acad Dermatol 2003;49:905-906.
4. Hartmann LC, Sellers TA, Frost MH, et al: Benign breast disease and the risk of breast cancer. N Engl J Med 2005;353:229-237.
5. Smith RL, Pruthi S, Fitzpatrick L: Evaluation and management of breast pain. Mayo Clin Proc 2004;79:353-372.

6. Santen RJ, Mansel RL: Benign breast disorders. N Engl J Med 2005;353:275-285.
7. Dijkstra PU, Rietman JS, Geertzen JHB: Phantom breast sensations and phantom breast pain: A 2-year prospective study and a methodological analysis of the literature. Eur J Pain 2007;11:99-108. Epub 2006, Feb. 17.
8. Department of Defense Congressionally Directed Medical Research Programs: Fact sheet: Breast Cancer Research Program. Available at http://cdmrp.army.mil/pubs/factsheets/bcrpfactsheet.htm.
9. Euhus DM: Breast cancer prevention in the 21st century: Defining the challenge. Breast J 2006;12:97-98.
10. Smith RA, Saslow D, Sawyer KA, et al: American Cancer Society guidelines for breast cancer screening: Update 2003. CA Cancer J Clin 2003;53:141-169.
11. Remennick L: The challenge of early breast cancer detection among immigrant and minority women in multicultural societies. Breast J 2006;12:S103-S110.
12. Becker C, Assouad J, Riquet M, Hidden G: Postmastectomy lymphedema: Long-term results following microsurgical lymph node transplantation. Ann Surg 2006;243:313-315.
13. Harper JL, Franklin LE, Jenretter JM, Aguero EG: Skin toxicity during breast irradiation: Pathophysiology and management. South Med J 2004;97:989-993.
14. Schierle C, Winograd JM: Radiation-induced brachial plexopathy: Review. Complication without a cure. J Recon Microsurg 2004:20:149-152.
15. Lloyd J, Flanagan AM: Mammary and extramammary Paget's disease. J Clin Pathol 2000;53:742-749.
16. Tewari M, Shukla HS: Breast tuberculosis: Diagnosis, clinical features and management. Indian J Med Res 2005;122:103-110.
17. Whitaker-Worth DL, Carlone V, Susser WS, et al: Dermatologic diseases of the breast and nipple. J Am Acad Dermatol 2000;43:733-751.
18. Versluijs-Ossewaarde FN, Roumen RMH, Goris RJA: Subareolar breast abscesses: Characteristics and results of surgical treatment. Breast J 2005;11:179-182.
19. Michie C, Lockie F, Lynn W: The challenge of mastitis. Arch Dis Child 2003;88:818-821.
20. American Academy of Pediatrics Committee on Drugs: The transfer of drugs and other chemicals into human milk. Pediatrics 2001;108:776-789.
21. Coutsoudis A: Breastfeeding and HIV. Best Pract Res Clin Obstet Gynaecol 2005;19:185-196.
22. Marotta JS, Widenhouse CW, Habal MB, Goldberg EP: Silicon gel breast implant failure and frequency of additional surgeries: Analysis of 35 studies reporting examination of more than 8000 explants. J Biomed Mater Res 1999;48:354-364.
23. Gabriel SE, Woods JE, O'Fallon M, Beard CM, et al: Complications leading to surgery after breast implantation. N Engl J Med 1997;336:677-382.

Chapter 125

Pediatric Gynecologic Disorders

Jennifer Anders

KEY POINTS

Prepubertal girls have thin, sensitive vaginal mucosa that is easily irritated.
If speculum examination is necessary in a young girl, examination under anesthesia should be considered.
Parents of young girls presenting to the ED with gynecologic complaints often are worried about the possibility of sexual abuse but may not verbalize this until appropriate questions are asked.
Most pediatric gynecologic complaints are not related to abuse.
Most sexually abused children have no abnormalities on examination.

Scope

Gynecologic concerns are common, but nonetheless anxiety-producing, in prepubertal girls. Many parents presenting to the ED have spoken or unspoken concerns about sexual abuse. A calm, professional, thoughtful approach is essential to allow parents to discuss their concerns, enable a physical examination, and appropriately treat the patient. Vulvovaginitis, for example, can cause vaginal discharge or bleeding, itching or pain, urinary retention, abnormal appearance noted by caregivers, and concerns about possible sexual abuse.

The approach to pediatric gynecologic problems must take into account the developmental and psychological state of the patient. Children zealously guard autonomy over their bodies. In addition, little girls are socialized to hide their genitals and will resist examination for various reasons throughout developmental stages—it is important to help them overcome their fear, embarrassment, or anxiety. It is helpful, when attempting to make the child comfortable with the examination, to speak directly to the child in language appropriate for her age (see Tips and Tricks box). In teaching hospitals, try to coordinate care so that the examination is performed only once.

Pediatric gynecologic problems differ from those of adult women chiefly because the vaginal mucosa is thin, dry, and sensitive in the absence of estrogen. This makes prepubertal girls more sensitive to a variety of chemical, physical, and microbiologic irritants. The normal hymen looks thin, with an average opening of about 4 mm. However, there is great variability in normal hymenal shape, ranging from imperforate to multiple small fenestrations to oval, round, or stellate openings (Fig. 125-1). Abnormal findings that may correlate with vaginal penetration include lacerations of the hymen or a thickened hymen with rolled edges. These are extremely difficult to differentiate from normal variations, and photos should always be taken if sexual abuse is suspected. Neonates have swollen labia and thick moist vaginal epithelium for several weeks after birth, but most prepubertal girls have smooth pink vaginal mucosa and pale vulva that barely cover the clitoris.

Tips and Tricks

PROMOTING BODY SAFETY WHILE ACCOMPLISHING THE NECESSARY GENITAL EXAMINATION

- State to the child that you are a doctor or nurse.
- Perform the non-threatening aspects of the physical examination first (listen to heart, palpate abdomen).
- Review and respect privacy and safe-touching rules.
- Stand back and let parent or other caregiver help the child with undressing.

Sample Conversation

"Hi, my name is Dr. Smith. I need to check you [begin with non-threatening parts of physical examination (even if not necessary)—listen to heart, palpate abdomen].

"Has anybody talked to you about your private parts? Most of the time, no one is allowed to look at or touch your private parts. But your parents or doctor can look if you need help. This is a time when a doctor needs to check because you are hurting.

"Mommy is going to be right here with you. Mommy will help you take your pants off, and then I will look at the outside."

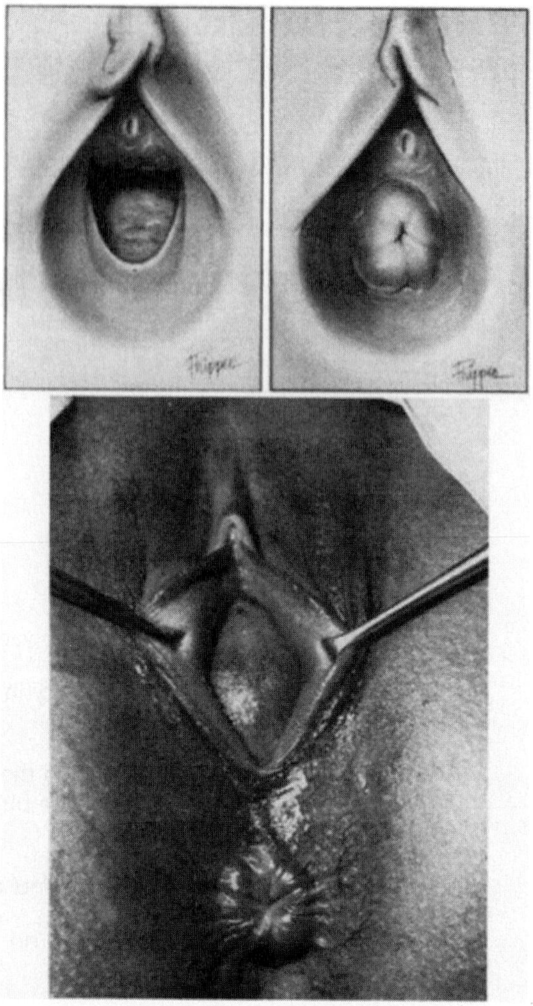

A B C

FIGURE 125-1 Types of hymens in prepubertal girls. **A,** Posterior rim of crescentic hymen. **B,** Fimbriated or redundant hymen. **C,** Imperforate hymen. (From Pokorny SF: Configuration of the prepubertal hymen. Am J Obstet Gynecol 157:950, 1987.)

Genital Examination

Infants and young toddlers can usually be examined easily if positioned supine in the "frog-leg" position (Fig. 125-2). Prepubertal girls can be examined placed in either the supine or the prone position. If the child is cooperative, she can lie in the supine position with feet together and the knees bent and placed apart in the frog-leg position. Visualization can be improved by applying labial traction in two directions—both "apart" and "apart and down" (Fig. 125-3).

Some children may be more comfortable hugging the knees to the chest (knee-chest position); labial traction will also be necessary when using this position. In a variation of the knee-chest position, the child rises on her hands and knees and then puts her head down on the examination table (see Fig. 125-2B).

If the child is uncooperative, it is a matter of clinical judgment whether the importance of the examination is worth the stress caused by it. Referral to a child sexual abuse center or examination under anesthesia should be considered.

The EP should avoid directly touching the sensitive mucosa.

Anatomic Problems

■ LABIAL ADHESIONS

In prepubertal girls, a small section or the entire labia majora may be fused in the midline (Fig. 125-4). Labial adhesion is a self-limited condition and will open with estrogenization at puberty. Although usually asymptomatic, some girls with labial adhesions may have an increased propensity for urinary tract infections. Occasionally, labial adhesions will be noted in the ED because they obscure the urethral meatus, making bladder catheterization difficult or impossible. In these cases, management options include a clean-catch midstream urine collection, a bagged urine specimen, or suprapubic aspiration.

If treatment for labial adhesion is necessary, an estrogen-containing cream may be applied to the fused area. In more than 90% of cases, adhesions will be released within a few weeks of treatment; however, fusion often recurs. A barrier cream such as Vaseline or zinc oxide should be applied to the labia after release of adhesions to prevent recurrence. Parents should be told that topical estrogen is easily absorbed and may cause vaginal hyperpigmenation or breast

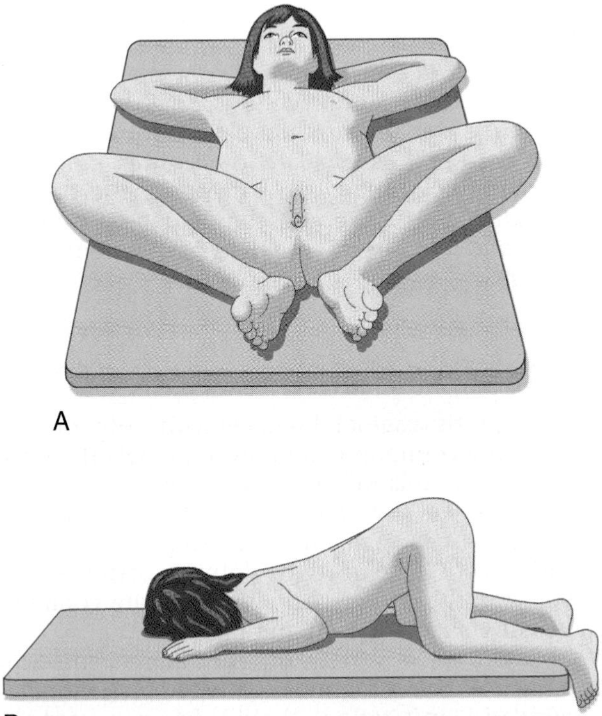

A

B

FIGURE 125-2 Pediatric gynecologic examination positions: frog-leg position **(A)** and knee-chest position **(B)**.

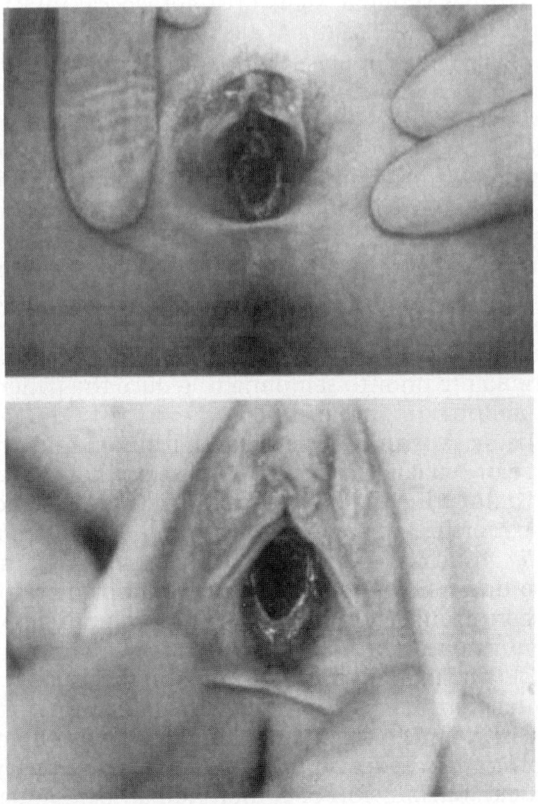

FIGURE 125-3 Examination of the vulva, hymen, and anterior vagina by gentle lateral retraction **(above)**, and gentle gripping of the labia and pulling anteriorly **(below)**. (From Emans SJ: Office evaluation of the child and adolescent. In Emans SJ, Laufer MR, Goldstein DP (eds): Pediatric and Adolescent Gynecology, 4th ed. Philadelphia, Lippincott-Raven, 1998.)

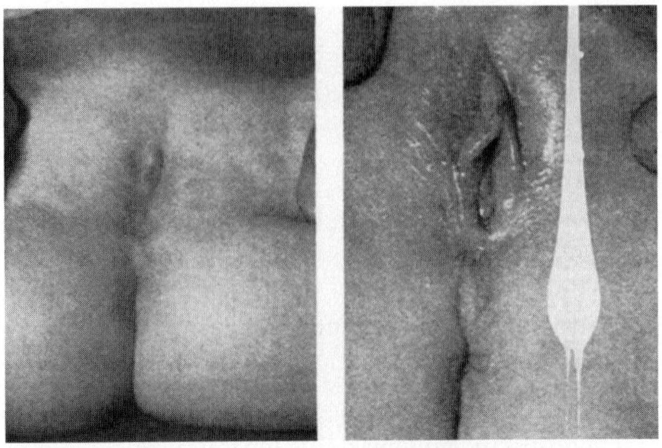

A B

FIGURE 125-4 **A,** Labial adhesions in a 2½-year-old girl. Two tiny openings exist—one beneath the clitoris and another near the middle line of fusion. **B,** Appearance in the same child after 10 days of local application of estrogen ointment. (From Dewhurst CJ: Gynaecological Disorders of Infants and Children, Philadelphia, FA Davis, 1963.)

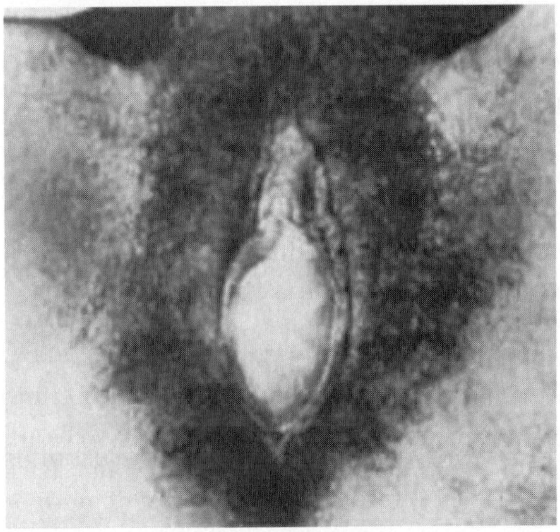

FIGURE 125-5 Imperforate hymen distended by hematocolpos. (From Baramki TA: Treatment of congenital anomalies in girls and women. J Reprod Med 29:376, 1984.)

swelling, which should resolve after discontinuation of the cream.

■ IMPERFORATE HYMEN

Imperforate hymen is a rare condition and may present at any age. Neonates and prepubertal girls may present with bulging hymen noted during diaper changing or bathing. More classically, pubertal or postpubertal girls present with abdominal pain and absence of menses despite development of breasts and pubic hair. The physical examination may be normal or may reveal a bulging hymen with dark (bloody) fluid collection behind it (Fig. 125-5). Ultrasonography will confirm the diagnosis of hydrometrocolpos (a fluid- and blood-filled uterus and vagina). A similar presentation may be seen with a transverse

BOX 125-1

Differential Diagnosis of Gynecologic Disorders in Children

Discharge

- Physiologic leukorrhea in newborns and early puberty
- Foreign body
- Sexually transmitted infection
- Sexual abuse

Pain or Itching

- Nonspecific vulvovaginitis (chemical or physical irritants)
- Group A *Streptococcus* infection
- *Shigella* infection
- Pinworm (*Enterobius vermicularis*) infestation
- Foreign body
- Genital warts
- Behçet's syndrome
- Lichen sclerosus et atrophicus
- Sexual abuse

Bleeding

- Trauma
- Urethral prolapse
- Foreign body
- Lichen sclerosus et atrophicus
- Sexual abuse
- Endocrine abnormalities
- Genital warts
- Genital tumor
- Withdrawal bleeding (newborn)

vaginal septum, but in this condition the hymen is patent. Referral should be made to a gynecologist for incision of the imperforate hymen or resection of the transverse septum.

Gynecologic Problems

The chief complaints of children with gynecologic problems include discharge or bleeding, itching or rubbing the genitals, dysuria or refusal to void, or foul genital odor noted by caregivers. The initial differential diagnosis can be guided by the predominant complaints (Box 125-1).

■ VAGINAL DISCHARGE WITHOUT ASSOCIATED SYMPTOMS

Physiologic leukorrhea is a manifestation of estrogen effect on the vaginal mucosa. Otherwise asymptomatic discharge may be seen in neonates and begins again 1 to 2 years before menarche. Many girls or their parents will complain of white or yellowish discharge found on the girls' underwear. Unlike vulvovaginitis, there is no irritation or pain. In sexually active girls, wet preparations and cultures may be necessary to rule out sexually transmitted infection. Treatment of physiologic leukorrhea consists only of reassurance. The EP should consider the possibility of a foreign body in the toddler even without other symptoms.

■ VULVOVAGINITIS

Vulvovaginitis (vaginal discharge with irritation and itching) is a common condition in prepubertal girls. Common complaints include vaginal discharge, itching, redness, dysuria, and bleeding (Fig. 125-6). The prepubertal vaginal mucosa is thin, dry, and very sensitive. Poor hygiene, tight clothing, perfumes and bubble baths, and overzealous wiping are common causes of vulvar irritation and inflammation.

In addition, a variety of infectious agents can also cause vulvovaginitis. Pinworm (*Enterobius vermicularis*) infestation should be suspected in girls with pronounced itching, particularly at night. Vulvovaginitis may be caused by group A beta-hemolytic streptococcal infection and should be suspected when the vulvar area is beefy red or if the patient has systemic signs of streptococcal infection (fever, scarletina rash). A retrospective study found that 21% of prepubertal girls with vulvovaginitis were culture-positive for group A streptococcal infection.[1] Streptoccocal infection is more likely in older girls (school-aged) and in those with recent exposure to other children with streptoccocal pharyngitis. Rarely, *Shigella* can cause a similar infectious vaginitis.

The EP should inquire about infectious contacts with pharyngitis or diarrhea and send culture swabs from the vagina for analysis when suspicion exists. The swabs should be moistened with nonbacteriostatic saline prior to sampling to reduce the patient's discomfort.

Rarely, vulvovaginitis may be caused by sexual abuse or sexually transmitted infection. If a sexually transmitted infection is suspected, culture specimens for gonorrhea (plated on chocolate agar) and *Chlamydia* (Dacron swab in viral transport medium) should be obtained, in addition to DNA-probe testing if warranted (in many areas, DNA-probe testing is not admissible in court).

Vulvar itching and bleeding can be caused by genital warts. If warts are seen on examination, this may suggest sexual abuse, but genital warts may result of nonsexual contact with common warts. Vertical transmission of genital human papillomavirus infection from the birth canal may give rise to condyloma acuminata after a period of several months. Yeast does not thrive in the dry mucosa of prepubertal girls, and vaginal candidiasis is extremely rare.

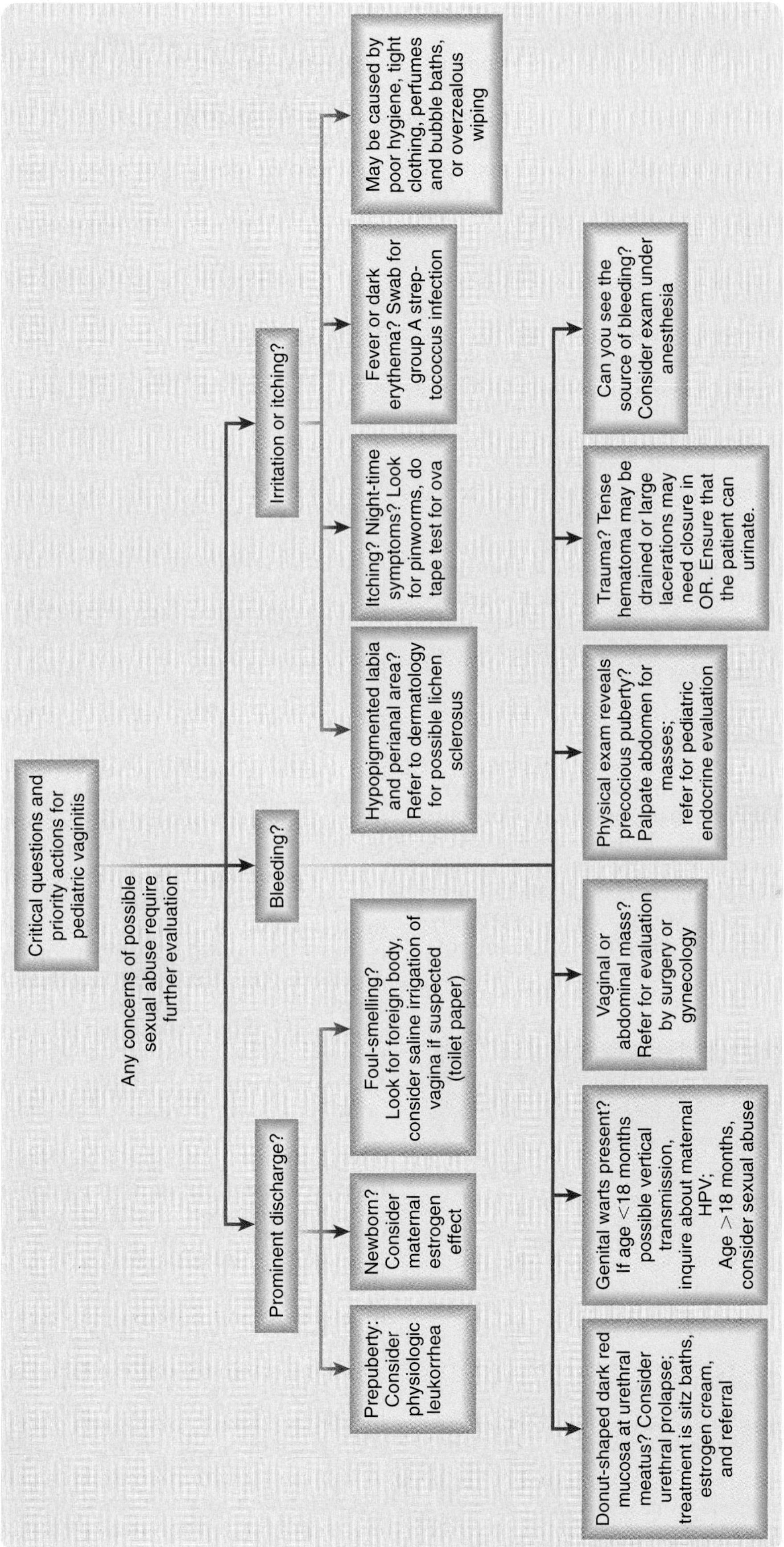
Critical questions and priority actions for pediatric vaginitis
Any concerns of possible sexual abuse require further evaluation
Prominent discharge?
Bleeding?
Irritation or itching?
Prepuberty: Consider physiologic leukorrhea
Newborn? Consider maternal estrogen effect
Foul-smelling? Look for foreign body, consider saline irrigation of vagina if suspected (toilet paper)
Hypopigmented labia and perianal area? Refer to dermatology for possible lichen sclerosus
Itching? Night-time symptoms? Look for pinworms, do tape test for ova
Fever or dark erythema? Swab for group A streptococcus infection
May be caused by poor hygiene, tight clothing, perfumes and bubble baths, or overzealous wiping
Donut-shaped dark red mucosa at urethral meatus? Consider urethral prolapse; treatment is sitz baths, estrogen cream, and referral
Genital warts present? If age <18 months possible vertical transmission, inquire about maternal HPV; Age >18 months, consider sexual abuse
Vaginal or abdominal mass? Refer for evaluation by surgery or gynecology
Physical exam reveals precocious puberty? Palpate abdomen for masses; refer for pediatric endocrine evaluation
Trauma? Tense hematoma may be drained or large lacerations may need closure in OR. Ensure that the patient can urinate.
Can you see the source of bleeding? Consider exam under anesthesia

FIGURE 125-6 Algorithm showing critical questions and priority actions for pediatric vaginitis. HPV, human papillomavirus; OR, operating room.

Lichen sclerosms et atrophicus is an autoimmune condition marked by thinned and bleeding labia. The classic finding is a figure-of-eight pattern of hypopigmentation and skin breakdown around the labia and anus. Often mistaken for trauma from sexual abuse, this is a potentially disfiguring condition. The patient should be referred to a dermatologist for evaluation and initiation of treatment, which usually consists of potent topical steroids or testosterone cream.

■ Treatment

Treatment of vulvovaginitis should be tailored to the underlying cause. For the majority of girls with nonspecific vulvovaginitis, sitz baths and education about hygiene will suffice. Girls with severe dysuria or urinary retention may be able to urinate in the tub during a sitz bath (see Patient Teaching Tips box). Streptococcal infection can be treated with oral penicillin, clindamycin, or a macrolide antibiotic for 10 days. *Shigella* infection can be treated with amoxicillin or trimethoprim/sulfamethoxazole. Pinworm infestation is easily treated with chewable mebendazole and a repeat dose in 2 weeks. Children with genital warts should be referred to dermatology or pediatric gynecology services for treatment.

■ VAGINAL FOREIGN BODIES

Patients with vaginal foreign bodies may present with complaints of itching, pain, and bloody or foul-smelling vaginal discharge. Toilet paper is overwhelmingly the most common type of vaginal foreign body. Insertion of other objects may be the result of exploratory play in very young, developmentally delayed, or sexually abused girls. Consider the possibility of sexual abuse in girls with vaginal foreign bodies other than toilet paper.[2,3]

Vaginal foreign bodies will often be visible on physical examination without the use of a speculum and can be removed under direct visualization or by irrigation.

To perform irrigation, instruct the patient to sit on a bedpan or absorbent pad. Insert a small catheter or feeding tube several centimeters into the vagina and flush warm saline through a large syringe until you are confident that no further foreign body remains. If you are unable to remove the foreign body by irrigation in the ED or if a speculum examination is required, it is advisable to schedule an examination under anesthesia and treatment by a pediatric gynecologist.

PATIENT TEACHING TIPS

PATIENT DISCHARGE INFORMATION FOR VULVOVAGINITIS

- It is normal for little girls to have sensitive skin in the vagina; this is nature's way of saying that they are not ready to be touched there.
- Sitz bath twice a day for 3 to 5 days—sit for 5 minutes in 2 inches of plain water.
- If it is too painful and difficult to urinate, urinate while in bath.
- Avoid irritants—bubble bath, lotions, perfumed toilet paper.
- Wear loose-fitting, cotton clothing and underwear.
- Practice proper hygiene—wipe gently front to back after using toilet.
- Take a complete course of antibiotic treatment for infections when indicated.

Vaginal Bleeding without Irritation

Precocious menarche is defined as cyclical bleeding before the age of 8 years. Precocious puberty should be suspected when vaginal bleeding is accompanied by breast swelling or growth of pubic hair. Most precocious puberty is idiopathic but occasionally may be a sign of hormone production by ovarian or pituitary tumors. The EP should document staging of pubertal development and palpation for abdominal masses. If an abdominal mass is palpated, ultrasonography or abdominal computed tomography should be performed. Girls with signs of precocious puberty should be referred to their primary care physician or a pediatric endocrinologist.

Urethral prolapse presents with dysuria and blood in the patient's underwear or on toilet paper. It is most commonly seen in prepubertal African-American girls. Examination reveals a donut-shaped eversion of dark red mucosa at the urethral meatus, which may cover the vaginal introitus. Conservative treatment with sitz baths should be initiated in the ED, with primary care follow-up to consider the need for estrogen cream or excision in recalcitrant cases.

Straddle injuries to the vulva and vagina result from falls onto playground equipment, bicycles, or furniture. Although straddle injuries require sensitive handling, they are no more likely than other traumatic injuries to be the result of sexual abuse. If the history does not correlate with physical examination findings, further investigation for child abuse is indicated. Frequent findings in straddle injury include abrasions or bruising of the labia, lacerations of the labia, posterior fourchette, tears of the vagina and hymen, and vulvar hematoma.[4] If there is any question about the extent of the internal injury, referral to a pediatric gynecologist or pediatric surgeon for examination under anesthesia should be considered. Other indications for referral include tense vulvar hematomas, which may require drainage to avoid tissue necrosis, and lacerations requiring surgical closure. For minor trauma not requiring further refer-

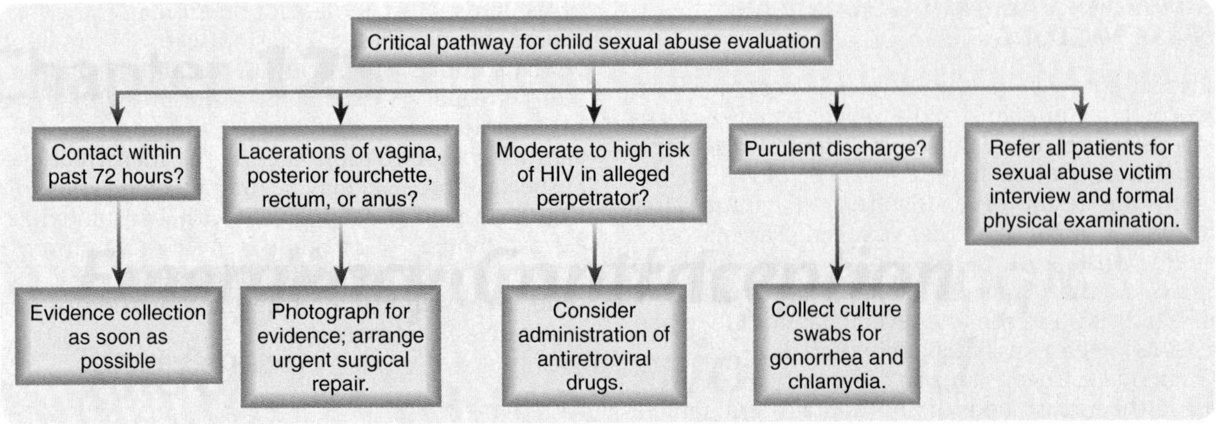
Critical pathway for child sexual abuse evaluation
Contact within past 72 hours?
Lacerations of vagina, posterior fourchette, rectum, or anus?
Moderate to high risk of HIV in alleged perpetrator?
Purulent discharge?
Refer all patients for sexual abuse victim interview and formal physical examination.
Evidence collection as soon as possible
Photograph for evidence; arrange urgent surgical repair.
Consider administration of antiretroviral drugs.
Collect culture swabs for gonorrhea and chlamydia.

FIGURE 125-7 Algorithm showing critical pathway for child sexual abuse evaluation. HIV, human immunodeficiency virus.

ral, ensure that the patient is able to urinate before she is discharged from the ED.

Sexual Abuse

The ED evaluation of possible sexual abuse should focus on identifying those patients who require urgent treatment, urgent evidence collection, or protective custody (Fig. 125-7). Open-ended questions by the EP will allow the parents to voice their concerns about possible molestation (this should be done away from the child). When interviewing the patient, history taking should be limited to open-ended questions phrased in child-appropriate language, such as "How did you get this owie?" Do not make suggestions that the child may follow in an attempt to please. Do not direct, lead, or ask questions with embedded information, because such information can appear in the child's later responses. Formal interviewing and complete examination is best minimized in the ED and carried out initially by trained personnel.

If abuse is alleged within the past 72 hours, evidence collection should be undertaken as soon as possible. In studies of forensic evidence collection in prepubertal sexual assault cases, the majority of usable evidence is found on clothing and linen. In one large study of prepubertal sexual assault victims, no swabs were positive for blood after 13 hours, or for semen/sperm after 9 hours.[5]

A brief physical examination of the vulva, vagina, and anal area should be undertaken, as described previously. The chief purpose of the initial physical examination is to discover injuries in need of urgent treatment (vaginal lacerations, anal tears) or injuries that may change over a short period of time and require documentation. Bruises or petechiae may fade quickly and the ED description of the fresh injuries may be important evidence in legal proceedings. If possible, photographs should taken for legal evidence. Areas of perineal erythema, abrasion, lacerations, bruising, and petechiae, as well as shape or tears of the hymen should be described in writing pictured in drawings.

Documentation

History—Duration of symptoms, description of any discharge, odor, itching, pain, dysuria, enuresis, or urinary retention; history of genital or urinary problems or trauma.

Physical examination—breast and pubic hair development; abdominal palpation for mass; genital examination including color (red or pale), discharge, odor, open sores, bleeding, lacerations, petechiae, or bruising, and tears of mucosa, hymen, posterior fourchette, and anal area; visualization of vaginal masses or foreign bodies; if necessary, rectal examination to palpate masses or large foreign bodies.

Studies—As indicated: urinalysis with microscopy and culture, bacterial culture, tape test for pinworm eggs, gonorrhea/*Chlamydia* cultures.

Medical decision-making—Concern or lack of concern for abuse; ability of child to tolerate gynecologic examination.

Procedures—Success of foreign body removal or suspicion of retained foreign body; document timing of sexual abuse evidence collection and transfer of evidence to police.

Photos—Photos should be taken of any abnormal findings or if there is a question of sexual abuse.

Patient instructions—Discussion of hygiene, education about warning signs of retained vaginal foreign body; record follow-up plan (phone or visit) for any cultures; if sexual abuse suspected, document referral to child protection services and sexual abuse evaluation center.

However, most children who have been molested have no physical findings related to abuse. The absence of physical findings should not be used to negate any statement or suspicions. All concerns must be thoroughly, supportively, and objectively explored by a trained interviewer.

NEWBORN VAGINAL DISCHARGE AND BREAST SWELLING

Maternal estrogen is the cause of most newborn gynecologic complaints. Physiologic leukorrhea appears as white or cream-colored vaginal discharge. Newborn girls often have a smear of blood on the diaper, the result of endometrial sloughing after withdrawal of the maternal estrogen. Parents occasionally mistake a peach-colored smear of urate crystals on the diaper for blood. Urate crystals are commonly seen in the first several days of life, when breast-fed babies are mildly dehydrated.

Maternal estrogen can also cause noticeable swelling of the breast buds in both male and female infants. Expression of milk on palpation (witch's milk) is possible, but manipulation of the swollen tissue should be discouraged, as it may cause infection. The swelling should be examined carefully for signs of infection; it should be mobile and without redness, warmth, or undue tenderness.

Neonatal mastitis is a potentially serious bacterial infection, and requires aggressive work-up and treatment like any other infection in this age group. Treatment consists of anti-staphylococcal antibiotic coverage. Neonatal mastitis can develop into an abscess, requiring incision and drainage. Consultation with a pediatric surgeon should be considered if incision near the breast bud is required, because damage to the breast bud can lead to poor cosmetic outcome of the breast in later life.

BREAST DISORDERS IN OLDER CHILDREN

Both male and female children and adolescents may experience some degree of breast bud swelling in early puberty, prior to the growth spurt and development of adult body hair. The physical examination should include palpation and description of breast swelling, description of axillary and pubic hair, and—in male patients—palpation of the testicles.

Normal breast tissue should be rubbery firm, smooth, mobile, and somewhat tender. Gynecomastia can be exceptionally distressing for boys, who should be told that this is a normal male response to hormonal surges and is not evidence of any developmental or sexual abnormality.

A breast mass in teenage girls is uncommon but causes considerable psychological distress. Although breast cancer is extraordinarily rare in adolescents, it is usually the prime concern of young girls with a breast mass. Most adolescent breast masses are cystic, caused by fibrocystic breast disease, as in adults. Fibroadenomas are the most common solid mass seen in teenagers. Most adolescent girls with a breast mass should be referred back to their primary physician for reexamination later in the menstrual cycle. Suspected abscesses may be drained by needle aspiration or treated conservatively with antistaphylococcal antibiotics. If imaging is necessary, ultrasonography is most helpful to differentiate cystic from solid masses and support needle aspiration of fibrocystic disease or abscesses.

Disposition

Nearly all children with gynecologic and breast problems can be treated as outpatients and referred to their primary care physician for follow-up. Newborns with mastitis and fever may require hospital admission for sepsis evaluation and IV antibiotic administration.

Older children may require admission for treatment under anesthesia for drainage of tense vulvar hematomas, repair of lacerations, incision of imperforate hymen, or removal of foreign bodies. Available surgical services vary, but care can be provided by pediatric general surgery, gynecology, or rarely urology. All prepubertal girls requiring internal pelvic examination should be referred to a pediatric specialty center for examination under anesthesia.

Suspicion of child sexual abuse mandates referral to child protective services and an experienced evaluation center. In cases of suspected abuse in which the home environment is not safe, children may require admission to the hospital or discharge to temporary foster care to ensure their safety pending investigation by child protective services.

REFERENCES

1. Cuadros J, Mazon A, Martinez R, et al: The aetiology of paediatric inflammatory vulvovaginitis. Eur J Pediatr 2004;163:105-107.
2. Stricker T, Navratil F, Sennhauser FH: Vaginal foreign bodies. J Paedriatr Child Health 2004;40:205-207.
3. Herman-Giddens ME: Vaginal foreign bodies and child sexual abuse. Arch Pediatr Adolesc Med 1994;148: 195-200.
4. Dowd MD, Fitzmaurice L, Knapp JF, Mooney D: The interpretation of urogenital findings in children with straddle injuries. J Pediatr Surg 1994;29:7-10.
5. Christian CW, Lavelle JM, De Jong AR, et al: Forensic evidence findings in pre-pubertal victims of sexual assault. Pediatrics 2000;106:100-104.

Chapter 126

Intimate Partner Violence

Beatrice D. Probst

KEY POINTS

Intimate partner violence (IPV) is violence committed by a spouse, ex-spouse, or current or former boyfriend or girlfriend.

IPV occurs among both heterosexual and same-sex couples and often is a repeated offense.

IPV occurs across all populations regardless of social, economic, religious, or cultural group.

Both men and women are victims of IPV, but the literature indicates that women are much more likely than men to suffer physical and probably psychological consequences from IPV.

Forty-four percent of women murdered by an intimate partner had visited an ED within 2 years of the homicide, 93% of whom had at least one visit for injury.

The consequences of IPV are physical, psychological, social, and economic.

IPV victims lose nearly 8 million days of paid work, and costs exceed $5.8 billion.

Positive change in the life of an IPV victim requires a multidisciplinary team approach and may not be felt acutely. Many attempts at intervention over several visits may be needed to effect a change.

Scope

IPV affects both genders; in the United States 5.3 million incidents occur each year among women older than 18 years of age, and 3.2 million occur among men.[1] There is some argument as to whether these statistics over- or underrepresent the magnitude of the problem, based on the lack of consensus and scope of the term "violence against women."[2,3]

In general, the term *intimate partner violence,* or domestic violence, refers to any behavior purposely inflicted by one person against another within an intimate relationship that causes physical, psychological, or sexual harm. These behaviors include acts of physical aggression and psychological or emotional abuse, including forced intercourse and other forms of sexual coercion. Because most incidents are not reported to the police, it is believed that the data greatly underestimate the magnitude of the problem.

Every year in the United States about 1.5 million women and more than 800,000 men are raped or physically assaulted by an intimate partner. This translates into about 47 and 32 IPV assaults per 1000 women and men, respectively. IPV results in nearly 2 million injuries and 1300 deaths nationwide every year.[1] According to one study, 44% of female homicide victims had presented to an ED within 2 years of the homicide, and 93% of the victims presented to the ED with injuries on at least one encounter.[3] Domestic violence is an increasingly burdensome public health issue that crosses racial, cultural, economic, and social borders.

According to ED survey studies, the incidence of domestic violence among women varies from 2.2% to 11.7%. Only a minority of women victims are either told or asked about domestic violence by ED professionals. Other studies report that the cumulative lifetime prevalence of exposure to domestic violence varies between 36.9% and 54.2%.[4,5] Certainly EPs have numerous occasions to treat victims and intervene if the problem is identified correctly.

Identification and Assessment

Statistics regarding the incidence and prevalence of violence in the ED population lends support for screening patients about domestic violence regardless of the presence of injury. The U.S. Preventive Services Task Force, however, evaluated available studies and found insufficient evidence to recommend either for or against routine screening of women for IPV.[6] No studies have assessed the effect of ED screening for domestic violence against measurable violence or health outcomes.[7,8] The American College of Emergency Physicians continues to encourage emergency personnel to screen patients for domestic violence and appropriately refer those patients in whom this may be a problem in their lives. However, screening tools have not been well validated in the ED setting and no agreement exists as to which screening tool to use in the ED.

The EP's role in caring for a potential victim of domestic violence must be that of facilitator in a nonjudgmental, respectful manner. Screening for domestic violence should be performed in a private setting, ensuring confidentiality. A summary of three potential screening devices (HITS, SAFE, and the Partner Violence Screen [PVC]) is shown in Table 126-1. These may aid in identifying victims of domestic violence. Although these tools demonstrate that only a limited number of questions are needed to identify a victim, a diagnosis of domestic violence should not be based on these questions alone, but they can increase the index of suspicion of violence and prompt further inquiry.

In a family practice setting, the four-question HITS scale showed good internal consistency and concurrent validity with the Conflict Tactics Scale (CTC), a tool widely used for identifying victims of domestic violence that consists of 78 questions and requires significantly more time to administer.[9]

The SAFE questions can identify a potential victim, alleviate her alienation, offer her an opportunity to validate her worth, assess her safety, and help her become aware of resources.[10] Two or three affirmative responses create a high index of suspicion for domestic violence. Certainly this tool can be applied easily to an ED setting.

When compared with the Index of Spouse Abuse (ISA) and the CTS,[11] the three-question partner violence screen (PVS) can detect a large number of

Table 126-1 SCREENING TOOLS USEFUL IN EVALUATING INTIMATE PARTNER VIOLENCE (IPV)

	HITS	SAFE	Partner Violence Screen (PVS)
Questions in the tool	How often does your partner: 1. physically ***H***urt you? 2. ***I***nsult you or talk down to you? 3. ***T***hreaten you with harm? 4. ***S***cream or curse at you?	***Stress/safety:*** What stress do you experience in your relationships? Do you feel safe in your relationships/marriage? Should I be concerned for your safety? ***Afraid/abused:*** Has your partner ever threatened or abused you? Have you been physically hurt or threatened by your partner? ***Friends/family:*** Are your friends aware that you have been hurt? Do your parents or siblings know about this abuse? ***Emergency plan:*** Do you have a safe place to go and the resources you need in an emergency? Would you like to talk to a social worker/counselor/me to develop an emergency plan?	1. Have you been hit, kicked, punched or otherwise hurt by someone within the past year? If so, by whom? 2. Do you feel safe in your current relationship? 3. Is there a partner from a previous relationship who is making you feel unsafe now?
Important information about the tool	Patients respond with the following 5-point frequency format: never, rarely, sometimes, fairly often, frequently; scores range from 4 to 20	Can identify a potential victim, alleviate her alienation, and offer her an opportunity to validate her worth, assess her safety, and become aware of resources; two or three affirmative responses create a high index of suspicion for domestic violence	When administered as one single question ("Have you been hit, kicked, punched, or otherwise physically hurt?"), the screen performed almost as well as the combined three-question PVS

women in the ED who have a history of partner violence. When faced with specific injuries or circumstances, the EP should have a high index of suspicion for violence (Box 126-1).[12] An astute physician also will observe the behaviors of the patient and/or partner as clues to identifying risks for domestic violence. A previously unrecognized victim may be evasive or embarrassed, may minimize concern over injuries, or may be unable to recall events accurately. The partner may appear calm, friendly, overly solicitous, and even answer questions for the patient. Alternatively, a partner may be openly hostile, defensive, or aggressive. Battering often increases during pregnancy as the abuser attempts to exert further control over the victim.

The EP also should be vigilant in identifying the victim who has no readily apparent injuries. Patients repeatedly seeking care in the ED, often with chronic complaints or complaints without abnormal physical findings, may be using the ED as a way of seeking assistance without the knowledge of the batterer.

Studies of risk factors for acute injury from domestic violence have found that victims are likely to be of a younger age, lower socioeconomic group, unmarried, abused as a child, and have a partner who abuses alcohol or drugs.[13-15] Although presence of these risk factors may heighten the index of suspicion for violence, other data have refuted the usefulness of any clinical presentation or demographic characteristic as a predictive indicator of domestic abuse.[16] EPs should be aware of the emotional, psychological, and social issues that can predispose individuals to abuse and limit the victim's willingness to volunteer historical information during an ED visit. Remaining open-minded and nonjudgmental and recognizing personal prejudices can facilitate identification and assistance of the victim.

BOX 126-1

Indications of Potential Domestic Violence

Injury Patterns
- Central—face, neck, chest, breasts, abdomen, genitalia
- Defensive—ulnar aspect of forearm, soles of feet, posterior head, back, legs, buttocks

Circumstances/Historical Information
- Injury inconsistent with history
- Delay from occurrence of injury to seeking care
- Increased battery during pregnancy
- Alcohol or drug abuse
- Suicide attempt
- Sexual assault
- Multiple ED visits for vague complaints

Victim
- Evasive
- Embarrassed
- Minimizes concern over injuries
- Unable to recall events accurately

Partner
- Calm, friendly, or overly solicitous
- Hostile, defensive, or aggressive
- Answers questions for the patient

Consequences

Patients with a history of IPV suffer from a broad range of consequences—ranging from physical and psychological to economic and social (Box 126-2). Women with a history of IPV have higher rates of all health problems than do women with no history of abuse. Victims also have chronic negative health problems such as chronic pain, gastrointestinal disorders, and irritable bowel syndrome. Abused girls and women often experience depression, anxiety, and low self-esteem. They have also been found to have a higher prevalence of sexually transmitted diseases, hysterectomy, and cardiovascular conditions. The more severe the abuse, the greater its impact on a woman's physical and mental health.

Women in violent relationships have been found to be restricted in their access to services, public life, and the ability to receive support from friends and relatives. Victims of IPV lose a total of nearly 8 million days of paid work and nearly 5.6 million days of household productivity each year as a result of vio-

BOX 126-2

Consequences of Domestic Violence

Physical
- Chronic pain—abdomen, chest, musculoskeletal, headache
- Gynecologic complaints, pelvic pain
- Sexually transmitted diseases
- Gastrointestinal—irritable bowel, peptic ulcer disease

Psychological
- Depression
- Suicidal ideations
- Substance abuse
- Anxiety
- Sleep disorders
- Posttraumatic stress disorder

Socioeconomic
- Abortions
- Lack of prenatal care

lence. The costs of IPV exceed an estimated $5.8 billion. These costs include nearly $4.1 billion for the direct costs of medical and mental health care.[17]

Management

Once a patient has been identified as a victim of domestic violence, impacting a positive change in her life requires a multidisciplinary team approach. EPs should recognize that their influence on a patient may not be felt acutely on the day-of-service but rather is cumulative and is an important part of the time and energies of multiple healthcare professionals, social workers, legal aids, and community support that the patient receives over time.

When caring for a victim of IPV, the EP should stabilize the patient medically and attend to any injuries of an emergent or urgent nature (Box 126-3). Hospital staff or ED security should be notified if the perpetrator or batterer is present in the ED.

A detailed history should be obtained in a nonjudgmental fashion. Information should be documented in the patient's actual words, and specific quotes, as well as names, dates, and places of alleged incidents, should be provided. Any history of abuse should be noted as well. Results of laboratory and other diagnostic procedures should be recorded.

Systemized documentation of an accurate history and physical exam is paramount as evidence in any civil or legal proceeding. Privacy of the medical records should be ensured to avoid risk of further abuse or inappropriate disclosure of the victim's health information.

All injuries should be accurately identified and defined. Body charts or injury maps can be used as visual aids. If the patient consents, injuries can be photographed; at least one photo of the patient's face should be included, and a ruler should be used as a reference point in the photos.

Once the patient is medically stable, the EP should discuss appropriate discharge plans with the patient, assessing both her physical and mental state, including possible homicidal or suicidal risk. The presence of a firearm at home may increase risk of serious injury to both the victim and the perpetrator. It is most important that the patient feels safe in returning home. "Safe" implies freedom of danger from physical and emotional abuse.

EPs should be aware of the resources available at their facility to provide patients with shelter, counseling, and legal assistance at all times of the day and night. Social services and advocacy organizations can assist in developing immediate and long-term plans for these patients. Patients should be given a written list of local and state agencies that support victims of domestic violence, including the national domestic violence hotline, 1-800-799-SAFE (7233) or 1-800-787-3224 (TTY).[18]

Laws governing reporting of domestic violence vary from state to state and change with legislative updates. Domestic violence is considered a crime in all states; cases may be considered misdemeanors or felony offenses, the majority being misdemeanors.[18,19] Approximately half of the states have reporting requirements for injuries resulting from crimes. Only seven states have statutes that specifically require healthcare providers to report injuries resulting from domestic violence. Reporting laws supersede the confidentiality of the patient-physician relationship. EPs should educate themselves about the reporting laws in the state in which they practice and contact their state legislature if they need more information.

BOX 126-3

Assessment and Treatment of Victims of Intimate Partner Violence (IPV)

1. Stabilize the patient medically:
   A. Attend to any injuries of an emergent or urgent nature
2. Notify ED security or local police if:
   A. Perpetrator or batterer is present in the ED
   B. You believe there is an immediate risk to patient or ED personnel
3. Screen in private setting; ask the following questions:
   A. Has anyone at home hit you or tried to injure you in any way?
   B. Do you ever feel unsafe at home?
4. Document findings:
   A. Accurately, legibly, and objectively use patient's own words
5. Photograph (with consent) evidence of abuse:
   A. Use 35-mm, digital (with security software), or instant color film
   B. Include measuring standard in photographs
6. Collect other evidence
7. Assure safety—consider the following:
   A. Does patient feel safe to return home?
   B. Are children at home safe?
   C. Is patient homicidal or suicidal?
   D. Is there a firearm in the home?
8. Contact the following referral services for immediate and long-term planning:
   A. Social worker
   B. Advocacy groups
   C. Shelters—housing, counseling, child care
   D. Legal assistance—orders of protection
   E. Domestic Violence Hotline: 1-800-799-SAFE
9. Report injuries to law enforcement agency:
   A. Find out if patient wants an official police report
   B. Know whether your state mandates reporting of domestic violence even though patient does not want the report made

Resources

- **Family Violence Prevention Fund (FVPF)** is a national nonprofit organization that focuses on domestic violence education, prevention, and public policy reform; website contains National Consensus Guidelines on Identifying and Responding to Domestic Violence Victimization in Health Care Settings. *Website:* www.endabuse.org/health.
- **National Domestic Violence Hotline** is open 24 hours and links individuals to resources for local assistance using a nationwide database that includes detailed information on shelters, legal advocacy, and assistance and social services programs. *Website:* http://www.ndvh.org.
- **National Women's Information Center** is a federal government source for women's health information aimed primarily at the lay population. *Website:* http://www.4woman.gov/violence.
- **Society of Academic Emergency Medicine (SAEM)** is a national organization advancing education in emergency medicine through case-based teaching modules on interpersonal violence. *Website:* http://www.saem.org.
- **National Center for Injury Prevention and Control** is a section of the Centers for Disease Control and Prevention (CDC) aimed at prevention of intimate partner violence. *Website:* http://www.cdc.gov/ncipc/factsheets/ipvfacts.htm.

REFERENCES

1. Tjaden P, Thoennes N: Extent, nature, and consequences of intimate partner violence: Findings from the National Violence Against Women Survey. Washington, Department of Justice (US), 2000a. Publication No. NCJ 181867. Accessed at www.ojp.usdoj.gov/nij/pubs-sum/181867.htm.
2. Wadman MC, Muelleman RL: Domestic violence homicides: ED use before victimization. Am J Emerg Med 1999;12:689-691.
3. Intimate Partner Violence Surveillance: Uniform Definitions and Recommended Data Elements. Accessed at www.cdc.gov/ncipc/pub-res/ipv_surveillance/intimate.htm.
4. Abbott J, Johnson R, Koziol-McLain J, Lowenstein SR: Domestic violence against women: Incidence and prevalence in an emergency department population. JAMA 1995;273:1763-1767.
5. Dearwater SR, Coben JH, Campbell JC, et al: Prevalence of intimate partner abuse in women treated at community hospital emergency departments. JAMA 1998;280:433-438.
6. U.S. Preventive Services Task Force: Screening for family and intimate partner violence: Recommendation statement. Ann Intern Med 2004;140:382-386.
7. Anglin D, Sachs C: Preventive care in the emergency department: Screening for domestic violence in the emergency department. Acad Emerg Med 2004;140:387-396.
8. Nelson HD, Nygren MA, Mcinerney Y, Klein J: Screening women and elderly adults for family and intimate partner violence: A review of the evidence for the U.S. Preventive Services Task Force. Ann Intern Med 2004;140:3887-3896.
9. Sherin KM, Sinacore JM, Li XQ, et al: HITS: A short domestic violence screening tool for use in a family practice setting. Fam Med 1998;30:508-512.
10. Ashur ML: Asking about domestic violence: SAFE questions [letter]. JAMA 1993;269:2367.
11. McFarlane J, Parker B, Soeken K, Bullock L: Assessing for abuse during pregnancy. JAMA 1992;267:3176-3178.
12. Easley J: Domestic violence. Ann Emerg Med 1996;27:762-763.
13. Kyriacou DN, McCabe F, Anglin D, et al: Emergency department–based study of risk factors for acute injury from domestic violence against women. Ann Emerg Med 1998;31:502-506.
14. Abbott J: Injuries and illnesses of domestic violence. Ann Emerg Med 1997;29:781-785.
15. Kyriacou DN, Anglin D, Taluaferro E, et al: Risk factors for injury to women from domestic violence. N Engl J Med 1999;341:1892-1898.
16. Zachary MJ, Mulvihill MN, Burton WB, Goldfrank LR: Domestic abuse in the emergency department: Can a risk profile be defined? Acad Emerg Med 2001;8:796-803.
17. National Center for Injury Prevention and Control: Costs of Intimate Partner Violence Against Women in the United States. Atlanta, Centers for Disease Control and Prevention, 2003.
18. National Consensus Guidelines on Identifying and Responding to Domestic Violence Victimization in Health Care Settings. www.endabuse.org/health (last accessed April 2006).
19. Houry D, Sachs CJ, Feldhaus KM, Linden J: Violence-inflicted injuries: Reporting laws in the fifty states. Ann Emerg Med 2002;39:56-60.

Chapter **127**

Sexual Assault

Matthew P. Lazio and Jamie Collings

KEY POINTS

- The history of the assault should be focused on details that affect management of the patient in the ED.
- General body trauma occurs in two thirds of sexual assault patients.
- Sexual assault nurse examiner (SANE) programs may increase the quality of evidence collection and result in more successful prosecutions.
- Treatment includes emergency contraception, prophylaxis for sexually transmitted diseases (STDs), infection risk assessment for nonoccupational post-exposure prophylaxis (nPEP) for human immunodeficiency virus (HIV) infection, and counseling.

Scope

Sexual assault requires the EP to competently evaluate and treat the physical, emotional, and legal needs of the patient. In this chapter, sexual assault is defined as the sexual contact or threat of contact of one person with another without appropriate legal consent. This definition encompasses the state and federal legal definitions of rape, sexual abuse, sexual assault, and sexual misconduct.[1]

Sexual assault is reported to affect one in three women in the course of her life. In 2005, 94,000 rapes were reported to law enforcement in the United States. This number is estimated to represent only 15% to 30% of the total number of rapes, because of underreporting[2]; 60% of offenders are well-known or casual acquaintances of their victims.[3]

Women comprise 94% of sexual assault victims. Sexual assault is the most common violent crime on college campuses; an estimated 25% of female college students are victims of sexual assault.[4] The peak incidence of sexual assault is in the 16- to 24-year-old age group. Statistics on male sexual assault have begun to be collected only recently.

Presenting Signs and Symptoms

Some patients may present to the ED immediately following the sexual assault. Others may delay their presentation because of the significant emotional trauma. The algorithm in Figure 127-1 outlines the scope of evaluation and treatment for sexual assault depending upon the timing of the presentation. If the patient presents less than 3 days after the assault, a complete work-up should be offered, including infection risk assessment for nonoccupational postexposure prophylaxis (nPEP) for HIV, evidence collection, and contraceptives. For patients presenting between 3 and 5 days after the assault, nPEP should not be offered because the side effects outweigh the potential benefits. The EP and the patient may consider evidence collection and contraceptives with the mutual understanding that efficacy will be low. If the patient presents more than 5 days after the assault, the

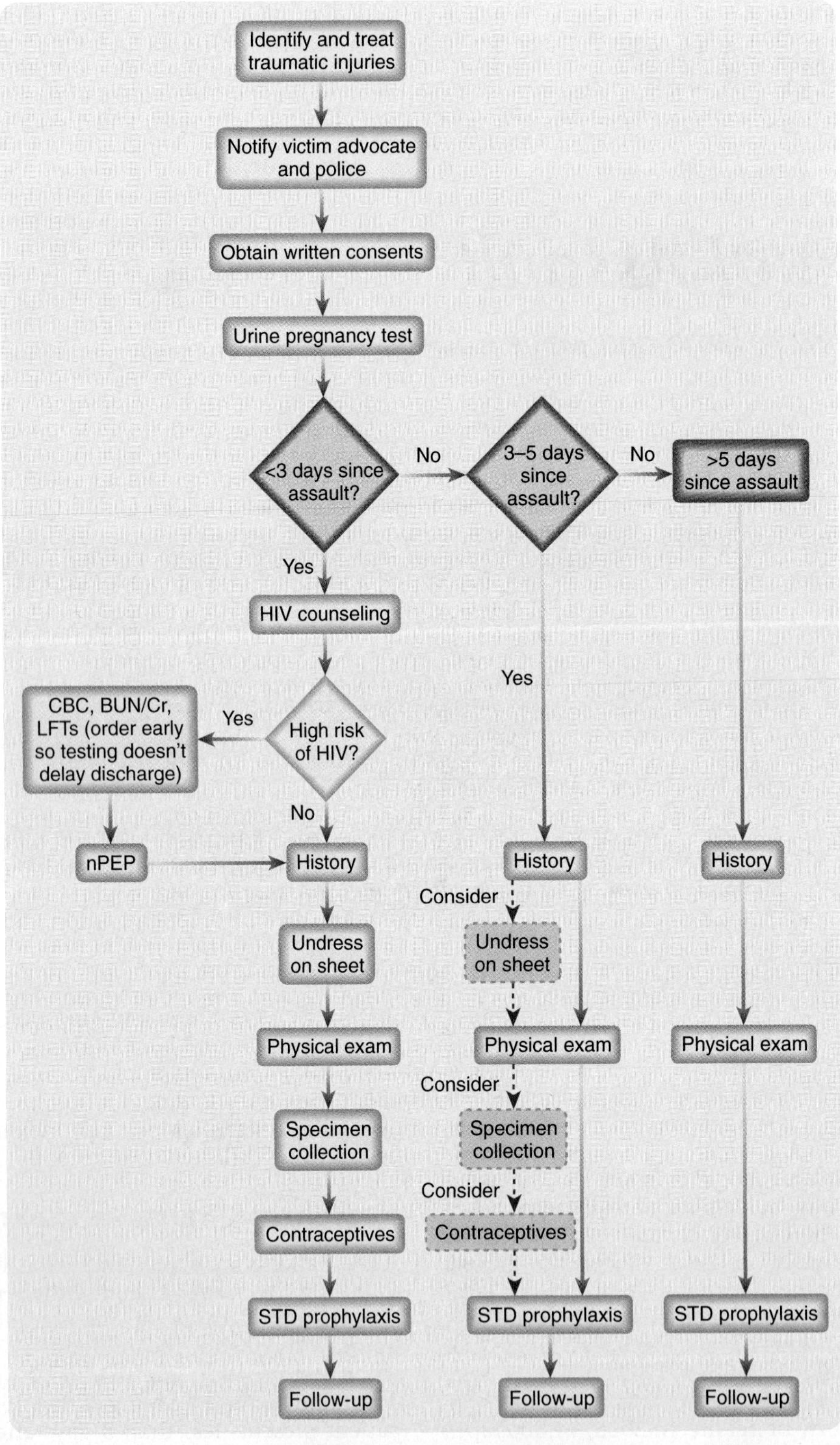
Identify and treat traumatic injuries
Notify victim advocate and police
Obtain written consents
Urine pregnancy test
<3 days since assault?
No
3–5 days since assault?
No
>5 days since assault
Yes
HIV counseling
Yes
CBC, BUN/Cr, LFTs (order early so testing doesn't delay discharge)
Yes
High risk of HIV?
No
nPEP
History
Undress on sheet
Physical exam
Specimen collection
Contraceptives
STD prophylaxis
Follow-up
History
Consider
Undress on sheet
Physical exam
Consider
Specimen collection
Consider
Contraceptives
STD prophylaxis
Follow-up
History
Physical exam
STD prophylaxis
Follow-up

FIGURE 127-1 Algorithm showing evaluation and management of sexual assault cases in the ED. BUN/Cr, blood urea nitrogen/creatinine; CBC, complete blood count; HIV, human immunodeficiency virus; LFTs, liver function tests; nPEP, nonoccupational post-exposure prophylaxis; STD, sexually transmitted disease.

work-up should include history, physical examination, prophylaxis against STDs, and follow-up.

Consent

Before proceeding with the history and physical examination, the EP should obtain the written consent of the patient. The EP or a multidisciplinary team should explain to the patient that they are mandatory reporters of the details of the evidence collection procedures; that the defense team may have access to the information obtained if the case goes to trial; and that consent may be withdrawn at any time.

History

After appropriate consent has been obtained, the EP should obtain a history of the assault as well the patient's pertinent past medical history. Salient features of the history that should be obtained are listed in Box 127-1. The history focuses on details that will help determine the risk of injuries, what types of evidence should be collected, and what treatment for STDs should be offered. Exhaustive histories of the assault acquired shortly after the event while the victim is under severe emotional stress have been shown to impede prosecution, because often there are discrepancies between the medical records and the police reports.

Additionally, a focused gynecologic history should be obtained. This includes last menstrual period, gravity, parity, last consensual sexual activity, contraceptive use, and history of sexually transmitted diseases. Finally, post-assault details should be elicited because they have implications for the forensic examination. Thus the EP should ask patients whether they have urinated, defecated, showered, inserted or removed a tampon or diaphragm, taken anything by mouth, vomited, or changed clothes since being assaulted.

BOX 127-1

Pertinent Historical Details of Sexual Assault

- Date, time, and location of the assault
- Patient description of events as they pertain to the sexual acts or trauma to the patient
- Loss of consciousness or amnesia by the patient
- Sexual acts described by the patient, including:
  - Vaginal penetration or contact by assailant's penis, finger, or a foreign object
  - Anal penetration or contact by assailant's penis, finger, or a foreign object
  - Receptive or insertive oral sex
  - Masturbation
  - Ejaculation inside or outside of body orifice
- Weapons, restraints, or foreign objects used
- Trauma sustained, especially to the mouth, breasts, vagina, or rectum
- Bleeding by either the assailant or victim
- Has the patient urinated, defecated, showered, inserted or removed a tampon or diaphragm, taken anything by mouth, vomited, or changed clothes since the assault?
- Focused gynecological history: last menstrual period, gravity, parity, last consensual sexual activity, contraceptive use, history of sexually transmitted diseases.

Physical Examination

The physical examination serves both to assess whether treatment is needed and to document findings that are consistent with the assault. Regardless of whether the patient decides to undergo a forensic evaluation, a thorough physical examination is necessary to evaluate for signs of trauma. General body trauma occurs in nearly two thirds of sexual assault victims and should be treated accordingly.[5] Some common injuries sustained by sexual assault patients are lacerations, abrasions, ecchymosis, and soft tissue swelling. Injuries of the oropharynx, breasts, vagina, anus, and rectum are especially common.

Interventions and Procedures

MULTIDISCIPLINARY APPROACH

Sexual assault response/resource teams (SARTs) are multidisciplinary teams designed to coordinate the medical, legal, and emotional aspects involved in treating sexual assault patients. These teams include sexual assault nurse examiners (SANEs), EPs, law enforcement officers, victim advocates, prosecutors, and forensic laboratory personnel. Sexual assault nurse examiners have education and training in the forensic examination of sexual assault victims. A coordinated, compassionate, timely evaluation may avoid the added trauma that victims often experience when arriving at the ED.[6]

PHYSICAL EXAMINATION ADJUNCTS

Anoscopy aids in the detection of trauma and should be used in all patients with rectal bleeding to determine the source. Colposcopy allows better detection of genital trauma, especially of the posterior fourchette. Toluidine blue can be applied to the vaginal mucosa externally at the introitus. Positive tests, signified by linear blue stains, suggest abrasions or lacerations because the dye is taken up by submucosal nuclei. A Wood's lamp may be used to visualize foreign debris or semen on the skin.

BOX 127-2

Specimens to Be Gathered for Forensic Evidence Collection

- Debris collection from sheet on which patient undressed
- Clothing (place in paper bag)
- Oral swabs
- Vaginal and cervical swabs *or* penile swabs
- Anal swabs
- Swabs of bite marks or of areas the assailant's mouth touched the patient
- Pubic hair combings
- Head hair combings
- Fingernail specimens
- Blood sample
- Photographs (3 views, 1 with ruler for scale) of any physical injuries—should be obtained by police photographer if available

BOX 127-3

Chain of Custody

- Label specimens with:
  - Hospital name, patient name, and patient medical record number
  - Date and time of collection
  - Description and location of body part from which the sample was obtained
  - Name and signature of person collecting the sample
- At every transfer of custody, record:
  - Name and signature of person receiving the sample
  - Date and time of transfer

■ STANDARDIZED EVIDENCE COLLECTION KITS

Most hospitals stock standardized evidence collection kits ("rape kits"). Commercial kits and state-specific kits are available; check with your local law enforcement officials to determine which is used in your locale. Traditionally, the use of evidence collection kits has been restricted for those patients who present within 72 hours of the assault. However, as specimen recovery technologies advance, this time limitation may be extended. Regardless of whether a forensic evidence collection is performed, the patient needs a full history and physical examination, treatment of medical issues, and prophylaxis against pregnancy and STDs.

The patient should undress while standing on the sheet provided in the kit. Specimens to be collected are listed in Box 127-2. All specimens collected should be placed in paper bags; plastic bags are more airtight and can cause samples to degrade. Clothing should be collected and placed in a brown paper bag. Since the clothing generally will not fit within the rape kit, the bag should be sealed and chain-of-custody precautions should be taken. Seminal fluid, as evidenced by spermatozoa, high levels of acid phosphatase, or p30 prostate-specific antigen, is recovered from 38% to 48% of sexual assault patients.[5]

■ CHAIN OF CUSTODY

Chain of custody, also referred to as chain of evidence, refers to the detailed documentation of the trail of the evidence from the time it is collected until it is exhibited during a legal trial. In order to comply with the chain of custody, EPs should clearly document the evidence collected and the transfer of that evidence as outlined in Box 127-3.

Furthermore, once opened, the evidence collection kit should never be left unguarded. If the EP is interrupted during the patient encounter and must leave the patient's room, the kit must remain in his/her possession.

All specimens collected should be sealed and labeled with the hospital name, patient name, and patient medical record number; date and time of collection; description and location of the body part from which the sample was obtained; and name and signature of person collecting the sample. Names, signatures, date, and time should be recorded each time that evidence is transferred from one person to another. When the EP has finished collecting evidence, the kit should be sealed. If the police are unavailable to collect the kit at that point, the kit should be locked up so as to not invalidate the evidence.

Diagnostic Testing

The choice of initial laboratory studies and imaging is guided by the trauma assessment. Box 127-4 outlines suitable diagnostic testing in sexual assault cases. All female sexual assault victims should undergo urine pregnancy testing. If nPEP for HIV is being considered, baseline complete blood count, blood urea nitrogen, creatinine, and serum liver enzyme tests should be ordered prior to the its initiation.

Drawing blood for these laboratory tests early in the patient encounter avoids making the patient wait for laboratory results after the history and physical examination are finished. Testing for syphilis, hepatitis B and C, and HIV can be performed on an outpatient basis in most cases. Instructions and follow-up arrangements should be discussed with the patient prior to discharge.

BOX 127-4

Diagnostic Testing in Sexual Assault Cases

- Basic laboratory evaluation and radiographic imaging is based on the history and physical examination.
- In addition, the following tests should be ordered for all sexual assault victims in the ED:
  - Urine test for β-hCG
  - Syphilis, HIV, hepatitis B and C serology (outpatient testing and counseling preferable to ensure follow-up)
- In patients in whom nPEP for HIV will be initiated, order:
  - Complete blood count
  - Blood urea nitrogen/creatinine assays
  - Serum liver enzymes
- Victims who decline antibiotic prophylaxis against STDs should also undergo the following:
  - Culture or polymerase chain reaction for *Neisseria gonorrhoeae* and *Chlamydia trachomatis*
  - Wet mount and culture for *Trichomonas vaginalis,* bacterial vaginosis, and candidiasis

β-hCG, beta-human chorionic gonadotropin; HIV, human immunodeficiency virus; nPEP, nonoccupational post-exposure prophylaxis.

Although the Centers for Disease Control and Prevention (CDC) recommends testing for sexually transmitted diseases, many EPs empirically offer antibiotic prophylaxis without testing; however, in the event that the victim declines prophylaxis, testing is important. Physicians should order cultures or polymerase chain reaction testing for *Neisseria gonorrhoeae* and *Chlamydia trachomatis* from specimens collected from any sites of penetration or attempted penetration. Wet mount and culture of vaginal swab specimens should be examined for *Trichomonas vaginalis,* bacterial vaginosis, and candidiasis.

Laws exist in every state that protect the victim's previous sexual history and previously acquired STDs from being admitted as evidence. Alcohol and drug screens should only be drawn if they affect medical management of the patient. Voluntary drug or alcohol use found incidentally on screening may ultimately be used by defense attorneys to weaken the victim's case. If the victim is amnestic, blood and urine samples testing for the presence of flunitrazepam (Rohypnol, the "date rape drug") and gamma-hydroxy butyrate (GHB) may be collected. Both drugs, however, have elimination half-lives of approximately 30 minutes; thus if more than a few hours have elapsed since the event, recovery is unlikely. These blood and urine samples should be treated as evidence with chain of custody maintained and tested in forensic, not hospital, laboratories.

Treatment and Disposition

Injuries related to the assault, such as fractures and soft tissue injuries, should be treated appropriately. Nearly 20% of sexual assault victims require medical procedures or interventions.[5] After treatment of physical injuries, treatment should then be focused on emergency contraception, prophylaxis for STDs, assessment of need for nPEP for HIV, and counseling. A summary of pharmacologic therapy for sexual assault victims is shown in Table 127-1.

■ EMERGENCY CONTRACEPTION

The overall risk of pregnancy following sexual assault is 5%; however, the risk of pregnancy varies throughout the menstrual cycle. The risk increases as the cycle approaches ovulation and is estimated to be 15% 3 days prior to ovulation; peaking at 30% 1 to 2 days before ovulation, declining to 12% the day of ovulation, and approaching 0% 1 to 2 days after ovulation (see Table 127-1).

Following a negative urine pregnancy test, emergency contraception should be offered to all victims of sexual assault. The preferred regimen is oral levonorgestrel (Plan B), 0.75 mg given once in the ED and repeated 12 hours later (Plan B may also be given as one combined dose). Although this regimen has the lowest incidence of nausea and vomiting, antiemetics should be prescribed concurrently. Because its efficacy decreases with time, levonorgestrel should be administered as quickly as possible in the ED. Regimens, options, and success rates are discussed in detail in Chapter 128.

■ PROPHYLAXIS FOR SEXUALLY TRANSMITTED DISEASES (STDS)

The most common STDs afflicting victims of sexual assault are trichomoniasis, bacterial vaginosis, gonorrhea, chlamydia, and hepatitis B. The risk of contracting individual STDs varies by geographic location. The estimated risks for various STDs are listed in Table 127-1. The risk of pelvic inflammatory disease from ascending infections with gonorrhea or chlamydia is estimated to be 11%. Given the difficulty in accurately assessing risk as well as the poor compliance of sexual assault victims with follow-up, many EPs empirically offer prophylaxis for victims.

Table 127-1 lists the CDC current recommended regimen for treatment of STDs in sexual assault victims.[7] A negative urine pregnancy test should be obtained before administering prophylaxis because pregnancy alters the preferred antibiotic regimen. For all nonpregnant victims of sexual assault, the recommended prophylactic antibiotic regimen is ceftriaxone, 125 mg intramuscularly (IM), in a single dose (for gonorrhea); azithromycin, 1 g orally in a single

Table 127-1 PROPHYLACTIC TREATMENT FOR THE SEXUAL ASSAULT VICTIM

	Risk	Indications	Treatment
Pregnancy		Offer to all victims	Levonorgestrel (Plan B), 0.75 mg PO q12h ×2
3 d before ovulation	15%		
1-2 d before ovulation	30%		
Day of ovulation	12%		
1-2 d after ovulation	~0%		
Gonorrhea	6-18%	Offer to all victims	Ceftriaxone, 125 mg IM ×1
Chlamydia infection	4-17%	Offer to all victims	Azithromycin, 1 g PO ×1
Trichomonas infection	7%	Offer to all victims	Metronidazole, 2 g PO ×1
Bacterial vaginosis	11%	Offer to all victims	Metronidazole, 2 g PO ×1
Syphilis	0.5-3%	Provide follow-up for outpatient testing	
Hepatitis B	<1%	Unimmunized or unsure of immunization status	Hepatitis B vaccine, 1.0 mL IM ×1; follow-up dose at 1 month; follow-up dose at 6 months
HIV Receptive anal intercourse Receptive vaginal intercourse	 0.5-3% 0.1-0.2%	Within 72 hr and any *one* of the following: Known HIV+ assailant Vaginal or anal penetration Ejaculation on mucous membranes Multiple assailants Mucosal lesions present	NNRTI-based (×28 d): Efavirenz *plus* lamivudine or emtricitabin *plus* zidovudine or tenofovir *or* PI-based (×28 d): Lopinavir/ritonavir (Kaletra) *plus* lamivudine or emtricitabine *plus* zidovudine

IM, intramuscularly; NNRTI, nonnucleoside reverse transcriptase inhibitor; PI, protease inhibitor; PO, orally.
From Centers for Disease Control and Prevention: Sexually transmitted diseases treatment guidelines 2006. MMWR Morb Mort Wkly Rep 2006; 55(RR-11).

Tips and Tricks

- Discuss HIV prophylaxis early and order the complete blood count, blood urea nitrogen/creatinine, and liver function tests so the patient will not have to remain in the ED waiting for baseline laboratory results after completion of the rape kit.
- Sexual assault nurse examiner (SANE) programs coordinate the treatment and improve evidence collection and prosecutions.
- Evidence collection kits vary according to location, and EPs should be familiar with the kit used in their jurisdiction.
- Plan B should be given in the ED as soon as possible; it can be given in one dose, rather than two, with equal efficacy and fewer complications.
- Care should be taken to maintain the chain of custody for all evidence collected in the evaluation of a sexual assault patient.

dose (for chlamydia); and metronidazole, 2 g orally in a single dose (for trichomoniasis and bacterial vaginosis). Additional regimens are discussed in detail in Chapter 123.

Postexposure hepatitis B vaccine, 1.0 mL IM, should be offered to all victims who have not been previously immunized or are unsure of their immunization status. Hepatitis B immune globulin is not recommended unless a patient has been previously immunized and antibody titers are inadequate. Follow-up doses of hepatitis B vaccine should be administered in 1 to 2 months and 4 to 6 months.

■ NONOCCUPATIONAL POST-EXPOSURE PROPHYLAXIS FOR HIV

The risk of contracting HIV infection following sexual assault is difficult to estimate but is thought to be low. Factors that influence the risk of HIV infection in sexual assault victims include the likelihood that the assailant is HIV-positive, the clinical status of the assailant if HIV-positive, body fluids and routes of exposure involved in the assault, number of discrete contacts, type and severity of physical trauma caused by the assault, and concurrent STDs in both the perpetrator and the victim.[8] Table 127-1 shows the risk of contracting HIV, assuming an HIV-positive source and consensual intercourse with various sexual practices.[9] The risk of contracting HIV after sexual assault is likely greater than that listed in Table 127-1 because of the frequency of concurrent genital trauma and the increased prevalence of STD in assailants compared with the general population.

nPEP should only be considered if the exposure occurred less than 72 hours previously. It has maximal efficacy when administered 2 hours post-exposure. The absolute indications for starting nPEP after a sexual assault are that the victim presents less than 72 hours post-exposure and the assailant is known to be HIV-positive. nPEP should be considered on a case-by-case basis when the victim presents less than 72 hours post-exposure and the probability of HIV

BOX 127-5

Initiation of Nonoccupational Post-Exposure Prophylaxis (nPEP) for HIV Infection

- Order the following baseline laboratory tests: complete blood count, blood urea nitrogen/creatinine, liver panel.
- Consult an infectious disease specialist to determine whether to perform NNRTI-based or PI-based prophylaxis.
- Prescribe NNRTI-based or PI-based prophylaxis to be given for 3 to 5 days.
  - NNRTI-based regimen:
    Efavirenz, 600 mg PO qhs
    plus
    Lamivudine, 150 mg PO bid, *or* emtricitabine, 200 mg PO qd
    plus
    Zidovudine, 300 mg PO bid, *or* tenofovir, 300 mg PO qd
  - PI-based regimen:
    Lopinavir/ritonavir, 400 mg/100 mg PO bid
    plus
    Lamivudine, 150 mg PO bid, *or* emtricitabine, 200 mg PO qd
    plus
    Zidovudine, 300 mg PO bid
- Arrange follow-up for confidential HIV antibody, syphilis, and hepatitis B and C serology testing.
- Arrange follow-up with infectious disease specialist in 3 to 5 days.

HIV, human immunodeficiency virus; NNRTI, nonnucleoside reverse transcriptase inhibitor; PI, protease inhibitor.

transmission is moderate or high (vaginal or anal penetration, ejaculation on mucous membranes, multiple assailants, presence of mucosal lesions). nPEP is contraindicated more than 72 hours post-exposure because the risks of treatment are greater than the benefits.[10]

If indicated, nPEP should be initiated in consultation with an infectious disease specialist. Baseline laboratory procedures, outlined in Box 127-5, should be ordered to monitor for toxicity. Box 127-5 also lists the CDC current recommendations for nPEP, which involves either nonnucleoside reverse transcriptase inhibitor based or protease inhibitor–based three-drug regimens for 28 days. The initial prescription should be for 3 to 5 days of nPEP, with follow-up thereafter.

■ DISPOSITION

Discharged patients require specific written instructions because victims of traumatic events frequently cannot remember the events immediately following a crisis. Many hospitals have multidisciplinary sexual assault response teams that coordinate medical, psychological, and legal aspects of follow-up. All patients should be given contact information for rape crisis counseling centers and 24-hour crisis phone numbers for psychological evaluation.

A follow-up appointment with a gynecologist in 1 to 2 weeks is important to ensure that emergency contraception and STD prophylaxis have been successful. Male victims and children should be scheduled for follow-up with a urologist and pediatrician, respectively. Victims started on HIV nPEP should be scheduled for follow-up with an infectious disease specialist in 3 to 5 days.

Patients should be discharged with a 3- to 5-day supply of all medications to save a trip to the pharmacy, thereby increasing compliance. Ideally, patients should be discharged with a friend or family member so that they do not go home alone.

PATIENT TEACHING TIPS

- Follow up in 3 to 5 days if patient is started on nPEP for HIV. Give the patient written information about the nPEP for HIV medications prescribed.
- Schedule consultation with gynecologist in 1 to 2 weeks for evaluation of treatment of STDs and emergency contraception, as well testing for syphilis, HIV, and hepatitis B and C.
- Provide rape hotline and rape advocate contact information.
- Provide psychiatric counseling contact information.
- Schedule follow-up for any traumatic injuries associated with the assault.

REFERENCES

1. Evaluation and Management of the Sexually Assaulted or Sexually Abused Patient. Dallas, TX, American College of Emergency Physicians, 1999.
2. United States Department of Justice, Federal Bureau of Investigation: Uniform Crime Reports. Crime in the United States, 2005: Forcible Rape. http://www.fbi.gov/ucr/05cius/offenses/violent_crime/forcible_rape.html
3. United States Department of Justice, Bureau of Justice Statistics: Criminal Victimization in the United States—Statistical Tables Index, Rape/Sexual Assault. http://www.ojp.usdoj.gov/bjs/abstract/cvus/rape_sexual_assault.htm
4. Sampson R: Acquaintance Rape of College Students. Washington, DC, United States Department of Justice, Office of Community Oriented Policing Services, 2002.
5. Riggs N, Houry D, Long G, et al: Analysis of 1,076 cases of sexual assault. Ann Emerg Med 2000;35:358-362.
6. Littel K: Sexual Assault Nurse Examiner Programs: Improving the Community Response to Sexual Assault Victims. Office for Victims of Crime Bulletin. Washington, DC, United States Department of Justice, 2001.

7. Centers for Disease Control and Prevention: Sexually transmitted diseases treatment guidelines 2006. MMWR Morb Mort Wkly Rep 2006;55(RR-11).
8. Bamberger JD, Waldo CR, Gerberding JL, Katz MH: Postexposure prophylaxis for human immunodeficiency virus (HIV) infection following sexual assault. Am J Med 1999;106:323-326.
9. Varghese B, Maher JE, Peterman TA, et al: Reducing the risk of HIV infection. Sex Transm Dis 2002;29:38-43.
10. Centers for Disease Control and Prevention: Antiretroviral postexposure prophylaxis after sexual, injection-drug use, or other nonoccupational exposure to HIV in the United States. MMWR Morb Mort Wkly Rep 2005; 54(RR-02):1-20.

Chapter **128**

Emergency Contraception

Tomer Begaz

KEY POINTS

Emergency contraception (EC) is more effective the sooner it is administered, and the effectiveness decreases with time. It can be administered up to 120 hours after intercourse with reasonable effectiveness.
Progestin-only EC (levonorgestrel, "Plan B") is more effective than combined estrogen/progestin and has fewer side effects.
Both levonorgestrel doses (1.5 mg total) can be administered as a single, one-time dose.
EC is not effective in pregnancy.
Hormonal EC can cause nausea. Antiemetics can help if administered 30 to 60 minutes before taking contraceptive pills.
Patients can still get pregnant for the remainder of the cycle after EC use. Alternative methods of contraception must still be used and patients should immediately resume taking their regular oral contraceptive pills.
A pelvic examination is not a prerequisite to providing EC.
More than half of pharmacies do not have Plan B available in a timely fashion; therefore it is prudent to give the pills directly to the patient, or call the pharmacy in advance.

Scope and Outline

Emergency contraception (EC) refers to methods of preventing pregnancy that are employed after sexual intercourse. Circumstances making ED necessary include rape, contraceptive failure (such as condom breakage), and failure to use a contraceptive.

Approximately 50% of women between the ages of 15 and 44 years have had at least one unwanted pregnancy, amounting to over 3 million unwanted pregnancies annually in the United States.[1] No contraceptive method is 100% effective, and the failure rates of contraceptives are surprisingly high (Table 128-1). Because contraceptive failure is so common, most EPs will deal with this issue on a regular basis, and they should be aware of the indications and complications of this treatment.

Methods of Emergency Contraception

Three regimens for EC are commonly used in the United States: combined estrogen/progesterone ("Yuzpe method"), progestin only (levonorgestrel), and the copper intrauterine device (IUD). A combined regimen of estrogen and progesterone pills for EC was first reported and popularized in the 1970s by Yuzpe et colleagues[3] and is often referred to as the Yuzpe method. The standard dosing in this regimen

Table 128-1 FAILURE RATES OF SELECTED CONTRACEPTIVE METHODS WITHIN 1 YEAR (%)[2]

Method	Perfect Use	Typical Use
Chance	85	85
Combination pill	0.1	5.0
Progestin-only pill	0.5	5.0
Male condom	3.0	14.0
Diaphragm	6.0	20
Spermicide	6.0	26
Periodic abstinence—calendar method	9.0	n/a
Hormonal emergency contraception	0.1	3.0
Copper IUD	0.1	n/a

IUD, intrauterine device; n/a, not available.

Table 128-2 COMMON HORMONAL METHODS OF EMERGENCY CONTRACEPTION

Method	Contains	Dosing
Combination oral (Yuzpe method)	0.1 mg ethinyl estradiol and 0.5 mg levonorgestrel	Two doses 12 hours apart
Progestin-only oral (Plan B)	0.75 mg levonorgestrel	Two doses 12 hours apart
Progestin-only oral, single-dose regimen*	1.5 mg levonorgestrel	One dose

*Recommended.

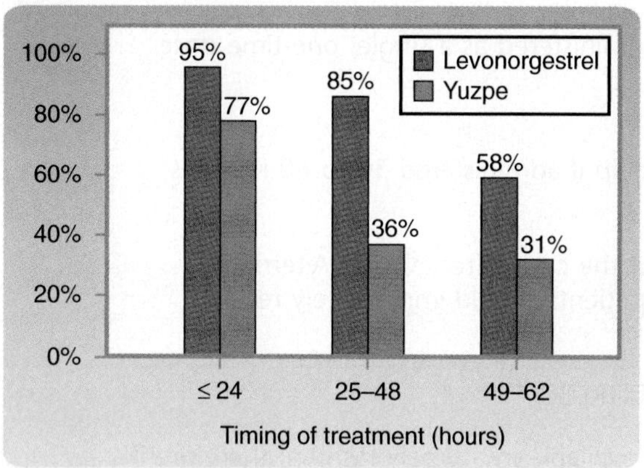
100%
80%
60%
40%
20%
0%
95%
77%
85%
36%
58%
31%
Levonorgestrel
Yuzpe
≤ 24
25–48
49–62
Timing of treatment (hours)

FIGURE 128-1 Proportion of pregnancies prevented by levonorgestrel versus Yupze by timing of treatment. (Adapted from Task Force on Postovulatory Methods of Fertility Regulation: Randomised controlled trial of levonorgestrel versus the Yuzpe regimen of combined oral contraceptives for emergency contraception. Lancet 1998;352:428-433. With permission.)

RED FLAGS

- Patients presenting immediately after coitus should have no symptoms.
- Patients requesting emergency contraception (EC) who are having medical symptoms (abdominal pain) should be evaluated for the cause of their symptoms.
- If there are signs or symptoms consistent with pregnancy, a pregnancy test should be done because EC is not effective in pregnant patients.
- Patients requesting EC may be at risk for sexually transmitted diseases and should be counseled and either tested or referred for outpatient follow-up/testing.

is two doses of 100 µg of ethinyl estradiol and 1 mg of norgestrel taken 12 hours apart. When taken within 72 hours of unprotected intercourse, this regimen will prevent approximately 75% of pregnancies.[4]

An alternative progestin-only method of EC has become popular and is marketed in the U.S. under the brand name "Plan B." Plan B consists of two doses of 0.75 mg of levonorgestrel given 12 hours apart. The recommended approach is to give the two doses simultaneously, which increases the compliance, decreases the side effects, and is equally effective. The EP should instruct the patient on this method because the packaging lists only the two-dose method (Table 128-2).

Of the hormonal EC methods, levonorgestrel is more effective and is recommended over the Yuzpe method. The difference in effectiveness varies with the timing of treatment (Fig. 128-1). Levonorgestrel is less likely to cause nausea and vomiting than combined estrogen/progestin formulations. Other hormonal methods have been employed for EC but are less popular either because of questionable efficacy (danazol) or because of a higher incidence of side effects (high-dose estrogens).

The IUD is the most effective postcoital contraceptive, preventing over 99% of pregnancies if inserted within 5 days of intercourse.[6] This can be an ideal form of EC in patients who prefer to continue using

Table 128-3 MYTHS AND FACTS ABOUT EMERGENCY CONTRACEPTION (EC)

Myth	Fact
EC causes a "medical abortion."	EC has no effect on an established pregnancy, and EC agents are not teratogenic. The primary mechanism of action of EC is the inhibition of ovulation. Estrogen/progestin combination EC may inhibit implantation of a fertilized egg.
If EC is too easily available, women will "abuse" it, using EC instead of regular forms of birth control.	Women who receive advance prescriptions for EC agents are not less likely to use regular forms of birth control.
EC agents contain high doses of hormones and are dangerous to use.	The small dose of hormones in EC agents is extremely safe and can be used by virtually any woman.
EC is readily available in the United States.	Although FDA approval for over-the-counter EC medications is an improvement, availability in EDs as well as pharmacies is variable. The EP must be a *patient advocate* and must ensure that the patient is able to obtain the medication that has been prescribed.
Prescriptions for EC should only be given when a woman presents after sexual intercourse when no contraceptive has been used or there was a failure of the contraceptive.	The ACOG recommends that all sexually active women of childbearing age are given a prescription for Plan B at their yearly medical examination.

ACOG, American College of Obstetrics and Gynecology; FDA, U.S. Food and Drug Administration.

the IUD as their contraceptive device for an extended period of time. IUDs should be avoided in patients with a history of sexually transmitted disease and in those with multiple sexual partners, because their use increases the likelihood of pelvic inflammatory disease. This makes the IUD unsuitable for patients presenting after rape and for adolescent patients. Other contraindications for copper IUD insertion are cervical or endometrial cancer, unexplained vaginal bleeding, and copper allergy. Patients should be informed of the marked superiority in effectiveness compared with other EC methods and referred for IUD insertion if they choose this method.

■ MIFEPRISTONE

Mifepristone (RU-486) is a progesterone antagonist that is effective in EC. It functions by inhibiting ovulation as well as endometrial maturation. In the United States, a 600-mg dose of mifepristone is approved as an abortifactant for pregnancies up to 49 days. Both the 600-mg dose and a lower, 10-mg dose are as effective as levonorgestrel for EC, with a very good side effect profile.[7] Currently, mifepristone administration is limited to registered providers who contract with the patient to schedule three office visits. This makes prescribing mifepristone in the ED impractical.

Mechanism of Action of EC Agents

The primary mechanism of action of estrogen/progestin EC is inhibition of ovulation. Additional possible contributing mechanisms include thickening of cervical mucus, altered sperm transport, and alteration of the endometrial lining.[8] Progestin-only methods (levonorgestrel) do not appear to have an effect on the endometrium. Once an embryo is implanted in the endometrium, hormonal EC has no effect on a pregnancy and does not cause abortion.[9]

It is important for the EP to understand the mechanism of action of EC in order to accurately address the concerns of individual patients. According to the American College of Obstetrics and Gynecology definition, pregnancy is established at the time of implantation of the embryo in the uterus.[10] By this definition, hormonal EC drugs are NOT abortifactants, as these medications do not interfere with already established (implanted) pregnancies. However, individual patients may have a different understanding of terms such as conception and abortion than the medical community. The known facts should be presented to patients simply and clearly so that they will be informed participants in their health care (Table 128-3 and Boxes 128-1 and 128-2).

Timing of EC Administration

Hormonal EC is effective when administered up to 120 hours after intercourse. There is an inverse linear relationship between time of administration of EC after unprotected intercourse and effectiveness; the sooner EC is started, the more effective it is.[13] For this reason, it is of the utmost importance to begin as soon as possible. Many EDs stock levonorgestrel; if it is available through the hospital pharmacy, it can be given directly to patient by the EP. If this is not possible, in addition to a prescription and instructions, the patient should be provided with a list of local 24-hour pharmacies that provide EC. It is advisable to call the pharmacies to confirm availability and expedite the preparation because as many as half of the pharmacies will not stock Plan B.[14]

Access to EC

On August 24, 2006, after contentious debate, the U.S. Food and Drug Administration approved over-the-counter sales of levonorgestrel, packaged as Plan B, for women 18 years of age or older. Men with proof of age could also buy Plan B for a partner. This ruling will likely go a long way in improving timely access to EC in a politically charged atmosphere. Over-the-counter availability is unlikely to change the reluctance of many pharmacies to stock Plan B and provide it in a timely fashion. Increased knowledge about the availability of EC method is likely to increase the number of adolescents under age 18 who access the ED for Plan B (Table 128-4).

Side Effects

Adverse effects of estrogen/progestin contraceptive drugs are primarily related to the estrogen component. The most common side effect is nausea, which affects half of women taking this regimen. Approximately 20% of women vomit as a result. Nausea and vomiting are significantly less common with progestin-only regimens (18% nausea and 4% vomiting).[15] The incidence and severity of nausea and vomiting can be decreased with the administration of an antiemetic 30 to 60 minutes before taking the EC agent. Meclizine (50 mg) has been used with success,[16] but any antiemetic can be used. If a patient vomits more than 1 hour after taking an EC drug, the dosage does not need to be repeated.[17]

A common side effect of both regimens is vaginal spotting; between 10 and 20% of patients report this

BOX 128-1

Sample Indications for Using Emergency Contraception (EC)[11,12]

- Failure to use a contraceptive method
- Dislodged, broken, or improperly used condom, diaphragm, or cervical cap
- Unprotected intercourse within 7 days of starting oral contraceptives
- Two or more missed estrogen/progestin birth control pills
- One or more missed progestin-only birth control pills
- Removal of a contraceptive skin patch or ring
- Unprotected intercourse within 14 days of first depot medroxyprogesterone (Depo-Provera) injection
- Ejaculation on the external genitalia without reliable contraception
- Sexual assault when the woman is not using reliable contraception
- Miscalculation of the periodic abstinence method

BOX 128-2

Contraindications to and Complications of Emergency Contraception (EC)

- There are no absolute contraindications to hormonal EC.
- EC agents are not abortifactants, and EC is not effective in pregnancy. A urine pregnancy test should be made before administering EC if the patient might be pregnant.
- Relative contraindications to estrogen-containing EC include smokers over age 35 and patients with a history of thrombophilia, stroke, heart attack, malignancy, deep vein thrombosis, and migraine with neurologic symptoms. In these cases, a progestin-only form of EC is recommended.
- An intrauterine device (IUD) should not be used by patients with multiple sexual partners or a risk of sexually transmitted diseases.

Table 128-4 COMMON AGENTS AND DOSAGES FOR EMERGENCY CONTRACEPTION (EC)[15]

Agent	Contains	EC Dosage
Plan B	0.75 mg levonorgestrel	1 pill q12h × 2 doses OR 2 pills once
Ovrette	0.75 mg levonorgestrel	20 pills q2h × 2 doses OR 40 pills once
Ovral, Ogestrel	100 μg Ethinyl estradiol, 0.5 mg levonorgestrel	2 pills q12h × 2 doses
Cryselle	120 μg Ethinyl estradiol, 0.6 mg levonorgestrel	4 pills q12h × 2 doses
Levora, Lo/Ovral, Low-Ogestrel, Levlen, Nordette, Portia, Seasonale	120 μg Ethinyl estradiol, 0.6 mg levonorgestrel	4 pills q12h × 2 doses
Trivora, Tri-Levlen, Triphasil, Enpresse	120 μg Ethinyl estradiol, 0.5 mg levonorgestrel	4 pills q12h × 2 doses
Alesse, Lessina, Levlite, Lutera, Aviane	100 μg Ethinyl estradiol, 0.5 mg levonorgestrel	5 pills q12h × 2 doses

symptom. Spotting should resolve without intervention and does not indicate failure of this method. Breast tenderness is another side effect of EC, particularly of estrogen/progestin methods and can be troublesome because it is also an early sign of pregnancy. Patients should be advised to have a pregnancy test if their next period is not normal and they have signs of pregnancy.

■ Patient Teaching and Discharge Instructions

Patients should be advised of common side effects of EC. More serious symptoms such as fever, severe abdominal pain, and heavy bleeding should NOT be attributed to EC, and patients should be advised to be reevaluated for serious symptoms.

Patients should be told to use barrier protection and/or resume taking oral contraceptive pills. If they have not been tested for sexually transmitted diseases in the ED, patients should follow up with a primary care provider for counseling and testing. For the majority of women, their next menstrual period should fall within 1 week of the time the menstrual period regularly is due. The patient should be instructed to have a pregnancy test if the menstrual cycle is delayed by more than 1 week.

Advise patients about the actual effectiveness of EC based on the timing of administration so that they understand that EC is not 100% effective even when taken as directed (see Table 128-3).

REFERENCES

1. Henshaw SK: Unintended pregnancies in the U.S. Fam Plann Perspec 1998;30:24-29.
2. Kafrissen M, Adashi E: Fertility control: Current approaches and global aspects. In Larsen PR, Kronenberg HM, Melmed S, Polonsky KS (eds): Williams Textbook of Endocrinology, 10th ed. Philadelphia, Saunders, 2003, pp 665-708.
3. Yuzpe AA, Thurlow HJ, Ramzy I, Leyshon JI: Post coital contraception—A pilot study. J Reprod Med 1974; 13:53-58.
4. WHO Task Force on Postovulatory Methods of Fertility Regulation: Randomised controlled trial of levonorgestrel versus the Yuzpe regimen of combined orel contraceptives for emergency contraception. Lancet 1998;352(9126): 428-433.
5. Task Force on Postovulatory Methods of Fertility Regulation: Randomised controlled trial of levonorgestrel versus the Yuzpe regimen of combined oral contraceptives for emergency contraception. Lancet 1998;352:428-433.
6. Cheng L, Gulmezoglu AM, Ezcurra E, Van Look PF: Interventions for emergency contraception. Cochrane Database Syst Rev 2004;(3):CD001324.
7. WHO Task Force on Postovulatory Methods of Fertility Regulation: Comparison of three single doses of mifepristone as emergency contraception: A randomised trial. Lancet 1999;353(9154):697-702.
8. Conard LA, Gold MA: Emergency contraceptive pills: A review of the recent literature. Curr Opin Obstet Gynecol 2004;16:389-395.
9. Croxatto HB, Ortiz ME, Muller AL: Mechanisms of action of emergency contraception. Steroids 2003;68:1095-1098.
10. Spinnato JA: Informed consent and the redefining of conception: A decision ill conceived? J Matern Fetal Med 1998;7:264-268.
11. Conard LA, Gold MA: Emergency contraception. Adolesc Med Clin 2005;16:585-602.
12. WHO Fact Sheet: Levonorgestrel for emergency contraception. October 2005. http://www.who.int/reproductive-health/family_planning/docs/ec_factsheet.pdf
13. Piaggio G, von Hertzen H, Grimes DA, Van Look PF: Timing of emergency contraception with levonorgestrel or the Yuzpe regimen. Task Force on Postovulatory Methods of Fertility Regulation. Lancet 1999;353(9154):721.
14. Harrison T: Availability of emergency contraception: A survey of hospital emergency department staff. Ann Emerg Med 2005;46:105-110.
15. American College of Obstetricians and Gynecologists: ACOG Practice Bulletin. Emergency contraception. Clinical Management Guidelines for Obstetrician-Gynecologists, Number 69, December 2005.
16. Raymond, EG, Creinin, MD, Barnhart, KT, et al: Meclizine for prevention of nausea associated with use of emergency contraceptive pills: A randomized trial. Obstet Gynecol 2000;95:271-277.
17. Hatcher RA: 10 common questions on emergency contraception. Contracept Technol Update 1998;19:6, 11-12.

SECTION XIII

Environmental Injuries

Chapter 129

Heat-Related Injuries

Catherine McLaren Oliver

KEY POINTS

Heat-related illness encompasses a continuum of disorders. Heat stroke is the most severe form.

Heat stroke is a life-threatening hyperthermic syndrome with central nervous system dysfunction. Additional organ dysfunction, due to the physiologic response to hyperthermia, cytotoxic effects of heat, and over-exuberant inflammatory and coagulation responses, is often present.

The height and duration of hyperthermia are the main determinants of mortality. Average mortality from heat stroke is 50%.

The main goal of therapy is rapid reduction of the patient's core temperature to about 39° C.

One of two methods—evaporative cooling or immersion—is recommended for lowering core body temperature.

Scope

Heat-related injury spans a wide spectrum from the unpleasant and transient conditions of heat cramps or prickly heat to the life-threatening multiorgan failure of heat stroke. Roughly 400 people die yearly of heat-related causes. An estimated half of the deaths are weather related, and 5% from being enclosed in motor vehicles, boiler rooms, or kitchens; in the remaining cases, the causes are unspecified.[1] Mortality from heat stroke is roughly 50%.[2]

Children and the elderly are at greater risk for severe heat illness because of their decreased physiologic ability to tolerate heat stress. Additionally, they may be less able to recognize or remove themselves from dangerously hot environments. Nonexertional heat stroke usually occurs in children enclosed in motor vehicles and in the chronically ill during heat waves. Other common settings for heat illness are the wilderness, athletics, and military or other physical occupations (e.g. miners, fire fighters), in which a combination of exertion and heat exposure induces heat stroke. The most important risk factors for heat illness are listed in Box 129-1.

Physiology

Thermoregulation is maintained by the anterior hypothalamus through information received from heat receptors (in the skin and core body) to balance the mechanisms of heat creation and dissipation. When the body's core temperature rises above the temperature set point, two methods of heat transfer are implemented: shunting of blood circulation to the skin and sweating. Heated blood is brought to the skin's surface to be transferred to the surrounding environment by sympathetic vasodilation and increased cardiac output. Skin blood flow can increase from 0.2 to 0.5 L/min in normothermia to 7 to

Table 129-1 ACCLIMATIZATION MECHANISMS

Cardiac	Increased cardiac performance: higher cardiac output
Vascular	Increases in Plasma volume Renal flow Shunting of blood away from visceral circulation
Endocrine	Enhanced renin-angiotensin-aldosterone system and improved salt retention by kidneys and sweat glands result in better fluid retention
Renal	Increased glomerular filtration rate
Sweat glands	Increased volume of sweat produced and more dilute sweat reduce salt loss and indirectly diminishes dehydration
Muscle	Improved ability to resist rhabdomyolysis from exertion
Cellular	Upregulation of transcription of heat shock proteins

BOX 129-1

Risk Factors for Severe Heat Illness

- Extremes of age
- Dehydration
- Inadequate fluid replacement during exertion or use of diuretics or alcohol
- Impaired cardiac function
  - Illness (e.g., heart failure)
  - Drug therapy (e.g., beta-blockers)
- Anhidrosis from use of anticholinergic agents or phenothiazines
- Intercurrent illness
  - Fever in children
  - Chronic obstructive pulmonary disease in the elderly
  - Mental illness
- Stimulant drugs that increase heat production
- Lack of air-conditioning in home

8 L/min in hyperthermia.[3] As a consequence, blood is shunted away from the central circulation, reducing perfusion of renal and gastrointestinal systems. Also, heated blood signals the thermal sweating response. The conversion of water to vapor absorbs heat and thereby cools the skin.[4]

The effectiveness of the thermoregulatory response depends on several environmental factors. A larger temperature gradient between the body and surrounding air temperature increases cooling. Additionally, wind assists with cooling through convection, and humidity hinders evaporation. Therefore an ideal environment for heat dissipation is cool, windy, and dry.

One last important physiologic concept is *acclimatization.* The body is able, over a period of weeks, to enhance its thermoregulatory mechanisms through multiple organ system and cellular modifications. Table 129-1 illustrates the mechanisms of acclimatization.

FACTS AND FORMULAS

In a hot, dry environment, evaporation can account for as much as 98% of the body's dissipated heat.[4]

Children are physiologically at greater risk for heat illness because of their larger body surface–to-volume ratio (greater absorption of heat from surroundings), smaller blood volume relative to body size, and lower sweating rate.

The main predictors of morbidity and mortality are duration and severity of hyperthermia.

Pathophysiology of Heat Stroke

Severe heat illness is thought to result from three main mechanisms: physiologic alterations in response to hyperthermia, direct cytotoxic effects of heat, and inflammatory and coagulation responses of the host. These mechanisms interact to create a spiraling deterioration resulting in circulatory collapse and multiorgan failure. The pathophysiology of heat stroke shares many features with that of sepsis.

Failure of thermoregulation often occurs when fluid and electrolyte replacement is not adequate. Dehydration hinders heat dissipation by diminishing cardiac output and also eventually leads to hypotension. Hyponatremia can result from perspiration but is more often seen when only free water replacement occurred during heat stress. Lack of salt repletion diminishes the kidney's ability to retain water.

In addition, prolonged shunting of blood away from splanchnic circulation leads to intestinal ischemia and acute renal failure. Intestinal ischemia appears to increase gut permeability and allow entrance of endotoxins, which may, along with ischemia, play a significant role in stimulating additional inflammatory mediators. Inflammation localized to the viscera would (1) cause local vasodilation and increase visceral circulation, inducing hypotension by increasing the vascular bed size, and (2) worsen hyperthermia by decreasing peripheral blood flow.

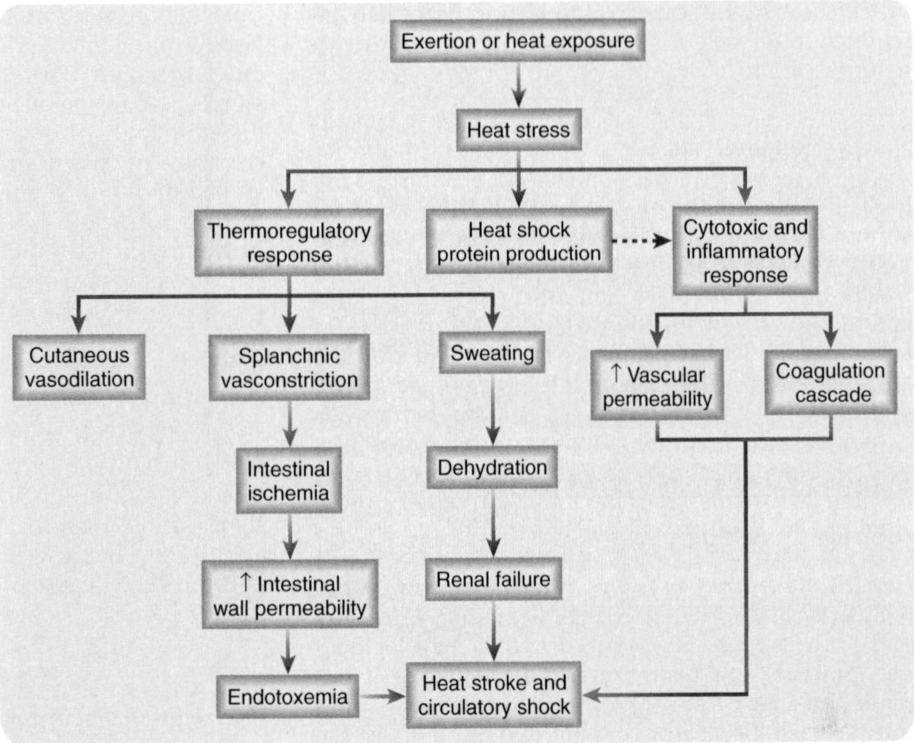
Exertion or heat exposure
Heat stress
Thermoregulatory response
Heat shock protein production
Cytotoxic and inflammatory response
Cutaneous vasodilation
Splanchnic vasconstriction
Sweating
↑ Vascular permeability
Coagulation cascade
Intestinal ischemia
Dehydration
↑ Intestinal wall permeability
Renal failure
Endotoxemia
Heat stroke and circulatory shock

FIGURE 129-1 Algorithm of the pathophysiology of heat stroke.

Heat itself has a direct cytotoxic effect. Cell death occurs over 45 minutes to 8 hours at body temperatures of 41.6° to 42° C.[5] Below these temperatures, cell death can still occur through apoptosis.[6] *Heat shock proteins* are the cell's defense against heat stress; they protect cells from direct damage by heat, ischemia, hypoxia, endotoxins, and inflammatory cytokines. Transcription of these proteins is upregulated during acute heat stress and during acclimatization.

Next, heat induces higher production of numerous inflammatory cytokines. These cytokines contribute to the neuronal injury and hypotension seen in heat stroke. Unlike the prior two mechanisms, cooling does not appear to suppress the inflammatory response once incited. Lastly, heat induces coagulation and endothelial cell injury, which can lead to disseminated intravascular coagulation and greater vascular permeability.

Figure 129-1 diagrams the current understanding of the pathophysiology of heat stroke.

Presenting Signs and Symptoms

■ MINOR HEAT-RELATED SYNDROMES

As stated earlier, heat-related illness is a continuum. Several conditions are mild and require simple or no treatment.

■ Heat Edema

Heat edema is a self-limited illness characterized by mild swelling in hands and feet from increased interstitial fluid after heat exposure. Treatment is not usually indicated because spontaneous resolution occurs in a period of a few days to 6 weeks. Elevation of extremities and use of compression hose may hasten recovery, but diuretics are not effective and may cause more serious heat illness through dehydration or electrolyte imbalance.

■ Prickly Heat

Clogging of the sweat glands leads to an erythematous, maculopapular, and pruritic rash commonly called "prickly heat." Treatment involves keeping the skin cool and dry with use of an antihistamine for the pruritus. Secondary staphylococcus infections can occur with heat rash, and patients with such infections should be treated for cellulitis by means of area-specific antistaphylococcal antibiotics (e.g., trimethoprim/sulfamethoxazole in areas with noted community-associated methicillin-resistant *Staphylococcus aureus*).

■ Heat Syncope

Heat syncope results from heat-induced volume depletion and peripheral vasodilation, which often occur in people with decreased vasomotor tone, such as the elderly, and in people poorly acclimated to the heat. It is important to regard heat syncope as a diagnosis of exclusion and to evaluate for other plausible causes of syncope. Also, the EP should remember to evaluate for any injuries sustained during a fall from syncope. Treatment involves removal of the patient from the hot environment, rest, and either oral or intravenous hydration. Hospitalization is not usually required, and patient should show rapid response to hydration.

Heat Cramps

Heat cramps are involuntary muscle spasms, most commonly of the calves, thighs, or shoulders, that occur either during or after vigorous physical activity. Cellular hyponatremia and hypokalemia are thought to cause this problem, and oral or intravenous hydration is effective management. Rhabdomyolysis is a very rare complication that can result from prolonged muscle spasm.

SEVERE HEAT-RELATED SYNDROMES

Heat Exhaustion

Heat exhaustion is a systemic illness occurring from heat stress and water and/or salt depletion. Common symptoms are extreme thirst, dizziness, lightheadedness, fatigue, weakness, syncope, headache, malaise, and vomiting. Usually the core body temperature is normal or slightly elevated (but often less than 40° C). Signs include tachycardia, orthostatic hypotension, tachypnea, and diaphoresis.

Neurologic assessment should be performed in all patients with presumed heat exhaustion to distinguish heat exhaustion from heat stroke. Heat exhaustion does not cause signs of central nervous system (CNS) dysfunction, such as delirium, ataxia, and seizures.

Most patients with heat exhaustion show good response to removal of their clothing, placement in a cool environment, and intravenous normal saline rehydration, and do not require hospitalization. Occasionally, a patient with severe hyponatremia and hypokalemia must be admitted. Therefore, the EP should check serum electrolyte levels and renal function in all but patients with the mildest cases. Discharge instructions should include advisement to continue to drink fluids and to avoid strenuous activity and heat for the next 1 to 2 days.

Heat Stroke

The classic definition of *heat stroke* was a core body temperature higher than 40° C, CNS dysfunction, and anhydrosis. However, there have been many cases of heat stroke in which sweating was present and the core temperature was not higher than 40° C. Therefore the definition is amended to a form of hyperthermia associated with a systemic inflammatory response leading to a syndrome of multiorgan dysfunction in which encephalopathy predominates.[7]

Heat stroke resulting from failure to stay normothermic in high environmental temperatures is usually termed *classic* or *nonexertional heat stroke,* as opposed to *exertional heat stroke,* in which a significant component of the heat is generated by the body's muscle tissue through strenuous work or exercise. Although both types of heat stroke are very similar, acute renal failure, rhabdomyolysis, and disseminated intravascular coagulation are more common in patients with exertional heat stroke.

The signs and symptoms of heat stroke are similar to those of heat exhaustion, except for the addition of CNS dysfunction in the form of delirium, hallucinations, ataxia, convulsions, or coma.

Differential Diagnosis

Many other conditions are associated with elevated core body temperature and altered mental status. Box 129-2 contains an extensive list. The EP should regard infection as a strong possibility in patients with these signs. In most cases, empirical antibiotic treatment is appropriate because infection is the most common and treatable cause of hyperthermia. Toxicologic, neurologic (e.g., hemorrhage or seizures), and endo-

Tips and Tricks

- Both neuroleptic malignant syndrome and heat stroke cause altered mental status and hyperthermia; unlike patients with heat stroke, however, all patients with neuroleptic malignant syndrome also have extrapyramidal rigidity.
- Hospital maintenance often has large fans used to dry hospital floors, which can be used to enhance evaporative cooling of a patient with heat illness.

BOX 129-2

Differential Diagnosis of Heat Stroke

- Sepsis
- Encephalitis
- Meningitis
- Brain abscess
- Malaria (cerebral falciparum)
- Typhoid fever
- Tetanus
- Alcohol withdrawal syndrome
- Neuroleptic malignant syndrome (see Tips and Tricks box)
- Anticholinergic toxicity
- Salicylate toxicity
- Phencyclidine hydrochloride (PCP), cocaine, or amphetamine toxicity
- Status epilepticus
- Cerebral hemorrhage
- Diabetic ketoacidosis
- Thyroid storm

crinologic (e.g., thyroid storm) etiologies should also be kept in mind.

Interventions and Procedures

■ Prevention

Informing patients about how to avoid severe heat illness when they present with mild heat illness may prevent future recurrence or more serious injury. The Patient Teaching Tips box lists information that can be given in the form of an educational handout to patients with heat illness.

■ FIELD MANAGEMENT

Morbidity and mortality are correlated with the duration and intensity of core body temperature elevation. Therefore field management that quickly identifies patients with possible heat stroke and immediately initiates cooling measures should have a significant positive effect on outcome. Intuitive measures include putting the patient in a cool, shaded environment and removing clothing. Next is to either immerse the patient in iced water (*immersion*) or wet the skin with water and use a fan to aid evaporation (*evaporative cooling*).

Continuous monitoring and assessment of core body temperature every 5 to 10 minutes are also recommended. Ability and resources to execute these measures will vary significantly according to the setting (wilderness vs. an ironman triathlon medical tent), but even simple measures recommended by the Israeli Defense forces—splashing 20 to 40 mL of water on the skin and fanning the person, and driving the person in an open car—effectively cool the core body temperature at a rate of 0.14°C/min.[8]

■ HOSPITAL MANAGEMENT

Initial treatment for heat stroke is identical to that for all patients in critical condition: assessment of the ABCs of respiration (airway, breathing, circulation), cardiac monitoring, establishment of intravenous access with administration of normal saline or lactated Ringer's solution, and liberal oxygen supplementation. Foley catheter placement with temperature monitoring capability will help guide management and determine whether the cooling measures are working. Liberal use of diagnostic studies to assess organ dysfunction and other potential diagnoses is important. However, these tests must not delay the initiation of cooling measures.

Diagnostic Testing

Heat stroke is a clinical diagnosis but may have associated multiorgan dysfunction. Therefore the EP must assess the patient for the severity of dysfunction in order to provide appropriate supportive manage-

PATIENT TEACHING TIPS

Heat Illness

- There are three main types of heat illness: heat cramps, heat exhaustion, and heat stroke.
- Heat cramps are painful muscle spasms and a mild form of heat illness that occur when you sweat too much or don't drink enough fluids.
- Heat exhaustion is due to dehydration and is more serious.
- Heat stroke is severe dehydration and confusion caused by overheating; it is life-threatening.

Prevention

During hot weather:

- Reschedule strenuous activities to cooler times of day.
- Reduce overall level of physical activity.
- Drink additional water or electrolyte solution (sports drink).
- Wear lightweight and light-colored clothing.
- Increase time spent in air-conditioned environments.
- Frequently check elderly, homebound, or disabled people, all of whom are at greater risk for heat illness.

Children

- Never leave children enclosed in motor vehicles. Yearly, 30 to 40 children die from heat stroke after being left in cars.

Athletics/Strenuous Labor

- Drink 500 mL of water/sports drink 2 hours prior to vigorous exercise/work.
- Continue to replace 250 mL of fluid for every 20 minutes of exertion and replace 150% of weight loss after exertion with fluids.
- Acclimatization takes at least 2 weeks, and gradual increase in activity is recommended to safely adjust to hotter environments.

Heat Illness Treatment

- If you have serious heat illness you may feel lightheaded, nauseated, tired, anxious, and confused.
- Get out of the heat into a cool, shaded place or air-conditioned building, and take off some clothing.
- Put cold water or cold wet towels on your skin, and drink cold liquids.
- If you are confused or lethargic or have a fever, seek medical attention immediately.

Table 129-2 METHODS OF CORE TEMPERATURE COOLING

Immersion	Placement of body into bath of cold or iced water
Immersion of extremities	Putting only hands and forearms in iced water
Evaporative cooling	Spraying tepid water or placing a wet sheet on skin with a fan to facilitate evaporation
Ice packing	Application of ice or cold packs to groin, axilla, and neck
Invasive measures	
Gastric lavage	Lavaging with iced water via nasogastric tube
Peritoneal lavage	Lavaging with sterile cold water
Dantrolene, 2-4 mg/kg	Decreases muscle contraction and, in theory, reduces heat production
Benzodiazepines	Theoretically, control shivering and heat production

BOX 129-3

Organ Dysfunction Seen in Heat Stroke

- Encephalopathy
- Rhabdomyolysis
- Acute renal failure
- Acute respiratory distress syndrome
- Myocardial injury
- Hepatocellular injury
- Intestinal ischemia/infarct
- Pancreatic injury
- Hemorrhagic complication (e.g., disseminated intravascular coagulation)

ment. Examples of multiorgan dysfunction seen in heat stroke are listed in Box 129-3.

Additionally, heat stroke often occurs in patients who have significant comorbidities, such as cardiac or respiratory diseases, or another concomitant acute illness, such as infection. Therefore, it is reasonable to assess cardiac function, perform a sepsis evaluation, and evaluate for any additional conditions that the EP suspects.

Treatment and Disposition

■ TREATMENT

Some experts liken treatment of heat stroke to that of trauma, for which there is a "golden hour" to effectively intervene and stabilize the patient. Often, after this time, aggressive measures cannot overcome the circulatory collapse and organ failure.

The EP's main goal is to cool the core body temperature to 38.5° or 39°C as quickly as possible. Active cooling is not continued to normothermic temperatures, so as to avoid the risk of overshooting and causing hypothermia. Usually a significant improvement is noted in the patient's cardiovascular stability and mental status immediately upon cooling. The methods of body cooling are defined in Table 129-2.

Debate and research continue about which cooling method is most effective and safest in treating heat stroke. Current research does not adequately answer the question whether water immersion or evaporative cooling is significantly more effective, but these are accepted as the two best options. Therefore the choice depends on which method can be instituted more quickly and effectively. Evaporative cooling with application of ice packs is more practical and effective. Ice packs, wet sheets, and a fan will provide rapid cooling. Table 129-3 lists advantages, disadvantages, and efficacy of various cooling methods.

■ Shivering and Vasoconstriction

Experts differ about whether shivering and vasoconstriction hinder cooling measures. Some believe that shivering and vasoconstriction require intervention, such as massage or a benzodiazepine, to prevent their negative effects on cooling. Others believe that shivering and vasoconstriction do not significantly slow the rate of cooling and may help prevent hypotension.

■ Hypotension

Hypotension is a common problem in heat stroke and should be treated aggressively with fluid boluses. If the patient's blood pressure remains unresponsive, vasopressors are indicated. One study used isoproterenol (beta-adrenergic agonist) to increase peripheral blood flow and cutaneous circulation, but this agent is infrequently used and is unlikely to result in significant blood pressure rise.[9] An alpha-adrenergic agent (e.g., dopamine, which is commonly used) may be more effective in raising blood pressure but has the theoretical disadvantage of causing peripheral vasoconstriction and hence diminishing cutaneous perfusion when given in higher doses.

■ DISPOSITION

All patients with heat stroke should be admitted to the intensive care unit for close monitoring and treatment. Occasionally for patients in whom heat stroke was initially suspected but assessment findings are more consistent with heat exhaustion, admission to a regular hospital bed is reasonable.

Table 129-3 ADVANTAGES, DISADVANTAGES, AND EFFICACY OF VARIOUS COOLING METHODS

Cooling Method	Advantages	Disadvantages	Effectiveness
Antipyretics		Can worsen liver or renal injury	Not effective (temperature set point is not elevated in hyperthermia) Not effective in controlling pathologic inflammation
Evaporative cooling	Noninvasive, easy to monitor, readily available	Labor intensive—requires constant moistening of skin	Comparison studies show cooling rate on average slightly slower than immersion Published rate range: 0.05° to 0.31°C/min
Immersion	Noninvasive, rapid	Cumbersome, poorly tolerated, safety questionable if comorbidities present, monitoring difficult, shivering and vasoconstriction	Comparison studies show cooling rate on average slightly faster than evaporation Published rate range: 0.04° to 0.23°C/min
Immersion of hands and forearms	Noninvasive, easy to perform in field	Shivering and vasoconstriction	Slower cooling but appropriate for mildly ill patients such as those with heat exhaustion
Ice packing	Noninvasive, readily available	Shivering and vasoconstriction, poorly tolerated	Less effective than immersion or evaporation Some authorities recommend using both evaporation and ice
Cold gastric or peritoneal lavage	Very rapid	Invasive, cumbersome (need for cold sterile saline for peritoneal lavage)	In canine studies, questionably faster than evaporation or immersion
Dantrolene	In theory, decreases heat production by inhibiting muscle contraction		No clear efficacy; it may be more effective in exertional than classic heat stroke
Benzodiazepines	Treatment of shivering to decrease heat production and heat-induced seizures	Sedation	Whether treatment increases cooling unknown, but may make cooling treatments tolerable Also effective for heat-related seizures

PRIORITY ACTIONS

- Use Advanced Cardiac Life Support principles to assess and monitor cardiac and respiratory stability.
- Obtain intravenous access as well as cardiac and core temperature monitoring, and place a Foley catheter for monitoring urine output and core temperature continuously.
- Start cooling measures immediately, preferably in the field if possible using either immersion or evaporative cooling.
- Actively cool the patient as quickly and safely as possible to a core temperature of 38.5° to 39°C.
- Continue monitoring for rebound hyperthermia.
- Assess for other organ dysfunction and intercurrent illness.
- Admit to the intensive care unit.

Documentation

Heat stroke is a life-threatening condition that requires intensive therapy and monitoring to treat effectively. Your documentation should demonstrate your efforts to monitor, resuscitate, and cool the patient as well as the patient's response to therapy. Because the definition of heat stroke involves encephalopathy, documentation should reflect a thorough neurologic assessment, including the patient's mental status.

REFERENCES

1. Heat-related deaths—four states, July-August 2001, and United States 1979-1999. MMWR Morb Mortal Wkly Rep 2002;51:567-570.
2. Ghaznawi HI, Ibrahim MA: Heat stroke and heat exhaustion in pilgrims performing the Haj (annual pilgrimage) in Saudi Arabia. Ann Saudi Med 1987;323-326.
3. Rowell LB: Human cardiovascular adjustments to exercise and thermal stress. Physiol Rev 1974;54:75-159.
4. Armstrong LE, Maresh CM: The exertional heat illness: A risk of athletic participation. Med Exer Nutr Health 1993;2:125-134.
5. Bynum GD, Pandolf KB, Schuette WH, et al: Induced hyperthermia in sedated humans and the concept of critical thermal maximum. Am J Physiol 1978;235:R228-R236.
6. Sakaguchi Y, Stephens LC, Makino M, et al: Apoptosis in tumors and normal tissues induced by whole body hyperthermia in rats. Cancer Res 1995;55:5459-5464.
7. Bouchama A, Knochel JP: Heat stroke. N Engl J Med 2002;346:1978-1988.
8. Hadad E, Rav-Acha M, Heled Y, et al: Heat stroke: A review of cooling methods. Sports Med 2004;34:501-511.
9. O'Donnell TF, Clowes GHA: The circulatory abnormalities of heat stroke. N Engl J Med 1972;287:734-737.

Chapter **130**

Hypothermia and Frostbite

Robert L. Stephen

KEY POINTS

Accidental (primary) hypothermia occurs when the ambient temperature outstrips a person's ability to thermoregulate (i.e., keep warm).

Secondary hypothermia is due to an underlying medical problem that alters thermoregulation (sepsis or endocrine disorders).

Treat *mild hypothermia* with passive external rewarming (blankets, dry clothes) and, subsequently, food and oral hydration.

Treat *moderate hypothermia* with a combination of passive and active external and active internal rewarming (warmed, humidified oxygen; forced-air heating blankets; heated blankets; heated intravenous fluids).

Treat *severe hypothermia* with active external and active internal rewarming. For patients without a pulse or blood pressure, pursue aggressive, invasive measures. For the patient with a pulse and blood pressure, warming blankets, heated oxygen, heated intravenous fluids, and continuous core temperature monitoring are sufficient. If the patient fails to warm or deteriorates, use invasive rewarming methods.

Hesitate to declare death in a hypothermic patient. Consider rewarming to a temperature of 32° to 35° C.

Hypothermia

■ SCOPE

Accidental hypothermia is responsible for approximately 700 deaths per year in the United States.[1] It primarily affects those least able to ward off the effects of cold weather: the very young, the very old, and the poor, disabled, pharmacologically inquisitive, environmentally adventurous, and mentally ill. Urban people are common victims. Hypothermia can occur in many latitudes, with episodes reported in Florida.[2] Not surprisingly, there is little strong scientific evidence for treatment recommendations, because trials cannot be conducted. The medical literature is mostly composed of animal experiments, case reports and series, and retrospective reviews. Still, rational approaches can be inferred from the extant literature for this uncommon but serious problem (Table 130-1).

■ PATHOPHYSIOLOGY

■ Mechanisms of Heat Loss

The mechanisms of heat loss are as follows:

Radiation of heat occurs when ambient temperature is less than body temperature and heat is lost directly to the environment via electromagnetic radiation.

Table 130-1 DEFINITIONS OF HYPOTHERMIA

Level of Hypothermia	Core Temperature (°C)
General	<35
Mild	32-35
Moderate	28-32
Severe	<28

Conduction is heat transfer from one (warmer) solid to another (cooler) when they are in contact.

Convection is heat loss from a surface to a (usually moving) gas or fluid, typically air or water. It can be considered an adjunct to conduction.

Evaporation causes heat loss through the energy required to vaporize water (i.e., sweat).

As a person cools, a fairly predictable procession of pathophysiologic changes occurs, as seen in Table 130-2 and Figure 130-1.

■ PRESENTING SIGNS AND SYMPTOMS

Patients with mild hypothermia are awake, occasionally drowsy, uncomfortable, and *shivering*. They simply need insulation (blanket), dry clothes, and food. They will recover completely and can be discharged when normothermic and feeling better.

Patients with moderate hypothermia are generally confused and lethargic, often have slurred speech, and are typically *not* shivering. They require more energetic rewarming measures, including heated blankets, resistive and hot air blankets (Bair Hugger), and close monitoring, including of core temperature. Although strictly considered active internal rewarming, the use of heated, humidified oxygen and warmed intravenous (IV) fluids is reasonable in this situation. Patients whose hypothermia responds to these measures may be discharged when normothermic, awake, alert, and ambulatory.

Patients with severe hypothermia require prompt intervention, close monitoring, and potentially aggressive, invasive rewarming therapies.

It is of the utmost importance to learn the circumstances that led to the patient's becoming hypothermic. The possibility of a causal drug overdose, trauma, infection, drowning, or decompensated comorbidities—to name but a few examples—must be considered, sought, and treated along with the hypothermia.

■ DIAGNOSTIC TESTING

The critical element of the diagnosis of hypothermia is the accurate measurement of core temperature. Several methods exist, all of which have potential

Table 130-2 PATHOLOGIC CHANGES SEEN IN HYPOTHERMIA

	LEVEL OF HYPOTHERMIA		
System	Mild	Moderate	Severe
Cardiovascular	↑ HR ↑ CO ↑ PVR	Progressive ↓ HR, ↓ CO, ↑ PVR Osborn waves possible on electrocardiogram	Profound ↓ HR, ↓ CO, ↓ PVR Ectopy (especially atrial fibrillation) Ventricular fibrillation Asystole
Central nervous system	Drowsiness, shivering	Confusion Lethargy Dysarthria Shivering cessation at <30°-32° C	Coma Muscular rigidity Pupils fixed and dilated Electroencephalogram flat at ~20° C
Hematologic	In general, hematocrit ↑ ~2% for every 1° C ↓ in temperature	Continuum	Coagulopathy Thrombocytopenia
Renal	Diuresis secondary to ↑ PVR with ↑ renal blood flow	Progressive loss of distal tubular resorption Resistance to antidiuretic hormone	Continued diuresis Limitation of clearance of electrolytes and glucose Acute renal failure
Respiratory	Tachypnea	Progressive bradypnea Loss of protective reflexes Bronchorrhea	Profound bradypnea Apnea Pulmonary edema (rare)
Gastrointestinal	Clinically silent	Progressive hepatic impairment	Decreased lactate clearance and detoxification and metabolism of drugs Pancreatitis in 20%-30% of cases
Acid-base		Can be either alkalotic or acidotic	
Endocrine		Patient usually hyperglycemic Thyroid, adrenal glands usually normal	Preexisting hypothyroidism or hypoadrenalism can impair rewarming

CO, cardiac output; HR, heart rate; PVR, peripheral vascular resistance.

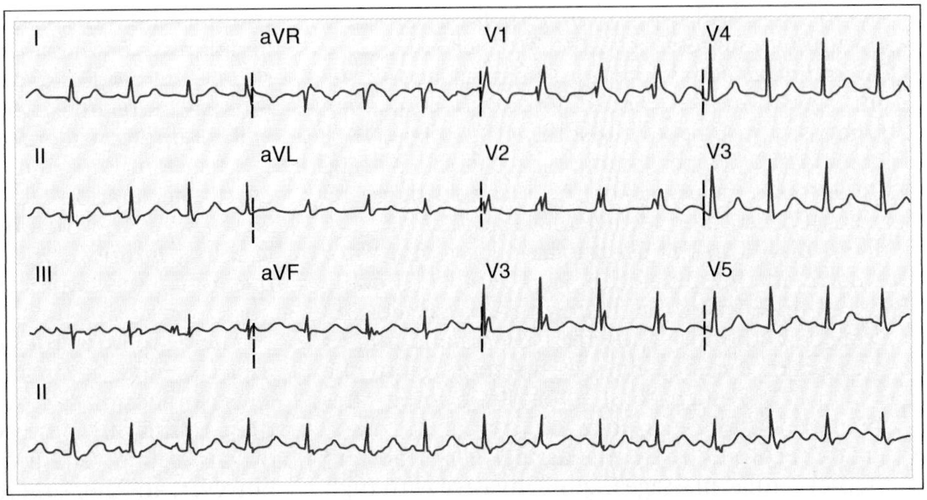
I
aVR
V1
V4
II
aVL
V2
V3
III
aVF
V3
V5
II

FIGURE 130-1 An Osborn wave in the electrocardiogram of a patient with hypothermia. The wave is usually seen at body temperatures less than 30° C; however, it is neither diagnostic nor prognostic in hypothermia and thus is of academic interest only.

drawbacks (Table 130-3). Laboratory and physiologic changes are correlated with the temperature. For example, a normal hematocrit value in a severely hypothermic patient should prompt a concern about hemorrhage because the hematocrit value should rise in a predictable fashion with ever-lowering temperature. Alternatively, the arterial blood gas values should be interpreted as if the patient is normothermic (the alpha-stat method) and not corrected for their actual core temperature (the pH-stat method). Evaluation for infection, metabolic derangement, and cardiac, neurologic, renal, and other organ system abnormality is important because comorbid conditions are common as a cause, a consequence, or coincidence of hypothermia.

TREATMENT

■ Mild Hypothermia

Patients with mild hypothermia may be treated with *passive external rewarming.* This treatment, which consists of the use of blankets, dry clothes, ambient warmth, oral hydration, and energy substrate (food), produces a rewarming rate of about 0.5° to 1°C per hour. The approach uses the patient's inherent ability to keep warm, primarily through shivering, and insulation.

■ Moderate Hypothermia

The patient with moderate hypothermia should undergo *active external rewarming.* Heat is actively supplied to the body via electric blankets, forced-air blankets, and space heaters. This method achieves rewarming rates of about 1° to 2°C per hour.

■ Severe Hypothermia

Active internal rewarming is needed for patients with moderate and severe hypothermia. Actions are directed toward heating the core preferentially over the periphery. This goal is accomplished via methods of variable invasiveness and complexity, as follows:

- Heated, humidified oxygen (40°-45° C) administered via face mask or endotracheal tube; primarily serves to prevent additional heat loss.
- Administration of heated IV fluids (40°-42° C) adds negligible heat overall but does aid in preventing further heat loss.
- Gastric and/or bladder lavage via nasogastric tube and Foley catheter is relatively easily accomplished; however, the small volume of these cavities limits the effectiveness of these modalities.
- Peritoneal lavage with prepackaged dialysate or standard crystalloid fluids heated to about 45°C. This method is quicker if two catheters, one for

Table 130-3 METHODS OF MEASURING CORE TEMPERATURE

Method	Comment(s)
Esophageal probe	Easy to insert Falsely high temperature readings possible with warmed oxygen via endotracheal tube
Rectal probe	Insert to 15-20 cm If probe is in/surrounded by cold stool, temperature recordings will lag behind true changes
Temperature-recording Foley catheter	Inflowing cold urine may falsely lower temperature recordings
Pulmonary artery catheter	Most accurate and most invasive method Higher iatrogenic injury potential, especially causing ventricular fibrillation in cold, irritable myocardium

afferent flow and one for efferent flow, are used. Rewarming rates average 2° to 3°C per hour.[3]

- Closed thoracic cavity lavage (pleural lavage) of the left hemithorax is done with two 36-French thoracostomy tubes with isotonic fluid heated to about 42°C. Large volumes are required. The afferent tube is placed in the second intercostal space (ICS) in the midclavicular line. The efferent tube is placed in the usual location, the fourth or fifth ICS in the midaxillary line. Fluid is literally poured in by hand, infused with a large (60-mL) syringe, or administered directly by a rapid infuser (the hub of the rapid infuser fits snugly into the bore of a 36-French chest tube). Rewarming rates average about 3°C per hour.[4-6]
- Left thoracotomy with mediastinal irrigation and internal cardiac massage is quite invasive with high attendant morbidity. It is very effective and self-explanatory and has rewarming rates as high as 5° to 6°C per hour.[7,8]
- Cardiopulmonary bypass (CPB) is the definitive method of rewarming. It is rapid, achieving rewarming rates of 9°C per hour or higher, and supports blood pressure; however, CPB also requires specialized equipment and personnel that are not readily available in most hospitals.[9,10]

The use of medications, particularly cardioactive medications and vasopressors, is theoretically unappealing and potentially dangerous in a patient with a core temperature lower than 30°C. This level of hypothermia causes a decrease in hepatic metabolism, resulting in potential accumulation of toxic concentrations that will have greater effect when the core temperature exceeds 30°C. Similarly, defibrillation is less likely to be effective at temperatures less than 30°C; therefore, the American Heart Association currently recommends a single shock for ventricular fibrillation in patients with core temperatures below this threshold, followed by CPR, sometimes prolonged, if cardioversion is unsuccessful. Once the temperature has exceeded 30°C, medications with a longer dosing interval and defibrillation can be administered.

The phenomenon of *core temperature after-drop* refers to the observation that a patient's temperature can fall after rewarming efforts have begun. It is believed to be due to a combination of temperature equilibration and the return of cold blood from the periphery to the patient's core as perfusion is restored and strengthened. The clinical importance of core temperature after-drop is keenly contested, and no consistent recommendations can be made regarding it. Certainly, attempts to rapidly rewarm a patient should not be delayed for fear of this consequence.

■ DISPOSITION

Patients with mild hypothermia and (most) patients with moderate hypothermia can be treated in the ED and released when normothermic. This statement relies on the assumption that there are no other complicating social or medical problems that must be addressed. All patients with severe hypothermia should be admitted to the hospital, usually to an intensive care unit. Successful revival of these patients will require considerable time and resources.

Clear, universally accepted criteria regarding death declaration for hypothermic patients are lacking, beyond the obvious recommendations as to terminal injuries, rigidity that precludes chest compressions, and physical blockage of the mouth or nose by ice.

There are numerous case reports of neurologically intact survival after prolonged, severe hypothermia with cardiac arrest.[6,11] A serum potassium level higher than 10 mmol/L has been postulated to be a marker of irreversible cell, and therefore patient, death[12,13]; however, another case report has called this approach into question.[14] The pronouncement of death in the severely hypothermic patient should be made with reluctance until the patient's core temperature has been warmed to more than 30° to 32°C and signs of life remain absent.

Frostbite

Frostbite is a freezing injury to soft tissues secondary to cold exposure that results in loss of circulation to, and therefore viability of, the affected area. The extremities, nose, ears, and male genitalia are the most commonly affected areas. Initial treatment consists of rapid rewarming in a controlled temperature bath, débridement of blisters, local wound care, and physical therapy. Additional treatment involves topical and systemic antiprostaglandin therapy. Definitive surgical excision is delayed for several weeks, until full demarcation of viability is established. Newer modalities to restore perfusion, such as thrombolytic agents, show promise in salvaging tissue.

■ SCOPE

In the United States, frostbite is often a disease of the indigent, the intoxicated, the mentally ill, and winter outdoor recreation enthusiasts. As for hypothermia, the literature on frostbite is primarily case reports, case series, and reviews.

■ PATHOPHYSIOLOGY

Frostbite is a freezing injury to tissues. During this process it is believed that deposits of ice crystals causing interstitial, cellular, and vascular endothelial cell damage are one part of the pathophysiologic process.[15] The vascular endothelial damage results in activation of the clotting cascade with resulting thrombosis, which leads to hypoperfusion, ischemia, and eventual tissue necrosis. The prominence of the clotting that can cause vascular occlusion can be seen on angiography and is the basis for the concept of treating selected patients with thrombolysis.

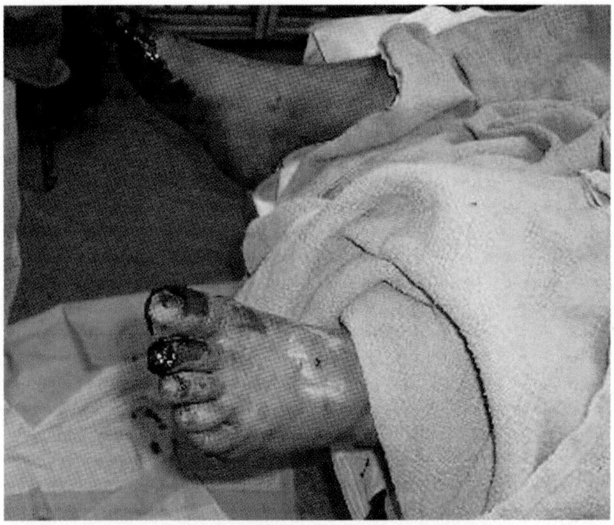

FIGURE 130-2 The frostbitten feet of a young man who had been running barefoot all night in winter secondary to a drug-induced paranoia.

■ PRESENTING SIGNS AND SYMPTOMS

The classic victim of frostbite presents with an either dusky or white affected area that is brawny to solid in texture, insensate, and without capillary refill. Variations are time dependent, and patients who delay presentation may have blisters that are either hemorrhagic or clear and even some tissue loss or frank necrosis already evident. Classification systems exist for frostbite but they are controversial and also are problematic for the EP, because the initial clinical appearance can be misleading and it takes time for the full extent of the damage to become clear. It is simpler and more realistic to start to treat the affected part and consult surgeons for ongoing wound care and treatment (Fig. 130-2).

■ DIFFERENTIAL DIAGNOSIS AND TREATMENT

Frostbite is a clinical diagnosis. Other cold-related tissue injuries to be considered are frostnip, pernio (chilblains), and trench foot. These, however, are nonfreezing injuries in distinction to frostbite. They are defined as follows:

Frostnip is a superficial freezing injury that appears pale and can be associated with discomfort. It resolves with rewarming without sequelae.

Pernio (chilblains) is due to repeated, intermittent exposure to wet, nonfreezing temperatures. Localized edema, erythema, nodules, plaques, cyanosis, and, possibly, vesicles and ulcerations appear up to 12 hours after exposure. Burning paresthesias and itching may be present, and rewarming can result in the formation of bluish nodules. Care is supportive, consisting of rewarming, bandaging, and elevation. Nifedipine, pentoxifylline, or limaprost has been advocated as potential therapy. Topical and oral corticosteroids may be useful.

Trench foot is direct soft tissue injury secondary to prolonged immersion in cold water. It develops slowly, but the damage, although initially reversible, may become permanent if not treated. Early on, paresthesias develop in a pale, mottled, insensate, and possibly pulseless foot. It becomes hyperemic after rewarming, with return of sensation (proximal more than distal) and severe burning pains. Edema and blisters can form, and in severe cases, tissue sloughing and gangrene can develop. Prevention is paramount, but when it does occur, trench foot is treated supportively much like chilblains.

Frostbite treatment in the field consists of application of dry sterile dressings separating the involved digits and elevation of the affected extremity. Avoid dry heat rewarming, such as with fires or heaters, and also assiduously prevent further cold injury. Rubbing the affected part with snow is soundly condemned. It is paramount to avoid a freeze-thaw-freeze cycle, which worsens tissue damage.

Once the patient is in the hospital, the mainstay of treatment is rapid rewarming with a circulating bath of water heated to 40° to 42°C for 10 to 30 minutes until the involved area is erythematous and pliable. Rewarming is extraordinarily painful, and liberal use of parenteral analgesics is usually necessary. Clear, large blisters should generally be débrided, but hemorrhagic ones should be left intact (their presence implies much deeper damage, and desiccation of the area is a concern). Débridement removes fluid that is rich in thromboxanes and prostaglandins, which are thought to be destructive to tissue. Aloe vera may be applied topically every 6 hours, and the wounds bandaged.

Prophylactic antibiotics are controversial. Penicillin G has been advocated. Additionally, ibuprofen, 400 mg by mouth twice daily is recommended to try to interrupt the arachidonic acid cascade.[16] Finally, both catheter-directed intraarterial and systemic thrombolytic therapies have been used with impressive success to prevent amputations (Figs. 130-3 and 130-4). This is a novel therapy that holds considerable promise but does have several limitations, including restriction to patients who present within 24 hours of injury and the risks of bleeding.[17]

Early surgical management is not indicated in frostbite because of the difficulty of ascertaining the full extent of tissue damage initially. Typically, the affected area is left to mummify and essentially autoamputate before the formal procedure is carried out. Some newer imaging modalities, such as nuclear scanning and magnetic resonance angiography, may be able to shorten the time to definitive surgery by delineating the viable tissue earlier than simple observation.[18]

Disposition

Because of the severity of frostbite, the need for daily hydrotherapy and wound care, and the often tenuous social circumstance of those afflicted, most patients

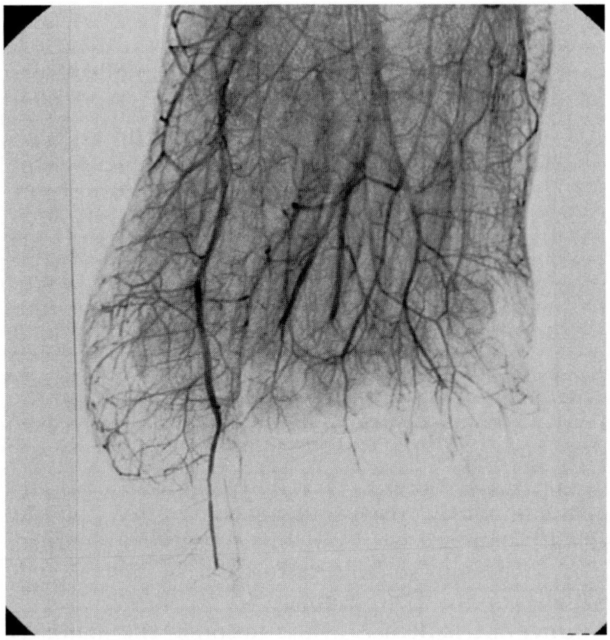

FIGURE 130-3 Angiogram of the left foot of a young female with frostbite after she wandered the desert all night under the influence of illicit drugs.

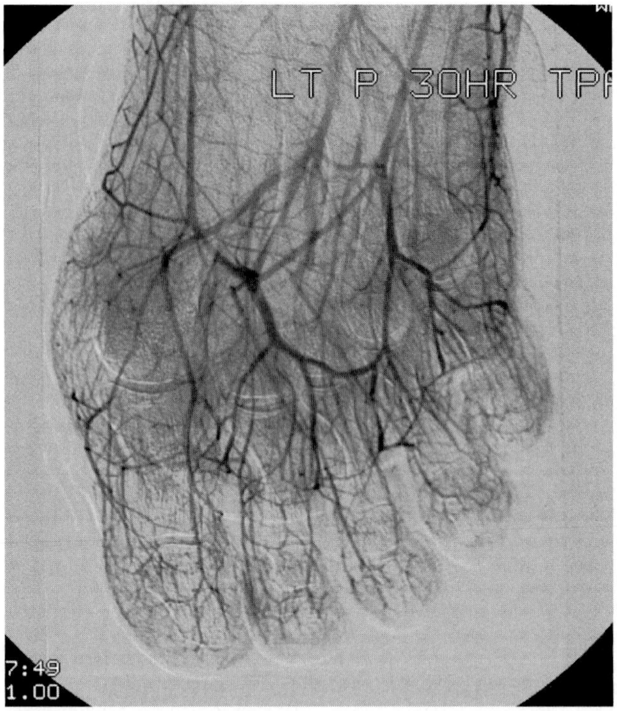
LT P 30HR TP
7:49
1.00

FIGURE 130-4 Angiogram of the foot shown in Fig. 130-3 after approximately 30 hours of tissue plasminogen activator infusion, showing restoration of perfusion. An amputation was averted with this therapy.

with frostbite should be admitted to the hospital under the care of a physician skilled in treating this illness. In many cases, burn centers are an excellent option.

REFERENCES

1. Centers for Disease Control and Prevention: Hypothermia-related deaths—Utah, 2000, and United States, 1979-1998. MMWR Morb Mortal Wkly Rep 2002;51:76.
2. Danzl DF, Pozos RS, Auerbach PS, et al: Multicenter hypothermia survey. Ann Emerg Med 1987;16:1042-1055.
3. Troelsen S, Rybro L, Knudsen F: Profound accidental hypothermia treated with peritoneal dialysis. Scand J Urol Nephrol 1986;20:221-224.
4. Hall KN, Syverud SA: Closed thoracic cavity lavage in the treatment of severe hypothermia in human beings. Ann Emerg Med 1990;19:204-206.
5. Walters DT: Closed thoracic cavity lavage for hypothermia with cardiac arrest. Ann Emerg Med 1991;20:439-440.
6. Winegard C: Successful treatment of severe hypothermia and prolonged cardiac arrest with closed thoracic cavity lavage. J Emerg Med 1997;15:629-632.
7. Brunette DD, Biros M, Mlinek EJ, et al: Internal cardiac massage and mediastinal irrigation in hypothermic cardiac arrest. Am J Emerg Med 1992;10:32-34.
8. Brunette DD, McVaney K: Hypothermic cardiac arrest: An 11 year review of ED management and outcome. Am J Emerg Med 2000;18:418-422.
9. Walpoth BH, Locher T, Leupi F, et al: Accidental deep hypothermia with cardiopulmonary arrest: Extracorporeal blood rewarming in 11 patients. Eur J Cardiothorac Surg 1990;4:390-393.
10. Walpoth BH, Walpoth-Aslan BN, Mattle HP, et al: Outcome of survivors of accidental deep hypothermia and circulatory arrest treated with extracorporeal blood warming. N Engl J Med 1997;337:1500-1505.
11. Pickering BG, Bristow GK, Craig DB: Case history number 97: Core rewarming by peritoneal irrigation in accidental hypothermia with cardiac arrest. Anesth Analg 1977; 56:574-577.
12. Hauty MG, Esrig BC, Hill JG, Long WB: Prognostic factors in severe accidental hypothermia: Experience from the Mt. Hood tragedy. J Trauma 1987;27:1107-1112.
13. Schaller MD, Perret CH: Hyperkalemia: A prognostic factor during severe hypothermia. JAMA 1990;264:18425-189445.
14. Dobson JA, Burgess JJ: Resuscitation of severe hypothermia by extracorporeal rewarming in a child. J Trauma 1996;40:483-485.
15. Murphy JV, Banwell PE, Roberts AH, McGrouther DA: Frostbite: Pathogenesis and treatment. J Trauma 2000; 48:171-178.
16. McCauley RL, Hing DN, Robson MC, Heggers JP: Frostbite injuries: A rational approach based on the pathophysiology. J Trauma 1983;23:143-147.
17. Twomey JA, Peltier G, Zera RT: An open-label study to evaluate the safety and efficacy of tissue plasminogen activator in treatment of severe frostbite. J Trauma 2005;59:1350-1354; discussion 1354-1355.
18. Barker JR, Haws MJ, Brown RE, et al: Magnetic resonance imaging of severe frostbite injuries. Ann Plast Surg 1997;38:275-279.

Chapter **131**

Lightning and Electrical Injuries

Christopher B. Colwell

KEY POINTS

In high-voltage electrical injuries, the internal damage the victim has suffered can be significantly greater than external damage or surface injury indicates.

Because of the potential direct effects of lightning on the eye, fixed, dilated pupils are not a reliable indicator of brain death in the victim of a lightning strike.

Oral burns in children can represent electrical injury from chewing on electrical wires. These injuries can result in delayed but very significant bleeding from the labial artery when the eschar separates.

In multiple or mass casualty situations, electrical or lightning injury victims in cardiac arrest should not be triaged as expectant deaths. Victims who are not in cardiac arrest often do not require immediate care, and those who are in cardiac arrest may respond quite well to defibrillation, so the latter group should receive highest priority for treatment at the scene.

Victims of electrical injuries who have any symptoms that raise concern about neurovascular compromise, or in whom evidence of neurovascular compromise is found on examination, are at high risk for compartment syndrome.

Blunt trauma can occur in up to one third of victims of lightning or high-voltage electrical injuries.

Scope and Outline

■ LIGHTNING

A strike of lightning in nature is a beautiful event that inspires both fear and amazement. The National Weather Service estimates that more than 100,000 thunderstorms occur in the United States each year, and lightning is present in all thunderstorms. Cloud-to-ground lighting strikes, the most destructive form of lightning, occur approximately 30 million times each year,[1] most often in Florida and along the southeastern coast of the Gulf of Mexico.[2] The danger may not be obvious or apparent, because lightning has struck more than 10 miles away from the rain of a thunderstorm.[1] Just as they have provided the skies with some of their more spectacular displays, such storms have also caused serious injury. Electrical injuries can be equally devastating. The spectrum of injuries from both can range dramatically from minor, localized injuries to death.

Although lightning injuries may be one of the most common injuries by natural phenomenon, the incidence of injury by lightning has not historically been accurately tracked. There were a total of 374 deaths from lightning injuries in the time period

Documentation

A large percentage of electrical injuries involve legal claims of some sort (worker's compensation, manufacturers, etc.), so the medical record should be complete with particular emphasis on available history, physical findings, and treatment rendered. The record should include the following:

- Whether loss of consciousness was involved
- Voltage of exposure, if known
- Presenting symptoms
- Skin findings
- Electrocardiogram findings
- Condition and symptoms at discharge

BOX 131-1

Definitions in Electrical Injuries

Alternating current (AC): Electrical source with changing direction of current flow

Current: The flow of electrons per second (measured in amperes)

Direct current (DC): Electrical source with unchanging direction of current flow

Frequency: The number of transitions from positive to negative per second in AC

Resistance: The tendency of a material to resist the flow of electrical current (measured in ohms)

Volt: Unit of electrical force

between 1995 and 2000. Incidence was higher in males and in people between 20 and 44 years of age, three of every four occurred in the South or Midwest, and one in four was work-related.[3] Sport- and travel-related activities also put people at higher risk for lightning injuries.

■ ELECTRICAL INJURY

Electrical injuries tend to occur in patients in three distinct age groups. The first group is toddlers, who encounter household electrical sockets, cords, and appliances. The second is adolescents, who engage in risky behavior. The third group comprises adults who work with electricity. Electrical burns account for between 3% and 7% of admissions to burn centers in the United States each year, many of which are occupational injuries. The annual occupational death rate from electrocution is 1 per 100,000; this type of death occurs more frequently in utility workers, miners, and construction workers.[4]

Pathophysiology

The definitions that should be familiar to those caring for patients with electrical injuries are listed in Box 131-1. Electrical current is the movement of electrical charge from one location to another. This movement occurs when there is a potential difference between two locations. Current strength is expressed in amperes. Materials that allow electrical current to flow easily (low-resistance) are referred to as *conductors*. Examples of conductors are metals such as copper and aluminum. Materials that do not allow electrical current flow are called *insulators*.

All body tissues conduct electricity to some extent, tissues with high fluid content conducting better than those with lower fluid content. Nerves tend to offer the least resistance, whereas bones offer the most. Table 131-1 lists body tissues according to level of resistance. Skin resistance can vary substantially,

Table 131-1 LEVEL OF RESISTANCE OF BODY TISSUES TO ELECTRICITY

Level of Resistance	Tissue(s)
Low	Nerves Blood vessels Mucous membranes Muscle
Intermediate	Skin
High	Tendon Fat Bone

with wet skin having the lowest resistance. This lower resistance allows more current to flow, and voltages that might not otherwise cause much damage can cause severe injury or even death. Skin that is callused provides the greatest resistance. The factors determining the severity of the injury caused by the electrical current are listed in Box 131-2.

Any electrical charge more than 1000 volts (V) is generally considered high voltage, although some authorities have argued that the risk for significant injury increases in charges exceeding 600 V. Typical household circuits in the United States are 110 V, with bigger appliances operating on 220 V circuits. Power lines in residential areas can have more than 7000 V.

Electricity causes injury in several ways, which are listed in Box 131-3. As current passes through the

FACTS AND FORMULAS

- Ohm's law: $V = I \times R$

  where V = potential (in volts); R = resistance (in ohms); I = current (an amperes)
- P = I2Rt

  where P = heat (in joules); I = current (in amperes); R = resistance (in ohms); t = time (in seconds)

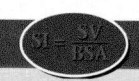

BOX 131-2

Factors Determining Severity of Electrical Injury

- Type of circuit
- Whether current was alternating or direct
- Duration of contact
- Voltage (electrical potential)
- Resistance of tissues
- Amperage (current intensity)
- Environmental circumstances
- Pathway of current

From Arrowsmith J, Usgaocar RP, Dickson WA: Electrical injury and the frequency of cardiac complications. Burns 1997;23: 576-578.

BOX 131-3

Mechanisms of Electrical Injury

- Direct tissue damage (entry and exit sites)
- Internal thermal heating
- Induced muscle contraction
- Flash burns
- Arc burns
- Blunt trauma

body, tissues through which it passes are heated, potentially causing significant damage. The EP must be aware of the potential for internal damage whenever caring for the victim of electrical injury; not all patients with significant internal injuries display significant external damage. When impressive external damage is encountered, significant internal damage should be assumed. Arc burns occur from an electrical source through the air and can cause significant damage. Temperatures can reach 2500° C and can ignite cloths or nearby material, causing thermal injuries. Flash burns occur when current strikes the body but does not enter the skin.

■ ALTERNATING CURRENT AND DIRECT CURRENT

The type of current involved contributes to the duration of exposure and therefore affects the degree of injury. *Direct current* (DC) is continuous in one direction, whereas current with periodic reversal of direction is *alternating current* (AC). AC is said to be three times more dangerous than DC, because it can cause continuous muscle contraction (tetany), which can prevent the victim from voluntarily terminating contact with the electrical source and result in prolonged contact. Alternatively, DC tends to evoke a single muscle spasm, often throwing the victim from the electrical source and resulting in a shorter duration of exposure but a greater risk for blunt trauma.

BOX 131-4

Mechanisms of Injury from Lightning Strikes

Direct strike

Contact strike: Lightning strikes an object the victim is touching.

Side flash: Lightning strikes a nearby object, and electrical current then traverses the air to strike the victim (can involve multiple victims).

Ground strike: Lightning hits the ground and is transferred to a person standing near the site of the strike. If there is a potential difference between the legs of the victim, lightning can enter one leg and exit the other, resulting in temporarily paretic, cold, insensate, and pulseless legs (keraunoparalysis).

Lightning delivers high-voltage direct current that tends to flow over the body rather than enter it. This event, often referred to as *flashover,* is one explanation for how people are able to sometimes survive an exposure to such a high voltage. Lightning current can also enter the victim and cause significant damage, particularly to the cardiac, respiratory, and neurologic systems. Blunt injury has been reported in up to one third of lightning victims,[6] from both the direct force of the strike and the rapid expansion of the surrounding air, often causing the victim to fall or be struck by flying debris. Lightning can also cause thermal injury (burns) by hot steam resulting from surrounding moisture or by metal objects heated by the electricity. Box 131-4 lists the mechanisms of injury from lightning strikes.

Anatomy

Although electrical and lightning injuries can affect any organ system, the cardiovascular and neurologic systems are principally affected. Cardiac arrest is the primary cause of immediate death in both electrical and lightning injuries. AC produces ventricular fibrillation, even at low voltages, whereas DC is more likely to cause asystole. Electrical injuries can result in virtually any type of dysrhythmia, although rhythm disturbances are unlikely if the exposure is to less than 120 V and water is not involved.[7] Lighting also causes a variety of cardiac rhythm disturbances. Although serum concentrations of creatinine kinase (CK), the MB fraction of CK (CK-MB), or troponin are often elevated, acute myocardial infarction is uncommon in both electrical and lightning injuries.

The nervous system can also be significantly affected by electrical or lightning injuries. Neurologic damage can be immediate or delayed. High-voltage electrical injuries can result in spinal cord injury from disruption of the spine (fracture or ligamentous injury).

The head is a common point of contact for high-voltage injuries, and skull and cervical spine injuries occur as the result of blunt trauma from lightning and electrical injuries.

Eye and ear injuries also happen with electrical or lightning injuries. A variety of initial eye findings or complaints have been described in both electrical and lightning injury victims. Delayed cataract formation is also described in both. Damage to the ear is rare in electrical injuries but relatively common in lightning injuries.

The skin is commonly affected by electrical or lightning injuries, primarily in the form of burns. Injury to the extremities occurs in both lightning and electrical injuries, but high-voltage electrical injuries are far more likely to result in compartment syndromes and the need for fasciotomy or even amputation.

Kidney damage or even acute renal failure can occur as the result of myoglobinemia, although this condition often responds well to fluid resuscitation. Gastrointestinal tract dysfunction, including bleeding and ulcer formation, has been described. Burns to the oral mucosa, seen more commonly in children, can be especially dangerous; these injuries can result in delayed but sometimes very significant bleeding from the labial artery when the eschar separates.

Presenting Signs and Symptoms

Victims of electrical or lightning injuries can present in virtually any fashion, from being apparently uninjured to being in cardiac arrest. Victims of high-voltage electrical injury typically have significant burns and present in dramatic fashion. Victims of low-voltage electrical injury or lightning injury may have very little evidence of injury. The most severe injuries are those affecting the cardiovascular and neurologic systems. As noted earlier, cardiac arrest is the most common cause of immediate death and generally manifests as asystole (DC) or ventricular fibrillation (AC).

Other than cardiac arrest, the most significant obvious injuries from electrical injuries are usually burns, which are most severe at the source of the electrical injury as well as at the exit point, which is commonly a ground contact point (usually the heel). Although significant external burns may indicate severe internal injuries, there can still be significant internal damage with minimal external findings, and one cannot predict internal damage from the extent of the external burns. The EP should assume significant underlying damage in all patients with electrical or lightning injuries. Lightning contact is usually instantaneous, leading to flashover burns that are often more superficial and minor. Extensive burns and deeper injury are more common in high-voltage electrical injuries, often owing to more prolonged contact.

Neurologic effects of electrical and lightning injuries can be immediate (which are often transient) or delayed (which are more likely to be progressive). Prognosis is usually better for patients with more immediate symptoms than for those with more delayed presentations. Initial presentations include altered mental status, which is often transient but can range from slightly agitated to comatose. As current passes through the skull, heat-induced coagulation can occur, resulting in subdural and epidural hematomas as well as intraventricular hemorrhage. Extremity weakness and paresthesias also occur and are more common in the lower than upper extremities. Seizures have also been described, and long-term seizure disorders may result.

Up to two thirds of victims of lightning strikes experience *keraunoparalysis,* a temporary paralysis specific to lightning injuries that is characterized by blue, mottled, and pulseless extremities (lower more commonly than upper). These findings are believed to be secondary to vascular spasm and often resolve within a few hours.[8] Permanent paresthesias can result but are unusual.

Vascular damage from electrical and lightning injuries has been well described. Thrombosis, hemorrhage, and ischemia can occur from direct damage to vessel walls, vasospasm, or burns. Small arteries to muscle are at particular risk.[9] Thrombosis and aneurysm formation are typically delayed.

Skin findings include feathering burns, flash burns, contact burns, punctate burns, blistering, and linear streaking. A specific type of burn associated with electrical injury is referred to as a "kissing burn," which occurs at the flexor creases of the knees, elbows, and axilla. Current causes flexion of the extremity, which in turn makes the flexor surfaces at the joint touch. This contact combined with a moist environment allows the current to arc across the flexor creases. Kissing burns indicate extensive underlying damage.

Contact with electrical current tends to produce burns that are discolored (often gray or yellow), painless, depressed, punctate areas of the skin. It is important to recognize that tissue damage under these burns can be massive.

Feathering burns (also known as Lichtenberg figures) are specific to lightning injuries and result from electron showers induced by the lightning, making a fern pattern on the skin. No permanent damage to the skin occurs, and no specific therapy is required. Punctate burns are full-thickness burns that look like multiple small burns from a cigarette. Deep burns are rare in lightning injuries.

Oral burns in children often represent electrical injury from chewing or sucking on electrical wires. These are particularly worrisome because of the possibility of delayed bleeding, which can be massive from the labial artery when the eschar separates, sometimes 5 days or more after the injury. Cosmetic defects also occur, particularly when the commissure is involved.

High-voltage electrical injuries and lightning injuries can both result in damage to the eye. Electrical injury is more likely to injure the eye if the exposure is to the head or neck, and injuries include corneal burns, retinal detachments, and intraocular hemorrhage. Delayed cataract formation has been described in up to 6% of patients.[10] Lightning injuries can also cause uveitis, iridocyclitis, mydriasis, anisocoria, or Horner's syndrome. It is for this reason that fixed, dilated pupils are not a reliable indicator of brain death in the lightning strike victim. As with high-voltage electrical injuries, delayed cataract formation is well described in lightning injuries.

Although uncommon in electrical injuries, damage to the ear is common in lightning injuries. Tympanic membrane rupture is the most common finding, and symptoms generally are transient hearing loss and vertigo. Patients usually recover without serious sequelae, although long-term hearing loss can occur.

Blunt trauma is common in the setting of electrical and lightning injuries, either from being thrown back from the source or from incidents resulting from the exposure, such as falls. Long bone fractures, dislocations, and solid internal organ injury have clearly been associated with electrical or lightning injuries.

Differential Diagnosis

Electrical injuries are generally more obvious than lightning injuries. With the exception of bathtub electrical injuries, in which burns may not be apparent, a good history and thorough physical examination usually reveal the cause of electrical injuries, ideally including the type of current, voltage, duration of contact, and symptoms immediately after the attack. Lightning injuries are not always as evident (lightning can strike when no rain or snow is present, and even on mostly sunny days) and may manifest as cardiac arrest, altered mental status, or paralysis. Recognition of classic patterns of lightning injury (such as feathering) may be the only way to initially distinguish these injuries from other causes of cardiac arrest, altered mentation, or acute neurologic injury. Some of the entities that should be included in the differential diagnosis of lightning injury or for the rare patient in whom high-voltage electrical injury is not obvious are listed in Box 131-5.

BOX 131-5

Differential Diagnosis of Lightning Injury

- Intracranial disease:
  - Cerebrovascular accident
  - Intracranial hemorrhage
- Seizure disorder
- Closed-head injury
- Spinal trauma
- Encephalopathy
- Primary cardiac dysrhythmia
- Toxic ingestion

Diagnostic Testing

Cardiac monitoring and electrocardiography (ECG) are indicated for all but the most benign electrical injuries and for virtually all lightning injuries. QT prolongation is a common finding. Complete blood counts are usually recommended but their results should be normal. The same may not be said of electrolyte, blood urea nitrogen (BUN), and creatinine values. Urinalysis should be obtained to look for evidence of myoglobinuria, the presence of which indicates rhabdomyolysis. The serum CK value may also show rhabdomyolysis. Elevation of the MB fraction of CK may be observed if a large amount of skeletal muscle is involved, so measurement of troponin or other cardiac markers would be more useful. The EP should remember that acute myocardial infarction is rare in either lightning or electrical injuries. Head CT should be performed in anyone with altered mental status or a significant headache, given the risk of intracranial bleeding from either direct contact (particularly lightning) or resulting head trauma. Radiographs of affected areas, in particular the spine, are indicated and should be performed on the basis of a thorough physical examination and appreciation of the likelihood of blunt trauma. Cervical spine films should be obtained in patients with altered mental status or significant cranial injuries, including burns. A pregnancy test should be performed in all women of childbearing age.

Treatment

Fasciotomy must be considered in patients with extremity burns from high-voltage electrical injuries in which compartment syndrome is a concern. Circumferential burns are more likely to result in compartment syndrome.

Prehospital providers must be particularly vigilant about scene safety. With electrical injuries involving a discrete electrical source other than intact electrical outlets, the power must be turned off before the victim is approached. Protective devices such as electrical gloves should not be used by medical providers in these situations as a way of bypassing the need to turn the power source off. Surrounding areas can be dangerous and should not be approached until provider safety is ensured. Any provider at the scene of a lightning injury must remember that lightning can strike in the same place twice. Also, both electrical injuries and lightning injuries should be considered to pose a high risk for concomitant blunt trauma,

PRIORITY ACTIONS

- Ensuring scene safety.
- Intravenous access; aggressive fluid resuscitation.
- Cardiac monitoring
- Electrocardiography in all victims of lightning or high-voltage electrical injuries
- Aggressive resuscitation of victims in cardiac arrest
- Fasciotomy:
  May be needed early in high-voltage electrical injuries
  Rarely, if ever, needed in lightning injuries

and spinal immobilization should be initiated unless clearly not indicated.

Lightning injuries are an exception to the general rule that in mass casualty or disaster situations, people in cardiac arrest should be categorized or tagged as "black" (or dead) and receive lowest priority for treatment on scene. Unlike in most other mass casualty situations, cardiac arrest in the setting of lighting or electrical injury may be quickly reversed with defibrillation. Also, victims with such injuries who are not in cardiac arrest are unlikely to die in the next several hours and generally do not require the immediate attention that victims without cardiac arrest victims at other scenes may demand. Triage for multiple victims of lightning injuries at one scene should concentrate on those in cardiorespiratory arrest, and the immediate treatment of those who are breathing can be delayed when necessary.

Intravenous access should be obtained in all victims of significant electrical injury or a lightning strike. Rhabdomyolysis can be effectively treated with aggressive fluid administration, with the goal of urine output higher than 1 mL/kg/hr. Alkalinization of the urine may raise the rate of clearance by increasing the solubility of myoglobin, although research has not shown a clear benefit of this approach. Formulas used to determine fluid resuscitation in burn victims cannot be used for electrical injuries. Because the damage to underlying tissue cannot be predicted from skin findings (damage is usually greater than skin findings suggest), formulas based on skin findings tend to underestimate fluid needs. Fluid resuscitation in lightning injuries does not have to be very aggressive unless there is hemodynamic compromise. Victims of lightning injury who do not experience cardiopulmonary arrest generally do well and do not need aggressive management. Fluid overload is a common iatrogenic complication in patients with lightning injuries.

CT of the head should be obtained in all victims of electrical injury with altered mental status because of the risk of intracranial bleeding. On the other hand, altered mental status in the form of confusion or amnesia is very common in lightning injuries and does not necessarily need further evaluation. Any patient with lightning or electrical injury whose mental status deteriorates after the exposure should have a head CT.

Tetanus boosters should be administered in patients whose immunization status is not up to date and even in those whose immunization status is current if they have significant muscle damage or there is contamination of the wounds, because electrical wounds are especially prone to tetanus. Burn wound care should be administered as appropriate for the apparent burns. Although clostridial infections are common, empirical penicillin therapy has not been shown to be effective.

RED FLAGS

- Do not underestimate the potential for significant underlying tissue damage, particularly with high-voltage electrical injury, even when skin findings appear minor.
- Traditional rules of triage do not apply to lightning victims. In this situation, care should be focused on, rather than withheld from, those in cardiopulmonary arrest.
- Do not miss compartment syndrome, particularly in high-voltage electrical injury.
- Consider the potential for rhabdomyolysis in all victims of high-voltage electrical injury, and provide adequate hydration. Beware of overaggressive hydration in lightning victims.
- Admit patients for cardiac monitoring who have lost consciousness, have any evidence of cardiac instability or dysrhythmia, or have a transthoracic injury pattern.
- Ensure good follow-up and careful instructions for parents of children with oral burns, who are at risk for both cosmetic defects and delayed labial artery bleed.
- Remember the risk of blunt trauma in victims of high-voltage electricity and lightning.
- Patients with neurologic complaints or deficits are at risk for permanent neurologic sequelae, particularly when symptoms are delayed.
- Remember to evaluate for tetanus immunization status and update as needed.

Disposition

Asymptomatic patients with normal physical findings who were victims of low-voltage electrical injury can be safely discharged without significant evaluation or observation. Patients with low-voltage injuries for whom risks are higher include those whose skin was wet during injury, those with tetany, and those in whom the current traversed the thorax. Patients with mild symptoms, normal ECG findings, and no evidence of myoglobinuria can be discharged after a period of observation (generally 4 to

PATIENT TEACHING TIPS

For Parents

- Hazards of unused sockets.
- Hazards of extension cords.
- Dangers of oral burns, in particular delayed labial artery bleed and cosmetic defect.

For Electrical Injuries

- Never work with electrical equipment alone.
- Sweaty or otherwise wet skin can decrease resistance significantly and turn a low-risk exposure into a higher-risk one.
- Insulation of electrical lines is meant to protect the lines from environmental challenges, NOT to protect humans from contact with the line.

For Lightning Injuries

- Seek shelter indoors or in a vehicle if lightning is anticipated.
- If shelter is not available, seek dense woods or a ditch to lie in.
- Lightning can strike even when the sun is out.
- Stay clear of metallic objects in a storm, particularly those that would elevate your height from the ground, because the highest object is generally struck by lightning.
- Get out of water and off small boats.
- Discard metallic objects such as golf clubs, umbrellas, and jewelry.
- A lightning strike is imminent when an individual's hair stands on end.
- Lightning CAN strike in the same place twice.
- Do not resume activity in the area of a storm until more than 30 minutes after the last flash of lighting or sound of thunder.

For the Patient with an Electrical or Lightning Injury

- Delayed neurologic symptoms can be serious and should prompt a return to the ED.
- Up to 74% of victims of lightning injuries suffer some sort of permanent sequela, such as sleep disturbance or chronic pain syndrome.

6 hours, although no research has confirmed this interval) and with recommendation for outpatient follow-up.

Any patient who experienced cardiac or respiratory arrest, or clear loss of consciousness or has abnormal or changed ECG findings, hypoxia, chest pain, dysrhythmia observed by a medical care provider, or serious concomitant injury should be admitted. Patients with known cardiac disease or multiple risk factors for cardiac disease should usually be admitted as well.

REFERENCES

1. Holle RL, Lopez RE, Howard KW, et al: Safety in the presence of lightning. Semin Neurol 1995;15:375-380.
2. Krider EP, Uman MA: Cloud-to-ground lightning: Mechanisms of damage and methods of protection. Semin Neurol 1995;15:227-232.
3. Adekoya N, Nolte KB: Struck-by-lightning deaths in the United States. J Environ Health 2005;67:45-50.
4. Ore T, Casini V: Electrical fatalities among US construction workers. J Occup Environ Med 1996;38:587-592.
5. Price TG, Cooper MA: Electrical and lightning injuries. In Marx JA (ed): Rosen's Emergency Medicine: Concepts and Clinical Practice, 6th ed. Philadelphia, Mosby, 2006.
6. Blount BW: Lightning injuries. Am Fam Physician 1990;42: 405-415.
7. Arrowsmith J, Usgaocar RP, Dickson WA: Electrical injury and the frequency of cardiac complications. Burns 1997;23: 576-578.
8. Duis HJ, Klasen HJ: Keraunoparalysis, a "specific" lightning injury. Burns 1985;12:54-57.
9. Hunt JL, McManus WF, Haney WP, Pruitt BA: Vascular lesions in acute electrical injuries. J Trauma 1974;14: 461-473.
10. Saffle JR, Crandall A, Warden GD: Cataracts: A long-term complication of electrical injury. J Trauma 1985;25:17-21.
11. Cooper MA, Andrews J, Holle RL, et al: Lightning injuries. In Auerbach P (ed): Wilderness Medicine, 4th ed. St. Louis, Mosby, 2001.
12. Cherington M, Yarnell P, Lammereste D: Lightning strikes: Nature of neurological damage in patients evaluated in hospital emergency departments. Ann Emerg Med 1992;21: 575-578.

Chapter **132**

Dysbarisms, Dive Injuries, and Decompression Illness

David Ulick and Heather Murphy-Lavoie

KEY POINTS

Decompression illness describes all types of diving injuries and includes decompression sickness and arterial gas embolism.

Decompression illness can manifest in a spectrum from mild constitutional symptoms to overt neurologic deficits.

Any severe symptoms that occur in a diver immediately upon or soon after resurfacing are highly suspicious for arterial gas embolism and need immediate medical attention. Delays in treatment are associated with worse outcomes.

The neurologic examination is the foundation of the diagnosis of decompression illness; history and physical examination alone are all that are needed to diagnose most dive injuries.

Dive injuries are best differentiated into the following categories: disorders of descent, disorders at depth, disorders of ascent, and disorders that occur upon resurfacing.

Decompression illness is treated on the scene by rapid implementation of high-flow oxygen and intravenous hydration, with definitive treatment being recompression with hyperbaric oxygen therapy.

One should delay flying after diving for at least 12 hours after a single dive and for 24 to 48 hours after multiple dives.

Consultation with a diving physician, hyperbaric specialist, and/or the Divers Alert Network is needed for a patient with *any* symptoms associated with a dive injury.

Perspective

Dysbarisms refers to medical conditions resulting from changes in ambient (surrounding) pressures on the body, while decompression illness (DCI) describes all types of diving injuries and includes decompression sickness (DCS) and arterial gas enbolism (AGE). DCI occurs during rapid ascent (decompression) when dissolved gases re-form bubbles and become lodged in various body cavities instead of being offloaded by the lungs with normal respiration. Diagnosis of decompression illness in the ED is important, because missed cases can have permanent sequelae, leading to potential litigation and malpractice suits for missed injuries (Box 132-1).

BOX 132-1

Typical Signs and Symptoms of Decompression Illness

Symptoms

- Dizziness
- Extreme fatigue
- Headache
- Itching
- Nausea
- Numbness
- Pain
- Personality changes

Signs

- Ataxia
- Hearing loss
- Paralysis
- Rash
- Sensory deficits
- Urinary retention

BOX 132-2

Fatality Statistics for Diving

- The annual fatality rate for DAN Members between 1997 and 2004 varied between 11 and 18 deaths per 100,000 members per year.
- Of the 160 reported dive fatalities in 2006, 88 of the victims were U.S. or Canadian residents.
- 42% of the fatalities in the United States occurred in the Southeast Region (North Carolina to Florida, Tennessee, and Alabama).
- Most fatalities occurred in people aged 50 to 59 years; 70% of the men and 80% of the women were 40 years or older. (*The age range for women was 30-69 years, with a median of 53 years; the range for men was 14-72 years, with a median age of 47 years.*)
- 74% of fatalities occurred in divers who were overweight or obese.
- 64% of fatalities were designated as drowning deaths.
- The initial triggering events that began the sequence leading to death, in order of occurrence, were insufficient gas (14%), rough seas and strong current (10%), heart disease (9%), entrapment (9%), and equipment problems (8%); 20% of cases had an unknown cause.
- 63% of deaths occurred during pleasure diving.
- Most deaths occurred during the summer months (May, June, July).
- 84% of deaths occurred during the daylight hours.
- 76% of deaths occurred in less than 90 feet of sea water (fsw).
- By far the greatest number of fatalities (37%) occurred with problems that evolved while the divers were on the bottom of the body of water, and 19% occurred after divers returned to the surface.

Data from Divers Alert Network: DAN Report on Decompression Illness, Diving Fatalities and Project Dive Exploration: 2006. Available at www.diversalertnetwork.org/

The annual report of the Divers Alert Network (DAN) states that there were 88 North American diving-related fatalities in 2006, a number that has been fairly stable for the last 2 or 3 years but has been as high as 147.[1] With the advent of "extreme sports" that involve more and more water contact, sport diving, and the increasing numbers of people engaging in breath-hold diving, there has been a sharp increase in the number of diving injuries seen in EDs (Box 132-2). In fact, the number of deaths from breath-hold diving alone has almost doubled in the last 5 years, further illustrating the potential for injury associated with this form of diving.[1]

With acute DCI, rapid assessment and treatment are the foundation of management. There are three keys to successful ED treatment: having a high index of suspicion, because the illnesses can be nonspecific; performing a thorough neurologic examination; and obtaining a hyperbaric medicine consultation when DCI is suspected.

Anatomy and Physiology

Dysbarism refers to the effects of variations in ambient (surrounding) pressure on the body. Hypobaric (low-pressure) exposures, such as those experienced by climbers, pilots, and astronauts, can result in symptoms and injuries similar to those found in divers with decompression illness, who are exposed to high pressures while at depth. Of the two, high-pressure (hyperbaric) exposures with decompression injuries are far more common.

■ DIVING PHYSIOLOGY

The evaluation of a diver or someone with a water-associated injury requires a basic understanding of dive physiology and the physics of pressures and gases. Different gases have different properties at depth and on the water surface. These properties allow gases to be used alone or in combination with each other for different types of diving. The gases that are used in both recreational and professional diving are air, oxygen, nitrogen, helium, and, occasionally, argon. Deep diving past 180 feet often requires helium-oxygen combinations (heliox) to mitigate the effects of nitrogen narcosis (discussed later), while nitrogen-oxygen combinations (nitrox) may be used to reduce decompression obligations (specific amounts of time spent at shallow depths that help divers offload nitrogen buildup in the body prior to exiting a dive).

In general, most recreational divers breathe compressed air and use a self-contained underwater breathing apparatus (SCUBA) when diving to depths less than 135 feet. Nitrogen, the inert gas in compressed air, represents about 78% of the gas that is inhaled with air diving. During diving, the nitrogen in the compressed air is dissolved and permeates body tissues because the increased outside hydrostatic pressure at depth effectively "pushes" nitrogen into the tissue. While the body is at depth, these gases remain saturated, and most divers experience minimal difficulties. Importantly, the greatest air volume changes happen in the first 33 feet of diving, which is why a large percentage of divers experience problems in shallower waters.

The deeper a diver goes and the longer he or she remains at depth, the more saturated the blood and tissues become with inspired inert gases. One of the tenets of diving is to ascend slowly when resurfacing. Doing so allows the dissolved gases to escape the tissues slowly during normal respiration. If a person ascends too fast, the dissolved gases are not offloaded by the lungs through respiration ("blown off") and are therefore free to travel in the blood, where they can cause damage downstream from where they were formed (emboli). They can also do local damage at the site of formation (*autochthonous bubbles*). When bubbles do become symptomatic, the disorder is called *decompression illness,* which has a variety of effects ranging from pain (most common presentation), numbness, and fatigue to severe neurologic symptoms such as seizure, paralysis, and loss of consciousness.

BUBBLE PHYSIOLOGY

Knowledge of the mechanism of bubble formation and the actions of bubbles in various body tissues is critical to understanding the pathophysiology and treatment of decompression illness. As discussed before, bubbles dissolved in the blood stream are not usually problematic because the lungs can filter a large gas load. It is when bubbles remain in tissues rather than being offloaded through respiration that they have damaging effects. Bubbles form in "nucleation sites" in the body tissues, such as the joint spaces, tendon sheaths, periarticular sheaths, and peripheral nerves.[2] Once inside these areas, bubbles can act as emboli that block distal tissue perfusion, act as foreign entities to the body, and cause vascular damage through compression of tissues and activation of inflammatory and clotting cascades.

PRINCIPLES OF GAS LAWS AND DYSBARISM

Decompression illness, as already described, involves bubble formation and the effects of gases on the body. Therefore, a basic understanding of some of the gas laws helps facilitate treatment and disposition of the dive-injured patient. The EP not only must be familiar with the gas laws that govern dive injuries but also must understand the units of measurement, abbreviations, and conversions that most commercial and recreational divers use daily. At sea level, the pressure of the atmosphere on the body (*ambient pressure*) is 760 mm Hg, which is said to equal *one atmosphere* (*1 ATM*). Furthermore, the term for the absolute pressure on a diver at sea level is called *atmospheres absolute* (*ATA*) and represents the total sum of pressures on a diver. Therefore, at sea level, a dive computer gauge reads zero, but sea level also represents one atmosphere of pressure (1 ATA). Knowing these facts helps the EP better comprehend the circumstances surrounding a dive injury.

Gas Laws

Although there are a large number of gas laws, the two that are the most important in diving medicine are Boyle's law and Dalton's law.

Boyle's Law

Boyle's law is important to understanding why a diver needs to exhale as he or she is ascending from depth and is the basis for many of the principles that diving physiology uses today. According to Boyle's law, the volume of a quantity of gas (V) varies inversely with the pressure upon that gas (P) if it is kept at a constant temperature. It is often represented by the following formula:

$$P_1V_1 = P_2V_2$$

where the subscripts *1* and *2* indicate two different combinations of pressure and volume; in other words, the *product of pressure and volume will always remain a constant.*

Usually, as a diver descends deeper into the water, the pressure surrounding the diver increases in a linear fashion. Water pressure at the surface is considered to be at 1 ATM. *In general, for every 33 feet of sea water (fsw) that the diver descends, there is an increase in pressure of 1 ATM.* Therefore, a descent to 33 fsw would be equivalent to 2 ATM, a descent to 66 fsw would be equivalent to 3 ATM, and so on. Furthermore, for every 1 ATM descended, the volume of gas present is reduced by *half of the original amount of gas at the surface,* a principle based on Boyle's law (Fig. 132-1).

Dalton's Law

Dalton's law of partial pressures describes the mechanism for decompression sickness ("the bends"), nitrogen narcosis, and oxygen toxicity. It is often represented by the following formula:

$$P_{total} = P_1 + P_2 + P_3$$

where P_{total} is the total pressure of the gases a diver breathes and the subscripts *1, 2,* and *3* indicate the partial pressures of each individual gas. This law

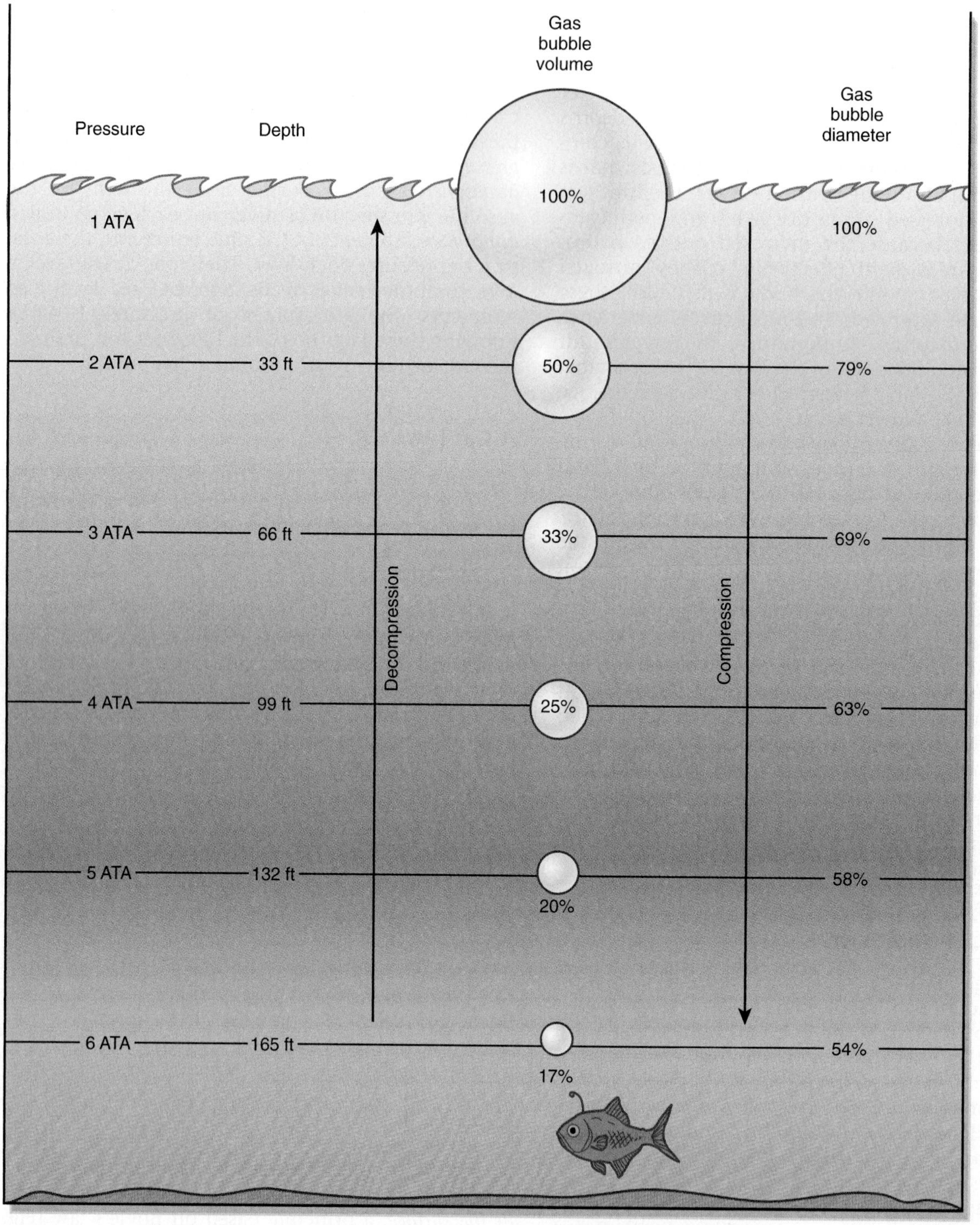
Gas
bubble
volume
Gas
bubble
diameter
Pressure
Depth
1 ATA
100%
100%
2 ATA
33 ft
50%
79%
3 ATA
66 ft
33%
69%
Decompression
Compression
4 ATA
99 ft
25%
63%
5 ATA
132 ft
20%
58%
6 ATA
165 ft
17%
54%

FIGURE 132-1 Boyle's law. ATA, atmospheres absolute.

explains how the side effects of gases occur as a diver goes deeper. Put simply, *as a diver descends while still breathing the same percentage of gases in the mixture, the amount of each gas inhaled increases proportionally with increasing depth.* When diving with air tanks, a diver is exposed to higher partial pressures of both oxygen and nitrogen the farther down he or she goes. This concept is important, because nitrogen at high concentrations has a narcotic effect (*nitrogen narcosis*), and oxygen at high concentrations can be toxic (*oxygen toxicity*). Both problems are described in further detail later in this chapter.

Clinical Presentation

Table 132-1 lists the differential diagnosis for dive injuries based on time of symptom onset.

■ BAROTRAUMA

Barotrauma is injury sustained from failure to equalize the pressure of an air-containing space with that of the surrounding environment. The most common examples of barotrauma occur in air travel and scuba diving. Although the pressure changes are much more dramatic during scuba diving, barotrauma is also possible during air travel.[3] An important fact to remember is that barotrauma occurs only in the gas-containing (and therefore *compressible*) spaces of the body. More than 95% of the body is composed of water, making most parts noncompressible. Typical gas-filled spaces in the body are the sinuses, the middle and inner ears, parts of the teeth, and the nonsolid organs of the body such as the intestines and lungs. Barotrauma incurred during descent is called a "squeeze," whereas barotrauma incurred during ascent is called "reverse squeeze," "reverse block," or expansion injury. In short, because all of these body spaces are air-filled cavities, they are all subject to Boyle's law and therefore to barotraumas.

Table 132-1 DIFFERENTIAL DIAGNOSIS OF DIVE INJURIES BASED ON PRESENTATION OF SYMPTOMS

Symptom Onset	Injuries to Consider
Descent	Ear or sinus barotrauma Trauma
Bottom	Nitrogen narcosis Oxygen toxicity Trauma
Ascent	Arterial gas embolism Pneumothorax Pneumomediastinum Subcutaneous emphysema Sever decompression sickness Ear or sinus barotrauma Trauma
Surfacing <15 min after	Arterial gas embolism Pneumothorax Pneumomediastinum Subcutaneous emphysema
15 min to 24 hrs after	Decompression sickness Trauma

■ EAR BAROTRAUMA

With greater participation in sport scuba diving and the increased use of hyperbaric chambers, the incidence of exposure to hyperbaric conditions with resultant ear and sinus injury is growing.[4] Injury to the middle or inner ear from equalization failure can consist of membranous damage, edematous change, rupture or hemorrhage of the eardrum, or trauma to the oval or round window, which can cause a perilymphatic fistula.[5] With an intact tympanic membrane, the only communication for pressure equilibration between the middle ear cleft and the ambient atmosphere is through the eustachian tube.[6] Table 132-2 summarizes the types of ear barotrauma.

■ *External Ear Barotrauma ("Squeeze")*

During diving, water normally replaces the air in the external ear canal. An obstruction such as wax, a bony growth, or earplugs can create an air-containing space that can change in volume in response to changes in ambient pressure, per Boyle's law. During descent, the increased pressure squeezes the volume of this space, causing the tympanic membrane to bulge outward toward the outer ear canal; this is simply called external ear "squeeze." It can cause pain, small hemorrhages in the eardrum, or blebs.[3] Treatment of external ear barotrauma consists of cleaning the external canal and removing foreign bodies.

■ *Middle Ear Barotrauma*

Middle ear barotrauma (middle ear "squeeze," barotitis media) is the most common disorder among divers and occurs principally during descent because of an inability to equalize pressure across the tympanic membrane. It is experienced by 30% of novice divers and 10% of experienced divers.[5] The mecha-

Table 132-2 BAROTRAUMA OF THE EAR

	Middle Ear Barotrauma	Inner Ear Barotrauma	Alternobaric Vertigo
Symptoms	Ear pain on descent Hearing loss Possible transient vertigo	Ear pain on descent Hearing loss Severe vertigo and nausea	Ear pain on ascent Transient hearing loss Nausea
Signs	Conductive hearing loss Tympanic membrane injury Unilateral face paralysis (rare)	Nystagmus Vomiting Ataxia Romberg's sign Neural hearing loss	Nystagmus Vomiting Tympanic membrane injury Abrupt relief with descent
Treatment	Decongestants	Refer to otorhinolaryngologist	None, if resolved

Modified from Shockley L: Scuba diving and dysbarism. In Hockberger RM, Walls JA, Marx RS (eds): Rosen's Emergency Medicine, 6th ed. St. Louis, CV Mosby, 2006.

nism involves the force of water pressure on the external part of the tympanic membrane, which pushes inward. Usually, a diver can equalize the pressure in the ears by means of a Valsalva maneuver or blowing against closed nostrils, swallowing, or yawning. However, a diver may be unable to clear the ears because of the anatomic variability of the eustachian tube, inflammation due to sinusitis, a viral infection, or other upper aerodigestive dysfunction. Without pressure equalization, either the eardrum ruptures, allowing air or water in to equalize the pressure, or blood vessel leakage occurs with rupture, which will equalize the pressure.[3] As little as 100 mm Hg (5 fsw) can create a differential large enough to rupture the tympanic membrane.[7]

Symptoms of middle ear barotrauma are ear pain, pressure, and muffled hearing; if the tympanic membrane is ruptured, vertigo can occur because of the effects of cold water on the middle ear or tympanic membrane. Very rarely, a patient can present with unilateral facial nerve palsy. Treatment consists of decongestants, rest from diving, and follow-up otorhinolaryngologic evaluation. In general, these injuries are self-limited. Sometimes, however, if a patient needs hyperbaric treatments, pressure equalization (PE) tubes must be placed or myringotomies must be performed. Any form of tympanic membrane rupture, PE tube placement, or myringotomy would therefore act as a contraindication to any form of diving in which water comes in direct contact with the tympanic membrane.

Alternobaric Facial Palsy

Another side effect of middle ear barotrauma is alternobaric facial palsy, which consists of unilateral facial nerve palsy, ataxia, vertigo, nausea, and vomiting after diving. Symptoms mimic those of AGE; however, the mechanism is elevated middle ear pressure pressing against the facial nerve and causing an ischemic neuropraxia.[7] Alternobaric palsy is also seen in divers who fly after diving, travelers flying at high altitude in unpressurized airplanes, and people who experience explosive decompression in flight.[7] Although uncomfortable, the symptoms usually resolve on their own in minutes once middle ear pressures equilibrate.

Reverse Middle Ear Barotrauma

Reverse middle ear barotrauma or "squeeze" is similar to middle ear squeeze but has to do with increased pressure in the middle ear pushing *outward* on the tympanic membrane. It is often due to eustachian tube obstruction and often occurs on *ascent*. The symptoms are similar to those of middle ear "squeeze," but reverse squeeze can rupture the round window as well.

Inner Ear Barotrauma

The inner ear is a complicated and delicate organ, and any diver complaining of hearing loss, vertigo, or ear pain might have inner ear barotrauma (IEBT). Although less common than middle ear squeeze, IEBT has a significantly higher morbidity because it often involves damage to the cochleovestibular organs of the ear. Separating the middle ear from the inner ear are the thin membranes of the round and oval windows, damage to which may cause a leakage of fluid from the inner to the middle ear. IEBT can occur in a diver because of difficulties with equalization during a dive. Performing a vigorous Valsalva maneuver or attempting to clear the ears on descent can cause a sudden change in pressure of the inner ear and damage to the round window. Symptoms can be quite significant; they include extreme dizziness, vertigo, nausea, and vomiting. The patient might also present with visual changes such as nystagmus, ataxia, and hearing loss. IEBT is considered an emergency and mandates *immediate* otolaryngologic evaluation.

Alternobaric Vertigo

Alternobaric vertigo is the result of difficulties that occur on *ascent* because of differences in pressure between the two middle ear spaces. This difference in turn causes asymmetrical stimulation of each vestibular organ, leading to vertigo. Symptoms are severe nausea and vomiting as well as transient hearing loss, and the patient reports abrupt relief with clearing of the ears or redescent.

Sinus Barotrauma

Sinus barotrauma (sinus squeeze) is the second most common disorder among divers. It manifests as sinus pain, pressure, and bleeding from sinuses but is significantly less common than middle ear barotrauma, affecting only 1% of divers.[6] Symptoms are sinus pain on descent and bloody nasal discharge on ascent.[3] Treatment consists of decongestants, anti-inflammatory agents, and rest from diving.

Pulmonary Barotraumas/Pulmonary Over-Pressurization Syndromes

Arterial Gas Embolism

AGE, the most lethal result of pulmonary barotrauma, is second only to drowning as the most common cause of death in recreational divers.[4] Considered an example of a pulmonary over-pressurization syndrome (POPS), AGE occurs when a diver resurfaces too rapidly while holding the breath. Ascending too fast without breathing out allows the rapidly expanding gases in the lungs to build up, stretching the lung. Without exhalation, the buildup of pressure overwhelms the lung parenchyma, which can rupture. Rupture of lung parenchyma allows gas into the lung interstitium and creates a pathway for bubbles to embolize to the brain. Sadly, this disorder is often seen in new or inexperienced divers who panic at depth and shoot to the surface without remembering to breathe slowly or complete their decompression stops.

The symptoms are usually dramatic and typically begin as a loss of consciousness immediately or within minutes of a diver's resurfacing. Death is not uncommon in affected divers. Although arterial emboli can travel anywhere, they are most deadly when they travel to the coronary or cerebral circulations. An air embolism that travels to the brain (cerebral artery gas embolism [CAGE]) manifests much like a stroke, resulting in headache, confusion, agitation, paralysis, severe vertigo, or sudden loss of consciousness. Air embolism can also block blood flow through the coronary circulation, heart, and large arteries, leading to shock, dysrhythmias, and death.

Definitive treatment for AGE consists of administration of high-flow oxygen on the site with immediate consultation for hyperbaric recompression. It is important for EPs to remember that an AGE can occur in as little as 2 to 4 feet of water (70-80 mm Hg) or during breath-hold diving when a diver takes a breath from another diver's tank—unlike DCS, which usually occurs only after deep diving.[8]

Pneumothorax

Pneumothorax is another severe and potentially life-threatening kind of pulmonary over-pressure syndrome. It can occur during a rapid ascent with breath-holding that causes a rupture of the pulmonary parenchyma. The rupture allows bubbles and gas into the pleural space and can place pressure on the lung itself. Symptoms vary greatly, depending on how much air enters the pleural space, how much of the lung collapses, and the patient's baseline lung function. They can range from dyspnea to shock and life-threatening cardiac arrest. The most common symptoms are sharp chest pain, shortness of breath, and, occasionally, a dry hacking cough that begins suddenly. Pain may also be felt in the shoulder, neck, or abdomen. Treatment is immediate administration of high-flow oxygen and emergency medical evaluation to determine the need for needle decompression and/or tube thoracostomy.

Pneumomediastinum/Mediastinal Emphysema

Pneumomediastinum occurs when alveolar rupture allows gas to enter the mediastinum through the perivascular sheath, causing chest and neck pain, shortness of breath, difficulty swallowing, and auditory crepitus that is appreciated with auscultation (*Hamman's sign*). Treatment is observation and diagnosis is made through chest radiograph and physical examination. Recompression is usually not necessary. Immediate high-flow oxygen may speed the resorption of gases in severe cases.

Subcutaneous Emphysema

Similar to pneumomediastinum, subcutaneous emphysema is due to alveolar rupture causing release of gas into the tissues that can track up into the neck and under the skin. Symptoms are palpable crepitus, a sensation of fullness in the chest, possible alteration of voice, and occasional dysphagia. Treatment consists of observation and administration of oxygen, and diagnosis is made through chest radiography and physical examination. Recompression is not usually necessary.

Tips and Tricks

- Inner ear barotrauma requires IMMEDIATE referral to an otolaryngologist.
- Difficulty in ascent + Severe vertigo + Abrupt relief with descent=Alternobaric vertigo.
- Sudden, severe neurologic symptoms upon resurfacing are assumed to be caused by arterial gas embolism until proven otherwise!

Other Barotrauma

Gastrointestinal Barotrauma

The stomach and intestine are both air-filled areas of the body and, although rarely affected, are also susceptible to barotrauma. Specifically, gas expansion occurring on ascent can cause symptoms of nausea, belching, flatulence, mild stomach pain, and reflux. Symptoms usually resolve fairly quickly after the diver resurfaces.

Tooth Barotrauma

Small air pockets can exist in teeth and are therefore susceptible to barotrauma (*barodontalgia*). The air can be due to cavity formation from tooth decay, or small amounts of air present after amalgam instillation, or other recent dental procedures. Most people experience pain only on ascent, but tooth fractures have been known to occur. Decompressions as mild as those experienced during commercial air flight pressurization (8000 ft or 0.75 ATA) are enough to cause these symptoms. The patient with barodontalgia should be referred for dental evaluation and treatment.

DECOMPRESSION SICKNESS

Decompression sickness is a type of DCI that usually occurs after diving at deeper depths (versus AGE, which can occur at shallow depths). DCS is due to the effects of bubble formation under increased pressure, by which tissues become more highly permeated with inspired inert gases. Also called "the bends," DCS can cause a spectrum of symptoms. Diagnosis can be very difficult because divers may complain of only mild to moderate symptoms, which they tend to ignore and attribute to other causes. Often, a diver complains, "I just don't feel right," or has limb pains without a history of trauma that he or she assumes are just muscular or due to overexertion during the dive. In general, symptoms rarely develop while the diver is in the water. The keys to diagnosing DCS

BOX 132-3

Diagnosis of Decompression Sickness (DCS)

Suspect DCS in all water-associated complaints.

Obtain a thorough dive history.

Know the risk factors for DCS.

Pinpoint exactly when symptoms began (before, during, or after dive):

- The median time to onset of DCS symptoms is within 30 minutes of ascent, with 90% of all cases presenting within the first 24 hours.[6]
- The longer the delay of symptom onset, the less likely the symptoms are due to DCS.

injuries are (1) timing of symptom onset (before, during, or after a dive), (2) knowing the dive-related risk factors for DCS, and (3) having a low threshold for suspicion of DCS in the first place (Box 132-3).

Decompression sickness is usually divided into two types according to the severity of illness and the location of symptoms. Some texts also refer to a third class of DCS (DCS type III), but it is not universally accepted and is still somewhat controversial. In reality, symptoms of DCS overlap because divers can present with both types of DCS at the same time. The important thing to remember is that treatment is usually the same for both types—recompression with hyperbaric oxygen.

■ Type I ("Mild" Symptoms)

Type I DCS describes "mild" symptoms such as joint pains, dermatologic manifestations, and lymphatics-associated swelling and edema, all of which are due to the effects of gas bubbles in the tissues (Box 132-4). The most common symptom of DCS, *pain* at the site of bubble formation (autochthonous bubbles), is thought to be due to the greater negative pressure that exists in joint spaces.[9] Pain is most often seen in the shoulders or knees but can appear in any joint, including the wrist, elbows, hips, or ankles. The pain is usually gradual in onset, aching in nature, and varies from mild to extreme in intensity but usually gets worse with time. Divers can also have brief, mild pains in their extremities ("niggles") that resolve within minutes. Usually, limb pain affects the upper extremities three times more often than the lower extremities, and distribution is often asymmetrical.[10] Caisson workers, however, are affected more often in their lower limbs.[4] One authority makes the point that DCS type I usually involves pain distal to the axilla or groin, whereas DCS type II usually involves areas proximal to these locations.[7]

Dermatologic manifestations of DCI ("skin bends") can have several manifestations. A diver can experience pure itching alone (without rash) in localized or

BOX 132-4

Type I Decompression Sickness (DCS)

Musculoskeletal Pain ("Limb Bends")

- Most common manifestation of DCS.
- Dull, aching pain often in the shoulder or elbow.
- Pain occurs both at rest and with movement (unlike in trauma).
- No evidence of joint inflammation on examination.
- Occurs within 24 hours of resurfacing (but almost never in the first 15 minutes).

Cutaneous DCS ("Skin Bends")

- Most common symptoms are itching and pruritus (self-resolving).
- Cutis marmorata (mottled appearance of skin); patient needs recompression!
- Peau d'orange (rindlike skin seen on truncal area).
- "Fleas" (formication-like symptoms of insects on skin).

Lymphatic Effects/Edema

- Swelling in the soft tissues or in areas of lymph nodes.
- Usually localized.
- Very uncommon.

Definitive Treatment

- *Definitive treatment is recompression.*
- All patients require oxygen. Remember to consult a hyperbaric medicine specialist *early* if the patient is being brought from a dive accident.

Adapted from Bove AA, Davis J: Bove and Davis' Diving Medicine, 4th ed. Philadelphia, WB Saunders, 2004; and reference 4.

generalized areas of the arms, legs, face, or trunk ("fleas"). This form is commonly thought to follow dry dives, appears shortly after resurfacing, and lasts only a few minutes to a few hours.[11] Other dermatologic manifestations of DCS are mottling (cutis marmorata) and rindlike skin (peau d'orange).

Least often seen are lymphatic effects of DCS type 1. In 2% of patients, DCS can manifest as localized lymphadenopathy due to bubble formation at the involved site or as a localized soft tissue swelling that usually resolves by itself.

■ Type II ("Severe" Symptoms)

Type II DCS causes more severe symptoms that have a high risk of leading to major disability or death. They consist of important cardiopulmonary, neurologic, and inner ear manifestations (Box 132-5). All patients with type II DCS manifestations require emergency hyperbaric recompression and immediate

BOX 132-5

Type II Decompression Sickness (DCS)

This condition is associated with a higher risk of permanent disability or death than Type I DCS.

Pulmonary DCS ("Chokes")

- Persistent, dry, nonproductive cough.
- Substernal, pleuritic chest pain.
- Seen more with high-altitude DCS and in tunnel and caisson workers.

Neurologic DCS

- Represents 60%-70% of DCS injuries.
- Spinal cord affected 3 times more often than the cerebrum.
- Seen more often in recreational divers.
- Symptoms occur minutes to hours after ascent:
  Tingling in trunk
  Progressive numbness and paresthesias
  Ascending motor weakness
  Bowel/bladder incontinence
  Severe cases can rarely manifest as loss of consciousness/paraplegia (although this usually represents arterial gas embolism)
  Memory impairment, aphasias, visual disturbances, personality changes

Vestibular DCS ("Staggers")

- Dizziness, nausea, vomiting, nystagmus, hearing loss, tinnitus.
- Not common in recreational divers.
- Confused with middle ear barotraumas.

Definitive Treatment

- Recompression.

medical evaluation. In general, recreational divers experience more neurologic symptoms, pulmonary barotrauma, and AGE than commercial or naval divers. The reasons are not only that commercial and naval divers are more experienced but also that they usually have decompression chambers on the boat deck or close by when they dive. On the other hand, commercial and naval divers experience more DCS type I pain and joint problems than recreational divers.[6]

Neurologic Decompression Sickness

Neurologic symptoms of DCS II include headache, loss of consciousness, seizures, personality changes, ataxia, progressive paresthesias, and paralysis. They occur within minutes to hours of ascent. A diver with spinal cord involvement (spinal DCS) can present with abdominal pain, urinary retention, incontinence, and pelvic or back pain. Pulmonary effects can often occur as well.

Tips and Tricks

- Limb pain due to decompression sickness (DCS) usually persists even at rest, whereas the pain of a traumatic injury often improves with rest or nonuse.
- Resolution of pain at a joint when an inflated blood pressure cuff is applied to it is a strong indicator of DCS at that site.
- The neurologic examination of the injured diver is best performed with the patient out of the stretcher or bed, to unmask any neurologic deficits.
- Diving injuries are much more common in recreational divers than in professional or naval divers.
- Abdominal pain may be an early signal of spinal cord injury in DCS.

Pulmonary Decompression Sickness

One form of potentially lethal decompression sickness occurs when a large number of bubbles enters the lungs and prevents gas exchange, thereby causing chest pain, cough, shortness of breath, sore throat, and wheezing ("chokes").

Vestibular Decompression Sickness

Divers with severe vertigo, ear pain, or nystagmus are also considered to have type II DCS ("staggers"). Typical symptoms are severe nausea, vomiting, and vestibular problems.

Neurologic Examination

The importance of performing a thorough neurologic examination with the patient out of the bed cannot be overstated. Many neurologic symptoms are missed when a neurologic examination is performed in a patient lying on a gurney. Unless obvious neurologic deficit is noted, many dive-injured patients do not realize that they have an injury and are surprised to discover during the examination that they have some level of deficit. However, if an obvious neurologic problem exists, *hyperbaric consultation should never be delayed to allow completion of a thorough neurologic examination*. If "hard" neurologic symptoms are observed, the patient needs immediate hyperbaric oxygen recompression (see Box 132-10).

The examination should begin with an evaluation of the diver's mental status and should include evaluations of balance and coordination, sensory testing, deep tendon reflexes, and both fine and gross motor skills. In general, it is a good idea to have a preprinted neurologic examination form that contains a list of key questions to ask any patient presenting with a suspected dive injury. Performing the examination in the same way with every patient enables the EP to maximize diagnosis and treatment as well as to standardize findings (Box 132-6).

BOX 132-6

ED Diagnostic Workup for the Dive-Injured Patient

Laboratory Tests

Basic laboratory evaluation should include the following tests:

- Complete blood count
- Measurement of serum electrolytes: magnesium, phosphorous, and calcium
- Oxygen saturation measurement

If patient has altered mental status, add the following tests:

- Urine and blood toxicologic tests with acetylsalicylic acid/acetaminophen and ethanol levels
- Arterial blood gas measurements, including a carboxyhemoglobin level (to look for alveolar-arterial gradient suggestive of embolism and to rule out carbon monoxide poisoning)

Imaging

The following evaluations are needed for suspicion of pulmonary barotrauma:

- Chest radiograph (to rule out pneumothorax, pneumomediastinum, and subcutaneous emphysema)
- Computed tomography of the chest (to look for blebs, small pneumothoraces, and other pulmonary problems)

BOX 132-7

Prehospital Treatment and Air Evacuation Instructions for Dive-Injured Patients

1. Maintain ABCs of resuscitation (airway, breathing, circulation) and evaluate serum glucose level with diabetic monitor (e.g., ACCU-CHEK), if possible.
2. Use Advanced Cardiac Life Support (ACLS) protocol to stabilize the patient.
3. Administer high-flow oxygen.
4. Establish intravenous (IV) lines and begin IV fluids.
5. Keep patient flat; *avoid* the Trendelenburg position. If aspiration is a risk, lay the patient on the left side or in the right lateral position.
6. If air evacuation is being used, ensure that the cabin of the airplane is *pressurized* or have the pilot fly at altitudes *below* 1000 feet.
7. Transport the patient with all of his/her gear (it will have to be examined later).
8. Remember that the other members of the diving party might also need transport and evaluation for decompression sickness; they should accompany the patient to the ED.
9. Alert the consultant dive physician/hyperbaric center ahead of time that a dive injury has occurred and the patient is being brought to the ED.

Treatment

■ PREHOSPITAL TREATMENT AND AIR EVACUATION FROM THE SITE

Prehospital treatment of a dive injury is similar to that given in the ED; however, for any diver being transported for a dive injury, pre-hospital hyperbarics should already have been consulted in order to minimize delay to needed decompression (Box 132-7).

■ ED EVALUATION AND TREATMENT

ED treatment of the dive-injured patient must follow a standard approach. In addition to the ordering of routine laboratory tests and administration of oxygen to those patients who need it, obtaining a thorough history is critical to diagnosis and direction of treatment (Boxes 132-8 and 132-9). Whether the EP rarely or routinely sees dive injuries, it is best, as previously recommended, to have a readily accessible list of questions to ask while interviewing the diver and all observers involved in a dive injury.

■ DIVER'S ALERT NETWORK

Many EDs have no associated hyperbaric facilities nearby or have no plan set up to deal with divers who need hyperbaric medicine consultations. The Diver's Alert Network (DAN) is available worldwide 24 hours a day, is able to put callers in direct communication with a diving physician to help guide patient treatment and arrange transfer, and can provide up-to-date listings of hyperbaric chambers worldwide (Boxes 132-10 and 132-11).

Disposition

Although each patient is unique, many patients with decompression illness can be safely discharged from the hospital. However, any diver with any serious DCS symptoms or barotrauma should be admitted. All patients who have experienced decompression or embolic dive injuries should be transferred immediately to the closest emergency hyperbaric facility. The EP should always err on the side of safety and caution: Any patient who has any concerning symptoms should not leave the ED until the EP has at least dis-

BOX 132-8

Dive History Interview: Questions to Ask the Dive-Injured Patient

1. Where did the dive occur (ocean, river, pool, etc.)?
2. When was the onset of the patient's symptoms (upon resurfacing, during descent or ascent, at the bottom)?
3. How deep did the patient go? Was he/she using a dive computer?
4. Was the patient intoxicated or dehydrated?
5. What type of diving equipment was used? What type of gas was used (compressed air, mixed gas, enriched air)? What was the source of the gas?
6. Did the patient perform heavy exertion or work during the dive?
7. Did the dive approach or exceed decompression limits?
8. How many dives did the patient perform, and what were the depth, bottom time, total time, and resurface intervals for all dives in the previous days preceding symptoms (the dive "profiles")?
9. Were decompression stops missed? Was in-water recompression attempted?
10. What was the time delay from the last dive to the time of air travel?
11. Has the patient experienced ear or sinus problems on this dive or in the past?
12. Does the patient have any other medical problems? What medications does the patient take?
13. Was oxygen given at the scene?

BOX 132-9

Emergency Medical Treatment for the Dive-Injured Patient

ABCs—First Priority

- Airway, breathing, circulation.
- Primary and secondary surveys.
- Intubate if necessary.
- Perform needle decompression/tube thoracostomy as needed for pneumothorax.

Immediate Administration of High-Flow Oxygen (100%)

- Creates a gradient for washout of inert gases (nitrogen, carbon monoxide, etc.).
- Perfuses ischemic tissues.

Hydration

- Decompression sickness can cause dehydration and decrease the circulating blood volume.
- Hydrate with intravenous fluids until urine output is 1-2 mL/min.

Position of Patient

- Keep the patient lying flat.
- Avoid the Trendelenburg position. (Previously thought to reduce cerebral embolization, the head-down position is now known to increase cerebral edema and intracranial pressure and facilitate coronary gas embolization.)

History and Physical Examination

- Perform a thorough history and physical examination.
- Ensure that the neurologic examination is performed with the patient out of the bed.

Definitive Treatment—Recompression with Hyperbaric Oxygen in a Chamber

- Counteracts new bubble formation.
- Reduces existing bubble size.
- Creates a strong gradient for nitrogen washout.
- Improves oxygenation of ischemic tissues.
- Reduces edema.
- Inhibits leukocyte-mediated reperfusion injuries.

BOX 132-9

Emergency Medical Treatment for the Dive-Injured Patient–cont'd

Other Therapies

Steroids

- Not routinely used.
- Considered only for certain spinal cord injuries (consult with neurosurgical and hyperbaric medicine specialists before using).
- Can worsen oxygen toxicity.

Prostaglandins and Platelet Inhibitors

- Nonsteroid anti-inflammatory drugs, aspirin.
- Inhibit inflammation and platelet formation.
- As pain medicines, should be used with caution because pain is an indicator of decompression sickness.

Heparin

- Not routinely used.
- Has been used for severe, life-threatening cerebral emboli.

BOX 132-10

Indications for Immediate Hyperbaric/Dive Medicine Consultation

A hyperbaric/dive medicine consultation should be sought immediately for the patient exhibiting:

- ANY alteration in mental status
- ANY neurologic deficit
- ANY loss of consciousness
- ANY worsening of symptoms during evaluation
- ANY worrisome sign, symptom, or behavior
- ANY limb pain after ascent from depth

PATIENT TEACHING TIPS

Diving Tips

- Avoid diving when you have any symptoms of upper respiratory infection.
- Do not drink alcohol and dive.
- Never dive alone.
- Do not dive and fly within the same 24 hours.
- Do not "push" dive tables or dive profiles.
- Do not perform heavy exercise before or after diving.
- Drink plenty of fluids, and get plenty of rest.
- Plan deeper dives at the beginning of a dive trip.

Follow-Up Tips

- If discharged after medical evaluation, the patient should be told to return *at any time* for worse, new, or nonimproving symptoms.

BOX 132-11

Using the Divers Alert Network (DAN) Emergency Hotline: +1-919-684-8111 or +1-919-684-4DAN (Collect)

DAN handles all diving emergencies, including decompression sickness, arterial gas embolism, pulmonary barotrauma, and other serious diving-related injuries. DAN's medical staff is on call 24 hours a day, 365 days a year. The phones are answered at the switchboard of Duke University Medical Center.

When calling, *tell the operator you have a diving emergency:*

- You will be connected directly with DAN or the operator will have someone call you back.
- DAN's staff may make immediate recommendations or call you back after making arrangements with a local physician or the DAN Regional Coordinator.
- DAN's staff may ask you to wait by the phone while they make arrangements, which may take 30 minutes or longer; this delay should not put the diver in any greater danger.

If the situation is life-threatening:

- Arrange to transport the diver immediately to the nearest local medical facility for immediate stabilization and assessment.
- Call DAN TravelAssist at 1-800-326-3822 at that time for consultation with the local medical provider.

cussed the case with a hyperbaric physician consultant. As already discussed, if no known hyperbaric facilities are located in the area, the Divers Alert Network (DAN) should be contacted.

Flying after Diving

One of the most important factors in the disposition of the diver is how long he or she should wait to fly after diving. This issue is also affected by whether a diver has had an injury and, if so, how severe the symptoms were. Forgetting to counsel the ED patient about flying limitations has the potential for injury to the patient and possible subsequent litigation for the EP.

A number of varying guidelines about flying are available, but for the most part, it is not a good idea to fly within 12 to 24 hours of diving. In general, a person should delay flying for at least 12 hours after diving if he or she has accumulated less than 2 hours of total dive time in the preceding 48 hours. A person who participates in multiple-day, unlimited diving should delay flying for at least 18 to 24 hours after the last dive. A diver who has had decompression sickness should be advised not to fly for 3 to 7 days after treatment for DCS type I, or for 4 weeks after recompression therapy for DCS type II.

REFERENCES

1. Divers Alert Network: DAN Report on Decompression Illness, Diving Fatalities and Project Dive Exploration, 2006. Available at www.diversalertnetwork.org/
2. Piantadosi C, Brown S: Diving medicine and near drowning. In Hall JB, Schmidt GA, Wood LDH (eds): Principles of Critical Care, 3rd ed. New York, McGraw-Hill, 2005.
3. Bookspan J: Diving and Hyperbaric Medicine Review for Physicians. Kensington, MD, Undersea and Hyperbaric Medical Society, 2000.
4. U.S. Department of Commerce: NOAA Navy Diving Manual, 5th ed. Flagstaff, AZ, Best Publishing Company, 2005.
5. Shockley L: Scuba diving and dysbarism. In Hockberger RM, Walls JA, Marx RS (eds): Rosen's Emergency Medicine, 6th ed. St. Louis, CV Mosby, 2006.
6. Bove AA, Davis J: Bove and Davis' Diving Medicine, 4th ed. Philadelphia, WB Saunders, 2004.
7. Merritt D: Mending the Bends—Assessment, Management, and Recompression Therapy. Flagstaff, AZ, Best Publishing Company, 2006.
8. Rutkowski D: UHMS Diving Accident and Management Manual. Undersea and Hyperbaric Medical Society. Flagstaff, AZ, Best Publishing Company, 1989.
9. Chandy D, Weinhouse G: Complications of scuba diving. UpToDate, 2007. Available at www.uptodate.com/
10. Barratt M, Harch P, Van Meter K: Decompression illness in divers: A review of the literature. Neurologist 2002;8: 186-202.
11. The London Diving Chamber and Hyperbarics website. Available at www.londondivingchamber.co.uk/

Chapter **133**

Submersion Injuries

Mohammed Abu Aish and Niranjan Kissoon

KEY POINTS
Drowning is the second leading cause of death in children.
Inadequate supervision is the main risk factor for drowning in children.
Some patients who present with relatively mild symptoms can deteriorate.
Cardiopulmonary resuscitation at the scene is the most important factor in improving survival.
Most drowning victims should be transferred to the ED regardless of the initial appearance at the scene.
Resuscitation efforts should be initiated in most patients.
The degree of hypoxia determines the outcome.
Cervical spine immobilization is unnecessary unless trauma is suspected.
Asymptomatic patients should be observed for at least 4 to 6 hours before being discharged.

Scope

Submersion simply means going under water. Different terms like drowning and near drowning were used in the past and created confusion, especially in reporting. In 2002 the World Congress on Drowning adopted a uniform definition of drowning, which is "the process resulting in primary respiratory impairment from submersion/immersion in a liquid medium."[1] Further expert opinions and recommendations from this organization are summarized in the drowning website (www.drowning.nl); the final report was published in 2004 as *Handbook on Drowning*.

Drowning is an important cause of childhood morbidity and mortality. It is the second leading cause of death in children 1 to 14 years, and the third leading cause of death in those younger than 1 year as well as people 15 to 34 years old. Drowning is estimated to kill 500,000 people every year worldwide. Eighty per cent of these episodes take place in low-income countries and low-income groups. About 80% of drowning episodes are deemed preventable.[2,3]

It is difficult to estimate the exact incidence of drowning events because there is no single registry and many deaths go unreported. In 2002, deaths from drowning in the United States accounted by the Centers for Disease and Control and Prevention (CDC) was 3447, of which 1019 victims were children (1-18 years). This number represents 10.6% of all accidental deaths in this age group (Table 133-1).

Table 133-1 UNINTENTIONAL INJURY DEATHS IN THE UNITED STATES, 2002

Age Group (yr)	Deaths from Other Causes	Drowning Deaths	Percentage
<1	946	63	6.7
1-4	1641	454	27.7
5-9	1176	159	13.5
10-14	1542	162	10.5
15-24	15,412	629	4.1
25-34	12,569	433	3.4
35-44	16,710	526	3.1
45-54	14,675	374	2.5
55-64	8345	212	2.5
65+	33,641	415	1.2

Adapted from National Center for Injury Prevention and Control, Centers for Disease Control and Prevention. Web-based Injury Statistics Query and Reporting System [database]. Available at http://www.cdc.gov/ncipc/wisgars/.

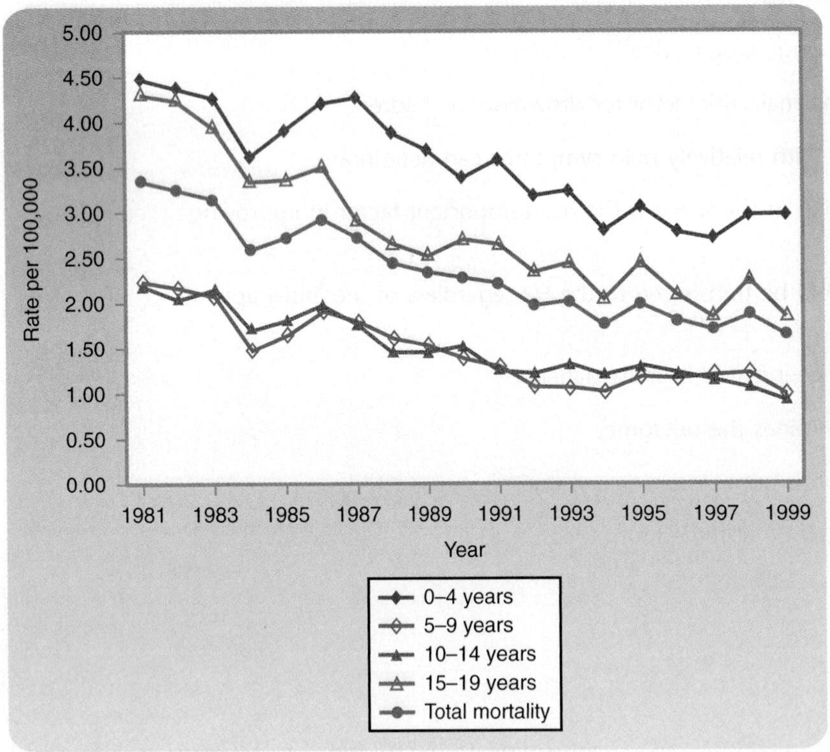
5.00
4.50
4.00
3.50
3.00
2.50
2.00
1.50
1.00
0.50
0.00
Rate per 100,000
1981
1983
1985
1987
1989
1991
1993
1995
1997
1999
Year
0–4 years
5–9 years
10–14 years
15–19 years
Total mortality

FIGURE 133-1 Drowning mortality by age group. (Adapted from Ibsen L, Koch T: Submersion and asphyxial injury. Crit Care Med 2002;11[Suppl]:S402-S408.)

Death is more common in black persons, almost double the rates in white persons older than 4 years. Overall rates of drowning have dropped in all age groups, probably reflecting improved awareness, use of preventive measures, and other factors (Fig. 133-1).

Most toddlers who drown do so in their own home pools, half within the first 6 months of pool exposure. Most infants drown in bathtubs, whereas adults and older children drown in fresh water. Fencing of private pools reduces the risk of drowning.[4]

Pathophysiology

Injuries from drowning result mainly from asphyxia leading to hypoxic-ischemic damage to vital organs.

The event starts with panic because of air hunger and, eventually, aspiration of fluids into the hypopharynx. Reflex laryngospasm occurs and is usually brief before the victim aspirates large amounts of fluids into the lungs. Further aspiration can occur if the victim vomits and aspirates gastric contents. Aspiration is the end result of all drownings, and the old terminology of dry and wet drowning should not be used.[5,6]

The *diving reflex* is one of the unique phenomena described in children. Due to vagal stimulation when the face is exposed to cold water (<10°C), this reflex is characterized by apnea, bradycardia, and intense vasoconstriction. It is presumed that this reflex can play a neuroprotective role in cold water submersions. Hypothermia slows cerebral metabolism when the body has time to cool before aspiration or with extremely cold water submersions and may also contribute to neuroprotection.

Hypoxia is the end result of drowning. If severe, it leads to multiorgan damage affecting mainly the lungs, heart, and brain. Brain injury is the major cause of death and disability from drowning.

Changes in intravascular volume, hematocrit, and electrolyte concentration due to aspiration are usually mild and not clinically significant. Both salt water and fresh water cause lung injury. The effect of tonicity on the intravascular compartment is minimal.[7,8]

ORGAN INVOLVEMENT

Lungs

Fluid aspiration causes surfactant loss, noncardiogenic pulmonary edema, and acute respiratory distress syndrome. Some patients present with mild respiratory symptoms and then deteriorate rapidly because of gradual leakage and influx of proteins and fluids into the alveoli as a result of surfactant loss and the effect of acidosis and hypoxia on the respiratory membranes.

Central Nervous System

Hypoxia and acidosis lead to neuronal injury, resulting in diffuse brain edema and eventually increased intracranial pressure.

Cardiac System

Arrhythmias due to hypoxia and hypothermia are common. Sinus bradycardia, atrial fibrillation, and, less commonly, asystole and ventricular fibrillation are reported to occur in patients who drown.

Other Organs

Acute tubular necrosis is uncommon. Significant electrolyte abnormalities are not seen unless drowning occurs in exceptionally concentrated media. Coagulopathy can occur with hypoxia but is uncommon.

Risk Factors

Inadequate supervision is the main risk factor for drowning in children.

PATIENT TEACHING TIPS

PREVENTION OF DROWNING

- Fencing private pools; use of personal flotation devices
- Minimizing alcohol and substance abuse in beaches and around water
- Counseling of new parents about importance of supervision as well as safety of bathtubs, buckets, and other vessels
- Educating parents about safe bathing of babies: A child can drown in just a few inches of water
- Recommending cardiopulmonary resuscitation courses for public
- Recommending swimming lessons with adult supervision

Other risk factors are as follows:

- Inability to swim
- Hyperventilation
- Trauma
- Use of alcohol and illicit drugs
- Intoxications
- Hypoglycemia
- Seizures
- Arrhythmias (long QT syndromes)
- Child abuse and neglect
- Vascular events (cerebrovascular accident, myocardial infarction)

Identifying these factors helps prevent a second incident if the victim survived.

Signs and Symptoms

Presentation varies from no symptoms to death. The severity of hypoxemia determines the presentation. Cervical spine injuries are uncommon with drowning unless trauma is suspected (e.g., diving and boating accidents, falls, and crashes).

Respiratory signs and symptoms can vary in severity. They result from aspiration of fluids and loss of surfactant, and they include shortness of breath, wheezing (rhonchi, crepitations), pulmonary edema, and acute respiratory distress syndrome. Symptoms of aspiration pneumonia may develop later from aspiration infected material.

Respiratory symptoms can be present early or can develop over time. It is important to observe drowned patients even if they are asymptomatic.

Neurologic symptoms also vary. Patients can be asymptomatic, irritable, confused, or comatose at initial presentation, depending on the degree of hypoxic insult to the brain. Deterioration can occur in asymptomatic patients and patients with mild symptoms. Seizures can also occur. Symptoms and signs of increased intracranial pressures appear late and are due to hypoxic brain injury.

Table 133-2 EXAMPLES OF SCORES PREDICTING OUTCOMES IN DROWNING PATIENTS

Score	Prognostic Factors	Interpretation
Orlowski*	Age <3 yrs Submersion time >5 min Time to initial resuscitation (no attempts for >10 min) Level of consciousness (coma) Acidosis (pH<7.10) in ED	2 or fewer factors predicted a 90% chance of full recovery; 3 or more predicted only a 5% chance of full recovery
Christensen†	Initial ED physical findings (apnea, coma) Need for cardiopulmonary resuscitation in the ED (pH < 7.0)	93% overall accuracy in predicting intact survivors (score predicted poor outcome in 5 intact survivors)

*Orlowski JP: Prognostic factors in pediatric cases of drowning and near-drowning. JACEP 1979;8:176-179.
†Christenser DW, Jansen P, Perkin RM: Outcome and acute care hospital costs after warm water near drowning in children. Pediatrics 1997;99: 715-721.

Arrhythmias can also manifest early or late and further compromise the cardiorespiratory status. Hypoxia, acidosis, and hypothermia can lead to bradycardia, tachycardia, hypotension, hypertension, arrhythmias, and asystole.

Differential Diagnosis

Although the diagnosis of drowning is obvious, it is important to rule out medical conditions that may predispose a person to submersion as well as the possibility of child abuse (see earlier list of risk factors).

■ DIAGNOSTIC INVESTIGATIONS

Investigations are not as important on initial presentation as clinical assessment and emergency therapy. Chest radiograph findings can be normal initially even in symptomatic patients. However, pulmonary edema (localized or diffuse) and various degrees of atelectasis may be present on initial presentation. The initial chest radiography will also help check endotracheal and gastric tube positions.

Measurement of arterial blood gas concentrations may be useful in guiding resuscitation efforts and in adjusting ventilator settings but should not be used as the sole predictor of outcome.

Neuroimaging has no role in the acute management but becomes important later to rule out unrecognized brain disease or to confirm hypoxic brain changes.

When major trauma is suspected, further imaging is determined by the severity of suspected injuries (e.g., head and cervical spine computed tomography [CT], abdominal CT).

BOX 133-1

Factors that May Help Predict Outcome of Drowning

Age
Duration of submersion
Cardiopulmonary resuscitation at the scene
Hypothermia
Fixed dilated pupils
Cardiopulmonary resuscitation in the ED
Glasgow Coma Scale score
pH<7
Respiratory status
Neurologic status

Prognostic Factors

■ AT THE SCENE

Performance of cardiopulmonary resuscitation (CPR) at the scene is documented to improve survival in some cases, especially for cold water submersion. Generally, hypothermia is a poor prognostic sign unless the victim has fallen into an extremely cold water (<10°C) or undergone rapid cooling. Several case reports of survival of victims with such circumstances were attributed to a protective effect of cooling on the brain through slowing of cerebral metabolism. This finding has led some authorities to recommend continuing CPR for hypothermic victims while actively rewarming them before declaring them dead.[9]

■ IN THE ED

Many factors were suggested as predictors for bad outcome, but none of them alone were consistently reliable across studies. A combination of these factors to make clinical scores may be better in predicting outcome, but without high predictive value (Box 133-1 and Table 133-2).

Prognostic factors such as low Glasgow Coma Scale (GCS) score and ineffective respiratory efforts become more predictive after resuscitation and stabilization and hence may be more useful in the intensive care unit. Such scoring systems can be used in disasters as triage tools and to initiate discussion with families about likely prognosis but should not used to guide decisions about initiating CPR in drowning victims. Because no single prognostic factor is reliable in the immediate postsubmersion period, it is recommended to perform CPR for most submersion victims until a patient's condition is fully assessed.

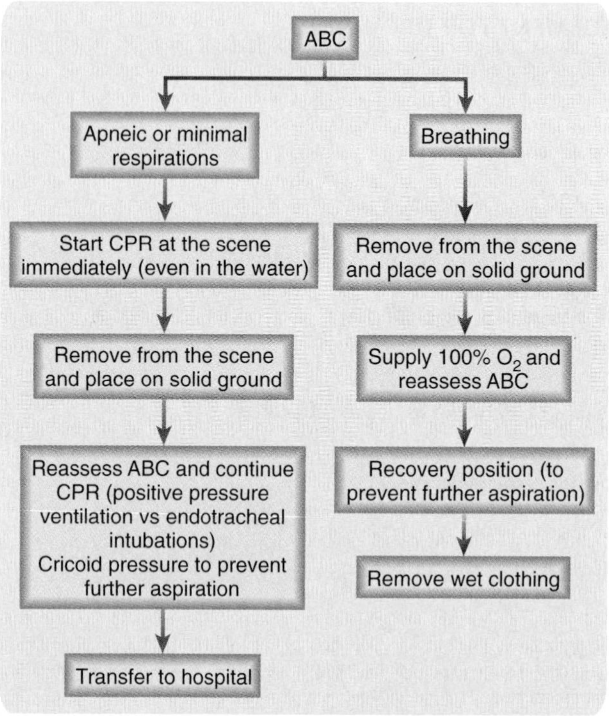
ABC
Apneic or minimal respirations
Breathing
Start CPR at the scene immediately (even in the water)
Remove from the scene and place on solid ground
Remove from the scene and place on solid ground
Supply 100% O_2 and reassess ABC
Reassess ABC and continue CPR (positive pressure ventilation vs endotracheal intubations) Cricoid pressure to prevent further aspiration
Recovery position (to prevent further aspiration)
Remove wet clothing
Transfer to hospital

FIGURE 133-2 Algorithm for prehospital treatment of drowning victims. ABC, airway-breathing-circulation (ABCs of resuscitation); CPR, cardiopulmonary resuscitation.

Documentation

Prehospital

- Patient demographics (age, sex, etc.)
- Description of the accident (rule out trauma, abuse, suicide)
- Nature of the fluid (temperature, level of cleanliness, etc)
- If drowning witnessed, estimated time of submersion
- Initial cardiorespiratory status
- Scene management (CPR, how long and by whom)
- Body temperature

Hospital

- Initial presentation (ABCDE; see Table 133-3)
- Cardiopulmonary resuscitation
- Glasgow Coma Scale score
- Temperature
- Other injuries (e.g., cervical spine)
- pH
- Serum glucose level
- Chest radiograph

Treatment

PREHOSPITAL TREATMENT

CPR at the scene is the most important initial step. It can be started even if the victim is still in the water. After the airway is secured and oxygenation and ventilation are ensured, the patient should be transferred to the nearest hospital. Further management at the scene depends on availability of experienced personnel in Advanced Life Support (Fig. 133-2). Most drowning victims should be transferred to an ED regardless of the initial appearance at the scene. Exceptions are obvious rigor mortis, lividity, and decay.

Emergency personnel dealing with a drowning victim should avoid the following:
- Maneuvers to try to get water out of the lung (i.e., abdominal thrusts).
- Cervical spine immobilization if there is no suspicion of trauma.
- Rough handling of a hypothermic patient (may induce arrhythmias).
- Delay in transport to hospital after optimizing respirations.

IN THE ED

The main aims of treatment of a drowning victim in the ED are to avoid further hypoxia and restore effective ventilation and circulation (Table 133-3). ED personnel should assume the triad of hypoxia, acidosis, and hypothermia to be present in every drowning victim until proven otherwise. The need for cervical spine immobilization should be assessed, but in atraumatic drowning, immobilization is not mandatory. Vomiting occurs frequently, so early airway protection should be considered in distressed patients.

Airway

- For breathing patients, keep FIO_2 value at 1.0.
- For patients in respiratory distress, there should be a low threshold for intubation. Treatment may start with positive-pressure and positive end-expiratory pressure (PEEP) ventilation with nasal cannula or a mask.
- Indications for intubation are as follows: unconscious patient, respiratory insufficiency, high O_2 requirements to keep the oxygen saturation value higher than 90% and/or PO_2 higher than 60 to 90 mm Hg.

Breathing

- Oxygen saturation value and respiratory status should be checked. The onset of respiratory distress can be delayed and progressive.
- In cases of trauma, life-threatening disorders (e.g., hemothorax, pneumothorax) should be ruled out.

Table 133-3 SUMMARY OF ED MANAGEMENT FOR DROWNING

Aspect	Intervention
Airway	100% O_2 (mask) Bag-valve mask Positive end-expiratory pressure ventilation Endotracheal intubation
Breathing	Respiratory status O_2 status Signs of trauma
Circulation	Cardiac status (pulses, perfusion, blood pressure) Intravenous access (intraosseous if intravenous route difficult) Monitor Blood work Glucometer Fluid management (crystalloid boluses of 20 mL/kg as needed) to correct hypovolemia and acidosis Manage arrhythmias Inotropic agents (e.g., dobutamine for cardiogenic shock)
Disability	Glasgow Coma Scale score Focal signs Manage seizures
Exposure	Temperature External injuries Active rewarming if temperature <30°C Passive rewarming if temperature >30°C to aim for 30° to 33°C

■ Circulation

- Vascular access should be established, either intravenous or intraosseous.
- Arrhythmia, which can be the inciting event or a complication of hypoxia and hypothermia, should be ruled out.
- A blood specimen should be collected for complete blood count and crossmatch as well as measurements of arterial blood gas, serum electrolyte, liver enzyme, and serum glucose levels.
- Blood levels of drugs alcohol, and cardiac enzymes may be measured in selected cases.
- Both hypoglycemia and hyperglycemia should be avoided to prevent further brain damage.
- Internal hemorrhage should be considered if a significant drop in hematocrit is noted.
- Cardiorespiratory instability can result from significant myocardial hypoxia, worsening acidosis, and hypothermia.
- Fluid management and inotropic support are important to reverse depressed myocardial function, shock, and acidosis.

■ Disability

- The Glasgow Coma Scale score should be documented at baseline; it can be used to follow the patient's status over time, because all drowning victims are at risk of worsening brain edema.
- Seizures can occur with hypoxia, focal lesions, and worsening edema.

■ Exposure

- The patient's whole body should be exposed to check for injuries that might suggest trauma, abuse, suicide, and so on.
- Rectal temperatures should be recorded.
- Active rewarming should be started if the temperature is less than 30°C and continued until it reaches between 30° and 33°C.
- Hyperthermia should be avoided because it can worsen brain injury; active rewarming beyond a body temperature of 35°C should not be attempted.

Management of Hypothermia

Hypothermia is core body temperature less than 35°C. Depending on the temperature, hypothermia may be mild, moderate, or severe (Box 133-2). This condition should be anticipated and treated in drowning victims (Box 133-3). Notably, standard thermometers may not accurately measure low temperatures.

Important considerations when rewarming hypothermia patient are as follows:

1. Rewarming the extremities rather than trunk can lead to further drop in core body temperature because of vasodilation of peripheral vessels and flow of cold blood centrally.
2. Rewarming should not aim for normal body temperature, which would worsen the brain damage. Active rewarming should be performed only until the patient is mildly hypothermic, at which point warm blankets are sufficient.

BOX 133-2

Classification of Hypothermia

Mild Hypothermia (32-35° C)

Depressed mental status and shivering may be the only manifestations of hypothermia. Passive rewarming is usually sufficient.

Moderate Hypothermia (28-32° C)

Thermoregulatory mechanisms (shivering) fail. An unresponsive state ensues at temperatures below 30° C, and cyanosis, tissue edema, and rigidity develop.

Respirations and pulses may be difficult to detect. An electrocardiogram may show a J (Osborn) wave (a distinctive deflection occurring at the QRS-ST junction). Atrial fibrillation and other dysrhythmias may occur.

Active internal and/or active external rewarming should be used.

Severe Hypothermia (<28° C)

The patient may appear dead with no detectable vital signs and with dilated, unresponsive pupils. Ventricular fibrillation (spontaneous or induced by mechanical stimuli), extreme bradycardia, and asystole may occur.

Active internal and/or external rewarming should be used.

Adapted from Danzl DF, Pozos RS: Accidental hypothermia. N Engl J Med 1994;331:1756-1760.

3. ED personnel should be alert for cardiac arrhythmias. The myocardium may not respond to drugs and electrical stimulation in a patient with a low core body temperature. Aggressive fluid management is needed for hypothermic victims undergoing rewarming, because of vasodilation.

Further Management

■ OXYGENATION AND VENTILATION

Because of lung injury, surfactant loss, and pulmonary edema, some patients will need higher end-expiratory pressures for optimal oxygenation. As PEEP is increased, blood pressures and cardiac output should be monitored, because they can be compromised by high end-expiratory pressure. Intensive monitoring of cardiac status, respiratory status, neurologic status, and complications such as aspiration pneumonia is indicated.

Some reports recommend inducing hypothermia in drowning victims after restoring spontaneous circulation as a neuroprotective therapy. Further studies of this therapy are needed, especially of its use in children.

BOX 133-3

Rewarming Techniques

Passive Rewarming
- Remove wet, cold clothing.
- Use warm blankets to insulate the patient.

Active Rewarming

For active external rewarming:
- Hot packs
- Heat lamps
- Forced-air external rewarmers

For active internal rewarming:
- Warmed humidified oxygen (via mask or endotracheal tube)
- Warmed intravenous fluid (shortest possible length of intravenous tubing must be used to ensure efficacy of this method)
- Warm saline lavage (gastric, peritoneal, rectal, and mediastinal)
- Peritoneal dialysis
- Extracorporeal membrane rewarming techniques
- Extracorporeal membrane oxygenation/warming and cardiopulmonary bypass

Adapted from Zuckerbraun N, Saladino R: Pediatric drowning: Current management strategies for immediate care. Clin Pediatr Emerg Med 2005;6:49-56.

There is no evidence to support prophylactic antibiotics, corticosteroids, barbiturate therapy, or intracranial pressure monitoring in patients who have drowned.

Disposition

Patients who are completely asymptomatic in the emergency room and whose arterial blood gas levels and chest radiograph findings are normal can be discharged after being observed for 6 hours.

Patients should be admitted to the hospital if they demonstrate any of the following features:
- Adverse symptoms
- Increasing O_2 requirement
- Submersion for more than 1 minute
- Hypothermia
- Any abnormalities in acid-base balance, serum electrolyte levels, or hematocrit.

REFERENCES

1. Bierens JJ (ed): Handbook on Drowning: Prevention, Rescue, Treatment. Amsterdam, Springer, 2004. Available online at: http://www.drowning.nl/
2. National Center for Injury Prevention and Control, Centers for Disease Control and Prevention: Web-based Injury Statistics Query and Reporting System [database]. Available at: http://www.cdc.gov/ncipc/wisqars/

3. Zuckerbraun N, Saladino R: Pediatric drowning: Current management strategies for immediate care. Clin Pediatr Emerg Med 2005;6:49-56.
4. Brenner RA, Trumble AC, Smith GS, et al: Where children drown, United States, 1995. Pediatrics 2001;108:85-89.
5. Modell JH, Bellefleur M, Davis JH: Drowning without aspiration: Is this an appropriate diagnosis? J Forensic Sci 1999;44:1119-1123.
6. Olshaker J: Submersion. Emerg Med Clin North Am 2004;22:357-367, viii.
7. Bierens JJ, Knape JT, Gelissen HP: Drowning. Curr Opin Crit Care 2002;8:578286.
8. Ibsen L, Koch T: Submersion and asphyxial injury. Crit Care Med 2002;11(Suppl):S402-S408.
9. Modell J, Idris A, Pineda J, Silverstein J: Survival after prolonged submersion in freshwater in Florida. Chest 2004;125:1948-1951.

Chapter 134

Acute Radiation Emergencies

David A. Caro

KEY POINTS

Establish the nature and extent of the event.
Determine the level of response necessary.
Prepare for decontamination.
Implement medical triage, assessment, and treatment.

Radiation emergencies present a complex problem for the entire medical system. Multiple agencies are involved when a radiation disaster has been declared. Importantly, emergency medical personnel will be at the forefront of decision-making when a radiologic event occurs.

The first order of business is to *establish the veracity and type of the event.* The information received from the field is essential in planning a response in the ED and the hospital. Important information to get from the field, if possible, is listed in Box 134-1. The more information that can be gleaned by the field report, the better prepared the response by the hospital will be. Hospital planners should expect the information from the scene to change as the initial chaos is controlled and more accurate analysis occurs.

The next step is to *prepare the hospital* to receive these patients.[1,2] The appropriate level of disaster management response should be determined, and the hospital's disaster management plan activated accordingly.[3] Hospital disaster managers, including the radiation officer of the hospital, should be contacted quickly because multiple preparatory events must occur at the same time. Access to the hospital must immediately be limited and controlled.[1,2] An incident command center must be set up serve as the central site for information processing and decision-making. Separate decontamination and initial receiving areas must be arranged.[1] Because of the environmental impact of radioactive material, this area must be equipped with containment equipment; such an area has usually been identified by hospital disaster planners well before the event occurs. The ED must be prepared to receive patients with all triage levels, and emergency bed space must be rearranged to provide care. Importantly, *standard personal protective equipment (PPE) that is sufficient to protect the emergency personnel treating these patients in the decontamination area and in the ED must be used.*[2,4] Guidelines for personal protective equipment are available at the Oak Ridge Associated Universities website (www.orau.gov/reacts). No health care workers who have adhered to these guidelines have become contaminated from handling a radiation-contaminated patient.[3]

The EP must determine whether the patient is contaminated or irradiated.[5] The patient with external contamination has radioactive material on his or her body; this material is an alpha- or beta-emitter that must be washed off and will not penetrate clothing to any appreciable extent. Significant radiation injuries can occur from irradiation with or without contamination (contact of the substance directly with human tissue) (Box 134-2).

The *contaminated* patient will have been exposed to radioactive material that could still be on or inside

BOX 134-1

Important Information to Obtain from the Field for a Patient with Radiation Injury

- *The type of material involved.* Different types of radioactive material can expose patients in different ways. Important specifics include the type of radioactivity (α-, β-, γ-emitters, or neutrino)*; the form it was in when exposure occurred (did it make contact with the patient, was it aerosolized, did the patient ingest it, etc.); and what other injuries occurred with the exposure.
- The form of *decontamination* occurring at the scene.
- The *types of injuries* being seen.
- *The number of patients* needing evaluation.

BOX 134-2

Classification of Radiation Exposure

Contamination: The patient has particulate radioactive material on or in the body, and therefore experiences ongoing irradiation because of its apposition to the skin, open wounds, the gastrointestinal tract, or the respiratory tract.

Irradiation: The patient has been exposed but does not have radioactive material on the body. Such a patient is not "radioactive."

BOX 134-3

Radiologic Decontamination Principles

Remove the patient's clothing (removes 95% of contaminants).[2,5,7]

Wash the patient with soap, water, and washcloth. Repeat if needed. Use a Geiger counter to confirm whether radioactivity remains.[1-3,5,15]

Health care workers should wear standard personal protective equipment (PPE) while in the hospital.[2,5,9,16]

The decontamination team should wear N95 masks and Tyvek gowns along with boots and gloves.[2,5,9,16]

Ideally, decontamination should occur at a site away from the hospital, preferably upwind from a separate patient receiving area.[1]

the patient's body. *Irradiated patients without contamination* have been exposed but do not have radioactive material on them. Irradiated patients are not "radioactive." A radioactivity meter (most commonly a Geiger counter is the initial screening tool) and history should be used to determine the difference (Box 134-3).

Patients should be analyzed for thermal burns and impact injuries from the blast, even if it requires transport to the operating room for surgery. A routine history should be obtained and a standard physical examination performed. If decontamination can occur immediately, it should begin with skin washing, with all of the water effluent contained; this most likely will occur in a decontamination shower with a containment tank. If contamination remains, further washing is needed. ED personnel should check under the patient's fingernails and in the patient's hair; if contamination remains, the nails should be clipped and the hair cut.

The EP can *use the presenting physical findings to help predict the patient's course and subsequent treatment,* regardless of whether the patient has been contaminated or irradiated. In a mass casualty, these signs are used to divide patients into those expected to die quickly, those who might have had a significant exposure and will have severe effects, and those who can be watched for now and evaluated after the more seriously injured have been evaluated and treated.[4,5] Acute radiation syndrome (ARS) usually occurs after a significant exposure (higher than 0.7 Gy), and the severity of illness correlates with the amount of exposure.[4,6,7] Three ARS syndromes have been described: bone marrow, gastrointestinal, and neurologic (Box 134-4).[8]

Laboratory values that are helpful in symptomatic patients include a complete blood count with a differential count.[1,4] It is valuable to have a baseline white blood cell count and platelet count early in the course of care. Specifically, calculate the absolute lymphocyte count (ALC) and the absolute neutrophil count to indicate outcomes:

- An ALC at 48 hours after exposure that is less than 300 cells/μL is a critically low value and a prognosticator of poor outcome. It would encourage heroic measures, such as bone marrow transplantation.
- An ALC that is higher than 1200 cells/μL signifies a nonlethal radiation dose.
- An ALC between 300 and 1200 cells/μL indicates that the patient might have received a lethal dose.

PRIORITY ACTIONS

- Establish the nature and extent of the event.
- Determine the level of response necessary.
- Prepare for decontamination.
- Implement medical triage, assessment, and treatment.

BOX 134-4

Estimating Severity of Radiation Dosage for Rapid Triage

- Initially, use the presence or absence of vomiting to determine whether a significant exposure has occurred.[5]
- *Significant irradiation usually results in vomiting.* If vomiting has not occurred within 4 hours of an exposure, a patient can safely be referred for further evaluation in 24 to 72 hours.[5]
- In a patient who is vomiting, a complete blood count (CBC) should be performed at baseline. At 48 hours, a second CBC is performed. An absolute lymphocyte count (ALC)<1200 cells/μL might signal a significant exposure; an ALC<300 cells/μL at 48 hours indicates a lethal exposure.[1,3,4,7,8,14]
- Chromosomal analysis can also help identify patients with significant exposure, but is usually done after initial stabilization.
- Skin manifestations early in the course indicate at least moderate exposure.
- Neurologic signs are ominous. The patient should be treated and managed expectantly (pain control, comfort care measures).
- Severe radiation exposure: A radiation dose >10 Gy is uniformly lethal and is accompanied by severe gastrointestinal damage, pneumonitis, altered mental status, and cognitive dysfunction.[3]

Such a patient should be monitored for hematopoietic depression, among other organ system failures. A 50% drop in ALC within 24 hours also signals a significant radiation dose.[3,7]

In exposed patients, blood should also be held in case HLA typing is needed. Recommendations are to obtain this blood along with the initial complete blood count specimen, in case the absolute ALC does fall dramatically and blood products are required.

Symptomatic care should be started early, including antiemetics for nausea and vomiting, intravenous fluids for dehydration, and wound care as needed.

Patients with potential gastrointestinal ingestion of radioactive materials should be decontaminated by nasogastric lavage if the ingestion was recent (1-2 hours). Other options are the use of aluminum- or magnesium-based antacids in an attempt to bind radioactive material and help its elimination. Patients who have inhaled a radioactive material might require bronchoalveolar lavage, if resources are not overwhelmed.[5]

Treatment options are available if the radioactive contaminant is known and antidotes exist.[5] Poison control centers can provide help with the identification of potential antidotes. Importantly, with a nuclear detonation or a nuclear reactor incident, radioactive iodine is a specific concern.[2,5,9] Specific treatment might include potassium iodide (KI) for radioactive iodine contamination.[1,4,7,10,11] The decision to treat with radioactive iodine will probably involve multiple agencies, including the U.S. Centers for Disease Control and Prevention, the U.S. Food and Drug Administration, and the Department for Homeland Security, but might require quick action to treat as many victims or potentially exposed people as possible.[2,10,11] Of note, "KI should be administered before or immediately coincident with passage of the radioactive cloud, though KI may still have a substantial protective effect even if taken 3 or 4 hours after exposure"[11] (Table 134-1).

FACTS AND FORMULAS

$SI = \frac{SV}{BSA}$

- Standard personal protective equipment is sufficient to protect the emergency personnel treating these patients in the decontamination area and in the ED.
- Use the presenting physical findings to predict the patient's course and subsequent treatment.
- Significant irradiation typically results in vomiting.
- An absolute lymphocyte count at 48 hours after exposure of less than 300 cells/μL is a critically low value and prognosticates a poor outcome.

Other therapies are diethylenetriamine pentaacetic acid (DTPA) for exposure to americium, plutonium, and other transuranic compounds[12]; oral Prussian blue for gastrointestinal contamination with cesium and thallium[4,7,13]; and intravenous Ca- and Zn-DTPA, which are chelating agents used for gastrointestinal contamination with plutonium, americium, and curium (Table 134-2).[4,13]

Treatment at this point is usually transferred to other hospital services. Standard treatment should be continued for injuries incurred during the event as well as complications that arise. The ALC, absolute neutrophil count, and complete blood count values help treatment teams determine whether bone marrow transplantation is necessary. It is just as important to recognize when further resources will be unable to change a patient's course and comfort care measures should begin. These decisions become critical when resources are overwhelmed in the setting of a major event. Narcotic pain control, antiemetics, and other comfort care measures then become essential to humane treatment (Box 134-5).

Importantly, preparations must be made to deal with an influx of people who are concerned that they might have been exposed and demand evaluation.[3,5] Estimates made on the basis of prior radiologic accidents state that approximately 8 to 10 patients who arrive at the hospital for evaluation have no significant exposure for each one who needs treatment, although one source estimates that up to 100 to 500

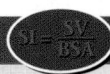

Table 134-1 THRESHOLD THYROID RADIOACTIVE EXPOSURES AND RECOMMENDED DOSE OF POTASSIUM IODIDE (KI) FOR DIFFERENT RISK GROUPS

Risk Group	Predicted Thyroid Exposure (cGy)	KI Dose (mg)	No. of 130-mg Tablets	No. of 65-mg Tablets
Adults >40 yrs	≥50	130	1	2
Adults <18 through 40 yrs	≥10	130	1	2
Pregnant or lactating women	≥5	130	1	2
Adolescents (>12 to 18 yrs)	≥5	65	½	1
Children >3 yrs through 12 yrs	≥5	65	½	1
Children >1 mo through 3 yrs	≥5	32	¼	½
Newborn through 1 mo	≥5	16	⅛	¼

From Potassium Iodide as a Thyroid Blocking Agent in Radiation Emergencies. Washington, DC, U.S. Department of Health and Human Services Food and Drug Administration Center for Drug Evaluation and Research (CDER), 2001.

Table 134-2 SPECIFIC THERAPIES FOR INTERNAL RADIATION CONTAMINATION

Radionuclide	Therapy
Tritium iodine-125 or -131	Dilution: Force fluids Blocking: Saturated solution of potassium iodide (SSKI) or potassium iodide Mobilization: Antithyroid drugs
Cesium-134 or -137	Decrease absorption Blocking: Strontium lactate Displacement: Oral phosphate Mobilization: Ammonium chloride or parathyroid extract
Plutonium and other transuranic compounds	Chelating: Zinc or calcium diethylenetriamine pentaacetatic acid (Zn-DTPA or Ca-DTPA; investigational)
Unknown ingestion	Reduce absorption: consider emetics, lavage, charcoal, laxatives

Modified from Koenig KL, Goans RE, Hatchett RJ, et al: Medical treatment of radiological casualties: Current concepts. Ann Emerg Med 2005;45:643-652.

BOX 134-5

What Is the Proper Disposition of Radiation-Exposed Patients after Stabilization?

- Asymptomatic patients: reassurance, information, and defined follow-up with the primary care doctor.[5]
- Mildly symptomatic patients: symptom control, baseline complete blood count (CBC), and 24- to 48-hour follow-up arranged before discharge.[1,4]
- Moderately symptomatic patients (continued emesis, lightheadedness, etc.): symptom control, a baseline CBC, and observation. Consideration should be given to empirical antibiotic therapy as well as colony-stimulating factor therapy. Dehydration from gastrointestinal fluid losses is a significant possibility.[4,6,7]
- Severely symptomatic patients (syncope; hypoxia, disseminated intravascular coagulation, shock): as much care as the situation will allow. In the setting of a mass casualty, these patients are managed expectantly, i.e., with comfort measures. With an isolated case, empirical antibiotic therapy, colon-stimulating factor therapy, transfusions, and search for bone marrow donors might ensue in a heroic attempt to save the patient's life.[4,7]

people concerned about exposure will present for each one who needs treatment.[14] Rapid, professional triage must occur so as to not delay care of those who have truly been exposed. Reassurance, informational handouts for patients, and recommendation for defined follow-up help improve the psychological care of patients who are not at risk but remain concerned. The psychological impact of a nuclear event can be overwhelming.[1] Early, consistent public information announcements can help inform the community of the nature and severity of the event as well as actions to take to protect themselves and their families. Box 134-6 lists sources of further information.

Summary

Acute radiation emergencies are thankfully infrequent but significantly strain the resources of any hospital system. Basic disaster principles apply with some significant caveats, including containment of

BOX 134-6

Suggested Readings and Websites

Readings

Generic Procedures for Medical Response during a Nuclear or Radiological Emergency. Vienna, International Atomic Energy Agency, 2005.

Military Medical Operations, Armed Forces Radiobiology Research Institute: Medical Management of Radiological Casualties Handbook, 2nd ed. Bethesda, MD, Armed Forces Radiobiology Research Institute, 2003.

Koenig KL, Goans RE, Hatchett RJ, et al: Medical treatment of radiological casualties: Current concepts. Ann Emerg Med 2005;45:643-652.

Waselenko JK, MacVittie TJ, Blakely WF, et al: Medical management of the acute radiation syndrome: Recommendations of the Strategic National Stockpile Radiation Working Group. Ann Intern Med 2004;140:1037-1051.

Champlin RE, Kastenberg WE, Gale RP: Radiation accidents and nuclear energy: Medical consequences and therapy. Ann Intern Med 1988;109:730-744.

Radiological Terrorism Emergency Management Pocket Guide for Clinicians. Washington, DC, Centers for Disease Control and Prevention, 2005.

Websites

Centers for Disease Control radiation homepage: http://www.bt.cdc.gov/radiation/

International Atomic Energy Agency: http://www.iaea.org/

Oak Ridge Institute for Science and Education: http://orise.orau.gov/reacts/

U.S. Armed Forces Radiological Research Institute: http://www.afrri.usuhs.mil/

U.S. Environmental Protection Agency: http://www.epa.gov/radiation/index.html/

U.S. Nuclear Regulatory Commission: http://www.nrc.gov/

any water or clothing that is contaminated and institution of certain treatments if the radioactive source is known.

Finally, in a radiologic exposure, it is important to remember to activate the emergency response plan designed to respond to such events.

REFERENCES

1. Smith JM, Spano MA: Interim Guidelines for Hospital Response to Mass Casualties from a Radiological Incident. Washington, DC, Centers for Disease Control and Prevention, 2003.
2. Generic Procedures for Medical Response during a Nuclear or Radiological Emergency. Vienna, International Atomic Energy Agency, 2005.
3. Waselenko JK, MacVittie TJ, Blakely WF, et al: Medical management of the acute radiation syndrome: Recommendations of the Strategic National Stockpile Radiation Working Group. Ann Intern Med 2004;140:1037-1051.
4. Koenig KL, Goans RE, Hatchett RJ, et al: Medical treatment of radiological casualties: Current concepts. Ann Emerg Med 2005;45:643-652.
5. Department of Homeland Security Working Group on Radiological Dispersal Device (RDD) Preparedness Medical Preparedness and Response Sub-Group: Radiological Medical Countermeasures. Washington, DC, Centers for Disease Control and Prevention, 2003.
6. Centers for Disease Control and Prevention: Acute Radiation Syndrome: A Fact Sheet for Physicians. Available at: http://www.bt.cdc.gov/radiation/
7. Military Medical Operations, Armed Forces Radiobiology Research Institute: Medical Management of Radiological Casualties Handbook, 2nd ed. Bethesda, MD, Armed Forces Radiobiology Research Institute, 2003.
8. Champlin RE, Kastenberg WE, Gale RP: Radiation accidents and nuclear energy: Medical consequences and therapy. Ann Intern Med 1988;109:730-744.
9. Centers for Disease Control and Prevention; Casualty Management after a Deliberate Release of Radioactive Material. Available at: http://www.bt.cdc.gov/radiation/
10. Potassium Iodide (KI). Washington, DC, Centers for Disease Control and Prevention, 2003.
11. Guidance: Potassium Iodide as a Thyroid Blocking Agent in Radiation Emergencies. U.S. Department of Health and Human Services Food and Drug Administration Center for Drug Evaluation and Research (CDER). December 2001.
12. DTPA. Washington, DC, Centers for Disease Control and Prevention, 2005.
13. Prussian blue. Washington, DC, Centers for Disease Control and Prevention, 2005.
14. Technology Assessment and Roadmap for the Emergency Radiation Dose Assessment Program. U.S. Department of Homeland Security, June 2005.
15. Centers for Disease Control and Prevention: Casualty Management after Detonation of a Nuclear Weapon in an Urban Area. Washington, DC, Centers for Disease Control and Prevention, 2005.
16. Radiological Terrorism: Emergency Management Pocket Guide for Clinicians. Centers for Disease Control and Prevention, 2005.

Chapter 135

Smoke Inhalation

Thomas Kunisaki and Andy Godwin

KEY POINTS

The majority (50%-80%) of deaths due to fire are caused by smoke inhalation rather than burns.
Smoke is a combination of heated particles and gases. The type of material that is burning, along with the amount of heat and oxygen, determines smoke composition.
Carbon monoxide is implicated in more smoke inhalation deaths than any other single compound.
In addition to inhalation of toxins, smoke inhalation can cause upper airway burns and pulmonary parenchymal injury.
The mainstay of treatment comprises ventilatory support, early intubation, optimized fluid resuscitation, pulmonary hygiene, and treatment for specific toxic inhalations.

Deaths from fires are most often caused by smoke inhalation.[1,2] Injury from smoke inhalation is from irritation, corrosion, and thermal injury of the airway and lung parenchyma as well as hypoxia and asphyxiation from toxic gases. The danger of toxic gases predominates. Smoke is a complex mixture of suspended small particles, fumes, and gases. As many as 400 toxic compounds have been demonstrated in the smoke of a house fire. Polyvinyl chloride, a component of many plastic goods, generates at least 75 different toxic products when burned, carbon monoxide being the most common fatal substance.[3,4]

Thermal inhalational injuries are usually localized to the upper airway. Irritant gases, depending on their water solubility, affect either the upper or lower airway. Highly water-soluble agents, such as ammonia, hydrogen chloride, and sulfur dioxide, predominantly affect the upper airway because their solubility rapidly causes adverse upper airway symptoms. Agents such as phosgene and nitrogen dioxide, which have low water solubility, create fewer immediate warning symptoms and so do more damage to the lower airway, that is, to the alveoli.[1] Phosgene, although originally manufactured as a weapon, is used in the manufacture of dyes, resins, and pesticides and is a product of the pyrolysis of chlorinated hydrocarbons (e.g., refrigerants). Nitrogen oxides are found in grain silos, engine exhaust, and gases commonly released from nitric or nitrous acid but also from burning of nitrocellulose and byproducts of explosions. Delayed onset of pulmonary edema is the classic presentation for these poorly water-soluble agents.

Asphyxiation further compounds the problem in smoke inhalation. Not only is there lack of oxygen in the smoke-filled environment, causing simple asphyxiation (i.e., the displacement of oxygen) but also certain byproducts of combustion, like cyanide and carbon monoxide, cause cellular asphyxiation at the level of the cytochrome oxidase system, specifically at the cytochrome aa_3, in the mitochondria. Cyanide is a common product of the combustion of wool, silk, plastics, and other synthetic polymers.

The toxic dose depends on the intensity and duration of the exposure. Despite the excellent warning properties of most smoke, the victim can quickly be overcome by the smoke if he or she is prevented from egress because of the condition of the building or is incapacitated by an injury.

Common, Dangerous Consequences of Smoke Inhalation

■ CARBON MONOXIDE

Carbon monoxide (CO) is a colorless, odorless, nonirritating gas produced by the incomplete combustion of hydrocarbons and petroleum distillates. In addition to smoke inhalation in fires, sources of carbon monoxide are kerosene or gas stoves, portable fuel generators, automobile exhaust, cigarette smoking, and the metabolism of methylene chloride, a solvent used for stripping paint from furniture.

■ Toxicity

One of the major mechanisms of the toxicity of carbon monoxide is that it avidly binds to hemoglobin, approximately 250 times as strongly as oxygen, resulting in the reduction of oxyhemoglobin. Furthermore, the impairment of oxygen delivery is exacerbated by displacement of the oxygen dissociation curve to the left. The impairment may also inhibit the cytochrome oxidase, further impairing cellular function. Carbon monoxide is known to bind to myoglobin as well, a feature that may contribute to any hemodynamic instability from impairment of myocardial contractility. Areas of the brain that are highly sensitive to hypoxia appear to sustain the most injury. Fetal hemoglobin is more sensitive to the binding of CO, with levels estimated to be approximately 10% higher than maternal level, and a half-life that is five times longer.

The carboxyhemoglobin will gradually dissociate, a process that can be enhanced with oxygen. In room air, the half-life of carboxyhemoglobin is approximately 4 to 6 hours. With 100% oxygen, the half-life decreases to approximately 90 minutes, and in the setting of hyperbaric oxygen therapy, it is about 20 minutes. The U.S. Occupational Safety and Health Administration (OSHA) has defined toxic levels of carbon monoxide in the workplace. Clinically, carboxyhemoglobin levels have not correlated with the severity of exposure, but it is generally accepted that levels around 25% to 30% is the threshold to consider hyperbaric oxygen therapy if available.

■ Evaluation

The main organ of concern with carbon monoxide poisoning is the brain. The clinical picture encompasses the entire spectrum of neurologic symptoms, from soft neurologic signs such as subtle memory deficits, to seizure, stroke, and coma. Persistent neurologic complications include stroke, neuropsychiatric sequelae, parkinsonism, and persistent vegetative state.

The pulse oximetry reading may be falsely elevated. The reason is that both oxyhemoglobin and carboxyhemoglobin absorb light in the same range. Because the pulse oximeter calibrates the oxygen saturation by the ratio of light absorption between the infrared and red wavelengths, the ratio remains the same, even with carboxyhemoglobin. Arterial blood gas (ABG) measurement with co-oximetry must be performed if information about acid-base disturbance is needed. However, if the only information needed is the carboxyhemoglobin level, a venous blood gas measurement is adequate because it seems to correlate with the ABG value. Although a carboxyhemoglobin level does not always correlate with the clinical severity of exposure, it will help in determining whether carboxyhemoglobin is a contributing factor.

■ Treatment

The treatment of carbon monoxide poisoning is administration of oxygen, preferably 100% and traditionally by occlusive mask. The use of hyperbaric oxygen remains controversial, but is classic, with case series arguing for a benefit.[5]

■ METHEMOGLOBIN

Methemoglobin is the oxidized form of hemoglobin that can occur from smoke inhalation.[6] Many chemicals, from many sources, can oxidize hemoglobin. In addition to a source in smoke from fires, chemical and munitions workers are at higher risk for acquiring methemoglobinemia. Children are susceptible to methemoglobinemia from well water contaminated with nitrates. Amyl nitrite and butyl nitrite are often abused recreationally, including for sexual enhancement. Oxides of nitrogen as products of combustion make smoke inhalation victims prime targets for methemoglobinemia.

■ Toxicity and Evaluation

Methemoglobin is incapable of carrying oxygen. Cyanosis becomes apparent when levels reach approximately 15% to 20%, although the patient may exhibit only mild distress. The cyanosis is characteristically noted in the periphery—nails, lips, and ears. Symptoms may range from mild headache and dizziness to seizure, coma, and hemodynamic instability. Levels of methemoglobin greater than 70% are usually considered lethal. As seen with carbon monoxide, the pulse oximeter reading is unreliable, inaccurately reflecting the level of hypoxia, but for a different reason. As the methemoglobin level rises, the ratio of light absorption between the red and infrared wavelengths approaches 1. The co-oximetry machine interprets a ratio of 1 as 85%. As the methemoglobin levels approach a dangerous high level, the pulse oximetry may give a falsely elevated value. Blood with methemoglobinemia greater than 15% is classically described as "chocolate brown."

The differential diagnosis is limited, including toxicants that cause cellular hypoxia, such as cyanide and hydrogen sulfide, as well as a condition known as sulfhemoglobinemia.

■ Treatment

Under normal physiologic condition, the methemoglobin is reduced by the enzyme system known as NAD (nicotinamide adenine dinucleotide) methemoglobin reductase. A minor pathway than can be induced and that is dependent on an intact glucose-6-phosphate dehydrogenase (G6PD) enzyme system, is the NADPH (NAD phosphate) methemoglobin reductase system. This latter system can be induced with the administration of a reducing agent called methylene blue. Thus, one contraindication for its use is in individuals with G6PD deficiency. In excess dosage, methylene blue may worsen the methemoglobinemia and possibly cause hemolysis. Other therapeutic options, for patients in whom methylene blue is a contraindication, are exchange transfusion and hyperbaric oxygen therapy.

■ CYANIDE

Cyanide is a highly toxic chemical. Hydrogen cyanide, a common byproduct of the pyrolysis of wool, silk, and plastics, is presumed to be a major cause of fatality in structural fires. Cyanide salts still remain an important method of homicide and suicide. Cyanogenic compounds are used in plastic and adhesive manufacture, and as solvents. The compounds are classified as nitriles. Unique to these compounds is that they are metabolized to cyanide. Acetonitrile, which is used to remove artificial nail glue, has caused significant pediatric poisonings, including fatalities.

■ Toxicity and Evaluation

By blocking the cytochrome aa_3 site on the electron transport system, located on the inner membrane of the mitochondria, cyanide causes rapid cellular asphyxia. The hallmark of clinical presentation of cyanide poisoning is a rapid and profound neurologic, cardiovascular, and metabolic deterioration. Syncope, seizure, coma, cardiovascular collapse, respiratory failure, and death quickly ensue in the absence of intervention. Delays in clinical signs and symptoms may be seen if a nitrile is involved owing to the need for the product to be metabolized.

The diagnosis is generally based on the history and the rapid deterioration. A severe lactic metabolic acidosis is usually present. The classic bitter almond odor noted in cyanide ingestion is detected in only 40% to 60% of cases. Indirectly, a small arterial-venous oxygen saturation gap less than 10% may strongly suggest cyanide. Specific cyanide measurements in body fluids or tissues are generally difficult to obtain in a timely manner.[2]

■ Treatment

Supportive care for a cyanide-poisoned patient is paramount. Currently, the only available antidote in the United States is the cyanide antidote kit (Taylor Pharmaceuticals, Akorn, Decatur, IL), which consists of amyl nitrite pearls, and ampoules of 10% sodium nitrite and 25% sodium thiosulfate. The nitrite is given to generate a controlled methemoglobinemia, which pulls the cyanide off the cytochrome oxidase, allowing the mitochondria to resume its aerobic respiration. The rhodanase enzyme system in the liver then utilizes the sodium thiosulfate as a substrate to convert the cyanomethemoglobin to thiocyanate. The danger of using this kit empirically on a victim of smoke inhalation from a fire is that it may severely compromise the available oxygen-carrying capacity of the patient with a preexisting significant carboxyhemoglobinemia or methemoglobinemia. A new, promising antidote that has been used in Europe is hydroxycobalamin. This agent combines with cyanide to produce cyanocobalamin, which is vitamin B_{12}. Once approved for use in the United States, this agent may be safer to use empirically at the scene of a fire.[7]

■ HYDROGEN SULFIDE

Hydrogen sulfide is produced naturally by decaying organic matter and sulfur hot springs, as well as being a byproduct of industries (paper pulp factories, petroleum refineries, and in dehairing hides). These products have the characteristic "rotten egg" odor that is easily detectible at levels estimated to be as low as 0.13 parts per million (ppm).

■ Toxicity

The danger of hydrogen sulfide arises when its detection is blunted by "olfactory fatigue," during which levels can reach 100 to 150 ppm. With this scenario, a person remains in a potentially dangerous environment. At levels of approximately 50 to 100 ppm, hydrogen sulfide is an irritant gas, causing blepharospasm, burning sensation of the eyes, dermatitis, bronchospasm, and, potentially, laryngeal edema. Its mechanism of action is inhibition of the cytochrome oxidase system, much like cyanide. Because the major route of exposure to hydrogen sulfide is inhalation, its absorption is rapid. Victims often experience a "rapid knockdown."

■ Evaluation and Treatment

Severe exposure to hydrogen sulfide causes immediate cardiovascular collapse and respiratory arrest. The diagnosis is based on the history, the rapid clinical deterioration, evidence of cellular asphyxiation and airway irritation, and the odor of rotten eggs. Measurement of serum levels is not available. Sulfhemoglobinemia is one product of hydrogen sulfide exposure thought to contribute to the systemic asphyxiation. It can also contribute to the hemoglobinopathy, although it is considered rather stable, and no known antidote is available.

As with cyanide, supportive care is paramount. Theoretically, nitrites from the cyanide antidote kit are potential antidotes because of a similar mechanism of action. However, the evidence is limited as to the effectiveness of their use. Animal data and limited human case reports suggest that hyperbaric oxygen therapy may be of some benefit if initiated early after exposure.

Differential Diagnosis

As a means of better understanding this complex problem, dividing smoke inhalation injury into toxidromes (toxic syndromes) may be more helpful in identifying the clinical presentations that one may encounter. Aside from the potential of concomitant thermal injuries associated with structural fires, the major toxidromes involving smoke inhalation are from the irritant gases, asphyxiants, and hydrocarbons.

Irritant gases can be divided into highly water-soluble and poorly water-soluble agents. Moderately water-soluble gases, such as chlorine gas, behave more like the highly water-soluble agents, and thus are grouped in that category for the purpose of this discussion.

Highly water-soluble gases, such as ammonia, hydrochloric acid, and sulfur dioxide, are very irritating substances and thus have excellent warning properties. An individual exposed to a highly water-soluble gas immediately experiences irritation of any mucous membrane and the upper airway. The clinical presentation consists of tearing, oral burns, bronchospasm, and shortness of breath, which rapidly progress to hoarseness, stridor, and acute airway obstruction. In general, if the victim can be removed from the exposure, symptoms should gradually improve. However, in situations in which the victim is incapacitated or confined, or perhaps the environment of exposure is so vast, the outcome may be fatal. A prime example is the incident in Bhopal, India, where approximately 20,000 pounds of isocyanate leaked from a storage tank. By the time the leak was discovered, the fumes covered an area of approximately 5 square miles. More than 200,000 individuals became victims of this accident. Nearly 2000 people died.

On the other hand, a poorly water-soluble gas has very poor warning properties and so is able to travel farther into the pulmonary system, affecting the alveoli. Examples of this type of gas are nitrogen dioxide and phosgene. The hallmark of inhalation injuries with these gases is the delayed pulmonary edema.

The asphyxiant toxidromes can be divided in simple and systemic asphyxiants. As asphyxiants, these substances affect the availability or utilization of oxygen to the tissues. The gases are generally inert (e.g., carbon dioxide), but they may be flammable (e.g., methane), creating an additional hazard. Simple asphyxiants displace oxygen and thus create a hypoxic environment. Symptoms depend on the severity of hypoxia and duration of exposure, ranging from central nervous system depression (lethargy to coma) to hypoxic seizure, metabolic acidosis, and death. Because the mechanism is deoxygenated hemoglobin, cyanosis may be present.

Systemic asphyxiants impair the body's ability to utilize oxygen, interfering with either the transport of oxygen (e.g., methemoglobinemia) or the utilization of oxygen at a cellular level (e.g., cyanide). Toxicants like carbon monoxide impair both transport and utilization of oxygen.

Methemoglobin-forming compounds affect the ability of hemoglobin to bind oxygen, thus affecting oxygen transport. Examples of such compounds are sodium nitrite and nitrobenzene. Substances that impair oxygen utilization are agents such as cyanide and hydrogen sulfide. These agents inhibit the utilization of oxygen at the cytochrome oxidase (i.e., electron transport system), effectively forcing the cells to undergo anaerobic metabolism. Central nervous system symptoms from lethargy to coma, seizures, metabolic acidosis, hypotension, and cardiac arrhythmias are common presentations. Carbon monoxide is unique in that it not only interferes with oxygen transport and with the formation of carboxyhemoglobin but also impairs oxygen utilization at the cytochrome oxidase.

Whether the etiology is lack of oxygen transport or impairment of oxygen utilization, however, the end result is cellular hypoxia. Therefore, the clinical presentation is a multisystem derangement. In sig-

Tips and Tricks

- Administer high-flow oxygen by face mask immediately to a person who has inhaled smoke.
- Intubate any patient who is exhibiting respiratory distress, even if that distress is apparently mild at first. Airway edema can rapidly develop.
- Closely observe the patient who is coughing and has sputum tinged with soot, and be prepared for intubation.
- After assurance of airway control and oxygenation, evaluate for the possibility of carbon monoxide, cyanide, and methemoglobinemia. Presumptive treatment for cyanide toxicity may be required, whereas laboratory evaluation for carbon monoxide and methemoglobin is indicated when the patient has a significant inhalation.

nificant intoxication, seizure, coma, cardiovascular collapse, respiratory distress or failure, and metabolic acidosis are common presentation. Cyanosis may not always be present, especially if the agent is a cellular asphyxiant, because the problem is with utilization and not transport of oxygen. The classic example is seen with cyanide. The clinical picture of cyanosis due to methemoglobinemia is different from that of cyanosis due to deoxyhemoglobin and hypoxemia. In the former, the patient appears clinically less symptomatic and more stable.

Hydrocarbons (e.g., methane, butane) are simple asphyxiants, displacing oxygen and resulting in hypoxia. These agents also sensitize the myocardium and thus predispose the exposed individual to cardiac arrhythmias. Furthermore, some hydrocarbons are flammable, posing an explosive danger as well.[3]

Diagnosis

The diagnosis of smoke inhalation injury should be suspected in any victim of a fire. The physical examination will suggest the severity of exposure. In general, the victim's vital signs, pulse oximetry value, chest radiography findings, and results of a basic metabolic panel and arterial blood gas measurement with co-oximetry (carboxyhemoglobin, methemoglobin) will be helpful. It should be emphasized that if carboxyhemoglobinemia or methemoglobinemia is being considered, the pulse oximetry reading will be unreliable. Another specific test that should be considered is a blood cyanide measurement. If obtaining such a measurement is impractical, determining the arterial-venous oxygenation saturation or P_{O_2} difference will help in the clinical determination of whether cyanide is involved. The principle behind this theory is based on the mechanism of cyanide. Because the cells are unable to utilize oxygen, the oxygen content in the venous system should theoretically be higher than normal. An arterial-venous oxygen saturation difference of less than 10% is highly suggestive of cyanide toxicity.

PATIENT TEACHING TIPS

- Once you are discharged, you should not have trouble breathing and should have only minor, uncomfortable symptoms such as tiredness and mild nausea.
- Seek treatment immediately if it becomes difficult to breathe in any way. Return to the ED if any of the following symptoms develop: wheezing, trouble breathing, a continuous cough, an upset stomach, or vomiting.
- Call 911 if you have confusion, irritability, or unusual sleepiness.

Treatment

Any patient in whom smoke inhalation injury is suspected should be started on high-flow supplemental oxygen. Aggressive airway management, including early endotracheal intubation, is necessary because of the potential for rapid deterioration. Good supportive care is critical, and pulmonary care must be optimized through ventilatory strategies. Antidotes should be considered early in the course. If the victim is hemodynamically stable, hyperbaric oxygen therapy should be considered.

REFERENCES

1. Young CJ, Moss J: Smoke inhalation: Diagnosis and treatment. J Clin Anesth 1989;1:377-386.
2. Heimbach DM, Waeckerle JF: Inhalation injuries. Ann Emerg Med 1988;17:1316-1320.
3. Orzel RA: Toxicological aspects of fire smoke: Polymer pyrolysis and combustion. Occup Med 1993;8:414-429.
4. Zhu BL, Ishikawa T, Michiue T, et al: Influence of inhaling carbon monoxide-containing gas in fire fatalities—an investigation of forensic autopsy cases. Chudoku Kenkyu 2007;20:37-44.
5. Weaver LK, Hopkins RO, Chan KJ, et al: Hyperbaric oxygen for acute carbon monoxide poisoning. N Engl J Med 2002;347:1057-1067.
6. Hoffman RS, Sauter D: Methemoglobinemia resulting from smoke inhalation. Vet Hum Toxicol 1989;31:168-170.

Chapter 136

Chemical and Nuclear Agents

Rick G. Kulkarni

KEY POINTS

For patients exposed to nerve agents, atropine in 2-mg increments should be administered until respiratory secretions have dried.

Prompt decontamination, preferably within minutes, with soap and water or 0.5% aqueous sodium hypochlorite solution is necessary in an exposure to a vesicating agent.

The extent of the drop in absolute lymphocyte count is prognostic in patients with radiation exposure.

Concomitant traumatic injury and exacerbation of underlying medical conditions should be considered in the evaluation of victims of nuclear attacks.

Scope and Outline

This chapter presents the basic approach to patients who have been exposed to chemical weapons, radiologic materials, and nuclear explosions. Although management is limited to supportive treatment for many types of exposure, specific agents and types of exposures demand aggressive and focused protective measures and therapy. The presentation and physical examination in several specific types of exposures can assist in a specific diagnosis. Medical and surgical emergencies arising from exacerbation of existing medical conditions and blunt trauma must also be considered.

Extensive resources are widely available. Following are some examples:

http://www.bt.cdc.gov/: Thorough information about chemical, radiation, biologic, and natural disasters, and even recent outbreaks and incidents.

http://www.osha-slc.gov/SLTC/emergencypreparedness/chemical_sub.html/: Information for first responders and emergency personnel.

http://sis.nlm.nih.gov/: The National Library of Medicine; compendium of high-quality web-based resources.

Chemical Weapons

■ NERVE AGENTS

■ Pathophysiology

Nerve agents are highly toxic organophosphate agents that were first synthesized in the 1930s and 1940s. Poisoning occurs by either inhalation or skin contact. There are several categories, according to the North Atlantic Treaty Organization (NATO) designation. The G-series is named for the German scientists who formulated them: Ga (Tabun), Gb (Sarin), Gd (Soman), and Gf (cyclosarin). Sarin, when exposed to air, is volatile and inhaled by the victims. The V series—Ve, Vg, Vm, and Vx—is far more potent than the G series and these agents are persistent, meaning they are not easily washed away. The most recently discovered group is the Novichok agent (Russian for "newcomer"), about which little is known.

Nerve agents act by binding and irreversibly inactivating acetylcholinesterase (AChE) receptors, leading to excessive acetylcholine. An excess of acetylcholine in the body leads to overstimulation of nicotinic and muscarinic receptors. The very earliest symptoms are runny nose, perhaps chest discomfort, and apprehension. Poisoning is evidenced by small pupils, hypersalivation, seizures, involuntary urination and defecation, and eventual death occurs from respiratory failure due either to bronchoconstriction or loss of respiratory muscle function.[1,2]

Presenting Signs and Symptoms

The presenting signs and symptoms of exposure to a nerve agent are as follows:

- Weakness
- Irritability
- Nausea
- Shortness of breath
- Cough
- Headache
- Blurry vision

Activation of muscarinic receptors leads to excessive salivation, lacrimation, vomiting, bronchoconstriction, diarrhea, and urinary and fecal incontinence. Activation of nicotinic receptors leads to sweating, muscle flaccidity, seizures, coma, and respiratory depression. Rapid loss of consciousness, paralysis, and respiratory failure can develop.

Diagnostic Testing

Erythrocyte cholinesterase activity should be measured to assess for decreased activity; this parameter is more specific and less variable than plasma cholinesterase activity. Arterial blood gas measurements may indicate the level of respiratory impairment. An electrocardiogram may demonstrate direct muscarinic receptor–mediated bradydysrhythmias or conduction defects.

Treatment and Disposition

All patients with suspected or known nerve agent exposure should be decontaminated by removal of all clothing, copious rinsing with water and washing of the skin with a solution of soap and water to neutralize the agent. Rescue and health care personnel can become victims from residual exposure. Personal protective equipment (PPE) should always be worn while treating exposure victims. Early aggressive endotracheal intubation and ventilatory support are essential in severely affected patients. Atropine in 2-mg increments should be administered until respiratory secretions have dried up. Pralidoxime chloride (2-PAM) prevents the permanent inactivation of AChE. It should be administered as soon as possible.

Exposures to other substances, such as insecticides (organophosphates), neostigmine or pyridostigmine (carbamates), nicotine, and mushrooms (muscarinic effects), can cause similar symptoms.

VESICATING AGENTS

Pathophysiology

The vesicating agents include the mustard agents, the organic arsenicals, and phosgene oxime; they range from oily substances to vapors that all easily penetrate clothing and skin. Named for their ability to cause vesicular lesions on the skin or blistering, these agents in fact damage any tissue with which they come in contact, including the lungs. Several countries have the ability to produce vesicating agents. This fact, combined with a relative economy of manufacturing cost compared with other potential mass casualty agents and a wide variety of delivery options, makes vesicating agents an attractive choice for potential terrorist activity.[3,4]

Presenting Signs and Symptoms

Specific symptoms of vesicating agents vary according to the exposure dose; they include the following:

- Eye irritation
- Pruritus
- Malaise
- Nausea
- Hoarseness
- Dysphonia
- Cough
- Shortness of breath
- Conjunctivitis
- Hemorrhagic keratitis
- Vesiculobullous rash
- Pseudomembranous pharyngitis
- Respiratory distress
- Vomiting
- Hematochezia
- Hypotension

Diagnostic Testing

The agents are metabolized or degraded within minutes of absorption, so no specific laboratory investigation can identify or quantify exposure. Baseline laboratory investigations, including a complete blood count along with a panel of basic metabolic tests, may assist in determining prognosis. Chest radiography may be consistent with a chemical pneumonitis.

Treatment and Disposition

Decontamination of exposed victims (unless carried out within minutes of exposure) does not prevent the tissue damage associated with these agents. Ongoing exposure can be prevented through removal of all clothing followed by chemical decontamination with plain soap and water. If a shower is not available or water is in short supply, decontamination may be performed using 0.5% aqueous sodium hypochlorite solution (prepared by diluting almost any commercially available household bleach in a solution of nine parts water to one part bleach) or an absorbent powder such as flour, talcum powder, or Fuller's earth. There is no specific antidote. Lubricant should be applied to the eyelids to prevent them from sticking together. Inhaled beta-agonists are indicated for patients with respiratory distress.

■ CYANIDE

■ Pathophysiology

Cyanogen chloride and hydrogen cyanide are the two volatile cyanide agents most likely to be used in a chemical attack. Both agents are colorless and gaseous with a pungent odor described as "bitter almond." Exposure leads to release of cyanide molecules, which act in the body on the cellular level by disrupting normal mitochondrial electron transport mechanisms involved in aerobic metabolism. The disruption of electron transport at the mitochondrial level means that the cell cannot aerobically produce adenosine triphosphate (ATP) for energy. The result is a shift to anaerobic metabolism with severe compromise of all organ systems, especially the brain and the heart because these are the systems most dependent on aerobic metabolism.

Hydrogen cyanide is produced by burning plastics that are made from acrylonitrile as well as combustion engines and cigarette smoke.[5] In addition, cyanide agents are used in bronze casting (potassium ferrocyanide creates a blue hue), jewelry making, photography, mining, and other industries and hobbies.

■ Presenting Signs and Symptoms

Specific symptoms of cyanide poisoning vary according to the exposure dose; they include the following:

- Bronchorrhea
- Lacrimation
- Vertigo
- Anxiety
- Nausea
- Respiratory distress
- Lightheadedness
- Seizures
- Apnea
- Cardiac arrest
- Cyanosis

■ Diagnostic Testing

Arterial and venous blood gas measurements will demonstrate a normal arterial oxygen level and an abnormally high venous oxygen level owing to impairment of cellular oxygen utilization. Severe acidemia may be present. High erythrocyte cyanide levels in the postmortem examination are diagnostic.

■ Treatment and Disposition

Administration of the cyanide antidote kit as soon as possible is the lifesaving intervention. Treatment must be initiated presumptively, because the inhalation of cyanide cannot be ascertained rapidly, or often at all. The Pasadena Cyanide Antidote Kit contains amyl nitrite, sodium nitrite, and sodium thiosulfate. The nitrite containing compounds oxidize hemoglobin into methemoglobin, creating a site for cyanide to bind and thus to dissociate from the cytochrome oxidase chain in mitochondria. The resultant cyanomethemoglobin is converted into thiocyanate by sodium thiosulfate or other naturally occurring enzymes (Table 136-1).

Radiologic Materials

■ DIRTY BOMB

■ Pathophysiology

A dirty bomb does not require a nuclear chain reaction, as occurs with traditional thermonuclear weapons. This device uses conventional explosives to widely disperse radioactive material. Injury can be caused through conventional trauma as well as through dispersal of ionizing radiation. Patients suffering blunt or penetrating trauma should be treated according to established trauma protocols. Ionizing radiation from a dirty bomb would likely be a small fraction of the amount released from a traditional nuclear device or as a result of compromise of a nuclear facility. Immediate or rapid death from ionizing radiation released from a dirty bomb is unlikely. Particulate material consisting of alpha particles, beta particles, and neutrons, as well as high-energy photons or gamma rays, would be released.[6] Gamma rays are responsible for most injury associated with acute radiation syndrome.

■ Presenting Signs and Symptoms

Signs and symptoms of radiation exposure from a dirty bomb are as follows:

- Nausea
- Weakness
- Abdominal cramping
- Confusion
- Headache
- Burn, skin
- Epilation
- Hematochezia
- Seizure
- Coma
- Hemodynamic collapse

Table 136-1 CYANIDE ANTIDOTE TREATMENT

	Medication	Dose	Mechanism	Precaution
First step	Oxygen	100%		
	Amyl nitrite	1 amp per 60 seconds of inhalation until intravenous (IV) access is established	Oxidizes hemoglobin to methemoglobin, which binds cyanide and reduces its effect on the electron transport chain	Can cause severe methemoglobinemia with overdose
	Sodium nitrite	300 mg IV over 5-20 min	Creates methemoglobin more effectively than amyl nitrite	Slower infusion if hypotension develops
Second step	Sodium thiosulfate	12.5 g IV over 10 min	Takes cyanide from cyanomethemoglobin and forms thiocyanate, which is less toxic	Rapid infusion may cause hypotension and electrocardiographic changes
Used outside the United States	Hydroxycobalamin	4 g IV over 30 min	Combines with cyanide to form nontoxic cyanocobalamin Large doses are needed for antidotal effect Only dilute formulations are available in the United States	Dose not to exceed 10 g

Diagnostic Testing

Baseline complete blood cell count and differential count should be obtained. The extent of the later drop in absolute lymphocyte count is prognostic.

Treatment and Disposition

All patients with radiation exposure from a dirty bomb should be thoroughly decontaminated. Removal of all clothing and rinsing and scrubbing of the patient remove approximately 80% of the contamination. All facilities should have a radiation safety plan with provisions for decontamination, personal protective gear, and equipment such as a Geiger counter available to evaluate for residual contamination. Conventional injuries from the blast should be attended to, but precautions must be taken for contaminated shrapnel. Chelating or blocking agents, such as potassium iodide for exposure to radioactive iodide, should be considered.

THERMONUCLEAR DEVICE

Pathophysiology

A thermonuclear device can cause injury through conventional trauma as well as dispersal of ionizing radiation. Patients suffering blunt or penetrating trauma should be treated according to established trauma protocols. Ionizing radiation from nuclear fallout is composed of particulate matter and pure energy. Particulate material consists of alpha particles, beta particles, and neutrons. Gamma rays, essentially high-energy photons, are responsible for most injury associated with nuclear events. The severity and rapidity of onset of acute radiation syndrome depends on several factors including exposure dose, age of the victim, pre-existing comorbidities, and portion of body exposed.

Presenting Signs and Symptoms

Signs and symptoms of radiation exposure from a thermonuclear device are as follows:

- Nausea
- Weakness
- Abdominal cramping
- Confusion
- Headache
- Burn, skin
- Epilation
- Hematochezia
- Seizure
- Coma
- Hemodynamic collapse

Diagnostic Testing

Baseline complete blood cell count and differential count should be obtained. The extent of the later drop in absolute lymphocyte count is prognostic.

Treatment and Disposition

All patients with radiation exposure should be thoroughly decontaminated. Removal of all clothing and rinsing and scrubbing of the patient removes approximately 80% of the contamination. All facilities should have a radiation safety plan with provisions for decontamination, personal protective gear, and equipment such as a Geiger counter available to evaluate for residual contamination. Conventional injuries from the blast should be attended to. Chelating or blocking agents, such as potassium iodide for exposure to radioactive iodide, should be considered.

Conventional Explosives

Pathophysiology

Conventional explosives can cause thermal and blast injuries. Traditionally, *blast injury* is divided into four categories. Primary injuries result from the pressurization of air on tissue. Secondary and tertiary injuries occur when flying objects strike the victim and an individual is thrown into another object, respectively. Miscellaneous injuries, the final category, include all other injuries, such as fire-related injuries and chemical exposures.[7] Explosions in enclosed spaces tend to cause more injury. Associated chemical, biological, and radiation contamination in persons involved in an explosion must be investigated. Decontamination is prudent if there is any suspicion of contamination.

Presenting Signs and Symptoms

Signs and symptoms of injury from a conventional explosive are as follows:

- Respiratory distress
- Decreased hearing
- Extremity pain
- Abdominal pain
- Hypoxia
- Hypotension
- Blunt trauma
- Penetrating trauma
- Asphyxiation
- Crush injury

Diagnostic Testing

The patient's carboxyhemoglobin level should be measured if the explosion was associated with smoke or fire exposure. Laboratory investigations such as a urinalysis, serial complete blood counts, coagulation profile, and a creatinine phosphokinase measurement should be performed. Chest radiography should be performed in victims who have respiratory symptoms or were exposed to high-pressure injury. Abdominal computed tomography is indicated in patients with abdominal pain or evidence of penetrating or blunt abdominal injury.

Treatment and Disposition

All patients involved in an explosion should undergo evaluation to rule out potential injury. Penetrating and blunt injuries should be managed according to established trauma protocols. The possibility of associated ionizing radiation, a biologic agent, or chemical agent exposure must be investigated.

REFERENCES

1. Holstege CP, Kirk M, Sidell FR: Chemical warfare: Nerve agent poisoning. Crit Care Clin 1997;13:923-942.
2. Sidell FR, Borak J: Chemical warfare agents. II: Nerve agents. Ann Emerg Med 199;21:865-781.
3. Pons P, Dart RC: Chemical incidents in the emergency department: If and when. Ann Emerg Med 1999;34:223-225.
4. Borak J, Sidell FR: Agents of chemical warfare: Sulfur mustard. Ann Emerg Med 1992;21:303-308.
5. Baud FJ, Barriot P, Toffis V, et al: Elevated blood cyanide concentrations in victims of smoke inhalation. N Engl J Med 1991;325:1761-1766.
6. Forrow L, Blair BG, Helfand I, et al: Accidental nuclear war—a post-cold war assessment. N Engl J Med 1998;338:1326-1331.
7. Wightman JM, Gladish SL: Explosions and blast injuries. Ann Emerg Med 2001;37:664-678.

SECTION **XIV**

Toxicologic Emergencies

Chapter **137**

General Approach to the Poisoned Patient

Victor Tuckler and Jorge Martinez

KEY POINTS

- Patient resuscitation and stabilization take priority over poison or drug detection.
- Observation is one of the most critical aspects in the management of poisoned patients.
- The most common toxicant class involved in poisoning deaths is analgesics, followed by antidepressants and street drugs.
- The most common lethal poison is carbon monoxide, which is not reflected in poison control data.
- All substances can be poisonous; toxicity usually depends on the dose and the duration of exposure.
- *Toxidromes* are symptom complexes that may provide clues to the identity of the offending agent on the basis of specific pharmacologic principles; they represent "physiologic fingerprints."
- Cocaine, amphetamines, and tricyclic antidepressants (TCAs) cause catecholamine depletion by releasing norepinephrine from storage sites in sympathetic nerve ending and blocking reuptake; therefore, norepinephrine is a more effective vasopressor in these cases.
- A drug-induced hypertensive emergency is often short-lived, and aggressive therapy is usually not needed.
- In the patient with an unknown ingestion, activated charcoal is the most efficacious decontamination method and has very few adverse side effects.

Scope

Toxicology and poisons have always been of great interest to the public. Mystery novels and plays by William Shakespeare, Agatha Christie, Sir Arthur Conan Doyle, and others have given toxicology a mysterious side that piques people's interest. Many famous celebrity deaths from overdoses have made the public even more aware of toxicology. The term toxicology is derived from two Greek terms: *toxikos,* meaning "bow," and *toxikon,* meaning "poison into which arrowheads are dipped." *Toxicology* is the study of harmful interactions between chemical and/or physical agents with biologic systems.

It is believed that about 5.3 million poisoning exposures take place every year in the United States, but only about half are reported to poison control centers. The American Association of Poison Control Centers reported 2,438,644 human poison exposure cases during 2004. Of these, 92.7% occurred at a residence, and only 2.0% occurred in the workplace. Children younger than 3 years were involved in 38.5% of reported poisonings, and half of the poisonings reported in 2004 occurred in children younger than 6 years. About 84% of the poisonings were unintentional, and suicide attempts accounted for only 8% of cases.

Clinical Presentation

The initial management of a poisoned patient is similar to that of any other patient requiring critical care in the ED. Patients with ingestions may not appear to be critically ill initially, but they all have the potential for clinical deterioration.

■ HISTORY

The history obtained from the patient may be unreliable.[1] It is crucial for ED personnel also to speak to family and friends. The paramedics who brought the patient can provide information about the scene where the overdose took place. What behavior did the patient have at the scene or prior to arrival? Were there seizures, emesis, changing vital signs? It is important to know whether any medicine bottles were found and, if so, whether any pills were missing from the bottles. The patient's private physician may provide important information. It is crucial to obtain an occupational history and to review past medical records for any poisoned patient. The initial work-up should determine whether a specific patient has been exposed to an agent for which an antidote (or other specific treatment) exists (Box 137-1).

BOX 137-1

Questions to Ask about a Poisoned Patient

Why?
Was the poisoning accidental or intentional?

Where?
Did the ingestion occur inside or outside? While the patient was alone, at a party, or at work?

What?
Question emergency medical services personnel and police as well as family and friends of the patient to learn what the substance is. What poisons/drugs were available?

When?
How long since the ingestion?

Who?
Who was at the scene who knows what occurred?

■ PRESENTING SIGNS AND SYMPTOMS

The toxic patient may present with many different clinical symptoms, including cardiac dysrhythmias, altered mental status, seizures, gastroenteritis, and respiratory depression. In many cases the offending agent is unknown. Vital signs, including pulse oximetry values, are important in the diagnosis of poisoning (Table 137-1) and should be measured often in the poisoned patient. All four vital signs (temperature, pulse, respirations, blood pressure) are important because they can provide clues to the type of poisoning. Physical findings such as pupil size, odors, seizure activity, and dermatologic changes can also provide clues as to the offending agent (Tables 137-2 through 137-4; Box 137-2). Hypertension with reflex bradycardia, for example, is characteristic of alpha-

Table 137-1 INGESTED SUBSTANCES ASSOCIATED WITH VITAL SIGN CHANGES

Vital Sign Change	Associated Substances
Bradycardia	Anticholinesterase drugs Beta-blockers Calcium channel blockers Clonidine Digoxin Ethanol/alcohols Opiates
Tachycardia	Amphetamines Anticholinergics Antihistamines Cocaine Solvent abuses Sympathomimetics Theophylline
Hypothermia	Carbon monoxide Ethanol Insulin Opiates Oral hypoglycemics Sedative-hypnotic agents
Hyperthermia	Anticholinergics Antidepressants Antihistamines Salicylates Sympathomimetics
Hypotension	Aminophylline Antidepressants Antihypertensive agents Opiates Sedative-hypnotic agents
Hypertension	Amphetamines Anticholinergics Caffeine Cocaine Nicotine Sympathomimetics Thyroid medications
Hypoventilation	Alcohols Marijuana Opiates Sedative-hypnotic agents
Hyperventilation	Phencyclidine Salicylates

Table 137-2 SPECIFIC SUBSTANCES ASSOCIATED WITH PUPIL CHANGES

Pupil Change	Associated Substances
Miosis	Carbamates Cholinergics Clonidine Opiates Organophosphates Phenothiazine Pilocarpine Sedative-hypnotic agents
Mydriasis	Anticholinergics Antidepressants Antihistamines Atropine Sympathomimetics (cocaine, amphetamines)

Table 137-3 SPECIFIC SUBSTANCES ASSOCIATED WITH SKIN CHANGES

Skin Change	Associated Substances
Diaphoresis	Organophosphates Phencyclidine Salicylates Sympathomimetics
Red skin	Anticholinergics Boric acid Carbon monoxide
Blue skin	Methemoglobin-forming agents (e.g., nitrates, nitrites, aniline dyes, dapsone, phenazopyridine)
Blisters	Barbiturates Carbon monoxide Sedative-hypnotic agents Venom (snake bites, spider bites)

Table 137-4 SPECIFIC SUBSTANCES ASSOCIATED WITH ODORS

Odor	Associated Substance(s)
Bitter almonds	Cyanide
Carrots	Water hemlock
Fruity	Ketones (from diabetic ketoacidosis) Isopropanol
Garlic	Arsenic Dimethyl sulfoxide Organophosphates
Gasoline	Hydrocarbons
Mothballs	Camphor
Peanuts	Rodenticide
Pears	Chloral hydrate
Rotten eggs	Hydrogen sulfide Sulfur dioxide
Wintergreen	Methylsalicylates

BOX 137-2

Causes of Seizures

Medical Causes

- Adrenergic stimulation
- Cholinergic inhibition
- Abrupt withdrawal from alcohol, benzodiazepines, barbiturates, gamma hydroxybutyrate
- Trauma
- Infections
- Hypoglycemia
- Hypoxia

Substances

- Amphetamines
- Anticholinergics
- Benzodiazepine withdrawal
- Botanicals
- Camphor
- Carbamates
- Carbon monoxide
- Cocaine
- Ethanol withdrawal
- Isoniazid
- Insulin
- Lead
- Lidocaine
- Lindane
- Lithium
- Methylxanthines (caffeine/theophylline)
- Organophosphates
- Phencyclidine (PCP)
- Propranolol
- Salicylates
- Sympathomimetics
- Tricyclic antidepressants

adrenergic syndrome, as seen with phenylpropanolamine, phenylephrine, ephedrine, mephentermine, metaraminol, methoxamine, and pseudoephedrine ingestions.

Toxidromes

Several drugs and toxins are associated with specific toxidromes (Table 137-5). *Toxidromes* are symptom complexes that may provide clues to the identity of the offending agent. They are based on specific pharmacologic principles and represent the "physiologic fingerprints" of the associated substances. An anticholinergic toxidrome, for example, is caused by parasympatholytic substances such as antihistamines, jimsonweed, tricyclic antidepressants (TCAs), and phenothiazines. Affected patients can have hypertension, fever, delirium, and mydriasis. Sympathomimetic toxidromes resemble anticholinergic

Table 137-5 TOXIDROMES AND THEIR CAUSES

Toxidrome	Presenting Features	Cause(s)
Anticholinergic: "Hot as a hare, dry as a bone, red as a beet, blind as a bat, mad as a hatter, fast as a cat, full as a tick"	Hyperthermia Dry, flushed skin Mydriasis Delirium Tachycardia Urinary retention	Amantadine Antihistamines Antiparkinsonian agents Antipsychotics Antispasmodics Belladonna alkaloids (atropine) Cyclic antidepressants Glycopyrrolate Phenothiazine Plants (jimsonweed, nightshade, *Amanita muscaria*) Scopolamine
Cholinergic: Muscarinic: "DUMBELS"	*D*iarrhea, diaphoresis *U*rination *M*iosis *B*radycardia, bronchosecretions *E*mesis *L*acrimation *S*alivation	Acetylcholine Betel nuts Carbamate Mushrooms (some species) Organophosphates Physostigmine Pilocarpine
Nicotinic	Tachycardia Hypertension Muscle fasciculations Muscle weakness	Black widow spider venom Carbamate Organophosphates Tobacco
Extrapyramidal	Ataxia Choreoathetosis Dystonic reactions Hyperreflexia Opisthotonos Rigidity Seizures Torticollis Tremor Trismus	Haloperidol Olanzapine Phenothiazines Risperidone
Hallucinogenic	Fever Hallucinations Hyperthermia Mydriasis Panic Psychosis	Amphetamines Cannabinoids Cocaine Lysergic acid diethylamide (LSD) Phencyclidine (PCP)
Narcotic/opiate	Bradycardia Coma Decreased bowel sounds Hypotension Hypothermia Hypoventilation Miosis	Dextromethorphan Opiates: codeine, diphenoxylate, fentanyl, heroin, hydrocodone, meperidine, methadone, morphine, oxycodone, pentazocine, propoxyphene*
Sedative-hypnotic	Abnormal gait Apnea Coma Confusion Decreased level of consciousness Hypoventilation Pulse slow or normal Sedation Slurred speech Stupor	Anticonvulsants Antipsychotics Barbiturates Benzodiazepines Ethanol Meprobamate Opiates
Serotonin	Diaphoresis Diarrhea Fever Flushing Hyperreflexia Irritability Myoclonus Tremor Trismus	Clomipramine Fluoxetine Meperidine Paroxetine Sertraline Trazodone

Table 137-5 TOXIDROMES AND THEIR CAUSES—cont'd

Toxidrome	Presenting Features	Cause(s)
Solvent	Confusion Depersonalization Derealization Headache Incoordination Lethargy Restlessness	Acetone Chlorinated hydrocarbons Hydrocarbons Naphthalene Toluene Trichloroethane
Sympathomimetic	Mydriasis Tachycardia Hypertension Hyperthermia Seizures (CNS excitation)	Aminophylline Amphetamines Caffeine Cocaine Dopamine Ephedrine Epinephrine Fenfluramine LSD Methylphenidate Phencyclidine Phenylpropanolamine Pseudoephedrine Theophylline
Withdrawal: Alcohol	Hallucinations Seizures Tremors	Abrupt cessation of the addictive substance
Antihypertensives	Hypertension Tachycardia	
Barbiturates	Agitation Seizures	
Benzodiazepines	Agitation Seizures	
Opioids	Cramps Diarrhea Mydriasis	
Delayed	Patients may not have any initial symptoms	Acetaminophen Cardiac medications Warfarin Oral hypoglycemic agents Sustained-release or delayed-release formulations†
Serotonin syndrome	Agitation Altered mental status Ataxia Diaphoresis Fever Hyperreflexia Incoordination Myoclonus Shivering Tremor	Citalopram Fluoxetine Fluvoxamine Paroxetine Sertraline

*Meperidine dilates the pupils; propoxyphene and pentazocine may not cause miosis.

†With transdermal patch–released medications, toxidromes may have slower onset.

toxidromes, except that parasympatholytic agents produce silent bowel sounds and dry skin.

Diagnostic Studies

The following diagnostic studies should be performed in poisoned patients: serum acetaminophen and ASA measurements, blood ethyl alcohol measurement, blood chemistry panel, electrocardiogram (ECG), pulse oximetry, and serum glucose measurement (Box 137-3). Toxicology screening may confirm a toxicant exposure but does not usually change management (see further discussion later). A blood chemistry profile can be extremely useful, especially in determining an anion gap.[2,3] The anion gap is calculated by the formula plasma sodium − (chloride + bicarbonate); the normal range of anion gap varies from 3 to 12 mEq/L. An increase in anion gap may indicate an intoxication, but the EP must be aware that a normal anion gap does not rule out a poison-

BOX 137-3

Key Points for Ordering Diagnostic Studies in a Poisoned Patient

- Treat the patient, not the laboratory results.
- Order laboratory tests according to the presenting signs and symptoms.
- The test results may not correlate with the toxidromes.
- Some drug screens lack clinical significance in some cases.
- A test may not be rapidly available; check with the laboratory about turnaround times.
- It is important to know what the specific laboratory drug panel covers.

ing. Conditions such as hypoalbuminemia can alter the anion gap. Every 1-g/L decrease in the plasma albumin leads in a drop in anion gap of 2.5 mEq/L. Multiple conditions can cause an elevated anion gap metabolic acidosis, and the mnemonic "A CAT MUD PILES" is an easy way to remember most of them (Boxes 137-4 and 137-5). Decreased anion gap can be seen with bromide and lithium poisonings.

Serum osmolality measurement can be useful for some toxin ingestions and should be ordered if toxic alcohols are suspected. The serum osmolality is calculated by the following formula:

$$\text{Serum osmolality} = 2(\text{Na}) + (\text{glucose}/18) + (\text{blood urea nitrogen}/2.8) + (\text{ethanol}/4.6)$$

The osmolar gap = measured osmol − calculated Osmol; normally it should be less than 10. An elevated osmolar gap suggests intoxication, although a low or no osmolar gap does not exclude intoxication. An elevated osmolar gap is seen with methanol, ethylene glycol, diruretics (mannitol), ethanol, and isopropyl alcohol.

Patients with possible poisoning should undergo cardiac monitoring. In cases of unknown ingestions or ingestions for which cardiac abnormalities are a known side effect, a 12-lead electrocardiogram should be evaluated for QRS and QT intervals, morphology, and rhythm. A wide QRS interval can be seen in ingestions of TCAs, cocaine, antihistamines, anticholinergics, and quinidine. Long QT interval can be seen in quinidine, procainamide, phenothiazine, and TCA ingestions. Variable atrioventricular block is associated with digoxin overdose, and ischemic changes can be the result of hypoxemia due to carbon monoxide poisoning.

BOX 137-4

Mnemonic for Causes of Elevated Anion Gap Metabolic Acidosis: A CAT MUD PILES

*A*lcoholic ketoacidosis
*C*yanide, carbon monoxide
*A*lcohol
*T*oluene
*M*ethanol
*U*remia
*D*iabetic ketoacidosis
*P*araldehyde
*I*ron, isoniazid
*L*actic acidosis
*E*thylene glycol
*S*alicylates, strychnine

BOX 137-5

Other Drugs Associated with an Elevated Anion Gap Metabolic Acidosis

Acetaminophen (>75 g)
Amiloride
Ascorbic acid
Chloramphenicol
Colchicine
Nitroprusside
Dapsone
Epinephrine
Ethanol
Formaldehyde
Hydrogen sulfide
Ketamine
Niacin
Nitroprusside
Nonsteroidal anti-inflammatory drugs
Papaverine
Phenformin
Propofol
Terbutaline
Tetracycline
Verapamil

■ TOXICOLOGY SCREENS

Toxicology screens are of variable utility, and not all drugs are detectable with the technologies used in toxicologic testing (Box 137-6). Urine screens are specifically designed for the drugs of abuse. False-negative results occur in urine screens at a rate of 10% to 30%, and false-positive results at a rate of about 10%. The single best specimen for a toxicology screen is urine (Box 137-7). Qualitative urine speci-

BOX 137-6

Indications for Performing a Drug Screen

- Medicolegal considerations
- Insight into a patient's personality
- Medical malpractice cases (ethanol and urinary drug screen)
- To establish a diagnosis (rarely) and satisfy a consulting service

BOX 137-7

Drug Detection on Routine Urinary Drug Screens

Drugs Detected

Amphetamines
Barbiturates
Benzodiazepines
Cannabinoids
Cocaine metabolites
Opiates
Propoxyphene
Phencyclidine (PCP)
Ethanol

Drugs Not Detected

Anabolic steroids
Azidothymidine (AZT)
Chloral hydrate
Diuretics
Gamma hydroxybutyrate (GHB)
Ketamine
Laxatives
Lysergic acid diethylamide (LSD)
Mescaline
Nonsteroidal anti-inflammatory drugs

mens are superior to blood specimens because drug metabolites can be detected days after exposure, but qualitative findings do not correlate with time of ingestion or severity of impairment (Table 137-6). Serum is useful only for quantitative levels of a specific drug (Box 137-8). To improve the chance of detection in a specimen, the toxicology laboratory should be informed when a particular drug or class of drug is suspected. A positive or negative screen result does not necessarily rule an overdose in or out, however, and treatment is based on the clinical presentations. Because blood testing accurately detects the presence of the drug or its metabolites at the time of testing, the results of this type of test are the best indication of current intoxication.

When drug metabolites are circulated in the blood, they enter the scalp's blood vessels and are filtered through the hair. These metabolites remain in the hair and provide a permanent record of drug use when tested. About 50 strands of hair can be collected and dissolved in a series of solvents. The laboratory then analyzes the liquefied sample by means of gas chromatography and mass spectrometry. This

Table 137-6 DETECTION PERIODS FOR TOXIC SUBSTANCES IN URINE

Substance	Detection Period*
Amphetamines	2-4 days
Ethanol	6-12 hrs
Barbiturates:	
Short-acting (e.g. secobarbital)	1 day
Long-acting (e.g. phenobarbital)	2-3 wks
Benzodiazepines	3-7 days
Cannabis:	
Single use	24-72 hrs
Habitual use	Up to 12 wks
Cocaine metabolite	2-4 days
Codeine/morphine	2-5 days
Euphorics (e.g., methylenedioxy-methamphetamine)	1-3 days
Heroin	8 hrs
Lysergic acid diethylamide	1-4 days
Methadone	3-5 days
Methaqualone	14 days
Opiates	2-4 days
Phencyclidine	2-4 days
Phenobarbital	10-20 days
Propoxyphene	6 hrs-2 days
Steroids (anabolic), used as performance enhancers:	
Oral	1 month
Parenterally	14 days

*Time after ingestion during which substance can be detected.

BOX 137-8

Serum Screening

Serum screening is useful only for quantitative levels of the following drugs:

Acetaminophen
Carbon monoxide
Digoxin
Dilantin
Ethanol
Ethylene glycol
Iron
Lithium
Methanol
Methemoglobin
Phenobarbital
Salicylates
Theophylline

Table 137-7 FALSE-POSITIVE RESULTS OF URINE DRUG SCREENINGS

Substance(s) for which False-Positive Result Occurs	Responsible Drug(s)
Tetrahydrocannabinol	Dronabinol (Marinol) Ibuprofen (Advil, Nuprin, Motrin, Excedrin) Ketoprofen (Orudis) Naproxen (Aleve) Promethazine (Phenergan, Promethegan) Riboflavin (vitamin B_2, hemp seed oil)
Amphetamines	Ephedrine, pseudoephedrine, propylephedrine, phenylephrine (Nyquil-D, Contac, Sudafed, Allerest, Tavist-D, Dimetapp, Phenergan-D, Robitussin Cold and Flu) Over-the-counter diet aids (Dexatrim, Accutrim) Over-the-counter nasal sprays (Vicks inhaler, Afrin) Asthma medications (Bronkaid tablets, Primatene tablets) Prescription medications—many (e.g., Ritalin, Selegiline, Dexedrine)
Phencyclidine	Diazepam
Cocaine	Some antibiotics like amoxicillin and ampicillin
Opiates	Poppy seeds Tylenol with codeine Most prescription pain medications Cough suppressants with dextromethorphan (DXM or DM) Nyquil-D Some antidepressants, including amitriptyline, can cause false-positive opiate results for up to 3 days after use Quinine in tonic water

is a highly sensitive evaluation, but its high cost and prolonged process prevent its everyday use. Saliva testing is limited to detection of very recent drug use, so it will probably be confined to detecting current intoxication only.

If an initial screening assay shows a sample as testing positive, a second method should be employed to confirm the initial result. Positive results from two different methods operating on different chemical principles greatly decrease the possibility that a methodologic problem or a "cross-reacting" substance could have created the positive result. A confirmation assay usually should be carried out with a method of comparable sensitivity and higher specificity (or selectivity) than a screening assay. Examples of confirmation methods are gas chromatography (GC), gas chromatography/mass spectrometry (GC/MS), and high-performance liquid chromatography (HPLC).

Many substances can cause false-positive results on toxicology screens (Table 137-7). Poppy seeds commonly used on bagels or other baked products contain sufficient amounts of morphine to produce detectable concentrations of morphine in urine, even though the amount of ingested morphine is insufficient to cause any behavioral effect in the individual. Caution must be exercised in interpreting such a positive result as an indicator of heroin use. One method of distinguishing true heroin use is to analyze the urine specimen for 6-monoacetylmorphine, a heroin metabolite that cannot come from poppy seeds. The assay requires use of GC/MS methods.

On the other hand, passive inhalation of marijuana smoke cannot lead to a positive urine test result for its metabolites. Inadvertent exposure to marijuana is commonly claimed as the basis for a positive urine drug screen result. Clinical studies have shown that it is unlikely that an individual who does not smoke marijuana could unknowingly inhale enough marijuana smoke passively for his or her urine to contain a drug concentration detectable at the cutoff used in current urinalysis methods.

Table 137-8 RADIOGRAPHIC FINDINGS ASSOCIATED WITH TOXIC INGESTIONS

Radiographic Finding	Cause(s)
Noncardiogenic pulmonary edema	Meprobamate Methadone Opiates Phenobarbital Propoxyphene Salicylates
Toxins appearing radiopaque on kidneys-ureters-bladder radiographs	Chloral hydrate Cocaine packets Iron and other heavy metals (e.g., lead, arsenic, mercury) Neuroleptic agents Opiate packets Sustained-release products and enteric-coated preparations
Concretions*	Barbiturates Extended-release theophylline Iron Salicylates Sedative-hypnotic agents

*Should be suspected if the patient's clinical/laboratory status waxes and wanes.

■ RADIOGRAPHIC EVALUATION

Table 137-8 summarizes the radiographic findings associated with toxic ingestions.

Management

The primary treatment for a poisoned patient is to stabilize the airway, breathing, and circulation. Initial management includes attention to the ABCDs of resuscitation for a toxic ingestion:

*A*irway
*B*reathing, oxygen
*C*irculation
*D*extrose, naloxone

After initial stabilization of a critically ill patient, specific antidote therapy is administered (Table 137-9) while a detailed history is elicited and a physical examination is performed. Patients who are externally contaminated with a toxicant that may injure staff must be immediately decontaminated to avoid incapacitation of health care staff and the facility. Patients should undergo skin and eye decontamination, including removal of all clothing and washing of the skin with soap and water if indicated. Care should be taken to protect health care providers from exposure.

Establishing and maintaining an airway with adequate breathing should occur first. Supplemental oxygen should be started with a nonrebreather mask. Death from an intoxication can occur with loss of airway-protective reflexes, and the patient should be intubated if the airway needs to be protected or the patient cannot be oxygenated or ventilated. Because it is hydrolyzed by plasma cholinesterase, succinylcholine can exacerbate cholinergic toxicity. Organophosphates can prolong the effects of succinylcholine. In drug-induced, hemodynamically significant bradycardia, atropine is usually not helpful but can be administered because it is not harmful. The major exception is in acute organophosphate or carbamate poisoning, in which the administration of atropine will be lifesaving. Electrical cardiac pacing is often effective in cases of mild to moderate drug-induced bradycardia. In patients with drug-induced cardiac arrest, electrical cardioversion or defibrillation is appropriate for those who are pulseless and have ventricular tachycardia or ventricular fibrillation.

Circulation should be maintained and hypotension treated aggressively. Intravascular volume should be restored with crystalloid fluid, and if the hypotension is not resolved after fluid administration, dopamine should be given to support the blood pressure. Dopamine is not the drug of choice for some cases of toxicant-induced hypotension, because it is a sympathomimetic amine vasopressor that must be converted into norepinephrine to be effective. This agent is not useful in treating the hypotension related to disulfiram (Antabuse) reactions, because the conversion of dopamine into norepinephrine is blocked. Cocaine, amphetamines, and TCAs cause catecholamine depletion by releasing norepinephrine from storage sites in sympathetic nerve endings and blocking reuptake; therefore, norepinephrine is a more effective vasopressor in these cases. Norepinephrine acts directly, not requiring any conversion. A new antidote for hypotension secondary to beta-blocker and calcium channel blocker overdoses is insulin. Regular insulin, given as a 10 to 20-unit bolus followed by 0.5 to 1 U/kg while euglycemia is maintained, improves myocardial contractility, cardiac output, and blood pressure. A drug-induced hypertensive emergency is often short-lived, and aggressive therapy is usually not needed. This is an important caution, because hypotension may occur later in cases of severe stimulant poisoning.

Benzodiazepines are first-line agents for toxicant-induced hypertension. Beta-blockers are contraindicated because they may block the β_2 receptors, leaving alpha-adrenergic stimulation unopposed and worsening hypertension. In patients with a drug-induced hypertensive emergency refractory to benzodiazepines, short-acting antihypertensive agents, such as nitroprusside, should be used. Labetalol is a third-line agent, effective at times for drug-induced hypertensive emergencies associated with sympathomimetic poisoning.

Treatment of drug-induced acute coronary syndromes is similar to the treatment recommended for drug-induced hypertensive emergencies. Catheterization studies have shown that (1) nitroglycerin and phentolamine (an alpha-blocker) reverse cocaine-induced vasoconstriction, (2) labetalol has no significant effect, and (3) propranolol worsens it. Therefore, benzodiazepines and nitroglycerin are first-line agents, phentolamine is a second-line agent, and propranolol is contraindicated for drug-induced coronary syndromes.[4,5]

In cases of poisoning, it is important to treat the patient, not the toxin. The EP should deal with the ABCDs of resuscitation, hypotension, seizures, and cardiac dysrhythmias aggressively. Such treatments can be started without knowledge of what the toxin is. Serial vital signs and physical examinations are crucial. Progressive neurologic deterioration must be caught early and dealt with appropriately. Observation is one of the most critical aspects of the management of poisoned patients.

■ "COMA COCKTAIL"

"Coma cocktail" is a slang term used to describe a combination of agents that has traditionally been given to poisoned patients with altered consciousness. It consists of dextrose, naloxone, thiamine, flumazenil, and oxygen. The use of the coma cocktail can be both therapeutic and diagnostic.

Hypoglycemia must be considered in all patients with an altered mental status or with active seizures. The overdosed patient can often be hypoglycemic because of the offending agent. Glucose, at a dosage of 1 g/kg (50% dextrose in water in adults, 25% dextrose in water in children, and 10% dextrose in water in neonates), should be given to patients with hypoglycemia unless a rapid finger-stick glucose measurement demonstrates euglycemia or hyperglycemia.

Naloxone reverses the coma and respiratory depression induced by opioids. A positive response may

Table 137-9 SPECIFIC TOXINS AND THEIR ANTIDOTES

Toxin(s)	Antidote(s)
Acetaminophen	*N*-acetylcysteine: 140 mg/kg PO, then 70 mg/kg every 4 hrs for up to 17 doses *OR* 150-mg/kg IV load over 1 hr with 50 mg/kg over 4 hrs followed by 100 mg/kg over 16 hrs
Anticholinergics	Physostigmine: 1-2 mg IV in adults or 0.5 mg in children over 2 min for anticholinergic delirium, seizures, or arrhythmias
Arsenic, lead, or mercury	Dimercaprol, 3-5 mg/kg IM only D-Penicillamine, 20-40 mg/kg/day or 500 mg tid in adults*
Benzodiazepines	Flumazenil: 0.2 mg, then 0.3 mg, then 0.5 mg; up to 5 mg†
Black widow spider bite	Latrodectus antivenin, 1 vial by slow IV infusion
Beta-blockers	Glucagon, 5-10 mg in adults, then infusion of same dose each hr Insulin and glucose, given as 10-20 U insulin with dextrose 25 g initially; then insulin 0.5-1.0 U/kg/hr with glucose 10-30 g/hr
Calcium channel blockers	Calcium, as 1 g calcium chloride IV in adults or 20-30 mg/kg/dose in children, over a few minutes with continuous monitoring Glucagon, 5-10 mg in adults followed by an infusion of the same dose each hour Insulin and glucose, given as 10-20 U insulin with dextrose 25 g initially; then insulin 0.5-1.0 U/kg/hr with glucose 10-30 g/hr
Cyanide, hydrogen sulfide	Sodium thiosulfate, 50 mL of 25% solution (12.5 g; 1 ampule) in adults or 1.65 mL/kg IV in children Sodium nitrate, 10 mL of 3% solution (300 mg; 1 ampule) in adults or 0.33 mL/kg slowly IV in children
Digitalis glycosides	Digoxin-specific Fab fragments, 10-20 vials if patient in ventricular fibrillation; dose is based on serum digoxin concentration or amount ingested
Ethylene glycol	Fomepizole: 15 mg/kg, then 10 mg/kg every 12 hrs×4, until serum ethylene glycol level <20 mg/dL; dose should be adjusted during dialysis Pyridoxine, 100 mg IV daily Thiamine, 100 mg IV
Hydrofluoric acid	Calcium gluconate
Iron	Deferoxamine, 15 mg/kg/hr IV
Isoniazid, hydrazine, and monomethylhydrazine	Pyridoxine, 5 g in adults, 1 g in children, if ingested dose is unknown
Lead, arsenic, and lead	Dimercaptosuccinic acid (succimer): one 100-mg capsule per 10-kg body weight tid for 1 wk; then bid, with chelation breaks Ethylenediaminetetraacetic acid, 75 mg/kg/day by continuous infusion
Methanol toxicity	Folate or leucovorin, 50 mg IV every 4 hrs in adults Ethanol: loading dose, 10 mL/kg of 10%; maintenance dose, 0.15 mL/kg/hr of 10% solution; rate should be doubled during dialysis Fomepizole: 15 mg/kg, then 10 mg/kg every 12 hrs×4, until serum methanol level <20 mg/dL; dose should be adjusted during dialysis
Methemoglobin-forming agents	Methylene blue, 1-2 mg/kg IV (one 10-mL dose of 10% solution [100 mg])
Opioids	Naloxone, 0.4 mg IV titrated to 2 mg initially; higher doses may be needed for synthetic opioids Nalmefene, 2 mg‡
Organophosphates and carbamates	Atropine 1-2 mg IV in adults, 0.03 mg/kg in children; titrate to drying of pulmonary secretions 2-PAM (2-pyridine aldoxime methylchloride): loading dose, 1-2 g IV in adults, 25-50 mg/kg in children; adult maintenance, 500 mg/hr or 1-2 g every 4-6 hrs
Rattlesnake bite	CroFab antivenin injection, 5 vials minimum dose by infusion in normal saline
Sulfonureas	Octreotide, 50 μg/12 hrs SC *OR* 5-10 μg/kg/24 hrs IV
Tricyclic antidepressants	Bicarbonate 44-88 mEq in adults, 1-2 mEq/kg in children; best used with IV "push" rather than slow infusion
Valproic acid	Carnitine: loading dose, 100 mg/kg IV *OR* PO; then 25 mg/kg every 6 hrs

IM, intramuscularly; IV, intravenously; PO, orally; SC, subcutaneously.
*May cross-react with penicillin in allergic patients.
†Should not be used if patient has signs of tricyclic antidepressant toxicity or a history of seizures.
‡Has much longer half-life than naloxone.

obviate the need for intubation. Patients should always be restrained prior to administration of naloxone, because they may become violent upon awakening. An initial dose of 0.2 to 0.4 mg is administered intravenously (IV), and if there is no response after 2 to 3 minutes, an additional 1 to 2 mg can be administered; doses can be repeated up to a total of 10 mg as required. More than 10 mg may be required and may have to be given as an intravenous drip with higher grades of heroin, pentazocine, diphenoxylate, meperidine, propoxyphene, and methadone overdose.[6] The naloxone is mixed with 5% dextrose in water (D_5W) and given at a rate that delivers two thirds of the initial reversal dose per hour.[7] Some opioid agonists, such as propoxyphene and pentazocine, may not produce the characteristic miosis of opioid intoxication. Naloxone has a short half-life (20-30 minutes), and its effect is not as long as the effects of some narcotics. Acute pulmonary edema, opioid withdrawal, and seizures have been reported with naloxone administration.[8-10]

Thiamine, 100 mg given intravenously, should be reserved for alcoholic, malnourished patients. Despite traditional belief, giving thiamine to every comatose patient to prevent Wernicke-Korsakoff syndrome is not well supported by the literature. There is no evidence that dextrose should be withheld until thiamine is administered.[11]

Flumazenil is a benzodiazepine reversal agent that can be used in a pure acute benzodiazepine overdose or when reversal of therapeutic conscious sedation is desired. It can reverse the seizure-protecting properties of benzodiazepines in mixed drug ingestions (TCAs).[12] Flumazenil can induce acute withdrawal symptoms in long-term benzodiazepine abusers; therefore, flumazenil is contraindicated in patients with a history of long-term benzodiazepine use, seizure disorder, and concomitant TCA ingestion. Flumazenil should not be used routinely to arouse an unconscious patient with overdose. Case reports have cautioned of the risk of precipitating seizures with flumazenil when there is a suspicion of benzodiazepine plus cyclic antidepressant overdose. In a large prospective trial of unconscious patients suspected of benzodiazepine overdose, investigators did not observe any significant side effects with flumazenil.[13] However, serious complications of flumazenil have now been reported, including seizures, ventricular arrhythmias, and benzodiazepine withdrawal in patients who are addicted.[14] Although flumazenil is successful in improving the Glasgow Coma Scale score, it has not had a dramatic impact on treatment of the unknown, unconscious overdose patient. Flumazenil does not appear to alter cost or major diagnostic or therapeutic interventions in patients presenting with decreased level of consciousness owing to an intentional unknown drug overdose. If partial reversal of benzodiazepine intoxication is necessary, the smallest possible dose of flumazenil, 0.05 to 0.1 mg, should be diluted in 10 mL saline or D_5W and given intravenously slowly, over several minutes. Goals are respiratory sufficiency and verbal responsiveness, not complete arousal.

DECONTAMINATION

Methods of decontamination include gastric emptying (syrup of ipecac administration and gastric lavage), activated charcoal, and whole-bowel irrigation. There is some controversy about, as well as little support in the medical literature for, the roles of gastric lavage, activated charcoal, and cathartics to decontaminate the poisoned patient. Studies have shown that after a delay of 60 minutes or more, very little of the ingested drug is removed by gastric lavage. In some circumstances, aggressive decontamination may be lifesaving, even more than 1 to 2 hours after ingestion. Examples are ingestion of highly toxic drugs as calcium channel blockers, of drugs not adsorbed by charcoal, and of sustained-release or enteric-coated products.

Use of syrup of ipecac to induce emesis is no longer part of the treatment of any ingestions. Persistent vomiting after ipecac use is likely to delay the administration of activated charcoal. There is no evidence from clinical studies that ipecac improves the outcome of poisoned patients, and its routine administration in the ED should be abandoned.[15]

Gastric lavage is a time-consuming procedure that also risks aspiration and other injury. The concept is to try to wash out stomach contents prior to absorption. It may still be useful when the toxin has not yet passed the pylorus. Gastric lavage should not be employed routinely in the management of poisoned patients, however. In general there is no advantage to gastric emptying more than 60 minutes since the ingestion. The method of gastric lavage is to place a 36F to 40F tube into the patient's stomach and "wash out" the stomach with 300-mL aliquots of normal saline until clear. Unless a patient is intubated, gastric lavage is contraindicated if airway protective reflexes are lost. It is also contraindicated if a hydrocarbon with high aspiration potential or a corrosive substance has been ingested. Gastric lavage should not be considered unless a patient has ingested a potentially life-threatening amount of a poison and the procedure can be undertaken within 60 minutes of the ingestion.[16] Multiple studies have shown no advantage of gastric emptying over activated charcoal in decreasing absorption.

Activated Charcoal

Activated charcoal is produced by heating wood pulp, washing it, and then activating it with steam or acid. It has a large surface area for direct adsorption of agents in the gastrointestinal tract. A cathartic such as sorbitol (5 mL/kg) can be used with the first dose of charcoal to prevent constipation. In the patient with an unknown ingestion, administration of activated charcoal is the most efficacious decontamination method, with very few adverse side effects. It is

BOX 137-9

Use of Activated Charcoal in Toxic Ingestions

Substances Poorly Adsorbed by Activated Charcoal

- Caustics and corrosives, cyanide.
- Heavy metals (arsenic, iron, lead, lithium, mercury)
- Alcohols (ethanol, methanol, isopropyl) and glycols (ethylene glycols)
- Rapid-onset or rapid-absorption cyanide and strychnine
- Chlorine and iodine
- Other substances that are insoluble in water (substances in tablet form)
- Aliphatic and poorly absorbed hydrocarbons (petroleum distillates)
- Laxatives (sodium, magnesium, and potassium based)

Contraindications to Use of Activated Charcoal

- Unprotected airway
- Intestinal obstruction
- Poor gastrointestinal tract function
- Decreased peristalsis
- Ileus
- Bowel obstruction
- Aspiration

Drugs with Enterohepatic Circulation

Multiple-dose activated charcoal (every 4 hrs) may be useful for some drugs with enterohepatic circulation, such as:

- Antidepressants
- Acetylsalicylic acid
- Aminophylline
- Barbiturates
- Carbamazepine
- Digitalis
- Dilantin
- Dapsone
- Phenobarbital
- Quinine

safe and inexpensive, and it adsorbs most toxins (Box 137-9). This agent should be administered in a dose of 1 to 2 g/kg.

Charcoal does not adsorb all poisons; it particularly does not absorb alcohols, metals, acids, alkalis, and hydrocarbons. Infrequent complications include intestinal obstruction and aspiration pneumonitis, which may result after repetitive dosing regimens. On the basis of volunteer studies, the effectiveness of activated charcoal decreases with time; the greatest benefit occurs within 1 hour of ingestion, and single-dose activated charcoal should not be administered routinely in the management of poisoned patients. The administration of activated charcoal may be considered if a patient has ingested a potentially toxic amount of a poison (which is known to be adsorbed to charcoal) up to 1 hour previously; there is insufficient data to support or exclude its use more than 1 hour after ingestion.[17]

Multiple-dose activated charcoal (every 4 hrs) may be useful in ingestions of some drugs with enterohepatic circulation (see Box 137-9). Studies have shown decreases in half-life of these drugs, however; clinical benefit of this approach has not been well established. Repetitive doses of charcoal are given as 1 g/kg every 4 to 6 hours. Although many studies in animals and volunteers have demonstrated that multiple-dose activated charcoal increases drug elimination significantly, this therapy has not yet been shown in a controlled study to reduce morbidity and mortality. On the basis of experimental and clinical studies, therefore, administration of multiple-dose activated charcoal should be considered only if a patient has ingested a life-threatening amount of carbamazepine, dapsone, phenobarbital, quinine, or theophylline.[18]

Cathartics

Cathartics include magnesium sulfate, sorbitol, and magnesium citrate. Not a single study has shown any benefit from use of cathartics in poisoned patients. Drugs and toxins are usually absorbed within 30 to 90 minutes, and cathartics/laxatives take hours to work. Serious fluid and electrolyte shifts can occur from cathartics, and a few infant deaths have been reported. Complications of cathartic use include electrolyte imbalance, dehydration, and hypermagnesemia. Contraindications include renal or cardiac failure, diarrhea, ileus, recent bowel surgery, electrolyte imbalance, and extremes of age. The administration of a cathartic alone has no role in the management of the poisoned patient and is not recommended as a method of gut decontamination.[19]

WHOLE-BOWEL IRRIGATION

Whole bowel irrigation consists of administration of a polyethylene glycol solution at a rate of 2 L/hr in adults until the rectal effluent is clear. Most of the time it requires the placement of a nasogastric tube for administration. Whole-bowel irrigation should be reserved for life-threatening intoxications from sustained-release (CR, SR, LA, XL) beta-blockers, calcium channel blockers, lithium, iron, and lead. Oral administration of charcoal followed by whole-bowel irrigation is the safest way to decontaminate people whose bodies have been packed and/or stuffed with packets of illegal drugs. The dose is 20 mL/kg/hr, which translates to about 2 L/hr for adults and about 0.5 L/hr for children. The endpoint is a clear rectal

BOX 137-10

Agents Removed by Hemodialysis

Barbiturates
Ethylene glycol
Isopropanol
Lithium
Methanol
Salicylates
Theophylline

effluent, which usually requires 4 to 6 hours of treatment.

Whole-bowel irrigation should not be used routinely in the management of the poisoned patient. Although some volunteer studies have shown substantial decreases in the bioavailability of ingested drugs with this method, no controlled clinical trials have been performed, and there is no conclusive evidence that whole-bowel irrigation improves outcome in the poisoned patient.[20]

■ ELIMINATION ENHANCEMENT

■ Alkalinization

Alkalinization traps weak acids in ionized state, thereby decreasing their reabsorption. Urine alkalinization increases the urine elimination of chlorpropamide, 2,4-dichlorophenoxyacetic acid, diflunisal, fluoride, mecoprop, methotrexate, phenobarbital, and salicylate. Sodium bicarbonate is given at 0.5 to 2 mEq/kg/hr in an intravenous drip after a bolus of 1 to 2 mEq/kg. Dosage should be titrated to keep urine pH at 7.5 to 8.0. Urine alkalinization should be considered first-line treatment for patients with moderately severe salicylate poisoning whose condition does not meet the criteria for hemodialysis. Urine alkalinization cannot be recommended as first-line treatment in cases of phenobarbital poisoning, for which multiple-dose activated charcoal is superior.[21]

■ Hemodialysis or Hemoperfusion

In the unstable overdosed patient, consultation with a nephrologist for emergency hemodialysis may be indicated before results of definitive diagnostic studies or drug level measurements are availability. Toxins for which hemodialysis may be useful should have the following features: low molecular weight (<500 d), water solubility, low protein binding (<70% to 80%), and small volume of distribution (<1 L/kg). Toxins for which hemodialysis may be required include methanol, ethylene glycol, boric acid, salicylates, and lithium (Box 137-10).

Disposition

All patients who are cleared from a toxicology standpoint should be evaluated by psychiatric services if there is any question of an intentional overdose. Any patient with symptoms should be admitted for observation, and a sitter should be provided if the patient is suicidal. Typically, patients with unknown ingestions can be observed for 6 hours; if asymptomatic, they can be released to home or psychiatric services as indicated. Parents of children who have been evaluated for an ingestion or potential ingestion should be counseled about poisoning precautions and given poison control center contact information. Specific recommendations are given in subsequent chapters related to specific toxin ingestions.

REFERENCES

1. Wright N: An assessment of the unreliability of the history given by self-poisoned patients. Clin Toxicol 1980;16:381-384.
2. Winter SD, Pearson R, Gabow PA, et al: The fall of the serum anion gap. Arch Intern Med 1990;150:311-313.
3. Gabow PA: Disorders associated with an altered anion gap. Kidney Int 1985;27:472-483.
4. Baumann BM, Perrone J, Hornig SE, et al: Randomized, double blind, placebo-controlled trial of diazepam, nitroglycerin, or both for treatment of cocaine-associated acute coronary syndromes. Acad Emerg Med 2000;7:878-885.
5. Honderick T: Lorazepam in the acute management of cocaine associated chest pain. Acad Emerg Med 2000;7:515.
6. Goldfrank LR: The several uses of naloxone. Emerg Med 1984;16:110-116.
7. Goldfrank LR, Weisman RS, Errick JK, et al: A dosing nomogram for continuous infusion intravenous naloxone. Ann Emerg Med 1986;15:566-570.
8. Schwartz JA, Koenigsberg MD: Naloxone-induced pulmonary edema. Ann Emerg Med 1987;16:1294-1296.
9. Goldfrank LR: Substance withdrawal. Emerg Med Clin North Am 1990;8:616-632.
10. Mariani PJ: Seizure associated with low-dose naloxone. Am J Emerg Med 1989;7:127-129.
11. Reuler JB, Girard DE, Cooney TG: Wernicke's encephalopathy. N Engl J Med 1985;312:1035-1039.
12. Mordel A, Winkler E, Almog S, et al: Seizures after flumazenil administration in a case of combined benzodiazepine and tricyclic antidepressant overdose. Crit Care Med 1992;20:1733-1734.
13. Weinbroum A, Rudick V, Sorkine P, et al: Use of flumazenil in the treatment of drug overdose: A double-blind and open clinical study in 110 patients. Crit Care Med 1996;24:199-206.
14. Gueye P, Hoffman J: Empiric use of flumazenil in comatose patients: Limited applicability of criteria to define low risk. Ann Emerg Med 1996;27:730-735.
15. American Academy of Clinical Toxicology; European Association of Poisons Centres and Clinical Toxicologists: Position paper: Ipecac syrup. J Toxicol Clin Toxicol 2004;42:133-143.
16. American Academy of Clinical Toxicology; European Association of Poisons Centres and Clinical Toxicologists: Position statement: Gastric lavage. J Toxicol Clin Toxicol 1997;35:711-719.
17. American Academy of Clinical Toxicology; European Association of Poisons Centres and Clinical Toxicologists: Position statement: Activated charcoal. J Toxicol Clin Toxicol 1997;35:721-741.
18. American Academy of Clinical Toxicology; European Association of Poisons Centres and Clinical Toxicologists: Position statement and practice guidelines on the use of

multi-dose activated charcoal in the treatment of acute poisoning. J Toxicol Clin Toxicol 1999;37:731-751.
19. American Academy of Clinical Toxicology; European Association of Poisons Centres and Clinical Toxicologists: Position statement: Cathartics. J Toxicol Clin Toxicol 1997;35:743-752.
20. American Academy of Clinical Toxicology; European Association of Poisons Centres and Clinical Toxicologists: Position paper: Whole bowel irrigation. J Toxicol Clin Toxicol 2004;42:843-854.
21. Proudfoot AT, Krenzelok EP, Vale JA: Position paper on urine alkalinization. J Toxicol Clin Toxicol 2004;42:1-26.

Chapter 138

Acetaminophen, Aspirin, and NSAIDs

Heather Long

ACETAMINOPHEN

KEY POINTS

- Acetaminophen (APAP) is available in numerous formulations, including cold, cough, and pain relief medications.
- Acetaminophen ingestion is the most commonly reported exposure to a potentially toxic pharmacologic agent.
- Acetaminophen toxicity is clinically silent up to 24 hours after ingestion. If any vital sign abnormalities or significant symptoms are present, co-ingestant should be suspected.
- Blood specimen for serum APAP determination should be collected 4 hours after ingestion.
- Serum APAP levels should be measured in cases of suspected suicidal ingestion.
- The serum APAP result should be applied to the APAP nomogram for determination of the patient's risk of toxicity.
- *N*-Acetylcysteine (NAC) is the antidote to APAP poisoning, and approach to treatment depends on timing of ingestion and of serum APAP level.
- NAC dose (oral): Loading dose 140 mg/kg; maintenance dose 70 mg/kg every 4 hours ×17 doses. An intravenous formulation of NAC is now approved for use and should be given when oral administration is not feasible.
- If there is any clinical suspicion of overdose, even if the patient does not admit to APAP ingestion or if the patient with an overdose exhibits altered mental status, the serum APAP level should be measured.

Scope

Acetaminophen (APAP) is widely available in single-agent preparations as well as in numerous cold, cough, and pain relief formulations. Although very safe at the recommended dosage, overdose and toxicity are common given its broad usage. More than 100,000 calls are made to poison control centers in the United States each year regarding APAP exposures, and there are more hospitalizations for APAP overdose than for overdose of any other pharmacologic agent.

Metabolism and Pathophysiology

After therapeutic ingestion of APAP, more than 90% is metabolized in the liver to inactive and nontoxic glucuronide and sulfate conjugates that are subsequently excreted in the urine. Less than 5% is metabolized by the cytochrome P-450 mixed-function oxidase system to form the highly reactive and toxic intermediate *N*-acetyl-para-benzo-quinone imine (NAPQI). Glutathione quickly reduces NAPQI to a nontoxic metabolite that is eliminated in the urine.

After overdose of APAP, the normal nontoxic glucuronidation and sulfation pathways of metabolism become saturated, allowing more APAP to be metabolized by the cytochrome P-450 system to the toxic metabolite NAPQI. Once available stores of glutathione are diminished, the highly reactive NAPQI binds to intracellular proteins, beginning the cascade of events that lead to cell death. Oxidative drug metabolism by the cytochrome P-450 system to NAPQI is concentrated in zone III (the centrilobular area of the hepatic lobule); hence the characteristic centrilobular necrosis described with APAP toxicity.

Clinical Presentation

Table 138-1 summarizes the four stages of APAP poisoning. Clinical manifestations of APAP overdose arise from the hepatotoxicity and resultant complications. Patients, even those who go on to have fulminant hepatic failure, are initially asymptomatic. Significant abnormalities of vital signs or clinical findings that manifest soon after ingestion should not be attributed to the acetaminophen alone; the EP should pursue diagnosis and treatment of a co-ingested agent.

Diagnostic Testing

The objective of diagnostic testing after overdose of APAP is to assist the clinician in determining which patients are at risk of hepatotoxicity and thus require further treatment. Laboratory evaluation is essential for all patients with potential risk because there are no reliable clinical manifestations early after APAP ingestion, when antidotal therapy is most effective. Risk is assessed through thorough history and physical examination as well as collection of a blood specimen for a serum APAP measurement 4 hours after ingestion—or as soon as possible in patients who present more than 4 hours after ingestion and application of the result to the acetaminophen nomogram (Fig. 138-1). For patients who present late after ingestion and already show signs and symptoms of hepatotoxicity or for whom the time of ingestion cannot readily be established, the serum aspartate transaminase (AST) level should also be measured. See Figures 138-2 and 138-3 for guidelines to assessing risk after acute and chronic APAP ingestions. *Acute ingestion* is defined as a single ingestion occurring over a single period shorter than 4 hours.

If there is any clinical suspicion of overdose, even if the patient does not admit to APAP ingestion or if the patient with overdose exhibits altered mental status, the serum APAP level should be measured.[1] Approximately 1 in 500 patients who present with overdose but do not admit to APAP ingestion have a potentially hepatotoxic serum APAP concentration.

Management and Treatment

Treatment with 50 g of activated charcoal should be considered in patients who present with large ingestions if APAP or co-ingestion of APAP and potentially toxic agents that bind to charcoal.[2] *N*-Acetylcysteine (NAC) is the antidote to APAP toxicity.[3] As long as it is given within 8 hours of ingestion, there is almost no risk of significant hepatotoxicity secondary to APAP toxicity. There does not appear to be a significant advantage to giving NAC within the first 2 or 3 hours after ingestion over giving it later as long as it

Table 138-1 FOUR STAGES OF ACETAMINOPHEN POISONING

Stage 1 (0-24 hours)	Asymptomatic	Patients are initially asymptomatic, with normal vital signs and no physical findings Laboratory results are normal Nonspecific complaints of nausea, vomiting, and malaise may start to develop near the end of this stage
Stage 2 (24-72 hours)	Onset of hepatotoxicity	Right upper quadrant abdominal pain may develop Levels of aspartate aminotransferase (AST), the most sensitive indicator of hepatotoxicity, and alanine aminotransferase (ALT) begin to rise Later, International Normalized Ratio (INR) values may begin to rise, and renal function to deteriorate
Stage 3 (72-96 hours)	Maximal hepatotoxicity	Patient exhibits clinical and laboratory manifestations of hepatic necrosis: varying degrees of hepatic encephalopathy, jaundice, renal failure, coagulation defects, and myocardial abnormalities AST and ALT levels peak, INR value rises, blood urea nitrogen (BUN) and creatinine levels rise, pH drops Death may occur, typically 3-5 days after overdose Death from fulminant hepatic failure may be characterized by cerebral edema, sepsis, multisystem organ failure, hemorrhage, and adult respiratory distress syndrome (ARDS)
Stage 4 (4 days to 2 wk)	Recovery phase	Patients who survive stage 3 undergo complete regeneration of the liver Laboratory abnormalities typically return to normal 5-7 days after overdose

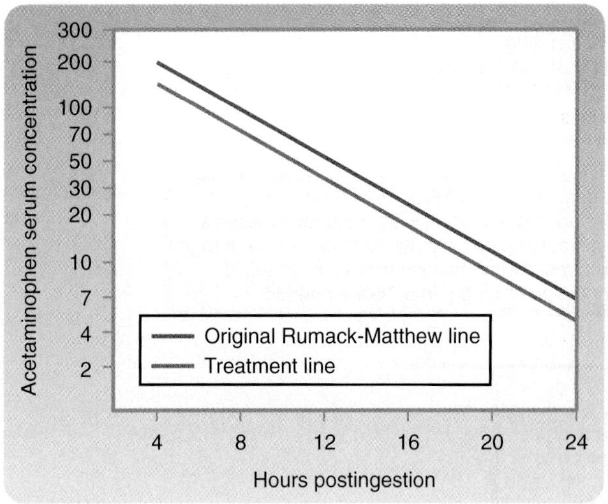
Acetaminophen serum concentration
300
200
100
70
50
30
20
10
7
4
2
Original Rumack-Matthew line
Treatment line
4
8
12
16
20
24
Hours postingestion

FIGURE 138-1 Treatment nomogram for acute acetaminophen overdose (From Marx JA, Hockberger RS, Walls RM [eds]: Rosen's Emergency Medicine: Concepts and Clinical Practice, 6th ed. Philadelphia, Mosby/Elsevier, 2006.)

is within the 8-hour window. See Figures 138-2 and 138-3 for guidelines in determining which patients should be given NAC after acute and chronic APAP ingestion and managing patient care. NAC is available in both oral and intravenous formulations.[4] See Table 138-2 for a comparison of the two formulations and Table 138-3 for dosing regimens.

Patients who present longer than 8 hours after ingestion should be treated with NAC upon presentation and their serum APAP and AST levels should be measured. If the APAP level is above the treatment threshold on the nomogram (see Fig. 138-1), treatment should continue. If not and the patient has no signs or symptoms consistent with hepatotoxicity, NAC should be discontinued. NAC improves morbidity and mortality even if given late after ingestion and even if given to patients who present with fulminant hepatic failure after APAP ingestion.[5] The EP should contact the regional poison control center for further assistance in managing patients with APAP overdose.

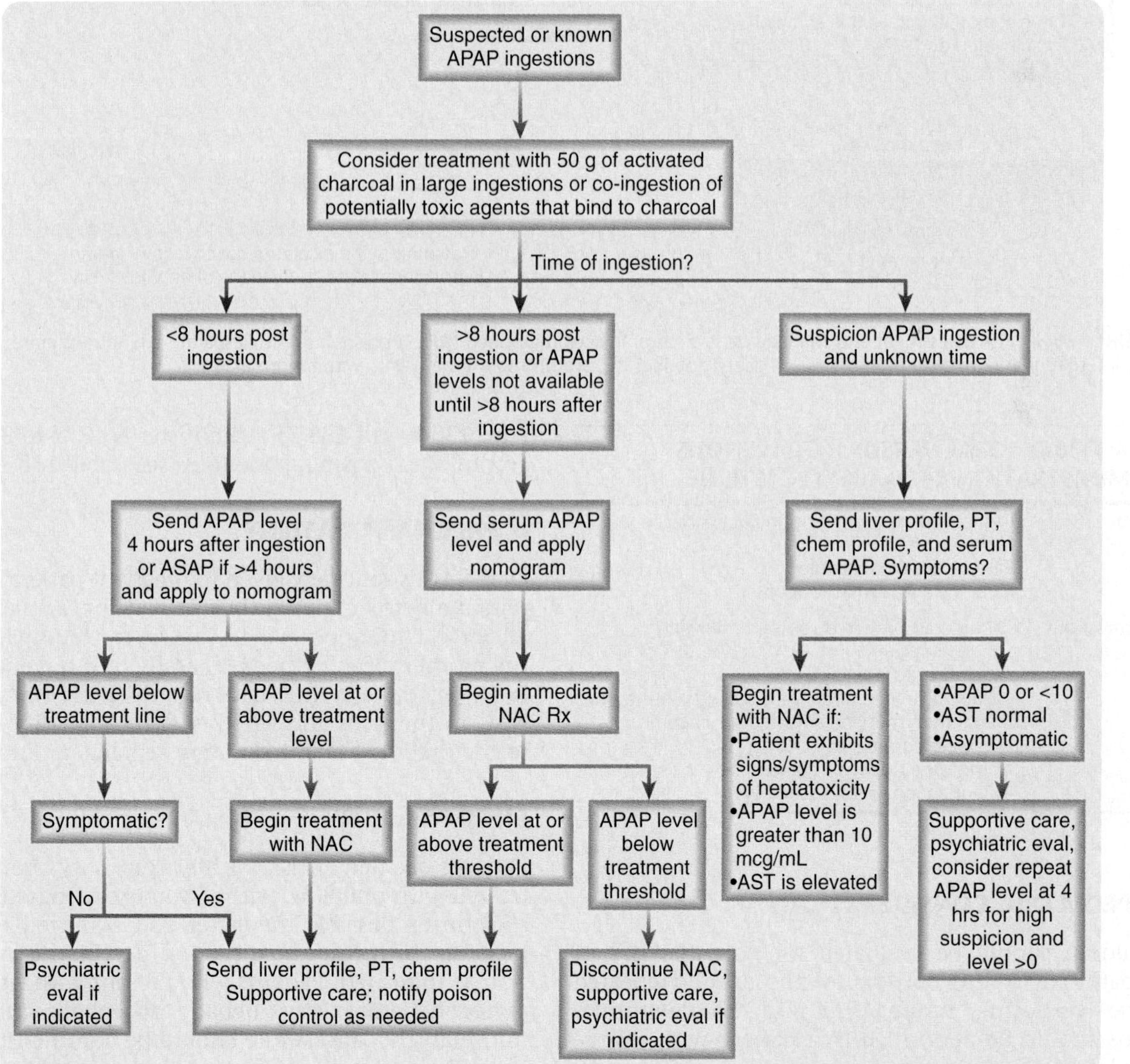
Suspected or known APAP ingestions
Consider treatment with 50 g of activated charcoal in large ingestions or co-ingestion of potentially toxic agents that bind to charcoal
Time of ingestion?
<8 hours post ingestion
>8 hours post ingestion or APAP levels not available until >8 hours after ingestion
Suspicion APAP ingestion and unknown time
Send APAP level 4 hours after ingestion or ASAP if >4 hours and apply to nomogram
Send serum APAP level and apply nomogram
Send liver profile, PT, chem profile, and serum APAP. Symptoms?
APAP level below treatment line
APAP level at or above treatment level
Begin immediate NAC Rx
Begin treatment with NAC if:
•Patient exhibits signs/symptoms of heptatoxicity
•APAP level is greater than 10 mcg/mL
•AST is elevated
•APAP 0 or <10
•AST normal
•Asymptomatic
Symptomatic?
Begin treatment with NAC
APAP level at or above treatment threshold
APAP level below treatment threshold
Supportive care, psychiatric eval, consider repeat APAP level at 4 hrs for high suspicion and level >0
No
Yes
Psychiatric eval if indicated
Send liver profile, PT, chem profile Supportive care; notify poison control as needed
Discontinue NAC, supportive care, psychiatric eval if indicated

FIGURE 138-2 Risk assessment and management of acute acetaminophen (APAP) poisoning. AST, asparate aminotransferase; NAC, *N*-acetylcysteine; PT, prothrombin time.

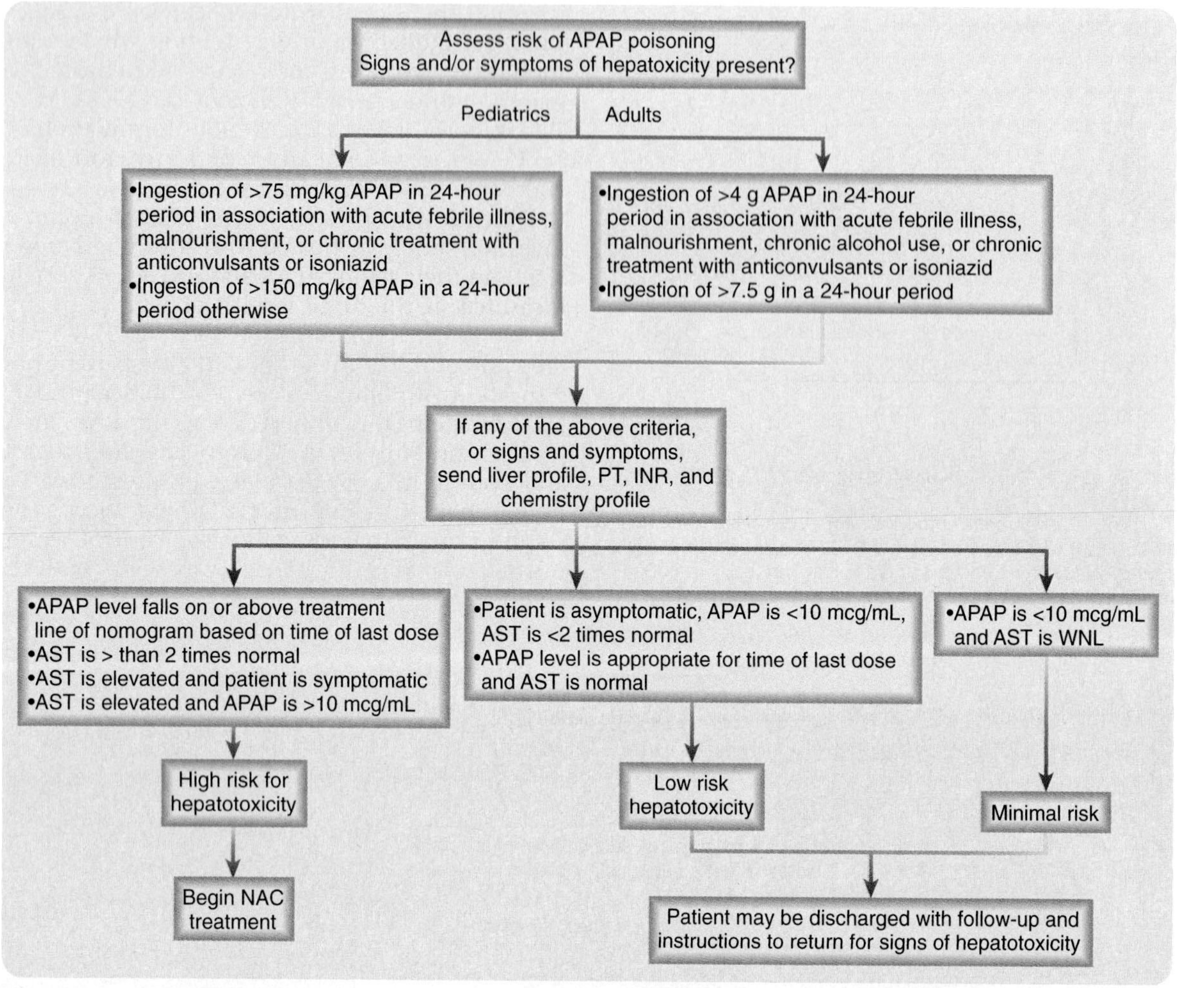
Assess risk of APAP poisoning
Signs and/or symptoms of hepatoxicity present?
Pediatrics
Adults
•Ingestion of >75 mg/kg APAP in 24-hour period in association with acute febrile illness, malnourishment, or chronic treatment with anticonvulsants or isoniazid
•Ingestion of >150 mg/kg APAP in a 24-hour period otherwise
•Ingestion of >4 g APAP in 24-hour period in association with acute febrile illness, malnourishment, chronic alcohol use, or chronic treatment with anticonvulsants or isoniazid
•Ingestion of >7.5 g in a 24-hour period
If any of the above criteria, or signs and symptoms, send liver profile, PT, INR, and chemistry profile
•APAP level falls on or above treatment line of nomogram based on time of last dose
•AST is > than 2 times normal
•AST is elevated and patient is symptomatic
•AST is elevated and APAP is >10 mcg/mL
•Patient is asymptomatic, APAP is <10 mcg/mL, AST is <2 times normal
•APAP level is appropriate for time of last dose and AST is normal
•APAP is <10 mcg/mL and AST is WNL
High risk for hepatotoxicity
Low risk hepatotoxicity
Minimal risk
Begin NAC treatment
Patient may be discharged with follow-up and instructions to return for signs of hepatotoxicity

FIGURE 138-3 Risk assessment and management of chronic acetaminophen (APAP) poisoning. AST, asparate aminotransferase; INR, international normalized ratio; NAC, *N*-acetylcysteine; PT, prothrombin time; WNL, within normal limits.

Table 138-2 ORAL VERSUS INTRAVENOUS ADMINISTRATION OF *N*-ACETYLCYSTEINE

Oral	Induces nausea/vomiting in over 50% Inexpensive Ease of dosing schedule Safer than IV administration
Intravenous	Considered preferred route in following settings: Fulminant hepatic failure Patient unable to tolerate oral administration Preparation must be adjusted for children weighing less than 40 kg Complicated dosing regimen Risk of anaphylactoid reactions

■ PEDIATRIC CONSIDERATIONS

Children should be evaluated for potential risk of hepatotoxicity after both acute exposure and repeated excessive dosing. Serum APAP and AST determinations should be performed in a patient with a large single ingestion or ingestion of more than 75 mg/kg of APAP in a 24-hour period as well as in any child with signs or symptoms of hepatotoxicity (see Figs. 138-2 and 138-3). Administer NAC if indicated according to dosing guidelines (see Table 138-3).

■ PREGNANT PATIENT

Oral NAC is routinely given to pregnant patients after potentially toxic APAP exposure and appears safe and effective. NAC appears to be safe for the fetus whether the mother receives the NAC orally or intravenously; however, there is little data regarding the efficacy of NAC in the fetus and whether there is an advantage to the oral or IV administration remains unknown.

Disposition

Patients deemed at risk for hepatotoxicity should be treated with oral NAC within 8 hours of ingestion or as soon as possible thereafter and admitted to the hospital for further medical and psychiatric evaluation as indicated. Patients who present with signs of severe hepatotoxicity, hepatic encephalopathy, or fulminant hepatic failure should be admitted to the intensive care unit (ICU), and early contact should be made with both the poison control center and the liver transplantation center (Box 138-1).

Table 138-3 DOSING SCHEDULE FOR *N*-ACETYLCYSTEINE (NAC)

Oral (adult and pediatric)	Loading dose (adult and pediatric): 140 mg/kg Maintenance dose: 70 mg/kg every 4 hr ×17 doses (next 68 hr) May be chilled and/or diluted with water, soda, or juice to ease administration
Intravenous (IV):	
Adult	Loading dose: 150 mg/kg in 200 mL of 5% dextrose in water (D_5W) over 15 min First maintenance dose: 50 mg/kg in 500 mL D_5W over 4 hr Second maintenance dose: 100 mg/kg in 1 L D_5W over 16 hr
Pediatric (<40 kg)	IV NAC is formulated as a 20% solution and must be diluted to a 2% solution: Remove 50 mL from a 500-mL bag of D_5W; add 50 mL IV NAC (20%) to 450 mL D_5W to create a 2% solution Loading dose: 7.5 mL/kg (150 mg/kg) of 2% solution over 1 hr First maintenance dose: 2.5 mL/kg (50 mg/kg) of 2% solution over 4 hr Second maintenance dose: 5 mL/kg (100 mg/kg) of 2% solution over 16 hr

BOX 138-1

Indications for Intensive Care Unit Admission or Transfer to Liver Transplantation Center for a Patient with Hepatotoxicity

Severe hepatotoxicity:

- Elevated aspartate transaminase (AST) and alanine transferase (ALT) values
- Prolonged prothrombin time
- Elevated blood urea nitrogen/creatinine value
- Metabolic acidosis
- Hypoglycemia

Signs of hepatic encephalopathy

ASPIRIN (SALICYLATES)

KEY POINTS

Aspirin (acetylsalicylic acid) is found in numerous single-agent preparations and in cold, cough, and pain relief formulations.

Methyl salicylate is found in topical liniments and in oil of wintergreen.

Aspirin toxicity in adults is characterized by a mixed respiratory alkalosis and metabolic acidosis.

Acute toxicity is characterized by tachypnea/hyperpnea, tachycardia, nausea, vomiting, and progressive central nervous system (CNS) deterioration.

Chronic aspirin toxicity is seen most commonly in the elderly and is frequently misdiagnosed as sepsis or dementia.[6]

Aspirin toxicity is treated with multiple-dose activated charcoal, fluid resuscitation, urine alkalinization, and hemodialysis.

Scope

Aspirin (acetylsalicylic acid [ASA]) is found in single-agent preparations, in numerous cold, cough, and pain relief formulations, and in topical ointments and topical wart removal agents. Bismuth salicylate is found in the antidiarrheal medicine Pepto Bismol, and methyl salicylate is used in varying concentrations in liniments (30%) and oil of wintergreen (up to 100%). The incidence of unintentional salicylate poisoning has diminished with the growing use of acetaminophen and nonsteroidal anti-inflammatory drugs (NSAIDs) and with the increasing use of acetaminophen rather than aspirin in children with viral illnesses to avoid Reye's syndrome.

Pathophysiology

Salicylate toxicity in adults is characterized by a mixed respiratory alkalosis and metabolic acidosis. Salicylates stimulate the respiratory center in the brainstem, causing hyperventilation and a primary respiratory alkalosis. Also, salicylates cause an anion gap metabolic acidosis, probably through several mechanisms.[7] They uncouple oxidative phosphorylation, leading to an accumulation of hydrogen ions, blocking the production of ATP and favoring the production of lactate. Salicylate toxicity interferes with renal elimination of sulfuric and phosphoric acids and induces fatty acid metabolism, generating β-hydroxybutyric acid and acetoacetic acid.

Among children, the primary metabolic alkalosis is commonly not seen, either because they do not sustain the hyperventilation adults do or they come to medical care later. In adults, the primary respiratory alkalosis may be blunted or absent because of salicylate-induced acute lung injury (noncardiogenic pulmonary edema), respiratory fatigue (a sign of severe toxicity), or concomitant ingestion of a CNS depressant.

Salicylate toxicity may induce acute lung injury, classically described as "noncardiogenic pulmonary edema." The mechanisms are unclear. Hypoxia is presumed to contribute to pulmonary hypertension and the release of vasoactive factors, resulting in greater capillary permeability and more exudate in the interstitial and alveolar spaces.

The increased metabolic state associated with salicylate poisoning results in hypoglycemia and ketosis.

Ototoxicity, characterized by hearing loss and tinnitus, is a predictable manifestation of salicylate toxicity that occurs with serum ASA concentrations of 25 to 40 mg/dL. The cause is unknown; it is postulated that salicylate's effects on glucose and protein metabolism affect the endolymph and perilymph and alter nerve transmission.

Presenting Signs and Symptoms

See Table 138-4 for clinical manifestations of salicylate toxicity, and Table 138-5 for comparison of acute and chronic salicylate toxicity.

Table 138-4 CLINICAL MANIFESTATIONS OF SALICYLATE TOXICITY

Central nervous system	Tinnitus/decreased hearing Confusion/agitation Lethargy Coma Seizure Syndrome of inappropriate antidiuretic hormone secretion (SIADH)
Gastrointestinal system	Nausea, vomiting Abdominal pain/gastritis Decreased motility
Cardiovascular system	Tachycardia (usually secondary to hypovolemia, hyperpyrexia)
Pulmonary	Tachypnea/hyperpnea Acute lung injury
Hematologic	Prolongation of prothrombin time Platelet dysfunction
Acid-base/electrolyte abnormalities	Respiratory alkalosis Metabolic acidosis Respiratory acidosis Hypokalemia Hyponatremia or hypernatremia
Metabolic changes	Hyperthermia/diaphoresis Hypoglycemia or hyperglycemia Hypoglycorrhachia Ketonemia/ketonuria

Table 138-5 COMPARISON OF ACUTE AND CHRONIC SALICYLATE TOXICITY

Acute	Chronic
Seen in toddlers and suicidal adults	Seen primarily in elderly
Typically due to intentional overdose in suicidal adults or unintentional ingestion by children	Typically due to unintentional overdose by elderly in treatment of chronic pain
Acute onset	Insidious onset
Gastrointestinal (GI) symptoms common	GI symptoms uncommon Central nervous symptoms predominate Typically misdiagnosed as altered mental status
Significant toxicity associated with high serum salicylate value	Significant toxicity associated with low to moderately elevated salicylate value

Table 138-6 DIAGNOSTIC TESTING IN SALICYLATE TOXICITY

Test	Findings and Significance
Serum acetylsalicylic acid (ASA) measurement	Check every 2-4 hr Therapeutic value: 15-30 mg/dL >30 mg/dL: clinical manifestations evident >90-100 mg/dL: severe toxicity (acute) Chronic toxicity: patient may have significant toxicity with mild to moderately elevated ASA value
Urinalysis	Ketonuria Glucosuria pH abnormality
Electrolytes	Elevated anion gap Hyperglycemia or hypoglycemia Hypokalemia
Arterial blood gas measurement	Initial respiratory alkalosis: pH>7.4 (rarely seen in pediatric patients) Metabolic acidosis: pH still >7.4; mixed metabolic acidosis and respiratory alkalosis Worsening metabolic acidosis with acidemia: pH<7.4; indicates severe toxicity
Chest radiograph	Acute lung injury
Electrocardiogram	Sinus tachycardia

Diagnostic Criteria

See Table 138-6 for laboratory and diagnostic tests useful in evaluating salicylate toxicity.

Management

The mainstays of therapy after salicylate ingestion are multiple-dose activated charcoal, fluid and electrolyte replenishment, urine alkalinization, and, in cases of severe toxicity, hemodialysis. Table 138-7 lists guidelines for managing and treating patients with salicylate toxicity, instructions on urine alkalization, and indications for hemodialysis. The EP should contact the renal service early in cases of severe toxicity and should consult with the regional poison control center for continued assistance soon after patient presentation.

Disposition

Patients who present with signs or symptoms of salicylate toxicity should be admitted to the hospital for continued monitoring of clinical condition and serial laboratory evaluations. Patients with signs and symptoms of serious toxicity should be admitted to the ICU and evaluated early by the renal service for possible hemodialysis.

Table 138-7 MANAGEMENT AND TREATMENT OF SALICYLATE TOXICITY

Gastric decontamination	Multidose activated charcoal: typically 1-2 g/kg every 4-6 hours up to 50 g for 2-3 doses Do not administer with sorbitol more than once[8]
Fluid replacement	Patients often significantly dehydrated due to vomiting, hyperthermia, diaphoresis, and tachypnea/hyperpnea Increasing fluids beyond resuscitation needs ("forced diuresis") not recommended
Urine alkalinization ("ion trapping")[9] Goal is to alkalinize blood and urine to "trap" ionized salicylate, keep it out of the brain, and enhance urinary elimination Acetazolamide administration is **NOT** recommended; it alkalinizes urine but acidifies blood and may increase brain salicylate concentration[9]	Indications: Patient has signs/symptoms of salicylate toxicity Serum acetylsalicylic acid (ASA) level >40 mg/dL Technique: IV bolus 1-2 mEq/kg sodium bicarbonate Sodium bicarbonate infusion: 132 mEq sodium bicarbonate (3 ampules)+40 mEq potassium chloride in 1 L 5% dextrose in water (D_5W) to run at 2×maintenance fluid requirements Goals: Serum pH 7.45-7.55 Urine pH 7.5-8.0 Need to replenish/maintain serum potassium to achieve urine alkalinization Monitor serum calcium and replenish as necessary during sodium bicarbonate therapy
Airway management	Avoid exacerbating acidemia during endotracheal intubation Important to maintain hyperventilation during mechanical ventilation
Hemodialysis	Indications: Signs/symptoms of end-organ toxicity (altered mental status, acute lung injury, metabolic acidemia despite treatment) Progressive clinical deterioration despite adequate supportive care Renal failure Serum ASA level (acute) >90-100 mg/dL

NONSTEROIDAL ANTI-INFLAMMATORY DRUGS

KEY POINTS

Nonsteroidal anti-inflammatory drugs (NSAIDs) are a large class of drugs that include the over-the-counter drugs ibuprofen, naproxen, and ketoprofen.

Nausea, vomiting, epigastric pain, and mild CNS depression are the most common clinical manifestations of NSAID poisoning.

NSAID toxicity is usually mild and should be managed with gastrointestinal decontamination and supportive care.

Scope

Nonsteroidal anti-inflammatory drugs (NSAIDs) are a large class of drugs; exposures to and overdoses of NSAIDs are common given their widespread use. Ibuprofen, naproxen, and ketoprofen are available over the counter. Ibuprofen accounts for 70% to 80% of all NSAID exposures reported to U.S. poison control centers.

Pathophysiology

All NSAIDs competitively inhibit cyclooxygenase (COX), preventing the formation of prostaglandins, prostacyclins, and thromboxane.[10] (Unlike salicylates, NSAIDs reversibly bind to COX.) There are two isoforms, COX-1 and COX-2. The analgesic and anti-inflammatory properties are attributed to COX-2 inhibition. Therapeutic use of COX-2–specific inhibitors has been associated with cardiotoxicity. Most of the adverse effects and the acute toxicity of NSAIDs are attributed to COX-1 inhibition.

NSAIDs directly irritate gastrointestinal mucosa; COX-1–mediated prostaglandin inhibition further contributes to gastrointestinal irritation, ulceration, and perforation.

Rarely, NSAID toxicity induces an anion gap metabolic acidosis associated with a serum lactate

Table 138-8 CLINICAL MANIFESTATIONS OF NONSTEROIDAL ANTI-INFLAMMATORY DRUG TOXICITY

Gastrointestinal	Nausea, vomiting, abdominal pain Gastritis, peptic ulcer disease Gastrointestinal bleeding
Renal[12]	Sodium, potassium, water retention Acute renal failure Chronic interstitial nephritis Papillary necrosis
Central nervous system	Headache Confusion, delirium, hallucinations (especially in the elderly) Tinnitus/hearing loss Coma
Pulmonary	Bronchospasm Pneumonitis
Hematologic	Platelet dysfunction Thrombocytopenia Hemolytic anemia, immune-mediated Aplastic anemia
Acid-base abnormality	Metabolic acidosis (associated with large ibuprofen overdose)
Hepatic	Elevated liver enzyme values

elevation. This condition is attributed to NSAID metabolites that are weak acids rather than to COX inhibition and is favored by relative hypotension and hypoxia.

NSAID-induced renal toxicity is due to prostaglandin inhibition and occurs in the setting of low intravascular volume such as occurs with hypovolemia, congestive heart failure, cirrhosis, or intrinsic renal disease.

Via inhibition of thromboxane A_2, NSAIDs decrease platelet aggregation. Other idiosyncratic reactions associated with some NSAIDs are hemolytic anemia, aplastic anemia, agranulocytosis, and thrombocytopenia.

NSAID-induced COX inhibition is associated with anaphylactoid reactions. Acute bronchospasm may develop within minutes to hours of NSAID ingestion in adult patients with asthma and chronic urticaria or nasal polyps. Agents that block 5-lipoxygenase or leukotriene receptors may prevent adverse reactions.

Presenting Signs and Symptoms

See Table 138-8 for clinical manifestations of NSAID toxicity. Gastrointestinal manifestations are the most common; rare manifestations after large ibuprofen ingestions include metabolic acidosis, coma, bradycardia, and hypotension.[11]

Diagnostic Testing

Serum NSAID concentrations are not readily available from hospital laboratories and are not clinically useful. After a large overdose or in symptomatic patients, serum electrolyte, blood urea nitrogen/creatinine, serum bicarbonate, and arterial blood gas measurements should be performed.

BOX 138-2

Management of NSAID Ingestion

- Gastric decontamination with activated charcoal
- Fluid and electrolyte replacement
- Supportive care

Management

Life-threatening complications after NSAID overdose are rare. Asymptomatic patients should receive one dose of activated charcoal and should be observed for 6 hours after ingestion. Patients who remain asymptomatic may be further evaluated by the psychiatric service or may be discharged with arrangements for follow-up and instructions to return if signs and symptoms of gastrointestinal or central nervous symptoms develop. For symptomatic patients, the diagnostic tests already described should be performed and the patients should be admitted to the hospital for further observation and evaluation. (See Box 138-2 for management guidelines).

Tips and Tricks

- Measure serum acetaminophen in all patients with suspected overdose.
- Initiate treatment with *N*-acetylcysteine (NAC) in patients who present late after acetaminophen overdose.
- Initiate early contact with the poison control center and liver transplant center for patients with severe acetaminophen toxicity.
- Consider chronic salicylate poisoning in elderly patients who present with altered mental status.
- Initiate treatment with sodium bicarbonate and contact the renal service for potential hemodialysis in patients with salicylate poisoning.
- Beware of the risk of worsening acidemia during intubation of patients with severe salicylate poisoning, and ensure adequate ventilation.

REFERENCES

1. Lucanie R, Chiang WK, Reilly R: Utility of acetaminophen screening in unsuspected suicidal ingestions. Vet Hum Toxicol 2002;44:171-173.
2. Renzi FP, Donovan JW, Martin TG, et al: Concomitant use of activated charcoal and *N*-acetylcysteine. Ann Emerg Med 1985;14:568-572.
3. Smilkstein MJ, Knapp GL, Kulig KW, et al: Efficiency of oral *N*-acetylcysteine in the treatment of acetaminophen overdose. Analysis of the National Multicenter Study (1976-1985). N Engl J Med 1988;319:1557-1562.
4. Prescott LF, Illingworth RN, Critchley JA, et al: Intravenous *N*-acetylcysteine: The treatment of choice for paracetamol poisoning. Br Med J 1979;2(6198):1097-1100.
5. Harrison PM, Wendon JA, Gimson AE, et al: Improvement by acetylcysteine of hemodynamics and oxygen transport in fulminant hepatic failure. N Engl J Med 1991; 324:1852-1857.
6. Anderson RJ, Potts DE, Gabow PA, et al: Unrecognized adult salicylate intoxication. Ann Intern Med 1976;85: 745-748.
7. Gabow PA, Anderson RJ, Potts DE, et al: Acid-base disturbances in the salicylate-intoxicated adult. Arch Intern Med 1978;138:1481-1484.
8. Barone JA, Raia JJ, Huang YC: Evaluation of the effects of multiple-dose activated charcoal on the absorption of orally administered salicylate in a simulated toxic ingestion model. Ann Emerg Med 1988;17:34-37.
9. Prescott LF, Balali-Mood M, Critchley JA, et al: Diuresis or urinary alkalinisation for salicylate poisoning? Br Med J (Clin Res Ed) 1982;285:1383-1386.
10. Hall AH, Smolinske SC, Stover B, et al: Ibuprofen overdose in adults. J Toxicol Clin Toxicol 1992;30:23-37.
11. Cryer B, Kimmey MB: Gastrointestinal side effects of non-steroidal anti-inflammatory drugs. Am J Med 1998;105: 20S-30S.
12. Clive DM, Stoff JS: Renal syndromes associated with non-steroidal antiinflammatory drugs. N Engl J Med 1984;310: 563-572.

Chapter 139

Anticholinergics

Jessica A. Fulton and Lewis S. Nelson

KEY POINTS

Antimuscarinic poisoning syndrome is a more appropriate description than *anticholinergic overdose* because only the muscarinic receptors, not the nicotinic acetylcholine receptors, are involved.

Anticholinergic (antimuscarinic) agents antagonize the neurotransmitter acetylcholine at both central and peripheral muscarinic acetylcholine receptors, leading to altered mental status, mydriasis, tachycardia, urinary retention, ileus, and dry, flushed skin.

Although patients with both adrenergic (sympathomimetic) and anticholinergic (antimuscarinic) poisoning may present with similar symptoms, the two syndromes may be differentiated by skin and mental status findings. Diaphoresis, agitation, paranoid hallucinations, and violent behavior are associated with sympathomimetic agents. Dry skin and mucous membranes, mumbling speech, delirium, and tactile or visual hallucinations are associated with anticholinergics.

The anticholinergic (antimuscarinic) syndrome can be caused by many agents, including atropine, diphenhydramine, and scopolamine.

Diagnosis of the anticholinergic (antimuscarinic) syndrome is largely clinical and should include a physical examination, fingerstick serum glucose measurement, and an electrocardiogram.

The anticholinergic syndrome is a key clinical finding leading to the diagnosis of poisoning by tricyclic antidepressants (a subset of antimuscarinic agents).

Basic treatment involves supportive care of vital signs, activated charcoal, benzodiazepines for agitation, sodium bicarbonate for QRS >100 msec or a wide-complex tachycardia, and physostigmine for central and peripheral anticholinergic (antimuscarinic) manifestations, if appropriate.

Scope

Anticholinergic agents hold a notable place in world history. In ancient times, anticholinergic agents were used as components in folk medicines to treat epilepsy and psychoses. *Datura stramonium* (containing atropine and scopolamine) was purportedly used by Cleopatra to woo Caesar. Marc Anthony's troops ate *Datura* as they left Parthia in 38 AD and thereafter became stuporous and confused, leading to their defeat. In 1676, British soldiers during a confrontation in Jamestown, Virginia, inadvertently consumed *Datura* in a salad. A witness described the result as "a very pleasant Comedy, for they turn'd natural Fools upon it for several Days: One would blow up a Feather in the Air; another wou'd dart Straws at it with much

Fury; and another, stark naked, was sitting up in a Corner like a Monkey, grinning and making Mows at them; a Fourth would fondly kiss and paw his Companions, and sneer in their faces. . . . [A] thousand such simple tricks they played, and after Eleven Days return'd themselves again, not remembering anything that had pass'd."[1] As a result of the victory for the burgeoning American nation, *Datura* became commonly known as Jamestown weed or jimsonweed.

Datura was used as a therapy for asthma in the early 20th century, and medications with anticholinergic effects are still in use today. Some effects are therapeutically intended by the prescriber, and others are undesired. Still other effects, such as hallucinations, are sought by recreational users.

The syndrome of anticholinergic toxicity is common, making the recognition of its associated signs and symptoms a necessary clinical skill (Table 139-1).

Table 139-1 AGENTS THAT PRODUCE THE ANTICHOLINERGIC (ANTIMUSCARINIC) POISONING SYNDROME

Plants	*Atropa belladonna* (deadly nightshade) *Datura stramonium* (jimsonweed) *Mandragora officinarum* (mandrake) *Hyoscyamus niger* (henbane)
Belladonna alkaloids and related synthetic compounds	Atropine Homatropine Scopolamine Glycopyrrolate (peripheral effects only)
Antispasmodics	Clidinium bromide (Librax) Cyclobenzaprine (Flexeril) Dicyclomine (Bentyl) Propantheline bromide (Pro-Banthine) Methantheline bromide (Banthine) Orphenadrine (Norflex) Flavoxate (Urispas) Oxybutynin (Ditropan)
Antiparkinsonian medications	Benztropine mesylate (Cogentin) Biperiden (Akineton) Trihexyphenidyl (Artane)
Topical mydriatics (ocular)	Cyclopentolate (Cyclogyl) Homatropine (Isopto Homatropine) Tropicamide (Mydriacyl)
Antihistamines	Brompheniramine (Dimetane) Chlorpheniramine (Ornade, Chlor-Trimeton) Cyclizine (Marezine) Dimenhydrinate (Dramamine) Diphenhydramine (Benadryl, Caladryl) Hydroxyzine (Atarax, Vistaril) Meclizine (Antivert) Doxylamine (Unisom) Promethazine (Phenergan)
Antipsychotics	Clozapine (Clozaril) Chlorpromazine (Thorazine) Prochlorperazine (Compazine) Thiothixene (Navane) Thioridazine (Mellaril) Trifluoperazine (Stelazine) Perphenazine (Trilafon)
Others	Amantadine (Symmetrel) Disopyramide (Norpace) Glutethimide (Doriden) Procainamide (Pronestyl) Quinidine (Quinidex)

Pathophysiology and Pharmacology

Acetylcholine is a neurotransmitter released from cholinergic nerve endings in the central (brain and spinal cord) and the peripheral (autonomic and somatic) nervous systems. In the autonomic (sympathetic and parasympathetic) nervous system, acetylcholine is released from all preganglionic neurons as well as postganglionic parasympathetic neurons. Its degradation by the enzyme acetylcholinesterase occurs in the synapse between the presynaptic and postsynaptic membranes.

There are two types of postsynaptic acetylcholine receptors, nicotinic and muscarinic. Nicotinic acetylcholine receptors are ion channels. Found throughout the central nervous system (CNS) (most abundantly in the spinal cord), they are the postsynaptic receptors in the preganglionic sympathetic and parasympathetic neurons. Additionally, these receptors are found in the somatic nervous system at postganglionic skeletal neuromuscular junctions that mediate muscle contraction as well as in the postganglionic neurons of the adrenal medulla, which are subsequently responsible for the release of epinephrine and norepinephrine.

Muscarinic acetylcholine receptors are G protein–linked. They are found primarily in the CNS (most abundantly in the brain). They are also found at effector organs innervated by postganglionic parasympathetic neurons. Stimulation of these end organs, either pharmacologically or through enhanced neuronal output, results in miosis, lacrimation, salivation, bronchospasm, bronchorrhea, bradydysrhythmias, urination, and increased gastrointestinal motility (Table 139-2). Finally, muscarinic receptors are located in sweat glands innervated by postsynaptic sympathetic neurons and cause diaphoresis when stimulated.

Muscarinic acetylcholine receptor antagonists competitively inhibit muscarinic acetylcholine receptors. These agents cause the classic "anticholinergic poisoning syndrome," which perhaps may be more appropriately named the *antimuscarinic poisoning syndrome,* because nicotinic acetylcholine receptors are not involved. Muscarinic receptors in different organs are not equally sensitive to antimuscarinic agents.

Tricyclic antidepressants are a unique subset of antimuscarinic agents that deserve special attention. Their antidepressant effect is achieved pharmacologically through blockade of the reuptake of norepinephrine, dopamine, and serotonin in the CNS. Additionally, tricyclic antidepressants interact with many other receptors, causing cardiovascular and CNS toxicity in overdose. Adverse effects of tricyclic antidepressant overdose include competitive inhibition at both central and peripheral muscarinic

Table 139-2 PATHOPHYSIOLOGY OF ANTICHOLINERGIC ("ANTIMUSCARINIC POISONING SYNDROME") SYMPTOMS

Anticholinergic Effect	Symptoms
Central inhibition of muscarinic acetylcholine receptors	Confusion, disorientation, psychomotor agitation, ataxia, myoclonus, tremor, picking movements, abnormal speech, visual/auditory hallucinations, psychosis, seizures, cardiovascular collapse, coma
Inhibition of postsynaptic sympathetic muscarinic acetylcholine receptors in the sweat glands as well as vasodilation of peripheral blood vessels	Dry, flushed skin
Inhibition of post-synaptic parasympathetic muscarinic acetylcholine receptors in the:	
Salivary glands	Dry mucous membranes
Eye	Paralysis of the sphincter muscle of the iris and the ciliary muscle of the lens, resulting in mydriasis, cycloplegia, and blurred vision
Heart (vagus nerve)	Tachycardia
Bladder	Urinary retention and overflow incontinence
Bowel	Adynamic ileus

Table 139-3 PATHOPHYSIOLOGY OF TRICYCLIC ANTIDEPRESSANTS AND ASSOCIATED SYMPTOMS

Effect	Symptoms
Blockade of reuptake of norepinephrine, dopamine, and serotonin in the central nervous system	Mood elevation
Competitive inhibition at both central and peripheral muscarinic acetylcholine receptors	"Antimuscarinic poisoning syndrome"
Histamine receptor antagonism	Sedation
Sodium channel blockade in the myocardium	QRS complex widening/wide-complex dysrhythmias, atrioventricular block, QT prolongation and rightward shift of the terminal 40-msec QRS axis on electrocardiogram as well as negative inotropy leading to hypotension
Alpha-adrenergic receptor antagonism on vascular smooth muscle	Vasodilation leading to hypotension
Gamma-aminobutyric acid (GABA) antagonism	Seizures

acetylcholine receptors (antimuscarinic poisoning syndrome); histamine receptor antagonism (sedation); sodium channel blockade in the myocardium (QRS complex widening/wide-complex dysrhythmias, atrioventricular block, QT prolongation, and rightward shift of the terminal 40-msec QRS axis on an electrocardiogram [ECG] as well as negative inotropy leading to hypotension); alpha-adrenergic receptor antagonism on vascular smooth muscle (vasodilation leading to hypotension); and, although the mechanism of this effect is unclear, gamma-aminobutyric acid (GABA) antagonism (seizures). The anticholinergic syndrome is a key clinical finding leading to the diagnosis of tricyclic antidepressant poisoning (Table 139-3).

Presenting Signs and Symptoms

■ CLASSIC

Central inhibition of muscarinic acetylcholine receptors results in confusion, disorientation, psychomotor agitation, ataxia, myoclonus, tremor, picking movements, abnormal speech, visual/auditory hallucinations, psychosis, seizures, cardiovascular collapse, and coma.

Inhibition of postsynaptic sympathetic muscarinic acetylcholine receptors in the sweat glands as well as vasodilation of peripheral blood vessels gives rise to dry, flushed skin. Inability to sweat, particularly in the presence of altered CNS regulation, may lead to hyperthermia. Inhibition of these receptors in the salivary glands results in dry mucous membranes. Inhibition of such receptors in the eye (which normally cause pupillary constriction) leads to paralysis of the sphincter muscle of the iris and the ciliary muscle of the lens, resulting in mydriasis, cycloplegia, and blurred vision. Tachycardia is caused by inhibition of postsynaptic parasympathetic muscarinic acetylcholine receptors on the vagus nerve. Dysrhythmias may be caused by antimuscarinic agents that possess additional pharmacologic effects. For example, agents that produce sodium channel blockade in the myocardium (i.e., tricyclic antidepressants, diphenhydramine, pheniramine, orphenadrine, pyrilamine) cause QRS complex widening/wide-

Documentation

History

- Any history of psychiatric illness or prior suicidal ingestions
- Time lapse since ingestion, if known
- History of renal or cardiac disease or other illnesses

Physical Examination

- Does the patient look ill? Pale? Febrile? What is mental status?
- Cardiac status (blood pressure, arrhythmias)
- Respiratory and airway status
- Urine output

Physical examination should be repeated while patient is in the ED.

Diagnostic Studies

- Electrocardiogram, blood chemistry panel, and serum glucose, serum creatine phosphokinase, and urine myoglobin measurements
- Acetaminophen and aspirin levels if there is concern about co-ingestion

Medical Decision-Making

- Decision to begin treatment or delays in starting treatment?
- Consultations desired and times of calls to consulting services

Treatment

Response to treatment (especially for sodium bicarbonate, magnesium, or physostigmine)

Patient Instructions

- Document discussion with patient regarding diagnosis, warning signs, what to do, follow-up, and when to return.
- With pediatric unintentional ingestions, document poison prevention counseling and assessment of home situation.
- The regional poison control center can be contacted by telephone at 1-800-222-1222. All poison emergencies should be reported by the patient to the local poison control center.
- A dose of medication other than what was prescribed by the patient's physician should never be taken or given unless it has been approved by the ordering physician.
- A second medication or herbal supplement should never be added to a previously taken medication without approval from the physician.

complex dysrhythmias, atrioventricular block, QT prolongation, and rightward shift of the terminal 40-msec QRS axis on an ECG as well as negative inotropy, leading to hypotension. Inhibition of postsynaptic parasympathetic muscarinic acetylcholine receptors in the bladder results in urinary retention and overflow incontinence, and in the bowel it causes adynamic ileus.

■ VARIATIONS

Often, patients with anticholinergic (antimuscarinic) poisoning do not present with all of the previously mentioned characteristics of the classic syndrome. This is especially true in the elderly and in patients with organic brain syndrome, in which the central anticholinergic (antimuscarinic) poisoning syndrome often is more pronounced than or outlasts the peripheral syndrome.

Differential Diagnosis

After an overdose of an anticholinergic (antimuscarinic) agent, a patient often presents with sufficient manifestations of the classic anticholinergic toxidrome and a compatible history, making the diagnosis apparent. However, the symptoms and signs in others may be less overt, forcing the clinician to broaden the differential diagnosis.

Although in both adrenergic (sympathomimetic) and anticholinergic (antimuscarinic) poisoning, patients may present with confusion, disorientation, psychomotor agitation, seizures, flushed skin, hyperthermia, mydriasis, and tachycardia, the two syndromes may be differentiated through examination of the skin and observation of the symptoms associated with altered mental status. Patients with anticholinergic (antimuscarinic) poisoning have dry skin and mucous membranes, and the alteration in mental status is characterized by mumbling speech, delirium, and tactile or visual hallucinations. Alternatively, patients poisoned by sympathomimetic agents, such as cocaine toxicity, are typically diaphoretic with agitated or violent behavior and hallucinations that are more typically paranoid.

Multiple toxicologic entities in addition to anticholinergic (antimuscarinic) poisoning may be associated with autonomic dysfunction (i.e., dysregulation of heart rate, blood pressure, temperature, gastrointestinal secretion, and metabolic and endocrine responses to stress). Acute withdrawal syndromes may be differentiated from the anticholinergic (antimuscarinic) syndrome by a history of recent cessation of ethanol or another sedative-hypnotic agent; serotonin syndrome may be differentiated by a history of recent (minutes to hours) exposure to a serotonergic agent; and neuroleptic malignant syndrome may be differentiated by a history of exposure (within 3 to 9 days) to an agent capable of producing central dopamine blockade. Drug-induced psychosis mimicking the central anticholinergic syndrome may be due to hallucinogens, phencyclidine, amphetamines, or corticosteroids.

Medical diseases that produce confusion, seizures, and tachycardia, such as hypoxia, hypoglycemia, and heat stroke, or those that cause hyperthermia, hypertension, tachycardia, and mydriasis, such thyrotoxicosis and pheochromocytoma, may also be confused with anticholinergic toxicity.

Finally, diseases that may manifest similarly to a central anticholinergic syndrome include schizophrenia and other psychotic disorders, cerebral vasculitis, CNS infection (e.g., encephalitis), sepsis, and psychiatric disease.

Diagnostic Testing

In the setting of anticholinergic (antimuscarinic) poisoning, results of the finger-stick serum glucose test and pulse oximetry analysis should be normal.

The ECG typically demonstrates sinus tachycardia. Some agents with anticholinergic (antimuscarinic) effects also have type IA antidysrhythmic effects, resulting in blockade of myocardial sodium channels. The blockade is seen on the ECG as prolongation of the QRS interval. Such agents are diphenhydramine, cyclobenzaprine, carbamazepine, and the tricyclic antidepressants.

With tricyclic antidepressant overdose in particular, the extent of QRS interval prolongation on an ECG is especially useful in predicting the severity of toxicity. A QRS interval shorter than 100 msec is not associated with toxicity; a QRS interval longer is 100 msec is associated with a 30% chance of seizures; and a QRS interval longer than 160 msec is associated with a 50% chance of ventricular dysrhythmias.[2] Additionally, an R wave in lead aVR greater than or equal to 3 mm[3] or a terminal 40-msec right axis deviation between 130 and 270 degrees[4] is a predictor of tricyclic antidepressant–induced toxicity.

Prolonged agitation and seizures can lead to the development of rhabdomyolysis. Measurement of serum creatine phosphokinase and urine myoglobin aids in the recognition of patients at risk for the development of acute renal failure.

Treatment

Most patients with anticholinergic (antimuscarinic) toxicity can be adequately treated with general supportive care of the airway, breathing, and circulation followed by frequent reassessment and close observation (Fig. 139-1). To avoid the risk of aspiration, activated charcoal (1 gm/kg) is recommended only for a patient who is capable of spontaneously drinking and of protecting his or her own airway. It may also be administered cautiously via a nasogastric tube in patients who are endotracheally intubated. Because anticholinergic (antimuscarinic) agents may slow gastrointestinal transit, activated charcoal may be useful hours after ingestion.[5] The specific role of activated charcoal in most of these poisonings is unstudied.

The initial therapy for cardiovascular toxicity due to sodium channel blockade is hypertonic sodium bicarbonate in 1-2 mEq/kg boluses.[6] Treatment with sodium bicarbonate is indicated in the presence of a QRS complex longer than 100 to 120 msec or of a wide-complex/ventricular tachycardia until the abnormality is reversed or the serum pH reaches 7.55. The ECG should be repeated within 60 seconds after a bolus of sodium bicarbonate to check for narrowing of the QRS complex. If narrowing has occurred, a continuous infusion at 1.5 times the maintenance IV fluid rate (3 ampules [132 mEq] sodium bicarbonate in 1 L of 5% dextrose in water [D_5W]) should be administered. Profound cardiovascular toxicity may require more aggressive interventions, such as the initiation of vasopressors or use of an intra-aortic balloon pump.

Agitation should be aggressively addressed to prevent the development of more serious sequelae, such as hyperthermia, acidosis, and rhabdomyolysis. It is best controlled with benzodiazepines. The ED should start with standard doses (i.e., diazepam 5-10 mg IV) and repeat until sedation (relief of agitation, myoclonus, tremor, picking movements, abnormal speech, and hallucinations)—but not stupor or coma—is achieved. Administration of physostigmine should also be considered for the treatment of agitation caused by an anticholinergic (antimuscarinic) agent (see later).

Anticholinergic (antimuscarinic) agent–induced seizures should also be treated with standard doses of benzodiazepines (i.e., lorazepam 2 mg IV) or with physostigmine. If this therapy fails, barbiturates or other GABAergic anticonvulsants should be administered. Phenytoin is rarely useful in toxin-induced seizures.

Patients with rhabdomyolysis should receive intravenous saline at a rate sufficient to maintain a brisk urine output (generally 3-5 mL/kg/hr after any lost intravascular volume is repleted). If urinary pH is less than 6.0, urine alkalinization is necessary and is achieved with the use of a sodium bicarbonate infusion at 1.5 times the maintenance IV fluid rate (3 ampules [132 mEq] sodium bicarbonate in 1 L of D_5W). Serum pH must be monitored during the sodium bicarbonate infusion and should be stopped if the serum pH is 7.55 or higher.

■ ANTIDOTAL THERAPY—PHYSOSTIGMINE

Physostigmine is a tertiary amine carbamate that penetrates into the CNS. It reversibly inhibits cholinesterases in both the central and peripheral nervous systems, thereby allowing acetylcholine to accumulate within the synapse. Accumulation of acetylcholine directly antagonizes the anticholinergic effects of antimuscarinic agents.

In the setting of a clear diagnosis of anticholinergic toxicity, physostigmine should be administered. It is beneficial in the treatment of agitation and delirium and also shortens the period to recovery after agitation. This agent should not be given once a benzodiazepine has been given, because the endpoint of a clear mental status has been lost.[7]

After administration of physostigmine, patients must be monitored for early signs of cholinergic tox-

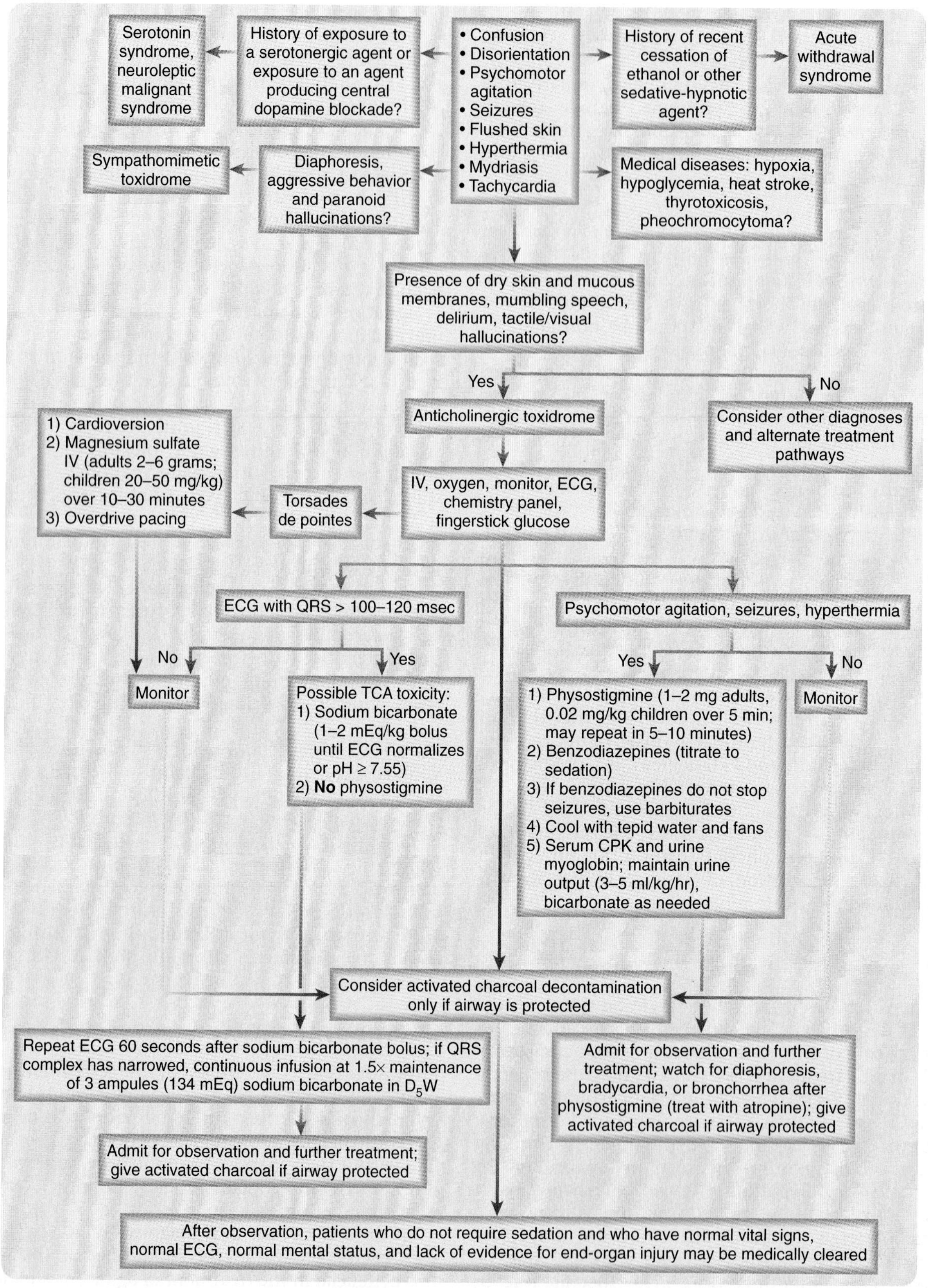
Serotonin syndrome, neuroleptic malignant syndrome
History of exposure to a serotonergic agent or exposure to an agent producing central dopamine blockade?
• Confusion
• Disorientation
• Psychomotor agitation
• Seizures
• Flushed skin
• Hyperthermia
• Mydriasis
• Tachycardia
History of recent cessation of ethanol or other sedative-hypnotic agent?
Acute withdrawal syndrome
Sympathomimetic toxidrome
Diaphoresis, aggressive behavior and paranoid hallucinations?
Medical diseases: hypoxia, hypoglycemia, heat stroke, thyrotoxicosis, pheochromocytoma?
Presence of dry skin and mucous membranes, mumbling speech, delirium, tactile/visual hallucinations?
Yes
No
Anticholinergic toxidrome
Consider other diagnoses and alternate treatment pathways
1) Cardioversion
2) Magnesium sulfate IV (adults 2–6 grams; children 20–50 mg/kg) over 10–30 minutes
3) Overdrive pacing
Torsades de pointes
IV, oxygen, monitor, ECG, chemistry panel, fingerstick glucose
ECG with QRS > 100–120 msec
Psychomotor agitation, seizures, hyperthermia
No
Yes
Yes
No
Monitor
Possible TCA toxicity:
1) Sodium bicarbonate (1–2 mEq/kg bolus until ECG normalizes or pH ≥ 7.55)
2) No physostigmine
1) Physostigmine (1–2 mg adults, 0.02 mg/kg children over 5 min; may repeat in 5–10 minutes)
2) Benzodiazepines (titrate to sedation)
3) If benzodiazepines do not stop seizures, use barbiturates
4) Cool with tepid water and fans
5) Serum CPK and urine myoglobin; maintain urine output (3–5 ml/kg/hr), bicarbonate as needed
Monitor
Consider activated charcoal decontamination only if airway is protected
Repeat ECG 60 seconds after sodium bicarbonate bolus; if QRS complex has narrowed, continuous infusion at 1.5× maintenance of 3 ampules (134 mEq) sodium bicarbonate in D5W
Admit for observation and further treatment; watch for diaphoresis, bradycardia, or bronchorrhea after physostigmine (treat with atropine); give activated charcoal if airway protected
Admit for observation and further treatment; give activated charcoal if airway protected
After observation, patients who do not require sedation and who have normal vital signs, normal ECG, normal mental status, and lack of evidence for end-organ injury may be medically cleared

FIGURE 139-1 Algorithm for the recognition and treatment of anticholinergic toxicity. CPK, creatine phosphokinase; D_5W, 5% dextrose in water; ECG, electrocardiogram; IV, intravenous; TCA, tricyclic antidepressant.

RED FLAGS

- Physostigmine is contraindicated in the presence of tricyclic antidepressant overdose and in patients with a QRS interval >100 msec because it may cause asystole.
- Flumazenil generally should not be administered to patients with anticholinergic (antimuscarinic) toxicity because it may cause seizures or other complications.
- Failure to become cholinergic (bradycardia, bronchorrhea, muscle weakness, etc.) after administration of physostigmine is essentially diagnostic of anticholinergic toxicity.
- When other cholinergic agents are used concurrently with physostigmine, their effects may be additive; therefore, caution should be used when choosing a paralytic agent for intubation. Physostigmine will prolong the action of drugs metabolized by plasma cholinesterases such as succinylcholine. A nondepolarizing agent should be used instead.

icity, such as diaphoresis and slowing heart rate. Atropine should be kept at the bedside and should be given in titrated doses if needed for cholinergic toxicity (development of bronchorrhea, hypoxia, bradycardia).

Physostigmine is indicated in the presence of central (and perhaps peripheral) anticholinergic manifestations. It is contraindicated in patients with a QRS interval longer than 100 msec or a suspected history of tricyclic antidepressant ingestion. The latter contraindication is based on two case reports of patients with tricyclic antidepressant overdose in whom asystole developed after the administration of physostigmine. The cause of asystole is theorized to be secondary to physostigmine-induced bradycardia that resulted in cardiac conduction defects and decreased cardiac output in the presence of tricyclic antidepressant–induced sodium channel blockade.[8] Other contraindications to the use of physostigmine are bronchospastic disease, peripheral vascular disease, intestinal or bladder obstruction, intraventricular conduction defects, and atrioventricular block.

Physostigmine is administered intravenously over 5 minutes, 1 to 2 mg in adults and 0.02 mg/kg (maximum 0.5 mg) in children. Onset of action occurs within minutes.[9] This initial dose can be repeated in 5 to 10 minutes if an adequate response is not achieved and muscarinic effects are not noted. Failure of the patient to become cholinergic after administration of physostigmine is essentially diagnostic of anticholinergic toxicity. Although the total effective dose of physostigmine depends on the individual as well as the dose and duration of action of the anticholinergic (antimuscarinic) agent, 4 mg is usually a sufficient dose for most patients.[10] Physostigmine's half-life is 16 minutes and its usual duration of action exceeds 1 hour.[11]

Adverse effects may occur if physostigmine is administered rapidly, in excess, or in the absence of an anticholinergic (antimuscarinic) agent. In all of these instances, an excess of acetylcholine at various sites within the body has various effects as follows:

At nicotinic receptors: muscle fasciculations, weakness, and paralysis

At muscarinic receptors: bronchospasm, bronchorrhea, bradycardia, salivation, lacrimation, urination, defecation, and emesis

At CNS sites: anxiety, dizziness, tremors, confusion, ataxia, coma, and seizures

Accordingly, overdoses of physostigmine may require atropine to control the bronchial secretions, and mechanical ventilation may be needed for neuromuscular weakness because there is no specific antidote for the excess nicotinic activity.

Additionally, it is important to note that when other cholinergic agents are used concurrently with physostigmine, the effects may be additive. Examples of such agents are pilocarpine, carbamates, organophosphates, pyridostigmine, and depolarizing neuromuscular blocking agents. Because physostigmine is an acetylcholinesterase inhibitor, it also prolongs the action of drugs metabolized by plasma cholinesterases, such as cocaine, succinylcholine, and mivacurium.

Disposition

Patients in whom there is resolution of anticholinergic (antimuscarinic) toxicity, who therefore do not require intervention for a period of 6 hours, and who have no evidence of complications of toxicity (e.g., aspiration pneumonia, rhabdomyolysis) may be medically cleared. All patients with suspected intentional overdose of any agent should be evaluated by a psychiatrist or otherwise appropriately cleared prior to hospital discharge according to local practice.

In patients with anticholinergic (antimuscarinic) toxicity, admission to a critical care setting should be arranged for those who have altered mental status, cardiac dysrhythmias or drug-related conduction abnormality, hyperthermia, or respiratory compromise requiring mechanical ventilation.

REFERENCES

1. Labianca DA, Reeves WJ: Scopolamine: A potent chemical weapon. J Chem Educ 1984;61:678.
2. Boehnert MT, Lovejoy FH: Value of the QRS duration versus the serum drug level in predicting seizures and ventricular arrhythmias after an overdose of tricyclic antidepressants. N Engl J Med 1985;313:474-479.
3. Leibelt EL: ECG lead aVR versus QRS interval in predicting seizures and arrhythmias in acute tricyclic antidepressant overdose. Ann Emerg Med 1995;26:195-201.
4. Niemann JT, Bessen HA, Rothstein RJ, Laks MM: Electrocardiographic criteria for tricyclic antidepressant cardiotoxicity. Am J Cardiol 1986;57:1154-1159.

5. Green R, Sitar DS, Tenenbein M: Effect of anticholinergic drugs on the efficacy of activated charcoal. Clin Toxicol 2004;42:267-272.
6. Sharma AN, Hexdall AH, Chang EK, et al: Diphenhydramine-induced wide complex dysrhythmia responds to treatment with sodium bicarbonate. Am J Emerg Med 2003;21: 212-215.
7. Burns MJ, Linden CH, Graudins A, et al: A comparison of physostigmine and benzodiazepines for the treatment of anticholinergic poisoning. Ann Emerg Med 2000; 35:374-381.
8. Pentel P, Peterson CD: Asystole complicating physostigmine treatment of tricyclic antidepressant overdose. Ann Emerg Med 1980;9:588-590.
9. Holzgrate RE, Vondrell JJ, Mintz SM: Reversal of postoperative reactions to scopolamine with physostigmine. Anesth Analg 1973;52:921-925.
10. Forrer GR, Miller JJ: Atropine coma—a somatic therapy in psychiatry. Am J Psychiatry 1958;115:455-458.
11. Asthana S, Greig NH, Hegedus L, et al: Clinical pharmacokinetics of physostigmine in patients with Alzheimer's disease. Clin Pharmacol Ther 1995;58:299-309

Chapter **140**

Insecticides, Herbicides, and Rodenticides

Robert Cannon and Anne-Michelle Ruha

KEY POINTS

Insecticides

Organophosphorus and carbamate poisonings cause excessive stimulation of muscarinic and nicotinic receptors by acetylcholine, potentially leading to life-threatening bronchorrhea and bronchospasm.

Aggressive airway management and liberal use of atropine are important to the management of both organophosphorus and carbamate poisonings.

Only a nondepolarizing neuromuscular blocker, such as vecuronium or rocuronium, should be used for intubation. Succinylcholine is metabolized by plasma cholinesterase, and prolonged paralysis may result if it is used in the setting of organophosphate poisoning.

The timely administration of pralidoxime is key to the treatment of organophosphorus poisoning, but pralidoxime is not indicated for carbamate poisoning.

Rodenticides

Unintentional pediatric ingestions of 4-hydroxycoumarins (superwarfarins) account for the vast majority of rodenticide exposures and rarely result in toxicity.

Anticoagulant rodenticide ingestion should be considered when a child younger than 6 years is presented with elevated prothrombin time and/or bleeding without another explanation.

Prothrombin time should be measured at 24 and 48 hours after large ingestions of 4-hydroxycoumarins.

INSECTICIDES

Organophosphorus Compounds and Carbamates

■ SCOPE

Organophosphate (OP) compounds and carbamates are used extensively worldwide for agricultural, industrial, and domestic pest control and, as a result, represent a significant public health issue in the developing world. An estimated 3 million poisonings and more than 200,000 deaths occur from OP compounds each year worldwide.[1] In the United States in 2004, 5874 exposures to OP compounds and 2935 exposures to carbamates were reported to the American Association of Poison Control Centers Toxic Exposure Surveillance System (TESS).[2]

Table 140-1 EFFECTS OF ORGANOPHOSPHORUS (OP) AND CARBAMATE INSECTICIDES

Receptor	Target Tissue	Clinical Effect
Autonomic nervous system:		
Postganglionic muscarinic (parasympathetic)—"DUMBBELS" (defecation, urination, miosis, bronchorrhea, bradycardia, emesis, lacrimation, salivation) or "SLUDGE" (salivation, lacrimation, urination, defecation, gastric secretions, emesis)	Gastrointestinal tract	Vomiting, diarrhea, cramping
	Genitourinary tract	Urination
	Heart	Bradycardia
	Lungs	Bronchorrhea, bronchospasm
	Eye	Miosis, lacrimation
Postganglionic muscarinic (sympathetic)	Salivary glands	Salivation
Preganglionic nicotinic	Sweat glands	Diaphoresis
	Adrenal glands	↑ Catecholamines—tachycardia
Central nervous system (nicotinic/muscarinic)	Brain	Agitation, seizures, coma (OP > carbamates)
Neuromuscular junction (nicotinic)	Skeletal muscle	Weakness, fasciculations, paralysis

The clinical severity and toxicodynamics vary according to the agent, the route of absorption, and whether or not the exposure was intentional. Regardless of these factors, the toxicologic mechanism of acetylcholinesterase (AChE) inhibition remains consistent. The end result is an excess of the neurotransmitter acetylcholine (ACh), resulting in overstimulation of muscarinic and nicotinic receptors and production of a cholinergic toxidrome.

Treatment focuses on aggressive airway management, liberal use of atropine for the control of excessive airway secretions and, in the case of OP compounds, early administration of the antidote pralidoxime. Prompt recognition of toxicity and early intervention usually result in complete recovery.

■ PATHOPHYSIOLOGY

Under normal circumstances, ACh is hydrolyzed by AChE to yield acetic acid and choline. In the presence of OP insecticides, AChE is phosphorylated, whereas in the presence of carbamate insecticides, the enzyme is carbamylated. As a result, the rate of regeneration of the active AChE is slowed, and its function is inhibited. Within 24 to 72 hours of OP poisoning, an alkyl group may dissociate from the AChE-OP complex, resulting in "aging" of the AChE. Once aging occurs, reactivation of the AChE is no longer possible, and only synthesis of new enzyme can restore activity. In the case of carbamate poisoning, breakdown of the carbamate-AChE complex occurs much more rapidly and aging does not occur (Box 140-1).[3]

ACh accumulates in the autonomic nervous system at postganglionic muscarinic (parasympathetic and sympathetic) receptors and preganglionic nicotinic (sympathetic) receptors. It also accumulates at the neuromuscular junction and in the central nervous system (CNS). Overstimulation of these receptors is responsible for the cholinergic toxidrome seen with OP and carbamate insecticide poisoning (Table 140-1).

BOX 140-1

Effects of Organophosphate and Carbamate on Acetylcholinesterase (AChE)

Organophosphate + AChE = phosphorylated AChE

Carbamate + AChE = carbamylated AChE

These complexes inactivate AChE and allow acetylcholine to sit on the nicotinic and muscarinic receptors producing the symptoms of toxicity.

Three things can happen to the phosphorylated or carbamylated AChE:

- Breakdown of the complex (occurs more rapidly with carbamate) to release active AChE
- Complete binding and inactivation (aging), which occurs within 24-72 hours (with organophosphates), requiring that new AChE be produced
- Reactivation by a strong nucleophile such as pralidoxime (2-PAM)

■ CLINICAL PRESENTATION

The onset of symptoms can occur within minutes after massive exposure and intentional ingestions or may be delayed up to 12 hours after accidental dermal, inhalational, or oral exposure in the occupational arena. Clinical effects may also be somewhat delayed owing to the need for bioactivation of some OP insecticides after absorption (for example, malathion). The mnemonic SLUDGE (salivation, lacrimation, urination, defecation, gastric secretions, emesis) has traditionally been used to describe the cholinergic toxidrome. However, the mnemonic DUMBBELS (defecation, urination, miosis, bronchorrhea, bradycardia, emesis, lacrimation, salivation) is probably more appropriate because it includes the life-threatening conditions bronchorrhea and bradyarrhythmias as well as the distinguishing feature miosis.

The clinical effects are summarized in Table 140-1; only the caveats in the clinical presentation are emphasized here. Bronchorrhea occurs commonly in moderate to severe poisonings[4] and can progress to pulmonary edema and respiratory failure. Miosis in the setting of cholinergic symptoms is fairly specific for OP and carbamate insecticides and may help make the diagnosis. Unfortunately, it is not consistently present.

Although the parasympathetic muscarinic effects are most often emphasized, certain sympathetic effects may predominate. Sinus tachycardia is more common than bradycardia,[4,5] and mydriasis may even be seen.[5] Nicotinic effects often predominate in mild cases and occur early on in severe cases. Excess nicotinic stimulation at the neuromuscular junction resembles the actions of a depolarizing neuromuscular blocking agent. Therefore, patients with OP or carbamate insecticide poisoning may present with muscle fasciculations and weakness. Paralysis occurs as toxicity worsens, and the primary cause of death in acute poisonings is probably respiratory arrest secondary to paralysis and bronchorrhea.

One to 3 days after apparent resolution of symptoms, patients may experience profound weakness and paralysis of proximal muscles, neck flexor muscles, and cranial nerves. This development, termed the *intermediate syndrome,*[6] is likely explained by ongoing AChE inhibition (Box 140-2).

Finally, carbamates produce peripheral effects similar to those of OP compounds, but generally to a much lesser extent. A distinguishing clinical feature of carbamate toxicity is the paucity of central effects which is secondary to their poor penetration of the CNS.

■ DIFFERENTIAL DIAGNOSIS

A detailed history in a patient presenting with signs and symptoms of cholinergic excess often elucidates an exposure to OP or carbamate insecticides. The diagnosis of OP or carbamate insecticide poisoning is therefore usually straightforward; however, certain clinical aspects may be mimicked by other entities. Table 140-2 is a partial list of other agents or diagnoses to consider.

■ DIAGNOSTIC TESTING

All patients with potential OP poisoning should undergo erythrocyte (red blood cell [RBC], or true) cholinesterase and plasma (pseudo) cholinesterase

BOX 140-2

Paralysis Seen after Organophosphate Poisoning

Type I

- Acute paralysis secondary to constant depolarization at the neuromuscular junction

Type II (Intermediate Syndrome)

- Develops 1 to 3 days after resolution of acute organophosphate poisoning symptoms
- Manifests as paralysis and respiratory distress secondary to weakness of proximal muscles, neck flexor muscles (with relative sparing of distal muscle groups), and cranial nerve palsies
- Lasts for 4-18 days and may require mechanical ventilation
- Results from ongoing acetylcholinesterase (AChE) inhibition or suboptimal treatment

Type III (Organophosphate-Induced Delayed Polyneuropathy [OPIDP])

- Manifests 2-3 weeks after exposure
- Results from inhibition of target esterase
- Characterized by distal muscle weakness with relative sparing of the neck muscles, cranial nerves, and proximal muscle groups
- Recovery can take up to 12 months

Table 140-2 DIFFERENTIAL DIAGNOSIS OF ORGANOPHOSPHORUS AND CARBAMATE POISONING

Other acetylcholinesterase inhibitors	Physostigmine, neostigmine, pyridostigmine
Other organophosphorus cholinesterase inhibitors (chemical weapon nerve agents)	Sarin, tabun, soman, Vx
Cholinomimetics	Pilocarpine, carbachol, methacholine, bethanechol, muscarine-containing mushrooms
Nicotinic alkaloids	Nicotine, coniine, lobeline
Other (symptom-based)	Coma, miosis, paralysis: Pontine hemorrhage Salivation, fasciculations: Bark scorpion (*Centruroides spp*) Vomiting, diarrhea: Gastroenteritis Respiratory failure: Any cause of pulmonary edema; status asthmaticus Weakness: Myasthenic crisis, electrolyte disturbance, botulism

measurement from specimens obtained upon presentation. Though not often useful or necessary for making a diagnosis in the ED, the results of this measurement may help guide continued therapy. RBC cholinesterase hydrolyzes acetylcholine and correlates with toxicity, whereas plasma cholinesterase is the first to decline and may be a more sensitive marker of exposure.[7] Both substances should be measured, because one may exhibit greater inhibition than the other, depending on the specific OP to which the patient was exposed. Box 140-3 summarizes the tests that may be helpful in evaluating a patient with moderate to severe toxicity.

Cholinesterase values may prove useful in diagnosing OP toxicity if the history or physical findings are unclear. The values must be interpreted with caution, however. There is great interindividual and intraindividual variation in baseline cholinesterase values. A patient may have a 50% depression in cholinesterase activity yet the level still falls within the "normal" reference range. This makes cholinesterase measurements of limited value in initial diagnosis of poisoning. The levels are helpful in confirming poisoning only if they are extremely low or undetectable upon presentation. The finding of "normal" levels does not necessarily rule out poisoning if the history and clinical picture are otherwise supportive.

TREATMENT

The treatment algorithm for OP and carbamate insecticide poisoning is summarized in Figure 140-1. The first step is adequate decontamination of the patient by removal of wet clothing and washing of contaminated skin with soap and water. ED personnel should wear gowns, gloves, and masks to prevent exposure to contaminated body fluids.[8]

As the patient is decontaminated, the EP should focus on the ABCs of respiration (airway, breathing circulation), paying particular attention to early airway management for copious secretions, seizures, coma, severe weakness, and paralysis. If intubation is necessary, only a nondepolarizing neuromuscular blocking agent, such as vecuronium or rocuronium, should be used. Succinylcholine is metabolized by plasma cholinesterase, so prolonged paralysis may result if this agent is used a patient with OP poisoning.[9]

Treatment should next be directed at controlling muscarinic activity. Atropine is the drug of choice and should be administered intravenously at a dose of 2 to 5 mg (pediatric dose 0.05 mg/kg) every 3 to 5 minutes, with the end point being control of respiratory secretions. Tachycardia is not a contraindication to atropine administration. Mild poisonings may resolve with just 1 to 2 mg of atropine, and severe poisonings may require more than 1000 mg.[10] Large doses of atropine may lead to antimuscarinic CNS toxicity. If this occurs, glycopyrrolate (1-2 mg; pediatric dose, 0.025 mg/kg) can be used in place of atropine.

Pralidoxime is the antidote to OP insecticide poisoning. Although its efficacy may vary according to the structure of the OP compound, it should be given to all OP-poisoned patients. It works by increasing the rate of AChE regeneration. It is a common belief that pralidoxime is not beneficial if given after 24 hours because of the "aging" of AChE. However, OP insecticides have been detected in blood weeks after exposure. Their presence may be secondary to redistribution from fat. Therefore, late oxime therapy may still be of benefit. The adult dose is 1 to 2 g via the intravenous (IV) route over 15 to 30 minutes followed by a continuous infusion of 500 mg/hr. Pediatric dosing is 25 to 50 mg/kg load followed by 10 to 20 mg/kg/hr infusion. Pralidoxime is not indicated in carbamate poisoning, which is usually mild and self-limited.

PRIORITY ACTIONS

Organophosphates

- Protect the airway in patients with increased secretions from organophosphates or carbamates.
- Administer atropine early and often to control airway secretions.
- Give intravenous fluids to replace gastrointestinal losses.
- Administer pralidoxime early in the course of organophosphate poisoning.
- Treat seizures with benzodiazepines.

BOX 140-3

Ancillary Studies in the Management of Organophosphate or Carbamate Poisoning

Laboratory tests:
- Red blood cell cholinesterase concentration
- Plasma cholinesterase concentration
- Complete blood count
- Electrolytes
- Blood urea nitrogen and creatinine levels
- Liver enzyme levels
- Arterial blood gas values

Electrocardiography
Chest radiograph

Organochlorines

SCOPE

Organochlorines are heavily chlorinated aromatic compounds that are nonvolatile and poorly water soluble. They are divided into four classes on the basis of their structural characteristics, and they vary

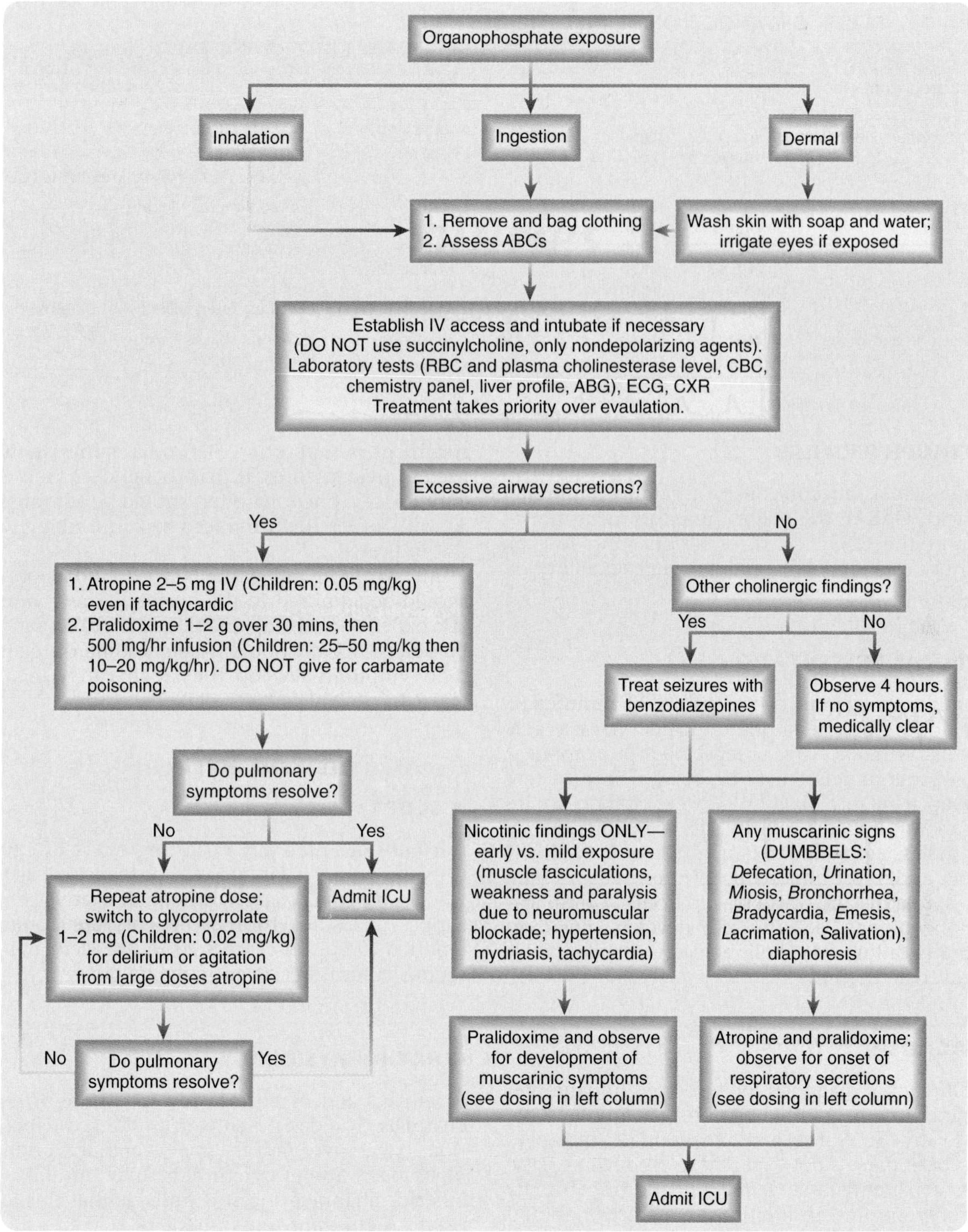
Organophosphate exposure
Inhalation
Ingestion
Dermal
1. Remove and bag clothing
2. Assess ABCs
Wash skin with soap and water; irrigate eyes if exposed
Establish IV access and intubate if necessary
(DO NOT use succinylcholine, only nondepolarizing agents).
Laboratory tests (RBC and plasma cholinesterase level, CBC, chemistry panel, liver profile, ABG), ECG, CXR
Treatment takes priority over evaulation.
Excessive airway secretions?
Yes
No
1. Atropine 2–5 mg IV (Children: 0.05 mg/kg) even if tachycardic
2. Pralidoxime 1–2 g over 30 mins, then 500 mg/hr infusion (Children: 25–50 mg/kg then 10–20 mg/kg/hr). DO NOT give for carbamate poisoning.
Other cholinergic findings?
Yes
No
Treat seizures with benzodiazepines
Observe 4 hours. If no symptoms, medically clear
Do pulmonary symptoms resolve?
No
Yes
Repeat atropine dose; switch to glycopyrrolate 1–2 mg (Children: 0.02 mg/kg) for delirium or agitation from large doses atropine
Admit ICU
Nicotinic findings ONLY—early vs. mild exposure (muscle fasciculations, weakness and paralysis due to neuromuscular blockade; hypertension, mydriasis, tachycardia)
Any muscarinic signs (DUMBBELS: Defecation, Urination, Miosis, Bronchorrhea, Bradycardia, Emesis, Lacrimation, Salivation), diaphoresis
No
Do pulmonary symptoms resolve?
Yes
Pralidoxime and observe for development of muscarinic symptoms (see dosing in left column)
Atropine and pralidoxime; observe for onset of respiratory secretions (see dosing in left column)
Admit ICU

FIGURE 140-1 Treatment algorithm for organophosphorus insecticide poisoning. ABCs (of respiration), airway, breathing, and circulation; ABG, arterial blood gas determination; CBC, complete blood count; CXR, chest radiograph; ECG, electrocardiography; ICU, intensive care unit; IV, intravenous; RBC, red blood cell.

tremendously with respect to dermal absorption, lipid solubility, and toxic doses. The clinical toxicity, which is similar for each of the classes, is summarized in Table 140-3.

Most organochlorines have been banned in North America from concerns about their environmental persistence and bioconcentration. The only organochlorine still in common use in the United States is lindane (Kwell). It is used in agriculture as a seed treatment and medicinally as a topical scabicide in a 1% formulation. Toxicity from therapeutic lindane application is exceedingly rare, and most clinically relevant toxicity events occur from inappropriate dermal application or ingestion.[11-13]

Table 140-3 MAJOR ORGANOCHLORINE INSECTICIDES

Class	Product	Dermal Absorption	Oral Toxicity	Characteristics
Hexachlorocyclohexane	Lindane	High	Moderate	Central nervous system (CNS) excitation, seizures
Dichlorodiphenylethanes	DDT	Low	Moderate	CNS excitation
	Methoxychlor	Low	Low	Less toxic than dichlorodiphenyltrichloroethane (DDT)
Cyclodienes	Aldrin	High	High	Metabolized to dieldrin
	Dieldrin	High	High	Seizures
	Endrin	High	Highest	Rapid onset seizures
	Chlordane	High	Moderate	Early and late seizures
	Endosulfan	High	High	Sulfur odor
	Toxaphene	Low	Moderate-high	Seizures, often mixed with parathion
Chlordecone and mirex	Chlordecone	High	Moderate	"Kepone shakes," no seizures
	Mirex	High	Low	Same as above

■ PATHOPHYSIOLOGY

Lindane acts as an antagonist of gamma-aminobutyric acid (GABA), the major inhibitory neurotransmitter in the CNS.[14] Toxicity results from loss of inhibitory tone and subsequent hyperexcitability of the CNS.

■ CLINICAL PRESENTATION

Symptoms, which can occur within 30 minutes of ingestion of lindane,[12] often include nausea and vomiting. With excessive or repeated topical applications, symptom onset may be delayed from a few hours up to 4 to 5 days.[11,14] CNS excitation is the hallmark of lindane toxicity. It is manifested by paresthesias, agitation, tremor, myoclonus, hallucinations, and, most important, seizures. Seizures may occur suddenly and without prodrome. Complications of prolonged seizures may develop, including respiratory failure, metabolic acidosis, rhabdomyolysis, and hyperthermia.

■ DIAGNOSIS

The differential diagnosis for suspected lindane poisoning is extremely broad because it can potentially include any cause of seizures. Appropriate, therapeutic use of lindane is not expected to produce toxicity. Unless a patient has ingested lindane prior to the onset of symptoms, an alternative explanation should be sought to explain seizures. Although measurement of lindane levels can be performed by some laboratories, results are not immediately available to the EP. Therefore, the diagnosis is primarily clinical.

■ TREATMENT

There is no specific antidote for lindane toxicity. Although activated charcoal can be considered early after ingestion, it may be dangerous in a patient who may have seizures without warning. The mainstay of treatment is supportive. Benzodiazepines should be used to treat seizures. If that therapy is unsuccessful, barbiturates (phenobarbital) should be administered. As with other toxin-induced seizures, phenytoin is not indicated.

All symptomatic patients with lindane toxicity should be admitted to the hospital. The asymptomatic patient presenting after ingestion of lindane may be observed for 6 hours from the time of ingestion; if no symptoms develop, the patient can be medically cleared.

Pyrethrins and Pyrethroids

■ SCOPE

Pyrethrins are naturally occurring esters of chrysanthemum resin that possess insecticidal activity, whereas *pyrethroids* are synthetic derivatives of pyrethrins. Exposures to these agents are commonly reported to poison centers. Most are accidental, and serious clinical effects are rare.[2]

■ PATHOPHYSIOLOGY

Pyrethrins and pyrethroids delay closure of sodium channels. The delay results in prolonged depolarization, repetitive firing, and eventual conduction blockade.[15] Some pyrethroids may inhibit GABA chloride channels, but it is unlikely that this feature plays a significant role in toxicity.

■ CLINICAL PRESENTATION

Most cases of clinically relevant toxicity from pyrethrins result from pulmonary allergic reactions rather than direct toxic effects. The presentation is clinically similar to that of asthma exacerbations, with wheezing, cough, dyspnea, and chest pain. Most reactions are mild and easily treated. However, fatal status asthmaticus has been reported with exposure to pyrethrin-containing shampoo.[16,17]

Accidental or occupational exposure to pyrethroids usually produces minimal, if any, toxicity. The most common symptoms reported are facial paresthesias, dizziness, headache, nausea, anorexia, and fatigue.[18] Massive exposures or large intentional ingestions may lead to the more serious manifestations: seizures, altered mental status, coma, respiratory failure, and death.

■ TREATMENT

Activated charcoal may be given to a patient who presents within 1 hour of a large oral ingestion of pyrethrin or pyrethroid. Skin decontamination is accomplished with soap and water. Pyrethrin-induced bronchospasm is treated with oxygen, beta-adrenergic agonists, and corticosteroids as needed. There is no specific antidote, and symptoms resolve with supportive care.

Tips and Tricks

INSECTICIDES

- Use glycopyrrolate in patients who need more atropine but show signs of central nervous system antimuscarinic toxicity, such as delirium and agitation.
- Do not rely on pupils to rule the diagnosis in or out.
- Presence of tachycardia should not prevent administration of atropine to a patient with bronchorrhea or wheezing.
- Base treatment on clinical signs and symptoms, not acetylcholinesterase (AChE) levels.

RED FLAGS

Insecticides

- Miosis in the setting of cholinergic symptoms, although not consistently present, is fairly specific for organophosphate and carbamate insecticides and may help make the diagnosis.
- Although the parasympathetic muscarinic effects are most often emphasized, certain sympathetic effects may predominate (sinus tachycardia is more common than bradycardia, and mydriasis may be seen).
- Nicotinic effects often predominate in mild cases and occur early on in severe cases.
- "Normal" cholinesterase levels do not necessarily rule out poisoning if the history and clinical picture are otherwise indicative.
- Symptoms can occur within 30 minutes of ingestion of lindane, but with excessive or repeated topical applications, symptom onset may be delayed from a few hours to 4-5 days.

HERBICIDES

Paraquat and Diquat

■ SCOPE

Paraquat and diquat belong to the bipyridyl class of herbicides. They are both commonly used worldwide for weed control in the agricultural, horticultural, and forestry industries, and paraquat is marketed in more than 130 countries. Both compounds are available for home and commercial use in varying concentrations. Paraquat is commonly sold as a 0.2% solution for home use but can be found in 10% to 24% concentrated commercial solutions.

Paraquat and diquat account for only 4.9% of herbicide poisonings but are responsible for over 50% of herbicide-related deaths.[19] This fact points to the extremely toxic nature of these compounds. Most serious toxicity events and deaths are secondary to intentional ingestions.[20]

■ PATHOPHYSIOLOGY

Paraquat is rapidly absorbed after ingestion and is concentrated in type I and type II alveolar epithelial cells. It is then reduced to a free radical, which then reacts with oxygen to form a superoxide anion (O_2^-). This anion then may form H_2O_2, which in the presence of Fe^{++} will generate highly reactive species such as the hydroxyl radical (OH). These reactive molecules cause lipid peroxidation and cellular destruction.[21] Initially, acute alveolitis may occur. Later, proliferative changes and pulmonary fibrosis are seen. Although paraquat is most concentrated in the lungs, it also distributes throughout the entire body, causing cellular destruction of multiple organs.

Diquat's pathophysiologic mechanism is similar to that of paraquat. Diquat is not concentrated in the lungs, however, and does not produce pulmonary fibrosis.[22]

■ CLINICAL PRESENTATION

Paraquat poisoning can be classified as mild, moderate, or severe according to the amount ingested.[20] Physical findings are summarized in Table 140-4. Mild poisonings, which occur when small amounts of dilute preparations are ingested, are characterized by development of gastrointestinal symptoms without other organ toxicity. As the amount of paraquat or diquat ion ingested rises, worsening gastrointestinal effects are seen, including severe oropharyngeal, esophageal, and gastric ulcerations. Large ingestions produce renal and hepatic failure within a few days. Paraquat toxicity results in pulmonary fibrosis and refractory hypoxemia several days to weeks after ingestion, and death usually

Table 140-4 CLINICAL MANIFESTATIONS OF PARAQUAT POISONING

Degree	Amount Ingested	Clinical Features
Mild	<20 mg/kg paraquat ion	Asymptomatic or gastrointestinal symptoms Patients recover fully
Moderate-severe	20-40 mg/kg	Oropharyngeal erythema and ulcerations may occur Vomiting and diarrhea Acute renal failure and hepatic dysfunction within 24 hours Pulmonary fibrosis in all patients, but may be delayed days to weeks Most die within 2-3 weeks
Fulminant	>40 mg/kg	Definite ulceration of oropharynx Rapid development of multiorgan failure Severe lung injury, cerebral edema, seizures, renal failure, hepatic necrosis, pancreatic necrosis, cardiovascular collapse 100% mortality Death occurs 24 hours to a few days after the overdose

occurs within a few weeks. Massive ingestions cause multiorgan failure and death within a few days. Diquat toxicity does not produce pulmonary fibrosis. Diquat ingestion has been associated with brainstem infarcts.[22] Effects from dermal exposure to paraquat and diquat are usually mild, but ulcers and blistering can occur with highly concentrated formulations.

■ DIAGNOSIS

A qualitative urine test can be performed to aid in diagnosis of paraquat or diquat poisoning. When alkaline sodium dithionate is added to urine, the color turns blue when paraquat is present and blue-green in the presence of diquat. Quantitative plasma measurements may also be obtained for confirmation of exposure and determining prognosis. Neither of these tests may be readily available in the emergency setting. Therefore, the diagnosis is often based on history alone. The differential diagnosis of paraquat and diquat poisoning is wide and includes exposure to other caustic substances.

■ TREATMENT

No specific antidote or pharmacologic intervention has been proven to affect outcome for paraquat or diquat poisoning. Early decontamination is the most important step in initial management and may be futile after large ingestions because of rapid absorption. There is little clinical or experimental evidence for the use of gastric lavage, and the procedure may even worsen oral or esophageal ulcerations. Therefore, activated charcoal (1-2 g/kg) is the agent of choice for gastric decontamination. Other agents, such as diatomaceous Fuller's earth (1-2 g/kg in 30% aqueous solution) and bentonite (1-2 g/kg of 7% aqueous solution), have been used but are not as likely to be available to the EP, nor do they provide any advantage over charcoal. Gastric decontamination should be initiated as soon as possible.

Supportive care should be provided, with airway protection and ventilation paramount. Supplemental oxygen may worsen toxicity by accelerating damage by oxygen radicals. It is generally accepted that supplemental oxygen be withheld until the PaO_2 falls below 40 to 50 mm Hg. IV fluids should be given to ensure normal urine output, and analgesics provided for the pain associated with mucosal ulcerations. Many other pharmacologic treatments for paraquat poisoning have been investigated, but none has proved useful.[21] Hemoperfusion and hemodialysis are effective at removing paraquat from the blood, but neither improves prognosis.

Chlorphenoxy Herbicides

■ SCOPE

Chlorphenoxy herbicides are widely used to control the growth of broad-leaved weeds in pastures and crop fields and along public streets. Poisoning is uncommon, and most emergency department encounters consist of accidental dermal or inhalational exposure, for which serious systemic toxicity is rare. However, intentional ingestion of these compounds carries high morbidity and mortality. From 1962 to 2004, there have been 69 cases reported of ingestion of chlorphenoxy herbicides alone (excluding other pesticides as co-ingestants). One third of the patients in these reports died.[23]

■ PATHOPHYSIOLOGY

The pathophysiology of chlorphenoxy herbicide toxicity involves three mechanisms. First, a dose-dependent disruption of cell membranes is thought to be responsible for mediation of CNS toxicity through disruption of the blood-brain barrier. Second, these compounds may form analogues of acetyl coenzyme A (CoA), disrupting its role in cellular metabolism. Because acetyl CoA is involved in the formation of the neurotransmitter acetylcholine, false cholinergic transmitters may be formed. A third mechanism of toxicity results from uncoupling of oxidative phosphorylation, which leads to depletion of cellular adenosine triphosphate (ATP).[24]

CLINICAL FEATURES

Vomiting is common early after ingestion and may be accompanied by abdominal pain and diarrhea. Hypotension may occur secondary to volume loss, peripheral vasodilation, and direct myocardial toxicity. Severe ingestions are often associated with rapid onset of coma. Other neurologic features that have been reported are hyperreflexia, hypertonia, seizures, hallucinations, clonus, and ataxia.[23,24] Peripheral neuromuscular effects include weakness, loss of deep tendon reflexes, and fasciculations. Common metabolic effects are acidosis, hyperthermia, and rhabdomyolysis.

> **Tips and Tricks**
>
> **HERBICIDES**
>
> - Withhold oxygen administration until $PaO_2 < 40$ mm Hg in paraquat poisoning because it may worsen toxicity through acceleration of damage by oxygen radicals.
> - Consider urinary alkalinization in severe chlorphenoxy herbicide poisoning.
> - Early decontamination with activated charcoal takes priority in paraquat and diquat ingestions.

DIAGNOSIS

The diagnosis is made by obtaining a history of ingestion or exposure to these agents. Plasma levels can be measured but results are not available in the emergency setting. When the history is lacking, the diagnosis is difficult because the differential diagnosis includes any potential cause of metabolic acidosis, myopathy, mental status changes, and gastroenteritis.

TREATMENT

Most patients can be managed with supportive care alone. Activated charcoal should be given if the patient presents within 1 hour of a large ingestion. Other supportive measures are airway protection, IV fluids, and benzodiazepines for seizures, fasciculations, hyperreflexia, or clonus.

Alkaline diuresis has been reported to reduce the half-life of 2,4-dichlorophenoxyacetic acid (2,4-D).[25] Although hemodialysis and resin hemoperfusion enhance elimination of 2,4-D, no controlled trials have been done to assess whether these measures change outcome. These modalities should be considered only in severe poisonings.

Glyphosate

Glyphosate is a widely used herbicide with formulations that range from a 1% household concentration to a 41% concentrate for commercial use. In addition, many of the commercial formulations are mixed with surfactants, which themselves produce toxicity by destroying mitochondrial cell walls and interfering with cellular energy production. The amine surfactants are also highly alkaline and corrosive, contributing to much of glyphosate's toxicity.

Unintentional or small ingestions of glyphosate typically produce only mild gastrointestinal symptoms. An exception occurs with glyphosate-trimesium (Touchdown), which has produced rapid death after small ingestions.[26] Most cases of significant toxicity result from intentional ingestion of the concentrated formulation of Roundup (41% glyphosate and 15% polyoxyethyleneamine surfactant). Common features are corrosive effects, such as oropharyngeal ulcers, dysphagia, abdominal pain, and vomiting. Significant laryngeal injury may lead to aspiration and lung injury. Metabolic acidosis is common with large ingestions of concentrated formulations. Hypovolemia and hypoperfusion may lead to secondary hepatic and renal insufficiency.[27]

Management is primarily supportive. Airway protection takes priority in patients presenting with signs of oral and gastrointestinal corrosive effects. IV fluids should be given to normalize urine output. In the rare severe poisoning, acidosis and hypotension may be refractory to IV fluids, necessitating sodium bicarbonate and vasopressors, respectively.

Glufosinate

Glufosinate is a nonselective herbicide used worldwide and marketed under the trade names BASTA, Ignite, Challenge, and Harvest. A glutamic acid analogue, glufosinate is combined with surfactants. As with glyphosate, ingestion of these products can lead to symptoms attributable to surfactants, such as corrosive injury, gastrointestinal symptoms, and acidosis. However, glufosinate is unique in that it may cause delayed onset of CNS toxicity. Ataxia, depressed level of consciousness, coma, and central apnea can be seen 4 to 12 hours after ingestion.[28,29] Delayed-onset seizures have been reported 29 hours after ingestion and may last for days.[29]

Treatment is supportive. Activated charcoal may be considered for patients presenting within 1 hour after a large ingestion, but vomiting will likely limit its utility.

RODENTICIDES

Rodenticides vary greatly with respect to pathophysiology, clinical presentation, degree of toxicity and management. Because these poisonings are rarely encountered by EPs, a detailed discussion on each one is beyond the scope of this text. Some of the characteristics can be found in Table 140-5. Instead we focus on the anticoagulant rodenticides warfarin

Table 140-5 CHARACTERISTICS OF SOME RODENTICIDES

Compound	Clinical Characteristics	Treatment
Sodium monofluoroacetate, fluoroacetamide	Vomiting 2-20 hours after exposure; acidosis, coma, seizures, hypokalemia, hypocalcemia	Supportive; intravenous fluids (IVF), benzodiazepines for seizures, bicarbonate for refractory acidosis
Zinc phosphide	Gastrointestinal distress within 30 minutes, cough, dyspnea, acidosis, seizures, coma	Supportive; IVF, benzodiazepines for seizures, bicarbonate for refractory acidosis
Yellow phosphorus	Dermal burns, "smoking" vomitus, diarrhea, and cardiovascular collapse in severe cases	Supportive; gastric lavage with 0.1% potassium permanganate suggested
ANTU (α-naphthyl-thiourea)	Possible pulmonary edema	Supportive; observe for development of pulmonary edema

and superwarfarin and the compound strychnine, which can be found in some rodenticides today.

Anticoagulants

■ SCOPE

Anticoagulant rodenticides can be categorized as warfarins or superwarfarins. The warfarins were the first anticoagulant rodenticides introduced, and their toxicity to rodents and humans depended on repeated ingestions. They are virtually nontoxic after a single small ingestion. This characteristic made them attractive from a safety standpoint but rendered them poor rodenticides.

In the 1980s, the 4-hydroxycoumarins and indanediones were developed (see Table 140-6 for a listing of brands and concentrations). These potent, long-acting "superwarfarins" are lethal to rodents and toxic to humans after a single acute ingestion. These compounds are now responsible for the majority of exposures to anticoagulant rodenticides. Of the 19,432 rodenticide exposures reported to poison control centers in 2004, 16,054 involved superwarfarins. Most were unintentional ingestions in children younger than 6 years.[2]

■ PATHOPHYSIOLOGY

The warfarins and superwarfarins inhibit the synthesis of vitamin K_1–dependent clotting factors (II, VII, IX, X) by blocking the conversion of inactive vitamin K to the active form (Fig. 140-2). Bleeding may occur when factor levels fall to 25% of baseline. Because factor VII has the shortest half-life (about 5 hours), a rise in the prothrombin time may be seen in three to four half-lives (15-20 hours after ingestion) and certainly will be seen within 48 hours.[30]

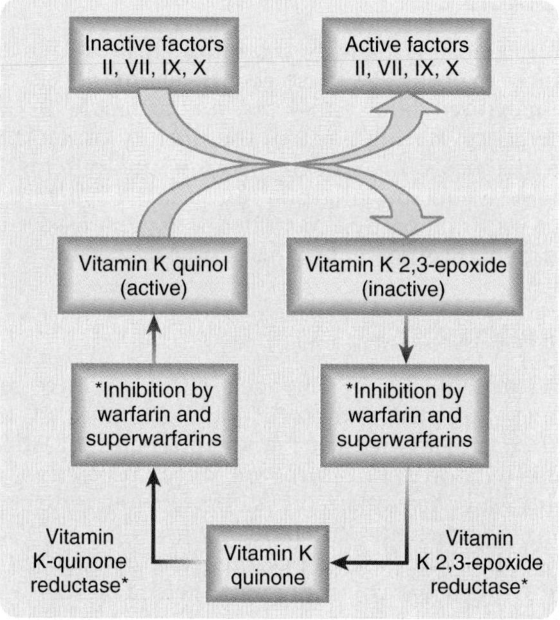
Inactive factors
II, VII, IX, X
Active factors
II, VII, IX, X
Vitamin K quinol
(active)
Vitamin K 2,3-epoxide
(inactive)
*Inhibition by
warfarin and
superwarfarins
*Inhibition by
warfarin and
superwarfarins
Vitamin
K-quinone
reductase*
Vitamin K
quinone
Vitamin
K 2,3-epoxide
reductase*

FIGURE 140-2 Mechanism of action of warfarin and superwarfarin.

Table 140-6 ANTICOAGULANT RODENTICIDE (SUPERWARFARIN) BRANDS AND CONCENTRATIONS

Rodenticide	Concentrations	Selected Brand Names
4-hydroxycoumarins:		
Brodifacoum	0.005	D-Con Mouse, Talon, Talon G, Havoc
Bromadiolone	0.005	Bromone, Super-Caid, Ratimus
Difenacoum	0.005	Endox, Endrocid, Racumin, Rodentin
Indanediones:		
Chlorophacinone	0.005, 0.25, 2.5	Caid, Drat, Liphadione, Microzul, Rozol
Diphacinone	0.005-2.0	Diphacin, Promar, Ramik
Pindone	0.025-2.0	Pival, Pivacin, Pivalyn

BOX 140-4

Initial Emergency Laboratory Tests in the Evaluation of Coagulopathy

- Prothrombin time, partial thromboplastin time, International Normalized Ratio
- Complete blood count
- Liver enzyme measurements
- Serum fibrinogen and fibrin split product tests
- Measurements of coagulation factors (II, VII, VIII, IX, X)
- 50:50 mixing test

■ CLINICAL PRESENTATION

When a child is presented immediately after an unintentional ingestion, he or she is asymptomatic without signs of bleeding; 24 to 48 hours after a large ingestion, however, patients may have any manifestation of a coagulopathy, including, in order of decreasing frequency, ecchymosis, hematuria, uterine bleeding, gastrointestinal bleeding, epistaxis, spontaneous hematoma, gingival bleeding, hemoptysis, and hematemesis.[31]

■ DIAGNOSIS

Anticoagulant rodenticide ingestion should be considered when a patient presents with elevated prothrombin time and/or bleeding without other explanation. The differential diagnosis includes vitamin K deficiency, hemophilia or other factor deficiencies, and disseminated intravascular coagulation. The myriad of causes of liver failure must also be considered, including viral hepatitis, alcoholic cirrhosis, hepatotoxic ingestions (e.g., acetaminophen, iron), and Wilson's disease. A thorough laboratory evaluation aimed at sorting out these processes should be obtained (Box 140-4). Brodifacoum and difenacoum measurements may be performed but results are not immediately available to the EP.

■ TREATMENT

Figure 140-3 summarizes management of warfarin or superwarfarin poisoning, which depends on the timing, amount ingested, and symptomatology. Accidental ingestions of less than one box of 4-hydroxycoumarin are unlikely to result in clinically significant toxicity and may be managed without gastric decontamination or laboratory evaluation unless signs of bleeding occur.[32] Patients who ingest one or more boxes should be given activated charcoal if they present within 1 hour of ingestion. Acute hemorrhage is managed with oxygen and IV crystalloids to replace volume losses. Fresh frozen plasma should be administered to patients with active bleeding and coagulopathy. Vitamin K_1 is given at doses of 1-5 mg in children and 10 mg in adults. It may be administered intravenously at no more than 1 mg/min to reduce the likelihood of anaphylactoid reactions. Oral or subcutaneous administration is also acceptable.

■ DISPOSITION

All patients with signs and symptoms of bleeding should be admitted to the hospital for reversal of coagulopathy and control of bleeding. Those with severe or life-threatening hemorrhage warrant intensive care unit admission. Asymptomatic patients who present soon after ingestion can be discharged with arrangements to have blood specimens obtained for prothrombin time measurements on an outpatient basis in 24 and 48 hours.

Strychnine

■ SCOPE

Strychnine is a naturally occurring alkaloid derived from the seeds of the tree *Strychnos nux vomica*. Although rarely used as a rodenticide today, it is still available in some gopher, mouse, and rat poisons. It also has been found in some traditional Cambodian home remedies. Strychnine is an odorless crystalline white powder with a bitter taste that is well absorbed in the gastrointestinal tract.

■ PATHOPHYSIOLOGY

Strychnine blocks the postsynaptic binding of glycine in the spinal cord and brainstem. Because glycine is the major inhibitory neurotransmitter in these areas, disinhibition results in excess stimulation of motor neurons.[33]

■ CLINICAL PRESENTATION

Symptom onset is usually within 15 to 30 minutes of ingestion. Initial symptoms include a heightened sense of awareness and muscle spasms. As toxicity progresses, muscular hyperexcitability worsens. Minimal stimuli can produce severe muscle spasms, opisthotonos, and trismus, which can be indistinguishable from seizures. Patients usually maintain a clear sensorium before and after these episodes, an effect unique to strychnine ingestion.[33] The complications of strychnine poisoning are secondary to muscle spasms. They include hyperthermia, metabolic acidosis, and rhabdomyolysis. Death is usually the result of respiratory failure from spasm of the respiratory muscles.

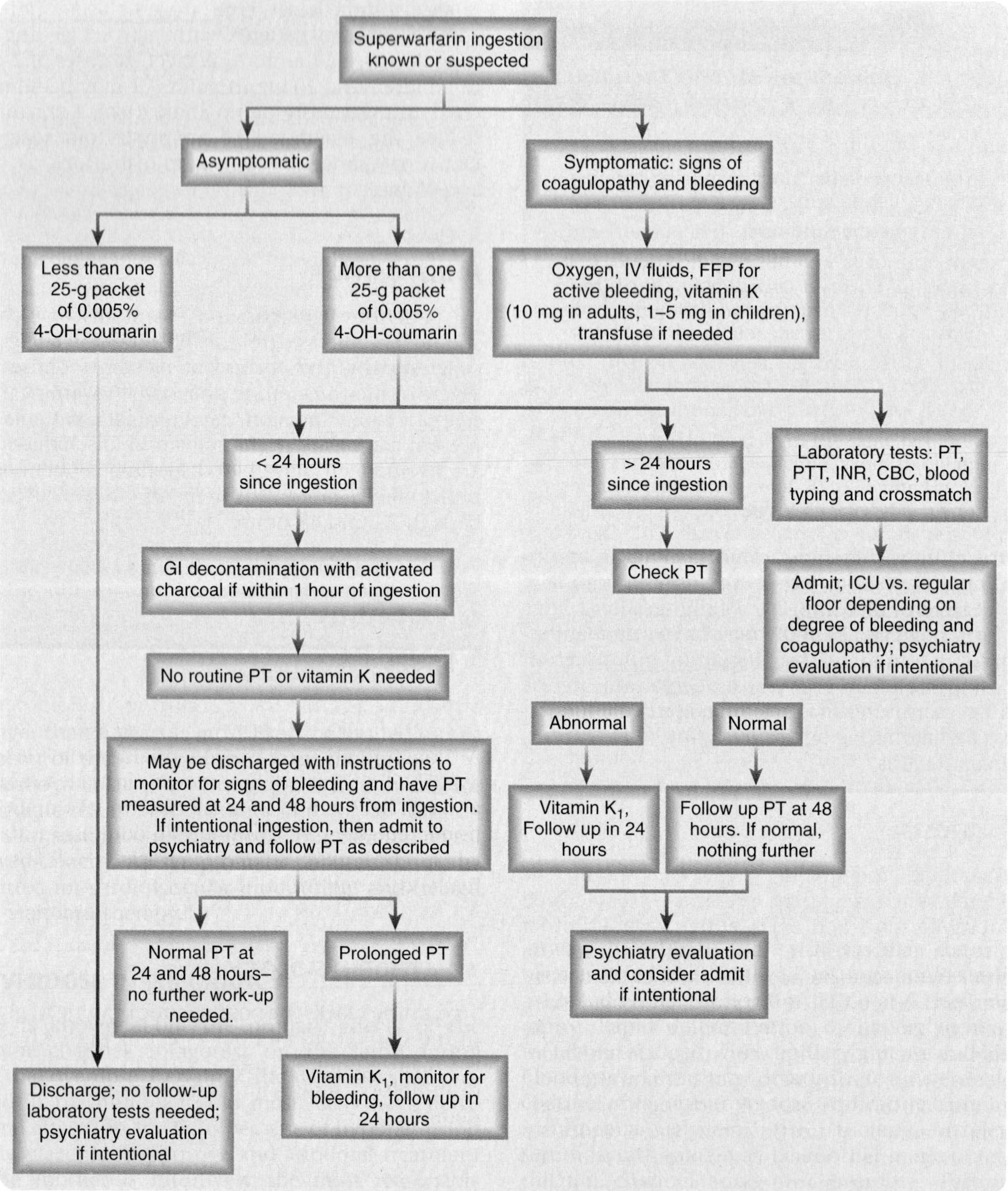
Superwarfarin ingestion known or suspected
Asymptomatic
Symptomatic: signs of coagulopathy and bleeding
Less than one 25-g packet of 0.005% 4-OH-coumarin
More than one 25-g packet of 0.005% 4-OH-coumarin
Oxygen, IV fluids, FFP for active bleeding, vitamin K (10 mg in adults, 1–5 mg in children), transfuse if needed
< 24 hours since ingestion
> 24 hours since ingestion
Laboratory tests: PT, PTT, INR, CBC, blood typing and crossmatch
GI decontamination with activated charcoal if within 1 hour of ingestion
Check PT
Admit; ICU vs. regular floor depending on degree of bleeding and coagulopathy; psychiatry evaluation if intentional
No routine PT or vitamin K needed
Abnormal
Normal
May be discharged with instructions to monitor for signs of bleeding and have PT measured at 24 and 48 hours from ingestion. If intentional ingestion, then admit to psychiatry and follow PT as described
Vitamin K1, Follow up in 24 hours
Follow up PT at 48 hours. If normal, nothing further
Normal PT at 24 and 48 hours– no further work-up needed.
Prolonged PT
Psychiatry evaluation and consider admit if intentional
Discharge; no follow-up laboratory tests needed; psychiatry evaluation if intentional
Vitamin K1, monitor for bleeding, follow up in 24 hours

FIGURE 140-3 Algorithm for management of superwarfarin ingestions. CBC, complete blood count; FFP, fresh frozen plasma; GI, gastrointestinal; ICU, intensive care unit; INR, international normalized ratio; PT, prothrombin time; PPT, partial thromboplastin time.

■ DIAGNOSIS AND TREATMENT

Diagnosis is based on a history of exposure in a patient presenting with the preceding signs and symptoms. If the history is unknown, the differential diagnosis includes stimulant intoxication, alcohol or benzodiazepine withdrawal, neuroleptic malignant syndrome, serotonin syndrome, salicylate intoxication, encephalitis, meningitis, and tetanus.

The treatment is largely supportive, with focus on airway protection and management of muscle spasms with benzodiazepines. Activated charcoal is unlikely to be of benefit, given the rapid absorption and onset of symptoms. For mild symptoms, the patient should be given diazepam or lorazepam and placed in a dark quiet environment to avoid stimuli. Airway and ventilatory status must be monitored closely and continually, because sudden deterioration can occur. The

Documentation

History

- Any history of psychiatric illness or prior suicide ingestions.
- Name, manufacturer, and concentration of active ingredient.
- Amount ingested.
- Time lapse since ingestion if known.
- History of renal or cardiac disease or other illnesses that might exacerbate the complications of toxins.

Physical Examination

- Does the patient look ill? Pale? Febrile? What is mental status? Is there bleeding?
- Cardiac status (blood pressure, arrhythmias).
- Respiratory and airway status.
- Physical examinations should be repeated while the patient is in the ED.

Studies

- Laboratory tests and time specimens were obtained.

Medical Decision-Making

- Decision to begin treatment or delays.
- Consultations and time of contact.

Treatment

- Availability of antidotes, time antidote was ordered, and any delays to treatment.

Patient Instructions

- Document discussion with patient regarding diagnosis, warning signs, what to do, follow-up, and when to return.
- With pediatric accidental ingestions, document poison prevention counseling for parents.
- For superwarfarin poisoning, instructions on where to return for prothrombin time measurements and who will monitor the results.

patient with severe symptoms should be intubated and paralyzed with a nondepolarizing neuromuscular blocker. The patient should then be aggressively sedated with benzodiazepines, propofol, or barbiturates. If this approach fails to control the muscle activity, continuous neuromuscular paralysis is an option. All symptomatic patients should be admitted to the intensive care unit.

REFERENCES

1. Jeyaraatnam J: Acute pesticide poisoning: A major global health problem. World Health Stat Q 1990;43:139-144.
2. Watson WA, Litovitz TL, Rodgers GC Jr, et al: 2004 Annual report of the American Association of Poison Control Centers Toxic Exposure Surveillance System. Am J Emerg Med 2005;23:589-666.
3. Kwong TC: Organophosphate pesticides: Biochemistry and clinical toxicology. Ther Drug Monit 2002;24:144-149.
4. Lee P, Tai DY: Clinical features of patients with acute organophosphate poisoning requiring intensive care. Intensive Care Med 2001;27:694-699.
5. Sungur M, Guven M: Intensive care management of organophosphate insecticide poisoning. Crit Care 2001;5: 211-215.
6. Senanayake N, Karalliedde L: Neurotoxic effects of organophosphorous insecticides: An intermediate syndrome. N Engl J Med 1987;316:761-763.
7. Lotti M: Cholinesterase inhibition: Complexities in interpretation. Clin Chem 1995;41:1814-1818.
8. Geller RJ, Singleton KL, Tarantino ML, et al: Nosocomial poisoning associated with emergency department treatment of organophosphate toxicity—Georgia, 2000. J Toxicol Clin Toxicol 2001;39:109-111.
9. Selden BS, Curry SC: Prolonged succinylcholine-induced paralysis in organophosphate insecticide poisoning. Ann Emerg Med 1987;16:215-217.
10. Du Toit PW, Muller FO, Van Tonder WM, Ungerer MJ: Experience with intensive care management of organophosphate insecticide poisoning. S Afr Med J 1981;60: 227-229.
11. Fischer TF: Lindane toxicity in a 24-year old woman. Ann Emerg Med 1994;24:972-974.
12. Aks SE, Krantz A, Hryhorczuk DO, et al: Acute accidental lindane ingestion in toddlers. Ann Emerg Med 1995;26:647-651.
13. Centers for Disease Control and Prevention: Unintentional topical lindane ingestions—United States, 1998-2003. MMWR Morbid Mortal Wkly Rep 2005;54:533-535.
14. Narahashi T, Frey JM, Ginsburg KS, Roy ML: Sodium and GABA-activated channels as the targets of pyrethroids and cyclodienes. Toxicol Lett 1992;64/65:429-436.
15. Tenenbein M: Seizures after lindane therapy. J Am Geriatr Soc 1991;39:394-395.
16. Wax PM, Hoffman RS: Fatality associated with inhalation of a pyrethrin shampoo. Clin Toxicol 1994;32:457-460.
17. Wagner SL: Fatal asthma in a child after use of an animal shampoo containing pyrethrin. West J Med 2000;173: 86-87.
18. He F, Wang S, Liu L, et al: Clinical manifestations and diagnosis of acute pyrethroid poisoning. Arch Toxicol 1989;63:54-58.
19. Klein Schwartz W, Smith GS: Agricultural and horticultural chemical poisonings: Mortality and morbidity in the United States. Ann Emerg Med 1997;29:232-238.
20. Vale JA, Merideth TJ, Buckley BM: Paraquat poisoning: Clinical features and immediate general management. Hum Toxicol 1987;6:41-47.
21. Bismuth C, Garnier R, Baud FJ, et al: Paraquat poisoning: An overview of the current status. Drug Saf 1990;5: 243-251.
22. Jones GM, Vale JA: Mechanisms of toxicity, clinical features, and management of diquat poisoning: A review. Clin Tox 2000;38:123-128.
23. Bradberry SM, Watt BE, Proudfoot AT, Vale JA: Mechanims of toxicity, clinical features, and management of acute chlorphenoxy herbicide poisoning: A review. Clin Tox 2000;38:111-122.
24. Bradberry SM, Proudfoot AT, Vale JA: Poisoning due to chlorphenoxy herbicides. Toxicol Rev 2004;23;65-73.
25. Prescott LF, Park J, Darrien I: Treatment of severe 2,4-D and mecoprop intoxication with alkaline diuresis. Br J Clin Pharmacol 1979;7:111-116.
26. Sorensen FW, Gregersen M: Rapid lethal intoxication caused by the herbicide glyphosate-trimesium (Touchdown). Human Exp Toxicol 1999;18:735-737.
27. Bradberry SM, Proudfoot AT, Vale JA: Glyphosate poisoning. Toxicol Rev 2004;23:159-167.
28. Koyama K, Andou Y, Saruki K, Matsuo H: Delayed and severe toxicities of a herbicide glufosinate and a surfactant. Vet Human Toxicol 1994;36:17-18.

29. Tanaka J, Yamashita M, Yamashita M, et al: Two cases of glufosinate poisoning with late onset convulsions. Vet Human Toxicol 1998;40:219-222.
30. Smolinske SC, Scherger DL, Kearns PS, et al: Superwarfarin poisoning in children: A prospective study. Pediatrics 1989;84:490-494.
31. Katona B, Wason S: Superwarfarin poisoning. J Emerg Med 1989;7:627-631.
32. Ingels M, Lai C, Manning BH, et al: A prospective study of acute, unintentional pediatric superwarfarin ingestions managed without decontamination. Ann Emerg Med 2002;40:73-78.
33. Smith BA: Strychnine poisoning. J Emerg Med 1990;8: 321-325.

Chapter 141

Antidepressants and Antipsychotics

Sean M. Bryant

KEY POINTS

Central nervous system depression is the most common symptom of antidepressant and antipsychotic overdose.

Tachycardia, hypotension, seizures, and ventricular dysrhythmias can also occur, especially after tricyclic antidepressant (TCA) overdose.

Airway intervention, benzodiazepines, intravenous fluids, and cooling measures (especially for serotonin syndrome and/or neuroleptic malignant syndrome) are the mainstays of supportive care and treatment.

Specific treatment options include sodium bicarbonate for TCA ingestion, and crystalloid fluids or hemodialysis for lithium ingestion.

Controversial treatment modalities include dantrolene for toxin-induced hyperthermia, cyproheptadine for serotonin syndrome, bromocriptine for neuromuscular malignant syndrome, and prophylactic magnesium for long QTc intervals without evidence of torsades de pointes.

Scope

According to data from United States poison control centers, the trend for toxic exposures from antidepressants and antipsychotic agents continues to climb (Figs. 141-1 and 141-2). Tricyclic antidepressant (TCA) and monoamine oxidase inhibitor (MAOI) overdoses have historically resulted in the most significant morbidity and mortality. Currently, however, these agents are prescribed much less frequently than selective serotonin reuptake inhibitors (SSRIs), atypical antipsychotics, and lithium.

Pathophysiology

Because the prevailing theory of depression remains neurotransmitter level fluctuations, therapy is prescribed in attempts to rectify a balance. Whether it is decreased serotonin neuronal storage, increased serotonin receptor sensitivity, serotonin hyperactivity resulting in depressed dopamine transmission, or destruction of serotonin neurons by some exogenous or genetic factor, targeting this imbalance has positive effects in treating depression. Overdose of antidepressant medications results in adverse central nervous system (CNS) effects.

■ TRICYCLIC ANTIDEPRESSANTS

TCAs, or "cyclic antidepressants," have similar ring structures and, with only a few exceptions, result in related toxicity. Examples are amitriptyline (Elavil), imipramine (Tofranil), and doxepin (Sinequan). The

Table 141-1 FIVE MAJOR PHARMACOLOGIC EFFECTS OF TRICYCLIC ANTIDEPRESSANTS

Pharmacologic Effect	Symptoms
Blockade of sodium conductance through fast channels in the myocardium	Prolonged phase 0 of the cardiac action potential, which results in a widened QRS complex on an electrocardiogram
Blockade of potassium efflux	Prolonged phase 3 of the cardiac action potential results in an increased QTc interval, which lends itself to the development of torsades de pointes
Peripheral α_1 receptor blockade	Vasodilation, decreased perfusion, and hypotension
Serotonin and norepinephrine reuptake inhibition	Agitation, delirium, or seizure activity
Anticholinergic activity	Range of physical findings (coma, delirium, urinary retention, mydriasis, seizures, tachycardia, flushing, hyperthermia, dry skin) "Hot as a hare, dry as a bone, red as a beet, blind as a bat, mad as a hatter, fast as a cat, full as a tick"

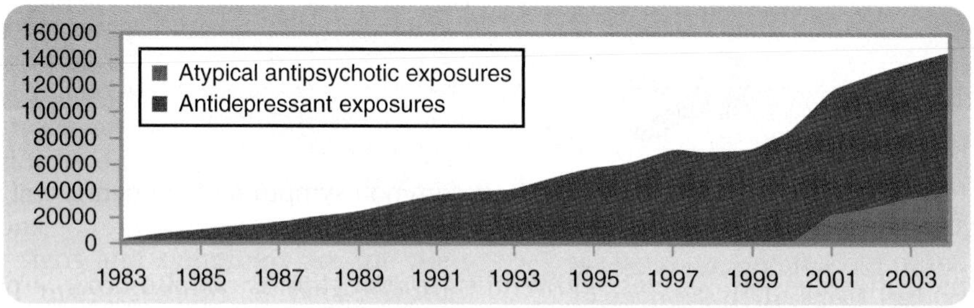
160000
140000
120000
100000
80000
60000
40000
20000
0
Atypical antipsychotic exposures
Antidepressant exposures
1983 1985 1987 1989 1991 1993 1995 1997 1999 2001 2003

FIGURE 141-1 Trends in exposure to atypical antipsychotics and antidepressants. (Compiled from the Toxic Exposure Surveillance System Data, 1983-2004.)

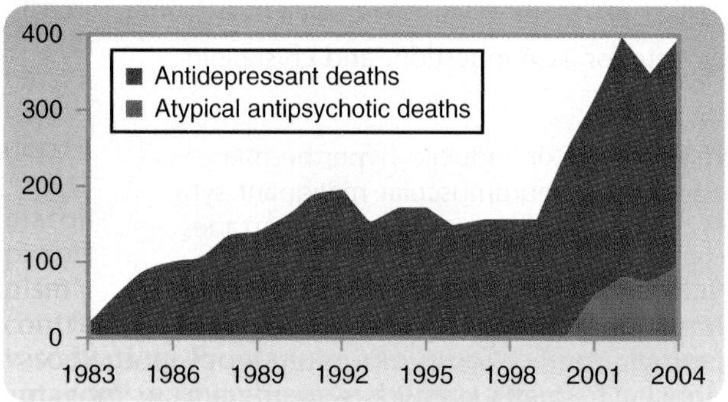
400
300
200
100
0
Antidepressant deaths
Atypical antipsychotic deaths
1983 1986 1989 1992 1995 1998 2001 2004

FIGURE 141-2 Trends in deaths related to atypical antipsychotics and antidepressants. (Compiled from the Toxic Exposure Surveillance System Data, 1983-2004.)

five major pharmacologic effects of TCAs are listed in Table 141-1.

■ MONOAMINE OXIDASE INHIBITORS

The two most commonly prescribed MAOIs marketed in the United States, phenelzine (Nardil) and tranylcypromine (Parnate), account for the majority of toxicity from this class of agent. The pharmacologic effects of MAOIs are listed in Box 141-1; each of these effects in overdose may result in overactive sympathomimetic manifestations. Although overdose is certainly concerning, interactions with food and beverages or drugs are just as important.

BOX 141-1

Pharmacologic Effects of Monamine Oxidase Inhibitors

- Inhibition of monoamine oxidase isoenzymes, which results in excessive activity of epinephrine, norepinephrine, serotonin, and tyramine
- Effects on exogenous amphetamines and methamphetamine
- Depletion of norepinephrine stores
- Inhibition of pyridoxine-containing enzymes

■ SELECTIVE SEROTONIN REUPTAKE INHIBITORS

SSRI antidepressants commonly prescribed are sertraline (Zoloft), paroxetine (Paxil), fluoxetine (Prozac), and citalopram (Celexa). The clinically beneficial effects of SSRIs in the CNS are commonly thought to occur as a result of blockade of presynaptic reuptake of serotonin at 5-hydroxytryptamine type 1 (5-HT_1) receptors. The blockade leads to higher synaptic serotonin levels and, hence, has positive effects on mood. Overdoses of these agents are much safer than overdoses of TCAs, although significant morbidity/mortality may occur with significant overdose or, more commonly, with ingestion of an SSRI in combination

BOX 141-2

Examples of Atypical Antipsychotic Medications

- Clozapine (Clozaril)
- Risperidone (Risperdal)
- Quetiapine (Seroquel)
- Ziprasidone (Geodon)
- Aripiprazole (Abilify)
- Paliperidone (Invega)
- Olanzapine (Zyprexa; also Symbyax when combined with fluoxetine [Prozac])

with ingestion of agents possessing pro-serotonergic activity.[1]

■ ATYPICAL ANTIPSYCHOTICS

Atypical antipsychotic agents have largely replaced the older, "typical" agents because of the newer agents' ability to effectively reduce hallucinations, restructure thinking, and control agitation while assisting with the negative effects of psychotic disorders (flattened affect, avolition, social withdrawal). Also, movement disorders such as dystonia, akathisia, tardive dyskinesia, and neuroleptic malignant syndrome occur less often with atypical antipsychotics than with the typical agents. The pharmacologic mechanism of action of atypical agents includes blockade at dopamine (D_2) receptors and serotonin ($5\text{-}HT_{2A}$) receptors.[2] These agents can also cause repolarization abnormalities by blocking potassium efflux in the myocardium, setting the stage for risk of torsades de pointes (Box 141-2).

■ LITHIUM

The lightest metal known, lithium has many similarities to sodium and potassium. Since the early 1970s, lithium has been a mainstay of treatment for bipolar disorder. Its mechanism of action is still debated. Lithium may affect the synthesis and turnover of serotonin in the CNS. In addition, it may downregulate $5\text{-}HT_{1A}$ receptors and alpha- and beta-adrenergic receptors. Serving as a "false ion" and affecting second messenger systems (inositol triphosphate) in the CNS may also play a part in both the therapeutic and toxicologic manifestations of lithium.

Presenting Signs and Symptoms

■ TRICYCLIC ANTIDEPRESSANTS

Serious toxicity is usually seen within 6 hours of ingestion. Signs and symptoms include obtundation, seizures, hypertension (early), hypotension (late), tachycardia (supraventricular or ventricular), and respiratory depression. Patients can deteriorate rapidly and usually do so within an hour of ingestion.[3] Seizures and cardiovascular collapse can occur.[4-6] In addition, profound hemodynamic instability follows seizure activity in 13% of patients who have been poisoned with TCAs. Seizures result in further acidemia, which contributes to cardiovascular poisoning.

Cardiac monitoring helps discern the severity of toxicity. Maximal limb-lead QRS interval duration is a sensitive indicator of illness.[7] Generally, QRS inter-

Documentation

History

- Any history of psychiatric illness or prior suicide ingestions
- Time lapse since ingestion if known
- History of renal or cardiac disease or other illnesses

Physical Examination

- Does the patient look ill? Febrile? What is mental status?
- Cardiac status (blood pressure, arrhythmias)
- Respiratory and airway status

Physical examination should be repeated while patient is in the ED.

Diagnostic Studies

- Electrocardiogram, serum glucose measurement, blood chemistry panel
- Acetaminophen and aspirin concentration should be checked if there is concern about co-ingestion

Medical Decision-Making

- Decision to begin specific treatment or delay it
- Consultations desired and times of phone calls to consulting services

Treatment

- Response to treatment (especially for sodium bicarbonate, cooling measures, and seizure treatment)

Patient Instructions

- Document discussion with patient regarding diagnosis, warning signs, what to do, follow-up, and when to return.
- With pediatric accidental ingestions, document poison prevention counseling and assessment of home situation.
- The regional poison control center can be contacted by telephone at 1-800-222-1222. All poison emergencies should be reported by the patient to the local poison control center.
- A dose of medication other than what was prescribed by the patient's physician should never be taken or given unless it has been approved by the ordering physician.

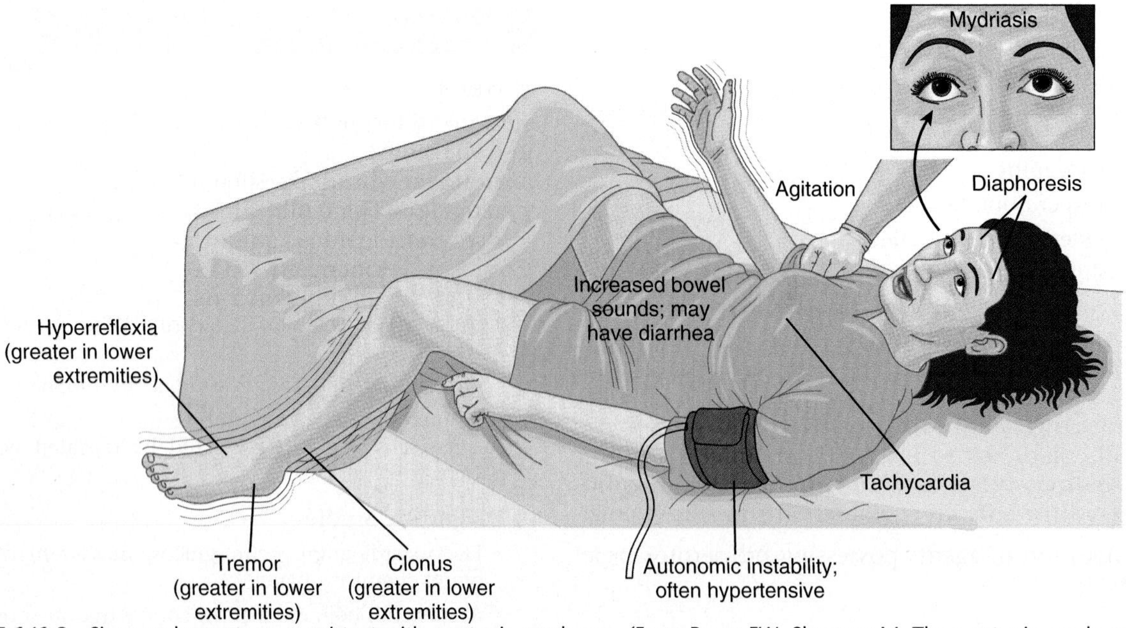
Mydriasis
Agitation
Diaphoresis
Increased bowel sounds; may have diarrhea
Hyperreflexia (greater in lower extremities)
Tachycardia
Tremor (greater in lower extremities)
Clonus (greater in lower extremities)
Autonomic instability; often hypertensive

FIGURE 141-3 Signs and symptoms consistent with serotonin syndrome. (From Boyer EW, Shannon M: The serotonin syndrome. N Engl J Med 2005;17:1112.)

val longer than 100 msec is associated with a 33% incidence of seizure activity, and QRS interval longer than 160 msec with a 50% incidence of ventricular dysrhythmia. One study has shown that the sensitivity of a QRS interval longer than 100 msec can be matched by two other parameters: the terminal 40 msec of lead aVR measuring longer than 3 mm (R wave in aVR > 3 mm), and an R-wave to S-wave amplitude ratio in the aVR lead greater than 0.7.[8]

■ MONOAMINE OXIDASE INHIBITORS

Overdose of an MAOI results in sympathomimetic overdrive. However, several phases have been described.[9,10] The phases can be classified as follows:

1. Asymptomatic phase.
2. Sympathetic hyperactivity.
3. CNS depression and/or cardiovascular collapse (hypotension and bradycardia).
4. Subsequent complications.

Onset of action occurs within 8 hours but may not manifest until 24 hours and then may last for several days. Agitation, delirium, seizures, coma, and muscular rigidity predominate. Significant late poisonings result in asystole because of depletion of catecholamines. In the presence of increased sympathetic tone, rhabdomyolysis can occur.

MAOI interactions with foods or beverages (aged cheeses, fava beans, ales, wines) produce rapid onset of signs and symptoms within minutes to hours.[10] Because of tyramine's short-lived action on the adrenal medulla (to increase endogenous amines), these interactions last only several hours. Interactions of MAOIs with other drugs (sympathomimetics, methylxanthines, SSRIs, meperidine) lead to elevated sympathetic tone as well; this effect manifests within minutes to hours and can last several hours to days.

■ SELECTIVE SEROTONIN REUPTAKE INHIBITORS

Overdose of SSRIs cause CNS abnormalities (sedation, agitation, delirium), peripheral alterations (tremor, hyperreflexia, rigidity), cardiovascular changes (tachycardia, bradycardia), and nausea, vomiting, and lightheadedness.[11-13] The patient with citalopram overdose should be observed for seizures and QTc and/or QRS interval lengthening. Although isolated SSRI ingestions frequently result in only mild toxicity, severe overdose or concomitant ingestion of proserotonergic medications can lead to serotonin excess and serotonin syndrome (Fig. 141-3). A history of ingestion of serotonergic agents, altered mental status, autonomic instability, and peripheral signs of rigidity or hyperreflexia are usually present.

■ ATYPICAL ANTIPSYCHOTICS

Patients usually present within a few hours of atypical antipsychotic overdose with signs of CNS depression (sedation, confusion, coma). Hypotension and reflex tachycardia from peripheral vasodilation may occur as well. Miosis may lead the examiner to consider opioid poisoning. QTc prolongation has been shown during therapeutic use of as well as overdose with these agents. Other adverse effects that are less commonly seen with newer agents than with the older typical agents are acute dystonias, akathisia, and tardive dyskinesia.

The most significant extrapyramidal effect is *neuromuscular malignant syndrome* (NMS).[14] It results when dopamine blockade agents act to cause "dopamine depleting" activity at D_2 receptors in the CNS. Although the history yields an ingestion of antipsychotic medications, NMS usually arises out of in-

Table 141-2 COMPARISON OF THE MANIFESTATIONS OF SEROTONIN SYNDROME AND NEUROMUSCULAR MALIGNANT SYNDROME

Feature	Serotonin Syndrome	Neuromuscular Malignant Syndrome
History	Drug(s) with serotonergic activity	Dopamine-blocking agents
Time of onset	Hours	Days
Mental status	Agitation to coma	Agitation to coma
Tone	Rigidity, greater in lower than in upper extremities	"Lead-pipe" rigidity
Vital signs	Hypertension, tachycardia, and hyperthermia	Hypertension, tachycardia, and hyperthermia

creased dosing or the addition of agents with similar activity (e.g., lithium which inhibits dopamine secretion). Manifestations of NMS include CNS abnormalities (sedation, agitation, delirium), peripheral alterations (tremor, hyperreflexia, rigidity), and cardiovascular changes with autonomic instability (tachycardia, bradycardia, hyperthermia) much like those in serotonin syndrome. Unlike serotonin syndrome, in which onset of symptoms is normally rather quick, NMS occurs more insidiously. Historical information and medication lists are often needed to enable differentiation between the two conditions (Table 141-2).

■ LITHIUM

The clinical effects of lithium overdose are gastrointestinal (nausea, vomiting, and diarrhea), neurologic (tremor, confusion, ataxia, weakness), and cardiovascular (QTc prolongation, bradycardia, T wave flattening or inversion, bundle branch blocks). Adverse effects include nephrogenic diabetes insipidus, polyuria, psoriasis, alopecia, edema, and leukocytosis. Gastrointestinal distress is usually one of the first manifestations of lithium toxicity. Many presentations are "chronic" in nature, arising out of continued dosing in the presence of dehydration (decreased fluid intake or vomiting and diarrhea). Lithium is recognized like sodium is and is retained by the kidney in patients with dehydration. In light of this feature, persistent dosing results in greater CNS levels and subsequent toxicity. Additionally, changes in a patient's renal status may decrease lithium clearance.

Differential Diagnosis

Any sedating agent (e.g., opioids, ethyl alcohol, benzodiazepines) should be considered in the differential diagnosis of most antidepressant and antipsychotic overdoses. The differential diagnosis for TCA overdose should be broader and should include anticholinergic/antihistamine products (e.g., diphenhydramine) and agents that can poison fast sodium channels, thereby lengthening the QRS interval (e.g., type I antidysrhythmics, cocaine, diphenhydramine, propoxyphene, carbamazepine, cyclobenzaprine, and phenothiazines). Life-threatening features are hyperthermia associated with mental status changes, autonomic instability, and tremors, clonus, or rigidity. Serotonin syndrome (e.g. SSRIs, ecstasy, meperidine, lithium, dextromethorphan, L-tryptophan), neuroleptic malignant syndrome (e.g., antipsychotics like phenothiazines), malignant hyperthermia (e.g., anesthetic agent use), sympathomimetic overdrive (e.g., cocaine, amphetamines), and MAOI overdose or drug/food interaction should also be considered (Box 141-3).

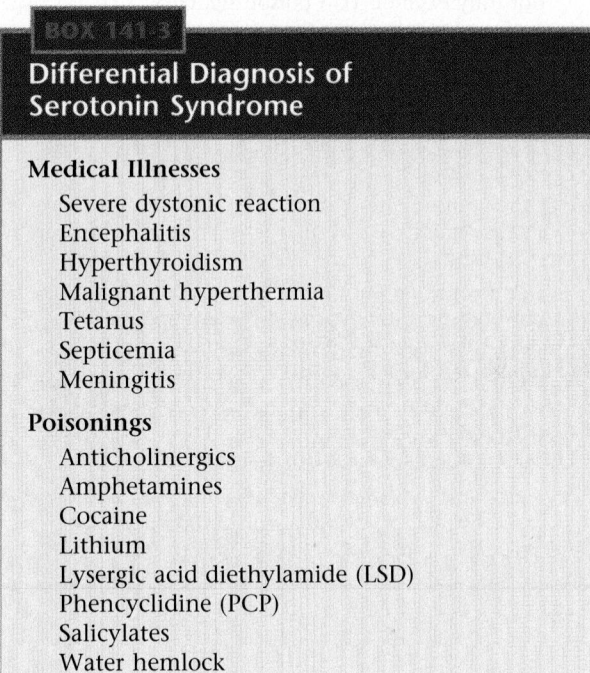

BOX 141-3

Differential Diagnosis of Serotonin Syndrome

Medical Illnesses
- Severe dystonic reaction
- Encephalitis
- Hyperthyroidism
- Malignant hyperthermia
- Tetanus
- Septicemia
- Meningitis

Poisonings
- Anticholinergics
- Amphetamines
- Cocaine
- Lithium
- Lysergic acid diethylamide (LSD)
- Phencyclidine (PCP)
- Salicylates
- Water hemlock

Diagnostic Testing

■ TRICYCLIC ANTIDEPRESSANTS

Life-threatening toxicity should be anticipated in an adult who has ingested TCA doses of 10 mg/kg or greater. Qualitative urine screens for TCAs are of no diagnostic benefit. Although quantitative serum levels of TCAs greater than 1000 ng/mL (therapeutic 50-300 ng/mL) have been correlated with severe toxicity, quantitative testing may not be available in a timely fashion. In addition, depending on the time from ingestion, type of TCA taken, and the chronicity of dosing, patients may be very ill with serum

Tips and Tricks

- Generally, QRS duration longer than 100 msec is associated with a 33% incidence of seizure activity, and a QRS greater than 160 msec with a 50% incidence of ventricular dysrhythmia. Cardiac monitoring is a valid way of discerning the severity of toxicity in tricyclic antidepressant (TCA) poisoning.
- Lithium toxicity is often precipitated by dehydration or worsening renal function.
- Although normal electrocardiographic findings do not fully exclude TCA poisoning, QRS prolongation to more than 100 to 120 msec should be a threshold for treatment.
- A serum lithium value obtained less than 6 hours after the last dose may result in excessively elevated concentrations (therapeutic 0.6-1.2 ng/mL).
- Devastating hemodynamic instability follows seizure activity in 13% of patients with TCA poisoning.
- Significant, late monoamine oxidase inhibitor poisoning results in asystole from depletion of catecholamines, so affected patients should be monitored for 24 hours.
- Atypical antipsychotic toxicity can be associated with sedation or coma and miosis and therefore can be confused with opiate intoxication.
- Rightward deviation of the terminal 40-msec QRS axis (R wave in aVR > 3 mm) should be a cause for concern in a patient with TCA overdose.

levels much lower than 1000 ng/mL. An electrocardiogram (ECG) is the diagnostic test of choice.[15] Normal ECG findings do not fully exclude TCA poisoning, but QRS prolongation greater than 120 msec should be a threshold for treatment (Fig. 141-4).[8] Additionally, rightward deviation of the terminal 40 msec of the QRS axis (R wave in aVR >3 mm) should be a cause for concern (Fig. 141-5).

■ MONOAMINE OXIDASE INHIBITORS

A clinical diagnosis (largely based on historical facts) is required for MAOI overdose. No laboratory (urine or blood) test is readily available to make a diagnosis of MAOI poisoning.

■ SELECTIVE SEROTONIN REUPTAKE INHIBITORS

Diagnosis of SSRI toxicity is purely clinical. The criteria for serotonin syndrome are met through focused elicitation of historical information and the finding of signs and symptoms consistent with the disorder (Table 141-3).[16]

■ ATYPICAL ANTIPSYCHOTICS

Blood or urine testing plays no role in diagnosis of atypical antipsychotic overdose. Although QTc prolongation can occur after both therapeutic and toxic ingestions, this finding is not specific for these agents. NMS is a clinical diagnosis coupled with diligent history taking.

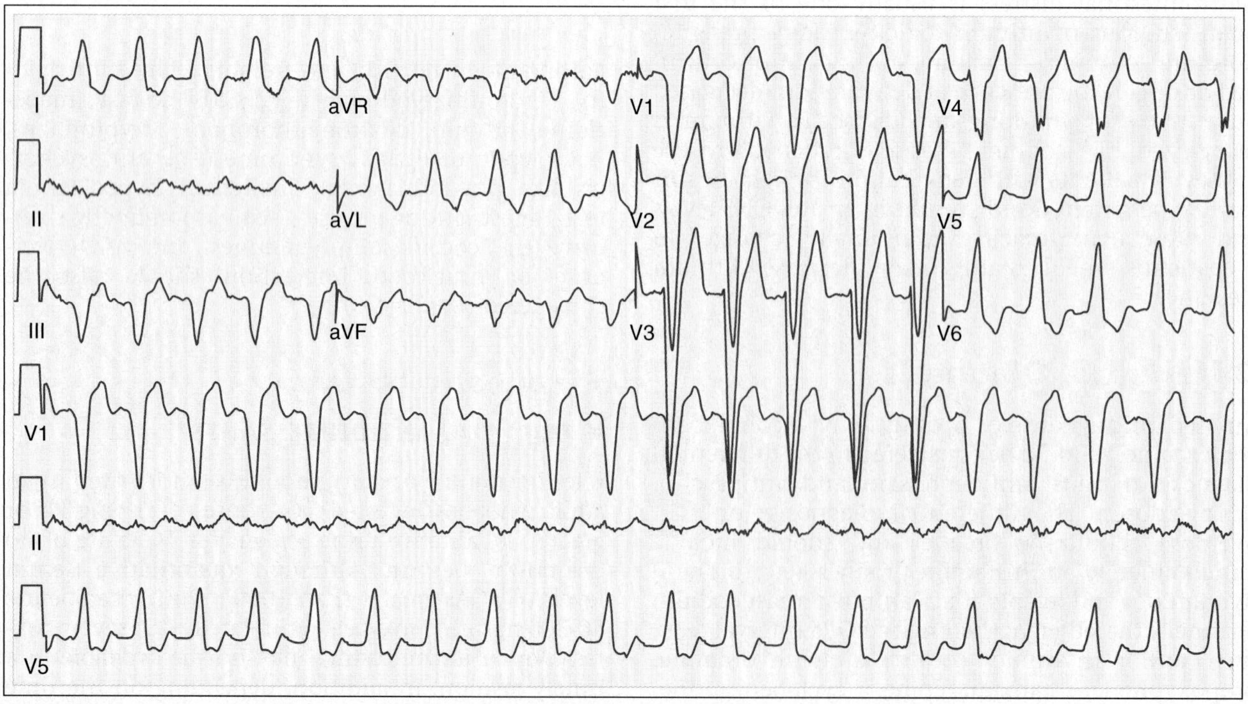
I
aVR
V1
V4
II
aVL
V2
V5
III
aVF
V3
V6
V1
II
V5

FIGURE 141-4 Electrocardiogram showing signs of poisoning by a tricyclic antidepressant. Tachycardia and severe sodium channel poisoning are evidenced by a significantly widened QRS interval.

■ LITHIUM

Clinical suspicion, historical features, and serum lithium concentrations form the basis of the diagnosis of lithium poisoning. Serum concentration values must be interpreted in the context of chronicity and timing of ingestion. Because long-term users of this drug have higher CNS levels, ill effects occur at lower serum levels. Additionally, lithium has a long distribution time after absorption. In light of this feature, measurement of a serum lithium level less than 6 hours after the last dose may yield an excessively elevated concentration (therapeutic 0.6-1.2 ng/mL). Generally, serum lithium levels greater than 4 ng/mL in an acute ingestion and greater than 2.5 ng/mL in a chronic poisoning are considered significant.

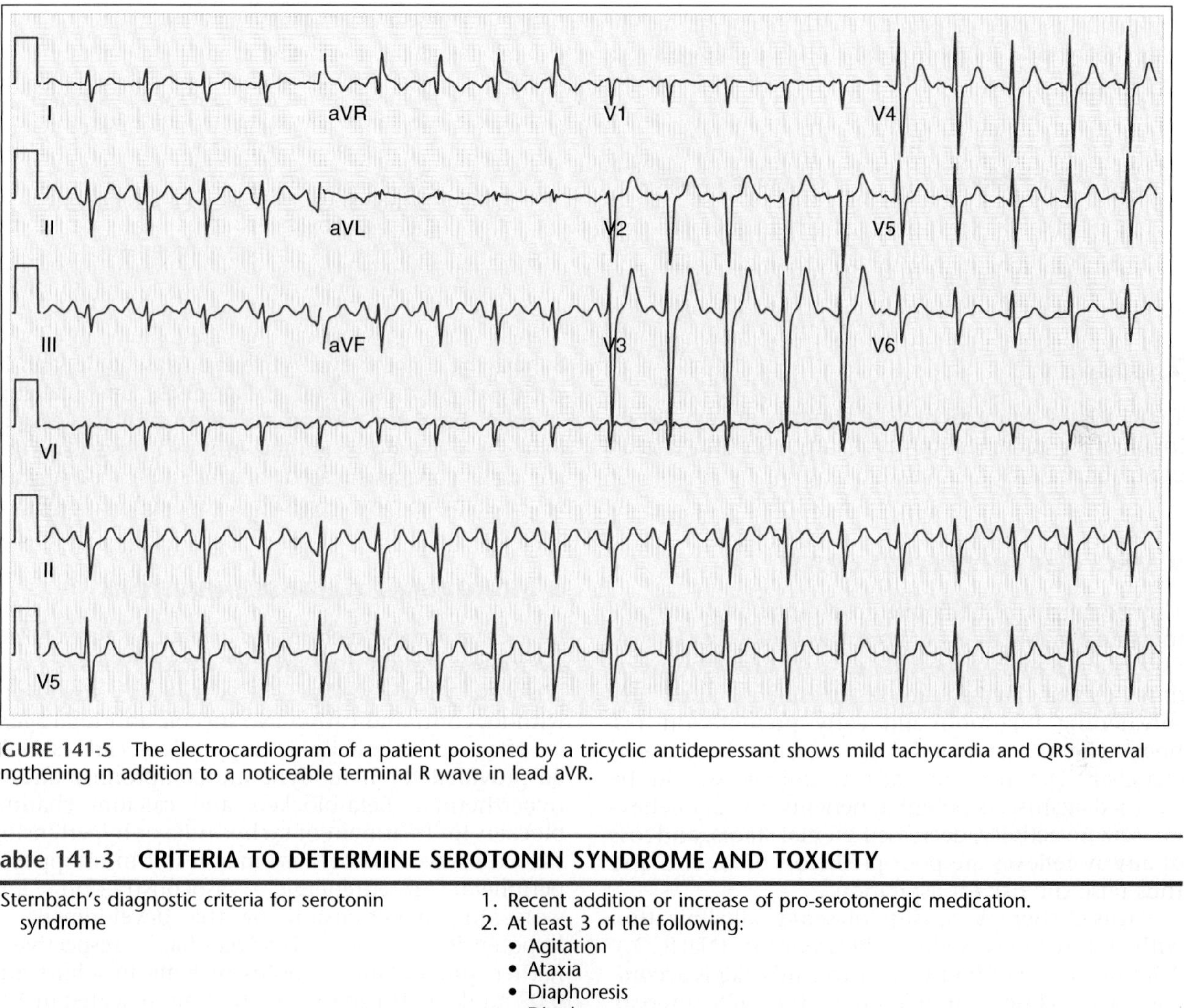
I
aVR
V1
V4
II
aVL
V2
V5
III
aVF
V3
V6
VI
II
V5

FIGURE 141-5 The electrocardiogram of a patient poisoned by a tricyclic antidepressant shows mild tachycardia and QRS interval lengthening in addition to a noticeable terminal R wave in lead aVR.

Table 141-3 CRITERIA TO DETERMINE SEROTONIN SYNDROME AND TOXICITY

Sternbach's diagnostic criteria for serotonin syndrome	1. Recent addition or increase of pro-serotonergic medication. 2. At least 3 of the following: • Agitation • Ataxia • Diaphoresis • Diarrhea • Hyperreflexia • Hyperthermia • Mental status changes • Myoclonus • Shivering • Tremor 3. Neuroleptic agent was not added or dose was increased prior to onset of symptoms. 4. Infections, withdrawal, and other poisoning or metabolic disruptions have been ruled out.
Hunter's criteria for serotonin toxicity (context of serotonergic medications)	1. If the patient has spontaneous clonus, serotonin toxicity is present. 2. If there is no spontaneous clonus, one of the following is needed for a diagnosis of serotonin toxicity: • Inducible clonus *and* agitation *or* diaphoresis • Ocular clonus *and* agitation *or* diaphoresis • Tremor *and* hyperreflexia • Hypertonic *and* temperature • Temperature >38°C *and* ocular clonus *or* inducible clonus

Table 141-4 **TREATMENT FOR NON–TRICYCLIC ANTIDEPRESSANT OVERDOSES**

Drug	Gastrointestinal Decontamination	Treatment
Lithium	Consider whole-bowel irrigation for sustained-release formulations (acute ingestions)	IV fluids at 1.5-2× maintenance levels Hemodialysis in severe cases
Monoamine oxidase inhibitors	Activated charcoal For significant ingestions, lavage prior to charcoal	For hypertension: phentolamine 2-5 mg IV over several minutes or nitroprusside 0.3 μg/kg/min titrated to effect For dysrhythmias: lidocaine Cooling with mist and fan Benzodiazepines for agitation
Selective serotonin reuptake inhibitors	Activated charcoal	Supportive care Aggressive cooling Benzodiazepines for cooling and/or agitation For life-threatening hyperthermia: sedation, paralysis, and ventilation
Atypical antipsychotics	Activated charcoal	Supportive care Benzodiazepines for agitation and/or rigidity Aggressive cooling Correction of electrolyte abnormalities

Treatment

Table 141-4 summarizes treatment of overdoses involving antidepressant and antipsychotic agents other than TCAs.

■ TRICYCLIC ANTIDEPRESSANTS

The treatment of TCA overdose depends on symptoms and is best judged from the ECG (Fig. 141-6). Decontamination is best done early after the overdose. Gastric lavage can be considered after life-threatening ingestion and early presentation (<1 hour). The mainstay of decontamination is activated charcoal. The risks of each technique should be weighed against its potential benefits. Unruly behavior, seizure activity, decreased mental status, and loss of airway reflexes are poor predictors of success and thus raise the risk for aspiration.

Focused therapy consists of serum alkalinization with intravenous sodium bicarbonate ($NaHCO_3$). Administration of boluses of 1 to 2 mEq/kg is accompanied by close examination of the QRS interval. Boluses should be repeated every 5 minutes until resolution of QRS widening resolves, dysrhythmias occur, or blood pH exceeds 7.55. Rarely, hypertonic saline can be considered for prolonged QRS intervals and severe alkalemia. Sodium bicarbonate drips—3 ampules added to 1 liter of 5% dextrose in water (D_5W) given at rates of 2 to 3 mL/kg/hr—and hyperventilation with ventilatory support are considered adjuncts to sodium bicarbonate bolus therapy. Serum potassium levels should be monitored with this therapy, and potassium losses replaced as necessary.

Seizure activity should be treated with sedatives such as benzodiazepines and barbiturates. If muscle paralysis is necessary, continuous electroencephalographic techniques should be used to measure seizure activity. Lidocaine is an alternative to sodium bicarbonate therapy for dysrhythmias. Class Ia, Ic, and III antidysrhythmics, beta antagonists, and calcium channel blockers are contraindicated in the patient with TCA overdose. Flumazenil and physostigmine are also contraindicated because they can cause seizure activity and asystolic arrest, respectively.

■ MONOAMINE OXIDASE INHIBITORS

Decontamination techniques in patients with MAOI overdoses should include activated charcoal and, possibly, gastric lavage for significant ingestions without contraindication. No specific antidotal agent is effective. Meticulous supportive care should be provided for hemodynamic compromise and/or hyperthermia. Beta-blockers and calcium channel blockers for treatment of tachycardia or hypertension should be avoided because may result in unopposed peripheral α_1-adrenergic vasoconstriction and worsening hypertension or the development of hypotension and bradycardia, respectively. Rather, phentolamine (bolus of 5 mg in adults and 0.02 mg/kg to 0.1 mg/kg in children, repeated in 5 to 10 minutes as needed) or nitroprusside (0.3 μg/kg/min titrated to effect) should be considered for hypertensive emergencies. Ventricular dysrhythmias should be treated with lidocaine. Controversy exists over the use of dantrolene for life-threatening hyperthermia in patients with MAOI overdose. Supportive cooling techniques (e.g., mist and fan) should be provided as well as intravenous fluids and judicious use of benzodiazepines for agitation.

■ SELECTIVE SEROTONIN REUPTAKE INHIBITORS

Standard activated charcoal decontamination should be employed for SSRI overdose. Supportive care of the airway, breathing, and circulation encompasses the

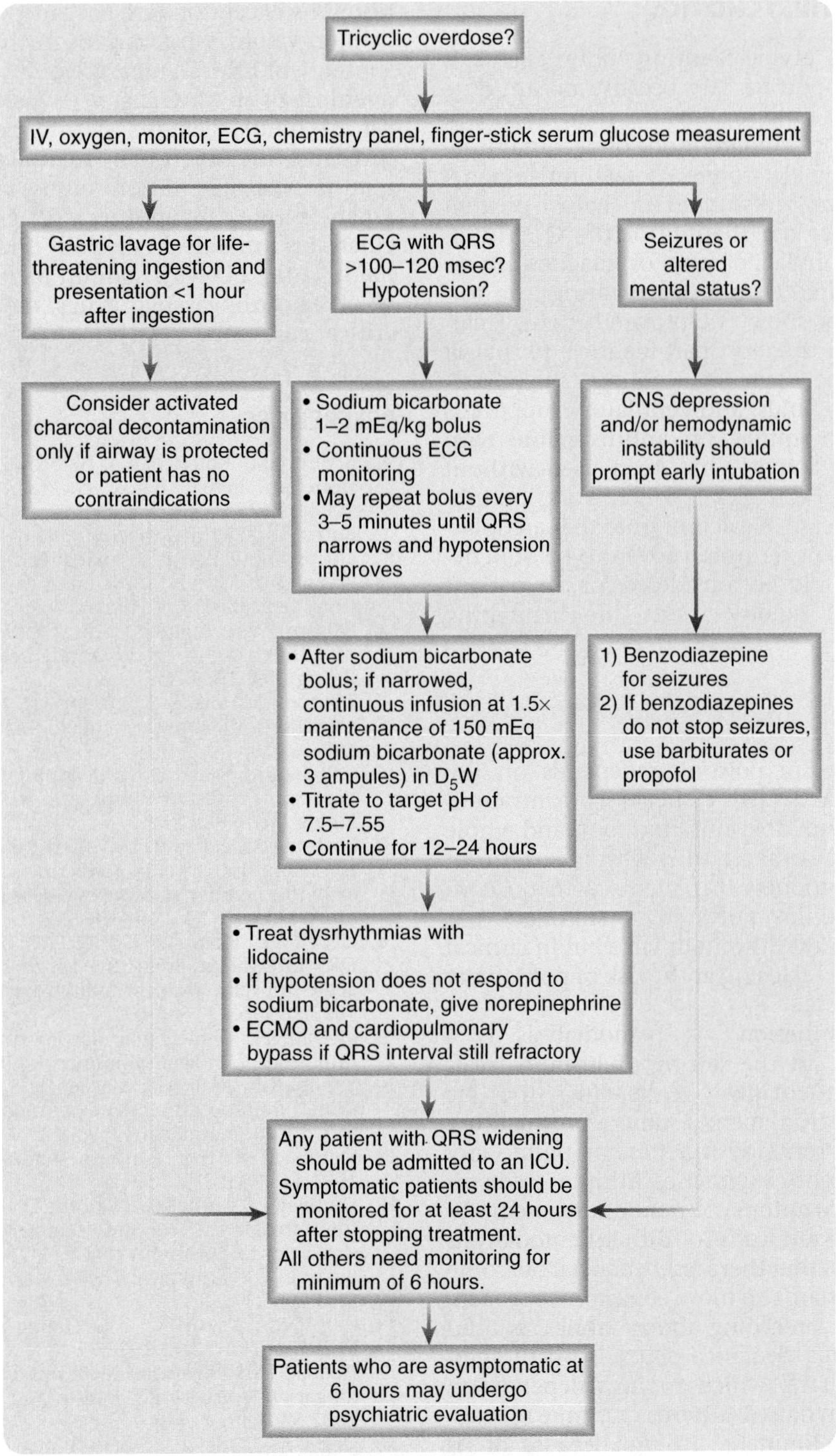
Tricyclic overdose?
IV, oxygen, monitor, ECG, chemistry panel, finger-stick serum glucose measurement
Gastric lavage for life-threatening ingestion and presentation <1 hour after ingestion
ECG with QRS >100–120 msec? Hypotension?
Seizures or altered mental status?
Consider activated charcoal decontamination only if airway is protected or patient has no contraindications
• Sodium bicarbonate 1–2 mEq/kg bolus • Continuous ECG monitoring • May repeat bolus every 3–5 minutes until QRS narrows and hypotension improves
CNS depression and/or hemodynamic instability should prompt early intubation
• After sodium bicarbonate bolus; if narrowed, continuous infusion at 1.5× maintenance of 150 mEq sodium bicarbonate (approx. 3 ampules) in D5W • Titrate to target pH of 7.5–7.55 • Continue for 12–24 hours
1) Benzodiazepine for seizures 2) If benzodiazepines do not stop seizures, use barbiturates or propofol
• Treat dysrhythmias with lidocaine • If hypotension does not respond to sodium bicarbonate, give norepinephrine • ECMO and cardiopulmonary bypass if QRS interval still refractory
Any patient with QRS widening should be admitted to an ICU. Symptomatic patients should be monitored for at least 24 hours after stopping treatment. All others need monitoring for minimum of 6 hours.
Patients who are asymptomatic at 6 hours may undergo psychiatric evaluation

FIGURE 141-6 Algorithm for treatment of tricyclic antidepressant overdoses. CNS, central nervous system; D_5W, 5% dextrose in water; ECG, electrocardiogram; ECMO, extracorporeal membrane oxygenation; ICU, intensive care unit; IV, intravenous.

majority of treatment. In cases of serotonin syndrome, aggressive cooling measures for hyperthermia, benzodiazepines for agitation, and intravenous fluids are usually the only measures required to decrease the risk of death. Life-threatening hyperthermia should be treated with sedation, neuromuscular paralysis, and ventilatory care. The use of cyproheptadine (8 mg by mouth; up to 24 mg per day) for serotonin syndrome has been described but remains controversial. Bromocriptine has been reported to worsen serotonin syndrome, and dantrolene (proven effective for malignant hyperthermia) should be considered only for life-threatening hyperthermia and significant rigidity.

ATYPICAL ANTIPSYCHOTICS

Acute overdose of atypical antipsychotic agents is managed with supportive care because no antidote exists. These agents bind to activated charcoal, use of which should be the standard mode of decontamination. Correction of electrolyte (potassium, magnesium, and calcium) disturbances helps prevent widening or further lengthening of the QTc interval.[15,17] The "prophylactic" use of magnesium to prevent a widened QTc from degenerating into torsades de pointes has shown no proven benefit. Treatment of NMS is for the most part identical to that of serotonin syndrome (aggressive cooling, benzodiazepines for agitation, fluids, and ventilatory support as warranted). Bromocriptine, an antihistamine with dopamine agonist activity, has been used without consistent benefit. Dantrolene, which works peripherally to inhibit release of calcium from the sarcoplasmic reticulum, has never been proven to be of benefit in NMS but should be considered for the patient with significant rigidity and life-threatening hyperthermia.[18]

LITHIUM

Treatment for lithium poisoning depends on the clinical context. Activated charcoal is contraindicated because lithium does not bind to it, and whole bowel irrigation is warranted only with ingestions of sustained-release products in patients with no contraindications. Sodium polystyrene sulfonate has been shown to bind to lithium in vitro but in clinical use requires excessive dosing at the risk of potentially causing hypokalemia.

Enhancing elimination via hemodialysis is a controversial topic in the setting of lithium treatment.[16,19,20] The patient likely to benefit is the one with an acute ingestion, mental status abnormalities, and/or significant renal dysfunction or pulmonary edema. Many patients experience lithium "redistribution" and an asymptomatic period after hemodialysis. This result often leads to further hemodialysis procedures, but whether there is a beneficial outcome remains controversial. The more common approach, barring any of the preceding abnormalities, is fluid hydration. Lithium's clearance depends on the glomerular filtration rate, which in turn depends on volume status. Dehydrated patients continue to reabsorb, rather than eliminate, lithium because of its physical characteristics. Crystalloids given at two times maintenance doses should suffice. There is no role for forced diuresis or diuretic therapy.

Disposition

Any patient with deliberate overdose of an antidepressant or antipsychotic medications or with clinical symptoms should be admitted to the hospital. Patients who are asymptomatic 6 hours after ingestion can be medically cleared for psychiatric evaluation. The exceptions are patients with elevated serum lithium values, who warrant further observation and subsequent lithium measurements, and patients with overdose of an MAOI agent, which may not manifest for 24 hours. Patients should be admitted to the intensive care unit for any mental status changes that require close observation for loss of airway reflexes or seizure activity. In addition, patients with cardiovascular abnormalities, especially those requiring treatment in the ED with sodium bicarbonate, lidocaine, or other cardiovascular drugs, merit disposition to a critical care unit.

REFERENCES

1. Bryant SM, Kolodchak J: Serotonin syndrome resulting from an herbal detox cocktail. Am J Emerg Med 2004;22:625.
2. Burns MJ: The pharmacology and toxicology of atypical antipsychotic agents. J Toxicol Clin Toxicol 2001;39:1.
3. Bryant SM, Mycyk MB: Human exposure to pet prescription medication. Vet Human Toxicol 2002;44:218.
4. Ellison DW, Pentel PR: Clinical features and consequences of seizures due to cyclic antidepressant overdoses. Am J Emerg Med 1989;7:5.
5. Shannon M, Merola J, Lovejoy FH: Hypotension in severe tricyclic antidepressant overdose. Am J Emerg Med 1988;6:439.
6. Callahan M, Kassel D: Epidemiology of fatal tricyclic antidepressant ingestion: Implications for management. Ann Emerg Med 1985;14:1.
7. Boehnert M, Lovejoy FH: Value of the QRS duration versus the serum drug level in predicting seizures and ventricular arrhythmias after an acute overdose of tricyclic antidepressants. N Engl J Med 1985;13:203.
8. Liebelt EL, Francis PD, Wolf AD: ECG lead aVR versus QRS interval in predicting seizures and arrhythmias in acute tricyclic antidepressant toxicity. Ann Emerg Med 1995;26:195.
9. McDaniel K: Clinical pharmacology of monoamine oxidase inhibitors. Clin Neuropharmacol 1986;9:207.
10. Shulman K, Walker S, Mackenzie S, et al: Dietary restrictions, tyramine, and the use of monoamine oxidase inhibitors. J Clin Pharmacol 1989;38:2.
11. Sternbach H: The serotonin syndrome. Am J Psychiatry 1991;148:705.
12. Dunkley EJ, Isbister GK, Sibbritt D, et al: The Hunter serotonin toxicity criteria: Simple and accurate diagnostic decision rules for serotonin toxicity. QJM 2003;96:635.
13. Boyer EW, Shannon M: The serotonin syndrome. N Engl J Med 2005;17:1112.
14. Caroff SN, Mann SC: Neuroleptic malignant syndrome. Med Clin North Am 1993;77:185.
15. Haddad PM, Anderson IM: Antipsychotic-related QTc prolongation, torsades de pointes and sudden death. Drugs 2002;62:1649.
16. Jaeger A, Sauder P, Kopferschmitt J, et al: When should dialysis be performed in lithium poisoning? A kinetic study in 14 cases of lithium poisoning. Clin Toxicol 1993;31:429.
17. Bryant SM, Zilberstein J, Cumpston KL, et al: A case series of ziprasidone overdoses. Vet Human Toxicol 2003;45:81.
18. Rusyniak DE, Sprague JE: Toxin-induced hyperthermic syndromes. Med Clin North Am 2005;89:1277.
19. Eyer F, Pfab R, Felgenhauer N, et al: Lithium poisoning: Pharmacokinetics and clearance during different therapeutic measures. J Clin Psychopharmacol 2006;26:325.
20. Bailey B, McGuigan M: Comparison of patients hemodialyzed for lithium poisoning and those for whom dialysis was recommended by PCC but not done: What lessons can we learn? Clin Nephrol 2000;4:388.

Chapter 142

Cardiovascular Drugs

Kirk Cumpston

KEY POINTS

Cardiovascular drugs are common and are responsible for many fatalities.

Beta-receptor antagonists, calcium channel antagonists, and digoxin primarily cause toxicity by disruption of intracellular calcium homeostasis and lead to hypotension and dysrhythmias.

With sustained-release forms of calcium channel antagonists, toxicity has a delayed peak and longer duration, which can lead to cardiovascular collapse and arrest if treatment is delayed or insufficient.

Diagnostic testing should include continuous cardiac monitoring, electrocardiogram, measurement of appropriate serum drug concentrations, electrolytes, and glucose, and investigation of co-ingestants.

Because significant toxicity can occur after a small overdose of a cardiovascular drug, aggressive gastric decontamination is warranted, with gastric lavage, activated charcoal, and whole-bowel irrigation when indicated and not contraindicated.

At this time there is no substantial evidence that methods of enhancing elimination of the cardiovascular drugs lead to clinical improvement.

The antidotes for calcium channel antagonists and beta-receptor antagonists are identical, except that hyperinsulinemia/euglycemia therapy has not been reported in single beta-receptor antagonist overdoses in humans, although it could be beneficial.

Administration of digoxin-specific Fab fragments is indicated as the definitive therapeutic option for the clinical, electrocardiographic, and laboratory manifestations of digoxin toxicity.

All symptomatic patients with cardiovascular drug overdose should be admitted for cardiovascular monitoring, diagnostic studies, and treatment.

The pervasiveness of hypertension, congestive heart failure, and coronary artery disease in the United States has led to an immense number of prescriptions for beta-blockers and calcium channel antagonists. The prevalence of digoxin as a therapy for atrial fibrillation and congestive heart failure has ostensibly diminished but it is still prescribed.

The 2004 Annual Report of the American Association of Poison Control Centers' Toxic Exposure Surveillance System (TESS) reported cardiovascular drugs as the sixth most common exposure in adults (46,470 exposures, or 5.6% of all exposures).[1] Cardiovascular drugs as a category were ranked as the fifth leading cause of death (162 total deaths, 25 from beta-

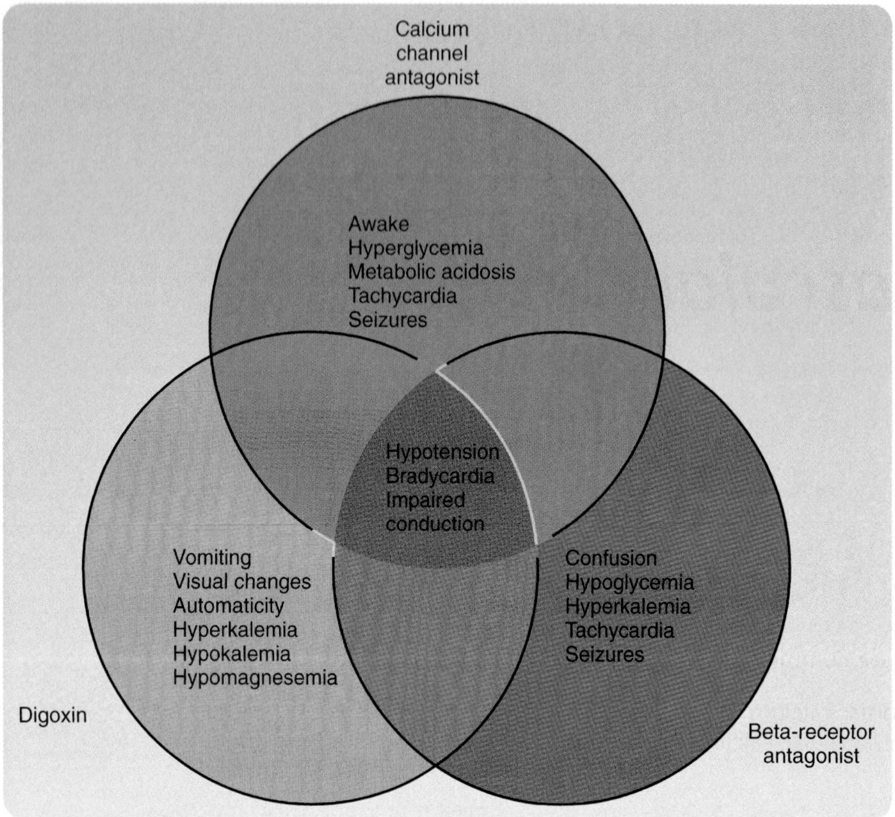
Calcium channel antagonist
Awake
Hyperglycemia
Metabolic acidosis
Tachycardia
Seizures
Hypotension
Bradycardia
Impaired conduction
Vomiting
Visual changes
Automaticity
Hyperkalemia
Hypokalemia
Hypomagnesemia
Confusion
Hypoglycemia
Hyperkalemia
Tachycardia
Seizures
Digoxin
Beta-receptor antagonist

FIGURE 142-1 Differential diagnosis of cardiovascular drug overdoses.

receptor antagonists, 62 from calcium channel antagonists, and 17 from cardiac glycosides). These specific cardiovascular drugs share the clinical effects of hypotension, bradycardia, and conduction disturbances. However, unique differences can help distinguish them in an unknown overdose (Fig. 142-1). Other pharmaceuticals included in the category of cardiovascular agents were angiotensin-converting enzyme inhibitors, antiarrhythmics, clonidine, and other antihypertensives; they are not discussed in this chapter.

Calcium Channel Antagonists

■ PATHOPHYSIOLOGY AND PHARMACOLOGY

Calcium channel antagonists block the intracellular flow of calcium ions through L-type voltage-gated calcium channels in myocardial, smooth muscle, and pancreatic beta-islet cells. These mechanisms of action result in cardiovascular toxicity both directly and indirectly. Depending on the selectivity of the calcium channel antagonist, the direct cardiovascular toxicity is a combination of the effects on the cardiac conduction system, myocardial contractility, and vascular smooth muscle vasodilation. The dihydropyridine class (e.g., amlodipine, nifedipine) preferentially acts on the peripheral vasculature, potentially leading to hypotension and reflex tachycardia. Verapamil operates on the sinoatrial and atrioventricular (AV) nodes and on the myocardium. Diltiazem acts to a lesser extent than verapamil on the cardiac tissue and nodes, and also dilates peripheral vasculature (Table 142-1). The size of the contribution of each mechanism of direct cardiovascular toxicity can be difficult to predict. Despite the differences in thera-

Table 142-1 CLASSIFICATION OF CALCIUM CHANNEL ANTAGONISTS

Class	Action(s)	Example(s)
Phenylalkylamines	Act on sinoatrial and atrioventricular nodes and the myocardium	Verapamil (Calan)
Benzothiazepines	Dilate peripheral vasculature and act to a lesser degree than verapamil on cardiac tissues and nodes	Diltiazem (Cardizem, Tiazac)
Dihydropyridines	Act on peripheral vasculature, leading to hypotension and reflex tachycardia	Nifedipine (Procardia) Isradipine (DynaCirc) Amlodipine (Norvasc) Felodipine (Plendil) Nimodipine (Nimotop) Nisoldipine (Sular) Nicardipine (Vascor)

peutic mechanisms, the distinctions between families of calcium channel antagonists are often blurred during an overdose, and the patient generally suffers from negative chronotropic, inotropic, and dromotropic effects.[2]

The indirect toxicity results from attenuation of the release of insulin from the pancreatic beta-islet cells. The attenuation leads to hyperglycemia and intracellular catabolism of fatty acids to create energy. The hypoinsulinemia contributes to impairment of cardiac function and shock by preventing the use of glucose as a metabolic substrate. Shock from negative inotropy, and diminished peripheral vascular resistance, leads to a metabolic acidosis similar to diabetic ketoacidosis.

The calcium channel antagonist families differ in volume of distribution, protein binding, and molecular weight. Efforts to enhance their elimination, such as dialysis, have proved to be clinically ineffective for all of these agents.

■ PRESENTING SIGNS AND SYMPTOMS

The potency of the calcium channel antagonists on the cardiovascular system is astounding. Significant cardiovascular toxicity can occur after supratherapeutic ingestion of calcium channel antagonists. Ingestion of double the therapeutic dose should instigate medical evaluation and treatment. Immediate-release calcium channel antagonists should have some clinical effect within 6 hours. Sustained-release calcium channel antagonists should result in clinical manifestations within 1 to 14 hours.[3]

Nearly all calcium channel antagonists are manufactured in modified-release formulation. This is convenient therapeutic dosing for the patient, but in overdose, the delayed peak and longer duration of toxicity can have disastrous consequences. The mistakes made by the physician are in finding reassurance in the patient's normal mental status despite hypotension and in not vigorously monitoring and treating the patient's hemodynamic condition. If close attention to hypotension is not maintained, the cardiovascular status of the patient will continue to deteriorate until cardiopulmonary arrest is imminent.

Because the calcium channel antagonists were developed to affect the cardiovascular system, the presenting signs and symptoms of overdose with such agents are primarily related to a malfunction of this system. A reduction in blood pressure is a hallmark of calcium channel antagonist toxicity. Cardiac output and peripheral vascular resistance determine systemic blood pressure. Cardiac output depends on two factors, heart rate and stroke volume. The pharmacologic effects of calcium channel antagonists can affect both components of cardiac output and can decrease peripheral vascular resistance.

Reflexive tachycardia can occur as a result of peripheral vasodilation after an overdose of a calcium channel antagonist in the dihydropyridine class, but this effect may be transient, and bradycardia usually develops in large overdoses. This tachycardia may prove fortuitous in maintaining organ perfusion by sustaining cardiac output when the stroke volume is depleted. Verapamil and diltiazem overdoses cause bradycardia and any number of conduction abnormalities in and below the AV node. The decreased cardiac output results in hypotension from vasodilation and from decreased cardiac contractility from the negative inotropic and chronotropic effects.[2]

Patients often complain of chest pain, dyspnea, dizziness, syncope, and palpitations. Other clinical manifestations are confusion, agitation, seizures, pulmonary edema (cardiogenic and noncardiogenic), hyperglycemia, and metabolic acidosis. Paradoxically, patients suffering severe hypotension and bradycardia from a calcium channel antagonist overdose often have a clear sensorium. There is no precise explanation for this occurrence, but it has been suggested that cerebrovascular vasodilation may be cerebroprotective, acting much like nimodipine does for subarachnoid hemorrhage.

■ PEDIATRIC OVERDOSE

In the 2004 TESS data, there were two pediatric deaths related to calcium channel antagonists (a 10-month-old child and a 15-month-old child).[1,4] The clinical manifestations, pathophysiology, and treatment of unintentional pediatric calcium channel antagonist ingestion mimic what is seen in the intentional adult ingestion. The clinical consequences of accidental pediatric calcium channel antagonist ingestions depend on the dose.

One must consider that the major flaw of studies attempting to demonstrate a dose response of accidental pediatric drug ingestions is that many of the reports are nonexposures. The caretaker of the child may report the exposure to a poison center if a pill is missing and the child is implicated by his or her presence in the vicinity. If the child did not take the drug, the case may be referred to as having a good outcome, and the "dose" considered safe.[4]

A guideline for prehospital triage of accidental pediatric ingestions of calcium channel antagonists states that immediate referral to a health care center is necessary if the dose exceeded the usual therapeutic dose or was considered equal to or greater than the lowest toxic dose (whichever is lower).[3] At these doses, significant bradycardia or hypotension may occur. Accidental single ingestions of calcium channel antagonists in children are considered lethal enough to be fatal.[5] Because many calcium channel antagonists are formulated in sustained-release preparations, there may be a delay in the peak concentration and clinical effects.

Realistically, administration of activated charcoal is prudent if the patient is presented within 1 hour of the ingestion. Whole-bowel irrigation may be considered for ingestion of a modified-release product but is technically difficult. Gastric lavage in a child

Tips and Tricks

CALCIUM CHANNEL ANTAGONIST TOXICITY

- The patient who presents with undifferentiated hypotension and bradycardia may paradoxically be relatively alert. This effect is more likely a result of calcium channel antagonist toxicity, which may cause a cerebrovascular vasodilation that is cerebroprotective, much like the effects of nimodipine in subarachnoid hemorrhage.
- Insulin is an ideal inotropic agent because it can increase the contractility of the heart without raising oxygen demand.
- Monitor electrolyte concentrations and excess intravenous fluid closely.
- An echocardiogram, central venous pressure monitor, and pulmonary artery catheter can be helpful for diagnosing and treating the multiple components of the shock that occurs during calcium channel antagonist toxicity.
- Continue to monitor serum glucose concentrations after the insulin infusion is discontinued until consistent euglycemia is achieved.

PRIORITY ACTIONS

Treatment Of Calcium Channel Antagonist Toxicity

- Intubate hemodynamically unstable patients electively, before emergency intubation is required because of cardiopulmonary arrest.
- Obtain central venous access for fluid resuscitation and administration of pharmaceutical infusions.
- Gastric decontamination is critical in the patient presenting with hemodynamic stability, but it should not be used if the patient is unstable.
- Use hyperinsulinemia/euglycemia (HIE) therapy early after intravenous boluses of normal saline, atropine, calcium, and glucagon have failed.
- Titrate the HIE therapy in the same fashion as other standard inotropic medicines to obtain a mean arterial pressure of 70 to 75 mm Hg. Unlike when HIE is used as goal-directed therapy for sepsis. Tight glucose control is not the target for treatment of calcium channel antagonist toxicity.
- Maintain the insulin infusion and taper and stop vasopressor therapy when the mean arterial pressure has achieved 70 to 75 mm Hg.
- If hypoglycemic episodes occur in the setting of hemodynamic stability, decrease the rate of the insulin infusion. If there is hemodynamic instability, increase the rate of the dextrose infusion.

younger than 6 years is most likely be limited by the diameter of the lumen of the lavage tubing.

Cardiovascular monitoring for 6 to 8 hours for immediate-release medications and for at least 24 hours for sustained-release medications should reveal delayed toxicity. All symptomatic children should be admitted for cardiovascular monitoring, and treated with standard therapy.[3]

OVERDOSE IN PREGNANCY

Little is known about the primary effects of the calcium channel antagonist on the fetus during maternal overdose. Certainly, the shocklike state produced in the mother would most likely have detrimental effects on the fetus because of hypoperfusion of the placenta. Supportive and antidotal treatment of the mother is intuitively the most reasonable approach to saving both patients. One must also consider the potential teratogenic effect of the antidotes on the fetus. The U.S. Food and Drug Administration (FDA) assigns glucagon, dopamine, and insulin to pregnancy category B, and calcium, atropine, epinephrine, inamrinone, and glucose to pregnancy category C. Norepinephrine can cause uterine ischemia or contractions.[6] For ingestion in the third trimester of pregnancy, emergency cesarean delivery may be indicated if maternal demise is imminent.

DIAGNOSTIC TESTS

Diagnostic testing is contingent on the necessity of treatment for hemodynamic instability. Once the airway, breathing, and cardiovascular status have been assessed and stabilized, testing should start with a 12-lead electrocardiogram (ECG) and chest radiography. Rapid determination of hyperglycemia and metabolic acidosis with capillary glucose and arterial blood gas analysis may demonstrate a severe calcium channel antagonist overdose, indicating early hyperinsulinemia-euglycemia (HIE) therapy. An elevated serum lactate value may be another marker of severe calcium channel antagonist overdose. Testing for serum concentrations of calcium channel antagonists is not clinically useful or available to guide treatment. Otherwise, standard laboratory testing for a general overdose is a good comprehensive approach.

TREATMENTS

Often, the lack of mental status impairment coinciding with hypotension can beguile the physician into believing that the patient is not suffering severe clinical effects of a calcium channel antagonist overdose. It is at this point that elective intubation should be considered, before emergency intubation has to be performed during cardiopulmonary arrest.

Gastrointestinal Decontamination

In the hemodynamically stable patient with a calcium channel antagonist overdose, aggressive gastric decontamination is warranted. It is reasonable to consider gastric lavage and activated charcoal to minimize intestinal absorption in a person who presents to the ED within 1 hour of the overdose.[7] Whole-bowel irrigation has been suggested for overdose of calcium channel antagonists because many are sustained-release preparations. Bowel irrigation is not indicated for a patient with hemodynamic instability because a significant amount of the drug has already been absorbed [8] and, therefore, the opportunity for prevention has passed. In addition, challenging a hypoperfused gastrointestinal system can have disastrous consequences, such as functional and physical obstruction by a calcium channel antagonist bezoar[9-11] and perforation.

Antidotes

The primary focus of antidotal treatment is the hypotension and the bradycardia/AV block usually improves when the hypotension improves. Antidotes for bradycardia/AV block and hypotension include atropine, but this agent is frequently ineffective because the bradycardia/AV block is not related to increased vagal tone. Intrauenous crystalloid calcium, glucagon, and catecholamines with chronotropic and inotropic effects can be administered intravenously for refractory bradycardia/AV block. Unfortunately, severe bradycardia/AV block is often refractory to pharmaceutical treatment, and transcutaneous or transvenous pacing may be required.

An antidotal treatment regimen is provided in Figure 142-2. This regimen emphasizes elemental calcium, either as calcium gluconate (30 mL of a 10% solution, or 3 g of calcium gluconate; 14 mEq elemental calcium) or calcium chloride (10 mL of a 10% solution, or 1 g; 13.5 mEq of elemental calcium). Calcium chloride should be administered through central venous access because it is an acidifying salt, which could cause necrosis of peripheral vasculature. If the intravenous calcium boluses appear to have improved hemodynamic status, close monitoring for recrudescence of toxicity must be maintained, and further boluses given as necessary. An intravenous infusion of calcium is warranted only when it effectively treats the hypotension and further boluses are required to support the blood pressure (Table 142-2). The serum calcium concentration should be monitored, but antidotal treatment rarely gives rise to clinically significant hypercalcemia later.

Next, glucagon in 5-mg intravenous boluses for two doses may theoretically increase cardiac contractility by bypassing the antagonized calcium channels. When glucagon binds to its receptor, it activates

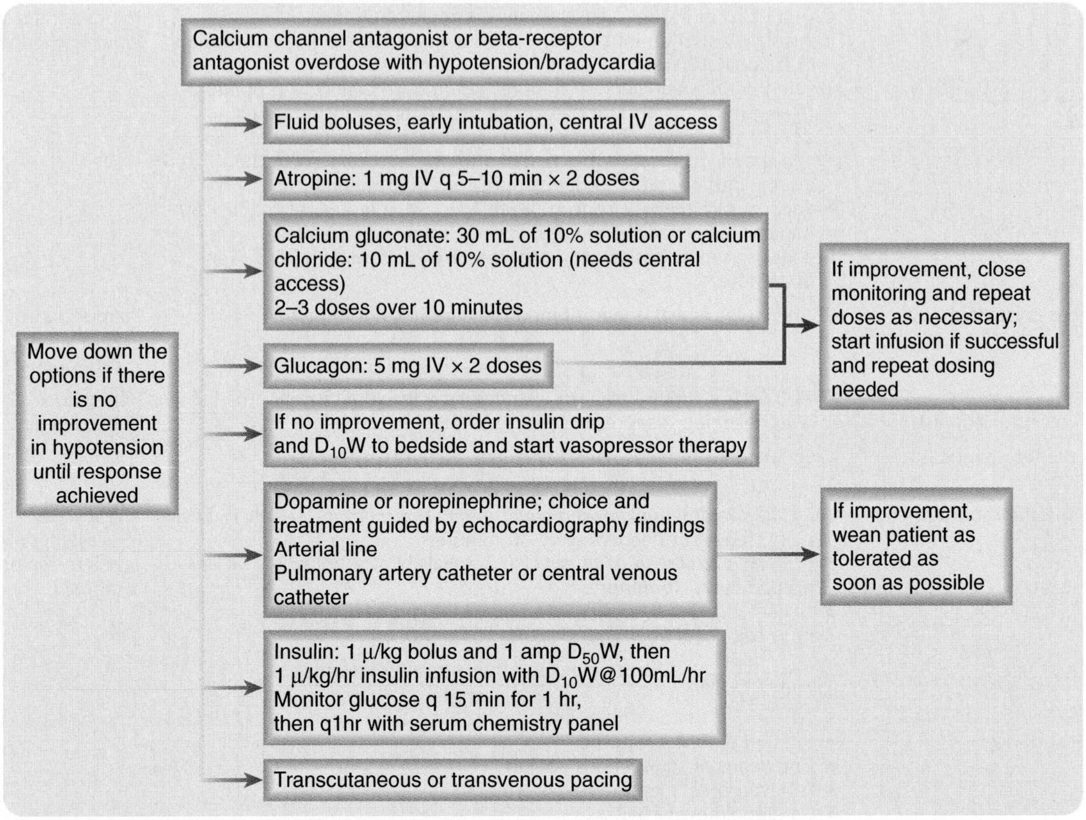
Calcium channel antagonist or beta-receptor antagonist overdose with hypotension/bradycardia
Fluid boluses, early intubation, central IV access
Atropine: 1 mg IV q 5–10 min × 2 doses
Calcium gluconate: 30 mL of 10% solution or calcium chloride: 10 mL of 10% solution (needs central access)
2–3 doses over 10 minutes
Glucagon: 5 mg IV × 2 doses
If improvement, close monitoring and repeat doses as necessary; start infusion if successful and repeat dosing needed
Move down the options if there is no improvement in hypotension until response achieved
If no improvement, order insulin drip and D10W to bedside and start vasopressor therapy
Dopamine or norepinephrine; choice and treatment guided by echocardiography findings
Arterial line
Pulmonary artery catheter or central venous catheter
If improvement, wean patient as tolerated as soon as possible
Insulin: 1 μ/kg bolus and 1 amp D50W, then
1 μ/kg/hr insulin infusion with D10W@100mL/hr
Monitor glucose q 15 min for 1 hr,
then q1hr with serum chemistry panel
Transcutaneous or transvenous pacing

FIGURE 142-2 Treatment of overdose with calcium channel antagonist or beta-receptor antagonist. $D_{10}W$, 10% dextrose in water; $D_{50}W$, 50% dextrose in water; IV, intravenous(ly).

Table 142-2 ANTIDOTES, TREATMENTS, FACTS, AND FORMULAS FOR CARDIOVASCULAR DRUGS

Antidote or Treatment	Dosing	Adverse Effects
Atropine	*Adult:* 1 mg IV bolus q5min as needed for symptomatic beta-receptor antagonist bradycardia (Maximum total dose: 0.04 mg/kg or 3 mg) *Pediatric:* 0.02 mg/kg total dose	Anticholinergic toxicity
Glucagon	*Adult:* 5 mg IV bolus over 2 min (Maximum total dose 10 mg) *Adult infusion:* 1-5 mg/hr; titrate to MAP of 70 mm Hg *Pediatric:* 0.05 mg/kg IV bolus over 2 minutes (Maximum total dose 10 mg) *Pediatric infusion:* 0.05 mg/kg/hr to 0.1 mg/kg/hr; titrate to MAP of 70 mm Hg	Emesis Hyperglycemia
Calcium chloride (10 mL of 10% solution=1 g=13.5 mEq elemental calcium)	*Adult:* 1-3 g IV (central line) over 10 min as needed for hypotension *Pediatric:* (27.7 mg/mL of elemental calcium) 5-7 mg/kg of elemental calcium or 0.2-0.25 mL/kg IV (central line) over 10 min as needed for hypotension *Infusion:* 20-50 mg/kg/hr	Sclerosis of veins Hypercalcemia
Calcium gluconate (10 mL of 10% solution=1 g=4.65 mEq elemental calcium)	*Adult:* 3-9 g IV (central line) over 10 min as needed for hypotension *Pediatric:* (9 mL/mL of elemental calcium) 5-7 mg/kg of elemental calcium or 0.6-0.8 mL/kg *Infusion:* 20-50 mg/kg/hr	Hypercalcemia
Norepinephrine (α_1 and β_1 agonist)	Start at 0.1 μg/kg/min; titrate to effect	Tachycardia Hypertension Arrhythmias Extravasation Anaphylaxis
Dopamine	For vasodilation of renal and splanchnic vasculature: 1-5 μg kg/min For β_1 agonist: 5-10 μg/kg/min For α_1 agonist 10-20 μg/kg/min	Same as for norepinephrine
Epinephrine (α_1, β_1, and β_2 agonist)	Start at 1 μg/min; titrate to effect	Same as for norepinephrine
Dobutamine (β_1 agonist)	2.5 μg/kg/min to 15 μg/kg/min	Same as for norepinephrine
Isoproterenol (β_1, β_2 agonist)	Not recommended because of β_2 agonist vasodilation and dysrhythmias at high doses Start at 0.02 μg/kg/min; titrate to effect	
Insulin (regular)	Consultation with a clinical toxicologist is recommended Give a bolus of 1.0 units/kg IV with 1 ampule of $D_{50}W$ Immediately start an infusion of 1.0 units/kg/hr with a glucose infusion of $D_{10}W$ at 100 mL/hr Titrate 0.5 units/kg every 30 minutes until desired effect; 1 ampule of $D_{50}W$ can be given during every increase in infusion; titrate to desired effect when blood pressure has reached desired value When the blood pressure has reached the desired value with the insulin infusion, taper and wean pressor agent therapy Monitor serum glucose concentration every 15 minutes for the first 60 minutes; when stable, monitor very 60 minutes thereafter Monitor serum potassium and other electrolyte concentrations every 60 minutes	Hypoglycemia Hypokalemia Volume overload
Intravenous crystalloid	20 mL/kg IV; repeat again it blood pressure has not improved	Pulmonary edema with severe cardiogenic shock
Vasopressin (V_1, V_2 receptor agonist)	0.01-0.04 units/min; titrate to effect along with administration of 1-2 catecholamine vasopressors	Ischemia Water intoxication
Phosphodiesterase inhibitor (Milrinone)	Give 50 μg/kg IV bolus over 2 minutes; then 1.0 μg/kg/min	
Digoxin-specific Fab fragments	*For acute overdose (unknown amount in adult or child):* 5-10 vials IV as a bolus; repeat as needed every 30 minutes *For chronic overdose in adult or child:* 1-2 vials IV as a bolus; repeat as needed every 30 minutes *If amount ingested is known:* 1 vial binds 0.5 mg of digoxin *Dosage calculated from serum digoxin concentration:* $\text{Number of vials} = \frac{\text{Serum concentration (ng/mL)} \times \text{weight (kg)}}{100}$	Anaphylaxis Increase in symptoms being treated by digoxin
Mechanical devices	• Intra-aortic balloon pump • Cutaneous or transvenous pacing • Extracorporeal membrane oxygenation • Cardiopulmonary bypass	—

$D_{10}W$, 10% dextrose in water; $D_{50}W$, 50% dextrose in water; MAP, mean arterial pressure.

cyclic adenosine monophosphate (cAMP). This may increase contractility by activating the phosphorylation cascade, which results in contraction of actin and myosin. Glucagon also stimulates release of endogenous insulin, a fortuitous side effect explained later. Like a calcium infusion, a glucagon infusion is warranted only if a beneficial effect is seen after several boluses have been given. Glucagon can cause emesis because of relaxation of the lower esophageal sphincter.

Catecholamines with inotropic and vasopressor activity are the next line of treatment for refractory hypotension in calcium channel antagonist overdose. There is no good evidence for the superiority of one agent over the others, but dopamine or norepinephrine is a good starting point. If clinically significant hypotension persists, adding more agents may be necessary. Cardiovascular data from diagnostic modalities such as transthoracic echocardiogram, pulmonary artery catheter, arterial catheter, and central venous catheter should dictate which cardiovascular agent is the most appropriate choice. Vasopressin has been used in human cases when peripheral vasoconstriction is indicated.[12] Worsening of the cardiac index has been demonstrated when vasopressin is used in an animal model to treat hypotension induced by calcium channel antagonist.[13]

In 1999, Yuan and colleagues[14] described the use of HIE therapy in four patients with verapamil overdose and one with amlodipine and atenolol overdose in 1999, but many questions remain about the use of this antidote for calcium channel antagonist toxicity. Consequently, scattered case reports, reviews, and HIE regimens have been published.[2,15-19] Insulin therapy has been described for multiple nontoxicologic conditions, such as acute myocardial infarction, post–cardiac surgery status, and septic shock.[20] The superiority of insulin therapy for cardiogenic shock due to calcium channel antagonist toxicity has also been demonstrated dramatically in animal models.[21-24] HIE promotes inotropy by improving myocardial energy production. In addition, insulin has anti-inflammatory attributes that protect against apoptosis and ischemic reperfusion injury.[2]

HIE therapy may be highly beneficial, but data are anecdotal. This approach seems to fail when used too late and for doses that are too small.[25] HIE therapy should be started when boluses of calcium, glucagon, atropine, and intravenous fluids have failed and the physician is considering a pressor agent to improve refractory hypotension. The call to the pharmacist to obtain the HIE infusion should be made when the dopamine and/or norepinephrine infusion is begun.

HIE therapy should start with a 1.0 unit/kg bolus of regular insulin followed by an intravenous injection of 1 ampule of 50% dextrose in water ($D_{50}W$). Immediately thereafter, an infusion of 1.0 unit/kg/hr of regular insulin should begin, along with an infusion of $D_{10}W$ at 100 mL/hr. Serum glucose levels should be monitored every 15 minutes during the first hour and then, if stable, every hour. A serum electrolyte analysis must be performed every hour to monitor serum potassium, glucose, and other electrolyte values. Clinically significant hypoglycemia has not been described with HIE therapy. The amount of intravenous fluid administered must be taken into consideration and the patient closely monitored for signs and symptoms of pulmonary edema because the calcium channel antagonist overdose can result in cardiogenic or noncardiogenic pulmonary edema. The clinician must also be cognizant of the limitations of HIE therapy for bradycardia and conduction abnormalities.

When hemodynamic stability has been achieved, the vasopressor therapy should be tapered and stopped because of these agents' potential detrimental effect on the myocardium from increased oxygen demand and metabolic acidosis. Consequently, HIE therapy can be gradually reduced when the patient becomes hemodynamically stable. After the insulin has been discontinued, the serum glucose concentration must be monitored continually for 4 to 6 hours.

Mechanical devices can also serve as adjunctive therapy in calcium channel antagonist poisoning. Transcutaneous or transvenous pacing is indicated when conduction is impaired beyond pharmacologic reversal. More invasive measures that can be used are the intra-aortic balloon pump, extracorporeal membrane oxygenation (ECMO), and cardiopulmonary bypass.

■ DISPOSITION

Asymptomatic patients who have ingested an immediate-release calcium channel antagonist can be monitored for 6 hours in the ED. After ingestion of a sustained-release calcium channel antagonist, the asymptomatic patient should have cardiovascular monitoring for 18 to 24 hours.[3] All symptomatic patients with cardiovascular instability after such an ingestion should be admitted to the intensive care unit until the effects have resolved.

Beta-receptor Antagonists

■ PATHOPHYSIOLOGY AND PHARMACOLOGY

As their name suggests, beta-receptor antagonists antagonize the effects of beta agonists by competing for beta-adrenergic receptors. The result within the cell is a decrease in cAMP, which inhibits the phosphokinase cascade, leading to decreased intracellular flow of calcium and actin/myosin contraction. The effects are bradycardia in the nodal cells and decreased contractility in the cardiac myocytes. Consequently, the attenuated stroke volume combined with a decreased heart rate elicits decline in cardiac output and promotion of a shocklike state.

Beta-receptor antagonism is not the only pharmacologic mechanism of toxicity seen after beta-receptor antagonist overdose. Depending on the type of beta-receptor antagonist, there may also be alpha-receptor antagonism, sodium or potassium channel antagonism, and sympathomimetic stimulation (Table 142-3).

The majority of the actively prescribed beta-receptor antagonists are first metabolized by hepatic enzymes and then processed by the kidney. One exception is atenolol, which is exclusively excreted in the urine. Atenolol also has a volume of distribution and protein-binding properties that permit hemodialysis as a method of enhancing elimination. Esmolol also has the unique metabolic characteristic of rapid metabolism in the serum by red blood cell esterases.

■ PRESENTING SIGNS AND SYMPTOMS

Immediate-release products should cause signs and symptoms within 6 hours. Unfortunately the majority of beta-receptor antagonists are of modified-release formulation. They have some pharmacologic effect during the first 6 hours after ingestion, but the peak serum concentration is delayed and the pharmacologic effect may last longer than with immediate-release formulations.[26]

Cardiovascular signs and symptoms are the predominant clinical manifestations of beta-receptor antagonist toxicity. As with the calcium channel antagonists, cardiogenic shock results primarily from a decrease in cardiac output secondary to diminished stroke volume and heart rate. Patients may complain of chest pain, shortness of breath, palpitations, and dizziness in relation to their bradycardia and hypotension. The ECG may demonstrate sinus arrest, sinus bradycardia, junctional bradycardia, and all degrees of AV block.

If the beta-receptor antagonist also possesses pharmacologic activity at other receptors, the clinical picture will be complicated. Alpha-receptor antagonism after ingestion of carvedilol or labetalol may contribute to hypotension by causing peripheral vasodilation. Propranolol can cause sodium channel antagonism (membrane-stabilizing effect). The addition of this pharmacologic activity may be exhibited clinically as a prolonged QRS complex on the cardiac monitor and hypotension, much as in a tricyclic antidepressant overdose. The cardiac rhythm can potentially degenerate into ventricular tachycardia.

Sotalol is infamous for antagonizing the delayed rectifier potassium channels in the myocardium. The result is a prolonged QT interval and a higher risk for torsades de pointes, monomorphic ventricular tachycardia, ventricular fibrillation, and asystole. These clinical effects can also be delayed and prolonged. In one case report, the onset of ventricular dysrhythmias occurred 4 to 9 hours after ingestion and did not normalize until 100 hours from the time of ingestion.[27] Observation of sympathomimetic effects after beta-receptor antagonist ingestion is rare because of the uncommon clinical use of beta-receptor antagonists with intrinsic sympathomimetic activity, such as acebutolol, oxprenolol, penbutolol, and pindolol. Patients who have ingested these agents may have tachycardia, hypertension, tremor, and, possibly, some antidotal efficacy, as some beta-antagonists can antagonize their own toxic effects.

Some of the beta-receptor antagonists, such as propranolol, are more lipophilic and can cross the blood-brain barrier. Symptoms of delirium, coma, and seizures have been reported in patients with overdose of highly lipophilic beta-receptor antagonists. Other less common clinical effects reported are respiratory depression, bronchospasm, hypoglycemia in children, and hyperkalemia.

Tips and Tricks

BETA-RECEPTOR ANTAGONIST TOXICITY

- Obtain a capillary blood glucose measurement to detect euglycemia or hypoglycemia.
- Identify the unique toxicity of each beta-receptor antagonist.
- Do not start infusions of glucagon or calcium until multiple boluses have successfully reversed the toxicity.
- Avoid isoproterenol as an antidotal agent.
- Remember that the hyperinsulinemia/euglycemia therapy may theoretically work to treat hypotension from beta-receptor antagonist toxicity, but there is very little experience with this antidote in human overdose.
- Atenolol has pharmacokinetic properties that allow the use of hemodialysis to enhance elimination.
- Monitor electrolyte concentrations and excess intravenous fluid closely.
- An echocardiogram, central venous pressure monitor, and pulmonary artery catheter can be helpful for diagnosing and treating the multiple components of the shock that occurs during beta-receptor antagonist toxicity.

■ PEDIATRIC OVERDOSE

In the 2004 TESS data, there were no pediatric deaths related to beta-receptor antagonists.[1,4] Children are more susceptible to the potential for hypoglycemia related to a beta-receptor antagonist overdose owing to their low hepatic glycogen stores.

Treatment involves the same supportive and antidotal measures as for a calcium channel antagonist ingestion. The general rules and limitations of pediatric gastric decontamination, mentioned earlier, apply in treatment of beta-receptor antagonist overdose.

The asymptomatic pediatric patient should be monitored for the same duration as the adult. Cardiovascular monitoring should continue for 6, 8, or 12 hours after ingestion of an immediate-release beta-receptor antagonist, a sustained-release beta-receptor antagonist, or sotalol, respectively.

Table 142-3 PHARMACOLOGY OF SELECTED BETA-RECEPTOR ANTAGONISTS

Agent	Receptor Activity	Agonist Activity	Membrane Stabilizing	Vasodilation?	Lipid Solubility	Protein Binding (%)	Half-life (hrs)	Metabolism	Volume of Distribution
Atenolol	β_1	No	No	No	No	<5	5-9	Renal	1
Carvedilol	α_1, β_1, β_2	No	No	Yes	Moderate	98	6-10	Hepatic	115
Esmolol	β_1, β_2	No	No	No	Low	50	8 min	Red blood cell esterases	2
Labetalol	α_1, β_1, β_2	No	Low	Yes	Moderate	50	4-8	Hepatic	9
Metoprolol	β_1	No	Low	No	No	10	3-4	Hepatic	4
Pindolol	β_1, β_2	Yes	Low	No	Moderate	50	3-4	Hepatic/renal	2
Propranolol	β_1, β_2	No	Yes	No	High	90	3-5	Hepatic	4
Sotalol	β_1, β_2	No	No	No	Low	0	9-12	Renal	2

Data from reference 32 and Brubacher JR: Beta adrenergic antagonists. In Goldfrank L, Flomenbaum N, Lewin N, et al: Goldfrank's Toxicologic Emergencies, 8th ed. New York, McGraw-Hill, 2006.

OVERDOSE IN PREGNANCY

The principles for treating the pregnant patient after a calcium channel antagonist overdose should be applied for a beta-receptor antagonist overdose. One must also consider the potential teratogenic effect of the antidotes on the fetus. As already mentioned, glucagon, dopamine, and insulin are FDA pregnancy category B; calcium, atropine, epinephrine, inamrinone, and glucose are FDA pregnancy category C; and norepinephrine can cause uterine ischemia or contractions.[6]

DIAGNOSTIC TESTS

Therapeutic interventions and patient stabilization are the priority. As resuscitation proceeds, a 12-lead ECG and cardiac monitoring may demonstrate bradycardia, AV conduction abnormalities, and prolonged QRS and QTc intervals. Rapid identification of hypoglycemia and hyperkalemia is prudent. Monitoring for hypocalcemia, and hypomagnesemia assists in treatment of coexisting cause of prolonged QTc intervals. Measurements of serum concentrations of beta-receptor antagonists are generally unavailable and unhelpful in the ED. Additional standard laboratory testing as for a general overdose is advisable.

TREATMENTS

Gastrointestinal Decontamination

In a hemodynamically stable patient who has overdosed on a beta-receptor antagonist, aggressive gastric decontamination is warranted. The rules for its use in calcium channel antagonist overdose apply to that in beta-receptor antagonist overdose.

ANTIDOTES

The end result of overdose with either beta-receptor or calcium channel antagonists is shock, despite their different mechanisms of action. Likewise, antidotal therapy is analogous. Treatment follows the same algorithm as shown in Figure 142-2. Atropine can be used initially, followed by intravenous calcium, glucagon, and catecholamines with chronotropic and inotropic effects for refractory bradycardia/AV block. Unfortunately, severe bradycardia/AV block is often refractory to pharmaceutical efforts, and transcutaneous or transvenous pacing may be required.

Theoretically, calcium reverses toxicity through circumvention of the beta-receptor antagonist by entering open L-type calcium channels and increasing the cytoplasmic concentration of calcium, leading to contraction of the myosin/actin apparatus. Fear of hypercalcemia should not prohibit the use of elemental calcium as antidotal treatment of beta-receptor antagonist toxicity.

Glucagon theoretically increases cardiac contractility by bypassing the antagonized beta receptors through activation of cAMP via agonism at the glucagon receptors. This activation increases contractility by activating the phosphorylation cascade, leading to contraction of actin and myosin. Glucagon also stimulates release of endogenous insulin, a fortuitous side effect. Unfortunately, glucagon is often ineffective at reversing beta-receptor antagonist toxicity.[28]

Vasopressin has been used in an experimental animal model poisoned by propranolol.[29] The investigators discovered equally dismal survival rates for treatment with glucagon and vasopressin.

HIE therapy is also regarded by some authorities as a therapeutic agent for beta-receptor antagonist toxicity. Animal models have demonstrated both the superiority of HIE therapy over glucagon, epinephrine, and saline and reversal of the toxic effects of propranolol.[30] Another animal study reported promising results of HIE therapy compared with vasopressin and epinephrine. There are no human case reports of the use of insulin to treat humans with only beta-receptor toxicity. Yuan and colleagues[14] reported effective reversal of the toxic effects of a beta-receptor and calcium channel antagonist co-ingestion with this treatment. Despite the absence of the diabetic ketoacidosis metabolic state produced by calcium channel antagonist, HIE therapy is believed to be just as effective in beta-receptor antagonist intoxication. Mechanistically, this antidote improves inotropy by stimulating myocardial glucose metabolism, inhibiting fatty-acid metabolism, lactate oxidation, increasing the oxygen-to-work ratio, hypokalemia, and improving the efficiency of intracellular use of calcium.[18]

The evidence is convincing that HIE is a remedy for a depressed inotropic state, but its reversal of the myriad of other toxicologic effects mediated by

PRIORITY ACTIONS

Treatment of Beta-Receptor Antagonist Toxicity

- Supportive care of airway, breathing, and circulation is the first critical step.
- Gastric decontamination is critical in the patient presenting with hemodynamic stability, but refrain from challenging the gastrointestinal system of a patient with hemodynamic instability.
- Administer doses of calcium and glucagon adequate to elicit a clinical response.
- If one antidote has failed, select another, and keep trying agents until the desired clinical response is demonstrated.
- Modify antidotal therapy according to the unique toxicity of the beta-receptor antagonist.
- Consider norepinephrine and dopamine as first choices for vasopressor therapy.
- Electrical pacing is an option for symptomatic beta-receptor antagonist bradycardia.

beta-receptor antagonists, such as bradycardia and conduction abnormalities, is unsubstantiated. The clinician must be aware of the limitations of HIE treatment and must treat other toxic effects appropriately. Vigilance in monitoring for the potential adverse effects of HIE therapy in this setting must be greater than for other uses of HIE therapy because of the lack of insulin resistance seen with the majority of beta-receptor antagonist intoxications.

■ DISPOSITION

The asymptomatic patient who has no cardiovascular effects from overdose with an immediate-release or sustained-release beta-receptor antagonist or sotalol can be discharged after 6, 8, or 12 hours of observation, respectively. All symptomatic patients should be admitted for intensive care monitoring of the hemodynamic effects. The duration of hospital stay depends on the clinical course of the individual patient.

Digoxin

Before considering digoxin toxicity, one must first define the different types of digoxin toxicity; they are as follows:

Acute digoxin toxicity: A patient who is naïve to the medication is exposed to a single acute ingestion.

Acute-on-chronic digoxin toxicity: The serum digoxin concentration increases owing to renal failure or an inadvertent increase in dose. The clinical presentations for this and acute toxicity are similar, so management will be similar.

Chronic digoxin toxicity: A patient has clinical signs of digoxin toxicity with a mildly elevated or therapeutic serum digoxin concentration.

■ PATHOPHYSIOLOGY AND PHARMACOLOGY

Digoxin is a cardiac glycoside that was historically used for the treatment of congestive heart failure and for rate control in atrial fibrillation. Calcium channel antagonists and beta-receptor antagonists have largely replaced digoxin. Despite a reduction in popularity, however, it is still clinically effective for many patients. Natural cardiac glycosides provide another possible exposure source (Box 142-1).

Digoxin pharmacologically alters inotropy and conduction. This agent has the additive effect of increasing automaticity. The result of digoxin therapy is an increase in the intracellular concentration of calcium and higher efficiency of its use by the contractile apparatus. This goal is achieved largely by inhibition of the Na^+,K^+ ATP-ase pump. The Na^+, K^+ ATP-ase pump regulates the intracellular and extracellular concentrations of sodium and potassium by increasing the intracellular potassium level and decreasing the intracellular sodium level. Digoxin inhibits this function, resulting in serum hyperkalemia and intracellular hypernatremia. This effect secondarily impairs the Na^+,Ca^{++} exchange pump, which exchanges extracellular sodium for intracellular calcium. The consequence of this sequence of events is an elevated intracellular calcium concentration, which leads to a dysfunction of intracellular calcium homeostasis and a tetany-like state of the cardiac myocyte. Without myocardial relaxation, an increase in left end-diastolic pressure proceeds to decreased filling and decreased cardiac output, culminating in cardiac failure.

Electrical conduction is prolonged in the sinoatrial and AV nodes. The prolongation occurs as a result of enhancement of vagally mediated parasympathetic tone and directly from digoxin. Automaticity is a reaction to alternating intracellular calcium concentrations, which delay ventricular repolarization. Frequently, delayed afterdepolarizations and premature ventricular contractions are seen.

A number of clinically important points must be remembered about the pharmacology of digoxin (Table 142-4). It is well absorbed, and the onset of action occurs within minutes to hours of administration. The serum digoxin concentration initially is supratherapeutic, until equilibrium between the serum and tissues has occurred. The optimum time for measurement of the serum digoxin concentration is at least 6 hours after ingestion. The volume of distribution is large and the enterohepatic circulation small, making methods for enhancing elimination clinically ineffective. These properties effectively make the elimination half-life approximately 36 to 48 hours.[31,32] The majority of digoxin is eliminated as the parent compound in the urine. Consequently, a decrease in renal function often leads to acute-on-chronic digoxin toxicity in the geriatric patient. The EP must keep in mind that these pharmacokinetic data are from controlled clinical scenarios. True toxicokinetic data are difficult to forecast in the patient with digoxin overdose because of inaccuracies about the timing and amount of the dose, comorbidities, drug interactions, and unpredictable variables in the human metabolism of digoxin.

BOX 142-1

Natural Cardiac Glycosides

Oleander (*Nerium oleander*), yellow oleander (*Thevetia peruviana*)
Lily of the valley (*Convallaria majalis*)
Foxglove (*Digitalis* spp.)
Red squill (*Urginea maritima*)
Dogbane (*Apocynum cannabinum*)
Skin secretions of *Bufo marinus* toad

Table 142-4 PHARMACOKINETICS OF DIGOXIN

Onset of action	Oral: 1.5-6 hr Intravenous: 5-30 min
Maximal effect	Oral: 4-6 hr Intravenous: 1.5-3 hr
Intestinal absorption (%)	40-90 Mean: 75
Metabolism	Small amount by bacteria in liver and gut
Plasma protein binding	25%
Volume of distribution (L/kg)	Neonates: 10 Infants: 16 Adults: 6-7 Adults with renal failure: 4-5
Routes of elimination	Renal: 50%-80% unchanged Hepatic: limited metabolism Enterohepatic circulation: 7%
Elimination half-life	Neonates: Premature: 61-170 hr Full-term: 35-40 hr Infants: 18-25 hr Children: 35 hr Adults: 38-48 hr Anephric patients: >4.5 days

Data from references 32 and 33.

■ PRESENTING SIGNS AND SYMPTOMS

Patients may be asymptomatic from minutes to hours after ingestion of digoxin. Gastrointestinal symptoms are common, and the patient has nausea and vomiting. There may be complaints of changes in vision, especially chromatopsia and xanthopsia. Some mild confusion, weakness, and dizziness also can occur from the direct effect of the digoxin. The cardiac effects are usually represented by symptoms such as palpitations, chest pain, dizziness, and dyspnea. The cardiac signs in acute toxicity are a mixture of bradydysrhythmias, tachydysrhythmias with conductive blockade, and hypotension. Cardiac conduction can be impaired anywhere along the pathway from the sinus node to the AV node and the His-Purkinje fibers. Commonly reported dysrhythmias are listed in Box 142-2.[33] Bidirectional ventricular tachycardia is considered pathognomonic for digoxin toxicity.

The patient with chronic digoxin toxicity is generally elderly and presents with nonspecific complaints, making diagnosis a challenge. Manifestations can be similar to those of acute digoxin toxicity patients, along with more neuropsychiatric complaints, such as delirium, confusion, drowsiness, and hallucinations, and the visual complaints. Ventricular tachydysrhythmias are more common in patients with chronic toxicity.

The patient with acute-on-chronic toxicity may have clinical manifestation of both of the other types of toxicity. In general, acute-on-chronic toxicity is clinically more like acute digoxin toxicity.

BOX 142-2

Dysrhythmias Associated with Digoxin Toxicity

- Atrial fibrillation
- Atrial flutter
- Atrial tachycardia with atrioventricular block
- Premature ventricular tachycardia
- Ventricular tachycardia
- Ventricular fibrillation
- Delayed after-depolarizations
- Bidirectional ventricular tachycardia (pathognomonic)
- Bigeminy
- Junctional tachycardia
- Sinus arrest
- Sinus bradycardia

Tips and Tricks

DIGOXIN TOXICITY

- Symptoms positive for digoxin toxicity are nausea and vomiting.
- Acute-on-chronic and acute digoxin toxicities have the same manifestations, but acute and chronic digoxin toxicities have distinct symptoms, dysrhythmias, and laboratory findings.
- The digoxin serum concentration may be only slightly elevated or normal in chronic digoxin toxicity.
- Digoxin toxicity can manifest as almost any dysrhythmia.
- The equilibrium concentration of serum digoxin occurs 6 hours after ingestion.
- The serum digoxin concentration is inaccurate after administration of digoxin-specific Fab fragments.
- Recurrence of toxicity is typically related to underdosing of digoxin-specific Fab fragments.
- The indications and treatment of digoxin toxicity and concomitant renal impairment are the same.
- No method of enhancing elimination, including hemodialysis, is effective in raising the rate of elimination in the digoxin-poisoned patient.

■ PEDIATRIC OVERDOSE

In the 2004 TESS data, there were no pediatric deaths related to digoxin.[1,4] Pediatric (age <6 years) exposure to digoxin occurs through either inadvertent ingestion or therapeutic error. The latter is seen in neonatal and pediatric intensive care units. This situation is complicated by dramatically higher volume of distribution and elimination half-life in neonates than in infants and adults (see Table 142-4).[34] Because the dosing for neonates is in fractions of milligrams or micrograms, a tenfold or greater dosing error can arise that, combined with prolonged elimination seen in neonates, makes such patients exceptionally susceptible to digoxin toxicity. The most common dysrhythmias are premature ventricular contractions, sinus bradycardia, and first-degree atrioventricular blockade.

As for adults, laboratory studies for children with digoxin toxicity should focus on serum concentrations of digoxin, potassium, and magnesium. Neonates (less than 1 week old) may have digoxin-like immunoreactive substances, which may cause a falsely elevated serum digoxin concentration.[34]

Treatment with digoxin-specific Fab fragments is indicated in the child who has ingested a dose greater than or equal to 0.3 mg/kg (or 4 mg) or who has underlying heart disease, a 6-hour serum digoxin concentration equal to or greater than 5 ng/mL or greater, life-threatening dysrhythmias, hemodynamic instability, serum potassium concentration greater than 5 mEq/L, or rapidly progressing toxicity.[35]

■ DIAGNOSTIC TESTS

An ECG and continuous cardiac monitoring are crucial initial steps in determining cardiovascular instability in a patient with digoxin toxicity. These tests will alert the clinician of dysrhythmias that require treatment with digoxin-specific Fab fragments and supportive care. A chest radiograph will demonstrate any evidence of cardiac failure related to the digoxin overdose.

Laboratory testing should be performed expeditiously in any digoxin overdose, with the focus on serum potassium, magnesium, and digoxin concentrations. Rapid assessment of serum potassium concentration will help determine the severity of the toxicity. In acute digoxin poisoning, the serum potassium value is elevated. If this value is 5 mEq/L or greater, digoxin-specific Fab fragment therapy should be considered.[36] In chronic digoxin toxicity, the serum potassium concentration is often low, usually because of concomitant ingestion of a diuretic. The hypokalemia, in effect, worsens the inhibition of the Na^+,K^+ ATP-ase pump.

Obviously, assessment of the serum digoxin concentration is essential. The therapeutic range is 0.5 to 2.0 ng/mL. The steady-state serum concentration is most accurate 6 hours after ingestion. It is generally accepted that a serum digoxin concentration of 10 ng/mL at steady state or 15 ng/mL at any time is an indication for digoxin-specific Fab fragment therapy. A serum digoxin concentration measured in blood collected after administration of digoxin-specific Fab fragments is clinically not useful and uninterpretable. The assay often measures the antidote, the drug, and the combination of the two, and interprets one or all of them as the serum digoxin concentration; the result may be above, below, or within the therapeutic range for serum digoxin.[37,38]

Screening for accompanying hypomagnesemia is important because this condition may lead to refractory hypokalemia, blockade of inward calcium channels and intracellular binding sites, blockade of extracellular movement of potassium, decrease in myocardial irritability, and a prolonged QT interval. Hypomagnesemia increases myocardial uptake of digoxin and worsens dysfunction of the Na^+,K^+-ATP-ase pump.[39]

■ TREATMENTS

■ Gastric Decontamination

It is reasonable to consider gastric lavage and activated charcoal to minimize intestinal absorption in a person presenting within 1 hour of digoxin overdose. Gastrointestinal decontamination may be limited by emesis induced by the digoxin, and although there is some enterohepatic circulation of digoxin, not enough evidence exists to recommend multiple doses of activated charcoal or cholestyramine to enhance elimination of digoxin.[40] Digitoxin has greater enterohepatic circulation, and multiple doses of charcoal or cholestyramine have been used to enhance its elimination. Whole-bowel irrigation is also not indicated because of rapid absorption of digoxin and the availability of other more practical options.

■ Antidotes

The successful use of digoxin-specific Fab fragments to treat digoxin intoxication was first described in 1976.[41] Since that time, multiple studies have demonstrated its safety and efficacy.[38,42,43] It is critical to understand that best antidote to administer for digoxin toxicity is digoxin-specific Fab fragments, whether for hypotension, dysrhythmias, serum digoxin concentration, or hyperkalemia.

Two commercial formulations of digoxin-specific Fab fragments are available, Digibind and DigiFab. Literature for both products warns against anaphylaxis and administration of the agents to people with papain, chymopapain, or papaya allergies. Other adverse events associated with administration of digoxin-specific Fab fragments occur from removal of the therapeutic benefit of the digoxin—for example, reoccurrence of congestive heart failure[42] or atrial fibrillation with a rapid ventricular response.

After an acute ingestion of digoxin, an empirical bolus of 5 to 10 vials (up to 10-20 vials) of digoxin-specific Fab fragments is indicated in the patient with life-threatening toxicity. When the clinical scenario allows determination of a serum digoxin concentration, the simple dosing calculation is as follows:

$$\text{Dosage} = \frac{\text{Serum concentration (ng/mL)} \times \text{Patient weight (kg)}}{100}$$

BOX 142-3

Indications for Administration of Digoxin-Specific Fab Fragments

Adult

- Ingestion of 10 mg of digoxin
- Serum digoxin concentration of 15 ng/mL at any time
- Serum digoxin concentration of 10 ng/mL at 6 hours after ingestion
- Serum potassium value ≥5 mEq/L
- Life-threatening dysrhythmia
- Hemodynamic instability

Pediatric

- Ingestion of 4 mg, or 0.3 mg/kg, of digoxin
- Pre-existing cardiac disease
- Serum potassium value ≥5 mEq/L
- Serum digoxin concentration >5 ng/mL
- Life-threatening dysrhythmia
- Hemodynamic instability

The number obtained is the number of vials needed to treat the patient.

When the amount ingested is known, the digoxin-specific Fab fragment dose can be calculated by dividing the dose ingested by 2 (1 vial binds 0.5 mg of digoxin) (see Table 142-4 for determining dose). In the noncritical patient, digoxin-specific Fab fragments should be reconstituted with 4 mL of saline, should be used immediately or within 4 hours if refrigerated, and should be infused over 30 minutes. Indications for digoxin-specific Fab fragments are listed in Box 142-3. A clinical response should be seen within 60 minutes.[42]

In patients with chronic digoxin toxicity, calculating dosage of digoxin-specific Fab fragments with the serum digoxin concentration often overshoots the amount needed to reverse toxicity. The concern is precipitating an exacerbation of hypokalemia, congestive heart failure,[42] or a rapid atrial fibrillation. It is prudent to administer 1 or 2 vials initially. If toxicity has resolved or an adverse effect has occurred, no further vials should be given. If no adverse effect has arisen and toxicity has not resolved, 1 or 2 vials more are indicated.

Many of the patients presenting with acute-on-chronic digoxin toxicity have renal failure. Digoxin-specific Fab fragments should not be withheld in these patients because of concern about the inability of the kidney to remove the digoxin-Fab complex. This complex cannot be removed by dialysis either. A mild recrudescence of toxicity has been reported when the Fab fragments become unbound and are eliminated faster than digoxin.[44] However, multiple studies cite inadequate dosing as a much greater risk factor for recrudescence, and the transient rise in serum digoxin concentration has been within the therapeutic range and not clinically significant.[37,42,43,45] Simply administering another dose of digoxin-specific Fab fragments or giving conscientious supportive care may be the only additional therapy required. These patients typically have transient renal impairment, and once it has resolved, the digoxin, Fab fragments, and Fab-digoxin complex will be removed. Finally, the use of digoxin-specific Fab fragments can be cost effective.[46]

Atropine may be effective in treating symptomatic bradycardia early in acute digoxin toxicity because it increases vagal tone. Treatment of bradycardia with atropine later in an acute presentation or in chronic digoxin toxicity is often unsuccessful because the bradycardia is directly mediated by digoxin.[33] The ultimate treatment of symptomatic bradycardia is administration of digoxin-specific Fab fragments.

Transcutaneous and transvenous pacing has been used to treat symptomatic bradycardia, but transvenous pacing must also be used with caution. One study reported a higher mortality rate in patients receiving transvenous pacing because of dysrhythmias.[33] Also, iatrogenic complications (36%) were seen in patients receiving transvenous pacing.

In the past, supraventricular dysrhythmias have been treated pharmacologically with lidocaine and phenytoin. The first-line agent is now digoxin-specific Fab fragments. Unstable supraventricular or ventricular dysrhythmias can be treated by electrical cardioversion. However, owing to the hyperexcitability of the digoxin-poisoned myocyte and nodal tissue, low current is recommended. The concern is that high voltages may induce refractive lethal ventricular tachycardia.

When treating the digoxin poisoned patient for hyperkalemia, the clinician must resist using intravenous calcium. Digoxin-specific Fab fragments should be delivered immediately. If they are not available immediately, the standard treatment of the hyperkalemic patient should be undertaken without intravenous calcium. This issue is admittedly controversial, but the concern about calcium administration in digoxin toxicity is an additive toxic effect. During digoxin toxicity, there already is a dysfunction in intracellular calcium regulation along with an elevated calcium concentration. If more calcium is added to this hypercontractile state, a condition referred to as "stone heart" is produced. Dysrhythmias, cardiac dysfunction, and cardiac arrest have occurred in experimental animal studies and human case series.[47-49] More recently, a case report and animal study found no synergistic effect of calcium and digoxin toxicity.[50,51] Digoxin-specific Fab fragments should be the first-line treatment of hyperkalemia related to digoxin toxicity, and numerous noncontroversial therapies are available.

Treatment of hypotension should also include increasing the preload with intravenous fluids and pharmaceutical agents that have inotropic and vasopressor properties, such as dopamine and norepi-

PRIORITY ACTIONS

Treatment of Digoxin Toxicity

- Supportive care of airway, breathing, and circulation is the first critical step.
- Gastric decontamination is critical in the patient presenting with hemodynamic stability, but refrain from challenging the gastrointestinal system of a patient with hemodynamic instability.
- Assess serum potassium and magnesium levels immediately.
- Digoxin-specific Fab fragments are the definitive treatment for all clinical manifestations of digoxin toxicity.
- Dosage of digoxin-specific Fab fragments can be (1) empirical (5-10 vials) in the hemodynamically unstable patient, (2) calculated according to the amount of digoxin bound by 1 vial, or (3) calculated from the serum digoxin concentration.
- Decrease the current for cardioversion in patients with digoxin toxicity.
- Use a small number of vials (1-2) to treat patients with chronic digoxin toxicity.

nephrine. Little is known about the effectiveness of other antidotes, such as glucagon, to treat hypotension or bradycardia. Hypomagnesemia should be treated in standard fashion, with 2 g of intravenous magnesium given over 20 minutes.

DISPOSITION

If the patient is asymptomatic, has no clinical findings of acute digoxin toxicity, with a serum digoxin concentration at 6 hours in the therapeutic range, it is probably safe to reclassify this patient medically as no longer having digoxin toxicity. Of course this decision depends on a reliable history. Six hours of monitoring is adequate because the latest peak effect from oral digoxin is 6 hours, and that from intravenous digoxin, 3 hours. Clinical effects should appear before this time.

All symptomatic patients with clinical evidence of acute or chronic digoxin toxicity should be admitted to a monitored setting. The symptomatic patient who has life-threatening signs of toxicity and has been treated with digoxin-specific Fab fragments should be admitted to the intensive care unit. The symptomatic patient with relatively stable vital signs and cardiac rhythm should be admitted to a unit with cardiac monitoring cepabilities with an adequate dose of digoxin-specific Fab fragments available at the bedside.

REFERENCES

1. Watson WA, Litovitz TL, Rodgers GC Jr, et al: 2004 Annual report of the American Association of Poison Control Centers Toxic Exposure Surveillance System. Am J Emerg Med 2005;23:589-666.
2. Shepherd G, Klein-Schwartz W: High-dose insulin therapy for calcium-channel blocker overdose. Ann Pharmacother 2005;39:923-930.
3. Olson KR, Erdman AR, Woolf AD, et al: Calcium channel blocker ingestion: An evidence-based consensus guideline for out-of-hospital management. Clin Toxicol (Phila) 2005;43:797-822.
4. Osterhoudt KC, Henretig FM: How much confidence that calcium channel blockers are safe? Vet Hum Toxicol 1998;40:239.
5. Belson MG, Gorman SE, Sullivan K, Geller RJ: Calcium channel blocker ingestions in children. Am J Emerg Med 2000;18:581-586.
6. AHFS Drug Information 2008. Bethesda, Md, American Society of Health-System Pharmacists, 2008.
7. Vale JA, Kulig K: Position paper: Gastric lavage. J Toxicol Clin Toxicol 2004;42:933-943.
8. Position paper: Whole bowel irrigation. J Toxicol Clin Toxicol 2004;42:843-854.
9. Wax PM: Intestinal infarction due to nifedipine overdose. J Toxicol Clin Toxicol 1995;33:725-728.
10. Sporer KA, Manning JJ: Massive ingestion of sustained-release verapamil with a concretion and bowel infarction. Ann Emerg Med 1993;22:603-605.
11. Fauville JP, Hantson P, Honore P, et al: Severe diltiazem poisoning with intestinal pseudo-obstruction: Case report and toxicological data. J Toxicol Clin Toxicol 1995; 33:273-277.
12. Leone M, Charvet A, Boyle WA: Terlipressin: A new therapeutic for calcium channel blocker overdose. J Crit Care 2005;20:114-115.
13. Sztajnkrycer MD, Bond GR, Johnson SB, Weaver AL: Use of vasopressin in a canine model of severe verapamil poisoning: A preliminary descriptive study. Acad Emerg Med 2004;11:1253-1261.
14. Yuan TH, Kerns WP 2nd, Tomaszewski CA, et al: Insulin-glucose as adjunctive therapy for severe calcium channel antagonist poisoning. J Toxicol Clin Toxicol 1999;37: 463-474.
15. Lheureux PE, Zahir S, Gris M, et al: Bench-to-bedside review: Hyperinsulinaemia/euglycaemia therapy in the management of overdose of calcium-channel blockers. Crit Care 2006;10:212.
16. Levine MD, Boyer E: Hyperinsulinemia-euglycemia therapy: A useful tool in treating calcium channel blocker poisoning. Crit Care 2006;10:149.
17. Ortiz-Munoz L, Rodriguez-Ospina LF, Figueroa-Gonzalez M: Hyperinsulinemic-euglycemic therapy for intoxication with calcium channel blockers. Bol Asoc Med P R 2005;97: 182-189.
18. Megarbane B, Karyo S, Baud FJ: The role of insulin and glucose (hyperinsulinaemia/euglycaemia) therapy in acute calcium channel antagonist and beta-blocker poisoning. Toxicol Rev 2004;23:215-222.
19. Boyer EW, Duic PA, Evans A: Hyperinsulinemia/euglycemia therapy for calcium channel blocker poisoning. Pediatr Emerg Care Feb 2002;18:36-37.
20. van den Berghe G, Wouters P, Weekers F, et al: Intensive insulin therapy in the critically ill patients. N Engl J Med 2001;345:1359-1367.
21. Kline JA, Leonova E, Raymond RM: Beneficial myocardial metabolic effects of insulin during verapamil toxicity in the anesthetized canine. Crit Care Med 1995;23: 1251-1263.
22. Kline JA, Leonova E, Williams TC, et al: Myocardial metabolism during graded intraportal verapamil infusion in awake dogs. J Cardiovasc Pharmacol 1996;27:719-726.
23. Kline JA, Raymond RM, Schroeder JD, Watts JA: The diabetogenic effects of acute verapamil poisoning. Toxicol Appl Pharmacol 1997;145:357-362.
24. Kline JA, Tomaszewski CA, Schroeder JD, Raymond RM: Insulin is a superior antidote for cardiovascular toxicity

induced by verapamil in the anesthetized canine. J Pharmacol Exp Ther 1993;267:744-750.
25. Cumpston KL, Mycyk M, Pallasch E, Manzanares M, et al: Failure of hyperinsulinemia/euglycemia therapy in a severe diltiazem overdose. Clin Toxicol (Phila) 2002;40:618.
26. Wax PM, Erdman AR, Chyka PA, et al: Beta-blocker ingestion: An evidence-based consensus guideline for out-of-hospital management. Clin Toxicol (Phila) 2005;43:131-146.
27. Neuvonen PJ, Elonen E, Vuorenmaa T, Laakso M: Prolonged Q-T interval and severe tachyarrhythmias, common features of sotalol intoxication. Eur J Clin Pharmacol 1981;20:85-89.
28. Boyd R, Ghosh A: Towards evidence based emergency medicine: Best BETs from the Manchester Royal Infirmary: Glucagon for the treatment of symptomatic beta blocker overdose. Emerg Med J 2003;20:266-267.
29. Holger JS, Engebretsen KM, Obetz CL, et al: A comparison of vasopressin and glucagon in beta-blocker induced toxicity. Clin Toxicol (Phila) 2006;44:45-51.
30. Kerns W 2nd, Schroeder D, Williams C, et al: Insulin improves survival in a canine model of acute beta-blocker toxicity. Ann Emerg Med 1997;29:748-757.
31. Smith TW, Antman EM, Friedman PL, et al: Digitalis glycosides: Mechanisms and manifestations of toxicity. Part I. Prog Cardiovasc Dis 1984;26:413-458.
32. Leikin JB, Paloucek F: Digoxin. In Leikin & Paloucek's Poisoning & Toxicology Handbook, 3rd ed. Hudson, Ohio, Lexicomp, 2002.
33. Hack JB, Levin N: Cardioactive steroids. In Goldfrank L, Flomenbaum N, Lewin N, et al: Goldfrank's Toxicologic Emergencies, 8th ed. New York, McGraw-Hill, 2006.
34. Leikin JB, Aks S: Digoxin. In Erickson TB (ed): Pediatric Toxicology: Diagnosis and Management of the Poisoned Child. New York, McGraw-Hill, 2005.
35. Woolf AD, Wenger TL, Smith TW, Lovejoy FH Jr: Results of multicenter studies of digoxin-specific antibody fragments in managing digitalis intoxication in the pediatric population. Am J Emerg Med 1991;(Suppl 1):16-20, discussion 33-14.
36. Bismuth C, Gaultier M, Conso F, Efthymiou ML: Hyperkalemia in acute digitalis poisoning: Prognostic significance and therapeutic implications. Clin Toxicol 1973;6:153-162.
37. Ujhelyi MR, Robert S: Pharmacokinetic aspects of digoxin-specific Fab therapy in the management of digitalis toxicity. Clin Pharmacokinet 1995;28:483-493.
38. Wenger TL, Butler VP Jr, Haber E, Smith TW: Treatment of 63 severely digitalis-toxic patients with digoxin-specific antibody fragments. J Am Coll Cardiol 1985;5(Suppl A):118A-123A.
39. French JH, Thomas RG, Siskind AP, et al: Magnesium therapy in massive digoxin intoxication. Ann Emerg Med 1984;13:562-566.
40. Kelly RA, Smith TW: Recognition and management of digitalis toxicity. Am J Cardiol 1992;69:108G-118G, discusion 118G-119G.
41. Smith TW, Haber E, Yeatman L, Butler VP Jr: Reversal of advanced digoxin intoxication with Fab fragments of digoxin-specific antibodies. N Engl J Med. 1976;294:797-800.
42. Antman EM, Wenger TL, Butler VP Jr, et al: Treatment of 150 cases of life-threatening digitalis intoxication with digoxin-specific Fab antibody fragments: Final report of a multicenter study. Circulation 1990;81:1744-1752.
43. Hickey AR, Wenger TL, Carpenter VP, et al: Digoxin immune Fab therapy in the management of digitalis intoxication: Safety and efficacy results of an observational surveillance study. J Am Coll Cardiol 1991;17:590-598.
44. Mehta RN, Mehta NJ, Gulati A: Late rebound digoxin toxicity after digoxin-specific antibody Fab fragments therapy in anuric patient. J Emerg Med 2002;22:203-206.
45. Mycyk MB, Bryant SM, Cumpston KL: Late rebound digoxin toxicity after digoxin-specific antibody Fab fragments therapy in anuric patient. J Emerg Med 2003;24:91.
46. Mauskopf JA, Wenger TL: Cost-effectiveness analysis of the use of digoxin immune Fab (ovine) for treatment of digoxin toxicity. Am J Cardiol 1991;68:1709-1714.
47. Bower JO, Mengle H: The additive effect of calcium and digitalis. JAMA 1936;106:1151-1153.
48. Gold H, Edwards D: The effects of ouabain on heart in the presence of hypercalcemia. Am Heart J 1927;3:45-50.
49. Smith PK, Winkler A, Hoff HE: L calcium and digitalis synergism: The toxicity of calcium salts injected intravenously into digitalized animals. Arch Intern Med 1939;64:322-328.
50. Van Deusen SK, Birkhahn RH, Gaeta TJ: Treatment of hyperkalemia in a patient with unrecognized digitalis toxicity. J Toxicol Clin Toxicol 2003;41:373-376.
51. Hack JB, Woody JH, Lewis DE, et al: The effect of calcium chloride in treating hyperkalemia due to acute digoxin toxicity in a porcine model. J Toxicol Clin Toxicol 2004;42:337-342.

Chapter 143

Sympathomimetics

Gar Ming Chan and Lewis S. Nelson

KEY POINTS

Sympathomimetic agents are components of many over-the-counter, prescription, and illicit drugs.

The sympathomimetic toxicologic syndrome (toxidrome) is a constellation of the following signs and symptoms: elevated mood, psychomotor agitation, diaphoresis, tremor, hypertension, tachycardia, and mydriasis.

The sympathomimetic toxidrome can mimic hypoglycemia, withdrawal syndromes, and the anticholinergic toxidrome.

Treatment, which is generally symptomatic and supportive, involves control of the patient's psychomotor agitation. Occasionally, specific correction of the patient's vital signs is necessary.

Scope

A sympathomimetic agent, by definition, emulates the clinical effects of the endogenous sympathetic catecholamines epinephrine and norepinephrine. The class of sympathomimetics comprises an exhaustive list of drugs ranging from over-the-counter (OTC) and prescription agents to drugs of misuse and abuse (Box 143-1).

Clinically, sympathomimetics were used to increase the level of arousal in patients with barbiturate overdose, as weight loss agents, and to treat depression. OTC preparations are available predominantly as decongestants and remain available as weight loss products. Ephedrine, a once popular dietary supplement for weight loss and arousal, has been banned by the U.S. Food and Drug Administration (FDA) for this use. Prescription and parenteral sympathomimetic agents are available for a myriad of medical illnesses, including hypersensitivity reactions, reactive airways disease, attention deficit–hyperactivity disorder (ADHD), and cardiovascular compromise. The misuse and abuse of licit and illicit agents constitute the remainder of sympathomimetic agents: cocaine, amphetamine derivatives (i.e., 3,4-methylenedioxymethamphetamine), and clenbuterol.

Pathophysiology

The biogenic amines are histamine, tyrosine, serotonin, and the catecholamines (epinephrine, norepinephrine, dopamine). These amines are found within the central nervous system (CNS), and their synthesis, release, and metabolism are very similar. Through several enzyme-linked steps, tyrosine can be converted into norepinephrine or dopamine; dopamine is made prior to entry into the vesicle, and norepinephrine is made within the vesicle. Serotonin, however, is made in the cytosol from tryptophan and resides in dissimilar vesicles. Despite the differences

BOX 143-1

Common Sympathomimetic Agents

Over-the-Counter Drugs and Dietary Supplements

Arousal Agents
- Caffeine

Weight Loss Products
- Ephedrine
- Synephrine
- Caffeine

Nasal Decongestants
- Pseudoephedrine
- Phenylpropanolamine (PPA)
- Phenylephrine

Prescription and Parenteral Agents

For Hypersensitivity
- Epinephrine (autoinjector)

For Reactive Airways Disease
- Albuterol
- Pirbuterol
- Salmeterol
- Levalbuterol
- Theophylline
- Ephedrine
- Epinephrine

Vasopressors
- Phenylephrine
- Epinephrine
- Norepinephrine
- Dopamine

For Weight Loss
- Dextroamphetamine
- Phentermine

For Attention Deficit–Hyperactivity Disorder
- Methylphenidate
- Dextroamphetamine

Inotropes
- Dobutamine
- Isoproterenol
- Milrinone

Illicit or Misused Drugs
- Cocaine

Amphetamine Derivatives
- Methamphetamine
- 3,4-Methylenedioxymethamphetamine (MDMA)
- 3,4-Methylenedioxyethamphetamine (MDEA)
- Para-methoxymethamphetamine (PMA)
- Methcathinone

For Sports Performance Enhancement
- Clenbuterol
- Caffeine
- Ephedrine

in synthesis and packaging, the stimulus for exocytosis is the same, being calcium dependent. After an amine is released into the synapse, reuptake can occur via transport proteins. Once within the cytoplasm, the biogenic amines are repackaged into vesicles or may undergo metabolism via monoamine oxidase (MAO). If released into the periphery, these amines may undergo metabolism extracellularly via catechol-*O*-methyltransferase (COMT).

To understand the pharmacology and pathophysiology of sympathomimetics, one must first understand the functions and roles of endogenous catecholamines (norepinephrine, epinephrine, dopamine). Within the autonomic nervous system, epinephrine and norepinephrine are released from the adrenal medulla via sympathetic stimulation. Norepinephrine, however, is also released into the circulation, resulting in much of the alpha-adrenergic stimulation. Dopamine is found within the CNS nerve terminals in areas where norepinephrine can be found and can also be found in the periphery. Excess dopamine results in findings of excess norepinephrine, because dopamine is converted to norepinephrine via dopamine β-hydroxylase. In the CNS, however, excess dopamine causes symptoms of psychosis. Similarly, serotonin can be found centrally and peripherally and has a broad spectrum of effects, on mood, appetite, sleep, and thermoregulation.

Pharmacotherapeutics can mimic increased catechol levels through various mechanisms, including inhibition of metabolism, impairment of reuptake, and increased release. The specific clinical effects of a sympathomimetic agent are related to the pharmacology of the agent. The relative effect of the agent on the two distinct adrenergic receptors, alpha and beta, can be used to predict the clinical response. Generally, from a cardiovascular perspective, alpha-adrenergic receptor agonism results in vasoconstriction, and beta-adrenergic receptor agonism results in tachycardia and hypotension. However, the other clinical effects (hypokalemia, hyperglycemia, and smooth muscle relaxation) are associated with beta-adrenergic agonism as well.

Sympathomimetics may act directly, indirectly, or, occasionally, in both ways to produce sympathomimesis. Direct-acting sympathomimetics act by introducing the catechol, norepinephrine or epinephrine, directly into the patient. Indirect-acting sympathomimetics are agents that increase the release of endogenous catecholamines or impair the uptake of endogenous catecholamines, with resultant adrenergic receptor stimulation. Additionally, indirect-acting sympathomimetics can lead to release of other biogenic amines, such as serotonin and dopamine. Serotonin excess results in euphoria and an elevated mood, whereas dopamine excess results in psychosis and hallucinations that clinically cannot be differentiated from primary psychosis.

Finally, mixed-acting sympathomimetics act as both direct- and indirect-acting sympathomimetics. These agents cause symptoms that emulate those of biogenic amine excess. Despite these underlying differences, however, the clinical presentation can be virtually indistinguishable. Clinical manifestations may also vary with the location of the neurotransmitter predominance within the CNS.

BOX 143-2

Clinical Manifestations of Sympathomimetic Exposure

Cardiovascular
- Hypertensive emergencies
- Acute coronary syndrome
- Cerebrovascular accident
- Tachycardias, dysrhythmias
- Vasospasm/ischemia of end-organs

Central Nervous System
- Altered mentation
- Anxiety
- Mania
- Psychosis
- Agitated delirium
- Seizures
- Intracerebral hemorrhage

Metabolic
- Hypokalemia
- Hyperglycemia

Other
- Rhabdomyolysis
- Muscle rigidity
- Hyperthermia

Unique
- 3,4-Methylenedioxymethamphetamine (MDMA)–associated (syndrome of inappropriate antidiuretic hormone secretion [SIADH])

Clinical Manifestations

Clinical manifestations of the sympathomimetic toxidrome consist of tachycardia, hypertension, diaphoresis, mydriasis, hyperthermia, and psychomotor agitation. This toxidrome can be further divided into alpha-adrenergic and beta-adrenergic receptor effects. Alpha-adrenergic subtype 1 receptor agonism results in vasoconstriction, whereas postsynaptic alpha-adrenergic subtype 2 receptor agonism results in sedation and hypotension, effects that have been seen with clonidine use. Beta-adrenergic receptors also have clinically significant subtypes, 1 and 2. β_1-receptor agonism results in chronotropy and thus increased cardiac output. β_2-receptor agonism results in vasodilation, and the nonspecific effects include hypokalemia, hyperglycemia, acidemia, and tremor. Exposure to methylxanthine is virtually indistinguishable from exposure to beta-adrenergic agonists because of the shared final pathway, an increase in intracellular cyclic adenosine monophosphate (cAMP). Methylxanthines also increase circulating catecholamines and inhibit adenosine receptors. Their potential effects are listed in Box 143-2.

■ CARDIOVASCULAR

As a result of hypertension and tachycardia, vascular events can occur during exposure to a sympathomimetic. Cocaine use is associated with myocardial infarction, coronary artery dissection, aortic dissection, cardiomyopathy, splanchnic infarction, cerebrovascular accidents, and cerebrovascular hemorrhage. Similar events are also associated with the use of amphetamine derivatives.

It is this hypertension and vasoconstriction that make beta-adrenergic blockade a precarious pharmacologic intervention. In the setting of cocaine-associated acute coronary syndrome, beta-adrenergic blockade is contraindicated despite the mortality benefit in patients with acute coronary syndrome not associated with cocaine. Even in the setting of a suspicious beta-adrenergic–specific agonist exposure, beta-blockade is rarely recommended because the underlying substrate is usually dependent on β-receptor agonism (e.g., the asthmatic patient who overdoses on albuterol).

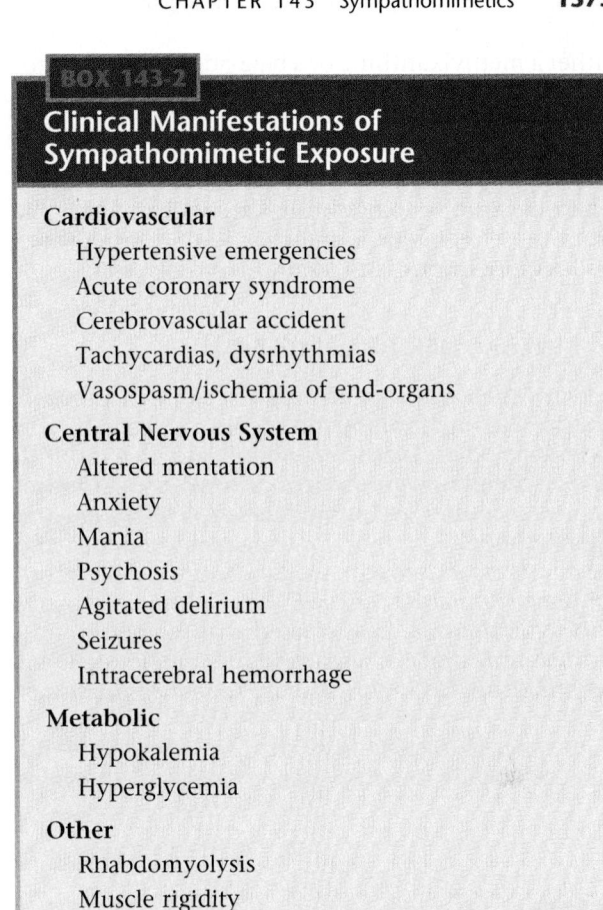

Methylxanthines and beta-adrenergic receptor agonists result primarily in β_2 stimulation. The β_2 stimulation produces diastolic hypotension secondary to vasodilation and systolic hypertension secondary to enhanced inotropy. The combination of diastolic hypotension and systolic hypertension manifests clinically as a widened pulse pressure. Beta-adrenergic agonism results in intracellular shuttling of serum potassium, producing hypokalemia. These nonspecific findings—a widened pulse pressure and hypokalemia—if present, may suggest exposure to either a methylxanthine or a beta-adrenergic receptor agonist.

A unique property of cocaine is its ability to block myocardial sodium channels. This manifests as a widened QRS complex on electrocardiogram (ECG). These electrophysiologic effects are indistinguishable from those seen with other class I antidysrhythmics and require immediate attention and reversal.

■ CENTRAL NERVOUS SYSTEM

As with the cardiovascular effects, some of the CNS effects of sympathomimetic agents are secondary to hypertension and vasoconstriction and may result in CNS ischemia, hemorrhage, and seizures. Central neurotransmitter excess produces elevated mood and altered thought content. Extreme bouts of mania and psychosis associated with hallucinations are common. Extreme stimulation of the CNS, resulting in seizures and hyperthermia, is associated with higher mortality in animal models. Aggressive therapy should focus on inhibiting CNS hyperactivity to reduce the risk of death.

Another CNS effect associated with amphetamine and cocaine use is withdrawal or "washout." It occurs with cessation of use of the agents and is associated with lethargy and depressed mood, both of which result from catecholamine depletion.

RED FLAGS

- Widened pulse pressure and hypokalemia, if present, may suggest exposure to either a methylxanthine or a beta-adrenergic receptor agonist.
- A unique property of cocaine is its ability to block myocardial sodium channels, which manifests as a widened QRS complex on electrocardiography. These electrophysiologic effects are indistinguishable from those of other class I antidysrhythmics and require immediate attention and reversal.
- Sympathomimetic stimulation of the central nervous system, resulting in psychomotor agitation and hyperthermia, is associated with high mortality and so should be aggressively treated.
- Psychomotor agitation can result in rhabdomyolysis, tremor, and muscle rigidity; if undetected, severe rhabdomyolysis may cause renal insufficiency or failure.
- The clinician should suspect cocaine body-packing in a patient whose symptoms recur or are prolonged, and when signs and symptoms of sympathomimetic exposure occur in a person who has recently flown into the country.
- Individuals already demonstrating signs and symptoms of cocaine packet leakage or rupture should receive urgent surgical consultation and invasive removal of remaining packages because the lethality of this much drug is high.

■ METABOLIC

Metabolic derangements during sympathomimetic exposure resemble the "flight or fight" response. The most common metabolic changes are hyperglycemia and hypokalemia, which result from a surge in epinephrine level. If the metabolic demands outstrip the ability to supply and clear energy constituents, a metabolic acidosis can occur as well. These metabolic effects usually do not require intervention, because when the vicious cycle of agitation and increased metabolic demand is halted, the body can achieve homeostasis through regulatory mechanisms.

Similarly, in combination with psychomotor agitation, these increases in demand and activity can result in rhabdomyolysis, tremor, and muscle rigidity. Severe rhabdomyolysis, if unrecognized, may lead to renal insufficiency or failure. Hyperthermia and metabolic acidosis in combination with rhabdomyolysis can produce another vicious cycle; affected patients should be sedated rapidly to halt the process.

Additionally, 3,4-methylenedioxymethamphetamine (MDMA) has been associated with syndrome of inappropriate antidiuretic hormone secretion (SIADH), reflected by hyponatremia and inappropriately concentrated urine in the setting of euvolemia. Patients with this syndrome typically have symptoms the day after exposure with either altered mental status or seizures. The condition responds well to fluid restriction; if symptoms are severe, hypertonic saline may be utilized.

Differential Diagnosis

The differential diagnosis for the patient with suspected sympathomimetic toxidrome is extensive (Box 143-3), ranging the spectrum from febrile illness to delirium.

Diagnostic Evaluation

Most individuals who misuse or abuse sympathomimetics do not present to the ED; those who do are usually symptomatic. While considering the extensive differential diagnosis and clinical effects, the EP should take aggressive measures (Fig. 143-1). In all patients, vital signs should be recorded and then continuously monitored, with close attention to core temperature. Supplemental oxygen should be administered owing to the increased metabolic demand. If the patient is too agitated to allow a thorough evaluation, a bedside glucose measurement should be obtained to exclude hypoglycemia-induced sympathomimetic response. An intravenous catheter should be placed and secured to allow parenteral administration of a sedative or hypnotic to control the patient's

BOX 143-3

Differential Diagnosis of Sympathomimetic Toxidromes

Toxic/Metabolic Problems
- Hyponatremia
- Anticholinergics
- Withdrawal syndromes

Endocrine Problems
- Hypoglycemia
- Hyperthyroidism/thyrotoxicosis
- Pheochromocytoma
- Pulmonary/cardiovascular
- Hypoxia

Neurologic Problems
- Cerebrovascular accident
- Intracranial hemorrhage
- Subarachnoid, subdural, or epidural hemorrhage

Infectious/Inflammatory
- Sepsis
- Meningitis/encephalitis

Environmental
- Heat stroke

Psychiatric
- Psychosis not otherwise specified
- Schizophrenia
- Mania

behavior and prevent further injury to patient and staff.

If the patient is well controlled or if the patient does not require sedation, a complete history and physical examination should be obtained, with close attention to the presence of a sympathomimetic toxidrome. Its presence supports the diagnosis of a sympathomimetic exposure but does not exclude the other possibilities.

A 12-lead ECG should be obtained in all patients with a potential exposure. Signs of ischemia, infarction, or electrolyte disturbance may be present despite the lack of patient endorsement of such exposure or when the patient's sensorium is too altered for a history to be obtained. Patients with suspected sympathomimetic toxidrome should undergo isotonic fluid resuscitation because most are volume depleted from agitation, increased metabolic demand, and diaphoresis. The only scenario in which fluid resuscitation should not be initiated before laboratory evaluation is in the individual in whom SIADH from MDMA use is suspected.

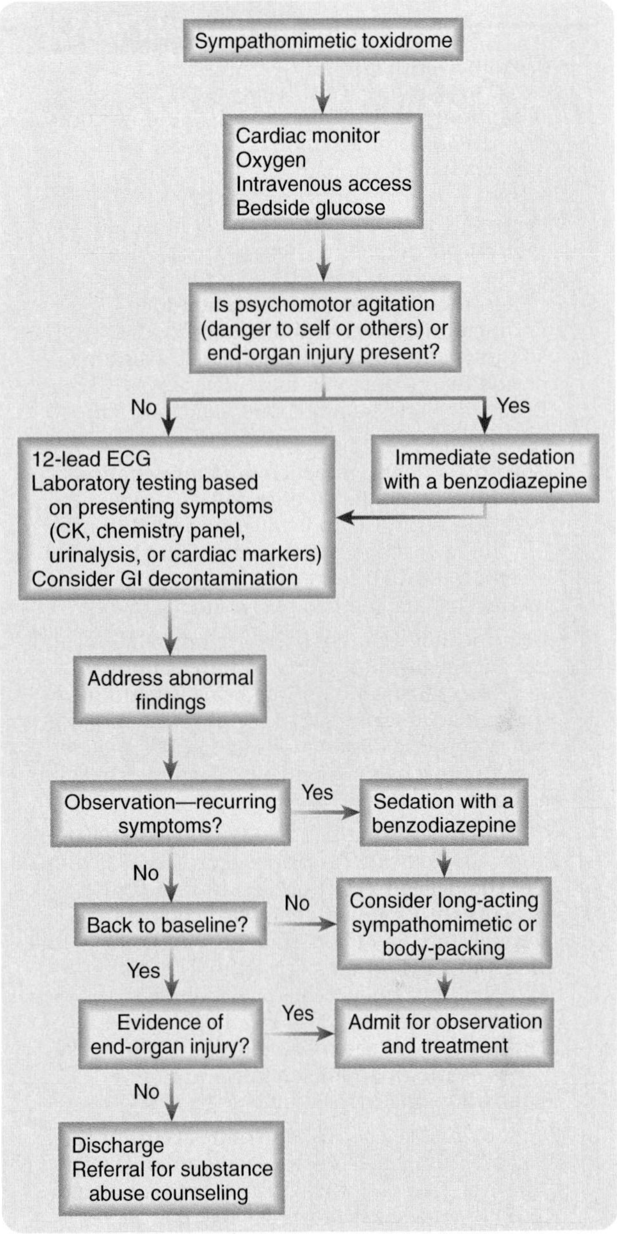

Sympathomimetic toxidrome
Cardiac monitor
Oxygen
Intravenous access
Bedside glucose
Is psychomotor agitation (danger to self or others) or end-organ injury present?
No
Yes
12-lead ECG
Laboratory testing based on presenting symptoms (CK, chemistry panel, urinalysis, or cardiac markers)
Consider GI decontamination
Immediate sedation with a benzodiazepine
Address abnormal findings
Observation—recurring symptoms?
Yes
Sedation with a benzodiazepine
No
Back to baseline?
No
Consider long-acting sympathomimetic or body-packing
Yes
Evidence of end-organ injury?
Yes
Admit for observation and treatment
No
Discharge
Referral for substance abuse counseling

FIGURE 143-1 Treatment algorithm for sympathomimetic toxidrome. CK, creatine kinase; ECG, electrocardiogram; GI, gastrointestinal.

A serum chemistry panel should be performed in all patients to evaluate for the presence of metabolic acidosis, hypokalemia, rhabdomyolysis, renal insufficiency, glucose derangement, and hyponatremia. In patients with suspected rhabdomyolysis, serum myoglobin marker evaluation as well as a urinalysis should be obtained for either myoglobinuria or inappropriately concentrated urine in the setting of hyponatremia. Patients who have symptoms of chest pain or anginal equivalent or in whom ECG findings are abnormal should undergo serum cardiac marker testing and perhaps emergency cardiac catheterization in the appropriate setting.

Individuals with headache, neurologic abnormalities, or persistent alteration in sensorium or cog-

Tips and Tricks

- The clinician should avoid neuroleptics (e.g., haloperidol) and antihistamines (e.g., diphenhydramine) to control the psychomotor agitation and psychosis associated with sympathomimetic overdose. Neuroleptics have anticholinergic properties, decrease seizure thresholds, and increase QT intervals, thus making them a poor choice to achieve sedation. Anticholinergic toxicity is within the diagnostic consideration for undifferentiated agitated delirium, so administration of an anticholinergic agent may be additive to potential morbidity. Benzodiazepines are the preferred choice for sedation.
- The only scenario in which fluid resuscitation should not be initiated prior to laboratory evaluation is in the individual suspected to have syndrome of inappropriate antidiuretic hormone secretion (SIADH) from use of 3,4-methylenedioxymethamphetamine (MDMA).
- Urine acidification has been demonstrated to enhance renal elimination of amphetamines; however, acidification of the urine is performed through acidification of the serum, which may worsen other manifestations of amphetamine toxicity such as rhabdomyolysis and metabolic acidosis.
- Owing to persistent tachycardia and extrapolation of data from acute coronary syndromes, EPs often feel compelled to control the heart rate in patients with sympathomimetic exposures through the use of beta-adrenergic receptor antagonists. However, such treatment has the potential for unopposed alpha-adrenergic agonism, which may lead to a hypertensive crisis. Therefore, these agents should be avoided in the patient with an undifferentiated sympathomimetic toxidrome.
- Amiodarone is listed as a first-line agent for the treatment of wide-complex tachycardia (WCT). However, because of its intrinsic beta-adrenergic receptor antagonist properties (see previous paragraph), amiodarone should not be used in the setting of cocaine toxicity.

nition should undergo emergency computed tomography (CT) of the brain to evaluate for injury, infarction, edema, and bleed. If CT findings are normal but the EP suspects a subarachnoid hemorrhage or an infectious etiology remains a possibility, a lumbar puncture should be obtained.

■ SPECIAL CONSIDERATIONS

■ Body-Packers

The possibility of concealment of illicit substances in pouches within the gastrointestinal tract in large quantities for the purposes of trafficking requires close and careful evaluation. Individuals who take part in this trafficking, known familiarly as "body-packers" or "mules," may be either asymptomatic or symptomatic when they present to the ED. If asymptomatic, a body-packer requires the evaluation as described previously but may need more intense and prolonged treatment and monitoring. Individuals with leaking or ruptured packets containing a sympathomimetic, most often cocaine, need to be identified quickly because they typically carry enough drug to exceed multiple median lethal doses of cocaine. Plain radiographs of the abdomen as well as CT scans of the abdomen after oral administration of a contrast agent have reasonable sensitivity in detecting packets within the gastrointestinal tract; however, in individuals already demonstrating signs and symptoms of packet leakage or rupture an urgent surgical consultation should be obtained and invasive removal of remaining packages should be performed because the lethality is high.[1]

■ Methylxanthines or Beta-Agonists

In patients who present with signs and symptoms consistent with methylxanthine or a beta-agonist exposure, the serum theophylline level should be measured. At-risk populations include individuals with a history of reactive airways disease and those with sinus tachycardia, diastolic hypotension, widened pulse pressure, nausea, vomiting, tremor, hypokalemia, or hyperglycemia.

■ Urine Testing and Toxicology Screening

Urine screening for sympathomimetics, with the exception of cocaine, is fraught with error and misinterpretation. The turnaround time for the screening tests limits their utility in the ED, because most patients would have been evaluated and treated before tests are completed. Additionally, a negative result does not exclude exposure to a sympathomimetic, and a positive result does not confirm that the patient is currently symptomatic from a sympathomimetic agent. Such tests are therefore not recommended in the evaluation of a potentially poisoned adult patient.

Treatment

■ GASTROINTESTINAL DECONTAMINATION

Patients who have ingested sympathomimetics orally should receive activated charcoal if it can be safely administered. Individuals who should receive aggressive multiple-dose activated charcoal (MDAC) include body-packers and patients who overdose on theophylline. Body-packers should receive MDAC in order to reduce drug burden. Use of MDAC for theophylline exposures has been shown to enhance elimination of the drug.

Owing to the large burden of drug and the risk of leakage or rupture in body-packers, whole-bowel irrigation should be utilized to hasten passage of the packets and drug through the gastrointestinal tract. This will require 2 L/hour of polyethylene glycol given orally to an adult patient; the dose should be adjusted for a child. The majority of patients require the placement of a nasogastric tube in order to maintain this rate of administration.

SEDATION

The focus of therapy in a patient with a toxic sympathomimetic exposure should revolve around the lowering of morbidity and mortality risks through reduction of psychomotor agitation or seizures and hyperthermia. Animal models show that benzodiazepines appear to be the most effective therapy for this purpose.

COOLING

Death related to cocaine use has been associated with elevation in core and ambient temperatures.[2] An ice bath that covers the largest surface area can effectively and quickly reduce core temperature. Other commonly employed modalities are use of mist and a fan and application of ice packs.

Most patients are hypovolemic from the increased metabolic demand, diaphoresis, and psychomotor agitation associated with sympathomimetic exposures. Fluid resuscitation to the point of euvolemia is recommended.

SPECIAL CONSIDERATIONS

Beta-Agonists

For known beta-agonist exposures, it would seem logical to administer a beta-adrenergic receptor antagonist. However, patients with such exposures usually overdose on their own medications and so have asthma; thus, the administration of beta-receptor adrenergic antagonist is contraindicated and potentially dangerous. However, if there is no contraindication to use of a beta-adrenergic receptor antagonist, careful administration and titration of agents such as esmolol and metoprolol can be performed.

Methylxanthines

Although not as common as in the past, theophylline overdoses can be treated aggressively with MDAC to enhance elimination as well as hemoperfusion or hemodialysis. Tachydysrhythmias associated with theophylline overdose can be suppressed with β_1-adrenergic receptor–selective antagonists. However, as mentioned previously, patients with this overdose usually have taken their own medications and therefore have asthma, making the use of beta-receptor antagonists precarious.

Cocaine

Multiple agents are available to treat cocaine's unique properties of vasoconstriction and sodium channel blockade. The first-line agent for cocaine toxicity is a benzodiazepine; however, a subset of cases does not respond to this therapy. Ongoing vasoconstriction or vasospasm can be treated with an alpha-adrenergic receptor antagonist, phentolamine. Another manifestation of cocaine toxicity may be a wide-complex tachydysrhythmia (WCT) resulting from sodium channel blockade. These dysrhythmias, like those seen with other sodium channel blockers, respond well to administration of sodium bicarbonate or lidocaine.

Cocaine Body-Packers

Symptomatic cocaine body-packers need urgent surgical removal of residual packets. In some cases, body-packers are not symptomatic and may be treated with whole-bowel irrigation. If the packets may cause mechanical obstruction, endoscopic removal has been reported as successful.

MDMA

MDMA-associated SIADH usually responds to conservative fluid restriction. However, the patient with severe CNS manifestations should receive hypertonic saline to rapidly correct a portion of the metabolic imbalance.

Vasopressors

Epinephrine and norepinephrine can extravasate within tissue compartments during infusions as well as during unintentional exposures from autoinjectors. Warm compresses should be placed topically for mild cases, with nitroglycerine paste added to generate vasodilation. For severe cases, intradermal phentolamine may be administered within the exposed tissue.

Disposition

Length of stay and disposition for patients with sympathomimetic exposures depend on the duration of the particular sympathomimetic agent, which is highly variable. Recreationally smoked or insufflated cocaine has a short duration of action, usually no more than 4 hours, and the patient can normally be discharged from the ED thereafter. Side effects such as rhabdomyolysis, heat stroke, and end-organ injury require ongoing monitoring and treatment. Prolonged effects may be seen in individuals who are body-packers and in people who use long-acting agents such as clenbuterol, a potent beta-adrenergic receptor agonist. These individuals require admission and prolonged treatment.

The evaluation and treatment of cocaine-associated chest pain has evolved and will vary by region. A short observation period with serial ECGs and serial measurements of cardiac-specific markers performed 6 to 8 hours apart can be used to exclude cocaine-associated myocardial infarction.[3] Even when the diagnosis of myocardial infarction has been excluded, all patients with such chest pain should undergo urgent outpatient evaluation for coronary artery disease and drug abuse counseling.

REFERENCES

1. Traub SJ, Hoffman RS, Nelson LS: Body packing—the internal concealment of illicit drugs. N Engl J Med 2003; 349:2519-2526.
2. Marzuk PM, Tardiff K, Leon AC, et al: Ambient temperature and mortality from unintentional cocaine overdose. JAMA 1998;279:1795-1800.
3. Weber JE, Shofer FS, Larkin GL, et al: Validation of a brief observation period for patients with cocaine-associated chest pain. N Engl J Med 2003;348:510-517.

Chapter 144

Hallucinogens and Drugs of Abuse

Mark B. Mycyk

KEY POINTS

The most common chief complaint when patients have hallucinogenic intoxication is altered mental status.

Substance abuse is common among all ED patients irrespective of demographic, age, race, or socioeconomic status.

Optimal treatment depends on *symptom-based* (rather than drug-based) diagnostic strategies and interventions.

An elevated temperature is the most important prognostic sign of poor outcome.

Most new drugs cannot be identified with hospital-based blood or urine tests, and results of urine drug screens should never be considered diagnostic.

Treatment for drug-induced hypertension should involve heavy doses of benzodiazepines before antihypertensive agents are considered.

Substance abuse counseling and referral are required for all patients before discharge.

Scope

Recreational abuse of hallucinogens and other drugs is common among ED patients and is directly responsible for many ED visits. Although the exact prevalence of drug abuse in ED patients is unknown because so much drug abuse goes undetected, various surveillance studies all indicate that ED visits related to drug use continue to rise yearly.[1-3]

Patients who present to an ED immediately after using a drug do so for a variety of reasons: for an unfavorable or unanticipated reaction to the drug, after an unintentional overdose, after sustaining a traumatic injury, for altered mental status, or for suicidal and other dangerous behavior. In addition to the acute complications directly related to drug use, many cardiovascular, neurologic, infectious, psychiatric, and social health problems treated in the ED are linked to chronic drug abuse. Because drug abuse is often not declared by the patient at the time of arrival, recognition and optimal treatment require vigilance from the EP as well as attention to historical, clinical, and laboratory clues.

It is important to understand that recreational drug use today knows no demographic, age, or socioeconomic boundaries. Drug use is just as common (but less frequently suspected) in white, employed, and insured individuals as in patients who are non-white, unemployed, or homeless.[1,4] In the last two decades, first-time drug use has become more common among adolescents, and the variety of drugs used has exploded.[5,6] Drug use is no longer limited to what can be identified on a standard hospital toxicology screen, and many of the drugs people abuse to get high are not illegal, such as cough and cold products and prescription medications.[7-10] The rampant growth of drug use is likely linked to the proliferation of the Internet and the wide availability of unregulated partisan drug sites that enable potential users to learn about drugs, to order the raw ingredients and supplies to manufacture their own drugs, or simply to purchase drugs online in the safety of their own homes.[6]

Pathophysiology

The drugs available for recreational abuse are countless and are constantly evolving. In the past, recreational drugs were categorized, for the purposes of discussion, identification, and treatment, somewhat arbitrarily on the basis of structural class, predominant biochemical or neurotransmitter activity (e.g., dopaminergic vs. serotonergic vs. gamma-aminobutyric acid [GABA]–ergic), or expected clinical effect (e.g., hallucinogen vs. stimulant vs. entactogen). In reality most drugs exhibit multiple biochemical effects of varying intensity that are not limited to a particular structural class, and clinical findings vary widely among different individuals even when they are exposed to the same drug. It is now recognized that clinical variability depends not only on the specific type of drug but also on the dose used, the form of drug (e.g., crystal vs. powder vs. liquid), the purity of the drug, the route of delivery (e.g., intranasal vs. ingestion vs. injection), the concomitant use of co-ingestants, individual genetic polymorphisms, and individual biochemical and physiologic adaptations from long-term exposure.

Most recreational drugs are highly lipophilic and easily cross the blood-brain barrier, so most result in some euphoria; otherwise there would be little reason to abuse them.[3] Although the exact mechanisms are still incompletely understood, modulation of central dopaminergic activity, which is responsible for pleasure seeking and reward reinforcement, is an important factor in the euphoric response and the development of drug addiction.[3] Recreational drugs also affect, to variable extents, peripheral and central norepinephrine, serotonin (5-HT), *N*-methyl-D aspartate (NMDA), and GABA activity.

Presenting Signs and Symptoms

The most common presenting feature in all patients with recreational drug use is some degree of altered mental status. It may range from seemingly benign giddiness to life-threatening agitation or obtundation. Drug-associated altered mental status may be associated with any kind of vital sign abnormalities or evidence of end-organ damage. Cardiovascular, neurologic, infectious, and psychiatric complaints are also common (Table 144-1). Because the predominant drugs seen in a particular ED vary depending on local geographic preferences and the types of drugs abused change far more quickly than published medical literature can keep up with, optimal treatment depends on *symptom-based* (rather than drug-based) diagnostic strategies and interventions.

The following paragraphs discuss some of the more common drugs of abuse prevalent in most EDs. Identifying previously undetected drug abuse requires some familiarity with these common drugs and the street slang associated with them (Table 144-2).

Table 144-1 SIGNS AND SYMPTOMS OF RECREATIONAL DRUG USE

Sign or Symptom	Responsible Drug(s)
Altered mental status	All
Agitation	Amphetamine Cocaine Dextromethorphan Jimsonweed MDMA Methamphetamine PCP Prescription medicines
Obtundation	GHB Opioids Prescription medicines
Hypothermia	Opiates GHB
Hyperthermia	Amphetamine Cocaine Jimsonweed MDMA Methamphetamine PCP
Tachycardia	Amphetamines Cocaine Jimsonweed Ketamine LSD Methamphetamine MDMA PCP Prescription medicines
Bradycardia	GHB Opioids Prescription medicines
Hypertension	Amphetamine Cocaine Jimsonweed Ketamine LSD Methamphetamine MDMA PCP Prescription medicines
Hypotension	GHB Opioids Prescription medicines
Seizures	Amphetamines Cocaine Dextromethorphan GHB Jimsonweed MDMA Methamphetamine Prescription medicines

GHB, gamma-hydroxybutyrate; LSD, D-lysergic acid diethylamide; MDMA, methylenedioxymethamphetamine; PCP, phencyclidine.

PRIORITY ACTIONS

Altered Mental Status, Seizures, or Behavioral Changes?

- Does the patient have a central nervous system infection, infarction, lesion, or mass?
- Consider brain imaging and lumber puncture if neurologic status is inconsistent with intoxication.

Apnea or Depressed Respirations?

- Consider treatment with naloxone to reverse potential narcosis or dextrose/thiamine for hypoglycemia.
- Intubation may be needed for persistent hypoxia or inability to protect airway.

Chest Pain?

- Evaluate the patient for myocardial ischemia with electrocardiography, telemetry, and cardiac enzyme measurements.

Fever?

- Does the patient have any history or evidence of intravenous drug use?
- Consider evaluation for endocarditis or epidural abscess.

Table 144-2 NEW DRUG SLANG

Dextromethorphan	DXM Robo Red hots Triple Cs
GHB (gamma-hydroxybutyrate)	Georgia home boy G Easy lay Liquid G
Ketamine	Vitamin K Special K Kitty Valium Cat tranquilizer
MDMA (methylenedioxymethamphetamine)	XTC X ADAM Hug drug
Methamphetamine	Meth Crystal Yaba Chicken feed Tweak White man's crack

■ AMPHETAMINE

Commonly referred to as "crank" or "speed," amphetamine is a specific drug first synthesized in 1887 and initially marketed as a decongestant and appetite suppressant. Many other drugs with a similar chemical structure, such as MDMA (methylenedioxymethamphetamine) and methamphetamine, are collectively called *amphetamines* even though their clinical effects vary. More precisely, these drugs are all derived from a phenylethylamine core and should be collectively called *phenylethylamines* (MDMA and methamphetamine are discussed separately). Amphetamines are currently available as tablets in the form of a prescription (e.g., Adderall) or in a designer form produced in a clandestine laboratory.[11] Onset of symptoms occurs within 15 minutes of ingestion and lasts 6 to 12 hours. The effects are primarily stimulant in nature because of amphetamine's activity at peripheral and central norepinephrine and dopamine sites.[3] Varying levels of tachycardia, hypertension, hyperthermia, diaphoresis, and agitation are commonly seen in the ED patient who has ingested an amphetamine, and cardiac and central nervous system (CNS) complications have been frequently reported.

■ COCAINE

Derived from *Erythroxylon coca,* a shrub indigenous to South America, cocaine is well absorbed by any mucosal route and thus is abused when snorted, smoked (crack), or injected intravenously. Effects typically occur within 5 to 15 minutes and last 1 to 4 hours. The effects are primarily stimulant in nature and related to its effect on the sympathetic nervous system—increasing the release of norepinephrine and blocking its reuptake.[3,12] Concomitant use of cocaine with alcohol results in cocaethylene, a byproduct with a clinical effect lasting longer than cocaine's and with direct myocardial depressant effects. After cocaine use, patients may present with chest pain, focal weakness, or altered mental status and typically exhibit tachycardia, hypertension, hyperthermia, diaphoresis, and agitation. Because of the intensity of the sympathomimetic stimulation, medical complications such as acute coronary syndrome, seizures, cerebral vascular accidents, intracranial hemorrhage, renal failure, and rhabdomyolysis are common.[12,13] *Cocaine washout syndrome* occurs after cocaine binging. Affected patients typically have a depressed mental status ranging from lethargy to obtundation that lasts up to 24 hours until depleted neurotransmitters are regenerated.

■ DEXTROMETHORPHAN

Also known as DXM, dextromethorphan is a common antitussive agent found in over-the-counter and prescription medications in liquid or tablet form. It is a synthetic analogue of codeine but does not have the same analgesic effect because its activity is primarily at NMDA and serotonin (5-HT) receptors.[7,10] Hallucinations are commonly reported, and in addition to some opioid features, patients may exhibit ataxia, slurred speech, nystagmus, tachycardia, hypertension, dystonia, and seizures.

GAMMA-HYDROXYBUTYRATE

Gamma-hydroxybutyrate (GHB), also known as "Georgia Home Boy" and "liquid G," has been variously used as an exercise supplement, for treatment of narcolepsy, for obtaining chemical submission of victims, and for euphoria. GHB works primarily at GABA receptors and the still poorly defined GHB receptor.[14,15] The analogues gamma-butyrolactone (GBL), 1.4-butanediol (1,4-BD), gamma-hydroxyvalerate methyl-GHB (GHV), and gamma-valerolactone 4-pentanolide (GVL) work similarly because they are all converted to GHB via various pathways after ingestion. GHB easily crosses the blood-brain barrier and produces loss of consciousness within 15 to 30 minutes of ingestion. Bradycardia, vomiting, myoclonic jerks, and hypothermia are commonly associated. Duration of unconsciousness lasts 2 to 6 hours in most cases.[16]

JIMSONWEED

Jimsonweed is the common name of plants in the *Datura* genera. Intoxication with jimsonweed was first reported in 1676. The plants grow throughout the United States, and all parts of it—the fruit, flower, and seeds—can be abused for their hallucinogenic properties. Because these plants contains the alkaloids atropine, scopolamine, and hyoscyamine, clinical effects associated with jimsonweed hallucinations include anticholinergic findings such as dilated pupils, dry mouth, warm and flushed skin, diminished bowel sounds, and urinary retention. Cardiovascular instability, hyperthermia, and seizures have been reported in large ingestions.[17]

KETAMINE

Also known as "vitamin K," "kitty Valium," and "kiddie Valium," ketamine is a structural and functional analogue of phencyclidine (PCP) and also works primarily at NMDA receptors.[18] Ketamine can be ingested or injected. Patients with ketamine abuse have symptoms similar to those of PCP intoxication, including rotatory nystagmus, excessive salivation, muscle rigidity, tachycardia, and hypertension, although the effects tend to last a shorter time.[5,18]

LSD

D-Lysergic acid diethylamide (LSD) was first synthesized in 1938. It is available in tablets, liquid, powder, and gelatin squares, although the most commonly abused form of LSD is "blotter" acid (sheets of paper sprayed with LSD, dried, and then perforated into small squares). Effects occur within 30 minutes, can last for 16 to 24 hours, and cause powerful hallucinations from serotonergic (5-HT) and dopaminergic activity. Time is distorted, and visual hallucinations of bright colors are common. Tachycardia, hypertension, anxiety, and paranoia are common in ED patients who seek treatment as a result of LSD use. Significant medical complications are uncommon.[18]

MARIJUANA

Also known as "grass," "weed," or "pot," marijuana is considered the most commonly used illegal substance in the United States. Marijuana is primarily smoked; its effects occur within 15 minutes and can last up to 4 hours. The psychoactive substance, delta-9-tetrahydrocannabinol (THC), is derived from the plant *Cannabis sativa*.[3] Clinical effects are variable and seem to occur as a result of cannabinoid receptor activity in the brain. Inappropriate laughter, excessive hunger, anxiety, paranoia, ataxia, and tachycardia are commonly seen. Acute medical complications associated with marijuana abuse alone are uncommon.[19]

METHYLENEDIOXYMETHAMPHETAMINE

MDMA is better known as "Ecstasy," "X," "XTC," and "ADAM." It was first synthesized in 1914 but became wildly popular at rave parties and on college campuses in the 1980s and 1990s.[4,5] Although it is a phenylethylamine like amphetamine, MDMA's strong serotonergic activity has clinical effects that are primarily hallucinogenic and entactogenic in nature.[3] Variable tachycardia and hypertension can occur from some stimulant activity as well. Hyperthermia has been reported as a complication from excessive dancing in warm rave clubs without adequate hydration, although other individual variabilities and drug contaminants are also likely responsible.[5] Hyponatremia, another common occurrence with MDMA use, results from excessive ingestion of water or from MDMA-induced syndrome of inappropriate antidiuretic hormone secretion (SIADH).

METHAMPHETAMINE

Also known as "meth," "yaba," "chicken feed," and "white man's crank," methamphetamine has become one of the most popular drugs of abuse in the 21st century.[20,21] Its popularity is related to its multiple forms (crystal, powder, liquid, and tablet), its ease of manufacture from decongestants like pseudoephedrine, and its low street cost (less than one-third the cost of cocaine). Methamphetamine has strong norepinephrine activity and, of all the phenylethylamines, is the most quickly addictive owing to its strong dopaminergic action.[3] It can be ingested, snorted, smoked, injected, or administered rectally. Clinical findings are similar to those associated with other stimulant intoxications, and acute coronary syndrome and cerebrovascular accident have been reported. Other hallmark features of methamphetamine are poor dentition, known as "meth mouth," from poor hygiene and bruxism and dermatologic lesions called "crank bugs" or "meth mites," from compulsive scratching that is likely delusional in etiology.

■ OPIOIDS

Naturally occurring or synthetic drugs with opium-like or morphine-like activity have always been popular. The poppy plant, *Papaver somniferum,* is the source of opium and contains the alkaloids morphine and codeine. Opioid effects are primarily modulated throughout the peripheral and CNS by interacting at three main opioid receptors: μ, κ, and δ.[3] The classic opioid toxidrome comprises CNS depression, respiratory depression, and miosis, although the intensity of each of those features varies among the different synthetic opioids. Prehospital deaths typically occur from untreated apnea.[22] Abuse of prescription opioids continues to rise, and recent data indicate that the abuse of combination acetaminophen-opioid analgesics is directly related to rising rates of acetaminophen-induced hepatic failure.[23]

■ PHENCYCLIDINE

First made available in 1957, phencyclidine is also known as the "PeaCe Pill." PCP can be ingested, smoked, snorted, or injected. Effects occur within 15 minutes and may last 6 to 16 hours. PCP binds to NMDA receptors and works as a dissociate anesthetic.[24] PCP intoxication has a wide spectrum of features, and depending on the dose, CNS excitation or depression may predominate. Common findings are disorientation, violent behavior, muscle rigidity, facial grimacing, and rotatory nystagmus. Patients seeking ED care often have tachycardia, hypertension, and agitation, as with other stimulant drugs.[3,25]

■ PSILOCYBIN

Also known as "magic mushrooms," psilocybin-containing mushrooms are found in cow pastures and were first used for religious ceremonies and for extrasensory perception (ESP) effects by Mexican Indians. The most desired mushroom is the *Psilocybe cubensis*. Because psilocybin resembles 5-HT, it primarily affects serotonin receptors and causes psychedelic hallucinations similar to those with LSD within 15 minutes of ingestion.[18] Effects typically last 2 to 6 hours. Medical complications are uncommon, although flashbacks have been reported.

■ PRESCRIPTION MEDICATIONS

Nonmedical abuse of prescription drugs has now been identified as a national epidemic. In 2005, nearly 15 million Americans abused prescription drugs, including prescribed opioids, sedatives, antidepressants, and stimulants.[1] One of the reasons for the rapid rise of prescription drug abuse is the perception that they are safer than traditional street drugs. The growing rates of prescriptions written for analgesia, for mood disorders, and for attention deficit–hyperactivity disorder (ADHD) have resulted in experimentation with easily available tablets by the family members or friends of the person for whom the agents were prescribed.[9,11]

Differential Diagnosis

Drug intoxication should always be considered in the differential diagnosis of any patient presenting to the ED with altered mental status. Infectious, metabolic, neurologic, endocrinologic, structural, and psychogenic causes should also be considered in the evaluation of the patient with suspected drug intoxication. The history of events immediately preceding onset of symptoms, if available to the clinician from the patient or witnesses, is most helpful in narrowing the diagnosis.

Diagnostic Testing

Asymptomatic patients with drug intoxication who have normal vital signs and normal physical findings do not require diagnostic testing. Patients with mild symptoms should undergo a rapid blood glucose

Documentation

- Amount ingested?
- Route of ingestion (oral, intravenous, subcutaneous dermal, sublingual, rectal)?
- Time of ingestion?
- Co-ingestants?
- History of trauma?
- Previous ED visits for drug abuse?
- Previous detoxification or other treatment programs?
- Referral for counseling, treatment program, or detoxification

RED FLAGS

- An elevated temperature is prognostic of poor outcomes.
- Focal neurologic findings are indicative of seizure activity or intracranial lesion.
- Rhabdomyolysis can occur in cases of agitation or prolonged obtundation.
- Renal insufficiency or creatine phosphokinase (CPK) elevation requires adequate fluid resuscitation to prevent renal failure.

Table 144-3 DIAGNOSTIC TESTING FOR SUSPECTED RECREATIONAL DRUG USE

Test	Indication
Rapid blood glucose measurement	Altered mental status
Blood chemistry panel	MDMA (methylenedioxymethamphetamine) intoxication or suspected rhabdomyolysis
Serum acetaminophen measurement	Prescription opioid ingestion
Blood alcohol evaluation	Suspected co-ingestant
Serum creatine phosphokinase (total) measurement	Agitation or suspected rhabdomyolysis
Urinalysis	Suspected rhabdomyolysis
Liver function tests	Prescription opioid ingestion
Electrocardiogram	Tachycardia, bradycardia, or dysrhythmia
Computed tomography of the head	Suspected trauma or mental status inconsistent with reported ingestion

measurement, because hypoglycemia or hyperglycemia may cause altered mental status. An ethanol measurement should be obtained if alcohol is suspected as a co-ingestant or to exclude it as a cause of altered mental status. Patients who are agitated, hyperthermic, or seizing or were found after prolonged obtundation are all at risk for development of rhabdomyolysis and should be evaluated with a basic metabolic profile, renal function tests, measurements of calcium, phosphorus, total creatine phosphokinase (CPK) levels, and urinalysis.[25]

Electrocardiography should be performed in all patients with tachycardia or bradycardia, and telemetry monitoring should be instituted. Patients with altered mental status inconsistent with their reported drug use, new-onset seizure, or signs of traumatic injury or suspected trauma should be evaluated with computed tomography of the head (Table 144-3).

The toxicology drug screen has limited utility in the ED setting and should be used only for a patient in whom mental status is altered and the diagnosis is not clear. Several studies confirm that a careful patient history and attention to clinical signs make toxicology screens unnecessary in most cases of drug intoxication.[26,27] For instance, a patient with depressed respirations, depressed mental status, and pinpoint pupils consistent with an opioid toxidrome who completely awakes after the administration of naloxone does not need a costly urine drug screen to confirm opioid toxicity. Furthermore, it is impractical to wait for the results of a urine drug screen before administering lifesaving naloxone in cases of severe intoxication.

The drug screens available in most hospitals have a limited panel, and many of the nontraditional, emerging, and web-based drugs (including prescription medications and club drugs) cannot be detected by such hospital screens. Toxicology screens are limited by what they cannot detect, and they can yield false-positive results owing to contaminants. For instance, over-the-counter decongestants used appropriately for an upper respiratory infection can yield in a falsely positive amphetamine screen result, and quinolones can result in falsely positive opioid screen results.[28] Finally, urine drug screen results are not forensically defensible, because most hospitals analyze urine with only one laboratory technique, and the chain of custody is not enforced from patient to laboratory (Box 144-1).

BOX 144-1

Hospital Urine Drug Screen

- Has limited utility and is never diagnostic.
- Primary use should be for altered mental status and unclear diagnosis.
- Does not indicate time or dose of exposure, because it identifies only the presence of drug metabolites from use within the last 72 to 96 hours.
- Can result in false-positive results owing to contaminants or cross-reactant medicines.
- Does not identify most *new* drugs used today.
- Does not meet basic forensic standards.
- Treatment decisions should be guided by clinical evaluation and never by a drug screen result.

Treatment and Disposition

Because the clinical presentation of drug intoxication varies widely, optimal treatment must be *symptom-based.* Attempts to confirm identification of the drug should be postponed until the patient is stabilized. As with any ED patient, attention to airway management is the top priority in all patients with drug intoxication. Obtunded patients with a poor respiratory effort should receive either naloxone in an effort to reverse potential narcosis or dextrose and thiamine for hypoglycemia. Intubation should be performed for persistent hypoxemia or the inability to protect a patient's airway. Intravenous fluids should be administered to treat hypotension. Dysrhythmias

Tips and Tricks

- Attempts to confirm or identify the drug should be postponed until the patient is stabilized.
- Attention to airway management is the top priority in all cases of drug intoxication.
- Close monitoring of the patient's core temperature is critical, because an elevated temperature is the only vital sign abnormality consistently associated with poor outcomes in cases of drug intoxication.
- Physical restraints might be needed temporarily for patient and staff safety; chemical sedation with benzodiazepines must be given high priority in order to minimize the duration of potentially harmful physical restraints.
- Drug-induced hypertension and tachycardia should also be treated first with benzodiazepines in very liberal doses.

should be treated according to standard Advanced Cardiac Life Support (ACLS) guidelines. A thorough examination must be completed to exclude concomitant traumatic injuries that require emergency management.

Patients who are agitated or difficult to control should receive liberal benzodiazepine treatment for their own safety as well as staff safety and to ensure a complete examination. Butyrophenones, such as haloperidol, may be considered if benzodiazepines do not successfully control the difficult patient. Although physical restraints might have to be used temporarily for patient and staff safety, chemical sedation with benzodiazepines must be given top priority to minimize the duration of potentially harmful physical restraints.[29]

Drug-induced hypertension and tachycardia should also be treated first with benzodiazepines, because these clinical findings primarily result from direct stimulant effects and are effectively managed in most cases with liberal benzodiazepine sedation. Short-acting antihypertensive agents with minimal beta-blocker activity may be considered only after sufficient doses of benzodiazepines have been administered.

Hyperthermia must be aggressively treated with external cooling measures, and if the patient is agitated, with liberal benzodiazepine therapy as well. Close monitoring of the patient's core temperature is critical, because an elevated temperature is the only vital sign abnormality consistently associated with poor outcomes in cases of drug intoxication.[29]

Renal insufficiency or an elevated creatine phosphokinase value requires adequate fluid resuscitation. Drug-induced rhabdomyolysis results in renal failure and hemodialysis in 10% of patients hospitalized for drug intoxication and associated rhabdomyolysis.[25,29]

Disposition

Most patients with single-drug intoxication have improved and can be safely discharged after 4 to 6 hours of ED observation. In patients with multiple drug ingestion, prolonged clinical effects from long-acting agents like methadone, or medical complications, admission to a monitored hospital bed is appropriate. Attention to signs of withdrawal is important before such a patient is discharged. Whether being discharged from the ED or from an inpatient bed, all patients with drug intoxication require substance abuse counseling and referral for support groups, detoxification, and other outpatient treatment.[30]

REFERENCES

1. Cherpital CJ: Trends in alcohol- and drug-related ER and primary care visits, 1995-2000: Are Healthy People 2000 objectives met? Am J Addict 2005;14:281-290.
2. Banken JA: Drug abuse trends among youth in the United States. Ann N Y Acad Sci 2004;1025:465-471.
3. Cami J, Farre M: Drug addiction. N Engl J Med 2003;349:975-986.
4. Patel MM, Wright DW, Ratcliff JJ, Miller MA: Shedding new light on the "safe" club drug: Methylenedioxymethamphetamine. Acad Emerg Med 2004;11:208-210.
5. Tong T, Boyer EW: Club drugs, smart drugs, raves, and circuit parties: An overview of the club scene. Pediatr Emerg Care 2002;18:216-218.
6. Wax PM: Just a click away: Recreational drug Web sites on the Internet. Pediatrics 2002;109:e96.
7. Nordt SP: "DXM": A new drug of abuse? Ann Emerg Med 1998;31:794-795.
8. Simoni-Wastila L, Strickler G: Risk factors associated with problem use of prescription drugs. Am J Public Health 2004;94:266-268.
9. McCabe SE, Teter CJ, Boyd CJ: The use, misuse and diversion of prescription stimulants among middle and high school students. Subst Use Misuse 2004;39:1095-1116.
10. Kirages TJ, Sule HP, Mycyk MB: Severe manifestations of Coricidin intoxication. Am J Emerg Med 2003;21: 473-475.
11. Anderson BB, Mycyk MB, DesLauriers C: Hospitalization for methylphenidate abuse is associated with concomitant abuse of other pharmaceutical products. Ann Emerg Med 2005;46:S78.
12. Lange RA, Hillis LD: Cardiovascular complications of cocaine use. N Engl J Med 2001;345:351-358.
13. Weber JE, Chudnofsky CR, Boczar M, et al: Cocaine-associated chest pain: How common is myocardial infarction? Acad Emerg Med 2000;7:873-877.
14. Li J, Stokes SA, Woeckener A: A tale of novel intoxication: A review of the effects of gamma-hydroxybutyric acid with recommendations for management. Ann Emerg Med 1998;31:729-736.
15. Zvosec DL, Smith SW, McCutcheon JR, et al: Adverse events, including death, associated with the use of 1,4-butanediol. N Engl J Med 2001;344:87-94.
16. Wong CG, Gibson KM, Snead OC 3rd: From the street to the brain: Neurobiology of the recreational drug gamma-hydroxybutyric acid. Trends Pharmacol Sci 2004;25: 29-34.
17. Boumba VA, Mitselou A, Vougiouklakis T: Fatal poisoning from ingestion of *Datura stramonium* seeds. Vet Hum Toxicol 2004;46:81-82.
18. McCambridge J, Winstock A, Hunt N, Mitcheson L: 5-Year trends in use of hallucinogens and other adjunct drugs among UK dance drug users. Eur Addict Res 2007; 13:57-64.

19. Gerberich SG, Sidney S, Braun BL, et al: Marijuana use and injury events resulting in hospitalization. Ann Epidemiol 2003;13:230-237.
20. Richards JR, Johnson EB, Stark RW, Derlet RW: Methamphetamine abuse and rhabdomyolysis in the ED: A 5-year study. Amer J Emerg Med 1999;17:681-685.
21. Tominaga GT, Garcia G, Dzierba A, Wong J: Toll of methamphetamine on the trauma system. Arch Surg 2004; 139:844-847.
22. Sporer KA: Acute heroin overdose. Ann Intern Med 1999;130:584-590.
23. Larson AM, Polson J, Fontana RJ, et al: Acetaminophen-induced acute liver failure: Results of a United States multicenter, prospective study. Hepatology 2005;42: 1364-1372.
24. McCarron MM, Schulze BW, Thompson GA, et al: Acute phencyclidine intoxication: Clinical patterns, complications, treatment. Ann Emerg Med 1981;10:290-297.
25. Curry SC, Chang D, Connor D: Drug- and toxin-induced rhabdomyolysis. Ann Emerg Med 1989;18:1068-1084.
26. Belson MG, Simon HK, Sullivan K, Geller RJ: The utility of toxicologic analysis in children with suspected ingestions. Pediatr Emerg Care 1999;15:383-387.
27. Langdorf MI, Rudkin SE, Dellota K, et al: Decision rule and utility of routine urine toxicology screening of trauma patients. Eur J Emerg Med 2002;9:115-121.
28. Baden LR, Horowitz G, Jacoby H, Eliopoulos GM: Quinolones and false-positive urine screening for opiates by immunoassay technology. JAMA 2001;286:3115-3119.
29. Roth D, Alarcon FJ, Fernandez JA, et al: Acute rhabdomyolysis associated with cocaine intoxication. N Engl J Med 1988;319:673-677.
30. Rockett IR, Putnam SL, Jia H, et al: Unmet substance abuse treatment need, health services utilization, and cost: A population-based emergency department study. Ann Emerg Med 2005;45:118-127.

Chapter **145**

Toxic Alcohols

Mark B. Mycyk

KEY POINTS
Toxic alcohol poisoning may initially be mistaken for simple inebriation.
Untreated ethylene glycol poisoning may result in renal failure.
Untreated methanol poisoning may result in blindness.
Acidemia from ethylene glycol or methanol may not be evident until several hours after exposure.
An osmol gap may not be evident in patients whose ED presentation is delayed.
An osmol gap measurement is only a screening test and is never diagnostic like a quantitative alcohol measurement.
Isopropanol poisoning classically results in an enlarged osmol gap without significant acidemia.
Treatment with ethanol or fomepizole should be considered in cases of a witnessed ingestion of a toxic alcohol, when such an ingestion is highly suspected from the history, in the presence of an enlarged osmol gap alone with appropriate clinical suspicion, in the patient with both an enlarged osmol gap and an anion gap acidosis, or when the serum concentration of a toxic alcohol exceeds 20 mg/dL.
Early alcohol dehydrogenase (ADH) inhibition minimizes metabolism of the toxic alcohol to organic toxic acids and reduces alcohol-specific complications.

Scope

Except for ethanol, no alcohols are fit for human consumption and are properly termed *toxic alcohols*. Ethylene glycol, methanol, and isopropanol are the most common toxic alcohols associated with human poisoning.[1] Less commonly reported but still clinically important toxic alcohols are propylene glycol, diethylene glycol, and other glycol ethers. Unintentional ingestion from a mislabeled or contaminated container occurs commonly in children, whereas intentional ingestion of a toxic alcohol as an ethanol substitute or for self-harm occurs more commonly in adults. If untreated, toxic alcohol poisoning can result in metabolic acidosis, renal failure, blindness, central nervous system (CNS) injury, pulmonary edema, or death.

Ethylene glycol is present in antifreeze solutions, deicing solutions, foam stabilizers, and chemical solvents.[2] Methanol is a component of windshield-washing solutions, gas-line antifreeze solutions, solvents, and brake cleaners.[3] Isopropanol is found in rubbing alcohol, aerosols, and other cosmetic products. Propylene glycol is commonly found as a diluent in parenteral medications such as phenytoin, diazepam, and lorazepam.[4] The other toxic glycols can be found in various household and industrial cleaners, paints, resins, and solvents.

More than 35,000 toxic alcohol exposures are reported yearly to the American Association of Poison Control Centers (AAPCC).[1] Most cases are individual poisonings. However, contamination of beverages or pharmaceutical products has resulted in epidemic poisonings, including two significant outbreaks, in India and in Haiti in the 1990s, from diethylene glycol that affected hundreds of victims.[5]

Definitive laboratory confirmation of toxic alcohol poisoning is usually not immediately available to the EP; however, early recognition of poisoning and ED-initiated interventions significantly improve patient outcomes and reduce the occurrence of alcohol-specific complications.[6]

Pathophysiology

Most toxic alcohol poisonings occur by oral ingestion. Significant methanol poisoning has also been reported to occur with inhalation of brake cleaning products, and isopropanol poisoning has occurred through transcutaneous absorption in children treated for fevers at home with rubbing alcohol baths.[7,8] Complete absorption is rapid by any route, each alcohol has a small volume of distribution (0.5 to 0.8 L/kg), and metabolism to toxic organic byproducts occurs via hepatic alcohol dehydrogenase (ADH) (Figs. 145-1 and 145-2).

Toxicity from the parent products is limited to local mucous membrane irritation and CNS depression. The term *toxic* is specifically related to the production of different toxic byproducts (oxalic acid and formic acid) by each of these alcohols. Ethylene glycol metabolism results in renal failure from deposition of oxalic acid in renal tubules.[2] Methanol metabolism to formic acid results in blindness from direct injury to the retinal and optic nerves.[3]

Because the rate of metabolism via ADH varies by alcohol type and by individual variability in cytochrome P-450 genetic expression, clinical onset of worrisome symptoms can be delayed by 1 to 36 hours.[2,3] Furthermore, the concomitant presence of ethanol may delay metabolism to the toxic byproducts, because ethanol has a higher affinity for ADH than the toxic alcohols and will competitively inhibit metabolism of these alcohols to toxic byproducts until the serum ethanol concentration drops well below 100 mg/dL.

Isopropanol is unlike ethylene glycol and methanol, in that it is not metabolized to an organic acid; instead, it is metabolized to acetone, an osmotically active CNS depressant, leading to profound inebriation (Fig. 145-3).[8]

Presenting Signs and Symptoms

■ CLASSIC OR TYPICAL

Most patients poisoned with a toxic alcohol demonstrate some level of CNS depression consistent with inebriation (Table 145-1). Patients who arrive in the ED either shortly after a large ingestion or later after an ingestion so that systemic accumulation of toxic metabolites has occurred may be obtunded on presentation or may become obtunded during ED evaluation. The level of inebriation does not correlate with peak serum concentrations of the parent product or the accumulation of metabolic byproducts.

Other clinical findings range from mild to life-threatening, depending on the type of alcohol and

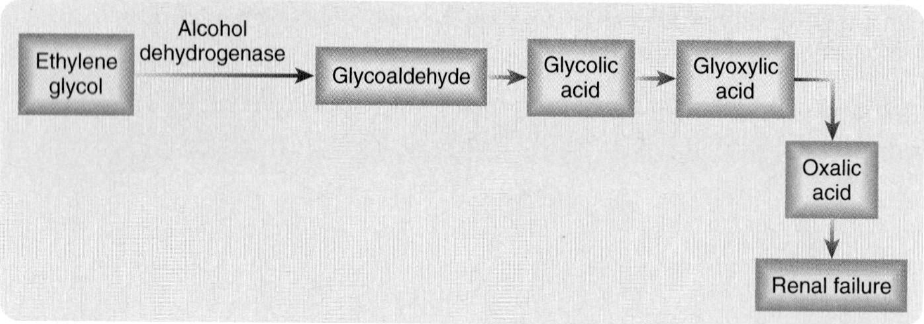
Ethylene glycol
Alcohol dehydrogenase
Glycoaldehyde
Glycolic acid
Glyoxylic acid
Oxalic acid
Renal failure

FIGURE 145-1 Ethylene glycol metabolism pathway.

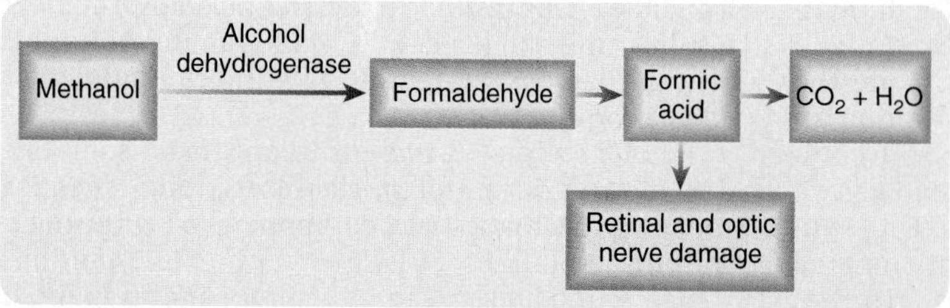
Methanol
Alcohol dehydrogenase
Formaldehyde
Formic acid
$CO_2 + H_2O$
Retinal and optic nerve damage

FIGURE 145-2 Methanol metabolism pathway.

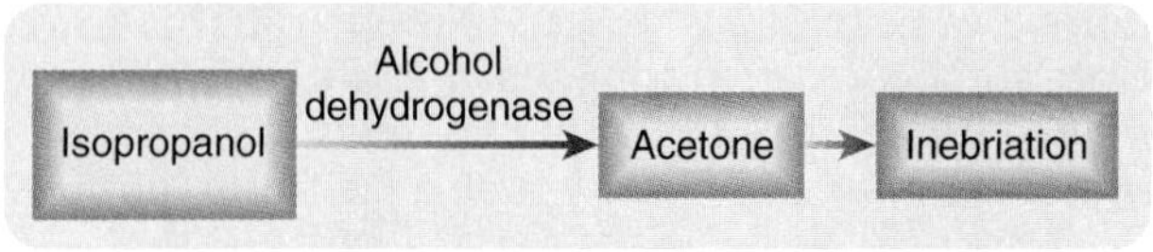
Isopropanol
Alcohol dehydrogenase
Acetone
Inebriation

FIGURE 145-3 Isopropanol metabolism pathway.

Table 145-1 SYMPTOMS AND SIGNS OF TOXIC ALCOHOL POISONING

Symptoms	Altered mental status
	Headache
	Nausea
	Vomiting
	Abdominal pain
	Weakness
	Unsteady gait
	Visual blurring
	Skin flushing
Signs	Hypotension
	Tachycardia
	Dysrhythmias
	Hyperventilation
	Hypoventilation
	Hypothermia
	Nystagmus
	Sluggish pupils
	Hyperemic optic disc
	Seizures
	Coma

BOX 145-1

Metabolic Acidosis with Elevated Anion Gap—"A CAT MUD PILES"

- Alcoholic ketoacidosis
- Cyanide, carbon monoxide
- Alcohol
- Toluene
- Methanol, metformin
- Uremia
- Diabetic ketoacidosis
- Paraldehyde
- Iron, isoniazid
- Lactic acidosis
- Ethylene glycol
- Salicylates, strychnine

the dose consumed. Because the clinical toxicity from these alcohols results from the accumulation of specific toxic metabolites, some patients might appear relatively asymptomatic before the manifestation of significant symptoms. Hypotension with a reflex tachycardia is common in significant ingestions because of the vasodilatory effects common to all alcohols. In patients with ethylene glycol or methanol poisoning, routine laboratory analysis classically shows an anion gap metabolic acidosis and an enlarged osmol gap. Patients with an isopropanol poisoning typically have only an enlarged osmol gap, because isopropanol is not metabolized to any organic acids. Patients poisoned with the other toxic alcohols have acidosis of varying degrees and inconsistently demonstrate an enlarged osmol gap.

■ TYPICAL VARIATIONS

Ethylene glycol poisoning that progresses to significant organic acid accumulation can cause Kussmaul's respirations from severe acidosis, cerebral edema, and seizures. Multiple reports have described various self-limited cranial nerve palsies associated with ethylene glycol. Tubular necrosis from local oxalate deposition and renal failure are common. Because oxalic acid precipitates calcium, dysrhythmias and tetanic spasms secondary to hypocalcemia have been reported.

Metabolism of methanol to formic acid gives rise primarily to neurologic and ophthalmologic findings. Patients who are not obtunded may have a severe headache, vomiting, dizziness, and amnesia. Cerebral edema, necrosis, and infarcts have been identified on intracranial imaging. Visual disturbances range from simple blurring to "snowstorm" vision to blindness. Worrisome eye findings include sluggish nonreactive pupils, papilledema, hyperemic optic disc, and retinal edema.

Isopropanol is associated with fruity breath odor from acetone accumulation and CNS depression that is reportedly two to four times more profound than would be expected from an equivalent dose of ethanol. Vomiting and hemorrhagic gastritis have also been reported in patients with isopropanol ingestion.

Propylene glycol is metabolized to lactic acid: This poisoning typically occurs iatrogenically from the diluent present in parenteral medications like phenytoin and various benzodiazepines. Accumulated lactate in these cases has been associated with profound hypotension and cardiac dysrhythmias.

Diethylene glycol and the other butyl ethers have been associated with renal tubular necrosis, hepatitis, and pancreatitis.

Differential Diagnosis

The differential diagnosis mnemonic "A CAT MUD PILES" should be used for any patient in whom ED evaluation demonstrates an anion gap acidosis (Box 145-1). Many of the possible conditions in the list can be easily excluded with a basic metabolic profile (e.g., uremia) and rapidly obtainable serum quantitative tests (e.g., salicylate). Although alcoholic ketoacidosis looks like toxic alcohol poisoning, it improves rapidly with only intravenous fluids and dextrose supplementation, whereas acidosis from a significant toxic alcohol exposure does not improve without antidotal treatment and/or enhanced elimination with hemodialysis. In children, disorders of organic acid metabolism should be considered when poisoning is unlikely or has been excluded.

Diagnostic Testing

Laboratory testing in all patients with potential poisoning should include a basic metabolic profile to determine baseline renal function and acid-base status and to calculate the anion gap and osmol gap. In calculation of the osmol gap, it is important that the measured osmolality be obtained at the same time as the basic metabolic panel (see "Facts and Formulas" box). The osmol gap value should be interpreted with caution. The traditionally accepted normal value for an osmol gap is less than 10 mOsm/L. Unfortunately, an individual's normal gap may range between −14 and +10 mOsm/L, so the osmol gap by itself is imperfect and not entirely diagnostic.[9,10]

Additional serum tests include (1) an ethanol measurement to enable accurate calculation of the osmol gap and determination of the need for additional ADH inhibition, and (2) measurement of the calcium level, which can be depressed in cases of ethylene glycol poisoning and may lead to prolonged QT, cardiac dysrhythmias, and tetany. Arterial blood gas measurements should also be obtained to determine the level of acidosis.

Urinalysis should be performed to look for crystals: Monohydrate (spindle-like) or dihydrate crystals

FACTS AND FORMULAS

$SI = \frac{SV}{BSA}$

ANION GAP

- Anion gap = $Na^+ - (HCO_3 + Cl^-)$ [normal anion gap = 8-12 mEq/L]
- Osmol gap = measured osmols—calculated osmols
- Calculated osmols = ($2Na^+BUN/2.8$ + glucose/18 + ethanol/4.6) [normal osmol gap <10 mEq/L]

RED FLAGS

- Urinalysis: The absence of crystals or fluorescence does *not* exclude poisoning.
- The absence of an osmol gap in patients with severe acidosis does *not* exclude toxic alcohol poisoning; it may be the result of a delayed presentation.
- The absence of an anion gap in patients who present early does *not* exclude toxic alcohol poisoning.
- Be prepared to have definitive laboratory confirmation delayed by 8 to 24 hours, depending on the individual hospital's access to an outside reference laboratory. Empirical treatment should be started if indicated.
- Renal specialists should be consulted early to prevent complications.
- Be wary of the potential for hypoglycemia in patients being treated with intravenous ethanol.
- *Do not* give ethanol with fomepizole—both agents compete for alcohol dehydrogenose and their use together may result in reduced antidotal effectiveness.
- Because metabolism varies by alcohol type and by individual variability, clinical onset of symptoms can be delayed by 1 to 36 hours.

Documentation

History

- Any history of psychiatric illness or prior suicide ingestions.
- Time lapse since ingestion if known.
- History of renal or cardiac disease or other illnesses that will exacerbate the complications of toxic alcohols.

Physical Examination

- Does the patient look ill? Pale? Febrile? Mental status? Cardiac status (blood pressure, arrhythmias)?
- Respiratory and airway status.
- Visual acuity if there is concern for methanol poisoning.
- Urine output.
- Examination should be repeated while patient is in the ED.

Studies

- Laboratory tests and time the samples were obtained (serum osmol should be done at the same time as blood chemistry panel).
- Availability of toxic alcohol levels.

Medical Decision-Making

- Decision to begin treatment or delays.
- Consultations and times that contacts were made.

Treatment

- Availability of antidotes, time antidote was ordered, and any delays to treatment.

Patient Instructions

- Document discussion with patient regarding diagnosis, warning signs, what to do, follow-up, and when to return.
- With accidental ingestions in children, document poison prevention counseling.

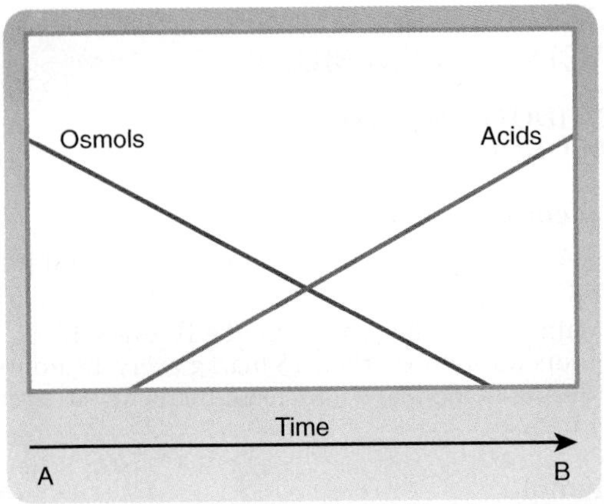
Osmols
Acids
Time
A
B

FIGURE 145-4 Mountain schematic. **A,** Patients who present early may have elevated osmols without an anion gap. **B,** Patients who present late may have an elevated anion gap without an elevation of osmol gap.

(envelope shaped) are present in 50% to 60% of cases of ethylene glycol poisoning and are suggestive of significant poisoning. However, the absence of these crystals does not reliably exclude poisoning. Some authorities have suggested examining the urine under a Wood's lamp for fluorescence, because antifreeze is commonly mixed with fluorescein. Unfortunately, urine may fluoresce in the presence or absence of ethylene glycol, so this maneuver has limited clinical utility.[11]

Although most clinicians are comfortable with considering ethylene glycol or methanol poisoning in patients with a concomitant anion gap acidosis and enlarged osmol gap, many patients do not arrive with those classic findings, and delays to definitive diagnosis and treatment are common.[6,12] Ethylene glycol and methanol are osmotically active and contribute to the enlarged osmol gap; the toxic metabolites are minimally osmotically active and primarily contribute to the anion gap. The Mountain Schematic is useful in helping one understand the time course of an acidosis and osmol gap without needing to memorize the kinetics of each intermediate step (Fig. 145-4).[12]

■ THE EARLY ARRIVAL

In a patient who arrives immediately after ingestion, as commonly occurs in children with an unintentional ingestion, an anion gap acid acidosis will not be present until enough time has elapsed for the parent product to be metabolized through ADH to produce laboratory evidence of acidosis. An enlarged osmol gap might be the only clue to potentially significant poisoning early after ingestion. In these cases, ADH inhibition with ethanol or fomepizole should be considered before acidosis develops (see Fig. 145-4A).

■ THE LATE ARRIVAL

In a patient who arrives with severe symptoms and significantly after ingestion, an abnormal osmol gap might not be present any longer despite a profound acidosis and other clinical findings suggestive of a treatable toxic alcohol (e.g., visual disturbances in methanol or renal failure in ethylene glycol). In these cases, the parent product has already been metabolized to the toxic organic acids via ADH, so the osmotically active parent product no longer contributes significantly to the osmol gap. The benefit of an ADH inhibitor (ethanol or fomepizole) in these cases is less important than the benefit achieved from rapid hemodialysis and cofactor supplementation (see Fig. 145-4B).

Although ED clinical decisions depend mostly on clinical suspicion and interpretation of imperfect laboratory data like the anion gap, osmol gap, and urinalysis, cases of suspected toxic alcohol poisoning require that measurements of serum concentrations of ethylene glycol, methanol, and isopropanol be ordered as soon as possible. These measurements are the only definitive means of confirming the diagnosis and guiding duration of both antidotal therapy and hemodialysis. Unfortunately, most hospital laboratories are not equipped to run these tests and need to send the specimens to an off-site reference laboratory.[12] Except in cases in which the patient arrives with the appropriately labeled product that was ingested in hand, a practical strategy is to initially order serum concentration measurements of all three of these alcohols, because patients often do not know exactly what they ingested. It is also important to confirm the units of measure when these results are available, because different laboratories use different units, and management decisions may be significantly affected if test results are interpreted incorrectly. Serum concentration measurements for toxic alcohols other than ethylene glycol, methanol, and isopropanol are not routinely available; even if obtainable, their results do not guide management decisions.[13]

In cases of ethylene glycol poisoning, baseline electrocardiography (ECG) should also be obtained because of the potential for dysrhythmias due to hypocalcemia.

Treatment

Treatment decision-making for the patient with toxic alcohol ingestion is easiest when the patient arrives with the ingested product in hand. Because this is an uncommon occurrence, definitive laboratory diagnosis is usually delayed by the need to send serum samples to off-site reference laboratories.[6,12] ED treatment in these cases should not be delayed and must be based on a presumptive clinical diagnosis. Attention to the airway in cases of CNS depression should be the first priority. Intravenous fluids should be administered to treat hypotension and maintain renal perfusion in all cases of toxic alcohol poisoning.

Tips and Tricks

- Consult your local poison center: 800-222-1222.
- Consult your local toxicologist.
- Refer to the Mountain Schematic (see Fig. 145-4) to help interpret anion gap and osmol gap results.
- If long delays until definitive laboratory confirmation of the ingested substance are expected, consider repeating the basic metabolic profile or measure arterial blood gases.
- If alcohol dehydrogenase (ADH) has not been blocked by ethanol or fomepizole, acidosis should worsen despite standard intravenous fluid resuscitation if ethylene glycol or methanol is present.
- Treatment difficulties associated with ethanol therapy are (1) iatrogenic inebriation and inability to monitor mental status, (2) potential occurrence of hypoglycemia in children, and (3) difficulty maintaining a therapeutic level because of individual variability in ethanol metabolism and clearance.

■ GASTRIC DECONTAMINATION

Because alcohols are so rapidly absorbed, there is no need to perform gastric emptying procedures in patients with toxic alcohol poisoning.

■ ANTIDOTE

In cases of suspected ethylene glycol or methanol poisoning, immediate ADH inhibition should be considered to block continued metabolism of the ethylene glycol to toxic acids.[6] ADH inhibition is most effective when administered as early as possible after exposure and before significant acidosis develops.[12] This treatment should be considered in cases of a witnessed ingestion, when this agent is highly suspected from the history, in the presence of an elevated osmol gap alone with appropriate clinical suspicion, in the patient with both an elevated osmol gap and an anion gap acidosis, or when the serum concentration of a toxic alcohol exceeds 20 mg/dL.

ADH inhibition can be achieved with either ethanol or fomepizole.[2,3] Until recently, ethanol was the only clinically available antidote. Its affinity for ADH is higher than that of ethylene glycol and methanol, it is inexpensive, and it is readily available. An ethanol level of 100 mg/dL has been the accepted goal for ensuring complete ADH inhibition; after IV loading, ethanol levels must be checked regularly until the measured ethylene glycol or methanol concentration is lower than 20 mg/dL. An ethanol load may be administered orally or with an IV infusion (see "Facts and Formulas" box). Treatment difficulties associated with ethanol therapy include (1) iatrogenic inebriation of the patient and inability to monitor mental status, (2) potential occurrence of hypoglycemia in pediatric patients, and (3) difficulty maintaining a therapeutic level because of individual variability in ethanol metabolism and clearance.[14]

Use of fomepizole, which was approved by the U.S. Food and Drug Administration (FDA) in 1999, is an easier form of ADH inhibition than use of ethanol.[15-17] Dosing is weight based and does not require a constant infusion like an ethanol drip (see "Facts and Formulas" box). Fomepizole is given every 12 hours in patients not receiving hemodialysis or every 4 hours in patients undergoing hemodialysis, does not cause inebriation, and does not require monitoring of serum levels to ascertain therapeutic efficacy.[14] Fomepizole should not be given in cases in which ethanol is significantly elevated, because ethanol works as an ADH inhibitor and fomepizole's higher affinity for ADH will prolong the half-life and the clinical inebriation by the ethanol. Fomepizole is not available in all hospitals because of its high cost.[6]

FACTS AND FORMULAS

ANTIDOTES FOR TOXIC ALCOHOLS

Fomepizole

- Loading dose: 15 mg/kg intravenously (IV) (up to 1 g)
- Maintenance therapy: 10 mg/kg IV every 12 hours for 4 doses, then 15 mg/kg every 12 hours (during hemodialysis, increase frequency to every 4 hours)

Ethanol

Goal: Maintain ethanol level of 100-150 mg/dL until ethylene glycol or methanol level is <20 mg/dL, pH normalizes, and patient is asymptomatic.

- 5% solution: 15 mL/kg IV load, then 2-4 mL/kg/hr
- 10% solution: 7.5 mL/kg IV load, then 1-2 mL/kg/hr
- 50% solution: 2 mL/kg oral load, then 0.2-0.4 mL/kg/hr

Cofactor Supplementation

- Folate: 50 mg (IV) every 6 hours until acidemia resolves (methanol only)
- Thiamine: 100 mg IV every 6 hours until acidemia resolves (ethylene glycol only)
- Pyridoxine: 50 mg IV every 6 hours until acidemia resolves (ethylene glycol only)

■ SODIUM BICARBONATE

In cases of poisoning with any of the toxic alcohols, the addition of sodium bicarbonate infusion should be initiated when acidosis is severe. Alkalinization of

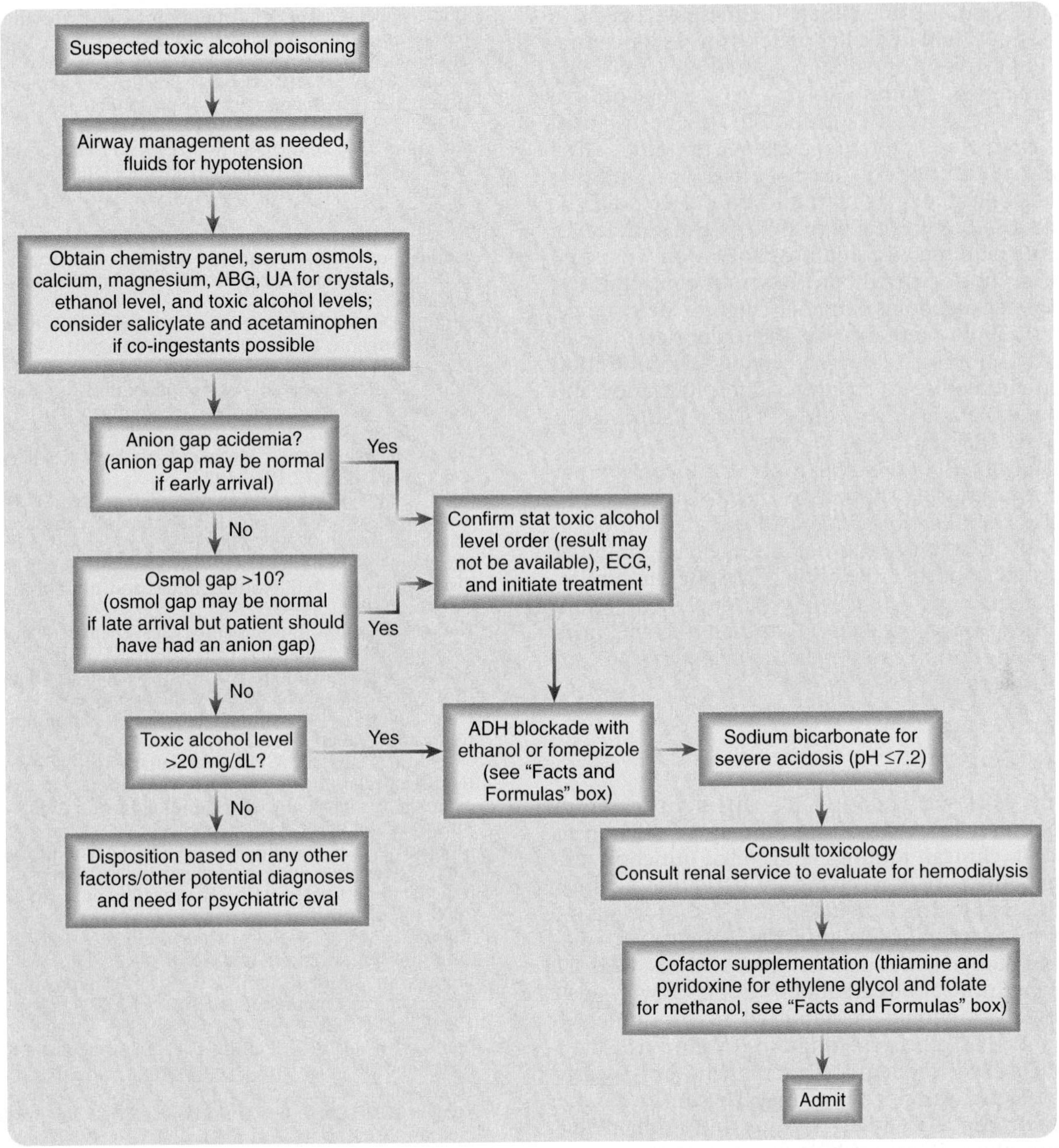
Suspected toxic alcohol poisoning
Airway management as needed, fluids for hypotension
Obtain chemistry panel, serum osmols, calcium, magnesium, ABG, UA for crystals, ethanol level, and toxic alcohol levels; consider salicylate and acetaminophen if co-ingestants possible
Anion gap acidemia? (anion gap may be normal if early arrival)
Yes
No
Confirm stat toxic alcohol level order (result may not be available), ECG, and initiate treatment
Osmol gap >10? (osmol gap may be normal if late arrival but patient should have had an anion gap)
Yes
No
Toxic alcohol level >20 mg/dL?
Yes
No
ADH blockade with ethanol or fomepizole (see "Facts and Formulas" box)
Sodium bicarbonate for severe acidosis (pH ≤7.2)
Disposition based on any other factors/other potential diagnoses and need for psychiatric eval
Consult toxicology
Consult renal service to evaluate for hemodialysis
Cofactor supplementation (thiamine and pyridoxine for ethylene glycol and folate for methanol, see "Facts and Formulas" box)
Admit

FIGURE 145-5 Treatment algorithm for toxic alcohol poisoning. ABG, arterial blood gas measurements; ECG, electrocardiography; UA, urinalysis.

serum is helpful in keeping acids in their ionic form. In patients with methanol poisoning, alkalinization of serum enhances the renal clearance of formate and may prevent formic acid from entering the CNS and affecting the optic nerves.

■ COFACTOR THERAPY

In cases of ethylene glycol poisoning, supplemental thiamine and pyridoxine should be administered to decrease the accumulation of oxalic acid (see "Facts and Formulas" box). In cases of methanol poisoning, supplemental folate should be given to enhance the elimination of formate by converting it to CO_2 and water. Although this approach is theoretically beneficial and has been found to be useful in some animal models, no human data demonstrate a clear benefit of cofactor administration.

■ ENHANCED ELIMINATION

Hemodialysis should be initiated in any patient with a significant ethylene glycol or methanol concentration and significant acidosis, because it will help remove both the parent product and the resultant toxic acids.[18-20] When a serum concentration is not immediately available, hemodialysis should be initiated in patients with clinical indicators of significant toxicity, such as pH less than 7.30 despite aggressive intravenous fluid resuscitation, creatinine concentration indicative of renal failure, or other electrolyte abnormalities unresponsive to conventional therapy.[2,3,18] Hemodialysis should also be initiated soon after presentation in patients in whom ADH inhibition cannot be used because of antidote unavailability or a contraindication. Hemodialysis should also be considered to shorten the duration of antidote requirements and hospitalization when acidosis has not occurred but the serum concentration of the toxic alcohol is extremely high.[18] For instance, the half-life of methanol has been reported to be as long as 54 hours in patients receiving ADH inhibition and might require several days of hospitalization and antidotal therapy if hemodialysis is not performed as well (Fig. 145-5).

Management of the other toxic alcohol poisonings requires aggressive supportive therapy, attention to medical complications from acidosis, and hemodialysis only if significant renal insufficiency or other electrolyte abnormalities occur.[13] Despite the similarity of its name to ethylene glycol, diethylene glycol does not produce oxalic acid, and any benefit from ADH inhibition in cases of diethylene glycol poisoning is uncertain.[21]

Disposition

Patients without acidosis and with a toxic serum alcohol level less than 20 mg/dL may be discharged home if clinical findings and renal function are normal. Any patient receiving an ADH antidote must be admitted to the hospital until a definitive serum alcohol concentration is available. Patients with significant mental status depression or acidosis, who are receiving intravenous ethanol infusion, or who need hemodialysis should be admitted to the intensive care unit (ICU), because laboratory values will have to be checked frequently. Patients who arrive early after a significant ingestion may be considered for treatment in a non-ICU setting with fomepizole therapy alone if no acidosis was detected prior to administration of the antidote.

In cases of intentional ingestion, appropriate psychiatric evaluation is warranted after the patient's medical issues are treated. In cases of unintentional poisoning, especially in children, appropriate poison prevention counseling for all caregivers is required before discharge.[22]

REFERENCES

1. Lai MW, Klein-Schwartz W, Rodgers GC, Abrams et al: 2005 Annual report of the American Association of Poison Control Centers' national poisoning and exposure database. Clin Toxicol 2006;44:803-932.
2. Barceloux DG, Krenzelok EP, Olson K, et al: American Academy of Clinical Toxicology Practice Guidelines on the treatment of ethylene glycol poisoning. Clin Toxicol 1999;37:537-560.
3. Barceloux DG, Bond GR, Krenzelok EP, et al: American Academy of Clinical Toxicology Practice Guidelines on the treatment of methanol poisoning. Clin Toxicol 2002;40:415-446.
4. Barnes BJ, Gerst C, Smith JR, et al: Osmol gap as a surrogate marker for serum propylene glycol concentrations in patients receiving lorazepam for sedation. Pharmacotherapy 2006;26:23-33.
5. Singh J, Dutta AK, Khare S, et al: Diethylene glycol poisoning in Gurgaon, India, 1998. Bull WHO 2001;79:88-95.
6. Mycyk MB, DesLauriers C, Metz J, et al: Compliance with poison center fomepizole recommendations is suboptimal in cases of toxic alcohol poisoning. Am J Ther 2006;13:485-489.
7. Frenia ML, Schauben JL: Methanol inhalation toxicity. Ann Emerg Med 1993;22:1919-1923.
8. Dyer S, Mycyk MB, Ahrens WR, Zell-Kanter M: Hemorrhagic gastritis from topical isopropanol exposure. Ann Pharmacother 2002;36:1733-1735.
9. Hoffman RS, Smilkstein MJ, Howland MA, Goldfrank LR: Osmol gaps revisted: Normal values and limitations. Clin Toxicol 1993;31:81-93.
10. Krahn J, Khajuria A: Osmolality gaps: Diagnostic accuracy and long-term variability. Clin Chem 2006;52:737-739.
11. Wallace KL, Suchard JR, Curry SC, Reagan C: Diagnostic use of physicians' detection of urine fluorescence in a simulated ingestion of sodium fluorescein–containing antifreeze. Ann Emerg Med 2001;38:49-54.
12. Mycyk MB, Aks SE: A visual schematic for clarifying the temporal relationship between the anion gap and the osmol gap in cases of toxic alcohol poisoning. Am J Emerg Med 2003;21:333-335.
13. McKinney PE, Palmer RB, Blackwell W, Benson BE: Butoxyethanol ingestion with prolonged hyperchloremic metabolic acidosis treated with ethanol therapy. Clin Toxicol 2000;38:787-793.
14. Shannon M: Toxicology reviews: Fomepizole—a new antidote. Pediatr Emerg Care 1998;14:170-172.
15. Brent J, McMartin K, Phillips S, et al: Fomepizole for the treatment of methanol poisoning. N Engl J Med 1999;340:832-838.
16. Brent J, McMartin K, Phillips S, et al: Fomepizole for the treatment of methanol poisoning. N Engl J Med 2001;344:424-429.
17. Mycyk MB, Leikin JB: Antidote review: Fomepizole for methanol poisoning. Am J Ther 2003;10:68-70.
18. Rydel JJ, Carlson A, Sharma J, Leikin J: An approach to dialysis for ethylene glycol intoxication. Vet Hum Toxicol 2002;44:36-39.
19. Moreau CL, Kerns W, Tomaszewski CA, et al: Glycolate kinetics and hemodialysis clearance in ethylene glycol poisoning. Clin Toxicol 1998;36:659-666.
20. Poldelski V, Johnson A, Wright S, et al: Ethylene glycol–mediated tubular injury: Identification of critical metabolites and injury pathways. Am J Kidney Dis 2001;38: 339-348.
21. Alfred S, Coleman P, Harris D, et al: Delayed neurologic sequelae resulting from epidemic diethylene glycol poisoning. Clin Toxicol 2005;43:155-159.
22. Schnitzer PG: Prevention of unintentional childhood injuries. Am Fam Physician 2006;74:1864-1869.

Chapter 146

Hydrocarbons

David D. Gummin

KEY POINTS

In assessing the patient with possible hydrocarbon exposure, important tasks are:
- Identification of the specific substance(s)
- Quantification of dose
- Determination of timing, duration, and course of exposure
- Identification of route(s) of exposure
- Consultation and/or referral, when indicated

Many hydrocarbons are acutely cardiotoxic and have a propensity to induce tachyarrhythmias by sensitizing the myocardium to the arrhythmogenic effects of catecholamines.

Recognition of hydrocarbon exposure can be challenging. When toxicity is recognized, intervention is crucial. Treatment is largely supportive.

Gaseous or volatilized hydrocarbons are likely to cause toxicity through inhalation.

Viscosity, surface tension, and volatility determine the aspiration potential and the risk of pulmonary toxicity.

Perspective

A hydrocarbon is an organic compound composed mainly of carbon and hydrogen atoms. In modern society, these compounds are virtually everywhere. Hydrocarbons are so common in our society that exposures—even illnesses related to exposures—are not usually documented. Hydrocarbons derive most commonly from distillation and processing of petroleum, but many derive from plants (pine oil, essential oils), animal fats, and natural gas. Most available hydrocarbon products are mixtures of individual chemical species, ranging from 1 to 60 carbon atoms in size. An example is gasoline, which is a mixture of alkanes, alkenes, naphthenes, and aromatic hydrocarbons. Most constituents contain 5 to 10 carbon atoms. Commercial gasoline, however, contains hundreds—up to 1500—individual chemical species.

The term *solvent* is often used to refer to an organic solvent—typically a hydrocarbon mixture—that is used to dissolve other substances. Occupational literature often uses the terms "solvent" and "hydrocarbon" interchangeably. Organic solvents are common in industry, and workers may suffer dermal or inhalational exposures. Children may suffer unintentional hydrocarbon exposures, often ingestions, with risk of pulmonary hydrocarbon aspiration. More concerning is a trend toward greater intentional abuse of volatile hydrocarbon inhalants by adolescents and young adults. This form of substance abuse, often termed *volatile substance abuse* (VSA), is a growing problem worldwide.

Structure and Function

One can predict many of the physical properties of hydrocarbons by knowing the molecular shape and size (number of carbon atoms in the molecule's chain). The nonpolar, covalent bonds between

Table 146-1 HYDROCARBON PROPERTIES AND ASPIRATION RISK

	Definition	Example	Value vs. Risk
Viscosity	Measure of a fluid's resistance to flow	Low-viscosity substances (<60 SUS [Saybolt universal seconds]), such as turpentine, gasoline, and naphtha, have higher tendency for aspiration in animal models	Lower value predicts higher risk
Surface tension	Indirectly measures dispersion forces between molecules, also the interaction with the surface that the fluid contacts	Adherence of the fluid along a surface ("the inability to creep")	Lower value predicts higher risk
Volatility	Tendency for a liquid to enter the gas phase	Hydrocarbons that are highly volatile have a high vapor pressure so tend to vaporize, get into the lungs, displace oxygen, and cause hypoxia	Higher value predicts higher risk

carbon-carbon and carbon-hydrogen atoms produce *dispersion forces,* which result in the attraction between hydrocarbon molecules. These same forces repel polar molecules (like water), making hydrocarbons generally hydrophobic. Once dissolved in aqueous solution, nonpolar hydrocarbons can transit rapidly through lipid membranes, including cell membranes and the blood-brain barrier. Small, light, aliphatic hydrocarbons with up to 4 carbons are gases at room temperature; those with 5 to 19 carbon molecules are liquids; and longer molecules form solids or *paraffins*. Branching in the molecule destabilizes intermolecular forces, so less energy is required to separate molecules. This makes it easier for a molecule to leave the liquid phase and enter the vapor phase (to *volatilize*). So, for a given molecular size, more branching means a lower boiling point, and the compound is typically more volatile. Gaseous or volatilized hydrocarbons are likely to cause toxicity by inhalation.

Aliphatic hydrocarbons contain carbon-carbon backbone chains, whereas aromatic hydrocarbons contain a benzene-like, unsaturated ring. Innumerable substitutions (for hydrogen atoms) can occur, including hydroxyl groups, multiple bonds, and the substitution of a halogen (like chlorine or fluorine) for hydrogen. Lipid-soluble solvents (aromatic, aliphatic, or halogenated hydrocarbons) are more likely than water-soluble hydrocarbons (alcohols, ketones, or esters) to cause acute central nervous system (CNS) effects. Clinicians are familiar with these effects from experience with inhaled anesthetic agents, which cause CNS sedation similar to that from other hydrocarbons. The Meyer-Overton hypothesis suggests that inhaled anesthetics dissolve into some critical lipid compartment of the CNS, causing generalized inhibition of neuronal transmission. This mechanism is probably oversimplified but helps to partly explain the nonspecific inhibition of neuronal transmission that hydrocarbons produce in the CNS. Specific membrane interactions may also contribute,[1] and a number of receptor-mediated interactions are known to occur.

Specific physical properties of ingested hydrocarbons help to predict the risk of pulmonary aspiration (Table 146-1). In particular, viscosity, surface tension, and volatility determine aspiration potential and the contribution to pulmonary toxicity.[2] *Viscosity* is a measure of a fluid's resistance to flow, commonly described in units of Saybolt universal seconds (SUS). This property is not the same as the fluid's density; in fact these two properties correlate poorly.

Low viscosity substances (<60 SUS), such as turpentine, gasoline, or naphtha, have higher tendency for aspiration in animal models. *A lower viscosity value predicts higher risk*. The U.S. Consumer Products Safety Commission now requires child-resistant packaging for products that contain 10% or more hydrocarbons and have a measured viscosity less than 100 SUS.

Surface tension indirectly measures dispersion forces between molecules in a fluid but also characterizes the interaction with the surface that the fluid contacts. This property can be quantified on a modified Wilhelmy balance, which measures adherence of the fluid along a surface ("the inability to creep"). In theory, the lower the surface tension, the higher the aspiration risk.[2] *A lower surface tension value predicts higher risk.*

Volatility is the tendency for a liquid to enter the gas phase. Hydrocarbons that are highly volatile have a high vapor pressure and so tend to vaporize, get into the lungs, displace oxygen, and cause hypoxia. *A higher volatility value predicts higher risk.*

Mechanisms of Toxicity

Route of exposure considerably influences the organs affected. The principal organ systems affected by hydrocarbons are the skin (from dermal contact), the gastrointestinal (GI) system (when ingested), the CNS, and lungs. Some classes of hydrocarbons are cardiotoxic. Certain agents may cause organ-specific toxicity to cranial or peripheral nerves, the liver, or the kidneys.

Although organ-specific pathophysiology is often unique to individual agents, much of the toxicity of hydrocarbons results from their ability to dissolve fats or, similarly, to diffuse across hydrophobic barriers intended to protect anatomical structures (e.g., lipid bilayers, myelin). Hydrocarbon solvents cause irritation of skin and mucous membranes. Recurrent or prolonged contact results in "defatting" of skin, dissolving lipid components and disrupting the normal architecture of the stratum corneum.[3]

Most hydrocarbons are flammable or combustible. Under appropriate conditions, most can explode. The widespread availability of hydrocarbons and their use as organic solvents account for the frequent finding of stored quantities of these solvents in clandestine illicit drug laboratories, among other places. Storage and use of these flammable agents appreciably contribute to the health hazards of these facilities.

Pathophysiology

■ SKIN

The skin is a common site of contact and a potential portal of entry for hydrocarbons. Skin is composed of both hydrophilic and hydrophobic elements. Agents that contain both hydrophobic and hydrophilic regions (glycol ethers, dimethylformamide, dimethylsulfoxide) are highly absorbed. But dermal absorption usually constitutes a small fraction of the hydrocarbon dose absorbed by other routes, such as inhalation. Absorbed dose depends on the surface area exposed, the duration of contact, and skin's integrity (e.g., cut, abraded).

Most hydrocarbons are nonspecific skin irritants. Prolonged exposure causes drying and cracking. Blistering and contact dermatitis may occur and, with continued or recurring exposure, may progress to partial or even full-thickness chemical burns.[4]

■ GASTROINTESTINAL

Ingested hydrocarbons typically cause local GI irritation. Abdominal pain and vomiting are common. Most hydrocarbons are poorly absorbed from the GI tract. Diarrhea is likely after ingestion, particularly of insoluble hydrocarbons (mineral oil, paraffins). Vomiting increases the risk of pulmonary aspiration.

■ PULMONARY

Gaseous or volatilized hydrocarbons can be inhaled, displacing alveolar oxygen and causing hypoxia. Contact with lung tissue results in interstitial inflammation, polymorphonuclear infiltration and exudate, intra-alveolar edema and hemorrhage, hyperemia, bronchial and bronchiolar necrosis, and vascular thrombosis. These results likely reflect both direct cytotoxicity and disruption of the surfactant layer, leading to poor oxygen exchange, atelectasis, and pneumonitis, with reductions in lung compliance and total lung capacity.

Severe hydrocarbon pneumonitis also results from intravenous (IV) injection of a hydrocarbon. In animals, intravascular hydrocarbons injure the first capillary bed encountered. The clinical course after IV hydrocarbon exposure mirrors that of aspiration injury.[5]

■ CARDIAC

Many hydrocarbons are acutely cardiotoxic. Especially important is their propensity to induce tachyarrhythmias. The mechanism by which hydrocarbons cause malignant rhythms is poorly characterized, but a number of these agents can precipitate ventricular tachycardia or fibrillation and can cause sudden death.

Endogenous or exogenous catecholamines (e.g., epinephrine) are pro-arrhythmic. Hydrocarbons enhance this potential and are said to "sensitize" the myocardium to the arrhythmogenic effects of catecholamines. Essentially every class of hydrocarbon compounds, including general anesthetic agents, can sensitize the heart. Some classes carry high risk, however, and others sensitize modestly if at all. Their ability to sensitize the heart constitutes an accepted system for grading halocarbon (e.g., Freon) toxicity. Unsaturated, aliphatic hydrocarbons (such as ethylene) as well as aliphatic ethers have been studied but do not appear to be sensitizers. Other unsaturated compounds, such as acetylene, are weak sensitizers. Aromatic hydrocarbons and, especially, halogenated hydrocarbons are often potent sensitizers.[6]

Sensitization appears to be mediated by slowed conduction velocity, possibly by chemical and functional changes in the membrane transport proteins at gap junctions. The major ventricular gap junction protein is composed of connexin 43. This protein is regulated by phosphorylation, such that the dephosphorylated state of the hexamers in the channel is associated with greater gap junction resistance. Halocarbons, in the presence of epinephrine, increase gap junction resistance in myocardial tissue, slowing conduction velocity.[7]

■ NERVOUS SYSTEM

The mechanism by which hydrocarbons depress consciousness is unknown. Diffusion across the blood-brain barrier with neuronal "membrane stabilization" provides the foundation of the Meyer-Overton hypothesis. To date, no specific receptor wholly explains this generalized effect. In cases of pulmonary toxicity, hypoxemia may contribute to depressed consciousness.[8]

Chronic solvent abuse leads to irreversible CNS toxicity, best described in the setting of toluene abuse. Volitional abusers demonstrate loss of cerebral white matter, with a characteristic syndrome of cognitive and motor deficits. Autopsied brains of long-term toluene abusers show profound atrophy and mottling of the white matter, as though the lipid-based myelin had been dissolved away. Microscopic examination shows a consistent pattern of demyelination, with relative preservation of axons. These pathologic features correlate with the clinical syndrome of subcortical dementia.[9] Mild cognitive deficits show improvement after 6 months of abstinence. With advanced disease, regardless of the exposure history, full recovery is unlikely.[10]

Exposure to n-hexane or to methyl n-butyl ketone (MnBK) can cause peripheral neuropathy. This toxic axonopathy appears to be due to 2,5-hexanedione, a metabolic intermediate common to both agents. The mechanism appears to involve decreased phosphorylation of neurofilament proteins, with disruption of the axonal cytoskeleton.[11]

■ HEPATIC

Chlorinated hydrocarbons are often hepatotoxic. Carbon tetrachloride is a prototype hepatotoxin, causing centrilobular necrosis, through a reactive intermediate metabolite. Other halogenated and nonhalogenated hydrocarbons have been associated with hepatic insult, including trichloroethylene, tetrachloroethylene, benzene, and even petroleum distillates. Vinyl chloride is a well-known hepatic carcinogen.

■ RENAL

Halogenated hydrocarbons may be nephrotoxic. Examples include chloroform, carbon tetrachloride, and ethylene dichloride. Further, recurrent or prolonged toluene exposure causes distal renal tubular acidosis. Sodium loss in the urine may transform the initial non-gap metabolic acidosis into an anion-gap positive metabolic acidosis. Toluene's principal metabolite, hippuric acid, contributes to the elevated anion gap. Renal potassium loss may be severe and can result in symptomatic hypokalemia. In one series, distal renal tubular acidosis was seen in 44% of hospitalized paint sniffers.[12]

■ OTHER EFFECTS

Methylene chloride and other halomethanes are metabolized to carbon monoxide by CYP 2E1 (a member of the cytochrome P-450 enzyme system). Significant and prolonged carboxyhemoglobin levels can be measured after inhalational or dermal exposures. This metabolic toxicant appears to be exclusively generated by halomethanes.

Some hydrocarbon agents contain nitrogenous moieties, and mixtures may contain coloring additives (such as aniline) that can induce methemoglobinemia. Benzene is directly hematotoxic, being associated with hemolysis, aplastic anemia, and acute myelogenous leukemia. Because of benzene's cancer risk, toluene has largely replaced benzene in many commercial products worldwide.

Clinical Presentation

A typical ED case involves a young child who is suspected to have unintentionally ingested a hydrocarbon mixture. Infrequently, a parent may have witnessed the ingestion; more typically, the situation was discovered shortly thereafter. The specific agent is often identified by the caregiver. A parent may report that the child was coughing, gagging, or vomiting, or that there is an odor of the suspected hydrocarbon. If the ingestion was unwitnessed, it may be difficult to quantify the amount ingested, but a "worst case scenario" can often be ascertained. History of coughing, choking, or vomiting should heighten the ED's suspicion for pulmonary aspiration. Respiratory findings include coughing, choking, gagging, grunting, tachypnea, retractions, fever, cyanosis or poor coloration, and abnormal sounds on chest auscultation. Mental status depression is common in larger ingestions but may not occur for 30 to 60 minutes after ingestion. In a prospective, multicenter study of 760 pediatric kerosene ingestions, there was no association between the age of the patient and the amount ingested. There was significantly higher risk of pulmonary toxicity and also of CNS depression in those who ingested more than 30 mL of kerosene (according to history). The incidence of pulmonary aspiration was higher in children who vomited after ingestion.[13]

Typical findings in hydrocarbon pneumonitis are audible abnormalities on chest auscultation, fever, leukocytosis, and abnormalities on chest radiograph (Fig. 146-1). These findings do not differ clinically from those of community-acquired pneumonia. Only the history differentiates the two entities. The elevated temperature initially noted in hydrocarbon aspiration often spikes at 8 to 12 hours, then declines

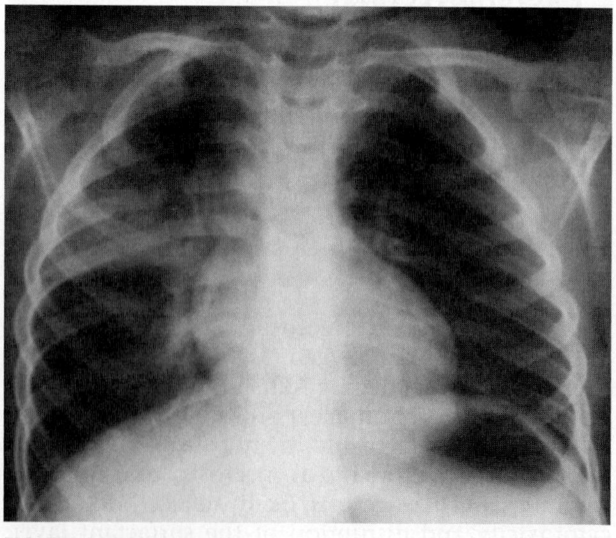

FIGURE 146-1 Aspiration pneumonitis in a child who ingested a hydrocarbon mixture. Note the early consolidation in the right upper lobe. Although 75% of cases demonstrate right-sided findings, upper lobe involvement is not common.

RED FLAGS

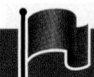

- History of coughing, choking, or vomiting should heighten the suspicion for pulmonary aspiration.
- "Sudden sniffing death syndrome" classically occurs after a sudden fright or physical exertion (e.g., running to avoid an authority), with sudden catecholamine surge and a sensitized heart.
- Volatile solvent abusers may leave telltale paint, shoeshine, or solvent stains on clothes or skin.
- Nonfreezing cold injury (frostbite) may occur on or about the face; it is caused by intentional release of liquid hydrocarbon propellant, which cools as it suddenly exits its container.
- Hypokalemia, with consequent muscle weakness or arrhythmia, may be the presenting complaint in volatile substance abusers in whom renal tubular acidosis develops from recurrent toluene exposure.
- Many hydrocarbons possess a characteristic odor similar to that of gasoline or lighter fluid. Solvents containing aldehyde or ketone groups smell sweet or fruity, and essential oils are characteristically pungent or aromatic. In acutely intoxicated patients, these odors are rarely missed.
- An adolescent or teen who presents to the ED with sudden death or a malignant tachyarrhythmia (especially ventricular tachycardia or ventricular fibrillation) must be considered to have been abusing hydrocarbons unless the EP is able to demonstrate otherwise.
- Hydrocarbons do not generally affect systemic vascular resistance, so co-ingestants should be considered in the persistently hypotensive patient.
- Hypotension may relate to excessive positive end-expiration pressure (PEEP), and reducing PEEP may improve hemodynamics.

over several days, unless bacterial superinfection intervenes.

The intentional inhalation in VSA can be more challenging to diagnose, because affected patients frequently withhold relevant history. Several common inhalational techniques have been identified. *Sniffing* involves inhaling vapor from an open container. *Huffing* involves placing a volatile hydrocarbon in a rag or cloth, then covering the nose and mouth with the cloth or rag and inhaling the agent through it. *Bagging* implies placing the substance inside a plastic (or other) bag, and then putting the bag over the face to inhale hydrocarbon vapor.

Respiratory findings are uncommon after inhalation, but the patient may manifest tachypnea or cyanosis or may suffer sudden cardiac arrest. Classically, arrest occurs after a sudden fright or physical exertion (e.g., running to avoid an authority), with sudden catecholamine surge and a sensitized heart. This is termed the *sudden sniffing death syndrome.*

Hydrocarbons cause CNS depression. Transient excitation may initially occur after inhalation or ingestion, but early sedation is more common. Initial findings include behavioral changes, impaired sense of smell, impaired concentration, and mildly unsteady movements or gait. As with alcohol or other sedatives, mild exposures produce euphoria, likely contributing to abuse potential. Further acute exposure leads to slurred speech and progressive incoordination. Physical signs are nystagmus, tremor, spasticity with hyperreflexia, abnormal plantar reflexes, hearing loss, impaired vision, and a broad-based, staggering gait. Pain inhibition explains why hydrocarbons were chosen as general anesthetic agents. Stupor, lethargy, or obtundation is seen in overdose. Coma and seizures occur in up to 3% of cases.[14]

Chronic CNS dysfunction occurs in recurrent volatile substance abusers, including reports of optic neuropathy, sensorineural hearing loss, equilibrium disorders, ataxia, and cognitive deficits. Occupational solvent exposures are also associated with persistent CNS abnormalities, although the exposures and the clinical findings are typically less impressive than those in habitual VSA. The majority of published reports involve exposure to toluene, a very common workplace and household hydrocarbon solvent. Neurologic deficits are tremor, ataxia, impaired fine-motor skills, and mild cognitive defects. Long-term occupational exposures are associated with a clinical syndrome consisting of fatigue, poor short-term memory, attention difficulties, visuospatial abnormalities, personality changes, and mood disorder. Clinically, this presentation has been dubbed *the painters' syndrome.*

Radiologically and histopathologically, prolonged, repeated exposures to toluene are associated with brain demyelination. Although the mechanism of this process is not fully understood, it is presumed to result from dissolution of myelin by the solvent. Toluene encephalopathy is characterized by a specific constellation of findings, alternatively described as "subcortical dementia," "white matter dementia," or "toxic leukoencephalopathy." Findings include loss of cortical gray matter–white matter differentiation, atrophic changes in the basal ganglia, cerebellum, pons, and thalamus, and thinning of the corpus callosum. Changes noted on magnetic resonance imaging appear to progress in a lifetime dose–dependent fashion.[15] Unfortunately, toluene is an addictive substance, and progression of abnormalities is likely with persistent use. Resolution of neurologic abnormalities has not been documented once white matter loss becomes radiographically evident. Complete recovery from solvent encephalopathy is not considered likely, even with abstinence or removal from exposure.[10]

Cutaneous findings may be the chief complaint, with dermal exposure to solvents from work or hobbies. Nonspecific skin irritation is most common but may progress to contact dermatitis with continued exposure. Drying, cracking, pitting, or eczematous lesions occur in up to 9% of workers who are

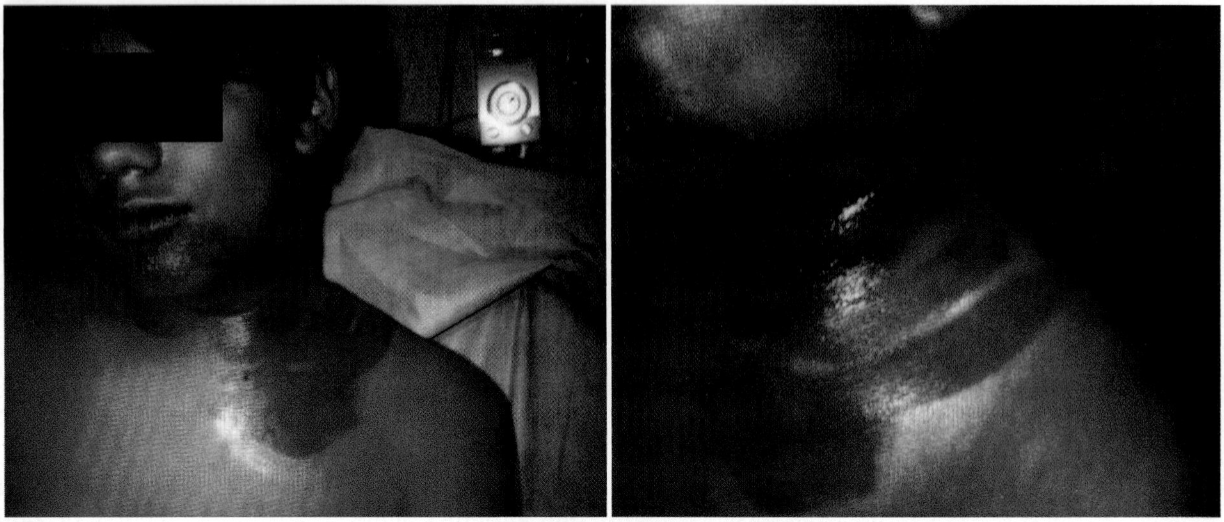

A B

FIGURE 146-2 **A** and **B,** "Huffer's rash" resulting from repeated "sniffing" of liquid propane. Both contact dermatitis and nonfreezing cold injury likely contribute to the skin findings in this characteristic distribution. (Courtesy of E. O'Connell, MD.)

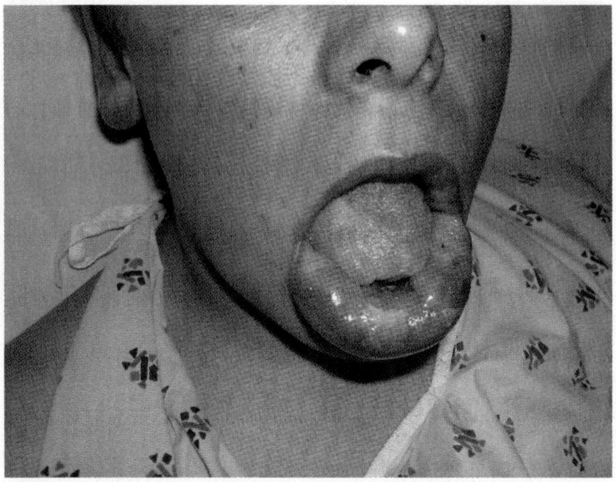

FIGURE 146-3 Nonfreezing cold injury resulting from intentional release and attempted inhalation of halocarbon propellant.

repeatedly exposed. Allergic reactions are uncommon but may be seen with exposure to a number of essential oils or to pine oil. Recurrent, prolonged, or protracted VSA may produce contact dermatitis in the areas exposed to solvent vapor. When it involves the skin surrounding the nose and mouth, the dermatitis has been dubbed "huffer's rash" (Fig. 146-2). Volatile solvent abusers may leave telltale paint, shoeshine, or solvent stains on clothes or skin. Nonfreezing cold injury (frostbite) may occur on or about the face because of intentional release of liquid hydrocarbon propellant, which cools as it suddenly exits its container (Fig. 146-3).

Variations

Hepatotoxicity and nephrotoxicity are uncommon in the setting of acute hydrocarbon toxicity from ingestion or inhalation. However, halogenated hydrocarbons can damage the liver, kidney, or both. Hypokalemia, with consequent muscle weakness or arrhythmia, may be the presenting complaint in volatile substance abusers in whom renal tubular acidosis develops from recurrent toluene exposure.

Seizures are uncommon in hydrocarbon toxicity, probably because of overwhelming anesthetic effects, and should raise suspicion of a co-ingestant. Exceptions are as follows:

- Seizures may occur after large ingestion of pine oil or essential oils such as oil of wormwood and fennel oil.
- Anoxic seizures may occur with hydrocarbon ingestion that results in respiratory depression or hypoxemia due to severe pulmonary insult.

Halomethanes, such as methylene chloride, are metabolized to carbon monoxide. Rarely, hydrocarbon mixtures cause methemoglobinemia. Benzene exposure can cause dyscrasias. Appropriate testing is necessary in the setting of toxicity related to these specific agents.

Chlorofluorocarbon and hydrochlorofluorocarbon refrigerants (Freon) can decompose in the presence of open flames or welding arcs, with liberation of toxic vapors, including fluorine or chlorine gas and phosgene. In this context, severe toxicity could result from one of these decomposition products.

Peripheral neuropathy (akin to that seen with n-hexane or MnBK), which has also been described in up to 40% of long-term toluene abusers, begins in the distal extremities and progresses proximally. With discontinuation of exposure, this neuropathy resolved over weeks to months. It is unclear whether the toluene in these early series may have been contaminated by n-hexane or MnBK. Trichloroethylene is associated with trigeminal nerve injury as well as other cranial and peripheral neuropathies. Pathologically, trichloroethylene appears to induce a myeli-

Table 146-2 SYMPTOMS ASSOCIATED WITH HYDROCARBON EXPOSURE

Symptom	Notes
Coughing, choking, or vomiting	Heightens suspicion for pulmonary aspiration
Behavioral changes, impaired sense of smell, impaired concentration, and mildly unsteady movements or gait	Transient excitation may initially occur after inhalation or ingestion, but early sedation is more common
Elevated temperature	Initially noted in hydrocarbon aspiration Often spikes at 8 to 12 hours then declines over several days, unless bacterial superinfection occurs
Drying, cracking, pitting, or eczematous lesions	Contact dermatitis or frostbite injury with intentional abuse
Muscle weakness	Renal tubular acidosis associated with hypokalemia, with consequent muscle weakness or arrhythmia, may be the presenting complaint
Seizures	Uncommon, probably because of overwhelming anesthetic effects, and should raise suspicion of a co-ingestant Exceptions: (1) seizures that occur after large ingestion of pine oil or essential oils such as oil of wormwood or fennel oil and (2) anoxic seizures
Persistent hypoxia	Methemoglobinemia, carbon monoxide toxicity, and blood dyscrasias are associated with specific ingestions
Peripheral neuropathy	Begins in distal extremities and progresses proximally

nopathy, often clinically distinguishable from the axonopathy that occurs with n-hexane or MnBK (Table 146-2).

Distinguishing Features and Clinical Presentations

Adolescents 12 to 17 years old are the most likely age group to abuse volatile substances, with a 15% lifetime prevalence among U.S. eighth grade students. Volatile substance use should be suspected in this population. The habitual volatile substance abuser may have paint stains or other telltale finding on the clothing or skin (see clinical presentation discussion).

Many hydrocarbons possess a characteristic odor similar to that of gasoline or lighter fluid. Solvents containing aldehyde or ketone groups smell sweet or fruity. Essential oils are characteristically pungent or aromatic. In acutely intoxicated patients, these odors are rarely missed.

Diagnostic Testing

The diagnostic evaluation of a patient with hydrocarbon exposure depends heavily on the known patterns of toxicity associated with specific hydrocarbon agents and the route of exposure. It is more crucial to obtain and verify the history, with particular attention to identifying the specific type and composition of the agent(s) involved. The route of exposure should direct the clinician to the anticipated target organ(s), which will direct testing.

Evaluation of renal function, serum electrolyte levels, and acid-base status should be performed in all patients with history of chronic or recurrent toluene exposure. Liver transaminases and bilirubin should be assayed in patients with significant exposure to halocarbons or to benzene. Electrocardiographic monitoring and a formal 12-lead electrocardiogram are indicated when there is significant exposure to "sensitizing" hydrocarbon agents. Cranial computed tomography and magnetic resonance imaging are valuable to assess the extent of brain involvement in chronic exposures. Pulse oximetry or arterial blood gas testing help assess the severity of pulmonary injury. Carboxyhemoglobin or methemoglobin measurements are indicated for exposures involving specific agents (see "Other Clinical Effects").

Early chest radiography may be indicated for severely symptomatic patients, to gauge the extent of pulmonary injury and guide the inpatient placement decision. For an asymptomatic hydrocarbon ingestion, however, early radiography does not help predict aspiration pneumonitis, and is not cost-effective. Patients who have been observed for 6 hours after an ingestion and demonstrate no abnormal pulmonary findings, have adequate oxygenation, are not tachypneic, and have normal chest radiography findings have a good prognosis with very low risk of subsequent deterioration.[16]

Results of bioassays and serum hydrocarbon levels are rarely available to the EP and have little to no value in management of hydrocarbon exposure. These measurements are available through reference laboratories for occupational monitoring or to document exposure in forensic cases.

▪ TREATMENT

An algorithm for the treatment of hydrocarbon exposure is shown in Figure 146-4. The first priority in managing toxicity is to protect rescuers. Personal protection is paramount at each level of health care delivery. Second, the exposure should be removed from the patient, and the patient from the exposure.

Tips and Tricks

- The EP should be aware of the intentional abuse of volatile hydrocarbon inhalants by adolescents and young adults, a growing problem worldwide.
- Hydrocarbons enhance the pro-arrhythmic potential of endogenous or exogenous catecholamines (like epinephrine) and are said to "sensitize" the myocardium to the arrhythmogenic effects of catecholamines, so these agents should be avoided in hydrocarbon exposure.
- Mental status depression is common in larger ingestions but may not occur for 30 to 60 minutes after ingestion.
- Typical findings in hydrocarbon pneumonitis are audible abnormalities on chest auscultation, fever, leukocytosis, and abnormalities seen on chest radiograph; these findings do not differ clinically from those of community-acquired pneumonia.
- Volitional abusers demonstrate loss of cerebral white matter, with a characteristic syndrome of cognitive and motor deficits.
- Dysrhythmias in the setting of hydrocarbon toxicity should prompt investigations into electrolyte and acid-base status, hypoxemia, hypotension, and hypothermia.
- The possibility of methemoglobinemia should be evaluated in any patient who remains cyanotic once arterial oxygenation is normalized.
- Patients with hydrocarbon exposure who have no symptoms at home or on initial evaluation generally do not require gastric emptying.

Contaminated clothing and external contamination must be removed prior to the patient's entry into any patient care or trafficked area. For most hydrocarbons, soap and water are all that are required for decontamination. Most hydrocarbons are flammable, and pose a fire risk to the hospital and staff. Personal protective equipment should be worn by anyone who will touch the patient or any articles brought with the patient. Once the patient is externally decontaminated, standard precautions generally suffice in the ED.

Several animal models show that prophylactic antibiotics have no role in hydrocarbon aspiration. Human studies are inconclusive. Nevertheless, antibiotics may be warranted in severely poisoned patients, because the clinical features do not differ from those of bacterial pneumonitis. Sputum culture results optimally guide antibiotic use. Empirical antibiotic therapy, if used, should cover the spectrum of community-acquired pathogens. Systemic corticosteroids do not improve the acute course of hydrocarbon pulmonary toxicity and are not recommended empirically.

Cyanosis is uncommon in hydrocarbon poisoning. When present, it is most commonly due to hypoxemia. Top priority should be given to oxygenating the arterial blood. The possibility of methemoglobinemia should be investigated in any patient who remains cyanotic once arterial oxygenation is normalized.

Dysrhythmias in the setting of hydrocarbon toxicity should prompt investigations into electrolyte and acid-base status, hypoxemia, hypotension, and hypothermia. Ventricular fibrillation is especially concerning, because resuscitation algorithms recommend epinephrine to treat this rhythm. If the dysrhythmia can be ascertained to emanate from myocardial sensitization by a solvent, catecholamines should be avoided. In this setting, lidocaine has been used successfully, as have beta-blockers.[17,18]

BOX 146-1

Mnemonic for Potent Hydrocarbon Toxicants

The clinician should consider gastric emptying/decontamination when these agents are ingested:

*C*amphor
*H*alogenated hydrocarbons
*A*romatic
*M*etal-containing hydrocarbons
*P*esticides

PROCEDURES

Gastric emptying may be useful when the hydrocarbon has severe toxicity (e.g., carbon tetrachloride), when a large volume of hydrocarbon is ingested (>30 mL), or when severe toxicity is predicted (Box 146-1). If gastric lavage is performed, a small (not large-bore) nasogastric tube should be used to reduce the risk of vomiting and aspiration. Activated charcoal has little ability to reduce GI absorption of hydrocarbons and may cause gastric distention and vomiting. Any role for activated charcoal in isolated hydrocarbon ingestion is limited, at best.

The vast majority of hydrocarbons cannot be removed by dialysis, but toxic agents that are water-soluble, small, highly polar molecules can be removed by dialysis. Examples are small alcohols and polyols, such as methanol and ethylene glycol. Small ketones (such as acetone) are also dialyzable. Chloral hydrate can be successfully removed by hemodialysis. Peritoneal dialysis has been employed to reduce the toxicity of both dichloroethane and trichloroethylene. Unfortunately, many hydrocarbon molecules are too large to be dialyzed. Most are lipophilic, so they dissolve into fat stores (with greater volume of distribution), reducing their availability in the central compartment.

Extracorporeal membrane oxygenation can successfully temporize the course of severe pulmonary

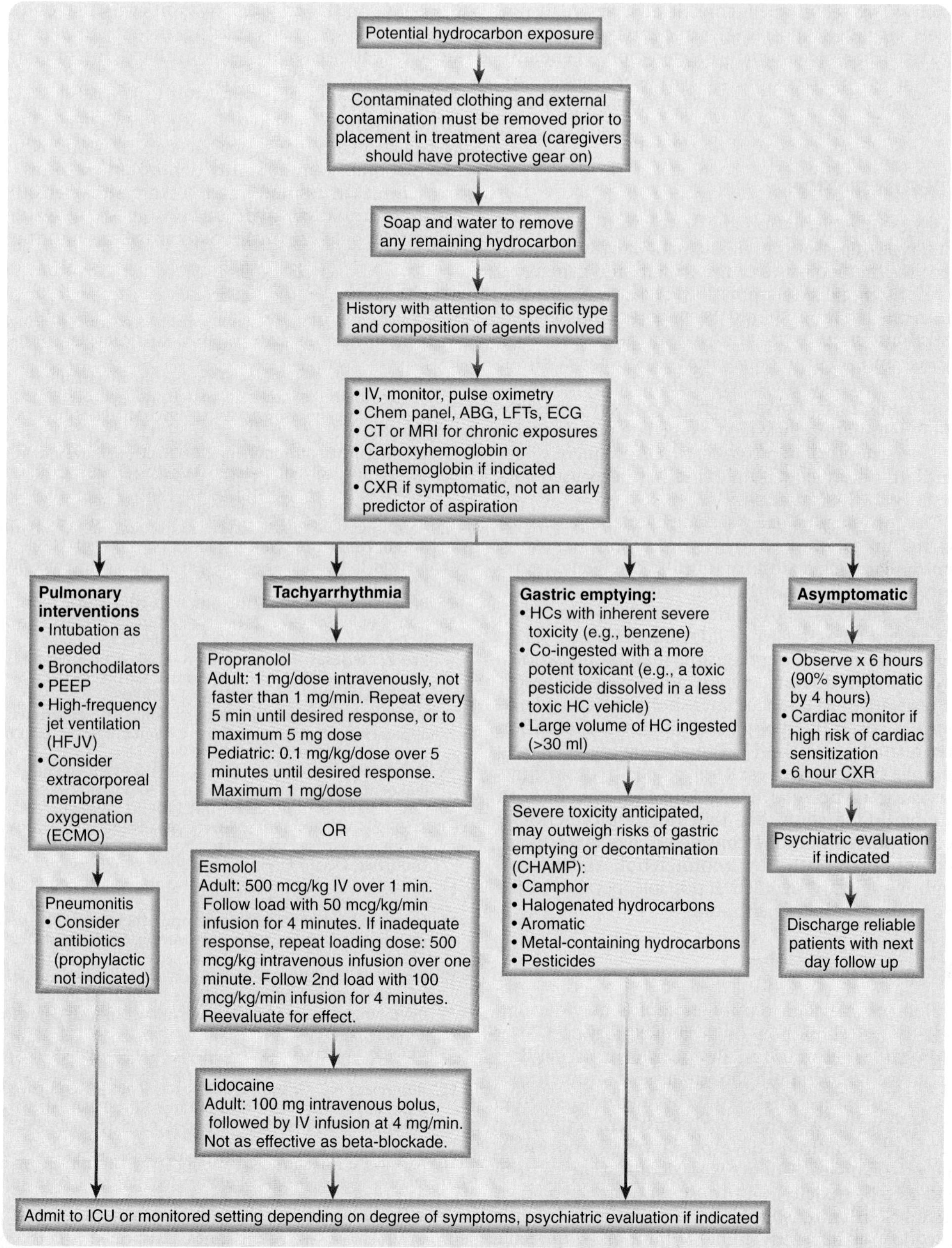
Potential hydrocarbon exposure
Contaminated clothing and external contamination must be removed prior to placement in treatment area (caregivers should have protective gear on)
Soap and water to remove any remaining hydrocarbon
History with attention to specific type and composition of agents involved
• IV, monitor, pulse oximetry
• Chem panel, ABG, LFTs, ECG
• CT or MRI for chronic exposures
• Carboxyhemoglobin or methemoglobin if indicated
• CXR if symptomatic, not an early predictor of aspiration
Pulmonary interventions
• Intubation as needed
• Bronchodilators
• PEEP
• High-frequency jet ventilation (HFJV)
• Consider extracorporeal membrane oxygenation (ECMO)
Pneumonitis
• Consider antibiotics (prophylactic not indicated)
Tachyarrhythmia
Propranolol
Adult: 1 mg/dose intravenously, not faster than 1 mg/min. Repeat every 5 min until desired response, or to maximum 5 mg dose
Pediatric: 0.1 mg/kg/dose over 5 minutes until desired response. Maximum 1 mg/dose
OR
Esmolol
Adult: 500 mcg/kg IV over 1 min. Follow load with 50 mcg/kg/min infusion for 4 minutes. If inadequate response, repeat loading dose: 500 mcg/kg intravenous infusion over one minute. Follow 2nd load with 100 mcg/kg/min infusion for 4 minutes. Reevaluate for effect.
Lidocaine
Adult: 100 mg intravenous bolus, followed by IV infusion at 4 mg/min. Not as effective as beta-blockade.
Gastric emptying:
• HCs with inherent severe toxicity (e.g., benzene)
• Co-ingested with a more potent toxicant (e.g., a toxic pesticide dissolved in a less toxic HC vehicle)
• Large volume of HC ingested (>30 ml)
Severe toxicity anticipated, may outweigh risks of gastric emptying or decontamination (CHAMP):
• Camphor
• Halogenated hydrocarbons
• Aromatic
• Metal-containing hydrocarbons
• Pesticides
Asymptomatic
• Observe x 6 hours (90% symptomatic by 4 hours)
• Cardiac monitor if high risk of cardiac sensitization
• 6 hour CXR
Psychiatric evaluation if indicated
Discharge reliable patients with next day follow up
Admit to ICU or monitored setting depending on degree of symptoms, psychiatric evaluation if indicated

FIGURE 146-4 Treatment algorithm for hydrocarbon (HC) exposure. ABG, arterial blood gases; CT, computed tomography; CXR, chest radiograph; ECG, electrocardiogram; LFTs, liver function tests; MRI, magnetic resonance imaging; PEEP, positive end-expiratory pressure.

toxicity. This technique is considered invasive, is not widely available, and requires special expertise. Use of extracorporeal membrane oxygenation is generally reserved for severe cases of hydrocarbon toxicity for which other available modalities have failed to achieve adequate oxygenation.

■ RESUSCITATION

Priorities of resuscitation are similar to those in any other type of poisoning. Nuances include the requirement to limit exposure of the patient and caregivers by prioritizing decontamination. The airway and systemic oxygenation should be restored and secured first. This should be achieved by any necessary means and may require high-flow oxygenation, endotracheal intubation, ventilation, and the use of bronchodilators. Positive end-expiratory pressure (PEEP) ventilation may help oxygenate patients who are persistently hypoxemic. High-frequency jet ventilation may be required and has been used successfully in this situation.

Caution must be exercised in the management of dysrhythmias induced by hydrocarbon exposure. Ventricular tachycardia or fibrillation likely represents myocardial sensitization. Exogenous catecholamines, such as epinephrine, should be avoided. Consider a beta-blocker or lidocaine instead.

Management of hypotension may be precarious. Hydrocarbons do not generally affect systemic vascular resistance, so co-ingestants should be considered in the persistently hypotensive patient. Hypotension may relate to excessive PEEP, and reducing PEEP may improve hemodynamics. Rarely, some hydrocarbons can cause myocardial depression; in a patient with this finding, an inotrope (but not isoproterenol or dobutamine) should be considered. Pressors such as dopamine, epinephrine, isoproterenol, and norepinephrine must be avoided, if possible, because of the risk of myocardial sensitization.[6]

Disposition

Radiographic evidence of pneumonitis may develop as early as 15 minutes or as late as 24 hours after hydrocarbon aspiration. Ninety percent of patients who have radiographic abnormalities do so within 4 hours.[19] After the initial episode of coughing, gagging, or choking, most patients with persistent respiratory signs and symptoms have pneumonitis and radiographic changes. Patients who demonstrate clinical evidence of toxicity, and those who are suicidal or intend self-harm, should be hospitalized. Patients who do not have any initial symptoms, who have normal chest radiograph findings 6 hours after ingestion, and in whom symptoms do not develop during a 6-hour observation can be safely discharged. Care may be individualized for asymptomatic patients with radiographic abnormalities as well as for patients who have initial respiratory symptoms but quickly become asymptomatic during medical evaluation. Reliable patients may be considered for discharge with next-day follow-up.

Special care should be given to patients who ingest, or who otherwise have significant toxicity from, agents known to cause cardiac sensitization, including gasoline. Mental status depression, seizures, or arrhythmias attributed to a known cardiac sensitizer (or to an unknown hydrocarbon ingestion) warrant at least 6 hours of continuous cardiac monitoring.

REFERENCES

1. Sikkema J, de Bont JA, Poolman B: Mechanisms of membrane toxicity of hydrocarbons. Microbiol Rev 1995;59: 201-222.
2. Gerarde HW: Toxicological studies on hydrocarbons. IX: The aspiration hazard and toxicity of hydrocarbons and hydrocarbon mixtures. Arch Environ Health 1963;6: 329-341.
3. Lupulescu AP, Birmingham DJ: Effect of protective agent against lipid-solvent–induced damages: Ultrastructural and scanning electron microscopical study of human epidermis. Arch Environ Health 1976;31:33-36.
4. Hansbrough JF, Zapata-Sirvent R, Dominic W, et al: Hydrocarbon contact injuries. J Trauma 1985;25:250-252.
5. Bratton L, Haddon JE: Ingestion of charcoal lighter fluid. J Pediatr 1975;87:633-636.
6. Brock WJ, Rusch GM, Trochimowicz HJ: Cardiac sensitization: Methodology and interpretation in risk assessment. Regul Toxicol Pharmacol 2003;38:78-90.
7. Jiao Z, De Jesus VR, Iravanian S, et al: A possible mechanism of halocarbon-induced cardiac sensitization arrhythmias. J Mol Cell Cardiol 2006;41:698-705.
8. Wolfsdorf J: Kerosene intoxication: An experimental approach to the etiology of the CNS manifestations in primates. J Pediatr 1976;88:1037-1040.
9. Kornfeld M, Moser AB, Moser HW: Solvent vapor abuse leukoencephalopathy: Comparison to adrenoleukodystrophy. J Neuropathol Exp Neurol 1994;53:389-398.
10. Triebig G, Hallermann J: Survey of solvent related chronic encephalopathy as an occupational disease in European countries. Occup Environ Med 2001;58:575-581.
11. Graham DG: Neurotoxicants and the cytoskeleton. Curr Opin Neurol 1999;12:733-737.
12. Voigts A, Kaufman CE: Acidosis and other metabolic abnormalities associated with paint sniffing. South Med J 1983; 76:443-477, 452.
13. Press E: Cooperative kerosene poisoning study: Evaluation of gastric lavage and other factors in the treatment of accidental ingestion of petroleum distillate products. Pediatrics 1962;29:648-674.
14. Kulig K, Rumack B: Hydrocarbon ingestion. Curr Top Emerg Med 1981;3:1-5.
15. Rosenberg NL, Grigsby J, Dreisbach J, et al: Neuropsychologic impairment and MRI abnormalities associated with chronic solvent abuse. J Toxicol Clin Toxicol 2002;40: 21-34.
16. Anas N, Namasonthi V, Ginsburg CM: Criteria for hospitalizing children who have ingested products containing hydrocarbon. JAMA 1981;246:840-843.
17. Moritz F, de La Chapelle A, Bauer F, et al: Esmolol in the treatment of severe arrhythmia after acute trichloroethylene poisoning [letter]. Intens Care Med 2000;26:256.
18. Zahedi A, Grant MH, Wong DT: Successful treatment of chloral hydrate cardiac toxicity with propranolol. Am J Emerg Med 1999;17:490-491.
19. Daeschner CW, Blattner RJ, Collins VP: Hydrocarbon pneumonitis. Pediatr Clin North Am 1957;4:243-253.

Chapter **147**

Inhaled Toxins

Trevonne M. Thompson and Steven E. Aks

KEY POINTS

Cyanide gas and hydrogen sulfide are rapid knock-down agents.
Cyanide is a cellular poison that inhibits the electron transport chain, reduces oxygen consumption, and converts aerobic to anaerobic metabolism.
The key characteristic of cyanide is a profound metabolic acidosis with a wide anion gap and elevation of serum lactate.
Clinical suspicion is paramount to the diagnosis of cyanide toxicity, and treatment may be required prior to confirmation.
Use the cyanide antidote kit early if poisoning is suspected; confirmatory blood cyanide measurements are not readily available.
Rescuers must wear adequate personal protective equipment, including self-contained breathing apparatus, in order to remove a victim from the source of exposure to hydrogen sulfide.
Patients who present alert, without altered mental status and with normal respiratory effort after exposure to hydrogen sulfide, should have a good outcome.
If administered shortly after severe hydrogen sulfide exposures, sodium nitrite may improve outcome.
The mainstays of treatment for hydrogen sulfide toxicity are 100% oxygen and meticulous supportive care.

Cyanide

■ SCOPE AND HISTORY

Cyanide poisoning is uncommon. It is also potentially rapidly fatal. Early recognition of poisoning, early administration of antidotal therapy, and aggressive supportive care are vital to patient survival.

Cyanide was first isolated in 1782. Since that time, it has been used widely. It is used today in precious metal extraction, electroplating, metal hardening, photography, and various other industries. Cyanide has also been used as an agent of chemical warfare and in judicial executions.[1]

Cyanide exists in several forms. The gaseous form is hydrogen cyanide (HCN); the salt forms are potassium cyanide and sodium cyanide. The inorganic salts release HCN gas when dissolved in water. *Cyanogens* are compounds that are metabolized to cyanide in vivo. The two clinically important cyanogens are amygdalin and

BOX 147-1

Cyanogen-Containing Plants

Prunus species (leaves, bark and seeds):
- Apricots
- Peaches
- Bitter almonds*
- Plums

Apple pits
Cassava beans and roots
Crab apple pits
Pear pits
Christmas berry
Linum species
Sorghum species

*Bitter almonds are not the common almonds eaten in the United States.
From Hall AH, Rumack BH: Clinical toxicology of cyanide. Ann Emerg Med 1986;15:1067-1074.

BOX 147-2

Combustion Sources of Cyanide

Wool
Silk
Nylon
Synthetic rubber
Polyurethane
Nitrocellulose
Polystyrene

From Jones J, McMullen MJ, Dougherty J: Toxic smoke inhalation: Cyanide poisoning in fire victims. Am J Emerg Med 1987;5:317-321.

acetonitrile. Amygdalin is a naturally occurring cyanogen found in the seeds of plants in the *Prunus* species and in the pits of other fruits (Box 147-1). Acetonitrile is found in some artificial nail removal products. Unlike other cyanide products, cyanogens may produce delayed cyanide toxicity because of the time required for their biotransformation.

Cyanide gas is also released during combustion of certain natural and synthetic materials (Box 147-2). Consequently, cyanide poisoning can occur in victims of structure fires.

■ PATHOPHYSIOLOGY

Cyanide is a potent cellular poison. The primary clinical effect occurs through the blockade of the electron transport chain in the mitochondrion, thereby shutting down oxidative phosphorylation. Cyanide binds to the ferric (Fe^{3+}) moiety of cytochrome oxidase aa_3, the last enzyme of the electron transport chain. The electron transport chain is responsible for oxygen consumption and the generation of the majority of cellular ATP. The net effects of cyanide poisoning are reduced oxygen consumption and conversion of aerobic to anaerobic metabolism.

The elevated serum lactate value seen in cyanide poisoning is directly related to the conversion from aerobic to anaerobic metabolism. The acidosis seen in cyanide poisoning occurs secondary to the production of hydrogen atoms (H^+) by the cellular use of adenosine triphosphate (ATP) without the concomitant consumption of H^+ by oxidative phosphorylation; the acidosis is not a result of the lactate production. The heart and brain are particularly sensitive to the effects of cyanide poisoning because of their high metabolic demand and dependence on ATP.

■ CLINICAL PRESENTATION

The clinical presentation of cyanide poisoning is protean and depends on the route of exposure and the cyanide compound involved. The early signs and symptoms are dyspnea, headache, weakness, nausea, vomiting, diaphoresis, hypotension, tachycardia, and altered mental status. The late signs and symptoms are bradycardia, atrioventricular heart block, ventricular dysrhythmias, asystole, seizures, and coma. Exposure to any form of cyanide can result in death.

Cyanide gas is a knock-down agent, causing those exposed to lose consciousness rapidly. Patients with exposure to 300 parts per million (ppm) of cyanide gas rapidly collapse and typically do not survive to ED admission. Exposure to 100 ppm for more than 30 minutes is considered life-threatening. An oral dose of 200 mg of potassium cyanide is considered a fatal ingestion. Features of cyanide poisoning typically develop 15 to 30 minutes after ingestion of cyanide salts. Exposure to cyanogens can result in delayed symptoms and signs because the parent compound must be metabolized before cyanide is produced.

■ DIFFERENTIAL DIAGNOSIS

Presentation of the patient with an unknown cyanide exposure leads to a broad differential diagnosis. All medical causes of altered mental status, hypotension, and acidosis must be considered. Without a history of cyanide exposure, the diagnosis is often difficult to make. The toxicologic differential diagnosis of cyanide poisoning is listed in Box 147-3, and a comparison of various gas exposures is shown in Table 147-1.

■ DIAGNOSTIC TESTING

A whole blood cyanide measurement is not readily available in the ED. The hallmark findings in cyanide

Table 147-1 COMPARISONS, DIAGNOSIS, AND TREATMENT OF VARIOUS GAS EXPOSURES

Exposure	Symptoms	Diagnostic Testing	Treatment
Cyanide	Depend on route of exposure and compound involved Dyspnea, headache, weakness, nausea, vomiting, diarrhea, hypotension, and altered mental status early Gas exposure is rapid knock-down	Nonspecific: ABGs (anion gap metabolic acidosis) Serum lactate (elevated) Electrocardiogram (arrhythmias)	Decontamination Supportive care Cyanide kit
Carbon monoxide	Generally, slow-onset alteration of mental status Coma with severe poisoning Nausea and vomiting, headache at low doses	Carbon monoxide level	Oxygen; hyperbaric in severe cases
Hydrogen sulfide	At high levels: rapid coma, collapse, seizures, respiratory arrest At lower levels: headache, dizziness, nausea, dyspnea, chest pain, altered mental status	ABGs (hypoxia) and serum lactate (elevated) suggest diagnosis	Oxygen Decontamination Sodium nitrite component of cyanide antidote kit Hyperbaric oxygen if readily available
Sodium azide	Similar to those in presentations of cyanide and hydrogen sulfide poisonings	None	Supportive care
Methane or butane	Alveolar hypoxia	None	Oxygen therapy with rapid improvement

ABGs, arterial blood gas measurements.

BOX 147-3

Differential Diagnosis of Cyanide and Hydrogen Sulfide Poisoning

Medical Conditions Mimicking Cyanide and Hydrogen Sulfide Poisoning

Acute myocardial infarction
Encephalitis/meningitis
Hyperglycemic coma
Hypoglycemic coma
Intracranial hemorrhage
Pneumonia
Pulmonary embolism
Shock
Stroke

Toxins Mimicking Cyanide and Hydrogen Sulfide Poisoning

Arsine gas
Asphyxiant gases
Carbon monoxide
Cyclic antidepressants
Irritant gases
Isoniazid
Phosphine gas
Salicylates
Sodium azide
Strychnine
Toxic alcohols

poisoning are a profound metabolic acidosis with a wide anion gap and an elevation of serum lactate. An arterial blood gas measurement defines the extent of the acidosis. An electrocardiogram (ECG) assesses for any potential dysrhythmias.

■ TREATMENT

Aggressive supportive care and early administration of the cyanide antidote kit are the mainstays of treatment (Fig. 147-1). Patients with cyanide exposure are often critically ill at presentation and may rapidly progress to respiratory and cardiovascular collapse. The EP must be prepared to provide ventilatory, inotropic, and pressor support for these patients.

The cyanide antidote kit contains three products—amyl nitrite, sodium nitrite, and sodium thiosulfate. The nitrates induce methemoglobinemia. Cyanide has a higher affinity for methemoglobin than cytochrome oxidase. Inducing methemoglobinemia allows cyanide to dissociate from cytochrome oxidase and preferentially bind to methemoglobin, forming cyanmethemoglobin. This process sequesters cyanide in the serum and allows cellular metabolism to resume. The sodium thiosulfate enhances the normal cyanide metabolic pathway. The small amount of cyanide present under normal circumstances is metabolized, in the presence of a sulfur donor, to thiocyanate by the enzyme rhodanese. Thiocyanate has minimal toxicity and is excreted in the urine. Sodium thiosulfate acts a sulfur donor and enhances the elimination of cyanide.

The amyl nitrite component of the cyanide antidote kit is contained in pearls meant to be crushed to produce a vapor that is inhaled. This component

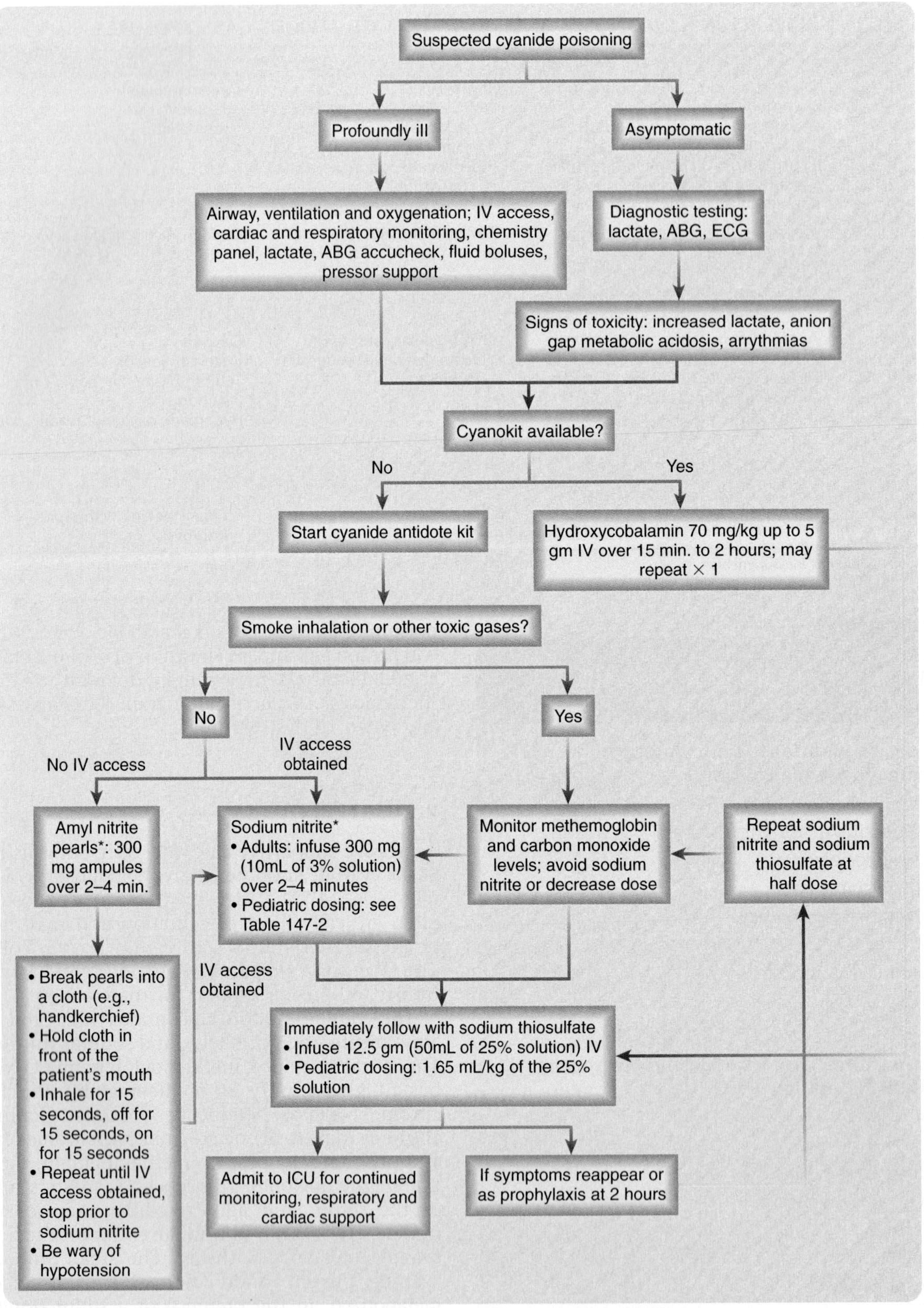
Suspected cyanide poisoning
Profoundly ill
Asymptomatic
Airway, ventilation and oxygenation; IV access, cardiac and respiratory monitoring, chemistry panel, lactate, ABG accucheck, fluid boluses, pressor support
Diagnostic testing: lactate, ABG, ECG
Signs of toxicity: increased lactate, anion gap metabolic acidosis, arrythmias
Cyanokit available?
No
Yes
Start cyanide antidote kit
Hydroxycobalamin 70 mg/kg up to 5 gm IV over 15 min. to 2 hours; may repeat × 1
Smoke inhalation or other toxic gases?
No
Yes
No IV access
IV access obtained
Amyl nitrite pearls*: 300 mg ampules over 2–4 min.
Sodium nitrite* • Adults: infuse 300 mg (10mL of 3% solution) over 2–4 minutes • Pediatric dosing: see Table 147-2
Monitor methemoglobin and carbon monoxide levels; avoid sodium nitrite or decrease dose
Repeat sodium nitrite and sodium thiosulfate at half dose
• Break pearls into a cloth (e.g., handkerchief) • Hold cloth in front of the patient's mouth • Inhale for 15 seconds, off for 15 seconds, on for 15 seconds • Repeat until IV access obtained, stop prior to sodium nitrite • Be wary of hypotension
IV access obtained
Immediately follow with sodium thiosulfate • Infuse 12.5 gm (50mL of 25% solution) IV • Pediatric dosing: 1.65 mL/kg of the 25% solution
Admit to ICU for continued monitoring, respiratory and cardiac support
If symptoms reappear or as prophylaxis at 2 hours

FIGURE 147-1 Diagnosis and treatment algorithm for cyanide poisoning. ABG, arterial blood gas measurement; ECG, electrocardiogram; ICU, intensive care unit; IV, intravenous(ly). *Nitrites are not given if hydroxycobalamin is available.

Table 147-2 PEDIATRIC NITRITE DOSING ACCORDING TO HEMOGLOBIN VALUE*

Hemoglobin Value (g/dL)	3% Sodium Nitrite Solution (mL/kg)
7.0	0.19
8.0	0.22
9.0	0.25
10.0	0.27
11.0	0.30
12.0	0.33
13.0	0.36
14.0	0.39

*Note: If giving sodium nitrite empirically to a patient with no history of anemia, do not wait for hemoglobin results; assume the hemoglobin level is 12 g/dL, and dose accordingly.

From Berlin CMJ: The treatment of cyanide poisoning in children. Pediatrics 1970;46:793-796.

is generally reserved for situations in which intravenous access is delayed or cannot be achieved. The sodium nitrite comes in 300-mg ampules meant to be infused over 2 to 4 minutes.

The patient's blood pressure must be monitored carefully because the nitrites can induce hypotension. Methemoglobin levels have to be monitored regularly with nitrite therapy because methemoglobin does not carry oxygen. The methemoglobin levels should be kept at less than 30%. Caution should be used in the administration of nitrites to fire victims, who may have carbon monoxide poisoning. Carboxyhemoglobin also does not carry oxygen. Inducing methemoglobinemia in these patients may worsen oxygen delivery to tissues. In such cases, a smaller dose of the nitrites or using only the sodium thiosulfate component of the cyanide antidote kit should be considered. In the case of anemia in the pediatric patient, the nitrite dose must be adjusted for the hemoglobin level; Table 147-2 provides dosing guidelines for such a situation.

The sodium thiosulfate dose is 12.5 g administered intravenously. There are no concerning adverse reactions to sodium thiosulfate. Both the sodium nitrite and sodium thiosulfate components of the cyanide antidote kit may be readministered as clinically indicated.

Hydroxycobalamin (also hydroxocobalamin, vitamin B_{12a}) is another antidote for cyanide poisoning. Marketed as the Cyanokit, it has now been approved in the United States as an antidote for cyanide poisoning. Hydroxycobalamin has a high affinity for cyanide and, via a nonenzymatic reaction, binds with cyanide to form cyanocobalamin (vitamin B_{12}), which is excreted in the urine. Transient hypertension and a self-limited reddish discoloration of the skin, mucous membranes, and urine are the only adverse effects of hydroxycobalamin. The adult dose is 5 g administered intravenously over 15 to 30 minutes up to 2 hours; the pediatric dose is 70 mg/kg. The dose may be repeated as clinically indicated up to a maximum of 10 g.[2]

If available, hydroxycobalamin replaces nitrites in the treatment of cyanide poisoning. Hydroxycobalamin can safely be administered with sodium thiosulfate, although the two agents cannot be given at the same time because sodium thiosulfate binds hydroxycobalamin and inactivates it. Hydroxycobalamin and sodium thiosulfate may be synergistic in cyanide elimination.[3] Finally, hydroxycobalamin does not induce methemoglobinemia, making it a better choice than the nitrites.

■ DISPOSITION

Cyanide-poisoned patients are critically ill. They should be admitted to an intensive care unit for continued respiratory and cardiovascular support and monitoring.

Hydrogen Sulfide

■ SCOPE AND HISTORY

Hydrogen sulfide is a known as a classic knock-down agent. It causes a patient to become comatose rapidly, with marked metabolic acidosis. The mechanism is similar to that of cyanide, and hydrogen sulfide inhibits cytochrome and the electron transport chain.

Hydrogen sulfide, also know by its rotten egg odor, is commonly referred to as "sewer gas" or "stink damp." The health hazard of the sewer is well illustrated by Victor Hugo in *Les Miserables*. He refers to the sewers of Paris as "a sarcophagus where asphyxia opens its claws in the filth and clutches you by the throat."[4]

In addition to being a well-known sewer hazard, hydrogen sulfide exposure can be seen in plumbing, mining, tanning, fisheries, drilling, and miscellaneous chemical manufacturing occupations. This agent can be produced by the decomposition of animal or organic material. It can also be produced by the addition of an acid to a metal sulfide. A clue to the presence of hydrogen sulfide is the blackening or tarnishing of silver coins, which results from the conversion of silver to silver sulfide upon exposure to hydrogen sulfide.

■ PATHOPHYSIOLOGY

Hydrogen sulfide is as potent as cyanide in inhibiting cytochrome *aa*$_3$.[5] Both hydrogen sulfide and cyanide form complexes with ferric iron at both the cytochrome and hemoglobin levels. Hydrogen sulfide dissociates into HS^- (hydrosulfide anion) and H^+ (hydrogen cation). When a victim is exposed to hydrogen sulfide, it is the HS^- that combines with methemoglobin to form sulfmethemoglobin. Sulfmethemoglobin has a half-life of approximately 2 hours.[5]

Table 147-3 HYDROGEN SULFIDE AIR CONCENTRATIONS AND THEIR CLINICAL EFFECTS*

Hydrogen Sulfide Concentration (ppm)	Clinical Effect(s)
30	Local irritation Sore throat Eye irritation "Rotten egg" odor
>30	Over time, olfactory fatigue
>40-200	Respiratory and mucous membrane irritation and respiratory distress
>200	Severe toxicity
700	Respiratory paralysis Asphyxia Death

*The U.S. Occupational Safety and Health Administration (OSHA) permissible exposure limit (PEL) is 20 ppm total, or 50 ppm for any 10-minute period. The National Institute for Occupational Safety and Health (NIOSH) recommended exposure limit (REL) is 10 ppm for 10 minutes, and evacuation is recommended for a reading of 50 ppm at any time.

Adapted from Agency for Toxic Substances and Disease Registry: Draft Toxicological Profile for Hydrogen Sulfide. Atlanta, Agency for Toxic Substances and Disease Registry, Department of Health and Human Services, 2004.

■ CLINICAL PRESENTATION

The classic feature of hydrogen sulfide exposure is the effect of the substance's being a rapid knock-down agent. If an individual is exposed to a large concentration of hydrogen sulfide, he or she can rapidly lose consciousness. At low levels of exposure, hydrogen sulfide can cause headache, dizziness, and nausea; at higher concentrations it can lead to shortness of breath, dyspnea on exertion, chest pain, and a decreased level of consciousness. At the highest concentrations it causes collapse, coma, and possibly seizures, respiratory arrest, and asphyxiation. See Table 147-3 for correlation of hydrogen sulfide air concentrations and clinical effect.

■ DIFFERENTIAL DIAGNOSIS

In formulating the differential diagnosis of hydrogen sulfide exposure, the clinician should consider the many causes of coma, including hypoglycemia and hyperglycemia. Severe cerebrovascular accident should be considered. Hydrogen sulfide can manifest as a shock state, and other causes of shock should be considered (sepsis, hemorrhage, etc.). Intoxication and coma in any patient should always prompt the consideration of meningitis, encephalitis, or intracranial hemorrhage. A hydrogen sulfide–intoxicated patient may present in a state of hypoxia, for which conditions such as pneumonia and pulmonary embolism should be considered. Some patients may complain of chest pain, which should prompt an investigation for myocardial ischemia.

Certain toxins can mimic hydrogen sulfide poisoning. The toxic syndromes produced by carbon monoxide and cyanide can look very similar. Carbon monoxide generally causes a slower onset in altered mental status, but can lead to coma with severe poisoning. Hydrogen sulfide exposure can also be associated with more upper respiratory irritation than seen with carbon monoxide exposure. Cyanide also causes a rapid knock-down and leads to a profound metabolic acidosis with lactic acid accumulation. The distinguishing features of cyanide poisoning are discussed in the part of the chapter on this agent. See Table 147-1 for differential diagnosis of cyanide and hydrogen sulfide poisoning.

Sodium azide can cause a toxic syndrome indistinguishable from that of cyanide and hydrogen sulfide. One should also beware of asphyxiant gases, such as methane and butane, which cause alveolar hypoxia by the direct displacement of oxygen. When a patient is removed from the source of exposure and with the correction of hypoxia, the patient will recover rapidly. Irritant gases, such as chlorine and chloramine, can also cause upper respiratory irritation but do not typically cause coma without profound pulmonary effects.

Finally one should consider other causes of coma and profound metabolic acidemia. The toxic alcohols methanol and ethylene glycol both cause coma and metabolic acidosis that progressively worsens without treatment. With hydrogen sulfide exposure, the patient who survives the initial insult should show progressive improvement. Salicylates are another commonly ingested toxin that can cause coma and profound metabolic acidemia in massive overdose.

■ DIAGNOSTIC TESTING

No single diagnostic test makes the diagnosis of hydrogen sulfide poisoning in real time. An arterial or venous blood gas measurement is useful to document acidemia. An arterial P_{O_2} measurement documents the level of hypoxia. A serum lactate measurement also suggests the diagnosis of hydrogen sulfide, but does not distinguish it from other cytochrome poisons (cyanide, sodium azide). Sulfide ion or thiosulfate measurements can be obtained, but they are not available on a "stat" basis, and their clinical correlation is very limited; they generally should not be ordered. Elevated urinary thiosulfate

BOX 147-4

Treatment of Hydrogen Sulfide Poisoning

- Rescue patient using self-contained breathing apparatus; remove patient from source
- Decontaminate with water
- Administer 100% oxygen
- Positive end-expiratory presssure (PEEP) if ventilation required
- Fluids and vasopressors for hypotension
- Sodium bicarbonate as needed for severe acidosis
- Sodium nitrite: 300 mg (10 mL of 3% solution) over 2 to 4 minutes in adults (measure methemoglobin concentration 30 minutes after infusion)
- Hyperbaric oxygen in severe cases when readily available

Tips and Tricks

- Hydrogen sulfide poisoning should be suspected whenever a person is found unconscious in an enclosed space, especially if an odor of rotten eggs is present.
- Hydroxycobalamin (Cyanokit) is associated with no risk for methemoglobinemia and should be given in place of the nitrite portions of the cyanide antidote kit when available.
- Hydrogen sulfide exposure is common at construction sites, and decontamination is important to prevent exposure of the health care team.
- Many cases of gas exposure respond rapidly to oxygenation; lack of response should raise the suspicion of cyanide or hydrogen sulfide poisoning.
- Hyperbaric therapy for hydrogen sulfide toxicity is indicated only when it is readily available on site.
- Patients who do not survive cyanide poisoning are still candidates for organ donation, including of the heart, liver, kidney, and pancreas.

values suggests exposure to hydrogen sulfide.[6] Some emergency medical services and industrial hygienists have the capability to measure hydrogen sulfide concentrations in air; this measurement can provide useful information at the scene and for clinical correlation.

TREATMENT

The most important way to ensure survival of a patient with hydrogen sulfide exposure is to remove the individual from the source of exposure. A significantly exposed individual should be immediately started on 100% oxygen. Comatose patients or those in respiratory distress should be intubated and given 100% oxygen. Principles of decontamination should be followed; the patient's clothes should be removed, and all chemicals irrigated off the patient's body. Ocular decontamination with fluorescein examination is appropriate to treat and address ocular chemical burns.

The sodium nitrite component of the cyanide antidote kit can be administered to patients presenting early after moderate to severe exposure to hydrogen sulfide. There is good animal evidence that nitrites are antidotal and, in fact, are superior to 100% oxygen.[5,7] Nitrites can be given intravenously in the same manner as described for cyanide. The animal models from which supporting data are taken are mostly pretreatment models, and the delayed clinical benefit is controversial. However, it is reasonable to give nitrites to severely exposed patients who present early after exposure.

Hyperbaric oxygen therapy (HBOT) has been utilized with anecdotal success in hydrogen sulfide poisoning.[8] Its use is based mostly on a theoretical benefit, and its indication is controversial. Transfer of an unstable patient to obtain HBOT is not justified by the published case reports. This therapy may be attempted if it is easily available at the receiving institution (Box 147-4).

DISPOSITION

Patients exposed to hydrogen sulfide who are asymptomatic on the scene can be safely monitored for a short observation period (approximately 4 hours). Significantly exposed patients and those with respiratory distress or altered mental status should be admitted to the intensive care unit for close monitoring and meticulous supportive care.

REFERENCES

1. Morocco AP: Cyanides. Crit Care Clin 2005;21:691-705.
2. Sauer SW, Keim ME: Hydroxocobalamin: Improved public health readiness for cyanide disasters. Ann Emerg Med 2001;37:635-641.
3. Hall AH, Rumack BH: Hydroxycobalamin/sodium thiosulfate as a cyanide antidote. J Emerg Med 1987;5:115-121.
4. Knight LD, Presnell SE: Death by sewer gas: Case report of a double fatality and review of the literature. Am J Forensic Med Pathol 2005;26:181-185.
5. Smith RP, Gosselin RE: Hydrogen sulfide poisoning. J Occup Med 1979;21:93-97.
6. Snyder JW, Safir EF, Summerville GP, Middleberg RA: Occupational fatality and persistent neurological sequelae after mass exposure to hydrogen sulfide. Am J Emerg Med 1995;13:199-203.
7. Smith RP, Kruszyna R, Kruszyna H: Management of acute sulfide poisoning: Effects of oxygen, thiosulfate, and nitrite. Arch Environ Health 1976;31:166-169.
8. Smilkstein MJ, Bronstein AC, Pickett HM, Rumack BH: Hyperbaric oxygen therapy for severe hydrogen sulfide poisoning. J Emerg Med 1985;3:27-30.

Chapter 148

Ethanol and Opioid Intoxication and Withdrawal

Michael J. Schmidt and Cynthia Galvan

KEY POINTS

Ethanol may have some beneficial cardiovascular effects in low doses; however, abuse, dependence, and withdrawal are common, often leading to related medical and societal complications.

Ethanol causes depressant effects, but abrupt cessation of its use in long-term users can cause potentially dangerous withdrawal syndromes.

Most organ systems in the body can be affected by ethanol consumption. Important associated disease states are electrolyte disturbances, traumatic injuries, infectious diseases, and primary central nervous system, gastrointestinal, and cardiovascular complications.

Alcohol withdrawal syndrome is a spectrum of disease ranging from minor signs and symptoms, such as anxiety and mild tremor, to severe withdrawal, including autonomic instability and delirium.

Supportive care is the mainstay of treatment for patients with acute intoxication and withdrawal. Benzodiazepines constitute the major form of pharmacotherapy for withdrawal syndromes.

Patients who have a history of major withdrawal, are currently in withdrawal, or have significant associated disease states should be admitted for further treatment. Substance disorders should be addressed with referral to outpatient therapy and proper follow-up.

Long-term opioid use may lead to dependency and predispose individuals to a withdrawal state after decreased intake or antidote reversal of an opioid overdose.

Opioid intoxication is marked by depressed central nervous system activity, respiratory depression, and miosis.

Opioid withdrawal syndrome is marked by yawning, piloerection, and mydriasis.

Ethanol

SCOPE

Ethanol use is a common part of our society, as evidenced by the fact that two thirds of adults in the United States consume ethanol-containing beverages during their lifetimes.[1] Mild to moderate consumption (up to 1 drink/day for women and 2 drinks/day for men) (Box 148-1)[2] has been shown to have beneficial cardiovascular effects, including decreased risk of myocardial infarction and stroke.[3,4] About 9% of adults, however, meet the diagnostic criteria for alcohol abuse and alcoholism.[5] This maladaptive behavior can lead to a number of individual medical complications as well as societal problems, including motor vehicle collisions, assaults, homicide, suicide, and domestic violence. More than 600,000 ED visits a year are related to uncomplicated ethanol intoxication,[6] and alcohol consumption has been found to be the third leading cause of preventable death in the United States.[7]

At the tail-end of the spectrum of alcohol-related problems is ethanol withdrawal syndrome. Almost half a million episodes of alcohol withdrawal, requiring pharmacologic treatment in the ED, occur each year in the United States.[8] Delirium tremens (DTs), a well-defined severe withdrawal syndrome marked by tremors, seizures, and delirium, has a mortality rate of up to 30%. Patients at risk for DTs include those with a previous history of DTs and those with tachycardia at presentation.[9] About 5% of patients at risk for ethanol withdrawal go on to have DTs.

BOX 148-1

Definition of One Standard Alcoholic Drink

A standard alcoholic drink can be defined as one of the following:

- 0.5 oz. ethanol
- 12 fluid oz. regular beer
- 5 fluid oz. wine
- 1.5 fluid oz. 80-proof distilled spirits

Adapted from U.S. Department of Health and Human Services and the U.S. Department of Agriculture (USDA): Dietary Guidelines for Americans, 2005 (6th ed). Washington, DC: U.S. Government Printing Office, 2005.

PATHOPHYSIOLOGY

Ethanol is readily absorbed from the gastrointestinal (GI) tract and primarily metabolized by the liver via the alcohol dehydrogenase pathway (Fig. 148-1). Metabolism of ethanol differs in men and women. Although alcohol dehydrogenase is found in the gastric mucosa and other tissues, women seem to have less ability to metabolize it via the gastric route.[10] Chronic ethanol users also utilize a second pathway, the microsomal ethanol-oxidizing system (MEOS). Ethanol is a central nervous system (CNS) depressant involving gamma-aminobutyric acid (GABA) neurotransmitters, α-receptors, β-receptors, and dopamine. The level of CNS depression depends on many factors affecting absorption and elimination, including age, weight, gender, presence of food, gastric motility, speed of consumption, and long-term alcohol use. Ethanol intoxication in most states is legally defined as a blood alcohol concentration (BAC) of 80 to 100 mg/dL (0.08 to 0.1 mg %). Elimination rates vary greatly, but a rate of 20 mg/dL/hr can be assumed for most intoxicated ED patients (chronic alcoholics may have a higher elimination rate, 30 to 40 mg/dl/hr, because of the alternate pathway).[11]

In chronic alcoholics who abruptly stop or significantly decrease their consumption of ethanol, the effect is pathologic CNS and autonomic excitation. GABA receptors are downregulated in chronic ethanol use, leading to decreased activity of the inhibitory

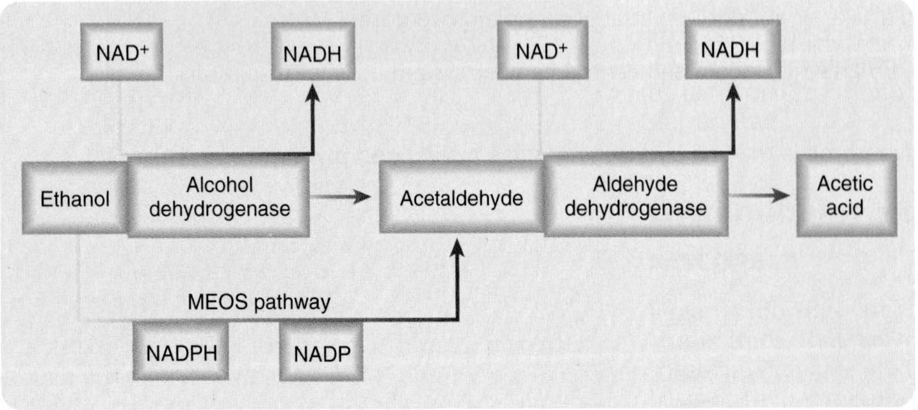
NAD+
NADH
NAD+
NADH
Ethanol
Alcohol dehydrogenase
Acetaldehyde
Aldehyde dehydrogenase
Acetic acid
MEOS pathway
NADPH
NADP

FIGURE 148-1 Alcohol dehydrogenase pathway, including the microsomal ethanol-oxidizing system (MEOS), the alternative metabolism seen in chronic alcoholics. NAD+, nicotinamide adenine dinucleotide; NADH, reduced nicotinamide adenine dinucleotide; NADP, nicotinamide adenine dinucleotide phosphate; NADPH, reduced nicotinamide adenine dinucleotide phosphate.

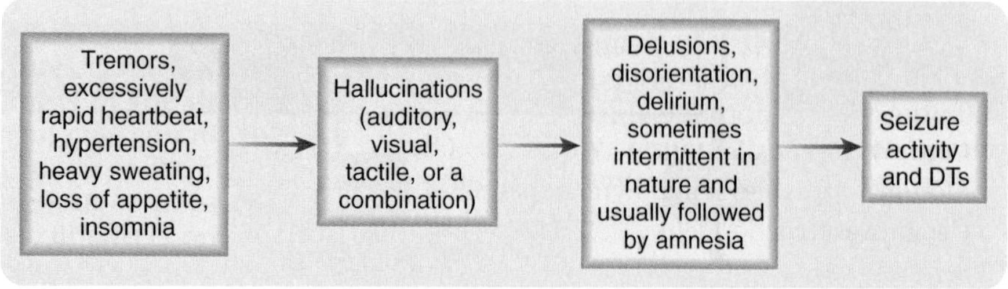
Tremors, excessively rapid heartbeat, hypertension, heavy sweating, loss of appetite, insomnia
Hallucinations (auditory, visual, tactile, or a combination)
Delusions, disorientation, delirium, sometimes intermittent in nature and usually followed by amnesia
Seizure activity and DTs

FIGURE 148-2 Progression of signs and symptoms of alcohol withdrawal. Symptoms on the *left* predominate during the first 24 hours without alcohol and progress over the next 48 hours. DTs, delirium tremers.

effects of GABA with abstention or with a significant decrease in ethanol consumption. Cessation of alcohol consumption may be inadvertent, as in the patient who is unable to tolerate oral intake because of vomiting or in the hospitalized patient whose access to ethanol is restricted. The excitatory glutamate neurotransmitter system, catecholamine levels, and catecholamine activity are also increased during withdrawal.[12]

■ CLINICAL PRESENTATION

Ethanol use is associated with many disease states affecting many organ systems in the body (Box 148-2). The Wernicke-Korsakoff syndrome bears special mention. This syndrome complex is composed of two disease processes, Wernicke's encephalopathy and Korsakoff's amnestic state, which can manifest individually or concomitantly. Classically, Wernicke's encephalopathy consists of ocular abnormalities (nystagmus, motor palsies), ataxia, and mental status changes (confusion), although presentations with this classic triad are rare. Korsakoff's amnestic state refers to the syndrome of memory deficits found in chronic alcohol abusers. Anterograde and retrograde amnesia are present, and confabulation is common. Thiamine deficiency is the cause, although ataxia and memory loss may persist despite treatment.

The CNS-depressive effects of ethanol range from diminished fine motor control to coma and respiratory depression The intoxicated patient often presents with the smell of ethanol on the breath, slurred speech, difficulty with coordination (including gait), and emotional lability (euphoria to agitation or even violence). Death can occur from respiratory depression and/or aspiration. Because of greater tolerance, chronic alcoholics may exhibit a high level of functioning despite a high BAC. Accidental injury is often associated with ethanol intoxication. Ethanol intoxication generally should not lower the Glasgow Coma Scale (GCS) score dramatically; whenever a low score is found, further CNS evaluation is warranted.[13]

Classically, the patient in ethanol withdrawal presents to the ED about 24 hours after a significant decrease or cessation of ethanol consumption. The patient is anxious, tremulous, tachycardic, hypertensive, and hyperreflexic and may complain of sleep and GI disturbances.

Alcohol withdrawal syndrome represents a spectrum of disease, ranging from minor to major. There is an accompanying time frame within this spectrum of disease, but there is significant overlap between timing and the signs and symptoms. Minor withdrawal begins within 6 to 24 hours and is characterized by the findings previously described. Major withdrawal syndrome begins after 24 hours and peaks at about 48 to 72 hours. It may have any or all of the following features: progression of signs and symptoms previously described, hyperpyrexia, seizures, altered mental status, hallucinations (visual, auditory, or tactile), and delirium. DTs are rare (although patients may mistakenly equate them with generalized withdrawal syndrome) and constitute the most severe form of withdrawal. DTs occupy the far end of the spectrum, consisting of substantial tremor, autonomic hyperactivity, profound confusion, fever, and hallucinations (Fig. 148-2).[14]

■ DIFFERENTIAL DIAGNOSIS

The diagnosis of ethanol intoxication is mainly one of exclusion, and a history consistent with ethanol consumption is important. The initial approach to the patient should be the same as for any patient with altered mental status. Traumatic injuries and co-ingestions (acetaminophen, illicit drugs, toxic

RED FLAGS

- Incorrectly assuming the patient is intoxicated
- Not suspecting ethanol abuse in an elderly patient
- Not recognizing concomitant head injury, intoxication, or associated diseases
- Not aggressively treating signs and symptoms of withdrawal
- Inappropriately discharging an acutely intoxicated patient
- Not managing the airway in a timely manner
- Not evaluating for other causes, including head trauma, infection, and cerebrovascular accident, after repeated doses of naloxone or continued altered consciousness in the patient with suspected intoxication or opioid overdose
- Not considering opioid withdrawal in patients with cancer and in other patients with long-term opioid use, and treating appropriately

BOX 148-2

Disease States Associated with Ethanol Use

Central Nervous System

Mononeuropathies and polyneuropathies
Cerebrovascular accident
Seizures
Wernicke-Korsakoff syndrome
Cerebellar degeneration

Cardiovascular

Alcohol-induced cardiomyopathy
Dysrhythmias ("holiday heart": atrial fibrillation, ventricular tachycardia)
Effects on coronary arteries (protective in low doses, damaging in high doses)

Pulmonary

Aspiration pneumonia
Concomitant tobacco use
Acute respiratory distress syndrome

Gastrointestinal

Gastritis/esophagitis
Upper gastrointestinal bleeding
Alcohol-induced hepatitis
Cirrhosis of liver
Acute and chronic pancreatitis

Musculoskeletal

Myopathies
Gout exacerbation

Fluids, Electrolytes, and Nutrition

Vitamin deficiencies (e.g. thiamine)
Hypoglycemia
Hypokalemia
Hypomagnesemia
Hypocalcemia
Hypophosphatemia
Alcoholic ketoacidosis

Hematologic/Oncologic

Cancers (gastric, oropharyngeal, laryngeal, esophageal)
Anemia
Thrombocytopenia

Infectious Diseases

Pneumonia
Tuberculosis
Spontaneous bacterial peritonitis (in those with ascites)

Trauma

All types of blunt and penetrating trauma

Psychiatric

Depression
Antisocial personality disorder
Increased risk of suicide

Table 148-1 MOST COMMON AND MOST THREATENING DIFFERENTIAL DIAGNOSES

	Most Common	Most Threatening
Intoxication	Acute, uncomplicated intoxication	Coma Respiratory depression Associated disease states (e.g., traumatic head injury) Drug co-ingestion
Withdrawal	Minor syndrome with anxiety Insomnia Mild tremor	Autonomic instability Altered mental status Delirium

BOX 148-3

Differential Diagnosis of Ethanol Intoxication and Withdrawal

Intoxication

Traumatic head injury
Cerebrovascular accident
Metabolic derangements (hypoglycemia)
Hypoxia
Drug ingestion
Central nervous system infections

Withdrawal

Infections (meningitis, encephalitis, sepsis)
Toxidromes (sympathomimetic, anticholinergic)
Thyrotoxicosis
Neuroleptic malignant syndrome
Heat stroke
Acute psychosis
Withdrawal from other sedative-hypnotic drugs (benzodiazepines, barbiturates) and those used to treat spasticity (baclofen)

alcohols) should be high on the differential diagnosis list (Box 148-3).

A history of previous ethanol withdrawal or alcohol abuse with decreased intake or cessation of alcohol is the key to the diagnosis of ethanol withdrawal. Withdrawal that is late in onset (>3 days) may be more consistent with sedative-hypnotic drug withdrawal. The differential diagnosis may also include possibilities considered in patients with delirium and seizures as well (Table 148-1).

■ DIAGNOSTIC STUDIES

Diagnostic testing for the acutely intoxicated patient should be guided by suspicion for concomitant disease states and potential traumatic injury. A blood alcohol measurement is necessary only to confirm a diagnosis or to guide treatment.[15]

Patients presenting in withdrawal may mandate a comprehensive evaluation, but the same guidelines apply as for the intoxicated patient. The laboratory tests will vary but may include a complete blood count, serum glucose measurement, blood chemistry panel with a full set of electrolyte measurements, urinalysis, toxicology screen, electrocardiogram (ECG), chest radiography, and head computed tomography (CT). Lumbar puncture for cerebrospinal fluid analysis may be indicated if subarachnoid hemorrhage or CNS infection is in the differential diagnosis.

■ TREATMENT

Supportive care is the mainstay of treatment for acute ethanol intoxication (Fig. 148-3). Airway and breathing must be assessed in the comatose patient, and endotracheal intubation, although rarely needed, should be used for airway protection if necessary. Circulation should be assessed, and isotonic intravenous (IV) fluids should be given initially for patients with hypotension or volume depletion. In the comatose patient, naloxone (0.8 mg) should be considered, and glucose (25 to 50 g IV) should be given to a hypoglycemic patient. If available, thiamine (100 mg IV) can be given prior to glucose administration to prevent or treat Wernicke's encephalopathy, but glucose administration need not be delayed.[16] Electrolyte and vitamin replacement can be achieved orally if the patient is tolerating oral intake, not at risk for aspiration, and is not being treated for active Wernicke's encephalopathy. For the rest, replacement can be given intravenously with use of a "banana bag" (Box 148-4). Concomitant disease states should be treated as necessary.

Patients who present to the ED with signs and symptoms of alcohol withdrawal should be evaluated to determine the severity of withdrawal. Treatment should focus on resuscitation with fluids, replacement of electrolyte and vitamin deficiencies, evaluation and treatment of concomitant diseases, and restoration of inhibitory tone to the CNS with long-acting benzodiazepines or barbiturates. Benzodiazepines are the mainstay of treatment for withdrawal itself. Lorazepam (1 to 4 mg) has an intermediate half-life and is easily used as either an oral, intramuscular (IM), or IV agent. The dose can be repeated every 10 minutes as necessary. Other benzodiazepines, such as diazepam, chlordiazepoxide, and midazolam, can also be used. Massive amounts of benzodiazepines have been known to be given to patients in major withdrawal and may be necessary

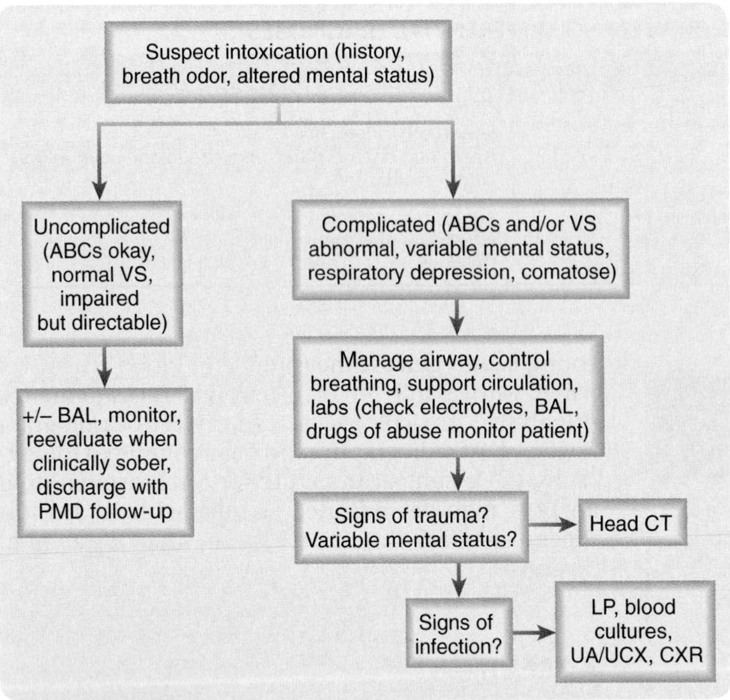
Suspect intoxication (history, breath odor, altered mental status)
Uncomplicated (ABCs okay, normal VS, impaired but directable)
+/– BAL, monitor, reevaluate when clinically sober, discharge with PMD follow-up
Complicated (ABCs and/or VS abnormal, variable mental status, respiratory depression, comatose)
Manage airway, control breathing, support circulation, labs (check electrolytes, BAL, drugs of abuse monitor patient)
Signs of trauma? Variable mental status?
Head CT
Signs of infection?
LP, blood cultures, UA/UCX, CXR

FIGURE 148-3 Treatment algorithm for ethanol intoxication. ABCs, airway, breathing, circulation; BAL, blood alcohol level; CT, computed tomography; CXR, chest radiograph; LP, lumbar puncture; PMD, primary-care physician; UA/UCX, urinalysis/urine culture; VS, vital signs.

BOX 148-4

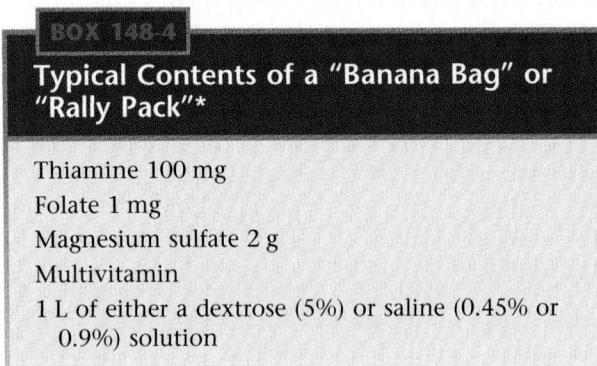

Typical Contents of a "Banana Bag" or "Rally Pack"*

Thiamine 100 mg
Folate 1 mg
Magnesium sulfate 2 g
Multivitamin
1 L of either a dextrose (5%) or saline (0.45% or 0.9%) solution

*Vitamins may be given orally if the patient can tolerate oral intake.

to control rapidly progressive symptoms, though a symptom-triggered approach has been shown to require less medication and shorter treatment.[17] Propofol, butyrophenones (haloperidol, droperidol), and barbiturates (phenobarbital, pentobarbital) are useful adjunct agents in patients not showing response to benzodiazepines. The airway must be closely monitored in these patients. Beta-blockers can also be used as adjuncts to decrease tachycardia in patients undergoing withdrawal from alcohol.

For patients being discharged from the ED and undergoing outpatient detoxification, a short course of benzodiazepines can be considered. Beta-blockers and clonidine may be useful additions to an outpatient treatment regimen for those with minor withdrawal.

Alcohol-related seizures can occur from withdrawal, precipitation of underlying epileptic disorder, acute toxicity, metabolic causes (hypoglycemia), trauma, or stroke. Benzodiazepines are first-line therapy for the treatment of acute seizure in the ED. Phenytoin is not recommended for treatment of an isolated, acute alcohol withdrawal seizure or as routine prophylaxis for patients with alcohol withdrawal and no history of seizures. Phenytoin can be continued in patients with alcohol withdrawal syndrome who are already taking it for seizures (either related or not related to withdrawal), and it can be given in the acute setting as deemed necessary for status epilepticus or for seizures resulting from other causes (e.g., stroke, trauma).[18,19]

■ DISPOSITION

The patient with uncomplicated ethanol intoxication may be discharged home after an evaluation for associated disease states if (1) the patient is not at risk of airway or breathing complications and (2) a responsible, sober adult is able to monitor the patient for the next 24 hours. Otherwise, the patient should be monitored in the ED until clinically and/or legally sober. Associated diseases complicating the intoxication guide admission.

Patients with major ethanol withdrawal require admission and may need an intensive care unit setting. Patients with minor withdrawal may be discharged after observation for 4 to 6 hours if the evaluation findings remain within normal limits (mental status, vital signs, and laboratory studies). A short course of benzodiazepines can be considered for the patient undergoing outpatient detoxification.

Referral to an outpatient treatment program is appropriate for all patients being discharged who are recognized as having a substance disorder. Options

Tips and Tricks

- Serum ethanol measurements are not needed in every patient.
- Obtain an ethanol measurement when needed for confirmation or to guide treatment.
- Reserve the "banana bag" (see Box 148-5) for patients who are ill and seem to be going into withdrawal; otherwise give the vitamins orally.
- Remember to rule out any other disease process in the patient with complicated ethanol intoxication.
- Discharge time can be guided by (1) a calculated sober time according to ethanol level, (2) an evaluation for clinical sobriety, or (3) whether the patient is awake and directable and will be in the care of a responsible sober adult.
- Calculate sober time as follows: (1) subtract 80 to 100 (legal limit) from the blood ethanol level; (2) divide the remainder by 20 to 30 (mg/dL/hr; estimate of ethanol metabolism every hour); the resulting number is the time to sobriety (sober time) in hours.
- Opioids may have a long half-life, so additional naloxone doses may be necessary if the patient seems to return to a depressed state after initially responding to naloxone.
- In patients with cancer or long-term pain medication use who present with symptoms of opioid withdrawal, treatment of nausea and vomiting and a dose of the prescribed opioid medications are appropriate.

include the use of inpatient versus outpatient treatment programs and/or referral to Alcoholics Anonymous (AA). Because of the high incidence of concomitant social and psychiatric problems,[20] referral to the ED's social or psychiatric worker (if available) may also be helpful.

Opioids

■ SCOPE

Opioids are a class of drugs that comprise natural, semisynthetic, and synthetic substances with analgesic and anesthetic properties. Opioids are related to opium, a narcotic resin from the poppy plant *Papaver somniferum* (Box 148-5). Opioids are used in short-term therapy for moderate to severe pain and to aid in sedation regimens in the ED. Long-term opioid therapy is used to treat pain and to aid in addiction therapy. National efforts to treat pain states more effectively has probably led to the fact that opioid-containing drugs are the now most prescribed medications in the United States, surpassing lipid-lowering drugs and antibiotics.[21,22]

Addiction to opioid drugs, considered narcotics, is not rare and can lead to significant morbidity and mortality. In 2004, 1.3 million ED visits were linked

BOX 148-5

Definition of Terms Commonly Related to Opioids

Opium: A resin from opium poppies (flowers) containing narcotic, morphine, codeine, and thebaine.

Opiate: Any of the narcotic alkaloids found in opium (morphine, codeine, thebaine).

Opioid: Natural, semisynthetic, and synthetic opium derivatives that bind opioid receptors and are reversed with naloxone.

Narcotic: Compounds with sedative properties; commonly include the opioids; in legal jargon, term refers to a controlled substance with illicit use.

Tolerance: Physiologic adaptation to opioid use with escalating doses required for similar effects.

Dependence: Continuous use despite negative impacts on life in addition to tolerance, withdrawal history, and compulsive use.

Withdrawal: Physiologic response to decreased intake of opioids in dependent individuals with behavioral, cognitive, and physical changes.

to drug misuse or abuse.[23] Unintentional drug overdoses, mainly opioid analgesics, account for the largest increase in drug-related deaths.[24] Opioid overdose can occur in several situations, including intentional self-injury, unintentional prescription, recreational or pediatric ingestion, and drug packing and stuffing.

■ PATHOPHYSIOLOGY

Opioids are a useful class of drugs used for sedation and analgesia, with morphine-like properties. The chemical structure of opioids is such that they bind several receptor types and act as partial and full opioid receptor agonists. Opioids bind receptors in the CNS, spinal cord, and GI system, being responsible for analgesia, anesthesia, and decreased GI motility. All opioids undergo hepatic metabolism and renal elimination; therefore, hepatic and renal functions play a large role in intoxication.

Long-term opioid use can result in physiologic tolerance and dependency via changes in opioid receptor structure, receptor trafficking, and mechanism of action. A withdrawal state can be precipitated in dependent individuals who decrease their opioid intake or are given the opioid receptor antagonist naloxone. The timing of withdrawal symptoms depends on the variable half-life of the particular opioid. Considered the opioid overdose antidote, naloxone is a competitive receptor antagonist that

Table 148-2 OPIOID INTOXICATION AND WITHDRAWAL SIGNS AND SYMPTOMS BY ORGAN SYSTEM

	Opioid Intoxication	Opioid Withdrawal
Central nervous system	Depression of activity Respiratory depression Increased parasympathetic activity	Excitation, restlessness, anxiety, seizures (rare) Tachypnea Adrenergic/sympathetic overdrive (lacrimation, piloerection, yawning, diaphoresis)
Head and neck	Miosis (pinpoint pupils) Antitussive	Mydriasis Rhinorrhea
Cardiovascular	Hypotension to normal blood pressure Bradycardia to normal heart rate	Normal blood pressure to hypertension Normal heart rate to tachycardia
Gastrointestinal	Constipation Nausea and vomiting	Diarrhea Nausea and vomiting
Genitourinary	Sphincter constriction/spasm	Sphincter relaxation
Musculoskeletal	Relaxed/flaccid	Myalgias
Psychiatric	Euphoria or dysphoria	Drug craving

can reverse opioid activity in dependent individuals. Naloxone is used to reverse the dangerous consequence of respiratory depression in opioid overdose and can be given intravenously, subcutaneously, intramuscularly, or endotracheally. Naloxone is not effective when given orally because of first-pass metabolism.

■ CLINICAL PRESENTATION

The hallmarks of opioid intoxication are CNS and respiratory depression, miosis, and constipation. Opioid overdose can lead to severe respiratory depression, apnea, and, if left untreated, cardiopulmonary arrest. History of opioid use is usually not readily available and should be considered in patients who are found unconscious, have a decreased respiratory rate, miosis, and lack a gag reflex. When antecedent history is available, it may include opioid use patterns such as multiple-drug substance abuse with or without methadone maintenance therapy, long-term prescription opioid use, and unknown poisoning. Patients with milder opioid intoxication may present with nausea, vomiting, constipation, miosis, depressed CNS level, and depressed respiratory status (Table 148-2).

The opioid withdrawel syndrome is classically marked by a generalized ill state. It may include yawning, rhinorrhea, mydriasis, piloerection, nausea, vomiting, diarrhea, myalgias, and abdominal pain. Withdrawal may be seen after administration of antidote in patients with unknown ingestion, whose history is later found to include chronic opioid use with elements of drug tolerance and dependence. Vital signs may include tachycardia, normal blood pressure to hypertension, and tachypnea. Another common picture of opioid withdrawal is seen in the patient who has cancer or uses an opioid for chronic pain and who misses a dose of medication; such a patient presents to the ED with nausea, vomiting, and abdominal cramping. The history usually uncovers a missed opioid dose.

■ Atypical Presentations

Opioid overdose may be complicated by unique opioid toxicities, trauma, environmental conditions, prolonged immobility, and co-ingestions. Opioid toxicity can also cause seizures, arrhythmias, pulmonary edema, serotonin syndrome, and co-ingestion toxicity (aspirin [ASA], acetaminophen, ethanol) with use of certain opioids (Table 148-3). Methadone, an agent used primarily for addiction therapy, is very-long-acting and can cause prolongation of corrected QT interval and torsades de pointes. Acute lung injury and aspiration pneumonia may add to the pulmonary issues in opioid overdose. Hypothermia may complicate resuscitation efforts, and prolonged immobility can contribute to rhabdomyolysis.

An atypical presentation of opioid withdrawal consists of repeated episodes of vomiting and diarrhea. Electrolyte abnormalities and dehydration may complicate withdrawal symptoms. Patients with high levels of tolerance may not experience some of the typical signs or symptoms; miosis should still be seen, even in patients with very high tolerance (Box 148-6).

Table 148-3 SPECIFIC OPIOID TOXICITIES

Compound	Toxicity
Morphine	Acute lung injury
Meperidine	Seizures
Methadone	QTc prolongation Torsades de pointes
Propoxyphene	QRS prolongation Seizures
Tramadol	Seizures

From Gutstein HB, Akil H: Opioid analgesia. In Brunton LL (ed): Goodman and Gilman's The Pharmalogical Basis of Therapentics, 11th ed. New York, McGraw-Hill, 2006.

BOX 148-6

Levels of Tolerance that May Develop to Some of the Effects of Opioids

High Tolerance
Analgesia
Euphoria, dysphoria
Mental clouding
Sedation
Respiratory depression
Antidiuresis
Nausea and vomiting
Cough suppression

Moderate Tolerance
Bradycardia

Minimal or No Tolerance
Miosis
Constipation
Convulsions

From Schumacher MA, Basbaum AI, Way WL: Opioid analgesics and antagonists. In Katzung BG (ed): Basic and Clinical Pharmacology, 10th ed., New York, McGraw-Hill, 2007.

BOX 148-7

Differential Diagnosis for Opioid Overdose and Opioid Withdrawal

Opioid Overdose
All components of differential diagnosis for a patient who is unconscious or in a coma
Ethanol intoxication/overdose
Benzodiazepine overdose
Clonidine overdose
Infection
Head trauma
Cerebrovascular accident

Opioid Withdrawal
Sympathomimetic overdose
Cholinergic overdose
Influenza

DIFFERENTIAL DIAGNOSIS

The differential diagnosis for opioid intoxication and overdose can be separated into the mantra of emergency medicine, "Sick or not sick?" The differential diagnosis for mild opioid intoxication includes hypoglycemia, ethanol intoxication, benzodiazepam use, clonidine use, drug co-ingestion, and poisoning; however, ethanol intoxication does not usually include miosis or decreased GI motility, and clonidine use causes hypotension and bradycardia. The differential diagnosis for the patient who is ill secondary to opioid overdose is similar to that for the patient in coma; infection, cerebrovascular accident, head trauma, and poisoning should be considered.

The diagnosis of opioid withdrawal is usually a diagnosis of exclusion unless withdrawal is induced by giving an antagonist in the ED. The differential diagnosis includes sympathomimetics, cholinergics, and influenza (Box 148-7).

DIAGNOSTIC TESTING

Diagnostic testing in opioid overdose usually does not guide treatment, given that the antidote is administered before test results are available. Tests are used to evaluate the complications of opioid toxicity, including arrhythmias, acute lung injury, pulmonary edema, and comorbid diseases. ECG and chest and abdominal radiographs can be useful as adjuncts in these cases. Urine drug testing aids in the overall picture of therapy but usually does not guide treatment in the acute setting of opioid overdose. Opiates can be detected for up to 36 hours in the urine, although false-positive results have been found with ingestion of poppy seeds. Acetaminophen, salicylate, and ethanol measurements should be included in evaluation for unknown ingestions. Findings of a serum chemistry panel and complete blood count can suggest a pattern of electrolyte disturbance and an etiology of infection. The serum creatinine kinase (CK) level may be elevated in patients with prolonged immobility and rhabdomyolysis. Many patients awaken after treatment with naloxone, admit to opioid overdose, and may not require any further testing.

Diagnostic testing in patients undergoing opioid withdrawal is guided by ruling out other causes of signs and symptoms. A comprehensive chemistry panel is useful when massive vomiting and diarrhea are present.

TREATMENT

Treatment of opioid intoxication and overdose should begin with assessment of the airway, breathing, and circulatory status of the patient. Airway adjuncts (oral or nasal airway) can be used to improve the viable airway, and with a decreased respiratory rate, bag-valve-mask ventilation may be necessary. If the patient lacks a gag reflex, endotracheal intubation may be warranted. Rapid administration of naloxone may prevent the need for intubation; if signs and symptoms are consistent with opioid intoxication, the antidote should be given immediately while preparations are being made for intubation. Naloxone should be administered IV, starting doses being 0.4 to 1 mg in apneic patients and 2 mg in those with

DOCUMENTATION

History

- How much alcohol or opioid was ingested, by what route, and over what period?
- Other drugs ingested?
- History of delirium tremens or alcohol-related seizures?
- Was there any trauma involved or loss of consciousness?
- Recent infections?
- Patterns of opioid use?
- Previous history of self-injury?

Physical Examination

- Stable or unstable vital signs (including repeat evaluation)?
- Does the patient look ill? Signs of trauma?
- Is the patient awake? Arousable? Does the patient have a gag reflex? What is Glasgow Coma Scale score?
- Cardiovascular status
- Respiratory and airway status
- Skin and musculoskeletal findings
- Eye examination—pinpoint pupils
- Findings of any repeat examinations made while the patient is in the ED
- Signs of intoxication at admission and discharge, especially if ethanol level was not measured

Laboratory Studies

- Levels of aspirin (ASA) and acetaminophen; urine drug screen results if needed
- Ethanol level if measured
- Electrocardiogram and chest radiograph in patients with abnormal physical findings
- Tests for electrolyte levels, anion gap, complete blood count, serum creatinine, creatine kinase

Medical Decision-Making

- Complex versus noncomplex alcohol intoxication
- Ruling out of concomitant diseases

Treatment

- Treatment strategy, including time monitored, fluid therapy, use of "banana bag," and any injuries addressed
- Decision to admit or discharge patient
- Time to administration of antidote, initial dose, redosing, or start of naloxone drip

Patient Instructions

- Discussion with patient regarding diagnosis, warning signs, what to do, follow-up, when to return
- Referral to outpatient treatment, if given
- For pediatric accidental ingestions: poison prevention counseling and child protective service notification if indicated

cardiopulmonary arrest. Naloxone can be repeated up to a total dose of 10 mg to reach the desired effect, which is increased respiratory rate.

Hypotension should be treated with intravenous fluids according to resuscitation protocols. Blood glucose levels should be checked at the bedside and patients with hypoglycemia should receive dextrose. When long-acting agents such as methadone are involved, the patient may require a naloxone drip and admission to an intensive care setting because of the prolonged risk of further symptoms. Care should be taken to reevaluate the patient frequently and observe him or her for a return of respiratory depression. Gastric lavage and use of activated charcoal are not routinely recommended in opioid overdose. Although activated charcoal will bind opioids, the aspiration risk precludes administration of charcoal. Hemodialysis is not indicated in opioid overdose because of the large and variable volume of distribution of these agents in the body.

Treatment of opioid withdrawal in the ED is aimed at stabilization of cardiopulmonary status and symptomatic therapy. Opioid replacement should be guided by the cause of the withdrawal—cessation of prescription medications, methadone therapy for addiction, decreased recreational intake. Administering missed doses of opioids and methadone replacement (20 mg PO or 10 mg IM) can be used to reverse withdrawal without overdose. If nonopioids are required, clonidine (0.1 to 0.3 mg IV every hour or in a sustained-release patch) can help with high blood pressure and decrease withdrawal symptoms. Benzodiazepines can also be used to aid in sedation and to temper withdrawal symptoms. Antiemetics can be given in the patient with nausea and vomiting.

■ DISPOSITION

Patients with opioid intoxication can probably be discharged from the ED after observation and evaluation of any active comorbid diseases at presentation. Patients with uncomplicated opioid overdose status after reversal can be monitored in the ED for 2 to 4 hours (the half-life of most opioids is in this range). While the patient is being monitored, special emphasis on relapse of opioid intoxication signs and symptoms should be noted. Additional doses of naloxone may be required to keep the patient from experiencing opioid re-intoxication. Any patient who requires a second dose of naloxone should be observed for an extended time, and intensive care unit admission should be considered. Patients with complicated opioid overdoses requiring respiratory assistance and maintenance and those with severe toxicity must be admitted to the hospital's critical care unit.

Unlike alcohol withdrawal, opioid withdrawal is not life-threatening. Most patients may be discharged for outpatient treatment.

REFERENCES

1. Dawson G: Subgroup variation in U.S. drinking patterns: Results of the 1992 national longitudinal alcohol epidemiologic study. J Subst Abuse 1995;7:331-344.
2. U.S. Department of Health and Human Services and the U.S. Department of Agriculture (USDA): Dietary Guidelines for Americans 2005 (6th ed). Washington, DC: U.S. Government Printing Office, 2005.
3. Thun MJ, Peto R, Lopez AD, et al: Alcohol consumption and mortality among middle-aged and elderly U.S. adults. N Engl J Med 1997;337:1705-1714.
4. Berger K, Ajani UA, Kase CS, et al: Light-to-moderate alcohol consumption and risk of stroke among U.S. male physicians. N Engl J Med 1999;341:1557-1564.
5. Grant BF: Alcohol consumption, alcohol abuse and alcohol dependence: The United States as an example. Addiction 1994;89:1357-1365.
6. Pletcher MJ, Maselli J, Gonzales R: Uncomplicated alcohol intoxication in the emergency department: An analysis of the National Hospital Ambulatory Medical Care Survey. Am J Med 2004;117:863-867.
7. Mokdad AH, Marks JS, Stroup DF, Gerberding JL: Actual causes of death in the United States, 2000. JAMA 2004;291:1238-1245.
8. Kosten TR, O'Connor PG: Management of drug and alcohol withdrawal. New Engl J Med 2003;348:1786-1795.
9. Lee JH, Jang MK, Lee JY, et al: Clinical predictors for delirium tremens in alcohol dependence. J Gastroenterol Hepatol 2005;20:1833-1837.
10. Frezza M, di Padova C, Pozzato G, et al: High blood alcohol levels in women: The role of decreased gastric alcohol dehydrogenase activity and the first-pass metabolism. New Engl J Med 1990;322:95-99.
11. Brennan DF, Bretzelos S, Reed R, Falk JL: Ethanol elimination rates in an ED population. Am J Emerg Med 1995;13:276-280.
12. Hall W, Zador D: The alcohol withdrawal syndrome. Lancet 1997;349:1897-1900.
13. Stuke L, Diaz-Arrastia R, Gentilello LM, Shafi S: Effect of alcohol on Glasgow Coma Scale in head-injured patients. Ann Surg 2007;245:651-655.
14. Turner RC, Lichstein PR, Peden JG Jr, et al: Alcohol withdrawal syndromes: A review of pathophysiology, clinical presentation, and treatment. J Gen Intern Med 1989; 4:432-444.
15. Gibb K: Serum alcohol levels, toxicology screens, and use of the breath alcohol analyzer. Ann Emerg Med 1986; 15:349-353.
16. Krishel S, SaFranek D, Clark RF: Intravenous vitamins for alcoholics in the emergency department: A review. J Emerg Med 1998;16:419-424.
17. Kahan M, Borgundvaag B, Borsoi D, et al: Treatment variability and outcome differences in emergency department management of alcohol withdrawal. Can J Emerg Med 2005;7:87-92.
18. American Society of Addiction Medicine Committee Practice Guidelines: ASAM Clinical Practice Guidelines: The role of phenytoin in the management of alcohol withdrawal syndrome. Available at www.asam.org/PracticeGuidelines.html.
19. Daeppen JB, Gache P, Landry U, et al: Symptom-triggered vs fixed-schedule doses of benzodiazepine for alcohol withdrawal: A randomized control treatment trial. Arch Intern Med 2002;27;162:1117-1121.
20. O'Connor PG, Schottenfield RS: Patients with alcohol problems. New Engl J Med 1998;338:592-602.
21. Kuehn BM: Opioid prescriptions soar. JAMA 2007; 297:249-251.
22. Haddox JD, Joranson D, Angarola RT, et al: Consensus Statement: The use of opioids for the treatment of chronic pain. Available at www.ampainsoc.org/advocacy/opioids.htm/
23. U.S. Department of Health and Human Services, Substance Abuse and Mental Health Services Administration, SAMSA Advisory: Data on drug-related emergency room visits released by SAMHSA. Available at www.samhsa.gov/news/newsreleases/060510_dawn2/
24. Paulozzi LJ, Budnitz DS, Xi Y: Increasing deaths from opioid analgesics in the United States. Pharmacoepidemiol Drug Safe 2006;15:618-627.

Chapter 149

Sedative-Hypnotic Agents

James W. Rhee and Timothy B. Erickson

KEY POINTS

Benzodiazepines account for the majority of overdoses with sedative-hypnotic drugs.
Benzodiazepines can induce cardiovascular and pulmonary toxicity, but fatalities resulting from pure benzodiazepine overdoses are rare.
Central nervous system depression is the primary symptom of a sedative-hypnotic toxicity.
Treatment should focus on supportive care with particular attention to airway patency and respiratory function.
Urinary alkalinization and multiple doses of activated charcoal can enhance the elimination of phenobarbital.
Flumazenil is a reversal agent for benzodiazepine toxicity, but it should be used cautiously to avoid the risk of seizures.
Other possible causes of altered mental status should always be considered.

Scope

Sedative-hypnotic agents are a heterogeneous group of agents that have tranquilizing (sedative) or sleep induction (hypnotic) properties. Since the beginning of this century, these agents have been among the top ten classes of poisoning exposures reported to the poison centers.[1-4] They are widely used in clinical settings but are also used for suicide, for illicit recreational activities, and for malicious endeavors such as homicide and facilitation of sexual assault ("date-rape"). Several high-profile deaths have been attributed to sedative-hypnotic overdoses. Toxicity may result from unintentional or intentional exposures, malicious exposures, and procedural sedation.

Pathophysiology

The sedative-hypnotic class of drugs contains many agents. However, there are no strict criteria to define this class other than sedative-hypnotic properties. Given such a broad definition, many other substances, such as opioids, some antipsychotics, antihistamines, and alcohol, would also be considered part of this class—except that these substances have other unique properties that set them apart.

■ BENZODIAZEPINES

Benzodiazepines, the most widely used sedative-hypnotic agents, have largely replaced the older sedative-hypnotic agents because of their efficacy and relative

Table 149-1 CLASSIFICATION OF BARBITURATES

Duration of Action	Barbiturate	Metabolism and Activity	Treatment
Ultrashort-acting	Methohexital (Brevital) Thiopental (Pentothal)	Highly lipid-soluble with rapid central nervous system (CNS) penetration	Supportive care Airway protection Activated charcoal
Short-acting	Pentobarbital (Nembutal) Secobarbital (Seconal)	Highly lipid-soluble with rapid CNS penetration	Supportive care Airway protection Activated charcoal
Intermediate-acting	Amobarbital (Amytal) Aprobarbital (Alurate) Butabarbital (Butisol) Butalbital (Fiorinal)	Intermediate CNS penetration (30-60 min)	Supportive care Airway protection Activated charcoal
Long-acting	Barbital (Veronal) Mephobarbital (Mebaral) Phenobarbital (Solfoton, Luminal) Primidone (Mysoline)	Metabolized slowly in liver; greater fraction excreted unchanged by kidney; undergoes enterohepatic recirculation	Multiple-dose activated charcoal (MDAC) for phenobarbital Urine alkalinization—use only if unable to give MDAC Hemodialysis in severe cases

safety. However, given their prevalence, benzodiazepines also account for the majority of sedative-hypnotic overdoses.[1-4] Although mostly used for sedation or anxiolysis, benzodiazepines have been also been used as recreational drugs, in suicide attempts, and to facilitate sexual assault.

Flunitrazepam (sometimes referred to as "roofies") is a potent benzodiazepine that has recently been popularized as a street drug of abuse and has been implicated as a "date-rape" drug.[5]

Benzodiazepines vary in onset and duration of action according to their lipid solubility and the presence or absence of active metabolites (Table 149-1). The more lipid-soluble the agent, the more rapidly it crosses the blood-brain barrier, yielding a faster onset of action. The duration of action depends largely on the elimination half-life of specific agents, which can range from hours to days. The duration of action is also affected by the metabolism of certain benzodiazepines because their active metabolites extend the duration of symptoms.

The benzodiazepines produce central nervous system (CNS) depression through effects mediated by gamma-aminobutyric acid (GABA)—a major inhibitory neurotransmitter. A specific benzodiazepine receptor exists on the $GABA_A$ receptor. When a benzodiazepine binds to this receptor, it subsequently promotes GABA binding to the $GABA_A$ receptor. Activation of the $GABA_A$ receptor results in influx of chloride into the neuronal cell, causing CNS inhibition. As such, benzodiazepines have anxiolytic, muscle relaxant, sedative, hypnotic, amnestic, and anticonvulsant properties.

Pure benzodiazepine overdoses cause mild to moderate CNS depression. Deep coma requiring assisted ventilation can occur, especially when benzodiazepine is used with other sedating drugs. In severe overdoses, these agents can induce cardiovascular and pulmonary toxicity, but fatalities resulting from pure benzodiazepine overdoses are rare.

■ BARBITURATES

Barbiturates were formally the primary sedative-hypnotic agents used for sedation or to induce and maintain sleep. They have largely been supplanted by the benzodiazepines both for these indications and in overdoses.[6] Currently, barbiturates are used as anticonvulsants and for induction of anesthesia.

The barbiturates are often classified according to their therapeutic duration of action (Box 149-1):

BOX 149-1

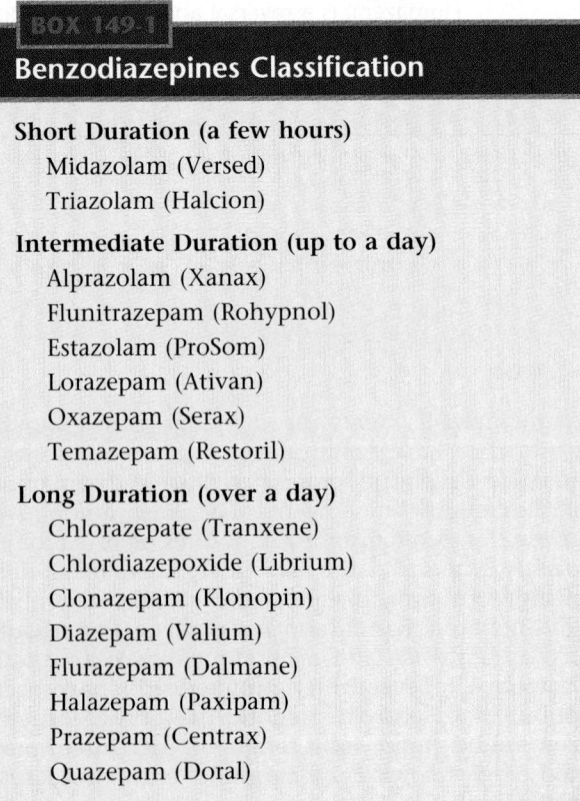

Benzodiazepines Classification

Short Duration (a few hours)
- Midazolam (Versed)
- Triazolam (Halcion)

Intermediate Duration (up to a day)
- Alprazolam (Xanax)
- Flunitrazepam (Rohypnol)
- Estazolam (ProSom)
- Lorazepam (Ativan)
- Oxazepam (Serax)
- Temazepam (Restoril)

Long Duration (over a day)
- Chlorazepate (Tranxene)
- Chlordiazepoxide (Librium)
- Clonazepam (Klonopin)
- Diazepam (Valium)
- Flurazepam (Dalmane)
- Halazepam (Paxipam)
- Prazepam (Centrax)
- Quazepam (Doral)

ultrashort-acting, short-acting, intermediate-acting, or long-acting. In overdoses, however, the duration of action varies with dose, rate of absorption, and rate of distribution and elimination. The ultrashort-acting and short-acting agents are highly lipid soluble and rapidly penetrate the CNS, so onset of symptoms is also rapid. In addition, the ultrashort-acting barbiturates are more highly protein bound, have higher acid-dissociation constant (pK_a), values, and have larger volumes of distribution. Long-acting agents like phenobarbital are metabolized more slowly in the liver, with a greater fraction of unchanged drug excreted in the kidney. These factors help explain why enhanced renal elimination through alkalinization may be more effective with phenobarbital, which also has a lower pKa than the other barbiturates, making it more sensitive to alkalinization. In addition, phenobarbital undergoes enterohepatic recirculation, making repetitive uses of activated charcoal potentially advantageous.

Barbiturates are primarily CNS depressants that mediate their effect through several mechanisms. The barbiturates promote GABA binding to the $GABA_A$ chloride channel complex. They can also bind directly to $GABA_A$ chloride ion channels in the CNS, and the influx of chloride into neuronal cells leads to greater CNS inhibition. Barbiturates may also reduce specific excitatory neurotransmission.

The reticular activating system and the cerebellum appear to be the most susceptible to the depressant effects of barbiturates. Toxicity can lead to suppression of skeletal, smooth, and cardiac muscles, leading to depressed myocardial contractility, bradycardia, vasodilation, and hypotension.

■ GAMMA-HYDROXYBUTYRATE

Gamma-hydroxybutyrate (GHB), which naturally occurs in the body, is an analogue of GABA and subsequently has sedative-hypnotic properties. In 1960, GHB was synthesized as an anesthetic agent. Although it had limited use as an anesthetic agent, GHB gained widespread acceptance in the body-building community as a purported anabolic agent. More recently this agent has been used as a recreational drug for its euphoric and intoxicating effects. It has also been implicated in "date-rape" owing to its "knockout" and amnestic properties. GHB is covered in more detail in Chapter 144.

■ NONBENZODIAZEPINE SEDATIVES

A few nonbenzodiazepine sedatives have been introduced for sleep induction. They are generally considered to have fewer side effects as well as to being less addictive than benzodiazepine. They can be divided into three general structural classes: imidazopyridines, pyrazolopyrimidines, and cyclopyrrones. However, their mechanisms of action are all similar—they all act selectively at the benzodiazepine receptor to enhance $GABA_A$ receptor activity. Therefore, they mimic benzodiazepine toxicity (Box 149-2).

BOX 149-2

Nonbenzodiazepine Sedatives

Imidazopyridines
- Zolpidem (Ambien)
- Alpidem

Pyrazolopyrimidines
- Zaleplon (Sonata)

Cyclopyrrones
- Eszopiclone (Lunesta)
- Zopiclone (Imovane)

■ OLDER SEDATIVE-HYPNOTIC AGENTS

■ Chloral Hydrate

Chloral hydrate has a long history. It has been used as a sedative since the 19th century. In the early 1900s, chloral hydrate was used maliciously, being added to alcoholic drinks that were consumed by unwary individuals in order to facilitate robberies. The drug-laced drink was referred to as a "Mickey Finn"—named after the owner of a Chicago bar who used these drinks to rob unsuspecting patrons.[7] Currently, chloral hydrate is used primarily for procedural sedation.

After being absorbed completely from the gastrointestinal tract, chloral hydrate is metabolized rapidly. One of its metabolites, trichloroethanol, is also pharmacologically active and produces sedation. In the presence of ethanol, the metabolism of trichloroethanol is inhibited, with resulting increase in sedation and prolongation of the sedative effects.

Although chloral hydrate has been used for over a century to induce sedation, its mechanism of action is still largely unknown. It probably works through effects at the GABA receptor, like the other sedative-hypnotic agents discussed. Chloral hydrate can also induce cardiac dysrhythmias, probably by increasing the sensitivity of the myocardium to catecholamines.[8]

■ Other Older Agents

Glutethimide, ethchlorvynol, meprobamate, and methaqualone are some older sedative-hypnotic agents that have fallen out of common use. In fact, of these drugs, only meprobamate is still available in the United States. All of these agents apparently act by enhancing GABA's effects.

Clinical Presentation

Although there are some variations from agent to agent, the hallmark of sedative-hypnotic overdoses is CNS depression (Box 149-3). The amount of CNS depression depends on the dose, specific agent, and coingestion(s).

Mild to moderate sedative-hypnotic overdoses may manifest as reduced level of consciousness, slurred speech, and ataxia. At high doses, sedative-hypnotic agents can cause hypothermia, hypotension, bradycardia, flaccidity, hyporeflexia, coma, and apnea. These severe symptoms are more commonly encountered in barbiturate overdoses. Patients with severe overdoses may appear to be dead, having no electroencelographic activity.

Differential Diagnosis

The differential diagnosis of any profound CNS depression should include other toxins that have sedative properties. However, care should be made to rule out other potential causes of the CNS depression. While sedative-hypnotic toxicity does well with just supportive care, other mimickers of a sedative-hypnotic overdose may need other acute interventions. Some other diagnoses that the clinician should consider include head trauma with subdural or epidural hematoma, intracerebral hemorrhage, embolic stroke, electrolyte abnormalities, hypoglycemia, hyperglycemic crisis, hypoxemia, hypothyroidism, liver or renal failure, CNS infection, seizures, and significant alterations in temperature.

Diagnostic Testing

Diagnostic testing should be utilized to help exclude other causes of altered mental status. Initially, a fingerstick blood sugar, cardiac monitoring, and pulse oximetry may help the clinician avoid the critical error of missing hypoglycemia, hypoxemia, or a dysrhythmia.

Further testing to help clarify the patient's presentation may include serum electrolytes, blood urea nitrogen, serum creatinine, serum ethanol, blood gas analysis, chest radiograph, computed tomography of the brain, cerebrospinal fluid analysis, complete blood count, serum transaminases, serum bilirubin, ammonia level, blood cultures, and a urinalysis. If the patient is female, a urine pregnancy test is warranted. Directed quantitative serum levels of some drugs should also be considered—this may include acetaminophen, salicylate, lithium, and anticonvulsant levels.

Most institutions have a qualitative urine drug screen that may be ordered. However, this screen may vary based on the institution. Most of the screens are immunoassays that detect the presence of certain drugs or metabolites in the urine. In the case of sedative-hypnotic agents, the commonly available screens will test for benzodiazepines. The other sedative-hypnotic agents are typically not included on most urine drug screens. The typical benzodiazepine screen identifies metabolites of 1,4-benzodiazepines such as oxazepam or desmethyldiazepam—benzodiazepines that are not metabolized or are metabolized to other compounds will remain undetected. Also, the detection cutoff may be set at a point where the assay may not detect certain agents that can induce effects in very small amounts. It is important for the clinician to recognize the limitations of this screen as a false negative screen is possible with certain benzodiazepines—these include alprazolam, clonazepam, and flunitrazepam.

BOX 149-3

Most Threatening and Most Common Presentations

Most Threatening

- Apnea
- Hypotension
- Acute lung injury
- Dysrhythmias
- Hypothermia

Most Common

- Sedation
- Ataxia
- Slurred speech

Tips and Tricks

- Pear-like odor is associated with chloral hydrate.
- Chloral hydrate overdoses may present with cardiac toxicity as well as CNS depression.
- Bullous lesions are sometimes associated with barbituate overdoses
- Consider rhabdomyolysis as a complication.
- A patient who appears brain dead after a severe sedative-hypnotic (barbiturate) overdose may not be brain dead.
- Use beta-blockers to treat chloral hydrate–induced cardiac dysrhythmias.
- Epinephrine and norepinephrine are relatively contraindicated in chloral hydrate overdose because the myocardium may have an increased sensitivity to these types of agents.
- The most common drug used to facilitate sexual assault is ethanol, not sedative-hypnotics.
- MDAC appears to be superior to urinary alkalinization in enhancing the elimination of phenobarbital, and there appears to be no apparent benefit to doing both procedures concurrently.

RED FLAGS

These signs, symptoms, and test results should prompt the clinician to search for other causes of CNS depression:

- Focal neurologic deficit
- Fever
- External evidence of trauma
- Seizure activity
- QRS prolongation on electrocardiogram (seen with agents that can block myocardial sodium channels such as tricyclic antidepressants)
- Electrolyte abnormalities
- Metabolic acidosis
- Hypoglycemia
- Dysrhythmias (except with chloral hydrate)

Quantitative benzodiazepine concentrations correlate poorly with pharmacological or toxicological effects, and are poor predictors of clinical outcome.

A quantitative serum phenobarbital level can be helpful to document the toxicity, but is not mandatory for definitive management. Therapeutic concentrations of phenobarbital range between 15 and 40 mg/L. Patients with levels >50 mg/L will exhibit mild toxicity, while those with levels >100 mg/L are typically unresponsive to pain and may suffer from respiratory and cardiac depression.

Treatment

Clinicians should manage the sedative-hypnotic overdose as they would any poisoned patient. A general approach to the poisoned patient has already been discussed earlier in this textbook. The mainstay of treatment for the sedative-hypnotic overdose consists of supportive care with particular attention to airway patency and respiratory status. Manage hypotension with fluid resuscitation and vasopressors as needed (Table 149-2).

Dysrhythmias that occur from chloral hydrate toxicity should be treated with beta-blockers as it is felt that myocardial catecholamine sensitivity induces the dysrhythmia.[8] Epinephrine and norepinephrine are relatively contraindicated given that chloral hydrate cardiac toxicity may be due to increased sensitivity of the myocardium to these types of agents.

■ GASTROINTESTINAL DECONTAMINATION

Patients who are stable with significant ingestions should receive activated charcoal as a means of preventing absorption of drugs still contained within the gastrointestinal tract. The efficacy of this procedure decays with time, so activated charcoal should be given expeditiously—ideally, within the first hour after the ingestion occurred. The initial dose of activated charcoal is typically 1 g/kg. Ideally, at least a 10:1 ratio of charcoal to drug should be achieved. Given the toxicity of sedative-hypnotics, careful attention should be directed to avoiding aspiration. If airway protective reflexes are not intact, then administration of activated charcoal should be withheld unless the airway is protected by some other means.

■ MULTIPLE-DOSE ACTIVATED CHARCOAL (MDAC)

Activated charcoal has a role in increasing the elimination of phenobarbital as well. Several investigations have demonstrated that repetitive dosing of activated charcoal will significantly reduce the serum half-life of certain drugs such as phenobarbital. This therapeutic procedure has been referred to as multiple-dose activated charcoal (MDAC) and has applications for a few other specific agents.

This process seems to work well for phenobarbital as it undergoes enterohepatic circulation and as phe-

Table 149-2 DIFFERENTIAL DIAGNOSIS OF SEDATIVE-HYPNOTIC TOXIDROMES AND PRIORITY ACTIONS

Diagnostic Consideration	Priority Action(s)
Airway/respiratory status?	Provide airway protection and respiratory support as needed
Trauma?	If trauma is suspected, maintain spinal immobilization Obtain computed tomography of the head
Cardiovascular status?	Start cardiac monitoring Establish intravenous access Administer vasopressors for refractory hypotension Administer intravenous bolus(es) of isotonic crystalloid solution for hypotension Avoid epinephrine and norepinephrine in known or suspected chloral hydrate overdose
Hypothermia/hyperthermia?	Actively rewarm severely hypothermic patients Use active cooling for hyperthermia, and evaluate for infectious causes
Overdose/toxicity?	Consider administering activated charcoal to patients with a secure airway Use multiple-dose activated charcoal (MDAC) in overdoses of long-acting barbiturates Perform primary alkalinization for overdoses of long-acting barbiturates in which MDAC is not advised Consider hemodialysis in severe cases

nobarbital is excreted into the gut, the activated charcoal present in the intestine binds to it before it gets reabsorbed more distally. Phenobarbital also has physical characteristics that allow it to diffuse from the blood into the intestinal lumen. During MDAC, activated charcoal avidly binds to the phenobarbital in the intestinal lumen effectively creating a concentration gradient into the intestine and subsequently enhancing the elimination of the phenobarbital.[9]

After the initial decontamination dose of activated charcoal, a reasonable dosing regimen for MDAC in adults can be accomplished by administering 25 grams of activated charcoal without a cathartic every two hours. In pediatrics, a dose 0.25 g/kg every two hours is reasonable. The activated charcoal can be administered orally or through a nasogastric or orogastric tube. If a feeding pump is available, the activated charcoal can be administered continuously instead of two-hour intervals.

Physicians must be aware that some charcoal preparations are premixed with a cathartic—usually sorbitol. The dose of sorbitol that is mixed with the charcoal varies based on the manufacturer. When performing MDAC, repeated doses of any cathartic agent are contraindicated in order to avoid dehydration and electrolyte imbalances. However, a small dose of sorbitol (0.2-0.5 g/kg) may be given with the first dose (the decontamination dose) of activated charcoal to prevent constipation.

MDAC is contraindicated in patients who do not have protective airway reflexes or an otherwise secure airway. MDAC is also contraindicated in patients who have evidence of ileus or who are hemodynamically unstable. It should be noted that MDAC has not been shown to change overall clinical outcome in phenobarbital toxicity.

■ URINARY ALKALINIZATION

Alkalinizing the urine with the intravenous administration of sodium bicarbonate can increase the elimination of phenobarbital. Urinary alkalinization with sodium bicarbonate to a pH of 7.5 to 8.0 can hasten the renal excretion of phenobarbital.[10]

Urinary alkalinization can be accomplished with an initial sodium bicarbonate bolus of 1 mEq/kg, followed by a continuous infusion. This infusion is made by adding 100 to 150 mEq of sodium bicarbonate to 850 mL of dextrose 5% in water, and titrating it to maintain a urine pH of greater than 7.5 with an arterial pH less than 7.5. The rate must be assessed hourly to avoid excessive administration of fluid or bicarbonate which can cause pulmonary or cerebral edema or electrolyte imbalance. While expediting the elimination of phenobarbital from the body has theoretical benefit, no clinical evidence exists that demonstrates improvement of patient outcome. Alkalinization does not increase excretion of short- and medium-acting agents, which are more lipid-soluble.

When compared with MDAC, MDAC appears to be superior to urinary alkalinization in enhancing the elimination of phenobarbital. Also, there appears to be no apparent benefit to doing both procedures concurrently.[11, 12] Urinary alkalinization may still be useful in a patient who cannot undergo MDAC.

■ HEMODIALYSIS

In unstable patients not responsive to standard therapeutic measures, or in those with renal failure, hemodialysis may be indicated for long-acting barbiturates. These agents are less protein bound and less lipid soluble that the shorter-acting barbiturates—these are characteristics that enhance the role of hemodialysis. Fortunately, extracorporeal elimination is rarely indicated since most barbiturate overdoses do well with supportive care alone.

While charcoal hemoperfusion has been advocated as being more efficacious than conventional hemodialysis, the availability of this procedure is very limited—conventional hemodialysis enhances drug removal effectively.[13] It appears that the high-efficiency dialyzers are just as efficacious with phenobarbital drug removal.[14]

Hemodialysis can enhance the elimination of chloral hydrate and its metabolites. However, supportive measure are generally all that is needed for chloral hydrate toxicity. There may be role for hemodialysis if a patient with chloral hydrate toxicity is not responding with conservative therapy.

■ FLUMAZENIL

Flumazenil is a specific antagonist for benzodiazepines (Box 149-4). It competitively binds at the benzodiazepine receptor thereby displacing benzodiazepines from the site and inhibiting GABA potentiation. Flumazenil is lipid-soluble so it readily crosses the blood-brain barrier to exert its effects quickly. Typically, benzodiazepine-induced sedation is

BOX 149-4

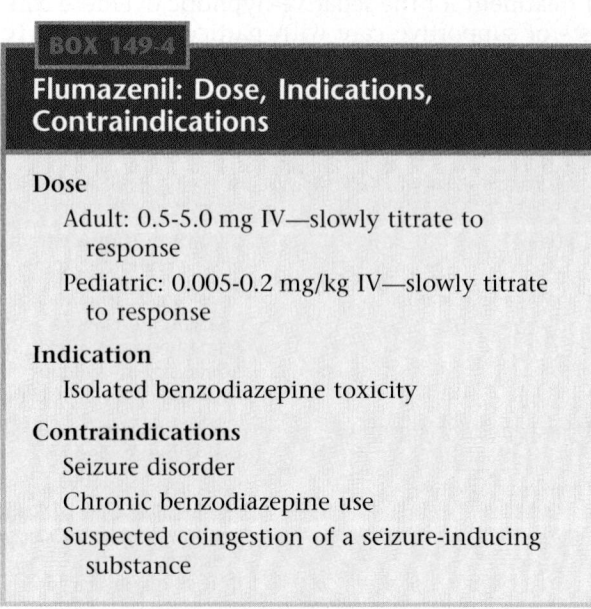

Flumazenil: Dose, Indications, Contraindications

Dose

- Adult: 0.5-5.0 mg IV—slowly titrate to response
- Pediatric: 0.005-0.2 mg/kg IV—slowly titrate to response

Indication

- Isolated benzodiazepine toxicity

Contraindications

- Seizure disorder
- Chronic benzodiazepine use
- Suspected coingestion of a seizure-inducing substance

Documentation

History

- Any history of psychiatric illness or prior suicide ingestions
- Time lapse since ingestion if known
- History of renal or cardiac disease or other illnesses that will exacerbate the complications
- Drug taken, dose, and quantity

Physical Examination

- Does the patient look ill? Febrile? Mental status? Respiratory and airway status? Signs of trauma?
- Cardiac status (blood pressure, arrhythmias)?
- Should include repeat exams while patient is in the ED

Laboratory Studies

For cases of alleged facilitated sexual assault, consult with local law enforcement regarding the handling of a patient's urine specimen as it may be tested at a forensic lab for the presence of "date-rape" drugs.

Medical Decision-Making

- Decision to begin treatment or delays
- Consults and time called

Treatment

- Interventions and timing

Patient Instructions

- Document discussion with patient regarding diagnosis, warning signs, what to do, follow-up, when to return.
- With pediatric accidental ingestions, document poison prevention counseling.
- Instruct patient to avoid combination with alcohol and antihistamines.

reversed within a couple of minutes. However, its effect on reversal of respiratory depression remains controversial.[15,16]

In the setting of procedural sedation, flumazenil is an excellent rescue agent for inadvertent supratherapeutic administrations of a benzodiazepine agent—flumazenil should always be readily available in this setting.

Flumazenil may also be helpful in the setting of an isolated known benzodiazepine overdose. Unfortunately, there is concern of coingestions in most overdoses—the use of flumazenil in the setting of a benzodiazepine overdose with other coningestions is less clear.

Overall, for the unknown overdose, the administration of flumazenil is not indicated for many reasons.[17] Flumazenil does not antagonize the CNS effects of alcohol, barbiturates, tricyclic antidepressants, or narcotics. There are also concerns regarding the precipitation of seizure activity in the setting of mixed tricyclic antidepressant–benzodiazepine overdose.[18] Flumazenil can also cause seizures and death in a rat model of mixed cocaine and diazepam intoxication.[19]

Flumazenil should not be given to patients who use benzodiazepines therapeutically to control seizures or who have raised intracranial pressure. The clinician should also be aware that benzodiazepine-dependent patients may acutely withdraw after flumazenil administration—this may manifest as acute agitation or seizures.

Disposition

Patients who are symptom-free from an isolated sedative-hypnotic overdose may be medically cleared after a six-hour observation period. However, the events leading to the exposure may preclude discharge home. Psychiatry consultation is necessary for those patients with intentional overdoses.

Patients with prolonged sedation or other evidence of toxicity should be admitted for further observation and treatment.

Admissions to a critical care setting are dictated by the severity of toxicity. Patients with hemodynamic instability, respiratory failure, coma, severe hypothermia, and need for hemodialysis are some conditions when a critical care admission is warranted.

REFERENCES

1. Litovitz TL, Klein-Schwartz W, Rodgers GCJ, et al: 2001 annual report of the American Association of Poison Control Centers Toxic Exposure Surveillance System. Am J Emerg Med 2002;20:391-452.
2. Watson WA, Litovitz TL, Rodgers GCJ, et al: 2002 annual report of the American Association of Poison Control Centers Toxic Exposure Surveillance System. Am J Emerg Med 2003;21:353-421.
3. Watson WA, Litovitz TL, Klein-Schwartz W, et al: 2003 annual report of the American Association of Poison Control Centers Toxic Exposure Surveillance System. Am J Emerg Med 2004;22:335-404.
4. Watson WA, Litovitz TL, Rodgers GCJ, et al: 2004 annual report of the American Association of Poison Control Centers Toxic Exposure Surveillance System. Am J Emerg Med 2005;23:589-666.
5. Waltzman ML: Flunitrazepam: A review of "roofies." Pediatr Emerg Care 1999;15:59-60.
6. Osselton MD, Blackmore RC, King LA, Moffat AC: Poisoning-associated deaths for England and Wales between 1973 and 1980. Hum Toxicol 1984;3:201-221.
7. Baum CR: A century of Mickey Finn—but who was he? J Toxicol Clin Toxicol 2000;38:683; author reply 685.
8. Sing K, Erickson T, Amitai Y, Hryhorczuk D: Chloral hydrate toxicity from oral and intravenous administration. J Toxicol Clin Toxicol 1996;34:101-106.
9. Berg MJ, Berlinger WG, Goldberg MJ, et al: Acceleration of the body clearance of phenobarbital by oral activated charcoal. N Engl J Med 1982;307:642-644.
10. Mawer GE, Lee HA: Value of forced diuresis in acute barbiturate poisoning. Br Med J 1968;2:790-793.
11. Frenia ML, Schauben JL, Wears RL, et al: Multiple-dose activated charcoal compared to urinary alkalinization for the enhancement of phenobarbital elimination. J Toxicol Clin Toxicol 1996;34:169-175.

12. Mohammed Ebid AH, Abdel-Rahman HM: Pharmacokinetics of phenobarbital during certain enhanced elimination modalities to evaluate their clinical efficacy in management of drug overdose. Ther Drug Monit 2001;23:209-216.
13. Jacobs F, Brivet FG: Conventional haemodialysis significantly lowers toxic levels of phenobarbital. Nephrol Dial Transplant 2004;19:1663-1664.
14. Palmer BF: Effectiveness of hemodialysis in the extracorporeal therapy of phenobarbital overdose. Am J Kidney Dis 2000;36:640-643.
15. Gross JB, Blouin RT, Zandsberg S, et al: Effect of flumazenil on ventilatory drive during sedation with midazolam and alfentanil. Anesthesiology 1996;85:713-720.
16. Shalansky SJ, Naumann TL, Englander FA: Effect of flumazenil on benzodiazepine-induced respiratory depression. Clin Pharm 1993;12:483-487.
17. Gueye PN, Hoffman JR, Taboulet P, et al: Empiric use of flumazenil in comatose patients: Limited applicability of criteria to define low risk. Ann Emerg Med 1996;27:730-735.
18. Mordel A, Winkler E, Almog S, et al: Seizures after flumazenil administration in a case of combined benzodiazepine and tricyclic antidepressant overdose. Crit Care Med 1992;20:1733-1734.
19. Derlet RW, Albertson TE: Flumazenil induces seizures and death in mixed cocaine-diazepam intoxications. Ann Emerg Med 1994;23:494-498.

Chapter 150

Anticonvulsant Drugs

Victor Tuckler and Michael Catenacci

KEY POINTS

Phenytoin intoxication causes ataxia, nystagmus, diplopia, and central nervous system depression.
Anticonvulsant hypersensitivity syndrome occurs between 2 and 12 weeks after initiation of therapy with the medication.
Valproate may cause hepatotoxicity, although early signs of toxicity may consist only of lethargy and weakness.

Anticonvulsant Hypersensitivity Syndrome

Anticonvulsant hypersensitivity syndrome is a drug-induced, multiple-organ syndrome that can be fatal. Phenytoin, carbamazepine, primidone, lamotrigine, and phenobarbital can all produce a hypersensitivity syndrome, which occurs between 2 and 12 weeks after drug therapy is started. Although the syndrome may occur with one anticonvulsant, it may also occur with change of therapy to another class. The hypersensitivity reaction is not dose dependent.

Patients with anticonvulsant hypersensitivity syndrome may experience mucocutaneous eruptions with fever, lymphadenopathy, and hemolytic anemia. They can also have exfoliative dermatitis, erythema multiforme, and toxic epidermal necrolysis. Eosinophilia, hepatitis, myositis, vasculitis, and rhabdomyolysis have been reported as well.[1]

Carbamazepine

Carbamazepine is an anticonvulsant prescribed for trigeminal neuralgia, partial seizures, and generalized tonic-clonic seizures. It has also been used in the treatment of bipolar-affective disorder, alcohol withdrawal syndrome, schizophrenia, pain syndromes, and restless legs syndrome. It is structurally and pharmacologically similar to tricyclic antidepressants and so can cause a false-positive result for these agents on a drug screen. Gastrointestinal absorption of carbamazepine is slow and erratic because this drug is a lipophilic compound that is insoluble in aqueous media. Peak plasma levels are reached in 6 to 24 hours but may occur up to 72 hours after overdose. Therapeutic serum levels are 4 to 12 mg/L. Carbamazepine has a large volume of distribution. It is metabolized by the liver cytochrome P-450 enzyme to an active metabolite called carbamazepine-epoxide. Because its metabolite is active, it may lengthen the duration of the toxidrome in overdoses.

Drug interactions may occur with carbamazepine because of its ability to induce the cytochrome P-450 system (Box 150-1). Carbamazepine may reduce concentrations of benzodiazepines, corticosteroids, cyclic antidepressants, cyclosporine, doxycycline, ethosuximide, haloperidol, oral contraceptives, phenobarbital, phenytoin, primidone, theophylline, valproic acid, and warfarin. Patients taking both lithium and carbamazepine have experienced neurotoxicity despite therapeutic levels of both drugs. When combined with other drugs, carbamazepine has also been

BOX 150-1

Drugs that Affect Carbamazepine Levels

Drugs that Raise Carbamazepine Levels

Cimetidine
Danazol
Diltiazem
Erythromycin
Isoniazid
Nicotinamide
Propoxyphene
Verapamil

Drugs that Reduce Carbamazepine Levels

Phenobarbital
Phenytoin
Primidone
Succinimides
Valproic acid

associated with neuroleptic malignant syndrome and serotonin syndrome.

Acute ingestion of more than 10 mg/kg of carbamazepine is potentially toxic. The first signs and symptoms appear after 1 to 3 hours after an overdose. Manifestations of toxicity may be delayed for several hours because of the erratic absorption of carbamazepine. Symptoms in overdose cases are those of central nervous system (CNS) depression. Patients may have cyclic coma because of the erratic absorption. Carbamazepine has sedative, anticholinergic, antidiuretic, muscle relaxant, and antidysrhythmic activities. Patients with carbamazepine toxicity can have ataxia, nystagmus, tachycardia, mydriasis, erythematous flushed skin, dry mucous membranes, urinary retention, hyperthermia, dystonia, and choreoathetosis. Ataxia, hallucinations, seizures, and tremors are also seen. Cardiovascular effects include arrhythmias and atrioventricular (AV) blocks. Carbamazepine may cause QRS and QT interval prolongation and myocardial depression. Levels do not correlate with clinical toxicity, but ataxia and nystagmus may take place at levels higher than 10 mg/L and cardiovascular effects are seen at levels higher than 12 mg/L.

Adverse effects of carbamazepine, such as bone marrow suppression, hepatitis, hyponatremia, cardiomyopathy, and exfoliative dermatitis, are not dose dependent. Aplastic anemia and agranulocytosis have been reported with this agent. The overall rates of these reactions in the general population are about 6 patients per 1 million population per year for agranulocytosis and 2 patients per 1 million population per year for aplastic anemia.

Gabapentin

Gabapentin is used as an add-on anticonvulsant agent in the treatment of refractory partial seizures. It also appears effective in generalized seizures.[2,3] The exact mechanism of action is unknown. Gabapentin is an amino acid structurally related to gamma-aminobutyric acid (GABA), but it does not act at the GABA receptor.

Peak serum levels occur 1 to 3 hours after ingestion.[4] The half-life is 5 to 7 hours. Adverse effects include peripheral edema, myalgia, ataxia, nystagmus, somnolence, Stevens-Johnson syndrome, seizure, mood swings, hostile behavior, and dizziness. Overdose symptoms are CNS depression, nystagmus, diplopia, and ataxia. Gabapentin can be removed by hemodialysis.

Phenytoin

Phenytoin is an antiepileptic drug. It is related to the barbiturates in chemical structure but has a five-member ring. Phenytoin is used to control tonic-clonic seizures and psychomotor seizures. It has many negative side effects, and the ratio between therapeutic and toxic levels is small. Therapeutic range is 10 to 20 μg/mL. Phenytoin is available in multiple formulations (oral, intravenous, extended-release). Fosphenytoin, the prodrug that is converted to phenytoin after administration, is used for intravenous or intramuscular use. Fosphenytoin has fewer side effects and is safer to administer parenterally than phenytoin.

Overdoses from phenytoin occur from chronic intoxications in patients with poorly controlled therapeutic regimens, from suicide, and from accidental poisonings in children. Phenytoin overdose causes nystagmus, ataxia, and drowsiness in the early stages. Overdoses are usually not fatal. There is no specific antidote, and treatment is discontinuation of the drug.

Phenytoin is a sodium channel blocker that stops the rapid transmission of excitatory impulses seen in seizures. A class IB antidysrhythmic, it increases AV conduction. It also induces cytochrome P-450 mixed-function oxidases and inhibits insulin release.

When phenytoin is given in therapeutic doses, the oral absorption is slow, because of the limited solubility of phenytoin, as well as erratic. In overdose cases, gastrointestinal absorption may occur as long as 60 hours after ingestion. Peak concentrations can occur as late as 24 hours with oral ingestion but in 10 minutes with intravenous administration. In therapeutic doses, the metabolism of phenytoin follows first-order kinetics; at toxic levels, it follows zero-order kinetics. The therapeutic half-life is 20 to 30 hours, but in overdose cases, the half-life can be from 24 hours to 200 hours. Steady-state therapeutic levels are achieved at least 7 to 10 days (5-7 half-lives) after initiation of therapy with recommended doses of 300 mg/day.

Protein binding of phenytoin is high, and there is an inverse relationship between plasma albumin and free phenytoin. Phenytoin level correction in hypoalbuminemia can be calculated as follows:

$$\text{Corrected level} = \frac{\text{Measured phenytoin level}}{(\text{albumin} \times 0.2) + 0.1}$$

■ CLINICAL PRESENTATIONS

The most common presenting symptoms of phenytoin intoxication are neurologic and are usually dose-related. The early signs are ataxia, nystagmus, diplopia, and CNS depression. Acute intoxication is usually seen at serum levels higher than 20 mg/dL. Nystagmus is the earliest sign of intoxication. Onset of symptoms usually occurs within 1 to 2 hours after an ingestion. Neurologic effects from toxicity include slurred speech, a resting tremor, decreased coordination, increased deep tendon reflexes, ankle clonus, extensor rigidity, opisthotonus, and seizures. Pupils may be dilated. A sensory peripheral polyneuropathy has been reported in patients undergoing long-term phenytoin therapy. Cardiac toxicity from phenytoin is due to the diluent, propylene glycol, which is used in the intravenous form. Too-rapid infusions of phenytoin may cause hypotension or dysrhythmias (bradycardia, AV blocks, asystole). Intravenous infusions of phenytoin should be administered at a rate no higher than 50 mg/min. Dysrhythmias from oral phenytoin overdose have not been reported in the literature.

Gastrointestinal effects of phenytoin intoxication include nausea, vomiting, and constipation. Toxic hepatitis and liver damage have been reported. Hyperglycemia may be seen in patients as a result of the drug's inhibitory effects on insulin release.

There is a correlation between serum phenytoin levels and clinical presentations (Table 150-1).

Phenobarbital

Phenobarbital is a barbiturate used primarily as a sedative hypnotic and also as an anticonvulsant in subhypnotic doses. Phenobarbital is a CNS depressant that exhibits GABA-like effects similar to those of the benzodiazepines and reversibly depresses activity of all excitable tissue. Peak serum levels usually occur 6 to 8 hours after ingestion. This drug's onset of action is 1 hour or longer, and the duration of action is 10 to 12 hours. The plasma half-life is about 100 hours.

Phenobarbital produces different degrees of depression of the CNS, from sedation to respiratory depression, at different doses. This agent depresses the sensory cortex, decreases motor activity, alters cerebellar function, and produces drowsiness, sedation, and hypnosis. CNS and respiratory depression are the more serious side effects in overdose cases. Dizziness, decreased level of consciousness, bradycardia, bradypnea, areflexia, hypothermia, hypotension, nystagmus, and ataxia are also seen. Overdose may lead to pulmonary edema and acute renal failure as a result of hypotension. In severe overdose, the electroencephalogram may show a marked decrease in electrical activity, to the point of mimicking brain death. This appearance is due to profound depression of the CNS, and its effect is usually fully reversible unless hypoxic damage has occurred.

Table 150-1 CORRELATION BETWEEN SERUM PHENYTOIN LEVELS AND CLINICAL PRESENTATIONS

Serum Phenytoin Level (μg/mL)	Clinical Presentation
>20	Nystagmus
>30	Ataxia
>40	Decrease mental status
>50	Coma
>100	Potentially lethal

Valproic Acid

Valproic acid is used in the treatment of epilepsy, migraine headaches, bipolar disorder, and schizophrenia. Valproic acid dissociates to the valproate ion in the gastrointestinal tract. The mechanisms by which valproate exerts its antiepileptic effects is unknown, but it is believed to affect the function of GABA.

Peak serum levels occur 1 to 4 hours after a single oral dose. However, in overdoses, peak serum concentrations can be seen after 17 hours. The therapeutic half-life of valproic acid is 6 to 16 hours, but after an overdose it may be 30 hours. Therapeutic serum levels are 50 to 100 μg/mL.

Valproic acid disrupts amino acid and fatty acid metabolism, and increased ammonia levels can occur. Hepatic failure resulting in death has occurred in patients taking valproic acid. These deaths have occurred during the first 6 months of treatment with valproic acid. Children younger than 2 years are at an increased risk for development of fatal hepatotoxicity with this agent; nonspecific symptoms, such as malaise, weakness, lethargy, anorexia, and vomiting, may be the presenting signs of this complication. Cases of life-threatening pancreatitis have also been reported in patients taking valproic acid.

The clinical symptom of valproic acid overdoses is usually CNS depression. Other symptoms are somnolence and coma. Patients may have hypotension, tachycardia, heart block, and hypoventilation. Serum concentrations higher than 180 μg/mL lead to CNS depression. Laboratory analysis may demonstrate hyperammonemia, hepatitis, pancreatic, anemia, and neutropenia.

Table 150-2 **MECHANISMS, SYMPTOMS, AND TREATMENT OF ANTICONVULSANT INTOXICATIONS**

Anticonvulsant	Therapeutic Levels	Mechanism	Toxic Symptoms	Treatment
Phenytoin	10-20 μg/mL	Blocks sodium channels in excitable cells	Central nervous system (CNS) depression Ataxia Nausea Nystagmus Diplopia	Multiple-dose activated charcoal (MDAC) decreases drug level Hemodialysis, hemoperfusion are ineffective
Valproic acid	50-100 μg/mL	Increases levels of the inhibitory neurotransmitter gamma-aminobutyric acid (GABA)	CNS depression Hyperammonemia	L-carnitine for hyperammonemia MDAC Hemodialysis, hemoperfusion are effective
Carbamazepine	4-12 mg/L	Stabilizes sodium channels	Choreoathetosis Dry mucous membranes Dystonia Hyperthermia Mydriasis Tachycardia Urinary retention	MDAC Charcoal hemoperfusion Hemodialysis is ineffective
Phenobarbital	10-30 μg/mL	Exhibits GABA-like effects similar to those of benzodiazepines, and reversibly depresses activity of all excitable tissue		MDAC Urine alkaline diuresis Hemodialysis is effective
Felbamate	25-104 μg/mL	Inhibits N-methyl-D-aspartate (NMDA) responses and potentiated GABA responses	Aplastic anemia Ataxia CNS depression Hepatic failure Nystagmus Tachycardia Nausea Vomiting Crystalluria	Activated charcoal (AC)
Gabapentin		Unknown mechanisms	Ataxia Diarrhea Slurred speech Diplopia Somnolence Dizziness Tachycardia Tremor	AC Hemodinlysis and hemoperfusion are effective but rarely required
Lamotrigine		Blocks sodium channels Inhibits the release of excitatory neurotransmitters	Ataxia Dizziness Fever Hepatitis Hypertonia Hypokalemia Lethargy Nausea/vomiting Nystagmus QRS prolongation Renal failure Seizures Stevens-Johnson syndrome	AC Electrocardiogram monitoring Sodium bicarbonate (1-2 mEq/kg) if QRS duration is >100 msec No data on the value of hemodialysis or hemoperfusion
Levetiracetam		Unknown mechanisms	Drowsiness	AC
Tiagabine		Enhances GABA activity	Agitation Dizziness Ataxia Confusion Depression Seizures Somnolence Tremor Weakness	AC

Table 150-2 MECHANISMS, SYMPTOMS, AND TREATMENT OF ANTICONVULSANT INTOXICATIONS—cont'd

Anticonvulsant	Therapeutic Levels	Mechanism	Toxic Symptoms	Treatment
Topiramate		Unknown mechanisms	Anxiety Confusion Nervousness Sedation Slurred speech Ataxia Tremor	
Vigabatrin		Prevents inactivation of GABA by irreversible inhibition of GABA transaminase	Agitation Coma Delirium Hallucinations Delusions Paranoia Sedation Confusion	
Zonisamide		Blocks sodium and calcium channels	Agitation Ataxia Bradycardia Hypotension Respiratory depression Somnolence	

Treatment

Table 150-2 summarizes the mechanisms and symptoms of anticonvulsant intoxications.

Most of the ED management of anticonvulsant overdoses consists of providing supportive care with attention to the airway. Usually there are no specific antidotes. It is important to maintain an open airway and assist ventilation if necessary. Patients should be given supplemental oxygen. Activated charcoal may be administered if the ingestion has occurred within 1 hour. Multiple-dose activated charcoal decreases serum levels of some of these medications, such as phenytoin, more rapidly but has not been shown to shorten the clinical course. Benzodiazepines should be used if the patient has agitation and delirium. Naloxone has been reported to reverse the CNS depressant effects of valproic acid overdoses.

Sodium bicarbonate is recommended for drug-induced prolongation of the QRS interval.

Hemodialysis is effective at removing gabapentin, phenobarbital, and topiramate.

Charcoal hemoperfusion is highly effective and may be indicated for severe intoxication in carbamazepine overdoses. Plasma exchange has been used in children with severe carbamazepine overdoses.

Asymptomatic patients with anticonvulsant overdose should be monitored for a minimum of 4 to 6 hours. Symptomatic patients should be admitted for at least 24 hours after ingestion of lamotrigine, felbamate, topiramate, or zonisamide.

REFERENCES

1. Silverman AK, Fairley J, Wong RC: Cutaneous and immunologic reactions to phenytoin. J Am Acad Dermatol 1988; 18:721-741.
2. Crawford P, Ghadiali E, Lane R, et al: Gabapentin as an antiepileptic drug in man. J Neurol Neurosurg Psychiatry 1987;50:682-686.
3. Sivenius J, Kälviäinen R, Ylinen A, Riekkinen P: Double-blind study of gabapentin in the treatment of partial seizures. Epilepsia 1991;32:539-542.
4. Gabapentin package insert. Morris Plains, NJ, Parke-Davis, 1994.

Chapter 151

Antimicrobial Drugs

Victor Tuckler

KEY POINTS

All medications, including antibiotic and antiviral agents, can have significant side effects, although most severe consequences are relatively uncommon.

Patients with true penicillin allergy have about a 5% to 10% likelihood of reacting to a first generation cephalosporin. The cross-reactivity rate is far lower with second- and third-generation cephalosporins.

Vancomycin, when rapidly infused, can cause "red man syndrome," which is characterized by generalized flushing and, at times, hypotension. This effect can be minimized by slow infusion.

Tetracycline can cause permanent staining of secondary teeth if used within the first 8 years of life.

Metronidazole and antifungal agents can have negative interactions with ethanol, causing reactions similar to those seen with disulfiram, including severe nausea and vomiting.

Macrolides, such as azithromycin, erythromycin, and clarithromycin, can have negative interaction with fluoroquinolones (cardiac dysrhythmias), statins (myopathy), and other medications such as warfarin (due to inhibition of cytochrome P-450).

Isoniazid overdose can cause seizures, nausea, vomiting, acidosis, and altered mental status. The seizures should be treated with pyridoxine.

The discovery of penicillin in 1928 by Sir Alexander Fleming marked the beginning of discovery, formulation, and eventual widespread application of antibiotics. In the 1950s the modern era of antibiotic utilization commenced as several antibiotic classes became widely available. The development of antibacterial, antifungal, and antiviral agents remains a top scientific and medical priority today, especially because organisms develop resistance and new diseases emerge. Diseases such as tuberculosis, pneumonia, and bacterial sepsis, once leading causes of death, have been replaced in the developed world by cardiovascular disease and cancer. Infectious threats continue to be prominent, however. The morbidity and mortality of infectious diseases remain high. The battle is not won, and the balance is precarious.

Aggressive and appropriate use of antibiotics can be lifesaving. Appropriate use of antibiotics has been shown to reduce mortality in sepsis from 43% to 33%.[1] For patients with pneumonia, hospital length of stay has been found to be shorter when antibiotics are delivered in the ED.[2]

Although early and appropriate use of antibiotics is critical, their overuse has a "downside." Just 4 years after the discovery of penicillin, the emergence of resistant *Staphylococcus aureus* was identified. Antibiotic resistance has been rapidly evolving ever since. For example, between 1979 and 1987, 0.02% of *Pneumococcus* species was penicillin-resistant, but by 1992, the resistance had increased 60-fold. In some locations, more than 30% of *Pneumococcus* species was resistant to penicillin.[3] Currently, some hospital-acquired staphylococcal infections are resistant to all antibiotics except vancomycin. More frighteningly, vancomycin resistance has emerged in *Enterococcus*, increasing the fear of vancomycin-resistant staphylococcal organisms. Bacterial resistance to antibiotics is widespread and significant. Discovery of new antibiotic types and classes may not be able to keep pace with bacterial adaptation. It is essential, then, that antibiotics be used prudently and, even better, that infections be prevented. The current emphasis on caregiver handwashing and clothing hygiene is well justified.

Fortunately, there is evidence that physicians are responding to the calls for prudent use of antibiotics. Prescriptions for antibiotics in patients with upper respiratory tract infections decreased from 55% in 1993 to 35% in 2004.[4] Still, the frequency of use appears to remain high.

Table 151-1 SIDE EFFECTS OF PENICILLINS

Agents	Toxicity/Adverse Effects
Penicillin V or G	Seizures in patients with renal dysfunction
Methicillin	Interstitial nephritis Leukopenia
Nafcillin	Neutropenia
Ampicillin, amoxicillin	Acute renal failure
Azlocillin Carbenicillin Mezlocillin Piperacillin Ticarcillin	Impaired platelet function Hypokalemia
Amoxicillin/clavulanic acid Ampicillin/sulbactam Benzathine penicillin Cloxacillin Dicloxacillin Flucloxacillin Oxacillin Piperacillin/tazobactam Procaine penicillin Ticarcillin/clavulanic acid	Angioedema Dermatitis Diarrhea Erythema Fever Nausea Oral and vaginal candidiasis Pseudomembranous colitis Rash Seizures Urticaria Vomiting

Antibacterial Agents

■ PENICILLINS AND CEPHALOSPORINS

The β-lactam antibiotics are a broad class of antibiotics comprising penicillin derivatives, cephalosporins, monobactams, carbapenems, and β-lactamase inhibitors. These antibiotics inhibit bacterial cell wall synthesis and are used in the treatment of infection with bacterial, rickettsial, mycoplasmal, and chlamydial organisms. Most overdoses of penicillins and cephalosporins are benign, with toxic effects being mild. Adverse effects have resulted from allergic reactions or iatrogenic intravenous overdose. Adverse reactions that have been seen with penicillins and cephalosporins include interstitial nephritis, bone marrow suppression, vasculitis, Stevens-Johnson syndrome, and seizures. Seizures are the result of gamma-aminobutyric acid (GABA) antagonism.[5]

Penicillins in use include penicillin V and G, amoxicillin, ampicillin, carbenicillin, cloxacillin, dicloxacillin, nafcillin, methicillin, oxacillin, piperacillin, procaine penicillin, benzathine penicillin, and ticarcillin. Large doses of amoxicillin or ampicillin may cause crystal formation in renal tubules, resulting in renal failure. Adverse reactions associated with the use of penicillins include angioedema, diarrhea, erythema, nausea and vomiting, rash, urticaria, and pseudomembranous colitis. Benzathine penicillin is given intramuscularly and is slowly absorbed into the circulation; it has a prolonged action, 2 to 4 weeks, after a single intramuscular dose. Cardiac conduction defects have been reported after rapid intravenous administration of potassium penicillin G (Table 151-1).

Cephalosporins are grouped into "generations" by their antimicrobial properties. The first cephalosporins were designated first-generation, and the later, more extended-spectrum cephalosporins are classified as second-, third-, and fourth-generation cephalosporins. Each newer generation of cephalosporins has significantly greater gram-negative antimicrobial properties than the preceding one. Cefamandole, cefazolin, cefmetazole, cefoperazone, cefotetan, and moxalactam have an *N*-methyltetrazolethiol side chain that inhibits aldehyde dehydrogenase to cause a disulfiram-like interaction with ethanol. Coagulopathy from inhibition of vitamin K_1 production has been seen with cephalosporin containing an *N*-methyltetrazolethiol side chain. Ceftriaxone use has been associated with pseudolithiasis (Table 151-2).

Allergic reactions to any β-lactam antibiotic may occur in up to 10% of patients. Anaphylaxis occurs in approximately 0.01% of patients. Patients with a true penicillin allergy have about a 5% to 10% incidence of hypersensitivity reactions to first-generation cephalosporins.[6] The second-, third-, and fourth-generation cephalosporins have a much lower rate of cross-reactivity with penicillin and no significantly higher risk for reactivity.

■ AMINOGLYCOSIDES

Aminoglycosides are used in the treatment of infections caused by gram-negative organisms such as *Pseudomonas, Acinetobacter,* and *Enterobacter.* Aminoglycosides currently in use are amikacin, gentamicin, kanamycin, neomycin, netilmicin, paro-

Table 151-2 CEPHALOSPORINS

Agents	Toxicity/Adverse Effects
Cefaclor	Coagulopathy
Cefadroxil	Convulsions
Cefamandole	Diarrhea
Cefazolin	Dizziness
Cefepime	Electrolyte disturbances
Cefixime	Eosinophilia
Cefmetazole	Fever
Cefoperazone	Headache
Cefotaxime	Nausea
Cefotetan	Neutropenia
Cefoxitin	Oral and vaginal candidiasis
Cefprozil	Proximal tubular necrosis
Ceftazidime	Pseudomembranous colitis
Ceftriaxone	Rash
Cefuroxime	Superinfection
Cephalexin	Vomiting
Cephaloridine	
Cephalothin	
Cephradine	
Moxalactam	

momycin, streptomycin, tobramycin, and apramycin. The agents derived from a *Streptomyces* genus of bacteria are named with the suffix *-mycin,* and those derived from Micromonospora are named with the suffix—*micin.* Aminoglycosides inhibit bacterial 30S ribosomal subunits and protein synthesis. Most toxic exposures to aminoglycosides involve iatrogenic administration, which can lead to ototoxicity and/or nephrotoxicity.

A single overdose of an aminoglycoside usually does not produce any toxic effects. Single daily therapeutic administration is efficacious and has no greater incidence of side effects than traditional 3 times-per-day dosing.[7,8] The risk for ototoxicity and/or nephrotoxicity is increased with high dosing, prolonged treatment, the volume status of the patient, renal damage, and extremes of age. Ototoxicity can occur to the vestibular and cochlear cells, with the damage being permanent in some cases. Nephrotoxicity manifests as proximal tubular damage and acute tubular necrosis. In addition to ototoxicity and nephrotoxicity, competitive neuromuscular blockade and inhibition of acetylcholine release at the neuromuscular junction can occur with aminoglycoside use. Aminoglycosides potentiate the effects of neuromuscular blocking drugs. This can also occur in patients receiving corticosteroids and in patients with myasthenia gravis (Table 151-3).

■ FLUOROQUINOLONES

Fluoroquinolones inhibit bacterial DNA replication and transcription. These agents inhibit potassium channels in the myocardium and rarely cause QTc prolongation/torsades de pointes. Peripheral neuropathy has been reported in patients taking fluoroquinolones.

Fetal hepatotoxicity has been reported with trovafloxacin.[9] Other adverse effects are acute renal failure, spontaneous tendon rupture with damage to growing cartilage, seizures, blood glucose alterations, pseudomembranous colitis, rhabdomyolysis, and Stevens-Johnson syndrome (Table 151-4).[10]

Table 151-3 AMINOGLYCOSIDES

Agents	Toxicity/Adverse Effects
Amikacin	Competitive neuromuscular blockade
Gentamicin	Nephrotoxicity
Kanamycin	Ototoxicity
Neomycin	
Streptomycin	
Tobramycin	

■ ISONIAZID

Isoniazid, which is used as a prophylaxis or in the treatment for *Mycobacterium tuberculosis,* inhibits synthesis of the mycobacterial cell wall. This agent produces pyridoxine deficiency by enhancing excretion of pyridoxine, direct binding of pyridoxine to form an inactive complex, and competitive inhibition of the enzyme that converts pyridoxine to its physiologically active form. Pyridoxine depletion causes decreased levels of gamma-aminobutyric acid, which can cause seizures. Isoniazid produces lactic acidosis by blocking the conversion of lactate to pyruvate. Toxicity in an acute overdose of isoniazid can manifest as nausea, vomiting, acidosis, and altered mental status. Most patients have symptoms within 2 hours after an overdose. Refractory seizures can be seen within 1 hour of an acute overdose (>30 mg/kg) of isoniazid. Long-term use of isoniazid may also cause peripheral neuropathy (Table 151-5).

■ MACROLIDES

The macrolides include azithromycin, clarithromycin, dirithromycin, erythromycin, and roxithromycin. Ketolides are a new class of antibiotics that are structurally related to the macrolides; they include telithromycin and cethromycin.

Macrolides inhibit bacterial protein synthesis by binding reversibly to the 50S subunit of the bacterial ribosome. Macrolides are used to treat infections caused by beta-hemolytic streptococci, pneumococci, staphylococci, enterococci, mycoplasma, mycobacteria, some rickettsiae, and chlamydia. Adverse effects of the macrolides as a group are abdominal pain, nausea, vomiting, cholestatic jaundice, ototoxicity,

Table 151-4 FLUOROQUINOLONES

Agents	Toxicity/Adverse Effects
Alatrofloxacin	Confusion
Ciprofloxacin	Hallucinations
Norfloxacin	Intracranial hypertension
Rifampin	Metabolic acidosis
Spectinomycin	Seizures
Trovafloxacin	Visual disturbances

Table 151-5 ANTIBACTERIAL AGENTS

Agent	Toxicity/Adverse Effects
Chloramphenicol	Gray baby syndrome Leukopenia Reticulocytopenia
Dapsone	Confusion Hallucinations Hemolysis Hepatitis Metabolic acidosis Methemoglobinemia Sulfhemoglobinemia
Ethambutol	Optic neuritis Peripheral neuropathy Red/green color blindness
Isoniazid (INH)	Seizures Hepatotoxicity with long-term use Metabolic acidosis Peripheral neuropathy with chronic use
Linezolid	Thrombocytopenia
Metronidazole	Disulfiram-like interaction with ethanol Seizures
Nitrofurantoin	Hemolysis in patients with glucose-6-phosphate dehydrogenase (G6PD) deficiency

thrombophlebitis, and ventricular dysrhythmia. These adverse effects are usually reversible upon discontinuation of use of the agent. Interaction with fluoroquinolones, cisapride, and disopyramide can cause QT prolongation and torsades de pointes. Administration of more than 4 g/day of a macrolide may cause tinnitus and ototoxicity.

Macrolides can inhibit cytochrome P-450 and raise levels of warfarin, theophylline, carbamazepine, and cyclosporine. They also induce P-glycoprotein–facilitated drug transport and, thus, can increase digoxin levels. The combination of macrolides and statins can lead to debilitating myopathy (Table 151-6).

■ METRONIDAZOLE

Metronidazole is an oral synthetic antiprotozoal and antibacterial agent. Adverse effects include gastrointestinal distress, reversible peripheral neuropathy, seizures, and disulfiram-like reactions with ethanol. Metronidazole has been reported to potentiate the anticoagulant effect of warfarin. The simultaneous administration of phenytoin or phenobarbital with metronidazole may accelerate the elimination of metronidazole.

Table 151-6 MACROLIDES

Agents	Toxicity/Adverse Effects
Azithromycin Clarithromycin Dirithromycin Erythromycin Roxithromycin	Abdominal pain Hepatotoxicity with estolate salt QT prolongation Torsade de pointes

Table 151-7 LINCOSAMIDES

Agents	Toxicity/Adverse Effects
Clindamycin Lincomycin	Agranulocytosis Glossitis Hypotension Leukopenia Nausea Neutropenia Pruritus ani Pseudomembranous colitis Stomatitis Thrombocytopenic purpura Tinnitus Vertigo Vomiting

■ LINCOSAMIDES

The lincosamides include lincomycin and clindamycin. These agents inhibit bacterial protein synthesis by binding to the 50S subunit of bacterial ribosomes. Hypotension and cardiopulmonary arrest can occur after rapid intravenous administration of a lincosamide. Adverse effects include pseudomembranous colitis, glossitis, stomatitis, nausea, vomiting, pruritus ani, neutropenia, leukopenia, agranulocytosis, thrombocytopenic purpura, tinnitus, and vertigo. Lincomycin has been shown to have neuromuscular blocking properties and may enhance the action of neuromuscular blocking drugs (Table 151-7).

■ POLYMYXINS

Polymyxins are antibiotics that disrupt the structure of the bacterial cell membrane by interacting with its phospholipids. Polymyxins have a bactericidal effect on gram-negative bacilli such as *Pseudomonas* and coliform organisms. Polymyxin antibiotics are highly neurotoxic and nephrotoxic. Neurotoxic reactions may manifest as irritability, weakness, drowsiness, ataxia, perioral paresthesia, numbness of the extremities, and blurring of vision. The neurotoxicity of a polymyxin can result in respiratory paralysis from neuromuscular blockade, especially when the drug is given soon after administration of a neuromuscular-blocking drug or muscle relaxant. Nephrotoxic reactions include albuminuria, azotemia, and cylindruria (Table 151-8).

■ SULFONAMIDES AND TRIMETHOPRIM

The sulfonamides (sulfa drugs) inhibit bacterial folate synthesis. Their adverse effects include hemolysis, methemoglobinemia, nephrotoxicity, bone marrow suppression, and a high incidence of allergic reactions. They also can increase the effects of warfarin

Table 151-8 POLYMYXINS

Agents	Toxicity/Adverse Effects
Polymyxin B Polymyxin E Pyrazinamide	Hepatotoxicity Hyperuricemia Nephrotoxicity Noncompetitive neuromuscular blockade

as well as the hypoglycemic effects of sulfonylurea medications.

Trimethoprim belongs to the class of drugs known as dihydrofolate reductase inhibitors. These agents inhibit bacterial folate synthesis. Trimethoprim is commonly used in combination with sulfamethoxazole (Table 151-9).

Trimethoprim-sulfamethoxazole act synergistically to block bacterial folate metabolism because they stop sequential steps in the process. Humans are less affected than the bacteria because folate is acquired in the diet and is not synthesized in the human body.

■ VANCOMYCIN

Vancomycin inhibits prevent bacterial cell wall synthesis by inhibiting bacterial glycopeptidase polymerase. Rapid intravenous infusion can cause an anaphylactoid reaction called "red man syndrome," which is characterized by generalized flushing and is sometimes accompanied by hypotension. Adverse effects of vancomycin include ototoxicity and nephrotoxicity (see Table 151-9).[11]

■ TETRACYCLINES

The tetracyclines inhibit the 30S and 50S subunits of bacterial ribosomes as well as protein synthesis. Their adverse effects include photosensitivity dermatitis, pseudotumor cerebri, and neuromuscular blockade in patients with myasthenia gravis. Another adverse effect of tetracyclines is permanent staining of secondary teeth if they are used in the first 12 weeks of gestation or given to children younger than 8 years (Table 151-10).

Table 151-9 SULFONAMIDES AND TRIMETHOPRIM

Agents	Toxicity/Adverse Effects
Sulfonamides	Acute renal failure Crystal deposition
Trimethoprim	Bone marrow depression Hyperkalemia Methemoglobinemia
Vancomycin	Ototoxicity and nephrotoxicity Hypertension Rash/flushing ("red man syndrome")

Table 151-10 TETRACYCLINES

Agents	Toxicity/Adverse Effects
Demeclocycline Minocycline Tetracycline	Benign intracranial hypertension Nephrogenic diabetes insipidus Vestibular symptoms

Antifungal Agents

There are three antifungal categories that can cause toxicity by different mechanisms (Table 151-11).

Polyene antifungals target the kidney and the cardiovascular system. Amphotericin B is an agent in this category. Synthetic nucleotide analogues like flucytosine interfere with DNA replication. Bone marrow and gastrointestinal mucosal cells are affected by this category. Imidazole antifungals such as ketoconazole and miconazole alter fungal cell membranes and interfere with the intracellular enzymes.

Acute toxicity from these agents is usually mild. Toxic doses have not yet been established. Adverse effects are numerous, but gastrointestinal distress is common. Antifungal agents decreased warfarin activity and the effects of oral contraceptives. Plasma concentrations of imidazole antifungal agents rise with concomitant use of digoxin, oral sulfonylurea, warfarin, and phenytoin. Fluconazole has been known to cause Stevens-Johnson syndrome.

Disulfiram-like reaction occurs as an interaction between ethanol and antifungal drugs.

Amphotericin B and other polyene antifungal agents act synergistically with other nephrotoxic agents. Amphotericin B binds to ergosterol, a component of fungal cell membranes, leading to disruptions in the membranes. Common adverse effects reported are fever, rigors, vomiting, and headache.

Amphotericin B can cause "red man syndrome"—erythema of the hands, soles, face, and neck—if infused too rapidly. Amphotericin B has been known to cause fever, hypokalemia, elevated liver function values, ventricular fibrillation, renal tubular acidosis,

Table 151-11 ANTIFUNGAL ANGENTS

Category	Agents	Toxicity/Adverse Effects
Polyenes	Amphotericin B Nystatin	Fever, chills, myalgias Nephrotoxicity
Antimetabolite	Flucytosine	Bone marrow suppression Peripheral neuropathies Seizures
Azoles	Butoconazole nitrate Clotrimazole Fluconazole Itraconazole Ketoconazole Miconazole nitrate Terconazole Tioconazole	Hepatotoxicity

Table 151-12 Antiviral Drugs

Agent	Toxicity/Adverse Effects
Acyclovir	Coma Confusion Crystalluria Hallucinations Leukopenia Renal failure Seizures
Foscarnet	Renal impairment Seizures
Ganciclovir	Hepatitis Increased serum creatinine Neutropenia Pancytopenia Seizure Thrombocytopenia
Trifluridine	Reversible bone marrow depression
Vidarabine	Ataxia Confusion Diarrhea Dizziness Hallucinations Nausea Psychosis Tremor Vomiting

agranulocytosis, and pulmonary hypertension. Synthetic nucleotide analogues are known to cause gastrointestinal distress and bone marrow depression.[12]

Flucytosine is metabolized to 5-fluorouracil (5-FU), resulting in disruption of fungal nucleic acid synthesis. Adverse effects reported are bone marrow suppression, peripheral neuropathies, and seizures.

Griseofulvin inhibits fungal microtubule formation. The common adverse effects reported for this agent are hypersensitivity reactions, headaches, and confusion.

Antiviral Agents

Serious toxicities that develop after short-term and long-term use of many antiviral agents are hepatic steatosis, bone marrow depression, diabetes mellitus, hepatotoxicity, lactic acidosis, lipodystrophy, lipoatrophy, pancreatitis, peripheral neuropathy, renal failure, nephrolithiasis, and seizures (Table 151-12).

Nucleoside (or nucleotide) reverse transcriptase inhibitors (NRTIs) can cause lactic acidosis, mitochondrial toxicity, and hepatotoxicity. Nonnucleoside reverse transcriptase inhibitors (NNRTIs) are associated with dermatitis and hepatotoxicity. Protease inhibitors (PIs) are associated with dyslipidemias, insulin resistance, hepatotoxicity, and osteoporosis.

■ ACYCLOVIR

Acyclovir is a synthetic purine nucleoside analogue with activity against herpes simplex virus type 1 (HSV-1) and type 2 (HSV-2) and varicella-zoster virus (VZV). This agent inhibits viral nucleic acid synthesis.[13]

Common adverse effects reported are nausea, vomiting, diarrhea, headache, and malaise. Other reported adverse effects are anaphylaxis, angioedema, fever, and peripheral edema. Dermatologic effects are alopecia, erythema multiforme, photosensitive rash, pruritus, Stevens-Johnson syndrome, toxic epidermal necrolysis, and urticaria. Nervous system effects are aggressive behavior, agitation, ataxia, coma, confusion, decreased consciousness, delirium, dizziness, dysarthria, encephalopathy, hallucinations, paresthesia, psychosis, seizure, somnolence, and tremors.

There are also case reports of anemia, leukocytoclastic vasculitis, leukopenia, lymphadenopathy, and thrombocytopenia with acyclovir. Elevated liver function values, hepatitis, hyperbilirubinemia, and jaundice may occur with therapeutic doses. Acyclovir causes crystal deposition in the renal tubular lumen, leading to an obstructive nephropathy. Renal failure, elevations of blood urea nitrogen and creatinine, and hematuria have been reported.

This drug is classified as a pregnancy category B agent (see later), and acyclovir concentrations have been documented in breast milk. Acyclovir should be administered to nursing mothers with caution and only when indicated.

Acute overdoses involving ingestion of up to 20 g have been reported. Agitation, coma, seizures, and lethargy have occurred with overdoses. Precipitation of acyclovir in renal tubules resulting in renal toxicity may occur with acute overdoses, and affected patients may benefit from hemodialysis until renal function is restored.

■ AMANTADINE

Amantadine is indicated for the prophylaxis and treatment of signs and symptoms of infection by various strains of influenza A virus. The mechanism by which amantadine exerts its antiviral activity is not clearly understood, but it appears to prevent the release of infectious viral nucleic acid into host cells by interfering with the viral penetration into the host cells. This agent enhances dopaminergic neurotransmission and has anticholinergic activity.

The commonly reported adverse reactions are nausea, dizziness, and insomnia. Other reported adverse reactions are depression, anxiety and irritability, hallucinations, confusion, psychosis, anorexia, dry mouth, constipation, ataxia, peripheral edema, orthostatic hypotension, headache, somnolence, nervousness, dream abnormality, visual disturbance, agitation, dry nose, diarrhea, and fatigue. Acute overdoses have resulted in cardiac, respiratory, renal, or central nervous system toxicity.

Acute overdose may lead to anticholinergic toxicity, QTc and QRS prolongation, and delirium. Deaths have been reported from overdose with amantadine. The lowest reported acute lethal dose was 2 g.[14]

Table 151-13 PREGNANCY CATEGORY CLASSIFICATIONS FOR PHARMACEUTICALS*

Pregnancy Category	Explanation/Definition
A	Adequate and well-controlled studies have failed to demonstrate a risk to the fetus in the first trimester of pregnancy (and there is no evidence of risk in later trimesters).
B	Animal reproduction studies have failed to demonstrate a risk to the fetus and there are no adequate and well-controlled studies in pregnant women *or* animal studies have shown an adverse effect, but adequate and well-controlled studies in pregnant women have failed to demonstrate a risk to the fetus in any trimester.
C	Animal reproduction studies have shown an adverse effect on the fetus and there are no adequate and well-controlled studies in humans, but potential benefits may warrant use of the drug in pregnant women despite potential risks.
D	There is positive evidence of human fetal risk based on adverse reaction data from investigational or marketing experience or studies in humans, but potential benefits may warrant use of the drug in pregnant women despite potential risks.
X	Studies in animals or humans have demonstrated fetal abnormalities and/or there is positive evidence of human fetal risk based on adverse reaction data from investigational or marketing experience and the risks involved in use of the drug in pregnant women clearly outweigh potential benefits.

*Classification has been determined by the U.S. Food and Drug Administration.

Table 151-14 PREGNANCY CATEGORIES FOR COMMONLY USED ANTIMICROBIAL AGENTS*

Agents	Pregnancy Category	Excreted in Breast Milk?	Comments
Aminoglycosides:			
Amikacin, gentamicin, and neomycin	C	Yes	
Kanamycin and tobramycin	D	Yes	
Antifungal agents:			Breastfeeding women should avoid these agents in oral form
Amphotericin B	B	Yes	All vaginal preparations are considered safe in pregnancy
Other antifungals	C	Yes	
Antiparasitic agents	C (in oral form)	Unknown	
Antiprotozoal agents:			
Metronidazole	B	Yes	
Chloroquine	D	Yes	
Antituberculous agents:			
Ethambutol	B	Yes	
Capreomycin and cycloserine	C	Yes	
Antiviral agents:			
Acyclovir	B	Yes	
Amantadine, rimantadine, cidofovir, famciclovir, foscarnet, ganciclovir, valacyclovir	C	Yes	
Chloramphenicol	C	Yes	
Clindamycin and lincomycin	B	Yes	
Fluoroquinolones	C	Yes	Breastfeeding women should avoid these agents
Macrolides:			
Azithromycin and erythromycin	B	Unknown	
Clarithromycin	C	Unknown	
Penicillins and cephalosporins	B	Yes	
Sulfonamides	C	Yes	
Vancomycin	C	Yes	

*Categories have been determined by the U.S. Food and Drug Administration.

Pregnancy Categories for Pharmaceutical Agents

The pregnancy category of a pharmaceutical agent is an assessment of the risk of fetal injury due to the agent if it is used by the mother during pregnancy (Table 151-13).[15] Table 151-14 lists the pregnancy categories for various antimicrobial agents.

REFERENCES

1. MacArthur, Miller M, Albertson T, et al: Adequacy of early empiric antibiotic treatment and survival in severe sepsis: Experience from the MONARCS trial. Clin Infect Dis 2004;38:284-288.
2. Battleman DS, Callahan M, Thaler HT: Rapid antibiotic delivery and appropriate antibiotic selection reduce length of hospital stay of patients with community-acquired pneumonia. Arch Intern Med 2002;162:682-688.
3. Breiman RF, Butler JC, Tenover FC, et al: Emergence of drug resistant pneumococcal infections in the United States. JAMA 1994;271:1831-1835.
4. Vanderweil SG, Pelletier AJ, Hamedani AG, et al: Declining antibiotic prescriptions for upper respiratory infections 1993-2004. Acad Emerg Med 2007;14:366-369.
5. Wynn M, Dalovisio JR, Tice AD, Jiang X: Evaluation of the efficacy and safety of outpatient parenteral antimicrobial therapy for methicillin-sensitive *Staphylococcus aureus*. South Med J 2005;98:590-595.
6. Cerny A, Pickler W: Allergy to antibacterials: The problem with beta-lactams and sulfonamides. Pharmacoepidemiol Drug Safety 1998;7:S23-S36.
7. Sifakis S, Angelakis E, Makrigiannakis A, et al: Chemoprophylactic and bactericidal efficacy of 80 mg gentamicin in a single and once-daily dosing. Arch Gynecol Obstet 2005;272(3):201-206.
8. Nordström L, Ringberg H, Cronberg S, et al: Does administration of an aminoglycoside in a single daily dose affect its efficacy and toxicity? J Antimicrob Chemother 1990;25:159-173.
9. Wlazlowski J, Krzyzanska-Oberbek A, Sikora JP, Chlebna-Sokól D: Use of the quinolones in treatment of severe bacterial infections in premature infants. Acta Pol Pharm 2000;57(Suppl):28-31.
10. Stahlmann R, Lode H: Toxicity of quinolones. Drugs 1999;58(Suppl 2):37-42.
11. Deresinski S: Vancomycin: Does it still have a role as an antistaphylococcal agent? Expert Rev Anti Infect Ther 2007;5:393-401.
12. Blau IW, Fauser AA: Review of comparative studies between conventional and liposomal amphotericin B (AmBisome) in neutropenic patients with fever of unknown origin and patients with systemic mycosis. Mycoses 2000;43:325-332.
13. Woo SB, Challacombe SJ: Management of recurrent oral herpes simplex infections. Oral Surg Oral Med Oral Pathol Oral Radiol Endod 2007;103(Suppl):S12e1-S12e18.
14. Lynch JP 3rd, Walsh EE: Influenza: Evolving strategies in treatment and prevention. Semin Respir Crit Care Med 2007;28:144-158.
15. Bertsche T, Haas M, Oberwittler H, et al: Drugs during pregnancy and breastfeeding: New risk categories-antibodies as a model. Dtsch Med Wochenschr 2006;131:1016-1022.

Chapter 152

Hypoglycemic Agent Overdose

Mark Su

KEY POINTS

Hypoglycemia may be defined either by serum glucose level or on the basis of symptoms.

Typically, an adult has enough glycogen to last about 6 to 8 hours.

Insulin treatment is the most common cause of hypoglycemia in adults with diabetes.

Extreme glucose values (either high or low) and hypoperfusion can cause a significant discrepancy in bedside glucose testing results.

Multiple-dose activated charcoal may enhance the elimination of the sulfonylurea glipizide.

Sodium bicarbonate administered to alkalinize the urine has been shown to reduce the half-life of the sulfonylurea chlorpropamide.

Patients with overdoses (intentional or unintentional) of insulin, sulfonylureas, and meglitinides should be admitted for inpatient observation because of the unpredictable kinetics.

Scope

Hypoglycemia is a common, potentially life-threatening occurrence in patients presenting to the ED with depressed mental status. The standard definition of hypoglycemia is based on Whipple's triad: decreased plasma glucose level, hypoglycemic symptoms, and improvement in hypoglycemic symptoms after administration of glucose. However, hypoglycemia may be defined either according to serum glucose level (numerically) or on the basis of symptomatology. It is usually defined as (1) serum glucose value lower than 50 to 60 mg/dL (2.8 to 3.0 mmol/L) in the absence of neuroglycopenic symptoms or (2) the presence of neuroglycopenic symptoms at any concentration of blood glucose. The development of symptoms from hypoglycemia varies among individuals. For the purposes of this chapter, the term *hypoglycemia* refers to the condition of blood glucose concentration for which medical intervention is usually necessary; it is occasionally referred to in the literature as *severe hypoglycemia*.[1]

Although hypoglycemia is usually a complication of diabetes mellitus (DM), nondiabetic patients may also have hypoglycemia from various disease states (e.g., sepsis) or drugs (e.g., ethanol), which are discussed in detail in Chapter 164. The exact incidence of hypoglycemia in nondiabetic persons is unknown. In patients with DM, the occurrence of hypoglycemia depends on factors such as whether the patient has type 1 or type 2 diabetes and what type of pharmacologic therapy the patient is undergoing (i.e., insulin or an oral antihyperglycemic agent). Hypoglycemia reportedly occurs at least one time per year in 10% to 30% of patients with type 1 DM.[2]

The diagnosis is often made empirically by prehospital care providers prior to the patient's arrival in the ED; however, death due to hypoglycemic coma still occurs if the condition is unrecognized.[3] A small subset of patients intentionally overdose, and treating them can be extremely difficult. This chapter discusses important factors in the evaluation and treatment of patients with toxicity secondary to hypoglycemic agent overdose.

Pathophysiology

The primary metabolic substrate for the central nervous system (CNS) is glucose. Usual sources of glucose are diet as well as endogenous production (via gluconeogenesis) and storage (via glycogenolysis). Serum glucose concentrations are relatively tightly controlled by physiologic mechanisms. After dietary sources of glucose are completely utilized, glycogenolysis is the major physiologic mechanism for maintaining euglycemia. Typically, an adult has enough glycogen to last about 6 to 8 hours. When glycogen stores are depleted, gluconeogenesis, which is fueled by amino acids from muscle, takes over. The CNS cannot make or store glucose, relying on the previously mentioned mechanisms to maintain normal metabolic activity during fasting periods. As glucose use exceeds glucose production and serum glucose concentrations decrease, various counterregulatory pathways are activated. Counterregulatory pathways triggered at the glycemic threshold are increases in glucagon, epinephrine, growth hormone, and cortisol. Glycemic thresholds are fairly reproducible in research studies on healthy subjects but can vary significantly among patients with both type 1 and type 2 DM; these thresholds also depend on other factors, such as tightness of glucose regulation, presence of chronic hyperglycemia, and recent episodes of hypoglycemia.[4]

Hypoglycemic agents induce hypoglycemia by various mechanisms. Insulins cause rapid transport of amino acids and glucose intracellularly. Sulfonylureas stimulate insulin secretion by binding to specific membrane receptors on the pancreatic beta-islet cell. They also benefit glucose homeostasis by decreasing hepatic glucose production and improving insulin sensitivity at the receptor and post-receptor levels.[5] Other drugs may induce hypoglycemia by inhibition of gluconeogenesis, glycogenolysis, counterregulatory hormones, or other unknown mechanisms. Ethanol, a toxin commonly encountered in the ED, inhibits gluconeogenesis by depleting nicotinamide adenine dinucleotide (NAD) and also inhibits the effects of cortisol, growth hormone, and epinephrine.[1]

Clinical Presentation

The symptoms of hypoglycemia can be divided into two basic groups, hyperadrenergic symptoms and neuroglycopenic symptoms (Box 152-1). Hyperadrenergic symptoms are more common with a rapid decrease in glucose and are due to autonomic nervous system stimulation (both sympathetic and cholinergic). The other clinical features of hypoglycemia are mediated through altered brain activity; the resulting constellation of signs and symptoms of hypoglycemia are termed *neuroglycopenia*.[6] Three neuroglycopenic syndromes are described: acute, subacute, and chronic.[7] *Subacute neuroglycopenia* is characterized by episodic disorientation, somnolence, slurring of speech, personality changes, amnesia, and loss of consciousness. Precipitous loss of consciousness may occur as the sole manifestation of subacute neuroglycopenia. Both subacute and acute forms of neuroglycopenia may manifest as acute neurologic deficits (e.g., transient hemiplegia), strabismus, hypothermia, hyperthermia, seizures, and automatism. *Chronic neuroglycopenia* is a rare condition that usually occurs in patients with insulinoma and in patients with DM who are treated with excessive insulin and demonstrate a gradual progressive mental illness similar to chronic psychiatric disorders.[7]

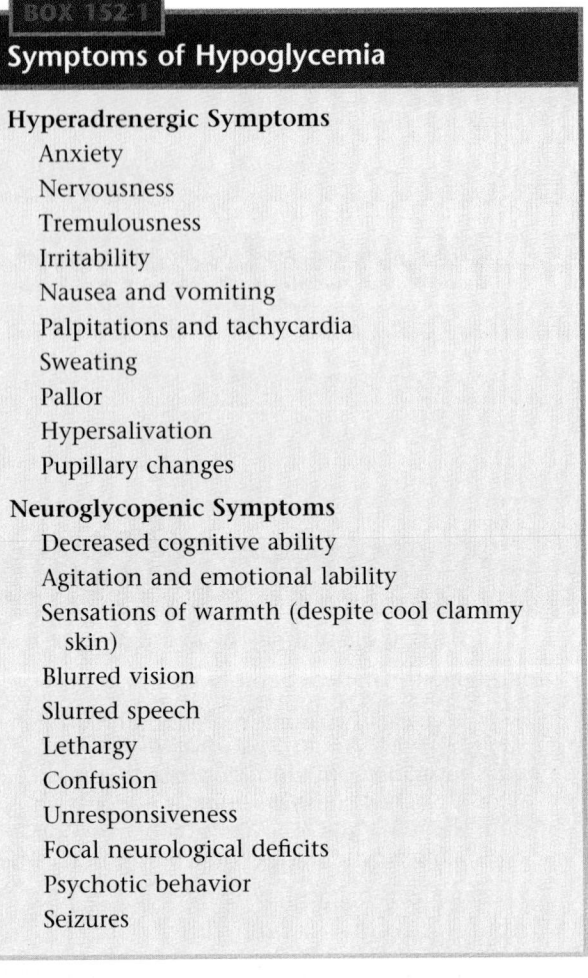

BOX 152-1
Symptoms of Hypoglycemia

Hyperadrenergic Symptoms
- Anxiety
- Nervousness
- Tremulousness
- Irritability
- Nausea and vomiting
- Palpitations and tachycardia
- Sweating
- Pallor
- Hypersalivation
- Pupillary changes

Neuroglycopenic Symptoms
- Decreased cognitive ability
- Agitation and emotional lability
- Sensations of warmth (despite cool clammy skin)
- Blurred vision
- Slurred speech
- Lethargy
- Confusion
- Unresponsiveness
- Focal neurological deficits
- Psychotic behavior
- Seizures

Differential Diagnosis

Hypoglycemia has numerous causes and may be classified into the following three categories: (1) postprandial, (2) fasting, and (3) drug- or toxin-induced (Table 152-1).[1] In healthy patients, fasting hypoglycemia is usually due to unintentional or intentional drug ingestion and insulinoma. In patients who are severely ill or hospitalized, hypoglycemia may be a complication of the illness, drug interactions, or other iatrogenic factors.

Hypoglycemic agents can be divided according to their route of administration (i.e., parenteral or oral). Insulins are the only medications for the treatment of DM that are given parenterally. A multitude of antidiabetic medications given orally, including the sulfonylureas (e.g., glyburide [Diabeta], glipizide [Glucotrol]), meglitinides (e.g., nateglinide [Starlix], repaglinide [Prandin]), biguanides (e.g., metformin), thiazolidinediones (e.g., rosiglitazone [Actos], pioglitazone [Avandia], troglitazone [Rezulin]), and α-glucosidase inhibitors (e.g., acarbose [Precose]). Of all of these antidiabetic drugs, only a few classes are commonly associated with hypoglycemia—the insulins, sulfonylureas, and meglitinides.

For adults with DM, insulin treatment is the most common cause of hypoglycemia. Factors associated with higher frequency of hypoglycemia in patients with type 1 DM include lower hemoglobin A_{1c} (HbA_{1c}), higher daily insulin requirements, longer duration of DM, and a previous history of hypoglycemia. About 25% of patients with DM are unable to recognize impending hypoglycemia owing to a lack of autonomic warning symptoms; this characteristic is also an important predictor of hypoglycemia.[1] Patients with insulin-dependent type 2 DM are also susceptible to hypoglycemia, especially if their disease has been treated with insulin for a long time and if their DM is tightly controlled.[8]

For patients who are taking oral agents rather than insulin, sulfonylureas are a common cause of hypoglycemia. According to the 2004 annual report of the American Association of Poison Control Centers Toxic Surveillance System, there were 4148 reported sulfonylurea exposures and 9 deaths in 2003.[9] The incidence of hypoglycemia secondary to these agents rises in elderly patients and with long-acting agents (e.g., chlorpropamide).[10] Consequently, independent risk factors for hypoglycemia include recent hospitalization, advanced age, and polypharmacy. Other risk factors for sulfonylurea-induced hypoglycemia are hepatic and renal dysfunction because of decreased metabolism (e.g., glyburide, glibenclamide, glipizide) and decreased elimination (e.g., chlorpropamide and glyburide). The most commonly used sulfonylureas have a duration of effect of at least 24 hours, and hypoglycemia in a patient taking such an agent can be prolonged, especially in the setting of overdose. In one case report, sulfonylurea-induced hypoglycemia was reported to last up to 27 days.[11] It should be noted that most other oral agents (e.g., thiazolidinediones, biguanides) used for the treatment of DM do not usually cause significant hypoglycemia.

Table 152-1 THREE CATEGORIES OF HYPOGLYCEMIA

Type of Hypoglycemia	Causes
Postprandial	Early diabetes Alcohol intake Post-gastrectomy status Renal failure Drugs such as salicylates, beta-blockers, pentamidine
Fasting	Conditions of excess insulin, including insulinoma and self-administration of insulin/oral hypoglycemic agents (diabetic insulin overdose) Alcohol abuse and liver disease (decreased gluconeogenesis) Pituitary or adrenal insufficiency
Drug- or toxin-induced	Ethanol Quinidine Beta-blocker Pentamidine Monoamine oxidase inhibitors Angiotensin-converting enzyme inhibitors Salicylates Haloperidol Disopyramide Akee fruit Trimethoprim-sulfamethoxazole

Diagnostic Testing

Hypoglycemia is a simple diagnosis to make provided that it is considered early on in a patient's presentation. In most cases, hypoglycemia is considered in a patient with altered sensorium or depressed mental status. Bedside blood glucose testing using a glucose meter in the patient with neuroglycopenic symptoms is generally the fastest as well as a fairly reliable technique to determine hypoglycemia. In general, there seems to be good correlation of capillary blood glucose levels (which are measured by a glucose meter) with venous or arterial glucose measurements.[12,13] However, at extreme values (either high or low) and in cases of systemic hypoperfusion, a clinically significant discrepancy may be apparent. In the setting of suspected hypoglycemia, confirmatory laboratory testing of a serum specimen is therefore necessary. Furthermore, because symptoms of hypoglycemia vary among individuals, hypoglycemia is still a possible diagnosis even in a patient with a glucose level categorized as "euglycemic."[14]

Additional diagnostic testing may be necessary, depending on the clinical scenario. For most patients with DM who present with hypoglycemia, routine testing of liver and renal function is indicated. Ethanol (or other alcohol) ingestion may also result in hypoglycemia, and measurement of serum ethanol concentration may be useful in the setting of "alcohol intoxication." Other tests that may be helpful are thyroid function tests and measurements of serum cortisol, insulin, and C peptide concentrations. Insulin and C peptide measurements are particularly useful in the setting of surreptitious exposure to insulin or sulfonylureas. Unlike endogenous insulin synthesized by the pancreas, exogenous insulin has no concomitant C peptide. In cases of intentional insulin poisoning, insulin concentrations will be high but C peptide concentrations will be normal. On the contrary, sulfonylurea ingestions cause elevations in both insulin and C peptide, the same findings in patients with insulinoma. Lastly, in patients with intentional self-harm, testing of a serum acetaminophen concentration is potentially useful.

Treatment

The EP must institute basic supportive measures, with particular attention to airway, breathing, and circulation, along with cardiorespiratory monitoring upon encountering the obtunded patient with hypoglycemia. Supplemental oxygen, intravenous (IV) thiamine, and naloxone are generally benign therapies that may be judiciously administered in a patient with depressed mental status of unknown etiology.

PRIORITY ACTIONS

Treatment of Hypoglycemic Agent Overdose

1. Basic support measures with attention to airway, breathing, circulation, and cardiopulmonary monitoring.
2. Bedside glucose testing and an immediate bolus of glucose. Hypoglycemia should be treated with intravenous (IV) glucose for severe episodes and when associated with obtundation: 0.5-1 g/kg of 50% dextrose in water ($D_{50}W$) for adults and of 25% dextrose in water ($D_{25}W$) for children.
3. Thiamine and naloxone should be considered for obtunded patients.
4. After initial euglycemia, continuous IV infusions of dextrose (D_5W or $D_{10}W$) should be started, and boluses repeated when indicated.
5. Decontamination with activated charcoal, either a single dose or multiple doses, for agents such as glipizide (enterohepatic circulation).
6. Enhanced elimination with IV sodium bicarbonate to alkalinize urine and reduce the half-life for long-acting sulfonylureas like chlorpropamide.
7. Observation and admission for signs of neuroglycopenia and repeated serum glucose checks every 1 to 2 hours. Monitoring of serum electrolyte levels every 4 hours.
8. Octreotide, 50 μg given subcutaneously every 6-8 hours, for at least 24 hours in cases of prolonged hypoglycemia secondary to long-acting sulfonylurea overdose.

After the primary survey has been performed and any needed measures taken, gastrointestinal decontamination should be considered for patients who have taken an intentional oral overdose of a hypoglycemic agent. The particular modality of decontamination implemented depends on the usual factors, such as time of ingestion, quantity of tablets, mental status of the patient, and potential harm to the patient. In general, emesis should not be induced in such patients because of the potential for aspiration of gastrointestinal contents. Activated charcoal has been shown to be very effective in binding to multiple sulfonylurea agents in vitro.[15] A single dose of activated charcoal may be beneficial in these ingestions; in theory, multiple-dose activated charcoal may enhance elimination of the sulfonylurea glipizide because glipizide undergoes enterohepatic circulation.[5] IV sodium bicarbonate administered to alkalinize the urine has been shown to reduce the half-life of the sulfonylurea agent chlorpropamide.[16] These and other forms of decontamination and enhanced elimination should be used on a case-by-case basis.

Patients who are documented to have hypoglycemia by rapid bedside glucose testing should be given glucose as soon as possible. If a patient is awake and is believed to have intact airway reflexes, oral carbohydrates in the form of flavored glucose tablets, juice, and soda may be given. The patient should show response within 10 to 15 minutes as he or she returns to a euglycemic state. After this initial therapy, the patient should be given additional nutrition in the form of a snack or meal for a sustained source of calories. If the patient does not show response to oral carbohydrates, parenteral therapy is required.

IV dextrose is the preferred treatment for severe hypoglycemia with obtundation and a patient's inability to take oral carbohydrates. The administration of 0.5 to 1 g/kg of IV dextrose rapidly reverses the clinical effects of hypoglycemia. Hypertonic dextrose solutions are commonly found in syringes containing 50 mL of 50% dextrose in water ($D_{50}W$), which is equivalent to 25 g of dextrose (4 calories per gram of glucose or 100 calories). An average man weighing 70 kg would therefore require 35 to 70 g of dextrose. Administration of hypertonic dextrose is fairly safe, and only a few cases of significant adverse effects such as seizures, hyperosmolar coma, and death have been reported.[17] A much more common effect is phlebitis, which can be mitigated by injection of the dextrose into a large vein followed by a saline flush.[1]

After initial euglycemia is achieved, patients should be given continuous IV infusions of dextrose. Dextrose-water solutions of 5% (D_5W) and 10% ($D_{10}W$) are usually used in this setting, dosage being titrated along with other therapies to maintain euglycemia. For patients with repeated episodes of hypoglycemia, higher concentrations of dextrose and repeated boluses of $D_{50}W$ may be required. In this setting, hypertonic dextrose solutions should be administered via central line access because of their irritant venous effects.

It should be noted that the treatment of overdose with a specific hypoglycemic agent depends the agent. Some hypoglycemic agents, such as the meglitinides, are very short-acting, and the resulting hypoglycemia is unlikely to be prolonged. For longer-acting insulins and the sulfonylureas, intensive therapy may be necessary for 1 or 2 days or even longer. The previously described approach to management is a general guideline to patients with hypoglycemia. Regardless of the etiology of the hypoglycemia, patients should be frequently observed for signs of neuroglycopenia, bedside glucose checks should be performed every 1 to 2 hours at minimum, and serum electrolyte levels should be monitored every 4 hours. Some patients may also require specific antidotal therapy as described later.

Glucagon may also be administered by the subcutaneous, intramuscular, or IV route to stimulate hepatic glycogenolysis. It is most beneficial if given soon after the onset of hypoglycemic coma and to treat hypoglycemia in type 1 DM.[1,17] Glucagon is less effective in patients with type 2 DM because it causes the release of insulin.[18] These patients are also likely to already have depleted glycogen stores, thus limiting the efficacy of glucagon. Furthermore, glucagon administration may cause nausea and vomiting, which impair the ability to give oral carbohydrate therapy. Hypertonic IV dextrose is therefore the preferred initial therapy in the setting of acute hypoglycemia.

In patients with sulfonylurea-induced hypoglycemia, the same supportive measures as previously described are initially implemented. Occasionally, prolonged hypoglycemia may occur after a sulfonylurea overdose, especially with the long-acting agents. Antidotal therapy with octreotide should be considered in such refractory cases. A synthetic somatostatin analogue, octreotide inhibits the secretion of several neuropeptides, including insulin, and is used clinically to suppress excessive growth hormone secretion, inhibit thyrotropin-secreting pituitary adenomas, and treat certain gastrointestinal and pancreatic neuroendocrine tumors (e.g., carcinoid insulinomas).[17]

Previously, the antihypertensive diazoxide was the recommended agent of choice for refractory hypoglycemia due to a sulfonylurea because of its ability to inhibit insulin secretion by opening adenosine triphosphate (ATP)–sensitive potassium (K_{ATP}) channels in pancreatic beta-islet cells.[17] Although the use of octreotide for sulfonylurea-induced hypoglycemia is "off label" (i.e., the agent has not been approved by the U.S. Food and Drug Administration for this purpose), multiple case reports and research document its efficacy and safety. On the contrary, diazoxide has been shown to be less effective and has several undesirable properties.[20] It is usually administered by IV infusion, and its efficacy is limited in these situations because of associated hypotension, tachycardia, nausea, and vomiting. Adverse effects associated with octreotide are minimally significant; they include pain at the injection site, nausea, bloating, flatulence, diarrhea, and constipation. For these reasons, octreotide has supplanted diazoxide as the treatment of choice for sulfonylurea-induced hypoglycemia.

Octreotide has an IV half-life of 72 minutes, but when administered subcutaneously, it appears to be effective for approximately 6 hours.[17] Consequently, a reasonable dosing scheme for most sulfonylurea agents would be 50 μg subcutaneously every 8 to 12 hours (one noted textbook recommends every 8 hours[19]) for at least 24 hours.[20] After the octreotide is discontinued, an observation period for repetition of hypoglycemia is warranted for a minimum of 12 to 24 hours.

Tips and Tricks

- Ill-appearing patients may have sepsis, chronic liver or renal failure, endocrinopathy resulting in deficiencies of cortisol or thyroid hormone, or acute-on-chronic alcohol abuse superimposed on chronic liver disease with or without a state of chronic malnutrition.
- Hypoglycemia should be presumed to be present in *all* patients presenting to the ED with altered mental or psychiatric status, and hypoglycemia should be expeditiously excluded by rapid bedside glucose testing.
- For overdose with longer-acting insulins and the sulfonylureas, intensive therapy may be necessary for 1 or 2 days or even longer.
- Although the use of octreotide for sulfonylurea-induced hypoglycemia is "off label," multiple case reports and research document its efficacy and safety. On the contrary, diazoxide has been shown to be less effective and has several undesirable properties.

Disposition

The decision to admit patients after an episode of hypoglycemia is multifactorial and in all cases depends on the cause. Patients with systemic conditions, such as sepsis, hepatic or renal failure, drug-induced hypoglycemia, hypoglycemia of unknown etiology, and persistent neurologic signs and symptoms, usually require admission. Patients who present with overdoses (unintentional or intentional) of insulin, sulfonylureas, and meglitinides need inpatient observation because of their unpredictable kinetics in this setting. For diabetic patients in whom hypoglycemia develops despite therapeutic dosing and without a history of an overdose, admission depends on the expected duration of effect of the drugs, the severity and recurrence of hypoglycemia, and other possible toxic effects. Because most commonly used sulfonylureas have a duration of effect of at least 24 hours, admission is warranted even for a single episode of hypoglycemia, even though in theory it might be possible to observe these patients closely at home. Discharge is possible for patients with hypoglycemia if the likelihood of recurrence is minimal or the patient has a simple explanation for the episode of hypoglycemia (e.g., a missed meal). In patients who do not require any treatment with glucose, observation for 8 hours may be considered. In all patients with hypoglycemia, it is best for the EP to err on the side of caution and exercise good clinical judgment when deciding on disposition.

REFERENCES

1. Carroll MJ, Burge MR, Schade DS: Severe hypoglycemia in adults. Rev Endocr Metab Disord 2003;4:149-157.
2. The Diabetes Control and Complications Trial Research Group: Hypoglycemia in the Diabetes Control and Complications Trial. Diabetes 1997;46:271-286.
3. Klatt EC, Beatie C, Noguchi TT: Evaluation of death from hypoglycemia. Am J Forensic Med Pathol 1988;9:122-125.
4. Cryer PE, Davis SN, Shamoon H: Hypoglycemia in diabetes. Diabetes Care 2003;26:1902-1912.
5. Salas M, Caro JJ: Are hypoglycaemia and other adverse effects similar among sulphonylureas? Adv Drug React Toxicol Rev 2002;21:205-217.
6. Marks V: Recognition and differential diagnosis of spontaneous hypoglycemia. Clin Endocrinol 1992;37:309-316.
7. Griffiths MJ, Gama R: Adult spontaneous hypoglycemia. Hosp Med 2005;66:277-283.
8. Hepburn DA, MacLeod KM, Pell AC, et al: Frequency and symptoms of hypoglycemia experienced by patients with type 2 diabetes treated with insulin. Diabetic Med 1993;10:231-237.
9. Watson WA, Litovitz TL, Rodgers GC Jr, et al: 2004 Annual report of the American Association of Poison Control Centers Toxic Exposure Surveillance System. Am J Emerg Med. 2005;23:589-666.
10. Stahl M, Berger W: Higher incidence of severe hypoglycemia leading to hospital admission in type 2 diabetic patients treated with long-acting versus short-acting sulphonylureas. Diabet Med 1999;16:586-590.
11. Ciechanowski K, Borowiak KS, Potocka BA, et al: Chlorpropamide toxicity with survival despite 27 day hypoglycemia. J Toxicol Clin Toxicol 1999;37:869-871.
12. Boyd R, Leigh B, Stuart P: Capillary versus venous bedside glucose estimations. Emerg Med J 2005;22:177-179.
13. Kulkarni A, Saxena M, Price G, et al: Analysis of blood glucose measurements using capillary and arterial blood samples in intensive care patients. Intensive Care Med 2005;31:142-145.
14. Boyle PJ, Schwartz NS, Shah SD, et al: Plasma glucose concentrations at the onset of hypoglycemic symptoms in patients with poorly controlled diabetes and in nondiabetics. N Engl J Med 1988;318:1487-1492.
15. Kannisto H, Neuvoven PJ: Adsorption of sulfonylureas onto activated charcoal in vitro. J Pharm Sci 1984;73:253-256.
16. Nuevonen PF, Karkkainen S: Effects of charcoal sodium bicarbonate and ammonium chloride on chlorpropamide kinetics. Clin Pharm Ther 1983;33:386-393.
17. Shah A, Stanhope R, Matthew D: Hazards of pharmacological tests of growth hormone secretion in childhood. Br Med J 1992;304:173-174.
18. Lheureux PE, Zahir S, Penaloza A, et al: Bench-to-bedside review: Antidotal treatment of sulfonylurea-induced hypoglycemia with octreotide. Crit Care 2005;9:543-549.
19. Howland MA: Octreotide. In Goldfrank LR, Flomenbaum NE, Lewin NA, et al (eds): Goldfrank's Toxicologic Emergencies, 7th ed. New York, McGraw-Hill, 2002, pp 611-613.
20. Boyle PJ, Justice K, Krentz AJ, et al: Octreotide reverses hyperinsulinemia and prevents hypoglycemia induced by sulfonylurea overdoses. J Clin Endocrinol Metab 1993;76:752-756.

Chapter 153

Over-the-Counter Medications

Tri Chau Tong

KEY POINTS

Always consider additional acetaminophen and salicylate toxicity when a patient has multiple co-ingestants or has taken combination formulations.

Antihistamine medications antagonize cholinergic and alpha-adrenergic receptors and cause sodium channel blockade and can therefore cause seizures, cardiac dysrhythmias, and hypotension in addition to sedation.

Treatment for antihistamine poisoning is supportive care, but sodium bicarbonate and physostigmine can be helpful adjuncts.

Dextromethorphan poisoning manifests as sedation, movement abnormalities, and psychoactive dysphoria. Most of these effects are mediated by *N*-methyl-D-aspartate (NMDA) rather than opioid receptor activity.

In overdose, poisoning with oral decongestants may manifest as a sympathomimetic toxidrome.

Oxymetazoline (Afrin) and tetrahydrozoline (Visine) can cause significant sedation when ingested orally.

Over-the-counter loperamide (Imodium) is safer than diphenoxylate (Lomotil) for use in treating diarrhea.

Dietary supplements are mostly safe but are unregulated. Common conditions leading to poisoning include mislabeling, variations in concentration, and contamination with unintended agents such as heavy metals.

Hypervitaminosis A can cause increased intracranial pressure with associated symptoms. Treatment is with symptomatic care.

Antihistamines

■ SCOPE

Antihistamines are available throughout the world and most do not require a prescription. They are used for the symptomatic relief of cold and allergy symptoms and are also found in nonprescription sleeping aids. Because of widespread access, they are commonly ingested both intentionally, in suicide attempts, and unintentionally, particularly by children. More than 14,000 cases annually involve children younger than 6 years. Failure to recognize redundant ingredients in multiple combination preparations, overzealous self-treatment, and accidental dosing errors also contribute to the potential dangers of these agents.

PATHOPHYSIOLOGY

All histamine receptor antagonists (antihistamines, histamine H blockers) are reversible competitive inhibitors of histamine receptors. Therapeutically, histamine H_1 receptor blockers inhibit the response of smooth muscle to histamine. The inhibition reduces bronchoconstriction, vasoconstriction, and capillary permeability (the cause of edema and wheal). These agents also inhibit the more rapid vasodilatory effects caused by H_1 receptors on endothelial cells. In overdose, H_1 blockers inhibit additional receptor and ion channels, leading to muscarinic-type cholinergic receptor inhibition, alpha-adrenergic receptor inhibition, and fast sodium channel blockade.

Newer generation H_1 blockers (e.g., loratadine, fexofenadine) are advantageous in their selective binding to peripheral histamine sites. Unlike their first-generation counterparts (e.g., diphenhydramine, hydroxyzine), these newer agents do not cross the blood-brain barrier, resulting in less central nervous system (CNS) and anticholinergic toxicity.

H_2 receptors are primary regulators of gastric acid secretion. H_2 receptor antagonists are relatively benign in overdose, with sedation as the primary reaction. Of the H_2 blockers, only cimetidine is known to inhibit hepatic oxidative metabolism by many cytochrome P-450 enzymes, thereby reducing the clearance of a variety of drugs (Box 153-1).

PRESENTING SIGNS AND SYMPTOMS

With mixed ingestions and with ingestions in elderly or very young patients, physical findings may be variable and the clinical picture unclear. Sedation is the most common adverse effect in therapeutic use and overdose.[1] In severe cases of H_1 antihistamine poisoning, presenting symptoms of delirium and anticholinergic poisoning accompany sedation. This toxidrome is summarized by the classic expression "dry as a bone, red as a beet, hot as a hare, mad as a hatter, and blind as a bat," representing anhydrosis, cutaneous vasodilation, hyperthermia, delirium, and mydriasis, respectively (Fig. 153-1). Peripheral findings do not always accompany central findings. Thus, a confused patient may not always have tachycardia or anhydrosis. Severe clinical manifestations include convulsions and cardiac conduction abnormalities due to blockade of fast sodium channels, and hypotension from peripheral α_1-adrenergic receptor inhibition.

H_2 receptor antagonists (e.g., cimetidine, ranitidine) in either therapeutic usage or overdose amounts do not cause symptoms related to H_1 receptor or cholinergic receptor blockade. Central H_2 receptor blockade can cause CNS neurotransmission alteration and lead to delirium and agitation. Convulsions are rare.

BOX 153-1

Drugs with Decreased Clearance (Prolonged Effect) after Cimetidine Use

- Antibiotics (amoxicillin, metronidazole)
- Antidepressants (amitriptyline, paroxetine)
- Antidiabetics (glyburide, glipizide)
- Antidysrhythmics (digoxin, amiodarone)
- Anticoagulant (warfarin)
- Anticonvulsants (phenytoin, carbamazepine)
- Antiemetics (metoclopramide)
- Antifungals (fluconazole, ketoconazole)
- Aspirin
- Benzodiazepines (diazepam, alprazolam, chlordiazepoxide)
- Beta-blockers (metoprolol, propranolol)
- Calcium channel blockers (diltiazem, nifedipine)
- Immunologic agents (cyclosporine)
- Methylxanthines (theophylline)
- Opioids (meperidine, morphine)

DIFFERENTIAL DIAGNOSIS

Sedation and altered mental status are common findings in overdose, and thus, H_1 blocker poisoning without a clear history or secondary evidence of ingestion (e.g., an empty medicine bottle) can be elusive. Common sedative-hypnotic agents (e.g., benzodiazepines, barbiturates), opioids, and most antidepressants can cause sedation. Anticholinergic poisoning can be observed with tricyclic antidepressants, antipsychotic agents, and even plant poisonings (e.g., Jimsonweed). Sympathomimetic poisoning (e.g., with cocaine, methamphetamine) can mimic the agitation and tachycardia of anticholinergic poisoning.

In all cases of potential poisoning, the EP should consider nontoxic causes of altered mental status. Delirium and hyperthermia can represent anticholinergic poisoning but might also be harbingers of meningitis. Occult head trauma can be secondary to a depressed level of consciousness or the cause of it.

INTERVENTIONS AND PROCEDURES

Lumbar puncture and cerebrospinal fluid analysis are important for patients who have altered mental status and hyperthermia that does not rapidly clear or is not easily explainable unless the patient improves rapidly with observation.

DIAGNOSTIC TESTING

- Bedside blood glucose measurements should be performed early as indicated for altered sensorium.
- Serum electrolyte levels should be measured to rule out metabolic abnormalities in patients who are confused or exhibit evidence of cardiotoxicity.

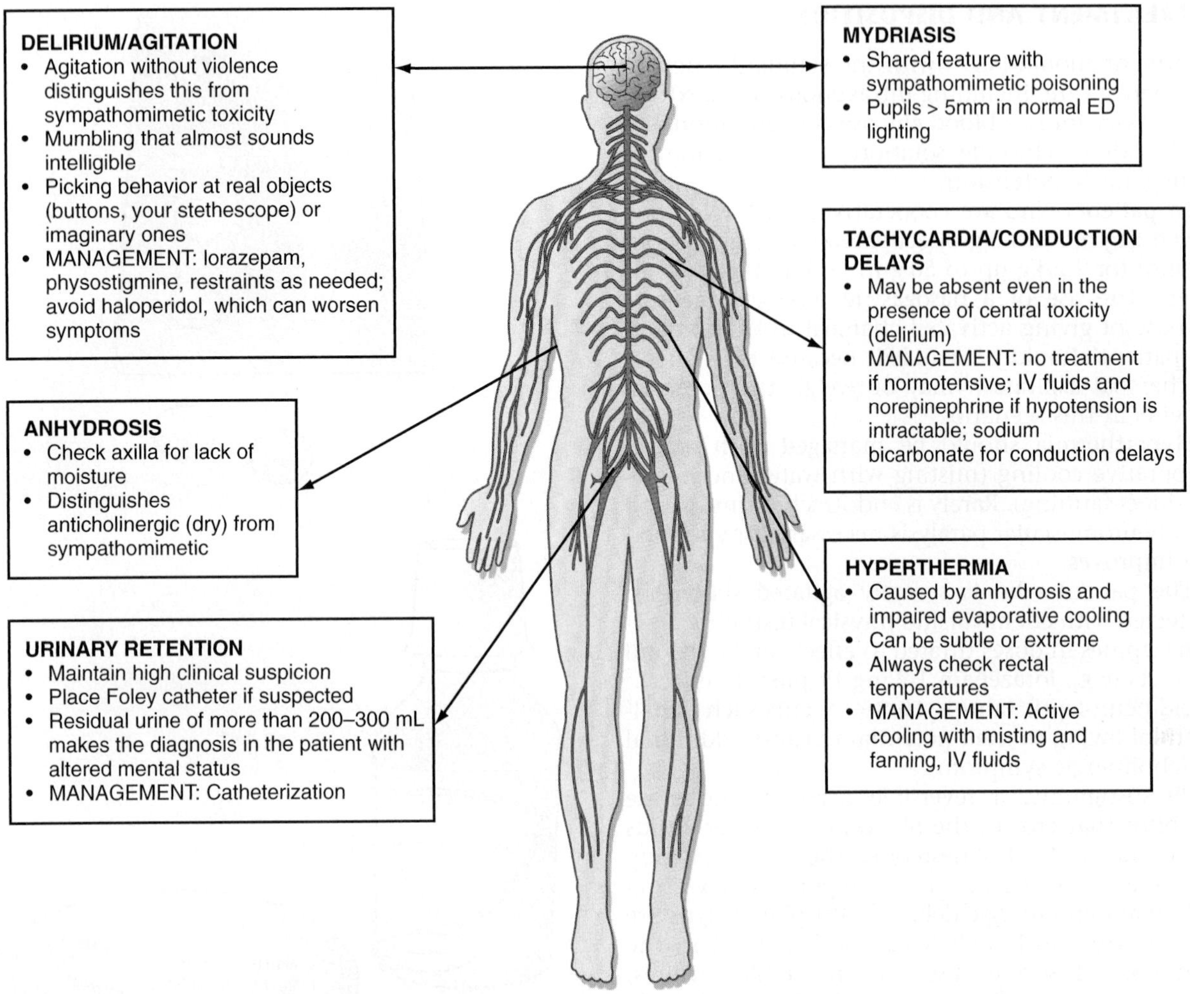
DELIRIUM/AGITATION
• Agitation without violence distinguishes this from sympathomimetic toxicity
• Mumbling that almost sounds intelligible
• Picking behavior at real objects (buttons, your stethescope) or imaginary ones
• MANAGEMENT: lorazepam, physostigmine, restraints as needed; avoid haloperidol, which can worsen symptoms
ANHYDROSIS
• Check axilla for lack of moisture
• Distinguishes anticholinergic (dry) from sympathomimetic
URINARY RETENTION
• Maintain high clinical suspicion
• Place Foley catheter if suspected
• Residual urine of more than 200–300 mL makes the diagnosis in the patient with altered mental status
• MANAGEMENT: Catheterization
MYDRIASIS
• Shared feature with sympathomimetic poisoning
• Pupils > 5mm in normal ED lighting
TACHYCARDIA/CONDUCTION DELAYS
• May be absent even in the presence of central toxicity (delirium)
• MANAGEMENT: no treatment if normotensive; IV fluids and norepinephrine if hypotension is intractable; sodium bicarbonate for conduction delays
HYPERTHERMIA
• Caused by anhydrosis and impaired evaporative cooling
• Can be subtle or extreme
• Always check rectal temperatures
• MANAGEMENT: Active cooling with misting and fanning, IV fluids

FIGURE 153-1 Recognizing the anticholinergic toxidrome.

Table 153-1 OVER-THE-COUNTER MEDICATIONS AND THE URINE IMMUNOASSAY ("URINE DRUG SCREEN")

OTC Medication Trigger	Drug Screen	Positive Screen Result?	Reason
Diphenhydramine (Benadryl)	Tricyclic antidepressants	Occasionally	Similar tricyclic chemical structure
Pseudoephedrine, ephedrine	Amphetamines	Yes	Shared phenylethylamine structure
Loperamide (Imodium), diphenoxylate (Lomotil)	Opiates	No	Different from morphine structure
Dextromethorphan	Opiates	No	Similar structure, but isomeric to codeine analogue
Dextromethorphan	PCP	Yes	Similar ring structure

- Serum salicylate and acetaminophen levels should be measured in all patients with intentional overdose, because many cough and cold preparations combine antihistamines with antipyretics and analgesics.
- An electrocardiogram should be obtained to assess the conduction abnormalities.
- A urine immunoassay (standard urine drug screen) should be performed to screen for exposure to opioids, benzodiazepines, or barbiturates. The EP should recognize, however, that a positive screening test result indicates only *exposure to* and not *active toxicity from* a compound. Qualitative testing for antihistamines is not useful and generally not readily available. Diphenhydramine may test false-positive as tricyclic antidepressants on the urine drug immunoassay (standard urine drug screen) (Table 153-1).

■ TREATMENT AND DISPOSITION

Treatment should begin with the standard tenets of emergency care, including intravenous (IV) dextrose if necessary for low blood glucose concentration and 0.9% sodium chloride solution (normal saline) in boluses for hypotension.

In patients who are cooperative and have a preserved gag reflex, 50 g of activated charcoal without sorbitol (or 1 g/kg up to 50 g in children) should be given. The use of a nasogastric tube for the sole purpose of giving activated charcoal in the combative patient should be avoided, because the dangers of charcoal aspiration may outweigh the potential benefits in this scenario.

Hyperthermia should be managed with active, evaporative cooling (misting with water and applying direct fanning). Rarely is endotracheal intubation with neuromuscular paralysis necessary if hyperthermia improves.

The patient who is severely agitated should be protected with chemical and physical restraints. Benzodiazepines in doses titrated to effect can be helpful adjuncts (e.g., lorazepam 1-2 mg IV push to effect).[2] Avoid neuroleptic (antipsychotic) agents such as haloperidol owing to their potential to cause additional anticholinergic symptoms.

Physostigmine, a reversible acetylcholinesterase inhibitor that crosses the blood-brain barrier, binds to central acetylcholinesterase, thereby increasing available acetylcholine and temporarily reversing central anticholinergic delirium. Peripheral signs are also reversed. Although it can be beneficial in the treatment of severe cases of intractable seizures, supraventricular tachycardias, and delirium, the role of physostigmine in the treatment of most anticholinergic poisonings with minor symptoms is debatable (see Chapter 139 for more details).

Sinus tachycardia from antihistamine poisoning (mostly secondary to anticholinergic effects) does not require pharmacologic treatment in patients with stable blood pressure. Severe cardiac conduction delays should be treated with sodium bicarbonate (1 mEq/kg slow IV push) to overcome impaired sodium conduction. Hypotension secondary to alpha-adrenergic receptor inhibition should be treated with intravenous fluids, and refractory hypotension with direct-acting alpha-agonists (e.g., norepinephrine 2-12 μg/min IV infusion).

Patients with evidence of ongoing cardiovascular or neurologic toxicity should be admitted. Completely asymptomatic patients who have been observed for several hours (4-6) after accidental ingestion may be medically cleared for discharge. Psychiatric evaluation should be obtained when appropriate.

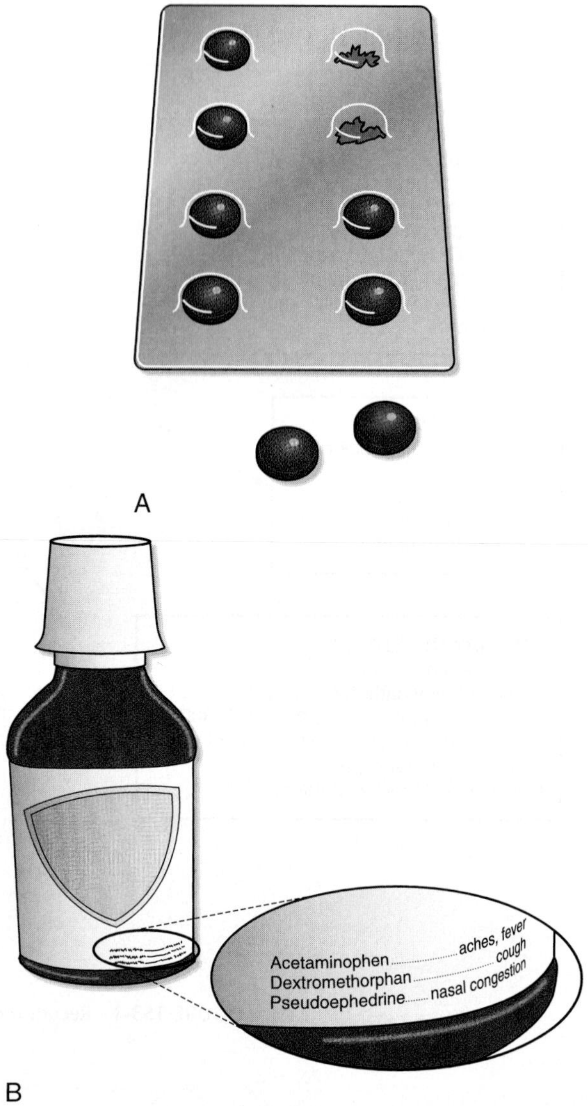
A
Acetaminophen
aches, fever
Dextromethorphan
cough
Pseudoephedrine
nasal congestion
B

FIGURE 153-2 **A**, Dextromethorphan, when combined with the antihistamine chlorpheniramine and marketed as Coricidin, is known popularly as "Skittles" for its candy-like appearance. **B**, Dextromethorphan is often formulated with other decongestants as well.

Antitussives: Dextromethorphan

■ SCOPE

Dextromethorphan was approved by the U.S. Food and Drug Administration (FDA) as an over-the-counter antitussive in response to the rampant abuse of codeine in cough preparations. It remains available without a prescription in cold preparations because of its perceived lack of addictive potential, although there is substantial recreational consumption of dextromethorphan-containing products. Recently, increased abuse of the decongestant preparation Coricidin (known on the streets as "Skittles") has highlighted dextromethorphan's abusive potential (Fig. 153-2). Other commonly used street names are "DXM," "dex," and "roboshots."

■ PATHOPHYSIOLOGY

Dextromethorphan is the structural isomer of the potent opioid analgesic levorphanol, but it is devoid of analgesic properties and its antitussive effects are not mediated through opioid receptors. Dextromethorphan binds to NMDA receptors at the phencyclidine (PCP) site and inhibits normal functioning of this excitatory receptor. Dopaminergic neurotransmission may also be altered. Associated psychoactive effects are attributed to the active metabolite dextrophan rather than to dextromethorphan itself. At very high doses, binding to opioid receptors does occur.

■ PRESENTING SIGNS AND SYMPTOMS

Sedation from NMDA receptor inhibition may be the sole finding in the initial presentation of dextromethorphan toxicity. Specific genetic differences in speed of metabolism to dextrophan govern a patient's disposition toward more sedation from the parent compound or more dysphoria from its metabolite. Contrary to the expectations of its abusers, who seek hallucination and euphoria, dysphoria often predominates. With large overdose, miosis can be present.

Because of altered dopaminergic neurotransmission, involuntary choreoathetoid-like movements may be present. This can accompany a shuffling gait, also referenced as a "robo-walk" in homage to the most common source of dextromethorphan (Robitussin DM) and to the "robotic-like" appearance of the gait. Finally, dextromethorphan may also cause blockade of presynaptic serotonin uptake, which can elicit serotonin syndrome in certain patients taking monoamine oxidase inhibitors. The development of autonomic lability, hyperthermia, and altered mental status suggests this condition.

■ DIFFERENTIAL DIAGNOSIS

Initial approach to patients with altered mental status includes ruling out potential emergency conditions such as trauma, CNS infection, and metabolic derangements. Other common CNS depressants, such as benzodiazepines, opioids, and ethanol, may also cause sedation. Recreational drugs of abuse with similar actions at the NMDA receptor, such as phencyclidine (PCP) and ketamine, may also cause dysphoria and psychoactive features. Anticholinergic poisoning does not result from dextromethorphan poisoning but can occur from combined H_1 antihistamines such as chlorpheniramine (found in Coricidin).

■ DIAGNOSTIC TESTING

Although structurally considered an opioid, dextromethorphan does not trigger the opiate screen on a standard urine immunoassay (see Table 153-1). However, exposure to dextromethorphan may result in a false-positive result for PCP. Thus, all patients with an unexpected positive finding of PCP in a urine immunoassay for drugs of abuse should be questioned about recent dextromethorphan exposure. Finally, dextromethorphan is often formulated as a hydrobromide salt; ingestions of such a formulation this may cause false elevations of chloride on an autoanalyzer test.

The EP should be mindful of potential coingestants, because many cough and cold preparations frequently contain aspirin and acetaminophen.

■ TREATMENT AND DISPOSITION

All cooperative patients should be decontaminated with activated charcoal, then observed and treated for symptomatic improvement. Severe delirium can be controlled with titrated dosages of benzodiazepines (lorazepam 1-2 mg IV, diazepam 5 mg IV, titrated to effect) or physical restraints. Naloxone (1-2 mg IV) should be given for significant sedation.[3] Patients with persistent altered mental status should be admitted.

Decongestants: Pseudoephedrine, Ephedrine, Phenylephrine, Oxymetazoline, and Tetrahydrozoline

■ SCOPE

Decongestants are sympathomimetic agents that act on alpha-adrenergic receptors to produce vasoconstriction and shrink swollen mucous membranes. Ephedrine, extractable from naturally growing herbaceous plants, was used in China for more than 2000 years before its introduction into Western markets. Modern society has seen the unapproved use of these agents to combat obesity and their abuse for stimulatory effects.

■ PATHOPHYSIOLOGY

Decongestants are applied topically or given orally. Pseudoephedrine, ephedrine, and phenylephrine are amphetamine-type oral agents that cause direct presynaptic catecholamine release, block catecholamine reuptake, and influence enzymes slowing catecholamine breakdown. Nasal congestion is reduced through the stimulation of α_1-adrenergic receptor sites on nasal smooth muscle vasculature. The resultant decrease in flow reduces nasal engorgement.

Imidazoline class decongestants are administered topically in the nose and the eyes, where they cause vasoconstriction through α_2-adrenergic stimulation on blood vessels. Common medications of this class are oxymetazoline hydrochloride (Afrin), tetrahydrozoline hydrochloride (Visine), and naphazoline (Clear Eyes, Naphcon). Binding to central imidazoline and α_2-adrenergic receptors generates sympatholytic effects.

■ PRESENTING SIGNS AND SYMPTOMS

After an oral decongestant overdose, patients commonly present with CNS stimulation, hypertension, and tachycardia (although occasionally, reflex bradycardia may develop as a result of pure α_1-adrenergic agonist–induced hypertension). Headache is the most common initial complaint in patients who later have more systemic toxicity. Increases in sinus dysrhythmias can be observed after ingestion of pseudoephedrine. Myocardial infarction and cerebral hemorrhage have been reported with ephedrine use, although vast majority of severe complications were related to phenylpropanolamine, a decongestant no longer available over the counter.

Imidazoline decongestants like oxymetazoline and tetrahydrozoline rarely cause systemic toxicity when taken topically. However, when these agents are ingested, potent peripheral and central α_2-adrenergic receptor stimulation (causing central sympatholytic effects) can lead to hypotension, bradycardia, respiratory depression, and severe CNS depression (as little as 2.5 to 5 mL of Visine has resulted in severe reactions in toddlers; see Chapter 154).[4] Imidazoline decongestants like Visine and Afrin have been implicated as potential date rape–type agents.

■ DIFFERENTIAL DIAGNOSIS

Other co-ingestants should be considered in the assessment for an unclear overdose. Antihistamines from other over-the-counter preparations may also cause significant tachycardia and agitation. Moderate toxicity from other sympathomimetic drugs of abuse such as methamphetamine and cocaine can also manifest as a similar clinical spectrum.

■ DIAGNOSTIC TESTING

For severe decongestant overdose with hyperactivity and agitation, the serum myoglobin level should be measured to assess for rhabdomyolysis. Cardiac creatinine phosphokinase and troponin I levels should also be measured to assess for cardiac ischemia in a patient with complaints of chest pain. An electrocardiogram should be performed to assess tachydysrhythmias.

■ TREATMENT AND DISPOSITION

Overdoses should be treated with typical methods of decontamination, including activated charcoal. Extreme agitation, tachycardia, and hypertension should be treated with benzodiazepines (lorazepam 1-2 mg IV, Valium 5-10 mg IV titrated to effect). For malignant hypertension, an alpha-adrenergic antagonist (e.g., phentolamine 5 mg IV) or a venous and arteriolar vasodilator (e.g., nitroprusside 0.3-10 μg/kg/min IV) should be given. In severe cases of CNS depression after imidazoline-type decongestant overdose, endotracheal intubation should be performed as indicated to support ventilation.

The majority of symptoms from decongestant exposure usually resolve within 8 to 16 hours. Patients with ongoing cardiovascular or neurologic symptoms should be admitted.

Antidiarrheals: Loperamide and Diphenoxylate

■ PATHOPHYSIOLOGY

Loperamide (Imodium) is a synthetic analogue of meperidine. Its systemic absorption is restricted by its insolubility, and only local μ-type opioid receptors in the gastrointestinal tract are affected, resulting in decreased intestinal motility. Diphenoxylate is also a meperidine derivative used for similar antidiarrheal purposes. It is combined in formulation with a small dose of atropine both to increase its antimotility effect and to discourage its abuse as an opioid (this combination is marketed as Lomotil). Diphenoxylate has a significantly worse adverse profile because it metabolizes to difenoxin, a compound with higher potency and longer serum half-life. Although diphenoxylate is not sold over the counter, it is often recommended interchangeably with loperamide.

■ PRESENTING SIGNS AND SYMPTOMS

Severe poisoning follows an opioid toxidrome. There are few reports of significant effects after the use of loperamide. Diphenoxylate use, however, has been associated with severe adverse outcomes. Toxicity can be delayed, prolonged, or recurrent owing to both the opioid effects of diphenoxylate and the anticholinergic effects of the atropine in Lomotil. Severe toxic effects include impairment of gastrointestinal motility, leading to intestinal ileus and profound sedation, particularly in children.[5] Effects in children are more pronounced, and ingestion of one adult dose of Lomotil has been documented to lead to death.

■ DIFFERENTIAL DIAGNOSIS

Manifestations of Lomotil poisoning are related to its opioid and anticholinergic effects. Therefore, unclear presentations of overdose must be evaluated for other potential agents in these drug classes.

■ DIAGNOSTIC TESTING

As a synthetic opioid, neither loperamide nor diphenoxylate reacts on the standard urine immunoassay for opiates. If a positive urine opiate test result occurs, the occult ingestion of other opioids (e.g., hydrocodone, oxycodone) should be considered. Qualitative testing for these agents with gas chromatography or mass spectrometry is neither timely nor useful in the ED.

■ TREATMENT AND DISPOSITION

Loperamide has a high safety profile and has been associated with very few adverse events, even in overdose. Decontamination begins with activated charcoal in the cooperative patient. Delayed decontamination can be useful, given the impairment of gastrointestinal motility with these agents. All patients with Lomotil overdose should be admitted for observation because of the potential for severe but delayed toxic effects. Naloxone (0.4-2 mg IV or subcutaneously every 2-3 min) is effective in reversing opioid toxicity, but recurrence of CNS and respiratory depression is common. Naloxone infusion ($^2/_3$ the initial reversal dose of naloxone per hr IV continuous) should be given if signs of toxicity recur.

Dietary Supplements

■ SCOPE

Any ingredient taken for the purpose of promoting health is considered a *dietary supplement.* Vitamins, minerals, herbs, and amino acids are included in this category. In 1994, the Dietary Supplement and Health Education Act diminished the role of the FDA in the oversight of these products. Unlike with prescription drugs, proof of safety and efficacy are not required for dietary supplements as long as the maker does not claim that they can treat a particular disease. To be removed from the market, a dietary supplement must be proven unsafe.

Severe toxicity from the vast majority of dietary supplements remains uncommon owing to low concentrations of specific agents in marketed products. Toxicity may arise not only from the product itself but also from unlisted active ingredients and from contaminants such as heavy metals.

■ PATHOPHYSIOLOGY; PRESENTING SIGNS AND SYMPTOMS

The term ephedra refers to several alkaloids of the plant genus *Ephedra.* These alkaloids include ephedrine, pseudoephedrine, and methylephedrine and are also known in traditional Chinese medicine as Ma Huang. The toxicity from ephedra alkaloids is similar to that from other sympathomimetic agents and is mediated through direct presynaptic catecholamine release and blockade of catecholamine reuptake.[6] Classic presenting signs and symptoms are related to vasoconstriction with greater chronotropy, mydriasis, headache, and nervousness. In 2004 the FDA banned the sale of ephedra after reports of significant adverse events even at very small doses; this ban was lifted and then upheld by the Federal Appeals Court. Ephedra remains available via the Internet at this time.

Ginkgo, St. John's wort, ginseng, and Echinacea are other top-selling supplements among the myriad available commercially (Table 153-2).

■ DIAGNOSTIC TESTING

Laboratory and diagnostic testing should be ordered according to either the individual clinical presentation or the expected symptoms for a known ingestion. For instance, for an individual who presents with chest tightness after ephedra overdose, cardiac enzymes should be measured to assess for myocardial injury. In most cases, however, the necessary testing should be based on regular clinical indications with an emphasis on screening diagnostics, such as electrocardiogram, cell blood count, serum chemistry profile, liver function tests, and coagulation studies. Additional diagnostic studies, such as computed tomography (CT) of the head and cerebrospinal fluid analysis, should be performed when warranted.

For the suspicion of ephedra overdose, a urine immunoassay screen often detects amphetamines as a class because of the phenylethylamine chemical backbone common to all amphetamines.

Table 153-2 EFFECTS OF TOP-SELLING OVER-THE-COUNTER DIETARY SUPPLEMENTS

Preparation	Scientific Name	Other Common Names	Popular Usage	Traditional or Adverse Effects
Ephedra (toxic or active ingredients: ephedrine, pseudoephedrine)	*Ephedra* spp	Ma-Huang, Mormon tea, yellow horse, desert tea	Stimulant, diet aid, bronchial disorders	Headache, dizziness, palpitations, convulsions, myocardial infarction, cerebral vascular accidents
Ginkgo	*Ginkgo biloba*	Maidenhair tree, Kew tree, Tebonin, tanakan, kaveri	Dementia, asthma, digestive aid, acute mountain sickness	Gastrointestinal distress, headache, skin reaction, allergic reaction, bleeding
St. John's wort	*Hypericum perforatum*	Klamath weed, goatweed, shogren-gyo	Anxiety, depression, gastritis, acquired immunodeficiency syndrome	Photosensitization, decreases levels of CYP 3A4–metabolized drugs (indinavir, oral contraceptives, cycloserine)
Ginseng	*Panax ginseng*	Ren shen	Respiratory illness, gastrointestinal disorders, fatigue, stress, impotence	Ginseng abuse syndrome (hypertension, nervousness, sleepiness, morning diarrhea)
Echinacea	*Echinacea purpurea*	American coneflower, purple coneflower, snakeroot	Infections, immunostimulant	Normally none Rarely: hepatitis, nausea, asthma, anaphylaxis

■ TREATMENT AND DISPOSITION

Dietary supplement exposures pose unique challenges owing to the lack of information about the toxicologic profiles, pharmacokinetics, and concentrations of their active ingredients. The vast majority of cases of toxicity from therapeutic use can be managed with supportive care and symptom-based therapy, appropriate follow-up, and discharge. In acute, intentional overdose, a single dose of activated charcoal should be given. In severe cases of metal poisoning, whole bowel irrigation and, possibly, appropriate chelating agents should be strongly considered.

Symptomatic patients should be admitted for observation and symptomatic therapy. A psychiatric consultation should be obtained when warranted. Patients who are asymptomatic 4 to 6 hours after an acute accidental overdosage of a known agent with known safety profiles can be discharged, with arrangement for follow-up in 48 to 72 hours.

Vitamins

■ SCOPE

Parents' concerns about their children's eating patterns result in routine vitamin over-supplementation.[7] The colorful appearance, fruity smells and flavors, and cartoon shapes of vitamins make these products attractive to children. Adults may take megavitamin therapy in the belief that more is better. All of these factors, added to the ready availability of vitamins, make them prime targets for potential toxic exposures. A wide range of vitamin products are involved in these exposures, including vitamins in pediatric and adult formulations, products with or without iron and/or fluoride, tablet and liquid preparations, and single-ingredient formulations.

■ PATHOPHYSIOLOGY

Vitamin A is transported by a retinol-binding protein to the liver, where it is primarily stored. Hypervitaminosis A occurs when this carrying system or the liver becomes saturated. Free vitamin A binds to lipoprotein membranes, resulting in greater permeability and instability of the cell and consequently to dermatologic and bone malformations. Deposition of excessive vitamin A in liver cells causes hepatotoxicity.[8] Hypervitaminosis A can also increase intracranial pressure by an unknown mechanism.

Acute ingestions of vitamin B_6 (pyridoxine) have few ill effects. Long-term use can produce a sensory neuropathy with as little as 200 mg/day. The exact mechanism of this effect is not known.

Vitamin C (ascorbic acid) is a water-soluble solid whose toxicity with excessive intake is mediated by its metabolism to oxalic acid. The results are excessive oxalate excretion and nephrolithiasis. Vitamin C has also been associated with hemolysis in patients with glucose-6-phosphate dehydrogenase deficiency through an un-elucidated mechanism.

Vitamin D is synthesized from a combination of cholesterol and exposure to sunlight. It is rare for toxicity to occur from acute ingestion; more likely, toxicity occurs from long-term over-supplementation. Ingestions of more than 2000 IU/day of vitamin D promote calcium absorption and mobilization from bone, leading to hypercalcemia.

■ PRESENTING SIGNS AND SYMPTOMS

The most serious effect of acute vitamin A ingestion is increased intracranial pressure. The patient should be evaluated for signs of headache, vomiting, lethargy, or anorexia. Long-term use of high doses of vitamin A may lead to alopecia, skin desquamation, pruritus, photophobia, and headache.

In long-term vitamin B_6 ingestion, sensory neuropathies are the primary manifestations of toxicity. Decrease or absence of deep tendon reflexes, poor muscle coordination, and decreased sensation to touch, pain, and temperature highlight the clinical findings. Muscular strength is preserved.

Large vitamin C ingestions may result in gastrointestinal symptoms with nausea and vomiting. Rarely, clinically significant nephrolithiasis, acute renal failure, hemolysis, anemia, and hemoglobinuria occur.

The toxicity of hypervitaminosis D reflects symptoms of general hypercalcemia. Gastrointestinal upset and headache are common, as are irritability, weakness, hypertension, renal tubular injury, and, occasionally, cardiac dysrhythmias.

■ DIFFERENTIAL DIAGNOSIS

Because of the relative infrequency of severe toxicity from hypervitaminosis, the more common causes of sensory neuropathies, increased intracranial pressure, and hypercalcemia must be explored first.

■ DIAGNOSTIC TESTING

The diagnosis of vitamin overdose is most often made from a history of ingestion. Because many vitamin preparations contain iron or fluoride, it is imperative that these agents be considered and evaluated as possible co-ingestants.

Plasma vitamin measurements, particularly for vitamin A, are available but not are useful in directing treatment or determining prognosis. In patients with hypervitaminosis A, elevations of aminotransferase, alkaline phosphatase, and bilirubin concentrations as well as of International Normalized Ratio values are indicators of hepatic toxicity. Computed tomography of the head or a lumbar puncture with measurement of the opening pressure should

Table 153-3 VITAMIN OVERDOSE RECOGNITION AND TREATMENT

Vitamin	Toxicity	Symptoms	Treatment
A	Deposits in liver cause hepatotoxicity Increased intracranial pressure	Headache, vomiting, lethargy, or anorexia Alopecia, desquamation, pruritus, photophobia	Rarely: mannitol, steroids, or hyperventilation for increased intracranial pressure
B_6 (pyridoxine)	Few ill effects Long-term use can produce sensory neuropathy	Decrease or absence of deep tendon reflexes, poor muscle coordination, and decreased sensation to touch, pain, and temperature	None needed
C (ascorbic acid)	Nephrolithiasis from oxalate excretion Hemolysis in patients with glucose-6-phosphate dehydrogenase deficiency	Nausea and vomiting, nephrolithiasis, hematuria, anemia	Treat symptoms with antiemetics, pain medications; stop vitamin C ingestion
D	Calcium mobilization from bone and hypercalcemia	Gastrointestinal upset, headache, irritability, weakness, hypertension, renal tubular injury, cardiac dysrhythmias	Check renal function; stop vitamin D ingestion; treat severe hypercalcemia with fluids and diuretics

be performed to confirm increased intracranial pressure.

With vitamin D oversupplementation, measurements of calcium and phosphate levels, blood urea nitrogen, and serum creatinine should be performed to rule out hypercalciuria-related renal injury.

Tips and Tricks

- Neuroleptic (antipsychotic) agents such as haloperidol should be avoided in antihistamine overdoses because of the agents' potential to cause additional anticholinergic symptoms.
- Many vitamin preparations contain iron or fluoride, so it is imperative that these agents be considered and evaluated as possible co-ingestants.
- In patients with mixed ingestion, elderly patients, or very young patients, physical findings may be variable and the clinical picture unclear.
- Peripheral findings do not always accompany central findings in antihistamine overdose; therefore, a confused patient may not always have tachycardia or anhydrosis.
- In all cases of potential poisoning, nontoxic causes of altered mental status should also be considered.
- With dextromethorphan ingestions, genetic differences in speed of metabolism of the drug to dextrophan can result in either more sedation or more dysphoria.

■ TREATMENT AND DISPOSITION

The mainstay of treatment consists of elimination of exposure and symptomatic therapy. In the vast majority of cases, improvement occurs with the cessation of exposure. Antiemetics should be given for nausea and vomiting in acute ingestions. Increased intracranial pressure from hypervitaminosis A generally resolves with discontinuation of its ingestion; only rarely is mannitol, corticosteroids, or hyperventilation required (Table 153-3).

REFERENCES

1. Koppel C, Ibe K, Tenczer J: Clinical symptomatology of diphenhydramine overdose: An evaluation of 136 cases, 1982-1985. J Tox Clin Toxicol 1987;25:53-70.
2. Burns MJ, Linden CH, Graudins A, et al: A comparison of physostigmine and benzodiazepines for the treatment of anticholinergic poisoning. Ann Emerg Med 2000;35: 374-381.
3. Shaul WL, Wandell M, Robertson WO: Dextromethorphan toxicity: Reversal by naloxone. Pediatrics 1977;59:117-118.
4. Higgins GL, Campbell B, Wallace K, et al: Pediatric poisoning from over-the-counter imidazoline-containing products. Ann Emerg Med 1991;20:6555-6658.
5. Rumack B, Temple A: Lomotil poisoning. Pediatrics 1974;52: 495-500.
6. Haller C, Benowitz NL: Adverse cardiovascular and central nervous system events associated with dietary supplements containing ephedra alkaloids. N Engl J Med 2000;343: 1833-1838.
7. Herbert V: The vitamin craze. Arch Intern Med 1980;140: 173-176.
8. Hatoff DE, Gertler SL, Miyai K, et al: Hypervitaminosis A unmasked by acute viral hepatitis. Gastroenterology 1982;82:124-248.

Chapter 154

Pediatric Overdoses

Jennifer E. McCain and Erica L. Liebelt

KEY POINTS

Young children (primarily less than 6 years of age) experience the majority of unintentional poisoning exposures and are also more susceptible to the toxicity.
Many over-the-counter medications, household substances, and prescription medications can cause toxicity in young children when ingested in small amounts—1 to 2 pills or 1 to 2 teaspoons.
Antidotal therapies for selective pediatric exposures resulting in clinical toxicities are the same as for adult exposures except for specific dosages of drugs.
Salicylate blood concentration should be measured earlier for methylsalicylate ingestions—within 1 hour—than for salicylate pill ingestion—2 to 4 hours.
With the potential of a caustic ingestion, the absence of burns in the mouth and oropharynx does not predict the absence of burns in the esophagus and stomach.

Scope

The peak incidence for exposures to potentially toxic substances in children occurs in those younger than 6 years, accounting for the majority of exposures (53%) in the United States. These are unintentional ingestions and result primarily from the children's developmental stage with hand to mouth behaviors. Fortunately, most of these ingestions are nontoxic or result in only mild sequelae, because the intent is exploration rather than self-harm. Cosmetics, personal care products, and plant exposures are the predominant ingested substances because they are readily available in the home.

The "one-pill" rule states that a single adult therapeutic dose would not be expected to produce significant toxicity in a child. This rule suggests that the ingestion of 1 or 2 tablets by a toddler is a benign act.[1] This may be true for most exposures, but some common agents have the potential to cause life-threatening toxicity or death despite the ingestion of only one or two tablets or sips. It is important for the EP to be aware of the substances that are toxic or occasionally lethal in very small amounts. In this chapter, we review the sources, pathophysiology, clinical presentation, diagnosis, and treatment for ingestions of the common medications and substances that have the potential for significant morbidity and mortality at small doses in young children.

Over-the-Counter Medications

(Table 154-1)

■ BENZOCAINE

■ Sources

Benzocaine is a local anesthetic that can cause methemoglobinemia, a specific dyshemoglobinemia that reduces oxygen delivery to the tissues. There are many sources of benzocaine, including teething gels,

Table 154-1 TOXICITY DOSES FOR COMMON OVER-THE-COUNTER MEDICATIONS

Product	Toxicity Dose and Example
Benzocaine	As little as ½ teaspoon or 2.5 mL of 10 % benzocaine has been reported to cause significant methemoglobinemia
Camphor	Clinically significant camphor toxicity has not been reported with ingestion of less than 30 mg/kg or 500 mg and is uncommon when less than 50 mg/kg of camphor is ingested: • 2-3 teaspoons of Vick's VapoRub (4.7% camphor) has central nervous system effects
Methylsalicylate	>150 mg/kg; ingestions of as little as 4 mL of methylsalicylate in a child have been fatal: • 1-oz tube of liniment containing 20% methyl salicylate would provide a fatal dose • 10 mL of oil of wintergreen (98% methylsalicylate) has caused death in a toddler (10 mL=44 adult aspirin)
Caustic agents	Toxicity dose varies by product; consult poison control center
Hydrofluoric acid	>50 mg fluoride and as little as 5 mL of 10% hydrofluoric acid solution can be lethal to a 10-kg child
Hydrocarbons	Aspiration risk is greatest for hydrocarbons with low viscosity and low surface tension

Table 154-2 COMMON OVER-THE-COUNTER PRODUCTS CONTAINING BENZOCAINE

Product	Benzocaine Content (%)
Baby Orajel	7.5
Baby Orajel Nighttime Formula	10.0
Baby Anbesol Gel	7.5
Anbesol Regular Strength	6.3
Anbesol Maximum Strength	20.0
Lanacane Spray	20.0
Americaine Topical Anesthetic First Aid Ointment	20.0
Vagisil Creme	20.0

Table 154-3 CLINICAL SYMPTOMS AND SEVERITY OF METHEMOGLOBINEMIA

Clinical Symptoms	Severity of Methemoglobinemia (%)
Cyanosis, chocolate brown blood, patient usually asymptomatic	15-20
Headache, dizziness, lethargy, syncope, dyspnea	20-45
Central nervous system depression	45-55
Coma, seizures, arrhythmias, shock	55-70
Death	>70

hemorrhoid creams, vaginal creams, first aid ointments, mouth rinses, and throat lozenges (Table 154-2). In February 2007 the U.S. Food and Drug Administration (FDA) sent out a Public Health Advisory warning of the dangers of topical anesthetic creams and gels containing benzocaine and the risk of methemoglobinemia.[2] Benzocaine is also found in Hurricaine and Cetacaine sprays, which are used to anesthetize the posterior oropharynx for insertion of nasogastric and orogastric tubes, endoscopy tubes, and transesophageal echocardiography probes.

■ Dose Causing Significant Toxicity

As little as ½ teaspoon or 2.5 mL of 10 % benzocaine has been reported to cause significant methemoglobinemia in a toddler.

■ Pathophysiology

Benzocaine is metabolized to methemoglobin-forming compounds (e.g., aniline). Methemoglobinemia results through oxidation of circulating hemoglobin from the ferrous form (Fe^{2+}) to the ferric form (Fe^{3+}). The process may be especially worse in infants younger than 4 months because they have a relative deficiency of methemoglobin reductase, one of the significant natural reduction pathways.

■ Clinical Presentation

Signs and symptoms of methemoglobinemia correlate somewhat with the percentage of methemoglobin in the blood (Table 154-3).

■ Diagnosis

Methemoglobin (MetHgb) percentage must be measured on a co-oximeter. The arterial blood is described characteristically as dark chocolate brown. The arterial blood gas values may be normal (falsely elevated calculated oxygen saturation) with a normal arterial partial pressure of oxygen. Oxygen saturation measured on a pulse oximeter is not helpful because this device does not measure the wavelength of MetHgb.

■ Treatment

Methylene blue is the specific antidote for benzocaine, increasing the conversion of methemoglobin

Table 154-4 COMMON CAMPHOR-CONTAINING PRODUCTS

Product	Camphor Content (%)
Camphorated oil	20.0
Campho-Phenique	10.8
Camphor spirits	10.0
Ben-Gay Children's Rub	5.0
Vicks VapoRub	4.81
Soltice Quick Rub (Children's)	3.75
Heet	3.60
Sloan's Liniment	3.35

to hemoglobin by reducing the oxidized hemoglobin. The dose is 1 to 2 mg/kg per dose (or 0.1-0.2 mL/kg of a 1% solution). Methylene blue should be administered if the MetHgb value is greater than 30% or if serious clinical toxicity is present. Gastrointestinal decontamination with charcoal is usually not necessary because the gels or lotions containing benzocaine are usually rapidly absorbed.[3] If the patient is asymptomatic or if the MetHgb value is less than 15%, the patient should be observed for 6 hours and then discharged. If discharged, the patient should follow up within 24 hours for any shortness of breath, increasing fatigue, or chest pain.

CAMPHOR

Sources

Camphor is used in topical liniments and in preparations designed to be applied externally for relief of muscle and joint aches. These topical rubefacients cause local hyperemia and warmth and are marketed as analgesics, antipruritics, and antitussives. In the past, camphor was also a primary constituent of mothballs (Table 154-4).

The FDA has banned all compounds containing camphor in concentrations higher than 11%. In some households, however, there may still be camphorated oil and camphor mothballs.

Dose Causing Significant Toxicity

A dose of 100 mg/kg of camphor in a toddler can result in death; 2 to 3 teaspoons of Vicks VapoRub (4.7% camphor) can have central nervous system (CNS) effects; 2 teaspoons of Campho-Phenique (10.8%) can cause symptoms. Clinically significant camphor toxicity has not been reported with ingestion of less than 30 mg/kg or 500 mg and is uncommon when less than 50 mg/kg of camphor is ingested. Acute camphor poisoning secondary to tasting or unintentional ingestion of small amounts—less than 1 teaspoon—is unlikely.

Pathophysiology

The exact mechanism by which camphor produces toxicity is unknown. The cyclic ketone of the hydroaromatic terpene group is hypothesized to be a neurotoxin.

Clinical Presentation

Clinical toxicity usually begins with generalized feelings of warmth followed by oral or epigastric burning, nausea, and vomiting. The onset of oral burning may occur within 5 to 15 minutes after ingestion. Symptoms may then progress rapidly to CNS effects (headache, confusion, vertigo, restlessness, seizure, delirium, and coma). CNS stimulation is exhibited first by hyperactivity followed quickly by depression. Death may result from respiratory failure or status epilepticus.

Diagnosis

There may be a characteristic odor on the breath. No specific tests are available to detect camphor ingestion.

Management

There is no specific therapy. If more than 30 mg/kg (or 500 mg) has been ingested, only observation and treatment of symptoms are needed. Administration of activated charcoal is not necessary because of the rapid absorption of camphor and the propensity for seizures. If asymptomatic at 4 hours, the patient may be discharged. Seizures should initially be treated with benzodiazepines. Phenobarbital should be used for recurrent or prolonged seizures. The patient who is asymptomatic or has ingested less than 30 mg/kg can be observed for 4 hours and then discharged if no symptoms develop.[4]

METHYLSALICYLATES

Sources

Methylsalicylates are concentrated forms of salicylates found in over-the-counter topical liniments, lotions, and oil of wintergreen (which is used both as a liniment and a food-flavoring additive). Examples are Pepto-Bismol, oil of wintergreen (98% methylsalicylate [1 tsp = 22 adult-strength [325-mg] aspirin]), Ben Gay Lotion (15%), Ben Gay Ointment (18%), Extra-Strength Arthritis Rub (30%), and Icy Hot Balm (29%).

Dose Causing Significant Toxicity

A dose greater than 150 mg/kg causes significant toxicity, and ingestions of as little as 4 mL of methylsalicylate in a child have been fatal. A 1-ounce tube of liniment containing 20% methyl salicylate would provide a fatal dose; 10 mL of oil of wintergreen has caused death in a toddler.

■ Pathophysiology

The pathophysiology for methylsalicylate is identical to that of the other salicylates. It uncouples oxidative phosphorylation and interrupts glucose and fatty acid metabolism, contributing to a metabolic acidosis (see Chapter 138 for further detail about pathophysiology, presentation, and treatment).

■ Clinical Presentation

The signs and symptoms of methylsalicylate poisoning are identical to those observed with poisoning by other salicylates except that they occur more rapidly (15-30 min). Acute intoxication manifests as vomiting, hyperpnea, tinnitus, and a mixed respiratory alkalosis and metabolic acidosis. Lethargy, confusion, seizures, and coma may ensue if the ingestion is severe.

■ Diagnosis

Salicylate blood concentration should be obtained earlier in methylsalicylate ingestions—within 1 hour, versus 2 to 4 hours for salicylate pill ingestion.

■ Treatment

Administration of activated charcoal in addition to urine and serum alkalinization and hemodialysis should be initiated, depending on clinical symptoms, salicylate concentration, and evidence of organ toxicity. If the patient is asymptomatic, the blood salicylate level should be measured at 1 hour; if the result is less than 20 mg/dL, the patient may be observed for 3 hours and then discharged home.[3]

Household Items

■ CAUSTICS

■ Sources

Many household products are caustic agents and can cause significant toxicity with small exposures. Caustic agents are classified as alkaline or acid corrosives depending on their pH (Table 154-5). In 1970 the Federal Hazardous Substances Act and Poison Prevention Packaging Act was passed, stating that caustic agents with a concentration higher than 10% must be placed in child-resistant containers. By 1973, the household product concentration limit for child-resistant packaging was lowered to 2%.

Table 154-5 HOUSEHOLD CAUSTIC AGENTS

Product	Caustic Ingredient(s)
Alkaline Corrosives	
Drain cleaners	Sodium hydroxide (lye)
Oven cleaners	Sodium hydroxide
Hair and permanent relaxers	Sodium hydroxide
Clinitest tablets	Sodium hydroxide
Automatic dishwasher detergents	Sodium tripolyphosphate Sodium metasilicate
Household ammonia cleaning solutions (glass cleaners, anti-rust products, floor strippers, toilet bowl cleaners, wax removers)	Ammonium hydroxide
Acidic Corrosives	
Drain cleaners	Sulfuric acid
Rust removers	Hydrofluoric acid Oxalic acid
Toilet bowl cleaners	Hydrochloric acid Sulfuric acid Phosphoric acid
Gun bluing agent	Selenious acid
Tire cleaning agent	Ammonium bifluoride

■ Dose Causing Significant Toxicity

The dose of a caustic agent causing significant toxicity varies by product and concentration. Information for specific agents can be obtained from a poison control center.

■ Pathophysiology

Alkaline corrosives cause liquefaction necrosis, which is characterized by protein dissolution, collagen destruction, fat saponification, cell membrane emulsification, and cell death. Damage continues after exposure because of the ability of corrosives to penetrate tissue. In contrast, acids cause coagulation necrosis, which leads to a desiccation of epithelial cells and produces an eschar, leading to edema, erythema, mucosal sloughing, ulceration, and necrosis of the tissues.

■ Clinical Presentation

Contact of caustic substances with mucosa causes immediate severe pain, usually limiting unintentional ingestions of large amounts. However, even a swallowed mouthful of a concentrated caustic substance could cause permanent injury. Severe pain of the lips, mouth, throat, chest, or abdomen may develop. Oropharyngeal edema and burns may lead to drooling and rapid airway compromise. Severity and rapidity of symptom development are limited by the type of agent, concentration, volume, viscosity, duration of contact, and pH.

■ Diagnosis

Depending on the substance ingested and the clinical presentation, chest and abdominal radiographs may be needed to evaluate for free air. Endoscopy should be performed within 12 hours and generally not later than 24 hours after ingestion to assess for the extent and severity of burns.

Treatment

Early intubation should be initiated for any patient with any symptom of airway compromise. Gastric lavage should not be performed, and activated charcoal should not be administered. Copious irrigation of the eyes and skin are indicated for dermal and eye exposures. Indications for endoscopy include vomiting, drooling, stridor, and dyspnea. The absence of burns in the mouth and oropharynx does not predict the absence of burns in the esophagus and stomach. The EP can consider observing the totally asymptomatic patient for 4 to 6 hours to ensure that he or she is able to take fluids orally without pain (see Chapter 189 for further details).

HYDROFLUORIC ACID

Sources

Hydrofluoric acid, a toxic agent found in many household products, can be toxic to children in very small amounts. Sources include rust removers, automobile wheel cleaners, toilet bowl cleaners, air conditioner coil cleaners, dentifrices, and insecticides.

Dose Causing Significant Toxicity

Exposure to more than 50 mg of fluoride and as little as 5 mL of 10% hydrofluoric acid solution can be lethal to a 10-kg child.

Pathophysiology

Because it is a weak acid, brief dermal exposure to hydrofluoric acid does not cause clinically apparent burns but may burn mucous membranes. The fluoride ion is highly toxic. It complexes with calcium and magnesium, and the complex then precipitates in tissues, causing tissue destruction and significant pain.

Clinical Presentation

Local injury may be minimal. A hallmark sign of dermal exposure to low concentrations of hydrofluoric acid is pain out of proportion to physical findings. Gastrointestinal symptoms are most common and include nausea, vomiting, and abdominal pain. After inhalation of low concentrations of hydrofluoric acid, acute respiratory distress syndrome may be noted. Ventricular arrhythmias resulting from hypocalcemia may occur suddenly and include ventricular fibrillation and torsades de pointes. Cardiac toxicity generally occurs within 6 hours. Nervous system manifestations include lethargy, obtundation, weakness, and loss of deep tendon reflexes. Onset of symptoms may occur immediately with pain from mucous membrane irritation. However, many patients have few effects early and then quickly progress to significant deterioration.

Diagnosis

Serum electrolyte levels should be measured to monitor for hypocalcemia, hypomagnesemia, and hyperkalemia from significant ingestions and dermal exposures. Electrocardiography should be performed to evaluate for prolonged QTc interval.

Treatment

Early intubation is necessary for any symptoms of airway compromise. Milk or milk of magnesia have been suggested to neutralize the acid for significant ingestions. For the asymptomatic patient, observation for at least 6 hours is warranted. For significant dermal exposures, topical use of calcium gluconate gel (in water-based jelly) can be very effective if applied immediately. Injection of calcium gluconate or arterial calcium gluconate may be needed for significant hand exposures (see Chapter 189).[5]

HOUSEHOLD HYDROCARBONS

Sources

Hydrocarbons are widely used as solvents, degreasers, fuels, and lubricants. Household hydrocarbons are aliphatic (or straight-carbon-chain hydrocarbons) and simple petroleum distillates such as gasoline, kerosene, lighter fluid, furniture polish, and lamp oil. They are poorly absorbed from the gastrointestinal tract and do not pose a significant risk of systemic toxicity after ingestion as long as they are not aspirated. Unintentional ingestions of these products occur frequently because they commonly are left around in the house with caps open or are transferred into "child-familiar" containers such as glass jars and soda bottles.

Dose Causing Significant Toxicity

The dose of a hydrocarbon causing significant toxicity varies according to the amount of and the specific hydrocarbon aspirated. Even a small amount of a low-viscosity aliphatic hydrocarbon may cause significant pulmonary toxicity. Aspiration risk is greatest for hydrocarbons with low viscosity and low surface tension (e.g., petroleum naphtha, mineral seal oil, kerosene, and turpentine).

Pathophysiology

Chemical pneumonitis is caused by direct tissue damage and destruction of surfactant in the alveoli and distal airways, leading to early airway closure, atelectasis, and pulmonary edema with subsequent ventilation-perfusion mismatching and hypoxia. Alveolitis occurs soon after aspiration, culminating in a chemical pneumonitis with frank necrosis of bronchial, bronchiolar, and alveolar tissues. If death does not ensue, these lesions usually heal over 3 to 8 days. Household hydrocarbons are aliphatic hydrocarbons and have little systemic effects.

■ Clinical Presentation

Initially, cough is due to local irritation and is very common but soon subsides. However, prolonged cough, gasping, or choking usually indicates aspiration. Mild physical examination abnormalities consist of coughing and tachypnea. Moderate signs, consist of grunting respirations, tachypnea, retractions, rales, wheezing, and hypoxemia that can worsen progressively over the course of 6 to 12 hours. When aspiration occurs, symptoms of respiratory distress usually, although not always, appear within 30 minutes of exposure and almost always within 2 to 6 hours. In symptomatic individuals, signs and symptoms progress over 24 hours, reach a plateau, and subside over 2 to 8 days.

■ Diagnosis

Diagnosis is based on a history of exposure and the presence of respiratory symptoms. If respiratory symptoms are not present within 6 hours of exposures, it is unlikely that chemical pneumonitis will occur. Chest radiograph and pulse oximetry may assist in the diagnosis, although chest radiographic findings may not appear for more than 6 hours.

■ Treatment

Basic supportive care, including oxygen and early intubation for respiratory failure, should be provided. There is no indication for gastric decontamination using either gastric lavage or activated charcoal. Corticosteroids and prophylactic antibiotics are of no proven value for chemical pneumonitis. Patient who remain completely asymptomatic for 4 to 6 hours may be discharged home.

Prescription Medications (Table 154-6)

■ CLONIDINE AND OTHER IMIDAZOLINES

■ Sources

Clonidine is an imidazoline used for the treatment of hypertension, opioid withdrawal, and attention deficit–hyperactivity disorder in children. It is available in a pill or patch form. Other imidazolines are over-the counter decongestants for the nose and eyes, such as oxymetazoline (Afrin), naphazoline (Clear Eyes), xylometazoline (Otrivin) and, tetrahydrozoline (Visine), as well as prescription medications for glaucoma, such as brimonidine and apraclonidine.

■ Dose Causing Significant Toxicity

As little as 1 clonidine tablet (0.1 mg) has produced a toxic effect in a toddler (0.3-mg dose in 21-month-old caused bradycardia, hypotension, and coma). Also, 2.5 to 5 mL of 0.05% tetrahydrozoline (Visine) has been reported to cause drowsiness, hypotension, and shock in toddlers.

■ Pathophysiology

The imidazolines are central α_2-adrenergic agonists and decrease sympathetic outflow. Clonidine, oxymetazoline, and tetrahydrozoline may also stimulate peripheral α_1-adrenergic receptors, resulting initially in vasoconstriction and transient hypertension.

■ Clinical Presentation

The clinical presentation of clonidine toxicity may appear similar to an opioid toxidrome, consisting of lethargy to coma, miosis, bradycardia, hypotension, hypothermia, decreased muscle tone, and respiratory depression. However, unlike opioid toxicity, clonidine toxicity may cause a transient period of hypertension prior to the hypotension and bradycardia, and the coma is stimulus-responsive. Symptoms usually appear in 30 to 90 minutes, and may last for 1 to 3 days, depending on the dose ingested.

■ Diagnosis

Poisoning should be suspected from the presentation of the clinical toxidrome. Clonidine and other imidazolines are not detected by screening or comprehensive urine toxicology testing.

■ Treatment

Patients with clonidine toxicity usually recover within 24 hours with supportive care. Symptomatic and hemodynamically significant bradycardia may be treated with atropine, but this treatment is rarely needed. Hypotension should be treated with fluids and dopamine. Naloxone usually does not improve CNS depression to a clinically significant degree. The risk of administering activated charcoal to a child with altered mental status, especially for 1- or 2-pill ingestions, is probably greater than the benefits received and should be considered carefully. Over-the-counter liquid imidazoline preparations are absorbed so rapidly from the stomach that there is little role for gastric decontamination.[6]

Table 154-6 DRUGS THAT CAN BE FATAL WITH ONE OR TWO DOSES

Drug	Potential Fatal Exposure	Major Toxic Effect	Treatment/Antidote(s)
Beta-blocker (propranolol)	1-2 tablets	Seizures, hypotension, bradycardia, hypotension	Glucagon Epinephrine[9]
Bupropion	1-2 tablets	Seizures, central nervous system (CNS) depression	Benzodiazepines Supportive care
Calcium channel antagonists (verapamil)	1-2 tablets	Bradycardia, hypotension	Calcium Glucagon Hyperinsulinemia/euglycemia[8]
Chloroquine	1 tablet	Seizures, arrhythmias	Epinephrine with high-dose diazepam Sodium bicarbonate (wide-complex arrhythmias)
Cyclic antidepressants	1-2 tablets	Seizures, arrhythmias, hypotension	Sodium bicarbonate Hypertonic saline
Methadone	1 tsp (10 mg/1 mL)	CNS depression, respiratory depression	Naloxone Supportive care
Phenothiazines (chlorpromazine)	1 tablet	Seizures, ventricular arrhythmias, CNS depression	Diphenhydramine Sodium bicarbonate (wide-complex arrhythmias) Supportive care
Quinidine	2 tablets	Seizures, ventricular arrhythmias, hypotension, CNS depression	Epinephrine with high-dose diazepam Sodium bicarbonate (wide complex arrhythmias)
Quinine	2-3 tablets	Seizures, ventricular arrhythmias, visual disturbances, cinchonism	Epinephrine with high-dose diazepam Sodium bicarbonate (wide-complex arrhythmias)

Data from Bar-Oz B, Levichek Z, Koren G: Medications that can be fatal for a toddler with one tablet or teaspoonful: A 2004 update. Paediatr Drugs 2004;6:123-126.

■ DIPHENOXYLATE WITH ATROPINE

■ Sources

Very small ingestions of diphenoxylate in a formulation with atropine (Lomotil) can be serious in small children. This agent is often prescribed for the relief of diarrhea symptoms. It is a unique opiate-anticholinergic combination; each tablet or 5 mL of liquid has 2.5 mg diphenoxylate and 0.025 mg atropine.

■ Dose Causing Significant Toxicity

The lowest toxic doses reported to be associated with signs and symptoms of opioid/atropine poisoning in children are ½ to 2 tablets. The lowest fatal dose is reportedly 1.2 mg/kg.

■ Pathophysiology

Diphenoxylate is an opiate, and atropine has anticholinergic properties. Lomotil prolongs the transit time of intestinal contents through its action on the smooth muscle of the gut. Diphenoxylate is metabolized to difenoxin, which is approximately five times more active than the parent compound and has an elimination half-life of 12 to 14 hours, leading to prolonged symptoms.

■ Clinical Presentation

Lomotil intoxication is classically described as having a biphasic onset of clinical symptoms. The first phase, attributed to atropine, lasts from 2 to 3 hours and is characterized by the anticholinergic toxidrome. The second or opioid phase, attributed to the diphenoxylate, is characterized by CNS and respiratory depression. However this classic pattern has been challenged by further reports; some patients have had only opioid symptoms, primarily coma and respiratory depression, which may be prolonged up to 30 hours because of delayed gastrointestinal motility. Recurrence of respiratory and CNS depression 12 to 24 hours after the ingestion may occur, presumably from an accumulation of the active long-acting opioid metabolite of diphenoxylate. Thus, the initial clinical manifestations of this overdose in children may be confusing until recognizable atropine or diphenoxylate effects occur. The onset of symptoms may be as early as 2 hours or as late as 24 to 30 hours after ingestion.

■ Diagnosis

Diagnosis of Lomotil toxicity is made from history and clinical presentation.

Management

All children with a history of Lomotil ingestion should be admitted to the hospital for 24 hours of observation and monitoring. Activated charcoal is indicated, even beyond 1 hour after ingestion, because of delayed gastrointestinal motility. Naloxone may be indicated for respiratory depression; higher than usual doses may be required to reverse the diphenoxylate toxicity.[3]

SULFONYLUREAS

Sources

Sulfonylureas are used for the treatment of non–insulin-dependent diabetes mellitus and can cause significant hypoglycemia with the ingestion of 1 or 2 pills by young children. Examples are chlorpropamide, glyburide, glimepiride, glipizide, tolazamide, and tolbutamide.

Dose Causing Significant Toxicity

Ingestion of a single tablet of chlorpropamide (250 mg), glipizide (5 mg), or glyburide (2.5 mg) has been reported to produce hypoglycemia in children younger than 4 years.

Pathophysiology

Sulfonylureas lower blood glucose primarily by stimulating endogenous insulin secretion and secondarily by enhancing peripheral insulin receptor sensitivity and reducing glycogenolysis.

Clinical Presentation

The clinical presentation of sulfonylurea toxicity is that of hypoglycemia: agitation, confusion, headache, lethargy, seizures, tachycardia, and diaphoresis. The onset of hypoglycemia may be delayed, depending on the agent, by 8 hours up to 16 hours.

Diagnosis

Diagnosis is made from the history, clinical presentation, and presence of hypoglycemia. Sulfonylureas are not detected on routine toxicology screens.

Management

The management of unintentional ingestions of oral hypoglycemics is somewhat controversial according to the literature. It is important to detect and treat hypoglycemia early. Fingerstick blood glucose measurements should be made every 1 to 2 hours for a minimum of 8 hours. Patients with normal glucose levels who are asymptomatic should not receive intravenous dextrose initially, because it might mask hypoglycemia. If hypoglycemia is detected (blood glucose <60 mg/dL) or the patient has clinical symptoms, a bolus of dextrose should be given, followed by a continuous infusion of 5% to 20% dextrose to keep the blood glucose value higher than 100 mg/dL. After starting dextrose, the patient may have subsequent rebound hypoglycemia. For significant and persistent hypoglycemia, octreotide should be administered. Octreotide is a somatostatin analogue that inhibits the secretion of insulin and may obviate the need for exogenous insulin. The dose is 1 to 2 µg/kg and can be administered subcutaneously.

The risk of administering activated charcoal to a child with altered mental status, especially for the ingestion of 1 or 2 sulfonylurea pills, is probably greater than the benefits received, and should be considered carefully. We recommend that all children with a history of ingestion of 1 or 2 sulfonylurea pills be monitored a minimum of 12 hours.

ATYPICAL ANTIPSYCHOTIC AGENTS

Sources

The atypical antipsychotics, or second- and third-generation antipsychotics, have been developed to decrease the long-term side effects (e.g., tardive dyskinesia) and minimize the extrapyramidal side effects of the older (first-generation) antipsychotics (thioridazine, trifluoperazine, fluphenazine, mesoridazine) as well to treat both the positive and negative effects of schizophrenia. These newer antipsychotics have been prescribed for bipolar disorder with growing frequency in children.

Dose Causing Significant Toxicity

One or two tablets of any of the atypical antipsychotic agents can cause toxicity in young children.

Pathophysiology

The atypical antipsychotics cause blockade of dopamine receptors as well as affect serotonin, histamine, α_2-adrenergic, and muscarinic receptors. They cause agonist as well as antagonist effects at serotonin and dopamine receptors, unlike the traditional neuroleptics, which are pure dopamine antagonists.

Clinical Presentation

Toxicity with any of the atypical antipsychotics can manifest as CNS effects, such as ataxia, slurred speech, agitation, sedation, and coma. Miosis, due to alpha-adrenergic antagonism, can also be seen. Other signs of clinical toxicity are listed in Table 154-7. QTc interval prolongation is seen with all except for aripiprazole (Abilify). Onset of symptoms can occur

Table 154-7 CLINICAL TOXICITY OF ATYPICAL ANTIPSYCHOTICS

Drug	Clinical Toxicity
Clozapine (Clozaril)	Agranulocytosis
Risperidone (Risperdal)	Lethargy, orthostatic hypotension, prolonged QTc interval
Olanzapine (Zyprexa)	Miosis, tachycardia, anticholinergic symptoms, prolonged coma, prolonged QTc interval
Ziprasidone (Geodon)	Central nervous system (CNS) depression, prolonged QTc interval
Quetiapine (Seroquel)	Seizures, tachycardia, CNS depression, prolonged QTc interval
Aripiprazole (Abilify)	Vomiting, lethargy, ataxia, tachycardia, drooling

as early as 1 to 2 hours after ingestion, and the effects typically peak at 6 hours. Although the atypical or newer antipsychotics have less pure dopaminergic antagonistic properties, extrapyramidal side effects, including acute dystonic reactions, still occur.

Diagnosis

Diagnosis is based on history and the finding of sedation, small pupils, hypotension, and QTc interval prolongation. Dystonias in children should suggest the possibility of antipsychotic medication exposures.

Treatment

Diphenhydramine or benztropine can reverse the signs and symptoms of acute dystonic reactions seen with atypical antipsychotic toxicity. Otherwise, there is no specific antidotal therapy. Supportive care, including airway management for significant CNS depression and benzodiazepines for seizures, may be necessary. The QTc interval prolongation usually resolves with discontinuation of the medication. The risk for torsades de pointes and prolongation of QTc intervals associated with the atypical antipsychotic cannot be extrapolated to young children with unintentional ingestions of these medications. The asymptomatic patient may be discharged after 6 hours of observation.

The risk of administering activated charcoal to a child with altered mental status and the ingestion of a drug with a propensity to cause seizures, especially for the ingestion of 1 or 2 pills (see Table 154-6),[7-9] is probably greater than the benefits received and should be considered carefully.[10]

Documentation

History

- Name and concentration of the drug ingestion.
- Time lapse, since ingestion if known.
- History of any other diseases that may complicate the ingestion.

Physical Examination

- Does the patient look ill? Pale? Febrile?
- Mental status.
- Cardiac status (blood pressure, arrhythmias).
- Respiratory and airway status.
- Physical examination should be repeated while the patient is in the ED.

Laboratory Studies

- Laboratory tests and time obtained.

Medical Decision-Making

- Calculation of the mg/kg ingested if possible.
- Decision to begin treatment or delays.
- Consultation(s) chosen and time(s) of request(s).
- If the patient is being discharged, documentation of medical reasons that the patient needs no further investigation or continuing care.

Treatment

- Availability of antidote, time antidote ordered, and any delays of treatment.

Patient Instructions

- Document discussion with patient or parent regarding diagnosis, warning signs, what to do, follow-up, and when to return.
- With pediatric accidental ingestions, document poison prevention counseling.
- Families should be given the phone number for their poison control center to address further concerns (1-800-222-1222).
- Any time there is concern about the situation surrounding the ingestion or an ingestion has occurred in an infant younger than 12 months, social services should be contacted.

REFERENCES

1. Michael JB, Sztajnkrycer MD: Deadly pediatric poisons: Nine common agents that kill at low doses. Emerg Med Clin North Am 2004;22:1019-1050.
2. U.S. Food and Drug Administration, Center for Drug Evaluation and Research: FDA Public Health Advisory: Life-Threatening Side Effects with the Use of Skin Products Containing Numbing Ingredients for Cosmetic Procedures. Available at http://www.fda.gov/cder/drug/advisory/topical_anesthetics.htm/
3. Liebelt EL, Shannon MW: Small doses, big problems: A selected review of highly toxic common medications. Pediatr Emerg Care 1993;9:292-297.

4. Love JN, Shannon M, Smereck J: Are one or two dangerous? Camphor exposure in toddlers. J Emerg Med 2004;27: 49-54.
5. Perry HE: Pediatric poisonings from household products: Hydrofluoric and methacrylic acid. Cur Opin Pediatr 2001;13:157-161.
6. Eddy O, Howell JM: Are one or two dangerous? Clonidine and topical imidazoline exposure in toddlers. J Emerg Med 2003;25:297-302.
7. Bar-Oz B, Levichek Z, Koren G: Medications that can be fatal for a toddler with one tablet or teaspoonful: A 2004 update. Paediatr Drugs 2004;6:123-126.
8. Boyer EW, Duic PA, Evans A: Hyperinsulinemia/euglycemia therapy for calcium channel blocker poisoning. Pediatr Emerg Care 2002;18:36-37.
9. Love JN, Sikka N: Are one or two tablets dangerous? Beta-blocker exposure in toddlers. J Emerg Med 2004;26:309-314.
10. Jacobs ES, Dickstein DP, Liebelt EL: Novel psychotropic medications in children: New toxicities to master. Pediatr Emerg Care 2001;17:226-231.

SECTION XV

Bites, Stings, and Injuries from Animals

Chapter 155

Mammalian Bites

Ashley Booth

KEY POINTS

Human bites, especially clenched-fist injuries (i.e., "fight bites") commonly cause septic joints, osteomylitis, tenosynovitis, and fractures.

Pasteurella species are the most common organisms present in wound infections from bites, specifically *Pasteurella multocida* in cat bites and *Pasteurella canis* in dog bites.

Wound infections caused by human bites are usually polymicrobial.

If there is any evidence that the patient has a human bite, the case should be considered as such.

When wounds are caused by mammalian bites, injury to deeper structures should be suspected.

When a patient presents with signs of infection, radiography should be considered to look for retained foreign bodies, gas in the tissues, and osteomyelitis.

The tetanus status of all patients sustaining mammalian (cat, dog, human, and other primates) bites must be ascertained.

Scope

Two to four million cat, dog, and human bites are reported by the Centers for Disease Control and Prevention (CDC) every year, as well as approximately 300,000 ED visits secondary to mammalian bites. The exact number of cases of mammalian bites is difficult to determine because many cases are not reported. Approximately 20 bites are fatal each year, and 20% to 80% of bites become infected. Cat, dog, and human bites account for over 100 million dollars a year in health care costs.[1-4]

Pathophysiology

Wounds infections from mammalian bites have a complicated microbiology profile. A majority of infections are polymicrobial with a mix of aerobic and anaerobic bacteria. Patients who present with acute cat bites (<24 hours from time of the bite) most often have wound cultures that grow *Pasteurella* organisms, especially *P. multocida*. Patients who present with subacute cat bites (>24 hours) or who return to the ED more than 24 hours after initial treatment for an acute bite typically have cultures that grow mixed aerobic and anaerobic species, with *Pasteurella*, *Staphylococcus*, and *Streptococcus* species as the predominant pathogens.[2,3,5]

Dog bites are the most common mammalian bite seen in the ED. Dog bites tend to cause more damage, injure deeper structures, and crush tissues because of the animal's powerful jaws, which can exert pressures of 200 to 450 pounds per square inch when biting.[1] Damage to deeper structures is more common with

Table 155-1 PATHOGENS IN MAMMALIAN BITES

Mammalian Bite	<24 Hours	>24 Hours
Human	Polymicrobial: *Streptococcus* sp., 60%-80% *Staphylococcus* sp., 37%-46% Anaerobic sp., 44%-60% (specifically *Eikenella corrodens*, 20%-25%)	Mixed aerobic/anaerobic *Staphylococcus* sp., *Streptococcus* sp.
Cat	*Pasteurella* sp.	Mixed aerobic/anaerobic *Pasteurella* sp. *Staphylococcus* sp. *Streptococcus* sp.
Dog	*Pasteurella* sp.	Mixed aerobic/anaerobic *Pasteurella* Sp. *Staphylococcus* sp. *Streptococcus* sp.

police dogs.[2] Dogs trained specifically for guard duty or for fighting, such as Pit bulls, Rottweilers, German shepherds, and Chows tend to cause a disproportionate number of bites resulting in serious injuries and death.[2]

Current research reveals that *Pasteurella* species are the most common organisms present in culture isolates from infected dog bite wounds, most commonly *P. canis*.[3] Other common aerobic pathogens in dog bite wound infections include *Staphylococcus* and *Streptococcus* species.[2,3,5] Aerobes less frequently associated with cat and dog bites wound infections include *Moraxella* and *Neisseria*. Causative anaerobic organisms include fusobacterium, bacteroides, porphyromonas and preveotella.[3]

Compared with cat bite victims, patients presenting with dog bites tend to present later after injury but have a lower infection rate. Conversely, patients whose injuries become infected secondary to cat bites tend to present earlier than dog bite patients with a mean time of 12 hours to presentation.[1] It is speculated that this higher infection rate occurs because the wounds from cats are more likely to be punctures, involve the hand, and become infected with *Pasteurella* species.[1,2]

Human bites have long been associated with high rates of infection and complications such as septic joints, osteomylitis, tenosynovitis, and fractures. However, recent studies show that human bites do not have a higher rate of infection compared with other bite wounds.[1,2,5]

There are two categories of human bites. The first category is referred to as *occlusional bites,* defined as intentional bites in which the teeth actually close down on the victim's skin. The second category is referred to as *clenched-fist injuries* (also called "fight bites"); these occur when the teeth hit or puncture the dorsum of the metacarpophalangeal region of a clenched hand. Clenched-fist injuries have a high propensity for causing injury to deep structures of the hand. Open fractures, joint involvement, and tendon injuries are common. Human bites to the hand, especially clenched-fist injuries, are at high risk for developing infection.[2,4,5]

Wound infections caused by human bites are usually polymicrobial. Streptococci are present in 60% to 80% of isolates. *Staphylococcus aureus* is present in 37% to 46% of isolates, and anaerobic species are present in 44% to 60% of isolates, specifically *Eikenella corrodens* (20%-25%). Herpes simplex virus can also be transmitted through infected saliva and can cause herpetic whitlow as well as wound infections (Table 155-1).[2]

Evaluation

■ HISTORY

A thorough history should be obtained (Fig. 155-1). This includes the timing of the bite incident, the circumstances surrounding the bite, and whether a report was filed with animal control officials. If the victim knows the animal, it may be possible to ascertain the immunization status of the bite source and whether the animal is going to be quarantined to observe for signs of rabies. This is especially important if the bite was unprovoked, if the animal was acting abnormal, or if the bite was caused by a wild animal. The patient's medical history (including a history of allergies, current medications, and immunization status) should also be obtained.

Patients who present with human bites, especially clenched-fist injuries, may not be forthcoming as to how their injury occurred. If the wound is on the extensor surface of the metacarpophalangeal joint, treat the patient as if the wound is a human bite. In patients with human bites, it is important to ascertain the human immunodeficiency virus (HIV) and hepatitis status of both the patient and the attacker.

■ PHYSICAL EXAMINATION

In major cases, when a patient suffers extensive injury, resuscitation from traumatic injury may be needed. Injury to deep structures, including major organs, and extensive blood loss is possible. It is usually apparent that a large animal has attacked the victim, but injuries from falls or other associated trauma can occasionally be occult. Disciplined, thorough evaluation of the patient's physical condition is warranted when associated injury may have

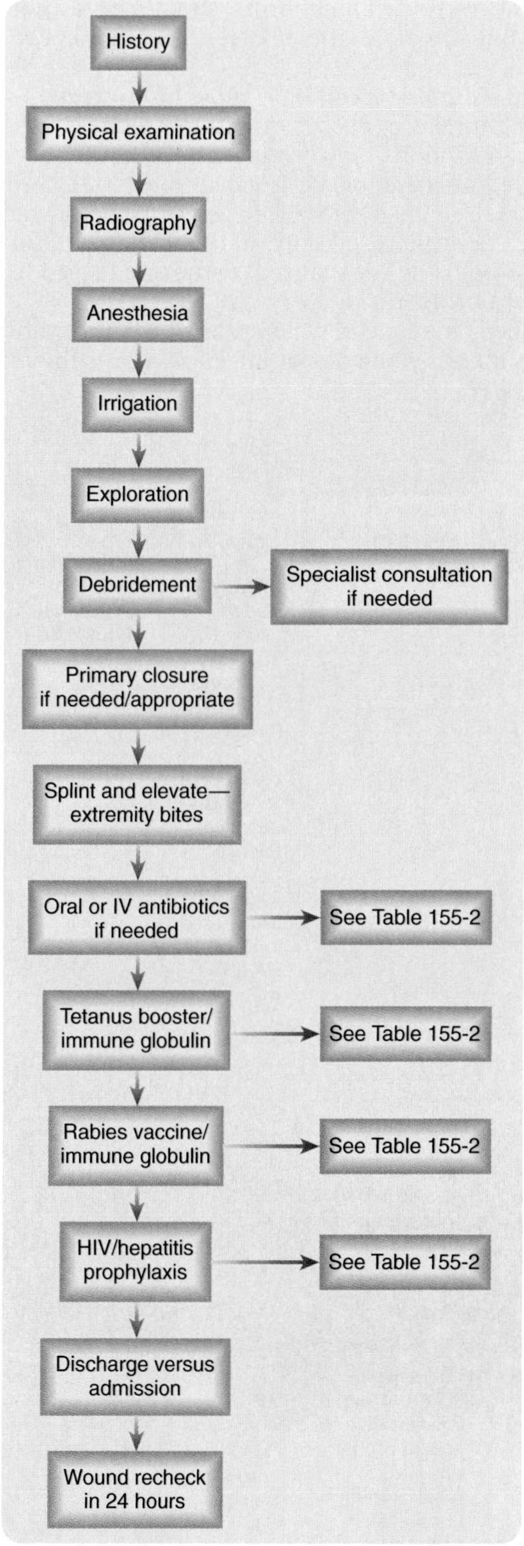
History
Physical examination
Radiography
Anesthesia
Irrigation
Exploration
Debridement
Specialist consultation if needed
Primary closure if needed/appropriate
Splint and elevate—extremity bites
Oral or IV antibiotics if needed
See Table 155-2
Tetanus booster/ immune globulin
See Table 155-2
Rabies vaccine/ immune globulin
See Table 155-2
HIV/hepatitis prophylaxis
See Table 155-2
Discharge versus admission
Wound recheck in 24 hours

FIGURE 155-1 Algorithm for management of human, cat, and dog bites. HIV, human immuunodeficiency virus.

occurred, especially since bite wounds draw the clinician's attention.

Vital signs should be obtained in all patients that present with bites since hypotension or tachycardia may be a sign of blood loss and fever may be a sign of infection. All bites mandate a full neurovascular exam including a thorough motor and sensory exam distal to the bite(s) as well as an exam of all the tendons and ligaments in the region of the bite. The physical examination should also include a thorough vascular examination and evaluation of any compartments involved.

If the patient presents with a deep puncture wound or small laceration and the ED clinician suspects possible injury to deeper structures but cannot visualize them he/she should extend the margins of the wound so that all possible injured structures can be visualized. Also keep in mind that tendons may retract proximally in the hand; thus a tendon injury may be missed on initial exam if the practitioner does not have a high level of suspicion.

The metacarpophalangeal joint and extensor tendons are covered by a thin layer of skin when the hand is clenched; therefore in human bites, especially clenched-fist injuries, the ED physician must have a high index of suspicion for tendon injuries as well as open fracture and open joints. Also if the patient has an extensor tendon laceration the tendon may often retract proximally when the hand is unclenched and the fingers extended.

If there is a risk of a retained foreign body such as a tooth or if there is a risk of deep structure injury such as a fracture a radiograph of the injured area must be obtained. Also if the patient presents with signs of infection consider obtaining a radiograph to look for retained foreign bodies, gas in the tissues, and osteomyelitis. If a vascular injury is suspected angiography may be needed to localize the injury or to determine the extent of the injury.

PRIORITY ACTIONS

Important Historical Questions To Ask

- Is the bite more or less than 12 hours old?
- Are you familiar with the animal or the owner of the animal that bit you?
- Was the bite provoked or unprovoked?
- Was a report filed with animal control/police?
- What is the immunization status of the bite source?
- Is/Can the animal be watched for the next 10 days for signs of rabies?
- Do you have any other medical problems? (especially diabetes, HIV infection, acquired immunodeficiency syndrome [AIDS], transplantation history)
- Are you taking any medications such as steroids or immunosuppressive agents?
- Are you allergic to any medications?
- When was your last tetanus shot? Have you had three doses of tetanus vaccine?
- Have you ever had the rabies vaccine?

Treatment (Table 155-2)

All bite wounds should undergo high-pressure irrigation of the wound with normal saline, dilute (<1%) povidone-iodine solution, or Fluronie F-68 (Shurclens). Recent studies have looked at the efficacy of tap water as an irrigation solution[2,6]; however, no conclusive data exist at present for bite wounds, and tap water as an irrigation solution for bite wounds cannot be supported at this time. Patients with larger or more complicated wounds may need to be anesthetized with lidocaine, bupivacaine, or another anesthetic agent prior to irrigation and exploration of the wound. Epinephrine should be avoided if the bite involves the fingers, toes, nose, ears, or penis.[2]

All wounds should be explored for foreign bodies and injuries to deeper structures such as arteries, nerves, tendons, and ligaments. All tendons in the injured area should be isolated and tested through their full range of motion to assess for partial lacerations or tears, especially if the hands or feet are involved. Any devitalized tissue or ragged edges should be débrided.

There is no clear evidence as to whether suturing bites increases the risk of infection, nor is there con-

Table 155-2 TREATMENT OF MAMMALIAN BITES

Type	Wound Care	Antibiotic Pr.	Tetanus Pr.	Rabies Pr.	HIV Pr.	Hepatitis Pr.
Human	High-pressure irrigation of wound with normal saline or dilute (<1%) povidone-iodine solution; débride devitalized tissue or ragged edges	Amoxicillin/clavulanate; second-generation cephalosporin with anaerobic activity; penicillin plus dicloxacillin; clindamycin plus ciprofloxacin or trimethoprim-sulfamethoxazole	Tetanus immune globulin (250 units IM) and tetanus toxoid (0.5 mg IM) if never had tetanus vaccine or have not had 3 doses of tetanus toxoid; tetanus toxoid (0.5 mg IM) if >5 yr since previous tetanus booster	None	HAART therapy started within the first 48-72 hr and continued for 28 days; or bite source tested HIV-negative; refer to hospital for specific drugs used in their HAART therapy	HBIG (0.06 mL/kg IM); HBV given at separate site from HBIG
Cat	High-pressure irrigation of wound with normal saline or dilute (<1%) povidone-iodine solution; débride devitalized tissue or ragged edges	Amoxicillin/clavulanate; second-generation cephalosporin with anaerobic activity; penicillin plus a first-generation cephalosporin; clindamycin plus a fluoroquinolone or trimethoprim-sulfamethoxazole	Tetanus immune globulin (250 units IM) and tetanus toxoid (0.5 mg IM) if never had tetanus vaccine or have not had 3 doses of tetanus toxoid; tetanus toxoid (0.5 mg IM) if >5 yr since previous tetanus booster	HRIG (20 IU/kg) injected IM and/or around bite site; rabies vaccine (1 mL IM), given in deltoid in adults/thigh in children, on days 0, 3, 7, 14, and 28	None	None
Dog	High-pressure irrigation of wound with normal saline or dilute (<1%) povidone-iodine solution; débride devitalized tissue or ragged edges	Amoxicillin/clavulanate; second-generation cephalosporin with anaerobic activity; penicillin plus a first-generation cephalosporin; clindamycin plus a fluoroquinolone or trimethoprim-sulfamethoxazole	Tetanus immune globulin (250 units IM) and tetanus toxoid (0.5 mg IM) if never had tetanus vaccine or have not had 3 doses of tetanus toxoid; tetanus toxoid (0.5 mg IM) if >5 yr since previous tetanus booster	HRIG (20 IU/kg) injected IM and/or around bite site; rabies vaccine (1 mL IM), given in deltoid in adults/thigh in children, on days 0, 3, 7, 14, and 28	None	None

Pr., prophylaxis; HAART, highly active antiretroviral therapy; HBIG, hepatitis B immune globulin; HBV, hepatitis B vaccine; HIV, human immunodeficiency virus; HRIG, human rabies immune globulin; IM, intramuscularly.

clusive data on which wounds can be safely sutured. The safest course of action is to leave most bite wounds open and have the patient return for delayed primary closure if the wound does not become infected; however, primary closure may be necessary for cosmetic or functional reasons.

Recent studies show that the infection rate of sutured bites initially may be lower in certain circumstances than historically predicted. Primary closure may be safe in the closure of simple bite wounds less than 6 hours old to the trunk and extremities (with the exception of hands and feet) and in the closure of simple bite wounds of the face and neck less than 12 hours old.[1,2]

The EP should leave wounds open or consider closure by secondary intention for all infected wounds and all wounds at increased risk for infection such as puncture wounds, hand and foot wounds, clenched- fist injuries, full-thickness wounds, wounds requiring débridement, wounds in patients older than 50 years or immunocompromised patients, wounds more than 12 hours old, and wounds involving damage to deep structures such as bones, joints, tendons, nerves, and blood vessels. Extremity wounds should be splinted and elevated.[2]

All patients sustaining mammalian (cat, dog, human, primates) bites should be given a dose of tetanus immune globulin and a dose of tetanus toxoid if they have never had the tetanus vaccine series or if they have not had three doses of tetanus toxoid. Patients who have had a full course of the tetanus vaccine series should be given a tetanus toxoid booster of 0.5 mg intramuscularly if it has been more than 5 years since their previous tetanus booster.

Patients who sustain dog, cat, or other animal bites should be evaluated for the potential need for rabies vaccination (see Chapter 181 on rabies). Patients who sustain high-risk bites in which the animal cannot be quarantined should receive 20 IU/kg of human rabies immune globulin (HRIG) injected around the bite site and/or intramuscularly and 1 mL of rabies vaccine given intramuscularly either in the deltoid in adults or in the thigh in children on days 0, 3, 7, 14, and 28. HRIG and rabies vaccine should be given at separate sites if both are given intramuscularly.[7]

Transmission of HIV and hepatitis B and C in human bites has been reported.[8] Patients who sustain human bites need to be evaluated and counseled about HIV infection and hepatitis B post-exposure prophylaxis (PEP) (PEP for hepatitis C does not exist). HIV PEP should be started as soon as possible within the first 48 to 72 hours after a high-risk bite and continued for 28 days. High-risk bites are those in which the assailant is known to be HIV- and/or hepatitis-positive and bites in which blood exposure is involved. Hepatitis B PEP should include hepatitis B immune globulin (HBIG) and the hepatitis B vaccine (HBV) if the patient has not been previously immunized. If the patient had previously undergone the hepatitis B vaccination series, a titer for anti-HBV should be drawn. If the patient has hepatitis B antibodies, no treatment is needed; if there are insufficient antibodies (anti-HBV <10 mIU/mL) the patient needs HBIG and an HBV booster.[8]

There is a lack of clinical evidence as to which cat and dog bites should receive prophylactic antibiotics. Cat bites—especially puncture wounds, wounds involving the hand and feet, wounds involving deeper structures, and wounds closed primarily—are considered high-risk bites, and the patient should receive prophylactic antibiotics. Prophylactic antibiotics for cat and dog bites, specifically those that present within the first 24 hours, should cover *Pasteurella, Staphylococcus, Streptococcus,* and anaerobic species. Options include amoxicillin/clavulanate, a second-generation cephalosporin with anaerobic activity, and penicillin plus a first-generation cephalosporin. Clindamycin plus a fluoroquinolone or trimethoprim-sulfamethoxazole may be used in penicillin-allergic patients.

Human bites are also considered high-risk bites. Prophylactic antibiotics should be considered for bites extending through the dermis, bites closed primarily, bites with significant crush injury or requiring significant débridement, puncture wounds, bites in elderly or immunocompromised patients, and bites that involve the hands, feet, or deeper structures. Human bite prophylaxis should cover *Staphylococcus, Streptococcus,* and anaerobes including *Eikenella corrodens*. Amoxicillin/clavulanate or penicillin plus dicloxacillin may be used. Clindamycin plus ciprofloxacin or trimethoprim-sulfamethoxazole may be used in penicillin-allergic patiens.

Disposition

Wounds with significant tissue loss may need plastic surgery or hand surgery consultation for skin grafting, depending on the location of the bite. Specialty consultation is also mandated for any hand or foot wound that involves a joint, tendon, artery, or nerve.

Most wounds, including infected wounds, can be managed on an outpatient basis; however, more severe infections, as well as wounds that fail outpatient therapy, may require hospital admission for parenteral antibiotic administration. Any patient discharged from the ED with a cat, dog, or human bite should be seen within 24 hours for a wound recheck either by the EP or by the patient's primary care physician.

REFERENCES

1. Broder J, Jerrard D, et al: Low risk of infection in selected human bites treated without antibiotics. Am J Emerg Med 2004;22:10-13.
2. Eilbert W: Dog, cat and human bites: Providing safe and cost-effective treatment in the ED. Emerg Med Pract 2003;5;1-20.
3. Talan D, Citron D, Abrahamiam FM, et al: Bacteriologic analysis of infected dog and cat bites. N Engl J Med 1999; 340:85-92.

4. Griego R, Rosen T, Orengo IF, Wolf JE: Dog, cat and human bites: A review. J Am Acad Derm 1995;33:1019-1029.
5. Brook I: Microbiology and management of human and animal bite wound infections. Prim Care Clin Office Pract 2003;30:25-39.
6. Bansal BC, Wiebe RA, Perkins SD, et al: Tap water for irrigation of lacerations. Am J Emerg Med 2002;20:469-472.
7. Human rabies prevention practices—United States. 1999, CDC MMWR. http://www.cdc.gov/mmwr/preview/mmwrhtml/00056176.htm.
8. Antiretroviral postexposure prophylaxis after sexual, injection-drug use, or other nonoccupational exposure to HIV in the United States. 2005, CDC MMWR. http://www.cdc.gov/mmwr/preview/mmwrhtml/rr5402al.htm.

Chapter **156**

Venomous Snakebites in North America

Robert L. Norris

KEY POINTS

Approximately 7000 to 8000 people are bitten by venomous snakes in the United States (U.S.) each year.

Mortality following venomous snakebites in the U.S. is less than 1%, especially when patients are treated with antivenom.

Permanent local sequelae following pit viper bites in the U.S. occurs in at least 10% of patients.

No field management (first aid) measure has been proved to be effective in pit viper bites other than expeditious transport to definitive medical care.

The key to management of venomous snakebite is the judicious and timely use of antivenom.

Hypotensive victims of snakebite are treated with an appropriate antivenom and IV fluids (beginning with crystalloid and switching to albumin if necessary). Vasopressors are a last resort.

All patients with suspected venomous snakebite and showing any signs or symptoms of envenomation are admitted to the hospital.

Fasciotomy is rarely needed following pit viper bites, and is only performed in the setting of objectively documented, sustained rises in intracompartmental pressures.

Scope

There are two families of dangerously venomous snakes in North America—the pit vipers (family Crotalidae, subfamily Crotalinae) and the elapids (family Elapidae). Pit vipers include the rattlesnakes (genera *Crotalus* and *Sistrurus*), cottonmouth water moccasins (*Agkistrodon piscivorus*), and copperheads (*Agkstrodon contortrix*). Pit vipers inflict approximately 99% of the 7000 to 8000 venomous snakebites that occur in the U.S. each year.[1,2] The only indigenous elapids in North America are the coral snakes, found in the southern and southwestern U.S. and Mexico. The coral snakes of the U.S. belong to two different genera—*Micrurus* (the eastern coral snake, *M. fulvius*, and the Texas coral snake, *M. tener*) and *Micruroides* (the Sonoran coral snake, *M. euryxanthus*).

Deaths due to snakebite are rare in the U.S., with only approximately 18 reported to the American Association of Poison Control Centers in the last 21 years.[1] Given that there is no requirement to report such cases, this is certainly an underestimate of the total number of deaths due to snake envenomation in the U.S. It does, however, illustrate the relatively low incidence of death due to this injury in the U.S. The case fatality rate following venomous snakebite in the U.S. when antivenom is used is less than 1%.[3] However, long-term complications, such as loss of some degree of function in the bitten extremity, are more likely. Approximately 10% of victims will be left with some functional disability following pit viper bites, and this does not include permanent dysfunction directly related to surgical procedures.[4] The incidence of disability may actually be higher if careful, delayed evaluation of extremity function is performed (e.g., using goniometry and precise sensory testing).[5] Given that the number of venomous snakes is reduced in the colder climate of Canada, the incidence of snakebites in that country is lower than in the U.S. In Mexico, however, as many as 150 people die each year from venomous snakebites.[4]

Pathophysiology

Snake venoms, particularly pit viper venoms, are complex mixtures of enzymes, low-molecular-weight (non-enzymatic) proteins, metallic ions, and other constituents.[6,7] There is great variability in venoms depending on the species of snake, its geographic origin, its age, health and diet, and the time of year.[8] Among the most important components found in pit viper venoms are phospholipase A_2 (PLA_2) enzymes, which cause cellular disruption and tissue damage; hyaluronidase, which facilitates distribution of venom within tissues; and thrombin-like enzymes, which affect various aspects of the coagulation cascade and lead to coagulation abnormalities.

Also of major importance in pit viper venom-induced coagulopathy are the metalloproteinases known as hemorrhagins, which increase vascular permeability and damage endothelial cells.[9,10] Some rattlesnakes, such as some Mohave rattlesnakes (*C. scutulatus*), possess neurotoxic components in their venoms. These are presynaptically acting toxins that prevent acetylcholine release at neuromuscular junctions. Depending on their geographic location, Mohave rattlesnakes may possess this component (Mohave toxin) and are termed "venom A–producing"[11,12] rattlesnakes.

Other rattlesnakes that may, based on their geographic origin, possess neurotoxic components closely related to Mohave toxin include the eastern diamondback rattlesnake (*C. adamanteus*), the timber rattlesnake (*C. horridus*), the southern Pacific rattlesnake (*C. oreganus helleri*), and the tiger rattlesnake (*C. tigris*).[13-17]

Coral snake venoms are less complex than pit viper venoms but are among the most toxic venoms of North America. The primary effects of coral snake venom are neurotoxic and are due to a component in the venom that blocks the postsynaptic endplates at neuromuscular junctions.[18,19]

Anatomy

Pit vipers get their name from the sensitive heat receptors (foveal organs) located on the anterior of their heads, slightly below and between the nostril and eye (Fig. 156-1). These organs aid the snake in finding prey, aiming its strike, and determining the volume of venom to be injected.

The presence of these pits can be used to identify a snake as a pit viper. Other characteristics typical of a pit viper include a triangular-shaped head (also found in many nonvenomous snakes), elliptic (cat-like) pupils, and, in the U.S., the presence of a single row of scales that spans the underside of its tail (Fig. 165-2). (Nonvenomous snakes in the U.S. generally have a double row of scales crossing the ventral aspect of the tail.) Rattlesnakes usually can also be identified by the keratin plates that make up their unique caudal rattle. Occasionally, however, these plates get broken off, and there is one species of rattlesnake (*C. catalinensis*) found on Catalina Island that has only a vestigial rattle.

Pit vipers range in size from the dimunitive pygmy rattlesnake (*S. miliarus*), typically 40 to 50 cm in length, to the massive eastern diamondback rattlesnake (*C. adamanteus*), which can attain lengths of over 1.5 m (Fig. 156-3).[20]

Coral snakes are identified in the U.S. by their characteristic color pattern—red, yellow, and black bands that completely encircle the body, with the red and yellow bands being contiguous. In harmless coral snake mimics, such as milksnakes, generally the red and yellow bands are separated by a band of black (Fig. 156-4). Color patterns cannot, however, be used outside of the U.S. to reliably identify coral snakes.

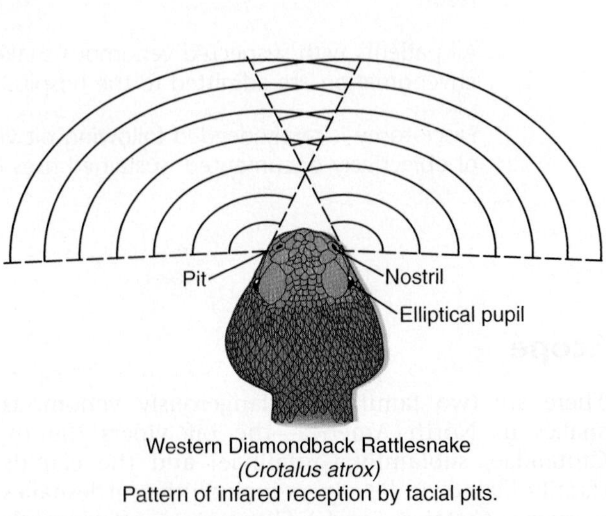
Pit
Nostril
Elliptical pupil
Western Diamondback Rattlesnake
(Crotalus atrox)
Pattern of infared reception by facial pits.

FIGURE 156-1 The heat-sensing pits or foveal organs of pit vipers. (Adapted from original drawing by Marlin Sawyer. With permission.)

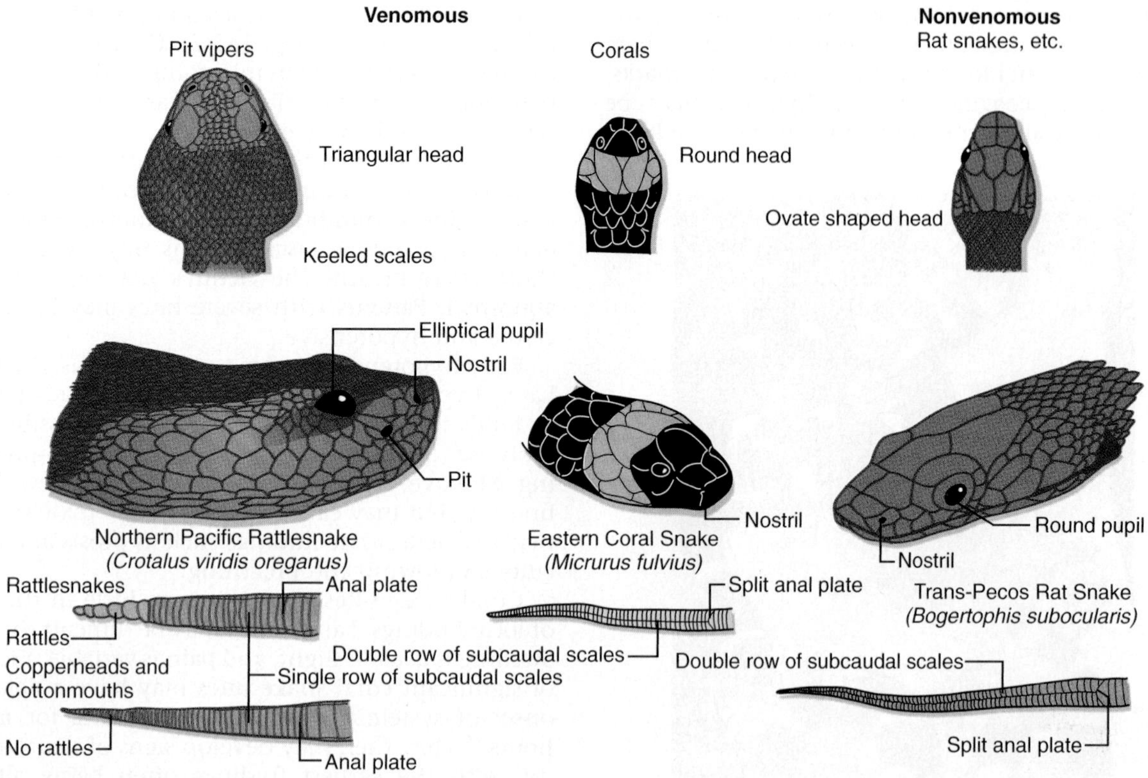
Venomous
Pit vipers
Triangular head
Keeled scales
Corals
Round head
Nonvenomous
Rat snakes, etc.
Ovate shaped head
Elliptical pupil
Nostril
Pit
Northern Pacific Rattlesnake
(Crotalus viridis oreganus)
Nostril
Eastern Coral Snake
(Micrurus fulvius)
Round pupil
Nostril
Trans-Pecos Rat Snake
(Bogertophis subocularis)
Rattlesnakes
Anal plate
Rattles
Copperheads and
Cottonmouths
Single row of subcaudal scales
No rattles
Anal plate
Split anal plate
Double row of subcaudal scales
Double row of subcaudal scales
Split anal plate

FIGURE 156-2 Anatomic comparison of pit vipers, coral snakes, and nonvenomous snakes of the United States. Pit vipers have a triangle-shaped head, elliptic pupils, heat-sensing pits, and a single row of subcaudal scales on the ventral aspect of the tail. Coral snakes are identified by their color pattern (see Figure 156-4), because they have round pupils and a single row of subcaudal scales, as do most harmless snakes in the United States. (Adapted from original drawing by Marlin Sawyer. With permission.)

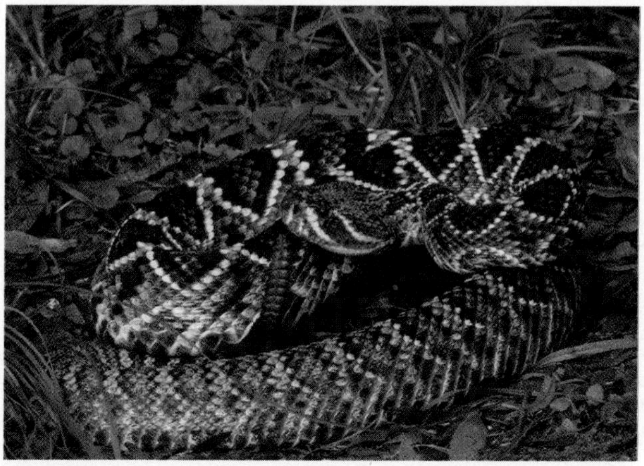

FIGURE 156-3 The eastern diamondback rattlesnake, found in the southeastern United States, is the largest of the rattlesnakes of North America. (Photo courtesy of Michael Cardwell/Extreme Wildlife Photography.)

Venomous snakes possess venom-producing glands in the upper jaw, behind the eyes (Fig. 156-5). These glands produce the venom that, at the time of a bite, is passed via a series of ducts to the hollow, needle-like fangs on the anterior maxillae. In pit vipers, these fangs range in length (proportional to the snake's overall length) from just a few millimeters to over 2.5 cm.[20] The fangs are quite mobile and are folded up against the roof of the snake's mouth when not in use. During a bite, the pit viper opens its mouth widely and swings the fangs into an upright position in order to drive them into the tissues of its target. Venom is then injected via a set of investing musculature. The speed of a pit viper's strike has been clocked at 8 feet per second[21]—faster than a human being can react.

The venom delivery apparatus of a coral snake is less sophisticated than that of a pit viper. Coral snakes have slightly enlarged, anterior, maxillary fangs, fixed in an erect position, with which they inject venom (Fig. 156-6). In order for a coral snake to effect an envenomation, it must chew on its victim for a matter of a few seconds. Bites by coral snakes almost always involve someone intentionally picking the snake up, often after misidentifying it as a harmless snake.[22]

Presenting Signs and Symptoms

The signs and symptoms of pit viper envenomation are broken down into local and systemic findings. Locally, the victim will have puncture wounds, although the pattern may be misleading and cannot be used to reliably differentiate between a venomous bite and a bite by a harmless snake. Generally the victim develops severe, burning pain at the bite site within minutes. This is followed shortly by local swelling that can progress over time to involve the entire bitten extremity and even the trunk. There may be persistent bloody oozing from the fang marks, indicative of coagulopathy. Ecchymosis may be present at the site, and more remotely, because hemorrhagins cause vascular leaks and loss of red blood cells into the tissues (Fig. 165-7). Over several hours to days, blisters and blebs may form on the extremity, particularly at the bite site. These are filled with clear serous fluid or bloody exudate.

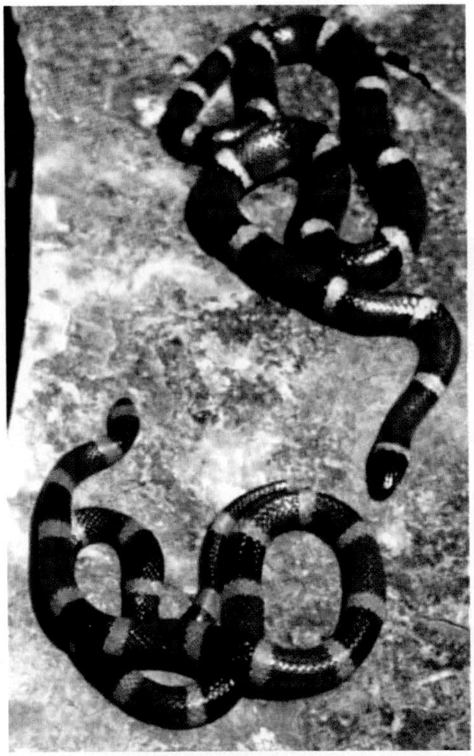

FIGURE 156-4 Venomous coral snakes in the United States can be identified by their color pattern, with the red and yellow bands being contiguous (**bottom,** *Micrurus tener*). Harmless mimics such as the milksnake (**top,** *Lampropeltis* sp.) have red and yellow bands separated by black bands. (Photo courtesy of Charles Alfaro.)

Systemically, victims present with a myriad of complaints, which can include nausea and vomiting and dizziness; numbness of the mouth, tongue, or extremities; muscle fasciculations (myokymia); and shortness of breath. The victim's vital signs may be abnormal. Patients with severe bites may be tachycardic and hypotensive.

Early hypotension is due to systemic vasodilation. Later, hypotension is compounded by third-spacing of fluids into the bitten extremity and possibly hemolysis.[21] Some pit vipers, such as venom A–producing Mohave rattlesnakes, may produce few local findings, but may cause more systemic toxicity, particularly neurotoxic findings such as ptosis and difficulty swallowing and breathing.

Coral snake bites generally have little in the way of local findings. Fang marks may be difficult to see.[23] Swelling is usually slight, and pain is variable. Victims of significant coral snake bites may have a delay in onset of systemic symptoms, sometimes for many hours.[24] They then may develop signs of neurotoxicity, with the earliest findings often being altered mental status and ptosis. Neurotoxicity can progress to frank skeletal muscle paralysis and respiratory failure.

Differential Diagnosis

The differential diagnosis in snakebite victims is generally limited. Most often, the victim can recount being bitten by a snake. On rare occasions, the victim may not have seen a snake, as when walking through

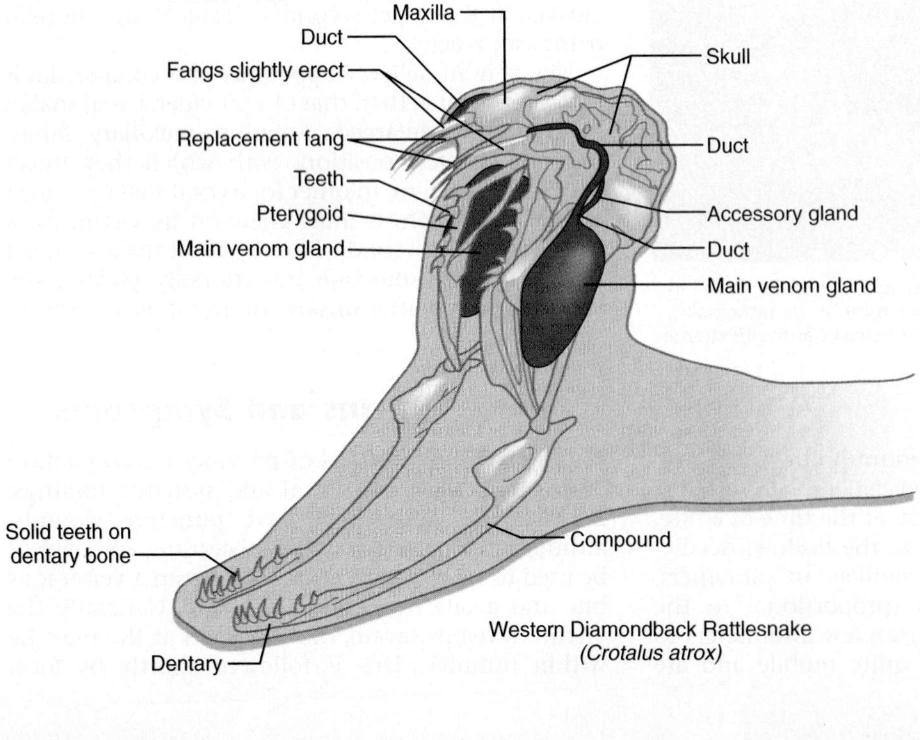
Maxilla
Duct
Fangs slightly erect
Replacement fang
Teeth
Pterygoid
Main venom gland
Skull
Duct
Accessory gland
Duct
Main venom gland
Solid teeth on dentary bone
Compound
Dentary
Western Diamondback Rattlesnake
(Crotalus atrox)

FIGURE 156-5 The venom apparatus of pit vipers. (Adapted from original drawing by Marlin Sawyer. With permission.)

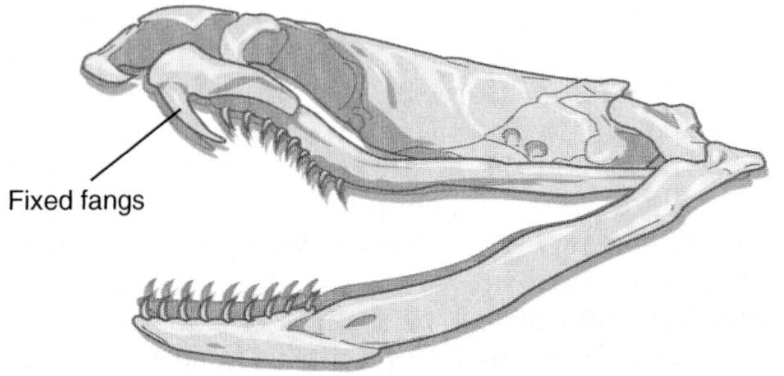
Fixed fangs
Skull
Texas Coral Snake
(*Micrurus fulvius tenere*)

FIGURE 156-6 Coral snake skull, demonstrating the smaller fixed anterior maxillary fangs of these reptiles. (Adapted from original drawing by Marlin Sawyer. With permission.)

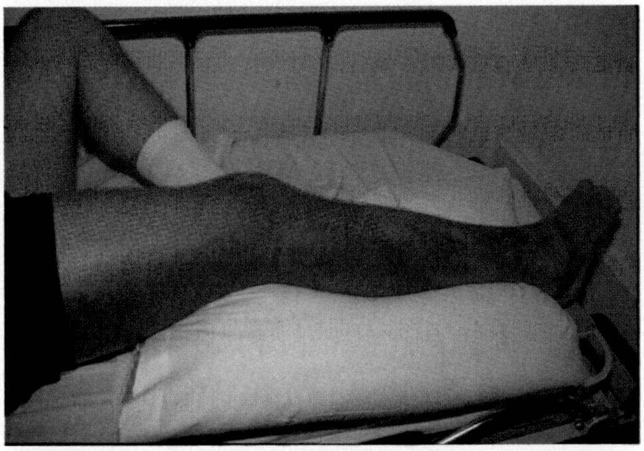

FIGURE 156-7 Extensive ecchymosis several days after a bite by a northern Pacific rattlesnake (*Crotalus oreganus*) to the victim's pretibial region. (Photo courtesy of Robert Norris.)

high grass when bitten. In such cases, the presence of at least one puncture wound and progression of local and systemic findings are usually diagnostic. If the victim saw the snake but cannot adequately describe it, careful observation over time will reveal whether envenomation has occurred. Having color photographs on hand of the snakes found locally can aid in proper identification of the offending reptile.

Victims of coral snake bite almost always see the snake owing to its need to actually chew on them to effect a significant bite. When a coral snake is implicated, the difficulty may be in differentiating the snake as a true coral snake versus a harmless coral snake mimic. Here again, color photos may help if the victim can recall the color pattern of the animal. All victims of coral snake bite should be observed carefully for at least 24 hours in the hospital because of the possible delay in onset of toxicity with these bites.

Young children have no innate fear of snakes and may be unable to describe precisely what bit them, particularly if they are pre-verbal. All children with possible venomous snakebites are admitted to the hospital for monitoring for at least 24 hours.

Diagnostic Testing

■ PIT VIPER BITES

Laboratory tests obtained in all potential victims of pit viper bite include a complete blood count, blood typing and screening, metabolic panel, and coagulation studies (prothrombin time [PT], activated partial thromboplastin time [aPTT], international normalized ratio [INR], fibrinogen level, and fibrin degradation products [FDP]). The white blood cell count may be elevated due to neutrophilic leukocytosis (demargination). The hematocrit may be elevated (due to volume contraction) or reduced (due to hemolysis or bleeding).

The metabolic panel is important to check renal and liver function. Victims of significant pit viper envenomation often develop laboratory-confirmed coagulopathies, with elevation of the PT, aPTT, INR, and FDP and decrease in fibrinogen level and platelet count. Fortunately, these victims rarely develop significant clinical bleeding, but coagulopathy is a marker of systemic envenomation and the need for antivenom therapy (see later). Blood typing and screening is important in the rare case of severe coagulopathy and bleeding that may require blood product replacement. Venom effects can, over time, interfere with blood crossmatching,[25] so it is important to draw a specimen for the lab early in the patient's course.

The victim's urine is checked for blood, myoglobin, and protein with each void. Arterial blood gases (ABGs) are obtained in victims with severe poisoning or with significant co-morbidities. ABGs provide information regarding the victim's respiratory status and the adequacy of resuscitation. An electrocardiogram is also obtained when the victim is severely ill, has a history of coronary artery disease, or is experiencing chest pain. A chest radiograph is obtained if the patient is experiencing respiratory distress, has a history of significant cardiopulmonary disease, or requires intubation. Laboratory assays are repeated at least every 6 hours until it is clear that the victim's condition is stabilized.

■ CORAL SNAKE BITES

Laboratory tests are of little benefit in cases of coral snake bites. These snakes do not cause coagulopathy. ABGs can be helpful if the victim demonstrates any evidence of respiratory embarrassment. Bedside pulmonary function testing can also be used to assess and monitor a coral snakebite victim's respiratory status.

Interventions and Procedures

Field management focuses on providing reassurance and rapid transport to a facility equipped with antivenom. If it is possible to do so safely, the snake is identified. No attempt should be made to capture or

PRIORITY ACTIONS

- Ensure an adequate airway, breathing, and circulation.
- Begin intravenous crystalloid infusion for patients that are volume-depleted or hypotensive.
- Assess the severity of envenomation and remain vigilant for signs of progression.
- Measure and record circumferences of the bitten extremity every 15 minutes during the early stages, to assess for progression of local findings.
- Send appropriate screening laboratory tests including blood typing and screening (see text).
- Begin the process of locating and obtaining an appropriate antivenom as soon as possible.
- To avoid delays in administration, begin reconstitution of antivenom as soon as it is clear that treatment is needed.
- Seek consultation with an expert in snake envenomation as needed.

kill the snake, although it may be possible to photograph the animal if a digital camera is available.

No first-aid measures have ever been proved to be beneficial in victims of pit viper bites. For victims of coral snake bite, the Australian pressure-immobilization technique is applied quickly in the field to limit venom spread. This involves wrapping the entire bitten extremity snuggly in an occlusive wrap followed by application of a splint (Fig. 156-8). Victims must then be carried from the field. Rescuers may have difficulty applying the technique in correct fashion, tending to underestimate the degree of pressure that needs to be exerted under the wrap.[26] Pressure-immobilization has been shown to significantly limit venom spread in elapid snakebites,[27] and was effective in one small animal study utilizing eastern coral snake (*Micrurus fulvius*) venom.[28] Although pressure-immobilization may limit spread of pit viper venom as well, it may actually exacerbate local tissue damage by severely restricting tissue-destroying venom access to the bite site and should therefore not be used.

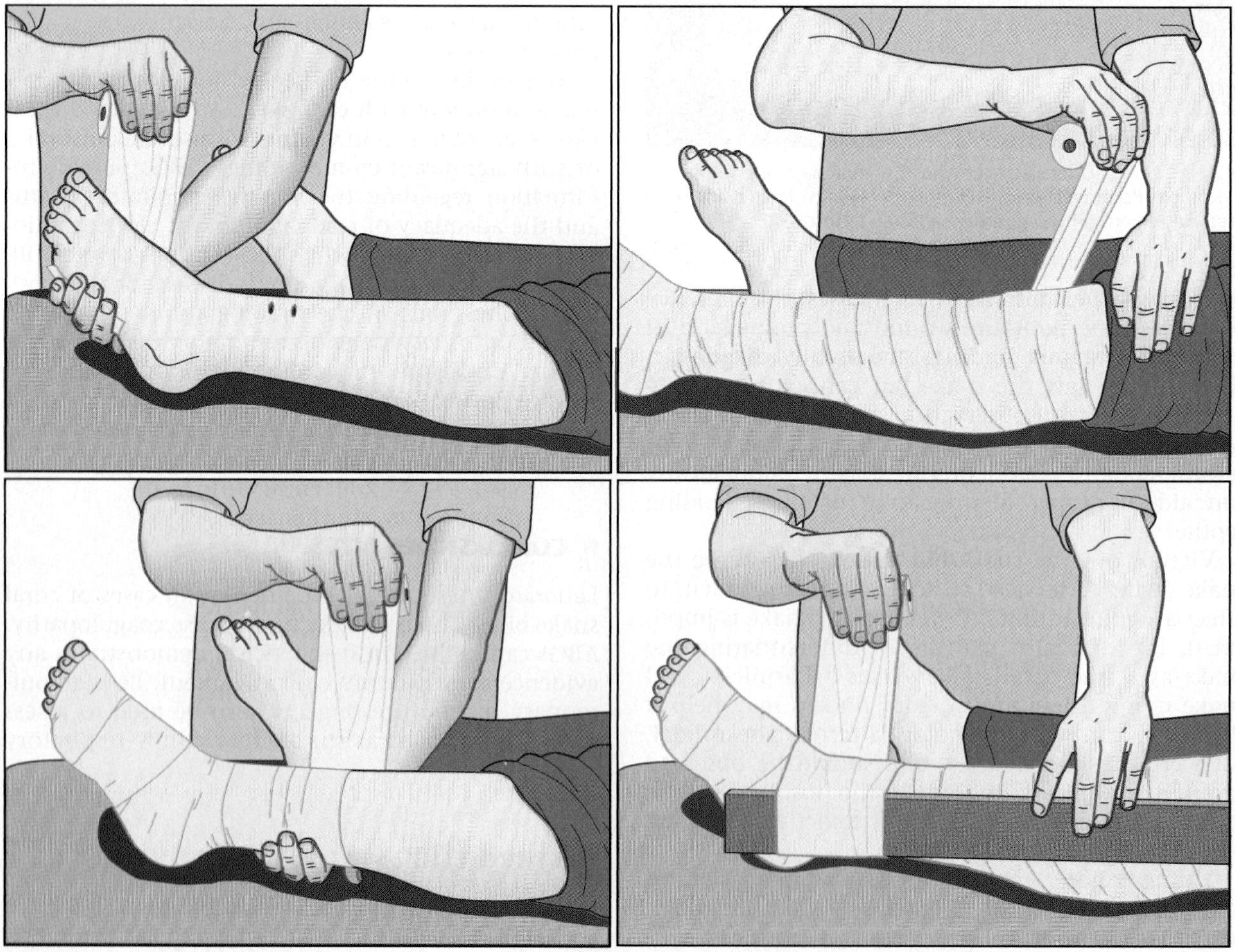

FIGURE 156-8 The Australian pressure-immobilization technique for field management of non-necrotizing elapid snakebites (e.g., coral snakes).

Treatment and Disposition

Hospital management of snakebite victims begins with an assessment of respiratory and circulatory status. The patient is initially placed on oxygen, and cardiac and pulse oximetry monitoring are begun while the EP takes a directed history and performs a focused physical examination. It is uncommon for snakebite victims in North America to present with significant respiratory compromise. Patients bitten by coral snakes or rattlesnakes with neurotoxic venoms can, however, develop difficulty with the airway and breathing.

If there are signs of neurotoxicity, and the victim develops any shortness of breath or difficulty speaking or swallowing, the airway should be promptly and definitively secured by endotracheal intubation to prevent aspiration. Two large-bore IV lines are established with normal saline. If the victim shows any signs of dehydration or shock, fluid resuscitation is begun with the administration of 1 to 2 liters of normal saline (20-40 mL/kg for children). If the blood pressure does not respond promptly to crystalloid infusion, albumin is added because it may remain in the leaky vasculature for a longer period of time. Vasopressors are used only as a last resort after adequate intravascular fluid repletion.[29] Inadequately treated hypotension is a key aspect in many cases of fatal snake envenomation.[30,31]

Once the ABCs (airway, breathing, and circulation) have been addressed, an attempt is made to identify the offending snake. If the victim has brought the snake to the hospital, extreme caution is used in examining it, even if it appears to be dead. A severed snake head can have a bite reflex for up to an hour following death and is capable of inflicting a serious bite.[32-34]

Circumferences of the bitten extremity are marked and measured at the bite site and at one or two sites more proximally every 15 minutes during the early stages of envenomation. This offers an objective measure of progression of local swelling. If the circumferences of the bitten extremity are increasing, severity of envenomation is progressing and antivenom will be needed.

The key to management of significant envenomation is antivenom administration. Initial decisions on antivenom administration (indication and dose) are guided by assessment of severity of envenomation (Table 156-1). Two antivenoms are currently available in the U.S. for pit viper bites: CroFab (Fougera, Melville, NY) and Antivenin (Crotalidae) Polyvalent (ACP) (Wyeth-Ayerst Laboratories, Philadelphia). Both products are produced by immunizing animals (CroFab—sheep; ACP—horses) with the venoms of four different pit vipers with a broad enough antigen spectrum in their venoms to allow protection against any pit viper found in North America. ACP consists largely of whole equine IgG antibodies (and a significant quantity of impurities such as horse albumin); CroFab is further refined by digesting the ovine IgG molecules with papain to yield Fc and Fab fragments. The Fc fragments—responsible for inducing many acute anaphylactoid reactions to antivenoms—are discarded, and the protective Fab fragments are isolated using affinity column chromatography. Both products are packaged in a lyophilized state and require reconstitution before administration. It is likely that ACP will no longer be available in the near future.

Antivenom administration is described in detail in Box 156-1.

Antivenom is effective in reversing most systemic and laboratory derangements seen following snake envenomation. However, its ability to reverse thrombocytopenia, rhabdomyolysis, or myokymia is variable.[11,35,36] Antivenom's efficacy in preventing local tissue damage has never been definitively demonstrated. If given very early in the course, it may reduce

Documentation

- Record a careful history in the patient's own words, including a description of the snake.
- Record thorough screening physical examination results.
- Have nursing staff measure and record circumferences of the bitten extremity every 15 minutes until swelling has ceased, then every hour for 24 hours.
- Note specifics of any discussion with consultants (e.g., poison control specialists).
- Measure and record intracompartmental pressures if concern arises about development of compartment syndrome.
- Document informed consent (for antivenom administration or fasciotomy).

Table 156-1 SEVERITY GRADING OF PIT VIPER ENVENOMATION*

Grade	Local Findings	Systemic Findings	Laboratory Abnormalities
Nonenvenomation ("dry bite")	Fang marks only	Absent	Absent
Mild envenomation	Present	Absent	Absent
Moderate envenomation	Present	Mild	Minor
Severe envenomation	Present	Significant	Significant

*This grading scale is only a rough guide and does not replace clinical judgment. Severity can increase rapidly and dramatically, and the patient should be closely monitored for worsening severity.

BOX 156-1

Pit Viper Antivenom Administration*

- Obtain informed consent if possible.
- Expand the patient's intravascular volume with normal saline (NS) if safe to do so (e.g., no history of congestive heart failure).
- Begin reconstitution of antivenom as soon as its need is evident, because this process takes 30 minutes or longer.
- Have epinephrine at the bedside, ready to administer immediately in the event of an acute reaction to the antivenom.

CroFab

- Dilute starting dose in 250 mL of NS.
- Starting dose (children receive same dose of antivenom as adults):
  - Nonenvenomation—0 vials
  - Mild bite—4 vials (indicated if there is any evidence of ongoing progression of local findings)
  - Moderate bite—46 vials
  - Severe bite—6+ vials
- Administer antivenom intravenously at a slow rate, with the EP at the bedside to intervene in the event of an acute (anaphylactoid) adverse reaction.
- If tolerated, after 5 to 10 minutes increase the rate of infusion to get the entire dose administered in 1 hour.
- Observe the patient for 1 hour after administration and repeat any abnormal laboratory tests.
- If findings of envenomation continue to worsen, repeat the starting dose (and continue this sequence until stable; generally no more than two "starting doses" are required).
- Once the patient's condition is stabilized, admit the patient (to an intensive care unit if the poisoning was severe, otherwise to a regular bed) for observation and further management (e.g., wound care; see text).
- After stabilized, repeat dosing of CroFab at 2 vials every 6 hours for 3 additional doses.

Antivenin (Crotalidae) Polyvalent (ACP)

- Although the manufacturer recommends a skin test for possible allergy to this product, such testing is very insensitive, does not accurately predict patients who will have an acute anaphylactoid reaction, wastes time, and should be omitted.
- Consider pretreating the patient with H_1- and H_2-blocking antihistamines in standard doses to mitigate a possible acute anaphylactoid reaction.
- Dilute starting dose in 1000 mL of NS (volume adjusted as appropriate for children).
- Starting dose (children receive the same dose of antivenom as adults):
  - Nonenvenomation—0 vials
  - Mild bite—0 or 5 vials (may be withheld if local findings are not progressing)
  - Moderate bite—10 vials
  - Severe bite—15 vials
- Administer antivenom intravenously at a slow rate, with the EP at the bedside to intervene in the event of an acute (anaphylactoid) adverse reaction.
- If tolerated, after approximately 10 minutes increase the rate of infusion to get the entire dose administered in 1 to 2 hours.
- Further ACP is given as needed for continued toxicity (in 5-10 vial increments with further dilution).
- Once the patient's condition is stabilized, admit the patient (to an intensive care unit if the poisoning was severe, otherwise to a regular bed) for observation and further management (e.g., wound care—see text).

*Administration of North American Coral Snake Antivenom (NACSA) proceeds in similar fashion to that of ACP, with dosing as per the package insert.

Tips and Tricks

- As soon as it is clear that antivenom is indicated, have the pharmacy or nursing staff begin reconstitution of the appropriate number of vials to be given. This is labor-intensive and it can take 30 minutes to prepare each vial.
- Warm diluent can be used to reconstitute lyophilized antivenom. Avoid excessive heat because it will denature antivenom proteins. Vials can be gently agitated under warm water to facilitate reconstitution.

BOX 156-2

Management of Acute Anaphylactoid Reactions to Antivenom

- Immediately stop the infusion.
- Treat signs and symptoms in standard fashion (airway management as needed, epinephrine, antihistamines [H_1- and H_2-blockers], steroids, fluids, vasopressors).
- Decide whether further antivenom is needed to treat envenomation.
- If antivenom is to be withheld, treat conservatively.
- If further antivenom is to be given:
  - If the reaction was to Antivenin (Crotalidae) Polyvalent (ACP), consider switching to CroFab if it is available.
  - Give additional doses of antihistamines.
  - Administer intravenous steroids.
  - Further dilute the antivenom (twofold if the volume can be tolerated by the patient).
  - Restart the antivenom at a slower rate, with the EP at the bedside.
- If the reaction persists, and antivenom treatment is necessary due to the severity of envenomation, admit the patient to the intensive care unit:
  - Establish full monitoring, including an arterial line (if there is no significant coagulopathy).
  - Establish an intravenous infusion of epinephrine (starting at 0.1 μg/kg/min).
  - Restart dilute antivenom at a slow rate.
  - Titrate epinephrine as the antivenom is administered, holding the reaction at bay (monitoring vital signs closely).

RED FLAGS

Cautions for the Physician

- Remain vigilant for worsening severity of venom poisoning; can progress rapidly and suddenly.
- Obtain consultation early from a clinician knowledgeable in snake envenomations (e.g., a regional poison control center specialist).
- Obtain informed consent whenever possible prior to giving antivenom.
- Give antivenom as soon as possible after its need is identified.
- Remain at the patient's bedside during the initiation of antivenom therapy in order to intervene if an acute anaphylactoid reaction occurs.
- Have epinephrine available at the bedside before beginning antivenom infusion.
- If a compartment syndrome is suspected, obtain objective measures of intracompartmental pressures.
- If a fasciotomy is indicated, obtain and document informed consent.
- Cases involving snake envenomation in the U.S. often end up in medical legal litigation. Document carefully.

or limit permanent local damage to some slight degree. After adequate antivenom administration, patients generally feel subjectively better, and there is improvement in local and systemic findings.

Adverse reactions to antivenom include early, acute reactions (that are likely anaphylactoid in nature) and delayed serum sickness, an immunoglobulin (IgG/IgM) immune complex–mediated disease. Anaphylactoid reactions may present with hives, wheezing, laryngeal edema, abdominal pain, vomiting, diarrhea, and hypotension (Box 156-2). The incidence of anaphylactoid reactions to ACP is approximately 25% to 50%,[3,37,38] and to CroFab approximately 15%.[38] Although there have been a few fatalities related to ACP-induced anaphylactoid reactions,[2,37] all acute reactions reported to date with CroFab have been relatively minor.[39]

Serum sickness occurs in approximately 3% of patients treated with CroFab, but in as many as 85% of those treated with ACP.[38] This illness presents approximately 1 to 2 weeks after antivenom administration with fever, urticaria, myalgias, arthralgias, renal dysfunction, and/or neuropathies. Serum sickness is easily treated with oral steroids (e.g., prednisone, 1-2 mg/kg orally per day) administered until the symptoms resolve, followed by a 2-week tapering of the dose. Oral antihistamines may provide additional symptomatic relief. Prior to discharge from the hospital, patients are warned to watch for signs and symptoms of serum sickness and told to return if they occur.

Currently an antivenom is available in the U.S. for bites by eastern and Texas coral snakes (*Micrurus* species)—North American Coral Snake Antivenin (NACSA) (Wyeth-Ayerst Laboratories). This product is administered to any victim with a confirmed bite by a *Micrurus* species snake, even in the absence of systemic findings, because progression of neurotoxicity may be difficult to halt once it begins. The likelihood of needing antivenom for a victim of Sonoran coral snakebite is very low because these snakes are quite small and inoffensive and have not been reported to cause a fatality.[40] There is no specific antivenom for Sonoran coral snakes (*Micruroides euryxanthus*). Adverse reactions to NACSA and their treatment are similar to those for pit viper antivenoms.

Given the rarity of coral snakebites in the U.S., it is likely that production of antivenom in this country against *Micrurus* species will be discontinued by the manufacturer. Should this occur, a mechanism for importing coral snake antivenoms from other countries (such as Mexico or Costa Rica) may be necessary. Otherwise, management of these patients will be limited to conservative therapy only (airway control, mechanical ventilation, hemodynamic support). Pit viper antivenom is of no benefit to victims of coral snake bite.

Blood products are rarely needed for victims of venomous snakebite, even with significant laboratory coagulopathy.[41] If a victim develops clinically significant bleeding (such as gastrointestinal hemorrhage or hemoptysis) or if blood counts (hematocrit or platelets) reach critically low levels, administration of packed red blood cells, platelets, and clotting factors may be necessary. Aggressive antivenom administration always precedes administration of any blood products in order to avoid feeding further substrate to an ongoing venom-induced consumptive coagulopathy.

Wound management of pit viper bites includes placing the extremity in a well-padded splint and elevating the extremity above heart level. Elevation, begun after starting antivenom therapy if indicated, helps to reduce swelling. Tetanus prophylaxis is given if needed, based on the patient's immunization history. Prophylactic antibiotics are not necessary unless misdirected first-aid measures included incisions into the bite wound or mouth suction. In such cases a broad-spectrum antibiotic (to cover both gram-positive and gram-negative bacteria) is administered in standard doses. Pit viper bites in the U.S. rarely become infected. When they do, however, antibiotic therapy is guided by wound culture testing. Tissue that is clearly necrotic is dibred after the patient is stabilized and once any attendant coagulopathy has been reversed. Intact blebs and blisters are left undisturbed, and those that rupture are conservatively dibred.

Physical therapy is started as early as possible in order to return the patient to an optimal level of functioning.

Some larger rattlesnakes have fangs long enough to penetrate deeply into muscle compartments.

FACTS AND FORMULAS

Antivenom Starting Doses (vials) for Pit Viper Bites

Severity:	Dry	Mild	Moderate	Severe
CroFab*	0	4	4-6	6+
ACP†	0	0 or 5	10	15

- If findings progress after the starting dose, give additional antivenom as needed (see text).

Intracompartmental Pressure (ICP) Measurements

- If <30-40 mm Hg, continue antivenom as indicated, with limb elevation and monitoring.
- If >30-40 mm Hg, give additional antivenom, keep the limb elevated, give mannitol (1 gm/kg, intravenously, if the patient's hemodynamic status will allow), and observe over 1 hour; then recheck ICP.
- If pressures fall below 30-40 mm Hg, continue nonoperative treatment. If ICP remains elevated, consider fasciotomy (with informed patient consent).

*CroFab (Fougera, Melville, NY).
†ACP, Antivenin (Crotalidae) Polyvalent (Wyeth-Ayerst Laboratories, Philadelphia).

Because many significant pit viper bites result in swollen extremities that are discolored and painful on any attempted range of motion, it can be difficult to determine when a compartment syndrome is imminent. This complication is actually rare following pit viper bites, but if there is concern about rising intracompartmental pressures, these can be objectively measured using any standard technique. If the pressures are elevated above 30 to 40 mm Hg, the limb is further elevated, more antivenom is administered, and mannitol is given (1.0 gm/kg IV over 30 minutes).[4] If the compartment pressure remains high 1 hour after these measures have been carried out, a fasciotomy should be considered. Although animal research has suggested an actual increase in myonecrosis following fasciotomy,[42] there is still a risk of ischemic neuropathy following unabated rises in compartment pressure. It is important to obtain informed consent, if possible, prior to proceeding with fasciotomy.

All patients with any evidence of envenomation are admitted to the hospital for further observation and management. If the poisoning is severe, the victim is admitted to an intensive care unit. If it appears that the snake did not inject any venom (i.e., there are no signs or symptoms of envenomation; simple puncture wounds only), the victim is observed in the ED for a minimum of 8 hours. After 8 hours, victims who remain asymptomatic, with normal vital signs and laboratory evaluations, are discharged in the care of a responsible adult and told to return if any evidence of envenomation occurs.

Nonenvenomation (so-called "dry bites") occurs in as many as 20% of pit viper bites, although the precise reason for this remains unclear.[8,43] Any child with a possible venomous snakebite is admitted to the hospital regardless of the presence or absence of signs or symptoms of poisoning. Likewise, victims of possible coral snake bite are admitted for observation because of the significant delay that can occur before any evidence of envenomation occurs.

■ RECURRENT COAGULOPATHY

Patients who develop coagulopathy during the initial stages of envenomation may develop delayed recurrence of abnormal coagulation studies for up to 2 weeks following the bite.[39,44] This is likely related to continued absorption of venom components from the depot site after all administered antivenom has been cleared from the body, particularly when a small molecular weight Fab antivenom is used. In most cases, delayed coagulopathy is benign, without evidence of clinically significant bleeding. Patients are warned of this possibility and instructed to avoid any elective surgery, contact sports, and other high-risk activities for a few weeks following the bite. Although antivenom administration for delayed coagulopathy may be effective, it is likely to be less effective than in the acute stages of envenomation, and its delayed use in the absence of clinical bleeding is controversial. Most such cases can be monitored on an outpatient basis without further antivenom administration.

Conclusion

Management of snake envenomation can be complicated. It requires the use of sound clinical judgment and careful initial evaluation of the patient with frequent monitoring for progression of severity. There are many available resources for assistance in managing these cases, including regional poison control centers, which usually maintain a list of snakebite experts on-call and available to assist in management of these cases. Consultation is obtained whenever necessary. A thoughtful approach to the victim of snakebite will yield the best possible outcome.

PATIENT TEACHING TIPS

- Never approach, torment, or attempt to catch or kill a venomous or unidentified species of snake.
- Do not keep any species of venomous snake as a "pet."
- Never handle a venomous snake that you believe is dead. These snakes may still have a bite reflex and can inflict a serious bite.
- If bitten by a venomous or unknown snake, proceed immediately to the nearest hospital for evaluation. No first-aid measures are effective or necessary following bites by pit vipers.
- If you have been treated for a venomous snakebite with antivenom, watch for signs of serum sickness (fever, muscle aches, joint aches, hives) in the first 2 weeks after you leave the hospital. If these occur, follow up immediately with your physician.
- Avoid any elective surgery, contact sports, or high-risk activities for 2 to 3 weeks after a pit viper bite, because your blood may not clot normally for this period of time

REFERENCES

1. Norris RL, Bush SP: Bites by venomous reptiles in the Americas. In Auerbach PS (ed): Wilderness Medicine, 5th ed. Philadelphia, Mosby, 2007, pp 1051-1085.
2. Russell FE: AIDS, cancer, and snakebite—what do these three have in common? West J Med 1988;148:84-85.
3. Dart RC, McNally J: Efficacy, safety, and use of snake antivenoms in the United States. Ann Emerg Med 2001;37:181-188.
4. Gomez HF, Dart RC: Clinical toxicology of snakebite in North America. In Meier J, White J (eds): Handbook of Clinical Toxicology of Animal Venoms and Poisons. Boca Raton, Fla, CRC Press, 1995.
5. Simon TL, Grace TG: Evenomation coagulopathy from snake bites. New Engl J Med 1981;305:1347-1348.
6. Dart RC, Gold BS: Crotaline snakebite. In Dart RC, Caravati EM, McGuigan MA, et al (eds): Medical Toxicology, 3rd ed. Philadelphia, Lippincott Williams & Wilkins, 2004, pp 1559-1565.
7. Kamiguti AS: Platelets as targets of snake venom metalloproteinases. Toxicon 2005;45:1041-1049.
8. Russell FE: Snake Venom Poisoning. New York, Scholium International, 1983.
9. Gutierrez JM, Rucavadoa R, Escalantea T, Diaz C: Hemorrhage induced by snake venom metalloproteinases: Biochemical and biophysical mechanisms involved in microvessel damage. Toxicon 2005;45:997-1011.
10. White J: Snake venoms and coagulopathy. Toxicon 2005;45:951-967.
11. Clark RF, Williams SR, Nordt SP, Boyer-Hassen LV: Successful treatment of crotalid-induced neurotoxicity with a new polyspecific crotalid Fab antivenom. Ann Emerg Med 1997;30:54.
12. Jansen PW, Perkin RM, Van Stralen D: Mojave rattlesnake envenomation: Prolonged neurotoxicity and rhabdomyolysis. Ann Emerg Med 1992;21:322.
13. Glenn JL, Straight RC: Venom characteristics as an indicator of hybridization between *Crotalus viridis viridis* and *Crotalus scutalatus scutulatus* in New Mexico. Toxicon 1990;28:857.
14. Glenn JL, Straight RC, Wolt TB: Regional variation in the presence of canebrake toxin in *Crotalus horridus* venom. Comp Biochem Physiol 1994;107C:337.
15. Hendon RA, Bieber AL: Presynaptic toxins from rattlesnake venoms. In Tu AT (ed): Rattlesnake Venoms: Their Actions and Treatment. New York, Marcel Dekker, 1982.
16. Weinstein SA, Minton SA, Wilde CE: The distribution among ophidian venoms of a toxin isolated from the venom of the Mojave rattlesnake (*Crotalus scutalatus scutulatus*). Toxicon 1985;23:825.
17. French WJ, Hayes WK, Bush SP, et al: Mojave toxin in venom of *Crotalus helleri* (southern Pacific rattlesnake): Molecular and geographic characterization. Toxicon 2004;44:781-791.
18. Chang CC: The action of snake venoms on nerve and muscle. In Lee CY (ed): Snake Venoms. New York, Springer-Verlag, 1979.
19. Van Mierop LHS: Poisonous snakebite: A review—snakes and their venom. J Fla Med Assoc 1976;63:191.
20. Klauber LM: Rattlesnakes: Their Habits, Life Histories, and Influence on Mankind, 2nd ed. Berkeley, University of California Press, 1997.

21. Wingert WA, Wainschel J: Diagnosis and management of envenomation by poisonous snakes. South Med J 1975;68:1015.
22. Pettigrew LC, Glass JP: Neurologic complications of a coral snake bite. Neurology 1985;35:589-592.
23. Norris RL, Dart RC: Apparent coral snake envenomation in a patient without fang marks. Am J Emerg Med 1989;7:402.
24. Kitchens CS, Van Mierop LHS: Envenomation by the eastern coral snake (*Micrurus fulvius fulvius*): A study of 39 victims. JAMA 1987;258:1615.
25. Van Mierop LH, Kitchens CS: Defibrination syndrome following bites by the eastern diamondback rattlesnake. J Fla Med Assoc 1980;67:21-27.
26. Norris RL, Ngo J, Nolan K, Hooker G: Physicians and lay people are unable to apply pressure immobilization properly in a simulated snakebite scenario. Wilderness Environ Med 2005;16:16-21.
27. Sutherland SK, Coulter AR, Harris RD: Rationalisation of first-aid measures for elapid snakebite. Lancet 1979;1:183-185.
28. German BT, Hack JB, Brewer K, Meggs WJ: Pressure-immobilization bandages delay toxicity in a porcine model of eastern coral snake (*Micrurus fulvius fulvius*) envenomation. Ann Emerg Med 2005;45(6):603-608.
29. Schaeffer RC, Carlson RW, Puri VK, et al: The effects of colloidal and crystalloidal fluids on rattlesnake venom shock in the rat. J Pharmacol Exp Ther 1978;206:687-695.
30. Dart RC, McNally JT, Spaite DW: The sequelae of pit viper poisoning in the United States. In Campbell JA, Brodie ED (eds): Biology of the Pitvipers. Tyler, TX, Selva, 1992.
31. Hardy DL, Bush SP: Pressure/immobilization as first aid for venomous snakebite in the United States. Herpetol Rev 1996;29:204.
32. Carroll RR, Hall EL, Kitchens CS: Canebrake rattlesnake envenomation. Ann Emerg Med 1997;30:45-48.
33. Kitchens CS, Hunter S, Van Mierop LHS: Severe myonecrosis in a fatal case of envenomation by the canebrake rattlesnake (*Crotalus horridus atricaudatus*). Toxicon 1987;25:455-458.
34. Suchard JR, LoVecchio F: Envenomations by rattlesnakes thought to be dead [letter]. N Engl J Med 1999; 340:1929.
35. Bond GR, Burkhart KK: Thrombocytopenia following timber rattlesnake envenomation. Ann Emerg Med 1997;30:40.
36. Bush SP, Wu VH, Corbett SW: Rattlesnake venom-induced thrombocytopenia response to Antivenin (Crotalidae) Polyvalent. Acad Emerg Med 2000;7:181-185.
37. Jurkovich GJ, Luterman A, McCuller K, et al: Complications of Crotalidae antivenin therapy. J Trauma 1988;28:1032-1037.
38. Gold BS, Dart RC, Barish RA: Bites of venomous snakes. New Engl J Med 2002;347:347-356.
39. Package insert. CroFab, Brentwood, TN, Protherics, Inc., 2006. http://www.fougera.com/products/crofab_digifab/crofab_packageinsert.pdf (accessed February 27, 2007).
40. Davidson TM, Eisner J: United States coral snakes. Wilderness Environ Med 1996;1:38.
41. Burgess JL, Dart RC: Snake venom coagulopathy: Use and abuse of blood products in the treatment of pit viper envenomation. Ann Emerg Med 1991;10:795.
42. Tanen DA, Danish DC, Grice GA, et al: Fasciotomy worsens the amount of myonecrosis in a porcine model of crotaline envenomation. Ann Emerg Med. 2004;44:99-104.
43. Parrish HM, Goldner JC, Silberg SL: Poisonous snakebites causing no venenation. Postgrad Med 1966;39:265-269.
44. Bogdan GM, Dart RC, Falbo SC, et al: Recurrent coagulopathy after antivenom treatment of crotalid snakebite. South Med J 2000;93:562-566.

Chapter 157

Arthropod Bites and Stings

Rais Vohra and Richard F. Clark

KEY POINTS

- Most envenomations and/or mechanical injuries due to arthropods can be treated with symptomatic medications for pain and pruritus.
- Anaphylaxis is a potential complication of hymenoptera stings and requires immediate diagnosis and treatment with epinephrine, steroids, and antihistamines. Patients should be discharged with a short course of steroids and an epinephrine auto-injector (Epi-Pen).
- Patients should be advised about the subacute or delayed development of infectious complications of insect bites/stings, particularly ticks, flies, fleas, and reduviid bugs.
- Patients bitten by black widow spiders can present with severe pain and hyperdynamic vital signs. The most important treatment for these conditions is adequate analgesia.
- Treatment for dermonecrotic arachnidism is controversial. In the ED setting, patients should be advised that the lesion may progress regardless of therapy because of ongoing venom effects within the skin.

Scope and Outline

Bites or stings from insects, spiders, and a variety of other arthropods are common complaints in the ED. One challenge in the approach to these injuries is that the perpetrating organism is often small and the initial encounter goes unnoticed; children especially are unable to provide details important for identification of the offending creature. Thus it is important to approach potential bites and stings with a keen grasp of the signs and symptoms expected to result from envenomation by arthropods endemic to the ED location. Furthermore, the EP must be familiar with not only the most common manifestations of these injuries, but also with the less common but serious complications of arthropod injuries that can mimic many other systemic disorders.

This chapter is a summary of common and medically important illnesses as they relate to arthropods. Acute features, diagnostic considerations, and therapeutic strategies of the bites or stings of insects, arachnids, and related arthropods are discussed. Common clinical effects of arthropod encounters are summarized in Table 157-1.

Patterns of human injury after encounters with arthropods can essentially be divided into four categories: traumatic, toxic, allergic, and infectious (typically via transmission of blood-borne pathogens that reside in insect salivary secretions). This chapter focuses on the first two types of illness, which usually result from mechanical trauma or the consequences of envenomation from bites or stings. A brief discussion of allergic reactions is included because anaphylactic reactions to hymenoptera envenomation are an important cause of mortality and morbidity. Infectious complications of insect and tick bites are discussed more fully in other chapters in this textbook.

Table 157-1 COMMON CLINICAL MANIFESTATIONS OF ARTHROPOD ENVENOMATION

Arthropod	Common Clinical Manifestations
Ants	Urticarial and papular dermatitis
Caterpillars	Painful papular dermatitis; ocular and mucosal irritation
Scabies	Severe, migratory pruritus; inflamed, scaly skin
Mites	Papular urticaria
Ticks	Local granulomatosis; paralysis; infectious complications
Reduviid bugs	Bullous dermal lesions; infectious complications
Bees	Urticarial eruptions; anaphylaxis risk; rhabdomyolysis, ARF, ARDS with massive envenomation burden
Wasps	Urticarial eruptions and anaphylaxis risk
Lice and fleas	Papular urticaria
Mosquitoes	Urticaria, pruritus, infectious complications
Black widow spiders	Severe muscular spasm and pain; hyperdynamic crisis
Recluse spiders	Progressive dermonecrosis; rarely hemolysis, DIC, ARDS
Tarantulas	Urticarial dermatitis, ocular irritation (hairs); pain (bites)
Scorpions	Pain, tingling, cranial neuropathy, ataxia; pancreatitis, DIC, ARDS (exotic species)
Centipedes	Pain
Millipedes	Pruritus; discoloration of skin due to oily excretions

ARDS, acute respiratory distress syndrome; ARF, acute renal failure; DIC, disseminated intravascular coagulation.

Anatomy and Pathophysiology

The arthropods represent a phylum that contains four fifths of all known organisms, including all insects, spiders, scorpions, and related creatures such centipedes and millipedes. Arthropods can be subdivided into classes; the most medically relevant include Insecta (bees, wasps, ants, lice, fleas, flies, butterflies, bedbugs, and mosquitoes), Arachnida (spiders, scorpions, ticks, and mites), Chilopoda (centipedes), and Diplopoda (millipedes). Although the anatomy of arthropod species seems bewilderingly diverse, it is useful to subdivide them into insects, arachnids, chilopods, and diplopods.

Insects have three body segments, three pairs of legs, one or two pairs of wings, and one pair of antennae. Considerable variability exists among the insects, resulting in fascinating anatomic adaptations that are beyond the scope of this chapter. Bites can be inflicted by certain creatures with developed mouth parts such as flies, fleas, and mosquitoes, whereas "stings" are delivered via modified (non–egg depositing) ovipositor or hairlike projections.

Arachnids (scorpions, spiders, ticks, and mites) have four pairs of legs, two body segments, and no wings or antennae. Scorpions have a stinging appendage in the shape of a bulbous sac (telson) in the caudal abdomen. All spiders can manufacture both venom and silk, but different species demonstrate considerable variability in their use of these adaptations. Medically relevant spiders include tarantulas, widows, recluse spiders, hobo spiders, and funnel web spiders. Mites and ticks are distinguished by a primitive oral orifice known as a gnathosoma, and fused abdomen and cephalothoracic segments. Mites and ticks can transmit a variety of infections because they generally feed on blood of host animals or humans, allowing transmission of bloodborne diseases.

Chilopods (centipedes) and diplopods (millipedes) are worm-like organisms with a large number of body segments. Centipedes have one pair of legs per body segment and are typically carnivorous, whereas millipedes have two pairs per segment and are usually herbivorous.[1]

Hymenoptera

■ ANATOMY AND PATHOPHYSIOLOGY

The order Hymenoptera contains insects with complex social organization and roles. In general they live in communities, so there is a risk of multiple stings with each encounter. The envenomation apparatus is a modified ovipositor located in the caudal abdominal segment. There are three families of medical relevance. Ants (Formicidae) are highly socially organized creatures, with each colony or mound potentially containing thousands of members. Wasps, hornets, and yellow jackets (Vespidae) are aggressive nest-builders, and each creature has the ability to sting multiple times. Bees (Apidae) can sting only once, because the ovipositor is barbed and once embedded into skin or clothing cannot be withdrawn. The domesticated (Italian) varieties in the United States generally are passive and avoid humans unless disturbed. In contrast, feral and aggressive colonies from South America have been found in Mexico and the southern United States since the 1990s. These bees, descended from strains of African species hybridized with domestic types in Brazil, have gradually migrated northward. They are difficult to distinguish morphologically from the domesticated bees, but in their behavior they are extremely

ing or nonhealing cases may require delayed reconstructive procedures once the destructive effect of the venom has halted.

An experimental *Loxosceles* antivenom has also been developed, but, based on data in animal models, it must be given within 24 hours in order to be effective. Because most patients present 2 to 3 days after being bitten, this type of antivenom is not a clinically useful adjunct in the treatment of *Loxosceles* spider bites.[8] Symptomatic and intensive supportive care is warranted in the rare cases of disseminated intravascular coagulation, hemolytic anemia, renal failure, and acute respiratory distress syndrome following the bites of recluse spiders.

■ TARANTULAS

Tarantulas are distributed worldwide and recognizable by their prominent hair-like projections. Large or aggressive species can bite, but the majority of human injuries result from the hairs. Effects of bites can range from relatively painless to deep, throbbing pain with a febrile reaction that requires analgesics and antipyretics.

By rubbing their hind legs against the abdominal wall, tarantulas can "flick" their hairs in the direction of perceived threats, and both dermal and ocular injuries have occurred from the highly irritating "urticating" hairs of tarantulas. The presence of urticaria, hives, intense pruritus, and mild erythema characterizes dermal lesions; ocular exposures to the urticating hairs have resulted in corneal abrasions, iritis, uveitis, and chronic granulomatous reactions (opthalmia nodosum).

■ Treatment

Therapy is essentially supportive with analgesics and antihistamines. Opthalmic antibiotics or steroids in conjunction with close follow-up or emergency ophthalmology consultation may be necessary in cases of ocular exposure to tarantula hairs.

■ SCORPIONS

The scorpion is easily recognized by a tail-like abdominal segment that forms into a venom-filled bulb (*telson*). In the United States, scorpions are commonly encountered hazards mainly in the southwest, where *Centruroides exilicauda* (formerly *C. sculpturatus*), or the bark scorpion, is endemic. They commonly hide in dark spaces such as closets and shoes; the exoskeleton's ability to fluoresce under ultraviolet light is sometimes helpful in localizing these creatures. Worldwide, species that represent significant hazards to human health include *Tityus* spp. in Trinidad and Brazil, and *Buthus* and *Parabuthus* spp. in India, Africa, and the Middle East. Most scorpion stings occur when the creature feels threatened or alarmed.

The venom of *C. exilicauda* is complex and targets excitable membranes. The result is abnormal prolonged opening of sodium channels at the neuromuscular junction and at both sympathetic and parasympathetic nerve endings. Dangerous varieties of scorpions from other countries can cause a massive release of catecholamines from nerve terminals, particularly norepinephrine and acetylcholine, leading to diverse effects.

■ Clinical Effects

Local effects of erythema and tingling may be present, but these may be quite subtle initially. Tapping the site of discomfort gently accentuates the reported symptoms, even in the absence of visible skin lesions. Systemic symptoms, which are more dramatic than local effects, peak around 5 hours after the sting; these commonly include hypertension, tachycardia, convulsions, cranial neuropathies, roving opthalmoplegia (also known as "oculogyric crisis"), ataxia, abdominal cramps, and respiratory failure from neuromuscular dysfunction.

The stings of other scorpion genera may produce unique syndromes. Tityus scorpions in Trinidad and South America can cause pancreatitis, and in India and Africa, the *Buthus* and *Parabissesuthus* varieties can cause pulmonary hemorrhage, gastrointestinal bleeding, and disseminated intravascular coagulation, presumably because of the presence of phospholipase in the venom.

■ Diagnostic Testing

Testing of serum electrolytes, creatinine phosphokinase (CPK), and cardiac isozymes, as well as chest radiography and electrocardiography should be considered in patients at high risk of cardiac ischemia. Neurologic testing such as computed tomography of the head and lumbar puncture may be required in cases in which other neurologic disease processes are suspected.

■ Treatment

The majority of patients respond to supportive care and aggressive pain management with analgesics and muscle relaxants.[9] Continuous infusion of benzodiazepines may be considered in well-monitored patients to decrease agitation and abnormal motor activity.[10] Short-acting antihypertensives such as esmolol or nitroprusside are also appropriate in the setting of severe hypertension and tachycardia.

Respiratory failure or fatigue warrant aggressive airway management and possibly intubation; this complication is especially concerning in the pediatric and elderly populations, which are most vulnerable to mortality from scorpion stings. Rarely, pancreatitis and coagulopathy require intensive supportive care with meticulous fluid management and transfusion of blood products.

Scorpion antivenom is not presently available in the United States.

Disposition

Patients with severe signs and symptoms require admission, and intensive care may be necessary for pediatric and elderly patients. Patients who are comfortable and have normal vital signs and diagnostic testing results can safely be discharged. Wounds from scorpion stings do not usually require specific therapy for infection.

TICK PARALYSIS

Several members of the *Dermacentor, Ixodes,* and *Amblyoma* genera of ticks can induce a rapidly progressive syndrome of ascending weakness and hyporeflexia. The lower extremities are affected first, similarly to Guillain-Barré syndrome. Careful physical examination is the key to diagnosis, since the tick remains attached to the skin while the paralytic neurotoxin is active. Removal of the offending tick rapidly leads to resolution of symptoms. Although the tick can be found attached to the skin in any anatomic location, well-protected areas such as the clothing waistline and the occipital scalp in victims with long hair are common sites of injury.

The condition is most common in the Rocky Mountain states and Pacific Northwestern United States. Although the pathogenesis is not fully elucidated, the neurotoxin is presumed to inhibit acetylcholine release at the neuromuscular junction. Respiratory failure is the most feared complication of a delayed diagnosis. In contrast to Guillain-Barré syndrome, cerebrospinal flluid analysis is normal in patients with tick paralysis.

SCABIES

Scabies is caused by the mite *Sarcoptes scabiei* var. *hominis,* an obligate parasite that resides in the epidermis. The adult female burrows and travels in the epidermal layers after impregnation, depositing several eggs daily. Males are smaller and die after copulation. Shedding and fecal droppings of the burrowing mite trigger a severely pruritic and mildly inflammatory reaction in the skin.

Most mites are transmitted via intimate interpersonal contact, but the adult forms of the mite can survive remote from human tissues for 24 to 36 hours in bedding, clothing, and furniture. Dogs and cats can host other variants of the scabies mite that cannot complete their life cycle in humans but are able to survive up to 96 hours in human skin. Contact with infected pets can cause humans to develop a self-limited illness characterized by itchy papules and urticaria.

Clinical Presentation

Severe nocturnal pruritus is the most characteristic symptom of scabies infestation. The typical skin findings are linear or curved burrows in the epidermal tissues, although excoriation can confound the appearance of these lesions. Nonspecific thickening and papules can result from long-standing cases that have prompted scratching of the skin surface.

Norwegian scabies is a severe, highly contagious form of the illness characterized by the presence of thousands of organisms and is seen most often in institutionalized or immunocompromised patients.

Diagnosis

Microscopy of the burrow contents can confirm the presence of organisms, egg casings, or fecal material from the ectoparasites. A specimen can be prepared by scraping the burrow with a scalpel lubricated with microscope oil and then smearing the blade onto a cover slip. Finger webspaces, wrists, elbows, and unscratched skin are the most productive sites of sampling. Patients with a large burden of organisms should be checked for underlying immunodeficiency.

Treatment

Treatment of scabies infestation consists of topical and oral antipruritic medications and antihistamines. Scabicidal therapy may include several weeks of topical permethrin cream (5%) or a single dose of oral ivermectin. Therapies no longer advocated include sulfur petrolatum balms and lindane, an organochlorine insecticide with the potential for neurotoxicity. Pretreatment with salicyclic acid ointments can help to soften scaled skin and allow better dermal penetration of topical scabicides.

All clothing and linens must be laundered and potential contacts must be treated simultaneously to avoid reinfection. Scabies-affected pets also should be treated with a scabicide.

MISCELLANEOUS MITES

Mites are small arachnids that reside in a wide variety of environments; approximately 50 species are known to cause skin lesions in people. Some species can also trigger anaphylactic reactions and transmit infectious diseases. Various mites thrive naturally in or on grains, pets, rodent pests, feathers, furniture, house floors, and straw. Upon inadvertent human contact, they can produce urticaria and pruritus.

Treatment is symptomatic and includes antihistamines and thorough cleansing of the skin and infested clothing and linens. Professional extermination may be necessary in cases of heavy infestation.

REFERENCES

1. Balit CR, Harvey MS, Waldock JM, et al: Prospective study of centipede bites in Australia. J Toxicol Clin Toxicol 2004; 42:41-48.
2. Betten DP, Richardson WH, Tong TC, et al: Massive honey bee envenomation-induced rhabdomyolysis in an adolescent. Pediatrics 2006;117:231.
3. Reisman RE: Unusual reactions to insect stings. Curr Opin Allergy Clin Immunol 2005;5:355-358.
4. Diaz JH: The evolving global epidemiology, syndromic classification, management, and prevention of caterpillar envenoming. Am J Trop Med Hyg 2005;72:347-357.
5. Hendrickson RG: Images in clinical toxicology: Millipede exposure. Clin Tox 2005;43:211-212.
6. da Silva PH, da Silveira RB, Appel MH, et al: Brown spiders and loxoscelism. Toxicon 2004;44:693-709.
7. Diaz JH: Global epidemiology, syndromic classification, management and prevention of *spider* bites. Am J Trop Med Hyg 2004;71:239-250.
8. Murray LM, Seger DL: Hemolytic anemia following a presumptive brown recluse spider bite. J Toxicol Clin Toxicol 1994;32:451-457.
9. Gateau T, Bloom M, and Clark R: Response to specific *Centuroides sculpturatus* antivenom in 151 cases of scorpion stings. Clin Toxicol 1994;32:165-171.
10. Gibly R, Williams M, Walter FG et al: Continuous intravenous midazolam infusion for *C. exilicauda* scorpion envenomation. Ann Emerg Med 1999;34:620-625.

Chapter 158

Non-Snake Reptile Bites

Troy E. Madsen and Stephen C. Hartsell

KEY POINTS

- Alligator and crocodile bites may inflict significant internal injury and should be managed as major traumas. Gila monsters and Mexican beaded lizards are the only non-snake venomous reptiles.
- Gila monster bites may leave teeth in the wound that are not visible by radiography.
- All patients with a Gila monster bite should be observed for 6 hours after the bite due to the risk of systemic toxicity.
- Komodo dragon bites carry a high risk of infection, due to the multiple flora carried in the reptile's mouth.
- Green iguanas and snapping turtles may carry Salmonella organisms.
- As with all animal bites, delayed wound closure should be considered, based on cosmetic considerations and the length of time from the bite to presentation.
- A 3- to 5-day course of prophylactic antibiotics is advisable, as well as careful follow-up to watch for signs of infection.

Scope

Although all reptiles have the potential to bite and to inflict some damage, this chapter focuses on several unique reptiles, excluding snakes, that can cause important complications. The prevalence of reptiles as pets increases the public's exposure to these animals, as well as to the potential harm associated with their bites.

Crocodilians

■ ANATOMY AND PATHOPHYSIOLOGY

Crocodilians comprise 23 species, but this section focuses on the two species most known for significant injury and potentially unprovoked attacks: the American alligator and the saltwater crocodile.

The American alligator (*Alligator mississippiensis*) is the largest reptile in North America; males average over 11 feet (3.5 m) in length, but may grow up to 16 feet (5 m) long and weigh almost 1000 pounds (450 kg). The alligator has a broader, more rounded snout than the crocodile. The American alligator may be found in the southeastern United States, from Florida to North Carolina. Sightings have been reported in other states, but these animals are presumed to be pets that were released. Approximately 400 alligator bites and 23 deaths from bites have been reported in United States since 1948.[1,2]

The saltwater crocodile (*Crocodylus porosus*) typically is found in more tropical climates, and much of the current information on attacks comes from Australia. Male saltwater crocodiles may reach lengths of greater than 23 feet (7 m). Between 1971 and 2004, 62 unprovoked crocodile attacks were reported in Australia, and 17 of these attacks were fatal. Nearly all of these attacks were on people swimming or wading in water.[3]

Other species of crocodilians (such as the black caiman, *Melanosuchus niger*) may inflict significant injury, but reports of unprovoked attacks by these species are rare. Evaluation and management of bites from these animals are similar to those from the American alligator and saltwater crocodile (Fig. 158-1).

■ PRESENTING SIGNS AND SYMPTOMS

Crocodilian bites are characterized by punctures and tears. Once the alligator or crocodile bites, it rotates on its long axis to tear the limbs and drown its victim; the animal's teeth are not designed for chewing but for grasping, while the strength of its body motion rips pieces from the victim. Crocodilians may also roll their entire body (known as the "death roll") to disorient and drown the victim, as well as to rip pieces from the victim's body.[3] The force of the alligator's massive jaws may lead to extensive internal injury.

■ ED EVALUATION

Victims of crocodilian bites often present with injuries comparable to those sustained in a severe motor vehicle collision. The EP should first make sure that there is adequate airway control, breathing, and circulatory support. Resuscitation with advanced life support measures may be appropriate. Individuals sustaining crocodilian bites may present after drowning or near-drowning events.

A secondary evaluation should be made to determine the extent of tendon, neurologic, and vascular

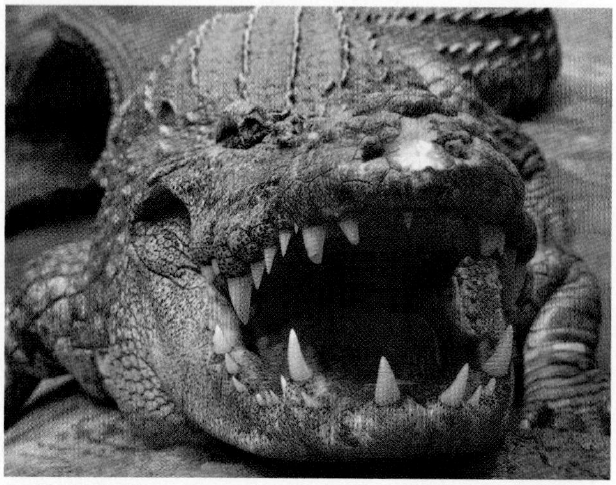

FIGURE 158-1 Crocodile. (Photo courtesy of Hogle Zoo, Salt Lake City, Utah.)

PRIORITY ACTIONS

Reptile Bite Wounds

- Evaluate for underlying vascular, tendon, nervous, or bony injury.
- Perform delayed wound closure or loosely approximate the wound, if possible.
- Facial wounds and others wounds with significant cosmetic concerns should be closed if the patients presents early and does not show signs of infection.
- Assure tetanus prophylaxis.
- Consider a 3- to 5-day course of prophylactic antibiotics with close outpatient follow-up to monitor for signs of infection.

injuries and possible internal organ damage. The crocodilian's bite may inflict significant internal injury, but even when bite wounds are not present, the force of the animal's movement, or even blunt trauma from its tail, may inflict massive internal injury.

Underlying bony injury should be considered, particularly in light of the force of the animal's bite, as well as more proximal injuries and dislocations, which may have been inflicted by the alligator's tearing motion.

■ DIAGNOSTIC TESTING

Depending on the nature and location of the bite, radiographs may aid in the physical examination. Computed tomography scanning may be useful to evaluate for internal injury, much as one would employ this diagnostic tool in the evaluation of a motor vehicle collision victim.

■ TREATMENT AND DISPOSITION

Specialists should be consulted to evaluate and treat internal injuries, tendon damage, fractures, and lacerations. Local wound care techniques are mandated to cleanse what are typically very contaminated wounds. Prophylactic broad-spectrum antibiotic therapy may be necessary to prevent wound infection. The patient's tetanus status should be checked and brought up to date.

Disposition is based on the extent of the injuries. If the patient is discharged, close follow-up is advisable for wound care and to evaluate for wound infection.

Gila Monster and Mexican Beaded Lizard

■ ANATOMY AND PATHOPHYSIOLOGY

The Gila monster (*Heloderma suspectum*) and the closely related Mexican beaded lizard (*Heloderma hor-*

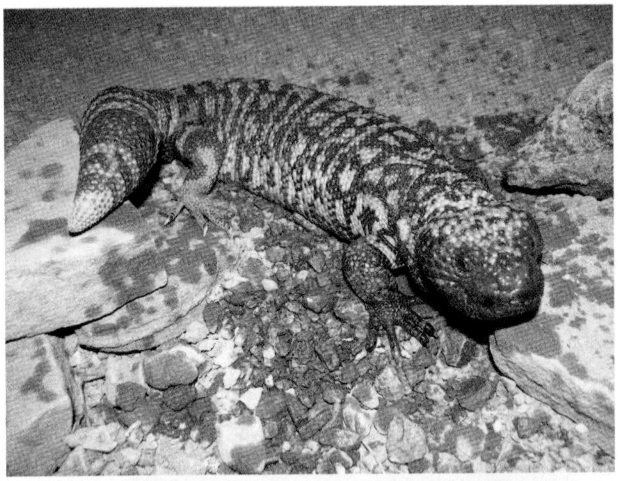

FIGURE 158-2 Gila monster. (Photo courtesy of Hogle Zoo, Salt Lake City, Utah.)

ridum) are characterized by yellow, orange, and pink scales mixed with bands of black scales and a thick, forked tongue. These reptiles typically range in length from 9 to 24 inches (22-60 cm); the Mexican beaded lizard is the larger of the two species.

These are the only two venomous lizards in the world; most envenomations are from captive animals. The animal has individual grooves in its teeth to deliver venom from anterior mandibular venom glands. A chewing motion augments the delivery of venom when attached to a victim.[4,5]

These reptiles are native to the southwestern United States and Mexico, but they may be found throughout the world in zoos and as illegal pets. The animals are most active during springtime, and they spend much of their lives underground, hibernating in the winter and staying hidden during hot summer months (Fig. 158-2).

■ PRESENTING SIGNS AND SYMPTOMS

Bite wounds are classically indurated and erythematous. Significant edema may develop at the site of the wound. Patients often describe excruciating pain associated with the bites. Patients may present with weakness, hypotension, and tachycardia, due to systemic effects of the animal's venom.

■ ED EVALUATION

The most important aspect of evaluation of the wound is physical examination for evidence of vascular or tendon injury and local wound exploration for retained teeth from the animal. Most reported cases of patients presenting to the ED for bites have associated systemic symptoms of hypotension, tachycardia, and weakness. Most patients also have significant pain and swelling associated with the wound.[4] Teeth have been found in wounds, and patients have presented with the animal still attached. The animal may also inflict damage to tendons and vascular structures.

The primary evaluation should focus on evidence of systemic symptoms associated with envenomation: hypotension, tachycardia, and weakness. Diagnostic testing may be necessary to rule out other potential causes of these symptoms.

PRIORITY ACTIONS

Envenomation by Gila Monster or Mexican Beaded Lizard

- Observe all patients for 6 hours to watch for the development of signs of envenomation.
- Initiate fluid therapy for hypotension and tachycardia.
- Initiate vasopressor therapy for hypotension and tachycardia unresponsive to fluids.
- Admit patients with systemic symptoms for observation and resolution of symptoms.
- Ensure tetanus prophylaxis.

■ DIAGNOSTIC TESTING

The most common reported laboratory abnormality in Gila monster bites is leukocytosis, although coagulopathy has also been reported in patients with envenomation.

Radiographs may be obtained to rule out associated fractures. However, retained teeth do not show up radiographically, and local wound exploration should be used to rule out this possibility.

■ TREATMENT AND DISPOSITION

If necessary, the animal must be removed from the patient. Increased time of the animal's bite increases the envenomation time. A flame placed under the animal's jaw usually will result in release within 3 to 5 seconds and decreases the possibility of leaving teeth in the wound while pulling or prying the animal loose. Other techniques, such as immersion in cold water, may be used as needed. Always take special care to prevent reattachment of the animal to the victim or subsequent attachment to the person removing the animal.

Envenomation may cause hypotension, tachycardia, and generalized weakness. These symptoms generally respond well to intravenous crystalloid administration. Refractory hypotension may require treatment with vasopressors such as dopamine. There is no commercially available antivenin for Gila monster or Mexican beaded lizard envenomation.

Patients should be observed for at least 6 hours to assess for signs of systemic toxicity. Hospitalize patients should be hospitalized as needed to treat systemic symptoms and for further resuscitation.

Tips and Tricks

ANIMAL REMOVAL

- Apply a flame under the animal's jaw.
- Immerse the animal in cold water.
- Use a handheld cast spreader to manually disengage the animal's mouth from the victim.
- Place a thin rod across the animal's mouth between the bite site and the jaw and push back on the jaw.
- Avoid pulling the animal off, if possible, as this may cause further tissue damage and release teeth into the wound.

Fractures, lacerations, and neurovascular function should be evaluated, as with any potentially penetrating wound. Teeth should be removed from the wound.

Pain typically requires large amounts of opiate analgesics; the few patients who have experienced both rattlesnake and Gila monster bites report much greater pain associated with the Gila monster bite. Pain generally peaks between 15 and 45 minutes following the bite and may last for days.

Although the use of prophylactic antibiotics in animal bites remain somewhat controversial, patients may benefit from treatment with broad-spectrum antibiotics, such as amoxicillin-clavulanate (Augmentin) for 3 to 5 days, with specific instructions to watch for signs of developing infection. Instruct in local wound care techniques. Delayed or loose wound closure should be considered to prevent early infection, and the patient should be instructed about local wound care techniques.

Tetanus prophylaxis is always necessary.[1]

Komodo Dragon

ANATOMY AND PATHOPHYSIOLOGY

The Komodo dragon (*Varanus komodoensis*) is the largest lizard in the world, reaching lengths of greater than 10 feet (3 m) and weighing as much as 360 pounds (165 kg). These lizards may run as fast as 13 miles per hour (20 km/hr). Komodo dragons' tooth serrations hold meat from their prey, which in turn nourishes multiple species of bacteria in the animal's mouth. If the initial bite does not kill the prey within 1 week, infections with these organisms usually will do so.

The Komodo dragons' natural habitat is the islands of Indonesia, but they are found in zoos throughout the world (Fig. 158-3).

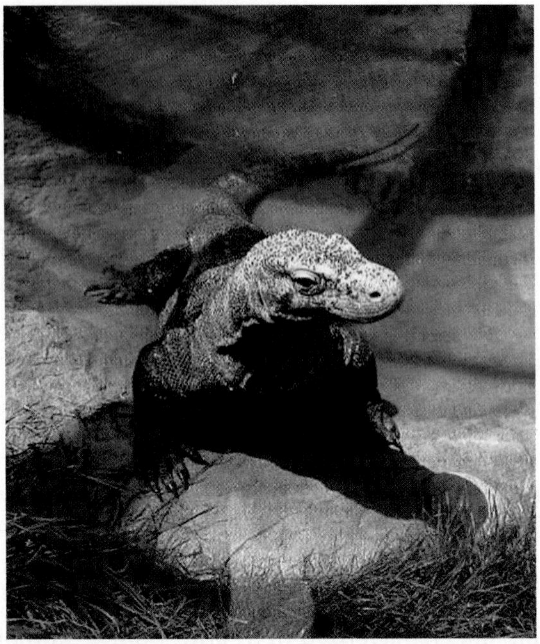

FIGURE 158-3 Komodo dragon. (Photo courtesy of Hogle Zoo, Salt Lake City, Utah.)

PRESENTING SIGNS AND SYMPTOMS

Most EP encounters with a Komodo dragon bite would expectedly come from an exposure at a zoo. Early bites typically demonstrate puncture wounds to the skin, with the potential for local tendon and vascular injury. Should patients delay presenting to the ED, these wounds may show signs of local or even systemic bacterial infection.

ED EVALUATION

EPs should be particularly aware of the potential for local and systemic wound infections with Komodo dragon bites, in light of the numerous bacteria harvested in the animal's mouth. Potential damage to tendons, nerves, vasculature, and underlying bony structures should be considered.

DIAGNOSTIC TESTING

Blood and local wound cultures may be useful to rule out other causes of hypotension and infection in the patient with system symptoms who may have delayed presentation to the ED. Radiography can identify underlying damage to bony structures.

TREATMENT AND DISPOSITION

Multiple bacteria have been isolated from the mouths of Komodo dragons; *Escherichia coli* is the most common organism in wild dragons, and *Staphylococcus* spp. are most common in captive animals.[6]

Treatment includes tetanus prophylaxis, broad-spectrum antibiotics, and close outpatient follow-up to monitor for signs of wound infection; hospitalization for IV antibiotics may be necessary even on initial presentation because of the high risk of significant infection in these wounds.

As with all bite wounds, delayed closure of the wound may be required, particularly because of the high risk of infection in the Komodo dragon bite wounds.

Green Iguana

■ ANATOMY AND PATHOPHYSIOLOGY

The green iguana (*Iguana iguana*) is native to Central and South America. It is the most common lizard sold in the United States as a pet, with over one million lizards imported each year (Fig. 158-4). There is no specific toxin associated with iguana bites.

■ PRESENTING SIGNS AND SYMPTOMS

Most reported damage from iguana bites is superficial soft tissue injury, although tendon injuries have been reported.[7] As with any bite, patients may present with infectious complications, particularly patients with delayed presentation.

■ ED EVALUATION

The physical examination should look for underlying tendon and vascular complications. Although associated bony damage is rare in iguana bites, this must be considered as well, as with all animal bites. Patients with delayed presentations should be evaluated for signs of developing infection.

When evaluating patients with an infected wound or septic-appearing patients, it is important to remember that green iguanas may carry *Salmonella*.

■ DIAGNOSTIC TESTING

Extensive diagnostic testing generally is not necessary in cases of iguana bites. Radiography may identify underlying bony injuries. Blood cultures and local wound cultures may be useful in wound infections with systemic signs and symptoms.

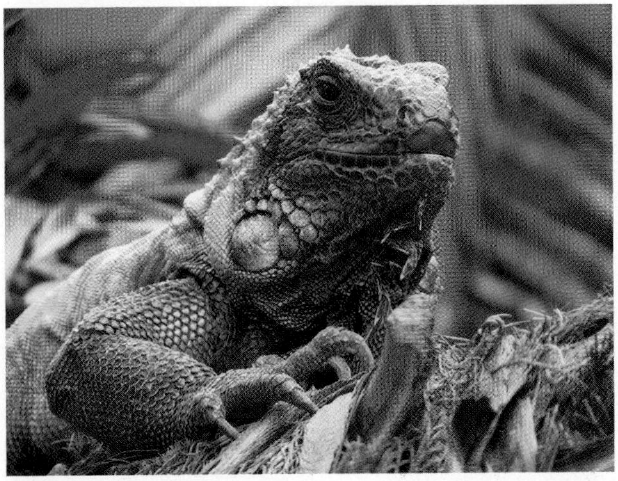

FIGURE 158-4 Iguana. (Photo courtesy of Hogle Zoo, Salt Lake City, Utah.)

■ TREATMENT AND DISPOSITION

As with any animal bite wounds, delayed wound closure should be carried out, if possible, and any underlying vascular, tendon, or bony injuries should be treated as appropriate. Prophylactic antibiotics remain somewhat controversial, but a 3- to 5-day course of ciprofloxacin, in light of the *Salmonella* typically carried by the green iguana, should be considered. In the septic-appearing patient or in one with developed wound infection requiring IV antibiotics, treatment with IV ceftriaxone may be beneficial. Tetanus prophylaxis is important.

Snapping Turtle

■ ANATOMY AND PATHOPHYSIOLOGY

The snapping turtle (*Chelydra serpentina*) has a powerful beak-like jaw and rigid shell. Turtles may be as long as 20 inches (50 cm) and are characterized by a long tail with spiky outgrowths, as well as a long neck that may extend up to two thirds the length of the body. These freshwater turtles live in habitats ranging from southeastern Canada to Mexico and Ecuador.

■ PRESENTING SIGNS AND SYMPTOMS

The snapping turtles' bite typically causes only soft tissue injury, but the force of its bite may lead to digit amputation, fractures, or damage to other underlying structures. Patients with delayed presentation to the ED may show signs of infection.

■ ED EVALUATION

When performing the physical examination, the ED should be aware of the potential for damage to nerve, vascular, and bony structures, because of the force of

FACTS AND FORMULAS $ST = \frac{SV}{BSA}$

ANTIBIOTIC THERAPY

- Crocodilian—multiple pathogens: Broad-spectrum coverage, such as amoxicillin-clavulanate (Augmentin)
- Gila monster—multiple pathogens: Broad-spectrum antibiotic coverage, such as amoxicillin-clavulate (Augmentin)
- Komodo dragon—multiple pathogens, including *Escherichia coli* and *Staphylococcus* spp.: Consider hospitalization for IV broad-spectrum antibiotics, such as ampicillin-sulbactam (Unasyn), because of high risk of infection
- Green lizard—may carry *Salmonella* spp.: *Salmonella* coverage, such as ciprofloxacin
- Snapping turtle—may carry *Salmonella* spp.: *Salmonella* coverage, such as ciprofloxacin

the snapping turtles' bite. Infection may occur in patients with delayed presentation.

■ DIAGNOSTIC TESTING

Radiography may be helpful to evaluate for underlying bony injury.

■ TREATMENT AND DISPOSITION

Underlying injuries should be repaired as appropriate. Delayed closure of wounds nay be necessary. Because snapping turtles may carry *Salmonella,* antibiotic prophylaxis with ciprofloxacin is advisable; in patients presenting with significant wound infections, treatment with IV ceftriaxone is recommended.

REFERENCES

1. Harding BE, Wolf BC: Alligator attacks in southwest Florida. J Forensic Sci 2006;51:674-677.
2. Langley RL: Alligator attacks on humans in the United States. Wilderness Environ Med 2005;16:119-124.
3. Caldicott DG, Croser D, Manolis C, et al: Crocodile attack in Australia: An analysis of its incidence and review of the pathology and management of crocodilian attacks in general. Wilderness Environ Med 2005;16:143-159.
4. Hooker KR, Caravati EM, Hartsell SC: Gila monster envenomation. Ann Emerg Med 1994;24:731-735.
5. Miller MF: Gila monster envenomation. Ann Emerg Med1995;25:720.
6. Montgomery JM, Gillespie D, Sastrawan P, et al: Aerobic salivary bacteria in wild and captive Komodo dragons. J Wildl Dis 2002;38:545-551.
7. Merin DS, Bush SP: Severe hand injury following a green iguana bite. Wilderness Environ Med. 2000;11:225-226.

Chapter 159

Marine Envenomation and Injuries

Christopher G. Jenson and Francis L. Counselman

KEY POINTS

Wounds that occur in fresh water may become infected by *Aeromonas* species. In salt water, *Vibrio* species can cause infection.

Ciprofloxacin and trimethoprim/sulfamethoxazole are effective against both *Aeromonas* and *Vibrio* species.

Ciguatera toxicity causes nausea, vomiting, and watery diarrhea followed by neurologic symptoms, including reversal of hot/cold sensation. Treatment includes mannitol, atropine for symptomatic bradycardia, and close follow-up since neurologic symptoms Scombroid poisoning is due to excess histamine, so it is treated like an allergic reaction, with antihistamines.

The pain of jellyfish stings diminishes with acetic acid treatment.

Scope and Outline

Hazardous aquatic organisms can be classified broadly into three categories based on their mechanism of injury: traumatic injuries, contact envenomation/bites and stings, and toxic marine ingestion (Fig. 159-1). Patients are not likely to remember "what" hurt them, but they usually remember "how" they were hurt; based on this limited information, logical assumptions may be made by the EP. Knowledge of these categories, combined with a rudimentary description by the patient, often provides sufficient information to treat the vast majority of injuries quickly and improve the morbidity and mortality of marine envenomation.

Traumatic Injuries

Most traumatic injuries in the water are caused by animals that are traditionally predators. Fortunately, it is exceedingly rare for these animals to hunt humans. When this does occur, the animal is usually searching for food or acting in self-defense. Perhaps the most infamous culprits are sharks. In 2006, 62 "unprovoked" shark attacks were documented, as well as numerous "provoked" encounters. Most of the reports come from Florida, with 23 incidents in 2006. This is a 50% increase from 1996.[1]

Other aquatic animals known to attack include barracudas, moray eels, giant groupers, sea lions, killer whales, and crocodiles. All of these animals can inflict traumatic wounds. The extent of injury is directly proportional to the size of the bite, exposure time to the offending agent, location of the inflicted wound, and power of the jaw or apparatus delivering the trauma.

Treatment of traumatic injuries depends upon the same thorough approach used for any other penetrating traumatic injury. After a primary survey is completed, resuscitative interventions are carried out,

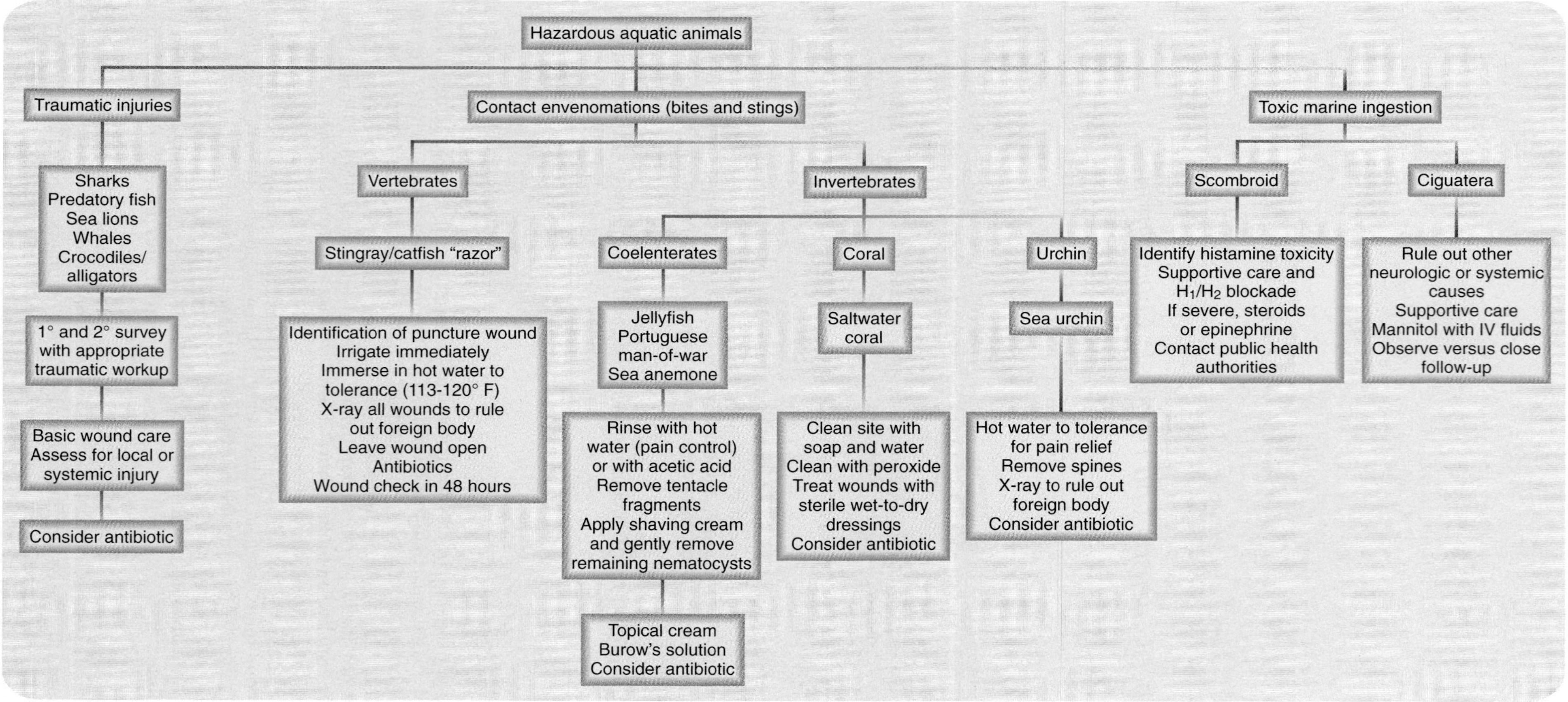

Hazardous aquatic animals
Traumatic injuries
Contact envenomations (bites and stings)
Toxic marine ingestion
Sharks
Predatory fish
Sea lions
Whales
Crocodiles/
alligators
1° and 2° survey
with appropriate
traumatic workup
Basic wound care
Assess for local or
systemic injury
Consider antibiotic
Vertebrates
Stingray/catfish “razor”
Identification of puncture wound
Irrigate immediately
Immerse in hot water to
tolerance (113-120° F)
X-ray all wounds to rule
out foreign body
Leave wound open
Antibiotics
Wound check in 48 hours
Invertebrates
Coelenterates
Jellyfish
Portuguese
man-of-war
Sea anemone
Rinse with hot
water (pain control)
or with acetic acid
Remove tentacle
fragments
Apply shaving cream
and gently remove
remaining nematocysts
Topical cream
Burow’s solution
Consider antibiotic
Coral
Saltwater
coral
Clean site with
soap and water
Clean with peroxide
Treat wounds with
sterile wet-to-dry
dressings
Consider antibiotic
Urchin
Sea urchin
Hot water to tolerance
for pain relief
Remove spines
X-ray to rule out
foreign body
Consider antibiotic
Scombroid
Identify histamine toxicity
Supportive care and
H_1/H_2 blockade
If severe, steroids
or epinephrine
Contact public health
authorities
Ciguatera
Rule out other
neurologic or systemic
causes
Supportive care
Mannitol with IV fluids
Observe versus close
follow-up

FIGURE 159-1 Algorithm for management of injuries caused by hazardous aquatic animals. 1° and 2°, primary and secondary.

Table 159-1 PHARMACOLOGIC TREATMENT OF DEEP LACERATIONS AND PUNCTURE WOUNDS

	INPATIENT	
Outpatient	Injuries from Salt Water Animals	Injuries from Fresh Water Animals
Bactrim Ciprofloxacin Tetracycline Doxycycline	Bactrim Ciprofloxacin Imipenem-cilastatin Aminoglycosides Cefoperazone Cefotaxime Ceftazidime Choramphenicol	Bactrim Ciprofloxacin Imipenem-cilastin Ceftazidime Gentamicin

wounds are identified, and imaging is completed if necessary; consideration can then be given to the specific nature of this injury.

Treatment of wounds requires exceptionally thorough local wound care. These injuries are at high risk for infection, including infection with *Aeromonas* bacteria, which are found in fresh water, and Vibrio bacteria, which occur in salt water. Antibiotics are often used for traumatic marine wounds.

All wounds should be irrigated with water or saline and investigated for the possibility of retained teeth, other biting implements, and foreign bodies. Standard dressings are employed. The wound should not be closed primarily, similar to other animal bites and wounds. Tetanus immunization should be provided if immunity is not otherwise assured.

Superficial lacerations or abrasions in the immunocompetent host do not need antibiotic prophylaxis, only wound care. Parmacologic medications for deep or complex wounds are listed in Table 159-1. Note that there is no role for the traditional combination of penicillin or first-generation cephalosporins that EDs often use for other types of cutaneous trauma.

Contact Envenomations (Bites and Stings)

Each year it is estimated that more than 40,000 envenomations occur from over eight different classes of fish. Most patients are unable to identify what injured them. However, a careful history may help establish the mechanism of injury.

Patients are usually able to recall that the injury was a contact envenomation. Further questioning may clarify whether the contact occurred with something floating, something swimming, or something fixed into coral/sea floor. The answer can help to quickly classify the injury as something that "stung them" or something that they "stepped on." These questions give insight into the likely organism and determine the course of action.

■ INVERTEBRATES

The casual observer may not identify many invertebrates as being alive. The beautiful coral and flora seen when ocean-diving tempts the observer to inspect closely. However, contact with the ocean floor provides quick and sometimes painful evidence that it is very much alive.

■ Coral

Coral is a common cause of invertebrae injury. Most corals possess a sharp, often razorlike, outer skeleton capable of causing "coral cuts." The mechanism of injury is simple but decisive. Any part of the patient that comes into contact with these edges can be lacerated. The resulting pain typically is immediate. It is common to later develop local erythema, swelling, and pruritic welts. In the next several hours to days, this can progress to cellulitis, ulceration, and necrosis.

Therapy includes cleaning the wound with soap and water followed by vigorous irrigation with sterile saline or peroxide. The wound may be covered with sterile wet-to-dry dressings. Antibiotics are not required unless the wound is major. A wound check in 48 hours is recommended.

■ Sea Urchins

Sea urchins have one of two defense mechanisms—either long, slender venom-bearing spines or triple-jawed pedicellariae. Both mechanisms cause essentially the same symptoms. Contact produces immediate pain described as burning. Local erythema and swelling develop quickly. Muscle cramps will commonly develop and last for 3 to 4 hours. Occasionally wounds caused by spines appear purple from injected dye.

Treatment for sea urchin stings is similar to that for coral cuts, with a few important additions. Soap and water may once again be used to clean the wound, but the water should be as hot as tolerable to neutralize the venom's burning sensation. All spines should be removed and a thorough investigation for foreign bodies should take place. Consider soft tissue radiographs, although all spines may not be easily visible. Standard wound care should be provided. Antibiotics usually are not needed but may be used for complex wounds.

Table 159-2 **CLINICAL MANIFESTATIONS OF JELLYFISH ENVENOMATION**

Mild Envenomation	Moderate Envenomation	Severe Envenomation
Skin irritation	All the findings of mild envenomation plus:	All the findings of moderate envenomation plus systemic manifestations such as:
Burning and paresthesia over contact area	Local edema	Arrhythmia
Whip-like pattern	Subepithelial hemorrhage	Bronchospasm
	Desquamation	Myalgia
	Potential ulceration	Nausea/vomiting
		Abdominal pain

■ Jellyfish and Related Species

Coelenterates, jellyfish and related species, injure through venomous nematocysts. There are more than 9000 species, collectively identified as "jellyfish," and about 100 of these species are hazardous to humans. The most notables are the Portuguese man-of-war, sea wasp, fire coral, and hell's fire sea anemone. These nematocysts are essentially clustered sacs of venom. One "sting" can be composed of hundreds to thousands of nematocysts discharging onto the target. The toxicity of these venoms highly variable. External factors such as the surface area of exposure, number of nematocysts, and number of times the victim is "stung" all come into play. Clinical manifestations range from local burning and paresthesia to myalgia, arrhythmia, and bronchospasm (Table 159-2).

Acetic acid is beneficial. Standard strength (5%) acetic acid or vinegar is applied to the wound for about 30 minutes. This helps inactivate the nematocysts and markedly decreases pain. If severe envenomation occurs, the patient may develop anaphylaxis to the venom. If a patient shows signs of cardiovascular collapse from envenomation, administration of histamine blockers, steroids, and epinephrine should be considered.

Once pain control has been established, the EP should double- or triple-glove for protection and attempt to remove all the tentacle fragments with a forceps. It is important to remove all the cysts because the toxic effect can last as long as they are in contact with the skin. Topical steroid or lotions may be applied. Patients will often need outpatient analgesia and should be encouraged to continue applying sterile dressings and Burow's solution daily until the wound is rechecked in 2 to 3 days.

■ Irukandji Jellyfish

The Irukandji jellyfish (*Carukia barnesi*) is worthy of special note because of its extreme toxicity. The natural habitat is in the northern waters of Australia.

Symptoms initially may appear mild but quickly progress. The manifestations are pain, sympathometic response, and cardiopulmonary collapse. The pain is usually localized to the chest, back, and abdomen regardless of where the victim was stung. It usually begins within 10 to 45 minutes and can last 4 to 30 hours after inoculation.[3] Sympathometic responses include delayed tachycardia, hypertension, and palpitations, often associated with vomiting.[4] Abnormal cardiac rhythms and myocardial damage may occur.

Occasionally, inotropic and pulmonary support with mechanical ventilation is required. There is some debate about the use of antivenin and IV verapamil, and aggressive supportive care is the primary treatment.

■ VERTEBRATES

Numerous vertebrates are capable of administering a sting. Patients usually relate that something "hurt them and then swam away." The ability of an organism to move under its own power usually provides an important clue to distinguish a vertebrate from an invertebrate. In all cases of injury from vertebrates, careful wound exploration and débridement of devitalized tissue are important.

■ Stingrays

The most notorious vertebrate offender is the stingray. Although there are numerous types of stingrays, all contain a whip-like tail with a venomous spine strategically located on the tail. Stingrays use this device to defend themselves from predators. Unfortunately, the occasional beach enthusiast walking along the sandy ocean floor can be on the receiving end.

Envenomation causes immediate local and intense pain in the spine. Usually about 10 minutes later, the deposited venom leads to further sharp, burning pain, with local edema and bleeding. This pain usually peaks at 30 to 60 minutes and may last for up to 48 hours.[5] Wounds often develop cellulitis in and in more serious cases the patient may develop systemic symptoms with gatrointestinal and neurologic complaints. Nausea, abdominal pain, diarrhea, seizures, paralysis, arrhythmias, and hypotension are not uncommon.

Treatment includes immediate wound irrigation and hot water (113-124°F) immersion to help with pain control. These wounds, due to the potential shattering of the spine, are at high risk for a retained foreign body. All patients should receive soft tissue radiography, and the wound should either be left open or be closed loosely. Additionally, because these wounds are from a puncture mechanism, prophylactic antibiotics are recommended.

Catfish and Related Species

Catfish and other "spiny" fish represent the other major class of vertebrate inoculations. These fish have razor-sharp dorsal and pectoral fins associated with venom glands. The venom is similar to that of the stingray, although usually with fewer systemic side effects. The mechanism of delivery is via contact with one of the fins, which produces immediate pain from the laceration. Within a matter of minutes, the pain spreads outward and often produces local swelling and erythema.

Therapy is similar to treatment of stingray injuries and once again, prophylactic antibiotics are recommended.

Toxic Marine Ingestion

Most EDs are familiar with the chief complaint of food poisoning. Rarely does the clinical presentation tend to be from a true toxin or poison. However, ocean cuisine is infamous for two types of envenomations—ciguatera toxicity and scombroid poisoning.

CIGUATERA

Ciguatera is one of the most commonly reported foodborne illness worldwide.[6] It is found in several hundred species of fish, but most often in predatory fish. Ciguatera is a heat-stable toxin produced by the dinoflagellate *Gambierdiscus toxicus*. This specific organism is found on algae attached to the coral reef. It is often consumed by small reef dwellers, which in turn are passed up the food chain to larger fish, which are consumed by humans. The toxin is not destroyed during cooking. Subsequently, the illness is due not to failure to prepare the fish properly but rather to chance, resulting in human inoculation.

Ciguatera toxicity is manifested as a bizarre constellation of gastrointestinal and neurologic symptoms because of sustained activation of sodium channels and additional cholinergic stimulation. Patients often complain of nausea, vomiting, and watery diarrhea within hours of ingestion. The captivating portion of ciguatera toxicity includes paresthesias and dysesthesias, especially the neurologic symptoms consisting of "loose teeth" and reversal of hot-cold sensation. This may progress to vertiginous symptoms and cardiac conduction abnormalities.

The severity of symptoms is difficult to predict, but symptoms often are more severe with increasing age. Life-threatening symptoms are usually restricted to those who were previously poisoned. These types of symptoms require an extensive work-up to rule out other possible causes. Once the diagnosis is established, supportive therapy may begin.

Mannitol at doses of 1 g/kg over 30 minutes often improves initial symptoms. Patients may require IV fluids for dehydration and atropine for symptomatic bradycardia. It is important to inform patients that the cholinergic toxicity may last for 8 to 9 days and the neurologic symptoms may linger for months. Further ingestion of reef fish and alcohol should be avoided for up to 6 months.

SCOMBROID

Scombroid is a toxin typically ingested with dark-meat fish such as tuna, mackerel, and mahi-mahi. Unlike ciguatera, this toxin can be avoided if fish are refrigerated properly. Scrombrotoxin forms when surface bacteria proliferate on the outer surface of the fish and degrade free histidine to histamine.[7] This produces the set-up for toxic ingestion. Patients that consume the scrombrotoxin often initially notice that the fish has a metallic or "peppery" taste. Within minutes, the histamine produces symptoms of excessive flushing, sweating, and a burning sensation in the mouth and throat. Sometimes, an impressive total body "sunburn-like" rash occurs. Symptoms may last up to 4 hours and should be treated aggressively.

Supportive care along with IV diphenhydramine and cimetidine should be given along with inhaled beta agonists for bronchospasm. In severe cases, steroids and epinephrine may be necessary. Once their condition is initially stabilized, patients tend to do well. It is important for patients to know this is not a fish allergy. The EP should contact public health authorities as well as the offending restaurant to limit further exposure.

REFERENCES

1. Burgess GH: Director, International Shark Attack File. http://www.flmnh.ufl.edu/fish/sharks/statistics/2006attack summary.htm
2. Fenner PJ: Dangers in the ocean: The traveler and marine envenomation. I. Jellyfish. J Travel Med 1998;5:135-141.
3. O'Reilly GM, Isbister GK, Lawrie PM, et al: Prospective study of jellyfish stings from tropical Australia, including the major box jellyfish *Chironex fleckeri*. Med J Aust 2001;175:652-655.
4. Grady JD, Burnett JW: Irukandji-like syndrome in South Florida divers. Ann Emerg Med 2003;42:763-766.
5. Fenner PJ: Dangers in the ocean: The traveler and marine envenomation. II. Marine vertebrates. J Travel Med 1998;5:213-221.
6. Morris PD,Campbell DS, Freeman JI: Ciguatera fish poisoning: An outbreak associated with fish caught from North Carolina coastal waters. South Med J 1990;83:371-372.
7. Morrow JD, Margolies GR, Rowland J, Roberts LJ: Evidence that histamine is the causative toxin of scombroid-fish poisoning. N Eng J Med 1991;324:716-720.

SECTION **XVI**

Metabolic and Endocrine Disorders

Chapter 160

Fluid Management

Alan C. Heffner and Matthew T. Robinson

KEY POINTS

The majority of ED patients who require resuscitation present in compensated shock with normal blood pressure.

Normal vital signs do not guarantee adequate systemic perfusion.

Volume expension with isotonic fluid is the most important immediate therapy for circutatory insufficiency.

Scope

Volume depletion is a direct consequence of acute fluid or blood loss. Relative and absolute hypovolemia complicates many clinical conditions. Severity ranges from mild compensated hypovolemia to shock and hypotension requiring aggressive, goal-directed resuscitation. Fluid therapy remains the cornerstone of macrocirculatory and microcirculatory support in most shock conditions. Timely aggressive therapy prevents disease progression and preserves organ function.

Pathophysiology

■ OXYGEN DELIVERY AND TISSUE PERFUSION

Cellular oxygen is delivered via the circulation as a function of red blood cell mass and cardiorespiratory function. Oxygen enables continuous production of cellular energy in the form of adenosine triphosphate (ATP). Poor oxygenation compromises cell energetics and function, resulting in the clinical manifestations of organ dysfunction and failure and, ultimately, death.

Cardiac output is the most important determinant of oxygen delivery, with the flexibility to compensate for reduced oxygen-carrying capacity and/or increased metabolic demands. The physiologic response to a decrease in cardiac output is catecholamine-induced peripheral vasoconstriction, tachycardia, and enhanced cardiac contractility.

Venoconstriction maintains intrathoracic blood volume (preload) while arterial vasoconstriction shunts perfusion to vital organs and maintains critical organ perfusion pressure. Hypovolemia induces swift sympathetic catecholamine release, resulting in enhanced heart rate and inotropy that maintain cardiac output in the face of decreasing stroke volume.

Effective circulating volume (ECV) conceptualizes the portion of intravascular volume contributing to organ perfusion. ECV decreases with hypovolemia but does not necessarily correlate with volume status, as organ perfusion is also dependent on cardiac output, arterial tone, and circulatory distribution. As an example, ECV may be compromised by limited cardiac output despite optimized volume status.

Cardiac output and organ perfusion vary dramatically under changing physiologic, pathologic, and pharmacologic stimuli. Organ blood flow is directly proportional to perfusion pressure in most vascular beds. In hypovolemia, protection of arterial (organ perfusion) pressure occurs by peripheral vasoconstriction at the expense of reduced flow to noncritical (hepatosplanchnic, renal, and cutaneous) circulations. As such, mean arterial pressure is maintained despite hypovolemia and organ hypoperfusion.

Table 160-1 **SIZE AND COMPOSITION OF BODY FLUID COMPARTMENTS***

Compartment	% Body wt	Volume (L)	H_2O (L)	Na (mmol/L)	K (mmol/L)	Cl (mmol/L)	HCO_3 (mmol/L)
Total body	60	45	42				
ICF	40	30	28 (60%)	16	150		10
ECF	20	15	14 (40%)	140	4	103	26
Interstitial	16	12					
Plasma	4	3					
Blood	7	5					

*Values based on male weighing 70 kg (154 lb).
ECF, extracellular fluid; ICF, intracellular fluid.

■ WATER

Water is the most abundant constituent of the body. An adult male weighing 70 kg (154 lb) contains approximately 45 liters of water, accounting for 60% of body mass (Table 160-1). Total body water (TBW) is proportional to lean body mass and affects maintenance fluid requirements. TBW is physiologically compartmentalized into intracellular and extracellular spaces. The extracellular compartment is anatomically and conceptually divided into vascular and interstitial spaces.

Water freely crosses cell membranes. Osmotic forces determine water distribution within the body. Intracellular and extracellular fluid environments remain iso-osmolar but physiochemically distinct via tight regulation of dissolved solutes and proteins. Membrane-bound Na^+-K^+ ATPase pumps compartmentalize sodium and potassium to the extracellular and intracellular spaces, respectively. Active restriction of sodium to the extracellular space is the foundation of isotonic sodium-based resuscitation solutions.

Starling's law describes the forces governing fluid flux across vascular endothelial membranes. In healthy persons, transcapillary hydrostatic force is nearly opposed by colloid oncotic pressure. Small net loss from the vascular space is ultimately returned to the systemic circulation via lymphatics. Albumin normally accounts for 80% of the colloid oncotic pressure, whereas large cellular moieties such as red blood cells and platelets contribute little oncotic pressure effect. Positive hydrostatic pressure, hypoalbuminemia, and pathologic endothelial permeability are common clinical conditions that enhance fluid extravasation from the vascular compartment. The clinical consequences include large and ongoing volume resuscitation requirements coupled with pulmonary and tissue edema.

Clinical Presentation

Volume depletion describes a state of contracted extracellular fluid with clinical implications of compromised ECV, tissue perfusion, and function. *Dehydration* implies an intracellular water deficit characterized by plasma hypernatremia and hyperosmolarity.[1]

Hypovolemia may occur as a consequence of blood loss, water and electrolyte loss, or primary water loss (Box 160-1). Patients with hypovolemia most often present with symptoms of reduced cardiac output such as fatigue, dyspnea, postural dizziness, and near-syncope or true syncope. Tolerance of hypovolemia is variable and depends on the acuity and severity of the hypovolemia, associated anemia, physiologic reserves, and primary etiology. Organ dysfunction is

BOX 160-1

Anatomic Sites of Nonhemorrhagic Volume Loss

Gastrointestinal
- Vomiting
- Diarrhea
- Drainage (ostomy, fistula, nasogastric)

Renal
- Diuresis (medication, osmotic)
- Salt wasting
- Diabetes insipidus

Skin
- Burn
- Wound
- Exfoliative rash
- Sweating

Third Space Sequestration
- Intestinal obstruction
- Peritonitis
- Crush injury
- Pancreatitis
- Ascites
- Pleural effusion
- Capillary leak
- Insensible loss

Respiratory
- Fever

BOX 160-2

Clinical Indicators of Hypoperfusion That Warrant Rapid, Monitored Fluid Challenge

- Mean arterial pressure (MAP) <65 mm Hg
- Systolic blood pressure <90 mm Hg
- Decrease in MAP >20 mm Hg from baseline
- Shock index >0.9
- Sinus tachycardia >100 beats per minute
- Serum lactate >4 mmol/L
- Oliguria (urine output <0.5 mL/kg/hr)
- Poor peripheral perfusion

PRIORITY ACTIONS

Prioritized Endpoints of Fluid Therapy

- Adequate intravenous access
- Mean arterial pressure >65 mm Hg
- Optimization of oxygen delivery and organ perfusion
- Clinical markers—cutaneous perfusion, urine output
- Systemic markers—central venous saturation ($S_{CV}O_2$), serum lactate
- Regional markers—gastric and sublingual PCO_2, tissue PO_2

often the heralding signal of hypovolemia and may occur in the absence of global hypoperfusion or hemodynamic instability.

Shock is defined as a state of inadequate tissue perfusion, in which oxygen delivery does not meet metabolic requirements. The term does not reflect perfusion pressure—shock may occur with low, normal, or elevated blood pressure. *Compensated shock* refers to inadequate perfusion in the setting of normal blood pressure. The term, "occult hypoperfusion" is sometimes used to describe hemodynamically stable patients with microvascular insufficiency. *Uncompensated shock* is characterized by hypotension and develops when physiologic attempts to maintain normal perfusion pressure are overwhelmed or exhausted. Sustained hypotension signifies a late stage of shock.

Volume status and perfusion should be evaluated during every ED examination (Box 160-2). Delayed capillary refill, dry axillae and mucous membranes, abnormal skin turgor, sunken eyes, and depressed fontanel are classic but imperfect hallmarks of hypovolemia.[2] Peripheral cyanosis, cool extremities, and cutaneous mottling (cutis marmorata) characterize hypovolemic, cardiogenic, and obstructive shock. In contrast, early hyperdynamic septic shock manifests peripheral vasodilation with warm extremities and brisk capillary refill. Generalized tissue edema reflects total body sodium and fluid excess but does not quantify intravascular status and may be accompanied by hypovolemia, especially in acute illness. Acute weight change implies loss of fluid rather than lean body mass and is helpful in patients with reliable comparison weight.

Circulatory failure is the final common pathway of many diseases. Inadequate circulating volume is the most common primary etiology of shock. Pathologic vasodilation compounds the fluid deficit in conditions such as sepsis, anaphylaxis, adrenal insufficiency, and neurogenic and toxin-induced shock. Acute cardiac decompensation and pulmonary embolus are two exceptional situations where limited volume resuscitation takes secondary priority to mechanical and inotropic resuscitation.

Treatment

Early recognition of hypovolemia and shock must be coupled with aggressive resuscitation to affect patients. The time window to reverse critical organ hypoperfusion is measured in hours and often occurs in the ED. Equivalent but delayed resuscitation yields greater morbidity and mortality.[3-5]

■ FLUID RESUSCITATION

Inadequate intravascular volume is the most common and easily reversible factor in acute circulatory failure. As such, fluid therapy is the cornerstone of the initial management of undifferentiated shock in the ED. The immediate goal of resuscitation is restoration of organ perfusion pressure with maintenance of mean arterial pressure greater than 65 mmHg.

Immediate volume expansion is achieved through rapid fluid administration under direct observation at the bedside. Serial aliquots of crystalloid (10-20 mL/kg) or colloid (5-10 mL/kg) solution should be infused over 15 to 30 minutes. Sequential boluses are titrated to sustain systemic perfusion pressure while monitoring for pulmonary congestion.

Total volume requirements are difficult to predict at the onset of resuscitation and are often underestimated. Classic hypovolemia such as occurs with acute hemorrhage or fluid loss may be rapidly stabilized with appropriate volume expansion. The 3:1 rule of hemorrhage resuscitation states that three volumetric units of crystalloid are required to replete the extracellular fluid deficit of one unit of blood loss.[6,7] However, experimental models confirm the experience in severely traumatized patients in whom isotonic fluid requirements vastly exceed those of the 3:1 rule.

Shock accompanied by pathologic vasodilation and capillary leak may also require substantial volume replacement. A transcapillary shift of up to 50% of circulating volume is observed within hours in experimentally induced sepsis and anaphylaxis. Crystalloid requirements average 40 to 60 mL/kg in the first hours of septic shock but may be as high as 200 mL/

kg to normalize perfusion parameters.[8,9] Early aggressive volume therapy improves patient outcome.

The clinical response to serial volume loading is the most common gauge of resuscitation. When available, dynamic respirophasic variations in arterial and central venous pressure waveforms are reliable signs to anticipate response to fluid loading. In the absence of conflicting data, a target central venous pressure of 8 to 12 mm Hg is recommended to maximize preload prior to instituting pressor and inotropic support.[5,7,10] Vasopressors should only be used after aggressive volume expansion, as they reduce tissue perfusion in under-resuscitated patients. Approximately 50% of hypotensive septic patients will be stabilized with volume resuscitation alone.[9]

■ FLUID SELECTION

The goal of fluid resuscitation is vascular expansion to maximize cardiac output and tissue oxygen delivery. Isotonic crystalloid and colloid solutions are effective volume expanders (Table 160-2). Fluid selection appears less important than volume dosage titrated to an appropriate therapeutic end point. Electrolyte disorders (including hypernatremia and hyponatremia) take secondary priority to isotonic volume loading in hypoperfused patients. Hypotonic solutions are ineffective and inappropriate for resuscitation.

Isotonic sodium-based crystalloids are distributed to the extracellular compartment, which includes the vascular space. Partitioning within the extracellular fluid leaves 20% of infused volume within the circulation. Normal saline and lactated Ringer's solution are two isotonic resuscitation solutions in common use. Lactated Ringer's solution, also known as Hartmann's solution, was developed as a more physiologic alkalinizing replacement solution (bicarbonate is generated by lactate metabolism via the Cori cycle).

Although the clinical superiority of any particular crystalloid remains unproved, fluid selection should be based on the source of hypovolemia, associated electrolyte derangements, and volume requirements. Normal saline provides a supraphysiologic chloride load that induces metabolic acidosis when administered in large volumes.[11] Lactated Ringer's solution is preferred for large-volume resuscitation and is a more physiologic replacement solution for most gastrointestinal fluid losses. Marked loss of gastric secretions (as occurs with profuse vomiting, gastric outlet obstruction, or nasogastric suctioning) presents an exception in which normal saline is preferred to correct volume and electrolyte disturbances (hypochloremic metabolic alkalosis). Lactated Ringer's solution is the recommended crystalloid solution for trauma resuscitation but is incompatible with blood.[6] Later generations of resuscitation crystalloids such as Ringer's ethyl pyruvate aim to ameliorate ischemia and reperfusion-induced organ dysfunction.[12]

Colloid solutions are composed of electrolyte preparations reinforced with macromolecules designed to preserve colloid oncotic pressure. Vascular retention of colloid makes these formulations efficient volume expanders. Although equally effective when titrated to the same clinical end points, crystalloid solutions require two to four times more volume for equivalent resuscitation. Dilutional hypoalbuminemia, transcapillary fluid shift, and interstitial and pulmonary edema are therefore limited with

Table 160-2 INTRAVENOUS FLUID COMPOSITION AND DISTRIBUTION

	ELECTROLYTES (mEq/L)									DISTRIBUTION	
Solution	Na	K	Ca	Mg	Cl	HCO_3	Lactate	mOsm/L	pH	ECF%	ICF%
Crystalloid											
0.9% NaCl	154				154			308	5	100	
Ringer's lactate	130	4	2.7		109		28	273	6.5		
D_5W with 3 amp HCO_3 (150 mEq)	130					130					
3% NaCl	513				513			1027	5		
7.5% NaCl								2400			
0.45% NaCl	77				77			154	5	67	33
0.20% NaCl	34				34			77	5		
D_5W								278	4	33	67
Colloid											
Hextend*	143	3	5	1	124		28	307	5.9		
Hespan†	154				154			310	5.5		
Human albumin 5%	145				95			300			

*Hetastarch 6% in lactated electrolyte injection.
†Hetastarch 6% in 0.9% sodium chloride injection.
ECF, extracellular fluid; ICF, intracellular fluid.

colloid use. However, endothelial integrity is incomplete following injury and illness such that macromolecules are not restricted to the vascular compartment.[13] Most important, randomized clinical trials of crystalloid versus colloid solutions failed to prove clinical superiority of one agent with comparable rates of mortality and lung dysfunction.[14-16] Crystalloid solutions remain the standard ED resuscitation fluids and confer significant cost advantage over colloid solutions.

Human albumin and hydroxyethyl starch are the colloids primarily used in clinical practice in the United States. Human albumin solutions are heat-sterilized derivatives of donor plasma. Isotonic 5% albumin is recommended for resuscitation of patients with severe hypoalbuminemia and cirrhotic ascites, but there is little outcome evidence to support this position.[10,17] Hydroxyethyl starch, a semisynthetic polymerized amylopectin compound, has supplanted dextran and gelatin-based colloids. A 6% solution provides volume expansion equivalent to 5% albumin. Renal dysfunction and coagulopathy that complicated early generation synthetic colloids do not appear clinically significant with current hydroxyethyl starch solutions.

■ HYPERTONIC SOLUTIONS

Hypertonic sodium solutions rapidly expand intravascular volume by mobilizing water from the interstitial and intracellular spaces. A small infusion expands plasma several times the infused volume. Used alone, the hemodynamic impact of hypertonic crystalloid is transient; hypertonic crystalloid is generally used in combination with hyperoncotic colloid (6% dextran or 10% hetastarch) to sustain vascular expansion. Animal resuscitation models have demonstrated additional benefits including enhanced cardiac output, improved microcirculatory flow, and attenuated inflammatory response. At present, hypertonic saline appears safe, but there is little evidence of outcome benefit over standard isotonic crystalloid resuscitation in human trauma trials. Patients with multitrauma and associated closed head injury are the sole exception in whom benefit is demonstrated. Limited use in non-trauma patients limits clinical extrapolation beyond this population.

■ SPECIAL TREATMENT CONSIDERATIONS

■ Minimal Volume Resuscitation of Hemorrhagic Shock

Traditional resuscitation of hemorrhagic shock prioritized rapid restoration of circulating blood volume with crystalloid and blood products. Strategic limited volume resuscitation for uncontrolled hemorrhage dates back to the early 1900s and re-emerged in the 1980s.

The rationale is that increased intravascular pressure and hemodilution resulting from aggressive fluid resuscitation compounds blood loss by precipitating rebleeding from hemostatic sites. Animal models of uncontrolled hemorrhage reveal that aggressive fluid administration reduces oxygen delivery and results in higher mortality. The widely recognized Houston experience showed mortality benefit for penetrating trauma victims, but the results have yet to be matched by other investigators.[18,19] Utilizing this strategy, hypotensive patients with a source of uncontrolled life-threatening hemorrhage receive IV fluids titrated to sustain critical organ flow until definitive surgical control (Box 160-3). Conventional resuscitation ensues once surgical hemostasis is achieved.

The degree and duration of permissive hypotension remain to be clarified, although current recommendations target a systolic blood pressure of 70 mm Hg. Patients with concomitant traumatic brain injury are not candidates for this strategy.

BOX 160-3

Conditions Warranting a Strategy of Limited Volume Resuscitation Pending Surgical Control of Hemorrhage

- Penetrating torso trauma
- Ruptured abdominal aortic aneurysm
- Major hemothorax
- Major hemoperitoneum
- Traumatic aortic injury
- Severe pelvic fracture
- Gastrointestinal bleeding
- Ectopic pregnancy
- Postpartum hemorrhage

■ Burn Resuscitation

Patients with partial-thickness and full-thickness burns exhibit marked fluid shifts related to denuded skin, injured tissue, and systemic inflammatory reaction. Early anticipation of these large fluid requirements prevents under-resuscitation. The Parkland formula remains the most commonly used guide for acute burn resuscitation. Formula calculations are based from time of injury, rather than time to medical attention and incorporate pre-hospital fluid administration. All burn formulas only estimate fluid requirement; thus modification and individualization must be based on patient response, because volume needs may substantially exceed formula approximation. Lactated Ringer's solution is the resuscitation crystalloid preparation of choice for acute burn management. In addition to burn formula replacement, maintenance fluid requirements should be allocated. Urine output greater than 1 mL/kg/hour is a traditional end point of acute burn resuscitation and may be augmented by perfusion end points discussed earlier.

Table 160-3 PEDIATRIC MAINTENANCE FLUID ESTIMATE FORMULAS*

Body Weight	Daily Maintenance (mL/day)	Hourly Maintenance (mL/hr)
1-10 kg	100 mL/kg	5 mL/kg
10-20 kg	1000 mL plus 50 mL/kg	40 mL plus 2 mL/kg
20-80 kg	1500 mL plus 20 mL/kg†	60 mL plus 1 mL/kg†

*Note that the following two formulas calculate disparate rates. The difference between these calculated rates is clinically insignificant. Sodium and chloride—2-3 mEq per 100 mL water; potassium—1-2 mEq per 100 mL water. D_5W normal saline with 20 mEq KCl is a common maintenance solution for most euvolemic pediatric patients and provides 20% of daily calories at a routine maintenance rate. Comorbid conditions and/or electrolyte abnormalities may require modification.

†To a maximum of 2400 mL/day or 100 mL/hr.

■ Oral Rehydration Therapy

Oral rehydration therapy is a valuable tool for maintenance and correction of mild to moderate dehydration due to gastroenteritis in children and adults. It remains underutilized in the United States despite worldwide success, guideline support, and controlled trial evidence.[20] Using published guidelines, oral rehydration therapy is comparable to IV therapy, with reduced hospitalizations and improved safety and expense. Small aliquots of fluid (as low as 5 mL, depending on patient size and tolerance) are administered by bottle, spoon, syringe, or nasogastric tube at regular 2- to 5-minute intervals to meet deficit and maintenance goals. Next to patient and family education, appropriate fluid selection is the most important factor in successful oral rehydration therapy.

Many common household fluids including fruit juice, sport drinks, carbonated beverages, and soups contain poorly tolerated concentrations of sugar and salt. Commercial (Rehydralyte, Pedialyte) and reconstituted liquids (oral rehydration salts or home recipe) are balanced, low-carbohydrate enteral solutions. One recipe for oral rehydration solution using home ingredients is made up of 1 liter of water, 8 teaspoons of sugar, and 1 teaspoon of salt.

■ Maintenance Fluid Therapy

In contrast to resuscitation therapy, the goal of maintenance fluid therapy is normal body fluid composition and volume. Fluid orders anticipate daily fluid requirements, ongoing losses, and coexisting electrolyte abnormalities. Although often ordered concurrently, the estimated physiologic fluid (true maintenance) should be consciously distinguished from therapy aimed to slowly replace an existing fluid deficit.

Routine water and electrolyte maintenance is based on normal energy expenditure, sensible loss from urine and stool, and insensible loss from the respiratory tract and skin. Calculations assume euvolemia and are adjusted for body mass. Greater per kilogram fluid requirements in children are proportionate to total body water and metabolism (Table 160-3).

All maintenance prescriptions should be individualized—energy expenditure, fluid losses, and electrolyte status vary with disease and dictate rate and electrolyte modifications. For example, exfoliative skin disease, increased work of breathing, and fever enhance insensible loss. Measurable nasogastric, fistula, ostomy, and urinary drainage can be estimated and replaced by drainage volume. Limitation of fluid and potassium is an important disease-specific modification for patients with renal insufficiency.

Hypotonic solutions (e.g., 0.45% and 0.2% sodium chloride) with or without dextrose and potassium are popular fixed-combination maintenance solutions. Hospitalized patients often suffer impaired free-water excretion due to nonosmotic antidiuretic hormone release, making them vulnerable to hyponatremia. Serum sodium concentration provides a simple and accurate marker of hydration status. Isotonic maintenance solutions should be considered in patients (including children) with serum sodium less than 138 mEq/L.[21,22] Glucose infusions are best formulated by adding dextrose to an electrolyte solution (e.g., lactated Ringer's solution, 0.45% or 0.2% normal saline) rather than using 5% dextrose (D_5W), which behaves as electrolyte-free water-upon-sugar metabolism.

REFERENCES

1. McGee S, Abernethy WB 3rd, Simel DL: Is this patient hypovolemic? JAMA 1999;281:1022-1029.
2. Steiner MJ, DeWalt DA, Byerley JS, et al: Is this child dehydrated? JAMA 2004;291:2746-2754.
3. Carcillo JA, Davis AL, Zaritsky A: Role of early fluid resuscitation in pediatric septic shock. JAMA 1991; 266:1242-1245.
4. Kern JW, Shoemaker WC: Meta-analysis of hemodynamic optimization in high risk patients. Crit Care Med 2002:30:1686-1692.
5. Rivers E, Nguyen B, Havstad S, et al: Early goal-directed therapy in the treatment of severe sepsis and septic shock. N Engl J Med 2001;345:1368-1377.
6. Advanced Trauma Life Support for Doctors, 7th Ed. Chicago, American College of Surgeons, 2004.
7. Moore FA, McKinley BA, Moore EE: The next generation in shock resuscitation. Lancet 2004;363:1988-1996.
8. Carcillo JA, Fields AI: Clinical practice parameters for hemodynamic support of pediatric and neonatal patients with septic shock. Crit Care Med 2002;30:1365-1378.
9. Hollenberg SM, Ahrens JT, Annane D, et al: Practice parameters for hemodynamic support of sepsis in adult patients: 2004 update. Crit Care Med 2004;32:1928-1948.
10. Dellinger RP, Carlet RP, Masur H, et al: Surviving Sepsis Campaign guidelines for management of severe sepsis and septic shock. Crit Care Med 2004;32:858-873.

11. Morgan TJ: Clinical review: The meaning of acid base abnormalities in the intensive care unit—effects of fluid administration. Crit Care 2005;9:204-211.
12. Sims CA, Wattanasirichaigoon S, Menconi MJ, et al: Ringer's ethyl pyruvate solution ameliorates ischemia/reperfusion-induced intestinal mucosal injury in rats. Crit Care Med 2001;29:1513-1518.
13. Fleck A, Raines G, Hawker G, et al: Increased vascular permeability: A major cause of hypoalbuminemia in disease and injury. Lancet 1985;1:781-784.
14. Finfer S, Bellomo R, Boyce N, et a:. A comparison of albumin and saline for fluid resuscitation in the intensive care unit. N Engl J Med 2004:350:2247-2256.
15. Alderson P, Schierhout G, Roberts F, Bunn E: Colloids versus crystalloids for fluid resuscitation in critically ill patients. Cochrane Database Syst Rev 2000(2);CD000567. Update in: Cochrane Database Syst Rev 2004;(4): CD000567.
16. Choi PT, Yip G, Quinonez LG, et al: Crystalloids vs. colloids in fluid resuscitation: A systematic review. Crit Care Med 1999;27:200-210.
17. Cook C, Guyatt G: Colloid use for fluid resuscitation: Evidence and spin. Ann Intern Med 2001:135:205-207.
18. Bickell WH, Wall MJ Jr, Pepe P, et al: Immediate versus delayed fluid resuscitation for patients with penetrating torso injuries. N Engl J Med 1994;331:1105-1109.
19. Dutton RP, Mackenzie CF, Scalea TM: Hypotensive resuscitation during active hemorrhage: Impact on in-hospital mortality. J Trauma 2002;52:1141-1146.
20. Fonseca BK, Holdgate A, Craig JC: Enteral vs. intravenous rehydration therapy for children with gastroenteritis: A meta-analysis of randomized controlled trials. Arch Pediatr Adolesc Med 2004;158:420-421.
21. Shafiee MA, Bohn D, Hoorn EJ, Halperin M: How to select optimal maintenance intravenous fluid therapy. QJM 2003;96:601-610.
22. Moritz ML, Ayus JC: Prevention of hospital-acquired hyponatremia: A case for using isotonic saline. Pediatrics 2003;111:227-230.

Chapter 161

Acid-Base Disorders

Matthew T. Robinson and Alan C. Heffner

KEY POINTS

Venous blood gas is a useful ED test because of the strong association between arterial and venous HCO_3^- and pH.

Correlation between venous PCO_2 and arterial PCO_2 is lacking, although venous PCO_2 levels may be used as a screening tool for hypercarbia.

Preresuscitation standard base excess is reliably linked to the degree of tissue acidosis and serves as an independent predictor of mortality in critically ill trauma patients.

The urine ketone dip test has been shown to have a sensitivity of 99% and a negative predictive value of 100% for detecting the presence of diabetic ketoacidosis.

Central venous measurements of serum lactate are highly correlated with arterial sampling.

Peripheral venous samples are sufficiently sensitive to screen for hyperlactatemia; however, lactate levels are significantly higher compared with arterial samples, producing poor specificity (57%). Elevations in venous lactate should be confirmed with arterial sampling.

The indiscriminate use of sodium bicarbonate infusions for the treatment of undifferentiated metabolic acidosis should be avoided.

Pathophysiology

■ REGULATION OF ACID-BASE BALANCE

Rigid control of free hydrogen ion (H^+) concentration is essential to life. Although the normal H^+ concentration in serum is approximately 1/1,000,000 the concentration of other major serum ions, the small size and high charge density of H^+ make it highly reactive, capable of inducing conformational and functional changes in the proteins that are necessary for organs to function.

The normal H^+ concentration is low, about 40 nanoequivalents/L. Less than 10 nanoequivalents/L variance is noted over the normal physiologic range, and less than 140 nanoequivalents/L variance is noted over the extremes of what is compatible with life.

Daily metabolism produces acid loads of about 150 mmol of nonvolatile acid and 12,000 mmol of volatile acid CO_2. Ingestions and endogenous production can increase the acid load. The system must have the capacity to rapidly accommodate these additional acid or alkali loads and maintain homeostasis.

The acute response to an acid or base load occurs in one of three general ways:

1. Chemical buffering
2. Alterations in alveolar ventilation
3. Alterations in renal hydrogen ion excretion

Chemical Buffering

Extracellular buffers include plasma proteins, phosphates, and bicarbonate—the earliest defenses against acidosis (onset within minutes). The most important extracellular buffer is bicarbonate, which not only is highly abundant but also acts as a dynamic buffer by independently regulating P_{CO_2} through changes in alveolar ventilation. Buffering also occurs within the intracellular compartment, delayed by approximately 2 to 4 hours, as H^+ equilibrates across the intracellular fluid space. Intracellular buffers including bone, inorganic phosphates, proteins, and hemoglobin are eventually responsible for providing more than 50% of overall chemical buffering.

Alterations in Alveolar Ventilation

Alterations in alveolar ventilation provide early compensation for acute acid-base disturbances, beginning within minutes through the stimulation of peripheral chemoreceptors. By altering the P_{CO_2} through variations in minute ventilation, the ratio remains relatively constant and alterations in pH are mitigated.

Alterations in Renal Hydrogen Ion Excretion

Renal compensation for acute acid-base disorders is immediate; however, the full effect is not appreciated for 5 or 6 days. Due to the inability of HCO_3^- to effectively buffer H_2CO_3 produced through acute CO_2 retention, renal compensation is centrally important in the response to primary respiratory disorders.

FACTS AND FORMULAS

- $pH = 6.1 + Log\ [HCO_3^-]\ /\ 0.0_3 \times P_{CO_2}$
- Anion gap = unmeasured anions – unmeasured cations = $Na^+ - [\ Cl^- + HCO_3^-]$
- Corrected anion gap = anion gap + 2.5 (normal albumin – measured albumin)
- Delta gap = Δ anion gap – Δ HCO_3^- = [calculated anion gap – 10] – [24 – measured serum HCO_3^-]
- Calculated Sosm (mOsm/Kg) = 2 (Na^+) + BUN/2.8 + glucose/18 + ethanol/4.8
- Osmolal gap = measured sosm – calculated Sosm
- Metabolic acidosis: $P_{CO_2} = 1.5\ (HCO_3^-) + 8$
- Metabolic alkalosis: Increase in $P_{CO_2} = 0.6 \times$ increa se in HCO_3^-
- Respiratory acidosis
  - Acute: [HCO_3^-] increases by 1 mEq/L for each 10 mm Hg increase in P_{CO_2}
  - Chronic: [HCO_3^-] increases by 4 mEq/L for each 10 mm Hg increase in P_{CO_2}
- Respiratory alkalosis
  - Acute: [HCO_3^-] decreases by 2 mEq/L for each 10 mm Hg decrease in P_{CO_2}
  - Chronic: [HCO_3^-] decreases by 5 mEq/L for each 10 m Hg decrease in P_{CO_2}

Diagnostic Testing

The normal range of serum pH is 7.40 to 7.44. When the serum pH falls below 7.40, the patient is described as *acidemic*. Likewise, when the serum pH rises above 7.44, the patient is described as *alkalemic*. In patients with mixed acid-base disorders, a normal pH does not exclude a significant acid-base disorder.

Processes may be divided into primary respiratory or metabolic disorders by examining the P_{CO_2} and the HCO_3^-. Primary elevations in the P_{CO_2} causes a respiratory acidosis, whereas decreased serum HCO_3^- causes metabolic acidosis.

Serum testing includes direct evaluation of the pH, P_{CO_2}, and HCO_3^- through arterial and venous blood sampling, calculation of the anion gap from serum chemistries, and additional measures (such as the standard base excess) that attempt to quantify the metabolic component of acid-base disorders (see "Facts and Formulas" for basic formulas used in this chapter).

ARTERIAL AND VENOUS BLOOD GASES

A strong association between arterial and venous HCO_3^- and pH has been demonstrated in diabetic ketoacidosis, tricyclic antidepressant overdose, acute respiratory disease, and uremia, with pH values varying by approximately 0.04 units and HCO_3^- values ranging from −1.72 to +1.88 mEq.[1]

Correlation between venous P_{CO_2} and arterial P_{CO_2} is lacking; however, venous P_{CO_2} levels may be used as a screening tool for hypercarbia. When using a value of greater than 45 mm Hg as a cutoff for venous P_{CO_2}, the sensitivity for detection of significant hypercarbia (defined as $P_{CO_2} > 50$ mm Hg) is 100%, with a specificity of 47%. Using this value as a screening tool for significant hypercarbia would have led to a 29% reduction in arterial sampling in one study.[2]

Arterial blood gas calculations cannot be abandoned because the poor association between arterial and venous P_{CO_2} does not allow for precise interpretation, although arterial sampling can be more judiciously employed.

ANION GAP

Within the serum, the requirement for electroneutrality dictates that the net serum cations must equal total anions. The calculated difference is the anion gap—the difference between unmeasured anions and unmeasured cations (Box 161-1).

The greatest utility of the anion gap is the assessment of the causes of metabolic acidosis by separating etiologies into anion gap and non–anion gap processes. When acids are added to the system, HCO_3^- is replaced by the acid anion (X) as follows:

$$HX + NaHCO_3 \rightarrow NaX + H_2O + CO_2$$

BOX 161-1

Etiologies for Measured Changes in the Anion Gap

Increased Anion Gap
- Increased anions
- Organic acids
- Albumin
- Decreased cations
- Ca, Mg, K, paraproteins

Decreased Anion Gap
- Decreased anions
- Hypoalbuminemia
- Increased cations
- Lithium
- Paraproteins (myeloma)
- Falsely elevated chloride
- Bromism
- Hyperlipidemia

The titration and replacement of HCO_3^- by the unmeasured organic acid produces an equimolar elevation in the anion gap. However, when HCl is added to the system, there is a millequivalent-for-millequivalent exchange of HCO_3^- for Cl^-, such that no change in the anion gap is observed.

$$HCl + NaHCO_3 \rightarrow NaCl + H_2CO_3 \rightarrow CO_2 + H_2O$$

Thus hyperchloremic metabolic acidosis produces no change in the anion gap because the acid anion (Cl^-) is included in the arterial blood gas calculation. Gastrointestinal and renal loss are the most common etiologies of non–anion gap acidosis because the loss of bicarbonate indirectly adds HCl to the system and NaCl is preferentially retained in an effort to maintain extracellular fluid volume.

Elevations in the anion gap do not always imply a metabolic acidosis, however; they may occur in both metabolic and respiratory alkalosis, because of an increase in the electronegative charge of albumin as the serum becomes more alkalemic, as well as through alkalemia-induced lactate production.

The classically accepted range for the anion gap has been defined as 12 ± 4 (8-16 mEq/L). However, with the advent of ion-specific electrodes, which measure chloride at a higher concentration than the older flame photometric techniques, the accepted range has been corrected to 6.6 ± 4 (2.6-10.6 mEq/L). Additionally, the anion gap (AG) must be corrected in the presence of hypoalbuminemia, which decreases the measured anion gap. The correction factor is calculated as follows:

$$\text{Corrected AG} = \text{Calculated AG} + 2.5\ (\text{normal albumin} - \text{measured albumin})$$

Using this correction factor improves the sensitivity of the anion gap by 66% for the detection of unmeasured anions within the serum.

The anion gap is also useful for investigating the presence of mixed acid-base disturbances. In a simple anion gap acidosis, HCO_3^- is titrated in a one-to-one fashion by organic acid. Therefore, one would expect the following relationship:

$$\text{Increase in anion gap} = \text{decrease in } HCO_3^-$$

The difference between the change in the anion gap and the change in the serum HCO_3^- is called the *delta gap,* or *delta/delta;* deviations from this relationship indicate a mixed acid/base disturbance. When the change (delta) in the anion gap is larger than the change in bicarbonate, an additional source of base from a metabolic alkalosis is present. Al ternatively, when the change in the anion gap is less than the change in the bicarbonate, an additional source of acid from a non–anion gap acidosis is present.

Specific Disorders

■ RESPIRATORY ACIDOSIS

Normal ventilatory control is regulated through central receptors that respond to elevated P_{CO_2} and peripheral chemoreceptors in the carotid bodies that respond to hypoxia. Because the ventilatory response to hypercapnea is much stronger than that of hypoxemia, only minor elevations in P_{CO_2} are required to increase minute ventilation. Because of this vigorous response and the ability to significantly increase minute ventilation, respiratory acidosis almost always develops as a consequence of impaired alveolar ventilation and not from increased production of CO_2.

Elevated P_{CO_2} causes a decrease in arterial pH and a variable increase in plasma HCO_3^-, acutely due to shifts in equilibrium reactions and chronically due to renal compensation through enhanced H^+ excretion and HCO_3^- retention. CO_2 functions as a volatile acid:

$$H^+ + HCO_3^- \rightarrow H_2CO_3 \rightarrow H_2O + CO_2$$

Under normal conditions, this acid load is immediately buffered by intracellular and extracellular nonbicarbonate buffers. The acute rise in P_{CO_2} elicits a similar elevation in HCO_3^- through a highly predictable relationship:

$$[HCO_3^-] \text{ increases by 1 mEq/L for each 10 mm Hg increase in } P_{CO_2}$$

In chronic respiratory acidosis, elevations in P_{CO_2} are partially protective, allowing larger amounts of CO_2 to be excreted at lower minute ventilations. The system also adapts to chronically elevated CO_2 by enhancing renal H^+ excretion and HCO_3^- retention, attenuating the ventilatory response to hypercapnea. The result of chronic respiratory acidosis is that ventilatory drive becomes dependent on hypoxic stimulus.

BOX 161-2

Acid-Base Interpretation Based on Clinical History

Case 1

A 65-year-old man with a history of chronic obstructive pulmonary disease presents with fever, increased shortness of breath, cough, and sputum production. The following arterial blood gas and serum HCO_3^- values are obtained:

pH = 7.27; $P{CO_2}$ = 65 mm Hg; HCO_3^- = 29 mEq/L; $P{O_2}$ = 70 mm Hg

Review shows a decreased pH and elevated $P{CO_2}$ indicative of respiratory acidosis. The chronicity of the acidosis can be evaluated by calculating the expected metabolic compensation:

Acute: $[HCO_3^-]$ increases by 1 mEq/L for each 10 mm Hg in $P{CO_2}$

$$\text{Expected } HCO_3^- = 24 + 2.5 = 26.5$$

Chronic: $[HCO_3^-]$ increases by 4 mEq/L for each 10 mm Hg in $P{CO_2}$

$$\text{Expected } HCO_3^- = 24 + 10 = 34$$

Comparing these values with the measured HCO_3^- reveals that the HCO_3^- falls between the two calculated levels. Based on the history, the clinical diagnosis is acute on chronic respiratory acidosis.

Case 2

A 65-year-old man with a history of chronic obstructive pulmonary disease has had diarrhea for 1 week and presents with a baseline $P{CO_2}$ of 65 mm Hg.

Based on the history, the patient's HCO_3^- is lower than predicted, representing an acute metabolic acidosis in the presence of a chronic respiratory acidosis.

Case 3

A 65-year-old man on chronic diuretic therapy presents with an acute exacerbation of asthma.

The history indicates an acute respiratory acidosis with an expected $P{CO_2}$ of 26.5 mm Hg. The elevated serum HCO_3^- indicates an acute respiratory acidosis with a concomitant metabolic alkalosis.

The clinical corollary is that the use of supplemental oxygen must be carefully monitored to avoid eliminating this hypoxic stimulus, which will produce relative hypoventilation, exacerbating the chronic respiratory acidosis. This is especially important in patients with chronic respiratory acidosis who suffer an acute respiratory acidosis through pulmonary insult (Box 161-2). The renal compensatory response in chronic respiratory acidosis requires 3 to 5 days to develop and may be predicted by the following equation:

$[HCO_3^-]$ increases by 4 mEq/L for each 10 mm Hg increase in $P{CO_2}$

▪ RESPIRATORY ALKALOSIS

Respiratory alkalosis is produced through alveolar hyperventilation, resulting in a decrease in the arterial $P{CO_2}$ and increased arterial pH. Plasma HCO_3^- is variably decreased, acutely due to shifts in equilibrium and later due to renal HCO_3^- wasting. The decreased $P{CO_2}$ causes a decreased volatile acid load, with secondary release of H^+ from nonbicarbonate buffers (Buf), as follows:

$$HCO_3^- + HBuf \rightarrow H_2CO_3 + Buf \rightarrow CO_2 + H_2O$$

The expected $[HCO_3^-]$ can be calculated from the following equation:

$[HCO_3^-]$ decreases by 2 mEq/L for each 10 mm Hg decrease in $P{CO_2}$

In chronic respiratory alkalosis, renal adaptive mechanisms result in diminished H^+ secretion and enhanced HCO_3^- excretion. This combined response begins within hours and is completed within 2 to 3 days. The expected response may be calculated as follows:

$[HCO_3^-]$ decreases by 5 mEq/L for each 10 mm Hg decrease in $P{CO_2}$

Ventilation is primarily controlled through peripheral, central, and pulmonary mechanical receptors. Peripheral chemoreceptors respond to changes in $P{CO_2}$ and O_2, and it is not surprising that many cases of hyperventilation stem from hypoxemia.

▪ METABOLIC ACIDOSIS

Metabolic acidosis is induced by the addition of H^+ ions or by the loss of HCO_3^-. Addition of H^+ may occur through exogenous administration or endogenous production of acids associated with pathologic states. The loss of bicarbonate occurs primarily through gastrointestinal or renal wasting, producing acidosis by driving the equilibrium reaction to the left:

$$H^+ + HCO_3^- \leftrightarrow H_2CO_3 \leftrightarrow CO_2 + H_2O$$

As previously discussed, the initial response to an acid is extracellular and intracellular buffering, combined with respiratory compensation through increasing alveolar ventilation. These protective mechanisms attempt to minimize the amount of free hydrogen ions within the system until a full renal response excretes the excess acid load.

It is important to remember that these compensatory responses do not fully normalize the pH. If a normal pH is seen in a patient with metabolic acido-

BOX 161-3

Metabolic Acidosis with Inadequate Respiratory Compensation

A 68-year-old woman presents with dyspnea and cough.

Vital signs:

Blood pressure, 100/50; heart rate, 120 beats/min; temperature, 101.3° F

Laboratory data:

$Na^+ = 142$; $Cl^- = 106$; $HCO_3^- = 6$ mEq/L; lactate = 8.8 mEq/L; pH = 7.08; $PCO_2 = 24$ mm Hg; $PO_2 = 70$ mm Hg

Review of the laboratory test results reveals an anion gap acidosis. Calculation of the expected respiratory compensation is as follows:

Expected $HCO_3^- = 1.5\ [HCO_3^-] + 8 = 1.5(6) + 8 = 17$

The expected PCO_2 is lower than the actual PCO_2, producing a relative respiratory acidosis and indicating a need for ventilatory assistance.

sis, then a second acid base disorder must be present. The typical laboratory pattern of a metabolic acidosis is decreased pH and bicarbonate with a compensatory decrease in PCO_2 (Box 161-3).

Alveolar ventilation is increased through pH-mediated stimulation of peripheral chemoreceptors, producing increased minute ventilation through enhanced tidal volumes that can normally be increased from 5 L up to 30 L/minute. This protective effect lasts only a few days, however, because the chronically diminished PCO_2 paradoxically signals renal bicarbonate wasting. The final effect is that the arterial pH in chronic metabolic acidosis is the same, with or without respiratory compensation. The expected PCO_2 is calculated by the equation:

$$PCO_2 = 1.5 \times (HCO_3^-) + 8 \pm 2$$

This equation assesses the adequacy of respiratory compensation. A PCO_2 that is significantly higher or lower than this calculated value signals the presence of a secondary respiratory acidosis or alkalosis, which may have profound impact on treatment decisions (Box 161-4).

Causes of metabolic acidosis are classified according to the presence or absence of an elevated anion gap. However, even in the absence of an anion gap, there may be accumulation of unmeasured anions.

Non–anion gap acidoses are those that add HCl to the system. The acid anion in these cases is chloride; because of its inclusion in the anion gap equation, no change in the gap is noted. The most common etiologies of non–anion gap acidosis include renal and gastrointestinal bicarbonate wasting (Box 161-5).

BOX 161-4

Diabetic Patient with Mixed Acid-Base Disorder

A 26-year-old woman with a history of diabetes mellitus presents with vomiting and generalized malaise for the past 3 days.

Laboratory evaluation shows the following:

$Na^+ = 134$; $K = 4.6$; $Cl^- = 94$; $HCO_3^- = 20$ mEq/L; pH = 7.38; $PCO_2 = 35$ mm Hg

Step 1: The patient is minimally acidemic on the arterial blood gas.

Step 2: Serum bicarbonate is less than 25 mEq/L, indicating a metabolic acidosis.

Step 3: The anion gap is elevated: $134 - 94 - 20 = 20 \pm 2 = [1.5 \times 20] + 8 = 38$ mm Hg

Step 5: Calculation of the delta gap reveals that the delta HCO_3^- (24 – 20 = 4 units) is significantly less than the delta anion gap (20 – 10 = 10 units). This indicates the presence of a concomitant metabolic alkalosis, masking the significant anion gap acidosis. These findings are explained by a vomiting-induced alkalosis in a patient with diabetic ketoacidosis.

■ METABOLIC ALKALOSIS

Metabolic alkalosis is characterized by the gain of base, reflected in the serum by an elevation in the measured plasma bicarbonate level. Direct H^+ loss from extracellular fluid produces an elevation in serum bicarbonate by shifting the following equilibrium reaction to the right:

$$H_2CO_3 \rightarrow H^+ + HCO_3^-$$

The elevated plasma pH produces a compensatory hypoventilatory response that elevates the serum PCO_2. Because the serum pH is determined by the ratio of HCO_3^- to PCO_2 and not by the absolute HCO_3^- level, this compensatory response acts to minimize the change in serum pH.

Metabolic alkalosis is the second most common acid base disorder, found in approximately one third of hospitalized patients. It can be caused by several processes: Increased H^+ loss, typically through renal or gastrointestinal wasting; increased bicarbonate resorption; infusion or ingestion of bicarbonate; intracellular shifts of H^+; or contraction of the extracellular fluid around a stable HCO_3^- pool.

Due to the kidneys' ability to excrete excess HCO_3^-, the maintenance of metabolic alkalosis requires impairment of this process. The majority of the filtered bicarbonate is reclaimed in the proximal tubule, with approximately 10% of HCO_3^- reabsorbed in the more distal segments. Type B intercalated cells in the cortical collecting tubule may also actively secrete

BOX 161-5

4-Year-Old Boy with Diarrhea for 5 Days

Physical examination reveals dry mucous membranes.

Vital signs:

Blood pressure, 80/50; heart rate, 170 beats/min; temperature, 99.1° F; respiratory rate, 44 breaths/min

Laboratory data:

$Na^+ = 134$; $K = 4.8$; $Cl^- = 114$; $HCO_3^- = 3$;
pH = 6.98; $PCO_2 = 13$ mm Hg; $PO_2 = 110$ mm Hg

Step 1: The patient is acidemic on examination of the arterial blood gases.

Step 2: Serum bicarbonate is less than 25 mEq, indicating the presence of a metabolic acidosis.

Step 3: The anion gap is elevated: $134 - 116 - 3 = 15$

Step 4: Respiratory compensation is appropriate: $1.5\ [HCO_3^-] + 8 \pm 2 = [1.5 \times 3] + 8 = 12.5$

Step 5: Calculation of the delta gap reveals that the delta HCO_3^- ($24 - 3 = 21$ units) is significantly greater than that of the delta anion gap ($15 - 10 = 5$ units). This indicates the presence of a concomitant non–anion gap acidosis that overshadows the anion gap acidosis. The mixed acidosis can be clinically explained by the presence of diarrhea (non–anion gap acidosis) with dehydration (anion gap acidosis).

excess HCO_3^-. Thus maintenance of metabolic alkalosis requires the failure of these mechanisms. This generally results from extracellular fluid volume contraction, which stimulates Na^+ retention and enhanced activity of the Na^+-H^+ antiporter in the proximal tubule, resulting in H^+ excretion.

Hyperaldosteronism, induced by extracellular fluid depletion, is also thought to play a role in maintaining alkalosis by increasing H^+ secretion in the distal nephron through activation of the H^+-ATPase. Hypokalemia, hypochloremia, and hyperaldosteronism maintain alkalosis through stimulation of proximal and distal bicarbonate resorption, transcellular exchange of K^+-H^+, and increased ammoniogenesis. The most frequent causes of metabolic alkalosis are loss of gastric secretions and diuretic use. Loss of gastric sections generates an equimolar gain of HCO_3^- for lost H^+. Likewise, loss of gastric secretion is associated with a contracted extracellular fluid, which maintains alkalosis through volume depletion and hyperaldosteronism. Diuretics also induce an alkalosis through secondary hyperaldosteronism associated with hypovolemia, hypokalemia, and enhanced distal H^+ secretion.

The respiratory compensation for metabolic alkalosis can be variable. On average, PCO_2 can be predicted as follows:

$$\text{Increase in } PCO_2 = 0.6 \text{ increase in } HCO_3^-$$

Compensation rarely results in a PCO_2 greater than 55 mm Hg. Significant deviations from this compensatory response indicate a superimposed respiratory acidosis or alkalosis.

Signs and symptoms of alkalosis are commonly related to the associated volume contraction. Weakness, fatigue, coma, seizure, carpopedal spasm, respiratory depression, and neuromuscular irritability are observed, likely related to decreased ionized calcium due to alkalemia. Neuromuscular signs and symptoms are not common in metabolic alkalosis because of the slow movement of charged HCO_3^- into the central nervous system.

Evaluation of urine chloride is helpful in determining the etiology and treatment of metabolic alkalosis. Urine chloride is more sensitive than urine Na^+ for assessing volume status in alkalotic states due to the variability in urine sodium measurements during the development of metabolic alkalosis. Excess urinary Na^+ may be seen early in alkalosis, because it is combined with filtered HCO_3^-. As volume depletion increases, increased proximal resorption of HCO_3^- and elevated aldosterone increase Na^+ resorption, thereby decreasing urine sodium. Urine chloride, which is not influenced in metabolic alkalosis, is a more reliable marker for hypovolemia. A urine chloride less than 25 mEq/L indicates hypovolemia, whereas a urine chloride greater than 40 mEq/L indicates adequate volume expansion.

Evaluation of Mixed Acid-Base Disorders

By applying the formulas for anion gap, delta gap, and expected physiologic compensation, a stepwise approach to the evaluation of simple and mixed acid-base problems can be developed. This process is summarized in Box 161-6.

■ METABOLIC ACIDOSIS

The initial treatment for metabolic acidosis includes assessing the adequacy of respiratory compensation and providing ventilatory support as needed. Respiratory exhaustion causes PCO_2 to increase, compounding the metabolic acidosis.

Alkali therapy is presumed to reverse acid-induced myocardial dysfunction and the pro-arrhythmic effects of acidosis. Sodium bicarbonate is most commonly used. However, the effects are complex. Indiscriminate use of sodium bicarbonate may be more deleterious than helpful.

Sodium bicarbonate infusions may introduce an additional volatile acid load because HCO_3^- produces CO_2:

BOX 161-6

Five-Step Approach to Acid-Base Disorders

Rule 1: Determine the pH status (alkalemia or acidemia: >7.44 or <7.40)

Rule 2: Determine whether the primary process is respiratory, metabolic, or both

- Alkalemia
- Respiratory alkalosis: If P_{CO_2} is substantially <40 mmHg
- Metabolic alkalosis: If HCO_3^- is >25 mEq/L
- Acidemia
- Respiratory acidosis: If P_{CO_2} is >44 mm Hg
- Metabolic acidosis: If HCO_3^- is <25 mEq/L

Rule 3: Calculate the anion gap*

- Anion gap = $Na^+ - (Cl^- + HCO_3^-)$
- Increased anion gap (>10 mEq/L) may indicate metabolic acidosis
- Increased anion gap (>20 mEq/L) always indicates metabolic acidosis

Rule 4: Check the degree of compensation

- Metabolic acidosis: $P_{CO_2} = 1.5\ [HCO_3^-] + 8$
- Metabolic alkalosis: Increase in P_{CO_2} = 0.6 increase in bicarbonate
- Respiratory acidosis
- Acute: $[HCO_3^-]$ increases by 1 mEq/L for each 10 mm Hg increase in P_{CO_2}
- Chronic: $[HCO_3^-]$ increases by 4 mEq/L for each 10 mm Hg increase in P_{CO_2}
- Respiratory alkalosis
- Acute: $[HCO_3^-]$ decreases by 2 mEq/L for each 10 mm Hg decrease in P_{CO_2}
- Chronic: $[HCO_3^-]$ decreases by 5 mEq/L for each 10 mm Hg decrease in P_{CO_2}

Rule 5: Determine whether there is a 1 : 1 relationship between the change in the anion gap and the change in the serum bicarbonate

- Each 1-point increase in the anion gap should be accompanied by a 1 mEq/L decrease in bicarbonate.
- If the bicarbonate is higher than predicted, a metabolic alkalosis is also present.
- If the bicarbonate is lower than predicted, a non–anion gap metabolic acidosis is present.

*For every 1 g/dL that albumin is less than normal (4.2 g/dL), add 2.5 to the calculated anion gap.
Modified from Whittier WL, Rutecki GW: Primer on clinical acid-base problem solving. Dis Mon 2004;50:122-162.

$$HBuf + P_{CO_2}HCO_3^- \rightarrow Buf + H_2CO_3 \rightarrow CO_2 + H_2O$$

The additional CO_2 produced must be excreted by the lungs. CO_2 freely diffuses across cell membranes, especially in the presence of inadequate respiration, paradoxically creating organ acidemia, including in the central nervous system and renal, cardiac, and muscle tissues.

Sodium bicarbonate has also been associated with complications such as hypertonicity, hypernatremia, hypervolemia, increased organic acid production, and impaired oxygen unloading.

The use of bicarbonate infusions is appropriate for bicarbonate wasting acidoses or toxic acidosis in which systemic alkalinization facilitates toxin removal through ion trapping. However, supplemental bicarbonate use in organic acidoses (lactic acidosis and ketoacidosis) has not been shown to be efficacious. In these states, therapy is aimed at addressing the underlying etiology of these acidoses and promoting regeneration of bicarbonate from the accumulated acid anions. In hyperchloremic acidosis, no anions exist for regeneration of bicarbonate; therefore infusions can promptly reverse acidemia and restore serum bicarbonate stores.

When used, the goal of bicarbonate infusion is an increase in pH of 7.1 to 7.2, restoration of buffering capacity (>8 mEq/L HCO_3^-), or reversal of cardiac dysrhythmias and hypotension. Bicarbonate infusions are prepared by combining 3 ampules of sodium bicarbonate (44.6-50 mEq/L) with 1 liter of D_5W, which creates an isotonic solution of approximately 150 mEq/L of $NaHCO_3$. Bicarbonate deficit may be calculated using the Henderson-Hasselbalch equation, or by estimating the deficit at 1 mEq/kg and infusing one half the amount over 20 to 30 minutes, with the remainder infused over the next 2 to 4 hours. During this time, the acid-base and volume status must be carefully monitored to avoid the complications listed previously.

■ METABOLIC ALKALOSIS

Metabolic alkalosis is best treated by correcting the underlying causes of the alkalosis. Examination of the urine chloride allows etiologies to be classified as saline-responsive or saline-resistant.

Saline-responsive etiologies are associated with volume depletion, such as vomiting, chloride-wasting diarrhea, and diuretic therapy. A urine chloride less than 20 mEq/L indicates volume depletion; therapy with intravenous saline will lower serum HCO_3^- by increasing renal HCO_3^- excretion. Assessment of the efficacy of therapy can be determined at the bedside by monitoring the urine pH after saline infusion, with the expectation that the pH will become greater than 7.0 with therapy as HCO_3^- is excreted in the urine.

Saline-resistant causes display excessive mineralocorticoid activity, such as hyperaldosteronism, Cushing syndrome, and renal artery stenosis. Treatment of saline-resistant causes (urine chloride

>20 mEq/L) is directed at the other causes of metabolic alkalosis. Potassium deficits should be corrected through supplementation or direct antagonism of aldosterone with agents such as spironolactone. In patients with metabolic alkalosis and concomitant edematous states (congestive heart failure, cirrhosis, nephritic syndrome), the use of acetazolamide beneficially increases renal $NaHCO_3$ excretion.

REFERENCES

1. Kelly AM, McAlpine R, Kyle E: Venous pH can safely replace arterial pH in the initial evaluation of patients in the emergency department. Emerg Med J 2001;18:340-342.
2. Kelly AM, Kerr D, Middleton P: Validation of venous PCO_2 to screen for arterial hypercarbia in patients with chronic obstructive pulmonary disease. J Emerg Med 2005;28:377-379.

Chapter 162

Alcoholic Ketoacidosis

Christopher R. Carpenter

KEY POINTS

Alcoholic ketoacidosis accounts for up to 20% of cases of ketoacidosis.
The characteristic presentation is that of an alcoholic person who abruptly abstains, with signs and symptoms such as vomiting, abdominal pain, malnutrition, and an anion gap metabolic acidosis, but no measurable alcohol levels.
Initial glucose levels may be low, normal, or high.
A ratio of beta-hydroxybutyrate to acetoacetate in excess of 10:1 is pathognomonic for alcoholic ketoacidosis.
Treatment emphasizes hydration with dextrose-containing solutions and thiamine; there usually is resolution of the acidosis in 6 to 12 hours.
Mortality from uncomplicated alcoholic ketoacidosis is less than 1%.

Scope

The diagnosis of alcoholic ketoacidosis is established when an alcoholic patient is found to have an anion gap metabolic acidosis without historical or laboratory evidence suggesting an alternative etiology. Malnourished, chronic alcoholics who consume a daily average of 200 g (about 7 oz) of ethanol typically present with alcoholic ketoacidosis following periods of protracted vomiting. Euglycemia is most common, but transient nondiabetic hyperglycemia and profound hypoglycemia also have been reported.

Pathophysiology

Alcoholic ketoacidosis generally occurs with equal frequency in adult men and women between 20 and 60 years of age. The exact incidence and prevalence remains undefined. Up to half of patients are likely to suffer recurrence. It is unclear whether these individuals have a genetic predisposition to alcoholic ketoacidosis or whether they repeatedly reproduce the hormonal milieu which precipitates ketoacidosis. Almost one fifth of ketoacidosis presentations are alcoholic ketoacidosis.[1-3]

The term *alcoholic acidosis* describes a syndrome of four types of metabolic acidosis that occur in alcoholics and vary in severity: ketoacidosis, lactic acidosis, acetic acidosis, and a loss of bicarbonate in the urine. Alcoholic ketoacidosis arises from a complicated interplay of the metabolic effects of alcohol in fasted, dehydrated alcoholics who abruptly stop their intake of ethanol.

Beta-hydroxybutyrate is the predominant ketoacid. Metabolism of ethanol to acetaldehyde is catalyzed by alcohol dehydrogenase in the liver and results in an accumulation of the reduced form of

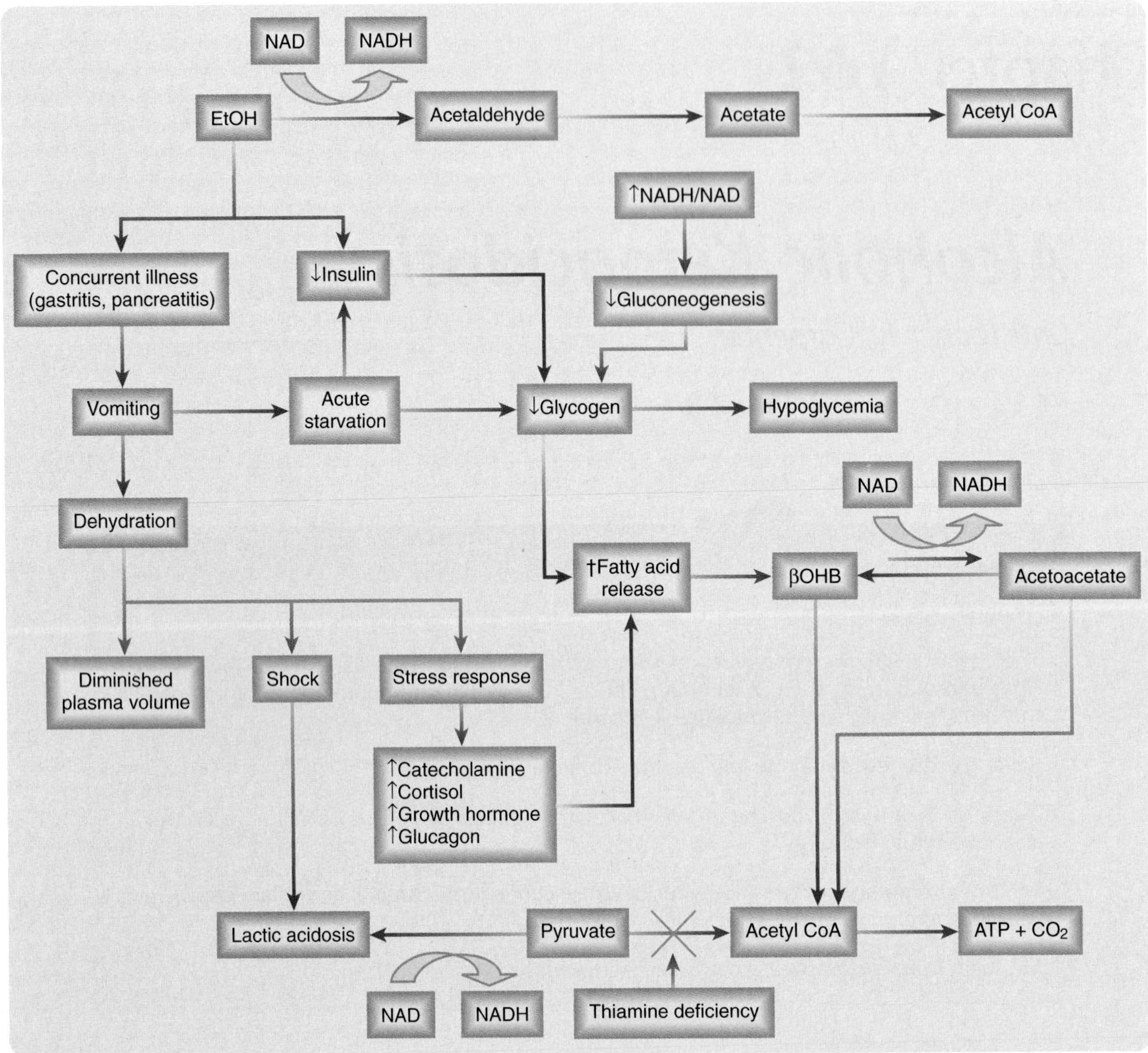
NAD
NADH
EtOH
Acetaldehyde
Acetate
Acetyl CoA
↑NADH/NAD
↓Gluconeogenesis
Concurrent illness (gastritis, pancreatitis)
↓Insulin
Vomiting
Acute starvation
↓Glycogen
Hypoglycemia
NAD
NADH
Dehydration
↑Fatty acid release
βOHB
Acetoacetate
Diminished plasma volume
Shock
Stress response
↑Catecholamine
↑Cortisol
↑Growth hormone
↑Glucagon
Lactic acidosis
Pyruvate
Acetyl CoA
ATP + CO2
NAD
NADH
Thiamine deficiency

FIGURE 162-1 The pathophysiology of alcoholic ketoacidosis. Alcohol dehydrogenase in hepatocyte cytosol metabolizes ethanol to acetaldehyde, which is then transported into the mitochondria for metabolism to acetate. Acetate is activated by adenosine triphosphate (ATP), co-enzyme A (CoA), and acetate thiokinase to form acetyl CoA, which can be (1) oxidized to carbon dioxide (CO_2) by the citric acid cycle, (2) form ketone bodies, or (3) be converted to fat.

Insulin depletion results from a number of influences, including endogenous suppression from malnutrition, the direct suppressive effects of ethanol, and α-adrenergic suppression from catecholamines. Volume depletion stimulates the counterregulatory release of catecholamines, cortisol, growth hormone, and glucagon. Glycogen depletion from malnutrition and alcoholic liver disease stimulates enhanced fatty acid release, which is further promoted by catecholamines. The relative increase of NADH over NAD resulting from the metabolism of ethanol drives several reactions to produce βOHB and lactate. Thiamine deficiency favors the conversion of pyruvate to lactate rather than acetyl CoA.

βOHB, beta-hydroxybutyrate; EtOH, ethyl alcohol; NAD, oxidized form of nicotinamide adenine dinucleotide; NADH, reduced form of nicotinamide adenine dinucleotide.

nicotinamide adenine dinucleotide (NADH) relative to the oxidized form nicotinamide adenine dinucleotide (NAD). The altered ratio of NADH/NAD is the rate-limiting step in alcohol metabolism and favors the conversion of acetoacetate to beta-hydroxybutyrate, as illustrated in Figure 162-1.

Impaired insulin effects, dehydration, and hormonal responses propagate ketoacid accumulation. Ethanol consumption, acute starvation, and catecholamine release cause a relative insulin insufficiency that acts to favor lipolysis and limit glycogen storage. The formation of ketone bodies is further promoted by a dehydration-induced stress response release of cortisol, growth hormone, glucagons, and catecholamines. It is unclear whether the elevated levels of cortisol and growth hormone observed in patients with alcoholic ketoacidosis initiate or sustain this process. Ketone bodies in the form of beta-hydroxybutyrate are produced as a result of the NADH/NAD ratio induced by ethanol metabolism, as well as the lipolytic effect of counterregulatory hormones. Renal excretion of ketone bodies becomes impaired due to dehydration, volume contraction, and diminished renal clearance. Ketoacid accumulation ensues.

Acetate formed by the metabolism of ethanol is converted to acetyl-CoA, which participates in one of three metabolic pathways:

1. Conversion to carbon dioxide and adenosine triphosphate via the citric acid cycle
2. Free fatty acid synthesis
3. Ketone body formation

Lactic acidosis is a common, concurrent acid-base disorder, in addition to ketoacidosis. Although lactic acidosis may result from another cause such as sepsis or seizures, the alcohol alone can cause a mild lactic acid accumulation by two distinct mechanisms. First, the elevated NADH/NAD ratio can shift the pyruvate–lactic acid equilibrium in favor of lactic acidosis. Second, the thiamine deficiency common in chronic alcoholics prohibits the alternative oxidation of pyruvate to acetyl-CoA, as thiamine is a co-enzyme in this reaction.[4-5]

Presenting Signs and Symptoms

Alcoholic ketoacidosis typically presents in severe alcoholics whose recent binge-drinking has abruptly and recently stopped. The sudden alcohol cessation is often due to an alcohol-related disease such as gastritis, pancreatitis, hepatitis, or pneumonia. Concurrent starvation, abdominal pain, and protracted vomiting are common presenting features.

Patients typically have a clear sensorium, are not confused, and are able to provide a complete history, though there are case reports of encephalopathic presentations. Box 162-1 summarizes the prevalence of signs and symptoms of alcoholic ketoacidosis.

Tachycardia and tachypnea are typically the most remarkable examination findings. Tachycardia results from volume depletion and early alcohol withdrawal, whereas tachypnea is generally a physiologic response to ongoing metabolic acidosis. Hypotension and hypothermia are rare. Fever usually indicates a separate, concurrent infectious process. Abdominal examination may reveal hepatomegaly, hepatic tenderness, epigastric discomfort, or severe and diffuse tenderness. The presence of hypotension, fever, peritoneal signs, bloody stools, trauma, or altered mental status mandates a search for alternative etiologies of the causes of these physical findings.

BOX 162-1

Prevalence of Signs and Symptoms of Alcoholic Ketoacidosis

- Nausea (76%)
- Vomiting (73%)
- Abdominal pain (62%)
- Dyspnea (20%)
- Heart rate >100 beats/minute (58%)
- Respiratory rate >20 breaths/minute (49%)
- Abdominal tenderness (43%)
- Altered mental status (18%)

Differential Diagnosis

Alcoholic patients are predisposed to a variety of complications that may precipitate alcoholic ketoacidosis, including gastritis, peptic ulcer disease, Boerhaave's syndrome, pancreatitis, and hepatitis. In addition, alcoholic patients are at increased risk of infectious complications such as aspiration pneumonia. Finally, patients with atypical acute coronary syndrome may present with nausea and abdominal pain and this should be considered in the differential diagnosis. Evaluation for alcohol-related conditions should occur in parallel with the evaluation and management of presumed alcoholic ketoacidosis.

Diagnostic Testing

Alcoholic ketoacidosis is one of the many conditions that cause an anion-gap metabolic acidosis, which is partly summarized by the mnemonic CAT-MUDPILES shown in the Tips and Tricks box. When an anion gap is present, an osmolar gap can help distinguish between these various entities. Additional rare etiologies of an anion-gap metabolic acidosis include sulfuric acidosis, short-bowel syndrome, formaldehyde, nalidixic acid, methenamine mandelate, rhubarb ingestion, and inborn errors of metabolism such as the methylmalonic acidemias.

The acid-base disorder in alcoholic ketoacidosis is usually a mixed anion-gap metabolic acidosis and respiratory alkalosis. pH ranges from 6.7 to 7.6, and the anion gap ranges from 20 to 40. Hypoalbumin-

Tips and Tricks

CAT-MUDPILES MNEMONIC

C = Carbon monoxide, Cyanide
A = Alcoholic ketoacidosis
T = Toluene
M = Methanol*
U = Uremia
D = Diabetic ketoacidosis
P = Paraldehyde, Phenformin
I = Iron, Isoniazid
L = Lactic acidosis
E = Ethylene glycol*
S = Salicylates, Strychnine, Starvation

*Osmolal gap >25 mosm/kg.

FACTS AND FORMULAS $SI = \frac{SV}{BSA}$

- Osmolar gap = Measured osmol – [2 (Na^+) + glucose + BUN + EtOH]
- Osmolar gap >25 mosm/kg is specific for methanol or ethylene glycol
- [Beta-hydroxybutyrate] >386 μmol/L has been proposed as a forensic pathology cut-off to identify "ketoalcoholic death." Levels >2500 μmol/L can be fatal.

BUN, blood urea nitrogen; EtoH, ethanol.

emia is common in alcoholics and may lower the observed anion gap.

Glucose levels may be low, normal, or elevated. Diabetic alcoholics with modest glucose elevations (above 250 mg/dL) pose a particular diagnostic challenge as they may present with diabetic ketoacidosis or concurrent diabetic ketoacidosis and alcoholic ketoacidosis. A useful distinguishing feature in these cases is the beta-hydroxybutyrate/acetoacetate ratio, which is 1:1 in normal individuals, 3:1 in diabetic ketoacidosis, and 10:1 in alcoholic ketoacidosis.

As the nitroprusside reaction utilized in a urine dipstick tests for diabetic ketoacidosis, a negative urine dipstick test for "ketones" does not exclude alcoholic ketoacidosis. In such instances, the dipstick may show a paradoxical worsening of urine ketones as alcoholic ketoacidosis resolves with treatment and beta-hydroxybutyrate is converted to acetoacetate.

Hypokalemia and hypophosphatemia are common in alcoholic ketoacidosis, particularly as treatment progresses. Alcohol levels are generally zero, although case reports have noted the presence of alcoholic ketoacidosis even when ethanol is detectable.[6-8]

Treatment

The treatment of alcoholic ketoacidosis is directed at correcting three deficits: volume depletion, glycogen depletion, and the elevated NADH/NAD ratio. Intravenous fluid and glucose are highly effective treatments. Dextrose-containing solutions in hypoglycemic or euglycemic patients stimulate NADH oxidation and replace glycogen stores, resulting in a more rapid correction of acidosis than with saline alone. Antiemetics should be provided.

Initially normal levels of magnesium, potassium, and phosphorus decrease during treatment and require repletion. IV thiamine supplementation (100 mg) provides a theoretical prophylaxis against Wernicke's encephalopathy and may help reverse lactic acidosis. Exogenous insulin and bicarbonate therapy are rarely indicated.[8-10]

Disposition

The mortality of patients from alcoholic ketoacidosis is less than 1%. Adverse outcomes are typically associated with concurrent alcohol-related complications rather than with the ketoacidosis itself. Admission for uncomplicated alcoholic ketoacidosis is indicated in cases of intractable vomiting or abdominal pain of unclear etiology.

If a thorough evaluation of the patient fails to reveal additional acute health issues, the acidosis can be treated and resolved within 6 to 12 hours. Discharged patients should have appropriate follow-up to address issues of chronic alcohol abuse. Patients may also benefit from an alcohol rehabilitation program. Discharge instructions should advise patients of their predisposition for recurrent episodes of alcoholic ketoacidosis, as well as the potentially detrimental effect of alcohol abuse on other aspects of their health. Return precautions should include intractable vomiting, caloric starvation, and increasing abdominal pain.

REFERENCES

1. Adams SL: Alcoholic ketoacidosis. Emerg Med Clin North Am 1990;8:749-760.
2. Adams SL, Matthews JJ, Flaherty JJ: Alcoholic ketoacidosis. Ann Emerg Med 1987;16:90-97.
3. Fulop M: Alcoholic ketoacidosis. Endocrinol Metab Clin North Am 1993;22:209-219.
4. Halperin ML, Hammeke M, Josse RG, et al: Metabolic acidosis in the alcoholic: A pathophysiologic approach. Metabolism 1983;32:308-315.
5. Iten PX, Meier M: Beta-hydroxybutyric acid—An indicator for an alcoholic ketoacidosis as cause of death in deceased alcohol abusers. J Forensic Sci 2000;45:624-632.
6. Umpierrez GE, DiGirolamo M, Tuvlin JA, et al: Differences in metabolic and hormonal milieu in diabetic- and alcohol-induced ketoacidosis. J Crit Care 2000;15:52-59.
7. Schelling JR, Howard RL, Winter SD, et al: Increased osmolal gap in alcoholic ketoacidosis and lactic acidosis. Ann Int Med 1990;113:580-582.
8. Hojer J: Severe metabolic acidosis in the alcoholic: Differential diagnosis and management. Human Exp Toxicol 1996;15:482-488.
9. Marinella MA: Alcoholic ketoacidosis presenting with extreme hypoglycemia. Am J Emerg Med 1997;15: 280-281.
10. Bakker SJL, Ter Maaten JC, Hoorntje SJ, et al: Protection against cardiovascular collapse in an alcoholic patient with thiamine deficiency by concomitant alcoholic ketoacidosis. J Int Med 1997;242:179-183.

Chapter **163**

Diabetes and Hyperglycemia

Matthew N. Graber

KEY POINTS

Type 1 insulin deficiency is defined as an absolute deficiency of insulin, and type 2 as a relative insulin deficiency. These terms replace older definitions.

The primary treatment modality for hyperglycemic emergencies is hydration with normal saline. In patients with diabetes, insulin therapy must follow evaluation of electrolyte levels.

Subcutaneous insulin is the preferred route for treatment of hyperglycemic emergencies. There is no role for IV bolus insulin. Continuous IV insulin infusion is warranted in patients with severe emergent conditions.

Patients with diabetic ketoacidosis have a significant potassium deficit and require supplementation.

IV administration of dextrose-containing fluid should be initiated in patients with diabetic ketoacidosis when the glucose level is at or below 250 mg/dL, in order to minimize the risk of hypoglycemia.

The majority of ketones in patients with diabetic ketoacidosis are beta-hydroxybutyrate, but standard laboratory tests evaluate for acetoacetate.

Diabetes Mellitis

■ SCOPE

Glucose is critical to the function of the central nervous system, as it is the primary fuel for these tissues. Plasma levels of glucose are strictly regulated, and even after a large oral glucose load or exercise they should not deviate from a range of 60 to 150 mg/dL.

■ EPIDEMIOLOGY

There are over 18 million patients with diabetes mellitus in the United States, and this number continues to increase at an accelerated rate, partially due to the worsening obesity epidemic in this country. In addition to the cost of life and morbidity associated with this disease, there is an enormous financial expense. In 2002, the estimated direct and indirect costs of treating diabetes mellitus in the United States were $92 billion and $40 billion, respectively.

■ STRUCTURE AND FUNCTION

Insulin is a 51–amino acid protein produced by the beta cells of the islet of Langerhans in the endocrine pancreas. After the initial protein, preproinsulin, is translated on the rough endoplasmic reticulum, it is

Table 163-1 COMPARISON OF THE FOUR TYPES OF DIABETES MELLITUS (DM)

	Type 1	Type 2	Gestational	Other
Insulin production	No	Yes	Yes	Dependent on degree of damage to pancreas; most often yes
Prior names	Type I DM, juvenile DM	Type II DM, adult-onset DM		
Usual onset	Sudden	Insidious	Insidious	Dependent on mechanism
Genetic predisposition	Moderate	Strong	Moderate	Dependent on mechanism

cleaved serially first to proinsulin and then to insulin and a C-peptide. Insulin along with its C-peptide is stored in a 1 : 1 ratio in secretory granules and released primarily in response to glucose and, to a lesser extent, amino acids. The release can be further potentiated or inhibited by a number of gastrointestinal and systemic hormones.

Upon release, insulin binds to its membrane-spanning receptor. This binding induces a conformational change in the structure of the receptor so that it becomes enzymatically active; it is now a functional tyrosine kinase that initiates anabolic pathways.

A newer classification system of diabetes mellitus reflects the pathophysiology of the disease and long-term treatment options. The new system identifies four types of diabetes mellitus: type 1, type 2, gestational diabetes, and "other" (Table 163-1).

Type 1 diabetes mellitus (note the Arabic numbering) has replaced older terms such as type I, insulin-dependent, and juvenile-onset diabetes mellitus. These older terms became confusing for a multitude of reasons. For example, a small subset of "type II" diabetics fail oral hypoglycemic treatment and must be treated with an insulin regimen; are these patients "insulin-dependent"? With increasing worldwide childhood obesity, more and more childhood diabetics are seen who are not "insulin-dependent,"and yet their disease cannot be classifed as "adult-onset."

Type 1 diabetes mellitus can best be defined as an absolute deficiency of insulin. The mechanism is complex and occurs in approximately 5% of all patients with diabetes mellitus. The process usually begins years before symptoms appear when the patient is exposed to an antigen (e.g., viral infection) that is similar in structure to a protein found in islet beta cells. The immune system begins to produce a humeral and cell-mediated assault upon those antigens, leading to progressive destruction of the beta cells. This leads to a progressive decrease in insulin levels, eventually reaching a critical point when insulin requirements are no longer being met and hyperglycemia ensues.

The other categories include patients with relative insulin deficiencies; it is important to note that the majority of hyperglycemic patients in the remaining groups do produce insulin, and thus it is easier to conceptualize their insulin deficiency as a balance.

Type 2 diabetes mellitus has replaced the older terms, including type II, non–insulin dependent, and adult-onset diabetes mellitus. The process leading to this type of diabetes also begins years prior to the onset of overt clinical symptoms. For a multitude of reasons, most commonly secondary to obesity, peripheral tissues become increasingly resistant to the effects of insulin. This leads to increased production of insulin by the beta cells, allowing years of relative glucose control. Eventually, the relative insulin resistance can no longer be met by increasing beta cell production, and the patient begins to experience hyperglycemia. Additionally, the beta cells begin to "burn out" and eventually produce progressively less and less insulin. The onset of clinical symptoms may be insidious in an otherwise healthy patient or abrupt when significant illness presents with a spike in counterreulatory hormones (e.g., epinephrine, glucagons, cortisol, growth hormone) that tends to increase plasma glucose levels. This abrupt onset occurs because the type 2 diabetic is not able to increase insulin production to counteract this rise, as would a non-diabetic.

The third category is gestational diabetes mellitus, which occurs in about 2% to 5% of all pregnancies, presenting most often in the second or third trimester. It is believed to occur in a manner similar to that of type 2 diabetes. Pregnancy induces increased levels of human placental lactogen, estrogen, and cortisol; all hormones that tend to increase plasma glucose levels. Pregnant women usually are able to produce insulin in sufficient quantities to combat this increase in glucose-elevating hormones; however, susceptible women cannot. This condition most often resolves postpartum but, as one would expect, these women are susceptible to developing type 2 diabetes later in life. There are fetal complications of this disease; mostly owing to increased fetal plasma glucose levels. In response to this elevated glucose derived via placental blood, the fetal pancreas increases plasma insulin levels, resulting in increased fetal birth weight.

The fourth category—"other"—is a catchall that contains all other causes of diabetes mellitus, including genetic anomalies causing malfunctioning insulin protein, insulin receptors, beta cells in general, and other immune-mediated causes. Any significant insult to the exocrine pancreas—be it trauma, chronic pancreatitis, or cystic fibrosis—may result in this type of diabetes. Many common drug-induced causes of diabetes mellitus fall into this category (Box 163-1), as well as endocrinopathies such as hyperthyroidism,

BOX 163-1

Drugs That May Cause Diabetes Mellitus*

- Pentamidine
- Nicotinic acid
- Glucocorticoids
- Thyroid hormone
- Diazoxide
- Beta-adrenergic agonists
- Thiazides
- Phenytoin
- Alfa-interferon

*"Other" category.

Cushing's syndrome, and pheochromocytoma. Infectious causes include congenital rubella and cytomegalovirus. Less common causes include genetic disorders that may be associated with diabetes mellitus including Down syndrome, Klinefelter's syndrome, Turner's syndrome, Prader-Willi syndrome, Huntington's chorea, and porphyria.

■ CLINICAL PRESENTATION

The clinical presentation of the diabetic patient can be quite varied. The classic presentations are discussed here, but it is important to note that many patients do not present with these symptoms. Typically, patients with type 1 diabetes have had years of progressively decreasing insulin secretion from beta cell destruction. However, most often an infection or other stressor acutely increases the levels of the counterregulatory hormones and the patient is unable to counter this spike with an insulin surge. Hyperglycemia (generally defined as a fasting glucose level >126 mg/dL) then ensues, and the patient suddenly presents to the ED.

As the plasma glucose level increases and eventually surpasses the threshold of the kidneys to reabsorb glucose, the patient begins to spill glucose into the urine. This leads to osmotic diuresis and ensuing polyuria and polydipsia.

■ TREATMENT

Patients who present with significant hyperglycemia, diabetic ketoacidosis, or hyperglycemic hyperosmolar state (HHS) are almost universally dehydrated and intravascularly depleted. While this is certainly more so in the latter two conditions, all conditions require hydration. The initial treatment is IV hydration with normal saline. Insulin is NOT the initial treatment for these diabetic complications.

■ DIAGNOSTIC TESTING

All diabetic patients who present with systemic complaints or complaints common to hyperglycemia require glucose testing at the time of first assessment. It is important to note that if serial tests are to be performed, there is a small but significant difference between capillary and venous blood glucose levels.[1] Additionally, any patient with altered mental status should also have glucose levels tested because patients with hypoglycemia or hyperglycemia may present with sensorium changes.

The purpose of laboratory testing in the hyperglycemic patient is to differentiate simple hyperglycemia from diabetic ketoacidosis and less commonly from HHS. It is important to note that there are no reliable physical examination findings that are sensitive or specific enough to rule in or rule out these acute and serious complications of diabetes. A bicarbonate level below 15 mmol/L with an elevated anion gap (varies depending on the laboratory, but the upper limit generally is about 16 mEq/L) strongly suggests diabetic ketoacidosis. A more complete laboratory evaluation for hyperglycemia includes venous pH, ketones, and plasma osmolality. Additional laboratory tests may be necessary as dictated by the clinical picture.

Hyperglycemia

■ PATHOPHYSIOLOGY

Hyperglycemia ensues when the endocrine pancreas cannot produce enough insulin to decrease plasma levels of glucose appropriately (<126 mg/dL in the fasting patient). In type 1 diabetes, this is due to an absolute deficiency; in the other types of diabetes, it is due to a relative deficiency of insulin compared with the levels of counterregulatory hormones. In this way, glucose levels increase in the plasma and eventually overwhelm the renal glucose threshold, resulting in the spilling of glucose into the urine. By osmosis, water is pulled into the urine, leading to increased urination and dehydration. This in turn leads to increased thirst and polydipsia. The degree of hyperglycemia and dehydration varies greatly from patient to patient and even in the same patient on different occasions.

■ DIAGNOSIS AND DIAGNOSTIC TESTING

The purpose of laboratory testing in the hyperglycemic patient is to differentiate simple hyperglycemia from diabetic ketoacidosis and less commonly from HHS.

It is important to ascertain the probable causes of hyperglycemia. Although dietary indiscretion and medicine non-compliance do play a role, these diagnoses should be considered only after ruling out more serious causes. The most concerning causes can be grouped into two classes: infection and infarction.

Diabetics have an increased rate of infection[2]; therefore a thorough search for an infection must be carried out. This includes a history and physical examination, including a thorough examination of the skin, and usually urinalysis. Chest radiography searching for pneumonia is indicated in patients with historical and physical examination findings suggesting pneumonia, patients in whom a thorough history and physical are not obtainable, clinically ill patients, and patients at the extremes of age. It is important to note that viral infection without any radiologic findings suggests hyperglycemia.

"Infarction" causes of hyperglycemia include acute coronary syndrome (acute myocardial infarction and unstable angina), pulmonary embolism, or cerebrovascular accident. It is important to note that acute coronary syndrome is very likely to present in an atypical manner in diabetic patients (e.g., new onset congestive heart failure without any history of chest pain or dyspnea without chest pain).[3] Any hyperglycemic patient with these "anginal equivalents" should have a complete ED evaluation for acute coronary syndrome. A computed tomography scan of the brain or chest may be required if there is any concern for cerebrovascular accident or pulmonary embolism.

■ TREATMENT

Hyperglycemia most often is associated with some degree of dehydration. Therefore the primary modality of treatment should be rehydration with normal saline. Early insulin therapy is contraindicated prior to obtaining electrolyte levels. After the patient is significantly rehydrated, laboratory studies have excluded additional complications such as diabetic ketoacidosis, and electrolytes have been repleted, subcutaneous insulin can be administered.

There is no role for the administration of IV bolus insulin in the treatment of hyperglycemia. The administration of insulin via a continuous drip is not indicated, except in very special circumstances where exceedingly tight glucose control is required (e.g., during progressing cerebral vascular accident) for the treatment of simple hyperglycemia. The dose of insulin depends upon the degree of hyperglycemia after hydration and on the patient's prior exposure to insulin therapy. Patients with known diabetes who are on insulin therapy may be given their usual dose after hydration. Patients new to insulin may be given low-dose subcutaneous insulin with the goal of decreasing glucose to acceptable levels at a rate of 100 mg/dL per hour.

A guideline for subcutaneous regular insulin dosing is shown in Table 163-2. This guideline is appropriate for hyperglycemic patients who have little to no previous experience with subcutaneous insulin. Those on insulin regimens may do better with a regimen approximating their typical dosage. Also, this guideline assumes that the patient has first been rehydrated and remains hyperglycemic.

Table 163-2 **REGULAR SUBCUTANEOUS INSULIN DOSING GUIDELINE***

Glucose Level	Dosage
>250 mg/dL	2 units
>300 mg/dL	4 units
>350 mg/dL	6 units
>400 mg/dL	8 units
>450 mg/dL	10 units
>500 mg/dL	12 units

*See text for discussion of modifications of this guideline.

It is important to note that euglycemia may not be a realistic or even appropriate goal in these patients while they are in the ED; longer-term (over days to weeks) personalization of an insulin or oral hypoglycemic regimen by the patient's primary care provider or inpatient physician is preferred. The ED goal may be simply to rehydrate the patient and then use subcutaneous insulin to decrease the patient's glucose level to less than 300 mg/dL. Targeting a "normal glucose" level in patients new to insulin therapy is fraught with risks, mostly notably hypoglycemia.

New-Onset Type 2 Diabetes

Box 163-2 summarizes the clinical and diagnostic findings in patients with new-onset diabetes. In the past, these patients were admitted without question and started on a new drug or insulin regimen. This

BOX 163-2

Diagnosis of New-Onset Diabetes Mellitus

- Patients with symptoms of uncontrolled diabetes including polyuria, polydipsia, and weight loss, with a random glucose level >200 mg/dL are diagnosed with diabetes mellitus.
- Patients with a fasting plasma glucose level of >125 mg/dL are diagnosed with diabetes mellitus.
- Fasting glucose levels >110 mg/dL suggest impaired glucose metabolism; these patients should be discharged and scheduled for follow-up with a primary care provider.
- Fasting glucose levels ≥95 mg/dL in pregnant patients ares consistent with the diagnosis of gestational diabetes mellitus.

Data from The American Diabetes Association: Diagnosis and classification of diabetes mellitus. Diabetes Care 2004;27: S5-S10; and Metzger BE, Coustan DR: Summary and recommendations of the Fourth International Workshop-Conference on Gestational Diabetes Mellitus. The Organizing Committee. Diabetes Care 1998;21(Suppl 2):B161-B167.

practice has changed in the last decade, as it is now recognized that these patients can be started on medications in the outpatient setting without exposing them to the inherent risks of hospitalization.

■ TREATMENT AND DISPOSITION

Initial medication for patients with new-onset diabetes most often is a low-dose sulfonylurea. A good choice is glyburide (1.25-2.5 mg orally once a day) or glipizide (2.5-5 mg orally once a day). These doses may not allow strict glucose control but are appropriate early therapy and pose little risk of hypoglycemia. When starting these medications, patients should be instructed to take them with an early meal or breakfast and to eat regular meals throughout the day. Metformin (850 mg orally once a day) is an appropriate choice for initiating diabetes therapy when a nonsulfonylurea drug is preferred. This drug, when used alone in initial therapy, poses a very low risk of hypoglycemia and may be a good choice for obese patients.[4]

All patients with new-onset diabetes should follow up in an expedited manner. Patients with comorbid conditions or acute disease should be admitted for inpatient evaluation and treatment.

Diabetic Ketoacidosis

The ED presentation of patients with diabetic ketoacidosis can be incredibly variable. For this reason it is important to remember that although there is a classic presentation of diabetic ketoacidosis, there is no typical presentation. The EP should not be lulled into a false sense of security by the hyperglycemic patient who "looks good." Diabetic ketoacidosis should be considered a spectrum of disease, and patients can progress from "looking good" to "being ill" very quickly. Thus any patient with hyperglycemia requires a laboratory evaluation.

■ EPIDEMIOLOGY

There are approximately 5 to 8 patients with diabetic ketoacidosis per 1000 diabetics per year. Mortality has remained approximately 1% to 2% for the last decade in patients who are diagnosed and begin treatment early in the disease course. Some mortality estimates for cases that are not diagnosed and treated early run as high as 14%.[5] Other estimates suggest that as many as 20% of patients with diabetic ketoacidosis are misdiagnosed and therefore have a significantly increased risk of death.

■ PATHOPHYSIOLOGY

The hyperglycemic patient has a deficiency in insulin; type 1 diabetics have an absolute deficiency and type 2 diabetics have a relative deficiency. When this deficiency is significant, they are unable to uptake glucose from the blood into cells and must rely on the metabolism of fat for energy. Fatty acids from the blood are metabolized in the liver to the three ketone bodies: acetoacetate (ACA), beta-hydroxybutyrate (BHB), and acetone. Acetone is a minor component and may be removed from the body via the lungs; this often presents as a fruity odor on the breath. The other ketone bodies are in an equilibrium whose ratio is determined by the redox state and relative levels of nicotinamide adenine dinucleotide (NAD) to NADH (the reduced form of NAD); because of this, the majority of ketones are in the form of BHB. The increasing level of BHB causes an acidosis and leads to significant electrolyte shifts. Increasing acidosis leads to a shift of potassium out of cells into the blood. Because of the continued hyperglycemia, the patient experiences hyperglycemic osmotic diuresis, leading to significant renal potassium losses and significant total body potassium depletion. The acidosis also causes a decrease in serum bicarbonate levels and eventually overwhelms this buffering system and leads to a decreased serum pH.

These changes result in the classic presentation of diabetic ketoacidosis, including dehydration, Kussmaul breathing (deep, sighing type of respiration caused by acidosis-induced stimulation of the central respiratory center that may be seen in other forms of acidosis), abdominal discomfort, vomiting, and often altered mental status.

■ CLINICAL PRESENTATION

The causes of diabetic ketoacidosis are many and are similar to those of hyperglycemia (Box 163-3). Initial presentation may be caused by infection or infarction or may be due to a deficiency of insulin, usually because the insulin dosage is insufficient, oral therapy is ineffective, or the patient is noncompliant with therapy. It is important to note that many diabetic patients have comorbid conditions—for example, patients with pneumonia may need increased insulin administration temporarily or they will develop diabetic ketoacidosis; in these cases the cause of the ketoacidosis is both infection and inadequate insulin administration.

BOX 163-3

Reasons Why Patients with Diabetic Acidosis Present to the ED*

- Infection (35%)
- Inadequate insulin (30%)
- Initial presentation (20%)
- Other illness (e.g., infarction) (10%)
- Unknown (5%)

*Percentage of approximate distribution is shown in parentheses.

BOX 163-4

Differential Diagnosis of Diabetic Ketoacidosis

- Hyperglycemic hyperosmolar state (HHS)
- Toxic alcohol ingestion
  - Methanol
  - Ethylene glycol
- Uremia
- Toxin overdose
  - Isoniazid
  - Iron
  - Salicylates
- Lactic acidosis
- Alcoholic ketoacidosis

BOX 163-5

Recommended Laboratory Work-up for Hyperglycemia

- Basic chemistry panel (Na, K, Cl, serum bicarbonate, blood urea nitrogen, creatinine, glucose)
- Venous pH
- Ketones (serum beta-hydroxybutyrate preferred)
- If diabetic ketoacidosis is suspected or confirmed: Add magnesium, phosphate, ECG
- If initial glucose level is >500 mg/dL or hyperglycemic hyperosmolar state is suspected: Add plasma osmolality
- As clinically indicated: Cardiac enzymes, serial ECG, lipase, ventilation/perfusion ratio, CTPA, CT head scan

ECG, electrocardiogram; CT, computed tomography; CTPA, computed tomography pulmonary angiography.

DIFFERENTIAL DIAGNOSIS, DIAGNOSTIC TESTING, AND TESTING PITFALLS

The differential diagnosis of diabetic ketoacidosis is summarized in Box 163-4. Any patient who may have diabetic ketoacidosis should have the laboratory evaluation shown in Box 163-5. There is no single standard laboratory diagnosis for diabetic ketoacidosis; however, any diagnosis should include the factors noted in Box 163-6. It should be stressed that the diagnosis of diabetic ketoacidosis is mainly based on clinical findings; although laboratory evaluation is important, common complicating factors often make laboratory diagnosis difficult. Each of the components of the laboratory diagnosis is fraught with limitations and qualifications.

BOX 163-6

Diabetic Ketoacidosis Diagnostic Test Findings*

- Glucose >250 mg/dL
- Elevated beta-hydroxybutyrate†
- At least two of the following:
  - pH>7.30
  - Serum bicarbonate <18 mmol/L‡
  - Anion gap >15 mEq/L‡

*The diagnosis of DKA ideally will be made using the above findings; however, it is important to note that the clinical scenario dictates the relative importance of each finding, as discussed in the text.
†Beta-hydroxybutyrate is the preferred ketone; however, most laboratories substitute blood (or less frequently, urine) acetoacetate.
‡These values may vary, depending on the laboratory.

Hyperglycemia commonly is considered the cornerstone of the work-up; however, diabetic ketoacidosis in the presence of "euglycemia" is not an uncommon finding. In fact, approximately 30% of patients with diabetic ketoacidosis have a glucose level higher than 300 mg/dL,[6] and some studies suggest that the longer patients are in a state of diabetic ketoacidosis, the more likely they are to be euglycemic. The reasons for this are manyfold. Patients with diabetic ketoacidosis often have gastrointestinal disturbances that cause vomiting and therefore limited oral intake, with the result that liver glycogen stores will be depleted, and gluconeogenesis will be the sole source of glucose production. It has been suggested that patients with poorly controlled diabetes do not store glucose as liver glycogen as readily or efficiently as nondiabetic individuals or patients whose disease is well controlled. Liver disease of any cause will also limit or prevent glycogen storage and gluconeogenesis.

Acidosis and decreased serum bicarbonate are basic components of the diagnosis. However, there have been reports of patients who otherwise fit the diagnosis of diabetic ketoacidosis but have alkalosis and/or have elevated serum bicarbonate levels. Patients with diabetic ketoacidosis often vomit considerably and lose acid through this mechanism. They also can become exceptionally dehydrated, leading to stimulation of the renin-angiotensin system, which promotes the loss of both potassium and the hydrogen ion in the distal tubule of the kidneys. Medications such as diuretics and antacids may also cause metabolic acidosis. A common presentation to the ED is the patient with a gastrointestinal disturbance, either as the result of diabetic ketoacidosis or as its primary cause, who has ingested a large amount of oral antacids to self-treat nausea and stomach upset.

Although the majority of patients have a low serum bicarbonate and pH, there are exceptions, due to the reasons just described, that may escape detection and therefore are not diagnosed and treated. It should be noted that a venous pH is perfectly acceptable, and there is no reason to obtain an arterial sample.[7]

The final component of the diagnosis is the presence of ketones. As discussed previously, the majority of ketones are in the form of BHB, but the standard laboratory urine and serum examinations assay for ACA. ACA levels may not be high enough to be detected, especially in the dilute urine of a patient experiencing hyperglycemic osmotic diuresis. However, as the patient is rehydrated and treatment begins, the serum BHB is converted to ACA. Thus, in a not-uncommon scenario, the hyperglycemic patient initially is negative for urine ketones but after rehydration and treatment begins to "suddenly spill" them, and the patient is falsely labeled as worsening and beginning to have diabetic ketoacidosis, when in fact the patient already had diabetic ketoacidosis, but the diagnosis was missed because the urine examination tested for the "wrong" ketone.

■ TREATMENT

A treatment plan for diabetic ketoacidosis is outlined in Box 163-7. Early treatment is similar to that for hyperglycemia. Patients usually are rather dehydrated and should receive normal saline. The average patient without a history of congestive heart failure or renal failure often requires 5 to 8 L of fluid. Potassium levels must be checked and hypokalemia corrected prior to the administration of insulin because patients may have significant (often hundreds of milliequivalents) total body potassium depletion. Insulin will drive extracellular potassium into cells and because of the total body depletion may cause an exaggerated serum hypokalemia that may lead to cardiac arrhythmia.

Other electrolytes such as magnesium and phosphorus are less crucial and may be repleted as usual. The correction of even moderate hypophosphatemia has not been shown to be beneficial in these patients. Therefore it is recommended that only severe hypophosphatemia (<1 mmol/L) or moderate hypophosphatemia with clinical findings such as respiratory muscle weakness or cardiomyopathy be corrected.[8] If necessary, potassium chloride may be replaced with potassium phosphate for this purpose. Hypomagnesemia may be corrected with IV magnesium sulfate.

Bicarbonate therapy rarely has a place in the treatment of patients with diabetic ketoacidosis. Although the administration of bicarbonate to a patient with a metabolic acidosis may seem logical, it is rarely helpful and may cause multiple, significant complications. Because bicarbonate cannot cross the blood-brain barrier but carbon dioxide can, the administration of bicarbonate may allow increased carbon dioxide to enter the cerebrospinal fluid and cause a paradoxical cerebrospinal fluid acidosis. Additionally, bicarbonate administration may worsen hypokalemia by driving potassium into cells. Studies have clearly shown that the administration of bicarbonate to a patient with diabetic ketoacidosis and a pH of at least 6.8 to be of no benefit.[9] No studies specifically support the administration of bicarbonate for any pH in patients with diabetic ketoacidosis. If there is any role for bicarbonate adminis-

BOX 163-7
Treatment Plan for Patients with Diabetic Ketoacidosis

This regimen is recommended for the average adult patient and must be tailored for the individual patient. Patients in whom volume overload is a concern (e.g., with a history of congenital heart failure or renal impairment) may need more gentle dehydration. Those with a greater degree of dehydration may require greater amounts of normal saline (NS).

Intravenous Fluids

- Administer 2 L NS over first 1 to 2 hours; a third liter may be administered over an additional hour.
- Change from NS to ½ NS after the patient's clinical hydration status begins to improve (usually after 2-3 L).
- Change from ½ NS to D_5 ½ NS when the patient's glucose level reaches 250 mg/dL.

Electrolytes

- No insulin should be given until the patient's potassium level is known.
- Potassium replacement (oral administration is preferred, but the IV route can be used if the patient cannot tolerate oral replacement) should be started as follows:
  - K>5.0 mEq/L—no acute replacement needed
  - K 3.5-5.0 mEq/L—give single oral dose of 40 mEq/L of KCl
  - K<3.5 mEq/L—give two oral doses of 40 mEq/L of KCl

Insulin

- There is no role for IV bolus insulin in the treatment of diabetic ketoacidosis.
- After the patient is hemodynamically stable, start a regular insulin drip at 0.05 to 0.1 unit/kg/hour.
- When the patient's anion gap has resolved to ≤15 mEq/L, administer subcutaneous regular insulin at the patient's usual dose or at a dose similar to those listed in Table 163-2. One hour later, the insulin drip can be discontinued.
- NOTE: The subcutaneous insulin and insulin drip should overlap by approximately 1 hour.

RED FLAGS

Pitfalls in the Treatment of Diabetic Ketoacidosis

- Insulin administration prior to correcting potassium deficiencies can lead to clinically significant hypokalemia and cardiac arrhythmias.
- Not performing regular (at a minimum of every 2 hours but every hour is preferred) laboratory testing to adjust the administration of fluids, insulin, and electrolytes. This should be continued at least for 2 hours after discontinuing the insulin drip.

tration, it may only be in a patient with shock and impending or present cardiovascular collapse.

The administration of insulin should begin only after the initial hydration and electrolyte correction. There is no role for IV bolus insulin. The administration of IV bolus insulin leads to a supraphysiologic serum insulin level that can cause a significant drop in plasma potassium levels and cardiac arrhythmias.[10] It may also cause hypoglycemia and cerebral and pulmonary edema, and it has been theorized to lead to changes in gene-regulated protein synthesis that may exert its effects for weeks.[11,12] Additionally, because IV regular insulin has a plasma half-life of less than 5 minutes, low-dose continuous infusion reaches a steady state level quickly.[13]

The standard insulin protocol has been to start a drip of regular insulin at 0.1 unit/kg. More recently it has been suggested that lower doses may work as well with less risk of hypokalemia, and some authors have even suggested the use of subcutaneous insulin.[14]

The patient on an insulin drip is at risk for hypoglycemia and hypokalemia, as mentioned previously, and therefore requires regular electrolyte and glucose assays. The author recommends alternating a bedside glucose assay with a basic chemistry panel every hour and charting a flow sheet as shown in Table 163-3. Potassium can then be supplemented as necessary. The patient's fluid should be changed to D_5 $^1/_2$ NS (5% dextrose solution in $^1/_2$ normal saline) when the glucose level reaches 250 mg/dL. When the anion gap has resolved to 15 mEq/L or less, the patient should be given subcutaneous regular insulin at the usual dose or at a dose similar to those listed in Table 163-2. One hour later, the insulin drip can be discontinued; this allows the subcutaneous insulin administration and the insulin drip to overlap by 1 hour.

It is not necessary nor should it be expected for the pH to return to normal before discontinuing the insulin drip. The treatment regimen by itself will often cause a hyperchloremic acidosis; therefore monitoring the anion gap is more helpful than monitoring the pH. In a patient with normally functioning kidneys, the chloride level and pH will then be slowly corrected over hours to days. In a patient who has otherwise recovered, a mild acidosis at this point should not prevent discharge.

■ DISPOSITION

Begin all discharged patients on an insulin regimen. Oral hypoglycemic medications are insufficient.

Patients on an insulin drip need to be closely monitored for all of the reasons discussed previously; for this reason they usually are admitted to an intensive care unit or other specialized unit that can closely monitor their glucose, electrolytes, and clinical status.

One last—but to the patient often critically important—comment. If patients with diabetic ketoacidosis are hungry and there is no other contraindication, there is no reason why they should not eat. They often are ravenous, and eating will act naturally to decrease the likelihood of hypoglycemia and hypokalemia.

Hyperglycemic Hyperosmolar State (HHS)

HHS is a comparatively uncommon but nonetheless serious complication of diabetes mellitus, with a mortality rate as high as 50%.[5] It has had many other names in the past, including hyperosmolar nonketotic coma, hyperglycemic hyperosmolar coma, and hyperosmolar nonacidotic diabetes mellitus. The term *hyperglycemic hyperosmolar state* is more appropriate because not all patients with HHS are nonke-

Table 163-3 TYPICAL FLOW SHEET FOR DIABETIC KETOACIDOSIS

		CHEM PANEL (MEQ/L)								
Time	Test	Na	K	Cl	HCO_3 (mmol/L)	Anion Gap (mEq/L)	pH	Glucose (mg/dL)	Current IVF	Current Tx
6:55	Accucheck							530		
7:00	Chem VBG	130	3.0	100	8	22	7.0	500	NS	KCl
8:00	Chem	132	3.4	106	8	18		402	NS	Insulin/KCl
9:00	Accucheck							312	$^1/_2$ NS	Insulin

Chem, chemistry; IVF, intravenous fluids; NS, normal saline; Tx, treatment; VBG, venous blood gases.

Table 163-4 COMPARISON OF TYPICAL LABORATORY TEST FINDINGS IN DIABETIC KETOACIDOS (DKA) AND HYPERGLYCEMIC HYPEROSMOLAR STATE (HHS)

Finding	DKA	HHS
Osmolarity (mOsm/L)	Normal	>320
Glucose (mg/dL)	Usually 250-600	>600
Insulin	Low to absent	Low to normal
Ketones	Present	Absent
pH	<7.35	7.35-7.45
HCO_3 (mmol/L)	<15	18-29
Onset	Variable	Usually slow onset over days to weeks

totic, and certainly not all are in a coma or have an altered mental status.[15]

■ PATHOPHYSIOLOGY

Like diabetic ketoacidosis, HHS is initiated by a relative lack of insulin; however, the insulin deficiency usually is significantly less profound than that of diabetic ketoacidosis. Very low levels of insulin (or a low ratio of insulin to counterregulatory hormones) are necessary to prevent ketoacidosis; as insulin levels increase, further gluconeogenesis and glycogen metabolism are sequentially switched off. Because only small amounts of insulin are needed to prevent ketosis, only limited amounts of ketones are made during HHS; however, the other factors present in the formation of diabetic ketoacidosis usually are diserved. The patient becomes successively more dehydrated secondary to the glucose-driven osmotic diuresis. This dehydration eventually may lead to an impaired renal function and the inability to excrete the continually produced glucose, resulting in severe hyperglycemia.[16]

■ CLINICAL PRESENTATION

Typically, these patients may state that they cannot or do not wish to drink liquids; thus patients with HHS may have an impaired thirst sensation or may be unable to obtain water (e.g., elderly or bed-ridden patients, psychiatric patients, jailed patients).

Although there are many similarities between diabetic ketoacidosis and HHS, they differ in some very important ways (Table 163-4). As discussed earlier in regard to diabetic ketoacidosis, patients with HHS may often present atypically. The diagnosis is associated with glucose levels higher than 600 mg/dL, but the average glucose level is approximately 900 mg/dL, and it is not uncommon for the glucose level to be well over 1000 mg/dL.

■ DIAGNOSTIC TESTING AND TESTING PITFALLS

Diagnostic criteria for HHS are summarized in Box 163-8. As with diabetic ketoacidosis, it needs to be stressed that the diagnosis is mainly based on clinical findings; although laboratory evaluation is important, common complicating factors often make laboratory diagnosis difficult.

When making the diagnosis, any treatment prior to the collection of samples for laboratory tests must be noted. These patients are severely dehydrated and hyperglycemic; any fluid administration—for example, by the emergency medical service—will significantly decrease their glucose level. In this context, it is not uncommon for HHS to be diagnosed in patients with an initial glucose of 450 to 500 mg/dL. Serum osmolarity may also decrease to a lesser degree with initial fluid resuscitation.

The absence of ketosis is required to differentiate pure HHS from pure diabetic ketoacidosis. However, many patients present within a spectrum between these two entities and may form a small amount of BHB. Additionally, because most laboratories actually assay for acetoacetate, as discussed earlier, mild ketoacidosis is common secondary to anorexia and vomiting. Another classic finding of HHS is a "normal pH." However, it is not uncommon to have a mild acidotic hyperosmolar state secondary to a lactic acidosis caused by a lack of perfusion to peripheral tissues from the severe dehydration. In fact, approximately one half of patients with HHS are believed to have a mild anion gap metabolic acidosis.[17] Also, the pH may temporarily decrease further during the

BOX 163-8

Diagnostic Testing Criteria for Patients with Hyperglycemic Hyperosmolar State (HHS)

- Glucose >600 mg/dL
- Normal pH
- No significant ketosis
- Serum osmolarity
  - >320 mOsm/L with any mental status changes or
  - >350 mOsm/L

initial fluid resuscitation as the peripherally produced lactic acid is returned to the liver for processing.

TREATMENT

A treatment plan for HHS is summarized in Box 163-9. As with simple hyperglycemia and diabetic ketoacidosis, the primary treatment is fluid resuscitation with normal saline. The average fluid deficit is 9 L.[18] Resuscitation includes administration of boluses of 1 to 2 L of normal saline initially, followed by administration of normal saline until there is improvement in vital signs that suggests improved hemodynamics, indicated by the onset of urine output and improved clinical hydration state. Fluids then can be changed to D_5 ½ NS.

Failure to change the fluid at this point is apt to lead to significant and clinically detrimental hypernatremia. Fluid administration can be further guided by the following:

1. Patients should have approximately 50% of their fluid deficit met in the first 12 hours of treatment.
2. Glucose levels should fall no faster than 100 mg/dL per hour after the initial resuscitation is completed.

Electrolytes also require aggressive monitoring and replacement. Total body deficits of potassium,

BOX 163-9

Treatment Plan for Patients with Hyperglycemic Hyperosmolar State (HHS)

This regimen is recommended for the average adult patient and must be tailored for the individual patient. Patients in whom volume overload is a concern (e.g., with a history of congenital heart failure or renal impairment) may need more gentle dehydration. Those with a greater degree of dehydration may require greater amounts of normal saline (NS).

Insulin

- There is no role for IV bolus insulin in the treatment of patients with HHS, and there is no role for insulin of any kind during the early resuscitation phase of treatment.
- After early fluid and electrolyte administration and when the patient is hemodynamically stable, start a regular insulin drip at 0.05 to 0.1 unit/kg/hour. Note that some authorities suggest significantly lower doses, starting around 2 units per hour in an average-sized adult and adjusting the rate based on the decrease in glucose levels.

Intravenous Fluids

- Administer 2 L of NS over the first 1 to 2 hours and continue until the patient is hemodynamically stable; change from NS to ½ NS when
  - Glucose levels are decreasing at a rate no higher than 100 mg/dL/hour
  - Approximately one half of the fluid deficit is replaced during the first 12 hours of treatment

Electrolytes

Patients with HSS have significant total-body depletion of potassium, phosphate, and magnesium; repletion should be started in the ED with the goal of reaching approximately normal blood levels during treatment, but the total-body repletion of these electrolytes may take days.

- Potassium replacement (oral administration is preferred, but the IV route can be used if the patient cannot tolerate oral replacement) should be started as follows:
  - K>5.0 mEq/L—no acute replacement needed
  - K 3.5-5.0 mEq/L—give single oral dose of KCl, 40 mEq/L
  - K<3.5 mEq/L—give two oral doses of KCl, 40 mEq/L
- Magnesium replacement—unless the patient is in renal failure and not able to produce urine, early administration of magnesium is mandatory:
  - Begin IV piggy-back (IVPB) administration of 2 g of $MgSO_4$ over 2 hours and continue administration over the course of treatment.
  - Magnesium must be supplemented along when administering phosphate to prevent the development of clinically significant hypocalcemia.
- Phosphate replacement
  - Potassium phosphate can be substituted for part of the potassium chloride.

Patients being treated for HHS are at risk for refeeding syndrome and should receive thiamine supplementation.

- An initial IVPB dose of 100 mg of thiamine in the ED is an appropriate early intervention.

magnesium, and phosphate cannot be accurately gauged from the initial laboratory assay and should be supplemented aggressively once urine output has been established. Note that although the initial measured potassium may be normal or even high, the patient is still severely potassium-depleted. Therefore, potassium supplementation must be started early in the treatment course and certainly prior to the initiation of any insulin therapy.

Phosphate and magnesium may be more essential in the management of HHS than in the treatment of diabetic ketoacidosis. Because HHS characteristically develops over days to weeks, total body stores of these electrolytes are more likely to have been significantly effected by the osmotic diuresis. Although compelling studies are lacking, it is likely of greater urgency to supplement these electrolytes early in the course of treatment.[19,20]

Insulin administration should begin only after the patient has been fluid-resuscitated to the point of hemodynamic stability and after potassium replacement has been started. *There is no role for insulin in the initial treatment of HHS—its early administration can lead to cardiovascular collapse.*

The effective osmolarity of the vasculature in patients with HHS is dependent on the high level of glucose present. This level may decrease slowly with the administration of normal saline as sodium begins to replace glucose in maintaining proper tonicity. However, if insulin is administered early before appropriate normal saline resuscitation is attained, this cannot happen. Insulin will drive glucose intracellularly, effectively, and quickly decreasing intravascular tonicity; this may lead to acute and catastrophic cardiovascular collapse. Additionally, early insulin administration will drive potassium intracellularly, risking the same hypokalemia-induced arrhythmias discussed earlier in the treatment of diabetic ketoacidosis.

RED FLAGS

Pitfalls in the Treatment of Hyperglycemic Hyperosmolar State (HHS)

- Hypernatremia may be caused by the failure to change normal saline to ½ normal saline after the resuscitation phase of treatment has concluded.
- The early administration of insulin may lead to:
  - Total cardiovascular collapse
  - Clinically significant hypokalemia, hypophosphatemia, and hypomagnesemia.
- Failure to replete electrolytes during fluid administration may lead to cellular and cerebral edema and cardiovascular instability.
- Seizures occurring in a patient with HHS should not be treated with dilantin because this drug is known to decrease endogenous insulin secretion.

After early fluid and electrolyte administration and when the patient is hemodynamically stable, insulin therapy can begin. Typically a drip of regular insulin is started at 0.05 to 1 unit/hour; many authorities suggest low doses of 2 to 4 units/hour. This is then titrated to control the rate of the decrease of glucose to approximately 50 to 100 mg/dL/hour. *As with diabetic ketoacidosis and hyperglycemia, there is no role for IV bolus administration of insulin in the treatment of HHS.*

DISPOSTION

Patients should be admitted to the intensive care unit because frequent neurologic examinations and regular laboratory studies are required during the first 24 hours of treatment. Electrolyte supplementation will need to be adjusted regularly based on the results of these laboratory tests. As with patients with diabetic ketoacidosis, if patients being treated for HHS are hungry, their mental status has returned to baseline, and there are no other contraindications, there is no reason why they should not eat. They often are ravenous and eating will act naturally to decrease the likelihood of hypoglycemia and acute electrolyte deficiencies.

REFERENCES

1. Boyd R, Leigh B, Stuart P: Capillary versus venous bedside blood glucose estimations. Emerg Med J 2005;22:177-179.
2. Joshi N, Caputo GM, Weitekamp MR, Karchmer AW: Infections in patients with diabetes mellitus. N Engl J Med 1999;341:1906-1902.
3. Singer DE, Moulton AW, Nathan DM: Diabetic myocardial infarction: Interaction of diabetes with other preinfarction risk factors. Diabetes 1989;38:350-357.
4. Lee A, Morley JE: Metformin decreases food consumption and induces weight loss in subjects with obesity with type II non–insulin-dependent diabetes. Obesity Res 1998;6:47-53.
5. Fishbein H, Palumbo PJ: Acute metabolic complications in diabetes. In National Diabetes Data Group (eds): Diabetes in America, 2nd ed. National Institutes of Health, 1995, pp 283-291.
6. Munro JF, Campbell IW, McCuish AC, et al: Euglycaemic diabetic ketoacidosis. BMJ 1973;2(866):578-580.
7. Kreshak A, Chen EH: Arterial blood gas analysis: Are its values needed for the management of diabetic ketoacidosis? Ann Emerg Med 2005;45:550-551.
8. Wilson HK, Keuer SP, Lea AS, et al: Phosphate therapy in diabetic ketoacidosis. Arch Intern Med 1982;142:517-520.
9. Morris LR, Murphy MB, Kitabchi AE: Bicarbonate therapy in severe diabetic ketoacidosis. Ann Intern Med 1986;105:836-840.
10. Fisher JN, Shahshahani MN, Kitabchi AE: Diabetic ketoacidosis: Low-dose insulin therapy by various routes. N Engl J Med 1977;297:238-241.
11. Schade DS, Eaton RP: Dose response to insulin in man: Differential effects on glucose and ketone body regulation. J Clin Endocrinol Metab 1977;44:1038-1053.
12. Carroll MF, Schade DS: Ten pivotal questions about diabetic ketoacidosis. Answers that clarify new concepts in treatment. Postgrad Med 2001;10:89-92, 95.
13. Fort P, Waters SM, Lifshitz F: Low-dose insulin infusion in the treatment of diabetic ketoacidosis: Bolus versus no bolus. J Pediatr 1980;96:36-40.

14. Umpierrez GE, Latif K, Stoever J, et al: Efficacy of subcutaneous insulin lispro versus continuous intravenous regular insulin for the treatment of patients with diabetic ketoacidosis. Am J Med 2004;117:291-296.
15. Carroll P, Matz R: Uncontrolled diabetes mellitus in adults: Experience in treating diabetic ketoacidosis and hyperosmolar nonketotic coma with low-dose insulin and a uniform treatment regimen. Diabetes Care 1983;6: 579-585.
16. Brodsky WA, Rapaport S, West CD: The mechanism of glycosuric diuresis in diabetic man. J Clin Invest 1950;29:1021-1032.
17. Matz R: Management of hyperosmolar hyperglycemic syndrome. Am Fam Physician 1999:60:1468-1476.
18. Siperstein M: Diabetic ketoacidosis and hyperosmolar coma. Endocrinol Metab Clin North Am 1992;21: 415-432.
19. Solomon SM, Kirby DF: The refeeding syndrome: A review. JPEN J Parenter Enteral Nutr 1990;14:90-97.
20. Matz R: Magnesium: Deficiencies and therapeutic uses. Hosp Pract (Off Ed) 1993;28:79-82, 85-87, 91-92.

Chapter **164**

Hypoglycemia

Wesley H. Self

KEY POINTS

Rapid bedside measurement of blood glucose concentration should be performed on patients with altered mental status. Hypoglycemia should be considered in patients with neurological abnormalities.

Exogenous insulin and sulfonylurea medications account for most cases of hypoglycemia, but low blood glucose can be the presenting feature of a large array of serious illnesses, including sepsis, liver disease, renal disease, and tumors.

A blood glucose concentration less than 60 mg/dL in a symptomatic patient should be immediately corrected with the administration of glucose, either orally or intravenously, or with intramuscular glucagon.

Only patients with a readily identifiable cause of hypoglycemia and negligible risk of recurrence may be discharged home safely.

Scope

Hypoglycemia is common, life-threatening, and readily treatable. Hypoglycemia often occurs in diabetic patients as a side effect of glucose-lowering therapy and can be easily identified and treated in this setting. However, hypoglycemia can sometimes be difficult to recognize, masquerading as psychosis, acute stroke, or even gastroenteritis. Etiologies of hypoglycemia can also be challenging to diagnose, as in the case of insulinomas that often require a 72-hour fasting study. Hypoglycemia may require complex management plans; for example, sulfonylurea overdose sometimes requires admission to the intensive care unit and continuous dextrose infusions.

Definition

Hypoglycemia is an abnormally low blood glucose concentration that causes symptoms—autonomic hyperactivity (anxiety, irritability, palpitations, trembling) and/or neurologic dysfunction (inattention, lethargy, altered consciousness, seizure, coma). A definitive diagnosis requires the fulfillment of *Whipple's triad:* symptoms consistent with hypoglycemia are present; the blood glucose concentration is low; and the symptoms resolve when the blood glucose recovers to the normal range. An exact threshold to define "low blood glucose" is not firmly established due to variations in the concentration at which individuals begin to experience symptoms. However, a blood glucose level less than 60 mg/dL is generally considered abnormally low.

Epidemiology

Patients who use insulin are at the greatest risk for hypoglycemia. In this population, mild hypoglycemic episodes are defined as symptomatic events that are self-treated; they occur about twice per week. Severe hypoglycemia, which requires the assistance of another person to regain euglycemia, is experienced at least once a year by 27% of patients on intensive insulin regimens.[1] Hypoglycemia is the cause of death of approximately 3% of insulin-dependent diabetic patients.

Patients who are treated with oral hypoglycemic agents also commonly experience hypoglycemia. Although these episodes generally manifest milder symptoms, they occur in more than 30% of patients each year. The incidence of hypoglycemia is expected to rise as tight glycemic control continues to be emphasized for the 17 million Americans with diabetes.

Hypoglycemia in nondiabetic patients is quite rare and should raise concern about the possibility of a severe underlying illness, alcohol ingestion, or inappropriate exposure to insulin or an oral hypoglycemic agent.

Normal Glycemic Control

■ INSULIN

Unlike many other organs, the brain cannot synthesize glucose or store a significant glycogen supply and therefore requires an uninterrupted flow of glucose from the blood for normal function and survival. Under normal physiologic conditions, the blood glucose concentration is maintained within a narrow range (70-110 mg/dL) through the balance of catabolic processes that increase blood glucose and anabolic processes that decrease blood glucose. Insulin, a protein released from the pancreatic beta-cells in response to an increasing blood glucose level, is the hormone responsible for initiating anabolic glucose metabolism. It promotes glycolysis, inhibits glycogenolysis and gluconeogenesis in the liver, inhibits proteolysis in skeletal muscle, and inhibits lipolysis and promotes lipogenesis in adipose tissue. Insulin secretion is inhibited during a fast in order to maintain euglycemia, essentially ceasing when the blood glucose concentration falls below 80 mg/dL.

■ COUNTERREGULATORY HORMONES

The hormones that promote catabolic glucose metabolism are called the *counterregulatory hormones* because they oppose the actions of insulin. These hormones include glucagon, epinephrine, cortisol, and growth hormone. Counterregulatory hormones inhibit the entry of glucose into cells, stimulate glycogenolysis and gluconeogenesis, mobilize amino acids to act as gluconeogenic precursors, activate lipolysis, and inhibit insulin secretion. Glucagon, secreted from pancreatic alpha-cells, and epinephrine, released from the adrenal medulla and sympathetic neurons, are released to protect against hypoglycemia when the blood glucose concentration drops below 65 to 70 mg/dL.

Glycogenolysis increases blood glucose within minutes and can maintain euglycemia in a well-nourished person for 24 hours. Gluconeogenesis requires several hours to raise blood glucose and is the principal mechanism responsible for maintaining euglycemia if fasting is extended beyond 24 hours. Secretion of cortisol from the adrenal cortex and growth hormone from the anterior pituitary gland are delayed responses to blood glucose falling below 60 to 65 mg/dL. Cortisol and growth hormone are not involved in the correction of acute hypoglycemia, but rather act to maintain euglycemia over a period of days to weeks.

A clinically important consequence of the counterregulatory system for insulin-dependent diabetics is the *Somogyi phenomenon.* A nighttime insulin dose that is too high causes hypoglycemia during sleep; the counterregulatory hormones respond to the hypoglycemia, increasing blood glucose and causing hyperglycemia during the morning glucose check. Increasing the nighttime insulin dose in response to morning hyperglycemia would cause dangerous overnight hypoglycemia and exacerbate the morning hyperglycemia. Paradoxically, decreasing the nighttime insulin dose in this case would lower morning blood glucose concentrations.

Many of the symptoms of hypoglycemia are caused by the acute increases in glucagon (which causes nausea, vomiting, and abdominal pain) and epinephrine (which causes anxiety, trembling, palpitations, tachycardia, and sweating). The hypoglycemic symptoms caused by epinephrine, termed *autonomic symptoms* or *hyperepinephrinemic symptoms,* function as a warning that mild hypoglycemia has developed. Most patients recognize autonomic symptoms and correct their hypoglycemia by eating, well before neurologic impairment ensues. *Hypoglycemia unawareness* is the development of hypoglycemia without autonomic symptoms to warn the patient, thus increasing the risk of severe hypoglycemia.

Patients with type 1 and advanced (insulin-dependent) type 2 diabetes may have an impaired counterregulatory reaction. In these patients, the glucagon response is often nonexistent and the epinephrine response is greatly attenuated.[2] This impaired counterregulatory response predisposes to severe hypoglycemia by blunting the glycemic response to falling blood glucose levels and masking the early warning symptoms of hypoglycemia. Furthermore, one hypoglycemic episode, even if asymptomatic, blunts the epinephrine response to future hypoglycemia, the so-called *hypoglycemia-associated autonomic failure.*[3] A vicious cycle of recurrent hypoglycemia can develop. Avoidance of hypoglycemia for only a few weeks improves hypoglycemia awareness and the epinephrine component of counterregulation.[2]

Causes of Hypoglycemia

Hypoglycemia occurs when there is a relative excess of insulin compared with the counterregulatory response; this can occur through the administration of exogenous insulin, an increase in endogenous insulin, or inhibition of the counterregulatory response. This section highlights the most important causes of hypoglycemia, their mechanisms of action, and the context in which they are likely to present in the ED (Table 164-1).

■ EXOGENOUS INSULIN AND ORAL HYPOGLYCEMIC AGENTS

Administration of insulin or an oral hypoglycemic agent is the most common cause of hypoglycemia. In a diabetic patient with an established regimen of insulin or oral hypoglycemic agent, hypoglycemia can develop for a number of reasons (Table 164-2).

Oral hypoglycemic agents include the sulfonylurea and meglitinide drug classes, both of which increase the endogenous pancreatic secretion of insulin. Sulfonylureas are more commonly used and more likely to cause hypoglycemia than the meglitinides. In 2004, 4148 sulfonylurea overdoses were reported to American poison control centers, of which 36% were in children less than 6 years of age, 21% required treatment for hypoglycemia, 2.5% were considered life-threatening, and 0.22% were fatal.[4]

Other classes of oral diabetes medications, including biguanides, alpha-glucosidase inhibitors, and thiazolidinediones, do not increase insulin levels and do not induce hypoglycemia. However, when used in addition to insulin or an oral hypoglycemic agent, these medicines can make hypoglycemia more refractory to treatment.

The time to peak effect and duration of action for insulin preparations and oral hypoglycemic agents are key features that dictate the management and disposition of the hypoglycemic patient (Table 164-3). Patients often cannot reliably recall which type of insulin they use; a helpful characteristic is that all rapid-acting and short-acting insulins (and glargine) are clear liquids, whereas NPH (neutral protamine Hagedorn) and Ultralente appear cloudy.

Diabetes caused by chronic pancreatitis has a concomitant deficiency of glucagon due to the loss of pancreatic alpha-cells, making these patients very susceptible to the hypoglycemic effects of insulin and oral hypoglycemic agents. Insulin and oral hypoglycemic agents can also cause hypoglycemia in a nondiabetic patient when taken accidentally, in a suicide attempt, as part of a factitious disorder, or Munchausen's by proxy. Factitious disorder and Munchausen's by proxy should be considered in cases of unexplained hypoglycemia in healthy patients, especially in female health care workers and family members of a diabetic person.

■ ADDITIONAL CAUSES OF HYPOGLYCEMIA

Alcohol ingestion (ethanol), the second most common cause of hypoglycemia in the ED, inhibits the counterregulatory response by suppressing hepatic gluconeogenesis. It has minimal effects on glycogenolysis. Therefore, alcohol use typically requires concomitant fasting to deplete glycogen stores before hypoglycemia ensues. The classic presentation of alcohol-induced hypoglycemia is a malnourished alcoholic who undertakes a prolonged binge. However, fasting for 6 hours before significant alcohol consumption in an otherwise healthy person can cause hypoglycemia. Hypoglycemia is rare (<1%) among intoxicated patients in the ED, but hypoglycemic episodes seen in the ED in lower socioeconomic areas involve alcohol nearly 50% of the time.[5]

Critical illness can cause hypoglycemia in both diabetic and nondiabetic patients. *Sepsis* is the third most common cause of hypoglycemia. The mechanism involves increased peripheral utilization of glucose and hepatic hypoperfusion impairing gluconeogenesis. Meanwhile, severe *liver disease* induces hypoglycemia via failure of hepatic gluconeogenesis and glycogenolysis. *Renal failure* can also cause hypoglycemia; the mechanism is not completely understood but probably involves delayed clearance of insulin and reduced mobilization of gluconeogenic precursors. The kidney is a minor contributor to gluconeogenesis, but loss of this function is not thought to play a significant role in renal failure–induced hypoglycemia. *Congestive heart failure* can also lead to hypoglycemia via hepatic vascular congestion impairing gluconeogenesis and glycogenolysis.

Starvation, such as with anorexia nervosa, depletes glycogen stores and gluconeogenic precursors and can eventually lead to hypoglycemia. Hypoglycemia as a complication of anorexia nervosa is a late finding that implies a poor prognosis.

Insulinomas are tumors of pancreatic beta-cell origin that secrete insulin without the normal mechanism of feedback regulation, thus producing hyperinsulinemia and hypoglycemia. Insulinomas are rare, with an incidence of 4/1,000,000/year. Early diagnosis is important, because these tumors are often curable with surgery before they lead to fatal hypoglycemia. Patients with insulinomas usually appear healthy and present with unexplained hypoglycemia. *Nesidioblastosis* is hypertrophied (not neoplastic) beta-cell tissue that oversecretes insulin and can also present with unexplained hypoglycemia.

Non–islet cell tumors, including hepatomas, carcinoids, sarcomas, and melanomas, can cause hypoglycemia by several diverse mechanisms: a paraneoplastic syndrome caused by secretion of insulin-like growth factors; multiple metastases to the liver with impaired hepatic function; massive tumor burden with increased metabolic demand for glucose; and produc-

Table 164-1 CAUSES OF HYPOGLYCEMIA

Cause (Examples)	Comment
Exogenous insulin (treatment of diabetes, factitious disorder, Munchausen's by proxy, total parenteral nutrition, hyperkalemia)	Hypoglycemia caused by excessive insulin administration; most common cause of hypoglycemia
Oral hypoglycemic agents (sulfonylureas, meglitinides)	Induce secretion of insulin from pancreatic beta-cells
Alcohol (ethanol)	Inhibition of hepatic gluconeogenesis; hypoglycemia usually requires concomitant fasting
Sepsis	Inhibition of hepatic gluconeogenesis and increased peripheral glucose utilization
Liver disease (hepatitis from infections or toxins, cirrhosis, Reye's syndrome, HELLP syndrome, hepatoma, metastatic tumors)	Inhibition of hepatic gluconeogenesis and glycogenolysis
Renal disease	Decreased clearance of insulin and reduced mobilization of gluconeogenic precursors
Congestive heart failure	Hepatic congestion causes inhibition of gluconeogenesis and glycogenolysis
Starvation (prolonged fasting, anorexia nervosa, pyloric stenosis, pediatric gastroenteritis)	Depletion of glycogen stores and gluconeogenic precursors
Hormone deficiency (cortisol, growth hormone, epinephrine, glucagon, hypopituitarism)	Failure of counterregulatory mechanism of glucose metabolism; the hormone deficiency may be either congenital or acquired
Medicines not used for treatment of diabetes mellitus (ACE inhibitors, acetaminophen, acetazolamide, aluminum hydroxide, beta-blockers, benzodiazepines, *Bordetella*-pertussis vaccine, chloroquine, chlorpromazine, cimetidine, ciprofloxacin, colchicine, diphenydramine, disopyramide, doxepin, ecstasy, EDTA, etomidate, ethionamide, fluoxetine, furosemide, haloperidol, imipramine, indomethacin, isoniazid, lidocaine, lithium, maprotiline, mefloquine, monoamine oxidase inhibitors, nefazodone, orphenadrine, pentamidine, phenytoin, propoxyphene, quinine, quinidine, ranitidine, ritodrine, selegiline, terbutaline, tetracyclines, trimethoprim-sulfamethoxazole, warfarin)	Induce hypoglycemia rarely and unpredictably, usually in otherwise healthy individuals
Insulinoma	Excessive, unregulated endogenous insulin secretion from a tumor of pancreatic beta-cell origin
Nesidioblastosis	Excessive insulin secretion by hypertrophic pancreatic beta-cells
Non–islet cell tumors (sarcoma, carcinoid, melanoma, leukemia, hepatoma, teratoma, colon, breast, prostate, stomach, mesothelioma)	Various mechanisms, including secretion of insulin-like growth factors, increased metabolic demand, production of insulin autoantibodies
Post gastric surgery (gastric bypass, gastrectomy, pyloroplasty)	Rapid dumping of glucose into small intestine causes exaggerated insulin response; nesidioblastosis may have a role
Inborn errors of metabolism (errors in glycogen synthesis, glycogenolysis, gluconeogenesis, mitochondrial beta-oxidation, amino acid metabolism)	Congenital defect prevents normal metabolism from maintaining euglycemia
Idiopathic ketotic hypoglycemia	Fasting intolerance, possibly due to deficiency of alanine as a gluconeogenic precursor
Autoimmune	Antibiodies against insulin or the insulin receptor augment the effects of insulin
Akee fruit	Unripe akee, a fruit found in Jamaica, contains toxins that inhibit hepatic gluconeogenesis
Vacor rat poison	Damages pancreatic beta-cells, initially causing release of insulin and hypoglycemia but eventually causing impaired insulin secretion and diabetes mellitus; banned in the United States
Transient neonatal hypoglycemia (prematurity, intrauterine growth retardation, severe infant distress syndrome, perinatal asphyxia, maternal hyperglycemia, erythroblastosis fetalis, beta-agonist tocolytic agents)	Presents in immediate newborn period; rarely seen in the ED
Persistent neonatal hypoglycemia (mutation in sulfonylurea receptor gene, glutamate dehydrogenase gene, glucokinase gene)	Presents in immediate newborn period; rarely seen in the ED

ACE, angiotensin-converting enzyme; EDTA, ethylenediaminetetraacetic acid; HELLP, *Hemolysis, Elevated Liver* enzymes, *Low Platelet* count.

Table 164-2 POTENTIAL CAUSES OF HYPOGLYCEMIA IN A DIABETIC PATIENT WITH AN ESTABLISHED REGIMEN OF INSULIN OR ORAL HYPOGLYCEMIC AGENT

Mechanism	Examples
Decreased glucose availability	Missed or unusually light meal Impaired gluconeogenesis Alcohol ingestion
Increased glucose usage	Unusually heavy exercise Illness, especially infection, with increased metabolic demands
Increased dose of drug	Patient/nursing mistake in delivering too much drug Patient with memory problem causing repeated doses Patient with seeing difficulty causing inaccurate dosing Inaccurate glucometer reading leading to excessive insulin dose Nursing change of shift and poor documentation Insulin pump malfunction or programming error Intentional overdose Suicide attempt Factitious disorder Munchausen's by proxy Pharmacy error Physician prescribing error
Increased availability of drug	Renal insufficiency (insulin and sulfonylureas are renally excreted) Liver failure (many sulfonylureas are hepatically metabolized) Drug interactions Warfarin inhibits metabolism of chlorpropamide and tolbutamide H_2 blockers inhibit metabolism of glipizide and glyburide Ciprofloxacin inhibits metabolism of glyburide Clarithromycin displaces glyburide from serum proteins

tion of autoantibodies to insulin or the insulin receptor. *Autoantibodies* that augment the effects of insulin can also occur in conjunction with autoimmune diseases, such as systemic lupus erythematosus and Graves' disease.

The condition of patients with vague autonomic symptoms after eating was once labeled "postprandial hypoglycemia," "alimentary hypoglycemia," or "functional hypoglycemia." This poorly understood mimic of hypoglycemic symptoms has never been linked to depressed blood glucose concentrations.[6] However, after gastric surgery (including gastric bypass surgery, gastrectomy, and pyloroplasty), patients may experience a true postprandial or alimentary hypoglycemia. Traditionally the mechanism was thought to be a rapid emptying of carbohydrates into the small intestines, causing an exaggerated insulin response (*dumping syndrome*). Recent evidence suggests that nesidioblastosis plays a role in postprandial hypoglycemia following gastric surgery.[7]

Medications other than those used for the treatment of diabetes have been associated with hypoglycemia (see Table 164-1).[8] Quinine/quinidine, pentamidine, and disopyramide stimulate insulin release from pancreatic beta-cells and have the potential to cause severe hypoglycemia. Commonly used drugs that rarely cause hypoglycemia include salicylates (mechanism unknown); acetaminophen (hypoglycemia only occurs in overdose with liver damage); angiotensin-converting enzyme (ACE) inhibitors (mechanism may involve increased insulin sensitivity); and beta-blockers (inhibit the counterregulatory response of epinephrine). ACE inhibitors and beta-blockers typically cause hypoglycemia only when used concomitantly with insulin or oral hypoglycemic agents. Non-selective beta-blockers (e.g., propranolol) have more hypoglycemic potential than selective $beta_1$-blockers (e.g., metoprolol) and can occasionally cause hypoglycemia in the absence of antidiabetic medicines, especially in children.

■ CAUSES OF HYPOGLYCEMIA IN PEDIATRIC POPULATIONS

Children are generally predisposed to hypoglycemia due to relatively small glycogen stores and a large brain-to-body mass ratio. Additionally, many inborn errors of metabolism, including glucose-6-phosphatase deficiency, galactosemia, and carnitine deficiency present with hypoglycemia. Neonates are at even greater risk for hypoglycemia due to developmental immaturity of gluconeogenesis and ketogenesis, as well as temporary impairment of glycogenolysis due to the stress of delivery. Neonates of mothers with poorly controlled diabetes are further predisposed to

Table 164-3 FEATURES OF INSULIN PREPARATIONS AND ORAL ANTI-DIABETIC AGENTS RELEVANT TO THE ED MANAGEMENT OF HYPOGLYCEMIA

Diabetic Agent	Risk of Hypoglycemia?	USUAL TIMING OF HYPOGLYCEMIC EFFECT IN ADULTS (HR)		
		Onset	Peak	Duration
Rapid-acting insulins	Yes			
Aspart (Novolog)		¼-½	1-2	3-5
Glulisine (Apidra)		¼-½	1	4-5
Lispro (Humalog)		¼-½	1-2	3-5
Short-acting insulins	Yes			
Regular		½-1	2-4	6-10
Semilente		1-2	3-8	10-16
Intermediate-acting insulins	Yes			
Lente		3-4	6-14	16-24
NPH		1-3	4-12	18-24
Long-acting insulins	Yes			
Glargine (Lantus)		2-4	none	24
Ultralente		4-8	8-12	18-36
Sulfonylureas, 1st generation	Yes			
Acetohexamide (Dymelor)			3	12-18
Chlorpropamide (Diabinase)			2-7	60
Tolazamide (Tolinase)			4-6	12-24
Tolbutamide (Orinase)			3-4	6-12
Sulfonylureas, 2nd-3rd generation	Yes			
Glimepiride (Amaryl)			2-3	16-24
Glipizide (Glucotrol)			1-3	12-24
Glipizide extended-release (Glucotrol XL)			6-12	24
Glyburide (Diabeta, Glycron, Glynase Prestab, Micronase)			2-6	12-24
Meglitinides	Yes			
Nateglinide (Starlix)			½-1	4-6
Repaglinide (Prandin)			½-1	4-6
Biguanides	No			
Metformin (glucophage)				
Alpha-glucosidase inhibitors	No			
Acarbose (Precose)				
Miglitol (Glyset)				
Thiazolidinediones	No			
Rosiglitazone (Avandia)				
Pioglitazone (Actos)				

NPH, neutral protamine Hagedorn insulin.

hypoglycemia due to hyperinsulinemia induced by maternal hyperglycemia.

Children with *gastroenteritis* are at risk for hypoglycemia because diarrhea decreases the intestinal absorption of carbohydrates and the illness increases metabolic demands for glucose. Reid and colleagues[9] found that 9% (18/196) of children aged 1 month to 5 years presenting to an ED with gastroenteritis and dehydration had hypoglycemia, although none of the children had altered mental status.

Idiopathic ketotic hypoglycemia is the most common cause of clinically significant hypoglycemia in nondiabetic children aged 7 months to 5 years. The syndrome is characterized by fasting intolerance and may be caused by a deficiency of alanine, an amino acid substrate for gluconeogenesis.[10] During a 10- to 16-hour fast, the counterregulatory response converts triglycerides to ketone bodies, resulting in a mild metabolic acidosis, ketonuria, and failure to maintain euglycemia. For example, a toddler awakening after an unusually long overnight fast may develop hypoglycemia that manifests as lethargy with or without seizures, as well as a ketotic state that induces anorexia, nausea, and vomiting. Most affected children are slender but not malnourished, with weight percentile below height percentile. These children often have a concurrent illness, present to the ED in the morning, and have a blood glucose concentration of 35 to 60 mg/dL, bicarbonate of 14 to 19 mMol/L, and ketonuria. The syndrome typically remits by age 6 because of increases in lean body mass and alanine levels.

Clinical Presentation

Signs and symptoms of hypoglycemia are divided into two categories: those caused by elevated levels of glucagon and epinephrine as part of the counterregulatory response (*autonomic* or *hyperepinephrinemic symptoms*) and those caused by insufficient supply of glucose to the brain (*neuroglycopenic symptoms*). Autonomic symptoms typically appear when the blood glucose concentration drops below 60 mg/dL and include anxiety, irritability, nausea, vomiting, palpitations, trembling, hunger, and sweating. Patients presenting to the ED with only autonomic symptoms not accompanied by neurologic impairment are unlikely to have hypoglycemia. Neuroglycopenic symptoms emerge when the blood glucose concentration falls below 50 mg/dL and include inability to concentrate, inattention, headache, lethargy, dizziness, blurry vision, agitation, confusion, and focal neurologic deficits. When the blood glucose concentration drops below 30 mg/dL, seizures and coma ensue. Permanent brain damage and death are rare, generally occurring when hypoglycemia is severe and left untreated. Predicting who will have permanent neurologic impairment is difficult in the ED, although elderly patients, hypoxic patients, and patients with a history of strokes are vulnerable to incomplete recovery.

All potential signs and symptoms are not uniformly present with each episode of hypoglycemia. Recurrent episodes in the same person tend to be symptomatically similar. However, hypoglycemia manifests differently among different individuals. Variations include the blood glucose threshold at which symptoms develop, the severity of symptoms at a given glucose concentration, the predominance of certain symptoms, and their order of appearance. The severity of neuroglycopenic symptoms depends on many factors other than the nadir of blood glucose, including general state of health, age, integrity of the counterregulatory response, and the severity, duration, timing, and number of previous hypoglycemic episodes. For example, Osoria and associates[11] showed that nondiabetic, neurologically normal subjects who were administered exogenous insulin to lower their blood glucose concentration to 30 mg/dL experienced only subtle neuroglycopenic symptoms and no alteration of consciousness. The rate at which the blood glucose declines does not appear to affect the severity of symptoms. As discussed previously, hypoglycemic episodes blunt the symptoms of future hypoglycemia. Therefore, lower blood glucose concentrations with recurrent episodes will be symptomatically silent, predisposing the patient to repeated severe hypoglycemia, which can cause cumulative cognitive decline.

Other than prior hypoglycemic episodes, additional features that increase the risk of hypoglycemia for diabetic patients include use of insulin, longer durations of insulin use, higher doses of insulin, initially high hemoglobin A1c (HbA1c) values that decrease rapidly with therapy, adolescence, and male gender.[1] Use of an insulin pump does not alter the risk of hypoglycemia compared with multiple daily insulin injections.

Differential Diagnosis

The clinical presentations for which hypoglycemia should be considered as part of the differential diagnosis, and the differential diagnosis of the causes of established hypoglycemia are both quite broad. Refer to Tables 164-1 and 164-2 for the causes of hypoglycemia.

Hypoglycemia should be considered in any patient with an acute neurologic abnormality, however gross or subtle, especially with an alteration in mental status. Classic examples include a diabetic patient who collapses during exercise, an alcoholic patient presenting with seizures, and a comatose patient who ingested unknown pills. More challenging presentations include a focal neurological deficit in an elderly patient, psychotic and combative behavior in a young adult, and hypotonia or lethargy in an infant. Hypoglycemia should be included in the differential diagnosis of each of the following diseases: stroke, transient ischemic attack, seizure disorder, traumatic brain injury, narcolepsy, multiple sclerosis, psychosis, and drug intoxication.

Blood glucose concentration should be checked in all patients requiring resuscitation, as critical illness can cause hypoglycemia. Losek[12] found that 18% (9/49) of pediatric patients undergoing nontraumatic ED resuscitation were hypoglycemic. Additionally, hypoglycemia should be considered in all patients with accidental and intentional drug ingestions, in children with prolonged vomiting and diarrhea, and in all diabetic patients presenting to the ED with any significant medical or surgical illness.

Diagnostic Testing

GLUCOMETRY

The optimal method for diagnosing hypoglycemia is the rapid determination of blood glucose concentration through point-of-care testing with a bedside glucometer. Bedside glucometers measure the concentration of glucose in whole blood, whereas laboratory tests measure the glucose concentration in plasma or serum. Due to the relative paucity of glucose in blood cells, whole blood concentrations of glucose are approximately 15% lower than plasma concentrations. Newer models of bedside glucometers calculate an estimated plasma glucose concentration based on measured whole blood concentration. Although bedside glucometers that undergo routine quality control have adequate accuracy to direct immediate therapy, laboratory tests of glucose concentration are more accurate than bedside glucometers, especially in the extreme high and low ranges; therefore abnormal glucose levels discovered at the bedside should be confirmed with laboratory testing.

Accuracy of bedside glucometry and laboratory tests of serum glucose concentration can be compromised by several mechanisms. An artificially high glucose concentration can be reported by bedside glucometry during acetaminophen overdose because of the interference of acetaminophen with the measuring technique. Bedside glucometers are less accurate with hematocrit levels above 55 or below 30, reflecting variations in the relative amounts of blood cells and plasma. Artificially low serum glucose measurements are seen with hemolytic anemia (nucleated red blood cells consume glucose in the collection tube), leukemia (leukocytes consume glucose), and when blood is collected in a tube lacking a glycolysis-suppressing agent such as fluoride.

■ URINALYSIS

Urinalysis occasionally is helpful. Urine ketones are expected in hypoglycemia when the counterregulatory hormones are in relative abundance compared with insulin, because the counterregulatory response induces ketone body production from lipolysis. Therefore, urine ketones typically are present in hypoglycemia not caused by hyperinsulinemia, and absent in hypoglycemia caused by hyperinsulinemia. An exception to this rule is hypoglycemia caused by an enzymatic defect in fatty acid oxidation, which prevents the synthesis of ketone bodies.

■ EXTENDED LABORATORY TESTING

Other diagnostic tests that are useful for the ill-appearing hypoglycemic patient include liver function tests, blood alcohol concentration, salicylate level, acetaminophen level, random cortisol level, chest radiology, urine culture, blood culture, electrocardiography, and cardiac enzyme measurement. Recent evidence suggests that hypoglycemia may be associated with cardiac ischemia. Desouza and co-workers[13] found that ischemic electrocardiographic changes were more common during hypoglycemia than during euglycemia or hyperglycemia in diabetic patients with coronary artery disease. Thus a work-up for ischemic heart disease is indicated for patients with hypoglycemia and coronary artery disease or significant risk factors for coronary artery disease that manifest electrocardiographic changes.

■ CRITICAL BLOOD SAMPLE

In nondiabetic patients who present with active symptoms suggesting hypoglycemia, a normal glucose reading on a bedside glucometer excludes hypoglycemia as the cause of the symptoms (Fig. 164-1). No further testing for hypoglycemia is indicated and other possible causes for the symptoms should be sought. However if a nondiabetic patient does have a low glucose level, a blood sample should be drawn (ideally before treating the hypoglycemia) for the following laboratory tests: glucose, insulin, c-peptide, proinsulin, glucagon, growth hormone, cortisol, beta-hydroxybutyrate, insulin antibodies, and sulfonylurea drug levels. This so-called *critical blood sample* is essential for determining the etiology of hypoglycemia. Treating the hypoglycemia before obtaining the critical blood sample limits its usefulness but may be necessary in life-threatening situations.

If a nondiabetic patient presents to the ED complaining of resolved symptoms consistent with transient or self-treated hypoglycemia, and the glucose level is normal, outpatient referral for a 72-hour fasting study to evaluate for insulinoma and other causes of hypoglycemia is appropriate.

In diabetic patients, all symptoms consistent with hypoglycemia should generally be assumed to be hypoglycemia caused by antidiabetic therapy; a critical blood sample and 72-hour fasting study are rarely indicated.

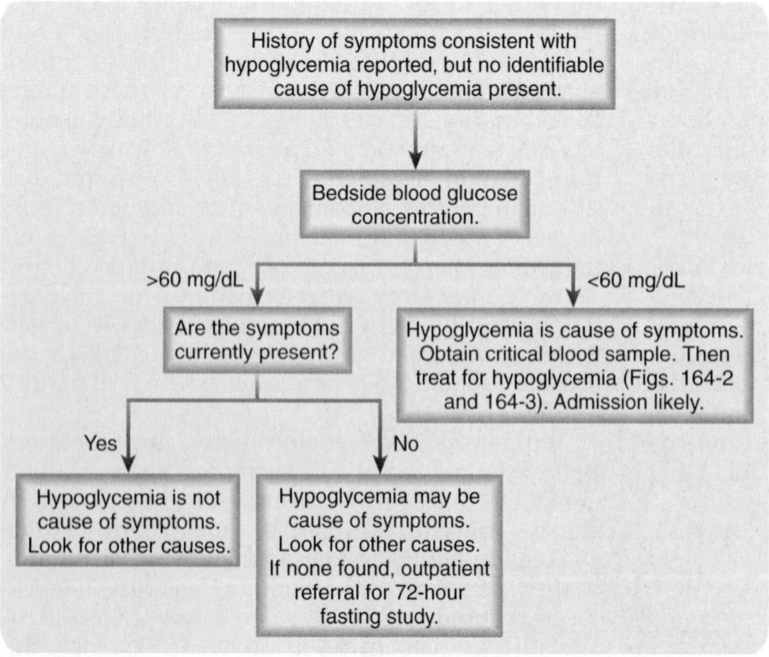
History of symptoms consistent with hypoglycemia reported, but no identifiable cause of hypoglycemia present.
Bedside blood glucose concentration.
>60 mg/dL
<60 mg/dL
Are the symptoms currently present?
Hypoglycemia is cause of symptoms. Obtain critical blood sample. Then treat for hypoglycemia (Figs. 164-2 and 164-3). Admission likely.
Yes
No
Hypoglycemia is not cause of symptoms. Look for other causes.
Hypoglycemia may be cause of symptoms. Look for other causes. If none found, outpatient referral for 72-hour fasting study.

FIGURE 164-1 Approach to determine if a nondiabetic patient's symptoms are the result of hypoglycemia.

Treatment

The treatment of hypoglycemia involves the repletion of blood glucose via oral or intravenous administration of exogenous glucose, or glucagon administration to stimulate endogenous glucose production. The specific treatment modality depends on the patient's age, whether the patient's mental status allows for safe oral ingestion, and whether an intravenous line can be established (Fig. 164-2).

METHODS OF ADMINISTRATION

Oral Administration

Oral repletion of glucose is appropriate if the patient can eat without a risk of aspiration. An initial oral dose is 15 g of a simple carbohydrate such as glucose, fructose (fruit juice), or sucrose (table sugar). Dextrose is the D-isomer of glucose, and for practical purpose can be considered synonymous with glucose. Commercially available oral glucose products include tablets (4-5 g/tablet), gels (15-45 g/tube), and nutritional bars (15-24 g/bar). Alternatively, the equivalent carbohydrate dose can be given as 6 ounces of regular soda or juice, or 1 tablespoon of honey, jelly, or table sugar.

Alpha-glucosidase inhibitors (acarbose, miglitol) interrupt the intestinal absorption of oral sucrose; therefore, if oral repletion is planned for a patient taking one of these medicines, sucrose products, including soda, candy, and table sugar, should be avoided in favor of glucose products. Oral repletion with simple carbohydrates increases blood glucose concentration within minutes and lasts about 20 minutes.

Intravenous Administration

If a patient's mental status prohibits oral repletion and IV access can be obtained, an IV dextrose bolus is the treatment of choice. The IV dose in adults is 1 ampule (amp) of 50% dextrose in water ($D_{50}W$), which can be repeated up to 3 amp (1 amp of $D_{50}W$ is a 50-mL solution that contains 25 g of glucose in water). The increase in blood glucose concentration in response to 1 amp of $D_{50}W$ is unpredictable, ranging from about 40 mg/dL to 350 mg/dL, and averaging about 160 mg/dL. The glycemic response to a bolus of dextrose peaks within 5 minutes and lasts about 30 minutes.

$D_{50}W$ should not be used in children younger than 8 years old due to the risk of hypertonicity sclerosing their small veins. The IV dextrose bolus dose in children is 2 to 4 mL/kg of $D_{25}W$; in infants it is 5 to 10 mL/kg of $D_{10}W$. These doses deliver 0.5 to 1 g of glucose per kilogram of body weight. As in adults, repeat boluses of dextrose are appropriate if there is an incomplete response.

The rare complications of dextrose administration include hypokalemia, hypophosphatemia, dilutional hyponatremia, and fluid overload. Electrolyte levels should be monitored if repeated boluses or continuous infusions are given.

Intramuscular Administration

If oral glucose repletion is not possible and IV access cannot be established, intramuscular (IM) or subcutaneous (SC) glucagon is indicated. IM or SC dosing is 1 mg of glucagon for adults, 0.5 mg for children younger than 8 years, and 50 μg/kg for infants. Glucagon stimulates glycogenolysis and reverses the

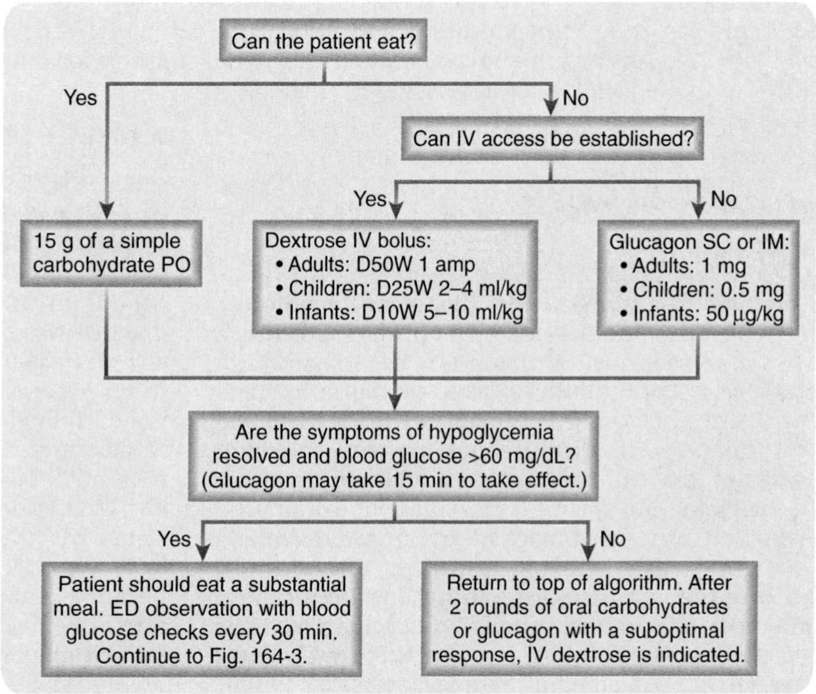
Can the patient eat?
Yes
No
Can IV access be established?
Yes
No
15 g of a simple carbohydrate PO
Dextrose IV bolus:
• Adults: D50W 1 amp
• Children: D25W 2–4 ml/kg
• Infants: D10W 5–10 ml/kg
Glucagon SC or IM:
• Adults: 1 mg
• Children: 0.5 mg
• Infants: 50 μg/kg
Are the symptoms of hypoglycemia resolved and blood glucose >60 mg/dL? (Glucagon may take 15 min to take effect.)
Yes
No
Patient should eat a substantial meal. ED observation with blood glucose checks every 30 min. Continue to Fig. 164-3.
Return to top of algorithm. After 2 rounds of oral carbohydrates or glucagon with a suboptimal response, IV dextrose is indicated.

FIGURE 164-2 Initial treatment of hypoglycemia.

symptoms of hypoglycemia after about 10 minutes, with a peak glycemic response in 30 minutes and 1- to 2-hour duration of action. Glucagon can be repeated after 10 minutes if neurologic recovery is incomplete, but dextrose is preferred if IV access can be established in the interim.

Glucagon is ineffective in patients with depleted glycogen stores, including alcoholic, malnourished, and elderly patients. Adverse effects include significant nausea and vomiting about 60 minutes after administration, so airway protection from vomiting and potential aspiration is a priority if mental status does not improve.

■ MONITORING AND REPEAT GLUCOSE ADMINISTRATION

The glycemic response to oral carbohydrates, intravenous dextrose, and glucagon is transient. It is essential to monitor for signs of recurrent hypoglycemia and recheck glucose levels every 30 minutes for 4 hours after euglycemia is achieved. The patient should also eat a substantial meal with protein, fat, and complex carbohydrates to rebuild glycogen stores and maintain euglycemia. If the glucose concentration falls toward hypoglycemic levels again, a continuous dextrose infusion (D_5W or $D_{10}W$) should be started. Patients with intact pancreatic insulin secretion, including nondiabetics and some patients with type 2 diabetes, are at risk for rebound hypoglycemia 1 to 2 hours after receiving dextrose boluses or glucagon because of the endogenous insulin response induced by these therapies.

Hypoglycemia caused by short-acting insulins, alcohol, and idiopathic ketotic hypoglycemia usually responds rapidly to initial replacement efforts and does not recur. Recurrent hypoglycemia is expected when the cause of hypoglycemia is ongoing, as with sulfonylureas, long-acting insulins, and critical illness. In these cases, initiating continuous dextrose infusion immediately after achievement of euglycemia is a reasonable approach.

■ ADJUNCTIVE TREATMENTS

■ Octreotide

Octreotide is a supplemental treatment for sulfonylurea- and insulinoma-induced hypoglycemia. It is a synthetic analogue of the hormone somatostatin and is a potent inhibitor of pancreatic insulin secretion. After euglycemia is initially achieved with dextrose boluses, octreotide can prevent recurrent hypoglycemia and reduce the amount of dextrose supplementation needed.[14] In sulfonylurea-induced hypoglycemia, continuous dextrose infusions and glucagon should be avoided in favor of octreotide, because they can stimulate further insulin secretion from the sulfonylurea-primed beta-cells. The most effective octreotide dose has not been established. One recommended adult dose is 50 to 100 µg of SC octreotide every 6 hours; continuous IV infusions of octreotide (100-125 µg/hour) have also been used successfully. A recommended pediatric dose is SC octreotide, 4 to 5 µg/kg/day divided every 6 hours. No significant side effects of octreotide have been demonstrated when used for hypoglycemia.

■ Diazoxide

Diazoxide, a rarely used antihypertensive medicine, also inhibits pancreatic insulin secretion and can be used for sulfonylurea-induced hypoglycemia. It is considered a second-line therapy to octreotide due to lower efficacy and greater risk of toxicity. Side effects include hypotension and sodium retention. The IV adult dose is 300 mg given over 1 hour; the IV pediatric dose is 1 to 3 mg/kg given over 1 hour. Doses can be repeated every 4 hours as needed.

■ Other Adjunctive Treatments

When hypoglycemia is caused by a severe overdose of subcutaneous insulin, one case report advocates needle aspiration or surgical excision of the subcutaneous reservoir to reduce the systemic absorption of the insulin.[15]

Early activated charcoal administration (1-2 g/kg) is indicated for sulfonylurea overdose and accidental pediatric sulfonylurea ingestions. Maximum efficacy is achieved if the charcoal is given within 1 hour of the ingestion. Glipizide undergoes enterohepatic circulation, and peak plasma concentrations may be mitigated by multiple doses of activated charcoal. Due to the delayed peak effects of extended-release glipizide, multiple doses of activated charcoal and whole bowel irrigation may be beneficial.

Urine alkalization can reduce the half-life of chlorpropamide from 49 hours to 13 hours through increased renal excretion but does not appear to be useful for other oral hypoglycemic agents.

■ RISKS OF PRESUMPTIVE TREATMENT

Classically, it was taught to administer dextrose to all patients with undifferentiated altered mental status as part of the "coma cocktail," which consists of oxygen plus IV administration of 1 amp of $D_{50}W$, 100 mg of thiamine, and 0.4 mg of naloxone. This practice was challenged in the 1980s when animal and retrospective human studies suggested that hyperglycemia may be detrimental to the injured brain, including injuries caused by acute stroke, cardiac arrest, hypotension, and head trauma. The true risk of administering a small glucose load to euglycemic or hyperglycemic patients with a brain injury has not been established, but is thought to be low. Hypoglycemia, on the other hand, is known to be detrimental, especially to the injured brain. Therefore, the current recommendation is to check a bedside glucose measurement in patients with altered mental status and only administer dextrose if the

Chapter 165

Sodium and Water Balance

Michael C. Wadman

KEY POINTS

Imbalances in sodium concentration may result in significant disability or death, from the causative disease, the direct effects of the sodium concentration, or as a complication of inappropriate treatment.

Signs and symptoms of hyponatremia reflect an increase in central nervous system cellular volume and subsequent cerebral edema. Symptoms are more pronounced with rapid decreases in sodium concentration.

Findings of hypernatremia are age-dependent and are directly correlated with serum sodium levels.

Alcoholics and malnourished patients are at the greatest risk for developing osmotic demyelination syndrome, the most serious treatment complication of hyponatremia.

Hypertonic saline should be administered to patients with hyponatremia who demonstrate severe neurologic signs.

Cerebral edema is the most concerning complication associated with the rapid correction of hypernatremia.

Scope

Water accounts for 60% of total body weight and is located in one of two spaces: the extracellular and intracellular compartments. Osmotic equilibrium between the extracellular and intracellular spaces depends on the free flow of water through a solute-impermeable/water-permeable cell membrane barrier. Water balance describes the normal state of equilibrium, using the concept of osmolality, the ratio of solute to free water, a constant between the two spaces when water freely diffuses across cell membranes. The predominant solute of the extracellular space is sodium.

Various disease states alter water balance, resulting in abnormally high or low sodium levels. Imbalances in sodium concentration may result in significant disability or death from either the causative disease or the direct effects of the sodium concentration or through the ill effects of inappropriate treatment. The presenting signs and symptoms of sodium imbalance range from subtle constitutional symptoms to seizure and coma. Suspicion for disorders of water balance depends on an assessment of existing risk factors and clinical information available at the time of presentation to the ED.

Hyponatremia is defined as a serum sodium level less than 135 mEq/L, although clinical manifestations most often occur when the sodium level falls below 130 mEq/L. Hyponatremia generally occurs in the very young and the very old; prevalence increases with advancing age.

Hypernatremia, defined as a plasma sodium level greater than 145 mEq/L, usually results from inadequate water intake. Hypernatremia is less common than hyponatremia but is associated with a much higher mortality rate. Hypernatremia will result in death in approximately 50% of patients, primarily from causative disease states in elderly patients or direct neurologic damage from the effects of high sodium concentration in the very young.[1]

Pathophysiology

Water balance is regulated through homeostatic mechanisms of thirst and renal excretion. High serum osmolality is detected by hypothalamic osmoreceptors, which lead to antidiuretic hormone secretion and stimulation of the thirst mechanism. Antidiuretic hormone also regulates plasma osmolality by increasing free water absorption in the kidney. Low levels of plasma osmolality result in the suppression of antidiuretic hormone and the production of dilute urine.

Hypovolemia causes a stimulation of thirst mechanisms, as well as the secretion of antidiuretic hormone and aldosterone. Aldosterone is synthesized in the adrenal cortex and is secreted in response to hypovolemia via the renin-angiotensin-aldosterone axis. Aldosterone acts by increasing sodium absorption at the distal tubule, leading to expansion of the intravascular volume.

■ HYPONATREMIA

Low osmolality of the intravascular space and the relative high osmolality of the intracellular space result in an osmotic gradient and the diffusion of water into the cell. Resulting cellular edema is generally well tolerated by most tissues, except when it occurs in a confined space such as the central nervous system. The initial, rapid response to an increase in central nervous system cellular volume is diffusion of electrolytes and water out of cells, leading to a partial reduction in neuronal cell volume. Continued hyponatremia over 48 to 72 hours generates slow diffusion of organic osmolytes out of cells, resulting in a further reduction in cell volume. These organic osmolytes consist primarily of large amino acids such as taurine.[2]

Treatment of hyponatremia with IV fluids may promote a state of relative hyperosmolality in the extracellular space, causing diffusion of water out of the cell and continued reduction in cellular volume. This cycle creates the most serious treatment complication of hyponatremia: osmotic demyelination syndrome.

■ HYPERNATREMIA

In hypernatremia, water diffuses out of the cell along the osmotic gradient, resulting in loss of cellular volume. In the acute phase, electrolytes and water rapidly diffuse into the cell to partially restore cellular volume. In ongoing hypernatremia, slow osmolyte redistribution occurs and water diffuses into the cell. With treatment, the relative hypo-osmolality of the infused IV fluid leads to an osmotic gradient that promotes further rapid water diffusion into the cell. The size of the larger organic osmolytes prevents diffusion out of the cell, causing the most serious treatment complication of hypernatremia: cerebral edema.[3,4]

Clinical Presentation

■ HYPONATREMIA

Most signs and symptoms of hyponatremia reflect an increase in central nervous system cellular volume and subsequent cerebral edema. The rapid compensatory mechanisms of the acute phase produce more obvious signs and symptoms, whereas the slow, adaptive phase of the chronic state results in minimal symptomatology.

The signs and symptoms of hyponatremia depend on both the rate of change and the absolute plasma sodium concentration. An acute decrease in the serum sodium level below 120 mEq/L almost always results in symptoms, whereas a more gradual decline to this level may be undetected.

Symptoms of hyponatremia include nausea, headache, and general malaise, with serum sodium levels between 125 and 130 mEq/L; lethargy, confusion, agitation, psychosis, and seizures occur as sodium levels fall to a range of 115 to 120 mEq/L; severe symptoms develop at 110 mEq/L regardless of the rate of change.

Concerning neurologic signs observed in patients with hyponatremia include a decreased level of alertness, cognitive impairment, focal or generalized seizure activity, and signs of brainstem herniation such as unilateral pupil dilation, posturing, and respiratory arrest.[5]

■ HYPERNATREMIA

Signs and symptoms of hypernatremia are age-dependent. Infants exhibit restlessness, tachypnea, alternating irritability and lethargy, hypotonia, and a characteristic high-pitched cry. Elderly patients with hypernatremia present with nausea, weakness, altered mental status, agitation, irritability, lethargy, stupor, coma, and seizures.[3,4] The severity of central nervous system symptoms correlates with serum sodium levels.[6]

Differential Diagnosis and Classification

■ HYPONATREMIA

The differential diagnosis of hyponatremia begins with a determination of the plasma (serum) osmolality (Fig. 165-1).[2] Osmolality is measured by osmometry in the laboratory or is calculated accord-

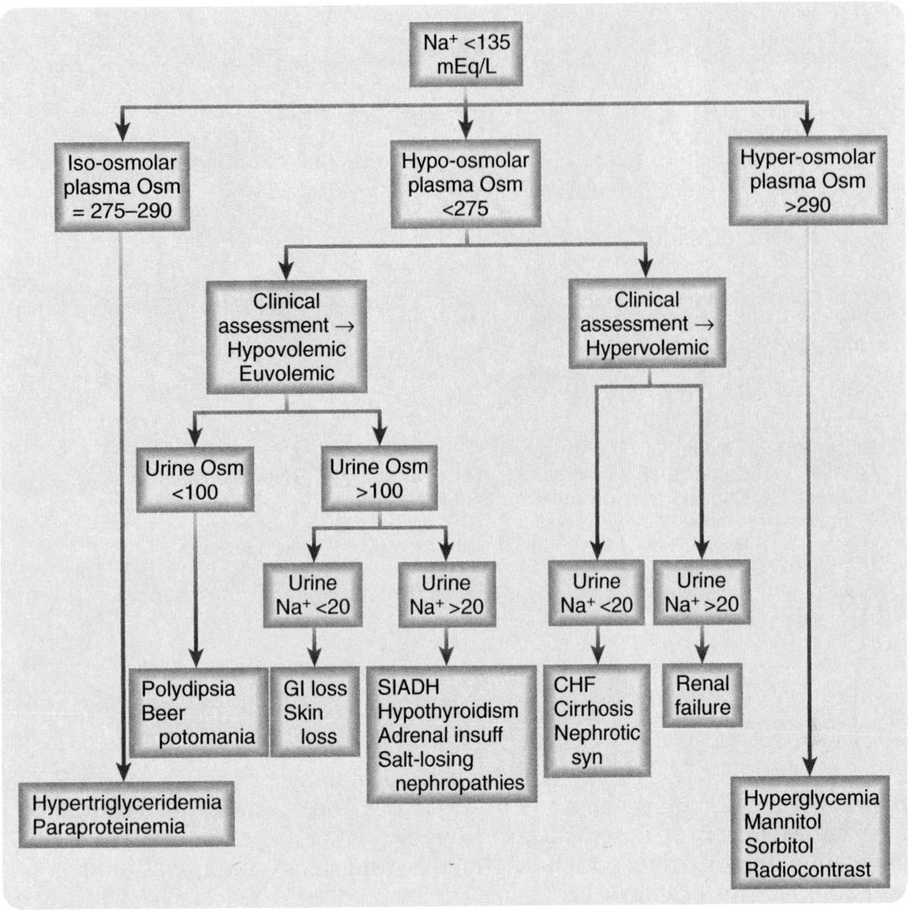
Na+ <135 mEq/L
Iso-osmolar plasma Osm = 275–290
Hypo-osmolar plasma Osm <275
Hyper-osmolar plasma Osm >290
Clinical assessment → Hypovolemic Euvolemic
Clinical assessment → Hypervolemic
Urine Osm <100
Urine Osm >100
Urine Na+ <20
Urine Na+ >20
Urine Na+ <20
Urine Na+ >20
Polydipsia Beer potomania
GI loss Skin loss
SIADH Hypothyroidism Adrenal insuff Salt-losing nephropathies
CHF Cirrhosis Nephrotic syn
Renal failure
Hypertriglyceridemia Paraproteinemia
Hyperglycemia Mannitol Sorbitol Radiocontrast

FIGURE 165-1 Diagnostic algorithm for hyponatremia. CHF, congestive heart failure; GI, gastrointestinal; Osm, osmolality; SIADH, syndrome of inappropriate antidiuretic hormone secretion. (Adapted from Kumar S, Berl T: Sodium. Lancet 1998;352:220-228.)

ing to the following formula (BUN=blood urea nitrogen):

$$\text{Plasma osmolality} = [2 \times Na^+ (\text{mEq/L})] + \text{glucose} (\text{mg/dL})/18 + \text{BUN} (\text{mg/dL})/2.8$$

Patients are classified as hypo-osmolar (plasma osmolality <275), iso-osmolar (plasma osmolality 275-290), or hyperosmolar (plasma osmolality >290). In hypo-osmolar patients, a clinical assessment of volume status further differentiates hyponatremic patients as hypovolemic, euvolemic, or hypervolemic.

Hypo-osmolar hypovolemic hyponatremia, the most common type of hyponatremia encountered in the ED,[7] is observed in patients with severe total body water (TBW) depletion in excess of sodium loss. Urine osmolality and sodium determinations allow further narrowing of the differential diagnosis. Dilute urine (urine osmolality >100 mOsm/kg) suggests polydipsia or beer potomania; in these patients, urine sodium levels less than 20 mEq/L indicate an extrarenal source of sodium and water loss, including gastrointestinal conditions such as vomiting or diarrhea. Urine sodium levels greater than 20 mEq/L suggest a renal source of sodium and water loss, such as sodium-losing nephropathy, hypoaldosteronism, diuretic excess, and osmotic diuresis.

BOX 165-1

Causes of Inappropriate Antidiuretic Hormone Secretion (SIADH)

- **Central nervous system disease—** meningitis, abscess, cerebrovascular accident
- **Drugs—**amiodarone, carbamazepine, chlorpromazine, theophylline, selective serotonin reuptake inhibitors (SSRIs), ecstasy (3,4-methylenedioxymethamphetamine)
- **Pulmonary disease—**pneumonia, empyema
- **Malignancy—**bronchogenic, central nervous system

Hypo-osmolar euvolemic hyponatremia is most commonly associated with the syndrome of inappropriate antidiuretic hormone secretion (SIADH) (Box 165-1). Antidiuretic hormone, or vasopressin, decreases free water excretion, resulting in an inappropriately concentrated urine, marked by urine osmololity greater than 100 mOsm/kg and urine sodium concentration less than 20 mEq/L. SIADH may be caused by various malignancies, pulmonary disorders, central nervous system diseases, and several

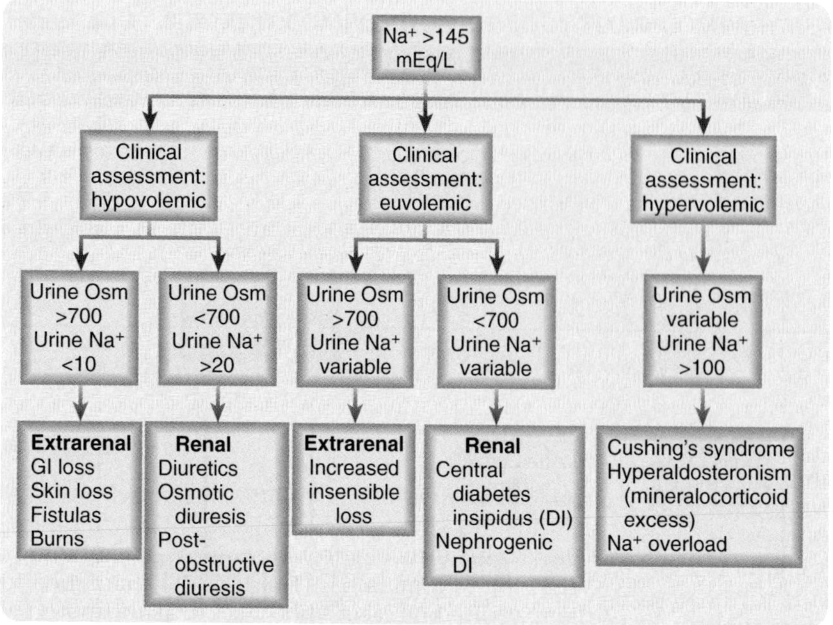
Na+ >145 mEq/L
Clinical assessment: hypovolemic
Clinical assessment: euvolemic
Clinical assessment: hypervolemic
Urine Osm >700 Urine Na+ <10
Urine Osm <700 Urine Na+ >20
Urine Osm >700 Urine Na+ variable
Urine Osm <700 Urine Na+ variable
Urine Osm variable Urine Na+ >100
Extrarenal GI loss Skin loss Fistulas Burns
Renal Diuretics Osmotic diuresis Post-obstructive diuresis
Extrarenal Increased insensible loss
Renal Central diabetes insipidus (DI) Nephrogenic DI
Cushing's syndrome Hyperaldosteronism (mineralocorticoid excess) Na+ overload

FIGURE 165-2 Diagnostic algorithm for hypernatremia. Osm, osmolality. (Adapted from Kumar S, Berl T: Sodium. Lancet 1998;352:220-228.)

drugs.[8,9] Diagnostic criteria include hypo-osmolar hyponatremia, inappropriately concentrated urine, and the exclusion of other causes of hypo-osmolar euvolemic hyponatremia such as hypothyroidism and adrenal insufficiency.

Iso-osmolar hyponatremia, or "pseudohyponatremia," is observed in the laboratory when the sodium concentration is affected by large molecules that increase the nonaqueous, sodium-free plasma fraction, leading to a corresponding decrease in the concentration of sodium per unit volume of serum. The large molecules responsible for pseudohyponatremia are usually from a paraproteinemia (as with multiple myeloma) or hyperlipidemia. Many newer laboratory methods for sodium determination measure only the aqueous serum component, eliminating the possibility of pseudohyponatremia.

Hyperosmolar hyponatremia commonly results from hyperglycemia. The high osmolality of the extracellular compartment that stems from elevated serum glucose drives water out of cells, diluting the concentration of sodium. In the evaluation of a patient with hyperosmolar hyponatremia, a decrease in plasma sodium of 1.6 mEq/L for every 100 mg/dL increase in serum glucose provides an estimate of the degree of hyponatremia present. A similar mechanism may also occur in patients receiving mannitol, sorbitol, or radiocontrast media.

■ HYPERNATREMIA

Figure 165-2 is an algorithm for the diagnosis of hypernatremia.[2] Hyponatremia may also be classified as hypovolemic, euvolemic, or hypervolemic.

Hypovolemic hypernatremia, the most common subtype observed in the ED, results from severe total body water depletion. Urine sodium measurement allows determination of an extrarenal or renal source of water loss. Levels less than 10 mEq/L suggest an extrarenal source of water loss, such as the skin (excessive sweating or severe burns) or gastrointestinal system (vomiting or diarrhea); levels greater than 20 Eq/L suggest renal causes such as excessive diuretic use, osmotic diuresis, postobstructive diuresis, and intrinsic renal disease.[3]

Euvolemic hypernatremia results from water loss without solute loss, such that most of the total water lost comes from the intracellular space. Water loss can have both extrarenal and renal sources. Extrarenal sources include insensible skin and respiratory loss coupled with a lack of water intake due to impaired thirst mechanism or an inability to procure fluids. Urine osmolality typically is high (U_{osm}>700 mOsm/kg) because of the secretion of antidiuretic hormone. Urine sodium levels vary. Renal losses of water occur secondary to diabetes insipidus of central or nephrogenic origin, resulting in a dilute urine (U_{osm}<700 mOsm/kg). Patients with central diabetes insipidus produce dilute urine due to a decrease in antidiuretic hormone secretion in the hypothalamus; those with nephrogenic diabetes insipidus exhibit a decreased response to antidiuretic hormone at the renal tubule itself.[3]

Hypervolemic hypernatremia stems from sodium overload and is the least common subtype encountered in ED patients. Hypervolemic hypernatremia usually results from iatrogenic causes during hospitalization.[10] Patients may present with hypervolemic hypernatremia due to high sodium intake from improperly prepared infant formula or home remedies, excessive salt tablet use, or hyperaldosteronism.

Diagnostic Testing

■ LABORATORY STUDIES

Accurate laboratory determination of serum sodium levels is critical to the diagnosis and treatment of hyponatremia and hypernatremia. Clinical information confirms laboratory results. The possibility of errors in laboratory analysis or serum sampling should be considered when serum sodium level and clinical information conflict. One common source of error may occur when a blood sample is obtained proximal to an IV line. When the results are in doubt, a repeat sample should be obtained to ensure diagnostic accuracy.

Key blood tests for the evaluation of sodium imbalance include plasma osmolality, sodium, potassium, BUN, glucose, and thyroid-stimulating hormone. Although most laboratories report a plasma osmolality measured by osmometry, determination of sodium, glucose, and BUN can also be used for the calculation of osmolality. Plasma osmolality allows the initial classification of hyponatremia as true hypo-osmolar, hyperosmolar, or iso-osmolar. In patients with hyponatremia, the diagnosis of true hypo-osmolar hyponatremia rules out paraproteinemia, hyperlipidemia, and hyperglycemia as causes of low laboratory sodium levels. Normal thyroid-stimulating hormone and potassium levels assist in the evaluation of euvolemic hypo-osmolar hyponatremia due to possible thyroid or adrenal etiologies.

Urine studies that impact the ED evaluation and management of patients with disorders of water balance include urine osmolality and urine sodium. High urine osmolality indicates the possibility of SIADH, whereas a low measurement suggests diabetes insipidus, excessive fluid intake, and hyperaldosteronism. Urine sodium levels obtained prior to the initiation of therapy provide valuable diagnostic information regarding the source of free water loss.

■ NEUROIMAGING

Patients presenting with hypernatremia may require neuroimaging for the evaluation of any observed alteration in consciousness. In the past, hypernatremia was theorized to cause intracranial hemorrhages and subdural hematomas due to brain shrinkage from cellular volume loss, with resultant traction on the bridging dural veins, and subsequent venous rupture. Recent studies suggest that hypernatremia most likely results from intracranial hemorrhage; there is no proof that hypernatremia is a direct cause of intracranial bleeding.

Treatment

■ HYPONATREMIA

Osmotic demyelination syndrome, the most serious complication of the treatment for hyponatremia, occurs when the administration of relatively hyperosmolar IV fluid causes intracellular water to rapidly diffuse out of central nervous system cells. Patients typically improve transiently after IV fluid administration, only to deteriorate a week after treatment. Signs and symptoms include altered mental status, dysarthria, vertigo, parkinsonism, pseudobulbar palsies, diffuse spastic hypertonia, quadriparesis, and coma. Risk factors for the development of osmotic demyelination syndrome include alcoholism and malnourishment—in the ED, close monitoring of IV fluid responses in alcoholic patients is critical.

The sodium deficit in *hypo-osmolar hypovolemic hyponatremia* is calculated by the following formula:

$$Na^+ \text{ deficit} = (\text{desired } Na^+ - \text{measured } Na^+) \times \text{TBW}$$

In patients with severe neurologic symptoms and laboratory-confirmed hyponatremia, the likelihood of cerebral edema outweighs the potential risk of treatment-related osmotic demyelination syndrome that develops due to rapid correction of the hyponatremic state. In patients with hyponatremia and neurologic symptoms, hypertonic saline is recommended for the first 2 to 4 hours; the patient's condition should improve with a maximum rate of sodium correction of 1.0 to 2.0 mEq/L/hour. Patients with acute hyponatremia of less than 48 hours' duration may tolerate a more rapid correction of sodium concentration. Hyponatremic patients with less severe symptoms usually have a more chronic condition. The risk for osmotic demyelination syndrome outweighs the benefits of rapid correction in these patients, and as such, the recommended rate of sodium correction is 0.5 mEq/L/hour.[5,11]

Most patients with *euvolemic and hypervolemic* hyponatremia require restriction of free water intake to 800 to 1000 mL per day. Patients with severe hyponatremia may need IV fluids to replace the total body sodium deficit.

■ HYPERNATREMIA

The ED management of hypernatremia requires restoration of plasma volume. IV fluid choice depends on the clinical situation. Lactated Ringer's solution or 0.9% saline (normal saline) is appropriate in the initial resuscitative treatment phase, with subsequent conversion to a hypotonic IV fluid such as 0.45% saline when euvolemia is attained. Patients with hypernatremia and a clinical picture consistent with hypovolemia may receive a 500-mL IV bolus of normal saline prior to laboratory confirmation of the diagnosis.

Once the serum sodium level is known, the goal rate of correction of the sodium concentration is 0.5 to 1.0 mEq/L/hour, not to exceed 10 mEq/L over 24 hours. One approach to correcting the water imbalance resulting in hypernatremia is to calculate the free water deficit and then replace the deficit over 48 hours, with the assumption that plasma sodium increases approximately 5 mEq/L for each liter of water replaced. The free water deficit is calculated as follows:

$$\text{Free water deficit (L)} = \text{TBW (L)} \times [(\text{plasma Na}^+/140) - 1]$$

$$\text{Total body water (TBW)} = \text{body mass factor} \times \text{weight (kg)}$$

Young men	0.6
Young women/elderly men	0.5
Elderly women	0.4

Another correction method is to calculate the effect of 1 liter of a given IV fluid (IVF) on the patient's sodium level, using the following formula and values described by Androgue and Madrias[4]:

Change in plasma Na^+ with 1 L IVF:

$$1\text{ L IVF} = [\text{IVF Na}^+ - \text{plasma Na}^+]/[\text{TBW}+1]$$

and the following values:

IVF	Na^+ mEq/L
D_5W	0
0.45% saline	77
0.9% saline	154
3% saline	513

A calculated decrease in serum sodium for each liter of IV fluid administered permits closer monitoring of the patient's response to therapy. This method facilitates changes during the course of therapy based on the current sodium levels.

The most serious complication of hypernatremia therapy is the development of cerebral edema secondary to excessively rapid rehydration (Box 165-2). In the chronic hypernatremic state, large organic osmolytes that slowly accumulated in neurons during the adaptive phase are unable to rapidly diffuse to the extracellular space when a relatively hypotonic treatment fluid is administered.

BOX 165-2

High-Risk Neurologic Complications Occurring in Hyponatremic Patients

Acute Cerebral Edema

- Postoperative menstruating patients
- Elderly women taking thiazide diuretics
- Pediatric patients
- Patients with psychiatric polydipsia
- Patients with hypoxemia

Osmotic Demyelination Syndrome

- Alcoholic patients
- Malnourished patients
- Patients with hypokalemia
- Patients with burns
- Elderly women taking thiazide diuretics

Adapted from Lauriat SM, Berl T: The hyponatremic patient: Practical focus on therapy. J Am Soc Nephrol 1997;8: 1599-1607.

REFERENCES

1. Mandal AK, Saklayen MG, Hillman NM, Markert RJ: Predictive factors for high mortality in hypernatremic patients. Am J Emerg Med 1997;15:130-132.
2. Kumar S, Berl T: Sodium. *Lancet* 1998;352:220-228.
3. Palevsky PM: Hypernatremia. Semin Nephrol 1998;18:20-30.
4. Adrogue HJ, Madias NE: Hypernatremia. N Engl J Med 2000;342:1493-1499.
5. Arieff AI: Central nervous system manifestations of disordered sodium metabolism. Clin Endocrinol Metab 1984;13(2):269-294.
6. Snyder Na, Feigal DW, Arieff AI: Hypernatremia in elderly patients. Ann Intern Med 1987;107:309-319.
7. Lee CT, Guo HR, Chen JB: Hyponatremia in the emergency department. Am J Emerg Med 2000;18:264-268.
8. Patel GP, Kasiar JB: Syndrome of inappropriate antidiuretic hormone–induced hyponatremia associated with amiodarone. Pharmacotherapy 2002;22:649-651.
9. Hartung TK, Schofield E, Short AI, et al: Hyponatremic states following 3,4-methylenedioxymethamphetamine (MDMA, "ecstasy") ingestion. QJM 2002;95:431-437.
10. Palevsky PM, Bhagrath R, Greenberg A: Hypernatremia in hospitalized patients. Ann Intern Med 1996;124(2): 197-203.
11. Adrogue HJ: Consequences of inadequate management of hyponatremia. Am J Nephrol 2005;25:240-249.

Chapter 166

Potassium

Sandy Sineff and Michael A. Gisondi

KEY POINTS

All potassium disorders result from one of three disturbances: impaired potassium intake, impaired distribution of potassium between intracellular and extracellular spaces, and impaired renal excretion of potassium.

Hypokalemia is more common than hyperkalemia. Most clinically significant cases are caused by diuretic therapy; other important etiologies in ED patients include metabolic acidosis and high-output diarrhea.

Hyperkalemia, a less common but more serious condition than hypokalemia, occurs almost exclusively in patients with renal insufficiency.

Small changes in extracellular potassium concentration can adversely affect the membrane potential in cardiovascular and neuromuscular tissues, accounting for the majority of symptoms and deaths caused by dyskalemic states.

Fatal arrhythmia is the most common cause of death in patients with severe hypokalemia or hyperkalemia.

Elevated serum potassium levels observed in patients with normal renal function and a normal electrocardiogram (ECG) should be rechecked before administering any treatment. Measurement error is the most common cause of an elevated potassium level in otherwise healthy patients.

The management of hyperkalemia focuses on three goals of care: cardiac stabilization, transcellular shift of potassium to the intracellular space, and elimination of excess potassium. Only potassium excretion is a definitive treatment step—other actions serve to temporarily stabilize the cell membrane in an effort to prevent hemodynamic collapse.

Hemodialysis is the most rapid method of potassium elimination for patients with persistent, symptomatic, or severe hyperkalemia.

Scope

Hypokalemia and hyperkalemia are electrolyte abnormalities common to both hospitalized and ED patients.[1] Hypokalemia is observed more frequently than hyperkalemia and affects a broader range of patients; diuretic therapy accounts for as much as 80% of clinically significant ED cases.[2] Although less common than hypokalemia, hyperkalemia is a potentially more serious condition that occurs almost exclusively in patients with underlying renal insufficiency.[1] Both disorders can result in cardiac dysfunction, arrhythmia, and death.

Physiology

Total body potassium (K) is approximately 50 mEq/kg, or 3500 to 4000 mEq, in a normal-sized adult. For conversion purposes, 1 mEq of potassium is equivalent to 39.09 mg. Potassium is the major intracellular cation, and more than 98% of total body potassium is stored in the intracellular space. Intracellular fluid concentrations of potassium range from 150 to 160 mEq/L, with the highest amounts sequestered either in muscle (75%) or in bones and cartilage (8%-10%).[2]

The daily minimum requirement of potassium is approximately 1600 to 2000 mg (40-50 mEq); actual potassium intake varies widely depending on diet, race, and ethnicity. Younger people whose diets are rich in fruits and vegetables may consume as much as 11,000 mg of potassium per day. Older, disabled, and poor patients generally have lower amounts of potassium in their diets.[3] In a balanced state, 80% of potassium intake is excreted by the kidneys, 15% is excreted in the gastrointestinal tract, and 5% is excreted in sweat.[3]

Extracellular potassium makes up less than 2% of total body stores, of which only two thirds is measurable in serum sampling. The normal plasma concentration range reported by most laboratory testing is 3.5 to 5 mEq/L; this small fraction is not reflective of total body potassium. Strict regulation of the ratio of intracellular to extracellular potassium (150 mEq/L to 4 mEq/L) maintains a critical voltage gradient across cell membranes and plays a crucial role in establishing membrane potential in cardiac and neuromuscular cells.[1] The Na^+,K^+-ATPase transmembrane pump continuously maintains this gradient by actively transporting potassium into and sodium (Na) out of the cells[1] (Fig. 166-1). Large changes in intracellular potassium concentration have little effect on the ratio of intra-to-extracellular potassium. Conversely, even small changes in extracellular concentration significantly affect this ratio, the transmembrane potential gradient, and the function of cardiac and neuromuscular tissues.[1]

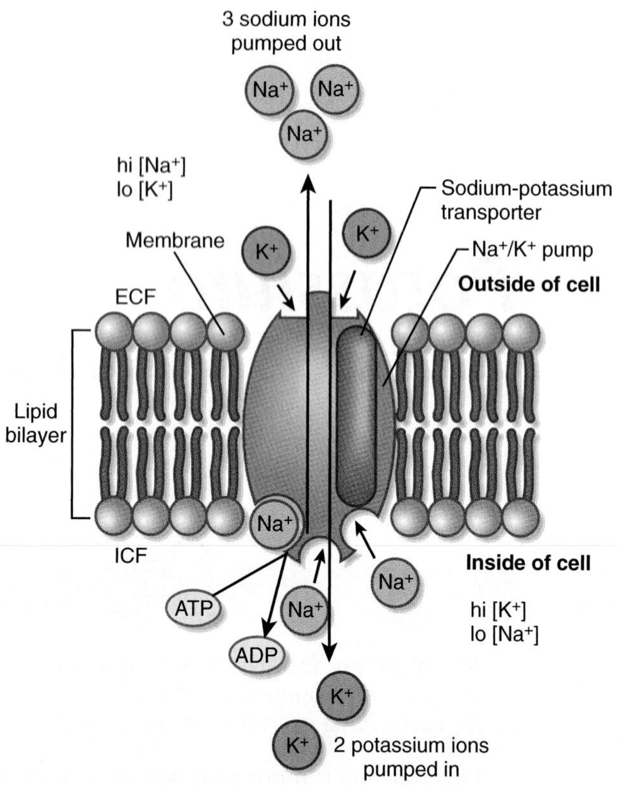
3 sodium ions
pumped out
Na+
Na+
Na+
hi [Na+]
lo [K+]
Sodium-potassium
transporter
Membrane
K+
K+
Na+/K+ pump
Outside of cell
ECF
Lipid
bilayer
Na+
ICF
Na+
Inside of cell
ATP
Na+
hi [K+]
lo [Na+]
ADP
K+
K+
2 potassium ions
pumped in

FIGURE 166-1 The Na^+,K^+-ATPase pump.

■ HOMEOSTASIS\

All potassium disorders result from one of three disturbances[4]: impaired potassium intake, impaired distribution of potassium between intracellular and extracellular spaces, and impaired renal excretion of potassium (Table 166-1; Fig. 166-2).

■ POTASSIUM INTAKE

Potassium can enter the extracellular fluid space in one of three ways: dietary ingestion, exogenous infusion, or massive release from traumatized muscle cells.

After ingestion, potassium is rapidly absorbed by passive diffusion through the upper gastrointestinal tract. Average dietary intake of potassium is roughly equal to the total potassium content of the extracellular compartment. Renal excretion is a slow phenomenon (requiring 4 to 6 hours) and does not autoregulate in response to an acute potassium load. To avoid meal-related hyperkalemic crises, potassium is transiently shifted to the intracellular fluid compartment for the first hour after intake.[2] By reverse compensatory mechanisms, short-term dietary potassium restriction does not result in hypokalemia.[1,2]

■ POTASSIUM DISTRIBUTION

■ Hormonal Control

The Na^+,K^+-ATPase pump actively exchanges two molecules of potassium for three molecules of sodium,

Table 166-1 REGULATORS OF POTASSIUM HOMEOSTASIS

Regulator	Mechanism
Insulin	Enhances activity of the Na^+,K^+-ATPase pump
β_2-agonist	β_2-receptor simulation enhances cellular uptake of potassium
Mineralocorticoids	Unknown
Serum osmolarity	Solvent drag
Acid-base changes	Exchange of H^+ for K

ATPase, adenosine triphosphate; H^+, hydrogen; K, potassium; Na, sodium.
Adapted from Gaffar M: Diagnosis and treatment of hyperkalemia. Med Clin North Am 2003;49:18-22.

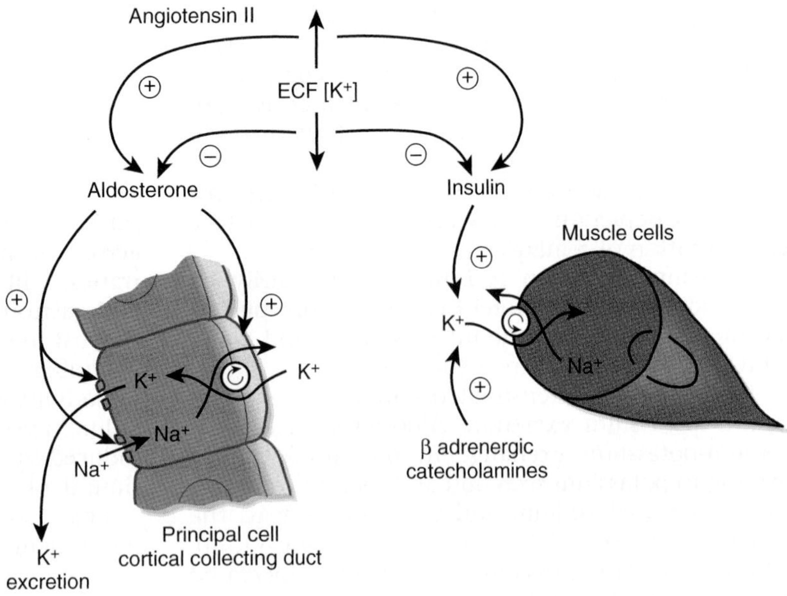

Angiotensin II
ECF [K+]
Aldosterone
Insulin
Muscle cells
K+
Na+
β adrenergic catecholamines
Principal cell cortical collecting duct
K+ excretion

FIGURE 166-2 Regulators of potassium homeostasis.

to counterbalance the passive effusion of potassium. The activity of this transmembrane pump is highly dependent on the interaction of certain hormones: insulin, β_2-adrenergic receptor agonists (e.g., catecholamines, exogenous albuterol), and aldosterone.

Insulin increases the activity of the Na^+,K^+-ATPase pump. An insulin feedback system exists such that hyperkalemia stimulates insulin secretion and hypokalemia inhibits secretion.[5] Patients with insulin deficiency disorders (e.g., diabetes mellitus) are predisposed to hyperkalemia because of impaired insulin feedback and subsequently poor intracellular potassium transfer.

β_2-adrenergic stimulation also promotes sodium-potassium exchange, although no feedback system has been identified for controlled catecholamine release. Thus asthmatic patients who receive bronchodilator therapy or epinephrine are predisposed to hypokalemia. For similar reasons, endogenous catecholamine release (as occurs with myocardial infarction or pain) promotes hypokalemia. Alpha-adrenergic agonists (antihypertensive drugs) and β_2-antagonists (beta-blockers) have an opposite effect on the transmembrane pump.[2]

Aldosterone also promotes an intracellular shift of potassium. In addition, aldosterone further decreases extracellular potassium by stimulating enhanced renal excretion.

Acid-Base Control

Acidemia causes hydrogen ions in the serum to shift into the intracellular fluid space along a concentration gradient. As hydrogen ions move into the cell, potassium ions exit into the plasma to maintain electroneutrality across the membrane. In alkalemia, the opposite exchange occurs: hydrogen ion efflux and potassium ion influx. With non–anion gap metabolic acidosis, for every 0.1 unit change in pH there is an opposite 0.6 mEq/L change in serum potassium concentration.[2]

Some variations in acid-base control exist. Organic acidotic states (e.g., lactic acidosis) are characterized by free movement of organic ions through the cell membrane without compensatory potassium efflux. Likewise, type I (distal) and type II (proximal) renal tubular acidosis produce a hypokalemic state.[3] Respiratory acid-base disorders elicit unpredictable although minimal changes in potassium concentration.

Miscellaneous Determinants of Potassium Distribution

Hypertonic conditions produced by hyperglycemia, diabetic ketoacidosis, or hypertonic (3%) saline infusions will create a concentration gradient that promotes potassium efflux and a resultant hyperkalemia. Transient hyperkalemia is observed during the initial phases of intense physical exercise, due to the effects of lactic acidosis.

Body temperatures below 86° F (30° C) will result in hyperkalemia. Elevated potassium is a predictor of mortality in severely hypothermic patients.[6]

Medications affect transmembrane potassium exchange. Drugs that promote hyperkalemia include succinylcholine (increases permeability of muscle cell membranes) and digitalis (toxic effect on the NA^+,K^+-ATPase pump). Barium bicarbonate inhibits potassium efflux from cells, thereby inducing hypokalemia.[2]

POTASSIUM EXCRETION

The excretion of potassium is almost entirely renal-dependent. Over 90% of filtered potassium is reabsorbed in the proximal nephron; excretion of potassium occurs primarily in the distal tubule and collecting duct, mediated by Na^+,K^+-ATPase exchange.[2] Normal kidneys can slowly compensate for a wide range of potassium intake by increasing or decreasing excretion in the urine.[1] With increases in total body potassium, the kidney can produce urinary potassium concentrations of 100 mEq/L. Chronic potassium depletion lowers urinary potassium to a concentration of 5 mEq/L.

Potassium excretion is influenced primarily by three factors: plasma protein concentration, plasma aldosterone, and the amount of sodium and water delivered to the distal collecting system.

The renin-angiotensin-aldosterone system increases potassium excretion. Aldosterone enhances sodium-potassium exchange in the distal tubule, leading to potassium secretion and sodium reabsorption.[2] Increased sodium and water delivery to the distal tubules stimulates the NA^+,K^+-ATPase pump, contributing to potassium excretion. Increased tubular flow (e.g., osmotic diuresis) causes potassium "washout" and elimination.[1]

In the ED, critical hyperkalemia is seen almost exclusively in patients with some degree of renal impairment.[2]

Hypokalemia

Hypokalemia is defined as a serum potassium level below 3.5 mEq/L. Hypokalemia is further classified as mild (3-3.5 mEq/L), moderate (2.5-2.9 mEq/L), and severe (<2.5 mEq/L).

Approximately 20% of hospitalized patients are found to have subtherapeutic serum potassium levels.[1] Despite this disease prevalence, most patients are asymptomatic, and only 5% of these patients have clinically significant hypokalemia.

In the outpatient setting, roughly 18% of patients have mild hypokalemia, which is generally asymptomatic. The vast majority of these cases (80%) are caused by potassium-wasting thiazide diuretic medications. Men and women are affected equally.

ETIOLOGIES (Box 166-1)

Hypokalemia is rarely suspected on the basis of clinical presentation; diagnosis is generally made based on measurement of the serum potassium as part of a screening chemistry panel. A low serum concentration indicates disruption of normal homeostasis from abnormal intake, abnormal losses, or an acute shift into the intracellular fluid compartment.

Potassium depletion induced by prescription drugs (e.g., thiazide diuretics) is the most frequent cause of hypokalemia. Other common etiologies include renal excretion induced by metabolic acidosis or potassium loss from high-output diarrhea.

CLINICAL PRESENTATION

Symptoms of hypokalemia are determined by the degree of hypokalemia, the cell or organ type affected, and the general health of the patient. Healthy patients with gradual-onset hypokalemia are usually asymptomatic with mild to moderate potassium depletion.

The effects of low serum potassium levels can range from vague myalgias to life-threatening paralysis or dysrhythmias. Because potassium is the major intracellular ion that maintains the charge gradient across cell membranes, any alteration in its concentration will have broad effects on muscle, cardiac, and gastrointestinal tissue. Skeletal muscle cells are the first to be affected, causing patients to experience cramping, fasciculations, and tetany. Patients with underlying ischemic heart disease or congestive heart failure are more likely to develop hypokalemia-induced dysrhythmias with mild to moderate potassium depletion.

Box 166-2 summarizes the clinical findings of hypokalemia.

Mild Hypokalemia (3-3.5 mEq/L)

Patients without significant comorbid conditions tolerate mild hypokalemia very well. Muscular symptoms generally are absent, although occasionally patients experience mild cramping or early muscle fatigue. Hypokalemia may affect smooth muscle function in the gastrointestinal tract with resultant constipation and/or abdominal cramping. Cardiac and neurologic symptoms are absent.

Moderate Hypokalemia (2.5-2.9 mEq/L)

Muscular symptoms become more pronounced as the degree of hypokalemia worsens; weakness is generalized, but proximal and lower-extremity muscle groups are affected.[2] Cardiac manifestations may include palpitations, non–life-threatening dysrhythmias (premature atrial contractions, premature ventricular contractions), and atrial fibrillation. ECG changes occur but do not correlate with the degree of hypokalemia (Box 166-3; Fig. 166-3).

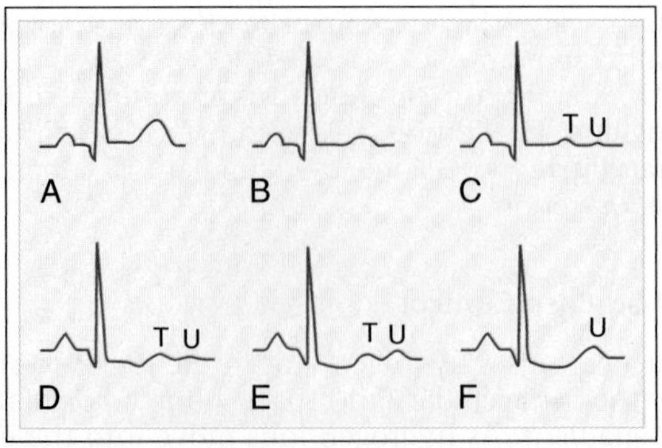
A
B
T U
C
T U
D
T U
E
U
F

FIGURE 166-3 Electrocardiogram findings in hypokalemia. **A,** Normal; **B,** Mild T-wave flattening (the earliest change); **C,** U wave associated with T-wave flattening; **D,** Slight ST depression and a "pseudo-P-pulmonale" pattern; **E,** ST depression is more noticeable, and the U wave increases in amplitude; **F,** The U wave overtakes the T wave—"Q-U" prolongation.

BOX 166-1

Etiologies of Hypokalemia

Inadequate Potassium Intake
- Malnutrition
  - Usually over prolonged periods of time
- Alcoholism
  - Multifactorial causes such as gastric loss through vomiting and renal loss from activation of the renin-angiotensin-aldosterone axis

Gastrointestinal Losses
- Pyloric stenosis, gastrointestinal suctioning
  - Emesis or removal of potassium in the setting of volume depletion and activation of the renin-angiotensin-aldosterone axis
- Diarrhea
- Ileal loop

Renal Losses
- Renal tubular acidosis (RTA)
  - Type I RTA—defective hydrogen secretion results in increased potassium secretion that facilitates sodium reabsorption
  - Type II RTA—increased delivery of bicarbonate to the distal tubule results in increased potassium excretion
- Primary hyperaldosteronism
  - Aldosterone-producing tumor
- Secondary hyperaldosteronism
  - Renal artery stenosis or renin-secreting tumor
- Magnesium depletion
  - Seen with thiazide diuretic use, malabsorption syndromes, and alcoholism/malnutrition

Malignancy
- Ectopic adrenocorticotropic hormone (ACTH) production
  - Tumors (e.g., small cell bronchogenic carcinoma) produce ACTH, which stimulates glucocorticoid and aldosterone production, which promotes renal potassium wasting
- Leukemia

Medications
- Diuretic therapy (thiazides, loop diuretics, carbonic anhydrase inhibitors)
  - Hypokalemia develops only after the total exchangeable body potassium has been depleted over several weeks; recently initiated diuretic therapy does not account for acute hypokalemia
- Antibiotics and antifungal agents
  - Penicillin, carbenicillin—large anionic antibiotics increase luminal electronegativity, caused by excretion of potassium in an effort to maintain electroneutrality
  - Gentamicin—damages renal tubular structure and function
  - Amphotericin B—induces Type I RTA
- Albuterol and theophylline—cause intracellular potassium shifts
- Steroids
- Laxative abuse
- Non-inhalational tobacco products
  - Chronic ingestion produces hypokalemia through stimulation of mineralocorticoids by glycyrrhizic acid (contained in these products)

Other
- Bartter's syndrome
  - Affects children and young adults
  - Features include hypokalemia, hyper-reninemia, hyperaldosteronism, and juxtaglomerular apparatus hyperplasia with normal blood pressure
- Liddle's syndrome
  - Opposite of Bartter's syndrome
  - Features include low renin activity, normal to low aldosterone, and elevated blood pressure
- Hypokalemic (familial) periodic paralysis
- Trauma
  - Hypokalemia seen in 50% to 60% of trauma patients
  - Serum potassium usually decreases within 1 hour of traumatic injury and returns to physiologic levels within 24 hours
- Immune-related (potassium-losing) nephropathy

Modified from Mandal AK: Hypokalemia and hyperkalemia: Med Clin North Am 1997;81:611-639.

Hypokalemia may precipitate or worsen encephalopathy in patients with severe liver disease. Potassium depletion increases renal production of ammonia, which readily crosses the blood-brain barrier in the setting of alkalosis.[2] Hypokalemia also inhibits the release of insulin and may cause hyperglycemia in patients with preexisting glucose intolerance or non–insulin-dependent diabetes mellitus. Renal complications of moderate hypokalemia reflect vasopressin resistance in the tubular reabsorption of

BOX 166-2

Clinical Findings in Hypokalemia

Gastrointestinal
- Ileus (nausea, vomiting, distention)

Vascular
- Postural hypotension (decreased peripheral resistance and autonomic dysfunction)

Cardiac
- Ventricular arrhythmias
- Cardiac arrest
- Bradycardia, tachycardia
- Premature ventricular contractions, premature atrial complexes
- ECG abnormalities (see Box 166-3)
- Enhanced digitalis toxicity

Respiratory
- Hypoventilation, respiratory distress
- Respiratory failure

Neurologic
- Lethargy
- Mental status changes
- Paralysis

Muscular
- Cramping, restless leg syndrome
- Decreased muscle strength, paralysis
- Fasciculations, tetany
- Decreased deep tendon reflexes
- Rhabdomyolysis

Renal
- Nephrogenic diabetes insipidus
- Metabolic alkalosis
- Impaired urinary concentrating ability (polyuria)
- Increased ammonia production and hydrogen ion excretion
- Hypokalemic nephropathy (interstitial renal disease)

Other
- Cushingoid appearance (edema)
- Inhibition of insulin release
- Aldosterone inhibition
- Negative nitrogen balance

Modified from Zull DN: Disorders of potassium metabolism. Emerg Med Clin North Am 1989;7:771-794.

BOX 166-3

ECG Abnormalities in Mild to Moderate Hypokalemia

- Low, flattened, or inverted T waves
- Potassium usually <3.5 mEq/L
- Decreased/depressed ST segment
- Increased P-R interval
- Increased QRS duration
- U waves
  - Taller than T wave
  - Seen in septal leads (V_2, V_3)
- Prominent R wave
- Atrial or ventricular arrhythmias

Adapted from Cohn JN, Kowey PR, Whelton PK, Prisant LM: New guidelines for potassium replacement in clinical practice. Arch Intern Med 2000;160:2429-243; and Zull DN: Disorders of potassium metabolism. Emerg Med Clin North Am 1989;7: 771-794.

water; symptoms include nocturia, polydipsia, and polyuria.[2]

Severe Hypokalemia (<2.5 mEq/L)

Alcoholics have the greatest risk of severe hypokalemia. Musculoskeletal symptoms include pronounced fasciculations, tetany, and rhabdomyolysis. Myolysis may cause a transient release of intracellular potassium that can mask the inciting hypokalemic state. In rare cases, life-threatening ascending paralysis and loss of deep tendon reflexes can result in quadriplegia.[2]

Cardiac manifestations of severe hypokalemia worsen the previously mentioned ECG abnormalities. Of great concern is the development of potentially life-threatening ventricular arrhythmias in patients with preexisting cardiac disease. Ventricular ectopy ranges from premature ventricular contractions to couplets, bigeminy, trigeminy, and episodes of ventricular tachycardia, torsades de pointes, and ventricular fibrillation. In the setting of myocardial infarction or digitalis toxicity, hypokalemia-induced ventricular dysrthythmias are directly proportional to the degree of potassium depletion.[2]

DIAGNOSTIC TESTING (Table 166-2)

Historical elements that may mandate serum potassium measurement include potential causes of inadequate intake (malnutrition, alcoholism) and excessive wasting (diarrhea, vomiting, polyuria). Longstanding use of diuretics, β_2-agonists, or laxatives should also prompt potassium screening.

In the ED, evaluation should focus on the identification of hypokalemia through laboratory testing, classification of disease severity, correlation with

Table 166-2 DIAGNOSTIC APPROACH TO HYPOKALEMIA IN THE ED

Laboratory Findings	Etiology
+ Normal acid-base profile+(Ur K/Ur Cr) <2	Transcellular shift (thyrotoxic periodic paralysis, familial periodic paralysis)
+ Non–anion gap metabolic acidosis +((Ur Na+Ur K)−Ur Cl)>−10	Gastrointestinal losses (diarrhea); bicarbonate loss
+ Non–anion gap metabolic acidosis +((Ur Na+Ur K)−Ur Cl)<−10 +(Ur K/Ur Cr)>2	Renal losses (renal tubular acidosis)
+ Metabolic alkalosis+Ur Cl <20 mEq/L	Diuretics; gastrointestinal losses (vomiting, nasogastric tube suctioning)
+ Metabolic alkalosis+Ur Cl >20 mEq/L	Diuretics; increased mineralocorticoid effects

K, potassium; Na, sodium; Cl, chloride; Cr, creatinine; Ur, urinary.
Adapted from Schaefer TJ, Wolford RW: Disorders of potassium. Emerg Med Clin North Am 2005;23:723-747.

physical examination findings, and correction or stabilization of potentially life-threatening conditions.

If hypokalemia is identified, screening for hypomagnesemia and hypophosphatemia is necessary; these coexistent entities are difficult to distinguish from hypokalemia by physical examination alone. Falsely elevated potassium levels occur with hemolysis caused by prolonged tourniquet application, improper collection, or mishandling of the blood sample. Repeat levels as necessary. A urine pH higher than 6 suggests type I renal tubular acidosis; urine electrolytes and a venous blood gas should be obtained to search for a corresponding metabolic alkalosis.

If the patient is taking digoxin, a serum digoxin level is indicated; hypokalemia potentiates digitalis toxicity and increases the likelihood of cardiac dysrthythmias.

Additional laboratory testing and imaging can be performed later in the inpatient or outpatient setting.

TREATMENT (Table 166-3)

Patients with Cardiovascular Disease

Optimal goals for serum potassium repletion are predicated on the underlying pathology. Patients with a history of congestive heart failure, coronary artery disease, or arrhythmias and hypertensive patients being treated with diuretic medications should have a serum potassium of at least 4 mEq/L. These patients require oral supplementation for even mild, asymptomatic hypokalemia, such as potassium chloride tablets (20-40 mEq daily for 1 to 2 weeks).[7] If the patient is taking a potassium-wasting diuretic, the dose should be decreased.

Asymptomatic Mild Hypokalemia

Healthy patients with asymptomatic, mild hypokalemia (3-3.5 mEq/L) do not require pharmacologic potassium supplementation. Treatment should be focused on minimizing further potassium loss and increasing oral intake. Patients should be encouraged to eat a diet rich in potassium (Box 166-4). Potassium-wasting diuretics should be decreased or eliminated, as blood pressure allows. The use of substances that contain glycyrrhizic acid (e.g., licorice, chewing tobacco, laxatives) should be avoided.[1,3]

Symptomatic Mild and Moderate Hypokalemia

Potassium supplementation is required for patients with symptomatic mild or moderate (<3 mEq/L) hypokalemia. Potassium supplements are available in several forms: potassium chloride, potassium phosphate, potassium citrate, potassium acetate, potassium gluconate, and potassium bicarbonate. Potassium chloride is the preferred formulation for most ED cases of hypokalemia. (Potassium phosphate may be beneficial in certain cases of diabetic ketoacidosis.)[3] Oral potassium supplements are available as tablets, powder, or elixir.

Dosing ranges from 20 to 80 mEq/day; doses greater than 40 mEq should be divided and given either two or three times a day. Oral therapy should

Table 166-3 TREATMENT OF HYPOKALEMIA

Formulation	Dosage Regimen	Indication
Oral KCl	20-80 mEq/day divided bid-tid	Non-urgent correction and/or maintenance therapy with diuretic use
Oral KCl liquid (recheck serum K in 24-72 hr)	40-60 mEq/dose	Rapid elevation for patients requiring urgent, but not emergent, correction
IV KCl	10-20 mEq/hour (recheck serum K after giving 60 mEq)	For patients with severe symptoms or inability to tolerate oral therapy

Adapted from Zull DN: Disorders of potassium metabolism. Emerg Med Clin North Am 1989;7:771-794; and Schaefer TJ, Wolford RW: Disorders of potassium. Emerg Med Clin North Am 2005;23:723-747.

BOX 166-4

Foods Rich in Potassium

Highest Content (>1000 mg/100 g)

- Figs
- Molasses

Very High Content (>500 mg/100 g)

- Dates, prunes
- Nuts
- Avocados
- Bran
- Wheat germ
- Lima beans

High Content (>250 mg/100 g)

- Vegetables—spinach, tomatoes, broccoli, beets, potatoes
- Fruits—bananas, cantaloupe, oranges, mangos
- Meat—beef, pork, veal, lamb

Adapted from Cohn JN, Kowey PR, Whelton PK, Prisant LM: New guidelines for potassium replacement in clinical practice. Arch Intern Med 2000;160:2429-2436.

be monitored daily, because serum potassium levels will rise within 48 to 72 hours.[3] Healthy patients that require daily oral supplementation can be safely discharged from the ED if repeat serum potassium measurements can be monitored by the primary care physician for 1 to 2 days. Patients who are elderly, have significant comorbidities, or poor access to follow-up should be admitted to the hospital for a 24-hour observation period.

Magnesium deficiency should be suspected in patients who fail to respond to oral potassium therapy within 96 hours. Magnesium promotes activity of the NA^+,K^+-ATPase pump, which will replenish intracellular fluid concentrations in the first days of potassium supplementation.[3]

■ Severe Hypokalemia

IV potassium replacement is indicated for patients with severe hypokalemia (<2.5 mEq/L) or moderate hypokalemia accompanied by cardiac arrhythmias, familial periodic paralysis, or severe myopathy.[3]

Replacement consists of 100 mEq of potassium chloride in 1 liter of normal saline (or D_5W) infused at a rate of 100 to 200 mL/hour (10-20 mEq/hour). If the patient has any form of heart block or renal insufficiency, the initial infusion rate should be reduced to 50 mL/hour (5 mEq/hour).

In rare instances of extreme hypokalemia or life-threatening clinical findings, potassium may be infused at 40 to 60 mEq/hour (400-600 mEq/L of normal saline at 100 mL/hour). Therapy should be monitored with great caution. Serum potassium levels should be rechecked after every 40 to 60 mEq infused.

IV potassium supplementation can cause excruciating phlebitis and cardiac arrest if directly injected into a vessel—never administer potassium as an IV push. Peripheral IV lines can be used for rates of 10 to 20 mEq/hour or less. To minimize the risk of phlebitis, a central line is necessary for infusion rates of greater than 20 mEq/hour. There is a theoretical concern for cardiac arrest when potassium is administered via central venous access—splitting the potassium infusion rate over two peripheral lines may be preferable.[2]

In general, patients receiving IV potassium supplementation require telemetry monitoring and frequent repeat potassium measurements (up to every 1 to 3 hours after the initial infusion begins). Significant potassium depletion may take days to correct. As serum potassium levels approach 3.5 mEq/L, patients should be converted to oral therapy if possible. IV potassium supplementation should be discontinued if any ECG signs of hyperkalemia are noted or if a single potassium measurement is higher than 3.5 mEq/L.

Unstable ventricular arrhythmias resulting from severe hypokalemia should be managed according to standard practice guidelines. Severe neuromuscular manifestations may endanger adequate respiratory effort and therefore mandate aggressive airway stabilization. Any volume depletion should be corrected, and co-existing medical conditions that may exacerbate the effects of hypokalemia should be addressed.[1]

Hyperkalemia

Hyperkalemia is defined as a potassium level above 5.0 mEq/L. Hyperkalemia is further classified as mild (5-6 mEq/L), moderate (6.1-7 mEq/L), and severe (>7 mEq/L).

Compared to hypokalemia, hyperkalemia is less common but more deadly. Even moderate hyperkalemia can present with life-threatening cardiac manifestations that require immediate treatment. As many as 8% of patients admitted to hospital are ultimately diagnosed with some degree of hyperkalemia; the vast majority of these cases are associated with renal insufficiency that impairs normal potassium clearance. Hyperkalemia affects men and women equally.

■ ETIOLOGIES (Box 166-5)

Hyperkalemia is predominately a condition associated with dialysis-dependent renal failure. In patients with moderate to severe renal insufficiency who are not anuric, clinically significant hyperkalemia rarely occurs. Potassium homeostasis is more difficult in these patients, however, such that relatively small changes in excretory function or exogenous supplementation will promote a hyperkalemic state. Causes

BOX 166-5

Etiologies of Hyperkalemia

Exogenous Potassium
- Potassium supplements (oral and intravenous)
- Dietary salt substitutes
  - Food indiscretion by dialysis-dependent patients
- Stored blood
- Potassium-containing penicillin preparations

Cellular Efflux of Potassium (Cell Injury)
- Rhabdomyolyis
- Severe intravascular hemolysis
- Acute tumor lysis syndrome
- Burns, crush injuries, trauma

Decreased Renal Excretion
- Glomerular filtration rate <10 mL/min
  - Acute renal failure
  - Chronic renal failure
- Hypoaldosteronism
  - Primary (Addison's disease)
  - Secondary—type IV RTA (hyporeninemic hypoaldosteronism), drug-induced
- NSAIDs
- ACE inhibitors
- Heparin
- Cyclosporin
- Tubular defects in potassium secretion
  - Renal transplant
  - Nephropathy
  - Sickle cell disease
  - Obstructive uropathy
  - Interstitial nephritis
  - Chronic pyelonephritis
  - Potassium-sparing diuretics (amiloride, triamterene, spironolactone)
  - Other (lead, lupus nephritis, pseudohypoaldosteronism)

Transcellular Shifts
- Acidosis
- Hypertonicity
- Insulin deficiency
- Hypoaldosteronism
- Drugs
  - Beta-blockers
  - Digitalis
  - Succinylcholine
- Exercise
- Hyperkalemic periodic (familial) paralysis

Pseudohyperkalemia
- Blood sample hemolysis
- Thrombocytosis (PLTs > 1,000,000
- Leukocytosis (WBCs > 100,000)
- Muscle exercise with tight clothing or tourniquet

ACE, angiotensin-converting enzyme; NSAIDs, nonsteroidal antiinflammatory drugs; PLTs, platelets; RTA, renal tubular acidosis; WBCs, white blood cells.
Adapted from Zull DN: Disorders of potassium metabolism. Emerg Med Clin North Am 1989;7:771-794; and Gennari FJ: Disorders of potassium homeostasis: Hypokalemia and hyperkalemia. Crit Care Clin 2002,18:273-288.

of hyperkalemia reflect impairments in normal potassium physiology.

Excessive Potassium Intake

Excessive potassium intake can overwhelm the excretory ability of the kidney. Although normal kidneys can generally compensate for brief yet massive oral potassium loads (through supplements or diet), patients with renal insufficiency may not be able to appropriately compensate.

Impaired Potassium Excretion

Impaired clearance of potassium occurs in patients with significant renal insufficiency. Worsening renal excretion of potassium results from a significant decrease in the glomerular filtration rate (acute or chronic), hypoaldosteronism, or a renal tubular defect causing excessive potassium secretion.

Pathologic Transcellular Shifts

Hyperkalemia may also arise from excess transcellular shifts or release from the intracellular space to the extracellular fluid compartment. Pathologic cellular release can result from cell injury (e.g., rhabdomyolysis, burns, trauma) or from metabolic changes that alter the activity of the Na^+,K^+-ATPase pump (e.g., acidosis, insulin deficiency).

Nonpathologic Hyperkalemia

"Pseudohyperkalemia" is a common presentation in the ED. Elevated serum potassium levels observed in patients with normal renal function and a normal ECG should be rechecked prior to any treatment. Measurement error is the most common cause of an elevated potassium level in otherwise healthy patients.

CLINICAL PRESENTATION

Hyperkalemia is often asymptomatic and only discovered on routine laboratory screening. When symptoms do occur, conduction abnormalities at the cellular level promote cardiac and neuromuscular findings. ECG abnormalities, usually the first nonlaboratory indicators of hyperkalemia, do not correlate with the degree of serum potassium elevation.

Mild Hyperkalemia (5-6 mEq/L)

Mild hyperkalemia is generally asymptomatic. Patients with underlying cardiac disease occasionally report palpitations or other well-tolerated rhythm disturbances.

Moderate Hyperkalemia (6.1-7 mEq/L)

Patients with moderate hyperkalemia may exhibit ECG abnormalities, including peaked T waves and prolongation of the P-R interval and QRS complex[8] (Fig. 166-4; Box 166-6).

Neuromuscular symptoms similar to those seen in hypokalemia can occur. Muscle cramps and weakness are the most commonly reported complaints.

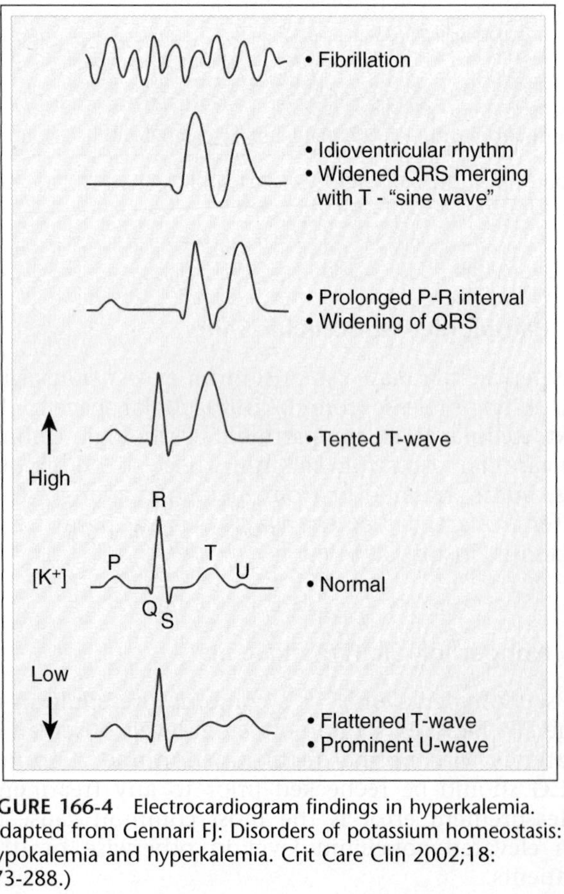
• Fibrillation
• Idioventricular rhythm
• Widened QRS merging with T - "sine wave"
• Prolonged P-R interval
• Widening of QRS
• Tented T-wave
High
R
P
T
U
[K+]
Q
S
• Normal
Low
• Flattened T-wave
• Prominent U-wave

FIGURE 166-4 Electrocardiogram findings in hyperkalemia. (Adapted from Gennari FJ: Disorders of potassium homeostasis: Hypokalemia and hyperkalemia. Crit Care Clin 2002;18: 273-288.)

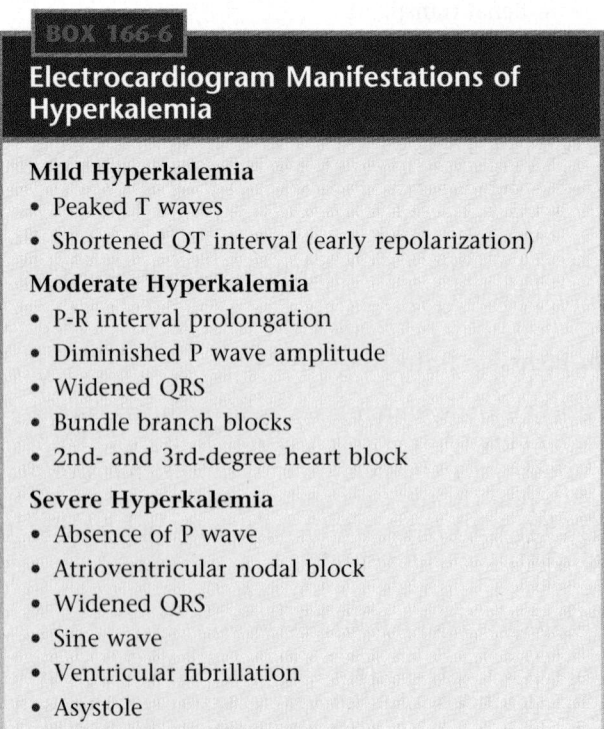

Severe Hyperkalemia (>7 mEq/L)

Progressively worsening hyperkalemia can result in significant conduction abnormalities, heart blocks, potentially life-threatening arrhythmias, and asystole. Symptoms such as palpitations, syncope, chest pain, and dyspnea (from left-sided heart failure) may be present. Ascending paralysis and tetany may result.

DIAGNOSTIC TESTING

The clinical diagnosis of hyperkalemia is difficult because patients either are asymptomatic or present with findings of hyperkalemia-induced cardiovascular disturbances. Historical features that should raise suspicion of hyperkalemia include known acute or chronic renal insufficiency, potassium supplementation, and ECG changes following an incomplete hemodialysis session. End-stage renal dialysis patients who have missed a scheduled dialysis session should be placed on a cardiac monitor and immediately screened for ECG abnormalities and electrolyte disturbances.

The first sign of hyperkalemia may be an abnormal ECG on arrival at the ED. If hyperkalemia is suspected in an asymptomatic renal patient with an abnormal ECG, obtain a complete serum chemistry panel and a whole blood potassium level measured by venous blood gas analysis. Arterial or venous blood gas sampling is generally the most efficient

BOX 166-6

Electrocardiogram Manifestations of Hyperkalemia

Mild Hyperkalemia
- Peaked T waves
- Shortened QT interval (early repolarization)

Moderate Hyperkalemia
- P-R interval prolongation
- Diminished P wave amplitude
- Widened QRS
- Bundle branch blocks
- 2nd- and 3rd-degree heart block

Severe Hyperkalemia
- Absence of P wave
- Atrioventricular nodal block
- Widened QRS
- Sine wave
- Ventricular fibrillation
- Asystole

Adapted from Mattu A, Brady WJ, Robinson DA: Electrocardiographic manifestations of hyperkalemia. Am J Emerg Med 2000;18:721-729.

method for obtaining an accurate measurement of potassium concentration.

Additional laboratory tests useful in the ED evaluation of hyperkalemia include serum calcium, creatinine, digoxin, and blood pH. Other testing can be deferred to the inpatient setting.

■ TREATMENT (Table 166-4)

The management of hyperkalemia focuses on three goals of care: cardiac stabilization, transcellular shift of potassium from extracellular fluid to intracellular fluid, and elimination of excess potassium. Only potassium excretion is a definitive treatment step—other actions serve to temporarily stabilize the cell membrane in an effort to prevent hemodynamic collapse.

■ Cardiac Stabilization: Calcium

IV calcium rapidly antagonizes the adverse effects of moderate to severe hyperkalemia on the cell membrane potential in cardiac myocytes. Calcium can be administered as IV calcium chloride or calcium gluconate, even in patients who are normocalcemic. IV preparations of calcium chloride contain three times more calcium per ampule than calcium gluconate formulations; calcium chloride is therefore the drug of choice for immediate cardiac stabilization in life-threatening hyperkalemia. Calcium normalizes ECG manifestations of hyperkalemia within minutes of administration; however, the clinical effects generally are short-lived. Repeat doses may be required within 30 minutes, or if no effects are observed within 5 to 10 minutes of the initial dose.

■ Transcellular Shift: Insulin and Albuterol

Potassium can be temporarily shifted from the extracellular to the intracellular compartment through stimulation of the Na^+,K^+-ATPase pump by insulin or a β_2-agonist such as albuterol. Although either of these agents can temporize moderate hyperkalemia when given alone, studies suggest that combination therapy using both agents may be more efficacious.

Insulin forces the transcellular shift of potassium into liver and muscle cells. Regular (short-acting) insulin administered as a 10-unit IV bolus will begin to lower serum potassium concentrations within 10 to 20 minutes, with a clinical effect that lasts several hours. An ampule of 50% dextrose solution ($D_{50}W$) should be given concurrently to prevent

RED FLAGS

Calcium Supplementation

- Calcium chloride may cause significant skin necrosis if extravasated.
- Calcium should not be administered with solutions that contain sodium bicarbonate, because calcium carbonate ($CaCO_3$) will precipitate.
- Avoid IV calcium boluses in hyperkalemic patients with suspected digoxin toxicity, due to the risk of cardiac tetany/fatal arrhythmia. Slow calcium infusions (over 30 minutes) require close monitoring in these patients.

Table 166-4 TREATMENT OF HYPERKALEMIA

Medication	Dosage Regimen	Onset	Duration
Cardiac Stabilization			
Calcium chloride	1 ampule IVP over 1-2 min	1-3 min	30-40 min
Calcium gluconate	10 mL of 10% solution	1-3 min	20-60 min
Transcellular Shift			
Insulin	10 units IV with 50 mL of 50% dextrose (one ampule of $D_{50}W$),		
	Or		
	10 units in 500 mL $D_{10}W$ over 1-hr infusion	10-20 min	2-4 hr
Albuterol nebulized over 20-60 min	10-20 mg in 4 mL NS	20-30 min	2-4 hr
Elimination			
Kayexalate	30 g PO 50 g PR	2 hr PO 1 hr PO	4-6 hr 4-6 hr
Lasix (furosemide)	20-40 mg IVP	variable	variable
Hemodialysis		minutes	variable

$D_{10}W$, 10% dextrose in water; IV, intravenously; IVP, intravenous push; NS, normal saline; PO, orally; PR, rectally.
Adapted from Zull DN: Disorders of potassium metabolism. Emerg Med Clin North Am 1989;7:771-794; and Schaefer TJ, Wolford RW: Disorders of potassium. Emerg Med Clin North Am 2005;23:723-747.

hypoglycemia; patients who are already hyperglycemic (>250 mg/dL) do not require supplemental dextrose.

Albuterol is the most readily available β_2-agonist used to treat hyperkalemia in the ED. Nebulized albuterol in 10- to 20-mg continuous treatments will decrease serum potassium by 1 mEq/L over 1 to 2 hours.[9] Although not approved for use in the United States, IV administration of albuterol shifts potassium into the intracellular fluid compartment even more rapidly.

Elimination: Resin Exchange (Kayexalate) and Dialysis

The definitive treatment of hyperkalemia is potassium elimination. For patients with renal insufficiency, resin exchange (Kayexalate), and dialysis are the mainstays of therapy. Potassium-wasting diuretics (thiazides, loop diuretics) may be taken by patients with normal renal function and mild asymptomatic hyperkalemia.

Sodium polystyrene sulfonate (Kayexalate) is an inert resin that exchanges sodium for potassium in the intestinal tract. One gram of Kayexalate removes approximately 0.5 to 1 mEq of potassium in exchange for 2 to 3 mEq of sodium.[9] The usual dose of Kayexalate is 30 to 60 g given orally or rectally. Oral Kayexalate begins to reduce total body potassium within several hours of administration, with a clinical effect of 4 to 6 hours. Rectal Kayexalate has a shorter time to onset than the oral formulation but is less efficacious. High-dose Kayexalate precipitates pulmonary edema by increasing extracellular sodium in fluid-overloaded patients.

Hemodialysis is the most rapid method of potassium elimination for patients with persistent, symptomatic, or severe hyperkalemia. If a potassium-free dialysate is used, serum potassium may decrease as much as 1.5 mEq/L per hour. Stable patients may be transferred to an inpatient hemodialysis unit for therapy under strict cardiac monitoring. Patients with ECG abnormalities, hypotension, significant volume overload, or respiratory distress should be dialyzed in the ED or intensive care unit. Cell membrane stabilization using IV calcium, IV insulin/glucose, and inhalational albuterol is necessary to prevent arrhythmia while awaiting emergency hemodialysis.

REFERENCES

1. Schaefer TJ, Wolford RW: Disorders of potassium. Emerg Med Clin North Am 2005;23:723-747.
2. Zull DN: Disorders of potassium metabolism. Emerg Med Clin North Am 1989;7:771-794.
3. Mandal AK: Hypokalemia and hyperkalemia. Med Clin North Am 1997;81:611-639.
4. Gaffar M: Diagnosis and treatment of hyperkalemia. Resid Staff Physician 2003;49:18-22.
5. Gennari FJ: Disorders of potassium homeostasis: Hypokalemia and hyperkalemia. Crit Care Clin 2002,18:273-288.
6. Schaller MD, Fischer AP, Perret CH: Hyperkalemia. A prognostic factor during acute severe hypothermia. JAMA 1990; 264:1842-1845.
7. Cohn JN, Kowey PR, Whelton PK, Prisant LM: New guidelines for potassium replacement in clinical practice. Arch Intern Med 2000;160:2429-2436.
8. Mattu A, Brady WJ, Robinson DA: Electrocardiographic manifestations of hyperkalemia. Am J Emerg Med 2000; 18:721-729.
9. Weiner ID, Wingo CS: Hyperkalemia: A potential silent killer. J Am Soc Nephrol 1998;9:1535-1543.

Chapter **167**

Calcium, Magnesium, and Phosphorus

Rawle A. Seupaul and Ryan Pursley

KEY POINTS

Patients at high risk for imbalances of calcium, magnesium, or phosphorus include those with alcohol addiction, renal failure, chronic obstructive pulmonary disease, diabetic ketoacidosis, shock, and poor nutrition.

Calcium, magnesium, and phosphorus homeostasis is interdependent. Abnormalities in the serum concentration of any of these electrolytes should initiate evaluation of the others.

Severe imbalances of calcium, magnesium, or phosphorus can be immediately life-threatening and require decisive, targeted therapy.

Fatal arrhythmias can occur with extreme elevation or depletion of any of these electrolytes.

Scope

Imbalances of calcium, magnesium, and phosphorus are frequently identified in the ED setting. A thorough understanding of these disorders and their treatment is essential for the EP.

Calcium plays a critical role in numerous metabolic reactions in the body including muscular contraction, platelet aggregation, cardiac contractility, neurotransmission, and immunomodulation. Disruption in calcium homeostasis can have significant clinical implications.

Magnesium is involved in many different enzymatic reactions that can seriously effect normal physiology and lead to significant morbidity and mortality. Because of its effects on hormonal regulation, adequate serum levels are a prerequisite for treating other electrolyte imbalances such as hypocalcemia and hypokalemia.

Clinically important disturbances in serum phosphate are rare but should be considered in patients with chronic obstructive pulmonary disease (COPD), alcoholism, malignancy, renal failure, and diabetic ketoacidosis.[1] Awareness of these high-risk groups and recognition of symptoms caused by either hyperphosphatemia or hypophosphatemia are critical to appropriate management and disposition of these patients.

CALCIUM

Pathophysiology

The body of an average-sized adult contains approximately 15 g/kg of calcium (about 1 kg total), the majority of which (98%) is stored in bone.

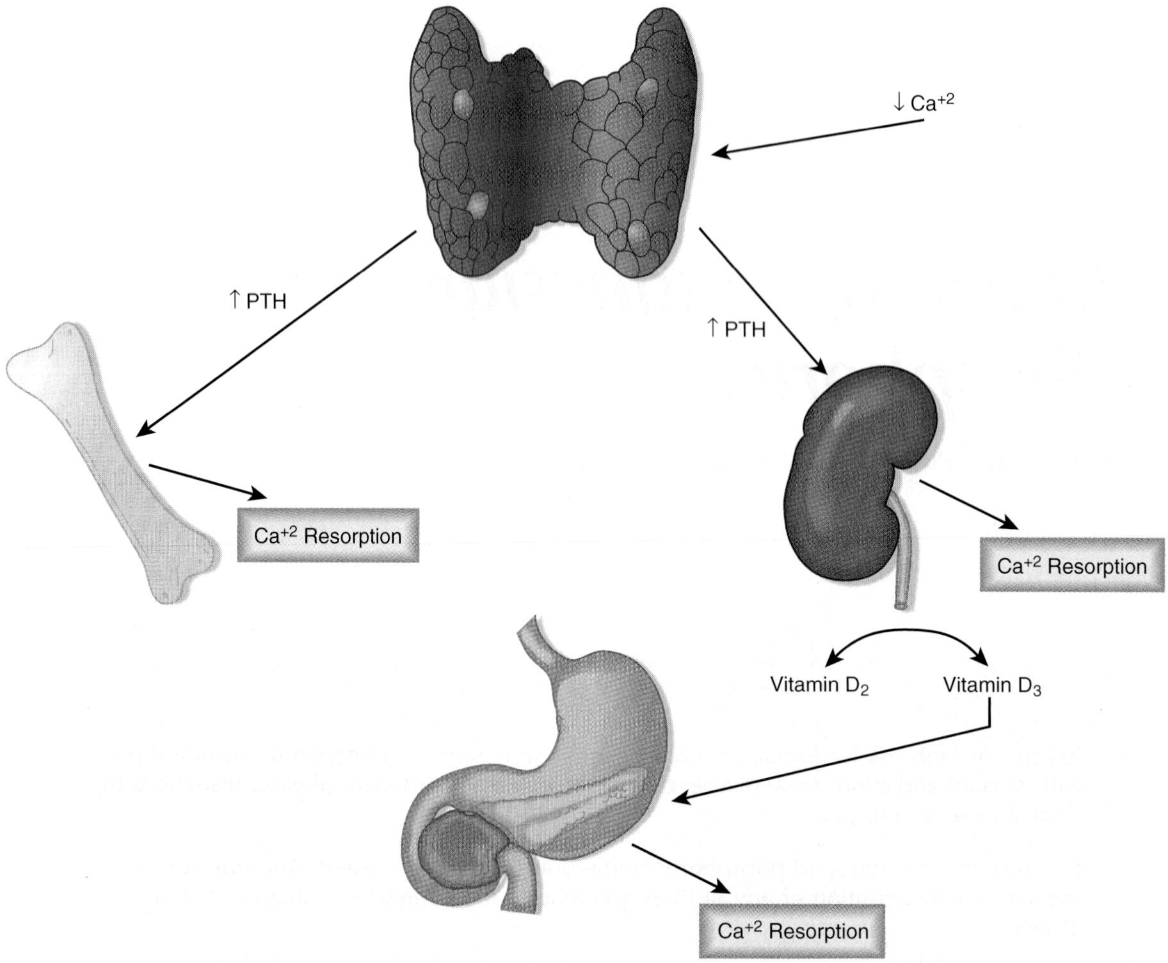
↓ Ca+2
↑ PTH
↑ PTH
Ca+2 Resorption
Ca+2 Resorption
Vitamin D2
Vitamin D3
Ca+2 Resorption

FIGURE 167-1 Summary of calcium homeostasis. PTH, parathyroid hormone.

Approximately 50% of the remaining calcium is present as physiologically active ionized calcium, 40% is protein-bound (mostly to albumin), and 10% is in complex with various anions.[2] Physiologic levels are maintained mainly by the actions of parathyroid hormone 1,25-dihydroxyvitamin D_3, calcitonin, phosphate, and calcium itself (serving as a negative feedback inhibitor on the kidney, gut, and bones) (Fig. 167-1).[2]

Disorders of calcium homeostasis are encountered when serum levels deviate from a narrow physiologic range (8.5-10.5 mg/dL).[2] The severity of symptoms is dependent on the rapidity and magnitude of change in serum levels.

Hypercalcemia is defined as a serum calcium level above 10.5 mg/dL. Althouth patients usually are not symptomatic at levels below 12 mg/dL, they may become critically ill once concentrations exceed 14 mg/dL (severe hypercalcemia). Patients with serum calcium concentrations above 14 mg/dL require immediate treatment.

Hypocalcemia is defined as a serum level below 8.5 mg/dL. Patients are rarely symptomatic until levels fall below 2.8 mg/dL.

Clinical Presentation

■ HYPERCALCEMIA

Patients with mild hypercalcemia (up to 12 mg/dL) usually are asymptomatic. As levels increase, patients may develop nonspecific complaints such as fatigue, weakness, anxiety, nausea and vomiting, and vague abdominal pain (Box 167-1).[2] Once serum levels rise above 14 mg/dL, symptoms become more pronounced and may include psychosis and coma. At these levels, patients may also develop pancreatitis, renal stones, and/or nephrocalcinosis. A classic memory aid for the presenting signs and symptoms of severe hypercalcemia is the following: *stones* (renal calculi), *bones* (osteolysis), *moans* (psychiatric disorders), and *groans* (constipation, peptic ulcer disease, and pancreatitis).

At levels above 14 mg/dL, cardiac manifestations of hypercalcemia may become evident, with electrocardiographic (ECG) findings of QT-interval shortening, T-wave inversions, and ST-segment elevations that can mimic acute myocardial infarction (Fig. 167-2). Cardiac irritability from severe hypercalcemia

BOX 167-1

Signs and Symptoms of Hypercalcemia*

Central Nervous System
- Fatigue
- Weakness
- Psychosis
- Coma

Cardiac
- P-R prolongation
- QT shortening
- QRS widening
- Dysrhythmias

Renal
- Renal stones
- Nephrocalcinosis renal failure

Gastrointestinal
- Vague abdominal pain
- Nausea and vomiting
- Constipation
- Peptic ulceration
- Pancreatitis

*Findings for each system are listed in order of increasing serum calcium levels. Note that as the serum levels increase (moving down the list), complications become more clinically significant in that system.

can also lead to bundle branch blocks, bradycardia, and cardiac arrest.

The most common renal effect of hypercalcemia is loss of the ability to concentrate urine. This reversible tubular defect begins a cycle of increasing serum calcium levels by causing polydipsia, polyuria, and volume depletion. Renal losses and volume contraction may be exacerbated by persistent vomiting, resulting in a severe volume deficit that can lead to oliguric renal failure, coma, and death.

■ HYPOCALCEMIA

Clinical manifestations of hypocalcemia are dependent on both the absolute serum level and the rapidity of decline (Box 167-2), which is influenced by acid-base status, degree of concurrent hypomagnesemia, and increased sympathetic activity.[2] Neuromuscular, psychiatric, and cardiac findings predominate. Neuromuscular symptoms include muscle weakness and cramps, perioral paresthesias, seizures, fasciculations, and tetany.

Chvostek's sign and Trousseau's sign are two physical examination findings seen in these patients. Chvostek's sign is defined by facial muscle twitching after tapping on the ipsilateral facial nerve. Trousseau's sign is characterized by carpal spasm (flexion at the wrist and metacarpophalangeal joints and spastically extended fingers) produced by applying a blood pressure cuff to the upper arm and maintaining a pressure above systolic pressure for 3 minutes.

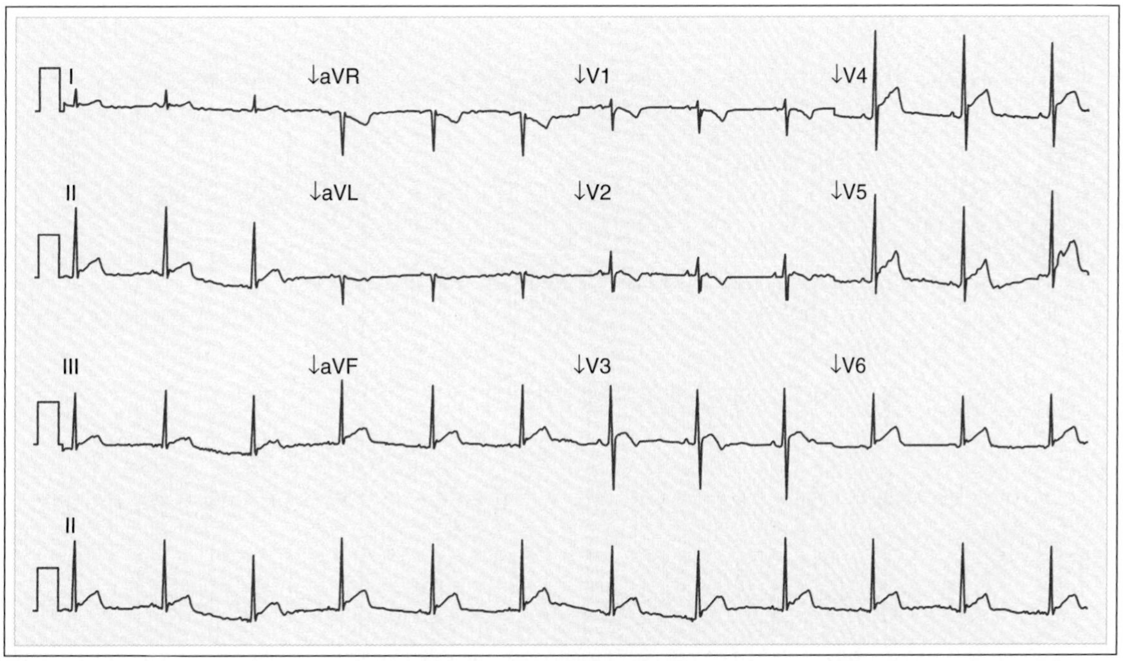
I
↓aVR
↓V1
↓V4
II
↓aVL
↓V2
↓V5
III
↓aVF
↓V3
↓V6
II

FIGURE 167-2 Electrocardiographic manifestations of hypercalcemia. Note the short QTc, terminal T-wave inversions, and ST-segment elevation. (Courtesy of Loren K. Rood, MD, Indiana University School of Medicine, Indianapolis, IN.)

Psychiatric symptoms include depression, confusion, and irritability.

Hypocalcemia may impair normal cardiovascular function as a negative inotrope. Severe hypocalcemia can precipitate congestive heart failure, bradycardia, and other dysrhythmias. The most common ECG finding is prolongation of the QT interval (Fig. 167-3).[3]

BOX 167-2

Signs and Symptoms of Hypocalcemia*

Neuromuscular
- Perioral paresthesias
- Cramps
- Muscle weakness
- Fasciculations
- Tetany
- Seizures

Cardiovascular
- Prolonged QT
- Bradycardia
- Congestive heart failure
- Dysrhythmias

Psychiatric
- Irritability
- Depression
- Confusion

*Findings for each system are listed in order of decreasing serum calcium levels. Note that as the serum levels decrease (moving down the table), complications become more clinically significant in that system.

Differential Diagnosis

■ HYPERCALCEMIA

The differential diagnosis for hypercalcemia is broad (Box 167-3). Primary hyperparathyroidism is the most common cause of hypercalcemia observed in outpatient populations. Of these cases, 80% are associated with a parathyroid adenoma, while small proportions are attributed to parathyroid hyperplasia, carcinoma, and familial endocrine tumor syndromes. The elevation in parathyroid hormone leads to increased bone resorption, increased intestinal absorption, and decreased renal calcium excretion (see Fig. 167-1).[4]

Malignancy accounts for most of the cases of hypercalcemia involving hospitalized patients. This can be attributed to both bony metastases and paraneoplastic syndromes. The most common sites of associated primary tumors include the lung, breast, and kidney. Hematologic malignancies such as multiple myeloma, lymphoma, and leukemia can also increase serum calcium levels.[5,6]

Thiazide diuretics commonly lead to hypercalcemia by increasing resorption of calcium in the distal convoluted tubule. Levels are usually only mildly elevated but can be exacerbated by hypovolemic states.

An emerging etiology for hypercalcemia is the milk-alkali syndrome. This syndrome has been observed after increased use of oral calcium supplements in the treatment of osteoporosis, peptic ulcer

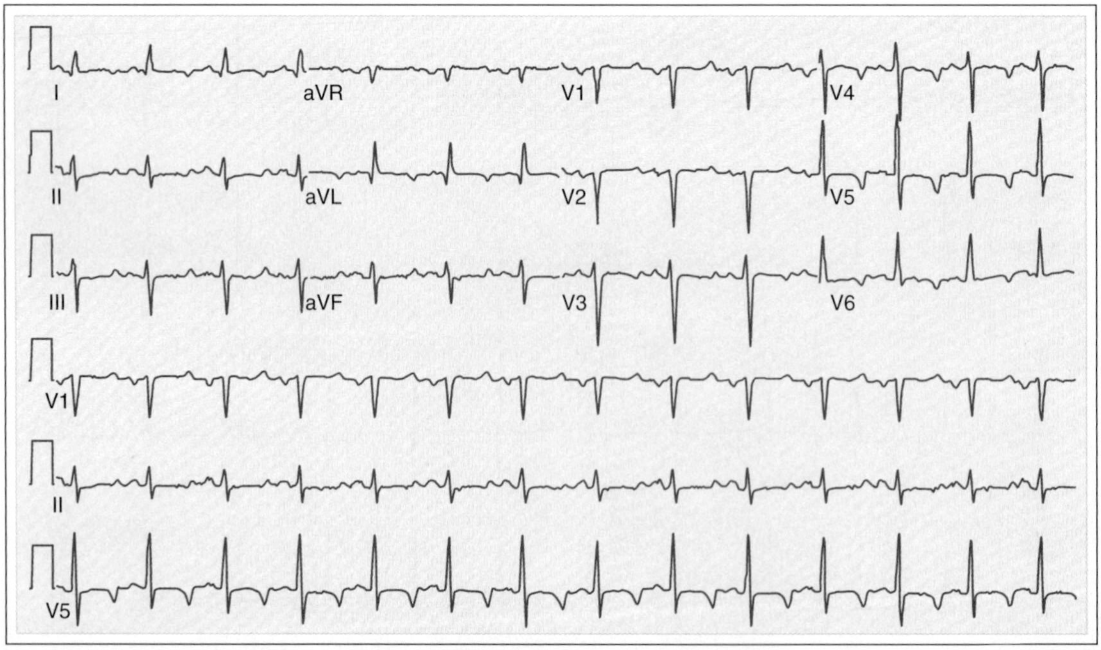
I
aVR
V1
V4
II
aVL
V2
V5
III
aVF
V3
V6
V1
II
V5

FIGURE 167-3 Electrocardiographic manifestations of hypocalcemia. Note the long QT segment with relatively normal T-wave morphology. (Courtesy of Richard Parks, MD, Indiana University School of Medicine, Indianapolis, IN.)

BOX 167-3

Common Causes of Hypercalcemia

Primary Hyperparathyroidism
- Gland hyperplasia
- Carcinoma
- Familial endocrine syndromes

Malignancy
- Bone metastases
- Paraneoplastic syndromes

Other
- Thiazide diuretics
- Milk-alkali syndrome
- Thyrotoxicosis
- Granulomatous disease

Rare
- Tuberculosis
- Sarcoid
- Leprosy

BOX 167-4

Common Causes of Hypocalcemia

Parathyroid Hormone Deficiency
- Gland removal
- Chronic renal insufficiency
- Infiltrative disorders
- Metastatic disease
- Medications
- Hypomagnesemia
- Congenital disorders

Vitamin D Deficiency
- Nutritional deficit
- Renal insufficiency
- Hepatic Insufficiency

Other
- Chelating agents
- Acute pancreatitis

disease, and hyperphosphatemia of chronic renal failure.[2,6,7]

■ HYPOCALCEMIA

Hypocalcemia has an extensive list of etiologies (Box 167-4). The majority of causes stem from deficiency of parathyroid hormone and/or vitamin D. The most common cause of parathyroid hormone insufficiency is accidental gland removal during neck surgery (secondary hypoparathyroidism). Other causes include infiltrative and metastatic diseases of the thyroid, magnesium abnormalities, and drugs that inhibit parathyroid hormone function. Primary hypoparathyroidism is rare and usually is the result of congenital disorders.

Tertiary hypoparathyroidism is seen in patients with chronic renal failure. In these patients, vitamin D deficiency, phosphate retention, and decreased responsiveness to parathyroid hormone results in hypocalcemia. This form of hypocalcemia is usually asymptomatic, due in part to the buffering effects of systemic acidosis. Conversely, rapid correction of the acidosis (e.g., with sodium bicarbonate) can precipitate profound hypocalcemia, tetany, and seizures.

Vitamin D deficiency results in diminished absorption of calcium from the gut (see Fig. 167-1). Although this disorder is rare in westernized societies, it is frequently observed in the developing world. Patients with hepatic and renal disease may also suffer from vitamin D deficiency despite adequate dietary intake, because vitamin D is hydroxylated to its active form in the liver and kidney.

Hypocalcemia can be found in patients treated with chelation agents, such as supplements containing phosphorus or bicarbonate. Patients also may become hypocalcemic as a result of elevated citrate levels after massive blood transfusion. This is a significant concern in traumatized patients, in patients with liver failure who require frequent transfusions, and in patients who are hypothermic.[8] Also, acute pancreatitis is a common disorder that can lead to hypocalcemia as a result of calcification (saponification) of this diseased organ.

Treatment

■ HYPERCALCEMIA

The mainstay of treatment for hypercalcemia is aggressive intravascular volume correction with normal saline. The use of central venous monitoring may be prudent in patients with compromised cardiac and renal function. Secondary treatment measures include the promotion of renal calcium excretion, reduction of osteoclastic activity, and identification and treatment of the underlying disorder.

Once intravascular volume has been replenished, furosemide or other loop diuretics may be required to stimulate renal elimination of calcium. Thiazide diuretics should be avoided as they enhance resorption of calcium from the renal tubules. Osteoclast inhibitors such as bisphosphonates, mithramycin, and calcitonin can also aid in decreasing serum calcium levels. Of these, calcitonin has the most rapid onset of action but leads to only a mild reduction in calcium levels.[9] Although mithramycin is a potent osteoclast inhibitor with a more rapid onset of action than bisphosphonates, it has significant side effects, including nausea, nephrotoxicity, and thrombocytopenia.[6]

Bisphosphonate analogues (etidronate and pamidronate) are the primary agents used in cases of severe hypercalcemia, due to effective enhancement of osteoclastic bone resorption and long half-lives.[6] For example, a single 90-mg dose of pamidronate effects normocalcemic levels within 1 week, with a duration of 1 month.[6]

The definitive treatment of hypercalcemia involves eliminating the underlying cause. Hyperparathyroidism is routinely treated surgically by parathyroidectomy. Therapies for malignancies and paraneoplastic syndromes depend on the particular tumor characteristics. If drug-induced hypercalcemia is diagnosed, the offending agent should be discontinued immediately.

■ HYPOCALCEMIA

The treatment of hypocalcemia depends on the severity of symptoms. Coincident hypomagnesemia, present in most cases, must be corrected before calcium replacement therapy will work. Asymptomatic patients with mildly low serum levels can be treated with oral supplementation. In severe cases, therapy should be initiated in the form of either calcium chloride or calcium gluconate (a 10-mL ampule of 10% calcium chloride contains 360 mg of elemental calcium; a 10-mL ampule of 10% calcium gluconate contains 93 mg of elemental calcium). The recommended dose for a normal adult is 100 to 300 mg of elemental calcium given intravenously. Unfortunately, this form of therapy increases levels for only 1 to 2 hours. A maintenance infusion of 0.5 to 2 mg/kg/hour or repeated doses is recommended to maintain therapeutic levels.[3]

The initial dose for neonates, infants, and children is 10 to 20 mg/kg of 10% calcium gluconate given intravenously over 5 minutes.[4]

MAGNESIUM

Pathophysiology

The body of an average adult contains approximately 2000 mEq of magnesium. The majority of total body magnesium is contained in bone (50%) and the intracellular space (40%-50%); only 1% to 2% is found in serum. Serum magnesium is maintained within a range of 1.8 to 3.0 mg/dL. This homeostasis is maintained by absorption in the gut and excretion by the kidneys. Common dietary sources of magnesium include green vegetables, meat, fish, beans, and grains. In the setting of hypomagnesemia, increased renal reabsorption of magnesium is modulated by parathyroid hormone. In the setting of hypermagnesemia, the opposite occurs (Fig. 167-4; Box 167-5).

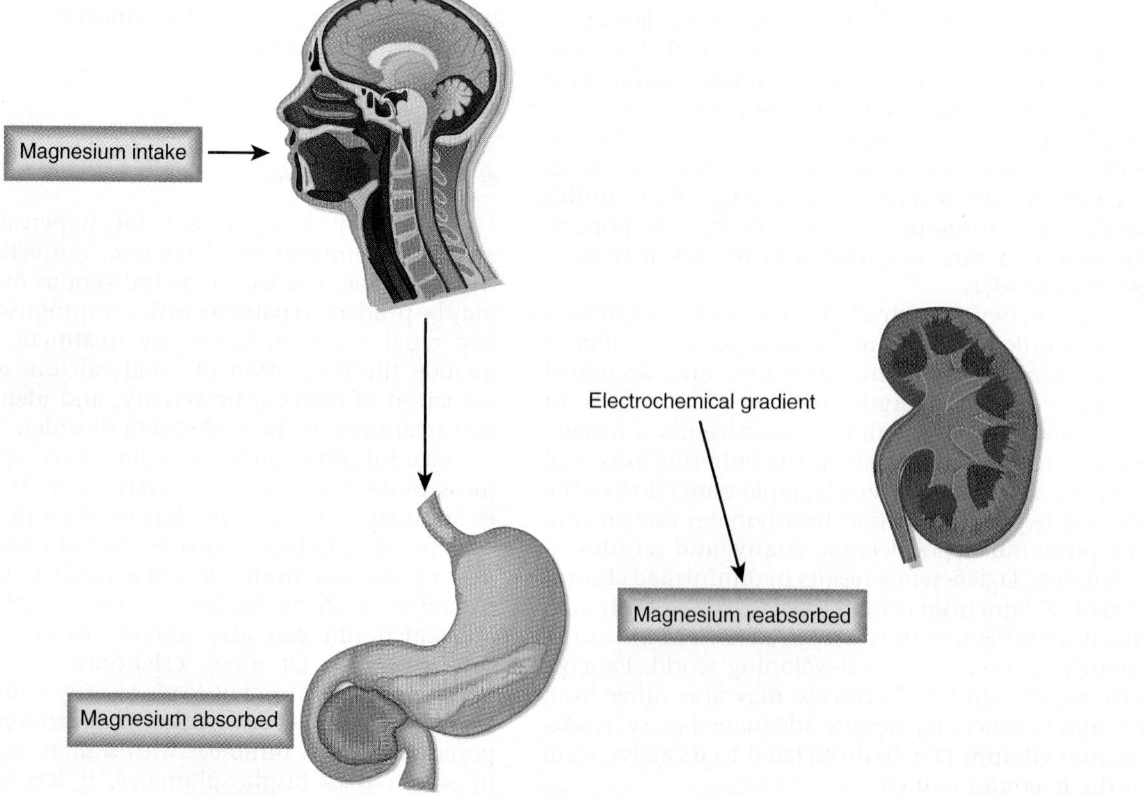
Magnesium intake
Electrochemical gradient
Magnesium reabsorbed
Magnesium absorbed

FIGURE 167-4 Summary of magnesium homeostasis. Magnesium is absorbed primarily in the ileum and excreted or reabsorbed passively across an electrochemical gradient.

BOX 167-5

Common Etiologies of Magnesium Dysregulation

Hypomagnesemia
- Malnutrition
- Alcoholism
- Total parenteral nutrition
- Human immunodeficiency virus/AIDS
- Cirrhosis
- Pancreatitis
- Gastrointestinal losses
- Diuretics

Hypermagnesemia
- Iatrogenic
- Rhabdomyolysis
- Diabetic ketoacidosis
- Hyperparathyroidism and hypoparathyroidism
- Tumor lysis syndrome
- Adrenal insufficiency
- Laxative abuse
- Antacid abuse
- Enema use

Clinical Presentation

HYPERMAGNESEMIA

Hypermagnesemia is rare and symptoms are usually nonspecific. Nausea, vomiting, weakness, and flushing occur with mildly elevated levels. Patients with significantly high magnesium levels can develop decreased deep tendon reflexes, hypotension, respiratory depression, and eventually cardiac arrest (Box 167-6). ECG manifestations of hypermagnesemia include QRS widening, prolonged QT and PR intervals, and conduction abnormalities.[10]

BOX 167-6

Signs and Symptoms of Hypermagnesemia*

- Nausea/vomiting, weakness, flushing
- Decreased deep tendon reflexes
- Hypotension
- Respiratory depression
- Cardiac arrest

*Findings are listed in order of increasing magnesium serum levels.

HYPOMAGNESEMIA

Hypomagnesemia presents in a similar fashion to hypocalcemia (see Box 167-2) with hyperreflexia, tetany, and convulsions. These patients may also exhibit Chvostek's sign or Trousseau's sign.

Dysrhythmia is a common and serious complication associated with hypomagnesemia. Atrial fibrillation, multifocal atrial tachycardia, paroxysmal supraventricular tachycardia, ventricular tachycardia, torsades de pointes (Fig. 167-5B), or ventricular fibrillation may be seen in hypomagnesemic patients. Patients who use diuretics or digitalis are at greater risk for developing arrhythmias. Common ECG changes include prolonged PR and QT intervals, widened QRS, ST-segment abnormalities, T-wave flattening or inversion, and U waves (see Fig. 167-5).

Differential Diagnosis

HYPERMAGNESEMIA

Hypermagnesemia is frequently iatrogenic in origin. This can be seen in patients with abnormal renal function who take massive doses of magnesium-coated laxatives, antacids, or enemas.[2] Common examples in patients with normal renal function include patients being treated with high doses of magnesium for preeclamsia/eclampsia and patients with rhabdomyolysis.[2] Under normal conditions, the kidney is able to excrete large amounts of magnesium to maintain physiologic serum levels.

HYPOMAGNESEMIA

Hypomagnesemia has numerous etiologies. Patients at risk for low serum magnesium levels include alcoholics, malnourished patients, and patients with cirrhosis, pancreatitis, and excessive gastrointestinal fluid losses.[6] Treatment of diabetic ketoacidosis without supplementing magnesium, especially in patients with underlying malnutrition, can lead to a sharp decline in magnesium levels. Magnesium can also be disproportionately excreted by the kidneys secondary to ketoacidosis or certain drugs (e.g., thiazide diuretics).[11]

Thiazide and loop diuretics can both cause magnesium wasting, which can be especially problematic in patients with underlying cardiac disease. Concomitant use of a potassium-sparing diuretic decreases the risk of hypomagnesemia.

Treatment

HYPERMAGNESEMIA

Treatment of hypermagnesemia involves the immediate discontinuation of any exogenous magnesium. If the patient remains symptomatic, normal saline is administered, followed by 20-80 mg of furosemide. Calcium supplementation may also be useful to directly antagonize the cellular effects of magnesium

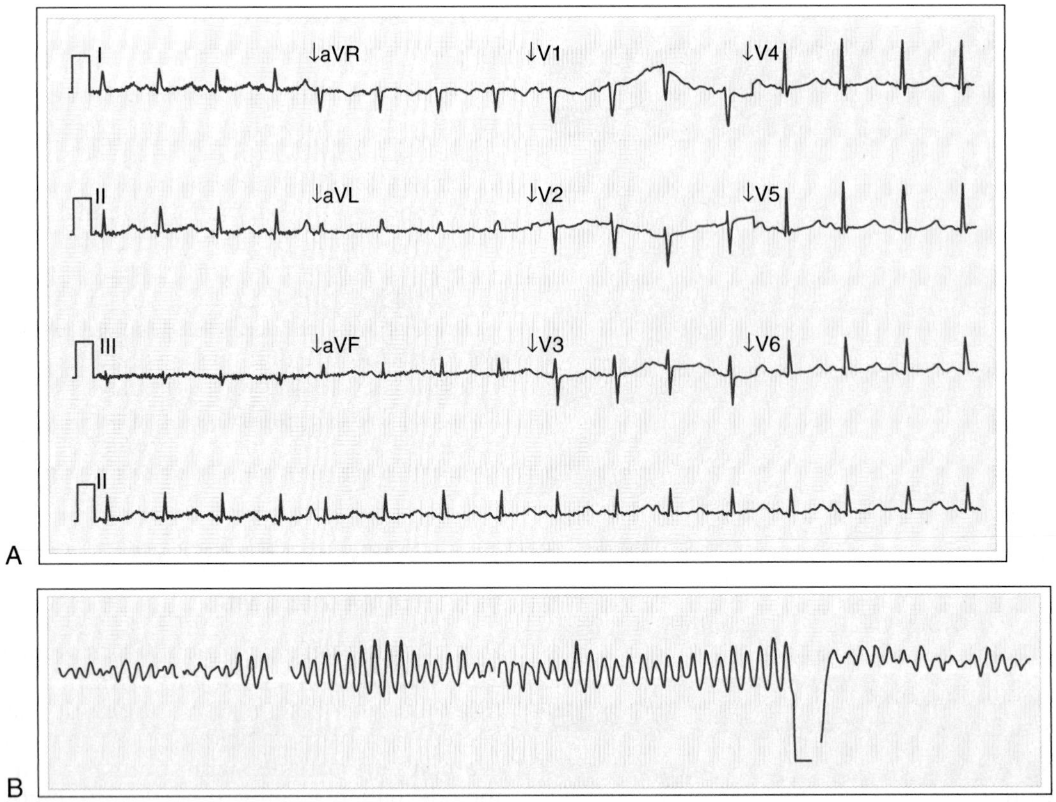
I
↓aVR
↓V1
↓V4
II
↓aVL
↓V2
↓V5
III
↓aVF
↓V3
↓V6
II
A
B

FIGURE 167-5 **A,** Example of prolonged QT in the setting of hypomagnesemia. **B,** Deterioration of the same patient's rhythm to torsades de pointes, which was corrected with IV magnesium. (Courtesy of Loren K. Rood, MD, Indiana University School of Medicine, Indianapolis, IN.)

and counteract hypotension, respiratory depression, and cardiac dysrhythmias. Either calcium chloride (360 mg per ampule) or calcium gluconate (93 mg per ampule) should be given at an initial dose of 100 to 200 mg. Critically ill patients require continuous infusions and/or hemodialysis.

■ HYPOMAGNESEMIA

Severe hypomagnesemia is corrected by administering 2 to 4 g of 50% magnesium sulfate initially, with a maximum dose of 2 to 8 g/day. Although this amount may seem aggressive, approximately half of the infused magnesium will be excreted renally.

PHOSPHORUS

Pathophysiology

An average daily diet consists of approximately 800 to 1400 mg of phosphorus, of which 60% to 80% is passively absorbed in the gut.[6] Serum calcium and phosphorus levels are inversely proportional, with a combined concentration of 30 to 40 mg/dL. The combined product of these electrolytes ([calcium] × [phosphate]) can be used as a clinical marker for therapy in the setting of hyperphosphatemia (defined as a product >70).

Phosphate excretion occurs primarily via the kidney, where more than 80% is reabsorbed in the proximal tubule. Phosphate reabsorption in the distal tubule is regulated by dietary intake and parathyroid hormone (Fig. 167-6).[6]

Normal serum phosphate levels decrease with age; normal ranges are 4.0 to 7.0 mg/dL in newborns, and 3.0 to 5.0 mg/dL in adults.

Hyperphosphatemia arises secondary to an increase in phosphate load or diminished renal excretion. Conditions that interfere with serum measurements can promote pseudohyperphosphatemia.

Hypophosphatemia occurs by cellular redistribution, decreased gut resorption, or renal wasting.[6]

Clinical Presentation

■ HYPERPHOSPHATEMIA

As hyperphosphatemia induces hypocalcemia, signs and symptoms reflect hypocalcemic states, neuromuscular hyperexcitability (paresthesias, tetany, and seizures) and cardiac dysfunction (see Hypocalcemia section) (Box. 167-7). Symptoms of hyperphosphate-

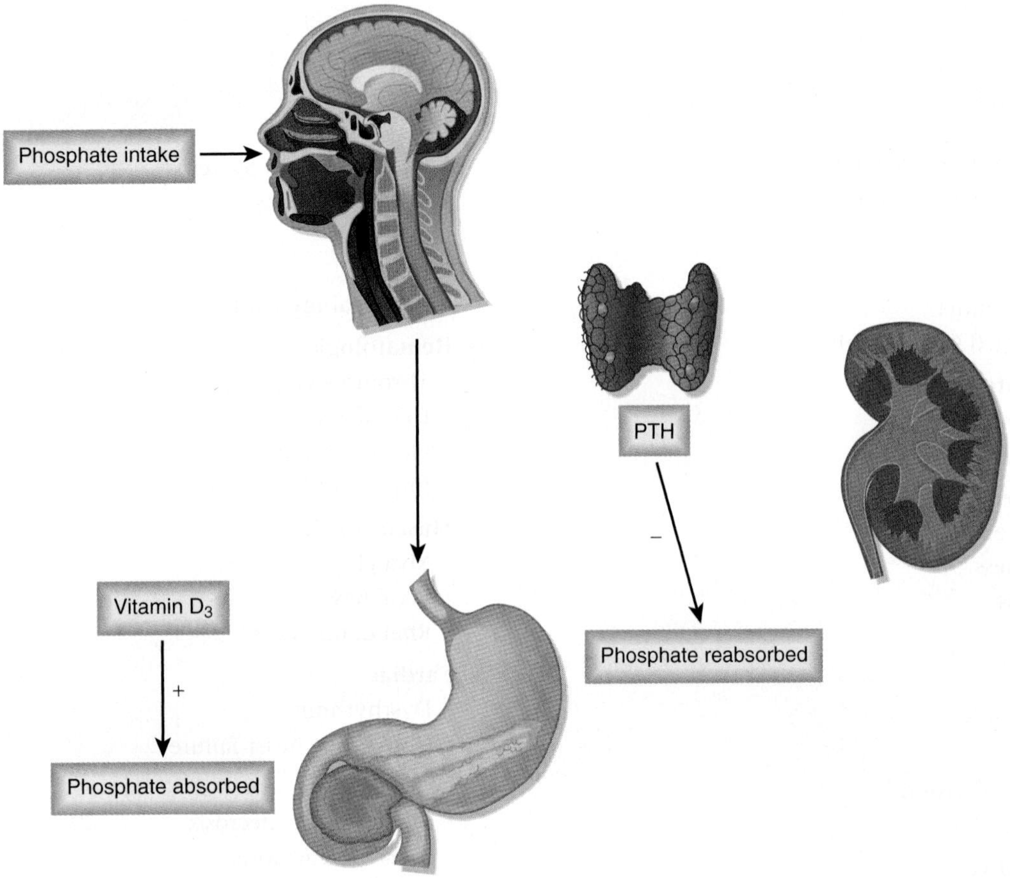
Phosphate intake
PTH
–
Vitamin D3
+
Phosphate reabsorbed
Phosphate absorbed

FIGURE 167-6 Summary of phosphate homeostasis. After oral intake, phosphate is absorbed via the gut and reabsorbed by the kidney. Vitamin D_3 stimulates this process, whereas parathyroid hormone acts as an inhibitor. PTH, parathyroid hormone.

mia usually occur when the calcium-phosphate product is greater than 70.

HYPOPHOSPHATEMIA

Hypophosphatemia does not typically manifest symptoms until levels are below 1.0 mg/dL. Patients at risk for hypophosphatemia include those with diabetic or alcoholic ketoacidosis, severe malnutrition, sepsis, primary hyperparathyroidism, vitamin D deficiency or resistance (e.g., rickets), malignancy, and prolonged severe dietary restriction (total parenteral nutrition with inadequate phosphate supplementation).

Almost any organ system can be affected by hypophosphatemia, resulting in a broad spectrum of signs and symptoms (Box 167-8). Decreased cardiac contractility, dysrhythmias, respiratory failure, seizure, and coma are all potential critical sequelae. Patients may develop rhabdomyolysis due to depletion of intracellular adenosine triphosphate.[12] Hematologic abnormalities include impaired phagocytosis, hemolysis, and thrombocytopenia. Additionally, diminished 2,2-diphosphoglycerate levels can lead to tissue hypoxia by increasing erythrocyte oxygen affinity.[6]

Differential Diagnosis

HYPERPHOSPHATEMIA

Hyperphosphatemia is most likely to occur in the presence of acute or chronic renal failure.[13] Rhabdomyolysis and tumor lysis syndrome can also lead to hyperphosphatemia. Pseudohyperphosphatemia occurs in the setting of hemolysis, hyperlipidemia, hyperbilirubinemia, and paraproteinemia.

HYPOPHOSPHATEMIA

Common ED presentations associated with hypophosphatemia include diabetic ketoacidosis, alcoholism, diuretic use, excessive antacid therapy, sepsis, and malnutrition. Processes that cause increased renal excretion, decreased gastrointestinal absorption, or intracellular shifts of phosphorus should also be considered.[6] In the setting of diabetic ketoacidosis, hypophosphatemia is precipitated by extracellular

BOX 167-7

Clinical Manifestations of Severe Hyperphosphatemia

Central Nervous System
- Altered mental status
- Seizures

Cardiac
- Dysrhythmia
- Prolonged QT interval

Gastrointestinal
- Anorexia
- Nausea and vomiting

Musculoskeletal
- Hyperreflexia
- Weakness
- Cramps
- Tetany

Renal
- Renal failure

Ocular
- Decreased vision
- Conjunctivitis

Dermatologic
- Papular eruptions

Data from Shiber JR, Mattu A: Serum phosphate abnormalities in the emergency department. J Emerg Med 2002;23:395-400, and Bushinsky DA, Monk RD: Electrolyte quintet: Calcium. Lancet 1998;352(9124):306-311.

BOX 167-8

Clinical Manifestations of Severe Hypophosphatemia

Central Nervous System
- Encephalopathy
- Seizures
- Coma
- Proximal myopathy

Hematologic
- Thrombocytopenia
- Hemolysis
- Platelet dysfunction
- Impaired phagocytosis

Musculoskeletal
- Myalgias
- Weakness
- Rhabdomyolysis

Cardiac
- Dysrhythmia
- Congestive heart failure

Renal
- Acute tubular necrosis
- Metabolic acidosis

Gastrointestinal
- Dysphagia
- Ileus

Pulmonary
- Respiratory failure
- Tissue hypoxia

Data from Shiber JR, Mattu A: Serum phosphate abnormalities in the emergency department. J Emerg Med 2002;23:395-400, and Bushinsky DA, Monk RD: Electrolyte quintet: Calcium. Lancet 1998;352(9124):306-311.

shifts secondary to metabolic acidosis and insulin deficiency (Box 167-9).[14]

Treatment

■ HYPERPHOSPHATEMIA

Hyperphosphatemia is corrected by treating the underlying cause, increasing the excretion of phosphorus, and/or restricting phosphorus intake. Excretion may be facilitated by IV infusion of normal saline and acetazolamide. Commonly used phosphate chelation agents include magnesium, aluminum, and calcium salts. Aluminum salts should be avoided in patients with chronic renal insufficiency due to the risk of long-term toxicity.[15]

■ HYPOPHOSPHATEMIA

Mild hypophosphatemia requires no therapy. Phosphorus is found in almost all food; cows' milk is an especially rich source (1 mg/mL). Symptomatic patients with mild to moderate hypophosphatemia can be safely treated with sodium or potassium phosphate salts. IV replacement should be reserved for patients with severe deficiency (<1 mg/dL), given at 0.08 to 0.16 mmol/kg over 6 hours. Because this form of therapy may induce severe hypocalcemia, these patients require close monitoring and immediate cessation of therapy once levels are satisfactorily elevated.

BOX 167-9

Etiologies of Serum Phosphate Imbalance

Hypophosphatemia

- Transcellular shift
  - Recovery from diabetic ketoacidosis
  - Medications (insulin, glucagons, epinephrine, steroids, xanthines, β-2 agonists)
  - Re-feeding syndrome
  - Hungry bone syndrome
- Decreased absorption
  - Chronic alcoholism
  - Anorexia or bulimia nervosa
  - Chronic diarrhea
  - Vitamin D deficiency
  - Antacid use
- Increased renal losses
  - Renal tubular abnormalities
  - Chronic alcoholism
  - Hyperparathyroidism
  - Metabolic acidosis
  - Vitamin D deficiency

Hyperphosphatemia

- Increased endogenous source
  - Rhabdomyolysis
  - Malignant hyperthermia
  - Tumor lysis syndrome
  - Hemolysis
  - Infarcted bowel
- Increased intake
  - Iatrogenic (infusions)
  - Cows' milk (in infants)
  - Phosphate-containing enemas
  - Vitamin D intoxication
- Decreased renal losses
  - Renal failure
  - Hypoparathyroidism
  - Acromegaly
  - Bisphosphonate therapy
  - Vitamin D intoxication

From Shiber JR, Mattu A: Serum phosphate abnormalities in the emergency department. J Emerg Med 2002;23:395-400.

REFERENCES

1. Shiber JR, Mattu A: Serum phosphate abnormalities in the emergency department. J Emerg Med 2002;23:395-400.
2. Weiss-Guillet E-M, Takala J, Jakob SM: Diagnosis and management of electrolyte emergencies. Best Pract Res Clin Endocrinol Metab 2003;17:623-651.
3. Reber PM, Heath H 3rd: Hypocalcemic emergencies. Med Clin North Am 1995;79:93-106.
4. Kainer G, Chan JC: Hypocalcemic and hypercalcemic disorders in children. Curr Probl Pediatr 1989;19:489-545.
5. Pimentel L: Medical complications of oncologic disease. Emerg Med Clin North Am 1993;11:407-419.
6. Bushinsky DA, Monk RD: Electrolyte quintet: Calcium. Lancet 1998;352(9124):306-311.
7. Beall DP, Scofield RH: Milk-alkali syndrome associated with calcium carbonate consumption. Report of 7 patients with parathyroid hormone levels and an estimate of prevalence among patients hospitalized with hypercalcemia. Medicine 1995;74:89-96.
8. Wilson RF, Binkley LE, Sabo FM Jr, et al: Electrolyte and acid-base changes with massive blood transfusions. Am Surg 1992;58:535-544.
9. Levine MM, Kleeman CR: Hypercalcemia: Pathophysiology and treatment. Hosp Pract (Office Ed) 1987;22:93-110.
10. Mosseri M, Porath A, Ovsyshcher I, Stone D: Electrocardiographic manifestations of combined hypercalcemia and hypermagnesemia. J Electrocardiol 1990;23:235-241.
11. Ramsay LE, Yeo WW, Jackson PR: Metabolic effects of diuretics. Cardiology 1994;84(Suppl 2):48-56.
12. Gravelyn TR, Brophy N, Siegert C, Peters-Golden M: Hypophosphatemia-associated respiratory muscle weakness in a general inpatient population. Am J Med 1988;84:870-876.
13. Peppers MP, Geheb M, Desai T: Endocrine crises. Hypophosphatemia and hyperphosphatemia. Crit Care Clin 1991;7:201-214.
14. Bohannon NJ: Large phosphate shifts with treatment for hyperglycemia. Arch Intern Med 1989;149:1423-1425.
15. Ghazali A, Ben Hamida F, Bouzernidj M, et al: Management of hyperphosphatemia in patients with renal failure. Curr Opin Nephrol Hypertens 1993;2:566-579.

Chapter 168

Thyroid Disorders

David Hackstadt and Frederick Korley

KEY POINTS

Hypothyroidism due to iodine deficiency is the most common endocrine disorder worldwide.

Primary hypothyroidism results from thyroid tissue dysfunction. Secondary hypothyroidism is a component of panhypopituitarism that results from pituitary disease.

Severe hypothyroidism is a rare condition characterized by altered mental status, hypothermia, and primary thyroid dysfunction. Myxedema is seen in most cases, true coma is not.

Patients with suspected severe hypothyroidism should receive empirical, low-dose IV levothyroxine.

Thyroid storm, the most extreme form of thyrotoxicosis, is a rapidly fatal condition.

Anti-thyroid medication should be given at least 1 hour prior to the administration of iodine in the treatment of thyroid storm.

ED testing for thyroid disease includes serum thyrotropin, or thyroid-stimulating hormone (TSH), and free thyroxine (FT_4) measurements.

Scope

Abnormal thyroid function is by far the most common endocrine disorder worldwide and is second only to diabetes mellitus in the United States. Hypothyroidism is a deficiency of thyroid hormones resulting in a hypometabolic state. Iodine deficiency accounts for most cases hypothyroidism and goiter in underdeveloped countries; Hashimoto's thyroiditis is a more commonly recognized cause in Westernized societies.

Thyrotoxicosis describes any condition in which there is an excess of free thyroid hormones in the circulation. The term is frequently used interchangeably with hyperthyroidism; however, hyperthyroidism refers only to disease states in which there is overproduction of thyroid hormones by the thyroid gland. Thyrotoxicosis is a rare condition that is 10 times more prevalent in women than in men (2% vs 0.2%).[1] It is uncommon before the age of 15 years.[2] Although most manifestations of thyrotoxicosis do not represent a true emergency, the extreme case of so-called thyroid storm does. Early detection and treatment of this condition may prevent progression to shock and death.

Anatomy

The thyroid gland derives its name from the shape of the nearby thyroid cartilage (from the Greek, meaning "shield"). Although this varies, the isthmus usually is centered over the third tracheal ring. Normal adult thyroid dimensions are height, 5 cm; thickness, 1.5 cm; isthmus thickness, 0.5 cm; volume, 10 cm; and weight, 12-20 g. Thyroid thickness greater than 2 cm is considered abnormal.

The thyroid gland is palpable on physical examination in nonobese patients; thyroid nodules and some cancers are sometimes noted on palpation. Rarely, ectopic thyroid gland tissue is found at the base of the tongue.

Physiology

Thyrotropin-releasing hormone (TRH) is synthesized in the hypothalamus and regulates the production of TSH, or thyrotropin, in the anterior pituitary gland. Principal cells in the thyroid bind TSH, which activates the production and release of thyroid hormones.

The thyroid is highly efficient in its absorption and extraction of iodine. Iodine is added twice to tyrosine to make up diiodotyrosine (DIT); two molecules of DIT combine to form thyroxine (T_4), much of which is stored in the thyroid gland. T_4 is released into the circulation largely bound by thyroid-binding globulin (TBG). Even though levels of TBG vary widely, this protein is seldom involved in a disease process.

Triiodothyronine (T_3) is formed by peripheral conversion of T_4 in tissues. Compared with T_4, T_3 is four to six times more active, has less affinity for TBG, and has a much shorter half-life (12 hours versus 6 days). T_3 and T_4 exert feedback on the hypothalamus and TRH levels, completing a regulatory loop.

T_3 and T_4 stimulate metabolic activity in tissues throughout the body. Both hormones are associated with growth and development early in life.

Goiter

Goiter refers to a visible enlargement of the thyroid gland that may result from euthyroid, hyperthyroid, or hypothyroid states. The presence of a goiter mandates a detailed review of systems and appropriate thyroid testing to determine the functional status of the tissue. The most common cause of goiter is iodine deficiency. Other causes include Hashimoto's thyroiditis, Grave's disease, nodules, cancers, and lithium therapy.

Goiters are usually benign, but thyroid malignancy must be considered in each case. Three rare but potentially life-threatening emergencies can result from continued enlargement of a malignant goiter. First, partial or complete obstruction of the jugular veins may occur, especially in patients who are hypercoagulable. Clot extension from a partially obstructed jugular vein can impede venous drainage from the brain. Second, invasive or extremely large goiters have been reported to cause airway compromise. Third, malignant involvement of the carotid sheath structures can result in devastating morbidity.

Hypothyroidism

■ PATHOPHYSIOLOGY

Primary hypothyroidism implies a condition of thyroid tissue dysfunction. Etiologies include Hashimoto's thyroiditis, surgical ablation, iodine I-131 ablation, and iodine deficiency. Idiopathic cases are frequently seen as well. The most common cause of hypothyroidism in industrialized countries is Hashimoto's thyroiditis, an autoimmune disease of unclear etiology.

Secondary hypothyroidism refers to pituitary dysfunction that results in a low TSH level and subsequent poor stimulation of otherwise normal thyroid tissue. Pituitary dysfunction generally affects more than one endocrine axis (panhypopituitarism); hypothyroidism is never the only resultant condition. Secondary hypothyroidism is seen with Sheehan's syndrome and space-occupying lesions (adenomas) of the pituitary gland.

Hypothyroidism is three to ten times more common in women than men. Incidence increases with age and obesity; 1% of young girls are affected, compared with 6% of older women. Smoking has been identified as an independent risk factor for hypothyroidism, but the reason for the observed association is unknown. Hypothryoidism has no racial or ethnic predilection. Symptoms of hypothyroidism are more apparent during winter months in moderate and cold climates.

Iodine deficiency is the major worldwide cause of both hypothyroidism and cretinism; the latter is characterized by growth and mental retardation. Selenium deficiency appears to worsen cretinism. Iodine deficiency is rare in the United States but affects approximately one in three persons worldwide, particularly in mountainous regions. Iodine deficiency has been decreasing due to supplementation programs sponsored by the World Health Organization. Excessive supplementation and high-seafood diets may contribute to thyroiditis.

■ CLINICAL PRESENTATION

Hypothyroidism is a deficiency of thyroid hormones that results in decreased metabolic activity. A hypometabolic state ensues, with a myriad of indolent symptomatology (Boxes 168-1 and 168-2).

Cold intolerance deserves special consideration in the history. The complaint of cold intolerance can be differentiated as "cold all over the body" versus a cold sensation in only the extremities or joints. If the former feeling lasts longer than several weeks, this often is a symptom of either marked anemia or hypothyroidism. Cold extremities and joints suggest rheumatologic and vascular diseases, which often overlap. Febrile illnesses and hypoglycemia usually produce

BOX 168-1

Symptoms of Hypothyroidism

- Fatigue
- Cold intolerance
- Weakness
- Weight gain
- Depression
- Decreased mental function
- Constipation
- Decreased libido
- Irritability
- Coarse hair
- Dry skin
- Myalgias
- Arthralgias
- Brittle fingernails
- Myxedema
- Menstrual irregularity
- Peripheral neuropathy

BOX 168-2

Signs of Hypothyroidism

- Prolonged reflexes
- Hypothermia
- Narrow eyebrows
- Peripheral neuropathy
- Hoarse voice
- Bradycardia
- Facial edema
- Periorbital edema
- Pale, dry skin
- Sparse axillary and pubic hair

chill feelings for much shorter periods of time. Persistent mild hypothermia, a few degrees less than the normal diurnal variation, is concerning for hypothyroidism.

Severe Hypothyroidism (Myxedema Coma)

Severe hypothyroidism is present in patients presenting with mild to moderate hypothermia, altered mental status, and laboratory abnormalities consistent with marked primary thyroid disease. *Myxedema coma* is a misnomer often used for severe hypothyroidism; not all patients with severe hypothyroidism are truly comatose, whereas most (but not all) patients with hypothyroid coma have myxedema. Myxedema coma best describes a patient in extremis secondary to a severe hypothyroid state (Box 168-3).

BOX 168-3

Presentation of Severe Hypothyroidism (Myxedema Coma)

- Decreased mentation
- Hypothermia
- Bradycardia
- Hypotension
- Periorbital edema
- Non-pitting edema
- Delayed or absent deep tendon reflexes
- Hypoglycemia
- Hyponatremia

DIAGNOSIS

Historical symptoms and physical signs suggestive of hypothyroidism justify testing. The incidence of disease is so high among elderly women that screening of these patients, even though they are asymptomatic, is performed by many primary care physicians.

Markers of primary hypothyroidism include a high serum TSH level and a low unbound, or FT_4, level, in the presence of classic signs and symptoms. Symptomatic patients with even minimally elevated TSH may benefit from low-dose thyroxine supplementation.

There is disagreement about the level of TSH and FT_4 measurements required to begin treatment in asymptomatic individuals. Several sources recommend thyroxine supplementation for asymptomatic patients with a serum TSH that is three times the upper limit of normal, regardless of a low or low-normal FT_4.

Secondary hypothyroidism, generally a component of panhypopituitarism, is marked by low TSH, low FT_4, and low serum cortisol levels. Both thyroid and steroid replacement are required, and further diagnostic evaluation (pituitary imaging, endocrine testing) is indicated.

Hypothyroid patients may also have low serum sodium levels and an elevated total cholesterol, both of which may resolve with thyroxine therapy.

TREATMENT

Mild Hypothyroidism

Treatment is initiated with levothyroxine, 0.05 mg/day. In patients with primary thyroid disease, TSH should be monitored every 30 days. Those on levothyroxine treatment do not require FT_4 monitoring. Although mild hypothyroidism is not an emergency

BOX 168-4

ED Treatment of Myxedema Coma

1. Provide airway support and supplemental oxygen as needed.
2. Obtain serum laboratory tests: CBC, CMP, TSH, FT_4, cortisol.
3. Obtain microbiology cultures: blood, urine, and spinal fluid.
4. Administer broad-spectrum antibiotics.
5. Support temperature with passive rewarming.
6. Administer 0.3 to 0.5 mg IV L-thyroxine; decrease to 0.1 mg in patients with suspected heart disease.
7. Give stress-dose steroid therapy as appropriate.

CBC, complete blood count, CMP, comprehensive medical panel; FT_4, free T_4; TSH, thyroid-stimulating hormone.

per se, initiating treatment for symptomatic patients is appropriate if the diagnosis is established in the ED. Routine follow-up is necessary.

Severe Hypothyroidism (Myxedema Coma)

The management of severe hypothyroidism includes standard ED resuscitation measures, including the consideration and empirical treatment of potential sepsis. The only treatment step specific for severe hypothyroidism is the IV administration of levothyroxine. Empirical administration of low dose L-thyroxine is appropriate for settings in which a serum TSH level cannot be obtained in a timely fashion. The ED treatment of myxedema coma is summarized in Box 168-4.

Note that previous studies have deemed T_3 supplementation to be unsafe; however, due to the low incidence of myxedema coma, large clinical trials of T_3 are not possible. Patients with severe hypothyroidism may suffer from this selection bias.

Thyrotoxicosis

Thyrotoxicosis is caused by at least one of four potential mechanisms: (1) overproduction of thyroid hormones by the thyroid gland, (2) unregulated release of thyroid hormones secondary to the destruction of thyroid cells (thyroiditis), (3) ingestion of thyroid hormones, and (4) production of thyroid hormones from ectopic foci (Fig. 168-1).

CAUSES

Graves' Disease

About 60% to 80% of cases of hyperthyroidism in the United States are caused by Graves' disease. It is the most common autoimmune disorder in North America. Patients with this condition produce thyroid-stimulating immunoglobulins that bind

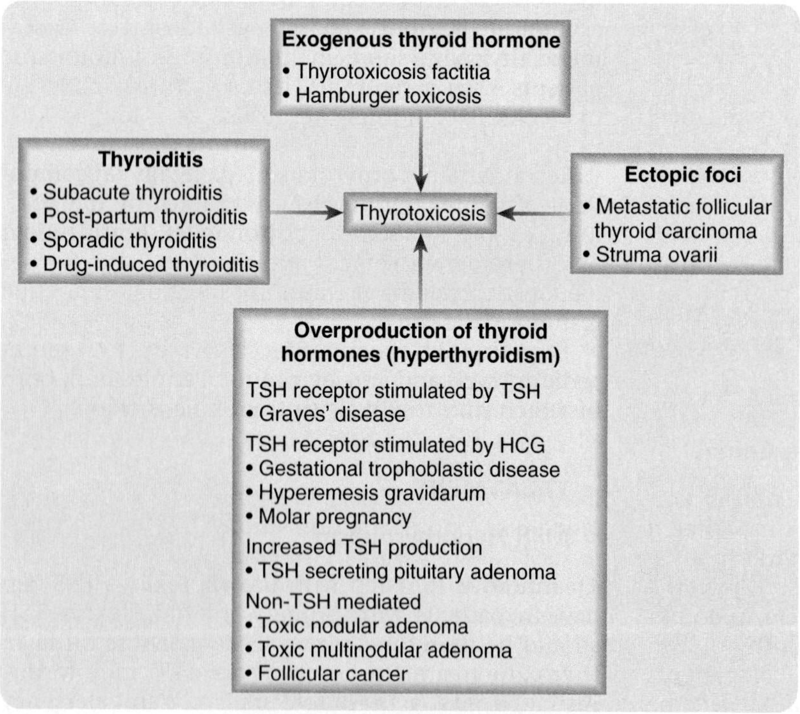
Exogenous thyroid hormone
• Thyrotoxicosis factitia
• Hamburger toxicosis
Thyroiditis
• Subacute thyroiditis
• Post-partum thyroiditis
• Sporadic thyroiditis
• Drug-induced thyroiditis
Thyrotoxicosis
Ectopic foci
• Metastatic follicular thyroid carcinoma
• Struma ovarii
Overproduction of thyroid hormones (hyperthyroidism)
TSH receptor stimulated by TSH
• Graves' disease
TSH receptor stimulated by HCG
• Gestational trophoblastic disease
• Hyperemesis gravidarum
• Molar pregnancy
Increased TSH production
• TSH secreting pituitary adenoma
Non-TSH mediated
• Toxic nodular adenoma
• Toxic multinodular adenoma
• Follicular cancer

FIGURE 168-1 Etiologies of thyrotoxicosis. HCG, human chorionic gonadotropin; TSH, thyroid-stimulating hormone.

to and activate thyrotropin-receptors on thyroid cells, leading to excessive production of thyroid hormones.

Thyroiditis

Thyroiditis describes conditions in which inflammatory changes lead to the destruction of thyroid cells, resulting in the release of excessive amounts of thyroid hormones. This is followed by depletion of thyroid hormones leading to euthyroid, and eventually hypothyroid states. Autoimmune destruction of thyroid cells is seen in Hashimoto's thyroiditis, painless sporadic thyroiditis, and painless postpartum thyroiditis.

Hashimoto's thyroiditis is characterized by high levels of serum anti-thyroid antibodies. This condition is the most common cause of hypothyroidism in the United States.

Painless postpartum thyroiditis occurs in up to 10% of American women. Its onset is usually 1 to 6 months after delivery. Approximately 80% of women recover normal thyroid function within a year. There is a 70% chance of recurrence with subsequent pregnancies.[3]

Painful subacute (de Quervain's) thyroiditis is the most common cause of thyroid pain. It is a self-limited disorder that is frequently preceded by an upper respiratory infection. Suppurative thyroiditis is a very rare condition. It is caused by a bacterial, fungal, or mycobacterial infection of the thyroid gland. It may be seen in severely immunocompromised patients. Amiodarone and lithium cause drug-induced thyroiditis.

Non-TSH Mediated Hyperthyroidism

Hyperthyroidism is sometimes caused by a benign, monoclonal autonomously-secreting thyroid nodule known as toxic adenoma (Plummer's disease). When more than one nodule is present, the condition is referred to as toxic multinodular goiter. In the United States, toxic multinodular goiter is seen in persons over 50 years old. Thyroid follicular cell cancer can also lead to excessive production of thyroid hormones.

Other Causes

Increased secretion of thyrotropin by a pituitary adenoma can cause thyrotoxicosis. Alternatively, thyroid hormones may be produced from sites outside the thyroid gland. This occurs in cases of metastatic follicular thyroid carcinoma and struma ovarii (an ovarian teratoma that has thyroid tissue).

Human chorionic gonadotropin can stimulate TSH receptors to produce excess thyroid hormones in gestational trophoblastic disease and hyperemesis gravidarum.

CLINICAL PRESENTATION

Thyrotoxicosis can be asymptomatic (subclinical hyperthyroidism), or feature mild, moderate, or severe symptoms that result from a surge in catecholamines. Patients with classic thyrotoxicosis may appear nervous, irritable, and tremulous. They may complain of unintentional weight loss, palpitations, exertional dyspnea, heat intolerance, thinning of their hair, irregular menses, increased frequency of bowel movements, and sleep disturbance. On physical examination, they may have a palpable goiter, warm moist skin, sinus tachycardia out of proportion to fever, or atrial fibrillation on electrocardiography.

Patients with Graves' disease may have the following physical findings: goiter, periorbital ecchymosis, chemosis, proptosis, lid retraction, and lower extremity edema.[4]

Patients with painful subacute thyroiditis may present with fever, malaise, myalgias, fatigue, and neck pain in addition to the symptoms of thyrotoxicosis mentioned previously.

Variations

Pregnancy

It may be difficult to distinguish between signs of thyrotoxicosis and normal physiologic changes of pregnancy. In addition to the symptoms mentioned previously, pregnant patients may have inappropriate weight gain for gestational age, fetal intrauterine growth retardation, and tachycardia that does not slow with Valsalva maneuver or with fluids.

Elderly Patients

Patients over 60 years of age may not exhibit signs of increased catecholamine levels. They may present with a small goiter, slow atrial fibrillation, weight loss, and severe depression. This presentation is termed *apathetic thyrotoxicosis*.[5] Other presentations in the elderly feature atrial fibrillation and congestive heart failure.

Thyroid Storm

Thyroid storm represents the extreme manifestation of thyrotoxicosis. Approximately 1% to 2% of patients with thyrotoxicosis progress to thyroid storm. Common precipitants of this condition are listed in Box 168-5. Patients in thyroid storm may present with fever, signs of congestive heart failure, agitation, psychosis, and coma. It is a rapidly fatal condition with a mortality rate of 20% to 30% in hospitalized patients.[6]

DIAGNOSTIC TESTING AND DIFFERENTIAL DIAGNOSIS

The most useful ED tests for diagnosing thyrotoxicosis are TSH and FT_4 measurements. The algorithm in

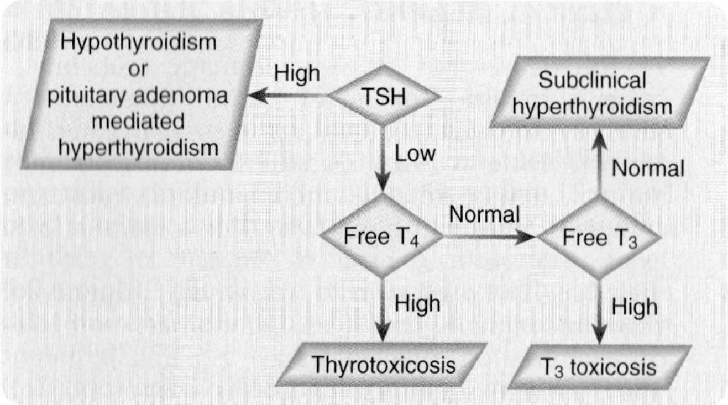
Hypothyroidism
or
pituitary adenoma
mediated
hyperthyroidism
High
TSH
Subclinical
hyperthyroidism
Low
Normal
Free T4
Normal
Free T3
High
High
Thyrotoxicosis
T3 toxicosis

FIGURE 168-2 Interpretation of thyroid-stimulating hormone (TSH), free T_4 (FT_4), and free T_3 (FT_3) levels.

BOX 168-5

Precipitants of Thyroid Storm

- Sepsis
- Surgery
- Iodinated contrast medium
- Withdrawal of antithyroid medications
- Myocardial infarction
- Cerebrovascular accident
- Trauma (e.g., strangulation)
- Ingestion of thyroid hormone

BOX 168-6

Differential Diagnosis of Thyroid Storm

- Sepsis
- Serotonin syndrome
- Malignant hyperthermia
- Neuroleptic malignant syndrome
- Sympathomimetic toxidrome
- Pheochromocytoma
- Panic attacks

BOX 168-7

ED Testing for Patients in Thyroid Storm

- Bedside serum glucose
- Complete blood count, chemistry panel
- Blood and urine cultures
- Chest radiograph
- Urinalysis
- Thyroid-stimulating hormone, free T_4

Figure 168-2 provides an interpretation of variable TSH, FT_4, and FT_3 levels. Box 168-6 lists conditions that should be considered in the differential diagnosis.

Patients with painful subacute thyroiditis will have elevated serum erythrocyte sedimentation rate and C-reactive protein levels. Box 168-7 lists the tests that should be obtained in the ED for patients in thyroid storm. If thyrotoxicosis is suspected, an endocrinologist may schedule further testing to confirm the diagnosis and determine the cause. These tests may include measurement of total T_3, thyroid autoantibodies, and radioactive iodine uptake; ultrasonography; and fine-needle biopsy.

■ TREATMENT

Patients with mild symptoms should be started on a beta-blocker to provide symptomatic relief from tremors, palpitations, tachycardia, and anxiety[7] (Fig. 168-3). It is important to withhold other treatment until the cause of the thyrotoxicosis is confirmed.[8] Treatment options include anti-thyroid medications, radioactive iodine ablation, and surgery. The risks and benefits of these treatments must be weighed by the patient and the endocrinologist.

Treatment of most forms of thyroiditis is supportive. Patients with persistent tachycardia should be given beta-blockers. Patients with painful subacute thyroiditis should be treated with nonsteroidal anti-inflammatory drugs, IV fluids, and beta-blockers.

■ Thyroid Storm

Medications are administered to stop the synthesis, release, and peripheral effects of thyroid hormones. The order in which anti-thyroid medications and iodide are given is very important.

First, the synthesis of new thyroid hormone is blocked by oral administration of 400 mg of propylthiouracil (PTU) or 25 mg of methimazole, every 6 hours. (PTU and methimazole should not be given together.) In addition to blocking the synthesis of new thyroid hormones, PTU also blocks the peripheral conversion of T_4 to T_3. Methimazole has a longer half-life than PTU and therefore can be administered less frequently to stable patients. There is currently no U.S. Food and Drug Administration–approved IV formulation of these medications. For patients who

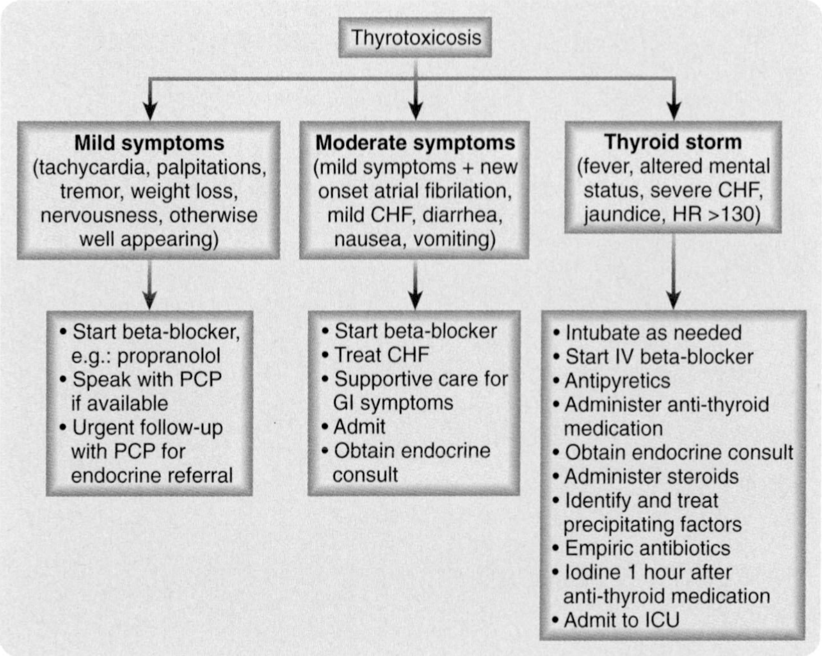
Thyrotoxicosis
Mild symptoms (tachycardia, palpitations, tremor, weight loss, nervousness, otherwise well appearing)
Moderate symptoms (mild symptoms + new onset atrial fibrilation, mild CHF, diarrhea, nausea, vomiting)
Thyroid storm (fever, altered mental status, severe CHF, jaundice, HR >130)
• Start beta-blocker, e.g.: propranolol
• Speak with PCP if available
• Urgent follow-up with PCP for endocrine referral
• Start beta-blocker
• Treat CHF
• Supportive care for GI symptoms
• Admit
• Obtain endocrine consult
• Intubate as needed
• Start IV beta-blocker
• Antipyretics
• Administer anti-thyroid medication
• Obtain endocrine consult
• Administer steroids
• Identify and treat precipitating factors
• Empiric antibiotics
• Iodine 1 hour after anti-thyroid medication
• Admit to ICU

FIGURE 168-3 ED treatment for thyrotoxicosis. CHF, congestive heart failure; PCP, primary-care physician. GI, gastrointestinal; HR, heart rate; ICU, intensive care unit.

cannot tolerate oral medications, PTU tablets should be dissolved in 60 mL of Fleet enema and administered rectally.

Next, the release of thyroid hormones is inhibited using iodine. This should be done no sooner than 1 hour after administering the antithyroid medications. Formulations of potassium iodide include Lugol's 10% solution (8 drops given orally every 6 hours) and saturated solution of potassium iodide (5 drops given orally every 5 hours), which is highly concentrated and more palatable.

Other supportive therapy that should be initiated includes beta-blockers (e.g., esmolol, metoprolol, propranolol), to counteract the catecholamine surge, and acetaminophen for fever; aspirin and other salicylates should be avoided because they decrease thyroid protein binding and increase the amount of free thyroid hormones in circulation.

Patients in thyroid storm may have concomitant adrenal insufficiency that may or may not lead to refractory hypotension. Treatment consists of hydrocortisone, 100 mg IV every 8 hours, or decadron, 8 mg given intravenously.[4,9,10]

■ DISPOSITION

Patients with mild symptoms of thyroid disease may be discharged with appropriate oral therapy and primary care follow-up instructions. Those with moderate symptoms should be admitted to the hospital for supportive care and endocrinology consultation. Patients with myxedema coma, thyroid storm, or other severe symptoms should be admitted to the intensive care unit.

REFERENCES

1. Tunbridge WM, Evered DC, Hall R, et al: The spectrum of thyroid disease in a community: The Whickham Survey. Clin Endocrinol (Oxf) 1977;7:481-493.
2. Lazarus JH: Hyperthyroidism. Lancet 1997;349(9048): 339-343.
3. Pearce EN, Farwell AP, Braverman LE: Thyroiditis. N Engl J Med 2003 ;348:2646-2655.
4. Weetman AP: Graves' disease. N Engl J Med 2000;343: 1236-1248.
5. Cooper DS, Greenspan FS, Ladenson PW: The thyroid gland. In Gardner DG, Shoback D (eds): Greenspan's Basic and Clinical Endocrinology, 8th ed. San Francisco, McGraw-Hill, 2007, pp 215-294.
6. Nayak B, Burman K: Thyrotoxicosis and thyroid storm. Endocrinol Metab Clin North Am 2006;35:663-686.
7. Geffner DL, Hershman JM: Beta-adrenergic blockade for the treatment of hyperthyroidism. Am J Med 1992;93: 61-68.
8. Singer PA, Cooper DS, Levy EG, et al: Treatment guidelines for patients with hyperthyroidism and hypothyroidism. JAMA 1995;273:808-812.
9. Cooper DS: Hyperthyroidism. Lancet 2003;362(9382): 459-468.
10. Ringel MD: Management of hypothyroidism and hyperthyroidism in the intensive care unit. Crit Care Clin 2001;17:59-74.

Chapter **169**

Adrenal Crisis

Brian K. Nelson

KEY POINTS

Adrenal crisis is an uncommon cause of shock.

Inappropriate adrenal response may contribute to shock in sepsis, trauma, myocardial infarction, and other conditions of extreme physiologic stress.

The diagnosis of acute adrenal crisis may be challenging, as symptoms are often nonspecific (e.g., weakness, fatigue, gastrointestinal symptoms, and abdominal, flank, or back pain).

Laboratory findings include hyponatremia, hyperkalemia, hypoglycemia, lymphocytosis, and eosinophilia.

Adrenal crisis may result from either primary adrenal insufficiency or secondary adrenal suppression from exogenous steroids or hypothalamic-pituitary-adrenal axis failure. In the latter, mineralocorticoid replacement is not necessary, but thyroid supplementation may be life-saving.

ED management includes aggressive fluid resuscitation, correction of electrolyte abnormalities, maintainance of euglycemia, and administration of glucocorticoids and mineralocorticoids.

Treatment should begin upon initial suspicion of adrenal crisis, not at the time of laboratory confirmation. Interventions are indicated when the cause of shock is obscure, the patient fails to respond to volume and pressors within 1 hour, or the diagnosis of adrenal insufficiency is confirmed.

Scope

Adrenal insufficiency is an uncommon disease with nonspecific manifestations, including fatigue, nausea, vomiting, hyperpigmentation, hypotension, and weight loss. Failure to recognize and treat the often subtle presentation of adrenal crisis can result in significant morbidity and mortality.

Most cases of adrenal insufficiency are autoimmune-mediated, but other common causes include infection and hemorrhage. Onset is generally subacute, although adrenal crisis accounts for approximately 25% of all cases. Primary adrenal insufficiency has an estimated incidence of 50 per 1 million persons. Secondary insufficiency due to chronic glucocorticoid administration is more common than primary insufficiency in the United States; 2% of the population is estimated to have relative insufficiency that becomes manifest only at times of physiologic stress.[1,2]

Acute adrenal crisis may complicate a variety of conditions that are related to an inadequate

Table 169-1 ACTIONS OF GLUCOCORTICOIDS

Function/Target System	Action
Metabolism	Stimulate gluconeogenesis Promote lipolysis Induce muscle protein catabolism Increase plasma glucose during stress
Endocrine	Inhibit insulin secretion; promote peripheral insulin resistance Increase epinephrine synthesis
Inflammatory	Cause demargination of granulocytes, suppress adhesion Reduce circulating eosinophils and lymphocytes Decrease production of inflammatory cytokines
Cardiovascular	Increase contractility and vascular response to vasoconstrictors
Renal	Increase glomerular filtration rate; pharmacologic doses act at mineralocorticoid receptors

neuroendocrine response to stress. Crisis may result from primary adrenal failure or may occur secondary to failure of the hypothalamic-pituitary-adrenal axis. Failure can result from a primary process or can be secondary to suppression by exogenous steroid administration.

Anatomy

The adrenal glands are retroperitoneal structures that lie within Gerota's fascia, superior and medial to the kidneys. Arterial blood supply arises from the aorta and renal and inferior phrenic arteries. Blood flows from the arteries through a sinusoidal system and collects into single veins draining into either the inferior vena cava or left renal vein, for the right and left adrenals respectively. The adrenal glands are encapsulated and divided into a cortex and a catecholamine-producing medullary zone. The cortex is further subdivided into the zona glomerulosa (which produces mineralocorticoids) and the zona fasciculata and reticularis (which secrete glucocorticoids and androgens).

Pathophysiology

■ ADRENAL PRODUCTS

Cholesterol is converted to pregnenolone, an adrenal precursor of more than 50 separate chemical pathways and by-products. Of these, the most clinically important glucocorticoid is cortisol, the most important androgen is dehydroepiandrosterone acetate (DHEA), and the most important mineralocorticoid is aldosterone.

Feedback Loops

Adrenocorticotropic hormone (ACTH) is the major regulator of cortisol and adrenal androgen production. ACTH is regulated by corticotropin-releasing hormone and antidiuretic hormone. Cortisol levels feed back on corticotropin-releasing hormone release. The renin-angiotensin system regulates aldosterone production.

■ CORTISOL PHYSIOLOGY

ACTH and cortisol levels vary by circadian rhythm. They both reach their nadir at about 4 AM and peak at about 8 AM. Serum levels also peak within minutes of stress-induced corticotropin-releasing hormone release in the central nervous system. Most circulating cortisol is protein-bound (75% to corticosteroid-binding globulin and 15% to albumin); only 10% is "free cortisol" (unbound).

■ TARGETS OF ACTION

Mineralocorticoids act at the renal tubules to maintain Na^+, K^+, and water balance. Glucocorticoid subunits enter various cell nuclei and modify expression of a wide range of genes in different organ systems (Table 169-1). Cortisol is capable of targeting the mineralocorticoid receptors at pharmacologic doses, although at physiologic levels it is converted to inactive cortisone upon entering the kidney.

■ CLINICAL APPLICATION

Adrenal insufficiency is classified as primary, secondary, or relative. Causes of primary insufficiency are enumerated in Table 169-2. Secondary insufficiency is most commonly due to exogenous steroid withdrawal. Relative adrenal insufficiency occurs in individuals who may have normal glucocorticoid levels but exhibit an inadequate hypothalamic-pituitary-adrenal axis response to major stress.

The most important type of adrenal insufficiency encountered in emergency medicine is relative adrenal insufficiency. It should be considered in any seriously ill patient who fails to respond to usual interventions. This condition is found most commonly among patients with severe sepsis but may be present in any hypotensive patient resistant to adequate fluid resuscitation and vasopressors.

Presenting Signs and Symptoms

Patients with primary and secondary adrenal insufficiency typically present with chronic complaints.

Table 169-2 CAUSES OF PRIMARY ADRENAL INSUFFICIENCY

Cause	Associated Factors
Autoimmune adrenal atrophy (80% of cases)	Hypoparathyroidism, hepatitis, candidiasis, type 1 diabetes mellitus, hypogonadism, hypothyroidism
Infections: disseminated tuberculosis, cytomegalovirus, histoplasmosis	Human immunodeficiency virus
Genetic diseases: congenital adrenal hyperplasia (CAH), adrenoleukodystrophy, familial glucocorticoid deficiency	Virilization in some forms of CAH
Metastatic malignancy or lymphoma	
Adrenal hemorrhage	Usually found on imaging of critically ill patients secondary to adrenal vein thrombosis; most patients either are predisposed to thrombosis (anti-phospholipid syndrome) or take anticoagulant medications for a coagulopathy
Infiltrative disorders	Amyloidosis, hemochromatosis
Drugs	Ketoconazole, suramin

Documentation

- History of steroid administration and withdrawal
- Risk factors for adrenal crisis: malignancy, tuberculosis, cytomegalovirus infection, human immunodeficiency virus infection, infiltrative disorders
- Record of initial serum glucose, sodium, potassium, and volume status

Those with primary disease may have weakness, fatigue, anorexia, nausea, vomiting, weight loss, hypotension, hyperpigmentation, hyponatremia, and hyperkalemia. Hyperpigmentation is initially generalized, later becoming manifest in the mucous membranes, palmar creases, nail beds, and nipples. Gastrointestinal disturbances are present in about half of patients with postural symptoms. Salt craving is a less common complaint. Associated endocrinopathies may complicate the initial presentation (see Table 169-2).

Patients with secondary adrenal insufficiency typically have normal mineralocorticoid levels and therefore do not present with volume or electrolyte abnormalities. The chronic presentation of secondary adrenal insufficiency is classically nonspecific in nature, consisting of weakness, lethargy, anorexia, and myalgias. Hyperpigmentation is not a feature of secondary adrenal insufficiency.

Types of Adrenal Insufficiency

■ ACUTE ADRENAL INSUFFICIENCY

Although most patients with subacute or chronic adrenal insufficiency are identified during outpatient evaluations, some undiagnosed patients will present to the ED with acute insufficiency. Such patients may have either primary or secondary insufficiency and present due to physiologic stress that cannot be met with appropriate rises in adrenal hormones. The majority of these patients will present with shock, nausea, vomiting, confusion, fever, and abdominal pain.

■ ACUTE ADRENAL HEMORRHAGE

Acute adrenal hemorrhage is a rare condition that should be suspected in patients who are seriously ill following surgery and in patients with antiphospholipid syndrome, severe sepsis, or shock. Such patients present with the general features of acute adrenal crisis and focal findings of abdominal, flank, or back tenderness. Abdominal examination may reveal a surgical abdomen.

Treatment should begin upon suspicion of this diagnosis. Early interventions have been shown to reduce mortality for postoperative patients and those with antiphospholipid syndrome; the timing of therapy does not appear to affect the usually high mortality of this condition in patients with sepsis or severe shock. Only a minority of patients will be found to have hyponatremia or hyperkalemia. Diagnosis is confirmed through imaging studies[3,4] (Fig. 169-1).

■ RELATIVE ADRENAL INSUFFICIENCY IN CRITICALLY ILL PATIENTS[5-16]

It is believed that about 2% of the U.S. population has inadequate adrenal response to stress. The incidence of relative adrenal insufficiency in the critically ill patient has been reported as low as 0 and as high as 77%.

The diagnosis and treatment of relative adrenal insufficiency is controversial. Disagreement exists about the incidence of disease; goal range of serum cortisol levels in response to stress or corticotropin testing; the dose of corticotropin to be administered for testing; and the indications for, optimal dosing of, and desired efficacy of steroids in the critically ill.

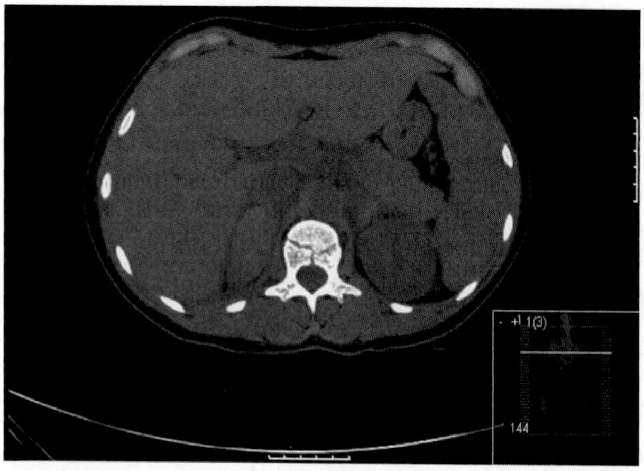
144

FIGURE 169-1 Bilateral adrenal hemorrhage in a patient with documented anti-phosphlipid syndrome and on coumadin for a recent deep venous thrombosis.

The use of steroids in sepsis has been explored. Well-designed trials of supraphysiologic doses of steroids have demonstrated no beneficial effect. Recent studies with new criteria have shown a reduction in mortality using physiologic doses of steroids in patients who do not respond to corticotropin.

For the purposes of immediate resuscitation before testing, a functional definition is used: a patient in shock who fails to respond to fluids and vasopressors within 1 hour should be treated for adrenal insufficiency.

■ DRUG-INDUCED ADRENAL INSUFFICIENCY

A number of medications may cause reversible adrenal insufficiency. Examples include ketoconazole, rifampin, phenytoin, and etomidate. The use of etomidate as an induction agent for rapid sequence intubation of critically ill patients is controversial. A single dose can cause a relative adrenal insufficiency for up to 24 hours. This reduction in adrenal activity may be of little clinical significance unless the administration of etomidate is repeated several times. The benefits of etomidate for rapid sequence intubation should be weighed against the necessary adrenal stress response. Alternative drugs should be considered for the induction of patients on chronic steroid therapies, such as a benzodiazepine used in combination with a muscle relaxant. Supplemental corticosteroids may be empirically administered for 24 hours if etomidate is used.[17-19]

Differential Diagnosis

The differential diagnosis of adrenal crisis includes most other conditions known to cause shock. Some common diseases that may be confused with adrenal insufficiency include gastroenteritis, sepsis, hypovolemia, myocardial infarction, and acute surgical pathology in the abdomen (Box 169-1). These same conditions may induce relative adrenal insufficiency, and as such, their diagnosis does not exclude a concurrent adrenal crisis.

BOX 169-1

Differential Diagnosis

Vomiting and Hypotension

Gastroenteritis with dehydration, sepsis, myocardial infarction, peptic ulcer disease, pancreatitis, cholecystitis, surgical disease

Weakness and Fatigue

Anemia, hypopituitarism, depression, neuromuscular disorders

Hyponatremia

See Chapter 165, Sodium and Water Balance.

RED FLAGS

- Conditions that promote shock may induce concurrent relative adrenal insufficiency; diagnosis of one condition does not exclude a second occult disease.
- Induction doses of etomidate may cause relative adrenal insufficiency for up to 24 hours after rapid sequence intubation in critically ill patients.

Diagnostic Testing

Empirical treatment of patients with suspected acute adrenal crisis should not be delayed for confirmatory laboratory testing. The initiation of glucocorticoid therapy should be accompanied by a concurrent, single measurement of serum cortisol. Levels below 15 μg/dL suggest adrenal crisis, although the interpretation may be difficult in seriously ill patients. The laboratory standards for adrenal function were established in normal subjects and are applied to populations with suspected chronic insufficiency.

Adrenal function testing begins with the administration of 250 μg of synthetic ACTH. A rise in serum cortisol to greater than 8 μg/dL within 30 minutes is considered a normal response. Such a finding excludes primary insufficiency but does not evaluate hypothalamic-pituitary-adrenal axis–related causes of secondary insufficiency. The hypothalamic-pituitary-adrenal axis is usually tested afterward with a metapyrone or an insulin-hypoglycemia challenge. Critically ill patients in whom the serum cortisol fails to rise by more than 9 μg in serial measurements should be considered nonresponders who require glucocorticoid therapy.

The classic finding of concurrent hyponatremia and hyperkalemia may indicate subacute or chronic

PRIORITY ACTIONS

Do:

- Use bedside glucometer, administer $D_{50}W$ as needed.
- Administer 20 mL/kg bolus of normal saline.
- Begin vasopressors when shock persists despite volume resuscitation.
- Check serum electrolytes, thyroid-stimulating hormone and free T_4 (thyroxine) levels.
- Check a random serum cortisol level.
- Administer 100 mg of hydrocortisone intravenously every 6 hours.
- Search for comorbid conditions, particularly causes of sepsis.

Do Not:

- Withhold glucocorticoids while awaiting laboratory results.
- Attempt endocrine stimulation testing in acutely ill patients.

adrenal insufficiency in the appropriate clinical setting.

Imaging studies may identify adrenal tumors or hemorrhage that can cause insufficiency. Incidental adrenal pathology is observed in approximately 2% of abdominal scans. Tumors may be benign or malignant, primary or metastatic.[20-21]

If Cushing's disease is suspected, a 24-hour urinary free cortisol should be checked. If pheochromocytoma is suspected, 24-hour urine metanephrine, vanillylmandellic acid, or catecholamine levels should be evaluated. Serum potassium may provide evidence of hyperaldosteronism.

Management

■ HYDROCORTISONE

Patients with adrenal crisis should receive IV hydrocortisone replacement. The initial adult dose is hydrocortisone 100 mg every 6 hours. In children, the dose can be given as 50 to 75 mg/m^2/day divided in four IV doses. The dose can be tapered as the patient's condition stabilizes. Severely ill patients, particularly those exhibiting septic shock, may require long durations of treatment.

■ DEXAMETHASONE

Stable patients should be given IV dexamethasone 4 mg every 6 hours. Dexamethasone allows a corticotropin stimulation test to be conducted because it does not immediately suppress hypothalamic activity. Dexamethasone has little mineralocorticoid activity, however, and therefore should be avoided in adrenal crisis.

PATIENT TEACHING TIPS

- Absolute lifelong compliance with outpatient medication regimens is mandatory.
- Double steroid doses during times of physiologic stress and minor illness.
- Seek medical attention if nausea and vomiting occur; these may be symptoms of adrenal crisis and may prevent tolerance of needed oral medications

■ FLUDOCORTISONE

Mineralocorticoid therapy is available only in oral form in the United States. Parenteral hydrocortisone, 100 mg given every 6 hours, has sufficient mineralocorticoid activity to adequately treat critically ill patients who cannot tolerate oral medications. As patients' condition stabilizes and they are able to take medications by mouth, hydrocortisone is tapered and oral fludocortisone, 0.05-0.1 mg, is added each morning. Patients with secondary adrenal insufficiency do not require mineralocorticoids.

■ OTHER TREATMENT

Patients with primary hypothalamic-pituitary-adrenal axis failure may have concurrent clinical hypothyroidism and require thyroxine supplementation. All patients with adrenal insufficiency should have prompt correction of volume status, electrolyte imbalance, and hypoglycemia.

Patients with incidental laboratory findings may be referred for outpatient management if there is no clinical evidence of acute adrenal insufficiency or excess, aldosterone excess, or pheochromocytoma. Adrenal masses larger than 6 cm will likely be removed, as well as those that demonstrate endocrine activity.

Disposition

Patients with shock or obtundation should be admitted to a critical care unit. Those who quickly respond to treatment may be considered for admission to an unmonitored floor. Patients with mild symptoms, known disease, and reliable follow-up can be treated in the ED and discharged to the care of their personal physician (see Tables 169-1 and 169-2).

REFERENCES

1. Levy A: Pituitary disease: Presentation, diagnosis, and management. J Neurol Neurosurg Psychiatry 2004;75(Suppl 3): iii47-iii52.

2. Silva Rdo C, Castro M, Kater CE, et al: [Primary adrenal insufficiency in adults: 150 years after Addison]. Arq Bras Endocrinol Metabol 2004;48:724-738.
3. Rao R H, Vagnucci AH, Amico JA: Bilateral massive adrenal hemorrhage: Early recognition and treatment. Ann Intern Med 1989;110:227-235.
4. Vella A, Nippoldt TB, Morris JC: Adrenal hemorrhage: A 25-year experience at the Mayo Clinic. Mayo Clin Proc 2001;76:161-168.
5. Annane D, Sebille V, Charpentier C, et al: Effect of treatment with low doses of hydrocortisone and fludrocortisone on mortality in patients with septic shock. JAMA 2002;288:862-871.
6. Briegel J, Schelling G, Haller M, et al: A comparison of the adrenocortical response during septic shock and after complete recovery. Intensive Care Med 1996;22:894-899.
7. Goodman S, Sprung CL: The International Sepsis Forum's controversies in sepsis: Corticosteroids should be used to treat septic shock. Crit Care 2002;6:381-383.
8. Keh D, Boehnke T, Weber-Cartens S, et al: Immunologic and hemodynamic effects of "low-dose" hydrocortisone in septic shock: A double-blind, randomized, placebo-controlled, crossover study. Am J Respir Crit Care Med 2003;167:512-520.
9. Manglik S, Flores E, Lubarsky L, et al: Glucocorticoid insufficiency in patients who present to the hospital with severe sepsis: A prospective clinical trial. Crit Care Med 2003; 31:1668-1675.
10. Minneci PC, Deans KJ, Banks SM, et al: Meta-analysis: The effect of steroids on survival and shock during sepsis depends on the dose. Ann Intern Med 2004;141:47-56.
11. Pizarro CF, Troster EJ, Damiani D, et al: Absolute and relative adrenal insufficiency in children with septic shock. Crit Care Med 2005;33:855-859.
12. Sessler CN: Steroids for septic shock: Back from the dead? Chest 2003;123(5 Suppl): 482S-489S.
13. Siraux V, De Backer D, Yalavatti G, et al: Relative adrenal insufficiency in patients with septic shock: Comparison of low-dose and conventional corticotropin tests. Crit Care Med 2005;33:2479-2486.
14. Soni A, Pepper GM, Wyrwinski PM, et al: Adrenal insufficiency occurring during septic shock: Incidence, outcome, and relationship to peripheral cytokine levels. Am J Med 1995;98:266-271.
15. Widmer IE, Puder JJ, König C, et al: Cortisol response in relation to the severity of stress and illness. J Clin Endocrinol Metab 2005;90:4579-4586.
16. Yildiz O, Doganay M, Aygen B, et al: Physiological-dose steroid therapy in sepsis [ISRCTN36253388]. Crit Care 2002;6:251-259.
17. Absalom A, Pledger D, Kong A, et al: Adrenocortical function in critically ill patients 24 h after a single dose of etomidate. Anaesthesia 1999;54:861-867.
18. De Coster R, Helmers JH, Noorduin H: Effect of etomidate on cortisol biosynthesis: Site of action after induction of anaesthesia. Acta Endocrinol (Copenh) 1985;110: 526-531.
19. Schenarts CL, Burton JH, Riker RR, et al: Adrenocortical dysfunction following etomidate induction in emergency department patients. Acad Emerg Med 2001;8:1-7.
20. Sanno N, Oyama K, Tahara S, et al: A survey of pituitary incidentaloma in Japan. Eur J Endocrinol 2003;149: 123-127.
21. Teramoto A, Hirakawa K, et al: Incidental pituitary lesions in 1,000 unselected autopsy specimens. Radiology 1994;193: 161-164.

Chapter **170**

Rhabdomyolysis

Bruce D. Adams and Jill A. Grant

KEY POINTS

- The most common causes of rhabdomyolysis include substance abuse, direct muscle injury, infection, strenuous physical activity, medications, and toxic ingestions.
- Only 50% of patients with rhabdomyolysis complain of specific muscle symptoms, and less than 10% have muscle tenderness on examination.
- Acute renal failure is the major complication of rhabdomyolysis.
- Slow or inadequate fluid resuscitation increases the likelihood of kidney damage.
- Crush injury is the strongest predictor of mortality from rhabdomyolysis.
- Rhabdomyolysis and crush syndrome often emerge as the leading causes of delayed mortality in mass casualty incidents involving building collapse.
- Early hemodialysis is indicated when severe hyperkalemia, refractory metabolic acidosis, or crush injury is present.
- The use of supplemental calcium or loop diuretics should be avoided in the setting of rhabdomyolysis.

Scope

Rhabdomyolysis afflicts more than 26,000 patients in the United States each year. Morbidity and mortality vary tremendously based on etiology, available treatment, time course, and comorbid factors. Acute renal failure, the major complication of rhabdomyolysis, occurs in 15% to 46% of cases. In the United States, approximately 5% to 7% of acute renal failure cases are caused by rhabdomyolysis. Mortality ranges from 3% to 10% but can be as high as 25% in mass casualty incidents that involve crush injuries.

Certain populations appear to be at increased risk of developing rhabdomyolysis. Alcohol and recreational drug abusers, patients taking numerous medications, military recruits, and athletes training well above their level of conditioning are of particular concern. Athletes with a predominance of type II fast twitch fibers (typically sprinters and weight lifters) are at higher risk for rhabdomyolysis than are those with a majority of type I slow twitch fibers (e.g., marathon runners). A large number of genetic disorders are linked to rhabdomyolysis as well.

Definitions

The pathologic definition of rhabdomyolysis is straightforward: acute injury or death of striated muscle cells, with subsequent release of cellular constituents into the systemic circulation. A clinical definition lacks widespread agreement, however, and both research and clinical care have been compromised by the absence of a widely accepted definition.

BOX 170-1

Suggested Definition of Clinical Rhabdomyolysis

- Absolute CK >15,000 U/L
  – or –
- CK >5000 U/L *and any* of these:
  - Crush injury
  - Acute renal insufficiency or failure
  - Myoglobinuria
  - Acidosis, disseminated intravascular coagulation, hypocalcemia, or hyperkalemia
  - Massive muscle injury
  - Prolonged extrication or delayed presentation >4 hrs

Authoritative thresholds for creatine kinase (CK) range between 1000 and 10,000 units per liter, but some definitions additionally mandate the presence of myoglobinuria (detection of free myoglobin in urine).[1] A consensus definition should be based on the criteria summarized in Box 170-1.

Pathophysiology

Rhabdomyolysis is a condition characterized by injury to skeletal muscle that alters the integrity of the cell membrane, resulting in release of muscle cell contents into the extracellular fluid and circulation.

Skeletal muscle is the largest internal organ in the human body, comprising more than 40% of its weight. The normal functioning of muscle depends on the maintenance of a healthy cell membrane, the sarcolemma, which is vital in the preservation of ionic gradients and the metabolic functioning of the cell. Despite the large number of causes of rhabdomyolysis, the final common pathway of muscle cell injury involves damage to the sarcolemma with loss of its intrinsic function. Injury to the muscle cell can be caused by direct muscle trauma or an altered relationship between energy production and energy consumption in the muscle.

Damage to the cell membrane results in loss of ionic gradients created by the Na^+, K^+-ATPase (adenosine triphosphatase) and Ca^{2+} pumps, with a resultant cascade of events leading to necrosis and death of the muscle cell. Immediately after cell injury there is an influx of Na^+, Cl^-, and water into the cell. The cell then begins to swell, promoting further muscle injury. Protein carriers that exchange Na^+ for Ca^{2+} ions promote an influx of calcium across the membrane, compounding muscle cell damage and overwhelming the capacity of the sarcoplasmic reticulum. With the continued influx of calcium ions, the mitochondria fail. Mitochondrial calcium loading becomes intolerable, and the excess calcium is released from the mitochondria back into the cytoplasm. The structural and functional damage to the mitochondria and resultant lack in energy production creates a vicious cycle, as less energy becomes available for pumping calcium out of the cell.

Calcium accumulates in the cytoplasm and activates phospholipase A, which results in accumulation of lysophospholipids in the muscle. This further raises the activity of neutral proteases to a level at which they become destructive to the muscle cell and cell membrane. The elevated cytoplasmic calcium level promotes a pathologic interaction of actin and myosin that ends in muscle destruction, fiber necrosis, and release of intracellular contents into the circulation. The most important products released include potassium, phosphorus, myoglobin, CK, aspartate aminotransferase, alanine aminotransferase, lactate dehydrogenase, urate, cytokines, and purines.

Causes of Rhabdomyolysis

Various categorizations of rhabdomyolysis have been proposed: traumatic vs. atraumatic, reversible vs. irreversible, endogenous vs. exogenous, and hereditary vs. acquired. Each classification has its limitations, and more than half of all rhabdomyolysis cases are multifactorial. Box 170-2 lists the many known causes of rhabdomyolysis. The most common causes include ethanol and drugs of abuse, direct muscle injury, infection, strenuous physical activity, and toxic ingestions.[2]

■ DRUGS OF ABUSE

Substance abuse is the most common medical cause of rhabdomyolysis, largely due to the high incidence of ethanol abuse and its direct toxicity to the myocyte membrane. Other drugs of abuse implicated in cases of rhabdomyolysis include cocaine, heroin, methamphetamine, phencyclidine hydrochloride; (PCP; "angel dust"), lysergic acid diethylamide (LSD), 3,4-methylenedioxymethamphetamine (MDMA; "ecstasy"), benzodiazepines, and barbiturates. Most abused drugs cause muscle damage through direct toxic effects or by immunologic reactions to the contaminants found mixed with the drug.

Ethanol, in addition to its direct toxicity, has multiple additional mechanisms by which it causes muscle damage. Its sedative and hypnotic properties may cause prolonged immobilization of a body part, with external compression of its blood supply leading to ischemia. Rhabdomyolysis can be induced by excessive motor activity when associated with alcohol-related seizures and delirium tremens. Poor nutrition inhibits the rate of ethanol metabolism, resulting in higher blood ethanol concentrations at the cell membrane for prolonged periods, leading to increased sarcolemmal damage.

Cocaine is also toxic to the sarcolemma and induces vasospasm resulting in ischemia. Cocaine

BOX 170-2

Causes of Rhabdomyolysis

Direct Muscle Injury
Trauma/crush/compression
Electrical injury
Lightning injury
Sickle cell disease
Burns

Ischemic injury
Compartment syndrome
Compression
Sickle cell disease
Vascular occlusion (embolism, thrombus)
Vasculitis

Excessive Muscular Activity
Acute dystonia
Contact sports
Delirium tremens
Isometric exercise
Lethal catatonia
Overexertion in untrained athletes
Psychosis
Seizures
Sports/basic training/marathon running
Status asthmaticus

Drugs of Abuse
Amphetamines
Caffeine
Cocaine
Methylenedioxymethamphetamine; "ecstasy" (MDMA)
Ethanol
Gasoline
Heroin
Lysergic acid diethylamide (LSD)
Marijuana
Mescaline
Methamphetamines
Opiates
Phencyclidine (PCP; "angel dust")
Polyweed
Toluene

Medications
Amphotericin B
Antihistamines
Azathioprine
Barbiturates
Benzodiazepines
Butyrophenones
Chlorpromazine
Cimetidine
Codeine
Clofibrate
Colchicine
Corticosteroids
Cotrimoxazole
Cyclosporins
Erythromycin
3-Hydroxy-3-methylglutaryl coenzyme A (HMG CoA) reductase inhibitors
Inhalation anesthetics
Isoniazid
Itraconazole
Lindane
Lithium
Lovastatin
Methadone
Monoamine oxidase inhibitors
Narcotics
Neuroleptic agents
Organic solvents
Pentamidine
Phenothiazines
Phenylpropanolamine
Phenytoin
Procainamide
Quinine
Salicylates
Serotonergic agents
Succinylcholine
Theophylline
Tricyclic antidepressants
Trimethoprim-sulfamethoxazole
Vasopressin
Total parenteral nutrition
Zidovudine

Metabolic Disorders
Diabetic ketoacidosis
Hyperaldosteronism
Hypernatremia
Hypokalemia
Hyponatremia
Hypophosphatemia
Hypothyroidism
Nonketotic hyperosmolar coma
Thyrotoxicosis
Renal tubular acidosis

Continued

BOX 170-2

Causes of Rhabdomyolysis—cont'd

Genetic Disorders

Affecting Carbohydrate Metabolism

Adenine deaminase deficiency
Alpha-glucosidase deficiency
Amylo-1,6-glucosidase deficiency
Cytochrome disturbances
Lactate dehydrogenase deficiency
Myophosphorylase deficiency (McArdle's disease)
Phosphofructokinase deficiency
Phosphoglycerate kinase deficiency
Phosphoglycerate mutase deficiency

Affecting Lipid Metabolism

Carnitine deficiency
Carnitine palmitoyltransferase deficiency
Short- and long-chain acyl-coenzyme A dehydrogenase deficiency

Affecting Purine Metabolism

Myoadenylate deaminase deficiency
Duchenne's muscular dystrophy

Immunologic Diseases

Dermatomyositis
Polymyositis

Infection

Bacterial

Gas gangrene
Group A beta-hemolytic streptococcus
Legionnaires' disease
Salmonella
Septic shock
Shigella
Staphylococcus aureus
Streptococcus pneumoniae
Tetanus

Viral

Adenovirus
Coxsackievirus
Cytomegalovirus
Echovirus
Epstein-Barr virus
Hepatitis
Herpes simplex virus
Human immunodeficiency virus
Influenza A and B
Parainfluenza
Rotavirus
Rickettsial—Rocky Mountain spotted fever
Parasites—trichinosis

Temperature-Related

Heat stroke
Hyperthermia
Hypothermia
Malignant hyperthermia
Neuroleptic malignant syndrome

Toxins

Brown spider bite
Carbon monoxide
Centipede bite
Ethylene glycol
Haff's disease
Hymenoptera sting
Quail ingestion
Isopropyl alcohol
Mercuric chloride
Methanol
Snake venom
Cyanide
Tetanus toxin
Typhoid toxin
Water hemlock
Toluene

increases energy demands of the cell that outstrip energy production.

■ DIRECT MUSCLE INJURY

Traumatic rhabdomyolysis is primarily the result of motor vehicle crashes, occupational injuries, or environmental tragedy (mine collapse, earthquakes, war). Muscle compression may also occur during torture and abuse, long-term confinement in the same position (as with orthopedic injuries), prolonged surgical interventions with improper positioning (high lithotomy or lateral decubitus), psychiatric conditions, and coma. Compression causes muscle ischemia as tissue pressure exceeds capillary perfusion pressure. Additionally, direct mechanical injury to the sarcolemma causes an incipient rise in intracellular calcium. Calcium activates destructive enzymes within the cell, facilitating necrosis and death of the myocyte.

■ INFECTION

Bacterial, viral, parasitic, and rickettsial infections have been associated with rhabdomyolysis. The most common viral etiology is influenza. Viruses cause rhabdomyolysis both by direct muscle invasion and by endotoxins and exotoxins that are responsible for skeletal muscle injury and subsequent release of myoglobin. *Legionella* is the most common bacterial cause, with its myotoxic effects mediated through an endotoxin. *Salmonella* and *Streptococcus* also induce rhabdomyolysis through direct myocyte invasion and inhibition of glycolytic enzymes.

■ EXCESSIVE MUSCULAR ACTIVITY

Strenuous muscular exercise in both trained and untrained athletes causes rhabdomyolysis. The degree of muscle injury is related to the duration and intensity of the exercise; damage is frequently confined to the lower extremities. Muscle injury is exacerbated by hot, humid conditions; lack of heat acclimatization; prolonged, profuse sweating; and an insufficient intake of salt. Patients at increased risk include athletes, marathon runners, new military recruits ("march myoglobinuria"), outdoor workers, and persons unused to strenuous exercise ("white collar rhabdomyolysis").

Pathologic causes of excessive muscle activity such as status epilepticus, myoclonus, dystonia, tetanus, chorea, and mania also lead to rhabdomyolysis. Additionally, patients suffering from a multitude of intoxications including isoniazid, strychnine, amoxapine, loxapine, theophyline, water hemlock, and lithium may experience excessive motor activity and seizures producing rhabdomyolysis.

Excessive muscle activity causes rhabdomyolysis through dehydration, increased activity of heat-sensitive degradative enzymes, and depletion of cellular energy (adenosine triphosphate [ATP]) with prolonged exercise. These insults lead to a failure of the sarcolemmal Na^+-K^+-ATPase and Ca^{2+} pumps, which results in increased intracellular calcium and cell necrosis.

■ MEDICATIONS

Drugs in almost every category have been implicated as a cause of rhabdomyolysis. The medications of most concern are the lipid-lowering agents, including the 3-hydroxy-3-methylglutaryl coenzyme A (HMG CoA) reductase inhibitors (lovastatin, simvastatin) and the fibric acid derivates that decrease triglyceride synthesis (gemfibrozil and clofibrate). HMG CoA reductase inhibitors block the production of coenzyme Q, which plays an important role in the production of ATP in the mitochondria. The resultant decrease in ATP production leads to cell death and subsequent rhabdomyolysis. Patients with preexisting renal dysfunction are at increased risk.

Immediate withdrawal of these drugs is mandatory if patients complain of muscle dysfunction or if their CK rises to more than three times normal. The risk of drug-induced muscle disease is aggravated by simultaneous administration of danazol, nicotinic acid, cyclosporine, itraconazole, or erythromycin. The combination of HMG CoA reductase inhibitors with gemfibrozil also carries a high rate of myotoxicity.

■ TOXINS

Toxins that cause direct myocyte damage include the venom from the European adder, the Australian tiger snake, the Australian king brown snake, the Death adder, and the North and South American rattlesnakes. These snakes deploy a single venom with multiple myocyte toxins (most likely phospholipases), causing direct muscle injury and rhabdomyolysis. Stings from Africanized bees (killer bees) and honey bees mediate rhabdomyolysis through myotoxins. Quail fed with hellebores or hemlock have also been associated with outbreaks of rhabdomyolysis (coturnism). Outbreaks of Haff's disease intermittently occur in the United States due to contaminated fish.

Toxins that act at the molecular level by interfering with the production of ATP are capable of producing damage to skeletal muscle. Carbon monoxide, cyanide, hydrogen sulfide, and phosphine inhibit electron transport in the mitochondria; salicylates and chlophenoxy herbicides uncouple oxidative phosphorylation; iodoacetate and sodium flouroacetate inhibit glycolysis in the Krebs cycle.

■ GENETIC DISORDERS

Rhabdomyolysis can result from genetic defects in glycolysis, glycogenolysis, fatty acid oxidation, and mitochondrial function. These disorders cause inappropriate use of carbohydrate and lipids leading to an imbalance between energy supply and demand in myocytes. Enzyme defects have been found in 23% to 47% of adult patients with rhabdomyolysis.

Genetic defects should be suspected in patients in whom the cause of rhabdomyolysis is obscure. Symptoms often begin before the age of twenty years, and attacks occur intermittently. Examples include patients with recurrent rhabdomyolysis after minimum to moderate exercise after viral infections starting in childhood, or patients with a family history of rhabdomyolysis. In glycogenolytic disorders, the mode of inheritance is usually autosomal dominant; phosphoglycerate kinase deficiency is X-linked.

Diagnostic Testing

Atypical symptoms are customary for rhabdomyolysis. Only 50% of patients complain of specific muscle symptoms, and less than 10% have muscle tenderness. Liberal testing for rhabdomyolysis is therefore warranted.

Consider rhabdomyolysis in patients with hyperkalemia, disseminated intravascular coagulation, sepsis, cardiovascular collapse, compartment syndrome, heat stroke, altered mental status, and acute renal failure. These patients may present with occult primary rhabdomyolysis or suffer from rhabdomyolysis as a complication of their primary disease process.

Though not consistently observed in all analyses, creatinine has at times been shown to rise faster with rhabdomyolysis than with other causes of acute renal failure. Markedly high creatinine levels or a relatively low ratio of blood urea nitrogen (BUN) to creatinine should raise suspicion of rhabdomyolysis (Box 170-3).

Diagnosis of an inherited muscle enzyme defect is based on muscle biopsy that demonstrates abnormally increased glycogen or lipid deposits, as well as histochemical staining that demonstrates a decrease or absence of specific enzymes.

■ CREATINE KINASE

Creatine kinase (CK) is the enzyme responsible for the reversible transfer of the terminal phosphate group of ATP to creatine to form phosphocreatine. Serum CK begins to rise 2 to 12 hours after the destruction of more than 200 g of muscle, with a peak measurement between 1 to 3 days. Levels decline within 3 to 5 days after muscle injury ceases. Serum CK levels remain elevated longer than those of myoglobin because of a relatively slow plasma clearance (serum $T_{1/2} = 1.5$ days). CK decreases at a steady rate of 39% per day.

A rise in serum CK follows the rise in serum myoglobin. Three isoenzymes of CK exist in human tissues: MM, MB, and BB. The predominant source of the CK-MM isoenzyme is skeletal and cardiac muscle; CK-BB is found in brain tissue, and CK-MB mainly in cardiac muscle. In rhabdomyolysis, the primary CK isoenzyme elevated is CK-MM. CPK (creatine phosphokinase) is a serum marker of CK-MM reported by many clinical laboratories.

■ MYOGLOBIN

Myoglobin is a small protein with a free circulating concentration that is very low under normal physiologic conditions. Myoglobin functions as an oxygen reservoir in muscles; serum myoglobin levels rise within 1 hour of skeletal muscle damage. Myoglobin levels become normal within 1 to 6 hours after cessation of muscle injury due to rapid clearing both by renal excretion and by metabolism to bilirubin.

When myoglobin levels reach 15 mg/L, it can be detected by urine dipstick; at 1 g/L it may cause the color of urine to appear dark, like cola. Myoglobinuria does not always result in dark urine, however; discoloration depends on (1) the amount of myoglobin released from muscle into the plasma, (2) the glomerular filtration rate, and (3) the urine concentration.

■ URINALYSIS

The urine dipstick is a commonly used screening test for rhabdomyolysis. The orthotoluidine test on the urine dipstick will react in the presence of either myoglobin or hemoglobin. A report of "large blood" on the urine dipstick and an absence of red blood cells on microscopic view classically suggest the presence of free myoglobin in the urine. Unfortunately, clinical data does not fully support this screening practice, as microscopic hematuria occurs in about 30% of rhabdomyolysis cases. Also, myoglobinuria may be transient and not present at the time of urinalysis despite the presence of significant clinical rhabdomyolysis. Dipstick testing will detect a urine myoglobin greater than 1.0 mg/dL, which correlates with a serum value of approximately 100 mg/dL.

Other common findings on urinalysis include the presence of tubular casts, proteinuria, and evidence of acute tubular necrosis.

Complications

Following sufficient muscle damage, cellular contents extruded into the general circulation cause several complications, including acute renal failure, metabolic derangements, disseminated intravascular coagulation, compartment syndrome, and peripheral neuropathy.

■ ACUTE RENAL FAILURE

Acute renal failure is the most important cause of morbidity in patients with rhabdomyolysis. There are three main pathophysiologic mechanisms by which rhabdomyolysis induces acute renal failure. First, the heme protein in myoglobin exerts direct toxicity on renal tubular cells by initiating lipid peroxidation. This toxicity is potentiated by an acidic pH (<5.6) in the tubular fluid. Second, myoglobin precipitates in the renal tubules causing intraluminal cast formation and tubular obstruction. The degradation of intratubular myoglobin results in the release of unbound iron, which catalyzes free radical production and further enhances ischemic damage. Third, renal vasoconstriction is promoted by platelet activating factor and endothelin.

Acute renal failure caused by rhabdomyolysis may be oliguric (most common) or nonoliguric. Rhabdomyolysis-induced acute renal failure results in a higher anion gap acidosis and higher uric acid levels. It is difficult to predict which patients will develop acute renal failure based on initial laboratory values at the time of presentation.[3]

BOX 170-3

Laboratory Abnormalities Observed with Rhabdomyolysis

Potassium
- Elevated, sometimes markedly so
- Risk of acute renal failure (ARF)

Bicarbonate
- Decreased
- Metabolic acidosis

Uric Acid
- Elevated
- Marker of ARF

Sodium
- Usually normal
- Can decrease with mannitol therapy
- Use serum osmolar values as guide

Phosphate
- High
- Risk of calcium phosphate precipitation
- May need phosphate binders if phosphate >7 mg/dL

Creatine kinase (CK)
- Elevated
- Associated with CK of 15-75,000

Blood urea nitrogen
- Elevated

Creatinine
- Elevated

Calcium
- Initially low, sometimes markedly so
- Rebound phase may demonstrate hypercalcemia

Liver function tests
- Sometimes elevated
- Serum glutamic oxaloacetic transaminase (SGOT), lactate dehydrogenase, aldolase, muscle enzyme levels elevated

Troponin
- Normal
- Suspect myocardial damage as cause (or effect) if elevated.
- 7% false-positive rate for troponin I.

Anion gap
- Sometimes elevated
- May be predictive of ARF

Prothrombin time/partial thromboplastin time/D-dimer
- Disseminated intravascular coagulation in up to 30% of severe cases
- Associated with higher mortality

■ METABOLIC AND ELECTROLYTE DERANGEMENTS

Hyperkalemia occurs in 10% to 40% of cases. It is the most serious electrolyte derangement observed with rhabdomyolysis because of its potential lethal effect on cardiac rhythm and function. More than 15 mmol of K^+ is released with necrosis of only 150 g of muscle, resulting in an acute increase in extracellular K^+ of 1.0 mmol/L. The degree of increase is further dependent on renal function, which is often concurrently impaired.

Hypocalcemia is the most common metabolic complication of rhabdomyolysis; low calcium levels are present early and are usually asymptomatic. Hypocalcemia results from deposition of calcium salts in necrotic muscle due to hypophosphatemia and decreased 1,25-dihydroxycholecalciferol. Soft tissue calcifications can be seen on radiographs of the involved limbs. Hypocalcemia should only be treated if severe symptoms or hyperkalemia develops, leading to cardiac arrhythmias, muscular contraction, and seizures. Later, as calcium is mobilized from the tissues, serum calcium levels rise and symptomatic hypercalcemia may develop. *Hypercalcemia* usually occurs in patients with acute renal failure during the diuretic phase, typically when urinary output is greater than 1500 mL/24 hours. Hypercalcemia also occurs more frequently if Ca^{2+} is supplemented in the hypocalcemic stage. Volume expansion and diuretics are adequate treatment.

Hyperphosphatemia is caused by leakage from injured myocytes and is higher in azotemic patients. Phosphate binders should be used when phosphate levels exceed 7 mg/dL. *Hypophosphatemia* may be seen later in the disease course but rarely requires treatment. *Hypermagnesemia* may occur in patients with renal insufficiency. Standard management is appropriate. *Hyperuricemia* is especially common in crush injury due to release of muscle adenosine nucleotides that are subsequently converted to uric acid in the liver. Uric acid levels typically correlate with serum CK levels.

Organic acids, especially lactic acid, are released from hypoxic, necrotic muscle cells and produce a pronounced anion gap acidosis.

■ COMPARTMENT SYNDROME

Most striated muscles are contained within rigid compartments formed by fascia and bones. When the muscle is traumatized, marked swelling and edema occur within a closed osteofascial compartment, reducing muscle perfusion to a level below that required for cellular viability. As intracompartmental pressures rise above 30 to 35 mm Hg, compartment syndrome develops and significant muscle ischemia ensues, requiring decompressive fasciotomy.

Classic signs and symptoms of compartment syndrome include pain, pallor, paresthesias, poikilothermia, paralysis, and pulselessness. Paresthesias are the most reliable sign—muscle edema exerts pressure on peripheral nerves, resulting in neuronal ischemia, paresthesias, and paralysis. Decompressive fasciotomy reverses peripheral neuropathies within a few days to weeks, although symptoms may be permanent in a minority of patients.

■ DISSEMINATED INTRAVASCULAR COAGULATION

Disseminated intravascular coagulation occurs in severe rhabdomyolysis when extensive injury results in multisystem organ failure. Although this disorder is more common with severe trauma and crush injury, rhabdomyolysis from medical causes may lead to disseminated intravascular coagulation. Severe bleeding is most pronounced on days 3 to 5 of illness. If severe bleeding does not occur, spontaneous improvement can be expected by days 10 to 14. When severe bleeding does occur, infusion of fresh frozen plasma (to replace coagulation factors) and transfusion of platelets may be indicated.

■ HEPATIC DYSFUNCTION

Hepatic dysfunction occurs in approximately 25% of patients with rhabdomyolysis. The proteases released from injured muscle may be implicated in hepatic inflammation.

■ CRUSH SYNDROME: DISASTER AND MASS CASUALTY CONSIDERATIONS

Delayed extrication from debris causes delayed resuscitation—rhabdomyolysis and crush syndrome often emerge as the leading causes of delayed mortality. Crush syndrome, perhaps the most dramatic presentation of rhabdomyolysis, results from both the initial blunt force trauma and even more so the reperfusion injury that appears after the release of the crushing pressure. Commonly, crush syndrome will present epidemically because of structural failure from earthquakes or warfare with resultant entrapment of victims beneath the debris. While acute renal failure is the most life threatening manifestation, crush syndrome can manifest with failure of any organ system, much like rhabdomyolysis. Often the obvious concomitant traumatic injuries can overshadow the emergency of crush syndrome due to the detriment of the patient.

Crush syndrome and compartment syndrome act synergistically on the degradation of muscle.[4] Acute musculoskeletal compartment syndrome can damage myocytes and induce rhabdomyolysis. Rhabdomyolysis in turn exacerbates the inflammatory cascade associated with crushing of the muscle compartment, worsening compartment pressures. Crush syndrome may worsen acute renal failure.[5]

During mass casualty situations in which crush injuries would be expected (earthquakes, building collapse, bombings), it is important to start IV volume

Tips and Tricks

MANAGEMENT OF CRUSH SYNDROME

Pre-hospital Phase:

- Begin high-volume IV fluid resuscitation before extrication from collapsed buildings.
- Remove constrictive jewelry and clothing.
- Flaccid paralysis may mimic spinal cord injury (but rectal tone will be normal).
- Pre-hospital amputation may be necessary to allow extrication of the victim.
- A "physiologic amputation" (the application of a tourniquet above the point of injury) may minimize release of toxic substances into the circulation, thereby reducing rates of rhabdomyolysis; ice or dry ice should be applied distal to the tourniquet.

Hospital Phase:

- Anticipate need for renal replacement therapy and hemodialysis resources.
- Decision for amputation can be aided by use of the Mangled Extremity Severity Score (MESS). A MESS score ≥ 7 is a 100% positive predictor of amputation.*
- Avoid early aggressive surgical débridement unless vascular compromise is obvious.

*Helfet DL, Howey T, Sanders R, Johansen K: Limb salvage versus amputation. Preliminary results of the Mangled Extremity Severity Score. Clin Orthop Relat Res 1990(250):80–86.

restoration in all survivors as quickly as possible (see Tips and Tricks: Management of Crush Syndrome). Emergency medical service and ED personnel should be instructed to begin IV resuscitation even before the victims are actually extricated from the scene. This may involve placing an IV line in a confined space on any free limb.

The International Society of Nephrology can be contacted to respond to a mass casualty incident with emergency renal therapy equipment through their Disaster Relief Task Force (www.nature.com/isn/society/committees/full/isn_051027_7.html).

Treatment

■ GENERAL MEASURES

Rhabdomyolysis is physiologically and clinically similar to cell degradation states such as tumor lysis syndrome and sepsis. An organized, aggressive treatment strategy should focus on clinical end points similar to those of other cell lysis conditions. The emergency treatment of rhabdomyolysis, in an early goal-directed fashion, is summarized in Figure 170-1.

The main goal of therapy is the prevention of acute renal failure through high-volume resuscitation.[6,7] The two most common reasons for the development of acute renal failure are slow fluid resuscitation and inadequate fluid resuscitation. Normal saline is superior to lactated Ringer's solution in the treatment of rhabdomyolysis because normal saline is not associated with a risk of phosphate toxicity. Over 10 liters of normal saline typically is administered in the first 24 hours of therapy, to maintain a high-volume dilute urine output.

Vital signs, cardiac rhythm, and urine output should be continuously monitored. Medication dosages should be adjusted to avoid affecting renal function, and drugs that are potentially nephrotoxic should be avoided.

■ PHARMACOLOGIC THERAPY

■ Mannitol

Mannitol exhibits several protective mechanisms. It is a potent diuretic, increasing myoglobin solubility and excretion in the renal tubules. It decreases sodium reabsorption in the kidney, which may promote renal conservation by decreasing the energy requirement of the renal medulla, and it is a potent oxygen free radical scavenger.

Mannitol also improves compartment pressures in compartment syndromes that result from crush injuries (though it is unknown whether mannitol reduces compartment pressures associated with ischemia or burns).

Animal literature supports the use of mannitol to promote the excretion of myoglobin and to increase intravascular volume in *non-oliguric* rhabdomyolysis. There are no randomized controlled studies of the use of mannitol for the treatment of rhabdomyolysis in humans.

Mannitol therapy can be given in both an intermittent or continuous fashion. Intermittent therapy is preferred, with a dose of 0.5 to 1 g/kg (with an average of 400 g over 60 hours) to achieve a urine output of 300 mL/hour. Serum sodium and osmolarity should be checked frequently to avoid a hyperosmolar state.

■ Sodium Bicarbonate

Patients with idiopathic rhabdomyolysis may not need bicarbonate therapy, but severely injured or hypotensive patients generate a tremendous organic acid load that probably requires treatment with supplemental sodium bicarbonate. Bicarbonate infusion of more than 500 mEq in 24 hours may be indicated. Caution should be exercised when administering large doses of bicarbonate, as treatment may exacerbate hypocalcemia, alkalemia, and related arrhythmias.

■ Acetazolamide

Acetazolamide prevents complications of serum alkalemia caused by bicarbonate therapy. It promotes

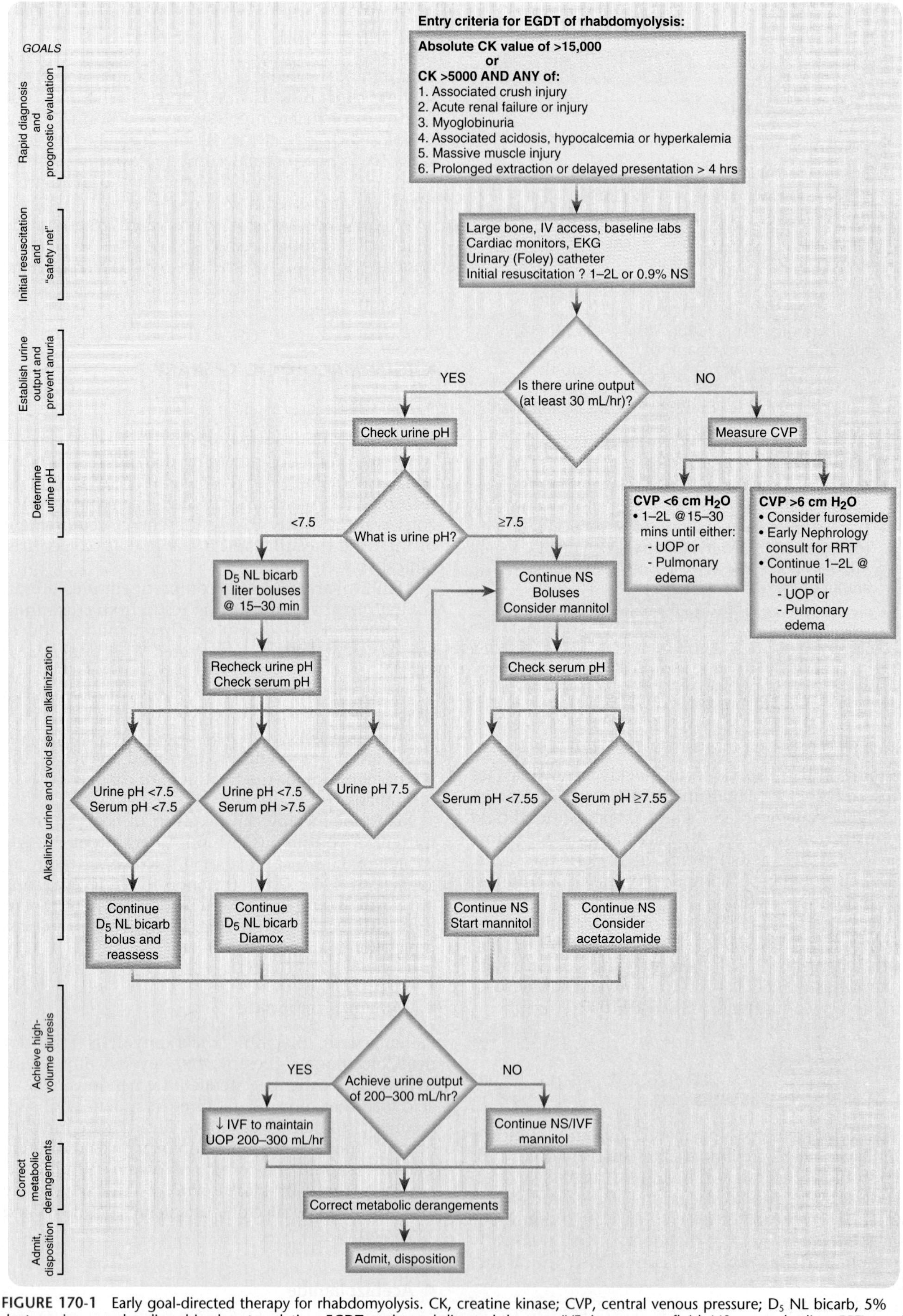
GOALS
Rapid diagnosis and prognostic evaluation
Initial resuscitation and "safety net"
Establish urine output and prevent anuria
Determine urine pH
Alkalinize urine and avoid serum alkalinization
Achieve high-volume diuresis
Correct metabolic derangements
Admit, disposition
Entry criteria for EGDT of rhabdomyolysis:
Absolute CK value of >15,000
or
CK >5000 AND ANY of:
1. Associated crush injury
2. Acute renal failure or injury
3. Myoglobinuria
4. Associated acidosis, hypocalcemia or hyperkalemia
5. Massive muscle injury
6. Prolonged extraction or delayed presentation > 4 hrs
Large bone, IV access, baseline labs
Cardiac monitors, EKG
Urinary (Foley) catheter
Initial resuscitation ? 1–2L or 0.9% NS
Is there urine output (at least 30 mL/hr)?
YES
NO
Check urine pH
Measure CVP
CVP <6 cm H_2O
• 1–2L @15–30 mins until either:
- UOP or
- Pulmonary edema
CVP >6 cm H_2O
• Consider furosemide
• Early Nephrology consult for RRT
• Continue 1–2L @ hour until
- UOP or
- Pulmonary edema
What is urine pH?
<7.5
≥7.5
D_5 NL bicarb 1 liter boluses @ 15–30 min
Continue NS Boluses Consider mannitol
Recheck urine pH Check serum pH
Check serum pH
Urine pH <7.5 Serum pH <7.5
Urine pH <7.5 Serum pH >7.5
Urine pH 7.5
Serum pH <7.55
Serum pH ≥7.55
Continue D_5 NL bicarb bolus and reassess
Continue D_5 NL bicarb Diamox
Continue NS Start mannitol
Continue NS Consider acetazolamide
Achieve urine output of 200–300 mL/hr?
YES
NO
↓ IVF to maintain UOP 200–300 mL/hr
Continue NS/IVF mannitol
Correct metabolic derangements
Admit, disposition

FIGURE 170-1 Early goal-directed therapy for rhabdomyolysis. CK, creatine kinase; CVP, central venous pressure; D_5 NL bicarb, 5% dextrose in normal sodium bicarborate solution; EGDT, early goal-directed therapy; IVF, intravenous fluid; NS, normal saline; RRT, renal replacement therapy; UOP, urinary output.

excretion of sodium bicarbonate in the renal tubules, thereby inhibiting cast formation. When the serum pH exceeds 7.50, a standard dose of acetazolamide (250 mg) may be administered.

■ RENAL REPLACEMENT THERAPY AND HEMODIALYSIS

Early hemodialysis is not necessary unless crush injuries or certain complications are present (e.g., severe hyperkalemia, refractory metabolic acidosis). Early consultation with a nephrologist is warranted. Myoglobin molecules can be removed by hemofiltration, but not by hemodialysis or peritoneal dialysis.[8]

Reductions in morbidity and mortality have been observed in victims of mass casualty incidents who received dialysis within 4 to 6 hours of injury.

■ SURGICAL THERAPY

Surgical therapy is a consideration for patients with rhabdomyolysis due to crush syndrome. Amputation removes damaged muscle that serves as the source of cellular toxins.

Physiologic amputation can act as temporizing measure when immediate surgical care is not available, particularly in the setting of disasters or military combat. To perform, firmly apply one or two tourniquets to the extremity above the level of injury or entrapment, with dry ice applied distal to the tourniquet. Combat surgery hospitals beginning in World War II through current conflicts have performed this procedure with success. Physiologic amputation rapidly reduces myoglobin and other intracellular toxins due to crushed, ischemic, or septic extremities. This can dramatically reduce myoglobinuria and reperfusion injury.[9] Physiologic tourniquets have allowed definitive surgery to be delayed for up to 32 days. *Be aware that physiologic amputation will inevitably result in the loss of the affected limb.*

Early prophylactic fasciotomy increases the need for transfusions and the risk of both sepsis and death. Fasciotomy is not indicated unless signs of compartment syndrome are observed.

■ EXPERIMENTAL THERAPY

Several promising experimental therapies for rhabdomyolysis have been studied in animal models but have not been well tested in humans. Nitric oxide may prevent acute renal failure by promoting renal vasodilation; lazaroids (21-aminosteroids) inhibit oxidant-induced lipid peridoxidation in animals. Other experimental treatment modalities include desferrioxamine (an iron chelator), glutathione, vitamin E, carvedilol, and dantrolene.

■ AVOID CALCIUM SUPPLEMENTATION AND LOOP DIURETICS

Patients with rhabdomyolysis often present with acute hypocalcemia. Supplemental calcium administration must be avoided because it can exacerbate cytoplasmic injury. During the rebound and recovery phases of rhabdomyolysis, calcium is remobilized and hypercalcemia becomes a true risk. Only in the settings of severe ventricular dysrhythmias should calcium be considered, and even then other measures to ameliorate hyperkalemia should be administered first.

Generally avoid loop diuretics (e.g., furosemide), which contribute to urine acidification and tubular cast formation. Forced diuresis is best conducted with mannitol.

Disposition

Patients with rhabdomyolysis should be admitted to a telemetry floor staffed by a physician or an intensive care unit. A nephrologist should be consulted early in the treatment course of any patient with crush injury or renal impairment.

REFERENCES

1. Gabow PA, Kaehny WD, Kelleher SP: The spectrum of rhabdomyolysis. Medicine 1982;61:141-152.
2. Allison RC, Bedsole DL: The other medical causes of rhabdomyolysis. Am J Med Sci 2003;326:79-88.
3. Fernandez WG, Hung O, Bruno GR, et al: Factors predictive of acute renal failure and need for hemodialysis among ED patients with rhabdomyolysis. Am J Emerg Med 2005; 23:1-7.
4. Gonzalez D: Crush syndrome. Crit Care Med 205;33(1 Suppl):S34-S41.
5. Bywaters E, Beall D: Crush injuries with impairment of renal function. J Am Soc Nephrol 1998;9:322-332.
6. Better OS, Stein JH: Early management of shock and prophylaxis of acute renal failure in traumatic rhabdomyolysis. N Engl J Med 1990;322:825-829.
7. Ron D, Taitelman U, Michaelson M, et al: Prevention of acute renal failure in traumatic rhabdomyolysis. Arch Intern Med 1984;144:277-280.
8. Zager RA: Studies of mechanisms and protective maneuvers in myoglobinuric acute renal injury. Lab Invest 1989;60: 619-629.
9. Slater MS, Mullins RJ: Rhabdomyolysis and myoglobinuric renal failure in trauma and surgical patients: A review. J Am Coll Surg 1998;186:693–716.

Chapter 171

Pituitary Apoplexy

Brian K. Nelson

KEY POINTS

Pituitary apoplexy is a rare but serious condition caused by hemorrhage or infarction of the pituitary gland.
Patients present acutely with severe headache, meningismus, visual field deficits, cranial nerve palsies, loss of visual acuity, and altered mental status.
Acute hypopituitarism may develop following pituitary apoplexy. Treatment for impending adrenal crisis is mandatory.
Emergent consultation of a neurosurgeon with expertise in pituitary surgery and management is required.

Scope

Pituitary adenomas are common, with a prevalence of 3% to 27% in various autopsy series. Apoplexy occurs in a minority of such lesions and occasionally can be seen with normal glands. Due to the relative rarity of this condition, pituitary apoplexy may be confused with more common entities such as subarachnoid hemorrhage. Delays in diagnosis and treatment may lead to blindness, permanent cranial nerve palsies, or death.[1,2]

Anatomy and Pathophysiology

The two lobes of the pituitary gland sit within an enclosed space known as the sella turcica. Blood supply to this gland is the richest of all mammalian tissues.

The anterior lobe receives the portal hypophyseal vessel from the hypothalamus. Differentiated cells in the anterior lobe secrete specific hormones. These include somatotrophs (growth hormone; GH), corticotrophs (adrenocorticotropic hormone; ACTH), lactotrophs (prolactin; PRL), thyrotrophs (thyroid-stimulating hormone or thyrotropin; TSH), and gonadotrophs (luteinizing hormone and follicle-stimulating hormone; LH and FH). Hormone secretion is controlled through the portal hypophyseal system arising from the hypothalamus.

The posterior lobe is an extension of the hypothalamus and secretes two hormones: antidiuretic hormone (or arginine vasopressin; ADH) and oxytocin. The pituitary stalk and the portal vessel pass through a small diaphragm that separates the sella turcica from the middle fossa. This anatomic position places the pituitary at risk for infarction or hemorrhage when a mass increases the pressure in the sella or compresses the stalk and vessels. Higher intrasellar pressures are associated with poor outcomes.

Pituitary tumors are common and many be asymptomatic. They are classified by size (microadenoma, <10 mm; macroadenoma, >10 mm) and by the hormone produced. Of those tumors that manifest clinical symptoms, the most commonly secreted hormones are PRL, leading to hypogonadism; GH, which promotes acromegaly; and ACTH, a cause of Cushing's disease.

Documentation

- Onset, location, and severity of headache
- Mental status
- Complete neurological examination, including visual acuity and confrontational visual fields
- Initial glucose, electrolytes, volume status
- Results of initial imaging studies

Tumors involved in apoplexy typically are nonfunctional and unsuspected macroadenomas. Patients receiving an endocrine stimulation test for hypogonadism, hypothyroidism, or adrenal insufficiency may occasionally develop apoplexy secondary to stimulation of a macroadenoma. Treatment of a pituitary tumor can also precipitate apoplexy, particularly in cases of surgery, irradiation, or bromocriptine administration. Other reported risk factors include pregnancy, head trauma, recent surgery, anticoagulation, hypertension, diabetic ketoacidosis, and ovarian stimulation medications.[3]

Most patients with pituitary apoplexy have no identifiable risk factor. Apoplexy may occur in normal glands.

Presenting Signs and Symptoms

CLASSIC

The presentation varies from mild headache to sudden collapse and coma. Most patients present with severe frontal or retro-orbital headache, vomiting, impaired visual acuity, visual field defects, hypopituitarism, and subsequent adrenal crisis. A minority have ocular palsies, obtundation, meningismus, blindness, or long track signs. The visual field deficit is classically a bitemporal upper quadrantopsia or hemianopsia. Associated cerebral infarction occasionally occurs secondary to vasospasm from subarachnoid hemorrhage or direct tumor compression of the internal carotid artery. Table 171-1 lists the frequency of signs and symptoms reported in four case series.

VARIATIONS

Hypopituitarism

Most cases of hypopituitarism are diagnosed in the outpatient setting due to their subacute or indolent presentation. Patients with hypopituitarism exhibit sequential signs and symptoms of growth hormone deficiency, hypogonadism, hypothyroidism, and adrenal insufficiency. They are typically weak, hypopigmented, and overweight, and appear chronically ill. Body hair and genitalia are diminished. Severe cases may be complicated by bradycardia and hypotension.

Table 171-1 SIGNS AND SYMPTOMS OF PITUITARY APOPLEXY

Sign or Symptom	Frequency (% incidence)
Headache	63-97
Visual field deficit	43-82
Hypopituitarism	81
Adrenal crisis	65
Vomiting	50
Visual impairment	60
Complete blindness	10
Ocular palsies	40-46
Meningismus	25
Altered mental status	13
Hyponatremia	12
Long tract signs	5

Data from references 1, 3, 5, 6.

RED FLAGS

These signal the need for immediate surgical decompression:

- Mental status changes
- Rapidly progressive course
- Severe vision loss

Asymptomatic Pituitary Tumors

Silent tumors are incidental microadenomas found during imaging studies ordered for an unrelated condition. Patients with silent tumors have no symptoms attributable to cell type.

Differential Diagnosis

Common neurologic emergencies are often confused with pituitary apoplexy (Box 171-1). The sudden onset of severe headache suggests subarachnoid hemorrhage. Obtundation and meningeal signs suggest meningitis, cerebral hemorrhage, or cerebral venous thrombosis. Cranial nerve findings in the setting of altered mental status may indicate cavernous sinus thrombosis or midbrain infarction. Rare hypothalamic and pituitary compressive or destructive processes may closely mimic apoplexy by presenting as headaches and visual field deficits. Two of these mimics are lymphocytic hypophysitis and Rathke cleft cysts. Pediatric craniopharyngiomas and several primary and metastatic lesions in adults may also compress the pituitary gland and mimic apoplexy. Generally, deficits in visual acuity and visual fields raise suspicion for apoplexy in the appropriate clinical setting.

BOX 171-1

Differential Diagnosis

- Sudden severe headache with or without mental status changes or long tract signs
- Subarachnoid hemorrhage, meningitis, cerebral hemorrhage, mass, infarction, intracranial venous thrombosis
- Severe headache with visual acuity, ocular palsies, or visual field changes
- Complicated migraine, cavernous sinus thrombosis, cerebellar hemorrhage, midbrain infarction
- Signs of hypogonadism, hypoadrenalism, or hypothyroidism
- Etiologies of hypopituitarism, including remote head injury, lymphocytic hypophysitis, iatrogenic surgical or radiation injury, and infections (particularly tuberculosis and mycotic infections); consider primary hypoadrenalism and hypothyroidism

Diagnostic Testing

Visual acuity and confrontational visual field testing should be performed when the diagnosis of pituitary apoplexy is considered. A noncontrast computed tomography scan of the head will exclude the diagnosis of acute subarachnoid hemorrhage. Serum cortisol, thyroxine, and TSH levels should be obtained. Endocrine simulation testing will worsen the condition and should be deferred.

Computed tomography is not sufficiently sensitive to exclude a pituitary process. Contrast-enhanced magnetic resonance imaging with diffusion-weighted imaging allows the best visualization of pituitary tumors and details of hemorrhage and infarction within them.[4]

Management

Parenteral hydrocortisone (100 mg every 6 hours) or dexamethasone (4 mg every 12 hours) is given to decrease tumor edema and to treat impending adrenal crisis. Obtunded or comatose patients should be intubated.

Definitive treatment is pituitary decompression, most often through a transsphenoidal approach. Patients with minimal or improving visual symptoms are sometimes medically managed. Outcome depends on symptom severity at presentation and prompt decompression of the sella turcica. Early diagnosis and treatment improve outcome and visual acuity; residual hypopituitarism generally persists.[5,6]

PRIORITY ACTIONS

Do:

- Fingerstick glucose; treat if hypoglycemic
- Draw serum cortisol, thyroid-stimulating hormone, and free T_4 (thyroxine)
- Administer parenteral hydrocortisone 100 mg qid or dexamethasone 4 mg bid
- Provide fluid and electrolyte support
- Computed tomography scan to exclude subarachnoid hemorrhage, followed by magnetic resonance imaging
- Early consultation with neurosurgeon with pituitary expertise
- Admit patient to neurologic critical care unit

Do Not:

- Withhold glucocorticoids while awaiting laboratory results
- Attempt endocrine simulation testing in the ED

Disposition

Patients with pituitary apoplexy require emergent consultation with a neurosurgeon experienced in pituitary surgery. Admission to a neurologic intensive care unit should be accompanied by consultation with a medical intensivist and an endocrinologist.

Patients presenting with subacute or chronic panhypopituitarism should be seen by an endocrinologist for further evaluation and initiation of therapy. Asymptomatic pituitary tumors can be safely managed in the outpatient setting, as such cases rarely progress to apoplexy.

REFERENCES

1. Semple PL, Webb MK, de Villiers JC, Laws ER: Pituitary apoplexy. Neurosurgery 2005;56:65-72.
2. Agrawal D, Mahapatra AK: Visual outcome of blind eyes in pituitary apoplexy after transsphenoidal surgery: A series of 14 eyes. Surg Neurol 2005;63:42-46.
3. Biousse V, Newman NJ, Oyesiku NM, et al: Precipitating factors in pituitary apoplexy. J Neurol Neurosurg Psychiatry 2001;71:542-545.
4. Pisaneschi M, Kapoor G: Imaging the sella and parasellar region. Neuroimaging Clin N Am 2005;15:203-219.
5. Ayuk J, McGregor EJ, Mitchell RD, Gittoes NJ: Acute management of pituitary apoplex—surgery or conservative management? Clin Endocrinol (Oxf) 2004;61:747-752.
6. Lubina A, Olchovsky D, Berezin M, et al: Management of pituitary apoplexy: Clinical experience with 40 patients. Acta Neurochir (Wien) 2005;147:151-157.

SECTION **XVII**

Infections

Chapte

Chil

James E.

KEY P

A *fever* is
Response fore shoul
The diagn group of t age).
The periph absence of

Scope

■ PERSPECTIVE

Developing an accura
forming an appropria
treatment and disposit
are not always straight
up varies dramatically,
tion and the age of the
a structured approach t
child based on pertine
and physical examin
patient age group. Fact
patient disposition and
are provided.

Before beginning a d
is critical to understar
commonly used terms (
Fever is defined as a tem
measured rectally in ch
and 39.0° C in children
body temperature highl
perature when the mea

Facts and Formulas

Fever: for ages 0 to 3 months, a temperature 38.0° C or higher measured rectally; for ages 3 to 36 months, a temperature of 39° C or higher measured rectally

Bacteremia: the presence of bacteria in the bloodstream

Occult bacteremia: the presence of bacteria in the bloodstream of a child who has a fever but who may not appear particularly sick and who has no apparent other source of infection

Serious bacterial illness: bacterial infection that poses a significant risk of progression if not treated

11.6%.[5,8] The prevalence of occult bacteremia in the post-Hib era has decreased by more than 90% to between 1.6% and 1.9%.[9,10] The current licensed pneumococcal vaccine is active against 7 of the 90 serotypes of *Streptococcus pneumoniae* and has an efficacy of 90% for reducing invasive infections from *S. pneumoniae*. Although preliminary investigations are promising, the effect of the pneumococcal vaccine on the rate of occult bacteremia is unclear. Given the paucity of data, management recommendations for children who have received the Hib and pneumococcal vaccines differ.[11,12] The growing body of literature will change the approach to the acutely febrile child in the near future. However, in what way and to what degree have yet to be determined.

Serious bacterial illness accounts for only 2% to 4% of fevers. Examples of serious bacterial illness include pneumonia, cellulitis, septic arthritis, osteomyelitis, urinary tract infection, meningitis, and sepsis.[6,13]

■ PATHOPHYSIOLOGY

Fever is the host's adaptive response to an invading microorganism. The microorganism comes into contact with cells of the immune system, including macrophages and leukocytes, and this contact leads to release of various cytokines, most notably interleukin-1, tumor necrosis factor, and interleukin-6. These cytokines circulate and come into contact with neuronal cell groups around the edges of the brain's ventricular system. Prostaglandin E_2 is then released and binds to receptors on neurons in the hypothalamus and brainstem, leading to upregulation of the hypothalamic thermostatic set-point.[14,15] Once the thermoregulatory center is reset, it maintains a higher body temperature through various mechanisms such as cutaneous vasoconstriction or shivering. The febrile response is not fully developed in young infants, and fever or even hypothermia may occur in response to infection. The physiologic limit of thermoregulation is estimated to be 41.1° C (106° F). According to McCarthy, children

BOX 172-1

Criteria Historically Used for Risk Stratification in Pediatric Fever

Rochester Criteria

Previously healthy term infants without perinatal complications who are less than 3 months of age and who are not found to have soft tissue, ear, or skeletal infection

Nontoxic appearance

No previous use of antimicrobials

Lack of a focus of infection on examination

Peripheral white blood cell count: 5000 to 15,000/µL

Band count: 1500/µL or higher

Stool white blood cell count: up to five white blood cells/high-power field in infants with diarrhea

Spun urine: up to 10 white blood cells/high-power field

Philadelphia Criteria

Infants 29 through 56 days of age with temperatures of 38.2°C

Observation score and diagnostic testing

Observation Score

Quality of cry (strong, whimpering, weak, high pitched)

Reaction to parent stimulation (cries briefly then stops, intermittent cry, continual cry)

State variation (awake, awake with stimulation, unarousable)

Color (pink, acrocyanosis, cyanotic)

Hydration (mucosal membranes: moist, slightly dry, dry)

Social responses (smile, brief smile, no smile)

Diagnostic Testing

White blood cell count: less than 15,000/mm^3

Spun urine: up to 10 white blood cells/high-power field and absence of bacteria on bright-field microscopy

Cerebrospinal fluid with a white blood cell count of less than eight/mm^3 and a negative Gram stain from a nonbloody sample

Chest radiograph demonstrating an infiltrate

with a fever of this degree have a high rate of central nervous system insult.[2]

Presenting Signs and Symptoms

When evaluating a febrile child, the clinician must obtain key information from the history and physical examination (Box 172-2 and see Documentation

BOX 172-2

Physical Examination Findings in the Evaluation of the Febrile Infant or Child

Vital Signs

General Appearance

Level of activity

Eye contact and tracking behaviors

Tone

Consolability

Color

Head, Ears, Eyes, Nose, and Throat

Meningeal signs (may not be present in children less than 1 year of age)

Otitis media (bulging tympanic membrane with decreased mobility)

Pharyngitis

Adenopathy

Respiratory System

Rate of respirations

Presence of increased work of breathing

- Grunting
- Nasal flaring
- Retracting
- Rales
- Rhonchi
- Wheezing
- Stridor
- Cough
- Decreased breath sounds

Cardiovascular System

Pulse rate

Presence of a murmur

Abdomen

Tenderness

Distention

Guarding

Rebound

Organomegaly

Costovertebral angle tenderness

Skin

Rash

Musculoskeletal System

Point tenderness to palpation of bone or joints

Swelling

Erythema

Range of motion of joints

Gait and ability to ambulate

box). According to McCarthy and colleagues, the sensitivity of the clinical evaluation for an infant less than 3 months and between 3 and 36 months of age is 78% and 89% to 92%, respectively.[2,16] After the history and physical examination, the source of fever remains inapparent in 20% of febrile children.[5,9]

Differential Diagnosis

The differential diagnosis of acute pediatric fever is vast (Box 172-3). It is imperative to become familiar with the myriad causes of pediatric fever. Defining characteristics of each diagnosis can be found elsewhere in this text.

■ DIAGNOSTIC TESTING

Diagnostic evaluation is based on the patient's age group.[1,5,17] Boxes 172-4 and 172-5 outline the indications for other common diagnostic tests in children with fever.

■ Urinalysis and Culture

Occult urinary tract infections occur in 2% to 3% of male infants less than 1 year of age. Most of these infections occur in uncircumcised boys and infants less than 6 months of age. Occult urinary tract infections occur in 8% to 9% of female children less than 2 years of age.[5] Girls between 2 months and 2 years of age can be risk stratified for urinary tract infection (see Box 172-5) with a sensitivity of 95% and specificity of 31%.[18]

Urine can be collected for testing in several different ways. Bag collection is a noninvasive, convenient method. However, it is not recommended because of the false-positive rate of nearly 85%.[16,19] Percutaneous bladder aspiration is another approach. Because this method is more invasive, it is also not the preferred approach except in male infants with severe phimosis.[8] Urethral catheterization is generally regarded as the preferred method of obtaining urine; it has a sensitivity and a specificity reported to be 95% and 99%, respectively.[8] Once a catheterized urine specimen has been obtained, it should be sent for testing. A negative urinalysis and a negative Gram stain are not sufficient to exclude a urinary tract infection. As many as 50% of patients with a urinary tract infection documented by urine culture have a false-negative urinalysis. Therefore, it is important to obtain a urine culture in conjunction with a urinalysis and Gram stain.[8,19]

The utility of an elevated peripheral white blood cell count in the evaluation of the febrile child is debatable. It has been shown to be an inaccurate screen for bacteremia and meningitis in febrile infants.[20,21] Thus, the decision to administer antibiotics, to perform or withhold lumbar puncture, or to admit or dismiss the patient should not be based

Documentation

Key Historical Findings in the Evaluation of the Febrile Infant or Child

Age of the child

Height and duration of the fever

Method of obtaining the temperature

Use, timing, and dose of antipyretics administered

Caretaker's Report of Well-Being

Level of activity

Consolability

Irritability

Lethargy

Playing

Smiling

Eating

Pitch of cry (a high-pitched cry may be indicative of a central nervous system infection)

Hydration Status

Fluid intake

Urinary output

Respiratory Symptoms

Cough

Work of breathing

- Nasal flaring
- Intercostal retractions
- Grunting

Gastrointestinal Symptoms

Vomiting

Diarrhea

Abdominal pain

Urinary Symptoms

Dysuria

Frequency

Urgency

Hematuria

Ear, Nose, and Throat Symptoms

Earache

Sore throat

Dermatologic Symptoms

Rash

Past Medical History

Birth history

- Length of gestation, mode of delivery, infections during pregnancy, antibiotics during pregnancy, mother's Group B *Streptococcus* status

Immunization status

Underlying medical illnesses

Prior hospitalizations

Social History

Ill contacts

Day care

Recent travel

solely on interpretation of the white blood cell count.[20-22]

Deciding when to perform a chest radiograph in the febrile child can also be challenging. Nearly 7% of all febrile children less than 2 years of age who have a temperature higher than 38° C have pneumonia.[23] In an investigation by Bachur and associates, occult pneumonia (defined as the presence of an infiltrate on a chest radiograph in a child without clear clinical evidence of pneumonia) was discovered in up to 26% of febrile children without a source and a white blood cell count greater than 20,000/mm^3.[24] Several criticisms of this study have been raised, including the high degree of interobserver variability in chest radiograph interpretation, the failure to perform a peripheral white blood count in more than half the infants with a temperature of 38° C of higher, and the performance of the majority of clinical assessments by physicians in training rather than by faculty physicians.[25-27] Nonetheless, data in the literature are sufficient to support the policy of the American College of Emergency Physicians that outlines the indications for obtaining a chest radiograph in children younger than 3 years[8] (Box 172-6).

Treatment and Disposition

The clinician should administer appropriate doses of antipyretics early in the evaluation of the febrile child (acetaminophen, 15 mg/kg, or ibuprofen, 10 mg/kg). The response to antipyretics is not a useful determinant of the presence of bacterial illness and should not influence clinical decision making.[28] Treatment and disposition for infants less than 90 days of age are outlined in Figures 172-1 and 172-2 and Box 172-4.[5] For infants managed on an outpatient basis, tests obtained in the ED occasionally come back positive after the patient has been discharged. If blood cultures are positive, the child should be admitted for sepsis evaluation and parenteral antibiotics, especially in the setting of persistent

BOX 172-3

Differential Diagnosis of Acute Pediatric Fever

Common Viral Infections

Central Nervous System

Meningitis
Encephalitis
Tumor
Brain abscess

Head, Ears, Eyes, Nose, and Throat

Pharyngitis
Retropharyngeal abscess
Peritonsillar abscess
Lateral pharyngeal wall abscess
Stomatitis
Influenza
Sinusitis
Parotitis
Viral stomatitis
Cervical adenitis
Periorbital cellulitis
Orbital cellulitis/abscess

Respiratory System

Bronchiolitis
Croup
Epiglottitis
Pneumonia
Upper respiratory infection

Cardiovascular System

Myocarditis
Pericarditis
Endocarditis

Genitourinary System

Urinary tract infection
Tubo-ovarian abscess

Gastrointestinal Tract

Acute viral gastroenteritis
Bacterial enteritis
Appendicitis

Focal Soft Tissue Infections

Cellulitis

Musculoskeletal System

Osteomyelitis
Septic arthritis

Rheumatologic Disorders

Acute rheumatic fever
Juvenile rheumatoid arthritis
Henoch-Schönlein purpura

Vasculitis

Behçet's syndrome

Malignancy

Leukemia
Lymphoma
Sarcoma

Systemic Illness

Bacteremia
Viremia
Sepsis
Kawasaki's disease
Toxic shock syndrome
Rocky Mountain spotted fever
Meningococcemia

Miscellaneous Disorders

Toxicologic
- Anticholinergic toxidromes
- Salicylate overdose
- Amphetamine
- Cocaine

Endocrine
- Thyrotoxicosis

fever.[5] For positive urine cultures, the patient's symptoms affect disposition. In the setting of persistent fever, the child should be admitted for sepsis evaluation and parenteral antibiotics. In the afebrile and well-appearing child, outpatient management with oral antibiotics is a reasonable management plan. Follow-up studies, including repeat cultures of the urine and blood as well as voiding cystourethrogram and renal ultrasound scanning, should be arranged.

In children 3 to 36 months of age, clinical impression and the patient's temperature guide management decisions. Toxic-appearing children with fever should be admitted and treated. Well-appearing children with a temperature lower than 39° C should be treated with antipyretics and may be discharged. Laboratory testing should be held in these patients, and parents should be provided with instructions to return if these patients have persistent fever or a deterioration in their condition. In the well-appearing child with a temperature higher than 39° C, the guidelines for urine testing and chest radiography outlined in Boxes 172-5 and 172-6 should

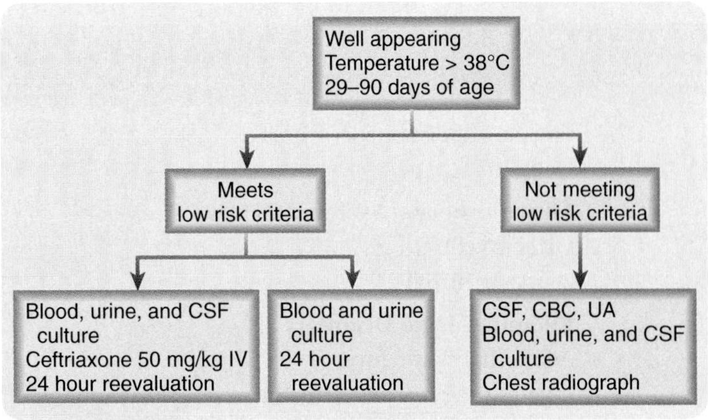
Well appearing
Temperature > 38°C
29–90 days of age
Meets low risk criteria
Not meeting low risk criteria
Blood, urine, and CSF culture
Ceftriaxone 50 mg/kg IV
24 hour reevaluation
Blood and urine culture
24 hour reevaluation
CSF, CBC, UA
Blood, urine, and CSF culture
Chest radiograph

FIGURE 172-1 Approach to the diagnosis of pediatric fever. CBC, complete blood count; CSF, cerebrospinal fluid; IV, intravenously; UA, urinalysis. (From Baraff LJ: Management of fever without source in infants and children. Ann Emerg Med 2000;36:605.

BOX 172-4

Low-Risk Criteria for Febrile Infants

Clinical Criteria

Term infant, previously healthy, without complications

Well appearing

Lack of focal bacterial infection on examination (except for otitis media)

Laboratory Criteria

White blood cell count 5 to 15,000/mm^3, 1500 bands/mm^3, or band-to-neutrophil ratio less than 0.2

Urine: Gram stain of unspun urine negative, or leukocyte esterase and nitrate negative, or fewer than 5 white blood cells/high-power field

Cerebrospinal fluid: fewer than 8 white blood cells/mm^3 and Gram stain negative

From Baraff LJ: Management of fever without source in infants and children. Ann Emerg Med 2000;36:605.

BOX 172-5

Indications for Common Diagnostic Tests in Children with Fever

Urinalysis, Gram Stain, and Culture

Circumcised male infants less than 1 year of age[5,8,12]

Uncircumcised male infants less than 2 years of age[5,8,12]

Female children between 2 months and 2 years of age with two or more of the following risk factors:

- Temperature 39°C of higher
- Fever for 2 days or longer
- White race
- Age less than 1 year
- Absence of another source of fever

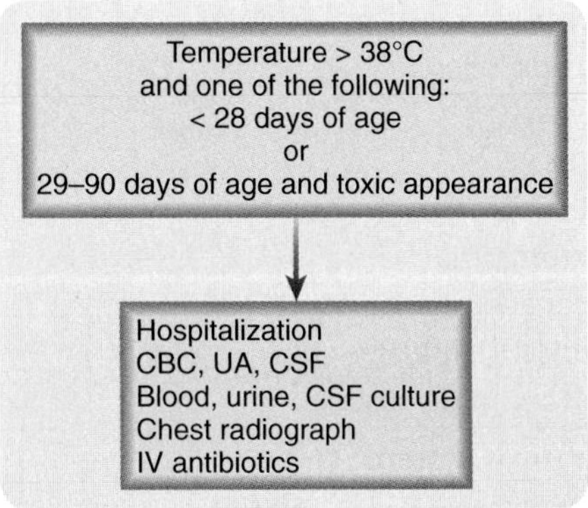
Temperature > 38°C
and one of the following:
< 28 days of age
or
29–90 days of age and toxic appearance
Hospitalization
CBC, UA, CSF
Blood, urine, CSF culture
Chest radiograph
IV antibiotics

FIGURE 172-2 Treatment approach in pediatric fever. CBC, complete blood count; CSF, cerebrospinal fluid; IV, intravenously; UA, urinalysis. (From Baraff LJ: Management of fever without source in infants and children. Ann Emerg Med 2000;36:605.)

BOX 172-6

Chest Radiograph

Should be obtained in children less than 3 months of age who have evidence of acute respiratory illness

Is usually not indicated in febrile children older than 3 months of age with a temperature lower than 39°C and a lack of significant clinical findings of acute pulmonary disease*

*Significant respiratory findings are defined as tachypnea, rales, rhonchi, retractions, grunting, wheezing, stridor, nasal flaring, cough, decreased breath sounds, and pulse oximetry less than 95% on room air.[17,23,29-30]

be followed. Regardless of the management approach chosen, close outpatient follow-up should be ensured, and the patient's parents should be provided with clear instructions that describe when to return to the ED for reevaluation. Box 172-7 provides information to provide the parent, and see also the Patient Teaching Tips, Tips and Tricks, and Red Flags boxes.

Fever is a common presenting complaint in the ED in children less than 36 months of age. Secondary to

BOX 172-7

Information for the Parent

GOALS FOR CARE AT HOME

1. Reduce the temperature
   a. Appropriate dosing and intervals of administration of antipyretics based on information written on the label and the child's weight
2. Maintain hydration
   a. Persistent or worsening vomiting and/or diarrhea
   b. Signs of dehydration
      i. Decreased urine output or tears
      ii. Sunken eyes
      iii. Dry diapers
3. Monitor for worsening or life-threatening illness and return immediately to the ED for
   a. Changes in level of alertness (lethargy, irritability, or inconsolability)
   b. Signs of increased work of breathing (grunting; retracting; nasal flaring; rapid, shallow, or difficult respirations)
   c. Bilious vomiting
   d. Seizure
   e. Purple or red rash
   f. Persistent headache

PATIENT TEACHING TIPS

Explain to the caretaker that a fever in the absence of a serious bacterial illness is not harmful.

Explain how to take a temperature properly.

It is best to take the infant's or toddler's temperature rectally.

Hold the child belly down on your lap.

Lubricate the thermometer with water-soluble jelly.

Spread the buttocks and insert the lubricated thermometer approximately 1 inch into the rectum.

Antipyretics

Explain that many formulations of acetaminophen are available and that parents should pay close attention to the dose and frequency on the label to ensure appropriate dosing.

Tips and Tricks

Perform most of the physical examination with the child in the parent's lap.

Begin with less noxious components of the examination and proceed gradually to those that may be upsetting to the child (i.e., the pulmonary, cardiac, and neurologic components of the physical examination are performed before the abdominal, tympanic, and pharyngeal components).

Attempt to calm the fussy or uncooperative child through feeding, the use of antipyretics, or the aid of the child life team.

RED FLAGS

Meningeal signs are not highly reliable in the first 12 to 16 months of life.

Remember to document the child's general appearance carefully.

Do not rely overly on the white blood cell count to determine the extent of an evaluation in an infant.

In cases in which the reliability of the caregiver is in question, it is safer to admit the patient. Indicators of unreliable follow-up are as follows:

- Young parents
- Parents without access to transportation
- Caretakers who do not feel their child is ill[31]

Close (next day) and reliable follow-up is important.

- Whenever possible consult with the infant's pediatrician to obtain information regarding parental reliability, to discuss evaluation, and to arrange close follow-up.
- In cases in which follow-up is uncertain, extensive evaluation and admission are reasonable.

PRIORITY ACTIONS

Administer appropriate doses of antipyretics early in the patient's evaluation (acetaminophen, 15 mg/kg, or ibuprofen, 10 mg/kg).

When indicated, antibiotics should be administered as early in the patient's evaluation as possible.

Ensure close, reliable follow-up. When follow-up is uncertain, consider more extensive evaluation and hospital admission.

the Hib and, more recently, the pneumococcal vaccines, the incidence of occult bacteremia has become less prevalent. As such, evaluation and management of the febrile infant and child are evolving. The rate and degree of evolution have yet to be determined.

REFERENCES

1. Baraff LJ, Bass JW, Fleischer GF, et al: Practice guideline for the management of infants and children 0 to 36 months of age with fever without source: Agency for Healthcare Policy and Research. Ann Emerg Med 1993;22:1198-1210.
2. McCarthy PL: Fever. Pediatr Rev 1998;19:401-407.
3. Petersen-Smith A, Barber N, Coody D, et al: Comparison of aural infrared with traditional rectal temperatures in children from birth to age three years. J Pediatr 1994;125: 83-85.
4. Grover G, Berkowitz CD, Lewis RJ, et al: The effects of bundling on infant temperature. Pediatrics 1994;94: 669-673.
5. Baraff LJ: Management of fever without source in infants and children. Ann Emerg Med 2000;36:602-614.
6. Dagan R, Powell KR, Hall CB, Menegus MA: Identification of infants unlikely to have serious bacterial infection although hospitalized for suspected sepsis. J Pediatr 1985;10:855-860.
7. Baker MD, Bell LM, Avner JR: Outpatient management without antibiotics of fever in selected infants. N Engl J Med 1993;329:1437-1441.
8. American College of Emergency Physicians Clinical Policies Committee: Clinical policy for children younger than three years presenting to the emergency department with fever. Ann Emerg Med 2003;42:530-545.
9. Lee G, Harper MD: Risk of bacteremia for febrile young children in the post-*Haemophilus influenzae* type B era. Arch Pediatr Adolesc Med 1998;152:624-628.
10. Alpern ER, Alessandrini EA, Bell LM, et al: Occult bacteremia from a pediatric emergency department: Current prevalence, time to detection, and outcome. Pediatrics 2000;106:505-511.
11. Lee GM, Fleisher GR, Harper MB: Management of febrile children in the age of the conjugate pneumococcal vaccine: A cost-effectiveness analysis. Pediatrics 2001;108:835-844.
12. Baraff LJ: Clinical policy for children younger than three years presenting to the emergency department with fever [editorial]. Ann Emerg Med 2003;42:4:546-549.
13. Kuppermann N: Occult bacteremia in young febrile children. Pediatr Clin North Am 1999;46:1073-1109.
14. Mackowiak PA: Concepts of fever. Arch Intern Med 1998;158:1870-1881.
15. Saper CB, Breder CDL: The neurologic basis of fever. N Engl J Med 1994;330:1880-1886.
16. McCarthy PL, Lembo RM, Fink HD, et al: Observation, history, and physical examination in diagnosis of serious illnesses in febrile children less than or equal to 24 months. J Pediatr 1987;110:26-30.
17. Steere M, Sharieff GQ, Stenklyft PH: Fever in children less than 36 months of age: Questions and strategies for management in the emergency department. J Emerg Med 2003;25:149-157.
18. Gorelick MH, Shaw KN: Clinical decision rule to identify febrile young girls at risk for urinary tract infection. Arch Pediatr Adolesc Med 2000;154:386-390.
19. American Academy of Pediatrics Committee on Quality Improvement, Subcommittee on Urinary Tract Infection: Practice parameter: The diagnosis, treatment, and evaluation of the initial urinary tract infection in febrile infants and young children. Pediatrics 1999;103:843-852.
20. Bonsu BK, Chb M, Harper MB: Identifying febrile young infants with bacteremia: Is the peripheral white blood cell count an accurate screen? Ann Emerg Med 2003;42: 216-225.
21. Bonsu BK, Harper MB: Utility of the peripheral blood white blood cell count for identifying sick young infants who need lumbar puncture. Ann Emerg Med 2003;41:206-214.
22. Bonsu BK, Harper MB: A low peripheral blood white blood cell count in infants younger than 90 days increases the odds of acute bacterial meningitis relative to bacteremia. Acad Emerg Med 2004;11:1297-1301.
23. Taylor JA, Del Beccaro M, Done S, et al: Establishing clinically relevant standards for tachypnea in febrile children younger than 2 years. Arch Pediatr Adolesc Med 1995;149:283-287.
24. Bachur R, Perry H, Harper MB: Occult pneumonias: Empiric chest radiographs in febrile children with leukocytosis. Ann Emerg Med 1999;33:166-173.
25. McCarthy PL, Spiesel SZ, Stashwick CA, et al: Radiographic findings and etiologic diagnosis in ambulatory childhood pneumonias. Clin Pediatr 1981;20:686-691.
26. Davies HD, Wang EE, Manson D, et al: Reliability of the chest radiograph in the diagnosis of lower respiratory infections in young children. Pediatr Infect Dis J 1996;15:600-604.
27. Kramer MS, Roberts-Brauer R, Williams RL: Bias and "overcall" in interpreting chest radiographs in young febrile children. Pediatrics 1992;90:11-13.
28. Baker MD, Fosarelli PD, Carpenter RO: Childhood fever: Correlation of diagnosis with temperature response to acetaminophen. Pediatrics 1987;80:315-318.
29. Bramson RT, Meyer TL, Silbiger ML, et al: The futility of the chest radiograph in the febrile infant without respiratory symptoms. Pediatrics 1993;92:524-526.
30. Leventhal JM: Clinical predictors of pneumonia as a guide to ordering chest roentgenograms. Clin Pediatr 1982;21: 730-734.
31. Scarfone RJ: Compliance with scheduled visits to a pediatric emergency department [abstract]. Acad Emerg Med 1994;1:41A.

Chapter 173

Meningitis, Encephalitis, and Brain Abscess

Amandeep Singh and Susan B. Promes

KEY POINTS

Acute bacterial meningitis is associated with a 20% mortality rate, and up to one third of survivors will experience permanent neurologic disability.

Prompt recognition and rapid diagnostic evaluation by the ED health care provider combined with appropriate and timely administration of parenteral antibiotics and adjunctive therapy are critical for treatment success.

Encephalitis refers to inflammation of the brain parenchyma and is typically characterized by cognitive deficits. Herpes simplex virus (HSV) is the most common cause of non-epidemic, acute focal encephalitis in the United States.

The most common causes of brain abscesses in immunocompetent adults are otitis media, mastoiditis, sinusitis, and odontogenic infection. Cyanotic congenital heart disease is a major risk factor for development of brain abscesses in infants and children.

Meningitis

■ EPIDEMIOLOGY

In the United States, several important epidemiologic changes in the nature of bacteria responsible for meningitis have been noted, including a decrease in the rate of infection from group B *Streptococcus* and *Listeria monocytogenes,* universal immunization against *Streptococcus pneumoniae, Haemophilus influenzae* type B (Hib), and *Neisseria meningitidis,* and the development of multidrug-resistant *S. pneumoniae* (MDRSP).

Two of the common pathogens responsible for early-onset neonatal meningitis have been targeted by the Centers for Disease Control and Prevention (CDC). In 2002, the CDC released revisions to the 1996 guidelines regarding maternal screening and intrapartum antibiotics for female patients colonized with group B *Streptococcus.* Early reports on the efficacy of improved surveillance and routine treatment resulted in a 65% decrease in the rate of early-onset neonatal group B *Streptococcus* disease.[1] Additionally, enhanced efforts aimed at prevention and improvements in food processing and food safety led to a decrease in the rate of listeriosis, a foodborne illness occurring as a result of *L. monocytogenes.*[2]

Routine immunization against the three most common bacterial agents responsible for meningitis in children and adults *(S. pneumoniae,* Hib, and *N. meningitidis)* resulted in a significant decrease in the rate of invasive infections with these organisms. *Invasive disease* is defined by the isolation of bacteria from a normally sterile site, such as sputum, blood, or cerebrospinal fluid (CSF). Before the widespread use of conjugate vaccines, Hib was the most common cause of bacterial meningitis in the United States. Routine clinical use of the Hib conjugate vaccine resulted in a 94% decrease in the rate of Hib meningitis among children less than 5 years of age.[3] Since the introduction of the Hib vaccine, bacterial meningitis has become primarily a disease of adults; the median age shifted from 15 months in 1986 to 25 years in 1995.

Like the Hib vaccine, the heptavalent conjugate pneumococcal vaccine, introduced in 2000, has been found to be highly effective in preventing invasive pneumococcal infection in young children. This newer vaccine has been associated with a 60% reduction in pneumococcal meningitis in children less than 5 years old.[4] In children less than 2 years old, vaccination has been reported to be greater than 90% effective in preventing invasive pneumococcal disease. An added benefit of this agent has been a decline in the incidence of invasive pneumococcal disease in other age groups, most likely the result of decreased transmission from infants and children, who may act as a reservoir for the organism.

The Food and Drug Administration has approved a more recently developed quadrivalent conjugate meningococcal vaccine for routine immunization of preteens and young adults. This vaccine offers protection against four of the five most common meningococcal serogroups that result in invasive disease in the United States, and it is projected to reduce the overall incidence of invasive meningococcal disease by 75% to 90%.[5] In 2005, the Advisory Committee on Immunization Practices to the CDC recommended routine immunization for children aged 11 and 12 years, teens entering high school, and college freshmen living in dormitories. Meningococcal vaccine has also been recommended for members of high-risk groups: military recruits living in barracks, immunocompromised individuals, and travelers to areas with endemic meningococcal disease.

The third important recent epidemiologic change in the bacteria responsible for meningitis has been the development of a strain of *S. pneumoniae* that is resistant to multiple antibiotics (i.e., MDRSP). A study conducted in 1999 through 2000 revealed that 35% of *S. pneumoniae* clinical isolates were penicillin resistant, and 20% were highly resistant.[6] This finding represented a 10% increase in the rate of MDRSP compared with data obtained just 5 years earlier. Concern regarding this organism prompted a change in the recommendations for empirical antibiotics to include vancomycin in children and adults with suspected meningitis. Although the rate of MDRSP has been reported to be increasing, in 2003 the rate of MDRSP in the United States returned to a level of 20%, possibly because of the efficacy of the heptavalent pneumococcal vaccine.[7]

■ TYPICAL PRESENTING SIGNS AND SYMPTOMS

The classic presentation of acute bacterial meningitis is rapid development of fever, accompanied by neck stiffness, severe headache, and mental confusion. However, this constellation of symptoms is seen in fewer than 50% of the patients presenting to the ED.[8,9] Although 95% of patients present with at least two of the four cardinal clinical features, more subtle presentations can be seen in infants, elderly patients, and immunocompromised patients.

Fever occurs in approximately 85% of patients.[8] The fever seen with meningitis is often higher than 38°C, but hypothermia has also been reported. In a large series of patients recorded with acute bacterial meningitis, the average temperature on presentation was 38.8±1.2°C.[9] The onset of acute bacterial meningitis is often quite rapid, with symptoms developing and progressing over the first 24 hours in nearly 50% of patients.[9] An extremely rapid progression of symptoms developing over a few hours can be seen in patients with meningococcal disease.

Although neck pain may be infrequently reported, the objective finding of neck stiffness is seen in more than 70% of patients.[8] Examining the neck for rigidity, during gentle forward flexion, with the patient in the supine position best assesses neck stiffness. Difficulty in lateral motion of the neck is a less reliable finding. Patients with severe meningeal irritation may spontaneously assume the tripod position with the knees and hips flexed, the back arched lordotically, the neck extended, and the arms brought back to support the thorax. Vladimir Kernig and Joseph Brudzinski signs may also indicate meningeal irritation. The *Kernig sign* is performed with the patient lying supine and the hip flexed to 90 degrees. A positive sign is present when extension of the knee from this position elicits resistance or pain in the lower back or posterior thigh. The classic *Brudzinski sign* refers to spontaneous flexion of the knees and hips during attempted passive flexion of the neck. A separate sign described by Brudzinski, the *contralateral reflex,* is present if passive flexion of one hip and knee causes flexion of the contralateral leg. The presence or absence of Kernig or Brudzinski signs has been shown to have little positive or negative predictive value in the diagnosis of meningitis, until severe meningeal inflammation is present.[10]

The headache associated with meningitis is often described as severe and generalized. It is frequently accompanied by nausea, vomiting, and photophobia. Worsening of the headache while the examiner rapidly turns the patient's head from side to side (at a rate of two to three times per second), the so-called *jolt accentuation test,* has been reported to have good sensitivity for CSF pleocytosis in patients who present with headache and fever without evidence of intracranial disease on a computed tomography (CT) scan.[11]

Nearly two thirds of patients ultimately diagnosed with acute bacterial meningitis will exhibit an alteration in mental status on presentation to the ED.[8] Most patients display some amount of mental confusion; however, up to 15% of patients will present with a Glasgow Coma Scale score lower than 8.[9] Subtle changes in the patient's mental status may be apparent to family and friends, but they may not be

Tips and Tricks

SEASONAL VARIATION IN MENINGITIS

- Summer/fall: Enterovirus, arbovirus
- Late winter/early spring: Mumps (95% reduction in incidence with routine immunization)
- Late fall/winter: Lymphocytic choriomeningitis virus

obvious to an unacquainted clinician. Focal neurologic deficits are seen in up to one third of patients on presentation, and 7% of patients present with hemiparesis. Aphasia is noted in nearly one fourth of patients on presentation.[9]

Although one or more of the classic findings on history (fever, altered mental status, headache) or physical examination (nuchal rigidity) may be absent in many patients with acute bacterial meningitis, virtually all patients have at least one of the findings of the classic triad of fever, neck stiffness, and altered mental status. The absence of all these findings is thought to exclude the diagnosis of acute bacterial meningitis.[9]

Other signs and symptoms associated with acute bacterial meningitis include papilledema, seizure, and rash. More than 90% of cases involving a rash, most often petechial or palpable purpura, are seen in patients with *N. meningitidis.*[9] Rarely, infection with *N. meningitidis* can manifest with signs of kidney or adrenal failure.

ATYPICAL PRESENTING SIGNS AND SYMPTOMS

Acute bacterial meningitis may manifest with more subtle signs and symptoms in infants, elderly persons, and immunocompromised patients. Infants can present with fever or hypothermia, hypoglycemia, poor sucking, or irritability (excessive crying), and they may have generalized body stiffness or bulging fontanelles on physical examination. Mothers of infants who develop these symptoms less than 1 month after delivery should be checked for group B *Streptococcus,* human immunodeficiency virus (HIV), and HSV-2.

Elderly and immunocompromised patients may also present atypically. These populations are associated with a higher rate of misdiagnosis, contributing to an increase in the morbidity and mortality following an episode of acute meningitis. A lower proportion of fever, headache, nausea, or vomiting is present in these groups. Neck stiffness has a lower sensitivity and specificity for meningitis in elderly patients. Finally, these populations may present to the ED with isolated altered mental status but without a fever.

DIAGNOSTIC TESTING

Although the CT scan is commonly obtained initially, it is an imperfect test to determine impending brain herniation. The 2004 Infectious Disease Society of America Practice Guidelines for the Management of Bacterial Meningitis recommended that a CT scan be performed before lumbar puncture (LP) in the following conditions: immunocompromised state (e.g., HIV infection or acquired immunodeficiency syndrome, immunosuppressive therapy, after organ transplantation), history of central nervous system (CNS) disease (mass lesion, stroke, focal infection), new-onset seizure (≤1 week of presentation), papilledema, abnormal level of consciousness, and focal neurologic deficit.[12]

LP with CSF analysis is the most important diagnostic test. If LP is delayed by the need for cranial imaging, blood cultures should be obtained without delay. Antibiotics and adjunctive dexamethasone should be administered empirically before the imaging study in high-risk patients.

The diagnosis of bacterial meningitis rests on CSF examination. However, CSF analysis cannot reliably distinguish bacterial meningitis from aseptic meningitis.[13] Analysis of the CSF should include Gram stain and culture, white blood cell (WBC) count and differential, and glucose and protein concentrations. In acute bacterial meningitis, the opening pressure is usually elevated to 200 to 500 mm H_2O (normal opening pressure, <170 mm H_2O), although values may be lower in neonates, infants, and children. Between 15% and 20% of adults with bacterial meningitis have a normal CSF opening pressure.[9] The appearance of the CSF can range from clear to cloudy, depending on the presence of significant concentrations of WBCs, red blood cells, bacteria, and protein. The CSF WBC count can be significantly elevated, usually in the range of 1000 to 5000 cells/mm^3, although this range can be quite broad (<100 to >10,000 cells/mm^3). Approximately 20% of adults with bacterial meningitis have CSF WBC counts lower than 1000 cells/mm^3, and one third of these adults have a CSF WBC count of less than 100 cells/mm^3.[9] Bacterial meningitis usually leads to a neutrophil predominance in CSF, typically between 80% and 95%; approximately 10% of patients with acute bacterial meningitis present with a lymphocyte predominance (defined as >50% lymphocytes or monocytes) in CSF, more commonly seen in *L. monocytogenes* and neonatal meningitides. A urinary reagent strip to determine the presence of leukocyte esterase can be used as a marker for the presence of WBCs in the CSF.

The CSF glucose concentration is lower than 40 mg/dL in 50% to 60% of patients; a ratio of CSF to serum glucose of 0.4 was 80% sensitive and 98% specific for the diagnosis of bacterial meningitis in children more than 2 months old. Because the ratio of CSF to serum glucose is higher in term neonates, a ratio of 0.6 is considered abnormal in this patient group. The CSF protein concentration is elevated to more than 50 mg/dL in virtually all patients with bacterial meningitis.

Gram stain of the CSF is useful because it may reveal the nature of the organism in 80% of culture-positive cases and in up to 10% of culture-negative specimens. Gram-positive diplococci suggest pneumococci; gram-negative diplococci suggest meningococci; small pleomorphic gram-negative coccobacilli suggest *H. influenzae;* gram-positive rods and coccobacilli suggest *L. monocytogenes.* The yield of positive CSF cultures falls to less than 50% in patients previously treated with antibiotics, although change in the CSF inflammatory indices is often insignificant.

Blood cultures are often positive, and cultures should be obtained whenever possible before administration of antibiotics. Approximately 50% to 75% of patients with bacterial meningitis have positive blood cultures. However, the yield of these cultures, similar to the yield of CSF cultures, decreases with time after antibiotic administration. Specific tests for tuberculosis, HIV infection, cryptococcosis, syphilis, and Lyme disease are indicated based on clinical suspicion.

Latex agglutination, enzyme immunoassay, enzyme-linked immunoassay, and, more recently, polymerase chain reaction (PCR), for detection of bacterial antigens may become useful to the EP, especially in cases associated with a negative Gram stain. Some of the latest experimental tests to help in distinguishing pyogenic from aseptic meningitis include CSF lactate, procalcitonin, and some cytokines or specialized stains such as ethidium bromide.

■ TREATMENT AND DISPOSITION

Infants less than 1 month of age are treated with the combination of ampicillin and cefotaxime. From 1 month to 50 years of age, a regimen of ceftriaxone, 50 mg/kg intravenously (IV) (maximum dose, 2 g) every 12 hours, in addition to vancomycin, 15 mg/kg IV (maximum dose, 500 mg) every 6 hours, is most commonly used. Adults older than 50 years of age and patients who have other debilitating associated disease or impaired cellular immunity are treated with ampicillin, 50 mg/kg IV (maximum dose, 3 g) every 6 hours, in addition to ceftriaxone and vancomycin. After neurosurgery, head trauma, or cochlear implantation, patients are treated with vancomycin in addition to cefepime, 50 mg/kg IV (maximum dose, 2 g) every 8 hours, or ceftazidime, 50 mg/kg IV (maximum dose, 2 g) every 8 hours. In patients in whom encephalitis cannot be ruled out based on history, physical examination, or CSF findings, empirical administration of acyclovir may be warranted.

Antibiotics should not be delayed for CT or LP in patients with high clinical suspicion of acute bacterial meningitis. Although no prospective clinical data are available on the relationship of the timing of antibiotics to clinical outcome in patients with bacterial meningitis, several retrospective reviews examined this issue and concluded that an association may exist between delayed administration of antibiotics and worse overall outcome.[14]

Treatment with high-dose dexamethasone (0.15 mg/kg IV, maximum dose 10 mg every 6 hours) before or concurrent with the first dose of antibiotics is thought to attenuate the inflammatory response and to lead to better outcome in children (excluding neonates) and adults with meningitis.[15] However, the clinical studies that argue for the routine use of dexamethasone were all conducted before the age of routine immunization against the three most common microbes responsible for acute bacterial meningitis.

Chemoprophylaxis is indicated for high-risk contacts (e.g., household, school, or work contacts) of patients with documented *N. meningitidis* or Hib infection, including health care providers who intubated the patient without first donning a face mask. Other health care providers do not require prophylaxis. First-line treatment is with rifampin 10 mg/kg IV (to a maximum of 600 mg per dose) every 12 hours for four doses. Alternatives are ceftriaxone, ciprofloxacin, and sulfisoxazole.

All patients with acute bacterial meningitis should be admitted to the hospital. In young, otherwise healthy, immunocompetent patients with viral meningitis, home management may be an option. Often, however, it is difficult to establish the diagnosis of viral meningitis definitively in the ED, and patients are admitted to the hospital pending CSF and blood culture results.

The overall prognosis of acute bacterial meningitis is poor. Mortality rates range from less than 5% for infection with *H. influenzae* to 10% with *N. meningitidis* to 20% with *S. pneumoniae.* Predictors of unfavorable outcome include the following: infection with *S. pneumoniae* (presence of otitis media or sinusitis, absence of rash, positive blood cultures), advanced age (>60 years); altered mental status, obtundation, or low Glasgow Coma Sale score on admission; heart rate greater than 120 beats per minute; hypotension; seizures within the first 24 hours of admission; a CSF WBC count lower than 1000 cells/mm^3, an elevated erythrocyte sedimentation rate; and a reduced platelet count.[9]

During hospitalization, focal neurologic deficits are seen in 50% of patients, and seizures occur in 15% of patients. Cardiopulmonary failure occurs in nearly 30% of patients and mechanical ventilation is required in almost 25% of patients. Two thirds of patients with acute bacterial meningitis have mild or no disability using a Glasgow outcome scale. Approximately 15% of patients have moderate to severe disability following infection. The most common neurologic findings on discharge are as follows: eighth nerve cranial palsy, which occurs in nearly 15% of survivors; hemiparesis, occurring in 4% of survivors; and sixth nerve cranial palsy, occurring in 3% of survivors.[9] Aphasia, quadriparesis, third nerve cranial palsy, and seventh nerve cranial palsy are all rare.

ETIOLOGY

The causes of meningitis are listed in Box 173-1.

Aseptic Meningitis

Aseptic meningitis, identified by the clinical syndrome of meningitis in the absence of positive bacterial cultures, is most often the result of viral infection. However, certain diseases other than viral meningitis can manifest with a clinical picture of meningitis and negative routine bacterial cultures, including mycobacterial and fungal meningitis, drug-induced meningitis, autoimmune or neoplastic processes, and parameningeal sources such as epidural abscess. Viral meningitis results in 36,000 hospitalizations per year. However, many cases go unrecognized or are underreported, and some patients are discharged home from an ED or a hospital clinic. Numerous viruses produce aseptic meningitis, the most common of which are enteroviruses (e.g., echovirus, coxsackievirus). As many as 75,000 cases (90% of cases of viral

BOX 173-1

Etiology of Meningitis

Medications

Immunosuppressive medications
Nonsteroidal anti-inflammatory drugs
Anticancer drugs

Parasites

Trichinella
Ascaris
Toxoplasma
Cysticercus
Toxocara

Bacteria

Viruses

Enterovirus (Coxsackievirus, Echovirus, Poliovirus)
Most common (>80%); summer
Incidence highest in children (age <15 years)
Often during epidemics
Associated signs: exanthemata, hand-foot-mouth disease, pleurodynia, myopericarditis, or hemorrhagic conjunctivitis
Diagnosis: CSF PCR

Arbovirus
Common; summer and early fall
Localized geographic epidemics
Transmitted by mosquitoes or ticks
Manifesting as viral meningitis or encephalitis; may mimic Lyme disease or Rocky Mountain spotted fever
Diagnosis: positive blood, stool, or CSF culture

Herpes Simplex Virus Type 2
Common; any time of year
Associated with primary HSV-2 genital infection in 35% of women and 11% of men
20% have recurrent attacks of HSV-2 meningitis
Onset may be preceded by genital or pelvic pain or associated with vesicular genital lesions
Rarely causes encephalitis, so acyclovir therapy not required?
Diagnosis: CSF PCR

Human Immunodeficiency Virus
Common; any time of year
Known HIV infection or HIV risk factors
Aseptic meningitis in 5% to 10% of primary infections
Often follows mononucleosis-like syndrome
Clues include rash, lymphadenopathy, mucous membrane lesions, splenomegaly
If HIV serology negative, assay for p24 antigen in serum or CSF

Lymphocytic Choriomeningitis Virus
Less common; fall and winter
Exposure to rodents
Rash, alopecia, parotitis, orchitis, myopericarditis
CSF: lymphocytosis, low glucose (30%)
Lab: leucopenia, thrombocytopenia, abnormal liver function tests
Pulmonary infiltrates
May have marked CSF pleocytosis (>1000 cells/mm^3)
CSF culture usually positive

Mumps
Less common; winter and spring
Nonvaccinated population
CSF: low glucose, high neutrophilic pleocytosis (25%)
Parotitis (50%), orchitis, oophoritis, pancreatitis
Elevated amylase and lipase (30%, nonspecific)
Diagnosis: with or without positive throat, urine, or CSF culture
Follow-up seroconversion

CSF, cerebrospinal fluid; HIV, human immunodeficiency virus; HSV-2, herpes simplex virus type 2; PCR, polymerase chain reaction.

meningitis) of enteroviral meningitis are estimated to occur each year in the United States. Bacterial meningitis cannot be differentiated from aseptic meningitis on clinical grounds alone.

- Specific diagnosis depends on the isolation of the virus or positive results on immunoassay of the CSF.
- It is difficult to distinguish early or partially treated bacterial meningitis from viral meningitis based on CSF alone.
- PCR for enterovirus has reported sensitivities greater than 85% in identifying a viral cause in viral meningitis.
- Depending on the diagnostic certainty, various practice ranges can be used in the management of presumed viral meningitis, from admission with empirical antibiotic therapy until culture results are known to discharge from the ED with 24-hour follow-up.

Encephalitis

EPIDEMIOLOGY

Encephalitis refers to inflammation of brain parenchyma that may coexist with inflammation of the meninges (meningoencephalitis) or spinal cord (encephalomyelitis). More than 20,000 identified cases of encephalitis occur in the United States annually, and many more cases are underreported or unrecognized. Viral infection is the most common identifiable cause of encephalitis, although infection with bacteria and other microbes has also been described, as well as noninfectious processes. The clinical presentation of encephalitis overlaps with that of meningitis, and it is often difficult to distinguish between the two entities because many patients have symptoms of both brain parenchymal and meningeal processes. Classically, patients with bacteriologically sterile CSF who present with a predominance of neuropsychiatric symptoms and a lack of signs of meningeal irritation are identified as having encephalitis.

Many viruses can result in infection of the brain parenchyma, and many can also cause aseptic meningitis. However, certain viruses are more likely to cause encephalitis and are responsible for the majority of cases. Most cases of encephalitis in the United States are caused by enteroviruses, HSV-1 and HSV-2, or arboviruses, which are transmitted from infected animals to humans through the bite of an infected tick, mosquito, or other blood-sucking insect.[16] Rare causes in the United States include human herpesvirus 6, respiratory viruses such as parainfluenza virus and respiratory syncytial virus, hepatitis viruses A and B, HIV-1, and rabies virus. Infection with *Borrelia burgdorferi* (Lyme disease) or *Rickettsia rickettsii* (Rocky Mountain spotted fever) can result in bacterial encephalitis.[17]

PATHOPHYSIOLOGY

At least three important viruses (rabies, HSV-1, and varicella-zoster virus) reach the CNS by traveling within axons from a distal site, where they gain access to nerve endings. Data from experimental cases using an animal model and from human cases suggest that the olfactory tract is one route of access of HSV to the brain. Rabies infection begins with transmission of the virus from the saliva within a bite from an infected animal to a human host. Following local viral replication within skin and muscle tissue, the virus is taken up by peripheral nerve cells. The virus is then transmitted in retrograde fashion by axoplasmic flow. Following a dormant period, the virus rapidly disseminates throughout the CNS.

SIGNS AND SYMPTOMS

Significant clinical overlap exists in the acute presentation of bacterial infection resulting in meningitis and of viral infection resulting in encephalitis. Both conditions can manifest with fever, headache, altered mental status, and focal neurologic deficits. In general, symptoms and signs of meningeal irritation (e.g., nuchal rigidity) are present in patients with acute meningitis and meningoencephalitis but are characteristically absent in encephalitis. The clinical course of symptoms with encephalitis may be slow or rapidly progressive. Encephalitis should be considered in patients presenting with the following clinical features, singly or in combination: new psychiatric symptoms, cognitive defects, and focal or diffuse neurologic signs such as hemiparesis or seizure. Patients with encephalitis usually have prominent cognitive and mental changes such as lethargy, aphasia, amnestic syndrome, confusion, stupor, or even coma. Seizures and postictal states can be seen in meningitis alone and should not be construed as

FACTS AND FORMULAS $SI = \frac{SV}{BSA}$

ENCEPHALITIS

Herpes simplex virus is the most common cause of nonepidemic, acute focal encephalitis in the United States.

RED FLAGS

Encephalitis

- Admit all patients with suspected meningoencephalitis.
- A primary psychiatric diagnosis should be considered in patients with bizarre behavior only after organic causes are excluded.

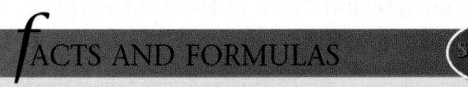

Tips and Tricks

ENCEPHALITIS

- The initial Gram stain can be used to tailor early treatment in patients with meningoencephalitis.
- Urine dipstick can be used to determine the presence of white blood cells in cerebrospinal fluid.
- An additional 2 to 3 mL of cerebrospinal fluid can be used for special viral studies in patients with meningoencephalitis and a negative Gram stain.

definitive evidence of encephalitis. Several historical, physical examination, imaging, or laboratory clues can help the practitioner to narrow the etiologic agent in patients with signs and symptoms of encephalitis.

DIAGNOSTIC TESTING

Routine blood tests, including a complete blood count, electrolytes, renal and liver function tests, and glucose concentrations, are not helpful in establishing the diagnosis of encephalitis and are performed to exclude alternative diagnoses. Tests for antinuclear antibodies and double-stranded DNA are obtained to exclude lupus cerebritis. Thyroid function tests and HIV and syphilis tests can be ordered if clinically indicated.

A noncontrast CT scan of the brain should be performed in patients suspected of having encephalitis with altered mental status or focal neurologic deficit before LP. Although it is often normal in this disease process, a CT scan may show diffuse cerebral edema or, in HSV encephalitis specifically, focal edema, with or without parenchymal hemorrhages, in the frontal and temporal lobe. Magnetic resonance imaging (MRI) is considered more sensitive and is the preferred imaging method in patients with suspected encephalitis.

The findings on CSF analysis of patients with encephalitis may be close to normal or similar to those see in viral infections causing aseptic meningitis (increased CSF WBC count, usually <250 cells/mm^3, normal or mildly elevated CSF protein <150 mg/dL, or normal or mildly reduced CSF glucose). CSF should be sent for routine analysis to exclude bacterial meningitis. In addition, viral cultures should be obtained and sent for analysis by PCR, if available. The yield of CSF viral cultures is often low; however, isolation and amplification of specific viral DNA by PCR are diagnostic. Electroencephalographic findings are usually abnormal in patients with encephalitis. HSV encephalitis produces a pathognomonic electroencephalographic pattern of periodic, usually asymmetrical sharp waves, in the setting of acute febrile encephalopathy.[18]

Documentation

ENCEPHALITIS

- Include the differential diagnosis of meningitis.
- Document consultations and review of initial lumbar puncture results.

TREATMENT AND DISPOSITION

Empirical treatment of HSV-1 infection with acyclovir (10 mg/kg IV every 8 hours) should be considered in patients with signs and symptoms of acute encephalitis and a negative CSF Gram stain. Before the advent of routine treatment with antiviral therapy, untreated mortality for HSV-1 encephalitis was greater than 70%, and only 2% to 5% of the survivors returned to a normal lifestyle. Current survival rates for HSV-1 encephalitis in children and adults treated with acyclovir is greater than 70%.[18]

A reasonable approach to immunocompetent patients with high suspicion for meningoencephalitis consists of empirical treatment with ceftriaxone, 50 mg/kg IV (maximum dose, 2 g) every 12 hours, in addition to vancomycin, 15 mg/kg IV (maximum dose, 500 mg) every 6 hours, and acyclovir, 10 mg/kg IV every 8 hours, along with adjunctive pretreatment with high-dose dexamethasone, 0.15 mg/kg IV (maximum dose, 10 mg) every 6 hours. These therapies should be initiated after blood cultures are obtained but before CT or LP is performed. Acyclovir can be discontinued in patients with a positive Gram stain for bacterial organisms, whereas dexamethasone can be discontinued for patients with a negative Gram stain for bacterial organisms.

The overall risks of death and morbidity from encephalitis are 3% to 4% and 7% to 10%, respectively. These rates are greatly influenced by the microbiology of the infectious organism and the immune response elicited by the infected host. Infections with rabies, the virus responsible for Eastern Equine encephalitis, HSV-1, and HSV-2 and infections in neonates, children, elderly persons, or immu-

PRIORITY ACTIONS

Encephalitis

- Consider immediate endotracheal intubation in patients with altered mental status.
- Patients with fever and altered mental status or focal neurologic deficit require a rapid diagnostic evaluation including computed tomography of the head and lumbar puncture.
- Obtain blood cultures before administering therapy.

PATIENT TEACHING TIPS

ENCEPHALITIS

- Prognosis of encephalitis depends on the specific etiologic agent and on the host (e.g., age, immunocompromise).
- Permanent neurologic sequelae (e.g., altered mental status, bizarre behavior, seizures, neurologic deficits) are common even in patients treated with acyclovir following herpes simplex virus encephalitis.
- Some encephalitides are associated with complete recovery without sequelae.
- Acute disseminated encephalomyelitis is a neurologic disorder that resembles multiple sclerosis in its presentation but can be distinguisted by associated encephalitis symptoms.

nocompromised patients are all associated with a poor outcome.

Significant lifelong morbidity may be present following acute encephalitis. In one series examining outcome after acyclovir-treated HSV encephalitis, 40% of surviving patients at 1 month had moderate to severe disability using the Glasgow outcome scale. Nearly 70% of the long-term survivors reported memory impairment, and 45% had a personality or behavioral abnormality. Severe anxiety, impaired concentration, insomnia, irritability, fatigue, poor motivation, and emotional lability were noted by 20% to 35% of the patients.[18]

Brain Abscess

EPIDEMIOLOGY

A *brain abscess* is a focal, intracerebral infection that begins as a localized area of cerebral inflammation and develops into a collection of pus surrounded by a well-vascularized capsule. These infections can occur in an age group, but they are relatively uncommon in infants younger than 2 years of age. Up until the last century, this diagnosis was nearly uniformly fatal; however, as a result of improvements in early recognition by cranial imaging, improved CNS penetration of antibiotics, and advanced neurosurgical drainage techniques, the current case fatality rate is less than 30%. The incidence of neurologic sequelae in patients who survive a brain abscess ranges from 30% to 60%.[19]

Bacterial species are the most common infectious agents responsible for brain abscesses. However, fungal and other atypical organisms can be seen in immigrants and immunocompromised patients. Most bacterial brain abscesses contain several mixed pathogens. Various aerobic and microaerophilic streptococcal species (e.g., *S. milleri, S. pneumoniae, S. pyogenes*), often in combination with *Haemophilus influenzae,* and anaerobes such as *Bacteroides* species and *Prevotella* species are cultured from brain abscess in patients with concurrent sinus or middle ear infections. *Staphylococcus aureus* is seen in patients with concurrent skin or soft tissue infection, endocarditis, or recent cranial trauma.[20]

PATHOPHYSIOLOGY

Microorganisms reach the brain by several different mechanisms. The most common pathogenic mechanism is spread from a contiguous focus of infection, such as otitis media, mastoiditis, sinusitis, meningitis, or odontogenic infection. Although by no means diagnostic, specific sites within the brain may give a clue to the site of infection. Frontal lobe abscess are often seen in patients with dental infections or paranasal sinus infection, whereas temporal lobe abscess are seen in patients with otitis or sphenoid sinus infection.

Brain abscesses may also develop following hematogenous seeding from a remote infection, such as lung abscess or empyema, infected heart valve, skin or soft tissue infection, osteomyelitis, or abdominal or pelvic infection. Cyanotic congenital heart disease, the most common predisposing risk factor in brain abscess in children, accounts for as much as 25% of the cases of brain abscesses in some pediatric case series. The new onset of a headache in these pediatric patients often requires imaging to exclude brain abscess. Brain abscesses are uncommonly associated with bacterial endocarditis.

The third mechanism by which bacteria can seed the brain parenchyma is through cranial trauma resulting from a penetrating or blunt mechanism with associated skull fracture or recent neurosurgical procedure. In 15% to 20% of all brain abscesses, the source of the infection remains unknown.

SIGNS AND SYMPTOMS

The presenting symptoms of a brain abscess are often nonspecific and vary according to multiple factors: abscess size, location, and number; age and past medical history of the patient (e.g., history of immunosuppression); host response and severity of edema; and virulence of infection. Typically, the diagnosis may be initially missed in the ED, and the patient may return for a subsequent visit when symptoms persist. On average, the diagnosis is made 13 to 14 days after the onset of symptoms, although symptoms can last from a few hours to several months. The most common signs and symptoms associated with brain abscess are headache, mental status change, focal neurologic deficit, and fever. The clinical triad of headache, fever, and focal deficit is present in less than 50% of cases.[19]

Headache is the most common presenting symptoms and is observed in approximately 70% of patients. The headache is described as constant, progressive in intensity, and moderately to severely painful; it may be hemicranial or generalized. Sudden worsening of the headache, accompanied by new onset of meningismus, may signify rupture of the abscess into the ventricular space, a life-threatening complication. Alteration in mental status or focal neurologic deficit may range in severity from confusion and drowsiness to obtundation and coma. Fever is absent in half the cases and is low grade (<101.5°F) in the other half. Other possible signs and symptoms include nausea, vomiting, seizures, nuchal rigidity, and papilledema.

■ DIAGNOSTIC TESTING

The routine use of CT and MRI scanning has dramatically affected the diagnosis and management of brain abscesses. Although CT scanning is not as sensitive as MRI, it is most often the initial imaging modality because it can more easily be obtained in the ED. In practice, an initial noncontrast head CT is often obtained, followed by a contrast-enhanced head CT for patients in whom the diagnosis is suspected.

Routine laboratory studies are not usually helpful in the diagnosis of brain abscess. Leukocyte counts are normal or only mildly elevated (<15,000 cells/mm^3) in 60% to 70% of cases. The erythrocyte sedimentation rate is elevated in up to 90% of patients, but it is nonspecific. Elevated C-reactive protein has been described as a method to distinguish brain abscess from brain tumor. Blood cultures are reported to be positive in 15% of cases.

■ TREATMENT AND DISPOSITION

Successful ED management of confirmed intracranial abscess involves parenteral antibiotic administration and neurosurgical consultation. The choice of initial antibiotics is based on the probability of specific pathogens, based on presumed mechanism of bacterial seeding within the cranium. The combination of a penicillin G (3 to 4 million units IV every 4 hours) or a third-generation cephalosporin (cefotaxime, 50 mg/kg IV [maximum dose, 2 g] every 4 to 6 hours, or ceftriaxone, 50 mg/kg IV [maximum dose, 2 g] every 12 hours) and metronidazole (15 mg/kg IV load, then 7.5 mg/kg IV every 6 to 8 hours) can be used in most patients presumed to have a contiguous source of infection (e.g., ear, sinus, or dental infection). Nafcillin, 50 mg/kg IV (maximum dose, 2 g) every 4 hours, or oxacillin, 50 mg/kg IV (maximum dose, 2 g) every 4 hours, should be added when *S. aureus* is a consideration (e.g., after surgery or trauma, concurrent skin or soft tissue infection). Vancomycin, 15 mg/kg IV (maximum dose, 500 mg) every 6 hours, should be substituted for nafcillin or oxacillin in areas with high rates of methicillin-resistant *S. aureus*.

The neurosurgeon needs to be contacted at the time of initial diagnosis of a brain abscess. Surgical drainage of the abscess generally is required for both diagnosis and for tailoring antibiotic therapy. Emergency neurosurgical drainage is considered in patients with signs of increased intracranial pressure; otherwise, patients may be observed for clinical response to parenteral antibiotics.

Corticosteroids (dexamethasone, 10 mg IV load followed by 4 mg IV every 6 hours) are beneficial in reducing edema and mass effect, but their use in the management of brain abscess is controversial. These agents may decrease antibiotic penetration into the CNS. However, some neurosurgeons believe that this treatment should be tried when substantial mass effect is thought to cause neurologic deficits or obtundation.[21]

Patients with the diagnosis of brain abscess should be admitted to the intensive care unit. Mortality rates from brain abscess currently range from 0% to 30%.[22] Poor prognostic factors for recovery include rapid progression of the infection before hospitalization, severe mental status changes on admission, stupor or coma, and abscess rupture into the ventricle. The most common neurologic sequelae are seizures, which are seen in up to 60% of survivors. Up to 50% of patients may suffer long-term neurologic deficit and disability depending on their age and the location of the abscess. Recurrence rates are 5% to 10% despite adequate treatment, and most recurrences are seen within 6 weeks.

REFERENCES

1. Centers for Disease Control and Prevention: Prevention of perinatal group B streptococcal disease: Revised guidelines from the CDC. MMWR Morb Mortal Wkly Rep 2002;51:1-22.
2. Centers for Disease Control and Prevention: Preliminary Foodnet data on the incidence of infection with pathogens transmitted commonly through food: 10 sites, United States, 2004. MMWR Morb Mortal Wkly Rep 2004;54: 352-356.
3. Schuchat A, Robinson K, Wenger JD, et al: Bacterial meningitis in the United States in 1995. Active Surveillance Team. N Engl J Med 1997;337:970-976.
4. Whitney CG, Farley MM, Hadler J, et al: Decline in invasive pneumococcal disease after the introduction of protein-polysaccharide conjugate vaccine. N Engl J Med 2003;348:1737-1746.
5. Mitka M: New vaccine should ease meningitis fears. JAMA 2005;293:1433-1434.
6. Bonthius DJ, Karacay B: Meningitis and encephalitis in children: An update. Neurol Clin North Am 2002;20: 1013-1038.
7. Kyaw MH, Lynfield R, Schaffner W, et al: Effect of introduction of the pneumococcal conjugate vaccine on drug-resistant *Streptococcus pneumoniae.* N Engl J Med 2006;354: 1455-1463.
8. Attia J, Hatala R, Cook DJ, Wong JG: The rational clinical examination: Does this adult patient have acute meningitis? JAMA 1999;282:175-181.
9. van de Beek D, de Gans J, Spanjaard L, et al: Clinical features and prognostic factors in adults with bacterial meningitis. N Engl J Med 2004;351:1849-1859.
10. Thomas KE, Hasbun R, Jekel J, Quagliarello VJ: The diagnostic accuracy of Kernig's sign, Brudzinski's sign, and nuchal rigidity in adults with suspected meningitis. Clin Infect Dis 2002;35:46-52.
11. Uchihara T, Tsukagosi H: Jolt accentuation of headache: The most sensitive sign of CSF pleocytosis. Headache 1991;31:167-171.

12. Tunkel AR, Hartman BJ, Kaplan SL, et al: Practice guidelines for the management of bacterial meningitis. Clin Infect Dis 2004;39:1267-1284.
13. Graham TP: Myth: Cerebrospinal fluid analysis can differentiate bacterial meningitis from aseptic meningitis. CJEM 2003;5:348-349.
14. Lepur D, Barsić B: Community-acquired bacterial meningitis in adults: antibiotic timing in disease course and outcome. Infection 2007;35:225-231.
15. van de Beek D, de Gans J, McIntyre P, Prasad K: Steroids in adults with acute bacterial meningitis: A systematic review. Lancet Infect Dis 2004;4:139-143.
16. Whitley RJ, Gnann JW: Viral encephalitis: Familiar infections and emerging pathogens. Lancet 2002;359:507-514.
17. Willoughby RE Jr: Encephalitis, meningoencephalitis, and postinfectious encephalomyelitis. In Long SS (ed): Principles and Practice of Pediatric Infectious Disease, 2nd ed. New York, Churchill Livingstone, 2003.
18. McGrath N, Anderson NE, Croxson MC, Powell KF: Herpes simplex encephalitis treated with acyclovir: Diagnosis and long-term outcome: J Neurol Neurosurg Psychiatry 1997;63:321-326.
19. Trunkel AR, Wispewey B, Scheld WM: Brain abscess. In Mandell GL, Bennett JE, Dolin R (eds): Principles and Practice of Infectious Diseases, 5th ed. New York, Churchill Livingstone, 2000.
20. Brook I: Microbiology and management of brain abscess in children. J Pediatr Neurol 2004;2:125-130.
21. Whitfield P: The management of intracranial abscess. ACNR 2005;5:12-15.
22. Goodkin HP, Harper MB, Pomeroy SL: Intracerebral abscess in children: Historical trends at Children's Hospital Boston. Pediatrics 2004;113:1765-1770.

Chapter 174

Sepsis

Michael J. Schmidt

KEY POINTS

Sepsis encompasses a spectrum of diseases: infection with signs of a systemic inflammatory response, severe sepsis, and septic shock.

Although most patients presenting with sepsis are usually ill, some may appear quite well. In the well-appearing patient, a lactate level may be more helpful than the clinical appearance.

Treatment in the ED includes early, presumptive administration of antibiotics and early, aggressive fluid resuscitation to optimize resuscitation.

Patients with severe sepsis and septic shock must be monitored closely and should be admitted to an intensive care unit setting.

Background

In the United States alone, more than 750,000 cases of sepsis occur, and approximately 215,000 deaths result from this disease annually.[1] Over the 25-year period between 1972 and 1997, essentially no change occurred in mortality rates (ranging from 40% to >60%) for patients with septic shock.[2] More recent advances in the early treatment of severe sepsis and septic shock have shown improvements in mortality and thus promise for patients and their treating physicians.[3-5]

Definitions of Sepsis

Sepsis is defined as a condition in which an identified or suspected source of infection leads to a systemic inflammatory process, known as the *systemic inflammatory response syndrome* (SIRS) (Box 174-1). *Severe sepsis* refers to sepsis that has progressed to cellular dysfunction and organ damage or evidence of hypoperfusion, whereas *septic shock* refers to sepsis with persistent hypotension despite adequate fluid resuscitation.

Pathophysiology

SIRS can develop when an exaggerated response of the body's immune system to infection occurs. As the immune cells encounter the organisms' endotoxins, inflammatory cytokines such as tumor necrosis factor-alpha, interleukin-1, and interleukin-6 are released.[6] Theses cytokines can lead to activation of the coagulation cascade with subsequent thrombosis and disseminated intravascular coagulation.[4] This cytokine cascade also leads to the release and activation of nitric oxide, thought to be the key mediator involved in vasodilation and shock.[7]

■ SOURCES OF INFECTION

The underlying cause of sepsis remains the infection itself. Several studies have shown similar results

BOX 174-1

Definition of Systemic Inflammatory Response Syndrome

The presence of two or more of the following four items constitutes sepsis:

Temperature lower than 36° C or higher than 38° C

Heart rate greater than 90 beats per minute

Respiratory rate greater than 20 breaths per minute or partial pressure of arterial carbon dioxide lower than 32 mm Hg

White blood cell count lower than 4000 or higher than 12,000 cells/mm^3 or more than 10% bands

BOX 174-2

Most Common Sites of Infection (in Order of Frequency)

Lung (pneumonia)

Abdominopelvic region

Urinary tract

Soft tissue (cellulitis)

Other (blood, central nervous system [meningitis], bone [osteomyelitis], joint, cardiac [endocarditis])

regarding the most common sites of infection (Box 174-2).[4,5,8]

Clinical Presentation

The classic patient with severe sepsis or septic shock will appear ill, with fever (less commonly hypothermic) and chills, an increased respiratory rate, and tachycardia. Patients may have cold skin showing outward signs of decreased perfusion (Fig. 174-1*A*), and they may have mental status changes.

The presentation may or may not direct the clinician to the potential source of infection. For example, a patient with dyspnea and crackles on a lung examination may point to pneumonia, or a patient with left lower quadrant tenderness on an abdominal examination may point to diverticulitis as the source. It may be difficult to determine the site of infection in the ED, and even retrospectively, an initial source is not determined in up to 15% of patients.[8]

More objective measures (SIRS criteria, lactate level) are used to determine whether a patient has sepsis because patients can sometimes appear surprisingly well even when they have severe sepsis or septic shock. Their only complaint may be fever, even though other SIRS criteria and hypotension may be present, especially in relatively younger, healthier, immunocompetent patients (Fig. 174-1*B*).

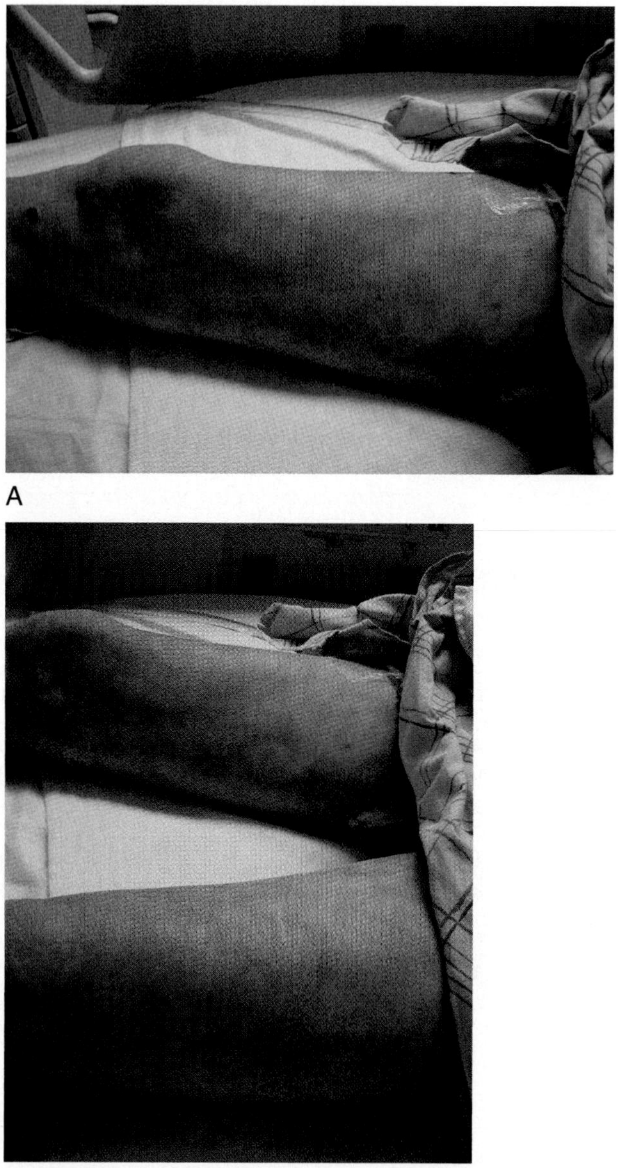

A

B

FIGURE 174-1 **A** and **B,** Skin mottling. This patient presented to the ED with septic shock and showed extreme signs of hypoperfusion. He underwent early-goal directed therapy and actually survived to discharge from the hospital.

Differential Diagnosis

The differential diagnosis of sepsis includes many other life-threatening emergencies, including toxidromes (sympathomimetic, anticholinergic), thyrotoxicosis or myxedema coma, neuroleptic malignant syndrome, heat stroke, withdrawal (ethanol, sedative-hypnotics), pulmonary embolism, and other causes of shock (anaphylactic, cardiogenic, hypovolemic).

Diagnostic Testing

The diagnostic work-up may vary among patients, but most require the following: blood cultures (before antibiotic administration), lactic acid level, complete blood count, chemistry panel, urinalysis, urine culture, chest radiograph, and prothrombin time/partial thromboplastin time (if concern exists about disseminated intravascular coagulation). Further work-up should be guided by the suspected source of infection. For example, concern about a possible abdominopelvic infection (e.g., diverticulitis or acute cholecystitis) may warrant a computed tomography scan of the abdomen or pelvis or a right upper quadrant ultrasound scan, whereas concern about a possible central nervous system infection (e.g., meningitis) may warrant lumbar puncture. The diagnostic evaluation is important, but aggressive treatment in advance of test results is essential.

Treatment Interventions, Procedures, and Resuscitation

Intubation may be necessary to provide airway protection (i.e., for decreased mental status) or to decrease the work of breathing and improve oxygenation. Etomidate causes measurable, but transient, adrenal suppression (see Chapter 169), but the use of a single dose of etomidate as an induction agent in the ED to facilitate rapid-sequence intubation remains clinically indicated.[9] Hydrocortisone or dexamethasone (4 mg intravenously) can be considered in patients with persistent hypotension unresponsive to fluids.

High-volume fluid resuscitation is required for patients with sepsis, even frail elderly patients, so two large-bore intravenous lines are required. Aggressive resuscitation with intravenous crystalloid (or colloid) fluids should be initiated immediately. The administration of 2 L of normal saline, or a 20 to 30 mL/kg bolus of fluids, is a good starting point.

Central venous access can be established to monitor central venous pressures, to administer intravenous fluids and medications such as vasopressors, and to obtain mixed venous oxygen saturation measurements. Foley catheterization should be performed to monitor urine output. All patients should have continuous cardiac monitoring and pulse oximetry.

Specific Therapies

■ SEPSIS BUNDLES

The Institute for Healthcare Improvement (IHI) has developed recommendations for early, initial treatment of the patient with severe sepsis or septic shock (Box 174-3).[10] These recommendations are based on the best current available evidence from the Surviving Sepsis Campaign's management guidelines.[11]

BOX 174-3

Institute for Healthcare Improvement Sepsis Resuscitation Bundle

A. Serum lactate measured
B. Blood cultures obtained before antibiotic administration
C. Antibiotics administered within 3 hours of ED presentation
D. In the event of hypotension or lactate greater than 4 mmol/L (36 mg/dL):
   1. Deliver an initial minimum of 20 mL/kg of crystalloid (or colloid equivalent).
   2. Apply vasopressors for hypotension not responding to initial fluid resuscitation to maintain mean arterial pressure higher than 65 mm Hg.
E. In the event of persistent hypotension despite fluid resuscitation or lactate greater than 4 mmol/L (36 mg/dL):
   1. Achieve central venous pressure higher than 8 mm Hg.
   2. Achieve central venous oxygen saturation greater than 70%.

From Institute for Healthcare Improvement: Sepsis (2006). Available at http://www.ihi.org/IHI/Topics/CriticalCare/Sepsis

■ ANTIMICROBIAL THERAPY

Patients should receive antibiotic coverage, early and presumptively. Coverage should be directed at the source, if known, but broad-spectrum antibiotics are generally advisable. Although the evidence used to support the timing of antibiotic administration is limited,[12,13] early administration likely favors improved outcomes.

■ EARLY GOAL-DIRECTED THERAPY

Early goal-directed therapy has generated great interest and is influencing treatment for patients with severe sepsis or septic shock.[3] Mortality is reduced by early identification of patients with severe sepsis (identified as patients with lactic acid >4 mmol/L) or septic shock (identified as systolic blood pressure <90 mm Hg after 20 to 30 mL/kg of fluid) and by early aggressive hemodynamic monitoring and optimization using specific resuscitation end points (central venous pressure, mean arterial pressure, mixed venous oxygen saturation). Early goal-directed therapy is summarized in Figure 174-2.

■ VASOPRESSORS

In patients with persistent hypotension (mean arterial pressure <65 mm Hg or systolic blood pressure

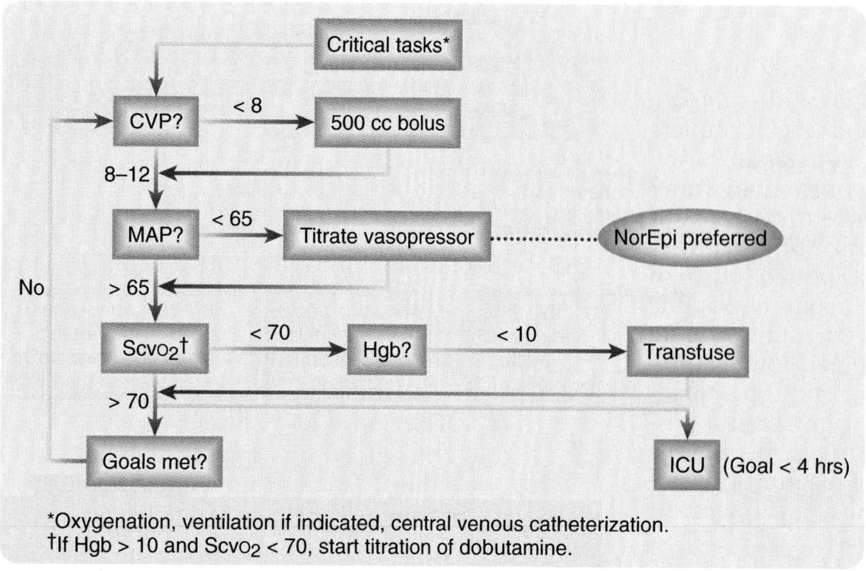
Critical tasks*
CVP?
< 8
500 cc bolus
8–12
MAP?
< 65
Titrate vasopressor
NorEpi preferred
No
> 65
Scvo2†
< 70
Hgb?
< 10
Transfuse
> 70
Goals met?
ICU (Goal < 4 hrs)
*Oxygenation, ventilation if indicated, central venous catheterization.
†If Hgb > 10 and Scvo2 < 70, start titration of dobutamine.

FIGURE 174-2 Early goal-directed therapy. CVP, central venous pressure; Hgb, hemoglobin; ICU, intensive care unit; MAP, mean arterial pressure; NorEpi, norepinephrine; $Scvo_2$, central venous oxygen saturation.

<90 mm Hg) despite initial fluid resuscitation (20 to 30 mL/kg), vasopressors should be used to help maintain organ perfusion. First-line agents include norepinephrine, at 2 to 20 µg/minute, or dopamine, at 5 to 20 µg/kg/minute.[11] Limited evidence indicates that norepinephrine (Levophed) may improve survival in patients with septic shock who require vasopressor therapy,[14,15] and that this agent may be better at correcting hypotension while avoiding the potential tachycardia seen with dopamine and epinephrine. Vasopressin, at 0.01 to 0.04 U/minute, can be considered as an additional agent in patients with hypotension refractory to initial vasoactive medications, because it appears to have synergistic effects.[16] Other second-line agents that can be considered include phenylephrine and epinephrine.

■ LOW-DOSE CORTICOSTEROIDS AND ACTIVATED PROTEIN C

Although these treatments are somewhat less conducive to administration in the ED, they have shown mortality benefit in randomized controlled trials.[4,5] Patients with septic shock who do not respond to a corticotropin stimulation test may benefit from intravenous hydrocortisone (200 to 300 mg/day as a continuous infusion or as 50-mg boluses). If adrenal suppression is highly suspected and an immediate corticotropin stimulation test is not practical or available, dexamethasone can be considered so as not to interfere with further testing.

Activated protein C promotes fibrinolysis and inhibits thrombosis and inflammation. Recombinant human activated protein C, or drotrecogin alfa (activated), can be considered in high-risk patients with severe sepsis or septic shock. Identification of appropriate patients (APACHE II ≥25), contraindications (risk of bleeding), and cost currently limit the utility of this agent in the ED.

Disposition

Patients with severe sepsis or septic shock warrant admission to an intensive care unit setting. An elevated lactate level is evidence of hypoperfusion. Patients without evidence of hypoperfusion, end-organ damage, or hypotension may be admitted to a medical ward. Close monitoring of all patients is warranted because signs and symptoms can progress.

REFERENCES

1. Angus DC, Linde-Zwirble WT, Lidicker J, et al: Epidemiology of severe sepsis in the United States: Analysis of incidence, outcome, and associated costs of care. Crit Care Med 2001;29:1303-1310.
2. Friedman G, Silva E, Vincent JL: Has the mortality of septic shock changed with time? Crit Care Med 1998;26: 2078-2086.
3. Rivers E, Nguyen B, Havstad S, et al: Early goal-directed therapy in the treatment of severe sepsis and septic shock. N Engl J Med 2001;345:1368-1377.
4. Bernard GR, Vincent JL, Laterre PF, et al: Efficacy and safety of recombinant human activated protein C for severe sepsis. N Engl J Med 2001;344:699-709.
5. Annane D, Sebille V, Charpentier C, et al: Effect of treatment with low doses of hydrocortisone and fludrocortisone on mortality in patients with septic shock. JAMA 2002;288:862-871.
6. Bone RC, Grodzin CJ, Balk RA: Sepsis: A new hypothesis for pathogenesis of the disease process. Chest 1997;112:235-243.
7. Vincent JL, Zhang H, Szabo C, Preiser JC. Effects of nitric oxide in septic shock. Am J Respir Crit Care Med 2000;161: 1781-1785.
8. Bernard GR, Reines HD, Halushka PV, et al: The effects of ibuprofen on the physiology and survival of patients with sepsis. N Engl J Med 1997;336:912-918.
9. Ray DC, McKeown DW: Effect of induction agent on vasopressor and steroid use, and outcome in patients with septic shock. Crit Care 2007;11:R56 [Epub ahead of print].
10. Institute for Healthcare Improvement. Sepsis (2006). Available at http://www.ihi.org/IHI/Topics/CriticalCare/Sepsis

11. Dellinger RP, Carlet JM, Masur H, et al: Surviving Sepsis Campaign guidelines for management of severe sepsis and septic shock. Intensive Care Med 2004;30:536-555.
12. Kumar A, Roberts D, Wood KE, et al: Duration of hypotension before initiation of effective antimicrobial therapy is the critical determinant of survival in human septic shock. Crit Care Med 2006;34:1589-1596.
13. Houck PM, Bratzler DW, Nsa W, et al: Timing of antibiotic administration and outcomes for Medicare patients hospitalized with community-acquired pneumonia. Arch Intern Med 2004;164:637-644.
14. Martin C, Viviand X, Leone M, Thirion X: Effect of norepinephrine on the outcome of septic shock. Crit Care Med 2000;28:2758-2765.
15. Martin C, Papazian L, Perrin G, et al: Norepinephrine or dopamine for the treatment of hyperdynamic septic shock? Chest 1993;103:1826-1831.
16. Landry DW, Levin HR, Gallant EM, et al: Vasopressin pressor hypersensitivity in vasodilatory septic shock. Crit Care Med 1997;25:1279-1282.

Chapter **175**

Infections in the Immunocompromised Host

Fredrick M. Abrahamian

KEY POINTS

Neutropenia is a significant risk factor for infections in patients with malignancies. Empirical antibiotic therapy should be administered to all neutropenic febrile patients and afebrile neutropenic patients who have signs and symptoms consistent with infection.

Neutropenia is defined as a neutrophil count of less than 500 cells/mm^3 or a count of less than 1000 cells/mm^3 with a predicted decrease to less than 500 cells/mm^3.

Splenectomized patients are at higher risk of fulminant infection by *Streptococcus pneumoniae, Haemophilus influenzae,* or *Neisseria meningitidis.*

Prolonged corticosteroid therapy (greater than 3 to 4 weeks) at doses of more than 20 mg per day places the patient at risk for hypothalamic-pituitary-adrenal suppression and infectious complications.

Malignant otitis externa, rhinocerebral mucormycosis, emphysematous pyelonephritis, emphysematous cholecystitis, and Fournier's gangrene occur predominantly in diabetic patients.

Scope

Immunocompromised patients frequently visit EDs for evaluation and treatment for a variety of conditions. Infectious complications are common, and they are a diagnostic priority because clinical presentations are often subtle and atypical. This chapter covers infections in patients with malignancies, patients receiving immunosuppressive and corticosteroid therapy, patients who have undergone solid organ or bone marrow transplantation, and diabetic patients. Human immunodeficiency virus infection is discussed in Chapter 177.

Malignancy

Patients with malignant diseases are predisposed to infections from a variety of organisms including bacterial, fungal, and viral pathogens. Patients with malignancy are more prone to infections because of impairment of normal host defenses (e.g., neutropenia associated with acute leukemia), complications associated with tumor growth and spread (e.g., bronchial obstruction from bronchogenic carcinoma resulting in pneumonia), the use of chemotherapeutic agents and corticosteroids, history of splenectomy, and infections associated with intravascular catheters or other implanted devices.[1]

Neutropenia is a significant risk factor for infections in patients with malignancies, and it can be a result of the condition itself (e.g., acute leukemia) or a consequence of the myelosuppressive effects of agents used in disease management. Fever associated with neutropenia is often a presenting sign in patients receiving cancer chemotherapy.

The 2002 guidelines by the Infectious Disease Society of America (IDSA) for the use of antimicrobial agents in neutropenic patients with cancer defined neutropenia as a neutrophil count of less than 500 cells/mm^3 or a count of less than 1000 cells/mm^3 with a predicted decrease to less than 500 cells/mm^3.[2] The frequency and severity of infection are inversely proportional to the neutrophil count, and susceptibility to infection increases when the neutrophil count falls to less than 1000 cells/mm^3.[3] In addition, vulnerability to infection increases with longer periods of neutropenia. The same guidelines also defined fever, in the absence of obvious environmental causes, as a single oral temperature measurement of 38.3° C (101° F) or higher or a temperature of 38.0° C (100.4° F) or higher for at least 1 hour.[2]

Because neutropenic patients may have fever as their only presenting feature of infection, and because they may lack other specific clinical manifestations, the initial evaluation often includes broad diagnostic testing, including serum chemistry, complete blood cell count, liver and renal function tests, urinalysis, blood and urine cultures, and radiographic evaluations (e.g., plain chest radiographs). Cellulitis, pustulation, or lymphadenopathy may be diminished. A pulmonary infiltrate may be absent on initial radiographs. Meningitis and urinary tract infection may cause minimal pleocytosis and pyuria, respectively. Pain at any site should heighten the suspicion of occult infection despite the absence of typical physical signs.

In addition to the neutrophils, other components of cell-mediated immunity such as lymphocytes, monocytes, or macrophages may also become deficient or defective in certain types of cancers (e.g., lymphoma, leukemia, Hodgkin's disease). Myriad organisms may be responsible for infections in patients with these types of cancers that impair cell-mediated immunity[1] (Box 175-1). These patients most often undergo an extensive work-up to establish the etiologic agent of infection. Special attention also needs to be paid to patients who have undergone splenectomy. These patients are at higher risk of developing fulminant infection by *Streptococcus pneumoniae, Haemophilius influenzae,* or *Neisseria meningitidis*.

Intravascular catheters are common in patients with cancer, especially those who are undergoing chemotherapy. When a catheter-related infection is suspected, blood cultures should be simultaneously drawn through the central venous catheter and the peripheral vein, and empirical intravenous antibiotic therapy with vancomycin should be promptly initiated[4] (Box 175-2). Peripheral venous catheters should be removed if the patient shows signs of infection at the exit site (e.g., drainage of pus, erythema) or evidence of septic shock with no other source of infection. Prompt removal of the catheter is also warranted when intravascular catheterization is complicated by septic thrombophlebitis.[4] The diagnosis can be made by ultrasonography with color Doppler imaging. EPs should involve the oncologist and the infectious disease specialist in the decision-making process when considering removal of a central line.

BOX 175-1

Organisms Often Associated with Infections in Patients with Impaired Cell-Mediated Immunity

Bacteria

Nocardia, Salmonella, Listeria, Legionella, Pseudomonas, Mycobacterium species

Fungi

Cryptococcus neoformans, Aspergillus, Candida species

Viruses

Cytomegalovirus, herpes simplex virus, varicella-zoster virus

Parasites

Toxoplasma gondii, Giardia lamblia

INITIAL EVALUATION

Initial laboratory and microbiologic evaluation should include a complete blood cell count and measurement of serum levels of creatinine, blood urea nitrogen, transaminases, and blood cultures. Blood cultures should be drawn before the initiation of antimicrobial therapy. In the presence of a central venous access device, at least one set of blood cultures should be obtained from the device lumen.[4] Urine cultures are indicated if the patient has signs and symptoms of urinary tract infection, if a urinary catheter is present, or if the urinalysis is abnormal. A chest radiograph is indicated if the patient has any respiratory abnormalities or chest discomfort. A negative chest radiograph does not rule out the presence of a pulmonary infection in a neutropenic patient. In this population of patients, multiple studies have shown that high-resolution computed tomography (CT) scanning of the chest is a better diagnostic test than plain chest radiographs for the early detection of pneumonia.[5-7] Unless clinically indicated, routine lumbar puncture and cerebrospinal fluid examination are not recommended.[8]

BACTERIAL INFECTIONS

Approximately 60% of bacterial infections are the result of gram-positive cocci and 35% are from gram-

BOX 175-2

Recommended Initial Antimicrobial Therapy for the Management of Febrile Neutropenic Patients[a]

Oral Therapy[b]

Ciprofloxacin *plus* amoxicillin-clavulanate

Intravenous Monotherapy[c,e,f]

Cefepime, ceftazidime, or carbapenem (e.g., imipenem, meropenem)

Intravenous Combination Therapy[d,e,f]

Aminoglycoside (e.g., gentamicin or tobramycin) *plus* antipseudomonal penicillin (e.g., ticarcillin-clavulanate or piperacillin-tazobactam)

Aminoglycoside (e.g., gentamicin or tobramycin) *plus* cefepime or ceftazidime

Aminoglycoside (e.g., gentamicin or tobramycin) *plus* carbapenem (e.g., imipenem, meropenem)

History of Immunoglobulin E–Mediated Beta-Lactam Allergy

Antipseudomonal aminoglycoside (e.g., gentamicin or tobramycin) or ciprofloxacin *plus* aztreonam with or without vancomycin[e]

[a] Selection of the empirical regimen should be based on knowledge of the local antibiotic susceptibility pattern, prevalence of methicillin-resistant *Staphylococcus aureus* (MRSA) and other resistant organisms within the community, and potential drug interactions and toxicities within each patient.
[b] This approach is indicated only for low risk adult patients (see text and Box 175-4).
[c] Monotherapy is preferred for uncomplicated cases.
[d] Combination therapy is preferred for complicated cases (e.g., shock).
[e] Include vancomycin if you clinically suspect catheter-related infections (e.g., bacteremia, cellulitis) or if the patient has known colonization or suspected infection with penicillin- and cephalosporin-resistant pneumococci or MRSA, hypotension or other evidence of cardiovascular impairment (e.g., septic shock, severe sepsis), a history of prophylaxis with quinolones (for afebrile neutropenic patients before the onset of fever), severe mucositis, and sudden elevation of temperature to more than 40°C.
[f] Add metronidazole if you suspect concomitant anaerobic infection (e.g., oral mucositis, perirectal or intra-abdominal infections).

negative bacilli.[1] Bacteremia complicates approximately 20% of the infections. The most common causes of bacteremia in febrile neutropenic patients are listed in Box 175-3.[2,8] Anaerobes are uncommon culprits of infections in neutropenic patients, except in the presence of clinical features of oral mucositis or perirectal or intra-abdominal infections.[1,9]

■ FUNGAL INFECTIONS

Fungal infections most commonly involve *Candida* and *Aspergillus* species and are typically encountered in patients with prolonged neutropenia, or they are present as secondary infections in patients who have received broad-spectrum antibiotics. Fungal infections can also cause fever following recovery from chemotherapy-induced neutropenia. Candidal infections commonly manifest with thrush and esophagitis, and less frequently with acute disseminated candidiasis. *Aspergillus* infections usually manifest with sinus and pulmonary infections. This organism may also infect catheter sites and the gastrointestinal tract and cause thrombosis and infarction of blood vessels. Both *Candida* and *Aspergillus* are often difficult to grow on blood cultures, and multiple blood cultures, as well as other diagnostic tests (e.g., nasal endoscopy, biopsy of lesions), are often necessary.

BOX 175-3

Most Common Causes of Bacteremia in Febrile Neutropenic Patients

Staphylococcus aureus
Staphylococcus epidermidis
Streptococcus pneumoniae
Streptococcus pyogenes
Viridans streptococci
Enterococcus faecalis
Enterococcus faecium
Corynebacterium species
Escherichia coli
Klebsiella species
Pseudomonas aeruginosa

■ EMPIRICAL TREATMENT

Empirical antibiotic therapy should be administered promptly to all neutropenic febrile patients as well as to afebrile neutropenic patients who have signs and symptoms consistent with infection. Box 175-2 depicts recommended initial antimicrobial therapy for the management of febrile neutropenic patients.[2,8,9] Although the trend has been more toward monotherapy, the 2002 IDSA guidelines[2] recommended combination therapy for complicated cases (e.g., shock). A recently conducted randomized, multicenter trial[10] revealed monotherapy with piperacillin-tazobactam to be efficacious and safe, when compared with monotherapy with cefepime for the empirical treatment of high-risk febrile neutropenic patients with cancer.

Antiviral agents should not be initiated empirically as initial therapy in the ED for all patients with neutropenic fever. However, the presence of lesions resulting from herpes simplex virus or varicella-zoster virus warrants the initiation of antiviral agents (e.g., acyclovir, valacyclovir), even if these pathogens are not suspected as the cause of fever.[2] Cytomegalovirus (CMV) is an uncommon cause of fever in neutropenic patients, unless these patients have undergone bone marrow transplantation. Empirical and routine use of granulocyte or granulocyte colony-stimulating factor transfusions is not recommended by the latest IDSA guidelines.[2]

Antifungal agents (e.g., amphotericin B) should not be initiated empirically in the ED as initial therapy for all patients with neutropenic fever. When considered, administration of an antifungal agent is best done in consultation with specialists. Empirical antifungal therapy is often initiated by the specialist in patients with persistent fever (5 days or more) despite adequate antimicrobial therapy, in whom no specific cause of infection has been found.[2]

BOX 175-4

Factors Associated with a Lower Risk for Complications and a Favorable Prognosis ($P < .001$) in Adult Patients Presenting with Neutropenic Fever

Absolute neutrophil and monocyte counts 100 cells/mm^3 or higher

Age less than 60 and more than 16 years

Cancer in partial or complete remission

No symptoms or only mild to moderate symptoms of illness

Outpatient status at the time of fever onset

Temperature lower than 39.0° C

Normal findings on chest radiographs

Absence of hypotension

Respiratory rate of up to 24 breaths per minute

Absence of chronic pulmonary diseases and diabetes mellitus

Absence of confusion or other signs of mental status alteration

Absence of blood loss and dehydration

No history of fungal infection or receipt of antifungal therapy during the 6 months before presentation with fever

■ ADMISSION

In general, almost all febrile neutropenic patients should be admitted to the hospital (in isolation) for intravenous antibiotic therapy and continued diagnostic work-up. Numerous studies, mostly in adult patients, have looked at the identification of variables and scoring indexes that predict a low risk of severe infection among febrile neutropenic patients[11-13] (Box 175-4). Because of the paucity of data in the pediatric population, the most current IDSA guidelines recommended consideration of oral therapy only in low-risk adults who can be vigilantly observed and who have timely access to continued medical care.[2] If outpatient therapy is considered, EPs should always involve the oncologist and the infectious disease specialist in the decision-making process.

Immunosuppressive and Corticosteroid Therapy

Chemotherapeutic agents induce variable degrees of myelosuppression. These agents can affect both the number and function of various cell lines such as neutrophils, lymphocytes, monocytes, and macrophages. The effect mostly depends on the type of agent and the duration of exposure. Immunosuppression can be prolonged even after completion of therapy. The potential organisms and treatment of neutropenic fever associated with treatment-induced immunosuppression are similar to those when the impairment results from the condition itself (see Boxes 175-1 to 175-3).

Like antitumor agents, corticosteroids can induce myelosuppression of various cell lines (e.g., lymphocytes, macrophages, immunoglobulins) and can increase the susceptibility to infections by various types of organisms. The risk of infection is directly related to the underlying condition, the dose of steroid, and the duration of therapy.[14] Prolonged treatment (greater than 3-4 weeks) at doses of more than 20 mg/day places the patient at risk for hypothalamic-pituitary-adrenal suppression and infectious complications.[14] In addition to pyogenic bacteria, infections can also involve *Mycobacterium*, *Aspergillus*, and *Listeria* species.[15] Because steroids can also suppress fever, the absence of fever does not exclude the possibility of infection. Fever in patients who are receiving long-term steroid therapy is infectious in origin until proven otherwise.

Solid Organ Transplantation

The two major complications of solid organ transplantation are infections and organ rejection. These two entities have similar clinical presentations and are impossible to differentiate with certainty based only on the initial signs and symptoms. When these complications are suspected, the patient should be isolated and admitted to the hospital. Initial evaluation in the ED includes the liberal use of blood tests (e.g., serum electrolytes, complete blood cell count, liver enzymes), urinalysis, cultures, arterial blood gases (especially for patients who have undergone lung transplantation), radiographic evaluations (e.g., plain chest radiographs), and drug levels (e.g., cyclosporine). The transplant team should be notified of the patient's clinical presentation and situation. The choice of antimicrobial therapy depends on the presenting clinical situation. After stabilization, the patient may require transfer to a transplant center for further evaluation.

All solid organ transplant recipients undergo similar immunosuppressive therapies after transplantation, and as a result of these standardized regimens, a predictive temporal pattern of infections (i.e., "timetable of infections") is recognized (Fig. 175-1).[16] This post-transplantation timetable is best divided into three periods: the first month, from 1 to 6 months, and more than 6 months after transplantation. Opportunistic pathogens (e.g., *Pneumocystis carinii, Aspergillus fumigatus, Listeria monocytogenes, Nocardia asteroides*) are more likely to cause infections during the period from 1 to 6 months after transplantation.

Of all the pathogens, CMV is the single most important infectious agent affecting solid organ transplant recipients.[16,17] The onset of infection is usually after the first month of transplantation. The clinical presentation is variable and can range from flulike illness (e.g., fever and myalgia) to pneumonitis and encephalitis. Laboratory abnormalities can include leukopenia, thrombocytopenia, mild atypical lymphocytosis, and mild hepatitis. The transplanted organ is more susceptible to infection by CMV than are native organs. CMV also has immunosuppressive properties that can render patients more susceptible to opportunistic infections.[16,17] The diagnosis is made by either tissue biopsy or demonstration of viremia. For a symptomatic patient with a confirmed diagnosis, the treatment of choice is intravenous ganciclovir.

In transplant recipients, unexplained fever or headache mandates exclusion of central nervous system (CNS) infection. Evaluation should include a CT scan of the head and lumbar puncture. Because of immunosuppression, these patients may not mount a high fever or have signs of meningeal inflammation. Common organisms that cause CNS infections include *A. fumigatus, L. monocytogenes, Cryptococcus neoformans,* herpes viruses (e.g., CMV, Epstein-Barr virus), and *Toxoplasma gondii.*

Aspergillus infections, most often caused by *A. fumigatus*, are associated with a high rate of mortality in solid organ transplantation. This pathogen can be associated with a variety of infections such as fungemia, wound infections, and sinus, pulmonary, and CNS infections. CNS infections caused by *Aspergillus* may be complicated by abscess or aneurysm formation. *Aspergillus* infection, especially the disseminated form, is more often seen in liver transplant recipients.

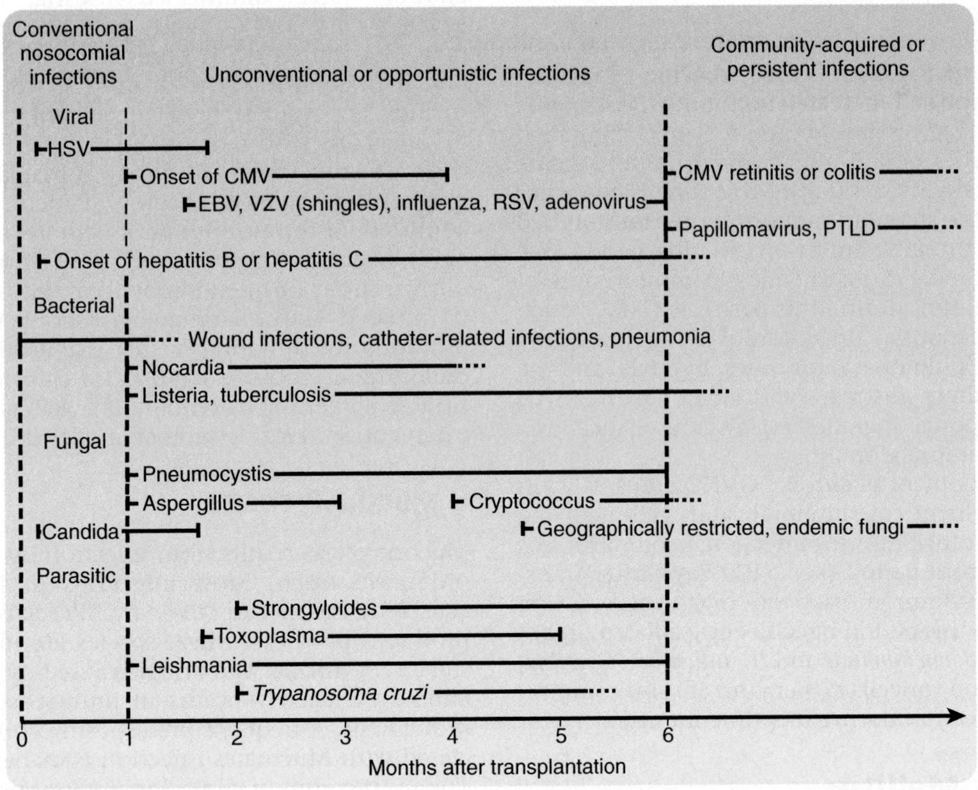
Conventional nosocomial infections
Unconventional or opportunistic infections
Community-acquired or persistent infections
Viral
HSV
Onset of CMV
CMV retinitis or colitis
EBV, VZV (shingles), influenza, RSV, adenovirus
Papillomavirus, PTLD
Onset of hepatitis B or hepatitis C
Bacterial
Wound infections, catheter-related infections, pneumonia
Nocardia
Listeria, tuberculosis
Fungal
Pneumocystis
Aspergillus
Cryptococcus
Candida
Geographically restricted, endemic fungi
Parasitic
Strongyloides
Toxoplasma
Leishmania
Trypanosoma cruzi
0
1
2
3
4
5
6
Months after transplantation

FIGURE 175-1 The usual temporal pattern of infections after organ transplantation. Exceptions to the usual sequence of infections after transplantation suggest the presence of unusual epidemiologic exposure or excessive immunosuppression. CMV, cytomegalovirus; EBV, Epstein-Barr virus; HSV, herpes simplex virus; PTLD, post-transplantation lymphoproliferative disease; RSV, respiratory syncytial virus; VZV, varicella-zoster virus. *Zero* indicates the time of transplantation. *Solid lines* indicate the most common period for the onset of infection; *dotted lines* and *arrows* indicate periods of continued risk at reduced levels. (From Fishman JA, Rubin RH: Infection in organ-transplant recipients. N Engl J Med 1998;338:1741-1751.)

Bone Marrow Transplantation

The risk of infection for the bone marrow transplant recipient depends on various factors such as the extent of immunosuppression before transplantation, the type of the transplant, the occurrence of graft-versus-host disease (GVHD), and the degree of immunosuppressive therapy. GVHD occurs when immunologically functioning cells in the graft attack antigens on the cells in the recipient. The clinical manifestation of GVHD is variable and involves organs such as the skin, the liver, and the gastrointestinal tract. GVHD is associated with profound immunosuppression that further adds to the risk of infectious complications.

As in solid organ transplantation, these patients also have a predictive temporal pattern of host defense defects and infectious complications after bone marrow transplantation. This timetable is also best divided into three periods: the first 30 days, from 31 to 100 days, and more than 100 days after transplantation.[18]

The first 30 days are associated with profound leukopenia, often coupled with absolute neutropenia and lymphocytopenia. During this period, bacteremia is the most common identifiable infectious complication. The bacterial causes, as well as the management of bacterial infections, are similar to those in other neutropenic patients (see Boxes 175-3 and 175-4). *Candida, Aspergillus,* and recurrent herpes infections are also common causes of infection during this period.[18]

The second period, from 31 to 100 days after bone marrow transplantation, is more notable for defects in humoral and cell-mediated immunity. Leukopenia during this stage is less profound when compared with the earlier period after transplantation. Acute GVHD typically occurs during this time frame, thus prolonging the state of immunosuppression. Myriad organisms can cause infections in this period (see Boxes 175-1 and 175-3). The most common cause of severe viral illness during this period is CMV, which can cause interstitial pneumonitis characterized by fever, diffuse pulmonary infiltrates, hypoxia, and the acute respiratory distress syndrome. Treatment of CMV pneumonia includes intravenous ganciclovir and CMV immunoglobulin.

The development of chronic GVHD and a delay in the development of humoral and cell-mediated immunity contribute to infectious complications during the third period (i.e., >100 days) after transplantation. Common bacterial organisms causing infections in this period include encapsulated organisms such as *S. pneumoniae* and *H. influenzae*. *Candida, Aspergillus,* and varicella-zoster virus are also common causes of infection during this time frame.[18]

Diabetes Mellitus

Diabetes mellitus affects several aspects of the immune system. Functional properties of polymorphonuclear leukocytes, monocytes, and lymphocytes such as adherence, chemotaxis, and phagocytosis are depressed in patients with diabetes. These effects are exaggerated with concomitant acidosis. Other alterations in the immune system can include reduced cell-mediated immune responses, impaired pulmonary macrophage function, and abnormal delayed-type hypersensitivity responses. No significant alternations are shown to occur with humoral immunity.[19,20]

Certain community-acquired infections are more common in patients with diabetes (e.g., lower respiratory tract infections, urinary tract infections, and skin and mucous membrane infections). The risk of recurrence of such infections is also higher in diabetic patients. Some specific types of infections also occur predominantly in diabetic patients (e.g., malignant otitis externa, rhinocerebral mucormycosis, emphysematous pyelonephritis and cholecystitis, and Fournier's gangrene).[19,20]

■ MALIGNANT OTITIS EXTERNA

Malignant otitis externa is primarily a disease of elderly diabetic patients. The infection involves the external auditory canal and adjacent temporal bone. It can also involve the cranial nerves (e.g., facial nerve) and vascular structures. The primary causative organism is *Pseudomonas aeruginosa.* Signs and symptoms of malignant otitis externa include severe otalgia, otorrhea, edema, and cellulitis of the external auditory canal, diminished hearing, and trismus. Fever is commonly absent. Initially, the condition may be confused with nonmalignant otitis externa and perichondritis. The diagnostic work-up should include an evaluation of the extent of soft tissue involvement with radiographic studies such as contrast CT scan (preferred at the initial diagnosis) or magnetic resonance imaging. Patients should be admitted for intravenous antimicrobial therapy (e.g., ciprofloxacin, ceftazidime, or imipenem). Simultaneously, topical antipseudomonal ear drops should also be initiated. The otolaryngologist should be consulted promptly for initiating further diagnostic tests (e.g., obtaining deep tissue samples for culture and exclusion of epidermal carcinoma) as well as for surgical intervention (e.g., débridement of necrotic tissue).

■ MUCORMYCOSIS

Mucormycosis results from infection by fungi of the order Mucorales. Most infections in humans are caused by the species *Mucor* and *Rhizopus*. The spores produced by these fungal species are ubiquitous in the environment. The disease caused by Mucoraceae almost exclusively occurs in immunocompromised individuals. A frequent predisposing condition associated with Mucorales infection is diabetes mellitus. The most common clinical manifestations are rhinocerebral and pulmonary mucormycosis.

Rhinocerebral mucormycosis involves infection of the sinuses with extension into the surrounding structures (e.g., bones, orbits, brain, cavernous sinus,

Table 177-3 CLASSIFICATION OF HUMAN IMMUNODEFICIENCY VIRUS INFECTION*

CD4 Cells	A Asymptomatic Persistent Generalized Lymphadenopathy or Acute Retroviral Syndrome	B Symptomatic Infection	C AIDS-Defining Conditions
>500/mm^3 (≥29%)	A1	B1	C1
200-499/mm^3 (14%–28%)	A2	B2	C2
<200/mm^3 (<14%)	A3	B3	C3

*AIDS: A3, B3, C1, C2, C3.
AIDS, acquired immunodeficiency syndrome.

■ RAPID ASSAYS

Rapid assays for detecting HIV-specific antibodies in serum can yield results in less that 30 minutes. These single-use diagnostic system tests can be as accurate as ELISA if they are properly performed. HIV-specific antibodies may also be detected in oral fluids, and several tests are currently available (e.g., OraQuick and OraSure). Many people find oral fluid testing more acceptable than blood testing. Unfortunately, single-use diagnostic system and oral tests suffer from the same limitation as ELISA in that they produce false-negative results during the window period. Positive results on both rapid assays require confirmation with the Western blot.[1]

Monitoring Infection and Treatment

Monitoring the progression of infection with HIV has been likened to a runaway train on railroad tracks that lead to the edge of a cliff. The CD4 cell count is analogous to the distance between the train and the cliff, and the viral load is analogous to the speed of the train.

Close monitoring of the level of viremia and of the CD4 cell counts is crucial in the management of the HIV-infected patient. PCR testing quantitatively measures the viral RNA in copies per milliliter of plasma, the *viral load.* Untreated patients typically have viral loads of up to 1,000,000 copies/mL of HIV-RNA. One goal of antiretroviral therapy is to decrease the viral load sufficiently to be undetectable, as occurs when fewer than 5 to 50 copies/mL of HIV-RNA are present. The CD4 cell counts provide prognostic information. Patients with CD4 cell counts higher than 200 cells/mL rarely develop opportunistic infections, and those with counts higher than 50 cells/mL rarely die of HIV/AIDS.

Viral resistance to antiretroviral medications is an emerging phenomenon that may require alteration of a particular antiretroviral regimen. Two types of test measure HIV resistance. The first is genotype testing, in which the sequences of the relevant viral genes are determined. The sequences reveal the presence or absence of mutations associated with antiretroviral resistance. Second, phenotypic tests excise relevant viral genes and insert them into a standard test virus. The test virus is then exposed to various antiretroviral medications to determine resistance.

Classification of Infection

Table 177-3 gives the classification of HIV infection.

Acute Infection

Acute HIV infection (also termed acute retroviral syndrome or primary HIV infection) is a self-limited stage that develops in the first few weeks following initial infection. During this period, viral replication is rapid and ongoing, leading to high viral loads. The CD4 cell count may decrease transiently during the acute phase. The signs and symptoms are nonspecific and most commonly include fever and rash (Box 177-1). The average duration of illness is 14 days, but this stage may last from a few days to more than 10 weeks.[2]

In time, the immune system recovers. CD8 cells proliferate, and the humoral immune system produces antibodies that lead to a diminishing of the viremia. With the falling viral load, symptoms also subside. Testing for HIV-specific antibodies (e.g., ELISA) during the early phase often produces false-negative results because of the low levels of antibodies. Testing for viral p24 antigen or PCR testing of HIV-RNA are options. The importance in establishing

BOX 177-1

Signs and Symptoms of Acute Human Immunodeficiency Virus Infection

- Fever
- Rash
- Headache
- Lymphadenopathy
- Pharyngitis
- Myalgias
- Nausea
- Vomiting
- Diarrhea

the diagnosis of acute HIV infection lies in early therapy. Many experts stress the need for early antiretroviral therapy. Early treatment may decrease the viral load set-point and may thus slow the progression to AIDS. If acute HIV infection is suspected, consultation with an infectious disease specialist is warranted to arrange proper testing, to assist with an initial antiretroviral regimen, and to prepare for future care of the patient.

Opportunistic Infections

Opportunistic infections continue to be responsible for considerable morbidity and mortality in people infected with HIV. The introduction of highly active antiretroviral therapy (HAART) has been profoundly beneficial in decreasing the number and severity of opportunistic infections. Unfortunately, not all HIV-infected people worldwide have access to HAART, and resistance to HAART continues to advance. The following sections discuss examples of opportunistic infections likely encountered in the ED.

■ CENTRAL NERVOUS SYSTEM INFECTIONS

■ Toxoplasmosis

The protozoan *Toxoplasmosis gondii* is capable of causing focal encephalitis in HIV-infected patients with severe immune suppression. This condition is rarely identified in patients with CD4 cell counts higher than 200 cells/μL, and it is most commonly found in those with CD4 cell counts lower than 50 cells/μL. Symptoms include headache, fever, and confusion. More advanced encephalitis may cause seizures and coma. Physical examination findings may include focal weakness or stupor.

The diagnosis is suggested with a contrast-enhanced computed tomography scan of the brain showing classic, multiple ring–enhancing lesions. Serologic testing for antitoxoplasmosis immunoglobulin G antibodies is helpful if it is positive, but a negative test cannot exclude the disease. The definitive diagnosis requires detection of the organism in a clinical sample (e.g., brain biopsy). Most patients are given empirical therapy based on a compatible clinical syndrome, typical radiographic appearance, and serologic results. Favorable response to therapy, both clinically and radiographically, supports the diagnosis. Brain biopsy is reserved for patients who fail to respond to treatment. A combination of pyrimethamine, sulfadiazine, and leucovorin (to prevent the hematologic toxicity of pyrimethamine) is the treatment of choice. Treatment is given for at least 6 weeks. Prophylactic anticonvulsants are not indicated in patients without seizures.

■ PULMONARY INFECTIONS

■ *Pneumocystis* pneumonia

Pneumocystis jiroveci (formerly *P. carinii*) is the organism causing PCP. Despite a decline in the incidence of PCP as a result of HAART and prophylaxis, many patients who are diagnosed with PCP are unaware of their underlying HIV infection. Infection is most likely to occur in patients with CD4 cell counts lower than 100 cells/μL.

Patients with PCP tend to experience a subacute illness with a dry cough, fever, and progressive dyspnea that worsens over the course of days to weeks. On physical examination, one may note tachycardia, tachypnea, and fine crackles on auscultation of the lungs. The patient may also have oropharyngeal candidiasis. Radiographs of the chest may be normal in the early stage of infection; however, the common findings are bilateral and diffuse interstitial infiltrates.

The definitive diagnosis is by recovery of the organism from the lung. Expectorated sputum samples have a very low diagnostic yield and are not recommended. Bronchoalveolar lavage is the preferred method of obtaining clinical specimens. Many patients are treated empirically based on the clinical presentation, presence of hypoxia, and elevation of lactate dehydrogenase level to more than 500 mg/dL (a common but nonspecific finding in PCP). The drug of choice is trimethoprim/sulfamethoxazole—orally for mild to moderate disease and intravenously for more severe infection. Those patients with severe disease, as defined by a room air oxygen pressure of less than 70 mm Hg, should receive additional treatment with corticosteroids that should be initiated in the ED. The current recommendations are for a regimen of prednisone, 40 mg orally twice daily for 5 days, then 40 mg orally once daily day for 5 days, then 20 mg orally once daily for an additional 11 days.

■ GASTROINTESTINAL INFECTIONS

■ Mucocutaneous Candidiasis

Candida species are frequent pathogens of the oral, pharyngeal, and esophageal mucosa. *C. albicans* is the most common culprit. Infection is most commonly found in patients with CD4 cell counts lower than 200 cells/μL. Infection limited to the oropharynx may be mild, without symptoms, and patients may be unaware of the disease. Esophageal candidiasis more likely produces symptoms of odynophagia, burning chest discomfort, and fever.

Clinically, candidiasis appears as patches of whitish lesions on the oropharyngeal mucosa. These lesions are painless and are easily scraped off. Scrapings from these lesions may be examined microscopically with the use of potassium hydroxide to search for yeast. Scrapings may also be cultured. However, the diagnosis is generally made based on clinical findings. The presence of oral candidiasis, in combination with symptoms of odynophagia, suggests the diagnosis of esophageal involvement. The definitive diagnosis of esophageal disease requires endoscopic visualization, and sampling, of the lesions.

Topical antifungal therapy, such as with nystatin oral suspension or clotrimazole troches for 5 to 7 days, may be adequate for mild cases of oropharyngeal candidiasis. Systemic therapy with oral fluconazole is indicated for patients with recurrent disease and esophageal involvement. The safety and convenience of fluconazole (200 mg orally on the first day and then 100 mg orally once daily for a total of 7 to 14 days) make it preferable to topical therapy.

■ DISSEMINATED INFECTION

■ *Mycobacterium avium* Complex

Organisms that comprise the *Mycobacterium avium* complex (MAC) are ubiquitous in the environment and are capable of causing disseminated and multiorgan disease in patients with profound immunosuppression. Patients at highest risk are those whose CD4 cell counts have fallen to less than 50 cells/μL. Early symptoms of disseminated MAC infection may be mild and intermittent. As the illness progresses, nonspecific symptoms of fever, diarrhea, weight loss, and fatigue develop. Some refer to these symptoms as "the dwindles." Physical examination reveals few clues. Patients may be cachectic. Lymphadenopathy may be present, and anemia may result in pallor. The diagnosis of disseminated MAC is confirmed by isolating the organism from cultures of blood or bone marrow. Treatment of disseminated MAC infection is with a combination of antimycobacterial agents. The agents of choice are clarithromycin and ethambutol.

■ OPHTHALMOLOGIC INFECTIONS

■ Cytomegalovirus Retinitis

It was once estimated that approximately one third of patients with AIDS would develop cytomegalovirus (CMV) retinitis, but with the introduction of potent HAART regimens, new cases of CMV retinitis have greatly declined. Retinitis is the most common form of CMV disease, although gastrointestinal and neurologic manifestations of CMV infection are not unusual. CMV disease is found primarily in patients with profound immunosuppression (i.e., CD4 cell counts <50 cells/μL). Patients with CMV retinitis may be asymptomatic, but typical symptoms include "floaters" (dark spots within the visual field that move), scotomata, or visual field defects. Symptoms primarily occur unilaterally. The diagnosis is suggested by findings on funduscopic examination, including the classic fluffy yellow-white retinal lesions. Hemorrhage into these retinal lesions leads to the appearance of "ketchup and mustard" lesions. Oral valganciclovir (900 mg orally twice daily for 21 days) is the initial treatment of choice for CMV retinitis.

Highly Active Antiretroviral Therapy

Medications that can control the reproduction of HIV and can slow the production of HIV-associated disease are called *antiretrovirals*. The United States Food and Drug Administration continues to approve newly developed antiretrovirals at a remarkable rate. Currently, more than 20 antiretrovirals are available, including combination formulations, and they fall within four classes (Box 177-2).

Antiretroviral medications are primarily prescribed by specialists in the field and are given in various combinations, referred to as HAART. Generally, two nucleoside reverse transcriptase inhibitors are prescribed with one protease inhibitor, or two nucleoside reverse transcriptase inhibitors are combined with one non-nucleoside reverse transcriptase inhibitor. The precise combination selected depends on the patient's previous antiretroviral exposure, the tolerability and side effects, and the possibility of viral resistance.

BOX 177-2

Antiretrovirals

Nucleoside Reverse Transcriptase Inhibitors
Abacavir (Ziagen)
Didanosine (ddI, Videx)
Emtricitabine (Emtriva)
Lamivudine (Epivir, 3TC)
Stavudine (Zerit, d4T)
Tenofovir (Viread)
Zalcitabine (Hivid, ddC)
Zidovudine (Retrovir, AZT)
Zidovudine/lamivudine (Combivir)
Zidovudine/lamivudine/abacavir (Trizivir)
Lamivudine/abacavir (Epzicom)
Emtricitabine/tenofovir (Truvada)

Non-nucleoside Reverse Transcriptase Inhibitors
Delavirdine (Rescriptor)
Efavirenz (Sustiva)
Nevirapine (Viramune)

Protease Inhibitors
Amprenavir (Agenerase)
Atazanavir (Reyataz)
Indinavir (Crixivan)
Nelfinavir(Viracept)
Ritonavir (Norvir)
Saquinavir (Invirase)
Lopinavir/Ritonavir (Kaletra)

Fusion Inhibitor
Enfuvirtide (Fuzeon)

ADVERSE EFFECTS

It has been estimated that approximately 25% of all patients discontinue HAART because of side effects. Adverse reaction may be mild to severe and potentially life-threatening (Table 177-4). It is often difficult for any clinician to distinguish between these adverse effects and possible symptoms from infection with HIV or opportunistic pathogens. Therefore, it is important for EPs to be familiar with the frequently encountered, and possibly deadly, adverse effects of HAART.

The severe adverse effects of HAART warrant discontinuation of the offending drug and of all antiretrovirals to prevent the development of resistance. Consultation with an infectious disease expert is prudent.

Prophylaxis against Common Opportunistic Infection

Patients infected with HIV and who are severely immunosuppressed are at risk for many opportunistic infections. Long-term antimicrobial prophylaxis has been demonstrated to be beneficial in preventing several common opportunistic infections (Table 177-5).

Postexposure Prophylaxis

HEALTH CARE WORKERS

Although the risk of occupational transmission of HIV to health care workers is quite small, it is not zero. Percutaneous exposure to blood from an HIV-infected patient carries an estimated risk of transmission of approximately 0.3%. Similar exposures to mucous membranes are associated with a 0.09% risk of transmission, whereas the risk of transmission following exposure to nonintact skin is even lower. The CDC provided an update to their recommendations for the management of health care workers exposed to HIV and for postexposure prophylaxis (PEP). The updated recommendations continue to be based on the severity of the exposure and the viral load of the source patient (Box 177-3). New recommendations include additional antiretrovirals that may be included in the PEP regimens. The duration of PEP is 4 weeks.[3]

Health care workers with high-risk exposures are recommended to take the expanded three-drug regimen of PEP (Box 177-4). Those with less severe exposures are recommended to take the basic two-drug regimens. A small-volume blood exposure to mucous membranes or nonintact skin from a source patient who is asymptomatic or who has a low viral load (<1500 RNA copies/mL) represents a very low risk of infection, and the recommendations are to "consider" the basic two-drug regimen. Less severe percutaneous exposure to a high-risk source patient

Table 177-4 ADVERSE EFFECTS OF ANTIRETROVIRAL AGENTS

Agents	Adverse Effects*
Nucleoside reverse transcriptase inhibitors	
Abacavir	Severe rash* Hypersensitivity* Lactic acidosis* Fever
Didanosine	Pancreatitis* Lactic acidosis* Neuropathy Transaminitis
Lamivudine	Lactic acidosis* Headache Insomnia Nausea
Stavudine	Lactic acidosis* Neuropathy Headache Transaminitis Enteritis
Zalcitabine	Neuropathy Rash Stomatitis
Zidovudine	Lactic acidosis* Headache Myalgias Anemia (elevated mean corpuscular volume)
Non-nucleoside reverse transcriptase inhibitors	
Nevirapine	Stevens-Johnson syndrome* Severe rash* Fever Headache Transaminitis Hepatitis*
Efavirenz	Severe rash Central nervous system effects Transaminitis Hepatitis*
Delavirdine	Severe rash* Headache Fatigue
Protease inhibitors	
Amprenavir (a sulfonamide)	Severe rash* Headache Enteritis
Indinavir	Nephrolithiasis Hyperbilirubinemia Enteritis
Lopinavir/ritonavir	Enteritis Headache Weakness
Ritonavir	Enteritis Headache Transaminitis Taste perversion
Saquinavir	Enteritis Transaminitis
Nelfinavir	Enteritis

*Severe adverse effect warrants discontinuation of all antiretrovirals.

Table 177-5 PROPHYLAXIS AGAINST OPPORTUNISTIC INFECTIONS

Opportunistic Infection	Indication	Recommended Antimicrobial
Pneumocystis pneumonia	CD4 cell count <200 cells/μL OR history of oropharyngeal candidiasis	TMP/SMX 1 DS/day PO
Toxoplasmosis	CD4 cell count <100 cells/μL	TMP/SMX 1 DS/day PO
Disseminated *Mycobacterium avium* complex	CD4 cell count <50 cells/μL	Azithromycin 1,200 mg/wk PO

DS, double strength; PO, orally; TMP/SMX, trimethoprim-sulfamethoxazole.

BOX 177-3

Occupational Transmission of Human Immunodeficiency Virus (HIV) to Health Care Workers

High Risk Exposure

Percutaneous exposure:
- Large, hollow bore needle
  - Deep puncture
  - Visibly bloody device
  - Needle from source patient's artery or vein

Source patient:
- Symptomatic HIV infection
- Acquired immunodeficiency syndrome
- Acute HIV infection
- High viral load

Large volume of blood/prolonged contact with mucous membranes or nonintact skin

Low Risk Exposure

Percutaneous exposure:
- Solid needle
- Superficial injury

Source patient:
- Asymptomatic HIV infection
- Viral load known to be <1500 RNA copies/mL

Small volume of blood (a few drops) in contact with mucous membranes or nonintact skin

BOX 177-4

Recommended Regimens for Postexposure Prophylaxis

Basic Two-Drug Regimen

Zidovudine plus lamivudine as Combivir
OR
Zidovudine plus emtricitabine
OR
Tenofovir plus lamivudine
OR
Tenofovir plus emtricitabine

Expanded Regimen

Basic regimen plus lopinavir and ritonavir as Kaletra

is considered to be a higher risk, and thus an expanded three-drug regimen is recommended.

No PEP is recommended for any type of exposure if the source patient is HIV negative. Available resources include PEPline (telephone, 888-448-4911; Internet, http://www.ucsf.edu.hivcntr/Holines/PEPline).

■ NONOCCUPATIONAL EXPOSURE

In 2005, the CDC published recommendations for antiretroviral PEP following sexual exposure, injection drug use, or other nonoccupational exposure to HIV. The recommendations are based on data accumulated from human, animal, and laboratory studies regarding the potential efficacy of nonoccupational PEP (nPEP). A 28-day course of HAART is now recommended for persons seeking care less than 72 hours after nonoccupational exposure to blood, genital secretions, or other potentially infectious bodily fluid from a source known to be HIV positive.

nPEP is not always effective, and antiretroviral medications may produce harmful adverse effects, so all persons should be evaluated on a case-by-case basis. For example, persons who engage in high-risk behaviors, resulting in frequent exposures to HIV and the use of multiple and repeated courses of antiretrovirals, should not take nPEP. They should instead be counseled on risk reductions strategies. All persons should be tested for baseline HIV infection using ELISA. Additionally, they should be evaluated for other sexually transmitted diseases because their presence may increase the risk of transmission of HIV.[4]

nPEP is currently recommended for persons with an exposure event within 72 hours, to a source known to be HIV positive, with a substantial risk for infection. The timing is based on available data indicating that nPEP is less likely to be effective after 72 hours. If the source's HIV status is unknown, the source should be tested. The first dose of nPEP may be given initially, and no further doses are given if the source is determined to be HIV negative.

Substantial exposure risk is defined as exposure of vagina, eyes, rectum, mouth or other mucous membranes, or nonintact skin, or percutaneous contact, with blood, semen, vaginal secretions, rectal secre-

BOX 177-5

Recommendations for Nonoccupational Postexposure Prophylaxis

Negligible Risk

nPEP not recommended regardless of source's HIV status

Substantial Risk

Source HIV positive: nPEP recommended

Source HIV status unknown: nPEP determined on a case-by-case basis

*nPEP, nonoccupational postexposure prophylaxis.

BOX 177-6

Preferred Nonoccupational Postexposure Prophylaxis Regimens

1. Efavirenz PLUS lamivudine OR emtricitabine PLUS zidovudine OR tenofovir
2. Lopinovir/ritonavir PLUS lamivudine OR emtricitabine PLUS zidovudine

tions, breast milk, or any bodily fluid that is visibly contaminated with blood from a source that is HIV positive. *Negligible exposure risk* is defined as exposure of vagina, eyes, rectum, mouth, or other mucous membranes, or nonintact skin, or percutaneous contact, with urine, nasal secretions, saliva, sweat, or tears if not visibly contaminated with blood, regardless of the known or suspected HIV status of the source. The CDC makes no recommendations if the source's HIV status cannot be determined and the person seeking care has been perceived to have a "substantial risk" exposure. The decision to initiate nPEP must be made on a case-by-case basis (Box 177-5).

Once the decision has been made to initiate nPEP, antiretroviral agents should be administered promptly. No data support any optimal nPEP regimen, and the recommendations are based on the experience of treating HIV-infected individuals. Preferred nPEP regimens are listed in Box 177-6. All regimens are administered for 28 days. Efavirenz should be avoided in pregnant women or in women of childbearing years because of the potential teratogenic effects of this drug.

Persons who are given nPEP must be counseled regarding potential adverse effects, in particular nausea, vomiting, and diarrhea, and must be offered symptomatic therapy such as antiemetics or antimotility drugs. All persons receiving nPEP should also have prompt follow-up medical care provided by their primary care practitioners or an infectious disease specialist.

REFERENCES

1. Greenwald JL, Burstein GR, Pincus J, Branson B: A rapid review of rapid HIV antibody tests. Curr Infect Dis Rep 2006;8:125-131.
2. Kahn JO, Walker BD: Acute human immunodeficiency virus type 1 infection. N Engl J Med 1998;339:33-39.
3. Centers for Disease Control and Prevention: Updated U.S. Public Health Services guidelines for the management of occupational exposures to HIV and recommendations for postexposure prophylaxis. MMWR Morb Mortal Wkly Rep 2005;54:RR-9.
4. Centers for Disease Control and Prevention: Antiretroviral postexposure prophylaxis after sexual, injection-drug use, or other nonoccupational exposure to HIV in the United States. MMWR Morb Mortal Wkly Rep 2005;54:RR-2.

Chapter **178**

Fungal Infections

Richard Paula

KEY POINTS

Fungi can cause significant human disease.

Human infection is overwhelmingly represented by the following organisms: *Aspergillus, Blastomyces, Candida, Coccidioides, Cryptococcus, Histoplasma, Paracoccidioides, Sporothrix,* and Zygomycetes.

Fungal infection rates have dramatically increased in the past 2 decades as a result of improved diagnostic capabilities and a growing immunosuppressed patient population.

Invasive fungal infections carry an extremely high mortality rate, and recognition with rapid treatment by an observant EP will prevent morbidity.

General Epidemiology

The risk of fungal infections is tied to both geography and immune status. Immunocompromised individuals are exponentially more likely to suffer from fungal infection. Immunocompetent patients do acquire significant, often invasive fungal disease, especially in endemic areas. In three counties in the southwestern United States, for example, coccidioidomycosis in immunocompetent patients occurred with an incidence of 40 of 100,000 in patients more than 65 years old. In addition to the best-known endemic areas, smaller areas in Africa and Asia are also known to harbor pockets of high rates of infection. Fungal infections are a scourge in hospitals, and they account for significant numbers of nosocomial infections. Previously published data showed that 10% of all nosocomial infections were fungal,[1] and *Candida* was responsible for 85% of those infections.[2]

■ GENERAL RISK FACTORS

Outside of endemic areas of concern, the significant risk factor for fungal infection is immune dysfunction. One of the reasons for the extended life expectancy of immunocompromised patients is the ability to recognize the increased susceptibility of these patients to fungal disease. Patients with selective specific immune deficiency often contract specific fungal infection. Different holes in immune-mediated host defense allow varying types of infection. Candidal infections offer a clear example of this point. Granulocytes primarily prevent bloodborne candidiasis, and this becomes apparent in neutropenic patients who develop *Candida*-induced fungemia and sepsis. Contrast this situation to T-cell–mediated defense that prevents mucosal *Candida* proliferation, which explains why almost 90% of patients with human immunodeficiency virus (HIV) infection have oropharyngeal colonization, and more than half develop clinical thrush. To stymie host defenses further, some fungal organisms, such as *Histoplasma capsulatum* and *Coccidioides immitis,* change form during active infection of the host, whereas others remain exclusively in the yeast form. This adaptation allows *Histoplasma* and *Coccidioides* to infect healthy individuals.

ANATOMY

Fungal disease may occur in any organ system (central nervous system [CNS], cardiovascular system, respiratory system, skin, eyes); no system is spared. The type of infection is often associated with a specific risk factor or endemic exposure. The anatomic location of infection may be noted by the presenting symptoms, as with other infections. A particular area of infection may help to identify a specific deficiency in a patient's immune system. Certain immune deficiencies are associated with specific fungal disease manifestations.

Presenting Signs and Symptoms

No specific presenting signs or symptoms are pathognomonic of fungal infection. However, certain patient populations are more likely to contract fungal infections (Table 178-1).

Depending on the site of infection, presenting symptoms vary. The important signs of fungal infection are indicated by indirect evidence found in the patient's history. Patients who have a history that lends itself to greater risk for fungal infection should be evaluated and treated more extensively. For example, if a patient with acquired immunodeficiency syndrome (AIDS) who was just discharged from the hospital after being treated for pneumonia returns to the ED with recurrent symptoms of pneumonia, the likelihood that the source is fungal, specifically *Candida,* is much higher. The patient needs cultures specifically for *Candida* and requires prompt antifungal therapy in the ED in addition to broad spectrum antibiotics covering health care–associated pneumonia (HCAP).

ORGAN-SPECIFIC CLINICAL FINDINGS

Pulmonary Disorders

Patients with fungal pneumonia present similarly to patients with other types of pneumonia. They have fever, dry or productive cough, fatigue, shortness of breath, or hemoptysis. The chest radiographic appearance also resembles that of other pneumonia types. No specific finding is associated with particular fungal infections; lobar and interstitial infiltrates are both common. Certain fungal infections occasionally manifest with visible masslike lesions (e.g., blastomycosis or aspergillosis), and others form cavitary lesions (e.g., sporotrichosis). However, these are the exception and not the rule. Fungal pneumonia causes varying symptoms and radiologic appearances. In a recent review,[3] aspergillosis was the most common fungal cause of pneumonia in patients with cancer. Other reviews have reported aspergillosis as the most common cause of pneumonia in immunocompromised patients. Healthy, immunocompetent individuals are overwhelmingly more likely to have one of the endemic fungal infections.

Central Nervous System Disorders

Almost all the common fungal pathogens can cause CNS infection. The best known is *Cryptococcus* because of its propensity to cause meningitis in 50% to 60% of infected, immunocompromised patients. CNS infections may also be seen in much lower proportions in healthy individuals. Histoplasmosis leads to meninigitis in approximately 1% of symptomatic individuals. Almost all patients with fungal meningitis present after known fungal infections and are hospitalized patients with severe immunodeficiency. Such is not the case in many HIV-infected patients with cryptococcal meninigitis. Patients with cryptococcal meningitis have varying presentations, often including a headache for weeks, fever, nausea, or frank mental status decline. Such patients require lumbar puncture and prompt antifungal therapy.

Sepsis

Fungal sepsis is rare, but it is highly fatal. The recent PROWESS trial[4] demonstrated a mortality rate of nearly 56% that was more than double the nonfungal mortality rate of 28% to 30%. Suspicion is necessary to identify these patients early. A patient with a history of recent hospitalization, immunosuppres-

Table 178-1 PREDISPOSING FACTORS IN FUNGAL INFECTIONS

Patient Risk Factor	Common Fungal Infection
Human immunodeficiency virus infection (acquired immunodeficiency syndrome)	Candidiasis, cryptococcosis, aspergillosis
Recent organ transplantation	Candidiasis, aspergillosis
Neutropenia	Candidiasis, aspergillosis
High-dose steroids	Zygomycosis, candidiasis
Recent antibiotic treatment	Candidiasis
Diabetes	Candidiasis, zygomycosis
Recent or ongoing hospitalization	Candidiasis, aspergillosis
Recent abdominal surgery or burns (especially with intensive care unit stay)	Candidiasis
Travel to endemic area	Histoplasmosis, blastomycosis, coccidioidomycosis

sion from organ transplants, or abdominal surgery has a dramatically increased risk for disseminated fungal infection causing sepsis. Cultures with specific fungal organism media should be sent, followed by initiation of antifungal therapy.

■ Ear, Nose, and Throat Disorders

Fungal infections in the craniofacial area may be progressive and often fatal (e.g., zygomycosis), or they may be chronic and need referral for eventual diagnosis and treatment (e.g., allergic fungal sinusitis). Zygomycosis is rare, but it is also extremely invasive and may manifest as facial pain and swelling. Patients with diabetes, especially those with diabetic ketoacidosis, require a thorough craniofacial examination to look for the characteristic black exudate. Craniofacial computed tomography (CT) scanning hastens the diagnosis when zygomycosis is suspected. Most patients with fungal sinusitis present with common sinusitis symptoms: facial pressure, congestion or drainage, swelling, and allergic "shiners." Although most of these patients may be treated conservatively, patients with ongoing symptoms, nasal polyps, or evidence of facial deformity or bone erosion on CT will need rapid ear, nose, and throat follow-up and evaluation for débridement and antifungal therapy.

■ Rheumatic Disorders

Patients with disseminated fungal infections often complain of polyarthritis. Specifically, sporotrichosis spreads to the elbow or knee, and blastomycosis spreads to the weight-bearing joints or spine. Patients with cutaneous evidence of sporotrichosis or blastomycosis who have joint pain and swelling need aspiration and specific fungal analysis of the synovial fluid.

■ Cutaneous Disorders

The most common fungal infections in humans are the superficial cutaneous fungal infections (e.g., tinea), which are detailed in Chapter 187. However, certain fungal species may start as cutaneous lesions and disseminate to invasive disease or may start as pulmonary disease and disseminate to form cutaneous lesions. The latter is a form of blastomycosis that can form a primary pulmonary infection and spread, leading to cutaneous lesions in 75% of patients with disseminated disease. Sporotrichosis behaves similarly, but in an opposite fashion, because most patients with disseminated disease have cutaneous lesions first. Both infections manifest as raised verrucous lesions with irregular borders that are painless and are often seen on the face or neck. Either infection can develop into the verrucous form or can become an extremity ulcer. Potassium hydroxide (KOH) scraping identifies these lesions as fungal.

■ Vulvovaginal Disorders

Candida is well known to cause vulvovaginal infection that is common among sexually active women. It is often seen after a course of antibiotics, or it may appear spontaneously. Patients describe itching, burning of the labia, and a thick, white discharge. The incidence is increased in women taking oral contraceptives and in patients with diabetes. Adequate treatment is usually provided by over-the-counter antifungal creams; however, patients may require oral medication if the infection is recurrent or severe.

Diagnostic Testing

Fungi are usually visible in a tissue or fluid sample with the aid of KOH solution, which destroys nonfungal cell structures. This approach identifies only fungi that are easy to sample. In cases of pneumonia or fungemia, this type of testing is not usually possible. Most fungi can be cultured, and species such as *Coccidioides* and *Candida* grow readily on most agar. Other species, such as *Histoplasma* and *Aspergillus,* are much more difficult to grow and require antigen testing such as enzyme-linked immunosorbent assay to confirm infection. Zygomycetes requires special stains and is often a laboratory contaminant. It may be erroneously discarded if the laboratory is not told that it is a possible pathogen. It is important to call your particular hospital or outpatient microbiology laboratory to determine the best method of identification.

Specific Fungal Infections

■ BLASTOMYCOSIS

Blastomycosis is caused by the fungus *Blastomyces dermatitidis.* It occurs primarily in healthy individuals who are exposed in one of the endemic areas (Table 178-2). Pulmonary infections are typical, especially in the acute phase, and are contracted though inhalation of the dormant form. After attaining body temperature, the organism transforms into the yeast form and develops a greater ability to infect. Many patients acquire the infection and have chronic pneumonia for years, often diagnosed as reactive airway disease before the infection is discovered. Patients with chronic pulmonary infections often develop extrapulmonary manifestations of the

Table 178-2 ENDEMIC AREAS OF COMMON FUNGI

Fungus	Endemic Area
Coccidioides	Southwestern United States
Blastomyces	Mississippi, St. Lawrence, and Ohio River valleys
Histoplasma	Mississippi and Ohio River valleys

PRIORITY ACTIONS

Differential Diagnosis

Shortness of Breath or Productive Cough?

Does the patient have evidence of pneumonia that did not respond to antibiotics?

Does the patient have a noninfectious cause for the infiltrate such as pulmonary embolism or congestive heart failure?

If not, fungal pneumonia should be suspected and treated. Although some controversy exists regarding treatment of mild fungal pneumonia with antifungal therapy, initiating therapy in the ED is prudent and recommended.

Headache or Mental Status Changes?

Does a patient with poorly controlled HIV infection have a significant or prolonged headache? Are mental status changes associated with this headache?

Does the patient have a normal brain CT scan?

If so, a lumbar puncture with the patient in the lateral decubitus position should be performed. The opening pressure should be recorded and the cerebrospinal fluid examined for evidence of fungal infection along with bacterial and viral causes.

Organ or Bone Graft Transplant Patient with a Fever?

Is there another cause for the fever? Is the patient hemodynamically stable?

If a transplant recipient has a fever while taking antibiotics or appears to have sepsis, it is appropriate and important to initiate antifungal therapy after obtaining appropriate cultures.

Difficult or Painful Swallowing?

Does the patient have evidence of an esophageal foreign body or a bacterial infection such as with streptococci?

If not, *Candida* esophagitis should be suspected in patients with HIV or other immunocompromised states and in healthy individuals after recent antibiotic exposure.

Patients who are not tolerating oral fluids need to be admitted for hydration and evaluation for esophagogastroduodenoscopy.

Verrucous Lesion or Extremity Ulcer?

Does the patient work with plant material such as roses or moss?

If so, scrape the lesions and send sample for a KOH preparation. If the patients has no sign of systemic disease, discharge on oral fluconazole with follow-up.

disease; they frequently have cutaneous lesions, and frank meninigitis occurs in 10% of disseminated cases. If CNS involvement is suspected, a simple lumbar puncture is inadequate, because it is routinely negative; ventricular fluid collection is required to confirm the diagnosis.

Patients with pulmonary blastomycosis present with pneumonia: cough, fever, chills, malaise, and classic pneumonia symptoms. The chest radiographic findings can be an infiltrate or a masslike structure. This masslike appearance explains why blastomycosis is regularly diagnosed at bronchoscopy. Therefore, patients from endemic areas with symptoms resembling pneumonia who present with mass lesions on radiography should be treated for blastomycosis in addition to appropriate antibiotics. The organism can be identified by sputum smear or culture. Identification of the organism is considered to be diagnostic of infection because colonization does not occur, as it may with other fungi such as *Candida*. Blastomycosis does not generally clear without treatment, and untreated patients have mortality rates higher than 50%. Treating pulmonary blastomycosis is best done with the azoles, either itraconazole or ketoconazole for immunocompetent hosts. If the patient has life-threatening, disseminated disease or is immunocompromised, amphotericin B remains the most recommended therapy.

■ HISTOPLASMOSIS

Histoplasmosis is caused by the fungus *Histoplasma capsulatum*. Infections regularly occur in healthy, immunocompetent individuals. The disease is prevalent in endemic areas, but it has a much greater geographic spread than blastomycosis and it is found in caves, chicken coops, and ships hulls all over the world. Pulmonary infections are typical, and infection is often contracted through inhalation of the dormant mold form. This mold form is then activated by increased body temperatures, thus causing proliferation. Histoplasmosis has a much greater affinity for extrapulmonary symptoms than blastomycosis; spreading infection causes pericarditis, rheumatologic symptoms, and CNS involvement. Active infection depends on the load of inoculation. Lighter exposures do not produce disease; published rates of infections higher than 50% occur in endemic areas without evidence of symptoms.

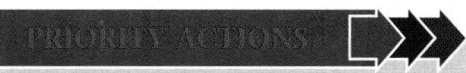

The common presentation of symptomatic histoplasmosis-induced pneumonia is indolent, with flulike symptoms, malaise, fever, and headache seen in almost 100% of patients. Chest radiography is highly variable and may be normal, but patchy alveolar infiltrates and hilar adenopathy are common. Disease disseminates in approximately 10% of patients, mostly immunocompromised persons, and it leads to pericarditis in 10%, arthritis and arthralgias in 10%, and meningitis in 10%. Disseminated symptoms are associated with pancytopenia with significant elevations in lactate dehydrogenase, and this condition must be differentiated from thrombotic thrombocytopenic purpura.

Identification of histoplasmosis is complicated. Culture is difficult because the organism is dangerous to laboratory personnel and must be held more than a month before being reported as negative. Antigen testing is helpful, but large numbers of individuals have been exposed, and complement fixation rates as high as 5% may suggest the diagnosis when it is not present. The polysaccharide antigen test is preferred, although it has problems because it cross-reacts with blastomycosis and coccidioidomycosis.

When treatment is discussed, it is important to remember that most healthy patients without chronic or disseminated infections recover without any treatment. Current literature still suggests a period of observation for otherwise healthy patients with symptomatic histoplasmosis. In making the decision to treat, side effects of therapy versus the high likelihood of spontaneous recovery must be considered. Admittedly, this was much more of an issue before azole therapy because the side effects of treatment with amphotericin B ("Amphoterrible") were sometimes worse than the infection itself.

Recommendations are to initiate treatment with oral itraconazole for a minimum of 6 weeks in patients who are hypoxic or who have not improved after 3 weeks of observation. Infected immunocompromised patients or patients with disseminated or life-threatening infections are treated best with amphotericin B, with a steroid taper added if pulmonary involvement is severe. Itraconazole has been used in patients with HIV who have not developed AIDS, with good results.

■ COCCIDIOIDOMYCOSIS

Coccidioidomycosis is caused by the soil fungus *Coccidioides immitis* endemic to the southwestern North American continent. Famously responsible for San Joaquin Valley fever, this organism regularly infects healthy persons. A dramatic increase in infections has been observed, with more than 100,000 annually in the United States alone. The increase mirrors population growth within the endemic geographic area. Infection occurs through inhalation of the mold form and subsequent transformation at body temperature into a more virulent spherule. Many infections are not symptomatic; estimates in the literature reflect that 40% to 70% of exposed individuals never show evidence of disease. Coccidioidomycosis disseminates in only 10% of cases, and much of the time only to the skin, where it frequently forms abscesses. Meningitis occurs in fewer than 5% of cases. Most complications are local; pulmonary cavitation and chronic pneumonia are responsible for the 20% of cases judged as severe.

Although primary infection usually remains in the lungs, extrapulmonary symptoms are common. Fever, chills, cough, pleuritic chest pain, and malaise are hallmarks of disease, and arthralgias and rash are also common, hence the designation "desert rheumatism." Only 50% of symptomatic patients have abnormal chest radiographs, thus making the diagnosis easy to overlook. When apparent, abnormal findings include hilar adenopathy, diffuse infiltrates, and pleural effusions. Cavitation occurs in 5% of untreated patients, and it often appears as a solitary, peripheral lesion.

Identification of coccidioidomycosis is significantly easier than detection of other fungi because of the rapid growth of this organism. Most growth media produce identifiable organisms in 2 to 3 days. Mature spherules may also been seen in tissue biopsies with special stains, and antibody detection is helpful as well. Unlike in histoplasmosis, colonization is rare. Complement immunoglobulin M identification is considered infection, and it disappears. Immunoglobulin G continues to remain positive in patients with chronic infection, but it also resolves when the infection clears.

Treatment for coccidioidomycosis is not always necessary because the infection often resolves without intervention. The Infectious Disease Society of America reported[5] that no evidence indicates that treating the mild form of pneumonia reduces morbidity or prevents chronic infection. Therefore, recommendations are to treat only the following groups: immunocompromised patients, patients with severe pneumonia, or patients with suspected high inoculum loads such as after laboratory accidents. The precise definition of severe pneumonia is left to the physician's judgment. Therapeutic options are similar to those in other fungi diseases, with azole therapy as first-line treatment. Some literature suggests a benefit of itraconazole over fluconazole.[3] Both drugs are associated with considerable relapse rates in chronic disease, and this is why a 3-month course of therapy is recommended. Disseminated disease may still be treated with the azoles if the patient is not immunocompromised. Patients with life-threatening cases require amphotericin. Patients with CNS involvement were traditionally treated with intrathecal amphotericin B. More recently, this approach was challenged by using high-dose azole therapy, and response rates were high, at 60% to 90%. However, cure was not observed, only suppression, and current thought is that a combination of intrathecal amphotericin B and intravenous azole therapy will work best.

■ ASPERGILLOSIS

The *Aspergillus* species that infects humans is most commonly *Aspergillus fumigatus,* and it is responsible for 90% of infections. *Aspergillus flavus* is less common, but it is much more likely to cause sinus disease. *Aspergillus* is a saprophyte, a soil-loving species found worldwide. Aspergillosis casts a wide spectrum of disease. It can benignly colonize immunocompetent hosts; it can cause chronic allergic symptoms, or it can devastatingly lead to overwhelming fungal sepsis in immunocompromised patients. Infection is usually contracted through inhalation of the conidia form that progresses to the hyphae form at increased body temperature. The hyphae form is much more aggressive and difficult for the human immune system to combat. Because of the pathogenicity of the hyphae form, infection occurs in normal and immunocompromised hosts.

Immunocompetent hosts who acquire aspergillosis frequently manifest disease in the form of sinusitis. The theory of the continuum of sinus disease termed *allergic fungal sinusitis* is controversial. *Aspergillus* was recovered from 13% of adults with allergic fungal sinusitis. The origin is obscured by the finding that the evidence points in both directions, toward the disease being either inflammatory or infectious. What are not debated are the secondary effects. The accumulation of mucinous debris leads to nasal polyps as well as possibly to more invasive disease, causing bone erosion and facial deformity. Patients with nasal polyps should be promptly referred to an ear, nose, and throat specialist because surgical débridement is currently thought necessary for cure. Because of the complex nature of the disease, therapy should not be initiated until ear, nose, and throat consultation has been obtained unless evidence of concomitant bacterial sinusitis is present. If clinical evidence of anatomic distortion is present, facial CT scanning is helpful in determining the extent of disease. Although sinusitis is the most common form of aspergillosis in immunocompetent hosts, pulmonary disease, particularly aspergilloma, often occurs in patients who are chronically diseased but not immunocompromised.

The long-recognized fungal ball or aspergilloma infects individuals with preexisting cavitary disease, such as tuberculosis, sarcoidosis, or bullous chronic obstructive pulmonary disease. These patients continue to have an infection rate of 10% to 15%. Symptoms, most commonly cough and hemoptysis, are difficult to discern from the chronic disease state in these patients. Aspergillomas are usually easily identified on plain chest radiography or on CT scans. Classic therapy involves surgical resection, and admission with surgical consultation is recommended.

Aspergilloma is the contained form of pulmonary aspergillosis. Invasive pulmonary aspergillosis is far more dangerous and needs to be addressed quickly. The immunocompromised patient, in particular the transplant recipient, is at great risk of contracting pulmonary aspergillosis. The incidence of *Aspergillus* in the bronchial tree of transplant recipients has been reported at 20% to 40%. Patients with AIDS have experienced an increase in invasive aspergillosis, and the current incidence has been reported at 1% to 2%. Symptoms of invasive pulmonary aspergillosis are variable, but they usually involve a combination of fever, cough, malaise, hemoptysis, and pleuritic chest pain. Heavily immunosuppressed patients present late and may have as their first symptom only fatigue, followed by massive hemoptysis or sepsis. Diagnosis in these patients is challenging, and no gold standard for diagnosis exists. Plain radiography may be normal. Chest CT is more helpful in identifying disease, but it is not specific for aspergillosis Serum culture for *Aspergillus* is highly specific, but it has a very low yield. Enzyme-linked immunosorbent assay may be better, although sensitivity has been reported to be as low as 60% and as high as 100%. Clinical suspicion is important, and even though no randomized study has proven the value of empirical therapy, initiating therapy before an official diagnosis has been confirmed prudent and may be lifesaving. Even treated patients have a 20% to 100% mortality rate.

Therapy for invasive aspergillosis was traditionally amphotericin B, but with cure rates reported as low as 40%, alternative treatments have been explored. In 2002, a randomized study comparing voriconazole with amphotericin B demonstrated a significantly higher survival rate of 71% versus 58%, respectively.[6] The study also reported the unfortunately high rate of adverse events that occur with amphotericin B therapy in 24% of the trial participants, almost double the 13% rate in the voriconazole-treated group. Although the authors of this study did not make any recommendations with regard to diseases other than aspergillosis, it is likely that patients with other invasive fungal diseases, especially life-threatening infection, may benefit from similar therapy.

▪ CRYPTOCOCCOSIS

Cryptococcus neoformans is an arboreal fungus found worldwide, with a predilection for the excrement of certain bird species, particularly pigeons. This disease was described in the 1950s to be similar to tuberculosis in terms of progression of disease in healthy individuals. Currently, *Cryptococcus* rarely infects immunocompetent individuals and is mainly linked to morbidity in HIV-infected individuals. Before the AIDS epidemic, infection rates were 0.8 per million in persons who were not infected with HIV. These rates spiked to 66 per 100,000 in patients with advanced HIV infection and then dropped again in that population with the advent of highly active antiretroviral therapy. Although *Cryptococcus* is not responsible for significant disease in otherwise healthy individuals, it is known to cause widespread asymptomatic colonization. Most adults have serum antibodies to *Cryptococcus*. A study of children in New York City demonstrated seroconversion before the age of 10 years.[7]

Infection is thought to occur through inhalation of contaminated propagules (microscopic plant material), although aerosolized pigeon dander has yielded a potentially infectious yeast form of the fungus. Patients who manifest pulmonary cryptococcosis have common pneumonia symptoms: cough, fever or chills, and pleuritic chest pain. *Cryptococcus* has a well-known predilection for CNS involvement, and even though infection may be through inhalation, 50% to 60% of patients with cryptococcosis have

CNS involvement. Patients with cryptococcal meningitis have varying presentations: often headache for weeks, fever, nausea, or frank mental status decline. Any HIV-infected patient with significant headache or mental status changes should be evaluated by lumbar puncture for cryptococcal meningitis.

Diagnosis is made with India ink examination of infected cerebrospinal fluid. Of HIV-infected patients with infected cerebrospinal fluid, 80% have organisms visible with India ink staining. Systemic involvement is often present in these patients and may be confirmed with either serum culture or latex agglutination, although the latter is more accurate, with a sensitivity and specificity of more than 90%. Latex agglutination should be added to the cerebrospinal fluid studies to increase the likelihood of diagnosis.

Treatment should begin immediately in ill-appearing patients, before lumbar puncture. The current literature points to combination therapy for CNS cryptococcosis in immunocompromised patients. Randomized trials have shown that flucytosine in combination with either amphotericin B or fluconazole is superior to any single agent. In less severe infection such as symptomatic pneumonia in healthy individuals, oral fluconazole as monotherapy is sufficient.

■ CANDIDIASIS

Candida is the most common fungal pathogen seen by physicians. It is common in healthy individuals and in immunocompromised patients, and it is a frequent cause of nosocomial infection. More than 100 species of *Candida* have been identified. *Candida albicans* remains the most common species, but there has been a rise of other species. The growth of non-*albicans* species is thought to be related to improved identification methods, the longer life span of immunocompromised patients, and a significant increase in the number of patients living with implantable devices.

Candida is a ubiquitous organism, existing as a yeast form and reproducing with buds and hyphae. It lives for long periods on surfaces, especially in hospital environments, but it is does not commonly cause laboratory contamination. *Candida* can infect any organ and is sometimes seen as having a commensal relationship with healthy humans. *Candida* infection is fought by multiple components of the immune system. T-cell–mediated attacks prevent mucosal overcolonization, and granulocytes help to prevent candidemia. Evidence of this is seen in the common occurrence of thrush in patients with AIDS and of *Candida* sepsis in neutropenic patients. However, the most common infection with *Candida* is vulvovaginal candidiasis. Although identification of vulvovaginal and oral candidiasis is almost always made clinically, identifying candidiasis in other disease states is a challenge.

Candidiasis may be diagnosed on sight, as is often the case with thrush or vulvovaginal infections. The diagnosis may be aided with a simple scraping and KOH preparation that will show the yeast or hyphae forms of the fungus. Culture is still the most common method of identification. *Candida* grows on most agars and is an unlikely contaminant. Unfortunately, the specificity of the culture is not matched by the sensitivity, and although the blood culture remains important, it can be misleading. In patients with autopsy-proven systemic candidiasis, the rate of recovery from blood cultures was only 40% to 60%. Because of the low sensitivity and increased incidence of invasive candidiasis, enzyme-linked immunosorbent assay and polymerase chain reaction testing are becoming more popular. Antigen testing should be pursued when invasive disease is suspected or identification of a particular species of *Candida* is important, such as in organ transplantation or in recent bone graft recipients. When patients develop invasive disease, treatment should be instituted when suspected, not when confirmed.

Treatment for invasive disease is much different than for mucocutaneous infection. *Candida* can infect any organ system and has become a deadly cause of sepsis. It is now one of the top five causative organisms for sepsis, and *Candida* sepsis has a mortality rate of 50%. Many of these cases are nosocomial, and *Candida* is responsible for approximately 9% of all nosocomial infections. Along with being immunocompromised, patients with burns, patients with recent abdominal surgery, newborns, and patients receiving total parental nutrition are at risk for invasive candidiasis. Traditional treatment of disseminated candidiasis has been with amphotericin B; however, intravenous fluconazole was equally effective in randomized trials in neutropenic patients. The IDSA guidelines stated that either drug may be used. No convincing studies exist to prove the value of initial treatment of septic immunocompromised patients with antifungal agents, although multiple guidelines have suggested that septic patients who are at high risk for candidemia may benefit from empirical antifungal therapy. Less invasive forms of candidiasis are much more prevalent and are commonly seen in EDs.

Oral candidiasis may occur in healthy individuals after antibiotic usage or in HIV-infected patients. Initial episodes should be treated with clotrimazole troches or nystatin. If this approach is not curative or if the condition recurs, oral azole therapy should be started. Oral fluconazole and itraconazole solutions are equivalent, and both are superior to other oral therapies. HIV-infected patients with oral thrush who complain of odynophagia or retrosternal chest pain likely have esophageal involvement and should be admitted for systemic azole therapy and culture of the *Candida* to check for resistance.

Vulvovaginal candidiasis is a common diagnosis, and 50% of women have received the diagnosis by the age of 25 years. This disorder is common after antibiotic use and is more frequent in women taking oral contraceptives. Infrequently, it can be the first sign of diabetes, and anyone who is diagnosed with vulvovaginal candidiasis for the first time should have a spot blood glucose check as a screening examination. Vulvovaginal candidiasis can be diagnosed by the combination of symptoms, visual inspection of the genitals, and KOH preparation of the scraping. Although coinfection may exist, if symptoms do not resolve, further evaluation is necessary. Patients often treat vulvovaginal candidiasis with over-the-counter agents before they see the physician. If treatment has not been attempted by patients, an over-the-counter cream should be suggested as first-line therapy. When over-the-counter treatment fails, a higher-concentration prescription azole cream is second-line therapy. An alternative is single-dose oral therapy with fluconazole or itraconazole.

SPOROTHRIX

Sporotrichosis, or rose cutter's disease, is caused by the fungal saprophyte *Sporothrix schenckii.* The fungus is found in the soil of tropical and subtropical environments, but it can be present in more austere areas, especially in greenhouses. Sporotrichosis is almost always identified as the cutaneous form in healthy individuals, although it can become disseminated through the pulmonary or cutaneous forms in immunocompromised patients. Outbreaks do occur occasionally, especially when heavy colonization is found in packed sphagnum moss that is used to protect plants (e.g., saplings, rose bushes) during transportation. More common is the sporadic case seen in plant workers, such as rose cutters.

The noninvasive form of the disease is caused by inoculation from a thorn or a skin tear during plant handling. Symptoms usually occur 3 to 4 weeks after exposure, and they begin with a small, erythematous area, usually on the forearm or hand. The lesion becomes indurated and often verrucous, and then it spreads locally to cause lymph node swelling. The lesions are not painful, but they may become superinfected with skin flora. In healthy individuals, the lesions grow very slowly and may appear the same for months. The reason for physician visits is often the cosmetic appearance. In immunocompromised patients, these skin lesions may spread. Disseminated sporotrichosis causes arthritis, often of the elbow or knee, and immunocompromised patients with suspicious skin lesions and joint effusions should be evaluated for fungal joint disease. Smaller numbers of patient with disseminated disease have pulmonary involvement, and symptoms in these patients are similar to those of other types of fungal pneumonia, commonly with productive cough and pleuritic chest pain. The chest radiograph is nonspecific; interstitial infiltrates, nodules, and cavitary lesions can be seen. Systemic illness causes constitutional symptoms such as fatigue, weight loss, and, uncommonly, fever.

The diagnosis is made with KOH examination of the cutaneous lesion scrapings. If a more specific diagnosis is required, or if extracutaneous disease is suspected, *S. schenckii* is easily cultured on a variety of media, and it is identified by latex agglutination. *Sporothrix* is not considered a contaminant, and its presence signifies disease.

Treatment for the cutaneous form of the disease has traditionally been with saturated solution of potassium iodide (SSKI). Although theories exist, it remains unknown exactly how this solution works to combat sporotrichosis. The main problem with this solution is the side effect profile. When used for more than a month, saturated solution of potassium iodide has a particular disabling effect on thyroid hormone production, especially in children. Itraconazole is more efficacious and produces fewer side effects, and other azoles may also be used. Therapy is long, often lasting 3 to 4 months, and should continue for a month after resolution of lesions. Patients with disseminated disease can also be treated with intravenous azoles.

ZYGOMYCOSIS

Zygomycosis is now the preferred term for the former mucormycosis. The preference stems from the use of zygomycosis to refer to an invasive form of disease produced by any of several Zygomycetes organisms: *Absidia corymbifera, Rhizomucor pugillus,* and *Rhizopus arrhizus.* Zygomycosis is rare, and it is almost always diagnosed in immunocompromised patients. In these patients, zygomycosis is invasive, rapidly progressive, and usually fatal. The rhinocerebral form has a mortality rate of 80% to 90%. The severity of disease is likely related to the particular affinity this group of fungi has for blood vessels. These fungi have been termed *angiotrophic* because of the widespread invasive blood vessel disease. This predilection for blood vessel invasion leads to ischemia, necrosis, and emboli.

Zygomycosis exists predominantly in the rhinocerebral, pulmonary, gastrointestinal, and cutaneous systems, and it may disseminate. The different forms are witnessed in particular subgroups of immunocompromised patients. The rhinocerebral form is seen in diabetic patients, especially during diabetic ketoacidosis, and in patients on high-dose or long-term steroids. Patients with leukemia or neutropenia often have the pulmonary form. Organ transplant recipients represent the group with the fastest growing incidence of disease; zygomycosis represented less than 1% of fungal disease in transplant recipients in 2001, and it now represents 20%.

Symptoms of the rhinocerebral form are insidious, consisting of local pain or swelling, nasal congestion, headache, fever, or epistaxis. *Rhizomucor* leaves a distinctive black exudate, "black pus," which is a foreboding sign of disease. Pulmonary involvement causes cough, fever, and occasional hemoptysis, and it is usually diagnosed in extremely ill-appearing patients. Gastrointestinal involvement is also seen in significantly ill patients, and it causes hematochezia, nausea, and emesis, eventually leading to intestinal ischemia.

Diagnosis is made by tissue biopsy with microscopic examination and culture. Special stains are often needed to identify the organism accurately, and it is vital that the laboratory be made aware that you are looking for Zygomycetes. Culture is available, but these organisms are common laboratory contaminants and are not considered diagnostic unless serial cultures are combined with direct tissue examination. Treatment should not wait for confirmation. The high mortality rate demands that treatment be initiated when the diagnosis is considered.

Rapid treatment may still not prevent death. Mortality of general zygomycosis is 50%, with a mortality of 80% to 90% in the rhinocerebral form. Amphotericin B is the recommended first-line therapy because the traditional azoles are not effective for zygomycosis. Members of a new class of extended-spectrum azoles, voriconazole and posaconazole, have achieved success in patients in whom amphotericin therapy has failed.

Medication

Antifungal therapy is the primary treatment for known or suspected fungal infections. Current therapy is transitioning from amphotericin B toward a more potent form of azole medications. Amphotericin B has been used for decades for nearly every type of fungal infection and is still recommended primarily in certain situations. Because of the large number of situations that call for antifungal therapy, it is impossible to recommend one particular drug over another. It is becoming increasingly apparent that a new generation of azole medications, the triazoles, is supplanting amphotericin. These medications, including voriconazole and fluconazole, have shown superior rates of improvement and cure compared with amphotericin B. In the most serious infections such as systemic aspergillosis and zygomycosis, voriconazole and posaconazole have been directly compared with amphotericin B and have had higher cure rates and lower side effects.[8] In less serious, but symptomatic infections, fluconazole is superior or equal to amphotericin B, with a dramatically lower side effect profile.

REFERENCES

1. Jarvis WR: Nosocomial outbreaks: The Centers for Disease Control's Hospital Infections Program experience, 1980-1990. Epidemiology Branch, Hospital Infections Program. Am J Med 1991;91:101S-106S.
2. Trick WE, Fridkin SK, Edwards JR, et al: Secular trend of hospital-acquired candidemia among intensive care unit patients in the United States during 1989-1999. Clin Infect Dis 2002;35:627-630.
3. Pound MW, Drew RH, Perfect JR: Recent advances in the epidemiology, prevention, diagnosis, and treatment of fungal pneumonia. Curr Opin Infect Dis 2002;15:183-194.
4. Bernard GR, Vincent JL, Laterre PF, et al: Efficacy and safety of recombinant human activated protein C for severe sepsis. N Engl J Med 2001;344:699-709.
5. Galgiani JN, Ampel NM, Blair JE, et al: Coccidioidomycosis. Clin Infect Dis 2005;41:1217-1223.
6. Denning DW, Ribaud P, Milpied N, et al: Efficacy and safety of voriconazole in the treatment of acute invasive aspergillosis. Clin Infect Dis 2002;34:563-571.
7. Goldman DL, Khine H, Abadi J, et al: Serologic evidence for *Cryptococcus neoformans* infection in early childhood. Pediatrics 2001;107:E66.
8. Aperis G, Mylonakis E: Newer triazole antifungal agents: pharmacology, spectrum, clinical efficacy and limitations. Expert Opin Investig Drugs 2006;15:579-602.

Chapter **179**

Helminths, Lice, and Scabies Infections

Kathleen J. Clem

KEY POINTS

Immigration and travel continue to increase the scope and variety of parasitic diseases seen in United States' emergency departments.

Parasitic diseases cause more death than cancer globally.[1]

The prevalence of endemic parasitic diseases in the southern part of the United States is significant, especially in rural areas.

Parasitic disease should be in the differential diagnosis for patients presenting with abdominal pain, diarrhea, unexplained fever, rash, or eosinophilia.

Approximately 20 species of helminths are natural parasites of humans, but many others cause zoonoses (infections of animals that also infect humans).

The helminthic parasites are multicellular organisms with three germ layers. The helminths of medical importance can be divided into two phyla: Platyhelminthes *(flat worms)* (classes Cestoidea and Trematoda) and Nemathelminthes *(roundworms)*. Trematodes have only an alimentary canal. In the cestode, neither an alimentary canal nor a body cavity is present. Nematodes have both an alimentary canal and a body cavity.

Modes of Transmission

Modes of transmission are described in Box 179-1.

Nematodes (Roundworms)

Roundworms are cylindrical, unsegmented white worms.

■ INTESTINAL ROUNDWORMS: *ASCARIS*

Ascariasis is the most prevalent helminthic infection in the world. Approximately one fourth of the world's population has ascariasis.[2] It is prevalent in warm countries and areas of poor sanitation. In developed countries, the incidence is much lower, but *Ascaris* is still endemic to the southern United States. The ova are resistant to dehydration and can survive up to 6 years under optimal conditions. They are sensitive to temperatures higher than 65° C or lower than –20° C, direct sunlight, and organic solvents.

Ascaris lumbricoides is the largest human nematode. Female adult worms measure between 20 and 35 cm in length and are characterized by a constricted area at the junction of the first and middle thirds of the body. Male worms are 15 to 30 cm in length and are identified by their coiled tail and two copulatory spicules. The eggs are ovoid and measure 60 by 40 μm, and they are golden brown.

■ Mode of Transmission

Ascariasis is transmitted by ingesting mature eggs from contaminated soil. Children frequently contract the disease by playing in dirt. Foods grown in contaminated soil and impure drinking water are also

BOX 179-1

Modes of Transmission of Parasitic Illness

Ingestion or inhalation: Usually, the eggs are ingested or inhaled in an infective form (e.g., *Enterobius vermicularis*), or the larvae, present in the intermediate host, are ingested (e.g., *Trichinella spiralis*).

Insect bite: The insect transmits the larvae into the host during a blood meal (e.g., filarial nematodes).

Skin penetration: The filariform larvae penetrate the skin directly (e.g., hookworms).

sources of infection. Fertilized eggs become infective in soil 3 to 4 weeks after excretion. When the eggs are swallowed, the larvae hatch in the duodenum, penetrate the intestinal wall, and migrate through the portal venous system to the liver. The larvae then migrate through the right side of the heart, the lungs, and into the tracheobronchial tree. They are then carried up the trachea to the larynx, where they move over the epiglottis and into the esophagus, and are swallowed a second time to reach the small intestine. This whole process takes approximately 2 weeks. The larvae mature in the small intestine. Female *Ascaris* worms begin to lay eggs 2 to 3 months after ingestion. The life span of the parasite is approximately 6 months to 1 year.[3] *Ascaris* coexists with *Trichuris trichiura* in the United States, predominately in the Appalachian Mountains and adjacent regions. The eggs of these two species require the same soil conditions for development of the infective state.

Presenting Signs and Symptoms

Many patients are asymptomatic or have mild symptoms, and the infection ends spontaneously within a few months after expulsion of the adult worms. However, ectopic migration can occur, and clinical manifestations can be severe. Approximately 5 to 6 days after ingestion, the larvae migrate to the lungs. This situation may cause fever, chills, dyspnea, paroxysmal cough associated with mucoid or bloody sputum, cyanosis, tachycardia, chest pressure, and, rarely, death. *Löffler's syndrome* is seen mainly in ascariasis, but it also may occur in other parasitic infections such as hookworm infestation and strongyloidiasis. The syndrome consists of radiographic evidence of infiltration of the lungs by eosinophils that may be seen on chest radiographs as a pulmonary infiltrate. Patients may present with pneumonia, cough, low-grade fever, and eosinophilia. Allergic reaction can occur with reinfection. Two to 3 months after ingestion, the parasite matures in the small intestine and can precipitate gastrointestinal signs and symptoms such as abdominal discomfort or pain, heartburn, nausea, vomiting anorexia, diarrhea, and constipation. Aggregate masses of worms can cause volvulus, intestinal obstruction, and intussusception. Liver abscesses can also occur when the female worm migrates up the common bile duct to release eggs in the liver. Rarely, patients have headaches, insomnia, and seizures. Protein malnutrition occurs in children with heavy infections and poor diets.

Diagnosis and Testing

A diagnosis can be made from the passage of worms in the stool or by finding eggs in the feces. The female worm produces 200,000 to 250,000 eggs daily. Therefore, a single stool specimen sent for ova and parasite examination is usually sufficient to make the diagnosis. Radiographic examination 4 to 6 hours after an opaque contrast meal displays the worms as cylindrical filling defects. Serologic antibodies can be used, including complement fixation, precipitin, agar-gel diffusion, immunoelectrophoresis, and the radioallergosorbent test.

Treatment

Treatment is effective only against the adult worms. Some commonly used drugs include albendazole, mebendazole, levamisole, and pyrantel pamoate. Unless complications result from ectopic migration, or severe malnutrition exists, patients can be given outpatient treatment for *Ascaris* infections.

NECATOR AMERICANUS (HOOKWORM)

Infestation with *Necator,* commonly known as hookworm disease, prevails in the southern United States and is frequently seen in immigrants from warmer climates. Soil-transmitted nematodes are of great importance in the health of many populations where the frequency of infection is a general indication of the local level of development of hygiene and sanitation.

Mode of Transmission and Life Cycle

Hookworm infection is contracted mainly by penetration of the skin or oral mucosa by the filariform larvae. Barefoot persons walking on contaminated soil or eating contaminated vegetables become infected. Transplacental infection and transmammary infection are alternative methods of transmission. Eggs are passed in the stools to the soil, where they hatch into larvae that undergo further development before they are ready to penetrate the skin. The filariform larvae penetrate the skin or mucosa directly. From the skin, the larvae move to the circulation, the lungs, and farther up the upper respiratory tract. The larvae then enter the esophagus and reach the small intestine, where they become adults. Infection is associated with the use of human feces as fertilizer. The wearing of shoes and the use of latrines are often the most important means of disease prevention.

Presenting Signs and Symptoms

Early signs and symptoms result from larval invasion of the skin. Patients develop pruritus and erythematous or vesicular papules. This condition may be known locally as "ground itch." As the larvae migrate, the tract becomes dry and then crusty. This manifestation is known as *cutaneous larva migrans,* an erythematous, serpiginous, linear skin lesion. During migration, the major symptoms are pulmonary. In severe cases, the migratory larvae may cause Löffler's syndrome. Each worm can withdraw 0.03 to 0.3 mL of blood a day, and even more blood is lost at the site of hookworm attachment. Severe infection often leads to chronic anemia. Loss of plasma protein results from malabsorption and increased intestinal permeability secondary to inflammation. Hypoalbuminemia may cause edema and anasarca. Pica and geophagy are often seen in infected children. Patients may present with cough, low-grade fever, abdominal pain, diarrhea, generalized weakness, weight loss, heme-positive stools, and eosinophilia.

Diagnosis and Testing

The stool should be sent for ova and parasite studies. In mild infections, multiple stool specimens or concentration techniques may be necessary. The parasite burden may be estimated using the Beaver stool or Kato slide smear method. Infections with fewer than 2100 eggs/g of feces (<50 adult worms) are usually not hematologically significant, whereas infections with more than 11,000 eggs/g result in significant anemia. Polymerase chain reaction technique can identify hookworm from a single egg. Hookworm infection may be confused with pneumonia, anemia, and malnutrition from other causes.

Treatment

Patients with hookworm infection are treated on outpatient basis with mebendazole, albendazole, or pyrantel pamoate. Occasionally, blood transfusion is needed to correct anemia.

ENTEROBIUS (PINWORMS)

Enterobiasis is worldwide in distribution and is more common in children than in adults. Because of its gross appearance, *Enterobius* is commonly known as pinworm. The adult worms are 6 to 12 mm in length and 0.3 to 0.5 mm in diameter. The eggs are 50 by 25 μm and are asymmetrically flattened on one side. Unlike other parasitic infections, pinworms are most common in developed countries with temperate or colder climates. The reasons are believed to be infrequent bathing and more frequent use of soiled underwear. Crowded conditions and lack of exposure to sunlight also favor transmission.[4]

Life Cycle and Mode of Transmission

The eggs are ingested by mouth, hatch in the stomach, and pass through to the intestine; here they invade the glandular crypts and mature. The adult worms live in the cecum and appendix. Adult pinworms are not infrequently found in the appendix following surgical removal of normal and inflamed appendices, but it is not known whether pinworm infestation is a cause of acute appendicitis. Unlike most worms that release their eggs within the intestine, the female migrates out through the rectum and onto the perianal skin to deposit her eggs. Rarely, the worms invade the abdominal cavity and cause threadworm granulomas of the liver, ovary, kidney, spleen, and lung.[5] Transmission of pinworms occurs by direct anus-to-mouth spread from contact with an infected person. It can also be caused by airborne eggs that are shaken free from contaminated clothing or bed linens. Autoinfection is common because patients scratch the pruritic anal area and then bite their nails or put their fingers in their mouth. The whole cycle takes 2 to 4 weeks.

Presenting Signs and Symptoms

Pruritus ani is the main symptom and varies from mild itching to acute pain. Pinworm disease is essentially an allergic reaction to the release of eggs and other secreted materials from the gravid female. The symptoms are generally worse at night. Associated scratching and excoriation can cause secondary infection. Vulvitis can occur when pinworms enter the vulva, thus causing a mucoid discharge and pruritus vulvae. Insomnia, restlessness, loss of appetite, weight loss, irritability, and enuresis may be associated with pinworm infection.

Diagnosis and Testing

The eggs are rarely seen in the feces, but they are usually seen when the adult worms migrate to the anus or vulvar area, particularly at night. The "Scotch tape test" is done by pressing a piece of clear sticky tape against the perianal region and then mounting the tape on a slide. The eggs are identified with light microscopy. Patients usually have no eosinophilia or associated anemia.

Treatment

The entire family should be treated simultaneously, to avoid reinfection. Medication must be combined with education and personal hygiene aimed at preventing autoinfection. All bedding and contaminated clothing should be washed. Fingernails should be kept short, and frequent hand washing and bathing may reduce reinfection. Eradication of the parasite may necessitate repeated courses of treatment. Albendazole, mebendazole, and pyrantel pamoate may be used, although pyrantel pamoate has significantly more associated adverse reactions. It is still the agent of choice for pregnant patients.

TRICHINELLA

Trichinosis has a worldwide distribution. Six species of *Trichinella* infect humans. *T. spiralis* is the most common species in the United States. The other five species (*T. nativa, T. nelsoni, T. britovi, T. pseudospiralis,* and *T. murrelli*) occur in other geographic regions.[6] Cases are often clustered because of the consumption of contaminated meat. Human infection results from ingestion of poorly cooked infected meat, particularly pork. Bear meat is becoming predominant as a source.[7]

Trichinosis occurs in two forms, adult and cystic. The adult is a white worm just visible to the naked eye that inhabits the small intestine. The cystic form is the larvae encysted in skeletal muscle. In the 1950s, it was estimated that 350,000 new *Trichinella* infections occurred in the United States annually.[8] As a result of enhanced public health efforts aimed at public education to cook meat well and federally mandated meat inspections, only approximately 40 cases of trichinellosis occur annually in the United States, but occasionally there are still associated deaths.[9]

Mode of Transmission and Life Cycle

Transmission is by mouth, from eating undercooked meat. The capsule of the infective larva is digested in the intestine; the larvae then penetrate the intestinal mucosa and thus cause symptoms of the enteric phase. After mating, the male worms die, and the female worms discharge larvae to the tissues that cause symptoms of the migratory stage after 5 to 7 days. After traveling through the circulation, the larvae encyst in the muscles of the diaphragm, the masseters, the intercostals, the laryngeal, tongue, and ocular muscles; the brain; and the heart. The cysts become calcified over time. The main methods of prevention are thorough cooking of all meat and regular meat inspection. *Trichinella* larvae in meat may be killed by heating to a temperature of 77°C, or freezing to –15°C for 3 weeks. Arctic species are known be to more resistant to freezing. Both encysted and free *Trichinella* larvae remain viable for years.

Signs and Symptoms

The presenting symptoms depend on the level of infection and the location of the larvae. Two phases are recognized: intestinal and muscular. The intestinal phase is marked by irritation and inflammation of the upper intestine and causes nausea, vomiting, diarrhea, abdominal pain, fever, headache, and diaphoresis. It occurs 2 to 7 days after infection. This phase is often confused with food poisoning. During the muscular phase, the larvae can invade any muscle.

The patient presents with high fever (seldom seen in other helminthic infections), myalgia, pleuritic pain, periorbital and facial edema, blurred vision, rash, and eosinophilia. The symptoms are caused by larval invasion, but they are primarily an allergic reaction to the parasite. In this phase, the cardinal clinical findings of trichinellosis develop. These include cachexia, edema, splinter hemorrhages, dehydration, ongoing fever, pruritus, congestive heart failure, hemiplegia, pain so severe as to limit all movement including breathing, psychiatric disturbances, and epilepsy. The patient can present with acute myocarditis, heart failure, bronchopneumonia, peritonitis, or nephritis. Death can occur during this phase. Eventually, the larvae encyst in skeletal muscles. Encystment is associated with resolution of clinical manifestations, although the larvae remain alive.

Trichinosis resembles many conditions: typhoid, encephalitis, myositis, and tetanus. Because of the association with eosinophilia, it resembles tissue stages of schistosomiasis, hookworm, *Strongyloides* infection, and other helminthic infections. Trichinosis may also be confused with collagen disorders such as periarteritis nodosa and rheumatoid arthritis. A high index of suspicion should be present in patients who present with periorbital edema, myositis, and eosinophilia, particularly if these patients have a history of eating inadequately cooked meat.

Diagnosis

Eosinophilia is a hallmark in clinical trichinellosis. However, there is no relationship between the level of eosinophilia and the clinical course of disease.[10] Other laboratory manifestations of trichinosis include leukocytosis and elevated creatine phosphokinase, lactate dehydrogenase, and myokinase levels. The diagnosis is made by identification of larvae and by serology. Because the location of infection is not always obvious, and muscle biopsy is invasive, serologic tests usually are used to make the diagnosis. Many different serologic assays are available, including enzyme-linked immunosorbent assay (ELISA), indirect immunofluorescence, and latex agglutination. Larvae have been isolated from the peripheral blood in the migration phase. The circulating antibody can be detected by serology between 2 and 4 weeks after infection. Immunofluorescence is positive 2 to 3 weeks after infection. The ELISA is very sensitive.[6] Larvae may be demonstrated in muscle by trichinoscopy. This procedure is performed during the muscular phase approximately 7 days from onset of symptoms. Muscle samples are taken from the deltoid, biceps, gastrocnemius, or pectoralis major muscle near a tendinous insertion.

PATIENT TEACHING TIPS

- Treating infected patients and avoiding contact with infected individuals or animal hosts help to control the spread of parasite related disease, but these measures are not enough. To control parasitic diseases adequately, the parasite's life cycle must be interrupted through hygienic and dietary practices.
- Patients with gastrointestinal and pulmonary symptoms who have traveled to or arrived from areas of the world where parasitic illnesses are endemic should be evaluated for possible parasitic illness. A travel history should be included for most patients seen in the ED.

■ Treatment

Most cases of trichinosis are self-limited, and patients require no treatment. Supportive care includes rest, analgesics, and antipyretics. For more severe cases, mebendazole, given in prolonged oral high doses, has proved effective, but the regimen may have to be repeated.[11] Albendazole is also used. In severe, life-threatening infections, such as central nervous system disease and myocarditis, corticosteroids are given and then tapered over 2 to 3 weeks. Corticosteroids are not indicated for mild disease because the use of these agents can increase the number of circulating larvae.

Taenia

The most distinctive feature of *Taenia* infection is that humans can serve as both the definitive host and the intermediary host. When humans are infected by the larval stage, the infection is known as *cysticercosis*. Infection with the adult tapeworm is associated with taeniasis. For *Taenia saginata* and *T. solium,* humans serve as the final obligatory host. Infection is uncommon in infants and in people who do not consume meat. Most human intestinal infections are with only one to a few adult tapeworms. *Taenia* has a worldwide distribution and is highly endemic in Latin America, Africa, Central Asia, and the Middle East.

■ *TAENIA SOLIUM* (PORK TAPEWORM)

■ Mode of Transmission and Life Cycle

Humans acquire the infection by ingestion of undercooked pork containing cysticerci (larval cysts). The cysts contain protoscolices. After ingestion, the protoscolices are released and attach to the intestinal wall. Each protoscolex can become an adult tapeworm. The head of the worm generally resides in the jejunum. Adult worms contain 800 to 900 proglottids. Maturation occurs over 2 to 4 months. The mature proglottids become gravid and contain 1000 to 2000 eggs. These eggs are passed in the stool. Pigs acquire the infection from soil contaminated with human feces.

■ Presenting Signs and Symptoms

Most patients are infected by a single worm. The symptoms are usually mild, or the patient may be asymptomatic. Because tapeworms can survive for years in an otherwise healthy host, symptomatic patients may have a protracted clinical course. Complaints are nonspecific and include indigestion, hunger or anorexia, diarrhea or constipation, and vague abdominal pain. Severe signs and symptoms may include intestinal obstruction, appendicitis, and perforation. The worms occasionally migrate to the biliary system, respiratory tract, uterine cavity, or nasopharynx.

■ Diagnosis and Testing

The diagnosis is suspected when a patient reports seeing mobile proglottid segments in the stool. Infection is confirmed by finding the eggs or proglottids in the feces. Because the eggs are often eliminated intermittently, several stool specimens may need to be obtained to confirm the diagnosis. ELISA, DNA probes, and co-proantigen assays are available in limited locations.

■ Treatment

Praziquantel is the classic treatment. Niclosamide is an alternative treatment; however, it is not currently available in the United States.

Trematodes (Flukes)

■ *SCHISTOSOMA*

Human schistosomiasis, also known as bilharziasis, remains a serious health threat for many nations. An estimated 200 million people are infected, mostly in Africa.[12] Schistosomiasis is a complex of acute and chronic parasitic infections caused by digenetic blood nematodes. Infection with *Schistosoma haematobium* (bladder fluke), *S. mansoni* (Manson's blood fluke), and *S. japonicum* causes illness in humans. Schistosomes have been documented to infect humans since earliest times and are associated with agricultural civilizations of the great river valleys. Hematuria, most likely caused by *S. haematobium,* occurred in ancient Egypt and Mesopotamia.

■ Mode of Transmission and Life Cycle

The life cycles of flukes are complex. The adult fluke lays eggs that leave the definitive host through the feces or urine, depending on the species and host location. A freshwater species of snail is required as an intermediate host for each species of fluke. In general, the miracidium (larval stage) emerges from the egg in fresh water, enters the snail host, and then undergoes multiplication. The cercaria (final larval state) leaves the snail. These larvae then penetrate the tissues of humans through contact in infested fresh water. The cercaria then loses its tail, becomes a schistosomula, and migrates to blood vessels to become an adult. The eggs leave the host in the feces for *S. mansoni* and *S. japonicum* and in the urine for *S. haematobium*. Behavioral interventions to limit contact with contaminated water are important.

Presenting Signs and Symptoms

Patients may be asymptomatic initially or may show mild maculopapular skin lesions within hours after exposure to cercariae. Granuloma formation in the bowel wall with *S. mansoni* or *S. japonicum* may cause bloody diarrhea, cramping, and colonic polyposis. Egg retention and granuloma formation in the urinary tract with *S. haematobium* can lead to hematuria, dysuria, and bladder polyps and ulcerations. This parasitic infection is also associated with an increased rate of squamous cell bladder cancer.

Acute schistosomiasis or *katakana fever* is an illness resembling serum sickness that develops in some, but not all patients. It is associated with a mortality rate of up to 25%. Patients present with fever, headache, malaise, arthralgias or myalgias, bloody diarrhea, and right upper quadrant abdominal pain.

Chronic schistosomiasis persisting months to years after primary exposure is more common than the acute form of the infection. Patients present with abdominal pain, hematemesis, ascites, hematuria, dysuria, vulvar or perianal lesions, dyspnea on exertion, fatigue, cough, chest pain, or seizures, depending on the site of infection and the involvement of the body system. Symptoms result from the body's immune response to invasion, not from the worms themselves. Eggs are highly immunogenic and induce an immune response as they travel to the liver, intestine, bladder, and (rarely) the brain or spinal cord. Complications include end-organ disease, pulmonary hypertension, cor pulmonale, portal hypertension, obstructive uropathy, and gastrointestinal bleeding.

Diagnosis and Testing

Diagnosis is by recovery of eggs in feces or urine; however, microscopy is not part of the standard ova and parasite evaluation and must be ordered specifically. Hatching assays on fresh stool specimens help to distinguish active from treated infection. Dead eggs may be shed for up to a year. Peripheral eosinophilia supports the diagnosis. Gross and microscopic hematuria is common in patients infected by *S. haematobium*.

Imaging techniques such as ultrasonography, echocardiography, and radiography can show body system involvement, when present. ELISA testing is available and confirms past exposure, although it cannot discriminate between acute and chronic infection. In some cases, colonic biopsy to visualize parasite eggs in the bowel wall is necessary to confirm enteric schistosomiasis.

Treatment

Antihelminthic medications for schistosomiasis include praziquantel and oxamniquine. Early treatment with cidal drugs may exacerbate Katayama's fever, and concomitant steroid therapy is recommended. Patients with long-term infection may necessitate procedures such as bladder stents, endoscopic treatment, or surgery, depending on the body system involved.

Ectoparasites

LOUSE INFESTATION

Scope

Lice are epidemic throughout the world, are very host specific, and are permanent ectoparasites. *Phthirus pubis* (crab louse) resembles a small crab and is 1 mm long.

Pediculus humanus var. *capitis* (head lice) and *Pediculus humanus* var. *corporis* (body lice) are 2 to 4 mm long. Infections are becoming more difficult to treat because of increasing resistance to common over-the-counter pediculicides.[13] The body louse is slightly larger, but similar in morphology to the head louse. Lice prevalence is estimated at least 6 million cases annually in the United States alone.[14] Head lice affect children most commonly.[15] Lice can transmit *Rickettsia* species, the causative agents of endemic typhus and trench fever. Louse-borne relapsing fever caused by *Borrelia recurrentis* is also transmitted by *Pediculus humanus*.

Pathophysiology

Lice live only on the host and survive only briefly in the environment. Eggs (nits) are deposited on hair shafts of the host. The order Anoplura consists of blood-sucking lice; the mouthparts are adapted for piercing the skin and sucking blood.

Mode of Transmission and Life Cycle

Lice are transferred directly from host to host. Eggs are transferred from louse-infested clothing or personal articles such as shared combs, headphones, beds, and hats. Pubic lice are usually transferred by sexual contact, but they may also be acquired in locker rooms from towels and gymnastic mats. The life span of the female louse is about one month. She lays up to 10 eggs per day and cements them to the shaft of a host hair. The nits are initially placed next to the scalp and move away from the scalp as the hair grows. Finding a nit a distance from the scalp may be evidence of an old infection.[16] It takes approximately 8 days for the louse to hatch into nymphs and another 8 days for the louse to mature. The mature forms feed on the scalp and adjacent areas of the face and neck. Head lice can live up to 55 hours without a host.[17] Body lice can live up to 30 days away from a host.

■ Presenting Signs and Symptoms

Signs and symptoms may include pruritus and pruritic papules at the site of infestation. Body lice cause skin changes concentrated around the waist and in the axillary folds. Saliva and fecal excretions of the louse may cause a local hypersensitivity reaction and inflammation. If a secondary bacterial infection occurs, the lesion may resemble mange. Patients often identify the presence of a parasite before they present for treatment.

■ Diagnosis

The diagnosis is made by identifying lice or nits on the patient. Using a fine-toothed comb and placing any removed lice or nits on a light-colored surface and viewing them with a magnifying device may assist in the identification. The head louse is a gray-white, 3- to 4-mm insect. *Phthirus pubis* is a round parasite 1 mm long. These parasites may be difficult to see except after a blood meal. The immature stages look like the adults. Finding nits without lice may not represent active infection because nits may persist for months after successful therapy.[16] Children can develop eyelash infestation (pediculosis ciliaris). The resulting blepharitis is usually bilateral. Crusting and matting of the eyelashes are present. The children complain of itching, burning, and eye irritation.

■ Treatment

Agents in use include pyrethrins, permethrin, lindane, ivermectin,[18] malathion, trimethoprim-sulfamethoxazole, and mechanical removal. Children can return to school immediately after completion of the first application of a topical insecticide.[16] Treatment of pediculosis ciliaris is with mechanical removal, as well as with physostigmine ophthalmic ointment.

Pyrethrins are natural flower extracts from chrysanthemums that are available over the counter. These extracts are usually combined with piperonyl butoxide. Pyrethrins are unstable in light and heat, do not kill unhatched eggs, and do not have residual activity. The extract is applied and then washed out after 10 minutes. A second treatment is needed approximately 7 days after the first. Treatment failures are becoming increasingly common.

Permethrin is an over-the-counter synthetic compound derived from natural pyrethrins. Permethrin is heat and light stable. It has residual activity for 2 or more weeks after application. It is more effective than pyrethrins, is poorly absorbed through the skin, and is rapidly metabolized to inactive compounds and excreted in the urine. Generally, it is sold as a 1% cream or rinse to be applied to clean, damp hair. Resistance to permethrin is increasing.[19] Five percent permethrin solutions may be used to treat head lice in patients who are more than 2 months old. This formula is left on overnight under a plastic cap. Resistance to the 5% solution has also been reported, and this 5% solution requires a prescription.

Lindane is a relatively expensive organochlorine, slow-killing insecticide. It is absorbed through the skin and is stored in adipose and nerve tissue. It was once the most common treatment for head lice, but over the last 2 decades it has become less effective than other treatments.[13] It is banned in some states out of concern for contamination of the water supply, and the Food and Drug Administration has issued a public health advisory on the use of lindane products as a result of potential neurotoxicity.

Ivermectin is an agent sometimes prescribed for body lice when other agents have failed.[20] It is not ovicidal, so repeat treatments may be needed. Because ivermectin does not treat reinfection, the source must also be addressed.

Malathion is a relatively expensive organophosphate pesticide irreversible cholinesterase inhibitor. It is the fastest killing and most ovicidal pediculicide currently available.[11] It has an objectionable odor and is flammable because of its alcoholic vehicle. Prescription instructions state an 8- to 12-hour application time; however, a more recent study by Meinking and colleagues showed that 0.5% malathion was 98% effective in one or two 20-minute applications.[21] Skin and eye irritations may occur, and the agent is contraindicated in infants. Malathion has been effective against lice resistant to permethrin.

Trimethoprim-sulfamethoxazole is used to treat *Phthirus pubis* infestation of the eyelashes and eyebrows. It has also been used (5 mg/kg oral twice daily for 10 days) to treat head lice in combination with 1% permethrin applied topically.[22] Resistance is a concern, so use of this agent should be reserved for severe or resistant cases.[11]

Mechanical removal should generally not be used as the sole therapy, except in children less than 2 years old, because it is very difficult to remove the entire infestation. Infested clothing and bed linen should be washed in hot water, dry cleaned, or discarded.

■ SCABIES

■ Scope

Scabies is a common parasitic infection caused by the mite *Sarcoptes scabiei* var. *hominis,* an arthropod of the order Acarina. Worldwide prevalence is estimated at 300 million. These obligate parasites complete their entire life cycle on humans. Scabies may mimic several diseases, including bullous pemphigoid, urticaria, chronic lymphocytic leukemia,

B-cell lymphoma, necrotizing vasculitis, and lupus erythematosus.[23]

Pathophysiology and Life Cycle

Scabies mites measure 0.4 by 0.3 mm in size, but they may be seen with the naked eye. Only the female mite burrows into the skin. The parasite completes its entire life cycle on humans. When fertilized, the mite burrows into the skin, where it tunnels at a rate of 2 mm/day. Each mite lays approximately 10 to 25 eggs and then dies in the stratum granulosum. Larvae hatch in 3 to 4 days, molt three times, then leave the burrow for the surface, copulate, and continue the cycle. It takes about 15 days for the parasite to mature. The number of mites infesting a person can range from five to hundreds and even millions in the case of crusted scabies. The skin eruption of classic scabies is a consequence of both the infestation and a hypersensitivity reaction to the mite. Symptoms of infestation usually manifest 3 to 6 weeks after the mite is acquired, but they may appear as soon as 1 day after the mire is acquired in cases of reinfestation, as a result of a hypersensitivity reaction.

Mode of Transmission

The primary mode of transmission is direct skin-to-skin contact. Transmission through shared clothing or other objects is rare, but it may occur with crusted scabies.[23] Mites crawl at a rate of 2.5 cm/minute on human skin. Mites can survive for 24 to 36 hours away from a human host and remain capable of infestation and epidermal burrowing. The greater the parasite load, the greater the chance of transmission will be. Sexual transmission also occurs.

Diagnosis

The diagnosis is primarily clinical. Patients complain of generalized and intense pruritus, usually sparing the face and head. Symptoms are often out of proportion to examination findings. Typically, itching is most intense at night. The chronic pruritus of scabies rapidly leads to scratching and explains why eczema is frequently observed. Classically, the burrow and associated lesions are located mostly in the finger webs, elbows, flexor surfaces of the wrists, in the axillae, breasts of women, and the buttocks and genitalia. The lesions are small, erythematous papules, often with associated excoriation and tipped with blood crusts. The burrow is a thin, grayish, reddish line 2 to 15 mm long. Burrows are not always identifiable because of associated excoriation resulting from scratching. Inflammatory pruritic papules are present. Although borrows and nodules are specific for scabies, they may be absent. The genitalia should be examined in all patients with suspected scabies. Nonspecific secondary lesions, excoriation, and associated impetigo may occur anywhere. Infestation in infants may involve the face, scalp, palms, and soles. Atypical papular scabies occurs in elderly patients. Immunocompromised patients develop crusted scabies and associated impetigo. Nail involvement is uncommon in classic scabies, but it occurs frequently in crusted scabies.

The definitive diagnosis is made by identification of mites, eggs, or mite fecal excretions. It is helpful to obtain multiple superficial skin samples from characteristic lesions. This is done by gently scraping laterally across the skin with a scalpel. The specimens are examined with a light microscope under low power. This technique is highly operator dependent. If the number of mites is low (as is common in classic scabies), mites may not be identified even in the presence of infestation. Skin biopsy may also be used. Definitive testing has relatively low sensitivity.

Treatment

Empirical treatment is not recommended in the absence of a history of prolonged skin-to-skin exposure, typical eruption, or both. Crusted scabies is very easily transmitted, and patients who have been even minimally exposed should be treated.

The infested patient and close physical contacts should be treated simultaneously, regardless of whether symptoms are present.[24] Topical or oral agents may be used. Permethrin and lindane are the classic topical treatments; however, lindane is no longer the preferred agent because of the potential of neurotoxicity, especially with repeated applications. Topical permethrin is a reasonable treatment in the United States. Patients should massage the cream thoroughly into the skin from the head to the soles of the feet. The cream is then washed away after 8 to 14 hours. Other topical treatments include benzyl benzoate (not currently available in the United States), crotamiton, and precipitated sulfur. Oral ivermectin may be prescribed for patients who are not able to tolerate topical treatment. A second treatment 2 weeks after the first may increase efficacy.[25] Data showing superiority over topical treatment are lacking. Clothes and bed linens should be washed in

PATIENT TEACHING TIPS

SCABIES

- Scabies is a benign, easily treated disease commonly called "the itch."
- It causes a pruritic rash and spreads rapidly among people in close proximity.
- Transmission among family members and within institutional settings is common.
- Itching can persist for up to 4 weeks after the completion of treatment.
- Schools do not ordinarily provide the level of contact necessary for transmission.

hot water and machine dried the day after treatment. Contaminated items may also be kept in a sealed plastic bag for 48 to 72 hours. Inanimate objects that cannot be treated with washing and drying or enclosure may be treatment with an insecticide.[26]

REFERENCES

1. Northrop-Clewes CA, Shaw C: Parasites. Br Med Bull 2000;56:193-208.
2. Giles HM: Ascaris. In Cook GC (ed): Manson's Tropical Diseases, 20th ed. London, WB Saunders, 1996, pp 1374-1381.
3. Sun T: Ascaris. In Parasitic Disorders: Pathology, Diagnosis, and Management, 2nd ed. Baltimore, Lippincott Williams & Wilkins, 1999, p 240.
4. Beaver PC, Jung RC, Cupp EW: Clinical Parasitology, 9th ed. Philadelphia, Lea & Febiger, 1984, p 302.
5. Daly JJ, Baker GF: Pinworm granulomas of the liver. Am J Trop Med Hyg 1984;33:62-64.
6. Murrell KD, Bruschi F: Clinical trichinellosis. Prog Clin Parasitol 1994;4:117-150.
7. Centers for Disease Control and Prevention: Trichinellosis associated with bear meat: New York and Tennessee, 2003. MMWR Morb Mortal Wkly Rep 2004;53:606-610.
8. Link VB: Trichinosis: A health and economic problem. Public Health Rep Wash 1953;68:417-418.
9. Moorhead A, Grunenwald PE, Dietz VJ, Schantz PM: Trichinellosis in the United States, 1991-1996: Declining but not gone. Am J Trop Med Hyg 1999;60:66-69.
10. Kociecka W: Trichinellosis: Human disease, diagnosis and treatment. Vet Parasitol 2000;93:365-383.
11. Abramowicz M (ed): Drugs for parasitic infections. Med Lett 1995;37:99-108.
12. Chitsulo L, Engels D, Montresor L: The global status of schistosomiasis and its control. Acta Trop 2000;77:41-51.
13. Meinking TL, Serrano L, Hard B, et al: Comparative in vitro pediculicidal efficacy of treatment in a resistant head lice population in the United States. Dermatology 2002;138:220-224.
14. Leventhal R, Cheadle R: Medical Parasitology: Programmed Instruction, 3rd ed. Philadelphia, FA Davis, 1989.
15. Ko CJ, Elston DM: Pediculosis. J Am Acad Dermatol 2004;50:1-12.
16. Roberts RJ: Clinical practice: Head lice. N Engl J Med 2002;346:1645-1650.
17. Chunge RN, Scott FE, Underwood JE, Zavarella KJ: A pilot study to investigate transmission of head lice. Can J Public Health 1991;82:207-208.
18. Burkhart CN, Burkhart CG: Oral ivermectin therapy for phthiriasis palpebrum. Arch Ophthalmol 2000;118: 134-135.
19. Lee SH, et al: Molecular analysis of KDR-like resistance in permethrin-resistant strains of head lice, *Pediculus capitis*. Pestic Biochem Physiol 2000;66:130.
20. Foucault C, Ranque S. Badiaga C, et al: Oral ivermectin in the treatment of body lice. J Infect Dis 2006;193:474-476.
21. Meinking TL, Vicaria M, Eyerdam DH, et al: Efficacy of a reduced application time of Ovide lotion (0.5% malathion) compared to Nix Crème Rinse (1% permethrin) for the treatment of head lice. Pediatr Dermatol 2004;21: 670-674.
22. Hipolito RB, Mallorca FG, Zuniga-Macaraig ZO, et al: Head lice infestation: Single drug versus combination therapy with one percent permethrin and trimethoprim/sulfamethoxazole. Pediatrics 2001;107:E30.
23. Chosidow O: Scabies. N Engl J Med 2006;354;1718-1727.
24. Chambliss ML: Treating asymptomatic bodily contacts of patients with scabies. Arch Fam Med 2000;9:473-474.
25. Centers for Disease Control and Prevention: Sexually Transmitted Diseases Treatment Guidelines. Atlanta, Centers for Disease Control and Prevention, 2002. Available at http://www.cdc.gov/mmwr/preview/mmwrhtml/rr5106a1.htm.
26. Elston DM: Controversies concerning the treatment of lice and scabies. J Am Acad Dermatol 2002;46:794-796.

Chapter 180

Tetanus

Lisa D. Mills

KEY POINTS

Puncture wounds pose the highest risk for tetanus. Tetanus also occurs following clean, minor wounds, abscesses, and cellulitis.

Keep current the tetanus status of patients with any injury, even minor, clean wounds.

Give tetanus immune globulin to patients with wounds, other than clean, simple wounds, who have never completed a primary tetanus immunization series.

Tetanus is a clinical diagnosis. Begin treatment when the diagnosis is suspected in any patient with unexplained rigidity.

Tetanus treatment consists of tetanus immune globulin, antibiotics, and local wound care.

Perspective

Tetanus is a rare disease in the United States, with only 20 cases reported in 2003. In 1990 to 2000, the average number of cases in the United States was 50 per year. The average annual incidence from 1995 to 2000 was approximately 0.16 cases per million population.[1,2] Tetanus is more common among people 60 years old or older (0.35 cases/million population), patients 60 years old or older who have diabetes (0.70 cases/million population), and Hispanic persons (0.37 cases/million population). Injecting drug users are at unique risk for tetanus. They accounted for 15% of cases of tetanus in 1998 to 2000.[1] Most (74%) injecting drug users who developed tetanus reported injecting heroin, and 100% reported "skin popping" rather than intravenous injection.[3]

Tetanus morbidity and mortality remain high, even with appropriate treatment. Current vaccination status decreases the severity of the disease and the likelihood of death from tetanus. In 1998 to 2000, 18% of patients with tetanus died. Of fatal cases, 75% occurred in patients who were 60 years old or older. No patients with up-to-date vaccination status died of tetanus.[1]

Although clinical cases are rare, EPs often are the first, and sometimes only, point of contact for patients. As a result, it is necessary for physicians to maintain an awareness of the clinical presentation of the disease. The diagnosis can be suspected but not confirmed in the ED.

In addition to recognizing the clinical presentation of tetanus, EPs play a vital role in the prevention of the disease. Primary pediatric vaccination and regular decennial booster vaccination are the mainstays of disease prevention and severity modulation.[4] Herd immunity does not occur with tetanus. Therefore, only people who receive the vaccination benefit from immunization. In the United States, the prevalence of tetanus immunity decreases by age, after 40 years of age. At 40 years of age, 80% of the population is immune to tetanus. By the age of 80 years, only 30% of the population remains immune. This is most striking in women and Mexican Americans.[5]

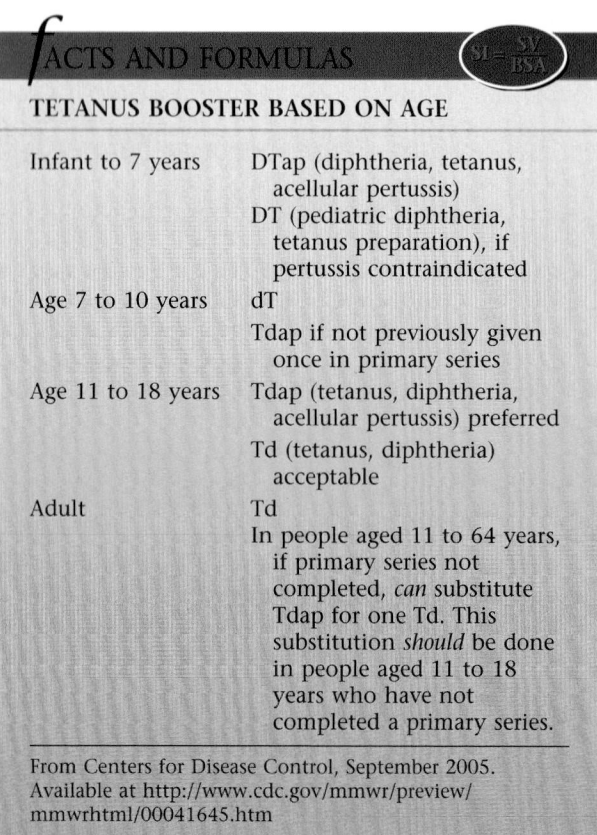

FACTS AND FORMULAS

TETANUS BOOSTER BASED ON AGE

Infant to 7 years	DTap (diphtheria, tetanus, acellular pertussis) DT (pediatric diphtheria, tetanus preparation), if pertussis contraindicated
Age 7 to 10 years	dT Tdap if not previously given once in primary series
Age 11 to 18 years	Tdap (tetanus, diphtheria, acellular pertussis) preferred Td (tetanus, diphtheria) acceptable
Adult	Td In people aged 11 to 64 years, if primary series not completed, *can* substitute Tdap for one Td. This substitution *should* be done in people aged 11 to 18 years who have not completed a primary series.

From Centers for Disease Control, September 2005. Available at http://www.cdc.gov/mmwr/preview/mmwrhtml/00041645.htm

Only 36% of person age 65 years old or older report receiving tetanus vaccination in the past 10 years.[6,7] Most cases of tetanus and fatalities resulting from tetanus are in patients who either have never been vaccinated or have not had a booster in the past 10 years.[8] EPs have the opportunity to provide booster vaccination at times of minor to severe injury and skin infection.

Anatomy

Most cases of tetanus are associated with acute trauma (Table 180-1). However, significant numbers of cases are associated with abscesses, cellulitis, chronic ulcers, dental infections, frostbite, and gangrene. In one study of injecting drug users with tetanus, 69% had an abscess at the injection site.[3] Tetanus affects postpartum women, with increased risk after unsanitary birth or abortion practices.[1]

Puncture wounds are the most frequent type of acute trauma associated with tetanus. Puncture wounds include nail injuries to the foot, splinters, barbed wire injuries, tattoos, drug injection, penetrating eye injuries, and spider bites. Crush injuries, burns, and eye injuries are also portals for tetanus infections. In patients with tetanus, approximately 50% of injuries are located on the lower extremity, 36% on the upper extremity, 10% on the head or trunk, and 5% on other areas.[1]

The occurrence of tetanus following minor or trivial wounds is well documented in the literature. Tetanus results from minor wounds and abrasions when proper wound care is not administered.[9-13] Nearly half of the wounds that resulted in tetanus in 1998 to 2000 occurred indoors.[1]

Table 180-1 TETANUS WOUND CHARACTERISTICS AND RISKS

	Most Threatening	Most Common
Location of injury	Face	Lower extremity Upper extremity Head and trunk
Type of injury	Puncture wound Crush injury Burn Chronic ulcer	Puncture wound Laceration Chronic wound Abrasion
Patients	Diabetics Age greater than 60 years Neonates No prior tetanus immunization	Intravenous drug users Age greater than 60 years Hispanic ethnicity Diabetics No prior tetanus immunization Last immunization more than 10 years ago

Pathophysiology

Clinical tetanus is caused by two exotoxins produced by *Clostridium tetani,* a gram-positive, anaerobic rod. The bacterium produces spores that are heat resistant, surviving autoclaving at 250°F for 10 to 15 minutes, and resistant to treatment with phenols and common chemical agents. The bacterium itself dies with heat or oxygen exposure. The bacterium and spores are widely disseminated in soil, intestines of farms animals and pets, and feces. Spores exist on human skin and contaminated heroin. In anaerobic conditions, such as puncture wounds and crush injuries, spores germinate.

RED FLAGS

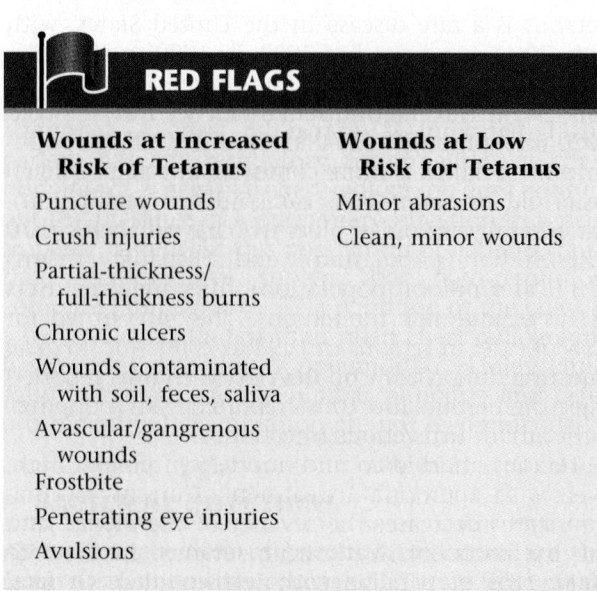

Wounds at Increased Risk of Tetanus	Wounds at Low Risk for Tetanus
Puncture wounds	Minor abrasions
Crush injuries	Clean, minor wounds
Partial-thickness/ full-thickness burns	
Chronic ulcers	
Wounds contaminated with soil, feces, saliva	
Avascular/gangrenous wounds	
Frostbite	
Penetrating eye injuries	
Avulsions	

C. tetani enters the body through a wound and produces two exotoxins, tetanolysin and tetanospasmin. Tetanolysin causes local cell death, creating an anaerobic environment in the wound site.[14] Tetanospasmin interferes with the transmission of inhibitory impulses in the central nervous system. It creates a presynaptic blockage of the inhibitory Renshaw cells and Ia fibers of alpha motor neurons that transmit gamma-aminobutyric acid (GABA) and glycine. Renshaw cells that transmit acetylcholine are not affected as strongly. Tetanospasmin binding prevents inhibitory signals in the central nervous system.

Tetanus becomes a systemic disease as the toxin spreads through the body. Tetanospasmin binds to nerve terminals, is internalized, and travels in retrograde fashion to the cell synapse. The toxin travels at 75 to 250 mm/day, and it affects synapses of shorter nerves before synapses of longer nerves.[15] The toxin also travels by lymphatic and blood flow to remote nerves. The toxin exhibits local effects first, then spinal motor effects. The autonomic system is the last to be affected because of the length of the nerves. Tetanospasmin also inhibits acetylcholine release, and the result is flaccid paralysis between episodes of spasticity.[16]

The result of the general loss of inhibitory signals is rigidity with periods of spasticity. The reflex inhibition of antagonizing muscles is lost, thus allowing agonist and antagonist muscle groups to contract simultaneously. Autonomic disinhibition occurs late in the disease. Toxin binding appears to be irreversible, requiring the growth of new nerve terminals to overcome the effects.[17]

Clinical Presentation

The average incubation period from time of injury to the onset of symptoms is 7 to 10 days, with a range of 1 to 60 days. Shorter incubation times are associated with more severe clinical presentation and a poor prognosis.[8,17] Tetanus is usually an afebrile disease until autonomic instability occurs late in the disease. Fever suggests coinfection of the wound or other infectious causes. *Generalized tetanus,* or tetanus affecting the whole body, is the most common form of tetanus.

In the first week of illness, the patient presents with rigidity and muscle spasms. Tetanus most commonly affects the cranial nerves first. The most common first symptoms and signs are trismus, neck stiffness, and dysphagia. Muscle spasm progresses diffusely to involve the facial muscles, causing the classic facial grimace *risus sardonicus.* Disinhibition of the neck muscles causes neck extension. Truncal rigidity follows head and neck involvement.

The general increased tone is interrupted by acute spastic events that can involve any muscle groups. These spastic events can be spontaneous or caused by tactile, visual, or auditory stimuli. Agonist and antagonist muscle groups can simultaneously contract. The contractions are painful and can be strong enough to break long bones and avulse tendons. Opisthotonos is a classic spastic event in tetanus. Abdominal rigidity can mimic acute abdomen. Spasticity of the trunk and diaphragm can interfere with respiration. Laryngeal spasm interferes with gag reflex or can occlude the airway.

Before modern mechanical ventilation, death resulted from respiratory failure or aspiration.[18] With modern mechanical ventilation, death is more commonly caused by autonomic events.[19,20]

The second week of illness involves autonomic instability in addition to the muscle spasms. The sympathetic system is more strongly affected. Sudden increased autonomic tone, with increased circulating catecholamine levels, increased vascular tone, hypertension, and tachycardia alternate with profound hypotension, bradycardia, and even cardiac arrest. Cardiac dysrhythmias occur, and the patient may develop hyperpyrexia at this point.[21-24]

Recovery begins in the third or fourth week. Muscle spasms decrease, but rigidity may persist. Recovery, in those who survive, ranges from 2 to 4 months, as new axon terminals grow. Most patients return to their baseline with no residual deficit.[8]

■ VARIATIONS

Local tetanus is an uncommon presentation of the disease in which only focal symptoms occur. Muscle spasticity is limited to the area adjacent to the wound. Local tetanus can progress to generalized tetanus, and the disease is generally milder. The exception is in cases of cephalic tetanus.

Cephalic tetanus is another rare form of disease. Cephalic tetanus follows a head or facial wound, or rarely, otitis media. The cranial nerves are initially affected. Spasticity or flaccid paralysis may be the presentation. Cephalic tetanus generally progresses rapidly to generalized tetanus and is associated with a severe course.[25]

Neonatal tetanus is generalized tetanus of the neonate. It occurs in infants born to mothers who are inadequately immunized. The port of entry is usually the umbilicus, with increased risk if the umbilicus is cut with a nonsterile instrument or is packed with contaminated material, such as soil, dung, or clay. Symptoms present on day 3 to 9 of life.[26]

The initial presentation is failure to feed in a child who previously fed normally. Neonatal tetanus progresses to generalized tetanus as described previously. The mortality for neonatal tetanus, when treated, is 25% to 90%.[27] Thirteen neonatal tetanus cases were diagnosed in the United States in 1992 to 2000. In these cases, 85% of the neonates had not been vaccinated because of parental religious or philosophic objections.[28]

Because tetanus is a rare disease in the United States, it is difficult to suspect and diagnose (Box 180-1). Tetanus should be considered in the differential of patients with rigidity or spasticity. It can be found in the setting of a minor or trivial injury that may not be remembered by the patient or family.[9-12] Tetanus is more common in patients without vaccination or without booster in the last 10 years. However, from 1998 to 2000, 6% of tetanus cases occurred in patients who reported being up to date on tetanus vaccination.[1]

Elderly patients and patients with chronic illness may have a decreased immune response to vaccination and therefore may lack protective antibody levels to tetanus in spite of appropriate vaccination. This is increasingly true in patients 65 years old or older.[29,30]

BOX 180-1

Differential Diagnosis of Tetanus

- Dystonic reaction
- Seizure
- Hysteria
- Craniofacial infection
- Meningitis
- Encephalitis
- Strychnine poisoning
- Hypocalcemia
- Black widow spider envenomation
- Intracranial hemorrhage
- Rabies
- Bell's palsy
- Ischemic stroke

Diagnostic Testing

The diagnosis of tetanus is clinical. The *Vaccine-Preventable Diseases Surveillance Manual* defines tetanus as "the acute onset of hypertonia or by painful muscular contraction (usually, initially of the jaw and neck) and generalized muscle spasms without other apparent medical cause."[28] No laboratory tests confirm or refute the diagnosis of tetanus. The organism is rarely recovered from wounds and can be cultured from patients without clinical tetanus. Serology to detect antitetanus antibody levels play a small role in the diagnosis of the disease. Patients can develop tetanus with "protective" levels of antibody.[28] The aim of testing is to rule out other causes of rigidity and spasticity. If tetanus is suspected, begin treatment immediately. Do not delay treatment, because no confirmatory test exists.

Check the patient's electrolytes, primarily to evaluate for hypocalcemia. Order a strychnine level if there is concern for exposure to strychnine, with

Documentation

History	Document the history of onset of symptoms and symptom progression and the history of trauma, even minor, healed wounds, including the location of the wound. Involve witnesses, especially if the patient is having difficulty with speech or breathing. Obtain an immunization history in as much detail as possible. Ascertain allergies or reactions to medications and immunizations.
Physical examination	Conduct a detailed neurologic examination. Evaluate the cranial nerves with motor function. Test for inducible spasticity (spatula test or other stimuli). Assess for compromise of respiration, ventilation, or airway protective reflexes.
Studies	Document review of any studies, even if normal. Exclusion of other disease is an important aspect of the diagnosis of tetanus.
Medical decision making	Document reasoning for excluding other, more common diagnoses or the reason for continued consideration of multiple diagnoses while concurrently treating the patient. Note findings in favor of tetanus. Document the choice of medications for spasticity, including those for deep sedation or muscle relaxation. Document the indications for intubation or assessment of adequate airway reflexes, ventilation, and respiration.
Procedures	Document wound care, including copious irrigation, incision and drainage, and débridement. Document rapid-sequence induction and intubation, the timing of consultation with the surgeon for extensive wounds, and the timing of the order for tetanus immune globulin.
Hospital course	Document the patient's response to treatment. Document the timing of interventions, including antibiotics, tetanus immune globulin, and intensive care consultation. Document the indications for change in care, including intubation, deeper sedation, and additional medications.

the understanding that illegally imported pesticides contain strychnine.[31-33] Ask patients about pesticide exposure and consider accidental ingestion in children.[34,35]

Obtain a computed tomography scan of the head if an acute intracranial event is considered. A lumbar puncture is necessary only if meningitis or encephalitis is included in the differential diagnosis. Examination of cerebrospinal fluid is noncontributory in tetanus, except to rule out other disorders. Because of unpredictable muscle spasms, performing a lumbar puncture on a patient with generalized tetanus may require intubation and deep sedation or muscle relaxation.

The *spatula test* has been used to distinguish tetanus from other forms of spasticity. In this test, a blunt instrument such as a tongue blade is used to touch the oropharynx. A patient without tetanus will gag and attempt to expel the instrument. In a patient with tetanus, the stimulus triggers masseter spasm, resulting in a reflex bite of the blade.[36] Although this test is reported to have a sensitivity of 94% and a specificity of 100%, the results may not be applicable to the United States, where tetanus is rare.

Management

Management of tetanus has two aspects, prevention and treatment. Each time an EP sees a patient with a wound, the opportunity for prevention exists. Treatment of tetanus is multifaceted and includes systemic treatment of the toxin, supportive treatment of the muscle spasms, and wound care.

PRIORITY ACTIONS

Suspect tetanus in patients with rigidity.
Control airway and ventilation.
Administer tetanus immune globulin.
Administer antibiotics.
Aggressively treat spasticity.
Débride wounds and incise abscesses.

PREVENTION

Prevention through vaccination and proper wound care remains the mainstay of therapy for tetanus. Update the patient's tetanus immunization, and administer tetanus immune globulin according to Centers for Disease Control and Prevention guidelines (Fig. 180-1). Maintain the patient's current tetanus immunization status for cellulitis, abscesses, eye injuries, chronic ulcers, burns, injecting drugs, and minor abrasions, as well as acute lacerations, punctures, and crush injuries (Figs. 180-2 to 180-4). Clean wounds to remove any contaminants.

Some patients have decrease in tetanus titers before 10 years. For this reason, patients with wounds that are not clean or are more than minor should receive a tetanus booster at 5 years after the last booster.[28] Clinical tetanus does not confer immunity. Therefore, survivors of tetanus require immunization when they are clinically stable. Pregnant women can receive

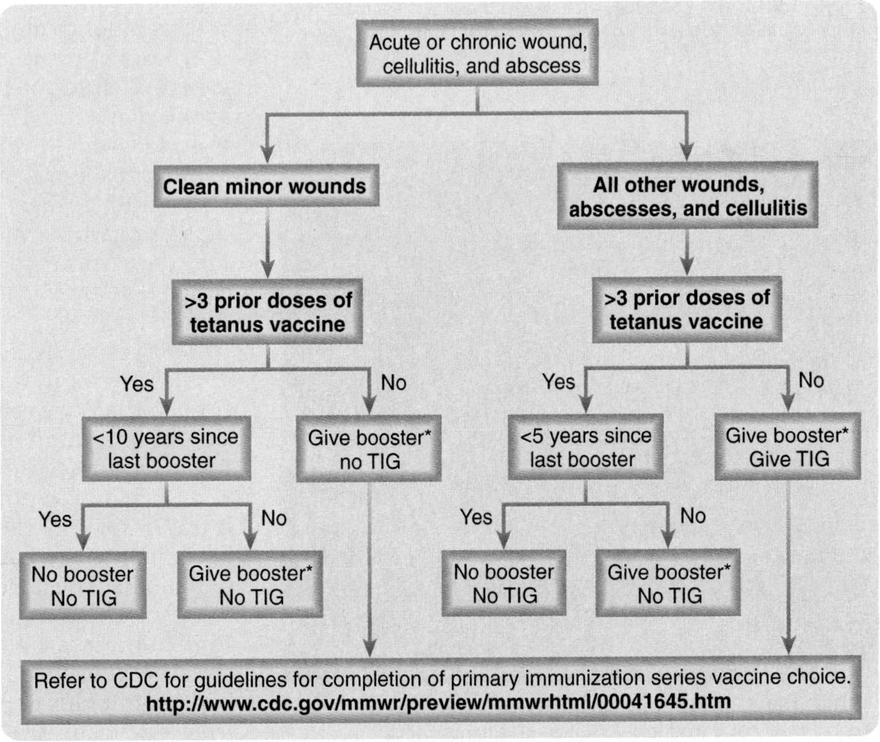
Acute or chronic wound, cellulitis, and abscess
Clean minor wounds
All other wounds, abscesses, and cellulitis
>3 prior doses of tetanus vaccine
>3 prior doses of tetanus vaccine
Yes
No
Yes
No
<10 years since last booster
Give booster* no TIG
<5 years since last booster
Give booster* Give TIG
Yes
No
Yes
No
No booster No TIG
Give booster* No TIG
No booster No TIG
Give booster* No TIG
Refer to CDC for guidelines for completion of primary immunization series vaccine choice.
http://www.cdc.gov/mmwr/preview/mmwrhtml/00041645.htm

FIGURE 180-1 Approach to tetanus prevention. TIG, tetanus immune globulin.

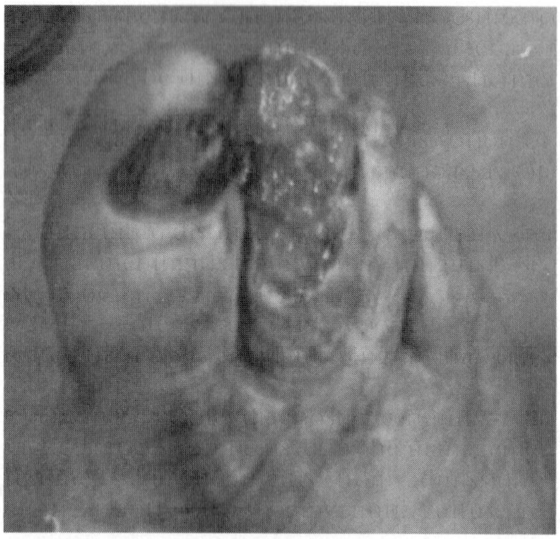

FIGURE 180-2 Chronic ulcers, especially in diabetic patients, pose an increased risk for tetanus.

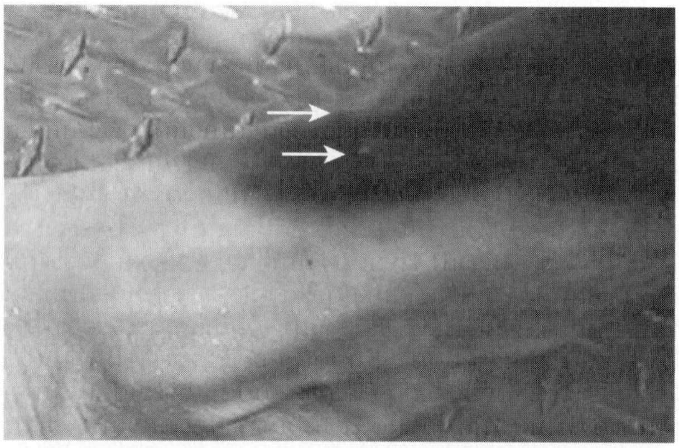

FIGURE 180-3 Two subtle puncture wounds *(arrows)* on this patient's ankle present an increased risk for tetanus.

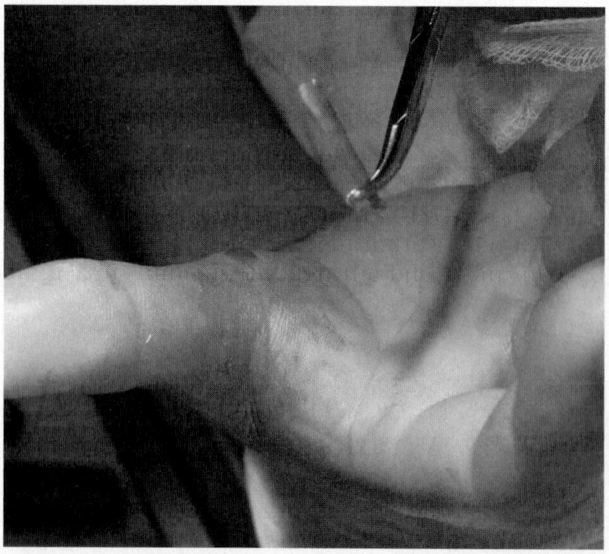

FIGURE 180-4 A puncture wound to the hand from this organic material introduces a significant tetanus inoculum.

tetanus prophylaxis, if indicated.[37-39] No confirmed risk to the fetus has been determined from tetanus-diphtheria or tetanus immune globulin.[37]

TREATMENT

Antitoxin Therapy

Administer tetanus immune globulin at a dose of 3000 to 5000 units intramuscularly to the pediatric or adult patient. Some sources recommend infiltration of some immune globulin around the wound site, if identified.[28] Intravenous immune globulin has tetanus antitoxin and may be administered if tetanus immune globulin is not available in a reasonable amount of time.

Antibiotic Therapy

Metronidazole is the drug of choice for tetanus. Administer intravenously, 1 g every 12 hours or 500 mg every 6 hours to adult patients. Administer intravenous metronidazole at 30 mg/kg/day, divided every 8 or 12 hours, for pediatric patients. Penicillin G is the second choice of antibiotics. Penicillin antagonizes GABA with unknown clinical significance. The dose of penicillin is 24 million U intravenously, divided every 4 to 6 hours for adults. The pediatric dose of penicillin G is 100,000 to 250,000 U/kg/day, divided every 6 hours.[41-44] Erythromycin, doxycycline, tetracycline, chloramphenicol, and clindamycin are alternatives if metronidazole and penicillin are contraindicated.[44,45]

Supportive Therapy

Muscle spasms are controlled with large doses of benzodiazepines to augment GABA activity. Continuous infusions improve effectiveness. Control pain with generous doses of morphine or another opiate, but avoid meperidine. If respiratory depression results from sedation, intubate the patient. Magnesium in a continuous intravenous infusion has been used as an adjunct to benzodiazepines in the treatment of muscle spasms. Magnesium contributes to respiratory depression.[46-49] Sedation with propofol at levels equivalent to those used during general anesthesia decreases muscle rigidity and spasm. Intubate the patient before using propofol.[50,51]

Closely monitor the patient's respiration, ventilation, and airway reflexes. Intubate patients with any sign of respiratory or ventilatory compromise resulting from truncal or laryngeal spasm. If deep sedation with benzodiazepines and opioids fails to control muscle spasm, intubate the patient. Intrathecal baclofen has been used with success in small numbers of patients. The large doses of baclofen required result in respiratory depression and coma necessitating intubation in a significant number of patients.[50,51] If intrathecal baclofen is not available on an emergency basis or if it fails to produce an improvement, administer a neuromuscular blocking muscle agent.

Tips and Tricks

Type of Wounds	Wound Care Tips
Puncture	Copiously irrigate. Remove foreign bodies as indicated.
Simple laceration	Copiously irrigate.
Complex laceration	Copiously irrigate. Débride nonviable tissue.
Abscess	Incise and drain. Débride avascular tissue.
Cellulitis	Débride any necrotic tissue.
Crush	Copiously irrigate. Débride avascular tissue.
Abrasion	Copiously irrigate.
Avulsion	Copiously irrigate. Débride nonviable tissue.

Patients with tetanus are at increased risk for aspiration because of the loss of laryngeal reflexes, atony of the stomach, and forceful contraction of the abdominal wall. Empty the patient's stomach to decrease the chances of aspiration. Autonomic instability is a late finding and will likely not be treated in the ED. Sedation, with morphine, and maintenance of a quiet, low-stimulus environment are critical in decreasing autonomic instability.[49,54,52] Esmolol has been used to control hyperadrenergic states. Propanolol and labetalol are both linked to increased mortality.[53,54]

Wound Therapy

Débride necrotic wounds with wide margins to remove the anaerobic environment and to arrest *C. tetani*. Incise and drain abscesses. Débride necrotic tissue at abscess sites. Do not delay débridement or incision and drainage. Perform these procedures on an emergency basis.

PATIENT TEACHING TIPS

- Inform all patients of the risk of tetanus for even minor, clean wounds.
- Recommend routine immunization every 10 years without injury.
- Encourage patients to record tetanus booster in their own records and to notify primary care doctor of vaccination booster.
- Update tetanus immunization before pregnancy and childbirth.
- The tetanus-diphtheria booster is believed to be safe in pregnancy, and is given, if an acute indication exists.

Disposition

Admit patients with tetanus to the intensive care unit. Consult a surgical service on an emergency basis if wound or abscess management requires surgical intervention.

REFERENCES

1. Pascual FB, McGinley EL, Zanardi LR, et al: Tetanus surveillance: United States, 1998-2000. MMWR Surveill Summ 2003;52:1-8.
2. Bardenheier B, Prevots DR, Khetsuriani N, Wharton M: Tetanus surveillance: United States, 1995-1997. MMWR CDC Surveill Summ 1998;47:1-13.
3. Centers for Disease Control and Prevention: Tetanus among injecting-drug users: California, 1997. JAMA 1998;279: 987.
4. Centers for Disease Control and Prevention: Update on adult immunization: Recommendations of the Immunization Practices Advisory Committee (ACIP). MMWR Recomm Rep 1991;40:1-94.
5. Gergen PJ, McQuillan GM, Kiely M, et al: A population-based serologic survey of immunity to tetanus in the United States. N Engl J Med 1995;332;761-766.
6. National Center for Health Statistics: National Health Interview Survey, 1995. Hyattsville, MD: National Health Interview Survey, 1995.
7. McQuillan GM, Kruszon-Moran D, Deforest A, et al: Serologic immunity to diphtheria and tetanus in the United States. Ann Intern Med 2002;136:660-666.
8. Atkinson W, Hamborsky J, McIntyre L, Wolfe S (eds): Centers for Disease Control and Prevention: Epidemiology and Prevention of Vaccine-Preventable Diseases, 9th ed. Washington, DC: Public Health Foundation, 2006.
9. Centers for Disease Control and Prevention: Tetanus: United States, 1982-1984. MMWR Morb Mortal Wkly Rep 1985;34:602, 607-611.
10. Bardenheier B, Prevots DR, Khetsuriani N, Wharton M: Tetanus surveillance: United States, 1995-1997. MMWR Surveill Summ 1998;47:1-13.
11. Centers for Disease Control and Prevention: Tetanus: United States, 1987 and 1988. MMWR Morb Mortal Wkly Rep 1990;39:37-41.
12. Centers for Disease Control and Prevention: Tetanus: Puerto Rico, 2002. MMWR Morb Mortal Whly Rep 2002; 51:613-615.
13. Rhee P, Nunley MK, Demetriades D, et al: Tetanus and trauma: A review and recommendations. J Trauma 2005;58: 1082-1088.
14. Rottem S, Cole RM, Habig WH, et al: Structural characteristics of tetanolysin and its binding to lipid vesicles. J Bacteriol 1982;152:888-892.
15. Davies J, Tongroach P: Tetanus toxin and synaptic inhibition in the substantia nigra and striatum of the rat. J Physiol (Lond) 1979;290:23-36.
16. Cook TM, Protheroe RT, Handel JM: Tetanus: A review of the literature. Br J Anaesth 2001;87:477-487.
17. Duchen LW, Tonge DA: The effects of tetanus toxin on neuromuscular transmission and on the morphology of motor end plates in slow and fast skeletal muscle of the mouse. J Physiol (Lond) 1973;228:157-172.
18. Trujillo MH, Castillo A, Espana J, et al: Impact of intensive care management on the prognosis of tetanus: Analysis of 641 cases. Chest 1987;92:63-65.
19. Tsueda K, Oliver PB, Richter RW: Cardiovascular manifestations of tetanus. Anesthesiology 1974;40:588-592.
20. Udwadia FE: Haemodynamics in severe in tetanus. In Udwadia FE (ed): Tetanus. New York: Oxford University Press, 1994.
21. Kerr JH, Corbett JL, Prys-Roberts C, et al: Involvement of the sympathetic nervous system in tetanus: Studies on 82 patients. Lancet 1968;2:236-241.

22. Kelty SR, Gray RC, Dundee JW, McCulloch H: Catecholamine levels in severe tetanus. Lancet 1968;2:195.
23. Kanarek DJ, Kaufman B, Zwi S. Severe sympathetic hyperactivity associated with tetanus. Arch Intern Med 1973;132:602-604.
24. Udwadia FE, Lall A, Udwadia ZF, et al: Tetanus and its complications: Intensive care and management experience in 150 Indian patients. Epidemiol Infect 1987;99: 675-684.
25. Jagoda A, Riggio S, Burguieres T: Cephalic tetanus: A case report and review of the literature. Am J Emerg Med 1988;6: 128-130.
26. World Health Organization: Neonatal tetanus. In Immunizations, Vaccines, and Biologicals. Available at http://www.who.int/vaccines/en/neotetanus.shtml
27. Stanfield JP, Galazka A: Neonatal tetanus in the world today. Bull World Health Organ 1984;62:647-669.
28. Nagachinta T, Cortese MM, Roper MH, et al: In Wharton M, Hughes H, Reilly M (eds): Vaccine-Preventable Diseases Surveillance Manual, 3rd ed. Atlanta: Centers for Disease Control and Prevention, 2002, pp 1-8.
29. Carson PJ, Nichol KL, O'Brien J, et al: Immune function and vaccine responses in healthy advanced elderly patients. Arch Intern Med 2001;160:2017-2024.
30. Solomonova K, Vizez S: Secondary response to boostering by purified aluminum-hydroxide–adsorbed tetanus in aging and aged adults. Immunobiology 1981;158: 312-319.
31. Cone J: 2005 NYC DOHMH Health Alert #16: Investigation of Possible Tainted Heroin [letter]. New York, New York City Department of Health and Mental Hygiene, 2005.
32. Centers for Disease Control and Prevention: Scopolamine poisoning among heroin users: New York City, Newark, Philadelphia, and Baltimore, 1995 and 1996. MMWR Morb Mortal Wkly Rep1996;45:457-460.
33. O'Callaghan WG, Joyce N, Counihan HE, et al: Unusual strychnine poisoning and its treatment: Report of eight cases. BMJ 1982;285:478.
34. Belson M, Kieszak S, Watson W, et al: Childhood pesticide exposures on the Texas-Mexico border: Clinical manifestations and poison center use. Am J Public Health 2003;93:310-315.
35. Centers for Disease Control and Prevention: Poisoning by an illegally imported Chinese rodenticide containing tetramethylenedisulfotetramine: New York City, 2002. MMWR Morb Mortal Wkly Rep 2003;52:199-201.
36. Apte NM, Karnad DR: Short report. The spatula test: A simple beside test to diagnose tetanus. Am J Trop Med Hyg 1995;53:386-387.
37. American College of Obstetricians and Gynecologists: ACOG committee opinion no. 282, January 2003: Immunization during pregnancy. Obstet Gynecol 2003;101: 207-212.
38. Demicheli V, Barale A, Rivetti A: Vaccines for women to prevent neonatal tetanus. Cochrane Database Syst Rev 2005;4:CD002959.
39. Centers for Disease Control and Prevention: General recommendations on immunization. MMWR Recomm Rep 2002;51(RR-2):1-35.
40. Ahmadsyah I, Salim A: Treatment of tetanus: An open study to compare the efficacy of procaine penicillin and metronidazole. BMJ 1985;291:648-650.
41. Yen LM, Dao LM, Day NPJ, et al: Management of tetanus: A comparison of penicillin and metronidazole. Symposium of antimicrobial resistance in southern Viet Nam. 1997.
42. Bleck TP: *Clostridium tetani*. In Mandell GL, Bennett JE, Dollin R (eds): Principle and Practice of Infectious Diseases, 4th ed, vol 2. New York: Churchill Livingstone, 1995; 2173-2178.
43. Bhatia R, Prabhakar S, Grover VK: Tetanus. Neurology India 2002;50:398-407.
44. Gilbert DV, Moillering RC, Eliopoulo GM, Sande MA (eds): The Sanford Guide to Antimicrobial Therapy 2005, 35th ed. Hyde Park, VT: Antimicrobial Therapy, 2005, p 30.
45. Edmondson RS, Flowers MW: Intensive care in tetanus: Management, complications and mortality in 100 cases. BMJ 1979;1:1401-1404.
46. Ceneviva GD, Thomas NJ, Kees-Folts D: Magnesium sulfate for control of muscle rigidity and spasms and avoidance of mechanical ventilation in pediatric tetanus. Pediatr Crit Care Med 2003;4:480-484.
47. Attygalle D, Rodrigo N: New trends in the management of tetanus. Expert Rev Anti Infect Ther 2004;2:73-84.
48. Thwaites CL, Farrar JJ: Magnesium sulphate as a first line therapy in the management of tetanus. Anaesthesia 2003;58:286.
49. Attagylle D, Rodrigo N: Magnesium sulphate for the control of spasms in severe tetanus. Anaesthesia 1999;54: 302-303.
50. Borgeat A, Dessibourg C, Rochani M, Suter PM: Sedation by propofol in tetanus: Is it a muscular relaxant? Intensive Care Med 1991;17;427-429.
51. Borgeat A, Popovic V, Schwander D: Efficiency of a continuous infusion of propofol in a patient with tetanus. Crit Care Med 1991;19:295-297.
52. Rie MA, Wilson RS: Morphine therapy controls autonomic hyperactivity in tetanus. Ann Intern Med 1978;88: 653-654.
53. Rocke DA, Wesley AG, Pather M, et al: Morphine in tetanus: The management of sympathetic nervous system overactivity. S Afr Med J 1986;70:666-668.
54. King WW, Cave DR: Use of esmolol to control autonomic instability of tetanus. Am J Med 1991;91:425-428.

Chapter 181

Rabies

Lisa D. Mills

KEY POINTS

Prevention of rabies through postexposure prophylaxis is the main treatment and the only one proven to be beneficial.

Once signs or symptoms of rabies manifest, the disease is nearly 100% fatal.

The postexposure prophylaxis regimen recommended by the World Health Organization should not be modified in any way.

Initiate prophylaxis for any high-risk exposure, even if the wound is healed and the event is remote.

Treatment of symptomatic rabies is experimental and requires consultation with the health department, the Centers for Disease Control and Prevention (CDC), or an infectious disease specialist. It may not begin in the ED.

Perspective

Rabies in humans remains rare in the United States. Only 36 cases were reported in the United States in the 20 years from 1980 to 2000.[1,2] However, rabies exposures in the United States require that approximately 40,000 people receive postexposure prophylaxis annually.[3] International travelers are at increased risk of exposure to rabies and may return to the United States to receive postexposure prophylaxis or rabies treatment. Rabies is a fatal disease.[1,2,4,5] Only six people are known to have survived the disease.[6-12]

Postexposure prophylaxis, if started before clinical sign of rabies, is highly effective. With strict adherence to protocol, including wound care, passive immunization, and vaccination with a cell culture vaccine, postexposure prophylaxis prevents rabies.[2,13-15] EPs should know when to begin rabies postexposure prophylaxis, when to delay it, and when postexposure prophylaxis is not indicated, and they should also know state and local resources for rabies information.

Anatomy

Rabies is transmitted when saliva or neural tissue from an infected host contacts open wounds or mucous membranes of a recipient. This transmission can occur through bites, aerosolized tissue, or tissue transplantation. Rabies virus is not transmitted by blood, feces, or urine. Rabies is not transmitted across intact skin.[2]

Once the virus is in a new host, it performs one of two actions. Some virus replicates at the site of the bite in non-nerve tissue. The virus then enters peripheral nerves and travels to the central nervous system

(CNS). Some virus does not replicate at the site, but rather immediately enters the peripheral motor and sensory nerves for transport to the CNS. During this time, the virus is in an eclipse phase and is difficult to detect with diagnostic tests.[16] The virus travels at speeds of 15 to 100 mm/day by retrograde axoplasmic flow.[5] When the virus enter the CNS, the incubation time ends. Incubation times range from 2 weeks to several years, and the average is 2 to 3 months.[5,16] Once in the CNS, the virus replicates and spreads by cell-to-cell transfer. The virus then travels by anterograde axoplasmic flow to nervous and non-nervous tissue. At the onset of clinical symptoms, the virus is disseminated throughout the body.

Pathophysiology

Rabies is caused by a negative-stranded RNA virus that belongs to the Lyssavirus family. The virus envelope fuses to the host cell membrane, and the virion penetrates the cell, where it replicates and buds new virus.

The virus causes inflammation in the CNS, both encephalitis and myelitis. Perivascular lymphocytic infiltration occurs with lymphocytes, polymorphonuclear leukocytes, and plasma cells. Cytoplasmic eosinophilic inclusion regions (Negri bodies) in neuronal cells are associated with rabies, but they are not sensitive or specific for the diagnosis of rabies.[16] Viral replication in dorsal root ganglia causes ganglionitis, which is responsible for the first clinical symptoms of the disease.[5]

Clinical Presentation

The first clinical symptoms of rabies are neuropathic pain, paresthesias, or pruritus at the inoculation site. These symptoms were present in 61% of cases in the United States.[4,17] A prodromal, flulike illness may mark the onset of clinical rabies. Brain involvement causes encephalitis, which manifests as delirium with periods of lucidity. Two major clinical forms of the disease exist: furious and paralytic.

Furious rabies is a manifestation of brainstem encephalitis. Hyperexcitability, autonomic dysfunction, and hydrophobia mark furious rabies. Spasms are induced with olfactory, visual, auditory, and tactile stimuli, causing aerophobia and hydrophobia. These spasms are painful, and the patient remains aware of the pain. Spasms are more prominent in the furious form of the disease. Focal neurologic signs are usually absent in furious rabies. The spasms are differentiated from tetanus by a lack of rigidity or trismus between spastic episodes. Involvement of the autonomic nervous system causes hypersalivation, profuse sweating, tachycardia, and hypertension.

Paralytic rabies results in quadriplegia.[18] It is more common after the bite of a vampire bat in South America. Peripheral neuropathy is responsible for the paralysis in paralytic rabies. Because peripheral nerves are involved, patients lose deep tendon reflexes. The paralysis occurs in an ascending pattern and is associated with pain and fasciculations. The anal sphincter is involved in the quadriplegia.[5] Death results from paralysis of bulbar and respiratory muscles.

Spontaneous inspiratory spasms occur in all patients with rabies at some point in the course of the disease. These painful inspiratory spasms can escalate to opisthotonos, generalized clonus, and respiratory arrest. Inspiratory spasms persist until death. Without treatment, clinical rabies is uniformly fatal in 2 to 10 days.

■ VARIATIONS

Consider rabies in patients with a clinical presentation of encephalitis.[19] Atypical presentation of disease is increasingly acknowledged, but it remains poorly described in the literature. Atypical presentations make the suspicion of rabies very difficult, especially if a clear history of rabies exposure is not presented.

Differential Diagnosis

The furious form of rabies is rapidly progressive and is fatal in 1 to 5 days (Table 181-1). The paralytic form of rabies is more slowly progressive, and patients live up to a month. However, clinical rabies is considered a fatal disease regardless of the clinical manifestation.

Diagnostic Testing

In the early stage of the disease, tests may show negative results.[5] The gold standard for the diagnosis of rabies is direct fluorescent antibody testing of the brain. Brain biopsy exclusively for the diagnosis of rabies is discouraged.[20,21]

Multiple testing techniques exist for the diagnosis of rabies during life. Discuss with the pathologist the preferred sample at your institution. Serum, saliva, and skin samples are commonly used, whereas cerebrospinal fluid, urine, and lacrimal fluid are occasionally tested.[5,22] Do not withhold empirical antirabies therapy to obtain diagnostic studies.

Perform a lumbar puncture for analysis of cerebrospinal fluid for meninigitis and encephalitis. Sedate the patient, if necessary, to control spasms. Send cere-

Table 181-1 DIFFERENTIAL DIAGNOSIS OF RABIES

Most Threatening Furious Rabies	Most Common Paralytic Rabies
Delirium tremens	Polio
Intoxication with stimulants/ hallucinogens	Guillain-Barré syndrome
Strychnine poisoning	Botulism
Tetanus	Tick paralysis
Encephalitis of other origin	Paralytic shellfish poisoning
Meningitis	Ciguatera toxin poisoning
African sleeping sickness	African sleeping sickness
	Herpes B virus encephalitis

Documentation

RABIES EXPOSURE

History	Exposure type: bite, nonbite Details of animal involved: species, vaccination history, domestic feral or wild, healthy or ill, provoked or nonprovoked in domestic animal, animal detained or escaped Animal control contacted or not Patient's rabies vaccination history
Physical examination	Neurovascular, tendons, wound size and depth, tenderness, visible contaminants, tattooing, discoloration, infection, masses, range of motion
Studies	Radiograph for tooth, if bite Urine pregnancy test in women of childbearing capacity
Medical decision making	Indication for rabies PEP or not, including type of exposure, likelihood of infection of animal, ability to observe animal; discussion with health department or CDC
Procedures	Wound care Wound infiltration with rabies immune globulin, if given Wound closure, if performed
Patient instructions	Documentation of discussion with patient regarding need for multiple vaccinations, if PEP initiated Documentation of discussion with patient regarding need to stay in contact with animal control for animal undergoing observation or for euthanized animal Wound care instructions

CDC, Centers for Disease Control and Prevention; PEP, postexposure prophylaxis.

brospinal fluid for diagnostic studies according to the patient's geographic exposure. Perform a toxicologic screen to evaluate for intoxication, but remember that intoxicants may be incidental findings.

Rabies Transmission

Rabies is transmitted only by mammals, both domestic and wild. Common wild animals known to contract and transmit rabies include foxes, skunks, raccoons, coyotes, and bats. Dogs, cats, cattle, and other domestic animals can also contract and transmit rabies.

Tips and Tricks

ZOONOTIC RABIES RESERVOIRS

Continent or Geographic Region	Primary Animal Reservoir
Africa	Dog, mongoose, antelope
Asia	Dog
Europe	Fox, bat
Middle East	Wolf, dog
North America	Fox, skunk, raccoon, bat (insectivorous)
South America	Dog, vampire bat

Patients commonly present after bites and scratches from small rodents, both wild and domestic. In these circumstances, wound care and reassurance are all that is required. Rats, mice, squirrels, chipmunks, hamsters, and guinea pigs do not transmit rabies. Rabbits and other lagomorphs have not been found to have rabies and have never been known to cause rabies.

Postexposure prophylaxis is virtually never indicated after a bite from or exposure to any rodent, so the health department should be consulted before initiating postexposure prophylaxis if the animal's behavior was suspicious and prophylaxis appears clinically indicated.

To assess the likelihood of rabies exposure, it is helpful to know the distribution of rabid animals in the area. The local or state health department can provide information about rabies prevalence and animal vectors. A list of state health department contact numbers is available through the CDC at http://www.cdc.gov/ncidod/dvrd/rabies/Links/Links.htm. Moreover, the CDC can be contacted at 877-554-4625 after hours or if the local or state health department is unavailable (http://www.cdc.gov/ncidod/dvrd/rabies/professional/professi.htm).

If the animal involved can carry rabies, determine whether the patient had an exposure (see the "Facts and Formulas" box). Consider any breech in the skin that was caused by teeth to be a bite exposure.[2,22] Exposure to aerosolized virus in a laboratory or cave setting constitutes a nonbite exposure. Saliva, neural tissue, or other infectious material contacting open wounds or mucous membranes constitutes an exposure. Contact of infectious material with intact skin does not constitute an exposure, nor does contact with noninfectious material, such as feces, blood, or urine, or petting a rabid animal. Do not provide postexposure prophylaxis to patients who have not had an nonexposure.[2]

If an exposure has occurred, the decision to begin postexposure prophylaxis is multifactorial. The type

FACTS AND FORMULAS

Exposure	Unlikely Exposure	Nonexposure
Bite Contamination of wound with saliva or infectious material Mucous membrane contact with saliva or infectious material Exposure to aerosolized virus Transplant of infected organ Bite, scratch, or mucous membrane contact with bat	Contact with dry secretions	Contact with intact skin Petting of rabid animal Contact with feces, blood, or urine

of animal, the epidemiology of rabies in the region of the exposure, and the health of the animal all contribute to the decision. Figure 181-1 provides an algorithm for the decision to start postexposure prophylaxis in humans. If an exposure involved a wild animal of a species that is a rabies vector, in a rabies-endemic area, begin postexposure prophylaxis immediately (see the "Tips and Tricks: Postexposure Prophylaxis" box). Do not await laboratory results. If the animal involved is an unlikely vector, postexposure prophylaxis can be withheld in consultation with the health department or CDC, as long as the animal can be tested for rabies with results available within 48 hours.[5]

If a wild animal that is a potential vector for rabies is responsible for an exposure but is unable to be captured, begin postexposure prophylaxis immediately (see the "Tips and Tricks: Postexposure Prophylaxis" box).[5] If a wild animal responsible for an exposure is caught, it should be immediately and humanely euthanized and tested. Wild animals should never be observed for signs of rabies because the time course of rabies in mammals other than dogs, ferrets, cats, and humans is not understood.[5]

Bats are common wildlife reservoirs of rabies in the United States, and prophylaxis is indicated even after seemingly trivial exposure. Rabies has been transmitted from unimportant or unrecognized exposures to bats.[2] Consider direct human-to-bat contact to be a likely exposure, even in the absence of a known bite. Begin rabies postexposure prophylaxis on all bites, scratches, and mucous membrane exposures to bats. Strongly consider postexposure prophylaxis in anyone who has had contact with a bat, even people who may be unaware of injury.[2] Strongly consider postexposure prophylaxis in a person who is near a bat and is uncertain whether contact has occurred, such as a person who awakens in a room with a bat.[23]

If the animal responsible for an exposure is a pet cat, dog, or ferret that is not currently showing signs of rabies, the animal can be observed for 10 days under the care of a veterinarian.[24,25] A currently vaccinated dog or cat is unlikely to have rabies, but vaccination failures have been reported. Therefore, even vaccinated animals should be reported to the health department for observation.[5]

Tips and Tricks

POSTEXPOSURE PROPHYLAXIS

Status	Postexposure Prophylaxis Regimen
Unvaccinated	Wash the wound thoroughly with soap and water. Treat the wound with a virucidal agent (povidone-iodine). Administer RIG, 20 IU/kg. Infiltrate as much as possible into wound and tissue immediately adjacent to the wound. Administer the remaining dose intramuscularly, remote from the tetanus vaccination site. Administer 1 mL tetanus vaccine intramuscularly. Use the deltoid in adults. Use the deltoid or anterior thigh in small children. Avoid the site of RIG administration. Instruct the patient to receive four more vaccination on days 3, 7, 14, and 28.
Previously vaccinated	Wash the wound thoroughly with soap and water. Treat the wound with a virucidal agent (povidone-iodine). Do NOT administer RIG. Administer 1 mL tetanus vaccine intramuscularly. Use the deltoid in adults. Use the deltoid or anterior thigh in small children. Instruct the patient to receive one more vaccination on day 3.

RIG, rabies immune globulin.

If the animal remains healthy, postexposure prophylaxis need not be started. If there is any suspicion that the animal is rabid, begin postexposure prophylaxis (see the "Tips and Tricks: Postexposure Prophylaxis" box). Postexposure prophylaxis can be terminated if laboratory results show that the animal does not have rabies. If the domestic animal is not

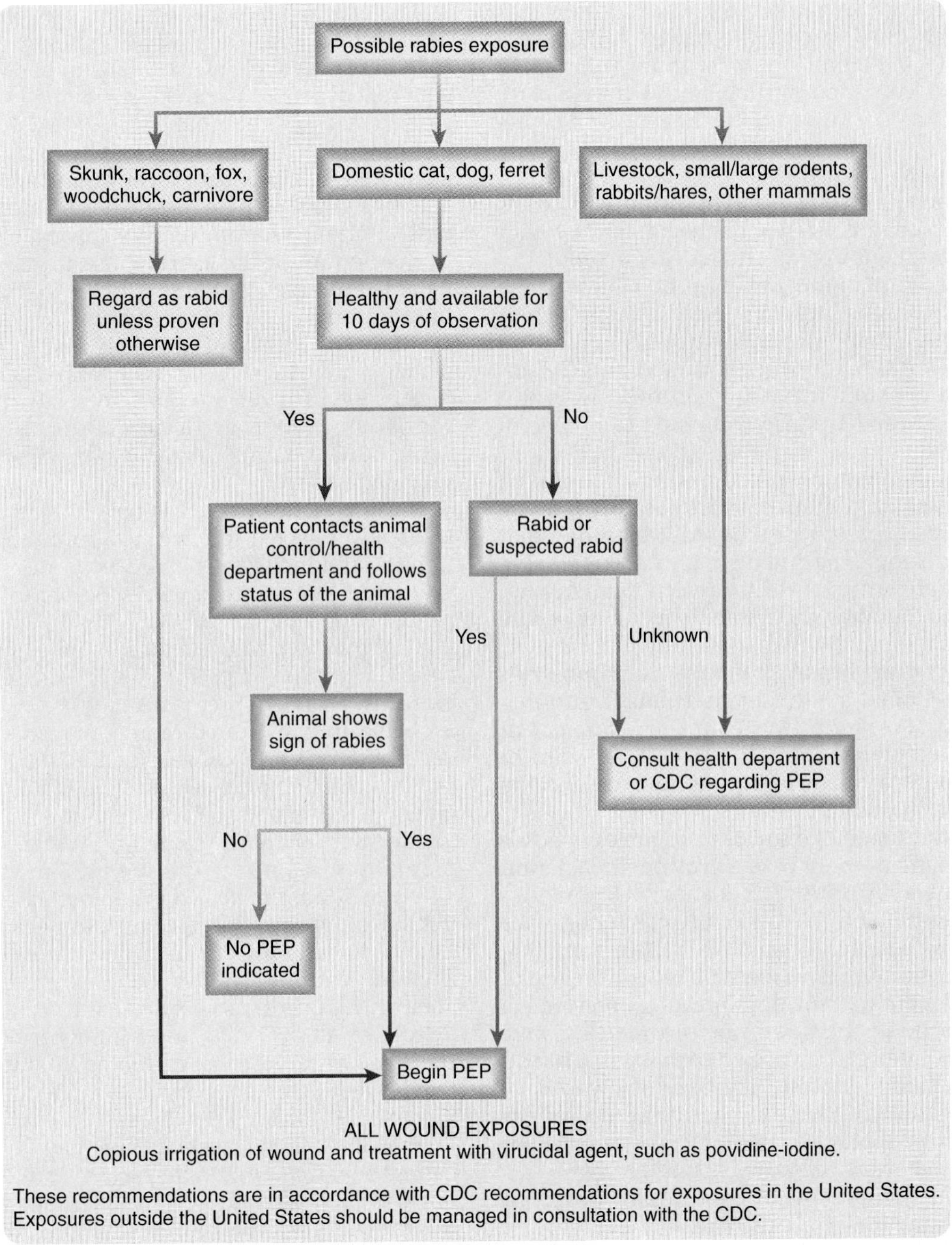
Possible rabies exposure
Skunk, raccoon, fox, woodchuck, carnivore
Domestic cat, dog, ferret
Livestock, small/large rodents, rabbits/hares, other mammals
Regard as rabid unless proven otherwise
Healthy and available for 10 days of observation
Yes
No
Patient contacts animal control/health department and follows status of the animal
Rabid or suspected rabid
Yes
Unknown
Animal shows sign of rabies
Consult health department or CDC regarding PEP
No
Yes
No PEP indicated
Begin PEP
ALL WOUND EXPOSURES
Copious irrigation of wound and treatment with virucidal agent, such as povidine-iodine.
These recommendations are in accordance with CDC recommendations for exposures in the United States.
Exposures outside the United States should be managed in consultation with the CDC.

FIGURE 181-1 Approach to assessing rabies exposure and initiating postexposure prophylaxis (PEP) in the United States. CDC, Centers for Disease Control and Prevention.

identifiable, contact the local health department to determine whether postexposure prophylaxis is indicated in your area.

In the case of a healthy, known pet that is not suspected of having rabies, provide the patient with information regarding the local health department and the need for animal quarantine by local animal control. The patient bears the responsibility of maintaining contact with the health department and animal control regarding the status of the animal. EPs are not expected to perform these functions for the patient. The CDC considers postexposure prophylaxis a medical urgency, not an emergency. Therefore, it is reasonable, in the low-risk exposures outlined in Figure 181-1, to delay postexposure prophylaxis. In this case, the patient will follow up with the health department or animal control and will return to a physician for postexposure prophylaxis, based on the finding in the animal.[2]

■ TRAVEL OUTSIDE THE UNITED STATES

Tens of thousands of people die of rabies worldwide, most commonly after being bitten by an infected dog. In developing countries of Africa, Asia, and

Latin America, rabies is common. Preexposure vaccination is indicated only if the patient will have a high likelihood of contact with animals, will remain for an extended period of time, and will have difficulty obtaining postexposure treatment. Even if preexposure prophylaxis is administered, postexposure treatment is still needed.

The World Health Organization (http://www.who.int/rabies/epidemiology) reports that rabies is present on every continent except Antarctica. Of 145 countries reporting, 45 note no cases of rabies. These rabies-free countries include selected islands such as New Zealand, Japan, Fiji, and Barbados, as well as certain developed European countries such as Greece, Portugal, and Scandinavian countries. In Latin America, Chile and Uruguay are noted to be free of rabies.

If a patient has had an exposure outside the United States, contact the CDC regarding the risk and the need for postexposure prophylaxis. Presume that prophylaxis should be initiated unless convincing evidence is present to the contrary. Initiate prophylaxis even if the wound is healed and the exposure was remote.

If a patient has begun postexposure prophylaxis outside the United States, obtain as much information as possible regarding the treatment before return to the United States. Contact the CDC or state or local health department regarding how to continue postexposure prophylaxis in this patient.

Human-to-human transmission of rabies is possible. Documented cases have involved inoculation through saliva by biting or kissing.[26] Human-to-human transmission has also occurred from the transplant of infected organs.[27,28] When providing routine healthcare to a person with rabies, the use of appropriate contact isolation practices prevents a rabies exposure in the healthcare provider.[2,29] There is no known case of transmission of rabies to a health care worker from a patient.[4] Treat persons who have been stuck with a contaminated needle from a patient with rabies as a rabies exposure. The concern is that the needle may contain neural tissue.

Incubation periods of up to 6 years have been reported for rabies.[16] For this reason, if exposure to rabies may have occurred, start postexposure prophylaxis regardless of the time from the exposure.[5] Adhere to the postexposure prophylaxis protocol as with any other exposure (see the "Tips and Tricks: Postexposure Prophylaxis" box).

Wound Treatment and Rabies Prevention

Postexposure prophylaxis consists of three steps: wound care, conferring of passive immunity, and active immunization. When World Health Organization guidelines for postexposure prophylaxis are followed, postexposure prophylaxis is effective. Postexposure prophylaxis failures have all involved deviation from the guidelines.[2]

The first step in rabies postexposure prophylaxis is local wound care. Copiously irrigate the wound with soap and water. Follow with treatment with a virucidal agent, such as povidone-iodine. Wound care alone decreases the chance of contracting rabies.[30] Failures of postexposure prophylaxis have been attributed to inadequate local wound care.[2]

The second step in postexposure prophylaxis is passive immunization. It takes approximately 7 days to develop an antibody response to rabies vaccine. Rabies immune globulin (RIG) provides passive immunization until the antibody response begins. Administer 20 IU/kg of RIG. This dose is the same for pediatric and adult patients. Infiltrate as much RIG as possible into the wound and tissue immediately surrounding the wound. Administer the remaining dose of RIG intramuscularly at a site remote from the vaccination site.

If the patient presents with a bite or wound that is already infected, clean the wound appropriately. Débride and incise the wound as needed. RIG can be infiltrated safely into an infected wound following proper local wound care.[5]

The third step in postexposure prophylaxis is vaccination (see the "Tips and Tricks: Postexposure Prophylaxis" box). Three cell culture vaccines are available in the United States: human diploid cell vaccine (HDCV), rabies vaccine adsorbed (RVA), and purified chick embryo cell vaccine (PCEC). These vaccines are all equally efficacious, and the dose and administration are the same for all three types.

Administer 1 mL of vaccine intramuscularly. The vaccine is administered intramuscularly into the deltoid of adults. The vaccine can be administered intramuscularly into the deltoid or anterior thigh of a child. Vaccine failures have been recorded for administration of vaccine into sites other than the deltoid of adults.[31] Do not administer vaccine into the same intramuscular region as RIG was administered. Do not use the same syringe to administer vaccine and RIG.

The first day of vaccination is day 0. Inform the patient that four additional vaccinations are required on days 3, 7, 14, and 28. The subsequent doses are the same, 1 mL intramuscularly. Postexposure prophylaxis should not be modified or discontinued unless the animal is found by laboratory testing to be free of rabies. If interruption of the postexposure prophylaxis schedule occurs, contact the local health department or the CDC to determine the new schedule.

Some people have been previously vaccinated against rabies. If they are exposed to rabies, previously vaccinated people undergo a modified vaccination regimen with two doses of vaccine, one dose on day 0 and one dose on day 3 (see the "Tips and Tricks: Postexposure Prophylaxis Vaccination" box). Administer a 1-mL intramuscular dose of vaccine in the deltoid. Instruct the patient to receive another dose of vaccine on day 3. Do NOT administer RIG to anyone who has been previously immunized. Provide local wound care, as with any exposure.

Because rabies is considered a fatal disease, postexposure prophylaxis is not withheld during pregnancy. Inform pregnant patients that no known fetal anomalies have been linked to rabies postexposure prophylaxis.[32-34] However, extensive testing in humans has not been performed. When possible, discuss the case with the patient's obstetrician.

Patients who are immunocompromised as a result of chronic illness or immune-modulating drugs require monitoring for immune response. Administer the same dose of vaccine and RIG, and provide appropriate wound care. If possible, discuss the case with the patient's primary physician or infectious disease specialist. Refer the patient to the patient's primary physician or infectious disease specialist for the remainder of the vaccination course and the appropriate antibody titers. Monitoring for immune response is outside the scope of emergency medicine.

Treatment

Rabies is considered a fatal disease.[4] Only six known cases of survivors of clinical rabies have been reported, and in five of these cases, patients had some form of rabies immunization before the onset of clinical disease. Four of the six survivors had neurologic devastation.[7-10]

■ TREATMENT OF SYMPTOMATIC RABIES

Once clinical signs or symptoms of rabies have begun, no reliably successful rabies treatment is known. Treatments are all considered experimental and have included antiviral therapy with ribavirin, vidarabine, and interferon alfa.[4,35,36] Rabies vaccine has not been demonstrated to have a beneficial effect in animal models when it is administered after the onset of clinical disease. RIG is of unknown benefit in clinical disease, but it is administered.[4] Ketamine has been used to induce coma and has been shown to decrease viral replication in rat models. It is of unknown clinical benefit in humans.[37] Corticosteroids are associated with increased mortality in laboratory studies. Avoid corticosteroids in patients suspected of having rabies encephalitis.[4] Because of the lack of an effective therapeutic regimen, the treatment of rabies involves consultation with local or state health departments and the CDC in conjunction with an infectious disease specialist and intensive care specialist, when available. The responsibility of the EP is to maintain a level of suspicion for rabies in a patient with signs of encephalitis, to consult for definitive diagnosis and management of rabies, and to provide supportive care while the patient is in the ED. The determination of an effective antiviral regimen for a patient with suspected or confirmed rabies is outside the scope of practice of emergency medicine.

When rabies is suspected, consult the local or state health department, the CDC, or an infectious disease specialist for emergency treatment guidance. Give RIG, 20 IU/kg intramuscularly, if significant delay in consultation is encountered. Provide supportive care to the patient. Spasms are painful, and the patient remains aware through much of the clinical course of the disease. When it is not contraindicated because of other comorbidities, administer ketamine by continuous intravenous infusion to sedate the patient and to alleviate the pain of rabies.[4] Intubate the patient if the patient has lost protective airway responses as a result of progression of the disease or because of sedation from medications. Unlike in bacterial infectious emergencies, delay in beginning antiviral agents is acceptable. Because of the lack of a standard of care in the treatment of rabies, the decision to begin antiviral therapy is best made in conjunction with consultants.

Documentation

CLINICAL RABIES

History	History of potential rabies exposure, including any bat or laboratory exposure Symptoms: onset, duration, progression Risk factors for other forms of encephalitis
Physical examination	Neurovascular features, tendons, wound size and depth, tenderness, visible contaminants, tattooing, discoloration, infection, masses, range of motion
Studies	Lumbar puncture: send routine studies and request that laboratory retain extra cerebrospinal fluid for encephalitis studies to be ordered by consultant If pathologist available, discuss preferred diagnostic tissues (if after hours, diagnostic studies can be sent during admission) screening for drugs of abuse
Medical decision making	Recommendations of infectious disease consultant, CDC, health department regarding treatment Indications for sedation Response to sedation Indication for intubation
Procedures	Lumbar puncture Rapid-sequence induction Intubation
Patient instructions	Documentation discussion with patient or family regarding suspicion of rabies and poor prognosis

CDC, Centers for Disease Control and Prevention.

PRIORITY ACTIONS

Clinical Rabies

Assess the patient for rabies exposure.

If exposure is likely or possible, contact the health department or the CDC for treatment recommendations.

Consult an infectious disease specialist, when available.

Consult an intensive care specialist.

Administer rabies immune globulin, 20 IU/kg intramuscularly, if there is delay in obtaining consultant recommendations.

Administer ketamine by intravenous infusion if the patient is in pain or is experiencing agitation.

Have the patient admitted by an intensive care specialist.

Defer vaccine administration and antiviral therapy to the health department or CDC or an infectious disease specialist.

CDC, Centers for Disease Control and Prevention.

PATIENT TEACHING TIPS

- Avoid contact with bats, including prevention of bat colonies.
- Seek medical care after exposure to bats.
- Avoid direct contact with wildlife.
- Avoid contact with any ill-appearing animal and with animals exhibiting bizarre behavior.
- Do not approach unknown cats or dogs.
- Seek medical attention for domestic animal bites.
- Any person bitten by a wild animal should seek medical attention.

Disposition

Patients who have had an exposure to a healthy pet that is undergoing 10 days of observation should be referred to animal control or to the health department. It is the patient's responsibility to stay in contact with animal control for information regarding the health of the animal.

Patients who have received the first treatment of postexposure prophylaxis are treated as outpatients. When possible, patients should continue the postexposure prophylaxis with a primary care physician or the health department, to ensure continuity of care. If not possible, the patient can return to the ED for the remainder of the postexposure prophylaxis. Patients with suspected clinical rabies require admission to the intensive care unit.

REFERENCES

1. Noah DL, Drenzek CL, Smith JS, et al: Epidemiology of human rabies in the United States, 1980-1996. Ann Intern Med 1998;128:922-930.
2. Centers for Disease Control and Prevention: Human Rabies Prevention: United States, 1999 Recommendations of the Advisory Committee on Immunization Practices (ACIP). MMWR Recomm Rep 1999;48:1-21.
3. Krebs JW, Long-Marin SC, Childs JE: Causes, costs and estimates of rabies postexposure prophylxis treatments in the United Sates. J Public Health Manage Pract 1998;4: 57-63.
4. Jackson AC, Warrell MJ, Rupprecht CE, et al: Management of rabies in humans. Clin Infect Dis 2003;36:60-63.
5. World Health Organization: WHO Expert Consultation on Rabies, 1st report. Geneva, World Health Organization, 2004, pp 1-121.
6. Gode GR, Raju AV, Jayalakshmi TS, et al: Intensive care in rabies therapy: Clinical observations. Lancet 1976;2:6-8.
7. Hattwick MAW, Weis TT, Stechschulte CJ, et al: Recovery from rabies: A case report. Ann Intern Med 1972;76: 931-942.
8. Tillotson JR, Axelrod D, Lyman DO: Rabies in a laboratory worker: New York. MMWR Morb Mortal Wkly Rep 1977;26:183-184.
9. Porras C, Barboza JJ, Fuenzalida E, et al: Recovery from rabies in man. Ann Intern Med 1976;85:44-48.
10. Alvarez L, Fajardo R, Lopez E, et al: Partial recovery from rabies in a nine-year-old boy. Pediatr Infect Dis J 1994;13:1154-1155.
11. Madhusudana SN, Nagaraj D, Uday M, et al: Partial recovery from rabies in a six-year-old girl [letter]. Int J Infect Dis 2002;6:85-86.
12. Centers for Disease Control and Prevention: Recovery of a patient from clinical rabies: Wisconsin, 2002. MMWR Morb Mortal Wkly Rep 2004;53:1171-1173.
13. Centers for Disease Control and Prevention: Rabies. Available at: http://www.cdc.gov/ncidod/dvrd/rabies/
14. Anderson LJ, Sikes RK, Langkop CW, et al: Postexposure trial of human diploid cell strain rabies vaccine. J Infect Dis 1980;142:133-138.
15. Bahmanyar M, Fayaz A, Nour-Salehi S, et al: Successful protection of humans exposed to rabies infection: Postexposure treatment with the new human diploid cell rabies vaccine and antirabies serum. JAMA 1976;236:2751-2754.
16. Centers for Disease Control and Prevention: Rabies: Natural history. Available at: www.cdc.gov/ncidod/dvrd/rabies/natural_history/nathist.htm.
17. Messenger SL, Smith JS, Rupprecht, CE: Emerging epidemiology of bat-associated cryptic cases of rabies in humans in the United States. Clin Infect Dis 2002;35:738-747.
18. Jackson AC: Human disease. In Jackson AC, Wunner WH (eds): Rabies. San Diego, Academic Press, 2002, pp 219-244.
19. Rupprecht CE, Hemachudha T: Rabies. In Scheld M, Whitley RJ, Marra C (eds): Infections of the Central Nervous System. Philadelphia, Lippincott Williams & Wilkins, 2004, pp 243-259.
20. Hemachudha T, Wacharapluesadee S: Ante-mortem diagnosis of human rabies. Clin Infect Dis 2004;39: 1085-1086.
21. Hanlon CA, Smith JS, Anderson GR: Recommendations of a national working group on prevention and control of rabies in the Unites States. Article II: Laboratory diagnosis of rabies. The National Working Group on Rabies Prevention and Control. J Am Vet Med Assoc 1999;215: 1444-1447.
22. Bourhy H, Rollin PE, Vincent J, Sureau P: Comparative field evaluation of the fluorescent-antibody test, virus isolation from tissue culture, and enzyme immunodiagnosis for rapid diagnosis of rabies. J Clin Microbiol 1989;27: 519-523.
23. Feder HM, Nelson R, Reiher HW: Bat bite? Lancet 1997;350:1300.

24. Centers for Disease Control and Prevention: Imported dog and cat rabies: New Hampshire, California. MMWR Morb Mortal Wkly Rep 1988;37:559-560.
25. Niezgoda M, Briggs DJ, Shaddock J, et al: Pathogenesis of experimentally induced rabies in domestic ferrets. Am J Vet Res 1997;58:1327-1331.
26. Fekadu M, Endshaw T, Wondimagegnehu A, et al: Possible human-to-human transmission of rabies in Ethiopia. Ethiop Med J 1996;34:123-127.
27. Centers for Disease Control and Prevention: Investigation of rabies infections in organ donor and transplant recipients: Alabama, Arkansas, Oklahoma, and Texas, 2004. MMWR Morb Mortal Wkly Rep 2004;53:1-3.
28. World Health Organization: Two rabies cases following corneal transplantation. Wkly Epidemiol Rec 1994;69:330.
29. Garner JS: Guidelines for isolation precautions in hospitals: The Hospital Infection Control Practices Advisory Committe. Infect Control Hosp Epidemiol 1996;17:53-80.
30. Kaplan MM, Cohen D, Koprowski H, et al: Studies on the local treatment of wounds for the prevention of rabies. Bull World Health Organ 1962;26:765-775.
31. Fishbein DB, Sawyer LA, Reid Sanden FL, Weir EH: Administration of human diploid-cell reabies vaccine in the gluteal area. N Engl J Med 1988;318:124-125.
32. Chutivonse S, Wilde H, Benjavongkulchai M, et al: Postexposure rabies vaccination during pregnancy: effect on 202 women and their infants. Clin Infect Dis 1995;20:818-820.
33. Varner MW, McGuinness GA, Galask RP: Rabies vaccination in pregnancy. Am J Obstet Gynecol 1982;143:717-718.
34. American College of Obstetricians and Gynecologists: ACOG committee opinion no. 282, January 2003: Immunization during pregnancy. Obstet Gynecol 2003;101:207-212.
35. Warrell MJ, White NJ, Looareesuwan S, et al: Failure of interferon alpha and ribavirin in rabies encephalitis. BMJ 1989;299:830-833.
36. Dolman CL, Charlton KM: Massive necrosis of the brain in rabies. Can J Neurol Sci 1987;14:162-165.
37. Lockhart BP, Tordo N, Tsiang H: Inhibition of rabies virus transcription in rat cortical neurons with the dissociative anesthetic ketamine. Antimicrob Agents Chemother 1992;36:1750-1755.

Chapter **182**

Tick-Borne Diseases

Jonathan A. Edlow

KEY POINTS

Tick-borne diseases (TBDs) most often can be diagnosed clinically and treatment initiated prior to definitive laboratory confirmation.

Many patients with TBDs will not recall a tick bite.

Some patients with TBDs will present with atypical findings.

Scope

Some tick-borne diseases (TBDs) are fatal if untreated; others are associated with significant morbidity. Curative treatments exist for most of them, and TBDs usually can be confidently diagnosed clinically based on pathognomonic or suggestive physical or laboratory findings that are available in the ED. Confirmatory laboratory testing is rarely available in real time. Therefore, physicians must understand both the classic and the atypical presentations and must be prepared to treat these illnesses based on clinical suspicion.

Because these illnesses frequently occur in the absence of a known tick bite, EPs must always consider TBDs when patients present in the correct epidemiologic context and with a recognizable syndrome. This chapter considers these diseases in syndromic groups, or patterns of presentation, rather than individually. Individual TBDs are listed in Table 182-1 (North America) and Table 182-2 (worldwide). Some travelers may return with these imported TBDs.

Epidemiologic context is a key principle in diagnosing TBDs. As in a criminal investigation, the practitioner must assess the tick's means, motive, and opportunity to transmit a TBD. The means has to do with tick anatomy—the ability to bite a mammal usually without the mammal's knowledge. This is crucial because most TBDs require many hours of tick attachment to transmit the infectious agent. The motive has to do with tick physiology; ticks require a blood meal from a host to live and transform to their next life stage. Opportunity relates to patient and geographic factors, that is, epidemiologic context. Taking a history that focuses on this epidemiologic context is absolutely crucial in the diagnosis of all TBDs. Ask whether the patient has been bitten by a tick, but remember that most patients with TBDs do *not* recall a tick bite. For example, only approximately 25% of patients with Lyme disease (smaller ticks) and only two thirds of patients with Rocky Mountain spotted fever (RMSF) (larger ticks) recall the bite. The more important issue is whether the patient *could* have been bitten by a tick. Physicians should therefore ask the following questions:

- How do you spend your time?
- What is your job?
- What hobbies and recreational activities do you enjoy?
- Where have you traveled recently?

With regard to season, although most TBDs are acquired from April through September, "tick season" depends on the stage of a disease and the local weather patterns for a given geographic area. For example, Lyme arthritis could manifest in January from a bite in July, and a warm spell in late fall in North Carolina could result in a case of RMSF that develops in November.

Table 182-1 TICK-BORNE DISEASES OF NORTH AMERICA

Disease	Pathogen or Agent	Major Tick Vector
Lyme disease	*Borrelia burgdorferi*	*Ixodes scapularis*, others
Babesiosis	*Babesia microti*	*Ixodes scapularis*
Ehrlichiosis, granulocytic	*Anaplasma phagocytophila*	*Ixodes scapularis*
Ehrlichiosis, monocytic	*Ehrlichia chaffeensis*	*Amblyomma americanum*
Rocky Mountain spotted fever	*Rickettsia rickettsiae*	*Dermacentor variabilis*
Tularemia	*Francisella tularensis*	*Dermacentor variabilis, Dermacentor andersoni, and Amblyomma americanum*
Relapsing fever	*Borrelia* species (various)	*Ornithodoros* species
Colorado tick fever	Coltivirus	*Dermacentor andersoni*
Tick paralysis	Neurotoxin	*Dermacentor variabilis*, others
Q fever	*Coxiella burnetii*	*Dermacentor variabilis*

Table 182-2 OTHER IMPORTANT TICK-BORNE DISEASES WORLDWIDE

Disease	Pathogen or Agent	Major Tick Vector
Mediterranean spotted fever	*Rickettsia connori*	*Rhipicephalus sanguineus*
Other spotted fevers	Other rickettsial species	Varies
Tick-borne encephalitis	Flavivirus	*Ixodes ricinus*, others
Relapsing fever	Various *Borrelia* species	Various *Ornithodoros* species

Table 182-3 COMMON TICKS RELATED TO HUMAN DISEASE

Tick Genus	Hard or Soft	Feeding Duration	Diseases Caused
Ixodes	Hard	Days	Lyme disease, babesiosis, human granulocytic ehrlichiosis
Amblyomma	Hard	Days	Human monocytic ehrlichiosis, Master's disease, tick paralysis
Dermacentor	Hard	Days	Rocky Mountain spotted fever, tularemia, tick paralysis, Colorado tick fever
Rhipicephalus	Hard	Days	Mediterranean spotted fever
Ornithodoros	Soft	Minutes to hours	Relapsing fever

Pathophysiology and Tick Anatomy

Two genera of ticks are important in human TBDs. Hard (Ixodidae) ticks tend to attach and feed for days, whereas soft ticks (Argasidae) feed in minutes to hours. Table 182-3 lists some characteristics of these different types of ticks. Because the hard ticks, which transmit most of the human TBDs, feed for so long, tick removal during the first 24 hours of attachment provides one strategy for disease prevention, a concept best studied in the context of Lyme disease. Figures 182-1 to 182-3 show various stages of *Ixodes scapularis, Dermacentor variabilis,* and *Amblyomma americanum* ticks.[1]

Presenting Signs and Symptoms

TBDs most commonly manifest as one of four syndromes (Table 182-4):

- Localized rash (with or without fever)
- Febrile illness without prominent rash
- Febrile illness with diffuse rash
- Acute neurologic symptoms.

Of course, other possible presentations are possible, especially with respect to atypical presentations of any of these diseases and, most notably, Lyme disease. The other signs and symptoms of Lyme disease are discussed separately.

Before discussing the individual syndromes and diseases, it is important to know that as often as 20%

Table 182-4 TICK-BORNE DISEASE SYNDROMES

Syndrome	Disease	Characteristics of Typical Cases
Localized rash (without or without fever)	Erythema migrans (Lyme disease) Tularemia (ulceroglandular)	Large, flat, red rash, sometimes with central clearing that occurs at the site of tick bite Shallow ulcer, usually acral at the site of tick bite, associated with regional lymphadenopathy
Febrile illness without rash	Ehrlichiosis Babesiosis Lyme disease Rocky Mountain spotted fever Tularemia Q fever Colorado tick fever	High fever, chills, headache, myalgias High fever, chills, headache, fatigue, myalgias Flulike illness without respiratory or gastrointestinal manifestations Severe headache, fever, myalgias High fever without localizing findings except respiratory symptoms in tularemic pneumonia Nonspecific febrile illness Fever (saddleback curve), headache, myalgias
Febrile illness with generalized rash	Rocky Mountain spotted fever Lyme disease Ehrlichiosis	As above with rash. Rash begins as maculopapular then may evolve into petechial and skin necrosis Multiple erythema migrans lesions (smaller, no punctum, less complexity than primary erythema migrans lesions) Nonspecific maculopapular rash
Acute neurologic illness	Tick paralysis	Generally occurs in young girls with the tick embedded in the scalp

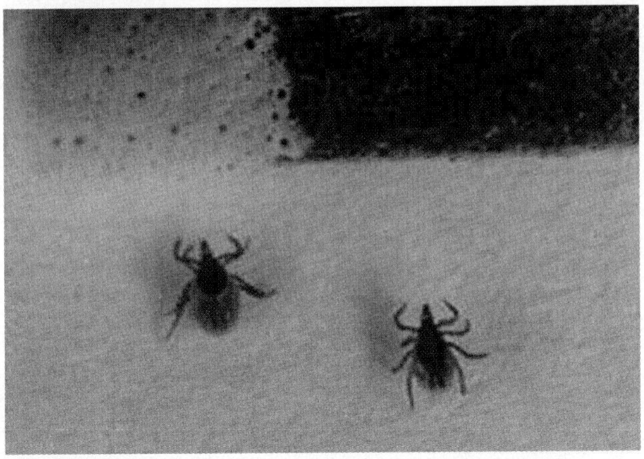

FIGURE 182-1 *Ixodes scapularis* ticks, nymphal stage. Two nymphal *I. scapularis* ticks are shown next to a common household match. The tick on the *left* has been feeding on a mouse for 48 hours and is larger than the unfed tick on the *right*. Seen in three dimensions, the fed tick is more spherical, whereas the unfed tick is flatter. (Photo by Darlyne Murawski.)

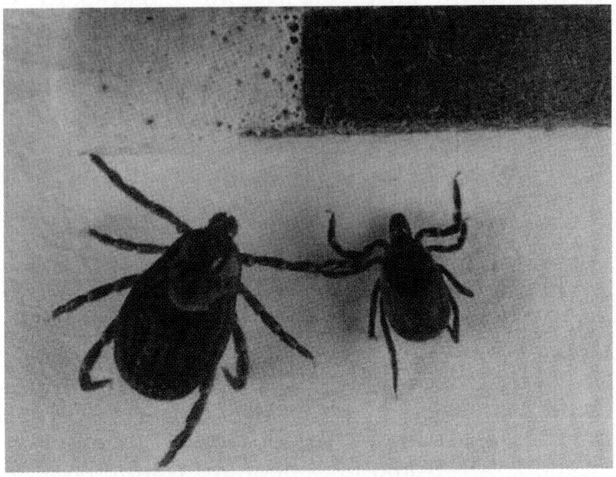

FIGURE 182-2 A *Dermacentor variabilis* tick next to an *Ixodes scapularis* tick. This photograph shows an adult *D. variabilis (left)* tick next to an adult *I. scapularis (right)* tick, both next to a common match for scale. In cases of Rocky Mountain spotted fever, even with this larger tick vector, 30% to 40% of patients are not aware of a tick bite. (Photo by Darlyne Murawski.)

of the time, a single tick bite results in multiple infections. Therefore, a patient may develop the rash of Lyme disease along with babesiosis or ehrlichiosis. This has implications with respect to the manifestations of the diseases and also the choice of antimicrobials.[2]

■ LOCALIZED RASH (WITH OR WITHOUT FEVER)

Localized rash from TBD occurs with early Lyme disease and ulceroglandular tularemia. Tularemia has multiple presentations, but the ulceroglandular form, which accounts for 80% of cases, usually starts with

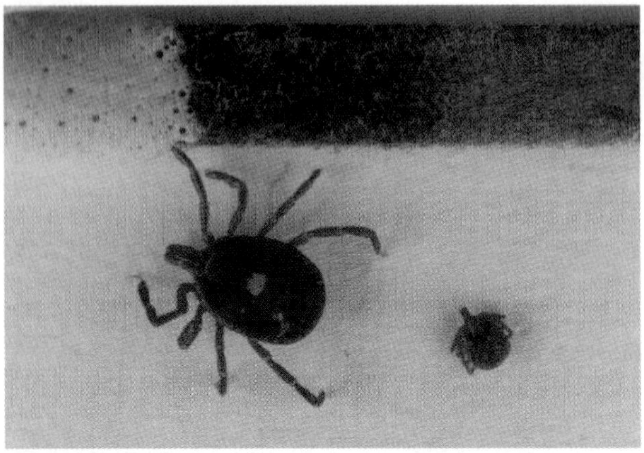

FIGURE 182-3 *Amblyomma americanum* tick. An adult female Lone Star tick next to a nymph of the same species. This tick is responsible for transmission of human monocytic ehrlichiosis and Master's disease. (Photo by Darlyne Murawski.)

a papule that evolves into an ulcer on an extremity at the site of a tick bite (or animal exposure). The lesion evolves into a necrotic eschar and is often associated with regional lymphadenopathy, fever, and other systemic signs.[2]

Erythema migrans (EM), the rash of early localized Lyme disease, is an important condition with which EPs ought to be familiar, because treatment with antibiotics at this stage almost always leads to excellent outcomes. Moreover, Lyme disease is by far the most common vector-borne illness in North America. EM develops at the site of the tick bite roughly 7 to 10 days later (range, 3 to 33 days), usually as a flat erythema that is neither pruritic nor painful (although it can be either). Although the "classic" form is described as having a target or bull's eye morphology, with central clearing, in fact, most EM rashes are uniformly red. Some are darker in the center, and still others are vesicular or necrotic. Know the spectrum of morphology of EM to avoid misdiagnosis of this infection[3,4] (Figs. 182-4 to 182-6).

The location of EM tends to be at the sites where ticks feed or experience an impediment to further movement (the groin, the popliteal fossa, the axilla, an elastic underwear strap, or the hairline in children). Although the rash can be anywhere, it tends not to occur acrally, and the torso is another common location. Size is another important feature because EM becomes large, 16 cm on average. Cellulitis, one of the more important diagnostic competitors, rarely attains this size in the absence of fever, significant tenderness, and other systemic findings.[3,4]

Some patients with EM have fever, headache, myalgias, neck pain or stiffness, and other systemic symptoms. However, the fever is usually low grade, and high fevers suggests coinfecting babesiosis or ehrlichiosis. Roughly 10% to 20% of patients with early Lyme disease have multiple cutaneous lesions (see later).

Finally, although EM has always been thought to be pathognomonic of Lyme disease, EM-like lesions have been reported in the southeastern and central

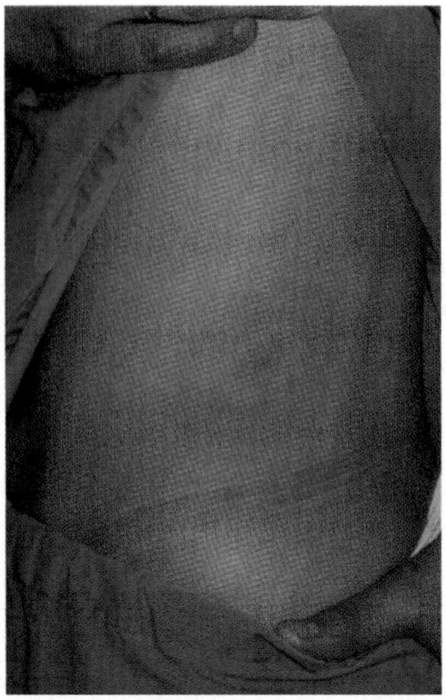

FIGURE 182-4 Classic erythema migrans. Note the location (torso) and the bull's eye appearance in this patient with fever and localized rash, which was flat and neither painful nor pruritic. There is a suggestion of a central punctum, the location of the tick bite.

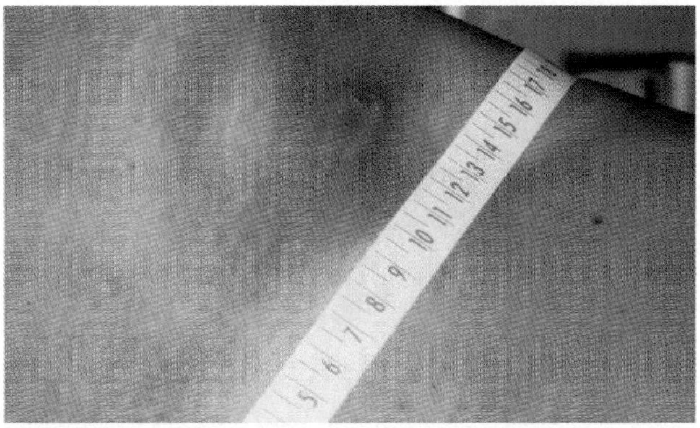

FIGURE 182-5 Erythema migrans with a raised, vesicular center. This patient presented in early July after having pulled a tick off himself 7 days earlier. Approximately 18 hours after starting doxycycline, the patient had a Jarisch-Herxheimer reaction (abrupt onset of chills, tachycardia, intensification of rash), which occurs with treatment of spirochetal diseases.

states. Although, as a group, these patients' rashes have some differences from classic EM in states endemic for Lyme disease, the rash in any individual patient is consistent with EM. This lesion is likely caused by one or more novel *Borrelia* species, and these patients should also be treated with antibiotics, similar to patients with Lyme disease.[5]

■ FEBRILE ILLNESS WITHOUT PROMINENT RASH

Most TBDs can manifest as a nonspecific febrile illness, specifically, babesiosis, ehrlichiosis, tularemia, Colorado tick fever, relapsing fever, and Q fever. Lyme disease can also manifest this way, although

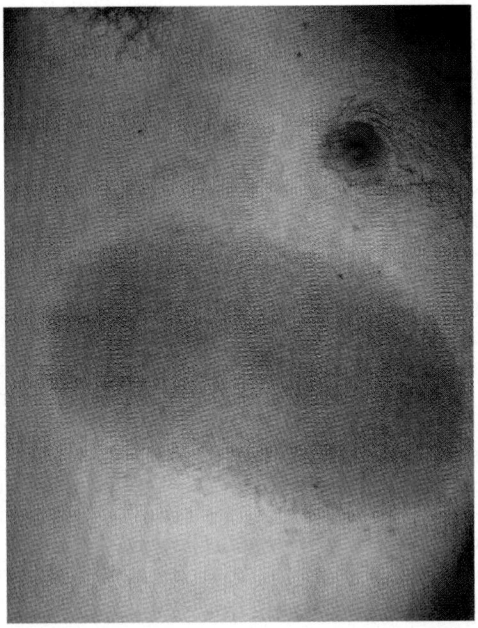

FIGURE 182-6 Erythema migrans with a homogeneous color. This young man had a rash that had been ascribed to a spider bite but was growing larger. It was painless, thus making a spider bite much less likely. The patient also had a tender, palpable lymph node in the right axilla.

the precise incidence is unclear. Typical patients with RMSF do not have a rash until the third to the sixth day of illness, and in as many as 15% of patients, a rash never appears. If RMSF is a real diagnostic possibility on epidemiologic grounds, treat with empirical antibiotics even in the absence of a rash. Finally, all these diseases that typically present without rash are sometimes associated with nonspecific, usually maculopapular rashes.[6]

Ehrlichiosis, a relatively newly described illness, has a presentation similar to that of RMSF but without the rash. (The nomenclature for ehrlichiosis has recently been changed to *anaplasmosis*.) The two most common forms in humans are granulocytic and monocytic (terms based on the predilection for which white blood cells of the organisms exhibit tropism). These patients complain of high fever, headache, and myalgias. The spectrum of disease is wide, and published series likely emphasize sicker patients. As in RMSF, some patients have prominent encephalitis, noncardiogenic pulmonary edema, and shock. First-line therapy for ehrlichiosis is doxycycline.[7]

Babesiosis, a malaria-like parasitic infection that is transmitted by *I. scapularis,* is another disease that is diagnosed with increasing frequency in areas of the country where this tick is active. The usual agent in North America is *Babesia microti*. Infection results in a wide spectrum of illness ranging from asymptomatic seroconversion to mild flulike illness, to malaria-like illness, or even overwhelming sepsis and death. Fever, fatigue, headache, sweats, and chills are the most common symptoms. Hepatosplenomegaly may be present. Complications include hemolysis and renal failure, noncardiogenic pulmonary edema, and coma. Patients with babesiosis can be ill for weeks to months and may have subacute or chronic illness. First-line treatment is clindamycin and quinine; atovaquone and azithromycin have also been used. Some patients with high circulating parasite levels and complications require exchange blood transfusion, and splenectomized patients have a particularly poor prognosis.[8,9]

Colorado tick fever is a viral illness that occurs in the Rocky Mountain states and southwestern Canada and is transmitted by *D. andersoni* at elevations of 1200 m to 3300 m. Only a few hundred cases are diagnosed annually in the United States. The presentation is nonspecific (fever, headache, and myalgias), but the fever often follows a characteristic "saddle-back" pattern (two periods of 2 to 3 days of fever, punctuated by an afebrile interval). Occasionally, a small, red, painless papule is seen, and less commonly, patients have nonspecific generalized rash. Pharyngitis, lower gastrointestinal symptoms, and central nervous system symptoms may also occur in some cases. Treatment is supportive.[10]

Q fever manifests as a nonspecific febrile illness sometimes associated with hepatitis or pneumonia. Hepatitis is particularly common. Other organ systems may be affected (i.e., heart and central nervous system), and a few patients also exhibit a nonspecific maculopapular rash. Q fever may become chronic, and in these patients, it often affects the heart (endocarditis), blood vessels, and liver. The diagnosis is established by serologic methods and polymerase chain reaction because the organism is very rarely cultured. First-line therapy consists of 2 weeks of doxycycline.

The typhoidal form of tularemia, which manifests as a nonspecific febrile illness and headache, is quite uncommon. Tularemic pneumonia may develop, and one outbreak of this form of the disease on Martha's Vineyard (an island off the coast of Massachusetts) likely resulted from inhalation of ticks aerosolized by power lawn mowers.

Relapsing fever is caused by various *Borrelia* species transmitted by *Ornithodoros* ticks, soft ticks that feed for very short times. This illness is characterized by intervals of fever interspersed with afebrile periods.[6] The explanation of these episodes is that the *Borrelia* organisms undergo antigenic shifting, thus presenting a new antigen to the patient's immune system. After an incubation period of approximately 1 week, patients develop fever, headache, myalgias, and chills. Abdominal pain and altered mental status are common. Untreated, most patients improve and then suffer a relapse from the new antigenic variety 1 week later. Complications include focal neurologic findings (including seventh nerve palsy), myocarditis, and ruptured spleen.

■ FEBRILE ILLNESS WITH GENERALIZED RASH

As noted earlier, most TBDs can manifest with fever and generalized rash, but this section deals with those illnesses in which the generalized rash is a prominent manifestation of the illness. RMSF is the most dramatic of these illnesses; patients present with fever, headache, myalgias, and rash. The classic triad of fever, headache, and rash in a patient with a recent tick bite is seen in a minority of patients. Even with the larger tick vector, only approximately two thirds of patients recall the tick bite. In addition, the rash of RMSF does not develop until the third to the sixth day of the illness. The rash begins as a maculopapular rash that becomes petechial and finally may evolve into frank ecchymosis. The classic description (begins acrally and spreads centrally) does not always apply. Thus, the rash can vary from nonexistent to frank skin necrosis. Because the organisms produce vasculitis, the manifestations are based on the particular organs affected. Patients can present with a surgical abdomen, an illness resembling meningitis, myocarditis, renal failure, or circulatory collapse. RMSF has an untreated mortality rate of 25% to 40%. Therefore, considering this diagnosis in any febrile patient with the correct epidemiologic context is important, because early antibiotic treatment (the first-line agent is doxycycline) reduces the mortality rate to less than 5%.[11-13]

Early disseminated Lyme disease with secondary EM is the other TBD that manifests as fever and generalized rash. Secondary lesions occur approximately 20% of the time and imply hematogenous spread of the organism. The secondary lesions differ from the primary EM lesion is several ways. They tend to be smaller, lack the central punctum, and exhibit less central clearing.

■ ACUTE WEAKNESS

The one TBD that is not caused by an infectious agent is tick paralysis. This illness can be caused by several tick species that produce neurotoxins. These patients present with gait instability, acute ascending weakness, and sometimes with cranial nerve findings that suggest Guillain-Barré syndrome. Typically, these patients are children, often girls, and the tick is found on the scalp, which must be very carefully inspected. The diagnosis is established by finding an engorged tick, the removal of which is also the treatment of this rare disease.[14]

Despite (or perhaps because of) the rarity of this disorder, consider this entity in all patients with acute onset of weakness. Recent cases have been reported in the Philadelphia area and another case occurred in Los Angeles (likely contracted in Montana). The neurologic findings resolve over 6 to 24 hours, and finding the tick will preclude the need for a more expensive and invasive evaluation and will prevent deaths. Patients have no fever and no alteration of consciousness.

Lyme disease can also manifest with different kinds of focal weakness resulting from meningoradiculitis; the deficit depends on which nerve roots are involved. Of course, any febrile illness can lead to overall and nonlocalizing malaise.

■ OTHER MANIFESTATIONS OF LYME DISEASE

Lyme disease has been traditionally divided into three phases (Table 182-5). Early localized disease is EM, although some authors include flulike illness in this stage. Early disseminated disease typically involves the skin, heart, joints, and nervous system. Late disseminated disease generally affects the joints, nervous system, and (in Europe) the skin. Although early disseminated Lyme disease has many potential manifestations, the common and important ones for EPs are cranial nerve palsy, meningitis, carditis, and arthritis.[5]

Any cranial nerve can be affected, but seventh nerve palsy is by far the most common. Bilateral facial involvement occurs more commonly with Lyme-induced facial palsy than in most other causes. Controversy exists regarding whether to perform lumbar puncture on these patients. The major ques-

Table 182-5 COMMON MANIFESTATIONS AND TREATMENT OF LYME DISEASE

Stage	Manifestation	Treatment
Early localized	Localized erythema migrans	Oral amoxicillin, doxycycline, or cefuroxine axetil for 10-30 days
Mild early disseminated	Disseminated erythema migrans Conjunctivitis Early arthritis Seventh nerve palsy with normal cerebrospinal fluid Carditis with PR interval <0.30	Ceftriaxone, cefotaxime, or penicillin G for 21-30 days
Severe early disseminated	Early neurologic manifestations with abnormal cerebrospinal fluid* Carditis with PR interval >0.30 or higher degrees of heart block	Ceftriaxone, cefotaxime, or penicillin G for 2-3 weeks
Late disseminated	Late neurologic manifestations (encephalopathy, peripheral neuropathy) Lyme arthritis	Intravenous antibiotics for 2-4 weeks Oral antibiotics for 30-60 days

*Manifestations include cranial neuropathy, lymphocytic meningitis (with or without radiculitis or plexitis), transverse myelitis, and cerebellitis. Controversy exists regarding parenteral antibiotics if seventh nerve palsy is the only manifestation (and cerebrospinal fluid pleocytosis).

tion is this: Should the presence of pleocytosis mandate parenteral therapy or not? Although this question has no definitive answer, I favor lumbar puncture, and I treat the patient parenterally if the cerebrospinal fluid shows abnormalities. Lyme meningitis (which can occur with or without other neurologic abnormalities) can be surprisingly "quiet" with respect to symptoms. Headache may be mild and intermittent, and meningeal signs are often absent.[2,5]

Carditis occurs in 5% to 10% of untreated patients, usually in young male patients. It has a predilection for the conduction system and often leads to complete heart block. Although temporary cardiac pacing is indicated, permanent pacers are rarely necessary. Arthritis is usually a late finding, but it can occur in the early disseminated phase as well.[5]

Diagnostic Testing

Physicians should diagnose early localized Lyme disease and tick paralysis by history and physical examination. Fifty percent of patients with EM have a negative Lyme serologic test; therefore, no testing is necessary because a negative result should not dissuade the physician from diagnosing EM and treating it. Physicians should also treat suspected RMSF empirically without waiting for diagnostic test confirmation. Table 182-6 gives clues to the diagnosis of TBDs.[2,15]

Physicians can often confidently diagnose babesiosis (Fig. 182-7), ehrlichiosis (Fig. 182-8), and relapsing fever (Fig. 182-9) on the basis of a blood smear. Numerous antigen and antibody tests are available for all these diseases, and the physician should talk to the clinical laboratory staff or infectious disease consultant to ascertain what tests are available at that hospital.

For later manifestation of Lyme disease, the Centers for Disease Control and Prevention currently recommends a two-step testing procedure (screening enzyme-linked immunosorbent assay followed by a confirmatory Western blot). Although this procedure remains the standard as of 2007, newer tests, especially the C-6 peptide, hold great promise for a single-tier test. In these patients, the physician must

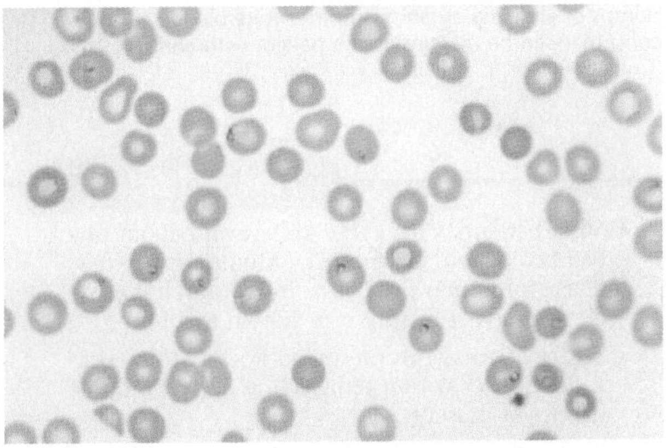

FIGURE 182-7 Blood smear showing babesiosis. This figure shows intraerythrocytic ring forms in multiple red blood cells from a patient with a high parasite count.

Table 182-6 CLUES ON HISTORY, PHYSICAL EXAMINATION, OR LABORATORY FINDINGS THAT SUGGEST THE DIAGNOSIS OF NORTH AMERICAN TICK-BORNE DISEASE MANIFESTING AS A NONSPECIFIC FEBRILE ILLNESS*

Disease	Clues
Ehrlichiosis	May have a faint rash Low white blood cell or platelet count Elevated hepatic transaminases
Babesiosis	Findings of hemolysis History of splenectomy Presence of faint rash, hepatomegaly, or splenomegaly
Lyme disease	Careful skin examination for any rash consistent with erythema migrans Bradycardia from heart block Associated seventh nerve palsy or lymphocytic meningitis
Colorado tick fever	Saddle-back fever curve
Rocky Mountain spotted fever	Maculopapular or petechial rash Normal white blood cell count or low platelet count Hyponatremia Peripheral edema
Relapsing fever	Recurring episodes of fever with afebrile intervals
Tularemia	Acrally located ulcer Regional lymphadenopathy Possible associated pneumonia

*Apart from an epidemiologic context suggesting a tick-borne disease.

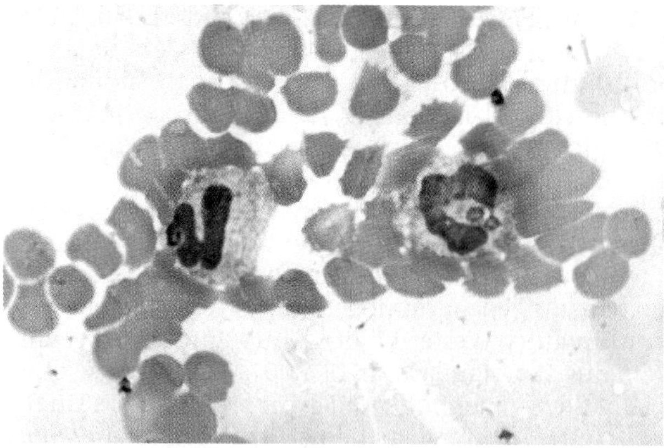

FIGURE 182-8 Blood smear showing a morula in a patient with ehrlichiosis. This blood smear shows two morulae (intracellular clumps of ehrlichia organisms in the white blood cell to the *right*) that can be diagnostic in a patient with ehrlichiosis. (Courtesy of Dr. J. S. Dumler.)

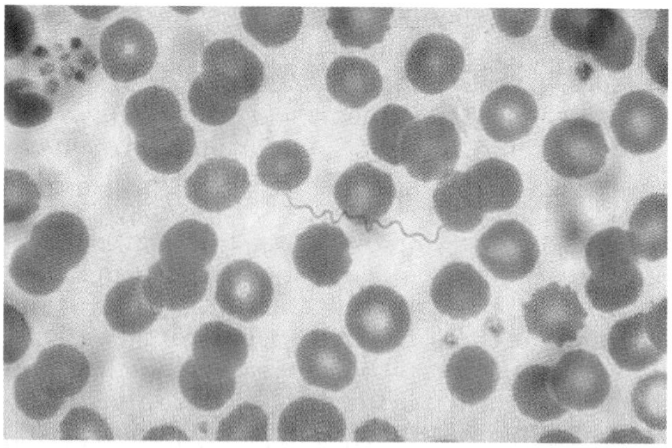

FIGURE 182-9 Blood smear showing relapsing fever *Borrelia*. This blood smear shows a spirochete in the blood from a patient with relapsing fever.

Tips and Tricks

- Most patients with Lyme disease and about one third of patients with Rocky Mountain spotted fever (for which the tick vector is much larger) do not have a history of a known tick bite.
- Treat patients with presumed Rocky Mountain spotted fever with a tetracycline even if a rash is not yet present.
- Remember that up to 20% of patients with tick-borne disease have more than one infection transmitted by the same tick bite.
- Examine the whole body, and particularly the scalp, in all patients presenting with acute significant weakness or a clinical picture resembling Guillain-Barré syndrome. This is especially important in young children and occurs most often in young girls.
- In early localized Lyme disease with erythema migrans, serologic testing in not indicated or helpful, unless the clinical findings and situation are very atypical or ambiguous. Serologic tests are normal approximately 50% of the time.
- In children, even those younger than 9 years of age, with life-threatening cases of Rocky Mountain spotted fever or ehrlichiosis, use intravenous doxycycline initially.

carefully interpret the serologic results in the context of the patient's symptoms, clinical course, and epidemiologic features.[15,16]

Interventions and Procedures

Tick removal is best accomplished by using fine forceps applied close to the skin and gradually pulling the tick up and outward. Because ticks use a cement-like substance to embed, this removal procedure may take steady gentle pressure over a minute or two. Try to remove the entire tick. Retained mouth parts may result in a foreign body reaction or a staphylococcal or streptococcal skin infection, but they have no implications in terms of TBD transmission. Occasionally, lumbar puncture and cardiac pacing may be indicated in selected patients.

Treatment and Disposition

No specific antimicrobial therapy exists for Colorado tick fever. For tick paralysis, the diagnosis and treatment are accomplished by removing the tick; improvement takes place over the ensuing 6 to 24 hours.

Treat patients with the remaining bacterial TBDs with specific antimicrobial therapy.[17-21] Again, the threshold to treat must be low, and frequently the decision to treat is based purely on presentation and epidemiologic context. In addition, although tetracyclines are generally contraindicated in children less than 9 years of age, in children with life-threatening manifestations of RMSF or ehrlichiosis, short courses of intravenous doxycycline can be used.

In most patients with TBDs, the diagnosis can be made and the illness can be treated on an outpatient basis with primary care follow-up. Patients with syndromes requiring intravenous antibiotics, cardiac pacing, or intensive care resulting from central nervous system, respiratory, renal, or circulatory failure should be admitted to an appropriate inpatient setting.

PATIENT TEACHING TIPS

- If you cannot avoid tick exposure, do daily tick checks and carefully remove any ticks found.
- If you become ill and have either been bitten by a tick or been exposed to ticks, be sure to mention this to you doctor, even if you develop new symptoms weeks or months later. It is possible that the tick bite could cause delayed problems.

REFERENCES

1. Anderson JF: The natural history of ticks. Med Clin North Am 2002;86:205-218.
2. Edlow JA: Lyme disease and related tick-borne illnesses. Ann Emerg Med 1999;33:680-693.
3. Edlow JA: Erythema migrans. Med Clin North Am 2002; 86:239-260.
4. Tibbles CD, Edlow JA: Does this patient have erythema migrans? JAMA 2007;297:2617-2627.
5. Dworkin MS, Schwan TG, Anderson DE Jr: Tick-borne relapsing fever in North America. Med Clin North Am 2002;86:417-433, viii-ix.
6. Steere AC: Lyme disease. N Engl J Med 2001;345:115-125.
7. Olano JP, Walker DH: Human ehrlichioses. Med Clin North Am 2002;86:375-392.
8. Krause PJ, Babesiosis. Med Clin North Am 2002;86: 361-373.
9. Krause PJ, Telford SR 3rd, Spielman A, et al: Concurrent Lyme disease and babesiosis: Evidence for increased severity and duration of illness. JAMA 1996;275:1657-1660.
10. Klasco R: Colorado tick fever. Med Clin North Am 2002; 86:435-440, ix.
11. Masters EJ, Olson GS, Weiner SJ, Paddock CD: Rocky Mountain spotted fever: A clinician's dilemma. Arch Intern Med 2003;163:769-774.
12. Sexton DJ, Kaye KS: Rocky Mountain spotted fever. Med Clin North Am 2002;86:351-360, vii-viii.
13. Demma LJ, Traeger MS, Nicholson WL, et al: Rocky Mountain spotted fever from an unexpected tick vector in Arizona. N Engl J Med 2005;353:587-594.
14. Greenstein P: Tick paralysis. Med Clin North Am 2002;86:441-446.
15. Aguero-Rosenfeld ME, Wang G, Schwartz I, Wormser GP: Diagnosis of Lyme borreliosis. Clin Microbiol Rev 2005;18: 484-509.
16. Philipp MT, Wormser GP, Marques AR, et al: A decline in C6 antibody titer occurs in successfully treated patients with culture-confirmed early localized or early disseminated Lyme borreliosis. Clin Diagn Lab Immunol 2005; 12:1069-1074.
17. Borg R, Dotevall L, Hagberg L, et al: Intravenous ceftriaxone compared with oral doxycycline for the treatment of Lyme neuroborreliosis. Scand J Infect Dis 2005;37: 449-454.
18. Dattwyler RJ, Luft BJ, Kunkel MJ, et al: Ceftriaxone compared with doxycycline for the treatment of acute disseminated Lyme disease. N Engl J Med 1997;337:289-294.
19. Klempner MS, Hu LT, Evans J, et al: Two controlled trials of antibiotic treatment in patients with persistent symptoms and a history of Lyme disease. N Engl J Med 2001; 345:85-92.
20. Nadelman RB, Nowakowski J, Fish D, et al: Prophylaxis with single-dose doxycycline for the prevention of Lyme disease after an *Ixodes scapularis* tick bite. N Engl J Med 2001;345:79-84.
21. Wormser GP, Ramanathan R, Nowakowski J, et al: Duration of antibiotic therapy for early Lyme disease: A randomized, double-blind, placebo-controlled trial. Ann Intern Med 2003;138:697-704.

Chapter 183

Tuberculosis

Jennifer L. Isenhour and D. Matthew Sullivan

KEY POINTS

Despite advances in diagnosis and therapy, tuberculosis (TB) remains a leading cause of death worldwide.

TB begins as a primary infection (usually in the lung, but other organ systems may be involved) that enters a latent period. Immunocompromised patients are at increased risk of reactivation of the disease and the development of active TB.

The presentation of TB can be very broad and should remain on the differential diagnosis for all patients who present with systemic signs of infection. Classic symptoms of pulmonary TB (fever, night sweats, and hemoptysis) may not be diagnostically accurate, given the high prevalence of immunocompromised patients in the world today.

Therapy for TB should include multiple drugs to which the mycobacterium is susceptible and should continue for at least 6 to 12 months.

Because of the risk of multidrug-resistant TB, an initial four-drug regimen with isoniazid (INH), rifampin (RIF), ethambutol (ETH), and pyrazinamide (PZA) is recommended by the Centers for Disease Control and Prevention, the American Thoracic Society, and the Infectious Diseases Society of America.

Pathophysiology

Mycobacterium tuberculosis is a small, slow-growing bacterium that is transmitted by inhalation of droplet nuclei. As infected persons talk, cough, or sneeze, numerous nuclei are expelled into the surrounding air. Only a few inhaled droplets are needed to infect, so an increased length of exposure to the pathogen and the number of bacilli present correlate with infectivity.[1]

Inhaled bacilli travel down the bronchi and lodge within an alveolus. Activated macrophages then ingest the bacilli, which replicate and ultimately cause lysis. Monocytes are attracted and differentiate into macrophages, which again consume the mycobacteria and form a tubercle. The tubercle travels through the lymphatic and hematogenous systems and lodges in apices of the lung, lymph nodes, meninges, vertebra, long bones, or kidney.

Two to 3 weeks after infection, cell-mediated immunity converts the tubercle to a granuloma by means of CD4 helper T cells. This process arrests the local infection for most immunocompetent hosts. At that time, the only sign of the disease may be a positive reaction to the purified protein derivative (PPD) skin test.

A delayed hypersensitivity response uses cytotoxic killer CD8 suppressor T cells to kill the other nonactivated macrophages with bacilli. This process creates local tissue destruction and the formation of a caseating granuloma. In immunocompromised patients, this caseous center may expand and then calcify to form a Ghon complex in the lung. If the infection is uncontrolled, primary tuberculous pneumonia may ensue, or infection may spread through blood and lymph, with resulting disseminated TB.[2]

Active TB develops months to years later in those patients with decreased capacity for cell-mediated immunity, such as patients with malnutrition, comorbidities, and immunosuppression. Patients with acquired immunodeficiency syndrome are especially prone to develop active disease. As the caseating granuloma liquefies and releases numerous bacilli, a delayed hypersensitivity response is initiated, and local tissue destruction follows. Ultimately, erosion through a bronchial wall creates a cavitary lesion and the development of pneumonia. The high oxygen tension of the cavity lends itself to replication of bacilli and persistent disease.

Classic Presentation

The symptom constellation of cough, night sweats, and hemoptysis, commonly associated with TB, is of little benefit in the early identification of disease because TB often has no early symptoms. Late symptoms are wide ranging and do not always involve the respiratory tract. Extrapulmonary manifestations of TB are seen in 20% of patients when the host is immunocompetent and are even more common when the host is immunocompromised.[3] In patients with one or more risk factors for TB (Table 183-1 and Box 183-1),[4] a detailed history helps to refine the pretest probability for the diagnosis of TB.

Early stages of infection are most often asymptomatic in the normal host. Unless cell-mediated immunity is impaired, symptoms may manifest only after reactivation of the infection. Patients may present with a combination of systemic symptoms including cough, fatigue, fever, anorexia, malaise, and weight loss. An indolent cough that has progressed over more than 2 weeks should raise the clinical suspicion for pulmonary TB.[5] Hemoptysis signifies erosion into the bronchial tree and is unlikely to be an early symptom of pulmonary TB. When the clinical suspicion is raised, the physical findings in pulmonary TB may include fever, pleural effusion, focal pneumonic ausculatory findings, and adenopathy.

Table 183-1 TUBERCULOSIS RATES (PER 100,000 POPULATION) AMONG FIVE RACIAL/ETHNIC POPULATIONS: UNITED STATES, 2003

Race/Ethnicity	Rate*
White, non-Hispanic	1.4
American Indian/Alaska Native	8.0 (5.7)
Hispanic	10.5 (7.5)
Black, non-Hispanic	11.5 (8.2)
Asian/Pacific Islander	29.4 (21.0)

*Numbers in parentheses represent risk for tuberculosis compared with white non-Hispanics.

From American Thoracic Society, et al: Treatment of tuberculosis [erratum appears in MMWR Recomm Rep 2005;53:1203; dosage error in text]. MMWR Recomm Rep 2003:52:1-77.

BOX 183-1

Populations at Risk for Contracting Tuberculosis

- Persons with human immunodeficiency infection
- Persons with exposure to a known case
- Persons of Asian, African, or Latin American descent
- Migrant farmers
- Homeless persons
- Persons of low income
- Elderly persons
- Nursing home residents
- Correctional facility residents
- Intravenous drug users
- Persons with occupational exposure

Adapted from American Thoracic Society/Centers for Disease Control and Prevention/Infectious Diseases Society of America: Controlling tuberculosis in the United States. Am J Respir Crit Care Med 2005;172:1169-1227.

■ VARIATIONS

Extrapulmonary manifestations clinically conform to the site of infection, and care should be taken to include TB in the differential diagnosis for patients who present with the following conditions:

- Diffuse adenopathy of the neck (scrofula)
- Recurrent urinary tract infections, scrotal mass, prostatitis, epididymitis, or orchitis (genitourinary TB)
- Headache, fever, meningeal signs, or altered mental status (TB meningitis)
- Focal neurologic deficits, cranial nerve abnormalities, cerebellar dysfunction, or seizure (central nervous system tuberculomas)
- Joint or spinal pain (Pott's disease)
- Chest pain or dullness to percussion (pleural TB)
- Multiple organ system disease (disseminated TB)

Differential Diagnosis

Depending on the clinical symptoms at presentation, TB may mimic numerous systemic diseases. Radiographic findings, sputum smears, and skin tests help in the diagnosis of TB. The gold standard diagnostic test, however, is culture, which may not be available for several weeks (Table 183-2).

Diagnostic Testing

Latent TB in asymptomatic patients is clinically difficult to identify. Targeted population screening has

Table 183-2 DIFFERENTIAL DIAGNOSIS

Pulmonary Tuberculosis	
Severe systemic symptoms?	Bacterial pneumonia
Geographic distribution for fungal infection?	Histoplasmosis Coccidioidomycosis Blastomycosis
HIV infection?	*Mycobacterium avium* infection *Mycobacterium kansasii* infection *Pneumocystis carinii* infection
Cavitary lesion?	*Klebsiella pneumoniae* infection *Staphylococcus pyogenes* infection Aspiration pneumonia Carcinoma Pulmonary infarction Wegener's granulomatosis Bullous disease
Mediastinal lymphadenopathy?	Lymphoma Sarcoidosis
Extrapulmonary Tuberculosis	
Is there lymphadenitis?	Scrofula Lymphoma Metastatic cancer Fungal disease Cat-scratch disease Sarcoidosis Toxoplasmosis Reactive or bacterial adenitis
Is there bone or joint infection?	Pott's disease Bacterial abscess Synovitis
Is there sterile pyuria?	Appendicitis Pelvic inflammatory disease Diverticulosis/diverticulitis Mesenteric adenitis
Is there headache and altered mental status?	Bacterial meningitis Viral meningitis Encephalitis

HIV, human immunodeficiency virus.

been advocated as a means to identify early disease while it is still in the more easily treated latent period. However, current recommendations are to perform a PPD skin test on patients who would benefit from therapy for latent TB and who are at high risk for developing active TB (Box 183-2).[6] Currently, the foundation of screening is skin testing with PPD in patients at risk for TB. Patients who harbor latent TB and who have intact cellular immunity demonstrate a hypersensitivity reaction at the site of PPD placement that can be graded and evaluated with a well-established scale reflecting positivity or negativity (Table 183-3).[6] However, this type of screening is not particularly sensitive in immunocompromised patients, elderly patients, newly infected patients, or very young children. Additionally, the test lacks the specificity to distinguish among other *Mycobacterium* infections.[7] Newer whole blood antigen-stimulated interferon-gamma release assays are available that have high sensitivity and specificity, are not affected by prior bacille Calmette-Guérin vaccination, and do not have a waning response over time.[4,7]

The advent of auscultation and radiography greatly advanced the diagnosis of TB in the 18th and 19th centuries.[8] Despite technical advances in diagnostic tests, the history, physical examination, and conventional radiography remain cornerstones in the diagnosis of TB in the ED. Frequently, patients who present to the ED with symptoms of pulmonary or extrapulmonary TB have limited prior access to care, and heightened suspicion is required. Once a history is obtained that suggests active pulmonary disease, patients should be isolated (in a negative-pressure room, if possible), and a chest radiograph should be obtained. The identification of an upper lobe infiltrate suggests the presence of active disease (Figs. 183-1 and 183-2). However, chest radiography is not highly sensitive, particularly in the immunocompromised patient, in whom reticulonodular and miliary patterns of disease may be present.[9] Moreover, the clinical syndrome of normal chest radiographs with sputum culture-positive TB is well described in patients with human immunodeficiency virus (HIV) infection and low CD4 counts.[10] Thus, a high clinical

Table 183-3 EVALUATION OF PURIFIED PROTEIN DERIVATIVE SKIN TESTING RESULTS

Induration Size	Considered Positive in
≥5 mm	Recent contact with TB-positive patient Chest radiographic findings consistent with prior TB HIV-infected patients Immunosuppressed patients Organ transplant recipients
≥10 mm	Recent immigrants from countries with a high prevalence of TB Intravenous drug users Homeless and low-income populations Residents or employees of nursing homes, hospitals, homeless shelters, correctional facilities Risk factors for reactivation TB (diabetes, renal failure, malignancy) Medically underserved populations Children <4 years old Children and adolescents exposed to TB-positive adult
≥15 mm	People with no risk factors

HIV, human immunodeficiency virus; TB, tuberculosis.
From Myers JP: New recommendations for the treatment of tuberculosis. Curr Opin Infect Dis 2005;18:133-140.

BOX 183-2

Indications for a Purified Protein Derivative Skin Test

- Increased risk of exposure to infectious cases
  - Close contacts of persons with known active TB
  - Health care workers where TB is treated
- Increased risk of TB infection
  - Foreign-born persons from a country with a high prevalence of TB
  - Homeless persons
  - Persons living or working in long-term care facilities
- Increased risk of active TB once infection has occurred
  - Persons infected with human immunodeficiency virus
  - Intravenous drug users
  - Persons receiving immunosuppressive therapy
  - Patients with end-stage renal disease
  - Patients with silicosis
  - Diabetic patients
  - Patients with hematologic malignancies
  - Patients with prior gastrectomies
  - Patients with prior jejunoileal bypass
  - Persons with severe malnutrition
  - Persons with recent TB infection

TB, tuberculosis.
From Myers JP: New recommendations for the treatment of tuberculosis. Curr Opin Infect Dis 2005;18:133-140.

suspicion for disease mandates that sputum studies be ordered.

Unfortunately, sputum Gram stain with carbolfuchsin and phenol or auramine O staining for the identification of acid-fast bacilli (AFB) is unreliable in the ED evaluation of patients suspected to have TB.

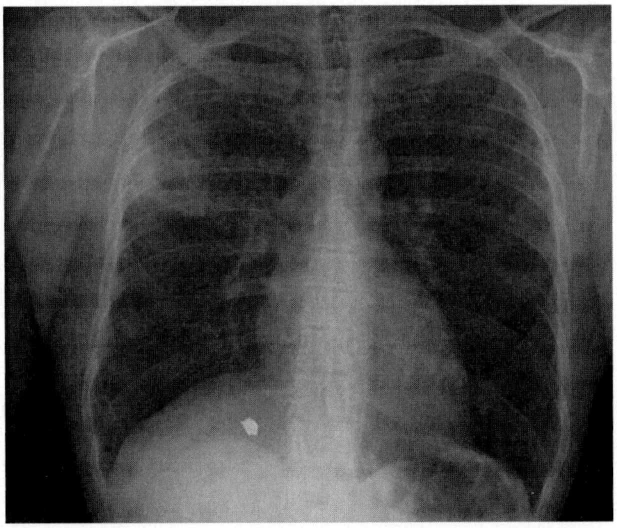

FIGURE 183-1 Right upper lobe cavitary lesion.

In addition to the variability in performance inherently linked to the skill of the laboratory technical staff, and the availability of rapid test results at all times of day, the sensitivity of a single AFB smear remains low (<50%), far too low for the safe discharge of the high-risk patient.[11] This situation necessitates further management by the inpatient team or close follow-up with the local health department for further sputum smears in those patients who are deemed safe for discharge. The additive value of three morning sputum smears is helpful for excluding the diagnosis of active pulmonary TB; however, when AFB smears are identified, it is not possible to distinguish which *Mycobacterium* species is present, and the definitive diagnosis should be confirmed with sputum culture.

Sputum culture is not part of the ED evaluation of a patient with suspected TB. Cultures traditionally take 4 to 8 weeks to grow; they are sensitive in more than 80% of cases of infiltrative pulmonary TB and in more than 90% of cases of cavitary TB.[12] Newer

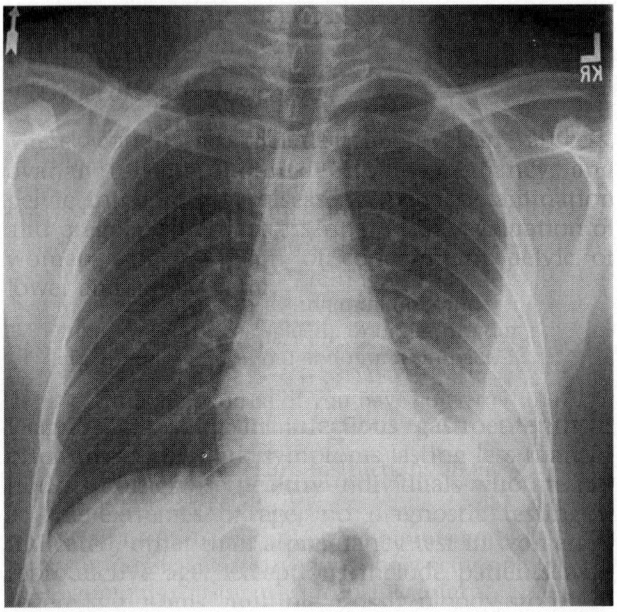

KR

FIGURE 183-2 Left lower lobe infiltrate with effusion.

methods of radiometric culture systems with radiolabeled carbon-14 yield faster results (1 to 3 weeks).

The advent of nucleic acid amplification tests and of polymerase chain reaction identification greatly increased the sensitivity (97% to 99%) for the diagnosis of TB from a single smear, and accurate results can be obtained in hours. Additional strain typing for *M. tuberculosis* with restriction fragment length polymorphism is available to identify the organism's DNA.[13] However, these tests are time and resource consuming, even for large centers, to perform on an as-needed basis and are thus impractical for use in the ED work-up of patients with suspected TB. The utility of these newer tests in smear-negative individuals has been called into question with reports of lower sensitivities (70%) in this population.[14]

Extrapulmonary TB is often confirmed by biopsy of affected lymph nodes. Blood culture, urine culture, and culture of other body fluids are used to aid in the diagnosis of extrapulmonary TB with varying sensitivities, depending on the host and the site of culture. The diagnosis of pleural TB is facilitated with pleural biopsy and culture; yields are 86% in immunocompetent patients and 47% in immunocompromised patients.[15]

Ultimately, the diagnosis of TB remains firmly grounded in the clinician's analysis. A high suspicion of disease, coupled with appropriate testing for the given presentation, will translate into clinical success (Fig. 183-3).[16]

Procedures

Historically, bleeding, leaches, cupping, application of animal excrement, "touching" by kings, pleurocentesis, and the isolation of patients in sanatoriums were used to treat TB. More modern medical times

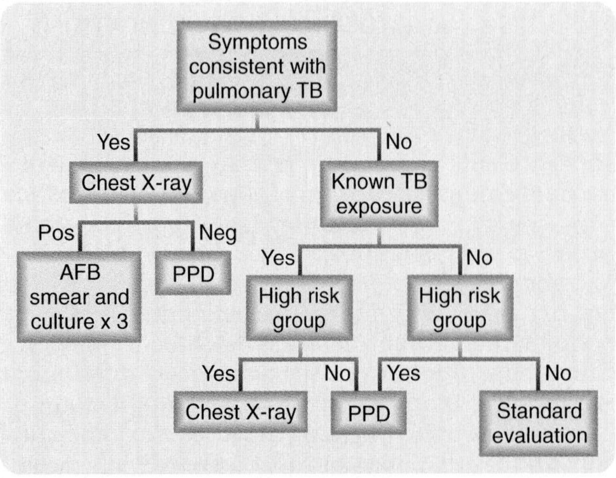

Symptoms consistent with pulmonary TB
Yes
No
Chest X-ray
Known TB exposure
Pos
Neg
AFB smear and culture x 3
PPD
Yes
No
High risk group
High risk group
Yes
No
Yes
No
Chest X-ray
PPD
Standard evaluation

FIGURE 183-3 Algorithm for patients suspected to have tuberculosis (TB). AFB, acid-fast bacillus; Neg, negative; Pos, positive; PPD, purified protein derivative.

have seen the use of surgical pneumonectomy, thoracoplasty, pneumothorax, and phrenic nerve interruption as potential therapeutic procedures.[8] The only procedure infrequently utilized today is surgical resection.

Treatment and Disposition

■ PULMONARY TUBERCULOSIS

Prevention of the spread of TB is paramount in the treatment regimen. Empirically in the ED, start patients with suspected TB on a drug regimen after obtaining sputum for AFB smears and cultures.

Treatment consists of two phases: the initiation (bactericidal) phase, lasting 2 months; and the continuation (sterilizing) phase, which is usually 4 to 7 months. Because of the risk of multidrug-resistant organisms, at least two drugs should be used. The American Thoracic Society, the Centers for Disease Control and Prevention, and the Infectious Diseases Society of America recommend an initial four-drug cocktail of INH, RIF, PZA, and ETH for 2 months (Table 183-4).[4] Directly observed therapy increases completion rates for pulmonary TB and prevents the spread of disease.[17-19]

Immunocompetent patients become noninfectious 2 to 4 weeks after initiating therapy if the organism is susceptible. If the initial treatment regimen fails, then at least two additional drugs should be added.[19] Usually, PZA or another first-line agent is coupled with a second-line agent such as ethionamide or a fluoroquinolone.[5]

■ Special Populations

Patients Infected with Human Immunodeficiency Virus

Because of specific drug interactions and resistance, HIV-infected patients present a challenge to standard treatment protocols. Many of the anti-TB drugs

Table 183-4 **ANTITUBERCULOSIS MEDICATIONS**

Drug	Mechanism	Daily Dose	Side Effects	Monitoring Needed
FDA-APPROVED FIRST-LINE AGENTS				
Isoniazid	Inhibition of cell wall synthesis	Adults: 5 mg/kg Peds: 10-15 mg/kg (max: 300 mg)	Hepatic; peripheral neuropathy	Prior liver disease; elevation in liver enzymes
Pyrazinamide	Sterilizing effect	Adults: 20-25 mg/kg Peds: 20-30 mg/kg (max: 2.0 g)	Hepatic; exacerbates gout	Prior liver disease; if used in combination with rifampin for latent tuberculosis
Rifampin	RNA synthesis interference	Adults: 10 mg/kg Peds: 10-20 mg/kg (max: 600 mg)	Orange body fluids; influenza-like syndrome	None needed; watch for drug interactions
Ethambutol	Inhibition of cell wall synthesis; possible increased permeability of cell wall	Adults: 15-20 mg/kg Peds: 15-25 mg/kg (max: 1.0 g)	Peripheral neuritis; optic neuritis	Baseline and monthly visual acuity and color discrimination test needed

Drug	Daily Dose
FDA-APPROVED SECOND-LINE AGENTS	
Cycloserine	Adults: 10-15 mg/kg; peds: 10-15 mg/kg (max: 1.0 g)
Ethionamide	Adults: 15-20 mg/kg; peds: 15-20 mg/kg (max: 1.0 g)
Rifapentine	Adults: 10 mg/kg/week dose; peds: not applicable (max: 600 mg)
Capreomycin	Adults: 15 mg/kg; peds: 15-30 mg/kg intramuscularly/intravenously (max: 1 g)
p-Aminosalicylic acid (PAS)	Adults: 8-12 g; peds: 200-300 mg/kg (peds max: 10 g)
Streptomycin	Adults: 15 mg/kg; peds: 20-40 mg/kg (max: 1 g)
NON–FDA-APPROVED DRUGS	
Rifabutin Aminoglycosides Fluoroquinolones	
DRUGS USED IN DRUG-RESISTANT TUBERCULOSIS TREATMENT	
Clarithromycin Amoxicillin/clavulanate Linezolid	

FDA, Food and Drug Administration; peds, pediatric patients.
Data from Sahbazian B, Weis SE: Treatment of active tuberculosis: Challenges and prospects. Clin Chest Med 2005;26:273-282; American Thoracic Society/Centers for Disease Control and Prevention/Infectious Diseases Society of America: Controlling tuberculosis in the United States. Am J Respir Crit Care Med 2005;172:1169-1227; and American Thoracic Society, CDC, Infections Diseases Society of America: Treatment of tuberculosis. MMWR Recomm Rep 2003;52(RR-11):1-77 [erratum in MMWR Recomm Rep 2005;53:1203; dosage error in text].
and CDC MMWR Treatment of Tuberculosis June 20, 2003/Vol 52/Norr-11 p. 4.

have overlapping toxicities with the antiretrovirals agents, and some anti-TB drugs may decrease the concentration of certain antiretroviral agents as a result of cytochrome system interactions.[20] HIV-infected patients should not receive once-weekly INH/RIF because of high relapse rates. Patients with CD4 counts lower than 100 cells/mL should receive the anti-TB regimen at least three times a week because of the potential for RIF resistance. If sputum cultures are still positive at 2 months, the continuation phase of treatment may need to be extended to 7 months.[19] Coordination with the patient's infectious disease specialist during treatment of these patients is important.

Multidrug-Resistant Organisms

By definition, *multidrug-resistant TB* is disease that is resistant to two or more first-line agents, usually INH and RIF. Multidrug-resistant TB results from improper treatment regimens, noncompliance with therapy, and spontaneous mutations of the mycobacterium (Box 183-3).[4] These patients should be treated with alternative drug regimens that include at least three drugs to which the organism is susceptible and that have not been previously administered. Ideally, one of these drugs should be injectable.[4]

Pregnancy

Pregnant patients may be treated with INH, RIF, and ETH. These drugs do cross the placenta, but they are not known to have any teratogenic effects.[4] Adjuvant pyridoxine should be given to decrease the potential for the development of peripheral neuropathy.[4]

Children

Disseminated TB occurs more frequently in children, so treatment of initial infection should be aggressive.

BOX 183-3

Risk Factors for Multidrug-Resistant Tuberculosis

Human immunodeficiency virus infection
Intravenous drug use
Recent immigration from a country with a prevalence of multidrug-resistant TB
Cavitary lung lesion
Homelessness
Incarceration
History of gastrectomy or ileal bypass
Prior failed TB treatment
Noncompliance with treatment regimen

TB, tuberculosis.
From American Thoracic Society/Centers for Disease Control and Prevention/Infectious Diseases Society of America: Controlling tuberculosis in the United States. Am J Respir Crit Care Med 2005;172:1169-1227.

Children may be treated with the same drug regimen as adults, with the exclusion of ETH. A regimen of 2 months of RIF, INH, and PZA, followed by 4 months of RIF and INH, has a treatment success of 95%. Children must have directly observed therapy. Children with disseminated TB, TB meningitis, and HIV infection may need an extended treatment period of 9 to 12 months.[4]

■ EXTRAPULMONARY TUBERCULOSIS

Most extrapulmonary TB infections may be treated with the same drug regimen as pulmonary TB. In patients with TB pericarditis or meningitis, add corticosteroids to prevent pericardial constriction and neurologic sequelae, respectively.[11] A regimen of 6 to 9 months of treatment is adequate for most infections; however, patients with meningeal infection require 9 to 12 months of therapy.[4]

■ LATENT TUBERCULOSIS TREATMENT

Patients with latent TB who are at high risk for developing active TB need empirial therapy. Before INH is initiated, patients need a chest radiograph and clinical evaluation to exclude active TB. The preferred treatment regimen for latent TB is daily INH for 9 months.[4]

■ MYCOBACTERIUM BOVIS BACILLE CALMETTE-GUÉRIN VACCINE

Bacille Calmette-Guérin is an attenuated strain of *Mycobacterium bovis* that is the only current vaccine for TB. It was developed by Albert Calmette and Camille Guérin in the early 20th century and remains the most commonly used vaccine in the world. Unfortunately, its efficacy may be waning as a result of mutations and deletions in the bacterium. There is renewed interest in creating alternative improved vaccines.[21]

Disposition

Most patients with TB may be treated as outpatients as long as directly observed therapy can be ensured, usually by the health department. Admit patients with significant comorbidities, severe disease, the need for parenteral therapy, HIV infection, multidrug-resistant TB, and social situations that would render outpatient therapy unsuccessful.

REFERENCES

1. Dye C, Watt CJ, Bleed DM, et al: Evolution of tuberculosis control and prospects for reducing tuberculosis incidence, prevalence, and deaths globally. JAMA 2005;293:2767-2775.
2. Dannenberg AM Jr: Delayed-type hypersensitivity and cell-mediated immunity in the pathogenesis of tuberculosis. Immunol Today 1991;12:228-233.
3. Frieden TR, Munsiff SS: The DOTS strategy for controlling the global tuberculosis epidemic. Clin Chest Med 2005;26:197-205.
4. American Thoracic Society/Centers for Disease Control and Prevention/Infectious Diseases Society of America: Controlling tuberculosis in the United States. Am J Respir Crit Care Med 2005;172:1169-1227.
5. Onyebujoh P, Zumla A, Ribeiro I, et al: Treatment of tuberculosis: Present status and future prospects. Bull World Health Organ 2005;83:857-865.
6. Myers JP: New recommendations for the treatment of tuberculosis. Curr Opin Infect Dis 2005;18:133-140.
7. Whalen CC: Diagnosis of latent tuberculosis infection: Measure for measure. JAMA 2005;293:2785-2787.
8. Rubin SA: Tuberculosis: Captain of all these men of death. Radiol Clin North Am 1995;33:619-639.
9. Perlman DC, el-Sadr WM, Nelson ET, et al: Variation of chest radiographic patterns in pulmonary tuberculosis by degree of human immunodeficiency virus-related immunosuppression: The Terry Beirn Community Programs for Clinical Research on AIDS (CPCRA). The AIDS Clinical Trials Group (ACTG). Clin Infect Dis 1997;25:242-246.
10. Smith RL, Yew K, Berkowitz KA, Aranda CP: Factors affecting the yield of acid-fast sputum smears in patients with HIV and tuberculosis. Chest 1994;106:684-686.
11. Woods GL, Petony E, Boxley MJ, Gatson AM: Concentration of sputum by cytocentrifugation for preparation of smears for detection of acid fast bacilli does not increase sensitivity of the fluorochrome stain. J Clin Microbiol 1995;33:1915-1916.
12. Van den Brande P: Revised guidelines for the diagnosis and control of tuberculosis: Impact on management in the elderly. Drugs Aging 2005;22:663-686.
13. Drobniewski FA, Caws M, Gibson A, Young D: Modern laboratory diagnosis of tuberculosis. Lancet Infect Dis 2003;3:141-147.
14. Lim TK, Zhu D, Gough A, et al: What is the optimal approach for using a direct amplification test in the routine diagnosis of pulmonary tuberculosis? A preliminary assessment. Respirology 2002;7:351-357.
15. Relkin F, Aranda CP, Garay SM, et al: Pleural tuberculosis and HIV infection. Chest 1994;105:1338-1341.
16. National Tuberculosis Controllers Association and Centers for Disease Control and Prevention: Guidelines for the investigation of contacts of persons with infectious tuberculosis: Recommendations from the National Tuberculosis Controllers Association and CDC. MMWR Morb Mortal Recomm Rep 2005;54:1-37.

17. Sahbazian B, Weis SE: Treatment of active tuberculosis: Challenges and prospects. Clin Chest Med 2005;26: 273-282.
18. Chaulk CP, Kazandjian VA: Directly observed therapy for treatment completion of pulmonary tuberculosis: Consensus Statement of the Public Health Tuberculosis Guidelines Panel [erratum appears in JAMA 1998;280:134]. JAMA 1998;279:943-948.
19. Blumberg HM, Leonard MK Jr, Jasmer RM: Update on the treatment of tuberculosis and latent tuberculosis infection [erratum appears in JAMA 2005;294:182; dosage error in text]. JAMA 2005;293:2776-2784.
20. Burman WJ, Gallicano K, Peloquin C: Therapeutic implications of drug interactions in the treatment of human immunodeficiency virus-related tuberculosis. Clin Infect Dis 1999;28:419-429.
21. Nor NM, Musa M: Approaches towards the development of a vaccine against tuberculosis: Recombinant BCG and DNA vaccine. Tuberculosis 2004;84:102-109.

Chapter 184

Epidemic Infections in Bioterrorism

Amer Aldeen

KEY POINTS

The anthrax bacillus is the agent considered most likely to be used in a bioterrorist attack.

Suspect a bioterrorism attack when large groups of patients present in a short period with respiratory or neurologic symptoms or when an index patient has characteristic findings.

Use isolation precautions and give antibiotics based on clinical suspicion, *before* diagnostic confirmation.

Always draw blood cultures and send Gram stains in suspicious cases.

Refer to the Centers for Disease Control and Prevention (CDC) Web site (www.bt.cdc.gov) for more detailed information on bioterrorism threats, and report any confirmed cases to the CDC.

Scope

Biologic agents have the potential to cause as many casualties in a densely populated area as a nuclear weapon. If used in a terrorist attack on civilian populations, biologic weapons could also result in widespread social disruption and complete exhaustion of health care resources.

The Centers for Disease Control and Prevention (CDC) has classified the major bioterrorist threats into three categories based on overall danger to the U.S. public. Category A agents are the most easily weaponized and disseminated, cause the highest mortality, produce extensive social disruption, and require special public health preparedness systems. Category B agents do not cause as high mortality as category A agents, but they still result in considerable morbidity and require enhancement of current surveillance systems. Category C agents are the third highest priority and comprise new and emerging agents that are of concern because of their potential to cause significant morbidity. The list of category A, B, and C agents is given in Table 184-1.

Bioterrorism agents are most dangerous to humans in aerosolized form. Particles smaller than 10 µg effectively reach the alveoli. Certain agents (e.g., the anthrax bacillus and botulinum toxin) are more resistant to environmental degradation than others (e.g., the plague bacillus). Certain diseases (e.g., plague and smallpox) may be transmitted from person to person, thus causing high rates of dissemination and requiring strict isolation measures. Until biologic contaminants are excluded, pulmonary isolation measures should be instituted in all these patients.

Surveillance and management protocols should be instituted at the hospital level for dealing with large numbers of patients presenting with respiratory complaints over a short period. If surveillance methods do indicate a bioterrorist attack, the community must work to prevent widespread contamination, to help curb the strain on health care resources. A joint report by the CDC and the U.S. Department of Health and

Table 184-1 CENTERS FOR DISEASE CONTROL AND PREVENTION CATEGORIES OF BIOTERRORISM AGENTS

Biologic Agent	Disease
Category A	
Variola major	Smallpox
Bacillus anthracis	Anthrax
Yersinia pestis	Plague
Clostridium botulinum	Botulism
Francisella tularensis	Tularemia
Filoviruses and arenaviruses	Viral hemorrhagic fevers
Category B	
Coxiella burnetii	Q fever
Brucella spp.	Brucellosis
Burkholderia mallei	Glanders
Burkholderia pseudomallei	Melioidosis
Alphaviruses (equine viruses)	Encephalomyelitis
Rickettsia prowazekii	Typhus fever
Toxins (e.g., ricin)	Toxic syndromes
Chlamydia psittaci	Psittacosis
Food threats *(Salmonella, Escherichia coli)*	Gastroenteritis
Water threats *(Vibrio, Cryptosporidium)*	Gastroenteritis
Category C	
Nipah virus	Encephalitis
Hantaviruses	Hanta pulmonary virus syndrome
Tickborne hemorrhagic fever viruses	Crimean-Congo hemorrhagic fever
Flaviviruses	Yellow fever
Multidrug-resistant *Mycobacterium tuberculosis*	Tuberculosis

CATEGORY A AGENTS: GENERAL INFORMATION

Disease	Pathogen	Incubation Period	Diagnosis	Characteristic Features
Anthrax	*Bacillus anthracis*	4-6 days	Gram stain, culture, ELISA	Hemorrhagic mediastinitis
Smallpox	*Variola major*	12-14 days	Clinical, culture	Same-stage vesicles
Plague	*Yersinia pestis*	2-8 days	Gram stain, culture, Wright's stain	Rapid respiratory failure
Tularemia	*Francisella tularensis*	1-14 days	Culture, direct fluorescent antibody	Extremely infectious, head, ear, eyes, nose, and throat, and pulmonary signs
Botulism	*Clostridium botulinum*	2 hr-8 days	Clinical, bioassays	Descending flaccid paralysis, cranial neuropathies
Viral hemorrhagic fevers	Lassa, Ebola, Marburg, Dengue, Crimean-Congo	2-21 days	ELISA, polymerase chain reaction	Nonspecific viral symptoms, rash, multi-organ dysfunction syndrome

CATEGORY A AGENTS: TREATMENT, PROPHYLAXIS, AND MORTALITY

Disease	Vaccine	Postexposure Prophylaxis	Treatment	Untreated Mortality
Anthrax	Yes	Ciprofloxacin 500 mg PO bid×60 days or Amoxicillin 500 mg PO tid×60 days or Doxycycline 100 mg PO bid×60 days	Ciprofloxacin 400 mg IV/500 mg PO×14 days or Doxycycline 100 mg IV bid×60 days or Penicillin 4 million units IV q4h×14 days	45%-90%

Documentation

History	General	Timing of symptoms, presence of viral prodrome, known exposure, travel to endemic area, close contacts, allergies to antibiotics, history of inflammatory skin disease
	Constitutional	Fever, chills, headache, myalgias, malaise
	Respiratory	Dyspnea, cough, hemoptysis, sputum color
	Gastrointestinal	Diarrhea, abdominal pain, hematochezia
	Neurologic	Weakness, paralysis, stiff neck
	Dermatologic	Rash, lesions, jaundice
Physical examination	General	Respiratory distress, handling of secretions, toxic appearance, coughing
	Head, ears, eyes, nose, and throat	Oropharyngeal lesions, drooling
	Lungs	Crackles, wheezes, decreased sounds, dullness to percussion
	Abdomen	Tenderness, distention, bowel sounds, hepatosplenomegaly, rectal examination
	Neurologic	Mental status, cranial nerves, meningismus, motor weakness
	Skin	Rash, lymphadenopathy, jaundice, necrosis
Studies	Chest radiograph Chest computed tomography Gram stain Vital capacity (if neurologic weakness is present)	
Medical decision making	CDC notification if diagnosis is confirmed Time of antibiotic order and administration	
Procedures	Intubation and mechanical ventilation: risks, benefits, rapid-sequence induction method, confirmation chest radiograph results, intensive care unit notification Lumbar puncture: risks, benefits, methods, cerebrospinal fluid results	
Patient instructions	Return instructions, warning signs, follow-up Recommendation for close contacts to seek evaluation Mandatory completion of postexposure prophylaxis CDC Web site for further information	

CDC, Centers for Disease Control and Prevention.

sions. Blood cultures are positive in 90% of cases, and gram-negative coccobacilli with bipolar stain uptake are seen in more than 70%. First-line treatment of pneumonic plague is with streptomycin or gentamicin. Without administration of antibiotics within 24 hours of overt signs of infection, mortality approaches 100%.

Botulism

Botulinum toxin is the most potent poison known. It is produced by the gram-positive, anaerobic, spore-forming bacillus, *Clostridium botulinum.* Food contamination and aerosolization are the likely mechanisms of a bioterrorist attack with botulinum toxin. Once absorbed, the agent causes irreversible inhibition of presynaptic acetylcholine release. The classic clinical picture starts with cranial neuropathies, followed by descending flaccid paralysis resulting in diaphragmatic weakness and requirement for mechanical ventilation. Mental status and sensation are usually preserved.

Although a specific bioassay exists to confirm the diagnosis, suspect botulism in any patient with descending flaccid paralysis. Treatment is with supportive care, mechanical ventilation, and antitoxin (available from the CDC). Antibiotic therapy does not improve outcomes in patients with aerosolized or food-borne botulism, and it does not play a role in this toxin-mediated bioterrorist threat.

Tularemia

Like anthrax and plague, tularemia occurs naturally as a zoonotic infection, transmitted by arthropods in rabbit, deer, and squirrel reservoirs. Tularemia is caused by *Francisella tularensis,* a gram-negative coccobacillus and a potential bioterrorism agent because of its extremely high infectivity, ease of spread, and significant morbidity. As few as 10 organisms can cause pulmonary illness. Six forms of tularemia exist: glandular, ulceroglandular, oculoglandular, oropharyngeal, typhoidal, and pneumonic.

Aerosolized bacteria causing pneumonic tularemia would be the primary threat in a bioterrorist attack. The clinical syndrome of pneumonic disease can resemble a nonspecific viral illness, meningitis, or pneumonia. Respiratory failure and shock are far less common in tularemia than in inhalational anthrax or pneumonic plague. Although mortality of tulare-

Table 184-2 CHARACTERISTICS OF VIRAL HEMORRHAGIC FEVERS

Illness	Vector/Reservoir	Human-to-Human Transmission	Mortality Rate	Vaccine
Dengue	Mosquito/monkey	No	1%-50%	No
Ebola/Marburg	Unknown/monkey	Yes	25%-90%	Experimental
Crimean-Congo	Tick/domestic animals	Yes	15%-30%	No
Rift Valley	Mosquito/sheep	No	<50%	Experimental
Lassa	Mice	Yes	15%-25%	Experimental
South American	Mice	Yes	15%-30%	No

mia is lower than that of other diseases caused by category A agents, and even though human-to-human transmission does not occur, the ability of *F. tularensis* to cause illness after seemingly insignificant exposures is prodigious. Treatment is with aminoglycosides or fluoroquinolones, and postexposure prophylaxis is with fluoroquinolones or doxycycline.

Viral Hemorrhagic Fevers

Viral hemorrhagic fevers represent a group of zoonotic RNA viruses that are currently geographically isolated to specific regions of the world. The dearth of vaccines, postexposure prophylaxis, and treatment options, combined with high mortality rates of these illnesses, would make these viruses especially dangerous if they were weaponized in a bioterrorist attack. The characteristics of the individual viruses are listed in Table 184-2. Clinical features common to all viral hemorrhagic fevers include fever, myalgias, headache, and rash (Table 184-3). Most patients exhibit

PATIENT TEACHING TIPS

- Use the Centers for Disease Control and Prevention Web site for further information about bioterrorism agents.
- Finish postexposure prophylaxis completely.
- Return immediately if you have worsening of the following:
  - Fever, chills, lightheadedness, fatigue
  - Shortness of breath, cough
  - Rash
  - Headache, stiff neck
- Tell your close contacts to be evaluated if they are symptomatic.
- Stay home from work or school until you are beyond the incubation period of the suspected agent or are no longer symptomatic.

Table 184-3 DIFFERENTIATION OF AEROSOLIZED BIOTERRORIST THREATS CAUSING RESPIRATORY ILLNESS

Finding	Anthrax (Inhalational)	Plague (Pneumonic)	Tularemia (Pneumonic)	Viral Hemorrhagic Fevers
Dyspnea	+	+	+	±
Odynophagia	–	–	+	±
Hemoptysis	±	+	–	±
Headache	±	–	±	+
Stiff neck	±	±	–	+
Rash	–	–	±	+
Fever	+	+	+	+
Leukopenia	–	–	–	+
Disseminated intravascular coagulation	±	+	±	+
Blood cultures	+ (always)	+	–	+ (viral culture)
Gram stain	Gram-positive bacilli	Gram-negative coccobacilli	Gram-negative coccobacilli	Not applicable
Chest radiograph	Widened mediastinum, pleural effusions	Patchy alveolar infiltrates, pleural effusions	Hilar adenopathy, pleural effusions	Patchy alveolar infiltrates (only when ARDS occurs)
Renal failure	±	±	–	±
Hepatic failure	–	–	–	±

+, present; ±, sometimes present; – absent; ARDS, acute respiratory distress syndrome.

thrombocytopenia, leukopenia, and either renal or hepatic failure. Diagnosis is made by serology or viral culture. Treatment is purely supportive, although ribavirin may provide some benefit. Mortality ranges from 1% for dengue hemorrhagic fever to almost 90% for Ebola.

SUGGESTED READINGS

1. Bronze MS, Huycke MM, Machado LJ, et al: Viral agents as biological weapons and agents of bioterrorism. Am J Med Sci 2002;323:316-325.
2. Cieslak TJ, Eitzen EMJ: Clinical and epidemiologic principles of anthrax. Emerg Infect Dis 1999;5:552-555.
3. Cunha BA: Anthrax, tularemia, plague, Ebola or smallpox as agents of bioterrorism: Recognition in the emergency room. Clin Microbiol Infect 2002;8:489-503.
4. Greenfield RA, Drevets DA, Machado LJ, et al: Bacterial pathogens as biological weapons and agents of bioterrorism. Am J Med Sci 2002;323:299-315.
5. Henderson DA: The looming threat of bioterrorism. Science 1999;283:1279-1282.
6. Karwa M, Currie B, Kvetan V: Bioterrorism: Preparing for the impossible or the improbable. Crit Care Med 2005;33: S75-S95.
7. Kyriacou DN, Stein AC, Yarnold PR, et al: Clinical predictors of bioterrorism-related inhalational anthrax. Lancet 2004;364:449-452.
8. O'Brien KK, Higdon ML, Halverson JJ: Recognition and management of bioterrorism infections. Am Fam Physician 2003;67:1927-1933.
9. Rotz LD, Khan AS, Lillibridge SR, et al: Public health assessment of potential biological terrorism agents. Emerg Infect Dis 2002;8:225-230.

Chapter **185**

Food- and Water-Borne Infections

David K. Zich

KEY POINTS

In patients who develop clinical illness from food-borne and water-borne pathogens, most symptoms resolve spontaneously without intervention.

Significant mortality does occur. Each year, thousands in the United States and millions of people in developing countries die of acute gastroenteritis.[1]

Proper treatment can lead to significant relief for the patient, but inappropriate medications may complicate the clinical picture, lengthen the carrier state, or trigger potentially life-threatening conditions.

Developing a systematic approach to gastrointestinal disease is essential to eliminate unnecessary testing and to restore health as quickly as possible while minimizing adverse and dangerous effects of intervention.

Structure and Function

The portion of the gastrointestinal tract affected by food- and water-borne illnesses depends on the pathogen. Staphylococcal food poisoning is caused by a toxin that has no effect on the intestinal mucosa. Instead, once absorbed, the toxin acts directly on nausea centers in the brain, thus causing severe nausea and vomiting.

Infections of the small intestine may disrupt ionic exchange and can result in increased chloride secretion and sodium retention within the bowel lumen. Water follows, thereby overwhelming absorption capacity, and diarrhea ensues. Viruses create diarrhea by distorting the epithelium and interfering with absorptive capabilities. This process results in loss of fluid, electrolytes, and in some cases fats and sugars.

Invasive organisms primarily affect the distal ileum and large intestine. Common invasive organisms include *Campylobacter, Salmonella, Shigella, Yersinia,* and *Entamoeba histolytica.* These pathogens penetrate the intestinal lining and create an intense inflammatory response. This results in loss of fluid and, in some cases, varying amounts of blood in the colonic lumen. Small bowel and large bowel are both susceptible to toxin-producing organisms that induce diarrhea through direct damage to the epithelium, thereby disrupting the regulation of fluid balance. Inflammation and exudates result in loss of large amounts of fluid into the lumen. Whereas bacterial toxin-induced diarrhea tends to be isotonic, virally induced diarrhea tends to lose primarily sodium, potassium, and bicarbonate. With large fluid losses, significant electrolyte disturbances and acidosis may occur.[2]

Presenting Signs and Symptoms

Presenting signs and symptoms vary widely, depending on the pathogen causing disease. Many parasites that infect the intestines cause no discernible symptoms. Asymptomatic chronic bacterial carrier states

Table 185-1 INCUBATION TIMES

Organism/Pathogen	Incubation
Scombroid fish (poisoning)	5-60 min, average 20-30 min
Staphylococcus	1-6 hr
Bacillus cereus	2-14 hr, average 2-4 hr
Ciguatera fish (poisoning)	2-6 hr, ≥24 hr
Clostridium perfringens enterotoxin	6-24 hr
Vibrio parahaemolyticus	4-48 hr, average 8-12 hr
Salmonella	8-48 hr
Shigella	24-48 hr
Plesiomonas shigelloides	24-48 hr
Cholera and noncholera *Vibrio* species	24-48 hr
Enterotoxigenic *Escherichia coli*	24-72 hr
Norovirus/rotavirus	24-72 hr
Campylobacter	2-5 days
Yersinia	1-14 days, average 2-4 days
Aeromonas hydrophila	1-5 days
Hemorrhagic *Escherichia coli* O157:H7	3-8 days
Cryptosporidium and *Isospora*	5-10 days
Clostridium difficile	Days to months, average 5-14 days
Giardia	1-3 wk
Entamoeba histolytica	1 wk-1 yr

can occur in otherwise healthy individuals. When symptoms do occur, they are limited in most patients to vomiting and diarrhea of varying degrees.

Although some food containing preformed toxins can cause illness within 1 to 6 hours, most acute gastroenteritis has at least a 12- to 48-hour incubation period (Table 185-1). Typically, the onset is gradual and is often noticed as mild dyspepsia after eating a meal. This is the meal often suspected by the patient to be the cause of the illness. However, the pathogen has usually been incubating for the last 1 to 2 days and is just starting to cause symptoms.

Within 1 to 2 hours after the initial dyspepsia, vomiting often begins. The vomitus is usually nonbloody. The most common cause of mild to moderate blood with vomiting is a Mallory-Weiss tear. This occurs when the forceful ejection of gastric contents creates a tear in the mucosa at the junction of the esophagus and the stomach. It rarely occurs with the first episode of vomiting, and treatment is almost always supportive. An initial presence of blood, or a persistent predominance of gross blood, should prompt a search for noninfectious causes of vomiting such as a bleeding peptic ulcer or esophageal varices.

Diarrhea can occur simultaneously with vomiting, or it may manifest with a delayed onset of up to 48 hours later. In some cases, diarrhea may be the only component of clinical illness. Gross diarrheal blood is more common than hematemesis and varies by pathogen (Box 185-1). Dysentery is, by definition, a diarrheal stool containing gross blood and can be accompanied by fever, abdominal pain, and tenesmus.

BOX 185-1

Infectious Causes of Bloody Diarrhea

Frequently
Campylobacter
Plesiomonas shigelloides
Hemorrhagic *Escherichia coli*
Entamoeba histolytica

Occasionally
Salmonella
Yersinia
Vibrio parahaemolyticus

Rarely
Shigella
Aeromonas hydrophila
Clostridium difficile

Atypical symptoms may occur with or without vomiting and diarrhea and are important to recognize because they may indicate a particular causative pathogen. Specifically, *Shigella* can cause seizures, or other neurologic symptoms may occur, especially in children. *Campylobacter* and *Yersinia* may cause focal right lower quadrant pain in the absence of vomiting

Documentation

History

- Onset/duration
- Amount of vomiting
- Amount of diarrhea
  - Presence of blood in either
- Associated symptoms
  - Fever
  - Headache
  - Neurologic symptoms
  - Pain
- Ingestion of suspicious foods in last 7 days
  - Raw or undercooked (sushi)
  - Well/wilderness water
  - Picnics
- Exposure to people with similar contacts
- Recent travel (consider traveler's diarrhea)
- Recent antibiotics or hospitalizations (consider *Clostridium difficile*)
- Past medical history
  - Abdominal surgical procedures (consider partial obstruction)
  - Irritable bowel syndrome/inflammatory bowel disease (consider flare)
  - Immunocompromised state (different causes)
  - Diabetes (look for ketoacidosis)
- Medications
  - Antibiotics (consider *Clostridium difficile*)
  - Warfarin (case reports of extreme international normalized ratio elevation in severe diarrhea have been published)
- Social history
  - Alcohol or illicit drugs (consider symptoms of withdrawal)
  - Sexual activity (consider pregnancy, gynecologic cause)
  - New pets in house (10% of dogs and cats excrete *Salmonella*)
- Family history
  - Irritable bowel syndrome/inflammatory bowel disease

Physical Examination

- Vital signs
  - Tachycardia
  - Hypotension/orthostasis
  - Fever
- Oropharynx examination
- Abdominal examination
  - Focal tenderness
  - Rebound/guarding
  - Distention
  - Bowel sounds

RED FLAGS

- Hemodynamic instability
  - Immediate intervention is required. Fluid resuscitate and consider other causes of illness in addition to simple gastroenteritis.
- Vomiting without diarrhea
  - Although diarrhea may begin later, vomiting alone should trigger consideration of ileus or obstruction, cardiac ischemia, or other noninfectious causes.
- Severe or sudden onset headache
  - Subarachnoid hemorrhage can trigger vomiting, and increased intracranial pressure from vomiting can rupture a cerebral aneurysm.
- Abdominal distention
  - Consider obstruction in patients with distention.
- Focal abdominal tenderness
  - Crampy or generalized mild abdominal pain is typical of acute gastroenteritis. Focal pain should elicit an evaluation for focal inflammation and irritation of noninfectious causes.
- Hunger despite vomiting
  - The symptoms of gastroenteritis almost always include profound anorexia. Hunger should indicate an extraintestinal trigger of vomiting such as a subarachnoid hemorrhage or pregnancy.
- Patients taking warfarin
  - In rare circumstances, profound coagulopathies have been reported in patients taking warfarin; these disorders are thought secondary to decreased bioavailability of vitamin K.
- Diabetic patients
  - They are at risk for rapid dehydration and ketoacidosis.
- Immunocompromised patients
  - This patient population has a greater incidence of complications, more aggressive disease, and greater difficulty resolving the illness without intervention.

or diarrhea; local cecitis may mimic acute appendicitis. *Bacillus anthracis* may cause minimal symptoms, but patients may have shallow oral ulcers, massive lymphadenopathy with tissue edema, and fulminant upper and lower gastrointestinal bleeding.

Differential Diagnosis

Vomiting and diarrhea can be from other pathologic states, some that are life-threatening. Maintaining a level of suspicion for other causes is essential to minimize the chance of missing a more dangerous cause.

The following subsections describe diagnoses to consider within broader categories of presentations.

VOMITING AND DIARRHEA

Toxic Ingestions and Overdoses

Accidental or intentional ingestion of toxic chemicals or medications frequently manifests with abdominal pain, nausea, vomiting, and sometimes diarrhea. Depending on the situation, patients may not be forthcoming with an accurate history unless they are specifically questioned.

Opiate Withdrawal

Nausea and vomiting are quite common in acute opiate withdrawal. In addition, a patient usually experiences agitation, diffuse aches, and diaphoresis. Although patients with acute gastroenteritis often have lower blood pressures because of dehydration and vagal stimulation, patients experiencing opiate withdrawal often have hypertension along with tachycardia and tachypnea. Patients may not always admit their illicit drug use, thus making the diagnosis more challenging.

VOMITING WITHOUT DIARRHEA

Vomiting is a symptom and not a diagnosis. Gastroenteritis can be diagnosed only if signs of gastritis or enteritis are clearly present, based on clinical evaluation. Vomiting can also be caused by many toxic and metabolic disorders and organ dysfunction. Ingestions, carbon monoxide, and other poisonings often incite vomiting, without other signs. Structural organ disorders, inside or outside the abdomen, can cause vomiting. Early hepatitis, biliary disease, and early appendicitis may cause vomiting with few other signs. Other important causes of vomiting include those discussed in the following paragraphs.

Obstruction

A history of abdominal surgery should raise suspicions of a possible intestinal obstruction. On physical examination, abdominal distention is common, and hypoactive bowel sounds are in contrast to hyperactive bowel sounds usually found in gastroenteritis.

Intracranial Disease

Headache is a common complaint that often accompanies acute gastroenteritis. However, vomiting also frequently accompanies headaches caused by an intracranial hemorrhage or tumor. When the history of a headache is elicited, it is imperative to determine the onset and quality of the pain so more dangerous disease is not overlooked. Headache that started before the onset of vomiting is concerning. Likewise, a sudden, severe headache occurring while vomiting may indicate an aneurysmal rupture resulting from increased intracranial pressure during the Valsalva maneuver.

Myocardial Infarction

Atypical presentations of myocardial infarction are important to recognize. Vomiting without diarrhea in a patient with significant risk factors should prompt consideration of a cardiac cause. Concomitant presence of shortness of breath and diaphoresis, with or without chest pain, increases the probability further.

Early Pregnancy

"Morning sickness" is most common within the first 13 weeks of gestation. However, pregnancy-associated nausea and vomiting may be more severe at other times besides the morning and may continue much past the first trimester. It is not unusual for vomiting to be the first symptom a woman experiences before she is aware of the pregnancy. Vomiting without diarrhea, symptoms spanning several days, and hunger between episodes should arouse suspicion of pregnancy as the cause. Inquiring about breast tenderness and missed or irregular menstrual periods can help to elicit the diagnosis. A pregnancy test should be standard in the evaluation of any woman of childbearing age who presents with symptoms of acute gastroenteritis.

FOCAL PAIN

Patients with acute gastroenteritis often complain of abdominal pain, but the quality tends to be crampy and fluctuating secondary to increased intestinal motility and spasm. Mild, constant midepigastric pain is also common after vomiting because of gastritis and abdominal wall muscle exertion. However severe, focal, unrelenting pain should prompt a search for other causes.

Focal Inflammation

Causes including gastritis, pancreatitis, cholecystitis, diverticulitis, or appendicitis are suspected when pain is isolated to their respective areas.

Perforated Viscus

A history of peptic ulcer disease, recent gynecologic or gastrointestinal instrumentation, or fever with peritoneal signs should raise the suspicion of perforated viscus.

Ischemic Bowel

In patients with risk factors for peripheral vascular disease, diffuse abdominal pain along with nausea and diarrhea after eating may indicate compromised blood flow to the intestines. The onset may be more gradual with slowly progressive atherosclerosis, or it may be abrupt from an embolic event to the intestinal vasculature. The physical examination is often unimpressive, given the severity of the stated discomfort (hence the finding "pain out of proportion to examination"). A high index of suspicion should be maintained, especially in the elderly population, because missing the diagnosis can lead to significant morbidity and even death.

Gynecologic Emergencies

These conditions include tubo-ovarian abscess, ovarian torsion, ruptured ectopic pregnancy, and pelvic inflammatory disease. A pelvic examination and pregnancy test are essential in the evaluation of women who complain of concomitant pelvic or lower abdominal pain.

Diagnostic Testing

Diagnostic testing in infectious gastroenteritis is often overused. With symptoms lasting less than 24 hours in otherwise healthy individuals who are not at the extremes of age, no diagnostic testing is indicated, other than a pregnancy test in women of reproductive age. Exceptions include patients with severe symptoms, multiple grossly bloody stools, or hemodynamic instability and testing for epidemiologic purposes if food poisoning or a bioterrorism event is suspected.[3,4]

Laboratory or radiologic evaluation may be helpful in the several situations. A bedside urine evaluation for ketones may be useful to document dehydration and to guide intravenous fluid management. In patients whose symptoms have persisted for more than 24 hours, electrolyte determinations and tests of kidney function may be indicated. If a chemistry panel is obtained, calculation of the anion gap should be done to prevent missing clues to diabetic or alcoholic ketoacidosis, toxic ingestions, or other serious conditions.

Although the diagnostic yield is generally low, stool culture in patients who have unrelenting diarrhea may detect a treatable cause that can significantly shorten the course of illness.[5] Typically, positive results take at least 2 to 3 days, and symptoms have often resolved by the time results return. For patients who develop diarrhea 3 days or more after being hospitalized, bacterial stool cultures have not been found to be helpful.[6] Testing for ova and parasites has not shown to be cost effective unless the patient is at identifiable risk. This group includes patients with diarrhea persisting for several days after international travel to endemic regions, persons who ingest untreated water while camping or hiking, those with exposure to daycare centers, men who have sexual contact with other men, or persons who have sexual contact with patients with acquired immunodeficiency syndrome.[7] *Clostridium difficile* testing should be performed for anyone with persistent diarrhea and a history of antibiotic use in the previous 6 months.

The recommended diagnostic work-up in patients with acquired immunodeficiency syndrome and in other patients who are severely immunocompromised is more aggressive. Studies in these cases tend to yield more positive results, and symptoms are less apt to resolve without intervention. Stool should be sent for culture and for analysis for ova, parasites, and *Mycobacterium*. Unlike in the immunocompetent patient, blood cultures may be positive in up to 40% of cases and may yield a diagnosis even in the absence of positive stool cultures.[8] In this population, if severe diarrhea persists despite negative evaluations, the patient will need endoscopic evaluation for mucosal biopsy and additional cultures.

For patients with severe abdominal pain or distention, an obstructive plain radiographic series or abdominal computed tomography scan with oral and intravenous contrast can help to differentiate other more serious causes of their symptoms. Abdominal computed tomography scans without contrast, or with oral contrast alone, may be sufficient, depending on the experience of the radiologist conducting the examination.

A complete blood count is usually of little value, with rare exceptions. The stress of vomiting often causes transient leukocytosis that does not correlate with the severity or cause of illness. The hemoglobin and hematocrit may be helpful in patients with hemorrhagic diarrhea for assessment of anemia. Eosinophilia may indicate an allergic or parasitic origin. Macrocytic anemia can occur with infection involving *Diphyllobothrium latum*.

In patients with an acute onset of vomiting and diarrhea, documentation of gross blood in the stool is helpful. Checking for occult blood has not been proven to be sensitive or specific. When gross blood is absent, Hemoccult testing provides little to no insight into the causative pathogen and should not be used to guide treatment. Similarly, fecal leukocyte testing has low sensitivity and specificity and should not be used to justify empirical antibiotic treatment.[9,10]

To reiterate, most cases are represented by young, otherwise healthy individuals who have had symptoms for less than 24 hours. In this population, minimal to no testing should be the rule.

Treatment and Disposition

The mainstays of treatment consist of rehydration and alleviation of symptoms through antiemetics (Fig. 185-1). The use of empirical antibiotics is not indicated in the majority of cases.

For those patients who are hemodynamically stable and whose vomiting can be controlled, oral rehydration is adequate and is often greatly underutilized. Ketonemia has been implicated in emetogenesis. In patients with significant dehydration, nausea and vomiting may continue because of circulating ketones long after the initial infectious cause has been eradicated by the body. In this circumstance, proper administration of intravenous fluids may be all that is required to resolve the patient's symptoms. If a patient is unable to tolerate oral intake, intravenous normal saline is adequate for initial hydration. For patients with significant ketosis, switching to dextrose-containing compounds after

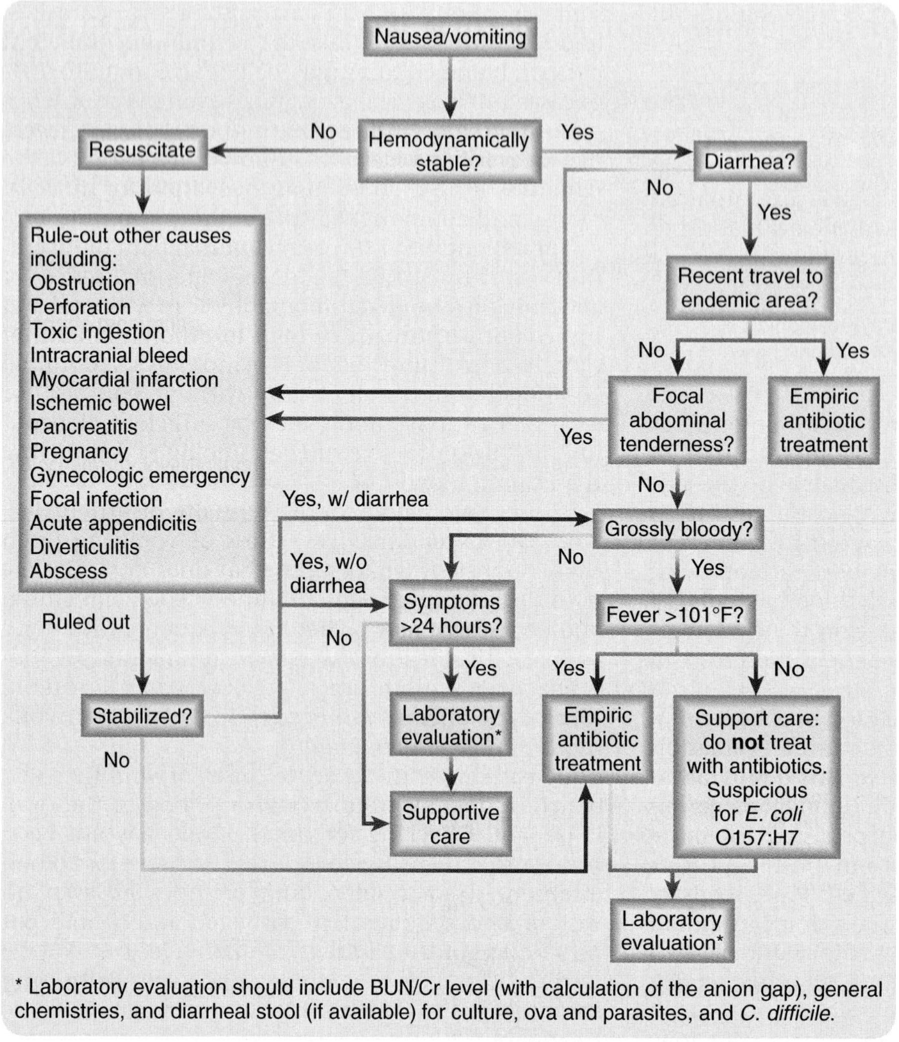
Nausea/vomiting
Hemodynamically stable?
No
Yes
Resuscitate
Diarrhea?
No
Yes
Rule-out other causes including:
Obstruction
Perforation
Toxic ingestion
Intracranial bleed
Myocardial infarction
Ischemic bowel
Pancreatitis
Pregnancy
Gynecologic emergency
Focal infection
Acute appendicitis
Diverticulitis
Abscess
Recent travel to endemic area?
No
Yes
Focal abdominal tenderness?
Empiric antibiotic treatment
Yes
No
Yes, w/ diarrhea
Grossly bloody?
No
Yes
Yes, w/o diarrhea
Symptoms >24 hours?
No
Fever >101°F?
Ruled out
Yes
Yes
No
Stabilized?
Laboratory evaluation*
Empiric antibiotic treatment
Support care: do **not** treat with antibiotics. Suspicious for *E. coli* O157:H7
No
Supportive care
Laboratory evaluation*
* Laboratory evaluation should include BUN/Cr level (with calculation of the anion gap), general chemistries, and diarrheal stool (if available) for culture, ova and parasites, and *C. difficile*.

FIGURE 185-1 Treatment algorithm for adults without significant comorbid illness. BUN, blood urea nitrogen; Cr, creatinine.

the initial rehydration may help to restore normal metabolic function more quickly.

Many choices of antiemetics and routes of administration are available. When choosing a medication, one should consider pregnancy class, cost, and side effects, particularly the extrapyramidal side effects of the phenothiazines and metoclopramide. Table 185-2 gives the characteristics of common antiemetic agents. If one agent fails, it is recommended to switch to a different class of agent rather than to repeat administration of an agent of the same class.

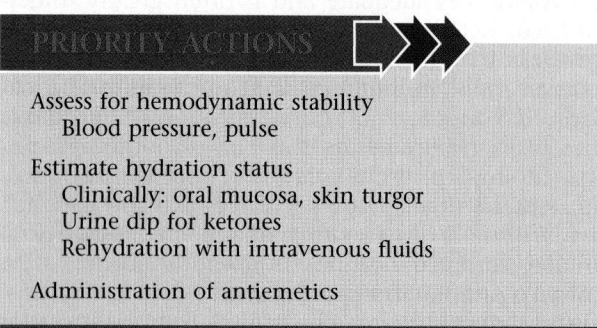

PRIORITY ACTIONS

Assess for hemodynamic stability
- Blood pressure, pulse

Estimate hydration status
- Clinically: oral mucosa, skin turgor
- Urine dip for ketones
- Rehydration with intravenous fluids

Administration of antiemetics

The hazards of using antidiarrheal agents in acute gastroenteritis appear to have been overstated. For afebrile patients without grossly bloody diarrhea or a high suspicion for *C. difficile* colitis from recent antibiotic use, antimotility agents such as loperamide or atropine/diphenoxylate can be safely administered. Use of these drugs is recommended for large-volume diarrhea that compromises hydration status or is otherwise hindering a patient's ability for self-care.

Antibiotics are rarely indicated in the empirical treatment of acute gastroenteritis, for many reasons. Viruses remain the most common causes of acute gastroenteritis in the general population, and these infections resolve without intervention. Most bacterial causes are self-limited and are eradicated by the host defenses in a short time. Common adverse reactions of most antibiotics are nausea or diarrhea, occurring in up to 10% of patients. Although certain antibiotics are more prone to causing *C. difficile* colitis, any antibiotic can predispose patients to this complication. Administering antibiotics to patients with non-*typhi Salmonella* infections is ineffective and may lead to a prolonged carrier state. If the patient has contracted illness from *Escherichia coli*

Table 185-2 COMMONLY USED ANTIEMETIC DRUGS

Generic Name	Brand Name	Pregnancy Class	Drug Class	Route	Cost	Common Side Effects
Prochlorperazine	Compazine	C	Phenothiazine	PO/PR/IM/IV	Inexpensive	Akathisia, drowsiness, extrapyramidal effects
Inapsine	Droperidol	C	Butyrophenone	IM/IV	Inexpensive	Akathisia, drowsiness, extrapyramidal effects
Promethazine	Phenergan	C	Nonselective antihistamine	PO/PR/IM/IV	Inexpensive	Extreme sedation, anticholinergic effects
Trimethobenzamide	Tigan	C	Nonselective antihistamine	PO/PR/IM/IV	Inexpensive	Extreme sedation, hypotension, anticholinergic effects
Metoclopramide	Reglan	B	Dopaminergic blocker	PO/IM/IV	Inexpensive	Restlessness, extrapyramidal effects
Ondansetron	Zofran	B	Selective 5-HT_3 antagonist	PO/ODT/IM/IV	Expensive	Less frequent: headache, dizziness, agitation
Granisetron	Kytril	B	Selective 5-HT_3 antagonist	PO/IV	Expensive	Less frequent: headache, drowsiness, taste changes
Dolasetron	Anzemet	B	Selective 5-HT_3 antagonist	PO/IV	Expensive	Less frequent: headache, dizziness, fatigue
Palonosetron	Aloxi	B	Selective 5-HT_3 antagonist	IV	Expensive	Less frequent: headache, prolonged QT interval

5-HT_3, 5-hydroxytryptamine 3; IM, intramuscular; IV, intravenous; ODT, orally disintegrating tablet; PO, oral; PR, rectal.

serotype O157:H7, antibiotics will have no effect on the symptoms but may lead to an increased incidence of hemolytic-uremic syndrome. Finally, empirical treatment with antibiotics contributes to the alarming development of resistant pathogens in the general patient population. Empirical antibiotics are usually ineffective, may complicate the picture, may even harm the patient, and contribute to the formation of resistant organisms.

The indications for empirical antibiotics are very narrow. If a patient appears toxic, has a fever higher than 101°F and bloody diarrhea, or is hemodynamically unstable, antibiotics may be helpful. Grossly bloody diarrhea alone is not an indication, and again, bloody diarrhea may be caused by *E. coli* O157:H7. This serotype does not usually cause a fever, and therefore empirical antibiotics for grossly bloody diarrhea in conjunction with a temperature greater than 101°F should not raise concerns of inducing hemolytic-uremic syndrome.

Another indication for empirical antibiotics involves acute gastroenteritis in the setting of travel to endemic areas for traveler's diarrhea. The most common pathogens include enterotoxigenic *E. coli, Shigella, Salmonella,* and *Campylobacter*. In many cases, prompt use of a fluoroquinolone can lead to relief of symptoms within hours. Unfortunately, resistance to this class of drugs and to many other antibiotics is rising throughout the world, and treatment failures are becoming more common. Of the foregoing pathogens, *Campylobacter* has a high enough resistance to fluoroquinolones that erythromycin is now the drug of choice in these infections. For continued empirical treatment of traveler's diarrhea in patients who do not respond to fluoroquinolones, azithromycin may be used. Sending stool cultures before the initiation of antibiotics can be helpful, given the high rates of resistance in anticipation of potential treatment failures. Table 185-3 gives specific antibiotic regimens for symptomatic patients in whom the pathogen is identified.

In general, patients who were hemodynamically unstable at any point in their stay, who have persistent pain, or who continue to vomit frequently should be admitted until oral intake can be tolerated and pain improves. If a noninfectious origin has not been ruled out and symptoms continue, admission should also be considered. Patients with severe comorbid illness and those who take multiple medications that would be affected by poor oral intake or malabsorption may also need to be admitted.

Diabetic patients may be particularly challenged by acute gastroenteritis. Infection combined with an inability to take hypoglycemic medications may increase their blood glucose and may exacerbate their dehydration. Diabetic patients may become hypoglycemic, given decreased intake in the setting of long-acting hypoglycemic medications, and it is prudent to have a low threshold for admitting diabetic patients. If an insulin-dependent patient is discharged, it is essential that a basal rate of insulin be continued. Halving the usual dose of insulin, or instructing the patient to take the long-acting insulin only and checking blood glucose levels regularly, may be sufficient. Discussion with the primary care physician before discharge facilitates outpatient management.

Patients with persistent nausea but no vomiting can usually be discharged with an antiemetic and careful instructions for maintaining hydration. Per-

Table 185-3 ANTIBIOTIC REGIMENS FOR IDENTIFIED PATHOGENS

Organism/Pathogen	Antibiotic Treatment	Comment
Unknown (if empirical therapy deemed necessary)	Ciprofloxacin 500 mg bid×3 days OR TMP-SMX DS bid×3 days	 Resistance high in tropics
Unknown with recent antibiotic exposure	Metronidazole 500 mg PO tid×10 days OR Vancomycin 125 mg PO qid×10 days	Also effective IV Not effective IV
Campylobacter	Erythromycin 500 mg bid×5 days OR Azithromycin 500 qd×3 days	Not fluoroquinolones because of resistance
Salmonella	Ciprofloxacin 500 mg bid×5 days OR Azithromycin 1 g then 500 mg qd×6 days OR Ceftriaxone IV	 Total 7 days For inpatient treatment
Shigella	Ciprofloxacin 500 mg bid×3 days OR TMP-SMX DS bid×3 days	
Yersinia	Ciprofloxacin 500 mg bid×3 days OR TMP-SMX DS bid×3 days	
Vibrio parahaemolyticus	Does not shorten the course	In vitro susceptibilities to ciprofloxacin
Hemorrhagic *Escherichia coli* O157:H7	Antibiotics not effective	
Aeromonas/Plesiomonas	TMP-SMX DS bid×3 days OR Ciprofloxacin 500 mg bid×3 days	
Staphylococcus	Antibiotics not effective	
Clostridium perfringens enterotoxin	Antibiotics not effective	
Bacillus cereus	Antibiotics not effective	
Cholera and noncholera *Vibrio* species	Ciprofloxacin 1 g×1 OR Doxycycline 300 mg×1 OR TMP-SMX DS bid×3 days	
Scombroid fish (poisoning)	Antihistamines; antibiotics not effective	
Ciguatera fish (poisoning)	Antibiotics not effective	
Enterotoxigenic *Escherichia coli*	Ciprofloxacin 750 mg×1 OR TMP-SMX DS bid×3 days OR Ciprofloxacin 500 mg bid×3 days	
Clostridium difficile	Metronidazole 500 mg PO tid×10 days OR Vancomycin 125 mg PO qid×10 days	Also effective IV Not effective IV
Norovirus/rotavirus	Antibiotics not effective	
Cryptosporidium	Antibiotics poorly effective	
Isospora/coccidia	TMP-SMX DS bid for 10 days OR Ciprofloxacin 500 mg×7 days	 87% effective
Giardia	Metronidazole 250 mg tid×5 days OR Paromomycin 500 mg qid×7 days	 In pregnancy
Entamoeba histolytica	Metronidazole 500 mg tid×10 days followed by Paromomycin 500 mg tid×7 days	
Enterobius vermicularis	Albendazole 400 mg×1 OR Mebendazole 100 mg chewed×1 OR Pyrantel pamoate 11 mg/kg (maximum, 1 g)×1	Repeat dose×1 in 2 wk Repeat dose×1 in 2 wk Repeat dose×1 in 2 wk
Taenia saginata/solium	Praziquantel 5-10 mg/kg PO×1 OR Niclosamide 2 g PO×1	
Diphyllobothrium latum	Praziquantel 5-10 mg/kg PO×1 OR Niclosamide 2 g PO×1	

bid, twice daily; DS, double strength; IV, intravenously; PO, orally; qd, once daily; qid, four times daily; tid, three times daily; TMP-SMX, trimethoprim-sulfamethoxazole.

FACTS AND FORMULAS

Homemade Oral Rehydration Solution

1/2 teaspoon salt
1/2 teaspoon baking soda
4 tablespoons sugar
All in 1 L of water

The most common cause of acute gastroenteritis is viral.

Of bacterial causes, the three most common are *Campylobacter, Salmonella,* and *Shigella.*

Escherichia coli O157:H7 is more common in patients with grossly blood stools.

Nonbloody bacterial stool cultures are positive 1% to 5% of the time in immunocompetent adults.

Grossly bloody bacterial stool cultures are positive up to 20% of the time in immunocompetent adults.[15]

A pathogen can be identified in 80% to 85% of patients with acquired immunodeficiency syndrome and diarrhea.[16]

PATIENT TEACHING TIPS

- Prevent transmission.
  - Wash hands well.
  - Separate drinking glasses, towels, and preferably bathrooms.
- Diet
  - Start drinking sips of liquids.
  - If tolerated, advance to full liquids.
  - Once hungry, eat small amounts of whatever sounds good, with the exception of alcohol and caffeine-containing foods and drinks because these may exacerbate the symptoms.
  - If dairy products exacerbate symptoms, avoid for 1 to 2 weeks as a temporary measure because lactose intolerance is not uncommon.
- Return to the emergency department if vomiting persists, if pain in the abdomen increases, if fever increases, or if signs of dehydration develop.

sistent diarrhea alone is not an indication for admission, unless the patient is immunocompromised and has significant dehydration on presentation.

Dietary recommendations are always of great concern to patients on discharge. There are many complex regimens involving significant dietary restrictions, based on limited scientific data. Patients should be advised that the number 1 priority is to stay hydrated. If solid foods do not sound appealing, then they should not be encouraged. For mild diarrhea or persistent nausea, water or commercially available sports drinks should be adequate. These drinks are not properly balanced for more severe dehydration. If the patient is having large volumes of diarrhea or fluid losses, a balanced glucose and electrolyte solution with or without starches is recommended. Oral rehydration solutions are available in many pharmacies. An effective solution can be made at home by adding one-half teaspoon of salt, one-half teaspoon of baking soda, and four tablespoons of sugar to 1 L of water.[11]

Once a patient becomes interested in solid foods, traditionally a bland diet of bananas, rice, apples, and toast (the BRAT diet) has been recommended. No data support the BRAT diet, and patients should be encouraged to eat small amounts of whatever appeals to them, with a few exceptions. Both caffeine and alcohol have direct stimulatory effects on the bowel and therefore may worsen symptoms. In addition, a few patients encounter temporary lactose intolerance after gastroenteritis. If dairy products exacerbate symptoms, then refraining from these products for 1 to 2 weeks should allow the intestines to restore their normal function.

Complications

Significant complications are fortunately quite rare following gastroenteritis. The most common minor complication is temporary lactose intolerance that usually resolves spontaneously. As symptoms of the primary infection improve, patients may ingest milk products. However, if dairy products result in worsening bloating and cramping symptoms, then patients are advised to avoid these products for 1 to 2 weeks. Rarely does the intolerance become more chronic. Likewise, steatorrhea, or fat malabsorption, may occur transiently, particularly after a rotavirus infection, but it also resolves spontaneously.

Case reports in patients taking warfarin have noted significant coagulopathies occurring with acute gastroenteritis. Although these disorders are usually associated with episodes lasting several days, one case occurred after a single day of diarrhea. The mechanism is presumed to be a decreased vitamin K level in the body, from both decreased oral intake and malabsorption within the intestine.[12,13] Prothrombin time and international normalized ratio should be checked in patients taking warfarin, and close follow-up with repeat blood tests can prevent potential bleeding complications.

Any patient who is forcefully retching may suffer a tear in the mucosal surface of the esophagus, called a *Mallory-Weiss tear,* and this can lead to blood in the vomitus. Patients usually have little to no associated pain, and bleeding almost always resolves spontaneously, but occasionally, endoscopic intervention is required to acquire hemostasis. A more serious complication results when complete transmural disruption occurs in the esophagus. Known as *Boerhaave's syndrome,* it is usually accompanied by significant pain and is associated with a high mortality. A chest radiograph is almost always positive for mediastinal or intra-abdominal free air. Surgical consultation and aggressive resuscitative management are essential.

Clostridium perfringens normally causes self-limited gastroenteritis. However, in rare cases, it can lead to enteritis necroticans, which rapidly progresses to shock and death.

Diabetic patients may become significantly dehydrated in combination with high blood glucose levels, especially if these patients are unable to take their usual oral hypoglycemic agents. In severe circumstances, acute gastroenteritis may lead to diabetic ketoacidosis, coma, and death. A low threshold for electrolyte testing and measurement of the anion gap can help to detect the patient in danger of this complication.

Although rare, invasive bacterial pathogens have been associated with systemic complications such as cholecystitis, pancreatitis, meningitis, endocarditis, and osteomyelitis. *Campylobacter* has been associated with a more severe form of Guillain-Barré syndrome, which occurs even in patients with asymptomatic infections who have no signs of gastroenteritis.[14]

E. coli 0157:H7 hemorrhagic colitis has been associated with the hemolytic-uremic syndrome and with thrombotic thrombocytopenic purpura. Using antibiotics to treating gastroenteritis caused by this pathogen does nothing to eradicate the disease, but it may increase the incidence of these complications.

REFERENCES

1. Mead PS, Slutsker L, Dietz V, et al: Food-related illness and death in the United States. Emerg Infect Dis 1999;5:607-625.
2. Field M, Rao MC, Chang EB: Intestinal electrolyte transport and diarrheal disease. Part II. N Engl J Med 1989;321: 879-883.
3. Guerrant RL, Van Gilder T, Steiner TS, et al: Practice guidelines for the management of infectious diarrhea. Clin Infect Dis 2001;32:331-351.
4. Thielman NM, Guerrant RL: Clinical practice: Acute infectious diarrhea. N Engl J Med 2004;350:38-47.
5. DuPont HL: Guidelines on acute infectious diarrhea in adults: The Practice Parameters Committee of the American College of Gastroenterology. Am J Gastroenterol 1997;92:1962-1975.
6. Rohner P, Pittet D, Pepey B, et al: Etiological agents of infectious diarrhea: Implications for requests for microbial culture. J Clin Microbiol 1997;35:1427-1432.
7. Siegel D, Edelstein P, Nachamkin I: Inappropriate testing for diarrheal diseases in the hospital. JAMA 1990;263: 979-982.
8. Smith PD, Quinn TC, Strober W, et al: NIH Conference: Gastrointestinal infections in AIDS. Ann Intern Med 1992;116:63-77.
9. Siegel D, Cohen PT, Neighbor M, et al: Predictive value of stool examination in acute diarrhea. Arch Pathol Lab Med 1987;111:715-718.
10. Herbert ME: Medical myth: Measuring white blood cells in the stools is useful in the management of acute diarrhea. West J Med 2000;172:414.
11. de Zoysa I, Kirkwood B, Feachem R, Lindsay-Smith E: Preparation of sugar-salt solutions. Trans R Soc Trop Med Hyg 1984;78:260-262.
12. Smith JK, Aljazairi A, Fuller SH: INR elevation associated with diarrhea in a patient receiving warfarin. Ann Pharmacother 1999;33:301-304.
13. Robert RJ, Rao P, Miske GR, et al: Diarrhea-associated over-anticoagulation in a patient taking warfarin: Therapeutic role of cholestyramine. Vet Hum Toxicol 2000; 42:351-353.
14. Allos M: *Campylobacter jejuni* infections: Update on emerging issues and trends. Clin Infect Dis 2001;32:1201.
15. Musher DM, Musher BL: Contagious acute gastrointestinal infections. N Engl J Med 2004;551:2417-2427.
16. Sanchez-Mejorada G, Ponce de Leon S: Clinical patterns of diarrhea in AIDS: Etiology and prognosis. Rev Invest Clin 1994;46:187-196.

Chapter 186

Skin and Soft Tissue Infections

Ellen M. Slaven

KEY POINTS

- Uncomplicated subcutaneous abscesses in otherwise healthy patients require incision and drainage alone without antibiotic therapy.
- Cellulitis with induration may harbor a deep purulent collection despite the lack of fluctuance on physical examination. Ultrasound or needle aspiration may be used to assist in the search for areas of pus that require incision and drainage.
- Diabetic foot infections that are mild may be treated with oral agents (e.g., cephalexin, dicloxacillin, or clindamycin) that target gram-positive organisms alone.
- EPs must always search for signs of necrotizing infection to exclude the deadly diagnosis early in the management of skin and soft tissue infections.
- Emergency consultation with a surgeon is mandated when a suspicion of necrotizing skin and soft tissue infection arises.

Superficial Skin Infections

■ IMPETIGO

Impetigo is most commonly encountered in preschool-aged children. It is a superficial infection involving the epidermis and is highly contagious. Impetigo is readily spread from one site to another on one child and just as easily from one child to another. Two types of impetigo are recognized. The classic *nonbullous impetigo* begins with a vesicular lesion that becomes purulent. The vesicle then ruptures and reveals the typical, honey-colored crusted lesion. The face and extremities are commonly involved. *Streptococcus pyogenes* is the pathogen. The infection is self-limited and heals without scarring. Treatment is aimed to speed resolution and to prevent transmission. The second type of impetigo, *bullous impetigo,* is caused by a toxin-producing strain of *Staphylococcus aureus*. The appearance of bullous impetigo is of a flaccid bullous lesion that may become filled with purulent fluid. Approximately 10% to 20% of all cases of impetigo are the bullous type.

Treatment with topical mupirocin is effective in patients with mild presentations of impetigo. Patients with more severe infections require systemic therapy with cephalexin for 7 days. Azithromycin (500 mg orally on day 1, then 250 mg orally on days 2 to 5) is an alternative for patients who are allergic to penicillin.

■ ERYSIPELAS

Group A streptococcus (*S. pyogenes*) is primarily responsible for the intradermal infections known as *erysipelas,* or Saint Anthony's fire. This infection also involves the lymphatic drainage of the skin and produces a bright, erythematous raised area of skin. It is very well demarcated. The diagnosis is based on clinical appearance. The rash is common in elderly persons and in young children. Seventy percent of infections occur on the lower leg, and approximately 20% occur on the face. The onset is quite sudden, fever may be present, and the rash is frequently very painful.

The drug of choice is penicillin. Admission to the hospital for intravenous antibiotics and supportive care may be indicated for patients who suffer from serious comorbidities or those who appear toxic. Azithromycin is an alternative agent.

Cellulitis

Cellulitis results from bacterial infection of the dermis and the subcutaneous fat. Infection may arise following the entry of bacteria into the dermis through small breaks in the skin, larger wounds, or preexisting dermatitis. Infection may be limited to a small patch, or it may spread to include extensive areas of skin. Cellulitis is manifested by erythematous, warm, tender regions of skin that frequently spread. Lymphangitis and lymphadenitis may be present. Fever, chills, and malaise are common associated symptoms.

The pathogens of cellulitis are rarely identified in any particular patient but are thought to be primarily *Streptococcus* species and *S. aureus*. Culture of material aspirated from the involved skin is not routinely performed because of the invasive nature of the procedure and the low diagnostic yield. Blood cultures are of little value because only approximately 2% to 5% of them yield results.

Patients with mild cases of cellulitis may be treated on an outpatient basis with an antibiotic effective against penicillinase-resistant *S. aureus*. Dicloxacillin and cephalexin are appropriate choices because these agents are also effective against *Streptococcus* species.[1] Patients with severe illness or comorbidities are likely to require admission to the hospital for intravenous antibiotics, such as oxacillin, nafcillin, or cefazolin. For patients allergic to penicillin, azithromycin or levofloxacin may be substituted.

In patients with cellulitis who require hospital admission (e.g., those with extensive disease or underlying immunocompromise and those who appear toxic), blood cultures are often obtained. Although the diagnostic yield of blood cultures is quite low, they may provide useful information for patients who are particularly ill. Radiography may provide valuable information about patients with cellulitis, in particular to establish the presence or absence of gas or foreign bodies.

Purulent Skin Infections

Small, superficial pustular infections arising from the hair follicle are usually caused by *S. aureus* and are referred to as *folliculitis*. The lesions of folliculitis tend to be approximately 2 to 5 mm in diameter, they are isolated to the epidermis, and they generally produce pruritus rather than pain. Treatment consists of warm, moist compresses and topical antibiotic ointment, such as mupirocin. If systemic therapy is desired (because of a lack of response to topical therapy, extensive infection, or the presence of underlying immunocompromising medical condition), an oral first-generation cephalosporin, such as cephalexin, or an antistaphylococcal penicillin, such as dicloxacillin, is recommended.

Furuncles begin as simple folliculitis and extend deeper into the subcutaneous tissue and surrounding dermis. Furuncles are also called boils or subcutaneous nodules. These painful lesions tend to erupt in areas with hairy skin, in particular the face, axilla, and buttock.

When multiple adjacent furuncles coalesce, a large, purulent mass develops in the subcutaneous tissues. This is a *carbuncle*. These lesions tend to occur in areas of overlying thick skin, such as the nape of the neck, back, and posterior thighs. Carbuncles appear as erythematous soft tissue masses, and they may contain several orifices capable of draining purulent material. Diabetes is a risk factor for the development of carbuncles. These lesions are quite painful and are frequently associated with fever.

Incision and drainage are required for both furuncles and carbuncles. Carbuncles generally require drainage in the operating room to provide sufficient analgesia and complete drainage. Antibiotics are indicated for patients with furuncles that are complicated by surrounding cellulitis and for all patients with carbuncles (Table 186-1).

Subcutaneous abscesses are collections of purulent material in the subcutaneous tissues, and they may occur anywhere on the body. The overlying skin may be uninvolved and may appear intact, or it may be erythematous and indurated. A pustule may be noted, or the overlying skin may be thin and in various stages of breakdown as the purulence drains spontaneously. Cellulitis of the surrounding dermis may also be noted around a subcutaneous abscess. Puru-

Table 186-1 ANTIBIOTICS FOR PURULENT SKIN INFECTIONS

Condition	Antibiotic Regimen
Folliculitis	Topical: mupirocin ointment tid×5-7 days Oral: cephalexin 500 mg PO qid×5-7 days Dicloxacillin 500 mg PO qid×5-7 days Azithromycin 500 mg PO day 1, then 250 mg PO qd×4 Clindamycin 300 mg PO qid×5-7 days
Furuncle	Cephalexin 500 mg PO qid×5-7 days Dicloxacillin 500 mg PO qid×5-7 days Azithromycin 500 mg PO day 1, then 250 mg PO qd×4 Clindamycin 300 mg PO qid×5-7 days
Carbuncle	Cefazolin 1 g IV q6h Oxacillin/nafcillin 1 g IV q4h Azithromycin 500 mg IV qd Clindamycin 600 mg IV q8h

IV, intravenously; PO, orally; q, every; qd, once daily; qid, four times daily; tid, three times daily.

Table 186-2 INDICATIONS FOR ANTIBIOTIC THERAPY FOR SUBCUTANEOUS ABSCESSES

Clinical Manifestation	Associated Conditions
Abscesses in patients with compromised immune systems	Diabetes Acquired immunodeficiency syndrome Liver disease Organ transplantation Medications, such as long-term corticosteroid therapy Chemotherapy
Abscesses complicated with other conditions	Cellulitis Lymphangitis Fever Sepsis
Abscesses located on the central face	

lent material must be sought out in patients who have cellulitis with moderate induration because pus may lie deep beneath the surface, without any signs of pustules or fluctuance. Ultrasound scanning or aspiration with a large-gauge needle (following local anesthesia) may reveal occult purulent collections. Incision and drainage are required for all subcutaneous abscesses. Antibiotics are not indicated for uncomplicated subcutaneous abscesses in healthy patients. The indications for antibiotics are listed in Table 186-2.

Community-Associated Methicillin-Resistant *Staphylococcus aureus*

Since the late 1990s, an epidemic of skin and soft tissue infections has been caused by community-acquired methicillin-resistant *S. aureus* (CA-MRSA). Currently, in the United States, CA-MRSA is the most common cause of skin and soft tissue infection in patients presenting to EDs. Patients who develop these infections have been previously healthy, and most have not been exposed to health care settings or prior antibiotic therapy.[2]

CA-MRSA is distinguished from hospital-acquired MRSA (HA-MRSA) not only by the location of acquisition, but also by the type of infection produced. HA-MRSA causes wound infections, sepsis, endocarditis, and metastatic infections, whereas CA-MRSA causes predominantly purulent skin infections. HA-MRSA rarely carries the Panton-Valentine leukocidin that is believed to be a potent virulence factor found in most CA-MRSA strains. In addition, HA-MRSA is generally resistant to many antibiotics, whereas CA-MRSA tends to be resistant predominantly to beta-lactams and remains susceptible to many other antibiotics, such as trimethoprim-sulfamethoxazole and the tetracyclines.

Although patients requiring antibiotic therapy for CA-MRSA skin infections would logically be better served by a non–beta-lactam antibiotic, no studies have demonstrated the lack of effect of cephalexin or oxacillin. On the contrary, several studies observed that outcomes of patients with CA-MRSA skin infections were equivalent when these patients were treated with either beta-lactams (e.g., cephalexin) or antibiotics to which the CA-MRSA strains were susceptible (e.g., trimethoprim-sulfamethoxazole).[2,3] Despite these findings, it is prudent to treat patients with purulent skin infections with antimicrobials that are effective in vitro against CA-MRSA (Table 186-3). Although most (>85%) infections caused by CA-MRSA are skin and soft tissue infections, rare cases of more severe infections have been reported, including pyomyositis, necrotizing fasciitis, and necrotizing pneumonia.

Table 186-3 ANTIBIOTICS FOR COMMUNITY-ACQUIRED METHICILLIN-RESISTANT STAPHYLOCOCCUS AUREUS SKIN INFECTIONS

Degree of Infection	Antibiotic Regimen
Mild	Trimethoprim-sulfamethoxazole (double strength) 1 PO bid Clindamycin 300 mg PO qid Doxycycline 100 mg PO bid
Moderate to severe	Vancomycin 1 g IV q12h Clindamycin 600-900 mg IV q8h Linezolid 400-600 mg IV q12h Daptomycin 4 mg/kg IV q24h

bid, twice daily; IV, intravenously; PO, orally; q, every; qid, four times daily.

Diabetic Foot Infections

With more than 16 million diabetic patients in the United States and a 3-year incidence of foot ulceration of 6% among them, EPs are likely to treat many patients with diabetic foot infections. The ulcers may begin as small lesions; however, these lesions are prone to infection and are associated with great morbidity and mortality. Fifteen percent of diabetic patients with foot ulcerations require amputation, and the 3-year mortality is almost 30%.[4]

Diabetic foot infections are diagnosed by their clinical appearance. Laboratory testing and radiography may be helpful to support the presence of infection or to define complications. The white blood cell count and erythrocyte sedimentation rate may be elevated in the presence of infection; however, these tests are neither sufficiently sensitive nor definitively specific. Blood glucose testing is important because infections often lead to hyperglycemia. Uremia is known to impair healing. Radiographs may reveal the bony changes of osteomyelitis or subcutaneous gas produced by a necrotizing infection.

Obtaining a sample for microbiologic testing is worthwhile, particularly in the setting of severe infection. However, simply swabbing the surface of an infected ulcer, or capturing purulent material as it makes its way to the surface, is likely to result in culture of contaminating bacteria, not necessarily the

Table 186-4 EMPIRICAL ANTIMICROBIAL THERAPY FOR INFECTIONS OF THE DIABETIC FOOT

Degree of Infection	Antibiotic Regimen
Mild	Cephalexin 500 mg PO qid×7 days Dicloxacillin 500 mg PO qid×7 days Clindamycin 300 mg PO qid×7 days
Moderate to severe	Ampicillin-sulbactam 3 g IV q6h Piperacillin-tazobactam 4.5 g IV q6h Levofloxacin 500 mg IV qd AND clindamycin 900 mg IV q8h
Limb- or life-threatening infections	Imipenem 500 mg IV q6h AND Vancomycin 1 g IV q12h OR Aztreonam 2 g IV q8h AND Metronidazole 7.5 mg/kg IV q8h AND Vancomycin 1 g IV q12h

IV, intravenously; PO, orally; q, every; qd, once daily; qid, four times daily.

offending pathogen. Aspiration of deep-lying purulent material and sampling of tissue obtained during débridement are superior methods of acquiring material for microbiologic testing. The management of diabetic foot infections is directed by the severity of infection; therefore, the EP must assess for the extent and depth of infection and for the presence of foreign bodies or necrosis.

Aerobic gram-positive cocci, in particular *S. aureus,* are the most predominant pathogens in diabetic foot infections. Patients with *mild infections,* defined as superficial when they have less than 2 cm of surrounding cellulitis and are lacking abscess or necrosis, may be treated with antibiotics targeting *S. aureus.* Examples of such agents are cephalexin, dicloxacillin, or clindamycin. Moderate to severe infections tend to be caused by gram-positive cocci in addition to gram-negative bacilli and anaerobes. *Moderate infections* are defined as those with cellulitis extending more than 2 cm, lymphangitis, spread to deep tissues, or the presence of abscess or necrosis. *Severe infections* cause systemic toxicity, including features such as fever, hypotension, confusion, acidosis, or azotemia. Empirical therapy for these polymicrobial infections requires a broad-spectrum regimen initially until the results of microbiologic culture are available. When a limb- or life-threatening infection is present, imipenem and vancomycin are recommended (Table 186-4).

Necrotizing Infections

Necrotizing skin and soft tissue infections comprise a group of potentially limb- and life-threatening diseases caused by various virulent pathogens or combinations of such. The common theme is infection leading to ischemia and necrosis of skin, subcutaneous tissue, fat, fascia, and even muscle. These infections are also characterized by their capacity to progress frighteningly rapidly. During the initial presentation of patients with necrotizing skin and soft tissue infections, EPs will not be able to discern the depth of the infection precisely, nor will they be capable of identifying the particular pathogen or pathogens. The most important component of the EP's initial evaluation is to detect, or at least suspect, the presence of necrosis based on clinical findings alone. Be cautious when intense, localized pain is otherwise unexplainable. An infection may be present. Early use of antibiotics and consultation with surgeons may allow for lifesaving surgical débridement.[5]

Gas gangrene, or clostridial myonecrosis, is the classic necrotizing skin and soft tissue infection. It often develops after a wound is contaminated with soil containing *Clostridium perfringens.* Another virulent bacterium, *Vibrio vulnificus,* is also capable of causing necrotizing soft tissue infections. *V. vulnificus* causes infections in patients who suffer wounds that are exposed to salt or brackish waters containing *Vibrio* species during warm months when the bacteria are abundant. Additionally, *S. pyogenes* is capable of causing necrotizing soft tissue infections frequently encountered in previously healthy patients.

Many patients with necrotizing skin and soft tissue infections are found to be infected with multiple pathogens. An example is *Fournier's gangrene.* This highly lethal infection of the perineum is commonly diagnosed in men with diabetes. These infections tend to be "mixed" owing to the recovery of several pathogens from culture such as *Streptococcus* species, Enterobacteriaceae, and anaerobes (e.g., *Bacteroides* species).

When a necrotizing skin and soft tissue infection is suspected, no diagnostic testing, in particular imaging studies, should delay consultation with a surgeon. Although many imaging studies have been employed in attempts to diagnose, and exclude, necrotizing skin and soft tissue infections, including plain radiographs, ultrasound scanning, computed tomography, and magnetic resonance imaging, none is superior to surgical exploration. A plain radiograph may demonstrate the presence of gas within the tissues, but it does not exclude necrosis. Ultrasound scanning and computed tomography may identify gas within the tissues in addition to deep-seated abscesses. Computed tomography and magnetic resonance imaging may show edema in the subcutaneous tissues or muscle and enhancement of inflamed fascia. None of these studies is adequately sensitive to exclude the presence of necrosis.

The definitive diagnosis of necrotizing skin and soft tissue infection is done by surgical exploration with direct visualization of the affected tissues and histologic examination of a frozen section biopsy specimen. Early surgical débridement is the definitive therapy.

Patients with known, or suspected, necrotizing skin and soft tissue infections require emergency

BOX 186-1

Clinical Indicators of the Potential for Necrotizing Soft Tissue Infections

Cellulitis that is rapidly advancing
Cellulitis with the following features:
- "Pain out of proportion" to physical examination
- Pain-restricted limb movement
- Crepitus
- Hemorrhagic bullae
- Ecchymosis
- Necrotic or black tissue

medicine management appropriate for those acutely ill. Attention to airway, breathing, and fluid management must be adequately aggressive.

Microbiologic studies, including blood cultures and culture of purulent material aspirated from a deep source, are indicated. Simply obtaining a swab from an open wound is likely to yield only contaminating bacteria. Infected tissue and fluids obtained during surgical débridement should also be cultured.

Antimicrobial therapy is vitally important early in the management of necrotizing skin and soft tissue infections. However, antimicrobial therapy alone without surgical débridement leads to a mortality approaching 100%.

Surgical consultation must be obtained as soon as the presence of a necrotizing soft tissue infection is suspected. Box 186-1 lists common clinical indicators that mandate surgical consultation.

Early empirical antimicrobial regimens require broad-spectrum activity, including coverage for gram-positive, gram-negative, and anaerobic organisms. Options for monotherapy include the carbapenems (imipenem and meropenem) and piperacillin-tazobactam. Multidrug regimens include high-dose penicillin with high-dose clindamycin and gentamicin (or levofloxacin). Vancomycin, or linezolid, should be added to all regimens until MRSA can be excluded (Table 186-5). Clindamycin inhibits protein synthesis and may be beneficial by blocking toxin production in several organisms responsible for necrotizing skin and soft tissue infections, in particular streptococcal and clostridial infections. All patients with necrotizing skin and soft tissue infections, even those with unproven infections, should be admitted to the hospital for intravenous antibiotic therapy and close observation for signs of clinical deterioration.

Table 186-5 ANTIMICROBIAL REGIMENS FOR THE EMPIRICAL TREATMENT OF NECROTIZING SKIN AND SOFT TISSUE INFECTIONS

Type of Therapy	Antibiotic Regimen
Monotherapy*	Imipenem 500 mg IV q6h OR Meropenem 1 g IV q8h OR Piperacillin/tazobactam 4.5 g IV q6h
Combination therapy*	Penicillin G 2 MU IV q6h AND Clindamycin 900 mg IV q8h AND Gentamicin 5 mg/kg IV q24h OR Penicillin G 2 MU IV q6h AND Clindamycin 900 mg IV q8h AND Ciprofloxacin 400 mg IV q12h

*Add vancomycin 1 g IV q12h or linezolid 600 mg in q12h until methicillin-resistant *Staphylococcus aureus* can be excluded.
IV, intravenously; q, every.

REFERENCES

1. Stevens DL, Bisno AL, Chambers HF, et al: Practice guidelines for the diagnosis and management of skin and soft tissue infections. Clin Infect Dis 2005;41:1373-1406.
2. Friedkin SK, Hageman JC, Morrison M, et al: Methicillin-resistant *Staphylococcus aureus* in three communities. N Engl J Med 2005;352:1436-1444.
3. Moran GJ, Krishnadasan A, Gorwitz RJ, et al: Methicillin-resistant *S. aureus* infections among patients in the emergency department. N Engl J Med 2006;355:666-674.
4. Lipsky BA, Berendt AR, Deery G, et al: Diagnosis and treatment of diabetic foot infections. Clin Infect Dis 2004;39:885-910.
5. Anaya DA, Dellinger P: Necrotizing soft-tissue infection: Diagnosis and management. Clin Infect Dis 2007;44:705-710.

SECTION **XVIII**

Wounds and Skin Injuries

Chapter 187

Wound Repair

E. Parker Hays, Jr.

KEY POINTS

List, consider, and document host and wound factors.

Evaluation, choice of the method of repair, and preparation are equally important as closure of the wound itself.

Antibiotics are not substitutes for adequate wound cleansing, irrigation, and exploration.

Proper skin eversion and suture placement actually make a difference and take no more time.

Address tetanus status in all patients.

Immobilization, a clean, moist environment, elevation, and sun avoidance are key elements of aftercare.

The pressure of the irrigating stream must be sufficient to overcome the adhesive forces of bacteria (≈5 to 12 psi).

The overall risk of infection and the likelihood of complications can be predicted by considering host and wound factors.

Record keeping should include description of the mechanism, history, prior home care of the wound, documentation of surrounding functions before and after any medical maneuvers, description of the steps taken to reduce infection, the search for foreign bodies, and closure of the wound.

Scope

Few things are as germane to emergency medicine as lacerations and wounds, both in practice and the public mindset. Approximately 12 million wounds are seen in EDs in the United States each year.[1] Although commonplace, each wound represents a personal and permanent event to the patient. To the practitioner, each wound represents an opportunity to alter the natural course of wound healing directly, ideally toward improved conditions and outcomes.

How a wound occurs, on whom, what is done to it before presentation, our management techniques, and wound aftercare all affect the end result. Most wounds heal themselves. However, think in terms of *creating optimal conditions* in which the wound does its own healing (Box 187-1).

Pathophysiology

Skin, the largest organ in the body, provides the varied functions of protection, heat exchange,

BOX 187-1

Goals of Wound Management

- Prevent impaired healing or infection.
- Preserve function of the injured part.
- Form an aesthetically acceptable scar.

prevention of infection, and tactile interface with the environment. The layers of skin—epidermis, dermis, and connective tissue—all play different roles in wounds and healing. The thickest and most important layer, the dermis, serves as structural integument, supports nutritional and waste product conveyances, and contains the cutaneous nerves (Fig. 187-1).

After injury, a continuum of coagulation, hemostasis, inflammation, tissue formation, and tissue remodeling ensues. Each of these steps can be influenced by the patient or the clinician. The aesthetic qualities of a scar are influenced by its thickness, color, and height or degree of depression. The thickness is most dependent on the width of the healing wound and on whether additional granulation tissue is necessary to fill gaps (secondary intention). The color results from the vascularity and pigmentation of the scar compared with surrounding tissue. Melanocytes do not necessarily produce pigment at the same even rate in injured and healing tissue or in scars as they do in normal tissue. The height of a scar is altered by the alignment and apposition of healing skin edges as well as by tensile and shear forces across the wound and the amount of inflammation preceding the formation of scar tissue. The increased height of a *hypertrophic* scar is the result of redundant tissue. If it extends beyond the original margins of the wound, it is called a *keloid*. Depressed scars create shadowing (consider the visibility of age-associated wrinkles) that make them appear darker than the neighboring reflective surfaces.

All these factors in scar formation vary among individuals. Some patients heal very well, and others invariably produce hypertrophic keloids. However, steps to improve outcomes remain generally the same in emergency management.

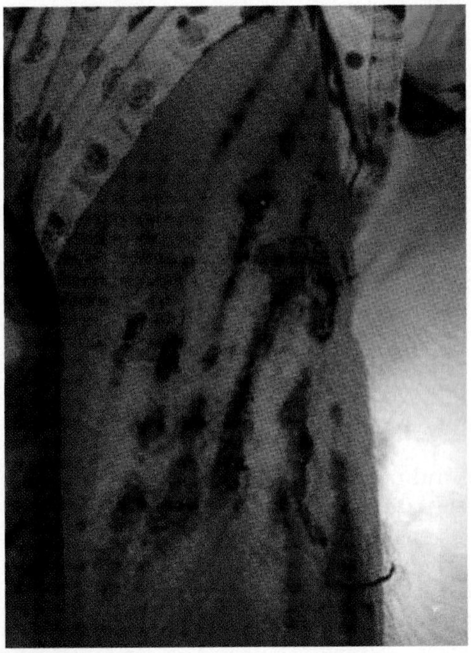

FIGURE 187-1 Skin anatomy. The layers of skin-epidermis, dermis, and connective tissue all play important roles in wound healing. The dermis is most important and thickest, but it thins with age or steroid use. Note the tearing appearance of the skin of this elderly patient, who fell on an escalator.

BOX 187-2

Host Factors

- Age
- Steroids
- Disease
- Tetanus status
- Latex allergy

Clinical Presentation

■ WOUND EVALUATION

A wound represents the entry point of an injurious force on the body. As such, a careful evaluation of the patient as a whole is critical. How was the patient injured? What was the implement or mechanism (shear, abrasion, compression)? What was the patient's functional level before and after injury? What characteristics of the patient (host) and the wound itself portend risk or advantage? A major pitfall of wound management is fixation on the wound, without sufficient attention to the functional person harboring it.

The overall risk of infection and the likelihood of complications can be predicted by considering host and wound factors. For example, a 4-cm linear laceration on the arm of a healthy 18-year-old patient has a different prognosis than the same wound on the shin of a 73-year-old diabetic patient with peripheral vascular disease.

■ Host Factors

With an infinite variety of medical conditions and health status, each patient has his or her own unique environment for wound healing (Box 187-2). Hosts also change over time, with thinning of the dermis, varying degrees of vascular compromise, increased likelihood of fractures, and medication use.

BOX 187-3

Wound Factors

- Location
- Mechanism
- Degree and type of contamination
- Proximity to underlying structures
- Timing of closure
- Antibiotics

■ Wound Factors

In terms of wound factors, patients have often attended to the injury themselves with therapies ranging from placing the cut finger in the mouth to using comprehensive irrigation and pressure dressings. The major wound factors are location, including proximity to other structures, contamination, and timing to presentation (Box 187-3).

Differential Diagnosis

■ FOREIGN BODIES

Various mechanisms carry varying possibilities of foreign body introduction into wounds. Common situations include shattered glass in motor vehicle accidents, vegetative material in wounds during outdoor pursuits, and puncture wounds through footwear. Foreign bodies increase infection risk and may prevent healing. For a complete discussion of foreign body evaluation and management, see Chapter 188.

■ UNDERLYING STRUCTURE INJURY

If sufficiently breached, skin can fail in its protective role and can allow underlying tendon, nerves, muscle, bone, or other structures to be injured. A diligent assessment of the functional aspects surrounding a wound site can be overlooked, yet it remains crucial to good emergency care.

Assess tendon function throughout a range of motion. It may help to ask the patient to estimate the position of a body part at the time of injury, especially in hand injuries. Tendons may be partially lacerated and range of motion may remain intact, thus potentially misleading the practitioner. Patients often complain of pain or decreased range of motion with movement of a partially injured tendon, and this finding should raise suspicion.

Nerves can be injured by the wounding mechanism itself or by iatrogenic maneuvers, especially indiscriminate ones. Clamping, blind probing, and injudicious débridement all can worsen the trauma to adjacent nerves. The hands and the face are at greatest risk because nerves run in close proximity to vasculature; zealous attempts to control bleeding vessels can result in damage to adjacent nerves. Injected anesthetics also may injure nerves through pressure necrosis in finite spaces. Examples include injections in the olecranon grooves or foramina in the hard palate of the mouth (Fig. 187-2).

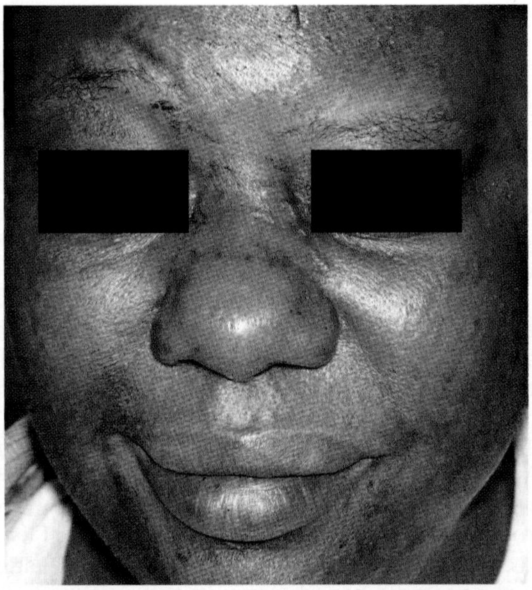

FIGURE 187-2 Underlying structure injury. Missing associated nerve, tendon, vascular, or bony injury is a significant pitfall in wound care. This patient had partial facial nerve palsy from injury, exacerbated slightly by anesthesia, but it resolved almost completely over time.

Muscles are highly vascular tissue and are often involved in deep wounds. Because muscles are dynamic units, subsequent hematomas, scars, or infection can result in dysfunction. Avoid unnecessary débridement, and control bleeding with direct pressure. Muscle can usually be repaired by securing the surrounding structures and thereby placing the cut surfaces of muscle in direct apposition. Repair muscle tissue directly only when the foregoing maneuver is insufficient.

Occasionally, a wound is the first sign of an underlying fracture, either because the skin was injured with the force carried onto the bone or because the broken bone edges tore the skin from inside.

Treatment

■ WOUND PREPARATION

To meet the goals of reducing infection risk, minimizing underlying structure damage, and forming a functional and cosmetically acceptable scar, preparation of the wound can be tantamount to or may surpass closure in importance. The prepared wound has been anesthetized, has been decontaminated of large particles or foreign bodies, has minimized bacterial counts, and has edges amenable to optimal repair.

Sterile Technique

Aseptic and *antiseptic* techniques revolutionized surgery in the latter part of the 19th century. *Aseptic technique* is the prevention of further bacterial contamination into a wound. The simple hand washing advocated by Semmelweis found vehement detractors at the time, yet it remains a famous early instance of commonly accepted aseptic practice today. The spray pump of carbolic acid that soaked both the patient and Lister during procedures resulted in lower infection rates and represents a dramatic example of *antiseptic technique,* which is the prevention of infection by reducing bacterial counts with extrinsic applications.

The use of sterile fields, gloves, cap, and mask and gowns is *de rigueur* in operating room surgery, but the use of each of these maneuvers as aseptic techniques in routine wound closure is no longer as well established. Studies have shown that the use of sterile versus nonsterile boxed gloves in the routine wound may not have a significant effect on infection rate.[2] However, infection is not the only factor to consider in choosing gloves. For example, the gloves packaged in sterile format may be of higher quality and the fit may be better than those of boxed nonsterile models. Avoid powdered gloves because of their association with granuloma formation, and be aware of possible latex allergy.

Anesthesia

In general, anesthesia should precede significant efforts at cleansing, irrigation, exploration, and closure. In spite of long-held dogma, lidocaine with epinephrine can be used in most areas of the body, including most hand wounds and digital blocks.[3] For a complete discussion of local and regional anesthesia, please see Chapter 12.

Wound Cleansing and Irrigation

The goals of wound cleansing and irrigation are to remove gross contaminants and particulate matter, to reduce bacterial counts in the wound, and to avoid impeding the host's responses and natural defenses. In general, ideal wound irrigation requires sufficient pressure and volume while providing drainage and preventing operator exposure. If large particles are present, perform gross decontamination before pressure irrigation. A sink, an intravenous infusion set, or holes made in the plastic top of a saline solution bottle can be used to make a spray of water for removing leaves, dirt, and other large contaminants. At some point, the pressure of the irrigating stream must be sufficient to overcome the adhesive forces of bacteria (≈5 to 12 psi). This pressure can be produced with a 35-mL syringe and a 19-gauge catheter or a commercial device with an integrated splash cup.[4] The volume of irrigant sufficient to decontaminate wounds is unknown. However, because bacteria may be present in all sections of a wound, expose all surfaces of a wound to the irrigating stream.

The composition of irrigating fluid has been debated and occasionally studied. Antiseptics such as povidone kill bacteria in wounds, but they can also kill fibroblasts and harm normal tissue in the process, especially if the antiseptics are not diluted from their typical 10% preparations. Anecdotally, some clinicians reserve diluted povidone irrigation for grossly contaminated or high-risk wounds, and they use saline solution for other wounds, but no good evidence supports this approach.[5] At the other end of the spectrum, studies demonstrated favorable results using irrigation with tap water versus sterile water or saline solution.[6] These investigators cited the ease of use, drainage, and some modest cost savings. Use tap water irrigation for wounds on body parts well suited to it (e.g., the hand), either alone or as an adjunct to subsequent pressure irrigation, depending on the risks associated with the individual wound and host. In summary, the composition of the fluid is much less important than its mechanical action in decontaminating a wound.

Wound Edge Preparation

Hair does not generally need removal. Shaving has been shown to increase the infection rate. Hair that directly and substantially interferes with proper suture placement can be clipped near the wound edge with scissors.

In general, do not débride any more than is absolutely necessary to remove clearly devitalized tissue. The irregular, undulating wound may be superior to the straight linear excised wound because the longer surface area results in better tensile strength across the healing wound, and it maintains the natural contours and marks of the original skin. If débridement is necessary, use high-quality forceps and a number 15 blade scalpel.

WOUND CLOSURE TECHNIQUES

Planning the Repair

The first decision to be made is whether to close a wound primarily. The time to presentation, the degree of contamination, host factors, and wound factors all play a role in deciding the best option. *Primary closure* refers to mechanical apposition of wound edges with subsequent wound healing. *Delayed primary closure* is the same technique but carried out 4 to 5 days after injury.[7] At this point, the host's defenses against infection have been mustered locally, and the risk of subsequent infection with primary closure declines significantly. *Secondary closure (secondary intention)* is the body's filling of gaps between wound edges with granulation tissue and subsequent reepithelialization.

No well-accepted studies have established firm guidelines for timing of closure on different portions of the body. However, clinicians agree that certain

Tips and Tricks

- Always place the patient supine.
- Measure wounds using premeasured parts of your hands.
- Remove as much gross contamination as possible before pressure irrigation.
- Assemble all your equipment before going into the room for the repair.
- Prebuffer and warm your lidocaine, and use the smallest-diameter needle.
- Use longitudinal traction on a wound to see how it aligns, and put together what you *know* goes together first.
- If you place a suture that you do not like, use it (to place another) or lose it.
- Remove sutures at the earliest safe time, especially on the face or in infection-prone areas.
- It may help to ask the patient to estimate the position of a body part at the time of injury, especially in hand injuries.
- Muscle can usually be repaired by securing the surrounding structures; repair muscle tissue directly only when this approach is insufficient.
- In spite of long-held dogma, lidocaine with epinephrine can be used in most areas of the body, including most hand wounds and digital blocks.
- Composition of the irrigating fluid is much less important than its mechanical action in decontamination.
- Ask patients about their preferred sleeping position and whether or not they wear headgear in sport or work because staples can be uncomfortable if direct pressure is applied against them during the wound healing.
- Hair does not generally need removal, and shaving has been shown to increase infection rate.
- Avoid placing deep sutures in a high-risk wound.
- The goal is to achieve a trapezoidal cross-section stitch with a wider base than top.
- Do not use staples on facial lacerations, on fine skin, or in other areas where cosmesis is of particular importance because the closure is less meticulous and tends to leave punctate marks alongside the linear scar.

wounds on the face and head, especially in pediatric patients, have such a low infection risk that they may be closed after protracted times from injury, including up to 1 to 2 days later. However, wounds of the same size on the hand or forearm in adults probably do have a higher infection risk after an increased amount of time from injury.[8]

If the decision is made to close a wound primarily, then various options are available. As in almost all decisions in wound management, more than one answer may be correct, but one answer is often best. The methods available for closure include sutures, staples, tissue adhesives, and wound tapes or strips.

Table 187-1 SUTURE CHOICES

Factor	Suture Choice
Tissue edema	Polybutester (PBE)
Keloid former	Polypropylene (PP or PBE)
Pediatric face	Polypropylene (PP) or nylon; consider polyglactin 910

Suture Repair

Sutures offer the most detailed and meticulous closure option, arguably the greatest tensile strength across the wound, and the best choice in characteristics such as the amount of time they remain present in the body. However, sutures can be time consuming to place, they require the discomfort of anesthesia, and they may need removal later. Further, a suture is a foreign body with attendant infection and inflammation risk. In particular, avoid placing deep sutures in a high-risk wound. Monofilament, braided, absorbable, and nonabsorbable sutures also connote varying infection risk as well as raise other considerations.

Select sutures for a wound based on size, absorbability, tissue reactivity, infection risk, and ease of use. In general, nonabsorbable and monofilament sutures are easiest to use and have the least tissue reactivity and infection risk. They are best for percutaneous closures. Traditionally, absorbable sutures are used for subcutaneous closures. However, some cutaneous closures can be done with absorbable sutures, thus obviating the need for suture removal.[9,10]

Choosing Suture

Table 187-1 gives possible suture choices.

Placing Sutures

At least four basic suture patterns should be at the command of EPs: simple interrupted suture, corner stitch, and two mattress suture techniques. Master the simple interrupted pattern first, then move to the others and then the more advanced subcuticular and plastic techniques as required.

Simple Interrupted Suture

Although it is simple in name, proper placement of an interrupted suture requires fastidious practice. Effecting proper wound apposition with regard to the height of each plane of skin and eversion of the closed product will result in more exact healing and a flatter scar. The angle of entry is often suggested at 90 degrees; however, the goal is to achieve a trapezoidal cross-section stitch with a wider base than top. As such, the angle of entry can exceed 90 degrees.

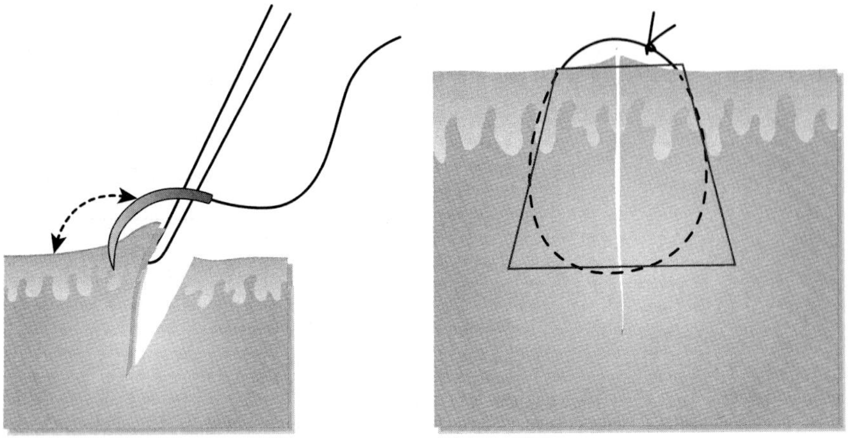

A B

FIGURE 187-3 **A** and **B,** Simple interrupted suture. This is easy to do, harder to master. Enter the skin pointing away from the wound edge and exit the skin pointing toward it, resulting in a trapezoidal cross section and slightly everted skin edges.

Simply, the needle should enter the skin pointing away from the wound edge and should exit the skin on the opposite side of the wound, pointed toward the wound edge (Fig. 187-3).

Running Suture

The tenets of eversion and aligning skin planes are the same if the suture is continued in running fashion. After starting at one end with a simple interrupted pattern, continue with the needle end of suture to run along its length. The suture is finished by tying the needle end of suture to the last-placed loop.

Deep Sutures

Subcutaneous or deep sutures are useful to eradicate a large dead space that could accumulate hematoma and to give structural support to the wound and skin. By drawing the skin edges closer together, these sutures also reduce tension needed to close the wound percutaneously or may allow tissue adhesive closure of the skin (Fig. 187-4).

Corner Stitch

Consider a corner suture when a Y- or V-shaped incision is encountered. Assess the shape of the wound for the most advantageous flap to secure into an apex. The corner suture encompasses both percutaneous and subcutaneous portions, but as the single first stitch it can achieve excellent overall wound alignment, thus facilitating subsequent interrupted sutures to finish the wound (Fig. 187-5).

Mattress Sutures

Both horizontal and vertical mattress sutures have, as a single benefit, better wound edge eversion than other sutures. The horizontal mattress pattern has the additional benefit of some added speed by cover-

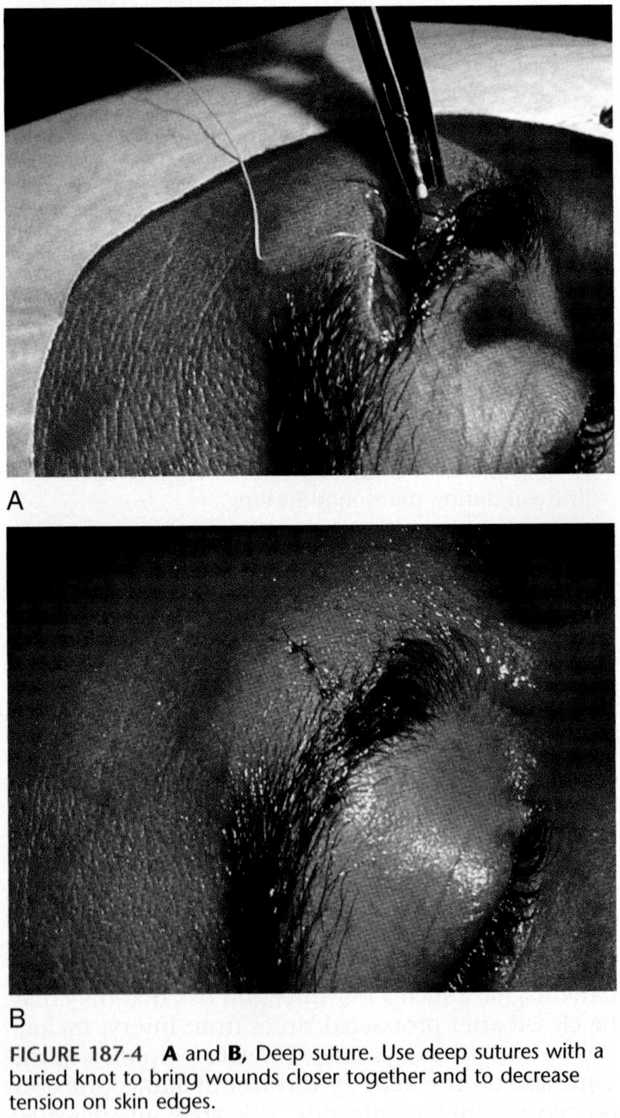

A

B

FIGURE 187-4 **A** and **B,** Deep suture. Use deep sutures with a buried knot to bring wounds closer together and to decrease tension on skin edges.

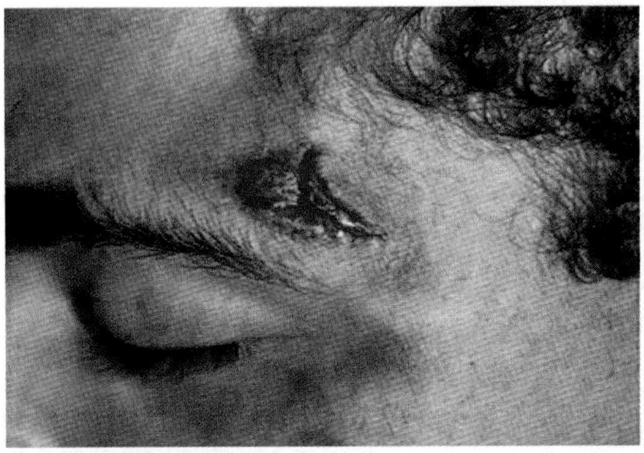

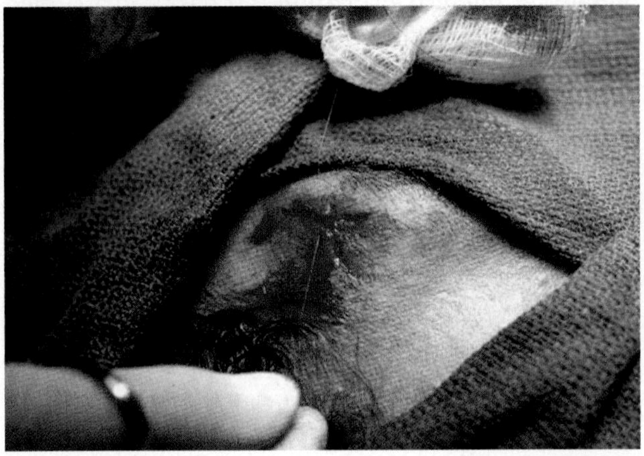

FIGURE 187-5 **A** and **B**, Corner suture. Use this stitch to secure a triangular flap into an apex, allowing rapid reapproximation of wound architecture.

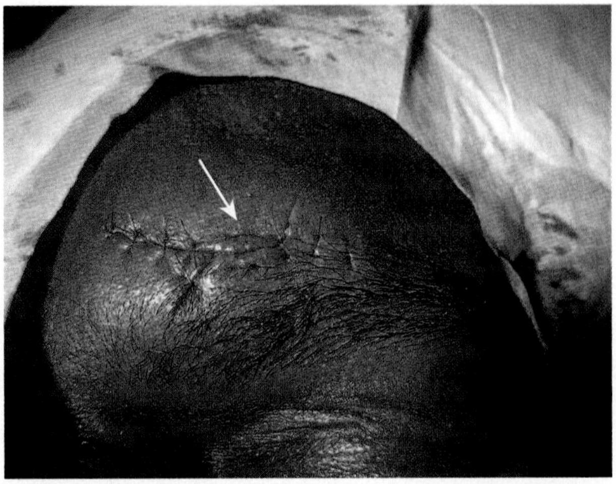

FIGURE 187-6 Mattress sutures. When wound sections are difficult to evert properly, consider a mattress suture. A single horizortal mattress suture (*arrow*) corrected a depressed area of the laceration.

ing more linear wound length with each knot tie. However, it does result in more suture material pressure on the epidermis, and this can have cosmetic effects. Horizontal mattress sutures may be useful to evert a problematic section of wound that has a tendency to roll inward (Fig. 187-6). It may then either be replaced with interrupted sutures holding it in place or left as is with timely suture removal. Similarly, an isolated vertical mattress suture may be useful to effect better skin eversion.

Running Subcuticular Sutures

Subcuticular sutures are more difficult to master. They are useful in that the entire suture remains under the skin surface and typically does not need to be removed because absorbable sutures are used. However, many wounds that were previously closed with subcuticular running suture and were of low tension and of some cosmetic importance are now amenable to tissue adhesive closure.

Staples

Staples can be used in many places where sutures would also be appropriate. Staples also have the benefits of speed and ease in placement and of removal. Staples may offer somewhat less meticulous closure and do have a tendency to leave punctate marks alongside the linear scar. For this reason, do not use them on facial lacerations, on fine skin, or in other areas where cosmesis is of particular importance. Although staples are frequently used to close scalp wounds, it is wise to ask patients about their preferred sleeping position and whether or not they wear headgear in sport or work because staples can be uncomfortable if direct pressure is applied against them during wound healing. Staples are most often used to close wounds on the proximal extremities.

Tissue Adhesives

Tissue adhesives have been approved for use in the United States since 1998 (Box 187-4). Tissue adhesives were originally thought to replace suture closure in 25% to 32% of wounds, but it is unclear how often they are currently employed in lieu of suture closure. The most common use of tissue adhesives is on low-tension, nongaping wounds on the face, particularly in pediatric patients. These adhesives are also useful for small avulsion injuries with

BOX 187-4

Tissue Adhesive Application Tips

- Have two sets of hands involved.
- Beware of eye run-down. Apply an ointment or gauze barrier, and position the patient so run-off follows gravity (i.e., Trendelenburg position for forehead lacerations).
- Hold the wound in place long enough.
- Avoid gluing gloves to the patient.

flaps and occlusion over abrasion injuries as a protective barrier. Various preparations by different manufacturers are in use, and they have slightly different chemical compositions. These adhesives are all similar to cyanoacrylate, commonly known as "Super Glue," although additional modifications to the chemical composition have been made in effort to reduce tissue reactivity, to increase pliability of the finished bond, and make the substance more suitable for use on human skin. Tissue adhesives should not be used in areas of high tension (e.g., across joint surfaces) or to close significantly gaping wounds (Fig. 187-7).

Wound Tapes and Strips

Wound tapes or strips may be an option in wounds in which foreign body placement (i.e., suture) may be disadvantageous, in initial management of wounds that may undergo delayed primary closure, or in wounds with a protracted time to presentation. Many wounds that were previously closed with wound tapes or strips are now amenable to tissue adhesive closure. Examples of wounds and their preferred and alternative closure methods are shown in Table 187-2.

Special Locations and Puncture Wounds

Table 187-3 gives recommendations for special locations and considerations.

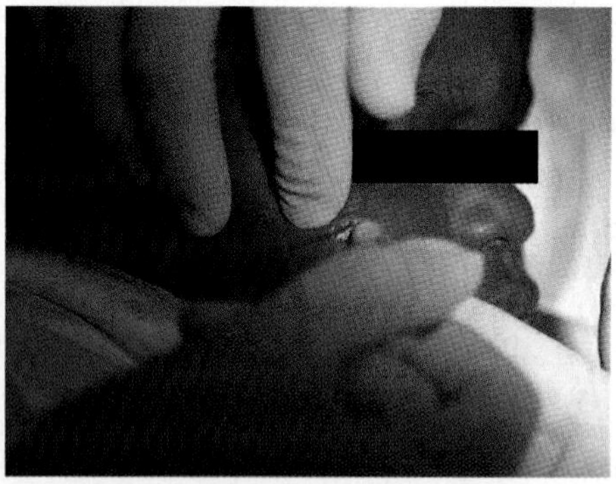

FIGURE 187-7 Tissue adhesive placement. Proper adhesive application has a learning curve. Typically, more than two hands are needed.

Puncture Wounds

By their nature, puncture wounds are different from other lacerations in mechanism, risk, and prognosis. No definitive studies exist to guide evaluation, acute management, or risk stratification in puncture wounds. Despite years of publications, the available data are largely retrospective and observational. What is clear is that plantar puncture wounds, in particular, are commonplace, and many patients do not present to the ED for evaluation. One self-reporting survey indicated that 44% of persons had experienced a plantar puncture wound at some time during their life. However, perhaps only half of those wounded present for medical evaluation.[11] It has been assumed that puncture wounds may have a higher rate of complication or infection than other wounds, but the true incidence is unknown. Wounds that do become infected on the plantar surface of the foot may have very serious types of complications including osteomyelitis, osteochondritis, and septic arthritis. The bones of the foot are in close proximity to the skin, and the mechanism of injury typically includes the weight of the body on the penetrating object with significant force.

Evaluation of plantar wounds includes the same delineation of host and wound factors as mentioned previously. Mechanisms associated with puncture wounds often include the penetration of a sock and shoe by a nail or by objects of varying degrees of contamination.

Many authors believe that the timing of presentation also guides initial evaluation and treatment. Patients who present within 24 hours of injury tend to have lower rates of cellulitis at the time of evaluation, but they may also have greater possibility of useful manipulative intervention. Patients who present after 24 hours may have concerns about infection and may be more likely to need invasive quests for foreign material in the wound.[12] One study indicated that 3% of plantar puncture wounds had a foreign body after initial cleansing without exploration.[13]

Reasonable recommendations in the management of plantar puncture wounds include a consideration for enlargement of the wound and tissue exploration or excision when the puncture wound mechanism was significant. Concerning mechanisms include puncturing of protective footwear in a sock, wounds

Table 187-2 WOUND CLOSURE METHODS

Location	Preferred Closure Method	Alternative Method
Face	Sutures (absorbable or nonabsorbable)	Tissue adhesive
Hand	Sutures (nonabsorbable)	No closure, wound tapes
Intraoral areas	Sutures (absorbable)	
Lower extremities	Staples	Sutures
Trunk	Sutures (nonabsorbable) or staples	
Scalp	Staples or sutures (nonabsorbable)	

Chapter **188**

Soft Tissue Injury

Matthew R. Levine and Jill F. Lehrmann

KEY POINTS

- Retained foreign bodies (FBs) can cause pain, infection, nerve/tendon injury, and other persistent problems.
- Specific injuries, such as those caused by broken glass or surfaces with gravel, are particularly prone to retained FBs.
- Explore wound for FBs after controlling bleeding.
- Plain radiographs are useful in FB evaluation and should be ordered commonly.
- Plain films may miss wood, plastic, and vegetative matter.
- Ultrasound scans and portable fluoroscopic studies may aid in localization and removal of foreign bodies. Computed tomography and magnetic resonance imaging are rarely indicated.
- Neither exploration nor imaging alone can rule out an FB. The two should be used in combination in most instances. No wound is too small or superficial to harbor a FB.
- Careful discharge instructions are crucial and can minimize the morbidity and medicolegal risk associated with retained FBs.
- Direct exploration of wounds, with visualization of tendons through full range of motion, is necessary for proper evaluation of tendon injuries.
- A detailed neurovascular examination is required, to identify possible nerve lacerations.
- Most tendon and nerve lacerations can be repaired on an outpatient basis. Ensuring appropriate and timely follow-up is important.

RETAINED FOREIGN BODY

The most common anatomic sites for wound FBs are the hands and feet. However, any wound, regardless of its size or location, can harbor an FB. For instance, the head is a common site for retained glass in motor vehicle collisions.[1,2,3]

A retained FB can lay harmlessly dormant for a long period and then can react with surrounding tissue. When a tissue reaction occurs, several sequelae are possible. An infection may occur. The patient's body may dissolve, extrude, or encapsulate the FB and form a granuloma. Subsequent granuloma rupture from minor trauma can cause delayed infection. The extent of tissue reactions depends primarily

BOX 188-1

Inert and Reactive Foreign Bodies

Inert Foreign Bodies
Glass
Most metals
Plastic

Reactive Foreign Bodies
Wood
Thorns
Other vegetative matter
Clothing
Skin fragments

BOX 188-2

Scenarios Suggestive of Wound Foreign Bodies

History of having stepped on glass
History of having punched through window
Motor vehicle collision wounds
Wounds on the sole of the foot
Puncture wounds
Head wounds from glass
Objects that fragment while in one's hand
Fall into gravel or soil
Pain at a site of intravenous drug use
Foot laceration while walking in a stream
Wound infection, especially if persistent
Perioral wounds in the presence of broken teeth
Persistent wound pain
Failure to heal

on the chemical composition of the material. Inert material causes less tissue inflammation, whereas reactive material can cause intense tissue reactions (Box 188-1), rarely even allergic reactions. Even when an FB does not cause a tissue reaction, it can have other effects. The FB may cause local compression on neighboring structures such as nerve, tendons, joints, or vessels, thereby causing pain or structural damage. Local migration or, more rarely, distant embolization can also occur.

Clinical Presentation

The classic presentation of a wound FB is the patient who sees or knows that foreign material is present in a wound, such as the patient who presents with a splinter, glass in the sole of the foot that the patient cannot remove, or an obviously soiled wound. Alternatively, it is also common for a patient to present with a wound and not to know that foreign material is present. Some mechanisms are highly suggestive of wound FBs (Box 188-2).[4-7] Neither the presence nor the lack of an FB sensation on the part of the patient can confidently rule in or exclude an FB. In a series of 164 wounds caused by glass, 41% that contained glass caused an FB sensation, with a positive predictive value of 31% and a negative predictive value of 89%.[4]

■ VARIATIONS

Frequently, patients do not know that an FB is present. Their chief complaint is simply that they have a wound. No wound is too small or superficial to harbor an FB. Therefore, the possibility of an FB must be considered for all wounds. Some unique wound FB presentations include shrapnel, fishhooks, bullets and BBs, cactus spines, and marine material (Table 188-1). Some patients may present with the sequelae of a retained FB from the near or distant past, such as a mass, persistent pain, infection, functional impairment from nerve or tendon injury, arthritis, vascular injury, or embolization.

Most wound FBs are wood, glass, and metal. The most threatening FBs are reactive. Wood is especially toxic to soft tissue and virtually always requires removal. FBs causing infection and pain and FBs that are near vital structures such as nerves, tendons, vessels, and joints are also potentially dangerous. Hand FBs tend to migrate locally but rarely embolize, whereas proximal forearm FBs are more likely to embolize.

Diagnostic Testing

The most important aspects of FB diagnosis are wound examination and the judicious use of imaging. The wound should be explored in a bloodless field. This may require tourniquets or lidocaine with epinephrine infiltration if direct pressure is insufficient. Adequate anesthesia is crucial. The wound should be visualized completely and with range of motion of the involved digit. The wound can be probed with an instrument. Sometimes, an FB is detected only by the grating sound of a metal probe against it. Probing the wound with the examiner's finger exposes the examiner to puncture wounds and should not be done. The wound can be palpated through the skin with two hands, one stationary as a "stabilizer" and the other mobile as a "mover." Palpate puncture wounds for exquisite tenderness that may be elicited in the presence of an FB. It is prudent to irrigate before imaging, in an attempt to remove foreign material.

Exploration alone is insufficient to rule out an FB,[4,8,9] even when the entire wound is thought to be visualized. Therefore, imaging should be used liber-

Table 188-1 SPECIAL CIRCUMSTANCES

Type of Foreign Body	Tips and Comments
Fishhooks	Anesthetize the area, advance the tip of the fishhook through the skin, cut the barb, and withdraw the hook.
Splinters	Do not pull long splinters out because they tend to fragment. Instead, excise along the long axis or elliptically.
Needle tips	Removal may require excision of a block of tissue.
Shrapnel	When extensive, ED removal of all shrapnel may not be feasible or indicated. Remove as much as reasonably possible, with a focus on dangerous locations, and refer the patient for further treatment.
Bullets, BBs	These are often left in situ, but objects larger than 4.5 mm in diameter tend to track skin and clothing into wounds, so visualize, irrigate, and leave open when possible. Remove these objects only if they are easily accessible or in the pleura (risk of lead poisoning).
Cactus spines	Use fine-tipped forceps or glue to remove them.
Marine envenomations	Treatment (hot water immersion, vinegar, shaving) depends on the type of spine or nematocyst.
Traumatic tattooing	Sources include pencils and blacktop. Débride with a scrub brush. Management is difficult. Consider referral to dermatology or plastic surgery for dermabrasion or laser treatment.

ally. Selecting proper imaging modalities requires knowledge of the radiographic properties of the material (Box 188-3 and Figs. 188-1 through 188-3). Even when a suspected FB is not radiopaque, plain film radiographs with underpenetrated soft tissue technique should be ordered initially because there may be other useful soft tissue or bony findings and reactions. Furthermore, failure to order radiographs has been associated with unsuccessful legal defense in cases of retained FBs.[10] Ultrasound scanning is particularly useful for nonradiopaque FBs (Fig. 188-4).[6] Low-power portable fluoroscopy, when available, is useful to aid removal of radiopaque FBs. Computed tomography and magnetic resonance imaging are rarely indicated. However, computed tomography may be useful for ocular or periorbital FBs (Table 188-2).[11,12]

PRIORITY ACTIONS

- Maintaining a high index of suspicion for foreign bodies in all wounds and for tendon or nerve injury
- Appropriate use of imaging
- Decision whether or not to attempt removal of foreign body in the ED
- High-pressure irrigation/wound cleansing
- Exploration of wound with visualization of wound base
- Exploration of wound with visualization of tendon through complete range of motion
- Decision whether to consult a specialist in the ED or refer as outpatient
- Appropriate use of antibiotics
- Specialty referrals/consultations for repair of injured structures
- Proper discharge instructions

BOX 188-3

Radiopaque and Nonradiopaque Foreign Bodies

Radiopaque Foreign Bodies

Glass
Metal
Bone
Teeth
Pencil tips/graphite
Gravel

Nonradiopaque Foreign Bodies

Wood (only 15% seen on radiographs)
Most plastic
Thorns
Cactus spines
Vegetative matter

Treatment

■ INTERVENTIONS AND PROCEDURES

After an FB is diagnosed, the next step is to decide whether to attempt removal or to leave the FB in place. Not all FBs require removal. If an FB is deep, small, inert, away from vital structures, and asymptomatic, then attempted removal may be more destructive than helpful (Box 188-4). Irrigation is an important intervention that not only cleans the wound, but also often removes tiny FBs and particulate matter that would otherwise be difficult to localize.

Exploration is best done while the EP is seated comfortably under conditions with optimal anesthesia, hemostasis, lighting (even headlamps), and

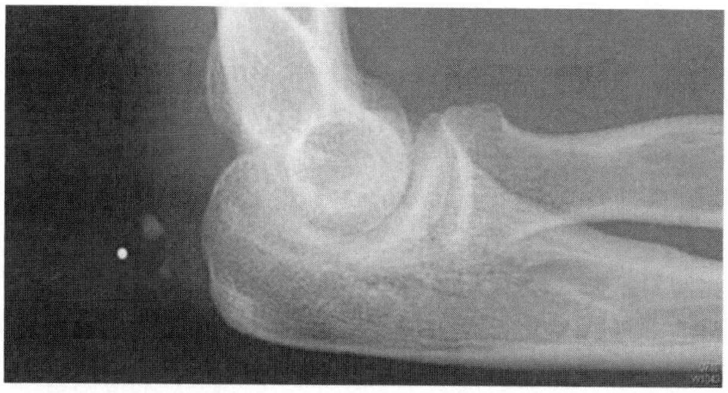

FIGURE 188-1 This patient had a laceration over the olecranon after a motor vehicle collision (the BB is a skin marker). Two retained glass fragments are present.

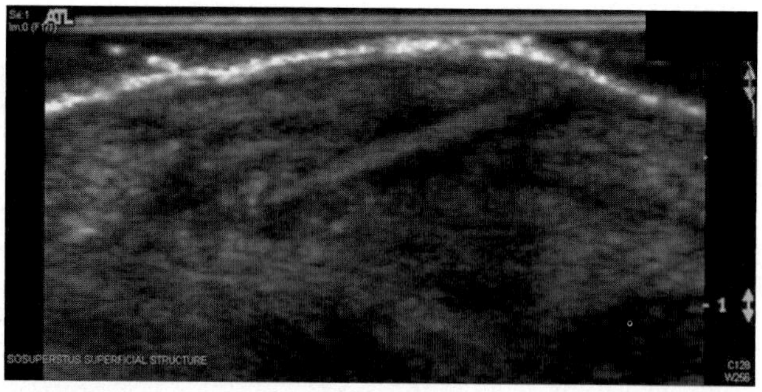

FIGURE 188-4 Ultrasound scan showing a wood foreign body with characteristic acoustic shadowing deep to the foreign body.

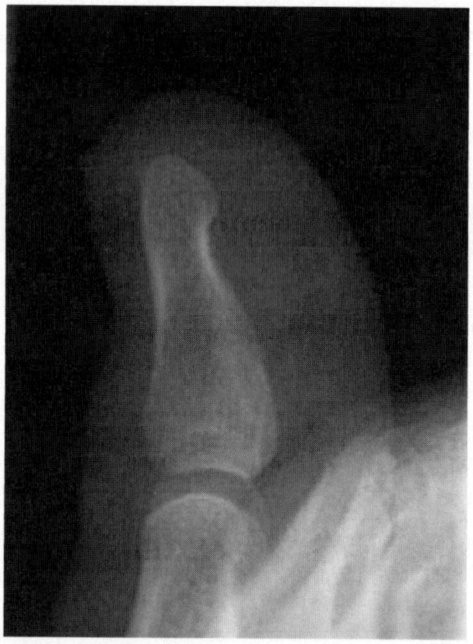

FIGURE 188-2 This patient sustained a laceration over the dorsum of her great toe when she moved a sharp-edged mirror while she was barefoot. She said the glass did not break. A pebble was recovered on exploration.

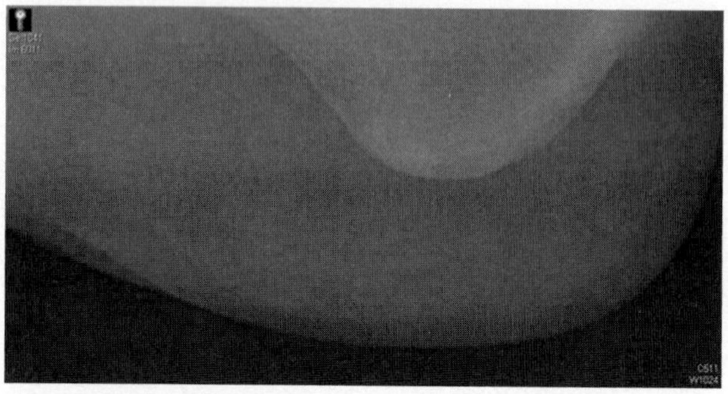

FIGURE 188-3 This patient had stepped on broken glass the previous night and had picked some glass out of the wound. She still felt as though there was a piece inside and had sharp pain when she bore weight on her foot. The fragment was unable to be recovered by exploration. Subsequent high-pressure irrigation, however, removed the foreign body and was documented on a repeat radiograph.

Tips and Tricks

Hemostasis

- Direct pressure
- Tourniquets
- Lidocaine with epinephrine when safe

Anesthesia

- Nerve blocks for difficult locations (sole of foot)

Irrigation

- High pressure: 30-mL syringe with 18-gauge angiocatheter generates 6 to 8 psi

Exploration

- Good lighting
- Equipment: loupes, fine-tipped forceps help
- Possible need to extend incision
- Incision perpendicular to long axis of long, thin foreign bodies (splinters, needles) to localize
- Bloodless field and adequate anesthesia required
- Listening for grating sounds of foreign body against probe
- Ultrasound or fluoroscopic guidance helpful
- Time limit needed

equipment. Fine-tipped forceps, retractors, special pick-ups, and magnifying loupes are particularly helpful. Many explorations require extending the incision for better exposure. Listen during probing for the grating sound of the FB against the instrument. Blind grasping is destructive to tissue and should be avoided. Consider using portable fluoroscopy or ultrasound scanning to facilitate removal, if these options are readily available. A time limit for the procedure should be set in advance because it is easy to become involved and determined to recover an FB that may be too difficult to remove in the ED setting. The patient should be aware of this time limit.

Wounds that are contaminated or may still contain FBs should be left open or packed. Antibiotics should probably be prescribed for these patients. Be sure to

Table 188-2 FEATURES OF AVAILABLE IMAGING TECHNIQUES

Imaging Modality	Positive Features	Negative Features
Radiography	Inexpensive Easy to obtain and read 99% sensitive for radiopaque objects >2 mm*	Misses nonradiopaque foreign bodies Sensitivity falls for objects <2 mm Two-dimensional still picture may not aid in removal
Ultrasound	Detects all materials[†] Live bedside images may aid removal Consider for wood, plastic No radiation exposure	Operator dependent Gel complicates use during foreign body removal Difficult in large open wounds, web spaces False-positive results: sesamoids, calcification False-negative results: gas, hematoma, near bone or scar
Portable fluoroscopy	Low radiation exposure Can aid in real-time removal For difficult removal of radiopaque foreign bodies	Misses nonradiopaque foreign bodies
Computed tomography	Good for periorbital, intraocular, intracranial foreign bodies May help in bony areas High resolution may enhance detection	Costly Impractical More radiation exposure
Magnetic resonance imaging	May help for some difficult plastic foreign bodies High resolution may enhance detection No radiation exposure	Costly Impractical Potential harm if metal foreign body

*Courter BJ: Radiographic screening for glass foreign bodies: What does a "negative" foreign body series really mean? Ann Emerg Med 1990;19: 997-1000.
[†]Horton LK, Jacobson JA, Powell A, et al: Sonography and radiography of soft-tissue foreign bodies. AJR Am J Roentgenol 2001;176:1155-1159.

BOX 188-4

Indications for Foreign Body Removal

- Significant pain
- Functional impairment/restriction of motion
- Reactive material: wood, thorn, other vegetative material, clothing
- Cause of infection
- Cause of psychological distress
- Contamination: tooth, soil
- Toxicity: venomous spines, lead poisoning from bullets
- Allergic reaction
- Impingement of nerve, tendon, vessel
- Intra-articular or periarticular location
- Intravascular location
- Location near fractured bone
- High potential to migrate toward anatomic structures or to embolize
- Cosmetic concerns: tattooing, masses

From Lammers RL, Magill T: Detection and management of foreign bodies in soft tissue. Emerg Med Clin North Am 1992;10:767-781.

pad or splint areas with retained FBs before patients are discharged. If all FBs have been removed and the wound has been thoroughly cleansed, closure may be appropriate. An algorithm for the approach to FBs is shown in Figure 188-5.

Disposition

If all FBs have been removed and the wound has been adequately cleaned, the patient is unlikely to require further referral. If concern still exists about a retained FB, the area should be padded or splinted, antibiotics should be prescribed, and the patient will require consultation or referral to a surgical specialty such as hand, orthopedic, plastic, or general surgery. This referral can almost always take place on an outpatient basis, unless severe infection or important structural damage is present.

TENDON AND NERVE LACERATIONS

Scope

Lacerations are one of the most common chief complaints of patients presenting to the ED. It is estimated that patients with a total of 6,400,000 open wounds presented to EDs in the United States in 2004, thereby making open wounds anywhere on the body the third leading primary diagnosis group. Approximately one third of all open wounds are located on the upper extremity (specifically the fingers, hand, or wrist).[13] An improperly functioning or insensate digit resulting from tendon or nerve injury in the fingers or arm can lead to markedly impaired function in fine motor control and significant subsequent morbidity. Wound claims including

Documentation

FOREIGN BODY

History	Detailed mechanism, timing, type of material, whether object broke on impact or was already broken, whether the wound was soiled, whether anything was pulled out of the wound, FB sensation, paresthesia, weakness, tetanus immunization status, medical conditions that may impair healing or compromise immune function, intravenous drug use, persistent pain/infection/drainage
Physical examination	Neurovascular, tendons, wound size and depth, tenderness, visible contaminants, tattooing, discoloration, infection, masses, range of motion
Studies	Document radiographic results before and after FB removal
Medical decision making	Reasons to pursue or not pursue FB work-up, factors to attempt FB removal or leave in place and refer/consult
Procedures	Document whether the entire extent of the wound base was visualized in a bloodless field with adequate anesthesia
Patient instructions	Document discussion with patient regarding possibility of retained FB, warning signs, what to do, when to return

FB, foreign body.

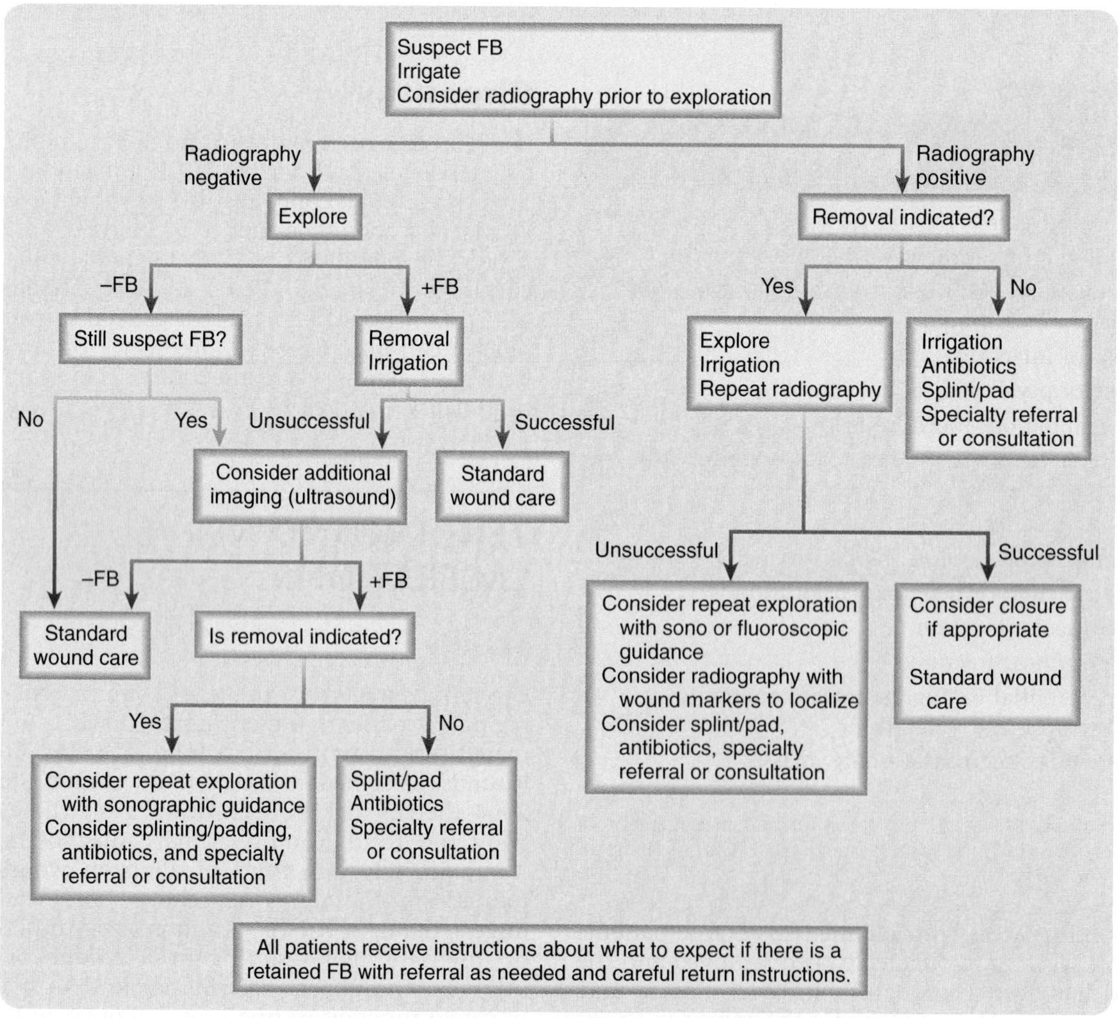
Suspect FB
Irrigate
Consider radiography prior to exploration
Radiography negative
Radiography positive
Explore
Removal indicated?
–FB
+FB
Yes
No
Still suspect FB?
Removal
Irrigation
Explore
Irrigation
Repeat radiography
Irrigation
Antibiotics
Splint/pad
Specialty referral or consultation
No
Yes
Unsuccessful
Successful
Consider additional imaging (ultrasound)
Standard wound care
Unsuccessful
Successful
–FB
+FB
Standard wound care
Is removal indicated?
Consider repeat exploration with sono or fluoroscopic guidance
Consider radiography with wound markers to localize
Consider splint/pad, antibiotics, specialty referral or consultation
Consider closure if appropriate
Standard wound care
Yes
No
Consider repeat exploration with sonographic guidance
Consider splinting/padding, antibiotics, and specialty referral or consultation
Splint/pad
Antibiotics
Specialty referral or consultation
All patients receive instructions about what to expect if there is a retained FB with referral as needed and careful return instructions.

FIGURE 188-5 Approach to detecting wound foreign bodies (FB).

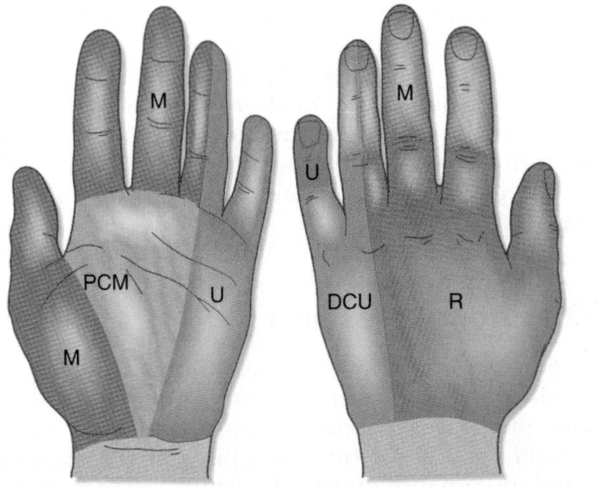
M
M
U
PCM
U
DCU
R
M

FIGURE 188-6 Cutaneous sensory innervation of the hand. DCU, dorsal cutaneous branch of ulnar nerve; M, median; PCM, palmar cutaneous branch of median nerve; R, radial; U, ulnar. (Redrawn from Lyn E, Antosia RE: Hand. In Rosen's Emergency Medicine, 6th ed. Philadelphia, Mosby, 2006, pp 576-621.)

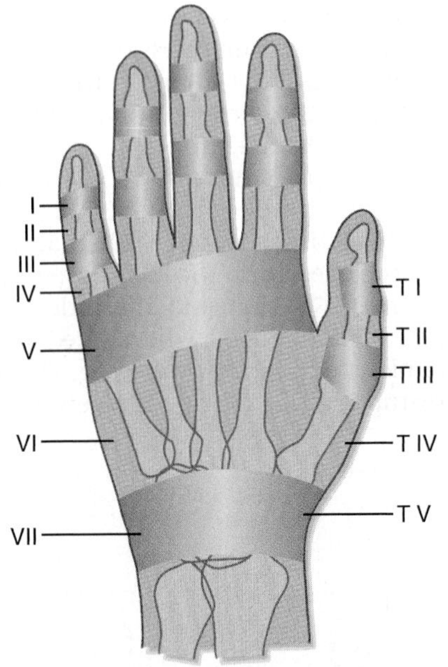
I
II
III
IV
V
VI
VII
T I
T II
T III
T IV
T V

FIGURE 188-7 Zone classification for extensor tendon injuries. (Redrawn from Lyn E, Antosia RE: Hand. In Rosen's Emergency Medicine, 6th ed. Philadelphia, Mosby, 2006, pp 576-621.)

missed tendon and nerve lacerations, particularly of the hand, are a leading cause of litigation.[2] Although lacerations about the foot and ankle are also relatively common, given the prevalence and importance of hand injuries, this chapter primarily focuses on tendon and nerve lacerations of the hand.

Pathophysiology

The hand is one the most multifaceted and complex musculoskeletal systems in the body. The precision and fine motor functions of the hand are the direct result of its intricate structure. The frequency and importance of hand injuries necessitate that EPs have a thorough understanding of the anatomic and functional complexity of the hand.

The nerve supply to the hand is provided by the radial, ulnar, and median nerves. The radial nerve is purely sensory in the hand (motor function of the radial nerve includes wrist extension). The median and ulnar nerves provide the entire motor function of the hand and some sensory function as well (Fig. 188-6). Each digit has two neurovascular bundles located near the palmar aspect of the finger, one on the radial side and the other on the ulnar side.

The extensor tendons are located on the dorsal surface of the forearm, wrist, and hand. Nine extensor tendons pass under the extensor retinaculum. The extensor tendons then join to become the extensor expansion and then separate into six fibro-osseous compartments. In each digit, the extensor expansion then divides into a central slip attaching to the middle phalanx and two lateral bands joining with the tendons of the lumbricals and then continuing on to attach to the base of each distal phalanx. See Figure 188-7 for extensor tendon zone classification.

The flexor tendons are located on the volar side of the forearm, wrist, and hand. A single tendon (the flexor pollicis longus) inserts on the distal phalanx of the thumb, and two flexor tendons go to each of the remainder digits. Each digit has a superficial flexor tendon that inserts at the base of the middle phalanx and a deep flexor tendon that inserts at the base of the distal phalanx.

The superficial location of the tendons and nerves of the hand and the lack of overlying subcutaneous tissue predispose these structures to injury. Injuries to the tendons have been grouped into anatomic zones for easy understanding and classification. The most widely accepted classification system is that of Verdan. This system uses eight zones, from zone I at the distal interphalangeal joint level to zone VIII at the distal forearm level. This system has been modified to five zones for the flexor tendons (Fig. 188-8).[14] Although Verdan's system is no longer used to determine treatment options, knowledge of the zones is useful for prognosis.

Clinical Presentation

Any patient with a laceration about the hand or wrist may have sustained a tendon or nerve laceration no matter how superficial the wound may appear. In a study of 226 patients with upper extremity lacerations that were less than 2 cm in length, 59% were found to have at least one deep structure injury.[15] Depending on the degree of injury, the patient may have no obvious injury other than a laceration through the skin. Limited or painful movement, especially if it is more severe than would be expected with the laceration, suggests partial tendon involvement.

Patients with nerve lacerations typically present with the complaint of numbness or tingling distal to the laceration. In cases of injury to the radial, ulnar, or median nerves, the corresponding motor distribution is affected. Overall, unless a motor deficit is noted the clinical presentation of a nerve injury may easily be missed.

The normal resting position of the hand in which the fingers are flexed, with the little finger having the greatest degree of flexion and the index finger the least degree of flexion, may be altered in patients with a complete tendon laceration (Fig. 188-9). Flexor tendon disruption is indicated when the injured finger lies in complete extension while the others are in slight flexion. When the patient has an extensor tendon injury, the affected digit is held in full flexion while the others are held in slight extension or the normal position of function. Partial lacerations may not be evident based on the position of the finger, and a further, more detailed examination is needed.

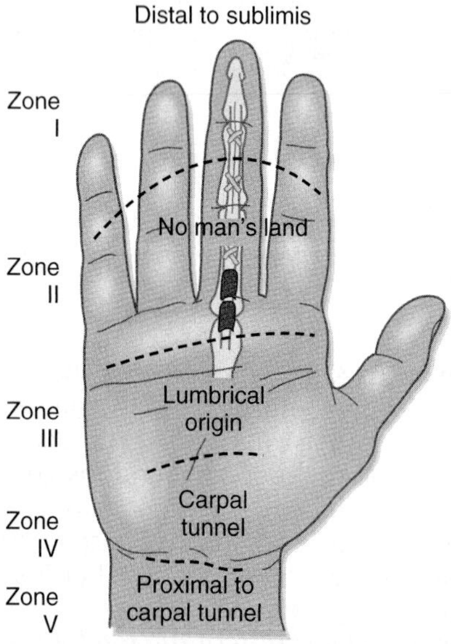
Distal to sublimis
Zone I
No man's land
Zone II
Lumbrical origin
Zone III
Carpal tunnel
Zone IV
Proximal to carpal tunnel
Zone V

FIGURE 188-8 Zones of classification for flexor tendon injuries. (From Canale ST [ed]: Campbell's Operative Orthopaedics, 10th ed. Philadelphia, Elsevier Mosby, 2003.)

Diagnostic Testing

The most important aspects of the diagnosis of tendon or nerve laceration are a thorough history and physical examination. Basic historical details should include the time of injury and the patient's hand dominance, medical history, tetanus status, allergies, previous hand injuries, and occupation and hobbies (musician or anyone requiring fine motor control). The mechanism of injury and the position of the hand when injured are both very important. Patients should be asked about loss of motion, weakness, pain, and any numbness or tingling.

Examine the hand beginning with an overall assessment of the position of the hand and fingers. Note pallor, gross deformity, or digits lying in abnormal positions compared with others or compared with the other hand. Next, assess the sensation and motor strength of the hand to detect nerve injury. As stated previously, the radial, ulnar, and median nerves provide sensation to the hand. Test for sensation of the median nerve at the palmar surface of the little finger, and test the radial nerve at the dorsal surface of the web space between the thumb and index finger.

Various stimuli can be used to test the sensory function of the hand. Gross touch with a blunt object

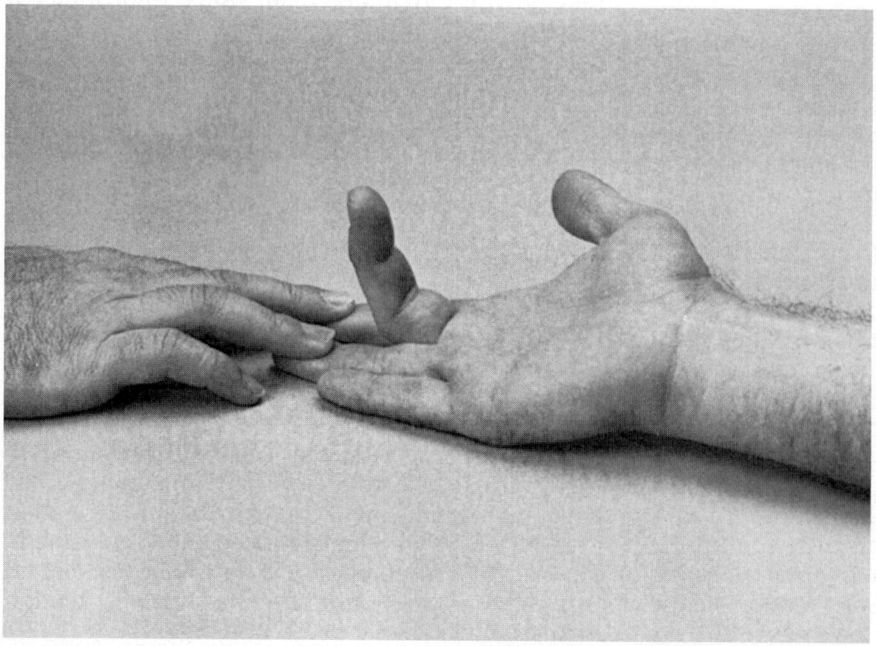

FIGURE 188-9 Examination to assess the function of the flexor digitorum superficialis. (From Lyn E, Antosia RE: Hand. In Rosen's Emergency Medicine, 6th ed. Philadelphia, Mosby, 2006, pp 576-621.)

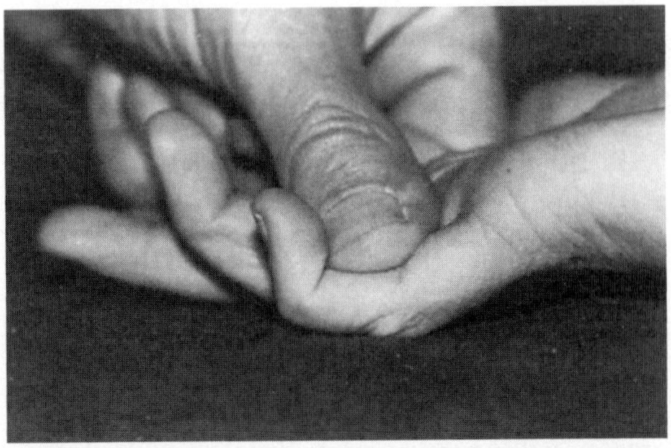

FIGURE 188-10 To test for an intact profundus tendon, the examiner maintains the digit in extension while the patient attempts to flex the terminal phalanx. (From Lyn E, Antosia RE: Hand. In Rosen's Emergency Medicine, 6th ed. Philadelphia, Mosby, 2006, pp 576-621.)

is the least specific. It can be useful for rapid screening to test for nerve injury, especially compared with the other hand. A more accurate method for assessing nerve function is two-point discrimination. A paper clip can be used. A patient with a normally innervated fingertip should be able to distinguish two simultaneously delivered stimuli 6 mm or more apart from each other. Most patients can detect a difference down to 3 mm. When identification of separate stimuli is not reported by the patient at 8 mm or more, the examination is clearly abnormal.

Objective documentation of digital nerve injuries is not always possible at the time of injury. The patient's pain and anxiety, as well as factors such as the presence of hand calluses, can interfere with two-point discrimination. Even though stimulus testing is inconsistent and may not clearly document nerve injury, any subjective "numbness" reported by the patient must be taken seriously, and consultation with a hand specialist should be considered. Under these circumstances, it is common to close the skin wound and refer the patient for evaluation within a few days of the initial injury.

A systematic primary and secondary examination of the hand and wrist includes assessment of active and passive range of motion of the wrists and digits and dynamic stability testing. To check specifically for extensor tendon injuries, have the patient actively extend each finger and then have the patient extend each finger against resistance. In evaluating the flexor tendons, the superficialis and profundus tendons should be tested independently, with the patient actively flexing individual proximal and distal interphalangeal joints (Fig. 188-10). Be sure to check tendon motion against resistance, because patients with partial tendon lacerations may have normal range of motion.

The next step is exploration of the wound, best done with the EP seated comfortably with optimal anesthesia, hemostasis, lighting, and equipment. Adequate anesthesia is crucial. Failure to provide adequate exposure of deeper wound structures because of the patient's discomfort often leads to missed injuries. The wound should be explored in a bloodless field. This may require tourniquets if direct pressure is insufficient to achieve hemostasis. The wound should be visualized completely and with full range of motion of the involved digit.

Additional studies or imaging techniques are indicated to evaluate for FBs, fractures, and avulsions, they are not useful in evaluating tendon or nerve lacerations. Ultrasonography may be a viable diagnostic tool in evaluating tendon injuries, although at this time it has not been studied in the ED.[16]

BOX 188-5

Indications for Immediate Consultation in the ED for Nerve or Tendon Laceration

Multiple or extensive lacerations
Inability to close wound
Contamination: tooth, soil
Joint involvement

Treatment

All motor branches of the ulnar and median nerve should be repaired. Both consultation in the ED or referral the following day after discussing with the referring physician are appropriate (Box 188-5). Digital nerve injuries proximal to the distal interphalangeal crease on the radial aspect of the index finger and middle fingers, the ulnar side of the little finger, and both sides of the thumb should be repaired. Timing of repair of simple, clean nerve injuries is somewhat controversial; some data show better results with repair in 6 to 12 hours, whereas other data show acceptable results with delayed repair.[17] Satisfactory return of function can occur after nerve repair or graft perforned within 3 months of injury.[18] In a study of 813 patients, 83 patients with nerve injury were treated other than by primary repair or elective delayed repair as a result of missed or uncertain diagnosis in the ED.[19] Any patient with a suspected nerve injury should be referred to a specialist for evaluation and possible repair.

Patients with tendon lacerations require early referral to a surgeon. Most surgeons recommend repairing complete lacerations primarily within 12 to 24 hours after the injury. The results of primary, delayed primary (<10 days), or early secondary (2 to 4 weeks) repair show little difference in outcomes.[20] In the past, knowledge of the anatomic zones guided the treatment of tendon lacerations. Overall, the zones of Verdan are useful to aid in prognosis, but they do not necessarily guide treatment (Tables 188-3 and 188-4).

Table 188-3 VERDAN'S EXTENSOR TENDON ZONES

Zone	Location
Zone I	Distal interphalangeal joint
Zone II	Between distal interphalangeal and proximal interphalangeal joints
Zone III	Proximal interphalangeal joint
Zone IV	Between proximal interphalangeal and metacarpophalangeal joints
Zone V	Metacarpophalangeal joints
Zone VI	Hand between metacarpophalangeal and wrist joints
Zone VII	Wrist joint
Zone VIII	Dorsal forearm

Table 188-4 VERDAN'S FLEXOR TENDON ZONES

Zone	Location
Zone I	Distal interphalangeal joint
Zone II	Proximal interphalangeal to metacarpophalangeal joints
Zone III	Lumbrical region
Zone IV	Wrist joint/carpal tunnel
Zone V	Proximal to carpal tunnel

Partial tendon laceration repair is still controversial, although most hand surgeons now repair only lacerations that involve more than 50% of the tendon surface. Whether the laceration is full or partial, primary coverage of the injured tendon by skin suturing after wound irrigation protects the tendon and retards infection, but it should be undertaken only after consultation with the referring physician who will perform the definitive repair.

Extensor tendon injuries are underestimated by EPs. Because of the superficial location and thin overlying subcutaneous tissue, these tendons are often injured. Their superficial location makes repair easier; in the past these injuries have been repaired by EPs, although it is generally best to coordinate with a surgeon willing to provide repair and follow-up. Zones VII and VIII are associated with significant retraction of tendons, and given the proximity of many tendons, multiple tendons may be injured. Therefore, injuries to tendons in these zones are more difficult to repair and may have worse outcomes.

BOX 188-6

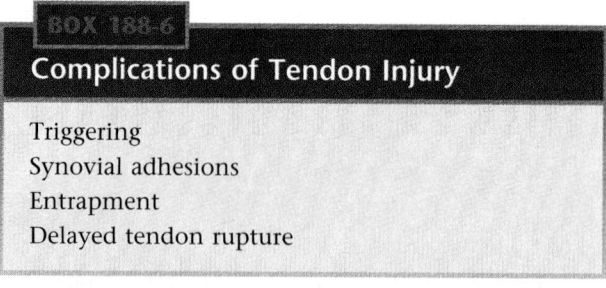

Complications of Tendon Injury

Triggering
Synovial adhesions
Entrapment
Delayed tendon rupture

Flexor tendon injuries are more difficult to repair. These injuries are more complicated because both superficial and deep tendons are present, and both may be injured (Box 188-6). Injuries in zones II and IV have a much worse prognosis as a result of a propensity to form adhesions within a confined space. Referral to a specialist is the most prudent course of action.

Disposition

Most patients with tendon and nerve lacerations can be safely discharged home from the ED. Educating the patient regarding expectations and the importance of follow-up is of utmost importance. All patients with documented lacerations of a tendon or nerve require evaluation by the appropriate surgeon. This can almost always be done on an outpatient basis, unless the patient has severe infection or important structural damage. The area should be appropriately splinted, antibiotics prescribed if indicated, and timely referral to a surgical specialty such

Documentation

TENDON AND NERVE LACERATIONS

History	Detailed hand dominance, mechanism, timing, whether the wound was soiled, whether anything was pulled out of the wound, paresthesias, weakness, tetanus immunization status, medical conditions that may impair healing or compromise immune function, persistent pain
Physical examination	Position of hand at rest, detailed neurovascular examination including two-point discrimination, ability for active range of motion, wound size and depth, tenderness, visible contaminants, infection
Medical decision making	Document reasons to refer to surgeon as outpatient, discuss case with referral physician
Procedures	Document whether the entire extent of the wound base was visualized in a bloodless field with adequate anesthesia and was tendon visualized through full range of motion
Patient instructions	Document discussion with patient regarding possibility of tendon or nerve injury, when follow-up should occur, when to return

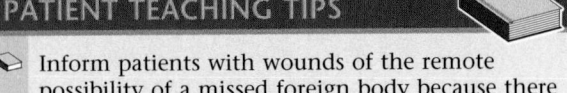

PATIENT TEACHING TIPS

- Inform patients with wounds of the remote possibility of a missed foreign body because there is no way to guarantee truly that all foreign material has been identified and removed.
- After the first couple days, a normal wound should have consistently gradual improvement in pain, swelling, and discoloration.
- Inform patients that a retained foreign body may result in persistent pain, loss or impairment of function, a mass, infection, or injury to a nerve, tendon, vessel, or joint. These complications may develop even months or years later.
- If any of the foregoing situations develop, the patient should know to return to the ED or should have received specialty referral.
- Warn patients who have documented partial tendon lacerations, depending on the degree of laceration and subsequent examination, that the referring physician may or may not repair the injury.
- Inform all patients of the possibility of tendon or nerve lacerations not visualized on examination.
- Warn the patient to return for signs of infection including redness, discharge, pain, and swelling.
- If there is a documented nerve or tendon laceration, ensure that the patient understands the importance of timely follow-up.

as hand, orthopedic, plastic, neurologic, or general surgery should be provided for the patient. A metal protective splint is recommended for patients who are going to return to work. All but very minor hand wounds are best followed up within 48 hours for dressing removal and inspection of the wound for signs of infection.

REFERENCES

1. McCaig LF, Burt CW: National Hospital Ambulatory Medical Care Survey: 2003 Emergency Department Summary. Advance data from vital and health statistics, no. 358. Hyattsville, MD, National Center for Health Statistics, 2005.
2. Karcz A, Korn R, Burke MC, et al: Malpractice claims against emergency physicians in Massachusetts: 1975-1993. Am J Emerg Med 1996;14:341-345.
3. Anderson MA, Newmeyer WL, Kilgore ES: Diagnosis and treatment of retained foreign bodies in the hand. Am J Surg 1982;144:63-67.
4. Steele MT, Tran LV, Watson WA: Retained glass foreign bodies in wounds: Predictive value of wound characteristics, patient perception, and wound exploration. Am J Emerg Med 1998;16:627-630.
5. Montano JB, Steele MT, Watson WA: Foreign body retention in glass-caused wounds. Ann Emerg Med 1992;21: 1360-1363.
6. Lammers RL, Magill T: Detection and management of foreign bodies in soft tissue. Emerg Med Clin North Am 1992;10:767-781.
7. Lammers RL: Soft tissue foreign bodies. Ann Emerg Med 1998;17:1336-1347.
8. Gron P, Andersen K, Vraa A: Detection of glass foreign bodies by radiography. Injury 1986;17:404-406.
9. Avner JR, Baker MD: Lacerations involving glass: The role of routine roentgenograms. Am J Dis Child 1992;146: 600-602.
10. Kaiser CW, Slowick T, Spurling KP, et al: Retained foreign bodies. J Trauma 1997;43:107-111.
11. Courter BJ: Radiographic screening for glass foreign bodies: What does a "negative" foreign body series really mean? Ann Emerg Med 1990;19:997-1000.
12. Horton LK, Jacobson JA, Powell A, et al: Sonography and radiography of soft-tissue foreign bodies. AJR Am J Roentgenol 2001;176:1155-1159.
13. McCraig LF, Burt CW: National Hospital Ambulatory Medical Care Survey: 2004 Emergency Department Summary. Advance data from vital and health statistics, no. 372. Hyattsville, MD, National Center for Health Statistics, 2006.
14. Steinberg DR: Flexor tendon lacerations in the hand. Univ Pa Orthop J 1997;10:5-11.
15. Tuncali D, Yavuz N, Terzioglu A, Aslan G: The rate of upper-extremity deep-structure injuries through small penetrating lacerations. Ann Plast Surg 2005;55:146-148.
16. Lee DH, Robbin ML, Galliott R, Graveman VA: Ultrasound evaluation of flexor tendon lacerations. J Hand Surg [Am] 2000;25:236-241.
17. Muller H, Grubel G: Long term results of peripheral nerve sutures: A comparison of micro-macrosurgical technique. Adv Neurosurg 1981;9:381-387.
18. Kotwal PP, Gupta V: Neglected tendon and nerve injuries of the hand. Clin Orthop Relat Res 2005;43:66-71.
19. McAllister RM, Gilbert SE, Calder JS, Smith PJ: The epidemiology and management of upper limb peripheral nerve injuries in modern practice. J Hand Surg [Br] 1996;21: 4-13.
20. Stone JF, Davidson JS: The role of antibiotics and timing of repair in flexor tendon injuries of the hand. Ann Plast Surg 1998;40:7-13.
21. Guly HR: Missed tendon injuries. Arch Emerg Med 1991;8:87-91.
22. Murphy BA: Zone 1 flexor tendon injuries. Hand Clin 2005;2:167-171.
23. Gaul JS Jr: Identifiable costs and tangible benefits resulting from the treatment of acute injuries of the hand. J Hand Surg [Am] 1987;12:966-970.
24. Clavero JA, Golano P, Farinas O, et al: Extensor mechanisms of the fingers: MR imaging and anatomic correlation. Radiographics 2003;23:593-611.
25. Thordarson DB, Shean CJ: Nerve and tendon lacerations about the foot and ankle. J Am Acad Orthop Surg 2005;13: 186-196.

Chapter 189

Thermal Burns

Jeffrey Druck

KEY POINTS

Many patients who initially appear to have a mild airway burn injury still require early intubation because critical edema will develop. Intubate; do not observe.
Large doses of narcotics are usually required to control pain in patients with severe burns.
Patients with severe burns have large fluid requirements, which are best determined initially by standard calculations.
The best measure of adequate fluid replacement is urine output.
Empirical oral antibiotics are not indicated, but topical antibiotics are.

Perspective

Approximately 500,000 patients sustain nonfatal burn injuries in the United States each year.[1] Only 6% of these patients require hospitalization, so most are treated as outpatients.

Serious burns are some of the most challenging critical care cases. Approximately 8% of all burns result in death. Further, care must be optimized because long-term disability can be moderated if initial resuscitation is adequate, infections are minimized, and specialty care by burn experts is promoted.

Structure and Function

■ ANATOMY

Knowing the anatomy of the skin is essential to understanding burn pathophysiology (Fig. 189-1). Burns are classified according to depth of injury (Table 189-1 and Fig. 189-2). First- and second-degree burns are partial-thickness burns and have a better prognosis. Full-thickness burns (third- and fourth-degree) are insensate and require skin grafts (unless <1 cm) or reconstruction as a result of the destruction of the epidermis and dermis. Based on the depth of the burn, the ability to heal can be predicted. Because the dermis itself is the living tissue, the depth of burn into the dermis determines how likely wounds are to heal and what degree of scarring can be expected.

■ PATHOPHYSIOLOGY

The severity of the burn depends on the duration of contact with the burn agent, the heat and conductivity of tissues, the heat of the burn agent, heat transfer (conduction, convection, or radiation), and the heat capacity of the burn agent.

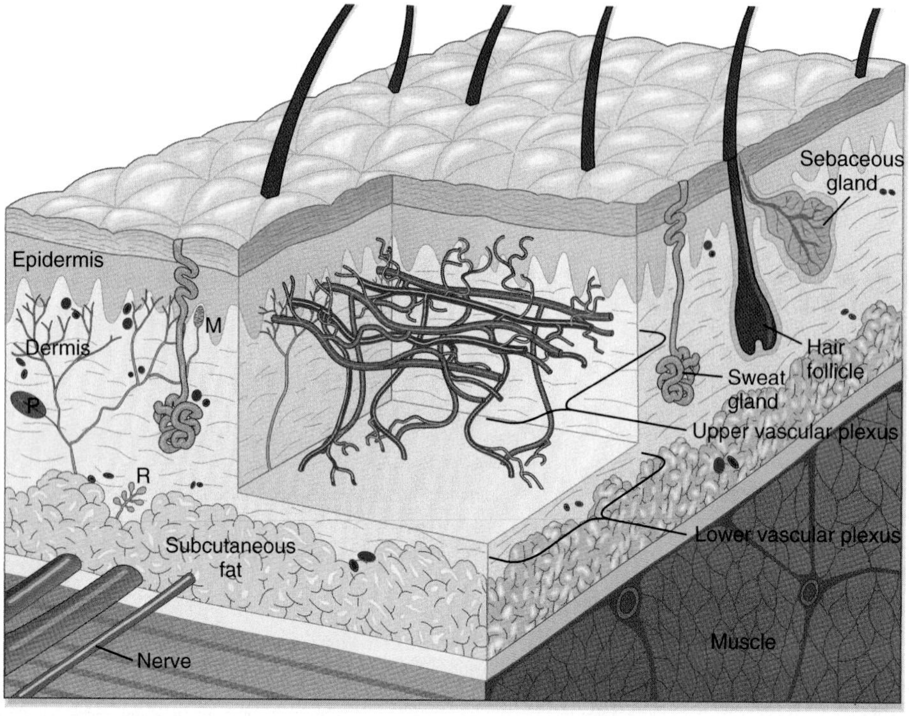
Epidermis
Dermis
M
P
R
Subcutaneous fat
Nerve
Sebaceous gland
Hair follicle
Sweat gland
Upper vascular plexus
Lower vascular plexus
Muscle

FIGURE 189-1 Structure of human skin. Schematic representation of skin cross-section. The two major layers of human skin, the epidermis and the dermis, overlie subcutaneous fat and muscle. Arterioles *(red)*, venules *(blue)*, and lymph vessels *(yellow-green)* of the dermis form a lower and an upper vascular plexus. Capillary loops extend toward the epidermis from the upper plexus of blood vessels into the dermal papillae, approximately one loop per dermal papilla. Sensory and autonomic nerves *(yellow fibers)* are also arranged in a lower and an upper plexus, at the junction of the dermis and subcutaneous fat and in the upper dermis. Sweat glands and hair follicles with their associated sebaceous glands are also integral components of the skin. (From Adkinson NF, Yunginger JW, Busse WW, et al [eds]: Middleton's Allergy: Principles and Practice, 6th ed. St. Louis, Mosby, 2003.)

Table 189-1 TYPES OF BURNS

Degree of Burn	Depth	Pain level	Blanching	Color	Example
First-degree	Epidermal	Painful	Blanches	Erythematous	Sunburn
Superficial second-degree	Superficial dermal	Painful	May blanch, usually blisters	Erythematous	Scald injury
Deep second-degree	Deep dermal	Painful to pinprick	Does not blanch	Pale and mottled	Hot grease burn
Third-degree	Full thickness	Insensate	Does not blanch	Hard, leathery eschar, often black	House fire (sustained burn)
Fourth-degree	Deep organ involvement	Insensate	Does not blanch	Burn to bone, fat or muscle apparent	Extensively sustained burn

Burns damage by two methods: first, by direct injury to the cellular structure of the tissue; and second, by the release of local mediators. Three zones are discussed with burn injuries: the zone of coagulation, the zone of stasis, and the zone of hyperemia. The *zone of coagulation* is the necrotic area of cell death from direct thermal injury. Surrounding this area is the *zone of stasis,* which has decreased blood flow and is at risk for cell death within 24 hours but may initially appear as living tissue. Cell mediators such as thromboxane A_2 are predominantly responsible for transforming this zone into the zone of coagulation. Outside this zone is the *zone of hyperemia.* The zone of hyperemia is defined as the outside area of tissue affected by the burn, usually blanching on touch, but with intact blood flow and a high potential to recover from the initial insult.

The secondary effects of burns, such as histamine release and edema, are thought to result from cellular mediators. Aggregated platelets from the burn release serotonin, whereas histamine derives from mast cells within the burned skin.

Clinical Presentation

Often, occupational exposures cause burns. Direct flame contact, scalds, injuries caused by heated equipment or arc welding, gasoline fires, and cooking acci-

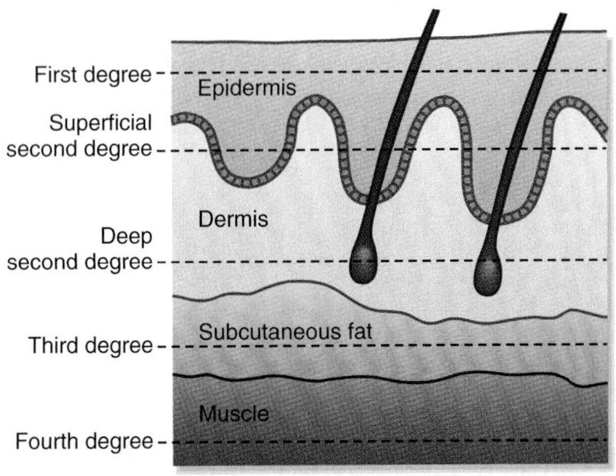
First degree
Superficial second degree
Deep second degree
Third degree
Fourth degree
Epidermis
Dermis
Subcutaneous fat
Muscle

FIGURE 189-2 Depths of burn. First-degree burns are confined to the epidermis. Second-degree burns are into the dermis (dermal burns). Third-degree burns are full-thickness burns through the epidermis and dermis. Fourth-degree burns involve injury to underlying tissue structures such as muscle, tendons, and bone. (From Townsend CM, Beauchamp RD, Evers BM, Mattox K [eds]: Sabiston Textbook of Surgery, 17th ed. Philadelphia, Saunders, 2004.)

RED FLAGS

Burns inconsistent with mechanism: concerning for nonaccidental trauma or abuse

Circular burns consistent with cigarette butt burns

Burns on the lower extremities without burns on the soles: consistent with forced immersion scald burns

Any perineal burn (area not exposed during normal activities)

dents are all common. In children or elderly patients presenting with burn injuries, the concern for abuse is always present.

In each patient presenting with a burn, airway is still the most important component. Burn victims are often also subject to smoke inhalation or thermal injury to the respiratory tissue from superheated air, and these injuries take priority over any others. Carbon monoxide, cyanide, and other inhaled toxins should be considered. The most threatening injuries are deep burns, burns covering a significant portion of body surface area, and respiratory burns (Box 189-1).

Diagnostic Testing

Aside from ABCs (airway, breathing, circulation), the most important aspect of burn assessment is estimation of burn depth and burn surface area. Burn depth can be assessed by evaluating the degree of blanching, noting the presence of blistering of the skin, and checking for the presence of pain. Total burn surface area is best assessed using a Lund and Browder chart (Fig. 189-3). Alternatively, a patient's palmar surface can be used as a crude measure of 1% of the patient's body surface area.

Children's body surface area is significantly different from that of adults. A child's head and torso comprise a much larger percentage of body surface area than in an adult. Patients with serious burns need specific burn unit care and require transfer if this care is unavailable in your institution.

In patients with severe burn injuries, burn shock can occur. Hypovolemic shock develops from capillary permeability alterations. Cell death can result in severe hyperkalemia, although this condition is usually a delayed finding.

BOX 189-1

American Burn Association Burn Unit Referral Criteria

1. Partial-thickness burns of greater than 10% total body surface area
2. Burns that involve the hands, face, feet, genitalia, perineum, or major joints
3. Third-degree (full-thickness) burns in any age group
4. Electrical burns, including lightning injury
5. Chemical burns
6. Inhalation injury
7. Burn injury in patients with preexisting medical disorders that could complicate management or recovery or could affect mortality
8. Patients with concomitant burn and trauma in which the burn injury poses the greatest risk of morbidity or mortality
9. Burned children in hospitals without qualified personnel or equipment for the care of children
10. Burn injury in patients who require special social, emotional, or long-term rehabilitative intervention

Adapted from the American Burn Association: Burn Unit Criteria. Available at http://www.ameriburn.org.

Treatment

The first intervention for burn victims is airway assessment. Smoke inhalation is a common issue, so all patients who do not need immediate intubation should be given 100% humidified oxygen by nonrebreather mask. Because edema can progress in minutes to hours and the full extent of respiratory damage may not become manifest until 12 hours after the initial injury, patients with evidence of

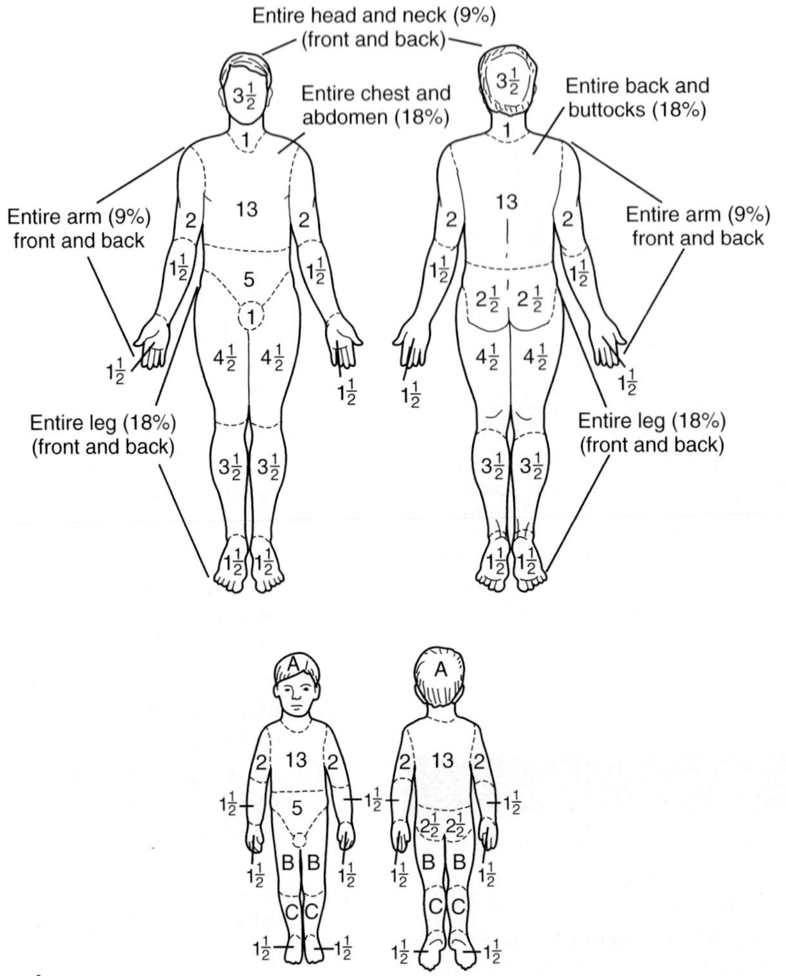
Entire head and neck (9%)
(front and back)
Entire chest and abdomen (18%)
Entire back and buttocks (18%)
Entire arm (9%) front and back
Entire arm (9%) front and back
Entire leg (18%) (front and back)
Entire leg (18%) (front and back)
3½
1
13
2
1½
5
4½
2½
3½
A
B
C

A

See chart for A, B, and C according to age

AGE	Birth–1 yr	1–4 yr	5–9 yr	10–14 yr	15 yr	Adult
Head	19	17	13	11	9	7
Neck	2					
Ant trunk	13					
Post trunk	13					
R. buttock	2½					
L. buttock	2½					
Genitalia	1					
R. U. arm	4					
L. U. arm	4					
R. L. arm	3					
L. L. arm	3					
R. hand	2½					
L. hand	2½					
R. thigh	5½	6½	8	8½	9	9½
L. thigh	5½	6½	8	8½	9	9½
R. leg	5	5	5½	6	6½	7
L. leg	5	5	5½	6	6½	7
R. foot	3½					
L. foot	3½					

Body area

B

FIGURE 189-3 **A,** The Lund and Browder charts are somewhat more accurate than the rule of nines in estimating the total body surface area burned. **B,** The proportion of total body surface area of individual areas, according to age. Compared with adults, children have larger heads and smaller legs. Other areas are relatively equivalent throughout life. The rule of nines is not accurate in determining the percentage of total body surface area burned in children. L, left or lower; R, right; U, upper. (From Roberts JR, Hedges J [eds]: Clinical Procedures in Emergency Medicine, 4th ed. Philadelphia, Saunders, 2004.)

Facts and Formulas

Parkland formula	Adults	Lactated Ringer's solution 4 mL × patient's weight (in kg) × percentage of TBSA	50% in first 8 hours; 50% divided over next 16 hours (goal mean arterial pressure >60 mm Hg and urine output >0.5 mL/kg/hour for adults)
Galveston formula	Pediatric patients	5% dextrose lactated Ringer's solution 5000 mL/TBSA burned (in m^2) + 2000 mL/TBSA (in m^2)/24 hours	50% in first 8 hours; 50% divided over next 16 hours (goal urine output 1 mL/kg/hour)

TBSA, total body surface area.

Priority Actions

- Address the patient's respiratory status, with a high suspicion for airway injury that will worsen; intubate if necessary, and supply supplemental oxygen otherwise.
- Assess burn injury size and depth.
- Provide anesthesia and pain management. Patients may require extremely high doses of narcotics.
- Start appropriate fluid management, and consider Foley catheter placement for fluid status assessment.
- Dress wounds appropriately.
- Evaluate for the need for escharotomies.
- Consider the need for burn unit referral.

airway damage should be intubated prophylactically, before the airway becomes edematous.

Because of the expected hypovolemic state of these patients, two large-bore intravenous lines should be placed. Although intravenous lines placed through burned skin are not optimal, given that they allow another portal for infection into an open wound, their placement is preferable to having no intravenous access at all.

Fluid requirements are a key facet in the management of the burn patient. Two specific formulas are most commonly used. The *Parkland formula* is used to estimate fluid replacement in adults. This formula gives suggested fluid replacement in addition to maintenance fluid amounts over a 24-hour period; half of this fluid should be given over the first 8 hours, with the remaining half over the following 16 hours. The original Parkland formula used lactated Ringer's solution as the fluid of choice.[2]

For children, the *Galveston formula* is recommended for fluid repletion calculations. The Galveston formula suggests that lactated Ringer's solution with 5% dextrose should be used for the fluid of choice because of the lack of glycogen stores in the pediatric population. Again, half of the total amount should be given in the first 8 hours, with the remainder within the next 16 hours. Maintenance fluid should be also added, and particular attention should be paid to maintaining body temperature (see Facts and Formulas box).

Despite these formulas, fluid resuscitation is more accurately based on appropriate urine output, which is 0.5 mL/kg/hour in adults, and up to 1 mL/kg/hour in children. When one is uncertain about the patient's fluid status, as may occur in congestive heart failure or pulmonary edema, a Swan-Ganz catheter may be necessary to provide guidance. Some controversy exists about the optimal fluid to use in burn patients. Although current guidelines specify crystalloid only initially, more recent studies suggest a likely role for colloid solutions.[3,4]

All burns should be gently cleansed of debris with normal saline solution. Superficial burns (superficial second- and first-degree burns) should be dressed with topical antimicrobial dressings, with frequent dressing changes planned (every 6 hours). A degree of controversy exists about the best antimicrobial dressing. No clearly superior agent has been reported in the literature.[5] One commonly used agent, silver sulfadiazine, should not be applied to the face because of concerns about staining. A good option, particularly for the face, is a simple, over-the-counter antibiotic ointment. For mild burns, aloe vera cream is also acceptable. Biosynthetic dressings are another option, but because of cost and availability, these dressings are usually limited to inpatient burn management.

Deeper burns may require débridement and grafting. Specific recommendations should be discussed with the local burn center. If burns are in areas that can be elevated, they should be; this approach decreases the amount of subsequent edema that develops in burn areas. Controversy also exists about whether burn blisters should be sterilely incised or left alone. No definitive data on the subject are available, but the general consensus appears to be that unless a blister prevents the application of a dressing, it should be left intact.

Pain management is beneficial to the patient and is important to address early. Third-degree (full-thickness) burns are insensate, but more superficial burns are exquisitely painful. Most burns vary in depth and are painful, so early use of intravenous morphine or

Table 189-2 ESCHAR TREATMENT

Type of Eschar	Recognition	Approach
Chest eschar	Burn across chest with difficulty of chest expansion, possible increased peak pressures if on the ventilator	Anesthetize, and cut to the subcutaneous fat on the chest in the anterior axillary lines from the clavicles to the inferior costal margins; connect these incisions superiorly and inferiorly, with possible other transverse incisions needed if ventilation is still not possible.
Extremity eschar	Burn of the extremity with vascular compromise in the extremity	Anesthetize, and cut to the subcutaneous fat on medial and lateral sides of the extremity from 1 cm proximal to the eschar to 1 cm distal to the eschar, with care taken where vascular or neurologic injury may occur.
Neck eschar	Circumferential burn of the neck	Anesthetize, and cut to the subcutaneous fat on the lateral and posterior aspects of the neck, to avoid carotid or jugular venous structures.
Penile eschar	Circumferential burn of the penis	Anesthetize, and cut to the subcutaneous fat on the midlateral portions of the penis to avoid the dorsal penile vein.
Hand eschar	Circumferential burn of the hand with evidence of vascular compromise	Anesthetize, and cut to the subcutaneous fat on the lateral side of each finger, the palmar crease, and between the metacarpals on the dorsum of the palm.
Abdominal wall eschar	Burn of the abdominal wall with evidence of increasing intra-abdominal pressures (elevated bladder pressures)	Anesthetize, and cut to the subcutaneous fat on the lateral sides of the abdominal wall.

Documentation

History	Circumstances of the burn, timing, type of material burning, presence of associated trauma, presence of other victims, presence of voice change, presence of pain or paresthesias, weakness, tetanus status, medical conditions that may impair healing or compromise immune function, family situation
Physical examination	Respiratory examination including signs of airway injury (soot in mouth, singed nasal hairs), neurovascular examination of all extremities, skin examination including wound size and depth, tenderness, neurologic examination, signs of concomitant trauma
Studies	None necessary; consideration of a chest radiograph for assessing pulmonary baseline status
Medical decision making	Reasons for intubation, reasons for transfer, initial cause of thermal injury, follow-up plan
Procedures	Documentation regarding the need for escharotomy; if necessary, documentation of reversal of signs for escharotomy after the procedure
Patient instructions	Documentation of discussion with the patient regarding the possibility of worsening injury and the warning signs of infection and vascular compromise; instructions on what to do and when to return

hydromorphone (Dilaudid) is indicated for patients with extensive or deep burns. First-degree burns can be managed with oral nonsteroidal anti-inflammatory medications. Superficial partial-thickness burns usually require oral narcotics for pain control.

Occasionally, a burn covers such a large area that it poses a risk for respiratory or vascular compromise. For example, a circumferential burn to an extremity can compromise the vascular supply to that extremity, whereas a near-circumferential full-thickness burn to the chest can prevent chest movement and can result in the inability to ventilate. Through escharotomies, these constricting bands of tissue can be released (Table 189-2). The basic method of performing an escharotomy is to incise the constricting band of tissue down to subcutaneous fat. Fasciotomies for compartment syndrome may also be required in thermal burns that cause edema with subsequent increased compartmental pressures.

Much discussion has centered around empirical antibiotics. No data support the use of empirical antibiotics for acute burn wounds, except in topical form, as is recommended for superficial burn wounds.[6]

■ COOLING

Applied cold inhibits lactate production, histamine and thromboxane release, and sequelae such as edema, microvascular congestion, and progressive ischemia. Cold should be used for small burns but

PATIENT TEACHING TIPS

- Inform all burn patients about the remote possibility that the burn may worsen over the next 24 hours, with tissue death possibly requiring grafts.
- After the first couple of days, a normal wound should have consistently gradual improvement in pain, swelling, size, and tissue color.
- Inform patients that a burn may result in a scar and probably will; the size and shape of the scar can be addressed by a plastic surgeon, who may need to do a scar revision to obtain the desired cosmetic result.
- If any of the foregoing situations develop, the patient should know to return to the ED or to follow up with specialty referral.
- Assure patients that if they follow these instructions, additional steps can then be taken to optimize recovery.
- Care of the partial thickness burn: Check the burn every day for signs of infection, such as increased pain, redness, swelling, or pus. If you see any of these signs, go to your doctor right away. To prevent infection, avoid breaking blisters. Change the dressing every day. First, wash your hands with soap and water. Then gently wash the burn and put antibiotic ointment on it. If the burn area is small, a dressing may not be needed during the day.
- Burned skin itches as it heals. Keep your fingernails cut short and do not scratch the burned skin. The burned area will be sensitive to sunlight for up to 1 year.

not for large burns because hypothermia can result. Ice should not be applied directly because frostbite can increase tissue injury. Cold water can help to relieve the pain of first- and second-degree burns, but patients with significant burns of more than 9% of their total body surface area should not have cold applied.

Disposition

Patients with major burns should receive care in a specialized burn center (see Box 189-1). Minor burns can be cared for on an outpatient basis, with close follow-up and instructions for assessing for infection.

Tips and Tricks

Escharotomy

- Consider local anesthesia (lidocaine).
- Pack wound with gauze with topical antibiotic.
- Treat the escharotomy wound as part of the burn.

Anesthesia

- Large doses of intravenous narcotics may be necessary.
- Intubated patients still have pain: address it.

Dressings

- First, ensure adequate anesthesia.
- Gently clean the wound with normal saline solution.
- Assess the depth of each wound individually.
- For superficial wounds, dress with a topical antibiotic and cover with gauze.
- For deep wounds, consider burn unit referral, surgical débridement, or dry dressing application.

All patients with concern for possible nonaccidental burns should be evaluated by both social services and law enforcement, and patients with self-inflicted injuries should be referred for psychiatric care. Any pediatric patient with suspected abuse should be admitted, even if the burn itself does not meet admission criteria, so social services can ensure the child's safety (see Tips and Tricks box).

REFERENCES

1. Centers for Disease Control and Prevention: Web-Based Injury Statistics Query and Reporting System. Available at www.cdc.gov/ncipc/wisqars.
2. Pham T, Gibran N: Thermal and electrical injuries. Surg Clin North Am 2007;87:185-206, vii-viii.
3. Fodor L, Fodor A, Ramon Y, et al: Controversies in fluid resuscitation of burn management: Literature review and our experience. Injury 2006;37:374-379.
4. Cooper AB, Cohn SM, Zhang HS, et al: Five percent albumin for adult burn shock resuscitation: Lack of effect on daily multiple organ dysfunction score. Transfusion 2006;46:80-89.
5. Costagliola M, Agrosi M: Second degree burns: A comparative, multicenter, randomized trial of hyaluronic acid plus silver sulfadiazine vs. silver sulfadiazine alone. Curr Med Res Opin 2005;21:1235-1240.
6. American College of Surgeons, Committee on Trauma: Resources for the Optimal Care of the Injured Patient. Chicago, American College of Surgeons, 1999.

Chapter 190

Chemical Burns

Jeffrey Druck

KEY POINTS

Copious, immediate irrigation is the most important treatment of chemical burns.
Elemental metal burns are the only chemical burns that should not be irrigated with water. Instead, wipe off the material with dry gauze, and protect yourself from contamination.
Identifying the cause of a chemical burn may be difficult, but the use of external resources (material safety data sheet [MSDS], paramedics, employers, poison center) will help to characterize the agents.
Patients who exhibit no further signs of systemic toxicity may require only a chemistry panel and an electrocardiogram to complete an assessment.
Patients with hydrofluoric acid burns require topical treatment with calcium gluconate gel, local infiltration of calcium gluconate, or, for the most severe cases, intra-arterial administration of calcium gluconate.

Perspective

Chemical burn is an unusual type of burn because the tissue injury is caused by the chemical reaction rather than by thermal damage. Chemical burns are common at work, at home, or in association with hobbies. With the recent concerns of terrorism, chemical agents have been emphasized as a possible method of attack, so knowledge of chemical burns is critical in the education of today's EPs. In addition, failure to recognize chemical burns or to treat them appropriately can have a detrimental impact not only on the patient but also on the care providers.

Structure and Function

■ ANATOMY

Most chemical burns occur to skin; as such, knowledge of skin anatomy is key to understanding the pathophysiology of various chemical burns because of the link to treatment. A direct injury results when the epidermis is penetrated. Systemic absorption is possible once the injury extends through the dermis.

■ PATHOPHYSIOLOGY

Different chemical burns affect tissue by different mechanisms. Table 190-1 provides different categories of chemical agents and their mechanism of tissue damage.

Clinical Presentation

A classic presentation of a chemical burn is an industrial worker who "got something" on his or her arm and developed pain and sloughing of the skin over the next few minutes. The burning may have

Table 190-1 CHEMICAL AGENTS AND THEIR MECHANISMS OF TISSUE DAMAGE

Type of Chemical Agent	Mechanism of Tissue Damage	Example of Agent
Acids	Coagulative necrosis	Sulfuric acid
Alkali agents	Saponification and liquefactive necrosis	Calcium hydroxide
Desiccants and vesicants	Dehydration of cells through exothermic reactions, release of amines within cells	Nitrogen mustards
Oxidizing and reducing agents	Denaturing of proteins and direct cytotoxic effects	Bleach
Protoplasmic poisons	Formation of salts with cellular proteins	Picric acid

RED FLAGS

Scenarios Suggestive of Specific Types of Chemical Burns

Scenario	Suspicious Agent
Circumferential lower extremity burns above sock line	Cement
Burn in a glass etcher	Hydrofluoric acid
Burn from fireworks	White phosphorus
Mass exposure (terrorist attack)	Nitrogen mustard

continued despite irrigation. An alternate presentation may be someone who got something on his or her clothes and noticed burning and a "rash" after touching the clothing.

■ VARIATIONS

In our modern times, chemical agents may be used in a terrorist attack, so multiple victims with similar burns and systemic toxicity should trigger the concern for a mass casualty event. In addition, burns that appear to worsen over short periods may not be thermal burns, as initially thought, but instead may be chemical.

Hazardous Materials

The United States Department of Transportation requires color-coded identification of the type of material transported. These identifying codes are widely used. Additionally, a standard four-number code should be present, to identify or characterize the agent more specifically. Figure 190-1 indicates the general categories and identifying colors, which include the following:

- Explosives (solid orange)
- Nonflammable gases (solid green)
- Flammable liquids (solid red)
- Flammable solids (white and red stripes)
- Oxidizers and peroxides (solid yellow)
- Poisons and biohazards (solid white)
- Radioactive materials (half white, half yellow, with black radiation symbol)
- Corrosives (half white, half black)
- Other (usually white)

Gowns and gloves that are readily available in the hospital are not sufficient for many substances. Most chemicals penetrate these materials immediately. Relatively inexpensive, chemical-resistant, multilayer suits are available. Further, respiratory precautions may be indicated for some agents. For these reasons, both hospital and community resources may be required for safe and expedient decontamination.

Diagnostic Testing

Along with irrigation, the most important task is to identify the offending agent. Various sources can be used, but the best source of information is usually patients themselves. The job site may provide clues, but the employer should also have the MSDS available. Paramedics or others can bring in bottles of the agent, which may have a list of ingredients. The presence of systemic symptoms may also suggest specific agents.

Although the specific agent may be difficult to identify without other information, further testing can assist in the diagnosis. pH paper can be used on the wound to determine the presence of acid or base. A chemistry panel may suggest acidosis, whereas hypocalcemia may suggest hydrofluoric acid exposure.

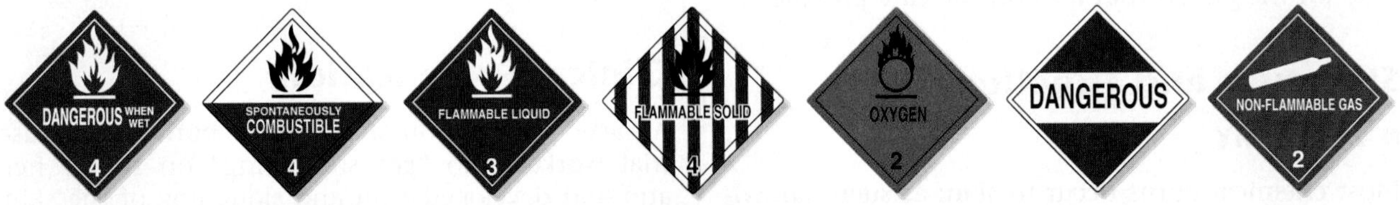
DANGEROUS WHEN WET
4
SPONTANEOUSLY COMBUSTIBLE
4
FLAMMABLE LIQUID
3
FLAMMABLE SOLID
4
OXYGEN
2
DANGEROUS
NON-FLAMMABLE GAS
2

FIGURE 190-1 The general categories and identifying colors for hazardous materials signs.

Tips and Tricks

Ocular Exposure

Ocular chemical burns are highly morbid injuries. The initial therapy of copious irrigation cannot be emphasized enough. Lid retraction with eversion is a key procedure to remove all chemical particles. Testing for the continued presence of chemicals can be accomplished using pH paper, but it is important to wait a minimum of 5 minutes after irrigation to make sure that you are not checking the pH of the irrigation fluid. Patients with burns caused by certain chemicals may require admission for continuous irrigation. Any patient with ocular exposure that results in corneal burns (identified by fluorescein examination) should have an ophthalmology consultation. Other elements of examination are similar to any eye examination, including visual acuity, slit-lamp examination, and visual field evaluation.

Ingestions

Although a discussion of the management of caustic chemical ingestion is beyond the scope of this chapter, two key concepts should be emphasized. First, the primary issue is airway maintenance. Second, the extent of burn is usually limited to the initial exposure, and decontamination of the gastrointestinal tract is difficult and not recommended; the only substance that has been suggested is water, but because of possible exothermic reactions resulting from attempted water irrigation, water decontamination of the gastrointestinal tract is controversial. Endoscopy is the only method of definitive assessment of the degree of injury, but the common complications of perforation and mediastinitis should also be assessed.[2]

Inhalational Injury

Again, the primary issue in patients with inhalational injury is airway maintenance. For a variety of chemicals, the initial chest radiograph and the absence of respiratory symptoms belie the serious pulmonary edema or tracheobronchitis that may develop even days later. Consultation with your local poison control center while supportive measures are instituted is the recommended pathway of care.

Treatment

Figure 190-2 is an algorithm for the management of patients with possible chemical burns.

INTERVENTIONS AND PROCEDURES

The first step in caring for patients with chemical burns is removal of the offending agent. This involves copious irrigation with several liters of either water or normal saline solution. All contaminated clothing should be removed, with care taken to ensure that health care providers are not exposed.

PRIORITY ACTIONS

Maintaining a high index of suspicion for chemical burns

Discovery of the offending agent

Appropriate decontamination or avoidance of self-contamination procedures

Irrigation

Appropriate use of laboratory testing and electrocardiographic monitoring

Specialty referrals or consultations for burns or specific area involvement

Proper discharge instructions

Elemental Metals: Do Not Irrigate

Regardless of the type of offending agent, copious irrigation is the first step, with one exception: elemental metals. Elemental sodium and potassium cause exothermic reactions when they are exposed to water, in addition to forming toxic alkali agents. Patients with these injuries should have specific decontamination and removal of the offending metal by brushing it off with gauze. The poison center may provide advice about proper disposal of the metal.

DIRECTED THERAPIES

Specific agents are known to cause specific toxicities. If the substance is known, therapy should be directed against that toxicity (Table 190-2).

Hydrofluoric Acid

Hydrofluoric acid is used in glass etching, automotive and industrial wheel cleaning, brick cleaning, semiconductor manufacturing, metal purification, and other industries. Immediate irrigation is indicated, as with other chemical injuries, but hydrofluoric acid can cause progressive tissue damage. Extensive exposure of an uncovered arm or leg can be fatal. Pain can be delayed but can subsequently continue for hours or days. The hydrofluoric acid ion does not dissociate, but rather penetrates tissues deeply and reacts with calcium and magnesium. Hypocalcemia can result.

Patients with mild, small, superficial exposures can be treated with topical calcium gluconate, which must usually be mixed in the ED by combining calcium gluconate powder with commonly available lubricant jelly. Affected fingers and hands can be placed in a medical glove that contains the solution.[1]

Subcutaneous infiltration of 10% calcium gluconate may help to relieve pain, but it also irritates the tissue. Slow infiltration with the smallest available needle, preferably 30 gauge, or dilution of the solution may minimize tissue damage. Intra-arterial

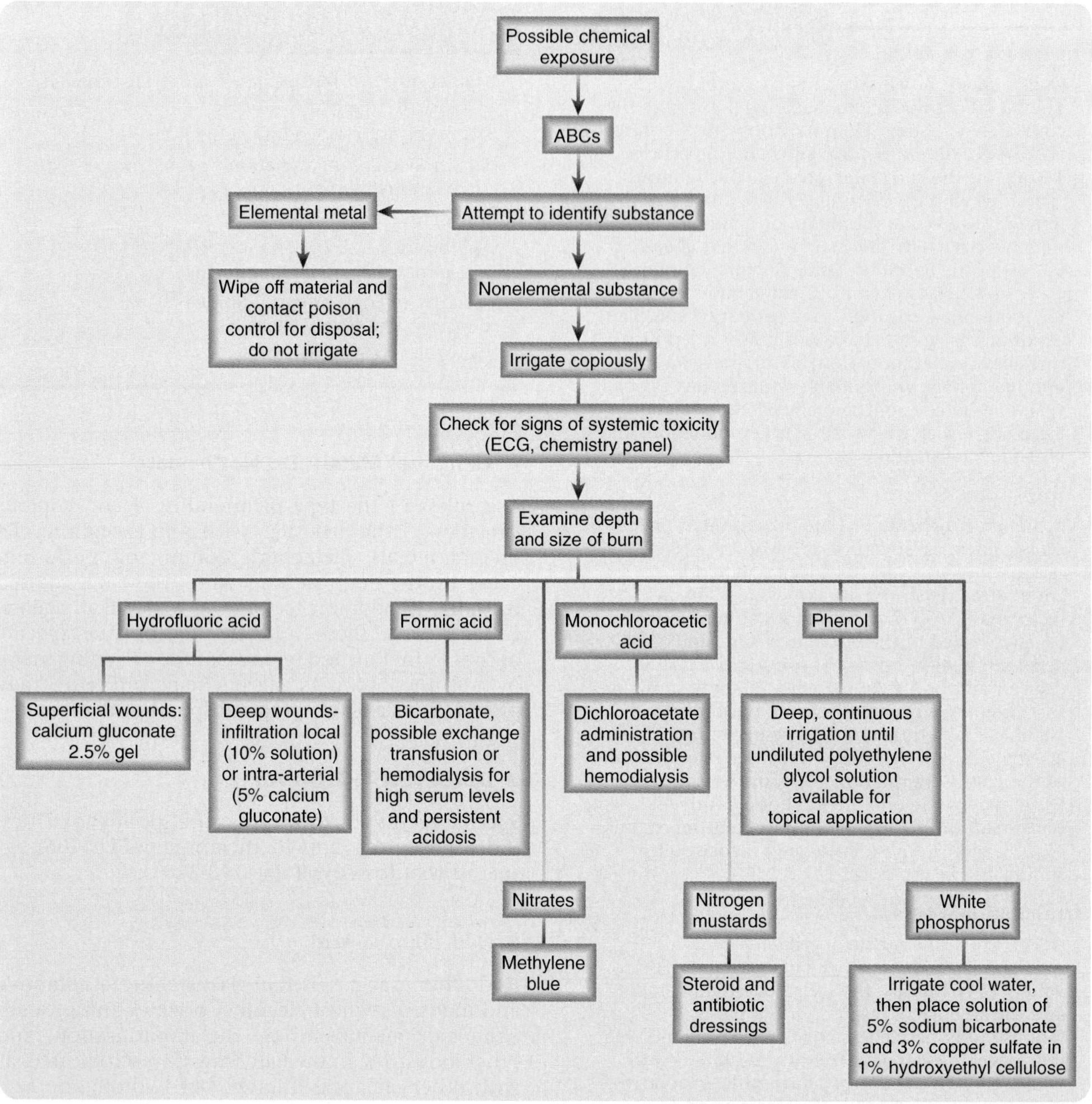
Possible chemical exposure
ABCs
Attempt to identify substance
Elemental metal
Wipe off material and contact poison control for disposal; do not irrigate
Nonelemental substance
Irrigate copiously
Check for signs of systemic toxicity (ECG, chemistry panel)
Examine depth and size of burn
Hydrofluoric acid
Formic acid
Monochloroacetic acid
Phenol
Superficial wounds: calcium gluconate 2.5% gel
Deep wounds-infiltration local (10% solution) or intra-arterial (5% calcium gluconate)
Bicarbonate, possible exchange transfusion or hemodialysis for high serum levels and persistent acidosis
Dichloroacetate administration and possible hemodialysis
Deep, continuous irrigation until undiluted polyethylene glycol solution available for topical application
Nitrates
Methylene blue
Nitrogen mustards
Steroid and antibiotic dressings
White phosphorus
Irrigate cool water, then place solution of 5% sodium bicarbonate and 3% copper sulfate in 1% hydroxyethyl cellulose

FIGURE 190-2 Algorithm of treatment for chemical burns.

Documentation

History	Type of chemical, physical form, concentration, duration of exposure before irrigation, duration and volume of irrigation, physical areas of contact, presence or absence of clothing, tetanus status, medical conditions that may impair healing or compromise immune function
Physical examination	Respiratory status, the location, size and depth of the burn, surrounding area skin changes, clues for occupational exposures, eye or mucous membrane involvement
Studies	Electrocardiogram and chemistry panel, including calcium and magnesium
Medical decision making	Reasons to pursue or not to pursue chemical burn concerns, indications for systemic toxicity requiring admission; time and amount of irrigation
Procedures	Documentation of whether the irrigation was successful in removing all the chemical, documentation of pH after irrigation
Patient instructions	Documentation of a discussion with the patient regarding the possibility of scar, cellulitis, need for graft, warning signs, as well as what to do and when to return

Table 190-2 SPECIFIC THERAPIES FOR CHEMICAL BURNS

Agent	Specific Toxicity	Additional Treatment
Hydrofluoric acid	Severe hypocalcemia and continued liquefactive necrosis	Superficial wounds: calcium gluconate 2.5% gel Deep wounds: infiltration locally (10% solution) or intra-arterial injection (5% solution) of calcium gluconate
Formic acid	Severe acidosis	Bicarbonate administration, possible exchange transfusions or hemodialysis for high serum levels and persistent acidosis
Cement (alkali burn)	Persistent burns when exposed to water if not irrigated completely away	Thorough irrigation
Phenol	Systemic absorption causing central nervous system depression, coma, and death	Because more dilute solution is more rapidly absorbed, deep, continuous irrigation until undiluted polyethylene glycol solution is available for topical application; all other treatment supportive for systemic symptoms
White phosphorus	Continued thermal burn, resulting from burns on exposure to oxygen; systemic absorption causing acidosis and electrocardiographic abnormalities, possibly sudden death	Removal of as much phosphorus as possible through irrigation with cool water, then placement of a solution of 5% sodium bicarbonate and 3% copper sulfate in 1% hydroxyethyl cellulose
Elemental metals (sodium, potassium)	Exothermic reaction when exposed to water	Wiping away of material and contacting poison control for disposal instructions
Nitrates	Methemoglobinemia	Methylene blue administration
Monochloroacetic acid	Systemic lactic acidosis	Dichloroacetate administration and possible hemodialysis
Nitrogen mustards	Vesicle formation	Steroid and antibiotic dressings after copious irrigation

administration, through the radial or ulnar artery, of 10 mL of calcium gluconate, mixed in 50 mL of 5% dextrose in water and administered through an arterial line over 4 hours, may be beneficial for severe exposures to the hand.

Cardiac dysrhythmias may result from systemic hypocalcemia and hypomagnesemia. The electrocardiogram should be monitored for QT prolongation. Calcium and magnesium should be administered as needed.

Disposition

After determination of the offending agent and copious irrigation until no further chemical remains (for acids and bases, this can be determined with pH paper), disposition of the patient should be based on the presence of systemic symptoms, the size and depth of the burn, the nature of the agent, and access to appropriate follow-up. All patients should be warned about scarring and the potential for infection. The circumstances of the exposure should be verified, and appropriate state and local authorities should be notified about exposures in industrial incidents.

PATIENT TEACHING TIPS

- Inform all patients with wounds that scars are possible and specialized care may be needed.
- After the first couple of days, a normal wound should have consistently gradual improvement in pain, swelling, and discoloration.
- If any of the foregoing situations develop, the patient should know to return to the ED or should have received specialty referral.
- Assure patients that if they follow these instructions, additional steps can then be taken to optimize recovery.

REFERENCES

1. Bethel CA, Krisanda TJ: Burn care procedures. In Roberts JR, Hedges J (eds): Clinical Procedures in Emergency Medicine, 4th ed. Philadelphia, Saunders, 2004.
2. Duncan M, Wong RKH: Esophageal emergencies: Things that will wake you from a sound sleep. Gastroenterol Clin North Am 2003;32:1035-1052.

SECTION **XIX**

Rashes

Chapter **191**

Rash in the Acutely Ill Patient

Guido F. Valdes

KEY POINTS

Infectious agents are by far the most common causes of rash, and early empirical antibiotic administration is crucial.
The morphology of a rash is the first step in determining the cause of illness.
In the ill or toxic-appearing patient, rapid identification of associated skin lesions narrows the differential diagnosis.
Particular attention should be taken and caution exercised with immunocompromised patients.
Travel history and occupational history are frequently overlooked, but they provide key information to make accurate diagnoses.
Petechiae and purpura signal diseases with rapid deterioration and high mortality.
Patients with extensive desquamation and blistering need care in a burn unit.
Admission to a monitored setting is indicated and necessary in the majority of cases.

Scope

The presence of skin lesions in an ill-appearing patient can be invaluable in both diagnosing and treating potentially life-threatening conditions. Rapid and accurate identification of particular rashes is facilitated through a simple classification scheme based on visual inspection and morphology.[1] The differential diagnosis is extensive and can be refined with the addition of history and physical examination.[2] The assumption of the presence of a life-threatening entity dictates and simplifies early management strategies and disposition, particularly in patients with fever or cardiorespiratory distress.[3] Most of these cases have an infectious cause. The primary focus is on early and aggressive respiratory and hemodynamic support, as well as antimicrobial therapy. Noninfectious causes must also be considered and can manifest with specific patterns of skin lesions. Autoimmune disorders and drug reactions are common causes of rash.

Anatomy

A rash is a collection of skin lesions that displays a particular distribution and morphology. The morphology of the lesion reflects the underlying histologic involvement and provides the most convenient way to categorize patients presenting with an acute illness and a rash.[4] Table 191-1 lists the morphologic features of each particular lesion. Rashes can be classified as petechial/purpuric, erythematous, maculopapular, vesicular/bullous, nodular, and urticarial.

Table 191-1 COMMON SKIN LESIONS

Lesion Type	Description
Macule	Circumscribed, flat discoloration of any size
Papule	Elevated, solid lesion ≤5 mm in diameter with variable color; confluent papules form plaques
Nodule	Circumscribed, elevated, solid lesion >5 mm in diameter
Vesicle	Circumscribed collection of free fluid ≤5 mm in diameter
Bulla	Same as vesicle but >5 mm in diameter
Pustule	Circumscribed collection of purulent fluid of variable size and color
Wheal	Firm, edematous plaque resulting from infiltration of the dermis with fluid
Petechia	Circumscribed deposit of blood <5 mm in diameter
Purpura	Same as petechia but >5 mm in diameter

Data from Habif TP: Clinical Dermatology: A Color Guide to Diagnosis and Therapy, 4th ed. Philadelphia, Mosby, 2004, p 1.

The distribution, the direction of spread of the lesions, and the timing of the onset of the rash relative to the appearance of signs of systemic illness are important diagnostic features.

Many of the rashes seen in ill patients manifest as exanthematous eruptions. Exanthems are characterized by widespread, symmetrical, erythematous macules and papules, resulting from systemic exposure to viruses, bacteria, or drugs.[5] Other lesions, such as pustules, vesicles, and petechiae, may appear subsequently. Lesions appearing on mucosal surfaces, such as the oral cavity and conjunctiva, are termed *enanthems*. They are less apparent and can be missed during physical examination. However, the presence of enanthems can be of significant diagnostic value.

Pathophysiology

The genesis of skin lesions at the tissue level is multifactorial. It is the result of inflammatory mediators synthesized in response to infectious agents, toxins, medications, or an autoimmune process. Bacteremia or viremia is common in acutely ill patients with rash and fever. Microorganisms can produce eruptions by means of local skin colonization, toxin production, and direct effects on blood vessels such as necrosis and vasodilation. Noninfectious causes, such as allergic and autoimmune disorders, are mediated by similar inflammatory processes.

Presenting Signs and Symptoms

Acute illness can be defined in a variety of ways. Terms such as "toxic" and "ill-appearing" are often used to describe a patient who may have fever, respiratory distress, hypotension, dehydration, or altered mental status. The clinical impression of acute illness is formed by a variety of factors. A distinctive rash can narrow a wide differential diagnosis.

History

A focused history includes the following elements:

- Contact with ill persons
- Recent travel
- Animal exposure
- Medication use
- Occupation
- Immunologic status
- Immunization status
- Onset and spread of rash

Physical Examination

Rapid clinical assessment, to ascertain the patient's stability and to identify the type of rash, is the priority. Particular attention should be given to the following conditions:

- Adenopathy
- Oral, conjunctival, or genital lesions
- Hepatosplenomegaly
- Arthritis
- Meningismus or neurologic dysfunction[1]

Skin Manifestations

Table 191-2 lists the most common causes of each morphologic category of rash.

■ PETECHIA/PURPURA

Petechial rashes in ill-appearing patients are true emergencies. Infectious causes are at the top of the differential diagnosis until proven otherwise. Meningococcemia, rickettsial infections, and bacteremia are important life-threatening diagnoses.[6]

■ Meningococcemia

Neisseria meningitidis is a gram-negative bacterium that causes fulminant septicemia and meningitis. The rapidly progressive form of disease is not usually associated with meningitis.[7] Infants, asplenic individuals, and immunosuppressed patients are at high risk. Patients may initially have a nonspecific prodrome of cough, headache, and sore throat that progresses rapidly to a toxic clinical picture.[8] In the early stages of disease, the skin manifestation may be a nonspecific maculopapular rash.[5] Within hours, these patients develop hypotension as well as a petechial eruption. Approximately 50% to 60% of patients present with a characteristic petechial rash.[9] Petechiae are first seen at the ankles, wrists, axillae, mucosal surfaces, and conjunctivae, with subsequent spread to the trunk and lower extremities.[7] Petechiae coalesce to form larger areas of discoloration (ecchymoses, purpura). *N. meningitidis* is the underlying

Table 191-2 CAUSES OF RASH BY MORPHOLOGY

Morphologic Type	Cause
Petechiae/Purpura	Meningococcemia Rocky Mountain spotted fever Ehrlichiosis Pneumococcemia Gonococcemia Staphylococcemia Gram-negative bacteremia Enterovirus infection Viral hemorrhagic fevers Henoch-Schönlein purpura Thrombotic thrombocytopenic purpura
Macules/Papules	Viral exanthems Typhoid fever Rickettsial infections Lyme disease *Mycoplasma* pneumonia Psittacosis Leptospirosis Acute HIV infection Epstein-Barr virus infection Erythema multiforme Dengue West Nile virus infection
Erythema	Exfoliative erythroderma Staphylococcal scalded skin syndrome Staphylococcal toxic shock syndrome Streptococcal toxic shock syndrome Scarlet fever Kawasaki's disease Toxic epidermal necrolysis Stevens-Johnson syndrome
Vesicles/Bullae	Herpes simplex Varicella Variola *Vibrio vulnificus* infection Bacteremia
Nodules	Disseminated fungal infections Bacillary angiomatosis Sweet's syndrome Erythema nodosum
Wheals/Urticaria	Allergic reaction/anaphylaxis *Mycoplasma* pneumonia Lyme disease Enterovirus infections HIV infection Hepatitis

HIV, human immunodeficiency virus.

cause in more than 90% of cases of sepsis with purpura.[10] These lesions can be seen in patients with symmetrical peripheral gangrene (purpura fulminans), consumptive coagulopathy, and shock.[3] Skin lesions can become pustular or nodular.[6] As soon as meningococcal infection is suspected, blood cultures should be obtained, and intravenous antibiotics should be administered. In patients with suspected meningitis, antibiotic administration may precede lumbar puncture because it takes at least an hour for these agents to arrive in the subarachnoid space, and putative bacterial agents may still be isolated and cultured.

■ Rocky Mountain Spotted Fever

Various rickettsial infections can present with fever and a petechial rash. Rocky Mountain spotted fever (RMSF) is the most common rickettsial infection in the United States.[11] It is caused by the gram-negative, intracellular bacterium *Rickettsia rickettsii,* which is transmitted through a tick bite.[9] The disease is highly endemic in the southeastern coastal states of North Carolina and Virginia, as well as in Oklahoma, and it occurs predominantly in the spring and early summer.[12] The onset of symptoms of RMSF usually begins 5 to 7 days after inoculation. The prodrome of fever, malaise, chills, myalgias, headache, and irritability mimics more common viral illnesses and delays diagnosis.[9] Maculopapular skin lesions may initially appear on the wrists, ankles, and forearms, with progression in 2 to 4 days to a petechial rash extending centripetally to the trunk and face and involving the palms and soles.[6] The classic petechial rash may not appear until 6 days or more after the initial symptoms occur.[9] A history of possible tick exposure in a patient with fever, headache, and rash suggests the diagnosis of RMSF. Most patients who develop RMSF do not manifest this classic triad of symptoms.[12] Of note, 20% of adults and 5% of children with RMSF display no rash (spotless fever).[9] Abdominal pain and focal neurologic symptoms ranging from seizures to meningismus may also be observed.[12] Meningococcemia is a more rapidly progressing and fulminant disease. Starting antibiotics on or before the fifth day of illness is important in decreasing mortality.[13] Patients with untreated infection have a mortality of 30%.[6]

Human ehrlichiosis is another tick-borne illness that may mimic RMSF, and differentiating between the two is difficult.[11] Involvement of the palms and soles is unusual in human ehrlichiosis.

■ Bacteremia

In addition to meningococcemia and RMSF, bacteremia of any origin can manifest with a petechial rash. *Streptococcus pneumoniae, Staphylococcus, Listeria,* and gram-negative enteric flora can cause petechial lesions and purpura in high-grade bacteremia, especially in susceptible patients (i.e., asplenic or neutropenic patients).[2] Patients with bacterial endocarditis may display small, red-brown petechiae on the extremities and mucous membranes.[14] Skin lesions are seen in 15% to 50% of cases, and petechiae are more common than subungual splinter hemorrhages, Osler's nodes, or Janeway lesions.[3]

Fever, polyarthritis, tenosynovitis, and petechial skin lesions suggest the diagnosis of gonococcemia. Skin lesions are found in 75% of patients with disseminated gonococcal infection. The skin eruption typically appears during the first day of symptoms, and it recurs with each febrile spike.[15] The rash is not as generalized, and the skin lesions tend to cluster in the extremities near symptomatic joints while sparing the scalp, face, trunk, and mucous membranes.[16] The lesions in gonococcemia are frequently polymorphic and may evolve through vesicular or pustular stages to develop a gray, necrotic center with a hemorrhagic base.

■ Viruses

Patients with viral infections can present with severe symptoms, and it is sometimes difficult to distinguish viral from bacterial infections acutely. Enterovirus infections and viral hemorrhagic fevers are associated with petechial rashes. Patients with coxsackievirus A9 and echovirus 9 infections can present with fever, pharyngitis, headache, and meningitis.[6] In addition to disseminated petechiae, maculopapular or vesicular lesions may also appear.

Infections with arenaviruses (Lassa fever, Venezuelan hemorrhagic fever), bunyaviruses (Rift Valley fever, hantavirus infection), filoviruses (Ebola and Marburg hemorrhagic fever), and flaviviruses (dengue hemorrhagic fever) result in the triad of fever, shock, and hemorrhage from mucosal surfaces and the gastrointestinal tract.[3] Early symptoms include conjunctival injection, flushing, petechial rash, and mild hypotension.[17]

■ Noninfectious Causes

Several noninfectious disorders cause acute illness and a petechial/purpuric eruption, but it is difficult to exclude an infectious process because many of these conditions are exacerbated by an underlying infection. Purpura and petechiae are seen in various vasculitides (hypersensitivity vasculitis, Henoch-Schönlein purpura) and, less commonly, in allergic reactions, acute rheumatic fever, and lupus.[2] The clinical acuity depends on underlying organ dysfunction, and these disorders do not always manifest acutely.

Patients with thrombotic thrombocytopenic purpura present clinically with fever, fluctuating neurologic symptoms, renal dysfunction with thrombocytopenia, and microangiopathic hemolytic anemia.[18] The most common presentation is thrombocytopenia with subsequent skin changes manifesting as petechial hemorrhages in the lower extremities.[19] Mortality is higher than 90% without treatment; plasma infusion and exchange transfusion reduce mortality to as low as 10%.[18]

■ ERYTHEMA

Erythema, with or without desquamation, is a worrisome finding in the acutely ill patient. *Toxic erythema* refers to a diffuse, red, blanchable rash.[4] Some causes of diffuse erythema may be rapidly fatal. As with petechial rashes, infectious causes are at the forefront of the differential diagnosis.

■ Staphylococcal Infections

Staphylococcus aureus causes a wide spectrum of systemic infections with skin manifestations. In addition to serious local infections such as abscesses, myositis, and fasciitis, certain strains of *S. aureus* elaborate toxins that lead to systemic syndromes.[3] Staphylococcal scalded skin syndrome manifests suddenly with diffuse, blanchable erythema, fever, irritability, and profound tenderness of the skin. This disorder is usually seen in small children following purulent conjunctivitis, otitis media, or nasopharyngeal infection.[4] Bullae subsequently develop, and light stroking causes rupture and separation of the upper portion of the epidermis, a feature known as *Nikolsky's sign*. Adult presentations are rare and are associated with renal impairment or immunosuppression.[6]

Staphylococcal toxic shock syndrome is an acute febrile illness manifesting with a generalized erythematous eruption, hypotension, and multiorgan system dysfunction (three or more organ systems).[8] After a nonspecific prodrome of malaise, the rash of toxic shock syndrome is almost always seen within 2 to 3 days, accompanied by conjunctival, oropharyngeal, and vaginal hyperemia.[20] Although this syndrome is classically associated with tampon use in menstruating female patients, more than 40% of cases occur in conjunction with postoperative wounds, skin infections, burn wounds, and postpartum status.[3] Desquamation may be seen after 7 to 10 days, usually in the hands and feet.[4]

■ Streptococcal Infections

Group A streptococci are the etiologic agents for several systemic syndromes associated with rash.[3] Scarlet fever usually follows a cutaneous or tonsillar infection.[6] Patients may appear acutely ill, with fever, sore throat, headache, chills, and nausea. Rash begins 2 to 3 days after the onset of illness and progresses from finely punctuate erythema on the head and neck to diffuse erythema covering the trunk and extremities.[20] The palms and soles are spared. Numerous small, papular elevations give the rash a "sandpaper" quality, and there is blanching to pressure.[20] Skin folds and pressure points may display petechiae (Pastia's lines).[6] The oral mucosa may have punctate erythema or petechiae, and the tongue may appear white with bright red papillae (strawberry tongue).[4]

Patients with group A streptococcal infection can present with a toxic shock–like syndrome with hypotension and multiorgan failure. Patients have an initial focus of pyogenic infection, usually on the skin; generalized erythema with diffuse desquamation and localized cellulitis are the principal skin manifestations.[3] Localized soft tissue necrosis as a result of streptococcal infection is part of the case definition for toxic shock syndrome.[20] The patient may complain only of localized pain, and physical findings may be limited to edema and erythema of the involved area.[7] As the disease progresses, the involved area develops increased swelling and hemorrhagic bullae that progress to frank necrosis with underlying fasciitis and myositis.[8] The mortality rate can reach 70% without prompt surgical intervention.[9]

■ Kawasaki's Disease

Kawasaki's disease, or mucocutaneous lymph node syndrome, tends to occur in young children, usually less than 5 years old.[2] The diagnosis is based on clinical criteria: fever lasting more than 5 days with conjunctival injection, cervical lymphadenopathy, oropharyngeal changes (injection, strawberry tongue, fissured lips), rash, erythema of the palms and soles, and periungual desquamation.[21] The rash usually appears within 3 days of the onset of fever and is variable. The rash is often scarlatiniform on the trunk and is accompanied by extremity erythema and desquamation.[4] Cardiovascular complications, most commonly coronary arteritis, develop in 20% to 25% of patients and are the major causes of morbidity and mortality.[6] A microbial pathogen is believed to be the etiologic agent, although no specific microorganism has been identified.

■ Toxic Epidermal Necrolysis/Stevens-Johnson Syndrome

Toxic epidermal necrolysis (TEN) and Stevens-Johnson syndrome (SJS) can be considered essentially the same disease.[9] They form a continuum of mucocutaneous reactions characterized by skin tenderness, erythema, epidermal necrosis, and desquamation.[8] Initial skin manifestations include widespread erythematous macules and targetoid lesions. Patients have involvement of more than one mucosal area (oral, conjunctival, anogenital), and conjunctival involvement may occur before the rash appears.[22] TEN affects more than 30% body surface area and SJS less than 10%; 10% to 30% involvement has been designated SJS/TEN overlap.[9] Although grossly similar to staphylococcal scalded skin syndrome, TEN involves the full thickness of the epidermis.[4] Nikolsky's sign is positive, but deeper involvement results in desquamation with removal of underlying pigmentation.[1] A prodromal phase of fever, nausea, malaise, headache, cough, and myalgia lasting up to 2 weeks may precede the skin eruption.[22] TEN/SJS is most commonly drug induced: sulfa-based antibiotics, penicillins, cephalosporins, fluoroquinolones, nonsteroidal anti-inflammatory drugs, and anticonvulsants have been implicated.[3] Infections with *Mycoplasma,* hepatitis viruses, Epstein-Barr virus, and coxsackievirus have also been discovered to be causative factors.[9] The incidence is increased up to 1000-fold in patients infected with human immunodeficiency virus (HIV).[3] The pathogenesis of TEN/SJS is thought to involve impaired capacity to detoxify drug metabolites and genetic susceptibility.[8]

SJS has a lower mortality rate (5%) than TEN, which has a mortality rate of up to 40%.[22] Loss of epithelial integrity, severe fluid loss, sepsis, and respiratory tract denudation are major complications.[22] Severe ophthalmic involvement may lead to permanent scarring and blindness.[8]

■ Exfoliative Erythroderma

Exfoliative erythroderma, or generalized exfoliative dermatitis, is a serious reaction associated with systemic toxicity.[1] It is a generalized, scaly, erythematous eruption involving more than 90% of the skin.[8] Patients present with generalized erythema and pruritus accompanied by fever and malaise.[4] The condition is associated with psoriasis, atopic dermatitis, cutaneous T-cell lymphoma ("red man syndrome"), and drug hypersensitivity reactions.[23] Scaling appears 2 to 6 days after the onset of erythema, usually starting on skin creases.[24] Thirty percent of cases are idiopathic.[24] Progression of the rash is related to the underlying cause: in patients with erythroderma attributed to psoriasis or dermatitis, the rash usually evolves slowly over months to years, whereas acute onset and rapid spread may be observed in patients with drug reactions or malignant diseases.[23] Fluid and protein loss through the skin can lead to hypotension, electrolyte losses, edema, and high-output cardiac failure.[8] These complications can cause significant morbidity, given that this disease is more prevalent in persons who are more than 40 years old.[24] Mortality varies according to the underlying illnesses precipitating the rash.

■ MACULES/PAPULES

Maculopapular rashes are perhaps the most commonly seen morphologic type encountered in clinical practice. These eruptions are most frequently seen in viral illnesses, immune complex–mediated syndromes, and drug eruptions.[3] Several life-threatening infections, such as acute meningococcemia, RMSF, and viral hemorrhagic fevers, can initially manifest with erythematous macules and papules that evolve into petechiae. Centrally distributed rashes, with truncal primary lesions, are the most common type of eruption.[1]

■ Typhoid Fever

Typhoid fever (or enteric fever), a nonrickettsial disease caused by *Salmonella typhi,* is usually acquired during travel outside the United States. The classic presentation includes fever, leukopenia, malaise, abdominal pain, constipation, and bradycardia.[2] Characteristic pink macules and papules that blanch under pressure, described as "rose spots," appear on the trunk and abdomen.[3] These lesions are usually oval or circular, sparse, and up to 1 cm in diameter.[2]

Rickettsial Infections

Many rickettsial infections manifest initially with a nonspecific macular eruption. RMSF is discussed earlier.

Patients with African tick bite fever *(Rickettsia africae)* and Mediterranean spotted fever *(R. conorii)* present with fever, headache, lymphadenitis, and myalgias, and approximately half these patients have a macular rash.[25] Multiple *inoculation eschars,* which are black crusts surrounded by a red halo at the site of a tick bite, are present in most cases but are easily missed.[26]

Classic epidemic typhus *(R. prowazekii)* presents with a macular rash beginning on the trunk and spreading to the extremities while sparing the face, palms, and soles.[2] The clinical onset is usually abrupt after an incubation period of approximately 14 days, and patients present with fever, severe headache, myalgias, and arthralgias.[27] Pulmonary complications are common and include interstitial pneumonia, noncardiogenic pulmonary edema, and secondary bacterial pneumonia.[27] Typhus typically occurs in situations that promote infestations with body lice, in which hygiene and sanitation practices are compromised, such as war, famine, or natural disasters.[1]

Lyme Disease

Lyme disease is the most common vector-borne infectious disease in the United States.[6] The pathognomonic skin manifestation of Lyme disease, *erythema chronicum migrans,* often occurs at or near the site of a tick bite and develops in almost 80% of affected patients 7 to 10 days after inoculation.[4] The lesion starts as a papule and expands to an erythematous annular lesion that may exhibit central clearing (bull's eye), averaging 15 cm in diameter but possibly reaching up to 50 cm.[1] The appearance of erythema chronicum migrans is part of stage 1 (early localized) of the disease, in conjunction with influenza-like symptoms of fever, malaise, arthralgia, headache, and cough.[11] Patients with early disseminated Lyme disease (stage 2) often exhibit multiple, smaller lesions in a more generalized distribution.[3] These lesions appear a few weeks after the initial infection, with fever, cough, pharyngitis, adenopathy, and central nervous system symptoms.[11]

Mycoplasma Pneumonia

Mycoplasma pneumoniae accounts for approximately 10% to 30% of cases of community-acquired pneumonia.[28] Infection can manifest in a variety of dermatologic manifestations. Patents commonly present with a generalized macular or morbilliform rash, as well as with urticarial variants.[2] SJS occurs in up to 7% of patients with pneumonia caused by *Mycoplasma.*[29]

Psittacosis

Infection with *Chlamydophila psittaci* should be suspected in a patient with atypical pneumonia and bird exposure.[2] Formerly labeled with the genus name *Chlamydia, C. psittaci* and *C. pneumoniae* occur with a prevalence of 3% to 20% of cases of community-acquired pneumonia.[28] Dermatologic findings include pink, blanching macules and papules called *Horder's spots,* which resemble the rose spots of typhoid fever. Psittacosis manifests with nonspecific symptoms initially, but after 1 week the systemic nature of the illness becomes evident, with rash, pericarditis/myocarditis, hepatitis, hemolytic anemia, arthritis, confusion, ataxia, and meningitis. Compared with *Mycoplasma pneumoniae* pneumonia, complications are more prevalent, and resolution times are longer.[28]

Leptospirosis

Leptospirosis is a zoonotic disease caused by the spirochete *Leptospira* and transmitted by exposure to water contaminated with the urine of infected mammals, particularly livestock. Almost 90% of exposed patients have a mild, anicteric, subclinical presentation. The diseased patient has an initial flulike illness that resolves in 4 to 7 days. Patients may present with a macular or maculopapular rash, conjunctivitis, abdominal pain, severe myalgias, and adenopathy. On resolution of this initial phase, profound jaundice, renal dysfunction, hepatic necrosis, pulmonary distress, and hemorrhagic diathesis may follow, a syndrome called *Weil's disease.*

Viruses

Many different viral infections manifest acutely with macules and papules. These infections include acute HIV infection, dengue fever, West Nile virus infection, parvovirus B19 infection, and the classic childhood exanthems rubeola (measles), rubella (German measles), and roseola. Primary HIV infection is characterized by fever, adenopathy, myalgias and arthralgias, diarrhea, nausea and vomiting, and weight loss with deep red macular/papular lesions appearing within the first 5 days of the acute illness.

Dengue fever, not the hemorrhagic presentation, manifests as a nonspecific viral syndrome with fevers, headaches, myalgias and arthralgias, cough, sore throat, and rash. Initially, diffuse skin flushing occurs, followed by a maculopapular rash that begins on the trunk and spreads to the extremities and the face.[25] Dengue, caused by a flavivirus, is found in most tropical and subtropical regions of the world and is transmitted by mosquito bites.

Another flaviviral mosquito-borne illness, West Nile fever, can manifest with an erythematous macular and papular eruption involving the neck, trunk, or the extremities in approximately 20% of affected patients. The diagnosis is based on a high index of suspicion in patients who are more than 50 years old and who have a sudden onset of febrile illness with a change in mental status during late summer.

Human parvovirus B19 infection (erythema infectiosum) is primarily a childhood illness characterized by mild, nonspecific symptoms of fever, coryza, and malaise, followed by bright, blanchable erythema on the face ("slapped cheeks") with a subsequent lacy, red eruption on the extremities and trunk. In adults, particularly immunosuppressed individuals, parvovirus infection can result in more severe symptoms.[25] The fever and constitutional symptoms tend to be worse in adults, and acute arthropathy often occurs, usually affecting the hands, wrists, knees, and ankles. The slapped-cheek feature is frequently absent, and only the lacy, macular rash is seen on the extremities.[3] Fetal hydrops and fetal loss can develop in pregnant women.[25] In patients with hemolytic anemia, hemoglobinopathy, or immunodeficiency, human parvovirus B19 infection can lead to transient aplastic crisis, persistent arthritis, and neurologic disease. A rare but noteworthy dermatologic manifestation is called *papular-purpuric gloves and socks syndrome.* This syndrome is characterized by rapidly progressive, painful, and pruritic symmetrical swelling and erythema of the hands and feet, with sharp margins at the wrists and ankles. Mucosal involvement has been described, with petechiae and pustules on the palate, buccal erosions, and lip swelling.[3] This syndrome usually clears within 2 weeks.

Of the classic pediatric viral exanthems manifesting with macular and papular lesions, rubeola (measles) usually causes more severe symptoms, particularly in unvaccinated children or in immunosuppressed patients. Worldwide, measles was the eighth leading cause of death in 1990.[1] It begins with a typical viral syndrome, followed by prominent cough, coryza, and conjunctivitis.[21] The rash begins around the fourth febrile day, with discrete lesions that become confluent spreading from the hairline caudally and sparing the palms and soles.[6] *Koplik's spots,* which are 1- to 3-mm, whitish or grayish elevations with an erythematous base seen on the buccal mucosa, are pathognomonic for measles and appear during the first 2 days of the illness. Morbidity and mortality result from respiratory and neurologic complications, including pneumonia, tracheobronchitis, and postinfectious encephalomyelitis.

Erythema Multiforme

Erythema multiforme is the most common papulomacular eruption with a peripheral distribution. This acute, self-limited rash is usually mild, with low morbidity and no mortality. The most characteristic features are so-called *target lesions,* round to oval macules and papules with central erythema surrounded by a narrow ring of normal-appearing skin that is, in turn, surrounded by another thin ring of erythema. Lesions are symmetrically distributed on the elbows, knees, palms, and soles. Most cases are secondary to prior infection with herpes simplex virus or drug reactions.[22] Presentations with blistering and mucosal involvement are referred to as *erythema multiforme major,* an entity thought to be indistinguishable from SJS.

VESICLES/BULLAE

Viruses, such as herpes viruses, varicella-zoster virus, and variola virus, are (or have been, in the case of variola) common causes of vesicles and bullae. Bullous and pustular lesions in septic patients are suggestive of bacteremia.

Herpes Simplex

Herpes simplex virus infection is the most common cause of vesiculobullous lesions. This infection is characterized by clusters of vesicles on an erythematous base.[3] Disseminated infection may occur in immunocompromised patients or in neonates with congenital infection.[6] Lesions are numerous and are not confined to a particular dermatome. Visceral dissemination, especially liver involvement, may occur in patients with only limited skin lesions.[1] Patients with underlying eczema may develop superinfection of skin lesions with herpes virus, a condition known as *eczema herpeticum.*[2]

Varicella

Varicella-zoster virus is responsible for varicella (chickenpox) and herpes zoster (shingles). Patients with primary infection present with chickenpox, a generally mild illness in children that can cause more severe features in adults and in immunocompromised patients.[6] A prodrome of fever and malaise precedes the appearance of pruritic, erythematous macules on the face and scalp that vesiculate and crust over. Any one area of the rash has lesions at various stages of development. Complications include meningitis, encephalitis, ataxia, pneumonia, myocarditis, and bacterial superinfection of skin lesions.

Variola

Smallpox is caused by the variola virus and no longer exists in the natural state; the last naturally occurring case was documented in 1977. However, there is increasing concern that smallpox may be used as a weapon of bioterrorism. The prodrome of smallpox includes high fever, malaise, myalgias, and headache.[3] Skin lesions appear 2 to 4 days later beginning as red macules on the oral mucosa and spreading to the face, followed by the extremities, including the palms and soles.[29] Within 1 to 2 days, the rash becomes vesicular and pustular. The pustules are round, firm, and deeply imbedded in the skin.[3] These pustules eventually crust over and heal with pitted scars. The prominent distribution of lesions on the face and extremities (including palms and soles) and the fact that they all appear at same stage of development help to differentiate smallpox from chickenpox.[1] Individuals receiving vaccinia virus immunization for smallpox prevention may rarely develop a widespread vesicular/pustular rash *(generalized vaccinia)* or dissemination of the virus within atopic skin lesions *(eczema vaccinatum)*.[3]

■ *Vibrio vulnificus* Infection

Vibrio vulnificus and other noncholera *Vibrio* bacteria can cause focal bullous skin lesions and sepsis in susceptible hosts, such as patients with underlying liver disease, renal dysfunction, or diabetes.[7] Septic patients present with fever, chills, hypotension, and hemorrhagic bullous lesions with associated cellulitis on the extremities. Infection is commonly acquired through the consumption of raw or undercooked shellfish, especially oysters, or exposure of exposed skin to contaminated seawater.[25] The time of onset of symptoms after exposure to the bacteria is short (hours to a couple of days), and progression of sepsis is rapid. Mortality is extremely high (~50%) despite timely antibiotic therapy.[1] *V. vulnificus* infection should be strongly considered in ill-appearing patients who have recently consumed raw seafood and who have a history of liver disease or other immunocompromising states.[3]

■ Bacteremia

In addition to *V. vulnificus*, bullous and pustular skin lesions associated with sepsis are suggestive of other disseminated bacterial infections. Staphylococcal bacteremia and gonococcemia may manifest with a widespread pustular eruption.[2] Group A streptococcal skin infection with fasciitis may also produce bullous lesions.[3] Scattered hemorrhagic vesicles and bullae can be seen in disseminated pseudomonal infection in approximately 15% to 40% of cases.[3] Another dermatologic manifestation of pseudomonal sepsis is *ecthyma gangrenosum:* hemorrhagic vesicles surrounded by a rim of erythema with central necrosis and ulceration that subsequently slough off and leave a gray-black eschar.[7] These lesions are most common in the axillary, groin, and perianal regions.[1] Ecthyma gangrenosum has also been associated with sepsis caused by other gram-negative bacteria *(Aeromonas, Serratia, Klebsiella)*, as well as with disseminated fungal infections.[3]

■ NODULES

Nodular lesions reflect disease of the dermal skin layer. Nodules may arise as a result of hypersensitivity reactions, infections, or malignant diseases. In immunocompromised hosts with acute illness, widespread nodules may represent disseminated fungal infections or bacillary angiomatosis.[1] Noninfectious conditions such as erythema nodosum and febrile neutrophilic dermatosis (Sweet's syndrome) can also manifest acutely with nodular lesions.

■ Disseminated Fungal Infections

Candidal sepsis may manifest with the appearance of subcutaneous nodules in an immunocompromised patient with fever and myalgia.[6] The rash is seen in up to 13% of affected patients and consists of discrete, firm, nontender subcutaneous nodules diffusely spread, with facial sparing.[3] Patients with histoplasmosis, blastomycosis, cryptococcosis, coccidioidomycosis, and sporotrichosis may also present with similar lesions in the setting of disseminated disease. Cryptococcal infection in patients with the acquired immunodeficiency syndrome may cause umbilicated nodules resembling molluscum contagiosum.[3] Necrotic nodules on the face and extremities can be seen in patients with mucormycosis and aspergillosis.[1]

■ Bacillary Angiomatosis

Bartonella species are gram-negative bacteria known to cause several clinical syndromes, particularly in immunocompromised patients. *Bartonella henselae* and *Bartonella quintana* cause bacteremia, endocarditis, and bacillary angiomatosis.[25] Cat-scratch disease is now known to be caused by *B. henselae*.[3] Bacillary angiomatosis is the most common manifestation of *Bartonella* infection in immunocompromised persons.[25] In patients with the acquired immunodeficiency syndrome, the infection causes fever, lymphadenopathy, abdominal pain, and cutaneous lesions.[3] The lesions may be elevated, friable, firm, bright red papules or subcutaneous nodules occurring anywhere on the body.[1] Bacteremia and hepatitis are common extracutaneous complications.[3]

■ Erythema Nodosum

Erythema nodosum is an acute inflammatory and immunologic process involving the panniculus adiposus (the fatty tissue layer underlying the skin), hence its alternative denomination panniculitis.[6] This condition is most likely a reaction to infections (especially streptococcal) and drugs (sulfonamides, oral contraceptives), and it has also been associated with autoimmune and malignant diseases.[22] It is more common in women, with a peak incidence between 15 and 30 years of age.[1] Systemic symptoms, including fever, myalgia, or arthralgia, may be present.[22] Skin lesions are painful red or brown nodules, varying in size between 2 and 6 cm and characteristically appearing on the anterior aspect of the legs and arms.[4] The course of the disease depends on the underlying cause, and the nodules may persist for up to 6 weeks.[6]

Sweet's Syndrome

Also known as febrile neutrophilic dermatosis, Sweet's syndrome is an unusual hypersensitivity disorder characterized by tender, red or blue edematous nodules, usually on the face, neck, and upper extremities.[4] A solitary, erythematous plaque with vesicular or pustular features may be seen initially. Patients may be febrile and appear ill with headache and arthralgia, and rare eye involvement such as conjunctivitis or episcleritis may be observed.[3] Most cases are idiopathic, but underlying malignant diseases, especially leukemia, are found to be the cause in 10% to 20% of patients.[1] Other causes include autoimmune disorders (inflammatory bowel disease, lupus, rheumatoid arthritis, thyroiditis) and pregnancy. The diagnosis of Sweet's syndrome is one of exclusion. Infections, neoplasia, and vasculitis must be excluded, and the lesions are difficult to distinguish from erythema nodosum. Patients with hematologic malignant diseases may present with anemia or thrombocytopenia with hemorrhagic skin lesions.[3] Patients with idiopathic cases respond to a 2-week tapering course of oral prednisone.

URTICARIA

Urticarial eruptions are very common and are usually hypersensitivity reactions without associated fever. Hives or wheals are red, raised, blanching, evanescent plaques caused by multiple factors.[4] Allergic reactions produce a spectrum of signs and symptoms that range from urticarial skin lesions and angioedema to bronchospasm, respiratory failure, and cardiovascular collapse. *Anaphylaxis* can be defined as the presence of allergic symptoms such as urticaria with either respiratory difficulty or hemodynamic instability (presyncope, syncope, hypotension) or both. Allergic urticaria usually resolves within 48 hours; longer-lasting or recurrent urticarial lesions accompanied by fever and constitutional symptoms are usually associated with an underlying infection, malignant disease, or autoimmune disorder.[1] *Mycoplasma* infection and Lyme disease may cause urticarial eruptions. Viral causes include enteroviruses, adenovirus, HIV, and hepatitis viruses.[2]

Differential Diagnosis

Several rapidly fatal diseases are associated with petechial rashes and purpuric lesions. Meningococcemia, RMSF, and bacterial septic shock are the main concerns and should be at the top of the differential diagnosis. Any febrile patient with a petechial rash should be suspected of having acute meningococcemia and should be treated promptly with antibiotics after blood cultures are obtained. A less fulminant course may be seen in septic shock from other bacterial sources. Patients with RMSF may not display skin lesions until the third or fourth day after the initial prodrome. Starting antibiotics on or before the fifth day of illness is an important factor in decreasing mortality: 3% to 7% versus 30% to 70%.[12] The presence of mucosal or gastrointestinal hemorrhage suggests a viral hemorrhagic fever. Finally, the diagnosis of thrombocytopenic thrombotic purpura should always be considered in the presence of thrombocytopenia, neurologic dysfunction, renal failure, and lower extremity petechiae or purpura because rapid diagnosis and treatment with plasma exchange transfusion are lifesaving.

The presence of generalized erythema is also a worrisome finding, particularly in the hypotensive patient. Toxic shock syndrome, both staphylococcal and streptococcal, is the initial working diagnosis. Hypotension develops rapidly, often within hours, after the onset of illness. Clinical evaluation confirms the diagnosis because toxic shock is defined by clinical criteria: fever, rash, hypotension, and multiorgan involvement. In streptococcal toxic shock, a pyogenic focus of infection is usually present and can result in necrotizing fasciitis, with localized swelling, tenderness, and erythema with subsequent formation of bullae. Scaling or desquamation is an important clinical feature accompanying generalized or localized erythema. TEN/SJS must be recognized quickly in patients with mucocutaneous involvement. Targetoid skin lesions and erythema with mucocutaneous involvement and subsequent desquamation warrant aggressive treatment. In pediatric patients with an infectious prodrome who present with a scarlatiniform rash, blistering skin lesions, or localized desquamation, streptococcal or staphylococcal infection should be suspected. Widespread erythema, scaling, and pruritus suggest exfoliative erythroderma in elderly patients.

Maculopapular rashes can be nonspecific signs in a variety of illnesses. Most patients presenting with these rashes and acute symptoms have a disorder of infectious origin, primarily viral. Acute HIV infection should be suspected. However, bacterial sepsis cannot be excluded. The presence of target-like lesions should elicit a search for mucous and conjunctival involvement as a harbinger of SJS.

Vesicular rashes are usually the result of disseminated viral infection, particularly in immunosuppressed individuals. Pustule formation can also be seen in these cases, but staphylococcemia and gonococcemia should be considered as well. Bullous lesions can be caused by local streptococcal infection or *V. vulnificus* sepsis. Generalized nodular eruptions suggest systemic fungal or *Bartonella* infections.

Generalized urticaria, hypotension, and respiratory distress are cardinal features of anaphylaxis. This condition should be recognized immediately because treatment with epinephrine is lifesaving.

Approach to the Acutely Ill Patient with Rash

Patients should be rapidly assessed for the presence of fever, toxic appearance, and abnormalities of vital signs. Any history of immunosuppression should be elicited, such as HIV infection, diabetes, malignant disease, chronic alcoholism, or organ transplantation. Isolation precautions should be instituted initially in all patients, and universal infection control precautions should be scrupulously taken by all personnel involved in the care of these patients. Once appropriate resuscitation measures are started, a quick and thorough skin inspection should be performed to identify the morphology and distribution of skin lesions. Petechiae/purpura should be identified quickly because their presence portends several rapidly fatal diseases. Similarly, anaphylaxis should be recognized rapidly, to allow expeditious treatment with epinephrine, antihistamines, and intravenous fluid administration. Infectious causes are otherwise the primary focus of diagnostic and therapeutic interventions. Sepsis is the initial working diagnosis in the majority of cases.

Cultures of blood, urine, cerebrospinal fluid, or wounds are obtained as clinically indicated. Broad-spectrum antimicrobial therapy is instituted early and empirically. This treatment should include antiviral and antifungal agents if the rash suggests a viral or fungal illness, particularly in immunosuppressed patients. Recognition of fasciitis is essential for early surgical consultation and aggressive débridement. Patients with extensive blistering and desquamation need close attention to fluid management, maintenance of electrolyte and temperature homeostasis, and infection control measures. Early dermatologic consultation is warranted in patients with TEN/SJS, adjunctive ophthalmologic evaluation is required for patients with ocular involvement.

Tips and Tricks

- Patients with fever and rash must be quickly evaluated for the presence of toxic appearance and vital sign abnormalities.
- Petechial rashes and purpuric lesions in ill patients constitute a true emergency.
- Thrombotic thrombocytopenic purpura should be suspected and aggressively treated in patients with thrombocytopenia, neurologic symptoms, and renal dysfunction.
- Bacteremia and sepsis are common causes of all morphologic types of rash.
- Tick-borne illnesses should always be part of the differential diagnosis in these patients, particularly patients with a suggestive travel or exposure history.
- Always look for mucosal involvement, especially in patients with target lesions suggestive of erythema multiforme.
- Do not forget to obtain ophthalmologic consultation in patients with Stevens-Johnson syndrome and ocular involvement.
- Treat patients with urticaria who have signs and symptoms of anaphylaxis aggressively, with epinephrine and hemodynamic support.

Disposition

Most, if not all, patients presenting with acute illness and rash need admission. Patients with frank sepsis need continued treatment and evaluation in a monitored setting, preferably the intensive care unit. Patients with extensive blistering and desquamation require care in a burn unit. A diagnosis of anaphylaxis mandates close observation for at least 24 hours because recurrences are common.

REFERENCES

1. Kaye ET, Kaye KM: Fever and rash. In Kasper DL, Braunwald E, Fauci AS, et al (eds): Harrison's Principles of Internal Medicine, 16th ed, vol 1. New York, McGraw-Hill, 2005, pp 108-116.
2. Schlossberg D: Fever and rash. Infect Dis Clin North Am 1996;10:101-110.
3. Weber DJ, Cohen MS, Rutala WA: The acutely ill patient with fever and rash. In Mandell GL, Bennett JE, Dolin R (eds): Mandell's Principles and Practice of Infectious Disease, 6th ed, vol 1. Philadelphia, Churchill Livingstone, 2005, pp 729-746.
4. Gropper CA: An approach to clinical dermatologic diagnosis based on morphologic reaction patterns. Clin Cornerstone 2001;4:1-14.
5. Habif TP: Clinical Dermatology: A Color Guide to Diagnosis and Treatment, 4th ed. Philadelphia, Mosby, 2004, pp 457-496.
6. McKinnon HD, Howard T: Evaluating the febrile patient with a rash. Am Fam Physician 2000;62:804-816.
7. Barlam TF, Kasper DL: Approach to the acutely ill infected febrile patient. In Kasper DL, Braunwald E, Fauci AS, et al (eds): Harrison's Principles of Internal Medicine, 16th ed, vol 1. New York, McGraw-Hill, 2005, pp 706-712.
8. Freiman A, Borsuk D, Sasseville D: Dermatologic emergencies. CMAJ 2005;173:1317-1319.
9. Buddin DA, Beddingfield FC: Recognizing emergent dermatologic conditions. Emerg Med 2004;3:26-35.
10. Hazelzet JA: Diagnosing meningococcemia as a cause of sepsis. Pediatr Crit Care Med 2005;6(Suppl):S50-S54.
11. Bratton RL, Corey G: Tick borne disease. Am Fam Physician 2005;71:2323-2330.
12. Sexton DJ, Kaye KS: Tick borne diseases. Med Clin North Am 2002;86:351-360.
13. Masters EJ: Rocky Mountain spotted fever: A clinician's dilemma. Arch Intern Med 2003;163:769-774.
14. Park MK: Cardiovascular Infections: In Park MK (ed): Pediatric Cardiology for Practitioners, 4th ed. Philadelphia, Mosby, 2002, pp 281-303.
15. Rice PA: Gonococcal arthritis (disseminated gonococcal infection). Infect Dis Clin North Am 2005;19:853-861.
16. Mehrany K, Kist JM, O'Connor WJ, et al: Disseminated gonococcemia. Int J Dermatol 2003;42:208-209.
17. Pigott DC: Hemorrhagic fever viruses. Crit Care Clin North Am 2005;21:765-783.
18. Tsai HM: Advances in the pathogenesis, diagnosis, and treatment of thrombotic thrombocytopenic purpura. J Am Soc Nephrol 2003;14:1072-1081.
19. Nabhan C, Kwaan HC: Current concepts in the diagnosis and management of thrombotic thrombocytopenic purpura. Hematol Oncol Clin North Am 2003;17:177-199.
20. Nelson C: Early recognition and treatment of staphylococcal and streptococcal toxic shock. J Pediatr Adolesc Gynecol 2004;17:289-292.

21. Blackwood CL: Rash and fever in an ill-appearing child. Am Fam Physician 2004;70:361-363.
22. McKenna JK, Leiferman KM: Dermatologic drug reactions. Immunol Allergy Clin North Am 2004;24:399-423.
23. Rothe MJ, Bialy TL, Grant-Kels JM: Erythroderma. Dermatol Clin North Am 2000;18:405-415.
24. Umar SH: Erythroderma (generalized exfoliative dermatitis). eMed Online Dermatol 2006. Available at www.emedicine.com.
25. Elston DM: New and emerging infectious diseases. J Am Acad Dermatol 2005;52:1062-1068.
26. Jensenius M, Fournier PE, Kelly P, et al: African tick bite fever. Lancet Infect Dis 2003;3:557-564.
27. Raoult D, Woodward T, Dumler JS: The history of epidemic typhus. Infect Dis Clin North Am 2004;18:127-140.
28. Weyers CM, Leeper KV: Nonresolving pneumonia. Clin Chest Med 2005;26:143-158.
29. Baum SG: Mycoplasma pneumonia and atypical pneumonia. In Mandell GL, Bennett JE, Dolin R (eds): Mandell's Principles and Practice of Infectious Disease, 6th ed., vol 2. Philadelphia, Churchill Livingstone, 2005, pp 2271-2280.

Chapter **192**

Localized Rashes, Generalized Rashes, and Pediatric Exanthems

David N. Zull, David Salzman, and Jamie Collings

KEY POINTS

Mucous membrane involvement in the form of ulcers and erosions suggests Stevens-Johnson syndrome, toxic epidermal necrolysis, or pemphigus, all of which are life-threatening conditions.

Many small or pinpoint ulcers suggest viral infections such as with coxsackievirus or varicella.

Drug reactions, contact dermatitis, and viral exanthems constitute the majority of diffuse rashes seen in an ED.

The distribution or geography of lesions provides valuable clues: dermatomal, herpes zoster; exposed areas, photodermatitis; palms and soles, erythema migrans, syphilis; well-demarcated, nondermatomal lesions, contact dermatitis; groin or crural lesions, tinea, intertrigo; scalp and ears, seborrheic dermatitis; following Langer's lines on the trunk, pityriasis rosea.

Drug reactions can follow many different patterns and may be associated with numerous conditions: generalized maculopapular, urticaria, erythema multiforme, acute generalized exanthematous pustulosis, drug rash with eosinophilia and systemic symptoms, acneiform, fixed, exfoliative erythroderma, Stevens-Johnson syndrome, and toxic epidermal necrolysis.[1]

Contact dermatitis can be allergic, from prior sensitization, or irritant, from chemical injury.

Purpura that is palpable suggests concomitant inflammation resulting from vasculitis.

Purpura with fever is always life-threatening (meningococcemia, Rocky Mountain spotted fever, thrombotic thrombocytopenic purpura).

Topical steroids are available in four strengths: mild (hydrocortisone), medium (triamcinolone), high (fluocinonide), ultrahigh (betamethasone, clobetasol).

Only low-potency steroids should be used on the face, but steroid creams should be avoided completely on the eyelids.

Seborrheic dermatitis is the only dermatitis in which topical steroids should be avoided.

High- and ultrahigh-strength steroid creams should be reserved for resistant lesions, lichenified areas, and hand lesions.

Systemic steroids are contraindicated in psoriasis and toxic epidermal necrolysis.

Pathophysiology

The skin is divided into three layers: the epidermis, the dermis, and the subcutaneous tissue. Most skin lesions involve one or more of the following alterations in skin anatomy: inflammation in the dermis (erythema), edema of the dermis (papular), death and separation of epidermal layers or the epidermal-dermal junction with exudation of fluid into the space (vesicular), hypertrophy of the epidermis with desquamation (papulosquamous), hemorrhage (purpuric), or vasculitis of dermal and subcutaneous arterioles.

Skin lesions result from injuries to the epidermal barrier (contact dermatitis), immune complex deposition, hypersensitivity reaction with cytokine release by T cells, vasculitis with vascular leaking, photosensitization, and hereditary disorders. The various types of skin lesions are described in Box 192-1.

Presenting Signs and Symptoms

Patients present with skin conditions as the primary complaint because of pruritus, pain, drainage, or unsightly appearance. Other presenting possibilities are systemic symptoms (fever, myalgias, arthralgias, headache) as primary complaints and skin conditions as secondary issues. The history and physical examination are extremely important, and Box 192-2 and the box "Red Flags: Identifying Potentially Life-Threatening Skin Eruptions" detail areas of focus.

RED FLAGS

Identifying Potentially Life-Threatening Skin Eruptions

- Does the patient appear sick or toxic? Is fever present? Does the patient have systemic symptoms such as fatigue, myalgia, arthralgia, malaise, nausea, or headache?
- Is mucous membrane involvement evident? Does the patient have oral erosions or ulcers? Does the patient have mucosal bleeding and crusted blood in the mouth or nose? Is the tongue swollen and red? Are the lips raw and pealing? Are the conjunctivae injected (Stevens-Johnson syndrome, toxic epidermal necrolysis)?
- Does the patient have vesicle or pustule formation? Does the skin slough easily with lateral pressure (Nikolsky's sign)? Is denuded skin present?
- Is the rash generalized and confluent, intensely erythematous, and indurated (early manifestation of exfoliative dermatitis, toxic epidermal necrolysis, Stevens-Johnson syndrome)?
- Does the patient have dry peeling of skin resembling sunburn on areas of intense erythema (exfoliative dermatitis, toxic shock syndrome)?
- Are petechiae or ecchymoses present? Do lesions evolve from macules and papules to purpura? Are skin lesions nonblanching? Is the purpuric lesion palpable or nonpalpable?

Adapted from Freiman A, Borsuk D, Sasseville D: Dermatologic emergencies. CMAJ 2005;173:1317-1319.

BOX 192-1
Types of Skin Lesions

Macule: Skin discoloration without elevation, not palpable; any shape, size, or margin

Papule: A lesion that is superficial, solid, raised, palpable, less than 1 cm in diameter

Maculopapular: Rash consisting of macules and papules that coalesce

Morbilliform: Generalized, intensely erythematous, macules and papules, tending to confluence, prominent on the trunk, head, and neck and resembling measles

Plaque: Confluence of papules forming a plateau-like elevation, well defined, larger than 1 cm in diameter

Nodule: Solid lesion with depth; larger, deeper, and better defined than a papule

Wheal: Erythematous lesions that are evanescent, flat-topped or rounded, raised, with serpiginous margins

Vesicles: Skin elevation containing serous fluid, less than 1 cm in diameter

Bullae: Vesicles greater than 1 cm in diameter

Herpetiform: Clustering to small vesicles resembling herpes simplex

Pustules: Skin elevations containing purulent fluid

Scales: Desquamation of epidermal cells forming flakes that can range in size from large membranes to fine, dustlike flecks

Papulosquamous: A rash consisting of papules with scales

Crusts: Dried serum, blood, or purulent exudate on the skin surface

Petechiae: Circumscribed deposits of blood less than 1 cm in diameter (usually 1 to 2 mm)

Purpura: Deposits of blood in the skin greater than 1 cm in diameter

Vasculitis: Palpable purpura with surrounding erythema

Fissure: A sharply defined crack in the skin extending into the dermis

Lichenification: Diffuse thickening and scaling of the skin resulting in accentuated skin markings and lines

Erythroderma: Generalized, intense erythema that is confluent, macular, or indurated

Infarct: A flat or depressed lesion that is firm or hard to the touch and black or brown

BOX 192-2

History and Physical Examination of the Patient with Rash

- Chief complaint
- Onset, rate of progression, and duration
- Exposure to medications (over-the-counter, prescription, or illicit agents)
- Food ingestion
- Exposure to animals, plants, chemicals, toxins, insects, or ill contacts
- Location of lesions and distribution (see Box 192-3)
- Pattern (dermatomal, linear, grouped, annular, arcuate, confluent, scattered, discrete, circular, or symmetrical; see Box 192-4)
- Lesion morphologic type (e.g., macule, papule, vesicle, purpura)
- Color (erythematous, violaceous, purple, or black)
- Margins and shape
- Consistency (palpable, indurated, flat, or atrophic)
- Variation in lesions or evolution noted
- Secondary lesions (excoriations, impetigo, or fissures)
- Signs of severe disease
- End-organ involvement (arthralgias, hematuria, jaundice, diarrhea, and photophobia)
- Angioedema of the lips, uvula, and palate

BOX 192-3

Differential Diagnosis by Location

Scalp: Seborrheic dermatitis, contact dermatitis, folliculitis, psoriasis, pediculosis

Face: Acne, seborrheic dermatitis, rosacea, contact dermatitis, lupus

Eyelids: Contact dermatitis, seborrheic dermatitis, atopic eczema, pediculosis, dermatomyositis

Ears: Contact dermatitis, seborrheic dermatitis, atopic eczema, lichen simplex chronicus

Neck: Atopic eczema, contact dermatitis, lichen simplex chronicus

Trunk: Drug eruption, pityriasis rosea, seborrheic dermatitis, psoriasis, contact dermatitis, secondary syphilis, tinea versicolor

Extensor areas: Psoriasis, eruptive xanthoma

Flexoral areas: Atopic dermatitis, candidiasis, intertrigo

Lower extremities: Erythema nodosum, Henoch-Schönlein purpura, pyoderma gangrenosum

Distal extremities: Photosensitivity, lichen planus, nummular eczema, contact dermatitis, Rocky Mountain spotted fever, lichen simplex chronicus, gonococcemia

Palms and soles: Erythema multiforme, secondary syphilis, Rocky Mountain spotted fever

Hands: Contact dermatitis, dyshidrotic eczema, erythema multiforme, secondary syphilis, psoriasis

Feet: Fungal infections, contact dermatitis (see Hands)

Penis: Contact dermatitis, fixed drug eruption, candidiasis, intertrigo, scabies, sexually transmitted disease

Groin: Tinea, candidiasis, intertrigo, scabies, pediculosis, contact dermatitis

Differential Diagnosis

In approaching a patient with a cutaneous eruption in the ED, the physician should first assess for potential life-threatening illness: systemic symptoms, mucosal involvement, total body involvement, diffuse desquamation or vesicle and pustule formation, and purpura (see box "Red Flags: Identifying Potentially Life-Threatening Skin Eruptions"). The next priority is narrowing the differential diagnosis. The most frequent cause of a generalized rash with or without fever is a drug eruption or allergic reaction. If a drug or allergy is not suspected and the patient is febrile, consider viral exanthems or bacterial toxin-mediated reactions. If the rash has well-demarcated margins that do not appear natural, contact reactions should be of primary concern. Most localized lesions either are contact reactions or are cellulitis or abscess. If the lesion is plaquelike with a fine scale (papulosquamous eruption), consider tinea corporis or early pityriasis rosea; a heavy scale suggests psoriasis. Clues to the differential diagnosis can be obtained by paying attention to the location and pattern (Boxes 192-3 and 192-4) combined with the type of lesion (Figs. 192-1 to 192-12, Boxes 192-5 and 192-6, and Table 192-1).

Diagnostic Studies

Patients with the potential for a life-threatening rash should undergo urinalysis, complete blood count, chemistry panel, and hepatic tests. Consider chest radiography and electrocardiography in elderly patients and in patients with severe systemic involvement. Leukocytoclastic vasculitis, serum sickness, and drug rash with eosinophilia and systemic symptoms can be associated with glomerulonephritis; therefore, urinalysis is an excellent screening tool, to

Text continued on p. 2019.

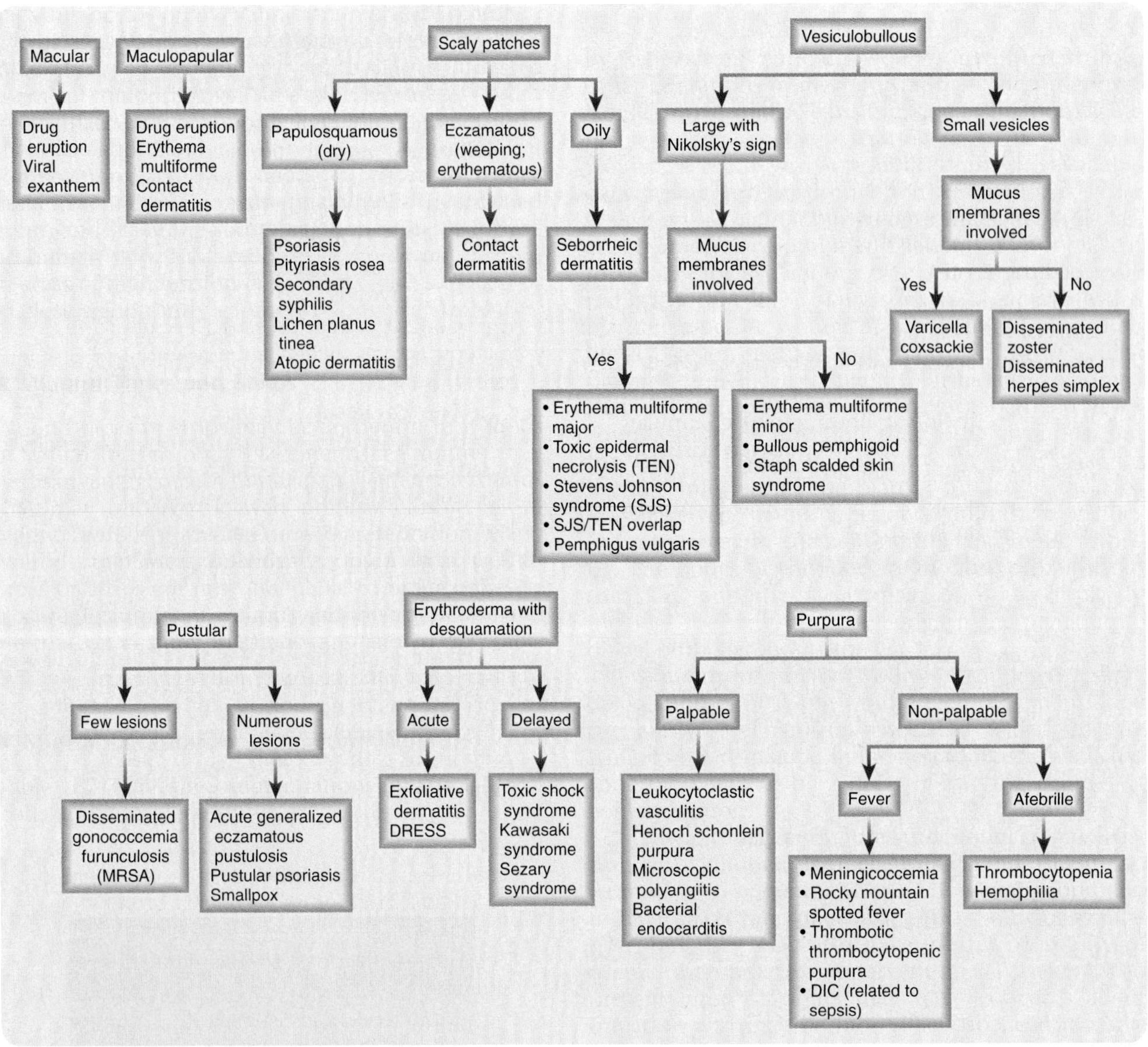
Macular
Drug eruption
Viral exanthem
Maculopapular
Drug eruption
Erythema multiforme
Contact dermatitis
Scaly patches
Papulosquamous (dry)
Psoriasis
Pityriasis rosea
Secondary syphilis
Lichen planus
tinea
Atopic dermatitis
Eczamatous (weeping; erythematous)
Contact dermatitis
Oily
Seborrheic dermatitis
Vesiculobullous
Large with Nikolsky's sign
Mucus membranes involved
Yes
No
• Erythema multiforme major
• Toxic epidermal necrolysis (TEN)
• Stevens Johnson syndrome (SJS)
• SJS/TEN overlap
• Pemphigus vulgaris
• Erythema multiforme minor
• Bullous pemphigoid
• Staph scalded skin syndrome
Small vesicles
Mucus membranes involved
Yes
No
Varicella coxsackie
Disseminated zoster
Disseminated herpes simplex
Pustular
Few lesions
Disseminated gonococcemia
furunculosis (MRSA)
Numerous lesions
Acute generalized eczamatous pustulosis
Pustular psoriasis
Smallpox
Erythroderma with desquamation
Acute
Exfoliative dermatitis
DRESS
Delayed
Toxic shock syndrome
Kawasaki syndrome
Sezary syndrome
Purpura
Palpable
Leukocytoclastic vasculitis
Henoch schonlein purpura
Microscopic polyangiitis
Bacterial endocarditis
Non-palpable
Fever
• Meningicoccemia
• Rocky mountain spotted fever
• Thrombotic thrombocytopenic purpura
• DIC (related to sepsis)
Afebrille
Thrombocytopenia
Hemophilia

FIGURE 192-1 Types of lesions.

BOX 192-4

Differential Diagnosis by Pattern of Lesions

Sun exposed: Phototoxic drug eruption, lupus
Dermatomal: Herpes zoster
Localized and demarcated: Contact reaction
Lesions in a row: Flea or bedbug bites
Streaks: Contact reactions (e.g., poison ivy or oak, jellyfish sting)
Cluster of vesicles: Herpes

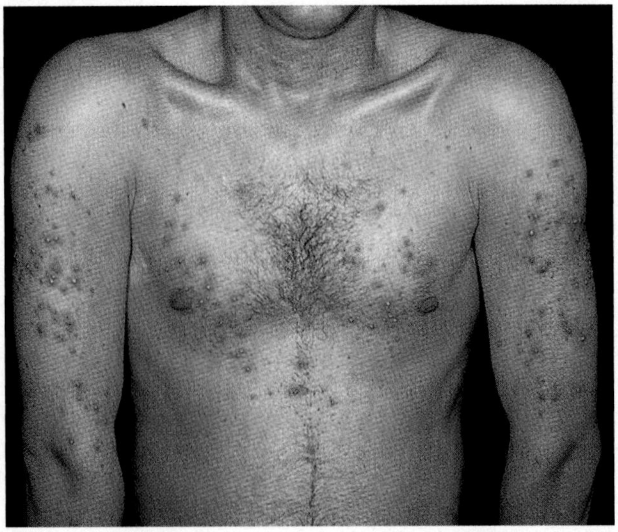

FIGURE 192-2 Acute generalized exanthematic pustulosis (AGEP), often the result of an immunologic reaction to ingested substances.

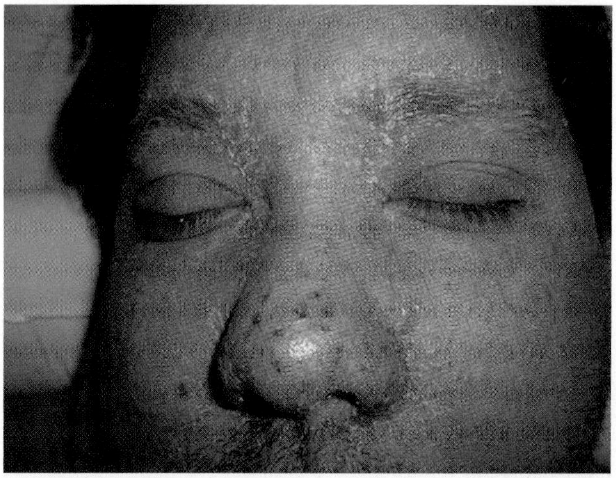

A

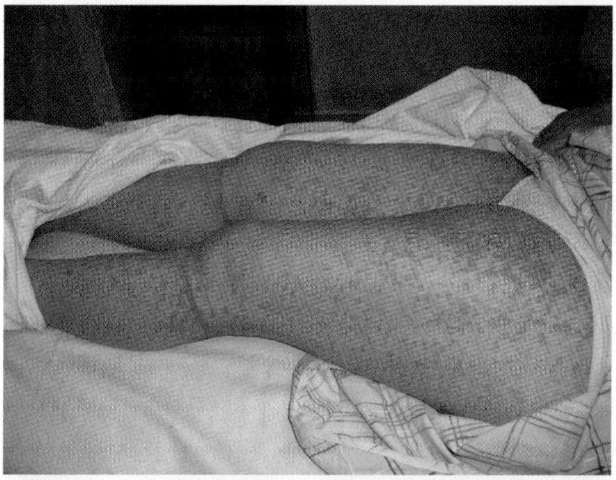

B

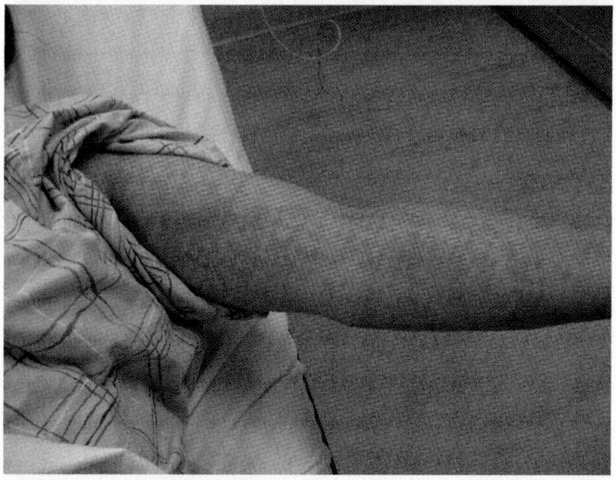

C

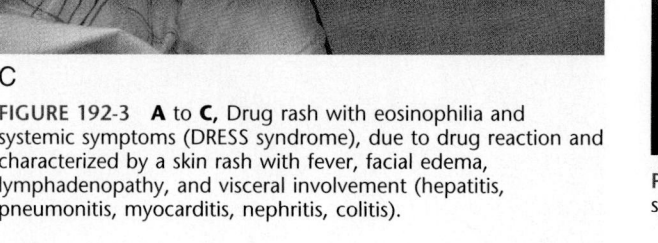

FIGURE 192-3 **A** to **C,** Drug rash with eosinophilia and systemic symptoms (DRESS syndrome), due to drug reaction and characterized by a skin rash with fever, facial edema, lymphadenopathy, and visceral involvement (hepatitis, pneumonitis, myocarditis, nephritis, colitis).

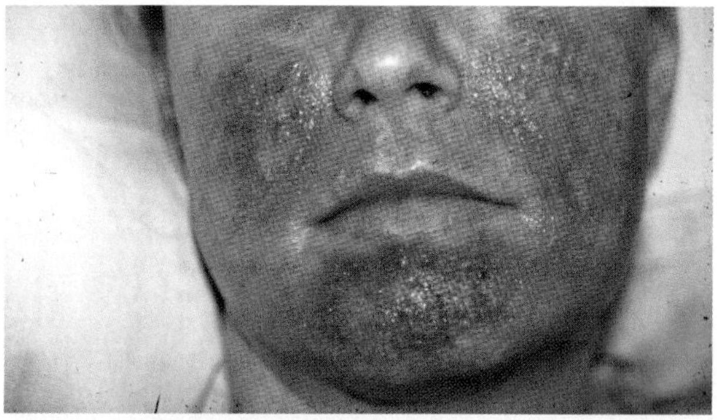

FIGURE 192-4 Eczema.

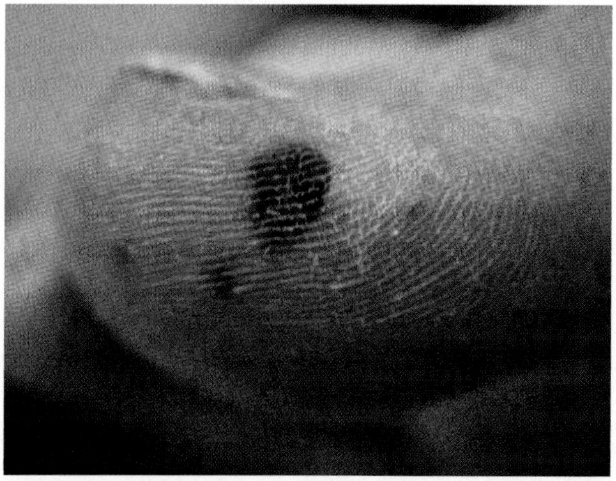

FIGURE 192-5 Endocarditis, causing microemboli.

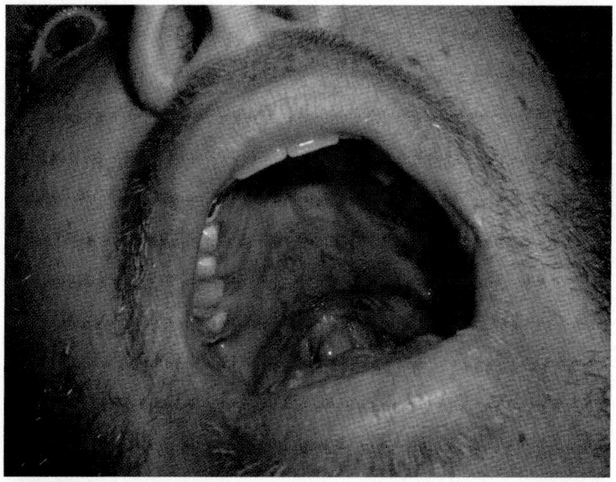

FIGURE 192-6 Erosion of the palate in Stevens-Johnson syndrome.

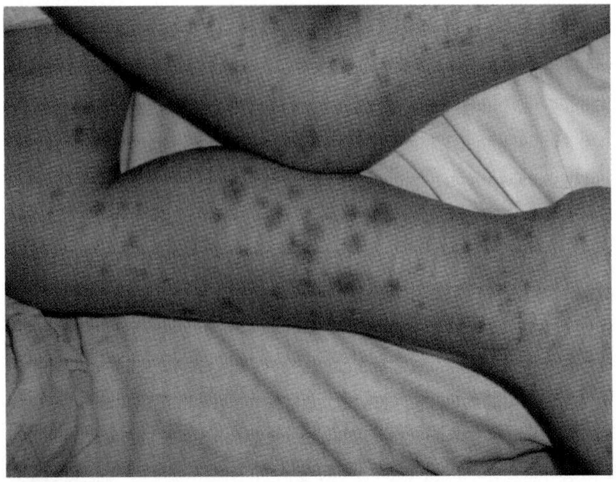

FIGURE 192-7 Henoch-Schönlein purpura, an immune-mediated disorder of unknown origin.

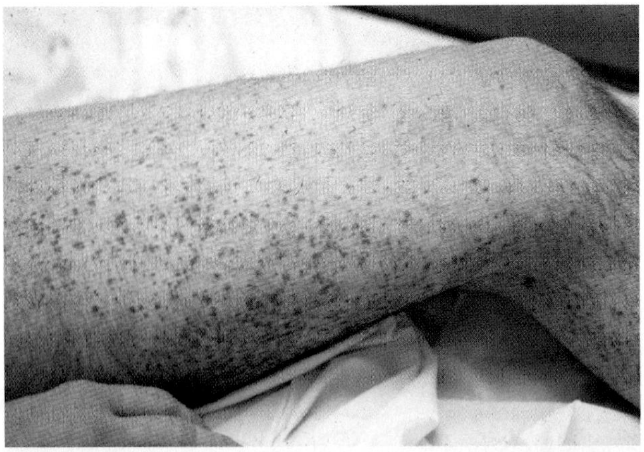

FIGURE 192-8 Leukocytoclastic reaction, immune mediated, of unknown origin.

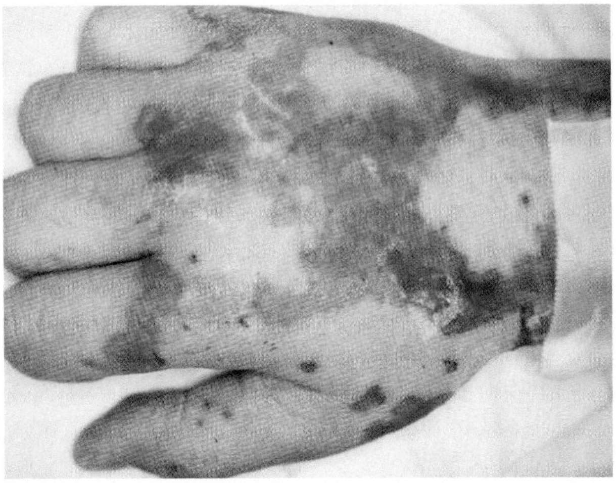

FIGURE 192-9 Meningococcal purpura fulminans in overwhelming meningococcal meningitis.

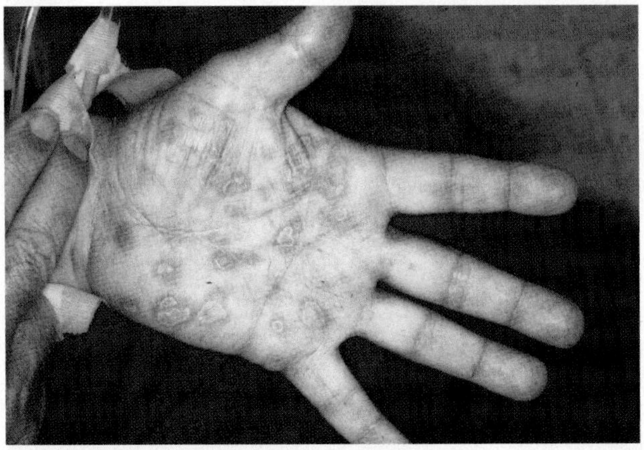

FIGURE 192-10 Secondary syphilis.

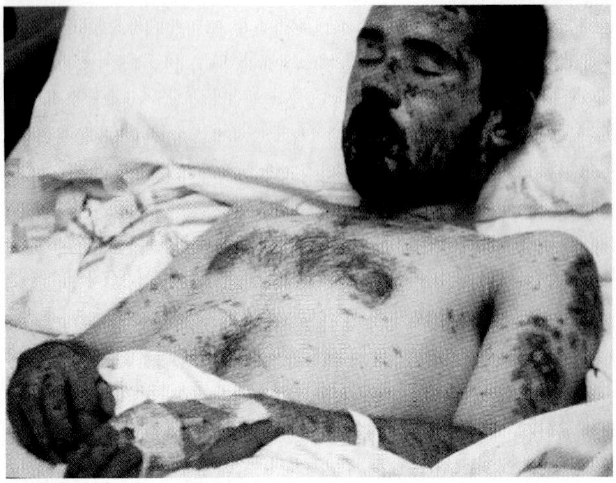

FIGURE 192-11 Toxic epidermal necrolysis.

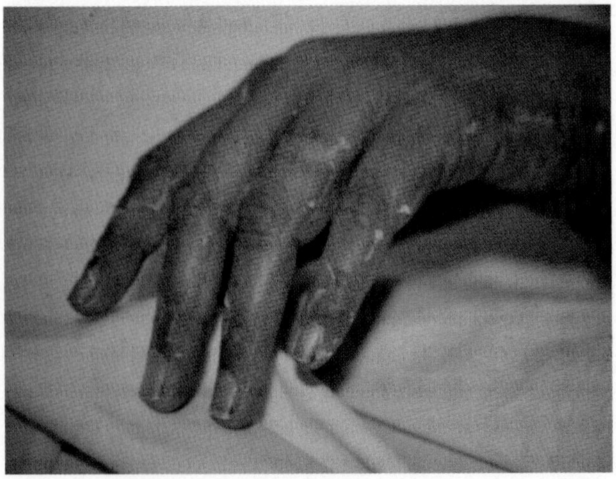

FIGURE 192-12 Toxic shock syndrome.

BOX 192-5

Mucous Membrane Involvement

Erosions or large bullae or ulcers
Pemphigus vulgaris
Stevens-Johnson syndrome
Toxic epidermal necrolysis
Small denuded vesicles
Coxsackievirus infection
Varicella
Hemorrhagic bullae
Thrombocytopenia
Angioedema of uvula, palate, tongue, or lip
Anaphylaxis
Erythema or strawberry tongue
Kawasaki's syndrome
Scarlet fever
Reticular whitish streaks
Lichen planus

look for hematuria and proteinuria. Low-grade hepatitis is often present in patients with drug rash with eosinophilia, systemic symptoms, and viral exanthems (e.g., mononucleosis); hence a hepatic panel may be reasonable in the toxic patient with generalized rash and fever. All patients with purpura should have a complete blood count and platelet count.

Treatment

Treatment of life-threatening diseases associated with rashes is discussed in more detail in specific chapters on those diseases. For the remaining illnesses, treatment frequently is aimed at the cause and the symptoms. The main goal of treatment is largely supportive and symptomatic, with relief of pain and pruritus. Usually, only those patients with severe systemic illness from overwhelming infection, fluid losses, and severe pain require inpatient care. Specific treatments for many diseases are listed in Table 192-1.

Symptomatic treatment is often focused on decreasing pruritus. Antihistamines (oral and topical) for symptomatic relief coupled with specific therapies of topical steroid agents or systemic corticosteroids, as indicated, provide the patient with significant relief. Older H_1 antihistamines (diphenhydramine) have significant associated side effects, mainly sedation. Newer forms, including loratadine, fexofenadine, and cetirizine, are considerably less sedating and should be considered in most cases where oral administration is sufficient. Concurrent use of H_2 antihistamines (cimetidine, famotidine, and ranitidine) may result in faster resolution of symptoms than the use of H_1 antihistamines alone. Topical treatment with topical antihistamines, oatmeal baths,

BOX 192-6

Drug Reaction Patterns

Maculopapular eruption: Antibiotics, NSAIDs
Exfoliative erythroderma: Antibiotics, anticonvulsants
Erythema multiforme: Antibiotics
Urticaria: Antibiotics, NSAIDs
Stevens-Johnson syndrome: Antibiotics (especially sulfonamides, amoxicillin), NSAIDs, anticonvulsants
Toxic epidermal necrolysis: Antibiotics (especially sulfonamides, amoxicillin), NSAIDs, anticonvulsants
Drug rash with eosinophilia sensitivity syndrome (DRESS): Anticonvulsants, allopurinol
Acute generalized exanthematous pustulosis (AGEP): Antibiotics
Serum sickness: Antibiotics
Leukocytoclastic vasculitis: Beta-lactam drugs, NSAIDs
Acneiform eruption: Steroids
Phototoxic eruption: Tetracyclines, quinolones
Fixed drug eruption: Tetracyclines, trimethoprim-sulfamethoxazole, phenolphthalein
Lichenoid pattern: Quinacrine, quinidine, NSAIDs
Toxic acral erythema: Cytarabine, docetaxel, 5-fluorouracil
Scleroderma-like pattern: Bleomycin, docetaxel
Drug-induced lupus: Procainamide, hydralazine
Porphyria-like pattern: Dapsone, naproxen
Pseudolymphoma: Phenytoin, carbamazepine, valproate
Hyperpigmentation: Amiodarone, imipramine, minocycline

NSAIDs, nonsteroidal anti-inflammatory drugs.

and other over-the-counter products may provide relief as well.

Several diseases that manifest with a rash have an associated component of pain. Nonsteroidal anti-inflammatory drugs and narcotics for pain control should be used judiciously. For example, adults with herpes zoster should be given high dose of nonsteroidal anti-inflammatory drugs and narcotics for pain and inflammation. Nonsteroidal anti-inflammatory drugs and aspirin are to be avoided in children with varicella or chickenpox because of the risk of Reye's syndrome. Each disease process must be closely studied for the appropriate use of pain medication.

The mainstay of therapy is frequently topical steroids. Their effects result in part from their ability to induce vasoconstriction of small vessels in the dermis, and this degree of vasoconstriction determines their

Text continued on p. 2032.

Table 192-1 SPECIFIC DISEASES

Diagnosis	Epidemiology	Symptoms and Signs of Rash	Work-up/Treatment
LOCALIZED ERYTHEMA			
Erysipelas	Can occur at any age Most frequent in children <3 yr and in older persons Commonly caused by group A streptococci	Characterized by red, hot, tender area of skin High fever and chills associated with group A streptococci Pus or clear discharge at skin entry site	Gram stain of discharge if present Blood cultures: very low yield Treatment with penicillin G, dicloxacillin, or equivalent
WHEALS			
Urticaria	Most common skin rash for which acute care sought; 15%-20% of population affected Caused by mast cell degranulation and release of histamine, which forms hives Majority of causes unknown; may result from infection, medications, foods, autoimmune diseases, and malignancies	Benign and self-limited Usually raised erythematous borders with serpiginous edges and blanched centers Diameter: few mm to 30 cm Pruritic Lasting few minutes to several hours	No laboratory tests usually indicated Consider streptococcal screen or culture Symptomatic treatment with antihistamines, both H_1 (diphenhydramine, loratadine, fexofenadine) and H_2 (cimetidine, famotidine) Steroids for severe or refractory cases (controversial in acute episodes) Epinephrine if severe associated reaction Most treated as outpatients
MACULAR AND MACULOPAPULAR RASHES			
Viral exanthem	Commonly caused by nonpolio enteroviruses (coxsackievirus, echovirus, enterovirus) and respiratory viruses (adenovirus, rhinovirus, parainfluenza virus, influenza, respiratory syncytial virus)	Nonspecific diffuse blanchable erythematous macules and papules on trunk and extremities	Clinical diagnosis Supportive care
Lyme disease	Tickborne illness Caused by spirochete *Borrelia burgdorferi* Predominantly seen in eastern United States in summer	Initial erythematous macule or papule expanding with distinct red border with central clearing (erythema migrans) Other symptoms: malaise, fever, chills, arthralgias, myalgias, sore throat, anorexia	Skin biopsy of erythema migrans shows spirochetes in ≤40% Serology studies *Borrelia* culture from skin biopsy Oral antibiotics (penicillin G, doxycycline, amoxicillin, or azithromycin) and close outpatient follow-up
Rubella (German measles)	Benign childhood infection of young adults Rarely seen in United States because of immunization Winter, spring	Pink maculopapules that start on forehead and spread to face, trunk, and extremities Characteristic 3-day course after which rash fades completely Infection during pregnancy can result in congenital fetal defects	Clinical diagnosis Laboratory tests not indicated Treatment usually only supportive Infection during pregnancy: therapeutic abortion or passive immunization

Table 192-1 SPECIFIC DISEASES—cont'd

MACULAR AND MACULOPAPULAR RASHES			
Diagnosis	**Epidemiology**	**Symptoms and Signs of Rash**	**Work-up/Treatment**
Measles	Highly contagious disease of childhood Rarely seen in children in the United States because of immunization Seen in third decade of life in the United States Winter, spring	Characterized by prodrome of fever, cough, coryza, and conjunctivitis Purple-red maculopapular rash spreads from hairline downward, confluent on face, neck, and shoulders Koplik's spots in mouth: bluish-white papules with erythema on buccal mucosa (pathognomonic)	Clinical diagnosis Laboratory tests not indicated Treatment usually only supportive Complications: otitis media, pneumonia, encephalitis (rare)
Roseola infantum	Infants ages 6-36 mo old Caused by HHV-6 and HHV-7 Spring, fall, summer	Characterized by sudden appearance of rash after defervescence of high fever (rash 3-4 days after fever) Infant usually appears well despite fever Rash: small rose-pink macules and papules that become confluent and fade	Clinical diagnosis Laboratory tests not indicated Treatment usually only supportive
Erythema infectiosum or fifth disease (parvovirus B19)	Childhood rash, primarily age 2-14 yr 50% of adults have serologic evidence of past infection Late winter, spring	Asymptomatic infection common, but severe complications possible in pregnancy, anemia, or immunocompromise Women (not men) can have acute polyarthropathy that can last 2 wk-yr First stage: Bright red erythema appears abruptly over the cheeks (slapped-cheek appearance) and marked by nasal, perioral, and periorbital sparing; typically fades over 2-4 days Second stage: Within 1-4 days, erythematous macular to morbilliform eruption on extremities; favors extensor surfaces and can involve palms and soles; pruritus rare Third stage: second stage eruption fades into lacy pattern, emphasis on proximal extremities; lasts 3 days-3 wk; after starting to fade, exanthem may recur over several weeks following physical stimuli (e.g., exercise, sun exposure, friction, bathing in hot water, or stress)	Clinical diagnosis Laboratory tests not indicated Treatment usually only supportive
Scarlet fever	Seen primarily in children with pharyngitis, usually 3-12 yr Winter, spring Usually caused by group A streptococci Rarely caused by *Staphylococcus aureus*	Rash appears 1-3 days after onset of infection Rash: finely punctate erythema on upper trunk, sandpaper feel Progresses to neck, back, groin, and axilla Spares palms and soles of feet Pharynx beefy red with "strawberry tongue"	Laboratory tests: rapid direct antigen test to screen for group A streptococci Oral swab for bacterial culture Antistreptolysin-O titer if diagnosis in question Treatment with penicillin G or equivalent

Continued

Table 192-1 **SPECIFIC DISEASES—cont'd**

SCALY PATCHES: PAPULOSQUAMOUS ERUPTIONS, ECZEMATOUS, OILY			
Diagnosis	**Epidemiology**	**Symptoms and Signs of Rash**	**Work-up/Treatment**
Lichen planus	Onset in middle age; high prevalence of hepatitis C Men and women affected equally Viral and bacterial agents and genetic predisposition possible causes Drugs may also precipitate similar eruption	Mucocutaneous lesions: violaceous, pruritic, flat-topped papules and plaques, often polygonal Six Ps: purple, pruritic, polygonal, planar, papules, plaques Most often on volar aspect of forearm, wrist, and shin, and often linear Oral lesions linear or reticular and usually on buccal surface Mucous membrane lesions may be painful with propensity for development of squamous cell carcinoma	Lesions often remit spontaneously in <1 yr, but topical steroids recommended for cosmetics and comfort Antihistamines for pruritus Referral to dermatologist for long-term care Consider testing for hepatitis C because of association
Pityriasis rosea*	Occurs between first and fourth decades of life More common in spring and fall Possibly caused by HHV-7	Begins with single truncal lesion or "herald" patch (2-5-cm diameter salmon-colored, single, oval scaly patch) Secondary eruption 1-2 wk later, usually on trunk and proximal aspects of extremities; erythematous macules or papules; "Christmas tree" pattern, following Langer's lines; lasts 4-6 wk Preceded by upper respiratory tract symptoms in two thirds of cases	Diagnosis made by skin biopsy and light microscopy Self-limited with spontaneous remission in 6-12 wk Treatment with oral antihistamines and topical steroid agents
Psoriasis	Peak incidence, 20-30 yr; second peak, 55-60 yr Genetic disorder Chronic disease without cure	Can be precipitated by trauma (Koebner's phenomenon) or infections Pruritus common Silver, scaly rash on erythematous base; located on scalp, extensor surfaces, and groin area Pitting and onycholysis of nails May produce arthritis in distal joints, asymmetrically	Should be managed by dermatologist because of need for "shifting" therapies Treatment with topical steroids, tar-based shampoos, and vitamin D analogues Moderate to severe cases need systemic treatment with methotrexate, cyclosporine, or phototherapy Avoid systemic steroids
Secondary syphilis	*Treponema pallidum* Called "great masquerader" because of varied rash presentations Rash starts 9-90 days after chancre (average, 3 wk)	Generalized painless and nonpruritic rash Distributed on skin and mucous membranes Follows skin cleavage lines Discrete, scaly, red-brown papules and plaques Associated with headache, sore throat, malaise, and generalized arthralgias ≤60% of patients do not remember chancre	Laboratory tests: VDRL or rapid plasma reagent necessary for diagnosis Dark-field examination of scrapings may be beneficial Treatment with penicillin G or equivalent

Table 192-1 SPECIFIC DISEASES—cont'd

SCALY PATCHES: PAPULOSQUAMOUS ERUPTIONS, ECZEMATOUS, OILY			
Diagnosis	**Epidemiology**	**Symptoms and Signs of Rash**	**Work-up/Treatment**
Tinea corporis	Occurs in all age groups Higher incidence in animal workers and individuals with pets Dermatophyte infection of the dermis	Characterized by small to large scaling, sharply demarcated plaques Lesions have peripheral enlargement and central clearing Most lesions have annular configuration	Diagnosis by potassium hydroxide slide preparation Wood's lamp can be used for diagnosis Treatment with topical azole cream usually efficacious Systemic antifungal treatment for large infections or if refractory to topical creams
Tinea pedis	20-50 yr olds More male than female patients affected Predisposing factors: hot, humid weather, occlusive footwear, excessive sweating	May be dry and scaly or macerated, peeling, and associated with fissures mostly between fourth and fifth toes Other forms include well-demarcated erythema with minute papules, vesicles or bullae, or ulceration	Scrapings to detect hyphae Wood's lamp Fungal culture Treatment with topical or oral antifungals (e.g., terbinafine, naftifine, fluconazole)
Tinea cruris	Predisposing factor warm, moist environment More male than female patients affected	Lesions often bilateral and beginning in skin folds Half moon–shaped plaque with well-defined scaly border	Treatment with topical antifungals (e.g., clotrimazole, miconazole, naftifine, terbinafine)
Tinea capitis	Mostly children 6-10 yr old Increased rural prevalence More black than white patients affected Risk factors: debilitation, malnutrition, chronic disease	Inflammatory type associated with pain, tenderness, and/or alopecia With noninflammatory infection, scaling, pruritus, diffuse or circumscribed alopecia, and lymphadenopathy Seborrheic type, black dot (stubs of broken hair), or discrete pustules	Wood's lamp Cultures Topical antifungals not effective; systemic treatment with griseofulvin, itraconazole, terbinafine, fluconazole, or ketoconazole Adjunctive selenium sulfide shampoo
Irritant contact dermatitis (ICD)	Reactions resulting from direct damage to epithelium with subsequent cytokine release Sensitization not required, thereby resulting in faster onset, depending on frequency and intensity of exposure Hands are most commonly affected Most cases caused by long-term exposure	Symptoms of itching, burning, stinging usually the only manifestations Dry skin with erythema and chapping common Severe cases: caustic burn with vesiculation Hands are primary site of involvement, and appearance is indistinguishable from allergic contact dermatitis	Patch testing can be done by dermatologist for possible allergic cause Avoidance of caustic agents is treatment of choice Topical corticosteroid creams and barrier creams effective
Allergic contact dermatitis (ACD)	Often associated with plants (allergic phytodermatitis); may result from allergic sensitization (may take 10 days) or chemical skin damage Reexposure to antigen results in reaction within hours to days, as sensitized T cells release inflammatory cytokines Poison ivy and poison oak most common causes Some allergic contact reactions IgE mediated (e.g., latex allergy and blepharitis from airborne allergens)	Primarily on hands and exposed extremities Skin appears erythematous and swollen, usually with papules, vesicles, and evidence of desquamation, often linear Involved skin sharply demarcated to area of exposure, providing strong evidence of contact origin Long-term exposure may lead to excoriation, scaling, or lichenification	For both allergic and irritant contact dermatitis, treatment is with topical steroids and avoidance of inciting agent Systemic steroids indicated for large areas of exposure or blisters; extensive contact reactions (poison ivy) often require systemic steroids for 7 to 10 days Weeping, excoriated areas can be treated with cool compresses and aluminum acetate or oatmeal bathing

Continued

Table 192-1 SPECIFIC DISEASES—cont'd

SCALY PATCHES: PAPULOSQUAMOUS ERUPTIONS, ECZEMATOUS, OILY			
Diagnosis	**Epidemiology**	**Symptoms and Signs of Rash**	**Work-up/Treatment**
Seborrheic dermatitis	Onset at puberty and peak in the 40s, but may recur in elderly patients; more common men Estimated to appear in ≈3% of healthy hosts, but ≤20% if dandruff sufferers included Related to abnormal immune response to normal skin fungus, *Malassezia,* limited to sebum-rich areas	Appears as inflamed skin with oily, flaking surface Predominates on scalp, nasolabial folds, eyebrows, postauricular folds, groin, and chest Infant form ("cradle cap") has dryer, more powdery scale Rash may worsen in winter and in patients with HIV or Parkinson's disease	Treatment focuses on frequent cleansing to reduce oil content of skin and shampoos containing selenium sulfide, sulfur, or coal tar for their keratolytic action Topical ketoconazole to reduce fungal load Topical steroids should be avoided because of risk of skin atrophy
Atopic dermatitis (eczema)	Begins in first year of life in 60% of patients; prevalence in children: 10%-20% Possible association with aeroallergens (dust mites) and foods (peanuts, milk, eggs) Exacerbated by skin dehydration from frequent showers and hand washing Chronic, remitting, and relapsing disease seen in patients with a personal or family history of atopy (asthma or allergic rhinitis)	Patients have dry skin Infants 3-6 mo old present with red, scaly areas on cheeks In contrast, children develop sharply demarcated, red, scaly areas on antecubital fossa, neck, wrists, and ankles Often remits in puberty, but over time these areas become lichenified and persist into adulthood; affected adults predisposed to hand dermatitis and unusually susceptible to contact reactions Pruritus is hallmark of atopic dermatitis Predilection for flexure surfaces, sides of neck, face, wrists, and dorsum of feet	Bacterial cultures for possible secondary infection with *S. aureus* Viral culture to rule out HSV in crusted lesions Check serum IgE levels Treatment: oral antihistamines, topical corticosteroids, limited bathing, and hydration of skin with emollient creams Sedating antihistamines at night may be beneficial

VESICULOBULLOUS DISEASES			
Diagnosis	**Epidemiology**	**Symptoms and Signs of Rash**	**Work-up/Treatment**
Erythema multiforme	Occurs at any age, but 50% <20 yr; more frequent in men than women; mortality 0% Associated primarily with HSV infection 50% of cases of unknown origin Minor and major forms Erythema multiforme minor limited to skin with mild systemic symptoms Erythema multiforme major involving mucous membranes and <10% dermal detachment	Erythema multiforme, as the name implies, can be macular, papular, urticarial, or vesicular, but maculopapular eruption with targeting is most characteristic Vesicle and bullae in center of papule Peripheral clearing produces distinct target lesion appearance Extremities involved more than trunk, with prominence on palms and soles; mucous membrane erosions absent	Clinical diagnosis Biopsy showing perivascular mononuclear infiltrate if absolute diagnosis needed Treatment supportive; may require large doses of pain medication Frequent recurrent episodes may be treated with oral acyclovir Stop any drugs that may be causative Resolves in 2-3 wk Steroids often used, but not proven effective

Table 192-1 SPECIFIC DISEASES—cont'd

VESICULOBULLOUS DISEASES			
Diagnosis	**Epidemiology**	**Symptoms and Signs of Rash**	**Work-up/Treatment**
Stevens-Johnson syndrome (SJS)	Occurs at any age but most common in adults >40 yr; mortality 5% 50% associated with drug exposure; most frequently implicated drugs: sulfonamides, aminopenicillins, carbamazepine, allopurinol Also caused by viral infections and *Mycoplasma pneumoniae* Significant overlap between TEN and SJS, with overlap syndrome described. If epidermal erosions are ≤10% of body surface area, disease is designated SJS	Prodrome with fever and flulike symptoms 1-3 days later, mucocutaneous lesions Skin rash: erythema multiforme, brightly erythematous with bullae Although mild cases may be manifested by maculopapular rash and minor mucosal erosions, more severe cases develop skin vesicular, sloughing, and necrosis; mucosal erosions dramatic Fever common Secondary infection may occur, making diagnosis more difficult Anemia, lymphopenia, and neutropenia possible	Diagnosis confirmed by biopsy Intravenous fluids critical to replace fluids lost from wounds Treatment similar to that of burn, mostly supportive Early diagnosis and withdrawal of suspected drugs critical Systemic steroids not proven to help
Toxic epidermal necrolysis (TEN)	Occurs at any age but most common in adults >40 yr 80% associated with drug exposure; drugs most frequently implicated: sulfonamides, aminopenicillins, carbamazepine, and allopurinol TEN has 25%-30% mortality attributed to sepsis and hypovolemia If epidermal detachment >30% of body surface area, defined as TEN; if 10%-30% of total body surface area involved, referred to SJS/TEN	TEN usually has prodromal phase of fevers, myalgias, malaise, and anorexia that may persist for several days, followed by rapid development of generalized, intense erythema Skin rash: erythema multiforme, brightly erythematous with bullae; erythema intense, pruritic, and often tender to touch. Although often starting as large macules, rash quickly confluent Within 24 hr, large flaccid vesicles in erythematous areas with subsequent sloughing, leaving denuded patches Fever common and typically higher than in SJS Secondary infection may occur, making diagnosis more difficult Nikolsky's sign present (with slight thumb pressure, skin wrinkles, slides laterally, and separates from dermis) Lip and mucous membrane erosions routine	Diagnosis confirmed by biopsy Intravenous fluids critical to replace fluids lost from wounds Treatment similar to that of burn; consider transfer to burn center Early diagnosis and withdrawal of suspected drugs critical Systemic steroids not proven to help Clinical course lasts 3-6 wk Complications related to secondary infection
Pemphigus vulgaris	Autoimmune disorder Occurs in fourth to sixth decade of life Caused by autoantibodies directed against surface of keratinocytes and resulting in intraepidermal separation and bulla formation Disease morbidity and mortality high, from secondary infection of lesions	Skin lesions round or vesicles and bullae with serous content Patient presents with painful oral lesions followed by development of diffuse, flaccid blisters that slough with gentle pressure (Nikolsky's sign) Found predominantly on scalp, face, chest, axilla, and groin	Immunofluorescence of skin biopsy reveals IgG deposits Intravenous fluid replacement necessary Treatment requires high-dose systemic steroids and immunosuppressive therapy

Continued

Table 192-1 **SPECIFIC DISEASES—cont'd**

VESICULOBULLOUS DISEASES			
Diagnosis	**Epidemiology**	**Symptoms and Signs of Rash**	**Work-up/Treatment**
Bullous pemphigoid	Autoimmune disorder Occurs in sixth to eighth decade of life Complement activation leading to inflammatory cascade response Lesions caused by autoantibodies directed at basement membrane and resulting in subepidermal blister formation Remissions ≤1-5 yr are common Overall prognosis good, depending on comorbidities	Blistering disease manifested by acute or subacute onset of generalized tense bullae with predilection for flexural surfaces Erythematous, papular, or urticarial-type lesions followed by bulla formation Bullae contain serous or hemorrhagic fluid Bleeding sometimes a problem Unlike pemphigus vulgaris, these blisters less prone to rupture, and mucosal involvement unusual Pruritus prominent; preexisting erythema or urticaria possible	Neutrophils at dermal-epidermal junction on light microscopy Serum tests for circulating autoantibodies Intravenous fluid replacement Azathioprine or dapsone Strong topical steroids and oral tetracycline preferred Systemic steroids reserved for more severe cases
Staphylococcal scalded skin syndrome (SSSS)	Seen almost exclusively in infants and small children Most common in neonates <3 mo old Caused by respiratory or skin infection with toxigenic *S. aureus* Infections of umbilical stump or nasal infection	Presenting with diffuse erythema followed by development of flaccid bullae that desquamate in large sheets Ranges from localized bullous impetigo to extensive epidermolysis Desquamation of affected area common Although sometimes confused with TEN, mucous membrane involvement absent, targeting not seen, course short, and prognosis good	Laboratory tests: CBC Blood cultures; bacterial cultures of wound not indicated Oral or intravenous antibiotics based on severity (erythromycins, penicillinase-resistant penicillins, or cephalosporins) Hospital admission for severe cases
Varicella (chickenpox)	>3 million cases/yr Most <10 yr Adults typically have more severe course Late winter, spring Decreased incidence secondary to vaccine Transmitted by both direct contact and airborne droplet	Highly pruritic Begins as macules, then papular eruption that evolves into vesicles; vesicles crust over in 12 hr Continual eruptions over 4-5 days Incubation 10-21 days; no longer infectious when crusted "Dewdrop-on-a-rose-petal" appearance Severe complications including pneumonia and meningitis or encephalitis, especially in adults	Diagnosis made by history of viral prodrome and recent exposure Laboratory tests not indicated Oral acyclovir may decrease severity of outbreak if started ≤24 hr of first eruptions Avoid aspirin and NSAIDs in children
Hand-foot-mouth disease (coxsackievirus)	Largely disease of childhood (1-4 yr) Coxsackievirus B Summer, fall	Characterized by ulcerative oral lesions, primarily on soft palate and rash on palms and soles of feet Rash: macular, with fast-developing pustular eruptions that crust over Resolves over 5-6 days	Diagnosis made clinically Laboratory tests not indicated Treatment usually only supportive

Table 192-1 SPECIFIC DISEASES—cont'd

Diagnosis	Epidemiology	Symptoms and Signs of Rash	Work-up/Treatment
VESICULOBULLOUS DISEASES			
Herpes zoster (shingles)	Reactivation of latent VZV virus in sensory ganglia Nearly 100% of U.S. adults seropositive for anti-VZV antibodies by third decade of life Two thirds of cases occur in patients >50 yr old	Rash erupts as papules and transforms to vesicles or bullae in 24 hr Vesicles become pustules in 48 hr and crusts by day 7 Erupts in dermatomal pattern (pathognomonic) Typically does not cross midline unless patient is immunocompromised	Diagnosis made by history and physical examination Tzanck smear if diagnosis in question Laboratory tests indicated only if severe secondary infection suspected Treatment with acyclovir or equivalent antiviral and pain medications Consult ophthalmology for ocular involvement
Herpes simpex virus (HSV) eruption	Two most common serotypes: 1 and 2 Most common in children (1-4 yr) and young adults	Grouped vesicles on erythematous base on keratinized skin and mucous membranes Usually on cheeks, lips, mouth, fingers, and genitalia Symptoms: 1-2 wk	Tzanck smear if diagnosis in question Viral cultures HSV antibody serologic studies Acyclovir or other antiviral used for both treatment and prevention of eruptions Prednisone may decrease acute pain, but increases complications Admit for urinary retention and disseminated infection
Scabies	Microscopic mite *Sarcoptes scabei* White-transparent creature <0.5-mm long Transmitted by close personal contact Incubation, life span 30 days	Highly contagious, pruritic, worse at night Papulovesicular dermatitis, can be papular or bullous also Distribution predominately volar wrists, medial palms, interdigital web spaces, and axillary folds Usually spares face and scalp, except in infants Skin burrows seen	Skin scrapings may demonstrate mites, eggs, or feces Treatment includes washing all clothes and bed linen Treat with lindane, permethrin, or crotamiton Pruritus may persist for 1-2 wk after treatment
PUSTULAR RASHES			
Disseminated gonococcal infection	Asymptomatic endocervical, urethral, rectal, or pharyngeal gonococcal infection Incidence higher in women and young and sexually active patients Onset often related to menses	Presenting with syndrome of fever, skin lesions, migratory arthritis, and tenosynovitis Skin lesions: small pustules on erythematous base, appearing near joints on extremities, often limited to 3-10 lesions (rarely ≤30)	Often a clinical diagnosis because cultures of skin, blood, or joint fluid usually negative (50%), and cultures of primary sites variable Response to antibiotics prompt and lends support to diagnosis
Impetigo	Primary infections most common in children Secondary infections in patients with underlying dermatoses Caused by *S. aureus* and group A streptococci Common during warm, humid summer months, temperate climates year-round	Classic or nonbullous in 70% Superficial bacterial infection of epidermal skin Rash appears as a golden yellow, crusted erosion after initial discrete papule or vesicle that erodes Commonly seen on face around mouth and on cheeks	Clinical diagnosis Laboratory tests not indicated Treatment with oral and/or topical antibiotics (e.g., 2% mupirocin ointment, dicloxacillin, first-generation cephalosporins, azithromycin)

Continued

Table 192-1 **SPECIFIC DISEASES—cont'd**

PUSTULAR RASHES			
Diagnosis	**Epidemiology**	**Symptoms and Signs of Rash**	**Work-up/Treatment**
Acute generalized exanthematous pustulosis (AGEP)†	Acute drug reaction (usually antibiotic related)	Presents with high fever and erythroderma Rash begins on face, axilla, and inguinal region and quickly becomes confluent Subsequently, small, white pustules develop in initial regions, which later undergo superficial desquamation Unlike TEN, targeting, large bullae, and Nikolsky's sign not seen In addition, mucous membrane involvement uncommon	Prognosis good, with resolution ≤2 wk Does not require steroid therapy
Ecthyma gangrenosum	Manifestation of gram-negative sepsis (especially *Pseudomonas*) in leukemia or other immunocompromised state	Lesion often starts as red macule or vesicle that becomes pustular or hemorrhagic, then sloughs and progresses to gangrenous ulcer or black eschar Lesions tend to be perineal or gluteal and are usually solitary or few	Treatment of infection with antibiotics Septic symptoms treated accordingly
Pyoderma gangrenosum	About one half of patients have associated inflammatory bowel disease or myeloproliferative disorder; remainder idiopathic	Begins as red papule or pustule that ulcerates then extends circumferentially Patient remains afebrile while borders become raised, smooth, and violaceous and ulcer bed develops purulent exudates Patients often treated for presumptive wound infection, but with no response	Lesions respond dramatically to oral prednisone Débridement should be avoided

ERYTHRODERMA WITH DESQUAMATION WHEALS			
Diagnosis	**Epidemiology**	**Symptoms and Signs of Rash**	**Work-up/Treatment**
Toxic shock syndrome	Most common in women 20-30 yr old Primarily caused by toxin-producing *S. aureus* Risk factors: vaginal tampons, surgical packing, postpartum wounds Wound and nasopharyngeal sources of staphylococci more common now than tampons in pathogenesis	Patients present with abrupt onset of high fever, hypotension, vomiting, diarrhea, and generalized macular rash that is often deep red and more intense on hands and feet Generalized scarlatiniform erythroderma most intense around infected area Erythema without ulceration seen on mucous membranes Sunburn-like peel of distal extremities typical, but occurs during recovery Edema of face, hands, and feet common Criteria for diagnosis: fever >38.9°C, erythroderma, mucous membrane involvement, signs of sepsis, particularly hypotension	Blood cultures and wound cultures (often negative) Laboratory tests: CBC, chemistries, LFTs Intravenous antibiotics with staphylococcal coverage (e.g., oxacillin, cefoxitin, vancomycin, clindamycin) Hospitalization and fluid resuscitation

Table 192-1 SPECIFIC DISEASES—cont'd

ERYTHRODERMA WITH DESQUAMATION WHEALS			
Diagnosis	**Epidemiology**	**Symptoms and Signs of Rash**	**Work-up/Treatment**
Streptococcal toxic shock syndrome	Group A beta-hemolytic streptococci Increasing frequency in recent years Mortality may be ≤30%	Generalized erythroderma with or without bullae either before or concomitant with onset of full syndrome May have fever, hypotension, cerebral dysfunction, renal failure, respiratory distress syndrome, toxic cardiomyopathy, hepatic dysfunction, and hypocalcemia Desquamation follows rash Infection of soft tissues or skin and bacteremia often present	Blood and wound cultures Intravenous antibiotics (e.g., oxacillin, cefoxitin, vancomycin, clindamycin) May require operative débridement
Kawasaki's disease	Peak onset at 1 yr; mean age, 2.5 yr Slight male and Asian predominance Acute febrile illness of infants and children Unknown origin Systemic vasculitis of microvessels 2000-4000 annual cases	Cutaneous and mucosal erythema and edema with subsequent desquamation Lesions appear 1-2 days after onset of fever Rash first noted on palms and soles then spreading to trunk and extremities Edema of hands and feet develops after rash Oropharynx becomes erythematous Complications predominately coronary including aneurysms, congestive heart failure, myocardial infarction, dysrhythmias, and valvular insufficiency; also gallbladder hydrops	Diagnosis clinical and includes fever for ≥5 days and skin changes Laboratory tests: CBC, leukocytosis >18,000 common LFTs abnormal Thrombocytosis and elevated ESR after tenth day of illness Urine may show sterile pyuria Treatment with high-dose aspirin and intravenous immunoglobulin Admission to hospital required
Exfoliative dermatitis (erythroderma)‡	Drugs, contact allergens, and malignancy often implicated 1% of hospitalizations for skin disease Mortality ≤30% May be marker for HIV infection Male-to-female ratio 2:1; usually >40 yr	Exfoliative dermatitis presents abruptly as generalized erythema or morbilliform eruption that tends to flake and scale early on Pruritus and sense of skin tightness common Low-grade fever common, but unlike DRESS, high fever, lymphadenopathy, hepatitis, or nephritis not seen Unlike TEN, vesiculation and sloughing not seen Unlike SJS, mucous membrane involvement rare Other skin disorders may also progress thus (e.g., cutaneous T-cell lymphoma; mycosis fungoides and Sézary's syndrome can be confused)	Evaluate for cardiac failure, renal abnormalities, and intestinal dysfunction Laboratory tests: CBC, LFTs, UA, chemistry profile, serum albumin, ESR Biopsy shows nonspecific findings Admit for supportive care including stopping inciting medications, fluid replacement, skin care May benefit from burn center care Steroids may worsen condition

Continued

Table 192-1 **SPECIFIC DISEASES—cont'd**

ERYTHRODERMA WITH DESQUAMATION WHEALS			
Diagnosis	**Epidemiology**	**Symptoms and Signs of Rash**	**Work-up/Treatment**
Drug rash with eosinophilia sensitivity syndrome (DRESS)*	Hypersensitivity response to a drug; phenytoin, carbamazepine, allopurinol, and sulfonamides most common precipitants 1 in 5000-10,000 exposures to phenytoin, carbamazepine, and phenobarbital Mortality 10%	Patients present with severe exfoliative dermatitis with high fever and evidence of hepatitis, nephritis, pneumonitis, myocarditis, pericarditis, nephritis, or lymphadenopathy Widespread and long-lasting papulopustular or erythematous skin eruption often progressing to exfoliative dermatitis Typically starts 2-6 wk after starting drug	Laboratory tests: CBC, chemistry panel, LFTs, chest radiograph, ECG Stop potential drug cause Systemic steroids rapidly improve symptoms and laboratory tests, but long-term impact unknown Relapses of rash and hepatitis may occur with tapering of steroids Supportive care: warming skin, local antiseptics, and topical steroids

PURPURA			
Diagnosis	**Epidemiology**	**Symptoms and Signs of Rash**	**Work-up/Treatment**
Rocky Mountain spotted fever	Incidence highest in 5-9 yr olds, 600 cases/yr Fatality highest in male patients *Rickettsia rickettsii* Transmitted by ticks Occurs mainly in northern climates in spring, later in southern climates	Symptoms begin about 1 wk after tick bite with sudden onset of fever, myalgias, nausea, and headache After ≈4 days of symptoms, maculopapular erythematous rash appears on wrists and ankles and spreads to the palms and soles, then progresses centrally to proximal extremities, trunk, and face Early lesions are 2-6-mm pink, blanchable macules that evolve to deep red papules and then become hemorrhagic over 1-4 days Over next 2-4 days, lesions become purpuric, and signs of encephalitis often follow Rash can start on the first day (14%) up to sixth day (20%) or may not appear at all (13%)	Diagnosis depends on clinical symptoms and history of potential or confirmed tick exposure because laboratory confirmation cannot occur before 10-14 days Associated with hyponatremia, thrombocytopenia, and hypoalbuminemia with or without increased WBC Treatment with tetracycline, doxycycline, chloramphenicol
Meningococcemia	Occurs at any age Meningococcemia is rapidly progressive, fulminant infection in school-age children, usually in high school and college 50%-88% develop meningitis	Brief prodrome of high fever, myalgias, headache, and gastrointestinal symptoms, followed by progressive signs of toxicity, altered mental status, and hypotension Petechial or fine maculopapular rash on trunk and extremities first clue of meningococcemia Progression of purpura with skin necrosis and infarction of distal extremities may occur Patients appear acutely ill with marked prostration	Immediate antibiotic treatment that penetrates CSF blood-brain barrier (penicillin G, ceftriaxone, cefotaxime, ampicillin, or chloramphenicol) Laboratory tests: CBC, basic metabolic panel, clotting studies Blood cultures CSF cultures Isolation and admission to hospital

Table 192-1 SPECIFIC DISEASES—cont'd

PURPURA			
Diagnosis	**Epidemiology**	**Symptoms and Signs of Rash**	**Work-up/Treatment**
Henoch-Schönlein purpura	Most patients 2-11 yr old, peak at 5 yr Male-to-female ratio, 2:1 Peaks in winter No clear origin Some association with group A beta-hemolytic streptococci and viruses Small vessel vasculitis often following upper respiratory infection Acute vasculitis with IgA deposits	Hallmark is maculopapular rash that predominates on lower extremities and buttocks, but may be seen on perineum, lower trunk, or diffusely; may begin as urticaria Lesions become palpable and purpuric early on and are histologically leukocytoclastic vasculitis; in severe cases, hemorrhagic vesicles Joint pain and inflammation with low-grade fever common Associated with arthritis in two third of cases Gastrointestinal involvement may occur with abdominal pain and heme-positive stool May be associated with intussusception Most serious complication is renal involvement manifested by hematuria with or without proteinuria, progressing to nephritic syndrome and chronic renal failure in ≈1% Disease generally self-limited in small children, but may be more severe in older children and young adults	Laboratory tests: increased WBC and mild anemia, thrombocytopenia possible; 40% have proteinuria and hematuria Blood cultures may be necessary to rule out sepsis Supportive care and NSAIDs, hydration, and prednisone
Thrombotic thrombocytopenic purpura (TTP)	Twice as often in women as in men Peaks in fourth to fifth decade Often associated with drugs (e.g., clopidogrel, cyclosporine, quinine)	Classic pentad includes thrombocytopenic purpura, fever, neurologic symptoms, microangiopathic hemolytic anemia, and nephritis Purpura resembles that seen in other causes of thrombocytopenia, manifested by showers of petechiae on distal extremities and at sites of pressure, as well as ecchymoses in areas of minor trauma Purpura not palpable because not associated with vasculitis	

Continued

Table 192-1 **SPECIFIC DISEASES—cont'd**

PURPURA			
Diagnosis	**Epidemiology**	**Symptoms and Signs of Rash**	**Work-up/Treatment**
Leukocytoclastic vasculitis	Small vessel vasculitis About one half of cases idiopathic; remainder attributed to drug reactions, viral infections, and collagen vascular disorders (microscopic polyangiitis, cryoglobulinemia)	Begins as maculopapular eruption in which hemorrhages into lesions make them palpable Lesions may coalesce, producing large areas of purpura Lower extremities below knees most prominently involved, but disease can be diffuse Prodromal symptoms of fever, myalgias, arthralgias, and malaise typical Lesions often itch and may be painful; often recurrent, with crops developing every 1-4 wk	Short courses of prednisone effective in most patients, but colchicine preferred for chronic disease

*Data from Gonzalez LM, Allen R: Pityriasis rosea: An important papulosquamous disorder. Int J Dermatol 2005;44:757-764.

†Data from Sidoroff A, Halevy S, Bayinck JN, et al: Acute generalized exanthematous pustulosis (AGEP): A clinical reaction pattern. J Cutan Pathol 2001;28:113-119.

‡Data from Rothe MJ, Bernstein ML, Grant-Kel JM: Life-threatening erythroderma. Clin Dermatol 2005;23:206-217; and Akhyani M, Ghodsi ZS, Toosi S, et al: Erythroderma: A clinical study of 97 cases. BMC Dermatol 2005;5:5.

CBC, complete blood count; CSF, cerebrospinal fluid; DRESS, drug rash with eosinophilia sensitivity syndrome; ECG, electrocardiogram; ESR, erythrocyte sedimentation rate; HIV, human immunodeficiency virus; HSV, herpes simplex virus; IgA, immunoglobulin A; IgE, immunoglobulin E; IgG, immunoglobulin G; LFT, liver function test; NSAIDs, nonsteroidal anti-inflammatory drugs; SJS, Stevens-Johnson syndrome; TENS, toxic epidermal necrolysis; UA, urinalysis; VDRL, Venereal Disease Research Laboratory [test]; VZV, varicella-zoster virus; WBC, white blood cell count.

category. Topical steroids are available in four strengths: mild (hydrocortisone), medium (triamcinolone), high (fluocinonide), and ultrahigh (betamethasone, clobetasol). Only low-potency steroids should be used on the face, but even the 1% form of hydrocortisone should be avoided on the eyelids, because of the risk of glaucoma. Medium-strength steroid creams are useful for most skin areas except the face, and therefore, triamcinolone 0.1% cream is the default prescription for most ED uses. High- and ultrahigh-strength steroid creams should be reserved for resistant lesions, lichenified areas, and hand lesions. Triamcinolone can be used in these latter groups, but occlusion with plastic food wrap helps to increase effectiveness.

Lowering the concentration of the drug does not necessarily decrease the vasoconstriction; may drugs have the same vasoconstriction despite different concentrations (0.25%, 0.5%, 1%). Generic substitutes are not necessarily equivalent (most important for potent steroids), and adequate potency and treatment length are important considerations when prescribing. Physicians should avoid prescribing a weaker, "safe" preparation that fails to give the desired anti-inflammatory effect and prolongs the disease, thus often leading to secondary infection. The base determines the rate at which the active ingredient is absorbed through the skin. Creams are somewhat greasy, can be used in most areas, are cosmetically most acceptable, dry with extended use, and are best for intertriginous areas. Ointments are translucent, greasy, more lubricating, more penetrant than creams, and too occlusive for use in acute eczematous inflammation or intertriginous areas. Gels are clear and are useful for acute exudative inflammation, such as poison ivy, and in the hair because they "mat" the hair less. Lotions are clear or milky, most useful for the scalp, and may result in stinging and drying when applied to intertriginous areas. The amount of cream dispensed is important: 1 g of cream covers 10×10 cm of skin; 20 to 30 g will cover the entire skin of most adults. For ointments, the amount that fits on your fingertip typically covers the equivalent of the front and back of the hand.

A systemic steroid is usually indicated for patients with any generalized eruption or when more than 10% of body surface area is involved. If the epidermis is denuded to a significant extent, steroids should be avoided. The spectrum of dermatologic diagnoses in which systemic steroids are recommended includes Stevens-Johnson syndrome, drug rash with eosinophilia and systemic symptoms, urticaria, maculopapular drug eruptions, serum sickness, and large contact reactions.

Little evidence is available with reference to dosage or course of steroid treatment in these entities, but by convention, patients are prescribed prednisone (40 to 60 mg/day for 5 to 7 days). Higher doses and the parenteral route are reserved for patients with Stevens-Johnson syndrome and drug rash with eosinophilia and systemic symptoms. Patients with autoimmune-mediated disorders may require the use of immunosuppression. Immunosuppressant medications should be given only after consultation with the appropriate specialist. Such medications carry with them severe adverse effects and often need close monitoring to prevent iatrogenic disease states.

Emollient creams and lotions restore water and lipids to the epidermis. Preparations that contain urea or lactic acid have special lubricating properties and may be the most effective. Creams are thicker and more lubricating than lotions. Because petroleum jelly and mineral oil contain no water, water should be added to the skin before these substances are applied.

Viral exanthems do not require antibiotics, nor are these drugs helpful in relieving symptoms. However, the use of antiretrovirals in varicella, herpes zoster, and other herpetic eruptions may change the duration of symptoms, decrease the incidence of postherpetic neuralgia, or decrease future outbreaks. For bacterial infections, antibiotics such as topical ointments in superficial cutaneous infections or intravenous antibiotics in patients with systemic infections are necessary. Antibiotics should be targeted to cover the likely bacterial pathogens.

The newest class of antifungal agents, the allylamines (e.g., terbinafine cream), have been shown to produce higher cure rates and faster responses in dermatophyte infections than older agents. Some of the oral medications (fluconazole) are effective in weekly dosing patterns that may increase compliance. Because most fungal infections require long antibiotic courses (≥2 to 12 weeks), lack of compliance is frequently associated with treatment failure. Other side effects such as hepatic injury have been associated with ketoconazole and, less frequently, with griseofulvin, so monitoring of liver enzymes is advised.

Very dry, scaly, or lichenified skin lesions do better with ointments. If a steroid is not required, emollients such as Eucerin or Aquaphor are often recommended. Dry skin should not become wet, and soaps should be avoided because they dry the skin further. Wet, weeping skin lesions should be kept wet to facilitate drying; thus, frequent rinsing and wet-dry dressings are in order. Aluminum acetate or oatmeal baths may also facilitate drying.

Denuded skin, as may occur in vesiculating eruptions such as toxic epidermal necrolysis, should be treated as you would a large surface area burn. Occlusive, sterile dressings, aggressive fluid resuscitation, and the avoidance of topical or systemic steroids are indicated. Finally, always maintain a high index of suspicion regarding a possible drug reaction, and stop the potentially offending drug if indicated (see Tips and Tricks box).

Tips and Tricks

- The most frequent cause of generalized rash with or without fever is drug eruption or allergic reaction.
- Medium-strength steroid creams are useful for most skin areas except the face; therefore, triamcinolone 0.1% cream is the default prescription for most ED uses.
- Warn patients that when treating scabies, repeated doses of lindane are neurotoxic, and pruritus may persist for 1 to 2 weeks, so repeat doses may not be necessary.
- Consider burn unit admission for patients with desquamation covering more than 10% of body surface area.
- Toxic epidermal necrolysis and staphylococcal scalded skin syndrome look similar, but they require different treatments (stopping the suspected drug versus instituting antibiotic therapy).
- Early in meningococcemia, the rash can be macular, maculopapular, or petechial.
- Syphilis is known as the "great masquerader," and the clinician should always have a low index of suspicion.
- Purpura can be the result of a drug reaction, and a careful history should be obtained.
- Urticaria can be the first sign of infection, lupus, pemphigoid, vasculitis, dermatitis herpetiformis, and occult malignancy.

Disposition

Most dermatologic conditions can be treated on an outpatient basis. Patients with life-threatening dermatologic diseases, especially those associated with desquamation, should be admitted. Consideration for admission or transfer to a burn unit is necessary when 10% or more of the skin is desquamated. Referral to dermatology may be indicated, but most patients are unable to make an appointment for many weeks to months. The patient should be given clear instructions on when to return to the ED and should be warned that they may have to wait several weeks to see a dermatologist. Follow-up with the primary care physician in the meantime should be recommended, and the patient should be given sufficient medication to last until follow-up (see Tips and Tricks).

REFERENCE

1. Roujeau JC: Clinical heterogeneity of drug hypersensitivity. Toxicology 2005;209:123-129.

SECTION XX

Emergency Psychiatric Disorders

Chapter **193**

The Emergency Psychiatric Assessment

Douglas M. Char

KEY POINTS

The primary goal of the emergency psychiatric evaluation is to distinguish between acute medical and psychiatric conditions.

Primary mental disorders include disturbances of thought, mood, or personality. *The onset is generally at younger ages.*

Delirium and dementia are causes of global cognitive impairment that may be mistaken for psychiatric disease in elderly patients.

Approximately 50% of patients seeking emergency psychiatric services have a poorly treated or undiagnosed medical illness contributing to their presentation.

Provisional diagnoses should drive the need for and extent of diagnostic testing.

Acute interventions should improve the patient's cooperation, reduce agitation, prevent secondary harm, and initiate treatment of the primary mental disorder.

Scope

The primary goal of the emergency psychiatric evaluation is to distinguish between medical and psychiatric causes of disturbed behaviors and thoughts. Comorbid medical conditions must be addressed to ensure the appropriate and safe admission of patients to a psychiatric facility. Controversy surrounds many aspects of this medical clearance process, because limited evidence is available to guide EPs' practice.

Definitions

The fourth edition of the *Diagnostic and Statistical Manual of Mental Disorders* (DSM-IV) distinguishes "mental disorders that are due to a general medical condition" from "primary mental disorders."[1] The terms *organic* and *functional* are no longer used to differentiate between illnesses of medical and psychiatric origin (Table 193-1).

Primary mental disorders include disturbances in thought, mood, or personality. Memory impairment, disorientation, and inattention are rarely features of primary mental disorders.

Delirium and dementia are medical conditions characterized by a global impairment in cognitive function. Patients with delirium or dementia may be mistakenly diagnosed with a primary mental disorder. It is important to differentiate between these conditions and other psychiatric disorders.

■ DELIRIUM

Delirious patients have impaired attention and concentration. They demonstrate alterations in consciousness that fluctuate over time. The delirious patient may become acutely agitated or lethargic because of disturbances in the sleep-wake cycle. Abnormal cognition and speech may be apparent. Sensory perceptions, delusions, and hallucinations

Table 193-1 MEDICAL CAUSES OF DISTURBED BEHAVIOR VERSUS PRIMARY MENTAL DISORDERS

Medical Causes of Disturbed Behavior	Primary Mental Disorders
Delirium	Cognitive disorders (thought)
Dementia	Affective disorders (mood)
Intoxication	Somatoform disorder
Addiction	Hysteria
Developmental disorders	Dissociative states

are prominent. The onset of delirium is usually acute, evolving over hours to days. The determination of a patient's baseline cognitive function and onset of symptoms is critical to distinguishing delirium from dementia.

■ DEMENTIA

Pervasive disturbance of cognitive function is the hallmark of dementia. Deficits commonly involve memory, judgment, personality, and language. Patients have no clouding of consciousness. The earliest sign of dementia is subtle memory loss, which may promote anxiety, depression, and psychosis. Patients with dementia may experience an acute worsening of symptoms when stressors overwhelm their intellectual and physiologic reserves. As the disease progresses, patients become less capable of recognizing concomitant medical illnesses.

Clinical Presentation

Most patients requiring emergency psychiatric care exhibit some form of altered mental status, psychosis, or self-harm. Common psychiatric problems seen in the ED include substance abuse and addiction, affective disorders, anxiety disorders, antisocial personality disorders, and severe cognitive impairment.

Primary mental disorders usually manifest in patients between 12 and 40 years of age. In older patients, various causes of delirium and dementia are more common than primary mental disorders.

The prevalence of coexisting medical illness in psychiatric patients has been reported to be as high as 50%. Untreated medical illness often causes deterioration of baseline cognitive function in patients with a known psychiatric disorder. The prevalence of medical disease in patients presenting to the ED with an acute exacerbation of an existing mental illness may be as high as 80%. Almost 50% of patients demonstrate a causal relationship between acute medical and psychiatric complaints.[2]

Differential Diagnosis

Patients with disturbed behavior or thought processes should be presumed to have a medical origin for their condition. Patients with chronic diseases such as diabetes mellitus, reactive airway disease, heart failure, stroke, thyroid disease, and dementia may present with a sudden and dramatic impairment in cognition or affect. Life-threatening causes of delirium should be considered in all patients with psychiatric disturbances. Primary mental disorders should be diagnosed only after medical conditions have been convincingly excluded (Box 193-1).

BOX 193-1

Life-Threatening Causes of Delirium

Hypoxia
Hypoglycemia
Hypertensive encephalopathy
Intracranial hemorrhage
Thyrotoxicosis
Sepsis
Arrhythmia
Wernicke's encephalopathy
Drug or alcohol intoxication or withdrawal
Meningitis or encephalitis
Status epilepticus
Poisonings
Hepatic failure
Renal failure

Diagnostic criteria such as those provided in the DSM-IV aid in the establishment of a provisional psychiatric diagnosis in the ED. Although standardized criteria are useful, interrater agreement among emergency psychiatrists is variable (correlation coefficient, 0.28 to 0.65).[3]

Multiaxial diagnoses serve to organize complex clinical information and acknowledge the interplay of medical and psychiatric disease. Axis I diagnoses reflect mental disorders, axis II diagnoses identify personality disorders, axis III diagnoses include general medical conditions, and axis IV and axis V diagnoses list psychosocial stressors and adaptive functioning (Fig. 193-1).

Assessment Methods

No standardized, widely accepted protocol exists for performing medical clearance of psychiatric patients in the ED. The differentiation between medical and psychiatric disease is best accomplished by a thorough history and physical examination. Laboratory tests, radiographs, and electrocardiograms are of limited diagnostic value.[4]

The following questions should guide every emergency psychiatric evaluation:

1. Is the patient stable or unstable?
2. Are the presenting behaviors the result of an underlying medical illness?

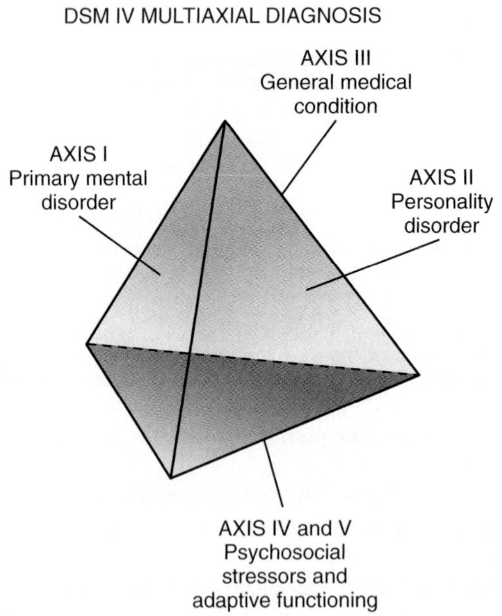
DSM IV MULTIAXIAL DIAGNOSIS
AXIS III
General medical
condition
AXIS I
Primary mental
disorder
AXIS II
Personality
disorder
AXIS IV and V
Psychosocial
stressors and
adaptive functioning

FIGURE 193-1 Multiaxial diagnoses data from fourth edition of the *Diagnostic and Statistical Manual of Mental Disorders* (DSM-IV).[1]

3. What is the severity of the primary mental disorder?
4. Is psychiatric consultation necessary?
5. Does the patient need to be detained to facilitate emergency treatment?

■ HISTORY

Obtain a focused history of the present illness that reviews current symptoms, elicits precipitating circumstances, assesses risk severity, and establishes a time course. Other necessary historical elements include past medical or psychiatric illnesses, medication use (Table 193-2), substance abuse or addiction, and a family history of psychiatric or pertinent medical illnesses.

Patients with cognitive or affective disorders are often unable to provide their complete clinical history. Friends, family members, and prehospital providers are useful sources for acquiring additional information. The patient's baseline cognitive function may be obtained from the medical record or solicited through discussion with the primary care provider.

■ PHYSICAL EXAMINATION

Perform an organized and thorough physical examination. Scrutinize the patient's vitals signs for evidence of shock, metabolic derangement, or infection. Search for signs of impaired organ and tissue perfusion. Check for hypoxia and abnormal respiratory effort. Look for abrasions or contusions that may represent recent trauma and unsuspected head injury. Identify subtle, focal weakness or neglect suggestive of possible neurologic impairment. Evaluate for other signs of neurologic disease including dysesthesias, apraxias, agnosia, left-right disorientation, aphasia, and an inability to follow commands. Sensory illusions can be associated with neurologic conditions or intoxications. Visual, tactile, and olfactory hallucinations are generally attributed to medical disease (Table 193-3).

The mental status examination should assess the patient's level of consciousness, appearance, behavior, mood, affect, language, thought form and content, perceptions, and cognition. Much of this information can be obtained indirectly by observing the patient during the interview. Brief, standardized assessment tools such as the Folstein Mini-Mental Status Examination or the Quick Confusional Scale allow for detection of subtle deficits (Table 193-4).

Cursory examinations of psychiatric patients are unacceptable. Uncooperative or fully dressed patients may hide evidence of physical abuse or medical illness; these same patients may conceal weapons or illicit drugs.

■ DIAGNOSTIC TESTING

Laboratory testing should be appropriate for the provisional diagnoses established through the history and the physical and mental status examinations. No standard, cross-specialty guidelines exist for laboratory testing as part of the emergency psychiatric evaluation. Many EDs have developed protocols based on local disease prevalence, common clinical presentations, the potential for needed treatment, and the likelihood of admission or extended monitoring.

Screening tests commonly ordered as part of the emergency psychiatric evaluation include pulse oximetry, complete blood count, serum chemistry panel with glucose, electrocardiogram, urine toxicology screen, urine pregnancy testing, and alcohol level assessment by serum or breath analysis. Testing of liver function and thyroid function, as well as computed tomography imaging of the head, may also be indicated. Chest radiography, lumbar puncture, arterial blood sampling, and electroencephalography should not be used as screening tests in the evaluation of patients with suspected psychiatric illness.

EPs and psychiatrists often disagree on the amount of diagnostic testing required for medical clearance in the ED.[5] One survey of EPs found that screening tests were required by 35% of psychiatric consultants or accepting institutions. At least one third of ED patients with a primary psychiatric complaint, past psychiatric history, and normal physical examination require no further ancillary testing.[6]

Diagnostic testing of psychiatric patients in the ED should accomplish one of the following goals: (1) detect or exclude the presence of a condition that has treatment consequences, (2) determine the relative safety or appropriate dose of potential alternative treatments, or (3) provide baseline information useful for monitoring treatment response.

Table 193-2 MEDICATIONS THAT CAUSE PSYCHIATRIC SYMPTOMS

Drug Class	Reactions
Amphetamines	Bizarre behavior, hallucinations, paranoia, agitation, anxiety, mania, nightmares
Antibiotics	Cephalosporins: euphoria, delusions, depersonalization, illusions Fluoroquinolones: psychosis, confusion, agitation, depression, hallucinations, paranoia, tics, mania Sulfonamides: confusion, disorientation, depression, euphoria, hallucinations
Anticholinergics	Confusion, memory loss, disorientation, depersonalization, delirium, auditory and visual hallucinations, fear, paranoia, incoherent speech, agitation, bizarre behavior, flushing, dry skin, retrograde amnesia
Antidepressants	Monoamine oxidase inhibitors: mania or hypomania Selective serotonin reuptake inhibitors: mania, hypomania, hallucinations Tricyclic antidepressants: mania or hypomania, delirium, hallucinations, paranoia, irritability, dysphoria
Antiepileptics	Agitation, confusion, delirium, depression, psychosis, aggression, mania, toxic encephalopathy, nightmares
Barbiturates	Hyperactivity, visual hallucinations, depression, confusion, dyskinesia
Benzodiazepines	Rage, hostility, paranoia, hallucinations, delirium, depression, nightmares, antegrade amnesia, mania, disinhibition
Antihypertensives	Angiotensin-converting enzyme inhibitors: mania, anxiety, hallucinations, depression, psychosis Beta-blockers: depression, psychosis, delirium, anxiety, nightmares, hallucinations Calcium-channel blockers: depression, delirium, confusion, psychosis, mania Thiazide diuretics: depression, suicidal ideation
Dopamine receptor agonists	Hallucinations, paranoia, delusions, confusion, mania, hypersexuality, anxiety, depression, nightmares
Histamine receptor antagonists	H_1-receptor antagonists: hallucinations H_2-receptor antagonists: delirium, confusion, psychosis, mania, aggression, depression, nightmares
Nonsteroidal anti-inflammatory agents	Depression, paranoia, psychosis, confusion, anxiety
Opioids	Nightmares, anxiety, agitations, euphoria, dysphoria, depression, paranoia, psychosis, hallucinations, dementia
Procaine derivatives	Fear of imminent death, anxiety, hallucinations, illusions, delusions, agitation, mania, depersonalization, psychosis
Salicylates	Agitation, confusion, hallucinations, paranoia
Statins (hepatic 3-methylglutaryl coenzyme A reductase inhibitors)	Anxiety, depression, obsessions, delusions
Steroids	Anabolic: psychosis, mania, depression, anxiety, aggressiveness, paranoia Corticosteroids: psychosis, delirium, mania, depression, hyperactivity, disinhibition

Adapted from Drugs that may cause psychiatric symptoms. Med Lett Drugs Ther 2002;44:59-62.

The utility of any recommended screening test depends on (1) the probability that the condition is currently present, (2) the probability that the test will detect the condition correctly, (3) the probability that the test will identify a condition that is not present incorrectly, and (4) the implications for treatment (Box 193-2).

Treatment

Acute behavioral disturbances mandate emergency care that is time and resource intensive. Treatment should be directed at the underlying cause of the disordered thought process or behavior, if known. Emergency psychiatric interventions are guided by three principles: (1) to improve patient cooperation, (2) to reduce agitation, and (3) to reduce the risk of secondary harm.

Patient safety and staff safety are of paramount importance. Suicidal patients need to be closely monitored and protected from self-harm. Agitated patients constitute a threat to themselves and to others. The rapid administration of psychotropic and anxiolytic medications is a safe and effective method for controlling potentially dangerous patients. Seclusion, sitters, and the use of physical and chemical restraints may be temporarily required. Chapters 194 to 196 provide specific treatment recommendations for psychotic, violent, and suicidal patients. Disease-appropriate treatments for the various causes of delirium and dementia are reviewed elsewhere in this text.

Table 193-3 PHYSICAL EXAMINATION FINDINGS AND MEDICAL CAUSES OF ABNORMAL BEHAVIOR

Organ System	Finding	Potential Medical Condition
General	Hyperthermia	Thyrotoxicosis, vasculitis, alcohol withdrawal, withdrawal from sedative-hypnotic agents, meningitis, inflammatory processes
	Hypothermia	Sepsis, dermal disease, endocrine disorders, central nervous system dysfunction, intoxication
	Hypotension	Shock, Addison's disease, hypothyroidism, adverse drug reactions, dehydration
	Hypertension	Hypertensive encephalopathy, stimulant abuse, anticholinergic excess
Gastrointestinal	Distention	Constipation, hepatic encephalopathy with ascites, obstruction, viscous perforation with sepsis
	Masses	Liver disease, cancer, obstruction
Cardiovascular	Bradycardia	Hypothyroidism, Stoke-Adams syndrome, elevated intracranial pressure
	Tachycardia	Hyperthyroidism, infection, heart failure, pulmonary embolism, alcohol intoxication or withdrawal
	Arrhythmias	Toxins, embolic strokes, electrolyte abnormalities
Neurologic	Confusion	Hypoxia, infection, toxins, electrolyte abnormalities, trauma, meningitis, encephalitis
	Seizures	Infections, head trauma, intoxication, poisonings, primary seizure disorder, meningitis
	Motor deficits	Stroke, encephalopathy, neuropathy, spinal trauma, movement disorders
	Aphasia	Stroke, head trauma, central nervous system disease
	Headache	Head trauma, meningitis, vasculitis, stroke, toxins, hypertensive emergencies
	Visual deficits	Head trauma, increased intracranial pressure, meningitis, cerebritis, ocular trauma, poisoning
Pulmonary	Tachypnea	Metabolic acidosis, pulmonary embolism, pneumonia, cardiac failure, fever
	Wheezing/stridor	Reactive airway disease, airway foreign body, hypoxia
	Rales	Pneumonia, pulmonary effusions, heart failure
Skin	Abrasions and contusions	Closed head injury, intracranial hemorrhage

Table 193-4 MINI-MENTAL STATUS EXAMINATION

Category	Test Behavior	Score
Orientation	What is the (year) (season) (date) (day) (month)?	5
	Where are we (state) (country) (town) (hospital) (floor)?	5
Registration	Name three objects (1 second to say each). Ask the patient to name all three after you have said them. Give one point for each correct answer. Repeat until he or she learns all three. Count and record trials __.	3
Attention and calculation	Serial 7s, backward from 100. Give one point for each correct answer. Stop after five answers. Alternatively, spell "world" backward.	5
Recall	Ask for the three objects named above. Give one point for each correct answer.	3
Language	Name a pencil and watch.	2
	Repeat the following: "No ifs, ands, or buts."	1
	Follow a three-stage command: "Take this paper in your hand, fold it in half, and put it on the floor."	3
	Read and obey the following: CLOSE YOUR EYES.	1
	Write a sentence.	1
	Copy the design shown (two intersecting pentagrams).	1

Maximum score = 30. Score <23 indicates cognitive impairment.

From Folstein M, Folstein SE, McHugh PR: "Mini-mental state": A practical method for grading the cognitive state of patients for the clinician. J Psychiatr Res 1975;12:189-198.

Disposition

The emergency psychiatric evaluation should result in one of four outcomes: (1) a medical cause of the chief complaint is identified, (2) a primary mental disorder is diagnosed, (3) the presenting symptom or condition was self-limited and resolved, or (4) the cause of the abnormal behavior or disordered thought process remains unclear and mandates medical admission (Box 193-3).

Patients without an apparent medical cause of their confusion, disordered thought, or bizarre behavior require psychiatric evaluation. Most of these patients need to be admitted to a psychiatric service

Table 193-5 **COMMON PITFALLS IN THE EMERGENCY PSYCHIATRIC EVALUATION**

Pitfall	Incorrect Rationale	Resultant Error
Inappropriate or premature referral to psychiatry	Bizarre, disruptive behavior is less urgent or serious than the medical complaints of other patients in the ED. Initial decisions are often based on a single symptom or historical feature.	Provider bias and faulty assumptions lead to incorrect diagnoses.
Bizarre behavior or thoughts as "diagnostic" of primary mental disorders	Delusions, hallucinations, and disorganized thoughts are usually signs of primary psychosis.	These symptoms are nonspecific and may reflect delirium.
Premature referral of violent patients to psychiatry	Violent patients place staff and others at risk and disrupt the flow of care in the ED.	Violent behavior may be the result of underlying medical illness.
Allowing biased staff to hinder evaluation and to guide care	Certain patients (alcoholic patients, drug abusers, suicidal individuals) create their own disease and do not deserve urgent intervention.	Blaming the patient for an illness does not correct the behavior or address the underlying psychiatric disease.
Provider convinced that the patient is insincere	The provider does not believe the threats or complaints of seemingly unreliable patients.	The provider underestimates the potential for serious or lethal outcomes.
Discharging elderly patients with "dementia"	Dementia cannot be treated.	The provider presumes that all elderly patients are permanently impaired (60% of dementias are treatable).

BOX 193-2

Rationale for Diagnostic Testing

1. The test detects or excludes the presence of a treatable condition.
2. The test determines the relative safety and appropriate dose of a potential therapy.
3. The test provides baseline information required for monitoring treatment response.

for extended observation and therapy. Some individuals may need to be held involuntarily according to individual state laws.

Discharge may be considered for those patients whose symptoms resolve rapidly after minimal treatment or after a short period of observation. Three discharge criteria must be met: (1) patients should be able to care for themselves or should have an appropriate caregiver at home, (2) patients cannot be actively suicidal or homicidal, and (3) patients should not have any unresolved symptoms of medical illness.

If subacute medical conditions are identified in patients requiring psychiatric admission, the accepting psychiatric service must be capable of providing appropriate care and follow-up. Untreated medical illnesses may complicate psychiatric interventions and may result in repeat presentations to the ED (Table 193-5).

BOX 193-3

Potential Outcomes of the Emergency Psychiatric Evaluation

1. A medical cause of the presenting abnormal behavior or thought process is identified, and treatment is initiated.
2. A primary mental disorder is diagnosed, and psychiatric consultation is obtained.
3. The patient's presenting condition is self-limited and resolved. Discharge criteria are met.
4. The cause of the abnormal behavior or disordered thought process remains unclear. Further evaluation mandates admission to a medical service with psychiatric consultation.

REFERENCES

1. First MB, Frances A, Pincus HA (eds): DSM-IV-TR Handbook of Differential Diagnosis. Arlington, VA, American Psychiatric Association, 2002.
2. Koran LM, Sox HC, Marton KI, et al: Medical evaluation of psychiatric patients. I. Results in a state mental health system. Arch Gen Psychiatry 1989;46:733-740.
3. Way BB, Allen MH, Mumpower JL, et al: Interrater agreement among psychiatrists in psychiatric emergency assessments. Am J Psychiatry 1998;155:1423-1428.
4. Kanich W, Brady WJ, Huff JS, et al: Altered mental status: evaluation and the etiology in the ED. Am J Emerg Med 2002;20:613-617.
5. Zun LS, Hernandez R, Thompson R, Downey L: Comparison of EPs' and psychiatrists' laboratory assessment of psychiatric patients. Am J Emerg Med 2004;22:175-180.
6. Korn CS, Currier GW, Henderson SO: "Medical clearance" of psychiatric patients without medical complaints in the emergency department. J Emerg Med 2000;18:173-176.

Chapter 194

Psychosis and Psychotropic Medication

Lynda Daniel-Underwood and Tae Eung Kim

KEY POINTS

Psychosis refers to symptoms that demonstrate impairments in thought content and process.
Schizophrenia, bipolar disease, substance abuse, and depression may all have psychotic features over time.
Most psychotic disorders initially manifest in adolescent and young adult populations.
Typical antipsychotic medications have a high affinity for dopamine receptors. Typical antipsychotic agents are useful in treating the "positive symptoms" of schizophrenia: hallucinations and delusions.
Atypical antipsychotic medications have a high affinity for serotonin receptors. These agents are better choices for the treatment of "negative" behavioral symptoms associated with psychosis.

Scope

Psychosis refers to a syndrome of symptoms demonstrating impairment of both thought content and thought process. Thought content disturbances include perceptions that are not reality based, whereas thought process is often disorganized and illogical in form. Psychotic symptoms include visual, tactile, or olfactory hallucinations, delusions, impairment of concentration and attention, and disorientation. Schizophrenia is the disorder that is most often associated with psychosis. Bipolar disorder, major depression, and substance abuse are examples of psychiatric diagnoses that can also cause symptoms of acute psychosis.

The 1-year prevalence of the schizophrenic disorders is 1.1%. One out of every 100 persons in the United States suffers from psychotic symptoms.[1] Episodes of psychosis are generally precipitated or exacerbated by psychosocial stressors. Psychosis may be acute or chronic. As is often the case with a first presentation of schizophrenia, acute psychotic episodes prompt patients to seek emergency care for their bizarre behavior or troubling perceptions.

Pathophysiology

The dominant theory used to explain the pathophysiology of psychotic thought is the *dopamine hypothesis*. This theory suggests that psychosis is likely the result of excess dopamine transmission in the mesolimbic pathway of the brain. Evidence offered for the behavioral influence of this neurotransmitter is based on the observed effects of antipsychotic medications on dopamine pathways of the brain. Dopamine receptor antagonists (D_2-receptor antagonists) improve disturbed thoughts in psychotic patients. The efficacy of the typical (first-generation) antipsychotic agents depends on the degree to which these drugs block D_2-receptor activity.

Competing theories that describe the pathophysiology of psychosis are also based on neurotransmitter activity. These theories generally cite the effects and interplay of serotonin and glutamate with dopamine.

Clinical Presentation

Most psychotic disorders initially manifest in adolescent and young adult populations. The median age for the onset of symptoms of a psychiatric disorder is 16 years. By the age of 38 years, more than 90% of patients with a mental disorder will have developed symptoms.[1] The typical presentation of a newly psychotic patient is that of a young person brought to the ED by family or friends who are concerned about the patient's bizarre behavior or unusual beliefs.

The key feature of psychotic symptoms is that perceptions and beliefs are not based in reality. These disturbances of thought content include hallucinations, illusions, and delusions.

Hallucinations are sensory perceptions that are apparent only to the patient experiencing them. Auditory hallucinations are most common, typically described as hearing voices of people who are not present. Hallucinations that involve other senses (visual, olfactory, or tactile) are less frequently reported. Patients who are hallucinating appear preoccupied or distracted as they respond to internal stimuli.

Illusions refer to misperceptions about a patient's surroundings, whereas hallucinations are wholly internal and are not prompted by an environmental stimulus.

Delusions are misinterpretations of events or perceptions that lead psychotic patients erroneously to attribute experiences to unlikely or bizarre beliefs. Unlike cultural beliefs that may be foreign to a provider, delusions are explanations that are not shared by others. Most delusions involve a sense of control. For example, patients with delusions of persecution may believe that they are under hostile surveillance or that people are plotting against them. Grandiose delusions cause other patients to believe that they are endowed with supernatural powers or are able to affect events outside of their sphere of influence.

Psychosis may also manifest as disorganization in thought process, in that patients express ideas and words that are not coherently linked. Thoughts are described as *tangential* when the patient switches from one topic to another without logical association. When thoughts become more disorganized, the patient may start using *neologisms,* or self-created "non-sense" words. Speech may later develop into an incomprehensible jumble of unassociated phrases, described as *word salad.*

Differential Diagnosis

First presentations of psychosis are uncommon in young children and older adults; do not confuse delirium or dementia with true psychotic behavior. Causes of delirium often manifest by abnormal vital signs or subtle physical examination findings, either of which should prompt a search for medical conditions that may mimic psychiatric disease. Medical causes of delirium that may be mistaken for psychosis include toxic ingestions, substance abuse, and brain tumors. Medical conditions may precipitate psychosis or exacerbate chronic mental disorders.

Diagnostic Testing

A detailed discussion of the emergency psychiatric evaluation can be found in Chapter 193.

Psychotropic Medications

■ TYPICAL (FIRST-GENERATION) ANTIPSYCHOTIC AGENTS

Typical antipsychotic medications have a high affinity for D_2 receptors, thus blocking dopamine overactivity in the mesocortical pathway. D_2 antagonism accounts for the clinical profile of these agents, which are useful in treating the "positive symptoms" of schizophrenia: hallucinations and delusions.[2] Haloperidol is the prototypical agent of this drug class (Table 194-1).

Typical antipsychotic agents also decrease dopaminergic activity in the nigrostriatal pathway at therapeutic doses. This adverse effect leads to increased cholinergic activity, promoting extrapyramidal symptoms (EPSs) and the presence of other movement disorders. Tardive dyskinesia is thought to arise from up-regulation (supersensitivity) of postsynaptic dopamine receptors in the nigrostriatal pathway after prolonged receptor blockade. Benztropine (Cogentin) administration can slow the development of EPSs.

■ ATYPICAL (SECOND-GENERATION) ANTIPSYCHOTIC AGENTS

Atypical antipsychotic medications have a high affinity for serotonin ($5\text{-}HT_{2A}$) receptors compared with the D_2 receptors. Serotonergic neurons in the dorsal raphe nuclei interact with the dopaminergic neurons in the nigrostriatal pathway and modulate clinical effects. Atypical antipsychotic agents are characterized by lower incidences of EPSs and show a diverse range of binding activities at other receptor sites as well. Serotonin and other neurotransmitter blockade may account for the beneficial effects of the atypical antipsychotic agents against "negative" behavioral

Table 194-1 TYPICAL ANTIPSYCHOTIC MEDICATIONS (DOPAMINE-2–RECEPTOR ANTAGONISTS)

Drug	Usual Dose	Comments
Haloperidol	5-10 mg IM or IV* 1-2.5 mg PO in elderly patients ≤20 mg PO per dose	Onset: 30-60 min Risk of adverse effects (extrapyramidal symptoms, akathisia)
Chlorpromazine	25 mg IM	Faster time to onset Prolonged sedation
Droperidol†	5-10 mg IM 2.5-5 mg IV	Onset: 3-5 min Arousal time: 2 hr Prolongation of QT interval reported at low doses†

*Administration of Haldol IV is off label because of the risk of QT prolongation and arrhythmia.
†A "black box" warning was mandated by the Food and Drug Administration in 2001, given the risk of fatal tachyarrhythmias.
IM, intramuscularly; IV, intravenously; PO, orally.

Table 194-2 ATYPICAL ANTIPSYCHOTIC MEDICATIONS (SEROTONIN AND DOPAMINE-2–RECEPTOR ANTAGONISTS)

Drug	Usual Dose	Comments
Clozapine	12.5 mg PO bid	Used for refractory schizophrenia Causes agranulocytosis, diabetes, weight gain
Risperidone	2 mg PO liquid or ODT	Causes weight gain, prolactin elevation, extrapyramidal symptoms
Olanzapine	10 mg IM, may repeat in 2 hr to maximum 30 mg/day 10-15 mg SL (ODT), maximum 20 mg/day	Strong antihistamine effect, sedating Controls positive, negative, and affective symptoms Promotes weight gain, diabetes Causes the least change in QT intervals
Ziprasidone	10 mg IM q2h or 20 mg IM q4h	Promotes the greatest QT prolongation of class

bid, twice daily; IM, intramuscularly; ODT, orally disintegrating tablet; PO, orally; q, every; SL, sublingually.

Table 194-3 PARTIAL RECEPTOR AGONIST

Drug	Usual Dose	Comments
Aripiprazole	10-30 mg PO daily	Low side effect profile

PO, orally.

symptoms by increasing dopamine activity in the prefrontal cortex (Table 194-2).

■ PARTIAL RECEPTOR AGONISTS

Partial receptor agonists demonstrate variable clinical effects, as influenced by the receptor binding affinity of the agent and the patient's endogenous levels of neurotransmitter. One available partial agonist, aripiprazole, appears to be an effective and possibly superior treatment option for patients with schizophrenia. It does not completely block the mesolimbic system (associated with negative symptoms and cognitive impairment), nor does it completely stimulate the nigrostriatal or tuberoinfundibular pathways responsible for EPSs and elevated prolactin levels[2] (Table 194-3).

■ BENZODIAZEPINES

Benzodiazepines are commonly used to treat psychotic agitation because of their efficacy and tolerability. These agents increase the effects of gamma-aminobutyric acid (GABA) on the chloride ionophore of the GABA-benzodiazepine receptor complex, thus causing sedation and sleepiness. Benzodiazepines are generally administered in combination with typical antipsychotic medications to sedate agitated or violent patients. Adverse effects, including oversedation and diminished respiratory drive, are minimal at low doses. Rare reports have noted "frontal disinhibition" leading to increased impulsive behavior with benzodiazepine use in patients with previous head injury or mental retardation[3] (Table 194-4).

Treatment

Pharmacologic management in the ED can be difficult because of the constellation of nonspecific behaviors observed in psychotic patients with an undifferentiated psychiatric or medical condition. Haloperidol remains the most accepted pharmacologic treatment for psychosis of uncertain origin. More recently, combination therapy using benzodiazepines with typical antipsychotic agents has been

Table 194-4 **BENZODIAZEPINES**

Drug	Usual Dose	Comment
Lorazepam	2-4 mg PO or 1-2 mg IM	Half-life: 6-20 hr Treats aggressive behavior
Clonazepam	1-2 mg IM	Rapid onset, long half-life
Diazepam	5-10 mg PO or 2-5 mg IM	Half-life: 20 hr IM

IM, intramuscularly; PO, orally.

shown to provide superior results. Combination therapy allows for rapid, safe sedation in addition to control of presenting psychotic features.

Any agitation or violent behavior associated with psychosis should be managed as soon as a patient arrives in the ED. Verbal warnings should precede the use of chemical or physical restraints. The least restrictive method of restraint is preferable, to facilitate a safe and complete diagnostic evaluation.[4,5]

Disposition

In many jurisdictions, patients may be held against their will by peace officers or attending medical staff if they are determined to be gravely disabled, a danger to themselves, or a danger to others because of a mental disturbance. The goal of such restraint is to provide treatment that may improve the patient's decision-making capacity and allow time for evaluation of any undiagnosed illnesses. Patients may be discharged from the ED if their psychotic behavior is well controlled, if medical and surgical concerns are addressed, if they have accompanying family or friends, and if aftercare is easily available.

REFERENCES

1. Norquist GS, Regier DA: The epidemiology of psychiatric disorders and the de facto mental health care system. Annu Rev Med 1996;47:473-479.
2. Lieberman J: Dopamine partial agonists: A new class of antipsychotic. CNS Drugs 2004;18:251-267.
3. Currier GW, Trenton A: Pharmacological treatment of psychotic agitation. CNS Drugs 2002;16:219-228.
4. Buckley PF, Noffsinger SG, Smith DA, et al: Treatment of the psychotic patient who is violent. Psychiatr Clin North Am 2003;26:231-272.
5. Yildiz A, Sachs GS, Turgay A: Pharmacological management of agitation in emergency settings. Emerg Med J 2003;20:339-346.

Chapter **195**

The Violent Patient

Eric Isaacs

KEY POINTS

Patient risk factors for violent behavior include evidence of agitation (e.g., pacing), substance abuse, a history of prior violence, arrival to the ED in police custody, and male gender.

Disarming protocols and de-escalation techniques are critical methods for violence prevention.

Agitated or violent behavior is frequently caused by medical conditions, such as hypoglycemia or intoxication.

Violent patients should be given a verbal warning before they are restrained. Physical restraint should be supplanted by chemical restraint when safety allows.

Medical complications of incorrect or prolonged physical restraint include hyperthermia, acidosis, rhabdomyolysis, and death.

Sedation is best achieved through a combination of intramuscular benzodiazepine (lorazepam) and butyrophenone (haloperidol).

Scope and Epidemiology

The goal of caring for a violent patient is first to protect everyone involved and also to diagnose and treat important medical and psychiatric conditions (see Priority Actions box). These goals are best achieved if warning signs of violence are recognized and the safest and most effective means of behavioral control are used.

The epidemiology of violence in the ED is inexact; past surveys suggest that as many as 80% of events are unreported.[1] Still, clear evidence indicates that most EDs experience violent patients routinely. Of greater concern, ED caregivers are often victims. More than 70% of ED nurses have reported being the victim of physical violence during their career.[2]

Violence may range from verbal threats to physical assaults. Of reported events in one survey, 90% of cases involved the patient and 10% involved family or visitors. A few staff members are confronted by former patients outside the ED, and ED staff may become the victims of stalking.

Nearly 60% of EDs in the United States have reported an armed threat on a staff member within 5 years.[3] Weapons may be carried by patients, family members, visitors, or even staff members. Patients most likely to carry weapons include those with schizophrenia or paranoid ideation and individuals who have been the victims of gunshot wounds. Many violent patients are intoxicated with alcohol or drugs.

Violence threatens the career longevity of ED staff. Violent events should be regularly reported to police and hospital administration to raise awareness of this societal problem and to encourage safer practice environments.

PRIORITY ACTIONS

Goals for the Care of the Violent Patient in the ED

- Recognize risk factors and warning signs before violence occurs.
- Use de-escalation (communication) techniques to prevent violent behavior.
- Control the patient and situation to minimize further violence.
- Diagnose and treat reversible causes of agitation.
- Protect the patient and others through appropriate restraint methods.

How to Predict Violence

Violent behavior rarely erupts without warning. Risk factors for violence include an escalating psychiatric illness (e.g. schizophrenia, personality disorders, or mania), alcohol and drug abuse, a history of prior violence, ED arrival in police custody, and male gender (Box 195-1). The use of risk factors to predict violent behavior has not been tested in cohorts of EPs; psychiatrists have been only 60% accurate in predicting violence when using risk factors alone.[4]

Verbal and nonverbal clues provide evidence of impending violence. As patients become more agitated, the level of their voice may rise and their hand gestures may be more pronounced and expressive. Patients may exhibit restlessness on their gurney or may pace. Providers should trust their instincts when they become uncomfortable with an agitated patient. Emotional stress, prolonged waiting times, and gaps in communication create a provocative and unsupportive environment.

BOX 195-1

Risk Factors for Concealed Weapon Use and Violent Behavior in the ED

Concealed Weapons

- Schizophrenia
- Paranoid ideation
- Victims of gunshot wounds

Violent Behavior

- Schizophrenia
- Personality disorders
- Mania
- Substance abuse or intoxication
- History of prior violent behavior
- Arrival in police custody
- Male gender

Interventions

Standardized methods to confiscate concealed weapons should be in place. Metal detectors are in use in some EDs and are recommended when weapons possession by patients or visitors is frequent. For patients, a policy of routine undressing and gowning, regardless of chief complaint, will minimize the likelihood of hidden weapon use and is unbiased.

Examination room preparation can facilitate safety. Remove as many objects as possible from examination rooms that routinely hold violent or agitated patients. Panic buttons should be present for use by staff in any room where agitated patients are interviewed. Ideally, examination rooms should have two exits so neither the clinician nor the patient feels trapped. Restless patients may become more agitated when physical outlets are constrained, so both the patient and caregiver must have unobstructed, rapid egress. Staff members should remove personal objects that could be used to cause injury by an assaultive patient. Such objects include neckties, large dangling earrings, and stethoscopes kept around the neck.

De-Escalation Techniques

Early attention and preferential treatment may defuse anger borne of impatience. If at triage, bring an agitated patient directly to a treatment room. Remove volatile patients from contact with other persons to decrease stimuli and to avoid tension.

Essential violence prevention techniques include interpersonal skills that convey respect and unconditional positive regard. Behaviors do not have to be accepted by ED staff, but no disrespect to the person should be conveyed. Start by stating explicitly that "this emergency department is a safe place" and the patient will be cared for well. Make the patient physically comfortable. Offer food or drink as both an expression of caring and also to minimize irritability. Do not surprise the patient; announce your arrival with a knock on the door or a verbal greeting. Ask permission to touch the patient before doing so. When speaking to the patient, use a calm and soothing voice. Listen attentively and intuitively to overt words and actions while attempting to assess underlying motivations and driving impulses. Additionally, the listening will reassure the patient, and it is a caring act. Use straightforward speech and always be honest.

Even as the person receives genuine, unconditional care, boundaries of acceptable behavior should be set, and consequences must be consistent. Inappropriate behavior is unacceptable, and patients should be told the ramifications. Some patients do not have the ability to cope with the stressful environment and become verbally or physically uncontrolled. Other patients respond to limit setting and rules. Most require anxiolytics. The early use of low-dose benzodiazepine often helps patients to cope and prevents later escalation. No action or treatment

Tips and Tricks

DE-ESCALATION TECHNIQUES USEFUL FOR VIOLENCE PREVENTION IN THE ED

Do

- Disrobe and gown all patients regardless of the chief complaint.
- Disarm all patients at triage through the use of metal detectors.
- Remove dangerous objects from the examination room.
- Remove personal objects that can be used as weapons (tie, stethoscope).
- Provide preferential, timely, and attentive care.
- Make the patient comfortable (offer food, blankets).
- Ask permission to enter the room and to examine or touch the patient.
- Use a calm voice.
- Explain anticipated waits, delays, and testing.
- Set limits and ramifications for inappropriate behaviors.

Do not

- Block exits from the examination room.
- Shout or yell at patients.
- Argue or challenge patients.
- Allow your emotions to overcome your judgment and behavior.

should ever be punitive. Chemical restraint, physical restraint, seclusion, and arrest are predictable consequences of inappropriate behavior, but early medical therapy is compassionate and usually prevents escalation.

Health care providers can escalate a patient's behavior through their own instinctive, impulsive, natural, human conduct.[5] Anger or frustration should never inspire professional behaviors or decisions. Physical and emotional distance may minimize the emotional reactions. A buffer zone of at least four body widths between you and the patient is recommended.

When a caregiver feels the urge to shout, argue, or engage in staring match with a patient, the caregiver is inadvertently reciprocating the violence of the patient. Controlling these natural instincts is an important professional skill that, for many, requires cultivation and practice. Other caregivers must cultivate a willingness to engage sufficiently because their instinct is to disengage. Too much distance can be equally detrimental. Finding the optimal emotional and physical distance to be effective and caring is a practiced art. If caregivers are too distant, they will be aloof, condescending, or disengaged. If caregivers are too close, they may become stimulated by the patient's disorder. The right distance enables control and effectiveness.

Medical Clearance

Agitated or violent behavior is frequently caused by treatable medical conditions. Reversible causes of altered mental status and violent behavior should be considered during the initial evaluation of the patient, including substance abuse, intoxication, glucose abnormalities, hypoxia, trauma, abnormal temperature (hypothermia and hyperthermia), infection, stroke, and seizures. Older adults with new agitated behavior, delirium, or psychosis should undergo an extensive inpatient medical evaluation before a first-time psychiatric unit admission.

Treatment

■ PHYSICAL RESTRAINT

■ Rationale

The use of restraint is indicated when verbal attempts have failed and action must be taken to prevent injury to the patient or staff. Restraint should be used only to facilitate diagnosis and treatment. It is inappropriate to use restraint as punishment or simply to quiet a disruptive patient.[6]

The Supreme Court case of *Youngberg v. Romero 1982* provided exception from assault statutes for physicians who restrained patients to protect the patient or others. This physician decision must be carefully made, as rarely as possible, and only under compelling circumstances to ensure safety.

The Joint Commission published clear guidelines regarding the monitoring, documentation, and application of physical restraint (Box 195-2). The protection of patients' rights, dignity, and well-being is of utmost importance. The decision to apply physical restraint should be assessment driven; the provider must evaluate the individual patient in some way before a restraint is applied. It is inappropriate to maintain standing protocols. The selection of restraint should be individualized, and the least restrictive method is preferred; for instance, it is not necessary to restrain an agitated elderly patient with dementia in the same manner as an aggressive, muscular patient with cocaine intoxication. Hospitals must provide adequate training such that competent staff members are available for the safe application of physical restraint at all times.

■ Documentation

Documentation differs for physicians and for nursing staff. A time-limited order for restraints must be on the chart before or shortly after restraints are applied. Providers must document why physical restraints were necessary and must cite that verbal techniques failed to calm the patient. Be specific about the patient's presentation and reasons for restraint, including the potential danger to the patient or others, the planned medical work-up or treatment, and an assessment of the patient's decision-making

Documentation

RESTRAINT*

Physician

- Document why physical or chemical restraint was chosen and necessary, and cite that verbal techniques failed to calm the patient.
- Record specific information about the patient's arrival, the reasons for restraint, the potential danger to self or others, the planned medical evaluation, and an assessment of the patient's decision-making capacity.
- Record the initial evaluation by a licensed, independent provider within 1 hour of the patient's arrival and restraint.
- A time-limited order should be charted within 1 hour of the patient's arrival.
- Update restraint orders every 4 hours for adults, 2 hours for adolescents aged 9 to 17 years, and 1 hour for children less than 9 years old.

Nursing

- Frequently reassess the patient's vital signs, condition, and personal needs.
- Patients should then be rechecked every 15 minutes for the following:
  1. Signs of injury associated with the application of restraint
  2. Nutrition and hydration
  3. Circulation and range of motion in the extremities
  4. Vital signs
  5. Hygiene and elimination
  6. Physical and psychological status and comfort
  7. Readiness for discontinuation of restraint

*Refer to www.jointcommission.org for more information.

capacity. Nursing responsibilities include the monitoring, frequent reassessment, and documentation of the patient's condition and personal needs.

■ Technique

The safe application of physical restraint is best achieved through systematic, consistent, protocol-driven techniques (Box 195-3). Many hospitals have a restraint team of at least five members that respond to the bedside when called by any provider. One staff member should lead the restraint team, which usually is comprised of nurses, medical assistants, and security personnel. Ideally, physician involvement in restraint is minimized in an effort to preserve the physician-patient relationship as much as possible. Physicians are held responsible for the negligent application of restraint, however, so they should limit their involvement only if there is another experienced team member to lead the restraint team.

BOX 195-2

Guidelines for the Application of Physical Restraint

- Protect the patient's rights, dignity, and well-being.
- The use of restraint is assessment driven.
- Use the least restrictive method.
- Trained, competent staff provides safe application of restraint.
- A time-limited order must be noted on the chart.
- Document why restraint is necessary—be specific.
- Protect yourself or others.
- Act in the best interests of the patient.
- Allow medical work-up or treatment.
- Nursing documentation is very thorough.
- Monitoring and reassessment of clinical condition and patient needs are essential.

Adapted from Joint Commission: 2006-2007. Corprehensive Accorditation Manual for Behavioral Health Care. Oakbrooh Terrace, IL, Joint Commission Resources, 2006.

It is important for the restraint team to enter the room together in a professional but nonthreatening manner. This "show of force" frequently defuses any patient resistance. The leader should be positioned at the head of the bed and should inform the patient that he or she is to be restrained as well as explaining the steps about to transpire. One member of the team is assigned to each limb and applies the restraint to that limb and to the solid frame of the bed or gurney. Limiting movement at major joints (elbow and knees) provides the most efficient and effective limb control.

BOX 195-3

Systematic Process for the Application of Physical Restraint

- Minimize physician involvement if possible.
- The restraint team consists of four members and an identified leader:
  - The restraint team enters together.
  - The restraint team is professional and nonthreatening.
  - The leader is at the head of the bed.
  - The leader explains the process to the patient.
  - Limbs are controlled by contact at the major joints.
- Restraints are attached to the solid frame of the gurney.

Once clinically appropriate, restraints should be removed one at a time in 5-minute intervals until two restraints are left. If the patient is cooperative, the last two restraints should be removed at the same time.

Types of Physical Restraints

The type of physical restraint used is frequently institution specific. Leather and soft cloth restraints are the types most commonly applied to the limbs. Leather restraints are difficult for the patient to remove and rarely compromise distal circulation; however, they require a special key to remove and are difficult to cut off in an emergency. Soft cloth restraints may tighten as the patient struggles against them, thus causing circulatory compromise. In contrast to leather restraint, soft cloth restraints are simpler for staff to remove by untying knots or cutting with trauma shears. Vest and waist restraints ("posies") are useful for elderly patients who are at risk of wandering or falls but who do not need their limbs restrained.

Positioning

Restraint position may be changed according to the patient's clinical status and the needs of the staff. Restraining a patient in the supine position is more comfortable for the patient and allows greater ease of examination. Patients with an increased risk of aspiration should be restrained on their side.

Agitated patients are able to generate significant force and momentum and have been known to overturn gurneys if they are not restrained in the proper position. If all four limbs are to be restrained, the patient should have one arm up and one arm down. When only two limbs are restrained, the contralateral arm and leg should be restrained. It is more difficult to generate enough force to overturn a gurney in these positions (Figs. 195-1 and 195-2).

Special situations may arise when additional or alternative restraint is indicated. A sheet may be placed across the patient's chest and tied to the gurney as a chest restraint when the movement of a patient's torso increases the risk of fall or injury, despite the use of four-point limb restraint. Extra attention should be paid to the patient's respiratory status if a chest restraint is added. A firm cervical collar, such as a Philadelphia collar, may be applied to patients who bite.

In the rare case of a patient who is loose in the ED or hospital with a knife or a needle-syringe assembly, a mattress may be used to push the patient into a wall, or two mattresses may be used to sandwich the patient and thus prevent injury to the patient, staff, or innocent bystanders.

Complications

Abrasions and bruising account for the majority of restraint complications.[7] However, serious complications and death can occur if restraints are inappropriately applied or the patient is not adequately monitored.

One small subset of physically restrained patients, usually accompanied by law enforcement, suffers cardiac arrest shortly before or after arrival in the ED. For many years, their demise was attributed to positional asphyxia related to the prone or hobble position.[8] Positional asphyxia results from an alteration in respiratory mechanics with ensuing decreased pulmonary function and increased cardiac output caused by the patient's position. This change in pulmonary function is not clinically relevant in normal volunteers subjected to prone restraint, however. More recent studies found that factors related to excited delirium are more likely to contribute to sudden death in these restrained individuals. Protracted struggle against physical restraint in patients with altered pain sensation may complicate or lead to hyperthermia, increased sympathetic tone with vasoconstriction, and lactic acid release from prolonged isotonic muscle contractions. Profound metabolic acidosis is associated with cardiovascular collapse in many restraint-associated deaths.[9] Cocaine and other sympathomimetic intoxications are frequently seen in this patient population.

Patients delivered to the ED who are restrained in a prone or hobble position should be turned onto their side. Patients who have been struggling against restraint should receive aggressive fluid resuscitation while evidence of associated metabolic acidosis or rhabdomyolysis is excluded. Aggressive chemical sedation should be administered to patients who continue to struggle against physical restraint.

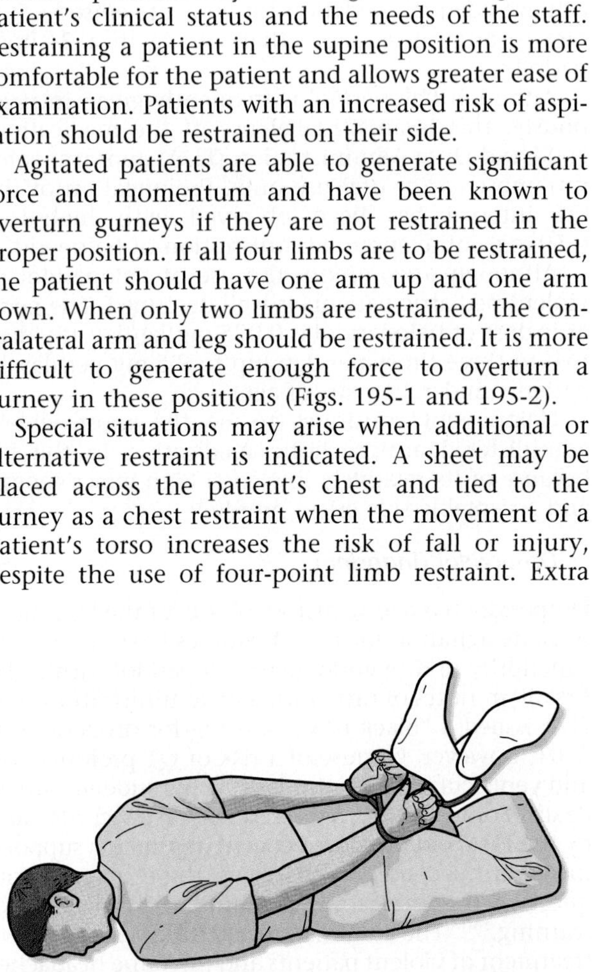

FIGURE 195-1 Correct method of patient restraint.

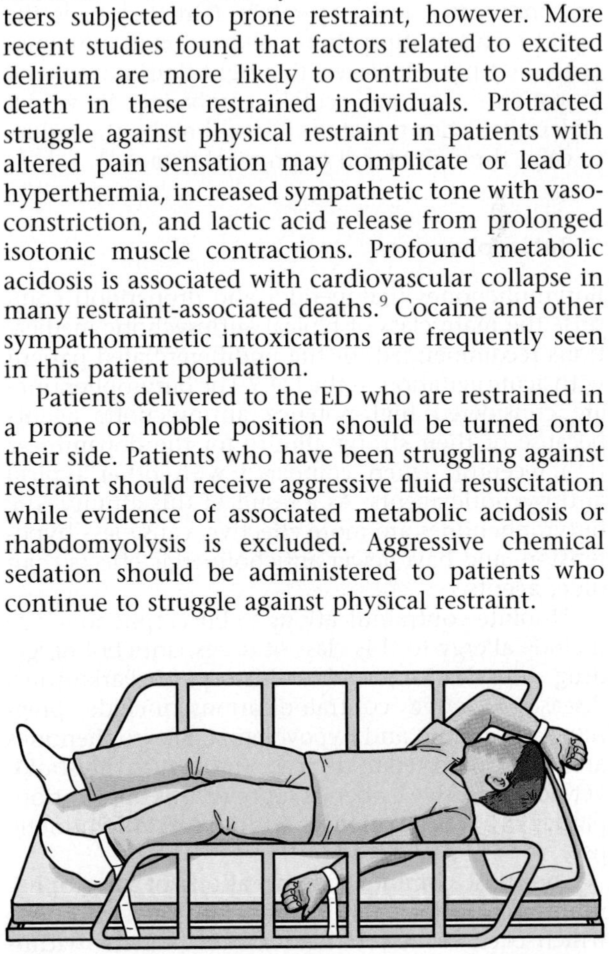

FIGURE 195-2 Proper attachment of restraints to the gurney.

CHEMICAL RESTRAINT, ANXIOLYSIS, AND SEDATION

Rationale

Chemical restraint is the administration, generally involuntarily, of medications to control a patient's dangerous behavior. Ideally, before violent behavior erupts, patients should be offered voluntary treatment with anxiolytics or sedatives, to prevent the need for acute, involuntary, behavioral control. Patients with the potential for violence often voluntarily present to the ED because they know they need help and treatment. Experienced, wise caregivers offer an anxiolytic when it is evident that patients have poor self-control and a propensity to violence. Early provision of benzodiazepines can maximize safety, patient comfort, and mutual trust. Chemical restraint is needed when verbal warnings and voluntary acceptance of low-dose anxiolytics are not prudent options. Chemical restraint is preferred over physical restraint to control a violent patient, but these methods are often properly used together for rapid control of dangerous behaviors. Physical restraint should be used for as brief a period as possible. Chemical restraint should be more broadly applied because sedation and anxiolysis are preferable.

Many patients with a history of chronic psychiatric conditions know, accurately, that they have the right to refuse antipsychotic medication in nonemergency settings. However, this right does not extend to patients who are acutely combative, in whom violent behavior threatens life or limb by the failure to calm through verbal or physical means.[10]

Butyrophenones

Butyrophenones (haloperidol and droperidol) comprise the main class of typical antipsychotic medications recommended for the undifferentiated patient with acute agitation in the ED.[11] The butyrophenones are considered high-potency antipsychotic agents because of their strong affinity for the dopamine-2 (D_2) receptor, when compared with other typical antipsychotic agents. As a result of this affinity, the butyrophenones are more effective, cause less hypotension, and have fewer anticholinergic effects than older agents.

Absolute contraindications to butyrophenone use include allergy to this class of drugs, anticholinergic drug intoxication, and a history of Parkinson's disease. Relative contraindications include pregnancy, lactation, and hypovolemia. Butyrophenones are widely reported to decrease the seizure threshold, yet no conclusive evidence supports this observation, particularly in patients with sympathomimetic use.[12]

The most common complications of butyrophenone use are related to extrapyramidal symptoms, which occur in fewer than 10% of patients within the first 24 hours of ED care. Dystonic reactions and akathisia are the most common manifestations of extrapyramidal symptoms requiring treatment in the ED. Akathisia is frequently misdiagnosed as psychiatric decompensation when it is manifested as restlessness, pacing, tension, and irritability. Extrapyramidal symptoms are treated with either benztropine (Cogentin), 2 mg, or diphenhydramine (Benadryl), 50 mg intramuscularly or intravenously. Doses may be repeated every 5 minutes up to three times. Relief is rapid and dramatic in most cases. Benzodiazepines may be added for patients who do not initially respond.

As with other neuroleptic agents, neuroleptic malignant syndrome has been reported with butyrophenone use (Table 195-1). This potentially fatal complex of autonomic instability is marked by high fever, muscle rigidity, and altered mental status. Aggressive symptomatic treatment includes cooling, benzodiazepines, dantrolene, and discontinuation of the offending agent.[13]

Haloperidol (Haldol)

Haloperidol may be given in 2.5- to 10-mg increments at 30- to 60-minute intervals for adults. The onset of action is between 15 and 30 minutes. Although a dosage ceiling has not been established, it is unusual to require more than three doses to achieve adequate sedation for an acute episode. It is rare to administer more than 60 mg in a 24-hour period.[14]

Although haloperidol is frequently given intravenously, this is an off-label use of the medication. Food and Drug Administration (FDA) approval is for intramuscular or oral use only. Prolongation of the QT interval has been observed with high-dose (>50 mg) intravenous administration of haloperidol.

Although uncommon, the use of haloperidol in violent pediatric patients is well described. The pediatric dose of haloperidol is 0.075 mg/kg/day, divided, two to three times per day (up to 2.5 mg per day in patients under 12 years of age).

Haloperidol continues to be the most widely administered antipsychotic medication in the ED because of its relatively low cost, high effectiveness, and acceptable side effect profile.[11]

Droperidol (Inapsine)

Droperidol has a long history of use for the treatment of acute agitation in the ED. Studies have shown the superiority of droperidol over haloperidol within the first 30 minutes of intramuscular administration. The FDA issued a "black box" warning for droperidol in 2001, however, because of a risk of QT prolongation and ventricular dysrhythmias causing sudden cardiac death. Some authors analyzed the case records cited by the FDA and presented cogent arguments supporting continued use of this drug; these investigators questioned the reasoning behind the "black box" warning.[16-18] The administration of droperidol for the treatment of violent patients and migraine headaches is now considered an off-label use of the drug.

Table 195-1 MANAGING ACUTE COMPLICATIONS OF SEDATION USING ANTIPSYCHOTIC AGENTS

Problem	Treatment
Acute dystonic reaction	Discontinue antipsychotic medication Benztropine (Cogentin) 2 mg IM Discharge with benztropine (Cogentin) 2 mg PO qd for 3 days OR Diphenhydramine (Benadryl) 50 mg IM Discharge with diphenhydramine (Benadryl) 25-50 mg PO qid for 3 days
Akathisia	Benztropine (Cogentin) 1-2 mg IM/IV/PO qd to bid OR Diphenhydramine (Benadryl) 50 mg IM/IV/PO tid to qid Lorazepam (Ativan) 1-2 mg PO
Hypotension Profound hypotension or cardiac arrest	Lie patient flat Normal saline bolus 250-500 mL (repeat as tolerated and clinically necessary) Phenylephrine (Neo-Synephrine) 0.005-0.02 mg/kg (0.35-1.4 mg for 70-kg adult) as bolus IV every 10-15 min as needed
Increased temperature without other signs of NMS	Discontinue antipsychotic medication
Increased temperature with signs of NMS ("lead pipe" rigidity, diaphoresis, labile blood pressure, tachycardia, urinary incontinence, altered mental status)	Monitor closely for signs of NMS Cool patient Add benzodiazepine for sedation Discontinue antipsychotic medication Active cooling measures Add benzodiazepine for sedation Consider neuromuscular blockade (paralysis) if temperature >40° C Aggressive hydration and alkalinization of urine to prevent renal failure from rhabdomyolysis *Dantrolene indicated for malignant hyperthermia, but of unproven clinical benefit in NMS*

bid, twice daily; IM, intramuscularly; IV, intravenously; NMS, neuroleptic malignant syndrome; PO, orally; qd, once daily; qid, four times daily; tid, three times daily.

Droperidol is still approved for intravenous administration to prevent and treat postoperative nausea and vomiting.

Droperidol may be given in 2.5- to 5-mg increments intravenously at 15-minute intervals for adults. The intramuscular dose is 5 to 10 mg. The onset of action is between 3 and 10 minutes. More than two doses are rarely required to achieve adequate sedation for an acute episode. The time to arousal is approximately 2 hours.[14]

Conduction abnormalities can occur with administration of butyrophenones in high doses. The FDA "black box" warning for droperidol also referred to some cases of conduction abnormalities at low doses. Experts recommend obtaining an electrocardiogram before administering droperidol to patients in the ED patients, a recommendation that is impractical for the acutely agitated or violent patient. Although many authors disagree with the conclusions of the FDA, it is prudent to avoid butyrophenone use in elderly patients in critical care or in patients with known preexisting heart disease.[13]

Benzodiazepines

Benzodiazepines are a preferred first-line choice for the acute management of agitation.[9] Benzodiazepines are particularly useful for agitation caused by sympathomimetic ingestions and alcohol withdrawal. Sedation and mild respiratory depression are the most prominent side effects of benzodiazepines. Therefore, these drugs are quite safe in patients with most medical comorbidities. Lorazepam and midazolam are the two prototypical benzodiazepines used for treatment of violent patients in the ED.

Lorazepam (Ativan)

Observational studies reported that lorazepam is at least as effective as haloperidol in treating patients with acute agitation. Lorazepam is given in 0.5- to 2-mg increments as frequently as every 15 minutes, depending on the patient's level of sedation and respiratory status. Intramuscular injection is the most common route of administration and is quite reliable. Lorazepam has a shorter half-life than some parenteral benzodiazepines and lacks active metabolites. Lorazepam may also be given intravenously, orally, and sublingually. The time of onset for intravenous or intramuscular injection is between 15 and 30 minutes, and the drug's effect lasts more than 3 hours. Sublingual or oral administration of lorazepam is a viable alternative route for the patient who is cooperative and would benefit from rapid relief of anxiety (Table 195-2). Lorazepam is classified as class D agent in pregnancy and thus should be avoided in pregnant and lactating women.

Midazolam (Versed)

Midazolam is particularly beneficial if rapid sedation is needed and prolonged sedation is less important.

Table 195-2 MEDICATION RECOMMENDATIONS FOR PATIENTS WILLING TO TAKE ORAL MEDICATION

Clinical Scenario	Recommended Oral Medication
No information on past history	Lorazepam
Psychosis in past; delirium or dementia	Risperidone
Cardiac arrhythmias or conduction defects	Lorazepam
Diabetes or hyperglycemia	Lorazepam and haloperidol, ziprasidone
Obesity	Lorazepam
Pediatric status	Haloperidol, lorazepam, atypical antipsychotic agents, antihistamines

The first ED study describing midazolam for this indication used a dose of 5 mg intramuscularly, thus providing rapid sedation with a mean time to onset of 18 minutes and arousal at a mean time of 82 minutes.[2] Another study reported the effective sedation time to be 45 minutes for midazolam and more than 2 hours for other agents.[19] Fewer cardiorespiratory effects are seen with the intramuscular administration of midazolam; most authors have reported no difference in vital signs or oxygen saturation compared with other agents used to sedate agitated or violent patients.[19,20] The intramuscular dose should be decreased by half in elderly patients or when midazolam is used in combination with opioid agents.

The treatment of oversedation and respiratory depression resulting from benzodiazepine use in agitated or violent patients is supportive care (Fig. 195-3). Supplemental oxygen, repositioning, and airway adjuncts such as nasal trumpets suffice in most cases. Active airway management, including jaw thrusts, use of bag-valve mask ventilation, or endotracheal intubation, is rarely necessary. It is prudent to avoid the use of flumazenil (Romazicon) because of the frequency of epileptogenic coingestions and the use of combination therapy with butyrophenones.

Combination Therapy

The combination of lorazepam, 2 mg, and haloperidol, 5 mg, for sedation of the agitated psychotic patient was found to be superior to either agent alone when investigators considered speed of sedation and frequency of side effects. The time of sedation was longer in the patients receiving combination therapy.[21] Lorazepam, haloperidol, and benztropine (Cogentin, 1 mg) can be administered in the same intramuscular syringe.

Atypical Antipsychotic Medications

The second-generation (atypical) antipsychotic drugs became feasible options for the treatment of agitated and violent patients in the ED with the approval of the first intramuscular formulation in 2001. Several such medications are now available in intramuscular or rapidly absorbable formulations indicated for the treatment of acute agitation in selected patient populations. This class of antipsychotics acts by blocking both D_2 and serotonin (5-HT) receptors and provides more tranquilization than sedation. The increased serotonin receptor activity allows for fewer extrapy-

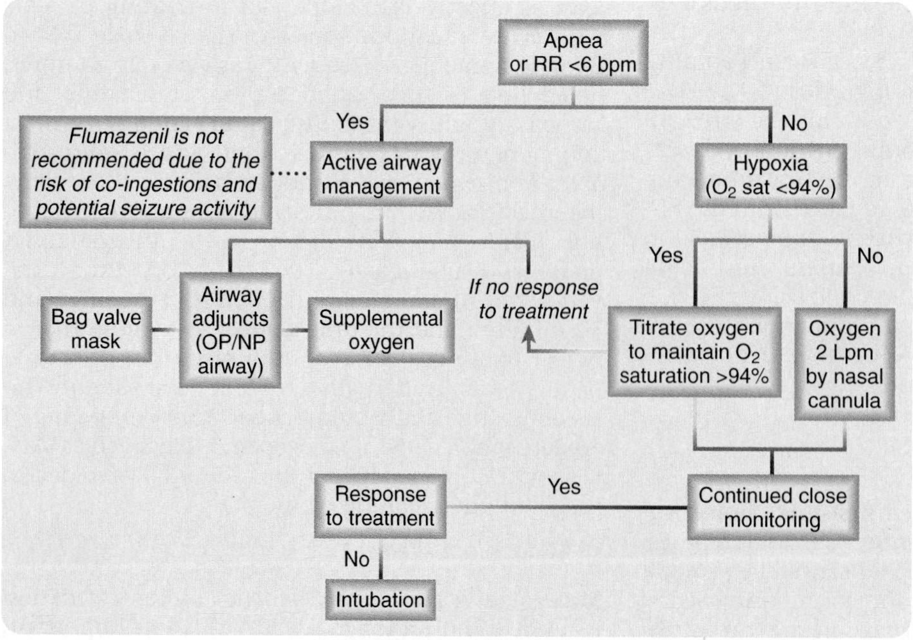
Apnea
or RR <6 bpm
Yes
No
Flumazenil is not recommended due to the risk of co-ingestions and potential seizure activity
Active airway management
Hypoxia
(O2 sat <94%)
Yes
No
Bag valve mask
Airway adjuncts (OP/NP airway)
Supplemental oxygen
If no response to treatment
Titrate oxygen to maintain O2 saturation >94%
Oxygen 2 Lpm by nasal cannula
Response to treatment
Yes
Continued close monitoring
No
Intubation

FIGURE 195-3 Respiratory depression after administration of sedative medication (respiratory rate [RR]<10 breaths per minute [bpm]). O_2, oxygen; OP/NP, oropharyngeal/nasopharyngeal.

ramidal effects. Second-generation antipsychotic agents are available in oral preparations that allow for easier conversion to long-term therapy when compared with the benzodiazepines and butyrophenones.

The atypical antipsychotic agents have been used in off-label fashion for the treatment of behavioral disorders in elderly patients for several years. In 2005, the FDA distributed an advisory describing a higher death rate in demented patients using atypical antipsychotic medications compared with placebo. It is unclear how this advisory applies to the limited use of these drugs in the ED for acutely agitated elderly patients.

Ziprasidone (Geodon)

Ziprasidone is approved for the treatment of acute agitation in schizophrenic and bipolar/manic patients. Ziprasidone has not been extensively studied in patients with undifferentiated causes of agitation in the ED. The typical dose is 10 mg intramuscularly every 2 hours or 20 mg intramuscularly every 4 hours. Ziprasidone is associated with the greatest change in QT interval of the atypical antipsychotics, comparable to the QT prolongation seen with haloperidol. No dosing information is available for ziprasidone use in children with agitation, but the drug is used for treatment of Tourette's syndrome at a dose of 5 to 40 mg/day.[19]

Olanzapine (Zyprexa)

Olanzapine is also approved for the treatment of acute agitation in schizophrenic and bipolar/manic patients in the ED. Olanzapine is available in either intramuscular or oral disintegrating tablet formulations at 5 to 10 mg. Olanzapine is strongly sedating and demonstrates 160 times the antihistamine potency of diphenhydramine. Olanzapine causes the smallest change in QT interval of the atypical antipsychotics. Long-term use of the drug is associated with weight gain and hyperglycemia. The manufacturer does not recommend the combination of intramuscular olanzapine with a parenteral benzodiazepine. Olanzapine has been approved for use in children at a dose of 2.5 to 20 mg/day or 0.12 to 0.29 mg/kg/day.[19]

Risperidone (Risperdal)

Risperidone is equivalent to haloperidol for the treatment of psychosis, and it is possibly more effective for treating aggressive behavior. Risperidone may be administered orally in the ED as a liquid formulation or as a rapidly disintegrating tablet at a dose of 1 to 3 mg. Although both methods of oral administration are easier with a cooperative patient, the liquid formulation can be mixed in a beverage or administered orally by syringe in resistant patients. Mean time to sleep was 43 minutes in one study. Risperidone has fewer anticholinergic properties, thus resulting in less confusion and sedation than with other atypical antipsychotic agents.

Tips and Tricks

Violence rarely erupts without warning.

- Primary prevention: Control factors leading to violence.
- Secondary prevention: Respond to previolent behavior.
- Tertiary prevention: Limit injury once violence is present.

Avoid the us versus them mentality: It is not just patients who start with an attitude.

R-E-S-P-E-C-T goes a long way toward helping patients regain their composure.

Be aware of your own reactions: You can make the situation worse.

GOT IVS: The seven *do not forget* reversible causes of altered metal status and violent behavior:

- *G*lucose
- *O*xygen
- *T*rauma/*T*emperature
- *I*nfection
- *V*ascular
- *S*eizure/*S*tatus epilepticus

Document, document, document: If restraint is the right thing to do, be sure to say why.

Different situations require different medications and treatment; one drug is not good for all circumstances, so tailor your treatment to the situation.

Disposition

Patients may demonstrate resolution of their agitation in the ED as a result of sleep or the metabolism of offending drugs and alcohol. Patients may be considered for discharge if they exhibit normal mental status without agitation on waking, presuming that other acute medical and psychiatric conditions have been addressed. Those patients who continue to exhibit violent or threatening behavior, abnormal vital signs, or evidence of psychiatric decompensation require further medical or psychiatric care.

Agitated or violent patients who elope from the ED before full evaluation or resolution of their symptoms represent a significant legal risk to providers, as well as a risk to the safety of themselves and other individuals. Notify legal authorities of the elopement of such patients.

REFERENCES

1. Lion JR, Snyder W, Merrill G: Under-reporting of assaults on staff in a state hospital. Hosp Community Psychiatry 1981;32:497-498.
2. Mahoney BS: The extent, nature and response to victimization of emergency nurses in Pennsylvania. J Emerg Med Nurs 1991;17:282-291.
3. Lavoie FW, Carter GL, Danzl DF, Berg RL: Emergency department violence in United States teaching hospitals. Ann Emerg Med 1988;17:1227-1233.
4. Beck JC, White KA, Gage B: Emergency psychiatric assessment of violence. Am J Psychiatry 1991;148:1562-1565.

5. Blanchard JC, Curtis KM: Violence in the emergency department. Emerg Med Clin North Am 1999;17: 717-731.
6. Annas GJ: The last resort: The use of physical restraints in medical emergencies. N Engl J Med 1999;341:1408-1412.
7. Zun LS: A prospective study of the complication rate of use of patient restraint in the emergency department. J Emerg Med 2003;24:119-124.
8. Chan TC, Vilke GM, Neuman T, Clausen JL: Restraint position and positional asphyxia. Ann Emerg Med 1997;30:578-586.
9. Hick JL, Smith SW, Lynch MT: Metabolic acidosis in restraint-associated cardiac arrest: A case series. Acad Emerg Med 1999;6:239-243.
10. Hill S, Petit J: The violent patient. Emerg Med Clin North Am 2000;18:301-315.
11. Allen MH, Currier GW, Carpenter D, et al: The expert consensus guideline series: Treatment of behavior emergencies 2005. J Psychiatr Pract 2005;11(Suppl 1):6-108.
12. Branney SW, Colwell CB, Aschbrenner JK, et al: Safety of droperidol for sedating out-of-control ED patients. Acad Emerg Med 1996;3:527.
13. Marco CA, Vaughan J: Emergency management of agitation in schizophrenia. Am J Emerg Med 2005;23:767-776.
14. Dubin WR, Feld JA: Rapid tranquilization of the violent patient. Am J Emerg Med 1989;7:313-320.
15. Sorrentino A: Chemical restraints for the agitated, violent, or psychotic pediatric patient in the emergency department: Controversies and recommendations. Curr Opin Pediatr 2004;16:201-205.
16. Chase PB, Biros MH: A retrospective review of the use and safety of droperidol in a large, high-risk, inner-city emergency department patient population. Acad Emerg Med 2002;9:1402-1410.
17. Kao LW, Kirk MA, Evers SJ, Rosenfeld SH: Droperidol, QT prolongation, and sudden death: What is the evidence? Ann Emerg Med 2003;41:546-548.
18. Van Zwieten Z, Mullins ME, Jang T: Droperidol and the black box warning. Ann Emerg Med 2004;43:139-140.
19. Martel M, Sterzinger A, Miner J, et al: Management of acute undifferentiated agitation in the emergency department: A randomized double-blind trial of droperidol, ziprasidone, and midazolam. Acad Emerg Med 2005;12:1167-1172.
20. Nobay F, Simon BC, Levitt MA, Dresden GM: A prospective, double-blind, randomized trial of midazolam versus haloperidol versus lorazepam in the chemical restraint of violent and severely agitated patients. Acad Emerg Med 2004;11:744-749.
21. Battaglia J, Moss S, Rush J, et al: Haloperidol, lorazepam, or both for psychotic agitation? A multicenter, prospective, double-blind, emergency department study. Am J Emerg Med 1997;15:335-340.

Chapter 196

Self-Harm and Danger to Others

Keith Borg

KEY POINTS

Risk factors that increase the likelihood of self-harm include psychiatric illnesses such as depression, schizophrenia, and substance abuse, as well as significant medical conditions such as human immunodeficiency virus (HIV) infection, cancer, and dialysis-dependent renal failure.

Psychiatric illness and substance abuse increase the likelihood of homicidal ideation.

Although adolescent and young adult female patients are more likely to present to the ED after a suicidal gesture, older men are more likely to commit suicide.

In the United States, all 50 states provide physicians the legal right to commit any patient who is a threat either to himself or herself or to others.

Health professionals are required to inform individuals directly if they are at risk of harm from a homicidal patient. Police should also be notified of such risk.

Any patient discharged from the ED after appropriate psychiatric evaluation should agree to seek immediate medical care if thoughts of violence or self-harm return.

Scope

Patients with suicidal or homicidal ideation frequently present to the ED. Suicidal patients account for approximately 0.4% of all ED visits in the United States, with an estimated 412,000 annual ED visits observed between 1997 and 2001. During that period, the mean age of a suicidal patient was 31 years, and the rate of attempted suicide was highest among female patients who were 15 to 19 years old. Of those patients presenting with evidence of self-harm, poisoning accounted for 68% of visits, and self-mutilation (by cutting or piercing) was observed in 20% of cases. One third of suicidal patients were admitted for inpatient management, one third were transferred to an off-site facility, and one fifth were referred to outpatient psychiatric services.[1] Suicide was the reported cause of death for 31,484 Americans in 2003.[2]

A focused risk assessment is the primary objective for the emergency provider caring for a patient who is threatening harm to himself or herself or others. Risk assessments vary widely, depending on the presenting circumstances of the patient, comorbid disease, mental status, and other social issues. The main challenge to effective risk assessment is the lack of a specific diagnostic test to stratify threat in suicidal or homicidal patients. No interventional test is currently available to determine who is at greatest risk of injury—data for risk stratification come from psychological autopsy, which is the study of patient characteristics in completed suicides. Predictive data for outcomes of these patients after ED evaluation are lacking. This chapter focuses on the directed examination and evaluation of patients who present with threats of harm to self or others.

Pathophysiology

Numerous factors influence the likelihood of self-harm. These include psychiatric conditions such as depression, schizophrenia, and substance abuse, as well as significant medical conditions such as HIV infection, cancer, and dialysis-dependent renal failure (see the Red Flags box). Besides the presence of risk factors, poorly understood biologic factors likely influence self-harm. Serotonin levels have been studied in suicidal patients, and data suggest that lower levels of cerebral 5-hydroxyindoleacetic acid (a serotonin metabolite) are noted in patients who attempt suicide.[3-5] Increasing serotonin levels through pharmacotherapy, with drug classes such as tricyclic antidepressants or selective serotonin reuptake inhibitors, is a common treatment for depression and suicidal ideation.

RED FLAGS

- Potentially lethal attempt
- Patient found accidentally
- Trauma incongruent with an accident (single-car motor vehicle crash, pedestrians struck by a vehicle)
- Intoxicated or altered patients
- Previous suicide attempts
- History of mental illness, especially depression or schizophrenia
- History of alcohol or substance abuse
- Male gender
- Widowed or divorced status
- Elderly status
- Family history of suicide
- Family history of child maltreatment
- Access to firearms
- Feelings of hopelessness
- Impulsive or aggressive tendencies
- Barriers to accessing mental health treatment
- Loss (relationship, work, financial)
- Physical illness (especially human immunodeficiency virus infection, cancer, end-stage renal disease)
- Easy access to lethal methods (stored pills, firearms)
- Unwillingness to seek help because of stigma attached to mental illness, substance abuse, and suicidal ideation
- Conflicting cultural or religious beliefs
- Local epidemics of suicide
- Isolation
- Presence of breast implants

Data from American Psychiatric Association: Practice Guideline for the Assessment and Treatment of Patients with Suicidal Behaviors, November 2003. Available at http://www.psych.org/psych_pract/treatg/pg/prac_guide.cfm; and Villeneuve P, Holowaty E, Brisson J, et al: Mortality among Canadian women with cosmetic breast implants. Am J Epidemiol 2006;164:334-341.

Clinical Presentation

Patients may present to the ED after considering or attempting to harm themselves or others. These presentations range from unsuccessful yet serious gestures to the use of suicidal ideation for secondary gain. Clinical suspicion should always be high, and patients' complaints must be taken seriously. Careful, open-ended, nonjudgmental questioning helps to discern the level of risk by understanding the patient's intent.

Injured patients with a concerning mechanism (ingestion, single-person car accident, fall) should be screened for suicidal ideation and intent. If an attempt is uncovered, the provider should solicit the patient's feelings about survival. It is important to understand why patients survived, as a predictor of immediate or ongoing risk of harm. Consider the following questions:

Was the patient accidentally found?

Did a low-risk gesture precede a phone call for help?

Is the patient sad to have survived?

Is the patient having increasing thoughts of suicide?

Does the patient have a plan? Has the patient gathered the means to act on that plan?

Is the patient feeling depressed or hopeless, or does he or she appear withdrawn?

A practice guideline of the American Psychiatric Association summarized large amounts of retrospective data regarding risk factors in patients who committed suicide.[6] The relative importance and clinical utility of such risk factors can be challenging, however. Seemingly innocuous patient data may represent significant risk, as evidenced by studies that demonstrated a higher suicide rate among women who received breast implants.[7] Such epidemiologic studies are difficult to translate into clinical practice, but they do provide an understanding of the complexity of risk stratification in suicidal and homicidal patients.

Differential Diagnosis

The differential diagnosis of self-harm includes minor depression, major depression, suicidal ideation, suicidal gestures, and suicidal attempts of varying lethality and intent. Other alternative diagnoses can be difficult to establish in the ED. One such alternative is the threat of suicide for secondary gain; very little is written or researched about patients who present

BOX 196-1

Most Threatening and Most Common Presentations

Most Threatening

Suicide attempt with potentially lethal means

Accidental discovery of a suicide attempt

Elderly men with suicidal ideation

Suicidal ideation with a clear plan or history of previous attempts

Homicidal ideation with a plan or means

Most Common

Depressive thoughts or expressions ("Life is not worth living")

Suicidal gestures such as nonlethal ingestions

Cutting

Threatening suicide for secondary gain

with such intents. The goal of secondary gain is often hospitalization, to avoid incarceration, legal prosecution, homelessness, or other social problems. A second alternative diagnosis is intentional self-mutilation, such as cutting or hair pulling. This is differentiated from suicidal ideation because of the nonlethal intent and frequency of behavior. Self-mutilation is believed to be a maladaptive response to stress.

■ MOST COMMON AND MOST THREATENING PRESENTATIONS

Common presentations of suicidality include minor threats or ideation of suicide by nonlethal means (Box 196-1). The most frequent ED presentations involve young female patients who report a recent ingestion. Depressive symptoms are also common.

Men are far more likely to complete suicide.[1] Threatening presentations include attempts with potentially lethal consequences, a history of previous attempts, traumatic attempts that are difficult to recognize (e.g., single-car motor vehicle crashes), and elderly men with suicidal ideation.

Diagnostic Testing

Diagnostic testing in patients who present with threats of harm to self should focus on the mechanism of the suicidal attempt and any significant comorbid disease (including alcohol and drug abuse). Specific testing may help to evaluate certain treatable ingestions, such as acetaminophen or salicylates; in many cases, no specific testing is required. Imaging should be appropriately ordered for patients whose presentations involve jumping, hanging, or other traumatic injuries. Screening laboratory tests may be required to arrange for transfer or admission to a

PRIORITY ACTIONS

- Evaluate for any immediate life threats from a suicide attempt or current ideation.
- Place the patient in a setting where he or she can be constantly monitored.
- Minimize the patient's risk to self, staff, and others.

psychiatric facility, although such testing has little diagnostic value in the ED evaluation and treatment of suicidal or homicidal patients.[8]

Treatment

Patients who have attempted suicide must be evaluated immediately to determine the lethality of the reported or suspected method of harm. Once the threat assessment is complete, the patient should be placed in a closely monitored setting. Physical or chemical restraints and suicide precautions may be required in certain circumstances. Suicide precautions include undressing and gowning the patient, removing potential weapons or harmful items, one-on-one or video supervision, and security escort for travel and transfer. Careful questioning and examination of the patient should establish the level of risk and cooperation.

All 50 states provide the physician the ability to commit any individual who is a threat either to himself or herself or to others or who is unable to care for himself or herself. This psychiatric hold is time limited (usually 72 hours), to permit emergency evaluation and treatment of the patient. Specific actions and documentation required to commit a patient vary by state jurisdiction. Adherence to process is very important, and the decision to act should be made with appropriate gravity. Documentation of the reason for committal should be provided in clear detail, and supplementary historical information from family, police, or others should also be included in the chart.

Tarasoff v. Regents of the University of California was a landmark legal decision in 1976 that established an obligation of the health care professional to warn a specific individual at identifiable risk of harm, thus overriding the patient's confidentiality. To fulfill this obligation, both the threatened individual and the police must be informed of the intentions of the homicidal patient. Patients who have an intention to hurt or kill an identifiable individual should be committed and evaluated by a psychiatrist. Discussions with legal and psychiatric colleagues should clarify who will perform any required notification.

Contracts for safety are pacts that include a patient's promise to seek immediate evaluation should he or she have increasing thoughts of violence or self-harm. Current American Psychiatric Association guidelines do not recommend contracts

Tips and Tricks

- Establish referral patterns with consultants and mental health services in advance.
- Know your local resources for inpatient and outpatient care.
- Patients need your care and compassion.
- Do not be judgmental or condescending. Despite being in crisis, patients perceive your degree of concern or lack of compassion.
- Do not allow staff to make pejorative comments in which they "instruct" patients how to complete a future suicide attempt.
- De-escalate the situation using calming mannerisms, voice, and tone.
- Be safe—stay between the door and the patient.
- Do not approach violent patients alone.
- Ask permission to sit down beside the patient and have a conversation. Be willing to listen.
- Involuntary commitment is frequently reportable on job applications and physician licensure. Voluntary commitment is seen as asking for help. This distinction can be used to persuade patients to agree to admission and to seek future help without long-term repercussions.

Documentation

- Document the patient's risk factors, psychiatric history, medical history, and discussions with supplemental historians (friends, family, police).
- Record the process of admission or discharge and make note of risk stratification and medical decision making.
  Example: "This patient is deemed stable for discharge because he has contracted for safety, has mental health follow-up tomorrow morning (which has been confirmed by telephone), is going home with family who are supportive, has no firearms or stockpile of pills at home, and has no concurrent medical or other high-risk social issues."
- Carefully document the reasons for psychiatric committal, and give specific examples.
- Document discussions and decision making with psychiatric consultants.

for safety in emergency situations,[6] although such understandings should be reinforced with any patient who is discharged after psychiatric evaluation in the ED.

Disposition

Once the initial challenges of medical assessment have been met, the practitioner should determine the safest and most appropriate disposition for the individual patient's social condition (Fig. 196-1). Psychiatric consultants often aid in the necessary evaluation, admission, or follow-up of at-risk patients. If the clinician has significant concern, then the patient should be admitted or transferred to an appropriately safe inpatient setting. Patients may need to be committed for involuntary psychiatric admission if they are not willing to sign in voluntarily.

One prospectively validated tool that is valuable for use in the ED is the Modified SAD PERSONS Scale developed by Hockberger and Rothstein in 1988 (Table 196-1). The scale uses a series of criteria that allow for an easy review of risk factors and assists in the identification of conditions that should prompt admission. Patients with a low score are less likely to have adverse events.[9]

Patients may be discharged home if they are deemed safe after medical evaluation and psychiatric consultation (Box 196-2). A treatment plan, return precautions, and conditions for safety should be clear, well documented, and understood by all parties involved (including friends and family of the patient).

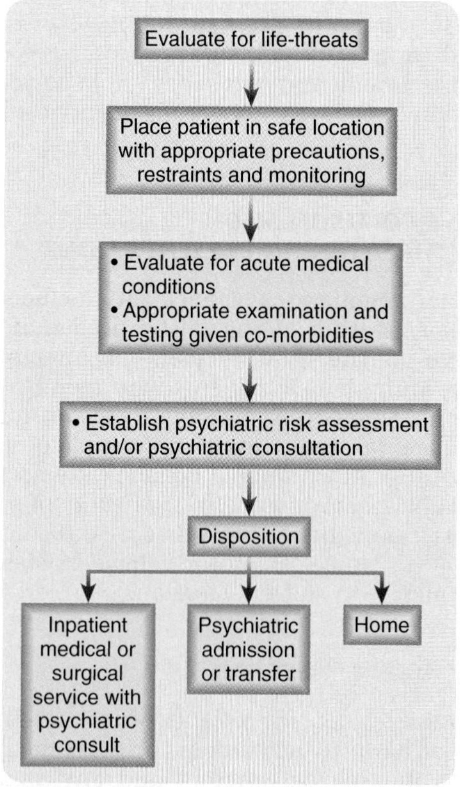
Evaluate for life-threats
Place patient in safe location with appropriate precautions, restraints and monitoring
• Evaluate for acute medical conditions
• Appropriate examination and testing given co-morbidities
• Establish psychiatric risk assessment and/or psychiatric consultation
Disposition
Inpatient medical or surgical service with psychiatric consult
Psychiatric admission or transfer
Home

FIGURE 196-1 Algorithm for evaluation and treatment of suicidal or homicidal patients.

Table 196-1 MODIFIED SAD PERSONS SCALE OF HOCKBERGER AND ROTHSTEIN: BASED ON THE SAD PERSONS MNEMONIC

Parameter	Finding	Points
Sex	Male Female	1 0
Age	<19 yr 19-45 yr >45 yr	1 0 1
Depression or hopelessness	Present Absent	2 0
Previous attempts or psychiatric care	Previous suicide attempts or psychiatric care Neither	1 0
Excessive alcohol or drug use	Excessive Not excessive or none	1 0
Rational thinking loss	Lost as a result of organic brain syndrome or psychosis Intact	2 0
Separated, divorced, or widowed	Separated divorced or widowed Married or always single	1 0
Organized or serious attempt	Organized, well-thought out, or serious Neither	2 0
No social support	None (no close family, friends, job, or active religious affiliation) Present	1 0
Stated future intent	Determined to repeat or ambivalent about the prospect No intent	2 0

Score=points for all 10 parameters
Interpretation:
Minimum score: 0
Maximum score: 14

The higher the score, the greater the risk of suicide.

A patient with a score ≤5 rarely requires hospitalization.

Score	Management
0-5	May be safe to discharge, depending on circumstances
6-8	Requires emergency psychiatric consultation
9-14	Probably requires hospitalization

Adapted from Hockberger RS, Rothstein RJ: Assessment of suicide potential by non-psychiatrists using the SAD PERSONS score. J Emerg Med 1988;99:6.

PATIENT TEACHING TIPS

- Patients who are going to be discharged must be sober.
- Contract for safety: Patients must state that they will not harm themselves and that they will return to the ED if thoughts of violence or self-harm return.
- Patients must be discharged to a safe environment, such as home with supportive friends or family who are able to offer needed assistance.
- It should be made clear that if patients' conditions change, they should return to the ED for re-evaluation. Patients should be made welcome to do so at any time.
- Resources for outpatient follow-up should be appropriate to the social situation.
- If possible, confirm that patients have a designated time and place for follow-up.

BOX 196-2

Reassuring Factors for Safe Discharge

- Established care for mental, physical, and substance abuse disorders
- Follow-up in 1 to 2 days
- Family and community support
- Problem-solving and conflict resolution skills
- Cultural and religious beliefs that discourage suicide and support the patient

From American Psychiatric Association: Practice Guideline for the Assessment and Treatment of Patients with Suicidal Behaviors, November 2003. Available at http://www.psych.org/psych_pract/treatg/pg/prac_guide.cfm.

REFERENCES

1. Doshi A, Boudreaux E, Wang N, et al: National study of US emergency department visits for attempted suicide and self-inflicted injury 1997-2001. Ann Emerg Med 2005;46:369-375.
2. Centers for Disease Control and Prevention: WISQARS (Web-based Injury Statistics Query and Reporting System), 2004. Available at www.cdc.gov/ncipc/wisqars/default.htm.
3. Roy A, De Jong J, Linnoila M, et al: Cerebrospinal fluid metabolites and suicidal behavior in depressed patients: A 5-year follow-up study. Arch Gen Psychiatry 1989;46:609-612.
4. Coccaro EF, Siever LJ, Klar HM, et al: Serotonergic studies in patients with affective and personality disorders: Correlates with suicidal and impulsive behaviors. Arch Gen Psychiatry 1989;46:587-599.
5. Mann JJ, Malone KM: Cerebrospinal fluid amines and higher-lethality suicide attempts in depressed patients. Biol Psychiatry 1997;41:162-171.
6. American Psychiatric Association: Practice Guideline for the Assessment and Treatment of Patients with Suicidal Behaviors, November 2003. Available at http://www.psych.org/psych_pract/treatg/pg/prac_guide.cfm.
7. Villeneuve P, Holowaty E, Brisson J, et al: Mortality among Canadian women with cosmetic breast implants. Am J Epidemiol 2006;164:334-341.
8. American College of Emergency Physicians: Clinical Policy: Critical Issues in the Diagnosis and Management of the Adult Psychiatric Patient in the Emergency Department. Availableat http://acep.org/webportal/PracticeResources/ClinicalPolicies.
9. Hockberger R, Rothstein R: Assessment of suicide potential by nonpsychiatrists using the sad persons score. J Emerg Med 1988;6:99-107.

Chapter 197

Anxiety and Panic Disorders

Christopher S. Kang and Benjamin P. Harrison

KEY POINTS

Anxiety disorders occur more frequently in women than in men, and they are the most common psychiatric illnesses diagnosed in children, adolescents, and older adults.

Potentially life-threatening medical disorders may feature somatic and cognitive symptoms that often mimic anxiety on initial presentation.

Most anxiety disorders have significant familial aggregation, with the inheritability of panic disorder approaching 40%.

Panic attack is a discrete episode of sudden, intense apprehension, fearfulness, or terror, often associated with feelings of impending doom.

Panic attack is not a billable ICD-9 (ninth edition of the International Classification of Diseases) diagnosis; rather, panic attacks should be considered the presenting feature of a specific anxiety disorder.

Benzodiazepines are the recommended first-line agents for the pharmacologic management of anxiety.

Scope

Anxiety is defined as an unpleasant emotional state consisting of psychological and physiologic responses to the anticipation of real or imagined danger.[1] Whether the observed disease prevalence is related to the escalating complexity and stresses of modern life, the changing access to medical care, the inherent nature of the ED, or an increased awareness of psychiatric disorders, anxiety is common among patients who seek emergency care.[2]

In the United States, anxiety disorders have a 12-month prevalence of 18% and a lifetime prevalence that approaches 25%. Anxiety-related conditions cost more than $42 billion in medical costs and lost worker productivity in 1990 alone.[3-5]

Anxiety disorders, particularly panic disorder, occur more frequently in women than in men.[6] These conditions are the most common psychiatric illnesses diagnosed in children, adolescents, and older adults.[7,8] Anxiety disorders may significantly affect a patient's quality of life and overall health. Anxiety is commonly associated with depression, other mood disorders, and substance abuse.

Numerous potentially life-threatening medical disorders feature symptoms that often mimic anxiety on initial presentation. EPs must be able to discern such serious medical conditions from the simply anxious patient.

Pathophysiology

Anxiety disorders are caused by a combination of biologic factors and environmental influences.[9] Despite increased basic science and clinical research, a specific explanatory mechanism or model to describe the exact causes of anxiety has yet to be identified.

The genetic epidemiology of anxiety disorders has been confirmed by numerous studies and meta-analysis. Most anxiety disorders have significant familial aggregation, and the inheritability of panic disorder approaches 40%.[10]

Several neurotransmitters play integral roles in the pathophysiology of stress and anxiety. Decreased gamma-aminobutyric acid and serotonin receptor sensitivity are common in most anxiety disorders. Overactivity of the central norepinephrine system and elevated sensitivities to lactate and carbon dioxide are prominent findings in panic disorder. Cholecystokinin and glutamate may contribute to the evolution of conditioned fear.[11] Evolving research suggests that corticotropin-releasing factor plays a role in both mood and anxiety disorders.[12]

Environmental factors are critical to the development of anxiety. Stressful childhood experiences, including divorce and abuse, contribute to generalized anxiety and panic disorders.[9] Caffeine and other socially accepted stimulants (e.g., taurine and ginseng), as well as recreational substance use (e.g., cocaine, methamphetamine, and gamma-hydroxybutyrate), often promote symptoms of anxiety.[13] Finally, increasing exposure to violence, natural disasters, and terrorism has caused greater numbers of people to suffer from acute stress reactions, anxiety, depression, and post-traumatic stress disorder.[14,15]

Clinical Presentation

Anxiety may manifest through many somatic and cognitive symptoms, as listed in Box 197-1.[7,8,16] Physical symptoms of acute anxiety are similar to those of excitation, such as chest pain, dry mouth, dyspnea, lightheadedness, and palpitations. Symptoms of subacute or chronic anxiety may not be innocuous, such as fatigue, insomnia, and menstrual abnormalities. The anxious patient may have a normal physical examination or may exhibit tachycardia, tachypnea, and diaphoresis.

Psychological symptoms of anxiety include distractibility, emotional lability, noncompliance, and recurrent or obsessive thoughts. The anxious patient may be easily startled, may demonstrate pressured speech, or may suffer repetitive behaviors.

Children may not be able to articulate their fear or anxiety. As a result, the anxious pediatric patient may present with seemingly disparate chief complaints, such as nonspecific abdominal pain and headache. During examination, anxious pediatric patients may have a temper tantrum or may appear more clingy or needy than expected.[7]

Although not a codable diagnosis itself, a panic attack may be the feature of most anxiety disorders.[17] A *panic attack* is a discrete episode of intense fear or discomfort in the absence of real danger that meets specific symptomatic criteria. The intensity of a panic

BOX 197-1

Symptoms and Signs of Anxiety

Somatic Symptoms
Lightheadedness
Headache
Dry mouth
Choking sensation
Chest tightness/pain
Palpitations
Dyspnea
Nausea
Abdominal pain
Increased flatulence
Frequent/loose stools
Frequent urination
Erectile dysfunction
Amenorrhea/dysmenorrhea
Paresthesias
Muscle tightness
Fatigue

Cognitive Symptoms
Amnesia
Apprehension
Depersonalization
Derealization
Distractibility
Emotional lability
Fear
Flashbacks/recurrent images
Intrusive thoughts
Irritability
Racing thoughts

Physical Signs
Atypical affect
Avoidance
Diaphoresis
Hyperkinesis
Hypervigilance
Pressured speech
Repetitive behavior
Restlessness
Startle response
Stiffness
Tachycardia
Tachypnea
Temper tantrum
Tremor

BOX 197-2

Definitions of Anxiety Disorders

Panic attack is a discrete period characterized by the sudden onset of intense apprehension, fearfulness, or terror, often associated with feelings of impending doom.

Agoraphobia is anxiety about, or avoidance of, places or situations from which escape may be difficult (or embarrassing), or in which help may not be available in the event of a panic attack or panic-like symptoms.

Panic disorder without agoraphobia is characterized by recurrent, unexpected panic attacks about which persistent concern exists.

Panic disorder with agoraphobia is characterized by both recurrent, unexpected panic attacks and agoraphobia.

Agoraphobia without history of panic disorder is characterized by the presence of agoraphobia and panic-like symptoms without a history of unexpected panic attacks.

Specific phobia is characterized by clinically significant anxiety provoked by exposure to a specific fear, object, or situation, often leading to avoidance behavior.

Social phobia is characterized by clinically significant anxiety produced by exposure to certain types of social or performance situations, often leading to avoidance behavior.

Obsessive-compulsive disorder is characterized by obsessions (that cause marked anxiety or distress) or compulsions (that serve to neutralize anxiety).

Post-traumatic stress disorder is characterized by the recurrent experiencing of an extremely traumatic event accompanied by symptoms of increased arousal and avoidance of stimuli associated with the trauma.

Acute stress disorder is characterized by symptoms similar to those of post-traumatic stress disorder that occur immediately after an extremely traumatic event.

Generalized anxiety disorder is characterized by at least 6 months of persistent and excessive anxiety and worry.

Anxiety disorder due to a general medical condition is characterized by prominent symptoms of anxiety that are judged to be a direct physiologic consequence of a general medical condition.

Substance-induced anxiety disorder is characterized by prominent symptoms of anxiety that are judged to be a direct physiologic consequence of a drug of abuse, medication use, or toxin exposure.

Anxiety disorder not otherwise specified is included for coding disorders with prominent anxiety or phobic avoidance that do not meet criteria for any of the specific anxiety disorders.

Data from American Psychiatric Association: Diagnostic and Statistical Manual of Mental Disorders, 4th ed, text rev. Washington, DC, American Psychiatric Association, 2000, pp 429-430.

attack usually peaks within 10 minutes and resolves within 30 minutes. Panic attacks are often accompanied by at least 4 of 13 discreet somatic and cognitive symptoms.[18]

Differential Diagnosis, Diagnostic Criteria, and Testing

As evidenced by the broad range of associated signs and symptoms, anxiety disorders are part of an extensive differential diagnosis. Anxiety may represent a primary psychiatric condition or may manifest secondary to medical illness. More than a dozen different anxiety disorders have similar physical symptoms and signs (Box 197-2).[18]

The first and most important step in the evaluation of an anxious patient is to eliminate potential medical causes of the patient's symptoms. As noted in Table 197-1, many different medical conditions and medications mimic, manifest, produce, or exacerbate anxiety.[19,20] A thorough history of all recent and past medical problems, current medications and supplements (including those available over the counter), family history, and social history (especially substance use and social stressors) may preclude an exhaustive and unnecessary medical evaluation. The onset of a new behavioral symptom at a late age or the report of any feature that is not typically associated with anxiety increases the likelihood of a medical cause.

An appropriate physical examination helps to identify or eliminate potential causes of anxiety. Abnormal vital signs and characteristic toxidromes often signal the presence of a medical illness or drug-induced condition. A focused neurologic examination, including mental status, is critical to the diagnosis of intracranial disease.[21]

Table 197-1 MEDICAL CONDITIONS ASSOCIATED WITH ANXIETY

System or Cause	Condition
Cardiac	Angina, arrhythmias, hypertensive urgency/emergency, mitral valve prolapse, myocardial ischemia, and Takotsubo syndrome
Endocrine	Addison's disease, carcinoid syndrome, Cushing's syndrome, diabetes, parathyroid disease, pheochromocytoma, postpartum depression, and thyroid disease
Exogenous	Caffeine/stimulant use, dietary supplement use, herbal remedies, acute intoxication (alcohol, amyl nitrate, cocaine, gamma-hydroxybutyrate, khat, lysergic acid diethylamide [LSD], methamphetamine, and yohimbine), monosodium glutamate, tyramine-containing foods in combination with monoamine oxidase inhibitors, and withdrawal (alcohol, benzodiazepine, heroin, and sedative)
Gastrointestinal	Dyspepsia, gastroesophageal reflux disease, irritable bowel syndrome, and liver failure
Immunologic	Allergic reaction and mastocytosis
Infectious	Acute/evolving infection, human immunodeficiency virus infection, and neurosyphilis
Medication	Amphetamine/dextroamphetamine (Adderall), albuterol, anticholinergics, digitalis, dystonic reaction, agents for erectile dysfunction, estrogen, histamine 1 and 2 blockers, selective serotonin reuptake inhibitors, and theophylline
Metabolic	Electrolyte abnormalities (calcium, glucose, magnesium, phosphorus, potassium, sodium, urea), nutritional deficiencies (vitamin deficiency such as B_{12} and folate), porphyrias, and Wilson's disease
Neurologic	Brain tumors, cerebrovascular accidents (including transient ischemia attack), degenerative disorders (Huntington's chorea, multiple sclerosis, and myasthenia gravis), delirium, dementia (Alzheimer's type), encephalitis, meningitis, and seizure disorder (nonconvulsive and temporal lobe)
Psychiatric	Conversion disorder, depression, insomnia/sleep disorders, mania, psychosis, schizophrenia, and stress disorder/stressors (e.g., abuse, finances, marital/relationship, trauma)
Pulmonary	Asthma, chronic obstructive pulmonary disease, pulmonary embolism, and upper respiratory infection

Myocardial infarction, angina pectoris, and dysrhythmias may have clinical presentations similar to those of a panic attack. Several studies have indicated that up to 30% of patients with chest pain who are evaluated in the ED meet diagnostic criteria for panic disorder. Alternatively, more than 40% of patients with panic disorder had documented coronary artery disease in a related study.[22]

Nearly 25% of medical conditions that cause symptoms of anxiety are endocrine disorders, such as hypoglycemia, hyperthyroidism, and hypoparathyroidism.[23] Approximately 30% to 50% of female hyperthyroid patients suffer from panic and generalized anxiety disorders.[24]

Transient ischemic attacks, temporal lobe seizures, and brain tumors may promote anxiety. Up to 50% of patients with intracranial tumors, such as pituitary adenomas and metastatic disease, may have psychiatric manifestations.[25]

Asthma and chronic obstructive pulmonary disease exacerbations may mimic the hyperventilation and respiratory distress observed during a panic attack. A patient with an acute pulmonary embolism may present with chest tightness, dyspnea, diaphoresis, and apprehension.

An appropriate screening evaluation with laboratory and ancillary tests should be considered for anxious patients whose presentation is not consistent with a past episode. At minimum, a chemistry panel, complete blood count, pregnancy test, prescription drug levels, and toxicology screen are often necessary. If indicated, additional tests such as an electrocardiogram, computed tomography of the brain, thyroid levels, or lumbar puncture may also be obtained (Box 197-3).

Treatment

Treatment of the anxious patient should begin with the creation of a calm, quiet clinical environment. An empathetic tone and willingness to listen will relieve some of the patient's anxiety as well as facilitate an appropriate medical evaluation. The presence of a trusted, supportive friend or family member may also be helpful.

Benzodiazepines are the recommended first line agents for pharmacologic management. If an anxious patient requires immediate treatment, lorazepam, diazepam, and midazolam may be administered intravenously. Lorazepam may be given in 0.5-mg doses, whereas diazepam and midazolam may be given in 2-mg increments. For milder, less urgent symptoms and limited outpatient use, the recommended dose of clonazepam and alprazolam is 0.25 to 0.50 mg.[17,26] Buspirone, monoamine oxidase inhibitors, and selective serotonin reuptake inhibitors are commonly used by psychiatrists for the outpatient treatment of anxiety disorders.[27,28]

Disposition

Most anxious patients may be discharged home after appropriate ED evaluation and stabilization. Immediate psychiatric consultation is recommended for anxious patients who report suicidal or homicidal

BOX 197-3

Laboratory and Ancillary Studies for Patients with Anxiety

Routinely Considered

Electrolytes
Calcium
Complete blood count
Glucose
Magnesium
Phosphorus
Pregnancy test
Prescription drug levels
Toxicology screen

If Indicated

Alcohol level
Ammonia level
Blood gas analysis
Cardiac enzymes
Electrocardiogram
Human immunodeficiency virus serology
Liver function tests
Lumbar puncture
Syphilis
Thyroid-stimulating hormone

ideation, who are severely depressed or unable to care for themselves, or who may not have reliable follow-up. Anxious patients discharged from the ED should be instructed to seek care from their primary physician or mental health provider as soon as possible.

REFERENCES

1. Dorland's Illustrated Medical Dictionary, 30th ed. Philadelphia, Saunders, 2003.
2. Larkin GL, Claasen CA, Emond JA, et al: Trends in U.S. emergency department visits for mental health conditions, 1992 to 2001. Psychiatr Serv 2005;56:671-677.
3. Kessler RC, Chiu WT, Demler O, et al: Prevalence, severity, and comorbidity of 12-month DSM-IV disorders in the National Comorbidity Survey replication. Arch Gen Psychiatry 2005;62:617-627.
4. Greenberg PE, Sisitsky T, Kessler RC, et al: The economic burden of anxiety disorders in the 1990s. J Clin Psychiatry 1999;60:427-435.
5. Kessler RC, McGonagle KA, Zhao S, et al: Lifetime and 12-month prevalence of DSM III-R psychiatric disorders in the United States: Results from the National Comorbidity Survey. Arch Gen Psychiatry 1994;51:8-19.
6. Weissman MM, Bland RC, Canino GJ, et al: The cross-national epidemiology of panic disorder. Arch Gen Psychiatry 1997;54:305-309.
7. Varley CK, Smith CJ: Anxiety disorders in the child and teen. Pediatr Clin North Am 2003;50:1107-1138.
8. Lauderdale SA, Sheikh JI: Anxiety disorders in older adults. Clin Geriatr Med 2003;19:721-741.
9. Hettema JM, Prescott CA, Myers JM, et al: The structure of genetic and environmental risk factors for anxiety disorders in men and women. Arch Gen Psychiatry 2005;62:182-189.
10. Hettema JM, Neale MC, Kendler KS: A review and meta-analysis of the genetic epidemiology of anxiety disorders. Am J Psychiatry 2001;158:1568-1578.
11. Krystal JH, D'Souza DC, Sanacora G, et al: Advances in the pathophysiology and treatment of psychiatric disorders: Implications for internal medicine. Med Clin North Am 2001;85:559-577.
12. Jetty PV, Charney DS, Goddard AW: Generalized anxiety disorder: Neurobiology of generalized anxiety disorder. Psychiatr Clin North Am 2001;24:75-97.
13. Zvosec DL, Smith SW: Agitation is common in gamma-hydroxybutyrate toxicity. Am J Emerg Med 2005; 23:316-320.
14. Ritchie EC, Owens M: Military issues. Psychiatr Clin North Am 2004;27:459-471.
15. Van Den Berg B, Grievink L, Stellato RK, et al: Symptoms and related functioning in a traumatized community. Arch Intern Med 2005;165:2402-2407.
16. Milner KK, Florence T, Glick RL: Emergency psychiatry: Mood and anxiety syndromes in emergency psychiatry. Psychiatr Clin North Am 1999;22:755-777.
17. Merritt TC: Psychiatric emergencies: Recognition and acute management of patients with panic attacks in the emergency department. Emerg Med Clin North Am 2000;18:289-300.
18. American Psychiatric Association: Diagnostic and Statistical Manual of Mental Disorders, 4th ed, text rev. Washington, DC, American Psychiatric Association, 2000.
19. Lagomasino I, Daly R, Stoudemire A: Medical assessment of patients presenting with psychiatric symptoms in the emergency setting. Psychiatr Clin North Am 1999;22: 819-850.
20. Geeraerts B, Vandenberghe J, van Oudenhove L, et al: Influence of experimentally induced anxiety on gastric sensorimotor function in humans. Gastroenterology 2005;129:1437-1444.
21. Talbot-Stern JK, Green T, Royle TJ: Psychiatric emergencies: Psychiatric manifestations of systemic illness. Emerg Med Clin North Am 2000;18:199-209.
22. Fleet RP, Dupuis G, Marchand A, et al: Panic disorder in emergency department chest pain patients: Prevalence, comorbidity, suicidal ideation, and physician recognition. Am J Med 1996;101:371-380.
23. Bazakis AM, Kunzler C: Altered mental status due to metabolic or endocrine disorders. Emerg Med Clin North Am 2005;23:901-908.
24. Bunevicius R, Velickiene D, Prange AJ: Mood and anxiety disorders in women with treated hyperthyroidism and ophthalmopathy caused by Graves' disease. Gen Hosp Psychiatry 2005;27:133-139.
25. Galasko D, Kwo-On-Yuen PF, Thal L: Intracranial mass lesions associated with late-onset psychosis and depression. Psychiatr Clin North Am 1988;11:151-166.
26. Currier GW, Allen MH, Bunney EB, et al: Standard therapies for acute agitation. J Emerg Med 2004;27(Suppl): S9-S12.
27. Kapczinski F, Lima MS, Souza JS, Schmitt R: Antidepressants for generalized anxiety disorder. Cochrane Database Syst Rev 2003;2:CD003592.
28. Otto MW, Tuby KS, Gould RA, et al: An effect-size analysis of the relative efficacy and tolerability of serotonin selective reuptake inhibitors for panic disorder. Am J Psychiatry 2001;158:1989-1992.

Chapter **198**

Conversion Disorder, Psychosomatic Illness, and Malingering

Robin A. C. Marshall

KEY POINTS

Somatization disorder, conversion disorder, and hypochondriasis are neither intentional nor planned, but rather they represent reactions to stressful circumstances.

Malingering and factitious disorders involve deliberate actions of deceit.

Somatoform conditions feature complaints and symptoms that are not attributable to medical illness.

The ED evaluation of patients with suspected somatoform disorders should focus on the exclusion of potential threats to life and a search for a medical cause of the reported symptom.

Identification and appropriate referral of somatoform illness are secondary objectives of the ED encounter.

As with other psychiatric and medical diagnoses, meticulous documentation is required when somatization is suspected.

Scope

Somatoform conditions include the following diagnoses: somatization disorder, conversion disorder, somatoform pain disorder, hypochondriasis, body dysmorphic disorder, and undifferentiated somatoform illness. Further classification of somatoform disorders is continually evolving as research better defines distinctive characteristics.[1]

The reported prevalence of somatoform conditions ranges from 50%[2] to 65%[3] in ambulatory settings. When definitions are narrowed to include only those patients meeting strict diagnostic criteria for somatization disorder, the lifetime prevalence drops to less than 3%.[4] Accurate classification is difficult because some patients exhibit somatoform findings in the presence of demonstrable medical illness.

True somatization disorder (or Briquet's syndrome, after Paul Briquet, who first described the illness in 1859) typically manifests in women before 30 years of age; somatization is less common in male patients. Although many patients somatize, few are ultimately diagnosed with somatization disorder.

Definitions

Conversion disorder is a condition in which patients complain of sensory or motor symptoms that cannot be attributed to a pathophysiologic process, as a manifestation of stress or unconscious conflict. Conversion disorder is more common among women and members of lower socioeconomic groups. It typically presents in adolescence and follows a discontinuous course. Conversion disorder has also been observed in military, mass casualty, and industrial accident settings,[5] in which the female predominance of the disorder is not found. Population prevalence varies considerably as a result of classifications and definitions of the disorder. Some authors have suggested that as the sophistication and medical knowledge of a patient population increase, the incidence of true conversion disorder drops, thus making the condition more common in developing parts of the world.

Body dysmorphic disorder is characterized by a preoccupation with an imagined defect in physical appearance. Although it is currently classified under somatoform disorders, body dysmorphic disorder more closely resembles an obsessive-compulsive disorder. This disorder is commonly encountered by primary care providers, plastic surgeons, and the body enhancement industry.

Hypochondriasis is a preoccupation with or excessive fear of illness despite negative testing and reassurance from a health care professional. Hypochondriasis is more common than somatization disorder and has a prevalence of 4% to 9% in general medical practice.[6] It peaks among men in their fourth decade and in women in their fifth, with no significant predilection by gender. Hypochondriasis is increasingly described in geriatric populations.[7]

Factitious disorders, including malingering, feature deliberate manufacturing of symptoms or illness. The term *Munchausen's syndrome* (after the famous 18th-century raconteur Baron von Munchausen) is reserved for chronic or "career" medical imposters, and it represents the extreme form of the disorder. The combined prevalence for all factitious disorders ranges from 1% to 5%, with a female predominance. Cases of Munchausen's syndrome tend to involve male patients.[8]

Malingering and symptom exaggeration are underreported. In one study, "39% of mild head injury, 35% of fibromyalgia/chronic fatigue, 31% of chronic pain, 27% of neurotoxic, and 22% of electrical injury claims resulted in diagnostic impressions of probable malingering."[9] Malingering is most often exhibited by patients who are either trying to avoid an unpleasant circumstance, such as military duty or a prison term, or attempting to secure some form of compensation, such as occupational health or personal injury plaintiff claims.[10] Malingering can result in criminal charges.[10]

Factitious disorder by proxy or *Munchausen's syndrome by proxy* deserves special mention because it represents a form of child abuse. It is defined as the intentional production or feigning of physical or psychiatric illness in a child by the child's guardian. Factitious disorder by proxy can be active (symptom producing) or passive (neglect). Munchausen's syndrome by proxy is rare, occurring roughly in 2.8 of 100,000 children less than 1 year old and in 0.5 of 100,000 children less than 16 years old.[11] As with the other factitious illnesses, the deceptive nature of the disorder makes it extremely difficult to detect and study.

Pathophysiology

Somatoform illnesses represent emotional stress experienced as physical symptoms. Both somatization and hypochondriasis are commonly associated with depression and anxiety, and somatization is classified as a potential presenting symptom of depression.[12] This strong association with depressive disorders has led to the practice of treating somatization with antidepressant medications. Hypochondriasis and depression coexist in roughly 40% of cases[13]; 20% of patients with hypochondria have a diagnosis of panic disorder, and 10% have obsessive-compulsive disorder. Not only does an association exist between somatoform illness and psychiatric comorbidity, but also, as the number of reported physical symptoms rises, the likelihood of an underlying psychiatric disorder rises proportionately.[14]

Unlike somatization and hypochondriasis, a significant correlation does not appear to exist between psychiatric illness and factitious disorder. Malingering is observed in individuals with antisocial and psychopathic personalities, but the nature of this association remains unclear.

Clinical Presentation

■ CLASSIC FEATURES

Somatization is exhibited by patients who are chronically and persistently "sick" with numerous, vague complaints and symptoms involving many organ systems; review of systems is often globally "positive." Patients maintain a very strong conviction of illness and tend to thrive on their "sick role" despite multiple negative diagnostic work-ups, hospital admissions, specialist referrals, and surgical procedures. An example of the breadth of symptoms associated with somatoform disorders can be seen in the diagnostic criteria listed in Box 198-1.

Conversion disorder, in contrast to somatoform disorder, is the acute, often episodic onset of one symptom or sign involving limited body parts or organ systems. Complaints are generally sensory or motor and often occur in response to an identified stressor. Unlike malingering or factitious disorders, the malady is not feigned or deliberate. Examples of conversion disorder typically seen in the ED include pseudoseizures, altered mental status, paralysis, and movement disorders.[15]

BOX 198-1

Diagnostic and Statistical Manual of Mental Disorders (Fourth Edition, Text Revision) Criteria for Somatization Disorder

1. Pain in at least four distinct locations or circumstances (e.g., headache, backache, chest pain, dysuria, dyspareunia)
2. Two or more gastrointestinal symptoms (e.g., nausea, vomiting, diarrhea, constipation, but not pain)
3. One or more sexual dysfunction symptoms (e.g., impotence, lack of libido, menorrhagia, but not pain)
4. One or more neurologic conversion symptoms (also see Box 198-2) (e.g., paresthesia, paralysis, ataxia, blindness, pseudoseizure)

Symptoms are not medically explainable or may represent an exaggeration of symptoms attributable to an organic illness.

Symptoms must not be deliberately produced.

Adapted from American Psychiatric Association: Diagnostic and Statistical Manual of Mental Disorders, 4th ed, text rev. Washington, DC, American Psychiatric Association, 2000.

BOX 198-2

Common Conversion Symptoms

Anesthesia
Paresthesia
Paralysis
Ataxia
Syncope
Seizure
Coma
Vertigo/dizziness
Diplopia
Blindness
Deafness
Tremor
Globus hystericus

Psychogenic or somatoform pain disorder, an important and particularly challenging subcategory of conversion disorder, features a conversion symptom that is limited to pain. Although listed as a distinct entity in the text revision of the fourth edition of the *Diagnostic and Statistical Manual of Mental Disorders,*[16] this disorder closely resembles a conversion reaction to stressful, often trauma-related events. Other common conversion symptoms appear in Box 198-2.

One of the more unusual conditions that deserves separate mention is *pseudocyesis* or "hysterical pregnancy," which includes the physical symptoms of pregnancy (even amenorrhea) in the absence of a gestation.

La belle indifference, a seemingly incongruous disinterest in one's illness, is classically associated with conversion reactions but has not been rigorously studied.

Patients with *hypochondria,* like somatizers, are convinced that they are gravely ill. Whereas the somatizer focuses on symptoms, the patient with hypochondria focuses on disease states and invests great personal energy seeking multiple extensive reassurances from the health care system at significant cost. Patients with hypochondria are typified by health anxiety leading to strong convictions of illness, fixation with the body and its functions in which ominous implications are often attributed to mundane or insignificant findings, and exaggerated symptoms out of proportion to actual organic illness.

Patients who *malinger* and those who have *factitious disorder* tend to limit themselves to exaggerations of symptoms of a previously diagnosed illness or to symptoms that are difficult to investigate and disprove; examples include pain of any variety, psychiatric conditions such as suicidality, and pseudoneurologic symptoms of tingling, amnesia, and seizures. Less commonly, patients with factitious disorder inflict injury or disease on themselves. Deliberate misuse of medications such as hypoglycemic agents has been described in health care workers.[8]

Unlike the somatoform disorders, malingering and factitious behaviors involve feigned illness. Even though they are aware of their deception, patients with factitious disorder (unlike malingerers) are helpless to control the behavior.[16] To illustrate the differences among somatoform disorder, factitious disorder, and malingering, one can use the example of pseudoseizures, which can be seen in each condition. The patient with a somatoform disorder suffers a nonvolitional seizure in response to a psychological stressor, the patient with factitious disorder has an uncontrollable compulsion to feign a seizure to gain attention and the sick role, whereas the patient who malingers feigns a seizure as part of ruse to achieve a specific end. What sets malingering apart from factitious disorder is an identifiable, tangible goal or gain.[17]

PRIMARY AND SECONDARY GAIN

Although EPs encounter somatoform behaviors, the brevity of the clinical encounter and a diagnostic focus on life threats make accurate identification of patients with a somatoform disorders difficult. Even when demonstrable medical disease is present, symptoms and severity are modulated by the psychological well-being of the patient. Whereas it stands to reason that many patients somatize to some degree, clearly a subset exists in whom such behavior represents a disorder.

A useful framework to understand somatoform illness is the concept of primary and secondary gain.[18] *Primary gain,* which is also known as *psychological gain* or *paranosic gain,* refers to a reduction of subconscious stress or anxiety by manifesting physical symptoms. *Secondary gain* is defined as an advantage or goal achieved through the expression of factitious illness. Examples of secondary gain include attention, pity, or sympathy, as well as deliberate or conscious gains such as opiate medications, money, or legal advantage.

■ Example

A patient experiences psychological stress as a result of an upsetting life event and derives primary gain by manifesting chest pain (the physical symptom gives the patient a focus and concrete context in which to deal with the stress). While seeking care for the chest pain, the patient experiences secondary gain in the form of attention from friends, family, and medical staff. The patient knows only that his or her chest hurts.

■ VICTIMS OF INTIMATE PARTNER VIOLENCE

Among patients who tend to use emergency care frequently, an important subgroup comprises victims of *intimate partner violence* (see Chapter 126). Intimate partner violence results in high levels of psychological stress for the victim. Many of these patients repeatedly present to the ED with somatoform behavior.[19] Physicians must screen for ongoing abuse when new or recurrent physical symptoms cannot be attributed to a medical condition. Just as with current abuse, patients with a past history of physical, sexual, or psychological abuse also tend to use medical services more frequently.

Differential Diagnosis and Testing

The goals when evaluating somatoform illness are identification of the condition and appropriate referral. In the ED, life-threatening conditions on a differential diagnosis are excluded first, other potential medical illnesses are excluded second, and somatoform causes are excluded last, if at all.

Classic presentations can make one suspect a somatoform illness; however, such behaviors are insufficient for psychiatric diagnostic criteria. Synopses of the characteristics of the somatoform disorders can be found in Table 198-1. It is useful to categorize these illnesses as *nondeliberate* (somatization, conversion, and hypochondriasis) and *deliberate* (factitious disorders and malingering).

The symptoms experienced by a patient with nondeliberate somatoform illness are perceived as very real. Diligent history taking often uncovers telling patterns. Useful questions to consider include the following: Are these complaints chronic? Do they correlate with identifiable stressors? Does the patient hold a conviction of a particular illness or imminent death? Does the patient have a lifelong history of "illness"? What has been done for this patient in previous visits, by previous providers? What is new today? Obtaining answers to these questions, along with careful physical examination, can help to direct the emergency evaluation while at the same time reassuring the patient that he or she is being taken seriously. Respect ultimately aids in disposition because these patients are far more likely to comply with a plan when they believe that a provider has their best interests at heart.

Table 198-1 CHARACTERISTICS OF SOMATOFORM DISORDERS

Disorder	Hallmarks
Somatization disorder	Multiple, chronic, vague symptoms occurring in differing organ systems Many past work-ups Associated psychiatric disorder
Conversion disorder	Acute, episodic Limited symptoms and body parts Motor or sensory complains predominant
Hypochondriasis	Health anxiety Fixation on diagnoses and body functions
Factitious disorder	Compulsive urge to feign illness by report or deed
Malingering	Feigned illness for the purpose of avoiding something unpleasant or to gain some reward

Concerns about making a diagnosis of somatoform illness should not preclude a thorough ED evaluation because many medical conditions can be mistaken for somatization, particularly when presentations are atypical. Box 198-3 provides examples of medical conditions that can mimic somatoform behavior.

As a general rule, patients presenting with nondeliberate somatoform illness acquiesce to invasive diagnostic testing, whereas patients with factitious disorders and malingerers are more reluctant. The presence of two or more of the following features suggests malingering behavior: mention of a medicolegal context of the visit, discrepancy between subjective and objective assessment of the degree of stress and disability, poor compliance with evaluation and treatment, and antisocial personality disorder.[16] Malingering is very difficult to prove, even in the presence of high clinical suspicion and deliberate investigation, and it often requires surveillance of the patient.[20] The determination of malingering is usually the purview of specialists such as neuropsychologists.

Various maneuvers are purported to assist in identifying factitious symptoms. Waddell's "behavioral

BOX 198-3

Medical Conditions That Can Mimic Somatization

Multiple sclerosis
Thyroid disorders
Guillain-Barré syndrome
Porphyria
Botulism
Myasthenia gravis
Parathyroid disorders
Insulin derangements
Uremia
Periodic paralysis
Lupus
Pituitary disorders
Addison's disease
Wilson's disease
Carbon monoxide exposure
Medication side effects

responses to examination," as applied to a chief complaint of back pain, are one example. Although *Waddell's signs* provide a compelling method of detecting feigned illness, the predictive value of such maneuvers is generally poor and correlates with unfavorable treatment outcome.[21]

Tests for factitious paralysis are somewhat more useful. *Hoover's test* involves placing the examiner's hand under a "weakened" lower extremity and asking the supine patient to raise the unaffected leg; downward pressure in the affected leg is considered positive for feigned paralysis. The *abductor test* is also useful: in true paresis, the unaffected leg abducts when the patient attempts to abduct the affected leg against resistance.[22]

Treatment

No specific treatment for nondeliberate somatoform illness exists. Psychiatric comorbidities such as depression, anxiety, and substance abuse should be addressed. Cognitive behavioral therapy has shown promise in the minority of patients willing to be referred.[23]

It is generally not recommended to confront a patient with a somatoform illness. Instead, reassure the patient that the symptoms do not represent an imminent threat. Even in cases of malingering, neuropsychologists rarely confront patients; most use descriptive terminology rather than the diagnosis "malingering."[24]

Whether to use medication to treat symptoms believed to be somatoform in origin is as much an ethical question as a medical one. This quandary often presents itself when considering analgesics for chronic pain syndromes. Applying the principles of beneficence and nonmalfeasance, one may want to spare a patient potential side effects and addiction; this is countered by the harm of leaving a patient in pain or consigning him or her to withdrawal if he or she is a chronic user of analgesics.

The final common pathway of pain is the perception of pain, and even imagined pain can be very real. Given that emergency providers do not primarily manage somatoform illness, it is not unreasonable to provide short-term "bridging" prescriptions on a case-by-case basis to patients with appropriate follow-up arrangements. Patients who present for care only to acquire narcotics are not considered to be suffering from somatoform illness; rather, they may have substance abuse, addiction, or illegal market motivations.

Good charting practices are critical when somatization is suspected. The history of present illness and review of systems should include liberal use of patient quotes to convey the character of the visit to subsequent providers. Physical examination findings also need to be carefully documented, because they may be the reason to pursue or defer diagnostic intervention. Discharge instructions must include times, dates, and names of follow-up visits; doses of medications; and specific return criteria.

The final discharge diagnosis should reflect the chief complaint (e.g., "leg pain"), rather than the suspected somatoform behavior. This is particularly true of feigned illness, because these diagnoses have criminal implications. Suspected or clear exceptions to this rule are intimate partner violence or Munchausen's syndrome by proxy, which deserve special consideration. In both these instances, a high index of suspicion and appropriate intervention are required.

REFERENCES

1. Mayou R, Kirmayer LJ, Simon G, et al: Somatoform disorders: Time for a new approach in DSM-V. Am J Psychiatry 2005;162:847-855.
2. Katon W, Walker EA: Medically unexplained symptoms in primary care. J Clin Psychiatry 1998;59(Suppl 20):15-21.
3. Kroenke K, Price RK: Symptoms in the community: Prevalence, classification, and psychiatric comorbidity. Arch Intern Med 1993;153:2474-2480.
4. Kirmayer LJ, Robbins JM: Three forms of somatization in primary care: Prevalence, co-occurrence, and sociodemographic characteristics. J Nerv Ment Dis 1991;179:647-655.
5. Ford C, Folks DG: Conversion disorders: An overview. Psychosomatics 1985;26:371-374, 380-383.
6. Fink P, Ornbol E, Toft T, et al: A new, empirically established hypochondriasis diagnosis. Am J Psychiatry 2004;161:1680-1691.
7. Monopoli J: Managing hypochondriasis in elderly clients. J Contemp Psychother 2005;35:285-300.
8. Krahn LE, Li H, O'Connor MK: Patients who strive to be ill: Factitious disorder with physical symptoms. Am J Psychiatry 2003;160:1163-1168.
9. Mittenberg W, Patton C, Canyock EM, Condit DC: Base rates of malingering and symptom exaggeration. J Clin Exp Neuropsychol 2002;24:1094-1102.
10. Mendelson G, Mendelson D: Malingering pain in the medicolegal context. Clin J Pain 2004;20:423-432.

11. McClure RJ, Davis PM, Meadow SR, Sibert JR: Epidemiology of Munchausen syndrome by proxy, non-accidental poisoning, and non-accidental suffocation. Arch Dis Child 1996;75:57-61.
12. Posse M, Hallstrom T: Depressive disorders among somatizing patients in primary health care. Acta Psychiatr Scand 1998;98:187-192.
13. Barsky AJ, Wyshak G, Klerman GL: Psychiatric comorbidity in DSM-III-R hypochondriasis. Arch Gen Psychiatry 1992;49:101-108.
14. Kroenke K, Spitzer RL, Williams JB, et al: Physical symptoms in primary care: Predictors of psychiatric disorders and functional impairment. Arch Fam Med 1994;9: 774-779.
15. Dula D, DeNaples L: Emergency department presentation of patients with conversion disorder. Acad Emerg Med 1995;2:120-123.
16. American Psychiatric Association: Diagnostic and Statistical Manual of Mental Disorders, 4th ed, text rev. Washington, DC, American Psychiatric Association, 2000.
17. Kalivas J: Malingering versus factitious disorder. Am J Psychiatry 1996;153:1108.
18. Hollifield MA: Somatization disorder. In Sadock BJ, Sadock VA (eds): Kaplan & Sadock's Comprehensive Textbook of Psychiatry, 8th ed. Philadelphia, Lippincott Williams & Wilkins, 2005.
19. Abbott J: Injuries and illnesses of domestic violence. Ann Emerg Med 1997;29:781-785.
20. LoPiccolo CJ, Goodkin K, Baldewicz TT: Current issues in the diagnosis and management of malingering. Ann Med 1999;31:166-174.
21. Fishbain DA, Cole B, Cutler RB, et al: A structured evidence-based review on the meaning of nonorganic physical signs: Waddell signs. Pain Med 2003;4:141-181.
22. Greer S, Chambliss L, Mackler L, Huber T: Clinical inquiries: What physical exam techniques are useful to detect malingering? J Fam Pract 2005;54:719-722.
23. Barsky AJ, Ahern DK: Cognitive behavior therapy for hypochondriasis: A randomized controlled trial. JAMA 2004;291:1464-1470.
24. Slick DJ, Tan JE, Strauss EH, Hultsch DF: Detecting malingering: A survey of experts' practices. Arch Clin Neuropsychol 2004;19:465-473.

Chapter 199

Addiction

Randall S. Jotte

KEY POINTS

Approximately 10% of ED visits are related to issues of substance abuse or dependence.

Addictive behaviors have devastating consequences on the personal life of the individual and the larger objectives of society.

Drug and alcohol abuse irrevocably changes brain physiology; addiction represents a brain disorder.

The acute presentations of substance abuse and dependency arise from drug-specific patterns of intoxication and withdrawal.

Acute pharmacologic detoxification is accomplished through the administration of a long-acting medication in the same category as the drug of dependence, thereby blocking withdrawal symptoms.

Anticraving medications are psychotropic agents that reduce the desire for drugs or alcohol in the detoxified patient and prevent relapse into compulsive substance abuse.

Scope

Addiction is a state of inner tyranny. Considerations of family, health, finances, and the law are incidental to one primal urge: obtaining the addictive agent. The destructive effects of drugs or alcohol on the individual addict are often easy to observe. Many physicians, however, are unaware of the cumulative consequences of addiction on society at large.

From most perspectives, the problem is vast. The U.S. Department of Health and Human Services reported that in 2003, 21.6 million Americans were classified with substance abuse or dependence, equal to 9.1% of the total U.S. population 12 years old or older.[1] Many of those abusing or dependent on drugs and alcohol disproportionately consume public health care resources, particularly emergency services. In 1998, alcohol-related ED visits totaled 8.13 million, more than 8% of all emergency visits.[2] In the same year, 326,500 patients presented to an ED with drug-related complaints.[3]

The societal burdens of substance abuse extend well beyond the hospital. In 1991, 18% of U.S. federal prison inmates convicted of violent offenses, including homicide, robbery, and sexual assault, committed their offense to obtain money to purchase drugs.[4] Once acquired, drugs often are associated with further violence. In 1995, 59% of persons arrested for homicide tested positive for drugs.[5]

The economic cost of substance abuse is alarming. In 1998, alcohol abuse in the United States cost the nation approximately $185 billion, and 47% of these costs were attributed solely to lost productivity at work.[6] In the same year, drug abuse in the United States cost $143 billion.[7] When adjusted to 2007 dollars, substance abuse of both drugs and alcohol totaled $420 billion—for comparison, this figure is double the cumulative nationwide expenditure for

BOX 199-1

Criteria for the Diagnosis of Substance Abuse

A. A maladaptive pattern of substance use leading to clinically significant impairment or distress, as manifested by one (or more) of the following, occurring within a 12-month period:
   1. Recurrent substance use resulting in a failure to fulfill major role obligations at work, school, or home (e.g., repeated absences or poor work performance related to substance use; substance-related absences, suspensions, or expulsions from school; neglect of children or household)
   2. Recurrent substance use in situations in which it is physically hazardous (e.g., driving an automobile or operating a machine when impaired by substance use)
   3. Recurrent substance-related legal problems (e.g., arrests for substance-related disorderly conduct)
   4. Continued substance use despite having persistent or recurrent social or interpersonal problems caused or exacerbated by the effects of the substance (e.g., arguments with spouse about consequences of intoxication, physical fights)

B. The symptoms have never met the criteria for substance dependence for this class of substance.

From First MB, Frances A, Pincus HA: Substance-related disorders. In DSM-IV-TR Guidebook. Washington, DC, American Psychiatric Publishing, 2004, p 133.

BOX 199-2

Criteria for the Diagnosis of Substance Dependence

A maladaptive pattern of substance use, leading to clinically significant impairment or distress, as manifested by three (or more) of the following, occurring at any time in the same 12-month period:

1. Tolerance, as defined by either of the following:
   a. A need for markedly increased amounts of the substance to achieve intoxication or desired effect
   b. Markedly diminished effect with continued use of the same amount of the substance
2. Withdrawal, as manifested by either of the following:
   a. The characteristic withdrawal syndrome for the substance
   b. The same (or a closely related) substance taken to relieve or avoid withdrawal symptoms
3. The substance is often taken in larger amounts or over a longer period than was intended.
4. There is a persistent desire or unsuccessful efforts to cut down or control substance use.
5. A great deal of time is spent in activities necessary to obtain the substance (e.g., visiting multiple doctors or driving long distances), use the substance (e.g., chain smoking), or recover from its effects.
6. Important social, occupational, or recreational activities are given up or reduced because of substance use.
7. The substance use is continued despite knowledge of having a persistent or recurrent physical or psychological problem that is likely to have been caused or exacerbated by the substance (e.g., current cocaine use despite recognition of cocaine-induced depression or continued drinking despite recognition that an ulcer was made worse by alcohol consumption).

From First MB, Frances A, Pincus HA: Substance-related disorders. In DSM-IV-TR Guidebook. Washington, DC, American Psychiatric Publishing, 2004, p 128.

prescription drugs and is 93% of the revenue allocated to fund public education for prekindergarten through 12th grades.[8,9] Substance abuse is as much a societal crisis for our nation as it is a personal crisis for the addict.

Definitions

Disorders related to substance abuse and dependence are defined not by the quantity of the cause, but rather by the effect on the individual. *Substance abuse* is characterized by the occurrence of adverse consequences related to alcohol or drug use, without a pattern or state of dependence (Box 199-1). More specifically, the American Psychiatric Association defined substance abuse as "a maladaptive pattern of substance use" revealed by the recurrent and significant problems arising from repeated use of the substance: failure to fulfill major role obligations, recurrent use in situations in which it is physically hazardous, multiple substance-related legal problems, and repeated social and interpersonal problems.[10] Consequences of use are significant, although a degree of control is present.

Substance dependence is defined by severe impairment or absence of control (Box 199-2). Use is compulsive, occurring under the ever-present threats of tolerance and withdrawal. The American Psychiatric Association more specifically defined substance dependence as a cluster of cognitive, behavioral, and physiologic symptoms that indicate the continued use of a substance despite significant adverse consequences.[11]

Tolerance is reflected by the "need for increasing amounts of the substance to achieve intoxication or desired effect . . . or diminished effect with continued use of the same amount of the substance."[12]

Withdrawal is a physiologic response manifested by characteristic signs and symptoms that occur with an acute decrease in use of a particular substance. Use of the same or a closely related substance relieves or prevents such symptoms.[11]

Addiction is a term of more general public reference that includes drug and alcohol dependence. However, the term also acknowledges other inherent self-destructive behavioral patterns, including eating disorders, compulsive gambling, and excessive sexual behaviors.

This chapter focuses on drug- and alcohol-related disorders. Although multiple agents of abuse exist, most substances of common clinical presentation can be classified as either central nervous system (CNS) depressants (alcohol, sedatives, hypnotics, and anxiolytics) or CNS stimulants (cocaine, amphetamines, and sympathomimetics).

Pathophysiology and Anatomy

Our understanding of the pathophysiology of substance-related disorders has progressed substantially in recent years. Neuropharmacologic animal studies and human brain imaging modalities have revealed anatomic structures and neurochemical processes that are altered by substance abuse. Addiction ultimately changes brain physiology and thus prompted the categorization of this condition as a brain disorder.[13]

Addictive substances alter dopamine neurotransmission within the mesolimbic system of the brain (Fig. 199-1). Projecting from the ventral tegmental area to the nucleus accumbens, olfactory tubercle, frontal cortex, and amygdala, the mesolimbic system is regarded as the reward center of the brain.[14] These neurocircuits presumably evolved to reward survival-enhancing behavior, such as reproduction and productive familial and social interactions. Some researchers believe that mesolimbic dopamine is a direct mediator of reward, whereas others emphasize that dopamine signals an interest in reward or the expectation that reward is forthcoming. Either way, evidence suggests that the common reinforcing and incentive effects of addictive substances are substantially mediated by increasing extracellular dopamine within the mesolimbic system. On an elementary level, this drug-induced efflux of dopamine is a pleasurable stimulant.[13]

As addicts and clinicians mutually recognize, these pleasant effects are accompanied by a grave physiologic shortcoming. Neurochemical pleasure circuits, overwhelmed by excessive stimulation, adapt through

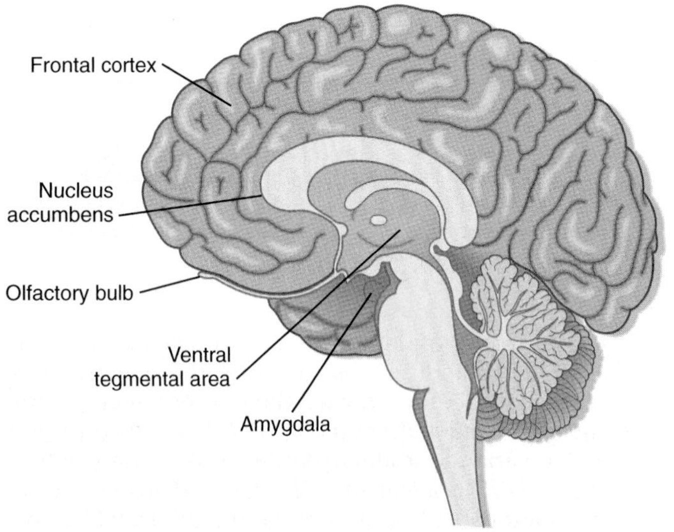
Frontal cortex
Nucleus accumbens
Olfactory bulb
Ventral tegmental area
Amygdala

FIGURE 199-1 Mesolimbic dopaminergic system.

desensitization.[15] Evaluations from multiple disciplines, including anatomic, behavioral, biochemical, and electrophysiologic studies, commonly show that dopamine neurons function insufficiently in the addict. A hypodopaminergic state develops.[13] The hypodopaminergic state associated with acute withdrawal is clinically demonstrated by dysphoria, depression, irritability, and anxiety. Neurochemically, baseline levels of the reward neurotransmitters are depressed.[14] Traditional social and behavioral stimulants of the mesolimbic system that function effectively in the nonaddictive state (e.g., positive affirmation from work or family) become inadequate to generate a significant perception of pleasure.

Drugs and alcohol are the sole stimuli sufficient to activate the impaired mesolimbic neurocircuits and to generate a sense of pleasure.[14] Although the baseline mesolimbic system remains hypodopaminergic in the addict, the system remains hyperresponsive to abused substances, thereby conferring long-lasting vulnerability even after extensive periods of abstinence.[13] The most promising avenues of treatment in the addict are pharmacologic agents aimed at restoring these dopaminergic neurocircuits.[13]

Not all individuals are equally susceptible. Those with risk-taking and novelty-seeking traits favor the use of addictive drugs. Psychiatric conditions, in particular schizophrenia, bipolar disorders, and attention-deficit/hyperactivity disorders, are associated with increased risk for substance abuse and dependency. A dual diagnosis of substance abuse and mental disorder has particularly unfavorable implications for both management and outcome.[16]

Genetic factors clearly enhance the risk of addiction. Men whose parents had alcoholism have an increased likelihood for alcoholism even when they were adopted at birth and raised by parents who did not have alcoholism.[16] Twin studies also provided clear evidence of a genetic predisposition to addiction.[17] Some of this genetic predilection is expressed through enzymatic variants. For example, highly

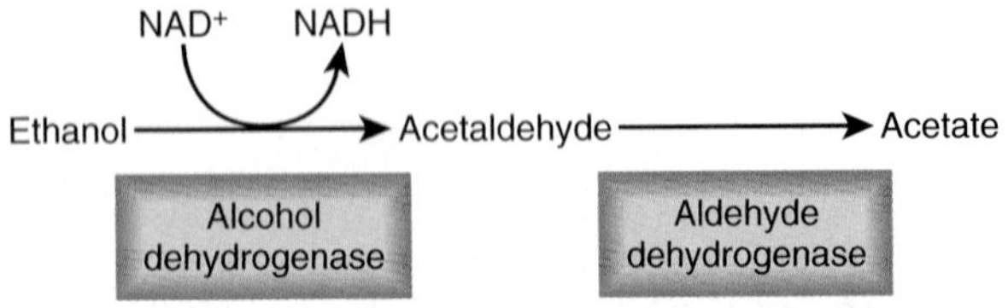
NAD+
NADH
Ethanol
Acetaldehyde
Acetate
Alcohol dehydrogenase
Aldehyde dehydrogenase

FIGURE 199-2 Metabolism of alcohol. NAD^+, oxidized form of nicotinamide adenine dinucleotide; NADH, reduced form of nicotinamide adenine dinucleotide.

active forms of aldehyde dehydrogenase increase alcohol metabolism and decrease the negative side effects of alcohol intake, thereby enhancing consumption and addiction (Fig. 199-2). In contrast, less active variants of aldehyde dehydrogenase (such as the *ALDH2*2* allele initially detected in East Asian populations) allow accumulation of acetaldehyde, the toxic intermediary byproduct of alcohol metabolism. Sensitivity to alcohol increases, with subsequent reduction in the rates of alcoholism.[18]

Genetic influence is also expressed through neurotransmitter variants. Neuropeptide Y, a 36-amino acid peptide neurotransmitter, regulates appetite, anxiety, and reward. A functional Lue7Pro polymorphism in the neuropeptide Y gene increases the risk for alcohol dependence by 7.3%, primarily among European Americans.[19]

Clinical Presentation

Signs and symptoms of substance abuse and dependency arise from acute states of intoxication and withdrawal. Although some manifestations are substance specific, common patterns exist.

■ CENTRAL NERVOUS SYSTEM DEPRESSANTS

Acute intoxication with CNS depressants manifests with dysfunctional behavioral and neurologic changes (Box 199-3). Individuals suffer mood swings and impaired social or occupational functioning. Poor judgment prevails, often reflected through inappropriate sexual behavior or aggression. Neurologic dysfunction occurs along a clinical spectrum determined by the degree of intoxication, ranging from slurred speech, incoordination, and unsteady gait to impairment in memory and attention, stupor, and coma.

In contrast, acute withdrawal from CNS depressants manifests with physiologic and behavioral agitation. Psychomotor distress can be significant, with transient visual, tactile, or auditory hallucinations. Patients experience autonomic hyperactivity, evident in tachycardia and diaphoresis. Nausea, vomiting, and hand tremors may be prevalent. Generalized seizures can occur. Patients become mentally, emotionally, and physically miserable—they are unable to perform and socialize as they once did.[20]

Opiate use manifests with somewhat unique situations of intoxication and withdrawal (Box 199-4).

BOX 199-3

Diagnostic Criteria for Intoxication with Alcohol, Sedatives, Hypnotics, or Anxiolytics

A. Recent use of a sedative, hypnotic, or anxiolytic
B. Clinically significant maladaptive behavioral or psychological changes (e.g., inappropriate sexual or aggressive behavior, mood lability, impaired judgment, impaired social or occupational functioning) that developed during or shortly after sedative, hypnotic, or anxiolytic use
C. One (or more) of the following signs, developing during or shortly after sedative, hypnotic, or anxiolytic use:
   1. Slurred speech
   2. Incoordination
   3. Unsteady gait
   4. Nystagmus
   5. Impairment in attention or memory
   6. Stupor or coma
D. Symptoms not the result of a general medical condition and not better accounted for by another mental disorder

From First MB, Frances A, Pincus HA: Substance-related disorders. In DSM-IV-TR Guidebook. Washington, DC, American Psychiatric Publishing, 2004, pp 141-142.

BOX 199-4

Diagnostic Criteria for Opioid Intoxication

A. Recent use of an opioid
B. Clinically significant maladaptive behavioral or psychological changes (e.g., initial euphoria followed by apathy, dysphoria, psychomotor agitation or retardation, impaired judgment, or impaired social or occupational functioning) that developed during or shortly after opioid use
C. Pupillary constriction (or pupillary dilation resulting from anoxia from severe overdose) and one (or more) of the following signs, developing during or shortly after opioid use:
   1. Drowsiness or coma
   2. Slurred speech
   3. Impairment in attention or memory
D. Symptoms not the result of a general medical condition and not better accounted for by another mental disorder

From First MB, Frances A, Pincus HA: Substance-related disorders. In DSM-IV-TR Guidebook. Washington, DC, American Psychiatric Publishing, 2004, pp 154-155.

BOX 199-5

Diagnostic Criteria for Cocaine and Amphetamine Intoxication

A. Recent use of cocaine or amphetamine
B. Clinically significant maladaptive behavioral or psychological changes (e.g., euphoria or affective blunting; changes in sociability; hypervigilance; interpersonal sensitivity; anxiety, tension, or anger; stereotyped behaviors; impaired judgment; or impaired social or occupational functioning) that developed during or shortly after use of cocaine or amphetamine
C. Two (or more) of the following, developing during or shortly after cocaine or amphetamine use:
    1. Tachycardia or bradycardia
    2. Pupillary dilation
    3. Elevated or lowered blood pressure
    4. Perspiration or chills
    5. Nausea or vomiting
    6. Evidence of weight loss
    7. Psychomotor agitation or retardation
    8. Muscular weakness, respiratory depression, chest pain, or cardiac arrhythmias
    9. Confusion, seizures, dyskinesias, dystonias, or coma
D. Symptoms not the result of a general medical condition and not better accounted for by another mental disorder

From First MB, Frances A, Pincus HA: Substance-related disorders. In DSM-IV-TR Guidebook. Washington, DC, American Psychiatric Publishing, 2004, pp 144-145.

Incremental doses are required to achieve euphoria, because of the rapid but variable degrees of tolerance that develop to most opiates. The unreliable concentration of opiates in street drugs complicates attempts by the addict to self-administer a specific dose. Overdosage frequently results in extreme drowsiness, coma, and death from respiratory depression.

Opiate withdrawal is an extremely unpleasant conscious experience. Patients experience severe dysphoria, diaphoresis, vomiting, and diarrhea.[21]

■ CENTRAL NERVOUS SYSTEM STIMULANTS

The clinical presentation of acute intoxication with CNS stimulants is determined by the specific agent, as well as the pattern, route, and amount of drug used (Box 199-5). Patients with intermittent "binge" uses often present with euphoria and heightened psychomotor and autonomic activity, causing tachycardia, hypertension, seizures, cardiac arrhythmias, and chest pain. Long-term daily users manifest a contrasting clinical picture. Psychomotor depression and affective blunting may be present, often in the setting of hypotension, bradycardia, and respiratory insufficiency.

Withdrawal from CNS stimulants occurs after a period of heavy and prolonged use. Withdrawal symptoms of dysphoria, suicidal ideation, extreme fatigue, and hypersomnia are the antithesis of symptoms of acute intoxication.[22]

BOX 199-6

Potential Drug-Seeking Behaviors

Overreporting of symptoms
Multiple somatic complaints
Vague symptom complexes
Insistence on specific medications
Refusal of generic equivalents
Arguments about pharmacology
Self-asserted high tolerance
Veiled threats
Flattery followed by prescription requests
Demands for polypharmacy

■ DRUG-SEEKING BEHAVIOR

EPs often encounter a particularly challenging clinical situation arising from addiction: drug-seeking activity (Box 199-6). Patients who seek drugs may engage in "doctor shopping" by visiting multiple outpatient clinics, EDs, and pain management clinics to obtain prescriptions for controlled substances. At times, false complaints are presented, such as chronic toothaches, lost or stolen prescriptions, and multiple drug allergies. While recognizing the need to evaluate each situation separately, the physician must be particularly vigilant when patients insist on specific controlled substances, self-assert a high tolerance to medications, or issue veiled threats. When in doubt, suspicion of drug-seeking behavior can often be substantiated through contact with the patient's personal physician, review of recently issued prescription drugs with the patient's pharmacist, or perusal of prior medical records.[23]

Differential Diagnosis

The differential diagnosis of substance-related disorders is limited (Box 199-7). Hypochondriasis and somatization disorders generally are difficult to distinguish from true addiction in a single ED encounter. *Pseudoaddiction* describes behavior similar to that of addiction but arising from mismanaged pain. Patients with pseudoaddiction are highly focused on obtaining medications, although usually through appropriate routes. They may be "clock-watchers," focused on the scheduled delivery of approved analgesics. When suspecting a disruption in the expected

BOX 199-7

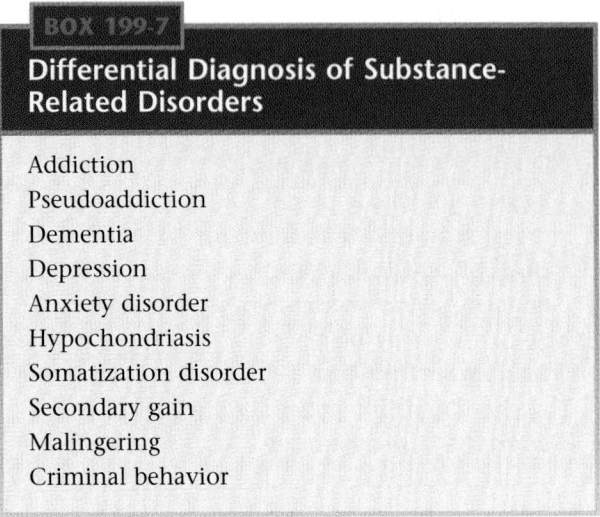

Differential Diagnosis of Substance-Related Disorders

Addiction
Pseudoaddiction
Dementia
Depression
Anxiety disorder
Hypochondriasis
Somatization disorder
Secondary gain
Malingering
Criminal behavior

regimen, the pseudoaddict may become deceptive or dramatic in attempts to ensure treatment. Distinguishing between the addict and the pseudoaddict is challenging in an isolated encounter. Pseudoaddicts generally function well once their pain is effectively treated, usually with long-acting opioids.[24]

Diagnostic Testing

The clinical interview remains the best tool for the diagnosis of substance-related disorders. Patients should be questioned about the quantity and frequency of use in an emphatic, nonjudgmental manner. Current and past symptoms should be solicited, as well as a family history of substance-related disorders. Various screening tools are available: CAGE, the Michigan Alcoholism Screening Test (MAST), the Alcohol Use Disorders Identification Test (AUDIT), and the Drug Abuse Screening Test (DAST). These interview tools are of variable length and require only several minutes to complete.[25]

When substance use is suspected, toxicologic analysis is recommended to establish or confirm a diagnosis. Qualitative analysis generally is sufficient to substantiate drug use, although quantitative levels are indicated for ethanol.

Treatment

Treatment goals for substance abuse and dependency are twofold: detoxification and prevention of relapse. These objectives are best accomplished through a combination of pharmacologic and behavioral therapies (Table 199-1).

■ DETOXIFICATION

The principles of pharmacologic detoxification are neither complex nor controversial. Patients should receive a long-acting medication in the same category as the drug of dependence, thereby blocking withdrawal symptoms. The dosage of treatment medication is gradually reduced under medical supervision.[26]

Patients with alcoholism are detoxified with benzodiazepines, commonly lorazepam, diazepam, or chlordiazepoxide. These medications act by decreasing the hyperautonomic state of alcohol withdrawal by facilitating inhibitory gamma-aminobutyric acid (GABA) transmission.[27] Patients who exhibit persistent signs of autonomic stimulation, such as tremor, tachycardia, or hypertension should be managed on an inpatient basis, with intravenous

Table 199-1 TREATMENT OPTIONS

Agent of Abuse	Detoxification Medications	Anticraving Medications
Ethanol	Benzodiazepines	Naltrexone Acamprosate Disulfiram Topiramate*
Opiates	Opioid agonists Methadone L-α-Acetyl-methadol Buprenorphine α_2-Agonists Clonidine Lofexidine†	Methadone Buprenorphine Naltrexone
Cocaine	Benzodiazepines	Topiramate‡ Modafinil‡ Vigabatrin‡ Disulfiram‡ Propranolol‡
Methamphetamine	Benzodiazepines	None

*Approved by the Food and Drug Administration (FDA) as an anticonvulsant but potentially effective in preventing alcohol relapse.
†Used in Britain; not currently FDA-approved for use in the United States.
‡FDA-approved for another indication.

benzodiazepines, often in large doses. Contemporaneous therapy is directed at frequently associated comorbid malnutrition states and includes supplementation with thiamine, multivitamins, folate, and magnesium.

Opiate detoxification is managed with opioid agonists and α_2-agonists. Opioid agonists stimulate mu receptors at durations that far exceed the 3- to 4-hour half-life of heroin. Examples of opioid agonists include methadone (24- to 36-hour half-life) and L-α-acetyl-methadol (LAAM, 72-hour half-life). Methadone may be prescribed only by maintenance programs approved by the Food and Drug Administration (FDA) and designated state authorities. LAAM is approved in the United States for opiate maintenance in patients in whom methadone maintenance fails. Buprenorphine, a partial mu-receptor agonist, has a half-life of 20 to 25 hours and may be prescribed by physicians who have received a waiver by the U.S. Drug Enforcement Agency.

α_2-Agonists are commonly used to treat mild to moderate opiate withdrawal symptoms in the ED. Activation of presynaptic α_2 receptors inhibits sympathetic outflow.[28] Clonidine is the only α_2-agonist currently available for treatment of opiate withdrawal in the United States; lofexidine, used in Britain, was approved for a phase III clinical trial in the U.S. in 2006.

Acute withdrawal from CNS stimulants, in particular cocaine and methamphetamine, is best managed with benzodiazepines. As noted earlier, benzodiazepines diminish the hyperautonomic withdrawal state by increasing inhibitory GABA transmission.

PREVENTION OF RELAPSE

Prevention of relapse is a critical component of treatment, and it significantly affects overall morbidity and mortality. Behavioral therapy should accompany any attempt at pharmacologic prevention.

Pharmacologic Prevention

Since the early 1980s, a new class of psychoactive medications emerged that showed substantial promise in the treatment of addiction disorders. These anticraving medications reduce desire for drugs or alcohol in the detoxified patient and prevent relapse into compulsive substance abuse.[26]

Alcohol

Three medications are FDA approved for the prevention of alcohol relapse: naltrexone, acamprosate, and disulfiram. Naltrexone, an opioid mu-receptor antagonist, blocks alcohol-induced dopamine release in the nucleus accumbens.[26,29] In a study of 99 men with alcoholism, those treated with naltrexone reported reduced alcohol craving, drinking, relapse, and alcohol-related euphoria. One challenge of naltrexone is that daily administration may result in limited long-term compliance. An injectable depot formulation, generating active blood levels for 30 to 40 days, may soon gain FDA approval.[26]

Acamprosate became available in 2004 for the maintenance of abstinence in detoxified alcohol-dependent patients. Although its precise mechanism of action is unclear, acamprosate appears to regulate the balance of glutamate and GABA neurotransmission.[26] Acamprosate is particularly useful when combined with naltrexone.[30]

Disulfiram blocks aldehyde dehydrogenase, an enzyme fundamental to alcohol metabolism. Acetaldehyde, an intermediate and relatively toxic byproduct, is produced at levels 5- to 10-fold those of normal metabolism. Acetaldehyde accumulation causes a disagreeable flushing known as the *disulfiram reaction*. Although disulfiram is effective for up to 14 days, poor compliance can be observed because of the unpleasantness of this reaction.[26]

Topiramate, approved by the FDA as an anticonvulsant, has shown promise in preventing alcohol relapse. Topiramate augments GABA neurotransmission and demonstrated efficacy in reducing drinking among alcoholic patients in a randomized, controlled trial.[26,31]

Opiates

Three medications are FDA approved for the prevention of relapse from opiates. Methadone and buprenorphine act as complete (methadone) or partial (buprenorphine) mu-receptor agonists. Conceptually, methadone and buprenorphine provide long-term replacement therapy in the brain disorder of addiction, comparable to the use of prednisone in adrenal insufficiency or levothyroxine in hypothyroidism. Naltrexone, which blocks the euphoric effects of opioids, has relatively poor long-term compliance.[26]

Methadone has been the mainstay of opiate pharmacotherapy since 1964. Studies have shown that moderate- to high-dose treatment with methadone (80 to 120 mg) reduced or eliminated opiate use in outpatient settings. One placebo-controlled, prospective study of methadone in 100 male narcotic-addicted subjects observed improved long-term treatment retention and decreased criminal activity.[32]

Cocaine

No FDA-approved drugs are available for the prevention of relapse from cocaine addiction, although five agents approved for other indications have been found to be effective in decreasing cocaine use. Topiramate, modafinil, and vigabatrin affect glutamate and GABA neurotransmission; the mechanisms of action of disulfiram and propranolol are unknown.[26]

Methamphetamine

Clinical trials have yet to demonstrate any preventive medication for relapse from methamphetamine abuse.[33]

■ Behavioral Therapy

Multiple behavioral therapies are available to decrease the likelihood of relapse from drug or alcohol abuse:

- *Contingency management* is based on the operant conditioning principle that behaviors that result in positive consequences are more likely to recur. Patients meeting specific drug-free goals receive incentives or rewards.
- *Cognitive behavior and skills training* emphasizes a functional analysis of substance use, with special consideration of the antecedents and consequences associated with periods of use. Addicts learn to identify situations at high risk for promoting relapse. Through rehearsal and role playing, they develop strategies either to avoid such situations or to cope effectively.
- *Motivational enhancement therapy* seeks to develop the individual's inner drive for change.
- *Couples or family treatment* acknowledges the familial and social systems in which substance use commonly occurs.
- *Alcoholics Anonymous* (AA) provides a facilitative form of behavioral therapy, consisting of a 12-step program based on self-assessment and fellowship activities.[34]

Pharmacologic and behavioral therapies are thought to be most effective when they are used in combination. To test this assumption, the National Institute on Alcohol Abuse and Alcoholism (NIAAA) initiated the nationwide clinical study COMBINE (Combining Medications and Behavioral Intervention). The efficacy of acamprosate, naltrexone, and placebo in combination with behavioral treatments has been compared among 1375 alcoholic patients in 11 treatment research centers across the United States since 2001. Longitudinal analysis may identify the most useful treatment regimen.[35]

Disposition

After treatment of withdrawal syndromes, patients with substance-related disorders should be referred to behavior-change programs. Success is determined by the pharmacologic anticraving therapy available to prevent relapse and the patient's intrinsic motivation for change.

REFERENCES

1. U.S. Substance Abuse and Mental Health Services Administration, Office of Applied Studies: Results from the 2003 National Survey on Drug Use and Health: National Findings. NSDUH Series H-25, DHHS Publication No. SMA 04-3964. Rockville, MD, U.S. Substance Abuse and Mental Health Services Administration, 2004.
2. McDonald A, Wang N, Camargo C: US Emergency department visits for alcohol-related diseases and injuries between 1992 and 2000. Arch Intern Med 2004;164:531-537.
3. U.S. Substance Abuse and Mental Health Services Administration, Office of Applied Studies: Year-End 1998 Emergency Department Data from the Drug Abuse Warning Network. Rockville, MD, U.S. Substance Abuse and Mental Health Services Administration, 1999.
4. Bureau of Justice Statistics: Comparing Federal and State Prison Inmates, 1991. NCJ-145864. Washington, DC, Bureau of Justice Statistics, 1994.
5. Stein JJ (ed): Substance Abuse: The Nation's Number One Health Problem. Princeton, NJ, Robert Wood Johnson Foundation, 2001.
6. Harwood H: Updating Estimates of the Economic Costs of Alcohol Abuse in the United States: Estimates, Update Methods, and Data. Report prepared by the Lewin Group for the National Institute on Alcohol Abuse and Alcoholism, 2000. Based on estimates, analyses, and data reported in Harwood H, Fountain D, Livermore G: The Economic Costs of Alcohol and Drug Abuse in the United States, 1992. Report prepared for the National Institute on Drug Abuse and the National Institute on Alcohol Abuse and Alcoholism, National Institutes of Health, Department of Health and Human Services. NIH Publication No. 98-4327. Rockville, MD, National Institutes of Health, 1998.
7. Office of National Drug Control Policy: The Economic Costs of Drug Abuse in the United States, 1992-1998. Publication No. NCJ-190636. Washington, DC, Executive Office of the President, 2001.
8. Smith C, Cowan C, Sensenig A, Catlin A: Health care spending slows in 2003. Health Aff (Millwood) 2005;4:185-194.
9. National Center for Education Statistics: Statistics in Brief: Revenues and Expenditures for Public Elementary and Secondary Education: School Year 1999-2000. NCES 2002-367. Washington, DC, National Center for Education Statistics, 2002.
10. First MB, Frances A, Pincus HA: Substance-related disorders. In DSM-IV-TR Guidebook. Washington, DC, American Psychiatric Publishing, 2004, p 133.
11. First MB, Frances A, Pincus HA: Substance-related disorders. In DSM-IV-TR Guidebook. Washington, DC, American Psychiatric Publishing, 2004, p 129.
12. First MB, Frances A, Pincus HA: Substance-related disorders. In DSM-IV-TR Guidebook. Washington, DC, American Psychiatric Publishing, 2004, p 128.
13. Melis M, Spiga S, Diana M: The dopamine hypothesis of drug addiction: Hypodopaminergic state. Int Rev Neurobiol. 2005;63:101-154.
14. Koob G: Neurobiology of addiction: Toward the development of new therapies. Ann N Y Acad Sci 2000;909:170-185.
15. Helmuth L: Addiction: Beyond the pleasure principle. Science 2001;294:983-984.
16. Camí J, Farré M: Drug Addiction. N Engl J Med 2003;349:975-986.
17. Crabbe J: Genetic contributions to addiction. Annu Rev Psychol 2002;53:435-462.
18. Nestler EJ: Genes and addiction. Nat Genet 2000;26:277-281.
19. Lappalainen J, Kranzler HR, Malison R, et al: A functional neuropeptide Y Leu7Pro polymorphism associated with alcohol dependence in a large population sample from the United States. Arch Gen Psychiatry 2002;59:825-831.
20. First MB, Frances A, Pincus HA: Substance-related disorders. In DSM-IV-TR Guidebook. Washington, DC, American Psychiatric Publishing, 2004, pp 141-142.
21. First MB, Frances A, Pincus HA: Substance-related disorders. In DSM-IV-TR Guidebook. Washington, DC, American Psychiatric Publishing, 2004, pp 154-155.
22. First MB, Frances A, Pincus HA: Substance-related disorders. In DSM-IV-TR Guidebook. Washington, DC, American Psychiatric Publishing, 2004, pp 144-145.
23. Parran T Jr: Prescription drug abuse: A question of balance. Med Clin North Am 1997;81:971-973.
24. Hansen GR: The drug-seeking patient in the emergency room. Emerg Med Clin North Am 2005;23:349-365.
25. Miller NS, Brady KT: Addictive disorders. Psychiatr Clin North Am 2004;27:xi-xviii.
26. O'Brien CP: Anticraving medications for relapse prevention: A possible new class of psychoactive medications. Am J Psychiatry 2005;162:1423-1431.

27. Chiang C, Wax PM: Withdrawal Syndromes: In Ford MD, Delaney KA, Ling LJ, et al (eds): Clinical Toxicology. Philadelphia, WB Saunders, 2001, p 585.
28. Gonzalez G, Oliveto A, Kosten TR: Combating opiate dependence: A comparison among the available pharmacological options. Expert Opin Pharmacother 2004;5: 713-725.
29. Roberts AJ, McDonald JS, Heyser CJ, et al: mu-Opioid receptor knockout mice do not self-administer alcohol. J Pharmacol Exp Ther 2000;293:1002-1008.
30. Kiefer F, Jahn H, Tarnaske T, et al: Comparing and combining naltrexone and acamprosate in relapse prevention of alcoholism: A double-blind, placebo-controlled study. Arch Gen Psychiatry 2003;60:92-99.
31. Johnson BA, Ait-Daoud N, Bowden CL, et al: Oral topiramate for treatment of alcohol dependence: A randomized controlled trial. Lancet 2003;361:1677-1685.
32. Kreek MJ, Vocci FJ: History and current status of opioid maintenance treatments: Blending conference session. J Subst Abuse Treat 2002;23:93-105.
33. Cretzmeyer M, Sarrazin MV, Huber DL, et al: Treatment of methamphetamine abuse: Research findings and clinical directions. J Subst Abuse Treat 2003;24:267-277.
34. Carroll KM, Onken LS: Behavioral therapies for drug abuse. Am J Psychiatry 2005;162:1452-1460.
35. National Institutes of Health: NIAAA Launches COMBINE Clinical Trial. National Institutes of Health News Release March 8, 2001. Available at http://www.nih.gov/news/pr/mar2001/niaaa-08.htm.

Chapter **200**

Anorexia Nervosa and Bulimia Nervosa

Jason E. Liebzeit

KEY POINTS

Anorexia nervosa and bulimia nervosa are increasing in both prevalence and incidence in Westernized societies.

Either disease may be associated with multiple somatic complaints.

Patients with anorexia or bulimia are at increased risk for life-threatening metabolic derangements and cardiac dysrhythmias that mandate hospital admission.

The most common cause of death from anorexia is cardiac arrest secondary to conduction delays or ventricular dysrhythmias.

Urgent outpatient psychiatric referral is appropriate for well-appearing patients who are able to adequately care for themselves.

Definitions

Anorexia nervosa ("anorexia") is a disturbance of body perception that results in a fear of gaining weight and a refusal to maintain a minimally normal body weight. *Bulimia nervosa ("bulimia")* is an obsessive self-evaluation of body shape and weight that leads to a characteristic cycle of binge eating and subsequent actions that prevent weight gain.

Although similar in their relationship with food, these diseases represent two separate psychiatric entities with distinct clinical sequelae. Distinguishing features include the body mass index (BMI) or height-matched weight and, in women, the presence of regular menstruation. Amenorrhea is a key finding of anorexia in postmenarchic women. Diagnosis requires fulfillment of all criteria listed in the text revision of the fourth edition of the *Diagnostic and Statistical Manual of Mental Disorders* (DSM-IV-TR) (Box 200-1). These diseases do not coexist in the same patient; a patient has *either* anorexia or bulimia, but never both simultaneously.[1]

Anorexia can be divided into the *restricting* or *binge eating/purging* subtypes. Restricting patients commonly eat only 300 to 700 calories each day, or they engage in excessive exercise to ward off weight gain. Binge/purging behavior involves intentional vomiting or the inappropriate use of laxatives, enemas, or diuretics in response to even small amounts of consumed food. Bulimia is similarly divided into purging and nonpurging. The subtypes are based on the behavior occurring at the time of diagnosis.[2]

Scope

Patients with eating disorders commonly present to the ED in a subtle manner. Those with anorexia or bulimia generally complain of symptoms related to associated disease states; they rarely seek primary treatment for their psychiatric illness. ED presentations provide an opportunity for both intervention and education. Recognition of these underdiagnosed diseases creates an opportunity for early initial

BOX 200-1

DSM-IV-TR Diagnostic Criteria Differentiating Anorexia and Bulimia

Anorexia Nervosa	Bulimia Nervosa
1. Refusal to maintain weigh greater than or equal to 85% of expected 2. Fear of gaining weight despite being underweight 3. Disturbance in body perception *or* excessive influence of body shape/weight on self-evaluation *or* denial of seriousness of current weight 4. In women of appropriate age, amenorrhea (defined as at least three consecutive missed menses) while not on hormones Subtype as either restrictive or binge-purge	1. Recurrent episodes of binge eating a) More food in a discreet period of time than most people would eat in similar circumstances b) Sense of lack of control over eating episode 2. Recurrent inappropriate compensatory behavior to prevent weight gain (vomiting, exercise, laxatives, diuretics) 3. Bingeing and compensatory behaviors occur at least twice a week for 3 months 4. Undue influence of body shape or weight on self-evaluation 5. This disturbance does not occur during an episode of anorexia

From American Psychiatric Association: Diagnostic and Statistical Manual of Mental Disorders, 4th ed, text rev (DSM-IV-TR). Washington, DC, American Psychiatric Association, 2000.

interventions. Medical care alone is often of transient utility. Successful cure of both anorexia and bulimia generally requires intensive individual or family psychotherapy.

Anorexia and bulimia are diseases nearly exclusively encountered in North America, Western Europe, and Japan. Childhood anxiety disorders may increase the likelihood of these disorders, although no clear cause has been identified for either illness. Women suffer from anorexia and bulimia more frequently than men. The lifetime prevalence of anorexia varies from 0.3% to 1% for women; men are estimated to have one tenth that prevalence. Bulimia is more common than anorexia, with a lifetime prevalence of 1% to 3% among women. Similarly, only 10% of bulimic patients are male; these men are more likely to suffer from premorbid obesity. The incidence is further increased among male wrestlers.[3]

Clinical Presentation

Concerned family members or friends usually accompany patients with anorexia or bulimia to the ED in those rare instances that these patients present for psychiatric treatment of their eating disorder. More commonly, patients complain of associated symptoms or complications of their restricting or purging behavior. An understanding of these symptom constellations speeds appropriate treatment and referral.

■ CLASSIC PRESENTATION

The typical patient with anorexia is an otherwise successful mid- to late-adolescent girl exhibiting marked cachexia. The patient may demonstrate a remarkable lack of insight regarding her appearance. Common complaints include fatigue, cold intolerance, abdominal pain, and amenorrhea. Weakness, especially symptomatic orthostasis, prominently features in the patient's review of systems. Emaciation is the most notable clinical feature. Bradycardia and hypotension are common findings. Lanugo, a fine body hair commonly seen on the extremities and trunk, may be present. Signs of nutritional deficiencies may be seen in patients with food restricting subtypes.

Patients with the purging subtypes of both bulimia and anorexia share physical findings, although bulimic patients may have a more normal-appearing body habitus. Purging through vomiting often results in erosion of dental enamel, particularly on the lingual ("back") side of the teeth. Manual induction of vomiting leads to calluses on the dorsal aspect of the fingers as a result of recurrent contact with the teeth, a finding known as *Russell's sign*. Benign parotid salivary enlargement is common.

■ ATYPICAL PRESENTATION

Advances in the management of severe anorexia and bulimia have extended life expectancy for those afflicted. Patients in their fifth or sixth decade of life continue to battle eating disorders by nontraditional means. Long-standing anorexia or bulimia affects normal physiology, as in any chronic disease. Notably, gastrointestinal motility may slow, leading to chronic nausea, gastroparesis, impaction, or obstruction. Rare complications of these eating disorders that may present to the ED are discussed in the following section.

Complications

- Arrhythmia: Disruption of normal cardiac conduction is the most life-threatening medical complication of anorexia. Prolongation of the QTc is ominous. Cardiac arrest resulting from conduction delays or ventricular dysrhythmias is the most common cause of death from anorexia.[4]
- Dehydration and renal insufficiency: Insufficient fluid intake may occur with anorexia. In bulimia, prerenal hypovolemia arises from fluid losses resulting from excessive vomiting or laxative abuse.
- Starvation and vitamin deficiency: These conditions result from inadequate caloric intake.
- Osteopenia: Pubescent anorexia or severe bulimia may cause hypoestrogenemia and resultant undermineralized bone. Bone pain or pathologic fractures may ensue.
- Electrolyte abnormality: This results from either insufficient intake or excessive gastrointestinal losses.
- Esophageal and gastric trauma: Repetitive, forceful vomiting may lead to Mallory-Weiss tears or Boerhaave's syndrome. Gastric distention occurs with binging.
- Nausea and constipation: Gastrointestinal motility decreases with starvation. Native colonic contraction decreases with laxative abuse, thus leading to colonic distention and constipation.
- Rectal prolapse: This results from muscle weakening secondary to laxative abuse.
- Congestive heart failure: Cardiomyopathy may be caused by starvation states or by ipecac abuse.
- Refeeding syndromes: Peripheral edema, hypophosphatemia, and dysrhythmias are common features associated with resumption of appropriate caloric intake.
- Inattention and mental status changes: Chronic disease may lead to decreases in both gray matter and white matter, with concurrent ventricular enlargement. Starvation-associated hypoglycemia or other electrolyte abnormalities may affect mental status.

Associated Comorbidities

- Anxiety disorders: The lifetime prevalence is 64% in eating-disordered patients versus 13% in the general population. Obsessive-compulsive disorder and social phobia are common.[5]
- Depression
- Substance abuse: This is often seen among patients with binge-type bulimia.

Differential Diagnosis

The evaluation of cachexia must be thorough. A notable lack of subjective complaints in an emaciated patient may be cause to suspect anorexia. The differential diagnosis of anorexia and bulimia is narrow, because the patient's behavior is an essential component of the disease. Catabolic states with increased caloric consumption, such as infection or hypermetabolism, should be differentiated from inadequate caloric intake (Box 200-2).

BOX 200-2

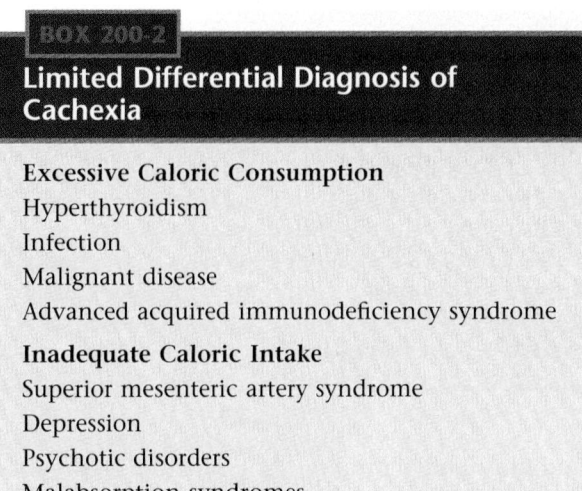

Limited Differential Diagnosis of Cachexia

Excessive Caloric Consumption
Hyperthyroidism
Infection
Malignant disease
Advanced acquired immunodeficiency syndrome

Inadequate Caloric Intake
Superior mesenteric artery syndrome
Depression
Psychotic disorders
Malabsorption syndromes

Diagnostic Testing

No ancillary tests are available to confirm the diagnosis of anorexia or bulimia. The diagnosis is made following the guidelines set forth in the DSM-IV-TR. Laboratory tests aid in the identification of potentially life-threatening physiologic abnormalities commonly seen in the eating-disordered patient. Serum electrolytes, including phosphorus, are critical in the evaluation of patients with suspected anorexia or bulimia. Hypokalemic, hypochloremic metabolic alkalosis is the most common finding of induced vomiting. Laxative abuse results in metabolic acidosis from the loss of intestinal bicarbonate. Endocrine abnormalities may be encountered in patients with chronic disease; insufficient thyroid hormone may cause hypotension, hypothermia, and bradycardia. An elevated serum amylase level may serve as useful evidence of surreptitious vomiting, although the increased level itself has little clinical significance (Table 200-1).

Electrocardiography should be performed. Although bradycardia is a common benign finding in anorexia, other arrhythmias are likely to result in

Table 200-1 DIAGNOSTIC LABORATORY FINDINGS

Laboratory Abnormality Diagnosis	Finding
Hypokalemia, hypochloremia, alkalosis (elevated HCO_3^- or pH); elevated amylase	Excessive vomiting
Hypokalemia, acidosis (decreased HCO_3^- or pH)	Diarrhea

HCO_3^-, bicarbonate.

PRIORITY ACTIONS

Primary survey
- Fluid resuscitation
- Cardiovascular stabilization

Obtain electrocardiogram

Laboratory evaluation: complete blood count, electrolytes, glucose, phosphorus

Chest radiography in cases of excessive vomiting or ipecac abuse

Do *NOT* initiate nutritional support in the ED

morbidity and mortality. Prolongation of the QTc interval is the most concerning electrocardiographic abnormality and may be present despite normal electrolytes.

Intracranial imaging reveals a loss of gray matter.[5] Such imaging studies are indicated only in patients with altered mental status or trauma.

Treatment

ED management should focus on correcting abnormalities detected during the medical evaluation. Cardiovascular compromise may require emergency intervention. Arrhythmias may be managed according to standard Advanced Cardiac Life Support guidelines. Electrolytes and glucose should be normalized, and body temperature should be regulated. Aggressive fluid resuscitation should be undertaken with caution and may result in sudden congestive heart failure. The mechanical sequelae of purging (esophageal rupture, Mallory-Weiss tears, or rectal prolapse) respond to conventional treatment discussed elsewhere in this text.

Nutritional support is not a priority in the ED. For outpatients, goal intake should be 1200 to 1500 kcal/day with weekly increases; weight gain should be limited to 0.5 to 0.9 kg (1 to 2 lb) each week. Inpatient feeding has been associated with life-threatening arrhythmias and transient edematous states; such refeeding is best managed in a monitored medical unit.

Sophisticated and concurrent psychological, social, dietary, and medical support is crucial for both inpatients and outpatients. Selective serotonin reuptake inhibitors, in particular fluoxetine, have been associated with increased compliance in the outpatient treatment of bulimia and may also address the anxiety states commonly encountered with eating disorders. Do not initiate antidepressants in the ED without the collaboration of the treating psychiatrist or primary physician.[6,7]

Disposition

Patients generally consent to hospital admission for treatment of symptomatic somatic disorders. Voluntary admission for psychiatric treatment is often more difficult to arrange. Lack of insight into disordered eating clouds a patient's appreciation of the severity of the disease. Adult patients whose weight is more than 25% less than that expected for their height are candidates for admission.

Telemetry monitoring is indicated when arrhythmias or QTc abnormalities are present. Additionally, refeeding may promote cardiovascular complications that require continuous monitoring. Critical care should be reserved for those patients with unstable vital signs or dangerous metabolic abnormalities.

Current guidelines suggest psychiatric or medical admission for any child or adolescent with rapid weight loss. Parents or guardians may request inpatient admission when outpatient management has failed. Psychiatric admission for minors is typically easier to accomplish than for adults. Early inpatient treatment is associated with a decreased risk of both arrhythmia and cortical volume loss. Advocate for admission in all patients who lack home support or who are otherwise at risk of outpatient management failure (Box 200-3).[8,9]

Barring clear impairment of decision-making capacity, involuntary admission of adults is rare. The judicial system in the United States generally recognizes that a patient's actions supersede stated intent. For example, an anorexic patient may deny suicidality, despite behaviors that clearly resulted in a life-threatening dysrhythmia. Consider involuntary admission in patients with such profound lack of insight, as well as those who lack decision-making capacity.[4,10]

BOX 200-3

Admission Guidelines

Medicine

Weight less than 25% expected

Electrolyte replacement

Gastrointestinal dysmotility

Heart failure

Telemetry

QT abnormality

Stable arrhythmia (i.e., premature ventricular contractions)

Intensive Care

Unstable vital signs

Life-threatening metabolic derangements

REFERENCES

1. American Psychiatric Association: Diagnostic and Statistical Manual of Mental Disorders, 4th ed, text rev. Washington, DC, American Psychiatric Association, 2000.
2. Yager J, Andersen AL: Anorexia nervosa. N Engl J Med 2005;353:1481-1488.

3. Kessler R, McGonagle K, Zhao S, et al: Lifetime and 12-month prevalence of DSM-III-R psychiatric disorders in the United States: Results from the National Comorbidity Survey. Arch Gen Psychiatry 1994;51:8-19.
4. Melamed Y, Mester R, Margolin J, Kalian M: Involuntary treatment of anorexia nervosa. Int J Law Psychiatry 2003;26:617-626.
5. Kaye W, Bulik C, Thornton L, et al: Comorbidity of anxiety disorders with anorexia and bulimia nervosa. Am J Psychiatry 2004;161:2215-2221.
6. Kaye W, Bailer U, Frank G, et al: Brain imaging of serotonin after recovery from anorexia and bulimia nervosa. Physiol Behav 2005;86:15-17.
7. Walsh B, Fairburn C, Mickley D, et al: Treatment of bulimia nervosa in a primary care setting. Am J Psychiatry 2004;161:556-561.
8. Keel P, Dorer D, Eddy K, et al: Predictors of mortality in eating disorders. Arch Gen Psychiatry 2003;60:179-183.
9. American Psychiatric Association Work Group on Eating Disorders: Practice guideline for the treatment of patients with eating disorders (revision). Am J Psychiatry 2000;157(Suppl):1-39.
10. Watson TL, Bowers WA, Andersen AE: Involuntary treatment of eating disorders. Am J Psychiatry 2000;157:1806-1810.

SECTION XXI

Hematology and Oncology Management

Chapter **201**

Introduction to Oncologic Emergencies

Jeremy D. Sperling

KEY POINTS

Fever in a neutropenic patient with cancer is assumed to be a life-threatening infection, so antibiotic therapy must be started immediately.

Hypercalcemia is common. Patients present with weakness, vomiting, and changes in mental status.

Tumor lysis syndrome (TLS) is a rare but life-threatening condition that occurs after chemotherapy. The syndrome causes acute renal failure, hyperkalemia, hyperphosphatemia, and hypocalcemia.

Adrenal insufficiency and pericardial tamponade are causes of hypotension.

Pleural effusions commonly cause dyspnea in the oncology patient. However, always exclude life-threatening causes (e.g., pulmonary embolism, pneumonia, pericardial tamponade) of dyspnea in this patient population.

Scope

As the population ages, the incidence of cancer is increasing. The American Cancer Society estimated that more than 1.3 million new cancer cases were diagnosed in the United States in 2005, and this number is estimated to double by 2050. At the same time, aggressive treatment strategies, whether involving surgery, chemotherapy, or radiation, are helping oncology patients to live longer. Overall, cancer death rates in the United States for all racial and ethnic populations decreased by 1.1% per year from 1993 through 2002.[1] Declines in cancer deaths are the result of many factors, including better screening, early detection strategies, public health risk reduction programs, and improved medical and surgical treatment. EPs routinely recognize and treat emergency complications. The interventions that the EP makes to keep a patient alive acutely may allow the patient's chemotherapy or radiation therapy to work for an overall cure. Today, oncology patients treated in the ED are increasingly more likely to survive to hospital discharge, even if they are admitted to an intensive care unit.[2]

Triage

Some oncologic emergencies require timely action. Specifically, a patient with fever and potential neutropenia requires rapid assessment and early antibiotic administration. Other major oncologic emergencies, such as airway or respiratory complications, spinal cord compression, or possible cerebral herniation, require more obvious immediate intervention.

Isolation and Infectious Control Issues

Each year, approximately 1.9 million nosocomial infections occur in U.S. hospitals, and approximately

88,000 patients die.[3] Immunocompromised patients with cancer, especially neutropenic patients and bone marrow transplant recipients, are at increased risk of contracting these infections. At-risk patients should be identified on ED arrival and should not be allowed to spend any significant amount of time in waiting rooms or busy ED hallways where they can be exposed to infections from other patients. Ideally, bone marrow transplant recipients and potentially neutropenic patients should be placed in single, positive air pressure rooms that have 12 or more air exchanges per hour. Positive airway pressure decreases the number of infectious particles that enter a patient's room. If such a room is unavailable, the next best option is to place the patient in an individual room with the door closed. Patients with a potential airborne illness (e.g., tuberculosis) are the exception; they should be placed in a negative pressure room to protect other patients and the ED staff.

As with all patients, careful hand washing is essential when dealing with the neutropenic patient. However, when providing noninvasive care, the use of sterile gowns, masks, and gloves does not provide any extra protection for these patients. Neutropenic patients should generally be offered only cooked food and bottled water to avoid bacterial contamination, although data supporting this type of "neutropenic diet" are quite limited.

Oncologic History

Although it is not always possible or necessary for the EP to obtain a complete past medical history from a patient with cancer, certain questions may prove crucial and are unique to the oncology patient. Pertinent information includes the type of cancer, the stage of the cancer (the extent of its spread), previous cancer-related complications, and previous cancer treatments including surgery, chemotherapy, and radiation therapy. Inquire about specific chemotherapeutic agents that have been used. Timing of recent treatments is especially important because the treatment may be the direct cause of the patient's current illness. Oncology patients may have complicated past medical histories; use reliable sources such as hospital records (if the patient has recently been admitted) or the patient's oncologist to obtain pertinent data quickly.

During your initial encounter with an oncology patient, ask the patient whether he or she has any specific wishes or advanced directives. Specifically, ask the patient whether he or she has a do not resuscitate or do not intubate order or a health care proxy. Many patients with cancer, especially those with late-stage disease, may have very defined treatment objectives in mind (e.g., intravenous hydration but no invasive procedures or tests). These objectives and wishes should be documented in the chart and respected. Early inquiry about the patient's wishes and expectations will help you to guide treatment appropriately.

Fever

■ SCOPE

Fever is a very common chief complaint for oncology patients who present to the ED, especially for patients undergoing chemotherapy. Fever can be the first sign of a life-threatening infectious process in this patient population. Neutropenic patients are highly susceptible to almost any type of bacterial or fungal infection. Assume that a fever in the setting of neutropenia (see the Facts and Formulas box) is a life-threatening bacterial infection, and start antibiotic therapy immediately.

Nearly 80,000 hospitalizations for neutropenic fever occur every year in the United States; the mean (median) length of stay is 11.5 (6) days, at a mean cost of more than $19,000 per case.[4] Besides the immediate infectious risks to the patient, an episode of neutropenic fever may delay or end future chemotherapy treatment and therefore may compromise the overall chances for a cancer cure.

Although the prudent approach in the ED is to assume and treat an oncology patient as if they had an infectious source, infection is not the only reason that oncology patients may have a fever. Fever can sometimes be a manifestation of the underlying malignant process itself or a side effect of a chemotherapeutic agent. For example, chemotherapeutic agents such as bleomycin and cytosine arabinoside have been noted to cause fevers. Lymphomas, leukemias, and renal cell carcinoma have been recognized as sources of fever without any concurrent infection; at times, fever can be the initial presenting symptom of these illnesses. Thrombophlebitis, drugs, and transfusion reactions can also be rare causes of fever.

■ PHYSIOLOGY

Chemotherapy can severely damage a patient's normal defense mechanisms, including both humoral and cellular immunity, thus leaving the patient defenseless to combat infection. Chemotherapy can destroy or weaken neutrophils, T lymphocytes, macrophages, monocytes, and immunoglobulin production. Radiation and chemotherapy also affect the patient's mechanical barriers against infection. In particular, they damage the integrity of the mucous membranes and skin. All this injury to the patient's immune system takes place in an individual who

FACTS AND FORMULAS $SI = \frac{SV}{BSA}$

Fever: Temperature >38.3° C or ≥38.0° C for ≥1 hour

Neutropenia: Absolute neutrophil count <500/mm³ or <1000/mm³ with a predicted decline to ≤500/mm³ already has cancer and therefore may already have either a weakened immune system or compromised physiologic factors.

■ DIAGNOSTIC TESTING

Search for the source of the infection. A minimum work-up should include at least two blood cultures, urinalysis and urine culture, a chest radiograph, a complete blood count with differential (to confirm neutropenia), and baseline chemistry studies of kidney and liver function. Obtain blood cultures from any indwelling catheters that are present, but draw at least one sample from a peripheral vein.

Further search should be dictated by the patient's specific complaints or symptoms. For example, send a throat culture if the patient complains of throat pain or order an abdominal or pelvic computed tomography (CT) scan if there is any possibility of an intra-abdominal source of the fever. Other sources to consider culturing in the appropriate clinical setting are cerebrospinal fluid, peritoneal fluid, pleural fluid, stool, and any skin lesions that contain purulent material. In general, long indwelling catheters should be left in place and not removed in the ED. Many catheters in this patient population are buried subcutaneously and are not easily removed. Consider removing the catheter in the ED if the tunnel is grossly infected or if the infected catheter has produced septic emboli or endocarditis.

■ TREATMENT AND DISPOSITION

Start empirical, broad-spectrum antibiotics as early as possible to patients who present to the ED with neutropenic fever. This strategy is the likely reason that the mortality rate for bacteremic patients with cancer has substantially decreased. In one study, mortality decreased from 21% to 7% in a 16-year period with the increased use of this approach.[5] Do not delay antibiotics while looking for the source; very often, an obvious source is not identifiable. Treat the patient empirically with antibiotics that reflect the resistance patterns and bacterial profiles of the institution where you practice. Most institutions have antibiotic protocols based on these bacterial patterns. Gram-positive organisms such as *Staphylococcus aureus, Staphylococcus epidermidis,* and *Streptococcus viridans* are currently more predominant than gram-negative organisms as the source of neutropenic fever. However, gram-negative organisms can be more virulent (e.g., *Pseudomonas*), and therefore the patient must always be empirically treated for these pathogens. Examples of antibiotic regimens include double-coverage regimens such as an antipseudomonal beta-lactam in addition to an aminoglycoside (e.g., piperacillin tazobactam and gentamicin or tobramycin), an antipseudomonal beta-lactam in addition to a fluoroquinolone (e.g., piperacillin tazobactam and levofloxacin), or a single antibiotic regimen such as cefepime or imipenem.

BOX 201-1

Characteristics of Lower-Risk Neutropenic Fever in Adult Patients with Cancer

- Age <65 years
- Neutropenia lasting <10 to 15 days
- >7 days from last cycle of chemotherapy
- No diarrhea, vomiting, dysphagia, sensory impairment, focal neurologic signs, or uncontrolled bleeding
- No history of diabetes mellitus or chronic pulmonary disease
- Absence of hypotension or hypertension
- No kidney, lung, or liver dysfunction
- Polymorphonuclear leukocyte count >100/μL and rising in the last 2 days
- Platelet count >75,000/μL and rising in the last 2 days
- Monocyte count >100/μL
- Hematocrit >15%
- C-reactive protein <50 mg/L
- Normal chest radiograph

From Viscoli C, Castagnola E: Treatment of febrile neutropenia: What is new? Curr Opin Infect Dis 2002;15:377-382.

Vancomycin should not be started empirically for neutropenic fever unless your institution has a high rate of methicillin-resistant *S. aureus* (MRSA) or resistant *S. viridans* strains. However, consider starting vancomycin if you suspect that the infection originates from the patient's indwelling central venous catheter or if a neutropenic patient presents in septic shock.

Not all patients with neutropenic fever require admission. Consider outpatient treatment in selected patients who are stable and at low risk for complications. See Box 201-1 for characteristics of the low-risk neutropenic patient who may be considered for outpatient management. Outpatient management should be undertaken in concert with the patient's oncologist to ensure very early and close follow-up. Ensure that appropriate cultures have been obtained and that the patient's oncologist will be able to obtain the results. If the patient does not have an oncologist who can be reached, it is most prudent to admit the patient.

In an effort to decrease the incidence of neutropenic episodes, many oncologists use a colony-stimulating factor (CSF; e.g., granulocyte CSF [G-CSF], granulocyte-macrophage CSF) with chemotherapy. The use of a G-CSF with chemotherapy has been shown to decrease the incidence, duration, and severity of neutropenic fever in patients with small-cell lung cancer.[6] Most commonly, G-CSF is used as prophylaxis against neutropenia with highly myelosuppressive chemotherapeutic regimens or when chemotherapy is administered to patients who had neutropenic fever during a previous treatment cycle. However, the use of G-CSF in the setting of neutropenic fever is controversial. One prospective randomized, multicenter clinical trial study found that G-CSF (5 μg/kg/day) added to standard antibiotic therapy decreased by 1 day the duration of severe neutropenia, antibiotic therapy, and hospital stay, but it did not reduce the rate of complications or mortality.[7] A meta-analysis of 13 studies with 1518 patients found that CSFs produced shorter hospitalizations, reduced neutrophil recovery times, and possibly reduced infection-related mortality.[8] Adverse side effects of CSF use include bone and joint pain and flulike symptoms.[8] Because it is not clear whether CSFs alter mortality and because these agents are very expensive, a CSF should not be given routinely in the setting of neutropenic fever in the ED. Rather, until more convincing evidence exists, CSFs should be given only after discussion with the patient's oncologist.

■ INFECTIOUS CAUSES OF FEVER UNIQUE TO THE PATIENT WITH CANCER

■ Typhlitis

Typhlitis (neutropenic enterocolitis) is an inflammatory process of the ileum and colon that affects neutropenic patients. Most commonly, typhlitis is a disease process associated with acute leukemia, but it can be seen with other malignant conditions. Additionally, although typhlitis most commonly occurs in patients who are undergoing chemotherapy, it occasionally occurs in patients who are not.[9] Presenting clinical symptoms may include fever, lower abdominal pain, and diarrhea, which can be bloody or watery. Other potential symptoms include abdominal distention and nausea or vomiting. On physical examination, the patient's abdomen may be generally tender, or the tenderness may be localized to the right lower quadrant. In at-risk patients, obtain a CT scan to make the diagnosis and to rule out other potentially dangerous abdominal processes (e.g., appendicitis, diverticulitis). If typhlitis is present, the CT scan will demonstrate diffuse submucosal thickening of the affected bowel wall (generally in the terminal ileum or ascending colon). Other CT scan findings may include paracolonic fluid and gas in the bowel wall. Treat patients who have uncomplicated cases with broad-spectrum antibiotics (covering aerobic and anaerobic pathogens, including *Pseudomonas aeruginosa*), bowel rest, and supportive care. Patients who present with perforation, obstruction, bleeding, or gangrenous bowel require prompt surgical consultation. The mortality rate of typhlitis is quite high; six out of nine patients died of sepsis in one case series.[9]

■ Fungal Infections

In neutropenic patients with cancer who are treated for long periods with broad-spectrum antibiotics, yeast infections increasingly become the likely source of infection and fever. *Candida albicans* is the most common fungal pathogen, but aspergillosis, cryptococcus, and other fungal infections can occur. Invasive candidiasis and aspergillosis are associated with high mortality rates (36.7% and 39.2%, respectively) in oncology patients with neutropenic fever.[4]

■ Invasive Fungal Sinusitis

Invasive fungal sinusitis affects immunocompromised patients and has a high mortality rate. Aspergillosis and species of the Mucoraceae family (usually *Rhizopus*) are the most common fungi involved; they can destroy both tissue and bone. Fungal infection of the paranasal sinuses becomes acute invasive fungal sinusitis as it spreads through tissues to the orbit or the central nervous system.

Patients with acute invasive fungal sinusitis may appear severely ill. Symptoms include fever, nasal congestion, headache, maxillary tenderness, periorbital swelling, and even mental status changes. Conversely, in an immunocompromised patient with cancer, symptoms may be subtle because the patient may not mount enough of an inflammatory response to produce clinical symptoms. Therefore, the clinician must maintain a high index of suspicion in this patient population. If the disease is suspected, consult an otorhinolaryngologist immediately for surgical débridement. Initiate intravenous antifungal therapy with amphotericin B. A CT scan of the sinuses may be helpful to define the extent of the disease, but it should not delay surgical consultation. Intravenous antifungal therapy is generally not effective without wide surgical débridement.

Electrolyte Disturbances in the Oncology Patient

■ TUMOR LYSIS SYNDROME

■ Scope

TLS is the constellation of metabolic abnormalities occurring in response to the rapid destruction of malignant cells, generally from the initiation of chemotherapy (Table 201-1). The sudden death of many malignant cells results in the release into the bloodstream of their intracellular contents, thus causing sudden increases in potassium, phosphorus, and uric acid levels. TLS is generally predictable. It usually occurs with the initiation of chemotherapy in a patient with newly diagnosed cancer. Acute lymphoblastic leukemia and non-Hodgkin's lymphoma (especially Burkitt's lymphoma) are the most common cancers associated with TLS.[10] Less commonly, TLS occurs in other leukemias, in multiple myeloma, or after the treatment of some solid tumors such as

Table 201-1 ELECTROLYTE DISTURBANCES IN TUMOR LYSIS SYNDROME AND TREATMENT

Disturbance	Treatment
Hyperkalemia	Sodium polystyrene sulfonate, insulin and glucose, calcium gluconate, dialysis if severe
Hyperphosphatemia	Aluminum hydroxide, dialysis if needed
Hypocalcemia	Calcium gluconate (if severe)
Uremia	IV hydration; consider IV sodium bicarbonate
Renal failure	Dialysis

IV, intravenous.

breast and lung cancer. Because chemotherapy is more likely to cause TLS with certain cancers, oncologists usually take measures to prevent it. At-risk patients are pretreated with aggressive hydration, diuresis, and allopurinol (in an attempt to decrease uric acid formation). Rarely, TLS develops spontaneously. When it does, it is usually in the setting of a relapsing or newly diagnosed (but untreated) malignant disease.

Structure and Function

TLS most frequently occurs when the patient has a high tumor burden that is very sensitive to chemotherapy. Chemotherapy rapidly destroys malignant cells; intracellular nucleic acids are released and are broken down into uric acid. Uric acid, which is renally excreted, precipitates in the renal tubules. The precipitation may obstruct flow and can result in renal failure. Clearly, patients with baseline renal dysfunction are at even greater risk. Potassium, found in high concentrations intracellularly, is also released with the destruction of the malignant cells. Because of worsening renal function secondary to uric acid precipitation, the kidneys are unable to clear all this excess potassium, and the result can be dangerously high potassium levels. Phosphorus is similar to potassium; it is concentrated intracellularly and is generally excreted in the kidney. Therefore, phosphorus levels also rise. The excess phosphorus congregates with available calcium to form calcium phosphate crystals and causes the calcium level to drop. These crystals may precipitate in the renal tubules and can thereby also worsen renal function.

Presenting Signs and Symptoms

TLS manifests with symptoms reflective of the metabolic abnormalities that are present (e.g., hyperkalemia, renal failure) and therefore may be nonspecific. Symptoms of hyperkalemia tend to be quite vague and may include palpitations, paresthesias, fatigue, and weakness; examination findings may include nonfocal reduced muscle strength or decreases in deep tendon reflexes. Mild hypocalcemia causes muscle cramps, paresthesias, and minor mental status changes. With severe hypocalcemia, the patient may have significant mental status changes, tetanic contractions, seizures, or hypotension. Classic physical examination findings include Chvostek's sign (twitching or spasms of the face with tapping over the facial nerve anterior to the ear) and Trousseau's sign (carpal spasm with inflation of a blood pressure cuff above the systolic blood pressure). Very high levels of phosphorus cause vomiting, diarrhea, lethargy, and even seizures.

Diagnostic Testing

Laboratory evaluation should include, at minimum, blood urea nitrogen, creatinine, potassium, calcium, magnesium, phosphorus, uric acid, albumin, and urinalysis. Consider performing an ionized calcium determination. Obtain an electrocardiogram (ECG) to look for signs of hyperkalemia or hypocalcemia. Obtain a chest radiograph if you are concerned about fluid overload secondary to renal failure.

Treatment

Despite the widespread practice of prophylaxis against TLS by oncologists to prevent this syndrome, the EP occasionally has to manage this potentially life-threatening syndrome. Keep a high index of suspicion for this clinical entity, especially in high-risk patients who recently started chemotherapy or who may have baseline renal insufficiency. Place patients with suspected TLS on continuous cardiac monitoring because they are at high risk for cardiac dysrhythmias. Focus your treatment on closely monitoring electrolytes and renal function, correcting electrolyte abnormalities, and ensuring appropriate hydration. If the patient does not have acute renal dysfunction, aggressively hydrate the patient. Hydration helps renal blood flow and the excretion of uric acid and phosphorus. Furosemide or mannitol may be added to increase urine output after adequate hydration.

Hyperkalemia and hyperphosphatemia should be treated. Treat only symptomatic hypocalcemia because infusing calcium to a hyperphosphatemic patient increases the risk of calcium phosphate formation and deposition throughout the body, including the renal tubules. Rasburicase (0.15 to 0.2 mg/kg/day), a recombinant form of urate oxidase, can be used in clinically significant TLS. Urate oxidase is an enzyme not found in humans that converts uric acid to allantoin, which is five times more soluble than uric acid. Consider rasburicase in patients with renal dysfunction, significant elevations in serum uric acid values, or large tumor burdens.[10] Allopurinol, which has been traditionally used in the prevention and treatment of TLS, works by decreasing uric acid production through competitive inhibition of the enzyme xanthine oxidase, which turns xanthine into uric acid. Once uric acid is present, allopurinol's effect is limited, and therefore this agent is not useful in the treatment of acute TLS. Finally, if renal failure develops and becomes severe (e.g., uncontrolled hyperkalemia, uncontrolled hypertension, fluid overload), emergency hemodialysis will be indicated.

Controversy exists regarding the practice of adding sodium bicarbonate to intravenous fluids in an effort to help excrete uric acid. The theory is that alkalinization (with a goal of achieving a urine pH of 7 to 7.5) decreases uric acid precipitation in the renal tubules and increases its excretion in the form of urate. Although a sodium bicarbonate infusion may help to eliminate uric acid, it may also worsen hypocalcemia. At an alkaline pH, phosphate and calcium may precipitate and worsen renal function. In patients with hyperphosphatemia, alkalinization may cause calcium phosphate deposition in organs such as the heart and kidney. Because hydration alone may achieve adequate uric acid excretion, urine alkalinization, if performed, should be done cautiously and discontinued as soon as normal uric acid levels are achieved.

HYPERCALCEMIA

Scope

Hypercalcemia is the most common metabolic abnormality found in patients with cancer; however, it is an underrecognized problem. At least 20% of patients with cancer have hypercalcemia at some point in their illness.[11] Because the symptoms of hypercalcemia are nonspecific, they are often attributed to other causes (e.g., chemotherapy, infection), and the hypercalcemia goes untreated. The malignant diseases most commonly responsible for hypercalcemia include lung cancer, breast cancer, renal cancer, head and neck cancers, and multiple myeloma.[11,12]

Structure and Function

In patients who do not have cancer, primary hyperparathyroidism is the most common cause of an elevated calcium level. In malignant disease, hypercalcemia is not related to parathyroid hormone activity, but rather to increased osteoclastic activity in bone. A few mechanisms are responsible for this increased osteoclastic activity. First, metastasis of solid tumors can cause extensive direct bone destruction. Some cancer cells release osteoclast-activating factors. In patients without metastasis, the cancer may produce a parathyroid-like hormone. This hormone acts on bone by increasing calcium uptake and on the kidneys by decreasing calcium excretion.

Presenting Signs and Symptoms

Symptoms of hypercalcemia are generally nonspecific. The severity of symptoms depends more on how rapidly the calcium level has escalated rather than on the actual calcium level. Symptoms include general weakness, constipation, nausea and vomiting, dehydration, polyuria and polydipsia, personality changes, and bone and muscle pains. Severe symptoms include confusion, drowsiness, and even coma. No physical examination findings are specific only to hypercalcemia. However, consider the diagnosis when evaluating an oncology patient with any degree of mental status alteration (from mild confusion to obtundation), hyporeflexia, or dehydration.

Diagnostic Testing

If hypercalcemia is suspected, perform an ECG and send laboratory tests for at minimum creatinine, potassium, calcium, phosphate, alkaline phosphatase, and albumin. Look for QT shortening on the ECG because this finding may provide the quickest method of diagnosing hypercalcemia. In patients with higher calcium levels, the ECG may demonstrate a prolonged PR or QRS interval, T-wave changes, bradycardia, or heart block. The calcium level reported in a basic metabolic profile reports the calcium concentration in serum, normally 9 to 11 mg/dL. Calcium levels greater than 12 mg/dL should generate concern, and levels higher than 14 mg/dL require immediate intervention. However, calcium levels correlate poorly with actual symptoms. Because calcium is present both in an ionized form and a protein bound form, the concentration of calcium depends on plasma protein concentrations. A total corrected calcium should be calculated to assess whether hypercalcemia is truly present. The corrected calcium is based on the albumin level. One formula used for this is the following:

$$\text{Corrected calcium (mg/dL)} = \text{measured calcium (mg/dL)} + 0.8 \times (4.4 - \text{measured albumin g/dL})$$

The average normal albumin level is 4.4 g/dL, and a normal range for corrected calcium is 9 to 10.6 mg/dL. If there is any uncertainty regarding the calcium level at this point, obtain an ionized calcium level.

Treatment and Disposition

Normalizing calcium not only improves symptoms, but it also decreases the risk of death during hospitalization.[12] For initial treatment of significant hypercalcemia, start aggressive intravenous hydration with normal saline. Hypercalcemic patients may be significantly fluid depleted and may require a few liters of fluid. Saline hydration dilutes the calcium concentration, promotes urinary excretion of calcium, and treats dehydration. Place patients with severe hypercalcemia on continuous cardiac monitoring and closely monitor their urine output (with a Foley catheter if necessary). Frequently repeat laboratory studies of electrolytes (e.g., at least every 4 hours) not only to monitor the calcium level but also to ensure that the saline hydration does not result in significant hypokalemia or hypomagnesemia. If the patient is in renal failure and will not tolerate aggressive saline hydration, dialysis may be needed to correct the calcium level. In addition to saline hydration, a bisphosphonate should be considered (e.g., pamidronate, zoledronic). Bisphosphonates work by inhibiting osteoclastic activity through prevention of osteoclast attachment to bone and interference with osteoclast recruitment; this process decreases bone reabsorption. Pamidronate, the most commonly used bisphosphonate, can be administered at 60 mg intravenously over 2 to 24 hours for moderate hypercalcemia and at 90 mg over 2 to 24 hours for severe hypercalcemia. Another bisphosphonate, zoledronic acid, 4 mg intravenously, may be more effective.[13] Calcitonin should be considered next. Calcitonin inhibits bone reabsorption and increases renal excretion of calcium. The effects of calcitonin are short-lived, but they can be seen within 4 hours. Calcitonin is administered at 4 to 8 U/kg either intramuscularly or subcutaneously. Even though loop diuretics (e.g., furosemide) are unlikely to lower the calcium level significantly, they may be useful if the patient starts to become volume overloaded and needs diuresis. Before administering a diuretic, ensure that the patient has already demonstrated adequate urine output; this will ensure that you are not worsening a volume-depleted state. Other possible treatments include gallium nitrate, mithramycin, and corticosteroids (e.g., hydrocortisone), and these agents should be initiated in consultation with the patient's oncologist.

Treat patients with mild calcium elevations or those who have minimal symptoms with oral hydration or initial intravenous hydration followed by oral hydration. Consider discharging patients with mild calcium elevations after hydration in the ED, if they have no other active issues and if close follow-up can be arranged with their oncologist. Patients with significant symptoms (e.g., dehydration, altered mental status) should be admitted, as should patients with baseline renal insufficiency, because they will be more difficult to treat.

■ HYPOTENSION

■ Scope

The causes of hypotension or shock in an oncology patient who presents to the ED vary somewhat from those seen in the general population (Box 201-2). Common causes of hypotension and shock such as sepsis and hypovolemia (e.g., secondary to gastrointestinal losses or bleeding) are also common in the oncology patient. Severe dehydration is a particular problem in this patient population because many cancers or cancer treatments make oral intake very difficult and may cause vomiting or diarrhea. Certain clinical entities such as pericardial tamponade and adrenal insufficiency appear with increased frequency in this patient population. Cardiac tamponade is discussed in Chapter 202, but it is essential always to consider tamponade in any patient with cancer who presents with hypotension, shock, or dyspnea. Some causes of hypotension are unique to the patient with cancer, such as myocardial dysfunction from a chemotherapeutic agent (e.g., doxorubicin). Because oncology patients are immunocompromised at baseline, they may require more intensive management and may suffer a worse outcome if hypotension is not addressed promptly in the ED.

BOX 201-2

Differential Diagnosis of Hypotension in the Patient with Cancer

- Sepsis
- Acute adrenal insufficiency
- Pericardial tamponade
- Severe dehydration
  - Secondary to chemotherapy-induced vomiting, diarrhea, hypercalcemia, anorexia, or mucositis
  - Secondary to an inability to tolerate oral intake as a result of obstruction or cancer
- Hemorrhage secondary to a tumor or thrombocytopenia
- Pulmonary embolism

■ ADRENAL INSUFFICIENCY

■ Scope

In the oncology patient, adrenal insufficiency is most commonly a result of previous treatment with high-dose steroids used in chemotherapy protocols. Metastatic infiltration of the adrenal glands is not uncommon because of the rich blood supply of these glands, but it rarely causes adrenal insufficiency. In one study, only 4.3% (20 of 464) of patients with cancer with metastasis to the adrenal glands on CT scan had or developed symptomatic adrenal insufficiency before they died.[14] Metastasis to the adrenal glands is most common in lung cancer, gastrointestinal malignant disease (stomach, esophagus, liver, pancreas, and bile duct), lymphoma, kidney cancer, and breast cancer.[14] Many patients with cancer may have subclinical or mild adrenal insufficiency that is not symptomatic until a significant stress (e.g., infection, dehydration) develops.

■ Presentation and Treatment

Adrenal insufficiency manifests with vague symptoms such as fatigue, weakness, nausea, vomiting, nonspecific abdominal pain, significant dehydration, and altered mental status. Laboratory analysis may show hyponatremia, hyperkalemia, or hypoglycemia. At a more severe stage, patients with acute adrenal insufficiency have significant hypotension secondary to distributive shock and may not respond to aggressive fluid resuscitation.

Administer a dose of dexamethasone, 4 to 10 mg intravenously. Dexamethasone is preferred over hydrocortisone because dexamethasone is less likely to interfere with a corticotropin-stimulation test, which can then be performed in the ED or later by the inpatient team to confirm the diagnosis. Obtain a serum cortisol level before initiating steroid therapy.

■ Diagnostic Testing

Isolated random cortisol levels are by themselves very unreliable; they predict increased mortality if they are either very high or very low.[15] If time permits, perform the short corticotropin-stimulation test in the ED. The test is performed by administering 250 μg of cosyntropin intravenously after a baseline cortisol level is obtained. Repeat the cortisol level 30 and 60 minutes later. If the patient has adrenal insufficiency, the response will be less than 9 μg/dL (the difference between the highest response to therapy and the patient's baseline level).[16] A multicenter, placebo-controlled, randomized double-blind study found that when septic patients who were nonresponders (<9 μg/dL response to the corticotropin-stimulation test) were treated with 7 days of hydrocortisone, 50 mg intravenously every 6 hours, and fludrocortisone, 50 μg/day orally, they significantly decreased their 28-day mortality, duration of vasopressor administration, and intensive care unit and hospital mortality versus placebo.[16] No significant effect on mortality was noted when responders to the corticotropin-stimulation test were treated with this protocol.[16] A more recent study compared performing the corticotropin-stimulation test with 1 μg of corticotropin with the traditional 250-μg dose and found a subgroup of patients who responded to the 250-μg dose but did not respond to the 1-μg dose. Nonresponders to the 1-μg dose had a higher mortality than the 1-μg responders; hence the authors concluded that the 1-μg stimulation test may be more sensitive for detecting patients with adrenal insufficiency. The mortality benefit of glucocorticoid replacement in this 1-μg nonresponder subgroup still needs to be prospectively evaluated.[17] If etomidate, which selectively inhibits 11-β-hydroxylase, is used in the ED course (specifically in the previous 4 hours), it may interfere with the cortisol response to corticotropin and thus may give a false-positive result to the corticotropin-stimulation test (may falsely conclude the patient is adrenally suppressed).[16,18]

Myocardial Dysfunction Secondary to Chemotherapy

As with the general population, the most common cause of cardiac dysfunction or cardiogenic shock in the oncology population is coronary artery disease.

Table 201-2 CHEMOTHERAPY AGENTS THAT CAUSE CARDIAC TOXICITY

Agent or Drug Class	Toxicity
Anthracyclines (e.g., doxorubicin, daunorubicin, epirubicin, idarubicin)	Myocardial cell death, fibrosis
5-Fluorouracil	Coronary vasospasm, ischemia
Cyclophosphamide	Acute hemorrhagic myopericarditis
Trastuzumab (Herceptin)	Decrease in left ventricular ejection fraction, congestive heart failure

Oncology patients, like any other patient who presents in congestive heart failure or cardiogenic shock, need to be evaluated for myocardial infarction. When treating oncology patients, recognize that a few chemotherapeutic agents, most notably the anthracyclines, can cause cardiomyopathies and congestive heart failure (Table 201-2). A newer drug, trastuzumab (Herceptin), which is a recombinant monoclonal antibody used in the treatment of breast cancer, has been associated with reductions in left ventricular ejection fraction and episodes of congestive heart failure.[19]

Dyspnea and Airway Issues in the Oncology Patient

■ AIRWAY MANAGEMENT

■ Scope

Airway management of the oncology patient differs only slightly from other emergency airway management approaches. The most challenging population consists of patients with certain head, neck, and laryngeal cancers or with cancers of the esophagus, thyroid, or lung whose tumor has impinged or distorted the airway. The major concern in these patients is that a typical rapid-sequence intubation protocol with a paralytic agent may turn a nonobstructing airway lesion into a lesion that, in a patient without any muscular tone, completely obstructs the airway and makes endotracheal intubation and bag-valve mask ventilation difficult or impossible.

■ Interventions and Procedures

Clues to a potentially hazardous airway may include complaints of dyspnea (especially if worse in the supine position), stridor, difficulty in handling secretions, hoarseness, or a recent change in voice. If there is concern regarding paralyzing the patient, a few options exist. One option is to give the patient topical lidocaine and a small dose of a sedative (e.g., midazolam or etomidate) and perform laryngoscopy. If the vocal cords can be visualized with this approach and there are no obvious concerns for airway obstruction, the patient should be either directly endotracheally intubated or can be intubated with typical rapid-sequence intubation utilizing a paralytic agent. If you have a few minutes before you have to establish an airway, an awake fiberoptic intubation may be the most prudent approach. Whatever method is taken, a cricothyroidotomy kit should be at the bedside, in case endotracheal intubation proves impossible. Even cricothyroidotomy may be difficult in the patient who has neck cancer or who had previous radiation to the neck because of significant alterations in neck anatomy.

Difficult airways may also be seen with oncology patients who have severe mucositis or bleeding disorders. Mucositis, especially, may make the tissues of the airway and oropharynx extremely friable, and the tissues may bleed easily with any manipulation; this problem makes standard endotracheal intubation more challenging. Many patients with cancer have significant thrombocytopenia. Special care must be taken with these patients because multiple or traumatic airway attempts may cause significant bleeding into the airway that may not be easily controlled. Rarely performed, nasotracheal intubation, which may cause trauma to the nasal passages, should be avoided in patients with mucositis or bleeding disorders.

Etomidate is one of the most commonly used sedatives in the management of airways by EPs. Etomidate reversibly blocks 11-β-hydroxylase, which blunts the normal cortisol response. Concern is often raised about using etomidate in a patient who is already immunocompromised (e.g., the patient with cancer). Studies show that the normal cortisol response returns by 12 hours after a single dose of etomidate, and no study has demonstrated a worse outcome after a single dose of etomidate.[18]

■ MALIGNANT PLEURAL EFFUSIONS

■ Presenting Signs and Symptoms

Pleural effusions are a common cause of dyspnea in the patient with cancer. Malignant pleural effusions are seen in patients with breast, lung, and ovarian cancers and in patients with lymphoma. The dyspnea is generally progressive and may occasionally be associated with cough or chest pain. The diagnosis is generally made with a chest radiograph, but it can also be diagnosed or confirmed by ultrasound. A chest CT scan can confirm the diagnosis and is especially useful because it can simultaneously rule out other life-threatening causes of dyspnea (e.g., pulmonary embolism, pneumonia).

■ Interventions and Procedures

Perform a thoracentesis in the ED for patients who are highly symptomatic. Removing pleural fluid may provide instant relief to some patients. Traditionally, a blind approach was incorporated. Today, however, bedside ultrasound scanning makes this procedure much simpler and safer. If it is the first presentation of a pleural effusion, sending the fluid for cytology may prove useful diagnostically. In general, unless a pleural effusion needs to be tapped for diagnostic purposes or to provide symptomatic relief, there is no need to tap the effusion in the ED. A chest radiograph should be performed at the completion of the procedure to ensure that a pneumothorax has not developed. More definitive treatment of the pleural effusion should be coordinated by the patient's oncologist. Treatment options include chemotherapy and sclerotherapy.

Emergency Side Effects of Oncology Treatment

Although some chemotherapeutic agents have unique side effects (Table 201-3), a few side effects are more universal. Bone marrow depression is a very common side effect of the majority of agents. Nausea and vomiting are also quite common, although some agents cause more severe symptoms than others.

Global Issues

■ PAIN

In a 1993 survey of physicians directly involved in cancer care (oncologists, hematologists, surgeons, and radiation therapists), 86% believed that most of their patients with cancer-related pain were being undermedicated, and 76% reported performing poor pain assessments for their patients.[20] After potentially dangerous causes of pain have been ruled out and the patient's pain is under control, usually in response to high doses of intravenous narcotics, a plan for outpatient pain control should be created with the patient and in consultation with the oncologist. Oncologists tend to use an escalating approach to outpatient pain management, starting with nonsteroidal anti-inflammatory drugs, then weaker opioids (e.g., codeine), and then stronger opioids (e.g., morphine, fentanyl). Because pain in the patient with cancer is ongoing, pain medication with longer half-lives or continuous action is preferred, such as very long-acting opioids or a transdermal opiate patch. Additional short-acting medication is also necessary for breakthrough pain. If you are prescribing a new opioid or escalating the dose, make sure to write a prescription for a laxative, because constipation is the most common side effect of opioid therapy.

■ NAUSEA AND VOMITING

Of all the side effects of chemotherapy, patients often consider nausea and vomiting to be the worst adverse effect. Nausea and vomiting can occasionally be severe enough to cause patients to discontinue their treatment. Poor antiemetic control with previous chemotherapy, female sex, low alcohol intake or

Table 201-3 **CHEMOTHERAPEUTIC AGENTS AND THEIR TOXICITIES***

Chemotherapy Agent	Drug Class	Common or Remarkable Toxicities	Indications for Use
5-Fluorouracil	Pyrimidine analogue	BMD, cerebellar problems, coronary vasospasm, ischemia, conjunctivitis, mucositis	Multiple cancers
6-Mercaptopurine	Purine analogue	BMD, pancreatitis, hepatotoxicity	Leukemia
Alemtuzumab	Monoclonal antibody	Neutropenia, anemia, thrombocytopenia, infusion-related reactions, immunosuppression	B-cell CLL
Anastrozole	Hormone (aromatase inhibitor)	Bone and joint pain, thrombophlebitis	Breast cancer
Asparaginase	Enzyme	Anaphylaxis, pancreatitis, acute renal failure, hyperglycemia, hyperthermia, seizure, altered mental status	Acute lymphoid leukemia
Bevacizumab	Monoclonal antibody	BMD, GI perforation, hemorrhage (GI, hemoptysis, epistaxis)	Colon, lung, and breast cancer
Bicalutamide	Hormone (antiandrogen)	Hepatotoxicity, GI hemorrhage	Prostate cancer
Bleomycin	Antibiotic	Pulmonary fibrosis, pneumonitis, fever, pericarditis, anaphylaxis, mucocutaneous reactions	Multiple cancers
Busulfan	Alkylating agent	Granulocytopenia, thrombocytopenia, addisonian symptoms, pulmonary fibrosis	Testicular, ovarian, and cervical cancer
Capecitabine	Pyrimidine analogue	BMD, ulcerations, diarrhea, mucositis	Breast and GI cancer
Carmustine (BCNU)	Nitrosourea (alkylating agent)	BMD, hepatotoxicity, pulmonary fibrosis, nephrotoxicity	Multiple cancers
Carboplatin	Alkylating agent (platinum)	BMD, anaphylactic-like reactions, peripheral neuropathy	Multiple cancers
Chlorambucil	Alkylating agent	BMD, erythema multiforme, hepatotoxicity, peripheral neuropathy	Leukemia and lymphoma
Cisplatin	Alkylating agent (platinum)	BMD, nephrotoxic, tinnitus, hearing loss, peripheral neuropathy, hypersensitivity reactions	Multiple cancers
Cladribine	Purine analogue	BMD, neurotoxicity, fever, nephrotoxicity	Leukemia and lymphoma
Cyclophosphamide	Alkylating agents	BMD, hemorrhagic cystitis, SIADH, fever, acute hemorrhagic myopericarditis	Brain and meningeal tumors
Cytarabine	Pyrimidine analogue	BMD, fever, hepatotoxicity, mucositis, peripheral neuropathy	Leukemia and lymphoma
Dacarbazine	Alkylating agent	BMD, hepatotoxicity, hepatic necrosis, flulike symptoms	Melanoma and Hodgkin's lymphoma
Dactinomycin (actinomycin D)	Anthracycline	BMD, fever, rash	Sarcomas
Daunorubicin	Anthracycline	Cardiac damage, CHF, BMD	Kaposi's sarcoma
Doxorubicin	Anthracycline	Cardiac damage, CHF, BMD	Multiple cancers
Epirubicin	Anthracycline	Cardiac damage, CHF, BMD	Multiple cancers
Etoposide	Podophyllotoxin	BMD, peripheral neuropathy, hypersensitivity reactions	Multiple cancers
Exemestane	Hormone (aromatase inhibitor)	CHF, MI, CVA, fractures, arthralgias, sweats	Breast cancer

Table 201-3 CHEMOTHERAPEUTIC AGENTS AND THEIR TOXICITIES—cont'd

Chemotherapy Agent	Drug Class	Common or Remarkable Toxicities	Indications for Use
Fludarabine	Purine analogue	BMD, autoimmune hemolytic anemia, neurotoxicity, blindness, edema, fever	CLL
Flutamide	Hormone (antiandrogen)	Hepatic failure, hepatotoxicity	Prostate cancer
Gemcitabine	Pyrimidine analogue	BMD, hemolytic-uremic syndrome	Multiple cancers
Gemtuzumab	Monoclonal antibody	Myelosuppression, severe hypersensitivity reactions (anaphylaxis), infusion-related reactions (often pulmonary symptoms), hepatotoxicity	Leukemia
Idarubicin	Anthracyclines	Cardiac damage, CHF, BMD	Leukemia
Ibritumomab tiuxetan	Monoclonal antibody	Fatal infusion reactions, cutaneous and mucocutaneous reactions, BMD	Lymphoma
Ifosfamide	Alkylating agent	BMD, nephrotoxicity, cystitis, metabolic acidosis	Multiple cancers
Letrozole	Hormone (aromatase inhibitor)	MI, DVT, PE, fractures, arthralgias, sweats	Breast cancer
Leuprolide	Hormone	Sweats	Prostate cancer
Lomustine (CCNU)	Nitrosourea (alkylating agent)	BMD, hepatotoxicity, pulmonary fibrosis, nephrotoxicity	Multiple cancers
Mechlorethamine (nitrogen mustard)	Alkylating agent	BMD, dermatitis, erythema multiforme	Leukemia
Megestrol	Hormone	PE, DVT, adrenal insufficiency, sweats	Breast and endometrial cancer
Melphalan	Alkylating agent	BMD, pulmonary fibrosis	Multiple cancers
Methotrexate	Folate antagonist	BMD, fever, conjunctivitis, pneumonitis, mucositis, hepatotoxicity, nephrotoxicity	Multiple cancers
Mitomycin	Antibiotic	BMD, hemolytic-uremic syndrome, nephrotoxicity	Multiple cancers
Mitoxantrone	Podophyllotoxin	Cardiotoxicity, CHF, BMD, hepatoxicity	Multiple cancers
Oxaliplatin	Alkylating agent (platinum)	BMD, anaphylactic-like reactions, peripheral neuropathy, neuropathic throat pain, abdominal pain, diarrhea, colitis	Colon cancer
Procarbazine	Alkylating agent	BMD, neurotoxicity, peripheral neuropathy	Hodgkin's lymphoma and multiple myeloma
Rituximab	Monoclonal antibody	BMD, fatal infusion reactions, severe mucocutaneous reactions, cardiac arrhythmias, hypersensitivity reactions	Lymphoma and leukemia
Tamoxifen	Hormone (antiestrogen)	CVA, PE, DVT	Breast cancer
Taxol (paclitaxel)	Plant (vinca) alkaloid	BMD, fever, cardiac arrhythmias, paresthesias, hypersensitivity reactions	Breast cancer
Temozolomide	Alkylating agent	BMD, headache, seizures, constipation	Brain malignancies
Teniposide	Podophyllotoxin	BMD, hypersensitivity reactions	Acute lymphoid leukemia and non-Hodgkin's lymphoma

Table 201-3 CHEMOTHERAPEUTIC AGENTS AND THEIR TOXICITIES—cont'd

Chemotherapy Agent	Drug Class	Common or Remarkable Toxicities	Indications for Use
Thioguanine (6-TG)	Purine analogue	BMD, hepatotoxicity, mucositis	Acute myeloid leukemia
Thiotepa	Alkylating agent	BMD, hypersensitivity reaction	Breast, bladder, and ovarian cancer
Tositumomab	Monoclonal antibody	BMD, fever	Lymphoma
Trastuzumab (Herceptin)	Monoclonal antibody	Cardiomyopathy (decrease in left ventricular ejection fraction), CHF, infusion reactions (anaphylaxis, angioedema, pneumonitis, ARDS), rash, abdominal pain, diarrhea	Breast cancer
Vinblastine	Plant (vinca) alkaloid	BMD, leukopenia, peripheral neuropathy, hypertension	Multiple cancers
Vincristine	Plant (vinca) alkaloid	SIADH, paresthesias, neuromuscular effects, peripheral neuropathy	Multiple cancers
Vindesine	Plant (vinca) alkaloid	BMD, neurotoxicity, peripheral neuropathy	Multiple cancers

*This chart is not meant to be all-inclusive. When dealing with a patient who is receiving a chemotherapeutic agent in the clinical setting, use an up-to-date on-line resource. Nausea and vomiting are common side effects of most chemotherapeutic agents and are not included in this table. See Box 201-3 for a list of chemotherapeutic agents that are particularly emetogenic.

ARDS, acute respiratory distress syndrome; BMD, bone marrow destruction/myelosuppression; CHF, congestive heart failure; CLL, chronic lymphocytic leukemia; CVA, cerebrovascular accident; DVT, deep venous thrombosis; GI, gastrointestinal; MI, myocardial infarction; PE, pulmonary embolism; SIADH, syndrome of inappropriate antidiuretic hormone.

Data from MICROMEDEX Healthcare Series (www. thomsonhc.com/hcs/librarian); Merck Manual Online Medical Library for Healthcare Professionals (www.merck.com/media/mmpe/pdf/Table_149_2.pdf); and Savarese D: Principles of cancer therapy. In Noble J (ed): Textbook of Primary Care Medicine, 3rd ed. St. Louis, Mosby, 2001, pp 1063-1073.

history, and younger age are all associated with a higher risk of emesis after chemotherapy.[21] In an effort to reduce the risk of emesis and to increase the tolerability of the treatment, chemotherapy regimens usually include an antiemetic drug. Chemotherapeutic agents with high emetogenic potential are listed in Box 201-3.[21]

Conversely, nausea and vomiting can be the initial symptoms of a potentially life-threatening issue. Nausea or vomiting can be the first sign of a neurologic condition (e.g., increase in central nervous system pressure, brain metastasis or bleeding), a gastroenterologic disorder (e.g., bowel obstruction), or even a metabolic problem (e.g., hypercalcemia).

Patients who complain of nausea or vomiting in the ED should be treated promptly with a strong antiemetic and appropriate hydration. Serotonin receptor antagonists (e.g., ondansetron, granisetron) are among the most commonly used antiemetics for patients with cancer. For example, ondansetron (Zofran), 8 to 12 mg over 15 to 30 minutes by intravenous piggyback infusion, can be used for severe postchemotherapy nausea and vomiting in the ED. Other commonly used antiemetics in this patient population include phenothiazines (e.g., prochlorperazine), benzamides (e.g., metoclopramide), corti-

BOX 201-3

Chemotherapeutic Agents with High Emetogenic Potential*

Carboplatin
Carmustine
Cisplatin
Cyclophosphamide
Cytarabine
Dacarbazine
Doxorubicin
Mechlorethamine
Methotrexate
Procarbazine
Streptozocin

*Emetogenic potential is generally dose dependent; antiemetics are generally coadministered with these agents to decrease the risk of emesis.

From Hesketh PJ: Defining the emetogenicity of cancer chemotherapy regimens: Relevance to clinical practice. Oncologist 1999;4:191-196.

costeroids (e.g., dexamethasone), and benzodiazepines (e.g., lorazepam).

MUCOSITIS

Scope

Mucositis is inflammation and ulceration of the mucous membranes. Most commonly, mucositis manifests in the mouth, but it can occur anywhere in the gastrointestinal, genitourinary, or respiratory tracts. Because mucositis is a breakdown of the normal integrity of mucous membranes, it is associated with an increased risk of infection. Oral mucositis is a side effect of chemotherapy or radiation, or it can result from certain cancers, such as oral cancers and leukemia. Mucositis is fairly prevalent; it occurs in up to 58% of cancer patients depending on their diagnosis.[22] Patients obtaining either radiation for head and neck cancers or chemotherapy with 5-fluorouracil, anthracyclines, or irinotecan, or are bone marrow transplant recipients, have high rates of mucositis.

Presenting Signs and Symptoms

Oral mucositis is quite painful and causes significant difficulties with swallowing. Oral mucositis can cause altered taste, halitosis, and dry mouth. Painful swallowing and altered taste may adversely affect the patient's oral intake and may result in dehydration. Oral mucositis can result in difficulty with speaking. In severe cases, mucositis can be secondarily infected with bacteria or fungi and can bleed.

Treatment

Patients who present to the ED with oral mucositis should be given proper pain control, which may include the use of opiates. Mouth wash rinses such as 2% viscous lidocaine can be helpful. Any secondary infections, such as oral candidiasis or herpes simplex, should be treated. A bland, soft diet is recommended, as well as ice chips or other cold products to keep the oral mucosa moist. Special attention to oral hygiene is essential for at-risk patients with cancer, including the use of a soft toothbrush, frequent saline or baking soda rinses, prophylactic anticandidal rinses (e.g., nystatin), and adequate general nutrition.

REFERENCES

1. Edwards BK, Brown ML, Wingo PA, , et al: Annual report to the nation on the status of cancer, 1975-2002, featuring population-based trends in cancer treatment. J Natl Cancer Inst 2005;97:1407-1427.
2. Kress JP, Christenson J, Pohlman AS, et al: Outcomes of critically ill cancer patients in a university hospital setting. Am J Respir Crit Care Med 1999;160:1957-1961.
3. Weinstein RA: Nosocomial infection update. Emerg Infect Dis 1998;4:416-420.
4. Kuderer NM, Dale DC, Crawford J, et al: Mortality, morbidity, and cost associated with febrile neutropenia in adult cancer patients. Cancer 2006;106:2258-2266.
5. Viscoli C, Castagnola E: Planned progressive antimicrobial therapy in neutropenic patients. Br J Haematol 1998;102:879-888.
6. Crawford J, Ozer H, Stoller R: Reduction by granulocyte colony-stimulating factor of fever and neutropenia induced by chemotherapy in patients with small-cell lung cancer. N Engl J Med 1991;325:164-170.
7. García-Carbonero R, Mayordomo JI, Tornamira MV, et al: Granulocyte colony-stimulating factor in the treatment of high-risk febrile neutropenia: A multicenter randomized trial. J Natl Cancer Inst 2001;93:31-38.
8. Clark O, Djulbegovic B, Dale DC, et al: Treatment with colony-stimulating factors improves clinical outcomes in patients with established febrile neutropenia: A meta-analysis of the randomized clinical trials [abstract 689]. Proc Am Soc Clin Oncol 2003;22:172.
9. Hsu TF, Huang HH, Yen DH, et al: ED presentation of neutropenic enterocolitis in adult patients with acute leukemia. Am J Emerg Med 2004;22:276-279.
10. Holdsworth MT, Nguyen P: Role of i.v. allopurinol and rasburicase in tumor lysis syndrome. Am J Health Syst Pharm 2003;60:2213-2222.
11. Vassilopoulou-Sellin R, Newman BM, Taylor SH, Guinee VF: Incidence of hypercalcemia in patients with malignancy referred to a comprehensive cancer center. Cancer 1993;71:1309-1312.
12. Lamy O, Jenzer-Closuit A, Burckhardt P: Hypercalcemia of malignancy: An undiagnosed and undertreated disease. J Intern Med 2001;250:73-79.
13. Major P, Lortholary A, Hon J, et al: Zoledronic acid is superior to pamidronate in the treatment of hypercalcemia of malignancy: A pooled analysis of two randomized, controlled clinical trials. J Clin Oncol 2001;19:558-567.
14. Lam KY, Lo CY: Metastatic tumours of the adrenal glands: A 30-year experience in a teaching hospital. Clin Endocrinol (Oxf) 2002;56:95-101.
15. Annane D, Sébille V, Troche G, et al: A 3-level prognostic classification in septic shock based on cortisol levels and cortisol response to corticotropin. JAMA 2000;283:1038-1045.
16. Annane D, Sebille V, Charpentier C, et al: Effect of treatment with low doses of hydrocortisone and fludrocortisone on mortality in patients with septic shock. JAMA 2002;288:862-871.
17. Siraux V, De Backer D, Yalavatti G, et al: Relative adrenal insufficiency in patients with septic shock: Comparison of low-dose and conventional corticotropin tests. Crit Care Med 2005;33:2479-2486.
18. Schenarts CL, Burton JH, Riker RR, et al: Adrenocortical dysfunction following etomidate induction in emergency department patients. Acad Emerg Med 2001;8:1-7.
19. Murray S: Trastuzumab (Herceptin) and HER2-positive breast cancer. CMAJ 2006;174:36-37.
20. Von Roenn JH, Cleeland CS, Gonin R, et al: Physician attitudes and practice in cancer pain management: A survey from the Eastern Cooperative Oncology Group. Ann Intern Med 1993;119:121-126.
21. Hesketh PJ: Defining the emetogenicity of cancer chemotherapy regimens: Relevance to clinical practice. Oncologist 1999;4:191-196.
22. Sonis ST, Elting LS, Keefe D, et al: Perspectives on cancer therapy-induced mucosal injury: Pathogenesis, measurement, epidemiology, and consequences for patients. Cancer 2004;100:1995-2025.

Chapter **202**

Cardiovascular and Neurologic Oncologic Emergencies

Jacob Ufberg and Manish Garg

KEY POINTS

Early symptoms of cardiac tamponade are tachypnea and dyspnea with exertion.

The superior vena cava (SVC) syndrome is caused by obstruction of blood flow through the SVC by compression or vascular thrombosis.

In patients with spinal cord compression from malignancy, pain may precede neurologic changes by several weeks. At the time of ED presentation, some motor weakness is usually evident.

Headaches from brain tumors are often described as tension-type headaches, but more frequently they have associated nausea and are sometimes worse with bending over.

Corticosteroids and radiation therapy are typical initial treatments for spinal cord compression from malignancy.

Cardiovascular Emergencies

■ CARDIAC TAMPONADE

■ Scope

Malignant cardiac involvement is common, occurring in 11% to 12% of patients with cancer. Of these patients, three fourths have epicardial involvement, and one third of these have an effusion.[1] The most common causative malignant primary tumor that progresses to involve the pericardium is lung cancer; breast cancer, gastrointestinal cancers, melanoma, sarcoma, lymphoma, and leukemia account for the majority of other cases. These tumors invade the pericardium through direct or metastatic spread. Less commonly, malignant primary pericardial tumors such as mesothelioma and sarcoma or benign tumors such as angioma, fibroma, or teratoma may occur.

■ Structure and Function

The pericardium is a fibroelastic sac surrounding the heart that normally contains a thin layer of fluid. When a larger amount of fluid accumulates and exceeds the elastic limit of the pericardium, the heart begins to compete for the now fixed amount of intrapericardial space. As more fluid accumulates, the cardiac chambers become compressed, and diastolic compliance lessens.

Throughout this process, the decline in intrathoracic pressure associated with inspiration continues to be transmitted through the pericardium to the heart. Thus, venous return to the heart is still increased with inspiration. However, the free wall of the right ventricle cannot expand to accommodate this increased volume, thus leading the intraventricular septum to bow to the left. The result is decreased left ventricular filling during inspiration. When the size of the effusion progresses further, total venous return diminishes, and cardiac output and blood pressure deteriorate.

Cardiac tamponade is generally classified as acute or subacute. In *acute* cardiac tamponade, the relatively stiff pericardium can become rapidly filled with blood, causing tamponade with only a small effusion. This generally occurs in the setting of trauma, myocardial or aortic rupture, or invasive medical interventions. In *subacute* cardiac tamponade, a much larger effusion accumulates slowly and allows the pericardium to stretch over time. This type of tamponade occurs most commonly in the setting of malignancy or renal failure, and it may not occur until the amount of pericardial fluid reaches 2 L or more. In either setting, very little additional fluid may cause cardiac tamponade once the limits of pericardial elasticity have been reached.

Presenting Signs and Symptoms

Classic

Cardiac tamponade is a physiologic continuum, from mild to severe. Classically, patients present with tachypnea and dyspnea on exertion. As the disease progresses, patients may have shortness of breath at rest, peripheral edema, or orthopnea. Patients with severe disease may be obtunded on presentation, thus obscuring the diagnosis of cardiac tamponade. A history of malignancy or symptoms and signs of malignant disease such as weight loss, fatigue, or anorexia may help to guide the clinician toward a diagnosis of malignant pericardial effusion.

Physical Findings

Patients with pericardiac tamponade most commonly present with some degree of shortness of breath, hypotension, and often with clear lungs. Unfortunately, physical examination holds little value for diagnosing the presence of a pericardial effusion. However, as a malignant effusion becomes large enough to cause cardiac tamponade, some distinct physical findings may become evident. Beck's triad, first described in 1935, consists of increased jugular venous pressure, hypotension, and muffled heart sounds. However, this triad is most useful in acute cardiac tamponade, and it may be uncommon or difficult to assess in patients with atraumatic cardiac tamponade.[2]

Sinus tachycardia is seen in most patients with cardiac tamponade. This physiologic response allows for maintenance of cardiac output despite decreased filling volumes. Patients may present with slightly lower heart rates if they are taking beta-blocking medications or if they suffer from hypothyroidism. Significant tamponade also manifests with absolute or relative hypotension. Patients with early tamponade may present with normotension or even hypertension, especially if they have preexisting hypertension.

Pulsus paradoxus is defined as a drop of more than 10 mm Hg in systolic blood pressure during normal inspiration. Most patients with moderate to severe cardiac tamponade have pulsus paradoxus, which is often palpable in the peripheral arteries. As cardiac output drops, however, pulsus paradoxus may be difficult to measure without invasive monitoring. Pulsus paradoxus results when effusion limits expansion of the free wall of the right ventricle as venous return increases during inspiration. The right ventricle is then forced to expand by bulging the intraventricular septum into the left ventricle, thus leading to greatly reduced filling and stroke volume during inspiration.

To quantify pulsus paradoxus noninvasively, a sphygmomanometer is used in the standard fashion. The cuff is inflated to more than the systolic blood pressure and then is slowly deflated until the first Korotkoff sounds are audible only during exhalation. This condition is typified by hearing Korotkoff sounds for several beats during exhalation, followed by silence during inspiration, followed by Korotkoff sounds for several beats during exhalation. The pressure is noted on the sphygmomanometer at this point, and then slow deflation is continued until all beats are audible. The amount of pulsus paradoxus is determined by subtracting the pressure at which all beats are heard from the pressure at which beats were heard only during exhalation.

Multiple conditions may alter the physiology of cardiac tamponade and may cause pulsus paradoxus to be absent. The most common conditions are elevated left ventricular diastolic pressures and increased heart rate. Others include severe hypotension, irregular rhythm, atrial septal defect, regional cardiac tamponade, and severe aortic regurgitation.

Electrocardiography

The electrocardiogram is abnormal in most, but not all, patients with pericardial effusion. The most common findings are nonspecific ST-segment and T-wave abnormalities and sinus tachycardia. The electrocardiogram may mimic that seen in acute pericarditis.

Low QRS voltage may be a sign of a large pericardial effusion, but it is more likely to be associated with tamponade physiology. In one small study, Bruch and colleagues studied 43 patients with a pericardial effusion. Of those patients, 14 of 23 with tamponade demonstrated low-voltage QRS complexes, as opposed to none of the 23 patients with effusion but without tamponade[3] (Fig. 202-1). Electrical alternans (Fig. 202-2), demonstrated as beat-to-beat alterations in the amplitude of the QRS

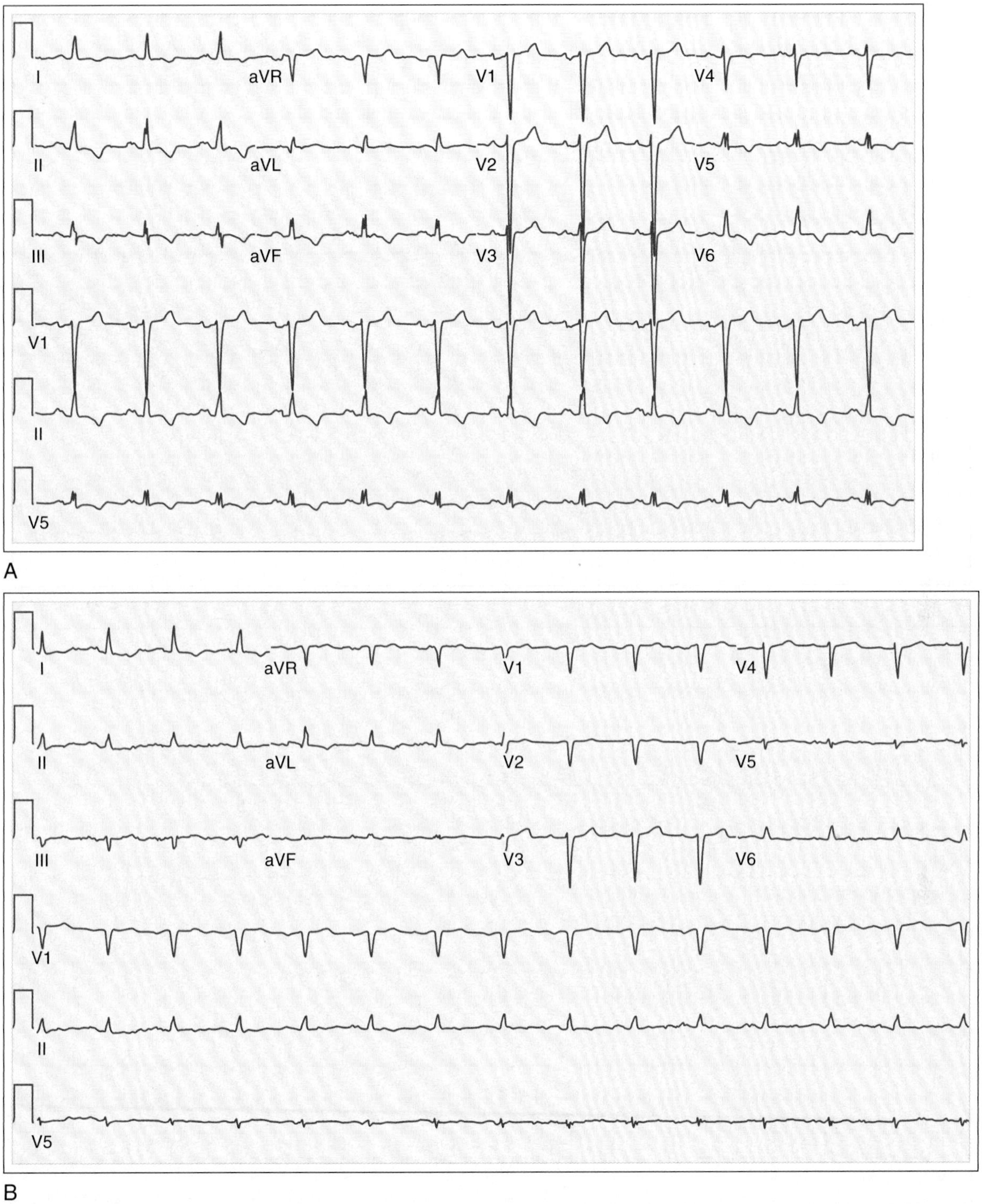
I
aVR
V1
V4
II
aVL
V2
V5
III
aVF
V3
V6
V1
II
V5
A
I
aVR
V1
V4
II
aVL
V2
V5
III
aVF
V3
V6
V1
II
V5
B

FIGURE 202-1 **A,** Patient's electrocardiogram on a prior ED visit. **B,** Patient's electrocardiogram on presentation to the ED with cardiac tamponade.

complex, is relatively specific, but not very sensitive for cardiac tamponade. It may also rarely occur in patients with very large effusions without tamponade. Electrical alternans is caused by swinging of the heart in the pericardial effusion, and it generally disappears after removal of even modest amounts of pericardial fluid.

Chest Radiography

The typical finding on chest radiograph is an enlarged cardiac silhouette (the "water bottle"–shaped heart), as seen in Figure 202-3. In most cases, the lung fields are clear unless preexisting lung disease (e.g., malignancy) is present. Cardiac tamponade may manifest

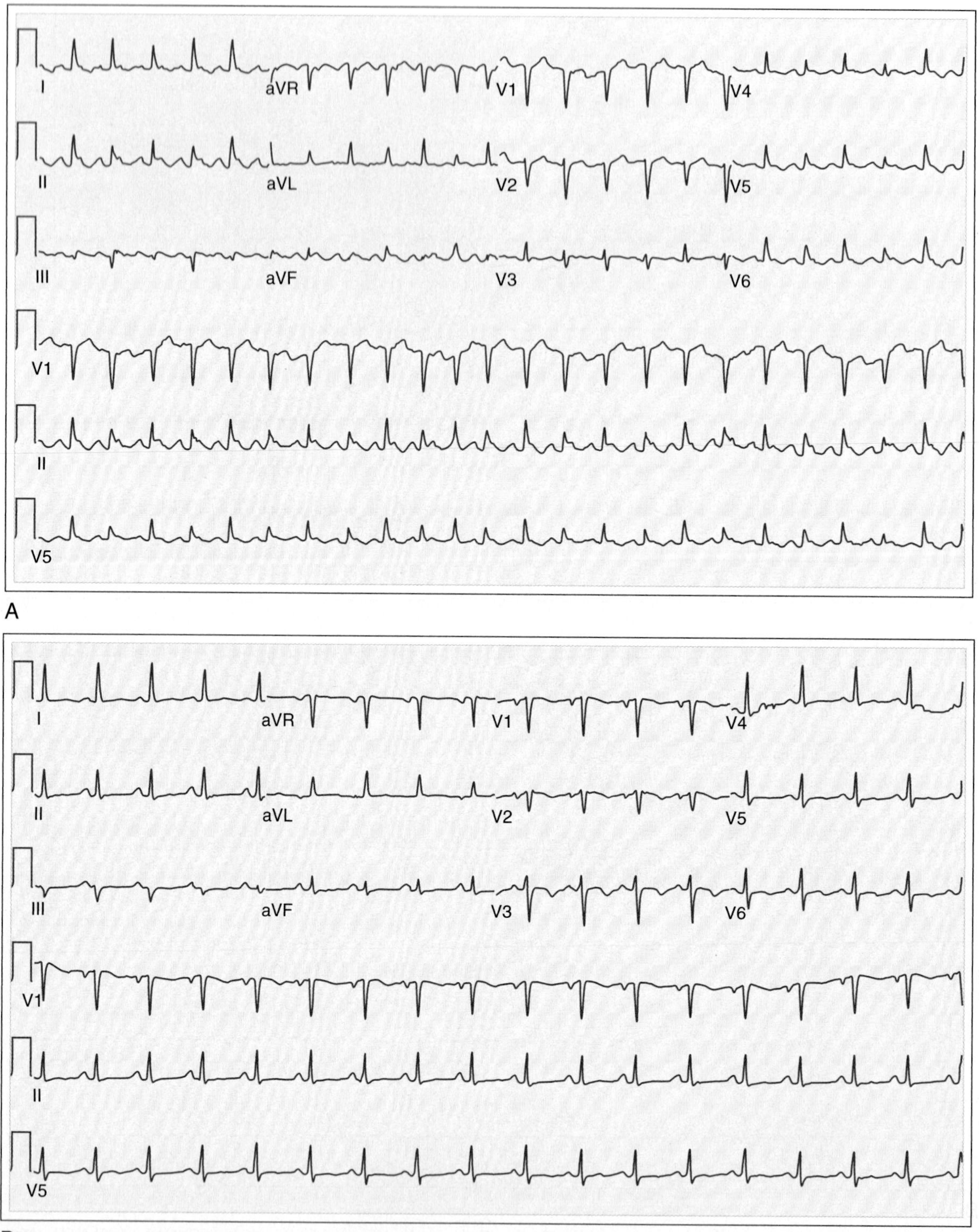
I
aVR
V1
V4
II
aVL
V2
V5
III
aVF
V3
V6
V1
II
V5
A
I
aVR
V1
V4
II
aVL
V2
V5
III
aVF
V3
V6
V1
II
V5
B

FIGURE 202-2 **A,** Electrocardiogram demonstrating electrical alternans most notable in lead II rhythm strip. This patient's electrocardiogram also has atrial flutter with 2:1 conduction. **B,** Electrocardiogram performed on the same patient several days after drainage of his pericardial effusion.

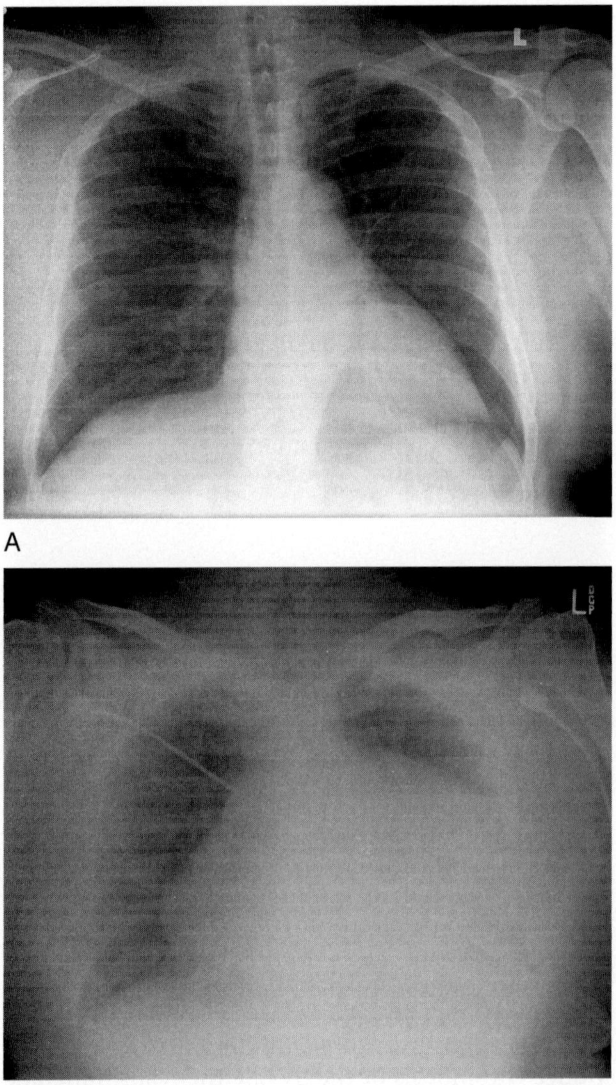

FIGURE 202-3 **A,** Patient's chest radiograph 1 year before presentation with cardiac tamponade. **B,** Same patient's chest radiograph on presentation to the ED with cardiac tamponade.

without an enlarged cardiac silhouette if a small, rapidly accumulating effusion is the cause.

Echocardiography and Emergency Medicine Bedside Ultrasound

Echocardiography and emergency medicine bedside ultrasound play crucial roles in the diagnosis of cardiac tamponade. The first steps are to suspect a problem and to perform a screening cardiac ultrasound examination[4] (Fig. 202-4).

Echocardiographic findings indicative of cardiac tamponade include the presence of pericardial fluid with accompanying diastolic collapse of the right atrium and right ventricle. During atrial relaxation at the end of diastole, pericardial pressure is maximal, whereas right atrial volume is minimal. This situation results in right atrial collapse that, if it lasts more than one third of the cardiac cycle, is sensitive and

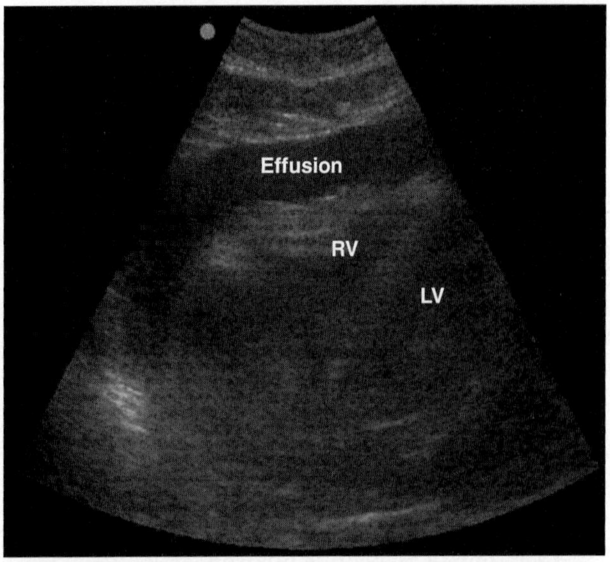
Effusion
RV
LV

FIGURE 202-4 Bedside ultrasound image showing large pericardial effusion. The patient subsequently had 2 L drained from this effusion.

specific for cardiac tamponade. Right ventricular diastolic collapse occurs early in diastole when ventricular volume is minimal. Left atrial collapse is less common, but it is also very specific for cardiac tamponade. Collapse of the left ventricle is uncommon because of its greater muscular thickness.

As discussed earlier, left- and right-sided volumes vary with the respiratory cycle. During inspiration, the atrial and ventricular septa bulge to the left. During expiration, the atrial and ventricular septa bulge rightward.

Treatment

Patients with mild hemodynamic compromise require urgent drainage of pericardial fluid. If the patient is sufficiently stable, cardiology and cardiothoracic surgery consultation may be appropriate to decide whether emergency catheter drainage or surgical creation of a pericardial window is the most appropriate therapy. In such cases, the EP should be prepared to perform emergency pericardial drainage if the patient's clinical condition should deteriorate.

Patients with severe hemodynamic compromise require immediate removal of pericardial fluid. Pericardiocentesis should be performed to remove as much of the pericardial effusion as possible. Percutaneous aspiration of even 50 to 100 mL has been demonstrated to reverse tamponade physiology temporarily.

Pericardiocentesis may be performed with electrocardiographic or echocardiographic guidance. Echocardiographic guidance is preferred when available, because it allows greater precision of procedure direction and needle angle. Placement of an indwelling catheter is advisable, to prevent reaccumulation of fluid. The technique used for pericardiocentesis can be found in Box 202-1. Fluid obtained from pericar-

BOX 202-1

Technique for Pericardiocentesis Using Ultrasound Guidance

- Using bedside ultrasound, locate the ideal site of skin puncture where the largest fluid collection lies closest to the skin surface. This is usually located on the left anterior chest wall. The clinician can choose either to mark the skin or to use the ultrasound device with a sterile sheath for dynamic guidance at this point
- Prepare the skin in sterile fashion, and anesthetize the skin if time permits.
- Attach a 20-mL syringe to an 18-gauge spinal needle.
- Insert the needle at the site and trajectory determined by bedside ultrasonogram. Take care to avoid the neurovascular bundle at the lower rib border and the internal mammary artery, which lies 3 to 5 cm lateral to the sternal border.
- Gently aspirate as the needle is advanced until fluid is obtained.
- Aspirate as much fluid as possible using the three-way stopcock.
- Alternately, use an over-the-needle catheter or the Seldinger technique if prolonged drainage is necessary. The Seldinger technique is performed using the same methods as outlined, but the clinician may use a thin-walled 18-gauge needle to pass a guidewire, followed by a catheter (e.g., a pigtail catheter) that may be left in place.

diocentesis should be sent for Gram's stain, culture, acid-fast stain and culture, cytology, carcinoembryonic antigen, and polymerase chain reaction evaluation. Complications of pericardiocentesis are listed in Box 202-2.

SUPERIOR VENA CAVA SYNDROME

Scope

The SVC may become obstructed either acutely or subacutely, thus causing the SVC syndrome. This condition may be caused by extrinsic mass, infiltration of the SVC by contiguous pathologic processes, or thrombosis. In the preantibiotic era, syphilitic aortic aneurysms, fibrosing mediastinitis, and complications of untreated infections were the most common causes of SVC syndrome.

Currently, malignant disease is the cause of the SVC syndrome in 85% of cases. Bronchogenic carcinomas account for the majority of cases, with small cell and squamous cell carcinomas by far the most

BOX 202-2

Complications of Pericardiocentesis

- Cardiac arrest (rare)
- Cardiac chamber laceration
- Coronary vessel laceration
- Cardiac tamponade
- Lung laceration with pneumothorax
- Dysrhythmia
- Postprocedure pulmonary edema
- "Dry tap"
- Pericardial-pleural shunt
- Air embolism or pneumopericardium
- Liver laceration

common. Although lung cancer is the leading cause of the SVC syndrome, the overall incidence of the SVC syndrome in patients with lung cancer is quite low. The next most common malignant cause of the SVC syndrome is non-Hodgkin's lymphoma, owing to its frequent presentation as a mediastinal mass. Metastatic cancers account for a small proportion of cases of the SVC syndrome. Patients with the SVC syndrome rarely experience immediately life-threatening complications in the absence of concurrent central airway obstruction.[5,6]

Benign causes of the SVC syndrome account for 10% to 15% of cases. In the patient with cancer, the most common benign cause is the presence of indwelling vascular devices such as hyperalimentation lines and chemotherapy ports or lines, which induce thrombosis of the SVC. Other causes include fibrosing mediastinitis resulting from histoplasmosis, as well as other infections.

Anatomy and Pathophysiology

The SVC syndrome is caused by one of several mechanisms. The first is direct compression by tumor or by enlarging lymph nodes (owing to inflammation or metastatic disease). The second is direct invasion of the SVC by tumor or other pathologic processes. The third is obstruction of the SVC by thrombus. Thrombus may additionally occur in up to 50% of patients with one of the other causes of SVC syndrome, and it may account for some treatment failures using therapy directed at the underlying malignancy.[7]

Clinical Presentation

The physical examination of the patient with SVC syndrome is often diagnostic. Most patients have facial edema or dilation of chest wall or neck veins. Some have cyanosis, arm edema, or plethora. It is rare to see a patient with the SVC syndrome who does

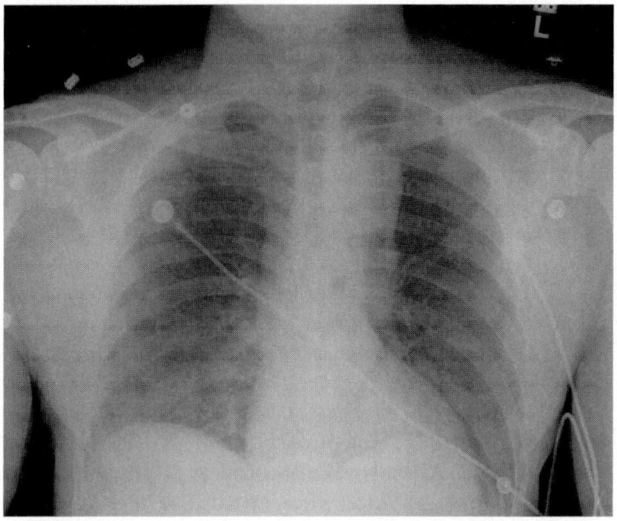
L

FIGURE 202-5 Chest radiograph showing widened mediastinum.

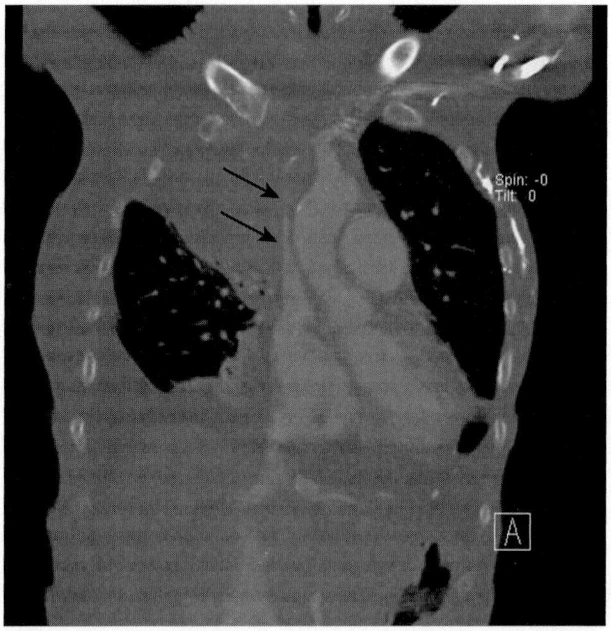
Spin: -0
Tilt: 0
A

FIGURE 202-6 Computed tomography scan showing blockage of the superior vena cava *(arrows).*

not have visible upper body venous dilation.[8] An indwelling central venous device may be a clue to the diagnosis in thrombotic causes of SVC syndrome.

Dyspnea, the most common symptom of the SVC syndrome, occurs in more than half of patients. Patients may complain of fullness or swelling of the face, trunk, or upper extremities that may be exacerbated by positional changes such as bending over or lying down. Contrary to previous beliefs, it appears that catastrophic neurologic events are quite rare.[5,6]

Diagnostic Testing

The initial test of choice when the SVC syndrome is suspected is chest plain film radiography. Most of these radiographs are abnormal; one series found 84% of films to be abnormal. The most common abnormal findings were mediastinal widening in 64% (Fig. 202-5) and pleural effusion in 26%.[8] A mass may also be seen in the superior mediastinum, right hilum or perihilum, or in the right upper lobe. Less commonly, right upper lobe collapse or rib notching may be apparent. However, a normal chest radiograph does not rule out the possibility of the SVC syndrome.[8]

The next test is a contrast-enhanced computed tomography (CT) scan (Fig. 202-6). CT is able to define the level and extent of blockage, provides detail on the amount of collateral flow, and is often able to identify the cause of obstruction.

Treatment

Symptomatic therapy should be instituted, including elevation of the head of the bed, oxygen, and bed rest. Diuretics and steroids have been used without clear evidence of efficacy. Anticoagulation may be of benefit in patients with thrombotic causes, after the origin is determined. Endovascular stenting has been successful in symptomatic improvement, and it has been steadily gaining favor as a treatment modality.

Disposition and Prognosis

All patients diagnosed with the SVC syndrome should be admitted to the hospital. The level of care should be chosen based on the clinical stability of the patient. Oncology specialists should be consulted to help begin the work-up necessary to establish a histologic diagnosis, if one is not already known.

Survival for patients with the SVC syndrome depends on the underlying diagnosis and the treatments chosen. Median survival is 6 months, but it may differ considerably based on the type of malignancy.

Neurologic Emergencies

CEREBRAL EMERGENCIES

Scope

The most important central nervous system (CNS) manifestations include altered mental status, elevated intracranial pressure (ICP), and seizures. Brain tumors represent a diverse group of neoplasms that can originate primarily from the CNS or metastatically through hematogenous spread from distant organs.

Although brain tumors account for only 2% of all tumors, they have significant sequelae. The 5-year survival rate for all ages and all races for malignant brain tumors is 33%; for children less than 14 years old, it is 62%; and for adults 65 years or older, it is 4.9%.[8] In children, brain tumors are the most common solid malignant tumors and the second

BOX 202-3

Approximate Differences in Primary Tumor Types between Adults and Pediatrics

Adults

50%	20%	15%	10%	4%	2%
Glioma >	Meningioma >	Pituitary tumor >	Astrocytoma >	CNS lymphoma >	Craniopharyngioma

Children

50%	25%	10%	10%	5%
Astrocytoma >	Medulloblastoma >	Ependymoma >	Glioma >	Craniopharyngioma

CNS, central nervous system.

leading cause of cancer death after leukemia. Box 202-3 illustrates the differences in primary tumor types between adults and pediatric patients.

Brain metastases are more common than primary tumors in adults and account for more than half of all intracranial brain tumors. In adults with systemic malignancies, brain metastases occur in 10% to 30% of patients. The most common primary tumors responsible for brain metastases in adults are carcinomas, and they include lung cancer, renal cell cancer, melanoma, breast cancer, and colorectal cancer. In children with systemic malignancies, brain metastases occur in 6% to 10% of patients. The most common primary tumors responsible for brain metastases in children are sarcomas, neuroblastomas, and germ cell tumors.

In general, there is a slight male predominance in the incidence of malignant brain tumor. Whites have the highest incidence, with descending incidence for Latinos and African Americans, and the lowest incidence for Native Americans and Asian Americans.[9] The rising incidence of brain tumors in industrialized countries is thought to be mostly a result of environmental exposures and improved detection using diagnostic imaging.

Although cancers typically are indolent in their evolution, the neurologic manifestations may be acute or chronic, and they may be local or distant from the primary source. Rapid diagnosis and treatment are imperative to prevent irreversible damage, primarily from cerebral hypoxia, inflammation, or swelling, which can have catastrophic consequences. The long-term prognosis of patients with cancer and significant neurologic complications is poor, and recurrence of illness is common despite optimal management.

Anatomy and Physiology

The pathogenesis of tumor-related neurologic dysfunction involves disruption of the blood brain barrier leading to vasogenic edema. This condition is caused primarily by factors that increase the permeability of the tumor vessels (vascular endothelial growth factor, glutamate, and leukotrienes) and by the absence of tight endothelial cell junctions in tumor blood vessels. This process culminates in leakage of protein-rich fluid into the extracellular space, predominantly in the white matter of the brain. When this peritumoral edema begins to accumulate, the synaptic transmission can be disrupted and thus can lead to altered neuronal excitability and neurologic sequelae (Fig. 202-7). Vasogenic edema is what causes patients to suffer from headaches, nausea or vomiting, seizures, cognitive dysfunction, focal neurologic deficits, encephalopathy, or increased ICP leading to syncope or fatal herniation. Intra-tumoral hemorrhage, obstructive hydrocephalus, and tumor embolization can also cause tumor-related consequences, but these entities are much less com-mon than vasogenic edema.

Brain metastases arrive through hematogenous spread. They are usually located in two places. The first is directly at the junction of the gray and white matter, where smaller vessels begin to trap tumor cells. The second is at terminal "watershed areas" of arterial circulation. Metastases distribute according to weight and blood flow and are seen in the cerebral hemispheres (80%), in the cerebellum (15%), and in the brainstem (5%). Pelvic (prostate and uterine) and gastrointestinal tumors commonly metastasize to the posterior fossa, whereas small cell lung carcinoma distributes equally through all regions of the brain.

Clinical Presentation

A classic presentation to the ED for a patient with brain metastasis is a patient with known cancer who has a sudden onset of a neurologic deficit or change in mental status, syncope, or seizure. Patients with primary or metastatic disease can present with either generalized or focal signs and symptoms. Generalized symptoms include headaches, nausea or vomiting, generalized seizures, cognitive dysfunction, and loss of consciousness. Focal symptoms include weakness, sensory loss, aphasia, focal seizures, and visual spatial dysfunction.

Headaches are the most common symptom of brain tumor, and they occur in approximately 40% to 50% of patients with primary or metastatic brain tumors. In one retrospective review, headaches were described variably, but most were described as

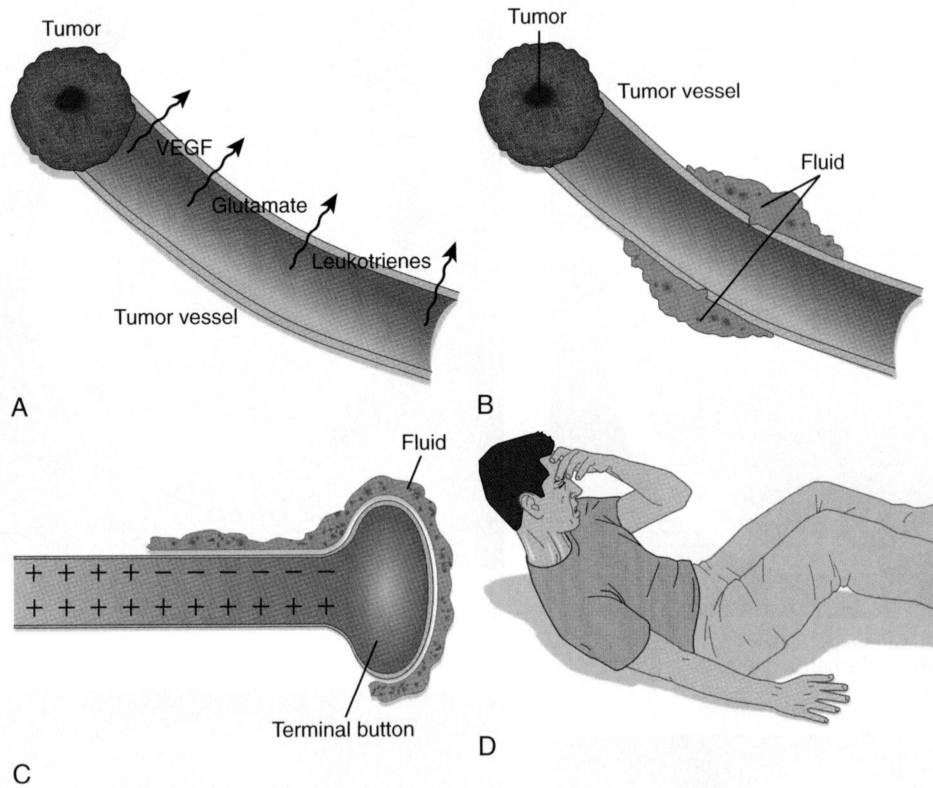
Tumor
VEGF
Glutamate
Leukotrienes
Tumor vessel
A
Tumor
Tumor vessel
Fluid
B
Fluid
+ + + + – – – – – –
+ + + + + + + + + + +
Terminal button
C
D

FIGURE 202-7 Pathophysiology of vasogenic edema. **A,** Tumor vessel with factors that increase vascular permeability. **B,** Protein-rich fluid leaking into extracellular spaces. **C,** Disruption of synaptic transmission. **D,** Neurologic sequelae.

tension-type headaches. The patients described the headaches as bifrontal and worsening ipsilateral to the lesion.[10] Tumor-related headaches were differentiated from tension headaches by complaints of nausea and vomiting or especially by worsening of the headache with changes in position such as bending over. Worsening of the headache typically occurred following maneuvers that increase intrathoracic pressure such as coughing, sneezing, or the Valsalva maneuver.

Tumor-related headaches tend to be worse at night because of small increases in the partial pressure of carbon dioxide, recumbency, and decreased cerebral venous return. Headaches related to increased ICP are thought to be mediated by the pain fibers of cranial nerve V in the dura and blood vessels. Headaches associated with increased ICP can be the result of large mass lesions or of restriction of cerebrospinal fluid outflow causing hydrocephalus. Classically, increased ICP is manifested by the classic triad of headache, nausea and vomiting, and papilledema. Thus, a careful ophthalmologic examination is requisite for all complaints of headache.

Seizures represent the most common presenting symptom of gliomas and cerebral metastases. In these tumor types, one study showed that seizure was the initial complaint in approximately 20% to 25% of patients.[11] Patients who present with seizure activity usually have smaller primary tumors or fewer metastatic lesions in the brain compared with other presenting symptoms, because the seizure will lead to earlier diagnostic imaging and diagnosis. Seizures can be generalized or focal, depending on the location in the brain of the tumor. Frontal lobe tumors may cause tonic-clonic movements in an extremity, and occipital lobe tumors may cause visual disturbances. Temporal lobe seizures may cause abrupt personality changes. Patients with a history of tumor-related seizures commonly present in a similar fashion on each visit, with or without a prodromal phase followed by a postictal period. If the seizures are generalized, the patient will be fatigued and sleepy; however, if the seizures are focal, the patient may have Todd's paralysis.

Acute mental status change describes a deficit in cognitive function and is a presenting complaint in approximately 30% to 35% of patients with brain metastases.[12] Cognitive dysfunction includes memory problems and mood or personality changes. Patients commonly present with fatigue, low energy, increased urge to sleep, and apathy toward daily activities.

■ Diagnostic Testing

Diagnostic neuroimaging is the standard for confirming brain tumors and subsequent neurologic manifestations of oncologic emergencies. For the EP, CT scanning is the initial test of choice because of its speed and availability. Contrast-enhanced magnetic

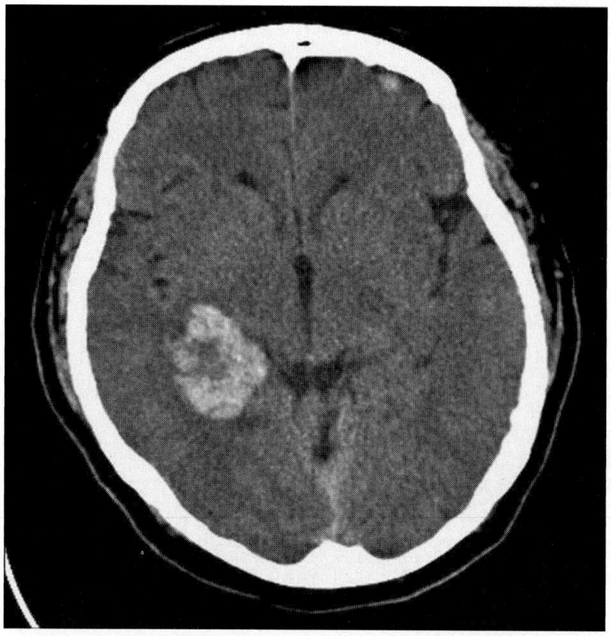

FIGURE 202-8 Noncontrast computed tomography scan of the head showing an intratumoral hemorrhage.

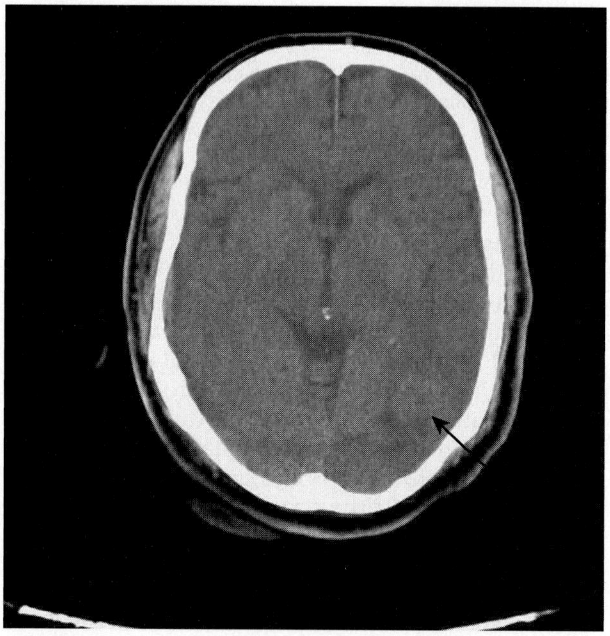

FIGURE 202-9 Noncontrast computed tomography scan of the head showing a brain tumor *(arrow).*

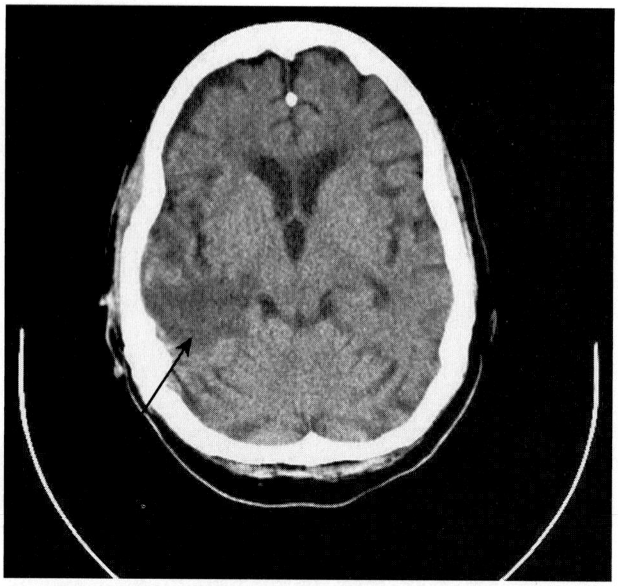

FIGURE 202-10 Noncontrast computed tomography scan of the head showing peritumoral edema *(arrow).*

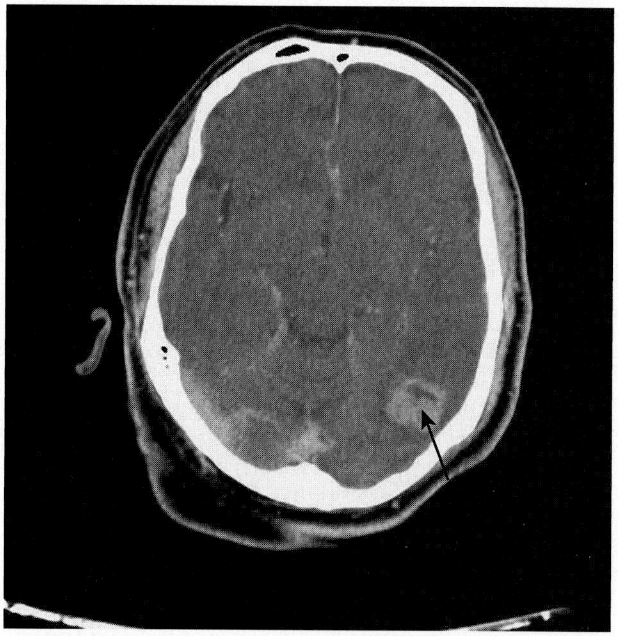

FIGURE 202-11 Contrast computed tomography scan of the head showing a brain tumor *(arrow).*

resonance imaging (MRI) is the preferred study for primary and metastatic brain tumors, but it does not need to be performed on an emergency basis (Figs. 202-8 through 202-12).

Treatment

The main goals of treatment for neurologic manifestations of oncologic emergencies are to preserve and maintain cerebral oxygenation and perfusion, to decrease inflammation and swelling, and to identify and correct the underlying condition. In the severely neurologically depressed patient with a declining Glasgow coma scale and an inability to protect the airway, rapid-sequence endotracheal intubation should be performed with supplemental oxygen to prevent cerebral hypoxia. Before intubation, care should be taken to prevent a rise in ICP, and appropriate choices for sedation and paralytic agents should be used.

Pretreatment with 1 to 1.5 mg/kg of lidocaine to blunt the rise in ICP from intubation has limited supporting evidence, but it can be used as an adjunct. Etomidate is the best choice for sedation, at a dose

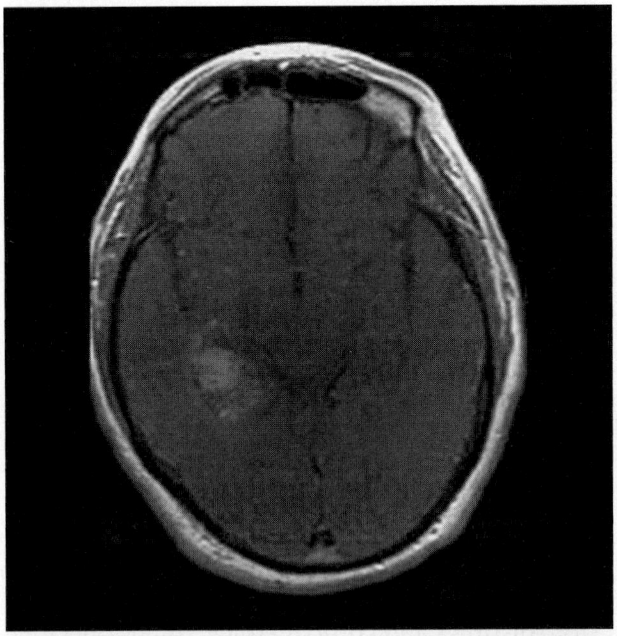

A

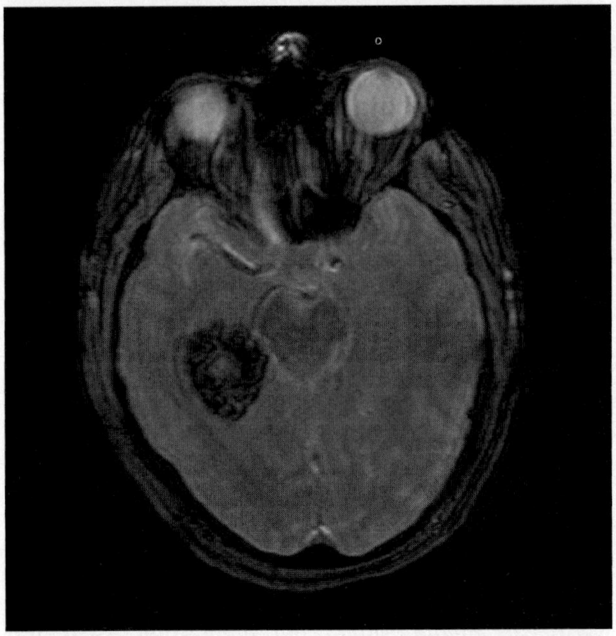

B

FIGURE 202-12 Magnetic resonance images showing brain tumor with hemorrhage and edema.

of 0.3 mg/kg, and it induces general anesthesia without raising ICP or dropping blood pressure. A defasciculating dose of a nondepolarizing agent (e.g., 0.01 mg/kg of vecuronium) may help to blunt the fasciculations caused by succinylcholine (1.5 mg/kg).

Diagnostic neuroimaging must be performed immediately following stabilization to ascertain the underlying cause of neurologic dysfunction. Once the patient is stabilized and the brain is adequately oxygenated, secondary treatments must be performed to protect the brain from further injury such as increasing edema or herniation.

Corticosteroids, specifically dexamethasone, help to reduce the inflammatory response by reducing the permeability of tumor capillaries and by clearing edema through transport of fluid into the ventricular system. Dexamethasone is the standard agent of choice because of its anti-inflammatory effects and its relative lack of mineralocorticoid activity, which may cause fluid retention. The initial dose is typically a 10-mg loading dose. If the drug is given orally, absorption is completed within 30 minutes. Tumor-related weakness is very responsive to dexamethasone treatment.

The reduction of ICP and improvement of neurologic symptoms usually begin within hours. The permeability of the blood-brain barrier has been found to improve within 6 hours, and changes in MRI demonstrating decreased edema have been shown within 2 to 3 days. The long-term side effects of corticosteroid use include gastrointestinal complications, steroid myopathy, and opportunistic infection.

If steroids alone cannot effect adequate reduction of ICP, increasing ICP can evolve into a medical emergency leading to herniation. The neurologic intensive care specialist will consider placement of a ventriculostomy to monitor the ICP and to drain cerebrospinal fluid to reduce ICP. The goal of ICP monitoring and treatment should be to keep ICP to less than 20 mm Hg and cerebral perfusion pressure (CPP) between 60 and 75 mm Hg. In the patient who has required intubation, the head of the bed should be elevated 30 degrees to decrease ICP.

Osmotic agents (e.g., mannitol, at a dose of 1 g/kg) reduce ICP 50% in 30 minutes, peak after 90 minutes, and last 4 hours. Loop diuretics (e.g., furosemide, 1 mg/kg) also decrease ICP without increasing serum osmolality. The use of mannitol or diuretics can be discussed with the neurologic intensive care specialist. Hyperventilation to reduce ICP is controversial; however, if it is performed after discussion with the neurologic intensive care specialist, all efforts should be made to keep the partial pressure of carbon dioxide between 30 and 35 mm Hg. Sedation should also be continued to reduce metabolic demand.

Blood pressure control should attempt to maintain CPP higher than 60 mm Hg, because systemic hypotension and resultant low CPP actually increase ICP. Pressors can be used safely without further increasing ICP if the blood pressure becomes too low. Hypertension should generally be treated only when CPP is higher than 120 mm Hg and the ICP is higher than 20 mm Hg, to prevent further damage. The patient should be kept euvolemic with 0.9% normal saline to ensure that no hypotension from hypovolemia or hydrocephalus from hypervolemia occurs. The patient should also be kept in the normal osmolarity range (295 to 305 mOsm); hyponatremia may be managed with hypertonic saline after discussion with the intensive care specialist because its use is controversial. Euglycemia (80 to 120 mg/dL) should be maintained for metabolic needs.

Antiemetic medications should be used so vomiting does not increase ICP. Barbiturate therapy can be

BOX 202-4

Treatment Alternatives for Patients with Acute Vasogenic Edema

Corticosteroids
- Dexamethasone (10-mg loading dose)

Osmotic agents/diuretics
- Consider mannitol (1 g/kg)
- Consider furosemide (1 mg/kg)

Antiemetics (*phenothiazine of choice* or ondansetron for refractory vomiting)

Euvolemia (0.9 normal saline)

Euglycemia (80 to 120 mg/dL)

Normal osmolarity (295 to 305 mOsm)
- Consider hypertonic saline after discussion with specialist

Blood pressure control (CPP > 60 mm Hg and CPP < 120 mm Hg when ICP > 20 mm Hg)
- Consider pressors for hypotension
- Consider calcium channel blockers or beta-blocking agents for hypertension

Airway protection with intubation if necessary
- Consider pretreatment with agent to blunt increased ICP (e.g., 1.5 mg/kg lidocaine)
- Choose sedative agent that does not increase ICP (e.g., etomidate 0.3 mg/kg)
- Consider defasciculating dose of nondepolarizing agent before depolarizing agent (e.g., 0.01 mg/kg vecuronium before 1.5 mg/kg succinylcholine)
- Elevate head of bed to 30 degrees
- Consider hyperventilation after discussion with specialist (ensure P_{CO_2} 30 to 35 mm Hg)
- Consider antiseizure medication or barbiturate therapy (i.e., lorazepam, 2 to 5 mg bolus, or pentobarbital, 5 to 20 mg/kg bolus, then 1 to 4 mg/kg/hour)

CPP, cerebral perfusion pressure; ICP, intracranial pressure; P_{CO_2}, partial pressure of carbon dioxide.

considered to reduce ICP based on the ability of these drugs to reduce brain metabolism and cerebral blood flow. Pentobarbital is generally the medication of choice, with a loading dose of 5 to 20 mg/kg as a bolus, followed by 1 to 4 mg/kg/hour. Treatment should be assessed based on ICP, CPP, and the presence of unacceptable side effects such as hypotension. Continuous electroencephalographic monitoring is generally used. Treatment alternatives to assist in the care of acute vasogenic edema are listed in Box 202-4.

The main goal of treatment in tumor-related seizures is to ensure adequate oxygenation and perfusion and to stop prolonged seizures or evolving status epilepticus. In addition to supplemental oxygenation and steps to ensure that the patient is not injured, the initial choice of medication is a benzodiazepine such as lorazepam (2 to 4 mg intravenous loading dose). If the seizure is refractory, and monotherapy with escalating doses of benzodiazepines is not working, consider the addition of phenytoin (18 mg/kg intravenous loading dose) or phenobarbital (20 mg/kg intravenous loading dose).

Prophylactic anticonvulsants are commonly considered in patients with diagnosed brain tumors but who have not had a seizure. Prophylactic anticonvulsants were reviewed by the Quality Standards Subcommittee of the American Academy of Neurology, and the summary recommendation stated that prophylaxis did not affect the frequency of subsequent seizures and should not be used in patients with either primary or metastatic brain tumors. Thus, the subcommittee believed the 5% to 25% subsequent seizure risk in brain tumors was outweighed by the deleterious interactions of anticonvulsants with cytotoxic drugs and corticosteroids. In postoperative seizure, the subcommittee recommended that anticonvulsants should be tapered and discontinued after the first postoperative week in patients who have not had a seizure, particularly in those who are medically stable and are experiencing anticonvulsant-related side effects.

Disposition

Once stabilized, patients presenting with neurologic complications of cancer require admission to the hospital. Patients with significantly depressed neurologic function require intubation, neuroprotective interventions, and intensive monitored care by a neurologic intensive care specialist. Patients who are awake, hemodynamically stable, and protecting their airway require admission to a general unit with neurology and medical oncology evaluation.

EPIDURAL SPINAL CORD COMPRESSION

Neoplastic *epidural spinal cord compression* (ESCC) is a common complication of metastatic cancer that has been documented to occur in 5% of patients with cancer.[13] The most widely accepted definition includes any radiographic indentation of the thecal sac. Although the cauda equina is not technically considered part of the spinal cord, the pathophysiology of compression of the cauda equina is the same as that of the spinal cord. Thus, compression of the thecal sac by malignancy at this level is also referred to as ESCC.

The most common primary tumors are prostate, breast, and lung cancer, which tend to metastasize to the vertebral column. Other important primary tumors are renal cell carcinoma, multiple myeloma, non-Hodgkin's lymphoma, and plasmacytoma, which make up the majority of the remaining cases. In children, the most common causes are sarcomas, neuroblastomas, Hodgkin's lymphoma, and germ cell tumors. Delays in diagnosis and treatment remain common, and reports from multiple countries describe poor neurologic outcome in half or more of patients diagnosed with ESCC, including motor weakness, bladder dysfunction, and inability to ambulate.[14-16]

Clinical Presentation

The most common presenting symptom of ESCC is back pain, occurring in more than 80% of patients.[13] In general, pain precedes the onset of neurologic symptoms by several weeks. The pain is generally slowly progressive, although abrupt worsening of pain may signal a pathologic compression fracture. The pain may worsen with recumbency, movement, or the Valsalva maneuver, or it may develop a radicular quality. The radicular pain may be bilateral, especially in thoracic lesions.

Motor weakness is present in the majority of patients with ESCC at the time of diagnosis. When the cauda equina is compressed, the deep tendon reflexes may also be depressed. Laterally situated tumors may cause isolated motor radiculopathy or radiculopathy superimposed on bilateral lower extremity weakness. Weakness tends to be most pronounced in patients with thoracic lesions.

Sensory findings are present in more than half the patients with ESCC. Patients often report ascending numbness or paresthesias. When a sensory level is present, it is generally several levels below the actual level of spinal cord compression. Cauda equina lesions result in saddle anesthesia, whereas higher lesions often spare these sacral dermatomes. Like motor symptoms, sensory symptoms can occur in a radicular pattern.

Bowel dysfunction and bladder dysfunction are often late findings, but these disorders are often present by the time of diagnosis of ESCC. The most common presenting symptom is urinary retention, which may be potentiated by the use of narcotic analgesics for the back pain. Other signs and symptoms of myelopathy that may indicate ESCC include diminished proprioception, ataxia, spasticity, reflex hyperactivity, and autonomic dysfunction.

Diagnostic Testing

Although plain radiography is easily accessible in the ED and is able to predict ESCC in the majority of patients with an evident lesion, it is still generally inadequate. Between 10% and 17% of patients will have ESCC without findings on plain radiography.[13]

MRI and myelography (or CT myelography) remain the cornerstones of diagnosis for ESCC. MRI holds several advantages in that it is accurate, reliable, noninvasive, and able to image the entire thecal sac regardless of whether myelographic block is present (Fig. 202-13).

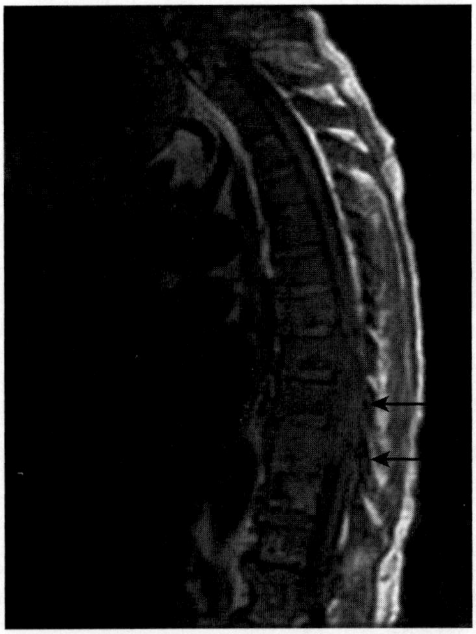

FIGURE 202-13 Magnetic resonance image demonstrating compression of the thecal sac *(arrows)*.

In general, definitive imaging is necessary when ESCC is suspected. Imaging should be performed on an emergency basis in any patient with evidence of neurologic dysfunction suspected to be caused by ESCC. In patients with cancer who have new or worsening back pain without any evidence of neurologic dysfunction and a normal plain radiograph, it is probably reasonable to allow urgent outpatient definitive imaging.

Treatment

When epidural metastatic lesions are found in the investigation for ESCC, therapy is indicated for any patients who have not had prolonged paraplegia (more than several days). The cornerstones of therapy are corticosteroids, radiation therapy, and, in some cases, surgery.

The value of corticosteroids to relieve edema contributing to spinal cord compression is well documented. What remains controversial is the dosage of dexamethasone. Initial bolus doses of anywhere from 10 to 100 mg have been used, with no clear answer on the most appropriate dosage. Subsequent lower doses may be given orally as directed by the consultant specialist. Steroids should be given immediately, even before MRI scanning if ESCC is strongly suspected, or if ESCC is suspected and appropriate imaging will be delayed for any reason.

Neurosurgery should be consulted immediately for cases of ESCC. The consultant will weigh the neurologic status of the patient and clinical variables such as life expectancy to tailor a treatment plan for the patient including radiation therapy or surgery.

Disposition and Prognosis

Patients with ESCC are admitted to the hospital, and they should have early ED consultation by a neurosurgeon. In general, the outcomes of patients following ESCC heavily depend on the neurologic status of the patient at the time of diagnosis. Although the median survival of patients diagnosed with ESCC is 6 months, the outcome is better in patients who are ambulatory at the time of diagnosis. Patients with lung cancer as the source of metastatic disease have poorer prognosis than those with breast or prostate cancer.

REFERENCES

1. Klatt EC, Heitz DR: Cardiac metastases. Cancer 1990;65:1456-1459.
2. Guberman BA, Fowler NO, Engel PJ, et al: Cardiac tamponade in medical patients. Circulation 1981;64:633-640.
3. Bruch C, Schmermund A, Dagres N, et al: Changes in QRS voltage in cardiac tamponade and pericardial effusion: Reversibility after pericardiocentesis and after anti-inflammatory drug treatment. J Am Coll Cardiol 2001;38:219-226.
4. Mandavia DP, Hoffner RJ, Mahaney K, Henderson SO: Bedside echocardiography by emergency physicians. Ann Emerg Med 2001;38:377-382.
5. Ahmann FR: A reassessment of the clinical implications of the superior vena caval syndrome. J Clin Oncol 1984;8:961-969.
6. Schraufnagel DE, Hill R, Leech JA, et al: Superior vena caval obstruction: Is it a medical emergency? Am J Med 1981;70:1169-1174.
7. Davenport D, Ferree C, Blake D, et al: Radiation therapy in the treatment of superior vena caval obstruction. Cancer 1978;42:2600-2603.
8. Parish JM, Marschke RF, Dines DE, et al: Etiologic considerations in superior vena cava syndrome. Mayo Clin Proc 1981;56:407-413.
9. Central Brain Tumor Registry of the United States (CBTRUS): Primary Brain Tumors in the United States, 1997-2001. CBTRUS Statistical Report. Chicago, Central Brain Tumor Registry of the United States, 2004.
10. Forsyth PA, Posner JB: Headaches in patients with brain tumors: A study of 111 patients. Neurology 1993; 43:1678-1683.
11. Coia LR, Aaronson N, Linggood R, et al: A report of the consensus workshop panel on the treatment of brain metastases. Int J Radiat Oncol Biol Phys 1992;23:223-227.
12. Clouston PD, DeAngelis LM, Posner JB: The spectrum of neurological disease in patients with systemic cancer. Ann Neurol 1992;31:268-273.
13. Bach F, Larsen BH, Rohde K, et al: Metastatic spinal cord compression: Occurrence, symptoms, clinical presentations, and prognosis in 398 patients with spinal cord compression. Acta Neurochir (Wien) 1990;107:37-43.
14. Husband DJ: Malignant spinal cord compression: Prospective study of delays in referral and treatment. BMJ 1998;317:18-21.
15. Helweg-Larsen S: Clinical outcome in metastatic spinal cord compression: A prospective study of 153 patients. Acta Neurol Scand 1996;94:269-275.
16. Milross CG, Davies MA, Fisher R, et al: The efficacy of treatment for malignant spinal cord compression. Australas Radiol 1997;41:137-142.

Chapter 203

White Blood Cell Disorders

Jay Lemery

KEY POINTS

Patients with hematologic malignancies often present to the ED with life-threatening, rapidly progressing diseases.

Immunocompromised patients often present with subtle signs and symptoms.

Rapid evaluation and intervention by the ED are essential to minimize morbidity and mortality.

The differential diagnoses of common ED complaints (dyspnea, abdominal pain) are much broader in these patients; an understanding of these diseases is essential for emergency diagnosis and management.

Scope

The National Cancer Institute has estimated that approximately 750,000 people are living with blood cancers in the United States, and an additional roughly 115,000 new cases were expected in 2006 (8% of all cancers diagnosed annually). With an estimated 55,000 deaths in 2005, the 5-year survival rates range from 32% (myeloma) to 85% (Hodgkin's lymphoma).[1] These numbers are expected to increase over the next few decades with the rising number of geriatric patients in the United States. In addition, the number of long-term survivors of cancer has increased dramatically, as has the number of patients living with treatment-related side effects from the increasing regimens of aggressive therapy.[2]

Epidemiology

Although rates vary among institutions, one epidemiologic study at a community teaching hospital with an annual ED census of 31,000 cited that roughly 5% of all patients presenting to the ED had a history of cancer, and of this subset, roughly 13% had a documented history of lymphoma or leukemia (≈1% of patients with a history of cancer presented with neutropenic fever).[3]

Structure and Function

Hematologic malignancies encompass a varied group of blood cell disorders, each with separate disease entities and different pathophysiologies and treatments. The treatment approach to these patients in the ED is less well understood by the histologic differences among these diseases than by their common systemic manifestations, such as fever, dyspnea, abdominal pain, or vague complaints of being "weak and dizzy." These diseases can manifest with emergency, life-threatening complications, and that presentation is the focus of this chapter (Boxes 203-1 to 203-8).

Presenting Signs and Symptoms

Signs and symptoms of leukemia result from anemia (fatigue, weakness, shortness of breath), thrombocy-

BOX 203-1

Hematologic Malignancies

- Chronic myelogenous leukemia (CML)
- Hairy cell leukemia
- Chronic lymphocytic leukemia (CLL)
- Acute lymphocytic leukemia (ALL)
- Acute myelogenous leukemia (AML)
- Hodgkin's disease
- Non-Hodgkin's lymphomas
- Plasma cell disorders
- Primary amyloidosis

BOX 203-2

Chronic Myelogenous Leukemia

- The patient presents with marked splenomegaly (>60%) and very high white blood cell counts (25,000 to 100,000/µL).
- The Philadelphia chromosome (Ph^1) is present in the basement membrane in more than 95% of cases.
- Fatigue, weight loss, early satiety, and left upper quadrant fullness are the most common symptoms.
- One third of patients develop a blast crisis over the course of the disease.

Adapted from Swenson K, Rose M, Ritz L, et al: Recognition and evaluation of oncology-related symptoms in the emergency department. Ann Emerg Med 1995;26:12-17.

BOX 203-3

Hairy Cell Leukemia

- This form of leukemia is uncommon (1% to 2% of all leukemias).
- Fatigue (secondary anemia), fever, weight loss, and splenomegaly are prominent.
- Patients may present only with infection (secondary granulocytopenia or monocytopenia).
- Gram-positive and gram-negative infections occur, as well as tuberculosis, atypical mycobacterial infection, and fungal infections.
- Pneumonia and septicemia are common causes of death.
- More than two thirds of patients have anemia, neutropenia, thrombacytopenia, and monocytopenia.
- Osteolytic bone lesions can also be seen.

Adapted from Swenson K, Rose M, Ritz L, et al: Recognition and evaluation of oncology-related symptoms in the emergency department. Ann Emerg Med 1995;26:12-17.

BOX 203-4

Chronic Lymphocytic Leukemia

- Most patients are asymptomatic; the disease is diagnosed with absolute lymphocytosis in peripheral blood.
- Nonspecific symptoms include fatigue, weight loss, anorexia, and lethargy.
- Many patients have predominantly cervical lymphadenopathy, which can progress to systemic lymphadenopathy causing luminal obstruction.
- Obstructive jaundice, uropathy, dysphagia, or partial small bowel obstruction may be noted.
- With disease progression, sinopulmonary infections can progress to gram-negative, fungal, and viral infections.

Adapted from Swenson K, Rose M, Ritz L, et al: Recognition and evaluation of oncology-related symptoms in the emergency department. Ann Emerg Med 1995;26:12-17.

topenia (easy bruising, petechiae), granulocytopenia (fever, infection), and leukemic infiltration of liver, spleen (abdominal pain), and superficial lymph nodes.

HEMORRHAGE

When the platelet count is less than 20,000/µL, bleeding from the gums, nose, gastrointestinal (GI) tract, or other location can occur. Petechiae or ecchymosis may be evident. Intracranial hemorrhage can result from clumping of blasts, causing hemorrhagic infarction, most commonly when the peripheral leukocyte count exceeds 150,000/µL.

Massive hemorrhage can occur in patients with acute promyelocytic leukemia. Between 5% and 8% of patients with leukemia have acute promyelocytic leukemia. The median age is younger than other subtypes (40 years versus 70 years). It is more frequently associated with disseminated intravascular coagulation and significant bleeding. The primary presentation to the ED may be a life-threatening bleeding episode. Early recognition is additionally important because of the unique sensitivity of acute promyelocytic leukemia to all-*trans*-retinoic acid (ATRA), a derivative of vitamin A. Treatment increases differentiation and thus promotes maturation of the granulocytes. Remission is possible in up to 90% of patients.

BOX 203-5

Acute Leukemias

- Anemia, infection, and bleeding are the most common complications secondary to myeloinvasive pancytopenia.
- ALL: No early peak occurs, and the incidence increases with age.
- AML: The maximal incidence is at 2 to 10 years of age, with a second peak later in life.
- ALL infiltrates normal organs more than AML.
- AML has greater incidence of life-threatening infections than ALL.
- Rapidly progressive, antileukemic therapy should be started as soon as possible (<48 hours).

ALL, acute lymphocytic leukemia; AML, acute myelogenous leukemia.
Adapted from Appelbaum FA: The acute leukemias. In Goldman L, Ausiello DA (eds): Cecil Textbook of Medicine, 22nd ed. Philadelphia, WB Saunders, 2004, pp 1161-1166.

BOX 203-6

Hodgkin's Disease

- This distinct malignant disorder of the lymphatic system primarily affects the lymph nodes.
- Bimodal incidence occurs, with the first peak in the third decade of life and a smaller peak in patients >50 years old.
- Regional lymphadenopathy is the rule:
  - >80% present with lymphadenopathy above the diaphragm
  - Often the anterior mediastinum is involved: cough, wheeze, chest pain
  - Cervical, supraclavicular, axillary, (uncommonly) inguinal lymphadenopathy
- Patients may present with systemic symptoms:
  - Chronic pruritus with excoriations
  - "B" symptoms: fever, night sweats, or weight loss
- Abnormal blood profile includes the following:
  - Leukocytosis with neutrophilia
  - Eosinophilia
  - Thrombocytosis
  - Pancytopenia

From Swenson K, Rose M, Ritz L, et al: Recognition and evaluation of oncology-related symptoms in the emergency department. Ann Emerg Med 1995;26:12-17.

BOX 203-7

Non-Hodgkin's Lymphomas

- Include B-cell and T-cell and NK cell lymphomas.
- Increased incidence past 4 decades:
  - Human immunodeficiency virus epidemic, aging population, improved diagnostic tools
  - Lymphadenopathy most common presentation
- Chest pain, cough, superior vena cava syndrome, abdominal pain, back pain, spinal cord compression, and renal insufficiency (ureteral compression)
- Systemic symptoms
  - Fevers, night sweats, weight loss
  - Organ failure involving any organ in the body
  - May present with immunogenic abnormalities
- Hemolytic anemia or thrombocytopenia

From Bierman P, Harris N, Armitage J, et al: Non-Hodgkin's lym-phomas. In Goldman L, Ausiello DA (eds): Cecil Textbook of Medicine, 22nd ed. Philadelphia, WB Saunders, 2004, pp 1174-1184.

BOX 203-8

Plasma Cell Disorders

- Proliferation of a single clone of immunoglobulin-secreting plasma cells
  - Homogenous monoclonal proteins
- Included conditions
  - Monoclonal gammopathies of undetermined significance (MGUS)
  - Multiple myeloma
  - Waldenström's macroglobulinemia
  - Heavy-chain diseases
  - Cryoglobulinemia
  - Primary amyloidosis
- Symptoms
  - Hyperviscosity syndromes
  - Bone pain (more than two thirds at diagnosis)
  - Pathologic fractures (>80% on radiograph)
  - Weakness and fatigue, often with anemia
  - Bleeding (Waldenström's macroglobulinemia), especially in oronasal areas
- Less common: acute infections, renal insufficiency, hypercalcemia
- Leukapheresis (with chemotherapy) for hyperviscosity complications

From Kyle RA, Rajkumar SV: Plasma cell disorders. In Goldman L, Ausiello DA (eds): Cecil Textbook of Medicine, 22nd ed. Philadelphia, WB Saunders, 2004, pp 1184-1195.

FEVER

Cancer treatment often hinders the immune system of a patient and causes an increased propensity for infection and a reduced ability to mount an immune response. Patients may appear well or toxic. *Fever* is defined as a temperature higher than 38.3°C (101°F) or higher than 38.0°C (100.4°F) over at least 1 hour. *Neutropenia* is defined as an absolute granulocyte count of less than 500/mm^3.[4]

Patients often have a history of recent chemotherapy, many approximately 1 week earlier, a timetable that places these patients in neutrophilic nadir. Chemotherapeutic agents disrupt chemotaxis and phagocytosis and interfere with the neutrophils' ability to disrupt intracellular microorganisms.

Although it is not technically neutropenia, patients with acute leukemia crisis or non-Hodgkin's lymphoma may suffer from functional neutropenia and should be considered neutropenic. Other causes, including radiation therapy and glucocorticoids, can also functionally impair neutrophils and diminish neutrophil recovery.

Patients may exhibit subtle findings, given their decrease in inflammatory response. Depending on the duration and severity of the condition and on the pathogen, the patient may have a varied clinical presentation. The potential for infection is proportional to the rate of neutrophil decline and the degree of granulocytopenia.[5] Between 48% and 60% of febrile neutropenic patients have an established or occult infection.[8]

The clinical should search for subtle signs of infection including a thorough examination of the head, ears, eyes, nose, and throat, including the gingiva, pharynx, and fundi. The perineal and anal areas should be examined, as well as the entire skin and vascular access sites (Fig. 203-1).

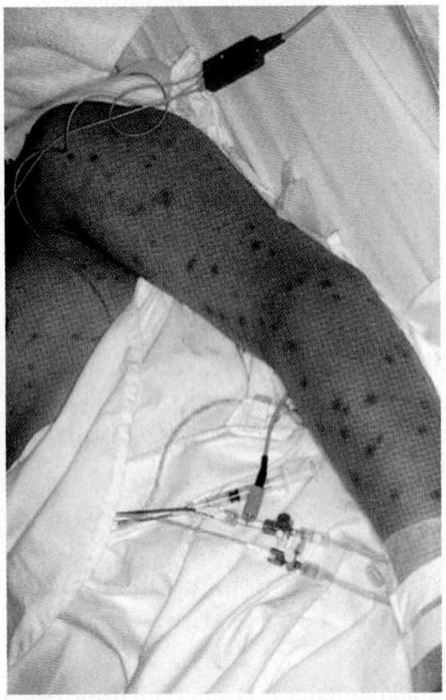

FIGURE 203-1 Disseminated candidiasis in a patient with chronic lymphocytic leukemia. (Courtesy of Jeff Groeger, M.D.)

ABDOMINAL PAIN

Abdominal pain is one of the most common symptoms in the patient with hematologic malignant disease, and it is one of the most difficult to diagnose by examination. Fortunately for the ED physician, CT and ultrasound imaging can determine life-threatening from chronic complications of leukemia.

Pain associated with nausea is commonly related to chemotherapeutic complications. The GI tract is one of the systems most sensitive to chemotherapy-induced mucosal damage. Although many patients can be appropriately treated with conservative management (antiemetics or fluid resuscitation or both), clinicians should have a low threshold for pursuing a radiographic work-up. After chemotherapy, patients often have a few-day history of nausea and anorexia, progressing to vomiting. These patients commonly present severely volume depleted and may have tachycardia, orthostatic hypotension, and dry mucous membranes. Patients may have a concomitant chief complaint of (pre)syncope. Many of these patients may be taking opioids for pain relief and may simply have constipation.

Although abdominal tenderness may help to pinpoint a focal diagnosis, these patients often have multisystemic disease, and clinicians should apply a broad diagnostic strategy, including abdominal CT imaging. As mentioned earlier, patients may have a diminished inflammatory response secondary to neutropenia and anti-inflammatory drug regimens. Therefore, abdominal examinations should not determine whether to obtain a CT scan or surgical consultation. Focal findings, when present, may be very helpful in tailoring a differential diagnosis. Obstructive adenopathy is a common problem in these patients and can affect the biliary tract, the renal collecting system, and the GI. Patients may present with an acute condition or with vague symptoms of chronic organ failure.

Patients with hematologic malignancies have a high incidence of splenomegaly, which may manifest as left upper quadrant discomfort. Although often resulting from myeloproliferation or lymphoproliferation, splenic vein thrombosis (hypercoagulable state of malignancy) must be considered an alternative diagnosis and excluded. Symptoms may include early satiety from compression of the stomach by the enlarged spleen. Physical examination findings of bruits may indicate inordinate blood return from a grossly enlarged spleen, thus increasing a concern for variceal bleeding. A left upper quadrant friction rub may indicate splenic infarction.

Veno-occlusive disease of the liver is a known complication of hematologic malignancies and consists of the triad of jaundice, painful hepatomegaly, and fluid retention or ascites. This disorder is often seen after stem cell transplantation. A rapid increase in intra-abdominal fluid may compromise respiratory effort with an upward displacement of the diaphragm, and these patients may present with respiratory failure.

■ Typhlitis

Mucosal damage to the GI tract can also occur. It may be secondary to leukemic infiltration, and it can cause GI bleeding and even perforation. Neutropenia in these patients can lead to perianal inflammation, abscesses, peritonitis, and necrotic enterocolitis, also known as *leukemic typhlitis*. Typhlitis is an inflammatory disease of the ascending colon that manifests with fever, abdominal pain (most commonly right lower quadrant), nausea, diarrhea, and hypotension[10] (Fig. 203-2). It is most common among pediatric patients undergoing high-dose chemotherapy for leukemia. Cecal distention in typhlitis may impair the blood supply and may thus lead to mucosal ischemia and ulceration. Classic findings on CT scans are circumferential low-attenuation colonic wall thickening and cecal distention. Inflammatory tissue appearing as mesenteric fat stranding is a common finding. High attenuation within the thickened colonic wall may represent hemorrhage. CT imaging may also detect potential surgical complications such as colonic wall hemorrhage, pneumatosis coli, pneumoperitoneum, and abscesses. Because of the myriad abdominal syndromes in patients with hematologic malignant disease, the diagnosis of common surgical emergencies can rarely be ascertained without CT imaging. Appendicitis and typhilitis have been shown to occur with similar frequency in children with leukemia and lymphoma.[11] Typhlitis may result in gram-negative bacteremia and, less commonly, candidemia, especially in patients who have not improved after administration of broad-spectrum antibiotics. Other causes of abdominal pain that are common in this group and that may not have pathologic radiologic features include hypercalcemia (see later), early zoster, and depression.

■ DYSPNEA

Patients presenting to the ED with dyspnea should be approached with a rapid assessment of respiratory status and should be given immediate resuscitative care in the form of supplemental oxygen, assisted ventilation, or intubation with mechanical ventilation. Despite this initial universal approach to the dyspneic patient, investigation of the broad differential diagnosis is essential to formulating an emergency care plan.

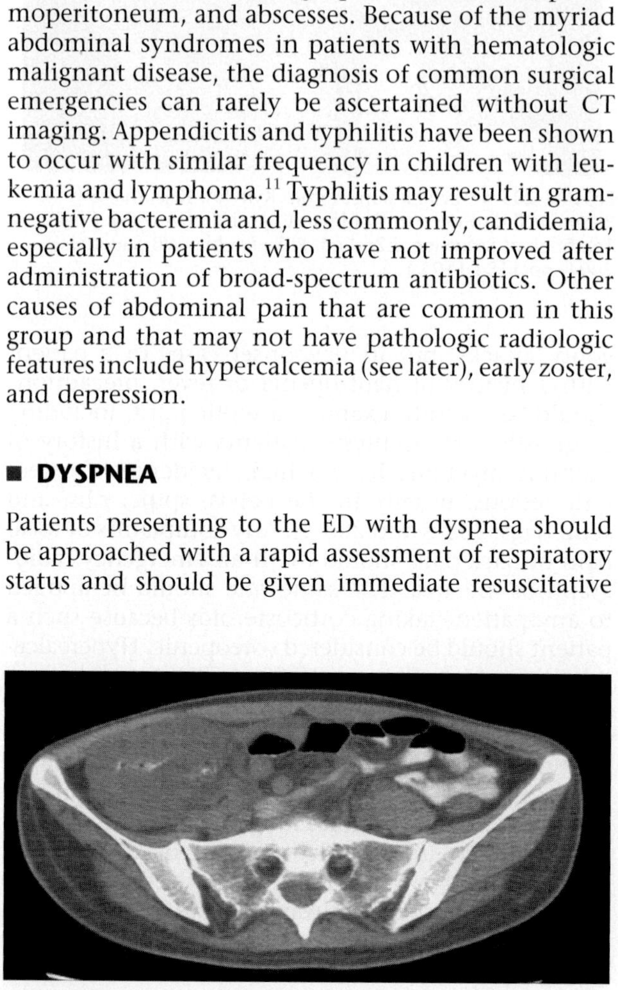

FIGURE 203-2 Computed tomography image of typhlitis. (Courtesy of Anita Price, M.D.)

Infection is one of the most common problems in patients with hematologic malignancies who present to the ED with dyspnea. These patients are especially predisposed to infection given their predisposition to neutropenia, frequent use of antibiotics or corticosteroids or both, prolonged hospital stays, asplenia, and defects in humoral immunity. Fever is generally present, but cough and sputum production are not always evident. Chest radiographs may initially be nondiagnostic. Encapsulated bacteria, *Pneumocystis jiroveci* (formerly *Pneumocystis carinii*), and *Mycoplasma pneumoniae* are common in patients with hematologic malignancies. Chemotherapy-induced neutropenia can give rise to *Staphylococcus aureus*, gram-negative bacilli, and fungi (*Aspergillus* and *Candida*).[12] Patients with tracheostomies, those who require assisted ventilation, and patients with swallowing difficulties may be at risk for aspiration pneumonia.

Pulmonary embolism remains an insidious and lethal complication in all patients with cancer. The hypercoagulable state of malignancy, the presence of indwelling catheters, a forced sedentary state of patients, and chemotherapeutic agents all contribute to this increased risk. Pulmonary emboli are notoriously difficult to diagnose on clinical presentation and are even less obvious in patients with cancer.[13] Symptoms of dyspnea, pleuritic chest pain, and palpitations and signs of tachycardia, tachypnea, and hypoxia should encourage the clinician to be aggressive about ruling out pulmonary embolism.

Pleural and pericardial effusions are common complications of malignant disease and should be rapidly excluded in any emergency work-up. Pericardial effusions can quickly lead to cardiac tamponade and circulatory collapse. These patients may present with subtle signs of dyspnea, hypoxia, or tachypnea. Often, they have recently been evaluated and treated for pneumonia, and they attribute their symptoms to "worsening pneumonia." Rapid evaluation can be made with ED cardiac ultrasonography. Lower lobe pleural effusions can similarly be seen on hepatorenal and splenorenal sonography views, respectively.

Patients with chemotherapy-related and radiation-induced lung injuries often present with nonspecific complaints such as fever, exertional dyspnea, and nonproductive cough, which may or may not correlate well with the timing of treatment. Often, these patients have diagnoses of exclusion, ascertained after extensive radiography, cultures, and even bronchoscopy or biopsy. Heart failure is a known complication of chemotherapy, but this too is a diagnosis of exclusion, and the patient in the ED should be approached with a broad differential diagnosis and treatment plan. Other postchemotherapeutic and radiation changes to the lung include pulmonary fibrosis, interstitial pneumonitis, and inflammatory syndromes such as bronchiolitis obliterans.

Blood count abnormalities can directly cause dyspneic events. Alveolar hemorrhage is common in patients with leukemia, multiple myeloma, and bone marrow transplantation, and it can occur in patients with platelet counts lower than $50{,}000/mm^3$.[12] Patients present with dyspnea, fever, and focal infiltrates on chest radiography that may be interpreted as a pneumonic process. They infrequently present with hemoptysis. Pulmonary leukostasis (leukocytes $>100{,}000/\mu L$) may manifest as hypoxemic respiratory failure because leukocytes aggregate in the small vessels of the lung. Patients with hyperleukocytic leukemia may have an artificially low partial pressure of arterial oxygen on arterial blood gas analysis despite the absence of pulmonary involvement. This is thought to result from oxygen metabolism by the leukocytes in the arterial blood gas syringe between blood draw and analysis. This process can be eliminated by rapid blood gas analysis on ice or by the addition of potassium cyanide to the blood gas syringe.[12]

Severely anemic patients can present with dyspnea on exertion and chest discomfort. Electrocardiographic ischemic changes may be seen in patient with underlying microvascular disease. Conversely, patients who have received recent transfusions with packed red blood cells or platelets may suffer from transfusion-related lung injury. This syndrome manifests with fever, hypoxemia, lung infiltrates, and noncardiogenic pulmonary edema.

Although mass effect airway obstruction is less likely in hematologic malignancies than in other cancers of the head and neck, patients with T-cell acute lymphocytic leukemia may suffer from an enlarged thymus gland that causes dyspnea and chest pain.

Although the EP may not have immediate access to a patient's medical records during the initial assessment, every effort should be made, particularly for patients with end-stage disease, to determine the patient's wishes regarding invasive procedures. Although this determination may not be possible in a critically ill patient, the ability to honor the care wishes of a patient or family is as important as any medical service we provide.

■ MALAISE AND BODY PAINS

Often, patients with hematologic malignancies present to the ED with vague symptoms of pain, malaise, and weakness. As discussed earlier, although a broad diagnostic approach should be applied to these patients, this discussion focuses on some of the unique conditions that may present as emergencies and that may affect initial therapy.

Musculoskeletal pain in the patient with hematologic malignancy can often be attributed to serologic abnormalities. The increased level of serum uric acid (caused by increased leukocyte turnover) can precipitate gouty attacks. Often, the patient has had prior gouty attacks, but in new-onset cases in a patient with a history of neutropenia or fever, precautions should be taken to examine a septic joint, including diagnostic arthrocentesis. Patients with a history of multiple myeloma have a high incidence of osteolytic lesions, usually in the pelvis, spine, ribs, and skull (Figs. 203-3 and 203-4). Any complaints of focal pain or back pain should merit an emergency radiograph of the area. The same rule should be applied to any patient taking corticosteroids because such a patient should be considered osteopenic. Hypercalcemia is common in cancer (10% to 20% of all known malignancies), and it often manifests with vague symptoms of nausea or vomiting, abdominal pain, and muscle or joint aches. In multiple myeloma, hypercalcemia results from bone destruction. In Hodgkin's disease or non-Hodgkin's lymphoma, it is caused by the increased conversion of 25-hydroxycholecalciferol to calcitriol by tumor cells.[14] An electrocardiogram should always be part of an initial work-up for evaluation of a short QT interval, which may progress to heart block.

Numerous soft tissue disorders are common in hematologic malignancies. *Oral mucositis* is

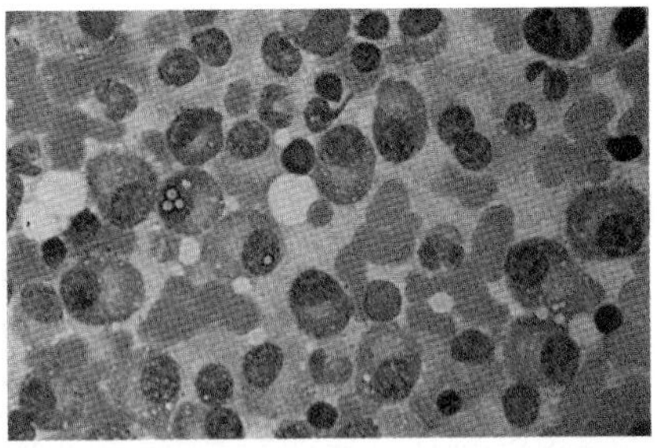

FIGURE 203-3 Multiple myeloma. (From Kyle RA, Rajkumar SV: Plasma cell disorders. In Goldman L, Ausiello DA (eds): Cecil Textbook of Medicine, 22nd ed. Philadelphia, WB Saunders, 2004, pp 1184-1195.)

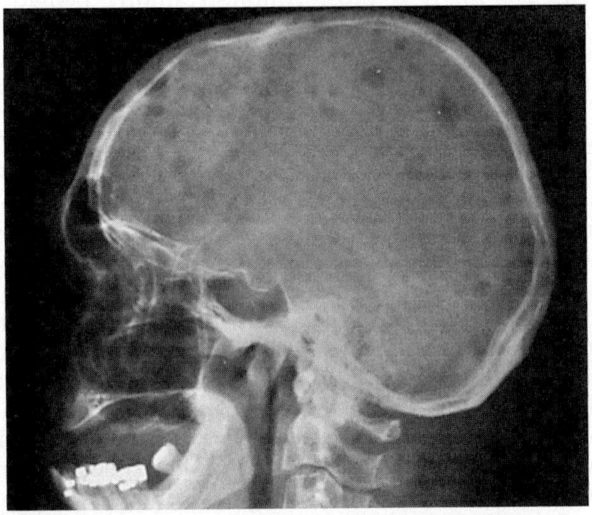

FIGURE 203-4 Lytic lesions. (From Kyle RA, Rajkumar SV: Plasma cell disorders. In Goldman L, Ausiello DA (eds): Cecil Textbook of Medicine, 22nd ed. Philadelphia, WB Saunders, 2004, pp 1184-1195.)

inflammation and ulceration of the oral mucous membranes, and it can be the result of disease (non-Hodgkin's lymphoma) or treatment (chemotherapy, radiation, or bone marrow transplantation). Patient can present with relatively minor symptoms of pain, ulcerations, and dry mouth, which can progress to infection, bleeding, and dysphasia and can culminate in sepsis complicated by poor nutritional status from anorexia. In extreme cases, bleeding from mucositis may present an airway risk, necessitating endotracheal intubation. *Skin lesions* that may suggest an underlying disease include cutaneous vasculitis in the form of palpable purpura (systemic [hairy cell] vasculitis) or the cutaneous nodules of leukemia cutis (neoplastic leukocyte infiltrates in the epidermis or dermis). Often, the latter condition manifests with local lymphadenopathy and a constellation of constitutional symptoms suggestive of systemic disease.

Leukostasis refers to the intravascular clumping of blast cells in the setting of an increased white blood cell count (Fig. 203-5). In addition to dyspnea and chest pain secondary to leukemic infiltration of the pulmonary vessels, an intravascular sludging effect may occur, manifesting as a pain crisis similar to that seen in sickle cell disease. Less commonly, patients have *central nervous system involvement,* which may manifest as headache, diplopia, cranial nerve palsies, or peripheral motor or sensory deficits. The *hyperviscosity syndrome of multiple myeloma* and *Waldenström's macroglobulinemia* are similar pathologic processes of increased serum viscosity from a proliferation of serum immunoglobulin. Classic clinical symptoms are the triad of mucosal bleeding (epistaxis, menorrhagias, rectal bleeding), visual changes, and varied neurologic symptoms including vertigo, paraesthesias, headaches, and ataxia.[15] Neuropathy can also be seen and is thought to be secondary to immunoglobulin M antibody reacting with a myelin-associated glycoprotein.[16]

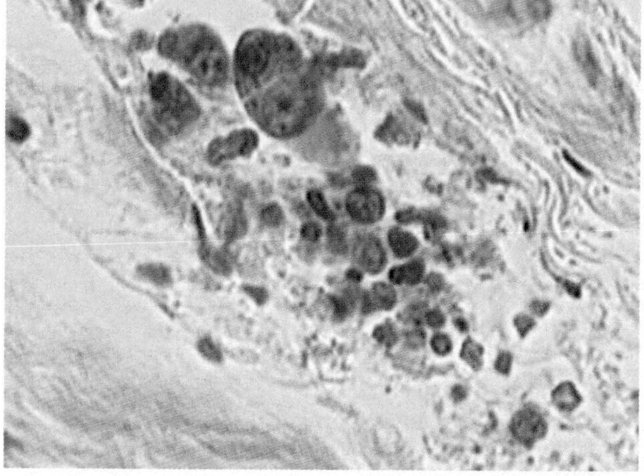

FIGURE 203-5 Leukostasis. (Courtesy Donald J. Innes, Jr., M.D., Professor of Pathology, University of Virginia School of Medicine, Charlottesville, VA.)

One of the pitfalls of the acute treatment of a lymphoproliferative crisis is the *tumor lysis syndrome*. It results from the rapid breakdown of malignant cells. This tumor cell lysis produces serologic increases in potassium, phosphate, and uric acid. Deposition of uric acid and calcium phosphate crystals at the renal tubules, combined with concomitant intravascular depletion, may precipitate acute renal failure.[17] A systemic inflammatory response may ensue that can mimic septic shock.

The EP must also be vigilant for constitutional complaints of malaise or diffuse pain (Box 203-9). *Renal failure* can often initially manifest with vague symptoms. Renal failure is a common complication of bone marrow transplantation. It can also result from chemotherapeutic toxicity, and it can have an iatrogenic cause, such as intravenous radiographic contrast media.

Interventions and Procedures

■ LEUKAPHERESIS

Leukapheresis is the definitive treatment of choice for patients with hyperviscosity leukostasis. This technique is a rapid and effective means of lowering high white blood cell counts in the setting of acute leukemic blast crises in patients with counts in the several hundreds or plasma cell disorders (multiple myeloma, Waldenström's macroglobulinemia).

Leukapheresis is indicated in patients with end-organ symptoms including visual disturbances ("sausage-like" hemorrhagic retinal veins are pathognomic), dizziness, cardiopulmonary symptoms, decreased consciousness, or bleeding diatheses.[16,19] Chemotherapy should be considered in conjunction with leukapheresis (alkylating agent–steroid combinations), to minimize malignant cell proliferation. A serum viscosity of more than 5 cP suggests hyperviscosity syndrome, and repeat leukapheresis may be needed to control refractory episodes.[19]

Because the effects of leukapheresis may be temporary, chemotherapy is considered the mainstay for achieving long-term cytoreduction. Other adjuncts include hydroxyurea, a ribonucleotide reductase inhibitor used to control leukocytosis that may be started in the ED in consultation with a hematologist.

Hypercalcemia of malignancy should be treated aggressively in the ED. Volume expansion with crystalloid is the initial preferred treatment, then followed by loop diuretics after adequate volume expansion. Other adjuncts to be considered are bisphosphonates (etidronate or pamidronate), which decrease efflux of calcium from bone and reduce bone pain.[20] Dialysis should be considered for any patient with severe hypercalcemia and renal failure.

The two therapeutic goals for patients who present to the ED with tumor lysis syndrome are aggressive hydration and treatment of hyperuricemia. Aggressive hydration facilitates renal excretion of uric acid

BOX 203-9

Differential Diagnosis

Fever (Nonlocalizing)
- Granulocytopenia
  - Bacterial → fungal → breakthrough fungemia
  - Great increase in the last 15 years of gram-positive organisms, often MRSA
- Cell-mediated immunodeficiency
  - Viral
  - Mycobacterial, fungal, nocardial, listerial
- Humoral immune deficiency
  - B-cell, splenectomy related

Abdominal Pain
- Chemotherapy-related nausea and dehydration
- Splenomegaly
- Obstructive adenopathy: jaundice/uropathy/small bowel obstruction
- Organ-specific pain
  - Ascites/spontaneous bacterial peritonitis
  - Portal vein thrombosis
- Mesenteric ischemia
- Typhlitis (neutropenic enterocolitis)
- Zoster
- Constipation (opioid)
- Hypercalcemia
- Psychogenic/depression

Dyspnea
- Pneumonia
- Pulmonary embolism
- Pleural effusion
- Pericardial effusion
- *Pneumocystis* pneumonia
- Acute respiratory distress syndrome
- Chemotherapeutic and radiographic toxicity
- Hyperviscosity leukostasis
- Paraneoplastic syndromes
- Heart failure
  - Chemotherapy related
- Adrenal insufficiency
- Thymus: pain and dyspnea with T-cell ALL infiltration
- Bronchiolitis obliterans organizing pneumonia
- Mass effect and obstruction
- Anemia
- Chronic obstructive pulmonary disease
- Anxiety disorder
- Superior vena cava syndrome

Malaise and Body Pains
- Elevated uric acid levels/gouty arthritis
- Osteolytic lesions
- Osteopenic fractures (corticosteroid induced)
- Hypercalcemia
- Oral mucositis
- Skin lesions
  - Systemic (hairy cell) vasculitis
  - Leukemia cutis
- Hyperviscosity leukostasis
- Tumor lysis syndrome
- Renal failure
- Anorexia of malignancy[17]
- Amyloidosis pains (accumulation of monoclonal plasma cells in tissues and organs, frequently the heart)[12]

ALL, acute lymphocytic leukemia; MRSA, methicillin-resistant *Staphylococcus aureus*.

and phosphate. Allopurinol is a xanthine oxidase inhibitor that acts to reduce levels of uric acid. Urinary alkalinization is another method used in emergencies to increase uric acid precipitation.[6] Hyperkalemia is often seen in tumor lysis syndrome and should be treated and monitored accordingly. Colchicine is generally not recommended in the ED because electrolyte imbalances may result from the potentially severe diarrheal side effects associated with this drug.

Disposition

Positive-pressure isolation rooms should be considered in patients with patients with prolonged neutropenia, in bone marrow transplant recipients, or in patients with other high-risk immunocompromised states (after intensive chemotherapy or solid organ transplantation). The question of inpatient or outpatient disposition is a matter of practicality for these patients. As with most patients in the ED, the disposition is based on clinical assessment, the ability to follow-up with a primary care physician, and the patient's home environment.

REFERENCES

1. National Cancer Institute: Surveillance, Epidemiology and End Results Program. Available at http://www.seer.cancer.gov/
2. Swenson K, Rose M, Ritz L, et al: Recognition and evaluation of oncology-related symptoms in the emergency department. Ann Emerg Med 1995;26:12-17.

3. Keating MJ, Kantarjian H: The chronic leukemias. In Goldman L, Ausiello DA (eds): Cecil Textbook of Medicine, 22nd ed. Philadelphia, WB Saunders, 2004, pp 1150-1160.
4. Appelbaum FA: The acute leukemias. In Goldman L, Ausiello DA (eds): Cecil Textbook of Medicine, 22nd ed. Philadelphia, WB Saunders, 2004, pp 1161-1166.
5. Portlock CS, Yahalom J: Hodgkin's disease. In Goldman L, Ausiello DA (eds): Cecil Textbook of Medicine, 22nd ed. Philadelphia, WB Saunders, 2004, pp 1166-1173.
6. Bierman P, Harris N, Armitage J: Non-Hodgkin's lymphomas. In Goldman L, Ausiello DA (eds): Cecil Textbook of Medicine, 22nd ed. Philadelphia, WB Saunders, 2004, pp 1174-1184.
7. Kyle RA, Rajkumar SV: Plasma cell disorders. In Goldman L, Ausiello DA (eds): Cecil Textbook of Medicine, 22nd ed. Philadelphia, WB Saunders, 2004, pp 1184-1195.
8. Hughes WT, Armstrong D, Bodey GP, et al: 1997 Guidelines for the use of antimicrobial agents in neutropenic patients with unexplained fever: Infectious Diseases Society of America. Clin Infect Dis 1997;25:551-573.
9. Chancock SJ, Pizzo PA: Infectious complications of patients undergoing therapy for acute leukemia: Current status and future prospects. Semin Oncol 1997;l24:132-140.
10. Hsu TF, Huang HH, Yen DH. ED presentation of neutropenic enterocolitis in adult patients with acute leukemia. Am J Emerg Med 2004;22:276-279.
11. Hobson MJ: Appendicitis in childhood hematologic malignancies: Analysis and comparison with typhilitis. J Pediatr Surg 2005;40:214-220.
12. Pastores SM: Acute respiratory failure in critically ill patients with cancer: Diagnosis and management. Crit Care Clin 2001;17:623-646.
13. Lee AYY, Levine MN: Management of VTE in cancer patients. Oncology 2000;14:409-421.
14. Kapoor M, Chan GZ: Fluid and electrolyte abnormalities. Crit Care Clin 2001;17:503-529.
15. Hussein M: Multiple myeloma: An overview of diagnosis and management. Cleve Clin J Med 1994;61:285-298.
16. Papadimitrakopoulou V, Weber D: Multiple Myeloma and Other Plasma-Cell Dyscrasias. Medical Oncology: A Comprehensive Review. Available at http://www.cancernetwork.com/textbook/morev08.htm.
17. Davidson MB, Thakkar S, Hix JK, et al: Pathophysiology, clinical consequences, and treatment of tumor lysis syndrome. Am J Med 2004;116:546-554.
18. Strasser F, Bruera E: Update on anorexia and cachexia. Hematol Oncol Clin North Am 2002;16:589-617.
19. Higdon M, Higdon J: Treatment of oncologic emergencies. Am Fam Physician 2006;74:1873-1880.
20. Berenson JR Lichtenstein A, Porter L, et al: Efficacy of pamidronate in reducing skeletal events in patients with advanced multiple myeloma. N Engl J Med 1996;335:1785-1791.

Chapter **204**

Emergency Management of Red Blood Cell Disorders

Ugo A. Ezenkwele

KEY POINTS

Anemia is the absolute reduction in the amount of oxygen-carrying pigment hemoglobin (Hgb) representing a relative decrease in the capacity of blood to carry oxygen to the tissues.

Anemia is not a diagnosis. It is an indication of an underlying disease, disorder, or deficiency.

Transfusion of red blood cells (RBCs) provides immediate correction of low Hgb levels helpful in the context of either severe anemia (in which the Hgb is <8.0 g/dL) or life-threatening anemia (in which the Hgb is <6.5 g/dL).

Most cases of anemia (chronic) do not require acute interventions and drug therapy in the ED. Patients can be referred for follow-up to their primary care physicians or gastroenterologists.

The cardinal features of acute chest syndrome are fever, pleuritic chest pain, referred abdominal pain, cough, lung infiltrates, and hypoxia.

Pneumococcal sepsis is a leading cause of death among infants with sickle cell anemia because a damaged spleen cannot clear pneumococci from the blood.

Transfusions are not needed for the usual anemia or episodes of pain associated with sickle cell disease.

Splenic sequestration is life-threatening and requires intensive care admission with transfusion and possibly splenectomy.

Patients with severe pain should be given an opiate parenterally at frequent, fixed intervals until the pain has diminished, at which time the dose of the opiate can be tapered, then stopped, and oral analgesic therapy can be instituted.

For polycythemia vera (PV), phlebotomy is the only therapy indicated for isolated erythrocytosis when its mechanism cannot be established.

ANEMIA

Scope

Anemia is more common than is generally realized. The World Health Organization defines *anemia* as a condition characterized by Hgb levels lower than 13 g/dL in men or lower than 12 g/dL in women.[1] Data from the National Center for Health Statistics that likely underestimate the frequency of anemia indicate that approximately 3.4 million Americans have anemia, and that the groups with the highest prevalence are women, African Americans, elderly persons, and those with the lowest incomes. Using laboratory data from the general U.S. population, the second National Health and Nutrition Survey reported anemia to be the most prevalent in infants, teenage girls, young women, and elderly men.[2] In persons 65 years old and older, anemia was present in 11.0% of men and 10.2% of women, and the prevalence rose to more than 20% in people 85 years and older. One third of the cases of anemia were the result of nutritional deficiencies, and one third were secondary to chronic illness, including but not limited to chronic renal disease.

Given the 120-day life span of a normal RBC, chronic anemias that are caused by RBC underproduction generally develop and progress slowly over weeks to months. In contrast, acute anemias that are caused by bleeding or hemolysis generally occur rapidly over days to weeks; the tempo of anemia development depends on the pace of bleeding or hemolysis in relation to RBC production.

Pathophysiology

Anemia is classified into three broad categories: (1) disorders of decreased RBC production, (2) disorders of increased RBC destruction, and (3) disorders resulting from RBC loss. Disorders in each of these categories may manifest differently and ultimately have their own management approaches (Table 204-1).

RBCs, or erythrocytes, contain fluid Hgb encased in a lipid membrane supported by a cytoskeleton and are the predominant cellular component of blood. RBCs make up 45% of the blood volume and are responsible for carrying oxygen from the lungs to the

Table 204-1 CLASSIFICATION OF ANEMIA

Category	Classification	Disease Process
Decreased red blood cell production (hypoproliferative)	Microcytic	Iron deficiency Thalassemia Sideroblastic anemia Chronic disease (neoplasm, infection, diabetes, uremia, thyroid disease, cirrhosis)
	Normocytic	Primary bone marrow problem (aplastic anemia, myeloid metaplasia, myelofibrosis, myelophthisic anemia, Diamond-Blackfan anemia) Secondary bone marrow problem (uremia, liver disease, endocrinopathy, chronic inflammation)
	Macrocytic	Folic acid deficiency Liver disease Vitamin B_{12} deficiency Scurvy Hypothyroidism Chemotherapy, immunosuppressive therapy
Increased red blood cell destruction (hemolytic)	Intrinsic	Membrane disorder (spherocytosis, sickle cell disease, stem cell disorder, elliptocytosis, spur cell)
	Extrinsic	Hemoglobin disorder (thalassemia, autoimmune disease, hemoglobinopathies) Infections (hepatitis and cytomegalovirus infection, Epstein-Barr virus infection, typhoid fever, *Escherichia coli* infection) Medications (penicillin, antimalarials, sulfa drugs, or acetaminophen) Leukemia or lymphoma Autoimmune disorders (systemic lupus erythematosus, rheumatoid arthritis, Wiskott-Aldrich syndrome, ulcerative colitis) Enzyme (glucose-6-phosphate dehydrogenase) defect
Red blood cell loss (hemorrhagic)	Acute or chronic	Gastrointestinal disorders Trauma Intraperitoneal disorders Extraperitoneal disorders Gynecologic disorders Urinary tract disorders Pelvic disorders Drug-related causes Epistaxis, hemoptysis

peripheral tissues. A 70-kg person has approximately 30 trillion RBCs, resulting in approximately 300 million in each drop of blood. The normal RBC is composed of three types of Hgb: Hgb A (97%), Hgb F (1%) or fetal Hgb, and Hgb A_2 (2%).[3] In utero, Hgb F predominates; it tightly binds oxygen and facilitates oxygen transfer from mother to fetus across the placenta. After birth, the amount of Hgb F decreases, and Hgb A is produced. The most abundant form of Hgb present after 1 year of life is Hgb A. Hgb A is composed of two beta-globin chains and two alpha-globin chains bonded to four iron-containing heme groups. Hgb production requires iron, the synthesis of the protoporphyrin ring, and the production of the globin chains. Reductions in any of these processes result in anemias. Furthermore, any alteration of the amino acid sequence that codes the production of the beta-globin chain results in one of the more than 600 different types of Hgb identified throughout the world. Common variants include sickle Hgb (result from substituting valine for glutamic acid in the sixth position of the beta chain, thus producing Hgb S) and Hgb C (substituting lysine for valine).

Inherited mutations resulting in deletions or dysfunctions of one or more of the alpha or beta gene decrease alpha- or beta-chain production and cause thalassemia.[4] If alpha chains are reduced, then alpha-thalassemia results, and if beta chains are reduced, then beta-thalassemia results, with compensatory increases in Hgb A_2 and Hgb F.

RBC precursors develop in bone marrow at rates usually determined by the body's demand for sufficient circulating Hgb to oxygenate tissues adequately. Once produced, the mature RBC remains in circulation for approximately 120 days before it is engulfed and destroyed. Consequently, anemia of any cause may manifest acutely or chronically, and the aggressiveness of intervention and management depends on the acuteness of onset and the severity of the clinical presentation.

Presenting Signs and Symptoms

Because anemia can be a primary disorder or can occur secondary to other systemic processes, a careful history and physical examination will provide valuable insight into the potential cause. All patients require a focused yet thorough history. For critically ill and noncommunicative patients, obtain the history from caretakers, paramedics, or primary care physicians. Relevant information should be obtained with the chief complaint and the presenting symptom in mind. For instance, information about injured patients should include the circumstances of the accident, the mechanism of the injury, the patient's initial vital signs, the estimated blood loss in the field, and the prehospital treatment initiated and the response to that treatment.

The extent of the symptoms, whether mild or life-threatening, depends on several contributing factors. If anemia develops acutely, there may not be enough time for compensatory adjustments to take place, and consequently, the patient may have more pronounced symptoms than if the anemia developed over weeks to months. Furthermore, underlying chronic comorbidities such as myocardial ischemia and transient cerebral ischemia may be unmasked in the presence of anemia.

ACUTE ANEMIA

Patients with anemia resulting from acute bleeding present with hypovolemia. The combined effects of hypovolemia and anemia may cause tissue hypoxia or anoxia through diminished cardiac output, resulting in decreased oxygen-carrying capacity (anemic hypoxia). When the Hgb concentration falls to less than 7.5 g/dL as a result of losses ranging from 5% to 15% in blood volume, the resting cardiac output rises significantly, with an increase in both heart rate and stroke volume. These patients are symptomatic at rest and may be aware of this hyperdynamic state; they often complain of palpitations, lightheadedness, or a pounding pulse. Larger losses cause progressive increases in heart rate and decreases in arterial blood pressure and evidence of organ hypoperfusion. Hypovolemic shock is seen when vital organ systems such as the kidneys, the central nervous system, and the heart are affected. In the ED, a source of blood loss may be readily apparent on evaluation (e.g., trauma with hemorrhage from the extremities, gastrointestinal bleeding, or menstrual blood loss); however, this may not be the case in, for example, aortic dissection or retroperitoneal hemorrhage.

Mild to moderate hypovolemia may be tolerated in the young patient. In elderly patients, however, these responses are modified by the rapidity of blood loss and by characteristics such as comorbid illnesses, preexisting volume status, Hgb values, and the use of medications that have cardiac or peripheral vascular effects (e.g., beta-blockers or antihypertensives). Therefore, it is important to elicit a thorough and focused history, including medications, while assessing the airway, stabilizing breathing, or initiating resuscitation as needed.

CHRONIC ANEMIA

Because anemia can be a primary disorder or can occur secondary to hypoproliferation or chronic blood loss, a careful history and physical examination will provide valuable insight into the potential cause. Individuals with mild anemia are often asymptomatic and are able to sustain a relatively normal level of function at significantly lower than normal Hgb levels. Other patients may present with myriad nonspecific symptoms (Box 204-1). Determining the concomitant presence of a systemic inflammatory disorder, infection, or malignant disease associated with fatigue may be critical in determining the underlying causes of anemia.

BOX 204-1

Chronic Anemia

- Fatigue
- Weakness
- Irritability
- Headache
- Dizziness (especially postural)
- Vertigo
- Headache

Past medical history is quite informative. For instance, a history of diabetes mellitus is associated with significantly impaired renal production of erythropoietin.[5] Certain medications are associated with bone marrow depression; therefore, all pharmacologic agents, both prescribed drugs and over-the-counter agents, including alternative medications, should be reviewed. Occupational history is relevant, as in the case of welders, who may have been exposed to lead or other agents potentially toxic to the bone marrow. Social history is important, because a history of intravenous drug use may suggest the possibility of human immunodeficiency virus infection, which can be associated with anemia.[6] Dietary history is relevant. For example, the finding of pica in adults (most commonly cornstarch) is well known to be associated with iron deficiency anemia, and the ingestion of paint chips may suggest the possibility of toxic lead ingestion. A family history of anemia is important; for example, adults with congenital hereditary spherocytosis may often develop symptoms later in life.

Physical findings are myriad, often nonspecific and may relate to the underlying disease process and the duration (Table 204-2). Pathognomonic findings are not the norm. Furthermore, patients with chronic anemia usually do not have the typical physical findings associated with acute anemia.

■ SPECIAL CONSIDERATIONS

Other signs may suggest more specific causes of anemia. Vitamin B_{12} deficiency may manifest as paresthesias and numbness resulting from peripheral neuropathy and lesions in the posterior and lateral columns of the spinal cord (subacute combined degeneration) and in the cerebrum. These lesions progress from demyelination to axonal degeneration and eventual neuronal death. Furthermore, vitamin B_{12} deficiency results in several abnormalities of the digestive tract, including atrophic glossitis, which manifests as a smooth and beefy red tongue.

Angular cheilitis (cracking at the edges of the lips) and koilonychia (spooning of the nails) may accompany iron deficiency anemia.[7] Splenomegaly may be present in patients with anemia arising from a wide variety of different causes. When present in childhood, splenomegaly suggests a congenital form of hemolytic anemia, such as thalassemia, sickle cell disease, or hereditary spherocytosis. When found for the first time later in life, splenomegaly may indicate an acquired disorder, such as autoimmune hemolytic anemia, lymphoproliferative disease, or agnogenic myeloid metaplasia.

Table 204-2 PHYSICAL FINDINGS IN ANEMIA

Organ or System	Finding
Skin	Pallor Usefulness limited by the color of the skin, hemoglobin concentration, and fluctuation of blood flow to the skin Color of palmar creases is a better indicator; if as pale as the surrounding skin, hemoglobin is usually <7 g/dL
Hematologic	Purpura, petechiae, and jaundice
Cardiovascular	Tachycardia Wide pulse pressure Orthostatic hypotension Hyperdynamic precordium Systolic ejection murmur over the pulmonic area
Respiratory	Tachypnea Rales
Gastrointestinal	Hepatomegaly or splenomegaly Ascites Masses Positive result on Hemoccult test
Ophthalmologic	Pale conjunctiva Scleral icterus Retinal hemorrhages
Neurologic	Peripheral neuritis or neuropathy Mental status changes

Differential Diagnosis and Diagnostic Testing

The differential diagnosis of anemia is myriad, as documented in Table 204-3. Once anemia is suspected, the initial diagnosis involves the complete blood count (CBC). The variables to focus on when examining the CBC are hematocrit (as a general indicator of anemia or polycythemia), mean corpuscular volume ([MCV] a key parameter for the classification of anemias), RBC distribution width (a relatively useful parameter in the differential diagnosis of anemia), RBC count (an increased RBC count associated with anemia is characteristic in the thalassemia trait), platelet count (to detect either thrombocytopenia or thrombocytosis), and white blood cell (WBC) count with differential (usually gives important clues for the diagnosis of acute leukemia and chronic lymphoid or myeloid disorders, as well as for the presence of leukopenia and neutropenia).[8]

The first step in approaching anemia is to classify the process as microcytic (MCV, <80 fL), normocytic (MCV, 80 to 100 fL), or macrocytic (MCV, >100 fL).

Table 204-3 DIFFERENTIAL DIAGNOSIS OF ANEMIA

Category	Differential	Complete Blood Count Clues
Microcytic	Iron deficiency anemia	Elevated RDW Thrombocytosis
	Thalassemia	Normal or elevated red blood cell count Normal or elevated RDW
	Anemia of chronic disease	Normal RDW
Normocytic	Hemolysis	Normal or elevated RDW Thrombocytosis
	Bleeding	Unchanged
	Nutritional anemia	Elevated RDW
	Anemia of chronic disease	Normal RDW
	Primary bone marrow disease	Elevated RDW Leukocytosis Thrombocytosis Monocytosis
Macrocytic	Alcohol use, liver disease	Normal RDW Thrombocytopenia
	Drug-induced condition	Elevated RDW
	Bone marrow disorder	Elevated RDW
	Hypothyroidism	Normal RDW
	Hemolysis	Normal or elevated RDW
	Nutritional disorders	Elevated RDW

RDW, red blood cell distribution width.

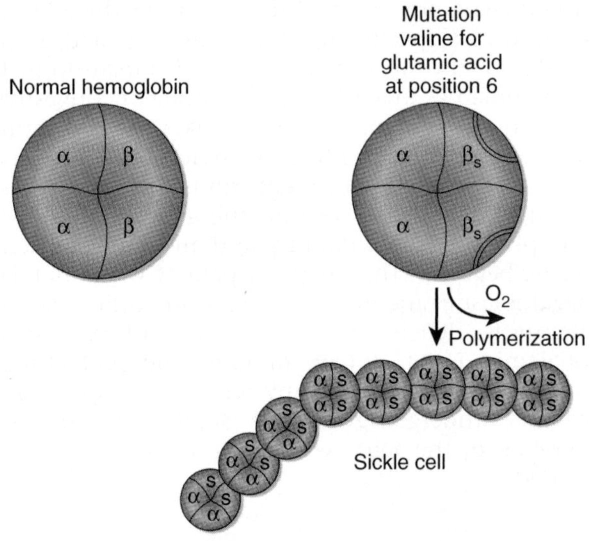
Normal hemoglobin
Mutation
valine for
glutamic acid
at position 6
α
β
β_s
O_2
Polymerization
Sickle cell

FIGURE 204-1 Sickle cell disease.

The three major diagnostic possibilities for microcytic anemia are iron deficiency anemia, thalassemia, and anemia of chronic disease. Clues to the diagnostic possibilities for the three major classes are listed in Table 204-3.

Along with anemia, another characteristic laboratory feature of hemolysis is reticulocytosis, the normal response of the bone marrow to the peripheral loss of RBCs. Patients with aplastic anemia or some other insult to the bone marrow from drugs or toxins have a reduced reticulocyte count. Some patients require special correction of their reticulocyte count (Fig. 204-1).

For instance, patients with hemolytic anemias require a *Finch reticulocyte count,* which corrects for the anemia and the expected maturation time. Generally, a 2-day life span (versus a 1-day life span, typically) is used for immature reticulocytes. The Finch count is the measured reticulocyte count, multiplied by the measured hematocrit level, divided by 45, and then divided by 2. Patients with sickle cell disease may utilize a simple corrected reticulocyte count. This is the *measured reticulocyte count,* multiplied by the measured hematocrit level, divided by 45. Normal reticulocyte counts are 0.5% to 1%. Blood type and cross should be sent to the blood bank so type-specific or type-matched and crossmatched blood can be readied.

Although this may not be readily available in the acute setting, review of the peripheral blood smear is a critical step in the evaluation of any anemia. Along with an assessment for pathognomonic RBC morphologies, such as spherocytes, helmet cells, basophilic stippling, sickled cells, Howell-Jolly bodies, or schistocytes, examination of the WBCs and platelets for coexisting hematologic or malignant disorders is essential.

Other tests to obtain are unconjugated bilirubin and lactate dehydrogenase. These values are increased when RBCs are destroyed. In patients with severe intravascular hemolysis, the binding capacity of haptoglobin is exceeded rapidly, and free Hgb is filtered by the glomeruli leading to decreased haptoglobin and increased hemoglobinuria or urobilinogen levels.

Additional diagnostic tests may be available in the ED, and although they aid with confirmation of the diagnosis, they are not helpful in the acute setting. These tests should be considered in the medical workup once inpatient care or outpatient referral has been initiated. For instance, patients with microcytic, hypochromic anemia require tests for serum iron, serum ferritin, and total iron binding capacity. Patients with macrocytic anemia require folate and vitamin B_{12} levels and thyroid function tests. Patients with hemolytic anemia require direct and indirect Coombs' tests, fractionated serum bilirubin, and serum and urine tests for free Hgb. Normocytic anemia in patients suspected of pica should prompt an evaluation of serum lead levels. Patients suspected of disseminated intravascular coagulation should have determinations of prothrombin time, activated partial thromboplastin time, fibrinogen, fibrin split products, and platelets. Classic findings in disseminated intravascular coagulation are elevated coagulation times, decreased platelets and fibrinogen, and the presence of fibrin split products. Further inpatient evaluations may be laboratory specific for certain disease states or may include a bone marrow biopsy.

Imaging studies are disease specific and depend on the patient's symptoms. Chest radiographs are indicated in all patients with significant anemia. Cardiomyopathy may be present in patients with chronic anemia. An electrocardiogram is required for older patients, those with chest pain, profound anemia, or those who have an underlying disease or increased risk factors for cardiac ischemia.

Patients with blood loss benefit from an ultrasound examination, which is a quick, noninvasive, and relatively simple bedside test useful for diagnosing intraperitoneal bleeding. The focused abdominal sonography for trauma (FAST) examination detects blood in the hepatorenal fossa, paracolic gutters, splenorenal area, and pelvis. It is also useful for detecting pregnancy-related bleeding, especially that emanating from a ruptured ectopic pregnancy. Stable patients with intra-abdominal blood loss benefit from computed tomography scanning. Computed tomography scanning has sensitivities similar to those of ultrasound, yet it better identifies causes, including retroperitoneal, pelvic, and subcapsular sites.

A nasogastric tube is indicated in the acute setting to diagnose and manage an ongoing upper gastrointestinal hemorrhage. Bile must be aspirated to rule out bleeding proximal to the ligament of Treitz. Once upper gastrointestinal bleeding is established, esophagogastroduodenoscopy is the study of choice for determining the source of bleeding and for treatment. Emergency esophagogastroduodenoscopy can be performed in the ED, and its use is indicated in the hemodynamically unstable patient. Consultation with a gastroenterologist is required.

Once the patient has been stabilized, other useful tests include tagged RBC studies and mesenteric angiography. The former is helpful in cases of gastrointestinal hemorrhage with an unidentified source, and the latter is used for diagnosing and treating hemorrhage from diverticula. Sigmoidoscopy or colonoscopy may be useful in diagnosing and treating lower gastrointestinal bleeding, but it is rarely helpful in the acute setting.

Treatment

After anemia is identified by a CBC determination in the ED, management is aided by an approach that categorizes anemia as a symptom caused by the decrease in Hgb, rather than as an isolated diagnosis. Like fever, anemia is a symptom of disease that requires investigation to determine the underlying origin.

The need for rapid intervention in the ED is determined by the patient's hemodynamic status and is often limited to those in hypovolemic shock. After immediate resuscitation and once patients are stabilized with crystalloids, blood transfusions are widely used as a rapid and effective therapeutic intervention. The transfusion of RBCs provides immediate correction of low Hgb levels and is particularly helpful in the context of either severe anemia (in which the Hgb is <8.0 g/dL) or life-threatening anemia (in which the Hgb is <6.5 g/dL), especially when the condition is aggravated by complications that involve bleeding.[9]

Patients with long-standing or chronic anemias are able to compensate and do not require transfusion, especially if the Hgb is greater than 9.0 g/dL. Patients who are expected to respond to the administration of a specific agent such as folic acid, iron, or vitamin B_{12} can usually be spared transfusions. If the anemia has precipitated an episode of congestive heart failure or myocardial ischemia, prompt administration of packed RBCs is indicated. For some patients in the ED, treatment can be begun without waiting for a definitive outpatient evaluation. For example, prenatal vitamins and iron replacement can be begun in the pregnant patient with anemia. Megaloblastic anemia resulting from folic acid or vitamin B_{12} deficiency can be treated with parenteral cobalamin (1000 μg/day) or oral folic acid (1 mg/day). Erythropoietin therapy remains an option for patients undergoing elective surgical procedures; however, in the acute setting, its role remains to be defined.

Disposition

Fortunately, most patients have chronic anemia without blood loss and can be managed conservatively. In many cases, acute interventions and drug therapy are not indicated in the ED, and patients can be referred for follow-up to their primary care physicians.

Emergency consultation and hospital admission are required for patients presenting with hypovolemia or active bleeding who demonstrate a considerable drop in Hgb and hematocrit values when compared with previous values. An Hgb value of less than 8.0 g/dL in a symptomatic patient is enough to warrant admission for replacement of blood products. Patients who have underlying disease such as cardiac ischemia or congestive heart failure and are now symptomatic and complaining of chest pain, tachypnea, or shortness of breath because of their anemia also require admission. Patients with new-onset or worsening pancytopenia require urgent consultation. Finally, admission is indicated for those patients who may not comply with follow-up or those in whom the clinician anticipates the need for an extensive work-up. Admission is to a ward bed, intermediate unit, or intensive care bed and depends on the patient's presenting symptoms.

SICKLE CELL ANEMIA

Scope

Sickle cell disease, characterized by lifelong hemolytic anemia and a wide variety of painful and debilitating vaso-occlusive events, occurs in 70,000 to 80,000 Americans of African, Mediterranean, or Middle Eastern descent. In the United States, the life expectancy for patients with sickle cell disease is shortened by approximately 30 years, whereas in Africa, where comprehensive medical care is less readily available, death in early childhood is usual.[10] Eight percent of black Americans are heterozygous carriers of the sickle cell trait; approximately 40% of their Hgb is Hgb S. They do not have anemia and need neither treatment nor occupational restrictions.

Pathophysiology

Sickle cell disease is an inherited condition caused by a point mutation in the beta-globin gene (Hgb B), resulting in the substitution of valine for glutamic acid at position 6 of the beta-globin chain (Glu6Val). This mutation results in the abnormal Hgb S[11] (Fig. 204-1). When deoxygenated, Hgb S polymerizes, thus damaging the sickle RBC. These sickle cells are short-lived and interact with endothelial cells, WBCs, platelets, and other plasma components to initiate the vaso-occlusive manifestations associated with sickle cell disease.[12] Among hemolytic anemias, the vaso-occlusive features of sickle cell disease are unique. By occluding small blood vessels and sometimes large vessels, sickle cells cause vascular injury (Fig. 204-2). No single mechanism explains the vaso-occlusion; its cause may be different from event to event, and its severity differs among patients.[13] Deoxygenation of sickle cells increases cell density and the tendency of Hgb S to polymerize. Sickle cell trait is benign, because the cellular concentration of Hgb S is too low for polymerization to occur under most conditions, and it is Hgb S polymers that cause the cellular injury responsible for the clinical manifestations of sickle cell disease.

Presenting Signs and Symptoms

Vaso-occlusion, which is responsible for most of the severe complications of sickle cell disease, can occur

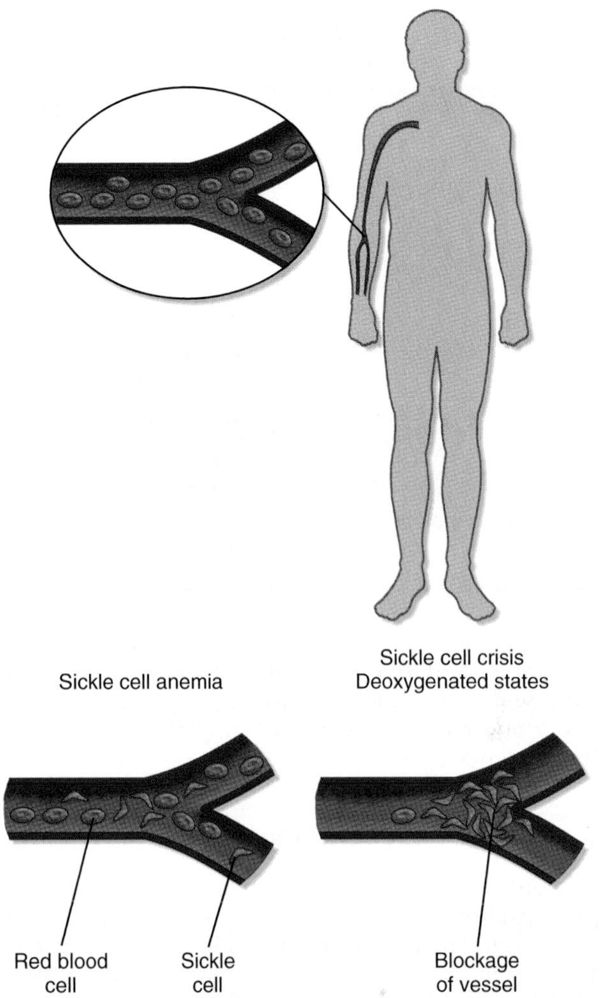

Sickle cell anemia
Sickle cell crisis
Deoxygenated states
Red blood cell
Sickle cell
Blockage of vessel

FIGURE 204-2 By occluding small blood vessels and sometimes large ones, sickle cells cause vascular injury.

wherever blood flows. The clinical features of sickle cell disease are outlined in Table 204-4.

■ PAINFUL EPISODES

Acute painful crisis in sickle cell disease is a frequent complication and considerably diminishes the quality of life of patients with this disease. Approximately 60% of patients have an episode of severe pain. A few patients have severe pain almost constantly. Episodes of pain are sometimes triggered by infection, extreme temperatures, or physical or emotional stress, but more often they are unprovoked and begin with little warning.

■ ACUTE CHEST SYNDROME

The *acute chest syndrome* is the leading cause of death and hospitalization among patients with sickle cell disease. Affecting approximately 40% of all patients with sickle cell anemia, it is a sometimes fatal complication. Its cardinal features are fever, pleuritic chest pain, referred abdominal pain, cough, lung

Table 204-4 CLINICAL COMPLICATIONS OF SICKLE CELL DISEASE

Type	Clinical Features
Vaso-occlusive complications	Pain crises Acute chest syndrome Splenic sequestration Cerebrovascular crisis Priapism Liver disease Leg ulcers Spontaneous abortion Osteonecrosis Renal crisis Retinopathy
Infectious complications	Osteomyelitis *Escherichia coli* sepsis *Streptococcus pneumoniae* sepsis
Hemolytic complications	Cholelithiasis Anemia Aplastic anemia

infiltrates, and hypoxia.[14] It is most common but least severe in children, can occur postoperatively, and when recurrent, can lead to chronic respiratory insufficiency.

■ CEREBROVASCULAR CRISIS

Cerebrovascular disease is the second leading cause of mortality and a common cause of morbidity in sickle cell anemia: approximately 10% of patients have a clinical stroke by age 20 years, and another 22% have evidence of silent infarction on magnetic resonance imaging. Manifestations of neurologic complications may include overt clinical stroke or subtler neuropsychological abnormalities often associated with subclinical stroke. The age distribution, pathophysiology, and type of stroke in sickle cell disease closely resemble those of moyamoya disease in Japanese patients. Risk factors for ischemic stroke presentation in sickle cell direase include prior transient ischemic attacks, a decrease in steady-state Hgb, a history of acute chest syndrome, and an increase in systolic blood pressure; risk factors for hemorrhagic stroke include a decrease in steady-state Hgb and an increase in steady-state WBC.

■ RIGHT UPPER QUADRANT SYNDROME

Right upper quadrant syndrome is manifested by any or all of the following features: hyperbilirubinemia, abdominal pain, fever, right upper quadrant abdominal tenderness, hepatomegaly, abnormalities on liver function testing, and hepatic failure. Possible causes include cholelithiasis, viral hepatitis, biliary cholestasis, and hepatic ischemia. Cholelithiasis occur in children as young as 3 to 4 years of age and is eventually found in approximately 70% of patients; this condition often necessitates cholecystectomy once right upper quadrant pain is identified.

The three acute hepatic syndromes seen in sickle cell disease are acute hepatic cell crisis, acute hepatic sequestration crisis, and sickle cell intrahepatic cholestasis. Intrahepatic cholestasis is benign and may be associated with severe hyperbilirubinemia that resolves in 7 to 10 days, especially in children.[15] A syndrome more common in adults is associated with fever, leukocytosis, abdominal pain, and deteriorating liver function, as indicated by measurement of liver enzymes. This hepatic crisis usually progresses to hepatic failure, coagulopathy, encephalopathy, and death.

■ PRIAPISM

Priapism is a sustained, painful, and unwanted erection of the penis that pathophysiologically is the result of an accumulation of sickled cells in the corpora cavernosa that cause ischemia or low flow. Approximately 30% of male patients with sickle cell disease who are less than 20 years old report at least one episode of priapism, whereas frequencies of 30% to 45% are estimated for adult men. The peak incidence is between the ages of 5 and 12 years, with a second peak between the ages of 20 and 30 years. This condition is most common in patients with the greatest amount of hemolysis. Postpubertal male patients tend to have more prolonged episodes of priapism and have a less favorable prognosis for future potency.[16] One sequela is impotence; therefore, for the EP, the utmost priority in these patients is detumescence, especially within the first 12 hours.

■ SPLENIC SEQUESTRATION

Splenic sequestration, caused by sickled cells trapped in the splenic circulation, causes precipitous decreases in Hgb concentration and rapid enlargement of the spleen. This condition may be life-threatening. It is common in infants and young children and is less common in older children and adults because the spleen is significantly fibrotic in these patients by the age of 5 years. *Acute splenic sequestration crisis* generally is defined as an acute drop in Hgb levels (>2 g/dL) associated with splenomegaly, reticulocytosis, and signs of intravascular volume depletion. Drops in Hgb levels greater than 4 g/dL are associated with 35% mortality. Splenic sequestration carries a 15% mortality and is the second leading cause of death among children. It may manifest as hypotension (caused by shock from worsening anemia) associated with an enlarged, tender spleen. Fatigue, listlessness, and pallor have also been described. An association between this crisis and acute viral infections exist, especially parvovirus B19 infection. In patients with increased destruction of RBCs and a high demand for the production of RBCs, acute parvovirus B19 infection can cause an abrupt cessation of RBC production that exacerbates or, in compensated states, provokes severe anemia.

■ TRANSIENT APLASTIC CRISIS

Aplastic crisis occurs in children with sickle cell anemia in response to transient suppression of erythropoiesis, most often because of infection with parvovirus B19, the same etiologic agent that causes erythema infectiosum ("fifth disease"). This crisis is usually a unique event in the life of a patient and suggests the induction of long-lasting, protective immunity. Although self-limited, aplastic crisis can cause severe, occasionally fatal, anemia that precipitates congestive heart failure, cerebrovascular accidents, and acute splenic sequestration. WBC and platelet counts may fall somewhat during transient aplastic crisis, especially in patients with functioning spleens. Aplastic crisis may be also be precipitated by other infections, including infections with *Streptococcus pneumoniae,* other streptococci, *Salmonella,* and Epstein-Barr virus. Children present with signs of severe anemia, such as tachycardia and pallor.

■ STREPTOCOCCUS PNEUMONIAE SEPSIS

The incidence of invasive *S. pneumoniae* infection is 20- to 100-fold higher in children with sickle cell disease than in the general population. Penicillin prophylaxis for children with sickle cell anemia reduces the incidence of invasive pneumococcal infection by 84%, independent of pneumococcal immunization status.

Differential Diagnosis and Diagnostic Testing

Patients with sickle cell disease frequently require immediate medical attention because of the severity of their disease and its potential complications. Understanding the various presenting symptoms and staying alert for severe manifestations of the disease are important for EPs (see the Priority Actions box). Diagnostic testing is often focused, depending on the presenting symptoms; however, in most patients a basic set of laboratory tests should be obtained. Baseline laboratory values are helpful, as well as knowledge of the patient's medication history, the severity and frequency of previous crisis, and any surgical complications.

If the diagnosis of sickle cell disease is suspected, especially in children, a Sickledex test can be obtained as an initial screening tool. This test does not differentiate between individuals who are homozygous and those who are heterozygous. All positive Sickledex tests should be confirmed with Hgb electrophoresis, which differentiates heterozygous from homozygous carriers. Given that these tests may not be readily available, it may be beyond the purview of the EP to confirm their suspicion of this disease.

Emergency management depends on clinical presentation and can be symptom specific. All patients with known sickle cell disease must be have a CBC and a reticulocyte count. These tests are necessary to help screen for severe anemia, aplastic crisis, sequestration crisis, and infection. A major drop in Hgb (e.g., >2 g/dL) from baseline values indicates a hematologic crisis. If the reticulocyte count is normal, splenic sequestration is the probable cause. If the reticulocyte count is low, bone marrow failure is the probable cause. An infection is indicated by major elevations in the WBC count (e.g., >15,000/mm^3) accompanied by a left shift and significant bandemia. In interpreting these values, it is important to know that most patients with sickle cell disease have chronic anemia (hematocrit of 20% to 30%), mild leukocytosis, elevated reticulocyte counts, and thrombocytosis.

Serum electrolytes, blood urea nitrogen, and creatinine levels are essential to determine when hydration status and metabolic function is of concern, However, these values are not always needed, especially in mild disease. Any toxic-appearing patient in respiratory distress requires arterial blood gas analysis, to establish a baseline and to diagnose acid-base abnormalities. Continuous pulse oximetry monitoring is warranted and reliable.

In some EDs, a peripheral smear can be obtained. Often, sickle-shaped RBCs are found along with target cells. Asplenia is indicated by the presence of Howell-Jolly bodies. Along with the peripheral smear, a type and cross-match are sent to the blood bank, in case transfusion is required. Measurement of prothrombin and partial thromboplastin times are indicated to evaluate for hypercoagulable states, especially in patients demonstrating evidence of thrombotic disease, including stroke and myocardial ischemia.

Patients with abdominal pain require liver function tests and serum lipase evaluations. An elevated baseline indirect bilirubin level may be normal because of chronic hemolysis. Extreme elevation may indicate cholelithiasis and cholecystitis. Patients with chest pain require an electrocardiogram to screen for myocardial ischemia.

The urine must be examined for evidence of infection if the patient has fever or signs of urinary tract infection. Hematuria and isosthenuria are often present in patients with sickle cell disease. If signs of urinary tract infection are present, obtain a urine Gram stain and culture. Patients with fever without clear evidence of pneumonia, cholecystitis, pyelonephritis, or apparent source require blood cultures, preferably two sets.

Imaging studies are also symptom specific. A chest radiograph is indicated in all patients with respiratory symptoms, including productive cough and tachypnea. Acute chest syndrome may be radiographically normal in the early stages of presentation. Bone radiographs are necessary in patients with localized bony pain if osteomyelitis is suspected. Although not readily available in the ED, bone scans may be used to confirm the diagnosis. Ultrasonography is necessary in patients with abdominal pain to rule out cholecystitis, cholelithiasis, hepatomegaly, and splenomegaly. Patients with new neurologic signs and symptoms require computed tomography

PRIORITY ACTIONS

Differential Diagnosis

Bony Pain?

Does the patient have evidence of trauma or infection?

If not, consider osteomyelitis. Although *Salmonella* is commonly described, *Staphylococcus aureus* is the predominant organism. Admit for intravenous antibiotics.

Diffuse or Isolated Pain?

Are there any identifiable triggers, such as infection, dehydration, hypoxia, pregnancy, cold exposure, acidosis, or recent flight in an unpressurized aircraft?

If yes, assess and treat the underlying cause. If not, consider whether this is a usual vaso-occlusive crisis, and inquire about the onset, duration, and location and about previous episodes. Treat with analgesics, preferably opiates.

Abdominal Pain, Nausea, and Vomiting?

Does the patient have pancreatitis, appendicitis, peptic ulcer disease, diverticulitis, colitis, or renal colic?

If not, consider symptomatic cholelithiasis, acute hepatic crisis, or splenic sequestration. Obtain a right upper quadrant ultrasound scan, check transaminases, and consider surgical consultation. Consider transfusion for severe anemia.

Focal Neurologic Deficits (Hemiplegia, Aphasia, Paresthesias) or Seizures?

Does the patient have hypertension, coronary artery disease, or atrial fibrillation with possible thromboembolic phenomena?

If not, consider vaso-occlusion in the cerebral circulation. Obtain an emergency computed tomography scan and a neurologic consultation, and consider red blood cell apheresis.

Productive Cough with Fever?

Does the patient have high fever, leukocytosis, positive gram stain, or evidence of pneumonia on radiographs?

If not, consider acute chest syndrome, especially if the patient has a low-grade fever and vaso-occlusive symptoms elsewhere. Obtain a chest radiograph and blood cultures. Admit for observation and possible exchange transfusion.

Child with Fever Greater Than 101.3° F?

Does the patient have pneumonia, pyelonephritis, cholangitis, cholecystitis, osteomyelitis, or meningitis?

If not, consider sepsis. Obtain a complete blood count, urinalysis, urine and blood cultures, chest radiograph, and lumbar puncture. Pneumococcal sepsis, a leading cause of childhood mortality, has a 14% mortality rate.

Pallor, Fatigue, Listlessness, Recent Viral Illness?

Consider aplastic anemia. Obtain a reticulocyte count. Treatment is supportive depends on the degree of anemia and hemodynamic instability

Abdominal Pain with Enlarged Spleen?

Splenic sequestration is life-threatening and requires intensive care admission with transfusion and possibly splenectomy.

Painful, Erect Penis?

Does the patient have paraphimosis, phimosis, or recent trauma?

If not, consider priapism. Obtain a urology consultation, and initiate oral terbutaline or pseudoephedrine. Intracavernosal injection with an alpha-adrenergic agonist is warranted. In addition, treat with hydration, analgesia, ice packs, and exchange transfusions.

scanning or magnetic resonance imaging of the head.

Treatment

Treatment of sickle cell disease is evolving. The description of barriers to effective pain management is interesting and has been well documented.[17] Health care providers tend to undertreat their patients because they fear patient dependence on pain medication, which in reality is present in only 1% to 3% of patients. In response, patients tend to hoard analgesics out of fear of pain. Patients with sickle cell disease who are in pain are also misunderstood because they display a different attitude to their severe pain than do trauma or oncology patients. While patients with sickle cell disease complain of severe pain, they may engage in activities that are inconsistent with the traditional image of the patient in severe pain, such as watching television or talking on the telephone. These patients are therefore often perceived as exaggerating their pain to receive additional narcotics, whereas these activities may actually be learned distractions or coping mechanisms. Another example is the sleeping patient who, when awakened, reports unrelenting pain. This situation may be the result of an imbalance between the sedative and analgesic effects of opiates or a need for sleep despite the pain. The result is a lack of trust between patients and health care providers. It follows that in centers specializing in sickle cell crises, the attitudes toward pain tend to be better understood and treatment outcomes are superior, compared with EDs. Patients in severe pain should be given an opiate parenterally at frequent, fixed intervals, not as needed, until the pain has diminished, at which time the dose of the opiate can be tapered and then stopped, and oral analgesic therapy can be instituted.[18] Oral analgesics suffice for treating mild to moderate pain. Patients with mild to moderate pain seem to find no difference between intravenous and oral morphine. Most opiates have comparable efficacy and safety profiles, but morphine is considered the drug of choice for treatment of acute sickle cell pain. The use of meperidine is discouraged because of the risk of seizures. Anti-inflammatory drugs and intravenous methylprednisolone may provide an opiate-sparing effect, but there is concern about their negative effects on bone healing. In addition, painful crises seem to recur frequently after treatment with methylprednisolone.

Patients with intracranial thrombosis and hemorrhage require treatment with partial exchange transfusions to attempt decrease of Hgb S to less than 30%. Although not tested in a clinical trial, long-term transfusion therapy was associated with a reduced recurrence rate as low as 10% and has become routine after stroke in children.

Urgent replacement of blood is often required for sudden severe anemia occurring in children when blood is sequestered in an enlarged spleen or when parvovirus B19 infection causes transient aplastic crisis. For aplastic crisis, clinical management is supportive and depends on the degree of anemia and cardiovascular compromise. Simple transfusions are administered to raise the Hgb to approximately 10 g/dL and the hematocrit to approximately 30% if the reticulocyte count is less than 1% to 2% with no signs of spontaneous recovery. For shock caused by splenic sequestration, emergency management is aimed at restoring circulating blood volume and hemodynamic stability through the infusion of crystalloids and volume expanders and by repeated simple or exchange blood transfusions. Ultimately, splenectomy may be performed because sequestration has been shown to recur in 50% of patients and represents a life-threatening event. Admission is required for patients with aplastic crisis and splenic sequestration. Transfusions are not needed for the usual anemia or episodes of pain associated with sickle cell disease.[18]

Hypoxia accompanying the acute chest syndrome necessitates transfusion and oxygen treatment. In practice, all patients with oxygen saturations of less than 85% on pulse oximetry or a drop of 5% from know baseline should receive oxygen. Pulse oximetry in sickle cell patients has been shown to correlate with arterial oxygen content. Antibiotics should be given to treat infections with *S. pneumoniae, Haemophilus influenzae,* and atypical organisms such as *Mycoplasma, Legionella,* and *Chlamydia.* Frequently, a macrolide with a third-generation cephalosporin is chosen.

Acute hepatic cell crisis manifests with tender hepatomegaly, worsening jaundice, and fever. This syndrome usually resolves within 3 to 14 days with supportive care alone, but it can progress to liver failure, which carries a dismal prognosis. Exchange transfusion should be considered for patients with signs of progressive liver dysfunction.

Sepsis is a leading cause of death, especially in younger children. Management incorporates (1) treatment of the infection with source control and antimicrobial agents; (2) rapid and targeted resuscitation from shock with administration of fluid (and, if appropriate, blood products), vasopressors, or inotropic agents; (3) adjuvant therapy with recombinant human activated protein C or corticosteroids in carefully selected patients; and (4) supportive measures such as lung-protective ventilation for acute respiratory distress syndrome. Appropriate cultures of blood and material from other sites should be quickly obtained, and broad-spectrum intravenous antibiotics should be started within the first hour after severe sepsis or septic shock is recognized. All patients who have high fevers and who are not receiving prophylactic penicillin should receive intravenous ceftriaxone as a precaution against meningitis from *S. pneumoniae* and *Neisseria meningitidis.* Patients with osteomyelitis should be treated for infection with *Salmonella* and *Staphylococcus aureus.* Patients with presumed urinary tract infections, especially pyelonephritis, should receive treatment for *Escherichia coli* infection.

Hydroxyurea increases the production of Hgb F in patients with sickle cell anemia and thus ameliorates their disease clinically. This agent selectively kills cells in the bone marrow, thereby increasing the number of erythroblasts that produce Hgb F. The only successful therapeutic strategy so far for sickle cell disease is based on the use of hydroxyurea to increase the RBC content of Hgb F. Substantial reductions in pain rate, acute chest crises, and transfusion requirements have been achieved with hydroxyurea therapy. Long-term follow-up (9 years) of hydroxyurea-treated patients showed a 40% reduction in mortality with this therapy. The use of this agent in the ED is limited. Other interventions as described previously should be initiated earlier.

Novel therapies may include dipyridamole (Persantine), which has been shown to be a powerful inhibitor of the deoxygenation-induced fluxes of sickled cell polymerization, especially in dehydrated cells in vitro. However, more clinical trials are needed to demonstrate this benefit in vivo. Low-dose, longer-acting glucocorticoids, especially dexamethasone, have shown a benefit in the management of acute chest syndrome. However, more research is also needed. More recent studies and ongoing clinical trials have hypothesized that inhaled nitric oxide may be beneficial in managing a variety of clinical conditions, including sickle cell anemia.[19] However, because the delivery of inhaled nitric oxide may have more limited applicability in the clinical setting as a result of inherent administration problems, the oral administration of L-arginine (precursor of nitric oxide) shows promise as a potential treatment for vaso-occlusive crises and acute chest syndrome.[20]

Disposition

Patients with sickle cell disease who have uncomplicated painful crises and who receive hydration and adequate pain relief in the ED can be discharged. Adequate pain relief can be achieved on a variable basis for different patients, and no set rule exists about when this occurs. Some practitioners advocate for either a temporal observation in the ED (6 hours) or a set amount of parenteral analgesics, most commonly opioids (two or three trials). Failure to achieve adequate pain relief requires inpatient admission (Box 204-2). In the absence of contraindications (temperature >38° C, respiratory signs/symptoms, low arterial oxygen saturation, tachycardia, or hypotension) and if adequate pain relief is attained, patients can be discharged home on a regimen of oral analgesics for 1 week, with continuity of care arranged. Patients who have minor infections can be discharged with oral antibiotics, more commonly amoxicillin/clavulanate, azithromycin, or levofloxacin. Primary care physicians should be contacted, and specialist care (hematology) referral should be arranged. Explicit instructions for immediate ED repeat visits are required, especially in the event of symptoms of fever, pleuritic chest pain, abdominal pain, cough, and painful crises (see Box 204-2).

Finally, counseling is indicated to prevent future crises, given the chronic nature of sickle cell disease. Preventive measures include advising the patient to adhere to an immunization schedule (especially pneumococcal, influenza, and hepatitis vaccines), to maintain biannual health care visits, and to take advantage of oral penicillin prophylaxis for patients with frequent infections.

BOX 204-2

Sickle Cell Anemia: Indications for Inpatient Evaluation

- Inability to control pain
- Inability to maintain adequate hydration
- Acute chest syndrome
- Bacterial infection with unexplained fever, leukocytosis
- Cerebrovascular crisis (new neurologic sign or symptom)
- Priapism
- Splenic sequestration
- Aplastic or hemolytic crisis
- Acute abdomen, especially right upper quadrant syndrome
- Noncompliance with follow-up schedules
- Uncertain diagnosis

POLYCYTHEMIA VERA

Scope

The Greek term *polycythemia* is synonymous with the word *erythrocytosis,* and it literally translates as "many cells in the blood." *Absolute polycythemia* is a condition with increased RBC mass. Numerous primary and secondary polycythemic disorders lead to absolute polycythemia.[21] Primary polycythemias are caused by a defect intrinsic to the erythroid progenitor cells. The best characterized primary polycythemia is the autosomal dominant primary familial and congenital polycythemia.

Polycythemia vera (PV) is traditionally classified as a myeloproliferative disorder, which is a broad category of clonal stem cell diseases that include myelofibrosis with myeloid metaplasia and chronic myeloid leukemia.[21] The true incidence and prevalence of PV are unknown. PV is relatively rare, occurring in 0.6 to 1.6 persons per million population. The disease has been around for more than 100 years, and the initial description as presented by Osler has not changed. Fortunately, PV has the survival characteristics of a benign disease, and much still needs to be learned. For the EP, understanding the complications of the disease ultimately aids in its management.

Pathophysiology

Primary polycythemias are characterized by an excessive response of erythroid progenitors to circulating cytokines, as a result of acquired mutations that are expressed within hematopoietic progenitors. Secondary polycythemias are caused by circulating factors that act on these progenitors, in most instances erythropoietin. Primary and secondary polycythemias can be either acquired or congenital. Congenital polycythemias may result from inherited appropriate responses to tissue hypoxia, acquired conditions characterized by autonomous erythropoietin production (secondary polycythemias), defects in hypoxia sensing (either primary or secondary polycythemia), or inherited intrinsic defects in RBC precursors that render erythroid progenitors hypersensitive to erythropoietin (primary familial and congenital polycythemia).[21]

Table 204-5 POLYCYTHEMIA VERA STUDY GROUP CRITERIA FOR THE DIAGNOSIS OF POLYCYTHEMIA VERA

Diagnostic Group	Criteria
Category A	Total red blood cell mass In male patients, ≥36 mL/kg In female patients, ≥32 mL/kg Arterial oxygen saturation ≥92% Splenomegaly
Category B	Thrombocytosis with platelet count >400,000/mL Leukocytosis with white blood cell count >12,000/mL Leukocyte alkaline phosphatase >100 U/L Serum vitamin B_{12} concentration >900 pg/mL or binding capacity >2200 pg/mL
Diagnosis	A1 plus A2 plus A3 A1 plus A2 plus any two criteria from category B

Data from Tefferi A, Solberg LA, Silverstein MN: A clinical update in polycythemia vera and essential thrombocythemia. Am J Med 2000;109:141-149.

PV, the most common primary polycythemia, is caused by the somatic change of a single hematopoietic stem cell, thus leading to clonal hematopoiesis. The molecular defects responsible for PV are unknown.

Presenting Signs and Symptoms

Symptoms of PV are related to hyperviscosity, sludging of blood flow, and thromboses, which lead to poor oxygen delivery and symptoms that include headache, dizziness, vertigo, tinnitus, visual disturbances, angina pectoris, and intermittent claudications. Hypertension is common in patients with PV.

Bleeding manifestations in PV involve primarily the skin and mucous membranes, a finding suggesting defective primary hemostasis, and include ecchymosis, epistaxis, menorrhagia, and gingival hemorrhage. Gastrointestinal hemorrhage occurs less frequently but can be severe, necessitating hospitalization and blood transfusion, and it is often associated with the use of aspirin.[22] This type of bleeding pattern is consistent with platelet defects (quantitative or qualitative) or von Willebrand's disease.

Thrombosis, hemorrhage, and systolic hypertension result from the hyperviscosity associated with RBC mass expansion. Historically, thrombosis, both venous and arterial, occurred in up to 40% of patients during the course of the illness.

Dyspepsia and gastric or peptic ulceration appear to be more common in patients with PV than in the general population. The most serious complication other than thrombosis is pruritus.

Physical findings in PV are the result of manifestations of the myeloproliferative process and include splenomegaly (present in 75% of patients) and hepatomegaly (present in ≈30% of patients). Plethora or a ruddy color results from the marked increase in total RBC mass. This manifests in the face, palms, nail beds, mucosa, and conjunctiva.

Differential and Diagnostic Testing

PV is a clinical diagnosis. Diagnostic tests are nonspecific, sometimes uninformative, and none establish clonality. The diagnosis is currently accomplished through the laboratory measurement of RBC mass, plasma volume, and arterial oxygen saturation and determination of oxygen pressure at 50% Hgb saturation. In the ED, RBC counts and hematocrit values (including Hgb levels) are used to make this diagnosis. Generally, Hgb concentrations of at least 20 g/dL or hematocrit values of at least 60% in male patients and 56% in female patients can be presumed to indicate a myeloproliferative disorder. Direct measurement of the RBC mass should show an increase, with a normal or slightly decreased plasma volume. However, this nuclear medicine test uses radiochromium-labeled RBCs to measure actual RBC and plasma volume and is not readily available. In fact, the chromium-51 isotope needed to perform the test is generally unavailable, and institutions are unwilling to perform the test because of the rarity of the disease and the lack of profitability. If RBC mass results are available, the Polycythemia Vera Study Group diagnostic criteria can be used (Table 204-5).

The arterial oxygen saturation and carboxyhemoglobin levels are important to rule out hypoxia as a secondary cause of erythrocytosis. Other tests have been described to assist in the diagnosis; however, none are relevant in the acute care setting. These include serum erythropoietin assays, karyotyping of PV bone marrow cells, and clonal assays using glucose-6-phosphate dehydrogenase markers.

Treatment

In the absence of other manifestations of disease, phlebotomy is the only therapy indicated for isolated erythrocytosis when the mechanism cannot be established. Phlebotomy can be initiated in the ED; however, a hematology consultation is required. Other agents such as aspirin, various antihistamines, synthetic androgens, and phototherapy have been described, and initiation of these therapeutic adjuncts can be carried out in the ward.

Hydroxyurea became the mainstay therapy for PV after several studies indicated its efficacy for myelosuppression; however, concerns have been raised regarding the long-term risks for leukemic transformation. Unfortunately, in some patients, suppression of hematopoiesis is required. Given that suppression of hematopoiesis by chemotherapy is not without significant potential toxicities, including acute leukemia, the approach to the alleviation of pruritus should exhaust all nonmutagenic remedies first, including interferon alfa.

Finally, splenectomy is an option for patients with painful splenomegaly or repeated episodes of thrombosis that cause splenic infarction. At this juncture, inpatient evaluation is warranted, and surgical consultation should be obtained.

Disposition

Patients requiring phlebotomy should be admitted. Bleeding and hemodynamically unstable patients require inpatient evaluation. In many patients with newly identified PV, drug administration and other interventions are not indicated in the ED setting. Asymptomatic patients can be referred to the hematologist for accurate determination of the underlying disease process, including measurements of RBC mass and karyotyping of bone marrow cells.

REFERENCES

1. DeMaeyer E, Adiels-Tegman M: The prevalence of anemia in the world. World Health Stat Q 1985;38:302-316.
2. Goodnough LT, Nissenson AR: Anemia and its clinical consequences in patients with chronic diseases. Am J Med 2004;116(Suppl 7A):1S-2S.
3. Weiss G, Goodnough LT: Anemia of chronic disease. N Engl J Med 2005;352:1011-1023.
4. Rund D, Rachmilewitz E: Beta-thalassemia. N Engl J Med 2005;353:1135-1146.
5. Thomas MC, Cooper ME, Tsalamandris C, et al: Anemia with impaired erythropoietin response in diabetic patients. Arch Intern Med 2005;165:466-469.
6. Saif MW: HIV-associated autoimmune hemolytic anemia: An update. AIDS Patient Care STDS 2001;15:217-224.
7. Skinner N, Junker JA, Flake D, et al: Clinical inquiries: What is angular cheilitis and how is it treated? J Fam Pract 2005;54:470-471.
8. Tefferi A, Hanson CA, Inwards DJ: How to interpret and pursue an abnormal complete blood cell count in adults. Mayo Clin Proc 2005;80:923-936.
9. Goodnough LT, Bach RG: Anemia, transfusion, and mortality. N Engl J Med 2001;345:1272-1274.
10. Scott RB: Sickle-cell anemia: High prevalence and low priority. N Engl J Med 1970;282:164-165.
11. Bunn HF: Pathogenesis and treatment of sickle cell disease. N Engl J Med 1997;337:762-769.
12. Ataga KI, Orringer EP: Hypercoagulability in sickle cell disease: A curious paradox. Am J Med 2003;115:721-728.
13. Wong WY, Elliott-Mills D, Powars D: Renal failure in sickle cell anemia. Hematol Oncol Clin North Am 1996;10:1321-1331.
14. Vichinsky EP, Neumayr LD, Earles AN, et al: Causes and outcomes of the acute chest syndrome in sickle cell disease: National Acute Chest Syndrome Study Group. [erratum appears in N Engl J Med 2000;343:824]. N Engl J Med 2000;342:1855-1865.
15. Edwards CQ: Anemia and the liver: Hepatobiliary manifestations of anemia. Clin Liver Dis 2002;6:891-907.
16. Molitierno JA Jr, Carson CC 3rd: Urologic manifestations of hematologic disease sickle cell, leukemia, and thromboembolic disease. Urol Clin North Am 2003;30:49-61.
17. Silbergleit R, Jancis MO, McNamara RM: Management of sickle cell pain crisis in the emergency department at teaching hospitals. J Emerg Med 1999;17:625-630.
18. Steinberg MH: Management of sickle cell disease. N Engl J Med 1999;340:1021-1030.
19. Griffiths MJD, Evans TW: Inhaled nitric oxide therapy in adults. N Engl J Med 2005;353:2683-2695.
20. Morris CR, Vichinsky EP, van Warmerdam J, et al: Hydroxyurea and arginine therapy: Impact on nitric oxide production in sickle cell disease. J Pediatr Hematol Oncol 2003;25:629-634.
21. Prchal JT: Polycythemia vera and other primary polycythemias. Curr Opin Hematol 2005;12:112-116.
22. Landolfi R, Marchioli R, Kutti J, et al: Efficacy and safety of low-dose aspirin in polycythemia vera. N Engl J Med 2004;350:114-124.

SECTION **XXII**

Leadership, Communication, and Administration

Chapter 205

Leadership and Emergency Medicine

J. Stephen Bohan

KEY POINTS
The value of leadership lies in its ability to form individuals into a group directed to a goal.
Even small groups benefit from a leader.
People seek leadership.
The soul of leadership is integrity.
The substrate of leadership is change.
Leadership and management are different.

Perspective

The library of books on leadership is extensive and heterogeneous, although most focus on large organizations, predominately businesses.[1-5] Most of these books describe general principles, whereas some are specific to gender or career stage or for chief executive officers or school principals. None are specific to emergency medicine, and few exist for physicians at all. This chapter isolates the characteristics possessed by recognized leaders and then applies them to the context of emergency medicine.

Scope

The nature of the practice of emergency medicine means that leadership is a constant requirement. Few patients can be managed by one person, and many require the simultaneous attention of multiple people. There is universal acknowledgment that better care is delivered when such a group works under effective leadership. This exact same phenomenon is present at the department level. Thus, leadership is an everyday requirement that is vital to the agreed mission of emergency medicine: respectful and good care for anyone, any time, irrespective of any restriction. The leader is an enabler in the goal of "always getting better" at this mission at every level: direct patient care, department operations and development, and national policy matters.

Leadership

Plato pointed out that it is difficult to say what quality is but that one recognizes it when one sees it. The same can be said, to a large extent, about leadership. Everyone recognizes an outstanding leader, but despite listing a variety of characteristics, it remains difficult to say what exactly makes that individual a leader worthy of note.

What is a leader? What do leaders do? Are leaders really managers, or is it the other way around? Can one learn leadership? Are leaders necessary? How big must a group be before it needs a leader?

Group Size and Leadership

Certainly, two people walking down a street do not need a leader, but observation tells us that 15 people walking down a street, as a group, do need leadership even for this simple task. It is the action as a group that makes leadership necessary. Whenever one person acts in concert with another and is recognized to do so by others, then that group, as small as two individuals, needs a leader if for no other purpose than to communicate the needs and wants of the pair to the outside world. Obviously, leading a pair is easier than leading a group of three, and so the complexity grows with each individual.

In large organizations, such as a university, or a firm such as General Electric or Wal-Mart, or the U.S. Navy, the leadership responsibility is divided at different levels. The chief executive officer is expected to lead on matters of policy and general direction of the institution or corporation. As one travels down the chain of responsibility, the ratio of leadership to managerial skill changes.

Manager Versus Leader

Managers direct processes, whereas leaders create change. Managers are given goals and are responsible for the tasks required to achieve that goal, whereas the responsibility of a leader is to make the organization better by creating goals.

> "The reasonable man adapts himself to the world; the unreasonable one persists in trying to adapt the world to himself. Therefore, all progress depends on the unreasonable man."
>
> *George Bernard Shaw*

The leader generates or adopts and then adapts the "better idea" to the needs of the organization. This process requires the leader to have a skill set for each of several roles (Box 205-1). All these roles (visionary, decision maker, informant, tone setter) require unfailing attention to interpersonal skills for the simple reason that someone else, and various others at various levels, will, of necessity, be executing the change.

BOX 205-1

Leadership Roles and Skill Sets

Visionary: The ability to see that options exist.

Decision maker: The ability to choose among options. These options may be self-generated or given to the leader by others, but decisions need to be explicit and timely, neither too early (insufficient data, inadequately prepared staff) or late (problem requiring change is now too large and with a different set of options prevailing). Making decisions is hazardous, but leaders cannot be averse to risk. Recognized leaders rarely revisit decisions and always look forward.

Informant: The ability to inform the members of the organization effectively of the nature of the change and the direction it will take them. This role involves informing related individuals outside the organization of how they will be affected.

Tone setter: Setting the tone (creating the atmosphere) that will allow the change to develop is actually more important than any policy that directs the change.

Character

The *primum non nocere* of interpersonal skills is character. Recognition by others that the leader is a person of character is the bedrock of the respect needed to take people to a goal.

> "He listens, he is honest and he always takes the high road."
>
> *Cheryl Kane, street nurse, Boston Health Care for the Homeless, about her boss, Robert Taube*

"Character" and selfishness are mutually exclusive. The leader must see and be seen to understand that the needs of the organization override individual interests and that "doing the right thing" is always in the interests of the organization. This includes recognizing that the needs of the organization are best served when the appropriate needs of the individual are properly served in the context of the community that is the organization. Character requires commitment, focus, and a willingness to undertake and exercise responsibility, including accepting responsibility for failures. There will always be failures as change proceeds. The absence of failures means that change is not happening.

> "Most things you try will fail."
>
> *Richard Pearle, M.D., chief executive officer, Kaiser Permanente Northern California*

> "If you are not succeeding, you need to double your failure rate."
>
> *Thomas Watson, founder, IBM*

Individuals of character rarely if ever complain, never gossip, and always follow through on what they said they would do. They are, and are seen to be, committed to making the organization and the individuals within it better. Persons of character hold themselves and others accountable while being loyal. Loyalty is a two-way street. The leader must be loyal to relevant external agents (the larger organization, the community, and its needs) while simultaneously acknowledging subordinates through recognition and by supporting them in time of personal need. Leaders are readily distinguishable from sycophants.

"Never complain, never explain."

Anonymous

"Take no credit; share no blame."

Anonymous

Communication

The person of character readily gains respect. This respect makes people willing to listen to what the individual has to say but, more importantly, makes them willing to talk to the leader because when integrity is recognized, trust exists. The individual telling his or her story is seeking, even demanding, attention and should receive it. That attention should be undivided because listening is the overarching virtue of a leader. The decision that follows is often viewed by the narrator as less important than the fact that the story was heard.

"Many a man would rather you heard his story than granted his request."

Lord Chesterfield

There is much to be learned in listening. Buried beneath the words are essential truths about the individual and the job that he or she does as well as the barriers faced while doing it.

Discerning the nature and number of barriers to success at each level is a hallmark of a leader. It also implies the intention and action to remove those barriers, thus allowing individuals to succeed in their tasks.

Over and over, when individuals in large organizations are asked what could be improved in both their work place and the organization as a whole, they reply "better communication." By this, they imply the need to be listened to and also to be told "what is going on." People left on the outside of the information stream feel powerless and neglected. Because a major purpose of any communication is to inform, the leader must be a successful informant. The message must be clear, so it must be simple and declarative. Avoidance of the passive voice enhances clarity. Jargon of any sort, whether medical, administrative, or managerial, should be avoided. The message must have a human touch to communicate not only the information but also sympathy with the recipient. To do this successfully in both written and oral forms takes practice and perhaps some coaching.

In the end, the whole purpose is to communicate the goal of the group and the way in which any change promotes that goal. The goal itself must be "a good," something that makes both the group and the community better, and it must be easily recognized as such. Effective communication aids in this recognition. The "good" is a reflection of the leader's beliefs, the underpinning of the leader's character. The beliefs are then known and are seen as the moral context in which goals and directives are enunciated. This sense of morality implies a sense of fairness and justice.

Fairness and Justice

Fairness and justice imply the absence of a special relationship between a leader and other individuals. Experience tells us that these relationships prevent us from viewing the object of our friendship or affection objectively, thus suggesting unequal regard among all individuals of the organization. The wise and successful leader develops successful acquaintanceships with members of his or her group, but rarely friendship and never affection. This dispassionate approach is absolutely necessary to treating members of the group fairly and justly.

"Get your luvin' at home."

Peter Rosen

Also necessary for developing a sense of equity and fairness is the willingness to abide by the rules, whatever those rules may be. If it is concluded that the rules are silly, counterproductive, or antiquated, then the successful leader will revise or remove them, but never ignore them.

Managing Leadership

Were one to posses and be able to exercise all the foregoing necessary virtues, one would be "the" natural leader, but such is only occasionally the case. Thus, one has to have the ability to recognize one's own weaknesses and to "staff them." This can be done by delegation. One may be excellent at decisional activities but a less than magnetic communicator. In that case, communication can, for some large part, be delegated, all the while taking precautions to ensure that the message is recognized as coming from the leader. The same holds for most activities, including fiscal, personnel management, and community affairs.

It is an unequivocal fact that some people possess leadership talent, whereas others do not. These other individuals may possess other talents that are useful for the organization, such as insight, salesmanship, or the ability to absorb and relate financial information. The successful organization places the individual with a particular talent needed in the position where that talent is useful, and the individual, once placed, will do the same all the way down through the organization. Having individuals in positions for which they have no talent is impairing both for the organization and for the individual, and if this position happens to be a leadership one, then the impairment reverberates widely. Having individuals succeed is a fundamental necessity to the success of the organization. Removing unsuccessful people from positions for which they have no talent is never a bad thing. Keeping these people in the position in which they are not succeeding does a substantive disservice both to the organization and to themselves because it perpetuates dysfunction and delays their placement into positions where they can succeed.

Learning and Knowledge in Leadership

Leaders must be knowledgeable. This requires being informed and trusting the informant. Thus, hiring trustworthy people is a key to success. This team of reliable informants helps the leader to "prepare relentlessly," to get the facts straight, and to "never assume anything." Each episode of "doing the right thing and doing it correctly" sets an example of the standard expected of others. Just as a single adverse headline in a newspaper, truthful or not, can undo decades of reputation building, being mistaken even once on factual matters can serve to diminish credibility, a virtue on which leadership rests. This fact supports the notion that, as in everything else, successful leadership comes from talent supplemented by hard work. One can learn important elements of leadership, or at least improve on them.

Preeminent musicians practice several hours per day, as do star athletes. The skills of leadership are as amenable to improvement as any other skill. Presentation skills can be improved through education and practice. Focusing on individuals, for instance, by learning and remembering names and personal facts of members of the team or work force, can alter the regard in which the leader is held, as can attendance at team social events. All these behaviors take initiative, time, and effort to learn and perform. Leadership is not a leisurely stroll in the park; attention can never lapse.

Effective Leadership

Leadership is about promoting and managing change. Changing people is more challenging than changing material. The effective leader is one who regularly succeeds in driving change. The methods for this entail all the previously mentioned characteristics and character traits. Communication must be regular but not frequent, simple, consistent, and persistent. It should antedate the effective date of the change by a period measured in months and should become more frequent as the date nears. The communication should be seen to be personal, should explain the value of the change to the group, and should continue well into the implementation period, until the change is stabilized in the culture of the institution or group. The use of e-mail is not an effective means of staff behavior change.

Leadership in Emergency Medicine

The scale of leadership in emergency medicine is usually small: the physician group, the department, the organization. The principles remain identical, however, irrespective of the size of the requirement. Leaders must be respected because without respect there is no willingness on the part of the group to listen and adopt the goals enunciated. The fundamental requisites for respect are character and then, not far behind, being good at the job. Technical skill (and "interpersonal skills" are actually a technique of the job) is necessary but not sufficient because it does not replace or make up for character deficiencies. Thus, anyone interested in being a leader in emergency medicine must devote a substantive amount of attention to becoming a respected clinician. This includes being completely knowledgeable about the core scientific knowledge as well as having sufficient interpersonal skills to be respected by both patients and other staff members. With character and clinical skill in place, a leader in emergency medicine usually has a record of academic accomplishment in addition to his or her record of administrative accomplishment (e.g., high-quality programs, emergency medical service activities, community outreach, fiscal management) that is needed in all emergency departments irrespective of size or mission.

> "Asking who the boss should be is like asking who should sing tenor in a quartet—it is the person who can sing tenor."
>
> *Henry Ford*

The record of accomplishment is the interface between the bedrock of character and clinical skill and the leadership position. Once a position of leadership is achieved, there is little difference in what successful leaders do in emergency medicine versus any other organization. An exception is that leaders in emergency medicine are more often expected to continue clinical activities, whereas in other organizations, most particularly large ones, there is no such expectation of "working on the shop floor." On a local level, leaders seek to move the organization forward, including the physician group and hospital activities, both internal and external, that affect the department. On a regional and national level, the principles remain the same; only the scale changes. Regional and national leaders in emergency medicine seek to initiate and manage change, be it through education, legislation, or new structures in national and state policy or new ways of thinking about processes. These leaders set and move toward goals by seeking to align talent and job requirements, to make the work place hospitable and just, thereby reducing costly employee turnover, and to inform peers, other members of the organization, the public, and politicians. These leaders listen, act, take responsibility, and pause and reflect often.

REFERENCES

1. Maxwell J: The 21 Indispensable Qualities of a Leader. Nashville, TN, Nelson Business, 1999.
2. Morrell M, Capparell S: Shackletons's Way. New York, Penguin, 2001.
3. Harvard Business Review: Harvard Business Review on Leadership. Boston, Harvard Business School Press, 1998.
4. Campbell MJ: Five Gifts of Insightful Leaders. Newton, MA, Charlesbank Press, 2006.
5. Gikley RW: The 21st Century Health Care Leader. San Francisco. Jossey-Bass, 1999.

Chapter **206**

The Quality Movement in Health Care: A Primer

Azita G. Hamedani and Elizabeth Mort

KEY POINTS

- The health care system in the United States is the most expensive in the world, yet it does not broadly provide superior patient outcomes.
- The great variability in regional and local clinical practice patterns indicates that Americans do not receive consistently high-quality health care.
- Quality problems in health care can grossly be divided into problems with overuse, underuse, and misuse of health care resources.
- The sources of quality problems in health care are not "bad apples" (i.e., incompetent providers), but rather "bad systems," specifically systems that promote, or at least do not mitigate, predictable human errors causing patient harm.
- Two watershed Institute of Medicine reports (*To Err is Human* and *Crossing the Quality Chasm*) brought the quality problem in health care to center stage. As a result, many different types of health care organizations are working on improving health care quality.
- Currently, the United States is experimenting with "public reporting" and "pay-for-performance" as two strategies by which to improve health care quality. The effectiveness of both these methods depends on valid performance measurement. Unfortunately, performance measurement in health care is in its infancy and has proven very controversial.
- As clinicians, the only way to translate the current energy of the quality movement into better care for our patients is to have a positive influence on the exploding number of quality initiatives through active involvement and leadership.

The United States has the most expensive health care system in the world. More than twice as much is spent per capita on health care than in the United Kingdom, France, Japan, and other developed countries, yet the United States ranks below other industrialized countries when comparing standard quality measures.[1,2] As such, it is appropriate that the Institute of Medicine (IOM) reported that "serious and widespread problems occur . . . in all parts of the country,"[3] that medical errors alone are a leading cause of death in the United States,[4] and that "in its current form, habits, and environment, American health care is incapable of providing the public with the quality health care it expects and deserves."[5] These IOM reports transformed a bubbling wave of quality improvement efforts in health care into an overwhelming quality movement tsunami that is dramatically changing the health care landscape. Although this landscape is continually changing, the two most notable streams to emerge from the movement are *public reporting* and *pay for performance*. The ED sits at a critical juncture between the inpatient and outpatient worlds. Although we can learn from failures and successes of acute care hospitals and ambulatory care practices in pursuing quality improvement, given our unique practice setting, we need to move forward on our own quality agenda.

Quality Is Not Optimal in Health Care

Perhaps most telling of our quality problem in health care is the incredible degree of variability that exists in clinical practice patterns. Wennberg and Gittelsohn[6] were the first to document geographic variation in clinical practice in their 1973 landmark *Science* article. As an example, 70% of women in one Maine county had had hysterectomies by the age of 70 years, as compared with 20% in a nearby county.[7] Since then, wide variability in all aspects of care, from testing to surgery to hospitalization, has been documented.[8-10] Disturbingly, supply is known to be a driving factor of the variability, as evidenced by Roemer's law (a hospital bed built is a hospital bed filled). Regardless of cause, the extent of variability in clinical practice pattern is too great to propose that its full range represents ideal care. Ironically, a 2003 study looking at regional variations in the number of services received by Medicare patients found that patients in higher spending areas received 60% more care, but the quality of care in those regions was no better, and at times worse, when key quality measures were compared.[11,12]

As an outgrowth of early work in variability, health care quality problems can be separated into three major categories: *overuse* problems (provision of services when potential for harm exceeds potential for benefit), *underuse* problems (failure to provide services when having done so would have produced a favorable outcome for the patient), and *misuse* problems (provision of appropriate services, complicated by a preventable error, such that the patient does not receive full benefit).[3] For example, in one study only 21% of Medicare patients with myocardial infarctions who were eligible for beta-blocker treatment received these drugs within 90 days of discharge. The adjusted mortality rate in patients in the study who were treated with beta-blockers was 43% less than in patients who did not receive this treatment.[13] In aggregate, Americans receive only 55% of recommended treatments, regardless of whether preventive, acute, or chronic care is examined.[14] (A listing of all articles since 1987 that document overuse, underuse, and misuse can be found in Appendix A of the IOM report, *Crossing the Quality Chasm*[5]).

Quality Is Not Optimal in Emergency Medicine

Before discussing examples of quality problems in emergency medicine, let us review factors that make the ED an extremely challenging work environment. Many different providers (e.g., physicians, nurses, technicians) work closely together to care simultaneously for multiple patients of varying medical acuity, who present with any imaginable chief complaint from the most life-threatening to the most poorly defined, with whom these providers have no prior relationship. Providers are bombarded with multiple interruptions and transfers, and they struggle with understaffing and overcrowding, while working through disruptive sleep cycles. That this setting predisposes to a higher error rate than other hospital settings is not surprising. That the error rate is not higher speaks to the dedication and vigilance of ED caregivers.

Despite the daily heroic efforts of ED caregivers, examples of overuse, underuse, and misuse are abundant. *Overuse* occurs when, for example, imaging is reordered because of a lack of access to outside facility films for a transferred patient or when a patient is admitted and exposed to nosocomial infections because timely outpatient follow-up cannot be arranged. *Underuse* occurs when, for example, a patient admitted for a pulmonary embolus or atrial fibrillation does not receive any anticoagulation despite boarding in the ED for many hours or when a septic patient is left underresuscitated or without appropriate antibiotic coverage until late in the ED stay because of competing demands. *Misuse* occurs when, for example, antibiotics are ordered for a patient with a known allergy to that medication, when succinylcholine is given for rapid-sequence intubation despite a documented high potassium level determined by laboratory tests earlier that day, or when outpatient follow-up is not arranged for a potentially sinister lesion found incidentally on imaging. Limited numbers of examples based on a limited definition of overuse, underuse, and misuse are provided here, but many more exist.

In addition to underuse, overuse, and misuse are the less clearly defined and less well-documented quality lapses that result from ED overcrowding. The significant increase in *waits*—wait times to be triaged, to be seen by a physician, to obtain a study, to be seen by a consultant, to obtain an inpatient bed—are but one means by which ED overcrowding influences the quality of health care we are able to provide. The full impact of ED overcrowding on the quality of emergency care, however, still needs to be fully investigated.

History of the Quality Movement in Health Care

For most of health care's history, quality was viewed as residing in the hands of physicians, and lapses were attributed to individual practitioners ("bad apples"). Efforts to assess quality in health care extend back to Ernest A. Codman. Codman, an early 20th-century surgeon at the Massachusetts General Hospital in Boston, was the first to advocate the tracking and public reporting of "end results" of surgical procedures. He believed outcomes should be made public so patients could choose among providers and surgeons could learn from each other. In 1913, the American College of Surgeons adopted Codman's proposal of an "end result system of hospital standardization." This system required hospitals to follow patients long enough to learn whether they benefited from their surgical procedures. The American College of Surgeons went on to develop the Minimum Standard for Hospitals and subsequently began on-site inspections. In 1951, the American College of Surgeons was joined by other medical specialty organizations to form the forerunner of today's Joint Commission (JC). Through the JC's accreditation process, and more locally through departmental case review processes, the medical profession was able to keep quality review of its activities internal to the industry for most of its history. The profession judged the quality of its own product and was held accountable only to itself.

In the 1980s, however, a shift occurred in health care from an implicit assumption of quality, as claimed by the profession, to a request for explicit evidence of quality by external validation. This shift was precipitated by ever increasing health care costs and news of the shocking variability in health care discussed earlier. The medical community's response was predominantly promulgation of clinical practice guidelines aimed at decreasing unexplained variability. The Agency for Healthcare Research and Quality took on a leadership role in generating guidelines and in funding related research. Despite enthusiasm for clinical practice guidelines as a means to reduce variability, physicians generally disparaged them as "cookbook medicine."

Given the failure of clinical practice guidelines to solve health care's quality problems, circumstances were ripe by the late 1980s for Donald Berwick, M.D., M.P.P., to enter the trickling health care quality movement. In his 1989 landmark *New England Journal of Medicine* article,[15] Berwick put forth two approaches to the problem of improving quality in U.S. health care: Theory of Bad Apples and Theory of Continuous Improvement. The Theory of Bad Apples relies on inspection to improve quality (i.e., find and remove the bad apples from the lot). In health care, those who subscribe to the Theory of Bad Apples seek outliers (deficient health care workers who need to be punished) and advocate a culture of blame and shame. The bad apple is often showcased in morbidity and mortality conference, in which he or she is publicly reprimanded to install fear of failure in others. The Theory of Continuous Improvement focuses on the average worker (not the outlier) and on systems problems (not on an individual's failure). Accordingly, for the average clinician, quality fails when systems fail.

Examples of bad systems leading to suboptimal human performance abound in medicine. One example provided by Berwick[16] is the reported deaths resulting from an inadvertent mix-up of racemic epinephrine and vitamin E. Newborns in a nursery received the former instead of the latter down their nasogastric tubes. Most of us would be appalled at the thought of any provider's mixing up a benign medication with a potentially toxic one. Through our training, we have come to view error as a character failure and surely as the result of negligence. Yet, when one notes that the two bottles look almost exactly alike, one can understand why the system "is perfectly designed to kill babies by ensuring a specific—low but inevitable—rate of mix-ups."[16] A more widely publicized example is that of oxygen and nitrous oxide in the operating room. In the past, a small number of patients died each year during surgery because the anesthesiologist inadvertently connected the nitrous oxide tank to the oxygen line. No amount of blame and shame during morbidity and mortality presentations reduced the rate of this error until the system was redesigned. Now connectors for nitrous oxide and oxygen have different and, more important, incompatible shapes. Such forcing of function is but one example of strategies used by human factor engineering to improve the safety of our systems in health care. The underlying principle is to "make it easy to do a task right and hard to do it wrong."[17]

Because "every system is perfectly designed to achieve the results it gets,"[16] to improve results, an improvement in system design is needed. As Berwick noted, the Theory of Continuous Improvement works "because of the immense, irresistible quantitative power derived from shifting the entire curve of production [or performance] upward even slightly, as compared with a focus on trimming the tails" (Fig. 206-1).[15]

To test his own hypothesis, Berwick spearheaded the National Demonstration Project on Quality Improvement in Health Care from 1987 to 1988. The project paired 21 health care organizations with 21 quality expert mentors from industries other than health care. The project was designed to test whether system improvement methodologies that helped turn around other industries could be applied successfully to health care. Many success stories emerged from the National Demonstration Project and are detailed in the book *Curing Health Care.*[7] It was not until nearly a decade later, however, that the Northern New England Cardiovascular Disease Study Group published their landmark *JAMA* article. This was the first publication in a major journal of a study whose design was most consistent with a plan-do-check-act (PDCA) cycle (Fig. 206-2).[18] Briefly, all regional cardiothoracic surgeons participated in an intervention aimed at improving coronary artery bypass grafting outcomes. The intervention included three parts: feedback of outcomes data, training in continuous quality improvement methodology, and site visits to other medical centers. Instead of ignoring or hiding their data and pursuing competitive behavior, the groups learned from each others' similarities and differences. The result was a dramatic 24% decline in perioperative mortality across all sites. In terms of improving the daily practice of medicine, PDCA cycles are more useful than both formal studies (e.g.,

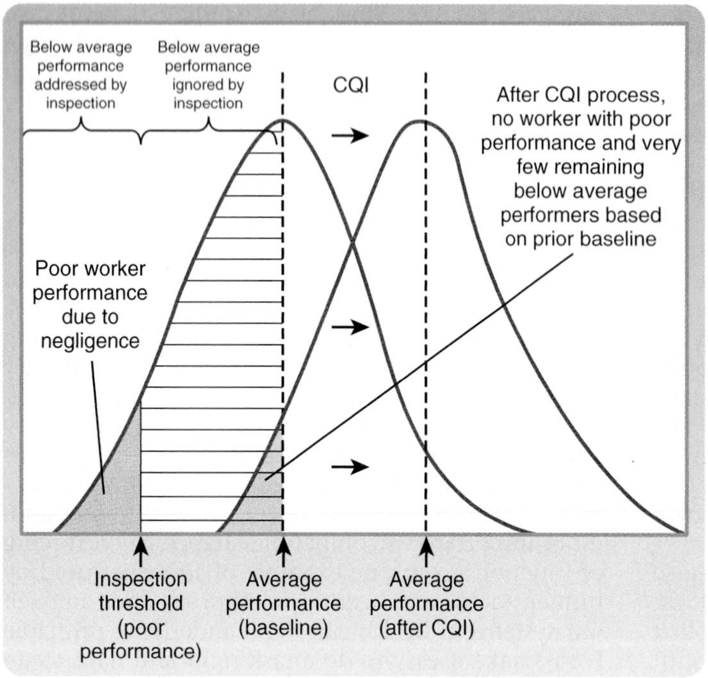
Below average performance addressed by inspection
Below average performance ignored by inspection
CQI
After CQI process, no worker with poor performance and very few remaining below average performers based on prior baseline
Poor worker performance due to negligence
Inspection threshold (poor performance)
Average performance (baseline)
Average performance (after CQI)

FIGURE 206-1 Inspection versus continuous quality improvement (CQI).

randomized trials) and erratic trial and error approaches. Indeed, most daily learning comes from a series of small PDCA cycles.

▪ INSTITUTE OF MEDICINE AND OTHER INFLUENTIAL ORGANIZATIONS FUEL THE QUALITY MOVEMENT

Although Berwick published his landmark paper in 1989, health care did not address its quality problems

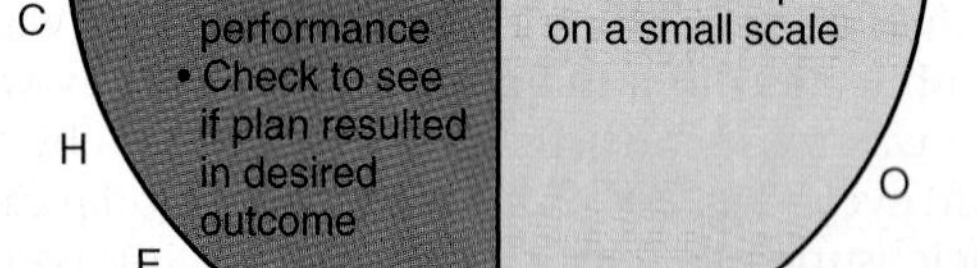
P
L
A
N
• Identify a problem
• Plan a solution
D
O
• Execute the plan on a small scale
C
H
E
C
K
• Measure performance
• Check to see if plan resulted in desired outcome
A
C
T
• Make changes to improve plan +/–
• Execute plan on large scale

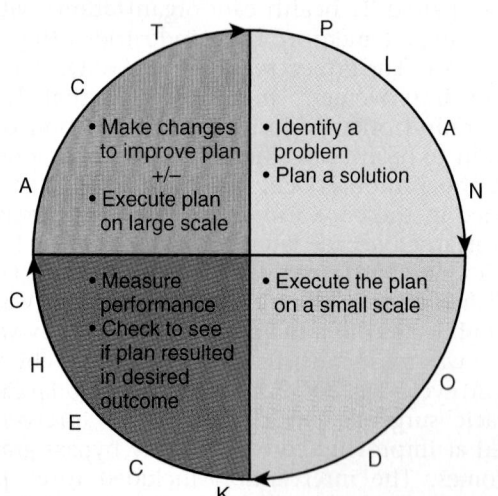

FIGURE 206-2 The PDCA (plan-do-check-act) cycle lays out the steps needed to engage in continuous quality improvement efforts. Although varying interpretations of this cycle have emerged, for the most part, the cycle encourages the following: *plan*—first identify a problem and plan a solution for improving the quality of a process; *do*—execute the plan on a small scale; *check/study*—determine whether the implemented plan has resulted in the desired outcome; and *act*—if successful, implement changes on a larger scale; if not successful, reevaluate by entering the planning stage again.

in any systematic manner until the later publication of two highly-publicized IOM reports: *To Err Is Human: Building a Safer Health System,*[4] in 1999, and *Crossing the Quality Chasm: A New Health System for the 21st Century,*[5] in 2001. The setting was right for the release of these reports. In 1998, the IOM's National Roundtable on Health Care Quality had issued a report documenting problems of overuse, underuse, and misuse. Similarly, the Advisory Commission on Consumer Protection and Quality in Health Care Industry, established by President Bill Clinton, released a report calling for a national commitment to improve quality. Finally, a literature review conducted by RAND Corporation documented significant shortcoming in the health care system.[19] The IOM formed the Committee on the Quality of Health Care in America this same year and charged the committee with developing a strategy to improve health care quality significantly over the next decade.

To Err is Human, the Committee's first report, focused on patient safety and medical errors.[4] This report is best known for its assertion that 44,000 to 98,000 deaths occur per year as a result of medical error, thus making hospital-based errors the eighth leading cause of death in the United States, ahead of breast cancer, acquired immunodeficiency syndrome, and motor vehicle crashes. These statistics were derived from two studies. The Harvard Medical Practice Study[20] reviewed more than 30,000 hospital records and found that adverse events occurred in 3.7% of hospitalizations. Of these adverse events, 13.6% were fatal, and 27.6% were caused by negligence. The Colorado-Utah study[21] reviewed 15,000 hospital records and found that adverse events occurred in 2.9% of hospitalizations. Negligent adverse events accounted for 27.4% of total adverse events in Utah and for 32.6% of those in Colorado.

Of these negligent adverse events, 8.8% were fatal. Extrapolation of results from these two studies provided the upper and lower limits for deaths associated with medical errors for the IOM report. In both studies, compared with other areas of the hospital, the ED had the highest proportion of adverse events resulting from negligence.

Crossing the Quality Chasm, the Committee's second report, focused more broadly on redesign of the health care delivery system to improve quality.[5] The report started out by stating: "The American health care delivery system is in need of fundamental change . . . Between the health care we have and the care we could have lies not just a gap, but a chasm." This chasm exists for preventive, acute, and chronic care.

The impact of the combined IOM reports was immense, even though these reports presented no new information. First, the reports publicized the problem of patient safety among the lay audience. As such, the report received extraordinary media attention, with coverage on all major television networks, newspapers, and talk shows. Second, the reports forced the medical community to acknowledge its quality problem. Initially, the community responded by questioning the accuracy of the numbers put forth in *To Err Is Human.* The sheer magnitude of the problem, however, forced the medical community eventually to come to terms with its quality lapses. Third, the reports solidified a key concept—quality problems are not the result of bad apples but of bad systems. In fact, good people are routinely defeated by bad systems, regardless of training, competence, and vigilance. As such, the *Chasm* report lists "Safety as a System Property" as one of 10 simple rules for the 21st-century health system. The IOM reports accelerated a frenzy of activity among diverse health care stakeholders, including government agencies, accrediting bodies, consumer groups, and other public and private entities.

▪ THE JOINT COMMISSION

The JC is the predominant health care accrediting body in the United States. Because the primary purpose of many hospital-based patient safety initiatives continues to be to meet JC requirements, some argue it is the most influential organization on the list. Over the past few years, the JC has steadily increased demands on hospitals. In 2002, the JC announced its National Patient Safety Goals (NPSG) program. Each year, a set of goals is identified from topics published in JC's *Sentinel Event Alert.* Although the goals are broad and nonprescriptive, the requirements are concrete, and failure to comply with them results in automatic conditional accreditation. The most significant addition to the fourth annual NPSGs (2006) for the ED is the requirement that "hand-offs" of patients among caregivers be standardized. Although the impact on quality of some NPSGs in the ED will invariably be favorable, the impact of others (e.g., medication reconciliation) remains to be seen. In addition to NPSGs, the JC has instituted tracer methodology. By following a hypothetical patient from admission to discharge, surveyors evaluate not only individual components of care but also how the system performs as a whole. In January of 2006, the JC implemented an unannounced hospital inspection policy to ensure that high-quality care is not limited to times of inspection. Very pertinent to the ED, the JC recently instituted a new Leadership Standard on Managing Patient Flow, which addresses ED overcrowding.

▪ CENTERS FOR MEDICARE AND MEDICAID SERVICES

The Centers for Medicare and Medicaid Services (CMS) has also been extremely active in promoting the quality agenda. In July of 2005, the centers released the CMS Quality Improvement Roadmap. Its vision is that of "the right care for every person every time." The CMS's goal is to implement five major systems strategies for improving care, including public reporting (strategy 2) and pay for performance (strategy 3). As such, CMS has been involved in numerous demonstration projects evaluating the impact of both types of initiatives.

▪ AGENCY FOR HEALTHCARE RESEARCH AND QUALITY

In 1999, the Agency for Health Care Policy and Research was reauthorized and renamed by Congress as the Agency for Healthcare Research and Quality, to expand its role to include quality and patient safety. The agency releases a congressionally mandated National Health Care Quality Report annually. This report includes data on more than 100 measures, thus making it the most comprehensive scorecard on health care quality produced. Although there has been modest improvement on all measures, substantial gaps between best possible care and average care still exist.[22] Other resources of the Agency for Healthcare Research and Quality include the Center for Quality Improvement and Patient Safety, the Patient Safety Improvement Corps, Quality Tools website, Indicators software (e.g., Preventive Quality Indicators, Inpatient Quality Indicators, and Patient Safety Indicators), Hospital Survey on Patient Safety Culture, and WebM&M (an online journal featuring expert analysis of medical error cases submitted by readers), to name a few.

▪ LEAPFROG GROUP

The Leapfrog Group was founded by the Business Roundtable and represents more than 150 public and private organizations that collectively buy health care for approximately 40 million people. The Leapfrog Group hopes to encourage quality improvement by rewarding higher-quality hospitals with increased business. To meet Leapfrog standards, hospitals must have a computerized order entry system for inpatient care, meet criteria for evidence-based hospital referral for five high-risk surgical procedures (coronary artery bypass grafting, percutaneous coronary intervention, repair of an abdominal aorta aneurysm, pancreatic resection, and esophagectomy), staff intensive care units with board-certified intensive care specialists, and implement the remaining 27 of 30 Safe Practices of the National Quality Forum (NQF). Initially, evidence-based hospital referral was purely a volume-based criterion. Based on some concern about the validity of volume as a proxy for quality, Leapfrog revised its criteria for evidence-based hospital referral to include an outcomes measure (risk-adjusted mortality for coronary artery bypass grafting and percutaneous coronary intervention) and a process measure (perioperative use of beta-blockers for patients undergoing repair of an abdominal aorta aneurysm). Hospital data are used for incentive programs designed either to affect consumers' selection of hospitals or to pay providers according to performance. For example, Boeing Company employees who choose hospitals that meet Leapfrog criteria have their coinsurance payments waived.[23]

▪ OTHER GROUPS

The National Committee for Quality Assurance is a private, not-for-profit organization, best known for its Health Plan Employer Data and Information Set, which provides comparative quality data (60 measures) for managed health plans. The NQF is a unique public-private venture whose mission is to improve health care by endorsing consensus-based national standards for measurement and public reporting of health care quality data. The CMS relies on the NQF to develop valid performance measures. The NQF has released a consensus report identifying 30 Safety Practices (e.g., using only standardized abbreviations and adhering to practices that prevent central venous catheter–associated bloodstream infections) that providers should use to reduce errors. In addition, the NQF has released a list of 27 Never Events, which are hospital errors that should never happen (including a patient's death from a fall, the suicide of a patient, and the abduction of a patient) but still sometimes occur.

The American Medical Association has also been involved in the quality movement, most notably by forming the National Patient Safety Foundation and by convening the Physician Consortium for Performance Improvement. The Consortium includes representatives from more than 70 national medical specialty and state medical societies, as well as the Agency for Healthcare Research and Quality and the CMS. The American College of Emergency Physicians/Emergency Medicine Workgroup of the American Medical Association Physician Consortium has developed seven emergency medicine–specific quality measures that are currently in process of review by the NQF (Box 206-1). Finally, the Institute for Healthcare Improvement, under Dr. Berwick's leadership, has been involved in innumerable quality improvement initiatives. The 100,000 Lives Campaign and its successor, the 5 Million Lives Campaign, have garnered the most recent attention. The initial initiative was launched in December of 2004, with the goal of saving lives of 100,000 hospitalized patients over the course of 1.5 years. Participating hospitals were asked to implement six interventions (rapid response teams, evidence-based care for acute myocardial infarction, measures to prevent adverse drug events through medication reconciliation, measures to prevent central line infections, measures to prevent surgical site infection, and measures to prevent ventilator-associated pneumonias). The most recent campaign, launched in December of 2006, promotes the adoption of 12 improvements that can save lives and improve patient care.

BOX 206-1

Subset of Quality Measures Specific to Emergency Medicine

- Electrocardiogram performed for nontraumatic chest pain
- Aspirin at arrival for acute myocardial infarction
- Electrocardiogram performed for syncope
- Vital signs for CAP
- Assessment for oxygen saturation for CAP
- Assessment of mental status for CAP
- Empirical antibiotics for CAP

CAP, community-acquired bacterial pneumonia.

▪ EMERGENCY MEDICINE

Of all disciplines, emergency medicine is one of the most eager to embrace the quality movement. Our specialty germinated from a desire to provide consistently high-quality emergency care in hospitals throughout the country. Our specialty was one of the first to develop a comprehensive curriculum (Model of the Clinical Practice of Emergency Medicine) and to develop a new model for Maintenance of Certification (Emergency Medicine Continuous Certification program). Shortly after the IOM *Err* and *Chasm* reports, the Society for Academic Emergency Medicine and the journal *Academic Emergency Medicine* sponsored conferences on Errors in Emergency Medicine (2000) and Assuring Quality in Emergency Care (2002). Quality—that quality emergency care, including patient safety, is ensured—is one of American College of Emergency Physicians' five college priorities. A Quality and Performance Committee has been formed, whose objectives include reviewing performance measures developed both internally and externally and monitoring CMS pay-for-performance initiatives. The Quality Improvement and Patient Safety section is also very active and sponsored the first quality course in emergency medicine in Spring of 2007. In addition, a substantial body of emergency medicine literature focuses on quality. Most of the key articles are listed in the reference sections of three outstanding articles in *Academic Emergency Medicine's* Special Consensus Issue on Assuring Quality in Emergency Care,[24-26] and the information not repeated here.

In addition to internal interest in the quality of emergency care, there is substantial external interest in our EDs. In June of 2006, the IOM's Committee on the Future of Emergency Care released a series of reports discussing the crisis in emergency care. The report concluded that the "nation's emergency medical system as a whole is overburdened, underfunded, and highly fragmented."[27] Specific areas of quality concern include overcrowding, ambulance diversions, and boarding of admitted patients. Similarly, Urgent Matters is a $6.4 million initiative of the Robert Wood Johnson Foundation that is focused on helping hospitals to eliminate ED crowding and helping communities to understand the challenges facing our health care safety net.

> ***Tips and Tricks***
>
> **QUALITY IN THE ED**
>
> - Do what is right for the patient regardless of timing (e.g., off hours) or circumstances (e.g., overcrowding).
> - At change of shift, briefly evaluate patients turned over to your care so you have a baseline in mind should an acute deterioration in a patient's condition occur.
> - Before discharge, make sure to review all laboratory results and radiographs even if you expect the results to be normal.
> - Explain diagnostic uncertainties at discharge so the patient will seek care if his or her condition deteriorates.
> - In general, think twice before:
>   - Discharging a patient against the preference or comfort of the patient or family.
>   - Discharging a patient against the advice of another physician.
>   - Discharging a patient who was seen in the past 48 hours for the same condition.
>   - Discharging a patient with narcotic pain medications without a clear diagnosis.
>   - Ruling out a critical diagnosis based on a negative result of a suboptimal test.

Future of the Quality Movement in Emergency Medicine

The only cure for our quality problem in health care is greater involvement of physicians with the rest of the care team. As a start, each ED should have a lead physician for quality (e.g., Director of Quality and Patient Safety). This leader should develop systems that allow easy reporting of quality concerns by any and all members of the ED and hospital staff. As an example, some hospitals have an e-mail (EDQA@hospital.edu) account that allows any provider throughout the hospital to submit cases for review. Providers should be encouraged to submit a variety of cases—bad outcomes, near misses, and saves. These cases should be reviewed, but not to identify bad apples. Instead, the goal is to discover systems issues that leave patients and providers vulnerable to unfavorable outcomes and to identify clinical practice patterns that may be suboptimal. Data from case reviews should be tracked for notable trends. Are most quality concerns raised on the night shift, with nursing home patients, with elderly trauma patients, with discharged patients, with radiology interpretations? A reminder to the group of high-risk situations (especially those specific to the institution or to the group's practice pattern) can be made periodically (see Tips and Tricks box). Targeted system fixes can be tested through the PDCA cycle.

Case review, even for identification of systems issues, is only one component of a quality program. In addition, a quality dashboard for the department would allow ED leadership to identify problem areas proactively. Most quality dashboards to date contain only a limited number of true quality measures and instead are filled with many proxy quality measures (e.g., rate of bounce-backs within 72 hours, rate of patients who left without being seen, number of floor admissions upgraded to the intensive care unit in the first 24 hours) and many operational measures (e.g., turnaround time for laboratory and diagnostic studies, emergency medical service divert time, and inpatient boarding hours). It could be successfully argued that in the ED, operational performance directly enhances or hinders patient quality. However, the time is also ripe to expand our catalog of quality measures to include those that reliably assess clinical care.

As early work in this area, Graff and associates[25] provided information on factors to be considered in selecting process measures and provided two tables of existing performance measures. Lindsay and colleagues[28] moved forward with measure development. They assembled an expert panel and used a modified-Delphi process that led to the identification of more than two dozen clinical indicators for use in the ED. More recently, American College of Emergency Physicians' Quality Improvement and Patient Safety section was granted funding for a Chief Compliant Based Quality Indicators project. The project chose to focus on chief complaints, rather than diagnoses, because patients present to the ED in an undifferentiated fashion. Six high-risk complaints (abdominal pain, altered mental status, chest pain, headache, shortness of breath, syncope) were chosen for measure development. Ultimately, if the emergency medicine

BOX 206-2

Hospital Compare Measures

Heart Attack Care Quality Measures

Percentage of patients given angiotensin-converting enzyme inhibitor or angiotensin-receptor blocker for left ventricular systolic dysfunction

Percentage of patients given aspirin at arrival

Percentage of patients given aspirin at discharge

Percentage of patients given beta-blocker at arrival

Percentage of patients given beta-blocker at discharge

Percentage of patients given percutaneous coronary intervention within 120 minutes of arrival

Percentage of patients given smoking cessation advice/counseling

Percentage of patients given thrombolytic medication within 30 minutes of arrival

Heart Failure Care Quality Measures

Percentage of patients given angiotensin-converting enzyme inhibitor or angiotensin-receptor blocker for left ventricular systolic dysfunction

Percentage of patients given assessment of left ventricular function

Percentage of patients given discharge instructions

Percentage of patients given smoking cessation advice or counseling

Pneumonia Care Quality Measures

Percentage of patients assessed and given pneumococcal vaccination

Percentage of patients assessed and given influenza vaccination

Percentage of patients given initial antibiotics within 4 hours after arrival

Percentage of patients given oxygenation assessment

Percentage of patients given smoking cessation advice or counseling

Percentage of patients given the most appropriate initial antibiotics

Percentage of patients having a blood culture performed before first antibiotic received in hospital

Surgical Infection Prevention Quality Measures

Percentage of surgical patients who received preventive antibiotics 1 hour before incision

Percentage of surgical patients whose preventive antibiotics are stopped within 24 hours postoperatively

BOX 206-3

Quality Web Sites of Interest

Agency for Healthcare Research and Quality

WebM&M (www.webmm.ahrq.gov)

QualityTools (www.qualitytools.ahrq.gov)

Quality Indicators (www.qualityindicators.ahrq.gov)

National Guideline Clearing House (www.guideline.gov)

Centers for Medicare and Medicaid Services

Hospital Compare (www.hospitalcompare.hhs.gov)

Quality initiatives (www.cms.hhs.gov/quality)

The Joint Commission

Quality Check (www.qualitycheck.org)

International Center for Patient Safety (www.jcipatientsafety.org)

Other Organizations

Veteran Affairs National Center for Patient Safety (www.patientsafety.gov)

Institute for Healthcare Improvement (www.ihi.org)

National Quality Forum (www.qualityforum.org)

Leapfrog (www.leapfroggroup.org)

Wisconsin Collaborative for Healthcare Quality (www.wchq.org)

Kaiser Family Foundation Quality of Care Reference Library (www.kaiseredu.org/topics_reflib.asp?id=139&parented=70&rID=1)

ED Benchmarking Alliance (www.edbenchmarking.org)

community does not continue to generate emergency medicine quality measures, we will be subject to measures developed by others. As the JC's pneumonia core measures have proven, this is not a theoretical assertion. The 4-hour antibiotic time in pneumonia has been called "ridiculous" and "silly," and the blood culture requirement has been labeled as having "essentially no clinical value" by emergency physicians in leadership roles.[29,30] Box 206-2 lists measures by which one can compare hospitals in terms of emergency care.

In addition to developing our own quality measures, we must continue to pursue the research agenda put forth on quality improvement in emergency care.[31] Box 206-3 provides a list of Web sites related to quality issues. Our overarching goal in the coming decade should be to redesign our EDs such that it will be easy for us to do the right thing at the right time and difficult to do the wrong thing at any time for our increasing numbers of patients.

Future of the Quality Movement in Health Care

The level of activity in the health care quality movement has accelerated significantly in the past decade. Despite focused attention, however, people do not feel safer. A 2004 survey revealed that 55% of respondents are dissatisfied with the quality of U.S. health care, and 40% believed that quality had worsened in the previous 5 years.[32] As such, there is some sense of disappointment about the results of the movement. Lack of adequate physicians' investment in the quality movement has been reported as one the major barriers to significant progress.[17] With respect to public reporting and pay-for-performance specifically, the lack of physician support could possibly lead to a backlash akin to that seen for utilization review, gatekeeping, and other managed care efforts.[33] Nonetheless, the quality movement is unlikely to recede. Physicians and other clinicians need to engage from this point forward. How the community of physicians responds will determine whether the quality movement will have the intended consequence of improving care or will only leave a legacy of increased regulatory and administrative burden.

REFERENCES

1. Blendon RJ, Kim M, Benson JM: The public versus the World Health organization on health system performance. Health Aff 2001;20:10-20.
2. World Health Organization: The World Health Report 2000: Health Systems, Improving Performance. Geneva, World Health Organization, 2000.
3. Chassin MR, Galvin RW: The urgent need to improve health care quality: Institute of Medicine National Roundtable on Health Care Quality. JAMA 1998;280:1000-1005.
4. Kohn LT, Corrigan JM, Donaldson MS (eds): To Err is Human: Building a Safer Health System. Washington, DC, National Academies Press, 1999.
5. Committee on Quality Health Care in America: Crossing the Quality Chasm: A New Health System for the 21st Century. Washington, DC, National Academies Press, 2001.
6. Wennberg JE, Gittelsohn A: Small area variations in health care delivery. Science 1973;182:1102-1108.
7. Berwick DM, Godfrey AB, Roessner J: Curing Health Care: New Strategies for Quality Improvement. San Francisco, Jossey-Bass, 2002.
8. Chassin MR, Brook RH, Park RE, et al: Variations in the use of medical and surgical services by the Medicare population. N Engl J Med 1986;314:285-290.
9. Wennberg JE, Freeman JL, Culp WJ: Are hospital services rationed in New Haven or over-utilized in Boston? Lancet 1987;1:1185-1190.
10. Welch WP, Miller ME, Welch HG, et al: Geographic variation in expenditures for physicians' services in the United States. N Engl J Med 1993;328:621-627.
11. Fisher ES, Wennberg DE, Stukel TA, et al: The implications of regional variations in Medicare spending. Part I: The content, quality, and accessibility of care. Ann Intern Med 2003;138:273-287.
12. Fisher ES, Wennberg DE, Stukel TA, et al: The implications of regional variations in Medicare spending. Part 2: Health outcomes and satisfaction with care. Ann Intern Med 2003;138:288-298.
13. Soumerai SB, McLaughlin TJ, Spiegelman D, et al: Adverse outcomes of underuse of beta-blockers in elderly survivors of acute myocardial infarction. JAMA 1997;277:115-121.
14. McGlynn EA, Asch SM, Adams J, et al: The quality of health care delivered to adults in the United States. N Engl J Med 2003;348:2635-2645.
15. Berwick DM: Continuous improvement as an ideal in health care. N Engl J Med 1989;320:53-56.
16. Berwick DM: Why the Vasa Sank: In Escape Fire. San Francisco, CA, Jossey-Bass, 2004.
17. Leape LL: Making health care safe: Are we up to it? J Pediatr Surg 2004;39:258-266.
18. O'Connor GT, Plume SK, Olmstead EM, et al: A regional intervention to improve the hospital mortality associated with coronary artery bypass graft surgery. JAMA 1996;275: 841-846.
19. Schuster MA, McGlynn EA, Brook RH: How good is the quality of health care in the United States? Milbank Q 1998;76:517-563.
20. Brennan TA, Leape LL, Laird NM, et al: Incidence of adverse events and negligence in the hospitalized patients: Results of the Harvard Medical Practice Study. N Engl J Med 1991;324:370-376.
21. Thomas EJ, Studdert DM, Burstin HR, et al: Incidence and types of adverse events and negligent care in Utah and Colorado. Med Care 2000;38:261-271.
22. Agency for Healthcare Research and Quality: 2004 National Healthcare Quality Report. Rockville, MD, Agency for Healthcare Research and Quality, 2004.
23. Galvsin RS, Delbanco S, Milstein A, et al: Has the Leapfrog Group had an impact on the health care market? Health Aff 2005;24:228-233.
24. Cone DC, Nedza SM, Augustine JJ, et al: Quality in clinical practice. Acad Emerg Med 2002;9:1085-1090.
25. Graff L, Stevens C, Spaite D, et al: Measuring and improving quality in emergency medicine. Acad Emerg Med 2002;9:1091-1107.
26. Sanders AB: Quality in emergency medicine: An introduction. Acad Emerg Med 2002;9:1064-1066.
27. Committee on the Future of Emergency Care in the United States Health System: Hospital-Based Emergency Care: At the Breaking Point. Washington, DC, National Academies Press, 2006.
28. Lindsay P, Schull M, Bronskill S, et al: The development of indicators to measure the quality of clinical care in the emergency departments following a modified-Delphi approach. Acad Emerg Med 2002;9:1131-1139.
29. Thompson D: The pneumonia controversy: Hospitals grapple with 4 hour benchmark. Ann Emerg Med 2006;47: 259-261.
30. Walls RM, Resnick JB: The CMS blood cultures for CAP program: The architects speak out. Editor's reply. J Watch Emerg Med 2005;April 27.
31. Magid DJ, Rhodes KV, Asplin BR, et al: Designing a research agenda to improve the quality of emergency care. Acad Emerg Med 2002;9:1124-1130.
32. Altman DE, Clancy C, Blendon RJ. Improving patient safety: Five years after the IOM report. N Engl J Med 2004;351:2041-2043.
33. Casalino LP, Alexander C, Jin L, et al: General internists' view on pay-for-performance and public reporting of quality scores: A national survey. Health Aff 2007;26:492-499.

Chapter 207

Patient Safety in Emergency Medicine

Cherri D. Hobgood

KEY POINTS

Underlying clinician behavior is a complex system that must be deliberately designed for safety.

Error, both active and latent, must first be recognized and studied before design changes can be made to enhance safety.

Eliminating ambiguity, minimizing work-arounds, reducing cognitive load, redesigning procedures, incorporating technology, and conducting simulations are strategies to prevent error.

High-reliability organizations are preoccupied with failure, reluctant to simplify event interpretation, sensitive to operations, resilient, defer to expertise, and have a common, clear mission and vision.

Scope

The Hippocratic oath's "Above all do no harm" principle defines our cultural standard for health care delivery.[1] Early in medical school and residency training, we are socialized to this principle and the belief that we are responsible for practicing error free. Thus, learning that medical errors are an unfortunate but inescapable part of medical practice can be disheartening.

Despite evidence that suggests error is a frequent occurrence in medical practice, malevolent providers, or "bad apples," are rarely at fault.[2] More often, problems inherent to systematic operations of the ED are the cause. Thus, practitioners, aware of the inevitability of errors and armed with the knowledge of how to create safer health care delivery systems, face a better chance of prevailing in a system that is designed to fail in many cases. This chapter is intended to give practitioners that awareness and knowledge.

Specifically, this chapter is designed to teach you how to

- Identify features of the ED that make it prone to errors.
- Recognize the cognitive limitations of practitioners that correlate highly with error rates.
- Use nomenclature recognized by the field when discussing medical errors.
- Understand error origins, to pinpoint variance arising from level of practitioner competence (skill based, rule based, knowledge based).
- Describe prevailing models of error development and analyses targeting errors.
- Build safety as a cornerstone into health care operations.
- Disclose errors to patients, other providers, and the public at large.
- Reduce errors by employing principles and practices that make the ED a safer place for all our patients.

Perspective

Patients should not be harmed by the very care that is intended to help them. The Institute of Medicine's *To Err is Human,* released in 2000, placed error in medicine at the forefront of the U.S. public health and health policy debate. Error was defined by the Institute of Medicine as "failure of a planned action to be completed as intended or the use of a wrong plan to achieve an aim." The report pointed out that errors in medicine were common, costly, and often disregarded by the medical community. Extrapolating outcome data from three large inpatient studies to the entire U.S. health care system, the report listed 44,000 and perhaps as many as 98,000 deaths annually as a result of medical error in the United States. Estimates of the costs to U.S. health care system ranged from 9 to 19 billion dollars and more than 100,000 human lives per year.[3]

The committee proposed six specific aims for improvement (Table 207-1). It concluded that if the current health system is to achieve these aims, fundamental changes in the way care is delivered will be necessary. Table 207-2 provides the Institute of Medicine's Patient Safety and Adverse Event Nomenclature, and Box 207-1 gives reasons for the complexities in documenting errors in health care.[4]

EDs rank among the top three hospital locations with the highest risk for error.[5] Notable similarities exist between EDs and the other high-risk clinical environments: operating rooms and intensive care units. Each environment serves patients who often are critically ill and who receive high-intensity, complex health care interventions provided by interdisciplinary teams of care providers.

Table 207-1 INSTITUTE OF MEDICINE'S SIX AIMS FOR QUALITY IMPROVEMENT

Aim	Definition
Health Care Should Be:	
Safe	"Avoiding injuries to patients from care that is intended to help"
Effective	"Providing services based on scientific knowledge (avoiding underuse and overuse)"
Patient centered	"Providing care that is respectful of and responsive to individual patient preferences, needs, and values and ensuring that patient values guide all clinical decisions"
Timely	"Reducing waits and sometimes harmful delays for both those who receive and those who give care"
Efficient	"Avoiding waste, in particular waste of equipment, supplies, ideas an energy"
Equitable	"Providing care that does not vary in quality because of personal characteristics such as gender, ethnicity, geographic location, and socioeconomic status"

Adapted from Committee on Quality Health Care In America: Crossing the Quality Chasm: A New Health System for the 21st Century. Washington, DC, National Academies Press, 2001.

Table 207-2 INSTITUTE OF MEDICINE'S PATIENT SAFETY AND ADVERSE EVENT NOMENCLATURE

Term	Definition
Safety	Freedom from accidental injury
Patient safety	Freedom from accidental injury; involves the establishment of operational systems and processes that minimize the possibility of error and maximize the probability of intercepting errors when they occur
Accident	An event that damages a system and disrupts the ongoing or future output of the system.
Error	The failure of a planned action to be completed as intended or the use of a wrong plan to achieve an aim
Adverse event	An injury caused by medical management rather than by the underlying disease or condition of the patient
Preventable adverse event	Adverse event attributable to error
Negligent adverse event	A subset of adverse event meeting the legal criteria for negligence
Adverse medication event	Adverse event resulting from a medication or pharmacotherapy
Active error	Error that occurs at the frontline and whose effects are felt immediately
Latent error	Error in design, organization, training, or maintenance that is often caused by management or senior level decisions; when expressed, these errors result in operator errors but may have been hidden, dormant in the system for lengthy periods before their appearance

Adapted from Kohn LT, Corrigan J, Donaldson MS, McKenzie D: To Err Is Human: Building a Safer Health System. Washington, DC, National Academies Press, 2000.

BOX 207-1

Complexities of Documenting Errors in Health Care

It has proven difficult to attain accurate counts of error in medicine, largely because many errors and safety issues are undetected or because those that are detected are either unrecognized or underreported.

Underreporting (failure to disclose errors) stems from numerous factors. The first factor, a prevailing cultural view that individuals should carry out health care flawlessly, is ingrained in practitioners and the public. This mindset causes providers, who fear criticism and personal embarrassment, not to disclose errors. The overall public perception that health care can be performed flawlessly has resulted in a nonforgiving liability system and a constant threat of malpractice.

Another notable cause for failure to report errors is a variability in interpretation that exists even for basic terms of patient safety, such as "incident," "error," and "mishap."[4] Practitioners are encouraged to review and use the nomenclature and the definitions provided by the Institute of Medicine to describe events within their clinical contexts.

Table 207-3 ACTIVE AND LATENT FAILURE TYPES

Failure Type	Characteristics
Active	Committed by those whose actions have immediate adverse consequences (e.g., direct patient care providers [sharp end]) Cognitive errors Slips Lapses Mistakes Rule based Knowledge based Violations Low morale Poor examples from senior staff Maladaptive decision styles Authority gradient Overconfidence or underconfidence
Latent	Resulting from the actions or decisions of those not directly involved in the work place (e.g., management or senior clinicians [blunt end]) Excessive workloads/inadequate staff Inadequate knowledge/experience/training Lack of supervision High-stress environment Poor communication systems Poor maintenance of work environment Rapid organizational change Conflict between institutional mission and values Production pressure Overcrowding Poor feedback Poor design characteristics

From Aghababian R (ed): Essentials of Emergency Care, 2nd ed. Sudbury, MA, Jones and Bartlett, 2006.

Three large inpatient studies provided some insight on ED error rates. In each of these studies, the ED was responsible for a small percentage of all adverse events (range, 1.5% to 3%), but it was always the clinical setting with the highest rate of preventable errors with serious consequences.[5]

Anatomy of an Error

Failures in the ED fall under two main failure types: active and latent (Table 207-3). This section discusses these two failure types, and later sections describe the various error types highlighted under each failure condition.

▪ ACTIVE AND LATENT FAILURE TYPES

Active failures are unsafe acts or omissions at the level of the front-line operator, such as the ED physician, nurse, or care provider, and the effects are felt almost immediately. This is sometimes called the *sharp end.*

Latent failures are failures of the system that can lie dormant, or latent, for years. Despite, or perhaps owing to, their obscurity, latent failures can cause multiple types of operator, or active, failures, thus posing the greatest threat to safety in the complex ED system. Masked as the cause of incidents, these failures are powerful in joining with other factors to breach the system's defenses and coalesce in errors. In large part, latent failures are the result of decisions affecting daily ED operations, often made by persons not directly involved in care delivery, for example, managers, designers, procedure writers, and drug manufacturers.

Problems arise when workers on the front line do not recognize or, even worse, when they learn to work around latent system failures. Imagine this situation. A nurse, intending to deliver drug X, picks up drug Y. Because these drugs are both colorless and share similar names, vial size, delivery method, and because they are side by side in the drug supply closet, they can easily be delivered incorrectly. When this is caught before it occurs, the potentially deadly error is termed a *near miss.* To guard against any future mix-ups, the nurse creates a mnemonic about the placement of each drug. This protects his or her patients from this potential error, but others are still at risk. Only by addressing the latent error at the root can we prevent this near miss from happening again and again.

As in this situation, when practitioners make a mistake, or nearly make one, they most often prevent it from harming the patient. They correct themselves quickly, almost reflexively, thus seldom drawing attention to the error. We need to draw attention to the error. Although quick fixes may meet patients' immediate needs, they do not resolve ambiguities (i.e., the latent failures). As a result, people confront "the same problem, every day, for years," regularly manifested as inefficiencies and irritations and, occasionally, as catastrophes.[6] We should not wait until a patient dies or suffers serious injury to subject all system lapses and their contributing factors to serious scrutiny.

■ COGNITIVE-BASED ERRORS

One of the most widely accepted error classification schemes is based on a model of cognitive performance originated by Rasmussen and Jensen in 1974[7] and elaborated on by Reason in 1990.[8] It uses three functional levels to describe three distinct types of errors: skill based, rule based, and knowledge based. Any of the three types can result in an active failure.

Consider the act of driving a car or putting on your shoes. At some point, most of us acquired the requisite skills to accomplish these tasks quickly and efficiently without having to think about them. *Skill-based cognitive performance* refers to such acts. In the clinical setting, experienced clinicians approach the tasks of preparing a wound, tying a suture, or starting a central line in like fashion; for them, such clinical actions require little conscious input, because their implementation is based on predefined schemata or preprogrammed instructions. Decisions about to how to proceed as well as technical performance in carrying out the course of action is virtually automatic.

Skill-based errors are known as slips and lapses. *Slips* arise when actions fail to proceed as planned, for example, when a physician chooses an appropriate medication and writes 10 mg when the intention was to write 1 mg. Slips are errors in execution resulting from a failure of attention or perception, often caused by interruptions or altered routines. In lay terms, slips are often equated with minor incidents. In the ED, patients can die as a result of slips. *Lapses* also result in failure to execute a plan, but whereas slips are observable, memory-based lapses are not. Turning the wrong knob on a piece of equipment because you are interrupted and lose your train of activity is a slip; not being able to *recall* something is a lapse.

Any task departure from skills-based processing requires either a rules-based or a knowledge-based approach. *Rules-based processing* occurs when the clinician applies a known rule to make a decision. Rules, typically applied in the form "if X, then Y," come from past experience, explicit instructions, or clinical guidelines. For example, to treat a patient with an ankle injury, the physician applies the Ottawa ankle rules, and this approach inherently leads to the decision about the need for a radiograph. *Knowledge-based processing* is when medical knowledge is applied and analytic processes are used to execute a plan of care.

Errors of rule-based and knowledge-based cognition are known as mistakes. In rules-based errors, the wrong rule is selected, applied, or linked to the situation. Rule-based errors increase as a new rule is applied until the fidelity of the application of the rule is refined, and then these substantially decline. Knowledge-based errors result when incomplete or incorrect knowledge is applied or flawed analytic processes are used, resulting in a poor plan of care. A mistake in medicine may involve selecting the wrong drug or treatment because of an incorrect diagnosis.

As clinicians gain experience, they engage to greater extent in skill-based and rule-based processing and to a lesser degree in knowledge-based processing. This shift in cognitive processing creates an interesting paradox with respect to the types of errors they are most likely to commit. Although the rate of their knowledge-based errors is substantially reduced, highly trained individuals are more likely to experience skill-based errors—errors that arise from processes requiring the least amount of cognitive function.

■ HIGH-RISK INTERFACES AND PATTERNS

Several high-risk interfaces and patterns are common in the emergency department. They cluster into two classification types: violation-producing behaviors (VPBs) and error-producing conditions (EPCs). Typical VPBs and EPCs are listed in Table 207-3. Errors arising from EPCs and VPBs occur continuously in most EDs. Some errors are inconsequential, whereas most of the significant errors are corrected continuously.

■ Violation-Producing Behaviors

Certain individual characteristics can lead to a high propensity to err in the ED. These characteristics are known as VPBs. These behaviors may be either intentional or erroneous (e.g., deliberately veering from protocols because of time pressure or veering from the protocol because they misunderstand or misinterpret the procedure). An individual's workplace behavior is influenced by his or her gender, personality factors (e.g., the willingness to take risks, underconfidence, and overconfidence), and style of decision making. Maladaptive decision making leads to impairments in performance. For example, *thematic vagabonding* is when clinicians move quickly between problems and thus avoid the pursuit of clinical closure. This indecisiveness is sometimes accomplished by the ordering of unnecessary tests or through other behaviors that stall a decision. *Encysting,* in contrast, is the tendency to focus unduly on minor clinical details of a case at the expense of more significant ones.

Decision making in the ER is often characterized by a reliance on heuristics. *Heuristics* are shortcuts, rules of thumb, or any kind of abbreviated thinking that accomplishes quick and efficient decision making. Although they often serve us well, heuristics sometimes fail, leading to poor outcomes. *Cognitive bias* is the term used most often to describe the failed application of a heuristic. The three most commonly applied heuristics are representativeness, availability, and anchoring.

The *representativeness heuristic* is applied when a clinician makes a subjective judgment of how similar an example is to its parent population. The more unrepresentative the patient's presentation, the greater is the chance that the diagnosis is delayed or missed. Representativeness errors appear most often in settings of high diagnostic uncertainty, such as that typifying the ED, and they are more likely to be committed by those with lower levels of experience.

Another heuristic that can lead to errors in decision making is *availability*. Certain encounters are more prevalent in our memories, perhaps because they have occurred more recently but, more often, because they are emotionally valent and salient. It is human nature when making diagnoses to place an overreliance on encounters that are vivid to us and to place less importance on those least salient. For example, if a physician has a particularly vivid experience of missing an acute myocardial infarction in a young person, the physician may become overcautious in managing all patients with chest pain, and this may lead to overconsultation and poor resource utilization. Availability may similarly be increased by indirect experience: a recent discussion with a colleague, a case presentation at rounds, or an article reviewing a particular case. In contrast, availability is decreased by long intervals since encountering, or never having previously seen, a particular disease.

Anchoring results when we commit early to a diagnosis and caught up in the momentum of the diagnosis, we fail to consider other possibilities. One way of avoiding anchoring is to ask ourselves "What else could this be?" We have a tendency to look for evidence that bolsters our original hypothesis. This is referred to as *confirmation bias*. Instead, we must look for disconfirming evidence that rejects our initial contention. If anchoring occurs early in a presentation and we operate under a strong confirmation bias, we are sure to miss diagnoses.

Awareness of such cognitive biases is crucial—simply knowing what they look like will help in overcoming them. Avoid reflexive thinking and action and taking the time to think about how we think can help us to minimize or avoid error.

■ Error-Producing Conditions

An EPC is any condition that increases the probability of human error in a given system. EPCs underlie latent failures; in other words, they are failures waiting to happen. In no other area of medicine does this combination of EPCs exist as it does in the ED. Table 207-3 highlights typical EPCs of the ED. The following factors also contribute to error.

■ *Diagnostic Uncertainty*

Indecisiveness about course of action can result in delayed or missed diagnoses. The ED physicians' primary roles are diagnosis and treatment in the undifferentiated patient. In conditions of high diagnostic uncertainty, delayed or missed diagnoses can occur. These absent or tardy diagnoses prevent the application of the correct treatment and are most likely to lead to disability and death. This failure or delay in diagnosis accounts for about half of all litigation brought against EPs.

■ *Low Signal-to-Noise Ratio*

Signals are bits of critical information that must not be missed. In the ED, signals are accompanied by noise—distracting stimuli or information reducing the likelihood of signal detection. Low signal-to-noise ratios occur when the incidence of the serious condition or diagnosis is low (e.g., cauda equina syndrome) and exceeded by the more common, usually benign diagnoses (musculoskeletal back pain). Problems in detection arise because signs and symptoms of both the signal and the noise can often be very similar. Unfortunately, low signal-to-noise ratios exist for all serious conditions that manifest in the ED.

■ *High Cognitive Load*

Cognitive load refers to the amount of thinking an EP must engage in at any moment. EPs are responsible for a variety of patients with a variety of illnesses, with a variety of acuities. This wide range requires varying degrees of memory, concentration, processing, and problem solving. In no other branch of medicine is cognitive load so high.

■ *Poor Feedback*

The efficient performance of any system depends on timely and reliable feedback for calibration. In the absence of feedback, EPs assume that their diagnoses and management are acceptable and see no need to change behavior or recalibrate. The reliability and timeliness of feedback in the ED are generally poor.

Initiatives designed to improve patient safety in the ED should focus on minimizing VPBs and EPCs and on improving the resilience of the system to manage the unexpected.

Error Analysis

When an organization experiences a sentinel event, defined as an "unexpected occurrence or variation involving death or serious physical or psychological injury or the risk thereof," the Joint Commission, formerly known as the Joint Commission on Accreditation of Healthcare Organizations, requires the organization to conduct a root cause analysis.[3] This technique has been criticized for its focus on the specific errors that "caused" the outcome and its neglect of the underlying vulnerabilities in the system (i.e., latent failures).[9] A focus on the immediate error makes detection and blocking of accident trajectories more difficult.

An alternative approach is systems analysis, wherein the incident acts as a "window" on the inadequacies in the health care system. The particular causes of the incident in question, now in the past, do not matter. Incident analysis instead looks to the future.[9]

A representation for such analysis is Reason's Swiss cheese model, which highlights how harmful events occur and how they can be prevented. According to the metaphor, in a complex system, hazards are prevented from causing human losses by a series of barriers (the cheese slice) that provide the safeguards against the realization of potential error (Fig. 207-1). Holes in the slices arise from *active failures* (mostly VPBs) in combination with *latent conditions* (mostly EPCs). In an ideal system, the slices would have no holes, but any ED will fall far short of the ideal. If conditions are such that the holes in the barriers align, this allows for accident trajectory through the system and results in a critical incident or catastrophe.

Vincent and colleagues proposed a safety analysis framework to evaluate adverse incidents in clinical medicine (Table 207-4). The framework for this analysis was based on a hierarchy of seven factors that influence clinical practice. Interventions designed to improve safety should be targeted at each level within this framework, yet interventions at the higher levels are more likely to be effective, and their effects are more likely to be long lasting. However, higher-level interventions are more difficult to implement than short-term, "quick fixes" at the lower levels.[10]

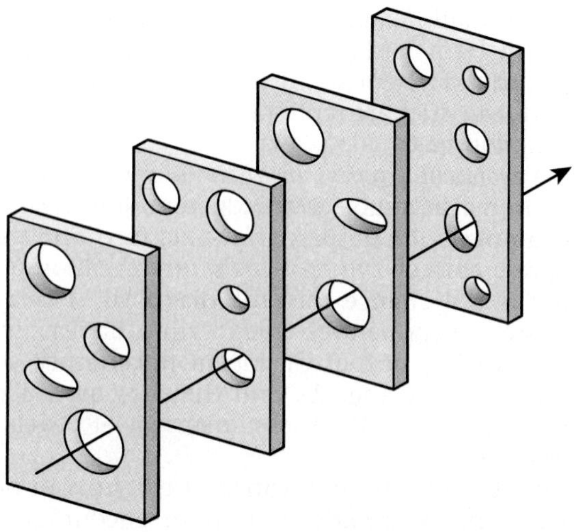

FIGURE 207-1 Reason's Swiss cheese model.

Integration of Knowledge from Other Disciplines

Knowledge from many other disciplines is insightful for critical incident and organizational analysis in health care. A few of the notable areas are as follows:

Cognitive engineering provides a foundation for modeling cognitive abilities such as perception, learning, language, memory, and problem solving.

Human factors evaluate the interface between human performance and the physical environment. System components, such as procedures, job designs,

Table 207-4 VINCENT'S HIERARCHY OF FACTORS INFLUENCING CLINICAL PRACTICE

Factor	Component Factors
Institutional context	Economic context: national, regional, and institutional Regulatory agenda (e.g., Joint Commission, Centers for Medicare and Medicaid Services) Legal constraints (malpractice)
Organizational and management factors	Organizational mission and values Organizational culture and administrative hierarchy Financial constraints and solvency
Work environment factors	Workload and staffing allocation Provider skills mix Administrative/managerial/leadership support Shift work and circadian pattern
Team factors	Communication both verbal and written Leadership Team work training and team structure
Individual (staff) factors	Skill level Training Individual health of providers
Task factors	Task design and clarity Protocol availability Accuracy of results
Patient factors	Complexity of presenting complaint Acuity of illness Language and communication skills Social and cultural traits

Adapted from Vincent C, Taylor-Adams S, Stanhope N: Framework for analysing risk and safety in clinical medicine. BMJ 1998;316:1154-1157.

equipment, communication, or information technology, are examined with respect to human factors such as fatigue, limitations on memory, and distraction, to make errors less common and less harmful.

Systems analysis models systems and organizations to understand their functions, including relationships with other systems and subsystems, more clearly. Errors can be prevented by designing systems that make it difficult for people to do the wrong thing and easy for people to do the right thing.

Integration of Knowledge from Other Industries

In the ED, we can learn from other industries that have developed and incorporated systems allowing for early error corrections or prevention. Such companies tightly couple the process of doing work with the process of learning to do it better as it is being done. Operations are expressly designed to reveal problems as they occur. When problems arise, no matter how trivial, they are addressed quickly.[6]

High-reliability organizations, exemplified by aviation, nuclear power, aircraft operators, and aircraft carrying operating systems, are similar to medicine in terms of operating characteristics and high hazard potential; yet they suffer far fewer mishaps. They share the following six traits:

1. Preoccupation with failure. These organizations are willing to examine any systems failure to identify causes. Even very small events are evaluated and valued as opportunities to remove systems errors before they coalesce to create large, catastrophic system failures.
2. Reluctance to simplify interpretations. Such organizations seek materials and accurate appraisals of any failure. They do not simply blame individual workers and then consider the case closed.
3. Sensitivity to operations. These organizations methodologically approach each task with an eye toward improvement, by probing the systems factors that contributed to the failure.
4. Commitment to resilience. These organizations continually address a deficit until resolution occurs.
5. Understanding of "expertise." These organizations defer decisions to the person who has the requisite knowledge rather than the requisite rank.
6. Clarity in mission and vision. A common view of the world allows team members to communicate accurately.

Design of Health Care Processes for Safety

Designing health care processes for safety involves a three-part strategy: (1) designing systems to prevent errors, (2) designing procedures to make errors overt and easy to recognize when they do occur, and (3) designing procedures that can mitigate the harm to patients from errors that are not detected or intercepted.[11]

PREVENTION

Prevention is the process of identifying latent errors in the system and eradicating these errors before they surface. An example could be reorganizing medications in the Pyxis system to prevent selection of a similar but fundamentally different agent or eradicating look-alike medication vials. The prevention strategies discussed in the following subsections lead to error reduction.

Eliminate Ambiguity and Work-arounds

When problems arise, it often seems that the most effective thing to do is to work around them as quickly as possible, particularly when lives are at risk. However, a systematic approach to eliminating problems often does not require more time than a temporary work-around.[6] For example, one hospital created a patient safety alert process that allows any employee immediately to halt, by means of a 24/7 hotline, any process likely to cause harm to a patient. Leadership follows a "drop and run" commitment, in that leaders immediately respond to reports and stop processes until they are fixed.

Reduce Cognitive Load

The volume and acuity in the ED reach dangerous levels. In such a setting, where cognitive loading is excessive, errors are inevitable. Strategies or devices that reduce the amount of cognitive work and cognitive time will, in turn, reduce cognitive load. Examples include avoiding reliance on memory and vigilance by instituting reminder systems and color coding, eliminating look-alike and sound-alike products, using checklists and protocols, and employing more complex automated systems.[12] Appropriate designation and delegation of tasks within the caregiver team distribute the cognitive load and reduce the individual burden. Other strategies and devices to reduce cognitive load are as follows:

- Mnemonics
- Hand-held computers
- Algorithms
- Decision rules
- Clinical practice guidelines and pathways
- Computerized physician order entry
- Computerized physician decision support

Redesign Jobs and Procedures

Jobs should be designed with safety in mind, including consideration of work hours, workloads, staffing ratios, appropriate training, and sources of distraction and their relation to fatigue. Standardization, simplification, and forcing functions are important practices that can prevent many errors.

Standardization ensures consistency. For example, all data displays should be expressed in the same units; on-off switches should be in consistent locations, as should supplies and equipment, and prescribing conventions should be adopted.

Simplification, defined as a reduction in the number of options, is almost as effective as standardization in reducing medication errors. The more steps in a process, the more likely it is that something in the process will go wrong, even if the individual steps are executed with a high degree of reliability. For example, in the clinical area, simplification of fibrinolytic dosing regimens has been shown to reduce dosing errors and has led to a 30% relative reduction in mortality.

Forcing functions involves the use of constraints. These constraints, designed into the system, make it difficult to do the wrong thing. For example, gas connectors on anesthesia machines are designed so oxygen and nitrous oxide tanks can be attached only to the proper ports, thus eliminating the chance of a gas mix-up with potentially fatal consequences. Bar-coded patient-identification bracelets prevent a surgical procedure intended for one patient from being performed on another. Prescriptions written on a computer can be forced to be legible and complete. Similarly, software applications can require constraints on clinicians' choices regarding the dose or route of administration of a potentially dangerous medication.

▪ Incorporate Technology

Many technologies are designed specifically to prevent error. Automated order entry systems, pharmacy software to alert about drug interactions, and decision support systems such as reminders, alerts, and expert systems are just a few. Electronic medical records can provide necessary medical history and can decrease diagnostic indecision. Automation and computerization, unfortunately, can cause systems to become more brittle; they fail less often, but their failures are more likely to be catastrophic. New technology should be introduced carefully, with an expectation that problems will arise and a readiness to face such issues promptly.

▪ Conduct Simulations

At times, acculturation to medical roles makes it difficult for members of a team to point out or admit to safety problems. Strong collaborative working relationships can improve patient safety, and effective teams have a culture that fosters openness, collaboration, teamwork, and learning from mistakes.

Simulation is a training and feedback method in which learners improve team skills by practicing tasks and implementing processes in lifelike circumstances, with feedback from observers, other team members, and video cameras. An example is a simulation of a resuscitation in which complex communication process, diagnostic difficulty, and multiple procedures often occur simultaneously. As the exercise proceeds, the team works through the clinical situation and then debriefs, discussing problems with the process and immediately developing and testing some kind of countermeasure.

The simulation exercise is designed to uncover vulnerabilities in the process rather than to affix blame; thus, when glitches are revealed, it is important to ask what specifics prevent the team from performing perfectly. Such impediments may include poor communication, lack of needed supplies or equipment, and failure to recognize a treatable condition. Having identified and developed a solution to the glitch, the providers are better prepared to face real-world conditions and to mitigate similar vulnerabilities in the empirical setting.

▪ RECOGNITION

Despite strategies to prevent errors, it is virtually certain that some will occur. Error is actually valuable in some contexts: frequent contact with small recoverable errors provides feedback about the boundaries of safe performance.[13]

Recognition is a defensive strategy designed to make mishaps easily visible so they can be corrected before they affect a patient. For example, Australian anesthetists have adopted a convention that paralytic agents are always drawn up in red-marked syringes; thus, it is obvious to everyone in the room when a paralytic agent is about to be given. If a worker inadvertently picks up the wrong syringe, it is more likely that someone will recognize the error in time to intervene. Similarly, the practice of repeating back verbal orders (check-back), or calling out medications when they are given, allows greater opportunity for failures to be recognized and handled quickly.

▪ MITIGATION

The third general strategy for designing safety into health care is *mitigation,* defined as enhancing the ability to recover from problems by preventing or minimizing their damage. An effective mitigation strategy is one in which errors are visible, operations can easily be reversed, and critical functions are duplicated. Examples of mitigation are having antidotes and up-to-date information available to clinicians, having equipment that is designed to default to the least harmful mode, and ensuring that teams are trained in effective recovery from crises (e.g., unexpected complications during procedures).

▪ Report Errors

To select or design corrective error interventions, it is necessary to have some form of reporting of incidents (near misses) and accidents (adverse events), coupled with in-depth investigation of selected episodes.

Currently, at least 20 states have mandatory adverse event reporting systems. Adverse events are deaths or serious injuries resulting from a medical intervention.[14] External reporting systems

- Ensure a response to specific reports of serious injury.
- Hold organizations and providers accountable for maintaining safety.
- Respond to the public's right to know.
- Provide incentives to health care organizations to implement internal safety systems that reduce likelihood of reoccurrence.

Voluntary reporting systems are intended to complement mandatory reporting systems. Unfortunately, fear of litigation is believed to contribute to underreporting of errors. Ideally, front-line practitioners report hazardous conditions that may or may not have resulted in patient harm. Voluntary reporting works best when it has minimal restrictions on acceptable content, includes descriptive accounts and stories, is confidential, and is accessible for contributions from all clinical and administrative staff. Health care organizations should establish nonpunitive systems for reporting errors and accidents within their organizations. One such environment is the morbidity and mortality (M&M) conference (Box 207-2).

BOX 207-2

Morbidity and Mortality Conferences

Morbidity and mortality (M&M) conferences investigate the reasons and responsibility for adverse outcomes of care. Mandated in 1983 by the Accreditation Council for Graduate Medical Education, M&M is a conference at which, under the moderation of a faculty member, residents and attendings present cases of all complications and deaths.

A study of emergency medicine residency programs found that all these programs have systems to track and report resident errors. However, resident participation varies widely among systems, as do resident remediation processes. In most programs performed monthly, the M&M conference is the most widely used (94%) error-based teaching conference. Case presentations are most often performed anonymously in an effort to enhance teaching, to avoid embarrassment, and to preclude individual blame. However, in other programs, residents are identified when presenting cases, to enhance teaching and to enforce personal responsibility for committing the error. The fact that many emergency medicine residency programs incorporate open discussion of errors may serve to educate residents that evaluating errors can be performed in an open manner.

Disclosure

In 2001, the Joint Commission required that hospitals document that "patients and, when appropriate, their families are informed about the outcomes of care, including unanticipated outcomes."[15] Most professional organizations, including the American College of Emergency Physicians,[16] have ethical standards that discuss disclosure of unintended medical outcomes to the patient. Physicians are ethically bound to disclose errors to a patient when disclosure furthers the patient's health, respects the patient's autonomy, or enables the patient to be compensated for serious irreparable harm. Legal duty requires a physician to disclose to the patient all medical information in the patient's best interest necessary to make an intelligent decision.

A study of patients' preferences for medical error disclosure (see the Tips and Tricks box) found that 88% of patients would wish to know everything about a mistake, whereas the remaining 12% would want to know about the mistake if it could or did affect their health.[17]

Tips and Tricks

**TELL THE TRUTH:
DISCLOSURE OF MEDICAL ERRORS**

Physicians may not be providing the information patients want about errors. Although physicians disclose the adverse event, they often avoid stating that an error occurred, why the error happened, or how recurrences could be prevented. Physicians should disclose the following minimal information about harmful errors regardless of whether the patients asks for

- An explicit statement that an error occurred.
- A basic description of the error, why the error happened, and how recurrences will be prevented.
- Emotional support, including an apology.[18]

Physicians experience powerful emotions after committing a medical error. For some, the emotional upheaval following an error leads to sleeplessness, difficulty with concentrating, and anxiety. Physicians feel upset and guilty about harming the patient, disappointed about failing to practice medicine to their own high standards, fearful about a possible lawsuit, and anxious about the error's repercussions on their reputation.[18]

Conclusion

Building a safer health care system means designing processes of care to ensure that patients are safe from

BOX 207-3

Containing and Reducing Error in the ED

- Design good human factors engineering interfaces.
- Improve detection and assessment of latent error.
- Improve detection and reporting systems for error.
- Discover, assess, and eliminate specific error-producing conditions.
- Conduct cultural and individual awareness training to reduce violation-producing behaviors.
- Recognize resource availability, continuous quality improvement trade-off, and the conditions that produce it.
- Improve awareness of error at departmental rounds.
- Train in containment and reduction of specific team errors.
- Train in the avoidance of procedural, affective, and cognitive errors.
- Improve response and support for individuals when adverse outcomes occur.

From Croskerry P, Wears RL: Safety errors in emergency medicine. In Markovchick VJ, Pons PT (eds): Emergency Medicine Secrets, 3rd ed. Philadelphia, Hanley and Belfus, 2003.

accidental injury. This chapter has focused on identifying common types of safety lapses in the ED and organizational efforts at error management in the ED, specifically with regard to containment and reduction of error. A review of these strategies is featured in Box 207-3.

REFERENCES

1. Leape LL: Error in medicine. JAMA 1994;272:1851-1857.
2. Weingart SN, Wilson RM, Gibberd RW, Harrison B: Epidemiology of medical error. West J Med 2000;172: 390-393.
3. Kohn LT, Corrigan J, Donaldson MS, McKenzie D: To Err Is Human: Building a Safer Health System. Washington, DC, National Academies Press, 2000.
4. Weingart SN: Beyond Babel: Prospects for a universal patient safety taxonomy. Int J Qual Health Care 2005;17: 93-94.
5. Thomas EJ, Studdert DM, Burstin HR, et al: Incidence and types of adverse events and negligent care in Utah and Colorado. Med Care 2000;38:261-271.
6. Spear SJ: Fixing health care from the inside, today. Harvard Bus Rev 2005;83:78-91, 158.
7. Rasmussen JA: Mental procedures in real-life tasks: A case study of electronic troubleshooting. Ergonomics 1974;17: 293-307.
8. Reason J: Human Error. Cambridge, Cambridge University Press, 1990.
9. Vincent CA: Analysis of clinical incidents: A window on the system not a search for root causes. Qual Saf Health Care 2004;13:242-243.
10. Vincent C, Taylor-Adams S, Stanhope N: Framework for analysing risk and safety in clinical medicine. BMJ 1998;316:1154-1157.
11. Nolan TW: System changes to improve patient safety. BMJ 2000;320:771-773.
12. Committee on Quality Health Care In America: Crossing the Quality Chasm: A New Health System for the 21st Century. Washington, DC, National Academies Press, 2001.
13. Wears RL: A different approach to safety in emergency medicine. Ann Emerg Med 2003;42:334-336.
14. Bates DW, Spell N, Cullen DJ, et al: The costs of adverse drug events in hospitalized patients: Adverse Drug Events Prevention Study Group. JAMA 1997;277:307-311.
15. Joint Commission: Standards. Available at http://www.jointcommission.org/Standards/
16. Moskop JC, Geiderman JM, Hobgood CD, Larkin GL: Emergency physicians and disclosure of medical errors. Ann Emerg Med 2006;48:523-531.
17. Hobgood C, Peck CR, Gilbert B, et al: Medical errors—what and when: What do patients want to know? Acad Emerg Med 2002;9:1156-1161.
18. Gallagher TH, Waterman AD, Ebers AG, et al: Patients' and physicians' attitudes regarding the disclosure of medical errors. JAMA 2003;289:1001-1007.

Chapter 208

Conflict Resolution in Emergency Medicine

Gus M. Garmel

KEY POINTS

Conflict is the result of differing expectations, agendas, personal needs, backgrounds, and communication styles among individuals.

Conflict in emergency medicine (EM) may occur with patients, nurses, consultants, family members, residents, students, hospital administrative staff, and agents inside and outside the ED.

The goal of effective conflict resolution is to optimize immediate outcomes and to improve subsequent interactions. Success depends on being aware of one's own communication style and the needs of the other party, along with insight into the other's psyche and an understanding of relationship dynamics.

EPs must remember that *at least* two perspectives exist for each situation. "Win or lose" thinking interferes with successful conflict resolution.

Not all conflict in EM can be resolved immediately, if at all. Some resolutions require the assistance of a neutral third party, such as a mediator. The immediate goal at the time of conflict is to set up the possibility of a successful, mediated solution at a later time and at an independent site.

Successful conflict resolution requires a systematic and structured approach. It is important to recognize each participant's principal interests and underlying positions. Whenever possible, one should try to prevent conflict before it happens.

The problem with conflict is not its existence, but rather its management.[1]

Conflict is unavoidable and occurs in all facets of life. The opportunities for conflict in EM are numerous because our practice involves the interaction of many individuals with varying backgrounds during times of great stress, pain, and anxiety. By nature, these interactions often result in tension and conflict. Many of these interactions occur between EPs and consultants or staff members who have differing agendas and with whom limited or no previous working relationship exists. As such, involved parties may not be able to reflect on past successful interactions that can decrease the likelihood of an intense exchange.

Controversy exists about the *value* of conflict. Many believe that, at its best, conflict is disruptive. Most agree that, at its worst, conflict is destructive to team harmony and patient safety. However, conflict also serves as a creative force, by providing both initiative and incentive to solve problems.

This chapter describes conflict in general, suggests many of its causes, and identifies contributing factors.

Several examples of conflict specific to EM are discussed. The role of effective communication in conflict resolution is presented, as well as its role in de-escalating, minimizing, and preventing conflict. Recommendations for decreasing conflict are offered, and this chapter guides EPs through the challenges of conflict resolution in situations in which it is necessary. The ultimate benefits of resolving conflict to the patient, staff, and EP are demonstrated, including optimizing patient care, decreasing patient morbidity, and maximizing an individual's or health care team's overall satisfaction. Finally, several strategies to facilitate conflict resolution are reviewed.

Communication, in the form of language and interaction, and *power,* in terms of how conflict is managed (or mismanaged), are tremendously important in the dynamics of groups. EM practice is all about groups, because physicians, nurses, and other staff members must consistently work well together to offer patients the best possible outcomes. Louise B. Andrew, M.D., J.D., shares how important communication is with respect to creating conflict, by stating ". . . conflict is often the result of miscommunication, and may be 'fueled' by ineffective communication."[2]

Many researchers identify three important sources of conflict: resources, psychological needs of individuals or groups, and values. *Resource-based* conflicts relate to limited resources, with the premise "I want what you have." *Psychological needs* include power, control, self-esteem, and acceptance. These needs often exist under the conflict's surface and may be difficult to identify and address. Finally, *values* (beliefs) are fundamental to conflict. "Core" values, such as religious, ethical, financial, or those involving patient care, may be difficult to change. Thus, these values generally have a large role in conflict. Value differences among people or groups (e.g., health care professionals and physicians having different training) may result in repeated conflicts. Two common examples of values serving as a source of conflict (perceived or real) in EM are the different work ethics and expectations of EPs and staff members. When conflict occurs, people feel as if their existence or integrity is being attacked. This is one reason that value-based conflicts are the most difficult to resolve (Box 208-1).

Conflict may be broken down into four general types. *Intrapersonal conflict* occurs when one individual has conflicting values or behaviors that cause difficulty for that individual (even though others have similar conflicting values). These are the character traits comprising personality that make conflict more likely. *Interpersonal conflicts* occur among individuals as a result of differences of opinion or beliefs, communication styles, or goals. These conflicts are the most common in EM and generally occur between EPs and patients, nurses, or consultants. *Intragroup* and *intergroup conflicts* occur within or among groups, when decision making is necessary (e.g., staff meetings, elections, hiring, scheduling, staffing) (Box 208-2).

It is relatively easy to understand conflict in medicine if you look at physicians' behavior. Physicians in general do not ask others for help, and they are encouraged by their training not to do so. They may have deficits in communication skills and social maturity, as well as a tendency to be perfectionists. These attributes are highly adaptive to doctoring, reinforced by training, and rewarded by society. However, these traits may be maladaptive in terms of communicating and interacting with nonphysicians. In fact, physicians tend to avoid unpleasant confrontations and typically have not developed the skills necessary to manage conflict.[3]

To assess interpersonal interactions in the health care environment, the responses of nearly 2100 health care providers were reported by the Institute for Safe Medication Practices in a 2003 survey on intimidating behaviors. Despite the inherent biases characteristic of survey research, 88% of respondents had been exposed to intimidating language or behavior and not just from physicians. Condescending language, voice intonation, impatience with questions, and a reluctance or refusal to answer questions or phone calls occurred far more frequently than the researchers expected. Nearly half of the respondents stated that they had been subjected to strong verbal abuse or threatening body language. Among the conclusions established by the Institute for Safe Medication Practices were that intimidation clearly affects patients' safety and that gender made little difference.[4]

However, not all conflict in medicine is the result of intimidation. The ED environment is particularly predisposed to conflict, and conflict occurs for many reasons. Differences in professional opinion and value systems among staff members and patients are only some of the contributing factors. EPs must interact with individuals from all areas of health care, at

BOX 208-1

General Sources of Conflict

1. Real or imagined differences in values
2. Dissimilar goals among individuals
3. Poor communication
4. Personalization of generic or organizational issues

BOX 208-2

General Types of Conflict

1. Intrapersonal
2. Interpersonal
3. Intragroup
4. Intergroup

all times of the day and night, and during periods of great stress. The results are often tension and conflict. Depending on the size of the hospital or medical staff, and the amount of turnover among health care personnel, it is likely that EPs will not know all the individuals with whom they must interact. This situation places a burden on EPs to identify differences in communication style preferences as well as a wide range of practice patterns among medical staff members, including personal idiosyncrasies. In many circumstances, the length of time that EPs and staff members have worked at the hospital precludes previous positive experiences among these individuals.

Examples of Conflict

Conflict in EM may also result from a mismatch of expectations on the part of the patient, family member, provider, or consultant, as well as the nurse, ED staff, or ancillary staff from outside the ED. Patients and family members may have unrealistic expectations about their ED experience, not to mention the pain or fear that brought them to the ED in the first place. Nurses may have unrealistic expectations of physicians, especially those they do not know, and all participants may have widely differing cultural backgrounds. Although gender representation of EPs has become more equal, older EPs tend to be male, whereas nurses remain predominantly female. Dr. John Grey's best-selling book *Men Are from Mars, Women Are from Venus* (HarperCollins, 1992) comments on the frequency of misunderstandings and communication difficulties that exist between genders. Research also clearly describes communication challenges in the workplace among individuals of differing ages. Consultants may be frustrated by the ED staff, based on previous unsatisfying experiences. Additionally, each consultation disrupts a consultant's practice, social life, or sleep and is likely to result in time away from the office or home. This increase in workload may ignite a spark for conflict.

Numerous additional factors further explain the high likelihood of conflict in EM. Diversity in training, experience, and physicians' perspective often result in differences of opinion between EPs and colleagues from other areas of medicine. This is true with nursing as well. For example, conflict arises simply from the fact that EPs do not want to send someone home who should not go home, whereas other specialists or hospital-based physicians prefer not to admit patients (and may be pressured not to) who do not require admission. Neither viewpoint is incorrect, but it is easy to see how these two opposing strategies create tension resulting in conflict.

EPs and ED staff members are expected to be patient advocates, although this role often creates conflict. Serving as a patient advocate may be contrary to a family member's interests or to what the patient ultimately desires from his or her ED visit. One common example from the ED occurs when a patient with chemical dependency wants narcotics for his or her addiction. How can this situation of declining to give narcotics not create conflict? Conflict is also common in EM over hospital admissions. A patient may desire admission to the hospital without a medical reason. His or her family may have this same desire. This results in conflict between the EP and the patient (or family members). At other times, an EP may believe that it is in the patient's best interest to be admitted to an inpatient medical service, even if hospitalization may not influence the ultimate outcome. This situation creates conflict between the EP and the admitting service. In other circumstances, conflict develops between two services over a patient's admission to the hospital when one service tries to influence the other to admit that patient. The EP must mediate the dispute between these two parties and must keep the patient's needs at the discussion's forefront.

Other areas in EM that predispose to conflict include the limited time and restricted availability of diagnostic testing. Conflict is inherent when a necessary test available at one period of the day is unavailable based on some arbitrary cutoff time, despite the full-service expectation of emergency care. Patients (and EPs) are frustrated by this situation and often take out their frustrations on EPs, other departments, or administrators involved in providing these tests or the decisions around their availability. Even consultative services and specialists are frustrated at these limitations, despite their own limited availability for providing patient care.

Perhaps the area most likely to create conflict centers on effective communication among involved parties. The importance of clarity in being understood, given the cultural and language nuances among patients, families, nurses, staff, and consultants, makes the cosmopolitan nature of the ED a setting primed for conflict. Frustrations and time demands, in addition to limited nursing, equipment, and testing in overcrowded spaces lacking privacy, may be overwhelming if communication is suboptimal or barriers to effective communication exist.

Because the specialty of EM is so complex and has tremendous liability associated with its challenging practice environment, many areas of potential conflict have been addressed at the federal, state, and local levels. Hospital policies and bylaws (especially those of the ED) attempt to address these issues by establishing guidelines to prevent conflict in certain areas. Despite these policies, common sources of conflict include patient care responsibilities of on-call consultants, minimum time standards for patients to be admitted and for hospital-based providers to see admitted patients, transfers of patients to or from outside hospitals, telephone treatment of private patients who present to the ED, and the use of the ED for directly admitting patients or various procedures. Many EM organizations have attempted to tackle these and other areas of potential conflict, based on the needs of emergency patients and professionals. Often, issues resulting in troublesome outcomes for patients, staff, or hospitals generate the greatest public attention and political awareness. As health policy and the specialty of EM continue to evolve, new challenges will be identified, and many more conflicting issues will require examination (Box 208-3).

As the specialty of EM has gained popularity since the 1980s, hospital administrators and medical staff members have increasingly come to recognize the importance of the ED and the EP's role in health care delivery. Multiple factors are responsible, including mandatory EM exposure in medical school curricula, which has increased student exposure to our specialty, greater public awareness and acceptance of our specialty, based in part on well-conducted outcomes research, and popular television series that represent our specialty in a positive light. Many of the challenging situations that result from the nature of our practice are less likely to create conflict than in previous decades, because hospital administrators seem more willing to collaborate with ED leadership to prevent conflict before it occurs. Many leaders in EM are honing special administrative skills to allow them to exchange ideas with hospital leaders. Any opportunity for communication and idea sharing to discuss and solve problems in important areas prone to conflict, especially during "business hours" and nonthreatening times, is in the best interest of patients, patient care, and the entire medical staff.

Effective communication is extremely important to the process of conflict resolution. For effective communication to take place, mutual respect and concern must exist among parties. This includes respect for an individual's professional and personal choices. Whether it is work ethic, practice style, or lifestyle, many physicians have difficulty (consciously or subconsciously) interacting and communicating with individuals who do not share similar behaviors and values.

Physicians have often witnessed and learned attitudes, communication patterns, and styles of interaction with staff from mentors, role models, or other authority figures dating back to medical school or training.[5] Yet successful conflict resolution often requires that parties demonstrate a willingness to listen fully to the concerns of the other party, without interrupting, planning a reply, or relying on old patterns of communication. Paraphrasing what is being said back to the concerned party, and expressing a willingness to find a common ground, may help to resolve conflict or at least attempt to de-escalate it.

Communication is often difficult, for various reasons. Many physicians do not have good listening skills. Data consistently demonstrate that physicians interrupt patients early and often; these patterns are likely present during communication with colleagues and team members, especially during stressful situations. However, this style of communication may be necessary for high-acuity situations. In the ED, time pressures make communication challenging, as does the fact that most communication occurs in a public area. Often this communication occurs by telephone, during which visual cues are not part of the equation. Furthermore, individuals often have unique or differing agendas that make it even more difficult to communicate efficiently, let alone effectively. Past interactions have a role in future communication attempts; previous negative interactions are far more likely to be remembered than are positive ones. The personalities of individuals practicing in different specialties are also likely to clash, which contributes to the likelihood of conflict.

Communication skills of physicians are not always developed with these concepts in mind. In fact, the *Model of the Clinical Practice of EM,* originally published in 2001 and updated in 2005, included an administrative section on communication and interpersonal issues that lists "conflict resolution" as one important subheading.[6,7] A subsequent publication by multiple educators in EM similarly described the importance of integrating communication and interpersonal skills as defined by the Accreditation Council for Graduate Medical Education competencies in the education of EM residents.[8] These essential documents guiding the training of future EPs emphasized the importance of acquiring and mastering these key skills.

A well-done three-part series of articles that focused on physician-patient communication in EM shared many pearls and problems inherent to our practice.[9-11] Other excellent references described the importance of the physician-patient relationship and EP communication.[12,13] The Association of American Medical Colleges, for instance, included communication in medicine as a central aspect of its Medical Schools Outcomes Project, which is intended to guide curricula in all U.S. medical schools. In 2004, the National Board of Medical Examiners began requiring all U.S. medical students to be evaluated in their communication skills as well as their clinical skills. The Accreditation Council for Graduate Medical Education now requires all U.S. residency programs to provide instruction in interpersonal and communication skills.[14] Medical licensing bodies have identified the importance of physician communication. As a result, instruction in this area (and that of conflict resolution) is now required in EM training programs.

In clinical practice, physicians characteristically spend much of their time listening and responding to patients' concerns. Studies have consistently found that clinicians' interpersonal skills are not always as good as patients or nurses desire. Research has demonstrated that poor communication skills and the lack of team collegiality and trust lead to lower patient satisfaction and worse patient outcomes.[15] Interestingly, when physicians and critical care nurses were surveyed to examine these behaviors, nearly all physicians did not consider their collaboration or communication with nurses to be problematic, whereas only 33% of nurse respondents rated the quality of these behaviors high or very high.[16]

BOX 208-3

Areas of Conflict Related to Emergency Medicine

1. The commitment to patient satisfaction is prone to create conflict. Limited resources and lack of consultant availability increase the likelihood of conflict. Additionally, patients' expectations for antibiotics, narcotics, or other drugs with abuse potential generate conflict. Conflict arises in emergency medicine when patients make unrealistic demands for medications, tests, consultation, return to work notices, or dispositions that are not appropriate. Additionally, long wait and throughput times often generate frustrations for patients and their families, because their time is valuable and the conditions are stressful. As a result, despite efforts to satisfy patients, conflict is common.
2. Final patient disposition may result in substantial disagreement between EPs and consultants or primary care physicians. Disposition is one of the most common areas for conflict among professionals in the ED setting. In EDs in which the final disposition is determined by hospital-based consultants who evaluate the patient in the ED, ill feelings may be generated on both sides: the EP feels powerless and unimportant, whereas the consultant feels as if he or she is doing the EP's work. The converse is true at hospitals in which the EP makes all final disposition decisions, as generally occurs in teaching institutions.
3. Occasionally, private physicians or specialty consultants mistreat EPs by not recognizing their vital role in health care delivery and its safety net. This situation may occur when these physicians do not acknowledge the knowledge base or skill set specific to an EP's training and experience. Conflict is likely when private physicians and consultants treat EPs as "extensions" of their own practices during evening, weekend, and holiday hours.
4. Timing of follow-up care for patients who are not admitted to the hospital, including the timing of necessary outpatient tests, often leads to disagreement between EPs serving as patient advocates and primary care or consultant physicians who may have limited access to subsequent testing.
5. In the ED, important telephone conversations about patient care often occur when one or both parties are not fully listening because of distractions, external noise, or interruptions. This unfortunate but common circumstance often leads to frustrations or conflict.
6. Conflict is likely to occur in emergency medicine as a result of differences in education, backgrounds, values, belief systems, and interpersonal styles of communication between EPs and nurses, consultants, patients and their families, and administrators. Often these interactions are deemed adversarial, simply by the nature of the patient's needs that the EP is trying to meet.
7. EPs are advocates for patients *and* for the medical staff. However, conflict is likely to arise if an EP is expected to be an advocate for both at the same time. Clearly, EPs have the primary duty of patient advocacy and not for staff physician or consultant advocacy if these outcomes are contradictory. Otherwise, this dual advocacy sets up a conflict of interest that may jeopardize patient safety.
8. Conflict between attending staff members and house staff members is prominent in teaching institutions. The attitudes toward patients or the ED of this training staff, the temporary nature of their positions (some for as little as 1 month or 1 year), and the fatigue, work demands, and personal difficulties that house staff members exhibit during training all contribute to conflict and interpersonal relationship difficulties. Furthermore, some house staff members in every institution take little pride in the manner of interaction they have with others. These same individuals may not feel that they are part of the hospital, they may not demonstrate hospital or patient "ownership," and they may have intrapersonal conflict about their career choice, thereby making conflict with others even more inevitable.
9. Conflict is common with respect to transfers and emergency care of patients with limited or no insurance (or ability to pay). Especially at hospitals that do not care for indigent or uninsured patients (unless the clinical situation mandates), arranging for transfer, consultation, and follow-up care may be extremely difficult. Often, it is downright contentious. Because differences of opinion are certain to exist, such situations almost always result in some form of disagreement or conflict.
10. Because of time limitations and the urgency of most interactions of EPs on behalf of their patients, disagreements among hospital colleagues often require EPs to move "up the ladder" and speak with higher authorities about patient care. In teaching hospitals, this means contacting an attending or teaching physician responsible for supervising a resident. These higher authorities also include specialty consultants, chiefs or chairpersons of divisions or departments, and nursing or hospital administrators. Contacting a house staff's supervisor or a staff member's superior results in unavoidable conflict with that initial individual, whether immediate or delayed. EPs who serve as passionate patient advocates therefore do not always have positive interactions with the entire medical or nursing staff.

Continued

BOX 208-3

Areas of Conflict Related to Emergency Medicine—cont'd

11. Conflict may arise with respect to differences in clinical practice between EPs and physicians from other specialties. Conflict may even occur among EPs within the same department. One example is when patient care is transferred at the end of a shift. This creates tension for the nurses as well as for the physicians involved. In addition, end-of-life decisions may result in conflicts, not only because these discussions typically take place during times of duress, but also because they are often time pressured, infrequently observed by staff, and rarely practiced.
12. Challenges inherent to the practice of emergency medicine commonly cause stress for EPs. These include, but are not limited to, time pressures, high patient acuity, issues of space and patient privacy, caring for patients with limited information and little or no previous relationship, federal and state mandates governing practice (Emergency Medical Treatment and Active Labor Act, emergency medical condition screening, mandatory reporting laws, and victim's rights), and hospital policies and regulations that change frequently. The seemingly endless influx of patients at uneven time intervals, regardless of the staff's ability to handle additional patients, adds to the challenges of our specialty and increases stress among physicians and staff members. This stress often results in conflict among individuals, even those generally not affected by it.
13. The nature of episodic care is likely to result in conflict between patients and EPs. Because EPs are unlikely to have previous relationships with patients or to maintain ongoing relationships with them, patients are more willing to "spar" with EPs if their expectations go unmet. It is unlikely that a patient with a 10-year relationship with his or her primary care provider, or planned future visits, would readily act in a hostile manner toward this physician or a referral consultant.

Interacting with consultants is equally challenging in terms of communication and other areas likely to result in conflict. A multicenter survey from London of 171 newly appointed senior house officers demonstrated the frequency and importance of communication problems, especially with reference to consultations in the ED. These authors concluded that senior house officers serving in EDs could benefit from consultation skills training in which they are taught communication skills.[17] It is not clear from this article how much communication training these individuals had before taking on their roles as senior house officers, or how much training or the type of training they would require. The challenges of interacting with consultants and the difficulties evaluating these interactions are described in the EM literature.[18,19]

A new era of patient care and physician training has developed. These changes are in part a response to the call by several medical organizations for improved training and competence in communication skills of physicians. The Patient's Bill of Rights, resident work hour (duty) restrictions, and the Institute of Medicine's Report on Medical Error released in 1999 all raised awareness of the importance of physician communication, interpersonal skills, and effective team functioning to improve patient safety. Although difficult to study, it will be interesting to see whether patient care outcomes and satisfaction within the medical profession improve over time as a result of these changes.

Many issues challenge communication in EM. Time urgency seems ubiquitous to all communication in the ED, even though many physicians and health care professionals are unaccustomed to this challenge. Disrupted sleep patterns, difficulties with challenging patients, and the uncertainty of high-risk presentations make simple communication even more difficult. As previously described, these interactions often occur over the telephone, thus obscuring facial expressions and body language that would otherwise reveal more accurate representations of events or "hidden agendas." As a result, telephone communications are often much more difficult to manage. Multiple distractions, frequent interruptions, background noise, concerns about other patients, and frustrations with the ED or the consultation process often result in fractured communication. This situation is likely to create strain in the relationships of colleagues and consultants over time, if not immediately. Therefore, an established communication style and rules (when possible) for unavoidable telephone consultations are integral to the smooth operation of the ED.

Rosenzweig defined *emergency rapport* as a "working alliance between two people," including recognizing each other's needs, sharing information, and setting common goals. He went on to write ". . . rapport implies mutuality, collaboration, and respect, and is built upon a groundwork of words and actions."[12] Although the rapport Rosenzweig referred to describes physician-patient interactions, it can just as easily (and perhaps more importantly) be used to describe interactions among physician colleagues or health care workers.

Finally, the role of stress on physician communication must not be overlooked. It is stressful for EPs to contact physicians about patient care issues, particularly in the middle of the night. It is especially difficult for EPs to contact physicians who have hospital leadership roles, reputations of demeaning behavior, or senior positions that may affect partnership opportunities or future employment. These situations may directly or indirectly result in less than optimal patient care when an EP's desire to avoid conflict becomes the first priority.

Costs of Conflict

With these issues in mind, what are the costs associated with conflict in EM? Some may be surprising, whereas others are likely intuitive. First, staff morale and staff retention are likely to be low in EDs with high levels of conflict. Staff turnover and dissatisfaction with the work environment are also likely to be high. Management must address an increasing number of complaints, not only from within the ED but also from other areas of the hospital. This takes up valuable administrative time that could instead be used for improving conditions in the ED. If conflict interferes with patient satisfaction, throughput, and efficient care, reimbursement may decrease, which affects salaries for ED staff members. Pride in the ED may decline, thus further reducing morale and creating a potentially debilitating negative spiral. Research has also shown other costs of conflict. In 1986, Knaus and associates demonstrated that predicted and observed patient death rates appeared related to the interaction and communication among physicians and nurses. In this prospective study from intensive care units at 13 tertiary care medical centers, controlled for APACHE II (Acute Physiology and Chronic Health Evaluation II) scores, patient mortality appeared related to the degree of intergroup conflict. The authors concluded that the "degree of coordination of intensive care significantly influences its effectiveness."[20] Although not studied directly, interpersonal or intergroup conflicts also likely result in decreased patient safety.

The impact of conflict (and poor conflict resolution) on EPs and ED staff members is also important. In addition to making the ED an unpleasant place to work during an EP's shifts, increased stress and decreased job security for the EP are possible. Reduced reimbursement compared with peers may occur, thus causing even greater professional dissatisfaction. These conditions may lead to isolation, withdrawal, or depression. Substance abuse and alcohol or chemical dependency are possible, as are marital strife and family or other personal difficulties common in physicians who repeatedly generate conflict with others. Not all stress is perceived or experienced in a similar manner; this is particularly true of staff members of different gender, culture, training, and generations. Medical errors are likely to occur more frequently, a situation that may compromise patient care and reduce patient care outcomes. Patients are likely to identify conflict among staff members, and the result may be lower patient satisfaction. The emotional and financial costs to patients, staff members (especially nurses), consultants, managers, and administrators are immeasurable if an EP frequently creates conflict and does not possess the skills to minimize it or to resolve it promptly.

Conflict Resolution

If conflict is a disruptive force in EM, conflict resolution and the skills necessary to achieve it are key factors for successful patient care. Simply stated, conflict management depends on effective communication among parties. In his popular book, *People Skills: How to Assert Yourself, Listen to Others, and Resolve Conflicts,*[21] Robert Bolton offers a simple three-step method for conflict resolution:

1. Treat the other person (party) with respect.
2. Listen until you "experience the other side" (reflect content, feelings, and meanings by restating the other parties' views to their satisfaction).
3. State your views, needs, and feelings.

Several additional methods specific to the practice of EM are described in this section, although Bolton's method breaks down this exigent process into these three essential components.

Conflict resolution has been defined many ways, but each definition comments on the importance of the present interaction and its impact on subsequent interactions during inevitable future conflict. The 2005 Nobel Prize in Economic Sciences was awarded to two researchers of *Game Theory* (a branch of applied mathematics) and its role in studying interactions and managing conflict among groups or people. This theory relates that the actions of one party in a conflict affect its adversaries' subsequent behavior. John Nash (the subject of the book *A Beautiful Mind*) and two other scholars brought public awareness to the concept of Game Theory when they received the Nobel Prize in Economics in 1994.

Individuals, groups, and organizations employ many responses to conflict (Fig. 208-1). Interestingly, styles of response have been described as related to

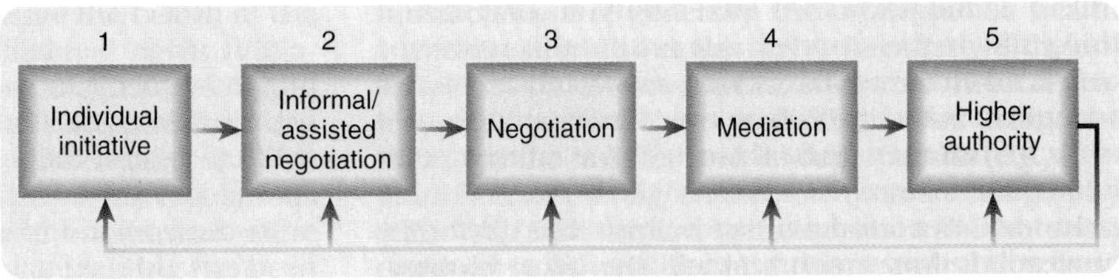
1
2
3
4
5
Individual initiative
Informal/ assisted negotiation
Negotiation
Mediation
Higher authority

FIGURE 208-1 Preferred pathway of conflict resolution. (Adapted from Ahuja J, Marshall P: Conflict in the emergency department: Retreat in order to advance. Can J Emerg Med 2003;5:429-433.)

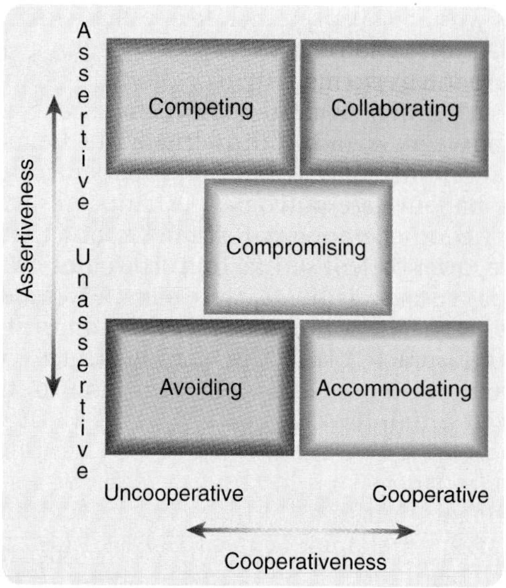
Assertive
Unassertive
Assertiveness
Competing
Collaborating
Compromising
Avoiding
Accommodating
Uncooperative
Cooperative
Cooperativeness

FIGURE 208-2 Thomas and Kilmann offered a matrix illustrating five distinct responses to conflict as they vary along the axes of *assertiveness* (the extent to which the individual attempts to satisfy his or her own concerns) and *cooperativeness* (the extent to which the individual attempts to satisfy the other person's concerns). (Adapted from Thomas-Kilmann Conflict Mode Instrument. Available at www.acer.edu.au/publications/acerpress/onlinetesting/documents/TKI.pdf.)

witnessed (or learned) behaviors of parents, childhood contacts, mentors, and role models. In other words, an individual's approach to managing conflict is likely to be adopted as a dominant approach that generally works for that individual (yet it may not work from other people's perspective). Difficulties with handling conflict may result in unhappiness or lack of success, as well as repeated problematic interactions with staff members and colleagues.

It is relatively easy to recognize that the conflict itself is not necessarily problematic, but the manner in which individuals (or organizations) deal with it may be. Thomas and Kilmann offered a matrix illustrating five distinct responses to conflict as they vary along the axes of *assertiveness* (the extent to which the individual attempts to satisfy his or her own concerns) and *cooperativeness* (the extent to which the individual attempts to satisfy the other person's concerns) (Fig. 208-2).[22] These five styles are as follows:

1. Avoiding
2. Accommodating
3. Compromising
4. Competing
5. Collaborating

Each of these methods for dealing with conflict has situations when it may be effective. The *avoiding* style uses the premise "I leave and you win" or "I'll think about it tomorrow." The goal in this style is to delay or walk away. This style is characterized by low assertiveness and low cooperativeness. Neither party's concerns are met when this style of conflict resolution is employed.

In the *accommodating* style, one party lets the other win ("It would be my pleasure" is the extreme). This style is characterized by low assertiveness and high cooperativeness, and it can be either an act of selflessness or one of obeying orders. The goal of this method is to yield or give in, typically by ignoring or neglecting one's own concerns to accommodate those of the other party. It may be useful for issues of little importance, or for creating good will and demonstrating reasonableness. Unfortunately, the accommodator can harbor ill will if this style becomes dominant and is abused by others. In the extreme, this style may result in poor patient outcomes.

In the *compromising* style of conflict resolution, both parties "win some and lose some." Made famous by television personality Monty Hall, "Let's make a deal" best describes this style's philosophy. This method has moderate assertiveness and cooperativeness and involves negotiating or splitting any differences of opinion. The goal is to find some middle ground, often expeditiously, and to exchange concessions, unlike the more time-consuming style of collaborating. The compromising method may be helpful in issues of moderate importance, especially when time constraints exist.

In the *competing* style, a conquest within the contest is the goal of the competitors. This style results in someone's winning and someone's losing ("my way or the highway"). High assertiveness and little cooperativeness dominate this interaction. This style may have utility when making unpopular decisions, especially for a leader or manager. This style tends to create quick results, and it may be used when bargaining is not an option or the position you support is undeniably correct. This style is, however, very one sided and is likely to be unpopular with others.

Collaborating, although the most complex style of conflict resolution, is ultimately the method to adopt when possible. Its outcome generally causes both sides to win. Collaboration is one of the main tenets of "win-win" negotiations, by taking on the philosophy that "two heads are better than one." Characterized by high assertiveness and high cooperativeness, this style is best used for learning, integrating solutions, and merging perspectives. Digging into the issues, exploring them in depth, and confronting differences are components of this method to manage conflict. This style often results in increased commitments and improved relationships among involved parties.

The distinct advantages to using the collaborating approach are that relationships are preserved for future interactions, and substantive outcomes may be achieved. This approach to dealing with conflict is the most challenging and perhaps takes the longest to negotiate. As such, the collaborating approach may be difficult in the time-pressured setting of the ED. However, ideal outcomes can be obtained if the willingness and the resources exist to pursue the collaborative method.

In the book *Gandhi's Way: A Handbook of Conflict Resolution,* Mahatma Gandhi examined the principles of moral action and conflict resolution, with the goal of finding satisfying and beneficial resolutions to all involved.[23] Gandhi used the term *satyagraha,* which means "grasping onto principles" or "truth force." The basic premise to Gandhi's approach to conflict is to redirect the focus of a fight from persons to principles. He assumed that behind any struggle lay a deeper clash, a confrontation between two views that were each in some measure true. Every fight, according to Gandhi, was on some level a fight between differing "angles of vision" illuminating the same truth.

A contemporary phrase used when dealing with two perspectives is that "the truth lies somewhere in the middle." Considering this concept, it is relatively easy to see why conflict is so prevalent in society, because opposing opinions are likely to exist in politics, health care, and interpersonal interactions, to name a few, and little effort is expended on finding the middle ground.

Conflict resolution in EM has a significant role with respect to effective patient care, as well as positive interpersonal and intragroup relations. Successful communication is integral to promoting positive interactions among individuals, in an effort to prevent (or minimize) conflict before it becomes detrimental. However, poor communication among individuals may provide the potential for ongoing conflict and misunderstanding.

Building alliances with colleagues may reduce the potential for and the amount of conflict. As a visitor to the internationally renowned Centre for Conflict Resolution in Capetown, South Africa, I learned that team building and the promotion of constructive, creative, and cooperative approaches to the resolution of conflict are key elements of this institution's success. Off-site exercises encourage input from the entire staff (at all levels) about their experiences. These meetings (referred to as "growth sessions") are regularly scheduled, yet they may occur when a particular need is present. These exercises allow all team members not only to be heard, but also to feel valued.

One team-building exercise done in our ED included a mandatory off-site meeting that included food, programs, and exercises. Led by non-EM professionals and supported by hospital administrators, this collaborative activity allowed ED staff members the opportunity to interact with each other outside the workplace in a relaxed setting. Throughout the day, opinions were solicited, voices were heard, hierarchies were eliminated, and friendships were kindled. Although the session was expensive, group dynamics improved dramatically following this event, including a reduction of animosity between staff members and a greater desire to work together and to solve problems to meet common workplace goals. It is difficult to measure the costs (direct and indirect) that resulted from interpersonal conflict in our ED on a daily basis, but staff members who remain years after this activity remember its value. It was wise of hospital administrators to recognize the importance of such a mandatory exercise to reunite the ED staff and to reestablish its patient-centered philosophy.

Challenges to Conflict Resolution

EPs interact with numerous individuals of varying backgrounds, interests, and goals on such a regular basis that this is part of our hospital experience. It is one we take for granted and generally do not find particularly difficult. However, other physicians on staff may not have a similar comfort level with these frequent interactions with such a diverse group of people. Successful EPs must be leaders within the ED (with respect to their clinical responsibilities), yet other staff members may not feel comfortable with their leadership style. This is particularly likely during stressful situations, when EPs gravitate toward the competing style of conflict resolution. Individuals who seldom use the ED (patients, families, consultants) may have even more difficulty being comfortable with the environment and the interactions related to it, because these "guests" of this unusually challenging environment are not familiar with its structure. Unfortunately, the ED does not always offer the kind of treatment that other health care professionals have come to expect. For example, in the operating suite, a surgeon is handed instruments in exactly the way he or she prefers by a designated individual who caters to that surgeon's personal style. This is done in both the patient's and the surgeon's best interests. In the ED, however, as a result of staffing shortages or more pressing cases, there is often no one available to cater to the consultant's needs. This situation often results in problems for staff members, who may inappropriately take their frustration out on EPs or the ED. Conflict is likely to result, and the patient and the ED staff members suffer. ED staff members may feel frustrated that they cannot do better in the eyes of the medical staff, but they are also frustrated by the challenges of staffing, the needs of patients, and the demands of multitasking that prevent them from being more accommodating.

With all this conflict occurring in the ED, what are some methods used by EPs to reduce or resolve it, to maintain the best possible patient and provider satisfaction, without compromising patient care? Drs. Marco and Smith developed 10 principles of conflict resolution in EM.[24] These principles seem quite reasonable to adopt into practice. On closer inspection, some are similar to the principles described by Robert Fulghum in his popular book (in its 15th edition) entitled *All I Really Need to Know I Learned in Kindergarten* (Ballantine Books, 2003) (Box 208-4).

Marco and Smith's last principle (be pleasant) is good to keep in mind during high-stress situations, when conflict is especially likely. Remember that kindness is contagious. Everyone benefits from a pleasant disposition, regardless of previous negative interactions. Dropping to a lower level of unpleasant or unprofessional interactions has no benefit; EPs

BOX 208-4

Principles of Conflict Resolution in Emergency Medicine

1. Establish common goals (e.g., to deliver the best or most appropriate patient care possible in a patient-centered fashion).
2. Communicate effectively.
3. Do not take conflict personally.
4. Avoid accusations and public confrontations.
5. Compromise.
6. Establish specific commitments and expectations (e.g., who will see the patient, and at what time?).
7. Accept differences of opinion.
8. Use ongoing communications (invest in future interactions).
9. Consider the use of a neutral mediator for situations that are not working and become disruptive or emotionally problematic.
10. Be pleasant!

should make it their "standard of care" to refrain from this behavior and to rise above it during conflict.

In a similar, well-written article, O'Mara focused on the interrelationship between communication and conflict resolution.[25] She stated that "each relationship presents its own potential for ongoing communication dynamics, which may include conflict and misunderstanding." She added that "appreciating alternative viewpoints and a willingness to adapt are prerequisites for managing interpersonal conflict."[25] Competent EPs are experts at adapting to many situations, and they should consider good communication a fundamental part of their skill set.

Relationships in the Emergency Department

Certain unique aspects of the EP-patient interaction may lead to conflict. First, the nature of this interaction is new, intense, unexpected, brief, and unselected. Neither the patient nor the EP chooses the other; instead, they become "connected" by schedule and circumstance. This is the nature of emergency care. Furthermore, despite how EPs at times may seem powerless and without control, the balance of power in any doctor-patient relationship is unequal. Each "side" has a different perspective on the nature of the emergency condition. Not only is the anxiety associated with the condition itself of great concern, but other concerns exist as well, including work, family, finances, disability, morbidity, and mortality. Furthermore, the timing of care—how long is appropriate to wait for tests, results, consultants, an admission bed, or discharge instructions—creates conflict and, often times, animus. In these situations, mismatches between patient and EP expectations and perspectives often result in conflict that can be intensified by social, cultural, ethnic, and language differences.

Perhaps the most intense interactions EPs have are with the nursing staff, not only because of the need for successful interaction at any given moment, but also because these interactions recur daily. Poor interactions between physicians and nurses are often remembered during subsequent interactions. Nurses are likely to interpret words, communication, and body language in the context of prior less than ideal interactions. The doctor-nurse relationship has been examined for years, because the ability of these two groups to communicate has a definite impact on patient care. In ground-breaking research examining these relationships, Stein and colleagues determined that one of the greatest negative influences on patient outcomes occurred when the nursing profession lacked the opportunity to communicate with physicians.[26,27] EDs that inadvertently encourage authoritarian behavior and attitudes in their EPs are at risk for lower morale among nursing staff. This appears to be true in EDs with training programs, in which the hierarchic nature of training may extend to communication efforts.[25] Enhanced relationship building between nurses and EPs includes improved communication styles and techniques aimed at conflict resolution.

Conflict resolution between EPs and consultants may be difficult to achieve, given the episodic nature of consultation, often occurring during inopportune times for both individuals. Although the immediate outcome of the interaction may seem appropriate to the EP (serving as patient advocate), the "scars" from this interaction may be deep. Suboptimal interactions may result in several responses, such as avoiding each other, harboring ill feelings toward that individual or department, sharing these feelings with others ("professional slander"), or reporting to administrators of respective departments. In all cases, the earlier that problem interactions are addressed, and the more directly, the better future outcomes are likely to be. Addressing these difficulties with the goal of conflict resolution is best done in a nonthreatening collegial environment. Taking the "personal" out of the problem is always wise, and seeking assistance from skilled, unbiased "outsiders" is a good idea if these problems are not easily handled. Given physician's temperaments and busy schedules, outside resources may be difficult to schedule, but they are necessary. These resources include chiefs or chairs of respective divisions or departments, ambassadors or communication experts selected by hospital administrators who specialize in interpersonal problems, ombudspersons, mediators, human resource managers, social workers, licensed therapists, and psychologists and other mental health professionals.

Effective communication among colleagues has been demonstrated to improve patient outcomes at many levels, and it is certain to improve subsequent interactions. Every effort should be made to have face-to-face meetings with consultants when they come to the ED. Shared educational activities with consulting colleagues are also important, whether it be journal review, didactic sessions such as Grand Rounds or other lectures, or question-and-answer opportunities, as long as there is a clear goal of education and not criticism. These opportunities allow colleagues with different training to communicate patient care principles, to discuss areas of changing or unclear practice, and to resolve potential conflict before it occurs. These interactions allow consultants the opportunity to recognize our knowledge and to see that EPs are interested in gaining skills to provide better patient care and to accommodate specialty consultants more readily. Furthermore, it is important for EPs to attend social activities within or outside the hospital, where they can get to know the medical staff members. Having positive personal interactions with non-EM colleagues away from the stressful environment of the ED is a wonderful opportunity for building alliances that may reduce the amount and intensity of conflict. This approach is also more likely to ensure faster conflict resolution in the future.

Some of the best-known writings about conflict resolution are from the business world. The Harvard Negotiation Project found that a working relationship depends on the ability to balance reason and emotion, and on the ability to understand each other's interests or position. Positive working relationships also require good communication, dependability, the use of persuasion rather than coercion, and mutual acceptance of each other's differences.[28]

In the seminal works *Getting to Yes* and *Getting Past No,* the authors discussed negotiation in terms of its being an everyday experience or a fact of life. These resources described the method of *principled negotiation,* which decides issues on their merit rather than through a haggling process focused on what each side says it will and will not do. This method suggests looking for mutual gains whenever possible. When interests conflict, individuals should insist that the result of negotiation be based on some fair standards independent of the will of the other side. This method of principled negotiation is therefore "hard on the merits, soft on the people"[29,30] (Box 208-5).

BOX 208-5

Strategies for Conflict Resolution from the Business World

1. Avoid positional bargaining.
2. Separate the people from the problem.
3. Move from positions to interests.
4. Avoid rushing to premature solutions.
5. Invent options for mutual gain.
6. Select and use objective criteria through which to evaluate the fairness of the options generated.
7. Use negotiation "jujitsu," wherein one negotiator embraces the other's positions rather than resisting them.

Data from references 29-31.

In his book *You Can Negotiate Anything,* Herb Cohen (self-proclaimed to be the world's best negotiator) offered three crucial variables for negotiations: power, time, and information.[31] *Power* is in the hands of the EP in the sense that he or she may use the phrase "I am not comfortable with that (advice)," or "I would like you to come in and see the patient now (let's discuss this at the bedside)." Power may, however, undermine negotiation and conflict resolution. Those with power have less to gain from negotiation, and they often walk away from the process (avoidance style of conflict resolution), because withholding participation may maximize their power (or at least not result in its loss). Many authors believe that a collaborative approach to conflict resolution minimizes the role of power in negotiations.

Time is not always on the side of the EP, and it may shift the balance of power to the consultant. Again, the EP must serve in the role of single advocacy for the patient; dual advocacy for both the patient and the consultant may result in a conflict of interest, thus jeopardizing patient care.

Information may be shared among parties. The EP has information about the patient's condition at the bedside in real time, and the consultant often has a special knowledge base or skill set to offer the patient or the EP. Parties may exchange information that benefits themselves, patients, or both, and it must be considered in the conflict resolution "equation."

Cohen's mantra for successful bargaining is to "be patient, be personal, (and) be informed."[31] Preparation, an important element before negotiations, is sometimes difficult or impossible in EM. However, several opportunities exist to increase preparation before consultation (which should be considered a negotiation). Efforts such as having the patient's identifying information immediately available at the time of the conversation, reviewing the laboratory and radiographic results before the call if possible, and clearly defining the specific goals of the contact ("I need you to come in and evaluate this patient," or "I need your input on testing, treatment, or follow-up care strategies for this patient") help to reduce conflict.

Fisher and colleagues' book *Getting to Yes* recommends that negotiators develop their best alternative to a negotiated agreement, which can serve as the basis for exploring and evaluating options.[29] This approach involves thinking carefully about what will happen if the parties cannot reach a negotiated agreement, and it simultaneously serves as an impetus to engage in a process to try to reach such an agreement (Box 208-6).

Several specific skills are effective in resolving conflict. Feedback and communication begin with

BOX 208-6

General Principles of Conflict Management

1. Creating trust: This occurs by understanding and being perceived as understanding the other party's issues.
2. Effective listening: This is the first step toward understanding the problem. Be careful not to project *your* understanding of the situation based on *your* experiences; the present situation and experiences are those of the individual. Successful responses after careful listening are neutral and without criticism. They allow concerns to be expressed, accepted, clarified, and perhaps validated. Empathy is a wonderful response to integrate at this stage of effective listening.
3. Eye communication: This allows the speaker to feel heard and to feel that what he or she is saying matters.
4. Focus on the issue, not the position: It is always best to bring the discussion or negotiation back to a level playing field by concentrating on the issue, not on the position.
5. Separate the individual or group of individuals from the problem: Effectiveness in dealing with conflict in part depends on this ability. Success requires the recognition that most people are not trying to create problems, but in fact are trying to meet their own needs. The key is to remember that others have different perceptions of reality from ours, and these perceptions are equally valid. Therefore, understanding their underlying or preexisting perceptions is important to resolving conflict.
6. Responding to emotion: Responding emotionally to an emotional situation reflects a loss of control. Maintaining composure and continuing to focus on the issue enhance the resolution process. Silence is an effective alternative response to an emotional interpersonal conflict. The power of silence is profound, and it often de-escalates heated situations.

Adapted from Strauss RW, Strauss SF: Conflict management. In Salluzzo RF, Mayer TA, Strauss RW, et al (eds): Emergency Department Management: Principles and Applications. St. Louis, Mosby, 1997.

careful, empathic listening. Avoiding negative comments or ridicule (especially public) and depersonalizing the conflict are healthy approaches to its management. This method allows the other party to maintain self-esteem and self-respect. Remaining objective while focusing on the issues is the best approach to dealing with the conflict.

Louise Andrew, M.D., J.D., an EP who is also an attorney-mediator, suggests "paraphrasing the communication back to the complainer" and "expressing a willingness to find a common ground."[2] This approach is of critical importance because conflict is often generated (and many times escalated) as a result of one side's fear that their concern will be neither heard nor validated. Andrew described four As to make her point:

1. *Acknowledge* the conflict ("I understand your concern. I can tell you are not pleased with what has taken place.").
2. *Apologize* (blamelessly) for the situation ("I'm sorry this situation occurred.").
3. *Actively* listen to the concern ("Please go on. I want to hear more about this.").
4. *Act* to amend ("I promise I will act to fix this situation and [try] to make certain it doesn't happen again to someone else.").[2]

Working together with others can create community, which affords the opportunity to develop creative solutions to resolve conflict. In this manner, conflict can be productive, rather than destructive. When possible, an attempt at solutions acceptable to all involved parties should be made. Addressing value differences resulting in the conflict (or making resolution difficult), establishing effective styles of communication (including active listening without interruption), and having all parties commit to the mutually satisfying resolution of these concerns are key factors to success. Given the challenging dynamics of EDs, and the instability of work groups, prompt conflict resolution is vital to the health of the system. It is especially important to acknowledge shared responsibilities for problems (and solutions) within the ED environment. In this manner, stakeholders have ownership, pride, and incentive to correct the situation. Prevention of potential conflict remains the superior approach to conflict resolution. When that is not possible, early intervention by trained and respected individuals in a safe haven for discussion is the next best approach.

Several models for conflict resolution exist in the literature, thus providing evidence that it is a much-needed skill. Box 208-7 combines ideas and protocols resulting in a detailed, logical, and multifaceted approach to conflict resolution.

Failure of Real-Time Conflict Resolution

When it is not possible to resolve conflict in real time, it may be necessary to have an outside mediator work with the parties. A well-written article on this topic in the *Canadian Journal of Emergency Medicine* reported that "... while early intervention through negotiation between conflicted parties is often the most desirable option, there may be situations where a dispute involves power imbalances, in which case resolution may be more achievable using the neutral facilitative approach provided by a third party media-

BOX 208-7

Comprehensive Approach to Conflict Resolution

1. Accept the existence of the conflict.
2. Focus on the big picture.
3. Separate the person from the problem.
4. Clarify and identify the nature of the problem creating conflict.
5. Deal with one problem at a time, beginning with the easiest.
6. Engage the respective parties in an environment of impartiality.
7. Listen with understanding and interest, rather than evaluation.
8. Validate issues and concerns.
9. Identify areas of agreement; focus on common interests, not on positions.
10. Attack data, facts, assumptions, and conclusions, but not individuals.
11. Brainstorm realistic solutions in which both parties benefit.
12. Use and establish objective criteria, when possible.
13. Do not prolong or delay the process.
14. Implement the plan.
15. Evaluate and assess the problem-solving process after implementing the plan (follow-up periodically).

tor or arbitrator."[1] Dr. Andrew defined mediation as a "process that takes negotiation to its highest level, employing a neutral party to help hurt and angry people communicate effectively and draft collectively a solution that is greater than the sum of the problems."[3] Mediation should be nonadversarial. Typically, it is scheduled at an unbiased location, away from the ED, at a time convenient for all parties. Scheduling the session takes time, and a good mediator meets with both parties privately before arranging a joint meeting. It is important that rules be established and agreed on before the meeting. Such rules may include treatment of the other party with respect, an agreement not to interrupt or use negative nonverbal communication, confidentiality, and allowance of time for each party to process ideas and information, because the conflict and this process are likely to create emotional intensity that may interfere with the ability to process information. Even if the parties do not like or respect each other, they should at least accept that they have different value systems. This seemingly small concession has a tremendous impact on resolving conflict. Finally, agreeing ahead of time to consider all ideas as valid, even if these ideas are not implemented, offers both parties

BOX 208-8

Positive Outcomes of Conflict Resolution

1. Improved communication with patients and colleagues
2. Lowered levels of stress
3. Increased productivity in the workplace
4. Promotion of healthy relationships with colleagues and staff
5. Improved patient and employee satisfaction
6. Decreased staff turnover (increased staff retention)
7. Prevention of future conflict, or at least resolution of future conflict more effectively and expeditiously
8. Improved overall patient care

more confidence that their ideas will be heard (see Fig. 208-1).

Benefits of Conflict Resolution

Skillful negotiating techniques embody an empowering, active, constructive, and positive approach to resolving difficulties and, as such, may yield successful outcomes or incremental change over time. Numerous benefits result from the successful resolution of conflict. Many of these are obvious, whereas others may not be readily identified (Box 208-8).

These positive outcomes of conflict resolution also have a definite long-term impact. Professional satisfaction increases, as do overall personal satisfaction and workplace harmony. These improve physician and staff longevity, patient safety, clinical outcomes, and cost savings, because less money will need to be diverted to grievance assistance, staff rehiring and retraining, medical-legal risk prevention, and litigation. The ultimate benefit of successful conflict resolution is the production of a more collaborative work environment, in which the ED runs more efficiently, with fewer frustrations and problems resulting from ineffective communication and inappropriate interpersonal or intragroup interactions.[28]

Red Flags Associated with Conflict and Inadequate Conflict Management

In several areas, conflict may result in problems for patients and staff. Some of these "red flag" areas of conflict and poor conflict management are described in Forte's article "The High Cost of Conflict."[32] Not all problems can be described in economic terms, however. Notably, the provision of suboptimal patient care, in part the result of decreased communication

RED FLAGS

1. Not being aware of personal feelings about conflict. This includes ignoring your "triggers" (words or actions that immediately provoke an emotional response, such as anger or fear). These triggers could be a facial expression, a tone of voice, a pointing finger, or a certain phrase. Once you are aware of your triggers, you are more likely able to control your emotions and responses.
2. Not listening to what the other party is saying, including what is not being said. Active listening goes beyond hearing words; it requires concentration and body language that says you are paying attention to the other party. Careful listening means avoiding thinking about what you are going to say next in response to what is being said.
3. Not acknowledging or understanding differing perspectives, backgrounds, agendas, or goals. This requires being flexible and open minded.
4. Not differentiating among positions, their meanings, needs, and facts. It is important to have accurate facts.
5. Not offering the other party room to admit to errors in judgment. This includes admitting to your own errors.
6. Not recognizing the importance for both sides to feel as if they "won" something ("win-win" collaboration); in other words, not allowing the other party to experience a winning feeling. Winning at another person's expense is not winning at all, and it has no role in conflict resolution. Thus, it is important to include more than one solution to conflict resolution.
7. Failing to learn from prior mistakes in conflict resolution. This process is difficult and takes practice.
8. Not having a plan to follow-up and monitor the agreed-on practices. It is important to decide who will be responsible for the specific actions of the plan and how these actions will be monitored (and enforced, if necessary).

and teamwork related to fear of approaching or interacting with staff members, is a tangible concern borne out in the literature.[28,33] An EP's desire to avoid conflict may place patients at risk by causing specific delays or inadequacies in care. For example, an EP may not consult a specialist based on some unresolved conflict with that consultant in an area outside his or her expertise. Clearly, this behavior jeopardizes patient care, and it does nothing to improve subsequent interactions (see Red Flags box).

Summary

Conflict has been described as a natural consequence of incompatible behaviors and unmet expectations.[34] The best way to manage conflict is to prevent it from occurring, which is not an easy task. Experts agree it is best to take action before these inevitable clashes spread beyond the source. Effective communication among individuals and within groups, in which parties are respected and listened to, produces an environment of trust. This situation is worth striving for because everyone, especially the patient, benefits.

A conflict resolution process should be in place before conflict occurs. Although stressful, conflict should not be considered a threatening situation if the environment has established rules, known to staff members, by which this process occurs. EPs should be aware of their behaviors and styles of interaction that increase conflict in an environment predisposed to conflict. Furthermore, EPs should strive to understand the principles of conflict management that may help them to achieve resolution. When neutral, outside parties are needed to address conflict, added time and stress are likely for the parties involved. When possible, mediators should encourage parties to agree to collaborate and should reach consensus decisions using interest-based negotiations that promote greater workplace harmony. If this process fails, arbitrators may be needed to make a unilateral decision, which may or may not afford mutual gain.

In their article on "Professionalism in Emergency Medicine," Finkel and Adams described the commitment that EM physicians must make to our profession: suspension of self-interest, honesty, authority, and accountability.[35] These elements are also essential for successful conflict resolution. These authors concluded that ". . . medicine can never succeed as a transaction; it can only succeed as a partnership, a trusting exchange with patients, which is the hallmark of professionalism."[35] Attitudes of and behaviors by EPs that enhance trust through placing the patient's needs above other interests serve as the operative definition of professionalism.[36] This philosophy, extended beyond patients to hospital staff members and consultants, suggests the approach physicians should take to resolve conflicts in EM. Effective communication and interpersonal skills promote a culture of teamwork, which, with professionalism and conflict management techniques, are essential components of successful EM practice.

Taoism has as its quintessential ideas guidelines for conflict resolution, which it describes as realizing harmony with one another and achieving consonance with nature. The *Art of War,* written 2400 years ago by the Chinese military philosopher Sun Tzu, is considered one of the most highly appreciated strategic texts in today's business world. Many translations of this work share important philosophic points, such as "winning without fighting" (no conflict) and "knowing your enemies and yourself" (to prevent conflict, or, if inevitable, to be more successful in its resolution). In conflict, one must consider the other party an equal, with real issues and needs, and not an adversary to be overcome. Winning at another's expense does not work if future collaboration is necessary, as is generally the case in EM practice. Successful conflict resolution requires collaboration in which both sides have at least some of their needs met, even if to varying degrees. If one side does not respect the other, or if judgment is passed, confrontation will continue and conflict will not likely be resolved. Truly collaborative solutions, such as those in which both parties feel supported, respected, and satisfied that their needs were met, should be the focus behind the resolution of any conflict.

Acknowledgments

I am grateful to Lou Binder, M.D., for generously sharing his materials, and Laura K. Kerr, M.S., M.A., Ph.D., for her thorough review of this chapter. I would also like to thank Doris Hayashikawa and Kandi Praska of the Kaiser Permanente Medical Center Health Sciences Library, Santa Clara, California, for their help in assembling literature for this research.

REFERENCES

1. Ahuja J, Marshall P: Conflict in the emergency department: Retreat in order to advance. Can J Emerg Med 2003;5: 429-433.
2. Andrew LB: Communication, conflict resolution, and negotiation. In Bintliff SS, Kaplan JA, Meredith JM (eds): Wellness Book for Emergency Physicians. Dallas, American College of Emergency Physicians, 2004, pp 48-50. Available at http://www.acep.org/NR/rdonlyres/A59F9CF2-E205-4A39-A470-D79D5E6F5600/0/WellnessBook.pdf.
3. Andrew LB: Conflict management, prevention, and resolution in medical settings. Physician Exec 1999;25:38-42.
4. Institute for Safe Medication Practices: Practitioners speak up about this unresolved problem. Part 1. Institute for Safe Medication Practices Newsletter, March 11, 2004. Available at http://www.ismp.org/MSAarticles/Intimidation.htm.
5. Garmel GM: Mentoring medical students in academic emergency medicine. Acad Emerg Med 2004;11: 1351-1357.
6. Hockberger RS, Binder LS, Graber MA, et al: The model of the clinical practice of emergency medicine. Ann Emerg Med 2001;37:745-770.
7. Thomas HA, Binder LS, Chapman DM, et al: The 2003 model of the clinical practice of emergency medicine: The 2005 update. Acad Emerg Med 2006:13:1070-1073.
8. Chapman DM, Hayden S, Sanders AB, et al: Integrating the Accreditation Council for Graduate Medical Education core competencies into the model of the clinical practice of emergency medicine. Acad Emerg Med 2004;11:674-685.
9. Knopp R, Rosenzweig S, Bernstein E, Totten V: Physician-patient communication in the emergency department. Part 1. Acad Emerg Med 1996;3:1065-1069.
10. Totten V, Knopp R, Rosenzweig S, et al: Physician-patient communication in the emergency department. Part 2: Communication strategies for specific situations. Acad Emerg Med 1996;3:1146-1153.
11. Rosenzweig S, Knopp R, Freas G, et al: Physician-patient communication in the emergency department. Part 3: Clinical and educational issues. Acad Emerg Med 1997;4: 72-77.
12. Rosenzweig S: Emergency rapport. J Emerg Med 1993;11:775-778.
13. Mahadevan SV, Garmel GM: The outstanding medical student in emergency medicine. Acad Emerg Med 2001;8: 402-403.
14. Lurie SJ: Raising the passing grade for studies of medical education. JAMA 2003;290:1210-1212.
15. Feiger SM, Schmitt MH: Collegiality in interdisciplinary health teams: Its measurement and its effects. Soc Sci Med 1979;13A:217-229.
16. Thomas EJ, Sexton JB, Helmreich RL: Discrepant attitudes about teamwork among critical care nurses and physicians. Crit Care Med 2003;31:956-959.
17. Williams S, Dale J, Glucksman E: Emergency department senior house officers' consultation difficulties: Implications for training. Ann Emerg Med 1998;31:358-363.
18. Holliman CJ: The art of dealing with consultants. J Emerg Med 1993;11:633-640.
19. Rosenzweig S, Brigham TP, Snyder RD, et al: Assessing emergency medicine resident communication skills using videotaped patient encounters: Gaps in inter-rater reliability. J Emerg Med 1999;17:355-361.
20. Knaus WA, Draper EA, Wagner DP, et al: An evaluation of outcome from intensive care in major medical centers. Ann Intern Med 1986;104:410-418.
21. Bolton R: People Skills: How to Assert Yourself, Listen to Others, and Resolve Conflicts. New York, Touchstone, Simon & Schuster, 1979.
22. Thomas-Kilmann Conflict Mode Instrument. Available at www.acer.edu.au/publications/acerpress/onlinetesting/documents/TKI.pdf.
23. Juergensmeyer M: Gandhi's Way: A Handbook of Conflict Resolution. Berkeley, CA, University of California Press, 2002.
24. Marco CA, Smith CA: Conflict resolution in EM. Ann Emerg Med 2002;40:347-349.
25. O'Mara K: Communication and conflict resolution. Emerg Med Clin North Am 1999;17:451-459.
26. Stein LI: The doctor-nurse game. Arch Gen Psychiatry 1967;16:699-703.
27. Stein LI, Watts DT, Howell T: The doctor-nurse game revisited. N Engl J Med 1990;323:201-203.
28. Gerardi DS, Morrison V: Manage conflict creatively. Crit Care Nurse 2005;25(Suppl):31-32.
29. Fisher R, Ury W, Patton B: Getting to Yes: Negotiating Agreement Without Giving In, 2nd ed. New York, Penguin Books, 1991.
30. Ury W: Getting Past No: Negotiating Your Way from Confrontation to Cooperation. New York, Bantam Books, 1993.
31. Cohen H: You Can Negotiate Anything. New York, Bantam Books, 1980.
32. Forte PS: The high cost of conflict. Nurs Econ 1997;15: 119-123.
33. Blickensderfer L: Nurses and physicians: Creating a collaborative environment. J Intraven Nurs 1996;19:127-131.
34. Strauss RW, Strauss SF: Conflict management. In Salluzzo RF, Mayer TA, Strauss RW, et al (eds): Emergency Department Management: Principles and Applications. St. Louis, Mosby, 1997.
35. Finkel MA, Adams JG: Professionalism in emergency medicine. Emerg Med Clin North Am 1999;17:443-450.
36. Adams JG, Schmidt T, Sanders A, et al: Professionalism in emergency medicine: SAEM Ethics Committee. Acad Emerg Med 1998;5:1193-1199.

Chapter 209

Informed Consent and Assessing Decision-Making Capacity in the Emergency Department

Diane B. Heller

KEY POINTS

To respect patient autonomy and abide by the law, the physician must obtain informed consent from a patient before examination and treatment.
To satisfy the informed consent requirement, three elements must be present: (1) disclosure of information by the physician must be adequate, (2) the patient's decision must be voluntary, and (3) the patient must possess decision-making capacity.
Decision-making capacity is a medical determination made by the treating physician and is specific to the clinical decision at issue.
The ED environment poses unique challenges to the determination of decision-making capacity.
To possess decision-making capacity, a patient must have the ability to (1) communicate a choice, (2) understand relevant information, (3) appreciate the significance of information to his or her own individual circumstances, and (4) use reasoning to arrive at a decision.

Whenever a patient presents to the ED for evaluation and treatment, the EP is bound by all the duties arising from the patient-physician relationship. Central among these duties is the EP's responsibility to ensure that the patient is fully informed and can participate in the decision-making process regarding his or her medical care. These duties form the core of the doctrine of informed consent and pose unique challenges for the EP.

Informed Consent

▪ BACKGROUND

The concept of *informed consent* is based on both ethical and legal obligations that have evolved over the past century. The ethical foundations of informed consent are that the physician must strive to balance the goals of acting in the best interest of the patient while respecting the patient's autonomy to decide what is best for his or her own body. Currently, informed consent requires an active role on the part of the patient as well as the physician's respect for the patient's wishes.

The legal foundation of informed consent centered initially on the protection of the patient from battery, or unwanted touching. In 1914, Justice Cardozo succinctly stated that, "Every human being of adult years and sound mind has a right to determine what shall be done with his own body."[1] When the patient is a minor, the general rule is that informed consent must be obtained from a parent before a physician may proceed with nonemergency treatment. Several broad exceptions exist to this general rule. For example, a married minor or one who is a parent can usually consent to all medical treatments on his or her own behalf. Many specific exceptions also exist; for example, a minor may have the ability to consent to treatment for sexually transmitted diseases or drug addiction. These exceptions vary from state to state, however, so it is important to be familiar with the local laws where you practice.

Today, in the absence of a recognized exception to the requirement of informed consent, failure to obtain consent properly may also result in liability under the legal theories of privacy or negligence. In the ED, we often find ourselves in a circumstance in which the so-called emergency exception applies. The *emergency exception* states that consent is implied in cases in which an immediate threat to the life or health of the patient exists, when the proposed treatment is necessary to address the emergency condition, and when one is unable to obtain the express consent of the patient or someone authorized to consent on the patient's behalf. In these instances, the EP may presume that the patient would consent to the emergency treatment if he or she were able, and the EP does not need to obtain express consent before proceeding with treatment.[2]

ELEMENTS

To satisfy the requirements of informed consent, three elements must be met. First, the physician must provide the patient with adequate disclosure of information to enable the patient to make an informed decision. Second, the patient must make the decision voluntarily. Finally, the patient must have the capacity to make the decision.

The scope of information to be disclosed is well established in theory but challenging in practice. The physician must disclose (1) the nature of the disease or problem and the nature and purpose of the proposed treatment or procedure, (2) the potential benefits and risks of the proposed treatment or procedure as well as the likelihood that they will occur, and (3) alternative approaches as well as the benefits and risks of such alternatives.[2] The amount of information that must be disclosed in each category, however, is only broadly established and is left to the individual physician to determine on a case-by-case basis. Depending on the state in which the physician practices, he or she is guided by one of two standards. The older standard, referred to as the *professional standard,* requires that a physician disclose information similar to the information that another physician would disclose to a patient under similar circumstances. The newer and more prevalent standard, known as the *objective patient standard,* requires that the physician disclose the information that a reasonable patient in similar circumstances would want or need to know to make an informed decision.[2]

Fulfilling the disclosure element in the ED poses several challenges. For example, time for patient-physician interaction is often limited in the ED. In addition, a quiet and private setting for the discussion is often unavailable. Furthermore, the EP is typically working with limited knowledge about the full scope of the patient's medical history, intellectual capabilities, and emotional state.[3] It is the EP's responsibility, however, to minimize the impact of these challenges and to provide information that will maximize the likelihood that the patient will participate effectively in the decision-making process.

The second element, that consent must be given voluntarily, is not as well delineated in the medical literature or by the courts. Although it is obvious that outright threats or forced treatments violate this tenet, there are subtle ways in which a physician may coerce a patient into making a decision that are also unacceptable. For example, if a physician tells a patient that pain medicine will be withheld until the patient agrees to have a CT scan, the voluntary nature of the patient's decision will be compromised. Additionally, the physician cannot withhold or distort information to alter a patient's decision. The physician must present information in a way that aids the patient in making the decision and leaves the patient feeling that he or she has an actual choice in the matter.

The final element, and the focus of the remainder of this chapter, is that the patient must possess decision-making capacity. *Decision-making capacity* refers to a patient's ability to participate in, and make a meaningful decision regarding, diagnosis and treatment. The treating physician must determine whether the patient is able to make a specific decision regarding his or her medical care. However, the physician must start with a presumption that an adult patient has the capacity to give informed consent, and, absent evidence to the contrary, health care decisions should be deferred to the patient. If the physician determines that the patient lacks capacity to make his or her own medical decisions, the physician must then determine how to proceed. If the patient has specifically expressed health care wishes through an advanced directive, those wishes should be honored. Similarly, if the patient has designated an individual to make health care decisions for him or her, that person should be contacted to make decisions on behalf of the patient. In other instances, family members should be contacted to help make health care decisions.

Although psychiatric consultation may be helpful when assessing decisional capacity in patients, it is not required. Formal legal procedures also exist to assist in the determination, but capacity evaluations are routinely made without recourse to the court system. The process is usually performed solely by the treating EP in the ED. Indeed, the EP assesses decision-making capacity as part of routine interactions with every patient treated.

Decision-Making Capacity

The term *decision-making capacity* is often used interchangeably with the term *competence.* In a strict sense, however, these terms are not the same. Competence is a legal term, and only a court of law can make the determination that a patient lacks competence. Competence is also a more global concept, and when a patient is found incompetent by a court of law, it often applies to many aspects of the person's life (e.g., financial matters, personal care). In contrast, decision-making capacity is a clinical term that is specific to the particular medical decision at issue. If the physician determines that the patient lacks decision-making capacity, the physician can deny the patient the right to make meaningful decisions regarding his or her medical care. Thus, although physicians do not have the authority to deem a patient incompetent as a matter of law, physicians often have the de facto authority to deprive patients of control over their decision making.

To possess decision-making capacity, the patient must exhibit the following four abilities: (1) to communicate a choice, (2) to understand relevant information as it is communicated, (3) to appreciate the significance of the information to his or her own individual circumstances, and (4) to use reasoning to arrive at a specific choice.[4] When the patient cannot demonstrate these abilities, he or she lacks the capacity to give informed consent for his or her medical care.

In all instances, the physician must balance the interests of protecting the patient from harm with respecting patient autonomy. The level of scrutiny that a physician applies to evaluating capacity therefore varies depending on the decision to be made and the risks and benefits of the proposed medical care. For example, if a patient with a superficial abrasion refuses the application of a bandage, the EP should exercise a very low level of scrutiny when assessing the patient's capacity to make decisions. If the same patient, however, refuses a computed tomography (CT) scan after head trauma with prolonged loss of consciousness, the EP should scrutinize the patient's capacity at a much higher level. This general approach to evaluating decision-making capacity is often referred to as the *sliding scale model.* The determination of capacity can be made only with reference to the particular facts surrounding an individual decision by the patient; as the risks associated with a decision increase, the level of capacity needed to consent to or refuse the intervention also increases.[5]

Just as decision-making capacity is not global in its application to all decisions made by a patient, it is also not global with respect to time. Depending on the patient's cognitive ability, clinical condition, treatment modalities, and other factors, a patient's capacity may fluctuate with time. Thus, a patient who has the capacity to make a health care decision at a specific time on one day may, indeed, lack the capacity to make the same decision on the following day or even at a different time the same day. For example, a patient who has just received conscious sedation for a procedure may lack the capacity to make further decisions regarding his or her care but may regain capacity to make the same decision when the medications wear off. In the ED, however, the patient's medical decisions are often time sensitive, and the EP may not be able to reevaluate the patient's capacity at a later time. If a diagnostic test or intervention can be safely postponed, the EP should discuss his or her concerns with the patient's primary care physician so appropriate follow-up and reevaluation of capacity can be arranged.

▪ WHEN TO EXERCISE ADDITIONAL CARE IN ASSESSING CAPACITY

Assessing a patient's decision-making capacity is an implicit part of every medical encounter in the ED (see Red Flags box). The process is generally spontaneous and straightforward and takes place as the EP examines and talks with the patient. The EP's starting point is always a presumption that the adult patient has the requisite capacity to consent to or refuse medical treatment. Under certain circumstances, however, a more detailed and direct inquiry into a patient's decision-making capacity must be performed. Although no accepted rules exist regarding when the EP must delve more deeply into this issue, certain situations should alert an EP to the need to assess a patient's decision-making capacity more carefully.[6]

The most common situation that triggers a more detailed inquiry into a coherent patient's decision-making capacity occurs when the patient chooses a course of treatment contrary to the one recommended by the EP or refuses treatment entirely.

RED FLAGS

Signs That a More Careful Evaluation of Capacity Might Be Warranted

- Patients who refuse recommended treatment (especially if they refuse to discuss their decision)
- Patients presenting with a change in mental status
- Patients with known risk factors for impaired decision making such as the following:
  - Chronic psychiatric or neurologic conditions
  - Cultural or language barriers
  - Educational level concern or developmental delay issues
  - Significant stress, anxiety, or untreated pain
  - Extremes of age: older than 80 years, because of increased risk of dementia; younger than 18 years, because of a potential need for parental involvement

Simple disagreement with an EP's recommendation, however, is not grounds for declaration of a lack of capacity. If the EP believes that the patient's choice is not reasonable, it may trigger the start of an inquiry, but it is not the end of the inquiry. As discussed earlier, refusal of treatment is more worrisome if the consequences of the patient's decision are great. Furthermore, if the patient is unwilling to discuss the reasons behind his or her refusal, the EP should be even more concerned about performing a careful evaluation of the patient's decision-making capacity before simply accepting the patient's choice.

A second general area that should raise the EP's concern regarding decision-making capacity is when a patient presents with an abrupt mental status change. Although the reasons for the mental status change may be as varied as infection, stroke, head trauma, or ingestion of mind-altering substances, the result is the same. The EP is under an obligation to conduct a more careful evaluation of the patient's capacity to participate in decisions regarding his or her medical care. The simple existence of a mental status change, however, does not automatically preclude a patient from possessing the requisite capacity. It is simply a situation that should trigger the EP to make a more detailed inquiry.

A third broad area that should prompt the EP to evaluate the patient's capacity more carefully is the presence of a known risk factor for impaired decision making. Risk factors may include known psychiatric conditions such as severe depression or schizophrenia. Although the presence of mental illness does not automatically preclude a patient from having the right to participate in his or her medical care, in such an instance it may be helpful to seek the opinion of a psychiatrist. If cultural or language barriers are present, or if concerns exist about a patient's level of education, the EP should also exercise heightened scrutiny of the patient's decision-making capacity. In these instances, the EP must take steps to compensate for these factors to ensure that the patient has the greatest opportunity to participate in his or her medical care. The EP should arrange for a translator when necessary and should take additional time to explain the issues in terms that the patient can more readily understand. Extremes of age are also known risk factors for impaired decision making. Although not every patient over a certain age exhibits dementia, the EP must be aware of the increased prevalence of such conditions in elderly patients. Other common risk factors in the ED are extreme pain, stress, and anxiety, each of which can impair a patient's ability to receive or process information.[7]

Although the foregoing situations are by no means all inclusive, they represent instances that should put an EP on notice that a more careful and detailed evaluation of capacity may be needed. Again, none of these circumstances will alter the presumption that an adult possesses the requisite capacity to participate in his or her medical care. They simply mark the need for a more detailed inquiry. In each of these instances, the EP should take additional care when documenting the care of the patient as well as his or her interactions with the patient (see the Documentation box).

Documentation

WHEN CAPACITY IS AT ISSUE

If any of the "red flag" situations exist, or if there are other reasons to have heightened concern regarding a patient's decision-making capacity, the EP should take care to document the following elements carefully:

- Whether or not the patient exhibits each of the elements of decision-making capacity
- The patient's medical condition
- The treatment or procedure and its necessity
- The urgent or emergency nature of the treatment or procedure
- Actions by the EP to maximize patient capacity
- Actions by the EP to minimize impediments to capacity
- Availability and involvement of family members or surrogate decision makers
- Psychiatric consultation when obtained

METHODS FOR EVALUATING CAPACITY

No absolute test scores or clear-cut rules on which clinicians can rely for a definitive determination of a patient's capacity are available. Physicians typically use some combination of three broad categories to evaluate decision-making capacity: (1) cognitive function testing, (2) specific capacity testing, and (3) general evaluation of capacity through a clinical interview.

Cognitive function testing, such as the Mini-Mental Status Examination, can be quick and easy for the EP to administer. Such tests may also be useful because they test functions such as attention and short-term memory, without which a patient cannot exercise decision-making capacity. The use of cognitive function testing to evaluate decision-making capacity has several drawbacks, however. First and foremost, it is unclear whether these tests truly have value for determining whether a patient has the capacity to consent to treatment. In addition, no minimum score has been identified as "passing" for purposes of a capacity determination. Furthermore, these tests do not evaluate upper-level functions, such as judgment and reasoning, that are clearly relevant to decision-making capacity.[8] Thus, although tests such as the Mini-Mental Status Examination may assist a physician in the assessment of a patient's capacity, they are neither sufficient nor necessarily reliable for this assessment.

An alternative set of evaluative tools falls under the category of specific capacity testing. These tests, such as the Aid to Decisional Capacity Evaluation, are detailed decisional aids designed to assist clinicians in carrying out specific capacity assessments.[9] Although these types of tests may have the strength of assessing the patient's functional ability to make clinical decisions more directly, they also have several drawbacks. For example, these tests are often time consuming and require specific training to perform. EPs are unlikely to be familiar with these tests and may not have the time to train for and perform these tests correctly. It is also difficult to use these tests to determine the reasons behind a patient's decisions. Further, the result of these tests is often inconclusive, yielding a "probably capable" or "probably incapable" result.[9] Again, although these tests are an option, many EPs may not find the option viable.

The final category, that of determining capacity by general impression with a directed clinical interview, is the method EPs should use given the challenges they face in the ED. However, this method can also be inaccurate because studies have shown that the results may not agree with expert assessments of capacity except at the extremes of "obviously capable" and "obviously incapable."[9] To increase the likelihood that informal testing will yield the correct result, the EP should address difficulties unique to the ED environment as well as those unique to individual patients. Noise and lack of privacy are difficult to overcome, but if there is a quiet room in the ED where the EP can discuss complex treatments or procedures, it should be used. The EP should obtain the aid of a translator when needed and should take care to avoid administering mind-altering substances or allow time for them to wear off when possible. Involving the patient's family and friends can also aid in making the patient feel supported and can help the patient through the decision-making process. Finally, asking questions specific to the four abilities of decision-making capacity will help the EP to focus the evaluation.

Tips and Tricks

QUESTIONS TO ASK PATIENTS TO FACILITATE THE DETERMINATION OF DECISION-MAKING CAPACITY

- The ability to communicate a choice:
  - Have you decided what you want to do?
  - We have discussed many things; have you made a decision?
- The ability to understand relevant information as it is communicated:
  - What is your understanding of your medical condition?
  - What are the possible diagnostic tests or treatments for your condition?
  - What are some of the risks of the options we have discussed?
  - How likely is it that you will have a bad outcome?
  - What could happen if you choose to do nothing at this time?
- The ability to appreciate the significance of the information to one's own individual circumstances:
  - Why do you think your doctor has recommended this specific test or treatment for you?
  - Do you think the recommended test or treatment is the best option for you?
  - Why do you think that this is the best option for you at this time?
  - What do you think will happen if you accept (or refuse) this option?
- The ability to use reasoning to arrive at a specific choice:
  - Why have you chosen the option you did?
  - What factors influenced your decision?
  - What weight did you give to these different factors?
  - How do you balance the positives and negatives (or risks and benefits)?

SUGGESTED QUESTIONS TO AID IN THE CAPACITY DETERMINATION

The final determination of a patient's decision-making capacity depends on whether the EP believes that the patient exhibits the four abilities required for capacity: (1) to communicate a choice, (2) to understand relevant information as it is communicated, (3) to appreciate the significance of the information to his or her own individual circumstances, and (4) to use reasoning to arrive at a specific choice. Thus, the EP's inquiry should ask focused questions to evaluate each of these areas (see the Tips and Tricks box).

The first requirement, communicating a choice, can be evaluated simply by asking the patient what he or she wants to do. Stability of the choice is also important. Although this may not be a factor given the urgency of many procedures in the ED, if the proposed treatment or procedure will not occur immediately, the EP should confirm that the patient's choice remains the same after some period of time. If, for example, Patient A agrees to a lumbar puncture for his headache, the EP can simply confirm the patient's decision after the preparations for the procedure have been made.

To test the patient's ability to understand relevant information, the EP may start out by simply asking the patient to paraphrase what he or she has been told. The EP can also ask pointed questions such as "What is your understanding of your condition and the options we have discussed?" The patient should be able to explain, in his or her own words, the nature of the condition, the available options, and the risks and benefits of these options. This includes his or her understanding of what will happen if the patient does nothing. In the foregoing example of a lumbar puncture, Patient A needs to understand the risks of the procedure as well as the possibility that a negative CT scan without a negative lumbar puncture may mean that he still has a life-threatening condition.

To satisfy the third element of decision-making capacity, the EP must be sure that the patient understands how the information discussed relates to him or her as an individual. The EP can ask the patient whether he or she thinks that the proposed option is the best option and why. The EP should also explore what the patient thinks will happen in the future if he or she chooses the proposed option. Using the foregoing example, this may be as simple as the fact that Patient A will need to spend several hours in the ED waiting for the lumbar puncture results or that he may experience a postprocedural headache that will interfere with work the following day.

To evaluate the patient's ability to reason, the EP should ask the patient why he or she has chosen a specific option. The EP can inquire what factors influenced the patient's decision and what weight was given to those factors. In the foregoing example, Patient A may tell the EP that he cannot wait for a lumbar puncture after the CT scan because he has to pick up his daughter after school or that he has had similar headaches in the past and therefore thinks that this headache is not serious. Alternatively, Patient A could tell the EP that he believes that when the procedure is performed, the EP will inject radioactive material into his body because the EP is trying to kill him. Sometimes simple questions yield very complex and interesting answers that can aid the EP's capacity determination.

In addition to asking focused questions relevant to capacity, the EP has the option of obtaining a consultation from a psychiatrist if time allows. Although no requirement mandates that a psychiatrist be involved, it may be helpful in certain circumstances. First, it can never hurt to obtain a second opinion when making a capacity determination. Second, psychiatrists are skilled at interviewing patients. Third, they are experts in diagnosing mental illnesses that may impair a patient's decision-making ability. The involvement of a psychiatrist does not relieve the EP of his or her responsibility to take part in the capacity determination. Decision-making capacity relies on the communication of adequate medical information that is unique to the patient's condition and proposed treatment. Only the treating EP can ensure adequate disclosure of this information, and the EP cannot delegate this task to a psychiatrist.

Conclusion

In every encounter in the ED, it is the treating EP's responsibility to ensure that the patient gives informed consent for his or her medical care. This consent must be given voluntarily in a patient with the requisite decision-making capacity, and the patient must receive adequate information to make the decision. Although an evaluation of decision-making capacity is usually an inherent part of every patient-physician encounter, certain situations should alert the EP to the need for a more detailed inquiry. To this end, the EP may use specific tools for testing or a more general impression as a result of the clinical interview in which questions specifically address the requisite elements of capacity.

REFERENCES

1. Schloendorff v. Society of New York Hospital. 1914;105 N.E. 92.
2. Bisbing S: Competency and capacity: A primer. In Baxter S (ed): Legal Medicine, 4th ed. St. Louis, Mosby, 1998.
3. Derse A: What part of "no" don't you understand? Patient refusal of recommended treatment in the emergency department. Mt Sinai J Med 2005;72:221-227.
4. Applebaum PS, Grisso T: Assessing patients' capacity to consent to treatment. N Engl J Med 1988;319:1635.
5. President's Commission for the Study of Ethical Problems in Medicine and Biomedical and Behavioral Research, Making Health Care Decisions: A Report on the Ethical and Legal Implications of Informed Consent in the Patient Practitioner Relationship. Washington, DC, U.S. Government Printing Office, 1982.
6. Tunzi M: Can the patient decide? Evaluating patient capacity in practice. Am Fam Physician 2001;64:299-306.
7. Grisso T, Applebaum P: Assessing Competence to Consent to Treatment: A Guide for Physicians and Other Health Professionals. New York, Oxford University Press, 1998, p 61.
8. Etchells E, Sharpe G, Elliott C, et al: Bioethics for clinicians: Part 3. Capacity. CMAJ 1996;155:657-661.
9. Etchells E, Darzins P, Silberfeld M, et al: Assessment of patient capacity to consent to treatment. J Gen Intern Med 1999;14:27-34.

Chapter **210**

Regulatory and Legal Issues in the Emergency Department

Paul D. Biddinger

KEY POINTS

Individual states have the authority to regulate the practice of emergency medicine within their borders. Oversight is generally granted to the state public health department.

Certain federal laws, such as the Emergency Medical Treatment and Active Labor Act (EMTALA) and the Health Insurance Portability and Accountability Act (HIPAA), create additional obligations and establish legal and financial peril for violations.

EMTALA requires EPs to provide appropriate screening and stabilization for all patients who present for emergency care. EMTALA further regulates access to on-call specialists as well as the transfer of patients among health care facilities.

HIPAA has changed the way in which physicians and hospitals collect, store, and share health information. Although the regulations are complex, physicians can best adhere to the regulations when they access or share health information only on a "need-to-know" basis and attempt to obtain the patient's permission for sharing information whenever possible.

Most states have special reporting requirements for victims of child abuse and certain infectious diseases. Some states establish additional reporting of violent crime victims, automobile drivers with a seizure disorder, or people with animal bites.

Background

ED treatment is highly regulated to advance individual and community goals. Regulations are intended to protect the vulnerable, to ensure the health of the community, and to respect individual rights. Violation of these regulations (especially EMTALA and HIPAA) may place both the physicians and the institution at significant financial and legal risk. This chapter highlights just a few of the many regulations that govern emergency care and emphasizes more recent developments.

Public Health Authority

Each state has the right to license and regulate the health care facilities and the providers within its jurisdiction, and generally the state public health authority administers this right. In other words, not only must physicians, nurses, and other medical professionals obtain their medical licenses from the state, but the hospital and its departments (e.g., hospital EDs, operating rooms, computed tomography scanners, and cardiac catheterization laboratories) must do so as well. Because this responsibility is so large, most states share, delegate, or "deem" some portions of this regulatory authority to national expert organizations to help them oversee the quality of health care delivered in their state.[1] The most visible of these expert organizations is the Joint Commission (JC), formerly known as the Joint Commission on Accreditation of Healthcare Organizations (JCAHO), which broadly manages the accreditation of health care institutions. Examples of other organizations to which states frequently delegate regulatory authority include the American College of Surgeons, which sets standards for trauma centers, and the American Burn Association, which sets standards for burn centers. In addition to delegating portions of their authority to national organizations, state departments of public health may also delegate portions of their authority over health care institutions to local public health officials. One example of this is the receipt of reports of suspected or confirmed cases of reportable communicable disease.

In no case does any sharing of authority supersede the state's ability to regulate and oversee health care quality. Indeed, although some states recognize JC accreditation as evidence of meeting acceptable standards, states can always perform their own inspections of facilities in addition to the JC surveys. Further, whenever a question or concern arises regarding specific care delivered, the state public health authority generally carries out the site inspection and investigation on its own.

BOX 210-1

2008 Joint Commission National Patient Safety Goals

- Improve the accuracy of patient identification.
- Improve the effectiveness of communication among caregivers.
- Improve the safety of using medications.
- Reduce the risk of health care–associated infections.
- Accurately and completely reconcile medications across the continuum of care.
- Reduce the risk of patient harm resulting from falls.
- Reduce the risk of influenza and pneumococcal disease in institutionalized older adults.
- Reduce the risk of surgical fires.
- Encourage patients' active involvement in their own care as a patient safety strategy.
- Prevent health care–associated pressure ulcers (decubitus ulcers).
- The organization identifies safety risks inherent in its patient population.
- Improve recognition and response to changes in a patient's condition.

From The Joint Commission: Facts about the 2008 National Patient Safety Goals. http://www.jointcommission.org/PatientSafety/NationalPatientSafetyGoals/08_npsg_facts.htm.

The Joint Commission

The JC is a private, not-for-profit, organization. Its mission is to "continually improve the safety and quality of care provided to the public through the provision of healthcare accreditation and related services that support performance improvement in healthcare organizations."[2] Broadly, the JC sets standards that hospitals must meet to receive accreditation (and sometimes, by extension, licensure from the state). These standards cover a broad range of subjects from patients' rights, to patient care, to infection control. The JC also integrates outcomes and other performance measures into its standards. To maintain their accreditation, health care organizations must undergo a site survey every 3 years. Laboratories must undergo a site survey every 2 years for the same accreditation.

Over the years, the JC has created special programs and work groups with particular relevance to the ED, including groups specifically examining ED overcrowding and hospital emergency preparedness. The most overarching of the programs related to the ED is the set of National Patient Safety Goals (Box 210-1). These goals have been revised and expanded over the years to reflect appropriately the changes in clinical care that have evolved as well as to address systemic sources of error in medicine as they are identified.

Two specific programs that institutions are required to use to help them achieve the national patient safety goals are the *do-not-use list* and the *universal protocol.* The universal protocol was developed by JC to prevent "wrong site, wrong person, and wrong procedure" surgery and is required of accredited institutions. Although the universal protocol has been generally interpreted to apply to EDs, its specific application in the ED may sometimes be unclear. Although it is difficult to conceive that a laceration repair or emergency intubation could be performed on the wrong limb or wrong patient, it is theoretically possible that a lumbar puncture or central venous cannulation (among other procedures) could be performed on the wrong patient, especially if transfer or communication breakdown among caregivers occurs.

The do-not-use list is a compilation of medical abbreviations that have been identified as the most likely sources of error found when orders are either miswritten or misinterpreted. The growing use of computerized order entry systems and computerized prescription writing programs is likely to decrease the numbers of these types of errors; however, physicians who write handwritten orders must be familiar with the prohibited abbreviations given in Table 210-1, and EDs should bar the use of these abbreviations in clinical practice.

Table 210-1 JOINT COMMISSION OFFICIAL "DO NOT USE" LIST OF ABBREVIATIONS

Do Not Use	Potential Problem	Use Instead
Official "Do Not Use" List*		
U (unit)	Mistaken for 0 (zero), the number 4 (four), or "cc"	Write "unit"
IU (International Unit)	Mistaken for IV (intravenous) or the number 10 (ten)	Write "International Unit"
Q.D., QD, q.d., qd (daily) Q.O.D., QOD, q.o.d., qod (every other day)	Mistaken for each other; period after the Q mistaken for "I" and the O mistaken for "I"	Write "daily"; write "every other day"
Trailing zero (X.0 mg)† Lack of leading zero (.X mg)	Decimal point is missed	Write "X mg"; write "0.X mg"
MS	Can mean morphine sulfate or magnesium sulfate	Write "morphine sulfate"; write "magnesium sulfate"
MSO_4, $MgSO_4$	Confused for one another	
Additional Abbreviations, Acronyms, and Symbols for Possible Future Inclusion in the Official "Do Not Use" List		
> (greater than), < (less than)	Misinterpreted as the number 7 (seven) or the letter L Confused for one another	Write "greater than"; write "less than"
Abbreviations for drug names	Misinterpreted due to similar abbreviations for multiple drugs	Write drug names in full
Apothecary units	Unfamiliar to many practioners Confused with metric units	Use metric units
@	Mistaken for the number 2 (two)	Write "at"
cc	Mistaken for U (units) when poorly written	Write "mL" or "milliliters"
µg	Mistaken for "mg" (milligrams), resulting in a 1000-fold overdose	Write "mcg" or "micrograms"

*Applies to all orders and all medication-related documentation that is handwritten (including free-text computer entry) or on preprinted forms.
†A trailing zero may be used only where required to demonstrate the level of precision of the value being reported, such as for laboratory results, imaging studies that report size of lesions, or catheter/tube sizes. It may not be used in medication orders or other medication-related documentation.
From The Joint Commission: The official "do not use" list. http://www.jointcommission.org/PatientSafety/DoNotUseList/

Emergency Medical Treatment and Active Labor Act

One of the most confusing, misinterpreted, and misquoted set of regulations in emergency medicine is EMTALA. Even the name itself can be confusing, because the regulations are sometimes inexactly referred to as "COBRA," referring to the broader Consolidated Omnibus Reconciliation Act in which the original EMTALA statutes were enacted. First enacted in 1986, and most recently revised in 2003, EMTALA originated as a response to several well-publicized allegations of patient "dumping" in which patients were reported to have been turned away or transferred from EDs without appropriate care. Broadly, EMTALA creates two major requirements for hospitals that have a dedicated ED and participate in Medicare. First, patients who come to the ED and request care must receive an appropriate medical screening examination. Second, for patients with an identified "emergency medical condition," the EP must either provide appropriate stabilization or arrange for transfer to another facility and meet several additional specific requirements pertaining to the transfer.[3]

The first requirement under EMTALA, the "medical screening examination," must be provided to all individuals who present to the ED and who requesting an evaluation for a medical condition. Although the specific components of this examination remain ill defined, it is generally agreed that an examination should be performed so the clinician can say with "reasonable clinical confidence" that a medical emergency does or does not exist. Further, this medical screening examination must be provided without regard to ability to pay, insurance status, race, citizenship, or gender.

The second requirement under EMTALA is to provide appropriate stabilization for an emergency medical condition, once identified. In general, this means that an appropriate level of medical care must be provided in the ED or in the hospital for the acute medical problem of the patient, again, without regard for ability to pay, insurance status, race, citizenship, or gender. This provision of EMTALA also has implications for on-call physicians. As part of Medicare, hospitals must maintain on-call physicians who are able to provide medical services necessary to treat an emergency medical condition after the medical screening examination. Although the list of on-call physicians is not required by Medicare to be comprehensive, the specialties represented in the on-call list must be appropriate to best meet the needs of the patients within the hospital's capability. If a hospital

Tips and Tricks

MEDICAL SCREENING EXAMINATION

- Must be performed on all patients without regard to ability to pay
- Must be performed before financial interview
- Not the same as triage
- Must be performed by a medical professional granted authority by hospital bylaws
- Must be sufficient to confirm or rule out an emergency medical condition

does not maintain an appropriate on-call roster, or if an on-call physician does not show up to care for a patient with an identified emergency medical condition within a reasonable amount of time, that hospital and the on-call physician may be liable under EMTALA.

In the event that the ED or hospital is unable to provide appropriate stabilization, EMTALA allows transfer of patients from one facility to another under certain very specific conditions. First, the patient must consent to the transfer, and a physician must state in writing that the medical benefits of the transfer outweigh its risks. Consent to the transfer may be considered to be implied if the patient is unconscious and no other legal representative for the patient is available. Second, the hospital that receives the transferred patient must be "appropriate," and it must have both the space and the qualified personnel to treat the emergency medical condition.[4]

Penalties for violations of EMTALA statutes can be significant for both the physician and the institution. Both physician and hospital can be liable for fines up to $50,000 per violation, and both can be excluded from future participation in the Medicare program. Malpractice insurance specifically excludes EMTALA violations. Further, hospitals that receive patients transferred in violation of EMTALA statutes may bring a civil suit against the transferring institution to recover the financial loss created by the inappropriate transfer (Box 210-2).

BOX 210-2

Key Provisions of the Emergency Medical Treatment and Active Labor Act

- Anyone who presents to the main hospital property with an emergency medical complaint must receive a medical screening examination and appropriate stabilization.
- Hospitals must maintain appropriate on-call lists of specialists to care for identified emergency medical conditions.
- Patients may not be transferred from a higher level of care to a lower level of care.
- All patients transferred from one facility to another must be accepted by a physician at the receiving facility before transfer.
- When transferring a patient to another hospital, the responsibility to choose the appropriate means of transport (e.g. private vehicle, Basic Life Support, Advanced Life Support, critical care transport) lies with the sending physician.
- Institutions with specialty care services must accept transfers from hospitals without such services, provided they have the space and capability at that time to deal with the patient's needs.
- Patients with an emergency condition must be stabilized before transport to another facility *except* if (a) the receiving facility has specialty services that the sending facility lacks and the benefits outweigh the risks of transfer and (b) the patient requests the transfer and understands the risks.
- Patients may refuse transfer from one facility to another.

Health Insurance Portability and Accountability Act

HIPAA was initially enacted in 1996 as an attempt to make it easier for individuals to transfer their medical records and health care coverage, as well as to provide greater accountability among providers to limit fraud.[5] Subsequent federal rules, implemented in 2000 and 2002, under HIPAA that defined privacy standards substantially changed the way in which health care providers and health plans collect, store, and share health information.

Health care providers, institutions, health plans, and health care clearinghouses are all required to conform to the HIPAA standards. As such, these organizations are all known as *covered entities*. Broadly, the HIPAA standards require that all covered entities have appropriate policies and procedures in place to ensure the privacy of all personally identifiable health information that they store and also that personally identifiable health information is shared only with the patient's permission and only in appropriate circumstances.[6] Being covered entities under HIPAA means that health care providers, institutions, and health plans may share health information with one another, when appropriate, without needing to verify each other's privacy protections. Each covered entity is assumed to have appropriate electronic and physical access controls to patient medical records and electronic data and to conduct routine audits of its data security procedures.

PATIENT TEACHING TIPS

THE HEALTH INSURANCE PORTABILITY AND ACCOUNTABILITY ACT

- Requires institutions and providers to develop policies and procedures to protect patients' unique health information
- Allows institutions and health care providers to use protected health information for treatment, payment, and normal health care operations with minimal restrictions as long as patients consent to its use
- Requires written permission for any use of protected health information outside of normal health care operations
- Gives patients the right to access, copy, and amend their health records
- Allows certain health information to be disclosed without the patient's consent only under very narrowly defined conditions (e.g., for public health reporting)
- Provides for significant penalties for violations

Tips and Tricks

REGULATORY AND LEGAL ISSUES

- Know the relevant public health regulations and reporting requirements in your area.
- Understand that patient safety initiatives and JC requirements generally improve care for patients, decrease the chance of error, and therefore decrease EPs' overall medicolegal risk.
- Develop mechanisms to perform medical screening examinations on all patients who present to the ED in a timely manner
- Ensure that patients transferred between health care institutions have (a) an accepting physician at the receiving institution, (b) a signed consent form for transfer when possible, (c) complete copies of their medical records and any relevant radiographic images with them, and (d) are transferred using staff with the appropriate level of training and monitoring capability.
- Access protected health information only when it is directly relevant to the medical care you provide.
- Be sure to obtain written permission whenever possible when sharing protected health information.

From the perspective of the EP, HIPAA means that personal health information should be obtained or accessed only when it is relevant to the immediate care of the patient. Further, personal health information should be disclosed only to other covered entities and only with the patient's permission. Sanctions for violating HIPAA standards include civil and criminal penalties with fines of up to $250,000 or imprisonment for up to 10 years, or both, for knowingly misusing a patient's identifiable health information.[7]

RED FLAGS

Emergency Medical Condition

- Acute symptoms
- May result in serious injury or impairment of function to organ or body part if not immediately treated
- Could jeopardize the health of the patient or unborn child
- Includes severe pain, psychiatric disturbance, active labor, and substance abuse, among others

Special Populations

Most state public health authorities have mandatory reporting requirements designed to protect vulnerable members of society. Some types of mandatory reporting have to do with the characteristics of the victim. The most common mandatory report of this type is a suspected case of child abuse or neglect. In addition, some states also mandate reporting of suspected elder abuse or abuse of the mentally handicapped.[8] Other types of mandatory reporting have to do with the characteristics of the event. The most common type of this mandatory report is the requirement that health care providers contact police when they treat victims of gun violence. Other examples of mandatory reporting may include knife injuries, animal bites, or major burns. Sexual assault represents a unique circumstance in which health care providers are frequently required to report that they treated the victim of such a crime, but they are not required to report the identity of the patient. This is because it is generally believed that mandatory reporting of individual identities would discourage some victims of sexual assault from seeking medical care.

REFERENCES

1. McNew R (ed): Emergency Department Compliance Manual. New York, Aspen Publishers, 2007.
2. The Joint Commission: Mission statement. Available at www.jointcommission.org.
3. Moy MM: The EMTALA Answer Book. New York, Aspen Publishers, 2007.
4. Kamoie B: EMTALA: Dedicating an emergency department near you. J Health Law 2004;37:41-60.
5. Beaver K, Herold R: The Practical Guide to HIPAA Privacy and Security Compliance. Boca Raton, FL, CRC Press, 2004.
6. Moskop JC, Marco CA, Larkin GL, et al: From Hippocrates to HIPAA: Privacy and confidentiality in emergency medi-

cine. Part I: Conceptual, moral, and legal foundations. Ann Emerg Med 2005;45:53-59.
7. Moskop JC, Marco CA, Larkin GL, et al: From Hippocrates to HIPAA: Privacy and confidentiality in emergency medicine. Part II: Challenges in the emergency department. Ann Emerg Med 2005;45:60-67.
8. Guldner G, Leinen A: Legal aspects of emergency care. In Mahadevan SV, Garmel G (eds): An Introduction to Clinical Emergency Medicine: Guide for Practitioners in the Emergency Department. New York, Cambridge University Press, 2005.

Chapter 211

Medical-Legal Issues in Emergency Medicine

Gregory L. Henry

KEY POINTS

Medicine is a business and is therefore covered under the usual concepts of business law.

Medical-legal considerations are an integral part of every doctor-patient interaction. The complete physician understands these aspects of care at the same level that he or she understands the science of such care.

Human interactive skills reduce lawsuits and improve patient satisfaction.

The chart is a physician's life boat in a sea of medical adversity.

The physician is not a bystander in the medical-legal process. The physician needs to be an active participant in the entire endeavor.

Specific medical-legal situations can be analyzed on a point-by-point basis. Specific actions and documentation programs can go a long way in reducing legal action.

Specific medical-legal problems dominate the lawsuit landscape in emergency medicine. Knowing the principal areas of risk and dealing with key points in advance are both good medicine and good risk management.

Scope

The nature of malpractice, what it is and what it is not, is often difficult for the medical mind to understand. Physicians are Apollonian in upbringing. They believe in science, they believe in what they can see, and they believe in proof. Malpractice is much more a societal concept. It is a battle that takes place in the arena of the court system. The usual concepts that dominate scientific thinking do not hold sway in court. The physician must come to grips with the idea that ordinary citizens will decide whether he or she has acted in the best interest of a patient. This never sits well in the hearts and minds of physicians. The general feeling in the medical community is that the medical community should police itself. That is not how the system is constructed, and the physician must become accustomed to the idea that issues that may seem trivial in the world of science are not in the world of human interaction.

Medicine is a profession. It is not a pure science. It is practiced on and with ordinary human beings. People respond both positively and negatively to our actions, and this response baffles physicians who have not analyzed the human interaction situation. To a large degree, physicians are in the business of comfort and reassurance. Only a doctor knows the difference between feeling bad and being sick. True professionals are those persons who do what they do to the best of their ability at any hour of the day or night with people with whom they would least like to do it. Pure science and emergency medicine have very little to do with each other. The truly skilled EPs can make patients want what they actually need. Part of the goal of every EP-patient interaction should be an elevation of the patient's understanding of the disease process and an appreciation for what was required for the diagnosis and treatment.

Be Service Oriented

It is a sign of maturity when an EP recognizes that he or she is in a service industry. In a service industry, perception is everything. Perception is the only reality. It makes very little difference whether the patient received excellent care if he or she believed it was substandard. Bringing the patient and family along in an understanding of the process is essential in proper risk management.

Looking for innate fairness in such a system is a waste of time. No one has ever guaranteed that the court system decides issues fairly. The court system is a mechanism for social conflict resolution. The courts set public policy and resolve disputes. This does not mean that disputes are always decided fairly or in a scientific context. Courts decide disputes based on human perceptions, and, knowing this, the physician can make intelligent decisions about how to practice. The intelligent physician understands that the patient's view of the situation needs to be brought in line with the dictates of science. Sometimes this is simple, and sometimes it is not. However, the physician who ignores the patient with indifference or arrogance will soon have a new name: the defendant physician. In general, to be named in a medical lawsuit is to lose. Physicians often have the gross misconception that if they are named in a suit and the suit is dropped or they win in court, they have won. The only way to win in the lawsuit game is not to play. Everything costs money. Evaluation of complaint letters, initial processing of legal suits, the deposition phase of discovery, and finally, going to court all have their costs. The actual dollar figure to defend lawsuits has risen rapidly since the late 1980s and may constitute up to half of the expenses of the insurance company in the handling of medical-legal actions.

The physician needs to understand the nonfinancial effects of lawsuits on his or her personality. Excellent information in the literature documents that a physician under suit is much more likely to become depressed. Physicians under the threat of suit also have a decrease in decision-making ability. They have a greater reported incidence of ulcers, divorce, and other social problems. This is understandable when one considers that a physician's image of self is integrally related to his or her medical degree. The physician has spent a life of study and hard work, from leaving high school to finishing a residency, a period of approximately 12 years, devoted to clinical excellence. When all this is challenged in the court of law, it hits home to the core of a physician's soul. The financial cost of malpractice is not the only cost. Any physician who has been sued understands the emotional stress and pain that comes with the process.

Emergency medicine is the ideal setup for poor doctor-patient interactions and malpractice problems. It is when one sees patients at the worst moments of their lives. We often have to make quick decisions on what is an incomplete database. We also have no long-term relationships to provide clues or insights into the nature of disease. Similarly, no long-term building of emotional bonds exists to prevent the patient from suing should the outcome be negative. In short, emergency medicine is the ideal climate for things that go wrong to be transferred into the legal arena as a means of retribution.

Human psychology leads us to understand that patients will behave as they would like and not as we would like. Residency training programs in the United States do not place a high value on interactive excellence. It is essentially antithetical to the university training program to spend more time on pleasing the patient than on understanding the science. A natural transition occurs when the resident finishes training and moves into a practice setting; a shift in priorities takes place. The young physician does not learn attitudes from books or meaningless statements mouthed at grand rounds. Young EPs learn how to behave and how to practice from watching their fellow, more senior residents and the attending staff who oversee patient care. It is at this level where malpractice will either be won or lost.

Small Things Count

It is often difficult for physicians to understand that small things count. How they are dressed, how they present themselves, how they introduce themselves to their patients, and their use of words may be a bigger factor in whether they are sued than their actual scientific thought processes. The art of medicine is not a "tack on" but is an essential fundamental base in creating a productive practice. The doctor who is a great communicator engenders better cooperation and has better results from patients. Such a physician has fewer complaint letters. He or she receives more help from emergency staff members and consultant physicians and consequently has a less stressful professional life.

Without question, the science of medicine concentrates on two principles: find it and fix it. Diagnosis and disposition are the principal, scientific elements of what we do. However, the physician should not underestimate his or her effect on the thought process of the patient in creating an atmosphere of caring. In emergency medicine, we are in the "bad outcome business." It is not whether something will go wrong, but rather when. The physician who has laid proper groundwork with the patient is in a much better position to avoid a medical-legal confrontation.

Barriers to Proper Care

The EP is often in the position of being emotionally hijacked. Information flows in from patients, their families, nurses, and emergency medical technicians, for example. Frequently, a physician's perception of a case can be altered by a word or phrase that sets off barriers to intelligent health care. This is the great problem of emergency medicine. Too many times, we are prejudiced before we see the patient. When one picks up a chart and the chief complaint says terminal fibromyalgia, recurrent back pain, or recurrent migraine headache, negative connotations and stereotypes often negatively color the doctor-patient interaction before it begins. Certain phrases and situations, again, set off irrational defense mechanisms in the physician that are difficult to overcome. As soon as the patient challenges the physician by asking "Did you call my doctor yet?" there is a strong tendency on the part of the physician to take offense.

Whenever a psychiatric diagnosis is written on the chart, beware. Physicians can ascribe virtually any other problem to mental health complaints. This approach is dangerous and can lead one to overlook obvious and treatable diseases. The concept of signal-to-noise ratio dominates information gathering in emergency medicine. We receive so many bits and fragments of information that are truly extraneous to the problem around us that it is often very difficult to focus on the actual patient and the possible disease entity. The physician needs to be aware that these natural human tendencies can manipulate thought processes to the detriment of both the patient and the doctor.

Establishing the Relationship

Good things happen only if they are planned; bad things happen all by themselves. It is important that the EP have a structured and stereotypic way of greeting the patient and gathering information. Some physicians object to this "acting" because they believe that it is somehow beneath their dignity. Nothing could be further from the case. The patient expects and deserves a compassionate physician who will dedicate at least some time to listening to his or her problem. A careful script is the best way of maintaining a sense of decorum and dignity in the interaction. Proper introductions and shaking hands go a long way to reassuring patient that the physician is there for their benefit. If there is one excellent risk management tool in the ED, it is the chair. EPs should sit down for at least a few moments if they can, to illustrate to the patient that they are sincerely interested in listening to the patient's problem. The physician, under our legal system, is the retained agent and servant of the patient. The degree to which a physician is comfortable with being a servant is the degree to which he or she is comfortable with being a doctor. Box 211-1 is a list of simple rules that should help to facilitate the doctor-patient interaction.

BOX 211-1

Rules for Physician-Patient Interactions

- It does not matter how long they waited; it was too long. Never argue with patients over the amount of time they waited.
- Never use excuses, such as you are working short staffed or "I've been here all day." The patient, quite frankly, does not care.
- Always apologize for the wait. As soon as you have apologized for the wait, you have at least acknowledged that the patient's time is as valuable as yours and you understand that waiting is not a comfortable situation. This is just common courtesy and goes a long way to making the doctor-patient interaction more desirable.
- Thank people for coming in. Business goes where it is invited and stays where it is appreciated. There is no reason not to thank people for using your institution. It is again common courtesy and is viewed as a sign of acceptance and reassurance by all.
- The trivialization of minor complaints can lead to major problems. Phrases such as "It's only a virus" are not terribly useful. Patients will listen to your discussion of why antibiotics are not going to be ordered and why further tests are not going to be done if the reasons are stated in a manner and context that they can understand. Most patients believe they have a legitimate reason to be in the ED. To be scolded because it is the doctor's perception that theirs is a minor illness never helps the doctor-patient interaction and really does not prevent further ED visits. This type of activity is not useful in the long run.

Medical-Legal System Organization and Problems

The legal world is divided into two major parts.

Part 1: Criminal acts: These activities are so heinous to the fabric of society that society acts to protect itself.

Part 2: Civil law: This part basically consists of dispute resolution in which the state acts as the forum for various parties to resolve conflicts.

The history of malpractice is long and varied. As early as the code of Hammurabi in 1760 BCE, a physician could have his hands amputated if a patient died at surgery. The code of Justinian in 600 CE also had laws governing physicians and pharmacy. The U.S. justice system is based on English law. Law courts from 1290 CE have records of resolving medical malpractice cases. A lawsuit is again the societal way of resolving a dispute. It is in the greater public and civic arena and is not under control of the medical system.

The EP should understand the various types of law. *Substantive law* states that specific activities are either allowed or not allowed within society. *Procedural law* dictates when to carry out various activities. Most malpractice falls under the realm of something called *common law*. Common law is case law. Judges make decisions based on what has happened in the past. This is the concept of *stare decisis*. This Latin phrase, meaning "what has been will be," states that courts are to decide cases based on the tradition of the law until new law is made. Because we have 50 states, there are 50 different collections of U.S. common law. Although the basic rules are similar, the details vary from state to state. It is essential that EPs know the law in the states in which they are practicing.

All English law is based on the concept of the standard of care. The term *standard of care* is often misunderstood. The standard of care is what an ordinary physician of like or similar training would do under like or similar circumstances. It is not just one action or one mode of care. There are often simultaneously multiple ways of treating a medical condition, and excellent physicians often disagree about the best mode of therapy for a particular problem. The standard of care is not the "best" care that may be available. It is what is reasonable. Acceptable care covers a large range of possibilities. In truth, the standard of care is constantly shifting as our knowledge base changes. The standard of care for a myocardial infarct in 1960 would certainly be below the standard of care in 2006.

▪ STRUCTURE OF A LAWSUIT

The structural base of a lawsuit has four components. The plaintiff is charged with showing that the physician has violated all these components in some way. First is *duty*. The duty is what is required by a physician practicing in an ED in the time frame specified by the case. The duty of emergency personnel, for example, to see all patients who present to the ED, has been clear since the passage of Emergency Medical Treatment and Active Labor Act/Consolidated Omnibus Reconciliation Act (EMTALA/COBRA) laws beginning in 1986. Your duty is to see everyone who presents to the ED and to treat patients up to your level of ability. The next aspect is *breach of that duty*. The injured party must show that the physician acted in such a way that the requirements for the performance of that duty were not met.

Harm done is what actually happened. Very often, no matter whether a physician practiced perfect care or did nothing at all, the outcome would be the same. The actual harm done to the patient is an aspect of the case that is often avoided, but it is truly what is compensated in a court of law. The award for malpractice is money, so financial damage must be presented as a part of the process.

Last is the concept of *proximate cause*. This is the relationship between the breach of duty and the harm actually done to the patient. The fact that a patient dies may not be in question. The question is whether the actions or inactions of the physician actually led to the patient's death. The proximate cause is precisely what expert testimony establishes as part of the civil process.

▪ ENGAGING A DEFENSE: FIRST STEPS

Physicians often take the position that they are merely injured victims in this system. Nothing could be further from the truth. The physician has the opportunity to participate in and to affect the outcome in every medical-legal situation. The biggest mistakes doctors make in the legal process are as follows:

- **Ignoring the claim and pretending it did not happen.** Nothing good comes through registered mail. A physician must notify his or her group and hospital whenever a legal summons is issued with regard to the question of malpractice. Physicians can be found guilty and can have money damages assessed against them under a default judgment if they do not respond in the proper time frame.
- **Going into a panic and talking to colleagues about the facts of the case.** A physician should not discuss a pending legal action except in the presence of the defense attorney or in the setting of a properly constituted quality assurance meeting. A physician must avoid the temptation to "try the case" with friends.
- **Contacting the patient.** Once a lawsuit has begun, it is absolutely forbidden for the physician to make any calls, write letters, or attempt to contact the patient who has brought the action. Once there is a specific legal action, all interaction between parties should be through their attorneys.
- **Failure to preserve the integrity of the chart.** Once a legal action has been commenced, the chart should be copied, and the original chart should be sealed and put in a secure place in hospital records. No physician should ever, in any way, alter a medical record after the fact.
- **Failure to assist counsel.** The physician's input is absolutely required and is mandated in the malpractice policy. Total candor is necessary and no lawyer likes a surprise. Failure to cooperate with a defense counsel may invalidate a physician's insurance policy.
- **Displaying an arrogant, hostile, or defensive attitude.** The physician must realize that he or she is in business. A lawsuit is a part of business. No juror wants to see a physician's God complex expressed in a deposition or from the stand. A simple, calm, and caring explanation of what actually happened goes best in court. It is important for the physician not to let pride or a sense of injury stand in the way of an intelligent defense.
- **Thinking the trial is a search for truth.** A trial is a dispute resolution process. No truth finding

is involved. Lawyers generally do not care about the truth; they care about winning and about the money. Everything in the trial matters: the dress and manner of the physician, the personality and politics of the judge, the quality of the lawyers, the degree of sympathy for the plaintiff and the family, and the quality of the experts. In this situation, the intelligent physician is an active participant who helps to obtain the best experts to help defend him or her in court.

- **Assuming the legal process will not affect you.** Physicians take the process seriously, even at a subconscious level. A physician should be prepared to seek emotional help as well as legal help when the strain of lawsuit hits.
- **Knowing when settlement is the right solution.** The physician should not ask a mediocre complaint expert to salvage the case. Not listening to medical and legal experts is a mistake. Certain cases are losers. The person least able to decide whether a case needs to be settled is the physician involved in the case. Other physicians with experience in medical malpractice and who know what wins and loses in court need to be involved in assessing the case. The effect of losing a lawsuit on the group, the hospital, and the emergency contract should not be underestimated.
- **Casually blaming another provider.** No physician should ever make casual, derogatory comments about anyone else's care. The physician is responsible for the care he or she has provided, not for the care of other physicians' patients. Physician in-fighting raises the cost of cases and does no one, including the patient, any good.
- **Expecting a quick resolution.** EPs, by nature, want a rapid resolution of a problem. Law moves in a time frame of its own. It often takes years to resolve a case. The physician needs to understand that such processes are not what a physician would want.

▪ CHARTING AND THE MEDICAL RECORD

A medical chart is produced for a reason. Health care workers have less than perfect memories, and as the time wanes from seeing a patient, the exact details also disappear. The principal document in any medical malpractice suit against an EP is the chart generated in the ED at the time of the visit in question. The only things that really go to court with a physician are the patient's medical record and the physician's credibility. The chart is the only document that the plaintiff attorney has to understand what happened and to be able to decide whether bringing a legal action is worthwhile.

Although the chart has multiple functions (e.g., billing, coding, and registration), to the EP it is important documentation of the care given. A patient can have received excellent care and have a poor chart, but it is rare that a patient receives poor care when charting is excellent. However, multiple issues with regard to a chart present themselves in every lawsuit.

▪ LEGIBILITY AND DECIPHERABILITY

Legibility and decipherability are different concepts. It is no longer adequate that a chart is decipherable. Handwritten entries to a chart must be legible to the average person. Actions can now be brought by hospitals against physicians for poor handwriting. Readability also becomes an issue when it comes to discharge instructions. Legibility-related errors in medications or in implementing other therapies are always potentially explosive for a jury.

▪ TIMELINESS OF MAKING A RECORD

All events and entries made on the chart should be timed. When a legal case is reconstructed years later in a courtroom, it is important for the defense to know what happened when. The function of the nursing notes, in particular, is to be a guide to the sojourn of the patient through the ED. When the patient arrives, when triage is performed, when the patient is first seen by the EP, and when various studies are ordered and carried out can become an issue in virtually any case.

▪ CHARTING USELESS INFORMATION

Do what you chart, but chart what you do. Comments on history and physical examination not performed will not go well in court. Vital signs should be taken as needed, but if they are taken and found to be abnormal, they should be answered. Unanswered vital signs are a significant problem in emergency medicine. Most vital signs do not need rapid reevaluation, but documentation that you have informed the patient that they have, for example, mildly elevated blood pressure that should be followed up by the family physician goes a long way in defending the EP should problems arise in the future.

▪ ALTERING THE MEDICAL RECORD

When medical records need adjustment, such corrections should be made in an obvious and straightforward manner. The EP should never cross out any other health care professional's note. All additions and corrections to the chart need to be dated and timed. A "doctored record" raises credibility questions. It is important that there be no devious attempt to correct or alter a chart. The nefarious correction of the medical chart is now a federal crime.

▪ DISCREPANCIES AMONG PROFESSIONALS

Legitimate reasons exist for discrepancies among various professions and what they record in the chart.

Histories are taken at different times, patients may refine their histories, and physical examination findings may change. For this reason, the nursing record needs to be available to the physician. The physician is responsible for nursing notes generated.

An absolute mistake is to have a negative nursing note written after the time of discharge. What good does it do a patient or a physician for a nurse to write "Patient still in pain at the time of discharge"? The rules should be obvious. If a negative nursing note is going to be recorded, the physician needs to be informed so an action can be taken. Conversely, the last nursing note does help to set the tone of the patient's condition at the time of discharge. A nursing note stating "Patient awake, alert, ambulatory, and improved at discharge" is excellent proof that the patient had received benefit from the ED visit.

▪ COMMENTS ON THE CHART

The chart is a legal document protected by both state and federal law. The chart is not a place where derogatory comments should ever be made. Rudeness and flippancy have no place in medical charting. The chart should reflect the objective observations of concerned health care personnel. Not only are rude generalizations about the patient inappropriate, but they may also prove deadly at the time of trial.

▪ DISCHARGE INSTRUCTIONS

Approximately half the lawsuits in emergency medicine revolve around discharge instructions and the discharge program given to patients. Box 211-2 gives a few paramount rules for discharge instructions.

Specific Medical-Legal Situations: Pearls

The function of this section is to delineate those areas where emergency medicine and the law come into direct contact on a regular basis. No practice of medicine brings the forces of the law, society, medical care, general inequities, and resource distribution problems together as does emergency medicine. The ED is under growing stress to solve all social problems. We are being asked to do more and more with less and less until finally we will be expected to do everything with nothing. No other specialty of medicine interacts with general society at the same level as in the ED.

- **Ownership of patients.** Patients own doctors; doctors do not own patients. The legal relationship of parties is that the physician is "the retained agent and servant of the patient." When a patient is in your department, he or she is your patient from a legal standpoint. The physician cannot abrogate responsibility by saying that the patient belongs to another physician.

BOX 211-2

Rules for Discharge Instructions

- All instructions are time specific. It rarely does a patient any good to have a bland statement such as "See your doctor if not better." That does not tell the patient when to act. Time-specific instructions such as "Return in 6 hours for reexamination of your abdomen or sooner if worse" are clear and to the point. The patient knows what to do and when to do it.
- Instructions must be action specific. It is not adequate to say "Ice a wound." Do you want it twice per day, three times per day? Should patients use ice directly on the skin or use an ice bag or pack? Patients must know where and when they are going to perform certain acts. The discharge instructions also need to be in plain language. If a fourth grader could not read the discharge instructions, the instructions are probably inadequate. They need to be brief and to the point. Overly complex and extensive discharge instructions are never read. Discharge instructions need to be separate from information sheets. The instructions are not everything the patient ever needs to know about a particular disease. They are a list telling the patient what to do, what to watch for, and when to return.
- Abbreviations in discharge instructions can be a serious problem. Most patients are not Latin scholars. They do not know the meaning of the terms *PRN* and *TID*. There is always room for confusion when a discharge instruction says "F/U in am."
- Whenever there is an untoward delay in patient care, the reason for that delay should be noted. The physician's memory will not maintain this type of information. If there is an unusually heavy crush of patients to use the computed tomography scanner or some other legitimate reason for delay in care, this should be noted on the chart, as well as any attempts to improve the situation. The physician will have little to no memory of such a situation in 5 years when the lawsuit comes to be tried, unless the situation is kept in perspective.

- **Combative patients.** The ED has not only the right to restrain, but also the duty to restrain when the patient constitutes a danger to self or others by virtue of a physical or mental condition (Box 211-3). The determination of competency is the key issue. Competent patients may refuse or accept any care they so chose. Patients who lack such competency will depend on the substitute judgment of the EP. Belligerent patients who are

BOX 211-3

Rules for Restraining Combative Patients

- Restraint methods must be appropriate, but both chemical and physical restraints are still commonly used to control patients who constitute a threat. The EP has obligations to the other patients in the ED and to the staff to make sure that a potentially combative or destructive patient does not hurt anyone else.
- When restraining a patient, the need for restraint needs to be documented, the specific mode of restraint needs to be written as an order, and the patient's basic personal needs require proper nursing care.
- All restrained patients require reevaluation at intervals to determine the continued need for restraints.
- EPs rarely become involved legally in restraint cases unless they (1) fail to document the reason for restraint and (2) fail to follow their own hospital ED's restraint policy.

competent require law enforcement to handle the situation.

- **Civil commitment.** In all 50 states, civil commitment is the act of the probate court. The role of the ED is again in securing the patient so he or she does not cause harm to self or others and in filling out a first certification detailing those behaviors and physical findings that justify civil commitment. The observations of the family and police, as well as those events seen by the physician, should be documented and used in the decision-making process. Most states require a second certification process to be done in a specified time frame by a mental health professional. In the ED, ruling out organic causes of disease and arranging for the patient to be reevaluated by mental health professionals are the primary goals of evaluation therapy. The authority for civil commitment of a patient is given over to the court system. It is up to the judge to decide on the continued suspension of civil liberties. The EP's proper documentation that the patient constitutes a danger to self or others by virtue of illness goes a long way in helping the court system to make such decisions.
- **Transfers.** EMTALA/COBRA is the law of the land. A transfer log is a high-profile document that must be maintained by federal law. Informed refusal can allow a patient to exempt himself or herself from EMTALA regulations. A refusal to be transferred should be carefully noted on the patient's chart by the EP and the nurse involved in the case. The transferring institution has strict legal responsibilities under the law. Stabilization is not an absolute process; stabilization is relative to the needs of the patient. The patient should be stabilized such that the acts of transfer and of moving the patient to a higher level of care have a reasonable probability of providing a better outcome for the patient. The appropriateness of transfer is left in the hands of the physician. The transferring institution needs to be able to send laboratory results, radiographs, and any other materials obtained from the patient. All these materials can be transferred by other means than direct travel, and there should be no unreasonable delays in transfer while awaiting laboratory studies. Similarly, records can be transferred by electronic means and should not delay the transfer of a critically ill patient. The receiving institution also has obligations under the EMTALA. A hospital that usually and customarily receives patients should accept those patients unless their capabilities, at that time, are overwhelmed and they are unable to find room. This fact should be noted on the records when trying to obtain a transfer of a patient.
- **Reportable illnesses.** The legal system and the ED function together as essentially an officer of the court. Legal reporting duties are mandated by law in every state. Other parts of the hospital (e.g., laboratory) also have obligations to report certain findings to public health authorities. Reporting statutes vary from state to state. The EP should be aware of the state in which he or she is practicing and should know the reporting requirements. In all 50 states, child abuse, elder abuse, and assaults are reportable illnesses. The EP also maintains a duty to third parties who may not be present in the ED. There is an obligation to protect third parties through reporting to the police. Therefore, when a patient has a gunshot or stab wound, other people may be at risk, and failure to report such injuries could place them in danger. This is a clear obligation of the ED and the EP to see that such reporting takes place.
- **Legal blood alcohol limits.** Legal blood alcohol limits have always been an area of controversy. This is a common problem, but the rules vary from state to state. Determinants for drawing blood and reportable blood alcohol levels are covered in each state under statute. The U.S. Supreme Court has spoken to this issue multiple times. With a court order (i.e., a signed warrant from a judge), the state does have a right to obtain blood alcohol levels. In most states, police officers alone have no authority to force a patient to have a blood alcohol determination made without a warrant. This does, however, vary from state to state because some states have given the police warrant authority to obtain blood. The U.S. Supreme Court ruled against forceful removal of stomach contents with a nasogastric tube. The Court viewed the taking of blood as a usual and customary medical procedure. The passing of a nasogastric tube was considered aggressive and offended the sensibilities of the Court. In no state can the police require the EP to pass nasogastric tubes to obtain samples. However,

once a patient has discarded bodily contents (e.g., vomitus, urine, or feces), such material then passes into the public domain, and the police have a right to discarded bodily materials.

- **Incident reports.** Incident reports are a part of the quality assurance system. In most states, incident reports are protected from both discovery and judicial admissibility. The function of this reporting is to improve care, not to point fingers. The important aspects of incident reports should be clear. The EP should not reference an incident report in the patient's chart. Medical information about a particular patient belongs in the patient's records, not in an incident report. Questions concerning the system of care are the proper subjects of incident reports. Incident reports should not be filed in a patient's chart. They are part of a separate system. If they are filed in the chart, they may inadvertently be discoverable should legal action take place.
- **Response to in-house emergencies.** The exact response capability of EPs to sick patients in the rest of the hospital varies from place to place. In large hospitals, this is rarely an issue. In many smaller or rural hospitals, the EP may be the only physician present. General rules should be followed if such care is given. The physician's contract with the hospital should not have the physician guarantee to be in two places at once. All contracts should be written such that the EP will respond if not required to remain in the ED by the acuity level of other patients. The hospital always has the alternative of putting a patient on a cot and bringing the patient to the ED. When the ED is extremely busy, this may be the only reasonable way of handling the situation. When an EP is called to see a sick patient in another part of the hospital, the attending physician should also be called. Someone will be required to rewrite the orders, and someone will be required to speak to the family. The EP should not be viewed as taking over continuing care of the case. In many states, response to in-house emergencies is considered part of an in-house Good Samaritan statute. This again varies from state to state and should not be assumed.
- **Writing orders for admitted patients.** This area is controversial and difficult. Without question, writing orders can potentially extend the liability of the EP to the in-house setting. Most EPs do not have in-hospital privileges, and so writing orders may not be justified. The EP's medical liability carrier may also have questions regarding orders written on already hospitalized patients. This issue should be explored and settled explicitly with the malpractice carrier. If in-house orders are to be written, specific parameters about when an EP's responsibility begins and ends should be determined between the ED and the medical staff through the medical executive committee. The best ways to limit exposure on the writing of inpatient orders are as follows:
    - Time limit all orders.
    - Write only true admitting orders and not continuing care orders.
    - Make it clear when Dr. X, the attending physician, assumes care of the patient.
- **Prescriptions from the ED.** Most medications written by EPs are for up to 10 days of antibiotics and usually for 4 to 5 days of pain medication. This type of prescription constitutes more than 90% of those written. For the EP to renew long-term prescriptions is generally considered inappropriate. Patients who are receiving medications for hypertension or seizures, for example, should be given only enough medication until they can see their own doctor. No long-term doctor-patient relationship is established in the ED, such patients are not monitored for side effects of drugs, and this monitoring is not be expected to be done through the ED. Any prescription requiring a Drug Enforcement Agency prescription number should have proper warnings documented on the discharge instructions, with a copy in the chart. Writing medications for third parties (i.e., enough medication to treat sexual contacts of patients with sexually transmitted diseases) is not a good idea until state laws change to cover EPs for any potential harm that may occur.
- **Doctor-to-doctor conflict resolution.** Conflicts on points of medical care are common in medicine: two doctors, two opinions. When an attending physician and an EP differ on certain issues, the problem must be resolved. Everyone's story changes in deposition. EPs can be left in a precariously dangerous situation if they have not followed their own instincts. It should be clear on the chart when patient care is managed by another physician. The ED requires a policy on conflict resolution. The ideal policy contains a reference to joint responsibility, obligations of the attending physician to see his or her patients, the ability to refer a case to a neutral third party, and review of all such cases by the executive committee. The EP should beware of the powerful, "big admitter" physician, who has unusual control of the executive committee. Such situations can lead to unhappy outcomes for both the patient and the physicians.
- **Patients who leave before examination, who elope, and who leave against medical advice.** Patients who leave before examination are always problematic. Someone must have seen them to register them in the ED. Capacity is everything. The question whether the patient had the mental capability to decide to go home is an issue. The last health care professional to see the patient should write a note about why the patient left and attesting that the patient had the mental capacity to make such a decision at that time. Elopement is a similar process in which the patient disappears in the middle of a work-up. In patients in whom we expect elopements, it is a good idea to take precautions. Placing armbands on these patients so

that they will be recognized by security, placing them in visible locations in the ED, and assigning a family member to watch them are all useful techniques. If a patient does elope from the ED, the following should be done:
  - Search the ED.
  - Have security check the parking and smoking areas.
  - Call the patient's contact phone number.
- Informed consent in emergency medicine is rarely an issue or a problem. Informed refusal is, however. Patients who leave against medical advice are using a form of informed refusal. Lawsuits concerning patients who leave against medical advice have a very stereotypic formula. It is claimed that the patient was not properly educated about the issues and therefore could not make an appropriate decision. Patients and families can claim that the patient's mental status was worse than initially presented or that the patient was, in some way, discouraged from seeking medical care. The largest mistake the EP can make is to believe that signing a piece of paper (i.e., the against medical advice form) is the same as following the legal process. It is not. The legal process contains the following:
  - Documentation of the capacity of the patient. Does the patient have the mental status and cognitive abilities to act in his or her own self-defense?
  - Have we provided the patient a diagnosis in a form that he or she can understand?
  - Does the patient understand the consequences of what can happen if he or she does not take the advice of health care workers?
  - Have we in some way tried to communicate with family or friends who are with the patient so that they may also be involved in persuading the patient to receive medical care?
  - Have we properly documented all the foregoing by both the EP and nursing personnel involved? It is also wise for the EP to have family or friends present sign the against medical advice form or the chart acknowledging that they have heard and witnessed the discussion with the patient and the patient is leaving of his or her own free will. If all the foregoing areas are covered, the EP is virtually suit proof on the issue.
- **Return visits.** In emergency medicine, the "bounce-back patient" is always difficult. Often, prejudice against such patients exists because they are perceived as not following orders or doctor shopping. In general, such patients have misunderstood instructions, or the disease entity has changed. Return visits have something that is always potentially dangerous—a diagnosis. The assumption is that the first physician was correct. Unscheduled revisits need to be evaluated as would any other new patient, to ensure that some obvious change or intellectual blockade in understanding the patient's health care condition has not occurred. In general, multiple bounce-backs constitute a serious problem. It is often stated that third visits should equal admission until proven otherwise. The possibility that the patient has been misdiagnosed or mismanaged increases with each revisit.
- **House staff, physician assistants, and medical students in the ED.** The functioning of house staff members can be problematic for many reasons. The actual care given to patients may not be at the same level as care given by the attending physicians. The expected standard of care under the law, however, is the same as would be given by a mature physician by virtue of attending level supervision. All resident work must be supervised if it is to be billed for under any federal program. Violations of this mandate are considered criminal violations of the federal law, and the current act has no exemptions. All training programs must follow the guidelines initially promulgated in 1969 and reestablished in 1995. What constitutes supervision has been defined for each specialty and is available and on public record. Ignorance of the law is no excuse. No EP should believe that merely signing the chart actually constitutes supervision of care. Unless the EP has been intimately involved in the examination and management of the patient, such care has not happened. The attending physician ultimately bears the responsibility for the acts and omissions of the resident. Off-service residents (i.e., residents called down from another service) are also under the supervision of their attending physicians. When conflict arises regarding what needs to be done with a patient, it should not be resolved among residents, but rather among attending physicians of the various services. The law expects this, and patients deserve it. Physician assistants constitute a different problem. Their payment depends on the level of supervision. Online direct supervision is generally reimbursed at 100% of professional charges. Off-site or added-distance supervision in many states constitutes a lower payment for the services rendered. EPs should be well aware of the laws within their states with regard to the amount of supervision required to bill for such cases.
- **Change of shift.** There are two dangerous times in an ED: July 1 and anytime a change of shift occurs. This is because the patient's care must be transferred from one doctor to another. Continuity of information or insight into the underlying problem is always difficult under these circumstances, and so a change of shift should be documented on the chart. A note should be made in the chart that the patient's care was transferred to another physician at a particular time and that discussion was held with this other physician so he or she is properly engaged in the continuing care of the patient. The discharging doctor—the second physician to see the patient—generally assumes the duty to make certain that the patient's care is complete.

- **Laboratory studies, radiographs, and electrocardiograms.** A general rule is that the physician should not ask a question to which he or she does not really want to know the answer. If you are going to order a test, then you must follow up on the results in some way. A system is required to detect what has been ordered and to account for the results received. Laboratory tests, radiographs, and electrocardiograms all must be interpreted with regard to the specific patient. Follow-up on these issues should be guaranteed. A system is needed in which each variance in laboratory or radiographic test should be handled within the ED. A general rule is that you should not order tests for which you have no follow-up system. Those patients who are admitted are not generally a problem. If tests are going to be ordered that must be followed up by an outside physician, however, this system needs to be guaranteed.
- **Release of information.** The doctor-patient relationship and patient records are protected under federal law. The information within the records is owned by the patient. The actual physical pieces of paper or materials on which the record is written are owned by the hospital, and the hospital has a duty to maintain such records. Release of information requires the expressed consent of the patient. A wife, contrary to popular belief, has no implied right to her husband's medical records. A parent, in the role of legal guardian, has a right to a child's records but no right when that child is emancipated or has reached the age of adulthood. The casual release of information over the telephone should be discouraged. The individual patient's right to protection of his or her record is a part of the duty of the EP.
- **Duty to a third party.** Duty to a third party is always a difficult question in an ED. Various therapies may render a patient incapacitated in some way and may thereby put the patient and others in danger. The very act of issuing a prescription requiring a Drug Enforcement Agency number means that the EP is accepting some responsibility to inform the patient about the drug's use. A patient who drives a car under the influence of heavy medication may injure himself or herself and others. Without proper warnings, the EP may be involved in litigation. Other devices that make the patient incapable of normal functioning (e.g., the use of crutches, eye patches, and various splints) also may put the patient and others at risk. Discussion of this situation on the chart is useful should the need to provide defense arise.
- **Minors.** State law varies to some extent regarding what constitutes a minor, particularly with regard to emancipation. Emancipated minors are those who live outside the home, provide their own financial support, and make their own life decisions. The true emancipation of a minor is the act of a probate court. Nonetheless, minors have rights. In most states, laws exempt certain disease entities from the purview of parents. In most states, children who present for treatment and who are more than 12 years old may have questions of child abuse, substance abuse, sexually transmitted disease, and pregnancy treated without parental consent. However, adolescents rarely know these legal rights.
- **Telephone orders and telephone advice.** In general, the ED should not give telephone advice. Telephone advice is not given out in any structured or competent way in most cases, and the EP is frequently unaware that such advice is given. In most cases, patient inquiries and calls for medical advice should be routed away from the EP and nursing staff. Answering machine devices that advise the patient to come into the ED or to call 911 are often the most useful.

Specific Medical Problems

Most suits in emergency medicine are based on the medical chief complaint. The Massachusetts Closed Claims study indicated that, since the early 1980s, the top diagnoses have not really changed. However, the causes of these claims (e.g., failure to diagnosis, failure to refer) may not be obvious from just looking at the raw statistics. Much of this section is a word association process. When you think wrist, think the navicular bone. This is from a teaching philosophy of automatic response. Associated with each type of chief complaint, very specific yes and no answers should be expressed on the chart to show that the physician has had correct, basic thought processes.

No single chapter of a textbook such as this, indeed no entire textbook, can cover a topic as broad as the intelligent practice of emergency medicine. What is attempted in this section is to alert the EP to those issues that have been found to be considerable malpractice problems over the last 25 years. This is not an attempt to teach medicine. That is the function of the residencies and continuing medical education. However, the physician should not make obvious errors. This is the low-hanging fruit. The following is a collection of warnings and aphorisms having to do with the practice of emergency medicine, which has caused considerable medical-legal consternation.

- **Orthopedics.** This field is still the most frequent area of lawsuit in emergency medicine, but it is relatively low as a cost-per-case situation (Box 211-4). The wrist and thumb are areas of higher dollar loss. Missed navicular fractures and gamekeeper's thumbs are still problematic only because they are frequently radiographically negative. Long bone fractures are rarely a problem. Smaller (i.e., radiographically negative) injuries are the major orthopedic problems in emergency medicine. The follow-up radiographic system should be airtight. If a reading is returned to the ED that discovers a fracture, proper notification of the patient should be guaranteed by the system. The total picture is what is important in emergency

BOX 211-4

Rules for Orthopedic Conditions

- There is no such thing as a sprained wrist, just an injury that is not recognized.
- If you think enough of an injury to radiograph it, you think enough of it to splint it.
- One radiograph does not rule out a fracture. The EP should never guarantee that something is not broken.
- A better approach is to say "Good news! No displaced or obvious fracture" and then explain the limitations of radiography.

medicine. Certain fractures indicate that other actions should be taken. Examples include the following:
  - Calcaneus fracture: Examination of the lumbar spine is indicated.
  - Spinal fractures in children: The thought process must include the possibility of child abuse.
  - Traumatic femur fracture: Other chest, abdominal, and cervical spine injuries must be considered.
- It is always wise for the EP to let patients know that this is the beginning of a process. Orthopedic management includes recognition, reduction, retention, and rehabilitation. The ED is only the first part of what may be a long and complex process.
- **High-risk ear, nose, and throat or airway.** Airway, in emergency medicine, is everything. Cases involving the airway are major problems because of serious neurologic injuries that result. As the disease spectrum in the country shifts, based on changes in immunizations, the incidence of severe conditions such as epiglottitis has markedly changed. However, because the disease is rare, it does not mean that it does not exist. The decision to control the airway is clinical and is not based on oxygen saturation or blood gas measurements. The proper management of the airway is a core skill required by EPs. Intubation is not necessarily the answer, however. Proper use of the laryngeal mask airway or bag-valve mask apparatus can frequently control and provide adequate ventilation for patients. The need for minute-to-minute intubation can be modified by other such airway controls. A much rarer, but still recognized complication in emergency medicine is that of nasal injury. The only condition that requires emergency intervention is septal hematoma. It should be a quality assurance standard that every patient with a nasal injury has a comment in the chart about the presence or absence of septal hematoma. Radiographs are rarely required in nasal injuries.
- **Wounds.** All wounds seen in the ED are potentially contaminated and have foreign material almost by definition (Box 211-5). Lawsuits in emergency medicine wound management are based on three things: foreign body, foreign body, and foreign body. The cosmetic appearance of a wound is rarely an issue in emergency medicine, unless a foreign body has been retained or infection has occurred.

BOX 211-5

Rules for Wound Care

- Never guarantee that no foreign bodies are left in a wound.
- Glass does show on radiographs. A liberal use of radiography in shattered glass–type wounds is advisable.
- A laceration chart that does not comment on foreign body is probably inadequate.

- **Tendon injuries.** Tendons, in the relevant area of a wound, should be tested independently to arrive at the most precise diagnosis possible. Deep wounds should be observed through a range of motion to make certain that the tendon injury is not hidden by soft tissue. There is essentially no reason to explore a tendon sheath in the ED. The repair of tendons is rarely an emergency procedure. These wounds can be properly irrigated and loosely closed, and tendon repair can be performed later, within a reasonable time period.
- **Nerve injuries.** Nerve injuries are like tendon injuries. There is essentially no reason for emergency repair of an injured nerve. It is very difficult to assess whether a nerve has actually been severed or merely has a functional contusion early in the injury. The need for proper follow-up is obvious, but immediate intervention is rarely, if ever, required.
- **Wound infections.** It is important to let the patient know that the wound has been cleaned. The sink is your ally. Once a wound is disinfected, it is perfectly reasonable to have patients wash out their own wounds. No evidence suggests that sterile saline is any better a wound irrigant than tap water.
- **Bite wounds.** Bite wounds are at higher risk for infection, but it depends on the organism involved. Dog bites tend to be less infective than most. Cat bites are highly infective. Human bites are even worse. The physician's judgment is crucial in all these specific wounds. For a wound you suspect will become infected, treat it as though you would on the patient's next visit. Immobilization, intravenous antibiotics, elevation, and short-term interval follow-up are essential.
- **Style points in wound management.** Style points in wound management are essential for patient satisfaction. Pain management is often key. Topical anesthetics placed on the wound are appreciated by the patient who has to wait before

being evaluated. Long-acting caine derivatives are now the anesthetic agents of choice. Sedation may be needed, particularly in children. Considering the safety profile, sedation should be used on a regular basis.

- **Follow-up and suture removal.** Arranging for follow-up and suture removal is important. Having the wound rechecked and arranging for proper interventions will essentially go a long way in preventing any legal actions concerning wound infections or retained foreign bodies.
- **Poisoning.** Poisoning falls into two general groups. The first group comprises cases of accidental poisoning, mostly involving children. Whenever an EP sees a child who has been seen more than once with "accidental poisoning," the possibility of child abuse or neglect should come to mind. It is not only reasonable, but also required that action be taken for the defense of the child. The second group in poisoning is overdose, which involves teens and adults. The science of treating poisonings has changed rapidly. It is generally wise for the physician to consult the poison control center or some other poison authority and to document such contacts to make certain that current, acceptable treatments are being used. It is just as important to tell the family that you are seeking such outside expertise in the management of the problem.
- **Psychiatry.** In emergency medicine, the major issue with psychiatry is that the physician must be able to delineate organic disease manifesting as abnormal behavior (Box 211-6). All psychiatric patients eventually die of some organic process, and thinking that it is easy to decide what is causing abnormal behavior is often wrong. It is certainly possible to have both a psychiatric diagnosis and an organic problem at the same time. Psychiatric consultation services are often not ideal. It is important to identify who is involved in the evaluation of a patient. Only another physician can truly relieve the EP of liability on the issue. A psychiatric worker from some community program can certainly be helpful and may give an opinion, but if the EP disagrees with that opinion, he or she has an obligation to protect the patient first. The largest single burden on the practice of emergency medicine is patients who are mentally ill or who have altered mental status, secondary to drugs and alcohol. There is really no way to dispute that these patients constitute a difficult and common part of emergency practice. When in doubt, the EP should wait until the proper resources are available. The need to restrain and reevaluate patients is a known part of the profession, and it often falls to the EP to perform these duties. Clearing patients for psychiatric admission is also wrought with danger. The EP cannot say that a patient is free of organic disease, only that the patient is capable of being evaluated by a psychiatric service. The rule, however, should be that if any doubt exists, the patient should be handled initially by a medical service. Abnormal vital signs should not be ascribed to psychiatric disease. No psychiatric diagnosis causes tachycardia, hyperthermia, or a decreased pulse oximetry measurement. Clues to organic disease include unexplained abnormal vital signs, tremors, and abnormal speech patterns.
- **Chest pain.** This condition is still the largest risk issue in emergency medicine. Between 20% and 25% of malpractice funds expended in emergency medicine are related to the complaint of chest pain. The groups of diseases that constitute most of these cases are acute coronary syndromes, aortic dissection, and pulmonary embolus. The reason that these entities are such large medical-legal problems is that they tend to attack patients in their most financially productive years and can manifest with diverse and complex symptoms. Coronary artery disease is a common but mysterious disease. Unfortunately, sudden death is often the next manifestation of this disease. No current systems can totally rule out coronary artery disease, but we can at least put the patient in a lower risk category. Pain is highly subjective. Many people describe this pain as a pressure sensation, or they may have no acute chest pain whatsoever but instead report pain in the neck, jaw, or arms. Patients frequently refer to their pain as heartburn. The physical examination in most patients with chest pain usually reveals nothing (Box 211-7). Only very unusual cases of nontraumatic chest pain have prominent physical findings. The electrocardiogram is important when it is positive and indecisive when it is negative. Cardiac markers are similar. An initial cardiac enzyme result, if positive, can prompt immediate therapeutic actions. A negative enzyme result is just that. It is often too early in the process to know the direction in which the patient is heading.
- **Pulmonary embolism.** Pulmonary embolism is also a difficult diagnosis in many cases. It can commonly be misdiagnosed as pleuritis, pneumonia, or unknown syncope. A psychiatric diagnosis, such as hyperventilation syndrome, is very difficult to defend in court when the patient has died of a pulmonary embolus. Work-up of pulmonary embolus has changed markedly in the last few years because of the use of D-dimer testing, Doppler testing of the extremities, and computed

BOX 211-6

Rules for Psychiatric Conditions

- Most psychiatric services want patients to be properly cleared and expect blood alcohol and drug screens to be done.
- It behooves the EP to adhere to the expected program so those issues are not impediments to the patient's admission.

BOX 211-7

Rules for Chest Pain

- There is no single description of the pain that rules out myocardial disease.
- One electrocardiogram and one cardiac marker are not adequate to rule out coronary artery disease, and this approach is a frequent loser in court.
- If you think enough to order one marker, finish the rule-out protocol.
- Do not be embarrassed to call the line widely. This is a major problem, and no one has the exact answer.
- The EP should not write prescriptions for nitroglycerin. Unstable chest pain is unstable angina until proven otherwise.
- A gastrointestinal cocktail response proves nothing. It is in no way related to being able to separate myocardial from esophageal disease.

tomography (CT) scanning. The age of ventilation-perfusion scanning has essentially come and gone.

- **Aortic dissection.** Aortic dissection is a relatively rare disease. There may be 300 to 500 times more myocardial infarctions in the United States than aortic dissections each year. The symptoms may overlap and may be difficult to diagnose. The EP may consider obtaining a chest radiograph before thrombolytic agents are given. The use of thrombolytic agents in aortic dissection should be discouraged.
- **Abdominal pain.** Lawsuits related to abdominal pain in emergency medicine are highly age and sex dependent because of difficulties in diagnosis. Excellent evidence suggests that up to 50% of the time, a patient with a complaint of abdominal pain leaves the ED without a specific diagnosis proven by testing. Short-term follow-up is the key because examination is merely a snapshot of a moving picture. Gastroenteritis is a frequent diagnosis on lawsuit charts. Entities such as missed appendicitis, arterial disease, and, in children, missed meningitis can often be described to gastroenteritis. In the ED, it is best to divide abdominal pains into either surgical or medical as general groupings, to guide reexamination and therapies. Often, we do not have the exact explanation, and this is perfectly acceptable if the patient has been properly instructed, and short-term interval follow-up care has been arranged. Abdominal CT scanning is useful, particularly in elderly patients with diffuse disease, but this method is not infallible. If a patient's examination shows peritonitis, remember that CT has a 5% to 8% error rate of appendicitis. Clinical judgment should rule (Box 211-8).

BOX 211-8

Rules for Abdominal Pain

- If the patient still has an appendix, it could be appendicitis. The EP should not avoid this discussion with the patient.
- Repeat evaluations may be the safest and single best test in abdominal pain.
- A few white blood cells in the urine do not equal a urinary tract infection; there may be some other cause for the problem.
- In elderly patients with new-onset abdominal or flank pain, think aortic disease as an important rule-out diagnosis.

- **Urologic issues.** In emergency medicine, urologic emergencies are few. With the advent of newer catheter types, the need for an EP to call a urologic specialist into the ED has become rare. However, some issues have caused considerable medical-legal consternation. Testicular pain needs a diagnosis. The 10-year-old boy with testicular pain has torsion until proven otherwise. Even in the sexually active male patient, the possibility of torsion should not be underestimated. In general, painful testes are best treated after examination and testing with a call to the urologist. A young male patient with testicular pain needs intervention in a timely manner. Overtesting can be a problem. Nuclear scans are not 100% accurate, nor are Doppler ultrasound scans. A young male patient with a painful testicle deserves the insight of the urologist. Sexually transmitted disease can also have long-term sociologic and medical-legal implications. A patient who is being treated for possible sexually transmitted diseases should be asked about partners and should be informed that these partners will also require evaluation and treatment. It is also fair to warn the patient that the public health department will be involved if cultures are positive. The health department has a duty to third parties who have been involved with the patient to seek them out and provide therapy. It may be best that the patient understand the need to inform contacts and to advise them that they may be at some risk.
- **Neurologic emergencies.** Headache is one of the most common chief complaints in emergency medicine (Box 211-9). The ED, in every patient with headache, must consider the possibility of subarachnoid hemorrhage, meningitis, or carbon monoxide poisoning. Although subarachnoid hemorrhages are relatively rare in the United States (≈50,000/year), they carry a high morbidity and mortality. The most important part of the patient's history in deciding the possibility of subarachnoid hemorrhage is the rate of onset of the pain. In all long-term studies, this is the key factor in headache

BOX 211-9

Rules for Neurologic Emergencies

- If you obtain a computed tomography scan for subarachnoid hemorrhage, do a spinal tap to confirm the negativity.
- If this is the sudden onset of the worst headache of the patient's life, it may be his or her last headache and the physician's worst headache.
- Sudden onset of neck pain can indicate a subarachnoid hemorrhage. One third of subarachnoid hemorrhages occur in the posterior fossa.

pain history. The CT scan is, by itself, not an adequate screen for subarachnoid hemorrhage. A positive CT scan is a positive indicator, but a negative CT scan is indeterminate. Meningitis is rarely confused with subarachnoid hemorrhage. In the patient in whom meningitis is a serious possibility, the timing of antibiotics is generally the issue at the time of a lawsuit. The EP should feel comfortable about starting therapy early.

- **Spinal cord injury.** Spinal cord injuries are relatively rare, but they carry a devastating societal and financial cost. Maintaining a quadriplegic patient costs enormous amounts of money. The ED should properly document immobilization, and there should be no hurry to remove such immobilization. Adequate films in patients seriously suspected of cervical spine injury are important. Plain radiographs are becoming less useful, and more and more physicians are advocating an immediate move toward CT of the neck, to delineate fractures clearly. The other end of the spectrum is also true. If a patient is awake, has no specific neck complaints, and has no obvious discomfort during examination of the neck, clinically clearing the cervical spine meets the standard of care. The various clinical trials looking at this study clearly point to the uselessness of radiologically pursuing patients whose findings are normal.
- **Seizures and syncope.** Seizures and syncope can be lethal from multiple perspectives. Injury to the patient is a real potential problem, particularly in patients with seizures. Warnings about driving and the operation of machinery are important for protection of the public in general. Such warnings should be indicated in some way on the patient's chart.
- **Transient ischemic attacks and stroke.** Transient ischemic attacks and stroke are becoming larger issues. The American College of Emergency Physicians has gone on record as specifically stating that tissue-type plasminogen activator is not the standard of care for stroke. Lack of rapid evaluation of patients with transient ischemic attack and the initial use of aspirin therapy have been the source of many ED lawsuits. Patients with transient ischemic attacks represent a high-risk group and require timely intervention.
- **Trauma.** The biggest issue in patients with trauma is too little, too late. Each ED should know what they can and cannot do and should move quickly to ensure that the patient receives the actual help needed. It is useless for a critically ill patient to be maintained in an ED and not moved toward needed surgical rescue. If necessary, the EP in a smaller hospital needs to hold the ambulance service, or other transfer service, to await rapid movement toward the facility of choice. The replacement of fluids and the giving of blood should not wait for the results of any particularly laboratory study. Administration of blood and treatment of shock are critical. Hemoglobin takes time to equilibrate, and patients who are in shock have no specific abnormal laboratory study early in the course of illness. In general, smaller hospitals should understand their capabilities. Excessive radiography is generally useless. Most limb injuries can be splinted, and radiographs can be performed at the receiving institution. Results of laboratory and radiographic studies can be sent after a patient has been transferred. The EP should beware admitting patients to a hospital that cannot care for these problems. Head-injured patients should not be merely admitted for observation, but sent to a center where intervention can take place if it is actually required.
- **Obstetric and gynecologic issues.** With regard to obstetric and gynecologic issues, it is important for the EP to realize that there may be two patients and not one. The right questions need to be asked. Patients can be inaccurate about the exact dates of their menstrual periods. The urine pregnancy test is an excellent screen, and if it is positive, it is correct at the 99% level. If any question exists, obtain a pregnancy test. Missed ectopic pregnancies have decreased dramatically in the United States as a medical-legal problem since the widespread use of beta-human chorionic gonadotropin testing and ultrasound scanning. Sudden loss of consciousness or shock in a young female patient should raise the possibility of a ruptured ectopic pregnancy until proven otherwise. Eclampsia is the second most common obstetric and gynecologic emergency. Believe the patient's blood pressure and follow it carefully. Protein in the urine, along with elevated blood pressure, means calling in the obstetrician to become involved with the management of the case. In postpartum febrile female patients, ultrasound scans to check for retained products of conception and infection within the uterus are as important as checking the urine. Women who are 5 months in gestation and who have sustained trauma to the abdomen should have a period of fetal monitoring. Some legitimate debates exist regarding the length of this monitoring, but most

authorities agree that a single reading of the fetal heart rate is not adequate. If a patient is hooked to a fetal monitor over a period of approximately 4 hours, most authorities would consider this a reasonable test to see whether there is fetal irritability.

- **Pediatrics.** The number of pediatric medical-legal cases in emergency medicine has actually decreased as the rates of immunization and the various diseases that can be immunized against have increased. The keys to pediatrics are examination and early reexamination. The major issues around febrile children have not changed. The ED needs a protocol for work-up of children at various ages to rule out infection. No single test can determine whether a child is ill. Important examinations on the chart should refer to the child's level of consciousness, playfulness, hydration, and activity. A term such as "lethargic child" should prompt reexamination to see whether this is correct. It is true that most adults are more anxious about their children than they are about themselves. The EP frequently needs to convince parents that the child will do well at home. In most well-appearing children, testing is generally useless. Very little evidence indicates that complete blood counts and blood cultures are of use. In particularly young children who are febrile, urinalysis has proven to be a more important screening laboratory study. Feeding of children is important. Offer popsicles or a balanced salt solution of some kind so the parents can actually observe the child eating and keeping food down. The ability to retain fluid is often the reason that children are either admitted or discharged home. Finally, child abuse is a serious social problem in EDs. In general, you never accuse anyone of abusing his or her child. You merely state that an investigative process is required because of the presenting findings. It is important to emphasize that "they" make us do this type of investigation in these situations. Abuse and neglect are often difficult to separate in the ED, and this distinction needs to be made through social service. When in doubt, however, the child's safety is paramount, and admitting a child for observation can certainly be a reasonable use of the hospital facility. Certain specific disease entities, such as sudden infant death syndrome, unusual burns, vaginal infections, certain types of fracture, and repeat toxic ingestions should always be considered suggestive of child abuse until further information is obtained.

Chapter 212

Coding and Billing

James K. Takayesu

KEY POINTS

The ED chart must be both adequate to support billing and accurate to prevent fraudulent claims against the EP.

Most reimbursement comes from the five levels of evaluation and management (E&M) codes and depends on a combination of historical and physical examination data, medical decision making (MDM), and diagnosis assignments.

Critical care billing requires more than 30 minutes of physician attention to a patient who is undergoing resuscitative treatment and obviates the level-specific E&M charting requirements.

Observation billing requires documentation separate from the ED chart and can increase ED billing on patients with anticipated hospital stays of less than 24 hours.

The EP is legally accountable for the claims made based on the ED chart, including the potential for criminal penalties in cases of up-coding such as assumption coding.

Scope

Documentation in the ED medical record serves three basic functions:

1. To provide a detailed record of a patient's medical conditions and treatments
2. To minimize the medical liability risk of EPs by documenting thought processes supporting treatment plans
3. To support the charges billed to the patient by clearly substantiating the services rendered

Documentation in the ED chart must be both adequate to support reimbursement claims and accurate to prevent claims of billing fraud. Providing excellent patient care correlates with appropriate reimbursement only if the EP documents the history, physical examination, and thought processes adequately. What is not documented is not reimbursed. Additionally, understanding the fundamentals of coding and billing from the ED chart is essential to ensuring a revenue stream on which any EP group's financial viability is based. This revenue, in turn, supports professional autonomy, continuing medical education, and improvements in ED patient care and technology.

Insurance agencies and the federal government require adequate documentation as proof of delivery of services to patients. Revenue from patient care is obtained through two parallel billing structures: hospital billing and professional billing. This chapter focuses primarily on professional billing. Reimbursement from professional billing comes from a variety of sources, including current procedural terminology (CPT) codes, E&M codes (including MDM), critical care services, observation services, and ambulatory payment classifications (APCs). These sources are covered sequentially in the following sections.

Current Procedural Terminology Codes

Before the publication of CPT codes, third-party payers had their own idiosyncratic list of physician services and their respective codes, thus making consistent and reliable procedural billing extremely difficult. Complicating matters was the lack of suggested values for these services. CPT coding was published by the American Medical Association in 1966 as an attempt to standardize reimbursement for medical procedures. These codes are used for reporting physician services for claims processing, as well as for local, regional, and national service utilization comparisons by the Centers for Medicare and Medicaid Services. CPT codes are reviewed annually by the American Medical Association CPT Editorial Committee with input from various specialty physician organizations to account for new procedures and changes in reimbursement patterns.

A CPT code is a unique five-digit code that represents a service in contemporary medical practice that is being performed by physicians.[1] Major code groupings include E&M services, anesthesia, surgery, radiology, pathology, and laboratory services. Some common examples of emergency procedures and physician fees are listed in Table 212-1. Appropriate documentation of care provided to a patient may include services that the EP may not consider billable, such as intravenous hydration (90760, 90761). Although certain procedures and services are not time oriented, others are. For example, procedural sedation, whether administered by the EP who is also performing the procedure (99143, 99144) or administered with the EP assisting a secondary physician (99148, 99149), is time oriented, not billable until a continuous block of 30 minutes is achieved.[2,3] Once the 30-minute period is surpassed, an additional code (99145 or 99150) may be used to account for each additional 15-minute increment.[2,4] In taking note of these fees, it becomes obvious why adequate visit and procedural documentation, including time increments for certain procedures such as conscious sedation, is essential to ensuring adequate reimbursement.

Once a CPT code is adopted or reviewed, the American Medical Association Relative Value Update Committee assigns a relative value unit to the code to account for that service's complexity relative to other services listed. This Resource-Based Relative Value Scale effectively ranks services provided based on three factors: (1) the relative work of the physician for the service (work value), (2) the cost of performing the service (practice expense value), and (3) the risk involved in the services to both patient and provider (professional liability insurance). Each of these factors is assigned a numeric value which, when added together, gives a total relative value unit for the service. This relative value unit is then multiplied by a monetary conversion factor to give an actual dollar amount for the services provided. These dollar figures are subsequently adjusted for different geographic regions based on a geographic adjustment factor to account for local practice costs.

Table 212-1 SAMPLE FEE SCHEDULE FOR BLUE CROSS/BLUE SHIELD OF MASSACHUSETTS EMERGENCY MEDICINE PROCEDURE AND PHYSICIAN FEES, EFFECTIVE SEPTEMBER 1, 2004

Procedure Code	Procedure	Fee
10060	Drainage of skin abscess	$102.98
10120	Remove foreign body	$78.37
12001	Repair of superficial wound(s)	$104.75
12032	Layer closure of wound(s)	$208.87
16020	Treatment of burn(s)	$68.77
23650	Shoulder dislocation	$308.73
29125	Apply forearm splint	$48.75
29130	Application of finger splint	$32.58
30901	Control of nosebleed	$73.45
31500	Insert emergency airway	$135.95
62270	Spinal fluid tap, diagnostic	$76.92
69210	Remove impacted earwax	$40.66
99235	Observation/hospital same date	$220.62
99236	Observation/hospital same date	$274.84
99281	ED visit (level 1)	$24.61
99282	ED visit (level 2)	$41.29
99283	ED visit (level 3)	$91.68
99284	ED visit (level 4)	$142.32
99285	ED visit (level 5)	$222.63
99291	Critical care first hour	$245.68
99292	Critical care, additional 30 min	$122.89

Evaluation and Management Codes

E&M codes are five CPT codes (see Table 212-1) that comprise approximately 80% of EP reimbursement.[1,5] These five codes are aimed at categorizing the complexity of the EP's thought process involved in a patient's care. As with the assignment of CPT codes, coders (and hence the payers) only see what is recorded on the chart after the services are rendered. Thus, they rely on the documentation of historical information, review of systems, past medical and surgical history, family and social history, physical examination, and MDM to determine the complexity of care delivered during the visit. The last digit of each CPT code is used to denote the level of service (Table 212-2). Each progressive level of service requires incrementally more documentation to support the

Table 212-2 EVALUATION AND MANAGEMENT CODE EXAMPLES

Visit Level	CPT Code	Description	Examples
Level 1	99281	Problem focused	Suture removal Tetanus-diphtheria immunization Insect bite
Level 2	99282	Expanded problem focused, low complexity	Sunburn Conjunctivitis Minor extremity trauma without radiograph indicated
Level 3	99283	Expanded problem focused, moderate complexity	Corneal foreign body Vaginal discharge without abdominal pain Extremity trauma with radiograph indicated Minor head injury
Level 4	99284	Detailed	Renal colic Hip fracture Abdominal pain Head injury with loss of consciousness Motor vehicle accident victim arriving by ambulance
Level 5	99285	Comprehensive	Acute myocardial infarction Chest requiring admission Gastrointestinal bleeding: active Transient ischemic attack Dyspnea Altered mental status Headache with stiff neck

CPT, current procedural terminology.

Table 212-3 CHARTING REQUIREMENTS FOR CHARTS BY LEVEL

Chart Billing Level	History of Present Illness	Review of Systems	Past Medical, Family, and Social History	Physical Examination
Level 1	1-3 elements	N/A	N/A	1 system
Level 2	1-3 elements	1 system	N/A	2-7 limited
Level 3	1-3 elements	1 system	N/A	2-7 limited
Level 4	4-8 elements	2-9 systems	1 of 3 areas	2-7 extensive
Level 5	4-8 elements	All systems	2 of 3 areas	8+

N/A, not applicable.

level of coding. The EP must be sure to document more thorough histories of present illness (HPI), review of systems (ROS), and past medical, family, social history (PMFSHx) to support level 4 and 5 charts (Table 212-3).

MDM is the section of E&M coding that is the most complex and, unfortunately, not clinically intuitive. MDM is intended to capture in text the complexity of the decision-making process involved in the care of a patient and thereby reflect the intellectual workload of the EP for that patient. In essence, the EP should include at minimum two of the three following elements:

1. Number of possible diagnoses or treatment options
2. Number and complexity of data and tests to review
3. The potential risk to the patient, including complications of treatment or possible morbidity or mortality

Because it is directed at assessing the complexity of thought rather than the procedures involved in a patient's care, MDM can maximize the reimbursement level of a chart regardless of whether any procedures are performed. The EP must capture the ED course by summarizing the testing and treatments provided to the patient. This must include any and all reevaluations, a review of test data, and discussion of potential life threats that the EP is considering. It is also important that the EP comment on whether the patient may become unstable during the course of the ED stay because this also gives a picture of the clinical severity of the case.

Some other helpful points to improve MDM are as follows:

- Mention all tests ordered and note additional work-ups planned.
- Mention all tests reviewed.
- Mention that nursing notes or old records were reviewed.

Table 212-4 MEDICAL DECISION MAKING CORRELATED WITH CHART BILLING LEVEL

	MEDICAL DECISION MAKING COMPLEXITY			
	Minimal	Low	Moderate	High
Diagnoses considered (number)	Minimum	Limited	Multiple	Extensive
Data or testing required/reviewed (number)	None/minimum	Limited	Moderate	Extensive
Clinical impression/potential risk to the patient	Minimum	Low	Moderate	High
Chart billing level	99281 or level 1	99282 or level 2	99283 or level 3; 99284 or level 4	99285 or level 5

- Mention that the EP has independently viewed a radiograph or study, not just a radiologist's report.
- List all major comorbid conditions that played a role in the decision making and work-up.
- Mention when discussion with others occurs or when consultations are requested.

The complexity of MDM in an ED encounter correlates with the level at which the chart can be billed (Table 212-4). Billing levels 3 and 4 for MDM are the same. Therefore, it is relatively easy to document a level 4 patient interaction by ensuring completeness of the history and physical requirements.

The final element is the diagnosis assignment of the chart. The chart should list all diagnoses applicable to the patient's current presentation, including abnormal vitals signs. The EP should avoid language that does not connote a specific diagnosis, such as "rule out," "probable," "motor vehicle accident," "possible," "chronic," or "mild." When applicable, two diagnoses should be listed. For example, a hypotensive patient with diverticulitis and fever should have the diagnosis assignments of "hypotension," "diverticulitis," and "pyrexia." As with the previous charting points discussed, the EP should include a breadth of diagnoses to paint a more thorough and accurate clinical picture of the patient's severity and the clinical workload involved.[6]

▪ CRITICAL CARE

Critical care (E&M code 99291) is the evaluation and management of an unstable, critically ill, or injured patient who required the EP's *constant cognitive attendance*.[1] The first 30 minutes, up until 1 hour of care, is billed with this code, after which additional increments of 30 minutes (code 99292) on a given patient may be billed. The physician need not be constantly at the bedside, but the EP must be engaged in physician-level work directly related to the individual patient's care. Because of the implied severity of the patient's condition, none of the foregoing history or physical examination requirements apply to a chart to qualify for critical care billing.

▪ "AFTER-HOURS" SERVICE

As of 2006, emergency services provided between the hours of 10 P.M. and 8 A.M. may be coded with an additional code, 99053.[2] This code is a supplement to the E&M codes for care levels 1 to 5.

▪ OBSERVATION CARE

Codes exist for E&M services provided to patients designated or admitted to "observation status" in a hospital. Observation charts may be billed at levels 1 to 3, based on the complexity of the history, physical examination, and MDM, much as the ED chart is billed (Table 212-5).[6] Observation services can create additional revenue by changing the focus of the ED from a "triage to service" unit to an acute diagnostic and treatment center. Observation status has many potential financial advantages that, given current problems of ED overcrowding, may provide EDs with limited inpatient capacity an additional revenue stream on a select group of patients with anticipated stays of less than 24 hours.

Whether this observation status occurs in a geographically separate ED observation unit or within the ED by placing a patient in observation status, these services are separate from the ED visit and hence require separate documentation in addition to the ED note. This additional documentation requires an admission order, a separate admission note that references the ED record, progress notes at specified time intervals during the patient's stay, a discharge note, and a discharge order on release of the patient. Physician extenders such as nurse practitioners may also be used to staff such a unit. However, for observational services to be billed under the attending physician's name as a "shared visit," the attending documentation must reference review of the nurse practitioner's note and must support the appropriate level of E&M service.

Hospital Billing and Capturable Revenue

In addition to the physician services provided to a patient during the ED visit, the hospital also generates a bill that covers the use of the physical plant and materials that the hospital provides, termed *hospital billing*. Hospital billing is accomplished through APCs. These are composed of Medicare groupings of more than 5800 CPT codes into approximately 540 APC code categories. Whereas historically the Medi-

Table 212-5 ED OBSERVATION CODES AND DESCRIPTIONS

Evaluation and Management Observation Service Level	History	Examination	Medical Decision Making
Level 1	Chief complaint 4 HPI 2-9 ROS 1 PFSHx	Extended examination of the affected body area or areas as well as other related organ systems Two to seven organ systems	Low complexity
Level 2	Chief complaint 4 HPI 10+ ROS 3 PFSHx	General multisystem examination (eight or more) Or Complete single examination of a single organ system	Moderate complexity
Level 3	Chief complaint 4 HPI 10+ ROS 3 PFSHx	General multisystem examination (eight or more) Or Complete single examination of a single organ system	High complexity

HPI, histories of present illness; PFSHx, past medical, family, social history; ROS, review of systems.

care reimbursement schedule paid for costs claimed by hospitals in providing care to give the patient, current APCs reimburse for units of outpatient services, and as such they are flat payments for taking care of patients with a particular diagnosis regardless of the cost incurred by the hospital in doing so. For example, a hospital involved in the treatment of a patient with pneumonia receives a flat payment regardless of the antibiotic given and the duration of the patient's stay in the hospital. Both nurse and physician documentations contribute to the number of APCs that may be billed on a given patient's stay based on how many diagnoses and services are documented.

Unfortunately, even after the ED chart has been coded and a bill has been submitted to the patient's insurer, the return on the dollar, or so-called *capturable billable revenue,* is approximately 40%.[6] In addition, this payment is sent out approximately 55 to 60 days after the bill is sent out, thus causing a significant delay in cash flow for the hospital or physician group, which has already provided and paid for the services rendered. The *payer mix* of a given ED contributes to the 40% of capturable revenue and is defined as the mix of insurance coverage sponsoring patient care for a given hospital or physician group that, in turn, ultimately determines the cash flow for that group.[6]

Billing Compliance

As mentioned at the beginning of the chapter, documentation must not only be adequate for billing purposes, but must also be accurate; it must reflect what is done for the patient and the complexity of care given. Accuracy is essential to avoid issues of fraud and abuse. Each EP is individually responsible and accountable for the correct processing of the claims associated with their charts. Therefore, it is incumbent on the EP to document the visit accurately, without underrepresenting or overrepresenting the encounter's complexity.[5,6]

Documentation is perhaps most important when it comes to protecting the EP from claims of fraud in providing care. Procedures or services that are billed for and not documented, regardless of whether they occurred, are considered fraudulent and are subject to criminal penalties. *Assumption coding* occurs when a chart is billed at a higher level than what the chart supports, based on what is assumed to have happened in view of the chief complaint or diagnosis assigned to a patient encounter. For example, a patient with chest pain who is admitted on intravenous heparin with electrocardiographic changes qualifies for a level 5 encounter. However, if the EP seeing this patient documents only a four-element history of present illness (HPI), five physical examination points, moderate-complexity MDM, and "rule out myocardial infarction" as the diagnosis, this note will provide inadequate evidence to support billing above a level 4. If this chart were billed as a level 5 encounter and was subsequently reviewed, the EP would be liable for filing a fraudulent claim. If nothing else, the potential for criminal investigation is a compelling argument for adequate and accurate documentation. To protect physicians from such pitfalls, physician groups or hospitals should have compliance review committees in place to review charts in a systematic fashion to ensure that services rendered and their medical necessity are being appropriately documented.[6]

REFERENCES

1. American Medical Association: Current Procedural Terminology 2004 Standard Edition. Chicago, American Medical Association, 2005.
2. Granovsky MA, Parker RB: 2006 CPT and ICD 9 changes impact emergency medicine coding and reimbursement. EM Today, December 19, 2005.

3. Reese S: 2007 Advanced Coding Education for Emergency Medicine. Gaithersburg, MD, Board of Medical Specialty Coding, 2007.
4. CPT Changes 2007: An Insider's View. Chicago, American Medical Association, 2007.
5. Siff JE: Fundamentals of physician billing, coding, and compliance. In Aghababian RV, Jackson E Jr, Allison MD (eds): Essentials of Emergency Medicine. Sudbury, MA, Jones and Bartlett, 2006, pp 1002-1003.
6. Eitel D: Advanced Business Life Support (personal communication).